Williams
OBSTETRICS

Williams OBSTETRICS

24TH EDITION

F. Gary Cunningham
Kenneth J. Leveno
Steven L. Bloom
Catherine Y. Spong
Jodi S. Dashe
Barbara L. Hoffman
Brian M. Casey
Jeanne S. Sheffield

Mc Graw Hill Education | Medical

New York Chicago San Francisco Lisbon London Madrid Mexico City
Milan New Delhi San Juan Seoul Singapore Sydney Toronto

Williams Obstetrics, Twenty-Fourth Edition

1 2 3 4 5 6 7 8 9 0 DOW/DOW 19 18 17 16 15 14

ISBN 978-0-07-179893-8
MHID 0-07-179893-5

This book was set in Adobe Garamond by Aptara, Inc.
The editors were Alyssa Fried and Peter J. Boyle.
The production supervisor was Richard Ruzycka.
Production management was provided by Indu Jawwad, Aptara, Inc.
The illustration manager was Armen Ovsepyan.
The designer was Alan Barnett.
The cover designer was Thomas De Pierro.
RR Donnelley was printer and binder.

This book was printed on acid-free paper.

Library of Congress Cataloging-in-Publication Data

Williams obstetrics / [edited by] F. Gary Cunningham, Kenneth J. Leveno, Steven L. Bloom, Catherine Y. Spong, Jodi S. Dashe, Barbara L. Hoffman, Brian M. Casey, Jeanne S. Sheffield. – 24th edition.
p. ; cm.
title: Obstetrics
Includes bibliographical references and index.
ISBN 978-0-07-179893-8 (hardcover : alk. paper) – ISBN 0-07-179893-5 (hardcover : alk. paper)
I. Cunningham, F. Gary, editor. II. Title: Obstetrics.
[DNLM: 1. Obstetrics. WQ 100]
RG524
618.2–dc23

2014007925

EDITORS

F. Gary Cunningham, MD
Beatrice and Miguel Elias Distinguished Chair in Obstetrics and Gynecology
Professor, Department of Obstetrics and Gynecology
University of Texas Southwestern Medical Center at Dallas
Parkland Health and Hospital System
Dallas, Texas

Kenneth J. Leveno, MD
Jack A. Pritchard Chair in Obstetrics and Gynecology
Professor, Department of Obstetrics and Gynecology
University of Texas Southwestern Medical Center at Dallas
Parkland Health and Hospital System
Dallas, Texas

Steven L. Bloom, MD
Mary Dees McDermott Hicks Chair in Medical Science
Professor and Chair, Department of Obstetrics and Gynecology
University of Texas Southwestern Medical Center at Dallas
Chief of Obstetrics and Gynecology
Parkland Health and Hospital System
Dallas, Texas

Catherine Y. Spong, MD
Bethesda, Maryland

Jodi S. Dashe, MD
Professor, Department of Obstetrics and Gynecology
University of Texas Southwestern Medical Center at Dallas
Medical Director of Prenatal Diagnosis and Genetics
Parkland Health and Hospital System
Dallas, Texas

Barbara L. Hoffman, MD
Associate Professor, Department of Obstetrics and Gynecology
University of Texas Southwestern Medical Center at Dallas
Parkland Health and Hospital System
Dallas, Texas

Brian M. Casey, MD
Professor, Department of Obstetrics and Gynecology
Director, Division of Maternal-Fetal Medicine
University of Texas Southwestern Medical Center at Dallas
Chief of Obstetrics
Parkland Health and Hospital System
Dallas, Texas

Jeanne S. Sheffield, MD
Alvin "Bud" Brekken Professor of Obstetrics and Gynecology
Professor, Department of Obstetrics and Gynecology
Fellowship Director, Maternal-Fetal Medicine
University of Texas Southwestern Medical Center at Dallas
Medical Director of Prenatal Clinics
Parkland Health and Hospital System
Dallas, Texas

ASSOCIATE EDITORS

Diane M. Twickler, MD
Dr. Fred Bonte Professorship in Radiology
Professor, Department of Radiology and Department of Obstetrics and Gynecology
University of Texas Southwestern Medical Center at Dallas
Medical Director of Obstetrics and Gynecology Ultrasonography
Parkland Health and Hospital System
Dallas, Texas

Mala S. Mahendroo, PhD
Associate Professor, Department of Obstetrics and Gynecology and Green Center for Reproductive Biological Sciences
University of Texas Southwestern Medical Center at Dallas
Dallas, Texas

CONTRIBUTING EDITORS

Kevin C. Worley, MD
Associate Professor, Department of Obstetrics and Gynecology
Associate Residency Program Director
University of Texas Southwestern Medical Center at Dallas
Parkland Health and Hospital System
Dallas, Texas

J. Seth Hawkins, MD, MBA
Assistant Professor, Department of Obstetrics and Gynecology
University of Texas Southwestern Medical Center at Dallas
Parkland Health and Hospital System
Dallas, Texas

Donald D. McIntire, PhD
Biostatistician
Professor, Department of Obstetrics and Gynecology
University of Texas Southwestern Medical Center at Dallas
Parkland Health and Hospital System
Dallas, Texas

Lewis E. Calver, MS, CMI, FAMI
Faculty Associate, Department of Obstetrics and Gynecology
University of Texas Southwestern Medical Center at Dallas

DEDICATION

These are trying times for academic medicine. They are especially vexing for departments of obstetrics and gynecology. Combined with draconian funding shortages, there is burdensome oversight with sometimes meaningless regulations as well as myriad forms and paperwork foisted upon us by an ever-increasing but already bloated bureaucracy. Despite these seemingly overwhelming challenges, the chairs of academic departments and the directors of residency training programs resiliently continue to emphasize the basics that are fundamental to academic training. It is to these stalwart individuals that we dedicate this 24th edition of *Williams Obstetrics*.

CONTENTS

SECTION 4

PRECONCEPTIONAL AND PRENATAL CARE

SECTION 5

THE FETAL PATIENT

SECTION 6

EARLY PREGNANCY COMPLICATIONS

SECTION 7

LABOR

SECTION 8

DELIVERY

SECTION 9

THE NEWBORN

SECTION 10

THE PUERPERIUM

SECTION 11

OBSTETRICAL COMPLICATIONS

SECTION 12

MEDICAL AND SURGICAL COMPLICATIONS

APPENDIX

PREFACE

This 24th edition of *Williams Obstetrics* has been extensively and strategically reorganized. Primarily writing for the busy practitioner—those "in the trenches"—we continue to present the detailed staples of basic obstetrics such as maternal anatomy and physiology, preconceptional and prenatal care, labor, delivery, and the puerperium, along with detailed discussions of obstetrical complications exemplified by preterm labor, hemorrhage, hypertension, and many more. Once again, we emphasize the scientific-based underpinnings of clinical obstetrics with special emphasis on biochemical and physiological principles of female reproduction. And, as was the hallmark of previous editions, these dovetail with descriptions of evidence-based practices. The reorganized format allows a greater emphasis on the fetus as a patient along with expanded coverage of fetal diagnosis and therapy. These changes are complemented by more than 100 new sonographic and magnetic resonance images that display normal fetal anatomy and common fetal anomalies. Finally, to emphasize the "M" in maternal–fetal medicine, we continue to iterate the myriad medical and surgical disorders that can complicate pregnancy.

To accomplish these goals, the text has been updated with more than 3000 new literature citations through 2014. Moreover, there are nearly 900 figures that include sonograms, MR images, photographs, micrographs, and data graphs, most in vivid color. Much of the original artwork was rendered by our own medical illustrators.

In this edition, as before, we continue to incorporate contemporaneous guidelines from professional and academic organizations such as the American College of Obstetricians and Gynecologists, the Society for Maternal–Fetal Medicine, the National Institutes of Health, and the Centers for Disease Control and Prevention, among others. Many of these data are distilled into almost 100 newly constructed tables, in which information has been arranged in a format that is easy to read and use. In addition, several diagnostic and management algorithms have been added to guide practitioners. While we strive to cite numerous sources to provide multiple evidence-based options for such management schemes, we also include our own clinical experiences drawn from a large obstetrical service. As usual, while we are convinced that these are disciplined examples of evidence-based obstetrics, we quickly acknowledge that they do not constitute the sole method of management.

This 24th edition shows a notable absence of four colleagues who provided valuable editorial assistance for prior volumes of *Williams Obstetrics*. From the University of Alabama at Birmingham, Dr. John Hauth, who served as an editor for the 21st through 23rd editions, has now directed his efforts to research endeavors. Dr. Dwight Rouse, an associate editor of the 22nd and an editor of the 23rd edition, has assumed a clinical and research role at Brown University. We will certainly miss their insightful wisdom concerning the vicissitudes of randomized controlled trials and their true meanings! Colleagues leaving us from the University of Texas Southwestern Medical Center include Dr. George Wendel, Jr.—associate editor for the 22nd and 23rd editions—who has now assumed the important role of overseeing development of Maintenance of Certification for the American Board of Obstetrics and Gynecology. And leaving for practice in Montana is Dr. Jim Alexander, who served as a contributing editor for the 23rd edition. These talented clinicians provided valuable knowledge, both evidence-based and from the bedside.

To fill the shoes of these departing stalwart colleagues, we have enlisted four new editors—all from UT Southwestern Medical Center—each of whom has expertise in important areas of contemporaneous obstetrics and maternal–fetal medicine. Dr. Jodi Dashe—who contributed extensively to the 21st through 23rd editions—joins us as editor and brings her extensive experiences and incredible skills with obstetrical sonography, fetal diagnosis, and prenatal genetics. Dr. Barbara Hoffman brings widespread clinical knowledge regarding general obstetrics and contraception as well as embryology, anatomy, and placental pathology. Dr. Brian Casey adds his in-depth obstetrical and research experience, with special interests in diabetes, fetal-growth disorders, and thyroid physiology. Dr. Jeanne Sheffield joins us with her knowledge and clinical acumen and research interests in maternal medical disorders, critical care, and obstetrical and perinatal infections.

There are also two returning associate editors who continue to add considerable depth to this textbook. Dr. Diane Twickler uses her fantastic experiences and knowledge regarding clinical and technological advances related to fetal and maternal imaging with ultrasonography as well as with x-ray and magnetic resonance techniques. Dr. Mala Mahendroo is a talented basic scientist who continues to perform a magnificent job of providing a coherent translational version of basic science aspects of human reproduction. Finally, four new contributing editors round out the editorial team that make this book possible. Drs. Kevin Worley and Seth Hawkins bring additional strengths to the areas of clinical and academic maternal–fetal medicine. Dr. Don McIntire provided much of the data garnered from the extensive database that chronicles the large obstetrical service at Parkland Hospital and UT Southwestern Medical Center. Mr. Lewis Calver continues to do an impeccable job of supervising and rendering new artwork for this and prior editions. In toto, the strength of each contributor has added to create the sum total of our academic endeavor.

F. Gary Cunningham
Kenneth J. Leveno
Steven L. Bloom

ACKNOWLEDGMENTS

During the creation and production of this textbook, we were fortunate to have the assistance and support of countless talented professionals both within and outside the Department of Obstetrics and Gynecology. To begin, we acknowledge that an undertaking of this magnitude would not be possible without the unwavering support provided by Dr. Barry Schwarz, whose financial and academic endorsement has been essential.

In constructing such an expansive academic compilation, the expertise of many colleagues was needed to add vital and contemporaneous information. It was indeed fortuitous for us to have access to a pantheon of contributors here as well as from other academic medical centers. From the University of Texas Southwestern Medical Center, Dr. April Bailey of the Departments of Radiology and Obstetrics and Gynecology added insights and provided illustrative maternal and fetal magnetic resonance images. These were further complimented by other visual contributions from Drs. Elysia Moschos, Michael Landay, Jeffrey Pruitt, and Douglas Sims. From the Department of Pathology, Drs. Kelley Carrick and Brian Levenson generously donated exemplary photomicrographs. From the Department of Dermatology, Dr. Amit Pandya provided a number of classic figures. From the Division of Urogynecology, our nationally known pelvic anatomist, Dr. Marlene Corton, prepared graphic masterpieces for the anatomy chapter. Drs. Claudia Werner and William Griffith lent valuable insight into the management of cervical dysplasia. Much of the Appendix of this textbook was originally compiled by Drs. Mina Abbassi-Ghanavati and Laura Greer. Finally, clinical photographs were contributed by many current and former faculty and fellows, including Drs. Patricia Santiago-Muñoz, Julie Lo, Lisa Halvorson, Kevin Doody, Michael Zaretsky, Judith Head, David Rogers, Sunil Balgobin, Manisha Sharma, Michael Hnat, Rigoberto Santos-Ramos, Shayzreen Roshanravan, April Bleich, and Roxane Holt.

Several contributions were made by our national and international colleagues. Experts in placental pathology who shared their expertise and images include Drs. Kurt Benirschke, Ona Marie Faye-Petersen, Mandolin Ziadie, Michael Conner, Jaya George, and Erika Fong. Input for hypertensive disorders was provided by Drs. Marshall Lindheimer and Gerda Zeeman and for operative vaginal delivery by Dr. Edward Yeomans. Seminal images were contributed by Drs. Timothy Crombleholme, Togas Tulandi, Edward Lammer, Charles Read, and Frederick Elder.

In addition to these contributors, we relied heavily on numerous other colleagues and coworkers for their intellectual and clinical input. Specifically, we cite the entire Division of Maternal–Fetal Medicine, whose faculty, in addition to providing expert content, graciously assisted us to cover clinical duties when writing and editing were especially time consuming. These include Drs. Scott Roberts, Oscar Andujo, Vanessa Rogers, Morris Bryant, Stephan Shivvers, Stephanie Chang, Robyn Horsager, Patricia Santiago-Muñoz, Julie Lo, Ashley Zink, Ed Wells, and Mark Peters.

We also note that production of *Williams Obstetrics* would not be feasible without the help of our maternal–fetal medicine fellows and residents in obstetrics and gynecology. Their insatiable curiosity serves to energize us to find new and effective ways to convey age-old truths, new data, and cutting-edge concepts. Their logical and critical questions lead us to weaknesses in the text, and thereby, always help us to improve our work. In addition, we sincerely thank them for their vigilance in capturing photographs of spectacular examples of both obstetrical pathology and normal findings. For example, included in this edition are photographs contributed by Drs. Elaine Duryea, Stacey Thomas, Jonathan Willms, Kara Ehlers, Nidhi Shah, Abel Moron, Kyler Elwell, Rebecca Stone, Angela Fields, Emily Adhikari, and Elizabeth Mosier.

Thanks to generous funding from the McGraw-Hill Companies, this 24th edition now contains more than 200 color illustrations. Most of these were crafted by several skilled medical illustrators, including Ms. Marie Sena, Ms. Erin Frederikson, Ms. Mollie Gove, Mr. Jordan Pietz, Ms. SangEun Cha, and Ms. Jennifer Hulsey. All of these talented artists trained here at UT Southwestern under the tutelage of Mr. Lewis Calver. Additional artistic support came from Mr. Joseph Varghese, Ms. Dharmesh Thakur, and their team at Thomson Digital, who provided the full-color graphs and line art used to enhance this edition. They were aided by medical-content expert Dr. Shetoli Zhimomi, who precisely translated our academic vision to each image. Their team tirelessly coordinated efforts between author and artist and graciously accommodated our numerous changes and tweaks.

Production of the 5000-page manuscript would not have been possible without a dedicated team to bring these efforts together. Once again, we are deeply indebted to Ms. Connie Utterback for her untiring efforts as production coordinator. She received able assistance with manuscript production from the Dallas group that included Ms. Melinda Epstein, Ms. Dawn Wilson, Ms. Marsha Zint, Ms. Minnie Tregaskis, Ms. Dina Trujillano, and Ms. Ellen Watkins. Information technology support was provided by the very knowledgeable and responsive Mr. Charles Richards and Mr. Thomas Ames. For these and many more that go unnamed, we could not have done our job without their expertise.

It again has been a privilege and a pleasure to work with the dedicated professionals from McGraw-Hill Education. Ms. Alyssa Fried has brought her considerable intelligence, energetic work ethic, and creativity to this edition of *Williams Obstetrics*. Her dedication to creating the best textbook possible equaled our efforts, and we are in awe of her unflappable, productive, and gracious style. Mr. Peter Boyle shepherded our book through production. We greatly appreciate his calm and efficient efforts. Mr. Richard Ruzycka served as production supervisor for this edition of the textbook. He skillfully kept our project on track through an array of potential hurdles. Last, we have had the pleasure to work with Mr. Armen Ovsepyan in coordinating the artwork for many of our editions. His organization and efficiency are unrivaled.

Our text took its final shape under the watchful care of our compositors at Aptara, Inc. We thank Ms. Indu Jawwad for her talents in skillfully coordinating and overseeing composition. Her dedicated attention to detail and organization were vital to completion of our project. Also at Aptara, Mr. Mahender Singh served a crucial task of quality control and assisted in creating beautiful chapter layouts to highlight our content aesthetically and informatively.

Finally—but certainly not last—we acknowledge our significant debt to the women who have allowed us to participate in their care. The clinical expertise and many graphic illustrations presented in this text would not have been possible without their collaborative spirit to help us advance obstetrical knowledge. We also offer enthusiastic and heartfelt appreciation to our families and friends. Without their patience, generosity, and encouragement, this task would have been impossible.

The Editors

SECTION 1

OVERVIEW

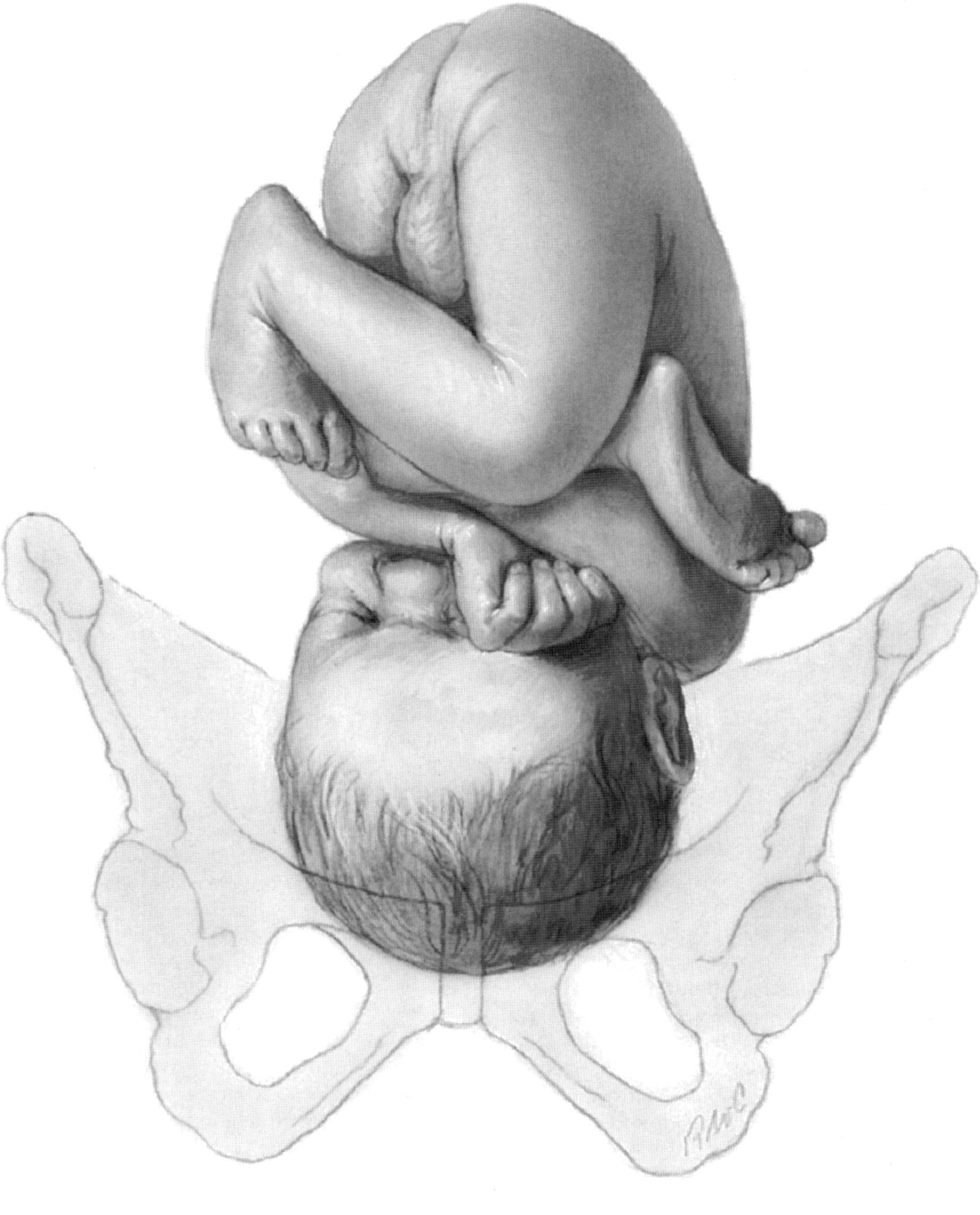

CHAPTER 1

Overview of Obstetrics

Obstetrics is concerned with human reproduction and as such is always a subject of considerable contemporary relevance. The specialty promotes health and well-being of the pregnant woman and her fetus through quality perinatal care. Such care entails appropriate recognition and treatment of complications, supervision of labor and delivery, ensuring care of the newborn, and management of the puerperium. Postpartum care promotes health and provides family planning options.

The importance of obstetrics is reflected by the use of maternal and neonatal outcomes as an index of the quality of health and life among nations. Intuitively, indices that reflect poor obstetrical and perinatal outcomes would lead to the assumption that medical care for the entire population is lacking. With those thoughts, we now provide a synopsis of the current state of maternal and newborn health in the United States as it relates to obstetrics.

VITAL STATISTICS

The National Vital Statistics System of the United States is the oldest and most successful example of intergovernmental data sharing in public health. The National Center for Health Statistics collects and disseminates official statistics through contractual agreements with vital registration systems. These systems that operate in various jurisdictions are legally responsible for registration of births, fetal deaths, deaths, marriages, and divorces. Legal authority resides individually with the 50 states; two regions—the District of Columbia and New York City; and five territories—American Samoa, Guam, the Northern Mariana Islands, Puerto Rico, and the Virgin Islands.

Standard certificates for the registration of live births and deaths were first developed in 1900. An act of Congress in 1902 established the Bureau of the Census to develop a system for the annual collection of vital statistics. The Bureau retained authority until 1946, when the function was transferred to the United States Public Health Service. It is presently assigned to the Division of Vital Statistics of the National Center for Health Statistics, which is a division of the Centers for Disease Control and Prevention (CDC). The standard birth certificate was revised in 1989 to include more information on medical and lifestyle risk factors and obstetrical practices.

In 2003, an extensively revised *Standard Certificate of Live Birth* was implemented in the United States to enhance collection of obstetrical and newborn clinical information. The enhanced data categories and specific examples of each are summarized in Table 1-1. By 2011, 36 states had implemented this revised birth certificate representing 83 percent of all births (Hamilton, 2012).

Definitions

The uniform use of standard definitions is encouraged by the World Health Organization as well as the American Academy of Pediatrics and the American College of Obstetricians and Gynecologists (2012). Such uniformity allows data comparison not only between states or regions of the country but also between countries. Still, not all definitions are uniformly applied. For example, the American College of Obstetricians and Gynecologists recommends that reporting include all fetuses and neonates born weighing at minimum 500 g, whether alive or dead. But not all states follow this recommendation. Twenty-eight states stipulate that fetal deaths beginning at 20 weeks' gestation should be recorded as such; eight states report all products of conception as fetal deaths;

TABLE 1-1. General Categories and Specific Examples of New Information Added to the 2003 Revision of the Birth Certificate

Risk Factors in Pregnancy—Examples: prior preterm birth, prior eclampsia
Obstetrical Procedures—Examples: tocolysis, cerclage, external cephalic version
Labor—Examples: noncephalic presentation, glucocorticoids for fetal lung maturation, antibiotics during labor
Delivery—Examples: unsuccessful operative vaginal delivery, trial of labor with prior cesarean
Newborn—Examples: assisted ventilation, surfactant therapy, congenital anomalies

and still others use a minimum birthweight of 350 g, 400 g, or 500 g to define fetal death. To further the confusion, the National Vital Statistics Reports tabulates fetal deaths from gestations that are 20 weeks or older (Centers for Disease Control and Prevention, 2009). This is problematic because the 50th percentile for fetal weight at 20 weeks approximates 325 to 350 g—considerably less than the 500-g definition. Indeed, a birthweight of 500 g corresponds closely with the 50th percentile for 22 weeks.

Definitions recommended by the National Center for Health Statistics and the Center for Disease Control and Prevention are as follows:

Perinatal period. The interval between the birth of an infant born after 20 weeks' gestation and the 28 completed days after that birth. When perinatal rates are based on birthweight, rather than gestational age, it is recommended that the perinatal period be defined as commencing at 500 g.

Birth. The complete expulsion or extraction from the mother of a fetus after 20 weeks' gestation. As described above, in the absence of accurate dating criteria, fetuses weighing < 500 g are usually not considered as births but rather are termed *abortuses* for purposes of vital statistics.

Birthweight. The weight of a neonate determined immediately after delivery or as soon thereafter as feasible. It should be expressed to the nearest gram.

Birth rate. The number of live births per 1000 population.

Fertility rate. The number of live births per 1000 females aged 15 through 44 years.

Live birth. The term used to record a birth whenever the newborn at or sometime after birth breathes spontaneously or shows any other sign of life such as a heartbeat or definite spontaneous movement of voluntary muscles. Heartbeats are distinguished from transient cardiac contractions, and respirations are differentiated from fleeting respiratory efforts or gasps.

Stillbirth or fetal death. The absence of signs of life at or after birth.

Early neonatal death. Death of a liveborn neonate during the first 7 days after birth.

Late neonatal death. Death after 7 days but before 29 days.

Stillbirth rate or fetal death rate. The number of stillborn neonates per 1000 neonates born, including live births and stillbirths.

Neonatal mortality rate. The number of neonatal deaths per 1000 live births.

Perinatal mortality rate. The number of stillbirths plus neonatal deaths per 1000 total births.

Infant death. All deaths of liveborn infants from birth through 12 months of age.

Infant mortality rate. The number of infant deaths per 1000 live births.

Low birthweight. A newborn whose weight is < 2500 g.

Very low birthweight. A newborn whose weight is < 1500 g.

Extremely low birthweight. A newborn whose weight is < 1000 g.

Term neonate. A neonate born any time after 37 completed weeks of gestation and up until 42 completed weeks of gestation (260 to 294 days). The American College of Obstetricians and Gynecologists (2013b) and the Society for Maternal-Fetal Medicine endorse and encourage specific gestational age designations. *Early term* refers to neonates born at 37 completed weeks up to $38^{6/7}$ weeks. *Full term* denotes those born at 39 completed weeks up to $40^{6/7}$ weeks. Last, *late term* describes neonates born at 41 completed weeks up to $41^{6/7}$ weeks.

Preterm neonate. A neonate born before 37 completed weeks (the 259th day).

Postterm neonate. A neonate born anytime after completion of the 42nd week, beginning with day 295.

Abortus. A fetus or embryo removed or expelled from the uterus during the first half of gestation—20 weeks or less, or in the absence of accurate dating criteria, born weighing < 500 g.

Induced termination of pregnancy. The purposeful interruption of an intrauterine pregnancy that has the intention other than to produce a liveborn neonate and that does not result in a live birth. This definition excludes retention of products of conception following fetal death.

Direct maternal death. The death of the mother that results from obstetrical complications of pregnancy, labor, or the puerperium and from interventions, omissions, incorrect treatment, or a chain of events resulting from any of these factors. An example is maternal death from exsanguination after uterine rupture.

Indirect maternal death. A maternal death that is not directly due to an obstetrical cause. Death results from previously existing disease or a disease developing during pregnancy, labor, or the puerperium that was aggravated by maternal physiological adaptation to pregnancy. An example is maternal death from complications of mitral valve stenosis.

Nonmaternal death. Death of the mother that results from accidental or incidental causes not related to pregnancy. An example is death from an automobile accident or concurrent malignancy.

Maternal mortality ratio. The number of maternal deaths that result from the reproductive process per 100,000 live births. Used more commonly, but less accurately, are the terms *maternal mortality rate* or *maternal death rate*. The term *ratio* is more accurate because it includes in the numerator the number of deaths regardless of pregnancy outcome—for example, live births, stillbirths, and ectopic pregnancies—whereas the denominator includes the number of live births.

Pregnancy-associated death. The death of a woman, from any cause, while pregnant or within 1 calendar year of termination of pregnancy, regardless of the duration and the site of pregnancy.

Pregnancy-related death. A pregnancy-associated death that results from: (1) complications of pregnancy itself, (2) the chain of events initiated by pregnancy that led to death, or (3) aggravation of an unrelated condition by the physiological or pharmacological effects of pregnancy and that subsequently caused death.

PREGNANCY IN THE UNITED STATES

Pregnancy Rates

Data from diverse sources have been used to provide the following snapshot of pregnancy in the United States during the first two decades of the 21st century. According to the Centers for Disease Control and Prevention, the fertility rate in the United States in 2011 of women aged 15 to 44 years was 63.2 live births per 1000 women (Sutton, 2011). As shown in Figure 1-1, this rate began slowly trending downward in 1990 and has now decreased below that for replacement births, indicating a population decline (Hamilton, 2012). There were 3.9 million births in 2011, and this constituted the lowest birth rate ever recorded for the United States of 12.7 per 1000 population. The birth rate decreased for all major ethnic and racial groups, for adolescents and unmarried women, and for those aged 20 to 24 years. For women older than 30 years, the birth rate was either unchanged or it increased slightly. Virtually half of newborns in 2010 in the United States were minorities: Hispanic—25 percent, African-American—14 percent, and Asian—4 percent (Frey, 2011).

The total number of pregnancies and their outcomes in 2008 are shown in Table 1-2. Of the 6,578,000 total pregnancies, most—65 percent—ended with live births. Of births in the United States, approximately 37 percent are unintended at the time of conception (Mosher, 2012). Importantly, the overall proportion of unintended births has not declined significantly since 1982. Unmarried women, black women, and women with less education or income are more likely to have unplanned pregnancies. That said, of the remaining pregnancies in 2008, 35 percent were almost equally divided into induced or spontaneous abortions. The induced abortion information is based on CDC abortion surveillance data from 45 states combined with Guttmacher Institute data on induced abortion. These data have been collected beginning in 1976. If the annual totals for 1976 to 2008 are tabulated, it can be estimated that approximately 46,657,000 women in the United States have elected induced abortions since *Roe v. Wade* legalization of abortion (Chap. 18, p. 363). Thus, legalized abortions have been chosen by more than 46 million American women. As discussed later, this provides a compelling argument for easily accessible family planning.

TABLE 1-2. Total Number of Pregnancies and Outcomes in the United States in 2008

Outcomes	Number (%)
Live births	4,248,000 (65)
Induced abortions	1,212,000 (18)
Spontaneous abortions	1,118,000 (17)
Total pregnancies	6,578,000 (100)

Data from Ventura, 2012.

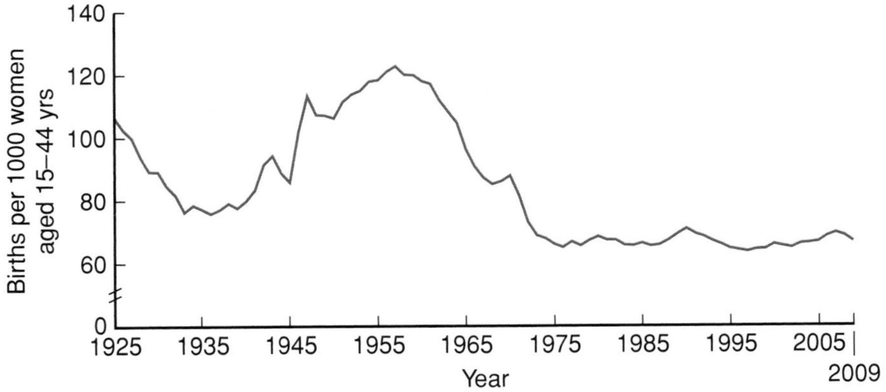

FIGURE 1-1 Fertility rate: United States, 1925–2009. (From Sutton, 2011.)

MEASURES OF OBSTETRICAL CARE

Perinatal Mortality

There are a number of indices—several among the vital statistic definitions described above—that are used as a yardstick of obstetrical and perinatal outcomes to assess quality of care.

As previously defined, the perinatal mortality rate includes the numbers of stillbirths and neonatal deaths per 1000 total births. According to the National Vital Statistics Reports by MacDorman and colleagues (2012a), the perinatal mortality rate in 2006 was 10.5 per 1000 births (Fig. 1-2). There were 25,972 fetal deaths in gestations 20 weeks or older. Fetal deaths at 28 weeks or more have been declining since 1990, whereas the rates for those between 20 and 27 weeks have been static (Fig. 1-3). By way of comparison, there were a total of 19,041 neonatal deaths in 2006—meaning that nearly 60 percent of the perinatal deaths in the United States were fetal. Thus, it is seen that fetal deaths have eclipsed neonatal deaths as a cause of perinatal mortality.

Infant Deaths

There were 6.1 infant deaths per 1000 live births in 2011 compared with 6.8 in 2001 (Hamilton, 2012). The three leading causes of infant death—congenital malformations, low birthweight, and sudden infant death syndrome—accounted for almost half of all deaths. Infants born at the lowest gestational ages and birthweights add substantively

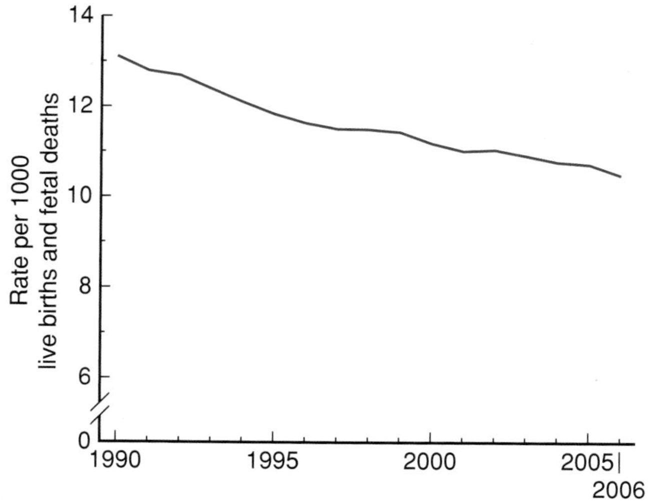

FIGURE 1-2 Perinatal mortality rate: United States, 1990–2006. *Perinatal* includes infant deaths under age 28 days and fetal deaths at 20 weeks or more. (From MacDorman, 2012a.)

to these mortality rates. For example, 55 percent of all infant deaths in 2005 were in the 2 percent of infants born before 32 weeks' gestation. Indeed, the percentage of infant deaths related to preterm birth increased from 34.6 percent in 2000 to 36.5 percent in 2005. When analyzed by birthweight, two thirds of infant deaths were in low-birthweight neonates. Of particular interest are those birthweights < 500 g, for which neonatal intensive care can now be offered. In 2001, there were 6450 liveborns weighing less than 500 g, but 86 percent of these newborns died during the first 28 days of life. Of the 1044 who survived the first 28 days of life, there were 934 who lived for at least 1 year. Thus, only 14 percent of all neonates weighing < 500 g survived infancy. Importantly, adverse developmental and neurological sequelae are common in the survivors (Chap. 42, p. 832).

More than a decade ago, St. John and associates (2000) estimated the total cost of initial newborn care in the United States to be $10.2 billion annually. Almost 60 percent of this

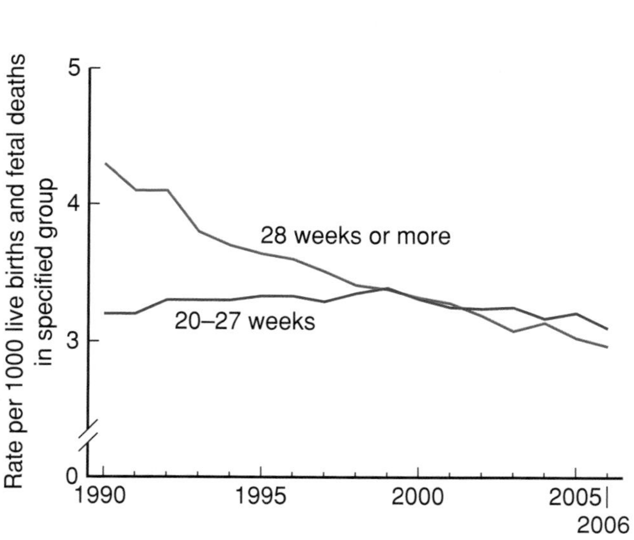

FIGURE 1-3 Fetal mortality rates by period of gestation: United States, 1990–2006. (From MacDorman, 2012a.)

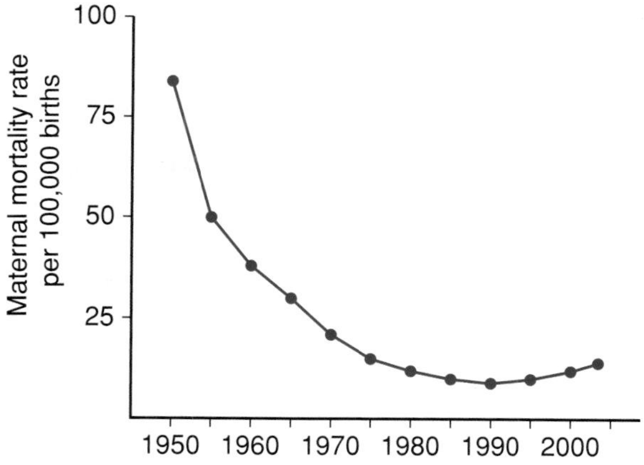

FIGURE 1-4 Maternal mortality rates for the United States, 1950–2003. (Data from Berg, 2010; Hoyert, 2007.)

expenditure is attributed to preterm births before 37 weeks, and 12 percent is spent on neonates born between 24 and 26 weeks.

Maternal Mortality

As shown in Figure 1-4, maternal mortality rates decreased precipitously in the United States during the 20th century. Pregnancy and childbirth have never been safer for women in this country. In fact, pregnancy-related deaths are so uncommon as to be measured per 100,000 births. The CDC since 1979 has maintained data on pregnancy-related deaths in its *Pregnancy Mortality Surveillance System* (Mackay, 2005). In the latest report, Berg and coworkers (2010) described 4693 pregnancy-related deaths during the 8-year period 1998 to 2005. Approximately 5 percent were early-pregnancy deaths due to ectopic gestation or abortive outcomes. The deadly obstetrical triad of hemorrhage, preeclampsia, and infection accounted for a third of all deaths (Table 1-3). Thromboembolism, cardiomyopathy, and other cardiovascular disease together accounted for another third (Fig. 1-5). Other significant contributors in this group were amnionic fluid

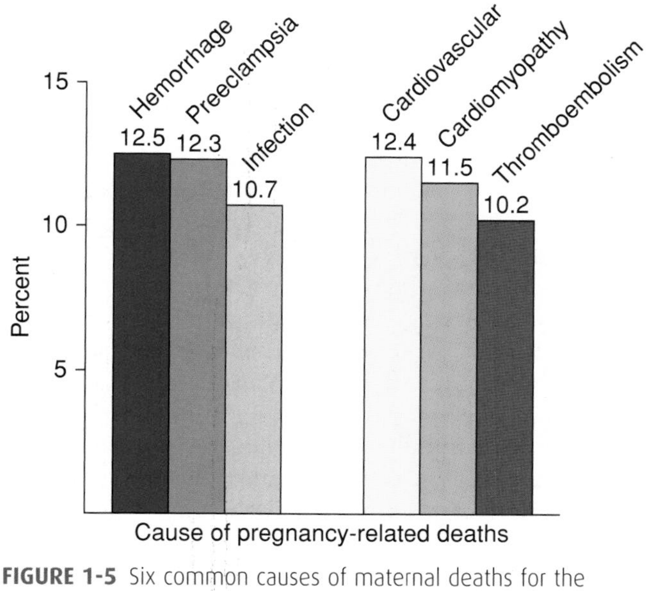

FIGURE 1-5 Six common causes of maternal deaths for the United States, 1998–2005. (Data from Berg, 2010.)

SECTION 1

TABLE 1-3. Causes of Pregnancy-Related Maternal Deaths in the United States[a,b] During Two Time Periods

Cause of Death	1991–1999[a,c] n = 4200 (%)	1998–2005[b,d] n = 4693 (%)
Embolism	19.6	10.2
Hemorrhage	17.2	12.5
Gestational hypertension	15.7	12.3
Infection	12.6	10.7
Other pregnancy-related	34.1	33.2
Cardiomyopathy	8.3	11.5
Stroke	5.0	6.3
Anesthesia	1.6	1.2
Others[e]	19.2	14.2
Unknown	0.7	2.1

[a]Data from Centers for Disease Control and Prevention reported by Chang, 2003.
[b]Data from the Centers for Disease Control and Prevention reported by Berg, 2010.
[c]Includes abortion and ectopic pregnancy.
[d]Excludes abortion and ectopic pregnancy.
[e]Includes cardiovascular, pulmonary, neurological, and other medical conditions.

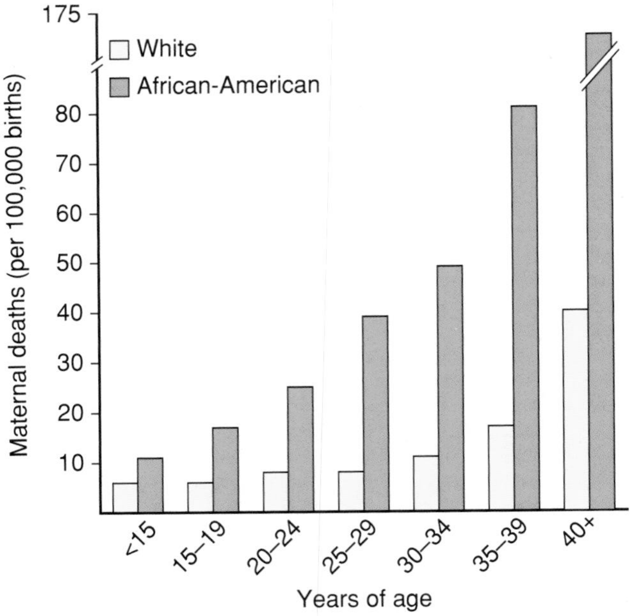

FIGURE 1-6 Maternal mortality ratio—deaths per 100,000 live births—by age and according to race for the United States, 1998–2005. (Data from Berg, 2010.)

embolism (7.5 percent) and cerebrovascular accidents (6.3 percent). Anesthesia-related deaths were at an all-time low of only 1.2 percent. It is also important to consider the role that the increasing cesarean delivery rate has on maternal mortality risks (Clark, 2008; Deneux-Tharaux, 2006; Lang, 2008).

The pregnancy-related mortality ratio for this 1998 to 2005 period of 14.5 per 100,000 live births is the highest during the previous 20 years (Berg, 2010). This simply may mean more women are dying, however, it may be due to improved reporting or to an artificial increase caused by the new International Statistical Classification of Diseases, 10th Revision (ICD-10), implemented in 1999. There is no doubt that maternal deaths are notoriously underreported, possibly by as much as half (Koonin, 1997).

A second important consideration is the obvious disparity of increased mortality rates in African-American compared with white women as shown in Figure 1-6. The disparity with indigent women is exemplified by the study of maternal deaths in women cared for in a third-party payer system, the Hospital Corporation of America. In this study of nearly 1.5 million pregnant women, Clark and associates (2008) reported an impressively low maternal mortality rate of 6.5 per 100,000.

The third important consideration is that many of the reported maternal deaths are considered preventable. In an earlier report, Berg and colleagues (2005) stated that this may be up to a third of pregnancy-related deaths in white women and up to half of those in African-American women. And even in the insured women described above and reported by Clark, 28 percent of 98 maternal deaths were judged preventable. Thus, although significant progress has been made, measures to prevent more deaths are imperative for obstetrics in the 21st century.

Severe Maternal Morbidity

Because maternal deaths have become so uncommon, the practice of analyzing severe maternal morbidity evolved as a surrogate to improve obstetrical and perinatal care. Because avoidance of medical errors serves to decrease the risks for maternal mortality or severe maternal morbidity, the concept of *near misses* or *close calls* was also introduced. These are defined by the Joint Commission and the Institution for Safe Medication and Practices (2009) as unplanned events caused by error that do not result in patient injury but have the potential to do so. These are much more common than injury events, but for obvious reasons, they are more difficult to identify and quantify. Systems designed to encourage reporting have been installed in various institutions and allow focused safety efforts. One example is the system described by Clark and associates (2012) and used for more than 200,000 annual deliveries within the Hospital Corporation of America (Table 1-4).

There are now a number of statistical data systems that measure indicators of unplanned events caused by errors that had potential to injure patients. This evolution followed inadequacies in how well hospitalization coding reflected the severity of maternal complications. Thus, coding indicators or modifiers are used to allow analysis of serious adverse clinical events (Clark, 2012; King, 2012). Such a system was implemented by the World Health Organization. It has been validated in Brazil and accurately reflects maternal death rates (Souza, 2012). Similar systems are in use in Britain as the *UK Obstetric Surveillance System—UKOSS* (Knight, 2005, 2008). Australia and New Zealand have also devised such a system—the

TABLE 1-4. Near-Miss Events in Labor and Delivery—Hospital Corporation of America, 2010

Error	Percent[a]
Medication	33
Patient identification	19
Failure/delay laboratory	11
Failure to respond	10
Failure to follow policy	9
Charting	6
Equipment failure	6
Slip/fall	5
Information transfer	5
Physician error	3
Others	~5

[a]Exceeds 100 percent because some events had multiple events.
Data from Clark, 2012.

Australasian Maternity Outcomes Surveillance System—AMOSS (Halliday, 2013). As emphasized by Tuncalp and coworkers (2012) after their systematic review, different locoregional approaches are needed to lower the rates of near misses.

In the United States, to study severe morbidity the CDC analyzed more than 50 million maternity records from the Nationwide Inpatient Sample from 1998 to 2009 (Callaghan, 2012). Selected International Classification of Diseases, 9th Revision, Clinical Modification (ICD-9-CM) codes were used to tabulate a number of severe morbidities. The frequencies of some of those most commonly encountered are listed in Table 1-5. These investigators reported that 129 per 10,000 of these nearly 50 million pregnant women had at least one indicator for severe morbidity. Thus, for every maternal death, approximately 200 women experience severe morbidity.

TABLE 1-5. Severe Obstetrical Morbidities Identified[a] During Nearly 50 Million Hospitalizations for Delivery—United States, 1998–2009

Category
Transfusions
Eclampsia
Hysterectomy
Cardiac surgery
Cerebrovascular disorders
Anesthesia complications
Pulmonary edema
Mechanical ventilation
Respiratory distress syndrome
Septicemia
Heart failure
Renal failure
Coagulopathy
Hemorrhagic shock

[a]Identified by International Classification of Diseases, 9th Revision, Clinical Modification (ICD-9-CM) codes.
Data from Callaghan, 2012.

TIMELY TOPICS IN OBSTETRICS

Health Care for Women and Their Infants

Various topics have been in the forefront for obstetrical providers in the 4 years since the last edition of this textbook. Of these, the ills of our health-care system are especially concerning for women's health (Hale, 2010). To cite but a few examples, uninsured women with breast cancer were up to 50 percent more likely than insured women to die from the disease. There were more than 17 million uninsured American women aged 18 to 64 years in 2008. Similarly, women without health-care insurance had a 60-percent greater risk of late-stage cervical cancer. Lack of medical insurance also has severe effects on pregnant women. Those without insurance have a 31-percent higher risk of adverse outcomes such as preterm delivery, neonatal death, and maternal mortality. Of American women aged 18 to 64 years in a recent study of 11 industrialized countries, 43 percent skipped seeing a doctor or did not take medicine due to costs (Robertson, 2012). This was the highest percentage of all 11 countries studied. By comparison, just 7 percent of British women and 17 percent of Canadian and French women refrained from seeking health care because of costs. Of the 11 countries studied, only the United States did not have universal health-care coverage.

There is also a geopolitical consequence of such increased adverse outcomes for American women. The World Health Organization analyzed neonatal mortality rates in 2009 for 193 countries (Oestergaard, 2011). The United States ranked 41st in 2009, dropping from 28th in 1990. The highest newborn death rate in the world was in Afghanistan, where one of every 19 babies died before their 1-month birthday. In comparison, one of every 233 newborns dies in the United States. This is far better than the rate in Afghanistan, but not as good as the rate in Japan—1 in 909, France—1 in 455, Lithuania—1 in 385, or Cuba—1 in 345. Some reasons given for the United States results include difficulty in accessing prenatal care, which contributes to the current high rate of preterm births.

There have been dramatic changes in women's health care regarding obstetrical and gynecological procedures during the past 30 years in the United States. Shown in Figure 1-7 are the rates per 1000 adult American women for the commonest gynecological procedures performed between 1979 and 2006. The rates are adjusted for age to correct for population changes over time. The dramatic decreases in the rates of gynecological procedures were thought largely due to changed criteria for these procedures. Changed criteria resulted from the health maintenance organization (HMO) movement of the 1980s. With this, health-care insurers of all types exercised increasing control over the indications for these procedures. Shown in Figure 1-8 are the rates per 1000 adult women for obstetrical procedures also from 1979 to 2006. Episiotomy use plummeted, as did operative vaginal delivery rates. Cesarean deliveries per 1000 women greatly increased. These rates changes are

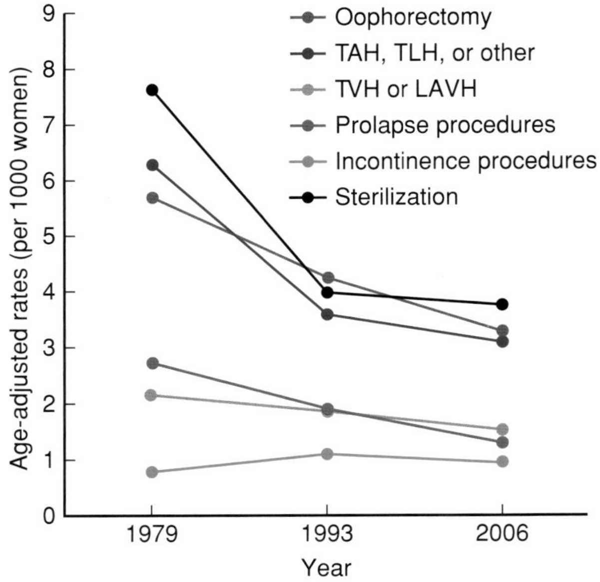

FIGURE 1-7 Age-adjusted rates of gynecological procedures in the United States, 1979–2006. (Data from Oliphant, 2010.)

discussed more fully in Chapters 27, 29, and 30, which cover these delivery routes.

There are only two federal programs dedicated solely to health care of women and their infants, and every obstetrician should know about these programs (Lu, 2012). The first is the Title V Maternal and Child Health Services Block Grant, which is the only federal program focused on improving the health of mothers, children, and their families. It was enacted by Congress in 1935 as part of the Social Security Act. Title V provides for state-level block grants in which states match with $3 every $4 in federal money. In 2009, states reported that 2.5 million primarily low-income

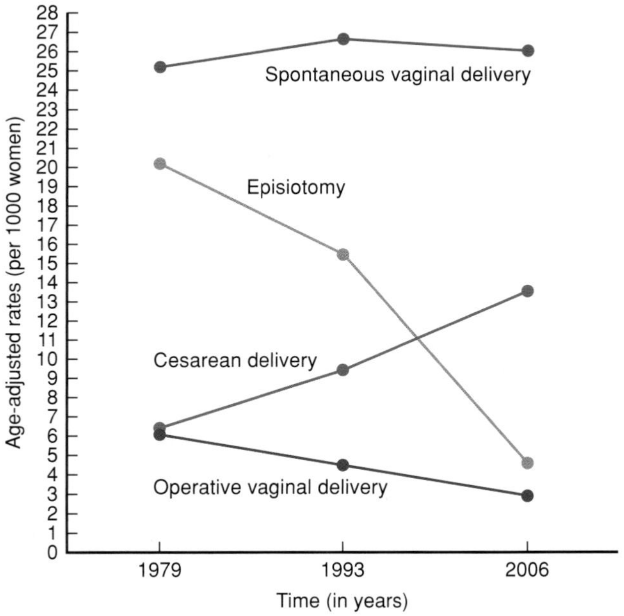

FIGURE 1-8 Age-adjusted rates of obstetrical procedures in the United States, 1979–2006. (Data from Oliphant, 2010.)

pregnant women and 35 million children were served by these state block grants.

The second federal program dedicated to women's health care is the Title X Family Planning Program. This is the only federal program focused on providing women with comprehensive family planning and related preventative health services. Title X was enacted in 1970, and in 2010, it served more than 5.2 million primarily low-income women.

Beginning with implementation of the 2003 United States Standard Birth Certificate described earlier, the principal source of payment for births was reported. In 2010, it was estimated that Medicaid financed 48 percent of the births in the United States (Markus, 2013). Importantly, Medicaid covered a disproportionate number of complicated births. Specifically, Medicaid paid for more than half of all hospital stays for preterm and low-birthweight infants and approximately 45 percent of infant hospital stays due to birth defects.

So, what is the "bottom line" for *obstetrical* health care in the United States for women and their infants? In 2008, the total national hospital bill was almost $1.2 trillion (Wier, 2011). These charges involved 39.9 million hospital stays but do not include outpatient care, emergency care for patients not admitted to the hospital, or physician fees. Medicare and Medicaid paid for 60 percent of the 2008 national hospital bill. Specifically, Medicare covered 46.2 percent and Medicaid 13.8 percent. The hospital bills for the mother's pregnancy and delivery plus care of the newborn exceeded $98 billion, representing 8 percent of all hospital bills. This bill for women and their infants is more than twice that of any other diagnosis across the entire spectrum of American health care and attests to the impact of health care for pregnant women in this country.

The Affordable Care Act

In the last edition of *Williams Obstetrics*, the Obama Administration was poised to pass universal health insurance—so-called Obamacare. This history-making legislation debuted on March 23, 2010, with passage into law of *The Patient Protection and Affordable Care Act—PPACA*. Although constitutional challenges followed, the Supreme Court upheld most aspects of the law in its ruling in 2012 of *National Federation of Independent Business v. Sebelius*. Implementation of this complex legislation began in 2010 and will continue over the current decade (Fig. 1-9). Indeed, initially registration began with a rocky start in late 2013.

As outlined by the Society for Maternal-Fetal Medicine, the act will expand obstetrical care of indigent women (Grande, 2013). The American College of Obstetricians and Gynecologists (2013a) estimates that nearly 20 million uninsured women aged 18 to 64 years have less than optimal access to prenatal care, family planning services, and breast and cervical cancer screening. Many of these women will have improved access to these services because of the expanded Medicaid coverage funded through the Act. The College encourages individual states to expand their Medicaid coverage and improve reimbursement rates.

One "fly in the ointment" of the Affordable Care Act is funding. Although it has been declared "budget neutral,"

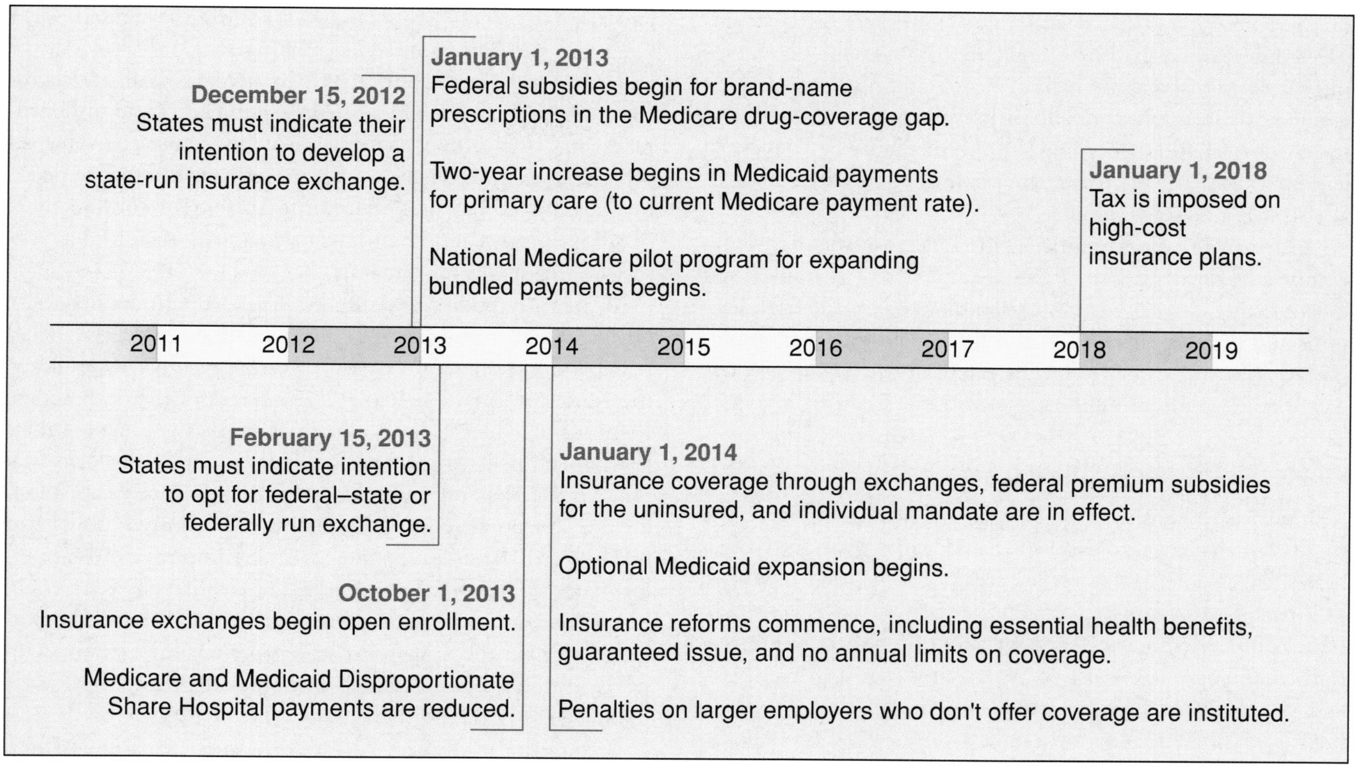

December 15, 2012
States must indicate their intention to develop a state-run insurance exchange.
January 1, 2013
Federal subsidies begin for brand-name prescriptions in the Medicare drug-coverage gap.
Two-year increase begins in Medicaid payments for primary care (to current Medicare payment rate).
National Medicare pilot program for expanding bundled payments begins.
January 1, 2018
Tax is imposed on high-cost insurance plans.
2011
2012
2013
2014
2015
2016
2017
2018
2019
February 15, 2013
States must indicate intention to opt for federal–state or federally run exchange.
January 1, 2014
Insurance coverage through exchanges, federal premium subsidies for the uninsured, and individual mandate are in effect.
Optional Medicaid expansion begins.
Insurance reforms commence, including essential health benefits, guaranteed issue, and no annual limits on coverage.
Penalties on larger employers who don't offer coverage are instituted.
October 1, 2013
Insurance exchanges begin open enrollment.
Medicare and Medicaid Disproportionate Share Hospital payments are reduced.

FIGURE 1-9 Timeline for implementation of provisions of the Patient Protection and Affordable Care Act. (From Oberlander, 2012, with permission.)

the Congressional Budget Office has calculated that 30 million Americans will remain uninsured. For these and a multitude of fiscal reasons—and we certainly do not profess to be economists—we, like Oberlander (2012) and others, remain nervous concerning costs and adequate funding for "universal health care."

Rising Cesarean Delivery Rate

In 2009, the cesarean delivery rate climbed to the highest level ever reported in the United States—32.9 percent (Centers for Disease Control and Prevention, 2013). After that, it appears to have stabilized. This rise in the total rate was a result of upward trends in both the primary and the repeat cesarean delivery rates. Indeed, more than 90 percent of women with a prior cesarean delivery now undergo a repeat procedure. The forces involved in these changes in cesarean delivery rates are multifactorial and complex. We cite a few examples:

1. The major indication for primary cesarean delivery is dystocia, and there is evidence that this diagnosis has increased. This is discussed in Chapter 23 (p. 455).
2. The sharp decline in vaginal births after cesarean (VBAC) delivery is closely related to the uterine rupture risk associated labor with a prior uterine incision. This is discussed throughout Chapter 31.
3. The controversial *cesarean delivery on maternal request (CDMR)* contributes to the rise. This is defined as a cesarean delivery at term for a singleton pregnancy on maternal request in the absence of any medical or obstetrical indication (Reddy, 2006). This is discussed in Chapter 30 (p. 589).
4. Near-term and term pregnancy labor induction is commonplace, and failed inductions contribute to the cesarean delivery rate. This is discussed in Chapter 26 (p. 524).

It is not possible to precisely measure the contribution of each of these components to the all-time-high cesarean delivery rate. The American College of Obstetricians and Gynecologists and the Maternal-Fetal Medicine Units Network have addressed these in an attempt to curtail the rising rate. The National Institute of Child Health and Human Development convened a State-of-the-Science Conference in 2006 to provide an in-depth evaluation of the evidence regarding cesarean delivery on maternal request. To date, there have been no evidence-based guidelines. Recognizing that repeat operations constitute a large percentage of cesarean deliveries, the National Institutes of Health (2010) convened a consensus conference entitled *Vaginal Birth after Cesarean: New Insights*. The findings are discussed in detail in Chapter 31 (p. 609), but to summarize, they supported a trial of labor for many selected women with a prior cesarean hysterotomy scar and recommended that this option be made more available. It is too early to conclude if this recommendation has significantly altered the cesarean delivery rate.

Genomic Technology

Recent breakthroughs in fetal testing and diagnosis are truly stunning. In one recent issue of the *New England Journal of Medicine,* there were three reports in which prenatal gene microarray techniques were used for clinical management (Dugoff, 2012). The advantages of these techniques are outlined in Chapters 13 and 14. Wapner and coworkers (2012) compared microarray analysis of maternal blood with karyotyping for chromosomal anomalies. Reddy and associates (2012) applied this technology to stillbirth evaluation and reported it to be superior to karyotyping. The third report by Talkowski and colleagues (2012) described whole-genome sequencing of a fetus using maternal blood.

Added to these possibilities is the specter of made-to-order embryos (Cohen, 2013). These are but a few examples that illustrate the power of genomic technology to pursue fetal diagnosis and possible therapy. At this juncture, there are complex obstacles to overcome, but with rapid advancement of these technologies, success is almost assured.

Electronic Health Records

Rising costs, inconsistent quality, and patient safety issues are significant challenges to the delivery of health care in the United States. Electronic health records (EHR) have been identified as a means of improving provider efficiency and effectiveness (Jha, 2009). Methods to speed the adoption of health information technology have received bipartisan support in Congress, and the *American Recovery and Reinvestment Act of 2009* has made such a system a national priority. This was soon followed by the *Health Information Technology for Economic and Clinical Health (HITECH) Act.* Recent surveys indicate that approximately half of outpatient practices and hospitals in the United States are now using EHR. This act also introduced the concept of "meaningful use" EHRs by providers. Classen and Bates (2011) appropriately note, however, that "meaningful use" does not necessarily equate with "meaningful benefits." According to the American College of Obstetricians and Gynecologists (2010), studies of effectiveness are critically needed to justify the safe implementation of these costly electronic computerized systems.

Health-Care Outcomes Research

Although per capita health-care expenditures in the United States are the highest in the world, health-care outcomes frequently lag behind those in nations spending far less. A major factor in this disparity is thought to be expenditure overuse, underuse, and misuse driven by rationale-based instead of evidence-based health care. Buried within the 2400 pages of the landmark health-care reform bill signed into law by President Barack Obama are several provisions that touch on clinical research (Kaiser, 2010). Two are aimed at determining which health-care interventions work best and identifying financial conflicts of researchers. A third provision funds acceleration of new drug development. Proponents hope these research studies will improve the quality and lower the cost of health care by identifying the best treatments. We applaud this effort. Indeed, we are of the view that systematic prospective measurement of health-care outcomes as related to treatments prescribed should be an on-going requirement for the practice of medicine.

Much publicity followed the report by the Institute of Medicine entitled *To Err Is Human* (Kohn, 2000). This report greatly increased interest in measuring health-care outcomes and adverse events (Grobman, 2006). Even the United States Congress has determined that reimbursements by Medicare and Medicaid should be indexed to selected health-care outcomes. Specifically, a wide, often dizzying spectrum of benchmarks has been proposed to measure the quality and safety of obstetrical care. In our view, the greatest impediment to deriving meaningful measures of obstetrical care is the continued use of administrative and financial data—instead of clinical data—to set benchmarks for outcomes.

Regulatory bodies typically evaluate hospital quality using obstetrical outcomes derived from administrative (financial) datasets not designed to measure clinical results. Accordingly, the Maternal-Fetal Medicine Units Network of the National Institute of Child Health and Human Development undertook an unprecedented and unparalleled study of obstetrical outcomes based on carefully collected *clinical data* (Bailit, 2013). The purpose was to establish risk-adjusted models for five obstetrical outcomes and then determine if hospital performance could be reliably measured so that hospitals could be compared. Outcomes studied included postpartum hemorrhage, peripartum infection, severe perineal laceration, neonatal morbidity, and venous thromboembolism. This study included 115,502 mother-infant pairs managed for 3 years at 25 hospitals. Clinical data were abstracted from medical records by specially trained research nurses using a prespecified manual of operations. The study clearly demonstrated that differences between obstetrical outcomes at different hospitals, when clinically adjusted for preexisting patient characteristics, *cannot* be used to accurately compare obstetrical care among hospitals.

So, what does this mean? It means that the widespread current practice of ranking obstetrical care at different hospitals based on single outcomes, such as third- or fourth-degree perineal lacerations, is useless when accurate data are used. Moreover, use of up to four obstetrical outcomes did not improve the ability to rank hospitals. Actually, use of more than one outcome greatly confused the ranking. A given hospital might rank number one out of 25 hospitals for one obstetrical outcome and 25 out of 25 for a second outcome. Thus, a given hospital could be both very good and very bad depending on the obstetrical outcome analyzed!

Medical Liability

Approximately 12 percent of obstetrician-gynecologists had at least one malpractice claim each year from 1991 through 2005 (Jena, 2011). The American College of Obstetricians and Gynecologists periodically surveys its fellows concerning the effect of liability on their practice. The 2012 Survey on Professional Liability is the 11th such survey since 1983 (Klagholz, 2012). The survey reflects experiences of more than 9000 members, and 58 percent of these fellows responded that some aspect(s) of the liability environment had caused them to alter their practice since the last survey. Undoubtedly not all of these changes were positive. Those cited included an increased cesarean delivery rate, fewer trials of labor after a prior cesarean delivery, and a decreased number of high-risk patients and total deliveries (Amon, 2014). Others have chosen to forego obstetrical practice entirely. Some of these changes have been linked to states with higher liability premiums (Zwecker, 2011).

Thus, by all accounts, there is still a "liability crisis," and the reasons for it are complex. Because it is largely driven by money and politics, a consensus seems unlikely. Although some interests are diametrically opposite, other factors contribute to the complexity of the crisis. For example, each state has its own laws and opinions of "tort reform." Meanwhile, liability claims remain a "hot button" in obstetrics because of their inherent adversarial nature and the sometimes outlandish plaintiff verdicts that contribute to increasing liability insurance premiums. In some states, annual premiums for obstetricians approach $300,000—expenses that at least partially are borne by the patient and certainly by the entire health-care system. Liability issues are daunting, and in 2008, all tort costs in the United States totaled nearly $255 billion. This is an astounding 1.8 percent of the gross domestic product and averages $838 per citizen (Towers Perrin, 2009). Annas (2013) has provided an interesting review of two centuries of malpractice law history. Interestingly, he compares medical malpractice litigation to the white whale in Melville's *Moby-Dick*—evil, ubiquitous, and seemingly immoral!

The American College of Obstetricians and Gynecologists has taken a lead in adopting a fair system for malpractice litigation—or *maloccurrence litigation*. The Committee on Professional Liability has produced several related documents that help fellows cope with the stresses of litigation, that provide advice for the obstetrician giving expert testimony, and that outline recommendations for disclosure of any adverse events (American College of Obstetricians and Gynecologists, 2013c,d,e).

National liability reform likely will come in some form with the push for universal medical insurance coverage. President Obama, in his 2009 address to the American Medical Association, indicated that national malpractice liability reform was negotiable. United States Congressman Michael Burgess—an obstetrician-gynecologist—asked the president to reaffirm this commitment. We applaud these efforts and wish for their success.

Home Births

Following a slight decline from 1990 through 2004, according to the National Center for Health Statistics, the percentage of home births in the United States increased from 0.56 to 0.72 percent—almost 70 percent—through 2009 (MacDorman, 2012b). But, as is so often the case with data analysis, the "devil is in the details." Only 62 percent of these 24,970 home births were attended by midwives—19 percent by certified nurse midwives and 43 percent by so-called lay midwives with minimal formal training. The remaining 38 percent of home births were *unplanned*—that is, the result of accidental delivery at home attended by a family member or emergency medical technician. So is home birth a good idea? Those currently conducted in the United States in which women are not attended by trained and certified personnel cannot be considered acceptable. There have been no randomized trials to test the safety of home deliveries (Olsen, 2012). Proponents of home births cite success from laudatory observational data from European countries such as England and The Netherlands (Van der Kooy, 2011). Data from the United States, however, are less convincing and indicate a higher incidence of perinatal morbidity and mortality (Grünebaum, 2013, 2014; Wasden, 2014; Wax, 2010). These findings have led Chervenak and coworkers (2013) to question the ethics of participation in planned home births.

Family Planning Services

Politics and religion over the years have led to various governmental interferences with the reproductive rights of women. These intrusions have disparately affected indigent women and adolescents. One example was the consideration by Congress in 1998 for the Title X Parental Notification Act. Reddy and colleagues (2002) estimated this bill would have dissuaded almost half of adolescents younger than 17 years from seeking contraceptive services and care for sexually transmitted disease.

Another example is the tug-of-war over emergency contraception, and more specifically over the *morning-after pill* (Chap. 38, p. 714). Efforts begun in 2004 by the Bush Administration to curtail *Plan B* for over-the-counter sales to women 17 years and younger was decried appropriately by editorials in the *New England Journal of Medicine* (Drazen, 2004; Steinbrook, 2004). This issue was not settled until April 2013 when a federal district court in New York ordered the Food and Drug Administration to make emergency contraception available for over-the-counter sales to all women regardless of age. The decision was quickly applauded by the American College of Obstetricians and Gynecologists (2013f). The decision was editorialized as "science prevails" in a subsequent issue of *Nature* (2013).

Perhaps the most egregious example of both federal and state governmental intrusion into women's reproductive rights is the often poor availability of federally funded family planning services for indigent women. This is despite all reports of the overwhelming success of such programs. According to the Guttmacher Institute, publicly funded family planning services in 2010 prevented nearly 2.2 million unintended pregnancies and 760,000 abortions in the United States. They concluded that without such funding the abortion rate would be nearly two-thirds higher for all women, and nearly 70-percent higher for adolescents (Frost, 2013). The American College of Obstetricians and Gynecologists (2012) has recently reviewed these and other barriers to emergency contraception access.

Abortion

It continues to be a preventable fact that up to a fifth of pregnancies in this country are terminated by elective abortion (see Table 1-1). According to the American College of Obstetricians and Gynecologists (2011): "The most effective way to reduce the number of abortions is to prevent unwanted and unintended pregnancies." Importantly, the negative attitudes, beliefs, and policies toward family planning services and sex education discussed above have helped to contribute to the more than 800,000 abortions performed yearly in the United States.

The history of legislative regulation and federal court decisions regarding abortions is considered in Chapter 18 (p. 363). The *Partial Birth Abortion Ban Act of 2003* has become law, and in 2007, the Supreme Court ruled that the ban—officially known as *Gonzales v. Carhart*—is constitutional. This again caused editorialists in the *New England Journal of Medicine* to decry the intrusion of government into medicine (Charo, 2007; Drazen, 2007; Greene, 2007). More ominous are restrictive state laws—many of which have been or will be ruled unconstitutional—which according to some will drive *Roe v. Wade* back to the Supreme Court.

REFERENCES

American Academy of Pediatrics and American College of Obstetricians and Gynecologists: Guidelines for perinatal care. 7th ed. Washington, 2012

American College of Obstetricians and Gynecologists: Patient safety and the electronic health record. Committee Opinion No. 472, November 2010

American College of Obstetricians and Gynecologists: Abortion policy. College Statement of Policy. September 2000. Reaffirmed July 2011

American College of Obstetricians and Gynecologists: Access to emergency contraception. Committee Opinion No. 542, November 2012

American College of Obstetricians and Gynecologists: Benefits to women of Medicaid expansion through the Affordable Care Act. Committee Opinion No. 552, January 2013a

American College of Obstetricians and Gynecologists: Definition of term pregnancy. Committee Opinion No. 579, November 2013b

American College of Obstetricians and Gynecologists: Disclosure and discussion of adverse events. Committee Opinion No. 520, March 2012, Reaffirmed 2013c

American College of Obstetricians and Gynecologists: Expert testimony. Committee Opinion No. 374, August 2007, Reaffirmed 2013d

American College of Obstetricians and Gynecologists: Coping with the stress of medical professional liability litigation. Committee Opinion No. 551, January 2013e

American College of Obstetricians and Gynecologists: Statement on FDA Approval of OTC Emergency Contraception. May 1, 2013f. Available at: http://www.acog.org/About_ACOG/News_Room/News_Releases/2013/Statement_on_FDA_Approval_of_OTC_Emergency_Contraception. Accessed October 24, 2013

Amon E, Bombard A, Bronsky G, et al: SMFM liability survey. Am J Obstet Gynecol 210:S242, 2014

Annas GJ: Doctors, patients, and lawyers—two centuries of health law. N Engl J Med 367(5):445, 2013

Bailit JL, Grobman WA, Rice MM, et al: Risk-adjusted models for adverse obstetric outcomes and variation in risk adjusted outcomes across hospitals. Am J Obstet Gynecol 209(5):446.e1, 2013

Berg CJ, Callaghan WM, Syverson C, et al: Pregnancy-related mortality in the United States, 1998 to 2005. Obstet Gynecol 116:1302, 2010

Berg CJ, Harper MA, Atkinson SM, et al: Preventability of pregnancy-related deaths. Results of a state-wide review. Obstet Gynecol 106:1228, 2005

Callaghan WM, Creanga AA, Kuklina EV: Severe maternal morbidity among delivery and postpartum hospitalizations in the United States. Obstet Gynecol 120(5):1029, 2012

Centers for Disease Control and Prevention: The challenge of fetal mortality. NCHS Data Brief No. 16, April 2009

Centers for Disease Control and Prevention: Changes in cesarean delivery rates by gestational age: United States, 1996–2011. NCHS Data Brief No. 124, June 2013

Chang J, Elam-Evans LD, Berg CJ, et al: Pregnancy-related mortality surveillance-United States, 1991–1999. MMWR 52(2):4, 2003

Charo RA: The partial death of abortion rights. N Engl J Med 356:2125, 2007

Chervenak FA, McCullough LB, Brent RL, et al: Planned home birth: the professional responsibility response. Am J Obstet Gynecol 208(1):31, 2013

Clark SL, Belfort MA, Dildy GA, et al: Maternal death in the 21st century: causes, prevention, and relationship to cesarean delivery. Am J Obstet Gynecol 199(1):36.e1, 2008

Clark SL, Meyers JA, Frye DR, et al: A systematic approach to the identification and classification of near-miss events on labor and delivery in a large, national health care system. Am J Obstet Gynecol 207(5):441, 2012

Classen DC, Bates DW: Finding the meaning in meaningful use. N Engl J Med 365:855, 2011

Cohen IG, Adashi EY, et al: Made-to-order embryos for sale—a brave new world? N Engl J Med 368(26):2517, 2013

Deneux-Tharaux C, Carmona E, Bouvier-Colle MH, et al: Postpartum maternal mortality and cesarean delivery. Obstet Gynecol 108:541, 2006

Drazen JM: Government in medicine. N Engl J Med 356:2195, 2007

Drazen JM, Greene MF, Wood AJJ: The FDA, politics, and Plan B. N Engl J Med 350:1561, 2004

Dugoff L: Application of genomic technology in prenatal diagnosis. N Engl J Med 367(23):2249, 2012

Frey WH: America reaches its demographic tipping point. 2011. Available at: http://www.brookings.edu/blogs/up-front/posts//2011/08/26-census-race-frey. Accessed September 24, 2013

Frost JJ, Zolna MR, Frohwirth L: Contraceptive Needs and Services, 2010. New York, Guttmacher Institute, 2013

Grande D, Srinivas SK, for the Society of Maternal-Fetal Medicine Health Care Policy Committee: Leveraging the Affordable Care Act to improve the health of mothers and newborns. Obstet Gynecol 121:1300, 2013

Greene MF: The intimidation of American physicians—banning partial-birth abortion. N Engl J Med 356:2128, 2007

Grobman WA: Patient safety in obstetrics and gynecology. The call to arms. Obstet Gynecol 108(5):1058, 2006

Grünebaum A, McCullough LB, Sapra KJ, et al: Apgar score of 0 at 5 minutes and neonatal seizures or serious neurologic dysfunction in relation to birth setting. Am J Obstet Gynecol 209(4):323, 2013

Grünebaum A, Sapra K, Chervenak F: Term neonatal deaths resulting from home births: an increasing trend. Am J Obstet Gynecol 210:S57, 2014

Hale RW, DiVenere L: Health care reform and your practice. ACOG Clinical Review 15(6–supplement):1S, 2010

Halliday LE, Peek MJ, Ellwood DA, et al: The Australasian Maternity Outcomes Surveillance System: an evaluation of stakeholder engagement, usefulness, simplicity, acceptability, data quality and stability. Aust N Z J Obstet Gynaecol 53(2):152, 2013

Hamilton BE, Martin JA, Ventura SJ: Births: Preliminary data for 2011. Natl Vital Stat Rep 61(5):1, 2012

Hoyert DL: Maternal mortality and related concepts. Vital Health Stat 3(33):1, 2007

Institute for Safe Medication Practices: ISMP survey helps define near miss and close call. Medication Safety Alert, September 24, 2009. Available at: https://www.ismp.org/newsletters/acutecare/articles/20090924.asp. Accessed October 25, 2013

Jena AB, Seabury S, Lakdawalla D, et al: Malpractice risk according to physician specialty. N Engl J Med 365(7):629, 2011

Jha AK, DesRoches CM, Campbell EG, et al: Use of electronic health records in US hospitals. N Engl J Med 360:1628, 2009

Kaiser J: Health bill backs evidence-based medicine, new drug studies. Science 327(5973):1562, 2010

King JC: Maternal mortality in the United States–why is it important and what are we doing about it? Semin Perinatol 36(1):14, 2012

Klagholz J, Strunk A: Overview of the 2012 ACOG survey on professional liability. Washington, American Congress of Obstetricians and Gynecologists, 2012

Knight M, UKOSS: Antenatal pulmonary embolism: risk factors, management and outcomes. BJOG 115:453, 2008

Knight M, Kurinczuk JJ, Tuffnell D, et al: The UK obstetric surveillance system for rare disorders of pregnancy. BJOG 112:263, 2005

Kohn LT, Corrigan JM, Donaldson MS (eds): To err is human: building a safer health system. Washington, National Academy Press, 2000

Koonin LM, MacKay AP, Berg CJ, et al: Pregnancy-related mortality surveillance—United States, 1987–1990. MMWR 46(4):17, 1997

Lang CT, King JC: Maternal mortality in the United States. Best Pract Res Clin Obstet Gynaecol 22(3):5117, 2008

Lu MC, Gee RE: What every obstetrician-gynecologist should know about Title V and Title X. Obstet Gynecol 120(3):513, 2012

MacDorman MF, Kirmeyer SE, Wilson EC: Fetal and perinatal mortality, United States, 2006. Natl Vital Stat Rep 60(8):1, 2012a

MacDorman MF, Mathews TJ, Declercq E: Home births in the United States, 1990–2009. NHCS Data Brief No. 84, January 2012b

MacKay AP, Berg CJ, Duran C, et al: An assessment of pregnancy-related mortality in the United States. Paediatr Perinat Epidemiol 19(3):206, 2005

Markus AR, Andrés E, West KD, et al: Medicaid covered births, 2008 through 2010, in the context of the implementation of health reform. Womens Health Issues 23(5):e273, 2013

Mosher WD, Jones, J, Abma JC: Intended and unintended births in the United States: 1982–2010. Natl Health Stat Report 55:1, 2012

National Institutes of Health: National Institutes of Health consensus development conference statement. Vaginal birth after cesarean: new insights March 8–10, 2010. Obstet Gynecol 115(6):1279, 2010

Nature Editorial: Science prevails. The US government gives up its fight to keep age restrictions on the morning-after pill. Nature 498:272, 2013
Oberlander J: The future of Obamacare. N Engl J Med 367(23):2165, 2012
Oestergaard MZ, Inoue M, Yoshida S, et al: Neonatal mortality levels for 193 countries in 2009 with trends since 1990: a systematic analysis of progress, projections, and priorities. PLoS Med 8(8):e1001080, 2011
Oliphant SS, Jones KA, Wang L, et al: Trends over time with commonly performed obstetrics and gynecologic inpatient procedures. Obstet Gynecol 116:926, 2010
Olsen O, Clausen JA: Planned hospital birth versus planned home birth. Cochrane Database Syst Rev 9:CD000352, 2012
Reddy DM, Fleming R, Swain C: Effect of mandatory parental notification on adolescent girls' use of sexual health care services. JAMA 288:710, 2002
Reddy UM, Page GP, Saade GR, et al: Karyotype versus microarray testing for genetic abnormalities after stillbirth. N Engl J Med 367(23):2185, 2012
Reddy UM, Spong CY: Introduction. Semin Perinatol 30(5):233, 2006
Robertson R, Squires D, Garber T, et al: Realizing health reform's potential. Oceans apart: the higher health costs of women in the US compared to other nations, and how reform is helping. Commonwealth Fund No. 1606, Vol. 19, 2012
Souza JP, Cecatti JG, Haddad SM, et al: The WHO maternal near-miss approach and the maternal severity index model (MSI): tools for assessing the management of severe maternal morbidity. PLoS One 7(8):e44129, 2012
Steinbrook R: Waiting for Plan B—the FDA and nonprescription use of emergency contraception. N Engl J Med 350:2327, 2004
St. John EB, Nelson KG, Cliver SP, et al: Cost of neonatal care according to gestational age at birth and survival status. Am J Obstet Gynecol 182:170, 2000
Sutton PD, Hamilton BE, Mathews TJ. Recent decline in births in the United States, 2007–2009. NCHS Data Brief No. 60, March 2011
Talkowski ME, Ordulu Z, Pillalamarri V, et al: Clinical diagnosis by whole-genome sequencing of a prenatal sample. N Engl J Med 367(23):2226, 2012
Towers Perrin: 2009 update on US tort cost trends. 2009. Available at: http://www.towersperrin.com/tp/getwebcachedoc?webc=USA/2009/200912/2009_tort_trend_report_12-8_09.pdf. Accessed October 25, 2013
Tuncalp O, Hindin MJ, Souza JP, et al: The prevalence of maternal near miss: a systematic review. BJOG 119(6):653, 2012
Van der Kooy J, Poeran J, de Graaf JP, et al: Planned home compared with planned hospital births in the Netherlands. Obstet Gynecol 118(5):1037, 2011
Ventura SJ, Curtin SC, Abma JC, et al: Estimated pregnancy rates and rates of pregnancy outcomes for the United States, 1990–2008. Natl Vital Stat Rep 60(7):1, 2012
Wapner RJ, Martin CL, Levy B, et al: Chromosomal microarray versus karyotyping for prenatal diagnosing. N Engl J Med 367(23):2175, 2012
Wasden S, Perlman J, Chasen S, et al: Home birth and risk of neonatal hypoxic ischemic encephalopathy. Am J Obstet Gynecol 210:S251, 2014
Wax JR, Lucas FJ, Lamont M, et al: Maternal and newborn outcomes in planned home birth vs planned hospital births: a metaanalysis. Am J Obstet Gynecol 203(3):243, 2010
Wier LM, Andrews RM: The national hospital bill: the most expensive conditions by payer, 2008. Healthcare Cost and Utilization Project Statistical Brief No. 107, March 2011
Zwecker P, Azoulay L, Abenhaim HA: Effect of fear of litigation on obstetric care: a nationwide analysis on obstetric practice. Am J Perinatol 28(4):277, 2011

SECTION 2

MATERNAL ANATOMY AND PHYSIOLOGY

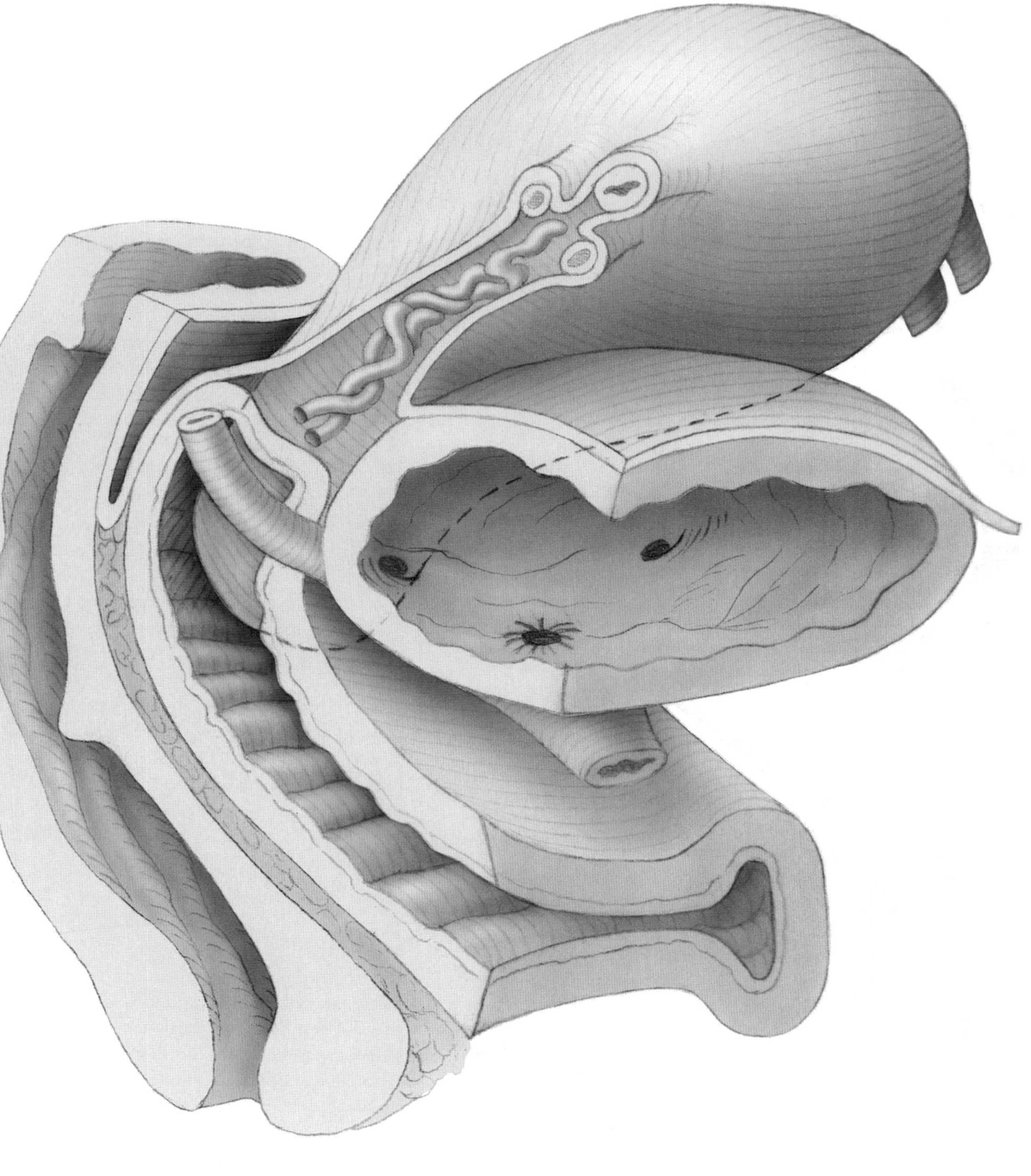

CHAPTER 2

Maternal Anatomy

An understanding of female pelvic and lower abdominal wall anatomy is essential for obstetrical practice. Although consistent relationships between these structures are the norm, there may be marked variation in individual women. This is especially true for major blood vessels and nerves.

ANTERIOR ABDOMINAL WALL

Skin, Subcutaneous Layer, and Fascia

The anterior abdominal wall confines abdominal viscera, stretches to accommodate the expanding uterus, and provides surgical access to the internal reproductive organs. Thus, a comprehensive knowledge of its layered structure is required to surgically enter the peritoneal cavity.

Langer lines describe the orientation of dermal fibers within the skin. In the anterior abdominal wall, they are arranged transversely. As a result, vertical skin incisions sustain increased lateral tension and thus, in general, develop wider scars. In contrast, low transverse incisions, such as the Pfannenstiel, follow Langer lines and lead to superior cosmetic results.

The subcutaneous layer can be separated into a superficial, predominantly fatty layer—Camper fascia, and a deeper membranous layer—Scarpa fascia. Camper fascia continues onto the perineum to provide fatty substance to the mons pubis and labia majora and then to blend with the fat of the ischioanal fossa. Scarpa fascia continues inferiorly onto the perineum as Colles fascia (p. 22). As a result, perineal infection or hemorrhage superficial to Colles fascia has the ability to extend upward to involve the superficial layers of the abdominal wall.

Beneath the subcutaneous layer, the anterior abdominal wall muscles consist of the midline rectus abdominis and pyramidalis muscles as well as the external oblique, internal oblique, and transversus abdominis muscles, which extend across the entire wall (Fig. 2-1). The fibrous aponeuroses of these three latter muscles form the primary fascia of the anterior abdominal wall. These fuse in the midline at the linea alba, which normally measures 10 to 15 mm wide below the umbilicus (Beer, 2009). An abnormally wide separation may reflect diastasis recti or hernia.

These three aponeuroses also invest the rectus abdominis muscle as the rectus sheath. The construction of this sheath varies above and below a boundary, termed the arcuate line (Fig. 2-2). Cephalad to this border, the aponeuroses invest the rectus abdominis bellies on both dorsal and ventral surfaces. Caudal to this line, all aponeuroses lie ventral or superficial to the rectus abdominis muscle, and only the thin transversalis fascia and peritoneum lie beneath the rectus (Loukas, 2008). This transition of rectus sheath composition can be seen best with a midline abdominal incision. Last, the paired small triangular pyramidalis muscles originate from the pubic crest, insert into the linea alba, and lie atop the rectus abdominis muscle but beneath the anterior rectus sheath.

Blood Supply

The superficial epigastric, superficial circumflex iliac, and superficial external pudendal arteries arise from the femoral artery just below the inguinal ligament within the femoral triangle. These vessels supply the skin and subcutaneous layers of the anterior abdominal wall and mons pubis. Of surgical importance, the superficial epigastric vessels, from their origin, course diagonally toward the umbilicus. With a low transverse

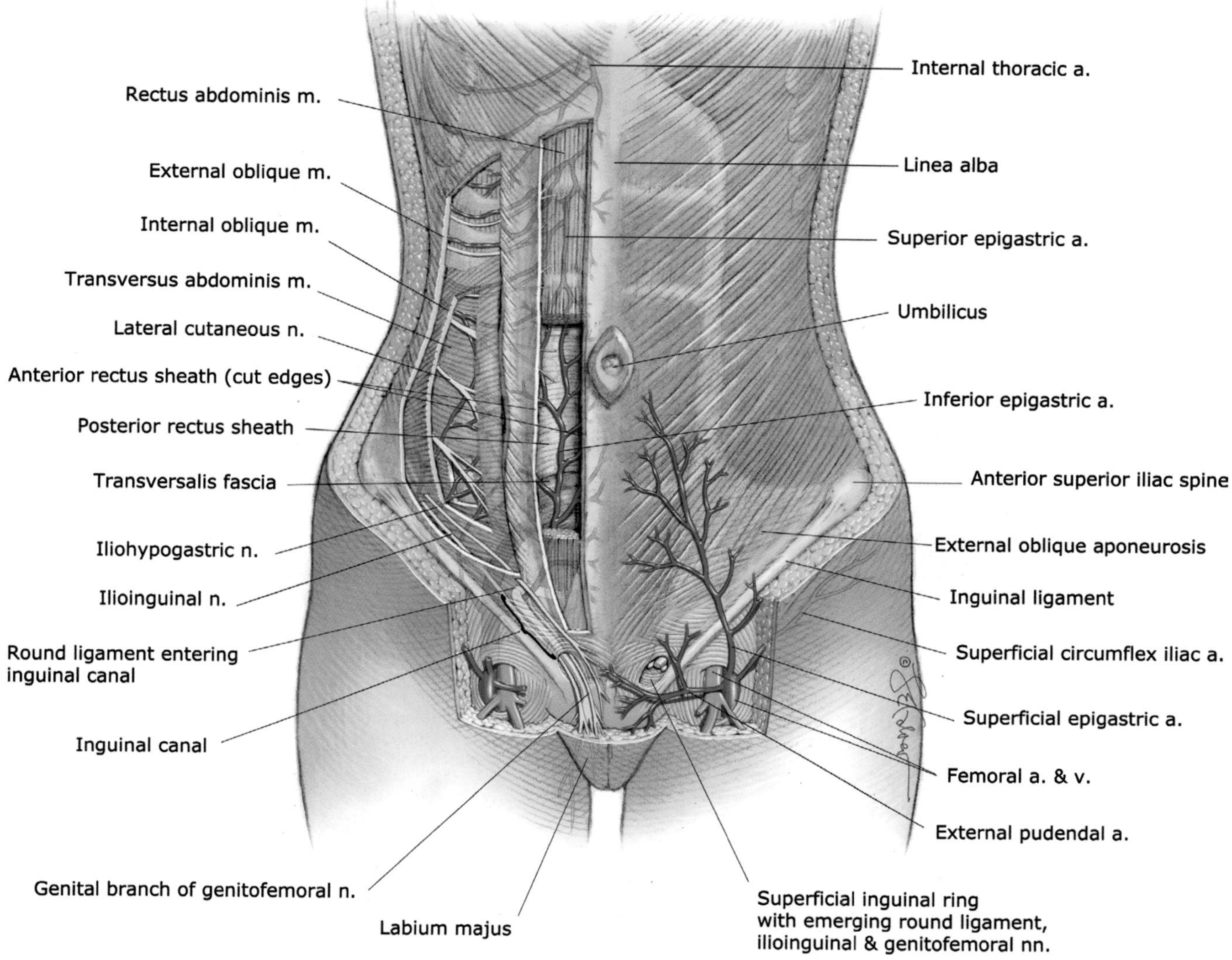

FIGURE 2-1 Anterior abdominal wall anatomy. (From Corton, 2012, with permission.)

skin incision, these vessels can usually be identified at a depth halfway between the skin and the anterior rectus sheath, above Scarpa fascia, and several centimeters from the midline.

In contrast, the inferior "deep" epigastric vessels and deep circumflex iliac vessels are branches of the external iliac vessels. They supply the muscles and fascia of the anterior abdominal wall. Of surgical relevance, the inferior epigastric vessels initially course lateral to, then posterior to the rectus abdominis muscles, which they supply. These vessels then pass ventral to the posterior rectus sheath and course between the sheath and the rectus muscles. Near the umbilicus, these vessels anastomose with the superior epigastric artery and veins, which are branches of the internal thoracic vessels. When a Maylard incision is used for cesarean delivery, the inferior epigastric artery may be lacerated lateral to the rectus belly during muscle transection. These vessels rarely may rupture following abdominal trauma and create a rectus sheath hematoma (Tolcher, 2010).

On each side of the lower anterior abdominal wall, Hesselbach triangle is the region bounded laterally by the inferior epigastric vessels, inferiorly by the inguinal ligament, and medially by the lateral border of the rectus muscle. Hernias that protrude through the abdominal wall in Hesselbach triangle are termed direct inguinal hernias. In contrast, indirect inguinal hernias do so through the deep inguinal ring, which lies lateral to this triangle, and then may exit out the superficial inguinal ring.

Innervation

The anterior abdominal wall is innervated by intercostal nerves (T_{7-11}), the subcostal nerve (T_{12}), and the iliohypogastric and the ilioinguinal nerves (L_1). Of these, the intercostal and subcostal nerves are anterior rami of the thoracic spinal nerves and run along the lateral and then anterior abdominal wall between the transversus abdominis and internal oblique muscles. This space is termed the transversus abdominis plane. Near the rectus abdominis lateral borders, these nerve branches pierce the posterior sheath, rectus muscle, and then anterior sheath to reach the skin. Thus, these nerve branches may be severed during a Pfannenstiel incision at the point in which the overlying anterior rectus sheath is separated from the rectus muscle.

In contrast, the iliohypogastric and ilioinguinal nerves originate from the anterior ramus of the first lumbar spinal nerve. They emerge lateral to the psoas muscle and travel retroperitoneally across the quadratus lumborum inferomedially

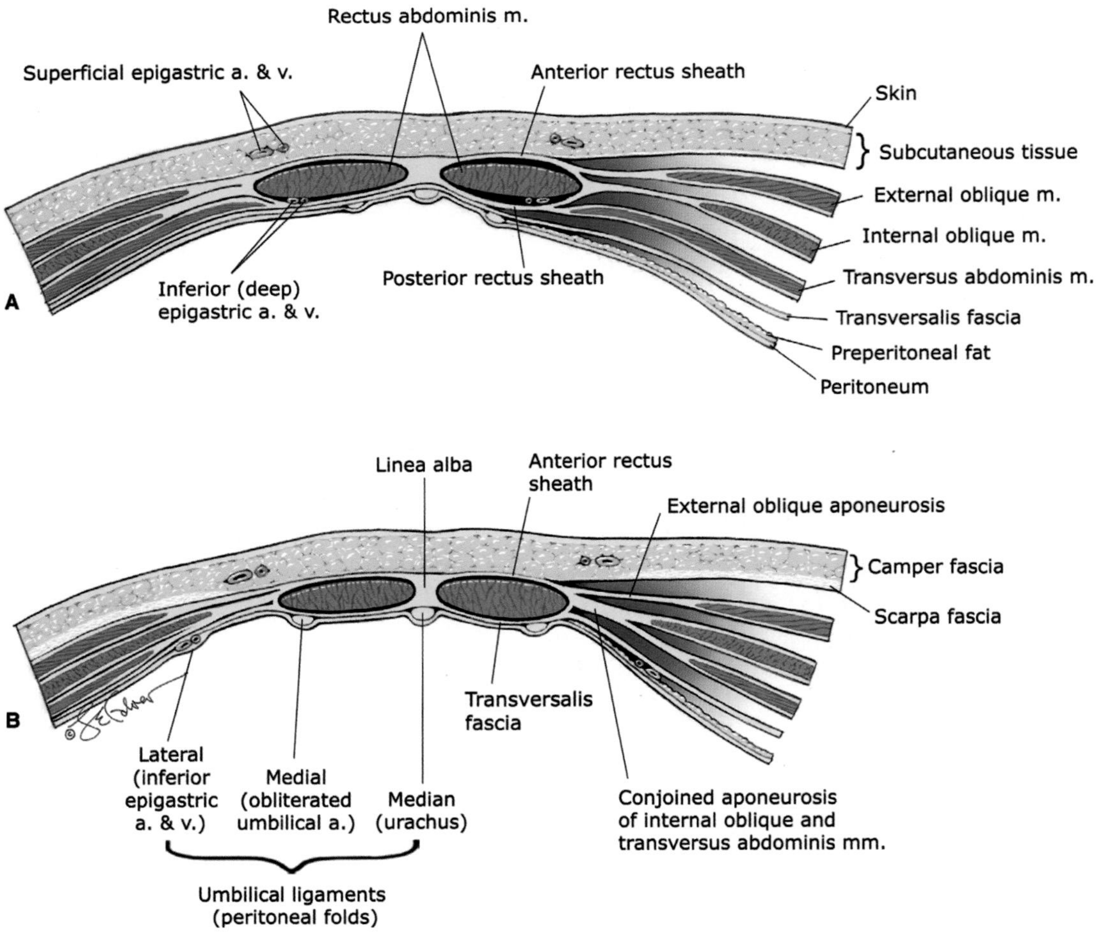

FIGURE 2-2 Transverse sections of anterior abdominal wall above **(A)** and below **(B)** the arcuate line. (From Corton, 2012, with permission.)

toward the iliac crest. Near this crest, both nerves pierce the transversus abdominis muscle and course ventrally. At a site 2 to 3 cm medial to the anterior superior iliac spine, the nerves then pierce the internal oblique muscle and course superficial to it toward the midline (Whiteside, 2003). The iliohypogastric nerve perforates the external oblique aponeurosis near the lateral rectus border to provide sensation to the skin over the suprapubic area. The ilioinguinal nerve in its course medially travels through the inguinal canal and exits through the superficial inguinal ring, which forms by splitting of external abdominal oblique aponeurosis fibers. This nerve supplies the skin of the mons pubis, upper labia majora, and medial upper thigh.

The ilioinguinal and iliohypogastric nerves can be severed during a low transverse incision or entrapped during closure, especially if incisions extend beyond the lateral borders of the rectus muscle (Rahn, 2010). These nerves carry sensory information only, and injury leads to loss of sensation within the areas supplied. Rarely, however, chronic pain may develop.

The T_{10} dermatome approximates the level of the umbilicus. As discussed in Chapter 25 (p. 511), regional analgesia for cesarean delivery or for puerperal sterilization ideally blocks T_{10} through L_1 levels. In addition, a transversus abdominis plane block can provide broad blockade to the nerves that traverse this plane and may be placed postcesarean to reduce analgesia requirements (Mishriky, 2012). There are also reports of rectus sheath block or ilioinguinal-iliohypogastric nerve block to decrease postoperative pain (Mei, 2011; Sviggum, 2012; Wolfson, 2012).

EXTERNAL GENERATIVE ORGANS

Vulva

Mons Pubis, Labia, and Clitoris

The pudenda—commonly designated the vulva—includes all structures visible externally from the symphysis pubis to the perineal body. This includes the mons pubis, labia majora and minora, clitoris, hymen, vestibule, urethral opening, greater vestibular or Bartholin glands, minor vestibular glands, and paraurethral glands (Fig. 2-3). The embryology of the external genitalia is discussed in Chapter 7 (p. 144), and its innervations and vascular support are described with the pudendal nerve (p. 24).

The mons pubis, also called the mons veneris, is a fat-filled cushion overlying the symphysis pubis. After puberty, the mons pubis skin is covered by curly hair that forms the escutcheon. In women, hair is distributed in a triangle, whose base covers the upper margin of the symphysis pubis and whose tip ends at the clitoris. In men and some hirsute women, the escutcheon is not so well circumscribed and extends onto the anterior abdominal wall toward the umbilicus.

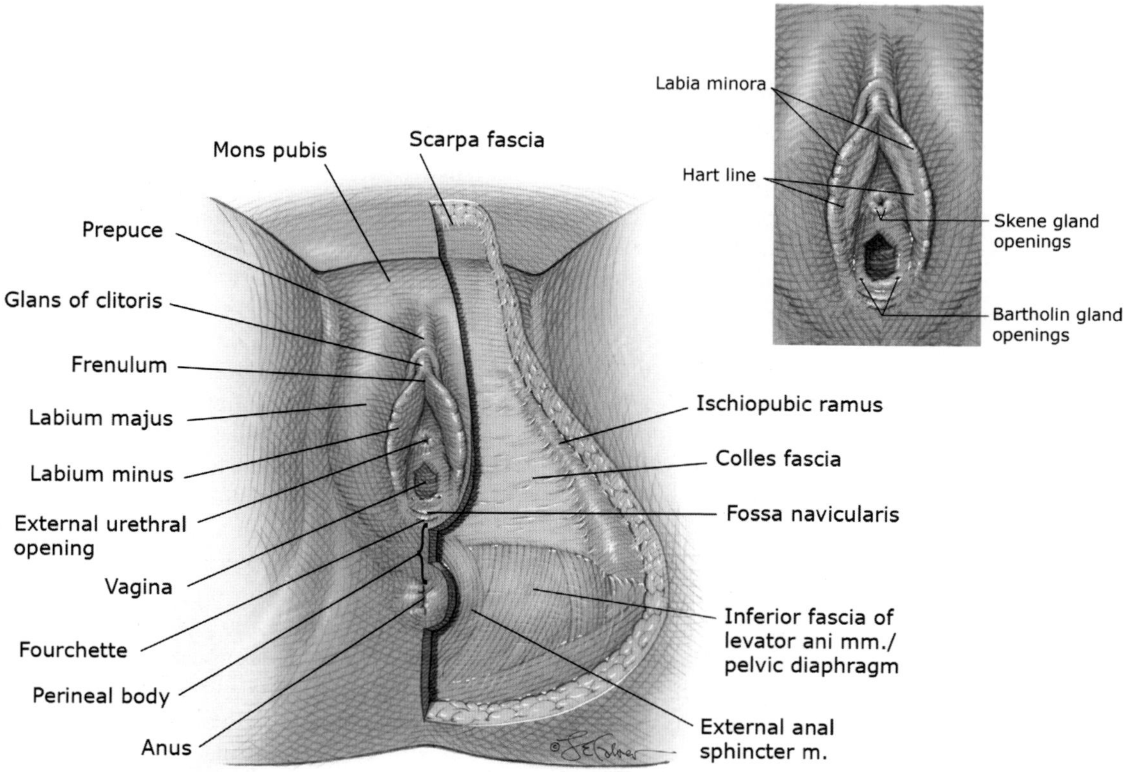

FIGURE 2-3 Vulvar structures and subcutaneous layer of the anterior perineal triangle. Note the continuity of Colles and Scarpa fasciae. Inset: Vestibule boundaries and openings onto the vestibule. (From Corton, 2012, with permission.)

Embryologically, the labia majora are homologous with the male scrotum. Labia vary somewhat in appearance, principally according to the amount of fat they contain. They are 7 to 8 cm in length, 2 to 3 cm in depth, and 1 to 1.5 cm in thickness. They are continuous directly with the mons pubis superiorly, and the round ligaments terminate at their upper borders. Posteriorly, the labia majora taper and merge into the area overlying the perineal body to form the posterior commissure.

Hair covers the labia majora outer surface but is absent on their inner surface. In addition, apocrine, eccrine, and sebaceous glands are abundant. Beneath the skin, there is a dense connective tissue layer, which is nearly void of muscular elements but is rich in elastic fibers and adipose tissue. This mass of fat provides bulk to the labia majora and is supplied with a rich venous plexus. During pregnancy, this vasculature commonly develops varicosities, especially in parous women, from increased venous pressure created by the enlarging uterus. They appear as engorged tortuous veins or as small grapelike clusters, but they are typically asymptomatic.

Each labium minus is a thin tissue fold that lies medial to each labium majus. In males, its homologue forms the ventral shaft of the penis. The labia minora extend superiorly, where each divides into two lamellae. From each side, the lower lamellae fuse to form the frenulum of the clitoris, and the upper merge to form the prepuce. Inferiorly, the labia minora extend to approach the midline as low ridges of tissue that join to form the fourchette. The size of the labia minora varies greatly among individuals, with lengths from 2 to 10 cm and widths from 1 to 5 cm (Lloyd, 2005).

Structurally, the labia minora are composed of connective tissue with numerous vessels, elastin fibers, and very few smooth muscle fibers. They are supplied with many nerve endings and are extremely sensitive (Ginger, 2011a). The epithelia of the labia minora vary with location. Thinly keratinized stratified squamous epithelium covers the outer surface of each labium. On their inner surface, the lateral portion is covered by this same epithelium up to a demarcating line—Hart line. Medial to this line, each labium is covered by squamous epithelium that is nonkeratinized. The labia minora lack hair follicles, eccrine glands, and apocrine glands. However, there are many sebaceous glands (Wilkinson, 2011).

The clitoris is the principal female erogenous organ and is the erectile homologue of the penis. It is located beneath the prepuce, above the frenulum and urethra, and projects downward and inward toward the vaginal opening. The clitoris rarely exceeds 2 cm in length and is composed of a glans, a corpus or body, and two crura (Verkauf, 1992). The glans is usually less than 0.5 cm in diameter, is covered by stratified squamous epithelium, and is richly innervated. The clitoral body contains two corpora cavernosa. Extending from the clitoral body, each corpus cavernosum diverges laterally to form a long, narrow crus. Each crus lies along the inferior surface of its respective ischiopubic ramus and deep to the ischiocavernosus muscle. The clitoral blood supply stems from branches of the internal pudendal artery. Specifically, the deep artery of the clitoris supplies the clitoral body, whereas the dorsal artery of the clitoris supplies the glans and prepuce.

Vestibule

This is the functionally mature female structure derived from the embryonic urogenital membrane. In adult women, it is an almond-shaped area that is enclosed by Hart line laterally, the external surface of the hymen medially, the clitoral frenulum anteriorly, and the fourchette posteriorly. The vestibule usually is perforated by six openings: the urethra, the vagina, two Bartholin gland ducts, and at times, two ducts of the largest paraurethral glands—the Skene glands. The posterior portion of the vestibule between the fourchette and the vaginal opening is called the fossa navicularis. It is usually observed only in nulliparas.

The bilateral Bartholin glands, also termed greater vestibular glands, are major glands that measure 0.5 to 1 cm in diameter. On their respective side, each lies inferior to the vascular vestibular bulb and deep to the inferior end of the bulbocavernosus muscle. The duct from each measures 1.5 to 2 cm long and opens distal to the hymeneal ring—one at 5 and the other at 7 o'clock on the vestibule. Following trauma or infection, either duct may swell and obstruct to form a cyst or, if infected, an abscess. In contrast, the minor vestibular glands are shallow glands lined by simple mucin-secreting epithelium and open along Hart line.

The paraurethral glands are a collective arborization of glands whose multiple small ducts open predominantly along the entire inferior aspect of the urethra. The two largest are called Skene glands, and their ducts typically lie distally and near the urethral meatus. Clinically, inflammation and duct obstruction of any of the paraurethral glands can lead to urethral diverticulum formation.

The lower two thirds of the urethra lie immediately above the anterior vaginal wall. The urethral opening or meatus is in the midline of the vestibule, 1 to 1.5 cm below the pubic arch, and a short distance above the vaginal opening.

Vagina and Hymen

In adult women, the hymen is a membrane of varying thickness that surrounds the vaginal opening more or less completely. It is composed mainly of elastic and collagenous connective tissue, and both outer and inner surfaces are covered by nonkeratinized stratified squamous epithelium. The aperture of the intact hymen ranges in diameter from pinpoint to one that admits one or even two fingertips. Imperforate hymen is a rare malformation in which the vaginal orifice is occluded completely, causing retention of menstrual blood (Chap. 3, p. 38). As a rule, the hymen is torn at several sites during first coitus. However, identical tears may occur by other penetration, for example, by tampons used during menstruation. The edges of the torn tissue soon reepithelialize. In pregnant women, the hymeneal epithelium is thick and rich in glycogen. Changes produced in the hymen by childbirth are usually readily recognizable. For example, over time, the hymen transforms into several nodules of various sizes, termed hymeneal or myrtiform caruncles.

Proximal to the hymen, the vagina is a musculomembranous tube that extends to the uterus and is interposed lengthwise between the bladder and the rectum (Fig. 2-4). Anteriorly, the vagina is separated from the bladder and urethra by connective tissue—the vesicovaginal septum. Posteriorly, between the

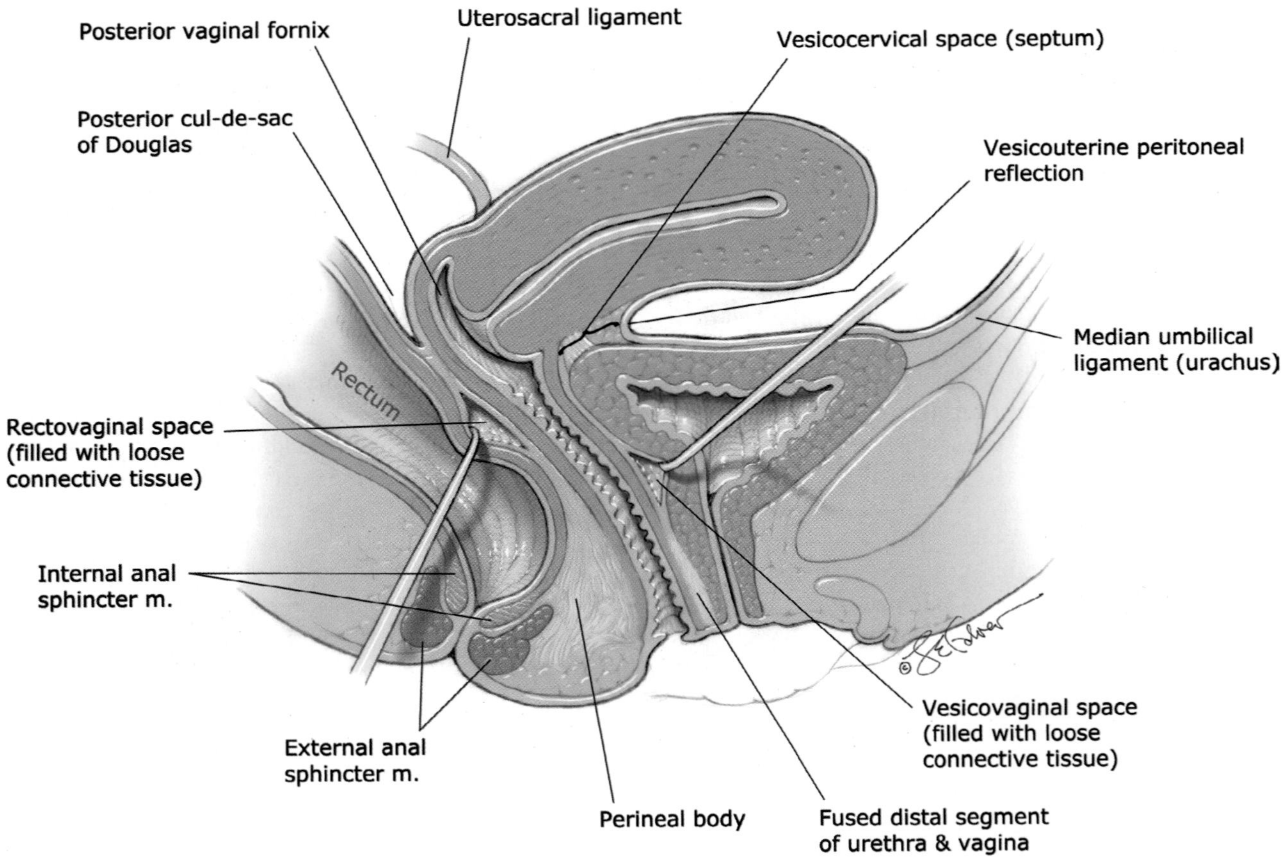

FIGURE 2-4 Vagina and surrounding anatomy. (From Corton, 2012, with permission.)

lower portion of the vagina and the rectum, there are similar tissues that together form the rectovaginal septum. The upper fourth of the vagina is separated from the rectum by the rectouterine pouch, also called the cul-de-sac or pouch of Douglas.

Normally, the anterior and posterior walls of the vaginal lumen lie in contact, with only a slight space intervening at the lateral margins. Vaginal length varies considerably, but commonly, the anterior wall measures 6 to 8 cm, whereas the posterior vaginal wall is 7 to 10 cm. The upper end of the vaginal vault is subdivided into anterior, posterior, and two lateral fornices by the cervix. These are of considerable clinical importance because the internal pelvic organs usually can be palpated through the thin walls of these fornices. Moreover, the posterior fornix provides surgical access to the peritoneal cavity.

At the midportion of the vagina, its lateral walls are attached to the pelvis by visceral connective tissue. These lateral attachments blend into investing fascia of the levator ani. In doing so, they create the anterior and posterior lateral vaginal sulci. These run the length of the vaginal sidewalls and give the vagina an H shape when viewed in cross section.

The vaginal lining is composed of nonkeratinized stratified squamous epithelium and underlying lamina propria. In premenopausal women, this lining is thrown into numerous thin transverse ridges, known as rugae, which line the anterior and posterior vaginal walls along their length. Deep to this, there is a muscular layer, which contains smooth muscle, collagen, and elastin. Beneath this muscularis lies an adventitial layer consisting of collagen and elastin (Weber, 1997).

There are no vaginal glands. Instead, the vagina is lubricated by a transudate that originates from the vaginal subepithelial capillary plexus and crosses the permeable epithelium (Kim, 2011). Due to increased vascularity during pregnancy, vaginal secretions are notably increased. At times, this may be confused with amnionic fluid leakage, and clinical differentiation of these two is described in Chapter 22 (p. 448).

After birth-related epithelial trauma and healing, fragments of stratified epithelium occasionally are embedded beneath the vaginal surface. Similar to its native tissue, this buried epithelium continues to shed degenerated cells and keratin. As a result, firm epidermal inclusion cysts, which are filled with keratin debris, may form and are a common vaginal cyst.

The vagina has an abundant vascular supply. The proximal portion is supplied by the cervical branch of the uterine artery and by the vaginal artery. The latter may variably arise from the uterine or inferior vesical or directly from the internal iliac artery. The middle rectal artery contributes supply to the posterior vaginal wall, whereas the distal walls receive contributions from the internal pudendal artery. At each level, blood supply from each side forms anastomoses on the anterior and posterior vaginal walls with contralateral corresponding vessels.

An extensive venous plexus immediately surrounds the vagina and follows the course of the arteries. Lymphatics from the lower third, along with those of the vulva, drain primarily into the inguinal lymph nodes. Those from the middle third drain into the internal iliac nodes, and those from the upper third drain into the external, internal, and common iliac nodes.

Perineum

This diamond-shaped area between the thighs has boundaries that mirror those of the bony pelvic outlet: the pubic symphysis anteriorly, ischiopubic rami and ischial tuberosities anterolaterally, sacrotuberous ligaments posterolaterally, and coccyx posteriorly. An arbitrary line joining the ischial tuberosities divides the perineum into an anterior triangle, also called the urogenital triangle, and a posterior triangle, termed the anal triangle.

The perineal body is a fibromuscular mass found in the midline at the junction between these anterior and posterior triangles (Fig. 2-5). Also called the central tendon of the perineum, the perineal body measures 2 cm tall and wide and

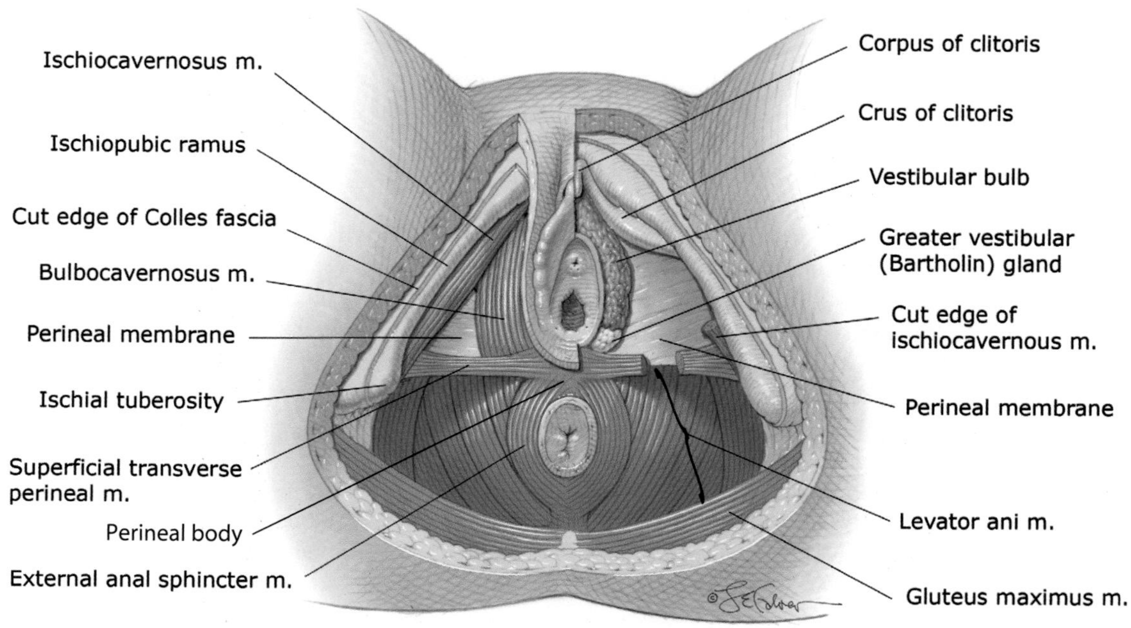

FIGURE 2-5 Superficial space of the anterior triangle and posterior perineal triangle. Structures on the left side of the image can be seen after removal of Colles fascia. Those on the right side are noted after removal of the superficial muscles of the anterior triangle. (From Corton, 2012, with permission.)

1.5 cm thick. It serves as the junction for several structures and provides significant perineal support (Shafik, 2007; Woodman, 2002). Superficially, the bulbocavernosus, superficial transverse perineal, and external anal sphincter muscles converge on the central tendon. More deeply, the perineal membrane, portions of the pubococcygeus muscle, and internal anal sphincter contribute (Larson, 2010). The perineal body is incised by an episiotomy incision and is torn with second-, third-, and fourth-degree lacerations.

Superficial Space of the Anterior Triangle

This triangle is bounded by the pubic rami superiorly, the ischial tuberosities laterally, and the superficial transverse perineal muscles posteriorly. It is divided into superficial and deep spaces by the perineal membrane. This membranous partition is a dense fibrous sheet that was previously known as the inferior fascia of the urogenital diaphragm. The perineal membrane attaches laterally to the ischiopubic rami, medially to the distal third of the urethra and vagina, posteriorly to the perineal body, and anteriorly to the arcuate ligament of the pubis.

The superficial space of the anterior triangle is bounded deeply by the perineal membrane and superficially by Colles fascia. As noted earlier, Colles fascia is the continuation of Scarpa fascia onto the perineum. On the perineum, Colles fascia securely attaches laterally to the pubic rami and fascia lata of the thigh, inferiorly to the superficial transverse perineal muscle and inferior border of the perineal membrane, and medially to the urethra, clitoris, and vagina. As such, the superficial space of the anterior triangle is a relatively closed compartment, and expanding infection or hematoma within it may bulge yet remains contained.

This superficial pouch contains several important structures, which include the Bartholin glands, vestibular bulbs, clitoral body and crura, branches of the pudendal vessels and nerve, and the ischiocavernosus, bulbocavernosus, and superficial transverse perineal muscles. Of these muscles, the ischiocavernosus muscles each attach on their respective side to the medial aspect of the ischial tuberosity inferiorly and the ischiopubic ramus laterally. Anteriorly, each attaches to a clitoral crus and may help maintain clitoral erection by compressing the crus to obstruct venous drainage. The bilateral bulbocavernosus muscles overlie the vestibular bulbs and Bartholin glands. They attach to the body of the clitoris anteriorly and the perineal body posteriorly. The muscles constrict the vaginal lumen and aid release of secretions from the Bartholin glands. They also may contribute to clitoral erection by compressing the deep dorsal vein of the clitoris. The bulbocavernosus and ischiocavernosus muscles also pull the clitoris downward. Last, the superficial transverse perineal muscles are narrow strips that attach to the ischial tuberosities laterally and the perineal body medially. They may be attenuated or even absent, but when present, they contribute to the perineal body (Corton, 2012).

Embryologically, the vestibular bulbs correspond to the corpora spongiosa of the penis. These almond-shaped aggregations of veins are 3 to 4 cm long, 1 to 2 cm wide, and 0.5 to 1 cm thick and lie beneath the bulbocavernosus muscle on either side of the vestibule. The bulbs terminate inferiorly at approximately the middle of the vaginal opening and extend upward toward the clitoris. Their anterior extensions merge in the midline, below the clitoral body. During childbirth, veins in the vestibular bulbs may be lacerated or even rupture to create a vulvar hematoma enclosed within the superficial space of the anterior triangle.

Deep Space of the Anterior Triangle

This space lies deep to the perineal membrane and extends up into the pelvis (Fig. 2-6) (Mirilas, 2004). In contrast to the superficial perineal space, the deep space is continuous superiorly with the pelvic cavity (Corton, 2005). It contains portions of urethra and vagina, certain portions of internal pudendal artery branches, and the compressor urethrae and urethrovaginal sphincter muscles, which comprise part of the striated urogenital sphincter complex.

Pelvic Diaphragm

Found deep to the anterior and posterior triangles, this broad muscular sling provides substantial support to the pelvic viscera. The pelvic diaphragm is composed of the levator ani and the coccygeus muscle. The levator ani is composed of the pubococcygeus, puborectalis, and iliococcygeus muscles. The pubococcygeus muscle is also termed the pubovisceral muscle and is subdivided based on points of insertion and function. These include the pubovaginalis, puboperinealis, and puboanalis muscles, which insert into the vaginal, perineal body, and anus, respectively (Kearney, 2004).

Vaginal birth conveys significant risk for damage to the levator ani or to its innervation (DeLancey, 2003; Weidner, 2006). Of these muscles, the pubovisceral muscle is more commonly damaged (Lien, 2004; Margulies, 2007). Evidence supports that these injuries may predispose women to greater risk of pelvic organ prolapse or urinary incontinence (DeLancey, 2007a,b; Rortveit, 2003). For this reason, current research efforts are aimed at minimizing these injuries.

Posterior Triangle

This triangle contains the ischioanal fossae, anal canal, and anal sphincter complex, which consists of the internal anal sphincter, external anal sphincter, and puborectalis muscle. Branches of the pudendal nerve and internal pudendal vessels are also found within this triangle.

Ischioanal Fossae. Also known as ischiorectal fossae, these two fat-filled wedge-shaped spaces are found on either side of the anal canal and comprise the bulk of the posterior triangle (Fig. 2-7). Each fossa has skin as its superficial base, whereas its deep apex is formed by the junction of the levator ani and obturator internus muscle. Other borders include: laterally, the obturator internus muscle fascia and ischial tuberosity; inferomedially, the anal canal and sphincter complex; superomedially, the inferior fascia of the downwardly sloping levator ani; posteriorly, the gluteus maximus muscle and sacrotuberous ligament; and anteriorly, the inferior border of the anterior triangle.

The fat found within each fossa provides support to surrounding organs yet allows rectal distention during defecation and vaginal stretching during delivery. Clinically, injury to vessels in the posterior triangle can lead to hematoma formation

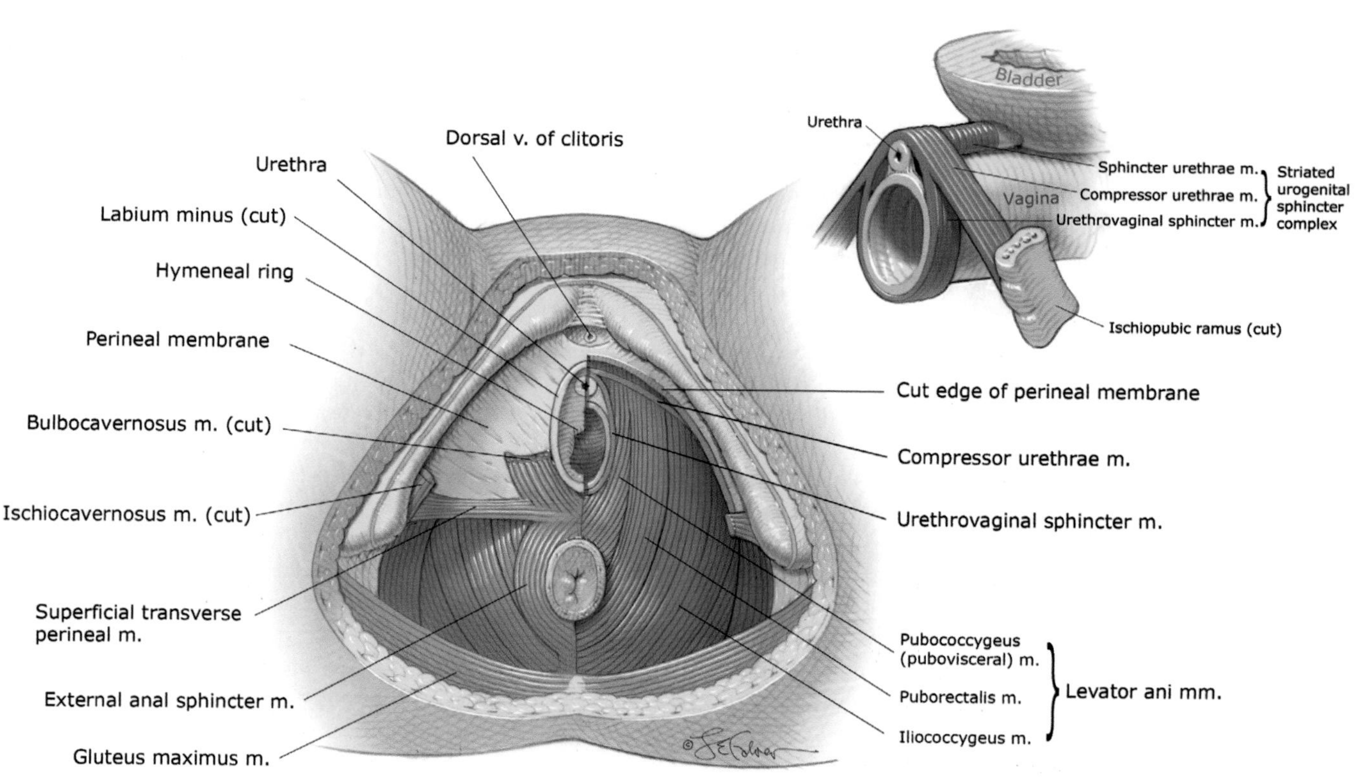

FIGURE 2-6 Deep space of the anterior triangle of the perineum. Structures on the right side of the image can be seen after removal of the perineal membrane. Also shown are structures that attach to the perineal body: bulbocavernosus, superficial transverse perineal, external anal sphincter, and puboperinealis muscles as well as the perineal membrane. (From Corton, 2012, with permission.)

in the ischioanal fossa, and the potential for large accumulation in these easily distensible spaces. Moreover, the two fossae communicate dorsally, behind the anal canal. This can be especially important because an episiotomy infection or hematoma may extend from one fossa into the other.

Anal Canal. This distal continuation of the rectum begins at the level of levator ani attachment to the rectum and ends at the anal skin. Along this 4- to 5-cm length, the mucosa consists of columnar epithelium in the uppermost portion, but at the dentate or pectinate line, simple stratified squamous epithelium begins and continues to the anal verge. Here, keratin and skin adnexa join the squamous epithelium.

The anal canal has several lateral tissue layers. Inner layers include the anal mucosa, the internal anal sphincter, and an intersphincteric space that contains continuation of the rectum's

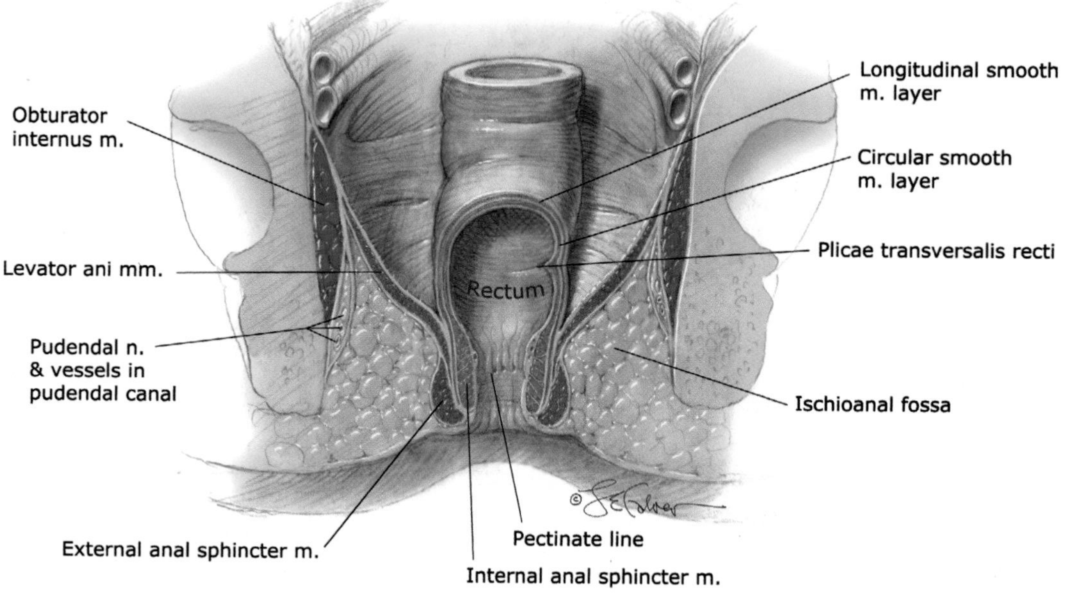

FIGURE 2-7 Anal canal and ischioanal fossa. (From Corton, 2012, with permission.)

longitudinal smooth muscle layer. An outer layer contains the puborectalis muscle as its cephalad component and the external anal sphincter caudally.

Within the anal canal, three highly vascularized submucosal arteriovenous plexuses termed anal cushions aid complete closure of the canal and fecal continence when apposed. Increasing uterine size, excessive straining, and hard stool create increased pressure that ultimately leads to degeneration and subsequent laxity of the cushion's supportive connective tissue base. These cushions then protrude into and downward through the anal canal. This leads to venous engorgement within the cushions—now termed hemorrhoids. Venous stasis results in inflammation, erosion of the cushion's epithelium, and then bleeding.

External hemorrhoids are those that arise distal to the pectinate line. They are covered by stratified squamous epithelium and receive sensory innervation from the inferior rectal nerve. Accordingly, pain and a palpable mass are typical complaints. Following resolution, a hemorrhoidal tag may remain and is composed of redundant anal skin and fibrotic tissue. In contrast, internal hemorrhoids are those that form above the dentate line and are covered by insensitive anorectal mucosa. These may prolapse or bleed but rarely become painful unless they undergo thrombosis or necrosis.

Anal Sphincter Complex. Two sphincters surround the anal canal to provide fecal continence—the external and internal anal sphincters. Both lie proximate to the vagina, and one or both may be torn during vaginal delivery. The internal anal sphincter (IAS) is a distal continuation of the rectal circular smooth muscle layer. It receives predominantly parasympathetic fibers, which pass through the pelvic splanchnic nerves. Along its length, this sphincter is supplied by the superior, middle, and inferior rectal arteries. The IAS contributes the bulk of anal canal resting pressure for fecal continence and relaxes prior to defecation. The IAS measures 3 to 4 cm in length, and at its distal margin, it overlaps the external sphincter for 1 to 2 cm (DeLancey, 1997; Rociu, 2000). The distal site at which this overlap ends, called the intersphincteric groove, is palpable on digital examination.

In contrast, the external anal sphincter (EAS) is a striated muscle ring that anteriorly attaches to the perineal body and that posteriorly connects to the coccyx via the anococcygeal ligament. The EAS maintains a constant resting contraction to aid continence, provides additional squeeze pressure when continence is threatened, yet relaxes for defecation. Traditionally, the EAS has been described as three parts, which include the subcutaneous, superficial, and deep portions. However, many consider the deep portion to be composed fully or in part by the puborectalis muscle (Raizada, 2008). The external sphincter receives blood supply from the inferior rectal artery, which is a branch of the internal pudendal artery. Somatic motor fibers from the inferior rectal branch of the pudendal nerve supply innervation. Clinically, the IAS and EAS may be involved in fourth-degree laceration during vaginal delivery, and reunion of these rings is integral to defect repair (Chap. 27, p. 548).

Pudendal Nerve

This is formed from the anterior rami of S_{2-4} spinal nerves (Fig. 2-8). It courses between the piriformis and coccygeus muscles and exits through the greater sciatic foramen at a location posterior to the sacrospinous ligament and just medial to the ischial spine (Barber, 2002). Thus, when injecting local anesthetic for a pudendal nerve block, the ischial spine serves

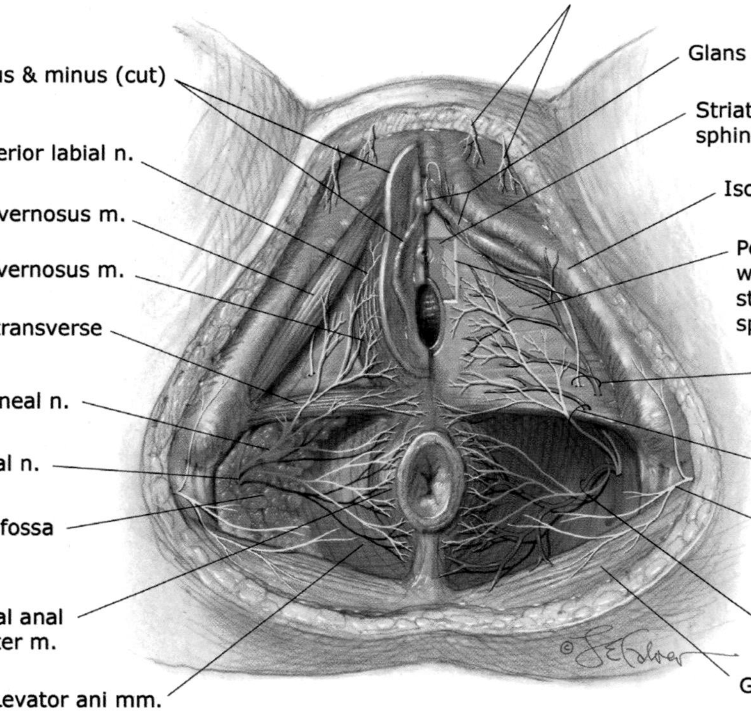

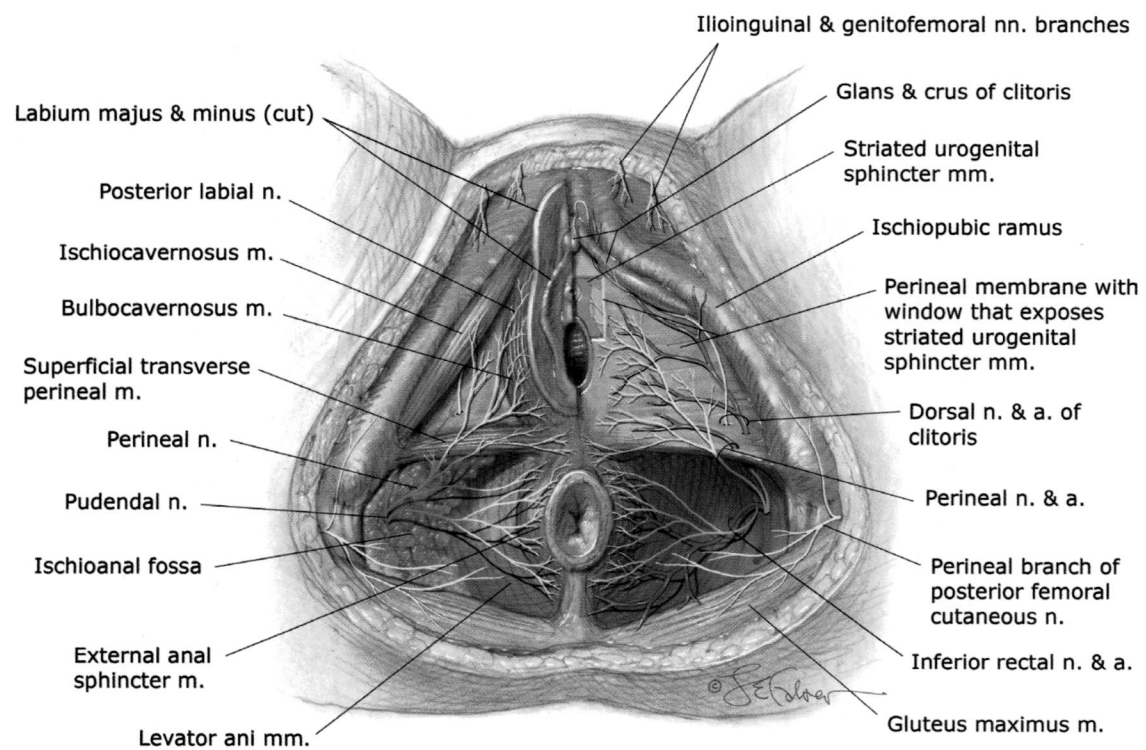

FIGURE 2-8 Pudendal nerve and vessels. (From Corton, 2012, with permission.)

an identifiable landmark (Chap. 25, p. 508). The pudendal nerve then runs beneath the sacrospinous ligament and above the sacrotuberous ligament as it reenters the lesser sciatic foramen to course along the obturator internus muscle. Atop this muscle, the nerve lies within the pudendal canal, also known as Alcock canal, which is formed by splitting of the obturator internus investing fascia (Shafik, 1999). In general, the pudendal nerve is relatively fixed as it courses behind the sacrospinous ligament and within the pudendal canal. Accordingly, it may be at risk of stretch injury during downward displacement of the pelvic floor during childbirth (Lien, 2005).

The pudendal nerve leaves this canal to enter the perineum and divides into three terminal branches. Of these, the dorsal nerve of the clitoris runs between the ischiocavernosus muscle and perineal membrane to supply the clitoral glans (Ginger, 2011b). The perineal nerve runs superficial to the perineal membrane (Montoya, 2011). It divides into posterior labial branches and muscular branches, which serve the labial skin and the anterior perineal triangle muscles, respectively. The inferior rectal branch runs through the ischioanal fossa to supply the external anal sphincter, the anal mucosa, and the perianal skin (Mahakkanukrauh, 2005). The major blood supply to the perineum is via the internal pudendal artery, and its branches mirror the divisions of the pudendal nerve.

INTERNAL GENERATIVE ORGANS

Uterus

The nonpregnant uterus is situated in the pelvic cavity between the bladder anteriorly and the rectum posteriorly. Almost the entire posterior wall of the uterus is covered by serosa, that is, visceral peritoneum (Fig. 2-9). The lower portion of this peritoneum forms the anterior boundary of the rectouterine cul-de-sac, or pouch of Douglas. Only the upper portion of the anterior wall of the uterus is so covered. The peritoneum in this area reflects forward onto the bladder dome to create the vesicouterine pouch. The lower portion of the anterior uterine wall is united to the posterior wall of the bladder by a well-defined loose connective tissue layer—the vesicouterine space. Clinically, during cesarean delivery, the peritoneum of the vesicouterine pouch is sharply incised, and the vesicouterine space is entered. Dissection caudally within this space lifts the bladder off the lower uterine segment for hysterotomy and delivery (Chap. 30, p. 593).

The uterus is pear shaped and consists of two major but unequal parts. There is an upper triangular portion—the body or corpus, and a lower, cylindrical portion—the cervix, which projects into the vagina. The isthmus is the union site of these two. It is of special obstetrical significance because it forms the lower uterine segment during pregnancy. At each superolateral margin of the body is a uterine cornu, from which a fallopian tube emerges. Also in this area are the origins of the round and uteroovarian ligaments. Between the points of fallopian tube insertion is the convex upper uterine segment termed the fundus.

The bulk of the uterine body, but not the cervix, is muscle. The inner surfaces of the anterior and posterior walls lie almost in contact, and the cavity between these walls forms a mere slit. The nulligravid uterus measures 6 to 8 cm in length compared with 9 to 10 cm in multiparous women. The uterus averages 60 g and typically weighs more in parous women (Langlois, 1970; Sheikhazadi, 2010). In nulligravidas, the fundus and cervix are approximately equal in length, but in multiparas, the cervix is only a little more than a third of the total length.

Pregnancy stimulates remarkable uterine growth due to muscle fiber hypertrophy. The uterine fundus, a previously flattened convexity between tubal insertions, now becomes dome shaped. Moreover, the round ligaments appear to insert at the

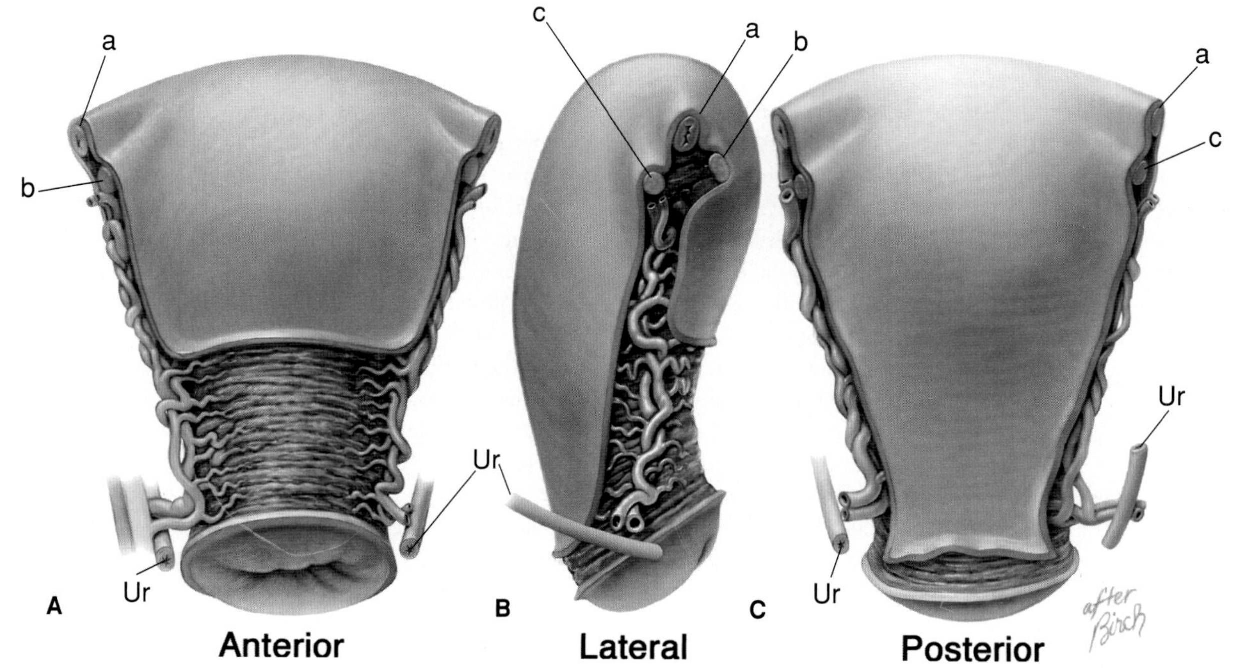

FIGURE 2-9 Anterior **(A)**, right lateral **(B)**, and posterior **(C)** views of the uterus of an adult woman. a = fallopian tube; b = round ligament; c = uteroovarian ligament; Ur = ureter.

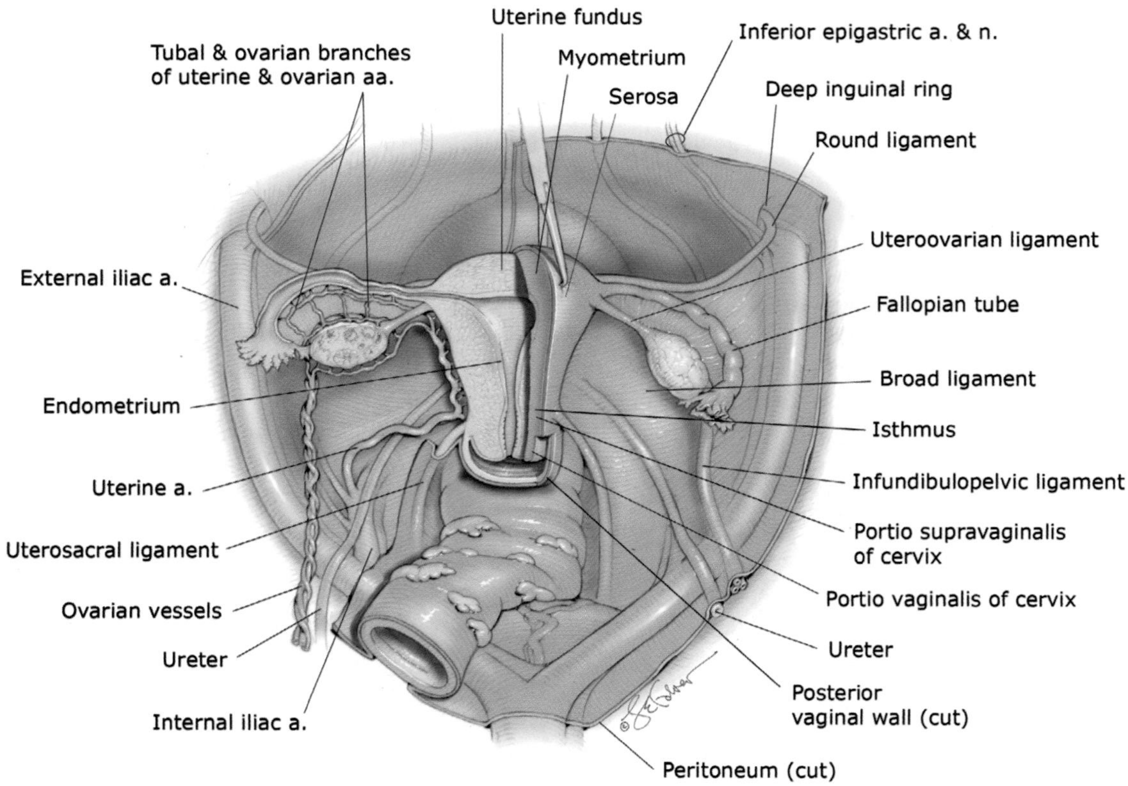

FIGURE 2-10 Uterus, adnexa, and associated anatomy. (From Corton, 2012, with permission.)

junction of the middle and upper thirds of the organ. The fallopian tubes elongate, but the ovaries grossly appear unchanged.

Cervix

The cervical portion of the uterus is fusiform and open at each end by small apertures—the internal and external cervical ora. Proximally, the upper boundary of the cervix is the internal os, which corresponds to the level at which the peritoneum is reflected up onto the bladder. The upper cervical segment—the portio supravaginalis, lies above the vagina's attachment to the cervix (Fig. 2-10). It is covered by peritoneum on its posterior surface, the cardinal ligaments attach laterally, and it is separated from the overlying bladder by loose connective tissue. The lower cervical portion protrudes into the vagina as the portio vaginalis. Before childbirth, the external cervical os is a small, regular, oval opening. After labor, especially vaginal childbirth, the orifice is converted into a transverse slit that is divided such that there are the so-called anterior and posterior cervical lips. If torn deeply during labor or delivery, the cervix may heal in such a manner that it appears irregular, nodular, or stellate.

The portion of the cervix exterior to the external os is called the ectocervix and is lined predominantly by nonkeratinized stratified squamous epithelium. In contrast, the endocervical canal is covered by a single layer of mucin-secreting columnar epithelium, which creates deep cleftlike infoldings or "glands." Commonly during pregnancy, the endocervical epithelium moves out and onto the ectocervix in a physiological process termed eversion (Chap. 4, p. 48).

The cervical stroma is composed mainly of collagen, elastin, and proteoglycans, but very little smooth muscle. Changes in the amount, composition, and orientation of these components lead to cervical ripening prior to labor onset. In early pregnancy, increased vascularity within the cervix stroma beneath the epithelium creates an ectocervical blue tint that is characteristic of Chadwick sign. Cervical edema leads to softening—Goodell sign, whereas isthmic softening is Hegar sign.

Myometrium and Endometrium

Most of the uterus is composed of myometrium, which is smooth muscle bundles united by connective tissue containing many elastic fibers. Interlacing myometrial fibers surround myometrial vessels and contract to compress these. As shown in Figure 2-11, this anatomy is integral to hemostasis at the placental site during the third stage of labor.

The number of myometrial muscle fibers varies by location (Schwalm, 1966). Levels progressively diminish caudally such that, in the cervix, muscle makes up only 10 percent of the tissue mass. In the uterine body inner wall, there is relatively more muscle than in outer layers. And, in the anterior and posterior walls, there is more muscle than in the lateral walls. During pregnancy, the upper myometrium undergoes marked hypertrophy, but there is no significant change in cervical muscle content.

The uterine cavity is lined with endometrium, which is composed of an overlying epithelium, invaginating glands, and a supportive, vascular stroma. As discussed in Chapter 5 (p. 84), the endometrium varies greatly throughout the menstrual cycle and during pregnancy. This layer is divided into a functionalis layer, which is sloughed with menses, and a basalis layer, which serves to regenerate the functionalis layer following each menses.

Ligaments

There are several ligaments that extend from the uterine surface toward the pelvic sidewalls and include the round, broad, cardinal, and uterosacral ligaments (Figs. 2-9 and 2-12). The round ligament corresponds embryologically to the male gubernaculum testis (Acién, 2011). It originates somewhat below and anterior to the origin of the fallopian tubes. Clinically, this orientation can aid in fallopian tube identification during puerperal sterilization. This is important if pelvic adhesions limit tubal mobility and thus, limit fimbria visualization prior to tubal ligation. Each round ligament extends laterally and downward into the inguinal canal, through which it passes, to terminate in the upper portion of the labium majus. Sampson artery, a branch of the uterine artery, runs within this ligament. In nonpregnant women, the round ligament varies from 3 to 5 mm in diameter and is composed of smooth muscle bundles separated by fibrous tissue septa (Mahran, 1965). During pregnancy, these ligaments undergo considerable hypertrophy and increase appreciably in both length and diameter.

The broad ligaments are two winglike structures that extend from the lateral uterine margins to the pelvic sidewalls. With vertical sectioning through this ligament proximate to the uterus, a triangular shape can be seen, and the uterine vessels and ureter are found at its base. The broad ligaments divide the pelvic cavity into anterior and posterior compartments. Each broad ligament consists of a fold of peritoneum termed the anterior and posterior leaves. This peritoneum drapes over structures extending from each cornu. Peritoneum that overlies the fallopian tube is

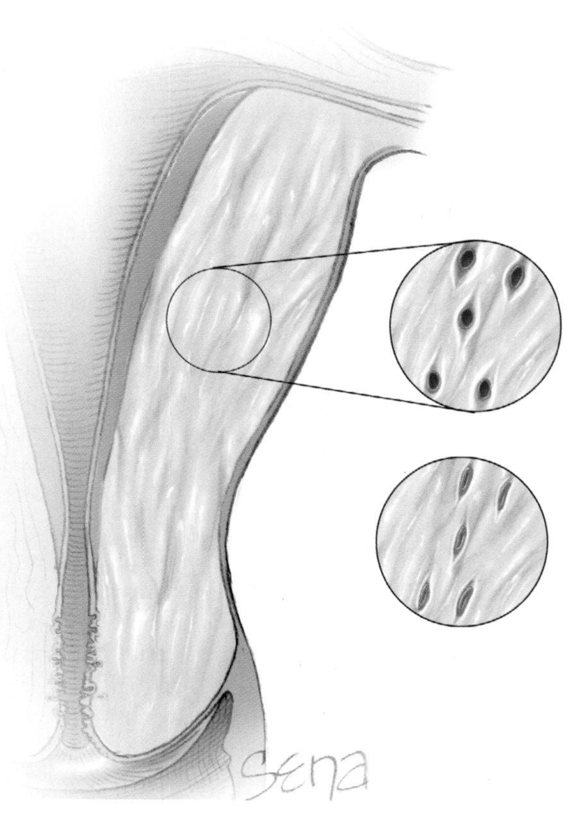

FIGURE 2-11 Smooth muscle fibers of the myometrium compress traversing blood vessels when contracted.

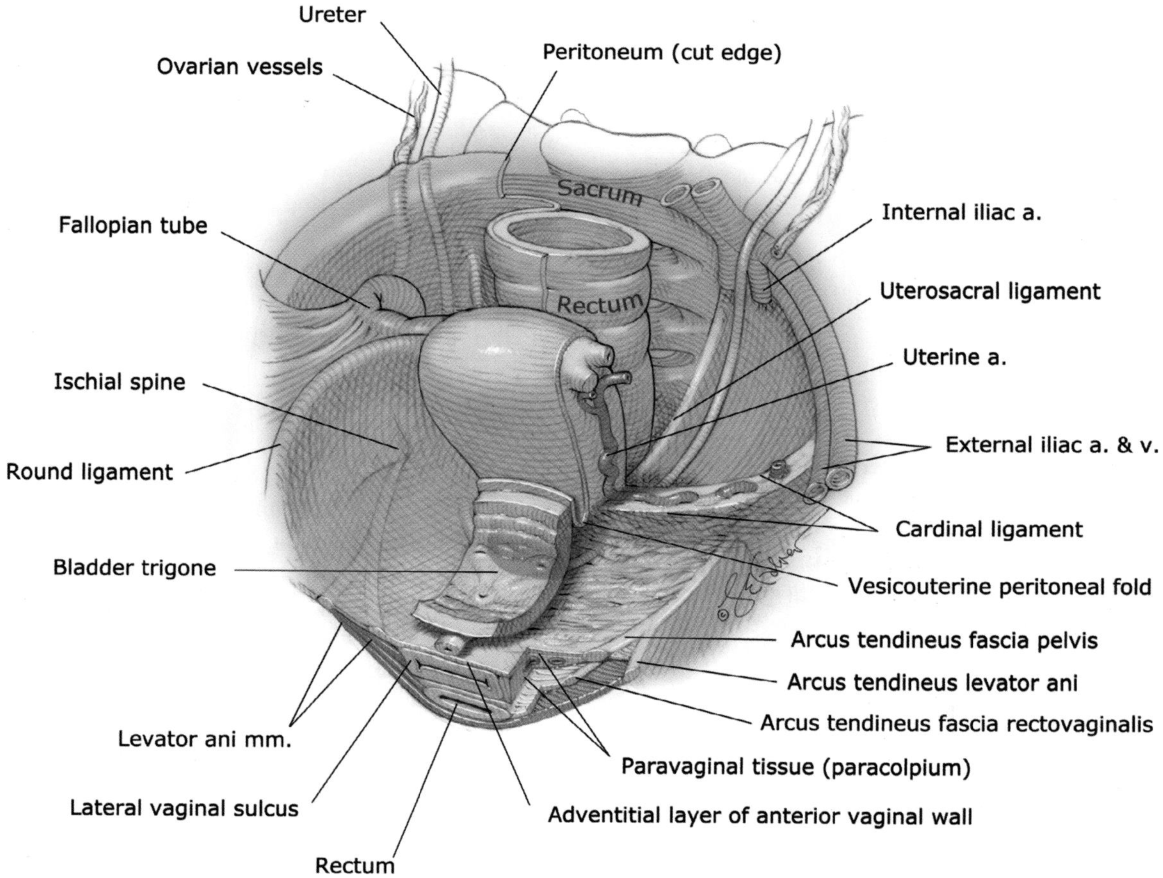

FIGURE 2-12 Pelvic viscera and their connective tissue support. (From Corton, 2012, with permission.)

termed the mesosalpinx, that around the round ligament is the mesoteres, and that over the uteroovarian ligament is the mesovarium. Peritoneum that extends beneath the fimbriated end of the fallopian tube toward the pelvic wall forms the infundibulopelvic ligament or suspensory ligament of the ovary. This contains nerves and the ovarian vessels, and during pregnancy, these vessels, especially the venous plexuses, are dramatically enlarged. Specifically, the diameter of the ovarian vascular pedicle increases from 0.9 cm to reach 2.6 cm at term (Hodgkinson, 1953).

The cardinal ligament—also called the transverse cervical ligament or Mackenrodt ligament—is the thick base of the broad ligament. Medially, it is united firmly to the uterus and upper vagina.

Each uterosacral ligament originates with a posterolateral attachment to the supravaginal portion of the cervix and inserts into the fascia over the sacrum, with some variations (Ramanah, 2012; Umek, 2004). These ligaments are composed of connective tissue, small bundles of vessels and nerves, and some smooth muscle. Covered by peritoneum, these ligaments form the lateral boundaries of the pouch of Douglas.

The term parametrium is used to describe the connective tissues adjacent and lateral to the uterus within the broad ligament. Paracervical tissues are those adjacent to the cervix, whereas paracolpium is that tissue lateral to the vaginal walls.

Blood Supply

During pregnancy, there is marked hypertrophy of the uterine vasculature, which is supplied principally from the uterine and ovarian arteries (see Fig. 2-9). The uterine artery, a main branch of the internal iliac artery—previously called the hypogastric artery—enters the base of the broad ligament and makes its way medially to the side of the uterus. Approximately 2 cm lateral to the cervix, the uterine artery crosses over the ureter. This proximity is of great surgical significance as the ureter may be injured or ligated during hysterectomy when the vessels are clamped and ligated.

Once the uterine artery has reached the supravaginal portion of the cervix, it divides. The smaller cervicovaginal artery supplies blood to the lower cervix and upper vagina. The main branch turns abruptly upward and extends as a highly convoluted vessel that traverses along the lateral margin of the uterus. A branch of considerable size extends into the upper portion of the cervix, whereas numerous other branches penetrate the body of the uterus to form the arcuate arteries. These encircle the organ by coursing within the myometrium just beneath the serosal surface. These vessels from each side anastomose at the uterine midline. From the arcuate arteries, radial branches originate at right angles, traverse inward through the myometrium, enter the endometrium, and branch there to become basal arteries or coiled spiral arteries. The spiral arteries supply the functionalis layer. These vessels respond—especially by vasoconstriction and dilatation—to a number of hormones and thus serve an important role in menstruation. Also called the straight arteries, the basal arteries extend only into the basalis layer and are not responsive to hormonal influences.

Just before the main uterine artery vessel reaches the fallopian tube, it divides into three terminal branches. The ovarian branch of the uterine artery forms an anastomosis with the terminal branch of the ovarian artery; the tubal branch makes its way through the mesosalpinx and supplies part of the fallopian tube; and the fundal branch penetrates the uppermost uterus.

In addition to the uterine artery, the uterus receives blood supply from the ovarian artery. This artery is a direct branch of the aorta and enters the broad ligament through the infundibulopelvic ligament. At the ovarian hilum, it divides into smaller branches that enter the ovary. As the ovarian artery runs along the hilum, it also sends several branches through the mesosalpinx to supply the fallopian tubes. Its main stem, however, traverses the entire length of the broad ligament and makes its way to the uterine cornu. Here, it forms an anastomosis with the ovarian branch of the uterine artery. This dual uterine blood supply creates a vascular reserve to prevent uterine ischemia if ligation of the uterine or internal iliac artery is performed to control postpartum hemorrhage.

Uterine veins accompany their respective arteries. As such, the arcuate veins unite to form the uterine vein, which empties into the internal iliac vein and then the common iliac vein. Some of the blood from the upper uterus, the ovary, and the upper part of the broad ligament is collected by several veins. Within the broad ligament, these veins form the large pampiniform plexus that terminates in the ovarian vein. From here, the right ovarian vein empties into the vena cava, whereas the left ovarian vein empties into the left renal vein.

Blood supply to the pelvis is predominantly supplied from branches of the internal iliac artery. These branches are organized into anterior and posterior divisions, and subsequent branches are highly variable between individuals (Fig. 2-13). The anterior division provides blood supply to the pelvic organs and perineum and includes the inferior gluteal, internal pudendal, middle rectal, vaginal, uterine, and obturator arteries, as well as the umbilical artery and its continuation as the superior vesical artery. The posterior division branches extend to the buttock and thigh and include the superior gluteal, lateral sacral, and iliolumbar arteries. For this reason, during internal iliac artery ligation, many advocate ligation distal to the posterior division to avoid compromised blood flow to the areas supplied by this division (Bleich, 2007).

Lymphatics

The endometrium is abundantly supplied with lymphatic vessels that are confined largely to the basalis layer. The lymphatics of the underlying myometrium are increased in number toward the serosal surface and form an abundant lymphatic plexus just beneath it. Lymphatics from the cervix terminate mainly in the internal iliac nodes, which are situated near the bifurcation of the common iliac vessels. The lymphatics from the uterine corpus are distributed to two groups of nodes. One set of vessels drains into the internal iliac nodes. The other set, after joining certain lymphatics from the ovarian region, terminates in the paraaortic lymph nodes.

Innervation

As a brief review, the peripheral nervous system is divided in a somatic division, which innervates skeletal muscle, and an

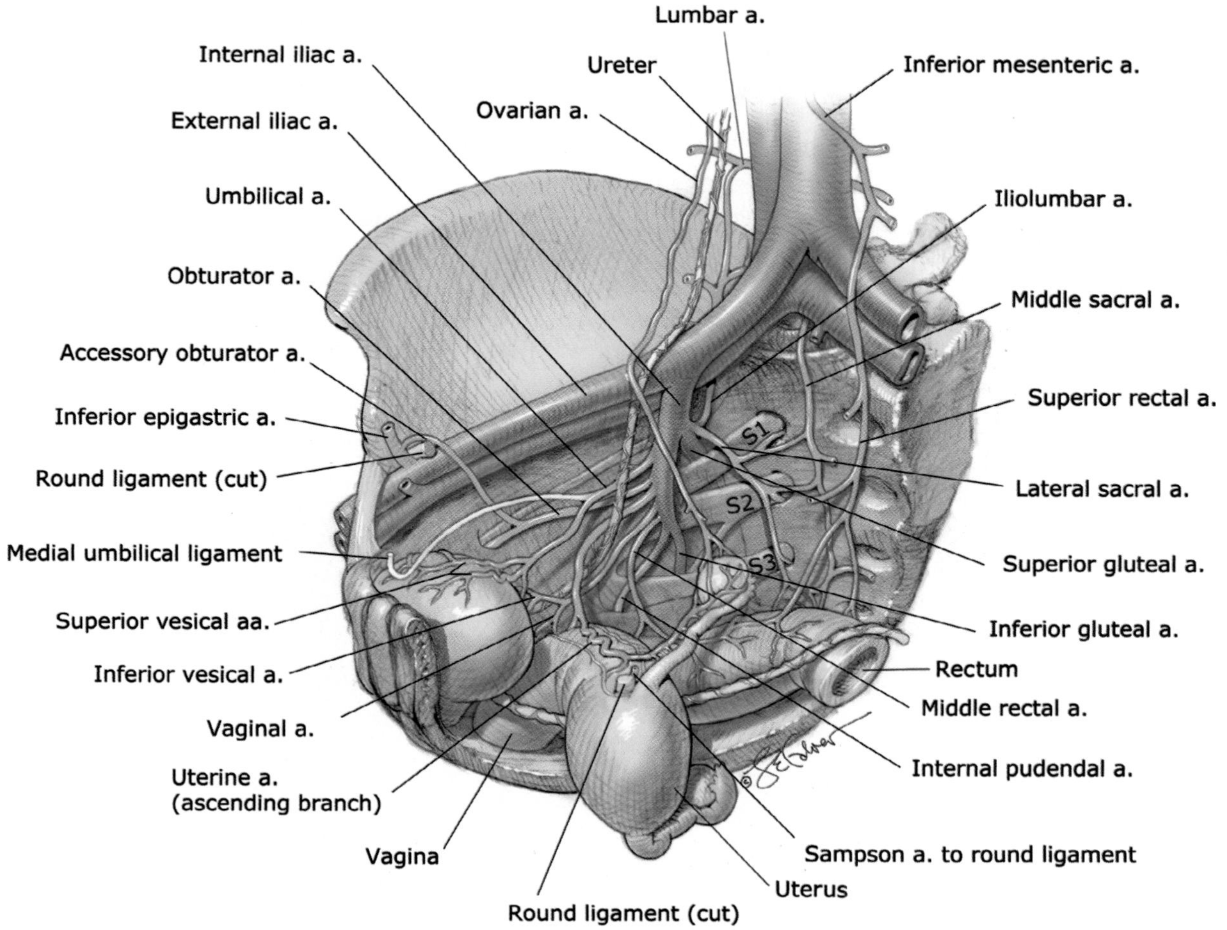

FIGURE 2-13 Pelvic arteries. (From Corton, 2012, with permission.)

autonomic division, which innervates smooth muscle, cardiac muscle, and glands. Pelvic visceral innervation is predominantly autonomic. The autonomic portion is further divided in sympathetic and parasympathetic components.

Sympathetic innervation to pelvic viscera begins with the superior hypogastric plexus, also termed the presacral nerve (Fig. 2-14). Beginning below the aortic bifurcation and extending downward retroperitoneally, this plexus is formed by sympathetic fibers arising from spinal levels T_{10} through L_2. At the level of the sacral promontory, this superior hypogastric plexus divides into a right and a left hypogastric nerve, which run downward along the pelvis side walls (Açar, 2012; Moszkowicz, 2011).

In contrast, parasympathetic innervation to the pelvic viscera derives from neurons at spinal levels S_2 through S_4. Their axons exit as part of the anterior rami of the spinal nerves for those levels. These combine on each side to form the pelvic splanchnic nerves, also termed nervi erigentes.

Blending of the two hypogastric nerves (sympathetic) and the two pelvic splanchnic nerves (parasympathetic) gives rise to the inferior hypogastric plexus, also termed the pelvic plexus. This retroperitoneal plaque of nerves lies at the S_4 and S_5 level (Spackman, 2007). From here, fibers of this plexus accompany internal iliac artery branches to their respective pelvic viscera. Thus, the inferior hypogastric plexus divides into three plexuses. The vesical plexus innervates the bladder and the middle rectal travels to the rectum, whereas the uterovaginal plexus, also termed Frankenhäuser plexus, reaches the proximal fallopian tubes, uterus, and upper vagina. Extensions of the inferior hypogastric plexus also reach the perineum along the vagina and urethra to innervate the clitoris and vestibular bulbs (Montoya, 2011). Of these, the uterovaginal plexus is composed of variably sized ganglia, but particularly of a large ganglionic plate that is situated on either side of the cervix, proximate to the uterosacral and cardinal ligaments (Ramanah, 2012).

Most afferent sensory fibers from the uterus ascend through the inferior hypogastric plexus and enter the spinal cord via T_{10} through T_{12} and L_1 spinal nerves. These transmit the painful stimuli of contractions to the central nervous system. The sensory nerves from the cervix and upper part of the birth canal pass through the pelvic splanchnic nerves to the second, third, and fourth sacral nerves. Those from the lower portion of the birth canal pass primarily through the pudendal nerve. As described earlier (p. 24), anesthetic blocks used in labor and delivery target this innervation.

Ovaries

Compared with each other, as well as between women, the ovaries differ considerably in size. During childbearing years, they measure 2.5 to 5 cm in length, 1.5 to 3 cm in breadth, and 0.6 to 1.5 cm in thickness. Their position also varies, but they usually lie

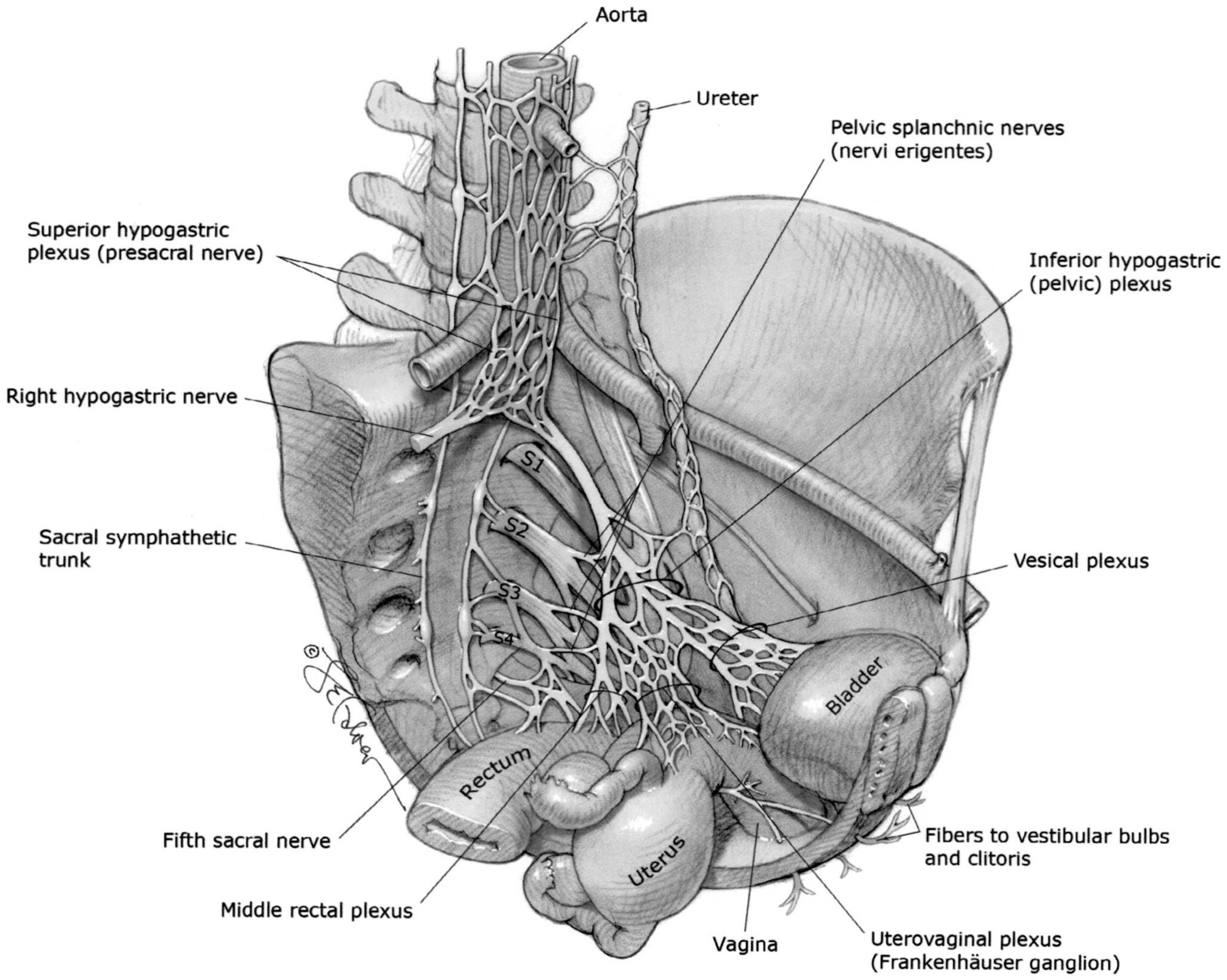

FIGURE 2-14 Pelvic innervation. (From Corton, 2012, with permission.)

in the upper part of the pelvic cavity and rest in a slight depression on the lateral wall of the pelvis. This ovarian fossa of Waldeyer is between the divergent external and internal iliac vessels.

The uteroovarian ligament originates from the lateral and upper posterior portion of the uterus, just beneath the tubal insertion level, and extends to the uterine pole of the ovary. Usually, this ligament is a few centimeters long and 3 to 4 mm in diameter. It is made up of muscle and connective tissue and is covered by peritoneum—the mesovarium. As described on page 28, blood supply traverses to and from the ovary through this double-layered mesovarium to enter the ovarian hilum.

The ovary consists of a cortex and medulla. In young women, the outermost portion of the cortex is smooth, has a dull white surface, and is designated the tunica albuginea. On its surface, there is a single layer of cuboidal epithelium, the germinal epithelium of Waldeyer. Beneath this epithelium, the cortex contains oocytes and developing follicles. The medulla is the central portion, which is composed of loose connective tissue. There are a large number of arteries and veins in the medulla and a small number of smooth muscle fibers.

The ovaries are supplied with both sympathetic and parasympathetic nerves. The sympathetic nerves are derived primarily from the ovarian plexus that accompanies the ovarian vessels and originates in the renal plexus. Others are derived from the plexus that surrounds the ovarian branch of the uterine artery. Parasympathetic input is from the vagus nerve. Sensory afferents follow the ovarian artery and enter at T_{10} spinal cord level.

Fallopian Tubes

Also called oviducts, these serpentine tubes extend 8 to 14 cm from the uterine cornua and are anatomically classified along their length as an interstitial portion, isthmus, ampulla, and infundibulum (Fig. 2-15). Most proximal, the interstitial portion is embodied within the uterine muscular wall. Next, the narrow 2- to 3-mm isthmus adjoins the uterus and widens gradually into the 5- to 8-mm, more lateral ampulla. Last, the infundibulum is the funnel-shaped fimbriated distal extremity of the tube, which opens into the abdominal cavity. The latter three extrauterine portions are covered by the mesosalpinx at the superior margin of the broad ligament.

In cross section, the extrauterine fallopian tube contains a mesosalpinx, myosalpinx, and endosalpinx. The outer of these,

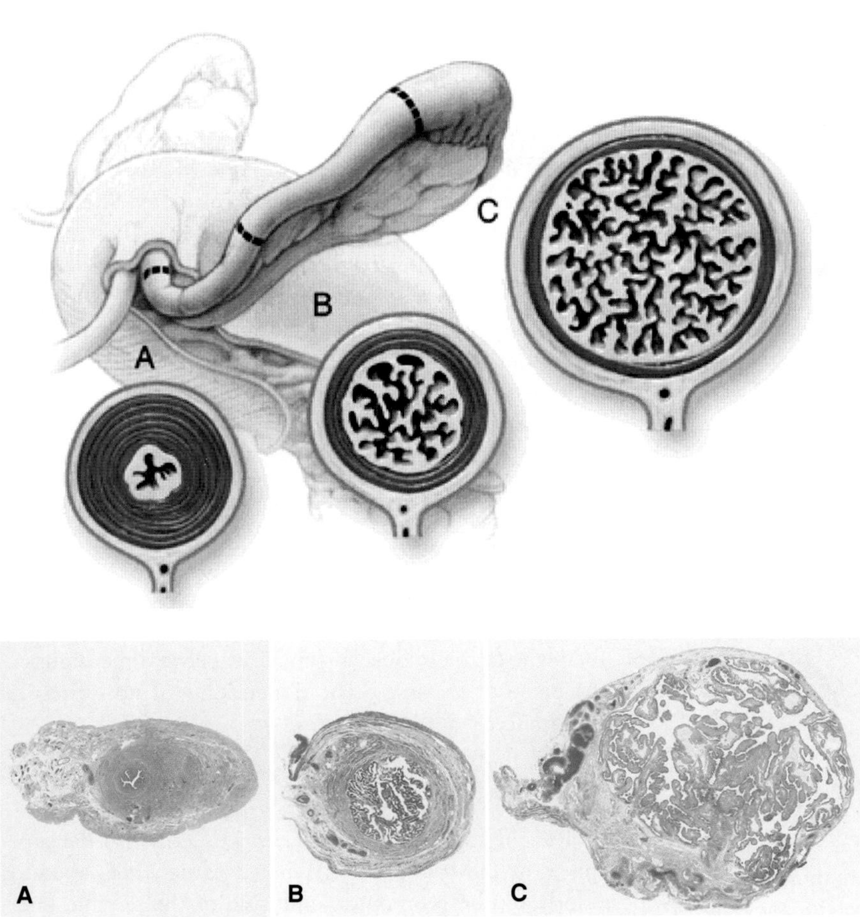

FIGURE 2-15 The fallopian tube of an adult woman with cross-sectioned illustrations of the gross structure in several portions: **(A)** isthmus, **(B)** ampulla, and **(C)** infundibulum. Below these are photographs of corresponding histological sections. (Photographs contributed by Dr. Kelley S. Carrick.)

the mesosalpinx, is a single-cell mesothelial layer functioning as visceral peritoneum. In the myosalpinx, smooth muscle is arranged in an inner circular and an outer longitudinal layer. In the distal tube, the two layers are less distinct and are replaced near the fimbriated extremity by sparse interlacing muscular fibers. The tubal musculature undergoes rhythmic contractions constantly, the rate of which varies with cyclical ovarian hormonal changes.

The tubal mucosa or endosalpinx is a single columnar epithelium composed of ciliated and secretory cells resting on a sparse lamina propria. It is in close contact with the underlying myosalpinx. The ciliated cells are most abundant at the fimbriated extremity, but elsewhere, they are found in discrete patches. There also are differences in the proportions of these two cell types in the different ovarian cycle phases. The mucosa is arranged in longitudinal folds that become progressively more complex toward the fimbria. In the ampulla, the lumen is occupied almost completely by the arborescent mucosa. The current produced by the tubal cilia is such that the direction of flow is toward the uterine cavity. Tubal peristalsis created by cilia and muscular layer contraction is believed to be an important factor in ovum transport (Croxatto, 2002).

The tubes are supplied richly with elastic tissue, blood vessels, and lymphatics. Sympathetic innervation of the tubes is extensive, in contrast to their parasympathetic innervation. This nerve supply derives partly from the ovarian plexus and partly from the uterovaginal plexus. Sensory afferent fibers ascend to T_{10} spinal cord levels.

MUSCULOSKELETAL PELVIC ANATOMY

Pelvic Bones

The pelvis is composed of four bones—the sacrum, coccyx, and two innominate bones. Each innominate bone is formed by the fusion of three bones—the ilium, ischium, and pubis (Fig. 2-16). Both innominate bones are joined to the sacrum at the sacroiliac synchondroses and to one another at the symphysis pubis.

The pelvis is conceptually divided into false and true components. The false pelvis lies above the linea terminalis, and the true pelvis is below this anatomical boundary (Fig. 2-17). The false pelvis is bounded posteriorly by the lumbar vertebra and laterally by the iliac fossa. In front, the boundary is formed by the lower portion of the anterior abdominal wall.

The true pelvis is the portion important in childbearing and can be described as an obliquely truncated, bent cylinder with its greatest height posteriorly. The linea terminalis serves as the superior border, whereas the pelvic outlet is the inferior margin. The posterior boundary is the anterior surface of the sacrum, and the lateral limits are formed by the inner surface of the ischial bones and the sacrosciatic notches and ligaments. In front,

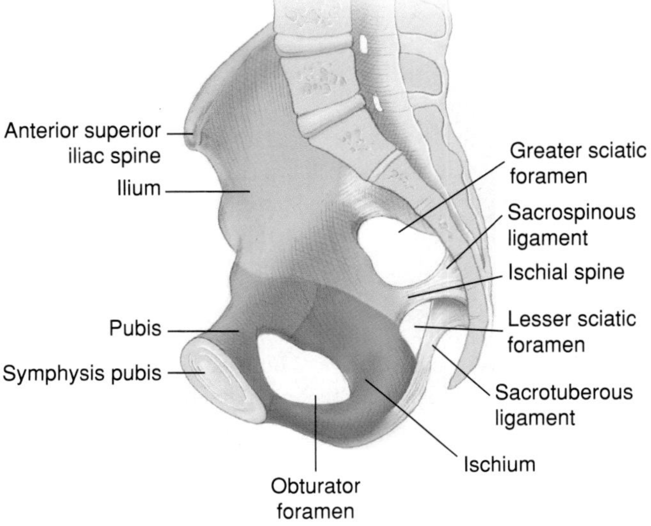

FIGURE 2-16 Sagittal view of the pelvic bones.

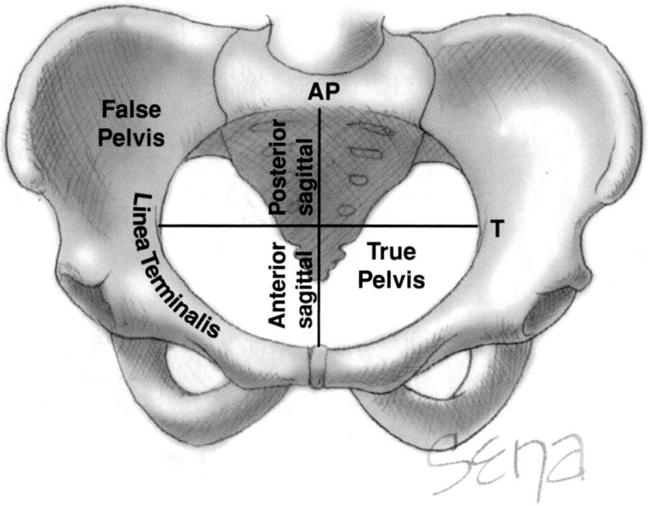

FIGURE 2-17 Anteroposterior view of a normal female pelvis. Anteroposterior (AP) and transverse (T) diameters of the pelvic inlet are illustrated.

the true pelvis is bounded by the pubic bones, by the ascending superior rami of the ischial bones, and by the obturator foramina.

The sidewalls of the true pelvis of an adult woman converge somewhat. Extending from the middle of the posterior margin of each ischium are the ischial spines. These are of great obstetrical importance because the distance between them usually represents the shortest diameter of the true pelvis. They also serve as valuable landmarks in assessing the level to which the presenting part of the fetus has descended into the true pelvis (Chap. 22, p. 449). Last, as described earlier, these aid pudendal nerve block placement.

The sacrum forms the posterior wall of the true pelvis. Its upper anterior margin corresponds to the promontory that may be felt during bimanual pelvic examination in women with a small pelvis. It can provide a landmark for clinical pelvimetry. Normally, the sacrum has a marked vertical and a less pronounced horizontal concavity, which in abnormal pelves may undergo important variations. A straight line drawn from the promontory to the tip of the sacrum usually measures 10 cm, whereas the distance along the concavity averages 12 cm.

Pelvic Joints

Anteriorly, the pelvic bones are joined together by the symphysis pubis. This structure consists of fibrocartilage and the superior and inferior pubic ligaments. The latter ligament is frequently designated the arcuate ligament of the pubis. Posteriorly, the pelvic bones are joined by articulations between the sacrum and the iliac portion of the innominate bones to form the sacroiliac joints.

These joints in general have a limited degree of mobility. However, during pregnancy, there is remarkable relaxation of these joints at term, caused by upward gliding of the sacroiliac joint (Borell, 1957). The displacement, which is greatest in the dorsal lithotomy position, may increase the diameter of the outlet by 1.5 to 2.0 cm. This is the main justification for placing a woman in this position for a vaginal delivery. But this pelvic outlet diameter increase occurs only if the sacrum is allowed to rotate posteriorly. Thus, it will not occur if the sacrum is forced anteriorly by the weight of the maternal pelvis against the delivery table or bed (Russell, 1969, 1982). Sacroiliac joint mobility is also the likely reason that the McRoberts maneuver often is successful in releasing an obstructed shoulder in a case of shoulder dystocia (Chap. 27, p. 541). These changes have also been attributed to the success of the modified squatting position to hasten second-stage labor (Gardosi, 1989). The squatting position may increase the interspinous diameter and the pelvic outlet diameter (Russell, 1969, 1982). These latter observations are unconfirmed, but this position is assumed for birth in many societies.

Planes and Diameters of the Pelvis

The pelvis is described as having four imaginary planes:

1. The plane of the pelvic inlet—the superior strait.
2. The plane of the pelvic outlet—the inferior strait.
3. The plane of the midpelvis—the least pelvic dimensions.
4. The plane of greatest pelvic dimension—of no obstetrical significance.

Pelvic Inlet

Also called the superior strait, the pelvic inlet is also the superior plane of the true pelvis. As noted earlier, it is bounded posteriorly by the promontory and alae of the sacrum, laterally by the linea terminalis, and anteriorly by the horizontal pubic rami and the symphysis pubis. During labor, fetal head engagement is defined by the fetal head's biparietal diameter passing through this plane. To aid this passage, the inlet of the female pelvis—compared with the male pelvis—typically is more nearly round than ovoid. Caldwell (1934) identified a nearly round or gynecoid pelvic inlet in approximately half of white women.

Four diameters of the pelvic inlet are usually described: anteroposterior, transverse, and two oblique diameters. Of these, distinct anteroposterior diameters have been described using specific landmarks. Most cephalad, the anteroposterior diameter, termed the true conjugate, extends from the uppermost margin of the symphysis pubis to the sacral promontory. The clinically important obstetrical conjugate is the shortest distance between the sacral promontory and the symphysis pubis. Normally, this measures 10 cm or more, but unfortunately, it cannot be measured directly with examining fingers. Thus, for clinical purposes, the obstetrical conjugate is estimated indirectly by subtracting 1.5 to 2 cm from the diagonal conjugate, which is determined by measuring the distance from the lowest margin of the symphysis to the sacral promontory (Fig. 2-18).

The transverse diameter is constructed at right angles to the obstetrical conjugate and represents the greatest distance between the linea terminalis on either side. It usually intersects the obstetrical conjugate at a point approximately 5 cm in front of the promontory and measures approximately 13 cm. Each of the two oblique diameters extends from one sacroiliac synchondrosis to the contralateral iliopubic eminence. Each eminence

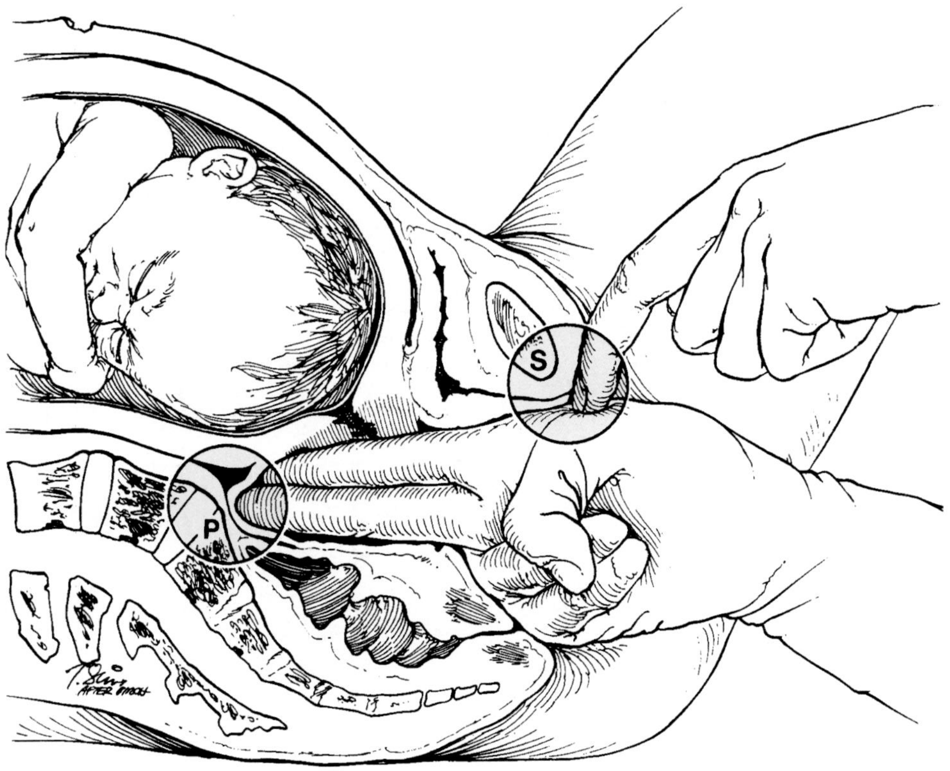

FIGURE 2-18 Vaginal examination to determine the diagonal conjugate. P = sacral promontory; S = symphysis pubis.

is a minor elevation that marks the union site of the ilium and pubis. These oblique diameters average less than 13 cm.

Midpelvis and Pelvic Outlet

The midpelvis is measured at the level of the ischial spines, also called the midplane or plane of least pelvic dimensions (Fig. 2-19). During labor, the degree of fetal head descent into the true pelvis may be described by station, and the midpelvis and ischial spines serve to mark zero station. The interspinous diameter is 10 cm or slightly greater, is usually the smallest pelvic diameter, and, in cases of obstructed labor, is particularly important. The anteroposterior diameter through the level of the ischial spines normally measures at least 11.5 cm.

The pelvic outlet consists of two approximately triangular areas whose boundaries mirror those of the perineal triangle described earlier (p. 21). They have a common base, which is a line drawn between the two ischial tuberosities. The apex of the posterior triangle is the tip of the sacrum, and the lateral boundaries are the sacrotuberous ligaments and the ischial tuberosities. The anterior triangle is formed by the descending inferior rami of the pubic bones. These rami unite at an angle of 90 to 100 degrees to form a rounded arch under which the fetal head must pass. Clinically, three diameters of the pelvic outlet usually are described—the anteroposterior, transverse, and posterior sagittal. Unless there is significant pelvic bony disease, the pelvic outlet seldom obstructs vaginal delivery.

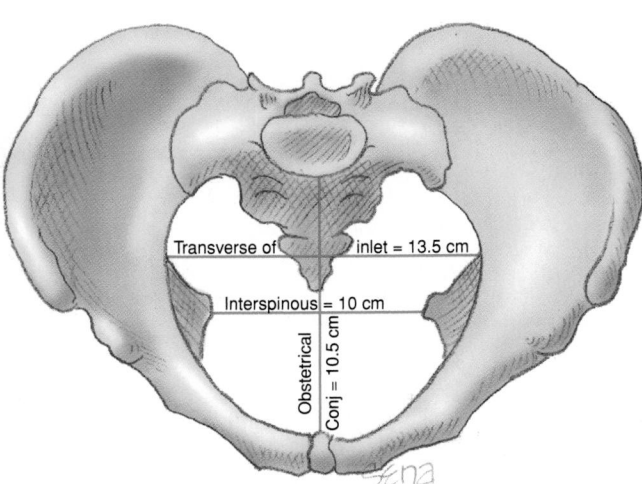

FIGURE 2-19 Adult female pelvis demonstrating the interspinous diameter of the midpelvis. The anteroposterior and transverse diameters of the pelvic inlet are also shown.

Pelvic Shapes

The Caldwell-Moloy (1933, 1934) anatomical classification of the pelvis is based on shape, and its concepts aid an understanding of labor mechanisms. Specifically, the greatest transverse diameter of the inlet and its division into anterior and posterior segments are used to classify the pelvis as gynecoid, anthropoid, android, or platypelloid. The posterior segment determines the type of pelvis, whereas the anterior segment determines the tendency. These are both determined because many pelves are not pure but are mixed types. For example, a gynecoid pelvis with an android tendency means that the posterior pelvis is gynecoid and the anterior pelvis is android shaped.

From viewing the four basic types in Figure 2-20, the configuration of the gynecoid pelvis would intuitively seem

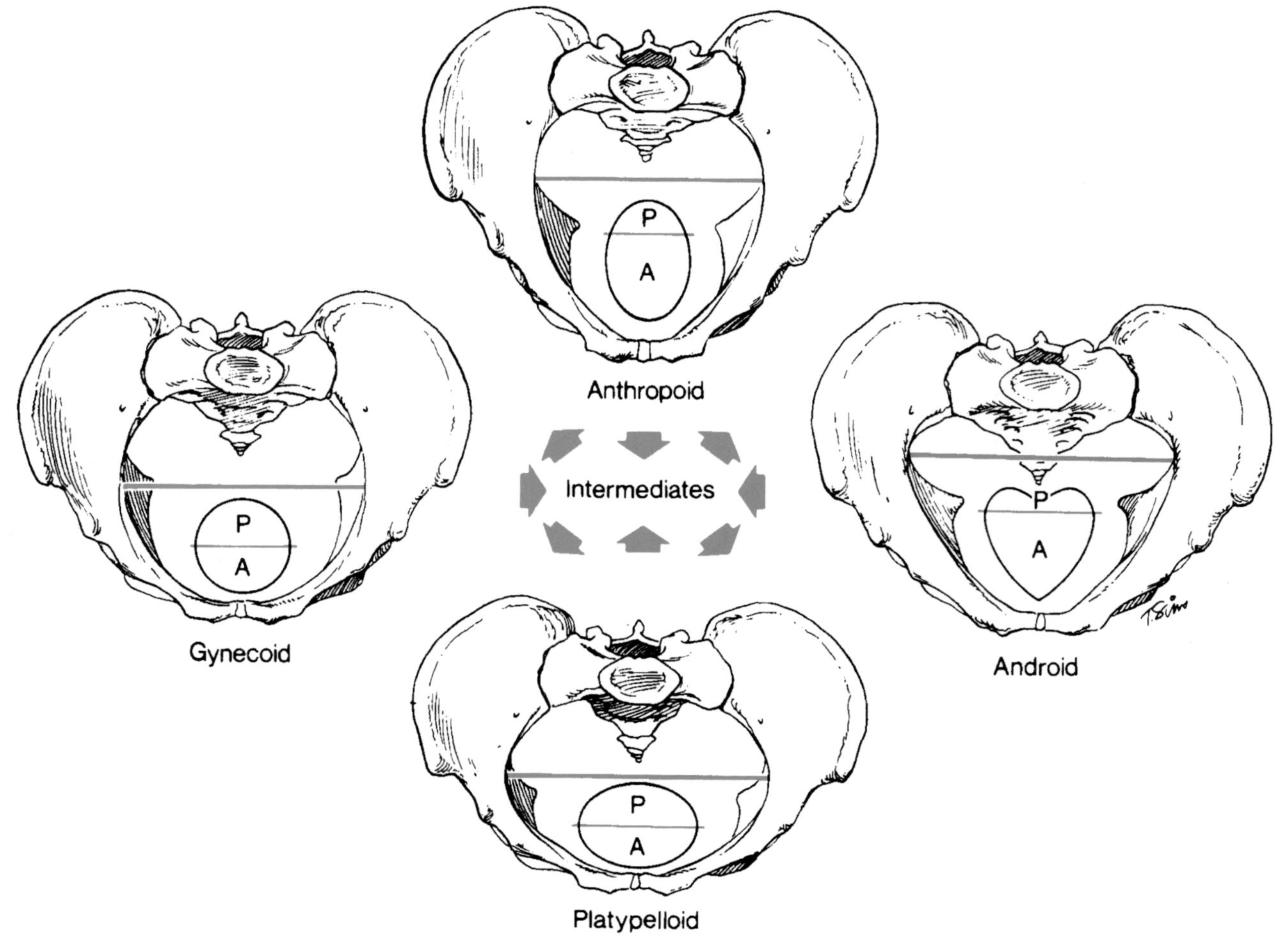

FIGURE 2-20 The four parent pelvic types of the Caldwell–Moloy classification. A line passing through the widest transverse diameter divides the inlets into posterior (P) and anterior (A) segments.

suited for delivery of most fetuses. Indeed, Caldwell (1939) reported that the gynecoid pelvis was found in almost half of women.

REFERENCES

Açar HI, Kuzu MA: Important points for protection of the autonomic nerves during total mesorectal excision. Dis Colon Rectum 55(8):907, 2012

Acién P, Sánchez del Campo F, Mayol MJ, et al: The female gubernaculum: role in the embryology and development of the genital tract and in the possible genesis of malformations. Eur J Obstet Gynecol Reprod Biol 159(2): 426, 2011

Barber MD, Bremer RE, Thor KB, et al: Innervation of the female levator ani muscles. Am J Obstet Gynecol 187:64, 2002

Beer GM, Schuster A, Seifert B, et al: The normal width of the linea alba in nulliparous women. Clin Anat 22(6):706, 2009

Bleich AT, Rahn DD, Wieslander CK, et al: Posterior division of the internal iliac artery: anatomic variations and clinical applications. Am J Obstet Gynecol 197:658.e1, 2007

Borell U, Fernstrom I: Movements at the sacroiliac joints and their importance to changes in pelvic dimensions during parturition. Acta Obstet Gynecol Scand 36:42, 1957

Caldwell WE, Moloy HC: Anatomical variations in the female pelvis and their effect in labor with a suggested classification. Am J Obstet Gynecol 26:479, 1933

Caldwell WE, Moloy HC, D'Esopo DA: Further studies on the pelvic architecture. Am J Obstet Gynecol 28:482, 1934

Caldwell WE, Moloy HC, Swenson PC: The use of the roentgen ray in obstetrics, 1. Roentgen pelvimetry and cephalometry; technique of pelviroentgenography. Am J Roentgenol 41:305, 1939

Corton MM: Anatomy of the pelvis: how the pelvis is built for support. Clin Obstet Gynecol, 48:611, 2005

Corton MM, Cunningham FG: Anatomy. In Hoffman BL, Schorge JO, Schaffer JI, et al (eds): Williams Gynecology, 2nd ed. New York, McGraw-Hill, 2012, p 943

Croxatto HB: Physiology of gamete and embryo transport through the fallopian tube. Reprod Biomed Online 4(2):160, 2002

DeLancey JO, Miller JM, Kearney R, et al: Vaginal birth and de novo stress incontinence: relative contributions of urethral dysfunction and mobility. Obstet Gynecol 110:354, 2007a

DeLancey JO, Morgan DM, Fenner DE, et al: Comparison of levator ani muscle defects and function in women with and without pelvic organ prolapse. Obstet Gynecol 109:295, 2007b

DeLancey JO, Toglia MR, Perucchini D: Internal and external anal sphincter anatomy as it relates to midline obstetric lacerations. Obstet Gynecol 90:924, 1997

DeLancey JOL, Kearney R, Chou Q, et al: The appearance of levator ani muscle abnormalities in magnetic resonance images after vaginal delivery. Obstet Gynecol 101:46, 2003

Gardosi J, Hutson N, Lynch CB: Randomised, controlled trial of squatting in the second stage of labour. Lancet 2:74, 1989

Ginger VA, Cold CJ, Yang CC: Structure and innervation of the labia minora: more than minor skin folds. Female Pelvic Med Reconstr Surg 17(4):180, 2011a

Ginger VA, Cold CJ, Yang CC: Surgical anatomy of the dorsal nerve of the clitoris. Neurourol Urodyn 30(3):412, 2011b

Hodgkinson CP: Physiology of the ovarian veins during pregnancy. Obstet Gynecol 1(1):26, 1953

Kim SO, Oh KJ, Lee HS, et al: Expression of aquaporin water channels in the vagina in premenopausal women. J Sex Med 8(7):1925, 2011

Kearney R, Sawhney R, DeLancey JO: Levator ani muscle anatomy evaluated by origin-insertion pairs. Obstet Gynecol 104:168, 2004

Langlois PL: The size of the normal uterus. J Reprod Med 4:220, 1970
Larson KA, Yousuf A, Lewicky-Gaupp C, et al: Perineal body anatomy in living women: 3-dimensional analysis using thin-slice magnetic resonance imaging. Am J Obstet Gynecol 203(5):494.e15, 2010
Lien KC, Mooney B, DeLancey JO, et al: Levator ani muscle stretch induced by simulated vaginal birth. Obstet Gynecol 103:31, 2004
Lien KC, Morgan DM, Delancey JO, et al: Pudendal nerve stretch during vaginal birth: a 3D computer simulation. Am J Obstet Gynecol 192(5):1669, 2005
Lloyd J. Crouch NS, Minto CL, et al: Female genital appearance: "normality" unfolds. BJOG 112(5):643, 2005
Loukas M, Myers C, Shah R, et al: Arcuate line of the rectus sheath: clinical approach. Anat Sci Int 83(3):140, 2008
Mahakkanukrauh P, Surin P, Vaidhayakarn P: Anatomical study of the pudendal nerve adjacent to the sacrospinous ligament. Clin Anat 18:200, 2005
Mahran M: The microscopic anatomy of the round ligament. J Obstet Gynaecol Br Commonw 72:614, 1965
Margulies RU, Huebner M, DeLancey JO: Origin and insertion points involved in levator ani muscle defects. Am J Obstet Gynecol 196:251.e1, 2007
Mei W, Jin C, Feng L, et al: Bilateral ultrasound-guided transversus abdominis plane block combined with ilioinguinal-iliohypogastric nerve block for cesarean delivery anesthesia. Anesth Analg 113(1):134, 2011
Mirilas P, Skandalakis JE: Urogenital diaphragm: an erroneous concept casting its shadow over the sphincter urethrae and deep perineal space. J Am Coll Surg 198:279, 2004
Mishriky BM, George RB, Habib AS: Transversus abdominis plane block for analgesia after Cesarean delivery: a systematic review and meta-analysis. Can J Anaesth 59(8):766, 2012
Montoya TI, Calver L, Carrick KS, et al: Anatomic relationships of the pudendal nerve branches. Am J Obstet Gynecol 205(5):504.e1, 2011
Moszkowicz D, Alsaid B, Bessede T, et al: Where does pelvic nerve injury occur during rectal surgery for cancer? Colorectal Dis 13(12):1326, 2011
Rahn DD, Phelan JN, Roshanravan SM, et al: Anterior abdominal wall nerve and vessel anatomy: clinical implications for gynecologic surgery. Am J Obstet Gynecol 202(3):234.e1, 2010
Raizada V, Mittal RK: Pelvic floor anatomy and applied physiology. Gastroenterol Clin North Am 37(3):493, 2008
Ramanah R, Berger MB, Parratte BM, et al: Anatomy and histology of apical support: a literature review concerning cardinal and uterosacral ligaments. Int Urogynecol J 23(11):1483, 2012
Rociu E, Stoker J, Eijkemans MJC, et al: Normal anal sphincter anatomy and age- and sex-related variations at high-spatial-resolution endoanal MR imaging. Radiology 217:395, 2000
Rortveit G, Daltveit AK, Hannestad YS, et al: Vaginal delivery parameters and urinary incontinence: the Norwegian EPINCONT study. Am J Obstet Gynecol 189:1268, 2003
Russell JGB: Moulding of the pelvic outlet. J Obstet Gynaecol Br Commonw 76:817, 1969
Russell JGB: The rationale of primitive delivery positions. Br J Obstet Gynaecol 89:712, 1982
Schwalm H, Dubrauszky V: The structure of the musculature of the human uterus—muscles and connective tissue. Am J Obstet Gynecol 94:391, 1966
Shafik A, Doss SH: Pudendal canal: surgical anatomy and clinical implications. Am Surg 65:176, 1999
Shafik A, Sibai OE, Shafik AA, et al: A novel concept for the surgical anatomy of the perineal body. Dis Colon Rectum 50(12):2120, 2007
Sheikhazadi A, Sadr SS, Ghadyani MH, et al: Study of the normal internal organ weights in Tehran's population. J Forensic Leg Med 17(2):78, 2010
Spackman R, Wrigley B, Roberts A, et al: The inferior hypogastric plexus: a different view. J Obstet Gynaecol 27(2):130, 2007
Sviggum HP, Niesen AD, Sites BD, et al: Trunk blocks 101: transversus abdominis plane, ilioinguinal-iliohypogastric, and rectus sheath blocks. Int Anesthesiol Clin 50(1):74, 2012
Tolcher MC, Nitsche JF, Arendt KW, et al: Spontaneous rectus sheath hematoma pregnancy: case report and review of the literature. Obstet Gynecol Surv 65(8):517, 2010
Umek WH, Morgan DM, Ashton-Miller JA, et al: Quantitative analysis of uterosacral ligament origin and insertion points by magnetic resonance imaging. Obstet Gynecol 103:447, 2004
Verkauf BS, Von Thron J, O'Brien WF: Clitoral size in normal women. Obstet Gynecol 80(1):41, 1992
Weber AM, Walters MD: Anterior vaginal prolapse: review of anatomy and techniques of surgical repair. Obstet Gynecol 89:311, 1997
Weidner AC, Jamison MG, Branham V, et al: Neuropathic injury to the levator ani occurs in 1 in 4 primiparous women. Am J Obstet Gynecol 195:1851, 2006
Whiteside JL, Barber MD, Walters MD, et al: Anatomy of ilioinguinal and iliohypogastric nerves in relation to trocar placement and low transverse incisions. Am J Obstet Gynecol 189:1574, 2003
Wilkinson EJ, Massoll NA: Benign diseases of the vulva. In Kurman RJ, Ellenson LH, Ronnett BM (eds): Blaustein's Pathology of the Female Genital Tract, 6th ed. New York, Springer, 2011, p 3
Wolfson A, Lee AJ, Wong RP, et al: Bilateral multi-injection iliohypogastric-ilioinguinal nerve block in conjunction with neuraxial morphine is superior to neuraxial morphine alone for postcesarean analgesia. J Clin Anesth 24(4):298, 2012
Woodman PJ, Graney DO: Anatomy and physiology of the female perineal body with relevance to obstetrical injury and repair. Clin Anat 15:321, 2002

CHAPTER 3

Congenital Genitourinary Abnormalities

Integral to successful reproduction is a normally functioning genital tract, both anatomically and physiologically. A number of developmental abnormalities can lead to infertility, subfertility, spontaneous abortion, or midpregnancy and preterm delivery. To care for affected women, it is imperative that the clinician have a working knowledge of genitourinary system development.

GENITOURINARY TRACT DEVELOPMENT

Embryologically in females, the external genitalia, gonads, and müllerian ducts each derive from different primordia and in close association with the urinary tract and hindgut. Abnormal embryogenesis of these is thought to be multifactorial and can lead to sporadic anomalies. Normal genitourinary development is summarized in Figure 3-1 and also discussed in Chapter 7 (p. 144).

Embryology of the Urinary System

Between the 3rd and 5th gestational weeks, an elevation of intermediate mesoderm on each side of the fetus–the urogenital ridge–begins development into the urogenital tract. This further divides into the gonadal or genital ridge, which will become the ovary, and into the nephrogenic cord, which is subsequently described. The müllerian ducts become the fallopian tubes, uterus, and upper vagina and derive from coelomic epithelium covering the nephrogenic cord. It is because of this separate gonadal and müllerian derivation that women with müllerian defects typically have functionally normal ovaries and are phenotypic females.

The urinary tract develops from the mesonephros or wolffian ducts situated within each nephrogenic cord and connects the mesonephric kidney to the cloaca (Fig. 3-1A). Recall that evolution of the renal system passes sequentially through the pronephric and mesonephric stages to reach the permanent metanephric system. Between the 4th and 5th weeks, each mesonephric duct gives rise to a ureteric bud, which grows cephalad toward its respective mesonephros (Fig. 3-1B). As each bud lengthens, it induces differentiation of the metanephros, which will become the final kidney (Fig. 3-1C). Each mesonephros degenerates near the end of the first trimester, and without testosterone, the mesonephric ducts regress as well.

The cloaca begins as a common opening for the embryonic urinary, genital, and alimentary tracts. By the 7th week it becomes divided by the urorectal septum to create the rectum and the urogenital sinus (Fig. 3-1D). The urogenital sinus is considered in three parts: (1) the cephalad or vesicle portion, which will form the urinary bladder; (2) the middle or pelvic portion, which creates the female urethra; and (3) the caudal or

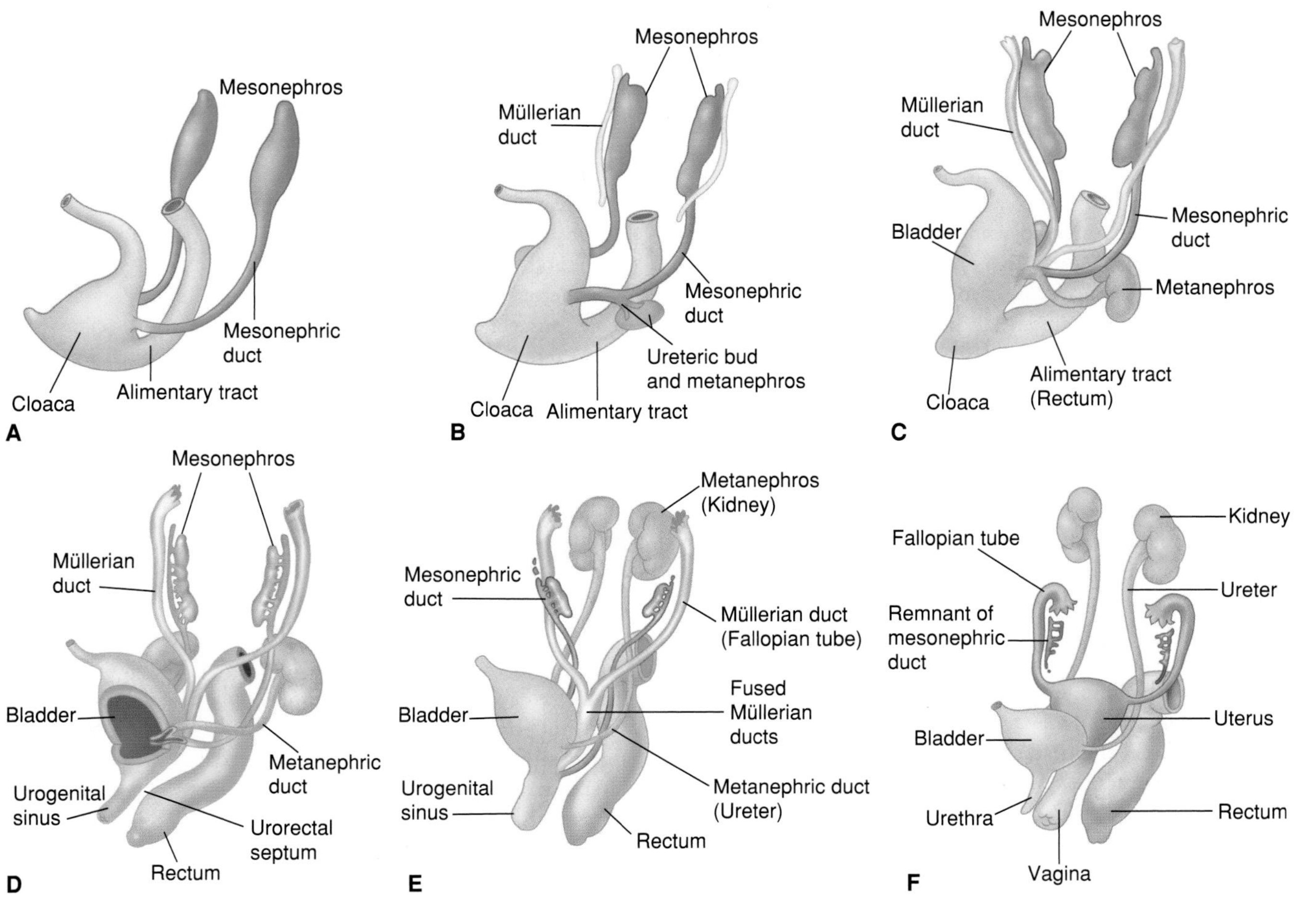

FIGURE 3-1 Embryonic development of the female genitourinary tract **(A-F)**. (From Bradshaw, 2012, with permission.)

phallic part, which will give rise to the distal vagina and to the greater vestibular (Bartholin) and paraurethral (Skene) glands.

Embryology of the Genital Tract

Development of the genital tract begins as the müllerian ducts, also termed paramesonephric ducts, form lateral to each mesonephros. These ducts extend downward and then turn medially to meet and fuse together in the midline. The uterus is formed by this union of the two müllerian ducts at approximately the 10th week (Fig. 3-1E). Fusion begins in the middle and then extends caudally and cephalad. With cellular proliferation at the upper portion, a thick wedge of tissue creates the characteristic piriform uterine shape. At the same time, dissolution of cells at the lower pole forms the first uterine cavity (Fig. 3-1F). As the upper wedge-shaped septum is slowly reabsorbed, the final uterine cavity is usually shaped by the 20th week. If the two müllerian ducts fail to fuse, then there are separate uterine horns. In contrast, resorption failure of the common tissue between them results in various degrees of persistent uterine septum.

As the distal end of the fused müllerian ducts contacts the urogenital sinus, this induces endodermal outgrowths termed the sinovaginal bulbs. These bulbs proliferate and fuse to form the vaginal plate, which later resorbs to form the vaginal lumen. This vaginal canalization is generally completed by the 20th week. However, the lumen remains separated from the urogenital sinus by the hymeneal membrane. This membrane further degenerates to leave only the hymeneal ring.

The close association of the mesonephric (wolffian) and paramesonephric (müllerian) ducts explains why there are commonly simultaneous abnormalities involving these structures. In an older study, Kenney and colleagues (1984) showed that up to half of females with uterovaginal malformations have associated urinary tract defects. Anomalies most frequently associated with renal defects are unicornuate uterus, uterine didelphys, and agenesis syndromes, whereas arcuate and bicornuate are less commonly linked (Reichman, 2010). When these are identified, the urinary system can be evaluated with magnetic resonance (MR) imaging, sonography, or intravenous pyelography (Hall-Craggs, 2013). Finally, in these cases, ovaries are functionally normal but have a higher incidence of anatomical maldescent into the pelvis (Allen, 2012; Dabirashrafi, 1994).

MESONEPHRIC REMNANTS

As discussed, the mesonephric ducts usually degenerate, however, persistent remnants may become clinically apparent. Mesonephric or wolffian vestiges can persist as Gartner duct cysts. These are typically located in the proximal anterolateral vaginal wall but may be found at other sites along the vaginal length. They can be further characterized by magnetic resonance (MR) imaging. Most are asymptomatic and benign, and although they may measure up to 7 cm in diameter, they usually do not require surgical excision. An infected cyst occasionally requires marsupialization.

Intraabdominal wolffian remnants in the female include a few blind tubules in the mesovarium—the epoöphoron—as well as similar ones adjacent to the uterus—collectively the paroöphoron (Moore, 2013). The epoöphoron or paroöphoron may develop into clinically identifiable cysts and are included in the differential diagnosis of an adnexal mass (Chap. 63, p. 1226).

BLADDER AND PERINEAL ABNORMALITIES

Very early during embryo formation, a bilaminar cloacal membrane lies at the caudal end of the germinal disc and forms the infraumbilical abdominal wall. Normally, an ingrowth of mesoderm between the ectodermal and endodermal layers of the cloacal membrane leads to formation of the lower abdominal musculature and pelvic bones. Without reinforcement, the cloacal membrane may prematurely rupture, and depending on the extent of the infraumbilical defect, *cloacal exstrophy, bladder exstrophy*, or *epispadias* may result. Of these, cloacal exstrophy is rare and includes the triad of omphalocele, bladder exstrophy, and imperforate anus.

Bladder exstrophy is characterized by an exposed bladder lying outside the abdomen. Associated findings commonly include a widened symphysis pubis, caused by outward innominate bone rotation, and abnormal external genitalia. For example, the urethra and vagina are typically short, and the vaginal orifice is frequently stenotic and displaced anteriorly. The clitoris is duplicated or bifid, and the labia, mons pubis, and clitoris are divergent. At the same time, however, the uterus, fallopian tubes, and ovaries are typically normal except for occasional müllerian duct fusion defects.

Pregnancy with bladder exstrophy is associated with greater risk for antepartum pyelonephritis, urinary retention, ureteral obstruction, pelvic organ prolapse, and breech presentation. Due to the extensive adhesions from prior repair and altered anatomy typically encountered, some recommend planned cesarean delivery at a tertiary center (Deans, 2012; Greenwell, 2003).

Epispadias without bladder exstrophy includes anomalies that include a widened, patulous urethra; absent or bifid clitoris; nonfused labial folds; and flattened mons pubis. Vertebral abnormalities and pubic symphysis diathesis are also common.

Clitoral anomalies are unusual. One is clitoral duplication or bifid clitoris, which is rare and usually develops in association with bladder exstrophy or epispadias. With female phallic urethra, the urethra opens at the clitoral tip. Last, clitoromegaly noted at birth is suggestive of fetal exposure to excessive androgens (Chap. 7, p. 148). In some preterm neonates, the clitoris may appear large, but then regresses as the infant grows. Other causes of newborn clitoromegaly include breech presentation with vulvar swelling, chronic severe vulvovaginitis, and neurofibromatosis (Dershwitz, 1984; Greer, 1981).

DEFECTS OF THE HYMEN

Hymeneal anomalies include imperforate, microperforate, cribriform (sievelike), navicular (boatshaped), and septate hymens. They result from failure of the inferior end of the vaginal plate—the hymeneal membrane—to canalize. Their incidences approximate one in 1000 to 2000 females (American College of Obstetricians and Gynecologists, 2013). During the neonatal period, significant amounts of mucus can be secreted due to maternal estrogen stimulation. With an imperforate hymen, secretions collect to form a bulging, translucent yellow-gray mass, termed hydro- or mucocolpos, at the vaginal introitus. Most are asymptomatic and resolve as mucus is reabsorbed and estrogen levels decrease, but occasionally they must be differentiated from a hymeneal cyst (Breech, 2009; Nazir, 2006). Problems with imperforate hymen are uncommon in neonates, and most become apparent during adolescence with classic findings of amenorrhea, cyclic abdominal pain, and a bulging bluish introital membrane.

MÜLLERIAN ABNORMALITIES

There are four principal deformities that arise from defective müllerian duct embryological steps: (1) agenesis of both ducts, either focally or along the entire duct length; (2) unilateral maturation of one müllerian duct with incomplete or absent development of the opposite side; (3) absent or faulty midline fusion of the ducts; or (4) defective canalization. Various classifications of these have been proposed, and shown in Table 3-1 is the one used by the American Fertility Society as derived by Buttram and Gibbons (1979).

TABLE 3-1. Classification of Müllerian Anomalies

- **I. Segmental müllerian hypoplasia or agenesis**
  - a. Vaginal
  - b. Cervical
  - c. Uterine fundal
  - d. Tubal
  - e. Combined anomalies
- **II. Unicornuate uterus**
  - a. Communicating rudimentary horn
  - b. Noncommunicating horn
  - c. No endometrial cavity
  - d. No rudimentary horn
- **III. Uterine didelphys**
- **IV. Bicornuate uterus**
  - a. Complete—division to internal os
  - b. Partial
- **V. Septate uterus**
  - a. Complete—septum to internal os
  - b. Partial
- **VI. Arcuate**
- **VII. Diethylstilbestrol related**

Adapted from the American Fertility Society, 1988.

It separates anomalies into groups with similar clinical characteristics, prognosis for pregnancy, and treatment. It also includes one for abnormalities associated with fetal exposure to diethylstilbestrol (DES).

Initially, müllerian anomalies may be suspected by symptoms or clinical findings. First, these defects are frequently identified during pelvic examination. Sonography is initially done to search for associated lesions. However, MR imaging is often required to more fully delineate anatomy, especially with obstructive lesions requiring surgery. Amenorrhea may be an initial complaint for those with agenesis of a müllerian component. For those with complete agenesis, karyotyping is typically indicated to exclude XY disorders of sex development, which were formerly termed male pseudohermaphroditism (Hughes, 2006). Last, pelvic pain due to occult blood accumulation may arise from functioning endometrium with outlet obstruction.

Müllerian Agenesis

Class I segmental defects can be caused by müllerian hypoplasia or agenesis as shown in Figure 3-2. These developmental defects can affect the vagina, cervix, uterus, or fallopian tubes and may be isolated or may coexist with other müllerian defects.

Vaginal Abnormalities

In addition to vaginal agenesis, there are two types of congenital septa. One is a longitudinal septum, which arises from a fusion or resorption defect. The other, a transverse septum, results either from incomplete canalization or from vertical fusion failure between the down-growing müllerian duct system and the up-growing urogenital sinus. All of these defects may be isolated or associated with other müllerian anomalies. One example is the Mayer-Rokitansky-Küster-Hauser (MRKH) syndrome, in which upper vaginal agenesis is typically associated with hypoplasia or uterine agenesis. This syndrome may also display abnormalities of the renal, skeletal, and auditory systems. This triad is known by the acronym MURCS–müllerian duct aplasia, renal aplasia, and cervicothoracic somite dysplasia (Duncan, 1979).

The obstetrical significance of vaginal anomalies depends greatly on the degree of obstruction. For example, complete vaginal agenesis, unless corrected operatively, precludes pregnancy by vaginal intercourse. With MRKH syndrome, a functional vagina can be created, but childbearing is impossible. In these women, however, ova can be retrieved for in vitro fertilization (IVF) in a surrogate mother.

With longitudinal septa, most are complete. When partial, they are high in the vagina. Septa are typically associated with

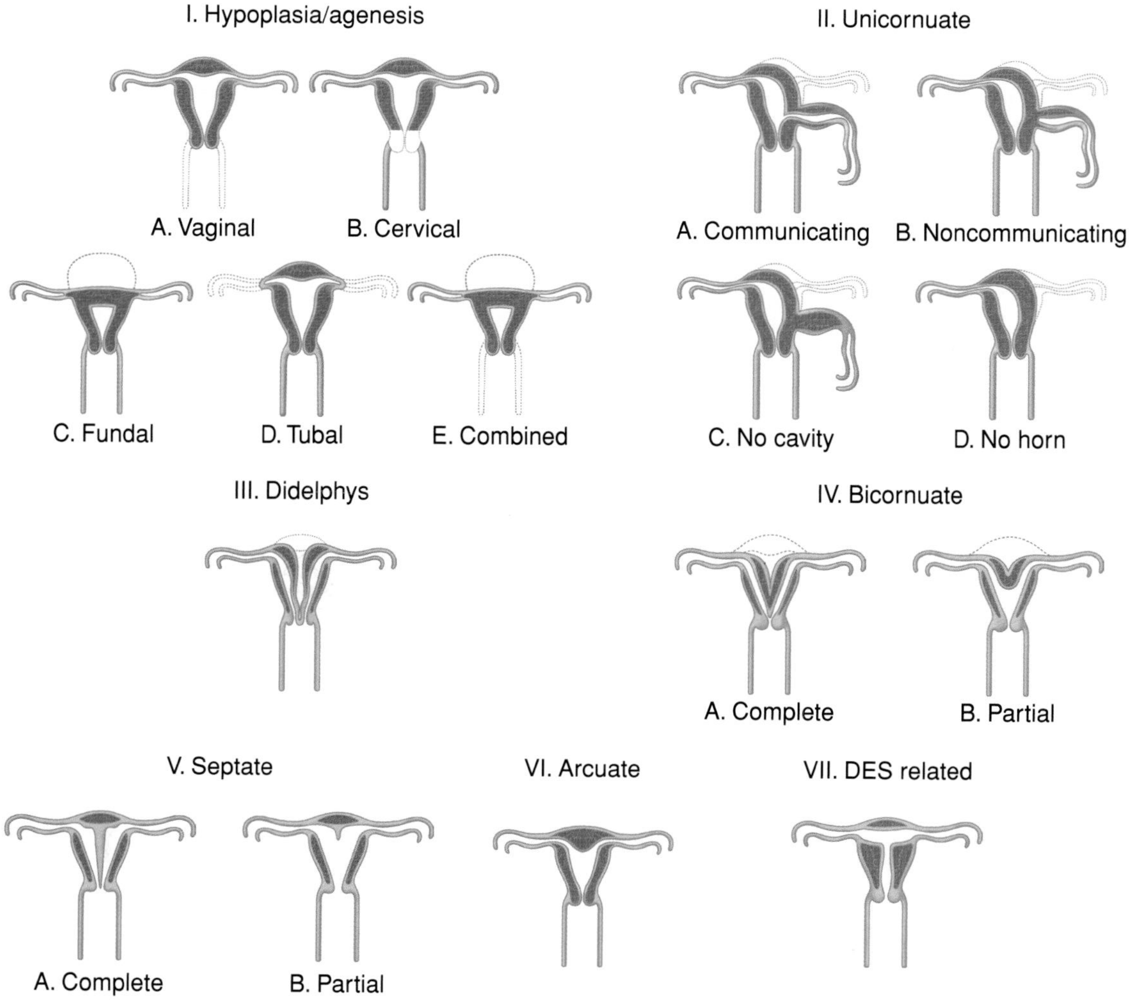

FIGURE 3-2 Classification of müllerian anomalies. (Redrawn from American Fertility Society, 1988.)

other müllerian anomalies (Haddad, 1997). A complete longitudinal vaginal septum usually does not cause dystocia because the vaginal side through which the fetus descends dilates satisfactorily. An incomplete or partially obstructed longitudinal septum, however, may interfere with descent.

A transverse septum causes an obstruction of variable thickness, and it may develop at any depth within the vagina. Occasionally, the upper vagina is separated from the rest of the canal by a septum with a small opening. Gibson (2003) reported this in association with miscarriage and described dilatation of the septal opening to permit evacuation of products. In labor, such strictures may be mistaken for the upper limit of the vaginal vault, and the septal opening is misidentified as an undilated cervical os. If encountered during labor, and after the external os has dilated completely, the head impinges on the septum and causes it to bulge downward. If the septum does not yield, slight pressure on its opening usually leads to further dilatation, but occasionally cruciate incisions are required to permit delivery (Blanton, 2003). If there is a thick transverse septum, however, cesarean delivery may be necessary.

Cervical Abnormalities

Developmental abnormalities of the cervix include partial or complete agenesis, duplication, and longitudinal septa. Uncorrected complete agenesis is incompatible with pregnancy, and IVF with gestational surrogacy is an option. Surgical correction by uterovaginal anastomosis has resulted in successful pregnancy (Deffarges, 2001; Fedele, 2008). There are significant complications with this corrective surgery, and the need for clear preoperative anatomy delineation has been emphasized by Rock (2010) and Roberts (2011) and their colleagues. For this reason, they recommend hysterectomy for complete cervical agenesis and reserve reconstruction attempts for carefully selected patients with cervical dysgenesis.

Uterine Abnormalities

From a large variety, a few of the more common congenital uterine malformations are shown in Table 3-1. Accurate population prevalences of these are difficult to assess because the best diagnostic techniques are invasive. The reported population prevalence ranges from 0.4 to 5 percent, and rates in women with recurrent miscarriage are significantly higher (Acién, 1997; Byrne, 2000; Chan, 2011b). In a review of 22 studies with more than 573,000 women who were screened for these malformations, Nahum (1998) reported the distribution of uterine anomalies as follows: bicornuate, 39 percent; septate, 34 percent; didelphic, 11 percent; arcuate, 7 percent; unicornuate, 5 percent; and hypo- or aplastic, 4 percent.

Müllerian anomalies may be discovered at routine pelvic examinations, cesarean delivery, during laparoscopy for tubal sterilization, or during infertility evaluation. Depending on clinical presentation, diagnostic tools may include hysterosalpingography, sonography, MR imaging, laparoscopy, and hysteroscopy. Each has limitations, and these may be used in combination to completely define anatomy. In women undergoing fertility evaluation, hysterosalpingography (HSG) is commonly selected for uterine cavity and tubal patency assessment. That said, HSG poorly defines the external uterine contour and can delineate only patent cavities. It is contraindicated during pregnancy.

In most clinical settings, sonography is initially performed. Transabdominal views may help to maximize the viewing field, but transvaginal sonography (TVS) provides better image resolution. For this indication, the pooled accuracy for TVS is 90 to 92 percent (Pellerito, 1992). Saline infusion sonography (SIS) improves delineation of the endometrium and internal uterine morphology, but only with a patent endometrial cavity. Also, SIS is contraindicated in pregnancy. Three-dimensional (3-D) sonography is more accurate than 2-D sonography because it provides uterine images from virtually any angle. Thus, coronal images can be constructed, and these are essential in evaluating both internal and external uterine contours (Olpin, 2009). Both 2-D and 3-D sonography are suitable for pregnancy. In gynecological patients, these are ideally completed during the luteal phase when the secretory endometrium provides contrast from increased thickness and echogenicity (Caliskan, 2010).

Several investigators have reported very good concordance between 3-D TVS and MR imaging of müllerian anomalies, although MR imaging is currently preferred for imaging such defects (Bermejo, 2010; Ghi, 2009). MR imaging provides clear delineation of both the internal and external uterine anatomy and has a reported accuracy of up to 100 percent in the evaluation of müllerian anomalies (Fedele, 1989; Pellerito, 1992). Moreover, complex anomalies and commonly associated secondary diagnoses such as renal or skeletal anomalies can be concurrently evaluated. Precautions with MR imaging in pregnancy are discussed in Chapter 46 (p. 934).

In some women undergoing an infertility evaluation, hysteroscopy and laparoscopy may be selected to assess for müllerian anomalies; screen for endometriosis, which is often coexistent; and exclude other tubal or uterine cavity pathologies (Puscheck, 2008; Saravelos, 2008). However, hysteroscopy is contraindicated in pregnancy.

Unicornuate Uterus (Class II)

With this anomaly, the underdeveloped or rudimentary horn may be absent. If present, it may or may not be communicating and may or may not contain an endometrium-lined cavity (see Fig. 3-2). General population estimates cite that a unicornuate uterus develops in 1 in 4000 women (Reichman, 2009). It may be detected during fertility evaluation by HSG. Although this study can define the primary cavity contour, noncommunicating or noncavitary rudimentary horns may not fill with dye. Conventional sonography may be difficult for less-experienced sonographers as the smaller size and lateral deviation of an isolated unicornuate uterus or a rudimentary horn may not be appreciated. If suspected, 3-D sonography increases diagnostic accuracy, but MR imaging is often preferred (Fig. 3-3). Importantly, 40 percent of affected women will have renal anomalies, and evaluation for these is indicated (Fedele, 1996a).

This müllerian anomaly carries significant obstetrical risks, including first- and second-trimester miscarriage, malpresenta-

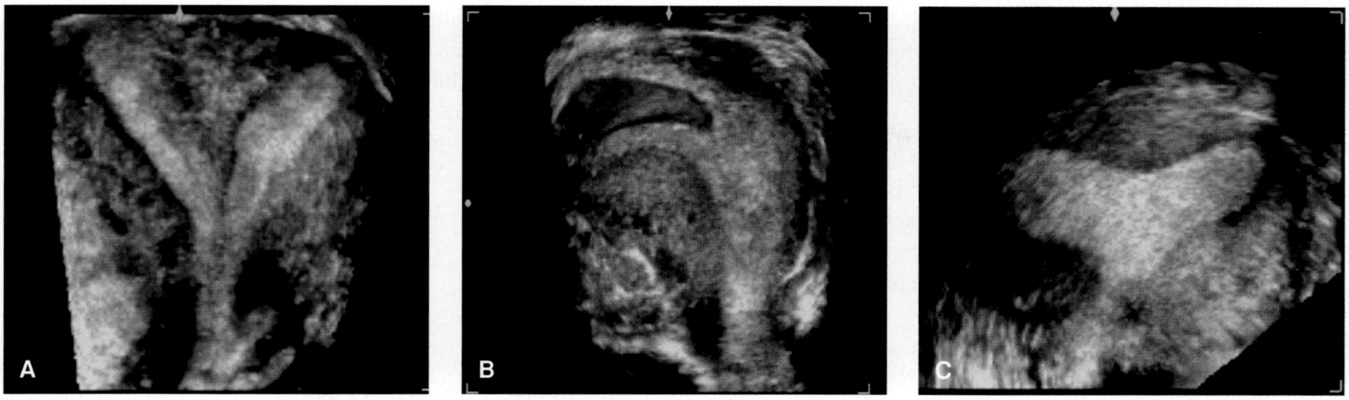

FIGURE 3-3 Three-dimensional transvaginal sonographic images. **A.** A nongravid septate uterus characteristically has a flat external fundal contour but a deep cleft that separates the hyperechoic endometrial cavities. **B.** This gravid unicornuate uterus illustrates the classic "banana" configuration. (A & B modified from Moschos, 2012, with permission.) **C.** A nongravid arcuate uterus characteristically has a flat external fundal contour and a shallow indentation into the hyperechoic endometrial cavity. (Modified from Werner, 2012, with permission.)

tion, fetal-growth restriction, fetal demise, prematurely ruptured membranes, and preterm delivery (Chan, 2011a; Hua, 2011; Reichman, 2009). Abnormal uterine blood flow, cervical incompetence, and diminished cavity size and muscle mass of the hemiuterus are postulated to underlie these risks (Donderwinkel, 1992).

Rudimentary horns also increase the risk of an ectopic pregnancy within the remnant, which may be disastrous. This risk includes noncommunicating cavitary rudiments because of transperitoneal sperm migration (Nahum, 2004). In a report of 70 such pregnancies, Rolen and associates (1966) found that the rudimentary uterine horn ruptured prior to 20 weeks in most. Nahum (2002) reviewed the literature from 1900 to 1999 and identified 588 rudimentary horn pregnancies. Half had uterine rupture, and 80 percent did so before the third trimester. Of the total 588, neonatal survival was only 6 percent.

Imaging allows an earlier diagnosis of rudimentary horn pregnancy so that it can be treated either medically or surgically before rupture (Edelman, 2003; Khati, 2012; Worley, 2008). If diagnosed in a nonpregnant woman, most recommend prophylactic excision of a horn that has a cavity (Fedele, 2005; Rackow, 2007).

Uterine Didelphys (Class III)

This interesting müllerian anomaly arises from a complete lack of fusion that results in two entirely separate hemiuteri, cervices, and usually two vaginas (see Fig. 3-2). Most women have a double vagina or a longitudinal vaginal septum (Heinonen, 1984). Uterine didelphys may be isolated or part of a triad that has an obstructed hemivagina and ipsilateral renal agenesis (OHVIRA), also known as Herlyn-Werner-Wunderlich syndrome (Smith, 2007; Tong, 2013). Didelphys derives from the Greek *di*—two + *delphus*—uterus. The term was once used to refer to all marsupials, but now only to one genus that includes the American possum—*Didelphys virginiana*—one of several mammalian species in which the female has a double uterus, cervix, and vagina.

These anomalies may be suspected on pelvic examination by identification of a longitudinal vaginal septum and two cervices. During HSG for fertility evaluation, contrast shows two separate endocervical canals. These open into separate noncommunicating fusiform endometrial cavities that each ends with a solitary fallopian tube. In women without fertility issues, sonography is a logical initial imaging tool, and separate divergent uterine horns with a large intervening fundal cleft are seen. Endometrial cavities are uniformly separate. MR imaging may be valuable in cases without classic findings.

Adverse obstetrical outcomes associated with uterine didelphys are similar but less frequent than those seen with unicornuate uterus. Increased risks include miscarriage, preterm birth, and malpresentation (Chan, 2011a; Grimbizis, 2001; Hua, 2011). Metroplasty for either uterine didelphys or bicornuate uterus involves resection of intervening myometrium and fundal recombination. These are uncommon surgeries and chosen for highly selected patients with otherwise unexplained miscarriages. Unfortunately, there is no evidence-based support to confirm efficacy of such surgical repair.

Bicornuate Uterus (Class IV)

This relatively common anomaly forms as lack of fundal fusion results in two hemiuteri, with only one cervix and vagina (see Fig. 3-2). As with uterine didelphys, a coexistent longitudinal vaginal septum is not uncommon. Radiological discrimination of bicornuate uterus from the septate uterus can be challenging. However, it is important because septate uterus can be treated with hysteroscopic septal resection. Widely diverging horns seen on HSG may suggest a bicornuate uterus. An intercornual angle greater than 105 degrees suggests bicornuate uterus, whereas one less than 75 degrees indicates a septate uterus. However, MR imaging is necessary to define fundal contour. With this, an intrafundal downward cleft measuring 1 cm or more is indicative of bicornuate uterus, whereas a cleft depth less than 1 cm indicates a septate uterus. Use of 3-D sonography also allows internal and external uterine assessment.

There are increased risks for adverse obstetrical outcomes with bicornuate uterus that include miscarriage, preterm birth, and malpresentation. As discussed earlier, surgical correction by metroplasty is reserved for highly selected patients.

Septate Uterus (Class V)

This anomaly is caused when a resorption defect leads to a persistent complete or partial longitudinal uterine cavity septum (see Fig. 3-2). In rare cases, a complete vaginocervicouterine septum is found (Darwish, 2009). Many septate uteri are identified during evaluation of infertility or recurrent pregnancy loss. Although an abnormality may be identified with HSG, MR imaging or 3-D sonography is typically required to differentiate this from a bicornuate uterus (see Fig. 3-3).

Septate anomalies are associated with diminished fertility as well as increased risks for adverse pregnancy outcomes that include miscarriage, preterm delivery, and malpresentation. The poorly vascularized uterine septum likely causes abnormal implantation or defective early embryo development and miscarriage (Fedele, 1996b). Hysteroscopic septal resection has been shown to improve pregnancy rates and outcomes (Grimbizis, 2001; Mollo, 2009; Pabuçcu, 2004). From their metaanalysis, Nouri and colleagues (2010) reported a 60-percent pregnancy rate and 45-percent live birth rate in those so treated.

Arcuate Uterus (Class VI)

This malformation is a mild deviation from the normally developed uterus (see Fig. 3-3). Although some studies report no increased adverse associated outcomes, others have found excessive second-trimester losses, preterm labor, and malpresentation (Chan, 2011a; Mucowski, 2010; Woelfer, 2001).

Treatment with Cerclage

Some women with uterine anomalies and repetitive pregnancy losses may benefit from transvaginal or transabdominal cervical cerclage (Golan, 1992; Groom, 2004). Some women with partial cervical atresia or hypoplasia may also benefit (Hampton, 1990; Ludmir, 1991; Mackey, 2001). Candidacy for cerclage is determined by the same criteria used for women without such defects, which is discussed in Chapter 18 (p. 361).

Diethylstilbestrol Reproductive Tract Abnormalities (Class VII)

During the 1960s, a synthetic nonsteroidal estrogen–diethylstilbestrol (DES)–was used to treat pregnant women for threatened abortion, preterm labor, preeclampsia, and diabetes. The treatment was remarkably ineffective. In addition, it was later discovered that women exposed as fetuses had increased risks of developing a number of specific reproductive-tract anomalies. These included vaginal clear cell adenocarcinoma, cervical intraepithelial neoplasia, small-cell cervical carcinoma, and vaginal adenosis. A fourth of affected women had identifiable structural variations in the cervix and vagina to include transverse septa, circumferential ridges, and cervical collars. Even more anomalies were smaller uterine cavities, shortened upper uterine segments, T-shaped and other irregular cavities, and fallopian tube abnormalities (see Fig. 3-2) (Barranger, 2002).

These women also had fertility issues that included impaired conception rates and higher rates of miscarriage, ectopic pregnancy, and preterm delivery, especially in those with structural abnormalities (Goldberg, 1999; Palmer, 2001). Now, more than 50 years after DES use was proscribed, most affected women are past childbearing age, but higher rates of earlier menopause and breast cancer have been reported in exposed women (Hatch, 2006; Hoover, 2011).

Fallopian Tube Abnormalities

The fallopian tubes develop from the unpaired distal ends of the müllerian ducts. Congenital anomalies include accessory ostia, complete or segmental tubal agenesis, and several embryonic cystic remnants (Woodruff, 1969). The most common is a small, benign cyst attached by a pedicle to the distal end of the fallopian tube—the hydatid of Morgagni (Zheng, 2009). In other cases, benign paratubal cysts may be of mesonephric or mesothelial origin. Last, in utero exposure to DES has been associated with various tubal abnormalities. Of these, short, tortuous tubes or ones with shriveled fimbria and small ostia have been linked to infertility (DeCherney, 1981).

UTERINE FLEXION

Anteflexion

This is defined by anterior flexion of the uterine fundus relative to the cervix in the sagittal plane. Mild or moderate flexion is typically without clinical consequence, but congenital or acquired extremes may lead to pregnancy complications. Exaggerated degrees of anteflexion usually pose no problem in early pregnancy. Later, however, particularly when the abdominal wall is lax such as with diastasis recti or ventral hernia, the uterus may fall forward. This may be so extreme that the fundus lies below the lower margin of the symphysis. Sometimes this abnormal uterine position prevents proper transmission of labor contractions, but this is usually overcome by repositioning and application of an abdominal binder.

Retroflexion

This is posterior uterine fundal flexion in the sagittal plane. A growing retroflexed uterus will occasionally become incarcerated in the hollow of the sacrum. Symptoms include abdominal discomfort, pelvic pressure, and voiding dysfunction that may include urinary frequency or retention. On bimanual pelvic examination, the cervix will be anterior and behind the symphysis pubis, whereas the uterus is appreciated as a mass wedged in the pelvis. Sonography or MR imaging may be necessary to confirm the clinical diagnosis (Gardner, 2013; Grossenburg, 2011; van Beekhuizen, 2003).

The incarcerated uterus must be repositioned to its normal anatomical position. After bladder catheterization, the uterus can usually be pushed out of the pelvis when the woman is placed in the knee-chest position. Often, this is best accomplished by digital pressure applied through the rectum. Conscious sedation, spinal analgesia, or general anesthesia may be necessary. Following repositioning, the catheter is left in place until bladder tone returns. Insertion of a soft pessary for a few weeks usually prevents reincarceration. Lettieri and colleagues (1994) described seven cases of uterine incarceration

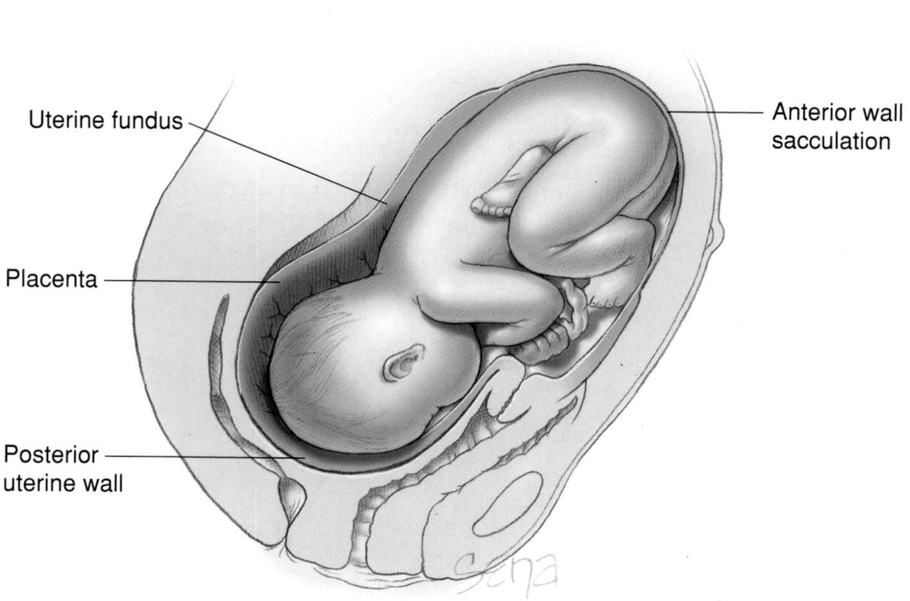

FIGURE 3-4 Anterior sacculation of a pregnant uterus. Note the markedly attenuated anterior uterine wall and atypical location of the true uterine fundus.

not amenable to these simple procedures. In two women, laparoscopy was used at 14 weeks to reposition the uterus using the round ligaments for traction. Alternatively, in two case series, colonoscopy was used to dislodge an incarcerated uterus (Dierickx, 2011; Seubert, 1999).

Sacculation

Persistent entrapment of the pregnant uterus in the pelvis may lead to extensive lower uterine segment dilatation to accommodate the fetus. An example of *anterior sacculation* is shown in Figure 3-4. In these extreme cases, sonography and MR imaging are typically required to define anatomy (Gottschalk, 2008; Lee, 2008). Cesarean delivery is necessary when there is marked sacculation, and Spearing (1978) stressed the importance of identifying the distorted anatomy. An elongated vagina passing above the level of a fetal head that is deeply placed into the pelvis suggests a sacculation or an abdominal pregnancy. The Foley catheter is frequently palpated above the level of the umbilicus! Spearing (1978) recommended extending the abdominal incision above the umbilicus and delivering the entire uterus from the abdomen before hysterotomy. This will restore correct anatomical relationships and prevent inadvertent incisions into and through the vagina and bladder. Unfortunately, this may not always be possible (Singh, 2007).

Friedman and associates (1986) described a rare case of posterior sacculation following aggressive treatment for intrauterine adhesions. Finally, uterine retroversion and a true uterine diverticulum have been mistaken for uterine sacculations (Hill, 1993; Rajiah, 2009).

Uterine Torsion

It is common during pregnancy for the uterus to rotate to the right side. Rarely, uterine rotation exceeds 180 degrees to cause torsion. Most cases of torsion result from uterine leiomyomas, müllerian anomalies, fetal malpresentation, pelvic adhesions, and laxity of the abdominal wall or uterine ligaments. Jensen (1992) reviewed 212 cases and reported that associated symptoms may include obstructed labor, intestinal or urinary complaints, abdominal pain, uterine hypertonus, vaginal bleeding, and hypotension. Both maternal and fetal complications were more common with early gestation and with greater degrees of torsion.

Most cases of uterine torsion are found at the time of cesarean delivery. In some women, torsion can be confirmed preoperatively with MR imaging, which shows a twisted vagina that appears X-shaped rather than its normal H-shape (Nicholson, 1995). As with uterine incarceration, during cesarean delivery, a severely displaced uterus should be repositioned anatomically before hysterotomy. In some cases, an inability to reposition may require that a posterior hysterotomy incision be done (Albayrak, 2011; De Ioris, 2010; Picone, 2006).

REFERENCES

Acién P: Incidence of Müllerian defects in fertile and infertile women. Hum Reprod 12(7):1372, 1997

Albayrak M, Benian A, Ozdemir I, et al: Deliberate posterior low transverse incision at cesarean section of a gravid uterus in 180 degrees of torsion: a case report. J Reprod Med 56(3–4):181, 2011

Allen JW, Cardall S, Kittijarukhajorn M, et al: Incidence of ovarian maldescent in women with mullerian duct anomalies: evaluation by MRI. AJR Am J Roentgenol 198(4):W381, 2012

American College of Obstetricians and Gynecologists: Müllerian agenesis: diagnosis, management, and treatment. Committee Opinion No. 562, May 2013

American Fertility Society: The American Fertility Society classifications of adnexal adhesions, distal tubal occlusion, tubal occlusion secondary to tubal ligation, tubal pregnancies, Müllerian anomalies and intrauterine adhesions. Fertil Steril 49:944, 1988

Barranger E, Gervaise A, Doumerc S, et al: Reproductive performance after hysteroscopic metroplasty in the hypoplastic uterus: a study of 29 cases. Br J Obstet Gynaecol 109:1331, 2002

Bermejo C, Martinez, Ten P, et al: Three-dimensional ultrasound in the diagnosis of Müllerian duct anomalies and concordance with magnetic resonance imaging. Ultrasound Obstet Gynecol 35: 593, 2010

Blanton EN, Rouse DJ: Trial of labor in women with transverse vaginal septa. Obstet Gynecol 101:1110, 2003

Bradshaw KB: Anatomical disorders. In Schorge JO, Schaffer JI, Halvorson LM, et al (eds): Williams Gynecology. New York, McGraw-Hill, 2008, p 413

Bradshaw KB: Anatomical disorders. In Hoffman BL, Schorge JO, Schaffer JI, et al (eds): Williams Gynecology, 2nd ed. New York, McGraw-Hill, 2012, p 483, 484, 494, 500, 501

Breech LL, Laufer MR: Müllerian anomalies. Obstet Gynecol Clin North Am 36(1):47, 2009

Brooks A, Hoffman BL: Pelvic mass. In Hoffman BL, Schorge JO, Schaffer JI, et al (eds): Williams Gynecology, 2nd ed. New York, McGraw-Hill, 2012, p 272

Buttram VC, Gibbons WE: Müllerian anomalies: a proposed classification (an analysis of 144 cases). Fertil Steril 32:40, 1979

Byrne J, Nussbaum-Blask A, Taylor WS, et al: Prevalence of Müllerian duct anomalies detected at ultrasound. Am J Med Genet 94(1):9, 2000

Caliskan E, Ozkan S, Cakiroglu Y, et al: Diagnostic accuracy of real-time 3D sonography in the diagnosis of congenital Mullerian anomalies in high-risk

CHAPTER 3

patients with respect to the phase of the menstrual cycle. J Clin Ultrasound 38(3):123, 2010

Chan YY, Jayaprakasan K, Tan A, et al: Reproductive outcomes in women with congenital uterine anomalies: a systematic review. Ultrasound Obstet Gynecol 38(4):371, 2011a

Chan YY, Jayaprakasan K, Zamora J, et al: The prevalence of congenital uterine anomalies in unselected and high-risk populations: a systematic review. Hum Reprod Update 17(6):761, 2011b

Dabirashrafi H, Mohammad K, Moghadami-Tabrizi N: Ovarian malposition in women with uterine anomalies. Obstet Gynecol 83:293, 1994

Darwish AM, Elsaman AM: Extended resectoscopic versus sequential cold knife-resectoscopic excision of the unclassified complete uterocervicovaginal septum: a randomized trial. Fertil Steril 92(2):722, 2009

Deans R, Banks F, Liao LM, et al: Reproductive outcomes in women with classic bladder exstrophy: an observational cross-sectional study. Am J Obstet Gynecol 206(6):496.e1, 2012

DeCherney AH, Cholst I, Naftolin F: Structure and function of the fallopian tubes following exposure to diethylstilbestrol (DES) during gestation. Fertil Steril 36(6):741, 1981

Deffarges JV, Haddad B, Musset R, et al: Utero-vaginal anastomosis in women with uterine cervix atresia: long-term follow-up and reproductive performance. Hum Reprod 16:1722, 2001

De Ioris A, Pezzuto C, Nardelli GB, et al: Caesarean delivery through deliberate posterior hysterotomy in irreducible uterine torsion: case report. Acta Biomed 81(2):141, 2010

Dershwitz RA, Levitsky LL, Feingold M: Picture of the month. Vulvovaginitis: a cause of clitorimegaly. Am J Dis Child 138(9):887, 1984

Dierickx I, Van Holsbeke C, Mesens T, et al: Colonoscopy-assisted reposition of the incarcerated uterus in mid-pregnancy: a report of four cases and a literature review. Eur J Obstet Gynecol Reprod Biol. 158(2):153, 2011

Donderwinkel PF, Dörr JP, Willemsen WN: The unicornuate uterus: clinical implications. Eur J Obstet Gynecol Reprod Biol 47(2):135, 1992

Duncan PA, Shapiro LR, Stangel JJ, et al: The MURCS association: Mullerian duct aplasia, renal aplasia. J Pediatrics 95(3):399, 1979

Edelman AB, Jensen JT, Lee DM, et al: Successful medical abortion of a pregnancy within a noncommunicating rudimentary uterine horn. Am J Obstet Gynecol 189:886, 2003

Fedele L, Bianchi S, Agnoli B, et al: Urinary tract anomalies associated with unicornuate uterus. J Urol 155:847, 1996a

Fedele L, Bianchi S, Frontino G, et al: Laparoscopically assisted uterovestibular anastomosis in patients with uterine cervix atresia and vaginal aplasia. Fertil Steril 89:212, 2008

Fedele L, Bianchi S, Marchini M, et al: Ultrastructural aspects of endometrium in infertile women with septate uterus. Fertil Steril 65:750, 1996b

Fedele L, Bianchi S, Zanconato G, et al: Laparoscopic removal of the cavitated noncommunicating rudimentary uterine horn: surgical aspects in 10 cases. Fertil Steril 83(2):432, 2005

Fedele L, Dorta M, Brioschi D, et al: Magnetic resonance evaluation of double uteri. Obstet Gynecol 74:844, 1989

Friedman A, DeFazio J, DeCherney A: Severe obstetric complications after aggressive treatment of Asherman syndrome. Obstet Gynecol 67:864, 1986

Gardner CS, Jaffe TA, Hertzberg BS, et al: The incarcerated uterus: a review of MRI and ultrasound imaging appearances. AJR Am J Roentgenol 201(1):223, 2013

Ghi T, Casadio P, Kuleva M, et al: Accuracy of three-dimensional ultrasound in diagnosis and classification of congenital uterine anomalies. Fertil Steril 92(2):808, 2009

Gibson ED: Transverse upper vaginal septum presenting in pregnancy: a case report and review of the literature. Aust N Z J Obstet Gynaecol 43(5):381, 2003

Golan A, Langer R, Neuman M, et al: Obstetric outcome in women with congenital uterine malformations. J Reprod Med 37:233, 1992

Goldberg JM, Falcone T: Effect of diethylstilbestrol on reproductive function. Fertil Steril 72:1, 1999

Gottschalk EM, Siedentopf JP, Schoenborn I, et al: Prenatal sonographic and MRI findings in a pregnancy complicated by uterine sacculation: case report and review of the literature. Ultrasound Obstet Gynecol 32(4):582, 2008

Greenwell TJ, Venn SN, Creighton SM, et al: Pregnancy after lower urinary tract reconstruction for congenital abnormalities. BJU Int 92:773, 2003

Greer DM Jr, Pederson WC: Pseudo-masculinization of the phallus. Plast Reconstr Surg 68(5):787, 1981

Grimbizis GF, Camus M, Tarlatzis BC, et al: Clinical implications of uterine malformations and hysteroscopic treatment results. Hum Reprod Update 7(2):161, 2001

Groom KM, Jones BA, Edmonds DK, et al: Preconception transabdominal cervicoisthmic cerclage. Am J Obstet Gynecol 191(1):230, 2004

Grossenburg NJ, Delaney AA, Berg TG: Treatment of a late second-trimester incarcerated uterus using ultrasound-guided manual reduction. Obstet Gynecol 118(2 Pt 2):436, 2011

Haddad B, Louis-Sylvestre C, Poitout P, et al: Longitudinal vaginal septum: a retrospective study of 202 cases. Eur J Obstet Gynecol Reprod Biol 74(2):197, 1997

Hall-Craggs MA, Kirkham A, Creighton SM: Renal and urological abnormalities occurring with Mullerian anomalies. J Pediatr Urol 9(1):27, 2013.

Halvorson LM: Evaluation of the infertile couple. In Schorge JO, Schaffer JI, Halvorson LM, et al (eds): Williams Gynecology. New York, McGraw-Hill, 2008, p 437

Hampton HL, Meeks GR, Bates GW, et al: Pregnancy after successful vaginoplasty and cervical stenting for partial atresia of the cervix. Obstet Gynecol 76:900, 1990

Hatch EE, Troisi R, Wise LA, et al: Age at natural menopause in women exposed to diethylstilbestrol in utero. Am J Epidemiol 164:682, 2006

Heinonen PK: Uterus didelphys: a report of 26 cases. Eur J Obstet Gynecol Reprod Biol 17:345, 1984

Hill LM, Chenevey P, DiNofrio D: Sonographic documentation of uterine retroversion mimicking uterine sacculation. Am J Perinatol 10:398, 1993

Hoffman BL, Hoggatt Krumwiede K: Embryologic development (update) in Cunningham FG, Leveno KL, Bloom SL, et al (eds), Williams Obstetrics Online. Available at: http://www.accessmedicine.com/williamsVideoPlayer.aspx?file=embryo_dev_flv/embryo_dev_flv.accessmedicine.com. New York, McGraw-Hill, 2010.

Hoover RN, Hyer M, Pfeiffer RM, et al: Adverse health outcomes in women exposed in utero to diethylstilbestrol. N Engl J Med 365:1304, 2011

Hua M, Odibo AO, Longman RE, et al: Congenital uterine anomalies and adverse pregnancy outcomes. Am J Obstet Gynecol 205(6):558.e1–5, 2011

Hughes IA, Houk C, Ahmed SF, et al: Consensus statement on management of intersex disorders. J Pediatr Urol 2:148, 2006

Jensen JG: Uterine torsion in pregnancy. Acta Obstet Gynecol Scand 71:260, 1992

Kenney PJ, Spirt BA, Leeson MD: Genitourinary anomalies: radiologic-anatomic correlations. Radiographics 4(2):233, 1984

Khati NJ, Frazier AA, Brindle KA: The unicornuate uterus and its variants: clinical presentation, imaging findings, and associated complications. J Ultrasound Med 31(2):319, 2012

Lee SW, Kim MY, Yang JH, et al: Sonographic findings of uterine sacculation during pregnancy. Ultrasound Obstet Gynecol 32(4):595, 2008

Lettieri L, Rodis JF, McLean DA, et al: Incarceration of the gravid uterus. Obstet Gynecol Surv 49:642, 1994

Ludmir J, Jackson GM, Samuels P: Transvaginal cerclage under ultrasound guidance in cases of severe cervical hypoplasia. Obstet Gynecol 78:1067, 1991

Mackey R, Geary M, Dornan J, et al: A successful pregnancy following transabdominal cervical cerclage for cervical hypoplasia. Br J Obstet Gynaecol 108:1111, 2001

Mollo A, De Franciscis P, Colacurci N, et al: Hysteroscopic resection of the septum improves the pregnancy rate of women with unexplained infertility: a prospective controlled trial. Fertil Steril 91(6):2628, 2009

Moore KL, Persaud TVN, Torchia MG: The urogenital system. In The Developing Human. Philadelphia, Saunders, 2013, p 272

Moschos E, Twickler DM. Techniques used for imaging in gynecology. In Hoffman BL, Schorge JO, Schaffer JI, et al (eds): Williams Gynecology, 2nd ed. New York, McGraw-Hill, 2012, p 45, 46

Mucowski SJ, Herndon CN, Rosen MP: The arcuate uterine anomaly: a critical appraisal of its diagnostic and clinical relevance. Obstet Gynecol Surv 65(7):449, 2010

Nahum G, Stanislaw H, McMahon C: Preventing ectopic pregnancies: how often does transperitoneal transmigration of sperm occur in effecting human pregnancy? Br J Obstet Gynaecol 111:706, 2004

Nahum GG: Rudimentary uterine horn pregnancy: the 20th-century worldwide experience of 588 cases. J Reprod Med 47:151, 2002

Nahum GG: Uterine anomalies. How common are they, and what is their distribution among subtypes? J Reprod Med 43(10):877, 1998

Nazir Z, Rizvi RM, Qureshi RN, et al: Congenital vaginal obstructions: varied presentation and outcome. Pediatr Surg Int 22(9):749, 2006

Nicholson WK, Coulson CC, McCoy MC, et al: Pelvic magnetic resonance imaging in the evaluation of uterine torsion. Obstet Gynecol 85(5 Pt 2):888, 1995

Nouri K, Ott J, Huber JC, et al: Reproductive outcome after hysteroscopic septoplasty in patients with septate uterus-a retrospective cohort study and systematic review of the literature. Reprod Biol Endocrinol 8:52, 2010

Olpin JD, Heilbrun M: Imaging of Müllerian duct anomalies. Clin Obstet Gynecol 52(1):40, 2009

Pabuçcu R, Gomel V: Reproductive outcome after hysteroscopic metroplasty in women with septate uterus and otherwise unexplained infertility. Fertil Steril 81:1675, 2004

Palmer JR, Hatch EE, Rao RS, et al: Infertility among women exposed prenatally to diethylstilbestrol. Am J Epidemiol 154:316, 2001

Pellerito JS, McCarthy SM, Doyle MB, et al: Diagnosis of uterine anomalies: relative accuracy of MR imaging, endovaginal sonography, and hysterosalpingography. Radiology 183:795, 1992
Picone O, Fubini A, Doumerc S, et al: Cesarean delivery by posterior hysterotomy due to torsion of the pregnant uterus. Obstet Gynecol 107(2 Pt 2):533, 2006
Puscheck EE, Cohen L: Congenital malformations of the uterus: the role of ultrasound. Semin Reprod Med 26(3):223, 2008
Rackow BW, Arici A: Reproductive performance of women with müllerian anomalies. Curr Opin Obstet Gynecol 19(3):229, 2007
Rajiah P, Eastwood KL, Gunn ML, et al: Uterine diverticulum. Obstet Gynecol 113(2 Pt 2):525, 2009
Reichman D, Laufer MR: Congenital uterine anomalies affecting reproduction. Best Pract Res Clin Obstet Gynaecol 24(2):193, 2010
Reichman D, Laufer MR, Robinson BK: Pregnancy outcomes in unicornuate uteri: a review. Fertil Steril 91(5): 1886, 2009
Roberts CP, Rock JA: Surgical methods in the treatment of congenital anomalies of the uterine cervix. Curr Opin Obstet Gynecol 23(4):251, 2011
Rock JA, Roberts CP, Jones HW Jr: Congenital anomalies of the uterine cervix: lessons from 30 cases managed clinically by a common protocol. Fertil Steril 94(5):1858, 2010
Rock JA, Zacur HA, Dlugi AM, et al: Pregnancy success following surgical correction of imperforate hymen and complete transverse vaginal septum. Obstet Gynecol 59(4):448, 1982
Rolen AC, Choquette AJ, Semmens JP: Rudimentary uterine horn: obstetric and gynecologic implications. Obstet Gynecol 27:806, 1966
Saravelos SH, Cocksedge KA, Li TC: Prevalence and diagnosis of congenital uterine anomalies in women with reproductive failure: a critical appraisal. Hum Reprod Update 14(5):415, 2008
Seubert DE, Puder KS, Goldmeier P, et al: Colonoscopic release of the incarcerated gravid uterus. Obstet Gynecol 94:792, 1999
Singh MN, Payappagoudar J, Lo J: Incarcerated retroverted uterus in the third trimester complicated by postpartum pulmonary embolism. Obstet Gynecol 109:498, 2007
Smith NA, Laufer MR: Obstructed hemivagina and ipsilateral renal anomaly (OHVIRA) syndrome: management and follow-up. Fertil Steril 87(4):918, 2007
Spearing GJ: Uterine sacculation. Obstet Gynecol 51:11S, 1978
Thompson M, Kho K: Minimally invasive surgery. In Hoffman BL, Schorge JO, Schaffer JI, et al (eds): Williams Gynecology, 2nd ed. New York, McGraw-Hill, 2012, p 1174
Tong J, Zhu L, Lang J: Clinical characteristics of 70 patients with Herlyn-Werner-Wunderlich syndrome. Int J Gynaecol Obstet 121(2):173, 2013
Van Beekhuizen HJ, Bodewes HW, Tepe EM, et al: Role of magnetic resonance imaging in the diagnosis of incarceration of the gravid uterus. Obstet Gynecol 102:1134, 2003
Werner CL, Moschos E, Griffith WF, et al: Williams Gynecology Study Guide, 2nd ed. New York, McGraw-Hill, 2012, p 35
Wilson EE: Pediatric gynecology. In Hoffman BL, Schorge JO, Schaffer JI, et al (eds): Williams Gynecology, 2nd ed. New York, McGraw-Hill, 2012, p 385
Woelfer B, Salim R, Banerjee S, et al: Reproductive outcomes in women with congenital uterine anomalies detected by three-dimensional ultrasound screening. Obstet Gynecol 98:1099, 2001
Woodruff JC, Pauersteine CJ: The Fallopian Tube: Structure, Function, Pathology and Management. Williams and Wilkins, Baltimore, 1969, p 18
Worley KC, Cunningham GC: Case report: rupture of pregnancy in a noncommunicating rudimentary uterine horn (update) in Cunningham FG, Leveno KL, Bloom SL, et al (eds), Williams Obstetrics, 22nd ed. Online. Available at: http://www.accessmedicine.com/updatesContent.aspx?aid=1001178. accessmedicine.com. New York, McGraw-Hill, 2007
Worley KC, Hnat MD, Cunningham FG: Advanced extrauterine pregnancy: diagnostic and therapeutic challenges. Am J Obstet Gynecol 198:287.e1, 2008
Zheng W, Robboy SJ: Fallopian tube. In Robboy SJ, Mutter GL, Prat J (eds): Robboy's Pathology of the Female Reproductive Tract. London, Churchill Livingstone, 2009, p 509

CHAPTER 4

Maternal Physiology

The anatomical, physiological, and biochemical adaptations to pregnancy are profound. Many of these remarkable changes begin soon after fertilization and continue throughout gestation, and most occur in response to physiological stimuli provided by the fetus and placenta. Equally astounding is that the woman who was pregnant is returned almost completely to her prepregnancy state after delivery and lactation. Many of these physiological adaptations could be perceived as abnormal in the nonpregnant woman. For example, cardiovascular changes during pregnancy normally include substantive increases in blood volume and cardiac output, which may mimic thyrotoxicosis. On the other hand, these same adaptations may lead to ventricular failure during pregnancy if there is underlying heart disease. Thus, physiological adaptations of normal pregnancy can be misinterpreted as pathological but can also unmask or worsen preexisting disease.

During normal pregnancy, virtually every organ system undergoes anatomical and functional changes that can alter appreciably criteria for disease diagnosis and treatment. Thus, the understanding of these pregnancy adaptations remains a major goal of obstetrics, and without such knowledge, it is almost impossible to understand the disease processes that can threaten women during pregnancy.

REPRODUCTIVE TRACT

Uterus

In the nonpregnant woman, the uterus weighs approximately 70 g and is almost solid, except for a cavity of 10 mL or less. During pregnancy, the uterus is transformed into a relatively thin-walled muscular organ of sufficient capacity to accommodate the fetus, placenta, and amnionic fluid. The total volume of the contents at term averages approximately 5 L but may be 20 L or more. By the end of pregnancy, the uterus has achieved a capacity that is 500 to 1000 times greater than in the nonpregnant state. The corresponding increase in uterine weight is such that, by term, the organ weighs nearly 1100 g.

During pregnancy, uterine enlargement involves stretching and marked hypertrophy of muscle cells, whereas the production of new myocytes is limited. Accompanying the increase in myocyte size is an accumulation of fibrous tissue, particularly in the external muscle layer, together with a considerable increase in elastic tissue content. This network adds strength to the uterine wall.

Although the walls of the corpus become considerably thicker during the first few months of pregnancy, they then begin to thin gradually. By term, the myometrium is only 1 to 2 cm thick. In these later months, the uterus is changed into a muscular sac with thin, soft, readily indentable walls through which the fetus usually can be palpated.

Uterine hypertrophy early in pregnancy probably is stimulated by the action of estrogen and perhaps progesterone. The hypertrophy of early pregnancy does not occur entirely in response to mechanical distention by the products of conception, because similar uterine changes are observed with ectopic pregnancy (Chap. 19, p. 379). But after approximately 12 weeks, the uterine size increase is related predominantly to pressure exerted by the expanding products of conception.

Uterine enlargement is most marked in the fundus. In the early pregnancy months, the fallopian tubes and the ovarian and round ligaments attach only slightly below the apex of the fundus. In later months, they are located slightly above the middle of the uterus. The position of the placenta also influences the extent of uterine hypertrophy. The portion of the uterus surrounding the placental site enlarges more rapidly than does the rest.

Myocyte Arrangement

The uterine musculature during pregnancy is arranged in three strata. The first is an outer hoodlike layer, which arches over the fundus and extends into the various ligaments. The middle layer is composed of a dense network of muscle fibers perforated in all directions by blood vessels. Last is an internal layer, with sphincter-like fibers around the fallopian tube orifices and internal cervical os.

Most of the uterine wall is formed by the middle layer. Each cell in this layer has a double curve so that the interlacing of any two gives approximately the form of a figure eight. This arrangement is crucial because when the cells contract after delivery, they constrict penetrating blood vessels and thus act as ligatures (Fig. 2-11, p. 27).

Uterine Size, Shape, and Position

For the first few weeks, the uterus maintains its original piriform or pear shape. But, as pregnancy advances, the corpus and fundus become more globular and almost spherical by 12 weeks' gestation. Subsequently, the organ increases more rapidly in length than in width and assumes an ovoid shape. By the end of 12 weeks, the uterus has become too large to remain entirely within the pelvis. As the uterus enlarges, it contacts the anterior abdominal wall, displaces the intestines laterally and superiorly, and ultimately reaches almost to the liver. With uterine ascent from the pelvis, it usually rotates to the right. This dextrorotation likely is caused by the rectosigmoid on the left side of the pelvis. As the uterus rises, tension is exerted on the broad and round ligaments.

With the pregnant woman standing, the longitudinal axis of the uterus corresponds to an extension of the pelvic inlet axis. The abdominal wall supports the uterus and, unless it is quite relaxed, maintains this relation between the long axis of the uterus and the axis of the pelvic inlet. When the pregnant woman is supine, the uterus falls back to rest on the vertebral column and the adjacent great vessels.

Uterine Contractility

Beginning in early pregnancy, the uterus undergoes irregular contractions that are normally painless. During the second trimester, these contractions may be detected by bimanual examination. Because attention was first called to this phenomenon in 1872 by J. Braxton Hicks, the contractions have been known by his name. Such contractions appear unpredictably and sporadically and are usually nonrhythmic. Their intensity varies between approximately 5 and 25 mm Hg (Alvarez, 1950). Until the last several weeks of pregnancy, these *Braxton Hicks contractions* are infrequent, but their number increases during the last week or two. At this time, the uterus may contract as often as every 10 to 20 minutes and with some degree of rhythmicity. Correspondingly, studies of uterine electrical activity have shown low and uncoordinated patterns early in gestation, which become progressively more intense and synchronized by term (Garfield, 2005). Late in pregnancy, these contractions may cause some discomfort and account for so-called false labor (Chap. 21, p. 409).

Uteroplacental Blood Flow

The delivery of most substances essential for fetal and placental growth, metabolism, and waste removal is dependent on adequate perfusion of the placental intervillous space (Chap. 5, p. 96). Accurate estimation of actual uteroplacental blood flow is technically challenging. Placental perfusion is dependent on total uterine blood flow, and simultaneous measurement of uterine, ovarian, and collateral vessels is currently not possible, even using magnetic resonance angiography (Pates, 2010). Using indirect measures, such as clearance rates of androstenedione and xenon-133, uteroplacental blood flow was found to increase progressively during pregnancy. Estimates range from 450 to 650 mL/min near term (Edman, 1981; Kauppila, 1980). These estimates are remarkably similar to those obtained with invasive methods—500 to 750 mL/min (Assali, 1953; Browne, 1953; Metcalfe, 1955). Putting this remarkable rate of blood flow in context, one recalls that the blood flow in the entire circulation of a nonpregnant woman is approximately 5000 mL/min.

The results of studies conducted in rats by Page and colleagues (2002) show that the uterine veins also significantly adapt during pregnancy. Specifically, their remodeling includes reduced elastin content and adrenergic nerve density. This creates increased venous caliber and distensibility. Logically, such changes are necessary to accommodate the massively increased uteroplacental blood flow.

Studying the effects of labor on uteroplacental blood flow, Assali and coworkers (1968) placed electromagnetic flow probes directly on a uterine artery in sheep and dogs at term. They found that uterine contractions, either spontaneous or induced, caused a decrease in uterine blood flow that was approximately proportional to the contraction intensity. They also showed that a tetanic contraction caused a precipitous fall in uterine blood flow. Harbert and associates (1969) made a similar observation in pregnant monkeys. In humans, uterine contractions appear to affect fetal circulation much less (Brar, 1988).

Uteroplacental Blood Flow Regulation. Maternal-placental blood flow progressively increases during gestation principally by means of vasodilation. Palmer and associates (1992) showed that uterine artery diameter doubled by 20 weeks and that concomitant mean Doppler velocimetry was increased eightfold. Recall that blood flow within a vessel increases in proportion to the fourth power of the radius. Thus, slight diameter increases in the uterine artery produces a tremendous blood flow capacity increase (Guyton, 1981). As reviewed by Mandala and Osol (2011), the vessels that supply the uterine corpus widen and elongate while preserving contractile function. In contrast, the spiral arteries, which directly supply the placenta, widen but completely lose contractility. This presumably results from endovascular trophoblast invasion that destroys the intramural muscular elements (Chap. 5, p. 93).

The vasodilation during pregnancy is at least in part the consequence of estrogen stimulation. For example, 17β-estradiol has been shown to promote uterine artery vasodilation and reduce uterine vascular resistance (Sprague, 2009). Jauniaux and colleagues (1994) found that estradiol and progesterone, as well as relaxin, contribute to the downstream fall in vascular resistance in women with advancing gestational age.

The downstream fall in vascular resistance leads to an acceleration of flow velocity and shear stress in upstream vessels. In turn, shear stress leads to circumferential vessel growth, and nitric oxide—a potent vasodilator—appears to play a key role regulating this process (p. 61). Indeed, endothelial shear stress, estrogen, placental growth factor (PlGF), and vascular endothelial growth factor (VEGF)—a promoter of angiogenesis—all augment endothelial nitric oxide synthase (eNOS) and nitric oxide production (Grummer, 2009; Mandala, 2011). As an important aside, VEGF and PlGF signaling is attenuated in response to excess placental secretion of their soluble receptor—*soluble FMS-like tyrosine kinase 1 (sFlt-1)*. As detailed in Chapter 40 (p. 735), increased maternal sFlt-1 levels inactivate and decrease circulating PlGF and VEGF concentrations and have been shown to be an important factor in preeclampsia pathogenesis.

Normal pregnancy is also characterized by vascular refractoriness to the pressor effects of infused angiotensin II and norepinephrine (p. 61). This insensitivity also serves to increase uteroplacental blood flow (Rosenfeld, 1981, 2012). Recent studies also suggest that relaxin may help mediate uterine artery compliance (Vodstrcil, 2012). Moreover, Rosenfeld and associates (2005, 2008) have discovered that large-conductance potassium channels expressed in uterine vascular smooth muscle also contribute to uteroplacental blood flow regulation through several mediators, including estrogen and nitric oxide. In contrast, uterine blood flow and placental perfusion in sheep significantly decline following nicotine and catecholamine infusions (Rosenfeld, 1976, 1977; Xiao, 2007). The placental perfusion decrease likely results from greater uteroplacental vascular bed sensitivity to epinephrine and norepinephrine compared with that of the systemic vasculature.

Cervix

As early as 1 month after conception, the cervix begins to undergo pronounced softening and cyanosis. These changes result from increased vascularity and edema of the entire cervix, together with hypertrophy and hyperplasia of the cervical glands (Straach, 2005). Although the cervix contains a small amount of smooth muscle, its major component is connective tissue. Rearrangement of this collagen-rich connective tissue is necessary to permit functions as diverse as maintenance of a pregnancy to term, dilatation to aid delivery, and repair following parturition so that a successful pregnancy can be repeated (Timmons, 2007; Word, 2007). As detailed in Chapter 21 (p. 410), the cervical ripening process involves connective tissue remodeling that decreases collagen and proteoglycan concentrations and increases water content compared with the nonpregnant cervix. This process appears to be regulated in part by localized estrogen and progesterone metabolism (Andersson, 2008).

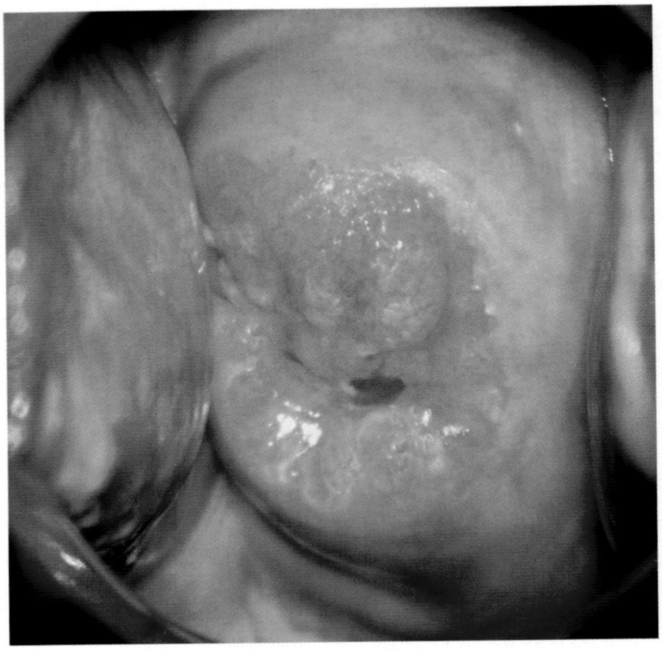

FIGURE 4-1 Cervical eversion of pregnancy as viewed through a colposcope. The eversion represents columnar epithelium on the portio of the cervix. (Photograph contributed by Dr. Claudia Werner.)

As shown in Figure 4-1, the cervical glands undergo marked proliferation, and by the end of pregnancy, they occupy up to one half of the entire cervical mass. This contrasts with their rather small fraction in the nonpregnant state. These normal pregnancy-induced changes represent an extension, or *eversion*, of the proliferating columnar endocervical glands. This tissue tends to be red and velvety and bleeds even with minor trauma, such as with Pap smear sampling.

The endocervical mucosal cells produce copious tenacious mucus that obstruct the cervical canal soon after conception. As discussed on page 56, this mucus is rich in immunoglobulins and cytokines and may act as an immunological barrier to protect the uterine contents against infection (Hein, 2005). At the onset of labor, if not before, this *mucus plug* is expelled, resulting in a *bloody show*. Moreover, the cervical mucus consistency changes during pregnancy. Specifically, in most pregnant women, as a result of progesterone, when cervical mucus is spread and dried on a glass slide, it is characterized by poor crystallization, or

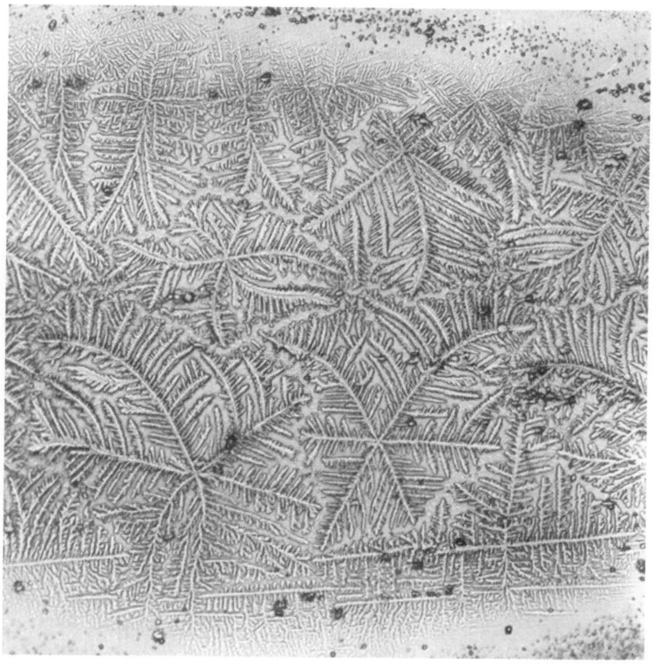

FIGURE 4-2 Cervical mucus arborization or ferning. (Photograph contributed by Dr. James C. Glenn.)

beading. In some women, an arborization of crystals, or *ferning*, is observed as a result of amnionic fluid leakage (Fig. 4-2).

During pregnancy, basal cells near the squamocolumnar junction are likely to be prominent in size, shape, and staining qualities. These changes are considered to be estrogen induced. In addition, pregnancy is associated with both endocervical gland hyperplasia and hypersecretory appearance—the *Arias-Stella reaction*—which makes the differentiation of these and atypical glandular cells on Pap smear particularly difficult (Connolly, 2005).

Pelvic Organ Prolapse

As a result of apical prolapse, the cervix, and occasionally a portion of the uterine body, may protrude variably from the vulva during early pregnancy. With further growth, the uterus usually rises above the pelvis and may draw the cervix up with it. If the uterus persists in its prolapsed position, symptoms of incarceration may develop at 10 to 14 weeks. As a prevention measure, the uterus can be replaced early in pregnancy and held in position with a suitable pessary.

In contrast, attenuation of fascial support between the vagina and the bladder can lead to prolapse of the bladder into the vagina, that is, a cystocele. Urinary stasis with a cystocele predisposes to infection. Pregnancy may also worsen associated *urinary stress incontinence* because urethral closing pressures do not increase sufficiently to compensate for the progressively increased bladder pressure (Iosif, 1981). Attenuation of rectovaginal fascia results in a rectocele. A large defect may fill with feces that occasionally can be evacuated only manually. During labor, a cystocele or rectocele can block fetal descent unless they are emptied and pushed out of the way. In rare instances, an enterocele of considerable size may complicate pregnancy. If symptomatic, the protrusion should be replaced, and the woman kept in a recumbent position. If the mass interferes with delivery, it should be pushed up or held out of the way.

Ovaries

Ovulation ceases during pregnancy, and maturation of new follicles is suspended. The single corpus luteum found in pregnant women functions maximally during the first 6 to 7 weeks of pregnancy—4 to 5 weeks postovulation—and thereafter contributes relatively little to progesterone production. These observations have been confirmed by surgical removal of the corpus luteum before 7 weeks—5 weeks postovulation. Removal results in a rapid fall in maternal serum progesterone levels and spontaneous abortion (Csapo, 1973). After this time, however, corpus luteum excision ordinarily does not cause abortion, and even bilateral oophorectomy at 16 weeks does not cause pregnancy loss (Villaseca, 2005). Interestingly in such cases, follicle-stimulating hormone (FSH) levels do not reach perimenopausal levels until approximately 5 weeks postpartum.

An extrauterine *decidual reaction* on and beneath the surface of the ovaries is common in pregnancy and is usually observed at cesarean delivery. These elevated patches of tissue bleed easily and may, on first glance, resemble freshly torn adhesions. Similar decidual reactions are seen on the uterine serosa and other pelvic, or even extrapelvic, abdominal organs (Bloom, 2010). These areas arise from subcoelomic mesenchyme as a result of progesterone stimulation and histologically appear similar to progestin-stimulated intrauterine endometrial stroma described in Chapter 5 (p. 86)(Russell, 2009).

The enormous caliber of the ovarian veins viewed at cesarean delivery is startling. Hodgkinson (1953) found that the diameter of the ovarian vascular pedicle increased during pregnancy from 0.9 cm to approximately 2.6 cm at term. Again, recall that flow in a tubular structure increases exponentially as the diameter enlarges.

Relaxin

As discussed in Chapter 5 (p. 105), this protein hormone is secreted by the corpus luteum as well as the decidua and the placenta in a pattern similar to that of human chorionic gonadotropin (hCG). It is also expressed in a variety of nonreproductive tissues, including brain, heart, and kidney. It is mentioned here because its secretion by the corpus luteum appears to play a key role in facilitating many maternal physiological adaptations (Conrad, 2013). One of its biological actions appears to be remodeling of reproductive-tract connective tissue to accommodate parturition (Park, 2005). Relaxin also appears important in the initiation of augmented renal hemodynamics, decreased serum osmolality, and increased uterine artery compliance associated with normal pregnancy (Conrad, 2011a,b). Despite its name, serum relaxin levels do not contribute to increasing peripheral joint laxity during pregnancy (Marnach, 2003).

CHAPTER 4

Theca-Lutein Cysts

These benign ovarian lesions result from exaggerated physiological follicle stimulation—termed *hyperreactio luteinalis.* These usually bilateral cystic ovaries are moderately to massively enlarged. The reaction is usually associated with markedly elevated serum levels of hCG. Thus not surprisingly, theca-lutein cysts are found frequently with gestational trophoblastic disease (Chap. 20, p. 398). They are also more likely found with a large placenta such as with diabetes, anti-D alloimmunization, and multifetal gestations (Tanaka, 2001). Theca-lutein cysts have also been reported in chronic renal failure as a result of reduced hCG clearance and in hyperthyroidism as a result of the structural homology between hCG and thyroid-stimulating hormone (Coccia, 2003; Gherman, 2003). However, they also are encountered in women with otherwise uncomplicated pregnancies and are thought to result from an exaggerated response of the ovaries to normal levels of circulating hCG (Langer, 2007).

Although usually asymptomatic, hemorrhage into the cysts may cause abdominal pain (Amoah, 2011). Maternal virilization may be seen in up to 30 percent of women, however, virilization of the fetus has not yet been described (Kaňová, 2011). Maternal findings including temporal balding, hirsutism, and clitoromegaly are associated with massively elevated levels of androstenedione and testosterone. The diagnosis typically is based on sonographic findings of bilateral enlarged ovaries containing multiple cysts in the appropriate clinical settings. The condition is self-limited, and resolution follows delivery. Their management was reviewed by Phelan and Conway (2011) and is discussed further in Chapter 63 (p. 1228).

Fallopian Tubes

Fallopian tube musculature undergoes little hypertrophy during pregnancy. However, the epithelium of the tubal mucosa becomes somewhat flattened. Decidual cells may develop in the stroma of the endosalpinx, but a continuous decidual membrane is not formed. Rarely, the increasing size of the gravid uterus, especially in the presence of paratubal or ovarian cysts, may result in fallopian tube torsion (Batukan, 2007).

Vagina and Perineum

During pregnancy, increased vascularity and hyperemia develop in the skin and muscles of the perineum and vulva, with softening of the underlying abundant connective tissue. Also, Bartholin gland duct cysts of 1-cm size are common (Berger, 2012). Increased vascularity prominently affects the vagina and results in the violet color characteristic of *Chadwick sign.* The vaginal walls undergo striking changes in preparation for the distention that accompanies labor and delivery. These changes include a considerable increase in mucosal thickness, loosening of the connective tissue, and smooth muscle cell hypertrophy. The papillae of the vaginal epithelium undergo hypertrophy to create a fine, hobnailed appearance. Studies in pregnant mice have shown that vaginal distention results in increased elastic fiber degradation and an increase in the proteins necessary for new elastic fiber synthesis. In the absence of this synthesis, rapid progression of vaginal wall prolapse ensues (Rahn, 2008a,b).

The considerably increased volume of cervical secretions within the vagina during pregnancy consists of a somewhat thick, white discharge. The pH is acidic, varying from 3.5 to 6. This results from increased production of lactic acid from glycogen in the vaginal epithelium by the action of *Lactobacillus acidophilus.* As discussed in Chapter 65 (p. 1276), pregnancy is associated with a 10- to 20-fold increase in the prevalence of vulvovaginal candidiasis (Farage, 2011).

BREASTS

In the early weeks of pregnancy, women often experience breast tenderness and paresthesias. After the second month, the breasts increase in size, and delicate veins become visible just beneath the skin. The nipples become considerably larger, more deeply pigmented, and more erectile. After the first few months, a thick, yellowish fluid—*colostrum*—can often be expressed from the nipples by gentle massage. During the same months, the areolae become broader and more deeply pigmented. Scattered through the areolae are a number of small elevations, the *glands of Montgomery,* which are hypertrophic sebaceous glands. If the increase in breast size is extensive, striations similar to those observed in the abdomen may develop. Rarely, breast enlargement may become so pathologically extensive—referred to as *gigantomastia* as shown in Figure 4-3—that it requires postpartum surgical intervention (Antevski, 2011; Pasrija, 2006; Shoma, 2011; Vidaeff, 2003).

For most normal pregnancies, prepregnancy breast size and volume of milk production do not correlate (Hytten, 1995). Histological and functional changes of the breasts induced by pregnancy and lactation are further discussed in Chapter 36 (p. 672).

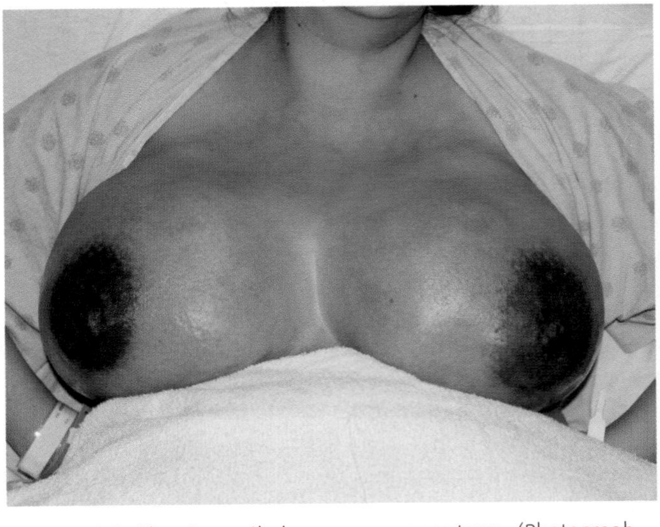

FIGURE 4-3 Gigantomastia in a woman near term. (Photograph contributed by Dr. Patricia Santiago-Muñoz.)

SKIN

There are several changes in the skin during pregnancy. These sometimes are noticeable and may provoke anxiety in some women. Skin changes are common, and Rathore and coworkers (2011) conducted a detailed dermatological examination of 2000 randomly selected asymptomatic women attending a prenatal clinic in India. They found at least one physiological cutaneous change in 87 percent of the women.

Abdominal Wall

Beginning after midpregnancy, reddish, slightly depressed streaks commonly develop in the abdominal skin and sometimes in the skin over the breasts and thighs. These are called *striae gravidarum* or *stretch marks.* In multiparous women, in addition to the reddish striae of the present pregnancy, glistening, silvery lines that represent the cicatrices of previous striae frequently are seen. In a study of 110 primiparous patients, Osman and colleagues (2007) reported that 48 percent developed striae gravidarum on their abdomen; 25 percent on their breasts; and 25 percent on their thighs. The strongest associated risk factors were weight gain during pregnancy, younger maternal age, and family history. The etiology of striae gravidarum is unknown, and there are no definitive treatments (Soltanipoor, 2012).

Occasionally, the muscles of the abdominal walls do not withstand the tension to which they are subjected. As a result, rectus muscles separate in the midline, creating *diastasis recti* of varying extent. If severe, a considerable portion of the anterior uterine wall is covered by only a layer of skin, attenuated fascia, and peritoneum to form a ventral hernia.

Hyperpigmentation

This develops in up to 90 percent of women. It is usually more accentuated in those with a darker complexion (Muallem, 2006). The midline of the anterior abdominal wall skin—*linea alba*—takes on dark brown-black pigmentation to form the *linea nigra.* Occasionally, irregular brownish patches of varying size appear on the face and neck, giving rise to *chloasma* or *melasma gravidarum*—the so-called *mask of pregnancy.* Pigmentation of the areolae and genital skin may also be accentuated. These pigmentary changes usually disappear, or at least regress considerably, after delivery. Oral contraceptives may cause similar pigmentation (Sheth, 2011).

Little is known of the etiology of these pigmentary changes. However, levels of melanocyte-stimulating hormone, a polypeptide similar to corticotropin, are elevated remarkably throughout pregnancy. Estrogen and progesterone also are reported to have melanocyte-stimulating effects.

Vascular Changes

Angiomas, called *vascular spiders,* develop in approximately two thirds of white women and approximately 10 percent of black women. Particularly common on the face, neck, upper chest, and arms, these are minute, red skin elevations, with radicles branching out from a central lesion. The condition is often designated as nevus, angioma, or telangiectasis. *Palmar erythema* is encountered during pregnancy in approximately two thirds of white women and one third of black women. These two conditions are of no clinical significance and disappear in most women shortly after pregnancy. They are most likely the consequence of hyperestrogenemia.

In addition to these discrete lesions, increased cutaneous blood flow in pregnancy serves to dissipate excess heat generated by increased metabolism.

METABOLIC CHANGES

In response to the increased demands of the rapidly growing fetus and placenta, the pregnant woman undergoes metabolic changes that are numerous and intense. Certainly no other physiological event induces such profound metabolic alterations. By the third trimester, maternal basal metabolic rate is increased by 10 to 20 percent compared with that of the nonpregnant state. This is increased by an additional 10 percent in women with a twin gestation (Shinagawa, 2005). Viewed another way, an analysis by the World Health Organization (2004) estimates that the additional total pregnancy energy demands associated with normal pregnancy are approximately 77,000 kcal or 85 kcal/day, 285 kcal/day, and 475 kcal/day during the first, second, and third trimester, respectively (Table 4-1). In addition to the corresponding increased caloric requirements, Löf (2011) found that the increased energy demands were also compensated for, in part, by normal pregnant women gravitating to less physically demanding activities.

Weight Gain

Most of the normal increase in weight during pregnancy is attributable to the uterus and its contents, the breasts, and increases in blood volume and extravascular extracellular fluid. A smaller fraction results from metabolic alterations that increase accumulation of cellular water, fat, and protein—so-called *maternal reserves.* Hytten (1991) reported that the average weight gain during pregnancy is approximately 12.5 kg or 27.5 lb (Table 4-2). Maternal aspects of weight gain are considered in greater detail in Chapter 9 (p. 177).

Water Metabolism

Increased water retention is a normal physiological alteration of pregnancy. It is mediated, at least in part, by a fall in plasma osmolality of approximately 10 mOsm/kg induced by a resetting of osmotic thresholds for thirst and vasopressin secretion (Heenan, 2003; Lindheimer, 1995). As shown in Figure 4-4, this phenomenon is functioning by early pregnancy.

At term, the water content of the fetus, placenta, and amnionic fluid approximates 3.5 L. Another 3.0 L accumulates from increases in maternal blood volume and in the size of the uterus and breasts. Thus, the minimum amount of extra water that the

TABLE 4-1. Additional Energy Demands During Normal Pregnancy[a]

	Rates of Tissue Deposition			
	1st Trimester g/d	2nd Trimester g/d	3rd Trimester g/d	Total Deposition g/280 d
Weight gain	17	60	54	12,000
Protein deposition	0	1.3	5.1	597
Fat deposition	5.2	18.9	16.9	3741

Energy Cost of Pregnancy Estimated from Basal Metabolic Rate and Energy Deposition					
	1st Trimester kJ/d	2nd Trimester kJ/d	3rd Trimester kJ/d	Total Energy Cost MJ	Total Energy Cost Kcal
Protein deposition	0	30	121	14.1	3370
Fat deposition	202	732	654	144.8	34,600
Efficiency of energy utilization[b]	20	76	77	15.9	3800
Basal metabolic rate	199	397	993	147.8	35,130
Total energy cost of pregnancy	**421**	**1235**	**1845**	**322.6**	**77,100**

[a]Assumes an average gestational weight gain of 12 kg.
[b]Efficiency of food energy utilization for protein and fat deposition estimated as 0.90.
Adapted from the World Health Organization, 2004.

average woman accrues during normal pregnancy is approximately 6.5 L. Clearly demonstrable pitting edema of the ankles and legs is seen in most pregnant women, especially at the end of the day. This fluid accumulation, which may amount to a liter or so, is caused by increased venous pressure below the level of the uterus as a consequence of partial vena cava occlusion. A decrease in interstitial colloid osmotic pressure induced by normal pregnancy also favors edema late in pregnancy (Øian, 1985).

Longitudinal studies of body composition have shown a progressive increase in total body water and fat mass during pregnancy. Both initial maternal weight and weight gained during pregnancy are highly associated with birthweight. It is unclear, however, what role maternal fat or water have in fetal growth. Studies in well-nourished women suggest that maternal body water, rather than fat, contributes more significantly to infant birthweight (Lederman, 1999; Mardones-Santander, 1998).

TABLE 4-2. Weight Gain Based on Pregnancy-Related Components

Tissues and Fluids	Cumulative Increase in Weight (g) 10 Weeks	20 Weeks	30 Weeks	40 Weeks
Fetus	5	300	1500	3400
Placenta	20	170	430	650
Amnionic fluid	30	350	750	800
Uterus	140	320	600	970
Breasts	45	180	360	405
Blood	100	600	1300	1450
Extravascular fluid	0	30	80	1480
Maternal stores (fat)	310	2050	3480	3345
Total	**650**	**4000**	**8500**	**12,500**

Modified from Hytten, 1991.

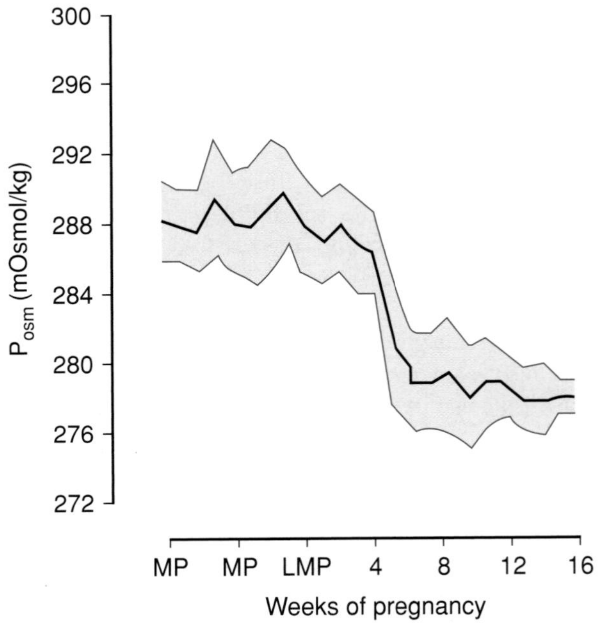

FIGURE 4-4 Mean values (*black line*) ± standard deviations (*blue lines*) for plasma osmolality (P_{osm}) measured at weekly intervals in nine women from preconception to 16 weeks. LMP = last menstrual period; MP = menstrual period. (Redrawn from Davison, 1981, with permission.)

Protein Metabolism

The products of conception, the uterus, and maternal blood are relatively rich in protein rather than fat or carbohydrate. At term, the fetus and placenta together weigh about 4 kg and contain approximately 500 g of protein, or about half of the total pregnancy increase (Hytten, 1971). The remaining 500 g is added to the uterus as contractile protein, to the breasts primarily in the glands, and to maternal blood as hemoglobin and plasma proteins.

Amino acid concentrations are higher in the fetal than in the maternal compartment (Cetin, 2005; van den Akker, 2009). This increased concentration is largely regulated by the placenta. The placenta not only concentrates amino acids into the fetal circulation, but also is involved in protein synthesis, oxidation, and transamination of some nonessential amino acids (Galan, 2009).

Mojtahedi and associates (2002) measured *nitrogen balance* across pregnancy in 12 healthy women. It increased with gestational age and thus suggested a more efficient use of dietary protein. They also found that urinary excretion of 3-methylhistidine did not change, indicating that maternal muscle breakdown is not required to meet metabolic demands. Further support that pregnancy is associated with nitrogen conservation comes from Kalhan and coworkers (2003), who found that the turnover rate of nonessential serine decreases across gestation. The daily requirements for dietary protein intake during pregnancy are discussed in Chapter 9 (p. 179).

Carbohydrate Metabolism

Normal pregnancy is characterized by mild fasting hypoglycemia, postprandial hyperglycemia, and hyperinsulinemia (Fig. 4-5).

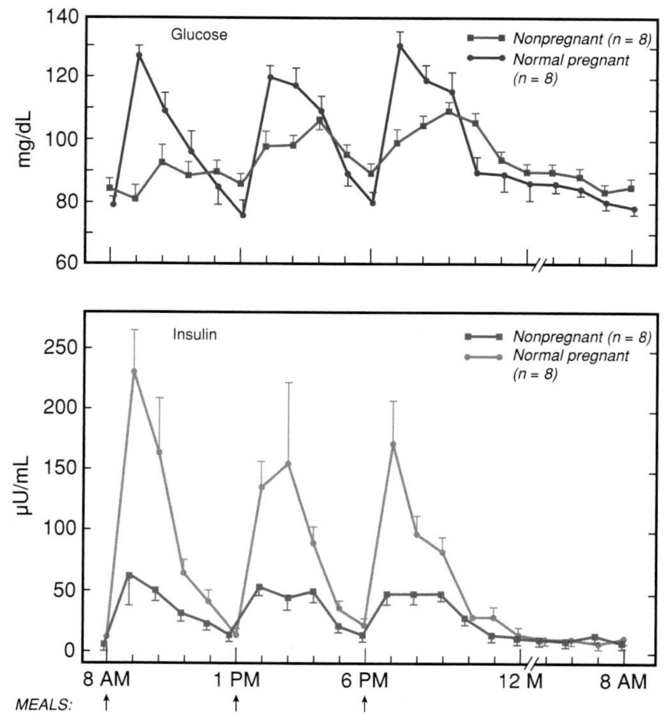

FIGURE 4-5 Diurnal changes in plasma glucose and insulin in normal late pregnancy. (Redrawn from Phelps, 1981.)

This increased basal level of plasma insulin in normal pregnancy is associated with several unique responses to glucose ingestion. For example, after an oral glucose meal, gravid women demonstrate prolonged hyperglycemia and hyperinsulinemia as well as a greater suppression of glucagon (Phelps, 1981). This cannot be explained by an increased metabolism of insulin because its half-life during pregnancy is not changed (Lind, 1977). Instead, this response is consistent with a pregnancy-induced state of peripheral insulin resistance, the purpose of which is likely to ensure a sustained postprandial supply of glucose to the fetus. Indeed, insulin sensitivity in late normal pregnancy is 45 to 70 percent lower than that of nonpregnant women (Butte, 2000; Freemark, 2006).

The mechanism(s) responsible for insulin resistance is not completely understood. Progesterone and estrogen may act, directly or indirectly, to mediate this insensitivity. Plasma levels of placental lactogen increase with gestation, and this protein hormone is characterized by growth hormone–like action. Higher levels may increase lipolysis and liberation of free fatty acids (Freinkel, 1980). The increased concentration of circulating free fatty acids also may aid increased tissue resistance to insulin (Freemark, 2006).

The pregnant woman changes rapidly from a postprandial state characterized by elevated and sustained glucose levels to a fasting state characterized by decreased plasma glucose and some amino acids. Simultaneously, plasma concentrations of free fatty acids, triglycerides, and cholesterol are higher. Freinkel and colleagues (1985) have referred to this pregnancy-induced switch in fuels from glucose to lipids as *accelerated starvation.* Certainly, when fasting is prolonged in the pregnant woman, these alterations are exaggerated and ketonemia rapidly appears.

Fat Metabolism

The concentrations of lipids, lipoproteins, and apolipoproteins in plasma increase appreciably during pregnancy (Appendix, p. 1291). Increased insulin resistance and estrogen stimulation during pregnancy are responsible for the maternal hyperlipidemia. As reviewed by Ghio and associates (2011), increased lipid synthesis and food intake contribute to maternal fat accumulation during the first two trimesters. In the third trimester, however, fat storage declines or ceases. This is a consequence of enhanced lipolytic activity, and decreased lipoprotein lipase activity reduces circulating triglyceride uptake into adipose tissue. This transition to a catabolic state favors maternal use of lipids as an energy source and spares glucose and amino acids for the fetus.

Maternal hyperlipidemia is one of the most consistent and striking changes of lipid metabolism during late pregnancy. Triacylglycerol and cholesterol levels in very-low-density lipoproteins (VLDLs), low-density lipoproteins (LDLs), and high-density lipoproteins (HDLs) are increased during the third trimester compared with those in nonpregnant women. During the third trimester, average total serum cholesterol, LDL-C, HDL-C, and triglyceride levels are approximately 267 ± 30 mg/dL, 136 ± 33 mg/dL, 81 ± 17 mg/dL, and 245 ± 73 mg/dL, respectively (Lippi, 2007). After delivery, the concentrations of these lipids, as well as lipoproteins and apolipoproteins, decrease. Lactation speeds the change in levels of many of these (Darmady, 1982).

Hyperlipidemia is theoretically a concern because it is associated with endothelial dysfunction. From their studies, however, Saarelainen and coworkers (2006) found that endothelium-dependent vasodilation responses actually improve across pregnancy. This was partly because increased HDL-cholesterol concentrations likely inhibit LDL oxidation and thus protect the endothelium. Their findings suggest that the increased cardiovascular disease risk in multiparous women may be related to factors other than maternal hypercholesterolemia.

Leptin

In nonpregnant humans, this peptide hormone is primarily secreted by adipose tissue. It plays a key role in body fat and energy expenditure regulation. Leptin deficiency is associated with anovulation and infertility, however, pregnancy in a woman with a leptin-receptor mutation has been reported (Maguire, 2012; Nizard, 2012).

Maternal serum leptin levels increase and peak during the second trimester and plateau until term in concentrations two to four times higher than those in nonpregnant women. This increase is only partially due to pregnancy weight gain, because leptin also is produced in significant amounts by the placenta (Maymó, 2011). Moreover, and as discussed in Chapter 5 (p. 106), placental weight is significantly correlated with leptin levels measured in umbilical cord blood (Pighetti, 2003).

Hauguel-de Mouzon and associates (2006) have hypothesized that increased leptin production may be critical for the regulation of increased maternal energy demands. As discussed in Chapter 48 (p. 961), leptin and adiponectin—a cytokine involved with energy homeostasis and lipid metabolism—may also help to regulate fetal growth (Henson, 2006; Karakosta, 2010; Nakano, 2012). As reviewed by Miehle and colleagues (2012), abnormally elevated leptin levels have been associated with preeclampsia (Chap. 40, p. 729) and gestational diabetes (Chap. 57, p. 1136).

Ghrelin

This peptide is secreted principally by the stomach in response to hunger. It cooperates with other neuroendocrine factors, such as leptin, in energy homeostasis modulation. It is also expressed in the placenta and likely has a role in fetal growth and cell proliferation (Chap. 5, p. 105). Maternal serum ghrelin levels increase and peak at midpregnancy and then decrease until term (Fuglsang, 2008). This is explicable in that ghrelin levels are known to be decreased in other insulin-resistant states such as metabolic syndrome and gestational diabetes mellitus (Baykus, 2012; Riedl, 2007). Muccioli and coworkers (2011) have provided an excellent review of the many functions of ghrelin in the regulation of reproductive function.

Electrolyte and Mineral Metabolism

During normal pregnancy, nearly 1000 mEq of *sodium* and 300 mEq of *potassium* are retained (Lindheimer, 1987). Although the glomerular filtration of sodium and potassium is increased, the excretion of these electrolytes is unchanged during pregnancy as a result of enhanced tubular resorption (Brown, 1986, 1988). And although there are increased total accumulations of sodium and potassium, their serum concentrations are decreased slightly because of expanded plasma volume (Appendix, p. 1289). Still, these levels remain very near the normal range for nonpregnant women (Kametas, 2003a).

Total serum *calcium* levels, which include both ionized and nonionized calcium, decline during pregnancy. This reduction follows lowered plasma albumin concentrations and, in turn, a consequent decrease in the amount of circulating protein-bound nonionized calcium. Serum ionized calcium levels, however, remain unchanged (Power, 1999). The developing fetus imposes a significant demand on maternal calcium homeostasis. For example, the fetal skeleton accretes approximately 30 g of calcium by term, 80 percent of which is deposited during the third trimester. This demand is largely met by a doubling of maternal intestinal calcium absorption mediated, in part, by 1,25-dihydroxyvitamin D_3 (Kovacs, 2006). In addition, dietary intake of sufficient calcium is necessary to prevent excess depletion from the mother (Table 9-6, p. 179). This is especially important for pregnant adolescents, in whom bones are still developing (Repke, 1994).

Serum *magnesium* levels also decline during pregnancy. Bardicef and colleagues (1995) concluded that pregnancy is actually a state of extracellular magnesium depletion. Compared with nonpregnant women, they found that both total and ionized magnesium concentrations were significantly lower during normal pregnancy. Serum *phosphate* levels lie within the nonpregnant range (Kametas, 2003a). The renal threshold for inorganic phosphate excretion is elevated in pregnancy due to increased calcitonin levels (Weiss, 1998).

Iodine requirements increase during normal pregnancy for several reasons (Leung, 2011; Zimmermann, 2012). First, maternal thyroxine (T_4) production increases to maintain maternal euthyroidism and to transfer thyroid hormone to the fetus early in gestation before the fetal thyroid is functioning (Chap. 58, p. 1147). Second, fetal thyroid hormone production increases during the second half of pregnancy. This contributes to increased maternal iodine requirements because iodide readily crosses the placenta. Third, the primary route of iodine excretion is through the kidney. Beginning in early pregnancy, the iodide glomerular filtration rate increases by 30 to 50 percent. Thus, because of increased thyroid hormone production, the iodine requirement of the fetus, and greater renal clearance, dietary iodine requirements are higher during normal gestation. Moreover, Burns and associates (2011) have reported that the placenta has the ability to store iodine. Whether placental iodine functions to protects the fetus from inadequate maternal dietary iodine, however, is currently unknown. Iodine deficiency is discussed later in this chapter (p. 69) as well as in Chapter 58 (p. 1155).

With respect to most other minerals, pregnancy induces little change in their metabolism other than their retention in amounts equivalent to those needed for growth (Chap. 7, p. 134 and Chap. 9, p. 179). An important exception is the considerably increased requirement for *iron,* which is discussed subsequently.

HEMATOLOGICAL CHANGES

Blood Volume

The well-known hypervolemia associated with normal pregnancy averages 40 to 45 percent above the nonpregnant blood volume after 32 to 34 weeks (Pritchard, 1965; Zeeman, 2009). In individual women, expansion varies considerably. In some there is only a modest increase, whereas in others the blood volume nearly doubles. A fetus is not essential for this because increased blood volume develops in some women with hydatidiform mole.

Pregnancy-induced hypervolemia has several important functions. First, it meets the metabolic demands of the enlarged uterus and its greatly hypertrophied vascular system. Second, it provides abundant nutrients and elements to support the rapidly growing placenta and fetus. Increased intravascular volume also protects the mother, and in turn the fetus, against the deleterious effects of impaired venous return in the supine and erect positions. Last, it safeguards the mother against the adverse effects of parturition-associated blood loss.

Maternal blood volume begins to increase during the first trimester. By 12 menstrual weeks, plasma volume expands by approximately 15 percent compared with that of prepregnancy (Bernstein, 2001). As shown in Figure 4-6, maternal blood volume expands most rapidly during the second trimester. It then rises at a much slower rate during the third trimester to plateau during the last several weeks of pregnancy.

Blood volume expansion results from an increase in both plasma and erythrocytes. Although more plasma than erythrocytes is usually added to the maternal circulation, the increase in erythrocyte volume is considerable and averages 450 mL (Pritchard, 1960). Moderate erythroid hyperplasia is present in the bone marrow, and the reticulocyte count is elevated slightly during normal pregnancy. As discussed in Chapter 56 (p. 1101), these changes are almost certainly related to an elevated maternal plasma erythropoietin level. This peaks early during the third trimester and corresponds to maximal erythrocyte production (Clapp, 2003; Harstad, 1992).

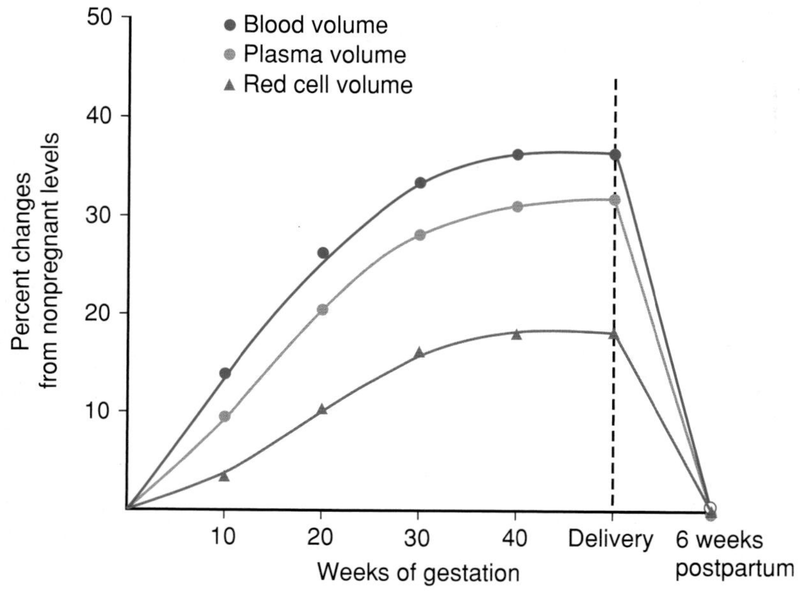

FIGURE 4-6 Changes in total blood volume and its components (plasma and red cell volumes) during pregnancy and postpartum. (Redrawn from Peck, 1979, with permission.)

Hemoglobin Concentration and Hematocrit

Because of great plasma augmentation, hemoglobin concentration and hematocrit decrease slightly during pregnancy (Appendix, p. 1287). As a result, whole blood viscosity decreases (Huisman, 1987). Hemoglobin concentration at term averages 12.5 g/dL, and in approximately 5 percent of women, it is below 11.0 g/dL (Fig. 56-1, p. 1102). Thus, a hemoglobin concentration below 11.0 g/dL, especially late in pregnancy, should be considered abnormal and usually due to iron deficiency rather than pregnancy hypervolemia.

Iron Metabolism

Storage Iron

The total iron content of normal adult women ranges from 2.0 to 2.5 g, or approximately half that found normally in men. Most of this is incorporated in hemoglobin or myoglobin, and thus, iron stores of normal young women are only approximately 300 mg (Pritchard, 1964).

Iron Requirements

Of the approximate 1000 mg of iron required for normal pregnancy, about 300 mg are actively transferred to the fetus and placenta, and another 200 mg are lost through various normal excretion routes, primarily the gastrointestinal tract. These are obligatory losses and accrue even when the mother is iron deficient. The average increase in the total circulating erythrocyte volume—about 450 mL—requires another 500 mg. Recall that each 1 mL of erythrocytes contains 1.1 mg of iron. Because most iron is used during the latter half of pregnancy, the iron requirement becomes large after midpregnancy and averages 6 to 7 mg/day (Pritchard, 1970). In most women, this amount is usually not available from iron stores. Thus, without supplemental iron, the optimal increase in maternal erythrocyte volume will not develop, and the hemoglobin concentration and hematocrit will fall appreciably as plasma volume increases. At the same time, fetal red cell production is not impaired because the placenta transfers iron even if the mother has severe iron deficiency anemia. In severe cases, we have documented maternal hemoglobin values of 3 g/dL, and at the same time, fetuses had hemoglobin concentrations of 16 g/dL. The complex mechanisms of placental iron transport and regulation have recently been reviewed by Gambling (2011) and Lipiński (2013) and all of their coworkers.

It follows that the amount of dietary iron, together with that mobilized from stores, will be insufficient to meet the average demands imposed by pregnancy. If the nonanemic pregnant woman is not given supplemental iron, then serum iron and ferritin concentrations decline after midpregnancy. The early pregnancy increases in serum iron and ferritin are likely due to minimal early iron demands combined with the positive iron balance from amenorrhea (Kaneshige, 1981).

The Puerperium

Generally, not all the maternal iron added in the form of hemoglobin is lost with normal delivery. During vaginal delivery and the first postpartum days, only approximately half of the added erythrocytes are lost from most women. These normal losses are from the placental implantation site, episiotomy or lacerations, and lochia. On average, maternal erythrocytes corresponding to approximately 500 to 600 mL of predelivery whole blood are lost with vaginal delivery of a single fetus (Pritchard, 1965; Ueland, 1976). The average blood loss associated with cesarean delivery or with the vaginal delivery of twins is approximately 1000 mL (Fig. 41-1, p. 781).

Immunological Functions

Pregnancy is thought to be associated with suppression of various humoral and cell-mediated immunological functions to accommodate the "foreign" semiallogeneic fetal graft (Redman, 2014; Thellin, 2003). This is discussed further in Chapter 5 (p. 97). In reality, pregnancy is both a proinflammatory and antiinflammatory condition, depending upon the stage of gestation. Indeed, Mor and colleagues (2010, 2011) have proposed that pregnancy can be divided into three distinct immunological phases. First, early pregnancy is proinflammatory. During implantation and placentation, the blastocyst must break through the uterine cavity epithelial lining to invade endometrial tissue. Trophoblast must then replace the endothelium and vascular smooth muscle of the maternal blood vessels to secure an adequate blood supply for the placenta (Chap. 5, p. 90). All these activities create a veritable "battleground" of invading cells, dying cells, and repairing cells. And, an inflammatory environment is required to secure cellular debris removal and adequate repair of the uterine epithelium. In contrast, midpregnancy is antiinflammatory. During this period of rapid fetal growth and development, the predominant immunological feature is induction of an antiinflammatory state. Last, parturition is characterized by an influx of immune cells into the myometrium to promote recrudescence of an inflammatory process.

An important antiinflammatory component of pregnancy appears to involve suppression of T-helper (Th) 1 and T-cytotoxic (Tc) 1 cells, which decreases secretion of interleukin-2 (IL-2), interferon-γ, and tumor necrosis factor-β (TNF-β). There is also evidence that a suppressed Th1 response is requisite for pregnancy continuation. It also may explain pregnancy-related remission of some autoimmune disorders such as rheumatoid arthritis, multiple sclerosis, and Hashimoto thyroiditis—which are Th1-mediated diseases (Kumru, 2005). As discussed in Chapter 40 (p. 733), failure of Th1 immune suppression may be related to preeclampsia development (Jonsson, 2006).

In contrast to suppression of Th1 cells, there is upregulation of Th2 cells to increase secretion of IL-4, IL-6, and IL-13 (Michimata, 2003). In cervical mucus, peak levels of immunoglobulins A and G (IgA and IgG) are significantly higher during pregnancy. Similarly, the amount of interleukin-1β found in cervical and vaginal mucus during the first trimester is approximately tenfold greater than that in nonpregnant women (Anderson, 2013).

Leukocytes

Beginning in the second trimester and continuing throughout pregnancy, some polymorphonuclear leukocyte chemotaxis and adherence functions are depressed (Krause, 1987). Although incompletely understood, this activity suppression may be partly related to the finding that relaxin impairs neutrophil activation (Masini, 2004). It is possible that these depressed leukocyte functions also account in part for the improvement of some autoimmune disorders.

As shown in the Appendix (p. 1287), leukocyte count ranges during pregnancy are higher than nonpregnant values, and the upper values approach 15,000/μL. During labor and the early puerperium, values may become markedly elevated, attaining levels of 25,000/μL or even more. However, values average 14,000 to 16,000/μL (Taylor, 1981). The cause for this marked increase is not known, but the same response occurs during and after strenuous exercise. It probably represents the reappearance of leukocytes previously shunted out of active circulation.

In addition to normal variations in the leukocyte count, the distribution of cell types is altered significantly during pregnancy. Specifically, during the third trimester, the percentages of granulocytes and CD8 T lymphocytes are significantly increased, along with a concomitant reduction in the percentages of CD4 T lymphocytes and monocytes. Moreover, circulating leukocytes undergo significant phenotypic changes including, for example, the upregulation of certain adhesion molecules (Luppi, 2002).

Inflammatory Markers

Many tests performed to diagnose inflammation cannot be used reliably during pregnancy. For example, *leukocyte alkaline phosphatase* levels are used to evaluate myeloproliferative disorders and are increased beginning early in pregnancy. The concentration of *C-reactive protein,* an acute-phase serum reactant, rises rapidly in response to tissue trauma or inflammation. Anderson (2013), Watts (1991), and all their associates measured C-reactive protein levels across pregnancy and found that median values were higher than for nonpregnant women. In the latter study, levels were also found to be elevated further during labor. Of nonlaboring women, 95 percent had levels of 1.5 mg/dL or less, and gestational age did not affect serum levels. Another marker of inflammation, the *erythrocyte sedimentation rate (ESR),* is increased in normal pregnancy because of elevated plasma globulins and fibrinogen (Hytten, 1971). *Complement factors C3* and *C4* also are significantly elevated during the second and third trimesters (Gallery, 1981; Richani, 2005). Last, levels of *procalcitonin,* a normal precursor of calcitonin, increase at the end of the third trimester and through the first few postpartum days (p. 70). Procalcitonin levels are elevated in severe bacterial infections but remain low in viral infections and nonspecific inflammatory disease. Based on their longitudinal study, Paccolat and colleagues (2011) concluded that a threshold of 0.25 μg/L can be used during the third trimester and peripartum to exclude infection.

Coagulation and Fibrinolysis

During normal pregnancy, both coagulation and fibrinolysis are augmented but remain balanced to maintain hemostasis (Appendix, p. 1288). They are even more enhanced in multifetal gestation (Morikawa, 2006). Evidence of activation includes increased concentrations of all clotting factors except factors XI and XIII (Table 4-3). The clotting time of whole blood, however, does not differ significantly in normal pregnant women. Considering the substantive physiological increase in plasma volume in normal pregnancy, such increased concentrations represent a markedly augmented production of these procoagulants (Kenny, 2014). In a longitudinal study of 20 healthy nulligravid women, for example, McLean and coworkers (2012) demonstrated progressive increases in the level and rate of thrombin generation throughout gestation. These returned to preconceptional levels by 1 year after pregnancy.

In normal nonpregnant women, plasma fibrinogen (factor I) averages 300 mg/dL and ranges from 200 to 400 mg/dL. During normal pregnancy, fibrinogen concentration increases approximately 50 percent. In late pregnancy, it averages 450 mg/dL, with a range from 300 to 600 mg/dL. The percentage of high-molecular-weight fibrinogen is unchanged (Manten, 2004). This contributes greatly to the striking increase in the *erythrocyte sedimentation rate* as discussed previously. Some of the pregnancy-induced changes in the levels of coagulation factors can be duplicated by the administration of estrogen plus progestin contraceptive tablets to nonpregnant women.

The end product of the coagulation cascade is fibrin formation, and the main function of the fibrinolytic system is to remove excess fibrin. Tissue plasminogen activator (tPA) converts plasminogen into plasmin, which causes fibrinolysis and produces fibrin-degradation products such as D-dimers. Studies of the fibrinolytic system in pregnancy have produced conflicting results, but most evidence suggests that fibrinolytic activity is actually reduced in normal pregnancy (Kenny, 2014). For example, tPA activity gradually decreases during normal pregnancy. Moreover, plasminogen activator inhibitor type 1 (PAI-1) and type 2 (PAI-2), which inhibit tPA and regulate fibrin degradation by plasmin, increase during normal pregnancy (Hui, 2012; Robb, 2009). As reviewed by Holmes and Wallace (2005), these changes—which may indicate that the fibrinolytic system is impaired—are countered by increased levels of plasminogen and decreased levels of another plasmin inhibitor, α_2 antiplasmin. Such changes serve to ensure hemostatic balance during normal pregnancy.

TABLE 4-3. Changes in Measures of Hemostasis During Normal Pregnancy

Parameter	Nonpregnant	Term Pregnant
Activated PTT (sec)	31.6 ± 4.9	31.9 ± 2.9
Fibrinogen (mg/dL)	256 ± 58	473 ± 72[a]
Factor VII (%)	99.3 ± 19.4	181.4 ± 48.0[a]
Factor X (%)	97.7 ± 15.4	144.5 ± 20.1[a]
Plasminogen (%)	105.5 ± 14.1	136.2 ± 19.5[a]
tPA (ng/mL)	5.7 ± 3.6	5.0 ± 1.5
Antithrombin III (%)	98.9 ± 13.2	97.5 ± 33.3
Protein C (%)	77.2 ± 12.0	62.9 ± 20.5[a]
Total protein S (%)	75.6 ± 14.0	49.9 ± 10.2[a]

[a]$p < .05$.
Data shown as mean ± standard deviation.
PTT = partial thromboplastin time; tPA = tissue plasminogen activator.
Data from Uchikova, 2005.

Platelets

Normal pregnancy also involves platelet changes. In a study of almost 7000 healthy women at term, Boehlen and colleagues (2000) found that the average platelet count was decreased slightly during pregnancy to 213,000/μL compared with 250,000/μL in nonpregnant control women. Thrombocytopenia defined as below the 2.5th percentile corresponded to a platelet count of 116,000/μL. Decreased platelet concentrations are partially due to hemodilutional effects. There likely also is increased platelet consumption, leading to a greater proportion of younger and therefore larger platelets (Valera, 2010). Further supporting this concept, Hayashi and associates (2002) found that beginning in midpregnancy, production of thromboxane A_2, which induces platelet aggregation, progressively increases. Because of splenic enlargement, there may also be an element of "hypersplenism" (Kenny, 2014).

Regulatory Proteins

There are several natural inhibitors of coagulation, including proteins C and S and antithrombin. Inherited or acquired deficiencies of these and other natural regulatory proteins—collectively referred to as *thrombophilias*—account for many thromboembolic episodes during pregnancy. They are discussed in detail in Chapter 52 (p. 1029).

Activated protein C, along with the cofactors protein S and factor V, functions as an anticoagulant by neutralizing the procoagulants factor Va and factor VIIIa (Fig. 52–1, p. 1030). During pregnancy, resistance to activated protein C increases progressively and is related to a concomitant decrease in free protein S and increase in factor VIII levels. Between the first and third trimesters, activated protein C levels decrease from 2.4 to 1.9 U/mL, and free protein S concentrations decline from 0.4 to 0.16 U/mL (Walker, 1997). Oral contraceptives also decrease free protein S levels. Levels of *antithrombin* remain relatively constant throughout gestation and the early puerperium (Delorme, 1992).

Spleen

By the end of normal pregnancy, the spleen enlarges by up to 50 percent compared with that in the first trimester (Maymon,

2007). Moreover, in a study of 77 recently delivered gravidas, Gayer and coworkers (2012) found that splenic size was 68-percent larger compared with that of nonpregnant controls. The cause of this splenomegaly is unknown, but it might follow the increased blood volume and/or the hemodynamic changes of pregnancy, which are subsequently discussed. Sonographically, the echogenic appearance of the spleen remains homogeneous throughout gestation.

CARDIOVASCULAR SYSTEM

During pregnancy and the puerperium, the heart and circulation undergo remarkable physiological adaptations. Changes in cardiac function become apparent during the first 8 weeks of pregnancy (Hibbard, 2014). Cardiac output is increased as early as the fifth week and reflects a reduced systemic vascular resistance and an increased heart rate. Compared with prepregnancy measurements, brachial systolic blood pressure, diastolic blood pressure, and central systolic blood pressure are all significantly lower 6 to 7 weeks from the last menstrual period (Mahendru, 2012). The resting pulse rate increases approximately 10 beats/min during pregnancy. Between weeks 10 and 20, plasma volume expansion begins, and preload is increased.

Ventricular performance during pregnancy is influenced by both the decrease in systemic vascular resistance and changes in pulsatile arterial flow. Multiple factors contribute to this overall altered hemodynamic function, which allows the physiological demands of the fetus to be met while maintaining maternal cardiovascular integrity (Hibbard, 2014). These changes during the last half of pregnancy are graphically summarized in Figure 4-7.

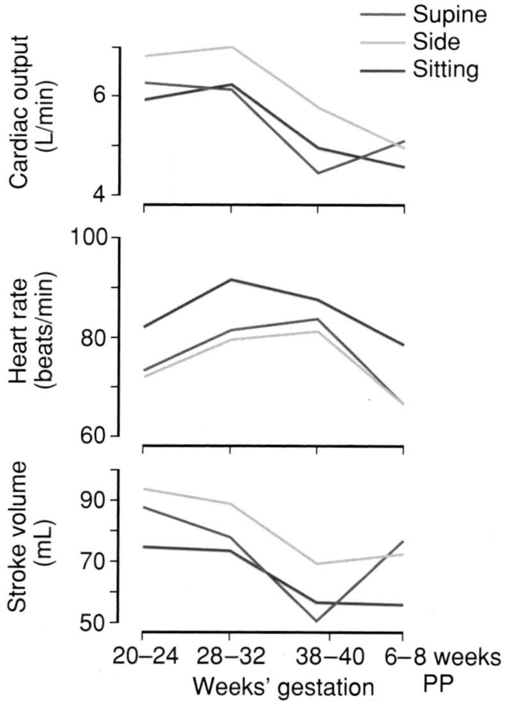

FIGURE 4-7 Effect of maternal posture on hemodynamics. PP = postpartum. (Redrawn from Ueland, 1975.)

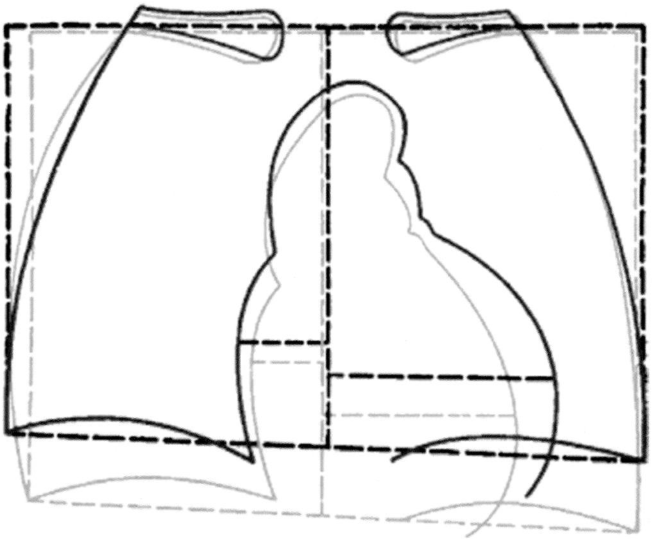

FIGURE 4-8 Change in cardiac radiographic outline that occurs in pregnancy. The blue lines represent the relations between the heart and thorax in the nonpregnant woman, and the black lines represent the conditions existing in pregnancy. These are based on radiographic findings in 33 women. (Redrawn from Klafen, 1927.)

The important effects of maternal posture on hemodynamics are also illustrated.

Heart

As the diaphragm becomes progressively elevated, the heart is displaced to the left and upward and is rotated on its long axis. As a result, the apex is moved somewhat laterally from its usual position and produces a larger cardiac silhouette in chest radiographs (Fig. 4-8). Furthermore, pregnant women normally have some degree of benign pericardial effusion, which may increase the cardiac silhouette (Enein, 1987). Variability of these factors makes it difficult to precisely identify moderate degrees of cardiomegaly by simple radiographic studies. Normal pregnancy induces no characteristic electrocardiographic changes other than slight left-axis deviation due to the altered heart position.

Many of the normal *cardiac sounds* are modified during pregnancy. Cutforth and MacDonald (1966) used phonocardiography and documented: (1) an exaggerated splitting of the first heart sound and increased loudness of both components, (2) no definite changes in the aortic and pulmonary elements of the second sound, and (3) a loud, easily heard third sound (Fig. 49-2, p. 975). In 90 percent of pregnant women, they also heard a systolic murmur that was intensified during inspiration in some or expiration in others and that disappeared shortly after delivery. A soft diastolic murmur was noted transiently in 20 percent, and continuous murmurs arising from the breast vasculature in 10 percent.

Structurally, the increasing plasma volume seen during normal pregnancy is reflected by enlarging cardiac end-systolic and end-diastolic dimensions. At the same time, however, there is no change in septal thickness or in ejection fraction. This is because the dimensional changes are accompanied by substantive ventricular remodeling, which is characterized by eccentric left-ventricular mass expansion averaging 30 to 35 percent near term. In the nonpregnant state, the heart is capable of remodeling in response to stimuli such as hypertension and exercise. Such cardiac *plasticity* likely is a continuum that encompasses physiological growth, such as that in exercise, as well as pathological hypertrophy—such as with hypertension (Hill, 2008).

And although it is widely held that there is physiological hypertrophy of cardiac myocytes as a result of pregnancy, this has never been absolutely proven. Hibbard and colleagues (2014) concluded that any increased mass does not meet criteria for hypertrophy.

Certainly for clinical purposes, ventricular function during pregnancy is normal, as estimated by the *Braunwald ventricular function* graph depicted in Figure 4-9. For the given filling pressures, there is appropriate cardiac output so that cardiac function during pregnancy is eudynamic. Despite these findings, it remains controversial whether myocardial function per se is normal, enhanced, or depressed. In nonpregnant subjects with a normal heart who sustain a high-output state, the left ventricle undergoes *longitudinal remodeling,* and echocardiographic functional indices of its deformation provide normal values. In pregnancy, there instead appears to be *spherical remodeling,* and these calculated indices that measure longitudinal deformation are depressed (Savu, 2012). Thus, these normal indices are likely inaccurate when used to assess function in pregnant women because they do not account for the spherical eccentric hypertrophy characteristic of normal pregnancy.

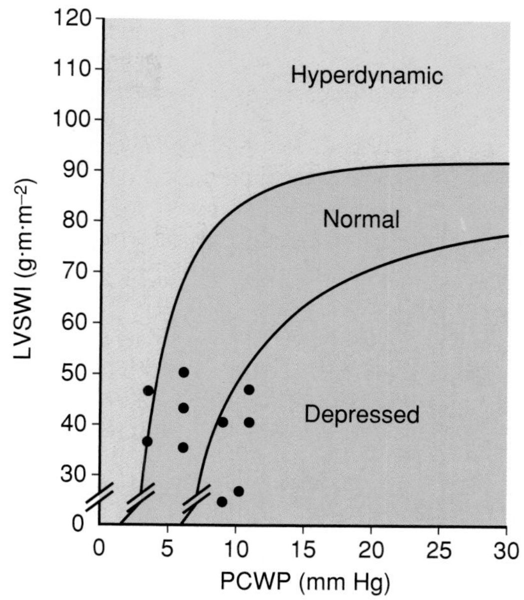

FIGURE 4-9 Relationship between left ventricular stroke work index (LVSWI), cardiac output, and pulmonary capillary wedge pressure (PCWP) in 10 normal pregnant women in the third trimester. (Data from Clark, 1989.)

In multifetal pregnancies, compared with singletons, maternal cardiac output is augmented further by almost another 20 percent because of a greater stroke volume (15 percent) and heart rate (3.5 percent). Left atrial diameter and left ventricular end-diastolic diameter are also increased due to augmented preload (Kametas, 2003b). The increased heart rate and inotropic

Cardiac Output

During normal pregnancy, mean arterial pressure and vascular resistance decrease, while blood volume and basal metabolic rate increase. As a result, cardiac output *at rest,* when measured in the lateral recumbent position, increases significantly beginning in early pregnancy (Duvekot, 1993; Mabie, 1994). It continues to increase and remains elevated during the remainder of pregnancy (Fig. 4-10).

During late pregnancy in a supine woman, the large uterus rather consistently compresses venous return from the lower body. It also may compress the aorta (Bieniarz, 1968). In response, cardiac filling may be reduced and cardiac output diminished. Specifically, Bamber and Dresner (2003) found cardiac output at term to increase 1.2 L/min—almost 20 percent—when a woman was moved from her back onto her left side. Moreover, in the supine pregnant woman, uterine blood flow estimated by Doppler velocimetry decreases by a third (Jeffreys, 2006). Of note, Simpson and James (2005) found that fetal oxygen saturation is approximately 10 percent higher if a laboring woman is in a lateral recumbent position compared with supine. Upon standing, cardiac output falls to the same degree as in the nonpregnant woman (Easterling, 1988).

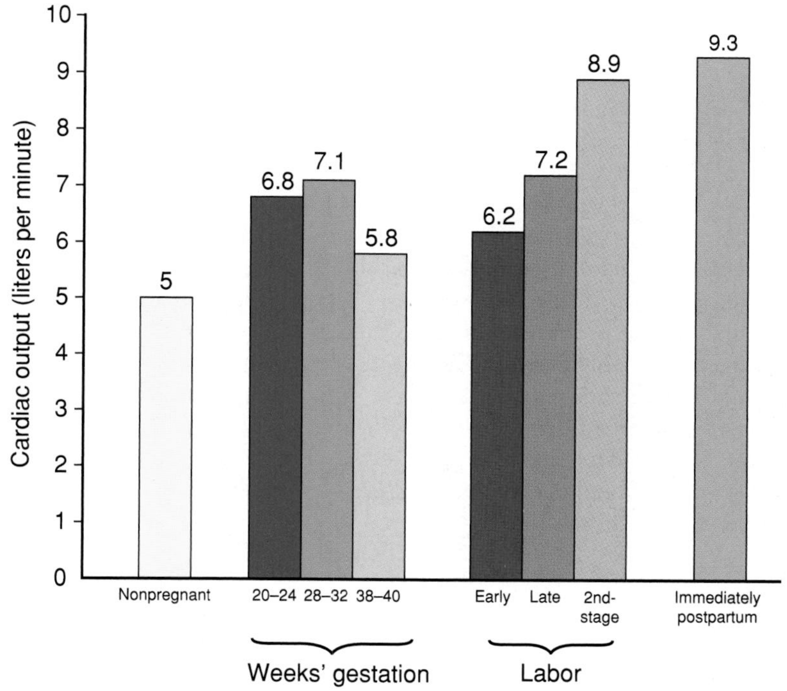

FIGURE 4-10 Cardiac output during three stages of gestation, labor, and immediately postpartum compared with values of nonpregnant women. All values were determined with women in the lateral recumbent position. (Adapted from Ueland, 1975.)

TABLE 4-4. Central Hemodynamic Changes in 10 Normal Nulliparous Women Near Term and Postpartum

	Pregnant[a] (35–38 wk)	Postpartum (11–13 wk)	Change[b]
Mean arterial pressure (mm Hg)	90 ± 6	86 ± 8	NSC
Pulmonary capillary wedge pressure (mm Hg)	8 ± 2	6 ± 2	NSC
Central venous pressure (mm Hg)	4 ± 3	4 ± 3	NSC
Heart rate (beats/min)	83 ± 10	71 ± 10	+17%
Cardiac output (L/min)	6.2 ± 1.0	4.3 ± 0.9	+43%
Systemic vascular resistance (dyn/sec/cm^{-5})	1210 ± 266	1530 ± 520	−21%
Pulmonary vascular resistance (dyn/sec/cm^{-5})	78 ± 22	119 ± 47	−34%
Serum colloid osmotic pressure (mm Hg)	18.0 ± 1.5	20.8 ± 1.0	−14%
COP-PCWP gradient (mm Hg)	10.5 ± 2.7	14.5 ± 2.5	−28%
Left ventricular stroke work index (g/m/m^2)	48 ± 6	41 ± 8	NSC

[a]Measured in lateral recumbent position.
[b]Changes significant unless NSC = no significant change.
COP = colloid osmotic pressure; PCWP = pulmonary capillary wedge pressure.
Adapted from Clark, 1989.

contractility imply that cardiovascular reserve is reduced in multifetal gestations.

During the first stage of labor, cardiac output increases moderately. During the second stage, with vigorous expulsive efforts, it is appreciably greater (see Fig. 4-10). The pregnancy-induced increase is lost after delivery, at times dependent on blood loss.

Hemodynamic Function in Late Pregnancy

To further elucidate the net changes of normal pregnancy-induced cardiovascular changes, Clark and associates (1989) conducted invasive studies to measure hemodynamic function late in pregnancy (Table 4-4). Right heart catheterization was performed in 10 healthy nulliparous women at 35 to 38 weeks, and again at 11 to 13 weeks postpartum. Late pregnancy was associated with the expected increases in heart rate, stroke volume, and cardiac output. Systemic vascular and pulmonary vascular resistance both decreased significantly, as did colloid osmotic pressure. Pulmonary capillary wedge pressure and central venous pressure did not change appreciably between late pregnancy and the puerperium. Thus, as shown earlier in Figure 4-9, although cardiac output is increased, left ventricular function as measured by stroke work index remains similar to the nonpregnant normal range. Put another way, normal pregnancy is not a continuous "high-output" state.

Circulation and Blood Pressure

Changes in posture affect arterial blood pressure. Brachial artery pressure when sitting is lower than that when in the lateral recumbent supine position (Bamber, 2003). Arterial pressure usually decreases to a nadir at 24 to 26 weeks and rises thereafter. Diastolic pressure decreases more than systolic (Fig. 4-11).

Antecubital venous pressure remains unchanged during pregnancy. In the supine position, however, femoral venous pressure rises steadily, from approximately 8 mm Hg early in pregnancy to 24 mm Hg at term. Wright and coworkers (1950) demonstrated that venous blood flow in the legs is retarded during pregnancy except when the lateral recumbent position is assumed. This tendency toward blood stagnation in the lower extremities during latter pregnancy is attributable to occlusion of the pelvic veins and inferior vena cava by the enlarged uterus. The elevated venous pressure returns to normal when the pregnant woman lies on her side and immediately after delivery (McLennan, 1943). These alterations contribute to the dependent edema

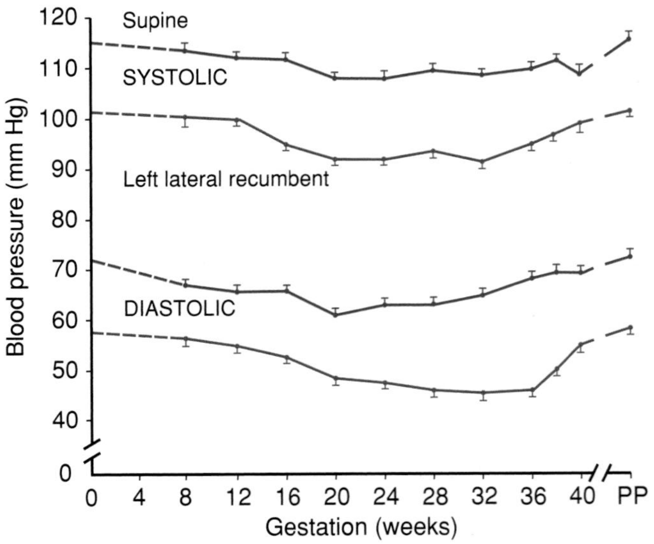

FIGURE 4-11 Sequential changes (±SEM) in blood pressure throughout pregnancy in 69 women in supine (*blue lines*) and left lateral recumbent positions (*red lines*). PP = postpartum. (Adapted from Wilson, 1980.)

frequently experienced and to the development of varicose veins in the legs and vulva, as well as hemorrhoids. These changes also predispose to deep-vein thrombosis (Chap. 52, p. 1035).

Supine Hypotension

In approximately 10 percent of women, supine compression of the great vessels by the uterus causes significant arterial hypotension, sometimes referred to as the *supine hypotensive syndrome* (Kinsella, 1994). Also when supine, uterine arterial pressure—and thus blood flow—is significantly lower than that in the brachial artery. As discussed in Chapter 24 (p. 494), this may directly affect fetal heart rate patterns (Tamás, 2007). These changes are also seen with hemorrhage or with spinal analgesia (Chap. 25, p. 511).

Renin, Angiotensin II, and Plasma Volume

The renin-angiotensin-aldosterone axis is intimately involved in blood pressure control via sodium and water balance. All components of this system are increased in normal pregnancy (Bentley-Lewis, 2005). Renin is produced by both the maternal kidney and the placenta, and increased renin substrate (angiotensinogen) is produced by both maternal and fetal liver. Elevated angiotensinogen levels result, in part, from increased estrogen production during normal pregnancy and are important in first-trimester blood pressure maintenance (August, 1995).

Gant and associates (1973) studied vascular reactivity to angiotensin II throughout pregnancy. Nulliparas who remained normotensive became and stayed refractory to the pressor effects of infused angiotensin II. Conversely, those who ultimately became hypertensive developed, but then lost, this refractoriness. Follow-up studies by Gant (1974) and Cunningham (1975) and their colleagues indicated that increased refractoriness to angiotensin II stemmed from individual vessel refractoriness. Said another way, the abnormally increased sensitivity was an alteration in vessel wall refractoriness rather than the consequence of altered blood volume or renin-angiotensin secretion.

The vascular responsiveness to angiotensin II may be progesterone related. Normally, pregnant women lose their acquired vascular refractoriness to angiotensin II within 15 to 30 minutes after the placenta is delivered. Moreover, large amounts of intramuscular progesterone given during late labor delay this diminishing refractoriness. And although exogenous progesterone does not restore angiotensin II refractoriness to women with gestational hypertension, this can be done with infusion of its major metabolite, 5α-dihydroprogesterone.

Cardiac Natriuretic Peptides

At least two species of these—*atrial natriuretic peptide (ANP)* and *B-type natriuretic peptide (BNP)*—are secreted by cardiomyocytes in response to chamber-wall stretching. These peptides regulate blood volume by provoking natriuresis, diuresis, and vascular smooth-muscle relaxation (Clerico, 2004). In nonpregnant and pregnant patients, levels of BNP and of amino-terminal pro-brain natriuretic peptide (Nt pro-BNP) may be useful in screening for depressed left ventricular systolic function and determining chronic heart failure prognosis (Jarolim, 2006; Tanous, 2010).

During normal pregnancy, plasma ANP and BNP levels are maintained in the nonpregnant range despite increased plasma volume (Lowe, 1992; Yurteri-Kaplan, 2012). In one study, Resnik and coworkers (2005) found median BNP levels to be stable across pregnancy with values < 20 pg/mL. BNP levels are increased in severe preeclampsia, and Tihtonen and colleagues (2007) concluded that this was caused by cardiac strain from increased afterload. It would appear that ANP-induced physiological adaptations participate in extracellular fluid volume expansion and in the increased plasma aldosterone concentrations characteristic of normal pregnancy.

A third species, *C-type natriuretic peptide (CNP),* is predominantly secreted by noncardiac tissues. Among its diverse biological functions, this peptide appears to be a major regulator of fetal bone growth. Walther and Stepan (2004) have provided a detailed review of its function during pregnancy.

Prostaglandins

Increased prostaglandin production during pregnancy is thought to have a central role in control of vascular tone, blood pressure, and sodium balance. Renal medullary prostaglandin E_2 synthesis is increased markedly during late pregnancy and is presumed to be natriuretic. Prostacyclin (PGI_2), the principal prostaglandin of endothelium, also is increased during late pregnancy and regulates blood pressure and platelet function. It also has been implicated in the angiotensin resistance characteristic of normal pregnancy (Friedman, 1988). The ratio of PGI_2 to thromboxane in maternal urine and blood has been considered important in preeclampsia pathogenesis (Chap. 40, p. 735). The molecular mechanisms regulating prostacyclin pathways during pregnancy have recently been reviewed by Majed and Khalil (2012).

Endothelin

There are several endothelins generated in pregnancy. Endothelin-1 is a potent vasoconstrictor produced in endothelial and vascular smooth muscle cells and regulates local vasomotor tone (Feletou, 2006; George, 2011). Its production is stimulated by angiotensin II, arginine vasopressin, and thrombin. Endothelins, in turn, stimulate secretion of ANP, aldosterone, and catecholamines. As discussed in Chapter 21 (p. 427), there are endothelin receptors in pregnant and nonpregnant myometrium. Endothelins also have been identified in the amnion, amnionic fluid, decidua, and placenta (Kubota, 1992; Margarit, 2005). Vascular sensitivity to endothelin-1 is not altered during normal pregnancy. Ajne and associates (2005) postulated that vasodilating factors counterbalance the endothelin-1 vasoconstrictor effects and reduce peripheral vascular resistance.

Nitric Oxide

This potent vasodilator is released by endothelial cells and may have important implications for modifying vascular resistance during pregnancy. Moreover, nitric oxide is one of the most important mediators of placental vascular tone and development (Krause, 2011; Kulandavelu, 2013). As discussed in Chapter 40 (p. 735), abnormal nitric oxide synthesis has been linked to preeclampsia development (Baksu, 2005; Teran, 2006).

RESPIRATORY TRACT

As shown in Figure 4-12, the diaphragm rises about 4 cm during pregnancy. The subcostal angle widens appreciably as the transverse diameter of the thoracic cage lengthens approximately 2 cm. The thoracic circumference increases about 6 cm, but not sufficiently to prevent reduced residual lung volumes created by the elevated diaphragm. Even so, diaphragmatic excursion is greater in pregnant than in nonpregnant women.

Pulmonary Function

The physiological changes in lung function during pregnancy are illustrated in Figure 4-13. *Functional residual capacity (FRC)* decreases by approximately 20 to 30 percent or 400 to 700 mL during pregnancy. This capacity is composed of *expiratory reserve volume*—which decreases 15 to 20 percent or 200 to 300 mL—and *residual volume*—which decreases 20 to 125 percent or 200 to 400 mL. FRC and residual volume decline due to diaphragm elevation, and significant reductions are observed by the sixth month with a progressive decline across pregnancy. *Inspiratory capacity*, the maximum volume that can be inhaled from FRC, increases by 5 to 10 percent or 200 to 250 mL during pregnancy. *Total lung capacity*—the combination of FRC and inspiratory capacity—is unchanged or decreases by less than 5 percent at term (Hegewald, 2011).

The respiratory rate is essentially unchanged, but *tidal volume* and *resting minute ventilation* increase significantly as pregnancy advances. In a study of 51 healthy pregnant women, Kolarzyk and coworkers (2005) reported significantly greater mean tidal volumes—0.66 to 0.8 L/min—and resting minute ventilations—10.7 to 14.1 L/min—compared with those of nonpregnant women. The increased minute ventilation is caused by several factors. These include enhanced respiratory drive primarily due to the stimulatory action of progesterone, low expiratory reserve volume, and compensated respiratory alkalosis, which is discussed in more detail subsequently (Wise, 2006).

Regarding pulmonary function, Grindheim and associates (2012) found in 75 healthy pregnant women that *peak expiratory flow rates* increase progressively as gestation advances. *Lung compliance* is unaffected by pregnancy. *Airway conductance* is increased and *total pulmonary resistance* reduced, possibly as a result of progesterone. The *maximum breathing capacity* and *forced* or *timed vital capacity* are not altered appreciably. It is unclear whether the critical *closing volume*—the lung volume

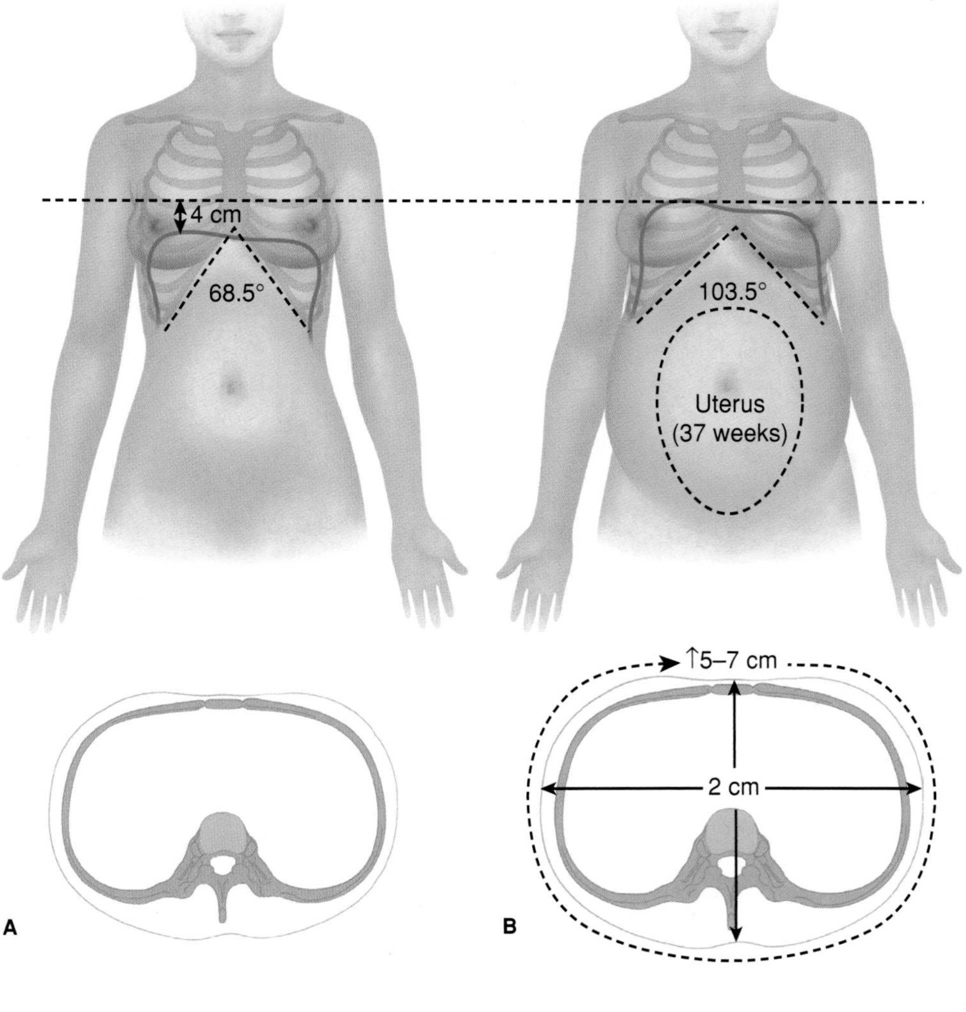

FIGURE 4-12 Chest wall measurements in nonpregnant **(A)** and pregnant women **(B)**. With pregnancy, the subcostal angle increases, as does the anteroposterior and transverse diameters of the chest wall and chest wall circumference. These changes compensate for the 4-cm elevation of the diaphragm so that total lung capacity is not significantly reduced. (Redrawn from Hegewald, 2011, with permission.)

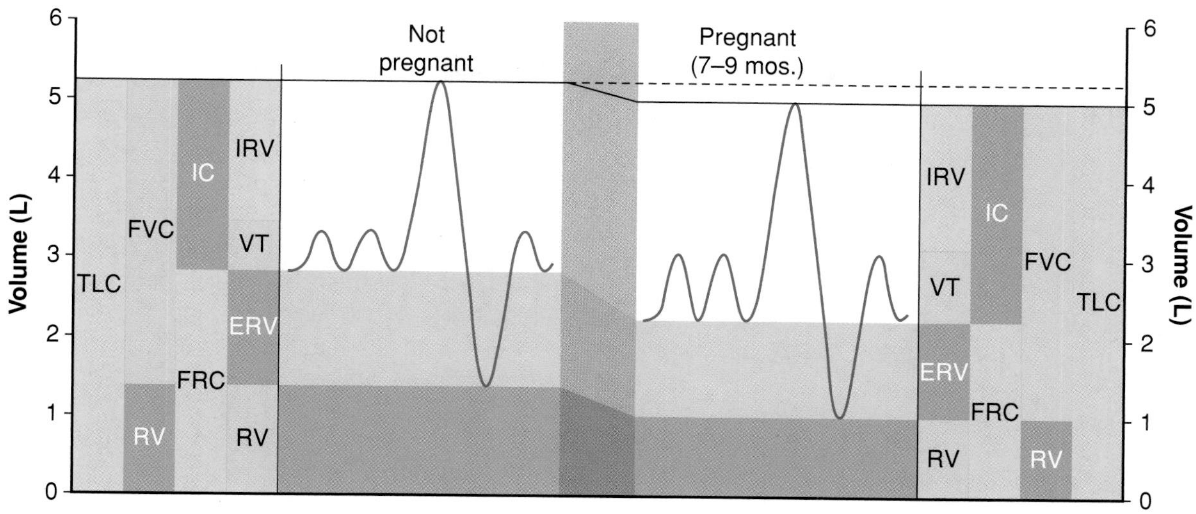

FIGURE 4-13 Changes in lung volumes with pregnancy. The most significant changes are reduction in functional residual capacity (FRC) and its subcomponents, expiratory reserve volume (ERV) and residual volume (RV), as well as increases in inspiratory capacity (IC) and tidal volume (VT). (Redrawn from Hegewald, 2011, with permission.)

at which airways in the dependent parts of the lung begin to close during expiration—is higher in pregnancy (Hegewald, 2011). The increased oxygen requirements and perhaps the increased critical closing volume imposed by pregnancy make respiratory diseases more serious.

McAuliffe and associates (2002) compared pulmonary function in 140 women with a singleton pregnancy with that in 68 women with twins. They found no significant differences between the two groups.

Oxygen Delivery

The amount of oxygen delivered into the lungs by the increased tidal volume clearly exceeds oxygen requirements imposed by pregnancy. Moreover, the total hemoglobin mass, and in turn, total oxygen-carrying capacity, increases appreciably during normal pregnancy, as does cardiac output. Consequently, the *maternal arteriovenous oxygen* difference is decreased. Oxygen consumption increases approximately 20 percent during pregnancy, and it is approximately 10 percent higher in multifetal gestations. During labor, oxygen consumption increases 40 to 60 percent (Bobrowski, 2010).

Acid–Base Equilibrium

An increased awareness of a desire to breathe is common even early in pregnancy (Milne, 1978). This may be interpreted as dyspnea, which may suggest pulmonary or cardiac abnormalities when none exist. This physiological dyspnea, which should not interfere with normal physical activity, is thought to result from increased tidal volume that lowers the blood P_{CO_2} slightly and paradoxically causes dyspnea. The increased respiratory effort during pregnancy, and in turn the reduction in P_{CO_2}, is likely induced in large part by progesterone and to a lesser degree by estrogen. Progesterone appears to act centrally, where it lowers the threshold and increases the sensitivity of the chemoreflex response to CO_2 (Jensen, 2005).

To compensate for the resulting respiratory alkalosis, plasma bicarbonate levels normally decrease from 26 to approximately 22 mmol/L. Although blood pH is increased only minimally, it does shift the oxygen dissociation curve to the left. This shift increases the affinity of maternal hemoglobin for oxygen—the *Bohr effect*—thereby decreasing the oxygen-releasing capacity of maternal blood. This is offset because the slight pH increase also stimulates an increase in 2,3-diphosphoglycerate in maternal erythrocytes. This shifts the curve back to the right (Tsai, 1982). Thus, reduced P_{CO_2} from maternal hyperventilation aids carbon dioxide (waste) transfer from the fetus to the mother while also aiding oxygen release to the fetus.

URINARY SYSTEM

Kidney

Several remarkable changes are observed in the urinary system as a result of pregnancy (Table 4-5). *Kidney size* increases approximately 1.5 cm (Bailey, 1971). Both the *glomerular filtration rate (GFR)* and *renal plasma flow* increase early in pregnancy. The GFR increases as much as 25 percent by the second week after conception and 50 percent by the beginning of the second trimester. This hyperfiltration appears to result from two principal factors. First, hypervolemia-induced hemodilution lowers the protein concentration and oncotic pressure of plasma entering the glomerular microcirculation. Second, renal plasma flow increases by approximately 80 percent before the end of the first trimester (Conrad, 2014; Cornelis, 2011). As shown in Figure 4-14, elevated GFR persists until term, even though renal plasma flow decreases during late pregnancy. Primarily as a consequence of this elevated GFR, approximately 60 percent of women report urinary frequency during pregnancy (Sandhu, 2009).

During the puerperium, a marked GFR persists during the first postpartum day principally from the reduced glomerular capillary oncotic pressure. A reversal of the gestational hypervolemia and hemodilution, still evident on the first postpartum day, eventuates by the second week postpartum (Hladunewich, 2004).

TABLE 4-5. Renal Changes in Normal Pregnancy

Parameter	Alteration	Clinical Relevance
Kidney size	Approximately 1 cm longer on radiograph	Size returns to normal postpartum
Dilatation	Resembles hydronephrosis on sonogram or IVP (more marked on right)	Can be confused with obstructive uropathy; retained urine leads to collection errors; renal infections are more virulent; may be responsible for "distension syndrome"; elective pyelography should be deferred to at least 12 weeks postpartum
Renal function	Glomerular filtration rate and renal plasma flow increase ~50%	Serum creatinine decreases during normal gestation; > 0.8 mg/dL (> 72 μmol/L) creatinine already borderline; protein, amino acid, and glucose excretion all increase
Maintenance of acid-base	Decreased bicarbonate threshold; progesterone stimulates respiratory center	Serum bicarbonate decreased by 4–5 mEq/L; Pco_2 decreased 10 mm Hg; a Pco_2 of 40 mm Hg already represents CO_2 retention
Plasma osmolality	Osmoregulation altered; osmotic thresholds for AVP release and thirst decrease; hormonal disposal rates increase	Serum osmolality decreases 10 mOsm/L (serum Na ~5 mEq/L) during normal gestation; increased placental metabolism of AVP may cause transient diabetes insipidus during pregnancy

AVP = vasopressin; IVP = intravenous pyelography; Pco_2 = partial pressure carbon dioxide.
Modified from Lindheimer, 2000.

Studies suggest that relaxin may be important for mediating both increased GFR and renal blood flow during pregnancy (Conrad, 2014; Helal, 2012). Relaxin increases endothelin and nitric oxide production in the renal circulation. This leads to renal vasodilation and decreased renal afferent and efferent arteriolar resistance, with a resultant increase in renal blood flow and GFR. Relaxin may also increase vascular gelatinase activity during pregnancy, which leads to renal vasodilation, glomerular hyperfiltration, and reduced myogenic reactivity of small renal arteries (Conrad, 2005).

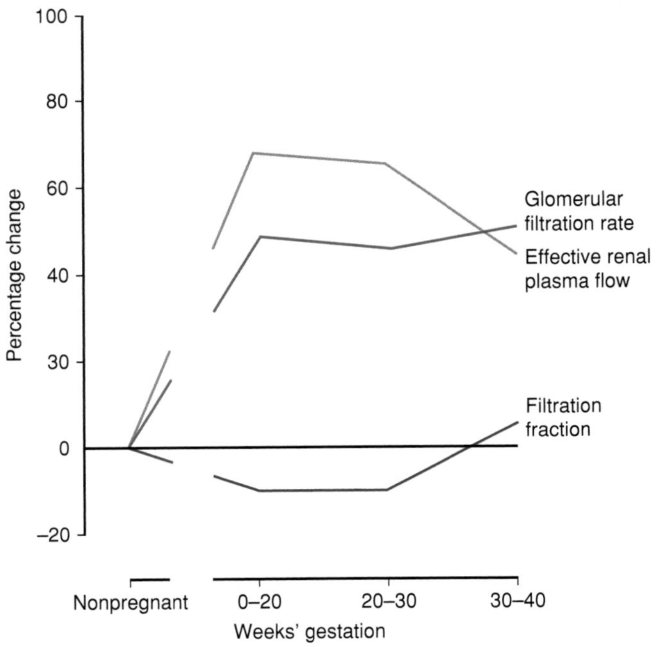

FIGURE 4-14 Relative changes in measures of glomerular filtration rate (GFR), effective renal plasma flow (ERPF), and filtration fraction during normal pregnancy. (Redrawn from Davison, 1980, with permission.)

As with blood pressure, maternal posture may have a considerable influence on several aspects of renal function. Late in pregnancy, for instance, urinary flow and sodium excretion average less than half the excretion rate in the supine position compared with that in the lateral recumbent position. The impact of posture on GFR and renal plasma flow is more variable.

One unusual feature of the pregnancy-induced changes in renal excretion is the remarkably increased amounts of various nutrients lost in the urine. Amino acids and water-soluble vitamins are excreted in much greater amounts (Hytten, 1973; Powers, 2004).

Renal Function Tests

The physiological changes in renal hemodynamics induced during normal pregnancy have several implications for the interpretation of renal function tests (Appendix, p. 1292). *Serum creatinine* levels decrease during normal pregnancy from a mean of 0.7 to 0.5 mg/dL. *Values of 0.9 mg/dL or greater suggest underlying renal disease and should prompt further evaluation.*

Creatinine clearance in pregnancy averages 30 percent higher than the 100 to 115 mL/min in nonpregnant women (Lindheimer, 2000). This is a useful test to estimate renal function, provided that complete urine collection is made during an accurately timed period. If either is done incorrectly, results are misleading (Lindheimer, 2010). During the day, pregnant women tend to accumulate water as dependent edema, and at night, while recumbent, they mobilize this fluid with diuresis. This reversal of the usual nonpregnant diurnal pattern of urinary flow causes nocturia, and urine is more dilute than in nonpregnant women. Failure of a pregnant woman to excrete concentrated urine after withholding fluids for approximately 18 hours does not necessarily signify renal damage. In fact, the kidney in these circumstances functions perfectly normally by excreting mobilized extracellular fluid of relatively low osmolality.

Urinalysis

Glucosuria during pregnancy may not be abnormal. The appreciable increase in GFR, together with impaired tubular reabsorptive capacity for filtered glucose, accounts for most cases of glucosuria (Davison, 1974). For these reasons alone, Chesley (1963) calculated that about a sixth of pregnant women should spill glucose in the urine. That said, although common during pregnancy, when glucosuria is identified, the possibility of diabetes mellitus should not be ignored.

Hematuria is often the result of contamination during collection. If not, it most often suggests urinary tract disease. Hematuria is common after difficult labor and delivery because of trauma to the bladder and urethra.

Proteinuria is typically defined in nonpregnant patients as a protein excretion rate of more than 150 mg/day. Because of the aforementioned hyperfiltration and possible reduction of tubular reabsorption, significant proteinuria during pregnancy is usually defined as a protein excretion rate of at least 300 mg/day (Hladunewich, 2011). Higby and coworkers (1994) measured protein excretion in 270 normal women throughout pregnancy (Fig. 4-15). Their mean 24-hour excretion for all three trimesters was 115 mg, and the upper 95-percent confidence limit was 260 mg/day without significant differences by trimester. These investigators also showed that albumin excretion is minimal and ranges from 5 to 30 mg/day. Interestingly, however, Cornelis and colleagues (2011) noted that proteinuria is greater in the second half of pregnancy, which does not correspond precisely to the earlier peak in GFR (see Fig. 4-14). Alternative explanations might include alterations in tubular reabsorptive capacity or the presence of other proteinaceous material that might be detected in the urine of pregnant women. A recent study in normal gravidas also showed proteinuria levels greater than established thresholds (Phillips, 2014).

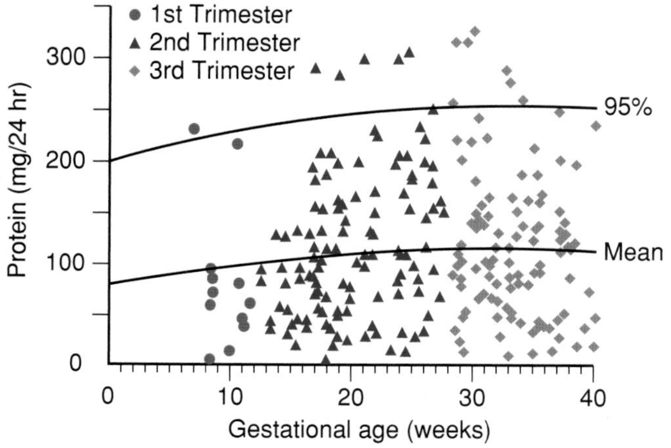

FIGURE 4-15 Scatter plot of women showing 24-hour urinary total protein excretion. Mean and 95-percent confidence limits are outlined. (Redrawn from Higby, 1994, with permission.)

Measuring Urine Protein

The three most commonly employed approaches for assessing proteinuria are the qualitative classic dipstick, the quantitative 24-hour collection, and the albumin/creatinine or protein/creatinine ratio of a single voided urine specimen. The pitfalls of each approach have recently been reviewed by Conrad and colleagues (2014). The principal problem with dipstick assessment is that renal concentration or dilution of urine is not accounted for. For example, with polyuria and extremely dilute urine, a negative or trace dipstick could actually be associated with excessive protein excretion.

The 24-hour urine collection is affected by urinary tract dilatation, which is discussed subsequently. The dilated tract may lead to errors related both to retention—hundreds of milliliters of urine remaining in the dilated tract—and to timing—the remaining urine may have formed hours before the collection. To minimize these pitfalls, Lindheimer and Kanter (2010) recommend that the patient first be hydrated and positioned in lateral recumbency—the definitive nonobstructive posture—for 45 to 60 minutes. After this, she is asked to void, and this specimen is discarded. Immediately following this void, her 24-hour collection begins. During the final hour of collection, the patient is again placed in the lateral recumbent position. But, at the end of this hour, the final collected urine is incorporated into the total collected volume.

The protein/creatinine ratio is a promising approach because data can be obtained quickly and collection errors are avoided. Disadvantageously, the amount of protein per unit of creatinine excreted during a 24-hour period is not constant, and there are various thresholds that have been promulgated to define abnormal. Nomograms for urinary microalbumin and creatinine ratios during uncomplicated pregnancies have been developed by Waugh and coworkers (2003).

Ureters

After the uterus completely rises out of the pelvis, it rests on the ureters, which laterally displaces and compresses them at the pelvic brim. Above this level, increased intraureteral tonus results (Rubi, 1968). Ureteral dilatation is impressive, and Schulman and Herlinger (1975) found it to be greater on the right side in 86 percent of women (Fig. 4-16). Unequal dilatation may result from cushioning provided the left ureter by the sigmoid colon and perhaps from greater right ureteral compression exerted by the dextrorotated uterus. The right ovarian vein complex, which is remarkably dilated during pregnancy, lies obliquely over the right ureter and may contribute significantly to right ureteral dilatation.

Progesterone likely also has some effect. Van Wagenen and Jenkins (1939) described continued ureteral dilatation after removal of the monkey fetus but with the placenta left in situ. The relatively abrupt onset of dilatation in women at midpregnancy, however, seems more consistent with ureteral compression.

Ureteral elongation accompanies distention, and the ureter is frequently thrown into curves of varying size, the smaller of which may be sharply angulated. These so-called kinks are poorly named, because the term connotes obstruction. They are usually single or double curves that, when viewed in a radiograph taken in the same plane as the curve, may appear as acute angulations. Another exposure at right angles nearly always identifies them

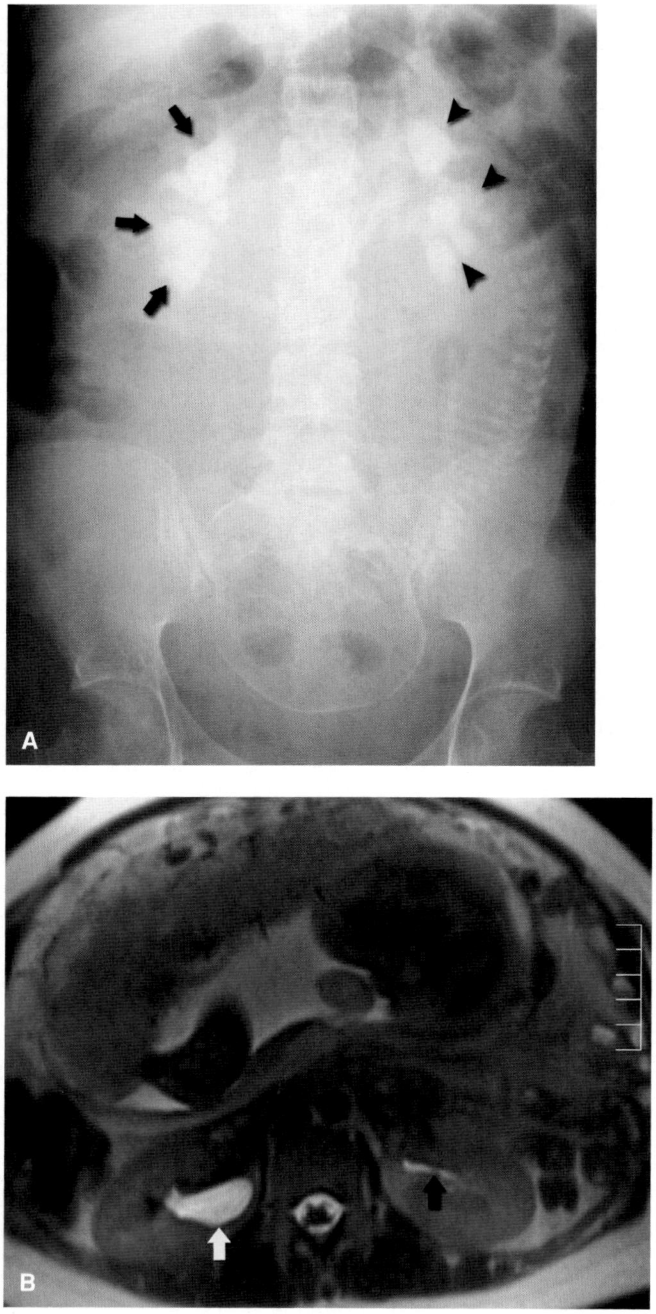

FIGURE 4-16 Hydronephrosis. **A.** Plain film from the 15-minute image of an intravenous pyelogram (IVP). Moderate hydronephrosis on the right (*arrows*) and mild hydronephrosis on the left (*arrowheads*) are both normal for this 35-week gestation. **B.** Axial magnetic resonance (MR) image from a study performed for a fetal indication. Moderate hydronephrosis on the right (*white arrow*) and mild on the left (*black arrow*) are incidental findings.

to be more gentle curves. Despite these anatomical changes, Semins and associates (2009) concluded, based on their review, that complication rates associated with ureteroscopy in pregnant and nonpregnant patients do not differ significantly.

Bladder

There are few significant anatomical changes in the bladder before 12 weeks. From that time onward, however, increased uterine size, the hyperemia that affects all pelvic organs, and the hyperplasia of bladder muscle and connective tissues elevate the trigone and cause thickening of its posterior, or intraureteric, margin. Continuation of this process to the end of pregnancy produces marked deepening and widening of the trigone. There are no mucosal changes other than an increase in the size and tortuosity of its blood vessels.

Using urethrocystometry, Iosif and colleagues (1980) reported that bladder pressure in primigravidas increased from 8 cm H_2O early in pregnancy to 20 cm H_2O at term. To compensate for reduced bladder capacity, absolute and functional urethral lengths increased by 6.7 and 4.8 mm, respectively. At the same time, maximal intraurethral pressure increased from 70 to 93 cm H_2O, and thus continence is maintained. Still, at least half of women experience some degree of urinary incontinence by the third trimester (van Brummen, 2006; Wesnes, 2009). Indeed, this is always considered in the differential diagnosis of ruptured membranes.

Toward the end of pregnancy, particularly in nulliparas in whom the presenting part often engages before labor, the entire base of the bladder is pushed forward and upward, converting the normal convex surface into a concavity. As a result, difficulties in diagnostic and therapeutic procedures are greatly increased. In addition, pressure from the presenting part impairs blood and lymph drainage from the bladder base, often rendering the area edematous, easily traumatized, and possibly more susceptible to infection.

GASTROINTESTINAL TRACT

During pregnancy, the gums may become hyperemic and softened and may bleed when mildly traumatized, as with a toothbrush. This *pregnancy gingivitis* typically subsides postpartum. A focal, highly vascular swelling of the gums, a so-called epulis gravidarum, is a pyogenic granuloma that occasionally develops but typically regresses spontaneously after delivery. Most evidence indicates that pregnancy does not incite tooth decay.

As pregnancy progresses, the stomach and intestines are displaced by the enlarging uterus. Consequently, the physical findings in certain diseases are altered. The appendix, for instance, is usually displaced upward and somewhat laterally as the uterus enlarges. At times, it may reach the right flank.

Pyrosis (heartburn) is common during pregnancy and is most likely caused by reflux of acidic secretions into the lower esophagus (Chap. 54, p. 1072). Although the altered stomach position probably contributes to its frequency, lower esophageal sphincter tone also is decreased. In addition, intraesophageal pressures are lower and intragastric pressures higher in pregnant women. At the same time, esophageal peristalsis has lower wave speed and lower amplitude (Ulmsten, 1978).

Gastric emptying time appears to be unchanged during each trimester and compared with nonpregnant women (Macfie, 1991; Wong, 2002, 2007). During labor, however, and especially after administration of analgesic agents, gastric emptying time may be appreciably prolonged. As a result, one danger of general anesthesia for delivery is regurgitation and aspiration of either food-laden or highly acidic gastric contents (Chap. 25, p. 519).

Hemorrhoids are common during pregnancy (Avsar, 2010). They are caused in large measure by constipation and elevated pressure in veins below the level of the enlarged uterus.

Liver

Unlike in some animals, there is no increase in liver size during human pregnancy (Combes, 1971). Hepatic arterial and portal venous blood flow, however, increase substantively (Clapp, 2000). Histological evaluation of liver biopsies, including examination with the electron microscope, has shown no distinct morphological changes in normal pregnant women (Ingerslev, 1946).

Some laboratory test results of hepatic function are altered during normal pregnancy, and some would be considered abnormal for nonpregnant patients (Appendix, p. 1289). Total alkaline phosphatase activity almost doubles, but much of the increase is attributable to heat-stable placental alkaline phosphatase isozymes. Serum aspartate transaminase (AST), alanine transaminase (ALT), γ-glutamyl transpeptidase (GGT), and bilirubin levels are slightly lower compared with nonpregnant values (Girling, 1997; Ruiz-Extremera, 2005).

The serum albumin concentration decreases during pregnancy. By late pregnancy, albumin concentrations may be near 3.0 g/dL compared with approximately 4.3 g/dL in nonpregnant women (Mendenhall, 1970). Total body albumin levels are increased, however, because of pregnancy-associated increased plasma volume. Serum globulin levels are also slightly higher.

Leucine aminopeptidase is a proteolytic liver enzyme whose serum levels may be increased with liver disease. Its activity is markedly elevated in pregnant women. The increase, however, results from a pregnancy-specific enzyme(s) with distinct substrate specificities (Song, 1968). Pregnancy-induced aminopeptidase has oxytocinase and vasopressinase activity that occasionally causes transient diabetes insipidus (Chap. 58, p. 1162).

Gallbladder

During normal pregnancy, gallbladder contractility is reduced and leads to increased residual volume (Braverman, 1980). Progesterone potentially impairs gallbladder contraction by inhibiting cholecystokinin-mediated smooth muscle stimulation, which is the primary regulator of gallbladder contraction. Impaired emptying, subsequent stasis, and an increased bile cholesterol saturation of pregnancy contribute to the increased prevalence of cholesterol gallstones in multiparas.

The pregnancy effects on maternal serum bile acid concentrations have been incompletely characterized. This is despite the long-acknowledged propensity for pregnancy to cause intrahepatic cholestasis and pruritus gravidarum from retained bile salts. Intrahepatic cholestasis has been linked to high circulating levels of estrogen, which inhibit intraductal bile acid transport (Simon, 1996). In addition, increased progesterone levels and genetic factors have been implicated in the pathogenesis (Lammert, 2000). Cholestasis of pregnancy is described further in Chapter 55 (p. 1084).

ENDOCRINE SYSTEM

Some of the most important endocrine changes of pregnancy are discussed elsewhere, especially in Chapters 57 and 58.

Pituitary Gland

During normal pregnancy, the pituitary gland enlarges by approximately 135 percent (Gonzalez, 1988). Although it has been suggested that this size increase may sufficiently compress the optic chiasma to reduce visual fields, impaired vision from this is rare (Inoue, 2007). Pituitary enlargement is primarily caused by estrogen-stimulated hypertrophy and hyperplasia of the lactotrophs (Feldt-Rasmussen, 2011). And, as discussed subsequently, maternal serum prolactin levels parallel the increasing size. Gonadotrophs decline in number, and corticotrophs and thyrotrophs remain constant. Somatotrophs are generally suppressed due to negative feedback by the placental production of growth hormone. Peak pituitary size may reach 12 mm on magnetic resonance (MR) imaging in the first days postpartum, but the gland involutes rapidly thereafter and reaches normal size by 6 months postpartum (Feldt-Rasmussen, 2011). According to Scheithauer and coworkers (1990), the incidence of pituitary prolactinomas is not increased during pregnancy. When these tumors are large before pregnancy—a macroadenoma measuring ≥ 10 mm—then growth during pregnancy is more likely (Chap. 58, p. 1162).

The maternal pituitary gland is not essential for pregnancy maintenance. Many women have undergone hypophysectomy, completed pregnancy successfully, and entered spontaneous labor while receiving compensatory glucocorticoids, thyroid hormone, and vasopressin.

Growth Hormone

During the first trimester, growth hormone is secreted predominantly from the maternal pituitary gland, and concentrations in serum and amnionic fluid are within nonpregnant values of 0.5 to 7.5 ng/mL (Kletzky, 1985). As early as 8 weeks' gestation, growth hormone secreted from the placenta becomes detectable (Lønberg, 2003). By approximately 17 weeks, the placenta is the principal source of growth hormone secretion (Obuobie, 2001). Maternal serum values increase slowly from approximately 3.5 ng/mL at 10 weeks to plateau after 28 weeks at approximately 14 ng/mL. Growth hormone in amnionic fluid peaks at 14 to 15 weeks and slowly declines thereafter to reach baseline values after 36 weeks.

Placental growth hormone—which differs from pituitary growth hormone by 13 amino acid residues—is secreted by syncytiotrophoblast in a nonpulsatile fashion (Fuglsang, 2006). Its regulation and physiological effects are incompletely understood, but it appears to have some influence on fetal growth as well as preeclampsia development (Mittal, 2007; Pedersen, 2010). Placental growth hormone is a major determinant of maternal insulin resistance after midpregnancy. And, maternal serum levels correlate positively with birthweight but negatively with fetal-growth restriction and uterine artery resistance (Chellakooty, 2004; Schiessl, 2007). That said, fetal growth still progresses in the complete absence of this hormone. Freemark (2006) concluded that, although not absolutely essential, the hormone may act in concert with placental lactogen and other somatolactogens to regulate fetal growth.

Prolactin

Maternal plasma prolactin levels increase markedly during normal pregnancy, and concentrations are usually tenfold greater at term—about 150 ng/mL—compared with those of nonpregnant women. Paradoxically, plasma concentrations decrease after delivery even in women who are breast feeding. During early lactation, there are pulsatile bursts of prolactin secretion in response to suckling.

The physiological basis of the marked prolactin level increase before parturition is still unclear. As mentioned earlier, it is known is that estrogen increases the number of anterior pituitary lactotrophs and may stimulate their release of prolactin (Andersen, 1982). Thyroid-releasing hormone also acts to increased prolactin levels in pregnant compared with nonpregnant women, but this response decreases as pregnancy advances (Miyamoto, 1984). Serotonin also is believed to increase prolactin levels. In contrast, dopamine—previously known as prolactin-inhibiting factor—inhibits its secretion.

The principal function of maternal prolactin is to ensure lactation. Early in pregnancy, prolactin acts to initiate DNA synthesis and mitosis of glandular epithelial cells and presecretory alveolar cells of the breast. Prolactin also increases the number of estrogen and prolactin receptors in these cells. Finally, prolactin promotes mammary alveolar cell RNA synthesis, galactopoiesis, and production of casein, lactalbumin, lactose, and lipids (Andersen, 1982). A woman with isolated prolactin deficiency described by Kauppila and colleagues (1987) failed to lactate after two pregnancies. This established prolactin as a requisite for lactation but not for pregnancy.

Prolactin is present in amnionic fluid in high concentrations. Levels of up to 10,000 ng/mL are found at 20 to 26 weeks' gestation. Thereafter, levels decrease and reach a nadir after 34 weeks. There is convincing evidence that the uterine decidua is the synthesis site of prolactin found in amnionic fluid (Chap. 5, p. 88). Although the exact function of amnionic fluid prolactin is unknown, suggestions are that this prolactin impairs water transfer from the fetus into the maternal compartment, thus preventing fetal dehydration.

A possible pathological role has been proposed for a prolactin fragment in the genesis of peripartum cardiomyopathy (Chap. 49, p. 988) (Cunningham, 2012).

Oxytocin and Antidiuretic Hormone

These two hormones are secreted from the posterior pituitary. The role of oxytocin in parturition and lactation is discussed in Chapters 21 (p. 426) and 36 (p. 672), respectively. Brunton and Russell (2010) have reviewed the complex mechanisms that promote quiescence of oxytocin systems during pregnancy. Levels of antidiuretic hormone, also called *vasopressin*, do not change during pregnancy. As discussed in Chapter 58 (p. 1162), vasopressin deficiency is associated with diabetes insipidus.

Thyroid Gland

Physiological changes of pregnancy cause the thyroid gland to increase production of thyroid hormones by 40 to 100 percent to meet maternal and fetal needs (Smallridge, 2005). To accomplish this, there are several pregnancy-induced changes. Anatomically, the thyroid gland undergoes moderate enlargement during pregnancy caused by glandular hyperplasia and increased vascularity. Glinoer and colleagues (1990) reported that mean thyroid volume increased from 12 mL in the first trimester to 15 mL at delivery. Total volume was inversely proportional to serum thyrotropin concentrations. Such enlargement is not pathological, but normal pregnancy does not typically cause significant thyromegaly. Thus, any goiter should be investigated.

Several alterations in thyroid physiology and function during pregnancy are outlined in Figure 4-17. Early in the first trimester, levels of the principal carrier protein—*thyroxine-binding globulin (TBG)*—increase, reach their zenith at about 20 weeks, and stabilize at approximately double baseline values for the remainder of pregnancy. The increased TBG concentrations result from both higher hepatic synthesis rates—due to estrogen stimulation—and lower metabolism rates due to increased TBG sialylation and glycosylation. These elevated TBG levels increase total serum thyroxine (T_4) and triiodothyronine (T_3) concentrations, but do not affect the physiologically important serum free T_4 and T_3 levels. Specifically, total serum T_4 increases sharply beginning between 6 and 9 weeks and reaches a plateau at 18 weeks. *Free serum T_4* levels rise slightly and peak along with hCG levels, and then they return to normal. The rise in total T_4 is more pronounced up to 18 weeks, and thereafter, it plateaus. As detailed in Chapter 58 (p. 1147), the fetus is reliant on maternal thyroxine, which crosses the placenta in small quantities to maintain normal fetal thyroid function. Recall that the fetal thyroid does not begin to concentrate iodine until 10 to 12 weeks' gestation. The synthesis and secretion of thyroid hormone by fetal pituitary thyroid-stimulating hormone ensues at approximately 20 weeks. At birth, approximately 30 percent of the T_4 in umbilical cord blood is of maternal origin (Leung, 2012).

Thyrotropin-releasing hormone (TRH) is secreted by the hypothalamus and stimulates thyrotrope cells of the anterior pituitary to release *thyroid-stimulating hormone* (*TSH*) or *thyrotropin*. TRH levels are not increased during normal pregnancy. However, this neurotransmitter does cross the placenta and may serve to stimulate the fetal pituitary to secrete thyrotropin (Thorpe-Beeston, 1991).

Interestingly, T_4 and T_3 secretion is not similar for all pregnant women (Glinoer, 1990). Approximately a third of women experience relative hypothyroxinemia, preferential T_3 secretion, and higher, albeit normal, serum thyrotropin levels. Thus, there may be considerable variability in thyroidal adjustments during normal pregnancy.

The modifications in serum TSH and hCG levels as a function of gestational age are shown in Figure 4-17. As discussed in Chapter 5 (p. 101), the α-subunits of the two glycoproteins are identical, whereas the β-subunits, although similar, differ in their amino acid sequence. As a result of this structural similarity, hCG has intrinsic thyrotropic activity, and thus, high serum hCG levels cause thyroid stimulation. Indeed, thyrotropin levels decrease in more than 80 percent of pregnant women, whereas they remain in the normal range for nonpregnant women.

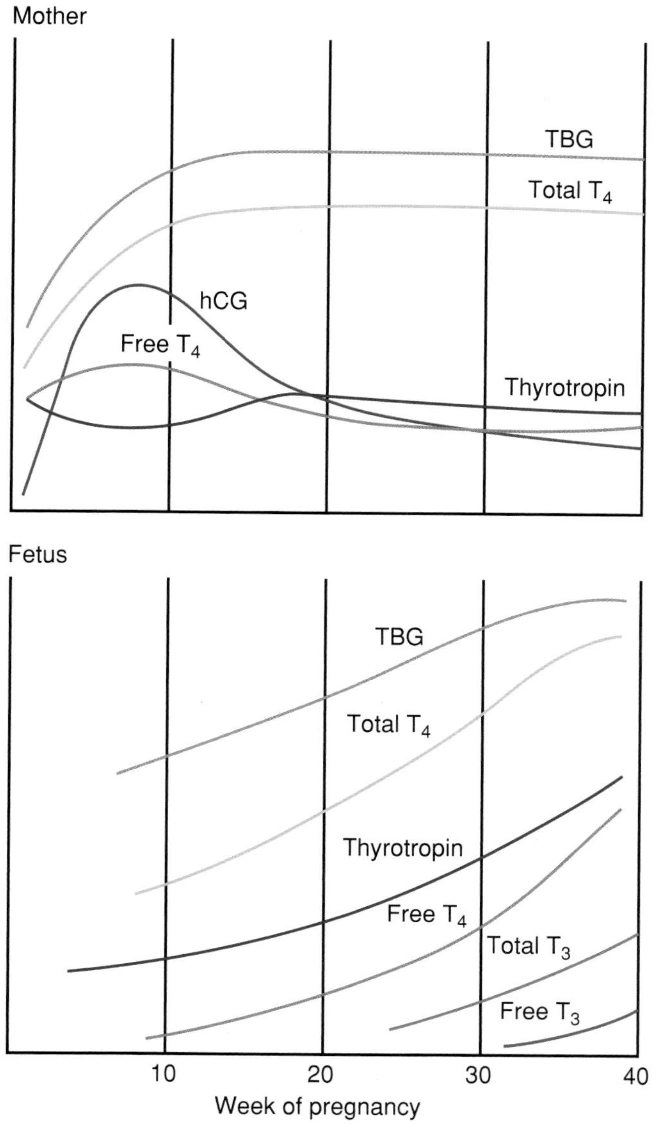

FIGURE 4-17 Relative changes in maternal and fetal thyroid-associated analytes across pregnancy. Maternal changes include a marked and early increase in hepatic production of thyroxine-binding globulin (TBG) and placental production of human chorionic gonadotropin (hCG). Increased thyroxine-binding globulin increases serum thyroxine (T_4) concentrations. hCG has thyrotropin-like activity and stimulates maternal free T_4 secretion. This transient hCG-induced increase in serum T_4 levels inhibits maternal secretion of thyrotropin. Except for minimally increased free T_4 levels when hCG peaks, these levels are essentially unchanged. Fetal levels of all serum thyroid analytes increase incrementally across pregnancy. Fetal triiodothyronine (T_3) does not increase until late pregnancy. (Modified from Burrow, 1994.)

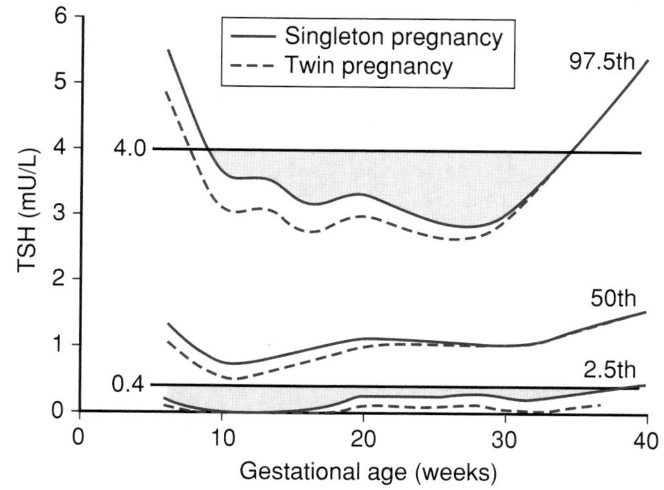

FIGURE 4-18 Gestational age-specific thyroid-stimulating hormone (TSH) normal curves derived from 13,599 singleton and 132 twin pregnancies. Singleton pregnancies are represented with solid blue lines and twin pregnancies with dashed lines. The nonpregnant reference values of 4.0 and 0.4 mU/L are represented as solid black lines. Upper shaded area represents the 28 percent of singleton pregnancies with TSH values above the 97.5th percentile threshold that would not have been identified as abnormal based on the assay reference value of 4.0 mU/L. Lower shaded area represents singleton pregnancies that would have been (falsely) identified as having TSH suppression based on the assay reference value of 0.4 mU/L. (From Dashe, 2005, with permission.)

As shown in Figure 4-18, normal suppression of TSH during pregnancy may lead to a misdiagnosis of subclinical hyperthyroidism. Of greater concern is the potential failure to identify women with early hypothyroidism because of suppressed TSH concentrations. To mitigate the likelihood of such misdiagnoses, Dashe and coworkers (2005) conducted a population-based study at Parkland Hospital to develop gestational-age-specific TSH normal curves for both singleton and twin pregnancies (Chap. 58, p. 1148). Similarly, Ashoor and associates (2010) have established normal ranges for maternal TSH, free T_4, and free T_3 at 11 to 13 weeks.

These complex alterations of thyroid regulation do not appear to alter maternal thyroid status as measured by metabolic studies. Although basal metabolic rate increases progressively by as much as 25 percent during normal pregnancy, most of this increase in oxygen consumption can be attributed to fetal metabolic activity. If fetal body surface area is considered along with that of the mother, the predicted and observed basal metabolic rates are similar to those in nonpregnant women.

Iodine Status

Iodine requirements increase during normal pregnancy. In women with low or marginal intake, deficiency may manifest as low thyroxine and increased TSH levels. Importantly, more than a third of the world population lives in areas where iodine intake is only marginal. For the fetus, early exposure to thyroid hormone is essential for the nervous system, and iodine deficiency is the most common preventable cause of impaired neurological development after famine (Kennedy, 2010). Severe deficiency leads to cretinism.

Parathyroid Glands

The regulation of calcium concentration is closely interrelated with magnesium, phosphate, parathyroid hormone, vitamin D, and calcitonin physiology. Any altered levels of one of these likely changes the others. In a longitudinal investigation of 20 women, More and associates (2003) found that all markers of bone turnover increased during normal pregnancy and failed to reach baseline level by 12 months postpartum. They concluded that the calcium needed for fetal growth and lactation may be drawn at least in part from the maternal skeleton.

Parathyroid Hormone

Acute or chronic decreases in plasma calcium or acute decreases in magnesium stimulate parathyroid hormone (PTH) release. Conversely, increased calcium and magnesium levels suppress PTH levels. The action of this hormone on bone resorption, intestinal absorption, and kidney reabsorption is to increase extracellular fluid calcium concentrations and decrease phosphate levels.

As reviewed by Cooper (2011), fetal skeleton mineralization requires approximately 30 g of calcium, primarily during the third trimester. Although this amounts to only 3 percent of the total calcium held within the maternal skeleton, the provision of calcium is still a challenge for the mother. In most circumstances, increased maternal calcium absorption provides the additional calcium. During pregnancy, the amount of calcium absorbed rises gradually and reaches approximately 400 mg/day in the third trimester. Increased calcium absorption appears to be mediated by elevated maternal 1,25-dihydroxyvitamin D concentrations. This occurs despite decreased levels during early pregnancy of PTH, which is the normal stimulus for active vitamin D production within the kidney. Indeed, PTH plasma concentrations decrease during the first trimester and then increase progressively throughout the remainder of pregnancy (Pitkin, 1979).

The increased production of active vitamin D is likely due to placental production of either PTH or a PTH-related protein (PTH-rP). Outside pregnancy and lactation, PTH-rP is usually only detectable in serum of women with hypercalcemia due to malignancy. During pregnancy, however, PTH-rP concentrations increase significantly. This protein is synthesized in both fetal tissues and maternal breasts.

Calcitonin

The known actions of calcitonin generally are considered to oppose those of PTH and vitamin D to protect maternal skeletal calcification during times of calcium stress. Pregnancy and lactation cause profound calcium stress, and during these times, calcitonin levels are appreciably higher than those in nonpregnant women (Weiss, 1998).

The C cells that secrete calcitonin are derived embryologically from the neural crest and are located predominantly in the perifollicular areas of the thyroid gland. Calcium and magnesium increase the biosynthesis and secretion of calcitonin. Various gastric hormones—gastrin, pentagastrin, glucagon, and pancreozymin—and food ingestion also increase calcitonin plasma levels.

Adrenal Glands

Cortisol

In normal pregnancy, unlike their fetal counterparts, the maternal adrenal glands undergo little, if any, morphological change. The serum concentration of circulating cortisol is increased, but much of it is bound by *transcortin*, the cortisol-binding globulin. The adrenal secretion rate of this principal glucocorticoid is not increased, and probably it is decreased compared with that of the nonpregnant state. The metabolic clearance rate of cortisol, however, is lower during pregnancy because its half-life is nearly doubled compared with that for nonpregnant women (Migeon, 1957). Administration of estrogen, including most oral contraceptives, causes changes in serum cortisol levels and transcortin similar to those of pregnancy (Jung, 2011).

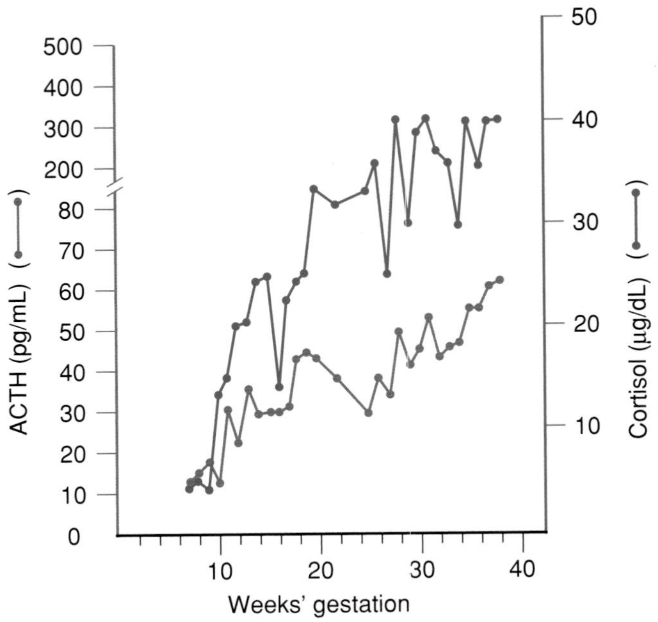

FIGURE 4-19 Serial increases in serum cortisol (*blue line*) and adrenocorticotropic hormone (ACTH) (*red line*) across normal pregnancy. (Redrawn from Carr, 1981, with permission.)

During early pregnancy, the levels of circulating *adrenocorticotropic hormone (ACTH)*, also known as *corticotropin*, are reduced strikingly. As pregnancy progresses, ACTH and free cortisol levels rise equally and strikingly (Fig. 4-19). This apparent paradox is not understood completely. Nolten and Rueckert (1981) suggest that the higher free cortisol levels observed in pregnancy result from a "resetting" of the maternal feedback mechanism to higher levels. They further propose that this might result from *tissue refractoriness* to cortisol. Keller-Wood and Wood (2001) later asserted that these incongruities may result from an antagonistic action of progesterone on mineralocorticoids. Thus, in response to elevated progesterone levels during pregnancy, an elevated free cortisol is needed to maintain homeostasis. Indeed, experiments in pregnant ewes demonstrate that elevated maternal cortisol and aldosterone secretion are necessary to maintain the normal increase in plasma volume during late pregnancy (Jensen, 2002).

Aldosterone

As early as 15 weeks' gestation, the maternal adrenal glands secrete considerably increased amounts of aldosterone, the principal mineralocorticoid. By the third trimester, approximately 1 mg/day is secreted. If sodium intake is restricted, aldosterone secretion is elevated even further (Watanabe, 1963). At the same time, levels of renin and angiotensin II substrate normally are increased, especially during the latter half of pregnancy. This scenario gives rise to increased plasma levels of angiotensin II, which acts on the zona glomerulosa of the maternal adrenal glands and accounts for the markedly elevated aldosterone secretion. It has been suggested that the increased aldosterone secretion during normal pregnancy affords protection against the natriuretic effect of progesterone and atrial natriuretic peptide. More recently, Gennari-Moser and colleagues (2011) provided evidence that aldosterone may play a role in modulating trophoblast growth and placental size.

Deoxycorticosterone

Maternal plasma levels of this potent mineralocorticosteroid progressively increase during pregnancy. Indeed, plasma levels of deoxycorticosterone rise to near 1500 pg/mL by term, a more than 15-fold increase (Parker, 1980). This marked elevation is not derived from adrenal secretion but instead represents increased kidney production resulting from estrogen stimulation. The levels of deoxycorticosterone and its sulfate in fetal blood are appreciably higher than those in maternal blood, which suggests transfer of fetal deoxycorticosterone into the maternal compartment.

Androgens

In balance, there is increased androgenic activity during pregnancy. Maternal plasma levels of both *androstenedione* and *testosterone* are increased during pregnancy. This finding is not totally explained by alterations in their metabolic clearance. Both androgens are converted to estradiol in the placenta, which increases their clearance rates. Conversely, increased plasma sex hormone-binding globulin in pregnant women retards testosterone clearance. Thus, the production rates of maternal testosterone and androstenedione during human pregnancy are increased. The source of this increased C_{19}-steroid production is unknown, but it likely originates in the ovary. Interestingly, little or no testosterone in maternal plasma enters the fetal circulation as testosterone. Even when massive testosterone levels are found in the circulation of pregnant women, as with androgen-secreting tumors, testosterone concentrations in umbilical cord blood are likely to be undetectable. This results from the near complete trophoblastic conversion of testosterone to 17β-estradiol (Edman, 1979).

Maternal serum and urine levels of *dehydroepiandrosterone sulfate* are decreased during normal pregnancy. As discussed in Chapter 5 (p. 107), this is a consequence of increased metabolic clearance through extensive maternal hepatic 16β-hydroxylation and placental conversion to estrogen.

MUSCULOSKELETAL SYSTEM

Progressive lordosis is a characteristic feature of normal pregnancy. Compensating for the anterior position of the enlarging uterus, lordosis shifts the center of gravity back over the lower extremities.

The sacroiliac, sacrococcygeal, and pubic joints have increased mobility during pregnancy. However, as discussed earlier (p. 49), increased joint laxity during pregnancy does not correlate with increased maternal serum levels of estradiol, progesterone, or relaxin (Marnach, 2003). Most relaxation takes place in the first half of pregnancy. It may contribute to maternal posture alterations and in turn create lower back discomfort. Although some symphyseal separation likely accompanies many deliveries, those greater than 1 cm may cause significant pain (Fig. 4-20) (Jain, 2005). Aching, numbness, and weakness also occasionally are experienced in the upper extremities. This may result from the marked lordosis and associated anterior neck flexion and shoulder girdle slumping, which produce traction on the ulnar and median nerves (Crisp, 1964).

Joint strengthening begins immediately following delivery and is usually complete within 3 to 5 months. Pelvic dimensions measured up to 3 months after delivery by MR imaging are not significantly different from prepregnancy measurements (Huerta-Enochian, 2006).

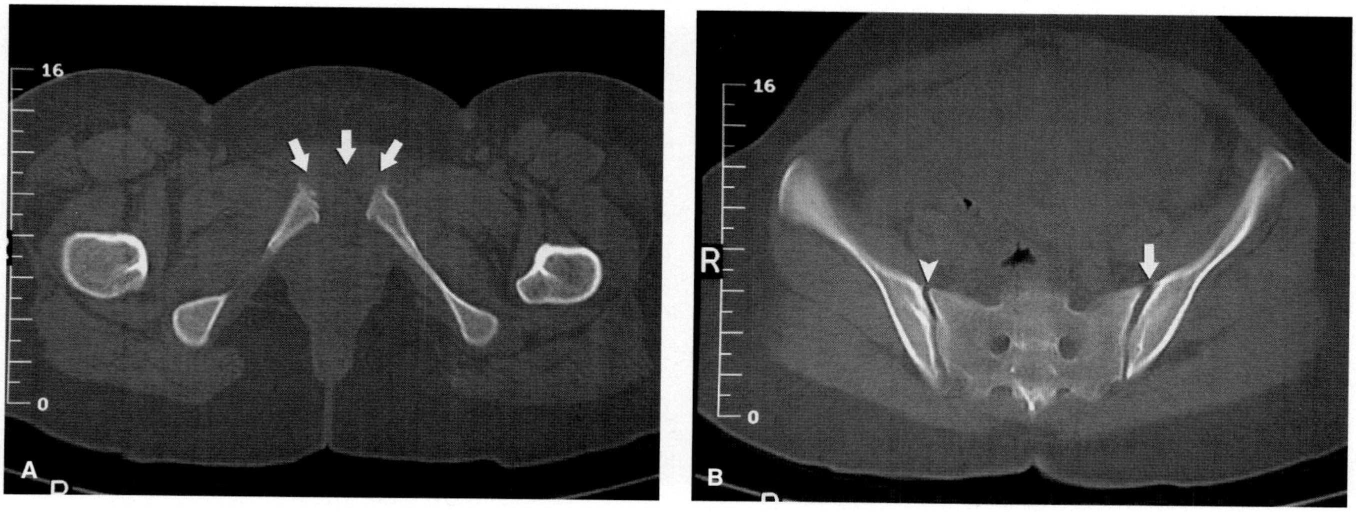

FIGURE 4-20 A. Symphyseal diastasis. Marked widening of the pubic symphysis (*arrows*) after vaginal delivery. **B.** Sacroiliac (SI) joint widening; left (*arrow*) greater than right (*arrowhead*). (Images contributed by Dr. Daniel Moore.)

CENTRAL NERVOUS SYSTEM

Memory

Changes in the central nervous center are relatively few and mostly subtle. Women often report problems with attention, concentration, and memory throughout pregnancy and the early puerperium. Systematic studies of memory in pregnancy, however, are limited and often anecdotal. Keenan and associates (1998) longitudinally investigated memory in pregnant women and a matched control group. They found pregnancy-related memory decline, which was limited to the third trimester. This decline was not attributable to depression, anxiety, sleep deprivation, or other physical changes associated with pregnancy. It was transient and quickly resolved following delivery. Henry and Sherwin (2012) also reported that pregnant women in late pregnancy performed significantly worse on tests of verbal recall and processing speed compared with matched nonpregnant controls. Interestingly, Rana and colleagues (2006) found that attention and memory were improved in women with preeclampsia receiving magnesium sulfate compared with normal pregnant women.

Zeeman and coworkers (2003) used magnetic resonance imaging to measure cerebral blood flow across pregnancy in 10 healthy women. They found that mean blood flow in the middle and posterior cerebral arteries decreased progressively from 147 and 56 mL/min when nonpregnant to 118 and 44 mL/min late in pregnancy, respectively. The mechanism and clinical significance of this decline is unknown. Pregnancy does not appear to affect cerebrovascular autoregulation (Bergersen, 2006; Cipolla, 2014).

Eyes

Intraocular pressure decreases during pregnancy and is attributed in part to increased vitreous outflow (Sunness, 1988). Corneal sensitivity is decreased, and the greatest changes are late in gestation. Most pregnant women demonstrate a measurable but slight increase in corneal thickness, thought to be due to edema. Consequently, they may have difficulty with previously comfortable contact lenses. Brownish-red opacities on the posterior surface of the cornea—*Krukenberg spindles*—have also been observed with a higher than expected frequency during pregnancy. Hormonal effects similar to those observed for skin lesions are postulated to cause this increased pigmentation. Other than transient loss of accommodation reported with both pregnancy and lactation, visual function is unaffected by pregnancy. These changes during pregnancy, as well as pathological eye aberrations, were recently reviewed by Grant and Chung (2013).

Sleep

Beginning as early as approximately 12 weeks' gestation and extending through the first 2 months postpartum, women have difficulty with going to sleep, frequent awakenings, fewer hours of night sleep, and reduced sleep efficiency (Pavlova, 2011). The frequency and duration of sleep apnea episodes were reported to be decreased significantly in pregnant women compared with those postpartum (Trakada, 2003). In the supine position, however, average Pa_{O_2} levels were lower. The greatest disruption of sleep is encountered postpartum and may contribute to *postpartum blues* or to frank depression (Chap. 61, p. 1205).

REFERENCES

Ajne G, Ahlborg G, Wolff K, Nisell H: Contribution of endogenous endothelin-1 to basal vascular tone during normal pregnancy and preeclampsia. Am J Obstet Gynecol 193:234, 2005

Alvarez H, Caldeyro-Barcia R: Contractility of the human uterus recorded by new methods. Surg Gynecol Obstet 91:1, 1950

Amoah C, Yassin A, Cockayne E, et al: Hyperreactio luteinalis in pregnancy. Fertil Steril 95(7):2429.e1, 2011

Andersen JR: Prolactin in amniotic fluid and maternal serum during uncomplicated human pregnancy. Dan Med Bull 29:266, 1982

Anderson BL, Mendez-Figueroa H, Dahlke J, et al: Pregnancy-induced changes in immune protection of the genital tract: defining normal. Am J Obstet Gynecol 208(4):321.e1, 2013

Andersson S, Minjarez D, Yost NP, et al: Estrogen and progesterone metabolism in the cervix during pregnancy and parturition. J Clin Endocrinol Metab 93(6):2366, 2008

Antevski B, Jovkovski O, Filipovski V, et al: Extreme gigantomastia in pregnancy: case report—my experience with two cases in last 5 years. Arch Gynecol Obstet 284(3):575, 2011

Ashoor G, Kametas NA, Akolekar R, et al: Maternal thyroid function at 11–13 weeks of gestation. Fetal Diagn Ther 27(3):156, 2010

Assali NS, Dilts PV, Pentl AA, et al: Physiology of the placenta. In Assali NS (ed): Biology of Gestation, Vol I. The Maternal Organism. New York, Academic Press, 1968

Assali, NS, Douglas RA, Baird WW: Measurement of uterine blood flow and uterine metabolism. IV. Results in normal pregnancy. Am J Obstet Gynecol 66(2):248, 1953

August P, Mueller FB, Sealey JE, et al: Role of renin–angiotensin system in blood pressure regulation in pregnancy. Lancet 345:896, 1995

Avsar AF, Keskin HL: Haemorrhoids during pregnancy. J Obstet Gynaecol 30(3):231, 2010

Bailey RR, Rolleston GL: Kidney length and ureteric dilatation in the puerperium. J Obstet Gynaecol Br Commonw 78:55, 1971

Baksu B, Davas I, Baksu A, et al: Plasma nitric oxide, endothelin-1 and urinary nitric oxide and cyclic guanosine monophosphate levels in hypertensive pregnant women. Int J Gynaecol Obstet 90:112, 2005

Bamber JH, Dresner M: Aortocaval compression in pregnancy: the effect of changing the degree and direction of lateral tilt on maternal cardiac output. Anesth Analg 97:256, 2003

Bardicef M, Bardicef O, Sorokin Y, et al: Extracellular and intracellular magnesium depletion in pregnancy and gestational diabetes. Am J Obstet Gynecol 172:1009, 1995

Batukan C, Tuncay-Ozgun M, Turkyilmaz C, et al: Isolated torsion of the fallopian tube during pregnancy: a case report. J Reprod Med 52:745, 2007

Baykus Y, Gurates B, Aydin S, et al: Changes in serum obestatin, preptin and ghrelins in patients with gestational diabetes mellitus. Clin Biochem 45(3):198, 2012

Bentley-Lewis R, Graves SW, Seely EW: The renin-aldosterone response to stimulation and suppression during normal pregnancy. Hypertens Pregnancy 24(1):1, 2005

Berger MH, Betschart C, Khandwala N, et al: Incidental Bartholin gland cysts identified on pelvic magnetic resonance imaging. Obstet Gynecol 120(4):798, 2012

Bergersen TK, Hartgill TW, Pirhonen J: Cerebrovascular response to normal pregnancy: a longitudinal study. Am J Physiol Heart Circ Physiol 290:1856, 2006

Bernstein IM, Ziegler W, Badger GJ: Plasma volume expansion in early pregnancy. Obstet Gynecol 97:669, 2001

Bieniarz J, Branda LA, Maqueda E, et al: Aortocaval compression by the uterus in late pregnancy, 3. Unreliability of the sphygmomanometric method in estimating uterine artery pressure. Am J Obstet Gynecol 102:1106, 1968

Bloom SL, Uppot R, Roberts DJ: Case 32–2010: a pregnant woman with abdominal pain and fluid in the peritoneal cavity. N Engl J Med 363(17):1657, 2010

Bobrowski RA: Pulmonary physiology in pregnancy. Clin Obstet Gynecol 53(2):286, 2010

Boehlen F, Hohlfeld P, Extermann P, et al: Platelet count at term pregnancy: a reappraisal of the threshold. Obstet Gynecol 95:29, 2000

Brar HS, Platt LD, DeVore GR, et al: Qualitative assessment of maternal uterine and fetal umbilical artery blood flow and resistance in laboring patients by Doppler velocimetry. Am J Obstet Gynecol 158:952, 1988

Braverman DZ, Johnson ML, Kern F Jr: Effects of pregnancy and contraceptive steroids on gallbladder function. N Engl J Med 302:362, 1980
Brown MA, Gallery EDM, Ross MR, et al: Sodium excretion in normal and hypertensive pregnancy: a prospective study. Am J Obstet Gynecol 159:297, 1988
Brown MA, Sinosich MJ, Saunders DM, et al: Potassium regulation and progesterone–aldosterone interrelationships in human pregnancy: a prospective study. Am J Obstet Gynecol 155:349, 1986
Browne JCM, Veall N: The maternal placental blood flow in normotensive and hypertensive women. J Obstet Gynaecol Br Emp 60(2):141, 1953
Brunton PJ, Russell JA: Endocrine induced changes in brain function during pregnancy. Brain Res 1364:198, 2010
Burns R, Azizi F, Hedayati M, et al: Is placental iodine content related to dietary iodine intake? Clin Endocrinol 75(2):261, 2011
Burrow GN, Fisher DA, Larsen PR: Maternal and fetal thyroid function. N Engl J Med 331:1072, 1994
Butte NF: Carbohydrate and lipid metabolism in pregnancy: normal compared with gestational diabetes mellitus. Am J Clin Nutr 7:1256S, 2000
Carr BR, Parker CR Jr, Madden JD, et al: Maternal plasma adrenocorticotropin and cortisol relationships throughout human pregnancy. Am J Obstet Gynecol 139:416, 1981
Cetin I, de Santis MS, Taricco E, et al: Maternal and fetal amino acid concentrations in normal pregnancies and in pregnancies with gestational diabetes mellitus. Am J Obstet Gynecol 192:610, 2005
Chellakooty M, Vangsgaard K, Larsen T, et al: A longitudinal study of intrauterine growth and the placental growth hormone (GH)–insulin-like growth factor I axis in maternal circulation. J Clin Endocrinol Metab 89:384, 2004
Chesley LC: Renal function during pregnancy. In Carey HM (ed): Modern Trends in Human Reproductive Physiology. London, Butterworth, 1963
Cipolla MJ, Zeeman GG, Cunningham FG: Cerebrovascular (patho)physiology in preeclampsia/eclampsia. In Taylor RN, Roberts JM, Cunningham FG (eds): Chesley's Hypertensive Disorders in Pregnancy, 4th ed. Amsterdam, Academic Press, 2014
Clapp JF III, Little KD, Widness JA: Effect of maternal exercise and fetoplacental growth rate on serum erythropoietin concentrations. Am J Obstet Gynecol 188:1021, 2003
Clapp JF III, Stepanchak W, Tomaselli J, et al: Portal vein blood flow—effects of pregnancy, gravity, and exercise. Am J Obstet Gynecol 183:167, 2000
Clark SL, Cotton DB, Lee W, et al: Central hemodynamic assessment of normal term pregnancy. Am J Obstet Gynecol 161:1439, 1989
Clerico A, Emdin M: Diagnostic accuracy and prognostic relevance of the measurement of cardiac natriuretic peptides: a review. Clin Chem 50:33, 2004
Coccia ME, Pasquini L, Comparetto C, et al: Hyperreactio luteinalis in a woman with high-risk factors: a case report. J Reprod Med 48:127, 2003
Combes B, Adams RH: Disorders of the liver in pregnancy. In Assali NS (ed): Pathophysiology of Gestation, Vol I. New York, Academic Press, 1971
Connolly TP, Evans AC: Atypical Papanicolaou smear in pregnancy. Clin Med Res 3:13, 2005
Conrad KP: Emerging role of relaxin in the maternal adaptations to normal pregnancy: implications for preeclampsia. Semin Nephrol 31(1):15, 2011a
Conrad KP, Baker VL: Corpus luteal contribution to maternal pregnancy physiology and outcomes in assisted reproductive technologies. Am J Physiol Regul Integr Comp Physiol 304(2):R69, 2013
Conrad KP, Gaber LW, Lindheimer MD: The kidney in normal pregnancy and preeclampsia. In Taylor RN, Roberts JM, Cunningham FG (eds): Chesley's Hypertensive Disorders in Pregnancy, 4th ed. Amsterdam, Academic Press, 2014
Conrad KP, Jeyabalan A, Danielson LA, et al: Role of relaxin in maternal renal vasodilation of pregnancy. Ann N Y Acad Sci 1041:147, 2005
Conrad KP, Shroff SG: Effects of relaxin on arterial dilation, remodeling, and mechanical properties. Curr Hypertens Rep 13(6):409, 2011b
Cooper MS: Disorders of calcium metabolism and parathyroid disease. Best Pract Res Clin Endocrinol Metab 25(6):975, 2011
Cornelis T, Odutayo A, Keunen J, et al: The kidney in normal pregnancy and preeclampsia. Semin Nephrol 31(1):4, 2011
Crisp WE, DeFrancesco S: The hand syndrome of pregnancy. Obstet Gynecol 23:433, 1964
Csapo AI, Pulkkinen MO, Wiest WG: Effects of luteectomy and progesterone replacement therapy in early pregnant patients. Am J Obstet Gynecol 115(6):759, 1973
Cunningham FG: Peripartum cardiomyopathy: we've com a long way, but . . . Obstet Gynecol 120(5):992, 2012
Cunningham FG, Cox K, Gant NF: Further observations on the nature of pressor responsivity to angiotensin II in human pregnancy. Obstet Gynecol 46:581, 1975
Cutforth R, MacDonald CB: Heart sounds and murmurs in pregnancy. Am Heart J 71:741, 1966
Darmady JM, Postle AD: Lipid metabolism in pregnancy. Br J Obstet Gynaecol 89:211, 1982
Dashe JS, Casey BM, Wells CE, et al: Thyroid-stimulating hormone in singleton and twin pregnancy: importance of gestational age-specific reference ranges. Obstet Gynecol 106:753, 2005
Davison JM, Dunlop W: Renal hemodynamics and tubular function in normal human pregnancy. Kidney Int 18:152, 1980
Davison JM, Hytten FE: Glomerular filtration during and after pregnancy. J Obstet Gynaecol Br Commonw 81:588, 1974
Davison JM, Vallotton MB, Lindheimer MD: Plasma osmolality and urinary concentration and dilution during and after pregnancy: evidence that lateral recumbency inhibits maximal urinary concentrating ability. Br J Obstet Gynaecol 88:472, 1981
Delorme MA, Burrows RF, Ofosu FA, et al: Thrombin regulation in mother and fetus during pregnancy. Semin Thromb Hemost 18:81, 1992
Duvekot JJ, Cheriex EC, Pieters FA, et al: Early pregnancy changes in hemodynamics and volume homeostasis are consecutive adjustments triggered by a primary fall in systemic vascular tone. Am J Obstet Gynecol 169:1382, 1993
Easterling TR, Schmucker BC, Benedetti TJ: The hemodynamic effects of orthostatic stress during pregnancy. Obstet Gynecol 72:550, 1988
Edman CD, Devereux WP, Parker CR, et al: Placental clearance of maternal androgens: a protective mechanism against fetal virilization. Abstract 112 presented at the 26th annual meeting of the Society for Gynecologic Investigation, San Diego, 1979. Gynecol Invest 67:68, 1979
Edman CD, Toofanian A, MacDonald PC, et al: Placental clearance rate of maternal plasma androstenedione through placental estradiol formation: an indirect method of assessing uteroplacental blood flow. Am J Obstet Gynecol 141:1029, 1981
Enein M, Zina AA, Kassem M, et al: Echocardiography of the pericardium in pregnancy. Obstet Gynecol 69:851, 1987
Farage MA, Maibach HI: Morphology and physiological changes of genital skin and mucosa. Curr Probl Dermatol 40:9, 2011
Feldt-Rasmussen U, Mathiesen ER: Endocrine disorders in pregnancy: physiological and hormonal aspects of pregnancy. Best Pract Res Clin Endocrinol Metab 25(6):875, 2011
Feletou M, Vanhoutte PM: Endothelial dysfunction: a multifaceted disorder (The Wiggers Award Lecture). Am J Physiol Heart Circ Physiol 291:H985, 2006
Freemark M: Regulation of maternal metabolism by pituitary and placental hormones: roles in fetal development and metabolic programming. Horm Res 65:41, 2006
Freinkel N: Banting Lecture 1980: Of pregnancy and progeny. Diabetes 29:1023, 1980
Freinkel N, Dooley SL, Metzger BE: Care of the pregnant woman with insulin-dependent diabetes mellitus. N Engl J Med 313:96, 1985
Friedman SA: Preeclampsia: a review of the role of prostaglandins. Obstet Gynecol 71:122, 1988
Fuglsang J: Ghrelin in pregnancy and lactation. Vitam Horm 77:259, 2008
Fuglsang J, Sandager P, Moller N, et al: Kinetics and secretion of placental growth hormone around parturition. Eur J Endocrinol 154:449, 2006
Galan HL, Marconi AM, Paolini CL, et al: The transplacental transport of essential amino acids in uncomplicated human pregnancies. Am J Obstet Gynecol 200(1):91.e1–7, 2009
Gallery ED, Raftos J, Gyory AZ, et al: A prospective study of serum complement (C3 and C4) levels in normal human pregnancy: effect of the development of pregnancy-associated hypertension. Aust N Z J Med 11:243, 1981
Gambling L, Lang C, McArdle HJ: Fetal regulation of iron transport during pregnancy. Am J Clin Nutr 94(6 Suppl):1903S, 2011
Gant NF, Chand S, Whalley PJ, et al: The nature of pressor responsiveness to angiotensin II in human pregnancy. Obstet Gynecol 43:854, 1974
Gant NF, Daley GL, Chand S, et al: A study of angiotensin II pressor response throughout primigravid pregnancy. J Clin Invest 52:2682, 1973
Garfield RE, Maner WL, MacKay LB, et al: Comparing uterine electromyography activity of antepartum patients versus term labor patients. Am J Obstet Gynecol 193:23, 2005
Gayer G, Ben Ely A, Maymon R, et al: Enlargement of the spleen as an incidental finding on CT in post-partum females with fever. Br J Radiol 85 (1014):753, 2012
Gennari-Moser C, Khankin EV, Schüller S, et al: Regulation of placental growth by aldosterone and cortisol. Endocrinology 152(1):263, 2011
George EM, Granger JP: Endothelin: key mediator of hypertension in preeclampsia. Am J Hypertens 24(9):964, 2011
Gherman RB, Mestman JH, Satis AJ, et al: Intractable hyperemesis gravidarum, transient hyperthyroidism and intrauterine growth restriction associated with hyperreactio luteinalis. A case report. J Reprod Med 48:553, 2003

Ghio A, Bertolotto A, Resi V, et al: Triglyceride metabolism in pregnancy. Adv Clin Chem 55:133, 2011

Girling JC, Dow E, Smith JH: Liver function tests in preeclampsia: importance of comparison with a reference range derived for normal pregnancy. Br J Obstet Gynaecol 104:246, 1997

Glinoer D, de Nayer P, Bourdoux P, et al: Regulation of maternal thyroid during pregnancy. J Clin Endocrinol Metab 71:276, 1990

Gonzalez JG, Elizondo G, Saldivar D, et al: Pituitary gland growth during normal pregnancy: an in vivo study using magnetic resonance imaging. Am J Med 85:217, 1988

Grant AD, Chung SM: The eye in pregnancy: ophthalmologic and neuro-ophthalmologic changes. Clin Obstet Gynecol 56(2):397, 2013

Grindheim G, Toska K, Estensen M-E, et al: Changes in pulmonary function during pregnancy: a longitudinal cohort study. BJOG 119(1):94, 2012

Grummer MA, Sullivan JA, Magness RR, et al: Vascular endothelial growth factor acts through novel, pregnancy-enhanced receptor signaling pathways to stimulate endothelial nitric oxide synthase activity in uterine artery endothelial cells. Biochem J 417(2):501, 2009

Guyton AC (ed): Textbook of Medical Physiology. Philadelphia, W. B. Saunders Company, 1981, p 218

Harbert GM Jr, Cornell GW, Littlefield JB, et al: Maternal hemodynamics associated with uterine contraction in gravid monkeys. Am J Obstet Gynecol 104:24, 1969

Harstad TW, Mason RA, Cox SM: Serum erythropoietin quantitation in pregnancy using an enzyme-linked immunoassay. Am J Perinatol 9:233, 1992

Hauguel-de Mouzon S, Lepercq J, Catalano P: The known and unknown of leptin in pregnancy. Am J Obstet Gynecol 194:1537, 2006

Hayashi M, Inoue T, Hoshimoto K, et al: The levels of five markers of hemostasis and endothelial status at different stages of normotensive pregnancy. Acta Obstet Gynecol Scand 81:208, 2002

Heenan AP, Wolfe LA, Davies GAL, et al: Effects of human pregnancy on fluid regulation responses to short-term exercise. J Appl Physiol 95:2321, 2003

Hegewald MJ, Crapo RO: Respiratory physiology in pregnancy. Clin Chest Med 32(1):1, 2011

Hein M, Petersen Ac, Helmig RB, et al: Immunoglobulin levels and phagocytes in the cervical mucus plug at term of pregnancy. Acta Obstet Gynecol Scand 84:734, 2005

Helal I, Fick-Brosnahan GM, Reed-Gitomer B, et al: Glomerular hyperfiltration: definitions, mechanisms and clinical implications. Nat Rev Nephrol 8(5):293, 2012

Henry JF, Sherwin BB: Hormones and cognitive functioning during late pregnancy and postpartum: a longitudinal study. Behav Neurosci 126(1):73, 2012

Henson MC, Castracane VD: Leptin in pregnancy: an update. Biol Reprod 74:218, 2006

Hibbard JU, Shroff SG, Cunningham FG: Cardiovascular alterations in normal and preeclamptic pregnancies. In Taylor RN, Roberts JM, Cunningham FG (eds): Chesley's Hypertensive Disorders in Pregnancy, 4th ed. Amsterdam, Academic Press, 2014

Higby K, Suiter CR, Phelps JY, et al: Normal values of urinary albumin and total protein excretion during pregnancy. Am J Obstet Gynecol 171:984, 1994

Hill JA, Olson EN: Cardiac plasticity. N Engl J Med 358:1370, 2008

Hladunewich MA, Lafayette RA, Derby GC, et al: The dynamics of glomerular filtration in the puerperium. Am J Physiol Renal Physiol 286(3):F496, 2004

Hladunewich MA, Schaefer F: Proteinuria in special populations: pregnant women and children. Adv Chronic Kidney Dis 18(4):267, 2011

Hodgkinson CP: Physiology of the ovarian veins in pregnancy. Obstet Gynecol 1:26, 1953

Holmes VA, Wallace JM: Haemostasis in normal pregnancy: a balancing act? Biochem Soc Transact 33:428, 2005

Huerta-Enochian GS, Katz VL, Fox LK, et al: Magnetic resonance—based serial pelvimetry: do maternal pelvic dimensions change during pregnancy? Am J Obstet Gynecol 194:1689, 2006

Hui C, Lili M, Libin C, et al: Changes in coagulation and hemodynamics during pregnancy: a prospective longitudinal study of 58 cases. Arch Gynecol Obstet 285(5):1231, 2012

Huisman A, Aarnoudse JG, Heuvelmans JHA, et al: Whole blood viscosity during normal pregnancy. Br J Obstet Gynaecol 94:1143, 1987

Hytten FE: Lactation. In The Clinical Physiology of the Puerperium. London, Farrand Press, 1995, p 59

Hytten FE: The renal excretion of nutrients in pregnancy. Postgrad Med J 49:625, 1973

Hytten FE: Weight gain in pregnancy. In Hytten FE, Chamberlain G (eds): Clinical Physiology in Obstetrics, 2nd ed. Oxford, Blackwell, 1991, p 173

Hytten FE, Leitch I: The Physiology of Human Pregnancy, 2nd ed. Philadelphia, Davis, 1971

Ingerslev M, Teilum G: Biopsy studies on the liver in pregnancy, 2. Liver biopsy on normal pregnant women. Acta Obstet Gynecol Scand 25:352, 1946

Inoue T, Hotta A, Awai M, et al: Loss of vision due to a physiologic pituitary enlargement during normal pregnancy. Graefe's Arch Clin Exp Ophthalmol 245:1049, 2007

Iosif S, Ingemarsson I, Ulmsten U: Urodynamic studies in normal pregnancy and in puerperium. Am J Obstet Gynecol 137:696, 1980

Jain N, Sternberg LB: Symphyseal separation. Obstet Gynecol 105:1229, 2005

Jarolim P: Serum biomarkers for heart failure. Cardiovasc Pathol 15:144, 2006

Jauniaux E, Johnson MR, Jurkovic D, et al: The role of relaxin in the development of the uteroplacental circulation in early pregnancy. Obstet Gynecol 84:338, 1994

Jeffreys RM, Stepanchak W, Lopez B, et al: Uterine blood flow during supine rest and exercise after 28 weeks of gestation. BJOG 113:1239, 2006

Jensen D, Wolfe LA, Slatkovska L, et al: Effects of human pregnancy on the ventilatory chemoreflex response to carbon dioxide. Am J Physiol Regul Integr Comp Physiol 288:R1369, 2005

Jensen E, Wood C, Keller-Wood M: The normal increase in adrenal secretion during pregnancy contributes to maternal volume expansion and fetal homeostasis. J Soc Gynecol Investig 9:362, 2002

Jonsson Y, Ruber M, Matthiesen L, et al: Cytokine mapping of sera from women with preeclampsia and normal pregnancies. J Reprod Immunol 70:83, 2006

Jung C, Ho JT, Torpy DJ, et al: A longitudinal study of plasma and urinary cortisol in pregnancy and postpartum. J Clin Endocrinol Metab 96(5):1533, 2011

Kalhan SC, Gruca LL, Parimi PS, et al: Serine metabolism in human pregnancy. Am J Physiol Endocrinol Metab 284:E733, 2003

Kametas N, McAuliffe F, Krampl E, et al: Maternal electrolyte and liver function changes during pregnancy at high altitude. Clin Chim Acta 328:21, 2003a

Kametas NA, McAuliffe F, Krampl E, et al: Maternal cardiac function in twin pregnancy. Obstet Gynecol 102:806, 2003b

Kaneshige E: Serum ferritin as an assessment of iron stores and other hematologic parameters during pregnancy. Obstet Gynecol 57:238, 1981

Kaňová N, Bičiková M: Hyperandrogenic states in pregnancy. Physiol Res 60(2):243, 2011

Karakosta P, Chatzi L, Plana E, et al: Leptin levels in cord blood and anthropometric measures at birth: a systematic review and meta-analysis. Paediatr Perinat Epidemiol 25(2):150, 2010

Kauppila A, Chatelain P, Kirkinen P, et al: Isolated prolactin deficiency in a woman with puerperal alactogenesis. J Clin Endocrinol Metab 64:309, 1987

Kauppila A, Koskinen M, Puolakka J, et al: Decreased intervillous and unchanged myometrial blood flow in supine recumbency. Obstet Gynecol 55:203, 1980

Keenan PA, Yaldoo DT, Stress ME, et al: Explicit memory in pregnant women. Am J Obstet Gynecol 179:731, 1998

Keller-Wood M, Wood CE: Pregnancy alters cortisol feedback inhibition of stimulated ACTH: studies in adrenalectomized ewes. Am J Physiol Regul Integr Comp Physiol 280:R1790, 2001

Kennedy RL, Malabu UH, Jarrod G, et al: Thyroid function and pregnancy: before, during and beyond. J Obstet Gynaecol 30(8):774, 2010

Kenny L, McCrae K, Cunningham FG: Platelets, coagulation, and the liver. In Taylor RN, Roberts JM, Cunningham FG (eds): Chesley's Hypertensive Disorders in Pregnancy, 4th ed. Amsterdam, Academic Press, 2014

Kinsella SM, Lohmann G: Supine hypotensive syndrome. Obstet Gynecol 83:774, 1994

Klafen A, Palugyay J: Vergleichende Untersuchungen über Lage und Ausdehrung von Herz und Lunge in der Schwangerschaft und im Wochenbett. Arch Gynaekol 131:347, 1927

Kletzky OA, Rossman F, Bertolli SI, et al: Dynamics of human chorionic gonadotropin, prolactin, and growth hormone in serum and amniotic fluid throughout normal human pregnancy. Am J Obstet Gynecol 151:878, 1985

Kolarzyk E, Szot WM, Lyszczarz J: Lung function and breathing regulation parameters during pregnancy. Arch Gynecol Obstet 272:53, 2005

Kovacs CS, Fuleihan GE: Calcium and bone disorders during pregnancy and lactation. Endocrin Metab Clin North Am 35:21, 2006

Krause BJ, Hanson MA, Casanello P: Role of nitric oxide in placental vascular development and function. Placenta 32(11):797, 2011

Krause PJ, Ingardia CJ, Pontius LT, et al: Host defense during pregnancy: neutrophil chemotaxis and adherence. Am J Obstet Gynecol 157:274, 1987

Kubota T, Kamada S, Hirata Y, et al: Synthesis and release of endothelin-1 by human decidual cells. J Clin Endocrinol Metab 75:1230, 1992

Kulandavelu S, Whiteley KJ, Bainbridge SA, et al: Endothelial NO synthase augments fetoplacental blood flow, placental vascularization, and fetal growth in mice. Hypertension 61(1):259, 2013

Kumru S, Boztosun A, Godekmerdan A: Pregnancy-associated changes in peripheral blood lymphocyte subpopulations and serum cytokine concentrations in healthy women. J Reprod Med 50:246, 2005

Lammert F, Marschall HU, Glantz A, et al: Intrahepatic cholestasis of pregnancy: molecular pathogenesis, diagnosis and management. J Hepatol 33:1012, 2000

Langer JE, Coleman BG: Case 1: diagnosis: hyperreactio luteinalis complicating a normal pregnancy. Ultrasound Q 23:63, 2007
Lederman SA, Paxton A, Heymsfield SB, et al: Maternal body fat and water during pregnancy: do they raise infant birth weight? Am J Obstet Gynecol 180:235, 1999
Leung AM: Thyroid function in pregnancy. J Trace Elem Med Biol 26(2–3): 137, 2012
Leung AM, Pearce EN, Braverman LD: Iodine nutrition in pregnancy and lactation. Endocrinol Metab Clin North Am 40(4):765, 2011
Lind T, Bell S, Gilmore E, et al: Insulin disappearance rate in pregnant and non-pregnant women, and in non-pregnant women given GHRIH. Eur J Clin Invest 7:47, 1977
Lindheimer MD, Davison JM: Osmoregulation, the secretion of arginine vasopressin and its metabolism during pregnancy. Eur J Endocrinol 132:133, 1995
Lindheimer MD, Grünfeld J-P, Davison JM: Renal disorders. In Barran WM, Lindheimer MD (eds): Medical Disorders During Pregnancy, 3rd ed. St. Louis, Mosby, 2000, p 39
Lindheimer MD, Kanter D: Interpreting abnormal proteinuria in pregnancy: the need for a more pathophysiological approach. Obstet Gynecol 115(2 Pt 1):365, 2010
Lindheimer MD, Richardson DA, Ehrlich EN, et al: Potassium homeostasis in pregnancy. J Reprod Med 32:517, 1987
Lipiński P, Styś A, Starzyński RR: Molecular insights into the regulation of iron metabolism during the prenatal and early postnatal periods. Cell Mol Life Sci 70(1):23, 2013
Lippi G, Albiero A, Montagnana M, et al: Lipid and lipoprotein profile in physiological pregnancy. Clin Lab 53:173, 2007
Löf M: Physical activity pattern and activity energy expenditure in healthy pregnant and non-pregnant Swedish women. Eur J Clin Nutr 65(12):1295, 2011
Lønberg U, Damm P, Andersson AM, et al: Increase in maternal placental growth hormone during pregnancy and disappearance during parturition in normal and growth hormone-deficient pregnancies. Am J Obstet Gynecol 188:247, 2003
Lowe SA, MacDonald GJ, Brown MA: Acute and chronic regulation of atrial natriuretic peptide in human pregnancy: a longitudinal study. J Hypertens 10:821, 1992
Luppi P, Haluszczak C, Trucco M, et al: Normal pregnancy is associated with peripheral leukocyte activation. Am J Reprod Immunol 47:72, 2002
Mabie WC, DiSessa TG, Crocker LG, et al: A longitudinal study of cardiac output in normal human pregnancy. Am J Obstet Gynecol 170:849, 1994
Macfie AG, Magides AD, Richmond MN, et al: Gastric emptying in pregnancy. Br J Anaesth 67:54, 1991
Maguire M, Lungu A, Gorden P, et al: Pregnancy in a woman with congenital generalized lipodystrophy. Obstet Gynecol 119(2 Pt 2):452, 2012
Mahendru AA, Everett TR, Wilkinson IB, et al: Maternal cardiovascular changes from pre-pregnancy to very early pregnancy. J Hypertens 30(11): 2168, 2012
Majed BH, Khalil RA: Molecular mechanisms regulating the vascular prostacyclin pathways and their adaptation during pregnancy and in the newborn. Pharmacol Rev 64(3):540, 2012
Mandala M, Osol G: Physiological remodeling of the maternal uterine circulation during pregnancy. Basic Clin Pharmacol Toxicol 110(1):12, 2011
Manten GTR, Franx A, Sikkema JM, et al: Fibrinogen and high molecular weight fibrinogen during and after normal pregnancy. Thrombosis Res 114: 19, 2004
Mardones-Santander F, Salazar G, Rosso P, et al: Maternal body composition near term and birth weight. Obstet Gynecol 91:873, 1998
Margarit L, Griffiths A, Tsapanos V, et al: Second trimester amniotic fluid endothelin concentration: a possible predictor for pre-eclampsia. J Obstet Gynaecol 25:18, 2005
Marnach ML, Ramin KD, Ramsey PS, et al: Characterization of the relationship between joint laxity and maternal hormones in pregnancy. Obstet Gynecol 101:331, 2003
Masini E, Nistri S, Vannacci A, et al: Relaxin inhibits the activation of human neutrophils: involvement of the nitric oxide pathway. Endocrinology 145: 1106, 2004
Maymó JL, Pérez Pérez A, Gambino Y, et al: Review: leptin gene expression in the placenta—regulation of a key hormone in trophoblast proliferation and survival. Placenta 32(Suppl B):S146, 2011
Maymon R, Zimerman AL, Strauss S, et al: Maternal spleen size throughout normal pregnancy. Semin Ultrasound CT MRI 28:64, 2007
McAuliffe F, Kametas N, Costello J, et al: Respiratory function in singleton and twin pregnancy. Br J Obstet Gynaecol 109:765, 2002
McLean KC, Bernstein IM, Brummel-Ziedins KE: Tissue factor-dependent thrombin generation across pregnancy. Am J Obstet Gynecol 207(2):135. e1, 2012
McLennan CE: Antecubital and femoral venous pressure in normal and toxemic pregnancy. Am J Obstet Gynecol 45:568, 1943
Mendenhall HW: Serum protein concentrations in pregnancy. 1. Concentrations in maternal serum. Am J Obstet Gynecol 106:388, 1970
Metcalfe J, Romney SL, Ramsey LH, et al: Estimation of uterine blood flow in normal human pregnancy at term. J Clin Invest 34(11):1632, 1955
Michimata T, Sakai M, Miyazaki S, et al: Decrease of T-helper 2 and T-cytotoxic 2 cells at implantation sites occurs in unexplained recurrent spontaneous abortion with normal chromosomal content. Hum Reprod 18:1523, 2003
Miehle K, Stephan H, Fasshauer M: Leptin, adiponectin and other adipokines in gestational diabetes mellitus and pre-eclampsia. Clin Endocrinol (Oxf) 76(1):2, 2012
Migeon CJ, Bertrand J, Wall PE: Physiological disposition of 4–^{14}C cortisol during late pregnancy. J Clin Invest 36:1350, 1957
Milne JA, Howie AD, Pack AI: Dyspnoea during normal pregnancy. Br J Obstet Gynaecol 85:260, 1978
Mittal P, Espinoza J, Hassan S, et al: Placental growth hormone is increased in the maternal and fetal serum of patients with preeclampsia. J Matern Fetal Neonatal Med 20:651, 2007
Miyamoto J: Prolactin and thyrotropin responses to thyrotropin-releasing hormone during the peripartal period. Obstet Gynecol 63:639, 1984
Mojtahedi M, de Groot LC, Boekholt HA, et al: Nitrogen balance of healthy Dutch women before and during pregnancy. Am J Clin Nutr 75:1078, 2002
Mor G, Cardenas I: The immune system in pregnancy: a unique complexity. Am J Reprod Immunol 63(6):425, 2010
Mor G, Cardenas I, Abrahams V, et al: Inflammation and pregnancy: the role of the immune system at the implantation site. Ann N Y Acad Sci 1221:80, 2011
More C, Bhattoa HP, Bettembuk P, et al: The effects of pregnancy and lactation on hormonal status and biochemical markers of bone turnover. Eur J Obstet Gynecol Reprod Biol 106:209, 2003
Morikawa M, Yamada T, Turuga N, et al: Coagulation-fibrinolysis is more enhanced in twin than in singleton pregnancies. J Perinat Med 34:392, 2006
Muallem MM, Rubeiz NG: Physiological and biological skin changes in pregnancy. Clin Dermatol 24:80, 2006
Muccioli G, Lorenzi T, Lorenzi, et al: Beyond the metabolic rate of ghrelin: a new player in the regulation of reproductive function. Peptides 32(12):2514, 2011
Nakano Y, Itabashi K, Nagahara K, et al: Cord serum adiponectin is positively related to postnatal body mass index gain. Pediatr Int 54(1):76, 2012
Nizard J, Dommergues M, Clément K: Pregnancy in a woman with a leptin-receptor mutation. N Engl J Med 366(11):1064, 2012
Nolten WE, Rueckert PA: Elevated free cortisol index in pregnancy: possible regulatory mechanisms. Am J Obstet Gynecol 139:492, 1981
Obuobie K, Mullik V, Jones C, et al: McCune-Albright syndrome: growth hormone dynamics in pregnancy. J Clin Endocrinol Metab 86:2456, 2001
Øian P, Maltau JM, Noddeland H, et al: Oedema-preventing mechanisms in subcutaneous tissue of normal pregnant women. Br J Obstet Gynaecol 92:1113, 1985
Osman H, Rubeiz N, Tamim H, et al: Risk factors for the development of striae gravidarum. Am J Obstet Gynecol 196:62.e1, 2007
Paccolat C, Harbarth S, Courvoisier D, et al: Procalcitonin levels during pregnancy, delivery and postpartum. J Perinat Med 39(6):679, 2011
Page KL, Celia G, Leddy G, et al: Structural remodeling of rat uterine veins in pregnancy. Am J Obstet Gynecol 187:1647, 2002
Palmer SK, Zamudio S, Coffin C, et al: Quantitative estimation of human uterine artery blood flow and pelvic blood flow redistribution in pregnancy. Obstet Gynecol 80:1000, 1992
Park JI, Chang CL, Hsu SY: New insights into biological roles of relaxin and relaxin-related peptides. Rev Endocr Metab Disord 6:291, 2005
Parker CR Jr, Everett RB, Whalley PJ, et al: Hormone production during pregnancy in the primigravid patients. II. Plasma levels of deoxycorticosterone throughout pregnancy of normal women and women who developed pregnancy-induced hypertension. Am J Obstet Gynecol 138:626, 1980
Pasrija S, Sharma N: Benign diffuse breast hyperplasia during pregnancy. N Engl J Med 355:2771, 2006
Pates JA, Hatab MR, McIntire DD, et al: Determining uterine blood flow in pregnancy with magnetic resonance imaging. Magn Reson Imaging 28(4): 507, 2010
Pavlova M, Sheikh LS: Sleep in women. Semin Neurol 31(4):397, 2011
Peck TM, Arias F: Hematologic changes associated with pregnancy. Clin Obstet Gynecol 22:785, 1979
Pedersen NG, Juul A, Christiansen M, et al: Maternal serum placental growth hormone, but not human placental lactogen or insulin growth factor-1, is positively associated with fetal growth in the first half of pregnancy. Ultrasound Obstet Gynecol 36(5):534, 2010

Phelan N, Conway GS: Management of ovarian disease in pregnancy. Best Pract Res Clin Endocrinol Metab 25(6):985, 2011
Phelps RL, Metzger BE, Freinkel N: Carbohydrate metabolism in pregnancy, 17. Diurnal profiles of plasma glucose, insulin, free fatty acids, triglycerides, cholesterol, and individual amino acids in late normal pregnancy. Am J Obstet Gynecol 140:730, 1981
Phillips J, McBride C, Hale S, et al: Examination of prepregnancy and pregnancy urinary protein levels in healthy nulligravidas. Abstract No. 356. Presented at the 34th Annual Meeting of the Society for Maternal-Fetal Medicine. February 3-8, 2014
Pighetti M, Tommaselli GA, D'Elia A, et al: Maternal serum and umbilical cord blood leptin concentrations with fetal growth restriction. Obstet Gynecol 102:535, 2003
Pitkin RM, Reynolds WA, Williams GA, et al: Calcium metabolism in normal pregnancy: a longitudinal study. Am J Obstet Gynecol 133:781, 1979
Power ML, Heaney RP, Kalkwarf HJ, et al: The role of calcium in health and disease. Am J Obstet Gynecol 181:1560, 1999
Powers RW, Majors AK, Kerchner LJ, et al: Renal handling of homocysteine during normal pregnancy and preeclampsia. J Soc Gynecol Investig 11:45, 2004
Pritchard JA: Changes in the blood volume during pregnancy and delivery. Anesthesiology 26:393, 1965
Pritchard JA, Adams RH: Erythrocyte production and destruction during pregnancy. Am J Obstet Gynecol 79:750, 1960
Pritchard JA, Mason RA: Iron stores of normal adults and their replenishment with oral iron therapy. JAMA 190:897, 1964
Pritchard JA, Scott DE: Iron demands during pregnancy. In Iron Deficiency-Pathogenesis: Clinical Aspects and Therapy. London, Academic Press, 1970, p 173
Rahn DD, Acevedo JF, Word RA: Effect of vaginal distention on elastic fiber synthesis and matrix degradation in the vaginal wall: potential role in the pathogenesis of pelvic organ prolapse. Am J Physiol Regul Integr Comp Physiol 295(4):R1351, 2008a
Rahn DD, Ruff MD, Brown SA, et al: Biomechanical properties of the vaginal wall: effect of pregnancy, elastic fiber deficiency, and pelvic organ prolapse. Am J Obstet Gynecol 198(5):590.e1, 2008b
Rana S, Lindheimer M, Hibbard J, Pliskin N: Neuropsychological performance in normal pregnancy and preeclampsia. Am J Obstet Gynecol 195:186, 2006
Rathore SP, Gupta S, Gupta V: Pattern and prevalence of physiological cutaneous changes in pregnancy: a study of 2000 antenatal women. Indian J Dermatol Venereol Leprol 77(4):402, 2011
Redman CWG, Sargent IL, Taylor RN: Immunology of normal pregnancy and preeclampsia. In Taylor RN, Roberts JM, Cunningham FG (eds): Chesley's Hypertensive Disorders in Pregnancy, 4th ed. Amsterdam, Academic Press, 2014
Repke JT: Calcium homeostasis in pregnancy. Clin Obstet Gynecol 37:59, 1994
Resnik JL, Hong C, Resnik R, et al: Evaluation of B-type natriuretic peptide (BNP) levels in normal and preeclamptic women. Am J Obstet Gynecol 193:450, 2005
Richani K, Soto E, Romero R, et al: Normal pregnancy is characterized by systemic activation of the complement system. J Matern Fetal Neonat Med 17:239, 2005
Riedl M, Maier C, Handisurya A, et al: Insulin resistance has no impact on ghrelin suppression in pregnancy. Intern Med 262:458, 2007
Robb AO, Mills NL, Din JN, et al: Acute endothelial tissue plasminogen activator release in pregnancy. J Thromb Haemost 7(1):138, 2009
Rosenfeld CR, Barton MD, Meschia G: Effects of epinephrine on distribution of blood flow in the pregnant ewe. Am J Obstet Gynecol 124:156, 1976
Rosenfeld CR, DeSpain K, Word RA, et al: Differential sensitivity to angiotensin II and norepinephrine in human uterine arteries. J Clin Endocrinol Metab 97(1):138, 2012
Rosenfeld CR, Gant NF Jr: The chronically instrumented ewe: a model for studying vascular reactivity to angiotensin II in pregnancy. J Clin Invest 67:486, 1981
Rosenfeld CR, Roy T, DeSpain K, et al: Large-conductance Ca^{2+} dependent K^+ channels regulate basal uteroplacental blood flow in ovine pregnancy. J Soc Gynecol Investig 12:402, 2005
Rosenfeld CR, West J: Circulatory response to systemic infusion of norepinephrine in the pregnant ewe. Am J Obstet Gynecol 127:376, 1977
Rosenfeld CR, Word RA, DeSpain K, et al: Large conductance Ca^{2+}-activated K^+ channels contribute to vascular function in nonpregnant human uterine arteries. Reprod Sci 15(7):651, 2008
Rubi RA, Sala NL: Ureteral function in pregnant women. 3. Effect of different positions and of fetal delivery upon ureteral tonus. Am J Obstet Gynecol 101:230, 1968
Ruiz-Extremera A, López-Garrido MA, Barranco E, et al: Activity of hepatic enzymes from week sixteen of pregnancy. Am J Obstet Gynecol 193:2010, 2005
Russell P, Robboy S: Ovarian cysts, tumor-like, iatrogenic and miscellaneous conditions. In Robboy SJ, Mutter GL, Prat J, et al (eds): Robboy's Pathology of the Female Reproductive Tract, 2nd ed. London, Churchill Livingstone, 2009, p 579
Saarelainen H, Laitinen T, Raitakari OT, et al: Pregnancy-related hyperlipidemia and endothelial function in healthy women. Circ J 70:768, 2006
Sandhu KS, LaCombe JA, Fleischmann N: Gross and microscopic hematuria: guidelines for obstetricians and gynecologists. Obstet Gynecol Surv 64(1):39, 2009
Savu O, Jurcuț R, Giușcă S, et al: Morphological and functional adaptation of the maternal heart during pregnancy. Circ Cardiovasc Imaging 5(3):289, 2012
Scheithauer BW, Sano T, Kovacs KT, et al: The pituitary gland in pregnancy: a clinicopathologic and immunohistochemical study of 69 cases. Mayo Clin Proc 65:461, 1990
Schiessl B, Strasburger CJ, Bidlingmeier M, et al: Role of placental growth hormone in the alteration of maternal arterial resistance in pregnancy. J Reprod Med 52:313, 2007
Schulman A, Herlinger H: Urinary tract dilatation in pregnancy. Br J Radiol 48:638, 1975
Semins MJ, Trock BJ, Matlaga BR: The safety of ureteroscopy during pregnancy: a systematic review and meta-analysis. J Urol 181(1):139, 2009
Sheth VM, Pandya AG: Melasma: a comprehensive update: part I. J Am Acad Dermatol 65(4):689, 2011
Shinagawa S, Suzuki S, Chihara H, et al: Maternal basal metabolic rate in twin pregnancy. Gynecol Obstet Invest 60:145, 2005
Shoma A, Elbassiony L, Amin M, et al: "Gestational gigantomastia": a review article and case presentation of a new surgical management option. Surg Innov 18(1):94, 2011
Simon FR, Fortune J, Iwahashi M, et al: Ethinyl estradiol cholestasis involves alterations in expression of liver sinusoidal transporters. Am J Physiol 271:G1043, 1996
Simpson KR, James DC: Efficacy of intrauterine resuscitation techniques in improving fetal oxygen status during labor. Obstet Gynecol 105:1362, 2005
Smallridge RC, Glinoer D, Hollowell JG, et al: Thyroid function inside and outside of pregnancy: what do we know and what don't we know? Thyroid 15:54, 2005
Soltanipoor F, Delaram M, Taavoni S, et al: The effect of olive oil on prevention of striae gravidarum: a randomized controlled clinical trial. Complement Ther Med 20(5):263, 2012
Song CS, Kappas A: The influence of estrogens, progestins and pregnancy on the liver. Vitam Horm 26:147, 1968
Sprague BJ, Phernetton TM, Magness RR, et al: The effects of the ovarian cycle and pregnancy on uterine vascular impedance and uterine artery mechanics. Eur J Obstet Gynecol Reprod Biol 144(Suppl 1):S170, 2009
Straach KJ, Shelton JM, Richardson JA, et al: Regulation of hyaluronan expression during cervical ripening. Glycobiology 15:55, 2005
Sunness JS: The pregnant woman's eye. Surv Ophthalmol 32:219, 1988
Tamás P, Szilágyi A, Jeges S, et al: Effects of maternal central hemodynamics on fetal heart rate patterns. Acta Obstet Gynecol Scand 86:711, 2007
Tanaka Y, Yanagihara T, Ueta M, et al: Naturally conceived twin pregnancy with hyperreactio luteinalis, causing hyperandrogenism and maternal virilization. Acta Obstet Gynecol Scand 80:277, 2001
Tanous D, Siu SC, Mason J, et al: B-type natriuretic peptide in pregnant women with heart disease. J Am Coll Cardiol 56(15):1247, 2010
Taylor DJ, Phillips P, Lind T: Puerperal haematological indices. Br J Obstet Gynaecol 88:601, 1981
Teran E, Escudero C, Vivero S, et al: NO in early pregnancy and development of preeclampsia. Hypertension 47:e17, 2006
Thellin O, Heinen E: Pregnancy and the immune system: between tolerance and rejection. Toxicology 185:179, 2003
Thorpe-Beeston JG, Nicolaides KH, Snijders RJM, et al: Fetal thyroid-stimulating hormone response to maternal administration of thyrotropin-releasing hormone. Am J Obstet Gynecol 164:1244, 1991
Tihtonen KM, Kööbi T, Vuolteenaho O, et al: Natriuretic peptides and hemodynamics in preeclampsia. Am J Obstet Gynecol 196:328.e1, 2007
Timmons BC, Mahendroo M: Processes regulating cervical ripening differ from cervical dilation and postpartum repair: insights from gene expression studies. Reprod Sci 14:53, 2007
Trakada G, Tsapanos V, Spiropoulos K: Normal pregnancy and oxygenation during sleep. Eur J Obstet Gynecol Reprod Biol 109:128, 2003
Tsai CH, de Leeuw NKM: Changes in 2,3-diphosphoglycerate during pregnancy and puerperium in normal women and in β-thalassemia heterozygous women. Am J Obstet Gynecol 142:520, 1982
Uchikova EH, Ledjev II: Changes in haemostasis during normal pregnancy. Eur J Obstet Gynecol Reprod Biol 119:185, 2005

Ueland K: Maternal cardiovascular dynamics, 7. Intrapartum blood volume changes. Am J Obstet Gynecol 126:671, 1976
Ueland K, Metcalfe J: Circulatory changes in pregnancy. Clin Obstet Gynecol 18:41, 1975
Ulmsten U, Sundström G: Esophageal manometry in pregnant and nonpregnant women. Am J Obstet Gynecol 132:260, 1978
Valera MC, Parant O, Vayssiere C, et al: Physiological and pathologic changes of platelets in pregnancy. Platelets 21(8):587, 2010
van Brummen H, Bruinse HW, van der Bom J, et al: How do the prevalences of urogenital symptoms change during pregnancy? Neurourol Urodyn 25:135, 2006
van den Akker CH, Schierbeek H, Dorst KY, et al: Human fetal amino acid metabolism at term gestation. Am J Clin Nutr 89(1):153, 2009
Van Wagenen G, Jenkins RH: An experimental examination of factors causing ureteral dilatation of pregnancy. J Urol 42:1010, 1939
Vidaeff AC, Ross PJ, Livingston CK, et al: Gigantomastia complicating mirror syndrome in pregnancy. Obstet Gynecol 101:1139, 2003
Villaseca P, Campino C, Oestreicher E, et al: Bilateral oophorectomy in a pregnant woman: hormonal profile from late gestation to post-partum: case report. Hum Reprod 20:397, 2005
Vodstrcil LA, Tare M, Novak J, et al: Relaxin mediates uterine artery compliance during pregnancy and increases uterine blood flow. FASEB J 26(10):4035, 2012
Walker MC, Garner PR, Keely EJ, et al: Changes in activated protein C resistance during normal pregnancy. Am J Obstet Gynecol 177:162, 1997
Walther T, Stepan H: C-type natriuretic peptide in reproduction, pregnancy and fetal development. J Endocrinol 180:17, 2004
Watanabe M, Meeker CI, Gray MJ, et al: Secretion rate of aldosterone in normal pregnancy. J Clin Invest 42:1619, 1963
Watts DH, Krohn MA, Wener MH, et al: C-reactive protein in normal pregnancy. Obstet Gynecol 77:176, 1991
Waugh J, Bell SC, Kilby MD, et al: Urinary microalbumin/creatinine ratios: reference range in uncomplicated pregnancy. Clin Sci 104:103, 2003
Weiss M, Eisenstein Z, Ramot Y, et al: Renal reabsorption of inorganic phosphorus in pregnancy in relation to the calciotropic hormones. Br J Obstet Gynaecol 105:195, 1998
Wesnes SL, Hunskaar S, Bo K, et al: The effect of urinary incontinence status during pregnancy and delivery mode on incontinence postpartum. A cohort study. BJOG 116(5):700, 2009
Wilson M, Morganti AA, Zervoudakis I, et al: Blood pressure, the renin-aldosterone system and sex steroids throughout normal pregnancy. Am J Med 68:97, 1980
Wise RA, Polito AJ, Krishnan V: Respiratory physiologic changes in pregnancy. Immunol Allergy Clin North Am 26:1, 2006
Wong CA, Loffredi M, Ganchiff JN, et al: Gastric emptying of water in term pregnancy. Anesthesiology 96:1395, 2002
Wong CA, McCarthy RJ, Fitzgerald PC, et al: Gastric emptying of water in obese pregnant women at term. Anesth Analg 105:751, 2007
Word RA, Li XH, Hnat M, et al: Dynamics of cervical remodeling during pregnancy and parturition: mechanisms and current concepts. Semin Reprod Med 25:69, 2007
World Health Organization: Human energy requirements. Food and nutrition technical report series 1. Rome, Food and Agriculture Organization of the United Nations, 2004, p 53
Wright HP, Osborn SB, Edmonds DG: Changes in rate of flow of venous blood in the leg during pregnancy, measured with radioactive sodium. Surg Gynecol Obstet 90:481, 1950
Xiao D, Huang X, Yang S, et al: Direct effects of nicotine on contractility of the uterine artery in pregnancy. J Pharmacol Exp Ther 322:180, 2007
Yurteri-Kaplan L, Saber S, Zamudio S: Brain natriuretic peptide in term pregnancy. Reprod Sci 19(5):520, 2012
Zeeman GG, Cunningham FG, Pritchard JA: The magnitude of hemoconcentration with eclampsia. Hypertens Pregnancy 28(2):127, 2009
Zeeman GG, Hatab M, Twickler DM: Maternal cerebral blood flow changes in pregnancies. Am J Obstet Gynecol 189:968, 2003
Zimmermann MB: The effects of iodine deficiency in pregnancy and infancy. Paediatr Perinat Epidemiol 26(Supp 1):108, 2012

SECTION 3

PLACENTATION, EMBRYOGENESIS, AND FETAL DEVELOPMENT

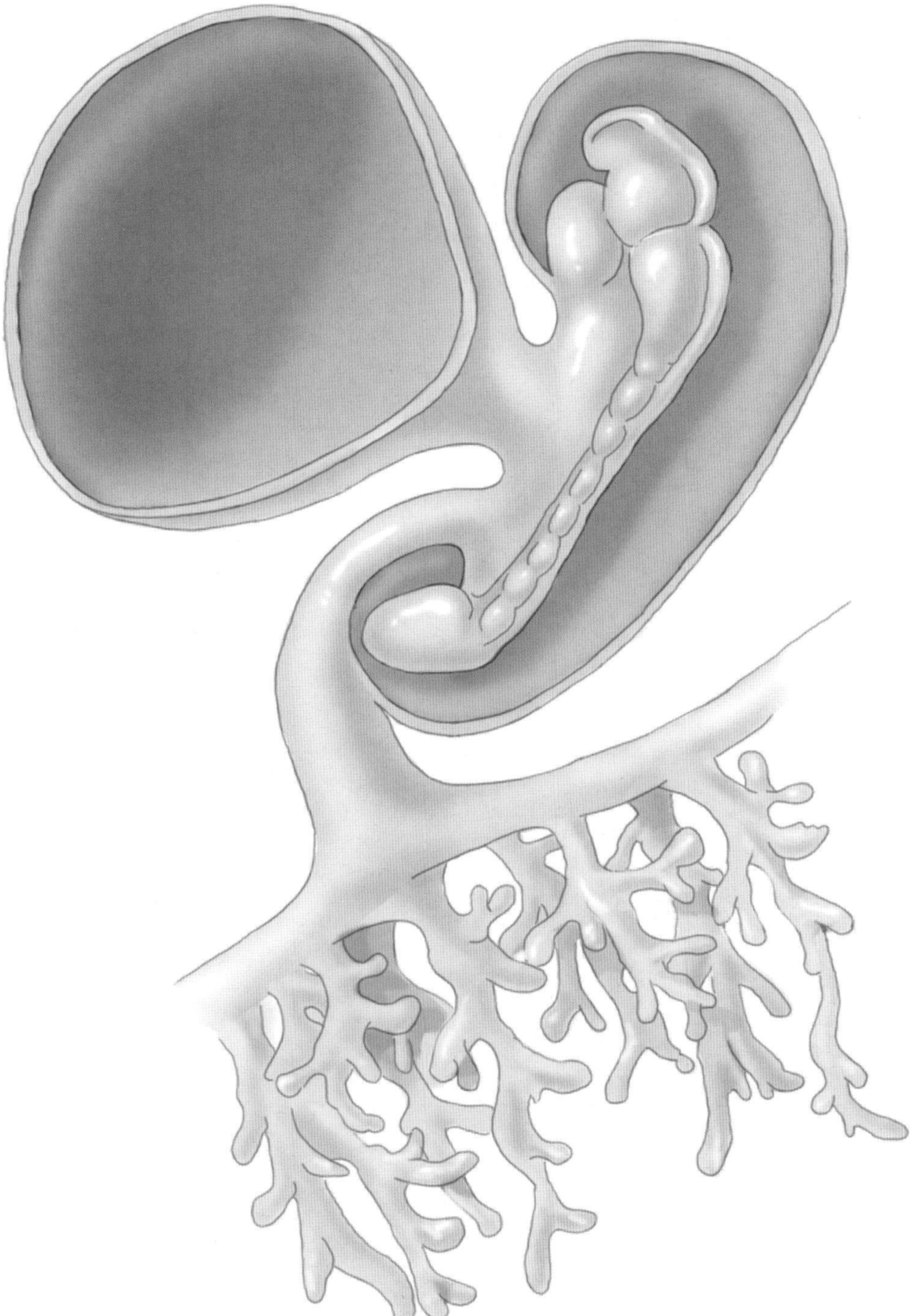

CHAPTER 5

Implantation and Placental Development

All obstetricians should be aware of the basic reproductive biological processes required for women to successfully achieve pregnancy. Several abnormalities can affect each of these and lead to infertility or pregnancy loss. In most women, spontaneous, cyclical ovulation at 25- to 35-day intervals continues during almost 40 years between menarche and menopause. Without contraception, there are approximately 400 opportunities for pregnancy, which may occur with intercourse on any of 1200 days—the day of ovulation and its two preceding days. This narrow window for fertilization is controlled by tightly regulated production of ovarian steroids. Moreover, these hormones promote optimal endometrial regeneration after menstruation in preparation for the next implantation window.

Should fertilization occur, events that begin after initial blastocyst implantation onto the endometrium and continue through to parturition result from a unique interaction between fetal trophoblasts and maternal endometrium-decidua. The ability of mother and fetus to coexist as two distinct immunological systems results from endocrine, paracrine, and immunological modification of fetal and maternal tissues in a manner not seen elsewhere. The placenta mediates a unique fetal–maternal communication system, which creates a hormonal environment that initially maintains pregnancy and eventually initiates events leading to parturition. The following sections address the physiology of the ovarian-endometrial cycle, implantation, placenta, and fetal membranes, as well as specialized endocrine arrangements between fetus and mother.

THE OVARIAN-ENDOMETRIAL CYCLE

Predictable, regular, cyclical, and spontaneous ovulatory menstrual cycles are regulated by complex interactions of the hypothalamic-pituitary axis, ovaries, and genital tract (Fig. 5-1). The average cycle duration is approximately 28 days, with a range of 25 to 32 days. The hormonal sequence leading to ovulation directs this cycle. Concurrently, cyclical changes in endometrial histology are faithfully reproduced. Rock and Bartlett (1937) first suggested that endometrial histological features were sufficiently characteristic to permit cycle "dating." In this scheme, the follicular-proliferative phase and the postovulatory luteal-secretory phase are customarily divided into early and late stages. These changes are detailed in Chapter 15 of *Williams Gynecology*, 2nd edition (Halvorson, 2012).

The Ovarian Cycle

Follicular or Preovulatory Ovarian Phase

The human ovary contains 2 million oocytes at birth, and approximately 400,000 follicles are present at puberty onset (Baker, 1963). The remaining follicles are depleted at a rate of approximately 1000 follicles per month until age 35, when

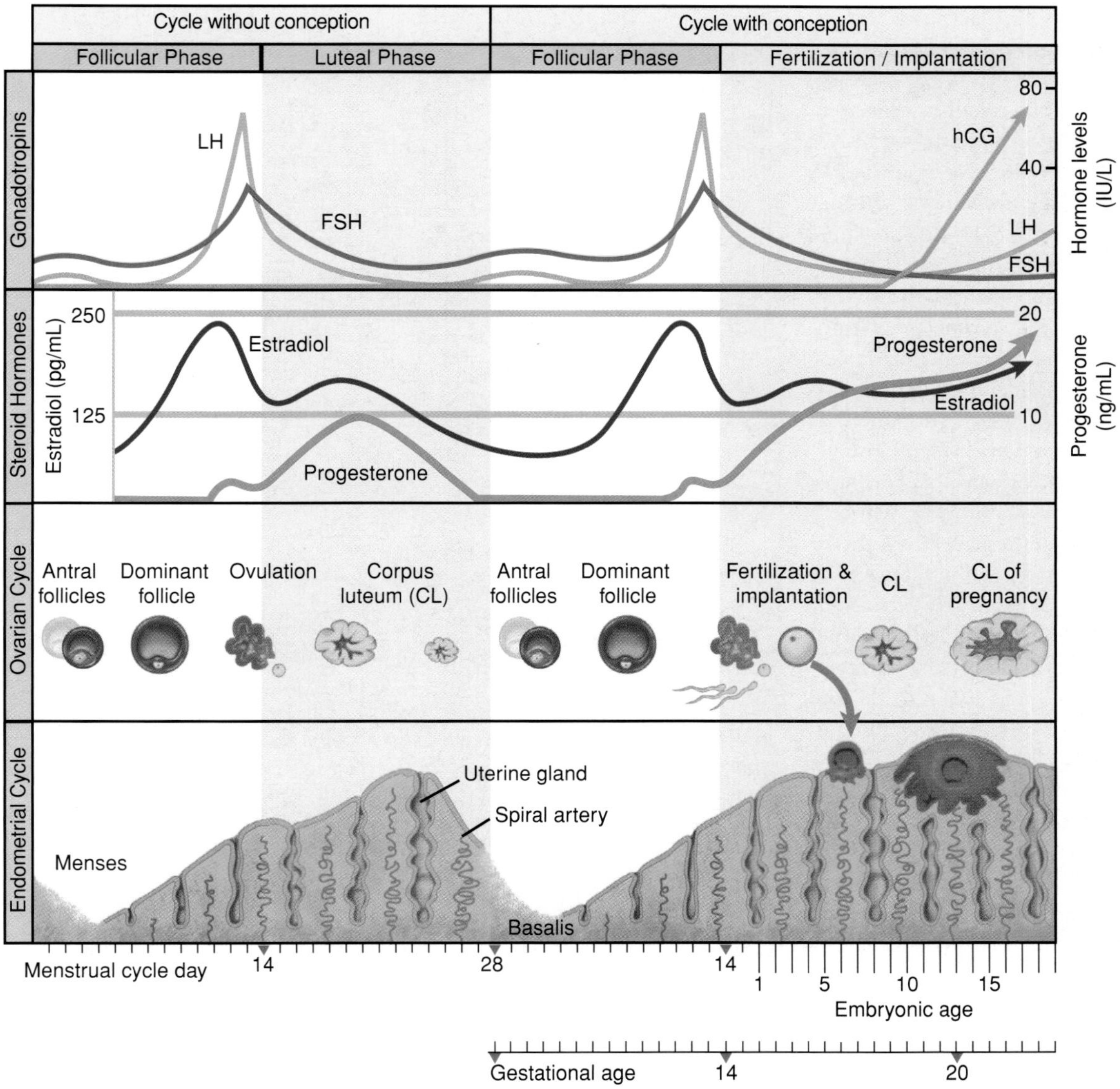

FIGURE 5-1 Gonadotropin control of the ovarian and endometrial cycles. The ovarian-endometrial cycle has been structured as a 28-day cycle. The follicular phase (days 1 to 14) is characterized by rising estrogen levels, endometrial thickening, and selection of the dominant "ovulatory" follicle. During the luteal phase (days 14 to 21), the corpus luteum (CL) produces estrogen and progesterone, which prepare the endometrium for implantation. If implantation occurs, the developing blastocyst begins to produce human chorionic gonadotropin (hCG) and rescues the corpus luteum, thus maintaining progesterone production. FSH = follicle-stimulating hormone; LH = luteinizing hormone.

this rate accelerates (Faddy, 1992). Only 400 follicles are normally released during female reproductive life. Therefore, more than 99.9 percent of follicles undergo atresia through a process of cell death termed apoptosis (Gougeon, 1996; Kaipia, 1997).

Follicular development consists of several stages, which include the gonadotropin-independent recruitment of primordial follicles from the resting pool and their growth to the antral stage. This appears to be controlled by locally produced growth factors. Two members of the transforming growth factor-β family—growth differentiation factor 9 (GDF9) and bone morphogenetic protein 15 (BMP-15)—regulate granulosa cell proliferation and differentiation as primary follicles grow (Trombly, 2009; Yan, 2001). They also stabilize and expand the cumulus oocyte complex in the oviduct (Hreinsson, 2002). These factors are produced by oocytes, suggesting that the early steps in follicular development are, in part, oocyte controlled. As antral follicles develop, surrounding stromal cells are recruited, by a yet-to-be-defined mechanism, to become thecal cells.

Although not required for early follicular maturation, follicle-stimulating hormone (FSH) is required for further development of large antral follicles (Hillier, 2001). During each ovarian cycle, a group of antral follicles, known as a cohort, begins a phase of semisynchronous growth based on their maturation state during the FSH rise in the late luteal phase of the previous cycle. This FSH rise leading to follicle development is called the *selection window* of the ovarian cycle (Macklon, 2001). Only the follicles progressing to this stage develop the capacity to produce estrogen.

During the follicular phase, estrogen levels rise in parallel to growth of a dominant follicle and to the increase in its number of granulosa cells (see Fig. 5-1). These cells are the exclusive site of FSH receptor expression. The rise of circulating FSH levels during the late luteal phase of the previous cycle stimulates an increase in FSH receptors and subsequently, the ability of cytochrome P_{450} aromatase within granulosa cells to convert androstenedione into estradiol. The requirement for thecal cells, which respond to luteinizing hormone (LH), and granulosa cells, which respond to FSH, represents the two-gonadotropin, two-cell hypothesis for estrogen biosynthesis (Short, 1962). As shown in Figure 5-2, FSH induces aromatase and expansion of the antrum of growing follicles. The follicle within the cohort that is most responsive to FSH is likely to be the first to produce estradiol and initiate expression of LH receptors.

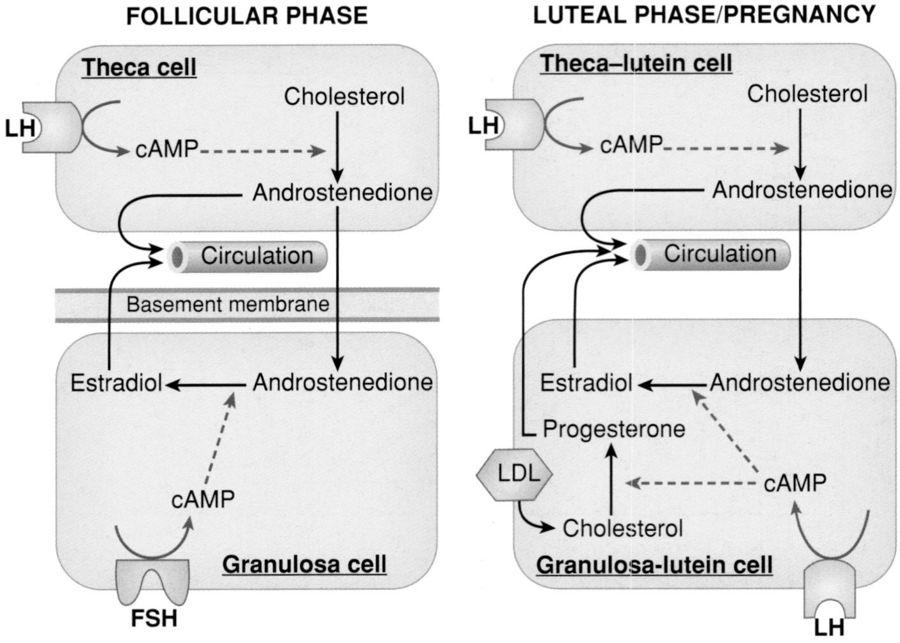

FIGURE 5-2 The two-cell, two-gonadotropin principle of ovarian steroid hormone production. During the follicular phase (*left panel*), luteinizing hormone (LH) controls theca cell production of androstenedione, which diffuses into the adjacent granulosa cells and acts as precursor for estradiol biosynthesis. The granulosa cell capacity to convert androstenedione to estradiol is controlled by follicle-stimulating hormone (FSH). After ovulation (*right panel*), the corpus luteum forms and both theca-lutein and granulosa-lutein cells respond to LH. The theca-lutein cells continue to produce androstenedione, whereas granulosa-lutein cells greatly increase their capacity to produce progesterone and to convert androstenedione to estradiol. LH and hCG bind to the same LH-hCG receptor. If pregnancy occurs (*right panel*), human chorionic gonadotropin (hCG) rescues the corpus luteum through their shared LH-hCG receptor. Low-density lipoprotein (LDL) is an important source of cholesterol for steroidogenesis. cAMP = cyclic adenosine monophosphate.

After the appearance of LH receptors, the preovulatory granulosa cells begin to secrete small quantities of progesterone. The preovulatory progesterone secretion, although somewhat limited, is believed to exert positive feedback on the estrogen-primed pituitary to either cause or augment LH release. In addition, during the late follicular phase, LH stimulates thecal cell production of androgens, particularly androstenedione, which are then transferred to the adjacent follicles where they are aromatized to estradiol (see Fig. 5-2). During the early follicular phase, granulosa cells also produce inhibin B, which can feed back on the pituitary to inhibit FSH release (Groome, 1996). As the dominant follicle begins to grow, production of estradiol and the inhibins increases and results in a decline of follicular-phase FSH. This drop in FSH levels is responsible for the failure of other follicles to reach preovulatory status—the Graafian follicle stage—during any one cycle. Thus, 95 percent of plasma estradiol produced at this time is secreted by the dominant follicle—the one destined to ovulate. Concurrently, the contralateral ovary is relatively inactive.

Ovulation

The onset of the gonadotropin surge resulting from increasing estrogen secretion by preovulatory follicles is a relatively precise predictor of ovulation. It occurs 34 to 36 hours before ovum release from the follicle (see Fig. 5-1). LH secretion peaks 10 to 12 hours before ovulation and stimulates resumption of meiosis in the ovum and release of the first polar body. Current studies suggest that in response to LH, increased progesterone and prostaglandin production by the cumulus cells, as well as GDF9 and BMP-15 by the oocyte, activates expression of genes critical to formation of a hyaluronan-rich extracellular matrix by the cumulus complex (Richards, 2007). As seen in Figure 5-3, during synthesis of this matrix, cumulus cells lose contact with one another and move outward from the oocyte along the hyaluronan polymer—this process is called expansion. This results in a 20-fold increase in the complex volume along with an LH-induced remodeling of the ovarian extracellular matrix to allow release of the mature oocyte and its surrounding cumulus cells through the surface epithelium. Activation of proteases likely plays a pivotal role in weakening of the follicular basement membrane and ovulation (Curry, 2006; Ny, 2002).

Luteal or Postovulatory Ovarian Phase

Following ovulation, the corpus luteum develops from the dominant or Graafian follicle remains in a process referred to as *luteinization*. The basement membrane separating the granulosa-lutein and theca-lutein cells breaks down, and by day 2 postovulation, blood vessels and capillaries invade the granulosa cell layer. The rapid neovascularization of the once-avascular granulosa may be due to angiogenic factors that include vascular endothelial growth factor (VEGF) and others

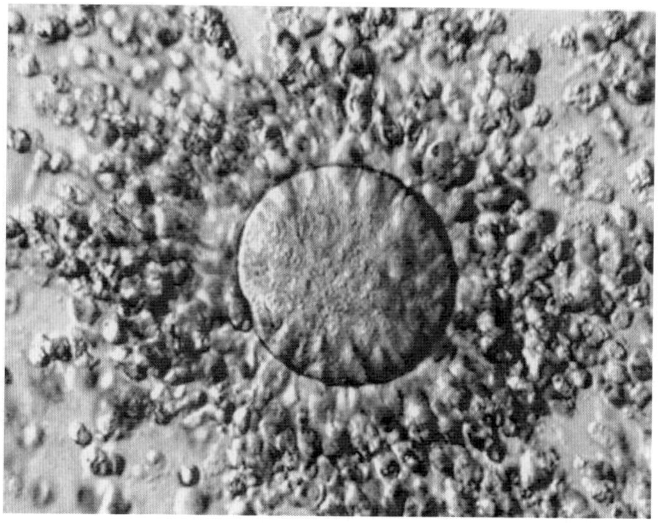

FIGURE 5-3 An ovulated cumulus-oocyte complex. An oocyte is at the center of the complex. Cumulus cells are widely separated from each other in the cumulus layer by the hyaluronan-rich extracellular matrix. (Photograph contributed by Dr. Kevin J. Doody.)

produced in response to LH by theca-lutein and granulosa-lutein cells (Albrecht, 2003; Fraser, 2001). During luteinization, these cells undergo hypertrophy and increase their capacity to synthesize hormones.

LH is the primary luteotropic factor responsible for corpus luteum maintenance (Vande Wiele, 1970). Indeed, LH injections can extend the corpus luteum life span in normal women by 2 weeks (Segaloff, 1951). In normal cycling women, the corpus luteum is maintained by low-frequency, high-amplitude LH pulses secreted by gonadotropes in the anterior pituitary (Filicori, 1986).

The hormone secretion pattern of the corpus luteum differs from that of the follicle (see Fig. 5-1). The increased capacity of granulosa-lutein cells to produce progesterone is the result of increased access to considerably more steroidogenic precursors through blood-borne low-density lipoprotein (LDL)-derived cholesterol as depicted in Figure 5-2 (Carr, 1981a). The important role for LDL in progesterone biosynthesis is supported by the observation that women with extremely low LDL cholesterol levels exhibit minimal progesterone secretion during the luteal phase (Illingworth, 1982). In addition, high-density lipoprotein (HDL) may contribute to progesterone production in granulosa-lutein cells (Ragoobir, 2002).

Estrogen levels follow a more complex pattern of secretion. Specifically, just after ovulation, estrogen levels decrease followed by a secondary rise that reaches a peak production of 0.25 mg/day of 17β-estradiol at the midluteal phase. Toward the end of the luteal phase, there is a secondary decline in estradiol production.

Ovarian progesterone production peaks at 25 to 50 mg/day during the midluteal phase. With pregnancy, the corpus luteum continues progesterone production in response to embryonic human chorionic gonadotropin (hCG), which binds to the same receptor as LH (see Fig. 5-2).

The human corpus luteum is a transient endocrine organ that, in the absence of pregnancy, will rapidly regress 9 to 11 days after ovulation via apoptotic cell death (Vaskivuo, 2002). The mechanisms that control luteolysis remain unclear. However, in part, it results from decreased levels of circulating LH in the late luteal phase and decreased LH sensitivity of luteal cells (Duncan, 1996; Filicori, 1986). The role of other factors is less clear, however, prostaglandin $F_{2\alpha}$ ($PGF_{2\alpha}$) appears to be luteolytic in nonhuman primates (Auletta, 1987; Wentz, 1973). The endocrine effects, consisting of a dramatic drop in circulating estradiol and progesterone levels, are critical for follicular development and ovulation during the next ovarian cycle. In addition, corpus luteum regression and decline in circulating steroid concentrations signal the endometrium to initiate molecular events that lead to menstruation.

Estrogen and Progesterone Action

The fluctuating levels of ovarian steroids are the direct cause of the endometrial cycle. Recent advances in the molecular biology of estrogen and progesterone receptors have greatly improved understanding of their function. The most biologically potent naturally occurring estrogen—17β-estradiol—is secreted by granulosa cells of the dominant follicle and luteinized granulosa cells of the corpus luteum (see Fig. 5-2). Estrogen is the essential hormonal signal on which most events in the normal menstrual cycle depend. Estradiol action is complex and appears to involve two classic nuclear hormone receptors designated estrogen receptor α (ERα) and β (ERβ) (Katzenellenbogen, 2001). These isoforms are the products of separate genes and can exhibit distinct tissue expression. Both estradiol-receptor complexes act as transcriptional factors that become associated with the estrogen response element of specific genes. They share a robust activation by estradiol. However, differences in their binding affinities to other estrogens and their cell-specific expression patterns suggest that ERα and ERβ receptors may have both distinct and overlapping function (Saunders, 2005). Both receptors are expressed in the uterine endometrium (Bombail, 2008; Lecce, 2001). Estrogens function in many cell types to regulate follicular development, uterine receptivity, or blood flow.

Most progesterone actions on the female reproductive tract are mediated through the nuclear hormone receptors, progesterone receptor type A (PR-A) and B (PR-B). Progesterone enters cells by diffusion and in responsive tissues becomes associated with progesterone receptors (Conneely, 2002). Both progesterone receptor isoforms arise from a single gene, are members of the steroid receptor superfamily of transcription factors, and regulate transcription of target genes. These receptors have unique actions. When PR-A and PR-B receptors are coexpressed, it appears that PR-A can inhibit PR-B gene regulation. The endometrial glands and stroma appear to have different expression patterns for progesterone receptors that vary during the menstrual cycle (Mote, 1999). In addition, progesterone can evoke rapid responses such as changes in intracellular free calcium levels that cannot be explained by genomic mechanisms. G-protein-coupled membrane receptors for progesterone have been identified, but their role in the ovarian-endometrium cycle remains to be elucidated (Peluso, 2007).

The Endometrial Cycle

Proliferative or Preovulatory Endometrial Phase

Fluctuations in estrogen and progesterone levels produce striking effects on the reproductive tract, particularly the endometrium. Epithelial—glandular cells; stromal—mesenchymal cells; and blood vessels of the endometrium replicate cyclically in reproductive-aged women at a rapid rate. The endometrium is regenerated during each ovarian–endometrial cycle. The superficial endometrium, termed the *functionalis layer*, is shed and regenerated from the deeper *basalis layer* almost 400 times during the reproductive lifetime of most women (Fig. 5-4). There is no other example in humans of such cyclical shedding and regrowth of an entire tissue.

Follicular-phase estradiol production is the most important factor in endometrial recovery following menstruation. Although up to two thirds of the functionalis endometrium is fragmented and shed during menstruation, reepithelialization begins even before menstrual bleeding has ceased. By the fifth day of the endometrial cycle—fifth day of menses, the epithelial surface of the endometrium has been restored, and revascularization is in progress. The preovulatory endometrium is characterized by proliferation of glandular, stromal, and vascular endothelial cells. During the early part of the proliferative phase, the endometrium is usually less than 2 mm thick. The glands are narrow, tubular structures that pursue almost a straight and parallel course from the basalis layer toward the endometrial cavity. Mitotic figures, especially in the glandular epithelium, are identified by the fifth cycle day. Mitotic activity in both epithelium and stroma persists until day 16 to 17, or 2 to 3 days after ovulation. Although blood vessels are numerous and prominent, there is no extravascular blood or leukocyte infiltration in the endometrium at this stage.

Clearly, reepithelialization and angiogenesis are important to endometrial bleeding cessation (Chennazhi, 2009; Rogers, 2009). These are dependent on tissue regrowth, which is estrogen regulated. Epithelial cell growth also is regulated in part by epidermal growth factor (EGF) and transforming growth factor α (TGFα). Stromal cell proliferation appears to increase through paracrine and autocrine actions of estrogen and increased local levels of fibroblast growth factor-9 (Tsai, 2002). Estrogens also increase local production of VEGF, which causes angiogenesis through vessel elongation in the basalis (Gargett, 2001; Sugino, 2002).

By the late proliferative phase, the endometrium thickens from both glandular hyperplasia and increased stromal ground substance, which is edema and proteinaceous material. The loose stroma is especially prominent, and the glands in the functionalis layer are widely separated. This is compared with those of the basalis layer, in which the glands are more crowded and the stroma is denser. At midcycle, as ovulation nears, glandular epithelium becomes taller and pseudostratified. The surface epithelial cells acquire numerous microvilli, which increase epithelial surface area, and cilia, which aid in the movement of endometrial secretions during the secretory phase (Ferenczy, 1976).

Dating the menstrual cycle day by endometrial histological criteria is difficult during the proliferative phase because of considerable phase-length variation among women. Specifically, the follicular phase normally may be as short as 5 to 7 days or as long

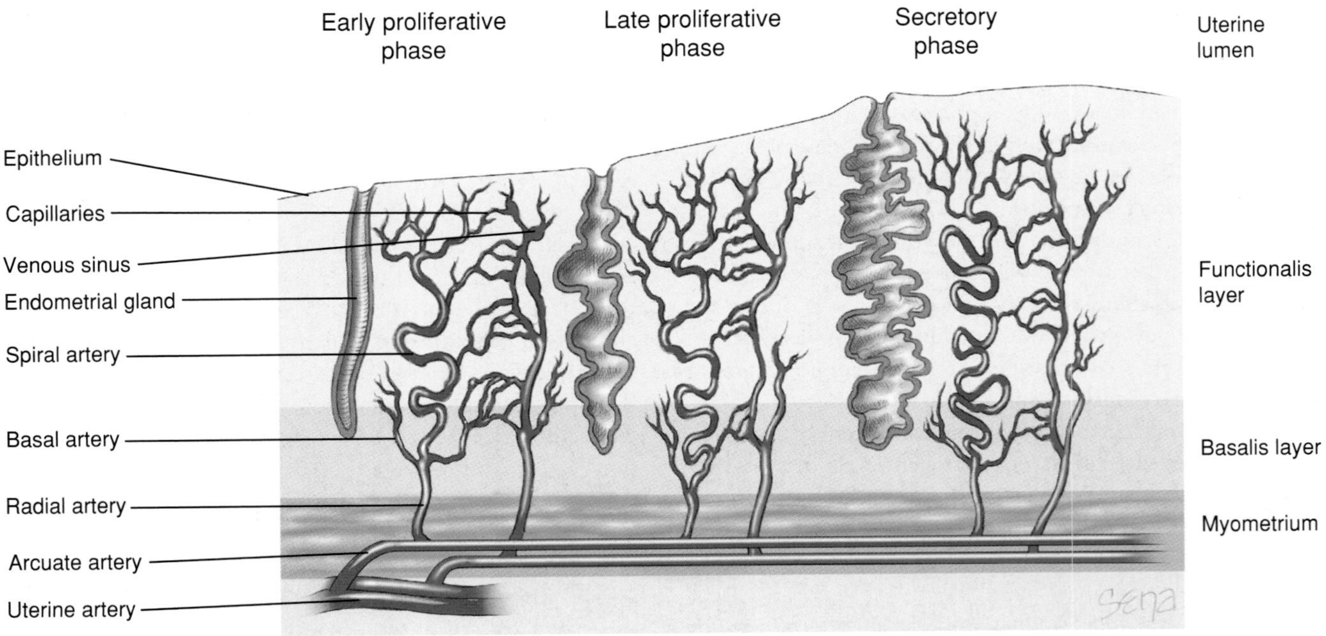

FIGURE 5-4 The endometrium consists of two layers, the functionalis layer and basalis layer. These layers are supplied by the spiral and basal arteries, respectively. Numerous glands also span these layers. As the menstrual cycle progresses, greater coiling of the spiral arteries and increased gland folding can be seen. Near the end of the menstrual cycle (day 27), the coiled arteries constrict, depriving the functionalis layer of its blood supply and leading to necrosis and sloughing of this layer.

as 21 to 30 days. In contrast, the luteal or secretory postovulatory phase of the cycle is remarkably constant at 12 to 14 days.

Secretory or Postovulatory Endometrial Phase

During the early secretory phase, endometrial dating is based on glandular epithelium histology. After ovulation, the estrogen-primed endometrium responds to rising progesterone levels in a highly predictable manner. By day 17, glycogen accumulates in the basal portion of glandular epithelium, creating subnuclear vacuoles and pseudostratification. This is the first sign of ovulation that is histologically evident. It is likely the result of direct progesterone action through receptors expressed in glandular cells (Mote, 2000). On day 18, vacuoles move to the apical portion of the secretory nonciliated cells. By day 19, these cells begin to secrete glycoprotein and mucopolysaccharide contents into the lumen (Hafez, 1975). Glandular cell mitosis ceases with secretory activity on day 19 due to rising progesterone levels, which antagonize the mitotic effects of estrogen. Estradiol action is also decreased because of glandular expression of the type 2 isoform of 17β-hydroxysteroid dehydrogenase. This converts estradiol to the less active estrone (Casey, 1996).

Dating in the mid- to late-secretory phase relies on endometrial stromal changes. On days 21 to 24, the stroma becomes edematous. On days 22 to 25, stromal cells surrounding the spiral arterioles begin to enlarge, and stromal mitosis becomes apparent. Days 23 to 28 are characterized by predecidual cells, which surround spiral arterioles.

An important feature of secretory-phase endometrium between days 22 and 25 is striking changes associated with predecidual transformation of the upper two thirds of the functionalis layer. The glands exhibit extensive coiling, and luminal secretions become visible. Changes within the endometrium also can mark the so-called window of implantation seen on days 20 to 24. Epithelial surface cells show decreased microvilli and cilia but appearance of luminal protrusions on the apical cell surface (Nikas, 2003). These pinopodes are important in preparation for blastocyst implantation. They also coincide with changes in the surface glycocalyx that allow acceptance of a blastocyst (Aplin, 2003).

The secretory phase is also highlighted by the continuing growth and development of the spiral arteries. Boyd and Hamilton (1970) emphasized the extraordinary importance of the endometrial spiral or coiled arteries. They arise from the radial arteries, which are myometrial branches of the arcuate and ultimately, uterine vessels (see Fig. 5-4). The morphological and functional properties of spiral arteries are unique and essential for establishing blood flow changes to permit either menstruation or implantation. During endometrial growth, spiral arteries lengthen at a rate appreciably greater than the rate of endometrial tissue thickening (Fig. 5-5). This growth discordance obliges even greater coiling of the already spiraling vessels. Spiral artery development reflects a marked induction of angiogenesis, consisting of widespread vessel sprouting and extension. Perrot-Applanat and associates (1988) described progesterone and estrogen receptors in the smooth muscle cells of the uterus and spiral arteries. Such rapid angiogenesis is regulated, in part, through estrogen- and progesterone-regulated synthesis of VEGF (Ancelin, 2002; Chennazhi, 2009).

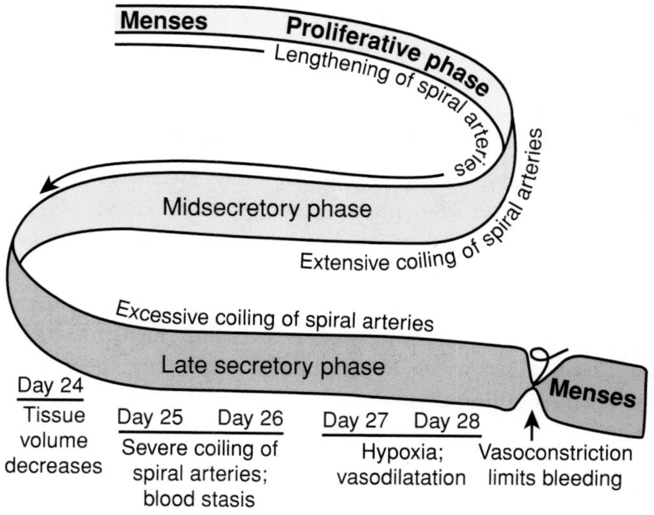

FIGURE 5-5 The spiral arteries of human endometrium are modified during the ovulatory cycle. Initially, blood flow changes through these vessels aid endometrial growth. Excessive coiling and blood flow stasis coincide with regression of corpus luteum function and lead to a decline in endometrial tissue volume. Finally, spiral artery coiling leads to endometrial hypoxia and necrosis. Before endometrial bleeding, intense spiral artery vasospasm serves to limit blood loss during menses.

Menstruation

The midluteal–secretory phase of the endometrial cycle is a critical branch point in endometrial development and differentiation. With corpus luteum rescue and continued progesterone secretion, the decidualization process continues. If luteal progesterone production decreases with luteolysis, events leading to menstruation are initiated (Critchley, 2006; Thiruchelvam, 2013).

A notable histological characteristic of late premenstrual-phase endometrium is stromal infiltration by neutrophils, giving a pseudoinflammatory appearance to the tissue. These cells infiltrate primarily on the day or two immediately preceding menses onset. The endometrial stromal and epithelial cells produce interleukin-8 (IL-8), a chemotactic–activating factor for neutrophils (Arici, 1993). Similarly, monocyte chemotactic protein-1 (MCP-1) is synthesized by endometrium and promotes monocyte recruitment (Arici, 1995).

Leukocyte infiltration is considered key to both endometrial extracellular matrix breakdown and repair of the functionalis layer. The term "inflammatory tightrope" refers to the ability of macrophages to assume phenotypes that vary from proinflammatory and phagocytic to immunosuppressive and reparative. These are likely relevant to menstruation, in which tissue breakdown and restoration occur simultaneously (Evans, 2012). Invading leukocytes secrete enzymes that are members of the matrix metalloprotease (MMP) family. These add to the proteases already produced by endometrial stromal cells and effectively initiate matrix degradation. This phenomenon has been proposed to initiate the events leading to menstruation (Dong, 2002). As tissue shedding is completed, microenvironment-regulated changes in macrophage phenotype promote repair and resolution (Evans, 2012; Thiruchelvam, 2013).

Anatomical Events During Menstruation. The classic study by Markee (1940) described tissue and vascular changes in endometrium before menstruation. First, there are marked changes in endometrial blood flow essential for menstruation. With endometrial regression, spiral artery coiling becomes sufficiently severe that resistance to blood flow increases strikingly, causing endometrial hypoxia. Resultant stasis is the primary cause of endometrial ischemia and tissue degeneration (see Fig. 5-5). Vasoconstriction precedes menstruation and is the most striking and constant event observed in the cycle. Intense spiral artery vasoconstriction also serves to limit menstrual blood loss. Blood flow appears to be regulated in an endocrine manner by sex steroid hormone–induced modifications of a paracrine-mediated vasoactive peptide system as described subsequently.

Prostaglandins and Menstruation. Progesterone withdrawal increases expression of cyclooxygenase 2 (COX-2), also called prostaglandin synthase 2, to synthesize prostaglandins. Withdrawal also decreases expression of 15-hydroxyprostaglandin dehydrogenase (PGDH), which degrades prostaglandins (Casey, 1980, 1989). The net result is increased prostaglandin production by endometrial stromal cells and increased prostaglandin-receptor density on blood vessels and surrounding cells.

A role for prostaglandins—especially vasoconstricting $PGF_{2\alpha}$—in menstruation initiation has been suggested (Abel, 2002). Large amounts of prostaglandins are present in menstrual blood. $PGF_{2\alpha}$ administration to nonpregnant women prompts menstruation and symptoms that mimic dysmenorrhea. Painful menstruation is common and likely caused by myometrial contractions and uterine ischemia. This response is believed to be mediated by $PGF_{2\alpha}$-induced spiral artery vasoconstriction that causes the uppermost endometrial zones to become hypoxic. The hypoxic environment is a potent inducer of angiogenesis and vascular permeability factors such as VEGF. Prostaglandins serve an important function in the event cascade leading to menstruation that includes vasoconstriction, myometrial contractions, and upregulation of proinflammatory responses.

Activation of Lytic Mechanisms. Following vasoconstriction and endometrial cytokine changes, protease activation within stromal cells and leukocyte invasion is required to degrade the endometrial interstitial matrix. Matrix metalloproteases—MMP-1 and MMP-3—are released from stromal cells and may activate other neutrophilic proteases such as MMP-8 and MMP-9.

Origin of Menstrual Blood. Menstrual bleeding is appreciably arterial rather than venous bleeding. Endometrial bleeding appears to follow rupture of a spiral arteriole and consequent hematoma formation. With a hematoma, the superficial endometrium is distended and ruptures. Subsequently, fissures develop in the adjacent functionalis layer, and blood and tissue fragments are sloughed. Hemorrhage stops with arteriolar constriction. Changes that accompany partial tissue necrosis also serve to seal vessel tips.

The endometrial surface is restored by growth of flanges, or collars, that form the everted free ends of the endometrial glands (Markee, 1940). These flanges increase in diameter very rapidly, and epithelial continuity is reestablished by fusion of the edges of these sheets of migrating cells.

Interval between Menses. The modal interval of menstruation is considered to be 28 days, but variation is considerable among women, as well as in the cycle lengths of a given woman. Marked differences in the intervals between menstrual cycles are not necessarily indicative of infertility. Arey (1939) analyzed 12 studies comprising approximately 20,000 calendar records from 1500 women. He concluded that there is no evidence of perfect menstrual cycle regularity. Among average adult women, a third of cycles departed by more than 2 days from the mean of all cycle lengths. In his analysis of 5322 cycles in 485 normal women, an average interval of 28.4 days was estimated.

THE DECIDUA

This is a specialized, highly modified endometrium of pregnancy. It is essential for *hemochorial placentation*, that is, one in which maternal blood contacts trophoblast. This relationship requires trophoblast invasion, and considerable research has focused on the interaction between decidual cells and invading trophoblasts. *Decidualization*, that is, transformation of secretory endometrium to decidua, is dependent on estrogen and progesterone and factors secreted by the implanting blastocyst. The special relationship that exists between the decidua and the invading trophoblast seemingly defies the laws of transplantation immunology. The success of this unique semiallograft not only is of great scientific interest but may involve processes that harbor insights leading to more successful transplantation surgery and perhaps even immunological treatment of neoplasia (Billingham, 1986; Lala, 2002).

Decidual Structure

The decidua is classified into three parts based on anatomical location. Decidua directly beneath blastocyst implantation is modified by trophoblast invasion and becomes the *decidua basalis*. The *decidua capsularis* overlies the enlarging blastocyst and initially separates the conceptus from the rest of the uterine cavity (Fig. 5-6). This portion is most prominent during the second month of pregnancy and consists of decidual cells covered by a single layer of flattened epithelial cells. Internally, it contacts the avascular, extraembryonic fetal membrane—the chorion laeve. The remainder of the uterus is lined by *decidua parietalis*. During early pregnancy, there is a space between the decidua capsularis and parietalis because the gestational sac does not fill the entire uterine cavity. By 14 to 16 weeks' gestation, the expanding sac has enlarged to completely fill the uterine cavity. The resulting apposition of the decidua capsularis and parietalis creates the *decidua vera*, and the uterine cavity is functionally obliterated.

In early pregnancy, the decidua begins to thicken, eventually attaining a depth of 5 to 10 mm. With magnification, furrows and numerous small openings, representing the mouths of uterine glands, can be detected. Later in pregnancy, the decidua becomes thinner, presumably because of pressure exerted by the expanding uterine contents.

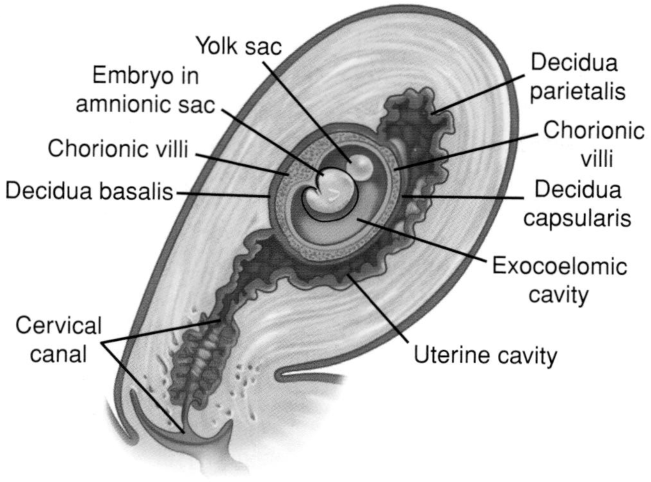

FIGURE 5-6 Three portions of the decidua—the basalis, capsularis, and parietalis—are illustrated.

The decidua parietalis and basalis are composed of three layers. There is a surface or compact zone—*zona compacta*; a middle portion or spongy zone—*zona spongiosa*—with remnants of glands and numerous small blood vessels; and a basal zone—*zona basalis*. The zona compacta and spongiosa together form the *zona functionalis*. The basal zone remains after delivery and gives rise to new endometrium.

Decidual Reaction

In human pregnancy, the decidual reaction is completed only with blastocyst implantation. Predecidual changes, however, commence first during the midluteal phase in endometrial stromal cells adjacent to the spiral arteries and arterioles. Thereafter, they spread in waves throughout the uterine endometrium and then from the implantation site. The endometrial stromal cells enlarge to form polygonal or round decidual cells. The nuclei become round and vesicular, and the cytoplasm becomes clear, slightly basophilic, and surrounded by a translucent membrane. Each mature decidual cell becomes surrounded by a pericellular membrane. Thus, the human decidual cells clearly build walls around themselves and possibly around the fetus. The pericellular matrix surrounding the decidual cells may allow attachment of cytotrophoblasts through cellular adhesion molecules. The cell membrane also may provide decidual cell protection against selected cytotrophoblastic proteases.

Decidual Blood Supply

As a consequence of implantation, the blood supply to the decidua capsularis is lost as the embryo-fetus grows. Blood supply to the decidua parietalis through spiral arteries persists. These arteries retain a smooth-muscle wall and endothelium and thereby remain responsive to vasoactive agents.

In contrast, the spiral arterial system supplying the decidua basalis directly beneath the implanting blastocyst, and ultimately the intervillous space, is altered remarkably. These spiral arterioles and arteries are invaded by cytotrophoblasts. During this process, the vessel walls in the basalis are destroyed. Only a shell without smooth muscle or endothelial cells remains. Importantly, as a result, these vascular conduits of maternal blood—which become the uteroplacental vessels—are not responsive to vasoactive agents. Conversely, the fetal chorionic vessels, which transport blood between the placenta and the fetus, contain smooth muscle and thus do respond to vasoactive agents.

Decidual Histology

Early in pregnancy, the zona spongiosa of the decidua consists of large distended glands, often exhibiting marked hyperplasia and separated by minimal stroma. At first, the glands are lined by typical cylindrical uterine epithelium with abundant secretory activity that contributes to blastocyst nourishment. As pregnancy progresses, the epithelium gradually becomes cuboidal or even flattened and later degenerates and sloughs to a greater extent into the gland lumens. With advanced pregnancy, the glandular elements largely disappear. In comparing the decidua parietalis at 16 weeks' gestation with the early proliferative endometrium of a nonpregnant woman, there is marked hypertrophy but only slight hyperplasia of the endometrial stroma during decidual transformation.

The decidua basalis contributes to formation of the placental basal plate (Fig. 5-7). It differs histologically from the decidua parietalis in two important respects. First, the spongy zone of the decidua basalis consists mainly of arteries and widely dilated veins, and by term, glands have virtually disappeared. Second,

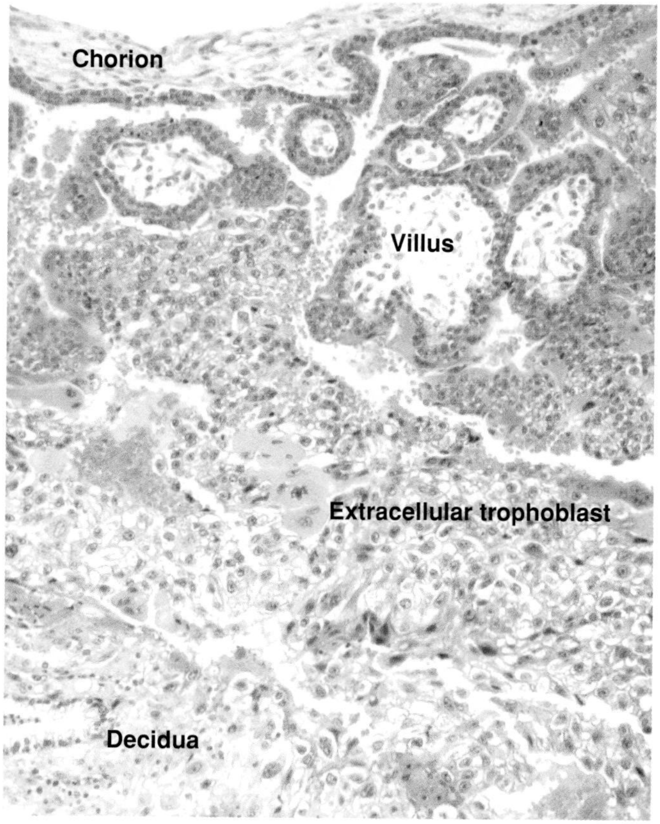

FIGURE 5-7 Section through a junction of chorion, villi, and decidua basalis in early first-trimester pregnancy. (Photograph contributed by Dr. Kurt Benirschke.)

the decidua basalis is invaded by many interstitial trophoblast cells and trophoblastic giant cells. Although most abundant in the decidua, the giant cells commonly penetrate the upper myometrium. Their number and invasiveness can be so extensive as to resemble choriocarcinoma.

The Nitabuch layer is a zone of fibrinoid degeneration in which invading trophoblasts meet the decidua basalis. If the decidua is defective, as in placenta accreta, the Nitabuch layer is usually absent (Chap. 41, p. 804). There is also a more superficial, but inconsistent, deposition of fibrin—*Rohr stria*—at the bottom of the intervillous space and surrounding the anchoring villi. McCombs and Craig (1964) found that decidual necrosis is a normal phenomenon in the first and probably second trimesters. Thus, necrotic decidua obtained through curettage after spontaneous abortion in the first trimester should not necessarily be interpreted as either a cause or an effect of the pregnancy loss.

Both deciduas contain numerous cell types whose composition varies with gestational stage (Loke, 1995). The primary cellular components are the true decidual cells, which differentiated from the endometrial stromal cells, and numerous maternal bone marrow–derived cells.

Early in pregnancy, a striking abundance of large, granular lymphocytes termed decidual natural killer (NK) cells are present in the decidua. In peripheral blood, there are two subsets of NK cells. Approximately 90 percent are highly cytolytic. Ten percent show less cytolytic ability but increased cytokine secretion. In contrast to peripheral blood, 95 percent of NK cells in decidua secrete cytokines, and about half of these unique cells also express angiogenic factors. These decidua NK cells likely play an important role in trophoblast invasion and vasculogenesis.

Decidual Prolactin

In addition to placental development, the decidua potentially provides other functions. The decidua is the source of prolactin that is present in enormous amounts in amnionic fluid (Golander, 1978; Riddick, 1979). *Decidual prolactin* is not to be confused with placental lactogen (hPL), which is produced only by syncytiotrophoblast. Rather, decidual prolactin is a product of the same gene that encodes for anterior pituitary prolactin. And although the amino-acid sequence of prolactin in both tissues is identical, an alternative promoter is used within the prolactin gene to initiate transcription in decidua (Telgmann, 1998). This may explain the different mechanisms that regulate expression in the decidua versus pituitary (Christian, 2002a,b).

Prolactin preferentially enters amnionic fluid, and little enters maternal blood. Consequently, prolactin levels in amnionic fluid are extraordinarily high and may reach 10,000 ng/mL at 20 to 24 weeks' gestation (Tyson, 1972). This compares with fetal serum levels of 350 ng/mL and maternal serum levels of 150 to 200 ng/mL. As a result, decidual prolactin is a classic example of paracrine function between maternal and fetal tissues.

The exact physiological roles of decidual prolactin are still unknown. Its action is mediated by the relative expression of two unique prolactin receptors and by the amount of intact or full-length prolactin protein compared with the truncated 16-kDa form (Jabbour, 2001). Receptor expression has been demonstrated in decidua, chorionic cytotrophoblasts, amnionic epithelium, and syncytiotrophoblast (Maaskant, 1996). There are several possible roles for decidual prolactin. First, most or all of this protein hormone enters amnionic fluid. Thus, it may serve in transmembrane solute and water transport and in amnionic fluid volume maintenance. Second, there are prolactin receptors in several bone marrow-derived immune cells, and prolactin may stimulate T cells in an autocrine or paracrine manner (Pellegrini, 1992). This raises the possibility that decidual prolactin may act in regulating immunological functions during pregnancy. Prolactin may play a role in angiogenesis regulation during implantation. Last, decidual prolactin has been shown in the mouse to have a protective function by repressing expression of genes detrimental to pregnancy maintenance (Bao, 2007).

Regulation of decidual prolactin is not clearly defined. Most agents known to inhibit or stimulate pituitary prolactin secretion—including dopamine, dopamine agonists, and thyrotropin-releasing hormone—do not alter decidual prolactin secretion either in vivo or in vitro. Brosens and colleagues (2000) demonstrated that progestins act synergistically with cyclic adenosine monophosphate on endometrial stromal cells in culture to increase prolactin expression. This suggests that the level of progesterone receptor expression may determine the decidualization process, at least as marked by prolactin production. Conversely, various cytokines and growth factors—endothelin-1, IL-1, IL-2, and epidermal growth factor—decrease decidual prolactin secretion (Chao, 1994; Frank, 1995). Studies in decidualized human endometrial cells in culture have led to identification of several transcription factors that regulate decidual prolactin (Jiang, 2011; Lynch, 2009).

IMPLANTATION AND EARLY TROPHOBLAST FORMATION

The fetus is dependent on the placenta for pulmonary, hepatic, and renal functions. These are accomplished through the unique anatomical relationship of the placenta and its uterine interface. Maternal blood spurts from uteroplacental vessels into the placental intervillous space and bathes the outer syncytiotrophoblast. This allows exchange of gases, nutrients, and other substances with fetal capillary blood within the villous core. Thus, fetal and maternal blood are not normally mixed in this hemochorial placenta. There is also a paracrine system that links mother and fetus through the anatomical and biochemical juxtaposition of the maternal decidua parietalis and the extraembryonic chorion laeve, which is fetal. This is an extraordinarily important arrangement for communication between fetus and mother and for maternal immunological acceptance of the conceptus (Guzeloglu-Kayisli, 2009).

Fertilization and Implantation

With ovulation, the secondary oocyte and adhered cells of the cumulus-oocyte complex are freed from the ovary. Although technically this mass of cells is released into the peritoneal cavity, the oocyte is quickly engulfed by the fallopian tube infundibulum. Further transport through the tube is accomplished by directional movement of cilia and tubal peristalsis. Fertilization, which normally occurs in the oviduct, must take place within a few hours, and no more than a day after ovulation. Because of this narrow opportunity window, spermatozoa must be present in the fallopian tube at the time of oocyte arrival. Almost all pregnancies result when intercourse occurs during the 2 days preceding or on the day of ovulation. Thus, postovulatory and postfertilization developmental ages are similar.

Steps of fertilization are highly complex. Molecular mechanisms allow spermatozoa to pass between follicular cells; through the zona pellucida, which is a thick glycoprotein layer surrounding the oocyte cell membrane; and into the oocyte cytoplasm. Fusion of the two nuclei and intermingling of maternal and paternal chromosomes creates the *zygote*. These steps are reviewed by Primakoff and Myles (2002).

Early human development is described by days or weeks postfertilization, that is, postconceptional. By contrast, in most chapters of this book, clinical pregnancy dating is calculated from the start of the last menses. As discussed earlier, the follicular phase length is more variable than the luteal phase. Thus, 1 week postfertilization corresponds to approximately 3 weeks from the last menstrual period in women with regular 28-day cycles.

The Zygote

After fertilization, the zygote—a diploid cell with 46 chromosomes—undergoes cleavage, and zygote cells produced by this division are called *blastomeres* (Fig. 5-8). In the two-cell zygote, the blastomeres and polar body continue to be surrounded by the zona pellucida. The zygote undergoes slow cleavage for 3 days while still within the fallopian tube. As the blastomeres continue to divide, a solid mulberry-like ball of cells—the *morula*—is produced. The morula enters the uterine cavity about 3 days after fertilization. Gradual accumulation of fluid between the morula cells leads to formation of the early *blastocyst*.

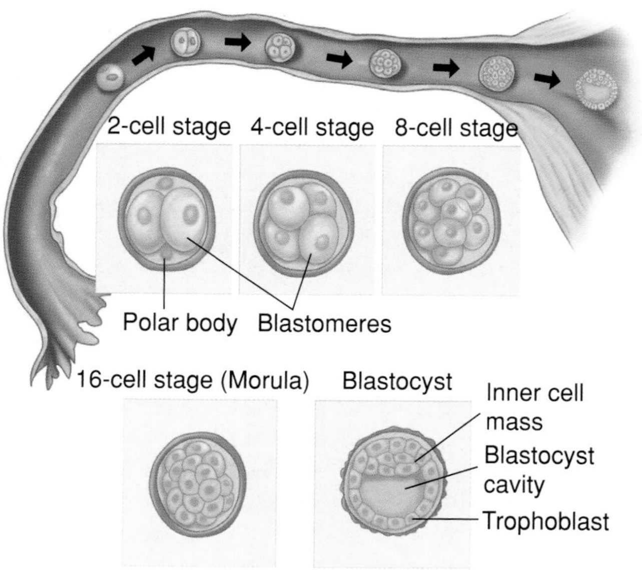

FIGURE 5-8 Zygote cleavage and blastocyst formation. The morula period begins at the 12- to 16-cell stage and ends when the blastocyst forms, which occurs when there are 50 to 60 blastomeres present. The polar bodies, shown in the 2-cell stage, are small nonfunctional cells that soon degenerate.

The Blastocyst

As early as 4 to 5 days after fertilization, the 58-cell blastula differentiates into five embryo-producing cells—the *inner cell mass*, and 53 cells destined to form *trophoblast* (Hertig, 1962). In a 58-cell blastocyst, the outer cells, called the *trophectoderm*, can be distinguished from the inner cell mass that forms the embryo (see Fig. 5-8).

Interestingly, the 107-cell blastocyst is found to be no larger than the earlier cleavage stages, despite the accumulated fluid. It measures approximately 0.155 mm in diameter, which is similar to the size of the initial postfertilization zygote. At this stage, the eight formative, embryo-producing cells are surrounded by 99 trophoblastic cells. And, the blastocyst is released from the zona pellucida secondary to secretion of specific proteases from the secretory-phase endometrial glands (O'Sullivan, 2002).

Release from the zona pellucida allows blastocyst-produced cytokines and hormones to directly influence endometrial receptivity (Lindhard, 2002). IL-1α and IL-1β are secreted by the blastocyst, and these cytokines likely directly influence the endometrium. Embryos also have been shown to secrete hCG, which may influence endometrial receptivity (Licht, 2001; Lobo, 2001). The receptive endometrium is thought to respond by producing leukemia inhibitory factor (LIF) and colony-stimulating factor-1 (CSF-1). These serve to increase trophoblast protease production. This degrades selected endometrial extracellular matrix proteins and allows trophoblast invasion. Thus, embryo "hatching" is a critical step toward successful pregnancy as it allows association of trophoblasts with endometrial epithelial cells and permits release of trophoblast-produced hormones into the uterine cavity.

Blastocyst Implantation

Six or 7 days after fertilization, the embryo implants the uterine wall. This process can be divided into three phases: (1) apposition—initial contact of the blastocyst to the uterine wall; (2) adhesion—increased physical contact between the blastocyst and uterine epithelium; and (3) invasion—penetration and invasion of syncytiotrophoblast and cytotrophoblasts into the endometrium, inner third of the myometrium, and uterine vasculature.

Successful implantation requires a receptive endometrium appropriately primed with estrogen and progesterone by the corpus luteum. Such uterine receptivity is limited to days 20 to 24 of the cycle. Adherence is mediated by cell-surface receptors at the implantation site that interact with blastocyst receptors (Carson, 2002; Lessey, 2002; Lindhard, 2002; Paria, 2002). If the blastocyst approaches the endometrium after cycle day 24, the potential for adhesion is diminished because antiadhesive glycoprotein synthesis prevents receptor interactions (Navot, 1991).

At the time of its interaction with the endometrium, the blastocyst is composed of 100 to 250 cells. The blastocyst loosely adheres to the endometrial epithelium by apposition. This most commonly occurs on the upper posterior uterine wall. Attachment of the blastocyst trophectoderm to the endometrial surface by apposition and adherence appears to be closely regulated by paracrine interactions between these two tissues.

Successful endometrial blastocyst adhesion involves modification in expression of cellular adhesion molecules (CAMs). The integrins—one of four families of CAMs—are cell-surface receptors that mediate cell adhesion to extracellular matrix proteins (Lessey, 2002). Great diversity of cell binding to several different extracellular matrix proteins is possible by differential regulation of the integrin receptors. Endometrial integrins are hormonally regulated, and a specific set of integrins is expressed at implantation (Lessey, 1996). Specifically, $\alpha V\beta 3$ and $\alpha 4\beta 1$ integrins expressed on endometrial epithelium are considered a receptivity marker for blastocyst attachment. Aberrant expression of $\alpha V\beta 3$ has been associated with infertility (Lessey, 1995). Recognition-site blockade on integrins for binding to extracellular matrix molecules such as fibronectin will prevent blastocyst attachment (Kaneko, 2013).

The Trophoblast

Human placental formation begins with the trophectoderm, which appears at the morula stage. It gives rise to a trophoblast cell layer encircling the blastocyst. From then until term, the trophoblast plays a critical part at the fetal-maternal interface. Trophoblast exhibits the most variable structure, function, and developmental pattern of all placental components. Its invasiveness promotes implantation, its nutritional role for the conceptus is reflected in its name, and its endocrine organ function is essential to maternal physiological adaptations and to pregnancy maintenance.

Trophoblast Differentiation

By the eighth day postfertilization, after initial implantation, the trophoblast has differentiated into an outer multinucleated syncytium—primitive *syncytiotrophoblast*, and an inner layer of primitive mononuclear cells—*cytotrophoblasts* (Fig. 5-9). The latter are germinal cells for the syncytium. Each cytotrophoblast has a well-demarcated cell border, a single nucleus, and ability to undergo DNA synthesis and mitosis (Arnholdt, 1991). These are lacking in the syncytiotrophoblast. It is so named because instead of individual cells, it has an amorphous cytoplasm without cell borders, nuclei that are multiple and diverse in size and shape, and a continuous syncytial lining. This configuration aids transport.

After implantation is complete, trophoblast further differentiate along two main pathways, giving rise to villous and extravillous trophoblast. As shown in Figure 5-10, both pathways create populations of trophoblast cells that have distinct functions (Loke, 1995). The *villous trophoblast* gives rise to the chorionic villi, which primarily transport oxygen, nutrients, and other compounds between the fetus and mother. Extravillous trophoblasts migrate into the decidua and myometrium and also penetrate maternal vasculature, thus coming into contact with various maternal cell types (Pijnenborg, 1994). Extravillous trophoblasts are thus further classified as *interstitial trophoblasts* and *endovascular trophoblasts*. The interstitial trophoblasts invade the decidua and eventually penetrate the myometrium to form placental bed giant cells. These trophoblasts also surround spiral arteries. The endovascular trophoblasts penetrate the spiral artery lumens (Pijnenborg, 1983). These are both discussed in greater detail in subsequent sections.

Early Trophoblast Invasion

After gentle erosion between epithelial cells of the surface endometrium, invading trophoblasts burrow deeper. By the 10th day, the blastocyst becomes totally encased within the endometrium. The mechanisms leading to trophoblast invasion are similar to those of metastasizing malignant cells and are discussed further on page 93.

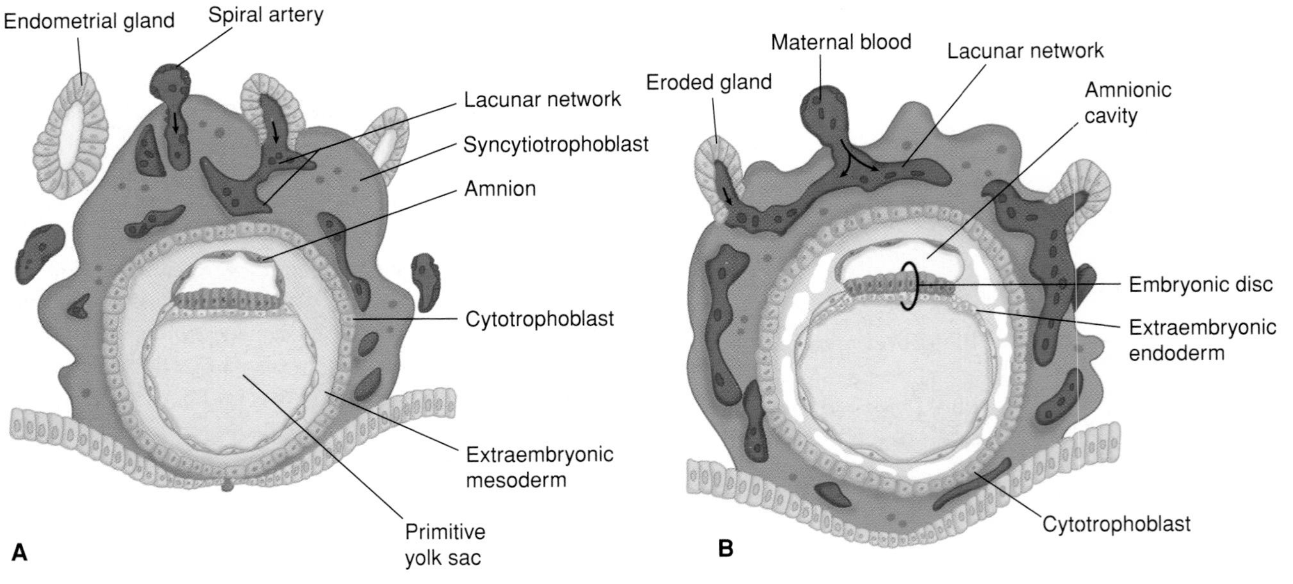

FIGURE 5-9 Drawing of sections through implanted blastocysts. **A.** At 10 days. **B.** At 12 days after fertilization. This stage is characterized by the intercommunication of the lacunae filled with maternal blood. Note in **(B)** that large cavities have appeared in the extraembryonic mesoderm, forming the beginning of the extraembryonic coelom. Also note that extraembryonic endodermal cells have begun to form on the inside of the primitive yolk sac. (Adapted from Moore, 1988.)

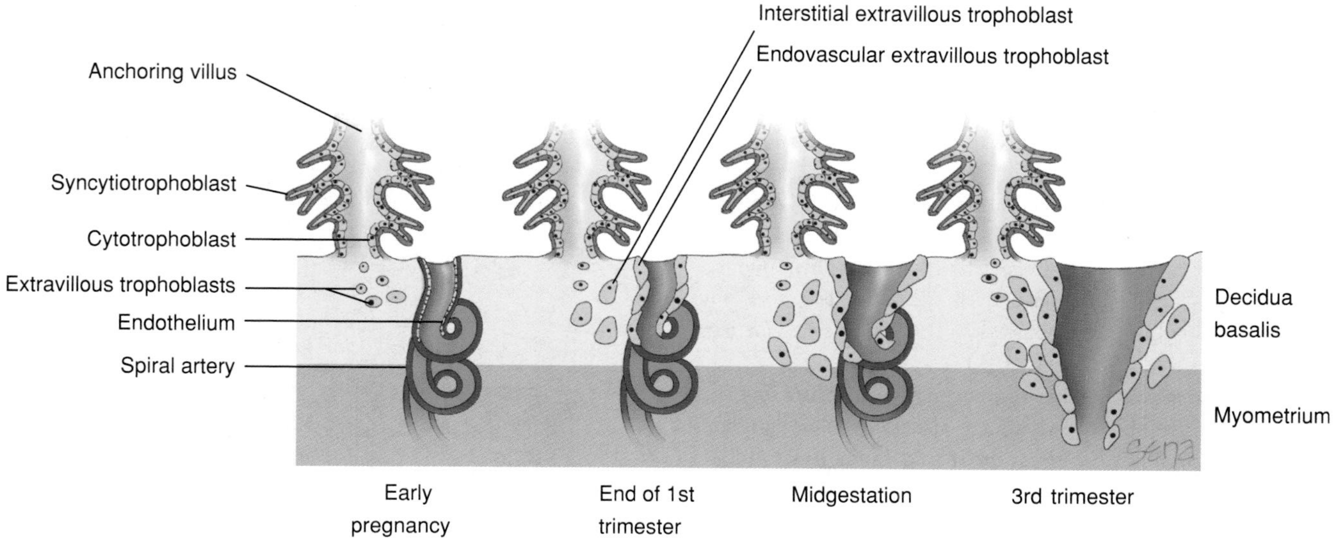

FIGURE 5-10 Extravillous trophoblasts are found outside the villus and can be subdivided into endovascular and interstitial categories. Endovascular trophoblasts invade and transform spiral arteries during pregnancy to create low-resistance blood flow that is characteristic of the placenta. Interstitial trophoblasts invade the decidua and surround spiral arteries.

At 9 days of development, the blastocyst wall facing the uterine lumen is a single layer of flattened cells (see Fig. 5-9A). The opposite, thicker wall comprises two zones—the trophoblasts and the embryo-forming inner cell mass. As early as 7½ days after fertilization, the inner cell mass or embryonic disc is differentiated into a thick plate of primitive ectoderm and an underlying layer of endoderm. Some small cells appear between the embryonic disc and the trophoblast and enclose a space that will become the amnionic cavity.

Embryonic mesenchyme first appears as isolated cells within the blastocyst cavity. When the cavity is completely lined with this mesoderm, it is termed the chorionic vesicle, and its membrane, now called the chorion, is composed of trophoblasts and mesenchyme. Some mesenchymal cells eventually will condense to form the body stalk. This stalk joins the embryo to the nutrient chorion and later develops into the umbilical cord. The body stalk can be recognized at an early stage at the caudal end of the embryonic disc (Fig. 7-4, 129).

Lacunae Formation within the Syncytiotrophoblast

As the embryo enlarges, more maternal decidua basalis is invaded by syncytiotrophoblast. Beginning approximately 12 days after conception, the syncytiotrophoblast is permeated by a system of intercommunicating channels called trophoblastic lacunae. After invasion of superficial decidual capillary walls, lacunae become filled with maternal blood (see Figs. 5-9B and 5-11). At the same time, the decidual reaction intensifies in the surrounding stroma. This is characterized by decidual stromal cell enlargement and glycogen storage.

Placental Organization

Chorionic Villi

With deeper blastocyst invasion into the decidua, the extravillous cytotrophoblasts give rise to solid primary villi composed of a cytotrophoblast core covered by syncytiotrophoblast. These arise from buds of cytotrophoblast that protrude into the primitive syncytium before 12 days postfertilization. As the lacunae join, a complicated labyrinth is formed that is partitioned by these solid cytotrophoblastic columns. The trophoblast-lined labyrinthine channels form the intervillous space, and the solid cellular columns form the *primary villous stalks*. The villi initially are located over the entire blastocyst surface. They later disappear except over the most deeply implanted portion, which is destined to form the placenta.

Beginning on approximately the 12th day after fertilization, mesenchymal cords derived from extraembryonic mesoderm

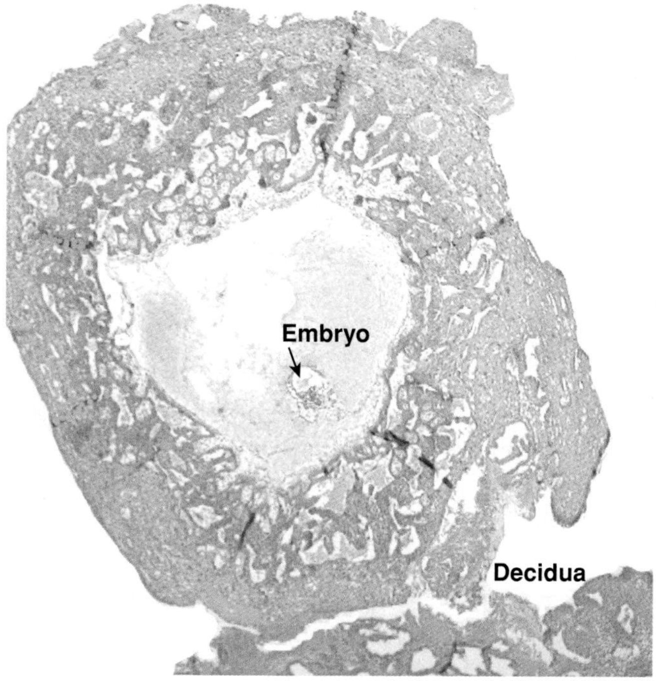

FIGURE 5-11 Early implantation of a conceptus. (Photograph contributed by Dr. Kurt Benirschke.)

invade the solid trophoblast columns. These form *secondary villi*. Once angiogenesis begins in the mesenchymal cores, *tertiary villi* are formed. Although maternal venous sinuses are tapped early in implantation, maternal arterial blood does not enter the intervillous space until around day 15. By approximately the 17th day, however, fetal blood vessels are functional, and a placental circulation is established. The fetal–placental circulation is completed when the blood vessels of the embryo are connected with chorionic vessels. In some villi, angiogenesis fails from lack of circulation. They can be seen normally, but the most striking exaggeration of this process is seen with hydatidiform mole (Fig. 20-1, p. 397).

Villi are covered by an outer layer of syncytium and an inner layer of cytotrophoblasts, which are also known as Langhans cells. Cytotrophoblast proliferation at the villous tips produces the trophoblastic cell columns that form anchoring villi. They are not invaded by fetal mesenchyme, and they are anchored to the decidua at the basal plate. Thus, the base of the intervillous space faces the maternal side and consists of cytotrophoblasts from cell columns, the covering shell of syncytiotrophoblast, and maternal decidua of the basal plate. The base of the chorionic plate forms the roof of the intervillous space. It consists of two layers of trophoblasts externally and fibrous mesoderm internally. The "definitive" chorionic plate is formed by 8 to 10 weeks as the amnionic and primary chorionic plate mesenchyme fuse together. This formation is accomplished by expansion of the amnionic sac, which also surrounds the connective stalk and the allantois and joins these structures to form the umbilical cord (Kaufmann, 1992).

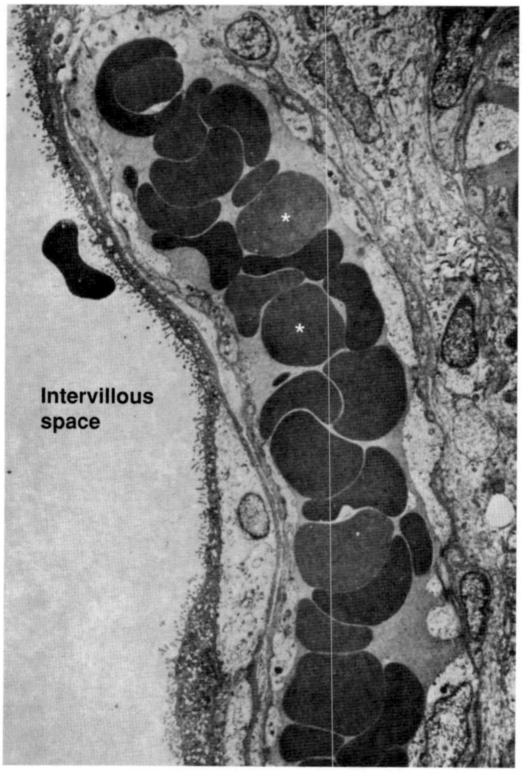

FIGURE 5-12 Electron micrograph of term human placenta villus. A villus capillary filled with red blood cells (*asterisks*) is seen in close proximity to the microvilli border. (From Boyd, 1970, with permission.)

Villus Ultrastructure

Interpretation of the fine structure of the placenta came from electron microscopic studies of Wislocki and Dempsey (1955). There are prominent microvilli on the syncytial surface that correspond to the so-called brush border described by light microscopy. Associated pinocytotic vacuoles and vesicles are related to absorptive and secretory placental functions. Microvilli act to increase surface area in direct contact with maternal blood. This contact between the trophoblast and maternal blood is the defining characteristic of a hemochorial placenta.

The human hemochorial placenta can be subdivided into hemodichorial or hemomonochorial (Enders, 1965). The dichorial type is more prominent during the first trimester of gestation. It consists of the inner layer of the cytotrophoblasts and associated basal lamina, covered by a syncytiotrophoblast layer. Later in gestation the inner layer of cytotrophoblasts is no longer continuous, and by term, there are only scattered cells present (Fig. 5-12). These create a narrower hemomonochorial barrier that aids nutrient and oxygen transport to the fetus.

PLACENTA AND CHORION DEVELOPMENT

Chorion and Decidua Development

In early pregnancy, the villi are distributed over the entire periphery of the chorionic membrane (Fig. 5-13). As the blastocyst with its surrounding trophoblasts grows and expands into the decidua, one pole faces the endometrial cavity. The

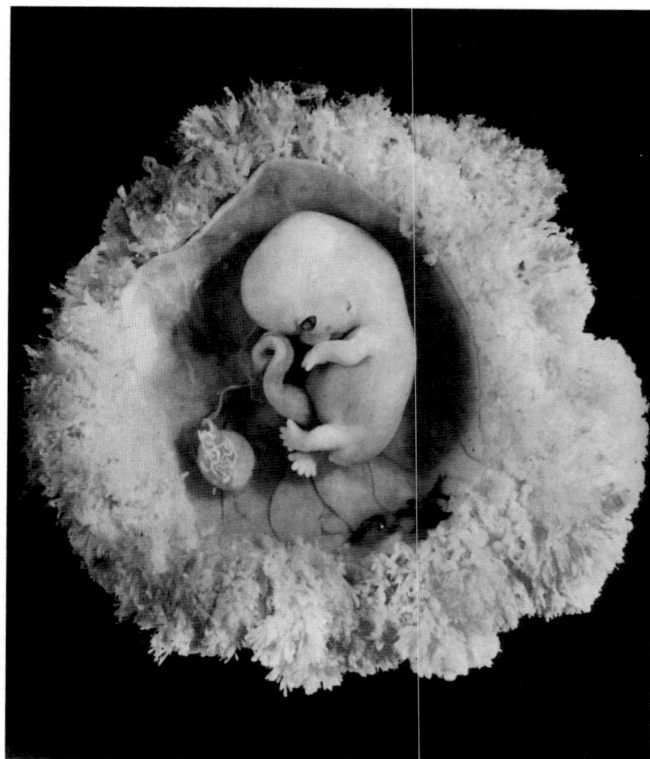
FIGURE 5-13 Photograph of an opened chorionic sac. An early embryo and yolk sac are seen. Note the prominent fringe of chorionic villi. (From Boyd, 1970, with permission.)

opposite pole will form the placenta from villous trophoblasts and anchoring cytotrophoblasts. Chorionic villi in contact with the decidua basalis proliferate to form the chorion frondosum—or leafy chorion—which is the fetal component of the placenta. As growth of embryonic and extraembryonic tissues continues, the blood supply to the chorion facing the endometrial cavity is restricted. Because of this, villi in contact with the decidua capsularis cease to grow and then degenerate. This portion of the chorion becomes the avascular fetal membrane that abuts the decidua parietalis, that is, the chorion laeve—or smooth chorion. This smooth chorion is composed of cytotrophoblasts and fetal mesodermal mesenchyme that survives in a relatively low-oxygen atmosphere.

Until near the end of the third month, the chorion laeve is separated from the amnion by the exocoelomic cavity. Thereafter, they are in intimate contact to form an avascular amniochorion. The chorion laeve is generally more translucent than the amnion and rarely exceeds 1-mm thickness. These two structures are important sites of molecular transfer and metabolic activity. Moreover, they constitute an important paracrine arm of the fetal–maternal communication system.

Maternal Regulation of Trophoblast Invasion and Vascular Growth

During the first half of pregnancy, decidual natural killer cells (dNK) accumulate in the decidua and are found in direct contact with trophoblasts. As described on page 88, these cells lack cytotoxic functions and are able to dampen inflammatory T(H)17 cells. These along with other unique properties distinguish dNK cells from circulating natural killer cells and from natural killer cells in the endometrium before pregnancy (Fu, 2013; Winger, 2013). Recent studies suggest that decidual macrophages play a regulatory role in inhibiting NK cell killing during pregnancy (Co, 2013). This importantly prevents them from recognizing and destroying fetal cells as "foreign." Hanna and colleagues (2006) have elucidated the ability of dNK cells to attract and promote trophoblast invasion into the decidua and promote vascular growth. Decidual NK cells express both IL-8 and interferon-inducible protein-10, which bind to receptors on invasive trophoblast cells to promote their decidual invasion toward the spiral arteries. Decidual NK cells also produce proangiogenic factors, including VEGF and placental growth factor (PlGF), which promote vascular growth in the decidua. In addition, trophoblasts secrete specific chemokines that attract the dNK cells to the maternal-fetal interface. Thus, both cell types simultaneously attract each other.

Trophoblast Invasion of the Endometrium

Extravillous trophoblasts of the first-trimester placenta are highly invasive. They form cell columns that extend from the endometrium to the inner third of the myometrium. Recall that hemochorial placental development requires invasion of endometrium and spiral arteries. This process occurs under low-oxygen conditions, and regulatory factors that are induced under hypoxic conditions contribute in part to invasive trophoblast activation (Soares, 2012). Invasive trophoblasts secrete numerous proteolytic enzymes that digest extracellular matrix and activate proteinases already present in the endometrium. Trophoblasts produce urokinase-type plasminogen activator, which converts plasminogen into the broadly acting serine protease, plasmin. This in turn both degrades matrix proteins and activates matrix metalloproteases. One member of the MMP family, MMP-9, appears to be critical for human trophoblast invasion. The timing and extent of trophoblast invasion is regulated by a balanced interplay between pro- and antiinvasive factors.

The relative ability to invade maternal tissue in early pregnancy compared with limited invasiveness in late pregnancy is controlled by autocrine and paracrine trophoblastic and endometrial factors. Trophoblasts secrete insulin-like growth factor II, which acts in an autocrine manner. It promotes invasion into the endometrium, whereas decidual cells secrete insulin-like growth factor binding-protein type 4, which blocks this autocrine loop. Thus, the degree of trophoblast invasion is controlled by matrix degradation regulation and by factors that cause trophoblast migration.

Low estradiol levels in the first trimester are critical for trophoblast invasion and remodeling of the spiral arteries. Recent studies in nonhuman primates suggest that the increase in second-trimester estradiol levels suppresses and limits vessel remodeling by reducing trophoblast expression of VEGF and specific integrin receptors (Bonagura, 2012). As the extravillous trophoblast differentiates, it gains expression of integrin receptors that recognize the extracellular matrix proteins collagen IV, laminin, and fibronectin. Binding of these extracellular matrix proteins to specific integrin receptors initiates signals that promote trophoblast cell migration and differentiation. As pregnancy advances, increasing estradiol levels repress and thus control the extent of uterine vessel transformation via downregulation of VEGF and integrin receptor expression.

Invasion of Spiral Arteries

One of the most remarkable features of human placental development is the extensive modification of maternal vasculature by trophoblasts, which are by definition of fetal origin. These events occur in the first half of pregnancy and are considered in detail because of their importance to uteroplacental blood flow. They are also integral to some pathological conditions such as preeclampsia, fetal-growth restriction, and preterm birth. Spiral artery modifications are carried out by two populations of extravillous trophoblast—interstitial trophoblasts, which surround the arteries, and endovascular trophoblasts, which penetrate the spiral artery lumen (see Fig. 5-10). Although earlier work has focused on the role of the endovascular trophoblast, interstitial trophoblast function has more recently been investigated (Benirschke, 2012; Pijnenborg, 1983). These interstitial cells constitute a major portion of the placental bed and penetrate the decidua and adjacent myometrium. They aggregate around spiral arteries, and their functions may include vessel preparation for endovascular trophoblast invasion.

Hamilton and Boyd (1966) report that Friedlander in 1870 first described structural changes in spiral arteries. Endovascular trophoblasts first enter the spiral-artery lumens and initially form cellular plugs. They then destroy vascular endothelium via an apoptosis mechanism and invade and modify the vascular media. Thus, fibrinoid material replaces smooth muscle and connective tissue of the vessel media. Spiral arteries later regenerate endothelium. Invading endovascular trophoblasts can extend several centimeters along the vessel lumen, and they must migrate against arterial flow. These vascular changes are not observed in the decidua parietalis, that is, in decidual sites removed from the invading cytotrophoblasts. Of note, invasion by trophoblasts involves only the decidual spiral arteries and not decidual veins.

In their summary of uteroplacental vasculature, Ramsey and Donner (1980) described uteroplacental vessel development as proceeding in two waves or stages. The first wave occurs before 12 weeks' postfertilization and consists of invasion and modification of spiral arteries up to the border between the decidua and myometrium. The second wave is between 12 and 16 weeks and involves some invasion of the intramyometrial segments of spiral arteries. Remodeling converts narrow-lumen, muscular spiral arteries into dilated, low-resistance uteroplacental vessels. Molecular mechanisms of these crucial events, and their significance in the pathogenesis of preeclampsia and fetal-growth restriction, have been reviewed by Kaufmann (2003) and Red-Horse (2006).

Establishment of Maternal Blood Flow

Approximately 1 month after conception, maternal blood enters the intervillous space in fountain-like bursts from the spiral arteries. Blood is propelled outside of the maternal vessels and sweeps over and directly bathes the syncytiotrophoblast. The apical surface of the syncytiotrophoblast consists of a complex microvillous structure that undergoes continual shedding and reformation during pregnancy.

Villus Branching

Although certain villi of the chorion frondosum extend from the chorionic plate to the decidua to serve as anchoring villi, most villi arborize and end freely within the intervillous space. As gestation proceeds, the short, thick, early stem villi branch to form progressively finer subdivisions and greater numbers of increasingly smaller villi (Fig. 5-14). Each of the truncal or main stem villi and their ramifications (rami) constitutes a placental lobule, or cotyledon. Each lobule is supplied with a single truncal branch of the chorionic artery. And each lobule has a single vein so that lobules constitute functional units of placental architecture.

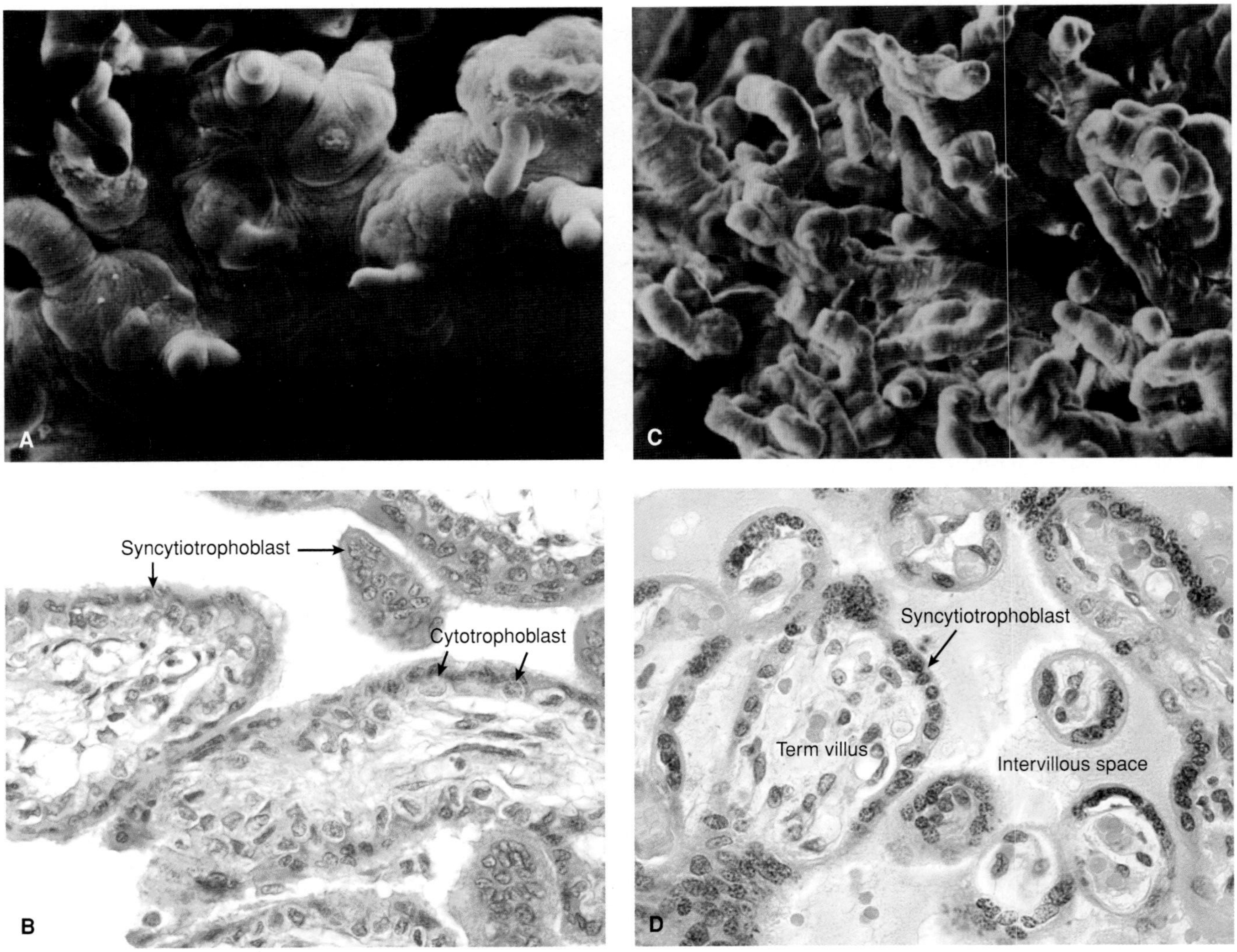

FIGURE 5-14 Electron micrographs **(A, C)** and photomicrographs **(B, D)** of early and late human placentas. **A** and **B.** Limited branching of villi is seen in this early placenta. **C** and **D.** With placenta maturation, increasing villous arborization is seen, and villous capillaries lie closer to the surface of each villus. (Photomicrographs contributed by Dr. Kurt Benirschke. Electron micrographs from King, 1975, with permission.)

Placental Growth and Maturation

Placental Growth

In the first trimester, placental growth is more rapid than that of the fetus. But by approximately 17 postmenstrual weeks, placental and fetal weights are approximately equal. By term, placental weight is approximately one sixth of fetal weight.

The mature placenta and its variant forms are discussed in detail in Chapter 6 (p. 116). Briefly, viewed from the maternal surface, the number of slightly elevated convex areas, called lobes, varies from 10 to 38 (Fig. 5-15). Lobes are incompletely separated by grooves of variable depth that overlie placental septa, which arise from folding of the basal plate. The total number of placental lobes remains the same throughout gestation, and individual lobes continue to grow—although less actively in the final weeks (Crawford, 1959). Although grossly visible lobes are commonly referred to as cotyledons, this is not accurate. Correctly used, lobules or cotyledons are the functional units supplied by each main stem villus.

Placental Maturation

As villi continue to branch and the terminal ramifications become more numerous and smaller, the volume and prominence of cytotrophoblasts decrease. As the syncytium thins, the fetal vessels become more prominent and lie closer to the surface. The villous stroma also exhibits changes as gestation progresses. In early pregnancy, the branching connective-tissue cells are separated by an abundant loose intercellular matrix. Later, the villous stroma becomes denser, and the cells more spindly and more closely packed.

Another change in the stroma involves the infiltration of Hofbauer cells, which are fetal macrophages. These are nearly round with vesicular, often eccentric nuclei and very granular or vacuolated cytoplasm. Hofbauer cells are characterized histochemically by intracytoplasmic lipid and by phenotypic markers specific for macrophages. They increase in numbers and maturational state throughout pregnancy and appear to be important mediators of protection at the maternal-fetal interface (Johnson, 2012). These macrophages are phagocytic, have an immunosuppressive phenotype, can produce various cytokines, and are capable of paracrine regulation of trophoblast functions (Cervar, 1999; Vince, 1996).

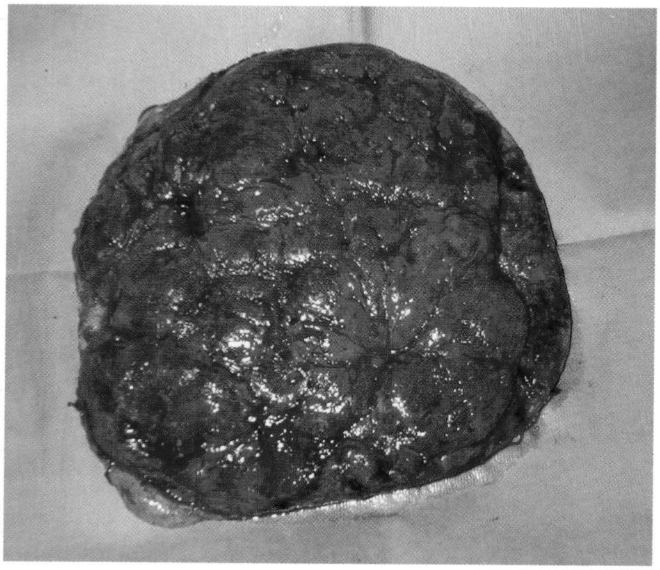

FIGURE 5-15 Photograph of the maternal surface of a placenta. Placental lobes are formed by clefts on the surface that originate from placental septa. (Photograph contributed by Dr. Judith J. Head.)

Some of the histological changes that accompany placental growth and maturation provide an increased efficiency of transport and exchange to meet increasing fetal metabolic requirements. Among these changes are decreased syncytiotrophoblast thickness, significantly reduced cytotrophoblast number, decreased stroma, and increased number of capillaries with close approximation to the syncytial surface. By 16 weeks, the apparent continuity of the cytotrophoblasts is lost. At term, villi may be focally reduced to a thin layer of syncytium covering minimal villous connective tissue in which thin-walled fetal capillaries abut the trophoblast and dominate the villi (see Fig. 5-14D).

There are some changes in placental architecture that can cause decreased placental exchange efficiency if they are substantive. As described in Chapter 6 (p. 119), these include thickening of the basal lamina of trophoblast or capillaries, obliteration of certain fetal vessels, increased villous stroma, and fibrin deposition on the villous surface.

Fetal and Maternal Blood Circulation in the Mature Placenta

Because the placenta is functionally an intimate approximation of the fetal capillary bed to maternal blood, its gross anatomy primarily concerns vascular relations. The fetal surface is covered by the transparent amnion, beneath which chorionic vessels course. A section through the placenta includes amnion, chorion, chorionic villi and intervillous space, decidual (basal) plate, and myometrium (Figs. 5-16 and 5-17).

Fetal Circulation

Deoxygenated venous-like fetal blood flows to the placenta through the two umbilical arteries. As the cord joins the placenta, these umbilical vessels branch repeatedly beneath the amnion and again within the villi, finally forming capillary networks in the terminal villous branches. Blood with significantly higher oxygen content returns from the placenta via a single umbilical vein to the fetus.

The branches of the umbilical vessels that traverse along the fetal surface of the placenta in the chorionic plate are referred to as the placental surface or chorionic vessels. These vessels are responsive to vasoactive substances, but anatomically, morphologically, histologically, and functionally, they are unique. Chorionic arteries always cross over chorionic veins. Vessels are most readily recognized by this interesting relationship, but they are difficult to distinguish by histological criteria. In 65 percent of placentas, chorionic arteries form a fine network supplying the cotyledons—a pattern of disperse-type branching. In the remaining 35 percent, the arteries radiate to the edge of the placenta without narrowing. Both types are end arteries that supply one cotyledon as each branch turns downward to pierce the chorionic plate.

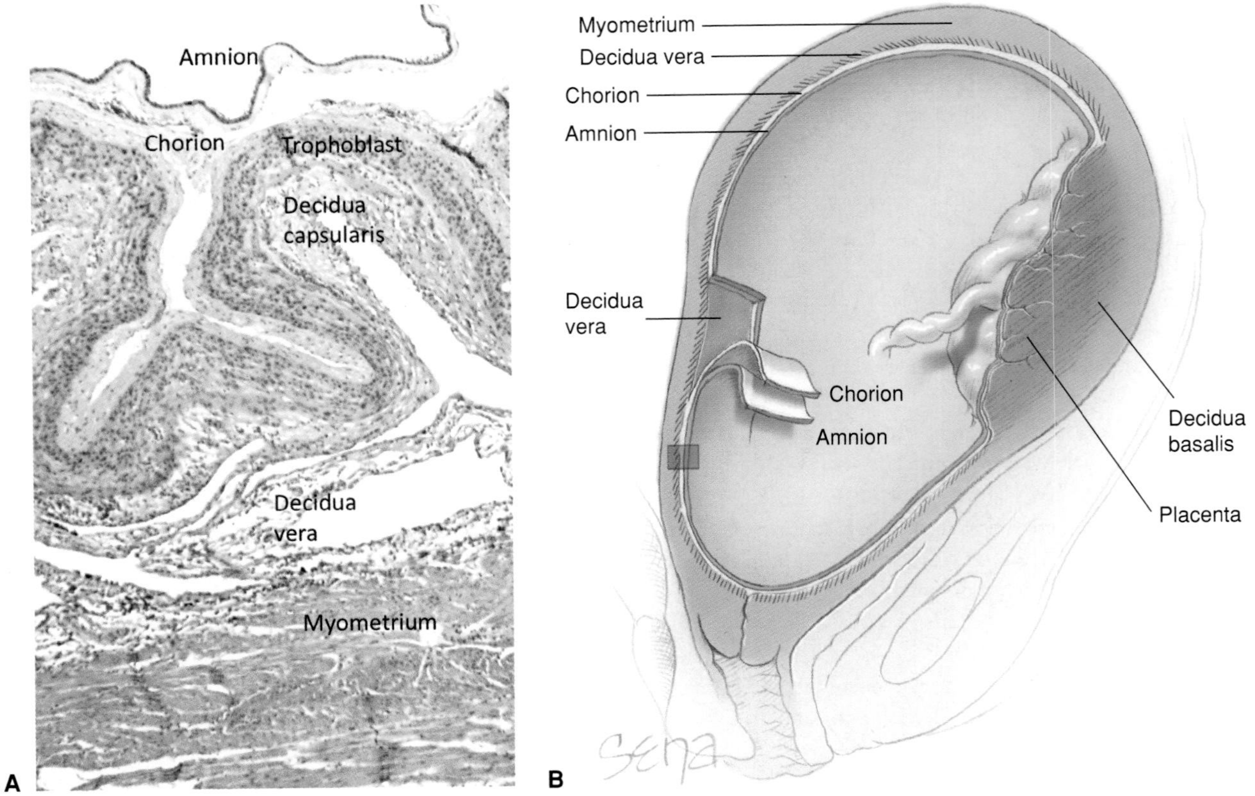

FIGURE 5-16 Uterus of pregnant woman showing a normal placenta in situ. **A.** Photomicrograph of a histologic section through amnion, chorion, and decidua vera that is depicted in **(B)** (*green slice*). (Photograph contributed by Dr. Kurt Benirschke.)

Truncal arteries are perforating branches of the surface arteries that pass through the chorionic plate. Each truncal artery supplies one main stem villus and thus one cotyledon. The amount of vessel wall smooth muscle decreases, and the vessel caliber increases as it penetrates the chorionic plate. The loss in muscle continues as the truncal arteries and veins branch into their smaller rami.

Before 10 weeks, there is no end-diastolic flow pattern within the umbilical artery at the end of the fetal cardiac cycle (Cole, 1991; Fisk, 1988; Loquet, 1988). After 10 weeks, end-diastolic flow appears and is maintained throughout normal pregnancy (Maulik, 1997). Clinically, these are studied with Doppler sonography to assess fetal well-being (Chap. 10, p. 219).

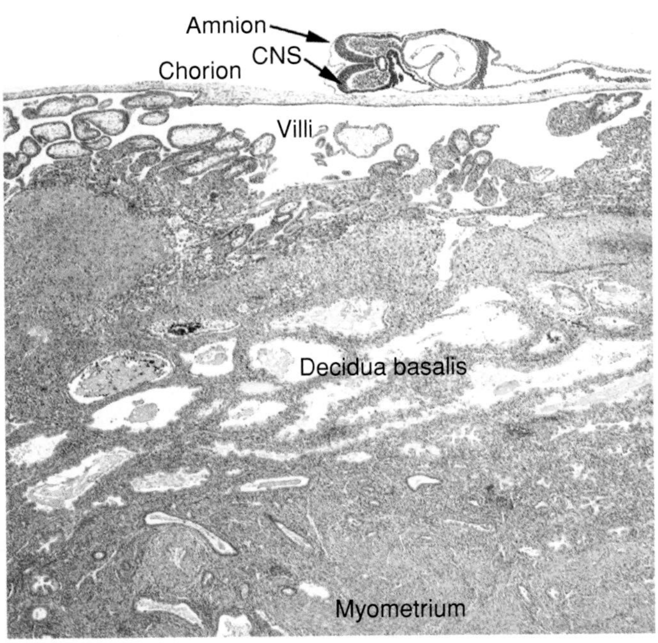

FIGURE 5-17 Photomicrograph of early implanted blastocyst. Trophoblasts are seen invading the decidua basalis. (Photograph contributed by Dr. Kurt Benirschke.)

Maternal Circulation

Because an efficient maternal–placental circulation is requisite, many investigators have sought to define factors that regulate blood flow into and from the intervillous space. An adequate mechanism must explain how blood can: (1) leave maternal circulation; (2) flow into an amorphous space lined by syncytiotrophoblast, rather than endothelium; and (3) return through maternal veins without producing arteriovenous-like shunts that would prevent maternal blood from remaining in contact with villi long enough for adequate exchange. Early studies of Ramsey and Davis (1963) and Ramsey and Harris (1966) provide a physiological explanation of placental circulation. These researchers demonstrated, by careful, low-pressure injections of radiocontrast material, that arterial entrances and venous exits are scattered randomly over the entire placental base.

The physiology of maternal-placental circulation is depicted in Figure 5-18. Maternal blood enters through the basal plate and is driven high up toward the chorionic plate by arterial pressure before laterally dispersing. After bathing the external microvillous surface of chorionic villi, maternal blood drains

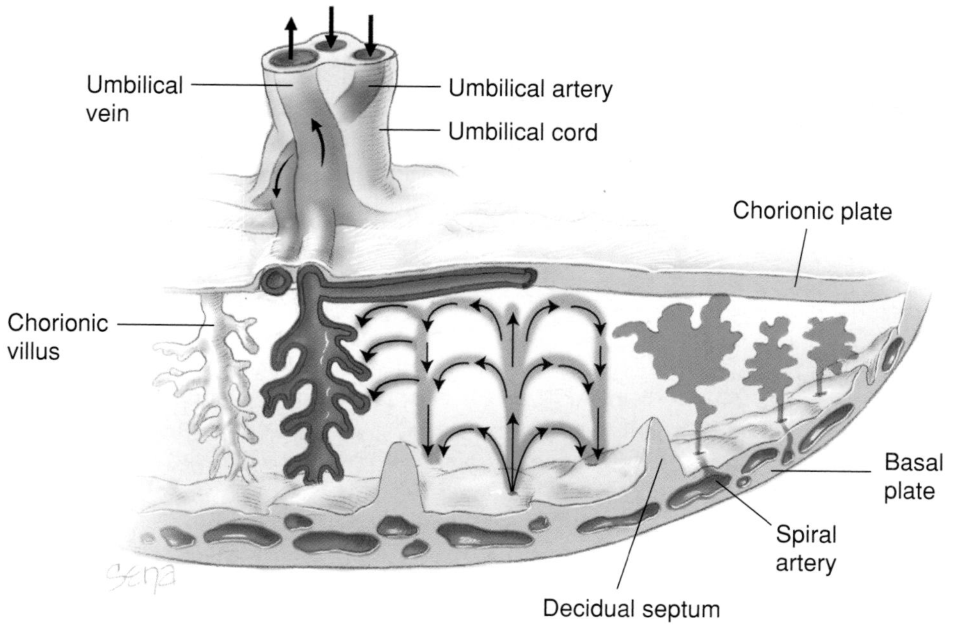

FIGURE 5-18 Schematic drawing of a section through a full-term placenta. Maternal blood flows into the intervillous spaces in funnel-shaped spurts. Exchanges occur with fetal blood as maternal blood flows around the villi. In-flowing arterial blood pushes venous blood into the endometrial veins, which are scattered over the entire surface of the decidua basalis. Note also that the umbilical arteries carry deoxygenated fetal blood to the placenta and that the umbilical vein carries oxygenated blood to the fetus. Placental lobes are separated from each other by placental (decidual) septa.

back through venous orifices in the basal plate and enters uterine veins. Thus, maternal blood traverses the placenta randomly without preformed channels. The previously described trophoblast invasion of the spiral arteries creates low-resistance vessels that can accommodate massive increase in uterine perfusion during gestation. Generally, spiral arteries are perpendicular to, but veins are parallel to, the uterine wall. This arrangement aids closure of veins during a uterine contraction and prevents the exit of maternal blood from the intervillous space. The number of arterial openings into the intervillous space becomes gradually reduced by cytotrophoblast invasion. According to Brosens and Dixon (1963), there are about 120 spiral arterial entries into the intervillous space at term. These discharge blood in spurts that bathes the adjacent villi (Borell, 1958). After the 30th week, a prominent venous plexus separates the decidua basalis from the myometrium and thus participates in providing a cleavage plane for placental separation.

As discussed, both inflow and outflow are curtailed during uterine contractions. Bleker and associates (1975) used serial sonography during normal labor and found that placental length, thickness, and surface area increased during contractions. They attributed this to distention of the intervillous space by impairment of venous outflow compared with arterial inflow. During contractions, therefore, a somewhat larger volume of blood is available for exchange even though the rate of flow is decreased. Similarly, Doppler velocimetry has shown that diastolic flow velocity in spiral arteries is diminished during uterine contractions. Thus, principal factors regulating intervillous space blood flow are arterial blood pressure, intrauterine pressure, uterine contraction pattern, and factors that act specifically on arterial walls.

Breaks in the Placental "Barrier"

The placenta does not maintain absolute integrity of the fetal and maternal circulations. There are numerous examples of trafficking cells between mother and fetus in both directions. This situation is best exemplified clinically by erythrocyte D-antigen alloimmunization and resulting erythroblastosis fetalis (Chap. 15, p. 307). Although fetal cell admixtures likely are small in most cases, occasionally the fetus exsanguinates into the maternal circulation (Silver, 2007).

It is indisputable that fetal cells can become engrafted in the mother during pregnancy and can be identified decades later. Fetal lymphocytes, CD34+ mesenchymal stem cells, and endothelial colony-forming cells reside in maternal blood, bone marrow, or uterine vasculature (Nguyen, 2006; Piper, 2007; Sipos, 2013). Termed *microchimerism*, such residual stem cells may participate in maternal tissue regeneration and have been implicated in the disparate female:male ratio of autoimmune disorders (Gleicher, 2007; Greer, 2011; Stevens, 2006). As discussed in Chapter 59 (p. 1168), they are associated with the pathogenesis of lymphocytic thyroiditis, scleroderma, and systemic lupus erythematosus.

Immunological Considerations of the Fetal–Maternal Interface

The lack of uterine transplantation immunity is unique compared with that of other tissues, and there have been many attempts to explain survival of the semiallogenic fetal graft. Some note the immunological peculiarity of cells involved in implantation and fetal-placental development. These include decidual natural killer cells with their inefficient cytotoxic abilities, decidual stromal cells, and invasive trophoblasts that populate the decidua (Hanna, 2006; Santoni, 2007; Staun-Ram, 2005). The trophoblasts are the only fetal-derived cells in direct contact with maternal tissues. Previous studies have suggested that maternal natural killer cells act to control the invasion of trophoblast, which have adapted to survive in an immunologically hostile environment (Thellin, 2000). Subsequently, Hanna and coworkers (2006) reported a "peaceful" model of trophoblast invasion and maternal vascular remodeling. In this scheme, decidual natural killer cells work in concert with stromal cells. They mediate angiogenesis through production of proangiogenic factors such as VEGF and control trophoblast chemoattraction toward spiral arteries by production of IL-8 and interferon inducible protein-10.

Immunogenicity of the Trophoblasts

More than 50 years ago, Sir Peter Medawar (1953) suggested that fetal semiallograft survival might be explained by immunological neutrality. The placenta was considered immunologically inert and therefore unable to create a maternal immune response. Subsequently, research was focused on defining expression of the major histocompatibility complex (MHC) antigens on trophoblasts. Human leukocyte antigens (HLAs) are the human analogue of the MHC. And indeed, MHC class I and II antigens are absent from villous trophoblasts, which appear to be immunologically inert at all gestational stages (Weetman, 1999). But invasive extravillous cytotrophoblasts do express MHC class I molecules, which have been the focus of considerable study.

Trophoblast HLA Class I Expression. The HLA genes are the products of multiple genetic loci of the major histocompatibility complex located within the short arm of chromosome 6 (Hunt, 1992). There are 17 HLA class I genes, including three classic genes, HLA-A, -B, and -C, that encode the major class I (class Ia) transplantation antigens. Three other class I genes, designated HLA-E, -F, and -G, encode class Ib HLA antigens.

Moffett-King (2002) reasoned that normal implantation depends on controlled trophoblastic invasion of maternal endometrium–decidua and spiral arteries. Such invasion must proceed far enough to provide for normal fetal growth and development, but there must be a mechanism for regulating its depth. She suggests that uterine decidual natural killer (uNK) cells combined with unique expression of three specific HLA class I genes in extravillous cytotrophoblasts act in concert to permit and subsequently limit trophoblast invasion.

Class I antigens in extravillous cytotrophoblasts are accounted for by the expression of classic HLA-C and nonclassic class Ib molecules of HLA-E and HLA-G. HLA-G antigen is expressed only in humans, with expression restricted to extravillous cytotrophoblasts contiguous with maternal tissues, that is, decidual and uNK cells. Indeed, HLA-G antigen expression is identified only in extravillous cytotrophoblasts in the decidua basalis and in the chorion laeve (McMaster, 1995). During pregnancy, a soluble major isoform—HLA-G2—has increased levels (Hunt, 2000a,b). Embryos used for in vitro fertilization do not implant if they do not express this soluble HLA-G isoform (Fuzzi, 2002). Thus, HLA-G may be immunologically permissive of the maternal-fetal antigen mismatch (LeBouteiller, 1999). HLA-G has a proposed role in protecting extravillous trophoblasts from immune rejection via modulation of uNK functions (Apps, 2011; Rajagopalan, 2012). Finally, Goldman-Wohl and associates (2000) have provided evidence for abnormal HLA-G expression in extravillous trophoblasts from women with preeclampsia.

Uterine Natural Killer Cells

These distinctive lymphocytes are believed to originate in bone marrow and belong to the natural killer cell lineage. They are the predominant population of leukocytes present in midluteal phase endometrium at the expected time of implantation (Johnson, 1999). These uNKs have a distinct phenotype characterized by a high surface density of CD56 or neural cell adhesion molecule (Manaster, 2008; Moffett-King, 2002). Their infiltration is increased by progesterone and by stromal cell production of IL-15 and decidual prolactin (Dunn, 2002; Gubbay, 2002).

Near the end of the luteal phase of nonfertile ovulatory cycles, uterine NK cell nuclei begin to disintegrate. But if implantation proceeds, they persist in large numbers in the decidua during early pregnancy. By term, however, there are relatively few uNK cells in the decidua. In first-trimester decidua, there are many uNK cells in close proximity to extravillous trophoblast, where it is speculated that they serve to regulate trophoblast invasion. These uNK cells secrete large amounts of granulocyte-macrophage–colony-stimulating factor (GM-CSF), which suggests that they are in an activated state. Jokhi and coworkers (1999) speculate that GM-CSF may function primarily to forestall trophoblast apoptosis and not to promote trophoblast replication. Expression of angiogenic factors by uNK cells also suggests a function in decidual vascular remodeling (Li, 2001). In this case, it is uNKs, rather than the T lymphocytes, that are primarily responsible for decidual immunosurveillance.

THE AMNION

At term, the amnion is a tough and tenacious but pliable membrane. This innermost avascular fetal membrane is contiguous with amnionic fluid and occupies a role of incredible importance in human pregnancy. The amnion provides almost all tensile strength of the fetal membranes. Thus, its resilience to rupture is vitally important to successful pregnancy outcome. Indeed, preterm rupture of fetal membranes is a major cause of preterm delivery (Chap. 42, p. 839).

Bourne (1962) described five separate amnion layers. The inner surface, which is bathed by amnionic fluid, is an uninterrupted, single layer of cuboidal epithelium (Fig. 5-19). This

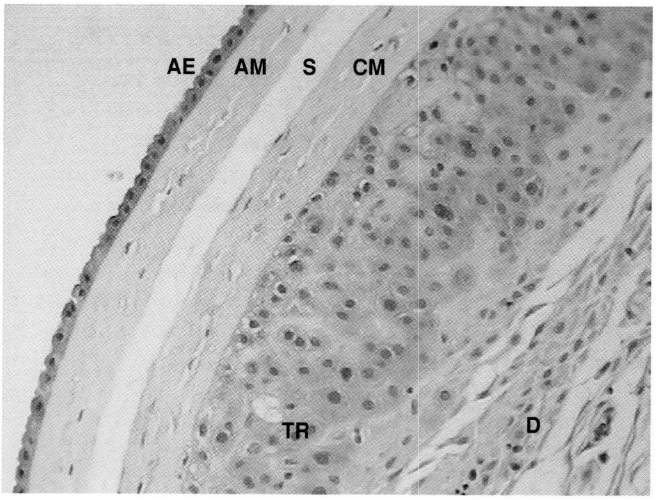

FIGURE 5-19 Photomicrograph of fetal membranes. From left to right: AE = amnion epithelium; AM = amnion mesenchyme; S = zona spongiosa; CM = chorionic mesenchyme; TR = trophoblast; D = decidua. (Photograph contributed by Dr. Judith R. Head.)

epithelium is attached firmly to a distinct basement membrane that is connected to an acellular compact layer composed primarily of interstitial collagens. On the outer side of the compact layer, there is a row of fibroblast-like mesenchymal cells, which are widely dispersed at term. There also are a few fetal macrophages in the amnion. The outermost amnion layer is the relatively acellular zona spongiosa, which is contiguous with the second fetal membrane, the chorion laeve. The human amnion lacks smooth muscle cells, nerves, lymphatics, and importantly, blood vessels.

Amnion Development

Early during implantation, a space develops between the embryonic cell mass and adjacent trophoblasts (see Fig. 5-9). Small cells that line this inner surface of trophoblasts have been called amniogenic cells—precursors of amnionic epithelium. The amnion is first identifiable the 7th or 8th day of embryo development. It is initially a minute vesicle, which then develops into a small sac that covers the dorsal embryo surface. As the amnion enlarges, it gradually engulfs the growing embryo, which prolapses into its cavity (Benirschke, 2012).

Distention of the amnionic sac eventually brings it into contact with the interior surface of the chorion laeve. Apposition of the chorion laeve and amnion near the end of the first trimester then causes an obliteration of the extraembryonic coelom. The amnion and chorion laeve, although slightly adhered, are never intimately connected and can be separated easily. Placental amnion covers the placenta surface and thereby is in contact with the adventitial surface of chorionic vessels. Umbilical amnion covers the umbilical cord. With diamnionic-monochorionic placentas, there is no intervening tissue between the fused amnions. In the conjoined portion of membranes of diamnionic-dichorionic twin placentas, fused amnions are separated by fused chorion laeve.

Amnion Cell Histogenesis

Epithelial cells of the amnion are thought to be derived from fetal ectoderm of the embryonic disc. They do not arise by delamination from trophoblasts. This is an important consideration from both embryological and functional perspectives. For example, HLA class I gene expression in amnion is more akin to that in embryonic cells than that in trophoblasts.

In contrast, the fibroblast-like mesenchymal cell layer previously described is likely derived from embryonic mesoderm. Early in human embryogenesis, the amnionic mesenchymal cells lie immediately adjacent to the basal surface of the amnion epithelium. At this time, the amnion surface is a two-cell layer with approximately equal numbers of epithelial and mesenchymal cells. Simultaneously with growth and development, interstitial collagens are deposited between these two cell layers. This marks formation of the amnion compact layer, which separates the two layers of amnion cells.

As the amnionic sac expands to line the placenta and then the chorion frondosum at 10 to 14 weeks, the compactness of the mesenchymal cells is progressively reduced and become sparsely distributed. Early in pregnancy, amnionic epithelium replicates at a rate appreciably faster than mesenchymal cells. At term, these cells form a continuous uninterrupted epithelium on the fetal amnionic surface. Conversely, mesenchymal cells are widely dispersed, being connected by a fine lattice network of extracellular matrix with the appearance of long slender fibrils.

Amnion Epithelial Cells. The apical surface of the amnionic epithelium is replete with highly developed microvilli. This structure reflects it function as a major site of transfer between amnionic fluid and amnion. This epithelium is metabolically active, and its cells synthesize tissue inhibitor of MMP-1, prostaglandin E_2 (PGE_2), and fetal fibronectin (fFN) (Rowe, 1997). In term pregnancies, amnionic expression of prostaglandin endoperoxide H synthase correlates with elevated fFN levels (Mijovic, 2000). Although epithelia produce fFN, recent studies suggest that fibronectin functions in the underlying mesenchymal cells. Here, fFN promotes synthesis of MMPs that break down the strength-bearing collagens and increases prostaglandin synthesis to prompt uterine contractions and cervical ripening (Mogami, 2013). This pathway is upregulated in premature rupture of membranes induced by infection.

Epithelial cells may respond to signals derived from the fetus or the mother, and they are responsive to various endocrine or paracrine modulators. Examples include oxytocin and vasopressin, both of which increase PGE_2 production in vitro (Moore, 1988). They may also produce cytokines such as IL-8 during labor initiation (Elliott, 2001).

Amnionic epithelium also synthesizes vasoactive peptides, including endothelin and parathyroid hormone-related protein (Economos, 1992; Germain, 1992). The tissue produces brain natriuretic peptide (BNP) and corticotropin-releasing hormone (CRH), which are peptides that invoke smooth-muscle relaxation (Riley, 1991; Warren, 1995). BNP production is positively regulated by mechanical stretch in fetal membranes and is proposed to function in uterine quiescence. Epidermal growth factor, a negative regulator of BNP, is upregulated in the membranes at term and leads to a decline in BNP-regulated uterine quiescence (Carvajal, 2013). It seems reasonable that vasoactive peptides produced in amnion gain access to the adventitial surface of chorionic vessels. Thus, the amnion may be involved in modulating chorionic vessel tone and blood flow. Amnion-derived vasoactive peptides function in both maternal and fetal tissues in diverse physiological processes. After their secretion, these bioactive agents enter amnionic fluid and thereby are available to the fetus by swallowing and inhalation.

Amnion Mesenchymal Cells. Mesenchymal cells of the amnionic fibroblast layer are responsible for other major functions. Synthesis of interstitial collagens that compose the compact layer of the amnion—the major source of its tensile strength—takes place in mesenchymal cells (Casey, 1996). These cells also synthesize cytokines that include IL-6, IL-8, and monocyte chemoattractant protein-1. Cytokine synthesis increases in response to bacterial toxins and IL-1. This functional capacity of amnion mesenchymal cells is an important consideration in amnionic fluid study of labor-associated accumulation of inflammatory mediators (Garcia-Velasco, 1999). Finally, mesenchymal cells may be a greater source of PGE_2 than epithelial cells, in particular in the case of premature membrane rupture (Mogami, 2013; Whittle, 2000).

Amnion Tensile Strength

During tests of tensile strength, the decidua and then the chorion laeve give way long before the amnion ruptures. Indeed, the membranes are elastic and can expand to twice normal size during pregnancy (Benirschke, 2012). The amnion tensile strength resides almost exclusively in the compact layer, which is composed of cross-linked interstitial collagens I and III and lesser amounts of collagens V and VI.

Collagens are the primary macromolecules of most connective tissues and are the most abundant proteins in the body. Collagen I is the major interstitial collagen in tissues characterized by great tensile strength, such as bone and tendon. In other tissues, collagen III is believed to contribute to tissue integrity and provides both tissue extensibility and tensile strength. For example, the ratio of collagen III to collagen I in the walls of a number of highly extensible tissues—amnionic sac, blood vessels, urinary bladder, bile ducts, intestine, and gravid uterus—is greater than that in nonelastic tissues (Jeffrey, 1991). Although collagen III provides some of the amnion extensibility, elastin microfibrils have also been identified (Bryant-Greenwood, 1998).

Amnion tensile strength is regulated in part by fibrillar collagen interacting with proteoglycans such as decorin, which promote tissue strength. Compositional changes at the time of labor include a decline in decorin and increase in hyaluronan. This leads to a loss of tensile strength and is further discussed in Chapter 42 (p. 840) (Meinert, 2007). Fetal membranes overlying the cervix have a reported regional decline in expression of matrix proteins such as fibulins. This change may contribute to tissue remodeling and tensile strength loss (Moore, 2009).

Amnion Metabolic Functions

From the foregoing, it is apparent that the amnion is more than a simple avascular membrane that contains amnionic fluid. It is metabolically active, is involved in solute and water transport for amnionic fluid homeostasis, and produces an impressive array of bioactive compounds. The amnion is responsive both acutely and chronically to mechanical stretch, which alters amnionic gene expression (Carvajal, 2013; Nemeth, 2000). This in turn may trigger both autocrine and paracrine responses to include production of MMPs, IL-8, and collagenase (Bryant-Greenwood, 1998; Maradny, 1996; Mogami, 2013). Such factors may modulate changes in membrane properties during labor.

Amnionic Fluid

Until about 34 weeks' gestation, the normally clear fluid that collects within the amnionic cavity increases as pregnancy progresses. After this, the volume declines. At term, the average volume is approximately 1000 mL, although this may vary widely in normal and especially abnormal conditions. The origin, composition, circulation, and function of amnionic fluid are discussed further in Chapter 11 (p. 231).

THE UMBILICAL CORD

Cord Development

The yolk sac and the umbilical vesicle into which it develops are prominent early in pregnancy. At first, the embryo is a flattened disc interposed between amnion and yolk sac. Its dorsal surface grows faster than the ventral surface, in association with the elongation of its neural tube. Thus, the embryo bulges into the amnionic sac, and the dorsal part of the yolk sac is incorporated into the embryo body to form the gut. The allantois projects into the base of the body stalk from the caudal wall of the yolk sac and later, from the anterior wall of the hindgut.

As pregnancy advances, the yolk sac becomes smaller and its pedicle relatively longer. By the middle of the third month, the expanding amnion obliterates the exocoelom, fuses with the chorion laeve, and covers the bulging placental disc and the lateral surface of the body stalk. The latter is then called the umbilical cord—or funis. A greater description of this cord and potential abnormalities is found in Chapter 6 (p. 121).

The cord at term normally has two arteries and one vein (Fig. 5-20). The right umbilical vein usually disappears early during fetal development, leaving only the original left vein. In sections of any portion of the cord near the center, the small duct of the umbilical vesicle can usually be seen. The vesicle is lined by a single layer of flattened or cuboidal epithelium. In sections just beyond the umbilicus, another duct representing the allantoic remnant is occasionally found. The intraabdominal portion of the duct of the umbilical vesicle, which extends from umbilicus to intestine, usually atrophies and disappears, but occasionally it remains patent, forming the Meckel diverticulum. The most common vascular anomaly is the absence of one umbilical artery, which may be associated with fetal anomalies (Chap. 6, p. 122).

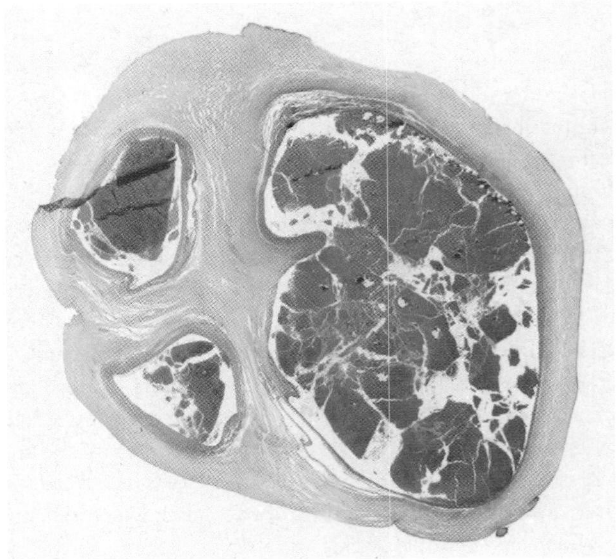

FIGURE 5-20 Cross section of umbilical cord. The large umbilical vein carries oxygenated blood to the fetus (*right*). To its left are the two smaller umbilical arteries, carrying deoxygenated blood from the fetus to the placenta. (Photograph contributed by Dr. Mandolin S. Ziadie.)

Cord Function

The umbilical cord extends from the fetal umbilicus to the fetal surface of the placenta, that is, the chorionic plate. Blood flows from the umbilical vein and takes a path of least resistance via two routes within the fetus. One is the ductus venosus, which empties directly into the inferior vena cava (Fig. 7–8, p. 136). The other route consists of numerous smaller openings into the hepatic circulation. Blood from the liver flows into the inferior vena cava via the hepatic vein. Resistance in the ductus venosus is controlled by a sphincter that is situated at the origin of the ductus at the umbilical recess and is innervated by a vagus nerve branch.

Blood exits the fetus via the two umbilical arteries. These are anterior branches of the internal iliac artery and become obliterated after birth. Remnants can be seen as the medial umbilical ligaments.

PLACENTAL HORMONES

The production of steroid and protein hormones by human trophoblasts is greater in amount and diversity than that of any single endocrine tissue in all of mammalian physiology. A compendium of average production rates for various steroid hormones in nonpregnant and in near-term pregnant women is given in Table 5-1. It is apparent that alterations in steroid hormone production that accompany normal human pregnancy are incredible. The human placenta also synthesizes an enormous amount of protein and peptide hormones as summarized in Table 5-2. It is understandable, therefore, that yet another remarkable feature of human pregnancy is the successful physiological adaptations of pregnant women to the unique endocrine milieu as discussed throughout Chapter 4 (p. 46).

TABLE 5-1. Steroid Production Rates in Nonpregnant and Near-Term Pregnant Women

	Production Rates (mg/24 hr)	
Steroid[a]	Nonpregnant	Pregnant
Estradiol-17β	0.1–0.6	15–20
Estriol	0.02–0.1	50–150
Progesterone	0.1–40	250–600
Aldosterone	0.05–0.1	0.250–0.600
Deoxycorticosterone	0.05–0.5	1–12
Cortisol	10–30	10–20

[a]Estrogens and progesterone are produced by placenta. Aldosterone is produced by the maternal adrenal in response to the stimulus of angiotensin II. Deoxycorticosterone is produced in extraglandular tissue sites by way of the 21-hydroxylation of plasma progesterone. Cortisol production during pregnancy is not increased, even though the blood levels are elevated because of decreased clearance caused by increased cortisol-binding globulin.

Human Chorionic Gonadotropin

This so-called pregnancy hormone is a glycoprotein with biological activity similar to luteinizing hormone. Both act via the same plasma membrane LH-hCG receptor. Although hCG is produced almost exclusively in the placenta, low levels are synthesized in the fetal kidney. Other fetal tissues produce either the β-subunit or intact hCG molecule (McGregor, 1981, 1983).

Various malignant tumors also produce hCG, sometimes in large amounts—especially trophoblastic neoplasms (Chap. 20, p. 396). Chorionic gonadotropin is produced in very small amounts in tissues of men and nonpregnant women, perhaps primarily in the anterior pituitary gland. Nonetheless, the detection of hCG in blood or urine almost always indicates pregnancy (Chap. 9, p. 169).

Chemical Characteristics

Chorionic gonadotropin is a glycoprotein with a molecular weight of 36,000 to 40,000 Da. It has the highest carbohydrate content of any human hormone—30 percent. The carbohydrate component, and especially the terminal sialic acid, protects the molecule from catabolism. The 36-hour plasma half-life of intact hCG is much longer than the 2 hours for LH. The hCG molecule is composed of two dissimilar subunits termed α and β subunits. These are noncovalently linked and are held together by electrostatic and hydrophobic forces. Isolated subunits are unable to bind the LH-hCG receptor and thus lack biological activity.

This hormone is structurally related to three other glycoprotein hormones—LH, FSH, and TSH. All four glycoproteins share a common α-subunit. The β-subunits, although sharing certain similarities, are characterized by distinctly different amino-acid sequences. Recombination of an α- and a β-subunit of the four glycoprotein hormones gives a molecule with biological activity characteristic of the hormone from which the β-subunit was derived.

Biosynthesis

Syntheses of the α- and β-chains of hCG are regulated separately. A single gene located on chromosome 6 encodes the α-subunit common to hCG, LH, FSH, and TSH. Seven genes on chromosome 19 encode for the β-hCG–β-LH family of subunits. Six genes code for β-hCG and one for β-LH (Miller-Lindholm, 1997). Both subunits are synthesized as larger precursors, which are then cleaved by endopeptidases. Intact hCG is then assembled and rapidly released by secretory granule exocytosis (Morrish, 1987). There are multiple forms of hCG in maternal plasma and urine that vary enormously in bioactivity and immunoreactivity. Some result from enzymatic degradation, and others from modifications during molecular synthesis and processing.

Before 5 weeks, hCG is expressed in both syncytiotrophoblast and cytotrophoblast (Maruo, 1992). Later, in the first trimester when maternal serum levels peak, hCG is produced almost solely in the syncytiotrophoblast (Beck, 1986; Kurman, 1984). At this time, mRNA concentrations of both α- and β-subunits in the syncytiotrophoblast are greater than at term (Hoshina,

TABLE 5-2. Protein Hormones Produced by the Human Placenta

Hormone	Primary Nonplacental Site of Expression	Shares Structural or Function Similarity	Functions
Human chorionic gonadotropin (hCG)	—	LH, FSH, TSH	Maintains corpus luteum function Regulates fetal testis testosterone secretion Stimulates maternal thyroid
Placental lactogen (PL)	—	GH, prolactin	Aids maternal adaptation to fetal energy requirements
Adrenocorticotropin (ACTH)	Hypothalamus	—	
Corticotropin-releasing hormone (CRH)	Hypothalamus	—	Relaxes smooth-muscle; initiates parturition? Promotes fetal and maternal glucocorticoid production
Gonadotropin-releasing hormone (GnRH)	Hypothalamus	—	Regulates trophoblast hCG production
Thyrotropin (TRH)	Hypothalamus	—	Unknown
Growth hormone-releasing hormone (GHRH)	Hypothalamus	—	Unknown
Growth hormone variant (hGH-V)	—	GH variant not found in pituitary	Potentially mediates pregnancy insulin resistance
Neuropeptide Y	Brain	—	Potential regulates CRH release by trophoblasts
Parathyroid hormone-releasing protein (PTH-rP)	—	—	Regulates transfer of calcium and other solutes; regulates fetal mineral homeostasis
Inhibin	Ovary/testis	—	Potentially inhibits FSH-mediated ovulation; regulates hCG synthesis
Activin	Ovary/testis	—	Regulates placental GnRH synthesis

GH = growth hormone; FSH = follicle-stimulating hormone; LH = luteinizing hormone; TSH = thyroid-stimulating hormone.

1982). This may be an important consideration when hCG is used as a screening procedure to identify abnormal fetuses.

Circulating free β-subunit levels are low to undetectable throughout pregnancy. In part, this is the result of its rate-limiting synthesis. Free α-subunits that do not combine with the β-subunit are found in placental tissue and maternal plasma. These levels increase gradually and steadily until they plateau at about 36 weeks' gestation. At this time, they account for 30 to 50 percent of hormone (Cole, 1997). Thus, α-hCG secretion roughly corresponds to placental mass, whereas secretion of complete hCG molecules is maximal at 8 to 10 weeks.

Concentrations of hCG in Serum and Urine

The combined hCG molecule is detectable in plasma of pregnant women 7 to 9 days after the midcycle surge of LH that precedes ovulation. Thus, hCG likely enters maternal blood at the time of blastocyst implantation. Plasma levels increase rapidly, doubling every 2 days in the first trimester (Fig. 5-21). Appreciable fluctuations in levels for a given patient are observed on the same day—evidence that trophoblast secretion of protein hormones is episodic.

Intact hCG circulates as multiple highly related isoforms with variable cross-reactivity between commercial assays. Thus, there is considerable variation in calculated serum hCG levels among the more than a hundred available assays. Peak maternal plasma levels reach approximately 100,000 mIU/mL between the 60th and 80th days after menses. At 10 to 12 weeks, plasma levels begin to decline, and a nadir is reached by approximately

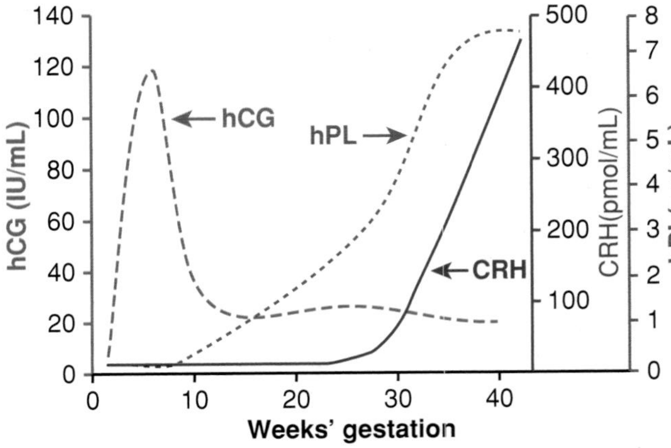

FIGURE 5-21 Distinct profiles for the concentrations of human chorionic gonadotropin (hCG), human placental lactogen (hPL), and corticotropin-releasing hormone (CRH) in serum of women throughout normal pregnancy.

16 weeks. Plasma levels are maintained at this lower level for the remainder of pregnancy (see Fig. 5-21).

The pattern of hCG appearance in fetal blood is similar to that in the mother. Fetal plasma levels, however, are only about 3 percent of those in maternal plasma. Amnionic fluid hCG concentration early in pregnancy is similar to that in maternal plasma. As pregnancy progresses, hCG concentration in amnionic fluid declines, and near term the levels are approximately 20 percent of those in maternal plasma.

Maternal urine contains the same variety of hCG degradation products as maternal plasma. The principal urinary form is the terminal degradation hCG product—the β-core fragment. Its concentrations follow the same general pattern as that in maternal plasma, peaking at about 10 weeks. It is important to recognize that the so-called β-subunit antibody used in most pregnancy tests reacts with both intact hCG—the major form in the plasma, and with fragments of hCG—the major forms found in urine.

Regulation of hCG Synthesis and Clearance

Placental gonadotropin-releasing hormone (GnRH) is likely involved in the regulation of hCG formation. Both GnRH and its receptor are expressed by cytotrophoblasts and syncytiotrophoblast (Wolfahrt, 1998). GnRH administration elevates circulating hCG levels, and cultured trophoblast cells respond to GnRH treatment with increased hCG secretion (Iwashita, 1993; Siler-Khodr, 1981). Pituitary GnRH production also is regulated by inhibin and activin. In cultured placental cells, activin stimulates and inhibin inhibits GnRH and hCG production (Petraglia, 1989; Steele, 1993).

Renal clearance of hCG accounts for 30 percent of its metabolic clearance. The remainder is likely cleared by metabolism in the liver (Wehmann, 1980). Clearances of β- and α-subunits are approximately 10-fold and 30-fold, respectively, greater than that of intact hCG.

Biological Functions of hCG

Both hCG subunits are required for binding to the LH-hCG receptor in the corpus luteum and the fetal testis. LH-hCG receptors are present in various other tissues, but their role there is less defined. The best-known biological function of hCG is the so-called rescue and maintenance of corpus luteum function—that is, continued progesterone production. Bradbury and colleagues (1950) found that the progesterone-producing life span of a corpus luteum of menstruation could be prolonged perhaps for 2 weeks by hCG administration. This is only an incomplete explanation for the physiological function of hCG in pregnancy. For example, maximum plasma hCG concentrations are attained well after hCG-stimulated corpus luteum secretion of progesterone has ceased. Specifically, progesterone luteal synthesis begins to decline at about 6 weeks despite continued and increasing hCG production.

A second hCG role is stimulation of fetal testicular testosterone secretion, which is maximum approximately when hCG levels peak. Thus, at a critical time in male sexual differentiation, hCG enters fetal plasma from the syncytiotrophoblast. In the fetus, it acts as an LH surrogate to stimulate Leydig cell replication and testosterone synthesis to promote male sexual differentiation (Chap. 7, p. 148). Before approximately 110 days, there is no vascularization of the fetal anterior pituitary from the hypothalamus. Thus, pituitary LH secretion is minimal, and hCG acts as LH before this time. Thereafter, as hCG levels fall, pituitary LH maintains modest testicular stimulation.

The maternal thyroid gland is also stimulated by large quantities of hCG. In some women with gestational trophoblastic disease, biochemical and clinical evidence of hyperthyroidism sometimes develops (Chap. 20, p. 399). This once was attributed to formation of chorionic thyrotropins by neoplastic trophoblasts. It was subsequently shown, however, that some forms of hCG bind to TSH receptors on thyrocytes (Hershman, 1999). And treatment of men with exogenous hCG increases thyroid activity. The thyroid-stimulatory activity in plasma of first-trimester pregnant women varies appreciably from sample to sample. Modifications of hCG oligosaccharides likely are important in the capacity of hCG to stimulate thyroid function. For example, acidic isoforms stimulate thyroid activity, and some more basic isoforms stimulate iodine uptake (Kraiem, 1994; Tsuruta, 1995; Yoshimura, 1994). Finally, the LH-hCG receptor is expressed by thyrocytes, which suggests that hCG stimulates thyroid activity via the LH-hCG receptor as well as by the TSH receptor (Tomer, 1992).

Other hCG functions include promotion of relaxin secretion by the corpus luteum (Duffy, 1996). LH-hCG receptors are found in myometrium and in uterine vascular tissue. It has been hypothesized that hCG may promote uterine vascular vasodilatation and myometrial smooth-muscle relaxation (Kurtzman, 2001). Chorionic gonadotropin also regulates expansion of uterine natural killer cell numbers during early stages of placentation, thus ensuring appropriate establishment of pregnancy (Kane, 2009).

Abnormally High or Low hCG Levels

There are several clinical circumstances in which substantively higher maternal plasma hCG levels are found. Some examples are multifetal pregnancy, erythroblastosis fetalis associated with fetal hemolytic anemia, and gestational trophoblastic disease. Relatively higher hCG levels may be found at midtrimester in women carrying a fetus with Down syndrome—an observation used in biochemical screening tests (Chap. 14, p. 290). The reason for this is not clear, but reduced placental maturity has been speculated. Relatively lower hCG plasma levels are found in women with early pregnancy wastage, including ectopic pregnancy (Chap. 19, p. 381).

Human Placental Lactogen

Prolactin-like activity in the human placenta was first described by Ehrhardt (1936). Because of its potent lactogenic and growth hormone-like bioactivity, as well as an immunochemical resemblance to human growth hormone (hGH), it was called human placental lactogen or chorionic growth hormone. Currently, human placental lactogen is used by most.

Grumbach and Kaplan (1964) showed that this hormone, like hCG, was concentrated in syncytiotrophoblast. It is detected as early as the second or third week after fertilization.

Also similar to hCG, hPL is demonstrated in cytotrophoblasts before 6 weeks (Maruo, 1992).

Chemical Characteristics and Synthesis

Human placental lactogen is a single, nonglycosylated polypeptide chain with a molecular weight of 22,279 Da. It is derived from a 25,000-Da precursor. The sequence of hPL and hGH is strikingly similar, with 96-percent homology. Also, hPL is structurally similar to human prolactin (hPRL), with a 67-percent amino-acid sequence similarity. For these reasons, it has been suggested that the genes for hPL, hPRL, and hGH evolved from a common ancestral gene—probably that for prolactin—by repeated gene duplication (Ogren, 1994).

There are five genes in the growth hormone–placental lactogen gene cluster that are linked and located on chromosome 17. Two of these—hPL2 and hPL3—encode hPL, and the amount of mRNA in the term placenta is similar for each.

Within 5 to 10 days after conception, hPL is demonstrable in the placenta and can be detected in maternal serum as early as 3 weeks. Maternal plasma concentrations are linked to placental mass, and they rise steadily until 34 to 36 weeks' gestation. The hPL production rate near term—approximately 1 g/day—is by far the greatest of any known hormone in humans. The half-life of hPL in maternal plasma is between 10 and 30 minutes (Walker, 1991). In late pregnancy, maternal serum concentrations reach levels of 5 to 15 μg/mL (see Fig. 5-21).

Very little hPL is detected in fetal blood or in the urine of the mother or newborn. Amnionic fluid levels are somewhat lower than in maternal plasma. Because hPL is secreted primarily into the maternal circulation, with only very small amounts in cord blood, it appears that its role in pregnancy is mediated through actions in maternal rather than in fetal tissues. Nonetheless, there is continuing interest in the possibility that hPL serves select functions in fetal growth.

Regulation of hPL Biosynthesis

Levels of mRNA for hPL in syncytiotrophoblast remain relatively constant throughout pregnancy. This finding supports the idea that the hPL secretion rate is proportional to placental mass. There are very high plasma levels of hCG in women with trophoblastic neoplasms, but only low levels of hPL in these same women.

Prolonged maternal starvation in the first half of pregnancy leads to increased hPL plasma concentrations. Short-term changes in plasma glucose or insulin, however, have relatively little effect on plasma hPL levels. In vitro studies of syncytiotrophoblast suggest that hPL synthesis is stimulated by insulin and insulin-like growth factor-1 and inhibited by PGE_2 and $PGF_{2\alpha}$ (Bhaumick, 1987; Genbacev, 1977).

Metabolic Actions

Placental lactogen has putative actions in several important metabolic processes. First, hPL promotes maternal lipolysis with increased circulating free fatty acid levels. This provides an energy source for maternal metabolism and fetal nutrition. In vitro studies suggest that hPL inhibits leptin secretion by term trophoblast (Coya, 2005).

Second, hPL may aid maternal adaptation to fetal energy requirements. For example, increased maternal insulin resistance ensures nutrient flow to the fetus. It also favors protein synthesis and provides a readily available amino-acid source to the fetus. To counterbalance the increased insulin resistance and prevent maternal hyperglycemia, maternal insulin levels are increased. Both hPL and prolactin signal through the prolactin receptor to increase maternal beta cell proliferation to augment insulin secretion (Georgia, 2010). Recent animal studies provide insight into the mechanism by which lactogenic hormones drive beta cell expansion. Specifically, prolactin and hPL upregulate serotonin synthesis via regulation of the rate-limiting enzyme, tryptophan hydroxylase-1, which in turn increases beta cell proliferation (Kim, 2010).

Last, hPL is a potent angiogenic hormone. It may serve an important function in fetal vasculature formation (Corbacho, 2002).

Other Placental Protein Hormones

The placenta has a remarkable capacity to synthesize numerous peptide hormones, including some that are analogous or related to hypothalamic and pituitary hormones. In contrast to their counterparts, the placental peptide/protein hormones are not subject to feedback inhibition. Examples include pro-opiomelanocortin-derived peptides, growth hormone variant V, and gonadotropin-releasing hormone.

Chorionic Adrenocorticotropin

Adrenocorticotropic hormone (ACTH), lipotropin, and β-endorphin—all proteolytic products of pro-opiomelanocortin—are recovered from placental extracts (Genazzani, 1975; Odagiri, 1979). The physiological action of placental ACTH is unclear. Placental corticotropin-releasing hormone stimulates synthesis and release of chorionic ACTH. Placental CRH production is positively regulated by cortisol, producing a novel positive feedback loop. As discussed later, this system may be important for controlling fetal lung maturation and parturition timing.

Growth Hormone Variant

The placenta expresses a growth hormone variant (hGH-V) that is not expressed in the pituitary. The gene encoding hGH-V is located in the hGH–hPL gene cluster on chromosome 17. Sometimes referred to as placental growth hormone, hGH-V is a 191 amino-acid protein that differs in 15 amino-acid positions from the sequence for hGH. Although hGH-V retains growth-promoting and antilipogenic functions similar to hGH, it has reduced diabetogenic and lactogenic functions relative to hGH (Vickers, 2009). Placental hGH-V presumably is synthesized in the syncytium. However, its pattern of synthesis and secretion during gestation is not precisely known because antibodies against hGH-V cross-react with hGH. It is believed that hGH-V is present in maternal plasma by 21 to 26 weeks' gestation, increases in concentration until approximately 36 weeks, and remains relatively constant thereafter. There is a correlation between the levels of hGH-V in maternal plasma and those of insulin-like growth factor-1. Also, hGH-V secretion by trophoblasts in vitro is inhibited by glucose in a dose-dependent manner (Patel, 1995). Overexpression of hGH-V in mice causes severe insulin resistance, and thus it is a likely candidate to mediate insulin resistance of pregnancy (Barbour, 2002).

Hypothalamic-Like Releasing Hormones

The known hypothalamic-releasing or -inhibiting hormones include GnRH, CRH, thyroid-releasing hormone (TRH), growth hormone-releasing hormone (GHRH), and somatostatin. For each, there is an analogous hormone produced in the human placenta (Petraglia, 1992; Siler-Khodr, 1988). Many investigators suggest this indicates a hierarchy of control in chorionic trophic-agent synthesis.

Gonadotropin-Releasing Hormone. There is a reasonably large amount of immunoreactive GnRH in the placenta (Siler-Khodr, 1978, 1988). Interestingly, it is found in cytotrophoblasts, but not syncytiotrophoblast. Gibbons and coworkers (1975) and Khodr and Siler-Khodr (1980) demonstrated that the human placenta could synthesize both GnRH and TRH in vitro. Placental-derived GnRH functions to regulate trophoblast hCG production, hence the observation that GnRH levels are higher early in pregnancy. Placental-derived GnRH is also the likely cause of elevated maternal GnRH levels in pregnancy (Siler-Khodr, 1984).

Corticotropin-Releasing Hormone. This hormone is a member of a larger family of CRH-related peptides that includes CRH, urocortin, urocortin II, and urocortin III (Dautzenberg, 2002). Maternal serum CRH levels increase from 5 to 10 pmol/L in the nonpregnant woman to approximately 100 pmol/L in the early third trimester of pregnancy and to almost 500 pmol/L abruptly during the last 5 to 6 weeks (see Fig. 5-21). Urocortin also is produced by the placenta and secreted into the maternal circulation, but at much lower levels than seen for CRH (Florio, 2002). After labor begins, maternal plasma CRH levels increase further by two- to threefold (Petraglia, 1989, 1990).

The biological function of CRH synthesized in the placenta, membranes, and decidua has been somewhat defined. CRH receptors are present in many tissues: placenta, adrenal gland, sympathetic ganglia, lymphocytes, gastrointestinal tract, pancreas, gonads, and myometrium. Some findings suggest that CRH can act through two major families—the type 1 and type 2 CRH receptors (CRH-R1 and CRH-R2). Trophoblast, amniochorion, and decidua express both CRH-R1 and CRH-R2 receptors and several variant receptors (Florio, 2000). Both CRH and urocortin increase trophoblast ACTH secretion, supporting an autocrine-paracrine role (Petraglia, 1999). Large amounts of trophoblast CRH enter maternal blood. That said, there also is a large concentration of a specific CRH-binding protein in maternal plasma, and the bound CRH seems to be biologically inactive.

Other proposed biological roles include induction of smooth-muscle relaxation in vascular and myometrial tissue and immunosuppression. The physiological reverse, however, induction of myometrial contractions, has been proposed for the rising CRH levels seen near term. One hypothesis suggests that CRH may be involved with parturition initiation (Wadhwa, 1998). Prostaglandin formation in the placenta, amnion, chorion laeve, and decidua is increased with CRH treatment (Jones, 1989b). This latter observation further supports a potential action in parturition timing.

Glucocorticoids act in the hypothalamus to inhibit CRH release, but in the trophoblast, glucocorticoids stimulate CRH gene expression (Jones, 1989a; Robinson, 1988). Thus, there may be a novel positive feedback loop in the placenta by which placental CRH stimulates placental ACTH to stimulate fetal and maternal adrenal glucocorticoid production with subsequent stimulation of placental CRH expression (Nicholson, 2001; Riley, 1991).

Growth Hormone-Releasing Hormone. The role of placental GHRH is not known (Berry, 1992). Ghrelin is another regulator of hGH secretion that is produced by placental tissue (Horvath, 2001). Trophoblast ghrelin expression peaks at midpregnancy and is a potential regulator of hGH-V production or a paracrine regulator of differentiation (Fuglsang, 2005; Gualillo, 2001).

Other Placental Protein Hormones

Relaxin

Expression of relaxin has been demonstrated in human corpus luteum, decidua, and placenta (Bogic, 1995). This peptide is synthesized as a single, 105 amino-acid preprorelaxin molecule that is cleaved to A and B molecules. Relaxin is structurally similar to insulin and insulin-like growth factor. Two of the three relaxin genes—H2 and H3—are transcribed in the corpus luteum (Bathgate, 2002; Hudson, 1983, 1984). Other tissues, including decidua, placenta, and membranes, express H1 and H2 (Hansell, 1991).

The rise in maternal circulating relaxin levels seen in early pregnancy is attributed to corpus luteum secretion, and levels parallel those of hCG. Relaxin, along with rising progesterone levels, may act on myometrium to promote relaxation and the quiescence of early pregnancy (Chap. 21, p. 421). In addition, the production of relaxin and relaxin-like factors within the placenta and fetal membranes may play an autocrine-paracrine role in postpartum regulation of extracellular matrix degradation (Qin, 1997a,b). One important relaxin function is enhancement of the glomerular filtration rate (Chap. 4, p. 64).

Parathyroid Hormone–Related Protein

In pregnancy, circulating parathyroid hormone-related protein (PTH-rP) levels are significantly elevated within maternal but not fetal circulation (Bertelloni, 1994; Saxe, 1997). Many potential functions of this hormone have been proposed. PTH-rP synthesis is found in several normal adult tissues, especially in reproductive organs that include myometrium, endometrium, corpus luteum, and lactating mammary tissue. PTH-rP is not produced in the parathyroid glands of normal adults. Based on insights from parathyroid hormone-related protein null mice, placental-derived PTH-rP may have an important function to regulate genes involved in transfer of calcium and other solutes. It also contributes to fetal mineral homeostasis in bone, amnionic fluid, and the fetal circulation (Simmonds, 2010).

Leptin

This hormone is normally secreted by adipocytes. It functions as an antiobesity hormone that decreases food intake through its hypothalamic receptor. It also regulates bone growth and immune function (Cock, 2003; La Cava, 2004). In the placenta, leptin also is synthesized by both cytotrophoblast and syncytiotrophoblast (Henson, 2002). Relative contributions of leptin from maternal adipose tissue versus placenta are currently not well defined. Maternal serum levels are significantly higher than those in nonpregnant women. Fetal leptin levels correlate positively with birthweight and likely play an important function in fetal development and growth. Studies suggest that leptin inhibits apoptosis and promotes trophoblast proliferation (Magarinos, 2007).

Neuropeptide Y

This 36 amino-acid peptide is widely distributed in brain. It also is found in sympathetic neurons innervating the cardiovascular, respiratory, gastrointestinal, and genitourinary systems. Neuropeptide Y has been isolated from the placenta and localized in cytotrophoblasts (Petraglia, 1989). There are receptors for neuropeptide Y on trophoblast, and treatment of placental cells with neuropeptide Y causes CRH release (Robidoux, 2000).

Inhibin and Activin

Inhibin is a glycoprotein hormone that acts preferentially to inhibit pituitary FSH release. It is produced by human testis and by ovarian granulosa cells, including the corpus luteum. Inhibin is a heterodimer made up of an α-subunit and one of two distinct β-subunits, βA or βB. All three are produced by trophoblast, and maternal serum levels peak at term (Petraglia, 1991). One function may be to act in concert with the large amounts of sex steroid hormones to inhibit FSH secretion and thereby inhibit ovulation during pregnancy. Inhibin may act via GnRH to regulate placental hCG synthesis (Petraglia, 1987).

Activin is closely related to inhibin and is formed by the combination of the two β-subunits. Its receptor is expressed in the placenta and amnion. Activin A is not detectable in fetal blood before labor but is present in umbilical cord blood after labor begins. Petraglia (1994) found that serum activin A levels decline rapidly after delivery. It is not clear if chorionic activin and inhibin are involved in placental metabolic processes other than GnRH synthesis.

Placental Progesterone Production

After 6 to 7 weeks' gestation, little progesterone is produced in the ovary (Diczfalusy, 1961). Surgical removal of the corpus luteum or even bilateral oophorectomy during the 7th to 10th week does not decrease excretion rates of urinary pregnanediol, the principal urinary metabolite of progesterone. Before this time, however, corpus luteum removal will result in spontaneous abortion unless an exogenous progestin is given (Chap. 63, p. 1227). After approximately 8 weeks, the placenta assumes progesterone secretion, resulting in a gradual increase in maternal serum levels throughout pregnancy (Fig. 5-22). By term, these levels are 10 to 5000 times those found in nonpregnant women, depending on the stage of the ovarian cycle.

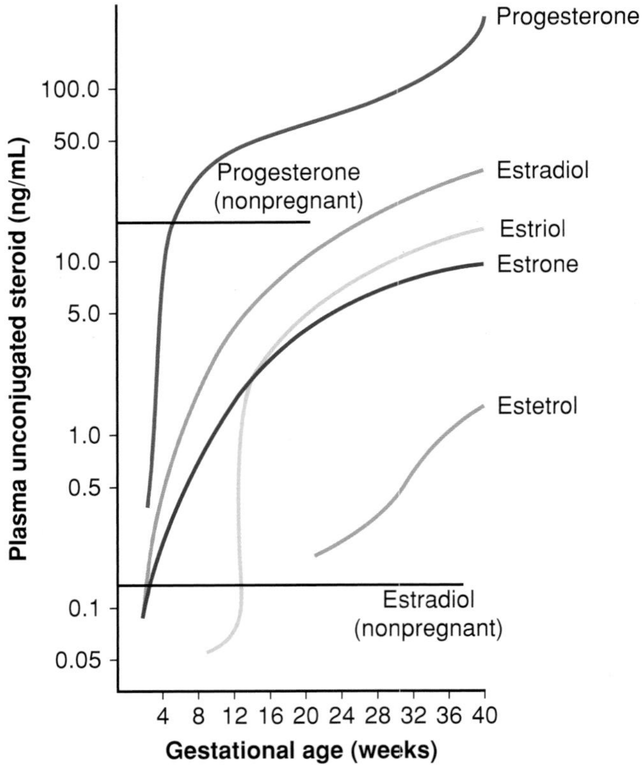

FIGURE 5-22 Plasma levels of progesterone, estradiol, estrone, estetrol, and estriol in women during the course of gestation. (Modified from Mesiano, 2009, with permission.)

Progesterone Production Rates

The daily production rate of progesterone in late, normal, singleton pregnancies is approximately 250 mg. In multifetal pregnancies, the daily production rate may exceed 600 mg/day. Progesterone is synthesized from cholesterol in a two-step enzymatic reaction. First, cholesterol is converted to pregnenolone within the mitochondria, in a reaction catalyzed by cytochrome P_{450} cholesterol side-chain cleavage enzyme. Pregnenolone leaves the mitochondria and is converted to progesterone in the endoplasmic reticulum by 3β-hydroxysteroid dehydrogenase. Progesterone is released immediately through a process of diffusion.

Although the placenta produces a prodigious amount of progesterone, there is limited capacity for trophoblast cholesterol biosynthesis. Radiolabeled acetate is incorporated into cholesterol by placental tissue at a slow rate. The rate-limiting enzyme in cholesterol biosynthesis is 3-hydroxy-3-methylglutaryl coenzyme A (HMG CoA) reductase. Because of this, the placenta must rely on exogenous cholesterol for progesterone formation. Bloch (1945) and Werbin and colleagues (1957) found that after intravenous administration of radiolabeled cholesterol to pregnant women, the amount of radioactivity of urinary pregnanediol was similar to that of plasma cholesterol. Hellig and associates (1970) also found that maternal plasma cholesterol was the principal precursor—as much as 90 percent—of progesterone biosynthesis. The trophoblast preferentially uses LDL cholesterol for progesterone biosynthesis (Simpson, 1979, 1980). In studies of pregnant baboons, when maternal serum LDL levels were reduced, there was a significant drop in placental progesterone production (Henson, 1997). Thus, placental progesterone is formed through the uptake and use of a maternal circulating precursor. This mechanism is unlike the placental production of estrogens, which relies principally on fetal adrenal precursors.

Progesterone Synthesis and Fetal Relationships

Although there is a relationship between fetal well-being and placental estrogen production, this is not the case for placental progesterone. Fetal demise, ligation of the umbilical cord with the fetus and placenta remaining in situ, and anencephaly are all conditions associated with very low maternal plasma levels and low urinary excretion of estrogens. In these circumstances, there is not a concomitant decrease in progesterone levels until some indeterminate time after fetal death. Thus, placental endocrine function, including the formation of protein hormones such as hCG and progesterone biosynthesis, may persist for long periods (weeks) after fetal demise.

Progesterone Metabolism During Pregnancy

The metabolic clearance rate of progesterone in pregnant women is similar to that found in men and nonpregnant women. During pregnancy, the plasma concentration of 5α-dihydroprogesterone disproportionately increases due to synthesis in syncytiotrophoblast from both placenta-produced progesterone and fetal-derived precursor (Dombroski, 1997). Thus, the concentration ratio of this progesterone metabolite to progesterone is increased in pregnancy. The mechanisms for this are not defined completely. Progesterone also is converted to the potent mineralocorticoid deoxycorticosterone in pregnant women and in the fetus. The concentration of deoxycorticosterone is increased strikingly in both maternal and fetal compartments (see Table 5-1). The extraadrenal formation of deoxycorticosterone from circulating progesterone accounts for most of its production in pregnancy (Casey, 1982a,b).

Placental Estrogen Production

The placenta produces huge amounts of estrogens using blood-borne steroidal precursors from the maternal and fetal adrenal glands. Near term, normal human pregnancy is a hyperestrogenic state. The amount of estrogen produced each day by syncytiotrophoblast during the last few weeks of pregnancy is equivalent to that produced in 1 day by the ovaries of no fewer than 1000 ovulatory women. The hyperestrogenic state of human pregnancy is one of continually increasing magnitude as pregnancy progresses, terminating abruptly after delivery.

During the first 2 to 4 weeks of pregnancy, rising hCG levels maintain production of estradiol in the maternal corpus luteum. Production of both progesterone and estrogens in the maternal ovaries decreases significantly by the 7th week of pregnancy. At this time, there is a luteal-placental transition. By the 7th week, more than half of estrogen entering maternal circulation is produced in the placenta (MacDonald, 1965a; Siiteri, 1963, 1966). These studies support the transition of a steroid milieu dependent on the maternal corpus luteum to one dependent on the developing placenta.

Placental Estrogen Biosynthesis

The estrogen synthesis pathways in the placenta differ from those in the ovary of nonpregnant women. Estrogen is produced during the follicular and luteal phases through the interaction of theca and granulosa cells that surround the follicles. Specifically, androstenedione is synthesized in ovarian theca cells and then is transferred to adjacent granulosa cells for estradiol synthesis. Estradiol production within the corpus luteum of nonpregnant women and in early pregnancy continues to require interaction between the luteinized theca and granulosa cells. However, in human trophoblast, neither cholesterol nor progesterone can serve as precursor for estrogen biosynthesis. A crucial enzyme necessary for sex steroid synthesis—steroid 17α-hydroxylase/17, 20-lyase (CYP17)—is not expressed in the human placenta. Consequently, the conversion of C_{21}-steroids to C_{19}-steroids—the latter being the immediate and obligatory precursors of estrogens—is not possible.

Dehydroepiandrosterone (DHEA) and its sulfate (DHEA-S) are C_{19}-steroids. Although these are often called adrenal androgens, these steroids can also serve as estrogen precursors (Fig. 5-23). Ryan (1959a) found that the placenta had an exceptionally high capacity to convert appropriate C_{19}-steroids to estrone and estradiol. The conversion of DHEA-S to estradiol requires placental expression of four key enzymes that are located principally in syncytiotrophoblast (Bonenfant, 2000; Salido, 1990). First, the placenta expresses high levels of steroid sulfatase (STS), which converts the conjugated DHEA-S to DHEA. DHEA is then acted upon by 3β-hydroxysteroid dehydrogenase type 1 (3βHSD) to produce androstenedione. Cytochrome P_{450} aromatase (CYP19) then converts androstenedione to estrone, which is then converted to estradiol by 17β-hydroxysteroid dehydrogenase type 1 (17βHSD1).

Plasma C_{19}-Steroids as Estrogen Precursors

Frandsen and Stakemann (1961) found that urinary estrogens levels in women pregnant with an anencephalic fetus were only about 10 percent of that found in normal pregnancy. The adrenal glands of anencephalic fetuses are atrophic because of absent hypothalamic-pituitary function, which precludes ACTH stimulation. Thus, it seemed reasonable that fetal adrenal glands might provide substance(s) used for placental estrogen formation.

In subsequent studies, DHEA-S was found to be a major precursor of estrogens in pregnancy (Baulieu, 1963; Siiteri, 1963). The large amounts of DHEA-S in plasma and its much longer half-life uniquely qualify it as the principal precursor for placental estradiol synthesis. There is a 10- to 20-fold increased metabolic clearance rate of plasma DHEA-S in women at term compared with that in men and nonpregnant women (Gant, 1971). This rapid use results in a progressive decrease in plasma DHEA-S concentration as pregnancy progresses (Milewich, 1978). However, maternal adrenal glands do not produce sufficient amounts of DHEA-S to account for more than a fraction of total placental estrogen biosynthesis. The fetal adrenal glands are quantitatively the most important source of placental estrogen precursors in human pregnancy. A schematic representation of the estrogen formation pathways in the placenta

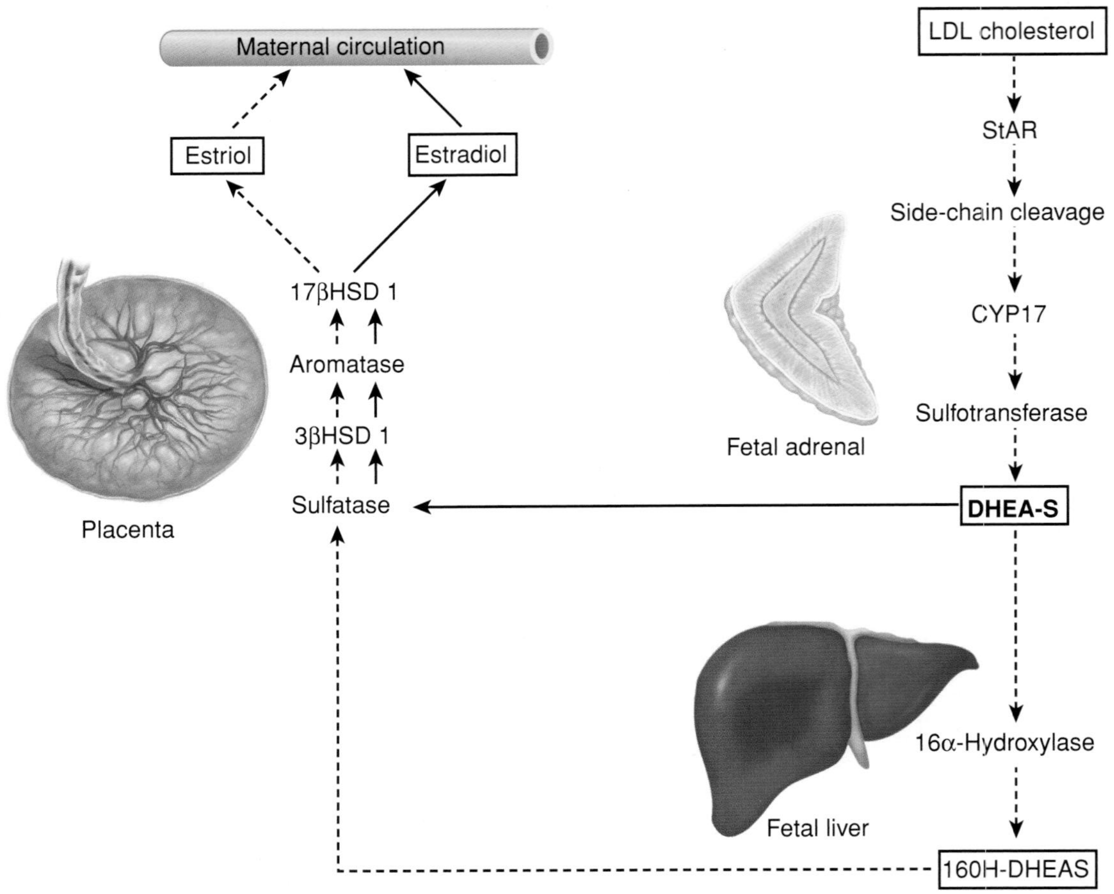

FIGURE 5-23 Schematic presentation of estrogen biosynthesis in the human placenta. Dehydroepiandrosterone sulfate (DHEA-S), secreted in prodigious amounts by the fetal adrenal glands, is converted to 16α-hydroxydehydroepiandrosterone sulfate (16αOHDHEA-S) in the fetal liver. These steroids, DHEA-S and 16αOHDHEA-S, are converted in the placenta to estrogens, that is, 17β-estradiol (E_2) and estriol (E_3). Near term, half of E_2 is derived from fetal adrenal DHEA-S and half from maternal DHEA-S. On the other hand, 90 percent of E_3 in the placenta arises from fetal 16αOHDHEA-S and only 10 percent from all other sources.

is presented in Figure 5-23. As shown, the estrogen products released from the placenta are dependent on the substrate available. Thus, estrogen production during pregnancy reflects the unique interactions among fetal adrenal glands, fetal liver, placenta, and maternal adrenal glands.

Directional Secretion of Steroids from Syncytiotrophoblast

More than 90 percent of estradiol and estriol formed in syncytiotrophoblast as shown in Table 5-1 enters maternal plasma (Gurpide, 1966). And 85 percent or more of placental progesterone enters maternal plasma, with little maternal progesterone crossing the placenta to the fetus (Gurpide, 1972).

The major reason for directional movement of newly formed steroid into the maternal circulation is the nature of hemochorioendothelial placentation. In this system, steroids secreted from syncytiotrophoblast can enter maternal blood directly. Steroids that leave the syncytium do not enter fetal blood directly. They must first traverse the cytotrophoblasts and then enter the stroma of the villous core and then fetal capillaries. From either of these spaces, steroids can reenter the syncytium. The net result of this hemochorial arrangement is that there is substantially greater entry of steroids into the maternal circulation compared with the amount that enters fetal blood.

FETAL ADRENAL GLAND–PLACENTAL INTERACTIONS

Morphologically, functionally, and physiologically, the fetal adrenal glands are remarkable organs. At term, the fetal adrenal glands weigh the same as those of the adult. More than 85 percent of the fetal gland is composed of a unique fetal zone, which has a great capacity for steroid biosynthesis. Daily steroid production of fetal adrenal glands near term is 100 to 200 mg/day. This compares with resting adult steroid secretion of 30 to 40 mg/day.

The fetal zone is lost in the first year of life and is not present in the adult. In addition to ACTH, fetal adrenal gland growth is influenced by factors secreted by the placenta. This is exemplified by the continued growth of the fetal glands throughout gestation, but rapid involution immediately after birth when placenta-derived factors dissipate. A discussion of the fetal adrenal and liver is warranted in this chapter, given the dependence of normal placental function on the unique fetal adrenal and vice versa.

Placental Estriol Synthesis

The estrogen products released from the placenta are dependent on the substrate available from the developing fetus. Estradiol is the primary placental estrogen secretory product at term. In addition, significant levels of estriol and estetrol are found in the maternal circulation, and they increase, particularly late in gestation (see Fig. 5-22). These hydroxylated forms of estrogen are produced in the placenta using substrates formed by the combined efforts of the fetal adrenal gland and liver.

There are important fetal-maternal interactions through the fetal liver (see Fig. 5-23). High levels of fetal hepatic 16α-hydroxylase act on adrenal-derived steroids. Ryan (1959b) and MacDonald and Siiteri (1965b) found that 16α-hydroxylated C_{19}-steroids, particularly 16α-hydroxydehydroepiandrosterone (16-OHDHEA), were converted to estriol by placental tissue. Thus, the disproportionate increase in estriol formation during pregnancy is accounted for by placental synthesis of estriol principally from plasma-borne 16-OHDHEA-sulfate. Near term, the fetus is the source of 90 percent of placental estriol and estetrol precursor in normal human pregnancy.

Thus, the placenta secretes several estrogens, including estradiol, estrone, estriol, and estetrol. Because of its hemochorial nature, most placental estrogens are released into the maternal circulation. Maternal estriol and estetrol are produced almost solely by fetal steroid precursors. Thus, levels of these steroids were used in the past as an indicator of fetal well-being. However, low sensitivity and specificity of such tests have caused them to be discarded.

Enzymatic Considerations

There is very low expression of the microsomal enzyme 3α-hydroxysteroid dehydrogenase, Δ^{5-4}-isomerase (3βHSD) in adrenal fetal zone cells (Doody, 1990; Rainey, 2001). This limits the conversion of pregnenolone to progesterone and of 17α-hydroxypregnenolone to 17α-hydroxyprogesterone, an obligatory step in cortisol biosynthesis. There is, however, very active steroid sulfotransferase activity in the fetal adrenal glands. As a consequence, the principal secretory products of the fetal adrenal glands are pregnenolone sulfate and DHEA-S. Comparatively, cortisol, which likely arises primarily in the neocortex and transitional zone of the fetal adrenal glands and not in the fetal zone, is a minor secretory product until late in gestation.

Fetal Adrenal Steroid Precursor

The precursor for fetal adrenal steroidogenesis is cholesterol. The steroid biosynthesis rate in the fetal gland is so great that its steroidogenesis alone is equivalent to a fourth of the total daily LDL cholesterol turnover in adults. Fetal adrenal glands synthesize cholesterol from acetate. All enzymes involved in cholesterol biosynthesis are elevated compared with that of the adult adrenal gland (Rainey, 2001). Thus, the de novo cholesterol synthesis rate by fetal adrenal tissue is extremely high. Even so, it is insufficient to account for the steroids produced by these glands. Therefore, cholesterol must be assimilated from the fetal circulation. Plasma cholesterol and its esters are present in the form of very-low-density lipoprotein (VLDL), LDL, and HDL.

Simpson and colleagues (1979) found that fetal glands take up lipoproteins as a source of cholesterol for steroidogenesis. LDL was most effective, HDL was much less, and VLDL was devoid of stimulatory activity. They also evaluated relative contributions of cholesterol synthesized de novo and that of cholesterol derived from LDL uptake. These authors confirmed that fetal adrenal glands are highly dependent on circulating LDL as a source of cholesterol for optimum steroidogenesis (Carr, 1980, 1981b, 1982).

Most fetal plasma cholesterol arises by de novo synthesis in the fetal liver (Carr, 1984). The low LDL cholesterol level in fetal plasma is not the consequence of impaired fetal LDL synthesis, but instead, results from the rapid use of LDL by the fetal adrenal glands for steroidogenesis (Parker, 1980, 1983). As expected, in the anencephalic newborn with atrophic adrenal glands, the LDL cholesterol levels in umbilical cord plasma are high.

Fetal Conditions That Affect Estrogen Production

Several fetal disorders alter the availability of substrate for placental steroid synthesis and thus highlight the interdependence of fetal development and placental function.

Fetal Demise

Fetal death is followed by a striking reduction in urinary estrogen levels. Similarly, after ligation of the umbilical cord with the fetus and placenta left in situ, placental estrogens production decline markedly (Cassmer, 1959). However, placental progesterone production was maintained. It was concluded that an important source of precursors of placental estrogen—but not progesterone—biosynthesis was eliminated upon fetal death.

Fetal Anencephaly

With absence of the adrenal cortex fetal zone, as seen with anencephaly, the placental estrogen formation rate—especially estriol—is severely limited because of diminished availability of C_{19}-steroid precursors. Therefore, almost all estrogens produced in women pregnant with an anencephalic fetus arise from placental use of maternal plasma DHEA-S. Furthermore, in such pregnancies, estrogen production can be increased by maternal administration of ACTH, which stimulates the DHEA-S secretion rate by the maternal adrenal gland. Because ACTH does not cross the placenta, there is no fetal adrenal stimulation. Finally, placental estrogen production is decreased in women pregnant with an anencephalic fetus when a potent glucocorticoid is given to the mother. This suppresses ACTH secretion and thus decreases the DHEA-S secretion rate from the maternal adrenal cortex (MacDonald, 1965a).

Fetal Adrenal Hypoplasia

Congenital adrenal cortical hypoplasia occurs in perhaps 1 in 12,500 births (McCabe, 2001). Estrogen production in these pregnancies is limited, which suggests the absence of C_{19}-precursors.

Fetal-Placental Sulfatase Deficiency

Placental estrogen formation is generally regulated by the availability of C_{19}-steroid prohormones in fetal and maternal plasma. Specifically, there is no rate-limiting enzymatic reaction in the placental pathway from C_{19}-steroids to estrogen biosynthesis. An exception to this generalization is placental sulfatase deficiency, which is associated with very low estrogen levels in otherwise normal pregnancies (France, 1969). Sulfatase deficiency precludes the hydrolysis of C_{19}-steroid sulfates, the first enzymatic step in the placental use of these circulating prehormones for estrogen biosynthesis. This deficiency is an X-linked disorder, and all affected fetuses are male. Its estimated frequency is 1 in 2000 to 5000 births and is associated with delayed onset of labor. It also is associated with the development of ichthyosis in affected males later in life (Bradshaw, 1986).

Fetal-Placental Aromatase Deficiency

There are a few well-documented examples of aromatase deficiency (Grumbach, 2011; Simpson, 2000). Fetal adrenal DHEA-S, which is produced in large quantities, is converted in the placenta to androstenedione, but in cases of placental aromatase deficiency, androstenedione cannot be converted to estradiol. Rather, androgen metabolites of DHEA produced in the placenta, including androstenedione and some testosterone, are secreted into the maternal or fetal circulation, or both, causing virilization of the mother and the female fetus (Belgorosky, 2009; Harada, 1992; Shozu, 1991).

Trisomy 21—Down Syndrome

Second-trimester maternal serum screening for abnormal levels of hCG, alpha-fetoprotein, and other analytes has become universal (Chap. 14, p. 290). As a result, it was discovered that serum unconjugated estriol levels were low in women with Down syndrome fetuses (Benn, 2002). The likely reason for this is inadequate formation of C_{19}-steroids in the adrenal glands of these trisomic fetuses.

Deficiency in Fetal LDL Cholesterol Biosynthesis

A successful pregnancy in a woman with β-lipoprotein deficiency has been described (Parker, 1986). The absence of LDL in the maternal serum restricted progesterone formation in both the corpus luteum and placenta. In addition, estriol levels were lower than normal. Presumably, the diminished estrogen production was the result of decreased fetal LDL formation, which limited fetal adrenal production of estrogen precursors.

Fetal Erythroblastosis

In some cases of severe fetal D-antigen alloimmunization, maternal plasma estrogen levels are elevated. A likely cause is increased placental mass from hypertrophy, which can be seen with such fetal hemolytic anemia (Chap. 15, p. 315).

Maternal Conditions That Affect Placental Estrogen Production

Glucocorticoid Treatment

The administration of glucocorticoids to pregnant women causes a striking reduction in placental estrogen formation. Glucocorticoids inhibit ACTH secretion from the maternal and fetal pituitary glands. This leads to decreased maternal and fetal adrenal secretion of the placental estrogen precursor DHEA-S.

Maternal Adrenal Dysfunction

In pregnant women with Addison disease, maternal urinary estrogen levels are decreased (Baulieu, 1956). The decrease principally affects estrone and estradiol. The fetal adrenal contribution to estriol synthesis, particularly in later pregnancy, is quantitatively much more important.

Maternal Ovarian Androgen-Producing Tumors

The extraordinary efficiency of the placenta in the aromatization of C_{19}-steroids may be exemplified by two considerations. First, Edman and associates (1981) found that virtually all androstenedione entering the intervillous space is taken up by syncytiotrophoblast and converted to estradiol. None of this C_{19}-steroid enters the fetus. Second, a female fetus is rarely virilized if there is a maternal androgen-secreting ovarian tumor. The placenta efficiently converts aromatizable C_{19}-steroids, including testosterone, to estrogens, thus precluding transplacental passage. Indeed, virilized female fetuses of women with an androgen-producing tumor may be cases in which a nonaromatizable C_{19}-steroid androgen is produced by the tumor—for example, 5α-dihydrotestosterone. Another explanation is that testosterone is produced very early in pregnancy in amounts that exceed the placental aromatase capacity at that time.

Gestational Trophoblastic Disease

With complete hydatidiform mole or choriocarcinoma, there is no fetal adrenal source of C_{19}-steroid precursor for trophoblast estrogen biosynthesis. Consequently, placental estrogen formation is limited to the use of C_{19}-steroids in the maternal plasma, and therefore the estrogen produced is principally estradiol (MacDonald, 1964, 1966). Great variation is observed in the rates of both estradiol and progesterone formation in molar pregnancies.

REFERENCES

Abel MH: Prostanoids and menstruation. In Baird DT, Michie EA (eds): Mechanisms of Menstrual Bleeding. New York, Raven, 2002, p 139

Albrecht ED, Pepe GJ: Steroid hormone regulation of angiogenesis in the primate endometrium. Front Biosci 8:D416, 2003

Ancelin M, Buteau-Lozano H, Meduri G, et al: A dynamic shift of VEGF isoforms with a transient and selective progesterone-induced expression of VEGF189 regulates angiogenesis and vascular permeability in human uterus. Proc Natl Acad Sci USA 99:6023, 2002

Aplin JD: MUC-1 glycosylation in endometrium: possible roles of the apical glycocalyx at implantation. Hum Reprod 2:17, 2003

Apps R, Sharkey A, Gardner L, et al: Ex vivo functional responses to HLA-G differ between blood and decidual NK cells. Mol Hum Reprod 17(9):577, 2011

Arey LB: The degree of normal menstrual irregularity: an analysis of 20,000 calendar records from 1,500 individuals. Am J Obstet Gynecol 37:12, 1939

Arici A, Head JR, MacDonald PC, et al: Regulation of interleukin-8 gene expression in human endometrial cells in culture. Mol Cell Endocrinol 94:195, 1993

Arici A, MacDonald PC, Casey ML: Regulation of monocyte chemotactic protein-1 gene expression in human endometrial cells in cultures. Mol Cell Endocrinol 107:189, 1995

Arnholdt H, Meisel F, Fandrey K, et al: Proliferation of villous trophoblast of the human placenta in normal and abnormal pregnancies. Virchows Arch B Cell Pathol Incl Mol Pathol 60:365, 1991

Auletta F: The role of prostaglandin F2a in human luteolysis. Contemp Obstet Gynecol 30:119, 1987
Baker T: A quantitative and cytological study of germ cells in human ovaries. Proc R Soc Lond B Biol Sci 158:417, 1963
Bao L, Tessier C, Prigent-Tessier A, et al: Decidual prolactin silences the expression of genes detrimental to pregnancy. Endocrinology 148:2326, 2007
Barbour LA, Shao J, Qiao L, et al: Human placental growth hormone causes severe insulin resistance in transgenic mice. Am J Obstet Gynecol 186:512, 2002
Bathgate RA, Samuel CS, Burazin TC, et al: Human relaxin gene 3 (H3) and the equivalent mouse relaxin (M3) gene. Novel members of the relaxin peptide family. J Biol Chem 277:1148, 2002
Baulieu EE, Bricaire H, Jayle MF: Lack of secretion of 17-hydroxycorticosteroids in a pregnant woman with Addison's disease. J Clin Endocrinol 16:690, 1956
Baulieu EE, Dray F: Conversion of 3H-dehydroepiandrosterone (3b-hydroxy-D5-androstene-17-one) sulfate to 3H-estrogens in normal pregnant women. J Clin Endocrinol 23:1298, 1963
Beck T, Schweikhart G, Stolz E: Immunohistochemical location of HPL, SP1 and beta-HCG in normal placentas of varying gestational age. Arch Gynecol 239:63, 1986
Belgorosky A, Guercio G, Pepe C, et al: Genetic and clinical spectrum of aromatase deficiency in infancy, childhood and adolescence. Horm Res 72(6): 321, 2009
Benirschke K, Burton GJ, Baergen RN: Pathology of the Human Placenta, 6th ed. Heidelberg, Springer, 2012
Benn PA: Advances in prenatal screening for Down syndrome: I. General principles and second trimester testing. Clin Chim Acta 323:1, 2002
Berry SA, Srivastava CH, Rubin LR, et al: Growth hormone-releasing hormone-like messenger ribonucleic acid and immunoreactive peptide are present in human testis and placenta. J Clin Endocrinol Metab 75:281, 1992
Bertelloni S, Baroncelli GI, Pelletti A, et al: Parathyroid hormone-related protein in healthy pregnant women. Calcif Tissue Int 54:195, 1994
Bhaumick B, Dawson EP, Bala RM: The effects of insulin-like growth factor-I and insulin on placental lactogen production by human term placental explants. Biochem Biophys Res Commun 144:674, 1987
Billingham RE, Head JR: Recipient treatment to overcome the allograft reaction, with special reference to nature's own solution. Prog Clin Biol Res 224:159, 1986
Bleker O, Kloostermans G, Mieras D, et al: Intervillous space during uterine contractions in human subjects: an ultrasonic study. Am J Obstet Gynecol 123:697, 1975
Bloch K: The biological conversion of cholesterol to pregnanediol. J Biol Chem 157:661, 1945
Bogic LV, Mandel M, Bryant-Greenwood GD: Relaxin gene expression in human reproductive tissues by in situ hybridization. J Clin Endocrinol Metab 80:130, 1995
Bombail V, MacPherson S, Critchley HO, et al: Estrogen receptor related beta is expressed in human endometrium throughout the normal menstrual cycle. Hum Reprod 23(12):2782, 2008
Bonagura TW, Babischkin JS, Aberdeen GC, et al: Prematurely elevating estradiol in early baboon pregnancy suppresses uterine artery remodeling and expression of extravillous placental vascular endothelial growth factor and $\alpha 1\beta 1$ integrins. Endocrinology 153(6):2897, 2012
Bonenfant M, Provost PR, Drolet R, et al: Localization of type 1 17beta-hydroxysteroid dehydrogenase mRNA and protein in syncytiotrophoblasts and invasive cytotrophoblasts in the human term villi. J Endocrinol 165:217, 2000
Borell U, Fernstrom I, Westman A: An arteriographic study of the placental circulation. Geburtshilfe Frauenheilkd 18:1, 1958
Bourne GL: The Human Amnion and Chorion. Chicago, Year Book, 1962
Boyd JD, Hamilton WJ: The Human Placenta. Cambridge, England, Heffer, 1970
Bradbury J, Brown W, Guay L: Maintenance of the corpus luteum and physiologic action of progesterone. Recent Prog Horm Res 5:151, 1950
Bradshaw KD, Carr BR: Placental sulfatase deficiency: maternal and fetal expression of steroid sulfatase deficiency and X-linked ichthyosis. Obstet Gynecol Surv 41:401, 1986
Brosens I, Dixon H: The anatomy of the maternal side of the placenta. Eur J Endocrinol 73:357, 1963
Brosens J, Hayashi N, White J: Progesterone receptor regulates decidual prolactin expression in differentiating human endometrial stromal cells. Eur J Obstet Gynaecol Surv 142:269, 2000
Bryant-Greenwood GD: The extracellular matrix of the human fetal membranes: structure and function. Placenta 19:1, 1998
Carr BR, Ohashi M, Simpson ER: Low density lipoprotein binding and de novo synthesis of cholesterol in the neocortex and fetal zones of the human fetal adrenal gland. Endocrinology 110:1994, 1982
Carr BR, Porter JC, MacDonald PC, et al: Metabolism of low density lipoprotein by human fetal adrenal tissue. Endocrinology 107:1034, 1980
Carr BR, Sadler RK, Rochelle DB, et al: Plasma lipoprotein regulation of progesterone biosynthesis by human corpus luteum tissue in organ culture. J Clin Endocrinol Metab 52:875, 1981a
Carr BR, Simpson ER: Cholesterol synthesis by human fetal hepatocytes: effect of lipoproteins. Am J Obstet Gynecol 150:551, 1984
Carr BR, Simpson ER: Lipoprotein utilization and cholesterol synthesis by the human fetal adrenal gland. Endocr Rev 2:306, 1981b
Carson DD: The glycobiology of implantation. Front Biosci 7:d1535, 2002
Carvajal JA, Delpiano AM, Cuello MA, et al: Mechanical stretch increases brain natriuretic peptide production and secretion in the human fetal membranes. Reprod Sci 20(5):597, 2013
Casey ML, Delgadillo M, Cox KA, et al: Inactivation of prostaglandins in human decidua vera (parietalis) tissue: Substrate specificity of prostaglandin dehydrogenase. Am J Obstet Gynecol 160:3, 1989
Casey ML, Hemsell DL, MacDonald PC, et al: NAD^+-dependent 15-hydroxyprostaglandin dehydrogenase activity in human endometrium. Prostaglandins 19:115, 1980
Casey ML, MacDonald PC: Extraadrenal formation of a mineralocorticosteroid: deoxycorticosterone and deoxycorticosterone sulfate biosynthesis and metabolism. Endocr Rev 3:396, 1982a
Casey ML, MacDonald PC: Metabolism of deoxycorticosterone and deoxycorticosterone sulfate in men and women. J Clin Invest 70:312, 1982b
Casey ML, MacDonald PC: The endothelin-parathyroid hormone-related protein vasoactive peptide system in human endometrium: modulation by transforming growth factor-beta. Hum Reprod 11 Suppl 2):62, 1996
Cervar M, Blaschitz A, Dohr G, et al: Paracrine regulation of distinct trophoblast functions in vitro by placental macrophages. Cell Tissue Res 295:297, 1999
Chao HS, Poisner AM, Poisner R, et al: Endothelin-1 modulates renin and prolactin release from human decidua by different mechanisms. Am J Physiol 267:E842, 1994
Chennazhi, Nayak NR: Regulation of angiogenesis in the primate endometrium: vascular endothelial growth factor. Semin Reprod Med 27(1):80, 2009
Christian M, Pohnke Y, Kempf R, et al: Functional association of PR and CCAAT/enhancer-binding protein beta isoforms: promoter-dependent cooperation between PR-B and liver-enriched inhibitory protein, or liver-enriched activatory protein and PR-A in human endometrial stromal cells. Mol Endocrinol 16:141, 2002a
Christian M, Zhang XH, Schneider-Merck T, et al: Cyclic AMP-induced forkhead transcription factor, FKHR, cooperates with CCAAT/enhancer-binding protein beta in differentiating human endometrial stromal cells. J Biol Chem 277:20825, 2002b
Co EC, Gormley M, Kapidzic M, et al: Maternal decidual macrophages inhibit NK cell killing invasive cytotrophoblasts during human pregnancy. Biol Reprod 88:155, 2013
Cock T-A, Auwerx J: Leptin: cutting the fat off the bone. Lancet 362:1572, 2003
Cole LA: Immunoassay of human chorionic gonadotropin, its free subunits, and metabolites. Clin Chem 43:2233, 1997
Cole LA, Kardana A, Andrade-Gordon P, et al: The heterogeneity of human chorionic gonadotropin (hCG). III. The occurrence and biological and immunological activities of nicked hCG. Endocrinology 129:1559, 1991
Conneely OM, Mulac-Jericevic B, DeMayo F, et al: Reproductive functions of progesterone receptors. Recent Prog Horm Res 57:339, 2002
Corbacho AM, Martinez DLE, Clapp C: Roles of prolactin and related members of the prolactin/growth hormone/placental lactogen family in angiogenesis. J Endocrinol 173:219, 2002
Coya R, Martul P, Algorta J, et al: Progesterone and human placental lactogen inhibit leptin secretion on cultured trophoblast cells from human placentas at term. Gynecol Endocrinol 21:27, 2005
Crawford J: A study of human placental growth with observations on the placenta in erythroblastosis foetalis. Br J Obstet Gynaecol 66:855, 1959
Critchley HO, Kelly RW, Baird DT, et al: Regulation of human endometrial function: mechanisms relevant to uterine bleeding. Reprod Biol Endocrinol 4 Suppl 1:S5, 2006
Curry TE Jr, Smith MF: Impact of extracellular matrix remodeling on ovulation and the folliculo-luteal transition. Semin Reprod Med 24(4):228, 2006
Dautzenberg FM, Hauger RL: The CRF peptide family and their receptors: yet more partners discovered. Trends Pharmacol Sci 23:71, 2002
Diczfalusy E, Troen P: Endocrine functions of the human placenta. Vitam Horm 19:229, 1961
Dombroski RA, Casey ML, MacDonald PC: 5-Alpha-dihydroprogesterone formation in human placenta from 5alpha-pregnan-3beta/alpha-ol-20-ones and 5-pregnan-3beta-yl-20-one sulfate. J Steroid Biochem Mol Biol 63:155, 1997

Dong JC, Dong H, Campana A, et al: Matrix metalloproteinases and their specific tissue inhibitors in menstruation. Reproduction 123:621, 2002
Doody KM, Carr BR, Rainey WE, et al: 3b-hydroxysteroid dehydrogenase/isomerase in the fetal zone and neocortex of the human fetal adrenal gland. Endocrinology 126:2487, 1990
Duffy DM, Hutchison JS, Stewart DR, et al: Stimulation of primate luteal function by recombinant human chorionic gonadotropin and modulation of steroid, but not relaxin, production by an inhibitor of 3 beta-hydroxysteroid dehydrogenase during simulated early pregnancy. J Clin Endocrinol Metab 81:2307, 1996
Duncan WC, McNeilly AS, Fraser HM, et al: Luteinizing hormone receptor in the human corpus luteum: lack of down-regulation during maternal recognition of pregnancy. Hum Reprod 11:2291, 1996
Dunn CL, Critchley HO, Kelly RW: IL-15 regulation in human endometrial stromal cells. J Clin Endocrinol Metab 87:1898, 2002
Economos K, MacDonald PC, Casey ML: Endothelin-1 gene expression and protein biosynthesis in human endometrium: potential modulator of endometrial blood flow. J Clin Endocrinol Metab 74:14, 1992
Edman CD, Toofanian A, MacDonald PC, et al: Placental clearance rate of maternal plasma androstenedione through placental estradiol formation: an indirect method of assessing uteroplacental blood flow. Am J Obstet Gynecol 141:1029, 1981
Ehrhardt K: Forschung und Klinik. Ober das Lacttazionshormon des Hypophysenvorderlappens. Muench Med Wochenschr 83:1163, 1936
Elliott CL, Allport VC, Loudon JA, et al: Nuclear factor-kappa B is essential for up-regulation of interleukin-8 expression in human amnion and cervical epithelial cells. Mol Hum Reprod 7:787, 2001
Enders AC: A comparative study of the fine structure in several hemochorial placentas. Am J Anat 116:29, 1965
Evans J, Salamonsen LA: Inflammation, leukocytes and menstruation. Rev Endocr Metab Disord 13(4):277, 2012
Faddy MJ, Gosden RG, Gougeon A, et al: Accelerated disappearance of ovarian follicles in mid-life: implications for forecasting menopause. Hum Reprod 7:1342, 1992
Ferenczy A: Studies on the cytodynamics of human endometrial regeneration. I. Scanning electron microscopy. Am J Obstet Gynecol 124:64, 1976
Filicori M, Santoro N, Merriam GR, et al: Characterization of the physiological pattern of episodic gonadotropin secretion throughout the human menstrual cycle. J Clin Endocrinol Metab 62:1136, 1986
Fisk NM, MacLachlan N, Ellis C, et al: Absent end-diastolic flow in first trimester umbilical artery. Lancet 2:1256, 1988
Florio P, Franchini A, Reis FM, et al: Human placenta, chorion, amnion and decidua express different variants of corticotropin-releasing factor receptor messenger RNA. Placenta 21:32, 2000
Florio P, Mezzesimi A, Turchetti V, et al: High levels of human chromogranin A in umbilical cord plasma and amniotic fluid at parturition. J Soc Gynecol Investig 9:32, 2002
France JT, Liggins GC: Placental sulfatase deficiency. J Clin Endocrinol Metab 29:138, 1969
Frandsen VA, Stakemann G: The site of production of oestrogenic hormones in human pregnancy: hormone excretion in pregnancy with anencephalic foetus. Acta Endocrinol 38:383, 1961
Frank GR, Brar AK, Jikihara H, et al: Interleukin-1 beta and the endometrium: an inhibitor of stromal cell differentiation and possible autoregulator of decidualization in humans. Biol Reprod 52:184, 1995
Fraser HM, Wulff C: Angiogenesis in the primate ovary. Reprod Fertil Dev 13:557, 2001
Fu B, Li X, Sun R, et al: Natural killer cells promote immune tolerance by regulating inflammatory TH17 cells at the human maternal-fetal interface. Proc Natl Acad Sci USA 110(3):E231, 2013
Fuglsang J, Skjaerbaek C, Espelund U, et al: Ghrelin and its relationship to growth hormones during normal pregnancy. Clin Endocrinol (Oxf) 62(5):554, 2005
Fuzzi B, Rizzo R, Criscuoli L, et al: HLA-G expression in early embryos is a fundamental prerequisite for the obtainment of pregnancy. Eur J Immunol 32:311, 2002
Gant NF, Hutchinson HT, Siiteri PK, et al: Study of the metabolic clearance rate of dehydroisoandrosterone sulfate in pregnancy. Am J Obstet Gynecol 111:555, 1971
Garcia-Velasco JA, Arici A: Chemokines and human reproduction. Fertil Steril 71:983, 1999
Gargett CE, Rogers PA: Human endometrial angiogenesis. Reproduction 121:181, 2001
Genazzani AR, Fraioli F, Hurlimann J, et al: Immunoreactive ACTH and cortisol plasma levels during pregnancy. Detection and partial purification of corticotrophin-like placental hormone: the human chorionic corticotrophin (HCC). Clin Endocrinol (Oxf) 4:1, 1975
Genbacev O, Ratkovic M, Kraincanic M, et al: Effect of prostaglandin PGE2alpha on the synthesis of placental proteins and human placental lactogen (HPL). Prostaglandins 13:723, 1977
Georgia S, Bhushan A: Pregnancy hormones boost beta cells via serotonin. Nat Med 16(7):756, 2010
Germain A, Attaroglu H, MacDonald PC, et al: Parathyroid hormone-related protein mRNA in avascular human amnion. J Clin Endocrinol Metab 75:1173, 1992
Gibbons JM Jr, Mitnick M, Chieffo V: In vitro biosynthesis of TSH- and LH-releasing factors by the human placenta. Am J Obstet Gynecol 121:127, 1975
Gleicher N, Barad DH: Gender as risk factor for autoimmune diseases. J Autoimmun 28:1, 2007
Golander A, Hurley T, Barrett J, et al: Prolactin synthesis by human chorion-decidual tissue: a possible source of prolactin in the amniotic fluid. Science 202:311, 1978
Goldman-Wohl DS, Ariel I, Greenfield C, et al: HLA-G expression in extravillous trophoblasts is an intrinsic property of cell differentiation: a lesson learned from ectopic pregnancies. Mol Hum Reprod 6:535, 2000
Gougeon A: Regulation of ovarian follicular development in primates: facts and hypotheses. Endocr Rev 17:121, 1996
Greer LG, Casey BM, Halvorson LM, et al: Antithyroid antibodies and parity: further evidence for microchimerism in autoimmune thyroid disease. Am J Obstet Gynecol 205(5):471.e1, 2011
Groome NP, Illingworth PJ, O'Brien M, et al: Measurement of dimeric inhibin B throughout the human menstrual cycle. J Clin Endocrinol Metab 81:1401, 1996
Grumbach MM: Aromatase deficiency and its consequences. Adv Exp Med Biol 707:19, 2011
Grumbach MM, Kaplan SL: On placental origin and purification of chorionic growth hormone prolactin and its immunoassay in pregnancy. Trans N Y Acad Sci 27:167, 1964
Gualillo O, Caminos J, Blanco M, et al: Ghrelin, a novel placental-derived hormone. Endocrinology 142:788, 2001
Gubbay O, Critchley HO, Bowen JM, et al: Prolactin induces ERK phosphorylation in epithelial and CD56(+) natural killer cells of the human endometrium. J Clin Endocrinol Metab 87:2329, 2002
Gurpide E, Schwers J, Welch MT, et al: Fetal and maternal metabolism of estradiol during pregnancy. J Clin Endocrinol Metab 26:1355, 1966
Gurpide E, Tseng J, Escarcena L, et al: Fetomaternal production and transfer of progesterone and uridine in sheep. Am J Obstet Gynecol 113:21, 1972
Guzeloglu-Kayisli O, Kayisli UA, Taylor HS: The role of growth factors and cytokines during implantation: endocrine and paracrine interactions. Semin Reprod Med 27(1):62, 2009
Hafez ES, Ludwig H, Metzger H: Human endometrial fluid kinetics as observed by scanning electron microscopy. Am J Obstet Gynecol 122:929, 1975
Halvorson LM: Reproductive endocrinology. In Hoffman BL, Schorge JO, Schaffer JI, et al (eds): Williams Gynecology, 2nd ed. McGraw-Hill, 2012
Hamilton W, Boyd J: Trophoblast in human utero-placental arteries. Nature 212:906, 1966
Hanna J, Goldman-Wohl D, Hamani Y, et al: Decidual NK cells regulate key developmental processes at the human fetal-maternal interface. Nat Med 12:1065, 2006
Hansell DJ, Bryant-Greenwood GD, Greenwood FC: Expression of the human relaxin H1 gene in the decidua, trophoblast, and prostate. J Clin Endocrinol Metab 72:899, 1991
Harada N, Ogawa H, Shozu M, et al: Biochemical and molecular genetic analyses on placental aromatase (P-450AROM) deficiency. J Biol Chem 267:4781, 1992
Hellig H, Gattereau D, Lefebvre Y, et al: Steroid production from plasma cholesterol. I. Conversion of plasma cholesterol to placental progesterone in humans. J Clin Endocrinol Metab 30:624, 1970
Henson MC, Castracane VD: Leptin: roles and regulation in primate pregnancy. Semin Reprod Med 20:113, 2002
Henson MC, Greene SJ, Reggio BC, et al: Effects of reduced maternal lipoprotein-cholesterol availability on placental progesterone biosynthesis in the baboon. Endocrinology 138:1385, 1997
Hershman JM: Human chorionic gonadotropin and the thyroid: Hyperemesis gravidarum and trophoblastic tumors. Thyroid 9:653, 1999
Hertig AT: The placenta: some new knowledge about an old organ. Obstet Gynecol 20:859, 1962
Hillier SG: Gonadotropic control of ovarian follicular growth and development. Mol Cell Endocrinol 179:39, 2001
Horvath TL, Diano S, Sotonyi P, et al: Minireview: ghrelin and the regulation of energy balance—a hypothalamic perspective. Endocrinology 142:4163, 2001

Hoshina M, Boothby M, Boime I: Cytological localization of chorionic gonadotropin alpha and placental lactogen mRNAs during development of the human placenta. J Cell Biol 93:190, 1982
Hreinsson JG, Scott JE, Rasmussen C, et al: Growth differentiation factor-9 promotes the growth, development, and survival of human ovarian follicles in organ culture. J Clin Endocrinol Metab 87:316, 2002
Hudson P, Haley J, John M, et al: Structure of a genomic clone encoding biologically active human relaxin. Nature 301:628, 1983
Hudson P, John M, Crawford R, et al: Relaxin gene expression in human ovaries and the predicted structure of a human preprorelaxin by analysis of cDNA clones. EMBO J 3:2333, 1984
Hunt JS, Jadhav L, Chu W, et al: Soluble HLA-G circulates in maternal blood during pregnancy. Am J Obstet Gynecol 183:682, 2000a
Hunt JS, Orr HT: HLA and maternal-fetal recognition. FASEB J 6:2344, 1992
Hunt JS, Petroff MG, Morales P, et al: HLA-G in reproduction: studies on the maternal-fetal interface. Hum Immunol 61:1113, 2000b
Illingworth DR, Corbin DK, Kemp ED, et al: Hormone changes during the menstrual cycle in abetalipoproteinemia: reduced luteal phase progesterone in a patient with homozygous hypobetalipoproteinemia. Proc Natl Acad Sci USA 79:6685, 1982
Iwashita M, Kudo Y, Shinozaki Y, et al: Gonadotropin-releasing hormone increases serum human chorionic gonadotropin in pregnant women. Endocr J 40:539, 1993
Jabbour HN, Critchley HOD: Potential roles of decidual prolactin in early pregnancy. Reproduction 121:197, 2001
Jeffrey J: Collagen and collagenase: pregnancy and parturition. Semin Perinatol 15:118, 1991
Jiang Y, Hu Y, Zhao J, et al: The orphan nuclear receptor Nur77 regulates decidual prolactin expression in human endometrial stromal cells. Biochem Biophys Res Commun 404(2):628, 2011
Johnson EL, Chakraborty R: Placental Hofbauer cells limit HIV-1 replication and potentially offset mother to child transmission (MTCT) by induction of immunoregulatory cytokines. Retrovirology 9:101, 2012
Johnson PM, Christmas SE, Vince GS: Immunological aspects of implantation and implantation failure. Hum Reprod 14(suppl 2):26, 1999
Jokhi P, King A, Loke Y: Production of granulocyte/macrophage colony-stimulating factor by human trophoblast cells and by decidual large granular lymphocytes. Hum Reprod 9:1660, 1999
Jones SA, Brooks AN, Challis JR: Steroids modulate corticotropin-releasing hormone production in human fetal membranes and placenta. J Clin Endocrinol Metab 68:825, 1989a
Jones SA, Challis JR: Local stimulation of prostaglandin production by corticotropin-releasing hormone in human fetal membranes and placenta. Biochem Biophys Res Commun 159:192, 1989b
Kaipia A, Hsueh AJ: Regulation of ovarian follicle atresia. Annu Rev Physiol 59:349, 1997
Kane N, Kelly R, Saunders PTK, et al: Proliferation of uterine natural killer cells is induced by hCG and mediated via the mannose receptor. Endocrinology 150(6):2882, 2009
Kaneko Y, Murphy CR, Day ML: Extracellular matrix proteins secreted from both the endometrium and the embryo are required for attachment: a study using a co-culture model of rat blastocysts and Ishikawa cells. J Morphol 2741(1):63, 2013
Katzenellenbogen BS, Sun J, Harrington WR, et al: Structure-function relationships in estrogen receptors and the characterization of novel selective estrogen receptor modulators with unique pharmacological profiles. Ann NY Acad Sci 949:6, 2001
Kaufmann P, Black S, Huppertz B: Endovascular trophoblast invasion: implications for the pathogenesis of intrauterine growth retardation and preeclampsia. Biol Reprod 69:1, 2003
Kaufmann P, Scheffen I: Placental development. In Polin R, Fox W (eds): Fetal and Neonatal Physiology. Philadelphia, Saunders, 1992, p 47
Khodr GS, Siler-Khodr TM: Placental luteinizing hormone-releasing factor and its synthesis. Science 207:315, 1980
Kim H, Toyofuku Y, Lynn FC; et al: Serotonin regulates pancreatic beta cell mass during pregnancy. Nat Med 16(7):804, 2010
King BF, Menton DN: Scanning electron microscopy of human placental villi from early and late in gestation. Am J Obstet Gynecol 122:824, 1975
Kraiem Z, Sadeh O, Blithe DL, et al: Human chorionic gonadotropin stimulates thyroid hormone secretion, iodide uptake, organification, and adenosine 3′, 5′-monophosphate formation in cultured human thyrocytes. J Clin Endocrinol Metab 79:595, 1994
Kurman RJ, Young RH, Norris HJ, et al: Immunocytochemical localization of placental lactogen and chorionic gonadotropin in the normal placenta and trophoblastic tumors, with emphasis on intermediate trophoblast and the placental site trophoblastic tumor. Int J Gynecol Pathol 3:101, 1984
Kurtzman JT, Wilson H, Rao CV: A proposed role for hCG in clinical obstetrics. Semin Reprod Med 19:63, 2001
La Cava A, Alviggi C, Matarese G: Unraveling the multiple roles of leptin in inflammation and autoimmunity. J Mol Med 82:4, 2004
Lala PK, Lee BP, Xu G, et al: Human placental trophoblast as an in vitro model for tumor progression. Can J Physiol Pharmacol 80:142, 2002
LeBouteiller P, Solier C, Proll J, et al: Placental HLA-G protein expression in vivo: where and what for? Hum Reprod Update 5:223, 1999
Lecce G, Meduri G, Ancelin M, et al: Presence of estrogen receptor beta in the human endometrium through the cycle: expression in glandular, stromal, and vascular cells. J Clin Endocrinol Metab 86:1379, 2001
Lessey BA, Castelbaum AJ: Integrins and implantation in the human. Rev Endocr Metab Disord 3:107, 2002
Lessey BA, Castelbaum AJ, Sawin SW, et al: Integrins as markers of uterine receptivity in women with primary unexplained infertility. Fertil Steril 63:535, 1995
Lessey BA, Ilesanmi AO, Lessey MA, et al: Luminal and glandular endometrial epithelium express integrins differentially throughout the menstrual cycle: implications for implantation, contraception, and infertility. Am J Reprod Immunol 35:195, 1996
Li XF, Charnock-Jones DS, Zhang E, et al: Angiogenic growth factor messenger ribonucleic acids in uterine natural killer cells. J Clin Endocrinol Metab 86:1823, 2001
Licht P, Russu V, Wildt L: On the role of human chorionic gonadotropin (hCG) in the embryo-endometrial microenvironment: implications for differentiation and implantation. Semin Reprod Med 19:37, 2001
Lindhard A, Bentin-Ley U, Ravn V, et al: Biochemical evaluation of endometrial function at the time of implantation. Fertil Steril 78:221, 2002
Lobo SC, Srisuparp S, Peng X, et al: Uterine receptivity in the baboon: Modulation by chorionic gonadotropin. Semin Reprod Med 19:69, 2001
Loke YM, King A: Human Implantation. Cell Biology and Immunology. Cambridge, Cambridge University Press, 1995
Loquet P, Broughton-Pipkin F, Symonds E, et al: Blood velocity waveforms and placental vascular formation. Lancet 2:1252, 1988
Lynch VJ, Brayer K, Gellersen B: HoxA-11 and FOXO1A cooperate to regulate decidual prolactin expression: towards inferring the core transcriptional regulators of decidual genes. PLoS One 4(9):e6845, 2009
Maaskant RA, Bogic LV, Gilger S, et al: The human prolactin receptor in the fetal membranes, decidua, and placenta. J Clin Endocrinol Metab 81:396, 1996
MacDonald PC: Placental steroidogenesis. In Wynn RM (ed): Fetal Homeostasis, Vol. I. New York, New York Academy of Sciences, 1965a, p 265
MacDonald PC, Siiteri PK: Origin of estrogen in women pregnant with an anencephalic fetus. J Clin Invest 44:465, 1965b
MacDonald PC, Siiteri PK: Study of estrogen production in women with hydatidiform mole. J Clin Endocrinol Metab 24:685, 1964
MacDonald PC, Siiteri PK: The in vivo mechanisms of origin of estrogen in subjects with trophoblastic tumors. Steroids 8:589, 1966
Macklon NS, Fauser BC: Follicle-stimulating hormone and advanced follicle development in the human. Arch Med Res 32:595, 2001
Magarinos MP, Sanchez-Margalet V, Kotler M, et al: Leptin promotes cell proliferation and survival of trophoblastic cells. Biol Reprod 76:203, 2007
Manaster I, Mizrahi S, Goldman-Wohl D, et al: Endometrial NK cells are special immature cells that await pregnancy. J Immunol 181:1869, 2008
Maradny EE, Kanayama N, Halim A, et al: Stretching of fetal membranes increases the concentration of interleukin-8 and collagenase activity. Am J Obstet Gynecol 174:843, 1996
Markee J: Menstruation in intraocular endometrial transplants in the rhesus monkey. Contrib Embryol 28:219, 1940
Maruo T, Ladines-Llave CA, Matsuo H, et al: A novel change in cytologic localization of human chorionic gonadotropin and human placental lactogen in first-trimester placenta in the course of gestation. Am J Obstet Gynecol 167:217, 1992
Maulik D: Doppler ultrasound in obstetrics. Williams Obstetrics, 20th ed. Stamford, Appleton & Lange, 1997, p 1
McCabe ERB: Adrenal hypoplasias and aplasias. In Scriver CR, Beaudet AL, Sly WE, et al (eds): The Metabolic and Molecular Bases of Inherited Disease. New York, McGraw-Hill, 2001, p 4263
McCombs H, Craig M: Decidual necrosis in normal pregnancy. Obstet Gynecol 24:436, 1964
McGregor WG, Kuhn RW, Jaffe RB: Biologically active chorionic gonadotropin: synthesis by the human fetus. Science 220:306, 1983
McGregor WG, Raymoure WJ, Kuhn RW, et al: Fetal tissue can synthesize a placental hormone. Evidence for chorionic gonadotropin beta-subunit synthesis by human fetal kidney. J Clin Invest 68:306, 1981
McMaster M, Librach C, Zhou Y, et al: Human placental HLA-G expression is restricted to differentiated cytotrophoblasts. J Immunol 154:3771, 1995

Medawar PB: Some immunological and endocrinological problems raised by the evolution of viviparity in vertebrates. Symp Soc Exp Biol 44:1953
Meinert M, Malmström E, Tufvesson E: Labour induces increased concentrations of biglycan and hyaluronan in human fetal membranes. Placenta 28:482, 2007
Mesiano S: The endocrinology of human pregnancy and fetoplacental neuroendocrine development. In Strauss JF, Barbieri RL (eds): Yen and Jaffe's Reproductive Endocrinology: Physiology, Pathophysiology, and Clinical Management, 6th ed. Philadelphia, Saunders, 2009, p 265
Mijovic JE, Demianczuk N, Olson DM, et al: Prostaglandin endoperoxide H synthase mRNA expression in the fetal membranes correlates with fetal fibronectin concentration in the cervico-vaginal fluids at term: evidence of enzyme induction before the onset of labour. Br J Obstet Gynaecol 107:267, 2000
Milewich L, Gomez-Sanchez C, Madden JD, et al: Dehydroisoandrosterone sulfate in peripheral blood of premenopausal, pregnant and postmenopausal women and men. J Steroid Biochem 9:1159, 1978
Miller-Lindholm AK, LaBenz CJ, Ramey J, et al: Human chorionic gonadotropin-beta gene expression in first trimester placenta. Endocrinology 138:5459, 1997
Moffett-King A: Natural killer cells and pregnancy. Nat Rev Immunol 2:656, 2002
Mogami H, Kishore AH, Shi H, et al: Fetal fibronectin signaling induces matrix metalloproteases and cyclooxygenase-2 (COX-2) in amnion cells and preterm birth in mice. J Biol Chem 288(3):1953, 2013
Moore JJ, Dubyak GR, Moore RM, et al: Oxytocin activates the inositol-phospholipid-protein kinase-C system and stimulates prostaglandin production in human amnion cells. Endocrinology 123:1771, 1988
Moore RM, Redline RW, Kumar D, et al: Differential expression of fibulin family proteins in the para-cervical weak zone and other areas of human fetal membranes. Placenta 30(4):335, 2009
Morrish DW, Marusyk H, Siy O: Demonstration of specific secretory granules for human chorionic gonadotropin in placenta. J Histochem Cytochem 35:93, 1987
Mote PA, Balleine RL, McGowan EM, et al: Colocalization of progesterone receptors A and B by dual immunofluorescent histochemistry in human endometrium during the menstrual cycle. J Clin Endocrinol Metab 84:2963, 1999
Mote PA, Balleine RL, McGowan EM, et al: Heterogeneity of progesterone receptors A and B expression in human endometrial glands and stroma. Hum Reprod 15(suppl 3):48, 2000
Navot D, Bergh P: Preparation of the human endometrium for implantation. Ann N Y Acad Sci 622:212, 1991
Nemeth E, Tashima LS, Yu Z, et al: Fetal membrane distention: I. Differentially expressed genes regulated by acute distention in amniotic epithelial (WISH) cells. Am J Obstet Gynecol 182:50, 2000
Nguyen H, Dubernard G, Aractingi S, et al: Feto-maternal cell trafficking: a transfer of pregnancy associated progenitor cells. Stem Cell Rev 2:111, 2006
Nicholson RC, King BR: Regulation of CRH gene expression in the placenta. Front Horm Res 27:246, 2001
Nikas G: Cell-surface morphological events relevant to human implantation. Hum Reprod 2:37, 2003
Ny T, Wahlberg P, Brandstrom IJ: Matrix remodeling in the ovary: regulation and functional role of the plasminogen activator and matrix metalloproteinase systems. Mol Cell Endocrinol 187:29, 2002
Odagiri E, Sherrell BJ, Mount CD, et al: Human placental immunoreactive corticotropin, lipotropin, and beta-endorphin: evidence for a common precursor. Proc Natl Acad Sci USA 76:2027, 1979
Ogren L, Talamantes F: The placenta as an endocrine organ: Polypeptides. In Knobil E, Neill JD (eds): The Physiology of Reproduction. New York, Raven, 1994, p 875
O'Sullivan CM, Liu SY, Karpinka JB, et al: Embryonic hatching enzyme strypsin/ISP1 is expressed with ISP2 in endometrial glands during implantation. Mol Reprod Dev 62:328, 2002
Paria BC, Reese J, Das SK, et al: Deciphering the cross-talk of implantation: advances and challenges. Science 296:2185, 2002
Parker CR Jr, Carr BR, Simpson ER, et al: Decline in the concentration of low-density lipoprotein-cholesterol in human fetal plasma near term. Metabolism 32:919, 1983
Parker CR Jr, Illingworth DR, Bissonnette J, et al: Endocrinology of pregnancy in abetalipoproteinemia: studies in a patient with homozygous familial hypobetalipoproteinemia. N Engl J Med 314:557, 1986
Parker CR Jr, Simpson ER, Bilheimer DW, et al: Inverse relation between low-density lipoprotein-cholesterol and dehydroisoandrosterone sulfate in human fetal plasma. Science 208:512, 1980
Patel N, Alsat E, Igout A, et al: Glucose inhibits human placental GH secretion, in vitro. J Clin Endocrinol Metab 80:1743, 1995
Pellegrini I, Lebrun JJ, Ali S, et al: Expression of prolactin and its receptor in human lymphoid cells. Mol Endocrinol 6:1023, 1992
Peluso JJ: Non-genomic actions of progesterone in the normal and neoplastic mammalian ovary. Semin Reprod Med 25:198, 2007
Perrot-Applanat M, Groyer-Picard MT, Garcia E, et al: Immunocytochemical demonstration of estrogen and progesterone receptors in muscle cells of uterine arteries in rabbits and humans. Endocrinology 123:1511, 1988
Petraglia F, Florio P, Benedetto C, et al: Urocortin stimulates placental adrenocorticotropin and prostaglandin release and myometrial contractility in vitro. J Clin Endocrinol Metab 84:1420, 1999
Petraglia F, Gallinelli A, De Vita D, et al: Activin at parturition: changes of maternal serum levels and evidence for binding sites in placenta and fetal membranes. Obstet Gynecol 84:278, 1994
Petraglia F, Garuti GC, Calza L, et al: Inhibin subunits in human placenta: localization and messenger ribonucleic acid levels during pregnancy. Am J Obstet Gynecol 165:750, 1991
Petraglia F, Giardino L, Coukos G, et al: Corticotropin-releasing factor and parturition: plasma and amniotic fluid levels and placental binding sites. Obstet Gynecol 75:784, 1990
Petraglia F, Sawchenko P, Lim AT, et al: Localization, secretion, and action of inhibin in human placenta. Science 237:187, 1987
Petraglia F, Vaughan J, Vale W: Inhibin and activin modulate the release of gonadotropin-releasing hormone, human chorionic gonadotropin, and progesterone from cultured human placental cells. Proc Natl Acad Sci USA 86:5114, 1989
Petraglia F, Woodruff TK, Botticelli G, et al: Gonadotropin-releasing hormone, inhibin, and activin in human placenta: Evidence for a common cellular localization. J Clin Endocrinol Metab 74:1184, 1992
Pijnenborg R: Trophoblast invasion. Reprod Med Rev 3:53, 1994
Pijnenborg R, Bland JM, Robertson WB, et al: Uteroplacental arterial changes related to interstitial trophoblast migration in early human pregnancy. Placenta 4:397, 1983
Piper KP, McLarnon A, Arrazi J, et al: Functional HY-specific CD8+ T cells are found in a high proportion of women following pregnancy with a male fetus. Biol Reprod 76:96, 2007
Primakoff P, Myles DG: Penetration, adhesion, and fusion in mammalian sperm-egg interaction. Science 296:2183, 2002
Qin X, Chua PK, Ohira RH, et al: An autocrine/paracrine role of human decidual relaxin. II. Stromelysin-1 (MMP-3) and tissue inhibitor of matrix metalloproteinase-1 (TIMP-1). Biol Reprod 56:812, 1997a
Qin X, Garibay-Tupas J, Chua PK, et al: An autocrine/paracrine role of human decidual relaxin. I. Interstitial collagenase (matrix metalloproteinase-1) and tissue plasminogen activator. Biol Reprod 56:800, 1997b
Ragoobir J, Abayasekara DR, Bruckdorfer KR, et al: Stimulation of progesterone production in human granulosa-lutein cells by lipoproteins: evidence for cholesterol-independent actions of high-density lipoproteins. J Endocrinol 173:103, 2002
Rainey WE, Carr BR, Wang ZN, et al: Gene profiling of human fetal and adult adrenals. J Endocrinol 171:209, 2001
Rajagopalan S, Long O: Cellular senescence induced by CD158d reprograms natural killer cells to promote vascular remodeling. Proc Natl Acad Sci USA 109(50):20596, 2012
Ramsey E, Davis R: A composite drawing of the placenta to show its structure and circulation. Anat Rec 145:366, 1963
Ramsey E, Harris J: Comparison of uteroplacental vasculature and circulation in the rhesus monkey and man. Contrib Embryol 38:59, 1966
Ramsey EM, Donner MW: Placental Vasculature and Circulation. Philadelphia, Saunders, 1980
Red-Horse K, Rivera J, Schanz A, et al: Cytotrophoblast induction of arterial apoptosis and lymphangiogenesis in an in vivo model of human placentation. J Clin Invest 116:2643, 2006
Richards JS: Genetics of ovulation. Semin Reprod Med 25(4):235, 2007
Riddick DH, Luciano AA, Kusmik WF, et al: Evidence for a nonpituitary source of amniotic fluid prolactin. Fertil Steril 31:35, 1979
Riley S, Walton J, Herlick J, et al: The localization and distribution of corticotropin-releasing hormone in the human placenta and fetal membranes throughout gestation. J Clin Endocrinol Metab 72:1001, 1991
Robidoux J, Simoneau L, St Pierre S, et al: Characterization of neuropeptide Y-mediated corticotropin-releasing factor synthesis and release from human placental trophoblasts. Endocrinology 141:2795, 2000
Robinson BG, Emanuel RL, Frim DM, et al: Glucocorticoid stimulates expression of corticotropin-releasing hormone gene in human placenta. Proc Natl Acad Sci USA 85:5244, 1988
Rock J, Bartlett M: Biopsy studies of human endometrium. JAMA 108:2022, 1937
Rogers PA, Donoghue JF, Walter LM, et al: Endometrial angiogenesis, vascular maturation, and lymphangiogenesis. Reprod Sci 16(2):147, 2009
Rowe T, King L, MacDonald PC, et al: Tissue inhibitor of metalloproteinase-1 and tissue inhibitor of metalloproteinase-2 expression in human amnion mesenchymal and epithelial cells. Am J Obstet Gynecol 176:915, 1997

Ryan KJ: Biological aromatization of steroids. J Biol Chem 234:268, 1959a
Ryan KJ: Metabolism of C-16-oxygenated steroids by human placenta: the formation of estriol. J Biol Chem 234:2006, 1959b
Salido EC, Yen PH, Barajas L, et al: Steroid sulfatase expression in human placenta: immunocytochemistry and in situ hybridization study. J Clin Endocrinol Metab 70:1564, 1990
Santoni S, Zingoni A, Cerboni C, et al: Natural killer (NK) cells from killers to regulators: distinct features between peripheral blood and decidual NK cells. Am J Reprod Immunol 58:280, 2007
Saunders PTK: Does estrogen receptor β play a significant role in human reproduction? Trends Endocrinol Metab 16:222, 2005
Saxe A, Dean S, Gibson G, et al: Parathyroid hormone and parathyroid hormone-related peptide in venous umbilical cord blood of healthy neonates. J Perinat Med 25:288, 1997
Segaloff A, Sternberg W, Gaskill C: Effects of luteotrophic doses of chorionic gonadotropin in women. J Clin Endocrinol Metab 11:936, 1951
Short R: Steroids in the follicular fluid and the corpus luteum of the mare. A "two cell type" theory of ovarian steroid synthesis. J Endocrinol 24:59, 1962
Shozu M, Akasofu K, Harada T, et al: A new cause of female pseudohermaphroditism: placental aromatase deficiency. J Clin Endocrinol Metab 72:560, 1991
Siiteri PK, MacDonald PC: Placental estrogen biosynthesis during human pregnancy. J Clin Endocrinol Metab 26:751, 1966
Siiteri PK, MacDonald PC: The utilization of circulating dehydroisoandrosterone sulfate for estrogen synthesis during human pregnancy. Steroids 2:713, 1963
Siler-Khodr TM: Chorionic peptides. In McNellis D, Challis JRG, MacDonald PC, et al (eds): The Onset of Labor: Cellular and Integrative Mechanisms. Ithaca, Perinatology Press, 1988, p 213
Siler-Khodr TM, Khodr GS: Content of luteinizing hormone-releasing factor in the human placenta. Am J Obstet Gynecol 130:216, 1978
Siler-Khodr TM, Khodr GS: Dose response analysis of GnRH stimulation of hCG release from human term placenta. Biol Reprod 25:353, 1981
Siler-Khodr TM, Khodr GS, Valenzuela G: Immunoreactive gonadotropin-releasing hormone level in maternal circulation throughout pregnancy. Am J Obstet Gynecol 150:376, 1984
Silver RM, Varner MW, Reddy U, et al: Work-up of stillbirth: a review of the evidence. Am J Obstet Gynecol 196:433, 2007
Simmonds CS, Karsenty G, Karaplis AD, et al: Parathyroid hormone regulates fetal-placental mineral homeostasis. J bone Miner Res 25(3):594, 2010
Simpson ER: Genetic mutations resulting in loss of aromatase activity in humans and mice. J Soc Gynecol Investig 7:S18, 2000
Simpson ER, Burkhart MF: Acyl CoA:cholesterol acyl transferase activity in human placental microsomes: inhibition by progesterone. Arch Biochem Biophys 200:79, 1980
Simpson ER, Carr BR, Parker CR, Jr, et al: The role of serum lipoproteins in steroidogenesis by the human fetal adrenal cortex. J Clin Endocrinol Metab 49:146, 1979
Sipos PI, Rens W, Schlecht H, et al: Uterine vasculature remodeling in human pregnancy involves functional macrochimerism by endothelial colony forming cells of fetal origin. Stem Cells 31:1363, 2013
Soares MJ, Chakraborty D, Renaud SJ, et al: Regulatory pathways controlling the endovascular invasive trophoblast cell linear. J Reprod Dev 58(3):283, 2012
Staun-Ram E, Shalev E: Human trophoblast function during the implantation process. Reprod Biol Endocrinol 3:56, 2005
Steele GL, Currie WD, Yuen BH, et al: Acute stimulation of human chorionic gonadotropin secretion by recombinant human activin-A in first trimester human trophoblast. Endocrinology 133:297, 1993
Stevens AM: Microchimeric cells in systemic lupus erythematosus: targets or innocent bystanders? Lupus 15:820, 2006
Sugino N, Kashida S, Karube-Harada A, et al: Expression of vascular endothelial growth factor (VEGF) and its receptors in human endometrium throughout the menstrual cycle and in early pregnancy. Reproduction 123:379, 2002
Telgmann R, Gellersen B: Marker genes of decidualization: Activation of the decidual prolactin gene. Hum Reprod Update 4:472, 1998
Thellin O, Coumans B, Zorzi W, et al: Tolerance to the foeto-placental "graft": ten ways to support a child for nine months. Curr Opin Immunol 12:731, 2000
Thiruchelvam U, Dransfield I, Saunders PTK, et al: The importance of the macrophage within the human endometrium. J Leukoc Biol 93(2):217, 2013
Tomer Y, Huber GK, Davies TF: Human chorionic gonadotropin (hCG) interacts directly with recombinant human TSH receptors. J Clin Endocrinol Metab 74:1477, 1992
Trombly DJ, Woodruff TK, Mayo KE: Roles for transforming growth factor beta superfamily proteins in early folliculogenesis. Semin Reprod Med 27(1):14, 2009
Tsai SJ, Wu MH, Chen HM, et al: Fibroblast growth factor-9 is an endometrial stromal growth factor. Endocrinology 143:2715, 2002
Tsuruta E, Tada H, Tamaki H, et al: Pathogenic role of asialo human chorionic gonadotropin in gestational thyrotoxicosis. J Clin Endocrinol Metab 80:350, 1995
Tyson JE, Hwang P, Guyda H, et al: Studies of prolactin secretion in human pregnancy. Am J Obstet Gynecol 113:14, 1972
Vande Wiele RL, Bogumil J, Dyrenfurth I, et al: Mechanisms regulating the menstrual cycle in women. Recent Prog Horm Res 26:63, 1970
Vaskivuo TE, Ottander U, Oduwole O, et al: Role of apoptosis, apoptosis-related factors and 17 beta-hydroxysteroid dehydrogenases in human corpus luteum regression. Mol Cell Endocrinol 194(1–2):191, 2002
Vickers MH, Gilmour S, Gertler A, et al: 20-kDa placental hGH-V has diminished diabetogenic and lactogenic activities compared with 22-kDa hGH-N while retaining antilipogenic activity. Am J Physiol Endocrinol Metab 297(3):E629, 2009
Vince GS, Johnson PM: Immunobiology of human uteroplacental macrophages—friend and foe? Placenta 17:191, 1996
Wadhwa PD, Porto M, Garite TJ, et al: Maternal corticotropin-releasing hormone levels in the early third trimester predict length of gestation in human pregnancy. Am J Obstet Gynecol 179:1079, 1998
Walker WH, Fitzpatrick SL, Barrera-Saldana HA, et al: The human placental lactogen genes: structure, function, evolution and transcriptional regulation. Endocr Rev 12:316, 1991
Warren W, Silverman A: Cellular localization of corticotrophin releasing hormone in the human placenta, fetal membranes and decidua. Placenta 16:147, 1995
Weetman AP: The immunology of pregnancy. Thyroid 9:643, 1999
Wehmann RE, Nisula BC: Renal clearance rates of the subunits of human chorionic gonadotropin in man. J Clin Endocrinol Metab 50:674, 1980
Wentz AC, Jones GS: Transient luteolytic effect of prostaglandin F2alpha in the human. Obstet Gynecol 42:172, 1973
Werbin H, Plotz EJ, LeRoy GV, et al: Cholesterol: a precursor of estrone in vivo. J Am Chem Soc 79:1012, 1957
Whittle WL, Gibb W, Challis JR: The characterization of human amnion epithelial and mesenchymal cells: the cellular expression, activity and glucocorticoid regulation of prostaglandin output. Placenta 21:394, 2000
Winger EE, Reed JL: The multiple faces of the decidual natural killer cell. Am J Reprod Immunol 70:1, 2013
Wislocki GB, Dempsey EW: Electron microscopy of the human placenta. Anat Rec 123:133, 1955
Wolfahrt S, Kleine B, Rossmanith WG: Detection of gonadotrophin releasing hormone and its receptor mRNA in human placental trophoblasts using in situ reverse transcription-polymerase chain reaction. Mol Hum Reprod 4:999, 1998
Yan C, Wang P, DeMayo J, et al: Synergistic roles of bone morphogenetic Protein 15 and growth differentiation Factor 9 in ovarian function. Mol Endocrinol 15:854, 2001
Yoshimura M, Pekary AE, Pang XP, et al: Thyrotropic activity of basic isoelectric forms of human chorionic gonadotropin extracted from hydatidiform mole tissues. J Clin Endocrinol Metab 78:862, 1994

CHAPTER 6

Placental Abnormalities

Obstetrical practice has always emphasized that gross examination of the placenta is integral following delivery. In some cases, findings prompt further action by the obstetrician or pediatrician. In addition, great strides have been made concerning the histopathological examination of placental tissue to provide clinically useful information. Pioneering efforts in this field include those of Benirschke, Driscoll, Fox, Naeye, Salafia, and Faye-Petersen.

HISTOPATHOLOGICAL EXAMINATION

We agree with most authorities that routine placental examination by a pathologist is not indicated, although there is still debate as to which placentas should be submitted. For example, the College of American Pathologists recommends routine examination for an extensive list of indications (Langston, 1997). However, data may be insufficient to support all of these. Certainly, the placenta and cord should be examined in the delivery room. As some correlation of specific placental findings with both short- and long-term neonatal outcomes is possible, the decision to request pathological examination should be based on clinical and placental findings (Redline, 2008; Roberts, 2008). Shown in Table 6-1 are indications used at Parkland Hospital to submit a placenta to the Pathology Department.

NORMAL PLACENTA

Placental abnormalities are better understood with knowledge of placental implantation, development, and anatomy presented in Chapter 5 (p. 88). At term, the "typical" placenta weighs 470 g, is round to oval with a 22-cm diameter, and has a central thickness of 2.5 cm (Benirschke, 2012). It is composed of a placental disc, extraplacental membranes, and three-vessel umbilical cord. The maternal surface is the basal plate, which is divided by clefts into portions—termed cotyledons. These clefts mark the site of internal septa, which extend into the intervillous space. The fetal surface is the chorionic plate, into which the umbilical cord inserts, typically in the center. Large fetal vessels that originate from the cord vessels then spread and branch across the chorionic plate before entering stem villi of the placenta parenchyma. In tracing these, fetal arteries almost invariably cross over veins. The chorionic plate and its vessels are covered by thin amnion, which can be easily peeled away from a postdelivery specimen.

Sonographically, the normal placenta is homogenous and 2 to 4 cm thick, lies against the myometrium, and indents into the amnionic sac. The retroplacental space is a hypoechoic area that separates the myometrium from the placenta's basal plate and measures less than 1 to 2 cm. During prenatal sonographic examinations, placental location and relationship to the internal cervical os are recorded. The umbilical cord is also imaged, its fetal and placental insertion sites examined, and its vessels counted.

TABLE 6-1. Some Indications for Placental Pathological Examination[a]

Maternal Indications
Abruption
Antepartum infection with fetal risks
Anti-CDE alloimmunization
Cesarean hysterectomy
Oligohydramnios or hydramnios
Peripartum fever or infection
Preterm delivery
Postterm delivery
Severe trauma
Suspected placental injury
Systemic disorders with known effects
Thick or viscid meconium
Unexplained late pregnancy bleeding
Unexplained or recurrent pregnancy complications
Fetal and Neonatal Indications
Admission to an acute care nursery
Birth weight ≤ 10th or ≥ 95th percentile
Fetal anemia
Fetal or neonatal compromise
Neonatal seizures
Hydrops fetalis
Infection or sepsis
Major anomalies or abnormal karyotype
Multifetal gestation
Stillbirth or neonatal death
Vanishing twin beyond the first trimester
Placental Indications
Gross lesions
Marginal or velamentous cord insertion
Markedly abnormal placental shape or size
Markedly adhered placenta
Term cord < 32 cm or > 100 cm
Umbilical cord lesions

[a]Indications are organized alphabetically.

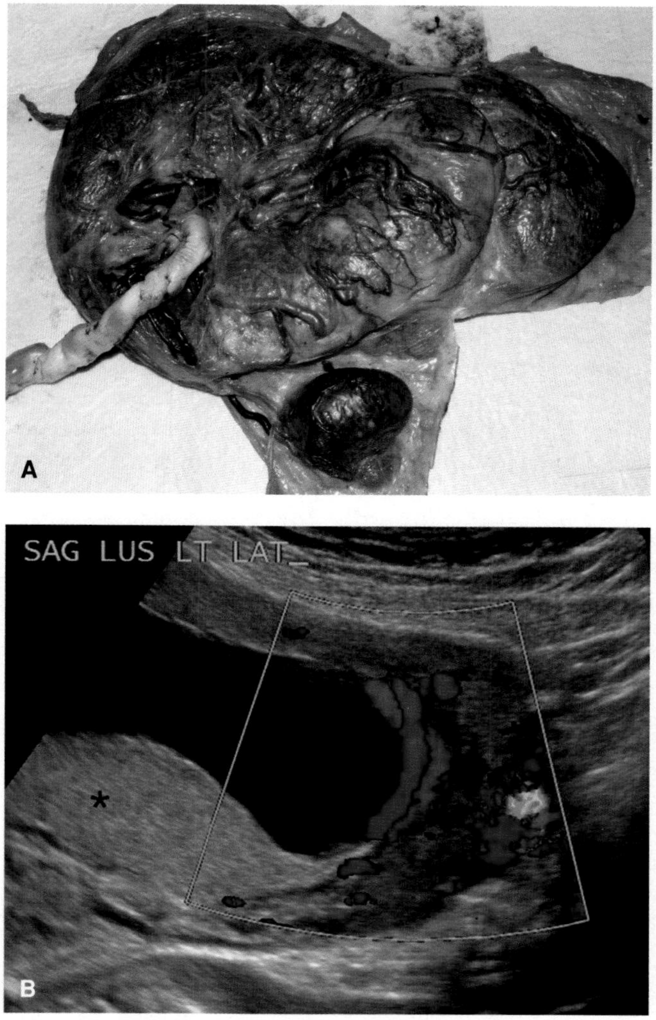

FIGURE 6-1 Succenturiate lobe. **A.** Vessels extend from the main placental disk to supply the small round succenturiate lobe located beneath it. (Photograph contributed by Dr. Jaya George.) **B.** Sonographic imaging with color Doppler shows the main placental disk implanted posteriorly (*asterisk*). The succenturiate lobe is located on the anterior uterine wall across the amnionic cavity. Vessels are identified as the long red and blue crossing tubular structures that travel within the membranes to connect these two portions of placenta.

Many placental lesions can be identified grossly or sonographically, but many abnormalities require histopathological examination for clarification. A detailed description of these is beyond the scope of this chapter, and interested readers are referred to textbooks by Benirschke (2012), Fox (2007), Faye-Petersen (2006), and their colleagues.

ABNORMALITIES OF THE PLACENTA

Shape and Size

In contrast to the normal architecture described earlier, placentas may infrequently form as separate, nearly equally sized discs. This is a bilobate placenta, but is also known as bipartite placenta or placenta duplex. In these, the cord inserts between the two placental lobes—either into a connecting chorionic bridge or into intervening membranes.

A placenta containing three or more equally sized lobes is rare and termed multilobate. However, more frequently, one or more small accessory lobes—succenturiate lobes—may develop in the membranes at a distance from the main placenta (Fig. 6-1). These lobes have vessels that course through the membranes. If these vessels overlie the cervix to create a vasa previa, they can cause dangerous fetal hemorrhage if torn (p. 123). An accessory lobe may also be retained in the uterus after delivery and cause postpartum uterine atony and hemorrhage.

Rarely, the portion of fetal membranes covered by functioning villi varies from the norm. With placenta membranacea, all or nearly all of the membranes are covered with villi. This placentation may occasionally give rise to serious hemorrhage because of associated placenta previa or accreta (Greenberg, 1991). A ring-shaped placenta may be a variant of placenta membranacea. The placenta is annular, and a partial or complete ring of placental tissue is present. These abnormalities appear to be associated with a greater likelihood of antepartum and postpartum bleeding and fetal-growth restriction (Faye-Petersen, 2006). With placenta fenestrata, the central portion of a placental disc is missing. In some instances there is an actual hole in the placenta, but more often, the defect involves only villous tissue, and the chorionic plate remains intact. Clinically, it may erroneously prompt a search for a retained placental cotyledon.

During pregnancy, the normal placenta increases its thickness at a rate of approximately 1 mm per week. Although not measured as a component of routine sonographic evaluation, this thickness typically does not exceed 40 mm (Hoddick, 1985). Placentomegaly defines those thicker than 40 mm and commonly results from striking villous enlargement. This may be secondary to maternal diabetes or severe maternal anemia, or to fetal hydrops or infection caused by syphilis, toxoplasmosis, or cytomegalovirus. Less commonly, villi are enlarged and edematous and fetal parts are present, such as in cases of partial mole or a complete mole that coexists with a normal twin (Chap. 20, p. 398). Cystic vesicles are also seen with placental mesenchymal dysplasia. Vesicles in this rare condition correspond to enlarged stem villi, but unlike molar pregnancy, there is not excessive trophoblast proliferation (Woo, 2011). And in some cases, rather than villous enlargement, placentomegaly may result from collections of blood or fibrin. Examples of this that are subsequently discussed on page 119 include massive perivillous fibrin deposition, intervillous or subchorionic thromboses, and large retroplacental hematomas.

Extrachorial Placentation

The chorionic plate normally extends to the periphery of the placenta and has a diameter similar to that of the basal plate. With extrachorial placentation, however, the chorionic plate fails to extend to this periphery and leads to a chorionic plate that is smaller than the basal plate (Fig. 6-2). In a circummarginate placenta, fibrin and old hemorrhage lie between the placenta and the overlying amniochorion. In contrast, with a circumvallate placenta the peripheral chorion is a thickened, opaque, gray-white circular ridge composed of a double fold of chorion and amnion. Sonographically, the double fold can be seen as a thick, linear band of echoes extending from one placental edge to the other. On cross section, it appears as a "shelf." This is important clinically because its location may help to differentiate this shelf from amnionic bands and amnionic sheets, which are described subsequently.

Clinically, most pregnancies with an extrachorial placenta have normal outcomes. In observational studies in which the diagnosis was made by placental examination, circumvallate placenta was associated with increased risk for antepartum bleeding and preterm birth (Lademacher, 1981; Suzuki, 2008a). In a prospective sonographic investigation, however, Shen and colleagues (2007a) found a circumvallate placenta—described as a placental "shelf"—in more than 10 percent of early second-trimester pregnancies. Importantly, they reported that these were transient and benign.

Placenta Accreta, Increta, and Percreta

These clinically important placental abnormalities develop when trophoblast invades the myometrium to varying depths to cause abnormal adherence. They are much more likely when there is placenta previa or when the placenta implants over a prior uterine incision or perforation. As discussed further in Chapter 41 (p. 804), torrential hemorrhage is a frequent complication.

Circulatory Disturbances

These are clinically important syndromes, and in most cases, the placenta is a target organ of maternal disease. Functionally, placental perfusion disorders can be grouped into: (1) those in which there is disrupted maternal blood flow to or within the intervillous space and (2) those with disturbed fetal blood flow through the villi. These lesions are frequently identified in the

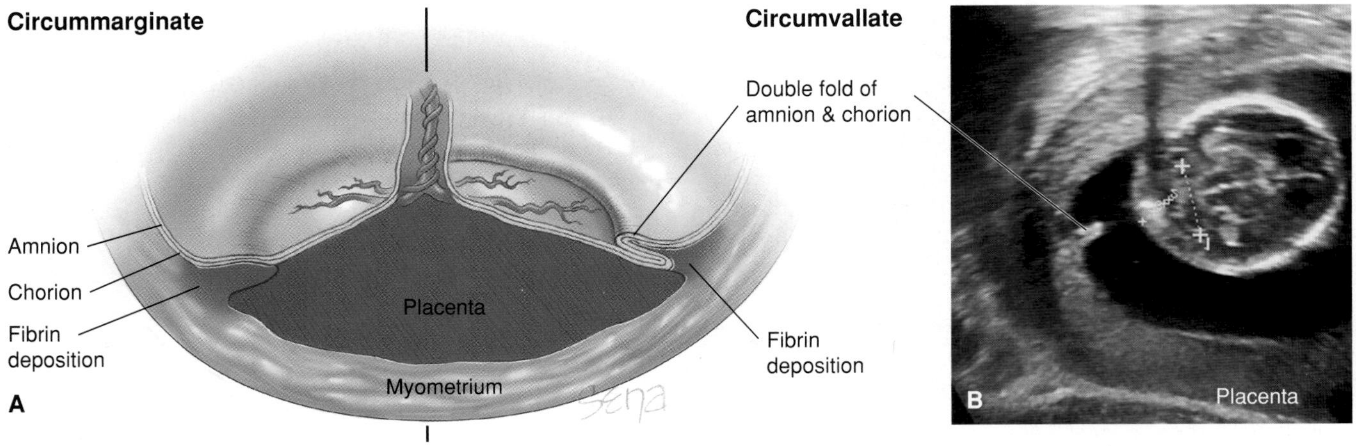

FIGURE 6-2 A. In this illustration, circummarginate (*left*) and circumvallate (*right*) varieties of extrachorial placentation are shown. A circummarginate placenta is covered by a single layer of amniochorion. **B.** This transabdominal gray-scale sonographic image shows a circumvallate placenta. The double fold of amnion and chorion creates a broad, opaque white ring and ridge on the fetal surface.

normal, mature placenta. Although they can limit maximal placental blood flow, placental functional reserve prevents harm in most cases. Indeed, some estimate that up to 30 percent of placental villi can be lost without untoward fetal effects (Fox, 2007). If extensive, however, these lesions can profoundly limit fetal growth.

Placental lesions that cause abnormal perfusion are frequently seen grossly or sonographically, whereas smaller lesions are seen only by microscopic examination. Sonographically, many of these lesions, such as subchorionic fibrin deposition, perivillous fibrin deposition, and intervillous thrombosis, may be appear as focal sonolucencies within the placenta. Importantly, in the absence of maternal or fetal complications, isolated placental sonolucencies are considered incidental findings.

Maternal Blood Flow Disruption

Subchorionic Fibrin Deposition. These are caused by slowing of maternal blood flow within the intervillous space with subsequent fibrin deposition. Blood stasis specifically occurs in the subchorionic area, and lesions that develop are commonly seen as white or yellow firm plaques on the fetal surface.

Perivillous Fibrin Deposition. Maternal blood flow stasis around an individual villus results in fibrin deposition and can lead to diminished villous oxygenation and syncytiotrophoblastic necrosis (Fig. 6-3). Within limits, these grossly visible small yellow-white placental nodules are considered to be normal placental aging.

Maternal Floor Infarction. This extreme variant of perivillous fibrinoid deposition is a dense fibrinoid layer within the placental basal plate and is erroneously termed an infarction. The lesion has a thick, white, firm, corrugated surface that impedes normal maternal blood flow into the intervillous space. These lesions are associated with miscarriage, fetal-growth restriction, preterm delivery, and stillbirths (Andres, 1990; Mandsager, 1994). These adverse outcomes occasionally recur in subsequent pregnancies. Their etiopathogenesis is not well defined, but some cases are associated with lupus anticoagulant (Sebire, 2002, 2003). Although unsettled, other cases may be associated with maternal thrombophilias (Gogia, 2008; Katz, 2002). These lesions are not reliably imaged with prenatal sonography, but they may create a thicker basal plate.

Intervillous Thrombus. This is a collection of coagulated maternal blood normally found in the intervillous space mixed with fetal blood from a break in a villus. Grossly, these round or oval collections vary in size up to several centimeters. They appear red if recent or white-yellow if older, and they develop at any placental depth. Intervillous thrombi are common and typically not associated with adverse fetal sequelae. Because there is potential for a communication between maternal and fetal circulations, they can cause elevated maternal serum alpha-fetoprotein levels (Salafia, 1988).

Infarction. Chorionic villi themselves receive oxygen solely from maternal circulation supplied to the intervillous space. Any uteroplacental disease that diminishes or obstructs this supply can result in infarction of individual villus. These are common lesions in mature placentas and are benign in limited numbers. If they are numerous, however, placental insufficiency can develop. When they are thick, centrally located, and randomly distributed, they may be associated with preeclampsia or lupus anticoagulant.

Hematoma. The maternal-placental-fetal unit can develop a number of hematoma types as depicted in Figure 6-3. These include: (1) retroplacental hematoma—between the placenta and its adjacent decidua; (2) marginal hematoma—between the chorion and decidua at the placental periphery—known clinically as subchorionic hemorrhage; (3) subchorial thrombosis—also known as Breus mole—along the roof of the intervillous space and beneath the chorionic plate; and (4) subamnionic

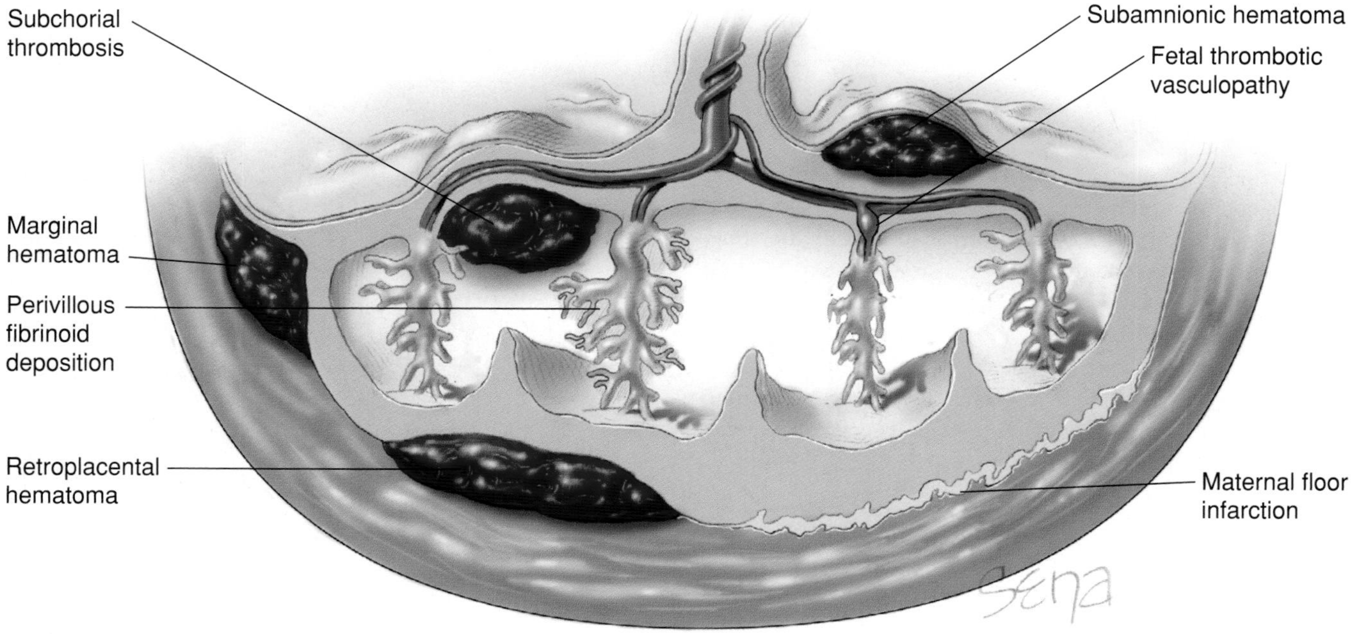

FIGURE 6-3 Potential sites of maternal- and fetal-related placental circulatory disturbances. (Adapted from Faye-Petersen, 2006.)

hematoma—these are of fetal vessel origin and found beneath the amnion but above the chorionic plate.

Sonographically, these hematomas may resemble a crescent-shaped fluid collection that is hyperechoic to isoechoic in the first week after hemorrhage, hypoechoic at 1 to 2 weeks, and finally, anechoic after 2 weeks. Most subchorionic hematomas visible sonographically are fairly small and of no clinical consequence. Extensive retroplacental, marginal, and subchorial collections have been associated with higher rates of miscarriage, placental abruption, fetal-growth restriction, preterm delivery, and adherent placenta (Ball, 1996; Madu, 2006; Nagy, 2003). In essence, placental abruption is a large clinically significant retroplacental hematoma (Chap. 41, p. 793)

Fetal Blood Flow Disruption

Placental lesions that arise from fetal circulatory disturbances are also depicted in Figure 6-3.

Fetal Thrombotic Vasculopathy. Deoxygenated fetal blood flows from the two umbilical arteries into arteries within the chorionic plate that divide and send branches out across the placental surface. These eventually supply individual stem villi, and their thrombosis will obstruct fetal blood flow. Distal to the obstruction, affected portions of the villus become infarcted and nonfunctional. Thrombi in limited numbers are normally found in mature placentas, but these may be clinically significant if many villi become infarcted.

Subamnionic Hematoma. As indicated earlier, these hematomas lie between the placenta and amnion. They most often are acute events during third-stage labor when cord traction ruptures a vessel near the cord insertion. Chronic lesions may cause fetomaternal hemorrhage or fetal-growth restriction (Deans, 1998). They also may be confused with other placental masses such as chorioangioma, which is discussed subsequently (Sepulveda, 2000; Van Den Bosch, 2000; Volpe, 2008). In most cases, Doppler interrogation will show absence of internal blood flow that permits differentiation of hematomas from other placental masses.

Placental Calcification

Calcium salts may be deposited throughout the placenta, but are most common on the basal plate. Calcification accrues with advancing gestation and is associated with nulliparity, smoking, higher socioeconomic status, and increasing maternal serum calcium levels (Fox, 2007). Calcifications can easily be seen sonographically, and Grannum and coworkers (1979) created a grading scale from 0 to 3 that reflected increasing calcification with increasing numerical grade. However, such grading criteria have not been found useful to predict neonatal outcome (Hill, 1983; McKenna, 2005; Montan, 1986; Sau, 2004).

Placental Tumors

Gestational Trophoblastic Disease

These pregnancy-related trophoblastic proliferative abnormalities are discussed in Chapter 20 (p. 396).

Chorioangioma

These benign tumors have components similar to blood vessels and stroma of the chorionic villus. Also called chorangioma, these placental tumors have an incidence of approximately 1 percent (Guschmann, 2003). In some cases, maternal serum alpha-fetoprotein (MSAFP) levels may be elevated with these tumors, an important diagnostic finding as discussed in Chapter 14 (p. 285). Their characteristic sonographic appearance has a well-circumscribed, rounded, predominantly hypoechoic lesion near the chorionic surface and protruding into the amnionic cavity. As shown in Figure 6-4, documenting increased blood flow by color Doppler helps to distinguish these lesions from

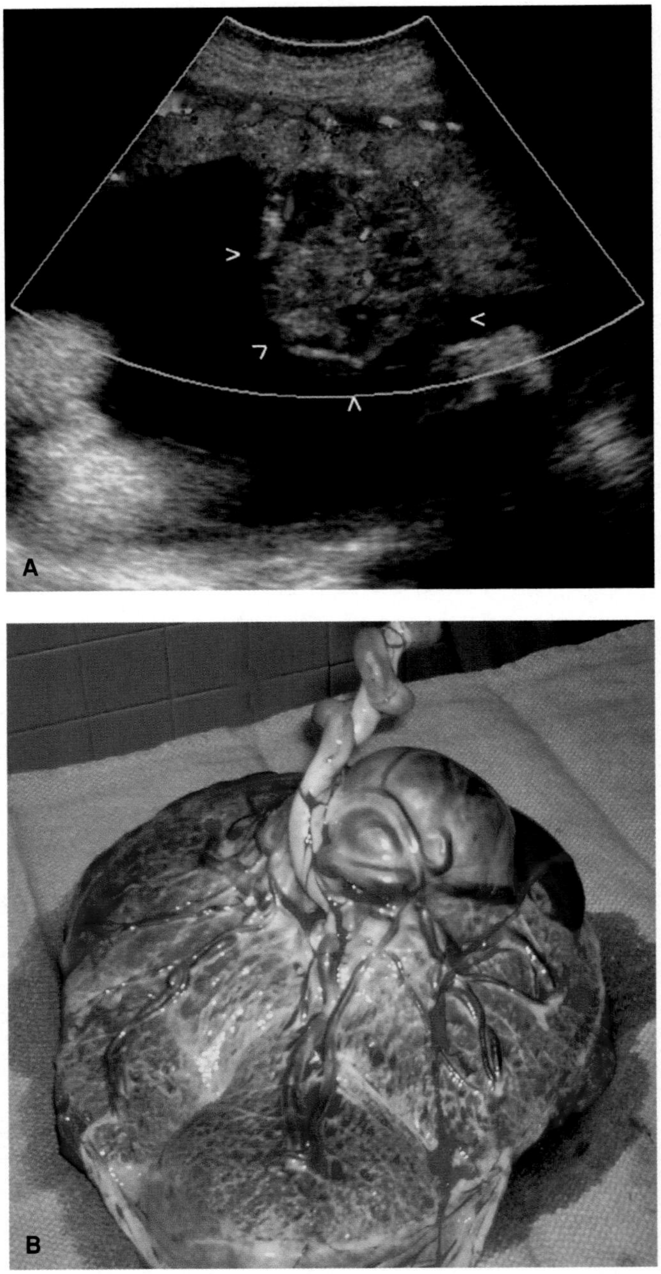

FIGURE 6-4 Placental chorioangioma. **A.** Color Doppler imaging displays blood flow through a large chorioangioma with its border outlined by white arrows. **B.** Grossly, the chorioangioma is a round, well-circumcised mass protruding from the fetal surface.

other placental masses such as hematoma, partial hydatidiform mole, teratoma, metastases, and leiomyoma (Prapas, 2000).

Small chorioangiomas are usually asymptomatic. Large tumors, typically those measuring > 5 cm, may be associated with significant arteriovenous shunting within the placenta that can cause fetal anemia and hydrops. Hemorrhage, preterm delivery, amnionic fluid abnormalities, and fetal-growth restriction may also complicate large tumors (Sepulveda, 2003a; Zalel, 2002). Because of this, some have treated large tumors by interdicting excessive blood flow using vessel occlusion or ablation (Lau, 2003; Nicolini, 1999; Quintero, 1996; Sepulveda, 2009).

Tumors Metastatic to the Placenta

Malignant tumors rarely metastasize to the placenta. Of those that do, melanomas, leukemias and lymphomas, and breast cancer are the most common (Al-Adnani, 2007a). Tumor cells usually are confined within the intervillous space. As a result, metastasis to the fetus is uncommon but is most often seen with melanoma (Alexander, 2003; Altman, 2003). These are discussed further in Chapter 63 (p. 1233).

ABNORMALITIES OF THE MEMBRANES

There are a few abnormalities of the fetal membranes that may be associated with adverse outcomes.

Meconium Staining

Fetal passage of meconium before or during labor is common with cited incidences that range from 12 to 20 percent (Ghidini, 2001; Oyelese, 2006; Tran, 2004). Importantly, staining of the amnion can be obvious within 1 to 3 hours, but its passage cannot be timed or dated accurately (Benirschke, 2012). This subject and its clinical implications are discussed in detail in Chapter 33 (p. 637).

Chorioamnionitis

Normal genital-tract flora can colonize and infect the membranes, umbilical cord, and eventually the fetus. Bacteria most commonly ascend after prolonged membrane rupture and during labor to cause infection. Organisms initially infect the chorion and adjacent decidua in the area overlying the internal os. Subsequently, progression leads to full-thickness involvement of the membranes—chorioamnionitis. Organisms may then spread along the chorioamnionic surface to colonize and replicate in amnionic fluid. Subsequently, inflammation of the chorionic plate and of the umbilical cord—funisitis—may follow (Al-Adnani, 2007b; Goldenberg, 2000; Redline, 2006).

Fetal infection may result from hematogenous spread if the mother has bacteremia, but more likely is from aspiration, swallowing, or other direct contact with infected amnionic fluid. Most commonly, there is microscopic or occult chorioamnionitis, which is caused by a wide variety of microorganisms. This is frequently cited as a possible explanation for many otherwise unexplained cases of ruptured membranes, preterm labor, or both as discussed in Chapter 42 (p. 838). In some cases, gross infection is characterized by membrane clouding and is sometimes accompanied by a foul odor that depends on bacterial species.

Other Membrane Abnormalities

The condition of amnion nodosum is characterized by numerous small, light-tan nodules on the amnion overlying the chorionic plate. These may be scraped off the fetal surface and contain deposits of fetal squames and fibrin that reflect prolonged and severe oligohydramnios (Adeniran, 2007).

There are at least two band-like structures that can be formed by the fetal membranes. Amnionic band sequence is an anatomic fetal disruption sequence caused by bands of amnion that entrap fetal structures and impair their growth and development. The most widely held theory concerning their etiology is that early rupture of the amnion results in adherence of part of the fetus to the underlying "sticky" chorion (Torpin, 1965). Amnionic bands commonly involve the extremities to cause limb-reduction defects and more subtle deformations. They may also affect other fetal structures such as the cranium, causing encephalocele.

In contrast, an amnionic sheet is formed by normal amniochorion draped over a preexisting uterine synechia. Generally these sheets pose little fetal risk, although slightly higher rates of preterm membrane rupture and placental abruption were recently described (Tuuli, 2012).

ABNORMALITIES OF THE UMBILICAL CORD

Length

Most umbilical cords are 40 to 70 cm long, and very few measure < 32 cm or > 100 cm. Cord length is influenced positively by both amnionic fluid volume and fetal mobility. Short cords may be associated with fetal-growth restriction, congenital malformations, intrapartum distress, and a twofold risk of death (Berg, 1995; Krakowiak, 2004). Excessively long cords are more likely to be linked with cord entanglement or prolapse and with fetal anomalies, acidemia, and demise.

Because antenatal determination of cord length is technically limited, cord diameter has been used as a predictive marker for fetal outcomes. Some have linked lean cords with poor fetal growth and large-diameter cords with macrosomia. However, the clinical utility of this parameter is still unclear (Barbieri, 2008; Cromi, 2007; Raio 1999, 2003).

Coiling

Although cord coiling characteristics have been reported, these are not currently part of standard sonography (Predanic, 2005a). Usually the umbilical vessels spiral through the cord in a sinistral, that is, left-twisting direction (Lacro, 1987). The number of complete coils per centimeter of cord length has been termed the umbilical coiling index (Strong, 1994). A normal antepartum index derived sonographically is 0.4, and this contrasts with a normal value of 0.2 derived postpartum by actual measurement (Sebire, 2007). Clinically, hypocoiling has been linked with fetal demise, whereas hypercoiling has been associated with fetal-growth restriction and intrapartum fetal acidosis. Both have been reported in the setting of trisomic fetuses and with single umbilical artery (de Laat, 2006, 2007; Predanic, 2005b).

Vessel Number

Occasionally, the usual arrangement of two thick-walled arteries and one thin, larger umbilical vein is altered. The most common aberration is that of a single umbilical artery, with a cited incidence of 0.63 percent in liveborn neonates, 1.92 percent with perinatal deaths, and 3 percent in twins (Heifetz, 1984).

The cord vessel number is a component of the standard prenatal ultrasound examination (Fig. 6-5). Identification of a single umbilical artery frequently prompts consideration for targeted sonography and possibly fetal echocardiography. As an isolated finding in an otherwise low-risk pregnancy with no apparent fetal anomalies, it does not significantly increase the fetal aneuploidy risk. But fetuses with major malformations frequently have a single umbilical artery. And when seen in an anomalous fetus, the aneuploidy risk is greatly increased, and amniocentesis is recommended (Dagklis, 2010; Lubusky, 2007). The most frequent anomalies described are cardiovascular and genitourinary. A single artery has also been associated with fetal-growth restriction in some but not all studies (Chetty-John, 2010; Hua, 2010; Murphy-Kaulbeck, 2010; Predanic, 2005c).

A rare anomaly is that of a fused umbilical artery with a shared lumen. It arises from failure of the two arteries to split during embryological development. The common lumen may extend through the entire cord, but if partial, is typically found near the placental insertion site (Yamada, 2005). In one report, these were associated with a higher incidence of marginal or velamentous cord insertion, but not congenital fetal anomalies (Fujikura, 2003).

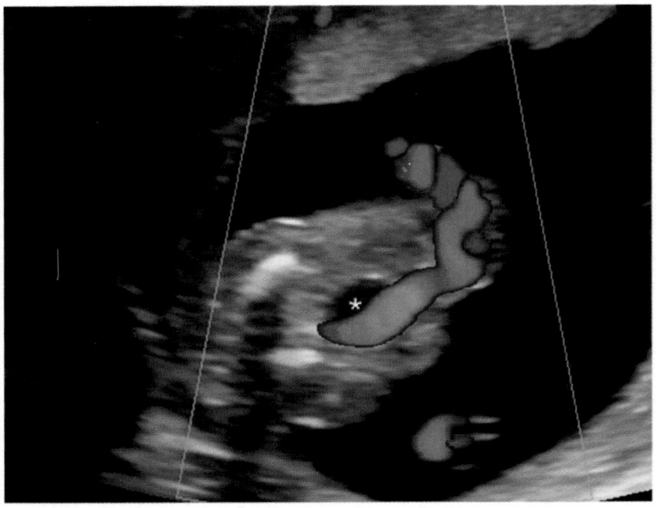

FIGURE 6-5 Two umbilical arteries are typically documented sonographically in the second trimester. They encircle the fetal bladder (*asterisk*) as extensions of the superior vesical arteries. In this color Doppler sonographic image, a single umbilical artery, shown in red, runs along the bladder wall before joining the umbilical vein (*blue*) in the cord. Below this, the two vessels of the cord, seen as a larger red and smaller blue circle, are also seen floating in a cross section of a cord segment.

Remnants and Cysts

A number of structures are housed in the umbilical cord during fetal development, and their remnants may be seen when the mature cord is viewed transversely. Recall that embryos in early development initially have two umbilical veins, and thus an umbilical vein remnant may be seen on careful inspection. Indeed, Jauniaux and colleagues (1989) sectioned 1000 cords, and in one fourth of the specimens, they found remnants of vitelline duct, allantoic duct, and embryonic vessels. These were not associated with congenital malformations or perinatal complications.

Cysts occasionally are found along the course of the cord. They are designated according to their origin. True cysts are epithelium-lined remnants of the allantoic or vitelline ducts and tend to be located closer to the fetal insertion site. In contrast, the more common pseudocysts form from local degeneration of Wharton jelly and occur anywhere along the cord. Both have a similar sonographic appearance. Single umbilical cord cysts identified in the first trimester tend to resolve completely, however, multiple cysts may portend miscarriage or aneuploidy (Ghezzi, 2003; Gilboa, 2011). Cysts persisting beyond this time are associated with a risk for structural defects and chromosomal anomalies (Bonilla, 2010; Zangen, 2010).

Insertion

The cord normally inserts centrally into the placental disc, but eccentric, marginal, or velamentous insertions are variants. The latter two are clinically important in that the cord or its vessels may be torn during labor and delivery. Of these, marginal insertion is a common variant—sometimes referred to as a battledore placenta—in which the cord anchors at the placental margin. These are more frequent with multifetal pregnancy, especially those conceived using assisted reproductive technology, and they may be associated with weight discordance (Delbaere, 2007; Kent, 2011). This common insertion variant rarely causes problems, but it occasionally results in the cord being pulled off during delivery of the placenta (Liu, 2002).

A velamentous insertion is a variant of considerable clinical importance. The umbilical vessels characteristically spread within the membranes at a distance from the placental margin, which they reach surrounded only by a fold of amnion (Fig. 6-6) As a result, vessels are vulnerable to compression, which may lead to fetal hypoperfusion and acidemia. The incidence of velamentous insertion is approximately 1 percent, but it is more commonly seen with placenta previa and multifetal gestations (Feldman, 2002; Fox, 2007; Papinniemi, 2007). When seen during prenatal sonography, cord vessels with velamentous insertion are seen traveling along the uterine wall before entering the placental disc.

Last, with the very uncommon furcate insertion, the topographic site of cord connection onto the placental disc is central, but umbilical vessels lose their protective Wharton jelly shortly before they insert. As a result, they are covered only

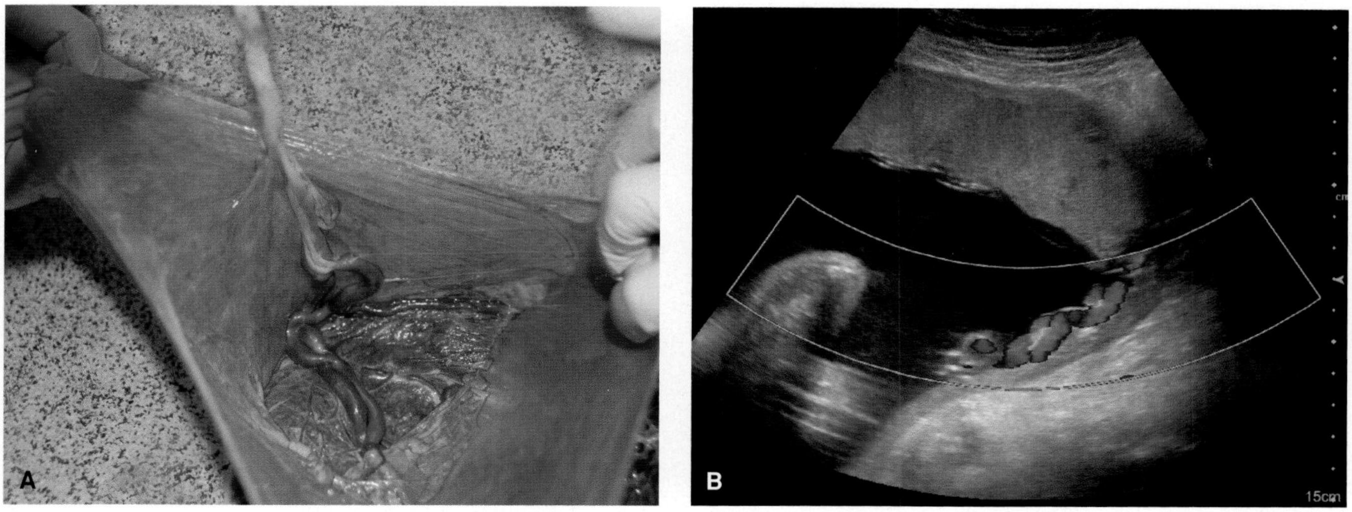

FIGURE 6-6 Velamentous cord insertion. **A.** The umbilical cord inserts into the membranes. From here, the cord vessels branch and are supported only by membrane until they reach the placental disk. **B.** When viewed sonographically and using color Doppler, the cord vessels appear to lie against the myometrium as they travel to insert marginally into the placental disk, which lies at the top of this image.

by an amnion sheath and prone to compression, twisting, and thrombosis.

Vasa Previa

This is a particularly dangerous variation of velamentous insertion in which the vessels within the membranes overlie the cervical os. The vessels can be interposed between the cervix and the presenting fetal part. Hence, they are vulnerable to compression and also to laceration or avulsion with rapid fetal exsanguination. Vasa previa is uncommon, and Lee and coworkers (2000) identified it in 1 in 5200 pregnancies. Risk factors include bilobate or succenturiate placentas and second-trimester placenta previa, with or without later migration (Baulies, 2007; Suzuki, 2008b). It is also increased in pregnancies conceived by in vitro fertilization (Schachter, 2003).

Because antepartum diagnosis has improved perinatal survival compared with intrapartum diagnosis, vasa previa would ideally be identified early (Oyelese, 2004). Unfortunately, this is not always possible. Clinically, an examiner is occasionally able to palpate or directly see a tubular fetal vessel in the membranes overlying the presenting part. With transvaginal sonography, cord vessels may be seen inserting into the membranes—rather than directly into the placenta—with vessels running above the cervical internal os (Fig. 6-7). Routine color Doppler interrogation of the placental cord insertion site, particularly in cases of placenta previa or low-lying placenta, may aid its detection.

Once vasa previa is identified, early scheduled cesarean delivery is planned. Bed rest apparently has no added advantage. Robinson and Grobman (2011) performed a decision analysis and recommend elective cesarean delivery at 34 to 35 weeks to balance the risks of perinatal exsanguination versus preterm birth morbidity. At delivery, the infant is expeditiously delivered after the hysterotomy incision in case a vessel is lacerated during uterine entry.

Whenever there is otherwise unexplained hemorrhage either antepartum or intrapartum, vasa previa with a lacerated fetal vessel should be considered. In many cases, bleeding is rapidly fatal, and infant salvage is not possible. With less hemorrhage, however, it may be possible to distinguish fetal versus maternal bleeding. Various tests may be used, and each relies on the characteristically increased resistance of fetal hemoglobin to denaturation by alkaline or acid reagents (Lindqvist, 2007; Oyelese, 1999).

Knots, Strictures, and Loops

Various mechanical and vascular abnormalities can impede cord vessel blood flow either toward or away from the fetus, and these sometimes cause fetal harm. True knots are caused by fetal movement and are seen in approximately 1 percent of births. They are especially common and dangerous in monoamnionic twins as described in Chapter 45 (p. 901). When true knots are associated with singleton fetuses, the stillbirth risk is increased four- to tenfold (Airas, 2002;

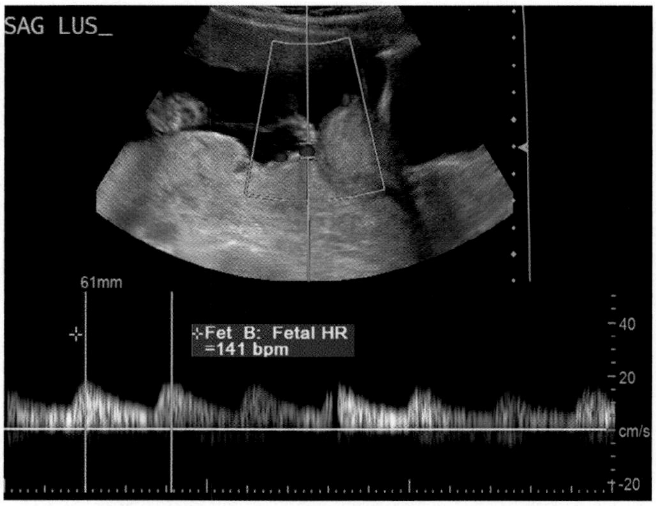

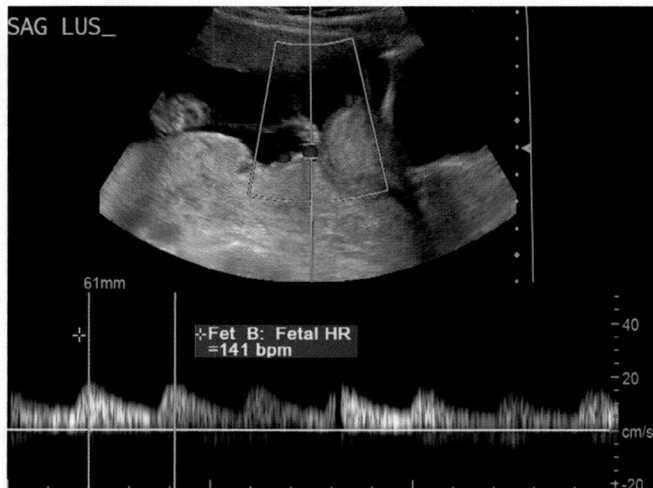

FIGURE 6-7 Vasa previa. Using color Doppler, an umbilical vessel (*red circle*) is seen overlying the internal os. At the bottom, the Doppler waveform seen with this vasa previa has the typical appearance of an umbilical artery, with a pulse rate of 141 beats per minute.

Sørnes, 2000). Abnormal fetal heart rate tracings are more often encountered during labor. However, cesarean delivery rates are not increased, and cord blood acid-base values are usually normal (Airas, 2002; Maher, 1996). False knots are of no clinical significance and appear as knobs protruding from the cord surface. These are focal redundancies of a vessel or Wharton jelly.

A cord stricture is a focal narrowing of its diameter that usually develops near the fetal cord insertion (Peng, 2006). Characteristic pathological features of strictures are absence of Wharton jelly and stenosis or obliteration of cord vessels at the narrow segment (Sun, 1995). In most instances, the fetus is stillborn (French, 2005). Even less common is a cord stricture caused by an amnionic band.

Cord loops are frequently encountered and are caused by coiling around various fetal parts during movement. As expected, they are more common with longer cords. A cord around the neck—a nuchal cord—is extremely common. One loop is reported in 20 to 34 percent of deliveries; two loops in 2.5 to 5 percent; and three loops in 0.2 to 0.5 percent (Kan, 1957; Sørnes, 1995; Spellacy, 1966). During labor these loops can result in fetal heart rate decelerations that persist during a contraction. Up to 20 percent of fetuses with a nuchal cord have moderate to severe variable heart rate decelerations, and these are associated with a lower umbilical artery pH (Hankins, 1987). Despite their frequency, nuchal cords are relatively uncommon causes of adverse perinatal outcome (Mastrobattista, 2005; Sheiner, 2006).

A funic presentation describes when the umbilical cord is the presenting part in labor. These are uncommon and most often are associated with fetal malpresentation. A funic presentation in some cases is identified with placental sonography and color flow Doppler (Ezra, 2003). Fetal heart rate abnormalities and overt or occult cord prolapse may complicate labor and lead to cesarean delivery.

Vascular

Cord hematomas are uncommon and have been associated with abnormal cord length, umbilical vessel aneurysm, trauma, entanglement, umbilical vessel venipuncture, and funisitis (Gualandri, 2008). They can follow varix rupture, which is usually of the umbilical vein. They are recognized sonographically as hypoechoic masses that lack blood flow.

Umbilical cord vessel thromboses are in utero events. Approximately 70 percent are venous, 20 percent are venous and arterial, and 10 percent are arterial thromboses (Heifetz, 1988). Compared with venous thromboses, those in the artery have higher perinatal morbidity and mortality rates and are associated with fetal-growth restriction, fetal acidosis, and stillbirths (Sato, 2006).

Another rare anomaly is an umbilical vein varix, which is a marked focal dilatation that can be within either the intraamnionic or fetal intraabdominal portion of the umbilical vein. The latter anomalies are associated with increased rates of fetal structural anomalies and aneuploidy (Byers, 2009; Mankuta, 2011). Complications may include rupture or thrombosis, compression of the umbilical artery, and fetal cardiac failure due to increased preload (Mulch, 2006). They may be visualized during sonography as a cystic dilatation of the umbilical vein. Continuity of the varix with a normal-caliber portion of the umbilical vein is confirmed using color-flow Doppler.

The rare umbilical artery aneurysm is caused by congenital thinning of the vessel wall with diminished support from Wharton jelly. Indeed, most form at or near the cord's placental insertion, where support is absent. These are associated with single umbilical artery, trisomy 18, amnionic fluid volume abnormalities, fetal-growth restriction, and stillbirth (Hill, 2010; Weber, 2007). At least theoretically, these aneurysms could cause fetal compromise and death by compression of the umbilical vein. These aneurysms may appear sonographically as a cyst with a hyperechoic rim. Within the aneurysm, color flow and spectral Doppler interrogation demonstrate either low-velocity or turbulent nonpulsatile flow (Olog, 2011; Sepulveda, 2003b; Shen, 2007b).

REFERENCES

Adeniran AJ, Stanek J: Amnion nodosum revisited: clinicopathologic and placental correlations. Arch Pathol Lab Med 131:1829, 2007

Airas U, Heinonen S: Clinical significance of true umbilical knots: a population-based analysis. Am J Perinatol 19:127, 2002

Al-Adnani M, Kiho L, Scheimberg I: Maternal pancreatic carcinoma metastatic to the placenta: a case report and literature review. Pediatr Dev Pathol 10:61, 2007a

Al-Adnani M, Sebire NJ: The role of perinatal pathological examination in subclinical infection in obstetrics. Best Pract Res Clin Obstet Gynaecol 21:505, 2007b

Alexander A, Samlowski WE, Grossman D, et al: Metastatic melanoma in pregnancy: risk of transplacental metastases in the infant. J Clin Oncol 21: 2179, 2003

Altman JF, Lowe L, Redman B, et al: Placental metastasis of maternal melanoma. J Am Acad Dermatol 49:1150, 2003

Andres RL, Kuyper W, Resnik R, et al: The association of maternal floor infarction of the placenta with adverse perinatal outcome. Am J Obstet Gynecol 163:935, 1990

Ball RH, Ade CM, Schoenborn JA, et al: The clinical significance of ultrasonographically detected subchorionic hemorrhages. Am J Obstet Gynecol 174:996, 1996

Barbieri C, Cecatti JG, Krupa F, et al: Validation study of the capacity of the reference curves of ultrasonographic measurements of the umbilical cord to identify deviations in estimated fetal weight. Acta Obstet Gynecol Scand 87:286, 2008

Baulies S, Maiz N, Muñoz A, et al: Prenatal ultrasound diagnosis of vasa praevia and analysis of risk factors. Prenat Diagn 27:595, 2007

Benirschke K, Burton GJ, Baergen R: Pathology of the Human Placenta, 6th ed. New York, Springer, 2012, p 908

Berg TG, Rayburn WF: Umbilical cord length and acid-base balance at delivery. J Reprod Med 40:9, 1995

Bonilla F Jr, Raga F, Villalaiz E, et al: Umbilical cord cysts: evaluation with different 3-dimensional sonographic modes. J Ultrasound Med 29(2):281, 2010

Byers BD, Goharkhay N, Mateus J, et al: Pregnancy outcome after ultrasound diagnosis of fetal intra-abdominal umbilical vein varix. Ultrasound Obstet Gynecol 33(3):282, 2009

Chetty-John S, Zhang J, Chen Z, et al: Long-term physical and neurologic development in newborn infants with isolated single umbilical artery. Am J Obstet Gynecol 203(4):368.e1, 2010

Cromi A, Ghezzi F, Di Naro E, et al: Large cross-sectional area of the umbilical cord as a predictor of fetal macrosomia. Ultrasound Obstet Gynecol 30:804, 2007

Dagklis T, Defigueiredo D, Staboulidou I, et al: Isolated single umbilical artery and fetal karyotype. Ultrasound Obstet Gynecol 36(3):291, 2010

Deans A, Jauniaux E: Prenatal diagnosis and outcome of subamniotic hematomas. Ultrasound Obstet Gynecol 11:319, 1998

de Laat MW, Franx A, Bots ML, et al: Umbilical coiling index in normal and complicated pregnancies. Obstet Gynecol 107:1049, 2006

de Laat MW, van Alderen ED, Franx A, et al: The umbilical coiling index in complicated pregnancy. Eur J Obstet Gynecol Reprod Biol 130:66, 2007
Delbaere I, Goetgeluk S, Derom C, et al: Umbilical cord anomalies are more frequent in twins after assisted reproduction. Hum Reprod 22(10):2763, 2007
Ezra Y, Strasberg SR, Farine D: Does cord presentation on ultrasound predict cord prolapse? Gynecol Obstet Invest 56:6, 2003
Faye-Petersen OM, Heller DS, Joshi VV: Handbook of Placental Pathology, 2nd ed. London, Taylor & Francis, 2006, pp 27, 83
Feldman DM, Borgida AF, Trymbulak WP, et al: Clinical implications of velamentous cord insertion in triplet gestations. Am J Obstet Gynecol 186:809, 2002
Fox H, Sebire NJ: Pathology of the Placenta, 3rd ed. Philadelphia, Saunders, 2007, pp 99, 133, 484
French AE, Gregg VH, Newberry Y, et al: Umbilical cord stricture: a cause of recurrent fetal death. Obstet Gynecol 105:1235, 2005
Fujikura T: Fused umbilical arteries near placental cord insertion. Am J Obstet Gynecol 188:765, 2003
Ghezzi F, Raio L, Di Naro E, et al: Single and multiple umbilical cord cysts in early gestation: two different entities. Ultrasound Obstet Gynecol 21:213, 2003
Ghidini A, Spong CY: Severe meconium aspiration syndrome is not caused by aspiration of meconium. Am J Obstet Gynecol 185:931, 2001
Gilboa Y, Kivilevitch Z, Katorza E, et al: Outcomes of fetuses with umbilical cord cysts diagnosed during nuchal translucency examination. J Ultrasound Med 30(11):1547, 2011
Gogia N, Machin GA: Maternal thrombophilias are associated with specific placental lesions. Pediatr Dev Pathol 11(6):424, 2008
Goldenberg RL, Hauth JC, Andrews WW: Intrauterine infection and preterm delivery. N Engl J Med 342:1500, 2000
Grannum PA, Berkowitz RL, Hobbins JC: The ultrasonic changes in the maturing placenta and their relation to fetal pulmonic maturity. Am J Obstet Gynecol 133:915, 1979
Greenberg JA, Sorem KA, Shifren JL, et al: Placenta membranacea with placenta increta: a case report and literature review. Obstet Gynecol 78:512, 1991
Gualandri G, Rivasi F, Santunione AL, et al: Spontaneous umbilical cord hematoma: an unusual cause of fetal mortality: a report of 3 cases and review of the literature. Am J Forensic Med Pathol 29(2):185, 2008
Guschmann M, Henrich W, Entezami M, et al: Chorioangioma—new insights into a well-known problem. I. Results of a clinical and morphological study of 136 cases. J Perinat Med 31:163, 2003
Hankins GD, Snyder RR, Hauth JC, et al: Nuchal cords and neonatal outcome. Obstet Gynecol 70:687, 1987
Heifetz SA: Single umbilical artery: a statistical analysis of 237 autopsy cases and a review of the literature. Perspect Pediatr Pathol 8:345, 1984
Heifetz SA: Thrombosis of the umbilical cord: analysis of 52 cases and literature review. Pediatr Pathol 8:37, 1988
Hill AJ, Strong TH Jr, Elliott JP, et al: Umbilical artery aneurysm. Obstet Gynecol 116(Suppl 2):559, 2010
Hill LM, Breckle R, Ragozzino MW, et al: Grade 3 placentation: incidence and neonatal outcome. Obstet Gynecol 61:728, 1983
Hoddick WK, Mahony BS, Callen PW, et al: Placental thickness. J Ultrasound Med 4(9):479, 1985
Hua M, Odibo AO, Macones GA, et al: Single umbilical artery and its associated findings. Obstet Gynecol 115(5):930, 2010
Jauniaux E, De Munter C, Vanesse M, et al: Embryonic remnants of the umbilical cord: morphologic and clinical aspects. Hum Pathol 20(5):458, 1989
Kan PS, Eastman NJ: Coiling of the umbilical cord around the foetal neck. Br J Obstet Gynaecol 64:227, 1957
Katz VL, DiTomasso J, Farmer R, et al: Activated protein C resistance associated with maternal floor infarction treated with low-molecular-weight heparin. Am J Perinatol 19:273, 2002
Kent EM, Breathnach FM, Gillan JE, et al: Placental cord insertion and birthweight discordance in twin pregnancies: results of the national prospective ESPRiT Study. Am J Obstet Gynecol 205(4):376.e1, 2011
Krakowiak P, Smith EN, de Bruyn G, et al: Risk factors and outcomes associated with a short umbilical cord. Obstet Gynecol 103:119, 2004
Lacro RV, Jones KL, Benirschke K: The umbilical cord twist: origin, direction, and relevance. Am J Obstet Gynecol 157(4 Pt 1):833, 1987
Lademacher DS, Vermeulen RCW, Harten JJVD, et al: Circumvallate placenta and congenital malformation. Lancet 1:732, 1981
Langston C, Kaplan C, Macpherson T, et al: Practice guideline for examination of the placenta. Arch Pathol Lab Med 121:449, 1997
Lau TK, Leung TY, Yu SC, et al: Prenatal treatment of chorioangioma by microcoil embolisation. BJOG 110:70, 2003
Lee W, Lee VL, Kirk JS, et al: Vasa previa: prenatal diagnosis, natural evolution and clinical outcome. Obstet Gynecol 95:572, 2000
Lindqvist PG, Gren P: An easy-to-use method for detecting fetal hemoglobin—a test to identify bleeding from vasa previa. Eur J Obstet Gynecol Reprod Biol 131:151, 2007
Liu CC, Pretorius DH, Scioscia AL, et al: Sonographic prenatal diagnosis of marginal placental cord insertion: clinical importance. Ultrasound Med 21:627, 2002
Lubusky M, Dhaifalah I, Prochazka M, et al: Single umbilical artery and its siding in the second trimester of pregnancy: relation to chromosomal defects. Prenat Diagn 27:327, 2007
Madu AE: Breus' mole in pregnancy. J Obstet Gynaecol 26:815, 2006
Maher JT, Conti JA: A comparison of umbilical cord blood gas values between newborns with and without true knots. Obstet Gynecol 88:863, 1996
Mandsager NT, Bendon R, Mostello D, et al: Maternal floor infarction of the placenta: prenatal diagnosis and clinical significance. Obstet Gynecol 83:750, 1994
Mankuta D, Nadjari M, Pomp G: Isolated fetal intra-abdominal umbilical vein varix: clinical importance and recommendations. J Ultrasound Med 30(2):273, 2011
Mastrobattista JM, Hollier LM, Yeomans ER, et al: Effects of nuchal cord on birthweight and immediate neonatal outcomes. Am J Perinatol 22:83, 2005
McKenna D, Tharmaratnam S, Mahsud S, et al: Ultrasonic evidence of placental calcification at 36 weeks' gestation: maternal and fetal outcomes. Acta Obstet Gynecol Scand 84:7, 2005
Montan S, Jörgensen C, Svalenius E, et al: Placental grading with ultrasound in hypertensive and normotensive pregnancies: a prospective, consecutive study. Acta Obstet Gynecol Scand 65:477, 1986
Mulch AD, Stallings SP, Salafia CM: Elevated maternal serum alpha-fetoprotein, umbilical vein varix, and mesenchymal dysplasia: are they related? Prenat Diagn 26:659, 2006
Murphy-Kaulbeck L, Dodds L, Joseph KS, et al: Single umbilical artery risk factors and pregnancy outcomes. Obstet Gynecol 116(4):843, 2010
Nagy S, Bush M, Stone J, et al: Clinical significance of subchorionic and retroplacental hematomas detected in the first trimester of pregnancy. Obstet Gynecol 102:94, 2003
Nicolini U, Zuliani G, Caravelli E, et al: Alcohol injection: a new method of treating placental chorioangiomas. Lancet 353(9165):1674, 1999
Olog A, Thomas JT, Petersen S, et al: Large umbilical artery aneurysm with a live healthy baby delivered at 31 weeks. Fetal Diagn Ther 29(4):331, 2011
Oyelese KO, Turner M, Lees C, et al: Vasa previa: an avoidable obstetric tragedy. Obstet Gynecol Surv 54:138, 1999
Oyelese Y, Catanzarite V, Prefumo F, et al: Vasa previa: the impact of prenatal diagnosis on outcomes. Obstet Gynecol 103:937, 2004
Oyelese Y, Culin A, Ananth CV, et al: Meconium-stained amniotic fluid across gestation and neonatal acid-base status. Obstet Gynecol 108:345, 2006
Papinniemi M, Keski-Nisula L, Heinonen S: Placental ratio and risk of velamentous umbilical cord insertion are increased in women with placenta previa. Am J Perinatol 24:353, 2007
Peng HQ, Levitin-Smith M, Rochelson B, et al: Umbilical cord stricture and overcoiling are common causes of fetal demise. Pediatr Dev Pathol 9:14, 2006
Prapas N, Liang RI, Hunter D, et al: Color Doppler imaging of placental masses: differential diagnosis and fetal outcome. Ultrasound Obstet Gynecol 16:559, 2000
Predanic M, Perni SC, Chasen ST, et al: Assessment of umbilical cord coiling during the routine fetal sonographic anatomic survey in the second trimester. J Ultrasound Med 24:185, 2005a
Predanic M, Perni SC, Chasen ST, et al: Ultrasound evaluation of abnormal umbilical cord coiling in second trimester of gestation in association with adverse pregnancy outcome. Am J Obstet Gynecol 193:387, 2005b
Predanic M, Perni SC, Friedman A, et al: Fetal growth assessment and neonatal birth weight in fetuses with an isolated single umbilical artery. Obstet Gynecol 105:1093 2005c
Quintero RA, Reich H, Romero R, et al: In utero endoscopic devascularization of a large chorioangioma. Ultrasound Obstet Gynecol 8:48, 1996
Raio L, Ghezzi F, Di Naro E, et al: Sonographic measurement of the umbilical cord and fetal anthropometric parameters. Eur J Obstet Gynecol Reprod Biol 83:131, 1999
Raio L, Ghezzi F, Di Naro E, et al: Umbilical cord morphologic characteristics and umbilical artery Doppler parameters in intrauterine growth-restricted fetuses. J Ultrasound Med 22:1341, 2003
Redline RW: Inflammatory responses in the placenta and umbilical cord. Semin Fetal Neonatal Med 11:296, 2006
Redline RW: Placental pathology: a systematic approach with clinical correlations. Placenta 29 Suppl A:S86, 2008
Roberts DJ: Placental pathology, a survival guide. Arch Pathol Lab Med 132(4):641, 2008

Robinson BK, Grobman WA: Effectiveness of timing strategies for delivery of individuals with vasa previa. Obstet Gynecol 117(3):542, 2011

Salafia CM, Silberman L, Herrera NE, et al: Placental pathology at term associated with elevated midtrimester maternal serum alpha-fetoprotein concentration. Am J Obstet Gynecol 158(5):1064, 1988

Sato Y, Benirschke K: Umbilical arterial thrombosis with vascular wall necrosis: clinicopathologic findings of 11 cases. Placenta 27:715, 2006

Sau A, Seed P, Langford K: Intraobserver and interobserver variation in the sonographic grading of placental maturity. Ultrasound Obstet Gynecol 23:374, 2004

Schachter M, Tovbin Y, Arieli S, et al: In vitro fertilization is a risk factor for vasa previa. Fertil Steril 79:1254, 2003

Sebire NJ: Pathophysiological significance of abnormal umbilical cord coiling index. Ultrasound Obstet Gynecol 30(6):804, 2007

Sebire NJ, Backos M, El Gaddal S, et al: Placental pathology, antiphospholipid antibodies, and pregnancy outcome in recurrent miscarriage patients. Obstet Gynecol 101:258, 2003

Sebire NJ, Backos M, Goldin RD, et al: Placental massive perivillous fibrin deposition associated with antiphospholipid antibody syndrome. Br J Obstet Gynaecol 109:570, 2002

Sepulveda W, Alcalde JL, Schnapp C: Perinatal outcome after prenatal diagnosis of placental chorioangioma. Obstet Gynecol 102:1028, 2003a

Sepulveda W, Aviles G, Carstens E, et al: Prenatal diagnosis of solid placental masses: the value of color flow imaging. Ultrasound Obstet Gynecol 16:554, 2000

Sepulveda W, Corral E, Kottmann C, et al: Umbilical artery aneurysm: prenatal identification in three fetuses with trisomy 18. Ultrasound Obstet Gynecol 21:213, 2003b

Sepulveda W, Wong AE, Herrera L, et al: Endoscopic laser coagulation of feeding vessels in large placental chorioangiomas: report of three cases and review of invasive treatment options. Prenat Diagn 29(3):201, 2009

Sheiner E, Abramowicz JS, Levy A, et al: Nuchal cord is not associated with adverse perinatal outcome. Arch Gynecol Obstet 274:81, 2006

Shen O, Golomb E, Lavie O, et al: Placental shelf—a common, typically transient and benign finding on early second-trimester sonography. Ultrasound Obstet Gynecol 29:192, 2007a

Shen O, Reinus C, Baranov A, et al: Prenatal diagnosis of umbilical artery aneurysm: a potentially lethal anomaly. J Ultrasound Med 26(2):251, 2007b

Sørnes T: Umbilical cord encirclements and fetal growth restriction. Obstet Gynecol 86:725, 1995

Sørnes T: Umbilical cord knots. Acta Obstet Gynecol Scand 79:157, 2000

Spellacy WN, Gravem H, Fisch RO: The umbilical cord complications of true knots, nuchal coils and cords around the body. Report from the collaborative study of cerebral palsy. Am J Obstet Gynecol 94:1136, 1966

Strong TH Jr, Jarles DL, Vega JS, et al: The umbilical coiling index. Am J Obstet Gynecol 170(1 Pt 1):29, 1994

Sun Y, Arbuckle S, Hocking G, et al: Umbilical cord stricture and intrauterine fetal death. Pediatr Pathol Lab Med 15:723, 1995

Suzuki S: Clinical significance of pregnancies with circumvallate placenta. J Obstet Gynaecol Res 34(1):51, 2008a

Suzuki S, Igarashi M: Clinical significance of pregnancies with succenturiate lobes of placenta. Arch Gynecol Obstet 277:299, 2008b

Torpin R: Amniochorionic mesoblastic fibrous strings and amnionic bands: associated constricting fetal malformations or fetal death. Am J Obstet Gynecol 91:65, 1965

Tran SH, Caughey AB, Musei TJ: Meconium-stained amniotic fluid is associated with puerperal infections. Am J Obstet Gynecol 191:2175, 2004

Tuuli MG, Shanks A, Bernhard L, et al: Uterine synechiae and pregnancy complications. Obstet Gynecol 119(4):810, 2012

Van Den Bosch T, Van Schoubroeck D, Cornelis A, et al: Prenatal diagnosis of a subamniotic hematoma. Fetal Diagn Ther 15:32, 2000

Volpe G, Volpe N, Fucci L, et al: Subamniotic hematoma: 3D and color Doppler imaging in the differential diagnosis of placental masses and fetal outcome. Minerva Ginecol 60:255, 2008

Weber MA, Sau A, Maxwell DJ, et al: Third trimester intrauterine fetal death caused by arterial aneurysm of the umbilical cord. Pediatr Deve Pathol 10:305, 2007

Woo GW, Rocha FG, Gaspar-Oishi M, et al: Placental mesenchymal dysplasia. Am J Obstet Gynecol 205(6):e3, 2011

Yamada S, Hamanishi J, Tanada S, et al: Embryogenesis of fused umbilical arteries in human embryos. Am J Obstet Gynecol 193:1709, 2005

Zalel Y, Weisz B, Gamzu R, et al: Chorioangiomas of the placenta: sonographic and Doppler flow characteristics. Ultrasound Med 21:909, 2002

Zangen R, Boldes R, Yaffe H, et al: Umbilical cord cysts in the second and third trimesters: significance and prenatal approach. Ultrasound Obstet Gynecol 36(3):296, 2010

CHAPTER 7

Embryogenesis and Fetal Morphological Development

Contemporary obstetrics includes physiology and pathophysiology of the fetus, its development, and its environment. An important result is that fetal status has been elevated to that of a patient who, in large measure, can be given the same meticulous care that obstetricians provide for pregnant women. Normal fetal development is considered in this chapter. Anomalies, injuries, and diseases that affect the fetus and newborn are addressed in Chapter 33 and others.

GESTATIONAL AGE VARIOUSLY DEFINED

Several terms are used to define pregnancy duration, and thus fetal age (Fig. 7-1). Gestational age or menstrual age is the time elapsed since the first day of the last menstrual period, a time that actually precedes conception. This starting time, which is usually about 2 weeks before ovulation and fertilization and nearly 3 weeks before blastocyst implantation, has traditionally been used because most women know their last period. Embryologists describe embryo-fetal development in *ovulation age,* or the time in days or weeks from ovulation. Another term is postconceptional age, nearly identical to ovulation age.

Clinicians customarily calculate gestational age as menstrual age. Approximately 280 days, or 40 weeks, elapse on average between the first day of the last menstrual period and the birth. This corresponds to 9 and 1/3 calendar months. A quick estimate of a pregnancy due date based on menstrual data can be made as follows: add 7 days to the first day of the last period and subtract 3 months. For example, if the first day of the last menses was July 5, the due date is 07–05 minus 3 (months) plus 7 (days) = 04–12, or April 12 of the following year. This calculation has been termed Naegele rule. Many women undergo first- or early second-trimester sonographic examination to confirm gestational age. In these cases, the sonographic estimate is usually a few days later than that determined by the last period. To rectify this inconsistency—and to reduce the number of pregnancies diagnosed as postterm—some have suggested assuming that the average pregnancy is actually 283 days long and that 10 days be added to the last menses instead of 7 (Olsen, 1998). The period of gestation can also be divided into three units, each 13 to 14 weeks long. These three trimesters are important obstetrical milestones.

EMBRYO-FETAL GROWTH AND DEVELOPMENT

The complexity of embryo-fetal development is almost beyond comprehension. Shown in Figure 7-2 is a schematic sequence of various organ systems as they develop. New information regarding organ development continues to accrue using modern technologies. For example, imaging techniques help evaluate the role of gene regulation and tissue interaction on eventual 3-dimensional organ morphology (Mohun, 2011). And, Williams and colleagues (2009) described the sequence of gene activation that underlies cardiac development.

Zygote and Blastocyst Development

During the first 2 weeks after ovulation and then fertilization, the zygote develops to the blastocyst stage, which undergoes implantation 6 or 7 days following fertilization. The 58-cell blastocyst differentiates into five embryo-producing cells—*the*

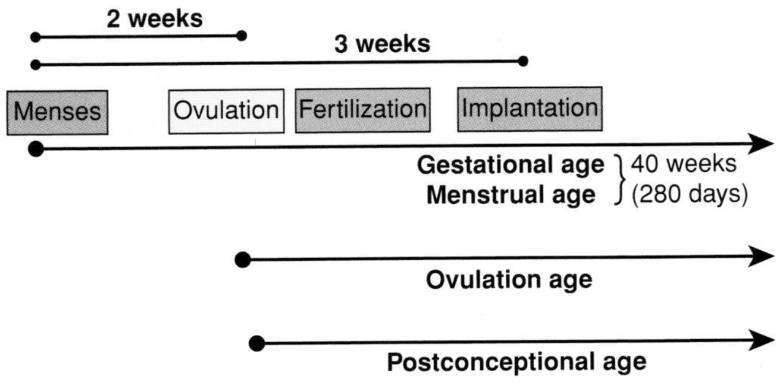

FIGURE 7-1 Terminology used to describe the pregnancy duration.

inner cell mass—and the remaining 53 cells form the placental trophoblast. Details of implantation and early development of the blastocyst and placenta are described in Chapter 5 (p. 88).

Embryonic Period

The conceptus is termed an embryo at the beginning of the third week after ovulation and fertilization. Primitive chorionic villi form, and this coincides with the expected day of menses. The embryonic period lasts 8 weeks, during which organogenesis takes place. The embryonic disc is well defined, and most pregnancy tests that measure human chorionic gonadotropin (hCG) become positive by this time. As shown in Figures 7-3 and 7-4, the body stalk is now differentiated, and the chorionic sac is approximately 1 cm in diameter. There are villous cores in which angioblastic chorionic mesoderm can be distinguished and a true intervillous space that contains maternal blood. During the third week, fetal blood vessels in the chorionic villi appear. In the fourth week, a cardiovascular system has formed, and thereby, a true circulation is established both within the embryo and between the embryo and the chorionic villi. By the end of the fourth week, the chorionic sac is 2 to 3 cm in diameter, and the embryo is 4 to 5 mm in length (Figs. 7-5 and 7-6). Partitioning of the primitive heart begins in the middle of the fourth week. Arm and leg buds are present, and the amnion is beginning to unsheathe the body stalk, which thereafter becomes the umbilical cord.

At the end of the sixth week, the embryo is 22 to 24 mm long, and the head is large compared with the trunk. The earliest synapses in the spinal cord develop at 6 to 7 weeks (Kadic, 2012). The heart is completely formed. Fingers and toes are present, and the arms bend at the elbows. The upper lip is complete, and the external ears form definitive elevations on either side of the head. Three-dimensional images and videos of human embryos from the MultiDimensional Human Embryo project are found at: http://embryo.soad.umich.edu/.

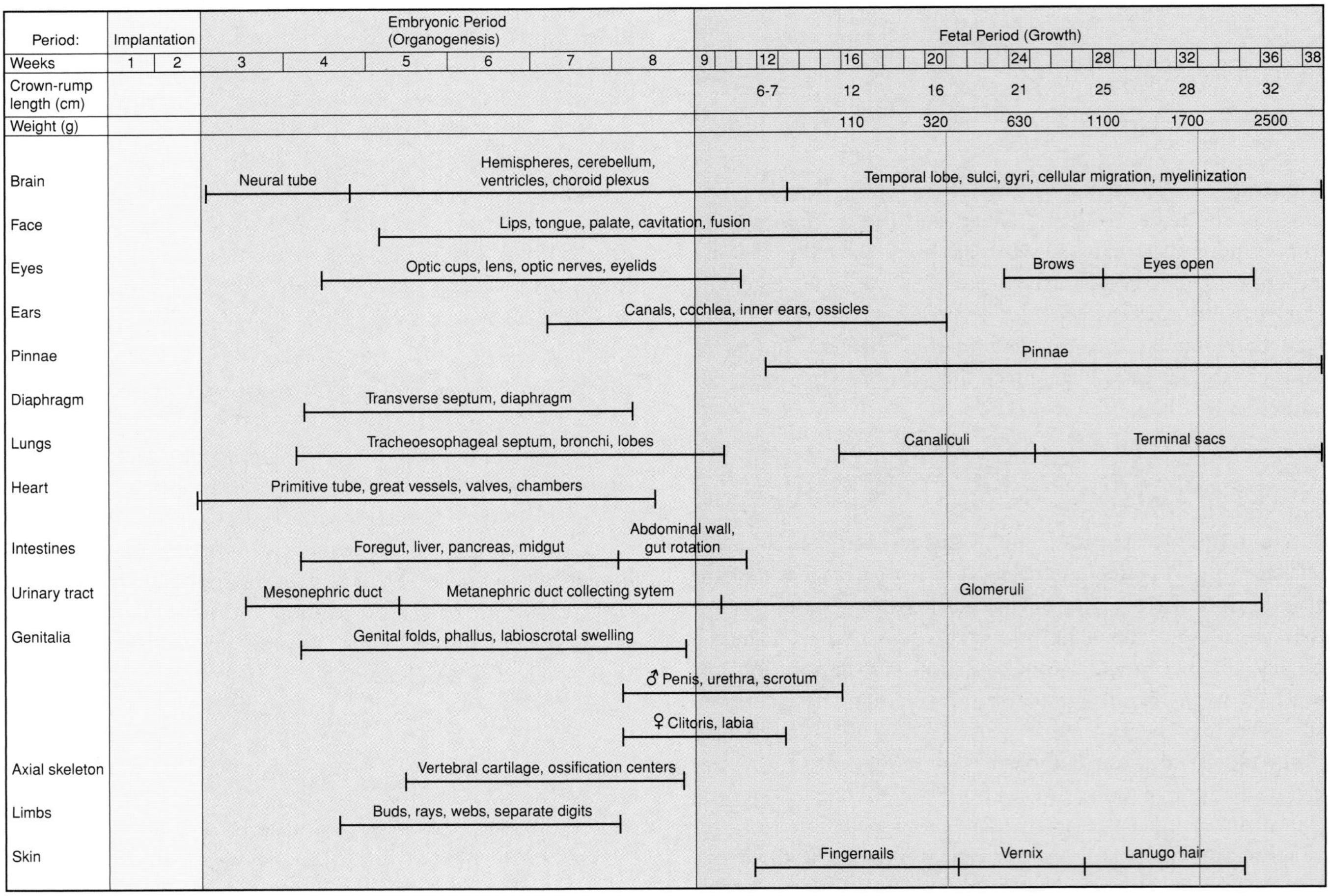

FIGURE 7-2 Embryo-fetal development according to gestational age determined by the first day of the last menses. Times are approximate.

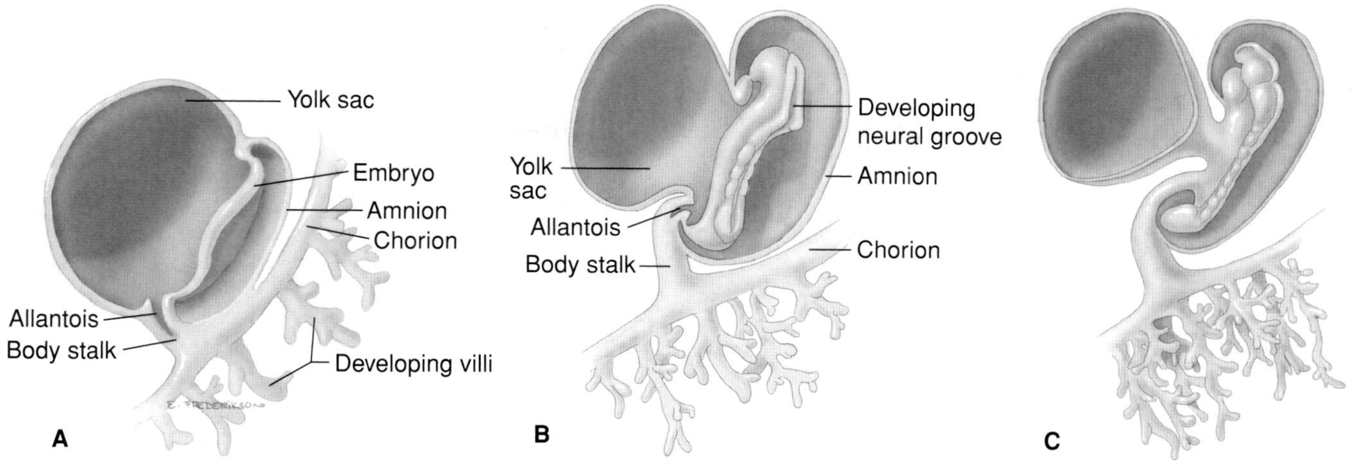

FIGURE 7-3 Early human embryos. Ovulation ages: **A.** 19 days (presomite). **B.** 21 days (7 somites). **C.** 22 days (17 somites). (After drawings and models in the Carnegie Institute.)

Fetal Period

Transition from the embryonic period to the fetal period is arbitrarily designated by most embryologists to begin 8 weeks after fertilization—or 10 weeks after onset of last menses. At this time, the embryo-fetus is nearly 4 cm long (see Fig. 7-6C).

Development during the fetal period consists of growth and maturation of structures that were formed during the embryonic period. Crown-to-rump measurements, which correspond to the sitting height, are most accurate for dating (Table 7-1).

12 Gestational Weeks

The uterus usually is just palpable above the symphysis pubis, and the fetal crown-rump length is 6 to 7 cm. Centers of ossification have appeared in most fetal bones, and the fingers and toes have become differentiated. Skin and nails have developed, and scattered rudiments of hair appear. The external genitalia are beginning to show definitive signs of male or female gender. The fetus begins to make spontaneous movements.

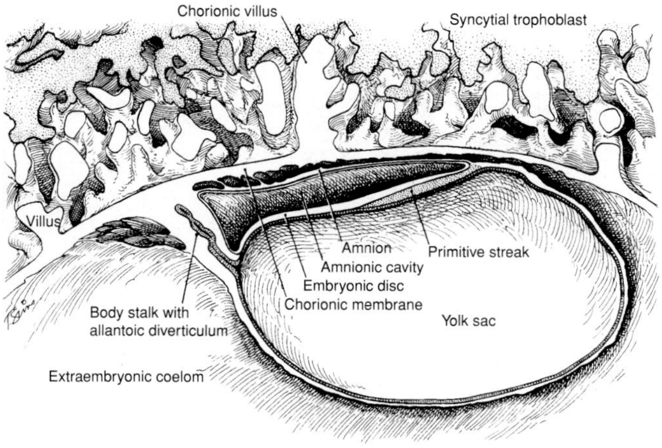

FIGURE 7-4 Drawing of an 18-day Mateer-Streeter embryo shows the amnionic cavity and its relations to chorion and yolk sac. (Redrawn from Streeter, 1920.)

16 Gestational Weeks

The fetal crown-rump length is 12 cm, and the weight is 110 g. By 14 weeks, gender can be determined by experienced observers by inspection of the external genitalia. Eye movements begin at 16 to 18 weeks, coinciding with midbrain maturation.

20 Gestational Weeks

This is the midpoint of pregnancy as estimated from the beginning of the last menses. The fetus now weighs somewhat more than 300 g, and weight increases in a linear manner. From this point onward, the fetus moves about every minute and is active 10 to 30 percent of the time (DiPietro, 2005). The fetal skin has become less transparent, a downy lanugo covers its entire body, and some scalp hair has developed. Cochlear function develops between 22 and 25 weeks, and its maturation continues for six months after delivery.

24 Gestational Weeks

The fetus now weighs approximately 630 g. The skin is characteristically wrinkled, and fat deposition begins. The head is still comparatively large, and eyebrows and eyelashes are usually recognizable. The canalicular period of lung development, during which the bronchi and bronchioles enlarge and alveolar ducts develop, is nearly completed. A fetus born at this time will attempt to breathe, but many will die because the terminal sacs, required for gas exchange, have not yet formed. By 26 weeks, nociceptors are present over all the body, and the neural pain system is developed (Kadic, 2012).

28 Gestational Weeks

The crown-rump length is approximately 25 cm, and the fetus weighs about 1100 g. The thin skin is red and covered with vernix caseosa. The pupillary membrane has just disappeared from the eyes. Isolated eye blinking peaks at 28 weeks. The otherwise normal neonate born at this age has a 90-percent chance of survival without physical or neurological impairment.

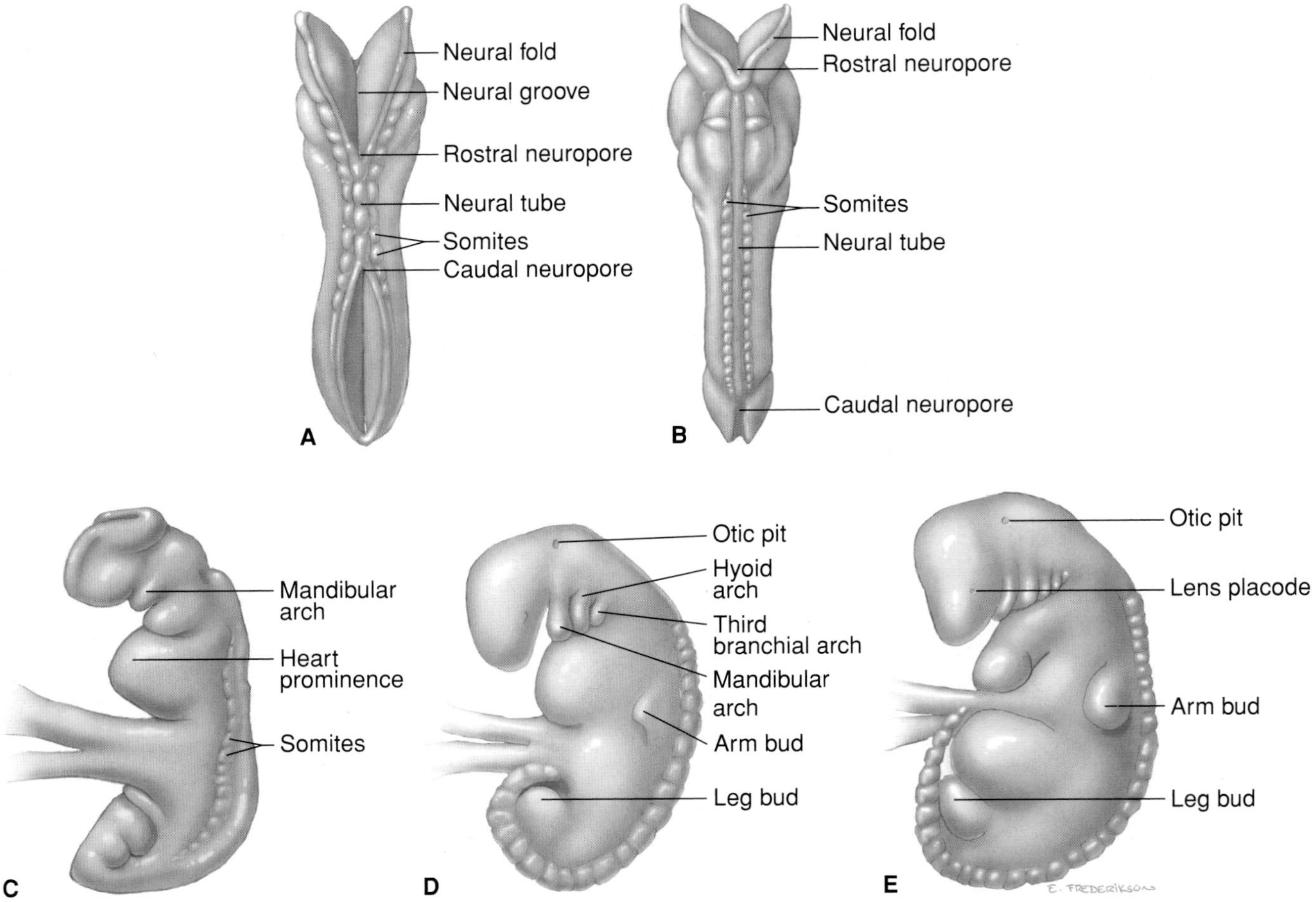

FIGURE 7-5 Three- to four-week-old embryos. **A, B.** Dorsal views of embryos during 22 to 23 days of development showing 8 and 12 somites, respectively. **C–E.** Lateral views of embryos during 24 to 28 days, showing 16, 27, and 33 somites, respectively. (Redrawn from Moore, 1988.)

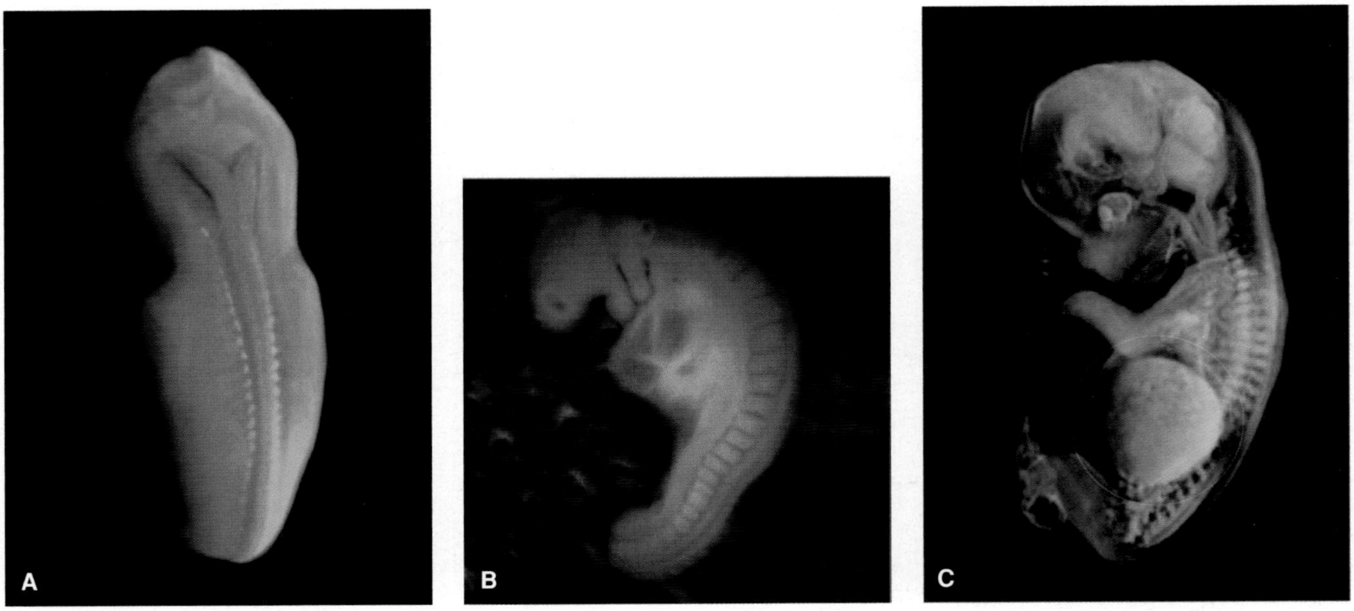

FIGURE 7-6 Embryo photographs. **A.** Dorsal view of an embryo at 24 to 26 days and corresponding to Figure 7-5C. **B.** Lateral view of an embryo at 28 days and corresponding to Figure 7-5E. **C.** Lateral view of embryo-fetus at 56 days, which marks the end of the embryonic period and the beginning of the fetal period. The liver is within the fine, white circle. (From Werth, 2002, with permission.)

TABLE 7-1. Criteria for Estimating Age During the Fetal Period

Age (weeks)		Crown-Rump Length (mm)[a]	Foot Length (mm)[a]	Fetal Weight (g)[b]	Main External Characteristics
Menstrual	Fertilization				
11	9	50	7	8	Eyes closing or closed. Head more rounded. External genitalia still not distinguishable as male or female. Intestines are in the umbilical cord.
12	10	61	9	14	Intestines in abdomen. Early fingernail development.
14	12	87	14	45	Sex distinguishable externally. Well-defined neck.
16	14	120	20	110	Head erect. Lower limbs well developed.
18	16	140	27	200	Ears stand out from head.
20	18	160	33	320	Vernix caseosa present. Early toenail development.
22	20	190	39	460	Head and body (lanugo) hair visible.
24	22	210	45	630	Skin wrinkled and red.
26	24	230	50	820	Fingernails present. Lean body.
28	26	250	55	1000	Eyes partially open. Eyelashes present.
30	28	270	59	1300	Eyes open. Good head of hair. Skin slightly wrinkled.
32	30	280	63	1700	Toenails present. Body filling out. Testes descending.
34	32	300	68	2100	Fingernails reach fingertips. Skin pink and smooth.
38	36	340	79	2900	Body usually plump. Lanugo hairs almost absent. Toenails reach toe tips.
40	38	360	83	3400	Prominent chest; breasts protrude. Testes in scrotum or palpable in inguinal canals. Fingernails extend beyond fingertips.

[a]These measurements are average and so may not apply to specific cases; dimensional variations increase with age.
[b]These weights refer to fetuses that have been fixed for approximately 2 weeks in 10-percent formalin. Fresh specimens usually weigh approximately 5 percent less.
Modified from Moore, 2013.

32 and 36 Gestational Weeks

At 32 weeks, the fetus has attained a crown-rump length of about 28 cm and a weight of approximately 1800 g. The skin surface is still red and wrinkled. In contrast, by 36 weeks, the fetal crown-rump length averages about 32 cm, and the weight is approximately 2500 g. Because of subcutaneous fat deposition, the body has become more rotund, and the previous wrinkled facial appearance has been lost.

40 Gestational Weeks

This is considered term from the onset of the last menstrual period. The fetus is now fully developed. The average crown-rump length is about 36 cm, and the weight is approximately 3400 g.

PLACENTAL PHYSIOLOGY AND FETAL GROWTH

The placenta is the organ of transfer between mother and fetus. At this maternal-fetal interface, there is transfer of oxygen and nutrients from the mother to the fetus and carbon dioxide and metabolic wastes from fetus to mother. There are no direct communications between fetal blood, which is contained in the fetal capillaries of the chorionic villi, and maternal blood, which remains in the intervillous space. Instead, bidirectional transfer depends on the processes that permit or aid the transport through the syncytiotrophoblast that line chorionic villi.

That said, there are occasional breaks in the chorionic villi, which permit escape of fetal cells into the maternal circulation. This leakage is the mechanism by which some D-negative women become sensitized by the erythrocytes of their D-positive fetus (Chap. 15, p. 306). It can also lead to chimerism from entrance of allogeneic fetal cells, including trophoblast, into maternal blood (Sunami, 2010). These are estimated to range from 1 to 6 cells/mL around midpregnancy, and some are "immortal" (Lissauer, 2007). A clinical corollary is that some maternal autoimmune diseases may be provoked by such chimerism (Bloch, 2011; Boyon, 2011). This is also discussed in Chapter 59 (p. 1168).

The Intervillous Space

Maternal blood within the intervillous space is the primary unit of maternal–fetal transfer. Blood from the maternal spiral arteries directly bathes the trophoblasts. Substances transferred from mother to fetus first enter the intervillous space and are then transported to the syncytiotrophoblast. Thus, the chorionic villi and intervillous space function together as the fetal lung, gastrointestinal tract, and kidney.

Circulation within the intervillous space is described in Chapter 5 (p. 95). Intervillous and uteroplacental blood flow increases throughout the first trimester of normal pregnancies (Mercé, 2009). At term, the residual volume of the intervillous space measures about 140 mL. Before delivery, however, the volume of this space may be twice this value (Aherne, 1966). Uteroplacental blood flow near term has been estimated to be 700 to 900 mL/min, with most of the blood apparently going to the intervillous space.

Active labor contractions reduce blood flow into the intervillous space. The degree of reduction depends on the contraction intensity. Blood pressure within the intervillous space is significantly less than uterine arterial pressure, but somewhat greater than venous pressure. The latter, in turn, varies depending on several factors, including maternal position. When supine, for example, pressure in the lower part of the inferior vena cava is elevated, and consequently, pressure in the uterine and ovarian veins, and in turn in the intervillous space, is increased.

Placental Transfer

Substances that pass from maternal to fetal blood must first traverse the syncytiotrophoblast, then villous stroma, and finally, the fetal capillary wall. Although this histological barrier separates maternal and fetal circulations, it is not a simple physical barrier. First, throughout pregnancy, syncytiotrophoblast actively or passively permits, facilitates, and adjusts the amount and rate of substance transfer to the fetus. The maternal-facing syncytiotrophoblast surface is characterized by a complex microvillous structure. The fetal-facing basal cell membrane is the site of transfer to the intravillous space. Finally, the villous capillaries are an additional site for transport from the intravillous space into fetal blood, or vice versa. In determining the effectiveness of the human placenta as an organ of transfer, at least 10 variables are important, as shown in Table 7-2 and described next.

TABLE 7-2. Variables of Maternal-Fetal Substance Transfer

Maternal plasma concentration and carrier-protein binding of the substance
Maternal blood flow rate through the intervillous space
Trophoblast surface area size available for exchange
Physical trophoblast properties to permit simple diffusion
Trophoblast biochemical machinery for active transport
Substance metabolism by the placenta during transfer
Fetal intervillous capillary surface area size for exchange
Fetal blood concentration of the substance
Specific binding or carrier proteins in the fetal or maternal circulation
Villous capillary blood flow rate

Mechanisms of Transfer

Most substances with a molecular mass less than 500 Da pass readily through placental tissue by simple diffusion. These include oxygen, carbon dioxide, water, most electrolytes, and anesthetic gases (Carter, 2009). Some low-molecular-weight compounds undergo transfer facilitated by syncytiotrophoblast. These are usually those that have low concentrations in maternal plasma but are essential for normal fetal development.

Insulin, steroid hormones, and thyroid hormones cross the placenta, but very slowly. The hormones synthesized in situ in the trophoblasts enter both the maternal and fetal circulations, but not equally (Chap. 5, p. 101). Examples are concentrations of chorionic gonadotropin and placental lactogen, which are much lower in fetal plasma than in maternal plasma. Substances of high molecular weight usually do not traverse the placenta, but there are important exceptions. One is immunoglobulin G—molecular weight 160,000 Da—which is transferred by way of a specific trophoblast receptor-mediated mechanism.

Transfer of Oxygen and Carbon Dioxide

Placental oxygen transfer is blood-flow limited. Using estimated uteroplacental blood flow, Longo (1991) calculated oxygen delivery to be approximately 8 mL O_2/min/kg of fetal weight. Normal values for oxygen, carbon dioxide, and pH in fetal blood are presented in Figure 7-7. Because of the continuous passage of oxygen from maternal blood in the intervillous space to the fetus, its oxygen saturation resembles that in maternal capillaries. The average oxygen saturation of intervillous blood is estimated to be 65 to 75 percent, with a partial pressure (Po_2) of 30 to 35 mm Hg. The oxygen saturation of umbilical vein blood is similar, but with a somewhat lower oxygen partial pressure.

The placenta is highly permeable to carbon dioxide, which traverses the chorionic villus by diffusion more rapidly than oxygen. Near term, the partial pressure of carbon dioxide (Pco_2) in the umbilical arteries averages about 50 mm Hg, or approximately 5 mm Hg more than in the maternal intervillous blood. Fetal blood has less affinity for carbon dioxide than does maternal blood, thereby favoring carbon dioxide transfer from fetus to mother. Also, mild maternal hyperventilation results in a fall in Pco_2 levels, favoring a transfer of carbon dioxide from the fetal compartment to maternal blood (Chap. 4, p. 63).

Selective Transfer and Facilitated Diffusion

Although simple diffusion is an important method of placental transfer, the trophoblast and chorionic villus unit demonstrate enormous selectivity in transfer. This results in different metabolite concentrations on the two sides of the villus. Importantly, the levels of many substances that are not synthesized by the fetus are several times higher in fetal than in maternal blood. Ascorbic acid is one example. This relatively low-molecular-weight substance might be expected to traverse the placenta by simple diffusion. The concentration of ascorbic acid, however, is two to four times higher in fetal plasma than in maternal plasma (Morriss, 1994). Another example is the unidirectional

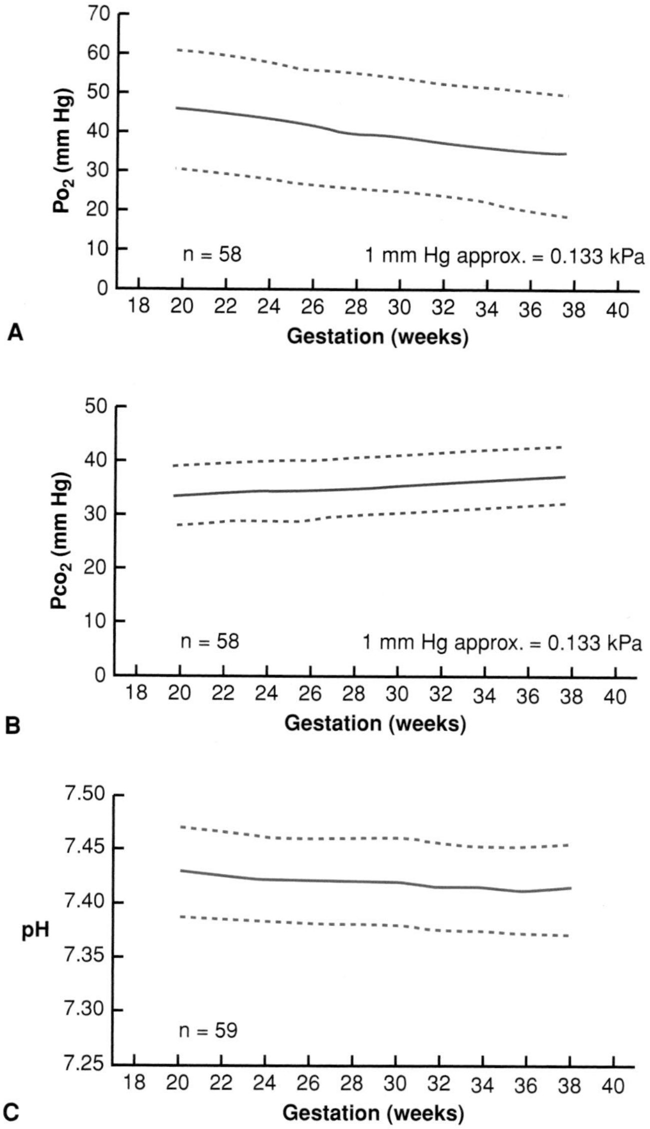

FIGURE 7-7 Umbilical venous oxygen pressure (Po_2) **(A)**; carbon dioxide pressure (Pco_2) **(B)**; and pH **(C)** from cordocentesis performed in fetuses being evaluated for possible intrauterine infections or hemolysis, but who were found to be healthy at birth and appropriately grown. (From Ramsay, 1996, with permission.)

transfer of iron. Typically, the mother's plasma iron concentration is much lower than that of her fetus. Even with severe maternal iron deficiency anemia, the fetal hemoglobin mass is normal.

FETAL NUTRITION

Because of the small amount of yolk in the human ovum, growth of the embryo-fetus is dependent on maternal nutrients during the first 2 months. During the first few days after implantation, blastocyst nutrition comes from the interstitial fluid of the endometrium and the surrounding maternal tissue.

Maternal adaptations to store and transfer nutrients to the fetus are discussed in Chapter 4 and summarized here. Three major maternal storage depots—the liver, muscle, and adipose tissue—and the storage-hormone insulin are intimately involved in the metabolism of the nutrients absorbed from the maternal gut.

Insulin secretion is sustained by increased serum levels of glucose and amino acids. The net effect is storage of glucose as glycogen primarily in liver and muscle, retention of some amino acids as protein, and storage of the excess as fat. Storage of maternal fat peaks in the second trimester and then declines as fetal energy demands increase in the third trimester (Pipe, 1979). Interestingly, the placenta appears to act as a nutrient sensor, altering transport based on the maternal supply and environmental stimuli (Fowden, 2006; Jansson, 2006b).

During times of fasting, glucose is released from glycogen, but maternal glycogen stores cannot provide an adequate amount of glucose to meet requirements for maternal energy and fetal growth. Augmentation is provided by cleavage of triacylglycerols, stored in adipose tissue, which result in free fatty acids and activation of lipolysis.

Glucose and Fetal Growth

Although dependent on the mother for nutrition, the fetus also actively participates in providing for its own nutrition. At midpregnancy, fetal glucose concentration is independent of and may exceed maternal levels (Bozzetti, 1988). Glucose is the major nutrient for fetal growth and energy. Logically, mechanisms exist during pregnancy to minimize maternal glucose use so that the limited maternal supply is available to the fetus. Human placental lactogen (hPL), a hormone normally abundant in the mother but not the fetus, is believed to block peripheral uptake and use of glucose, while promoting mobilization and use of free fatty acids by maternal tissues (Chap. 5, p. 104).

Glucose Transport

The transfer of D-glucose across cell membranes is accomplished by a carrier-mediated, stereospecific, nonconcentrating process of facilitated diffusion. There are 14 glucose transport proteins (GLUTs) encoded by the *SLC2A* gene family and characterized by tissue-specific distribution (Leonce, 2006). GLUT-1 and GLUT-3 primarily facilitate glucose uptake by the placenta and are located in the plasma membrane of the syncytiotrophoblast microvilli (Korgun, 2005). DNA methylation regulates expression of placental GLUT genes, with epigenetic modification across gestation (Novakovic, 2013). GLUT-1 expression is essential for decidualization. It increases as pregnancy advances and is induced by almost all growth factors (Frolova, 2011; Sakata, 1995).

Lactate is a product of glucose metabolism and is also transported across the placenta by facilitated diffusion. By way of cotransport with hydrogen ions, lactate is probably transported as lactic acid.

Glucose and Insulin Role in Fetal Macrosomia

The precise biomolecular events in the pathophysiology of fetal macrosomia are not defined. Nonetheless, it seems clear that fetal hyperinsulinemia is one driving force (Schwartz, 1994). As discussed in Chapter 44 (p. 872), insulin-like growth factor and fibroblast growth factor are important regulators of placental development and function (Forbes, 2010; Giudice, 1995). In addition, recent work has shown that placental corticotropin-releasing hormone (CRH) stimulates trophoblastic production of GLUT-1 and inhibits expression of GLUT-3 through interaction on the CRH-R1 receptor. This suggests a role for CRH in the nutritional regulation of fetal growth and development (Gao, 2012).

Leptin

This polypeptide hormone was originally identified as a product of adipocytes and a regulator of energy homeostasis. It also contributes to angiogenesis, hemopoiesis, osteogenesis, pulmonary maturation, and neuroendocrine, immune, and reproductive functions (Henson, 2006; Maymó, 2009). Leptin is produced by the mother, fetus, and placenta. It is expressed in syncytiotrophoblast and fetal vascular endothelial cells. Of placental production, 5 percent enters fetal circulation, whereas 95 percent is transferred to the mother (Hauguel-de Mouzon, 2006). As a result, the placenta greatly contributes to maternal leptin levels.

Fetal leptin levels begin rising at approximately 34 weeks and are correlated with fetal weight. Abnormal levels have been associated with growth disorders and preeclampsia. Postpartum, leptin levels decline in both the newborn and mother (Grisaru-Granovsky, 2008). Perinatal leptin is associated with the development of metabolic syndromes later in life (Granado, 2012).

Free Fatty Acids and Triglycerides

The newborn has a large proportion of fat, which averages 15 percent of body weight (Kimura, 1991). Thus, late in pregnancy, a substantial part of the substrate transferred to the human fetus is stored as fat. Although maternal obesity affects placental fatty acid uptake, it appears to have no effect on fetal growth (Dube, 2012). Neutral fat in the form of triacylglycerols does not cross the placenta, but glycerol does. There is preferential placental-fetal transfer of long-chain polyunsaturated fatty acids (Gil-Sanchez, 2012). Lipoprotein lipase is present on the maternal but not on the fetal side of the placenta. This arrangement favors hydrolysis of triacylglycerols in the maternal intervillous space while preserving these neutral lipids in fetal blood. Fatty acids transferred to the fetus can be converted to triacylglycerols in the fetal liver.

The placental uptake and use of low-density lipoprotein (LDL) is an alternative mechanism for fetal assimilation of essential fatty acids and amino acids (Chap. 5, p. 109). The LDL binds to specific receptors in the coated-pit regions of the syncytiotrophoblast microvilli. The large—about 250,000 Da—LDL particle is taken up by a process of receptor-mediated endocytosis. The apoprotein and cholesterol esters of LDL are hydrolyzed by lysosomal enzymes in the syncytium to give: (1) cholesterol for progesterone synthesis; (2) free amino acids, including essential amino acids; and (3) essential fatty acids, primarily linoleic acid. Indeed, the concentration of arachidonic acid, which is synthesized from linoleic acid in fetal plasma, is greater than that in maternal plasma. Linoleic acid or arachidonic acid or both must be assimilated from maternal dietary intake.

Amino Acids

The placenta concentrates many amino acids in the syncytiotrophoblast, which are then transferred to the fetal side by diffusion (Lemons, 1979). Based on data from cordocentesis blood samples, the amino acid concentration in umbilical cord plasma is greater than in maternal venous or arterial plasma (Morriss, 1994). Transport system activity is influenced by gestational age and environmental factors. These include heat stress, hypoxia, and under- and overnutrition, as well as hormones such as glucocorticoids, growth hormone, and leptin (Fowden, 2006). Trophoblastic mammalian target of rapamycin complex 1 (mTORC1) regulates placental amino acid transporters and modulates transfer across the placenta (Jansson, 2012). In vivo studies suggest an upregulation of transport for certain amino acids and an increased fetal delivery in women with gestational diabetes associated with fetal overgrowth (Jansson, 2006a).

Proteins

Placental transfer of larger proteins is limited, but there are exceptions. Immunoglobulin G (IgG) crosses the placenta in large amounts via endocytosis and trophoblast Fc receptors. IgG transfer depends on maternal levels of total IgG, gestational age, placental integrity, IgG subclass, and antigen nature (Palmeira, 2012). IgA and IgM of maternal origin are effectively excluded from the fetus (Gitlin, 1972).

Ions and Trace Metals

Iodide transport is clearly attributable to a carrier-mediated, energy-requiring active process. And indeed, the placenta concentrates iodide. The concentrations of zinc in the fetal plasma also are greater than those in maternal plasma. Conversely, copper levels in fetal plasma are less than those in maternal plasma. This fact is of particular interest because important copper-requiring enzymes are necessary for fetal development.

Placental Sequestration of Heavy Metals

The heavy-metal–binding protein metallothionein-1 is expressed in human syncytiotrophoblast. This protein binds and sequesters a host of heavy metals, including zinc, copper, lead, and cadmium. Lead enters the fetal environment at a level 90 percent of maternal concentrations, but placental transfer of cadmium is limited (Kopp, 2012). The most common source of environmental cadmium is cigarette smoke. Cadmium levels in maternal blood and placenta are increased with maternal smoking, but there is no increase in cadmium transfer into the fetus. In the rat, data suggest that cadmium reduces the number of trophoblasts, leading to poor placental growth (Lee, 2009).

Metallothionein also binds and sequesters copper (Cu^{2+}) in placental tissue. This accounts for the low levels of Cu^{2+} in cord blood (Iyengar, 2001). Several enzymes require Cu^{2+}, and its deficiency results in inadequate collagen cross-linking and, in turn, diminished tensile strength of tissues. This may be important because the concentration of cadmium in amnionic fluid is similar to that in maternal blood. The incidence of preterm membrane rupture is increased in women who smoke. It is possible that cadmium provokes metallothionein synthesis in the amnion. This may cause sequestration of Cu^{2+}, a pseudocopper deficiency, and in turn, a weakened amnion.

Calcium and Phosphorus

These minerals also are actively transported from mother to fetus. Calcium is transferred for fetal skeletal mineralization (Olausson, 2012). A calcium-binding protein is produced in placenta. Parathyroid hormone-related protein (PTH-rP), as the name implies, acts as a surrogate PTH in many systems (Chap. 5, p. 105). PTH is not demonstrable in fetal plasma. However, PTH-rP is present, suggesting that PTH-rP is the fetal parathormone. The expression of PTH-rP in cytotrophoblasts is modulated by the extracellular concentration of Ca^{2+} (Hellman, 1992). It seems possible, therefore, that PTH-rP synthesized in decidua, placenta, and other fetal tissues is important in fetal Ca^{2+} transfer and homeostasis.

Vitamins

The concentration of *vitamin A (retinol)* is greater in fetal than in maternal plasma and is bound to retinol-binding protein and to prealbumin. Retinol-binding protein is transferred from the maternal compartment across the syncytiotrophoblast. The transport of *vitamin C—ascorbic acid*—from mother to fetus is accomplished by an energy-dependent, carrier-mediated process. The levels of the principal *vitamin D—cholecalciferol*–metabolites, including 1,25-dihydroxycholecalciferol, are greater in maternal plasma than are those in fetal plasma. The 1β-hydroxylation of 25-hydroxyvitamin D_3 is known to take place in placenta and in decidua.

FETAL ORGAN SYSTEM DEVELOPMENT

Amnionic Fluid Formation

In early pregnancy, amnionic fluid is an ultrafiltrate of maternal plasma. By the second trimester, it consists largely of extracellular fluid that diffuses through the fetal skin and thus reflects the composition of fetal plasma (Gilbert, 1993). After 20 weeks, the cornification of fetal skin prevents this diffusion, and amnionic fluid is composed largely of fetal urine. Fetal kidneys start producing urine at 12 weeks, and by 18 weeks, they are producing 7 to 14 mL per day. Fetal urine contains more urea, creatinine, and uric acid than fetal plasma. Amnionic fluid also contains desquamated fetal cells, vernix, lanugo, and various secretions. Because these are hypotonic, the net effect is that amnionic fluid osmolality decreases with advancing gestation. Pulmonary fluid contributes a small proportion of the amnionic volume, and fluid filtering through the placenta accounts for the rest. Aquaporins 8 and 9 play a role in water flow via intramembranous absorption and placental water transfer (Jiang, 2012)

The volume of amnionic fluid at each week is variable (Chap. 11, p. 231). In general, the volume increases by 10 mL per week at 8 weeks and increases to 60 mL per week at 21 weeks, then peaks at 34 weeks (Brace, 1989).

Amnionic fluid serves to cushion the fetus, allowing musculoskeletal development and protecting it from trauma. It also maintains temperature and has a minimal nutritive function. Epidermal growth factor (EGF) and EGF-like growth factors, such as transforming growth factor-β, are present in amnionic fluid. Ingestion of fluid into the gastrointestinal tract and inhalation into the lung may promote growth and differentiation of these tissues. Animal studies have shown that pulmonary hypoplasia can be produced by draining amnionic fluid, by chronically draining pulmonary fluid through the trachea, or by physically preventing the prenatal chest excursions that mimic breathing (Adzick, 1984; Alcorn, 1977). Thus, intrapulmonary fluid formation and, at least as important, the alternating egress and retention of fluid in the lungs by breathing movements are essential to normal pulmonary development.

Cardiovascular System

The fetal circulation is substantially different from that of the adult and functions until birth, when it is required to change dramatically. For example, because fetal blood does not need to enter the pulmonary vasculature to be oxygenated, most of the right ventricular output bypasses the lungs. In addition, the fetal heart chambers work in parallel, not in series, which effectively supplies the brain and heart with more highly oxygenated blood than the rest of the body.

Oxygen and nutrient materials required for fetal growth and maturation are delivered from the placenta by the single umbilical vein (Fig. 7-8). The vein then divides into the ductus venosus and the portal sinus. The ductus venosus is the major branch of the umbilical vein and traverses the liver to enter the inferior vena cava directly. Because it does not supply oxygen to the intervening tissues, it carries well-oxygenated blood directly to the heart. In contrast, the portal sinus carries blood to the hepatic veins primarily on the left side of the liver, and oxygen is extracted. The relatively deoxygenated blood from the liver then flows back into the inferior vena cava, which also receives less oxygenated blood returning from the lower body. Blood flowing to the fetal heart from the inferior vena cava, therefore, consists of an admixture of arterial-like blood that passes directly through the ductus venosus and less well-oxygenated blood that returns from most of the veins below the level of the diaphragm. The oxygen content of blood delivered to the heart from the inferior vena cava is thus lower than that leaving the placenta.

In contrast to postnatal life, the ventricles of the fetal heart work in parallel, not in series. Well-oxygenated blood enters the left ventricle, which supplies the heart and brain, and less oxygenated blood enters the right ventricle, which supplies the rest of the body. These two separate circulations are maintained by the right atrium structure, which effectively directs entering blood to either the left atrium or the right ventricle, depending on its oxygen content. This separation of blood according to its oxygen content is aided by the pattern of blood flow in the inferior vena cava. The well-oxygenated blood tends to course along the medial aspect of the inferior vena cava and the less oxygenated blood flows along the lateral vessel wall. This aids their shunting into opposite sides of the heart. Once this blood enters the right atrium, the configuration of the upper interatrial septum—the *crista dividens*—preferentially shunts the well-oxygenated blood from the medial

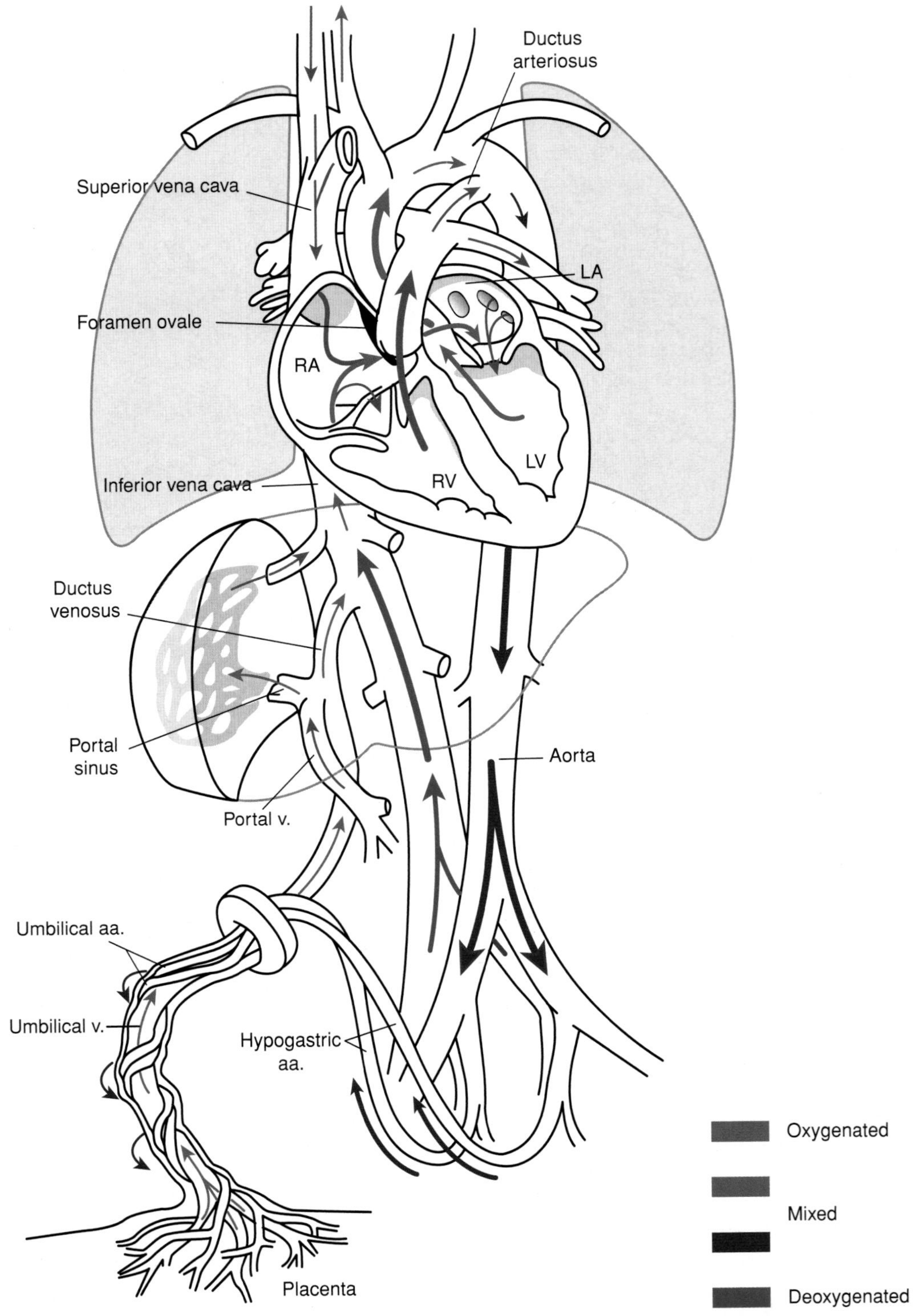

FIGURE 7-8 The intricate nature of the fetal circulation is evident. The degree of blood oxygenation in various vessels differs appreciably from that in the postnatal state. aa = arteries; LA = left atrium; LV = left ventricle; RA = right atrium; RV = right ventricle; v = vein.

side of the inferior vena cava through the foramen ovale into the left heart and then to the heart and brain (Dawes, 1962). After these tissues have extracted needed oxygen, the resulting less oxygenated blood returns to the right atrium through the superior vena cava.

The less oxygenated blood coursing along the lateral wall of the inferior vena cava enters the right atrium and is deflected through the tricuspid valve to the right ventricle. The superior vena cava courses inferiorly and anteriorly as it enters the right atrium, ensuring that less well-oxygenated blood returning from the brain and upper body also will be shunted directly to the right ventricle. Similarly, the ostium of the coronary sinus lies just superior to the tricuspid valve so that less oxygenated blood from the heart also returns to the right ventricle. As a result of this blood flow pattern, blood in the right ventricle is 15 to 20 percent less saturated than blood in the left ventricle.

Almost 90 percent of blood exiting the right ventricle is shunted through the ductus arteriosus to the descending aorta. High pulmonary vascular resistance and comparatively lower resistance in the ductus arteriosus and the umbilical–placental vasculature ensure that only about 15 percent of right ventricular output—8 percent of the combined ventricular output—goes to the lungs (Teitel, 1992). Thus, one third of the blood passing through the ductus arteriosus is delivered to the body. The remaining right ventricular output returns to the placenta through the two hypogastric arteries, which distally become the umbilical arteries. In the placenta, this blood picks up oxygen and other nutrients and is recirculated through the umbilical vein.

Circulatory Changes at Birth

After birth, the umbilical vessels, ductus arteriosus, foramen ovale, and ductus venosus normally constrict or collapse. With the functional closure of the ductus arteriosus and the expansion of the lungs, blood leaving the right ventricle preferentially enters the pulmonary vasculature to become oxygenated before it returns to the left heart. Virtually instantaneously, the ventricles, which had worked in parallel in fetal life, now effectively work in series. The more distal portions of the hypogastric arteries, which course from the level of the bladder along the abdominal wall to the umbilical ring and into the cord as the umbilical arteries, undergo atrophy and obliteration within 3 to 4 days after birth. These become the umbilical ligaments, whereas the intraabdominal remnants of the umbilical vein form the ligamentum teres. The ductus venosus constricts by 10 to 96 hours after birth and is anatomically closed by 2 to 3 weeks, resulting in formation of the ligamentum venosum (Clymann, 1981).

Hematological Development

Hemopoiesis

In the early embryo, hemopoiesis is demonstrable first in the yolk sac, followed by the liver and finally bone marrow. The first erythrocytes released into the fetal circulation are nucleated and macrocytic. Mean cell volumes are expressed in femtoliters (fL), and one femtoliter equals one cubic micrometer. The mean cell volume is at least 180 fL in the embryo and decreases to 105 to 115 fL at term. The erythrocytes of aneuploid fetuses generally do not undergo this maturation and maintain high mean cell volumes—130 fL on average (Sipes, 1991). As fetal development progresses, more and more of the circulating erythrocytes are smaller and nonnucleated. With fetal growth, both the blood volume in the common fetoplacental circulation and hemoglobin concentration increase. Hemoglobin content of fetal blood rises to approximately 12 g/dL at midpregnancy and to 18 g/dL at term (Walker, 1953). Because of their large size, fetal erythrocytes have a short life span, which progressively lengthens to approximately 90 days at term (Pearson, 1966). As a consequence, red blood cell production is increased. Reticulocytes are initially present at high levels, but decrease to 4 to 5 percent of the total at term. Fetal erythrocytes differ structurally and metabolically from those of the adult. They are more deformable, which serves to offset their higher viscosity. They also contain several enzymes with appreciably different activities (Smith, 1981).

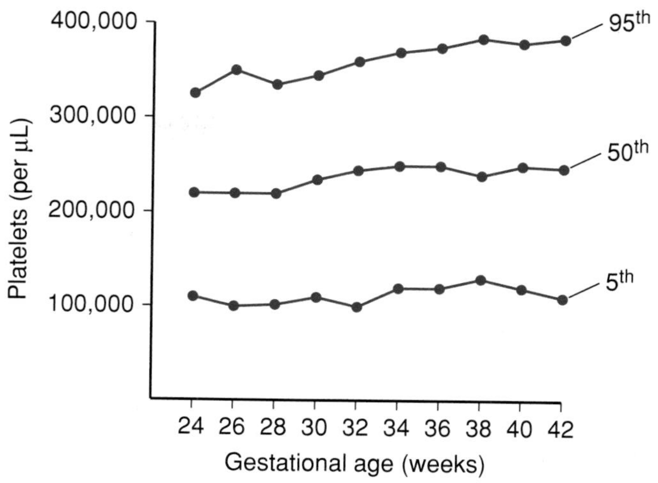

FIGURE 7-9 Platelet counts by gestational age obtained the first day of life. Mean values and 5th and 95th percentiles are shown. (Data from Christensen, 2012.)

Erythropoiesis is controlled primarily by fetal erythropoietin because maternal erythropoietin does not cross the placenta. Fetal hormone production is influenced by testosterone, estrogen, prostaglandins, thyroid hormone, and lipoproteins (Stockman, 1992). Serum erythropoietin levels increase with fetal maturity. Although the exact production site is disputed, the fetal liver appears to be an important source until renal production begins. There is a close correlation between the erythropoietin concentration in amnionic fluid and that in umbilical venous blood obtained by cordocentesis. After birth, erythropoietin normally may not be detectable for up to 3 months.

In contrast, platelet production reaches stable levels by midpregnancy, although there is some variation across gestation (Fig. 7-9). The fetal and neonatal platelet count is subject to various agents as discussed in Chapter 15 (p. 313).

Fetoplacental Blood Volume

Although precise measurements of human fetoplacental blood volume are lacking, Usher and associates (1963) reported values in term normal newborns to average 78 mL/kg when immediate cord clamping was conducted. Gruenwald (1967) found the fetal blood volume contained in the placenta after prompt cord clamping to average 45 mL/kg of fetal weight. Thus, fetoplacental blood volume at term is approximately 125 mL/kg of fetal weight.

Fetal Hemoglobin

This tetrameric protein is composed of two copies of two different peptide chains, which determine the type of hemoglobin produced. Normal adult hemoglobin A is made of α and β chains. During embryonic and fetal life, various α and β chain precursors are produced. This results in the serial production of several different embryonic hemoglobins. Genes for β-type chains are on chromosome 11 and for α-type chains on chromosome 16. This sequence is shown in Figure 7-10. Each of these genes is turned on and then off during fetal life, until the α and β genes, which direct the production of hemoglobin A, are permanently activated.

CHAPTER 7

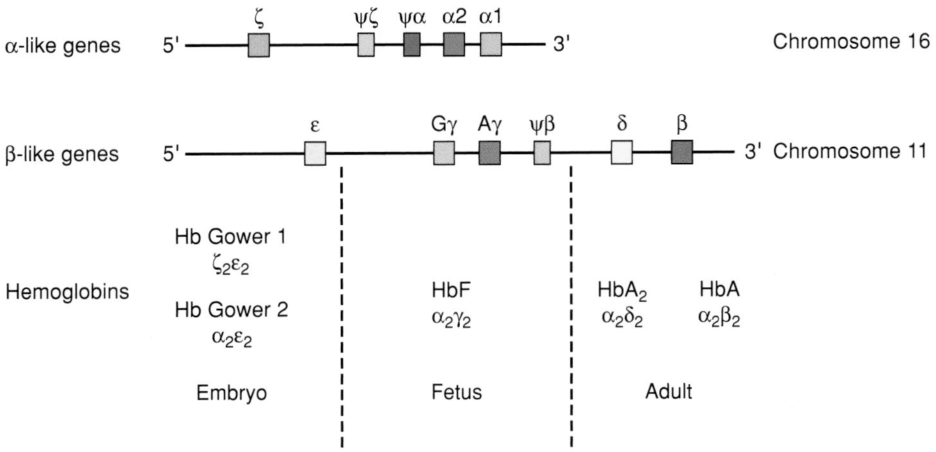

FIGURE 7-10 Schematic drawing of the arrangement of the α and β gene precursors on chromosomes 11 and 16 and the hemoglobin types made from them. (Modified after Thompson, 1991.)

The timing of the production of each of these early hemoglobins corresponds to the site of hemoglobin production. Fetal blood is first produced in the yolk sac, where hemoglobins Gower 1, Gower 2, and Portland are made. Erythropoiesis then moves to the liver, where fetal hemoglobin F is produced. When hemopoiesis finally moves to the bone marrow, adult-type hemoglobin A appears in fetal red blood cells and is present in progressively greater amounts as the fetus matures (Pataryas, 1972).

The final adult version of the α chain is produced exclusively by 6 weeks. After this, there are no functional alternative versions. If an α-gene mutation or deletion occurs, there is no alternate α-type chain that could substitute to form functional hemoglobin. In contrast, at least two versions of the β chain—δ and γ—remain in production throughout fetal life and beyond. In the case of a β-gene mutation or deletion, these two other versions of the β chain often continue to be produced, resulting in hemoglobin A_2 or hemoglobin F, which substitute for the abnormal or missing hemoglobin.

Genes are turned off by methylation of their control region, which is discussed in Chapter 13 (p. 272). In some situations, methylation does not occur. For example, in newborns of diabetic women, hemoglobin F may persist due to hypomethylation of the γ gene (Perrine, 1988). With sickle-cell anemia, the γ gene remains unmethylated, and large quantities of fetal hemoglobin continue to be produced (Chap. 56, p. 1108). Increased hemoglobin F levels are associated with fewer sickle-cell disease symptoms, and pharmacological modification of these levels by hemoglobin F-inducing drugs is one approach to disease treatment (Trompeter, 2009).

There is a functional difference between hemoglobins A and F. At any given oxygen tension and at identical pH, fetal erythrocytes that contain mostly hemoglobin F bind more oxygen than do those that contain nearly all hemoglobin A (Fig. 47-2, p. 945). This is because hemoglobin A binds 2,3-diphosphoglycerate (2,3-DPG) more avidly than does hemoglobin F, thus lowering the affinity of hemoglobin A for oxygen (De Verdier, 1969). During pregnancy, maternal 2,3-DPG levels are increased, and because fetal erythrocytes have lower concentrations of 2,3-DPG, the latter has increased oxygen affinity.

The amount of hemoglobin F in fetal erythrocytes begins to decrease in the last weeks of pregnancy. At term, approximately three fourths of total hemoglobin is hemoglobin F. During the first 6 to 12 months of life, the hemoglobin F proportion continues to decrease and eventually reaches the low levels found in adult erythrocytes. Glucocorticosteroids mediate the switch from fetal to adult hemoglobin, and the effect is irreversible (Zitnik, 1995).

Coagulation Factors

There are no embryonic forms of the various hemostatic proteins. With the exception of fibrinogen, the fetus starts producing normal, adult-type procoagulant, fibrinolytic, and anticoagulant proteins by 12 weeks. Because they do not cross the placenta, their concentrations at birth are markedly below the levels that develop within a few weeks of life (Corrigan, 1992). In normal neonates, the levels of factors II, VII, IX, X, and XI, as well as those of prekallikrein, protein S, protein C, antithrombin, and plasminogen, are all approximately 50 percent of adult levels. In contrast, levels of factors V, VIII, XIII, and fibrinogen are closer to adult values (Saracco, 2009). Without prophylactic treatment, the vitamin K-dependent coagulation factors usually decrease even further during the first few days after birth. This decline is amplified in breast-fed infants and may lead to newborn hemorrhage (Chap. 33, p. 644).

Fetal fibrinogen, which appears as early as 5 weeks, has the same amino acid composition as adult fibrinogen but has different properties (Klagsbrun, 1988). It forms a less compressible clot, and the fibrin monomer has a lower degree of aggregation (Heimark, 1988). Plasma fibrinogen levels at birth are less than those in nonpregnant adults, however, the protein is functionally more active than adult fibrinogen (Ignjatovic, 2011).

Levels of functional fetal factor XIII—fibrin-stabilizing factor—are significantly reduced compared with those in adults (Henriksson, 1974). Nielsen (1969) described low levels of plasminogen and increased fibrinolytic activity in cord plasma compared with that of maternal plasma. Platelet counts in cord blood are in the normal range for nonpregnant adults (see Fig. 7-9).

Despite this relative reduction in procoagulants, the fetus appears to be protected from hemorrhage because fetal bleeding is rare. Excessive bleeding does not usually occur even after invasive fetal procedures such as cordocentesis. Ney and coworkers (1989) have shown that amnionic fluid thromboplastins and a factor(s) in Wharton jelly combine to aid coagulation at the umbilical cord puncture site.

Various thrombophilias may cause thromboses and pregnancy complications in adults (Chap. 52, p. 1029). If the fetus inherits one of these mutations, thrombosis and infarction can develop in the placenta or in fetal organs. This is usually seen with homozygous inheritance.

Plasma Proteins

Liver enzymes and other plasma proteins are produced by the fetus, and these levels do not correlate with maternal levels (Weiner, 1992). Concentrations of plasma proteins, albumin, lactic dehydrogenase, aspartate aminotransferase, γ-glutamyl transpeptidase, and alanine transferase all increase, whereas prealbumin levels decrease with gestational age (Fryer, 1993). At birth, mean total plasma protein and albumin concentrations in fetal blood are similar to maternal levels (Foley, 1978).

Immunology

Infections in utero have provided an opportunity to examine mechanisms of the fetal immune response. Evidence of immunological competence has been reported as early as 13 weeks (Kohler, 1973; Stabile, 1988). In cord blood at or near term, the average level for most components is approximately half that of the adult values (Adinolfi, 1977).

In the absence of a direct antigenic stimulus such as infection, fetal plasma immunoglobulins consist almost totally of transferred maternal immunoglobulin G (IgG). Thus, antibodies in the newborn are most often reflective of maternal immunological experiences.

Immunoglobulin G

Maternal IgG transport to the fetus begins at approximately 16 weeks and increases thereafter. The bulk of IgG is acquired during the last 4 weeks of pregnancy (Gitlin, 1971). Accordingly, preterm neonates are endowed relatively poorly with protective maternal antibodies. Newborns begin to slowly produce IgG, and adult values are not attained until 3 years of age. In certain situations, the transfer of IgG antibodies from mother to fetus can be harmful rather than protective to the fetus. The classic example is hemolytic disease of the fetus and newborn resulting from D-antigen alloimmunization (Chap. 15, p. 306).

Immunoglobulin M and A

In the adult, production of immunoglobulin M (IgM) in response to an antigenic stimulus is superseded in a week or so predominantly by IgG production. In contrast, very little IgM is produced by normal fetuses, and that produced may include antibody to maternal T lymphocytes (Hayward, 1983). With infection, the IgM response is dominant in the fetus and remains so for weeks to months in the newborn. And because IgM is not transported from the mother, any IgM in the fetus or newborn is that which it produced. Increased levels of IgM are found in newborns with congenital infection such as rubella, cytomegalovirus infection, or toxoplasmosis. Serum IgM levels in umbilical cord blood and identification of specific antibodies may be useful in intrauterine infection diagnosis. In infants, adult levels of IgM are normally attained by age 9 months.

Immunoglobulin A (IgA) ingested in colostrum provides mucosal protection against enteric infections. This role as an immune barrier against infection may explain the small amount of fetal secretory IgA found in amnionic fluid (Quan, 1999).

Lymphocytes and Monocytes

The immune system develops early. B lymphocytes appear in fetal liver by 9 weeks and in blood and spleen by 12 weeks. T lymphocytes begin to leave the thymus at approximately 14 weeks. Despite this, the newborn responds poorly to immunization, and especially poorly to bacterial capsular polysaccharides. This immature response may be due to either deficient response of newborn B cells to polyclonal activators, or lack of T cells that proliferate in response to specific stimuli (Hayward, 1983). In the newborn, monocytes are able to process and present antigen when tested with maternal antigen-specific T cells. DNA methylation patterns are developmentally regulated during monocyte-macrophage differentiation and contribute to the antiinflammatory phenotype in macrophages (Kim, 2012).

Skull

Fetal head size is important because an essential feature of labor is the adaptation between the head and the maternal bony pelvis. The firm skull is composed of two frontal, two parietal, and two temporal bones, along with the upper portion of the occipital bone and the wings of the sphenoid. These bones are separated by membranous spaces termed sutures (Fig. 7-11).

The most important sutures are the frontal, between the two frontal bones; the sagittal, between the two parietal bones; the two coronal, between the frontal and parietal bones; and the two lambdoid, between the posterior margins of the parietal bones and upper margin of the occipital bone. The term fontanel describes the irregular space enclosed by a membrane at the junction of several sutures (see Fig. 7-11). The greater, or anterior, fontanel is a lozenge-shaped space situated at the junction of the sagittal and the coronal sutures. The lesser, or posterior, fontanel is a small triangular area at the intersection of the sagittal and lambdoid sutures. The localization of these fontanels gives important information concerning the presentation and position of the fetus during labor.

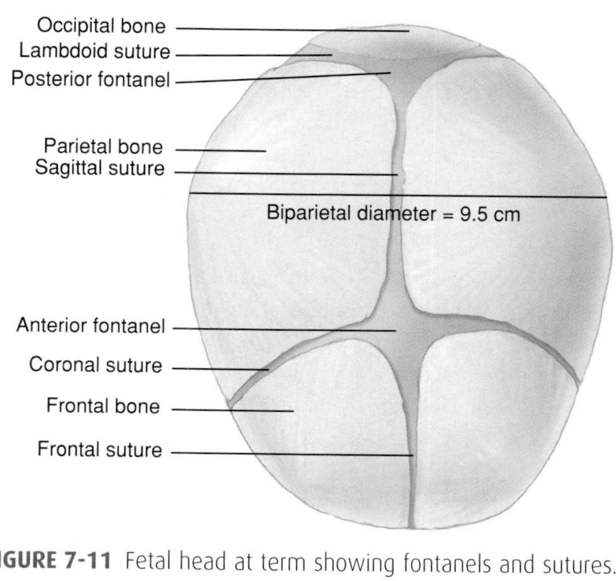

FIGURE 7-11 Fetal head at term showing fontanels and sutures.

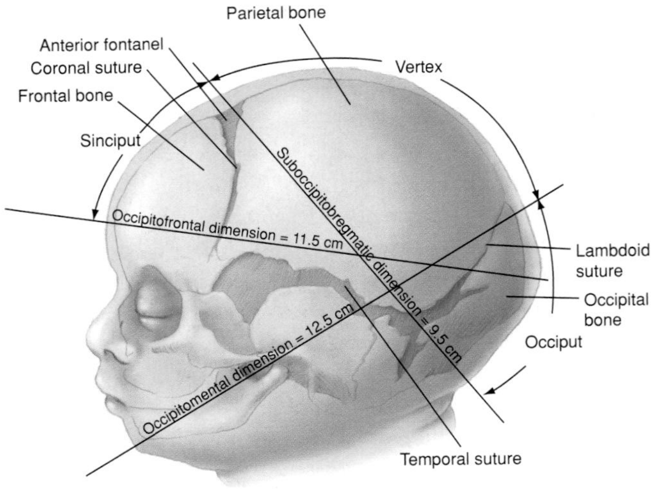

FIGURE 7-12

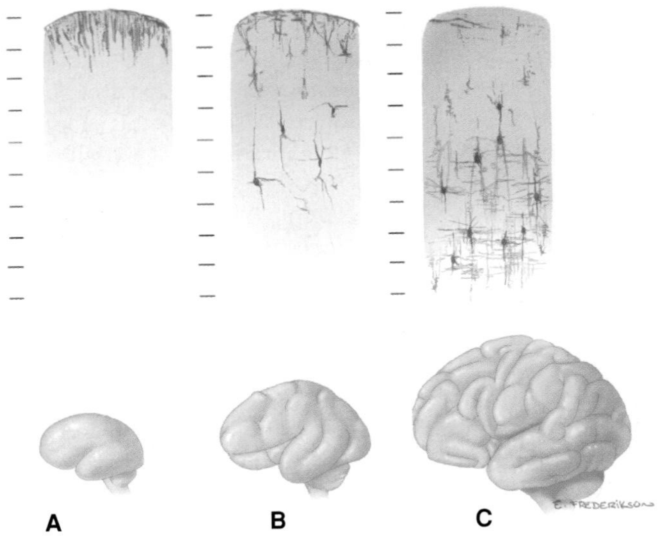

FIGURE 7-13 Neuronal proliferation and migration are complete at 20 to 24 weeks. During the second half of gestation, organizational events proceed with gyral formation and proliferation, differentiation, and migration of cellular elements. Approximate gestational ages are listed. **A.** 20 weeks. **B.** 35 weeks. **C.** 40 weeks.

It is customary to measure certain critical diameters and circumferences of the newborn head (Fig. 7-12). These include:

1. The occipitofrontal (11.5 cm), which follows a line extending from a point just above the root of the nose to the most prominent portion of the occipital bone.
2. The biparietal (9.5 cm), the greatest transverse diameter of the head, which extends from one parietal boss to the other.
3. The bitemporal (8.0 cm), which is the greatest distance between the two temporal sutures.
4. The occipitomental (12.5 cm), which extends from the chin to the most prominent portion of the occiput.
5. The suboccipitobregmatic (9.5 cm), which follows a line drawn from the middle of the large fontanel to the undersurface of the occipital bone where it joins the neck.

The greatest circumference of the head, which corresponds to the plane of the occipitofrontal diameter, averages 34.5 cm, a size too large to fit through the pelvis. The smallest circumference, corresponding to the plane of the suboccipitobregmatic diameter, is 32 cm. The cranial bones are normally connected only by a thin fibrous tissue layer. This allows considerable shifting or sliding of each bone to accommodate the size and shape of the maternal pelvis. This process is termed molding. The head position and degree of skull ossification result in a spectrum of cranial plasticity. In some cases, this contributes to fetopelvic disproportion, a leading indication for cesarean delivery (Chap. 23, p. 463).

Central Nervous System and Spinal Cord

Brain Development

There is a steady gestational-age-related change in the fetal brain appearance so that it is possible to identify fetal age from its external appearance (Dolman, 1977). Neuronal proliferation and migration proceed along with gyral growth and maturation (Fig. 7-13). Sequential maturation studies have characterized the developing fetal brain imaged using magnetic resonance (MR) imaging (Fig. 10-41, p. 224). (Manganaro, 2007). Recent studies also using MR imaging have quantified development of subcortical brain structures from 12 to 22 weeks (Meng, 2012). Myelination of the ventral roots of the cerebrospinal nerves and brainstem begins at approximately 6 months, but most myelination occurs after birth. This lack of myelin and incomplete skull ossification permit fetal brain structure to be seen with sonography throughout gestation.

Spinal Cord and Sensory Organs

The spinal cord extends along the entire length of the vertebral column in the embryo, but after that it grows more slowly. By 24 weeks, the spinal cord extends to S1, at birth to L3, and in the adult to L1. Spinal cord myelination begins at midgestation and continues through the first year of life. Synaptic function is sufficiently developed by the eighth week to demonstrate flexion of the neck and trunk (Temiras, 1968). During the third trimester, integration of nervous and muscular function proceeds rapidly.

The internal, middle, and external components of the ear are well developed by midpregnancy (see Fig. 7-2).

Gastrointestinal System

Swallowing begins at 10 to 12 weeks, coincident with the ability of the small intestine to undergo peristalsis and transport glucose actively (Koldovsky, 1965; Miller, 1982). Much of the water in swallowed fluid is absorbed, and unabsorbed matter is propelled to the lower colon (Fig. 7-14). It is not clear what stimulates swallowing, but the fetal neural analogue of thirst, gastric emptying, and change in the amnionic fluid composition are potential factors (Boyle, 1992). The fetal taste buds may play a role because saccharin injected into amnionic fluid increases swallowing, whereas injection of a noxious chemical inhibits it (Liley, 1972).

Fetal swallowing appears to have little effect on amnionic fluid volume early in pregnancy because the volume swallowed is small compared with the total. Late in pregnancy, however, amnionic fluid regulation is substantially affected by fetal swallowing. For example, if swallowing is inhibited, hydramnios is common (Chap. 11, p. 233). Term fetuses swallow between

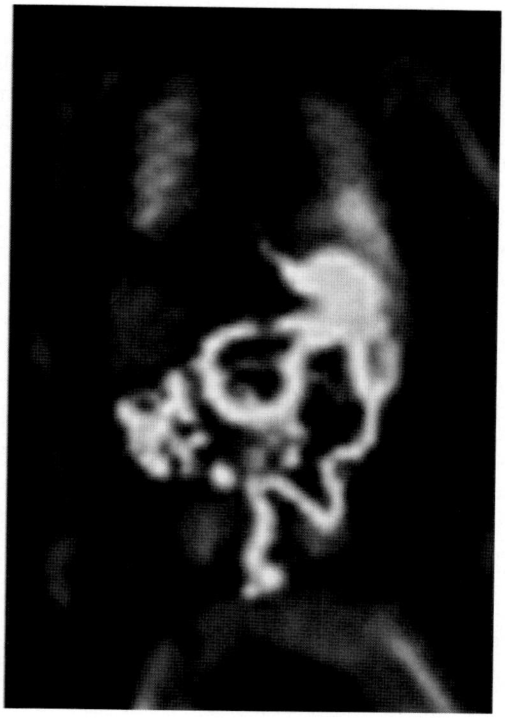

FIGURE 7-14 Radiograph of a 115-g fetus at about 16 weeks' gestational age showing radiopaque dye in the lungs, esophagus, stomach, and entire intestinal tract after injection into the amnionic cavity 26 hours before delivery. These reflect inhalation as well as active swallowing of amnionic fluid. (From Davis, 1946, with permission.)

200 and 760 mL per day—an amount comparable to that of the neonate (Pritchard, 1966).

Hydrochloric acid and some digestive enzymes are present in the stomach and small intestine in very small amounts in the early fetus. Intrinsic factor is detectable by 11 weeks, and pepsinogen by 16 weeks. The preterm neonate, depending on the gestational age when born, may have transient deficiencies of these enzymes (Lebenthal, 1983).

Stomach emptying appears to be stimulated primarily by volume. Movement of amnionic fluid through the gastrointestinal system may enhance growth and development of the alimentary canal. That said, other regulatory factors likely are involved because anencephalic fetuses, in whom swallowing is limited, often have normal amnionic fluid volumes and normal-appearing gastrointestinal tracts. Gitlin (1974) demonstrated that late in pregnancy, approximately 800 mg of soluble protein is ingested daily by the fetus.

Several anomalies can affect normal fetal gastrointestinal function. Hirschsprung disease—known also as congenital aganglionic megacolon, prevents the bowel from undergoing parasympathetic-mediated relaxation and thus from emptying normally (Watkins, 1992). It may be recognized prenatally by grossly enlarged bowel during sonography. Obstructions such as duodenal atresia, megacystis-microcolon syndrome, or imperforate anus can also prevent normal bowel emptying. Meconium ileus, commonly found with fetal cystic fibrosis, is bowel obstruction caused by thick, viscid meconium that blocks the distal ileum.

Meconium

Fetal bowel contents consist of various products of secretion, such as glycerophospholipids from the lung, desquamated fetal cells, lanugo, scalp hair, and vernix. It also contains undigested debris from swallowed amnionic fluid. The dark greenish-black is caused by pigments, especially biliverdin. Meconium can pass from normal bowel peristalsis in the mature fetus or from vagal stimulation. It can also pass when hypoxia stimulates arginine vasopressin (AVP) release from the fetal pituitary gland. AVP stimulates colonic smooth muscle to contract, resulting in intraamnionic defecation (DeVane, 1982; Rosenfeld, 1985).

Liver

Serum liver enzyme levels increase with gestational age. However, the fetal liver has a gestational-age-related diminished capacity for converting free unconjugated bilirubin to conjugated bilirubin (Chap. 33, p. 644). Because the life span of normal fetal macrocytic erythrocytes is shorter than that of adult erythrocytes, relatively more unconjugated bilirubin is produced. As noted, the fetal liver conjugates only a small fraction, and this is excreted into the intestine and ultimately oxidized to biliverdin. Most of the unconjugated bilirubin is excreted into the amnionic fluid after 12 weeks and transferred across the placenta (Bashore, 1969).

Importantly, placental transfer is bidirectional. Thus, a pregnant woman with severe hemolysis from any cause has excess unconjugated bilirubin that readily passes to the fetus and then into the amnionic fluid. Conversely, conjugated bilirubin is not exchanged to any significant degree between mother and fetus.

Most fetal cholesterol is from hepatic synthesis, which satisfies the large demand for LDL cholesterol by the fetal adrenal glands. Hepatic glycogen is present in low concentration during the second trimester, but near term there is a rapid and marked increase to levels two to three times those in the adult liver. After birth, glycogen content falls precipitously.

Pancreas

Insulin-containing granules can be identified by 9 to 10 weeks, and insulin is detectable in fetal plasma at 12 weeks (Adam, 1969). The pancreas responds to hyperglycemia by secreting insulin (Obenshain, 1970). Glucagon has been identified in the fetal pancreas at 8 weeks. In the adult rhesus monkey, hypoglycemia and infused alanine cause an increase in maternal glucagon levels. Although, similar stimuli do not evoke a fetal response in the human, by 12 hours after birth, the newborn is capable of responding (Chez, 1975). At the same time, however, fetal pancreatic α cells do respond to L-dopa infusions (Epstein, 1977). Therefore, nonresponsiveness to hypoglycemia is likely the consequence of failure of glucagon release rather than inadequate production. This is consistent with developmental expression of pancreatic genes in the fetus (Mally, 1994).

Most pancreatic enzymes are present by 16 weeks. Trypsin, chymotrypsin, phospholipase A, and lipase are found in the 14-week fetus, and their concentrations increase with gestation (Werlin, 1992). Amylase has been identified in amnionic fluid at 14 weeks (Davis, 1986). The exocrine function of the fetal pancreas is limited. Physiologically important secretion occurs only after stimulation by a secretogogue such as acetylcholine, which is released locally after vagal stimulation (Werlin, 1992). Cholecystokinin normally is released only after protein ingestion and thus ordinarily would not be found in the fetus.

Urinary System

Two primitive urinary systems—the pronephros and the mesonephros—precede the development of the metanephros, which forms the final kidney (Chap. 3, p. 36). The pronephros has involuted by 2 weeks, and the mesonephros is producing urine at 5 weeks and degenerates by 11 to 12 weeks. Failure of these two structures either to form or to regress may result in anomalous urinary system development. Between 9 and 12 weeks, the ureteric bud and the nephrogenic blastema interact to produce the metanephros. The kidney and ureter develop from intermediate mesoderm. The bladder and urethra develop from the urogenital sinus. The bladder also develops in part from the allantois.

By week 14, the loop of Henle is functional and reabsorption occurs (Smith, 1992). New nephrons continue to be formed until 36 weeks. In preterm neonates, their formation continues after birth. Although the fetal kidneys produce urine, their ability to concentrate and modify the pH is limited even in the mature fetus. Fetal urine is hypotonic with respect to fetal plasma and has low electrolyte concentrations.

Renal vascular resistance is high, and the filtration fraction is low compared with values in later life (Smith, 1992). Fetal renal blood flow and thus urine production are controlled or influenced by the renin-angiotensin system, the sympathetic nervous system, prostaglandins, kallikrein, and atrial natriuretic peptide. The glomerular filtration rate increases with gestational age from less than 0.1 mL/min at 12 weeks to 0.3 mL/min at 20 weeks. In later gestation, the rate remains constant when corrected for fetal weight (Smith, 1992). Hemorrhage or hypoxia generally results in a decrease in renal blood flow, glomerular filtration rate, and urine output.

Urine usually is found in the bladder even in small fetuses. The fetal kidneys start producing urine at 12 weeks. By 18 weeks, they are producing 7 to 14 mL/day, and at term, this increases to 27 mL/hr or 650 mL/day (Wladimiroff, 1974). Maternally administered furosemide increases fetal urine formation, whereas uteroplacental insufficiency, fetal-growth restriction, and other types of fetal disorders decrease it. Obstruction of the urethra, bladder, ureters, or renal pelves can damage renal parenchyma and distort fetal anatomy. With urethral obstruction, the bladder may become sufficiently distended that it ruptures or dystocia results. Kidneys are not essential for survival in utero, but are important in the control of amnionic fluid composition and volume. Thus, abnormalities that cause chronic anuria are usually accompanied by oligohydramnios and pulmonary hypoplasia. Pathological correlates and prenatal therapy of urinary tract obstruction are discussed in Chapter 16 (p. 330).

Lung Development

Lung maturation and the biochemical indices of functional fetal lung maturity are of considerable interest to the obstetrician. Morphological or functional immaturity at birth leads to the development of the respiratory distress syndrome (Chap. 34, p. 653). A sufficient amount of surface-active materials—collectively referred to as surfactant—in the amnionic fluid is evidence of fetal lung maturity. As Liggins (1994) emphasized, however, the structural and morphological maturation of fetal lung also is extraordinarily important to proper lung function.

Anatomical Maturation

Like the branching of a tree, lung development proceeds along an established timetable that apparently cannot be hastened by antenatal or neonatal therapy. The limits of viability appear to be determined by the usual process of pulmonary growth. There are four essential lung development stages as described by Moore (2013). First, the pseudoglandular stage entails growth of the intrasegmental bronchial tree between 6 and 16 weeks. During this period, the lung looks microscopically like a gland. Second, during the canalicular stage, from 16 to 26 weeks, the bronchial cartilage plates extend peripherally. Each terminal bronchiole gives rise to several respiratory bronchioles, and each of these in turn divides into multiple saccular ducts. Next, the terminal sac stage begins at 26 weeks. During this stage, respiratory bronchioles give rise to primitive pulmonary alveoli—the terminal sacs. Last, the alveolar stage begins at 32 weeks, although the exact transition from the terminal sac stage is unclear. During the alveolar stage, the alveolar epithelial lining thins to improve gas exchange. Simultaneously, an extracellular matrix develops from proximal to distal lung segments until term. An extensive capillary network is built, the lymph system forms, and type II pneumonocytes begin to produce surfactant. At birth, only approximately 15 percent of the adult number of alveoli is present. Thus, the lung continues to grow, adding more alveoli for up to 8 years.

Various insults can upset this process, and their timing determines the sequelae. With fetal renal agenesis, for example, there is no amnionic fluid at the beginning of lung growth, and major defects occur in all three stages. A fetus with membrane rupture before 20 weeks and subsequent oligohydramnios usually exhibits nearly normal bronchial branching and cartilage development but has immature alveoli. Membrane rupture after 24 weeks may have little long-term effect on pulmonary structure.

Pulmonary Surfactant

After the first breath, the terminal sacs must remain expanded despite the pressure imparted by the tissue-to-air interface, and surfactant keeps them from collapsing. Surfactant is formed in type II pneumonocytes that line the alveoli. These cells are characterized by multivesicular bodies that produce the lamellar bodies in which surfactant is assembled. During late fetal life, at a time when the alveolus is characterized by a water-to-tissue interface, the intact lamellar bodies are secreted from the lung and swept into the amnionic fluid during respiration-like movements that are termed fetal breathing. At birth, with the first breath, an air-to-tissue interface is produced in the lung alveolus. Surfactant uncoils from the lamellar bodies, and it then spreads to line the alveolus to prevent alveolar collapse during expiration. Thus, it is the capacity for fetal lungs to produce surfactant, and not the actual laying down of this material in the lungs in utero, that establishes lung maturity.

Surfactant Composition. Gluck and associates (1967, 1970, 1972) and Hallman and coworkers (1976) found that approximately 90 percent of surfactant dry weight is lipid. Proteins account for the other 10 percent. Approximately 80 percent of the glycerophospholipids are phosphatidylcholines (lecithins). The principal active component of surfactant is a specific lecithin—dipalmitoylphosphatidylcholine (DPPC or PC)—which accounts for nearly 50 percent. Phosphatidylglycerol (PG) accounts for another 8 to 15 percent. Its precise role is unclear because newborns without phosphatidylglycerol usually do well. The other major constituent is phosphatidylinositol (PI). The relative contributions of each component are shown in Figure 7-15.

Surfactant Synthesis. Biosynthesis takes place in the type II pneumocytes. The apoproteins are produced in the endoplasmic reticulum, and the glycerophospholipids are synthesized by cooperative interactions of several cellular organelles. Phospholipid is the primary surface tension-lowering component of surfactant, whereas the apoproteins aid the forming and reforming of a surface film. The surface properties of the surfactant phospholipids are determined principally by the composition and degree of saturation of their long-chain fatty acids.

The major apoprotein is surfactant A (SP-A), which is a glycoprotein with a molecular weight of 28,000 to 35,000 Da (Whitsett, 1992). It is synthesized in the type II cells, and its content in amnionic fluid increases with gestational age and fetal lung maturity. SP-A may also play a role in the onset of parturition (Mendelson, 2005). Synthesis of SP-A is increased by treatment of fetal lung tissue with cyclic adenosine monophosphate (AMP) analogues, epidermal growth factors, and triiodothyronine. Increased apoprotein synthesis precedes surfactant glycerophospholipid synthesis.

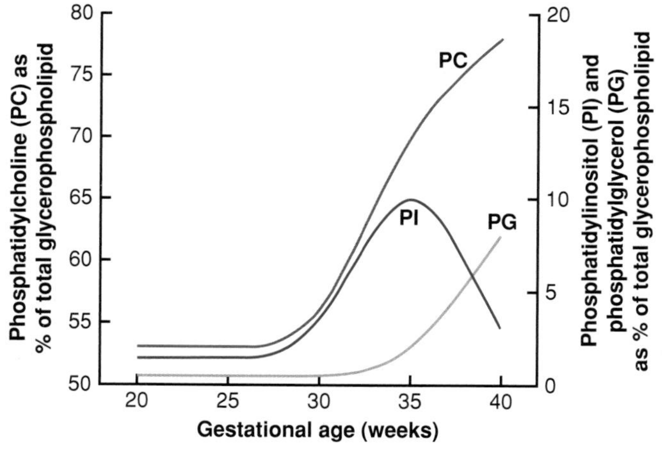

FIGURE 7-15 Relation between the levels of lecithin, or dipalmitoylphosphatidylcholine (PC), phosphatidylinositol (PI), and phosphatidylglycerol (PG) in amnionic fluid as a function of gestational age.

SP-A gene expression is demonstrable by 29 weeks (Snyder, 1988). There are two separate genes on chromosome 10. These are *SP-A1* and *SP-A2,* and their regulation is distinctive and different (McCormick, 1994). Specifically, cyclic AMP is more important in *SP-A2* expression, whereas dexamethasone decreases *SP-A2* expression.

Several smaller apoproteins such as SP-B and SP-C are likely important in optimizing the action of surfactant. For example, deletions in *SP-B* gene are incompatible with survival despite production of large amounts of surfactant.

Corticosteroids and Fetal Lung Maturation. Since Liggins (1969) first observed lung maturation in lamb fetuses given glucocorticosteroids before preterm delivery, many suggested that fetal cortisol stimulates lung maturation and surfactant synthesis. It is unlikely that corticosteroids are the only stimulus for augmented surfactant formation. There is evidence, however, that glucocorticosteroids administered at certain critical times during gestation improve fetal lung maturation. The use of betamethasone and dexamethasone to accelerate fetal lung maturity, as well as neonatal replacement surfactant therapy, is discussed in Chapter 34 (p. 653).

Breathing

Within a few minutes after birth, the respiratory system must provide oxygen as well as eliminate carbon dioxide. Respiratory muscles develop early, and fetal chest wall movements are detected by sonography as early as 11 weeks (Boddy, 1975). From the beginning of the fourth month, the fetus is capable of respiratory movement sufficiently intense to move amnionic fluid in and out of the respiratory tract.

Endocrine Gland Development

Pituitary Gland

The fetal endocrine system is functional for some time before the central nervous system reaches maturity (Mulchahey, 1987). The anterior pituitary gland develops from oral ectoderm—Rathke pouch, whereas the posterior pituitary gland derives from neuroectoderm.

Anterior and Intermediate Lobes. The adenohypophysis, or anterior pituitary, differentiates into five cell types that secrete six protein hormones: (1) lactotropes produce prolactin—PRL; (2) somatotropes produce growth hormone—GH; (3) corticotropes produce corticotropin—ACTH; (4) thyrotropes produce thyrotropin or thyroid-stimulating hormone—TSH; and (5) gonadotropes produce luteinizing hormone—LH and follicle-stimulating hormone—FSH.

ACTH is first detected in the fetal pituitary gland at 7 weeks, and GH and LH have been identified by 13 weeks. By the end of the 17th week, the fetal pituitary gland synthesizes and stores all pituitary hormones. Moreover, the fetal pituitary is responsive to hormones and is capable of secreting these early in gestation (Grumbach, 1974). The fetal pituitary secretes β-endorphin, and cord blood levels of β-endorphin and β-lipotropin increase with fetal P_{CO_2} (Browning, 1983).

There is a well-developed intermediate lobe in the fetal pituitary gland. The cells of this structure begin to disappear before term and are absent from the adult pituitary. The principal secretory products of the intermediate lobe cells are α-melanocyte–stimulating hormone (α-MSH) and β-endorphin.

Neurohypophysis. The posterior pituitary gland or neurohypophysis is well developed by 10 to 12 weeks, and oxytocin and arginine vasopressin (AVP) are demonstrable. Both hormones probably function in the fetus to conserve water by actions largely at the lung and placenta rather than kidney. AVP levels in umbilical cord plasma are strikingly higher than maternal levels (Chard, 1971; Polin, 1977). Elevated fetal blood AVP appears to be associated with fetal stress (DeVane, 1982).

Thyroid Gland

The pituitary–thyroid system is functional by the end of the first trimester. The thyroid gland is able to synthesize hormones by 10 to 12 weeks, and thyrotropin, thyroxine, and thyroxine-binding globulin (TBG) have been detected in fetal serum as early as 11 weeks (Ballabio, 1989). The placenta actively concentrates iodide on the fetal side, and by 12 weeks and throughout pregnancy, the fetal thyroid concentrates iodide more avidly than does the maternal thyroid. Thus, maternal administration of either radioiodide or appreciable amounts of ordinary iodide is hazardous after this time. Normal fetal levels of free thyroxine (T_4), free triiodothyronine (T_3), and thyroxine-binding globulin increase steadily throughout gestation (Ballabio, 1989). Compared with adult levels, by 36 weeks, fetal serum concentrations of TSH are higher, total and free T_3 concentrations are lower, and T_4 is similar. This suggests that the fetal pituitary may not become sensitive to feedback until late in pregnancy (Thorpe-Beeston, 1991; Wenstrom, 1990).

Fetal thyroid hormone plays a role in the normal development of virtually all fetal tissues, especially the brain. Its influence is illustrated by congenital hyperthyroidism, which occurs when maternal thyroid-stimulating antibody crosses the placenta to stimulate the fetal thyroid. These fetuses develop tachycardia, hepatosplenomegaly, hematological abnormalities, craniosynostosis, and growth restriction. As children, they have perceptual motor difficulties, hyperactivity, and reduced growth (Wenstrom, 1990). Neonatal effects of fetal thyroid deficiency are discussed in Chapter 58 (p. 1147).

The placenta prevents substantial passage of maternal thyroid hormones to the fetus by rapidly deiodinating maternal T_4 and T_3 to form reverse T_3, a relatively inactive thyroid hormone (Vulsma, 1989). Several antithyroid antibodies cross the placenta when present in high concentrations. Those include the long-acting thyroid stimulators (LATS), LATS-protector (LATS-P), and thyroid-stimulating immunoglobulin (TSI). It was previously believed that normal fetal growth and development, which occurred despite fetal hypothyroidism, provided evidence that T_4 was not essential for fetal growth. It is now known, however, that growth proceeds normally because small quantities of maternal T_4 prevent antenatal cretinism in fetuses with thyroid agenesis (Vulsma, 1989). The fetus with congenital hypothyroidism typically does not develop stigmata of cretinism until after birth. Because administration of thyroid hormone will prevent this, all newborns are tested for high serum levels of TSH (Chap. 32, p. 631).

Immediately after birth, there are major changes in thyroid function and metabolism. Cooling to room temperature evokes sudden and marked increase in TSH secretion. This in turn causes a progressive increase in serum T_4 levels that are maximal 24 to 36 hours after birth. There are nearly simultaneous elevations of serum T_3 levels.

Adrenal Glands

The fetal adrenal glands are much larger in relation to total body size than in adults. The bulk is made up of the inner or fetal zone of the adrenal cortex and involutes rapidly after birth. This zone is scant to absent in rare instances in which the fetal pituitary gland is congenitally absent. The function of the fetal adrenal glands is discussed in detail in Chapter 5 (p. 108).

DEVELOPMENT OF GENITALIA

Embryology of Uterus and Oviducts

The uterus and tubes arise from the müllerian ducts, which first appear near the upper pole of the urogenital ridge in the fifth week of embryonic development (Fig. 7-16). This ridge is composed of the mesonephros, gonad, and associated ducts. The first indication of müllerian duct development is a thickening of the coelomic epithelium at approximately the level of the fourth thoracic segment. This becomes the fimbriated extremity of the fallopian tube, which invaginates and grows caudally to form a slender tube at the lateral edge of the urogenital ridge. In the sixth week, the growing tips of the two müllerian ducts approach each other in the midline. One week later, they reach the urogenital sinus. At that time, the two müllerian ducts fuse to form a single canal at the level of the inguinal crest. This crest gives rise to the gubernaculum, which is the primordium of the round ligament.

Thus, the upper ends of the müllerian ducts produce the fallopian tubes, and the fused parts give rise to the uterus. The vaginal canal is not patent throughout its entire length until the sixth month (Koff, 1933). Because of the clinical importance of anomalies that arise from abnormal fusion and dysgenesis of these structures, their embryogenesis is discussed in detail in Chapter 3 (p. 37).

Embryology of the Ovaries

At approximately 4 weeks, gonads form on the ventral surface of the embryonic kidney at a site between the eighth thoracic and fourth lumbar segments. The coelomic epithelium thickens, and clumps of cells bud off into the underlying mesenchyme. This circumscribed area is called the *germinal epithelium*. By the fourth to sixth week, however, there are many large ameboid cells in this region that have migrated into the embryo body from the yolk sac (see Fig. 7-16). These primordial germ cells are distinguishable by their large size and certain morphological and cytochemical features.

When the primordial germ cells reach the genital area, some enter the germinal epithelium and others mingle with groups of cells that proliferate from it or lie in the mesenchyme. By the end of the fifth week, rapid division of all these

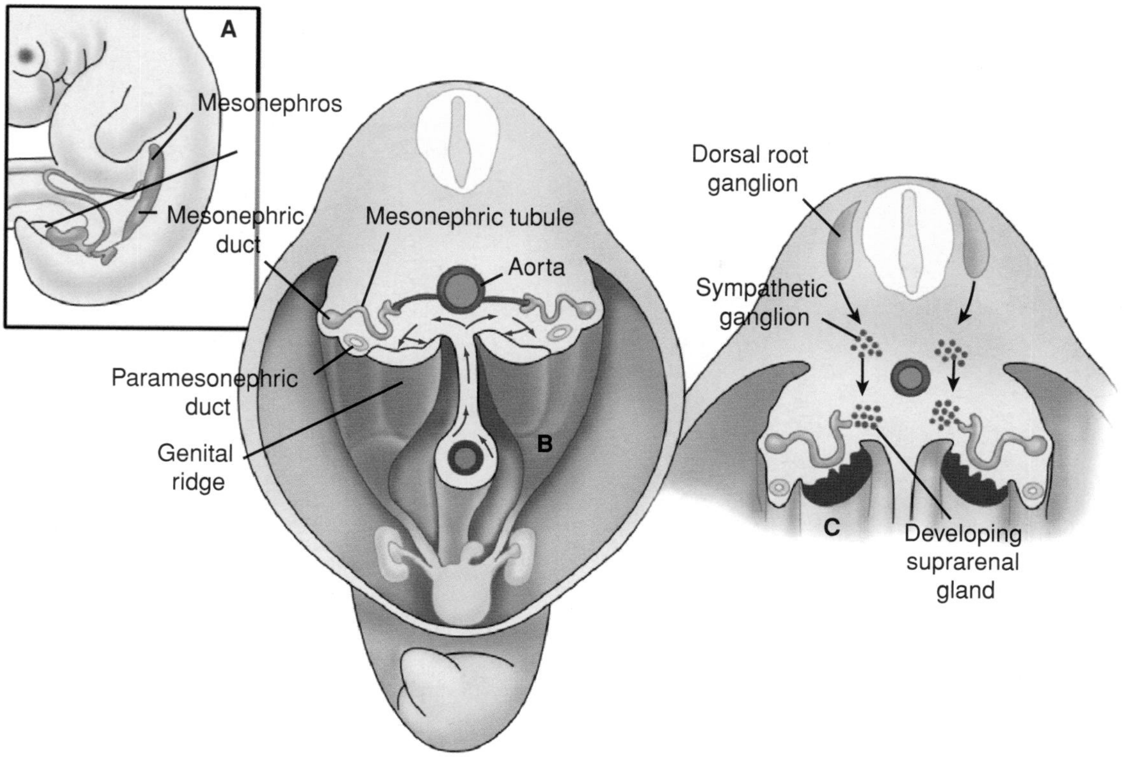

FIGURE 7-16 A. Cross section of an embryo at 4 to 6 weeks. **B.** Large ameboid primordial germ cells migrate (*arrows*) from the yolk sac to the area of germinal epithelium, within the genital ridge. **C.** Migration of sympathetic cells from the spinal ganglia to a region above the developing kidney. (Redrawn from Moore, 1988.)

cell types results in development of a prominent genital ridge. The ridge projects into the body cavity medially to a fold in which there are the mesonephric (wolffian) and paramesonephric (müllerian) ducts (Fig. 7-17). By the seventh week, this ridge is separated from the mesonephros except at the narrow central zone, the future hilum, where blood vessels enter. At this time, the sexes can be distinguished, because the testes can be recognized by well-defined radiating strands of cells termed sex cords. These cords are separated from the germinal epithelium by mesenchyme that is to become the tunica albuginea. The sex cords, which consist of large germ cells and smaller epithelioid cells derived from the germinal epithelium, develop into the seminiferous tubules and tubuli rete. The latter establishes connection with the mesonephric tubules that develop into the epididymis. The mesonephric ducts become the vas deferens.

In the female embryo, the germinal epithelium proliferates for a longer time. The groups of cells thus formed lie at first in the region of the hilum. As connective tissue develops between them, these appear as sex cords. These cords give rise to the medulla cords and persist for variable times (Forbes, 1942). By the third month, medulla and cortex are defined (see Fig. 7-17). The bulk of the ovary is made up of cortex, a mass of crowded germ and epithelioid cells that show some signs of grouping, but there are no distinct cords as in the testis. Strands of cells extend from the germinal epithelium into the cortical mass, and mitoses are numerous. The rapid succession of mitoses soon reduces germ-cell size to the extent that these no longer are differentiated clearly from the neighboring cells. These germ cells are now called oogonia.

By the fourth month, some germ cells in the medullary region begin to enlarge. These are called primary oocytes at the beginning of the growth phase that continues until maturity. During this cell growth period, many oocytes undergo degeneration, both before and after birth. A single layer of flattened follicular cells that were derived originally from the germinal epithelium soon surrounds the primary oocytes. These structures are now called primordial follicles and are seen first in the medulla and later in the cortex. Some follicles begin to grow even before birth, and some are believed to persist in the cortex almost unchanged until menopause.

By 8 months, the ovary has become a long, narrow, lobulated structure that is attached to the body wall along the line of the hilum by the mesovarium. The germinal epithelium has been separated for the most part from the cortex by a band of connective tissue—tunica albuginea. This band is absent in many small areas where strands of cells, usually referred to as cords of Pflüger, are in contact with the germinal epithelium. Among these cords are cells believed by many to be oogonia that resemble the other epithelial cells as a result of repeated mitosis. In the underlying cortex, there are two distinct zones. Superficially, there are nests of germ cells in meiotic synapsis, interspersed with Pflüger cords and strands of connective tissue. In the deeper zone, there are many groups of germ cells in synapsis, as well as primary oocytes, prospective follicular cells, and a few primordial follicles.

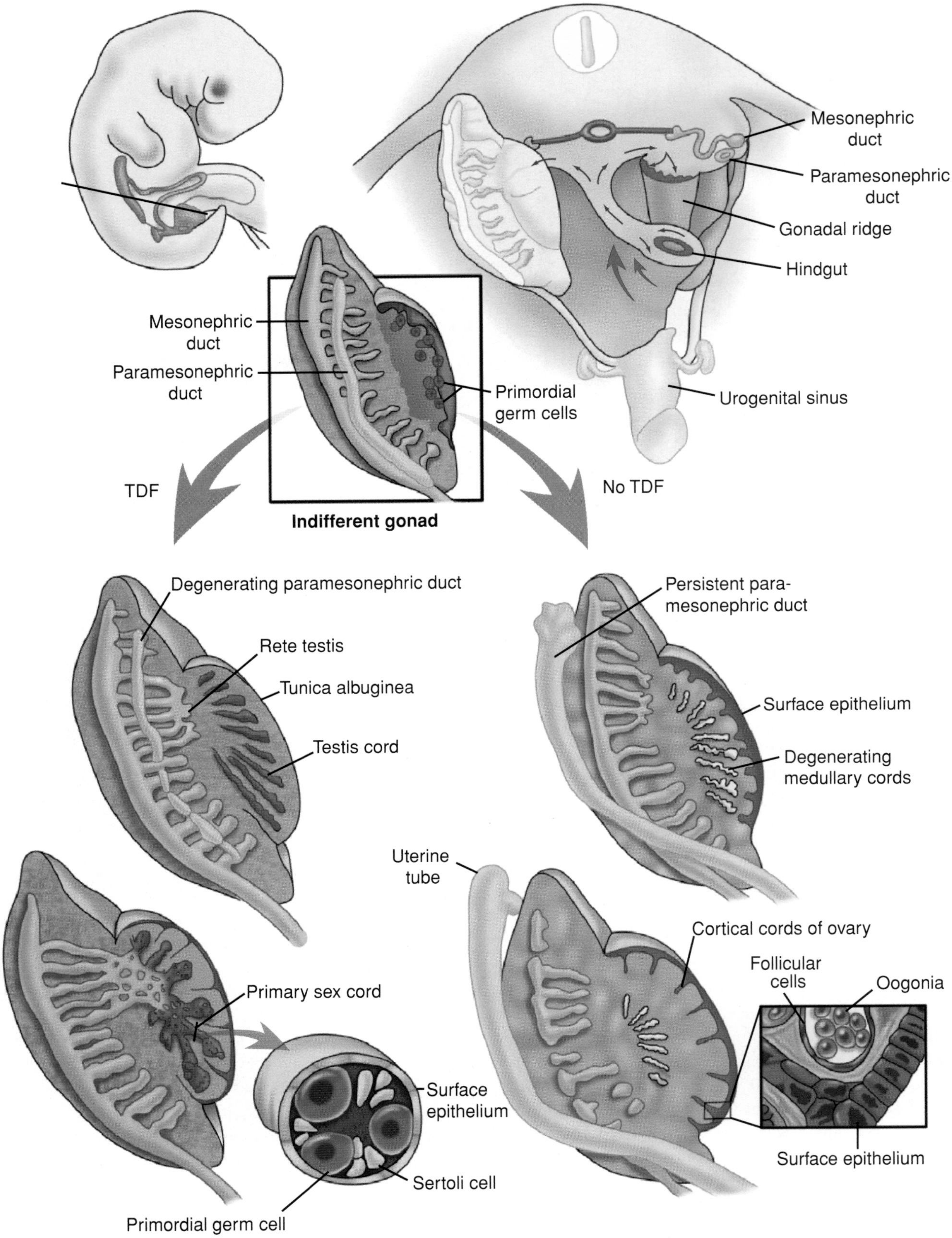

FIGURE 7-17 Continuation of embryonic sexual differentiation. TDF = testis-determining factor. (Redrawn from Moore, 1988.)

Fetal Gender

Theoretically, there should be a primary gender ratio of 1:1 at the time of fertilization because there are equal numbers of X- and Y-bearing spermatozoa. This is not the case, however, and many factors have been shown to contribute to gender ratios at conception. These include differential susceptibility to environmental exposures as well as medical disorders. Also, couples with a large age discrepancy are more likely to have a male offspring (Manning, 1997). Whatever the cause, it is impossible to determine the primary gender ratio because this would require gender assignment to zygotes that fail to cleave, blastocysts that fail to implant, and other early pregnancy losses.

The secondary gender ratio pertains to fetuses that reach viability and is usually held to be approximately 106 males to 100 females. The unbalanced secondary gender ratio is explicable by the loss of more female than male embryo-fetuses during early pregnancy. That said, Davis and colleagues (1998) report a significant decline in male births since 1950 in Denmark, Sweden, The Netherlands, the United States, Germany, Norway, and Finland. Similarly, Allan and associates (1997) reported that male births in Canada since 1970 dropped by 2.2 per 1000 live births.

Gender Assignment at Birth

In the delivery room, parents first want to know the gender of their newborn. If the external genitalia of the newborn are ambiguous, the obstetrician faces a profound dilemma. In these cases, assignment requires knowledge of the karyotypic sex, gonadal sex, hormonal milieu to which the fetus was exposed, exact anatomy, and all possibilities for surgical correction. In the past, newborns with a small or likely insufficient phallus were often assigned to the female gender. Based on what is now known of the role of fetal exposure to hormones in establishing gender preference and behavior, it can be seen why such a policy may have caused gender identity disorder (Slijper, 1998). Thus, it seems best to inform the parents that although their newborn appears healthy, the gender will need to be determined by a series of tests. To develop a plan that can assist in determining the cause of ambiguous genitalia, the mechanisms of normal and abnormal sexual differentiation must be considered.

Sexual Differentiation

Phenotypic gender differentiation is determined by the chromosomal complement acting in conjunction with gonadal development.

Chromosomal Gender

Genetic gender—XX or XY—is established at fertilization, but for the first 6 weeks, development of male and female embryos is morphologically indistinguishable. The differentiation of the primordial gonad into testis or ovary heralds the establishment of gonadal sex.

Gonadal Gender

As described earlier and shown in Figure 7-16, primordial germ cells that originate in the yolk sac endoderm migrate to the genital ridge to form the indifferent gonad. If a Y chromosome is present, at about 6 weeks after conception, the gonad begins developing into a testis (Simpson, 1997). Testis development is directed by a gene located on the short arm of Y—*testis-determining factor (TDF)*, also called sex-determining region (SRY). This gene encodes a transcription factor that acts to modulate the transcription rate of a number of genes involved in gonadal differentiation. The *SRY* gene is specific to the Y chromosome and is expressed in the human single-cell zygote upon ovum fertilization. It is not expressed in spermatozoa (Fiddler, 1995; Gustafson, 1994). In addition, testis development requires a *dose-dependent sex reversal (DDS)* region on the X chromosome, as well as other autosomal genes (Brown, 2005).

The contribution of chromosomal gender to gonadal gender is illustrated by several paradoxical conditions. The incidence of 46,XX phenotypic human males is estimated to be approximately 1 in 20,000 male births (Page, 1985). These infants apparently result from translocation of the Y chromosome fragment containing *TDF* to the X chromosome during meiosis of male germ cells (George, 1988). Similarly, individuals with XY chromosomes can appear phenotypically female if they carry a mutation in the *TDF/SRY* gene. There is evidence that genes on the short arm of the X chromosome are capable of suppressing testicular development, despite the presence of the *SRY* gene. Indeed, this accounts for a form of X-linked recessive gonadal dysgenesis.

The existence of autosomal sex-determining genes is supported by several genetic syndromes in which disruption of an autosomal gene causes, among other things, gonadal dysgenesis. For example, camptomelic dysplasia, localized to chromosome 17, is associated with XY phenotypic sex reversal. Similarly, male pseudohermaphroditism has been associated with a mutation in the Wilms tumor suppressor gene on chromosome 11.

Phenotypic Gender

Urogenital tract development in both sexes is indistinguishable before 8 weeks. Thereafter, development and differentiation of the internal and external genitalia to the male phenotype is dependent on testicular function. In the absence of a testis, female differentiation ensues irrespective of genetic gender. The fundamental experiments to determine the testis role in male sexual differentiation were conducted by the French anatomist Alfred Jost. Ultimately, he established that the induced phenotype is male and that secretions from the gonads are not necessary for female differentiation. Specifically, the fetal ovary is not required for female sexual differentiation. Jost and associates (1973) found that if castration of rabbit fetuses was conducted before differentiation of the genital anlagen, all newborns were phenotypic females with female external and internal genitalia. Thus, the müllerian ducts developed into uterus, fallopian tubes, and upper vagina.

If fetal castration was conducted before differentiation of the genital anlagen, and thereafter a testis was implanted on one side in place of the removed gonad, the phenotype of all fetuses was male. Thus, the external genitalia of such fetuses were masculinized. On the side of the testicular implant, the wolffian duct developed into the epididymis, vas deferens, and seminal vesicle. With castration, on the side without the implant, the müllerian duct developed but the wolffian duct did not.

Wilson and Gloyna (1970) and Wilson and Lasnitzki (1971) demonstrated that testosterone action was amplified by conversion to 5α-dihydrotestosterone (5α-DHT). In most androgen-responsive tissues, testosterone is converted by 5α-reductase to 5α-DHT. This hormone acts primarily and almost exclusively in the genital tubercle and labioscrotal folds.

Mechanisms of Gender Differentiation

Based on these observations, the physiological basis of gender differentiation can be summarized. Genetic gender is established at fertilization. Gonadal gender is determined primarily by factors encoded by genes on the Y chromosome, such as the *SRY* gene. In a manner not yet understood, differentiation of the primitive gonad into a testis is accomplished.

Fetal Testicles and Male Sexual Differentiation

The fetal testis secretes a proteinaceous substance called müllerian-inhibiting substance, a dimeric glycoprotein with a molecular weight of approximately 140,000 Da. It acts locally as a paracrine factor to cause müllerian duct regression. Thus, it prevents the development of uterus, fallopian tube, and upper vagina. Müllerian-inhibiting substance is produced by the Sertoli cells of the seminiferous tubules. Importantly, these tubules appear in fetal gonads before differentiation of Leydig cells, which are the cellular site of testosterone synthesis. Thus, müllerian-inhibiting substance is produced by Sertoli cells even before differentiation of the seminiferous tubules and is secreted as early as 7 weeks. Müllerian duct regression is completed by 9 to 10 weeks, which is before testosterone secretion has commenced. Because it acts locally near its site of formation, if a testis were absent on one side, the müllerian duct on that side would persist, and the uterus and fallopian tube would develop on that side. Female external genital differentiation is complete by 11 weeks, whereas male external genital differentiation is complete by 14 weeks (Sobel, 2004).

Fetal Testosterone Secretion

Apparently through stimulation initially by human chorionic gonadotropin (hCG), and later by fetal pituitary LH, the fetal testes secrete testosterone. This hormone acts directly on the wolffian duct to effect the development of the vas deferens, epididymis, and seminal vesicles. Testosterone also enters fetal blood and acts on the external genitalia anlagen. In these tissues, however, testosterone is converted to 5α-DHT to cause virilization of the external genitalia.

Genital Ambiguity of the Newborn

Ambiguity of the neonatal genitalia results from excessive androgen action in a fetus that was destined to be female or from inadequate androgen representation for one destined to be male. Rarely, genital ambiguity indicates true hermaphroditism. Several transcription factors—SOX9, SF1, and WT1, and disruptions of signaling molecules—hedgehog, WNT, cyclin-dependent kinase, and Ras/MAP kinase—cause disorders of sexual development. Examples are congenital adrenal hyperplasia and androgen insensitivity syndrome (Larson, 2012). Abnormalities of gender differentiation causing genital ambiguity can be assigned to one of four clinically defined categories: (1) female pseudohermaphroditism; (2) male pseudohermaphroditism; (3) dysgenetic gonads, including true hermaphroditism; and rarely (4) true hermaphroditism (Low, 2003).

Category 1: Female Pseudohermaphroditism

In this condition, müllerian-inhibiting substance is not produced. Androgen exposure is excessive, but variable, for a fetus genetically predestined to be female. The karyotype is 46,XX and ovaries are present. Therefore, by genetic and gonadal gender, all are predestined to be female, and the basic abnormality is androgen excess. Because müllerian-inhibiting substance is not produced, the uterus, fallopian tubes, and upper vagina develop.

If affected fetuses were exposed to a small amount of excess androgen reasonably late in fetal development, the only genital abnormality will be slight to modest clitoral hypertrophy, with an otherwise normal female phenotype.

With somewhat greater androgen exposure, clitoral hypertrophy will be more pronounced, and the posterior labia will fuse. If androgen levels increase earlier in embryonic development, then more severe virilization can be seen. This includes labioscrotal fold formation; development of a urogenital sinus, in which the vagina empties into the posterior urethra; and development of a penile urethra with scrotal formation—the empty scrotum syndrome (Fig. 7-18A).

Congenital Adrenal Hyperplasia. This is the most common cause of androgenic excess in fetuses with female pseudohermaphroditism. The hyperplastic glands synthesize defective enzymes that cause impaired cortisol synthesis. This leads to excessive pituitary ACTH stimulation of the fetal adrenal glands with secretion of large amounts of cortisol precursors, including androgenic prehormones. These prehormones, for example, androstenedione, are converted to testosterone in fetal extraadrenal tissues.

Mutations may involve any of several enzymes, but the most common are steroid 21-hydroxylase, 11β-hydroxylase, and 3β-hydroxysteroid dehydrogenase. Deficiency of the last prevents synthesis of virtually all steroid hormones. Deficiency of either 17β- or 11β-hydroxylase results in increased deoxycorticosterone production to cause hypertension and hypokalemic acidosis. These forms of congenital adrenal hyperplasia thus constitute medical emergencies in the newborn (Fritz, 2011). Currently, 21-hydroxylase deficiency can be diagnosed in utero through molecular fetal DNA analysis. Prenatal maternal dexamethasone administration has been used to reduce fetal genital virilization, however, this is controversial (Miller, 2013; New, 2012) This fetal therapy is discussed in Chapter 16 (p. 323).

Excessive Androgen from Maternal Sources. Transfer of androgen from the maternal compartment may arise from the ovaries with hyperreactio luteinalis or theca-lutein cysts or from Leydig cell and Sertoli-Leydig cell ovarian tumors (Chap. 63,

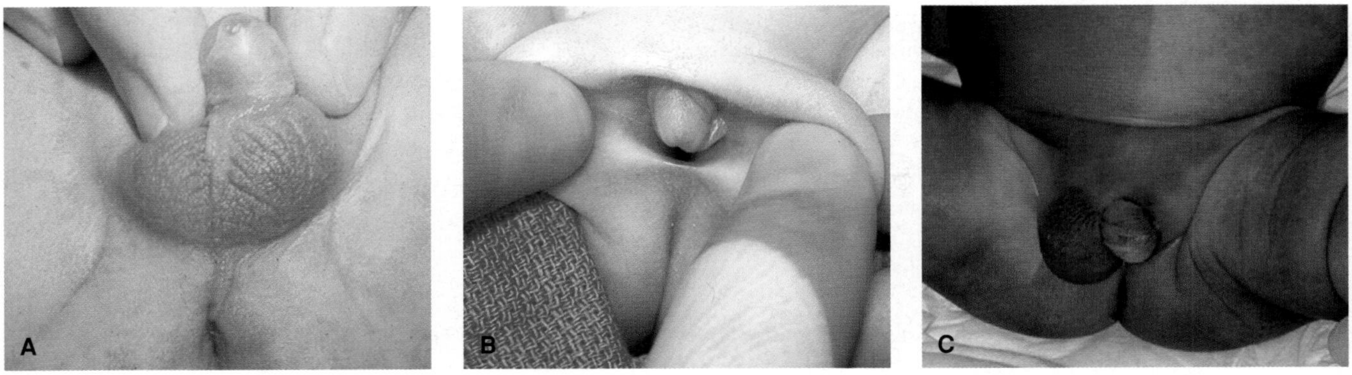

FIGURE 7-18 Ambiguous genitalia. **A.** Female pseudohermaphroditism caused by congenital adrenal hyperplasia. Infant was 46,XX and has severe virilization with scrotal formation without a testis and has a penile urethra. **B.** Male pseudohermaphroditism caused by incomplete androgen insensitivity syndrome. Infant is 46,XY with external genitalia demonstrating clitoral hypertrophy. **C.** True hermaphroditism in an infant with 46,XX/46,XY. A hemiscrotum is seen and there are different skin tones on each side. (Photographs contributed by Dr. Lisa Halvorson.)

p. 1228). In most of these conditions, the female fetus does not become virilized. This is because during most of pregnancy, the fetus is protected from excess maternal androgen by the extraordinary capacity of the syncytiotrophoblast to convert most C_{19}-steroids, including testosterone, to estradiol-17β. The only exception to this generalization is fetal aromatase deficiency, which produces both maternal and fetal virilization (Chap. 5, p. 110). Some drugs also can cause female fetal androgen excess. Most commonly, the drugs implicated are synthetic progestins or anabolic steroids (Chap. 12, p. 249). Importantly, except those with aromatase deficiency, all with female pseudohermaphroditism can be normal, fertile women if the proper diagnosis is made and appropriate and timely treatment initiated.

Category 2: Male Pseudohermaphroditism

This is characterized by incomplete and variable androgenic exposure of a fetus predestined to be male. The karyotype is 46,XY, and there are either testes or no gonads. In some cases, incomplete masculinization follows inadequate production of testosterone by the fetal testis. It also may arise from diminished responsiveness of the genital anlage to normal quantities of androgen—including failure of the in situ formation of 5α-DHT in androgen-responsive tissue. Because testes were present for at least some time in embryonic life, müllerian-inhibiting substance is produced. Thus, the uterus, fallopian tubes, and upper vagina do not develop.

Fetal testicular testosterone production may fail if there is an enzymatic defect of steroidogenesis that involves any one of four enzymes in the biosynthetic pathway for testosterone synthesis. Impaired fetal testicular steroidogenesis can also be caused by an abnormality in the LH-hCG receptor and by Leydig cell hypoplasia.

With embryonic testicular regression, the testes regress during embryonic or fetal life, and there is no testosterone production thereafter (Edman, 1977). This results in a phenotypic spectrum that varies from a normal female with absent uterus, fallopian tubes, and upper vagina, to a normal male phenotype with anorchia.

Androgen resistance or deficiencies in androgen responsiveness are caused by an abnormal or absent androgen receptor protein or by enzymatic failure of conversion of testosterone to 5α-DHT in appropriate tissues (Wilson, 1978).

Androgen Insensitivity Syndrome. Formerly called testicular feminization, this is the most extreme form of the androgen resistance syndrome, and there is no tissue responsiveness to androgen. More than 800 mutations that cause this syndrome have been reported in the androgen receptor, which is an eight-exon gene on the long arm of the X chromosome (Hughes, 2012; The Lady Davis Institute for Medical Research, 2013).

These result in a female phenotype with a short, blind-ending vagina, no uterus or fallopian tubes, and no wolffian duct structures. At the expected time of puberty, testosterone levels in affected individuals increase to values for normal men. Nonetheless, virilization does not occur, and even pubic and axillary hair does not develop because of end-organ resistance. Presumably, because of androgen resistance at the level of the brain and pituitary, LH levels also are elevated. In response to high concentrations of LH, there is increased testicular secretion of estradiol-17β compared with that in normal men (MacDonald, 1979). Increased estrogen secretion and absence of androgen responsiveness act in concert to cause feminization in the form of breast development.

Individuals with incomplete androgen insensitivity are slightly responsive to androgen. They usually have modest clitoral hypertrophy at birth (see Fig. 7-18B). And at the expected time of puberty, pubic and axillary hair develops but virilization does not occur. These patients also develop feminine breasts, presumably through the same endocrine mechanisms as in those with the complete form of the disorder (Madden, 1975). Insensitivity may also be due to germline missense mutations in the X-linked androgen-receptor gene in the highly structured DNA and ligand binding domains (Lagarde, 2012).

Another group has been referred to as familial male pseudohermaphroditism, type I (Walsh, 1974). Also commonly referred to as Reifenstein syndrome, it constitutes a spectrum of incomplete genital virilization. Phenotypes can vary from a phenotype similar to that of individuals with incomplete androgen insensitivity to that of a male phenotype with only a bifid scrotum, infertility, and gynecomastia.

The gene encoding the androgen-receptor protein is located on the X chromosome. More than 100 different mutations have been demonstrated. This accounts for the wide variability in androgen responsiveness among persons in whom the androgen-receptor protein is absent or abnormal and for the many different mutations associated with one disorder (McPhaul, 1991; Patterson, 1994).

An alternate form of androgen resistance is caused by 5α-reductase deficiency in androgen-responsive tissues. Because androgen action in the external genitalia anlagen is mediated by 5α-DHT, persons with this enzyme deficiency have external genitalia that are female but with modest clitoral hypertrophy. But because androgen action in the wolffian duct is mediated directly by testosterone, there are well-developed epididymides, seminal vesicles, and vas deferens, and the male ejaculatory ducts empty into the vagina (Walsh, 1974).

Category 3: Dysgenetic Gonads

In affected individuals, karyotype varies and is commonly abnormal. As the name describes, most have abnormally developed gonads, and streak gonads are typically found. As a result, müllerian-inhibiting substance is not produced and fetal androgen exposure is variable. The uterus, fallopian tubes, and upper vagina are present.

The most common form of gonadal dysgenesis is Turner syndrome (46,X). The phenotype is female, but secondary gender characteristics do not develop at the time of expected puberty, and genital infantilism persists. In some persons with dysgenetic gonads, the genitalia are ambiguous, a finding indicating that an abnormal gonad produced androgen, albeit in small amounts, during embryonic and fetal life. Generally, there is mixed gonadal dysgenesis—one example is a dysgenetic gonad on one side and an abnormal testis or dysontogenetic tumor on the other. Recombinant human growth hormone (hGH) is approved by the Food and Drug Administration for treatment of short stature in Turner syndrome (Chacko, 2012).

Category 4: True Hermaphroditism

In most cases, the guidelines for category 3 are met. External genitalia of such a case are shown in Figure 7-18C. In addition, true hermaphrodites have both ovarian and testicular tissues with germ cells for both ova and sperm in the abnormal gonads.

Preliminary Diagnosis of the Cause of Genital Ambiguity

A preliminary diagnosis of genital ambiguity can be made at the birth of an affected child. By history, during physical and sonographic examination of the newborn, an experienced examiner can ascertain a number of important findings. These include gonad location, phallus length and diameter, urethral meatus position, degree of labioscrotal fold fusion, and identification of a vagina, vaginal pouch, or urogenital sinus (Fritz, 2011). If the uterus is present, the diagnosis must be female pseudohermaphroditism, testicular or gonadal dysgenesis, or true hermaphroditism. A family history of congenital adrenal hyperplasia is helpful. If the uterus is not present, the diagnosis is male pseudohermaphroditism. Androgen resistance and enzymatic defects in testicular testosterone biosynthesis are often familial.

REFERENCES

Adam PAJ, Teramo K, Raiha N, et al: Human fetal insulin metabolism early in gestation: response to acute elevation of the fetal glucose concentration and placental transfer of human insulin-I-131. Diabetes 18:409, 1969

Adinolfi M: Human complement: onset and site of synthesis during fetal life. Am J Dis Child 131:1015, 1977

Adzick NS, Harrison MR, Glick PL, et al: Experimental pulmonary hypoplasia and oligohydramnios: relative contributions of lung fluid and fetal breathing movements. J Pediatr Surg 19:658, 1984

Aherne W, Dunnill MS: Morphometry of the human placenta. Br Med Bull 22:1, 1966

Alcorn D, Adamson TM, Lambert TF, et al: Morphological effects of chronic tracheal ligation and drainage in the fetal lamb lung. J Anat 3:649, 1977

Allan BB, Brant R, Seidel JE, et al: Declining sex ratios in Canada. Can Med Assoc J 156:37, 1997

Ballabio M, Nicolini U, Jowett T, et al: Maturation of thyroid function in normal human foetuses. Clin Endocrinol 31:565, 1989

Bashore RA, Smith F, Schenker S: Placental transfer and disposition of bilirubin in the pregnant monkey. Am J Obstet Gynecol 103:950, 1969

Bloch EM, Reed WF, Lee TH, et al: Male microchimerism in peripheral blood leukocytes from women with multiple sclerosis. Chimerism 2(1):6, 2011

Boddy K, Dawes GS: Fetal breathing. Br Med Bull 31:3, 1975

Boyle JT: Motility of the upper gastrointestinal tract in the fetus and neonate. In Polin RA, Fox WW (eds): Fetal and Neonatal Physiology. Philadelphia, Saunders, 1992, p 1028

Boyon C, Collinet P, Bovlanger L, et al: Is fetal microchimerism beneficial for the fetus or the mother. Gynecol Obstet Fertil 39(4):224, 2011

Bozzetti P, Ferrari MM, Marconi AM, et al: The relationship of maternal and fetal glucose concentrations in the human from midgestation until term. Metabolism 37:358, 1988

Brace RA, Wolf EJ: Normal amniotic fluid volume changes throughout pregnancy. Am Obstet Gynecol 161:382, 1989

Brown J, Warne G: Practical management of the intersex infant. J Pediatr Endocrinol Metab 18:3, 2005

Browning AJF, Butt WR, Lynch SS, et al: Maternal plasma concentrations of β-lipotropin, β-endorphin and α-lipotropin throughout pregnancy. Br J Obstet Gynaecol 90:1147, 1983

Carter AM: Evolution of factors affecting placental oxygen transfer. Placenta 30(Suppl A):19, 2009

Chacko E, Graber E, Regelmann MO: Update on Turner and Noonan syndromes. Endocrinol Metab Clin North Am 41(4):713, 2012

Chard T, Hudson CN, Edwards CRW, et al: Release of oxytocin and vasopressin by the human foetus during labour. Nature 234:352, 1971

Chez RA, Mintz DH, Reynolds WA, et al: Maternal-fetal plasma glucose relationships in late monkey pregnancy. Am J Obstet Gynecol 121:938, 1975

Christensen RD, Henry E, Antonio DV: Thrombocytosis and thrombocytopenia in the NICU: incidence, mechanisms and treatments. J Matern Fetal Neonat Med 25(54):15, 2012

Clymann RI, Heymann MA: Pharmacology of the ductus arteriosus. Pediatr Clin North Am 28:77, 1981

Corrigan JJ Jr: Normal hemostasis in the fetus and newborn: Coagulation. In Polin RA, Fox WW (eds): Fetal and Neonatal Physiology. Philadelphia, Saunders, 1992, p 1368

Davis DL, Gottlieb MB, Stampnitzky JR: Reduced ratio of male to female births in several industrial countries: a sentinel health indicator? JAMA 279:1018, 1998

Davis ME, Potter EL: Intrauterine respiration of the human fetus. JAMA 131:1194, 1946

Davis MM, Hodes ME, Munsick RA, et al: Pancreatic amylase expression in human pancreatic development. Hybridoma 5:137, 1986

Dawes GS: The umbilical circulation. Am J Obstet Gynecol 84:1634, 1962

DeVane GW, Naden RP, Porter JC, et al: Mechanism of arginine vasopressin release in the sheep fetus. Pediatr Res 16:504, 1982

De Verdier CH, Garby L: Low binding of 2,3-diphosphoglycerate to hemoglobin F. Scand J Clin Lab Invest 23:149, 1969

DiPietro JA: Neurobehavioral assessment before birth. MRDD Res Rev 11:4, 2005

Dolman CL: Characteristic configuration of fetal brains from 22 to 40 weeks gestation at two week intervals. Arch Pathol Lab Med 101:193, 1977

Dube E, Gravel A, Martin C, et al: Modulation of fatty acid transport and metabolism by maternal obesity in the human full-term placenta. Biol Reprod 87(1):14, 2012

Edman CD, Winters AJ, Porter JC, et al: Embryonic testicular regression. A clinical spectrum of XY agonadal individual. Obstet Gynecol 49:208, 1977

Epstein M, Chez RA, Oakes GK, et al: Fetal pancreatic glucagon responses in glucose-intolerant nonhuman primate pregnancy. Am J Obstet Gynecol 127:268, 1977

Fiddler M, Abdel-Rahman B, Rappolee DA, et al: Expression of SRY transcripts in preimplantation human embryos. Am J Med Genet 55:80, 1995

Foley ME, Isherwood DM, McNicol GP: Viscosity, hematocrit, fibrinogen and plasma proteins in maternal and cord blood. Br J Obstet Gynaecol 85:500, 1978

Forbes K, Westwood M: Maternal growth factor regulation of human placental development and fetal growth. J Endocrinol 207(1):1, 2010

Forbes TR: On the fate of the medullary cords of the human ovary. Contrib Embryol Carneg Inst 30:9, 1942

Fowden AL, Ward JW, Wooding FPB, et al: Programming placental nutrient transport capacity. J Physiol 572(1):5, 2006

Fritz MA, Speroff L (eds): Normal and abnormal sexual development. In: Clinical Gynecologic Endocrinology and Infertility, 8th ed. Philadelphia, Lippincott Williams & Wilkins, 2011, p 331, 382

Frolova AI, Moley KH: Quantitative analysis of glucose transporter mRNAs in endometrial stromal cells reveals critical role of GLUT1 in uterine receptivity. Endocrinology 152(5):2123, 2011

Fryer AA, Jones P, Strange R, et al: Plasma protein levels in normal human fetuses: 13–41 weeks' gestation. Br J Obstet Gynecol 100:850, 1993

Gao L, Lv C, Xu C, et al: Differential regulation of glucose transporters mediated by CRH receptor type 1 and type 2 in human placental trophoblasts. Endocrinology 153:1464, 2012

George FW, Wilson JD: Sex determination and differentiation. In Knobil E, Neill J (eds): The Physiology of Reproduction. New York, Raven, 1988, p 3

Gilbert WM, Brace RA: Amniotic fluid volume and normal flows to and from the amniotic cavity. Semin Perinatol 17:150, 1993

Gil-Sanchez A, Koletzko B, Larque E: Current understanding of placental fatty acid transport. Curr Opin Clin Nutr Metab Care 15(3):265, 2012

Gitlin D: Development and metabolism of the immune globulins. In Kaga BM, Stiehm ER (eds): Immunologic Incompetence. Chicago, Year Book, 1971

Gitlin D: Protein transport across the placenta and protein turnover between amnionic fluid, maternal and fetal circulation. In Moghissi KS, Hafez ESE (eds): The Placenta. Springfield, Thomas, 1974

Gitlin D, Kumate J, Morales C, et al: The turnover of amniotic fluid protein in the human conceptus. Am J Obstet Gynecol 113:632, 1972

Giudice LC, de-Zegher F, Gargosky SE, et al: Insulin-like growth factors and their binding proteins in the term and preterm human fetus and neonate with normal and extremes of intrauterine growth. J Clin Endocrinol Metab 80:1548, 1995

Gluck L, Kulovich MV, Eidelman AI, et al: Biochemical development of surface activity in mammalian lung. 4. Pulmonary lecithin synthesis in the human fetus and newborn and etiology of the respiratory distress syndrome. Pediatr Res 6:81, 1972

Gluck L, Landowne RA, Kulovich MV: Biochemical development of surface activity in mammalian lung. 3. Structural changes in lung lecithin during development of the rabbit fetus and newborn. Pediatr Res 4:352, 1970

Gluck L, Motoyama EK, Smits HL, et al: The biochemical development of surface activity in mammalian lung. 1. The surface-active phospholipids; the separation and distribution of surface-active lecithin in the lung of the developing rabbit fetus. Pediatr Res 1:237, 1967

Granado M, Fuente-Martín E, García-Cáceres C, et al: Leptin in early life: a key factor for the development of the adult metabolic profile. Obes Facts 5(1):138, 2012

Grisaru-Granovsky S, Samueloff A, Elstein D: The role of leptin in fetal growth: a short review from conception to delivery. Eur J Obstet Gynecol Reprod Biol 136(2):146, 2008

Gruenwald P: Growth of the human foetus. In McLaren A (ed): Advances in Reproductive Physiology. New York, Academic Press, 1967

Grumbach MM, Kaplan SL: Fetal pituitary hormones and the maturation of central nervous system regulation of anterior pituitary function. In Gluck L (ed): Modern Perinatal Medicine. Chicago, Year Book, 1974

Gustafson ML, Donahoe PK: Male sex determination: current concepts of male sexual differentiation. Annu Rev Med 45:505, 1994

Hallman M, Kulovich MV, Kirkpatrick E, et al: Phosphatidylinositol and phosphatidylglycerol in amniotic fluid: indices of lung maturity. Am J Obstet Gynecol 125:613, 1976

Hauguel-de Mouzon S, Lepercq J, Catalano P: The known and unknown of leptin in pregnancy. Am J Obstet Gynecol 193(6):1537, 2006

Hayward AR: The human fetus and newborn: development of the immune response. Birth Defects 19:289, 1983

Heimark R, Schwartz S: Cellular organization of blood vessels in development and disease. In Ryan U (ed): Endothelial Cells, Vol II. Boca Raton, CRC Press, 1988, p 103

Hellman P, Ridefelt P, Juhlin C, et al: Parathyroid-like regulation of parathyroid hormone related protein release and cytoplasmic calcium in cytotrophoblast cells of human placenta. Arch Biochem Biophys 293:174, 1992

Henriksson P, Hedner V, Nilsson IM, et al: Fibrin-stabilization factor XIII in the fetus and the newborn infant. Pediatr Res 8:789, 1974

Henson MC, Castracane VD: Leptin in pregnancy: an update. Biol Reprod 74(2):218, 2006

Hughes IA, Erner R, Bunch T: Androgen insensitivity syndrome. Semin Reprod Med 30(5):432, 2012

Ignjatovic V, Ilhan A, Monagle P: Evidence for age-related differences in human fibrinogen. Blood Coagul Fibrinolysis 22(2):110, 2011

Iyengar GV, Rapp A: Human placenta as a "dual" biomarker for monitoring fetal and maternal environment with special reference to potentially toxic trace elements. Part 3: Toxic trace elements in placenta and placenta as a biomarker for these elements. Sci Total Environ 280:221, 2001

Jansson T, Aye IL, Goberdhan DC: The emerging role of mTORC1 signaling in placental nutrient-sensing. Placenta 33(Suppl 2):e23, 2012

Jansson T, Cetin I, Powell TL, et al: Placental transport and metabolism in fetal overgrowth—a workshop report. Placenta 27:109, 2006a

Jansson T, Powell TL: Human placental transport in altered fetal growth: does the placenta function as a nutrient sensor? A review. Placenta 27:S91, 2006b

Jiang SS, Zhu XJ, Ding SD, et al: Expression and localization of aquaporins 8 and 9 in term placenta with oligohydramnios. Reprod Sci 19(12):1276, 2012

Jost A, Vigier B, Prepin J: Studies on sex differentiation in mammals. Recent Prog Horm Res 29:1, 1973

Kadic AS, Predojevic M: Fetal neurophysiology according to gestational age. Semin Fetal Neonatal Med 17(5):256, 2012

Kim ST, Romero R, Tarca AL: Methylome of fetal and maternal monocytes and macrophages at the feto-maternal interface. Am J Reprod Immunol 68(1):8, 2012

Kimura RE: Lipid metabolism in the fetal-placental unit. In Cowett RM (ed): Principles of Perinatal-Neonatal Metabolism. New York, Springer, 1991, p 291

Klagsbrun M: Angiogenesis factors. In Ryan U (ed): Endothelial Cells, Vol II. Boca Raton, CRC Press, 1988, p 37

Koff AK: Development of the vagina in the human fetus. Contr Embryol Carnegie Inst 24:59, 1933

Kohler PF: Maturation of the human complement system. J Clin Invest 52:671, 1973

Koldovsky O, Heringova A, Jirsova U, et al: Transport of glucose against a concentration gradient in everted sacs of jejunum and ileum of human fetuses. Gastroenterology 48:185, 1965

Kopp RS, Kumbartski M, Harth V, et al: Partition of metals in the maternal/fetal unit and lead-associated decreases of fetal iron and manganese: an observational biomonitoring approach. Arch Toxicol 86(10):1571, 2012

Korgun ET, Celik-Ozenci C, Seval Y, et al: Do glucose transporters have other roles in addition to placental glucose transport during early pregnancy? Histochem Cell Biol 123:621, 2005

Lagarde WH, Blackwelder AJ, Minges JT: Androgen receptor exon 1 mutation causes androgen insensitivity by creating phosphorylation site and inhibiting melanoma antigen-A11 activation of NH_2- and carboxyl-terminal interaction-dependent transactivation. J Biol Chem 287(14):10905, 2012

Larson A, Nokoff NJ, Travers S: Disorders of sex development: clinically relevant genes involved in gonadal differentiation. Discov Med 12(78)301, 2012

Lebenthal E, Lee PC: Interactions of determinants of the ontogeny of the gastrointestinal tract: a unified concept. Pediatr Res 1:19, 1983

Lee CK, Lee JT, Yu SJ, et al: Effects of cadmium on the expression of placental lactogens and Pit-1 genes in the rat placental trophoblast cells. Mol Cell Endocrinol 298(1–2):11, 2009

Lemons JA: Fetal placental nitrogen metabolism. Semin Perinatol 3:177, 1979

Leonce J, Brockton N, Robinson S, et al: Glucose production in the human placenta. Placenta 27:S103, 2006

Liggins GC: Fetal lung maturation. Aust N Z J Obstet Gynaecol 34:247, 1994

Liggins GC: Premature delivery of fetal lambs infused with glucocorticoids. J Endocrinol 45:515, 1969
Liley AW: Disorders of amniotic fluid. In Assali NS (ed): Pathophysiology of Gestation. New York, Academic Press, 1972
Lissauer D, Piper KP, Moss PA, et al: Persistence of fetal cells in the mother: friend or foe? BJOG 114:1321, 2007
Longo LD: Respiration in the fetal-placental unit. In Cowett RM (ed): Principles of Perinatal-Neonatal Metabolism. New York, Springer, 1991, p 304
Low Y, Hutson JM: Rules for clinical diagnosis in babies with ambiguous genitalia. J Paediatr Child Health 39:406, 2003
MacDonald PC, Madden JD, Brenner PF, et al: Origin of estrogen in normal men and in women with testicular feminization. J Clin Endocrinol Metab 49:905, 1979
Madden JD, Walsh PC, MacDonald PC, et al: Clinical and endocrinological characterization of a patient with syndrome of incomplete testicular feminization. J Clin Endocrinol 41:751, 1975
Mally MI, Otonkoski T, Lopez AD, et al: Developmental gene expression in the human fetal pancreas. Pediatr Res 36:537, 1994
Manganaro L, Perrone A, Savelli S, et al: Evaluation of normal brain development by prenatal MR imaging. Radiol Med 112:444, 2007
Manning JT, Anderton RH, Shutt M: Parental age gap skews child sex ratio. Nature 389:344, 1997
Maymó JL, Pérez Pérez A, Sánchez-Margalet V, et al: Up-regulation of placental leptin by human chorionic gonadotropin. Endocrinology 150(1):304, 2009
McCormick SM, Mendelson CR: Human SP-A1 and SP-A2 genes are differentially regulated during development and by cAMP and glucocorticoids. Am J Physiol 266:367, 1994
McPhaul MJ, Marcelli M, Tilley WD, et al: Androgen resistance caused by mutations in the androgen receptor gene. FASEB J 5:2910, 1991
Mendelson CR, Condon JC: New insights into the molecular endocrinology of parturition. J Steroid Biochem Mol Biol 93:113, 2005
Meng H, Zhang Z, Geng H, et al: Development of the subcortical brain structures in the second trimester: assessment with 7.0-T MRI. Neuroradiology 54(10):1153, 2012
Mercé LT, Barco MJ, Alcázar JL, et al: Intervillous and uteroplacental circulation in normal early pregnancy and early pregnancy loss assessed by 3-dimensional power Doppler angiography. Am J Obstet Gynecol 200(3):315.e1, 2009
Miller AJ: Deglutition. Physiol Rev 62:129, 1982
Miller WL, Witchel SF: Prenatal treatment of congenital adrenal hyperplasia: risks outweigh benefits. Am J Obstet Gynecol 208:354, 2013
Mohun TJ, Weninger WJ: Imaging heart development using high resolution episcopic microscopy. Curr Opin Genet Dev 21(5):573, 2011
Moore KL: The Developing Human: Clinically Oriented Embryology, 4th ed. Philadelphia, Saunders, 1988
Moore KL, Persaud TVN, Torchia MG: The Developing Human: Clinically Oriented Embryology, 9th ed. Philadelphia, Saunders, 2013, P 94
Morriss FH Jr, Boyd RDH, Manhendren D: Placental transport. In Knobil E, Neill J (eds): The Physiology of Reproduction, Vol II. New York, Raven, 1994, p 813
Mulchahey JJ, DiBlasio AM, Martin MC, et al: Hormone production and peptide regulation of the human fetal pituitary gland. Endocr Rev 8:406, 1987
New MO, Abraham M, Yuen T, et al: An update on prenatal diagnosis and treatment of congenital adrenal hyperplasia. Semin Reprod Med 30(5):396, 2012
Ney JA, Fee SC, Dooley SL, et al: Factors influencing hemostasis after umbilical vein puncture in vitro. Am J Obstet Gynecol 160:424, 1989
Nielsen NC: Coagulation and fibrinolysis in normal women immediately postpartum and in newborn infants. Acta Obstet Gynecol Scand 48:371, 1969
Novakovic B, Gordon L, Robinson WP, et al: Glucose as a fetal nutrient: dynamic regulation of several glucose transporter genes by DNA methylation in the human placenta across gestation. J Nutr Biochem 24(1):282, 2013
Obenshain SS, Adam PAJ, King KC, et al: Human fetal insulin response to sustained maternal hyperglycemia. N Engl J Med 283:566, 1970
Olausson H, Goldberg GR, Laskey A, et al: Calcium economy in human pregnancy and lactation. Nutr Res Rev 25(1):40, 2012
Olsen O, Clausen JA: Determination of the expected day of delivery—ultrasound has not been shown to be more accurate than the calendar method. Ugeskr Laeger 160:2088, 1998
Page DC, de la Chapelle A, Weissenbach J: Chromosome Y-specific DNA in related human XX males. Nature 315:224, 1985
Palmeira P, Quinello C, Silveira-Lessa AL, et al: IgG placental transfer in health and pathological pregnancies. Clin Dev Immunol 2012:985646, 2012
Pataryas HA, Stamatoyannopoulos G: Hemoglobins in human fetuses: evidence for adult hemoglobin production after the 11th gestational week. Blood 39:688, 1972
Patterson MN, McPhaul MJ, Hughes IA: Androgen insensitivity syndrome. Bailleres Clin Endocrinol Metab 8:379, 1994
Pearson HA: Recent advances in hematology. J Pediatr 69:466, 1966
Perrine SP, Greene MF, Cohen RA, et al: A physiological delay in human fetal hemoglobin switching is associated with specific globin DNA hypomethylation. FEBS Lett 228:139, 1988
Pipe NGJ, Smith T, Halliday D, et al: Changes in fat, fat-free mass and body water in human normal pregnancy. Br J Obstet Gynaecol 86:929, 1979
Polin RA, Husain MK, James LS, et al: High vasopressin concentrations in human umbilical cord blood—lack of correlation with stress. J Perinat Med 5:114, 1977
Pritchard JA: Fetal swallowing and amniotic fluid volume. Obstet Gynecol 28:606, 1966
Quan CP, Forestier F, Bouvet JP: Immunoglobulins of the human amniotic fluid. Am J Reprod Immunol 42:219, 1999
Ramsay, MM: Normal Values in Pregnancy. Ramsay MM, James DK, Steer PJ, et al (eds). London, Elsevier, 1996, p 106
Rosenfeld CR, Porter JC: Arginine vasopressin in the developing fetus. In Albrecht ED, Pepe GJ (eds): Research in Perinatal Medicine, Vol 4. Perinatal Endocrinology. Ithaca, Perinatology Press, 1985, p 91
Sakata M, Kurachi H, Imai T, et al: Increase in human placental glucose transporter-1 during pregnancy. Eur J Endocrinol 132:206, 1995
Saracco P, Parodi E, Fabris C, et al: Management and investigation of neonatal thromboembolic events: genetic and acquired risk factors. Thromb Res 123(6):805, 2009
Schwartz R, Gruppuso PA, Petzold K, et al: Hyperinsulinemia and macrosomia in the fetus of the diabetic mother. Diabetes Care 17:640, 1994
Simpson JL: Diseases of the gonads, genital tract, and genitalia. In Rimoin DL, Connor JM, Pyeritz RE (eds): Emery and Rimoin's Principles and Practice of Medical Genetics, Vol I, 3rd ed. New York, Churchill Livingstone, 1997, p 1477
Sipes SL, Weiner CP, Wenstrom KD, et al: The association between fetal karyotype and mean corpuscular volume. Am J Obstet Gynecol 165:1371, 1991
Slijper FM, Drop SL, Molenaar JC, et al: Long-term psychological evaluation of intersex children. Arch Sex Behav 27:125, 1998
Smith CM II, Tukey DP, Krivit W, et al: Fetal red cells (FC) differ in elasticity, viscosity, and adhesion from adult red cells (AC). Pediatr Res 15:588, 1981
Smith FG, Nakamura KT, Segar JL, et al: Renal function in utero. In Polin RA, Fox WW (eds): Fetal and Neonatal Physiology, 2nd ed. Philadelphia, Saunders, 1992, p 1187
Snyder JM, Kwun JE, O'Brien JA, et al: The concentration of the 35 kDa surfactant apoprotein in amniotic fluid from normal and diabetic pregnancies. Pediatr Res 24:728, 1988
Sobel V, Zhu YS, Imerato-McGinley J: Fetal hormones and sexual differentiation. Obstet Gynecol Clin North Am 31:837, 2004
Stabile I, Nicolaides KH, Bach A, et al: Complement factors in fetal and maternal blood and amniotic fluid during the second trimester of normal pregnancy. Br J Obstet Gynaecol 95:281, 1988
Stockman JA III, deAlarcon PA: Hematopoiesis and granulopoiesis. In Polin RA, Fox WW (eds): Fetal and Neonatal Physiology. Philadelphia, Saunders, 1992, p 1327
Streeter GL: A human embryo (Mateer) of the presomite period. Contrib Embryol 9:389, 1920
Sunami R, Komuro M, Tagaya H, et al: Migration of microchimeric fetal cells into maternal circulation before placenta formation. Chimerism 1(2):66 2010
Teitel DF: Physiologic development of the cardiovascular system in the fetus. In Polin RA, Fox WW (eds): Fetal and Neonatal Physiology, Vol I. Philadelphia, Saunders, 1992, p 609
Temiras PS, Vernadakis A, Sherwood NM: Development and plasticity of the nervous system. In Assali NS (ed): Biology of Gestation, Vol VII. The Fetus and Neonate. New York, Academic Press, 1968
The Lady Davis Institute for Medical Research, Jewish General Hospital, McGill University: The Androgen Receptor Gene Mutations Database World Wide Web Server. 2013. Available at: http://androgendb.mcgill.ca./ Accessed April 18, 2013
Thompson MW, McInnes RR, Willard HF: The hemoglobinopathies: models of molecular disease. In Thompson MW, McInnes RR, Huntington FW (eds): Thompson and Thompson Genetics in Medicine, 5th ed. Philadelphia, Saunders, 1991, p 247
Thorpe-Beeston JG, Nicolaides KH, Felton CV, et al: Maturation of the secretion of thyroid hormone and thyroid-stimulating hormone in the fetus. N Engl J Med 324:532, 1991
Trompeter S, Roberts I: Haemoglobin F modulation in childhood sickle cell disease. Br J Haematol 144(3):308, 2009

Usher R, Shephard M, Lind J: The blood volume of the newborn infant and placental transfusion. Acta Paediatr 52:497, 1963
Vulsma T, Gons MH, De Vijlder JJM: Maternal-fetal transfer of thyroxine in congenital hypothyroidism due to a total organification defect or thyroid agenesis. N Engl J Med 321:13, 1989
Walker J, Turnbull EPN: Haemoglobin and red cells in the human foetus and their relation to the oxygen content of the blood in the vessels of the umbilical cord. Lancet 2:312, 1953
Walsh PC, Madden JD, Harrod MJ, et al: Familial incomplete male pseudohermaphroditism, type 2: decreased dihydrotestosterone formation in pseudovaginal perineoscrotal hypospadias. N Engl J Med 291:944, 1974
Watkins JB: Physiology of the gastrointestinal tract in the fetus and neonate. In Polin RA, Fox WW (eds): Fetal and Neonatal Physiology. Philadelphia, Saunders, 1992, p 1015
Weiner CP, Sipes SL, Wenstrom K: The effect of fetal age upon normal fetal laboratory values and venous pressure. Obstet Gynecol 79:713, 1992
Wenstrom KD, Weiner CP, Williamson RA, et al: Prenatal diagnosis of fetal hyperthyroidism using funipuncture. Obstet Gynecol 76:513, 1990
Werlin SL: Exocrine pancreas. In Polin RA, Fox WW (eds): Fetal and Neonatal Physiology. Philadelphia, Saunders, 1992, p 1047
Werth B, Tsiaras A: From Conception to Birth: A Life Unfolds. New York, Doubleday, 2002
Whitsett JA: Composition of pulmonary surfactant lipids and proteins. In Polin RA, Fox WW (eds): Fetal and Neonatal Physiology. Philadelphia, Saunders, 1992, p 941
Williams AH, Liu N, vanRooij E, et al: MicroRNA Control of muscle development and disease. Curr Opin Cell Biol 21(3):461, 2009
Wilson JD, Gloyna RE: The intranuclear metabolism of testosterone in the accessory organs of reproduction. Recent Prog Horm Res 26:309, 1970
Wilson JD, Lasnitzki I: Dihydrotestosterone formation in fetal tissues of the rabbit and rat. Endocrinology 89:659, 1971
Wilson JD, MacDonald PC: Male pseudohermaphroditism due to androgen resistance: testicular feminization and related syndromes. In Stanbury JB, Wyngaarden JD, Frederickson DS (eds): The Metabolic Basis of Inherited Disease. New York, McGraw-Hill, 1978
Wladimiroff JW, Campbell S: Fetal urine-production rates in normal and complicated pregnancy. Lancet 1:151, 1974
Zitnik G, Peterson K, Stamatoyannopoulos G, et al: Effects of butyrate and glucocorticoids on gamma- to beta-globin gene switching in somatic cell hybrids. Mol Cell Biol 15:790, 1995

SECTION 4

PRECONCEPTIONAL AND PRENATAL CARE

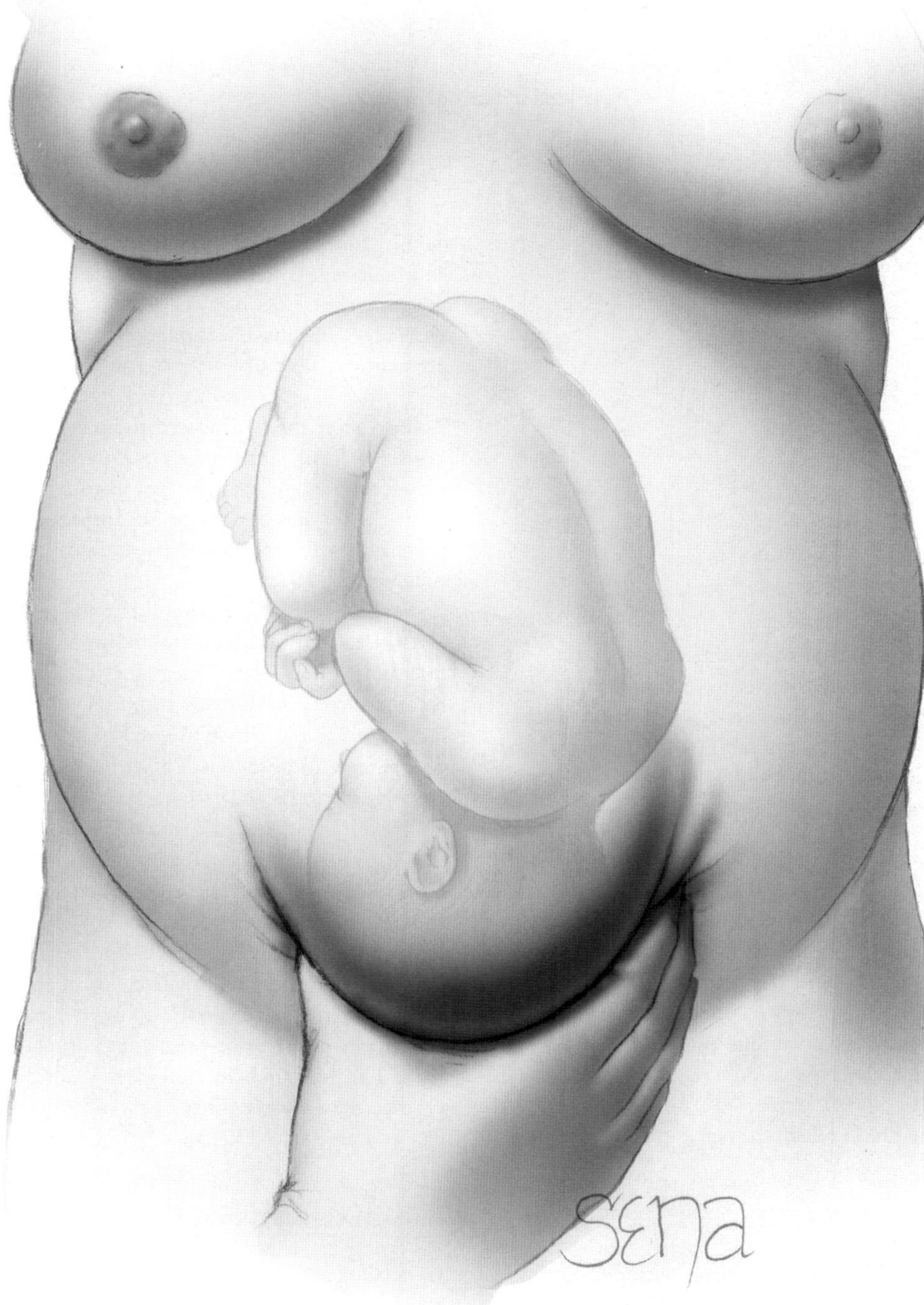

CHAPTER 8

Preconceptional Counseling

The Centers for Disease Control and Prevention defines preconceptional care as "a set of interventions that aim to identify and modify biomedical, behavioral, and social risks to a woman's health or pregnancy outcome through prevention and management" (Johnson, 2006). The following goals were established for advancing preconceptional care:

1. Improve knowledge, attitudes, and behaviors of men and women related to preconceptional health.
2. Assure that all women of childbearing age receive preconceptional care services—including evidence-based risk screening, health promotion, and interventions—that will enable them to enter pregnancy in optimal health.
3. Reduce risks indicated by a previous adverse pregnancy outcome through interconceptional interventions to prevent or minimize recurrent adverse outcomes.
4. Reduce the disparities in adverse pregnancy outcomes.

The American College of Obstetricians and Gynecologists (2012c) also has reaffirmed the importance of preconceptional and interpregnancy care.

To illustrate potentially modifiable conditions, data that describe the health status of women who gave birth to liveborn infants in the United States in 2004 are reviewed. Table 8-1 demonstrates the high prevalence of many conditions that may be amenable to intervention during the preconceptional and interpregnancy periods (D'Angelo, 2007). To be successful, however, preventative strategies that mitigate these potential pregnancy risks must be provided before conception. By the time most women realize they are pregnant—usually 1 to 2 weeks after the first missed period—the embryo has already begun to form. Thus, many prevention strategies—for example, folic acid to prevent neural-tube defects—will be ineffective if initiated at this time. Importantly, up to half of all pregnancies are unplanned, and often these are at greatest risk (Cheng, 2009).

Few randomized trials evaluate preconceptional counseling efficacy, in part because withholding such counseling would be unethical. Also, because pregnancy outcomes are dependent on the interaction of various maternal, fetal, and environmental factors, it is often difficult to ascribe salutary outcomes to a specific intervention (Moos, 2004). There are, however, prospective observational and case-control studies that demonstrate the successes of preconceptional counseling. Moos and coworkers (1996) assessed the effectiveness of a preconceptional counseling program administered during routine health care provision to reduce unintended pregnancies. The 456 counseled women had a 50-percent greater likelihood of subsequent pregnancies that they considered "intended" compared with 309 uncounseled women. Moreover, the counseled group had a 65-percent higher rate of intended pregnancy compared with women who had no health care before pregnancy. There are interesting ethical aspects of *paternal* lifestyle modification reviewed by van der Zee and associates (2013).

COUNSELING SESSION

Gynecologists, internists, family practitioners, and pediatricians have the best opportunity to provide preventive counseling during periodic health maintenance examinations. The

TABLE 8-1. Prevalence of Prepregnancy Maternal Behaviors, Experiences, Health Conditions, and Previous Poor Birth Outcomes in the United States in 2004

Factor	Prevalence (%)
Tobacco use	23
Alcohol use	50
Multivitamin use	35
Contraceptive nonuse[a]	53
Dental visit	78
Health counseling	30
Physical abuse	4
Stress	19
Underweight	13
Overweight	13
Obesity	22
Diabetes	2
Asthma	7
Hypertension	2
Heart problem	1
Anemia	10
Prior low-birthweight infant	12
Prior preterm infant	12

[a]Among women who were not trying to become pregnant.
Data from D'Angelo, 2007.

occasion of a negative pregnancy test is also an excellent time for education. Jack and colleagues (1995) administered a comprehensive preconceptional risk survey to 136 such women, and almost 95 percent reported at least one problem that could affect a future pregnancy. These included medical or reproductive problems—52 percent, family history of genetic disease—50 percent, increased risk of human immunodeficiency virus infection—30 percent, increased risk of hepatitis B and illegal substance abuse—25 percent, alcohol use—17 percent, and nutritional risks—54 percent. Counselors should be knowledgeable regarding relevant medical diseases, prior surgery, reproductive disorders, or genetic conditions and must be able to interpret data and recommendations provided by other specialists. If the practitioner is uncomfortable providing guidance, the woman or couple should be referred to an appropriate counselor.

Women presenting specifically for preconceptional evaluation should be advised that information collection may be time consuming depending on the number and complexity of factors that require assessment. The intake evaluation includes a thorough review of the medical, obstetrical, social, and family histories. Useful information is more likely to be obtained by asking specific questions regarding each history and each family member than by asking general, open-ended questions. Some important information can be obtained by questionnaires that address these topics. Answers are reviewed with the couple to ensure appropriate follow-up, including obtaining relevant medical records.

MEDICAL HISTORY

With specific medical conditions, general points include how pregnancy will affect maternal health and how a high-risk condition might affect the fetus. Afterward, advice for improving outcome is provided. Detailed preconceptional information regarding a few conditions is found in the next sections as well as in the other topic-specific chapters of this text.

Diabetes Mellitus

Because maternal and fetal pathology associated with hyperglycemia is well known, diabetes is the prototype of a condition for which preconceptional counseling is beneficial. Diabetes-associated risks to both mother and fetus are discussed in detail in Chapter 57 (p. 1125). Many of these complications can be avoided if glucose control is optimized before conception. The American College of Obstetricians and Gynecologists (2012b) has concluded that preconceptional counseling for women with pregestational diabetes is both beneficial and cost-effective and should be encouraged. The American Diabetes Association has promulgated consensus recommendations for preconceptional care for diabetic women (Kitzmiller, 2008). These guidelines advise that a thorough inventory of disease duration and related complications be obtained and clinical and laboratory examination for end-organ damage be completed. Perhaps most importantly, they encourage a preconceptional goal of the lowest hemoglobin A_{1c} level possible without undue hypoglycemic risk to the mother. In addition to assessing diabetic control during the preceding 6 weeks, hemoglobin A_{1c} measurement can also be used to compute risks for major anomalies (Fig. 8-1). Although these data are from women with severe overt diabetes, the incidence of fetal anomalies in women who have gestational diabetes with fasting hyperglycemia is increased fourfold compared with that in normal women (Sheffield, 2002).

Such counseling has been shown to be effective. In one review, Leguizamón and associates (2007) identified 12 studies that included more than 3200 pregnancies in women with insulin-dependent diabetes. Of the 1618 women without preconceptional counseling, 8.3 percent had a fetus with a

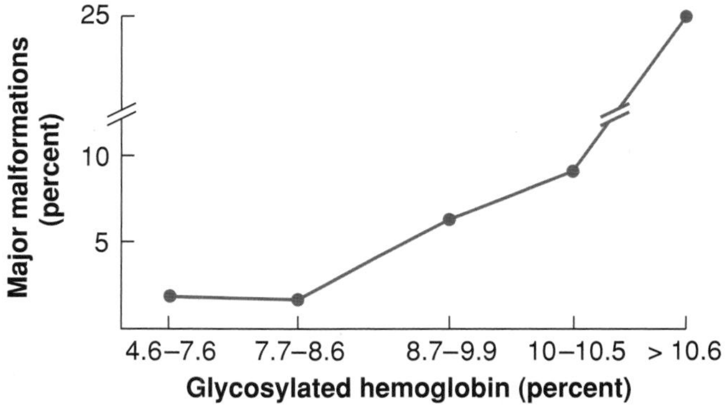

FIGURE 8-1 Relationship between first-trimester glycosylated hemoglobin values and risk for major congenital malformations in 320 women with insulin-dependent diabetes. (Data from Kitzmiller, 1991.)

major congenital anomaly, and this compared with a rate of 2.7 percent in the 1599 women who did have counseling. Tripathi and coworkers (2010) compared outcomes in 588 women with pregestational diabetes in whom about half had preconceptional counseling. Those women who received counseling had improved glycemic control before pregnancy and in the first trimester, had higher folate intake rates preconceptionally, and experienced lower rates of adverse outcomes—defined as a perinatal death or major congenital anomaly. These cited benefits are accompanied by reduced health-care costs in diabetic women. From their review, Reece and Homko (2007) found that each $1 expended for a preconceptional care program saved between $1.86 and $5.19 in averted medical costs. Despite such benefits, the proportion of diabetic women receiving preconceptional care is suboptimal. In their study of approximately 300 diabetic women in a managed-care plan, Kim and colleagues (2005) found that only about half had preconceptional counseling. Counseling rates are undoubtedly much lower among uninsured and indigent women.

Epilepsy

Women who have epilepsy have an undisputed two- to threefold risk of having infants with structural anomalies compared with unaffected women (Wide, 2004). Some early reports indicated that epilepsy conferred an increased a priori risk for congenital malformations that was independent of any effects of anticonvulsant treatment. Although more recent publications have largely failed to confirm this increased risk in untreated women, it is difficult to refute entirely because women who are controlled without medication generally have less severe disease (Cassina, 2013). Fried and associates (2004) conducted a metaanalysis of studies comparing epileptic women, both treated and untreated, with controls. In this study, increased malformation rates could only be demonstrated in the offspring of women who had been exposed to anticonvulsant therapy. Veiby and coworkers (2009) used the Medical Birth Registry of Norway to compare pregnancy outcomes in 2861 deliveries by epileptic women with 369,267 control deliveries. They identified an increased malformation risk only in women who were exposed to valproic acid (5.6 percent) and polytherapy (6.1 percent). Untreated women had anomaly rates that were similar to those of nonepileptic controls.

Ideally, seizure control is optimized preconceptionally. Vajda and colleagues (2008) reported data from the Australian Register of Antiepileptic Drugs in Pregnancy. The risk of seizures during pregnancy was decreased by 50 to 70 percent if there were no seizures in the year preceding pregnancy. There were no further advantages that accrued if the seizure-free period exceeded a year.

Efforts should attempt to achieve seizure control with monotherapy and with medications considered less teratogenic (Aguglia, 2009; Tomson, 2009). As discussed in detail in Chapter 60 (p. 1190) and shown in Table 8-2, some one-drug regimens are more teratogenic than others. Valproic acid, in particular, should be avoided if possible, as this medication has consistently been associated with a greater risk for major congenital malformations than other antiepileptic drugs (Jentink, 2010). According to Jeha and Morris (2005), the American Academy of Neurology recommends consideration of antiseizure medication discontinuation before pregnancy in suitable candidates. These are women who satisfy the following criteria: have been seizure-free for 2 to 5 years, display a single seizure type, have a normal neurological examination and normal intelligence, and show electroencephalogram results that have normalized with treatment.

TABLE 8-2. First-Trimester Antiepileptic Monotherapy and the Associated Congenital Malformation Risk

Antiepileptic (n)	Major Congenital Malformations n (%)	Relative Risk (95% CI)[a]
Unexposed controls (442)	5 (1.1)	Reference
Lamotrigine (1562)	31 (2.0)	1.8 (0.7–4.6)
Carbamazepine (1033)	31 (3.0)	2.7 (1.0–7.0)
Phenytoin (416)	12 (2.9)	2.6 (0.9–7.4)
Levetiracetam (450)	11 (2.4)	2.2 (0.8–6.4)
Topiramate (359)	15 (4.2)	3.8 (1.4–10.6)
Valproate (323)	30 (9.3)	9.0 (3.4–23.3)
Phenobarbital (199)	11 (5.5)	5.1 (1.8–14.9)
Oxcarbazepine (182)	4 (2.2)	2.0 (0.5–7.4)
Gabapentin (145)	1 (0.7)	0.6 (0.07–5.2)
Zonisamide (90)	0 (0)	NA
Clonazepam (64)	2 (3.1)	2.8 (0.5–14.8)

[a]Risk compared with that of the unexposed reference population of nonepileptic women.
NA = not applicable.
Data from Hernández-Díaz, 2012.

Epileptic women should be advised to take supplemental folic acid. However, it is not entirely clear that folate supplementation reduces the fetal malformation risk in pregnant women taking anticonvulsant therapy. In one case-control study, Kjær and associates (2008) reported that the congenital abnormality risk was reduced by maternal folate supplementation in fetuses exposed to carbamazepine, phenobarbital, phenytoin, and primidone. Conversely, from the United Kingdom Epilepsy and Pregnancy Register, Morrow and coworkers (2009) compared fetal outcomes of women who received preconceptional folic acid with those who did not receive it until later in pregnancy or not at all. In this study, a paradoxical *increase* in the number of major congenital malformations was observed in the group who received preconceptional folate. These investigators concluded that folate metabolism may be only a part of the mechanism by which malformations are induced in women taking these medications.

Immunizations

Preconceptional counseling includes assessment of immunity against common pathogens. Also, depending on health status, travel plans, and time of year, other immunizations may be indicated as discussed in Chapter 9 (Table 9-9, p. 186). Vaccines that contain toxoids—for example, tetanus, or that consist of killed bacteria or viruses—such as influenza, pneumococcus, hepatitis B, meningococcus, and rabies—have not been associated with adverse fetal outcomes and are not contraindicated preconceptionally or during pregnancy. Conversely, live-virus vaccines—including varicella-zoster, measles, mumps, rubella, polio, chickenpox, and yellow fever—are not recommended during pregnancy. Moreover, 1 month or longer should ideally pass between vaccination and conception attempts. That said, inadvertent administration of measles, mumps, rubella (MMR) or varicella vaccines during pregnancy should not generally be considered indications for pregnancy termination. Most reports indicate that the fetal risk is only theoretical. Immunization to smallpox, anthrax, and other bioterrorist diseases should be discussed if clinically appropriate (Chap. 64, p. 1258). Based on their study of approximately 300 women who received smallpox vaccination near the time of conception, Ryan and colleagues (2008) found that rates of pregnancy loss, preterm birth, and birth defects were not higher than expected.

GENETIC DISEASES

The Centers for Disease Control and Prevention (2013) estimate that 3 percent of neonates born each year in the United States will have at least one birth defect. Importantly, such defects are the leading cause of infant mortality and account for 20 percent of deaths. The benefits of preconceptional counseling usually are measured by comparing the incidence of new cases before and after initiation of a counseling program. Congenital conditions that clearly benefit from patient education include neural-tube defects, phenylketonuria, thalassemias, and other genetic diseases more common in individuals of Eastern European Jewish descent.

Family History

Pedigree construction using the symbols shown in Figure 8-2 is the most thorough method for obtaining a family history as a part of genetic screening. The health and reproductive status of each "blood relative" should be individually reviewed for medical illnesses, mental retardation, birth defects, infertility, and pregnancy loss. Certain racial, ethnic, or religious backgrounds may indicate increased risk for specific recessive disorders.

Although most women can provide some information regarding their history, their understanding may be limited. For example, several studies have shown that pregnant women often fail to report a birth defect in the family or they report it incorrectly. Thus, any disclosed defect or genetic disease should be confirmed by reviewing pertinent medical records or by contacting affected relatives for additional information.

Neural-Tube Defects

The incidence of neural-tube defects (NTDs) is 0.9 per 1000 live births, and they are second only to cardiac anomalies as the most frequent structural fetal malformation (Chap. 14, p. 283). Some NTDs, as well as congenital heart defects, are associated with specific mutations. One example is the 677C → T substitution in the gene that encodes methylene tetrahydrofolate reductase. For this and similar gene defects, the trial conducted by the Medical Research Council Vitamin Study Research Group (1991) showed that preconceptional folic acid therapy significantly reduced the risk for a recurrent NTD by 72 percent. More importantly, because more than 90 percent of infants with NTDs are born to women at low risk, Czeizel and Dudas (1992) showed that supplementation reduced the a priori risk of a first NTD occurrence. It is currently recommended, therefore, that all women who may become pregnant take 400 to 800 μg of folic acid orally daily before conception and through the first trimester (U.S Preventive Services Task Force, 2009). Folate fortification of cereal grains has been mandatory in the United States since 1998, and this practice has also resulted in decreased neural-tube defect rates (Mills, 2004). Despite the demonstrated benefits of folate supplementation, only half of women have taken folic acid supplementation periconceptionally (de Jong-van den Berg, 2005; Goldberg, 2006). The strongest predictor of use appears to be consultation with a health-care provider before conception.

Phenylketonuria

This inherited phenylalanine metabolism defect exemplifies diseases in which the fetus may not be at risk to inherit the disorder but may be damaged by maternal disease. Specifically, mothers with phenylketonuria (PKU) who eat an unrestricted diet have abnormally high blood phenylalanine levels. This amino acid readily crosses the placenta and can damage developing fetal organs, especially neural and cardiac tissues (Table 8-3). With appropriate preconceptional counseling and adherence to a phenylalanine-restricted diet before pregnancy, the incidence of fetal malformations is dramatically reduced (Guttler, 1990; Hoeks, 2009; Koch, 1990). It is recommended, therefore, that the phenylalanine concentration be normalized 3 months before conception and that these levels be maintained throughout pregnancy (American College of Obstetricians and Gynecologists, 2009b).

TABLE 8-3. Frequency of Complications in the Offspring of Women with Untreated Phenylketonuria[a] (Blood Phenylalanine > 1200 μmol/L)

Complication	Frequency in Affected Pregnancies (%)
Spontaneous abortion	24
Mental retardation	92
Microcephaly	73
Congenital heart disease	12
Fetal-growth restriction	40

[a]Blood phenylalanine level > 1200 μmol/L.
Adapted from Maillot, 2007.

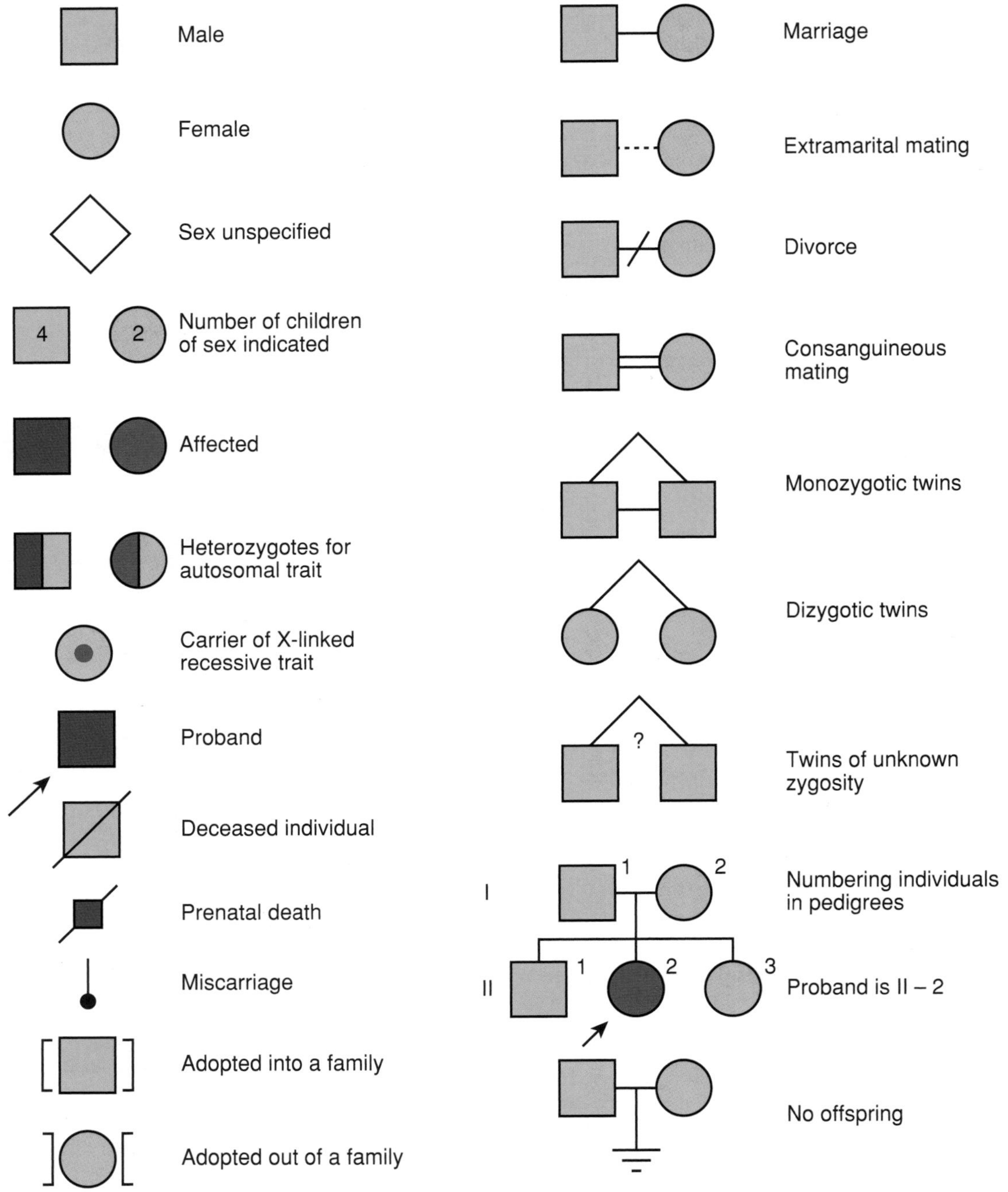

FIGURE 8-2 Symbols used for pedigree construction. (Redrawn from Thompson, 1991.)

Thalassemias

These disorders of globin-chain synthesis are the most common single-gene disorders worldwide. As many as 200 million people carry a gene for one of these hemoglobinopathies, and hundreds of mutations are known to cause thalassemia syndromes (Chap. 56, p. 1112). In endemic areas such as Mediterranean and Southeast Asian countries, counseling and other prevention strategies have reduced the incidence of new cases by up to 80 percent (Angastiniotis, 1998). For example, more than 25,000 students of Mediterranean origin were counseled and tested for β-thalassemia during a 20-year period (Mitchell, 1996). Within a few years of program initiation, all high-risk couples who requested prenatal diagnosis had completed the program, and remarkably, there were no affected children born during this period.

The American College of Obstetricians and Gynecologists (2013b) recommends that individuals of high-risk ancestry be offered carrier screening to allow them informed decision making regarding reproduction and prenatal diagnosis. One method—*preimplantation genetic diagnosis,* which is discussed in Chapter 14 (p. 301)—is available for patients at risk for certain thalassemia syndromes (Chen, 2008; Kuliev, 2011).

Individuals of Eastern European Jewish Descent

Most individuals of Jewish ancestry in North America are descended from Ashkenazi Jewish communities and are at increased risk for having offspring with one of several autosomal recessive disorders. These include Tay-Sachs disease, Gaucher disease, cystic fibrosis, Canavan disease, familial dysautonomia, mucolipidosis IV, Niemann-Pick disease type A, Fanconi anemia group C, and Bloom syndrome. The American College of Obstetricians and Gynecologists (2009c) recommends preconceptional counseling and screening for these in this population. Carrier frequency and features of these conditions are discussed in Chapter 14 (Table 14-11, p. 298).

REPRODUCTIVE HISTORY

During preconceptional screening, information should be sought regarding infertility; abnormal pregnancy outcomes that may include miscarriage, ectopic pregnancy, and recurrent pregnancy loss; and obstetrical complications such as preeclampsia, placental abruption, and preterm delivery (Stubblefield, 2008). As discussed in Chapter 35 (p. 664), details involving a prior stillbirth are especially important. For example, Korteweg and associates (2008) identified chromosomal abnormalities in 13 percent of stillborns who underwent karyotyping. More recently, Reddy and colleagues (2012) confirmed that chromosomal microarray analysis yielded better detection of genetic abnormalities than did standard karyotyping, primarily because nonviable tissue can be used for the analysis. Identification of a genetic abnormality in stillborns can help determine the recurrence risk and aid in the preconceptional or prenatal management in subsequent pregnancies.

PARENTAL AGE

Maternal Age

Women at both ends of the reproductive-age spectrum have unique outcomes to be considered. First, according to the Centers for Disease Control and Prevention, in 2010, 3.4 percent of births in the United States were in women between the ages of 15 and 19 years (Martin, 2012). This rate represents a historical low in the United States for teenage births with a 45-percent decline since 1991. That said, adolescents are at increased risk for anemia, preterm delivery, and preeclampsia compared with women aged 20 to 35 years (Usta, 2008). The incidence of sexually transmitted diseases—common in adolescents—is even higher during pregnancy (Niccolai, 2003). Unfortunately, because most of their pregnancies are unplanned, adolescents rarely seek preconceptional counseling.

In contrast, conceptions after age 35 currently comprise approximately 15 percent of pregnancies in the United States (Martin, 2012). The older woman is more likely to request preconceptional counseling, either because she has postponed pregnancy

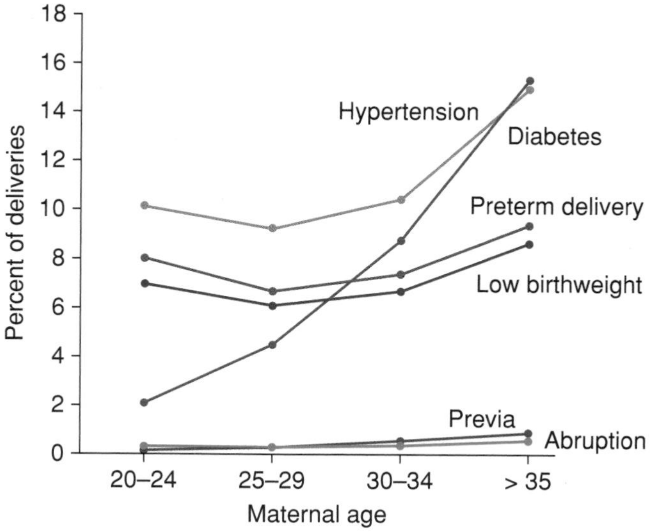

FIGURE 8-3 Incidence of selected pregnancy complications in relation to maternal age among 295,667 women delivered at Parkland Hospital, 1988–2012. (Courtesy of Dr. Donald McIntire.)

and now wishes to optimize her outcome, or because she plans to undergo infertility treatment. Some studies—including data from Parkland Hospital presented in Figure 8-3—indicate that after age 35, there is an increased risk for obstetrical complications as well as perinatal morbidity and mortality (Cunningham, 1995; Huang, 2008). The older woman who has a chronic illness or who is in poor physical condition usually has readily apparent risks. For the physically fit woman without medical problems, however, the risks are much lower than previously reported.

Overall, the maternal mortality rate is higher in women aged 35 and older (Chap. 1, p. 5). Compared with women in their 20s, women aged 35 to 39 are 2.5 times more likely and women aged 40 or older are 5.3 times more likely to suffer pregnancy-related mortality (Geller, 2006). According to Buehler and coworkers (1986), improved medical care may ameliorate these risks. They reviewed maternal deaths in the United States from 1974 through 1982. Through 1978, older women had a fivefold increased relative risk of maternal death compared with that of younger women. By 1982, however, the mortality rates for older women had decreased by 50 percent.

For the fetus, maternal age-related risks primarily stem from: (1) indicated preterm delivery for maternal complications such as hypertension and diabetes, (2) spontaneous preterm birth, (3) fetal-growth disorders related to chronic maternal disease or multifetal gestation, (4) fetal aneuploidy, and (5) pregnancies resulting from assisted reproductive technology.

Assisted Reproductive Technologies

Recall that older women have subfertility problems. And although the incidence of dizygotic twinning increases with maternal age, the more important cause of multifetal gestation in older women follows the use of *assisted reproductive technology (ART)* and *ovulation induction*. Indeed, according to the Centers for Disease Control and Prevention, 40 percent of all multifetal gestations in the United States in 2005 were conceived with the use of ART (Martin, 2010). Multifetal pregnancies account for much of the morbidity and mortality from preterm delivery. Other obstetrical morbidities, such as placenta previa and abruption, are also risks associated with ART (Fong, 2014).

During the past decade, experience has accrued that links ART to increased major congenital malformation rates. Davies and colleagues (2012) reported that of 308,974 births in South Australia, 8.3 percent of infants conceived by ART had major birth defects. In this analysis, after adjustment for maternal age and other risk factors, intracytoplasmic injection continued to be associated with a significantly increased risk for malformations, but in vitro fertilization did not.

Paternal Age

Although there is an increased incidence of genetic diseases in offspring caused by new autosomal-dominant mutations in older men, the incidence is still low (Chap. 13, p. 270). Accordingly, targeted sonographic examination performed solely for advanced maternal or paternal age is controversial.

SOCIAL HISTORY

Recreational Drugs and Smoking

Fetal risks associated with alcohol, marijuana, cocaine, amphetamines, and heroin are discussed in Chapter 12 (p. 253). The first step in preventing drug-related fetal risk is for the woman to honestly assess her use. Questioning should be nonjudgmental. Screening for at-risk drinking can be accomplished using a number of validated tools, like the well-studied TACE questions (American College of Obstetricians and Gynecologists, 2013a). This is a series of four questions concerning *tolerance* to alcohol, being *annoyed* by comments about their drinking, attempts to *cut down*, and a history of drinking early in the morning—the *eye opener*.

In a Canadian study of more than 1000 postpartum patients, Tough and coworkers (2006) found that a high percentage of women reported alcohol use concurrent with conceptional attempts. Specifically, nearly half of those planning for pregnancy reported a mean of 2.2 drinks daily during early gestation before they recognized their pregnancy. Of note, Bailey and associates (2008) found that rates of binge drinking and marijuana use by men were unaffected by their partner's pregnancy. The frequency and pattern of such behaviors clearly underscore the opportunity for preconceptional counseling.

In 2005, approximately 14 percent of women giving birth in the United States smoked cigarettes (Tong, 2009). This practice has been consistently associated with numerous adverse perinatal outcomes. These risks are largely mitigated by cessation before pregnancy, highlighting the importance of screening for tobacco use in the preconceptional period and during prenatal care as outlined in Chapter 9 (p. 172).

Environmental Exposures

Contact with environmental substances is inescapable. Thus, it is fortunate that only a few agents have been shown to cause adverse pregnancy outcomes (Windham, 2008). Exposures to infectious diseases have myriad deleterious effects, and these are detailed in Chapters 64 and 65 (p. 1239). Likewise, contact with some chemicals may impart significant maternal and fetal risks. As discussed in Chapters 8 and 12 (pp. 183 and 250), excess exposure to methyl mercury or lead is associated with neurodevelopmental disorders.

In the past, some concerns were raised over common everyday exposure to *electromagnetic fields* such as emanated by high-voltage power lines, electric blankets, microwave ovens, and cellular phones. Fortunately, there is no human or animal evidence that any of these cause adverse fetal effects (O'Connor, 1999; Robert, 1999). The effects of *electrical shock* are discussed in Chapter 47 (p. 956).

Diet

Pica is the craving for and consuming of ice, laundry starch, clay, dirt, or other nonfood items. It should be discouraged due to its inherent replacement of healthful food with nutritionally empty products (Chap. 9, p. 188). In some cases, it may represent an unusual physiological response to iron deficiency (Federman, 1997). Many *vegetarian diets* are protein deficient but can be corrected by increasing egg and cheese consumption. *Anorexia* and *bulimia* increase maternal risks of nutritional deficiencies, electrolyte disturbances, cardiac arrhythmias, and gastrointestinal pathology (Becker, 1999). With these, pregnancy-related complications include greater risks of low birthweight, smaller head circumference, microcephaly, and small for gestational age (Kouba, 2005).

In contrast, *obesity* is linked with several maternal complications. As discussed in Chapter 48 (p. 965), these include hypertension, preeclampsia, gestational diabetes, labor abnormalities, cesarean delivery, and operative complications (American College of Obstetricians and Gynecologists, 2013c). Obesity also appears to be associated with a range of structural fetal anomalies (Stothard, 2009). By comparing changes in prepregnancy body mass index (BMI), Villamor and Cnattingius (2006) found that modest increases in BMI before pregnancy could result in perinatal complications, even if a woman does not become overweight.

Exercise

Conditioned pregnant women usually can continue to exercise throughout gestation (American College of Obstetricians and Gynecologists, 2009a). As discussed in Chapter 9 (p. 182), there are no data to suggest that exercise is harmful during pregnancy. One caveat is that as pregnancy progresses, balance problems and joint relaxation may predispose to orthopedic injury. A woman should be advised not to exercise to exhaustion, and she should augment heat dissipation and fluid replacement. Further avoidances include supine positions, activities requiring good balance, and extreme weather conditions.

Intimate Partner Violence

Pregnancy can exacerbate interpersonal problems and is a time of increased risk from an abusive partner. According to the American College of Obstetricians and Gynecologists (2012a), approximately 324,000 pregnant women are abused each year. As discussed in Chapter 47 (p. 951), intimate partner violence has been associated with an increased risk for several pregnancy-related complications, including hypertension, vaginal bleeding, hyperemesis, preterm delivery, and low-birthweight infants (Silverman, 2006). Because domestic violence can escalate during pregnancy, even to the point of homicide, the preconceptional period provides an ideal time for screening, and if indicated, intervention (Cheng, 2010). As outlined in Chapter 9 (p. 174), the American College of Obstetricians and Gynecologists (2012a) has provided recommendations and resources for screening both pregnant and nonpregnant women for domestic violence.

SCREENING TESTS

Certain laboratory tests may be helpful in assessing the risk for and preventing some complications during pregnancy. These include basic tests that are usually performed during prenatal care and are discussed in Chapter 9. More specific tests may assist evaluation of women with certain chronic medical diseases. Examples of some, but certainly not all, chronic diseases that ideally would be assessed before conception are highlighted in Table 8-4. With several of these, optimizing maternal condition before conception will improve pregnancy outcomes. Cox and coworkers (1992) reviewed pregnancy outcomes in 1075 high-risk women who received such evaluation. They reported that the 240 women with hypertension, asthma, or renal, thyroid, or cardiac disease had better outcomes compared with the outcomes from their previous pregnancies.

TABLE 8-4. Selected Preconceptional Counseling Topics

Condition	Reference Chapter	Recommendations for Preconceptional Counseling
Environmental exposure	Chap. 9, p. 183 Chap. 12, p. 250	*Methyl mercury*: Avoid shark, swordfish, king mackerel, and tile fish. Ingest no more than 12 ounces or 2 servings of canned tuna and no more than 6 ounces of albacore per week. *Lead*: Blood lead testing if a risk factor is identified from Table 9-9; treat if indicated according to recommendations.
Abnormal weight	Chap. 48, p. 961	Calculate BMI yearly from Figure 48-1, p. 962 *BMI* $\geq$ *25 kg/m*^{2}: Counsel on diet. Test for diabetes and metabolic syndrome if indicated. Consider weight loss prior to conception. *BMI* $\leq$ *18.5 kg/m*^{2}: Assess for eating disorder.
Cardiovascular disease	Chap. 49, p. 973 Chap. 12, p. 247	Counsel on cardiac risks during pregnancy; discuss situations in which pregnancy is contraindicated. Optimize cardiac function. Discuss medication teratogenicity (warfarin, ACE inhibitor, ARB) and if possible, switch to less dangerous agent when conception planned. Offer genetic counseling to those with congenital cardiac anomalies (Table 49-4, p. 977).
Chronic hypertension	Chap. 50, p. 1000	Counsel on specific risks during pregnancy. Assess those with long-standing HTN for ventricular hypertrophy, retinopathy, and renal disease. Optimize blood pressure control. If medications indicated, select or switch to an agent appropriate for pregnancy.
Asthma	Chap. 51, p. 1011	Counsel on asthma risks during pregnancy. Optimize pulmonary function preconceptionally if possible. Treat women with pharmacological step therapy for chronic asthma based on ACOG-ACAAI (2000) recommendations.
Thrombophilia	Chap. 52, p. 1028	Question for personal or family history of thrombotic events or recurrent poor pregnancy outcomes. If a thrombophilia is found or known, counsel and offer least teratogenic appropriate anticoagulation regimen.
Renal disease	Chap. 53, p. 1051 Chap. 12, p. 247	Counsel on specific risks during pregnancy. Optimize blood pressure control before conception. Counsel women taking ACE inhibitors and ARBs on these drugs' teratogenicity and the need to switch agents before pregnancy if possible.
Gastrointestinal disease	Chap. 54, p. 1076 Chap. 12, p. 248	*Inflammatory bowel disease:* Counsel affected women on subfertility risks and risks of adverse pregnancy outcomes. Discuss teratogenicity of methotrexate and the other immunomodulators. Offer effective contraception during their use and switch agents, if possible, before conception.
Hepatobiliary disease	Chap. 55, p. 1090	*Hepatitis B*: Vaccinate all high-risk women before conception (Table 9-9, p. 185). Counsel chronic carriers on transmission prevention to partners and fetus. *Hepatitis C*: Screen high-risk women. Counsel affected women on risks of disease and transmission. If treatment indicated, discuss ramifications and appropriateness of pregnancy.

(continued)

TABLE 8-4. Continued

Condition	Reference Chapter	Recommendations for Preconceptional Counseling
Hematological disease	Chap. 56, p. 1101	*Iron deficiency anemia:* Iron supplementation if identified. *Sickle-cell disease:* Screen all black women. Counsel those with trait or disease. Test partner if desired. *Thalassemias:* Screen women of Southeast Asian or Mediterranean ancestry.
Diabetes	Chap. 57, p. 1125	Optimize glycemic control to minimize teratogenicity of hyperglycemia. Evaluate for end-organ damage such as retinopathy, nephropathy, hypertension, and others.
Thyroid disease	Chap. 58, p. 1147	Screen those with thyroid disease symptoms. Ensure iodine-sufficient diet. Treat overt hyper- or hypothyroidism before conception. Counsel on risks to pregnancy outcome.
Connective-tissue disease	Chap. 59, p. 1169 Chap. 12, p. 247	*RA*: Counsel on flare risk after pregnancy. Discuss methotrexate and leflunomide teratogenicity, as well as possible effects of other immunomodulators. Switch these agents before conception. Halt NSAIDs by 27 weeks' gestation. *SLE*: Counsel on risks during pregnancy. Optimize disease before conception. Discuss mycophenolate mofetil and cyclophosphamide teratogenicity as well as possible effects of newer immunomodulators. Switch these agents before conception..
Psychiatric disorders	Chap. 61, p. 1204	*Depression:* Screen for symptoms of depression. In those affected, counsel on risks of treatment and of untreated illness and the high risk of exacerbation during pregnancy and the puerperium.
Neurological disorders	Chap. 60, p. 1189	*Seizure disorder:* Optimize seizure control using monotherapy if possible. (p. 158 and Table 8-2).
Dermatological disease	Chap. 12, p. 251	Discuss isotretinoin and etretinate teratogenicity and effective contraception during their use; switch agents before conception.
Cancer	Chap. 63, p. 1219	Counsel on fertility preservation options before cancer therapy and on decreased fertility following certain agents. Discuss appropriateness of pregnancy balanced with need for ongoing cancer therapy and prognosis of the disease state.
Infectious diseases	Chap. 64, p. 1239	*Influenza:* Vaccinate all women who will be pregnant during flu season. Vaccinate high-risk women prior to flu season. *Malaria:* Counsel to avoid travel to endemic areas during conception. If unable, offer effective contraception during travel or provide chemoprophylaxis for those planning pregnancy. *Rubella:* Screen for rubella immunity. If nonimmune, vaccinate and counsel on the need for effective contraception during the subsequent month. *Tetanus:* Update vaccination, as needed, in all reproductive-aged women. *Varicella:* Question regarding immunity. If nonimmune, vaccinate.
STDs	Chap. 65, p. 1265	*Gonorrhea, syphilis, chlamydial infection:* Screen high-risk women and treat as indicated. *HIV:* Screen at-risk women. Counsel affected women on risks during pregnancy and on perinatal transmission. Discuss initiation of treatment before pregnancy to decrease transmission risk. Offer effective contraception to those not desiring conception. *HPV:* Provide Pap smear screening per guidelines. Vaccinate candidate patients. *HSV:* Provide serological screening to asymptomatic women with affected partners. Counsel affected women on risks of perinatal transmission and of preventative measures during the third trimester and labor.

ACAAI = American College of Allergy, Asthma, and Immunology; ACE = angiotensin-converting enzyme; ARB = angiotensin-receptor blocker; ACOG = American College of Obstetricians and Gynecologists; BMI = body mass index; HIV = human immunodeficiency virus; HPV = human papillomavirus; HSV = herpes simplex virus; HTN = hypertension; NSAID = nonsteroidal antiinflammatory drug; RA = rheumatoid arthritis; SLE = systemic lupus erythematosus; STD = sexually transmitted disease.
Adapted from Jack, 2008.

REFERENCES

Aguglia U, Barboni G, Battino D, et al: Italian consensus conference on epilepsy and pregnancy, labor and puerperium. Epilepsia 50:7, 2009

American College of Obstetricians and Gynecologists: Exercise during pregnancy and the postpartum period. Committee Opinion No. 267, January 2002, Reaffirmed 2009a

American College of Obstetricians and Gynecologists: Maternal phenylketonuria. Committee Opinion No. 449, December 2009b

American College of Obstetricians and Gynecologists: Preconception and prenatal carrier screening for genetic diseases in individuals of Eastern European Jewish descent. Committee Opinion No. 442, October 2009c

American College of Obstetricians and Gynecologists: Intimate partner violence. Committee Opinion No. 518, 2012a

American College of Obstetricians and Gynecologists: Pregestational diabetes mellitus. Practice Bulletin No. 60, March 2005, Reaffirmed 2012b

American College of Obstetricians and Gynecologists: The importance of preconception care in the continuum of women's health care. Committee Opinion No. 313, September 2005, Reaffirmed 2012c

American College of Obstetricians and Gynecologists: At-risk drinking and alcohol dependence: obstetric and gynecologic implications. Committee Opinion No. 496, August 2011, Reaffirmed 2013a

American College of Obstetricians and Gynecologists: Hemoglobinopathies in pregnancy. Practice Bulletin No. 78, January 2007, Reaffirmed 2013b

American College of Obstetricians and Gynecologists: Obesity in pregnancy. Committee Opinion No. 549, January 2013c

Angastiniotis M, Modell B: Global epidemiology of hemoglobin disorders. Ann NY Acad Sci 850:251, 1998

Bailey JA, Hill KG, Hawkins JD, et al: Men's and women's patterns of substance use around pregnancy. Birth 35:1, 2008

Becker AE, Grinspoon SK, Klibanski A, et al: Eating disorders. N Engl J Med 340:14, 1999

Buehler JW, Kaunitz AM, Hogue CJR, et al: Maternal mortality in women aged 35 years or older: United States. JAMA 255:53, 1986

Cassina M, Dilaghi A, Di Gianantonio E, et al: Pregnancy outcome in women exposed to antiepileptic drugs: teratogenic role of maternal epilepsy and its pharmacologic treatment. Reprod Toxicol 39:50, 2013

Centers for Disease Control and Prevention: Birth defects. 2013. Available at: http://www.cdc.gov/ncbddd/birthdefects/data.html. Accessed June 16, 2013

Chen SU, Su YN, Fang MY, et al: PGD of beta-thalassaemia and HLA haplotypes using OminiPlex whole genome amplification. Reprod Biomed Online 17:699, 2008

Cheng D, Horon IL: Intimate-partner homicide among pregnant and postpartum women. Obstet Gynecol 115(6):1181, 2010

Cheng D, Schwarz EB, Douglas E, et al: Unintended pregnancy and associated maternal preconception, prenatal and postpartum behaviors. Contraception 79:194, 2009

Cox M, Whittle MJ, Byrne A, et al: Prepregnancy counseling: experience from 1075 cases. Br J Obstet Gynaecol 99:873, 1992

Cunningham FG, Leveno KJ: Childbearing among older women—the message is cautiously optimistic. N Engl J Med 333:953, 1995

Czeizel AE, Dudas I: Prevention of the first occurrence of neural-tube defects by periconceptional vitamin supplementation. N Engl J Med 327:1832, 1992

D'Angelo D, Williams L, Morrow B, et al: Preconception and interconception health status of women who recently gave birth to a live-born infant—Pregnancy Risk Assessment Monitoring System (PRAMS), United States, 26 reporting areas, 2004. MMWR 56(10):1, 2007

Davies MJ, Moore VM, Willson KJ, et al: Reproductive technologies and the risk of birth defects. N Engl J Med 366(19):1803, 2012

de Jong-van den Berg LTW, Hernandez-Diaz S, Werler MM, et al: Trends and predictors of folic acid awareness and periconceptional use in pregnant women. Am J Obstet Gynecol 192:121, 2005

Federman DG, Kirsner RS, Federman GS: Pica: are you hungry for the facts? Conn Med 61:207, 1997

Fong A, Lovell S, Rad, S, et al: Obstetrical complications of deliveries conceived by assisted reproductive technology in California. Abstract No. 433. Presented at the 34th Annual Meeting of the Society for Maternal-Fetal Medicine. February 3-8, 2014

Fried S, Kozer E, Nulman I, et al: Malformation rates in children of women with untreated epilepsy: a meta-analysis. Drug Saf 27(3):197, 2004

Geller SE, Cox SM, Callaghan WM, et al: Morbidity and mortality in pregnancy: laying the groundwork for safe motherhood. Womens Health Issues 16:176, 2006

Goldberg BB, Alvarado S, Chavez C, et al: Prevalence of periconceptional folic acid use and perceived barriers to the postgestation continuance of supplemental folic acid: survey results from a Teratogen Information Service. Birth Defects Res Part A Clin Mol Teratol 76:193, 2006

Guttler F, Lou H, Andresen J, et al: Cognitive development in offspring of untreated and preconceptionally treated maternal phenylketonuria. J Inherit Metab Dis 13:665, 1990

Hernández-Díaz S, Smith CR, Shen A, et al: Comparative safety of antiepileptic drugs during pregnancy. Neurology 78:1692, 2012

Hoeks MP, den Heijer M, Janssen MC: Adult issues in phenylketonuria. J Med 67:2, 2009

Huang L, Sauve R, Birkett N, et al: Maternal age and risk of stillbirth: a systematic review. CMAJ 178:165, 2008

Jack BW, Atrash H, Coonrod DV, et al: The clinical content of preconception care: an overview and preparation of this supplement. Am J Obstet Gynecol 199(6 Suppl 2):S266, 2008

Jack BW, Campanile C, McQuade W, et al: The negative pregnancy test. An opportunity for preconception care. Arch Fam Med 4:340, 1995

Jeha LE, Morris HH: Optimizing outcomes in pregnant women with epilepsy. Cleve Clin J Med 72:928, 2005

Jentink J, Loane MA, Dolk H, et al: Valproic acid monotherapy in pregnancy and major congenital malformations. N Engl J Med 362(23):2185, 2010

Johnson K, Posner SF, Biermann J, et al: Recommendations to improve preconception health and health care—United States. A report of the CDC/ATSDR Preconception Care Work Group and the Select Panel on Preconception Care. MMWR Recomm Rep 55(6):1, 2006

Kim C, Ferrara A, McEwen LN, et al: Preconception care in managed care: the translating research into action for diabetes study. Am J Obstet Gynecol 192:227, 2005

Kitzmiller JL, Block JM, Brown FH, et al: Managing preexisting diabetes for pregnancy: summary of evidence and consensus recommendations for care. Diabetes Care 31(5):1060, 2008

Kitzmiller JL, Gavin LA, Gin GD, et al: Preconception care of diabetics. JAMA 265:731, 1991

Kjær D, Horvath-Puhó E, Christensen J, et al: Antiepileptic drug use, folic acid supplementation, and congenital abnormalities: a population-based case-control study. BJOG 115:98, 2008

Koch R, Hanley W, Levy H, et al: A preliminary report of the collaborative study of maternal phenylketonuria in the United States and Canada. J Inherit Metab Dis 13:641, 1990

Korteweg FJ, Bouman K, Erwich JJ, et al: Cytogenetic analysis after evaluation of 750 fetal deaths: proposal for diagnostic workup. Obstet Gynecol 111(4):865, 2008

Kouba S, Hällström T, Lindholm C, et al: Pregnancy and neonatal outcomes in women with eating disorders. Obstet Gynecol 105:255, 2005

Kuliev A, Pakhalchuk T, Verlinsky O, et al: Preimplantation genetic diagnosis for hemoglobinopathies. Hemoglobin 35(5–6):547, 2011

Leguizamón G, Igarzabal ML, Reece EA: Periconceptional care of women with diabetes mellitus. Obstet Gynecol Clin North Am 34:225, 2007

Maillot F, Cook P, Lilburn M, et al: A practical approach to maternal phenylketonuria management. J Inherit Metab Dis 30:198, 2007

Martin JA, Hamilton BE, Ventura SJ, et al. Births: final data for 2010. Natl Vital Stat Rep 61(1):1, 2012

Martin JA, Hamilton BE, Sutton PD, et al. Births: final data for 2007. Natl Vital Stat Rep 58(24):1, 2010

Medical Research Council Vitamin Study Research Group: Prevention of neural tube defects: results of the Medical Research Council vitamin study. Lancet 338:131, 1991

Mills JL, Signore C: Neural tube defect rates before and after food fortification with folic acid. Birth Defects Res A Clin Mol Teratol 70(11):844, 2004

Mitchell JJ, Capua A, Clow C, et al: Twenty-year outcome analysis of genetic screening programs for Tay-Sachs and beta-thalassemia disease carriers in high schools. Am J Hum Genet 59:793, 1996

Moos MK: Preconceptional health promotion: progress in changing a prevention paradigm. J Perinat Neonatal Nurs 18:2, 2004

Moos MK, Bangdiwala SI, Meibohm AR, et al: The impact of a preconceptional health promotion program on intendedness of pregnancy. Am J Perinatol 13:103, 1996

Morrow JI, Hunt SJ, Russell AJ, et al: Folic acid use and major congenital malformations in offspring of women with epilepsy: a prospective study from the UK Epilepsy and Pregnancy Register. J Neurol Neurosurg Psychiatry 80(5):506, 2009

Niccolai LM, Ethier KA, Kershaw TS, et al: Pregnant adolescents at risk: sexual behaviors and sexually transmitted disease prevalence. Am J Obstet Gynecol 188:63, 2003

O'Connor ME: Intrauterine effects in animals exposed to radiofrequency and microwave fields. Teratology 59:287, 1999

Reddy UM, Page GP, Saade GR, et al: Karyotype versus microarray testing for genetic abnormalities after stillbirth. N Engl J Med 367(23):2185, 2012

Reece EA, Homko CJ: Prepregnancy care and the prevention of fetal malformations in the pregnancy complicated by diabetes. Clin Obstet Gynecol 50:990, 2007

Robert E: Intrauterine effects of electromagnetic fields (low frequency, mid-frequency RF, and microwave): review of epidemiologic studies. Teratology 59:292, 1999

Ryan MA, Seward JF, for the Smallpox Vaccine in Pregnancy Registry Team: Pregnancy, birth, and infant health outcomes from the National Smallpox Vaccine in Pregnancy Registry, 2003–2006. Clin Infect Dis 46:S221, 2008

Sheffield JS, Butler-Koster EL, Casey BM, et al: Maternal diabetes mellitus and infant malformations. Obstet Gynecol 100:925, 2002

Silverman JG, Decker MR, Reed E, et al: Intimate partner violence victimization prior to and during pregnancy among women residing in 26 U.S. States: associations with maternal and neonatal health. Am J Obstet Gynecol 195:140, 2006

Stothard KJ, Tennant PW, Bell R, et al: Maternal overweight and obesity and the risk of congenital anomalies: a systematic review and meta-analysis. JAMA 301:636, 2009

Stubblefield PG, Coonrod DV, Reddy UM, et al: The clinical content of preconception care: reproductive history. Am J Obstet Gynecol 199(6 Suppl 2):S373, 2008

Thompson MW, McInnes RR, Huntington FW (eds): Genetics in Medicine, 5th ed. Philadelphia, Saunders, 1991

Tomson T, Battino D: Pregnancy and epilepsy: what should we tell our patients? J Neurol 256(6):856, 2009

Tong VT, Jones JR, Dietz PM, et al: Trends in smoking before, during, and after pregnancy-Pregnancy Risk Assessment Monitoring System (PRAMS), United States, 31 sites, 2000–2005. MMWR 58(4):1, 2009

Tough S, Tofflemire K, Clarke M, et al: Do women change their drinking behaviors while trying to conceive? An opportunity for preconception counseling. Clin Med Res 4:97, 2006

Tripathi A, Rankin J, Aarvold J, et al: Preconception counseling in women with diabetes: a population-based study in the North of England. Diabetes Care 33(3):586, 2010

U.S. Preventative Services Task Force: Recommendation statement: folic acid for the prevention of neural tube defects. Ann Intern Med 150:629, 2009

Usta IM, Zoorob D, Abu-Musa A, et al: Obstetric outcome of teenage pregnancies compared with adult pregnancies. Acta Obstet Gynecol 87:178, 2008

Vajda FJ, Hitchcock A, Graham J, et al: Seizure control in antiepileptic drug-treated pregnancy. Epilepsia 49:172, 2008

van der Zee B, de Wert G, Steegers EA, et al: Ethical aspects of paternal preconception lifestyle modification. Am J Obstet Gynecol 209(1):11, 2013

Veiby G, Daltveit AK, Engelsen BA, et al: Pregnancy, delivery, and outcome for the child in maternal epilepsy. Epilepsia 50(9):2130, 2009

Villamor E, Cnattingius S: Interpregnancy weight change and risk of adverse pregnancy outcomes: a population-based study. Lancet 368: 1164, 2006

Wide K, Winbladh B, Kallen B: Major malformations in infants exposed to antiepileptic drugs in utero, with emphasis on carbamazepine and valproic acid: a nation-wide population-based register study. Acta Paediatr 93:174, 2004

Windham G, Fenster L: Environmental contaminants and pregnancy outcomes. Fertil Steril 89:e111, 2008

CHAPTER 9

Prenatal Care

As described by the American Academy of Pediatrics and the American College of Obstetricians and Gynecologists (2012), "A comprehensive antepartum program involves a coordinated approach to medical care, continuous risk assessment, and psychological support that optimally begins before conception and extends throughout the postpartum period and interconceptional period." Optimizing the health and well-being of women before pregnancy should logically be an integral prelude to prenatal care. Adequate and appropriate preconceptional care, as discussed in detail in Chapter 8, has the potential to assist women by reducing risks, promoting healthy lifestyles, and improving readiness for pregnancy.

PRENATAL CARE IN THE UNITED STATES

Almost a century after its introduction, prenatal care has become one of the most frequently used health services in the United States. In 2001, there were approximately 50 million prenatal visits. The median was 12.3 visits per pregnancy, and many women had 17 or more total visits. This information is gathered from birth certificates, and a revised form was introduced in 2003. It is now used by 27 states and Puerto Rico, whereas the remaining 23 states continue to use a 1989 form. Unfortunately, data regarding the timing of prenatal care from these two systems are not directly comparable (Osterman, 2011).

Since the early 1990s, the largest gains in timely prenatal care have been among minority groups. As shown in Figure 9-1, however, disparity continues. Of the 27 states using the revised birth certificate, the percentage of non-Hispanic white, Hispanic, and African-American women who received no prenatal care in 2008 was 1.1, 2.7, and 3.3, respectively (Osterman, 2011). Some of the obstetrical and medical risk factors or complications identifiable during prenatal care are summarized in Table 9-1. Importantly, many of these complications are treatable.

Assessing Prenatal Care Adequacy

A commonly employed system for measuring prenatal care adequacy is the index of Kessner and colleagues (1973). This *Kessner Index* incorporates three items from the birth certificate: length of gestation, timing of the first prenatal visit, and number of visits. Although it does not measure the quality of care, the index remains a useful measure of prenatal care adequacy. Using this index, the National Center for Health Statistics concluded that 12 percent of American women who were delivered in 2000 received inadequate prenatal care (Martin, 2002a).

The Centers for Disease Control and Prevention (2000) analyzed birth certificate data for the years 1989 to 1997 and found that half of women with delayed or no prenatal care wanted to begin care earlier. Barriers to care varied by social and ethnic group, age, and payment method. The most common reason cited was late identification of pregnancy by the patient. The second most commonly cited barrier was lack of money or insurance. The third was inability to obtain an appointment.

Prenatal Care Effectiveness

Care designed during the early 1900s focused on lowering the extremely high maternal mortality rate. Such care undoubtedly contributed to the dramatic decline in this rate from

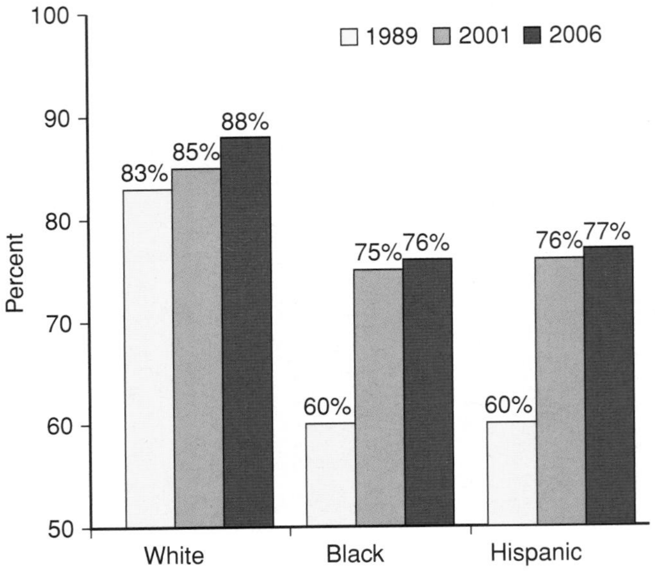

FIGURE 9-1 Percentage of women in the United States with prenatal care beginning in the first trimester by ethnicity in 1989, 2001, and 2006. (Adapted from Martin, 2002b, 2009.)

690 per 100,000 births in 1920 to 50 per 100,000 by 1955 (Loudon, 1992). As discussed in Chapter 1 (p. 5), the relatively low current maternal mortality rate of approximately 10 to 15 per 100,000 is likely associated with the high utilization of prenatal care (Xu, 2010). Indeed, in their analysis of data from 1998 to 2005 from the Pregnancy Mortality Surveillance System (PRAMS), Berg and associates (2010) identified a fivefold increased risk for maternal death in women who received no prenatal care.

There are other studies that attest to the efficacy of prenatal care. Herbst and colleagues (2003) found that lack of prenatal care was associated with more than a twofold increased risk of preterm birth. National Center for Health Statistics data showed that women with prenatal care had an overall stillbirth rate of 2.7 per 1000 compared with 14.1 per 1000 for women without prenatal care (Vintzileos, 2002a). These same investigators later reported that prenatal care was associated with lower rates of preterm birth as well as neonatal death associated with

TABLE 9-1. Obstetrical and Medical Risk Factors Detected During Prenatal Care in the United States in 2001

	Births	Percent
Total live births	4,025,933	100
Risk Factor		
Gestational hypertension	150,329	3.7
Diabetes	124,242	3.1
Anemia	99,558	2.5
Hydramnios/oligohydramnios	54,694	1.4
Lung disease	48,246	1.2
Others	139,860	< 1 each
Total	616,929	15.3

Data from Martin, 2002b.

placenta previa, fetal-growth restriction, and postterm pregnancy (Vintzileos, 2002b, 2003). Evaluating the format of care, Ickovics and associates (2007) compared individual prenatal care and group prenatal care. The latter provided traditional pregnancy surveillance in a group setting with special focus on support, education, and active health-care participation. Women enrolled in group prenatal care had significantly reduced preterm birth rates compared with those receiving individual care.

DIAGNOSIS OF PREGNANCY

Pregnancy is usually identified when a woman presents with symptoms and possibly a positive home urine pregnancy test result. Typically, such women receive confirmatory testing of urine or blood for human chorionic gonadotropin (hCG). Further, there may be presumptive or diagnostic findings of pregnancy during examination. Sonography is often used, particularly if miscarriage or ectopic pregnancy is a concern.

Signs and Symptoms

Amenorrhea

The abrupt cessation of menstruation in a healthy reproductive-aged woman who previously has experienced spontaneous, cyclical, predictable menses is highly suggestive of pregnancy. As discussed in Chapter 5 (p. 80), menstrual cycles vary appreciably in length among women and even in the same woman. Thus, amenorrhea is not a reliable pregnancy indicator until 10 days or more after expected menses. Occasionally, uterine bleeding occurs after conception and can be somewhat suggestive of menstruation. During the first month of pregnancy, such episodes are likely the consequence of blastocyst implantation. Still, first-trimester bleeding should generally prompt evaluation for an abnormal pregnancy.

Lower-Reproductive-Tract Changes

During pregnancy, the vaginal mucosa usually appears dark-bluish red and congested—*Chadwick sign,* popularized by him in 1886. Although presumptive evidence of pregnancy, it is not conclusive. Also, there is increased cervical softening as pregnancy advances. Other conditions, however, such as estrogen–progestin contraceptives, may cause similar softening. As pregnancy progresses, the external cervical os and cervical canal may become sufficiently patulous to admit a fingertip, but the internal os should remain closed.

The substantial increase in progesterone secretion associated with pregnancy affects the consistency and microscopic appearance of cervical mucus. Specifically, microscopic observation of a fernlike pattern of mucus, which is typically seen in the midportion of the menstrual cycle, makes pregnancy unlikely (Fig. 4-2, p. 49).

Uterine Changes

During the first few weeks of pregnancy, uterine size grows principally in the anteroposterior diameter. During bimanual examination, it feels doughy or elastic. At 6 to 8 weeks' menstrual age, the firm cervix contrasts with the now softer fundus and the compressible interposed softened isthmus—*Hegar sign*. Isthmic softening may be so marked that the cervix and uterine body seem to be separate organs. By 12 weeks' gestation, the uterine body is almost globular, with an average diameter of 8 cm.

In later pregnancy, using a stethoscope for auscultation, one may hear the *uterine souffle*. This is a soft, blowing sound that is synchronous with the maternal pulse. It is produced by the passage of blood through the dilated uterine vessels and is heard most distinctly near the lower portion of the uterus. In contrast, the *funic souffle* is a sharp, whistling sound that is synchronous with the fetal pulse. It is caused by the rush of blood through the umbilical arteries and may not be heard consistently. Fetal heart tones can also be heard and are described on page 176.

Breast and Skin Changes

Anatomical changes in the breasts that accompany pregnancy are characteristic during a first pregnancy (Chap. 4, p. 50). These are less obvious in multiparas, whose breasts may contain a small amount of milky material or colostrum for months or even years after the birth of their last child, especially if the child was breast fed.

Increased pigmentation and visual changes in abdominal striae are common to, but not diagnostic of, pregnancy. They may be absent during pregnancy and may also be seen in women taking estrogen-containing contraceptives.

Fetal Movement

Maternal perception of fetal movement depends on factors such as parity and habitus. In general, after a first successful pregnancy, a woman may first perceive fetal movements between 16 and 18 weeks' gestation. A primigravida may not appreciate fetal movements until approximately 2 weeks later. At about 20 weeks, depending on maternal habitus, an examiner can begin to detect fetal movements.

Pregnancy Tests

Detection of hCG in maternal blood and urine is the basis for endocrine assays of pregnancy. This hormone is a glycoprotein with high carbohydrate content. There are subtle hCG variants, and these differ by their carbohydrate moieties. The general structure of hCG is a heterodimer composed of two dissimilar subunits, designated α and β, which are noncovalently linked. As described in Chapter 5 (p. 101), the α-subunit is identical to those of luteinizing hormone (LH), follicle-stimulating hormone (FSH), and thyroid-stimulating hormone (TSH). HCG prevents involution of the corpus luteum, which is the principal site of progesterone formation during the first 6 weeks of pregnancy.

Syncytiotrophoblast produce hCG in amounts that increase exponentially during the first trimester following implantation. With a sensitive test, the hormone can be detected in maternal serum or urine by 8 to 9 days after ovulation. The doubling time of serum hCG concentration is 1.4 to 2.0 days. As shown in Figure 9-2, serum hCG levels increase from the day of implantation and reach peak levels at 60 to 70 days. Thereafter, the concentration declines slowly until a plateau is reached at approximately 16 weeks.

Measurement of hCG

As noted, hCG is composed of both an α- and a β-subunit, but the β-subunit is structurally distinct from that of LH, FSH, and TSH. With this recognition, antibodies were developed with high specificity for the hCG β-subunit. This specificity allows its detection, and numerous commercial immunoassays are available for measuring serum and urine hCG levels. Although each immunoassay detects a slightly different mixture of hCG variants, its free subunits, or its metabolites, all are appropriate for pregnancy testing (Cole, 1998).

One commonly employed technique is the *sandwich-type immunoassay*. With this test, a monoclonal antibody against the β-subunit is bound to a solid-phase support. The attached antibody is then exposed to and binds hCG in the serum or urine specimen. A second antibody is then added, binds to another site on the hCG molecule, and "sandwiches" the bound hCG between the two antibodies. In some assays, the second antibody is linked to an enzyme, such as alkaline phosphatase. When substrate for the enzyme is added, a color develops. The color intensity is proportional to the amount of enzyme and thus to the amount of the second antibody bound. This, in turn, is a function of the hCG concentration in the test sample. The sensitivity for the laboratory detection of hCG in serum is as low as 1.0 mIU/mL using this technique. With extremely sensitive immunoradiometric assays, the detection limit is even lower (Wilcox, 2001).

False-positive hCG test results are rare (Braunstein, 2002). A few women have circulating serum factors that may bind erroneously with the test antibody directed to hCG in a given assay. The most common factors are heterophilic antibodies. These are produced by an individual and bind to the animal-derived test antibodies used in a given immunoassay. Thus, women who have worked closely

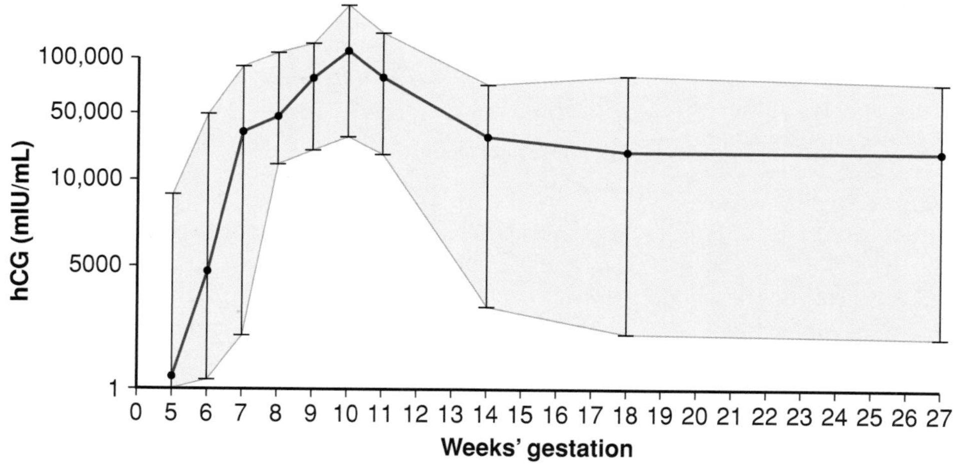

FIGURE 9-2 Mean concentration (95% CI) of human chorionic gonadotropin (hCG) in serum of women throughout normal pregnancy.

with animals are more likely to develop such antibodies, and alternative laboratory techniques are available (American College of Obstetricians and Gynecologists, 2013a). Elevated hCG levels may also reflect molar pregnancy and its associated cancers (Chap. 20, p. 396). Other rare causes of positive assays without pregnancy are: (1) exogenous hCG injection used for weight loss, (2) renal failure with impaired hCG clearance, (3) physiological pituitary hCG, and (4) hCG-producing tumors that most commonly originate from gastrointestinal sites, ovary, bladder, or lung (Montagnana, 2011).

Home Pregnancy Tests

Millions of over-the-counter pregnancy test kits are sold annually in the United States. In one study, Cole and associates (2011) found that a detection limit of 12.5 mIU/mL would be required to diagnose 95 percent of pregnancies at the time of missed menses. They noted that only one brand had this degree of sensitivity. Two other brands gave false-positive or invalid results. In fact, with an hCG concentration of 100 mIU/mL, clearly positive results were displayed by only 44 percent of brands. As such, only about 15 percent of pregnancies could be diagnosed at the time of the missed menses. Some manufacturers of even newer home urine assays claim > 99-percent accuracy on the day of—and some up to 4 days before—the expected day of menses. But, careful analysis suggests that these assays are often not as sensitive as advertised (Cole, 2011).

Sonographic Recognition of Pregnancy

Transvaginal sonography has revolutionized early pregnancy imaging and is commonly used to accurately establish gestational age and confirm pregnancy location. A *gestational sac*—a small anechoic fluid collection within the endometrial cavity—is the first sonographic evidence of pregnancy. It may be seen with transvaginal sonography by 4 to 5 weeks' gestation. A fluid collection, however, can also be seen within the endometrial cavity with an ectopic pregnancy and is termed a *pseudogestational sac* or *pseudosac* (Fig. 19-5, p. 382). Thus, further evaluation may be warranted if this is the only sonographic finding, particularly in a patient with pain or bleeding. A normal gestational sac implants eccentrically in the endometrium, whereas a pseudosac is seen in the midline of the endometrial cavity. Other potential indicators of early intrauterine pregnancy are an anechoic center surrounded by a single echogenic rim—the *intradecidual sign*—or two concentric echogenic rings surrounding the gestational sac—the *double decidual sign* (Fig. 9-3) (Chiang, 2004). If sonography yields equivocal findings—the so-called *pregnancy of unknown location*, then serial serum hCG levels can also help differentiate a normal intrauterine pregnancy from an extrauterine pregnancy or an early miscarriage (Chap. 19, p. 381).

Visualization of the *yolk sac*—a brightly echogenic ring with an anechoic center—confirms with certainty an intrauterine location for the pregnancy and can normally be seen by the middle of the fifth week. As shown in Figure 9-3, after 6 weeks, an embryo is seen as a linear structure immediately adjacent to the yolk sac, and cardiac motion is typically noted at this point. Up to 12 weeks' gestation, the crown-rump length is predictive of gestational age within 4 days (Chap. 10, p. 195).

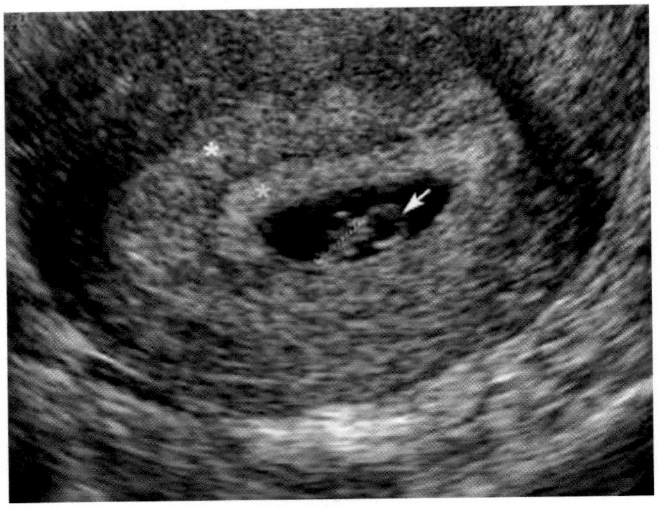

FIGURE 9-3 Transvaginal sonogram of a first-trimester intrauterine pregnancy. The double decidual sign is noted surrounding the gestational sac and is defined by the decidua parietalis (*white asterisk*) and the decidua capsularis (*yellow asterisk*). The arrow notes the yolk sac, and the crown-rump length of the embryo is marked with measuring calipers. (Image contributed by Dr. Elysia Moschos.)

INITIAL PRENATAL EVALUATION

Prenatal care should be initiated as soon as there is a reasonable likelihood of pregnancy. Major goals are to: (1) define the health status of the mother and fetus, (2) estimate the gestational age, and (3) initiate a plan for continuing obstetrical care. Typical components of the initial visit are summarized in Table 9-2. The initial plan for subsequent care may range from relatively infrequent routine visits to prompt hospitalization because of serious maternal or fetal disease.

Prenatal Record

Use of a standardized record within a perinatal health-care system greatly aids antepartum and intrapartum management. Standardizing documentation may allow communication and care continuity between providers and enable objective measures of care quality to be evaluated over time and across different clinical settings (Gregory, 2006). A prototype is provided by the American Academy of Pediatrics and the American College of Obstetricians and Gynecologists (2012) in their *Guidelines for Perinatal Care, 7th edition.*

Definitions

There are several definitions pertinent to establishment of an accurate prenatal record.

1. *Nulligravida*—a woman who currently is not pregnant nor has ever been pregnant.
2. *Gravida*—a woman who currently is pregnant or has been in the past, irrespective of the pregnancy outcome. With the establishment of the first pregnancy, she becomes a *primigravida,* and with successive pregnancies, a *multigravida.*
3. *Nullipara*—a woman who has never completed a pregnancy beyond 20 weeks' gestation. She may not have been pregnant or may have had a spontaneous or elective abortion(s) or an ectopic pregnancy.

TABLE 9-2. Typical Components of Routine Prenatal Care

	Text Referral	First Visit	Weeks 15–20	Weeks 24–28	Weeks 29–41
History					
Complete	Chap. 9, p. 172	•			
Updated			•	•	•
Physical examination					
Complete	Chap. 9, p. 174	•			
Blood pressure	Chap. 40, p. 729	•	•	•	•
Maternal weight	Chap. 9, p. 177	•	•	•	•
Pelvic/cervical examination	Chap. 9, p. 174	•			
Fundal height	Chap. 9, p. 176	•	•	•	•
Fetal heart rate/fetal position	Chap. 9, p. 176	•	•	•	•
Laboratory tests					
Hematocrit or hemoglobin	Chap. 56, p. 1101	•		•	
Blood type and Rh factor	Chap. 15, p. 307	•			
Antibody screen	Chap. 15, p. 307	•		A	
Pap smear screening	Chap. 63, p. 1221	•			
Glucose tolerance test	Chap. 57, p. 1137			•	
Fetal aneuploidy screening	Chap. 14, p. 288	B[a] and/or	B		
Neural-tube defect screening	Chap. 14, p. 283		B		
Cystic fibrosis screening	Chap. 14, p. 295	B or	B		
Urine protein assessment	Chap. 4, p. 65	•			
Urine culture	Chap. 53, p. 1053	•			
Rubella serology	Chap. 64, p. 1243	•			
Syphilis serology	Chap. 65, p. 1265	•			C
Gonococcal screening	Chap. 65, p. 1269	D			D
Chlamydial screening	Chap. 65, p. 1270	•			C
Hepatitis B serology	Chap. 55, p. 1090	•			D
HIV serology	Chap. 65, p. 1276	B			D
Group B streptococcus culture	Chap. 64, p. 1249				E
Tuberculosis screening[b]	Chap. 51, p. 1020				

[a]First-trimester aneuploidy screening may be offered between 11 and 14 weeks.
[b]Screening can be done with either the Mantoux tuberculin skin test or a tuberculosis blood test as clinically indicated at any visit.
A Performed at 28 weeks, if indicated.
B Test should be offered.
C High-risk women should be retested at the beginning of the third trimester.
D High-risk women should be screened at the first prenatal visit and again in the third trimester.
E Rectovaginal culture should be obtained between 35 and 37 weeks.
HIV = human immunodeficiency virus.

4. *Primipara*—a woman who has been delivered only once of a fetus or fetuses born alive or dead with an estimated length of gestation of 20 or more weeks. In the past, a 500-g birthweight threshold was used to define parity. As discussed in Chapter 1 (p. 2), this threshold is now controversial because many states still use this weight to differentiate a stillborn fetus from an abortus. However, the survival of neonates with birthweights < 500 g is no longer uncommon.
5. *Multipara*—a woman who has completed two or more pregnancies to 20 weeks' gestation or more. Parity is determined by the number of pregnancies reaching 20 weeks. It is not increased to a higher number if multiples are delivered in a given pregnancy. Moreover, stillbirth does not lower this number. In some locales, the obstetrical history is summarized by a series of digits connected by dashes. These refer to the number of term infants, preterm infants, abortuses younger than 20 weeks, and children currently alive. For example, a woman who is para 2–1–0–3 has had two term deliveries, one preterm delivery, no abortuses, and has three living children. Because these are nonconventional, it is helpful to specify the outcome of any pregnancy that did not end normally.

Normal Pregnancy Duration

The mean duration of pregnancy calculated from the first day of the last normal menstrual period is very close to 280 days or 40 weeks. In a study of 427,581 singleton pregnancies from the Swedish Birth Registry, Bergsjø and coworkers (1990) found that the mean pregnancy duration was 281 days with a standard deviation of 13 days.

It is customary to estimate the expected delivery date by adding 7 days to the date of the first day of the last normal menstrual period and counting back 3 months—*Naegele rule.* For example, if the last menstrual period began September 10, the expected date of delivery is June 17. However, a *gestational age* or *menstrual age* calculated in this way assumes pregnancy to have begun approximately 2 weeks before ovulation, which is not always the case.

Clinicians use this gestational age to mark temporal events during pregnancy. In contrast, embryologists and other reproductive biologists more often employ *ovulatory age* or *fertilization age,* both of which are typically 2 weeks earlier. Somewhat related, Bracken and Belanger (1989) tested the accuracy of various "pregnancy wheels" provided by three pharmaceutical companies and found that such devices predicted incorrect delivery dates in 40 to 60 percent of estimates, with a 5-day error being typical. As physicians and hospitals increasingly transition to electronic medical records, however, such errors should be largely obviated by more precise estimates of gestational age produced by calculator software applications.

Trimesters

It has become customary to divide pregnancy into three equal epochs of approximately 3 calendar months. Historically, the first trimester extends through completion of 14 weeks, the second through 28 weeks, and the third includes the 29th through 42nd weeks of pregnancy. Thus, there are three periods of 14 weeks each. Certain major obstetrical problems tend to cluster in each of these time periods. For example, most spontaneous abortions take place during the first trimester, whereas most women with hypertensive disorders due to pregnancy are diagnosed during the third trimester.

In modern obstetrics, the clinical use of trimesters to describe a specific pregnancy is imprecise. For example, it is inappropriate in cases of uterine hemorrhage to categorize the problem temporally as "third-trimester bleeding." Appropriate management for the mother and her fetus will vary remarkably depending on whether bleeding begins early or late in the third trimester (Chap. 41, p. 782). Because precise knowledge of fetal age is imperative for ideal obstetrical management, the clinically appropriate unit is *weeks of gestation completed.* And more recently, clinicians designate gestational age using completed weeks and days, for example, $33^{4/7}$ weeks or 33 + 4, for 33 completed weeks and 4 days.

Previous and Current Health Status

For the most part, the same essentials go into appropriate history taking from the pregnant woman as elsewhere in medicine. In addition to queries concerning medical or surgical disorders, detailed information regarding previous pregnancies is essential as many obstetrical complications tend to recur in subsequent pregnancies.

The *menstrual history* is also important. The woman who spontaneously menstruates approximately every 28 days is most likely to ovulate at midcycle. Thus, gestational or menstrual age is the number of weeks since the onset of the last menstrual period. If her menstrual cycles were significantly longer than 28 to 30 days, ovulation more likely occurred well beyond 14 days. If the intervals were much longer and irregular, chronic anovulation is likely to have preceded some of the episodes identified as menses. Thus, without a history of regular, predictable, cyclic, spontaneous menses that suggest ovulatory cycles, accurate dating of pregnancy by history and physical examination is difficult.

It is also important to ascertain whether or not steroidal contraceptives were used before the pregnancy. Because ovulation may not have resumed 2 weeks after the onset of the last withdrawal bleeding and instead may have occurred at an appreciably later and highly variable date, using the time of ovulation for predicting the time of conception in this circumstance may be erroneous. Use of sonography in early pregnancy will clarify gestational age in these situations.

Psychosocial Screening

The American Academy of Pediatrics and the American College of Obstetricians and Gynecologists (2012) define psychosocial issues as nonbiomedical factors that affect mental and physical well-being. Women should be screened regardless of social status, education level, race, or ethnicity. Such screening should seek barriers to care, communication obstacles, nutritional status, unstable housing, desire for pregnancy, safety concerns that include intimate partner violence, depression, stress, and use of substances such as tobacco, alcohol, and illicit drugs. This screening should be performed on a regular basis, at least once per trimester, to identify important issues and reduce adverse pregnancy outcomes. Coker and colleagues (2012) compared pregnancy outcomes in women before and after implementation of a universal psychosocial screening program and found that screened women were less likely to have preterm or low-birthweight newborns. Although this study was observational, these investigators also reported decreased rates of gestational diabetes, premature rupture of membranes, and vaginal bleeding in women who underwent universal screening.

Cigarette Smoking

There are unequivocal adverse perinatal sequelae for smoking (United States Department of Health and Human Services, 2000). Such data have been included on the birth certificate since 1989. The number of pregnant women who smoke continues to decline. From 2000 to 2010, the prevalences were 12 to 13 percent (Tong, 2013). Based on the Pregnancy Risk Assessment Monitoring System (PRAMS), 13 percent of women admitted to smoking. These women were more likely younger, had less education, and were either Alaska Natives or American Indians (Centers for Disease Control and Prevention, 2012b).

Numerous adverse outcomes have been linked to smoking during pregnancy. Potential teratogenic effects are reviewed in Chapter 12 (p. 255). There is a twofold risk of placenta previa, placental abruption, and premature membrane rupture compared with nonsmokers. Further, neonates born to women who smoke are more likely to be preterm, have lower birthweights, and are more likely to die of sudden infant death syndrome (SIDS) than infants born to nonsmokers (Tong, 2009). In 2005, the incidence of low-birthweight infants born to American women who smoked during pregnancy was 11.9 percent compared with 7.5 percent born to nonsmokers (Martin, 2007). Risks for spontaneous abortion, fetal death, and fetal digital anomalies are also increased (Man, 2006). Finally, children who were exposed to smoking in utero are at increased risk for asthma, infantile colic, and childhood obesity (American College of Obstetricians and Gynecologists, 2013i).

Several pathophysiological mechanisms have been proposed to explain these adverse outcomes. They include fetal hypoxia from increased carboxyhemoglobin, reduced uteroplacental blood flow, and direct toxic effects of nicotine and other compounds in smoke (Jazayeri, 1998). Nicotine transfer is so efficient that fetal nicotine exposure is greater than that of the mother (Luck, 1985). Exposed fetuses have decreased heart rate variability due to impaired autonomic regulation (Zeskind, 2006).

Smoking Cessation. The United States Department of Health and Human Services recommends that clinicians offer counseling and effective intervention options to pregnant smokers at the first and subsequent prenatal visits. Although benefits are greatest if smoking ceases early in pregnancy or preferably preconceptionally, quitting at any stage of pregnancy can improve perinatal outcomes (England, 2001; Fiore, 2008).

Person-to-person psychosocial interventions are significantly more successful in achieving smoking abstinence in pregnancy than are simple advisements to quit (Fiore, 2008). One example is a brief counseling session covering the "5As" of smoking cessation (Table 9-3). This approach to counseling can be accomplished in 15 minutes or less and has been proven to be effective when initiated by health-care providers (American College of Obstetricians and Gynecologists, 2013i).

Nicotine replacement products have not been sufficiently evaluated to determine their effectiveness and safety in pregnancy. Trials evaluating such therapy have yielded conflicting evidence. Wisborg and colleagues (2000) randomly assigned 250 women who smoked at least 10 cigarettes per day to receive a nicotine or placebo patch beginning after the first trimester. There were no significant differences in birthweights or in smoking cessation or preterm delivery rates between the two groups. Pollak and associates (2007) randomized 181 pregnant smokers to cognitive-behavioral therapy alone versus this therapy plus nicotine replacement. They identified significantly improved smoking cessation rates in the women with nicotine replacement at 7 weeks after randomization and at 38 weeks' gestation. The trial was terminated early due to an increased rate of negative birth outcomes in the nicotine replacement arm. Some of these included neonatal intensive care unit admission, small-for-gestational age, and placental abruption. Because of limited available evidence to support pharmacotherapy for smoking cessation in pregnancy, the American College of Obstetricians and Gynecologists (2013i) has recommended that if nicotine replacement therapy is used, it should be done with close supervision and after careful consideration of the risks of smoking versus nicotine replacement.

TABLE 9-3. Five A's of Smoking Cessation

ASK about smoking at the first and subsequent prenatal visits. To improve assessment accuracy, a patient should choose the following statement that best describes her smoking status:
- I smoke regularly now; the same as before pregnancy.
- I smoke regularly now, but I've cut down with pregnancy. I smoke every once in a while.
- I have quit smoking since pregnancy.
- I wasn't smoking before pregnancy, and I do not currently smoke.
- If smoking abstinence has already begun, then reinforce her decision to quit, congratulate her on success, and encourage her continued abstinence. For persistent smokers, proceed to the following steps:

ADVISE with clear, strong statements that explain the risks of continued smoking to the woman, fetus, and newborn.

ASSESS the patient's willingness to attempt cessation.

ASSIST with pregnancy-specific, self-help smoking cessation materials. Offer a direct referral to the smoker's quit line (1-800-QUIT NOW) to provide ongoing counseling and support.

ARRANGE to track smoking abstinence progress at subsequent visits.

Adapted from Fiore, 2008.

Alcohol

Ethyl alcohol or ethanol is a potent teratogen that causes a fetal syndrome characterized by growth restriction, facial abnormalities, and central nervous system dysfunction (Chap. 12, p. 245). Women who are pregnant or considering pregnancy should abstain from using any alcoholic beverages. The Centers for Disease Control and Prevention (2012a) analyzed data from the Behavioral Risk Factor Surveillance System from 2006 to 2010 and estimated that 7.6 percent of pregnant women used alcohol and 1.4 percent reported binge drinking. By comparison, in 1999, rates of alcohol use and binge drinking were estimated to be 12.8 and 2.7 percent, respectively (Centers for Disease Control and Prevention, 2002). Among pregnant women, those most likely to use alcohol were aged 35 to 44 years, white, college graduates, or employed. The American College of Obstetricians and Gynecologists (2008), in their committee opinion on this topic, has reviewed methods for screening women during pregnancy for alcohol abuse and for illicit drug use.

Illicit Drugs

It is estimated that 10 percent of fetuses are exposed to one or more illicit drugs (American Academy of Pediatrics and the American College of Obstetricians and Gynecologists, 2012). Agents may include heroin and other opiates, cocaine, amphetamines, barbiturates, and marijuana. Chronic use of large quantities is harmful to the fetus (Chap. 12, p. 253). Well-documented sequelae include fetal-growth restriction, low birthweight, and drug withdrawal soon after birth. Women who use such drugs frequently do not seek prenatal care, or if they do, they may not admit to substance abuse. El-Mohandes and associates (2003) reported that when women who use illicit drugs receive prenatal care, the risks for preterm birth and low birthweight are reduced.

For women who abuse heroin, methadone maintenance can be initiated within a registered methadone treatment program to reduce complications of illicit opioid use and narcotic withdrawal, to encourage prenatal care, and to avoid drug culture risks (American College of Obstetricians and Gynecologists, 2012c). Available programs can be found through the treatment locator of the Substance Abuse and Mental Health Services Administration at www.samhsa.gov. Methadone dosages usually are initiated at 10 to 30 mg daily and titrated as needed. Although less commonly used, buprenorphine alone or in combination with naloxone may also be offered and managed by physicians with specific credentialing.

Intimate Partner Violence

This term refers to a pattern of assaultive and coercive behaviors that may include physical injury, psychological abuse, sexual assault, progressive isolation, stalking, deprivation, intimidation, and reproductive coercion (American College of Obstetricians and Gynecologists, 2012a). Such violence has been recognized as a major public health problem. Unfortunately, most abused women continue to be victimized during pregnancy. With the possible exception of preeclampsia, domestic violence is more prevalent than any major medical condition detectable through routine prenatal screening (American Academy of Pediatrics and the American College of Obstetricians and Gynecologists, 2012). The prevalence during pregnancy is estimated to be between 4 and 8 percent. As discussed in Chapter 47 (p. 951), intimate partner violence is associated with an increased risk of several adverse perinatal outcomes including preterm delivery, fetal-growth restriction, and perinatal death.

The American College of Obstetricians and Gynecologists (2012a) has provided methods for domestic violence screening and recommends their use at the first prenatal visit, then again at least once per trimester, and again at the postpartum visit. Such screening should be done privately and away from family members and friends. Patient self-administered or computerized screenings appear to be as effective for disclosure as clinician-directed interviews (Ahmad, 2009; Chen, 2007). Physicians should be familiar with state laws that may require reporting of intimate partner violence. Coordination with social services can be invaluable in such cases. The National Domestic Violence Hotline (1–800–799-SAFE [7233]) is a nonprofit telephone referral service that provides individualized information regarding city-specific women's shelter locations, counseling resources, and legal advocacy.

Clinical Evaluation

A thorough, general physical examination should be completed at the initial prenatal encounter. Many of the expected changes that result from normal pregnancy are addressed throughout Chapter 4 (p. 46).

Pelvic examination is performed as part of the evaluation. The cervix is visualized employing a speculum lubricated with warm water or water-based lubricant gel. Bluish-red passive hyperemia of the cervix is characteristic, but not of itself diagnostic, of pregnancy. Dilated, occluded cervical glands bulging beneath the ectocervical mucosa—*nabothian cysts*—may be prominent. The cervix is not normally dilated except at the external os. To identify cytological abnormalities, a Pap smear is performed according to current guidelines noted in Chapter 63 (p. 1221). Specimens for identification of *Chlamydia trachomatis* and *Neisseria gonorrhoeae* are also obtained when indicated (p. 175).

Bimanual examination is completed by palpation, with special attention given to the consistency, length, and dilatation of the cervix; to uterine and adnexal size; to the bony pelvic architecture; and to any vaginal or perineal anomalies. Later in pregnancy, fetal presentation often can also be determined. Lesions of the cervix, vagina, or vulva should be further evaluated as needed by colposcopy, biopsy, culture, or dark-field examination. The perianal region should be visualized, and digital rectal examination performed as required for complaints of rectal pain, bleeding, or mass.

Gestational Age Assessment

Precise knowledge of gestational age is one of the most important aspects of prenatal care because several pregnancy complications may develop for which optimal treatment will depend on fetal age. Gestational age can be estimated with considerable precision by appropriately timed and carefully performed clinical uterine size examination that is coupled with knowledge of the last menses. Uterine size similar to a small orange roughly correlates with a 6-week gestation; a large orange, with an 8-week pregnancy; and a grapefruit, with one at 12 weeks (Margulies, 2001). That said, a first-trimester crown-rump length is the most accurate tool for gestational age assignment and is performed as clinically indicated. As described in Chapter 10 (p. 198), later sonographic interrogation can also provide an estimated gestational age, but with declining accuracy.

Laboratory Tests

Recommended routine tests at the first prenatal encounter are listed in Table 9-2. Initial blood tests include a complete blood count, a determination of blood type with Rh status, and an antibody screen. The Institute of Medicine recommends universal human immunodeficiency virus (HIV) testing, with patient notification and right of refusal, as a routine part of prenatal care. The Centers for Disease Control and Prevention (2006) as well as the American Academy of Pediatrics and the American College of Obstetricians and Gynecologists (2012) continue to support this practice. If a woman declines testing, this should be recorded in the prenatal record. All pregnant women should also be screened for hepatitis B virus, syphilis, and immunity to rubella at the initial visit. Based on their prospective investigation of 1000 women, Murray and coworkers (2002) concluded that in the absence of hypertension, routine urinalysis beyond the first prenatal visit was not necessary. A urine culture is performed because treating asymptomatic bacteruria significantly reduces the likelihood of developing symptomatic urinary tract infections in pregnancy (Chap. 53, p. 1053).

Cervical Infections

Chlamydia trachomatis is isolated from the cervix in 2 to 13 percent of pregnant women. The American Academy of Pediatrics and the American College of Obstetricians and Gynecologists (2012) recommend that all women be screened for chlamydia during the first prenatal visit, with additional third-trimester testing for those at increased risk. Risk factors include unmarried status, recent change in sexual partner or multiple concurrent partners, age younger than 25 years, inner-city residence, history or presence of other sexually transmitted diseases, and little or no prenatal care. Following treatment, a second testing—a so-called *test of cure*—is recommended in pregnancy 3 to 4 weeks after treatment completion (Chap. 65, p. 1270).

Neisseria gonorrhoeae is the gram-negative diplococcal bacteria responsible for causing gonorrhea. Risk factors for gonorrhea are similar for those for chlamydial infection. The American Academy of Pediatrics and the American College of Obstetricians and Gynecologists (2012) recommend that pregnant women with risk factors or those living in an area of high *N gonorrhoeae* prevalence be screened at the initial prenatal visit and again in the third trimester. Treatment is given for gonorrhea as well as possible coexisting chlamydial infection, as outlined in Chapter 65 (p. 1269). Test of cure is also recommended following treatment.

Pregnancy Risk Assessment

Many factors exist that can adversely affect maternal and/or fetal well-being. Some are evident at conception, but many become apparent during the course of pregnancy. The designation of "high-risk pregnancy" is overly vague for an individual patient and probably should be avoided if a more specific diagnosis has been assigned. Some common risk factors for which consultation is recommended by the American Academy of Pediatrics and the American College of Obstetricians and Gynecologists (2012) are shown in Table 9-4. Some conditions may require the involvement of a maternal-fetal medicine subspecialist, geneticist, pediatrician, anesthesiologist, or other medical specialist in the evaluation, counseling, and care of the woman and her fetus.

TABLE 9-4. Conditions for Which Maternal-Fetal Medicine Consultation May Be Beneficial

Medical History and Conditions
Cardiac disease—including cyanotic, prior myocardial infarction, moderate to severe valvular stenosis or regurgitation, Marfan syndrome, prosthetic valve, American Heart Association class II or greater
Diabetes mellitus with evidence of end-organ damage or uncontrolled hyperglycemia
Family or personal history of genetic abnormalities
Hemoglobinopathy
Chronic hypertension if uncontrolled or associated with renal or cardiac disease
Renal insufficiency if associated with significant proteinuria ($\geq$ 500 mg/24 hour), serum creatinine $\geq$ 1.5 mg/dL, or hypertension
Pulmonary disease if severe restrictive or obstructive, including severe asthma
Human immunodeficiency virus infection
Prior pulmonary embolus or deep-vein thrombosis
Severe systemic disease, including autoimmune conditions
Bariatric surgery
Epilepsy if poorly controlled or requires more than one anticonvulsant
Cancer, especially if treatment is indicated in pregnancy
Obstetrical History and Conditions
CDE (Rh) or other blood group alloimmunization (excluding ABO, Lewis)
Prior or current fetal structural or chromosomal abnormality
Desire or need for prenatal diagnosis or fetal therapy
Periconceptional exposure to known teratogens
Infection with or exposure to organisms that cause congenital infection
Higher-order multifetal gestation
Severe disorders of amnionic fluid volume

SUBSEQUENT PRENATAL VISITS

Subsequent prenatal visits have been traditionally scheduled at 4-week intervals until 28 weeks, then every 2 weeks until 36 weeks, and weekly thereafter. Women with complicated pregnancies often require return visits at 1- to 2-week intervals. For example, in twin pregnancies, Luke and colleagues (2003) found that a specialized prenatal care program emphasizing nutrition and education and requiring return visits every 2 weeks resulted in improved outcomes.

In 1986, the Department of Health and Human Services convened an expert panel to review the content of prenatal care. This report was subsequently reevaluated and revised in 2005 (Gregory, 2006). The panel recommended, among other things, early and continuing risk assessment that is patient specific. It also endorsed flexibility in clinical visit spacing; health promotion and education, including preconceptional care; medical and psychosocial interventions; standardized documentation; and expanded prenatal care objectives—to include family health up to 1 year after birth.

The World Health Organization (WHO) conducted a multicenter randomized trial with almost 25,000 women comparing routine prenatal care with an experimental model designed to minimize visits (Villar, 2001). In the new model, women were seen once in the first trimester and screened for certain risks. Those without anticipated complications—80 percent of those screened—were seen again at 26, 32, and 38 weeks. Compared with routine prenatal care, which required a median of eight visits, the new model required a median of only five. No disadvantages were attributed to the regimen with fewer visits, and these findings were consistent with other randomized trials (Clement, 1999; McDuffie, 1996).

Prenatal Surveillance

At each return visit, the well-being of mother and fetus are assessed (see Table 9-2). Fetal heart rate, growth, amnionic fluid volume, and activity are evaluated. Maternal blood pressure and weight and their extent of change are assessed. Symptoms such as headache, altered vision, abdominal pain, nausea and vomiting, bleeding, vaginal fluid leakage, and dysuria are sought. Uterine examination measures size from the symphysis to the fundus. In late pregnancy, vaginal examination often provides valuable information that includes confirmation of the presenting part and its station, clinical estimation of pelvic capacity and its general configuration, amnionic fluid volume adequacy, and cervical consistency, effacement, and dilatation (Chap. 22, p. 438).

Fundal Height

Between 20 and 34 weeks, the height of the uterine fundus measured in centimeters correlates closely with gestational age in weeks (Calvert, 1982; Jimenez, 1983; Quaranta, 1981). This measurement is used to monitor fetal growth and amnionic fluid volume. It is measured as the distance along the abdominal wall from the top of the symphysis pubis to the top of the fundus. Importantly, the bladder must be emptied before fundal measurement. Worthen and Bustillo (1980) demonstrated that at 17 to 20 weeks, fundal height was 3 cm higher with a full bladder. Obesity or the presence of uterine masses such as leiomyomata may also limit fundal height accuracy. In such cases, sonography may be necessary for assessment. Moreover, using fundal height alone, fetal-growth restriction may be undiagnosed in up to a third of cases (American College of Obstetricians and Gynecologists, 2013b).

Fetal Heart Sounds

Instruments incorporating Doppler ultrasound are often used to easily detect fetal heart action, and in the absence of maternal obesity, heart sounds are almost always detectable by 10 weeks with such instruments (Chap. 24, p. 474). The fetal heart rate ranges from 110 to 160 beats per minute and is typically heard as a double sound.

Using a standard nonamplified stethoscope, the fetal heart may be audible as early as 16 weeks in some women. Herbert and coworkers (1987) reported that the fetal heart was audible by 20 weeks in 80 percent of women, and by 22 weeks, heart sounds were heard in all. Because the fetus moves freely in amnionic fluid, the site on the maternal abdomen where fetal heart sounds can be heard best will vary.

Sonography

As described in detail in Chapter 10 (p. 199), sonography provides invaluable information regarding fetal anatomy, growth, and well-being, and most women in the United States have at least one prenatal sonographic examination during pregnancy (American College of Obstetricians and Gynecologists, 2011b). Recent trends suggest that the number of these examinations performed per pregnancy is increasing. Siddique and associates (2009) reported that the average number of sonographic evaluations per pregnancy increased from 1.5 in 1995 through 1997 to 2.7 almost 10 years later. This trend was noted in both high- and low-risk pregnancies. The actual clinical utility of increasing sonography use in pregnancy has not been demonstrated, and it is unclear that the cost-benefit ratio is justified (Washington State Health Care Authority, 2010). The American College of Obstetricians and Gynecologists (2011b) has concluded that sonography should be performed only when there is a valid medical indication under the lowest possible ultrasound exposure setting. The College further indicates that a physician is not obligated to perform sonography without a specific indication in a low-risk patient, but that if she requests sonographic screening, it is reasonable to honor her request.

Subsequent Laboratory Tests

If initial results were normal, most tests need not be repeated. Fetal aneuploidy screening may be performed at 11 to 14 weeks and/or at 15 to 20 weeks, depending on the protocol selected as described in Chapter 14. Serum screening for neural-tube defects is offered at 15 to 20 weeks (Chap. 14, p. 284). Hematocrit or hemoglobin determination, along with syphilis serology if it is prevalent in the population, should be repeated at 28 to 32 weeks (Hollier, 2003; Kiss, 2004). For women at increased risk for HIV acquisition during pregnancy, repeat testing is recommended in the third trimester, preferably before 36 weeks' gestation (American College of Obstetricians and Gynecologists, 2011a). Similarly, women who engage in behaviors that place them at high risk for hepatitis B infection should be retested at the time of hospitalization for delivery (American Academy of Pediatrics and the American College of Obstetricians and Gynecologists, 2012). Women who are D (Rh) negative and are unsensitized should have an antibody screening test repeated at 28 to 29 weeks, with administration of anti-D immune globulin if they remain unsensitized (Chap. 15, p. 311).

Group B Streptococcal Infection

The Centers for Disease Control and Prevention (2010b) recommend that vaginal and rectal group B streptococcal (GBS) cultures be obtained in all women between 35 and 37 weeks' gestation, and the American College of Obstetricians and Gynecologists (2013g) has endorsed this recommendation. Intrapartum antimicrobial prophylaxis is given for those whose cultures are positive. Women with GBS bacteriuria or a previous infant with invasive disease are given empirical intrapartum prophylaxis. These infections are discussed in detail in Chapter 64 (p. 1249).

Gestational Diabetes

All pregnant women should be screened for gestational diabetes mellitus, whether by history, clinical factors, or routine laboratory testing. Although laboratory testing between 24 and 28 weeks' gestation is the most sensitive approach, there may be pregnant women at low risk who are less likely to benefit from testing (American Academy of Pediatrics and the American College of Obstetricians and Gynecologists, 2012). Gestational diabetes is discussed in Chapter 57 (p. 1136).

Selected Genetic Screening

Selected screening for certain genetic abnormalities should be offered to those at increased risk based on family history, ethnic or racial background, or age (American College of Obstetricians and Gynecologists, 2009c, 2011c, 2013h). These are discussed in greater detail in Chapters 13 (p. 275) and 14 (p. 294). Some examples include testing for Tay-Sachs disease for persons of Eastern European Jewish or French Canadian ancestry; β-thalassemia for those of Mediterranean, Southeast Asian, Indian, Pakistani, or African ancestry; α-thalassemia for individuals of Southeast Asian or African ancestry; sickle-cell anemia for people of African, Mediterranean, Middle Eastern, Caribbean, Latin American, or Indian descent; and trisomy 21 for those with advanced maternal age.

NUTRITIONAL COUNSELING

Weight Gain Recommendations

For the first half of the 20th century, it was recommended that weight gain during pregnancy be limited to less than 20 lb or about 9 kg. It was believed that such restriction would prevent gestational hypertension and fetal macrosomia. By the 1970s, however, women were encouraged to gain at least 25 lb or 11 to 12 kg to prevent preterm birth and fetal-growth restriction, a recommendation supported by subsequent research (Ehrenberg, 2003). The Institute of Medicine and National Research Council (2009) revised its guidelines for weight gain in pregnancy and continues to stratify suggested weight gain ranges based on prepregnancy body mass index (BMI) (Table 9-5). BMI can easily be calculated with commonly available graphs (Fig. 48-1, p. 962). Of note, the new guidelines include a specific, relatively narrow range of recommended weight gains for obese women. Also, the same recommendations apply to adolescents, short women, and women of all racial and ethnic groups. The American Academy of Pediatrics and the American College of Obstetricians and Gynecologists (2012) have endorsed these guidelines.

As emphasized by Catalano (2007), when the Institute of Medicine guidelines were formulated, concern focused on low-birthweight newborns. Current emphasis now, however, is on the obesity epidemic. This likely explains renewed interest in *lower* weight gains during pregnancy. As discussed in Chapter 48 (p. 965), obesity is associated with significantly increased risks for gestational hypertension, preeclampsia, gestational diabetes, macrosomia, cesarean delivery, and other complications. The risk appears "dose related" to prenatal weight gain. In a population-based cohort of more than 120,000 obese pregnant women, Kiel and associates (2007) found that those who gained *less than 15 pounds* had the lowest rates of preeclampsia, large-for-gestational age neonates, and cesarean delivery. Among 100,000 women with normal prepregnancy BMI, DeVader and colleagues (2007) found that those who gained less than 25 pounds during pregnancy had a lower risk for preeclampsia, failed induction, cephalopelvic disproportion, cesarean delivery, and large-for-gestational age infants. This cohort, however, had an increased risk for small-for-gestational age newborns.

There is irrefutable evidence that maternal weight gain during pregnancy influences birthweight. Martin and coworkers (2009) studied this using birth certificate data for 2006. As shown in Figure 9-4, 60 percent of pregnant women gained 26 lb or more. Maternal weight gain had a positive correlation with birthweight. Moreover, women with the greatest risk—14 percent—for delivering an infant weighing < 2500 g were those with weight gain < 16 lb. Nearly 20 percent of births to women with such low weight gains were preterm.

TABLE 9-5. Recommendations for Total and Rate of Weight Gain During Pregnancy, by Prepregnancy BMI[a]

Category (BMI)	Total Weight Gain Range (lb)	Weight Gain in 2nd and 3rd Trimesters Mean in lb/wk (range)
Underweight (< 18.5)	28–40	1 (1–1.3)
Normal weight (18.5–24.9)	25–35	1 (0.8–1)
Overweight (25.0–29.9)	15–25	0.6 (0.5–0.7)
Obese (≥ 30.0)	11–20	0.5 (0.4–0.6)

[a]Empirical recommendations for weight gain in twin pregnancies include: normal BMI, 37–54 lb; overweight women, 31–50 lb; and obese women, 25–42 lb.
BMI = body mass index.
Modified from the Institute of Medicine and National Research Council, 2009.

Severe Undernutrition

Meaningful studies of nutrition in human pregnancy are exceedingly difficult to design because experimental dietary deficiency is not ethical. In those instances in which severe nutritional

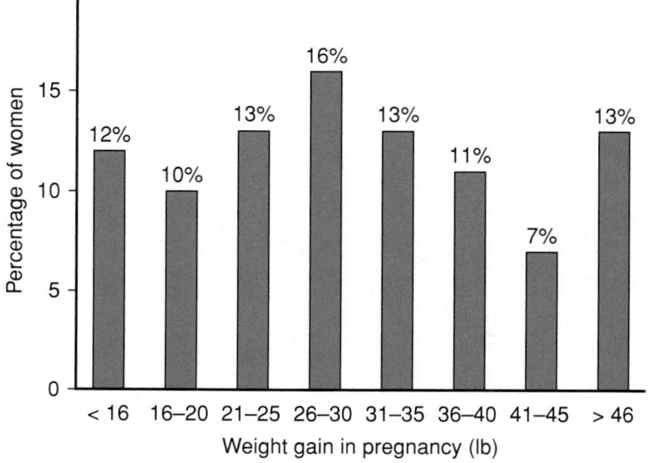

FIGURE 9-4 Percentage distribution of maternal weight gain in the United States reported on 2006 birth certificates. (From Martin, 2009.)

deficiencies have been induced as a consequence of social, economic, or political disaster, coincidental events have often created many variables, the effects of which are not amenable to quantification. Some past experiences suggest, however, that in otherwise healthy women, a state of near starvation is required to establish clear differences in pregnancy outcome.

During the severe European winter of 1944 to 1945, nutritional deprivation of known intensity prevailed in a well-circumscribed area of The Netherlands occupied by the German military (Kyle, 2006). At the lowest point during this *Dutch Hunger Winter,* rations reached 450 kcal/day, with generalized rather than selective malnutrition. Smith (1947) analyzed the outcomes of pregnancies that were in progress during this 6-month famine. Median infant birthweights decreased approximately 250 g and rose again after food became available. This indicated that birthweight can be influenced significantly by starvation during later pregnancy. The perinatal mortality rate, however, was not altered, nor was the incidence of malformations significantly increased. Interestingly, the frequency of pregnancy "toxemia" declined.

Evidence of impaired brain development has been obtained in some animal fetuses whose mothers had been subjected to intense dietary deprivation. Subsequent intellectual development was studied by Stein and associates (1972) in young male adults whose mothers had been starved during pregnancy in the Hunger Winter. The comprehensive study was made possible because all males at age 19 underwent compulsory examination for military service. It was concluded that severe dietary deprivation during pregnancy caused no detectable effects on subsequent mental performance.

Several studies of the long-term consequences to this cohort of children born to nutritionally deprived women have been performed and have been reviewed by Kyle and Pichard (2006). Progeny deprived in mid to late pregnancy were lighter, shorter, and thinner at birth, and they had a higher incidence of subsequent diminished glucose tolerance, hypertension, reactive airway disease, dyslipidemia, and coronary artery disease. Early pregnancy deprivation was associated with increased obesity in adult women but not men. Early starvation was also linked to increased central nervous system anomalies, schizophrenia, and schizophrenia-spectrum personality disorders.

These observations, as well as others, have led to the concept of *fetal programming* by which adult morbidity and mortality are related to fetal health. Known widely as the *Barker hypothesis*, as promulgated by Barker and colleagues (1989), this concept is discussed in Chapter 44 (p. 876).

Weight Retention after Pregnancy

Not all the weight gained during pregnancy is lost during and immediately after delivery (Hytten, 1991). Schauberger and coworkers (1992) studied prenatal and postpartum weights in 795 women. Their average weight gain was 28.6 lb or 4.8 kg. As shown in Figure 9-5, most maternal weight loss was at delivery—approximately 12 lb or 5.5 kg—and in the ensuing 2 weeks—approximately 9 lb or 4 kg. An additional 5.5 lb or 2.5 kg was lost between 2 weeks and 6 months postpartum. Thus, average total weight loss resulted in an average retained

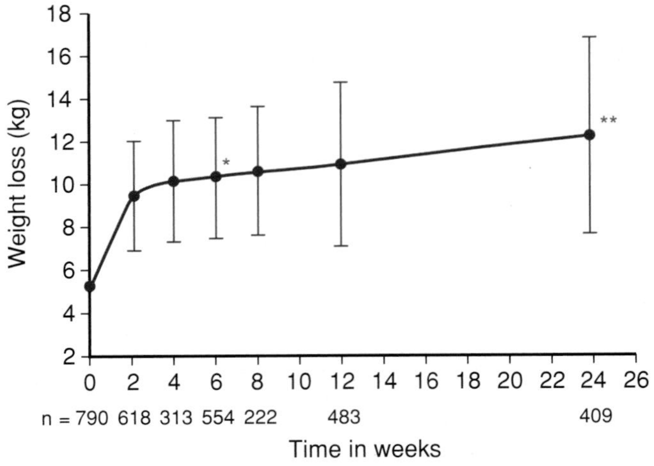

FIGURE 9-5 Cumulative weight loss from last antepartum visit to 6 months postpartum. *Significantly different from 2-week weight loss; **Significantly different from 6-week weight loss. (Redrawn from Schauberger, 1992, with permission.)

pregnancy weight of 3 lb or 1.4 kg. Overall, the more weight that was gained during pregnancy, the more that was lost postpartum. Interestingly, there is no relationship between prepregnancy BMI or prenatal weight gain and weight retention (American Academy of Pediatrics and the American College of Obstetricians and Gynecologists, 2012). Accruing weight with age—rather than parity—is considered the main factor affecting weight gain over time.

Recommended Dietary Allowances

Periodically, the Institute of Medicine (2006, 2011) publishes recommended dietary allowances, including those for pregnant or lactating women. The latest recommendations are summarized in Table 9-6. Certain prenatal vitamin–mineral supplements may lead to intakes well in excess of the recommended allowances. Moreover, the use of excessive supplements, which often are self-prescribed, has led to concern regarding nutrient toxicities during pregnancy. Those with potentially toxic effects include iron, zinc, selenium, and vitamins A, B_6, C, and D. In particular, excessive vitamin A—more than 10,000 IU per day—may be teratogenic (Chap. 12, p. 252). Vitamin and mineral intake more than twice the recommended daily dietary allowance shown in Table 9-6 should be avoided.

Calories

As shown in Figure 9-6, pregnancy requires an additional 80,000 kcal, mostly during the last 20 weeks. To meet this demand, a caloric increase of 100 to 300 kcal per day is recommended during pregnancy (American Academy of Pediatrics and the American College of Obstetricians and Gynecologists, 2012). This intake increase, however, should not be divided equally during the course of pregnancy. The Institute of Medicine (2006) recommends adding 0, 340, and 452 kcal/day to the estimated nonpregnant energy requirements in the first, second, and third trimesters, respectively. Calories are necessary for energy. Whenever caloric intake is inadequate, protein is

TABLE 9-6. Recommended Daily Dietary Allowances for Adolescent and Adult Pregnant and Lactating Women

	Pregnant		Lactating	
Age (years)	14–18	19–50	14–18	19–50
Fat-Soluble Vitamins				
Vitamin A	750 µg	770 µg	1200 µg	1300 µg
Vitamin D[a]	15 µg	15 µg	15 µg	15 µg
Vitamin E	15 mg	15 mg	19 mg	19 mg
Vitamin K[a]	75 µg	90 µg	75 µg	90 µg
Water-Soluble Vitamins				
Vitamin C	80 mg	85 mg	115 mg	120 mg
Thiamin	1.4 mg	1.4 mg	1.4 mg	1.4 mg
Riboflavin	1.4 mg	1.4 mg	1.6 mg	1.6 mg
Niacin	18 mg	18 mg	17 mg	17 mg
Vitamin B_6	1.9 mg	1.9 mg	2 mg	2 mg
Folate	600 µg	600 µg	500 µg	500 µg
Vitamin B_{12}	2.6 µg	2.6 µg	2.8 µg	2.8 µg
Minerals				
Calcium[a]	1300 mg	1000 mg	1300 mg	1000 mg
Sodium[a]	1.5 g	1.5 g	1.5 g	1.5 g
Potassium[a]	4.7 g	4.7 g	5.1 g	5.1 g
Iron	27 mg	27 mg	10 mg	9 mg
Zinc	12 mg	11 mg	13 mg	12 mg
Iodine	220 µg	220 µg	290 µg	290 µg
Selenium	60 µg	60 µg	70 µg	70 µg
Other				
Protein	71 g	71 g	71 g	71 g
Carbohydrate	175 g	175 g	210 g	210 g
Fiber[a]	28 g	28 g	29 g	29 g

[a]Recommendations measured as adequate intake.
From the Institute of Medicine, 2006, 2011.

metabolized rather than being spared for its vital role in fetal growth and development. Total physiological requirements during pregnancy are not necessarily the sum of ordinary nonpregnant requirements plus those specific to pregnancy. For example, the additional energy required during pregnancy may be compensated in whole or in part by reduced physical activity (Hytten, 1991).

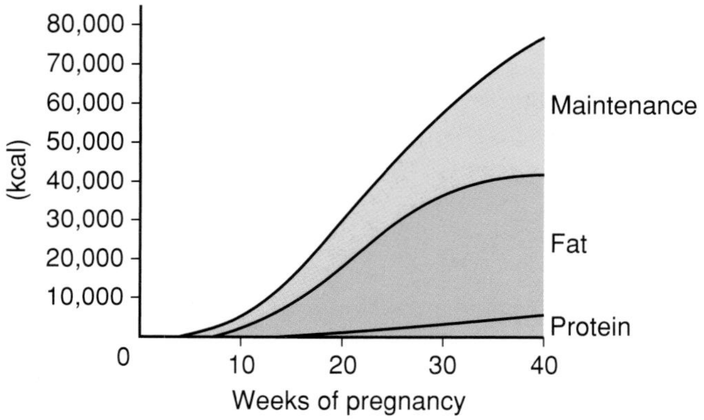

FIGURE 9-6 Cumulative kilocalories required for pregnancy. (Redrawn from Chamberlain, 1998, with permission.)

Protein

To the basic protein needs of the nonpregnant woman are added the demands for growth and remodeling of the fetus, placenta, uterus, and breasts, as well as increased maternal blood volume (Chap. 4, p. 53). During the second half of pregnancy, approximately 1000 g of protein are deposited, amounting to 5 to 6 g/day (Hytten, 1971). Most amino-acid levels in maternal plasma fall markedly, including ornithine, glycine, taurine, and proline (Hytten, 1991). Exceptions during pregnancy are glutamic acid and alanine, the concentrations of which rise.

Preferably, most protein should be supplied from animal sources, such as meat, milk, eggs, cheese, poultry, and fish. These furnish amino acids in optimal combinations. Milk and dairy products have long been considered nearly ideal sources of nutrients, especially protein and calcium, for pregnant or lactating women. Ingestion of specific fish and potential methylmercury toxicity are discussed on page 183.

Minerals

Iron

The intakes recommended by the Institute of Medicine (2006) for various minerals are presented in Table 9-6. With the exception of iron and iodine, practically all diets that supply sufficient calories for appropriate weight gain will contain enough minerals to prevent deficiency.

The reasons for substantively increased iron requirements during pregnancy are discussed in Chapter 4 (p. 55). Of the approximately 300 mg of iron transferred to the fetus and placenta and the 500 mg incorporated into the expanding maternal hemoglobin mass, nearly all is used after midpregnancy. During that time, iron requirements imposed by pregnancy and maternal excretion total approximately 7 mg per day (Pritchard, 1970). Few women have sufficient iron stores or dietary iron intake to supply this amount. Thus, the American Academy of Pediatrics and the American College of Obstetricians and Gynecologists (2012) endorse the recommendation by the National Academy of Sciences that at least 27 mg of elemental iron supplement be given daily to pregnant women. This amount is contained in most prenatal vitamins.

Scott and coworkers (1970) established that as little as 30 mg of elemental iron, supplied as ferrous gluconate, sulfate, or fumarate and taken daily throughout the latter half of pregnancy, provides sufficient iron to meet pregnancy requirements and to protect preexisting iron stores. This amount will also provide for iron requirements of lactation. The pregnant woman may benefit from 60 to 100 mg of elemental iron per day if she is large, has twin fetuses, begins supplementation late in pregnancy, takes iron irregularly, or has a somewhat depressed hemoglobin level. The woman who is overtly anemic from iron deficiency responds well to oral supplementation with iron salts (Chap. 56, p. 1102).

Because iron requirements are slight during the first 4 months of pregnancy, it is *not necessary* to provide supplemental iron during this time. Withholding iron supplementation during the first trimester of pregnancy also avoids the risk of aggravating nausea and vomiting (Gill, 2009). Ingestion of iron at bedtime or on an empty stomach aids absorption and appears to minimize the possibility of an adverse gastrointestinal reaction.

Since 1997, the Food and Drug Administration (FDA) has required that iron preparations containing 30 mg or more of elemental iron per tablet be packaged as individual doses, such as in blister packages. This regulation is targeted at preventing accidental iron poisoning in children.

Iodine

The recommended daily iodine allowance is 220 μg (Table 9-6). The use of iodized salt and bread products is recommended during pregnancy to offset the increased fetal requirements and maternal renal losses of iodine. Despite this, iodine intake has declined substantially in the last 15 years, and in some areas, it is probably inadequate (Chap. 58, p. 1155). Interest in increasing dietary iodine was heightened by reports linking subclinical maternal hypothyroidism to adverse pregnancy outcomes and possible neurodevelopmental defects in children (Casey, 2005; Haddow, 1999). Severe maternal iodine deficiency predisposes offspring to endemic cretinism, characterized by multiple severe neurological defects. In parts of China and Africa where this condition is common, iodide supplementation very early in pregnancy prevents some cretinism cases (Cao, 1994). To obviate this, many prenatal supplements now contain various quantities of iodine.

Calcium

As discussed in Chapter 4 (p. 54), the pregnant woman retains approximately 30 g of calcium. Most of this is deposited in the fetus late in pregnancy (Pitkin, 1985). This amount of calcium represents only approximately 2.5 percent of total maternal calcium, most of which is in bone and can readily be mobilized for fetal growth. Moreover, Heaney and Skillman (1971) demonstrated increased calcium absorption by the intestine and progressive retention throughout pregnancy. Efforts to prevent preeclampsia using routine calcium supplementation have not proven efficacious (Chap. 40, p. 748).

Zinc

Severe zinc deficiency in a given person may lead to poor appetite, suboptimal growth, and impaired wound healing. During pregnancy, the recommended daily intake is approximately 12 mg. But, the safe level of zinc supplementation for pregnant women has not been clearly established. Goldenberg and colleagues (1995) randomly assigned 580 indigent women to daily 25-mg zinc supplementation or placebo beginning at midpregnancy. Plasma zinc levels were significantly higher in women who received supplements. Infants born to zinc-supplemented women were slightly larger—mean increase 125 g—and had a slightly larger head circumference—mean 4 mm. Later, Osendarp and associates (2001) randomly assigned 420 women in Bangladesh to receive either daily 30-mg zinc supplementation or placebo from 12 to 16 weeks' gestation until delivery. Supplementation did not improve birthweight. However, low-birthweight infants of mothers who received zinc had reduced risks of acute diarrhea, dysentery, and impetigo. In a follow-up study of these infants at 13 months, zinc supplementation did not benefit their developmental outcome (Hamadani, 2002).

Magnesium

Deficiency of this mineral as a consequence of pregnancy has not been recognized. Undoubtedly, during prolonged illness with no magnesium intake, the plasma level might become critically low, as it would in the absence of pregnancy. We have observed magnesium deficiency during pregnancies in some with previous intestinal bypass surgery. Sibai and coworkers (1989) randomly assigned 400 normotensive primigravid women to 365-mg elemental magnesium supplementation or placebo tablets from 13 to 24 weeks' gestation. Supplementation did not improve any measures of pregnancy outcome.

Trace Metals

Copper, selenium, chromium, and manganese all have important roles in certain enzyme functions. In general, most are provided by an average diet. A severe geochemical selenium deficiency has been identified in a large area of China. Deficiency is manifested by a frequently fatal cardiomyopathy in young children and reproductive-aged women. Conversely, selenium toxicity resulting from oversupplementation also has been observed. There is no reported need to supplement selenium in American women.

Potassium

The concentration of potassium in maternal plasma decreases by approximately 0.5 mEq/L by midpregnancy (Brown, 1986). Potassium deficiency develops in the same circumstances as in nonpregnant individuals.

Fluoride

There is no evidence that supplemental fluoride during pregnancy is beneficial (Institute of Medicine, 1990). Maheshwari and colleagues (1983) found that fluoride metabolism is not altered appreciably during pregnancy. Horowitz and Heifetz (1967) concluded that there were no additional benefits from maternal ingestion of fluoridated water if the offspring ingested such water from birth. Sa Roriz Fonteles and associates (2005) studied microdrill biopsies of deciduous teeth and concluded that prenatal fluoride provided no additional fluoride uptake compared with postnatal fluoride alone. Supplemental fluoride ingested by lactating women does not increase the fluoride concentration in breast milk (Ekstrand, 1981).

Vitamins

The increased requirements for most vitamins during pregnancy shown in Table 9-6 usually are supplied by any general diet that provides adequate calories and protein. The exception is folic acid during times of unusual requirements, such as pregnancy complicated by protracted vomiting, hemolytic anemia, or multiple fetuses. That said, in impoverished countries, routine multivitamin supplementation reduced the incidence of low-birthweight and growth-restricted fetuses, but did not alter preterm delivery or perinatal mortality rates (Fawzi, 2007).

Folic Acid

The Centers for Disease Control and Prevention (2004) estimated that the number of pregnancies affected by neural-tube defects has decreased from 4000 pregnancies per year to approximately 3000 per year since mandatory fortification of cereal products with folic acid in 1998. Perhaps more than half of all neural-tube defects can be prevented with daily intake of 400 μg of folic acid throughout the periconceptional period. Putting 140 μg of folic acid into each 100 g of grain products may increase the folic acid intake of the average American woman of childbearing age by 100 μg per day. Because nutritional sources alone are insufficient, however, folic acid supplementation is still recommended (American College of Obstetricians and Gynecologists, 2013f). Likewise, the United States Preventive Services Task Force (2009) has issued a Level-A recommendation that all women planning or capable of pregnancy take a daily supplement containing 0.4 to 0.8 mg of folic acid. Using data from 15 international registries, Botto and associates (2006) demonstrated a significant reduction in neural-tube defect rates only in countries with folic acid fortification programs. There was no rate decrease in areas with supplementation recommendations alone.

A woman with a prior child with a neural-tube defect can reduce the 2- to 5-percent recurrence risk by more than 70 percent with daily 4-mg folic acid supplements the month before conception and during the first trimester. As emphasized by the American Academy of Pediatrics and the American College of Obstetricians and Gynecologists (2012), this dose should be consumed as a separate supplement and not as multivitamin tablets. This practice avoids excessive intake of fat-soluble vitamins. Unfortunately, surveys continue to suggest that many women, especially among minorities, remain unaware of the recommendations regarding folic acid supplementation (Perlow, 2001; Rinsky-Eng, 2002). This important relationship between folic acid deficiency and neural-tube defects is further discussed in Chapter 14 (p. 284).

Vitamin A

Although essential, this vitamin has been associated with congenital malformations when taken in higher doses (> 10,000 IU per day) during pregnancy. These malformations are similar to those produced by the vitamin A derivative isotretinoin—*Accutane*—which is one of the most potent teratogens (Chap. 12, p. 251). Beta-carotene, the precursor of vitamin A found in fruits and vegetables, has not been shown to produce vitamin A toxicity. Most prenatal vitamins contain vitamin A in doses considerably below the teratogenic threshold. Dietary intake of vitamin A in the United States appears to be adequate, and additional supplementation is not routinely recommended.

Vitamin A deficiency is an endemic nutritional problem in the developing world. It is estimated that 6 million pregnant women suffer from night blindness secondary to vitamin A deficiency (West, 2003). In a study from India, Radhika and coworkers (2002) found overt deficiency manifested as night blindness in 3 percent of 736 women in their third trimester. Another 27 percent had subclinical vitamin A deficiency defined as a serum retinol concentration below 20 μg/dL. Vitamin A deficiency, whether overt or subclinical, was associated with an increased risk of maternal anemia and spontaneous preterm birth.

Vitamin B_{12}

Maternal plasma vitamin B_{12} levels decrease in normal pregnancy mostly as a result of reduced plasma levels of their carrier proteins—*transcobalamins*. Vitamin B_{12} occurs naturally only in foods of animal origin, and strict vegetarians may give birth to infants whose B_{12} stores are low. Likewise, because breast milk of a vegetarian mother contains little vitamin B_{12}, the deficiency may become profound in the breast-fed infant (Higginbottom, 1978). Excessive ingestion of vitamin C also can lead to a functional deficiency of vitamin B_{12}. Although its role is still controversial, low levels of vitamin B_{12} preconceptionally, similar to folate, may increase the risk of neural-tube defects (Molloy, 2009; Thompson, 2009).

Vitamin B_6—Pyridoxine

Limited clinical trials in pregnant women have failed to demonstrate any benefits of vitamin B_6 supplements (Thaver, 2006). For women at high risk for inadequate nutrition—for example, substance abusers, adolescents, and those with multifetal gestations—a daily 2-mg supplement is recommended. As discussed on page 187 and in Chapter 54 (p. 1072), vitamin B_6, when combined with the antihistamine *doxylamine,* is helpful in many cases of nausea and vomiting of pregnancy (Boskovic, 2003; Staroselsky, 2007).

Vitamin C

The recommended dietary allowance for vitamin C during pregnancy is 80 to 85 mg/day—approximately 20 percent more than when nonpregnant (see Table 9-6). A reasonable diet should readily provide this amount. The maternal plasma level declines during pregnancy, whereas the cord-blood level is higher, a phenomenon observed with most water-soluble vitamins.

Vitamin D

This is a fat-soluble vitamin that, after being metabolized to its active form, increases the efficiency of intestinal calcium absorption and promotes bone mineralization and growth. Unlike most vitamins that are obtained exclusively from dietary intake, vitamin D is also synthesized endogenously with exposure to sunlight. There is increasing recognition that vitamin D deficiency is common during pregnancy. This is especially true in high-risk groups such as women with limited sun exposure, ethnic minorities—particularly those with darker skin, and vegetarians (Bodnar, 2007). Such maternal deficiency can cause disordered skeletal homeostasis, congenital rickets, and fractures in the newborn (American College of Obstetricians and Gynecologists, 2011d). The Food and Nutrition Board of the Institute of Medicine (2011) established that an adequate intake of vitamin D during pregnancy and lactation was 15 μg per day (600 IU per day). In women suspected of having vitamin D deficiency, serum levels of 25-hydroxyvitamin D can be obtained. Even then, the optimal levels in pregnancy have not been established (American Academy of Pediatrics and the American College of Obstetricians and Gynecologists, 2012).

Pragmatic Nutritional Surveillance

Although researchers continue to study the ideal nutritional regimen for the pregnant woman and her fetus, basic tenets for the clinician include:

1. In general, advise the pregnant woman to eat what she wants in amounts she desires and salted to taste.
2. Ensure that food is amply available for socioeconomically deprived women.
3. Monitor weight gain, with a goal of approximately 25 to 35 lb in women with a normal BMI.
4. Explore food intake by dietary recall periodically to discover the occasional nutritionally errant diet.
5. Give tablets of simple iron salts that provide at least 27 mg of elemental iron daily. Give folate supplementation before and in the early weeks of pregnancy. Provide iodine supplementation in areas of known dietary insufficiency.
6. Recheck the hematocrit or hemoglobin concentration at 28 to 32 weeks' gestation to detect significant decreases.

COMMON CONCERNS

Employment

More than half of the children in the United States are born to working mothers. Federal law prohibits employers from excluding women from job categories on the basis that they are or might become pregnant (Annas, 1991). The Family and Medical Leave Act requires that covered employers must grant up to 12 workweeks of unpaid leave to an employee for the birth and care of a newborn child. In the absence of complications, most women can continue to work until the onset of labor (American Academy of Pediatrics and the American College of Obstetricians and Gynecologists, 2012).

Some types of work, however, may increase pregnancy complication risks. Mozurkewich and colleagues (2000) reviewed 29 studies that involved more than 160,000 pregnancies. With physically demanding work, women had a 20- to 60-percent increase in rates of preterm birth, fetal-growth restriction, or gestational hypertension. In a prospective study of more than 900 healthy nulliparas, Higgins and associates (2002) found that women who worked had a fivefold risk of preeclampsia. Newman and coworkers (2001) reported outcomes in 2929 women with singleton pregnancies studied by the Maternal-Fetal Medicine Units Network. Occupational fatigue—estimated by the number of hours standing, intensity of physical and mental demands, and environmental stressors—was associated with an increased risk of preterm premature membrane rupture. For women reporting the highest degrees of fatigue, the risk was 7.4 percent.

Thus, any occupation that subjects the pregnant woman to severe physical strain should be avoided. Ideally, no work or play should be continued to the extent that undue fatigue develops. Adequate periods of rest should be provided. It seems prudent to advise women with previous pregnancy complications that are at risk to recur—for example, preterm birth—to minimize physical work.

Exercise

In general, pregnant women do not need to limit exercise, provided they do not become excessively fatigued or risk injury. Clapp and associates (2000) randomly assigned 46 pregnant women who did not exercise regularly to either no exercise or to weight-bearing exercise beginning at 8 weeks' gestation. Exercise consisted of treadmill running, step aerobics, or stair stepper use for 20 minutes three to five times each week. They did this throughout pregnancy at an intensity level between 55 and 60 percent of the preconceptional maximum aerobic capacity. Both placental size and birthweight were significantly greater in the exercise group. Duncombe and coworkers (2006) reported similar findings in 148 women. In contrast, Magann and colleagues (2002) prospectively analyzed exercise behavior in 750 healthy women and found that working women who exercised had smaller infants and more dysfunctional labors, and they had more frequent upper respiratory infections.

The American College of Obstetricians and Gynecologists (2009b) advises a thorough clinical evaluation before recommending an exercise program. In the absence of contraindications listed in Table 9-7, pregnant women should be

TABLE 9-7.

Absolute Contraindications to Aerobic Exercise During Pregnancy
• Hemodynamically significant heart disease
• Restrictive lung disease
• Incompetent cervix/cerclage
• Multiple gestation at risk for preterm labor
• Persistent second- or third-trimester bleeding
• Placenta previa after 26 weeks of gestation
• Preterm labor during the current pregnancy
• Ruptured membranes
• Preeclampsia/pregnancy induced hypertension
Relative Contraindications to Aerobic Exercise During Pregnancy
• Severe anemia
• Unevaluated maternal cardiac arrhythmia
• Chronic bronchitis
• Poorly controlled type 1 diabetes
• Extreme morbid obesity
• Extreme underweight (BMI < 12)
• History of extremely sedentary lifestyle
• Intrauterine growth restriction in current pregnancy
• Poorly controlled hypertension
• Orthopedic limitations
• Poorly controlled seizure disorder
• Poorly controlled hyperthyroidism
• Heavy smoker

From Exercise during pregnancy and the postpartum period. ACOG Committee Opinion No. 267. American College of Obstetricians and Gynecologists. Obstet Gynecol 2002;99:171–173; reaffirmed 2009b.

encouraged to engage in regular, moderate-intensity physical activity for 30 minutes or more day. Each activity should be reviewed individually for its potential risk. Pregnant women should refrain from activities with a high risk of falling or abdominal trauma. Similarly, scuba diving is avoided because the fetus is at increased risk for decompression sickness.

In the setting of certain pregnancy complications, it is wise to abstain from exercise and even limit physical activity. For example, some women with pregnancy-associated hypertensive disorders, preterm labor, placenta previa, or severe cardiac or pulmonary disease may gain from being sedentary. Also, those with multiple or suspected growth-restricted fetuses may be served by greater rest.

Seafood Consumption

Fish are an excellent source of protein, are low in saturated fats, and contain omega-3 fatty acids. Because nearly all fish and shellfish contain trace amounts of mercury, pregnant and lactating women are advised to avoid specific types of fish with potentially high methylmercury levels. These include shark, swordfish, king mackerel, and tile fish. It is further recommended that pregnant women ingest no more than 12 ounces or two servings of canned tuna per week and no more than 6 ounces of albacore or "white" tuna (United States Environmental Protection Agency, 2004). If the mercury content of locally caught fish is unknown, then overall fish consumption should be limited to 6 ounces per week (American Academy of Pediatrics and the American College of Obstetricians and Gynecologists, 2012). The Avon Longitudinal Study of Parents and Children, however, reported beneficial effects on pregnancy outcomes in women who consumed 340 g or more of seafood weekly (Hibbeln, 2007).

Lead Screening

Maternal lead exposure has been associated with several adverse maternal and fetal outcomes across a range of maternal blood lead levels (Bellinger, 2005). These include gestational hypertension, spontaneous abortion, low birthweight, and neurodevelopmental impairments in exposed fetuses (American College of Obstetricians and Gynecologists, 2012b). The exposure levels at which these risks increase remains unclear. But, recognizing that such exposure remains a significant health issue for reproductive-aged women, the Centers for Disease Control and Prevention (2010a) has issued guidelines for screening and managing exposed pregnant and lactating women. These guidelines, which have been endorsed by the American College of Obstetricians and Gynecologists (2012b), recommend blood lead testing only if a risk factor is identified (Table 9-8). If the levels are > 5 μg/dL, then counseling is completed, and the lead source is sought and removed. Subsequent blood levels should be obtained. Blood lead levels ≥ 45 μg/dL are consistent with lead poisoning, and women in this group may be candidates for chelation therapy. Such pregnancies should be managed in consultation with lead poisoning treatment experts. National and state resources are available at the CDC website: www.cdc.gov/nceh/lead.

TABLE 9-8. Risk Factors for Lead Exposure in Pregnant and Lactating Women

Recent immigration from or residency in areas of high ambient lead contamination
Living near a point source of lead
Working with lead or living with someone who does
Using lead-glazed ceramic pottery
Eating nonfood substances (pica)
Using alternative or complementary medicines, herbs, or therapies
Using imported cosmetics or certain food products
Renovating or remodeling older homes without implementing lead hazard controls
Consuming lead-contaminated drinking water
Having a prior lead-exposure history or evidence of an elevated body burden of lead
Living with someone identified with an elevated lead level

Adapted from Centers for Disease Control and Prevention, 2010a.

Automobile and Air Travel

The American College of Obstetricians and Gynecologists (2010) has formulated guidelines for automobile passenger restraints use during pregnancy (Chap. 47, p. 951). Women should be encouraged to wear properly positioned three-point restraints throughout pregnancy while riding in automobiles. The lap portion of the restraining belt should be placed under the abdomen and across her upper thighs. The belt should be comfortably snug. The shoulder belt also should be firmly positioned between the breasts. Available information suggests that airbags should not be disabled for the pregnant woman.

In general, air travel in a properly pressurized aircraft has no harmful effect on pregnancy (Aerospace Medical Association, 2003). Thus, in the absence of obstetrical or medical complications, the American Academy of Pediatrics and the American College of Obstetricians and Gynecologists (2009a, 2012) have concluded that pregnant women can safely fly up to 36 weeks' gestation. It is recommended that pregnant women observe the same precautions for air travel as the general population. These include seatbelt use while seated and periodic lower extremity movement and at least hourly ambulation to lower venous thromboembolism risks. Significant risks with travel, especially international travel, are infectious disease acquisition and development of complications remote from adequate resources (Ryan, 2002).

Coitus

In healthy pregnant women, sexual intercourse usually is not harmful. Whenever abortion, placenta previa, or preterm labor threatens, however, coitus should be avoided. Nearly 10,000 women enrolled in a prospective investigation by the Vaginal Infection and Prematurity Study Group were interviewed regarding sexual activity (Read, 1993). They reported a decreased frequency of sexual intercourse with advancing gestation. By 36 weeks, 72 percent had intercourse less than once weekly. According to Bartellas and colleagues (2000), the decline is attributed to decreased desire in 58 percent and fear of harm to the pregnancy in 48 percent.

Intercourse late in pregnancy specifically has not been found to be harmful. Grudzinskas and coworkers (1979) found no association between gestational age at delivery and coital frequency during the last 4 weeks of pregnancy. Sayle and colleagues (2001) found no increased—and actually a decreased— risk of delivery within 2 weeks of intercourse. Tan and associates (2007) studied women scheduled for nonurgent labor induction and found that spontaneous labor ensued at equal rates in groups either participating in or abstaining from intercourse.

Oral-vaginal intercourse is occasionally hazardous. Aronson and Nelson (1967) described a fatal air embolism late in pregnancy as a result of air blown into the vagina during cunnilingus. Other near-fatal cases have been described (Bernhardt, 1988).

Dental Care

Examination of the teeth should be included in the prenatal examination, and good dental hygiene is encouraged. Indeed, periodontal disease has been linked to preterm labor. Unfortunately, although its treatment improves dental health, it has not prevented preterm birth (Michalowicz, 2006). Dental caries are not aggravated by pregnancy. Importantly, pregnancy is not a contraindication to dental treatment including dental radiographs (Giglio, 2009).

Immunization

Current recommendations for immunization during pregnancy are summarized in Table 9-9. Well-publicized concerns regarding a causal link between childhood exposure to the thimerosal preservative in some vaccines and neuropsychological disorders has led to some parental prohibition. Although controversy continues, these associations have proven groundless (Sugarman, 2007; Thompson, 2007; Tozzi, 2009). Thus, many vaccines may be used in pregnancy. The American College of Obstetricians and Gynecologists (2013c) stresses the importance of integrating an effective vaccine strategy into the care of both obstetrical and gynecological patients. The College further emphasizes that information on the safety of vaccines given during pregnancy is subject to change and recommendations can be found from the Centers for Disease Control and Prevention website at: www.cdc.gov/vaccines.

The frequency of pertussis infection has substantially increased in the United States. This resulted in updated recommendations for use of the three-agent Tdap vaccine—tetanus toxoid, reduced diphtheria toxoid, and acellular pertussis (Centers for Disease Control and Prevention, 2013a). Young infants are at increased risk for death from pertussis and are entirely dependent on passive immunization from maternal antibodies until the vaccine series is initiated at 2 months of age. As demonstrated by Healy and coworkers (2013), maternal antipertussis antibodies are relatively short-lived, and Tdap administration before pregnancy—or even in the first half of the current pregnancy—is not likely to provide a high level of newborn antibody protection. The Advisory Committee on Immunization Practices, therefore, has recommended that a dose of Tdap be given to women during each pregnancy, optimally between 27 and 36 weeks' gestation to maximize passive antibody transfer to the fetus (Centers for Disease Control and Prevention, 2013a). The American College of Obstetricians and Gynecologists supports this recommendation (2012j).

All women who will be pregnant during influenza season should be offered vaccination, regardless of gestational age. Those with underlying medical conditions that increase the risk for complications should be provided the vaccine before flu season starts (American Academy of Pediatrics and the American College of Obstetricians and Gynecologists, 2012). Zaman and colleagues (2008) showed that prenatal maternal vaccination reduced the infant influenza incidence in the first 6 months of life by 63 percent in infants born to these treated women. Moreover, it reduced all febrile respiratory illnesses in these infants by a third.

Women who are susceptible to rubella during pregnancy should receive MMR—measles, mumps, rubella—vaccination postpartum. Although this vaccine is not recommended during pregnancy, congenital rubella syndrome has never resulted from its inadvertent use. There is no contraindication to MMR vaccination while breast feeding (Centers for Disease Control and Prevention, 2011).

Biological Warfare and Vaccines

The ongoing threat of bioterrorism requires familiarity with smallpox and anthrax vaccines during pregnancy. The smallpox vaccine is made with live attenuated vaccinia virus, which is related to smallpox and cowpox viruses. Fetal vaccinia infection is rare, but it may result in abortion, stillbirth, or neonatal death. Thus, in nonemergency circumstances, vaccination is contraindicated during pregnancy and in women who might become pregnant within 28 days of vaccination (Centers for Disease Control and Prevention, 2013c). But, if vaccination is inadvertently administered in early pregnancy, this is not an indication for termination (Suarez, 2002). If the pregnant woman is at risk because of exposure to smallpox—either as a direct victim of a bioterrorist attack or as a close contact of an individual case—the risks from clinical smallpox substantially outweigh any potential risk from vaccination.

Anthrax vaccination has been limited principally to individuals who are occupationally exposed, such as special veterinarians, laboratory workers, and military personnel. The vaccine contains no live bacteria and thus would not be expected to pose significant fetal risk. Wiesen and Littell (2002) studied the reproductive outcomes of 385 women in the United States Army who became pregnant after vaccination and reported no adverse effects on fertility or pregnancy outcome. Smallpox, anthrax, and other infections related to bioterrorism are discussed in Chapter 64 (p. 1258).

TABLE 9-9. Recommendations for Immunization During Pregnancy

Immunobiological Agent	Indications for Immunization During Pregnancy	Dose Schedule	Comments
Live Attenuated Virus Vaccines			
Measles	Contraindicated—see immune globulins	Single dose SC, preferably as MMR[a]	Vaccinate susceptible women postpartum. Breast feeding is not a contraindication
Mumps	Contraindicated	Single dose SC, preferably as MMR	Vaccinate susceptible women postpartum
Rubella	Contraindicated, but congenital rubella syndrome has never been described after vaccine	Single dose SC, preferably as MMR	Teratogenicity of vaccine is theoretical and not confirmed to date; vaccinate susceptible women postpartum
Poliomyelitis Oral = live attenuated; injection = enhanced-potency inactivated virus	Not routinely recommended for women in the United States, except women at increased risk of exposure[b]	Primary: Two doses of enhanced-potency inactivated virus SC at 4–8 week intervals and a 3rd dose 6–12 months after 2nd dose Immediate protection: One dose oral polio vaccine (in outbreak setting)	Vaccine indicated for susceptible women traveling in endemic areas or in other high-risk situations
Yellow fever	Travel to high-risk areas	Single dose SC	Limited theoretical risk outweighed by risk of yellow fever
Varicella	Contraindicated, but no adverse outcomes reported in pregnancy	Two doses needed: 2nd dose given 4–8 weeks after 1st dose	Teratogenicity of vaccine is theoretical. Vaccination of susceptible women should be considered postpartum
Smallpox (vaccinia)	Contraindicated in pregnant women and in their household contacts	One dose SC, multiple pricks with lancet	Only vaccine known to cause fetal harm
Other			
Influenza	All pregnant women, regardless of trimester during flu season (October–May)	One dose IM every year	Inactivated virus vaccine
Rabies	Indications for prophylaxis not altered by pregnancy; each case considered individually	Public health authorities to be consulted for indications, dosage, and route of administration	Killed-virus vaccine
Human papillomavirus	Not recommended	Three-dose series IM at 0, 1, and 6 months	Quadrivalent or bivalent vaccines; both are inactivated virus. No teratogenic effects have been observed with either
Hepatitis B	Preexposure and postexposure for women at risk of infection	Three-dose series IM at 0, 1, and 6 months	Used with hepatitis B immune globulin for some exposures. Exposed newborn needs birth-dose vaccination and immune globulin as soon as possible. All infants should receive birth dose of vaccine
Hepatitis A	Preexposure and postexposure if at risk (international travel)	Two-dose schedule IM, 6 months apart	Inactivated virus

(*continued*)

TABLE 9-9. Continued

Immunobiological Agent	Indications for Immunization During Pregnancy	Dose Schedule	Comments
Inactivated Bacterial Vaccines			
Pneumococcus	Indications not altered by pregnancy. Recommended for women with asplenia; metabolic, renal, cardiac, or pulmonary diseases; immunosuppression; or smokers	In adults, one dose only; consider repeat dose in 6 years for high-risk women	Polyvalent polysaccharide vaccine; safety in the first trimester has not been evaluated
Meningococcus	Indications not altered by pregnancy; vaccination recommended in unusual outbreaks	One dose; tetravalent vaccine	Antimicrobial prophylaxis if significant exposure
Typhoid	Not recommended routinely except for close, continued exposure or travel to endemic areas	Killed Primary: 2 injections IM 4 weeks apart Booster: One dose; schedule not yet determined	Killed, injectable vaccine or live attenuated oral vaccine. Oral vaccine preferred
Anthrax	See text	Six-dose primary vaccination, then annual booster vaccination	Preparation from cell-free filtrate of *B anthracis.* No dead or live bacteria. Teratogenicity of vaccine theoretical
Toxoids			
Tetanus-diphtheria-acellular pertussis (Tdap)	Recommended in every pregnancy, preferably between 27 and 36 weeks to maximize passive antibody transfer	Primary: Two doses IM at 1–2 month interval with 3rd dose 6–12 months after the 2nd Booster: Single dose IM every 10 years, as a part of wound care if ≥ 5 years since last dose, or once per pregnancy	Combined tetanus-diphtheria toxoids with acellular pertussis (Tdap) preferred. Updating immune status should be part of antepartum care
Specific Immune Globulins			
Hepatitis B	Postexposure prophylaxis	Depends on exposure (Chap. 55, p. 1090)	Usually given with hepatitis B virus vaccine; exposed newborn needs immediate prophylaxis
Rabies	Postexposure prophylaxis	Half dose at injury site, half dose in deltoid	Used in conjunction with rabies killed-virus vaccine
Tetanus	Postexposure prophylaxis	One dose IM	Used in conjunction with tetanus toxoid
Varicella	Should be considered for exposed pregnant women to protect against maternal, not congenital, infection	One dose IM within 96 hours of exposure	Indicated also for newborns or women who developed varicella within 4 days before delivery or 2 days following delivery

TABLE 9-9. Continued

Immunobiological Agent	Indications for Immunization During Pregnancy	Dose Schedule	Comments
Standard Immune Globulins			
Hepatitis A: Hepatitis A virus vaccine should be used with hepatitis A immune globulin	Postexposure prophylaxis and those at high risk	0.02 mL/kg IM in one dose	Immune globulin should be given as soon as possible and within 2 weeks of exposure; infants born to women who are incubating the virus or are acutely ill at delivery should receive one dose of 0.5 mL as soon as possible after birth

[a]Two doses necessary for students entering institutions of higher education, newly hired medical personnel, and travel abroad.
[b]Inactivated polio vaccine recommended for nonimmunized adults at increased risk.
ID = intradermally; IM = intramuscularly; MMR = measles, mumps, rubella; PO = orally; SC = subcutaneously.
Adapted from the Centers for Disease Control and Prevention, 2013a,b,c.

Caffeine

Whether adverse pregnancy outcomes are related to caffeine consumption is somewhat controversial. As summarized from Chapter 18 (p. 353), heavy intake of coffee each day—about five cups or 500 mg of caffeine—slightly increases the abortion risk. Studies of "moderate" intake—less than 200 mg daily—did not report increased risk.

It is unclear if caffeine consumption is associated with preterm birth or impaired fetal growth. Clausson and coworkers (2002) found no association between moderate caffeine consumption of less than 500 mg daily and low birthweight, fetal-growth restriction, or preterm delivery. Bech and associates (2007) randomly assigned more than 1200 pregnant women who drank at least three cups of coffee per day to caffeinated versus decaffeinated coffee. They found no difference in birthweight or gestational age at delivery between groups. The CARE Study Group (2008), however, evaluated 2635 low-risk pregnancies and reported a 1.4-fold risk for fetal-growth restriction among those whose daily caffeine consumption was > 200 mg compared with those who consumed < 100 mg daily. The American College of Obstetricians and Gynecologists (2013d) has concluded that moderate consumption of caffeine—less than 200 mg per day—does not appear to be associated with miscarriage or preterm birth, but that the relationship between caffeine consumption and fetal-growth restriction remains unsettled. The American Dietetic Association (2008) recommends that caffeine intake during pregnancy be limited to less than 300 mg daily, or approximately three 5-oz cups of percolated coffee.

Nausea and Vomiting

These are common complaints during the first half of pregnancy. Nausea and vomiting of varying severity usually commence between the first and second missed menstrual period and continue until 14 to 16 weeks' gestation. Although nausea and vomiting tend to be worse in the morning—thus erroneously termed *morning sickness*—both symptoms frequently continue throughout the day. Lacroix and coworkers (2000) found that nausea and vomiting were reported by three fourths of pregnant women and lasted an average of 35 days. Half had relief by 14 weeks, and 90 percent by 22 weeks. In 80 percent of these women, nausea lasted all day.

Treatment of pregnancy-associated nausea and vomiting seldom provides complete relief, but symptoms can be minimized. Eating small meals at more frequent intervals but stopping short of satiation is valuable. Borrelli and colleagues (2005) performed a systematic literature search and reported that the herbal remedy ginger was likely effective. Mild symptoms usually respond to vitamin B_6 given along with doxylamine, but some women require phenothiazine or H_1-receptor blocking antiemetics (American College of Obstetricians and Gynecologists, 2013e). In some, *hyperemesis gravidarum* develops—vomiting so severe that dehydration, electrolyte and acid-base disturbances, and starvation ketosis become serious problems. Its management and that of less severe nausea are described in Chapter 54 (p. 1072).

Backache

Low back pain to some extent is reported by nearly 70 percent of pregnant women (Wang, 2004). Minor degrees follow excessive strain or significant bending, lifting, or walking. It can be reduced by squatting rather than bending when reaching down, by using a pillow back support when sitting, and by avoiding high-heeled shoes. Back pain complaints increase with progressing gestation and are more prevalent in obese women and those with a history of low back pain. In some cases, troublesome pain may persist for years after the pregnancy (Norén, 2002).

Severe back pain should not be attributed simply to pregnancy until a thorough orthopedic examination has been conducted. Severe pain also has other uncommon causes, such as pregnancy-associated osteoporosis, disc disease, vertebral osteoarthritis, or septic arthritis (Smith, 2008). More commonly, muscular spasm and tenderness are classified clinically as acute strain or fibrositis. Although evidence-based clinical research directing care in pregnancy is limited, such low back pain usually responds well to analgesics, heat, and rest. Tylenol may be used chronically as needed. Nonsteroidal anti-inflammatory drugs may also be beneficial but are used only in short courses to avoid fetal effects (Chap. 12, p. 247). Muscle relaxants that include cyclobenzaprine (Flexeril) or baclofen may be added when needed. Once acute pain is improved, stabilizing and strengthening exercises provided by physical therapy improve spine and hip stability, which is essential for the increased load of pregnancy. For some, a sacroiliac joint stabilizing support belt may be beneficial. There may also be a role for chiropractic manipulation in selected women. George and associates (2013) randomized 169 women with low back pain at 24 to 28 weeks' gestation to standard obstetrical care or standard care plus multimodal therapy—a combination of manual chiropractic therapy, exercises, and patient education. The patients who received the multimodal therapy experienced significantly less pain, less disability, and greater global improvement in daily activities.

Varicosities and Hemorrhoids

Venous leg varicosities have a congenital predisposition and accrue with advancing age. They can be aggravated by factors that cause increased lower extremity venous pressures. As discussed in Chapter 4 (p. 60), femoral venous pressures in the supine pregnant woman increase from 8 mm Hg early to 24 mm Hg at term. Thus, susceptible women develop leg varicosities that typically worsen as pregnancy advances, especially with prolonged standing. Symptoms vary from cosmetic blemishes and mild discomfort at the end of the day to severe discomfort that requires prolonged rest with feet elevation. Treatment is generally limited to periodic rest with leg elevation, elastic stockings, or both. Surgical correction during pregnancy generally is not advised, although rarely the symptoms may be so severe that injection, ligation, or even stripping of the veins is necessary.

Vulvar varicosities frequently coexist with leg varicosities, but they may appear without other venous pathology. Uncommonly, they become massive and almost incapacitating. If these large varicosities rupture, blood loss may be severe. Treatment is with specially fitted pantyhose that will also minimize lower extremity varicosities. With particularly bothersome vulvar varicosities, a foam rubber pad suspended across the vulva by a belt can be used to exert pressure on the dilated veins.

Hemorrhoids are rectal vein varicosities and may first appear during pregnancy as pelvic venous pressures increase. Commonly, they are recurrences of previously encountered hemorrhoids. Pain and swelling usually are relieved by topically applied anesthetics, warm soaks, and stool-softening agents. With thrombosis of an external hemorrhoid, there can be considerable pain. This may be relieved by incision and removal of the clot under local analgesia.

Heartburn

This symptom is one of the most common complaints of pregnant women and is caused by gastric content reflux into the lower esophagus. The increased frequency of regurgitation during pregnancy most likely results from upward displacement and compression of the stomach by the uterus, combined with relaxation of the lower esophageal sphincter (Chap. 4, p. 66). In most pregnant women, symptoms are mild and are relieved by a regimen of more frequent but smaller meals and avoidance of bending over or lying flat. Antacids may provide considerable relief. Aluminum hydroxide, magnesium trisilicate, or magnesium hydroxide alone or in combination are given. Management for symptoms that do not respond to these simple measures is discussed in Chapter 54 (p. 1072).

Pica and Ptyalism

The craving of pregnant women for strange foods is termed *pica*. At times, nonfoods such as ice—pagophagia, starch—amylophagia, or clay—geophagia may predominate. This desire has been considered by some to be triggered by severe iron deficiency. Although such cravings usually abate after iron deficiency correction, not all pregnant women with pica are iron deficient. Indeed, if strange "foods" dominate the diet, iron deficiency will be aggravated or will develop eventually.

Patel and coworkers (2004) from the University of Alabama at Birmingham prospectively completed a dietary inventory on more than 3000 women during the second trimester. The prevalence of pica was 4 percent. The most common nonfood items ingested were starch in 64 percent, dirt in 14 percent, sourdough in 9 percent, and ice in 5 percent. The prevalence of anemia was 15 percent in women with pica compared with 6 percent in those without it. Interestingly, the rate of spontaneous preterm birth before 35 weeks was twice as high in women with pica.

Women during pregnancy are occasionally distressed by profuse salivation—*ptyalism*. Although usually unexplained, ptyalism sometimes appears to follow salivary gland stimulation by the ingestion of starch.

Sleeping and Fatigue

Beginning early in pregnancy, many women experience fatigue and need increased amounts of sleep. This likely is due to the soporific effect of progesterone but may be compounded in the first trimester by nausea and vomiting and in the latter stages of pregnancy by general discomforts, urinary frequency, and dyspnea. Moreover, sleep efficiency appears to progressively diminish as pregnancy advances. Wilson and associates (2011) performed overnight polysomnography in 27 women in the third trimester, in 21 women in the first trimester, and in 24 nonpregnant control women. Women in the third trimester had poorer sleep efficiency, more awakenings, and less of both stage 4 (deep) and rapid-eye movement sleep. Women in the first trimester were also affected but to a lesser extent. Subjective assessments of sleep quality have yielded similar findings. Facco and colleagues (2010) prospectively evaluated 189 healthy nulliparous women with a sleep survey completed once before midpregnancy and again in the third trimester. They found that women in the third trimester had significantly shorter sleep durations and were more likely to snore and meet criteria for restless leg syndrome. Most women experience some degree of sleep disturbance by the third trimester. Daytime naps and mild sedatives at bedtime such as diphenhydramine (Benadryl) can be helpful.

Leukorrhea

Pregnant women commonly develop increased vaginal discharge that in many instances is not pathological. Increased mucus secretion by cervical glands in response to hyperestrogenemia is undoubtedly a contributing factor. Occasionally, troublesome leukorrhea is the result of vulvovaginal infection. In the adult woman, most of these are bacterial vaginosis, candidiasis, or trichomoniasis, which are reviewed in Chapter 65 (p. 1276).

Cord Blood Banking

Since the first successful cord blood transplantation in 1988, more than 25,000 umbilical cord blood transplantations have been performed to treat hemopoietic cancers and various genetic conditions (Butler, 2011). There are two types of cord blood banks. Public banks promote allogeneic donation, for use by a related or unrelated recipient, similar to blood product donation. Private banks were initially developed to store stem cells for future autologous use and charged fees for initial processing and annual storage. The American College of Obstetricians and Gynecologists (2012d) has concluded that if a woman requests information on umbilical cord banking, information regarding advantages and disadvantages of public versus private banking should be explained. Some states have passed laws that require physicians to inform patients about cord blood banking options. Importantly, few transplants have been performed by using cord blood stored in the absence of a known indication in the recipient (Thornley, 2009). The likelihood that cord blood would be used for the child or family member of the donor couple is considered remote and estimated to be about 1 in 2700 individuals (American College of Obstetricians and Gynecologists, 2008). It is recommended that directed donation be considered when an immediate family member carries the diagnosis of a specific condition known to be treatable by hemopoietic transplantation.

REFERENCES

Aerospace Medical Association, Medical Guidelines Task Force: Medical guidelines for airline travel, 2nd ed. Aviat Space Environ Med 74:5, 2003

Ahmad F, Hogg-Johnson S, Stewart D, et al: Computer-assisted screening for intimate partner violence and control. Ann of Intern Med 151(2):94, 2009

American Academy of Pediatrics and American College of Obstetricians and Gynecologists: Guidelines for perinatal care. 7th ed. Washington, DC, 2012, p 301

American College of Obstetricians and Gynecologists: At-risk drinking and illicit drug use: ethical issues in obstetric and gynecologic practice. Committee Opinion No. 422, December 2008

American College of Obstetricians and Gynecologists: Air travel during pregnancy. Committee Opinion No. 443, October 2009a

American College of Obstetricians and Gynecologists: Exercise during pregnancy and the postpartum period. Committee Opinion No. 267, January 2002, Reaffirmed 2009b

American College of Obstetricians and Gynecologists: Preconception and prenatal carrier screening for genetic diseases in individuals of Eastern European Jewish descent. Committee Opinion No. 442, October 2009c

American College of Obstetricians and Gynecologists: Obstetric aspects of trauma management. Educational Bulletin No. 251, September 1998, Reaffirmed 2010

American College of Obstetricians and Gynecologists: Prenatal and perinatal human immunodeficiency virus testing: expanded recommendations. Committee Opinion No. 418, September 2008, Reaffirmed 2011a

American College of Obstetricians and Gynecologists: Ultrasonography in pregnancy. Practice Bulletin No. 101, December 2009, Reaffirmed 2011b

American College of Obstetricians and Gynecologists: Update on carrier screening for cystic fibrosis. Committee Opinion No. 486, April 2011c

American College of Obstetricians and Gynecologists: Vitamin D: screening and supplementation during pregnancy. Committee Opinion No. 495, July 2011d

American College of Obstetricians and Gynecologists: Intimate partner violence. Committee Opinion No. 518, February 2012a

American College of Obstetricians and Gynecologists: Lead screening during pregnancy and lactation. Committee Opinion No. 533, August 2012b

American College of Obstetricians and Gynecologists: Opioid abuse, dependence, and addiction in pregnancy. Committee Opinion No. 524, May 2012c

American College of Obstetricians and Gynecologists: Umbilical cord blood banking. Committee Opinion No. 399, February 2008, Reaffirmed 2012d

American College of Obstetricians and Gynecologists: Avoiding inappropriate clinical decisions based on false-positive human chorionic gonadotropin test results. Committee Opinion No. 278, November 2002, Reaffirmed 2013a

American College of Obstetricians and Gynecologists: Fetal growth restriction. Practice Bulletin No. 134, May 2013b

American College of Obstetricians and Gynecologists: Integrating immunization into practice. Committee Opinion No. 558, April 2013c

American College of Obstetricians and Gynecologists: Moderate caffeine consumption during pregnancy. Committee Opinion No. 462, August 2013d

American College of Obstetricians and Gynecologists: Nausea and vomiting of pregnancy. Practice Bulletin No. 52, April 2004, Reaffirmed 2013e

American College of Obstetricians and Gynecologists: Neural tube defects. Practice Bulletin No. 44, July 2003, Reaffirmed 2013f

American College of Obstetricians and Gynecologists: Prevention of early onset group B streptococcal disease in newborns. Committee Opinion No. 485, April 2013g

American College of Obstetricians and Gynecologists: Screening for fetal chromosomal abnormalities. Practice Bulletin No. 77, January 2007, Reaffirmed 2013h

American College of Obstetricians and Gynecologists: Smoking cessation during pregnancy. Committee Opinion No. 471, November 2010, Reaffirmed 2013i

American College of Obstetricians and Gynecologists: Update on immunization and pregnancy: tetanus, diphtheria, and pertussis vaccination. Committee Opinion No. 566, June 2013j

American Dietetic Association: Position of the American Dietetic Association: nutrition and lifestyle for a healthy pregnancy outcome. J Am Diet Assoc 108:553, 2008

Annas GJ: Fetal protection and employment discrimination—the Johnson Controls case. N Engl J Med 325:740, 1991

Aronson ME, Nelson PK: Fatal air embolism in pregnancy resulting from an unusual sex act. Obstet Gynecol 30:127, 1967

Barker DJ, Osmond C, Law CM: The intrauterine and early postnatal origins of cardiovascular disease and chronic bronchitis. J Epidemiol Community Health 43:237, 1989

Bartellas E, Crane JMG, Daley M, et al: Sexuality and sexual activity in pregnancy. Br J Obstet Gynaecol 107:964, 2000

Bech BH, Obel C, Henriksen TB, et al: Effect of reducing caffeine intake on birth weight and length of gestation: randomized controlled trial. BMJ 335:409, 2007

Bellinger DC: Teratogen update: lead and pregnancy. Birth Defects Research 73:409, 2005

Berg CJ, Callaghan WM, Syverson C, et al: Pregnancy-related mortality in the United States, 1998 to 2005. Obstet Gynecol 116(6):1302, 2010

Bergsjø P, Denman DW III, Hoffman HJ, et al: Duration of human singleton pregnancy. A population-based study. Acta Obstet Gynecol Scand 69:197, 1990
Bernhardt TL, Goldmann RW, Thombs PA, et al: Hyperbaric oxygen treatment of cerebral air embolism from orogenital sex during pregnancy. Crit Care Med 16:729, 1988
Bodnar LM, Simhan HN, Powers RW, et al: High prevalence of vitamin D insufficiency in black and white pregnant women residing in the northern United States and their neonates. J Nutr 137(2):447, 2007
Borrelli F, Capasso R, Aviello G, et al: Effectiveness and safety of ginger in the treatment of pregnancy-induced nausea and vomiting. Obstet Gynecol 105:849, 2005
Boskovic R, Einarson A, Maltepe C, et al: Dilectin therapy for nausea and vomiting of pregnancy: effects of optimal dosing. J Obstet Gynaecol Can 25:830, 2003
Botto LD, Lisi A, Bower C, et al: Trends of selected malformations in relation to folic acid recommendations and fortification: an international assessment. Birth Defects Res A Clin Mol Teratol 76:693, 2006
Bracken MB, Belanger K: Calculation of delivery dates. N Engl J Med 321:1483, 1989
Braunstein GD: False-positive serum human chorionic gonadotropin results: causes, characteristics, and recognition. Am J Obstet Gynecol 187:217, 2002
Brown MA, Sinosich MJ, Saunders DM, et al: Potassium regulation and progesterone-aldosterone interrelationships in human pregnancy: a prospective study. Am J Obstet Gynecol 155:349, 1986
Butler MG, Menitove JE: Umbilical cord blood banking: an update. J Assist Reprod Genet 28:669, 2011
Calvert JP, Crean EE, Newcombe RG, et al: Antenatal screening by measurement of symphysis–fundus height. BMJ 285:846, 1982
Cao XY, Jiang XM, Dou ZH, et al: Timing of vulnerability of the brain to iodine deficiency in endemic cretinism. N Engl J Med 331:1739, 1994
CARE study group: Maternal caffeine intake during pregnancy and risk of fetal growth restriction: a large prospective observational study. BMJ 337:a2332, 2008
Casey BM, Dashe JS, McIntire DD, et al: Subclinical hypothyroidism and pregnancy outcomes. Obstet Gynecol 105:239, 2005
Catalano PM: Increasing maternal obesity and weight gain during pregnancy: the obstetric problems of plentitude. Obstet Gynecol 110:743, 2007
Centers for Disease Control and Prevention: Entry into prenatal care—United States, 1989–1997. MMWR 49:393, 2000
Centers for Disease Control and Prevention: Alcohol use among women of childbearing age—United States, 1991–1999. MMWR 51(13):273, 2002
Centers for Disease Control and Prevention: Spina bifida and anencephaly before and after folic acid mandate—United States, 1995–1996 and 1999–2000. MMWR 53(17):362, 2004
Centers for Disease Control and Prevention: Revised recommendations for HIV testing of adults, adolescents, and pregnant women in health-care settings. MMWR 55(14):1, 2006
Centers for Disease Control and Prevention: Guidelines for the identification and management of lead exposure in pregnant and lactating women. November, 2010a. Available at: http://www.cdc.gov/nceh/lead/publications/leadandpregnancy2010.pdf. Accessed June 26, 2013
Centers for Disease Control and Prevention: Prevention of perinatal group B streptococcal disease: revised guidelines from CDC, 2010. MMWR 59(10):1, 2010b
Centers for Disease Control and Prevention: General recommendations on immunization—recommendations of the Advisory Committee on Immunization Practices (ACIP). MMWR 60(2):1, 2011
Centers for Disease Control and Prevention: Alcohol use and binge drinking among women of childbearing age—United States, 2006–2010. MMWR 60(28):534, 2012a
Centers for Disease Control and Prevention: PRAMS and smoking. 2012b. Available at: http://www.cdc.gov/prams/TobaccoandPrams.htm. Accessed June 26, 2013
Centers for Disease Control and Prevention: Advisory Committee on Immunization Practices (ACIP) recommended immunization schedule for adults aged 19 years and older—United States, 2013. MMWR 62(1):9, 2013a
Centers for Disease Control and Prevention: Guidelines for vaccinating pregnant women. 2013b. Available at: http://www.cdc.gov/vaccines/pubs/downloads/b_preg_guide.pdf. Accessed June 26, 2013
Centers for Disease Control and Prevention: Updated recommendations for use of tetanus toxoid, reduced diphtheria toxoid, and acellular pertussis vaccine (Tdap) in pregnant women—Advisory Committee on Immunization Practices (ACIP), 2012. MMWR 62(7):131, 2013c
Chamberlain G, Broughton-Pipkin F (eds): Clinical Physiology in Obstetrics, 3rd ed. Oxford, Blackwell Science, 1998
Chen PH, Rovi S, Washington J, et al: Randomized comparison of 3 methods to screen for domestic violence in family practice. Ann Fam Med 5(5):430, 2007
Chiang G, Levine D, Swire M, et al: The intradecidual sign: is it reliable for diagnosis of early intrauterine pregnancy. AJR 183:725, 2004
Clapp JF III, Kim H, Burciu B, et al: Beginning regular exercise in early pregnancy: effect on fetoplacental growth. Am J Obstet Gynecol 183:1484, 2000
Clausson B, Granath F, Ekbom A, et al: Effect of caffeine exposure during pregnancy on birth weight and gestational age. Am J Epidemiol 155:429, 2002
Clement S, Candy B, Sikorski J, et al: Does reducing the frequency of routine antenatal visits have long term effects? Follow up of participants in a randomised controlled trial. Br J Obstet Gynaecol 106:367, 1999
Coker AL, Garcia LS, Williams CM, et al: Universal psychosocial screening and adverse pregnancy outcomes in an academic obstetric clinic. Obstet Gynecol 119(6):1180, 2012
Cole LA: HCG, its free subunits and its metabolites: roles in pregnancy and trophoblastic disease. J Reprod Med 43:3, 1998
Cole LA: The utility of six over-the-counter (home) pregnancy tests. Clin Chem Lab Med 49(8): 1317, 2011
DeVader SR, Neeley HL, Myles TD, et al: Evaluation of gestational weight gain guidelines for women with normal prepregnancy body mass index. Obstet Gynecol 110:745, 2007
Duncombe D, Skouteris H, Wertheim EH, et al: Vigorous exercise and birth outcomes in a sample of recreational exercisers: a prospective study across pregnancy. Aust N Z J Obstet Gynaecol 46:288, 2006
Ehrenberg HM, Dierker L, Milluzzi C, et al: Low maternal weight, failure to thrive in pregnancy, and adverse pregnancy outcomes. Am J Obstet Gynecol 189:1726, 2003
Ekstrand J, Boreus LO, de Chateau P: No evidence of transfer of fluoride from plasma to breast milk. Br Med J (Clin Res Ed) 283:761, 1981
El-Mohandes A, Herman AA, Kl-Khorazaty MN, et al: Prenatal care reduces the impact of illicit drug use on perinatal outcomes. J Perinatol 23:354, 2003
England LJ, Kendrick JS, Wilson HG, et al: Effects of smoking reduction during pregnancy on the birth weight of term infants. Am J Epidemiol 154(8):694, 2001
Facco FL, Kramer J, Ho KH, et al: Sleep disturbances in pregnancy. Obstet Gynecol 115(1): 77, 2010
Fawzi WW, Msamanga GI, Urassa W, et al: Vitamins and perinatal outcomes among HIV-negative women in Tanzania. N Engl J Med 356:14, 2007
Fiore MC, Jaen CR, Baker TB, et al: Treating tobacco use and dependence: 2008 update. Clinical practice guideline. 2008. Available at: http://www.ahrq.gov/professionals/clinicians-providers/guidelines-recommendations/tobacco/clinicians/treating_tobacco_use08.pdf. Accessed June 26, 2013
George JW, Skaggs CD, Thompson PA, et al: A randomized controlled trial comparing a multimodal intervention and standard obstetrics care for low back and pelvic pain in pregnancy. Am J Obstet Gynecol 208:295.e1, 2013
Giglio JA, Lanni SM, Laskin DM, et al: Oral health care for the pregnant patient. J Can Dent Assoc 75(1):43, 2009
Gill SK, Maltepe C, Koren G: The effectiveness of discontinuing iron-containing prenatal multivitamins on reducing the severity of nausea and vomiting of pregnancy. J Obstet Gynaecol 29(1):13, 2009
Goldenberg RL, Tamura T, Neggers Y, et al: The effect of zinc supplementation on pregnancy outcome. JAMA 274:463, 1995
Gregory KD, Johnson CT, Johnson TRB, et al: The content of prenatal care. Women's Health Issues 16:198, 2006
Grudzinskas JG, Watson C, Chard T: Does sexual intercourse cause fetal distress? Lancet 2:692, 1979
Haddow JE, Palomaki GE, Allan WC, et al: Maternal thyroid deficiency during pregnancy and subsequent neuropsychological development of the child. N Engl J Med 341:549, 1999
Hamadani JD, Fuchs GJ, Osendarp SJ, et al: Zinc supplementation during pregnancy and effects on mental development and behaviour of infants: a follow-up study. Lancet 360:290, 2002
Healy CM, Rench MA, Baker CJ: Importance of timing of maternal combined tetanus, diphtheria, and acellular pertussis (Tdap) immunization and protection of young infants. Clin Infect Dis 56(4):539, 2013
Heaney RP, Skillman TG: Calcium metabolism in normal human pregnancy. J Clin Endocrinol Metab 33:661, 1971
Herbert WNP, Bruninghaus HM, Barefoot AB, et al: Clinical aspects of fetal heart auscultation. Obstet Gynecol 69:574, 1987
Herbst MA, Mercer BM, Beazley D, et al: Relationship of prenatal care and perinatal morbidity in low-birth-weight infants. Am J Obstet Gynecol 189:930, 2003
Hibbeln JR, Davis JM, Steer C, et al: Maternal seafood consumption in pregnancy and neurodevelopmental outcomes in childhood (ALSPAC study): an observation cohort study. Lancet 369:578, 2007

Higginbottom MC, Sweetman L, Nyhan WL: A syndrome of methylmalonic aciduria, homocystinuria, megaloblastic anemia and neurologic abnormalities in a vitamin B_{12}-deficient breast-fed infant of a strict vegetarian. N Engl J Med 299:317, 1978
Higgins JR, Walshe JJ, Conroy RM, et al: The relation between maternal work, ambulatory blood pressure, and pregnancy hypertension. J Epidemiol Community Health 56:389, 2002
Hollier LM, Hill J, Sheffield JS, et al: State laws regarding prenatal syphilis screening in the United States. Am J Obstet Gynecol 189:1178, 2003
Horowitz HS, Heifetz SB: Effects of prenatal exposure to fluoridation on dental caries. Public Health Rep 82:297, 1967
Hytten FE, Chamberlain G (eds): Clinical Physiology in Obstetrics, 2nd ed. Oxford, Blackwell, 1991, pp 152, 173
Hytten FE, Leitch I: The Physiology of Human Pregnancy, 2nd ed. Oxford, Blackwell, 1971
Ickovics JR, Kershaw TS, Westdahl C, et al: Group prenatal care and perinatal outcomes. Obstet Gynecol 110(2):330, 2007
Institute of Medicine: Dietary Reference Intakes: The Essential Guide to Nutrient Requirements. Washington, DC, The National Academies Press, 2006, p 529
Institute of Medicine: DRI Dietary Reference Intakes for Calcium and Vitamin D. Washington, DC, The National Academies Press, 2011
Institute of Medicine: Nutrition During Pregnancy, 1. Weight Gain; 2. Nutrient Supplements. Washington, DC, National Academy Press, 1990
Institute of Medicine and National Research Council: Weight Gain During Pregnancy: Reexamining the Guidelines. Washington, DC, The National Academic Press, 2009, p 2
Jazayeri A, Tsibris JCM, Spellacy WN: Umbilical cord plasma erythropoietin levels in pregnancies complicated by maternal smoking. Am J Obstet Gynecol 178:433, 1998
Jimenez JM, Tyson JE, Reisch JS: Clinical measures of gestational age in normal pregnancies. Obstet Gynecol 61:438, 1983
Kessner DM, Singer J, Kalk CE, et al: Infant death: an analysis by maternal risk and health care. In: Contrasts in Health Status, Vol 1. Washington, Institute of Medicine, National Academy of Sciences, 1973, p 59
Kiel DW, Dodson EA, Artal R, et al: Gestational weight gain and pregnancy outcomes in obese women: how much is enough. Obstet Gynecol 110:752, 2007
Kiss H, Widham A, Geusau A, et al: Universal antenatal screening for syphilis: is it still justified economically? A 10-year retrospective analysis. Eur J Obstet Gynecol Reprod Biol 112:24, 2004
Kyle UG, Pichard C: The Dutch Famine of 1944–1945: a pathophysiological model of long-term consequences of wasting disease. Curr Opin Clin Nutr Metab Care 9:388, 2006
Lacroix R, Eason E, Melzack R: Nausea and vomiting during pregnancy: a prospective study of its frequency, intensity, and patterns of change. Am J Obstet Gynecol 182:931, 2000
Loudon I: Death in Childbirth. New York, Oxford University Press, 1992, p 577
Luck W, Nau H, Hansen R: Extent of nicotine and cotinine transfer to the human fetus, placenta and amniotic fluid of smoking mothers. Dev Pharmacol Ther 8:384, 1985
Luke B, Brown MB, Misiunas R, et al: Specialized prenatal care and maternal and infant outcomes in twin pregnancy. Am J Obstet Gynecol 934, 2003
Magann EF, Evans SF, Weitz B, et al: Antepartum, intrapartum, and neonatal significance of exercise on healthy low-risk pregnant working women. Obstet Gynecol 99:466, 2002
Maheshwari UR, King JC, Leybin L, et al: Fluoride balances during early and late pregnancy. J Occup Med 25:587, 1983
Man LX, Chang B: Maternal cigarette smoking during pregnancy increases the risk of having a child with a congenital digital anomaly. Plast Reconstr Surg 117:301, 2006
Margulies R, Miller L: Fruit size as a model for teaching first trimester uterine sizing in bimanual examination. Obstet Gynecol 98(2):341, 2001
Martin JA, Hamilton BE, Sutton PD, et al: Births: final data for 2005. Natl Vital Stat Rep 56(6):1, 2007
Martin JA, Hamilton BE, Sutton PD, et al: Births: final data for 2006. Natl Vital Stat Rep 57(7):1, 2009
Martin JA, Hamilton BE, Ventura SJ, et al: Births: final data for 2000. Natl Vital Stat Rep 50:1, February 12, 2002a
Martin JA, Hamilton BE, Ventura SJ, et al: Births: final data for 2001. Natl Vital Stat Rep 51:2, December 18, 2002b
McDuffie RS Jr, Beck A, Bischoff K, et al: Effect of frequency of prenatal care visits on perinatal outcome among low-risk women. A randomized controlled trial. JAMA 275:847, 1996
Michalowicz BS, Hodges JS, DiAngelis AJ, et al: Treatment of periodontal disease and the risk of preterm birth. N Engl J Med 355;1885, 2006
Molloy AM, Kirke PN, Troendle JF, et al: Maternal vitamin B_{12} status and risk of neural tube defects in a population with high neural tube defect prevalence and no folic acid fortification. Pediatrics 123(3):917, 2009
Montagnana M, Trenti T, Aloe R, et al: Human chorionic gonadotropin in pregnancy diagnostics. Clin Chim Acta 412(17–18):1515, 2011
Mozurkewich EL, Luke B, Avni M, et al: Working conditions and adverse pregnancy outcome: a meta-analysis. Obstet Gynecol 95:623, 2000
Murray N, Homer CS, Davis GK, et al: The clinical utility of routine urinalysis in pregnancy: a prospective study. Med J Aust 177:477, 2002
Newman RB, Goldenberg RL, Moawad AH, et al: Occupational fatigue and preterm premature rupture of membranes. Am J Obstet Gynecol 184: 438, 2001
Norén L, Östgaard S, Johansson G, et al: Lumbar back and posterior pelvic pain during pregnancy: a 3-year follow-up. Eur Spine J 11:267, 2002
Osendarp SJ, van Raaij JM, Darmstadt GL, et al: Zinc supplementation during pregnancy and effects on growth and morbidity in low birthweight infants: a randomised placebo controlled trial. Lancet 357:1080, 2001
Osterman MJ, Martin JA, Mathews TJ, et al: Expanded data from the new birth certificate, 2008. Natl Vital Stat Rep 59(7):1, 2011
Patel MV, Nuthalapaty FS, Ramsey PS, et al: Pica: a neglected risk factor for preterm birth. Obstet Gynecol 103:68S, 2004
Perlow JH: Comparative use and knowledge of preconceptional folic acid among Spanish- and English-speaking patient populations in Phoenix and Yuma, Arizona. Am J Obstet Gynecol 184:1263, 2001
Pitkin RM: Calcium metabolism in pregnancy and the perinatal period: a review. Am J Obstet Gynecol 151:99, 1985
Pollak KI, Oncken CA, Lipkus IM, et al: Nicotine replacement and behavioral therapy for smoking cessation in pregnancy. Am J Prev Med 33(4):297, 2007
Pritchard JA, Scott DE: Iron demands during pregnancy. In Hallberg L, Harwerth HG, Vannotti A (eds): Iron Deficiency: Pathogenesis, Clinical Aspects, Therapy. New York, Academic Press, 1970
Quaranta P, Currell R, Redman CWG, et al: Prediction of small-for-dates infants by measurement of symphysial-fundal height. Br J Obstet Gynaecol 88:115, 1981
Radhika MS, Bhaskaram P, Balakrishna N, et al: Effects of vitamin A deficiency during pregnancy on maternal and child health. Br J Obstet Gynaecol 109:689, 2002
Read JS, Klebanoff MA: Sexual intercourse during pregnancy and preterm delivery: effects of vaginal microorganisms. Am J Obstet Gynecol 168:514, 1993
Rinsky-Eng J, Miller L: Knowledge, use, and education regarding folic acid supplementation: continuation study of women in Colorado who had a pregnancy affected by a neural tube defect. Teratology 66:S29, 2002
Ryan ET, Wilson ME, Kain KC: Illness after international travel. N Engl J Med 347:505, 2002
Sa Roriz Fonteles C, Zero DT, Moss ME, et al: Fluoride concentrations in enamel and dentin of primary teeth after pre- and postnatal fluoride exposure. Caries Res 39:505, 2005
Sayle AE, Savitz DA, Thorp JM Jr, et al: Sexual activity during late pregnancy and risk of preterm delivery. Obstet Gynecol 97:283, 2001
Schauberger CW, Rooney BL, Brimer LM: Factors that influence weight loss in the puerperium. Obstet Gynecol 79:424, 1992
Scott DE, Pritchard JA, Saltin AS, et al: Iron deficiency during pregnancy. In Hallberg L, Harwerth HG, Vannotti A (eds): Iron Deficiency: Pathogenesis, Clinical Aspects, Therapy. New York, Academic Press, 1970
Sibai BM, Villar MA, Bray E: Magnesium supplementation during pregnancy: a double-blind randomized controlled clinical trial. Am J Obstet Gynecol 161:115, 1989
Siddique J, Lauderdale DS, VanderWeele TJ, et al: Trends in prenatal ultrasound use in the United States. Med Care 47:1129, 2009
Smith CA: Effects of maternal undernutrition upon the newborn infant in Holland (1944–1945). Am J Obstet Gynecol 30:229, 1947
Smith MW, Marcus PS, and Wurtz LD: Orthopedic issues in pregnancy. Obstet Gynecol Surv 63:103, 2008
Staroselsky A, Garcia-Bournissen F, Koren G: American Gastroenterological Association Institute medical position statement on the use of gastrointestinal medication in pregnancy. Gastroenterology 132:824, 2007
Stein Z, Susser M, Saenger G, et al: Nutrition and mental performance. Science 178:708, 1972
Suarez VR, Hankins GD: Smallpox and pregnancy: from eradicated disease to bioterrorist threat. Obstet Gynecol 100:87, 2002
Sugarman SD: Cases in vaccine court—legal battles over vaccines and autism. N Engl J Med 257:1275, 2007
Tan PC, Yow CM, Omar SZ: Effect of coital activity on onset of labor in women scheduled for labor induction. Obstet Gynecol 110:820, 2007
Thaver D, Saeed MA, Bhutta ZA: Pyridoxine (vitamin B_6) supplementation in pregnancy. Cochrane Database Syst Rev 2:CD000179, 2006

Thompson MD, Cole DE, Ray JG: Vitamin B_{12} and neural tube defects: the Canadian experience. Am J Clin Nutr 89(2):697S, 2009
Thompson WW, Price C, Goodson B, et al: Early thimerosal exposure and neuropsychological outcomes at 7 to 10 years. N Engl J Med 257:1281, 2007
Thornley I, Eapen M, Sung L, et al: Private cord blood banking: experiences and views of pediatric hematopoietic cell transplantation physicians. Pediatrics 123(3):1011, 2009
Tong VT, Dietz PM, Morrow B, et al: Trends in smoking before, during, and after pregnancy—pregnancy risk assessment monitoring system, United States, 40 sites, 2000–2010. MMWR 62(6):1, 2013
Tozzi AE, Bisiacchi P, Tarantino V, et al: Neuropsychological performance 10 years after immunization in infancy with thimerosal-containing vaccines. Pediatrics 123(2):475, 2009
United States Department of Health and Human Services: Reducing tobacco use: a report of the Surgeon General. Atlanta, U.S. Department of Health and Human Services, Centers for Disease Control and Prevention, National Center for Chronic Disease Prevention and Health Promotion, Office on Smoking and Health, 2000
United States Environmental Protection Agency: What you need to know about mercury in fish and shellfish. 2004. Available at: www.epa.gov/waterscience/fish/advice./ Accessed July 1, 2013
U.S. Preventive Services Task Force: Recommendation statement: clinical guidelines: folic acid for the prevention of neural tube defects. Ann Intern Med 150:626, 2009
Villar J, Báaqeel H, Piaggio G, et al: WHO antenatal care randomised trial for the evaluation of a new model of routine antenatal care. Lancet 357:1551, 2001
Vintzileos AM, Ananth CV, Smulian JC, et al: Prenatal care and black-white fetal death disparity in the United States: heterogeneity by high-risk conditions. Obstet Gynecol 99:483, 2002a
Vintzileos AM, Ananth CV, Smulian JC, et al: The impact of prenatal care on neonatal deaths in the presence and absence of antenatal high-risk conditions. Am J Obstet Gynecol 186:1011, 2002b
Vintzileos AM, Ananth CV, Smulian JC, et al: The impact of prenatal care on preterm births among twin gestations in the United States, 1989–2000. Am J Obstet Gynecol 189:818, 2003
Wang SM, Dezinno P, Maranets I, et al: Low back pain during pregnancy: prevalence, risk factors, and outcomes. Obstet Gynecol 104:65, 2004
Washington State Health Care Authority: Ultrasonography (ultrasound) in pregnancy: a health technology assessment. 2010. Available at: http://www.hta.hca.wa.gov/documents/final_report_ultrasound.pdf. Accessed July 1, 2013
West KP: Vitamin A deficiency disorders in children and women. Food Nutr Bull 24:S78, 2003
Wiesen AR, Littell CT: Relationship between prepregnancy anthrax vaccination and pregnancy and birth outcomes among US Army women. JAMA 287:1556, 2002
Wilcox AJ, Baird DD, Dunson D, et al: Natural limits of pregnancy testing in relation to the expected menstrual period. JAMA 286:1759, 2001
Wilson DL, Barnes M, Ellett L, et al: Decreased sleep efficiency, increased wake after sleep onset and increased cortical arousals in late pregnancy. Aust N Z J Obstet Gynaecol 51(1):38, 2011
Wisborg K, Henriksen TB, Jespersen LB, et al: Nicotine patches for pregnant smokers: a randomized controlled study. Obstet Gynecol 96:967, 2000
Worthen N, Bustillo M: Effect of urinary bladder fullness on fundal height measurements. Am J Obstet Gynecol 138:759, 1980
Xu J, Kochanek KD, Murphy SL: Deaths: final data for 2007. Nat Stat Vit Rep 58(19):1, 2010
Zaman K, Roy E, Arifeen SE, et al: Effectiveness of maternal influenza immunization in mothers and infants. N Engl J Med 359(15):1555, 2008
Zeskind PS, Gingras JL: Maternal cigarette-smoking during pregnancy disrupts rhythms in fetal heart rate. J Pediatr Psychology 31:5, 2006

SECTION 5

THE FETAL PATIENT

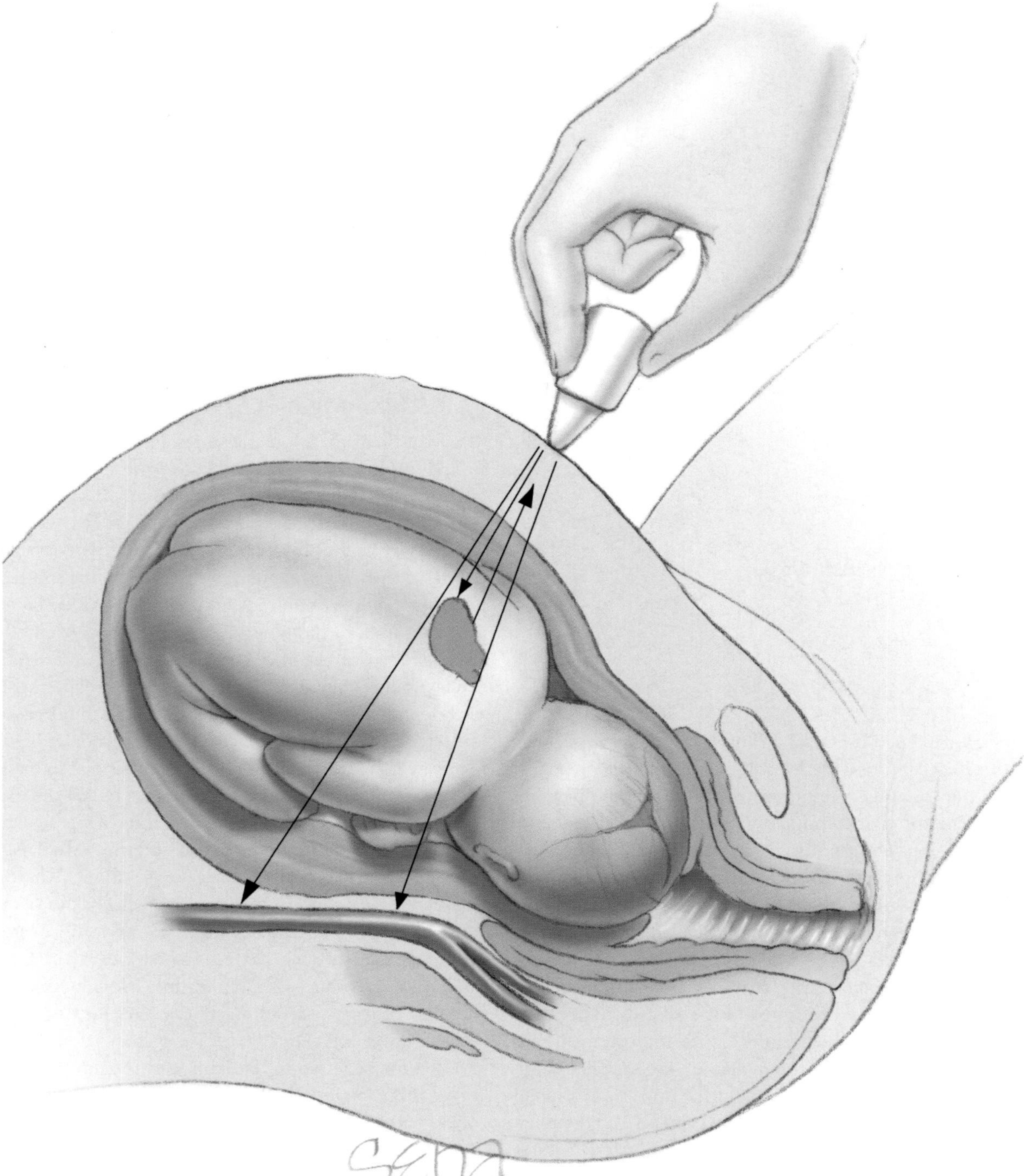

CHAPTER 10

Fetal Imaging

SONOGRAPHY IN OBSTETRICS

A great hallmark in obstetrical history began in the second half of the 20th century with the ability to image the pregnant uterus and its contents. Beginning with sonographic imaging and continuing through computed tomographic and magnetic resonance imaging, obstetrical practice was revolutionized and gave birth to the specialty of fetal medicine. Today's practitioner can hardly imagine obstetrical care without these technical advances, which have become commonplace and regarded almost as a sixth sense.

Sonography in prenatal care includes first- and second-trimester fetal anatomic evaluation and specialized studies performed to characterize abnormalities. With improvements in resolution and image display, anomalies are increasingly diagnosed in the first trimester. Applications for three-dimensional sonography and Doppler continue to expand. A sonographic examination performed with the exacting recommended standards of the American Institute of Ultrasound in Medicine (2013a) offers vital information regarding fetal anatomy, physiology, growth, and well-being. Indeed, a National Institute of Child Health and Human Development (NICHD) workshop concluded that "every fetus deserves to have a physical examination" (Reddy, 2008).

Technology and Safety

The real-time image on the ultrasound screen is produced by sound waves that are reflected back from fluid and tissue interfaces of the fetus, amnionic fluid, and placenta. Sector array transducers used in obstetrics contain groups of piezoelectric crystals working simultaneously in arrays. These crystals convert electrical energy into sound waves, which are emitted in synchronized pulses. Sound waves pass through tissue layers and are reflected back to the transducer when they encounter an interface between tissues of different densities. Dense tissue such as bone produces high-velocity reflected waves, which are displayed as bright echoes on the screen. Conversely, fluid generates few reflected waves and appears dark—or anechoic. Digital images generated at 50 to more than 100 frames per second undergo postprocessing that yields the appearance of real-time imaging.

Ultrasound refers to sound waves traveling at a frequency above 20,000 hertz (cycles per second). Higher-frequency transducers yield better image resolution, whereas lower frequencies penetrate tissue more effectively. Transducers use wide-bandwidth technology to perform over a range of frequencies. In the second trimester, a 4- to 6-megahertz abdominal transducer is often in close enough proximity to the fetus to provide precise images. By the third trimester, however, a lower frequency 2- to 5-megahertz transducer may be needed for penetration, but can lead to compromised resolution. This explains why resolution is often poor when imaging obese patients and why low-frequency transducers are needed to *reach* the fetus through maternal tissues. In early pregnancy, a 5- to 10-megahertz vaginal transducer may provide excellent resolution, because the early fetus is close to the transducer.

Fetal Safety

Sonography should be performed only for a valid medical indication, using the lowest possible exposure setting to gain necessary information—the ALARA principle—as low as reasonably achievable. It should be performed only by those trained to recognize medically important conditions such as fetal anomalies, artifacts that may mimic pathology, and techniques to avoid ultrasound exposure beyond what is considered safe for the fetus (American Institute of Ultrasound in Medicine, 2008a, 2013a). Prolonged ultrasound exposure may affect brain cell migration in fetal mice (Rakic, 2006). However, no causal relationship has been demonstrated between diagnostic ultrasound and recognized adverse effects in human pregnancy (American Institute of Ultrasound in Medicine, 2010).

All sonography machines are required to display two indices: the *thermal index* and the *mechanical index*. The thermal index is a measure of the relative probability that the examination may raise the temperature, potentially enough to induce injury. That said, it is extremely unlikely that fetal damage could occur using commercially available ultrasound equipment in routine practice. The potential for temperature elevation is higher with longer examination time and is greater near bone than in soft tissue. Also, theoretical risks are greater during organogenesis than later in gestation. The thermal index is higher with pulsed Doppler applications than with routine B-mode scanning (p. 219). In the first trimester, if pulsed Doppler is *needed* for a clinical indication, the thermal index should be ≤ 1.0, and exposure time should be kept as short as possible, usually no longer than 5 to 10 minutes (American Institute of Ultrasound in Medicine, 2011; Salvesen, 2011). To document the embryonic or fetal heart rate, M-mode imaging should be used instead of pulsed Doppler imaging (American Institute of Ultrasound in Medicine, 2013a).

The mechanical index is a measure of likelihood of adverse effects related to rarefractional pressure, such as cavitation—which is relevant only in tissues that contain air. Microbubble ultrasound contrast agents are not used in pregnancy for this reason. No adverse effects have been reported in mammalian tissues that do not contain gas bodies over the range of diagnostically relevant exposures. Because fetuses cannot contain gas bodies, they are not considered at risk (American Institute of Ultrasound in Medicine, 2008b).

The use of sonography for any nonmedical purpose, such as "keepsake fetal imaging," is considered *contrary to responsible medical practice* and is not condoned by the Food and Drug Administration (Rados, 2007), the American Institute of Ultrasound in Medicine (2012, 2013a), or the International Society of Ultrasound in Obstetrics and Gynecology (2011).

Operator Safety

The reported prevalence of work-related musculoskeletal discomfort or injury among sonographers and sonologists is as high as 70 to 80 percent (Janga, 2012; Magnavita, 1999; Pike, 1997). According to the National Institute for Occupational Safety and Health, the main risk factors for injury during transabdominal ultrasound are awkward posture, sustained static forces, and various pinch grips while maneuvering the transducer (Centers for Disease Control and Prevention, 2006). Another possible contributory factor is maternal habitus—as more force may be employed when imaging obese patients.

The following guidelines may help avert injury:

1. Position the patient on the examination table close to you, so that your elbow is close to your body, with less than 30 degrees shoulder abduction, keeping your thumb facing up.
2. Adjust the table or chair height so that your forearm is parallel to the floor.
3. If seated, use a chair with back support, support your feet, and keep ankles in neutral position. Do not lean toward the patient or monitor.
4. Face the monitor squarely and position it so that it is viewed at a neutral angle, such as 15 degrees downward.
5. Avoid reaching, bending, or twisting while scanning.
6. Frequent breaks may avoid muscle strain. Stretching and strengthening exercises can be helpful.

First-Trimester Sonography

Indications for sonography before 14 weeks' gestation are listed in Table 10-1. Early pregnancy can be evaluated using transabdominal or transvaginal sonography, or both. The components listed in Table 10-2 should be assessed. The crown-rump length (CRL) is the most accurate biometric predictor of gestational age (Appendix, p. 1294). The CRL should be obtained in a sagittal plane and include neither the yolk sac nor a limb bud. If carefully performed, it has a variance of only 3 to 5 days.

TABLE 10-1. Some Indications for First-Trimester Ultrasound Examination

Confirm an intrauterine pregnancy
Evaluate a suspected ectopic pregnancy
Define the cause of vaginal bleeding
Evaluate pelvic pain
Estimate gestational age
Diagnose or evaluate multifetal gestations
Confirm cardiac activity
Assist chorionic villus sampling, embryo transfer, and localization and removal of an intrauterine device
Assess for certain fetal anomalies such as anencephaly, in high-risk patients
Evaluate maternal pelvic masses and/or uterine abnormalities
Measure nuchal translucency when part of a screening program for fetal aneuploidy
Evaluate suspected gestational trophoblastic disease

Modified from the American Institute of Ultrasound in Medicine, 2013a.

SECTION 5

TABLE 10-2. Components of Standard Ultrasound Examination by Trimester

First Trimester	Second and Third Trimester
Gestational sac size, location, and number Embryo and/or yolk sac identification Crown-rump length Fetal number, including amnionicity and chorionicity of multifetal gestations Embryonic/fetal cardiac activity Assessment of embryonic/fetal anatomy appropriate for the first trimester Evaluation of the maternal uterus, adnexa, and cul-de-sac Evaluation of the fetal nuchal region, with consideration of fetal nuchal translucency assessment	Fetal number, including amnionicity and chorionicity of multifetal gestations Fetal cardiac activity Fetal presentation Placental location, appearance, and relationship to the internal cervical os, with documentation of placental cord insertion site when technically possible Amnionic fluid volume Gestational age assessment Fetal weight estimation Fetal anatomical survey, including documentation of technical limitations Evaluation of the maternal uterus, adnexa, and cervix when appropriate

Modified from the American Institute of Ultrasound in Medicine, 2013a.

First-trimester sonography can reliably diagnose anembryonic gestation, embryonic demise, ectopic pregnancy, and gestational trophoblastic disease. Multifetal gestation can be identified early, and this is the optimal time to determine chorionicity (Chap. 45, p. 896). The first trimester is also the ideal time to evaluate the uterus, adnexa, and cul-de-sac. Cervical length and the relationship of the placenta to the cervical os are best evaluated in the second trimester.

An intrauterine gestational sac is reliably visualized with transvaginal sonography by 5 weeks, and an embryo with cardiac activity by 6 weeks. The embryo should be visible transvaginally once the mean sac diameter has reached 20 mm—otherwise the gestation is *anembryonic* (Chap. 18, p. 355). Cardiac motion is usually visible with transvaginal imaging when the embryo length has reached 5 mm. If an embryo less than 7 mm is not identified to have cardiac activity, a subsequent examination is recommended in 1 week (American Institute of Ultrasound in Medicine, 2013a). At Parkland hospital, first-trimester demise is diagnosed if the embryo has reached 10 mm without cardiac motion, taking into consideration the standard error of the ultrasound measurements.

Nuchal Translucency (NT)

Nuchal translucency evaluation, a component of first-trimester aneuploidy screening, has had a major impact on the number of pregnancies receiving late first-trimester ultrasound examination. It represents the maximum thickness of the subcutaneous translucent area between the skin and soft tissue overlying the fetal spine at the back of the neck (Fig. 14-5, p. 290). It is measured in the sagittal plane between 11 and 14 weeks using precise criteria (Table 10-3). When the nuchal translucency is increased, the risk for fetal aneuploidy and various structural anomalies—including heart defects—is significantly elevated. Aneuploidy screening using nuchal translucency measurement in conjunction with assessment of maternal serum human chorionic gonadotropin and pregnancy-associated plasma protein A levels is discussed in Chapter 14 (p. 290).

First-Trimester Fetal Anomaly Detection

Assessment for selected fetal abnormalities in an at-risk pregnancy is another indication for first-trimester sonography (see Table 10-1). Research in this area has focused on anatomy visible at 11 to 14 weeks, to coincide with sonography performed as part of aneuploidy screening (Chap. 14, p. 289). *With current technology, it is not realistic to expect that all major abnormalities detectable in the second trimester may be visualized in the first trimester.* A study of systematic anatomy evaluation between 11 and 14 weeks in more than 40,000 pregnancies yielded a detection rate of approximately 40 percent for nonchromosomal abnormalities (Syngelaki, 2011). This detection rate is nearly identical

TABLE 10-3. Guidelines for Nuchal Translucency (NT) Measurement

The margins of NT edges must be clear enough for proper caliper placement
The fetus must be in the midsagittal plane
The image must be magnified so that it is filled by the fetal head, neck, and upper thorax
The fetal neck must be in a neutral position, not flexed and not hyperextended
The amnion must be seen as separate from the NT line
Electronic calipers must be used to perform the measurement
The + calipers must be placed on the inner borders of the nuchal space with none of the horizontal crossbar itself protruding into the space
The calipers must be placed perpendicular to the long axis of the fetus
The measurement must be obtained at the widest space of the NT

From the American Institute of Ultrasound in Medicine, 2013a, with permission.

to that from a review of more than 60,000 pregnancies from 15 studies and is also comparable with other reports (Pilalis, 2012; Syngelaki, 2011). Identification varies considerably according to the specific abnormality. For example, reported detection rates are extremely high for anencephaly, alobar holoprosencephaly, and ventral wall defects. However, only one-third of major cardiac anomalies have been identified, with *no* detected cases of microcephaly, agenesis of the corpus callosum, cerebellar abnormalities, congenital pulmonary airway malformations, or bowel obstruction (Syngelaki, 2011). Thus, as first-trimester sonography is unreliable for detection of many major abnormalities, it should not replace second-trimester anatomical evaluation.

Second- and Third-Trimester Sonography

The many indications for second- and third-trimester sonography are listed in Table 10-4. There are three types of examinations: *standard, specialized,* and *limited.*

1. *Standard* sonographic examination is the most commonly performed. Components are listed in Table 10-2. The fetal anatomical structures that should be evaluated during the examination, which are listed in Table 10-5, may be adequately assessed after approximately 18 weeks. When examining twins or other multiples, documentation also includes the number of chorions and amnions, comparison of fetal sizes, estimation of amnionic fluid volume within each sac, and fetal sex determination (Chap. 45, p. 912).
2. There are several types of *specialized* examinations. The *targeted* examination is a detailed anatomical survey performed when an abnormality is suspected on the basis of history, screening test result, or abnormal findings from a standard examination (American Institute of Ultrasound in Medicine, 2013a). A targeted examination is performed and interpreted by an experienced operator. It includes the anatomical structures listed in Table 10-5, along with additional views of the brain and cranium, neck, profile, lungs and diaphragm, cardiac anatomy, liver, shape and curvature of the spine, hands and feet, and any placental abnormalities. The physician performing the examination further determines whether other examination components will be needed on a case-by-case basis (American College of Obstetricians and Gynecologists, 2011). Other specialized examinations

TABLE 10-4. Indications for Second- or Third-Trimester Ultrasound Examination

Maternal Indications
Vaginal bleeding
Abdominal/pelvic pain
Pelvic mass
Suspected uterine abnormality
Suspected ectopic pregnancy
Suspected molar pregnancy
Suspected placenta previa and subsequent surveillance
Suspected placental abruption
Preterm premature rupture of membranes and/or preterm labor
Cervical insufficiency
Adjunct to cervical cerclage
Adjunct to amniocentesis or other procedure
Adjunct to external cephalic version
Fetal Indications
Gestational age estimation
Fetal-growth evaluation
Significant uterine size/clinical date discrepancy
Suspected multifetal gestation
Fetal anatomical evaluation
Fetal anomaly screening
Assessment for findings that may increase the aneuploidy risk
Abnormal biochemical markers
Fetal presentation determination
Suspected hydramnios or oligohydramnios
Fetal well-being evaluation
Follow-up evaluation of a fetal anomaly
History of congenital anomaly in prior pregnancy
Suspected fetal death
Fetal condition evaluation in late registrants for prenatal care

Adapted from the American Institute of Ultrasound in Medicine, 2013a.

TABLE 10-5. Minimal Elements of a Standard Examination of Fetal Anatomy

Head, face, and neck
Lateral cerebral ventricles
Choroid plexus
Midline falx
Cavum septum pellucidi
Cerebellum
Cisterna magna
Upper lip
Consideration of nuchal fold measurement at 15–20 weeks
Chest
Four-chamber view of the heart
Left ventricular outflow tract
Right ventricular outflow tract
Abdomen
Stomach—presence, size, and situs
Kidneys
Urinary bladder
Umbilical cord insertion into fetal abdomen
Umbilical cord vessel number
Spine
Cervical, thoracic, lumbar, and sacral spine
Extremities
Legs and arms
Fetal sex
In multifetal gestations and when medically indicated

Summarized from the American Institute of Ultrasound in Medicine, 2013a.

include fetal echocardiography and Doppler evaluation (discussed below), biophysical profile (Chap. 17, p. 341), and additional biometric measurements.

3. A *limited* examination is performed to address a specific clinical question. Examples include amnionic fluid volume assessment, placental location, or evaluation of fetal presentation or viability. In most cases, a limited examination is appropriate only when a prior standard or targeted examination has previously been performed (American Institute of Ultrasound in Medicine, 2009, 2013a).

Fetal Biometry

Equipment software derives the estimated gestational age from the crown-rump length. Formulas are similarly used to calculate estimated gestational age and fetal weight from measurements of the biparietal diameter, head and abdominal circumference, and femur length (Fig. 10-1). The estimates are most accurate when multiple parameters are used and when nomograms derived from fetuses of similar ethnic or racial background living at similar altitude are selected. Even the best models may over- or underestimate fetal weight by as much as 15 percent (American Institute of Ultrasound in Medicine, 2013a). Various nomograms for other fetal structures, including the cerebellum diameter, ear length, interocular and binocular distances, thoracic circumference, and kidney, long bones, and feet lengths, may be used to address specific questions regarding organ system abnormalities or syndromes. These nomograms may be found in the Appendix (p. 1298).

In the second trimester, the biparietal diameter (BPD) most accurately reflects the gestational age, with a variation of 7 to 10 days. The BPD is measured in the *transthalamic view*, at the level of the thalami and cavum septum pellucidum (CSP), from the outer edge of the skull in the near field to the inner edge of the skull in the far field (see Fig. 10-1A). The head circumference (HC) is also measured in the transthalamic view, either by placing an ellipse around the outer edge of the skull, or by measuring the occipital-frontal diameter (OFD) and calculating the circumference from the BPD and OFD. The *cephalic index*, which is the BPD divided by the OFD, is normally approximately 70 to 86 percent. If the head shape is flattened—*dolichocephaly,* or rounded—*brachycephaly,* the HC is more reliable than the BPD. Dolichocephaly and brachycephaly may be normal variants or may be secondary to positional changes or oligohydramnios. However, dolichocephaly can occur with neural-tube defects, and brachycephaly may be seen in fetuses with Down syndrome (Chap. 13, p. 262). Whenever the skull shape is abnormal, *craniosynostosis* and other craniofacial abnormalities are a consideration.

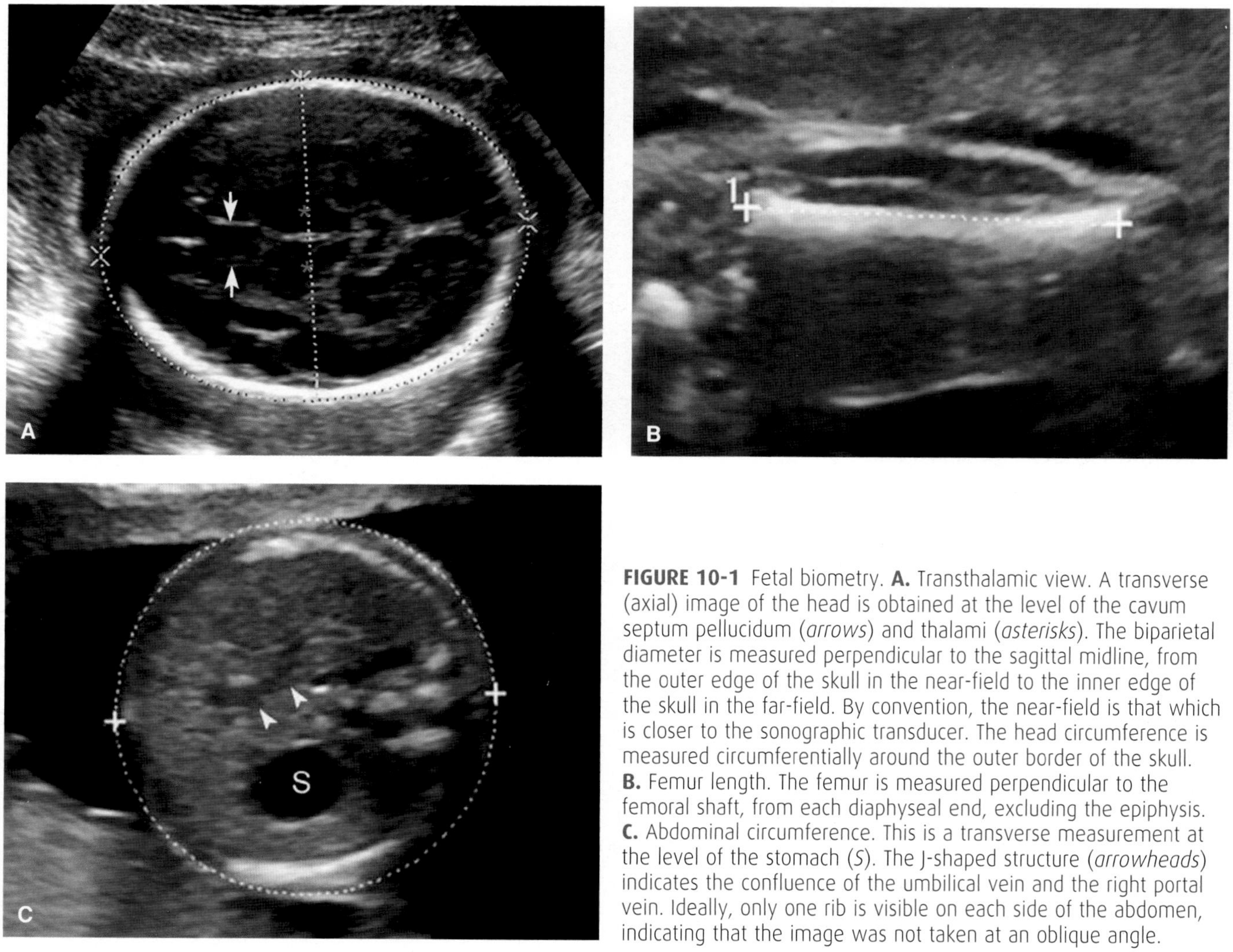

FIGURE 10-1 Fetal biometry. **A.** Transthalamic view. A transverse (axial) image of the head is obtained at the level of the cavum septum pellucidum (*arrows*) and thalami (*asterisks*). The biparietal diameter is measured perpendicular to the sagittal midline, from the outer edge of the skull in the near-field to the inner edge of the skull in the far-field. By convention, the near-field is that which is closer to the sonographic transducer. The head circumference is measured circumferentially around the outer border of the skull. **B.** Femur length. The femur is measured perpendicular to the femoral shaft, from each diaphyseal end, excluding the epiphysis. **C.** Abdominal circumference. This is a transverse measurement at the level of the stomach (*S*). The J-shaped structure (*arrowheads*) indicates the confluence of the umbilical vein and the right portal vein. Ideally, only one rib is visible on each side of the abdomen, indicating that the image was not taken at an oblique angle.

The femur length (FL) correlates well with both BPD and gestational age. It is measured with the beam perpendicular to the long axis of the shaft, excluding the epiphysis. For gestational age estimation, it has a variation of 7 to 11 days in the second trimester (see Fig. 10-1B). A mildly foreshortened femur—one that is 90 percent or less than that expected for gestational age—has been used as a minor marker for Down syndrome (Chap. 14, p. 292). A femur length that is dramatically foreshortened prompts an evaluation for a skeletal dysplasia, as discussed on page 217. In general, the normal range for the FL to abdominal circumference (AC) ratio is 20 to 24 percent. A FL/AC < 16 percent suggests a lethal skeletal dysplasia, particularly if other skeletal abnormalities are present (Rahemtullah, 1997; Ramus, 1998).

The abdominal circumference has the greatest variation, up to 2 to 3 weeks, for gestational age estimation. The AC is measured around the outer border of the skin. This is a transverse image at the level of the stomach and the confluence of the umbilical vein with the portal sinus (see Fig. 10-1C). Of the biometric parameters, AC is most affected by fetal growth. As discussed in Chapter 44 (p. 875), a small abdominal circumference has been used as an early indicator of fetal-growth restriction (Baschat, 2011).

Variability of the estimated gestational age and of fetal weight increases with advancing gestation. Individual measurements are least accurate in the third trimester. Although estimates are improved by averaging multiple parameters, if one parameter differs significantly from the others, consideration is given to excluding it from the calculation. The outlier could result from poor visibility, but it could also indicate a fetal abnormality or growth problem. Reference tables such as the one in the Appendix (p. 1296) are used to estimate fetal weight percentiles. Menstrual dates are generally considered confirmed if an estimated gestational age (EGA) based on a sonographic first-trimester crown-rump length is within 1 week or if the EGA from biometry at 14 to 20 weeks is within 10 days (American College of Obstetricians and Gynecologists, 2011). In the third trimester, the accuracy of sonography is only within 3 to 4 weeks. Sonographic evaluation performed to monitor fetal growth should typically be performed at least 2 to 4 weeks after a prior examination (American Institute of Ultrasound in Medicine, 2013a).

Amnionic Fluid

Amnionic fluid volume evaluation is a component of every second- or third-trimester sonogram. *Oligohydramnios* indicates that the volume is below normal range, and subjective crowding of the fetus is often noted. *Hydramnios*—also called *polyhydramnios*—is defined as amnionic fluid volume above normal (Fig. 11-3, p. 234). Although it is considered acceptable for an experienced examiner to assess the amnionic fluid volume qualitatively, fluid is usually assessed semiquantitatively (American Institute of Ultrasound in Medicine, 2013a). Measurements include either the single deepest vertical fluid pocket or the sum of the deepest vertical pockets from each of four equal uterine quadrants—the *amnionic fluid index* (Phelan, 1987). Reference ranges have been established for both measurements from 16 weeks' gestation onward (Fig. 11-1, p. 233). The single deepest vertical pocket is normally between 2 and 8 cm, and the amnionic fluid index normally ranges between 8 and 24 cm. Amnionic fluid volume is discussed further in Chapter 11 (p. 232).

Fetal Anatomical Evaluation

An important goal of second- and third-trimester sonography is to systematically evaluate fetal anatomy and determine whether specific anatomical components appear normal or abnormal. If a single ultrasound examination is planned for the purpose of evaluating fetal anatomy, the American College of Obstetricians and Gynecologists (2011) recommends that it be performed at 18 to 20 weeks. At this gestational age range, complex organs such as the fetal brain and heart can be imaged clearly enough to visualize many major malformations. Technical factors such as maternal habitus, abdominal wall scarring, fetal size, and fetal position may limit adequate visualization, and these limitations should be noted in the report. If imaging is suboptimal, a follow-up examination may be helpful. If an abnormality is identified or suspected during a standard examination of fetal anatomy, specialized sonography is indicated.

Second-Trimester Fetal Anomaly Detection. The sensitivity of sonography for detecting fetal anomalies varies according to factors such as gestational age, maternal habitus, fetal position, equipment features, examination type, operator skill, and the specific abnormality in question. For example, maternal obesity has been associated with a 20-percent reduction in the fetal anomaly detection rate, regardless of examination type (Dashe, 2009).

Imaging technological advances have contributed to dramatic improvements in anomaly detection. In a review of more than 925,000 pregnancies evaluated between 1978 and 1997, Levi (2002) identified an overall anomaly detection rate of 40 percent. The single largest trial, the EUROFETUS study, included 170,800 pregnancies and identified 55 percent with severe malformations before 24 weeks (Grandjean, 1999). The most recent data are available from a network of population-based registries from 21 European countries, termed EUROCAT, found at: www.eurocat-network.eu.

Between 2006 and 2010, EUROCAT prenatal detection rates for selected anomalies were as follows: anencephaly, 97 percent; spina bifida, 84 percent; hydrocephaly, 77 percent; cleft lip, 54 percent; hypoplastic left heart, 73 percent; diaphragmatic hernia, 59 percent; gastroschisis, 94 percent; omphalocele, 84 percent; bilateral renal agenesis, 91 percent; posterior urethral valves, 81 percent; limb-reduction defects, 52 percent; and clubfoot, 43 percent (EUROCAT, 2012). Importantly, however, the overall anomaly detection rate, excluding aneuploidy, was only *34 percent.* This reflects inclusion of anomalies with minimal or no sonographic detection, such as microcephaly, anotia, choanal atresia, cleft palate, bile duct atresia, Hirschsprung disease, anal atresia, and congenital skin disorders. These are mentioned because clinicians tend to focus on abnormalities amenable to sonographic detection, whereas families may find those not readily detectable no less devastating. *Every sonographic examination should include a frank discussion of examination limitations.*

The sensitivity of specialized sonography in experienced centers is considered to be at least 80 percent (American College of Obstetricians and Gynecologists, 2011). Most anomalous infants—approximately 75 percent—occur in pregnancies that are otherwise low-risk, that is, without an indication for specialized sonography. Thus, the quality of a standard screening sonogram greatly affects overall anomaly detection from a population perspective (Dashe, 2009; Levi, 2002). Practice guidelines and standards established by organizations such as the American Institute of Ultrasound in Medicine (2013a) and the International Society of Ultrasound in Obstetrics and Gynecology (Salomon, 2011) have undoubtedly contributed to improvements in anomaly detection rates.

NORMAL AND ABNORMAL FETAL ANATOMY

Many fetal anomalies and syndromes may be characterized with targeted sonography. Selected abnormalities of the anatomical components in Table 10-5 are discussed below. This list is not intended to be comprehensive but covers abnormalities that are relatively common and may be detectable with standard sonography, as well as those that are potentially amenable to fetal therapy. Sonographic features of chromosomal abnormalities are reviewed in Chapters 13 and 14, and fetal therapy is discussed in Chapter 16.

Brain and Spine

Standard sonographic evaluation of the fetal brain includes three transverse (axial) views. The *transthalamic view* is used to measure the BPD and HC and includes the midline falx, cavum septum pellucidum (CSP), and thalami (see Fig. 10-1A). The CSP is the space between the two laminae that separate the frontal horns. Inability to visualize a normal CSP may indicate a midline brain abnormality such as agenesis of the corpus callosum, lobar holoprosencephaly, or septo-optic dysplasia (de Morsier syndrome). The *transventricular view* includes the lateral ventricles, which contain the echogenic choroid plexus (Fig. 10-2). The ventricles are measured at their atrium, which is the confluence of their temporal and occipital horns. The *transcerebellar view* is obtained by angling the transducer back through the posterior fossa (Fig. 10-3). In this view, the cerebellum and cisterna magna are measured, and between 15 and about 20 weeks, the nuchal skinfold thickness may be measured (Chap. 14, p. 289). From 15 until 22 weeks, the cerebellar diameter in millimeters is roughly equivalent to the gestational age in weeks (Goldstein, 1987). The cisterna magna normally measures between 2 and 10 mm. Effacement of the cisterna magna is present in the *Chiari II malformation*, discussed on page 202.

Imaging of the spine includes evaluation of the cervical, thoracic, lumbar, and sacral regions (Fig. 10-4). Representative spinal images for record keeping are often obtained in the sagittal or coronal plane. However, real-time imaging should include evaluation of each spinal segment in the transverse plane, as this is more sensitive for abnormality detection. Transverse images demonstrate three ossification centers. The anterior ossification center is the vertebral body, and the posterior paired ossification centers represent the junction of vertebral laminae and pedicles. Ossification of the spine proceeds in a cranial-caudal fashion, such that ossification of the upper sacrum (S1-S2) is not generally visible sonographically before 16 weeks' gestation. Ossification of the entire sacrum may not be visible until 21 weeks (De Biasio, 2003). Thus, detection of some spinal abnormalities may be challenging in the early second trimester.

Examples of spinal abnormalities include spina bifida, caudal regression sequence, and sacrococcygeal teratoma. More subtle spinal abnormalities may be visible. These include *diastematomyelia*, which is a longitudinal cleft or splitting of the spinal cord itself, and *hemivertebrae*—a component of the

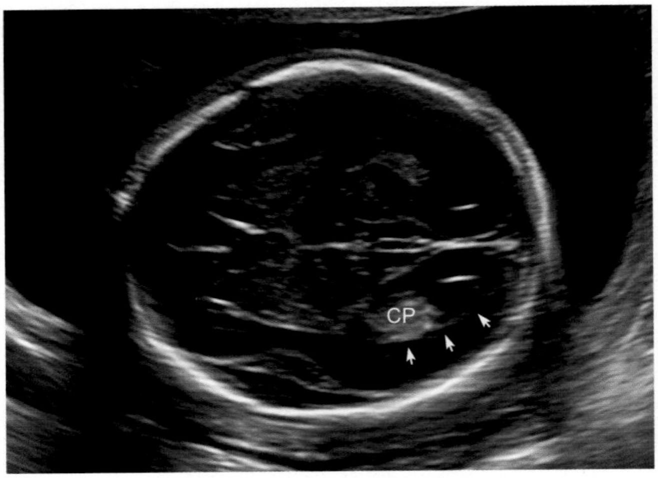

FIGURE 10-2 The transventricular view depicts the lateral ventricles, which contain the echogenic choroid plexus (*CP*). The lateral ventricle is measured at the *atrium* (*arrows*), which is the confluence of the temporal and occipital horns. A normal measurement is between 5 and 10 mm throughout the second and third trimesters. The atria measured 6 mm in this 21-week fetus.

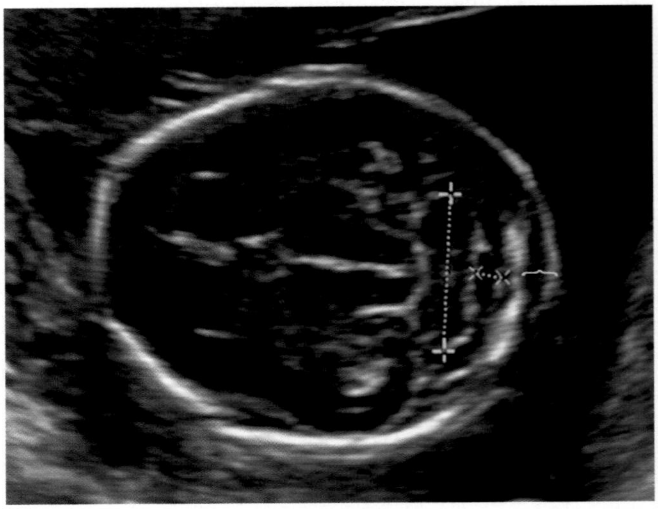

FIGURE 10-3 Transcerebellar view of the posterior fossa, demonstrating measurement of the cerebellum (+), cisterna magna (*X*), and nuchal fold thickness (*bracket*). Care is taken not to angle obliquely down the spine, which may artificially increase the nuchal fold measurement.

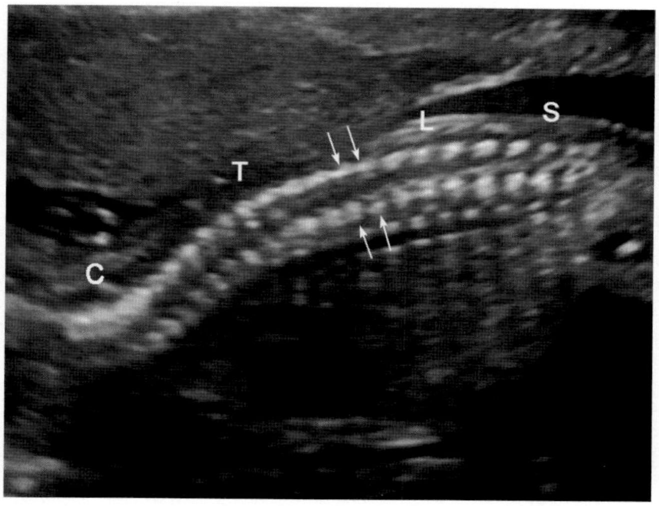

FIGURE 10-4 Normal fetal spine. In this sagittal image of a 21-week fetus, the cervical (*C*), thoracic (*T*), lumbar (*L*), and sacral spine (*S*) are depicted. Arrows denote the parallel rows of paired posterior ossification centers—representing the junction of vertebral lamina and pedicles.

vertebral, anal, cardiac, tracheo-esophageal fistula, renal, limb (VACTERL) association.

If a brain or spinal abnormality is identified, specialized sonography is indicated. The International Society of Ultrasound in Obstetrics and Gynecology (2007) has published guidelines for a "fetal neurosonogram." Fetal magnetic resonance (MR) imaging may be helpful in further characterizing central nervous system (CNS) abnormalities (p. 223).

Neural-Tube Defects

These result from incomplete closure of the neural tube by the embryonic age of 26 to 28 days. They are the second most common class of malformations after cardiac anomalies. Their prevalence was previously considered to be 1.4 to 2 per 1000 births. However, birth defect registries in the United States and Europe now report a prevalence of only 0.9 per 1000. In the United Kingdom, the prevalence is 1.3 per 1000 (Dolk, 2010). Neural-tube defects can be prevented with folic acid supplementation (Chap. 9, p. 181), and their prenatal diagnosis is discussed in Chapter 14 (p. 283). When isolated, neural-tube defect inheritance is multifactorial, and the defect recurrence risk without periconceptional folic acid supplementation is 3 to 5 percent.

Anencephaly is characterized by absence of the cranium and telencephalic structures, with the skullbase and orbits covered only by angiomatous stroma. *Acrania* is absence of the cranium, with protrusion of disorganized brain tissue. Both are generally grouped together, and anencephaly is considered to be the final stage of acrania (Bronshtein, 1991; McGahan, 2003). These lethal anomalies can be diagnosed in the late first trimester, and with adequate visualization, virtually all cases may be diagnosed in the second trimester (Fig. 10-5). An inability to view the biparietal diameter should raise suspicion. Hydramnios from impaired fetal swallowing is common in the third trimester.

Cephalocele is the herniation of meninges through a cranial defect, typically located in the midline occipital region (Fig. 10-6). When brain tissue herniates through the skull defect,

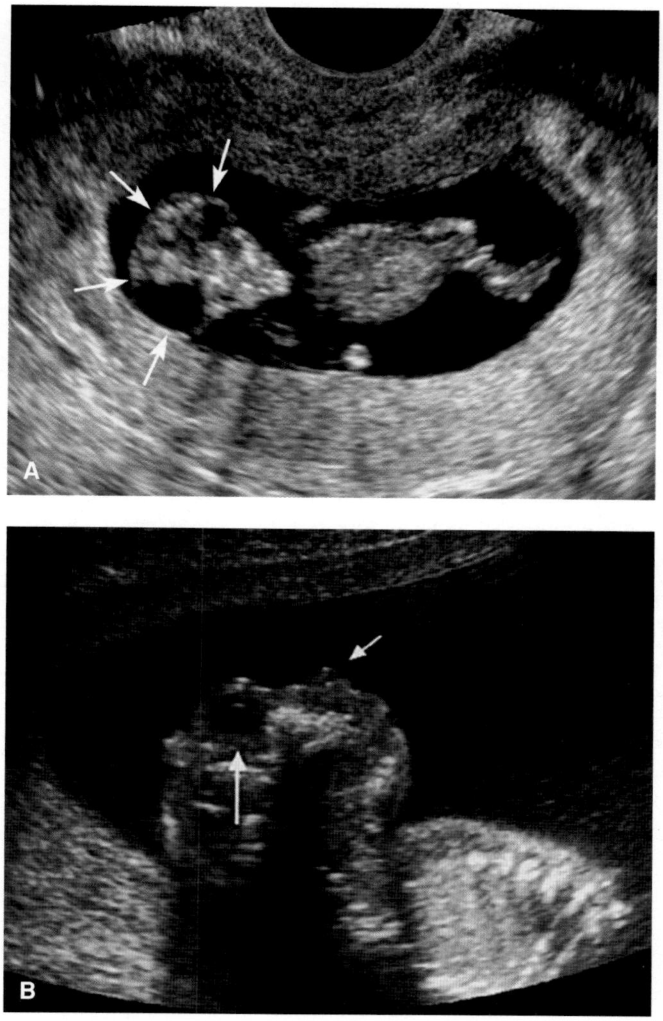

FIGURE 10-5 Anencephaly/acrania. **A.** Acrania. This 11-week fetus has absence of the cranium, with protrusion of a disorganized mass of brain tissue that resembles a "shower cap" (*arrows*) and a characteristic triangular facial appearance. **B.** Anencephaly. This sagittal image shows the absence of forebrain and cranium above the skull base and orbit. The long white arrow points to the fetal orbit, and the short white arrow indicates the nose.

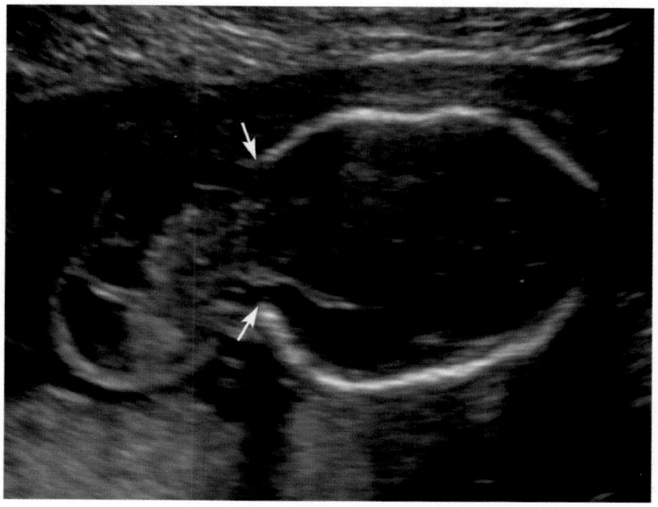

FIGURE 10-6 Encephalocele. This transverse image depicts a large defect in the occipital region of the cranium (*arrows*) through which meninges and brain tissue have herniated.

the anomaly is termed an *encephalocele*. Associated hydrocephalus and microcephaly are common. Surviving infants—those with smaller defects—have a high incidence of neurological deficits and developmental impairment. Cephalocele is an important feature of the autosomal recessive *Meckel-Gruber syndrome,* which includes cystic renal dysplasia and polydactyly. A cephalocele not located in the occipital midline raises suspicion for *amnionic-band sequence* (Chap. 6, p. 121).

Spina bifida is a defect in the vertebrae, typically the dorsal arch, with exposure of the meninges and spinal cord. The birth prevalence is approximately 1 per 2000 (Cragan, 2009; Dolk, 2010). Most cases are *open spina bifida*—the defect includes the skin and soft tissues. Herniation of a meningeal sac containing neural elements is termed a *myelomeningocele* (Fig. 10-7). When only a meningeal sac is present, the defect is a *meningocele.* Although the sac may be easier to image in the sagittal plane, transverse images more readily demonstrate separation or splaying of the lateral processes.

As discussed in Chapter 14 (p. 285), spina bifida may be reliably diagnosed with second-trimester sonography, often because of two characteristic cranial findings. These are scalloping of the frontal bones—the *lemon sign* (Fig. 14-4, p. 287), and anterior curvature of the cerebellum with effacement of the cisterna magna—the *banana sign* (Fig. 14-5) (Nicolaides, 1986). These findings are manifestations of the Chiari II malformation (also called Arnold-Chiari malformation), which occurs when downward displacement of the spinal cord pulls a portion of the cerebellum through the foramen magnum and into the upper cervical canal. *Ventriculomegaly* is another frequent sonographic finding, particularly after midgestation, and more than 80 percent of infants with open spina bifida require ventriculoperitoneal shunt placement. A small biparietal diameter is often present as well. Children with spina bifida require multidisciplinary care to address problems related to the defect, shunt, swallowing, bladder and bowel function, and ambulation. They are also at increased risk for latex allergy.

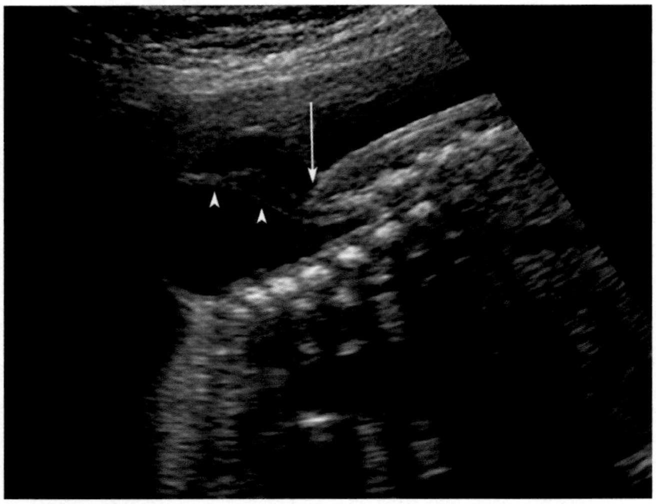

FIGURE 10-7 Myelomeningocele. In this sagittal image of a lumbosacral myelomeningocele, the arrowheads indicate nerve roots within the anechoic herniated sac. The overlying skin is visible above the level of the spinal defect but abruptly stops at the defect (*arrow*).

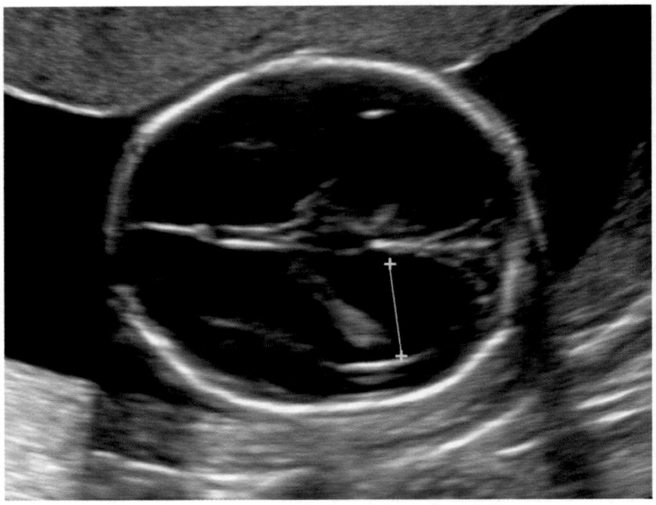

FIGURE 10-8 Ventriculomegaly. In this transverse view of the cranium, the yellow line depicts measurement of the atria, which measured 12 mm, consistent with mild ventriculomegaly.

Fetal surgery for myelomeningocele is discussed in Chapter 16 (p. 325).

Ventriculomegaly

This distention of the cerebral ventricles by cerebrospinal fluid (CSF) is a nonspecific marker of abnormal brain development (Pilu, 2011). The atrium normally measures between 5 and 10 mm from 15 weeks until term (see Fig. 10-2). Mild ventriculomegaly is diagnosed when the atrial width measures 10 to 15 mm, and overt or severe ventriculomegaly when it exceeds 15 mm (Fig. 10-8). CSF is produced by the choroid plexus, which is an epithelium-lined capillary core and loose connective tissue found in the ventricles. A *dangling choroid plexus* characteristically is found with severe ventriculomegaly.

Ventriculomegaly may be caused by various genetic and environmental insults, and prognosis is determined by etiology, degree, and rate of progression. In general, the larger the atrium, the greater the likelihood of abnormal outcome (Gaglioti, 2009; Joó, 2008). The finding of an enlarged ventricle may be due to another central nervous system abnormality—such as Dandy-Walker malformation or holoprosencephaly, due to an obstructive process—such as aqueductal stenosis, or secondary to a destructive process—such as porencephaly or an intracranial teratoma. Initial evaluation includes a specialized examination of fetal anatomy, fetal karyotyping, and testing for congenital infections such as cytomegalovirus and toxoplasmosis (Chap. 64, p. 1245).

Even when ventriculomegaly is mild and appears isolated, counseling may be a challenge because of the wide variability in prognosis. Devaseelan and colleagues (2010) conducted a systematic review of nearly 1500 pregnancies with apparently isolated mild ventriculomegaly. They found that 1 to 2 percent of cases were associated with congenital infection, 5 percent with aneuploidy, and 12 percent with neurological abnormality in the absence of infection or aneuploidy. Neurological abnormality was significantly more common if ventriculomegaly progressed, but asymmetry of ventricular size did not affect

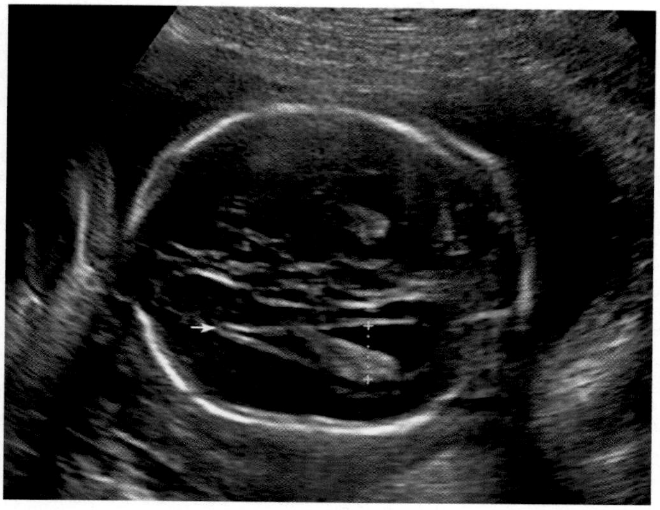

FIGURE 10-9 Agenesis of the corpus callosum. This image demonstrates a "teardrop" shaped ventricle with mild ventriculomegaly (*dotted line*) and laterally displaced frontal horns (*arrow*). A normal cavum septum pellucidum cannot be visualized.

prognosis. As abnormalities associated with mild ventriculomegaly may not be detectable sonographically, fetal MR imaging may be considered.

Agenesis of the Corpus Callosum

The corpus callosum is the major fiber bundle connecting reciprocal regions of the cerebral hemispheres. With complete agenesis of the corpus callosum, a normal cavum septum pellucidum cannot be visualized sonographically, and the frontal horns are displaced laterally. Also, there is mild enlargement of the atria posteriorly—such that the ventricle has a characteristic "teardrop" appearance (Fig. 10-9). Callosal dysgenesis can also occur, in which absence involves only the caudal portions—the body and splenium—and is consequently more difficult to detect prenatally.

In population-based studies, prevalence of agenesis of the corpus callosum is 1 in 5000 births (Glass, 2008; Szabo, 2011). In a recent review of apparently isolated cases of agenesis, fetal MR imaging identified additional brain abnormalities in more than 20 percent (Sotiriadis, 2012). If the anomaly was still considered isolated following MR imaging, normal developmental outcome was reported in 75 percent of cases, and severe disability in 12 percent. Agenesis of the corpus callosum is associated with other CNS and non-CNS anomalies, aneuploidy, and many genetic syndromes—more than 200—and thus genetic counseling can be challenging.

Holoprosencephaly

In early normal brain development, the prosencephalon or forebrain divides into the telencephalon and diencephalon. With holoprosencephaly, the prosencephalon fails to divide completely into two separate cerebral hemispheres and into underlying diencephalic structures. Main forms of holoprosencephaly are a continuum that contains, with decreasing severity, *alobar*, *semilobar*, and *lobar* types. In the most severe form—*alobar holoprosencephaly*—a single monoventricle, with or without a covering mantle of cortex, surrounds the fused central thalami (Fig. 10-10). In *semilobar holoprosencephaly*, partial separation of the hemispheres occurs. *Lobar holoprosencephaly* is characterized by a variable degree of fusion of frontal structures. Lobar holoprosencephaly should be considered when a normal cavum septum pellucidum cannot be visualized.

Differentiation into two cerebral hemispheres is induced by prechordal mesenchyme, which is also responsible for differentiation of the midline face. Thus, holoprosencephaly may be associated with anomalies of the orbits and eyes—hypotelorism, cyclopia, or micro-ophthalmia; lips—median cleft; or nose—ethmocephaly, cebocephaly, or arhinia with proboscis (see Fig. 10-10).

The birth prevalence of holoprosencephaly is only 1 in 10,000 to 15,000. However, the abnormality has been identified in nearly 1 in 250 early abortuses, which attests to the extremely high in-utero lethality of this condition (Orioli, 2010; Yamada 2004). The alobar form accounts for 40 to 75 percent of cases, and approximately 30 to 40 percent have a numerical chromosomal abnormality, particularly trisomy 13 (Orioli, 2010; Solomon, 2010). Conversely, two thirds of

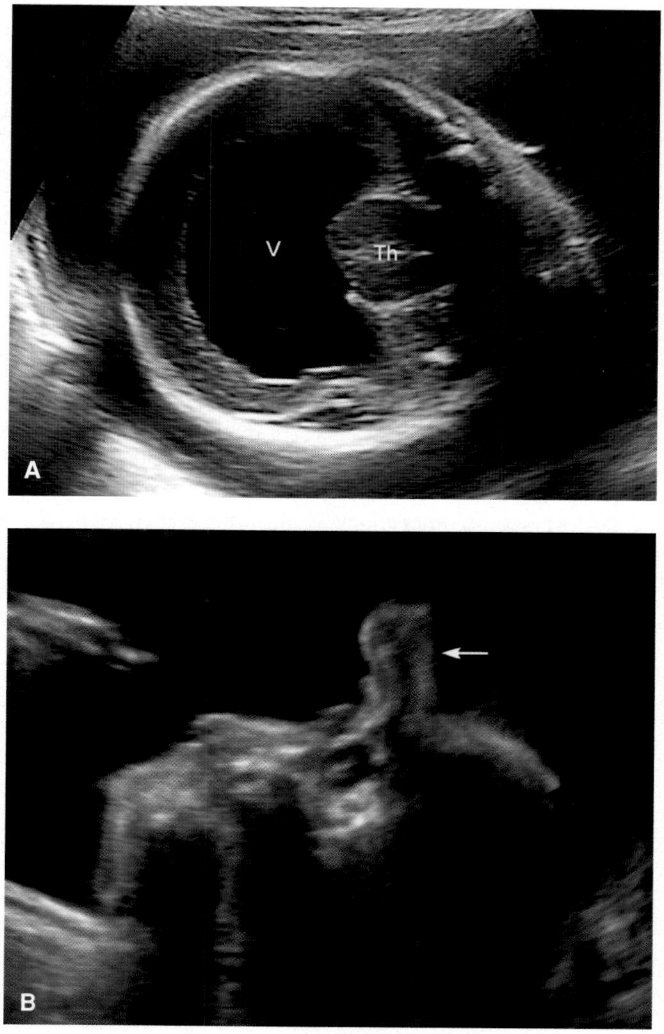

FIGURE 10-10 Alobar holoprosencephaly. **A.** Transverse cranial image of a 26-week fetus with alobar holoprosencephaly, depicting fused thalami (*Th*) encircled by a monoventricle (*V*). The midline falx is absent. **B.** In this profile view of the face and head, a soft tissue mass—a proboscis (*arrow*), protrudes from the region of the forehead.

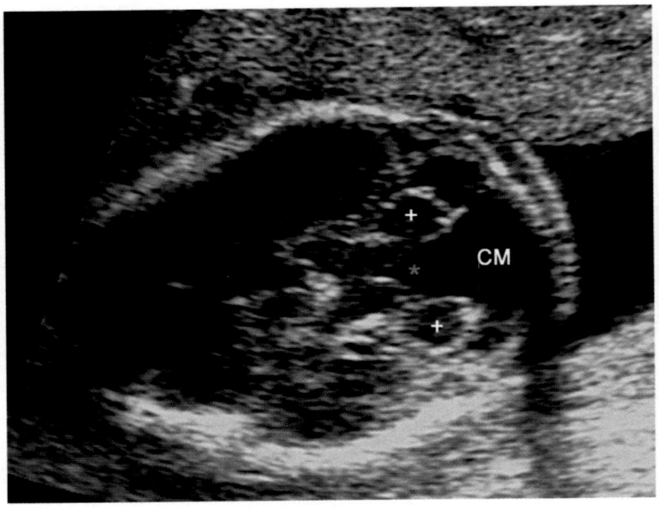

FIGURE 10-11 Dandy-Walker malformation. This transcerebellar image demonstrates agenesis of the cerebellar vermis. The cerebellar hemispheres (+) are widely separated by a fluid collection that connects the 4th ventricle (*red asterisk*) to the enlarged cisterna magna (*CM*).

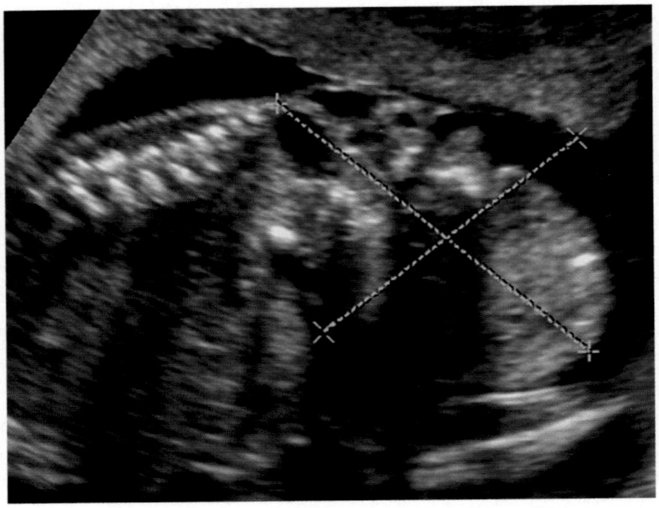

FIGURE 10-12 Sacrococcygeal teratoma. Sonographically, this tumor appears as a solid and/or cystic mass that arises from the anterior sacrum and tends to extend inferiorly and externally as it grows. In this image, a 7 × 6 cm inhomogeneous solid mass is visible below the normal-appearing sacrum. There is also an internal component to the tumor.

trisomy 13 cases are found to have holoprosencephaly. Fetal karyotyping should be offered when this anomaly is identified.

Dandy-Walker Malformation—Vermian Agenesis

Originally described by Dandy and Blackfan (1914), this posterior fossa abnormality is characterized by agenesis of the cerebellar vermis, posterior fossa enlargement, and elevation of the tentorium. Sonographically, fluid in the enlarged cisterna magna visibly communicates with the fourth ventricle through the cerebellar vermis defect, with visible separation of the cerebellar hemispheres (Fig. 10-11). The birth prevalence is approximately 1 in 12,000 (Long, 2006). Associated anomalies and aneuploidy are very common in prenatal series. These include ventriculomegaly in 30 to 40 percent, other anomalies in approximately 50 percent, and aneuploidy in 40 percent (Ecker, 2000; Long, 2006). Dandy-Walker malformation is also associated with numerous genetic and sporadic syndromes, congenital viral infections, and teratogen exposure, all of which greatly affect the prognosis. Thus, the initial evaluation mirrors that for ventriculomegaly (p. 202).

Inferior vermian agenesis, also called *Dandy-Walker variant*, is a term used when only the inferior portion of the vermis is absent. But, even when vermian agenesis appears to be partial and relatively subtle, there is a high prevalence of associated anomalies and aneuploidy, and the prognosis is often poor (Ecker, 2000; Long, 2006).

Sacrococcygeal Teratoma

This germ cell tumor is one of the most common tumors in neonates, with a birth prevalence of approximately 1 per 28,000 (Derikx, 2006; Swamy, 2008). It is believed to arise from the totipotent cells along Hensen node, anterior to the coccyx. The American Academy of Pediatrics–Surgical Section classification for sacrococcygeal teratoma (SCT) includes four types. Type 1 is predominantly external with a minimal presacral component; type 2 is predominantly external but with a significant intrapelvic component; type 3 is predominantly internal but with abdominal extension; and type 4 is entirely internal with no external component (Altman, 1974). The tumor may be mature, immature, or malignant. Sonographically, SCT appears as a solid and/or cystic mass that arises from the anterior sacrum and usually extends inferiorly and externally as it grows (Fig. 10-12). Solid components often have varying echogenicity, appear disorganized, and may grow rapidly with advancing gestation. Internal pelvic components may be more challenging to visualize, and fetal MR imaging should be considered. Hydramnios is frequent, and hydrops may develop from high-output cardiac failure, either as a consequence of tumor vascularity or secondary to bleeding within the tumor and resultant anemia. Fetuses with tumors > 5 cm often require cesarean delivery, and classical hysterotomy may be needed (Gucciaro, 2011). Fetal surgery for SCT is discussed in Chapter 16 (p. 327).

Caudal Regression Sequence—Sacral Agenesis

This rare anomaly is characterized by absence of the sacral spine and often portions of the lumbar spine. It is approximately 25 times more common in pregnancies with pregestational diabetes (Garne, 2012). Sonographic findings include a spine that appears abnormally short, lacks the normal lumbosacral curvature, and terminates abruptly above the level of the iliac wings. Because the sacrum does not lie between the iliac wings, they are abnormally close together and may appear "shield-like." There may be abnormal positioning of the lower extremities and lack of normal soft tissue development. Caudal regression should be differentiated from sirenomelia, which is a rare anomaly characterized by a single fused lower extremity in the midline.

Face and Neck

Normal fetal lips and nose are shown in Figure 10-13. A fetal profile is not a required component of standard examination

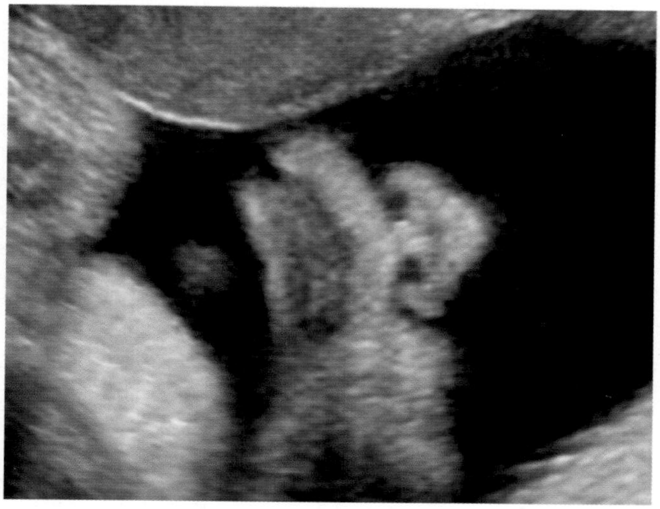

FIGURE 10-13 Midline face. This view demonstrates the integrity of the upper lip.

but may be helpful in identifying cases of *micrognathia*—an abnormally small jaw (Fig. 10-14). Micrognathia should be considered in the evaluation of hydramnios (Chap. 11, p. 235). Use of the *ex-utero intrapartum treatment (EXIT)* procedure for severe micrognathia is discussed in Chapter 16 (p. 331).

Facial Clefts

There are three main types of clefts. The first type, *cleft lip and palate*, always involves the lip, may also involve the hard palate, may be unilateral or bilateral, and has a birth prevalence of approximately 1 per 1000 (Cragan, 2009; Dolk, 2010). If isolated, the inheritance is multifactorial—with a recurrence risk of 3 to 5 percent for one prior affected child. If a cleft is visible in the upper lip, a transverse image at the level of the alveolar ridge may demonstrate that the defect also involves the primary palate (Fig. 10-15).

In a recent systematic review of low-risk pregnancies, cleft lip was identified sonographically in only about half of cases (Maarse, 2010). Approximately 40 percent of those detected in prenatal series are associated with other anomalies or syndromes, and aneuploidy is common (Maarse, 2011; Offerdal, 2008). The rate of associated anomalies is highest for bilateral defects that involve the palate. Using data from the Utah Birth Defect Network, Walker and associates (2001) identified aneuploidy in 1 percent with cleft lip alone, 5 percent with unilateral cleft lip and palate, and 13 percent with bilateral cleft lip and palate. It seems reasonable to offer fetal karyotyping when a cleft is identified.

The second type of cleft is *isolated cleft palate*. It begins at the uvula, may involve the soft palate, and occasionally involves the hard palate—but does not involve the lip. The birth prevalence is approximately 1 per 2000 (Dolk, 2010). Identification of isolated cleft palate has been described using specialized 2- and 3-dimensional sonography (Ramos, 2010; Wilhelm, 2010). However, it is not expected to be visualized during a standard ultrasound examination (Maarse, 2011; Offerdal, 2008).

A third type of cleft is *median cleft lip*, which is found in association with several conditions. These include agenesis of the primary palate, hypotelorism, and holoprosencephaly. Median clefts may also be associated with hypertelorism and frontonasal hyperplasia, formerly called the *median cleft face syndrome*.

Cystic Hygroma

This is a venolymphatic malformation in which fluid-filled sacs extend from the posterior neck (Fig. 10-16). Cystic hygromas may be diagnosed as early as the first trimester and vary widely in size. They are believed to develop when lymph from the head fails to drain into the jugular vein and accumulates instead in jugular lymphatic sacs. Their birth prevalence is approximately 1 in 5000, but given the high in-utero lethality of this condition, the incidence is much higher (Cragan, 2009).

Up to 70 percent of cystic hygromas are associated with aneuploidy. Of those diagnosed in the second trimester, approximately 75 percent of aneuploid cases are 45,X—*Turner syndrome*

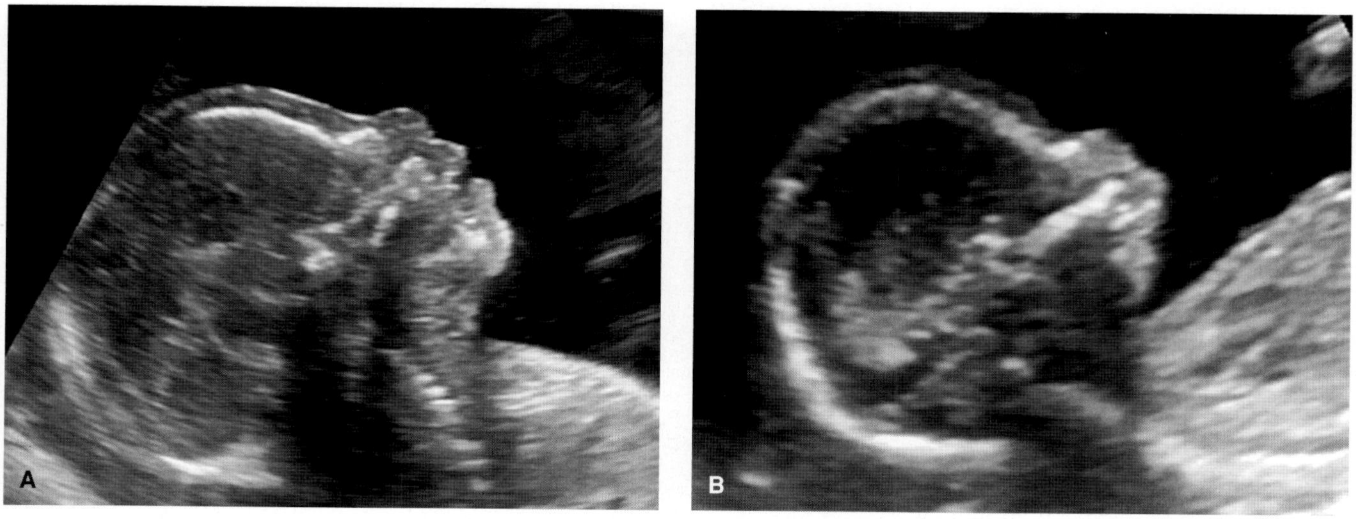

FIGURE 10-14 Fetal profile. **A.** This image depicts a normal fetal profile. **B.** This fetus has severe micrognathia, which creates a severely recessed chin.

(Johnson, 1993; Shulman, 1992). When cystic hygromas are diagnosed in the first trimester, trisomy 21 and 45,X are both common, followed by trisomy 18 in frequency (Kharrat, 2006; Malone, 2005). In a review of more than 100 cystic hygroma cases from the First And Second Trimester Evaluation of Risk (FASTER) trial, trisomy 21 was the single most common aneuploidy (Malone, 2005). First-trimester fetuses with cystic hygromas were five times more likely to be aneuploid than the fetuses with an increased nuchal translucency.

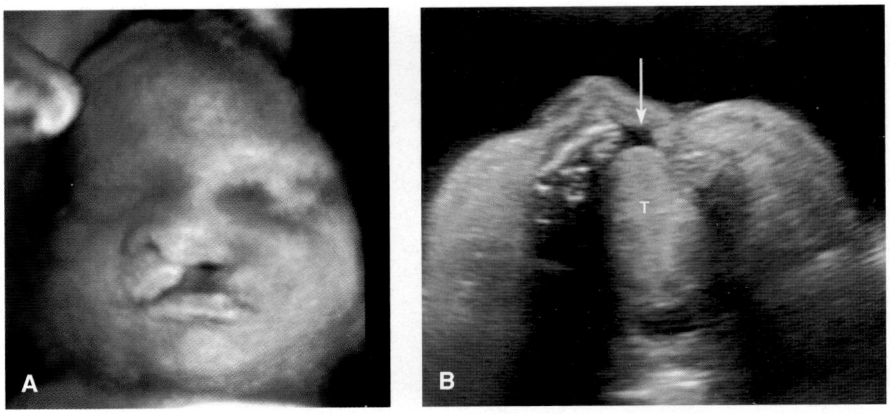

FIGURE 10-15 Cleft lip/palate. **A.** This fetus has a prominent unilateral (left-sided) cleft lip. **B.** Transverse view of the palate in the same fetus demonstrates a defect in the alveolar ridge (*arrow*). The tongue (*T*) is also visible.

In the absence of aneuploidy, cystic hygromas confer a significantly increased risk for other anomalies, particularly cardiac anomalies that are flow-related. These include hypoplastic left heart and coarctation of the aorta. Cystic hygromas also may be part of a genetic syndrome. One is *Noonan syndrome,* an autosomal dominant disorder that shares several features with Turner syndrome, including short stature, lymphedema, high-arched palate, and often pulmonary valve stenosis.

Large cystic hygromas are usually found with hydrops fetalis, rarely resolve, and carry a poor prognosis. Small hygromas may undergo spontaneous resolution, and provided that fetal karyotype and echocardiography results are normal, the prognosis *may* be good. The likelihood of a nonanomalous liveborn infant with normal karyotype following identification of first-trimester hygroma is approximately 1 in 6 (Kharrat, 2006; Malone, 2005).

Thorax

The lungs appear as homogeneous structures surrounding the heart and are best visualized after 20 to 25 weeks' gestation. In the four-chamber view of the chest, they comprise approximately two thirds of the area, with the heart occupying the remaining third. The thoracic circumference is measured at the skin line in a transverse plane at the level of the four-chamber view. In cases of suspected pulmonary hypoplasia secondary to a small thorax, such as with severe skeletal dysplasia, comparison with a reference table may be helpful (Appendix, p. 1299). Various abnormalities may be seen sonographically as cystic or solid space-occupying lesions. Fetal therapy for thoracic abnormalities is discussed in Chapter 16 (p. 329).

Congenital Diaphragmatic Hernia

This is a defect in the diaphragm through which abdominal organs herniate into the thorax. It is left-sided in approximately 75 percent of cases, right-sided in 20 percent, and bilateral in 5 percent (Gallot, 2007). The prevalence of congenital diaphragmatic hernia (CDH) is approximately 1 per 3000 to 4000 births (Cragan, 2009; Dolk, 2010; Gallot, 2007). Associated anomalies and aneuploidy occur in 40 percent of cases (Gallot, 2007;

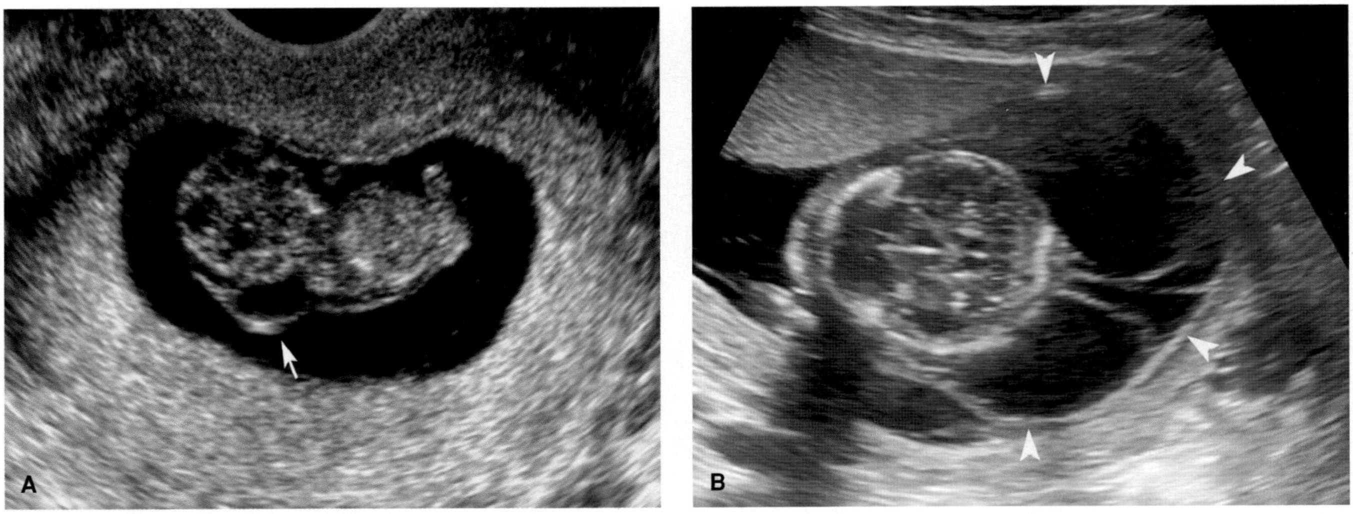

FIGURE 10-16 Cystic hygromas. **A.** This 9-week fetus with a cystic hygroma (*arrow*) was later found to have Noonan syndrome. **B.** Massive multiseptated hygromas (*arrowheads*) in the setting of hydrops fetalis at 15 weeks.

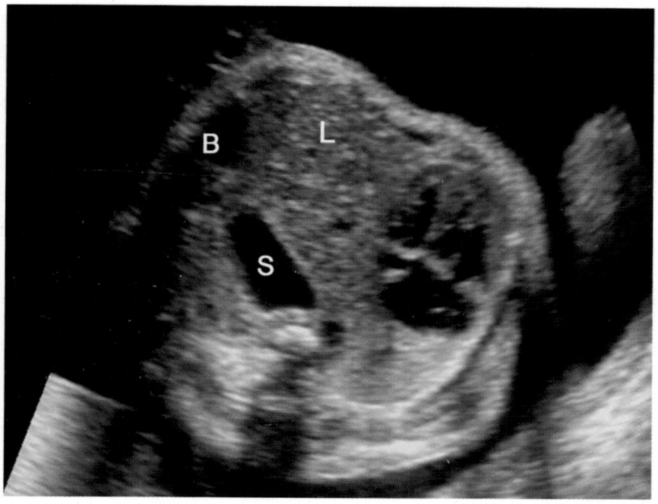

FIGURE 10-17 Congenital diaphragmatic hernia. In this transverse view of the thorax, the heart is shifted to the far right side of the chest by a left-sided diaphragmatic hernia containing stomach (*S*), liver (*L*), and bowel (*B*).

Stege, 2003). Targeted sonography and fetal echocardiography should be performed, and fetal karyotyping should be offered. Given the association with genetic syndromes, chromosomal microarray analysis is a consideration (Chap. 13, p. 277). In population-based series, the presence of an associated abnormality reduces the overall survival rate of neonates with diaphragmatic hernia from approximately 50 percent to about 20 percent (Colvin, 2005; Gallot, 2007; Stege, 2003). In the absence of associated abnormalities, the major causes of mortality are pulmonary hypoplasia and pulmonary hypertension.

Sonographically, the most frequent finding with a left-sided defect is repositioning of the heart to the mid or right hemithorax. With this, the axis of the heart points toward the midline (Fig. 10-17). Associated findings include the stomach bubble or bowel peristalsis in the chest and a wedge-shaped mass—the liver—located anteriorly in the left hemithorax. Liver herniation complicates at least 50 percent of cases and is associated with a 30-percent reduction in the survival rate (Mullassery, 2010). With large lesions, impaired swallowing and mediastinal shift may result in hydramnios and hydrops, respectively.

Efforts to predict survival have focused on indicators such as the sonographic lung-to-head ratio, MR imaging measurements of lung volume, and the degree of liver herniation (Jani, 2012; Mayer, 2011; Metkus, 1996; Worley, 2009). These and fetal therapy for CDH are reviewed in Chapter 16 (p. 328).

Congenital Cystic Adenomatoid Malformation

This abnormality represents hamartomatous overgrowth of terminal bronchioles that communicates with the tracheobronchial tree. It is also called *CPAM—congenital pulmonary airway malformation,* based on an understanding that not all histopathologic types are *cystic* or *adenomatoid* (Azizkhan, 2008; Stocker, 1977, 2002). The prevalence is estimated to be 1 per 6000 to 8000 births, and the reported prevalence appears to be increasing with improved sonographic detection of milder cases (Burge, 2010; Duncombe, 2002).

Sonographically, congenital cystic adenomatoid malformation (CCAM) is a well-circumscribed thoracic mass that may appear solid and echogenic or may have one or multiple variably sized cysts (Fig. 10-18). It usually involves one lobe and has blood supply from the pulmonary artery, with drainage into the pulmonary veins. When the mass is large, hydrops and pulmonary hypoplasia may result. Lesions with cysts ≥ 5 mm are generally termed *macrocystic*, and lesions with cysts < 5 mm are termed *microcystic* (Adzick, 1985).

In a review of 645 CCAM cases *without* hydrops, the overall survival rate was above 95 percent, and 30 percent of cases

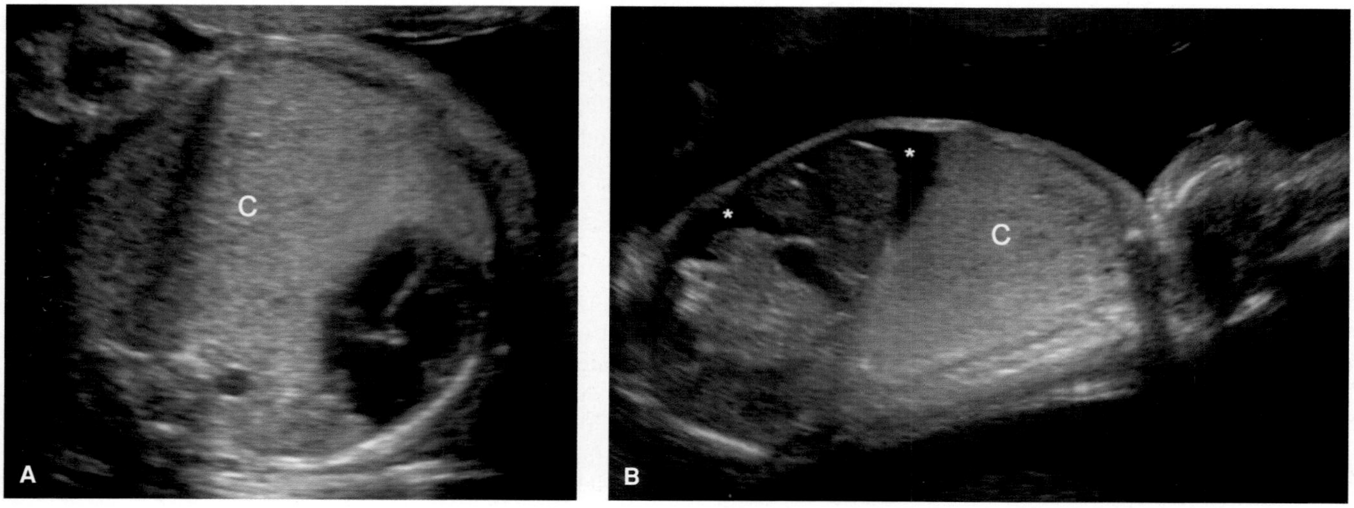

FIGURE 10-18 Transverse **(A)** and sagittal **(B)** images of a 26-week fetus with a very large left-sided microcystic congenital cystic adenomatoid malformation (CCAM). The mass (*C*) fills the thorax and has shifted the heart to the far right side of the chest, with development of ascites (*asterisks*). Fortunately, the mass did not continue to grow, the ascites resolved, and the infant was delivered at term and did well following resection.

demonstrated apparent prenatal resolution. In the 5 percent complicated by hydrops, there typically were very large lesions with mediastinal shift, and the prognosis was poor without fetal therapy (Cavoretto, 2008). A subset of CCAMs demonstrate rapid growth between 18 and 26 weeks' gestation, and a measurement called the *CCAM volume ratio,* discussed in Chapter 16 (p. 323), has been used to quantify size and hydrops risk. Corticosteroid therapy has been used for large microcystic lesions to forestall growth and potentially ameliorate hydrops (Curran, 2010). If a large dominant cyst is present, thoracoamnionic shunt placement may lead to hydrops resolution (Wilson, 2006). Fetal therapy for CCAM/CPAM is discussed in Chapter 16 (p. 323).

Extralobar Pulmonary Sequestration

Also called a *bronchopulmonary sequestration,* this abnormality is an accessory lung bud "sequestered" from the tracheobronchial tree, that is, a mass of nonfunctioning lung tissue. Most cases diagnosed prenatally are *extralobar,* which means they are enveloped in their own pleura. Overall, however, most sequestrations present in adulthood and are *intralobar*—within the pleura of another lobe. Extralobar pulmonary sequestration (ELS) is considered significantly less common than CCAM, and no precise prevalence has been reported. Lesions have a left-sided predominance and most often involve the left lower lobe. Approximately 10 to 20 percent of cases are located below the diaphragm, and associated anomalies have been reported in about 10 percent of cases (Yildirim, 2008).

Sonographically, ELS presents as a homogeneous, echogenic thoracic mass. Thus, it may resemble a microcystic CCAM. However, the blood supply to an ELS is from the systemic circulation—from the aorta rather than the pulmonary artery. In approximately 5 to 10 percent of cases, a large ipsilateral pleural effusion develops, and this may result in pulmonary hypoplasia or hydrops without treatment (Chap. 16, p. 329). Hydrops may also result from mediastinal shift or high-output cardiac failure due to the left-to-right shunt imposed by the mass (Chap. 15, p. 316). In the absence of a pleural effusion, the reported survival rate exceeds 95 percent, and 40 percent of cases demonstrate apparent prenatal resolution (Cavoretto, 2008).

Congenital High Airway Obstruction Sequence (CHAOS)

This rare anomaly usually results from laryngeal or tracheal atresia. The normal egress of lung fluid is obstructed, and the tracheobronchial tree and lungs become massively distended. Sonographically, the lungs appear brightly echogenic, and the bronchi are dilated with fluid (Fig. 10-19). Flattening and eversion of the diaphragm is common, as is compression of the heart. Venous return is impaired and ascites develops, typically followed by hydrops (Chap. 15, p. 316). In one series, associated anomalies were reported in three of 12 cases (Roybal, 2010). This anomaly is a feature of the autosomal recessive *Fraser syndrome.* In some cases, spontaneous perforation of the obstructed airway can occur, potentially conferring a better prognosis. The EXIT procedure has also been used to treat this anomaly, as discussed in Chapter 16 (p. 331).

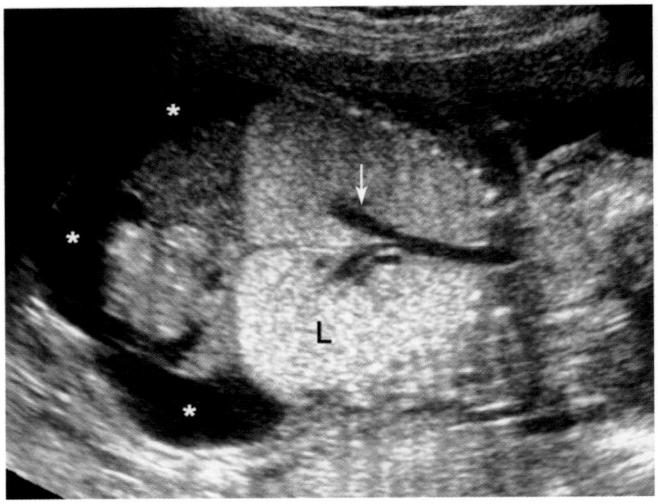

FIGURE 10-19 Congenital high airway obstruction sequence (CHAOS). The lungs appear brightly echogenic, and one is marked by an "L." The bronchi, one of which is noted by an arrow, are dilated with fluid. Flattening and eversion of the diaphragm is common, as is ascites (*asterisks*).

Heart

Cardiac malformations are the most common class of congenital anomalies, with an overall prevalence of 8 per 1000 births (Cragan, 2009). Almost 90 percent of cardiac defects are multifactorial or polygenic in origin; another 1 to 2 percent result from a single-gene disorder or gene-deletion syndrome; and 1 to 2 percent are from exposure to a teratogen such as isotretinoin, hydantoin, or maternal diabetes. Based on data from population-based registries, approximately 1 in 8 liveborn and stillborn neonates with a congenital heart defect has a chromosomal abnormality (Dolk, 2010; Hartman, 2011). The most frequent chromosomal abnormality found in those with a heart defect is trisomy 21. This accounts for more than half of cases and is followed by trisomy 18, 22q11.2 microdeletion, trisomy 13, and monosomy X (Hartman, 2011). Approximately 50 to 70 percent of aneuploid fetuses have extracardiac anomalies that are identifiable sonographically. Fetal karyotyping should be offered, and 22q11.2 microdeletion testing should be offered for conotruncal defects.

Traditionally, detection of congenital cardiac anomalies has been more challenging than anomalies of other organ systems. In recent series, routine second-trimester sonography identified approximately 40 percent of those with major cardiac anomalies before 22 weeks, and specialized sonography identified 80 percent (Romosan, 2009; Trivedi, 2012). There is evidence that prenatal detection of selected cardiac anomalies may improve neonatal survival rates. This may be particularly so with *ductal-dependent* anomalies—those requiring prostaglandin infusion after birth to keep the ductus arteriosus open (Franklin, 2002; Mahle, 2001; Tworetsky, 2001).

Basic Cardiac Examination

Standard cardiac assessment includes a four-chamber view (Fig. 10-20), evaluation of rate and rhythm, and evaluation of the left and right ventricular outflow tracts (Fig. 10-21)

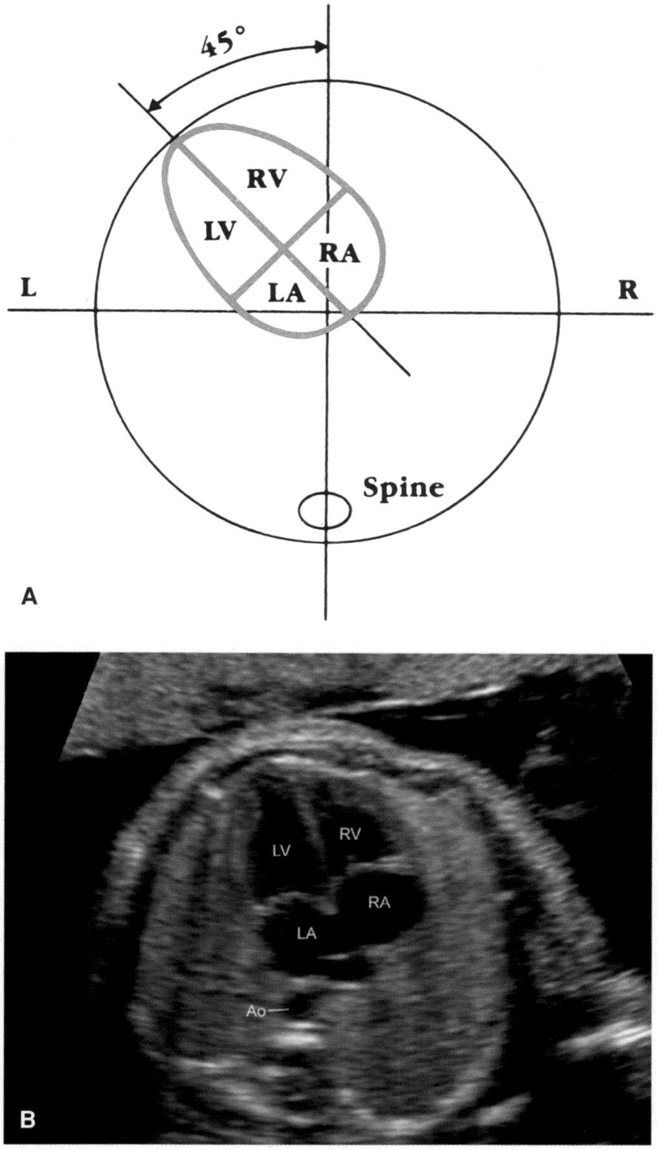

FIGURE 10-20 The four-chamber view. **A.** Diagram demonstrating measurement of the cardiac axis from the four-chamber view of the fetal heart. **B.** Sonogram of the four-chamber view at 22 weeks demonstrates the normal symmetry of the atria and ventricles, normal position of the mitral and triscuspid valves, pulmonary veins entering the left atrium, and descending aorta (*Ao*). L = left; LA = left atrium; LV = left ventricle; R = right; RA = right atrium; RV = right ventricle.

(American Institute of Ultrasound in Medicine, 2013a). Evaluation of the cardiac outflow tracts may aid in detection of abnormalities not initially appreciated in the four-chamber view. These may include tetralogy of Fallot, transposition of the great vessels, or truncus arteriosus.

Four-Chamber View. This is a transverse image of the fetal thorax at a level immediately above the diaphragm. It allows evaluation of cardiac size, position in the thorax, cardiac axis, atria and ventricles, foramen ovale, atrial septum primum, interventricular septum, and atrioventricular valves (see Fig. 10-20). The atria and ventricles should be similar in size, and the apex of the heart should form a 45-degree angle with the left anterior chest wall. Abnormalities of cardiac axis are frequently encountered with structural cardiac anomalies and occur in more than a third (Shipp, 1995). Smith and coworkers (1995) found that 75 percent of fetuses with congenital heart anomalies had an axis angle that exceeded 75 degrees.

Fetal Echocardiography

This is a specialized examination of fetal cardiac structure and function designed to identify and characterize abnormalities. Guidelines for its performance have been developed collaboratively by the American Institute of Ultrasound in Medicine (2013b), American College of Obstetrics and Gynecology, Society of Maternal-Fetal Medicine, American Society of Echocardiography, and American College of Radiology. Echocardiography indications include suspected fetal cardiac anomaly, extracardiac anomaly, or chromosomal abnormality; fetal arrhythmia; hydrops; increased nuchal translucency; monochorionic twin gestation; first-degree relative to the fetus with a congenital cardiac defect; in vitro fertilization; maternal anti-Ro or anti-La antibodies; exposure to a medication associated with increased cardiac malformation risks; and maternal metabolic disease associated with cardiac defects—such as pregestational diabetes or phenylketonuria (American Institute of Ultrasound in Medicine, 2013a). Components of the examination are listed in Table 10-6, and examples of the nine required gray-scale imaging views are shown in Figure 10-21. Examples of selected cardiac anomalies are reviewed below.

Ventricular Septal Defect. This is the single most common congenital cardiac anomaly and occurs in approximately 1 per 300 births (Cragan, 2009; Dolk, 2010). Even with adequate visualization, the prenatal detection rate of ventricular septal defect (VSD) is low. A defect may be appreciated in the membranous or muscular portion of the interventricular septum in the four-chamber view, and color Doppler demonstrates flow through the defect. Imaging of the left ventricular outflow tract may demonstrate discontinuity of the interventricular septum as it becomes the wall of the aorta (Fig. 10-22). Fetal VSD is associated with aneuploidy, particularly with coexistent other congenital abnormalities, and fetal karyotyping should be offered. That said, the prognosis for an isolated defect is good—more than a third of prenatally diagnosed VSDs close in utero, and another third close in the first year of life (Axt-Fliedner, 2006; Paladini, 2002).

Endocardial Cushion Defect. This is also called an *atrioventricular (AV) septal defect* or *AV canal defect*. It develops in approximately 1 per 2500 births and is associated with trisomy 21 in more than half of cases (Cragan, 2009; Dolk, 2010). The endocardial cushions are the crux of the heart, and defects jointly involve the atrial septum primum, interventricular septum, and medial leaflets of the mitral and tricuspid valves (Fig. 10-23). In addition to trisomy 21 and other aneuploidies, an endocardial cushion defect may develop with heterotaxy syndrome. In this condition, which is also called *atrial isomerism*, the heart and/or abdominal organs are on the incorrect side. Endocardial cushion defects associated with heterotaxy are more likely to have

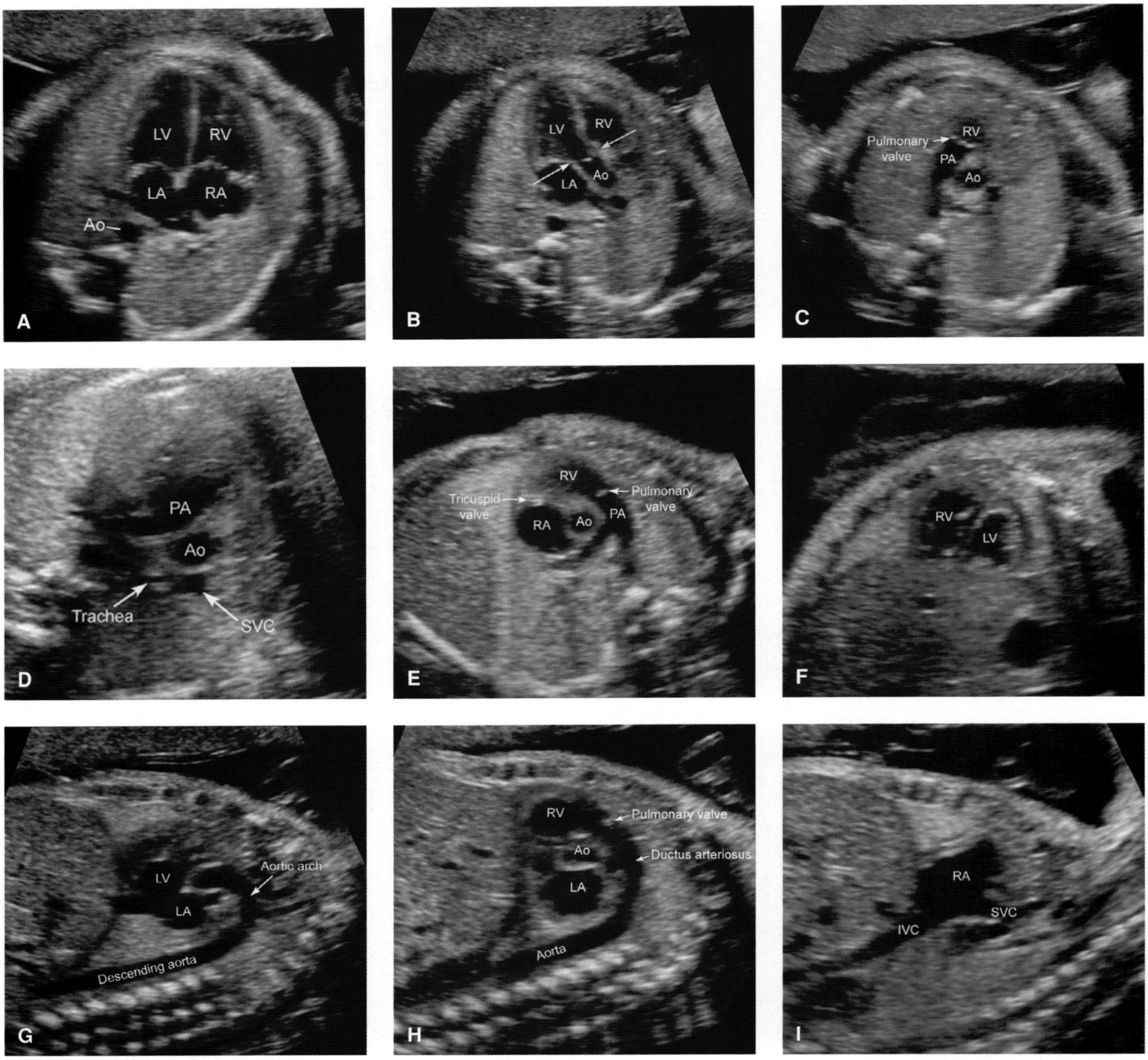

FIGURE 10-21 Fetal echocardiography gray-scale imaging planes. **A.** Four-chamber view. **B.** Left ventricular outflow tract view. The white arrow illustrates the mitral valve becoming the wall of the aorta. The yellow arrow marks the interventricular septum becoming the opposing aortic wall. **C.** Right ventricular outflow tract view. **D.** Three vessel and trachea view. **E.** High short-axis view (outflow tracts). **F.** Low short-axis view (ventricles). **G.** Aortic arch view. **H.** Ductal arch view. **I.** Superior and inferior vena cavae views. Ao = aorta; IVC = inferior vena cava; LA = left atrium; LV = left ventricle; PA = pulmonary artery; RA = right atrium; RV = right ventricle; SVC superior vena cava.

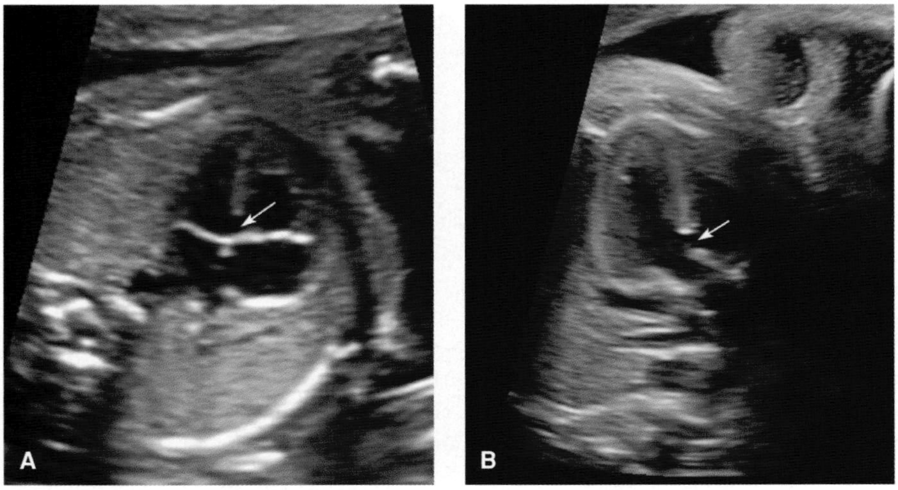

FIGURE 10-22 Ventricular septal defect. **A.** In this four-chamber view of a 22-week fetus, a defect (*arrow*) is noted in the superior (membranous) portion of the interventricular septum. **B.** The left-ventricular outflow tract view of the same fetus demonstrates a break (*arrow*) in continuity between the interventricular septum and the anterior wall of the aorta.

TABLE 10-6. Components of Fetal Echocardiography

Basic imaging parameters
Evaluation of atria
Evaluation of ventricles
Evaluation of great vessels
Cardiac and visceral situs
Atrioventricular junctions
Ventriculoarterial junctions
Scanning planes, gray scale
Four-chamber view
Left ventricular outflow tract
Right ventricular outflow tract
Three-vessel and trachea view
Short-axis view, low (ventricles)
Short-axis view, high (outflow tracts)
Aortic arch
Ductal arch
Superior and inferior vena cavae
Color Doppler evaluation
Systemic veins (vena cavae and ductus venosus[a])
Pulmonary veins
Foramen ovale
Atrioventricular valves[a]
Atrial and ventricular septae
Aortic and pulmonary valves[a]
Ductus arteriosus
Aortic arch
Umbilical artery and vein (optional)[a]
Cardiac rate and rhythm assessment

[a]Pulsed-wave Doppler sonography should be used as an adjunct to evaluate these structures.
Cardiac biometry and functional assessment are optional but should be considered for suspected structural/functional abnormalities.
Adapted from the American Institute of Ultrasound in Medicine, 2013b.

conduction system abnormalities resulting in third-degree AV block. As discussed in Chapter 16 (p. 322), this confers a poor prognosis.

Hypoplastic Left Heart Syndrome. This anomaly occurs in approximately 1 per 4000 births (Cragan, 2009; Dolk, 2010). Postnatal treatment consists of a three-stage palliative repair or a cardiac transplantation. Once considered a lethal prognosis, it is now estimated that 70 percent of infants may survive to adulthood (Feinstein, 2012). Morbidity remains high, and developmental delays are common. Sonographically, the left side of the heart may appear so small that it is difficult to appreciate a ventricular chamber. There may be no visible inflow or outflow and may be reversal of flow in the ductus arteriosus. Fetal therapy for hypoplastic left heart is discussed in Chapter 16 (p. 331).

Tetralogy of Fallot. This anomaly occurs in approximately 1 per 3500 births (Cragan, 2009; Dolk, 2010). It is characterized by four components: ventricular septal defect, an overriding aorta, pulmonary valve abnormality, and right ventricular hypertrophy. The last does not present before birth. Due to the location of the ventricular septal defect, it is often not visible in the four-chamber view, which may appear normal. The prognosis following postnatal repair is usually excellent, and 20-year survival rates exceed 95 percent (Knott-Craig, 1998). Cases with *pulmonary atresia* have a more complicated course, however. There is also a variant in which the pulmonary valve is *absent*. Affected fetuses are at risk for hydrops and for tracheomalacia from compression of the trachea by the enlarged pulmonary artery.

Cardiac Rhabdomyoma. This is the most common cardiac tumor. Approximately 50 percent of cases are associated with tuberous sclerosis, an autosomal dominant disease with multiorgan system manifestations caused by mutations in the hamartin (*TSC1*) and tuberin (*TSC2*) genes. Cardiac rhabdomyomas appear as well-circumscribed echogenic masses, usually within the ventricles or outflow tracts. There may be one or multiple; they may increase in size during gestation; and occasionally, inflow or outflow obstruction may result. In the absence of obstruction or very large size, the prognosis is relatively good from a cardiac standpoint. These tumors are largest

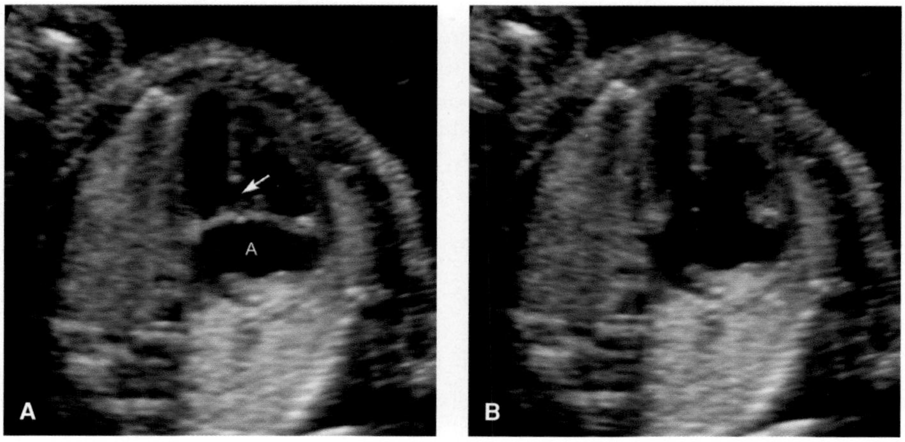

FIGURE 10-23 Endocardial cushion defect. **A.** During ventricular systole, the lateral leaflets of the mitral and triscuspid valves come together in the midline. But the atrioventricular valve plane is abnormal, a common atrium (*A*) is observed, and there is a visible defect (*arrow*) in the interventricular septum. **B.** During diastolic filling, opening of the atrioventricular valves more clearly demonstrates the absence of their medial leaflets.

in the neonatal period and tend to regress as children grow. It is problematic, however, that other findings of neurofibromatosis, including growth of benign tumors in the brain, kidney, and skin, may not be apparent prenatally or may develop later in gestation. If a fetal rhabdomyoma is identified, in the absence of a family history, evaluation of the parents for clinical manifestations of neurofibromatosis should be considered. Fetal MR imaging may be considered to evaluate CNS anatomy (p. 223).

M-Mode

Motion-mode or M-mode imaging is a linear display of cardiac cycle events, with time on the x-axis and motion on the y-axis. It is used frequently to measure fetal heart rate (Fig. 10-24). If there is an abnormality of heart rate or rhythm, M-mode imaging permits separate evaluation of atrial and ventricular waveforms. Thus, it is particularly useful for characterizing arrhythmias and their response to treatment, which is discussed in Chapter 16 (p. 321). M-mode can also be used to assess ventricular function and atrial and ventricular outputs.

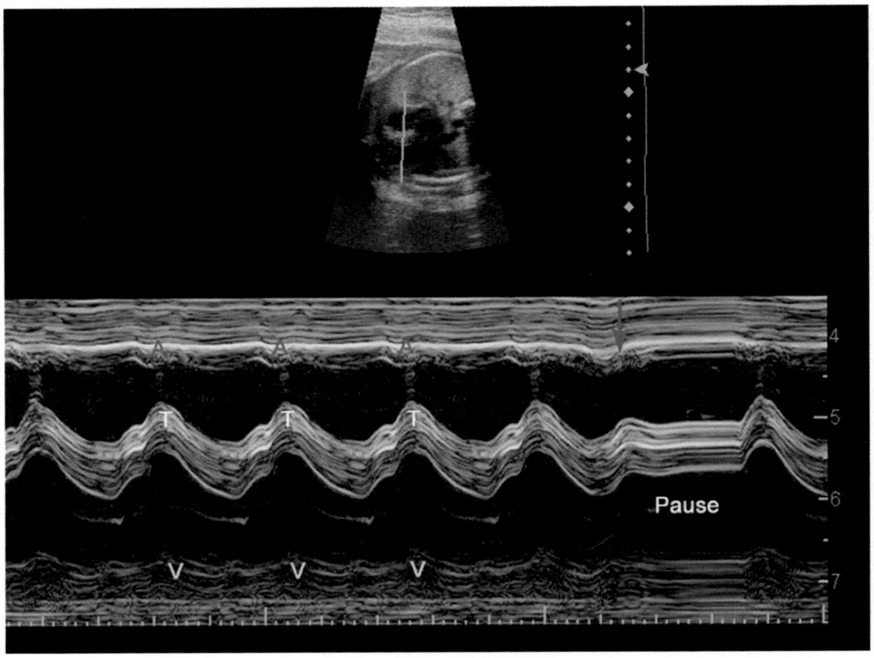

FIGURE 10-24 M-mode, or motion mode, is a linear display of the events of the cardiac cycle, with time on the x-axis and motion on the y-axis. M-mode is used commonly to measure the fetal heart rate. In this image, there is normal concordance between atrial (*A*) and ventricular contractions (*V*). Movement of the tricuspid valve (*T*) is also shown. There is also a premature atrial contraction (*arrow*) and a subsequent early ventricular contraction, followed by a compensatory pause.

Premature Atrial Contractions. Also called atrial extrasystoles, these are the most common fetal arrhythmia and a frequent finding. They represent cardiac conduction system immaturity and typically resolve later in gestation or in the neonatal period. Premature atrial contractions (PACs) may be conducted—and sound like an extra beat. However, they are more commonly blocked, and with handheld Doppler or fetoscope, they sound like a dropped beat. As shown in Figure 10-24, the dropped beat may be demonstrated with M-mode evaluation to be the compensatory pause that follows the premature contraction.

Premature atrial contractions are not associated with major structural cardiac abnormalities, although they sometimes occur with an atrial septal aneurysm. In case reports, they have been associated with maternal caffeine consumption and hydralazine (Lodeiro, 1989; Oei, 1989). In a small percentage of cases, about 2 percent, affected fetuses are later identified to have a *supraventricular tachycardia* (SVT) that requires urgent treatment (Copel, 2000). Given the importance of identifying SVT, pregnancies with fetal PACs are often followed with fetal heart rate assessment as often as every 1 to 2 weeks until ectopy resolution.

Abdominal Wall

The integrity of the abdominal wall at the level of the cord insertion is assessed during the standard examination (Fig. 10-25). *Gastroschisis* and *omphalocele*, collectively termed *ventral wall defects,* are relatively common fetal anomalies. As discussed in Chapter 14 (p. 285), both are associated with maternal serum alpha-fetoprotein elevation.

Gastroschisis

This is a full-thickness abdominal wall defect typically located to the right of the umbilical cord insertion. Bowel herniates through the defect into the amnionic cavity (Fig. 10-26). The prevalence is 1 per 2000 to 4000 pregnancies (Canfield, 2006; Dolk, 2010). Gastroschisis is the one major anomaly more common in fetuses of younger mothers, and the average maternal age is 20 years (Santiago-Muñoz, 2007). Bowel abnormalities such as *jejunal*

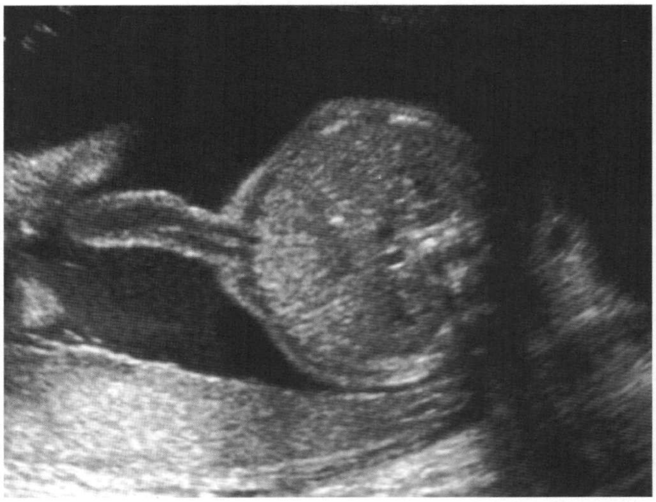

FIGURE 10-25 Normal ventral wall. Transverse view of the abdomen in a second-trimester fetus with an intact anterior abdominal wall and normal cord insertion.

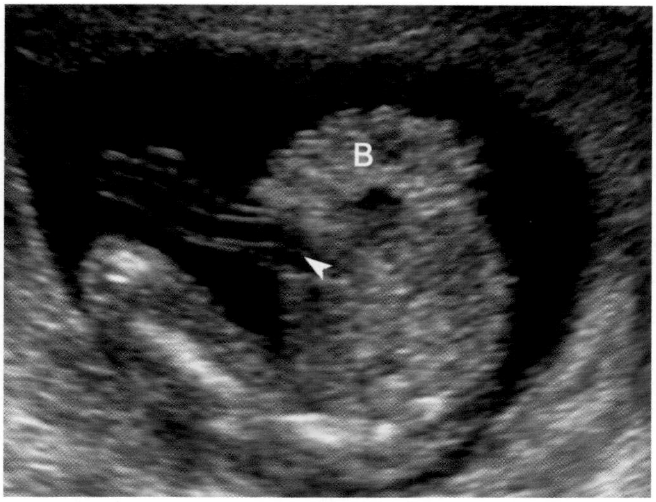

FIGURE 10-26 Gastroschisis. This 18-week fetus has a full-thickness ventral wall defect to the right of the cord insertion (*arrowhead*), through which multiple small bowel loops (*B*) have herniated into the amnionic cavity.

atresia are found in 15 to 30 percent of cases. Gastroschisis is not associated with an increased risk for aneuploidy, and the survival rate approximates 90 percent (Kitchanan, 2000; Nembhard, 2001; Santiago-Muñoz, 2007).

Fetal-growth restriction develops with gastroschisis in 15 to 40 percent of cases (Nicholas, 2009; Puligandla, 2004; Santiago-Muñoz, 2007). Whereas Nicholas and colleagues (2009) reported an association between growth restriction and adverse outcome with gastroschisis, Santiago-Muñoz and associates (2007) found that such newborns did not have increased mortality rates or longer hospitalizations compared with those of normally grown neonates. In a series of 75 infants with gastroschisis, Ergün and coworkers (2005) reported that the only risk factor associated with longer hospitalization was delivery before 36 weeks.

Omphalocele

This anomaly complicates approximately 1 per 3000 to 5000 pregnancies (Canfield, 2006; Dolk, 2010). It forms when the lateral ectomesodermal folds fail to meet in the midline, leaving the abdominal contents covered only by a two-layered sac of amnion and peritoneum into which the umbilical cord inserts (Fig. 10-27). In more than half of cases, omphalocele is associated with other major anomalies or aneuploidy. It also is a component of syndromes such as *Beckwith–Wiedemann, cloacal exstrophy,* and *pentalogy of Cantrell.* Smaller defects confer an even greater risk for aneuploidy (De Veciana, 1994). Like other major anomalies, identification of an omphalocele mandates a complete anatomical evaluation, and fetal karyotyping is recommended.

Body Stalk Anomaly

Also known as *limb-body-wall complex* or *cyllosoma,* this is a rare, lethal anomaly characterized by abnormal formation of the body wall. Typically, *no* abdominal wall is visible, and there is extrusion of the abdominal organs into the extraamnionic coelom. There is close approximation or fusion of the body to the placenta, and an extremely short umbilical cord. Acute-angle scoliosis is another feature. Amnionic bands are often identified.

Gastrointestinal Tract

The stomach is visible in nearly all fetuses after 14 weeks' gestation. The liver, spleen, gallbladder, and bowel can be identified in many second- and third-trimester fetuses. If the stomach is not seen on an initial evaluation, the examination should be repeated, and targeted sonography should be considered. Nonvisualization of the stomach may be secondary to impaired swallowing. And, underlying causes may include esophageal atresia, a craniofacial abnormality, or a CNS or musculoskeletal abnormality such as arthrogryposis. Fetuses with oligohydramnios or with severe illness from various causes—such as hydrops, may also have impaired swallowing.

Bowel appearance changes with fetal maturation. Occasionally, it may appear bright or echogenic, which may indicate small amounts of swallowed intraamnionic blood, particularly in the setting of maternal serum alpha-fetoprotein elevation. Bowel that appears as bright as fetal bone confers a slightly increased risk for underlying gastrointestinal malformations, cystic fibrosis, trisomy 21, and congenital infection such as cytomegalovirus.

Gastrointestinal Atresia

Bowel atresia is characterized by obstruction and proximal bowel dilatation. In general, the more proximal the obstruction, the more likely it is to be associated with hydramnios. The hydramnios associated with proximal small bowel obstruction may be severe enough to result in maternal respiratory compromise or preterm labor. This may at times necessitate large-volume amniocentesis, also termed amnioreduction (Chap. 11, p. 236).

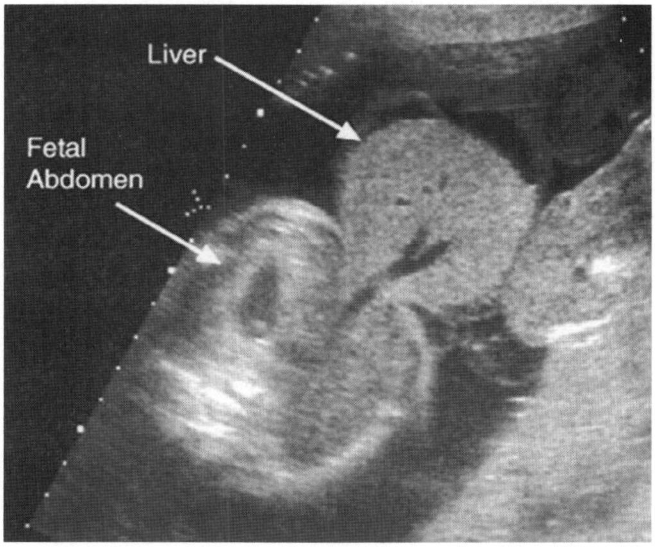

FIGURE 10-27 Omphalocele. Transverse view of the abdomen showing an omphalocele as a large abdominal wall defect with exteriorized liver covered by a thin membrane.

Esophageal atresia occurs in approximately 1 in 4000 births (Cragan, 2009; Pedersen, 2012). It may be suspected when the stomach cannot be visualized, and hydramnios is present. That said, in up to 90 percent of cases, a concomitant *tracheoesophageal fistula* allows fluid to enter the stomach, such that prenatal detection is problematic. More than half have associated anomalies and/or genetic syndromes. Specifically, multiple malformations are present in 30 percent, and aneuploidy are found in 10 percent, particularly trisomies 18 and 21 (Pedersen, 2012). Cardiac, urinary tract, and other gastrointestinal abnormalities are the most frequent. Approximately 10 percent of cases of esophageal atresia occur in the setting of the VACTERL association (p. 201) (Pedersen, 2012).

Duodenal atresia occurs in approximately 1 in 10,000 births (Best, 2012; Dolk, 2010). It is characterized by the sonographic *double-bubble sign,* which represents distention of the stomach and the first part of the duodenum (Fig. 10-28). This finding is usually not present before 22 to 24 weeks' gestation and thus would not be expected to be identified during an 18-week standard sonographic examination. Demonstrating continuity between the stomach and proximal duodenum confirms that the second "bubble" is the proximal duodenum. Approximately 30 percent of affected fetuses have an associated chromosomal abnormality or genetic syndrome, particularly trisomy 21. In the *absence* of a genetic abnormality, a third of cases have associated anomalies, most commonly cardiac defects and other gastrointestinal abnormalities (Best, 2012). Obstructions in the more distal small bowel usually result in multiple dilated loops that may have increased peristaltic activity.

Large bowel obstructions and anal atresia are less readily diagnosed by sonography, because hydramnios is not a typical feature, and the bowel may not be significantly dilated. A transverse view through the pelvis may show an enlarged rectum as a fluid-filled structure between the bladder and the sacrum.

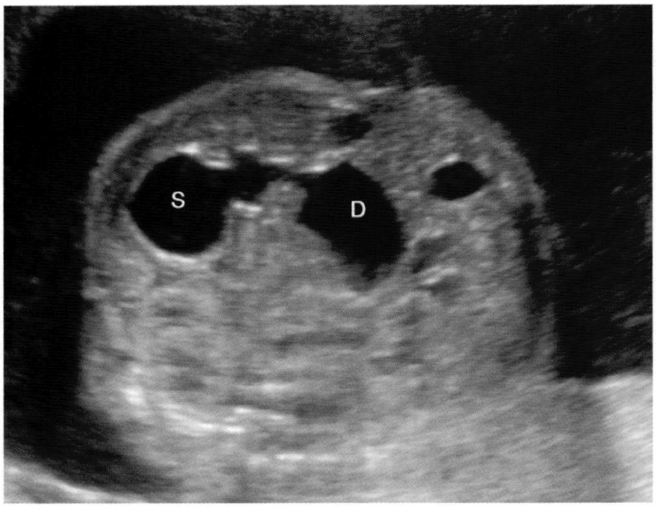

FIGURE 10-28 Duodenal atresia. The *double-bubble* sign represents distension of the stomach (*S*) and the first part of the duodenum (*D*), as seen on this axial abdominal image. Demonstrating continuity between the stomach and proximal duodenum confirms that the second "bubble" is the proximal duodenum.

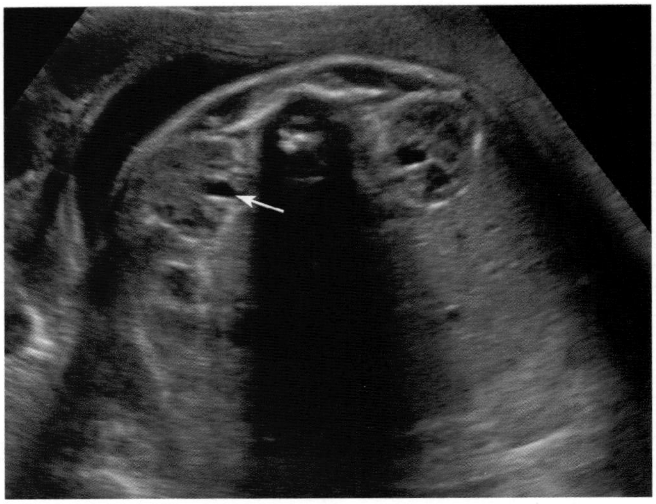

FIGURE 10-29 Normal fetal kidneys. The kidneys are visible adjacent to the fetal spine in this 29-week fetus. With advancing gestation, a rim of perinephric fat facilitates visualization of the margins of the kidney. A physiological amount of urine is visible in the renal pelves and is marked in one kidney by an arrow.

Kidneys and Urinary Tract

The fetal kidneys are visible adjacent to the spine, frequently in the first trimester and routinely by 18 weeks' gestation (Fig. 10-29). The length of the kidney is about 20 mm at 20 weeks, increasing by approximately 1.1 mm each week thereafter (Chitty, 2003). With advancing gestation, the kidneys become relatively less echogenic, and a rim of perinephric fat aids visualization of their margins.

The placenta and membranes are the major sources of amnionic fluid early in pregnancy. However, after 18 weeks' gestation, most of the fluid is produced by the kidneys (Chap. 11, p. 231). Fetal urine production increases from 5 mL/hr at 20 weeks to approximately 50 mL/hr at term (Rabinowitz, 1989). Unexplained oligohydramnios suggests a placental or urinary tract abnormality, whereas normal amnionic fluid volume in the second half of pregnancy suggests urinary tract patency with at least one functioning kidney.

Renal Pelvis Dilatation

This finding is present in 1 to 5 percent of fetuses. In 40 to 90 percent of cases, it is transient or physiological and does not represent an underlying abnormality (Ismaili, 2003; Nguyen, 2010). In approximately a third of cases, a urinary tract abnormality is confirmed in the neonatal period. Most frequently, this is either *ureteropelvic junction (UPJ) obstruction* or *vesicoureteral reflux (VUR).*

During evaluation, the renal pelvis is measured anterior-posterior in the transverse plane (Fig. 10-30). Although various thresholds have been defined, the pelvis is typically considered dilated if it exceeds 4 mm in the second trimester or 7 mm in the third trimester. Usually, the second-trimester threshold is used to identify pregnancies that warrant third-trimester evaluation.

Based on a metaanalysis of more than 100,000 screened pregnancies, the Society for Fetal Urology has categorized

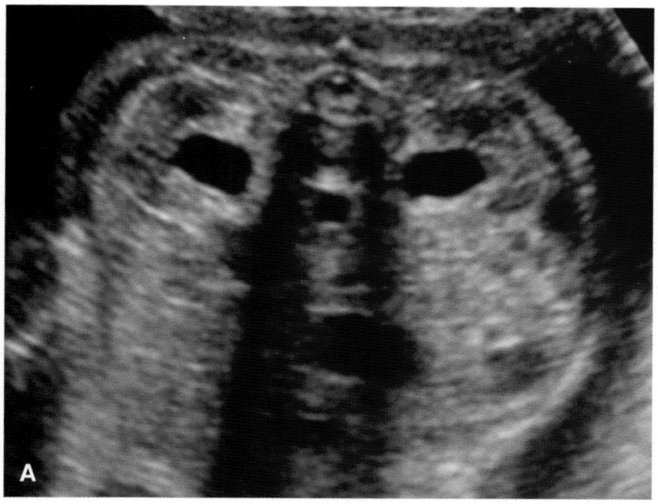

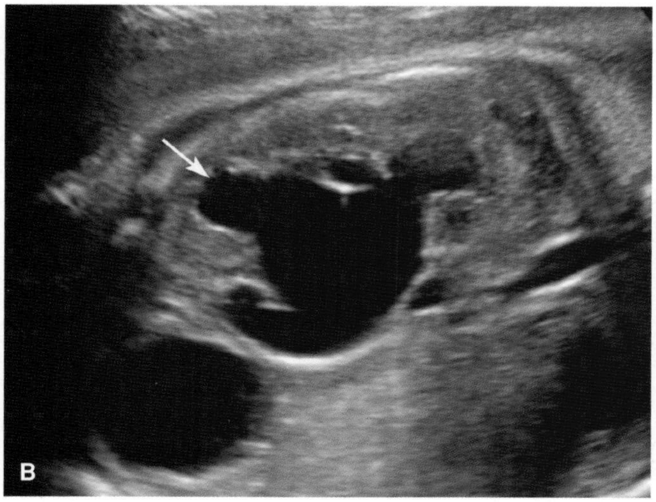

FIGURE 10-30 Renal pelvis dilatation. This common finding is identified in 1 to 5 percent of pregnancies. **A.** In this 34-week fetus with mild renal pelvis dilatation, the anterior-posterior diameter of the renal pelvis measured 7 mm in the transverse plane. **B.** Sagittal image of the kidney in a 32-week fetus with severe renal pelvis dilatation secondary to ureteropelvic junction obstruction. One of the rounded calyces is marked (*arrow*).

dilatation according to renal pelvis measurements and gestational age (Table 10-7) (Lee, 2006; Nguyen, 2010). The degree of renal pelvic dilatation correlates with the likelihood of underlying abnormality. Other findings that suggest pathology include calyceal dilatation, cortical thinning, or dilatation elsewhere along the urinary tract. Mild pyelectasis in the second trimester is associated with a slightly increased risk for Down syndrome (Chap. 14, p. 293).

Ureteropelvic Junction Obstruction. This condition is the most common abnormality associated with renal pelvis dilatation. The birth prevalence approximates 1 per 1000 to 2000, and males are affected three times more often than females (Williams, 2007; Woodward, 2002). Obstruction is generally functional rather than anatomical, and it is bilateral in up to a fourth of cases. The likelihood of UPJ obstruction increases from 5 percent with mild renal pelvis dilatation to more than 50 percent with severe dilatation (Lee, 2006).

TABLE 10-7. Risk for Postnatal Urinary Abnormality According to Degree of Renal Pelvis Dilatation[a]

Dilatation	Second Trimester	Third Trimester	Postnatal Abnormality
Mild	4 to < 7 mm	7 to < 9 mm	12%
Moderate	7 to ≤ 10 mm	9 to ≤ 15 mm	45%
Severe	> 10 mm	> 15 mm	88%

[a]Society for Fetal Urology Classification.
Modified from Lee, 2006; Nguyen, 2010.

Duplicated Renal Collecting System

This occurs when the upper and lower poles of the kidney—called moieties—are each drained by a separate ureter (Fig. 10-31). Duplication is more common in females and is bilateral in 15 to 20 percent of cases (Whitten, 2001). It is recognized in approximately 1 per 4000 pregnancies (James,

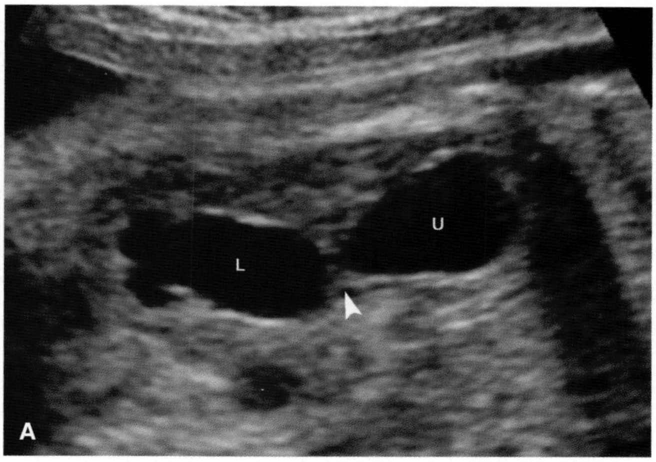

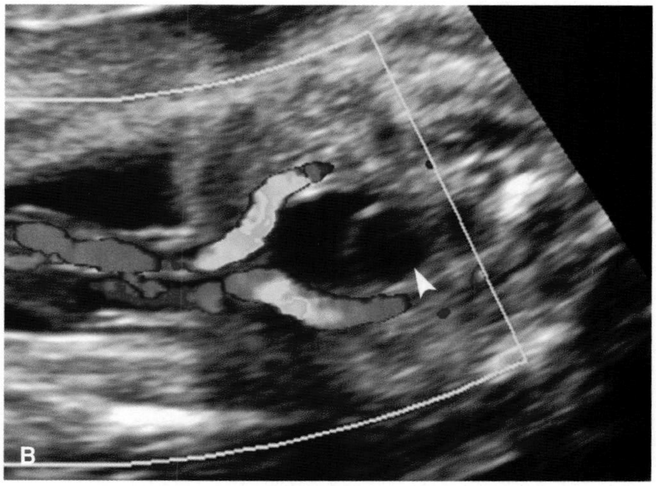

FIGURE 10-31 Duplicated renal collecting system. The upper and lower moieties of the kidney are each drained by a separate ureter. **A.** Renal pelvis dilation is visible in both the upper (*U*) and lower (*L*) pole moieties, which are separated by an intervening band of renal tissue (*arrowhead*). **B.** The bladder, encircled by the highlighted umbilical arteries, contains a ureterocele (*arrowhead*).

1998; Vergani, 1998). Sonographically, an intervening tissue band separates two distinct renal pelves. These are typically cases in which hydronephrosis and/or ureteral dilatation develops, due to abnormal implantation of one or both ureters within the bladder—a relationship described by the *Weigert-Meyer* rule. The upper pole ureter often develops obstruction from a ureterocele within the bladder, whereas the lower pole ureter has a shortened intravesical segment that predisposes to vesicoureteral reflux (see Fig. 10-31). Thus, both moieties may become dilated from different etiologies, and both are at risk for loss of function. In the neonatal period, additional testing such as voiding cystourethrography will determine whether antimicrobial treatment is needed to minimize urinary infections and will assist with follow-up or surgical intervention.

Renal Agenesis

The prevalence of bilateral renal agenesis is approximately 1 per 8000 births, whereas that of unilateral renal agenesis is 1 per 1000 births (Cragan, 2009; Dolt, 2010; Sheih, 1989; Wiesel, 2005). When a kidney is absent, the ipsilateral adrenal gland typically enlarges to fill the renal fossa, termed the *lying down adrenal sign* (Hoffman, 1992). In addition, color Doppler imaging of the descending aorta will demonstrate absence of the renal artery.

If renal agenesis is bilateral, no urine is produced. The resulting anhydramnios leads to pulmonary hypoplasia, limb contractures, and a distinctively compressed face. When this combination of abnormalities results from renal agenesis, it is called *Potter syndrome,* after Dr. Edith Potter who described it in 1946. When these abnormalities result from severely decreased amnionic fluid volume from another etiology, such as bilateral multicystic dysplastic kidney or autosomal recessive polycystic kidney disease, it is called *Potter sequence.*

Multicystic Dysplastic Kidney

This severe form of renal dysplasia results in a nonfunctioning kidney. The nephrons and collecting ducts do not form normally, such that primitive ducts are surrounded by fibromuscular tissue, and the ureter is atretic (Hains, 2009). Sonographically, the kidney contains numerous smooth-walled cysts of varying size that do not communicate with the renal pelvis and are surrounded by echogenic cortex (Fig. 10-32).

Unilateral multicystic dysplastic kidney (MCDK) has a prevalence of 1 per 4000 births. It is associated with contralateral renal abnormalities in 30 to 40 percent of cases—most frequently vesicoureteral reflux or ureteropelvic junction obstruction (Schreuder, 2009). Nonrenal anomalies have been reported in 25 percent of cases, and cystic dysplasia may occur as a component of many genetic syndromes (Lazebnik, 1999; Schreuder, 2009). If MCDK is isolated and unilateral, the prognosis is generally good.

Bilateral MCDK develops in approximately 1 per 12,000 births. It is associated with severely decreased amnionic fluid volume from early in gestation. This leads to *Potter* sequence and a poor prognosis (Lazebnik, 1999).

Polycystic Kidney Disease

Of the hereditary polycystic diseases, only the infantile form of *autosomal recessive polycystic kidney disease (ARPKD)* may be reliably diagnosed prenatally. ARPKD is a chronic, progressive disease that involves the kidneys and liver. It results in cystic dilatation of the renal collecting ducts and congenital hepatic fibrosis (Turkbey, 2009). The carrier frequency of a disease-causing mutation in the *PKHD1* gene approximates 1 in 70, and the disease prevalence is 1 in 20,000 (Zerres, 1998). ARPKD has wide phenotypic variability. This ranges from lethal pulmonary hypoplasia at birth to presentation in late childhood or even adulthood with predominantly hepatic manifestations. Infantile polycystic kidney disease is characterized by abnormally large kidneys that fill and distend the fetal abdomen and have a solid, ground-glass texture. Severe oligohydramnios confers a poor prognosis.

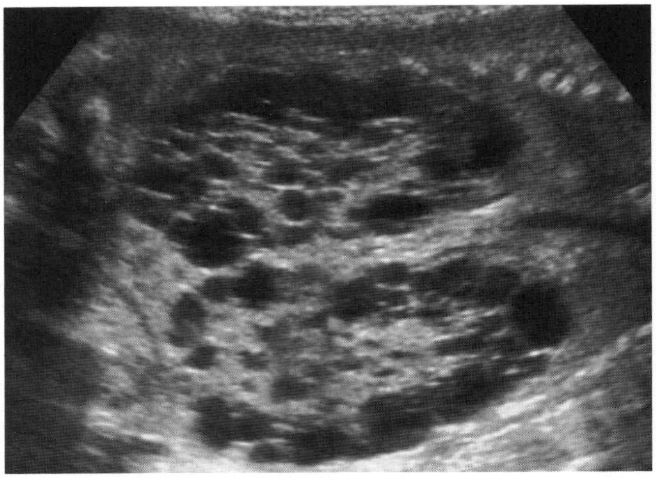

FIGURE 10-32 Multicystic dysplastic kidneys. Coronal view of the fetal abdomen demonstrates markedly enlarged kidneys containing multiple cysts of varying sizes that do not communicate with a renal pelvis.

As discussed in Chapter 53 (p. 1058), *autosomal dominant polycystic kidney disease (ADPKD),* which is far more common, usually does not manifest until adulthood. Even so, some fetuses with ADPKD have mild renal enlargement, increased renal echogenicity, and normal amnionic fluid volume. The differential diagnosis for these findings includes several genetic syndromes, aneuploidy, or normal variant.

Bladder Outlet Obstruction

Distal obstruction of the urinary tract is more frequent in male fetuses, and the most common etiology is *posterior urethral valves.* Characteristically, there is dilatation of the bladder and proximal urethra, termed the "keyhole" sign, and the bladder wall is thick (Fig. 10-33). Oligohydramnios, particularly before midpregnancy, portends a poor prognosis because of pulmonary hypoplasia. Unfortunately, the outcome may be poor even with normal amnionic fluid volume. Evaluation includes a careful search for associated anomalies, which may occur in 40 percent of cases, and for aneuploidy, which has been reported in 5 to 8 percent (Hayden, 1988; Hobbins, 1984; Mann, 2010). If neither are present, affected male fetuses with severe oligohydramnios who have fetal urinary electrolytes suggesting a potentially favorable prognosis may be fetal therapy candidates. Evaluation and treatment of fetal bladder outlet obstruction is discussed in Chapter 16 (p. 330).

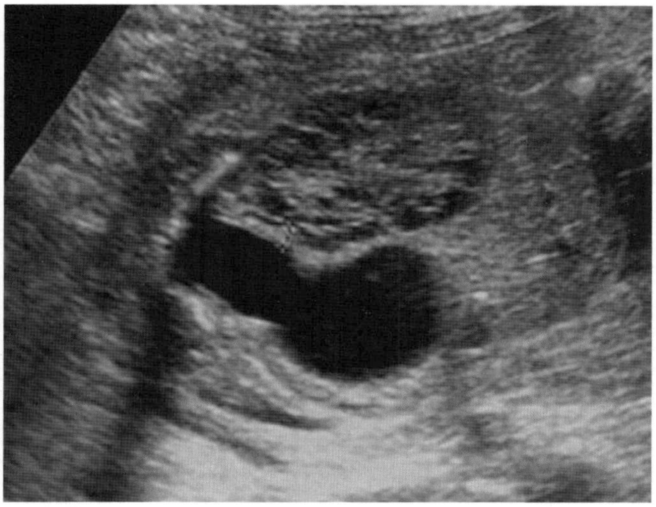

FIGURE 10-33 Posterior urethral valve. In this 19-week fetus with severe bladder outlet obstruction, the bladder is dilated and thick-walled, with dilatation of the proximal urethra that resembles a "keyhole." Adjacent to the bladder is an enlarged kidney with evidence of cystic dysplasia, conferring a poor prognosis.

Skeletal Abnormalities

The 2010 revision of the Nosology and Classification of Genetic Skeletal Disorders includes an impressive 456 skeletal abnormalities in 40 groups that are defined by molecular, biochemical, and/or radiographic criteria (Warman, 2011). There are two types of skeletal dysplasias: *osteochondrodysplasias*—the generalized abnormal development of bone and/or cartilage, and *dysostoses*—which are abnormalities of individual bones, for example, *polydactyly*. In addition to these *malformations*, skeletal abnormalities include *deformations*, as with some cases of clubfoot, and *disruptions* such as limb-reduction defects.

Skeletal Dysplasias

The prevalence of skeletal dysplasias approximates 3 per 10,000 births. Two groups account for more than half of all cases: the *fibroblast growth factor 3 (FGFR3) chondrodysplasia* group and the *osteogenesis imperfecta* and decreased bone density group. Each has a prevalence of approximately 0.8 per 10,000 births (Stevenson, 2012).

Evaluation of a pregnancy with suspected skeletal dysplasia includes a survey of every long bone, as well as the hands and feet, skull size and shape, clavicles, scapulae, thorax, and spine. Reference tables are used to determine which long bones are affected and ascertain the degree of shortening (Appendix, p. 1299). Involvement of all long bones is termed *micromelia,* whereas predominant involvement of only the proximal, intermediate, or distal long bone segments is termed *rhizomelia, mesomelia,* and *acromelia*, respectively. The degree of ossification should be noted, as should presence of bowing or fractures. Each of these may provide clues to narrow the differential diagnosis and occasionally suggest a specific skeletal dysplasia. Many, if not most, skeletal dysplasias have a genetic component, and knowledge of specific mutations has advanced rapidly (Warman, 2011).

Although precise characterization of a specific skeletal dysplasia may elude prenatal diagnosis, it is frequently possible to determine whether a skeletal dysplasia is lethal. Lethal dysplasias are frequently characterized by profound long bone shortening, with measurements below the 5th percentile and by femur length-to-abdominal circumference ratios < 16 percent (Appendix, p. 1299) (Rahemtullah, 1997; Ramus, 1998). Evidence of pulmonary hypoplasia includes a thoracic circumference < 80 percent of the abdominal circumference, thoracic circumference below the 2.5th percentile, and a cardiothoracic circumference ratio > 50 percent (Appendix, p. 1298). Affected pregnancies also may develop hydramnios and/or hydrops.

The FGFR3 chondrodysplasias include *achondroplasia* and *thanatophoric dysplasia.* Achondroplasia, also called *heterozygous achondroplasia,* is the most common nonlethal skeletal dysplasia. It is inherited in an autosomal dominant fashion, with 80 percent of cases resulting from a new mutation. An impressive 98 percent are due to one mutation in the *FGFR3* gene. Achondroplasia is characterized by long bone shortening that is predominantly *rhizomelic*, an enlarged head with frontal bossing, depressed nasal bridge, exaggerated lumbar lordosis, and a trident configuration of the hands. Intelligence is typically normal. Sonographically, the femur and humerus measurements may not be below the 5th percentile until the early third trimester. Thus, this condition is usually not diagnosed until late in pregnancy. In homozygotes, which represent 25 percent of the offspring of heterozygous parents, the condition is characterized by much more severe long bone shortening and is lethal.

The other major class of FGFR3 dysplasias, *thanatophoric dysplasia*, is the most common lethal skeletal disorder. It is characterized by severe micromelia, and affected fetuses—particularly those with type II—may develop a characteristic cloverleaf skull deformity (*kleeblattschädel*) due to craniosynostosis. More than 99 percent of cases may be confirmed with genetic testing.

Osteogenesis imperfecta represents a group of skeletal dysplasias characterized by hypomineralization. There are multiple types, and more than 90 percent of cases are characterized by a mutation in the *COL1A1* or *COL1A2* gene. Type IIa, also called the perinatal form, is lethal. It is characterized by profound lack of skull ossification, such that gentle pressure on the maternal abdomen from the ultrasound transducer results in visible skull deformation (Fig. 10-34). Other features include multiple in-utero fractures and ribs that appear "beaded." Inheritance is autosomal dominant, such that all cases result from either new mutations or gonadal mosaicism (Chap. 13, p. 269). Another skeletal dysplasia that results in severe hypomineralization is *hypophosphatasia*, which is inherited in an autosomal recessive fashion.

Clubfoot—Talipes Equinovarus

This disorder is notable for a deformed talus and shortened Achilles tendon. The affected foot is abnormally fixed and positioned with *equinus*—downward pointing, *varus*—inward rotation, and forefoot adduction. Most cases are considered malformations, with a multifactorial genetic component. However, an association with environmental factors and with early amniocentesis

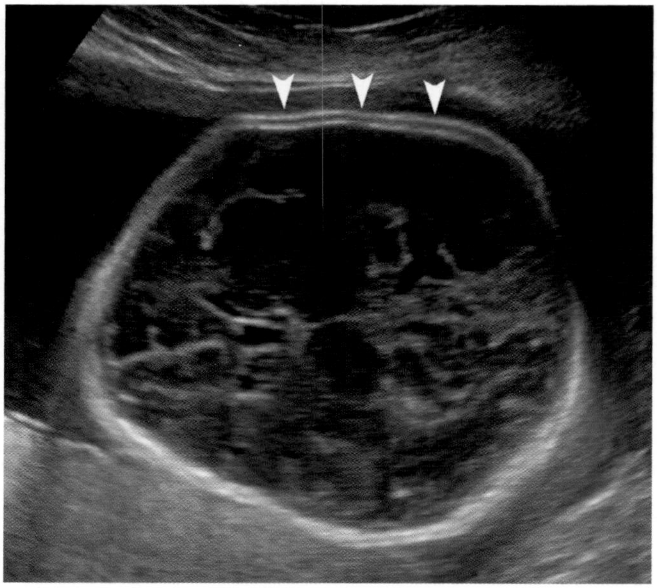

FIGURE 10-34 Osteogenesis imperfecta. Type IIa, which is lethal, is characterized by such profound lack of skull ossification that gentle pressure on the maternal abdomen from the ultrasound transducer results in visible deformation (flattening) of the skull (*arrowheads*).

suggests that deformation also plays a role (Tredwell, 2001). Sonographically, the footprint is visible in the same plane as the tibia and fibula (Fig. 10-35).

In population-based series, the prevalence of clubfoot is approximately 1 per 1000 births, with a male:female ratio of 2:1 (Carey, 2003; Pavone, 2012). Clubfoot is bilateral in approximately 50 percent of cases, and associated anomalies are present in at least 50 percent (Mammen, 2004; Sharma, 2011). Frequently associated anomalies include neural-tube defects, arthrogryposis, and myotonic dystrophy and other genetic syndromes. In the setting of associated anomalies, aneuploidy is present in approximately 30 percent, but it has been reported in less than 4 percent when clubfoot appears isolated (Lauson, 2010; Sharma, 2011). Thus, a careful search for associated anomalies is warranted, and fetal karyotyping may be considered.

Limb-Reduction Defects

Documentation of the arms and legs is a component of the standard examination. A limb-reduction defect is the absence of all or part of one or more extremities. Absence of an entire extremity is termed *amelia. Phocomelia,* associated with thalidomide exposure, is an absence of one or more long bones with the hands or feet attached to the trunk (Chap. 12, p. 252). Limb-reduction defects are associated with numerous genetic syndromes, such as *Roberts syndrome*, an autosomal recessive condition characterized by *tetraphocomelia.* A *clubhand deformity*, usually from an absent radius, is associated with trisomy 18 and is also a component of the *thrombocytopenia-absent radius syndrome.* Limb-reduction defects may occur in the setting of a disruption such as amnionic band sequence (Chap. 6, p. 121). They have also been associated with chorionic villus sampling when performed before 10 weeks' gestation (Chap. 14, p. 300).

THREE- AND FOUR-DIMENSIONAL SONOGRAPHY

During the last two decades, three-dimensional (3-D) sonography has gone from a novelty to a standard feature of most modern ultrasound equipment (Fig. 10-36). 3-D sonography is not *routinely* used during a standard examination nor considered a required modality. However, it may be a component of various specialized evaluations.

Most 3-D scanning uses a special transducer developed for this purpose. After a region of interest is identified, a 3-D volume is acquired that may be rendered to display images of any plane—axial, sagittal, coronal, or even oblique—within that volume. Sequential "slices" can be generated, similar to computed tomographic (CT) or MR images. Technique applications include evaluation of intracranial anatomy in the sagittal plane, for example, the corpus callosum, and imaging of the palate and skeletal system (Benacerraf, 2006; Pilu, 2008; Timor-Tritsch, 2000).

Unlike 2-D scanning, which appears to be in "real time," 3-D imaging is static and obtained by processing a volume of stored images. There is also *four-dimensional (4-D) sonography*, also known as real-time 3-D sonography. This enhancement allows rapid reconstruction of the rendered images to convey the impression that the scanning is in real time. One application of 4-D imaging has been to improve visualization of cardiac anatomy. Postprocessing algorithms and techniques take advantage of real-time image volumes, with and without color Doppler mapping. An example is *spatiotemporal image correlation—STIC*, used to evaluate complex cardiac anatomy and function (DeVore, 2003; Espinoza, 2008). Addition of an inversion-mode algorithm may aid imaging of blood flow within the heart and great vessels and may even permit measurement of ventricular blood volume (Goncalves, 2004). Systematic approaches or protocols for using these new techniques to evaluate cardiac anatomy and physiology are under development (Espinoza, 2007; Turan, 2009).

For selected anomalies, such as those of the face and skeleton, 3-D sonography may provide additional useful information

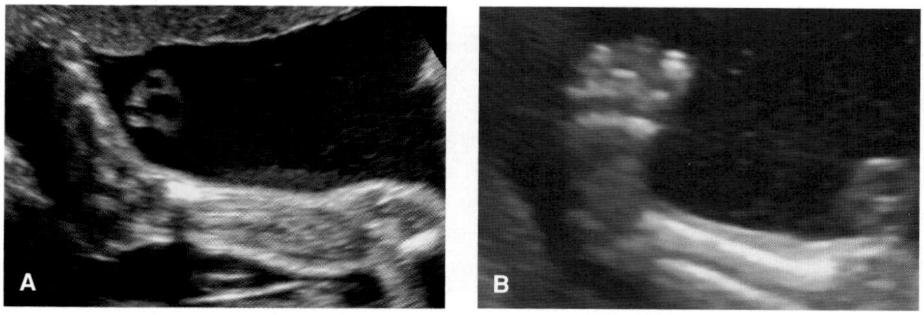

FIGURE 10-35 Foot position. **A.** Normal fetal lower leg, demonstrating normal position of the foot. **B.** With talipes equinovarus, the foot "print" is visible in the same plane as the tibia and fibula.

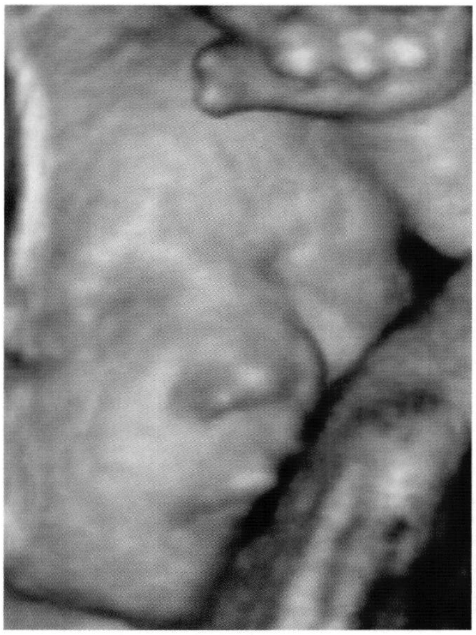

FIGURE 10-36 Fetal face. Surface rendered three-dimensional image of a normal fetal face and hand at 32 weeks.

(Goncalves, 2005). That said, comparisons of 3-D with conventional 2-D sonography for the diagnosis of most congenital anomalies have not demonstrated an improvement in overall detection (Goncalves, 2006; Reddy, 2008). The American College of Obstetricians and Gynecologists (2011) currently recommends that 3-D ultrasound be used only as an adjunct to conventional sonography.

DOPPLER

When sound waves strike a moving target, the frequency of the waves reflected back is shifted proportionate to the velocity and direction of that moving target—a phenomenon known as the *Doppler shift*. Because the magnitude and direction of the frequency shift depend on the relative motion of the moving target, Doppler can be used to evaluate flow within blood vessels. The Doppler equation is shown in Figure 10-37.

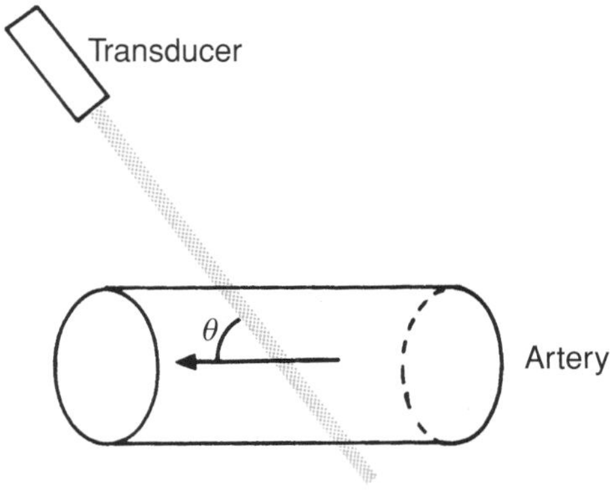

$$f_d = 2f_o \frac{v \cos \theta}{c}$$

FIGURE 10-37 Doppler equation. Ultrasound emanating from the transducer with initial frequency f_o strikes blood moving at velocity v. Reflected frequency f_d is dependent on angle θ between beam of sound and vessel.

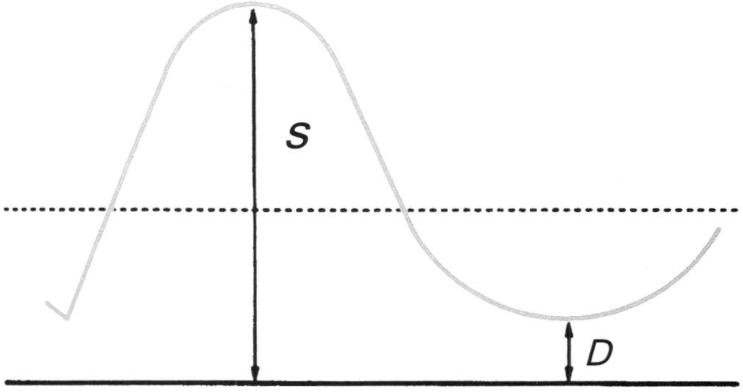

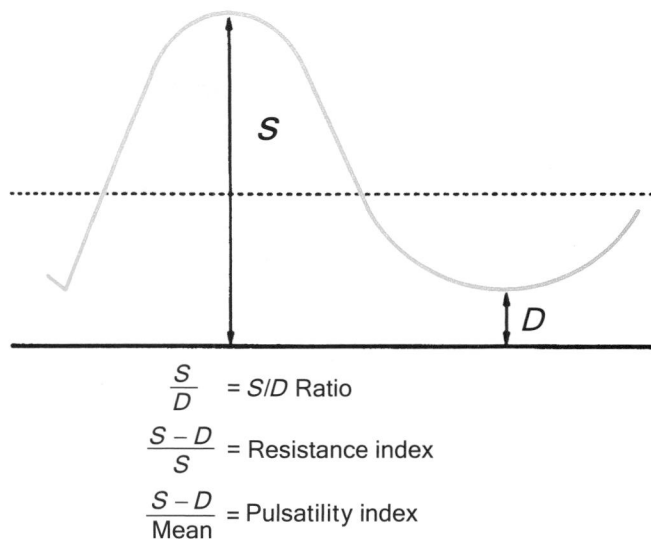

$$\frac{S}{D} = S/D \text{ Ratio}$$

$$\frac{S-D}{S} = \text{Resistance index}$$

$$\frac{S-D}{\text{Mean}} = \text{Pulsatility index}$$

FIGURE 10-38 Doppler systolic–diastolic waveform indices of blood flow velocity. S represents the peak systolic flow or velocity, and D indicates the end-diastolic flow or velocity. The mean, which is the time-average mean velocity, is calculated from computer-digitized waveforms.

An important component of the equation is the angle of insonation, abbreviated as theta (θ), which is the angle between the sound waves from the transducer and flow within the vessel. Measurement error becomes large when θ is not close to zero, in other words, when blood flow is not coming *directly* toward or away from the transducer. For this reason, ratios are often used to compare different waveform components, allowing cosine θ to cancel out of the equation. Figure 10-38 is a schematic of the Doppler waveform and describes the three ratios commonly used. The simplest is the *systolic-diastolic ratio (S/D ratio),* which compares the maximal (or peak) systolic flow with end-diastolic flow to evaluate downstream impedance to flow.

Continuous wave Doppler equipment has two separate types of crystals—one transmits high-frequency sound waves, and another continuously captures signals. In M-mode imaging, continuous wave Doppler is used to evaluate motion through time, however, it cannot image individual vessels.

Pulsed-wave Doppler uses only one crystal, which transmits the signal and then waits until the returning signal is received before transmitting another one. It allows precise targeting and visualization of the vessel of interest. Pulsed-wave Doppler can be configured to allow color-flow mapping—such that blood flowing toward the transducer is displayed in red and that flowing away from the transducer appears in blue. Various combinations of pulsed-wave Doppler, color-flow Doppler, and real-time sonography are commercially available.

Umbilical Artery

As discussed in Chapter 17 (p. 344), umbilical artery Doppler has been subjected to more rigorous assessment than has any previous test of fetal health. The umbilical artery differs from other vessels in that it normally has forward flow throughout the cardiac cycle. Moreover, the amount of flow during diastole increases as gestation advances—a function of decreasing placental impedance. *The S/D ratio normally decreases from approximately 4.0 at 20 weeks to 2.0 at term, and it is generally less than 3.0 after 30 weeks.* Because of downstream impedance to flow, *more* end-diastolic flow is observed at the placental cord insertion than at the fetal ventral wall. Thus, abnormalities such as absent or reversed end-diastolic flow will appear first at the fetal cord insertion site. The International Society of Ultrasound in Obstetrics and Gynecology recommends that umbilical artery Doppler measurements be made in a free loop of cord (Bhide, 2013). However, the Society for Maternal Fetal Medicine has recommended that assessment be performed close to the ventral wall insertion to optimize reproducibility (Berkley, 2012).

The waveform is considered abnormal if the *S/D* ratio is above the 95th percentile for gestational age. In extreme cases of growth restriction, end-diastolic flow may become absent or even reversed (Fig. 10-39). Such reversal of end-diastolic flow has been associated with greater than 70-percent obliteration of the small muscular arteries in placental tertiary stem villi (Kingdom, 1997; Morrow, 1989).

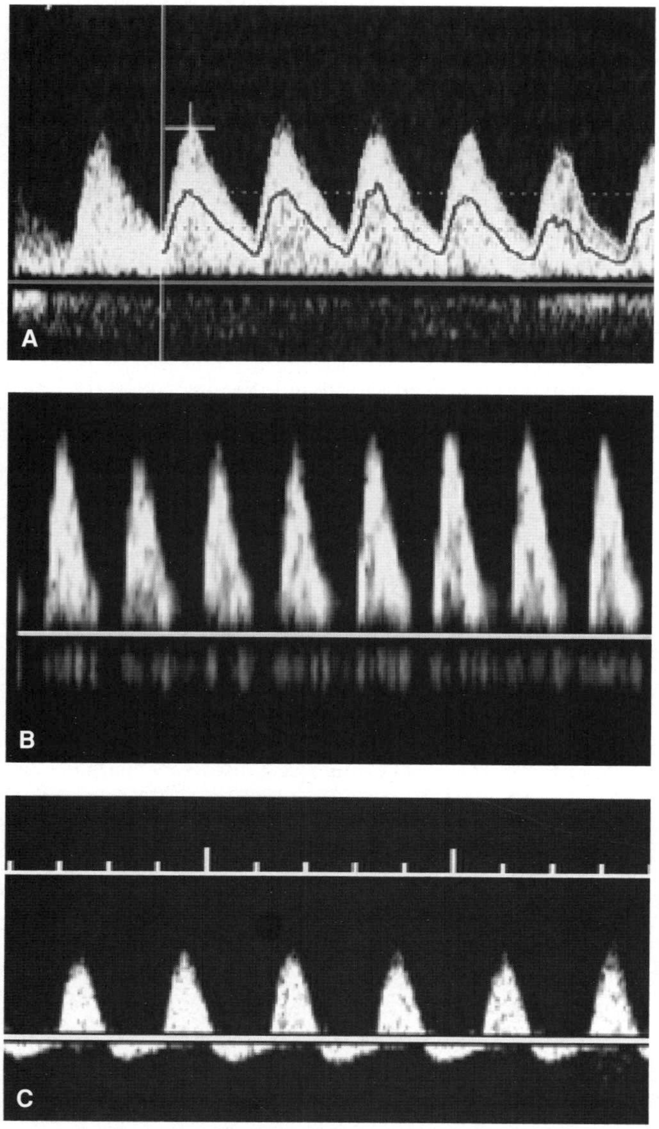

FIGURE 10-39 Umbilical artery Doppler waveforms. **A.** Normal diastolic flow. **B.** Absence of end-diastolic flow. **C.** Reversed end-diastolic flow.

Umbilical artery Doppler is a useful adjunct in the management of pregnancies complicated by fetal-growth restriction, and it has been associated with improved outcome in such cases (American College of Obstetricians and Gynecologists, 2013). It is not recommended for complications other than growth restriction. Similarly, it is not recommended as a screening tool for identifying pregnancies that will subsequently be complicated by growth restriction (Berkley, 2012). Abnormal umbilical artery Doppler findings should prompt a complete fetal evaluation if not already done, as such findings are associated with major fetal anomalies and aneuploidy (Wenstrom, 1991). The Society for Maternal Fetal Medicine has recommended that *so long as fetal surveillance remains reassuring*, pregnancies with fetal-growth restriction and absent end-diastolic flow in the umbilical artery may be managed expectantly until delivery at 34 weeks, and those with reversed end-diastolic flow managed expectantly until delivery at 32 weeks (Berkley, 2012).

Ductus Arteriosus

Doppler evaluation of the ductus arteriosus has been used primarily to monitor fetuses exposed to indomethacin and other nonsteroidal antiinflammatory agents (NSAIDs). Indomethacin, which is used by some for tocolysis, may cause ductal constriction or closure, particularly when used in the third trimester (Huhta, 1987). The resulting increased pulmonary flow may cause reactive hypertrophy of the pulmonary arterioles and eventual development of pulmonary hypertension. In a review of 12 randomized controlled trials involving more than 200 exposed pregnancies, Koren and colleagues (2006) reported that NSAIDs increased the odds of ductal constriction 15-fold. They also concluded that this was a low estimate because most of the pregnancies were exposed only briefly. Fortunately, ductal constriction is often reversible after NSAID discontinuation. Because ductal constriction is a potentially serious complication that should be avoided, the duration of NSAID administration is typically limited to less than 72 hours, and women taking NSAIDs are closely monitored so that these can be discontinued if ductal constriction is identified.

Uterine Artery

Uterine blood flow is estimated to increase from 50 mL/min early in gestation to 500 to 750 mL/min by term (Chap. 4, p. 47). The uterine artery Doppler waveform is characterized by high diastolic flow velocities and by highly turbulent flow. Increased resistance to flow and development of a diastolic *notch* are associated with later development of gestational hypertension, preeclampsia, and fetal-growth restriction. Zeeman and coworkers (2003) also found women with chronic hypertension who had increased uterine artery impedance at 16 to 20 weeks were at increased risk to develop superimposed preeclampsia. Even so, the predictive value of uterine artery Doppler testing is low, and screening is not recommended in either high-risk or low-risk pregnancies (Sciscione, 2009). The technique has not been standardized, frequency of assessment has not been

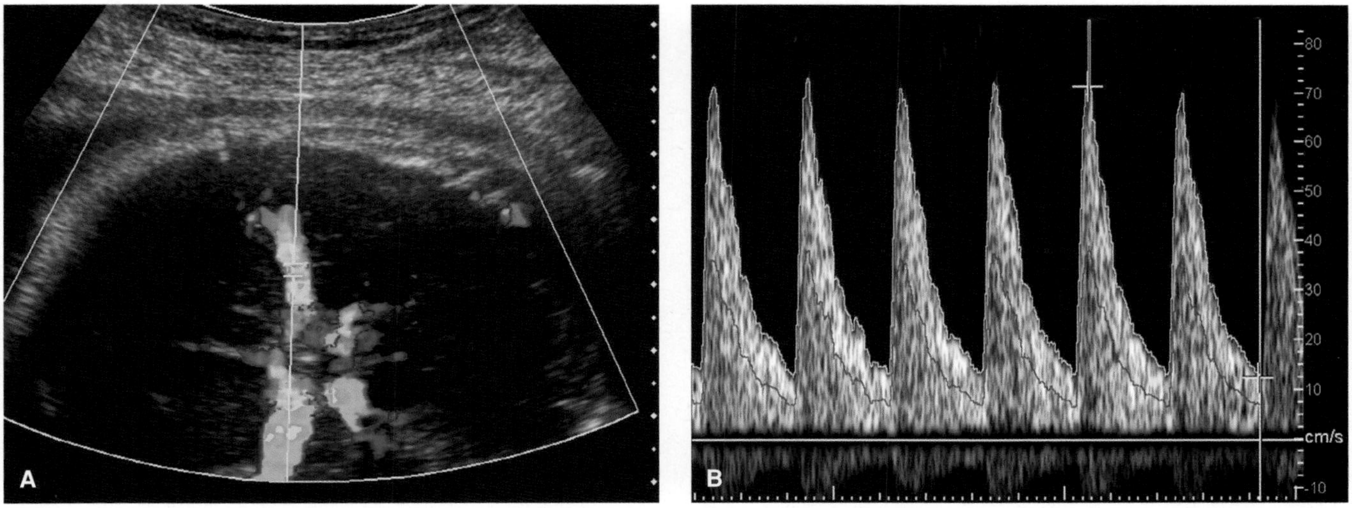

FIGURE 10-40 Middle cerebral artery (MCA) Doppler. **A.** Color Doppler of the circle of Willis, demonstrating the correct location to sample the MCA. **B.** The waveform demonstrates a peak systolic velocity exceeding 70 cm/sec in a 32-week fetus with severe fetal anemia secondary to Rh alloimmunization.

established, and criteria for an abnormal test have not been determined. In a report from a workshop on prenatal imaging held by the NICHD, Reddy and associates (2008) concluded that perinatal benefits of uterine artery Doppler screening have not yet been demonstrated.

Middle Cerebral Artery

Doppler interrogation of the middle cerebral artery (MCA) has been investigated and applied clinically for fetal anemia detection and fetal-growth restriction evaluation. Anatomically, the path of the MCA is such that flow often approaches the transducer "head-on," allowing for accurate determination of flow velocity (Fig. 10-40). The MCA is imaged in an axial view of the head at the base of the skull, ideally within 2 mm of the internal carotid artery origin. Velocity measurement is optimal when the insonating angle is close to zero, and no more than 30 degrees of angle correction should be used. In general, velocity assessment is not performed in other fetal vessels, because a larger insonating angle is needed and confers significant measurement error.

When fetal anemia is present, the *peak systolic velocity* is increased due to increased cardiac output and decreased blood viscosity (Segata, 2004). This has permitted the reliable, noninvasive detection of fetal anemia in cases of blood-group alloimmunization. More than a decade ago, Mari and colleagues (2000) demonstrated that an MCA peak systolic velocity threshold of 1.50 multiples of the median (MoM) could reliably identify fetuses with moderate or severe anemia. In most referral centers, MCA peak systolic velocity has replaced invasive testing with amniocentesis for fetal anemia detection (Chap. 15, p. 310).

MCA Doppler has also been studied as an adjunct in the evaluation of fetal-growth restriction. Fetal hypoxemia is believed to result in increased blood flow to the brain, heart, and adrenal glands, leading to increased end-diastolic flow in the MCA. This phenomenon, "brain-sparing," is actually a misnomer, as it is not protective for the fetus but rather is associated with perinatal morbidity and mortality (Bahado-Singh, 1999; Cruz-Martinez, 2011). The utility of MCA Doppler to aid the timing of delivery is uncertain. It has *not* been evaluated in randomized trials nor adopted as standard practice in the management of growth restriction (American College of Obstetricians and Gynecologists, 2013; Berkley, 2012).

Ductus Venosus

The ductus venosus is imaged as it branches from the umbilical vein at approximately the level of the diaphragm. Fetal position poses more of a challenge in imaging the ductus venosus than it does with either the umbilical artery or the middle cerebral artery. The waveform is biphasic and normally has forward flow throughout the cardiac cycle. The first peak reflects ventricular systole, and the second is diastolic filling. These are followed by a nadir during atrial contraction—termed the *a-wave*.

It is believed that there is a progression of Doppler findings in preterm fetuses with growth restriction, such that umbilical artery Doppler abnormalities occur first, followed by those in the middle cerebral artery and then the ductus venosus. However, there is wide variability in manifestation of these abnormalities (Berkley, 2012). When severe fetal-growth restriction is present, cardiac dysfunction may lead to flow in the a-wave that is decreased, absent, and eventually reversed, along with pulsatile flow in the umbilical vein (Reddy, 2008).

Thus, ductus venosus abnormalities have potential to identify preterm growth-restricted fetuses that are at greatest risk for adverse outcomes (Baschat, 2003, 2004; Bilardo, 2004; Figueras, 2009). As noted by the Society for Maternal-Fetal Medicine, however, they have not been sufficiently evaluated in randomized trials (Berkley, 2012). The American College of Obstetricians and Gynecologists (2013) recently concluded that Doppler assessment of vessels other than the umbilical artery has not been shown to improve perinatal outcome and that its role in clinical practice remains uncertain.

MAGNETIC RESONANCE IMAGING

The fetus was first studied with MR imaging in the mid-1980s, when image acquisition was slow and motion artifact was problematic (Lowe, 1985). Since then, technological advances that allow fast-acquisition MR protocols have been developed. These newer protocols permit image acquisition in 1 second or less, which significantly reduces motion artifact and eliminates the need for sedation.

Image resolution with MR is often superior to that with sonography because it is not as hindered by bony interfaces, maternal obesity, oligohydramnios, or an engaged fetal head. MR may be a useful adjunct to sonography in evaluating and further characterizing suspected fetal abnormalities. MR imaging, however, is not portable, it is time-consuming, and its use is generally limited to referral centers with expertise in fetal imaging. It may be helpful in the evaluation of complex abnormalities of the fetal CNS, thorax, gastrointestinal system, genitourinary system, and musculoskeletal system. MR has also been used in the evaluation of maternal pelvic masses, placental invasion, and abnormalities of the pelvic floor and cervix.

The American College of Radiology and Society for Pediatric Radiology (2010) have developed a practice guideline for fetal MR imaging. This guideline acknowledges that sonography is the screening modality of choice. Moreover, it recommends that fetal MR imaging be used for problem solving to ideally contribute to prenatal diagnosis, counseling, treatment, and delivery planning. Specific indications for fetal MR imaging are listed in Table 10-8 and are discussed subsequently.

Safety

MR imaging uses no ionizing radiation. Theoretical concerns include the effects of fluctuating electromagnetic fields and high sound-intensity levels. The strength of the magnetic field is measured in *tesla (T),* and all imaging studies during pregnancy are currently performed using 1.5 T or less.

Human studies and tissue studies support the safety of fetal MR imaging. Repetitive exposure of human lung fibroblasts to a static 1.5-T magnetic field has not been found to affect cellular proliferation (Wiskirchen, 1999). Fetal heart rate patterns have been evaluated before and during MR imaging, with no significant differences observed (Vadeyar, 2000). Children exposed to MR as fetuses have not been found to have an increased incidence of disease or disability when tested at age 9 months or 3 years (Baker, 1994; Clements, 2000).

Glover and associates (1995) attempted to mimic the sound level experienced by the fetal ear by having an adult volunteer swallow a microphone while the stomach was filled with a liter of fluid to represent the amnionic sac. There was at least 30-dB attenuation in intensity from the body surface to the fluid-filled stomach, reducing the sound pressure from 120 dB to below 90 dB. This level is considerably less than the 135 dB experienced from vibroacoustic stimulation (Chap. 17, p. 341). Cochlear function testing has been performed in infants who were exposed to 1.5-T MR imaging as fetuses. Such testing has not demonstrated evidence of hearing impairment (Reeves, 2010).

TABLE 10-8. Fetal Conditions for Which Magnetic Resonance Imaging May Be Indicated

Brain and spine
Ventriculomegaly
Agenesis of the corpus callosum
Holoprosencephaly
Posterior fossa abnormalities
Cerebral cortical malformations
Vascular malformations
Hydranencephaly
Infarctions
Monochorionic twin pregnancy complications
Neural-tube defects
Sacrococcygeal teratoma
Caudal regression sequence
Sirenomelia
Vertebral anomalies
Skull, face, and neck
Venolymphatic malformations
Hemangiomas
Goiter
Teratomas
Facial clefts
Other abnormalities with potential airway obstruction
Thorax
Congenital cystic adenomatoid malformation
Extralobar pulmonary sequestration
Congenital diaphragmatic hernia
Evaluation of pulmonary hypoplasia secondary to oligohydramnios, chest mass, or skeletal dysplasia
Abdomen, pelvis, and retroperitoneum
Assess the size and location of tumors (such as sacrococcygeal teratoma, neuroblastoma, suprarenal or renal masses)
Assess renal anomalies with oligohydramnios
Diagnose bowel anomalies
Complications of monochorionic twins
Determine vascular anatomy prior to laser treatment
Assess morbidity after death of a monochorionic cotwin
Evaluate conjoined twins
Fetal surgery assessment
Fetal brain anatomy before and after surgical intervention
Fetal anomalies for which surgery is planned

Adapted from American College of Radiology–Society of Perinatal Radiologists Practice Guideline, 2010.

The Expert Panel on MR Safety of the American College of Radiology (2013) has concluded that based on available evidence, there are no documented deleterious effects of MR imaging exposure on the developing fetus. Therefore, MR can be performed in pregnancy if the data are needed to care for the fetus or mother. Health-care providers who are pregnant may work in and around an MR unit, but it is recommended that they not remain in the MR scanner magnet room—known as Zone IV—while an examination is in progress (American College of Radiology, 2013).

Gadolinium-based MR contrast agents should be avoided during pregnancy because of the potential for dissociation of the chelate molecule in the amnionic fluid (American College of Radiology, 2013). These readily enter the fetal circulation and are excreted into the amnionic fluid via fetal urine. Here, they may remain for an indeterminate period before being reabsorbed. The longer the gadolinium-chelate molecule remains in a protected space such as the amnionic sac, the greater the potential for dissociation of the toxic gadolinium ion (American College of Radiology, 2013). In adults with renal disease, this contrast agent has been associated with development of nephrogenic systemic fibrosis, a potentially severe complication.

Technique

All women complete a written MR safety screening questionnaire before the examination. This includes information regarding metallic implants, pacemakers, or other metal- or iron-containing devices that may alter the study (American College of Radiology, 2013). Iron supplementation may cause artifact in the colon but does not usually affect the fetal resolution. In more than 2000 MR procedures in pregnancy performed at Parkland Hospital during the last 10 years, maternal anxiety secondary to claustrophobia and/or fear of the MR equipment has occurred in fewer than 1 percent of our patients. To reduce maternal anxiety in this small group, a single oral dose of diazepam, 5 to 10 mg, or lorazepam, 1 to 2 mg, is given.

Women are placed in the supine or left lateral decubitus position. A torso coil is used in most circumstances, with the occasional use of either the body or cardiac coil depending on maternal or fetal size and area of interest. A series of three-plane localizers are obtained relative to the maternal coronal, sagittal, and axial planes. The gravid uterus is imaged in the maternal axial plane (7-mm slices, 0 gap) with a T2-weighted fast acquisition. Typically, these may be a single-shot fast spin echo sequence (SSFSE), half-Fourier acquisition single-shot turbo spin echo (HASTE), or rapid acquisition with relaxation enhancement (RARE), depending on the brand of machine and manufacturer. Next, a fast T1-weighted acquisition such as spoiled gradient echo (SPGR) is performed (7-mm thickness, 0 gap). These acquisitions are particularly good for identifying fetal and maternal anatomy.

Orthogonal images of targeted fetal or maternal structures are then obtained. In these cases, 3- to 5-mm slice thickness, 0 gap T2-weighted acquisitions are performed in the coronal, sagittal, and axial planes. Depending on the anatomy and underlying suspected abnormality, T1-weighted images can be performed to evaluate for subacute hemorrhage, fat, or location of normal structures that appear bright on these sequences, such as liver and meconium in the colon (Brugger, 2006; Zaretsky, 2003b).

Short TI inversion recovery images (STIR) may provide differentiation in cases in which the water content of the abnormality is similar to the normal structure. An example is a thoracic mass compared with normal lung. Occasionally, *fluid attenuated inversion recovery (FLAIR)* images may be obtained for CNS abnormalities to evaluate the ventricular system and other CSF-containing spaces. Diffusion-weighted imaging may be employed to evaluate for restricted diffusion and ischemia (Brugger, 2006; Zaretsky, 2003b). Our series also includes an axial brain 3- to 5-mm T2-weighted sequence to obtain head biometry for gestational age estimation using the biparietal diameter and head circumference (Reichel, 2003).

Fetal Anatomical Evaluation

Whenever a fetal abnormality has been identified, findings from the affected organ as well as other organ systems should be thoroughly characterized. Accordingly, a fetal anatomical survey is generally completed during each MR examination. In a recent prospective study, nearly 95 percent of the anatomical components recommended by the International Society of Ultrasound in Obstetrics and Gynecology were visible at 30 weeks (Millischer, 2013). The aorta and pulmonary artery were the structures most difficult to evaluate. Zaretsky and coworkers (2003a) similarly found that with the exclusion of cardiac structures, fetal anatomical evaluation was possible in 99 percent of cases.

Central Nervous System

With MR imaging, the brain can be visualized in the axial, coronal, and sagittal planes, without the near-field attenuation caused by the fetal skull during sonography. This makes MR a valuable adjunct in the evaluation of selected intracranial anomalies. Very fast T2-weighted images produce excellent tissue contrast, and CSF-containing structures are hyperintense or bright. This allows exquisite detail of the posterior fossa, midline structures, and cerebral cortex. T1-weighted images are occasionally used to differentiate between fat and hemorrhage.

CNS biometry obtained with MR imaging has been found to be comparable with that obtained using sonography (Twickler, 2002). Nomograms have been published for multiple intracranial structures, including corpus callosum and cerebellar vermis lengths (Garel, 2004; Tilea, 2009).

Levine and colleagues (1999a) demonstrated that MR imaging accurately portrays cerebral gyration and sulcation patterns (Fig. 10-41). This is important because fetuses with a cerebral abnormality may have a significant lag in cortical development. Sonography permits limited evaluation of subtle migrational abnormalities, and MR imaging provides greater accuracy, particularly later in gestation.

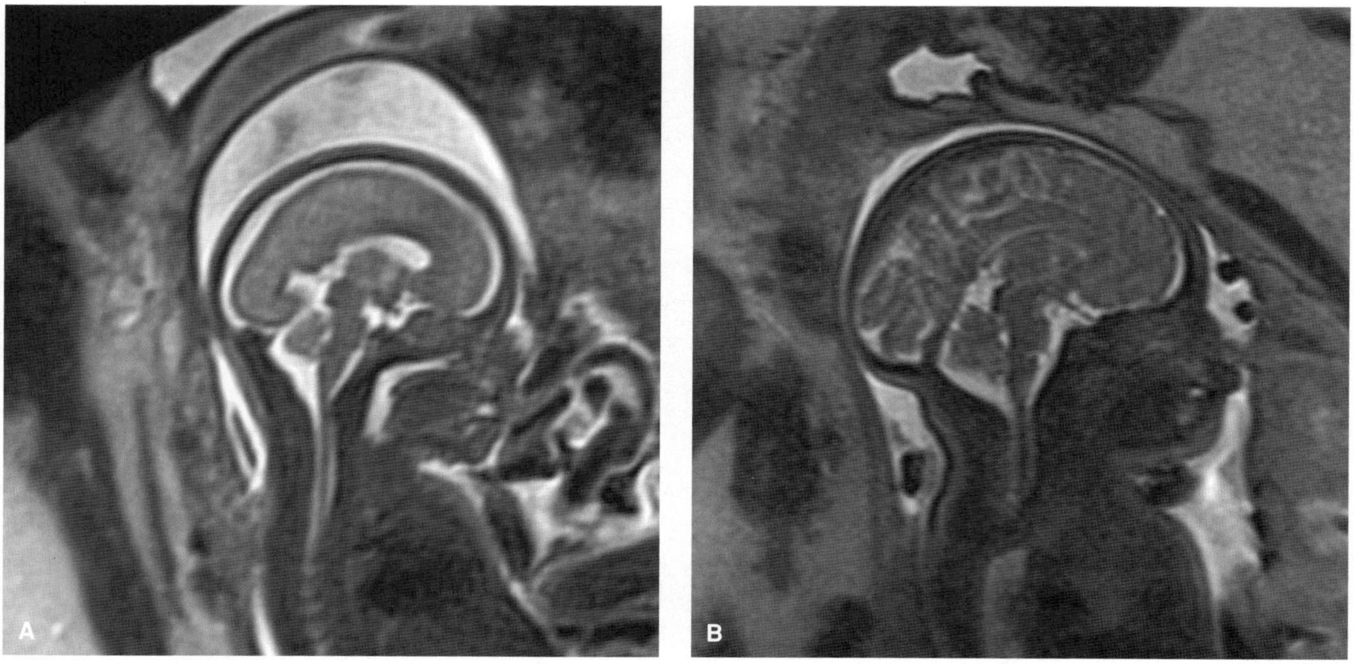

FIGURE 10-41 Sagittal images of the fetal brain at 25 weeks **(A)** and at 37 weeks **(B)** demonstrate the normal increase in gyration and sulcation that occurs during fetal development. These images were obtained using a Half Fourier Acquisition Single Shot Turbo Spin Echo (HASTE) sequence.

Indications. There have been numerous studies of second-opinion MR examination for a cerebral abnormality detected or suspected sonographically (Benacerraf, 2007; Li, 2012). Levine and associates (1999b) found that MR imaging changed the diagnosis in 40 percent of cases and affected management in 15 percent. Simon and coworkers (2000) reported that MR-imaging findings changed management in almost half of cases. Twickler and colleagues (2003) also reported that fetal CNS MR imaging changed the diagnosis in half of fetuses and altered clinical management in a third. Additional information was more likely to be gained when the examination was performed beyond 24 weeks' gestation.

Ventriculomegaly is a common fetal MR imaging indication, if used to determine whether this finding is truly isolated or associated with other CNS dysmorphology (p. 202). For example, MR may demonstrate that severe ventriculomegaly is secondary to aqueductal stenosis, shown in Figure 10-42, or that it is actually hydranencephaly. In the case of mild ventriculomegaly, MR may identify agenesis of the corpus callosum or migrational abnormalities (Benacerraf, 2007; Li, 2012; Twickler, 2003).

Another fetal MR imaging indication is the evaluation of possible intraventricular hemorrhage (IVH), such as shown in Figure 10-43. Fetal IVH risk factors may include an atypical appearance of ventriculomegaly, neonatal alloimmune thrombocytopenia, and a monochorionic multifetal gestation complicated by demise of one fetus or by severe twin-twin transfusion syndrome (Hu, 2006). If hemorrhage is identified, MR imaging characteristics may indicate which structures are involved and approximately when bleeding occurred.

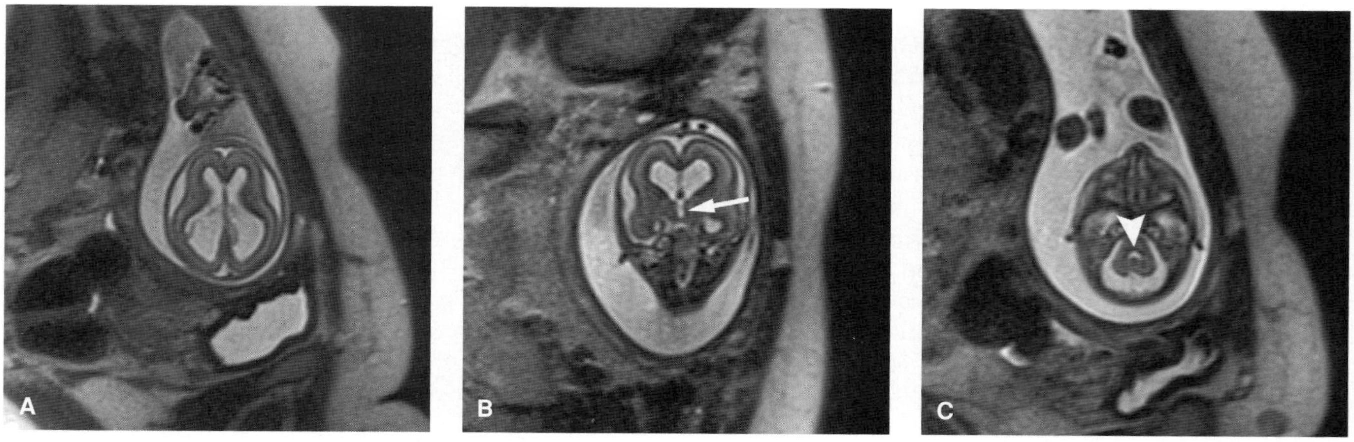

FIGURE 10-42 Aqueductal stenosis. **A.** An axial transventricular image at 22 weeks using a HASTE sequence demonstrates severe ventriculomegaly. **B.** A coronal image of the same fetus shows that the third ventricle (*arrow*) is dilated. **C.** An axial image at the level of the posterior fossa reveals that the fourth ventricle (*arrowhead*) appears normal, consistent with a diagnosis of aqueductal stenosis.

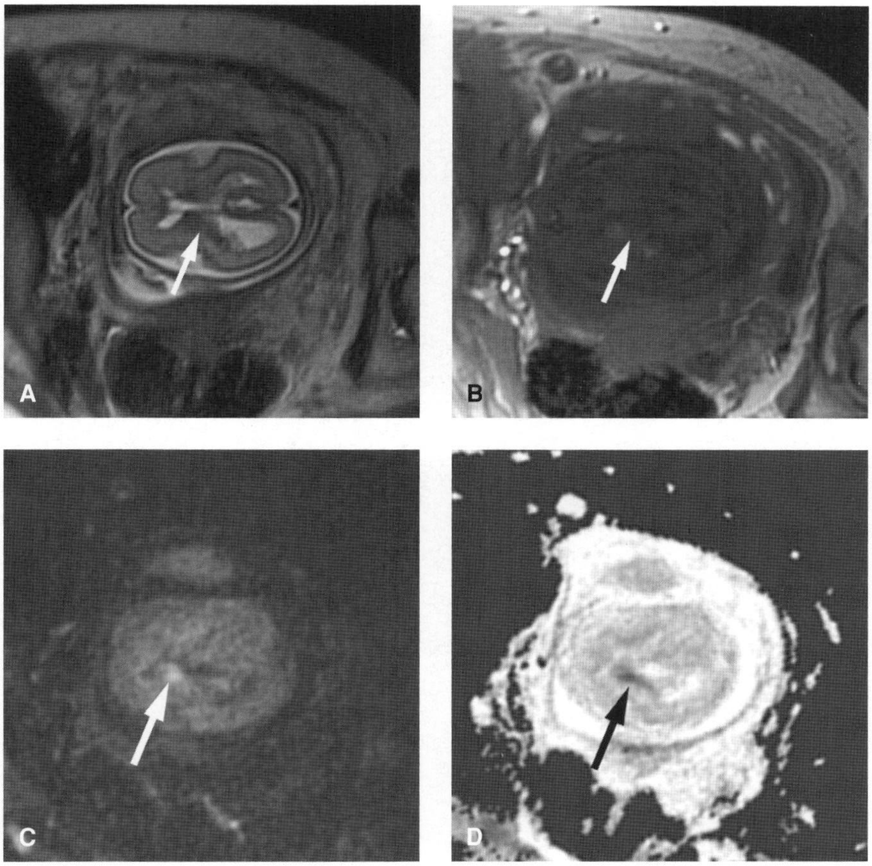

FIGURE 10-43 Intraventricular hemorrhage. Axial images through the brain a 24-week fetus. Arrows denote an area of abnormal signal in the left lateral ventricle. On the HASTE image **(A)**, the irregularity is well delineated but of nonspecific low signal intensity. The T1-weighted image **(B)** demonstrates increased signal intensity within this area of concern, suggesting an intraventricular hemorrhage. Diffusion-weighted image **(C)** and Apparent Diffusion Coefficient map **(D)** demonstrate true restricted diffusion associated with the hemorrhage.

Thorax

Thoracic abnormalities are readily visualized with targeted sonography. MR imaging, however, may help delineate the location and size of space-occupying thoracic lesions and quantify remaining lung tissue volumes. MR imaging may aid in characterizing the type of cystic adenomatoid malformation and in visualizing the blood supply of extralobar pulmonary sequestration (p. 208). With congenital diaphragmatic hernia, MR imaging may be used to verify and quantify the abdominal organs within the thorax. This includes the volume of herniated liver as well as compressed lung tissue volumes (Fig. 10-44) (Debus, 2013; Lee, 2011; Mehollin-Ray, 2012). MR imaging has also been used to identify other organ-system abnormalities in fetuses with diaphragmatic hernia. This may greatly clarify fetal prognosis (Kul, 2012). MR imaging similarly has been used for lung volume evaluation in cases of skeletal dysplasia and prolonged oligohydramnios secondary to renal disease or ruptured membranes (Messerschmidt, 2011; Zaretsky, 2005).

Abdomen

When sonographic visualization is limited by oligohydramnios or maternal obesity, MR imaging may be useful (Caire, 2003). Hawkins and associates (2008) found that

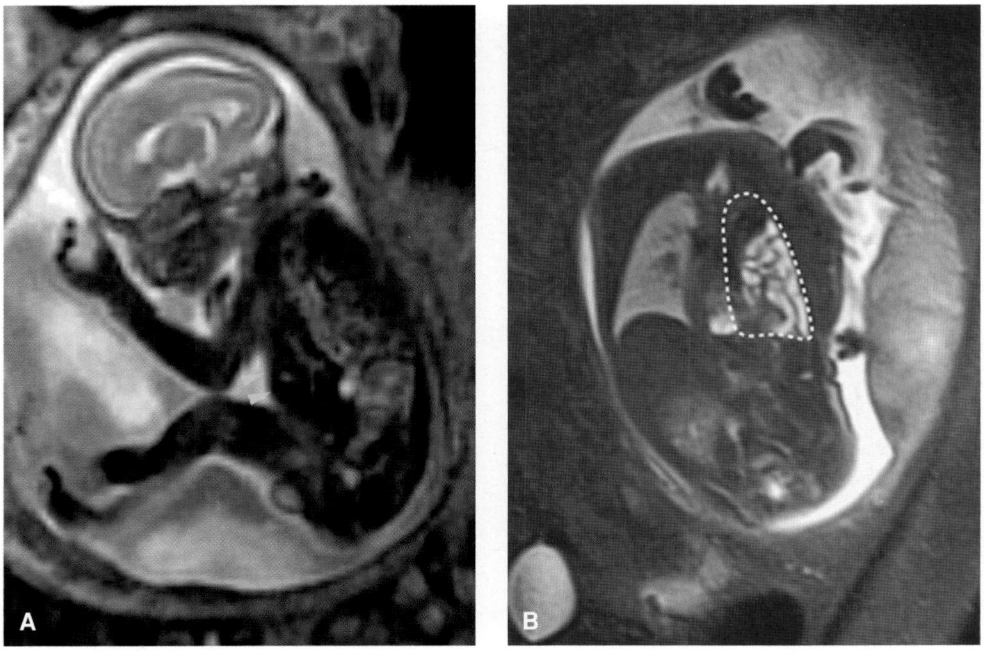

FIGURE 10-44 Congenital diaphragmatic hernia **A.** A HASTE image of a 26-week fetus with congenital diaphragmatic hernia involving the liver (*arrows*). **B.** Coronal STIR image through a 33-week fetal chest demonstrates multiple loops of bowel filling the left chest (*dashed lines*).

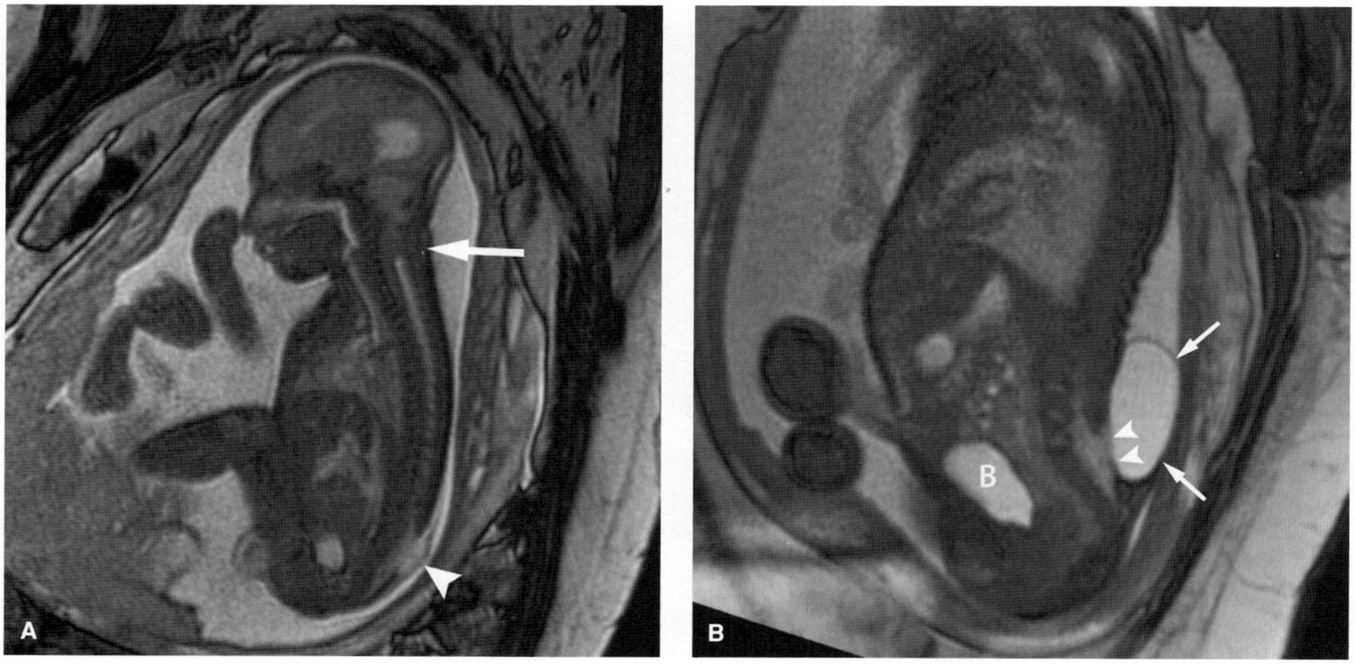

FIGURE 10-45 Myelomeningocele. **A.** A sagittal balanced TruFisp image at 32 weeks demonstrates herniation of the cerebellum into the cervical canal (*arrow*) and a small sacral neural-tube defect with a thin covering membrane (*arrowhead*). **B.** A sagittal TruFisp image of a different fetus demonstrates a neural-tube defect (*arrowheads*) and prominent myelomeningocele (*arrows*). B = fetal bladder.

lack of signal in a contracted fetal bladder on T2-weighted sequences was associated with lethal renal abnormalities. Differences in signal characteristics between meconium in the fetal colon and urine in the bladder may permit characterization of cystic abdominal abnormalities (Farhataziz, 2005).

Adjunct to Fetal Therapy

As indications for fetal therapy have increased, MR imaging has been become more routinely used to outline abnormalities preoperatively. At some centers, before laser ablation of placental anastomoses for twin-twin transfusion syndrome, MR imaging is performed to assess the brain for IVH or periventricular leukomalacia (Chap. 34, p. 656) (Hu, 2006; Kline-Fath, 2007). Because of its precision in visualizing brain and spine findings in cases of myelomeningocele, it is often used before fetal spina bifida surgery (Fig. 10-45). If fetal surgery is considered for sacrococcygeal teratomas, MR imaging may identify tumor extension into the fetal pelvis (Avni, 2002; Neubert, 2004). With a fetal neck mass for which an EXIT procedure is considered, MR imaging may help delineate the lesion extent and its effect on the oral cavity and hypopharynx (Hirose, 2003; Ogamo, 2005; Shiraishi, 2000). Finally, MR imaging has also been used when an EXIT procedure may be needed for severe micrognathia (MacArthur, 2012; Morris, 2009). Fetal therapy is discussed in Chapter 16 (p. 331).

Placenta

The clinical importance of identifying women with placenta accreta is discussed in Chapter 41 (p. 804). Sonography is generally used to identify placental invasion into the myometrium, however, MR evaluation has been used as an adjunct in indeterminate cases. Findings concerning for invasion include uterine bulging, dark intraplacental bands on T2-weighted images, and placental heterogeneity (Leyendecker, 2012). When used in a complementary role, MR imaging sensitivity for detection of placental invasion has been high, although the depth of invasion has been difficult to predict. Clinical risk factors and sonographic findings should be taken into account when interpreting MR placental images (Leyendecker, 2012). Identification of placenta percreta with bladder wall invasion has been a challenge, even when both sonography and MR imaging are used.

Emerging Concepts

As MR acquisition times improve and technology allows for better resolution of structures and movement, there are three potential directions that fetal imaging may proceed. One is volume acquisition and 3-D postprocessing. This would occur in a manner similar to spiral CT with multiple channel detectors, in which one large high-resolution image can be processed in any plane. Applying this to the fetal structure of interest would require faster acquisition times, the ability to correct for fetal motion, and improved field-of-view options—which are in development.

The second direction is real-time MR imaging for evaluation of the fetal heart and other moving structures. A feasibility study reviewed MR evaluations of the chest to ascertain specific fetal heart components (Gorincour, 2007). These authors found, among other things, that balanced fast imaging with steady-state precession (TruFISP) was helpful in defining atrial, ventricular, conotruncal, and venous relationships.

A third direction is further assessment of already established acquisitions of fetal physiological functions. This includes spectroscopy for brain maturity, which has been discussed in small series (Fenton, 2001; Kok, 2002). Other possibilities include diffusion-weighted imaging (DWI) and apparent diffusion coefficient (ADC) for fetal CNS evaluation (Chung, 2009; Garel, 2008). The latter has the added advantage of white matter tract imaging. These emerging technologies are still experimental and will require rigorous investigation before clinical application.

REFERENCES

Adzick NS, Harrison MR, Glick PL, et al: Fetal cystic adenomatoid malformation: prenatal diagnosis and natural history. J Pediatr Surg 20:483, 1985

Altman RP, Randolph JG, Lilly JR: Sacrococcygeal teratoma: American Academy of Pediatrics Surgical Section survey—1973. J Pediatr Surg 9:389, 1974

American College of Obstetricians and Gynecologists: Ultrasonography in pregnancy. Practice Bulletin No. 101, February 2009, Reaffirmed 2011

American College of Obstetricians and Gynecologists: Fetal growth restriction. Practice Bulletin No. 134, May 2013

American College of Radiology: Expert Panel on MR Safety: ACR guidance document on MR safe practices. J Magn Reson Imaging 37:501, 2013

American College of Radiology and Society for Pediatric Radiology: ACR-SPR practice guideline for the safe and optimal performance of fetal magnetic resonance imaging. Resolution No. 13, 2010. Available at: http://www.acr.org/~/media/ACR/Documents/PGTS/guidelines/MRI_Fetal.pdf. Accessed May 26, 2013

American Institute of Ultrasound in Medicine (AIUM): American Institute of Ultrasound in Medicine consensus report on potential bioeffects of diagnostic ultrasound. J Ultrasound Med 27:503, 2008a

American Institute of Ultrasound in Medicine (AIUM): Official statements. Conclusions regarding epidemiology for obstetric ultrasound. 2010a. Available at: http://www.aium.org/resources/viewStatement.aspx?id=16. Accessed May 10, 2013

American Institute of Ultrasound in Medicine (AIUM): Official statements. Limited obstetrical ultrasound. 2009. Available at: http://www.aium.org/resources/viewStatement.aspx?id=19. Accessed May 10, 2013

American Institute of Ultrasound in Medicine (AIUM): Official statements. Prudent use in pregnancy. 2012. Available at: http://www.aium.org/resources/viewStatement.aspx?id=33. Accessed May 10, 2013

American Institute of Ultrasound in Medicine (AIUM): Official statements. Statement on the safe use of Doppler ultrasound during 11–14 week scans (or earlier in pregnancy). 2011. Available at: http://www.aium.org/resources/viewStatement.aspx?id=42. Accessed May 10, 2013

American Institute of Ultrasound in Medicine (AIUM): Official statements. Statement regarding naturally-occurring gas bodies. 2008b. Available at: http://www.aium.org/resources/viewStatement.aspx?id=6. Accessed May 10, 2013

American Institute of Ultrasound in Medicine (AIUM): Practice guideline for the performance of fetal echocardiography. J Ultrasound Med 32(6):1067, 2013b

American Institute of Ultrasound in Medicine (AIUM): Practice guideline for the performance of obstetric ultrasound examinations J Ultrasound Med 32(6):1083, 2013a

Avni FE, Guibaus L, Robert Y, et al: MR imaging of fetal sacrococcygeal teratoma: diagnosis and assessment. Am J Roentgenol 178(1):179, 2002

Axt-Fliedner R, Schwarze A, Smrcek J, et al: Isolated ventricular septal defects dated by color Doppler imaging: evolution during fetal and first year of postnatal life. Ultrasound Obstet Gynecol 27:266, 2006

Azizkhan RG, Crombleholme TM: Congenital cystic lung disease: contemporary antenatal and postnatal management. Pediatric Surg Int 24:643, 2008

Bahado-Singh RO, Kovanci E, Jeffres A, et al: The Doppler cerebroplacental ratio and perinatal outcome in intrauterine growth restriction. Am J Obstet Gynecol 180(3):750, 1999

Baker PN, Johnson IR, Harvey PR, et al: A three-year follow-up of children imaged in utero with echo-planar magnetic resonance. Am J Obstet Gynecol 170:32, 1994

Baschat AA: Doppler application in the delivery timing of the preterm growth-restricted fetus: another step in the right direction. Ultrasound Obstet Gynecol 23:111, 2004

Baschat AA: Neurodevelopment following fetal growth restriction and its relationship with antepartum parameters of placental dysfunction. Ultrasound Obstet Gynecol 37:501, 2011

Baschat AA: Relationship between placental blood flow resistance and precordial venous Doppler indices. Ultrasound Obstet Gynecol 22:561, 2003

Benacerraf BR, Shipp TD, Bromley B, et al: Three-dimensional US of the fetus: volume imaging. Radiology 238:988, 2006

Benacerraf BR, Shipp TD, Bromley B, et al: What does magnetic resonance imaging add to the prenatal sonographic diagnosis of ventriculomegaly? J Ultrasound Med 26:1513, 2007

Berkley E, Chauhan SP, Abuhamad A: Society for Maternal-Fetal Medicine Clinical Guideline: Doppler assessment of the fetus with intrauterine growth restriction. Am J Obstet Gynecol 206(4):300, 2012

Best KE, Tennant PWG, Addor M, et al: Epidemiology of small intestinal atresia in Europe: a register-based study. Arch Dis Child Fetal Neonatal Ed 97(5):F353, 2012

Bhide A, Acharya G, Bilardo CM, et al: ISUOG Practice Guidelines: Use of Doppler ultrasonography in obstetrics. Ultrasound Obstet Gynecol 41(2):233, 2013

Bilardo CM, Wolf H, Stigter RH, et al: Relationship between monitoring parameters and perinatal outcome in severe, early intrauterine growth restriction. Ultrasound Obstet Gynecol 23:119, 2004

Bronshtein M, Ornoy A: Acrania: anencephaly resulting from secondary degeneration of a closed neural tube: two cases in the same family. J Clin Ultrasound 19(4):230, 1991

Brugger PC, Stuhr F, Lindner C, et al: Methods of fetal MR: beyond T2-weighted imaging. Euro J Radiol 57(2):172, 2006

Burge D, Wheeler R: Increasing incidence of detection of congenital lung lesions. Pediatr Pulmonol 45(1):103, 2010

Caire JT, Ramus RM, Magee KP, et al: MRI of fetal genitourinary anomalies. AJR Am J Roentgenol 181:1381, 2003

Canfield MA, Honein MA, Yuskiv N, et al: National estimates and race/ethnic-specific variation of selected birth defects in the United States, 1999–2001. Birth Defects Res A Clin Mol Teratol 76(11):747, 2006

Carey M, Bower C, Mylvaganam A, et al: Talipes equinovarus in Western Australia. Paediatr Perinat Epidemiol 17:187, 2003

Cavoretto P, Molina F, Poggi S, et al: Prenatal diagnosis and outcome of echogenic fetal lung lesions. Ultrasound Obstet Gynecol 32:769, 2008

Centers for Disease Control and Prevention: Workplace Solutions. Preventing work-related musculoskeletal disorders in sonography. DHHS (NIOSH) Publication No. 2006–148, 2006

Chitty LS, Altman DG: Charts of fetal size: kidney and renal pelvis measurements. Prenat Diagn 23:891, 2003

Chung R, Kasprian G, Brugger PC, et al: The current state and future of fetal imaging. Clin Perinatol 36(3):685, 2009

Clements H, Duncan KR, Fielding K, et al: Infants exposed to MRI in utero have a normal paediatric assessment at 9 months of age. B J Radiol 73(866):190, 2000

Colvin J, Bower C, Dickinson JE, et al: Outcomes of congenital diaphragmatic hernia: a population-based study in Western Australia. Pediatr 116:e356, 2005

Copel JA, Liang R, Demasio K, et al: The clinical significance of the irregular fetal heart rhythm. Am J Obstet Gynecol 182:813, 2000

Cragan JD, Gilboa SM: Including prenatal diagnoses in birth defects monitoring: experience of the Metropolitan Atlanta Congenital Defects Program. Birth Defects Res (Part A) 85:20, 2009

Cruz-Martinez R, Figueras F, Hernandez-Andrade E, et al: Fetal brain Doppler to predict cesarean delivery for nonreassuring fetal status in term small-for-gestational-age fetuses. Obstet Gynecol 117:618, 2011

Curran PF, Jelin EB, Rand L, et al: Prenatal steroids for microcystic congenital adenomatoid malformations. J Pediatr Surg 45:145, 2010

Dandy WE, Blackfan KD: Internal hydrocephalus: An experimental, clinical, and pathological study. Am J Dis Child 8:406, 1914

Dashe JS, McIntire DD, Twickler DM: Effect of maternal obesity on the ultrasound detection of anomalous fetuses. Obstet Gynecol 113(5):1001, 2009

De Biasio P, Ginocchio G, Aicardi G, et al: Ossification timing of sacral vertebrae by ultrasound in the mid-second trimester of pregnancy. Prenat Diagn 23:1056, 2003

Debus A, Hagelstein C, Kilian A, et al: Fetal lung volume in congenital diaphragmatic hernia: association of prenatal MR imaging findings with postnatal chronic lung disease. Radiology 266(3):887, 2013

Derikx JPM, De Backer A, Van De Schoot L, et al: Factors associated with recurrence and metastasis in sacrococcygeal teratoma. Br J Surg 93:1543, 2006

Devaseelan P, Cardwell C, Bell B, et al: Prognosis of isolated mild to moderate fetal cerebral ventriculomegaly: a systematic review. J Perinat Med 38:401, 2010

De Veciana M, Major CA, Porto M: Prediction of an abnormal karyotype in fetuses with omphalocele. Prenat Diagn 14:487, 1994

DeVore GR, Falkensammer P, Sklansky MS, et al: Spatio-temporal image correlation (STIC): New technology for evaluation of the fetal heart. Ultrasound Obstet Gynecol 22:380, 2003

SECTION 5

Dolk H, Loane M, Garne E: The prevalence of congenital anomalies in Europe. Adv Exp Med Biol 686:349, 2010

Duncombe GJ, Dickinson JE, Kikiros CS: Prenatal diagnosis and management of congenital cystic adenomatoid malformation of the lung. Am J Obstet Gynecol 187(4): 950, 2002

Ecker JL, Shipp TD, Bromley B, et al: The sonographic diagnosis of Dandy-Walker and Dandy-Walker variant: associated findings and outcomes. Prenat Diagn 20:328, 2000

Ergün O, Barksdale E, Ergün FS, et al: The timing of delivery of infants with gastroschisis influences outcome. J Pediatr Surg 40:424, 2005

Espinoza J, Gotsch F, Kusanovic JP, et al: Changes in fetal cardiac geometry with gestation: implications for 3- and 4-dimensional fetal echocardiography. J Ultrasound Med 26:437, 2007

Espinoza J, Romero R, Kusanovic JP, Gotsch F, et al: Standardized views of the fetal heart using four-dimensional sonographic and tomographic imaging. Ultrasound Obstet Gynecol 31:233, 2008

EUROCAT: Prenatal detection rates. 2012. Available at: http://www.eurocat-network.eu/prenatalscreeninganddiagnosis/prenataldetection(pd)rates. Accessed May 24, 2013

Farhataziz N, Engels JE, Ramus RM, et al: Fetal MRI of urine and meconium by gestational age for the diagnosis of genitourinary and gastrointestinal abnormalities. AJR Am J Roentgenol 184:1891, 2005

Feinstein JA, Benson DW, Dubin AM, et al: Hypoplastic left heart syndrome: current considerations and expectations. J Am Coll Cardiol 59 (1 Suppl):S1, 2012

Fenton BW, Lin CS, Macedonia C, et al: The fetus at term: in utero volume-selected proton MR spectroscopy with a breath-hold technique—a feasibility study. Radiology 219(2):563, 2001

Figueras F, Benavides A, Del Rio M, et al: Monitoring of fetuses with intrauterine growth restriction: longitudinal changes in ductus venosus and aortic isthmus flow. Ultrasound Obstet Gynecol 33(1):39, 2009

Franklin O, Burch M, Manning N, et al: Prenatal diagnosis of coarctation of the aorta improves survival and reduces morbidity. Heart 87:67, 2002

Gaglioti P, Oberto M, Todros T: The significance of fetal ventriculomegaly: etiology, short-and long-term outcomes. Prenat Diagn 29(4):381, 2009

Gallot D, Boda C, Ughetto S, et al: Prenatal detection and outcome of congenital diaphragmatic hernia: a French registry-based study. Ultrasound Obstet Gynecol 29:276, 2007

Garel C: Development of the fetal brain. In MRI of the Fetal Brain: Normal Development and Cerebral Pathologies. New York, Springer, 2004

Garel C: Fetal MRI: what is the future? Ultrasound Obstet Gynecol 31(2):123, 2008

Garne E, Loane M, Dolk H, et al: Spectrum of congenital anomalies in pregnancies with pregestational diabetes. Birth Defects Res A Clin Mol Teratol 94(3):134, 2012

Glass HC, Shaw GM, Ma C, et al: Agenesis of the corpus callosum in California 1983–2003: a population-based study. Am J Med Genet A 146A:2495, 2008

Glover P, Hykin J, Gowland P, et al: An assessment of the intrauterine sound intensity level during obstetric echo-planar magnetic resonance imaging. Br J Radiol 68:1090, 1995

Goldstein I, Reece EA, Pilu G, et al: Cerebellar measurements with ultrasonography in the evaluation of fetal growth and development. Am J Obstet Gynecol 156:1065, 1987

Goncalves LF, Espinoza J, Lee W, et al: Three- and four-dimensional reconstruction of the aortic and ductal arches using inversion mode: a new rendering algorithm for visualization of fluid-filled anatomical structures. Ultrasound Obstet Gynecol 24:696, 2004

Goncalves LF, Lee W, Espinoza J, et al: Three- and 4-dimensional ultrasound in obstetric practice: does it help? J Ultrasound Med 24:1599, 2005

Goncalves LF, Nien JK, Espinoza J, et al: What does 2-dimensional imaging add to 3- and 4-dimensional obstetric ultrasonography? J Ultrasound Med 25:691, 2006

Gorincour G, Bourliere-Najean B, Bonello B, et al: Feasibility of fetal cardiac magnetic resonance imaging: preliminary experience. Ultrasound Obstet Gynecol 29(1):105, 2007

Grandjean J, Larroque D, Levi S, et al: The performance of routine ultrasonographic screening of pregnancies in the Eurofetus Study. Am J Obstet Gynecol 181:446, 1999

Gucciardo L, Uyttebroek A, de Wever I, et al: Prenatal assessment and management of sacrococcygeal teratoma. Prenat Diagn 31:678, 2011

Hains DS, Bates CM, Ingraham S, et al: Management and etiology of the unilateral multicystic dysplastic kidney: a review. Pediatr Nephrol 24:233, 2009

Hartman RJ, Rasmussen SJ, Botto LD, et al: The contribution of chromosomal abnormalities to congenital heart defects: a population-based study. Pediatr Cardiol 32:1147, 2011

Hawkins JS, Dashe JS, Twickler DM: Magnetic resonance imaging diagnosis of severe fetal renal anomalies. Am J Obstet Gynecol 198:328.e1, 2008

Hayden SA, Russ PD, Pretorius DH, et al: Posterior urethral obstruction. Prenatal sonographic findings and clinical outcome in fourteen cases. J Ultrasound Med 7:371, 1988

Hirose S, Sydorak RM, Tsao K, et al: Spectrum of intrapartum management strategies for giant fetal cervical teratoma. J Pediatr Surg 38(3):446, 2003

Hobbins JC, Robero R, Grannum P, et al: Antenatal diagnosis of renal anomalies with ultrasound: I. Obstructive uropathy. Am J Obstet Gynecol 148:868, 1984

Hoffman CK, Filly RA, Callen PW: The "lying down" adrenal sign: a sonographic indicator of renal agenesis or ectopia in fetuses and neonates. J Ultrasound Med 11:533, 1992

Hu LS, Caire J, Twickler DM: MR findings of complicated multifetal gestations. Obstet Gynecol 36(1): 76, 2006

Huhta JC, Moise KJ, Fisher DJ, et al: Detection and quantitation of construction of the fetal ductus arteriosus by Doppler echocardiography. Circulation 75:406, 1987

International Society of Ultrasound in Obstetrics & Gynecology: Sonographic examination of the fetal central nervous system: guidelines for performing the "basic examination" and the "fetal neurosonogram." Ultrasound Obstet Gynecol 29:109, 2007

Ismaili K, Hall M, Donner C, et al: Results of systematic screening for minor degrees of fetal renal pelvis dilatation in an unselected population. Am J Obstet Gynecol 188:242, 2003

James CA, Watson AR, Twining P, et al: Antenatally detected urinary tract abnormalities: changing incidence and management. Eur J Pediatr 157:508, 1998

Janga D, Akinfenwa O: Work-related repetitive strain injuries amongst practitioners of obstetric and gynecologic ultrasound worldwide. Arch Gynecol Obstet 286(2):353, 2012

Jani JC, Peralta CFA, Nicolaides KH: Lung-to-head ratio: a need to unify the technique. Ultrasound Obstet Gynecol 39:2, 2012

Johnson MP, Johnson A, Holzgreve W, et al: First-trimester simple hygroma: cause and outcome. Am J Obstet Gynecol 168:156, 1993

Joó JG, Tóth Z, Beke A, et al: Etiology, prenatal diagnoses and outcome of ventriculomegaly in 230 cases. Fetal Diagn Ther 24(3):254, 2008

Kharrat R, Yamamoto M, Roume J, et al: Karyotype and outcome of fetuses diagnosed with cystic hygroma in the first trimester in relation to nuchal translucency thickness. Prenat Diagn 26:369, 2006

Kingdom JC, Burrell SJ, Kaufmann P: Pathology and clinical implications of abnormal umbilical artery Doppler waveforms. Ultrasound Obstet Gynecol 9:271, 1997

Kitchanan S, Patole SK, Muller R, et al: Neonatal outcome of gastroschisis and exomphalos: a 10-year review. J Paediatric Child Health 36:428, 2000

Kline-Fath BM, Calvo-Garcia MA, O'Hara SM, et al: Twin-twin transfusion syndrome: cerebral ischemia is not the only fetal MR imaging finding. Ped Radiol 37(1):47, 2007

Knott-Craig CJ, Elkins RC, Lane MM, et al: A 26-year experience with surgical management of tetralogy of Fallot: risk analysis for mortality or late reintervention. Ann Thorac Surg 66:506, 1998

Kok RD, van den Berg PP, van den Bergh AJ, et al: Maturation of the human fetal brain as observed by 1 H MR spectroscopy. Magn Reson Med 48(4)611, 2002

Koren G, Florescu A, Costei AM, et al: Nonsteroidal antiinflammatory drugs during third trimester and the risk of premature closure of the ductus arteriosus: a meta-analysis. Ann Pharmacother 40(5):824, 2006

Kul S, Korkmaz HA, Cansu A, et al: Contribution of MRI to ultrasound in the diagnosis of fetal anomalies. J Magn Reson Imaging 35:882, 2012

Lauson S, Alvarez C, Patel MS, et al: Outcome of prenatally diagnosed isolated clubfoot. Ultrasound Obstet Gynecol 35:708, 2010

Lazebnik N, Bellinger MF, Ferguson JE, et al: Insights into the pathogenesis and natural history of fetuses with multicystic dysplastic kidney disease. Prenat Diagn 19:418, 1999

Lee RS, Cendron M, Kinnamon DD, et al: Antenatal hydronephrosis as a predictor of postnatal outcome: a meta-analysis. Pediatrics 118:586, 2006

Lee TC, Lim FY, Keswani SG, et al: Late gestation fetal magnetic resonance imaging-derived total lung volume predicts postnatal survival and need for extracorporeal membrane oxygenation support in isolated congenital diaphragmatic hernia. J Pediatr Surg 46(6):1165, 2011

Levi S: Ultrasound in prenatal diagnosis: polemics around routine ultrasound screening for second trimester fetal malformations. Prenat Diagn 22:285, 2002

Levine D, Barnes PD: Cortical maturation in normal and abnormal fetuses as assessed with prenatal MR imaging. Radiology 210:751, 1999a

Levine D, Barnes PD, Madsen JR, et al: Central nervous system abnormalities assessed with prenatal magnetic resonance imaging. Obstet Gynecol 94:1011, 1999b

Leyendecker JR, DuBose M, Hosseinzadeh K, et al: MRI of pregnancy-related issues: abnormal placentation. AJR Am J Roentgenol 198(2):311, 2012

Li Y, Estroff JA, Khwaja O, et al: Callosal dysgenesis in fetuses with ventriculomegaly: levels of agreement between imaging modalities and postnatal outcome. Ultra Obstet Gynecol 40(5): 522, 2012
Lodeiro JG, Feinstein SJ, Lodeiro SB: Fetal premature atrial contractions associated with hydralazine. Am J Obstet Gynecol 160:105, 1989
Long A, Moran P, Robson S: Outcome of fetal cerebral posterior fossa anomalies. Prenat Diagn 26:707, 2006
Lowe TW, Weinreb J, Santos-Ramos R, et al: Magnetic resonance imaging in human pregnancy. Obstet Gynecol 66(5):629, 1985
Maarse W, Berge SJ, Pistorius L, et al: Diagnostic accuracy of transabdominal ultrasound in detecting prenatal cleft lip and palate: a systematic review. Ultrasound Obstet Gynecol 35:495, 2010
Maarse W, Pistorius LR, Van Eeten WK, et al: Prenatal ultrasound screening for orofacial clefts. Ultrasound Obstet Gynecol 38:434, 2011
MacArthur CJ: Prenatal diagnosis of fetal cervicofacial anomalies. Curr Opin Otolaryngol Head Neck Surg 20(6):482, 2012
Magnavita N, Bevilacqua L, Mirk P, et al: Work-related musculoskeletal complaints in sonologists. J Occup Environ Med 41:981, 1999
Mahle WT, Clancy RR, McGaurn SP, et al: Impact of prenatal diagnosis on survival and early neurologic morbidity in neonates with the hypoplastic left heart syndrome. Pediatrics 107:1277, 2001
Malone FD, Ball RH, Nyberg DA, et al: First-trimester septated cystic hygroma: prevalence, natural history, and pediatric outcome. Obstet Gynecol 106:288, 2005
Mammen L, Benson CB: Outcome of fetuses with clubfeet diagnosed by prenatal sonography. J Ultrasound Med 23:497, 2004
Mann S, Johnson MP, Wilson RD: Fetal thoracic and bladder shunts. Semin Fetal Neonatal Med 15:28, 2010
Mari G, Deter RL, Carpenter RL, et al: Noninvasive diagnosis by Doppler ultrasonography of fetal anemia due to maternal red-cell alloimmunization. Collaborative group for Doppler assessment of the blood velocity in anemic fetuses. N Engl J Med 342:9, 2000
Mayer S, Klaritsch P, Petersen S, et al: The correlation between lung volume and liver herniation measurements by fetal MRI in isolated congenital diaphragmatic hernia: a systematic review and meta-analysis of observational studies. Prenat Diagn 31:1086, 2011
McGahan JP, Pilu G, Nyberg DA: Neural tube defects and the spine. In: Nyberg DA, McGahan JP, Pretorius DH, et al (eds): Diagnostic Imaging of Fetal Anomalies. Lippincott Williams & Wilkins, 2003, p 293
Mehollin-Ray AR, Cassady CI, Cass DL, et al: Fetal MR imaging of congenital diaphragmatic hernia. Radiographics 32(4):1067, 2012
Messerschmidt A, Pataraia A, Helber H, et al: Fetal MRI for prediction of neonatal mortality following preterm premature rupture of the fetal membranes. Pediatr Radiol 41:1416, 2011
Metkus AP, Filly RA, Stringer MD, et al: Sonographic predictors of survival in fetal diaphragmatic hernia. J Pediatr Surg 31:148, 1996
Millischer AE, Sonigo P, Ville Y, et al: Standardized anatomical examination of the fetus at MRI. A feasibility study. Ultrasound Obstet Gynecol 42(5):553, 2013
Morris LM, Lim F-Y, Elluru RG, et al: Severe micrognathia: indications for EXIT-to-Airway. Fetal Diagn Ther 26(30:162, 2009
Morrow RJ, Abramson SL, Bull SB, et al: Effect of placental embolization of the umbilical artery velocity waveform in fetal sheep. Am J Obstet Gynecol 151:1055, 1989
Mullassery D, Ba'ath ME, Jesudason EC, et al: Value of liver herniation in prediction of outcome in fetal congenital diaphragmatic hernia: a systematic review and meta-analysis. Ultrasound Obstet Gynecol 35:609, 2010
Nembhard WN, Waller DK, Sever LE, et al: Patterns of first-year survival among infants with selected congenital anomalies in Texas, 1995–1997. Teratology 64:267, 2001
Neubert S, Trautmann K, Tanner B, et al: Sonographic prognostic factors in prenatal diagnosis of SCT. Fetal Diagn Ther 19(4): 319, 2004
Nguyen HT, Herndon CDA, Cooper C, et al: The Society for Fetal Urology consensus statement on the evaluation and management of antenatal hydronephrosis. J Pediatr Urol 6:212, 2010
Nicholas SS, Stamilio DM, Dicke JM, et al: Predicting adverse neonatal outcomes in fetuses with abdominal wall defects using prenatal risk factors. Am J Obstet Gynecol 201:383.e1, 2009
Nicolaides KH, Campbell S, Gabbe SG, et al: Ultrasound screening for spina bifida: cranial and cerebellar signs. Lancet 2:72, 1986
Oei SG, Vosters RP, van der Hagen NL: Fetal arrhythmia caused by excessive intake of caffeine by pregnant women. BMJ 298:568, 1989
Offerdal K, Jebens N, Swertsen T, et al: Prenatal ultrasound detection of facial cleft: a prospective study of 49,314 deliveries in a non-selected population in Norway. Ultrasound Obstet Gynecol 31:639, 2008
Ogamo M, Sugiyama T, Maeda T, et al: The ex utero intrapartum treatment (EXIT) procedure in giant fetal neck masses. Fetal Diagn Ther 20(3):214, 2005
Orioli IM, Catilla EE: Epidemiology of holoprosencephaly: prevalence and risk factors. Am J Med Genet Part C Semin Med Genet 154C:13, 2010
Paladini D, Russo M, Teodoro A, et al: Prenatal diagnosis of congenital heart disease in the Naples area during the years 1994–1999—the experience of a joint fetal-pediatric cardiology unit. Prenatal Diagn 22(7):545, 2002
Pavone V, Bianca S, Grosso G, et al Congenital talipes equinovarus: an epidemiological study in Sicily. Acta Orthop 83(3):294, 2012
Pedersen RN, Calzolari E, Husby S, et al: Oesophageal atresia: prevalence, prenatal diagnosis and associated anomalies in 23 European regions. Arch Dis Child 97:227, 2012
Phelan JP, Ahn MO, Smith CV, et al: Amnionic fluid index measurements during pregnancy. J Reprod Med 32:601, 1987
Pike I, Russo A, Berkowitz J, et al: The prevalence of musculoskeletal disorders among diagnostic medical sonographers J Diagn Med Sonography 13:219, 1997
Pilalis A, Basagiannis C, Eleftheriades M, et al: Evaluation of a two-step ultrasound examination protocol for the detection of major fetal structural defects. J Matern Fetal Neonatal Med 25(9):1814, 2012
Pilu G: Prenatal diagnosis of cerebrospinal anomalies. In: Fleischer AC, Toy EC, Lee W, et al (eds): Sonography in Obstetrics and Gynecology: Principles and Practice, 7th ed. New York, McGraw-Hill, 2011
Pilu G: Ultrasound evaluation of the fetal neural axis. In Callen PW (ed): Ultrasonography in Obstetrics and Gynecology, 5th ed. Philadelphia, Saunders, 2008, p 366
Puligandla PS, Janvier A, Flageole H, et al: The significance of intrauterine growth restriction is different from prematurity for the outcome of infants with gastroschisis. J Pediatr Surg 39:1200, 2004
Rabinowitz R, Peters MT, Vyas S, et al: Measurement of fetal urine production in normal pregnancy by real-time ultrasonography. Am J Obstet Gynecol 161:1264, 1989
Rados C: FDA cautions against ultrasound "keepsake" images. FDA Consumer Magazine 38(1):9, 2007
Rahemtullah A, McGillivray B, Wilson RD: Suspected skeletal dysplasias: femur length to abdominal circumference ratio can be used in ultrasonographic prediction of fetal outcome. Am J Obstet Gynecol 177:864, 1997
Rakic P: Ultrasound effects on fetal brains questioned. RSNA News 16(11):8, 2006
Ramos GA, Romine LE, Gindes L, et al: Evaluation of the fetal secondary palate by 3-dimensional sonography. J Ultrasound Med 29:357, 2010
Ramus RM, Martin LB, Twickler DM: Ultrasonographic prediction of fetal outcome in suspected skeletal dysplasias with use of the femur length-to-abdominal circumference ratio. Am J Obstet Gynecol 179(5):1348, 1998
Reddy UM, Filly RA, Copel JA: Prenatal imaging: ultrasonography and magnetic resonance imaging. Obstet Gynecol 112:145, 2008
Reeves MJ, Brandreth M, Whitby EH, et al: Neonatal cochlear function: measurement after exposure to acoustic noise during in utero MR imaging. Radiology 257(3):802, 2010
Reichel TF, Ramus RM, Caire JT, et al: Fetal central nervous system biometry on MR imaging. Am J Roentgenol 180(4): 1155, 2003
Romosan G, Henriksson E, Rylander A, et al: Diagnostic performance of routine ultrasound screening for fetal malformations in an unselected Swedish population 2000–2005. Ultrasound Obstet Gynecol 34:526, 2009
Roybal JL, Liechty KW, Hedrick HL, et al: Predicting the severity of congenital high airway obstruction syndrome. J Pediatr Surg 45(8):1633, 2010
Salomon LJ, Alfirevic Z, Berghella V, et al: Practice Guidelines for performance of the routine mid-trimester fetal ultrasound scan. Ultrasound Obstet Gynecol 37(1):116, 2011
Salvesen K, Lees C, Abramowicz J, et al: ISUOG statement on the safe use of Doppler in the 11 to 13+6-week fetal ultrasound examination. Ultrasound Obstet Gynecol 37:625, 2011
Santiago-Munoz PC, McIntire DD, Barber RG, et al: Outcomes of pregnancies with fetal gastroschisis. Obstet Gynecol 110:663, 2007
Schreuder MF, Westland R, van Wijk JA: Unilateral multicystic dysplastic kidney: a meta-analysis of observational studies on the incidence associated urinary tract malformations and the contralateral kidney. Nephrol Dial Transplant 24:1810, 2009
Sciscione AC, Hayes EJ, Society for Maternal-Fetal Medicine: Uterine artery Doppler flow studies in obstetric practice. Am J Obstet Gynecol 201(2):121, 2009
Segata M, Mari G: Fetal anemia: new technologies. Curr Opin Obstet Gynecol 16:153, 2004
Sharma R, Stone S, Alzouebi A, et al: Perinatal outcome of prenatally diagnosed congenital talipes equinovarus. Prenat Diagn 31:142, 2011
Sheih CP, Liu MB, Hung CS, et al: Renal abnormalities in schoolchildren. Pediatrics 84:1086, 1989
Shipp TD, Bromley B, Hornberger LK, et al: Levorotation of the fetal cardiac axis: a clue for the presence of congenital heart disease. Obstet Gynecol 85:97, 1995

Shiraishi H, Nakamura M, Ichihashi K, et al: Prenatal MRI in a fetus with a giant neck hemangioma: a case report. Prenat Diagn 20(12):1004, 2000
Shulman LP, Emerson DS, Felker RE, et al: High frequency of cytogenetic abnormalities in fetuses with cystic hygroma diagnosed in the first trimester. Obstet Gynecol 80:80, 1992
Simon EM, Goldstein RB, Coakley FV, et al: Fast MR imaging of fetal CNS anomalies in utero. Am J Neuroradiol 21:1688, 2000
Smith RS, Comstock CH, Kirk JS, et al: Ultrasonographic left cardiac axis deviation: a marker for fetal anomalies. Obstet Gynecol 85:187, 1995
Solomon BD, Rosenbaum KN, Meck JM, et al: Holoprosencephaly due to numeric chromosome abnormalities. Am J Med Genet Part C Semin Med Genet 154C:146, 2010
Sotiriadis A, Makrydimas G: Neurodevelopment after prenatal diagnosis of isolated agenesis of the corpus callosum: an integrative review. Am J Obstet Gynecol 206(4):337.e1, 2012
Stege G, Fenton A, Jaffray B: Nihilism in the 1990s: the true mortality of congenital diaphragmatic hernia. Pediatr 112:532, 2003
Stevenson DA, Carey JC, Byrne JLB, et al: Analysis of skeletal dysplasias in the Utah population. Am J Med Genet 158A:1046, 2012
Stocker JT: Congenital pulmonary airway malformation: a new name and expanded classification of congenital cystic adenomatoid malformation of the lung. Histopathology 41(Suppl):424, 2002
Stocker JT, Madewell JE, Drake RM: Congenital cystic adenomatoid malformation of the lung: classification and morphologic spectrum. Hum Pathol 8:155, 1977
Swamy R, Embleton N, Hale J, et al: Sacrococcygeal teratoma over two decades: birth prevalence, prenatal diagnosis and clinical outcomes. Prenat Diagn 28:1048, 2008
Syngelaki A, Chelemen T, Dagklis T, et al: Challenges in the diagnosis of fetal non-chromosomal abnormalities at 11–13 weeks. Prenat Diagn 31:90, 2011
Szabo N, Gergev G, Kobor J, et al: Corpus callosum abnormalities: birth prevalence and clinical spectrum in Hungary. Pediatr Neurol 44:420, 2011
Tilea B, Alberti C, Adamsbaum C, et al: Cerebral biometry in fetal magnetic resonance imaging: new reference data. Ultrasound Obstet Gynecol 33(2):173, 2009
Timor-Tritsch IE, Monteagudo A, Mayberry P: Three-dimensional ultrasound evaluation of the fetal brain: the three horn view. Ultrasound Obstet Gynecol 16:302, 2000
Tredwell SJ, Wilson D, Wilmink MA, et al: Review of the effect of early amniocentesis on foot deformity in the neonate. J Pediatr Orthol 21:636, 2001
Trivedi N, Levy D, Tarsa M, et al: Congenital cardiac anomalies: prenatal readings versus neonatal outcomes. J Ultrasound Med 31:389, 2012
Turan S, Turan O, Baschat AA: Three- and four-dimensional fetal echocardiography. Fetal Diagn Ther 25:361, 2009
Turkbey B, Ocak I, Daryanani K, et al: Autosomal recessive polycystic kidney disease and congenital hepatic fibrosis Pediatr Radiol 39:100, 2009
Twickler DM, Magee KP, Caire J, et al: Second-opinion magnetic resonance imaging for suspected fetal central nervous system abnormalities. Am J Obstet Gynecol 188:492, 2003
Twickler DM, Reichel T, McIntire DD, et al: Fetal central nervous system ventricle and cisterna magna measurements by magnetic resonance imaging. Am J Obstet Gynecol 187:927, 2002
Tworetzky W, McElhinney DB, Reddy VM, et al: Improved surgical outcome after fetal diagnosis of hypoplastic left heart syndrome. Circulation 103:1269, 2001
Vadeyar SH, Moore RJ, Strachan BK, et al: Effect of fetal magnetic resonance imaging on fetal heart rate patterns. Am J Obstet Gynecol 182:666, 2000
Vergani P, Ceruti P, Locatelli A, et al: Accuracy of prenatal ultrasonographic diagnosis of duplex renal system. J Ultrasound Med 18:463, 1998
Walker SJ, Ball RH, Babcook CJ, et al: Prevalence of aneuploidy and additional anatomic abnormalities in fetuses and neonates with cleft lip with or without cleft palate. A population-based study in Utah. J Ultrasound Med 20(11):1175, 2001
Warman ML, Cormier-Daire V, Hall C, et al: Nosology and classification of genetic skeletal disorders: 2010 revision. Am J Med Genet Part A 155:943, 2011
Wenstrom KD, Weiner CP, Williamson RA: Diverse maternal and fetal pathology associated with absent diastolic flow in the umbilical artery of high-risk fetuses. Obstet Gynecol 77:374, 1991
Whitten SM, Wilcox DT: Duplex systems. Prenat Diagn 21:952, 2001
Wiesel A, Queisser-Luft A, Clementi M, et al: Prenatal detection of congenital renal malformations by fetal ultrasonographic examination: an analysis of 709,030 births in 12 European countries. Euro J Med Genet 48:131, 2005
Wilhelm L, Borgers H: The "equals sign": a novel marker in the diagnosis of fetal isolated soft palate. Ultrasound Obstet Gynecol 36:439, 2010
Williams B, Tareen B, Resnick M: Pathophysiology and treatment of ureteropelvic junction obstruction. Curr Urol Rep 8:111, 2007
Wilson RD, Hedrick HL, Liechty KW, et al: Cystic adenomatoid malformation of the lung: review of genetics, prenatal diagnosis, and in utero treatment. Am J Med Genet 140A:151, 2006
Wiskirchen J, Groenewaeller EF, Kehlbach R, et al: Long-term effects of repetitive exposure to a static magnetic field 1.5 T on proliferation of human fetal lung fibroblasts. Magn Reson Med 41:464, 1999
Woodward M, Frank D: Postnatal management of antenatal hydronephrosis. BJU Int 89:149, 2002
Worley KC, Dashe JS, Barber RG, et al: Fetal magnetic resonance imaging in isolated diaphragmatic hernia: volume of herniated liver and neonatal outcome. Am J Obstet Gynecol 200(3):318.e1, 2009
Yamada S, Uwabe C, Fujii S, et al: Phenotypic variability in human embryonic holoprosencephaly in the Kyoto collection. Birth Defects Res Part A Clin Mol Teratol 70:495, 2004
Yildirim G, Gungorduk K, Aslan H, et al: Prenatal diagnosis of extralobar pulmonary sequestration. Arch Gynecol Obstet 278:181, 2008
Zaretsky M, Ramus R, McIntire D, et al: MRI calculation of lung volumes to predict outcome in fetuses with genitourinary abnormalities. AJR Am J Roentgenol 185:1328, 2005
Zaretsky MV, McIntire DD, Twickler DM: Feasibility of the fetal anatomic and maternal pelvic survey by magnetic resonance imaging at term. Am J Obstet Gynecol 189:997, 2003a
Zaretsky MV, Twickler DM: Magnetic imaging in obstetrics. Clin Obstet Gynecol 46:868, 2003b
Zeeman GG, McIntire DD, Twickler DM: Maternal and fetal artery Doppler findings in women with chronic hypertension who subsequently develop superimposed pre-eclampsia. J Matern Fetal Neonatal Med 14:318, 2003
Zerres K, Mucher G, Becker J, et al: Prenatal diagnosis of autosomal recessive polycystic kidney disease: molecular genetics, clinical experience, and fetal morphology. Am J Med Genet 6:137, 1998

CHAPTER 11

Amnionic Fluid

Amnionic fluid serves several roles during pregnancy. It creates a physical space for fetal movement, which is necessary for normal musculoskeletal development. It permits fetal swallowing—essential for gastrointestinal tract development, and fetal breathing—necessary for lung development. Amnionic fluid guards against umbilical cord compression and protects the fetus from trauma. It even has bacteriostatic properties. Amnionic fluid volume abnormalities may reflect a problem with fluid production or its circulation, such as underlying fetal or placental pathology. These volume extremes may be associated with increased risks for adverse pregnancy outcome.

NORMAL AMNIONIC FLUID VOLUME

Amnionic fluid volume increases from approximately 30 mL at 10 weeks to 200 mL by 16 weeks and reaches 800 mL by the mid-third trimester (Brace, 1989; Magann, 1997). This fluid is approximately 98-percent water. A full-term fetus contains roughly 2800 mL of water, and the placenta another 400 mL, such that the term uterus holds nearly 4 liters of water (Modena, 2004). Abnormally decreased fluid volume is termed *oligohydramnios,* whereas abnormally increased fluid volume is termed *hydramnios* or *polyhydramnios.*

Physiology

Early in pregnancy, the amnionic cavity is filled with fluid that is similar in composition to extracellular fluid. During the first half of pregnancy, transfer of water and other small molecules takes place across the amnion—*transmembranous flow*, across the fetal vessels on placental surface—*intramembranous flow*, and across fetal skin. Fetal urine production begins between 8 and 11 weeks, but it does not become a major component of amnionic fluid until the second trimester. This latter observation explains why fetuses with lethal renal abnormalities may not manifest severe oligohydramnios until after 18 weeks. Water transport across the fetal skin continues until keratinization occurs at 22 to 25 weeks. This explains why extremely preterm infants can experience significant fluid loss across their skin.

With advancing gestation, four pathways play a major role in amnionic fluid volume regulation (Table 11-1). First, fetal urination is the primary amnionic fluid source by the second half of pregnancy. By term, fetal urine production may exceed 1 liter per day—such that the entire amnionic fluid volume is recirculated on a daily basis. Fetal urine osmolality is significantly hypotonic to that of maternal and fetal plasma and similar to that of amnionic fluid. Specifically, the osmolality of maternal and fetal plasma is approximately 280 mOsm/mL, whereas that of amnionic fluid is about 260 mOsm/L. This hypotonicity of fetal urine—and thus of amnionic fluid—accounts for significant *intramembranous* fluid transfer across and into fetal vessels on the placental surface, and thus into the fetus. This transfer reaches 400 mL per day and is a second regulator of fluid volume (Mann, 1996). In the setting of maternal dehydration, the resultant increase in maternal osmolality favors fluid transfer from the fetus to the mother, and then from the amnionic fluid compartment into the fetus (Moore, 2010).

An important third source of amnionic fluid regulation is the respiratory tract. Approximately 350 mL of lung fluid is

TABLE 11-1. Amnionic Fluid Volume Regulation in Late Pregnancy

Pathway	Effect on Volume	Approximate Daily Volume (mL)
Fetal urination	Production	1000
Fetal swallowing	Resorption	750
Fetal lung fluid secretion	Production	350
Intramembranous flow across fetal vessels on the placental surface	Resorption	400
Transmembranous flow across amnionic membrane	Resorption	Minimal

Adapted from Magann, 2011; Modena, 2004; Moore, 2010.

produced daily late in gestation, and half of this is immediately swallowed. Last, fetal swallowing is the primary mechanism for amnionic fluid resorption and averages 500 to 1000 mL per day (Mann, 1996). Impaired swallowing, secondary to either a central nervous system abnormality or gastrointestinal tract obstruction, can result in an impressive degree of hydramnios. The other pathways—transmembranous flow and flow across the fetal skin—account for a far smaller proportion of fluid transport in the second half of pregnancy.

Measurement

From a practical standpoint, the actual volume of amnionic fluid is rarely measured outside of the research setting. That said, direct measurement and dye-dilution methods of fluid quantification have contributed to an understanding of normal physiology. These measurements have further been used to validate sonographic fluid assessment techniques. The dye-dilution method involves injection of a small quantity of a dye such as aminohippurate into the amnionic cavity under sonographic guidance. The amnionic fluid is then sampled to determine the dye concentration and hence to calculate the fluid volume in which it was diluted.

Brace and Wolf (1989) reviewed 12 studies done through the 1960s in which amnionic fluid volume was assessed using these measurement techniques. Although fluid volume increased across gestation, they found that the mean value did not change significantly between 22 and 39 weeks—it was approximately 750 mL. There was considerable variation at each week of gestation, particularly in the mid-third trimester. At this time, the 5th percentile was 300 mL, and the 95th percentile approximated 2000 mL. In contrast, Magann and colleagues (1997) used dye-dilution measurements and found that the amnionic fluid volume continues to increase with advancing gestation. Specifically, the average fluid volume was approximately 400 mL between 22 and 30 weeks, doubling thereafter to a mean of 800 mL. The volume remained at this level until 40 weeks and then declined by approximately 8 percent per week thereafter. The two reports differed in the regression methodology employed, and despite different conclusions, both identified a wide normal range at each week of gestation, particularly in the third trimester. This normal variation has also been identified using semiquantitative sonographic methods, described next.

Sonographic Assessment

Amnionic fluid volume evaluation is a component of every standard sonogram performed in the second or third trimester (Chap. 10, p. 199). Volume is typically assessed semiquantitatively, by measuring either a single pocket or the amnionic fluid index—AFI (Phelan, 1987). A qualitative or subjective estimate of amnionic fluid volume is also considered acceptable when performed by an experienced examiner (American College of Obstetricians and Gynecologists, 2011; American Institute of Ultrasound in Medicine, 2013). One limitation of subjective estimation, however, is that it does not permit a longitudinal assessment of trends in the amount or adequacy of fluid volume.

Single Deepest Pocket

This is also called the *maximum vertical pocket.* The ultrasound transducer is held perpendicular to the floor and parallel to the long axis of the pregnant woman. In the sagittal plane, the largest vertical pocket of fluid is identified. The fluid pocket may contain fetal parts or loops of umbilical cord, but these are not included in the measurement.

The normal range for single deepest pocket that is most commonly used is 2 to 8 cm, with values above and below this indicating hydramnios and oligohydramnios, respectively. These thresholds are based on data from Chamberlain and associates (1984) and correspond to the 3rd and 97th percentiles. This group also reported increased perinatal mortality rates among nonanomalous infants if the single deepest pocket was below the normal range. The fetal biophysical profile similarly uses a 2-cm single deepest vertical pocket threshold to indicate a normal amnionic fluid volume (American College of Obstetricians and Gynecologists, 2012). This is discussed in more detail in Chapter 17 (p. 341).

Other less commonly used thresholds to determine amnionic fluid volume adequacy involve measurement of a single pocket in both the vertical and transverse planes. Adequate fluid volume is defined as a 2 × 1 cm pocket, a 2 × 2 cm pocket, or a pocket that is at least 15 cm^2 (Gramellini, 2004; Magann, 2000; Manning, 1990, 1993).

When evaluating twin pregnancies and other multifetal gestations, a single deepest pocket of amnionic fluid is assessed in each gestational sac, again using a normal range of 2 to 8 cm (Hernandez, 2012; Society for Maternal-Fetal Medicine, 2013).

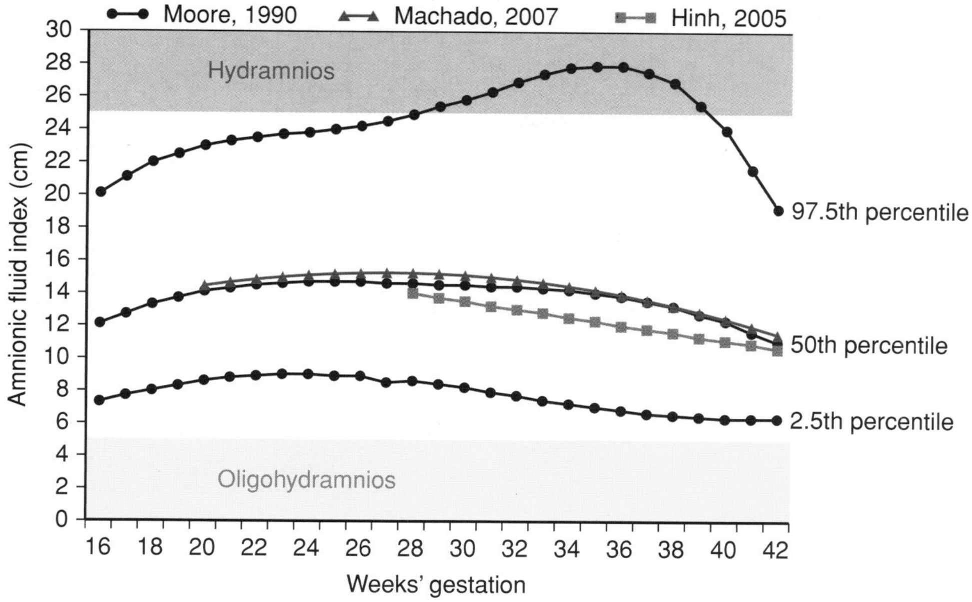

FIGURE 11-1 Amnionic fluid index (AFI) according to gestational-age-specific nomograms and threshold values. The blue curves represent the 2.5th, 50th, and 97.5th AFI percentile values, based on the nomogram by Moore (1990). Red and tan curves represent 50th percentile values for AFI from Machado (2007) and from Hinh and Ladinsky (2005), respectively. The light blue and yellow shaded bars indicate threshold values used to define hydramnios and oligohydramnios, respectively.

Amnionic Fluid Index (AFI)

This was described by Phelan and coworkers (1987) more than 25 years ago, and it remains one of the most commonly used methods of amnionic fluid volume assessment. As with the single deepest fluid pocket measurement, the ultrasound transducer is held perpendicular to the floor and parallel to the long axis of the pregnant woman. The uterus is divided into four equal quadrants—the right- and left-upper and lower quadrants, respectively. The AFI is the sum of the single deepest pocket from each quadrant. A fluid pocket may contain fetal parts or umbilical cord loops, but these are not included in the measurement. Color Doppler is generally used to verify that no umbilical cord is included in the measurement. This may result in greater consistency and in reduction of intraobserver variation (Callen, 2008; Hill, 2003). It has been reported, however, that color Doppler use results in a lower AFI measurement, thus potentially leading to overdiagnosis of oligohydramnios (Magann, 2001).

The intraobserver variability of the AFI is approximately 1 cm and the interobserver variability about 2 cm. There are larger variations when fluid volumes are above the normal range (Moore, 1990; Rutherford, 1987b). A useful guideline is that the AFI is approximately three times the single deepest pocket of fluid encountered (Hill, 2003).

Normal AFI. Determination of whether the AFI is normal—that is, the thresholds for defining oligohydramnios and hydramnios—may be based on either a static numerical cut-off or a gestational age-specific percentile reference range.

The normal range for AFI that is most commonly used is 5 to 24 cm, with values above and below this indicating hydramnios and oligohydramnios, respectively. Rutherford and colleagues (1987a) reported an increased risk for adverse pregnancy outcomes with indices outside of this range. Moore and Cayle (1990) published normal curves for AFI values based on a cross-sectional evaluation of nearly 800 uncomplicated pregnancies. As shown in Figure 11-1, the mean AFI was found to be between 12 and 15 cm from 16 weeks until 40 weeks. Other investigators have published nomograms with similar mean values (Hinh, 2005; Machado, 2007).

In the Moore (1990) nomogram, a threshold of 5 cm is < 2.5th percentile throughout the second and third trimesters. A value of 25 cm is > 95th percentile, but is not necessarily the 97.5th percentile, depending on gestational age. Using other published nomograms, a value of 25 cm exceeds the 97.5th percentile (Hinh, 2005; Machado, 2007). At this time, there is no consensus as to whether AFI nomogram use improves prediction of adverse outcome compared with use of a numerical threshold alone, and both are considered acceptable.

HYDRAMNIOS

This is an abnormally increased amnionic fluid volume, and it complicates 1 to 2 percent of pregnancies (Biggio, 1999; Dashe, 2000; Magann, 2007; Pri-Paz, 2012). Also termed *polyhydramnios*, hydramnios may be suspected if the uterine size exceeds that expected for gestational age. The uterus may feel tense, and palpating fetal small parts or auscultating fetal heart tones may be difficult. An extreme example is shown in Figure 11-2.

Hydramnios may be further categorized according to degree. Such categorization has been primarily used in research studies to stratify risks. Several groups have termed hydramnios as *mild* if the AFI is 25 to 29.9 cm, *moderate* if 30 to 34.9 cm, and *severe* if 35 cm or more (Dashe, 2002; Lazebnik, 1999; Pri-Paz, 2012). Mild hydramnios is the most common, comprising approximately two thirds of cases. Moderate hydramnios accounts for about 20 percent, and severe hydramnios approximately 15 percent. Using the single deepest pocket of amnionic fluid, criteria for mild is 8 to 9.9 cm, moderate is 10 to 11.9 cm, and severe hydramnios, ≥ 12 cm. An example of severe hydramnios seen sonographically is shown in Figure 11-3. These definitions fit the general rule that the AFI is approximately three times the measurement of the single deepest fluid pocket (Hill, 2003). *In general, severe hydramnios is far more likely to have an underlying etiology and to have consequences for the pregnancy than mild hydramnios—which is frequently idiopathic and benign.*

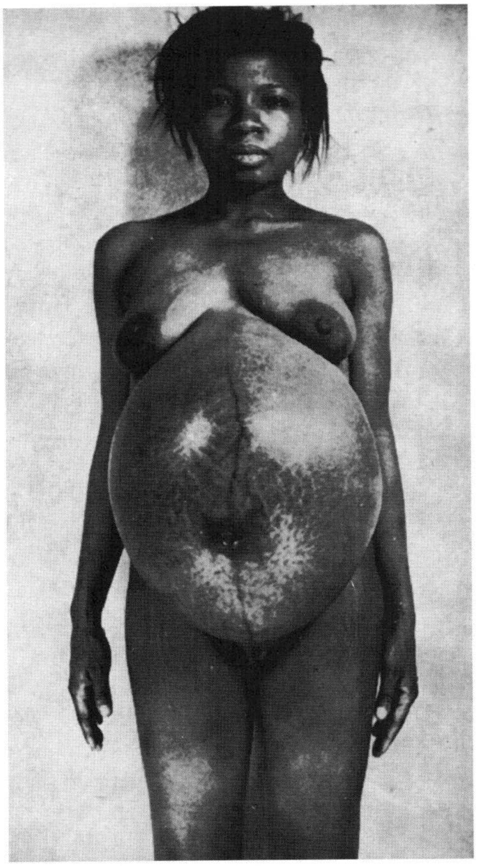

FIGURE 11-2 Severe hydramnios—5500 mL of amnionic fluid was measured at delivery.

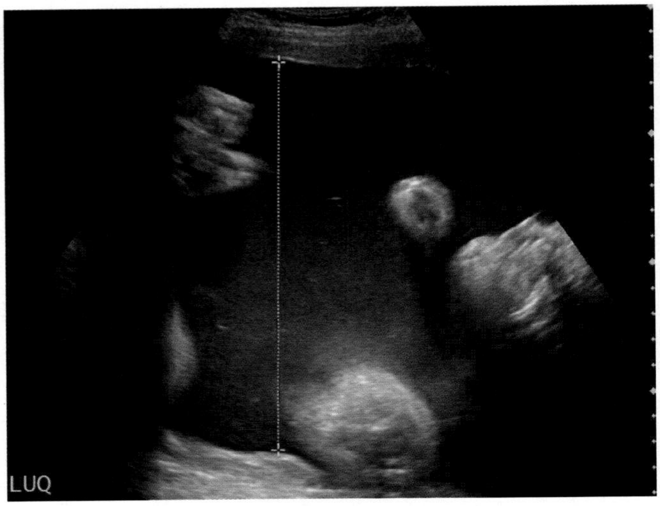

FIGURE 11-3 Sonogram of severe hydramnios at 35 weeks in a pregnancy complicated by fetal aqueductal stenosis. This pocket of amnionic fluid measures more than 15 cm, and the amnionic fluid index measured nearly 50 cm.

Etiology

Common underlying causes of hydramnios include fetal congenital anomalies in approximately 15 percent and diabetes in 15 to 20 percent (Table 11-2). Congenital infection and red blood cell alloimmunization are less frequent reasons. Infections that may present with hydramnios include cytomegalovirus, toxoplasmosis, syphilis, and parvovirus (Chaps. 64 and 65). Hydramnios is often a component of *hydrops fetalis*, and several of the above etiologies—selected anomalies, infections, and alloimmunization—may result in a hydropic fetus and placenta. The underlying pathophysiology in such cases is complex but is frequently related to a high cardiac-output state. Severe fetal anemia is the classic example. Because the etiologies of hydramnios are so varied, hydramnios treatment also varies and is tailored in most cases to the underlying cause. These etiologies are discussed further in Chapter 15 (p. 315) and in other chapters covering specific topics.

Diabetes Mellitus

The amnionic fluid glucose concentration is higher in diabetic women than in those without diabetes, and the amnionic fluid index may correlate with the amnionic fluid glucose concentration (Dashe, 2000; Spellacy, 1973; Weiss, 1985). Such findings support the hypothesis that maternal hyperglycemia causes fetal hyperglycemia, with resulting fetal osmotic diuresis into the amnionic fluid compartment.

TABLE 11-2. Hydramnios: Prevalence and Associated Etiologies—Values in Percent

	Golan (1993) n = 149	Many (1995) n = 275	Biggio (1999) n = 370	Dashe (2002) n = 672	Pri-Paz (2012) n = 655
Prevalence	1	1	1	1	2
Amnionic fluid index					
Mild 25–29.9 cm	—	72	—	66	64
Moderate 30–34.9 cm		20		22	21
Severe > 35 cm		8		12	15
Etiology					
Idiopathic	65	69	72	82	52
Fetal anomaly[a]	19	15[a]	8	11[a]	38[a]
Diabetes	15	18	20	7	18

[a]A significant correlation was identified between severity of hydramnios and likelihood of an anomalous infant.

Congenital Anomalies

Various anomalies may be found in the setting of hydramnios, and some are more characteristically linked with it than others. Because of this association, identification of hydramnios is an indication for targeted sonography. Many of the anomalies described next are displayed sonographically in Chapter 10 (p. 200).

Severe central nervous system abnormalities, such as anencephaly, hydranencephaly, or holoprosencephaly, can result in hydramnios due to impaired fetal swallowing. Fetal neuromuscular disorders such as myotonic dystrophy also may lead to excessive amnionic fluid. Obstruction of the fetal upper gastrointestinal tract—esophageal or duodenal atresia—is often associated with hydramnios. Other obstructive causes include clefts, micrognathia, congenital high-airway obstruction sequence, and fetal neck masses. Severe fetal thoracic abnormalities, such as diaphragmatic hernia, cystic adenomatoid malformation, and pulmonary sequestration, may be associated with hydramnios due to mediastinal shift and impaired swallowing, occasionally with development of hydrops. A common fetal renal anomaly, ureteropelvic junction obstruction, may at times result in *paradoxical hydramnios*. And although rare, tumors such as fetal sacrococcygeal teratoma, fetal mesoblastic nephroma, and large placental chorioangiomas are frequently accompanied by abnormally increased amnionic fluid volume.

The degree of hydramnios is associated with the likelihood of an anomalous infant (Many, 1995; Pri-Paz, 2012). For example, at Parkland Hospital, the prevalence of an anomalous infant was approximately 8 percent with mild hydramnios, 12 percent with moderate hydramnios, and more than 30 percent with severe hydramnios (Dashe, 2002). If no abnormality was detected with targeted sonography, the likelihood of a major anomaly identified at birth was 1 to 2 percent if the hydramnios was mild or moderate but exceeded 10 percent if hydramnios was severe. Dorleijn and associates (2009) have also reported an increased risk for abnormalities detected in the first year of life with apparent idiopathic hydramnios. The anomaly risk is particularly high with hydramnios coexistent with fetal-growth restriction (Lazebnik, 1999). If a fetal abnormality is encountered concurrent with hydramnios, amniocentesis should be considered, because the aneuploidy risk is significantly increased (Dashe, 2002; Pri-Paz, 2012).

Although amnionic fluid volume abnormalities are associated with fetal malformations, the converse is not usually the case. In the Spanish Collaborative Study of Congenital Malformations that included more than 27,000 anomalous infants, only 4 percent were complicated by hydramnios, and another 3 percent with oligohydramnios (Martinez-Frias, 1999).

Multifetal Gestation

Hydramnios is generally defined in multifetal gestations as a single deepest amnionic fluid pocket measuring 8 cm or more. It may be further characterized as moderate if the single deepest pocket is at least 10 cm and severe if this pocket is at least 12 cm. In monochorionic pregnancies, hydramnios of one sac and oligohydramnios of the other are diagnostic criteria for twin-twin transfusion syndrome, which is discussed in Chapter 45 (p. 904). In a review of nearly 2000 twin gestations, Hernandez and coworkers (2012) identified hydramnios in 18 percent of both monochorionic and dichorionic pregnancies. As in singletons, severe hydramnios was more strongly associated with fetal abnormalities. In the absence of an abnormality, pregnancy risks were not generally increased compared with twins with normal amnionic fluid volume.

Idiopathic Hydramnios

When there is no obvious cause of hydramnios it is considered *idiopathic*. As shown in Table 11-2, this accounts for up to 70 percent of cases (Golan, 1993; Many, 1995; Panting-Kemp, 1999). Pregnancies with idiopathic hydramnios have been reported to have at least twice the likelihood of infant birthweight exceeding 4000 g (Lazebnik, 1999; Magann, 2010; Maymon, 1998). A rationale for this association is that larger infants have higher urine output, by virtue of their increased volume of distribution, and fetal urine is the largest contributor to amnionic fluid volume. Mild, idiopathic hydramnios is most commonly a benign finding, and associated pregnancy outcomes are usually good.

Complications

Unless hydramnios is severe or develops rapidly, maternal symptoms are infrequent. With chronic hydramnios, fluid accumulates gradually, and a woman may tolerate excessive abdominal distention with relatively little discomfort. Acute hydramnios, however, tends to develop earlier in pregnancy. It may result in preterm labor before 28 weeks or in symptoms that become so debilitating as to necessitate intervention.

Symptoms may arise from pressure exerted within the overdistended uterus and upon adjacent organs. When distention is excessive, the mother may suffer dyspnea and orthopnea to such a degree that she may be able to breathe comfortably only when upright (see Fig. 11-2). Edema may develop as a consequence of major venous system compression by the enlarged uterus, and it tends to be most pronounced in the lower extremities, vulva, and abdominal wall. Rarely, oliguria may result from ureteral obstruction by the enlarged uterus (Chap. 53, p. 1064). Maternal complications such as these are typically associated with severe hydramnios from an underlying etiology.

Maternal complications associated with hydramnios include placental abruption, uterine dysfunction, and postpartum hemorrhage. Placental abruption is fortunately infrequent. It may result from the rapid decompression of an overdistended uterus that follows fetal-membrane rupture or therapeutic amnioreduction. With prematurely ruptured membranes, a placental abruption occasionally occurs days or weeks after amniorrhexis. Uterine dysfunction consequent to overdistention may lead to postpartum atony and, in turn, postpartum hemorrhage.

Pregnancy Outcomes

Some outcomes that have been reported to be increased with hydramnios include cesarean delivery rate, birthweight > 4000 g, and importantly, perinatal mortality rate. The cesarean delivery rate is increased approximately threefold when hydramnios has been identified, and the perinatal mortality rate rises approximately fourfold (Biggio, 1999; Hill, 1987; Maymon, 1998). Pri-Paz and colleagues (2012) found that pregnancies with severe hydramnios were at particular risk, but reported no perinatal deaths with *idiopathic* hydramnios.

Risks appear to be compounded when a growth-restricted fetus is identified with hydramnios. Erez and associates (2005) reported that this combination was independently associated with a 20-fold increase in the perinatal mortality rate. The combination also has a recognized association with trisomy 18 (Sickler, 1997).

Considering that uterine distention from hydramnios may result in uterine size approaching that of a term gestation, preterm delivery is a logical concern. Somewhat surprisingly, studies of *idiopathic* hydramnios have generally found no association with preterm birth (Magann, 2010; Many, 1995; Panting-Kemp, 1999). Conversely, severe hydramnios and hydramnios concurrent with recognized fetal abnormalities have been linked with preterm birth (Many, 1995; Pri-Paz, 2012).

Management

As noted previously, hydramnios etiologies are varied, and treatment is directed in most situations to the underlying cause. Occasionally, severe hydramnios may result in early preterm labor or the development of maternal respiratory compromise. In such cases, large-volume amniocentesis—termed *amnioreduction*—may be needed. The needle insertion technique is the same as for amniocentesis, described in Chapter 14 (p. 297). However, either an evacuated container bottle or a larger syringe is connected to the needle via sterile intravenous tubing with a stopcock. In general, approximately 1000 to 1500 mL of fluid is slowly withdrawn during approximately 30 minutes, depending on the severity of hydramnios and gestational age. The goal is to restore amnionic fluid volume to upper normal range (p. 232). Hydramnios severe enough to necessitate amnioreduction almost invariably has an underlying etiology, and subsequent amnioreduction procedures may be required as often as weekly or even semiweekly. Importantly, amnioreduction is typically performed later in gestation and carries additional risks of membrane rupture, preterm labor or its exacerbation, and placental abruption.

OLIGOHYDRAMNIOS

This is an abnormally decreased amount of amnionic fluid. Oligohydramnios complicates approximately 1 to 2 percent of pregnancies (Casey, 2000; Petrozella, 2011). Unlike hydramnios, which is often mild and confers a benign prognosis in the absence of an underlying etiology, oligohydramnios is a cause for concern. When no measurable pocket of amnionic fluid is identified, the term *anhydramnios* may be used.

The sonographic diagnosis of oligohydramnios is usually based on an AFI ≤ 5 cm or on a single deepest pocket of amnionic fluid ≤ 2 cm (American College of Obstetricians and Gynecologists, 2012). The diagnosis also may be based on an AFI below the 5th or 2.5th percentile determined by a gestational-age-specific nomogram. Or, it may be based on subjective assessment of decreased amnionic fluid volume. In the Moore nomogram, a threshold of 5 cm is below the 2.5th percentile throughout the second and third trimesters (see Fig. 11-1). When evaluating twin pregnancies for twin-twin transfusion syndrome, a single deepest pocket ≤ 2 cm is used to define oligohydramnios (Society for Maternal-Fetal Medicine, 2013).

In general, no one criterion is considered superior to the others. As discussed subsequently, however, use of AFI rather than single deepest pocket will identify more pregnancies as having oligohydramnios, albeit without evidence of pregnancy outcome improvement (Nabhan, 2010).

Etiology

Pregnancies complicated by oligohydramnios include those in which the amnionic fluid volume has been severely decreased since the early second trimester and those in which the fluid volume was normal until near-term or even full-term. The prognosis depends heavily on the underlying etiology and is variable. Whenever oligohydramnios is diagnosed, it becomes an important consideration in management decisions.

Early-Onset Oligohydramnios

When amnionic fluid volume is abnormally decreased from the early second trimester, it may reflect a fetal abnormality that precludes normal urination, or it may represent a placental abnormality severe enough to impair perfusion. In either circumstance, the prognosis is poor. Second-trimester rupture of the fetal membranes may result in oligohydramnios—and should be excluded. More commonly, membrane rupture presents with fluid leakage, vaginal bleeding, or uterine contractions. With early-onset oligohydramnios, targeted sonography should be offered to assess for fetal abnormalities.

Oligohydramnios after Midpregnancy

When amnionic fluid volume becomes abnormally decreased in the late second or in the third trimester, it more likely is associated with fetal-growth restriction, a placental abnormality, or a maternal complication such as preeclampsia or vascular disease (Table 11-3). In such cases, the underlying etiology is often presumed to be uteroplacental insufficiency, which can impair fetal growth and reduce fetal urine output. Exposure to selected medications has also been linked with oligohydramnios as discussed subsequently. Investigation of third-trimester oligohydramnios generally includes evaluation for membrane rupture and sonography to assess growth. Umbilical artery Doppler studies may be performed if growth restriction is identified (Chap. 10, p. 219).

Oligohydramnios is commonly encountered in *postterm pregnancies* as discussed in Chapter 43 (p. 865). Magann and coworkers (1997) found that amnionic fluid volume decreased by approximately 8 percent per week beyond 40 weeks. In postterm pregnancies, oligohydramnios has been associated with nonreassuring fetal heart rate patterns and adverse pregnancy outcomes (Leveno, 1984).

TABLE 11-3. Pregnancy Outcomes in Women Diagnosed with Oligohydramnios between 24 and 34 Weeks

Factor	AFI ≤ 5 cm (n = 166)	AFI 8 to 24 cm (n = 28,185)	*p*-Value
Major malformation	42 (25)	634 (2)	< .001
Stillbirth	8 (5)	133 (< 1)	< .001
Gestational age at delivery[a]	35.1 ± 3.3	39.2 ± 2.0	< .001
Preterm birth, spontaneous[a]	49 (42)	1698 (6)	< .001
Preterm birth, indicated[a]	23 (20)	405 (2)	< .001
Cesarean delivery for non-reassuring fetal status[a]	10 (9)	1083 (4)	< .001
Birthweight < 10th percentile[a]	61 (53)	3388 (12)	< .001
< 3rd percentile[a]	43 (37)	1130 (4)	< .001
Neonatal death[a]	1 (1)	24 (< 1)	< .001[b]

[a]Analysis performed after exclusion of anomalous infants.
[b]This difference was no longer significant after adjustment for gestational age at delivery.
Data expressed as No. (%) and mean ± standard deviation.
Data from Petrozella, 2011.

Congenital Anomalies

By approximately 18 weeks, the fetal kidneys are the main contributor to amnionic fluid volume. Among those with fetal abnormalities, most cases of severely decreased amnionic fluid volume beginning early in gestation are secondary to genitourinary anomalies. Anomalies of other organ systems, aneuploidy, and other genetic syndromes also have the potential to cause oligohydramnios *indirectly*, either from fetal decompensation, fetal-growth restriction, or an accompanying placental abnormality. Overall, approximately 3 percent of newborns with congenital anomalies have oligohydramnios found during prenatal sonography (Martinez-Frias, 1999).

Selected renal abnormalities that lead to absent fetal urine production include bilateral *renal agenesis*, bilateral *multicystic dysplastic kidney*, unilateral renal agenesis with contralateral multicystic dysplastic kidney, and the infantile form of *autosomal recessive polycystic kidney disease*. Urinary abnormalities may also result in oligohydramnios because of fetal *bladder outlet obstruction*. Examples of this are *posterior urethral valves*, *urethral atresia* or *stenosis*, or the *megacystis microcolon intestinal hypoperistalsis syndrome*. Complex fetal genitourinary abnormalities such as *persistent cloaca* and *sirenomelia* similarly may result in lack of amnionic fluid. These renal abnormalities are also discussed and depicted in Chapter 10 (p. 216).

If there is bilateral renal agenesis, no urine is produced, and the resulting anhydramnios leads to limb contractures, a distinctively compressed face, and death from pulmonary hypoplasia (Fig. 11-4). When this combination of abnormalities results from renal agenesis, it is called *Potter syndrome*, after Dr. Edith Potter, who described it in 1946. When this constellation stems from another etiology of decreased amnionic fluid volume, it is generally called *Potter sequence*.

If no amnionic fluid is visible beyond the mid-second trimester due to a genitourinary etiology, the prognosis is extremely poor unless fetal therapy is an option. Fetuses with bladder-outlet obstruction may be candidates for vesicoamnionic shunt placement (Chap. 16, p. 330).

Medication

Oligohydramnios has been associated with exposure to drugs that block the renin-angiotensin system. These include angiotensin-converting enzyme (ACE) inhibitors and nonsteroidal antiinflammatory drugs (NSAIDs). When taken in the second or third trimester, ACE inhibitors and angiotensin-receptor blockers may create fetal hypotension, renal hypoperfusion, and

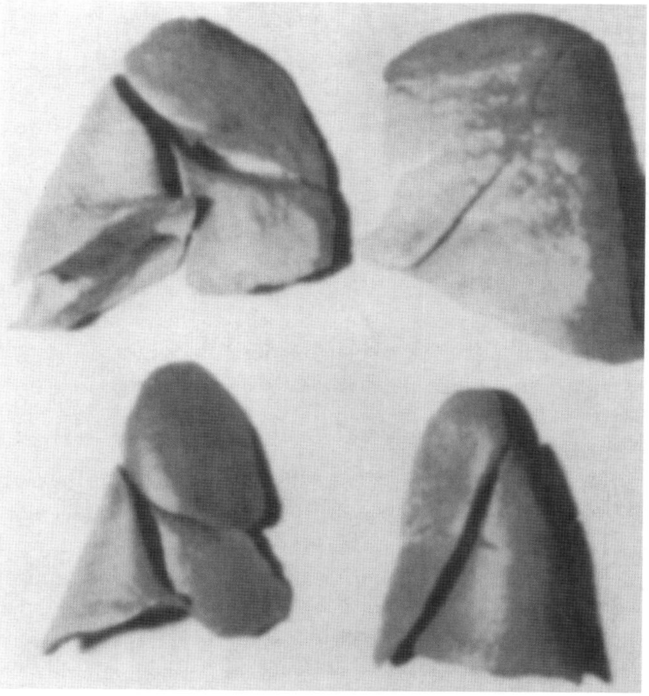

FIGURE 11-4 Normal-sized lungs (*top*) are shown in comparison with hypoplastic lungs (*bottom*) of fetuses at the same gestational age. (From Newbould, 1994, with permission.)

renal ischemia, with subsequent anuric renal failure (Guron, 2000; Pryde, 1993). These adverse outcomes appear to be more prevalent following exposure to angiotensin-receptor blockers, but both medication types are contraindicated in pregnancy (Bullo, 2012). NSAIDs have been associated with fetal ductus arteriosus constriction and with decreased fetal urine production. In neonates, their use may result in acute and chronic renal insufficiency (Fanos, 2011). All these agents are also discussed in Chapter 12 (p. 247).

Pregnancy Outcomes

Oligohydramnios is associated with increased risk of adverse pregnancy outcomes. Casey and colleagues (2000) found that an AFI ≤ 5 cm complicated 2 percent of pregnancies undergoing sonography at Parkland Hospital after 34 weeks. Newborns from pregnancies with oligohydramnios were more likely than those with AFIs > 5 cm to have malformations. Even in the absence of malformations, higher rates of fetal stillbirth, growth restriction, nonreassuring heart rate pattern, and meconium aspiration syndrome were noted. Petrozella and associates (2011) similarly reported that with an AFI ≤ 5 cm identified between 24 and 34 weeks, there was increased risk for stillbirth, spontaneous or medically indicated preterm birth, heart rate pattern abnormalities, and growth restriction (see Table 11-3). In a metaanalysis of 18 studies comprising more than 10,000 pregnancies, Chauhan and coworkers (1999) found that women with oligohydramnios had a twofold increased risk for cesarean delivery for fetal distress and a fivefold risk for an Apgar score < 7 at 5 minutes compared with pregnancies with normal AFI.

As noted earlier, there is evidence that if oligohydramnios is defined as an AFI ≤ 5 cm rather than a single deepest pocket ≤ 2 cm, more pregnancies will be classified as having oligohydramnios. However, this increased diagnostic frequency is not associated with improved pregnancy outcomes. Nabhan and Abdelmoula (2008) reviewed five randomized controlled trials involving more than 3200 pregnancies in which outcomes were compared according to which definition was used. The trials included both high-risk and low-risk pregnancies. There was no difference in the rates of cesarean delivery, neonatal intensive care unit admission, umbilical artery pH < 7.1, or Apgar score < 7 at 5 minutes. Using AFI criteria, however, twice as many pregnancies were diagnosed with oligohydramnios, along with a doubling of the labor induction rate, and a 50-percent increase in the cesarean delivery rate for fetal distress.

Pulmonary Hypoplasia

When decreased amnionic fluid is first identified before the mid-second trimester, particularly before 20 to 22 weeks, pulmonary hypoplasia is a significant concern. The underlying etiology is a major factor in the prognosis for such pregnancies. Severe oligohydramnios secondary to a renal abnormality generally has a lethal prognosis (see Fig. 11-4). If a placental hematoma or chronic abruption is severe enough to result in oligohydramnios—the *chronic abruption-oligohydramnios sequence*—it commonly also causes growth restriction (Chap. 41, p. 794). The prognosis for this constellation is similarly poor. Oligohydramnios that results from membrane rupture in the second trimester is reviewed in Chapter 42 (p. 848).

Management

As with hydramnios, management targets the underlying etiology when feasible. Initially, an evaluation for fetal anomalies and growth is essential. In a pregnancy complicated by oligohydramnios and fetal-growth restriction, close fetal surveillance is important because of associated morbidity and mortality. In many cases, evidence for fetal or maternal compromise will override potential complications from preterm delivery. But, oligohydramnios detected before 36 weeks in the presence of normal fetal anatomy and growth may be managed expectantly in conjunction with increased fetal surveillance.

Amnioinfusion, as discussed in Chapter 24 (p. 494), may be used intrapartum in the setting of variable fetal heart rate decelerations. It is not considered treatment for oligohydramnios per se, although the decelerations are presumed secondary to umbilical cord compression resulting from lack of amnionic fluid. Amnioinfusion is not the standard of care for other etiologies of oligohydramnios and is not generally recommended.

"Borderline" Oligohydramnios

The term *borderline AFI* or *borderline oligohydramnios* is somewhat controversial. It usually refers to AFIs between 5 and 8 cm (Baron, 1995; Magann, 2011; Petrozella, 2011). Through the mid-third trimester, an AFI value of 8 cm is below the 5th percentile on the Moore nomogram (see Fig. 11-1). Petrozella and colleagues (2011) found that pregnancies between 24 and 34 weeks with an AFI between 5 and 8 cm were not more likely than those with an AFI above 8 cm to be complicated by maternal hypertension, stillbirth, or neonatal death. However, higher rates of preterm delivery, cesarean delivery for a nonreassuring fetal heart rate pattern, and fetal-growth restriction were found. Study results evaluating pregnancy outcomes with borderline AFI have been mixed. A recent review by Magann and associates (2011) concludes that there is insufficient evidence to support fetal testing or delivery in this setting.

REFERENCES

American College of Obstetricians and Gynecologists: Ultrasonography in pregnancy. Practice Bulletin No. 101, February 2009, Reaffirmed 2011

American College of Obstetricians and Gynecologists: Antepartum fetal Surveillance, Practice Bulletin No. 9, October 1999, Reaffirmed 2012

American Institute of Ultrasound in Medicine (AIUM): Practice guideline for the performance of obstetric ultrasound examinations. J Ultrasound Med 32(6):1083, 2013

Baron C, Morgan MA, Garite TJ: The impact of amniotic fluid volume assessed intrapartum on perinatal outcome. Am J Obstet Gynecol 173:167, 1995

Biggio JR Jr, Wenstrom KD, Dubard MB, et al: Hydramnios prediction of adverse perinatal outcome. Obstet Gynecol 94:773, 1999

Brace RA, Wolf EJ: Normal amniotic fluid volume changes throughout pregnancy. Am J Obstet Gynecol 161(2):382, 1998

Bullo M, Tschumi S, Bucher BS: Pregnancy outcome following exposure to angiotensin-converting enzyme inhibitors or angiotensin receptor antagonists: a systematic review. Hypertension 60:444, 2012

Callen PW (ed): Amniotic fluid volume: its role in fetal health and disease. In Ultrasonography in Obstetrics and Gynecology, 5th ed. Philadelphia, Saunders Elsevier, 2008, p 764

Casey BM, McIntire DD, Bloom SL, et al: Pregnancy outcomes after antepartum diagnosis of oligohydramnios at or beyond 34 weeks' gestation. Am J Obstet Gynecol 182:909, 2000
Chamberlain PF, Manning FA, Morrison I, et al: Ultrasound evaluation of amniotic fluid. The relationship of marginal and decreased amniotic fluid volumes to perinatal outcome. Am J Obstet Gynecol 150:245, 1984
Chauhan SP, Sanderson M, Hendrix NW, et al: Perinatal outcome and amniotic fluid index in the antepartum and intrapartum periods: a meta-analysis. Am J Obstet Gynecol 181:1473, 1999
Dashe JS, McIntire DD, Ramus RM, et al: Hydramnios: anomaly prevalence and sonographic detection. Obstet Gynecol 100(1):134, 2002
Dashe JS, Nathan L, McIntire DD, et al: Correlation between amniotic fluid glucose concentration and amniotic fluid volume in pregnancy complicated by diabetes. Am J Obstet Gynecol 182(4):901, 2000
Dorleijn DM, Cohen-Overbeek TE, Groenendaal F, et al: Idiopathic polyhydramnios and postnatal findings. J Matern Fetal Neonatal Med 22(4):315, 2009
Erez O, Shoham-Vardi I, Sheiner E, et al: Hydramnios and small for gestational age are independent risk factors for neonatal mortality and maternal morbidity. Arch Gynecol Obstet 271(4):296, 2005
Fanos V, Marcialis MA, Bassareo PP, et al: Renal safety of Non Steroidal Anti Inflammatory Drugs (NSAIDs) in the pharmacologic treatment of patent ductus arteriosus. J Maternal Fetal Neonatal Med 24(S1):50, 2011
Golan A, Wolman I, Saller Y, et al: Hydramnios in singleton pregnancy: sonographic prevalence and etiology. Gynecol Obstet Invest 35:91, 1993
Gramellini D, Fieni S, Verrotti C, et al: Ultrasound evaluation of amniotic fluid volume: methods and clinical accuracy. Acta Bio Medica Ateneo Parmanese 75(Suppl 1):40, 2004
Guron G, Friberg P: An intact renin-angiotensin system is a prerequisite for normal renal development. J Hypertens 18(2):123, 2000
Hernandez JS, Twickler DM, McIntire DM, et al: Hydramnios in twin gestations. Obstet Gynecol 120(4):759, 2012
Hill LM, Breckle R, Thomas ML, et al: Polyhydramnios: ultrasonically detected prevalence and neonatal outcome. Obstet Gynecol 69:21, 1987
Hill LM, Sohaey R, Nyberg DA: Abnormalities of amniotic fluid. In Nyberg DA, McGahan JP, Pretorius DH, et al (eds): Diagnostic Imaging of Fetal Anomalies. Philadelphia, Lippincott Williams & Wilkins, 2003, p 62
Hinh ND, Ladinsky JL: Amniotic fluid index measurements in normal pregnancy after 28 gestational weeks. Int J Gynaecol Obstet 91:132, 2005
Lazebnik N, Many A: The severity of polyhydramnios, estimated fetal weight and preterm delivery are independent risk factors for the presence of congenital anomalies. Gynecol Obstet Invest 48:28, 1999
Leveno KJ, Quirk JG Jr, Cunningham FG, et al: Prolonged pregnancy, 1. Observations concerning the causes of fetal distress. Am J Obstet Gynecol 150:465, 1984
Machado MR, Cecatti JG, Krupa F, et al: Curve of amniotic fluid index measurements in low risk pregnancy. Acta Obstet Gynecol Scand 86:37, 2007
Magann EF, Bass JD, Chauhan SP, et al: Amniotic fluid volume in normal singleton pregnancies. Obstet Gynecol 90(4):524, 1997
Magann EF, Chauhan SP, Barrilleaux PS, et al: Ultrasound estimate of amniotic fluid volume: color Doppler overdiagnosis of oligohydramnios. Obstet Gynecol 98:71, 2001
Magann EF, Chauhan SP, Doherty DA, et al: A review of idiopathic hydramnios and pregnancy outcomes. Obstet Gynecol Surv 62:795, 2007
Magann EF, Chauhan CP, Hitt WC, et al: Borderline or marginal amniotic fluid index and peripartum outcomes: a review of the literature. J Ultrasound Med 30(4):523, 2011
Magann EF, Doherty D, Lutegendorf MA, et al: Peripartum outcomes of high-risk pregnancies complicated by oligo- and polyhydramnios: a prospective longitudinal study. J Obstet Gynaecol Res 36(2):268, 2010
Magann EF, Sanderson M, Martin JN, et al: The amniotic fluid index, single deepest pocket, and two-diameter pocket in normal human pregnancy. Am J Obstet Gynecol 182:1581, 2000
Mann SE, Nijland MJ, Ross MG: Mathematic modeling of human amniotic fluid dynamics. Am J Obstet Gynecol 175(4):937, 1996
Manning FA, Harman CR, Morrison I, et al: Fetal assessment based on fetal biophysical profile scoring. IV. An analysis of perinatal morbidity and mortality. Am J Obstet Gynecol 162(3):703, 1990
Manning FA, Snijders R, Harman CR, et al: Fetal biophysical profile score. VI. Correlation with antepartum umbilical venous fetal pH. Am J Obstet Gynecol 169(4):755, 1993
Many A, Hill LM, Lazebnik N, et al: The association between polyhydramnios and preterm delivery. Obstet Gynecol 86(3):389, 1995
Martinez-Frias ML, Bermejo E, Rodriguez-Pinilla E, et al: Maternal and fetal factors related to abnormal amniotic fluid. J Perinatol 19:514, 1999
Maymon E, Ghezzi F, Shoham-Vardi I, et al: Isolated hydramnios at term gestation and the occurrence of peripartum complications. Eur J Obstet Gynecol 77:157, 1998
Modena AB, Fieni S: Amniotic fluid dynamics. Acta Bio Medica Ateneo Parmanese 75(Suppl 1):11, 2004
Moore TR: Amniotic fluid dynamics reflect fetal and maternal health and disease. Obstet Gynecol 116(3):759, 2010
Moore TR, Cayle JE: The amniotic fluid index in normal human pregnancy. Am J Obstet Gynecol 162(5):1168, 1990
Nabhan AF, Abdelmoula YA: Amniotic fluid index versus single deepest vertical pocket as a screening test for preventing adverse pregnancy outcome. Cochrane Database Syst Rev 3:CD006953, 2008
Newbould MJ, Lendon M, Barson AJ: Oligohydramnios sequence: the spectrum of renal malformations. Br J Obstet Gynaecol 101:598, 1994
Panting-Kemp A, Nguyen T, Chang E, et al: Idiopathic polyhydramnios and perinatal outcome. Am J Obstet Gynecol 181(5):1079, 1999
Petrozella LN, Dashe JS, McIntire DD, et al: Clinical significance of borderline amniotic fluid index and oligohydramnios in preterm pregnancy. Obstet Gynecol 117 (2 pt 1):338, 2011
Phelan JP, Smith CV, Broussard P, et al: Amniotic fluid volume assessment with the four-quadrant technique at 36–42 weeks' gestation. J Reprod Med 32:540, 1987
Pri-Paz S, Khalek N, Fuchs KM, et al: Maximal amniotic fluid index as a prognostic factor in pregnancies complicated by polyhydramnios. Ultrasound Obstet Gynecol 39(6):648, 2012
Pryde PG, Sedman AB, Nugent CA, et al: Angiotensin-converting enzyme fetopathy. J Am Soc Nephrol 3(9):1575, 1993
Rutherford SE, Phelan JP, Smith CV, et al: The 4 quadrant assessment of amnionic fluid volume: an adjunct to antepartum fetal heart rate testing. Obstet Gynecol 70(3 pt 1):353, 1987a
Rutherford SE, Smith CV, Phelan JP, et al: Four-quadrant assessment of amniotic fluid volume. Interobserver and intraobserver variation. J Reprod Med 32(8):587, 1987b
Sickler GK, Nyberg DA, Sohaey R, et al: Polyhydramnios and fetal intrauterine growth restriction: ominous combination. J Ultrasound Med 16(9):609, 1997
Society for Maternal-Fetal Medicine Clinical Guidelines, Simpson LL: Twin-twin transfusion syndrome. Am J Obstet Gynecol 208(1):3, 2013
Spellacy WN, Buhi WC, Bradley B, et al: Maternal, fetal, amniotic fluid levels of glucose, insulin, and growth hormone. Obstet Gynecol 41: 323, 1973
Weiss PA, Hofmann H, Winter R, et al: Amniotic fluid glucose values in normal and abnormal pregnancies. Obstet Gynecol 65:333, 1985

CHAPTER 12

Teratology, Teratogens, and Fetotoxic Agents

Birth defects are common—2 to 3 percent of all newborns have a major congenital abnormality detectable at birth (Cragan, 2009; Dolk, 2010). By age 5, another 3 percent have been diagnosed with a malformation, and by age 18, another 8 to 10 percent have one or more apparent functional or developmental abnormalities. Importantly, nearly 70 percent of birth defects do not have an obvious etiology, and of those with an identified cause, it is far more likely to be genetic than teratogenic (Schardein, 2000; Wlodarczyk, 2011). The Food and Drug Administration (FDA) (2005b) estimates that less than 1 percent of all birth defects are caused by medications. Examples of medications considered teratogenic are shown in Table 12-1.

Although only a relatively small number of medications have proven harmful effects, there is significant concern surrounding medication use in pregnancy. This is because most pregnant women take medications and for most medications, available safety data are limited. In a review of more than 150,000 pregnancies, 40 percent of women were prescribed a medication other than multivitamins in the first trimester (Andrade, 2004). More recently, data from the National Birth Defects Prevention Study showed that women use an average of 2 to 3 medications per pregnancy and that 70 percent take medication in the first trimester (Mitchell, 2011).

Despite improvements in safety information, data are particularly limited for newer medications. For example, in a review of medications approved by the FDA between 2000 and 2010, the Teratogen Information System (TERIS) expert advisory board deemed the pregnancy risk "undetermined" for more than 95 percent (Adam, 2011).

TERATOLOGY

The study of birth defects and their etiology is termed teratology. The word teratogen is derived from the Greek *teratos,* meaning monster. Pragmatically, a teratogen may be defined as any agent that acts during embryonic or fetal development to produce a permanent alteration of form or function. Thus, a teratogen may be a drug or other chemical substance, a physical or environmental factor such as heat or radiation, a maternal metabolite such as in phenylketonuria or diabetes, a genetic abnormality, or an infection. Tightly defined, a teratogen causes structural abnormalities, whereas a hadegen—after the god Hades—is an agent that interferes with normal maturation and function of an organ. A trophogen is an agent that alters growth. Substances in the latter two groups typically affect development in the fetal period or after birth, when exposures are often more difficult to document. In most circumstances, teratogen is used to refer to all three types of agents.

Studies in Pregnant Women

The study of medication safety—or teratogenicity—in pregnant women is fraught with complications. Animal studies are considered necessary but insufficient, which is a lesson learned from the safety of thalidomide in several animal species. Rarely are medications approved by the FDA with the specific indication for their use being pregnancy. Between 1996 and 2011, for example, the only medication approved specifically for pregnancy was hydroxyprogesterone caproate for recurrent preterm birth prevention.

Pregnant women are generally considered a special population and excluded from trials. An obvious reason is to protect

TABLE 12-1. Selected Teratogens and Fetotoxic Agents

Acitretin	Lenalidomide
Alcohol	Lithium
Ambrisentan	Methimazole
Angiotensin-converting enzyme inhibitors	Mercury
	Methotrexate
Angiotensin-receptor blockers	Misoprostol
Androgens	Mycophenolate
Bexarotene	Paroxetine
Bosentan	Phenobarbital
Carbamazepine	Phenytoin
Chloramphenicol	Radioactive iodine
Cocaine	Ribavirin
Corticosteroids	Tamoxifen
Cyclophosphamide	Tetracycline
Danazol	Thalidomide
Diethylstilbestrol (DES)	Tobacco
Efavirenz	Toluene
Fluconazole	Topiramate
Isotretinoin	Trastuzumab
Lamotrigine	Tretinoin
Lead	Valproic acid
Leflunomide	Warfarin

the embryo and fetus from potentially harmful effects of a medication—its pharmacodynamic effect(s) on the body. Another reason is that pregnancy physiology affects the medication—its pharmacokinetics. Specifically, changes in volume of distribution, cardiac output, gastrointestinal absorption, hepatic metabolism, and renal clearance may each affect drug concentration and thus embryo-fetal exposure (Chap. 4, p. 51).

Case Reports and Series

Several major teratogens were first described by astute clinicians. Congenital rubella syndrome was identified in this way by Gregg (1941), an Australian ophthalmologist whose observations challenged the view that the uterine environment was impervious to noxious agents. Other teratogens identified through case series include thalidomide and alcohol (Jones, 1973; Lenz, 1962). Unfortunately, teratogens are less likely to come to attention through identification of clinical cases if the exposure is uncommon, if the defects are relatively nonspecific, or if abnormalities occur in only a small proportion of exposed infants. A major limitation of case series is that they lack a control group.

Pregnancy Registries

Potentially harmful agents may be monitored by clinicians who prospectively enroll exposed pregnancies in a registry. The FDA maintains a list of ongoing pregnancy registries on their website: www.fda.gov. Included are medication groups used to treat asthma, autoimmune disease, cancer, epilepsy, human immunodeficiency virus (HIV) infection, and transplant rejection. Similar to case series, exposure registries are limited by lack of a control group. To compare the prevalence of an abnormality identified among exposed infants with that expected in the general population, investigators use a birth defect registry. One example is the Metropolitan Atlanta Congenital Defects Program, which is an active surveillance program ongoing since 1967 for fetuses and infants with birth defects.

Case-Control Studies

In these studies, investigators retrospectively assess prenatal exposure to particular substances between affected infants and controls. Birth defect registries are ideal for ascertainment of cases. However, case-control studies have two inherent weaknesses. First, there is potential for recall bias, in which the mother of an affected infant may be more likely to recall exposure. Second, case-control studies can only evaluate associations, rather than causality, and are thus hypothesis-generating. For these reasons, Grimes and Schulz (2012) caution that unless odds ratios in case-control studies are above three- to fourfold, then observed findings may be incorrect.

The National Birth Defects Prevention Study. This population-based case-control study involves 10 states with active birth defects surveillance programs (www.nbdps.org). It represents an important collaborative effort by the Centers for Birth Defects Research and Prevention to evaluate medications as a cause of birth defects. Since 1997, each center has annually enrolled 300 or more cases—including live births, stillbirths, and terminated pregnancies that have one or more of 30 structural birth defects, along with 100 randomly selected controls. Clinical geneticists review each potential case, and standardized telephone interviews are conducted 6 weeks and 24 months after delivery to obtain information regarding medication exposure and medical risk factors (Mitchell, 2011). This large volume has considerable statistical power and permits identification of relatively small associations.

As of 2012, the National Birth Defects Prevention Study (NBDPS) had identified associations between individual birth defects and the following classes of medications: sulfonamides and nitrofurantoin, asthma medications, antiemetics, nonsteroidal antiinflammatory drugs, and opioids (Broussard, 2011; Crider, 2009; Hernandez, 2012; Lin, 2012; Munsie, 2011). For each, the authors discussed the possibility that the observed associations may have been due to chance alone or that the underlying medical disorder for which the drug was given may have caused the abnormality. Based on the degree of risk identified, if any of these medications is eventually deemed teratogenic, it would be considered a low-risk teratogen, as subsequently discussed. Thus, the American College of Obstetricians and Gynecologists (2013b) considers nitrofurantoin and sulfonamides appropriate for first-trimester use if no suitable alternative is available, and they remain the first-line agents for treatment and prevention of urinary infections beyond the first trimester (Chap. 53, p. 1052).

CRITERIA FOR DETERMINING TERATOGENICITY

The guidelines shown in Table 12-2, which were proposed by Shepard (1994) as a framework for discussion, have proven

TABLE 12-2. Criteria for Determining Teratogenicity

Essential Criteria:

1. Careful delineation of clinical cases, particularly if there is a specific defect or syndrome
2. Proof that exposure occurred at critical time during development (see Fig. 12-1)
3. Consistent findings by at least two epidemiological studies with:
   a. exclusion of bias,
   b. adjustment for confounding variables,
   c. adequate sample size (power),
   d. prospective ascertainment if possible, and
   e. relative risk (RR) of 3.0 or greater, some recommend RR of 6.0 or greater

or

For a rare environmental exposure associated with a rare defect, at least three reported cases. This is easiest if defect is severe

Ancillary Criteria:

4. The association is biologically plausible
5. Teratogenicity in experimental animals is important but not essential
6. The agent acts in an unaltered form in an experimental model

Modified from Shepard 1994, 2002a.

useful for more than 20 years. Although all criteria may not be required to establish teratogenicity, the following tenets must be considered (Shepard, 2002a):

- The defect has been completely characterized. This is preferably done by a geneticist or dysmorphologist because various genetic and environmental factors may produce similar anomalies. It is easiest to prove causation when a rare exposure produces a rare defect, when at least three cases with the same exposure have been identified, and when the defect is severe.
- The agent must cross the placenta. Although almost all drugs cross the placenta, transport must be of sufficient quantity to directly influence embryonic or fetal development or to alter maternal or placental metabolism to exert an indirect effect. Placental transfer depends on maternal metabolism; on specific characteristics of the drug, such as protein binding and storage, molecular size, electrical charge, and lipid solubility; and on placental metabolism such as the cytochrome P_{450} enzyme systems. In early pregnancy, the placenta also has a relatively thick membrane that slows diffusion.
- Exposure must occur during a critical developmental period:
  1. The preimplantation period is the 2 weeks from fertilization to implantation and is known as the "all or none" period. As the zygote undergoes cleavage, an insult damaging a large number of cells typically causes embryonic death. However, if only a few cells are injured, compensation may be possible, with normal development (Clayton-Smith, 1996). Based on animal data, insults that appreciably diminish the cell number in the inner cell mass may produce a dose-dependent diminution in body length or size (Iahnaccone, 1987).
  2. The embryonic period is from the second through the eighth week. It encompasses organogenesis and is thus the most crucial period with regard to structural malformations. Critical developmental periods for each organ system are illustrated in Figure 12-1.
  3. The fetal period, which is beyond 8 weeks, is characterized by continued maturation and functional development, and during this time, certain organs remain vulnerable. For example, brain development remains susceptible to environmental influences such as alcohol exposure throughout pregnancy.
- A biologically plausible association is supportive. Because birth defects and medication exposures are both common, they may be temporally but not causally related.
- Epidemiological findings must be consistent. Because initial evaluation of teratogen exposure is often retrospective, it may be hampered by recall bias, inadequate reporting, and incomplete assessment of the exposed population. Potential confounding factors include varying dosages, concomitant drug therapy, and maternal disease(s). Familial and environmental factors can also influence development of birth defects. Thus, an important criterion for teratogenicity is that two or more high-quality epidemiological studies report similar findings. Finally, a relative risk of 3.0 or greater is generally considered necessary to support the hypothesis, whereas a lesser risk is interpreted with caution (Khouri, 1992).
- The suspected teratogen causes a defect in animal studies. Human teratogenicity is more likely if an agent produces an adverse effect in different animal species. However, a major lesson was learned from the thalidomide tragedy in that its teratogenicity was not recognized because of reliance on animal data, in which thalidomide produced no defects in several animal species. Not until thousands of infants were affected by thalidomide embryopathy was it realized that this agent was a potent human teratogen.

Failure to employ these tenets and criteria has contributed to erroneous conclusions regarding the safety of some widely used drugs. The poster child for this is the medicolegal fiasco surrounding Bendectin. This antiemetic was a combination of doxylamine and pyridoxine that was both safe and effective for nausea and vomiting common in early pregnancy. More than 30 million women used this drug worldwide, and the 3-percent congenital anomaly rate among exposed fetuses was not different from the background rate (McKeigue, 1994). Despite evidence that the drug was not teratogenic, Bendectin was the target of numerous lawsuits, and the financial burden of defending these forced its withdrawal. As a consequence, hospitalizations for hyperemesis doubled (Koren, 1998). Ironically, the combination of doxylamine and pyridoxine has now been recently remarketed under the brand name Diclegis, which was FDA approved in 2013.

COUNSELING FOR TERATOGEN EXPOSURE

Questions regarding medication and illicit drug use should be part of routine preconceptional and prenatal care. Women

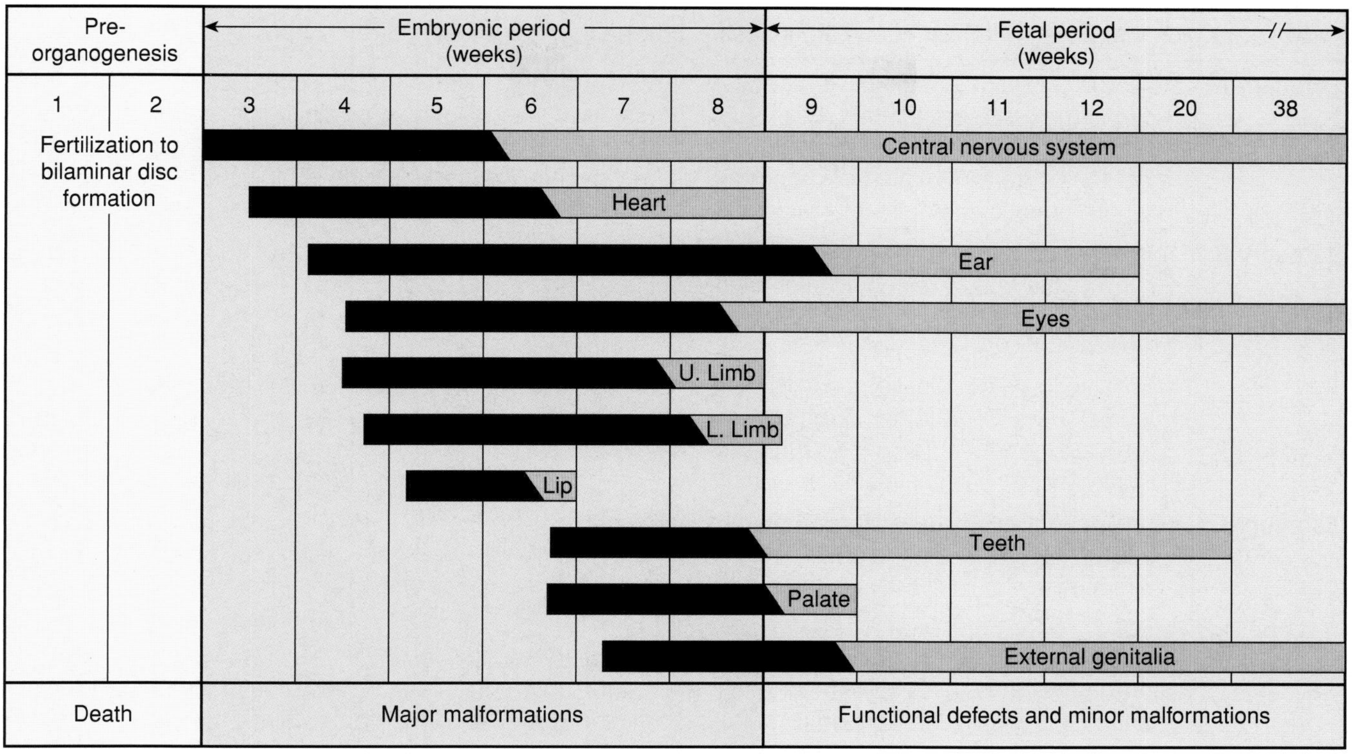

FIGURE 12-1 Timing of organogenesis during the embryonic period. (Redrawn from Sadler, 1990, with permission.)

who request counseling for prenatal drug exposure often have misinformation regarding their level of risk. Not uncommonly, they may underestimate the background risk for birth defects in the general population and exaggerate the potential risks associated with medication exposure. Koren and colleagues (1989) reported that a fourth of women exposed to nonteratogenic drugs thought they had a 25-percent risk for fetal anomalies. Misinformation may be amplified by inaccurate reports in the lay press. Knowledgeable counseling may allay anxiety considerably and in some situations may even avoid pregnancy termination.

The Food and Drug Administration Classification System

This system for evaluating drug safety in pregnancy was developed in 1979. It was designed to provide therapeutic guidance by using five categories—A, B, C, D, or X, shown in Table 12-3, to simplify risk-benefit information. In its present form, the system has important limitations, and these have been acknowledged by the FDA. One is that drugs in categories D and X, and some in category C, may pose similar risks but are in different categories because of different risk-benefit considerations. A higher letter grade does not necessarily confer an increased risk, and even drugs in the same category may have very different risks! And, despite the understanding that medications may affect human and animal development differently, the letter category is often based on animal data.

From the foregoing, it follows that it may be insufficient or even inappropriate to rely on this classification to make complex therapeutic decisions in pregnant women. Rather than simplifying counseling, the letter classification shifts responsibility to the clinician, who must interpret category information in the context of medication dosage, route and timing of exposure, other medications used, and underlying medical condition(s).

Because of the limitations of its current classification, the FDA (2011b) has proposed a new system for labeling drugs for use by pregnant and lactating women. Letter categories A through X are to be replaced with: (1) a fetal risk summary, (2) a section on clinical considerations—including inadvertent exposure, (3) a section on prescribing decisions for pregnant and lactating women, and (4) a detailed discussion of human and animal data. It is anticipated that this evidence-based rating system may soon become available (Gee, 2014).

The FDA has also expanded the information available on its website: www.fda.gov. The website includes updated, detailed information regarding potentially harmful medications—in the form of drug advisories, registries, and product information. It is an excellent resource for counseling. Current, accurate information is also available through online reproductive toxicity services such as Reprotox and TERIS.

Presenting Risk Information

In addition to potential embryonic and fetal risks from drug exposure, counseling should include a discussion of the risks and/or genetic implications of the underlying condition for which the drug is given, as well as risks associated with not treating the condition. Even the manner in which information is presented affects perception. Jasper and associates (2001) found that women given negative information—such as a 2-percent chance of a malformed infant—are more likely to

TABLE 12-3. Food and Drug Administration Categories for Drugs and Medications

Category A:	Studies in pregnant women have not shown an increased risk for fetal abnormalities if administered during the first (second, third, or all) trimester(s) of pregnancy, and the possibility of fetal harm appears remote. Fewer than 1 percent of all medications are in this category. Examples include levothyroxine, potassium supplementation, and prenatal vitamins, when taken at recommended doses.
Category B:	Animal reproduction studies have been performed and have revealed no evidence of impaired fertility or harm to the fetus. Prescribing information should specify kind of animal and how dose compares with human dose. ***or*** Animal studies have shown an adverse effect, but adequate and well-controlled studies in pregnant women have failed to demonstrate a risk to the fetus during the first trimester of pregnancy, and there is no evidence of a risk in later trimesters. Examples include many antibiotics, such as penicillins, most cephalosporins, and macrolides.
Category C:	Animal reproduction studies have shown that this medication is teratogenic (or embryocidal or has other adverse effect), and there are no adequate and well-controlled studies in pregnant women. Prescribing information should specify kind of animal and how dose compares with human dose. ***or*** There are no animal reproduction studies and no adequate and well-controlled studies in humans. Approximately two thirds of all medications are in this category. It contains medications commonly used to treat potentially life- threatening medical conditions, such as albuterol, zidovudine, and calcium-channel blockers.
Category D:	This medication can cause fetal harm when administered to a pregnant woman. If this drug is used during pregnancy or if a woman becomes pregnant while taking this medication, she should be apprised of the potential hazard to the fetus. This category also contains medications used to treat potentially life-threatening medical conditions, for example: corticosteroids, azathioprine, carbamazepine, and lithium.
Category X:	This medication is contraindicated in women who are or may become pregnant. It may cause fetal harm. If this drug is used during pregnancy or if a woman becomes pregnant while taking this medication, she should be apprised of the potential hazard to the fetus. There are a few medications in this category that have never been shown to cause fetal harm but should be avoided nonetheless, such as the rubella vaccine.

perceive an exaggerated risk than women given positive information—such as a 98-percent chance of a child without a malformation. Instead of citing an increased odds ratio, it may be helpful to provide the *absolute risk* for a particular defect or the *attributable risk*, which is the difference between prevalence in exposed and unexposed individuals (Conover, 2011). The association between oral corticosteroid medications and cleft lip sounds far more concerning when presented as a tripling or 200-percent increase in risk than when presented as an increase from 1 per 1000 to 3 per 1000, or a 99.7-percent likelihood of not developing a cleft following exposure.

With a few notable exceptions, most commonly prescribed drugs and medications can be used with relative safety during pregnancy. All women have an approximate 3-percent chance of having an infant with a birth defect. Although exposure to a confirmed teratogen may increase this risk, the magnitude of the increase is usually only 1 or 2 percent or at most, doubled or tripled. The concept of risk versus benefit is often central to counseling. Some untreated diseases pose a more serious threat to both mother and fetus than medication exposure risks.

There undoubtedly are a number of major teratogens. However, many drugs described in this chapter are low-risk teratogens, which are medications that produce defects in fewer than 10 per 1000 maternal exposures (Shepard, 2002a). Some examples include corticosteroids, lithium, trimethoprim, and methimazole. Because risks conferred by low-risk teratogens are so close to background, they may not be a major factor in deciding whether to discontinue treatment for an important condition (Shepard, 2002b). Obviously, clinicians and patients must carefully weigh risks and benefits in these instances.

GENETIC AND PHYSIOLOGICAL SUSCEPTIBILITY TO TERATOGENS

Teratogens act by disturbing specific physiological processes, which may in turn lead to abnormal cellular differentiation, altered tissue growth, or cell death. Because pathophysiological processes may be induced in various cell types and tissues, exposure may result in multiple effects, and because different teratogens may disturb similar processes, they may produce similar phenotypic abnormalities. But even the most potent teratogen induces birth defects in only a fraction of exposed embryos. Despite the numerous factors that influence exposure, teratogens appear merely to have potential to cause birth defects. The reasons why some infants are affected and others are not remains largely unknown.

Fetal Genome

In some cases, genetic composition has been linked to susceptibility to teratogenic effects of specific medications. For example, fetuses exposed to hydantoin are more likely to develop anomalies if homozygous for a gene mutation that results in abnormally low levels of epoxide hydrolase (Buehler, 1990). If activity of epoxide hydrolase enzyme is reduced, then hydantoin, carbamazepine, and phenobarbital are metabolized by microsomes to oxidative intermediates that accumulate in fetal tissues (Horning, 1974). These free oxide radicals have carcinogenic, mutagenic, and other toxic effects that are dose related and increase with multidrug therapy (Buehler, 1990; Lindhout, 1984).

Disruption of Folic Acid Metabolism

Fetal neural-tube defects, cardiac defects, and oral clefts can be a result of folic acid metabolic pathway disturbances. Folates are essential for methionine production, which is required for gene methylation and thus production of proteins, lipids, and myelin. Some anticonvulsants—phenytoin, carbamazepine, valproic acid, and phenobarbital—either impair folic acid absorption or act as folic acid antagonists. The resultant low periconceptional folic acid levels in some women with epilepsy may then cause fetal malformations (Dansky, 1987; Hiilesmaa, 1983). In one study of more than 5000 infants with birth defects, exposure to these folic acid antagonists was associated with a two- to threefold increased risk for oral clefts and cardiac abnormalities (Hernandez-Diaz, 2000).

Some congenital heart defects are related to interactions between folate-related genes and environmental or genetic factors. In a case-control study with more than 500 infants with a cardiac defect, maternal polymorphisms in three folate-related genes were found to increase the risk for cardiac anomalies when combined with maternal cigarette smoking, alcohol consumption, or obesity (Hobbs, 2010). Data from the National Down Syndrome Project demonstrated that trisomy 21 fetuses born to women not given periconceptional folic acid supplementation may be more likely to have endocardial cushion defects (Bean, 2011).

Paternal Exposures

In some cases, paternal exposures to drugs or environmental influences may increase the risk of adverse fetal outcome. Proposed mechanisms include induction of a gene mutation or chromosomal abnormality in sperm. Because of the 64 days in which male germ cells mature into functional spermatogonia, drug exposure during the 2 months before conception could cause gene mutations. It may be that epigenetic pathways suppress germ-cell apoptosis or interfere with imprinting (Cordier, 2008). Another possibility is that during intercourse the developing embryo is exposed to a teratogenic agent in seminal fluid.

There is some evidence to support these hypotheses. For example, ethyl alcohol, cyclophosphamide, lead, and certain opiates have been associated with an increased risk of behavioral defects in the offspring of exposed male rodents (Nelson, 1996). In humans, paternal environmental exposure to mercury, lead, solvents, pesticides, anesthetic gases, or hydrocarbons may be associated with early pregnancy loss (Savitz, 1994). In a 20-year study of Swedish university employees, paternal exposure to carcinogenic solvents resulted in offspring with more than a fourfold increase in neural-crest malformations (Magnusson, 2004). Other occupations associated with an increased risk for men to have anomalous offspring include janitors, woodworkers, firemen, printers, and painters (Olshan, 1991; Schnitzer, 1995). Risk attribution is limited because assessment of paternal exposure is often imprecise, and there is potential for simultaneous maternal exposure, particularly for environmental agents such as pesticides (Cordier, 2008).

KNOWN AND SUSPECTED TERATOGENS

The number of medications and other substances strongly suspected or proven to be human teratogens is small, as shown in Table 12-1. With few exceptions, in every clinical situation potentially requiring therapy with a known teratogen, alternative drugs can be given with relative safety. As a general rule, because there are no adequate and well-controlled studies in pregnant women for most medications, and because animal reproduction studies are not always predictive of human response, any medication in pregnancy must be carefully considered and only used if clearly needed.

Alcohol

Ethyl alcohol is a potent and prevalent teratogen. Alcohol is one of the most frequent nongenetic causes of mental retardation as well as the leading cause of preventable birth defects in the United States. According to the Centers for Disease Control and Prevention (CDC)(2012), 8 percent of women report drinking alcohol during pregnancy, and the NBDPS identified a prevalence as high as 30 percent (Ethen, 2009). Between 1 and 2 percent of pregnant women admit to binge drinking.

The fetal effects of alcohol abuse have been recognized since the 1800s. Lemoine (1968) and Jones (1973) and their coworkers are credited with describing the spectrum of alcohol-related fetal defects known as *fetal alcohol syndrome* (Table 12-4). The Institute of Medicine (1996) has estimated that prevalence of the syndrome ranges from 0.6 to 3 per 1000 births.

For every child with fetal alcohol syndrome, many more are born with neurobehavioral deficits from alcohol exposure (American College of Obstetricians and Gynecologist, 2013a). *Fetal alcohol spectrum disorder* is an umbrella term that includes the full range of prenatal alcohol damage that may not meet the criteria for fetal alcohol syndrome. Prevalence of this disorder is estimated to be as high as 1 percent of births in the United States (Centers for Disease Control, 2012; Guerri, 2009).

Clinical Characteristics

Fetal alcohol syndrome has specific criteria, listed in Table 12-4, and which include dysmorphic facial features, pre- or postnatal

TABLE 12-4. Fetal Alcohol Syndrome and Alcohol-Related Birth Defects

Fetal Alcohol Syndrome Diagnostic Criteria—all required
1. Dysmorphic facial features (all 3 are required)
   a. Small palpebral fissures
   b. Thin vermilion border
   c. Smooth philtrum
2. Prenatal and/or postnatal growth impairment
3. Central nervous system abnormalities (1 required)
   a. Structural: head size < 10th percentile, significant brain abnormality on imaging
   b. Neurological
   c. Functional: global cognitive or intellectual deficits, functional deficits in at least three domains

Alcohol-Related Birth Defects
1. Cardiac: atrial or ventricular septal defect, aberrant great vessels, conotruncal heart defects
2. Skeletal: radioulnar synostosis, vertebral segmentation defects, joint contractures, scoliosis
3. Renal: aplastic or hypoplastic kidneys, dysplastic kidneys, horseshoe kidney, ureteral duplication
4. Eyes: strabismus, ptosis, retinal vascular abnormalities, optic nerve hypoplasia
5. Ears: conductive or neurosensory hearing loss
6. Minor: hypoplastic nails, clinodactyly, pectus carinatum or excavatum, camptodactyly, "hockey stick" palmar creases, refractive errors, "railroad track" ears

Modified from Bertrand, 2005; Hoyme, 2005.

growth impairment, and central nervous system abnormalities that may be structural, neurological, or functional (Bertrand, 2005). The distinctive facial features are shown in Figure 12-2. Other alcohol-related major and minor birth defects include cardiac and renal anomalies, orthopedic problems, and abnormalities of the eyes and ears. An association has also been reported between periconceptional alcohol use and omphalocele and gastroschisis (Richardson, 2011). There are no established criteria for prenatal diagnosis of fetal alcohol syndrome, although in some cases, major abnormalities or growth restriction may be suggestive (Paintner, 2012).

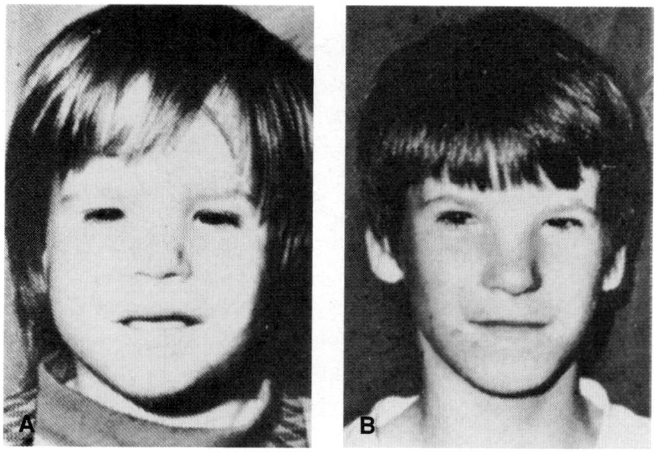

FIGURE 12-2 Fetal alcohol syndrome. **A.** At 2½ years. **B.** At 12 years. Note persistence of short palpebral fissures, epicanthal folds, flat midface, hypoplastic philtrum, and thin upper vermilion border. (From Streissguth, 1985, with permission.)

Dose Effect

Fetal vulnerability to alcohol is modified by genetic factors, nutritional status, environmental factors, coexisting maternal disease, and maternal age (Abel, 1995). The minimum amount of alcohol required to produce adverse fetal consequences is unknown. Binge drinking, however, is believed to pose particularly high risk for alcohol-related birth defects and has also been linked to an increased risk for stillbirth (Centers for Disease Control, 2012; Maier, 2001; Strandberg-Larsen, 2008).

Anticonvulsant Medications

Pragmatically, no anticonvulsant drugs are considered truly "safe" in pregnancy. This is because most medications used to treat epilepsy have been proven or suspected to confer an increased risk for fetal malformations. The North American Antiepileptic Drug (NAAED) Pregnancy Registry was established to improve counseling information. Providers are encouraged to enroll pregnant women treated with antiepileptic medication through the FDA website or 1–888–233–2334.

Management of epilepsy in pregnancy, including risks associated with individual anticonvulsants, is discussed in Chapter 60 (p. 1190). Traditionally, women with epilepsy were informed that their risk for fetal malformations was increased two- to threefold. More recent data suggest that the risk may not be as great as once thought, particularly for newer agents. In a recent population-based study involving more than 800,000 pregnancies, exposure to newer anticonvulsants was associated with a 3-percent major malformation risk, compared with a 2-percent risk in unexposed fetuses (Molgaard-Nielsen, 2011). Similarly, the United Kingdom Epilepsy and Pregnancy Registry reported a 3-percent risk for major malformations in pregnancies treated with a single anticonvulsant—monotherapy. This is the same malformation rate as for those with untreated epilepsy (Morrow, 2006). There is one important exception to these findings. Women treated with valproic acid are at significantly increased risk for malformations as subsequently discussed.

The most frequently reported anomalies are orofacial clefts, cardiac malformations, and neural-tube defects (Food and Drug Administration, 2009). Several older anticonvulsants produce a constellation of malformations similar to the fetal hydantoin syndrome (Fig. 12-3). Of agents in current use, valproic acid confers the greatest risk. The NAAED Pregnancy Registry reported that major malformations occurred in 9 percent of fetuses with first-trimester valproate exposure and included a 4-percent risk for neural-tube defects (Hernandez-Diaz, 2012). Moreover, children with in utero exposure to valproic acid are reported to have significantly lower intelligence quotient (IQ) scores at age 3 years compared with scores of those exposed to

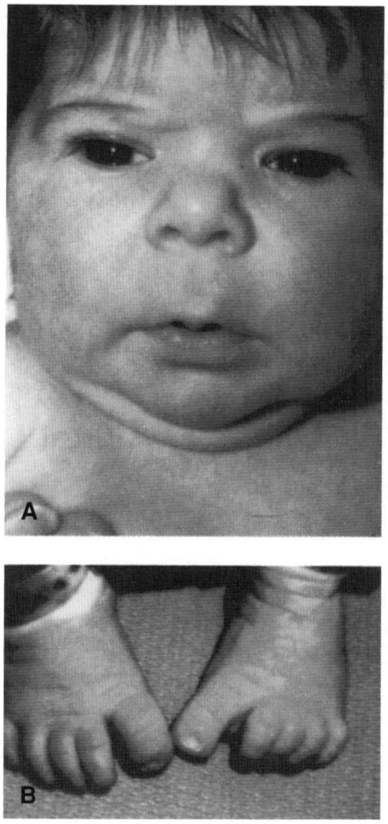

FIGURE 12-3 Fetal hydantoin syndrome. **A.** Facial features including upturned nose, mild midfacial hypoplasia, and long upper lip with thin vermilion border. **B.** Distal digital hypoplasia. (From Buehler, 1990, with permission.)

phenytoin, carbamazepine, or lamotrigine (Meador, 2009). Of the newer agents, topiramate has recently been reported by the NAAED Pregnancy Registry and the NBDPS to confer a risk for orofacial clefts at least fivefold higher than in unexposed pregnancies (Food and Drug Administration, 2011c; Margulis, 2012). Regardless of the anticonvulsant medication used, specialized sonography should be considered.

Angiotensin-Converting Enzyme Inhibitors and Angiotensin-Receptor Blocking Drugs

Angiotensin-converting enzyme (ACE) inhibitors are considered fetotoxic and result in ACE-inhibitor fetopathy. Normal renal development depends on the fetal renal-angiotensin system. ACE-inhibitor medication causes fetal hypotension and renal hypoperfusion, with subsequent ischemia and anuria (Guron, 2000; Pryde, 1993). Reduced perfusion may cause fetal-growth restriction and calvarium maldevelopment, whereas oligohydramnios may result in pulmonary hypoplasia and limb contractures (Barr, 1991). Because angiotensin-receptor blockers have a similar mechanism of action, concerns regarding fetotoxicity have been generalized to include this entire medication class.

The possible embryotoxicity of these two drug classes is less certain. Cooper and colleagues (2006) reported that first-trimester ACE-inhibitor exposure was associated with a two- to threefold increased risk for cardiac and central nervous system abnormalities, but these observations have not been corroborated. It is reasonable to offer specialized sonography for pregnancies with first-trimester exposure. Given the many therapeutic options for treating hypertension during pregnancy, discussed in Chapter 50 (p. 1006), it is recommended that ACE inhibitors and angiotensin receptor-blocking drugs be avoided.

Antifungal Medications

From this class of drugs, fluconazole has been associated with a pattern of congenital malformations resembling the autosomal recessive Antley-Bixler syndrome. Abnormalities include oral clefts, abnormal facies, and cardiac, skull, long-bone, and joint abnormalities. Such findings have been reported only with chronic, high-dose treatment in the first trimester—at doses of 400 to 800 mg daily. In a recent population-based cohort of more than 7000 pregnancies with first-trimester exposure to low-dose fluconazole, a threefold increased risk for tetralogy of Fallot was identified (Molgaard-Nielsen, 2013). However, risks for other birth defects were not increased. The FDA (2011e) lists fluconazole as pregnancy category D, but it states that a single 150-mg dose to treat vulvovaginal candidiasis does not appear to be teratogenic.

Antiinflammatory Agents

Nonsteroidal Antiinflammatory Drugs

This drug class includes both aspirin and traditional "NSAIDs" such as ibuprofen and indomethacin. They exert their effects by inhibiting prostaglandin synthesis. At least 20 percent of pregnant women report use of these drugs in the first trimester. But, based on data from the NBDPS, such exposure does not appear to be a major risk factor for birth defects (Hernandez, 2012). Aspirin is not considered to increase the overall risk for congenital malformations (Kozer, 2002). Low-dose aspirin, 100 mg daily or lower, does not confer an increased risk for constriction of the ductus arteriosus or for adverse infant outcomes (Di Sessa, 1994; Grab, 2000). As with other NSAIDs, however, high-dose aspirin use should be avoided, particularly in the third trimester.

Importantly, NSAIDs may cause adverse fetal effects when taken in late pregnancy (Parilla, 2004; Rebordosa, 2008). Indomethacin may cause constriction of the fetal ductus arteriosus, resulting in pulmonary hypertension. The drug may also decrease fetal urine production and thereby reduce amnionic fluid volume. This is presumed due to an increase in vasopressin levels and vasopressin responsiveness (Rasanen, 1995; van der Heijden, 1994; Walker, 1994). Fetal ductal constriction is more likely when the drug is taken in the third trimester for longer than 72 hours' duration. In a study of 60 exposed pregnancies, ductal constriction developed in 50 percent and was significantly more likely after 30 weeks (Vermillion, 1997). Fortunately, ductal flow velocity returned to normal in all fetuses following discontinuation of therapy. Other NSAIDs are assumed to confer similar risks.

Leflunomide

This is a pyrimidine-synthesis inhibitor used to treat rheumatoid arthritis (Chap. 59, p. 1177). It is considered contraindicated in pregnancy because when given at or below human-equivalent doses in several animal species, it is associated with multiple abnormalities. These include hydrocephalus, eye anomalies, skeletal abnormalities, and embryo death (sanofi-aventis, 2012). The active metabolite of leflunomide is detectable in plasma for up to 2 years following its discontinuation. Women of childbearing potential who discontinue this medication should consider cholestyramine treatment/washout, followed by verification that serum levels are undetectable on two tests performed 14 days apart. Guidelines are also available for cholestyramine treatment/washout for men who discontinue leflunomide and who are contemplating fatherhood (Brent, 2001).

Antimicrobial Drugs

Medications used to treat infections are among those most commonly administered during pregnancy. Over the years, experience has accrued regarding their general safety. With a few exceptions cited below, most of the commonly used antimicrobial agents are considered safe for the embryo/fetus.

Aminoglycosides

Preterm infants treated with gentamicin or streptomycin have developed nephrotoxicity and ototoxicity. Despite theoretical concern for potential fetal toxicity, no adverse effects have been demonstrated, and no congenital defects resulting from prenatal exposure have been identified.

Chloramphenicol

This antimicrobial is not considered teratogenic and is no longer routinely used in the United States. More than 50 years ago, a constellation of findings termed the gray baby syndrome was described in neonates who received the medication. Preterm infants were unable to conjugate and excrete the drug and manifested abdominal distention, respiratory abnormalities, an ashen-gray color, and vascular collapse (Weiss, 1960). Chloramphenicol was subsequently avoided in late pregnancy due to theoretical concerns.

Nitrofurantoin

As discussed on page 241, the NBDPS found an association between first-trimester nitrofurantoin exposure and selected birth defects. These include a fourfold increased risk for hypoplastic left heart syndrome and microphthalmia/anophthalmia and a twofold increased risk for clefts and atrial septal defects (Crider, 2009). For postexposure counseling purposes, the absolute risk of these defects remains quite low. For example, a fourfold increased incidence of hypoplastic left heart would result in a prevalence of less than 1 per 1000 exposed infants (Texas Department of State Health Services, 2012). Nitrofurantoin is a proven first-line treatment of urinary infections. The American College of Obstetricians and Gynecologists (2013b) has concluded that first-trimester nitrofurantoin use is appropriate if no suitable alternatives are available.

Sulfonamides

These drugs are often combined with trimethoprim and used to treat various infections during pregnancy. One example is treatment of methicillin-resistant *Staphylococcus aureus* (MRSA). The NBDPS found associations between first-trimester sulfonamide exposure and a threefold increased risk for anencephaly and left ventricular outflow tract obstruction, an eightfold increased risk for choanal atresia, and a twofold increased risk for diaphragmatic hernia (Crider, 2009). The American College of Obstetricians and Gynecologists (2013b) considers sulfonamides appropriate for first-trimester use if suitable alternatives are lacking. There are also theoretical concerns that because sulfonamides displace bilirubin from protein binding sites, they may worsen hyperbilirubinemia if given near the time of preterm delivery. However, a recent population-based review of more than 800,000 births from Denmark found no association between receiving sulfamethoxazole in late pregnancy and neonatal jaundice (Klarskov, 2013).

Tetracyclines

These drugs are no longer commonly used in pregnant women. They are associated with yellowish-brown discoloration of deciduous teeth when used after 25 weeks, although the risk for subsequent dental caries does not appear increased (Billing, 2004; Kutscher, 1966).

Antineoplastic Agents

Cancer management in pregnancy includes many chemotherapeutic agents generally considered to be at least potentially toxic to the embryo, fetus, or both. For the many novel polyclonal antibody therapies designated as antineoplastics, there are scant data concerning their safety. Some risks associated with cancer treatment with antineoplastic agents are discussed elsewhere—gestational trophoblastic neoplasia in Chapter 20 and cancer chemotherapy in Chapter 63. A few more common agents for which experience in pregnancy has accrued are considered below.

Cyclophosphamide

This alkylating agent inflicts a chemical insult on developing fetal tissues and leads to cell death and heritable DNA alterations in surviving cells. Pregnancy loss is increased, and reported malformations include skeletal abnormalities, limb defects, cleft palate, and eye abnormalities (Enns, 1999; Kirshon, 1988). Surviving infants may have growth abnormalities and developmental delays. Environmental exposure among health-care workers is associated with an increased risk for spontaneous abortion (Chap. 18, p. 354).

Methotrexate

This folic-acid antagonist is a potent teratogen. It is used for cancer chemotherapy, immunosuppression in conditions such as autoimmune diseases and psoriasis, nonsurgical treatment of ectopic pregnancy, and finally, as an abortifacient. It is similar in action to aminopterin, which is no longer in clinical use, and can cause defects known collectively as the fetal methotrexate-aminopterin syndrome. This includes craniosynostosis with "clover-leaf" skull, wide nasal bridge, low-set ears, micrognathia, and limb abnormalities (Del Campo, 1999). The critical developmental period of these abnormalities is believed to be 8 to 10 weeks, at a dosage of at least 10 mg/week, although this is not universally accepted (Feldcamp, 1993). As discussed in Chapter 19 (p. 384), the standard 50 mg/m^2 dose given to treat ectopic pregnancy or to induce elective abortion exceeds this threshold dose. Thus, ongoing pregnancies after treatment with methotrexate—especially if it is used in conjunction with misoprostol—raise serious concerns for fetal malformations (Creinin, 1994; Nurmohamed, 2011).

Tamoxifen

This nonsteroidal selective estrogen-receptor modulator (SERM) is used as an adjuvant to treat breast cancer (Chap. 63, p. 1231). Although it has not been associated with fetal malformations, it is fetotoxic and carcinogenic in rodents, inducing malformations similar to those caused by diethylstilbestrol (DES) exposure. Consequently, tamoxifen is pregnancy category D. It is recommended that women who become pregnant while either on therapy or within 2 months of its discontinuation be apprised of potential long-term risks of a DES-like syndrome. Exposed offspring should be monitored for carcinogenic effects for up to 20 years (Briggs, 2011).

Trastuzumab

This is a recombinant monoclonal antibody directed to the human epidermal growth factor receptor 2 (HER2) protein. It is used to treat breast cancers that over express HER2 protein (Chap. 63, p. 1230). This drug has not been associated with fetal malformations, but cases of oligohydramnios, anhydramnios, and fetal renal failure have been described (Beale, 2009; Sekar, 2007; Watson, 2005). Use may result in fetal pulmonary hypoplasia, skeletal abnormalities, and neonatal death.

Antiviral Agents

The number of drugs used to treat viral infections has increased rapidly during the past 20 years. For most, experience in pregnant women is limited.

Ribavirin

This nucleoside analogue is a component of therapy for hepatitis C infection, discussed in Chapter 55 (p. 1091). Ribavirin causes birth defects in multiple animal species at doses significantly lower than those recommended for human use. Reported malformations include skull, palate, eye, skeleton, and gastrointestinal abnormalities. The drug has a long half-life and persists in extravascular compartments following discontinuation of therapy. It is recommended that women use two forms of contraception while on therapy and delay childbearing for 6 months following drug discontinuation (Schering Corporation, 2012).

Efavirenz

This is a nonnucleoside reverse transcriptase inhibitor used to treat HIV infection (Chap. 65, p. 1279). Central nervous system and ocular abnormalities have been reported in cynomolgus monkeys treated with human-comparable doses. More worrisome are multiple case reports of central nervous system abnormalities following human exposure (Bristol-Meyers Squibb, 2010).

Endothelin-Receptor Antagonists

Two endothelin-receptor antagonists—bosentan and ambrisentan—are used to treat pulmonary arterial hypertension (Chap. 49, p. 986). Teratogenic concerns with these drugs stem from the fact that mice deficient in endothelin receptors develop abnormalities of the head, face, and large blood vessels. However, no human data are available (Clouthier, 1998). Bosentan and ambrisentan may be obtained only through restricted programs—the Tracleer Access Program for bosentan and the Letairis Education and Access Program (LEAP) for ambrisentan. Each program has stringent requirements for women, including contraception and monthly pregnancy tests (Actelion Pharmaceuticals, 2012; Food and Drug Administration, 2012).

Sex Hormones

Some of the functions and effects of male and female hormones on the developing fetus are discussed in Chapter 7 (p. 147). It is intuitive that exposure of female fetuses to excessive male sex hormones—and vice versa—might be detrimental.

Testosterone and Anabolic Steroids

Androgen exposure in reproductive-aged women is typically anabolic steroid use to increase lean body mass and muscular strength. Exposure of a female fetus may cause varying degrees of virilization and may result in ambiguous genitalia similar to that encountered in cases of congenital adrenal hyperplasia (Fig. 7-18A, p. 149). Findings may include labioscrotal fusion with first-trimester exposure and phallic enlargement from later fetal exposure (Grumbach, 1960; Schardein, 1985).

Danazol

This ethinyl testosterone derivative has weak androgenic activity. It is used to treat endometriosis, immune thrombocytopenic purpura, migraine headaches, premenstrual syndrome, and fibrocystic breast disease. In a review of inadvertent exposure during early pregnancy, Brunskill (1992) reported that 40 percent of exposed female fetuses were virilized. There was a dose-related pattern of clitoromegaly, fused labia, and urogenital sinus malformation.

Diethylstilbestrol

From 1940 until 1971, between 2 and 10 million pregnant women were given this synthetic estrogen. Subsequently, Herbst and associates (1971) reported a series of eight women exposed to DES in utero who developed an otherwise rare neoplasm, vaginal clear-cell adenocarcinoma. The absolute cancer risk in DES-exposed fetuses was approximately 1 per 1000, with no relationship to dosage. Women with in utero DES exposure also had a twofold increase in vaginal and cervical intraepithelial neoplasia (Vessey, 1989).

Diethylstilbestrol exposure has further been associated with genital tract abnormalities in exposed fetuses of both genders. Women may have a hypoplastic, T-shaped uterine cavity; cervical collars, hoods, septa, and coxcombs; and "withered" fallopian tubes, as described and illustrated in Chapter 3 (p. 42) (Goldberg, 1999; Salle, 1996). Later in life, women exposed in utero have slightly higher rates of earlier menopause and breast cancer (Hoover, 2011). Men may develop epididymal cysts, microphallus, hypospadias, cryptorchidism, and testicular hypoplasia (Klip, 2002; Stillman, 1982).

Immunosuppressant Medications

Some of the immune functions necessary for pregnancy maintenance are discussed in Chapter 5 (p. 97). Given these important interactions, it would be logical that immunosuppressant drugs might affect pregnancy.

Corticosteroids

These medications include glucocorticoids and mineralocorticoids, which have antiinflammatory and immunosuppressive actions. They are commonly used to treat serious disorders such as asthma and autoimmune disease. Corticosteroids have been associated with clefts in animal studies. In a metaanalysis of case-control studies by the Motherisk program, systemic corticosteroid exposure was associated with a threefold increase in clefts, an absolute risk of 3 per 1000 exposed fetuses (Park-Wyllie, 2000). A 10-year prospective cohort study by the same group, however, did not identify increased risks for major malformations. Based on these findings, corticosteroids are not considered to represent a major teratogenic risk. Unlike other corticosteroids, the active metabolite of prednisone, which is prednisolone, is inactivated by the placental enzyme 11-beta-hydroxysteroid dehydrogenase 2 and does not effectively reach the fetus.

Mycophenolate Mofetil

This inosine monophosphate dehydrogenase inhibitor, and a related agent, mycophenolic acid, are potent immunosuppressants used to prevent rejection in organ-transplant recipients. They are also used for treatment of autoimmune disease such as lupus nephritis (Chap. 59, p. 1172). The National Transplantation Pregnancy Registry reported that almost half of exposed pregnancies spontaneously aborted and a fifth of surviving infants had malformations—nearly half of which were ear abnormalities (Food and Drug Administration, 2008). A Risk Evaluation and Mitigation Strategy (REMS) is necessary before mycophenolate is prescribed. Providers receive a brochure detailing associated risks; acceptable protocols for contraception during therapy—because the medication may decrease oral contraceptive efficacy; importance of reporting pregnancies that are conceived while on therapy to the Pregnancy Registry; and finally, a patient-prescriber acknowledgement form.

Radioiodine

Radioactive iodine-131 is used in the treatment of thyroid cancer and thyrotoxicosis and for diagnostic thyroid scanning (Chap. 63, p. 1231). It is also a component of iodine-131 tositumomab therapy, which is employed to treat a type of non-Hodgkin lymphoma. Radioiodine is contraindicated during pregnancy because it readily crosses the placenta and is then concentrated in the fetal thyroid gland by 12 weeks. It causes irreversible fetal hypothyroidism and may increase the risk for childhood thyroid cancer (Chap. 58, p. 1149).

Lead

Prenatal lead exposure is associated with fetal-growth abnormalities and with childhood developmental delay and behavioral abnormalities. According to the CDC (2010), there is no lead exposure level that is considered safe in pregnancy. Care for at-risk pregnancies is discussed in Chapter 9 (p. 183).

Mercury

Environmental spills of methyl mercury in Minamata Bay, Japan, and rural Iraq demonstrated that the developing nervous system is particularly susceptible to this heavy metal. Prenatal exposure causes disturbances in neuronal cell division and migration and leads to a range of defects from developmental delay to microcephaly and severe brain damage (Choi, 1978). The principal concern for prenatal mercury exposure is the consumption of certain species of large fish (Chap. 9, p. 183). Pregnant women are advised to not eat shark, swordfish, king mackerel, or tilefish, and consumption of albacore tuna should be limited to 6 ounces per week (Food and Drug Administration, 2004).

Psychiatric Medications

Treatment of psychiatric illness in pregnancy, including a discussion of the risks and benefits of various psychiatric medications, is discussed in Chapter 61 (p. 1204). Selected birth defects and adverse effects associated with specific medications are presented here.

Lithium

This medication has been associated with Ebstein anomaly, a cardiac abnormality characterized by apical displacement of the tricuspid valve. Ebstein anomaly often results in severe tricuspid regurgitation and marked right atrial enlargement, which confer significant morbidity. Its prevalence in the absence of lithium is approximately 1 per 20,000 births. Although a report from the Lithium Baby Register initially suggested that the risk for Ebstein anomaly was as high as 3 percent, subsequent series have demonstrated that the attributable risk is only 1 to 2 per 1000 exposed pregnancies (Reprotox, 2012; Weinstein, 1977). Fetal echocardiography should be considered for pregnancies exposed to lithium in the first trimester.

Neonatal lithium toxicity from exposure near delivery has been well documented. Findings typically persist for 1 to 2 weeks and may include hypothyroidism, diabetes insipidus, cardiomegaly, bradycardia, electrocardiogram abnormalities, cyanosis, and hypotonia (American College of Obstetricians and Gynecologists, 2012b; Briggs, 2011).

Selective Serotonin- and Norepinephrine-Reuptake Inhibitors

As a class, these medications are not considered major teratogens (American College of Obstetricians and Gynecologists, 2012b; Hviid, 2013). The one exception is paroxetine, which has been associated with increased risk for cardiac anomalies, particularly atrial and ventricular septal defects. Three large databases—a Swedish national registry, a United States insurance claims database, and the Motherisk Program—all identified a similar 1.5- to twofold increased rate of cardiac malformations following first-trimester paroxetine exposure (Bar-Oz, 2007; Food and Drug Administration, 2005a). For these reasons, the American College of Obstetricians and Gynecologists (2012b) recommends that paroxetine be avoided in women planning pregnancy, and that fetal echocardiography be considered for those with first-trimester paroxetine exposure.

Neonatal effects have been associated with prenatal exposure to selective serotonin-reuptake inhibitors (SSRIs) and selective norepinephrine-reuptake inhibitors (SNRIs). Approximately 25 percent of infants exposed to SSRIs in late pregnancy have been found to manifest one or more nonspecific findings considered to represent poor neonatal adaptation (Chambers, 2006; Costei, 2002; Jordan, 2008). Collectively termed the *neonatal behavioral syndrome*, findings may include jitteriness, irritability, hyper- or hypotonia, feeding abnormalities, vomiting, hypoglycemia, thermoregulatory instability, and respiratory abnormalities. Fortunately, these neonatal effects are typically mild and self-limited, lasting only about 2 days. Jordan and coworkers (2008) reported that newborns of mothers whose depression was not treated with medication were not more likely to require a higher level of care or extended hospitalization than SSRI-exposed newborns. Rarely, infants exposed to SSRIs in late pregnancy may demonstrate more severe adaptation abnormalities, including seizures, hyperpyrexia, excessive weight loss, or respiratory failure. This has been reported in 0.3 percent and has been compared to manifestations of SSRI toxicity or withdrawal in adults (Levin, 2004).

Another concern with late-pregnancy exposure is the possible association of SSRI medications with persistent pulmonary hypertension of the newborn. Its baseline incidence is 1 to 2 per 1000 term infants and is characterized by high pulmonary vascular resistance, right-to-left shunting, and profound hypoxemia. Chambers and colleagues (2006) identified a sixfold increase in pulmonary hypertension among those infants exposed to SSRIs after 20 weeks. A population-based cohort study involving 1.6 million pregnancies from the five Nordic countries identified a twofold increased risk following late-pregnancy exposure, an attributable risk of approximately 2 per 1000 births (Kieler, 2012). Other investigators have not found any increased risk (Wilson, 2011).

Antipsychotic Medications

There are no antipsychotic medications that are considered teratogenic. Exposed neonates have manifested abnormal extrapyramidal muscle movements and withdrawal symptoms, including agitation, abnormally increased or decreased muscle tone, tremor, sleepiness, feeding difficulty, and respiratory abnormalities. These findings are nonspecific and transient, similar to the neonatal behavioral syndrome that has been described following SSRI exposure. An FDA (2011a) alert cited all medications in this class. These include older drugs such as haloperidol and chlorpromazine, as well as newer medications such as aripiprazole, olanzapine, quetiapine, and risperidone.

Retinoids

These vitamin A derivatives are among the most potent human teratogens. Three retinoids available in the United States are highly teratogenic when orally administered—isotretinoin, acitretin, and bexarotene. By inhibiting neural-crest cell migration during embryogenesis, they result in a pattern of cranial neural-crest defects—termed retinoic acid embryopathy—that involve the central nervous system, face, heart, and thymus (Fig. 12-4). Specific anomalies may include ventriculomegaly, maldevelopment of the facial bones or cranium, microtia or anotia, micrognathia, cleft palate, conotruncal heart defects, and thymic aplasia or hypoplasia.

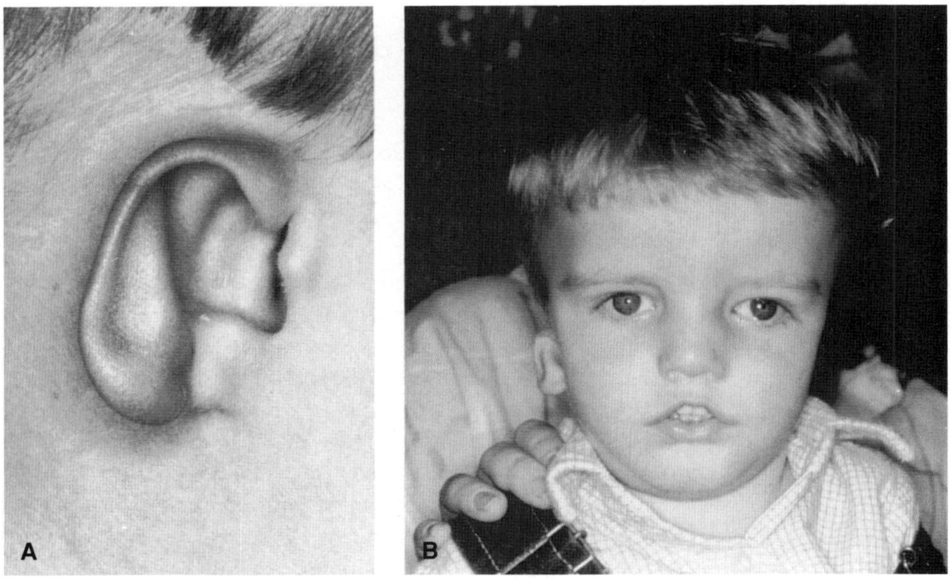

FIGURE 12-4 Isotretinoin embryopathy. **A.** Bilateral microtia or anotia with stenosis of external ear canal. **B.** Flat, depressed nasal bridge and ocular hypertelorism. (Photograph contributed by Dr. Edward Lammer.)

Isotretinoin

13-*cis*-Retinoic acid is a vitamin A isomer that stimulates epithelial cell differentiation and is used for dermatological disorders, especially cystic nodular acne. First-trimester exposure is associated with a high rate of pregnancy loss, and up to a third of fetuses have malformations (Lammer, 1985). The iPLEDGE program is an FDA-mandated REMS for isotretinoin and is found at: www.ipledgeprogram.com. This web-based restricted distribution program requires participation for all patients, physicians, and pharmacies to eliminate embryo-fetal exposure. Although other countries have instituted similar programs, inadvertent exposure remains a global concern (Crijns, 2011).

Acitretin

This retinoid is used to treat severe psoriasis. Acitretin was introduced to replace etretinate, a lipophilic retinoid with such a long half-life (120 days) that birth defects resulted more than 2 years after therapy was discontinued. Although acitretin has a short half-life, it is metabolized to etretinate, and thus remains in the body for prolonged periods (Stiefel Laboratories, 2011). To obviate exposure, the manufacturer of acitretin has developed a pregnancy risk management program called "Do Your P.A.R.T"–Pregnancy prevention Actively Required during and after Treatment, which is found at: www.soriatane.com. It promotes a delay of conception for at least 3 years following therapy discontinuation.

Bexarotene

This retinoid is used to treat cutaneous T-cell lymphoma. When given to rats in human-comparable doses, fetuses developed eye and ear abnormalities, cleft palate, and incomplete ossification (Eisai Inc., 2011). To receive this medication, the manufacturer requires two forms of contraception, beginning one month before therapy and continuing for one month after discontinuation, and monthly pregnancy tests during treatment (Eisai Inc., 2011). Males who have partners who could become pregnant are advised to use condoms during sexual intercourse while taking bexarotene and for one month after discontinuing therapy.

Topical Retinoids

These compounds, initially used to treat acne, have become so popular for the treatment of sun damage that they are called cosmeceuticals (Panchaud, 2011). Examples include topical tretinoin and tazarotene. Systemic absorption is low, and this argues against plausible teratogenicity. Still, the manufacturer of tazarotene cautions that application over a sufficient body surface area could be comparable with oral treatment, which causes cranial neural-crest defects in animals (Allergan, 2011). Isolated case reports have described malformations following topical tretinoin. However, a prospective study by the European Network of Teratology Information Services, which included more than 200 pregnancies with first-trimester exposure to topical retinoids, found no differences in the rate of spontaneous abortion or birth defects compared with that of nonexposed pregnancies (Panchaud, 2011).

Vitamin A

There are two natural forms of vitamin A. Beta-carotene, which is a precursor of provitamin A, is found in fruits and vegetables and has never been shown to cause birth defects (Oakley, 1995). Retinol is preformed vitamin A, which has been associated with cranial neural-crest defects when more than 10,000 IU per day were consumed in the first trimester (Rothman, 1995). It seems reasonable to avoid doses of preformed preparations that exceed the recommended 3000 IU daily allowance (American Academy of Pediatrics and American College of Obstetricians and Gynecologists, 2012).

Thalidomide and Lenalidomide

The drug thalidomide is likely the most notorious human teratogen. It causes malformations in 20 percent of fetuses exposed between 34 and 50 days menstrual age. The characteristic malformation is phocomelia—an absence of one or more long bones, which results in the hands or feet being attached to the trunk by a small rudimentary bone. Cardiac malformations, gastrointestinal abnormalities, and other limb reduction defects are also common following thalidomide exposure.

Thalidomide was marketed outside the United States from 1956 to 1960, before its teratogenicity was appreciated. The ensuing disaster, with thousands of affected children, was instructive of a number of important teratological principles:

1. The placenta is not a perfect barrier to the transfer of toxic substances from mother to fetus (Dally, 1998).
2. There is extreme variability in species susceptibility to drugs and chemicals. Because thalidomide produced no defects in experimental mice and rats, it had been assumed to be safe for humans.
3. There is a close relationship between exposure timing and defect type (Knapp, 1962). Upper-limb phocomelia developed with thalidomide exposure during days 27 to 30. This coincides with appearance of the upper-limb buds at day 27. Lower-limb phocomelia was associated with exposure during days 30 to 33, gallbladder aplasia at 42 to 43 days, duodenal atresia at 40 to 47 days.

Thalidomide was first approved in the United States in 1999, and currently it is used to treat leprosy and multiple myeloma (Celgene, 2013). The FDA has mandated an REMS for thalidomide called THALOMID REMS, which is found at: www.thalomidrems.com/. This web-based restricted distribution program is required before participation by patients, physicians, and pharmacies.

Lenalidomide is an analogue of thalidomide that is used to treat some types of myelodysplastic syndrome and multiple myeloma. Because of obvious teratogenicity concerns, an REMS has been developed similar to that used for thalidomide, called the Revlimid REMS and is found at: www.revlimidrems.com/.

Warfarin

Like other coumarin derivatives, warfarin is a vitamin K antagonist and a potent anticoagulant. It has a low molecular weight and readily crosses the placenta, causing embryotoxic and fetotoxic effects. Exposure between the 6th and 9th weeks may result in warfarin embryopathy. This is characterized by stippling of the vertebrae and femoral epiphyses and by nasal hypoplasia with depression of the nasal bridge as shown in Figure 12-5 (Hall, 1980). Affected infants may also have choanal atresia, resulting in respiratory distress. The syndrome is a phenocopy of chondrodysplasia punctata, a group of genetic diseases thought to be caused by defects in osteocalcin. In studies conducted before the mid-1980s, warfarin embryopathy was reported in approximately 10 percent of exposed pregnancies (Briggs, 2011). A more recent study by the European Network of Teratology Information Services involving more than 600 pregnancies exposed to vitamin K antagonists found that warfarin embryopathy occurred in less than 1 percent of

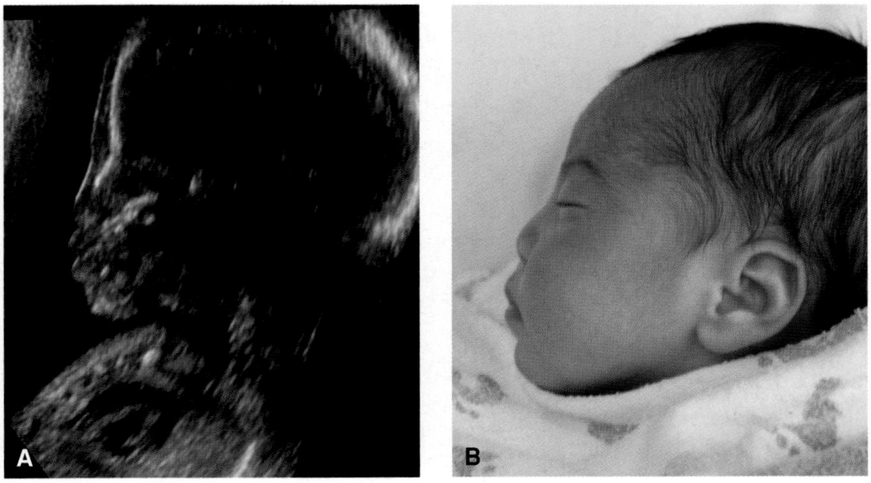

FIGURE 12-5 Warfarin embryopathy or fetal warfarin syndrome: nasal hypoplasia and depressed nasal bridge seen in a fetal sonographic image **(A)** and in the same newborn **(B)**.

cases. However, the overall rate of structural abnormalities was increased nearly fourfold (Schaefer, 2006). The risk of embryopathy may be greater in women who require more than 5 mg daily (Vitale, 1999).

When used beyond the first trimester, warfarin exposure may result in hemorrhage into fetal structures, which can cause abnormal growth and deformation from scarring (Warkany, 1976). Abnormalities may include agenesis of the corpus callosum; cerebellar vermian agenesis, which is the Dandy-Walker malformation; microphthalmia; and optic atrophy (Hall, 1980). Affected infants are also at risk for blindness, deafness, and developmental delays (Briggs, 2011).

Herbal Remedies

Risks associated with various herbal remedies are difficult to estimate because these compounds are not regulated by the FDA. Thus, the identity, quantity, and purity of each ingredient are usually unknown. Because animal studies have not been conducted, knowledge of complications may be limited to reports of acute toxicity (Hepner, 2002; Sheehan, 1998). Given these uncertainties, it seems prudent to counsel pregnant women to avoid these substances. A list of selected herbal compounds and their potential effects is shown in Table 12-5.

Recreational Drugs

At least 10 percent of fetuses are exposed to one or more illicit drugs (American Academy of Pediatrics and the American College of Obstetricians and Gynecologists, 2012). Assessment of outcomes attributable to illicit drugs may be confounded by factors such as poor maternal health, malnutrition, infectious disease, and polysubstance abuse. As discussed on page 245, alcohol is a significant teratogen, and because it is legally obtained and ubiquitous, its use also confounds that of illicit drugs. Moreover, illegal substances may contain toxic contaminants such as lead, cyanide, herbicides, and pesticides. Impurities added as diluents may independently have serious adverse perinatal effects. Some examples include fine glass beads, sawdust, strychnine, arsenic, antihistamines, and warfarin.

Amphetamines

These sympathomimetic amines are not considered to be major teratogens. Some are used to dilute other illicit drugs. Methamphetamine is prescribed to treat obesity, narcolepsy, and attention deficit disorders. In utero exposure to methamphetamine is associated with fetal-growth restriction and with behavioral abnormalities in both infancy and early childhood. Limited data are available regarding later development (LaGasse, 2011a,b; Little, 1988).

Cocaine

This central nervous system stimulant is derived from the leaves of the *Erythroxylum coca* tree. Most adverse outcomes associated with cocaine result from its vasoconstrictive and hypertensive effects. It can cause serious maternal complications such as cerebrovascular hemorrhage, myocardial damage, and placental abruption. Studies of congenital abnormalities in the setting of cocaine exposure have yielded conflicting results, but associations have been reported with cleft palate, cardiovascular abnormalities, and urinary tract abnormalities (Chasnoff, 1988; Chavez, 1989; Lipshultz, 1991; van Gelder, 2009). Cocaine use is also associated with fetal-growth restriction and preterm delivery. Children exposed as fetuses are at increased risk for behavioral abnormalities and cognitive impairments (Bada, 2011; Gouin, 2011; Singer, 2002).

Opioids–Narcotics

As a class, opioids are not considered to be major teratogens. That said, the NBDPS has identified a slightly increased risk for spina bifida, gastroschisis, and cardiac abnormalities in the setting of periconceptional exposure to therapeutic opioid medication (Broussard, 2011).

In contrast, opioid use is strongly associated with adverse fetal and neonatal effects. Heroin-addicted pregnant women are at increased risk for preterm birth, placental abruption, fetal-growth restriction, and fetal death—in part due to the effects of repeated narcotic withdrawal on the fetus and placenta (American College of Obstetricians and Gynecologists, 2012a; Center for Substance Abuse Treatment, 2008). Neonatal narcotic withdrawal, which is called the neonatal abstinence syndrome, may manifest in up to 90 percent of exposed infants (Blinick, 1973; Finnegan, 1975; Zelson, 1973). It is characterized by central nervous system irritability that may progress to seizures if untreated, along with tachypnea, episodes of apnea, poor feeding, and failure to thrive. At-risk neonates are closely monitored using a scoring system, and those severely affected are treated with opioids

TABLE 12-5. Pharmacological Actions and Adverse Effects of Some Herbal Medicines

Herb and Common Name	Relevant Pharmacological Effects	Concerns
Black cohosh	Smooth muscle stimulant	Causes uterine contractions; also has an estrogenic compound
Blue cohosh	Smooth muscle stimulant	Causes uterine contractions; contains compounds teratogenic in multiple animal species
Echinacea: *purple coneflower root*	Activates cell-mediated immunity	Allergic reactions; decreases immunosuppressant effectiveness; possible immunosuppression with long-term use
Ephedra: *ma huang*	Direct and indirect sympathomimetic; tachycardia and hypertension	Hypertension, arrhythmias, myocardial ischemia, stroke; depletes endogenous catecholamines; life-threatening interaction with monoamine oxidase inhibitors
Evening primrose oil	Contains linoleic acids, a prostaglandin precursor	Possible complications if used for labor induction
Garlic: *ajo*	Inhibits platelet aggregation; increased fibrinolysis; antihypertensive activity	Risk of bleeding, especially when combined with other platelet aggregation inhibitors
Ginger	Cyclooxygenase inhibitor	Increased risk of bleeding
Ginkgo biloba	Anticoagulant	Risk of bleeding; interferes with monoamine oxidase inhibitors
Ginseng	Lowers blood glucose; inhibition of platelet aggregation	Hypoglycemia; hypertension; risk of bleeding
Kava: *awa, intoxicating pepper, kawa*	Sedation, anxiolysis	Sedation; tolerance and withdrawal
Valerian: *all heal, garden heliotrope, vandal root*	Sedation	Sedation; hepatotoxicity, benzodiazepine-like acute withdrawal
Yohimbe		Hypertension, arrhythmias

Data from Ang-Lee, 2001; Briggs, 2011; Hall, 2012.

(Center for Substance Abuse Treatment, 2008; Finnegan, 1975). Data from the Birth Events Records Database from Washington state suggest that the proportion of exposed infants developing neonatal abstinence syndrome has increased in the past decade (Creanga, 2012).

Methadone is a synthetic opioid that has been routinely offered to pregnant heroin users since the 1970s to obviate uncontrolled narcotic withdrawal. It has a half-life of 24 to 36 hours and blocks narcotic cravings without producing intoxication. Women treated with methadone during pregnancy have been reported to be at increased risk for preterm birth and fetal-growth restriction (Cleary, 2010). Neonatal abstinence syndrome may occur in 40 to 70 percent of methadone-exposed infants and may be more protracted than with heroin exposure (Cleary, 2011; Dashe, 2002; Seligman, 2010). There is controversy as to whether a dose-response relationship exists between the maternal methadone dosage and neonatal withdrawal. At Parkland Hospital, pregnant opioid users are offered inpatient hospitalization for controlled methadone taper, with the goal of reducing the likelihood of neonatal abstinence syndrome (Dashe, 2002; Stewart, 2013). The American College of Obstetricians and Gynecologists (2012a) discourages withdrawal from methadone during pregnancy because of high relapse rates.

Miscellaneous Drugs

Marijuana use has not been associated with an increased risk for human fetal anomalies. Its active ingredient, delta-9-tetrahydrocannabinol, is teratogenic when given in high doses to animals. *Phencyclidine (PCP)* or angel dust is not associated with congenital anomalies. More than half of exposed newborns, however, experience withdrawal symptoms characterized by tremors, jitteriness, and irritability. *Toluene* is a common solvent used in paints and glue. Occupational exposure is reported to have significant fetal risks (Wilkins-Haug, 1997). It is abused by intentional inhalation, which produces lightheadedness, dizziness, and loss of consciousness. When abused by women in early pregnancy, it is associated with toluene embryopathy, which is phenotypically similar to fetal alcohol syndrome. Abnormalities include pre- and postnatal growth deficiency, microcephaly, and characteristic face and hand findings. These include midface hypoplasia, short palpebral fissures, wide nasal bridge, and abnormal palmar creases (Pearson, 1994). Up to 40 percent of exposed children have developmental delays (Arnold, 1994).

Tobacco

Cigarette smoke contains a complex mixture of nicotine, cotinine, cyanide, thiocyanate, carbon monoxide, cadmium, lead, and various hydrocarbons (Stillerman, 2008). In addition to being fetotoxic, many of these substances have vasoactive effects or reduce oxygen levels. Tobacco is not considered a major teratogen, although selected birth defects have been reported to occur with increased frequency among infants of women who smoke. It is plausible that the vasoactive properties of tobacco smoke could produce congenital defects related to vascular disturbances. For example, the prevalence of Poland sequence, which is caused by an interruption in the vascular supply to one side of the fetal chest and ipsilateral arm, is increased twofold (Martinez-Frias, 1999). An increased risk for cardiac anomalies has also been reported and may be dose-related (Alverson, 2011; Malik, 2008). A study using data from the National Vital Statistics System of more than 6 million births found an association between maternal smoking and hydrocephaly, microcephaly, omphalocele, gastroschisis, cleft lip and palate, and hand abnormalities (Honein, 2001).

The best-documented adverse reproductive outcome from smoking is a dose-response reduction in fetal growth. Newborns of mothers who smoke weigh an average of 200 g less than newborns of nonsmokers (D'Souza, 1981). Smoking doubles the risk of low birthweight and increases the risk of fetal-growth restriction two- to threefold (Werler, 1997). Growth disparity can be detected sonographically between 10 and 20 weeks (Mercer, 2008). Women who stop smoking early in pregnancy generally have neonates with normal birthweights (Cliver, 1995). Cigarette smoking has also been linked to subfertility and spontaneous abortions, to an increased risk for placenta previa and placental abruption, and to preterm delivery.

REFERENCES

Abel EL, Hannigan, JH: Maternal risk factors in fetal alcohol syndrome: provocative and permissive influences. Neurotoxicol Teratol 17(4):445, 1995

Actelion Pharmaceuticals: Tracleer (Bosentan) risk evaluation mitigation strategy. 2010. Available at: http://www.accessdata.fda.gov/drugsatfda_docs/label/2010/021290s018REMS.pdf. Accessed April 10, 2013

Adam MP, Polifka JE, Friedman JM: Evolving knowledge of the teratogenicity of medications in human pregnancy. Am J Med Genet Part C 157:175, 2011

Allergan: Tazorac. Available at: http://www.allergan.com/assets/pdf/tazorac_cream_pi.pdf. Accessed April 10, 2013

Alverson CJ, Strickland MJ, Gilboa SM, et al: Maternal smoking and congenital heart defects in the Baltimore-Washington Infant Study. Pediatrics 127:e647, 2011

American Academy of Pediatrics and American College of Obstetricians and Gynecologists: Guidelines for Perinatal Care, 7th ed. 2012

American College of Obstetricians and Gynecologists: Opioid abuse, dependence, and addiction in pregnancy. Committee Opinion No. 524, May 2012a

American College of Obstetricians and Gynecologists: Use of psychiatric medications during pregnancy and lactation. Practice Bulletin No. 92, April 2008, Reaffirmed 2012b

American College of Obstetricians and Gynecologists: At-risk drinking and alcohol dependence: obstetric and gynecologic implications. Committee Opinion No. 496, August 2013a

American College of Obstetricians and Gynecologists: Sulfonamides, nitrofurantoin, and risk of birth defects. Committee Opinion No. 494, June 2011, Reaffirmed 2013b

Andrade SE, Gurwitz JH, Davis RL, et al: Prescription drug use in pregnancy. Am J Obstet Gynecol 191:398, 2004

Ang-Lee MK, Moss J, Yuan CS: Herbal medicines and perioperative care. JAMA 286:208, 2001

Arnold GL, Kirby RS, Langendoerfer S, et al: Toluene embryopathy: clinical delineation and developmental follow-up. Pediatrics 93:216, 1994

Bada HS, Bann C, Bauer CR, et al: Preadolescent behavior problems after prenatal cocaine exposure: relationship between teacher and caretaker ratings. Neurotoxicol Teratol 33:78, 2011

Bar-Oz B, Einarson T, Einarson A, et al: Paroxetine and congenital malformations: meta-analysis and consideration of potential confounding factors. Clin Ther 29:918, 2007

Barr M, Cohen MM: ACE inhibitor fetopathy and hypocalvaria: the kidney-skull connection. Teratology 44:485, 1991

Beale JM, Tuohy J, McDowell SJ: Herceptin (trastuzumab) therapy in a twin pregnancy with associated oligohydramnios. Am J Obstet Gynecol 201(1):e13, 2009

Bean LJH, Allen EG, Tinker SW, et al: Lack of maternal folic acid supplementation is associated with heart defects in Down syndrome: a report from the National Down Syndrome Project. Birth Defects Res A Clin Mol Teratol 91:885, 2011

Bertrand J, Floyd RL, Weber MK: Guidelines for identifying and referring persons with fetal alcohol syndrome. MMWR 54(11):1, 2005

Billings RJ, Berkowitz RI, Watson G: Teeth. Pediatrics 113(4):1120, 2004

Blinick G, Jerez E, Wallach RC: Methadone maintenance, pregnancy, and progeny. JAMA 225:477, 1973

Brent RL: Teratogen update: reproductive risks of leflunomide (Arava), a pyrimidine synthesis inhibitor: counseling women taking leflunomide before or during pregnancy and men taking leflunomide who are contemplating fathering a child. Teratology 63(2):106, 2001

Briggs GG, Freeman RK, Yaffe SJ: Drugs in Pregnancy and Lactation, 9th ed. Philadelphia, Lippincott Williams & Wilkins, 2011

Bristol-Meyers Squibb: Efavirenz (Sustiva) prescribing information 2010. Available at: http://www.accessdata.fda.gov/drugsatfda_docs/label/2010/020972s035,021360s023lbl.pdf. Accessed April 10, 2013

Broussard CS, Rasmussen SA, Reefhuis J, et al: Maternal treatment with opioid analgesics and risk for birth defects. Am J Obstet Gynecol 204:e1, 2011

Brunskill PJ: The effects of fetal exposure to danazol. Br J Obstet Gynaecol 99:212, 1992

Buehler BA, Delimont D, van Waes M, et al: Prenatal prediction of risk of the fetal hydantoin syndrome. N Engl J Med 322:1567, 1990

Celgene Corporation: Thalomid: highlights of prescribing information. 2013. Available at: http://www.thalomid.com/pdf/Thalomid_PI.pdf. Accessed April 10, 2013

Center for Substance Abuse Treatment. Medication-assisted treatment for opioid addiction during pregnancy. In SAHMSA/CSAT (eds): Treatment Improvement Protocols. 2008. Available at: http://www.ncbi.nlm.nih.gov/books/NBK26113. Accessed April 10, 2013

Centers for Disease Control and Prevention: Alcohol use and binge drinking among women of childbearing age—United States, 2006–2010. MMWR 61(28):534, 2012

Centers for Disease Control and Prevention: Guidelines for the Identification and Management of Lead Exposure in Pregnant and Lactating Women. 2010. Available at: http://www.cdc.gov/nceh/lead/publications/leadandpregnancy2010.pdf. Accessed April 10, 2013

Chambers CD, Hernandez-Diaz S, Van Marter LJ, et al: Selective serotonin-reuptake inhibitors and risk of persistent pulmonary hypertension of the newborn. N Engl J Med 354(6):579, 2006

Chasnoff IJ, Chisum GM, Kaplan WE: Maternal cocaine use and genitourinary tract malformations. Teratology 37:201, 1988

Chavez GF, Mulinare J, Cordero JF: Maternal cocaine use during early pregnancy as a risk factor for congenital urogenital abnormalities. JAMA 262:795, 1989

Choi BH, Lapham LW, Amin-Zaki L, et al: Abnormal neuronal migration, deranged cerebellar cortical organization, and diffuse white matter astrocytosis of human fetal brain. A major effect of methyl mercury poisoning in utero. J Neuropathol Neurol 37:719, 1978

Clayton-Smith J, Donnai D: Human malformations. In Rimoin DL, Connor JM, Pyeritz RE (eds): Emery and Rimoin's Principles and Practice of Medical Genetics, 3rd ed. New York, Churchill Livingstone, 1996, p 383

Cleary BJ, Donnelly J, Strawbridge J, et al: Methadone dose and neonatal abstinence syndrome—systematic review and meta-analysis. Addiction 105:2071, 2010

Cleary BJ, Donnelly JM, Strawbridge JD, et al: Methadone and perinatal outcomes: a retrospective cohort study. Am J Obstet Gynecol 204:139.e1, 2011

Cliver SP, Goldenberg RL, Lutter R, et al: The effect of cigarette smoking on neonatal anthropometric measurements. Obstet Gynecol 85:625, 1995

Clouthier DE, Hosoda K, Richardson JA, et al: Cranial and cardiac neural crest defects in endothelin-A receptor-deficient mice. Development 235:813, 1998

Conover EA, Polifka JE: The art and science of teratogen risk communication. Am J Med Genet C Semin Med Genet 157:227, 2011
Cooper WO, Hernandez-Diaz S, Arbogast PG, et al: Major congenital malformation after first-trimester exposure to ACE inhibitors. N Engl J Med 354:2443, 2006
Cordier S: Evidence for a role of paternal exposures in developmental toxicity. Basic Clin Pharmacol Toxicol 102(2):176, 2008
Costei AM, Kozer E, Ho T, et al: Perinatal outcome following third trimester exposure to paroxetine. Arch Pediatr Adolesc Med 156:1129, 2002
Cragan JD, Giboa SM: Including prenatal diagnoses in birth defects monitoring: experience of the Metropolitan Atlanta Congenital Birth Defects Program. Birth Defects Res A Clin Mol Teratol 85(1)20, 2009
Creanga AA, Sabel JC, Ko JY, et al: Maternal drug use and its effect on neonates: a population-based study in Washington state. Obstet Gynecol 119:924, 2012
Creinin MD, Vittinghoff E: Methotrexate and misoprostol vs misoprostol alone for early abortion: a randomized controlled trial. JAMA 272:1190, 1994
Crider KS, Cleves MA, Reefhuis J, et al: Antibacterial medication use during pregnancy and risk of birth defects. National Birth Defects Prevention Study. Arch Pediatr Adolesc Med 163:978, 2009
Crijns HJMJ, Straus SM, Gispen-de Wied, et al: Compliance with pregnancy prevention programmes of isotretinoin in Europe: a systematic review. Br J Dermatol 164:238, 2011
Dally A: Thalidomide: was the tragedy preventable? Lancet 351:1197, 1998
Dansky LV, Andermann E, Rosenblatt D, et al: Anticonvulsants, folate levels, and pregnancy outcome: a prospective study. Ann Neurol 21:176, 1987
Dashe JS, Sheffield JS, Olscher DA, et al: Relationship between maternal methadone dosage and neonatal withdrawal. Obstet Gynecol 100:1244, 2002
Del Campo M, Kosaki K, Bennett FC, et al: Developmental delay in fetal aminopterin/methotrexate syndrome. Teratology 60:10, 1999
Di Sessa TG, Moretti ML, Khoury A, et al: Cardiac function in fetuses and newborns exposed to low-dose aspirin during pregnancy. Am J Obstet Gynecol 171(4):892, 1994
Dolk H, Loane M, Garne E: The prevalence of congenital anomalies in Europe. Adv Exp Med Biol 686:349, 2010
D'Souza SW, Black P, Richards B: Smoking in pregnancy: associations with skinfold thickness, maternal weight gain, and fetal size at birth. BMJ 282:1661, 1981
Eisai Inc.: Targretin (bexarotene) prescribing information. 2011. Available at: http://us.eisai.com/pdf_files/TargretinCaps_PI.pdf. Accessed April 9, 2013
Enns GM, Roeder E, Chan RT, et al: Apparent cyclophosphamide (Cytoxan) embryopathy: a distinct phenotype? Am J Med Genet 86:237, 1999
Ethen MK, Ramadhani TA, Scheurele AE, et al: National Birth Defects Prevention Study. Alcohol consumption by women before and during pregnancy. Matern Child Health J 13(2):274, 2009
Feldcamp M, Carey JC: Clinical teratology counseling and consultation case report: low dose methotrexate exposure in the early weeks of pregnancy. Teratology 47:533, 1993
Finnegan LP, Kron RE, Connaughton JF, et al: Assessment and treatment of abstinence in the infant of the drug dependent mother. Int J Clin Pharmacol Biopharm 12:19, 1975
Food and Drug Administration: Antipsychotic drug labels updated on use during pregnancy and risk of abnormal muscle movements and withdrawal symptoms in newborns. 2011a. Available at: http://www.fda.gov/Drugs/DrugSafety/ucm243903.htm. Accessed April 9, 2013
Food and Drug Administration: EPA and FDA advice for women who might become pregnant, women who are pregnant, nursing mothers, young children. 2004. Available at: http://www.fda.gov/Food/FoodborneIllnessContaminants/BuyStoreServeSafeFood/ucm110591.htm. Accessed April 9, 2013
Food and Drug Administration: FDA approves Diclegis for pregnant women experiencing nausea and vomiting. 2013. http://www.fda.gov/NewsEvents/Newsroom/PressAnnouncements/ucm347087.htm. Accessed April 9, 2013
Food and Drug Administration: Information for healthcare professionals: mycophenolate mofetil (marketed as Cellcept) and mycophenolic acid (marketed as Myfortic), 2008. Available at: http://www.fda.gov/Drugs/DrugSafety/PostmarketDrugSafetyInformationforPatientsandProviders/ucm124776.htm. Accessed April 9, 2013
Food and Drug Administration: Information for healthcare professionals: risk of neural tube birth defects following prenatal exposure to valproate. 2009. Available at: http://www.fda.gov/Drugs/DrugSafety/PostmarketDrugSafetyInformationforPatientsandProviders/DrugSafetyInformationforHeathcareProfessionals/ucm192649.htm. Accessed April 9, 2013
Food and Drug Administration: Letairis (ambrisentan) safety information. 2012. Available at: http://www.fda.gov/Safety/MedWatch/SafetyInformation/ucm233391.htm. Accessed April 9, 2013
Food and Drug Administration: Pregnancy and lactation labeling. 2011b. Available at: http://www.fda.gov/Drugs/DevelopmentApprovalProcess/DevelopmentResources/Labeling/ucm093307.htm. Accessed April 9, 2013
Food and Drug Administration: Pregnancy categories for prescription drugs. FDA Bulletin, 1979
Food and Drug Administration: Public health advisory: paroxetine. 2005a. Available at: http://www.fda.gov/Drugs/DrugSafety/PostmarketDrugSafetyInformationforPatientsandProviders/DrugSafetyInformationforHeathcareProfessionals/PublicHealthAdvisories/ucm051731.htm. Accessed April 9, 2013
Food and Drug Administration: Reviewer guidance: evaluating the risks of drug exposure in human pregnancies. 2005b. Available at: http://www.fda.gov/downloads/ScienceResearch/SpecialTopics/WomensHealthResearch/UCM133359.pdf. Accessed April 9, 2013
Food and Drug Administration: Risk of oral clefts in children born to mothers taking Topamax (topiramate). 2011c. Available at: http://www.fda.gov/Drugs/DrugSafety/ucm245085.htm. Accessed April 9, 2013
Food and Drug Administration: Use of long-term, high-dose Diflucan (fluconazole) during pregnancy may be associated with birth defects in infants. 2011e. Available at: http://www.fda.gov/Drugs/DrugSafety/ucm266030.htm. Accessed April 9, 2013
Gee RE, Wood SF, Schubert KG: Women's Health, Pregnancy, and the U.S. Food and Drug Administration. Obstet Gynecol 2014 123(1):161, 2014
Goldberg JM, Falcone T: Effect of diethylstilbestrol on reproductive functions. Fertil Steril 72:1, 1999
Gouin K, Murphy K, Shah PS, et al: Effects of cocaine use during pregnancy on low birthweight and preterm birth: systematic review and meta-analyses. Am J Obstet Gynecol 204:340.e1, 2011
Grab D, Paulus WE, Erdmann M, et al: Effects of low-dose aspirin on uterine and fetal blood flow during pregnancy: results of a randomized, placebo-controlled, double-blind trial. Ultrasound Obstet Gynecol 15:19, 2000
Gregg NM: Congenital cataract following German measles in the mother. Trans Ophthalmol Soc 3:35, 1941
Grimes DA, Schulz KF. False alarms and pseudo-epidemics: the limitations of observational epidemiology. Obstet Gynecol 120:920, 2012
Grumbach MM, Ducharme JR: The effects of androgens on fetal sexual development. Androgen-induced female pseudohermaphrodism. Fertil Steril 11:157, 1960
Guerri C, Bazinet A, Riley EP: Foetal alcohol spectrum disorders and alterations in brain and behaviour. Alcohol 44(2):108, 2009
Guron G, Friberg P: An intact renin-angiotensin system is a prerequisite for normal renal development. J Hypertension 18:123, 2000
Hall JG, Pauli RM, Wilson K: Maternal and fetal sequelae of anticoagulation during pregnancy. Am J Med 68:122, 1980
Hall HG, McKenna LG, Griffiths DL: Complementary and alternative medicine for induction of labor. Women Birth 25(3):142, 2012
Hepner DL, Harnett M, Segal S, et al: Herbal medicine use in parturients. Anesth Analg 94:690, 2002
Herbst AL, Ulfelder H, Poskanzer DC: Adenocarcinoma of the vagina. Association of maternal stilbestrol therapy. N Engl J Med 284:878, 1971
Hernandez RK, Werler MM, Romitti P, et al: Nonsteroidal antiinflammatory drug use among women and the risk of birth defects. Am J Obstet Gynecol 206:228.e1, 2012
Hernandez-Diaz S, Smith CR, Shen A, et al: Comparative safety of antiepileptic drugs during pregnancy. Neurology 78:1692, 2012
Hernandez-Diaz S, Werler MM, Walker AM, et al: Folic acid antagonists during pregnancy and the risk of birth defects. N Engl J Med 343:1608, 2000
Hiilesmaa VK, Teramo K, Granstrom ML, et al: Serum folate concentrations in women with epilepsy. BMJ 287:577, 1983
Hobbs CA, Cleves MA, Karim MA, et al: Maternal folate-related gene environment interactions and congenital heart defects. Obstet Gynecol 116:316, 2010
Honein MA, Paulozzi LJ, Watkins ML: Maternal smoking and birth defects: validity of birth certificate data for effect estimation. Public Health Rep 116:327, 2001
Hoover RN, Hyer M, Pfeiffer RM, et al: Adverse health outcomes in women exposed in utero to diethylstilbestrol. N Engl J Med 365:1304, 2011
Horning MG, Stratton C, Wilson A, et al: Detection of 5-(3,4)-diphenylhydantoin in the newborn human. Anal Lett 4:537, 1974
Hoyme HE, May PA, Kalberg WO, et al: A practical clinical approach to diagnosis of fetal alcohol spectrum disorders: clarification of the 1996 Institute of Medicine Criteria. Pediatrics 115:39, 2005
Hviid A, Melbye M, Pasternak B: Use of selective serotonin reuptake inhibitors during pregnancy and the risk of autism. N Engl J Med 369:2406, 2013
Iahnaccone PM, Bossert NL, Connelly CS: Disruption of embryonic and fetal development due to preimplantation chemical insults: a critical review. Am J Obstet Gynecol 157:476, 1987

Institute of Medicine, National Academy of Sciences: Fetal Alcohol Syndrome: Diagnosis, Epidemiology, Prevention and Treatment. Washington, DC, National Academies Press, 1996

Jasper JD, Goel R, Einarson A, et al: Effects of framing on teratogenic risk perception in pregnant women. Lancet 358:1237, 2001

Jones KL, Smith DW, Ulleland CN, et al: Pattern of malformation in offspring of chronic alcoholic mothers. Lancet 1:1267, 1973.

Jordan AE, Jackson GL, Deardorff D, et al: Serotonin reuptake inhibitor use in pregnancy and the neonatal behavioral syndrome. J Matern Fetal Neonatal Med 21(10):745, 2008

Khouri MI, James IM, Flanders WD, et al: Interpretation of recurring weak association obtained from epidemiologic studies of suspected human teratogens. Teratology 46:69, 1992

Kieler H, Artama M, Engeland A, et al: Selective serotonin reuptake inhibitors during pregnancy and risk of persistent pulmonary hypertension in the newborn: population based cohort study from the five Nordic countries. BMJ 344:d8012, 2012

Kirshon B, Wasserstrum N, Willis R, et al: Teratogenic effects of first trimester cyclophosphamide therapy. Obstet Gynecol 72:462, 1988

Klarskov P, Andersen JT, Jimenez-Solem E, et al: Short-acting sulfonamides near term and neonatal jaundice. Obstet Gynecol 122(1):105, 2013

Klip H, Verloop J, van Gool JD, et al: Hypospadias in sons of women exposed to diethylstilbestrol in utero: a cohort study. Lancet 359:1102, 2002

Knapp K, Lenz W, Nowack E: Multiple congenital abnormalities. Lancet 2:725, 1962

Koren G, Bologa M, Long D, et al: Perception of teratogenic risk by pregnant women exposed to drugs and chemicals during the first trimester. Am J Obstet Gynecol 160:1190, 1989

Koren G, Pastuszak A, Ito S: Drugs in pregnancy. N Engl J Med 16;338(16):1128, 1998

Kozer E, Nikfar S, Costei A, et al: Aspirin consumption during the first trimester of pregnancy and congenital anomalies: a meta-analysis. Am J Obstet Gynecol 187:1623, 2002

Kutscher AH, Zegarelli EV, Tovell HM, et al: Discoloration of deciduous teeth induced by administration of tetracycline antepartum. Am J Obstet Gynecol 96:291, 1966

LaGasse LL, Derauf C, Smith LM, et al: Prenatal methamphetamine exposure and childhood behavior problems at 3 and 5 years of age. Pediatrics 129:681, 2012

LaGasse LL, Wouldes T, Newman E, et al: Prenatal methamphetamine exposure and neonatal neurobehavioral outcome in the USA and New Zealand. Neurotoxicol Teratol 33:166, 2011

Lammer EJ, Chen DT, Hoar RM, et al: Retinoic acid embryopathy. N Engl J Med 313:837, 1985

Lemoine P, Harouusseau H, Borteyru JP, et al: Les enfants de parents alcooliques: anomalies observées, a propos de 127 cas. Ouest Med 21:476, 1968

Lenz W, Knapp K: Thalidomide embryopathy. Arch Environ Health 5:100, 1962

Levin R: Neonatal adverse events associated with in utero SSRI/SNRI exposure. 2004. Available at: www.fda.gov/ohrms/dockets/ac/04/slides/2004-4050S1_11_Levin.ppt. Accessed April 9, 2013

Lin S, Munsie JW, Herdt-Losavio ML: Maternal asthma medication use and the risk of selected birth defects. Pediatrics 129:317, 2012

Lindhout D, Rene JE, Hoppener A, et al: Teratogenicity of antiepileptic drug combinations with special emphasis on epoxidation of carbamazepine. Epilepsia 25:77, 1984

Lipshultz SE, Frassica JJ, Orav EJ: Cardiovascular abnormalities in infants prenatally exposed to cocaine. J Pediatr 118:44, 1991

Little BB, Snell LM, Gilstrap LC: Methamphetamine abuse during pregnancy: outcome and fetal effects. Obstet Gynecol 72:541, 1988

Maier SE, West JR: Drinking patterns and alcohol-related birth defects. Alcohol Res Health 25:168, 2001

Magnusson LL, Bonde J, Olsen J, et al: Paternal laboratory work and congenital malformations. J Occup Environ Med 46:761, 2004

Malik S, Cleves MA, Honein MA, et al: Maternal smoking and congenital heart defects. Pediatrics 121(4):e810, 2008

Margulis AV, Mitchell AA, Gilboa SM, et al: Use of topiramate in pregnancy and the risk of oral clefts. Am J Obstet Gynecol 207:292.405.e1, 2012

Martinez-Frias ML, Czeizel AE, Rodriguez-Pinilla E, et al: Smoking during pregnancy and Poland sequence: results of a population-based registry and a case-control registry. Teratology 59:35, 1999

McKeigue PM, Lamm SH, Linn S, et al: Bendectin and birth defects: I. A meta-analysis of the epidemiologic studies. Teratology 50:27, 1994

Meador KJ, Baker GA, Browning N, et al: Cognitive function at 3 years of age after fetal exposure to antiepileptic drugs. N Engl J Med 360:1597, 2009

Mercer BM, Merlino AA, Milluzzi CJ, et al: Small fetal size before 20 weeks' gestation: associations with maternal tobacco use, early preterm birth, and low birthweight. Am J Obstet Gynecol 198(6):673, 2008

Mitchell AA, Gilboa SM, Werler MM, et al: Medication use during pregnancy, with particular focus on prescription drugs: 1976–2008. Am J Obstet Gynecol 205(1)51:e1, 2011

Molgaard-Nielsen D, Hviid A: Newer-generation antiepileptic drugs and the risk of major birth defects. JAMA 305:1996, 2011

Molgaard-Nielsen D, Pasternak B, Hviid A: Use of oral fluconazole during pregnancy and the risk of birth defects. N Engl J Med 369(9):830, 2013

Morrow JI, Russell A, Guthrie E, et al: Malformation risks of antiepileptic drugs in pregnancy: a prospective study from the UK Epilepsy and Pregnancy Register. J Neurol Neurosurg Psych 77:193, 2006

Munsie JW, Lin S, Browne ML, et al: Maternal bronchodilator use and the risk of oral clefts. Hum Reprod 26:3147, 2011

Nelson BK, Moorman WJ, Schrader SM: Review of experimental male-mediated behavioral and neurochemical disorders. Neurotoxicology 18:611, 1996

Nurmohamed L, Moretti ME, Schechter T, et al: Outcome following high-dose methotrexate in pregnancies misdiagnosed as ectopic. Am J Obstet Gynecol 205(6):533.e1, 2011

Oakley GP, Erickson JD: Vitamin A and birth defects. N Engl J Med 333:1414, 1995

Olshan AF, Teschke K, Baird PA: Paternal occupation and congenital anomalies. Am J Ind Med 20:447, 1991

Paintner A, Williams AD, Burd L: Fetal alcohol spectrum disorders—implications for child neurology, Part 2: Diagnosis and management. J Child Neurol 27:355, 2012

Panchaud A, Csajka C, Merlob P, et al: Pregnancy outcome following exposure to topical retinoids: a multicenter prospective study. J Clin Pharmacol 52:1844, 2012

Parilla BV: Using indomethacin as a tocolytic. Contemp Ob/Gyn 49:90, 2004

Park-Wyllie L, Mazzota P, Pastuszak A, et al: Birth defects after maternal exposure to corticosteroids: prospective cohort study and meta-analysis of epidemiological studies. Teratology 62(6):385, 2000

Pearson MA, Hoyme HE, Seaver LH, et al: Toluene embryopathy: delineation of the phenotype and comparison with fetal alcohol syndrome. Pediatrics 93:211, 1994

Pryde PG, Sedman AB, Nugent CE, et al: Angiotensin converting enzyme inhibitor fetopathy. J Am Soc Nephrol 3:1575, 1993

Rasanen J, Jouppila P: Fetal cardiac function and ductus arteriosus during indomethacin and sulindac therapy for threatened preterm labor: a randomized study. Am J Obstet Gynecol 173:20, 1995

Rebordosa C, Kogevinas M, Horváth-Puhó E, et al: Acetaminophen use during pregnancy: effects on risk for congenital abnormalities. Am J Obstet Gynecol 198(2):178, 2008

Reprotox-Micromedex 2.0: Lithium. Available at: http://www.reprotox.org/Search/result.aspx?txtSearch=lithium. Accessed November 3, 2013

Richardson S, Browne ML, Rasmussen SA et al: Associations between periconceptional alcohol consumption and craniosynostosis, omphalocele, and gastroschisis. Birth Defects Res A Clin Mol Teratol 91:623, 2011

Rothman KJ, Moore LL, Singer MR, et al: Teratogenicity of high vitamin A intake. N Engl J Med 333:1369, 1995

Sadler TW (ed): Langman's Medical Embryology, 6th ed. Baltimore, Williams & Wilkins, 1990, p 130

Salle B, Sergeant P, Awada A, et al: Transvaginal ultrasound studies of vascular and morphological changes in uteri exposed to diethylstilbestrol in utero. Hum Reprod 11:2531, 1996

Sanofi-aventis: Arava tablets: prescribing information. 2012. Available at: http://products.sanofi.us/arava/arava.html. Accessed April 10, 2013

Savitz DA, Sonnenfeld N, Olshan AF: Review of epidemiological studies of paternal occupational exposure and spontaneous abortion. Am J Ind Med 25:361, 1994

Schaefer C, Hannemann D, Meister R, et al: Vitamin K antagonists and pregnancy outcome—a multicenter prospective study. Thromb Haemost 95(6):949, 2006

Schardein JL (ed): Chemically Induced Birth Defects, 3rd ed. New York, Marcel Dekker, 2000

Schardein JL: Congenital abnormalities and hormones during pregnancy: a clinical review. Teratology 22:251, 1985

Schering Corporation: PegIntron Medication Guide. 2012. Available at: http://www.fda.gov/downloads/Drugs/DrugSafety/UCM133677.pdf. Accessed April 10, 2013

Schnitzer PG, Olshan AF, Erickson JD: Paternal occupation and risk of birth defects in the offspring. Epidemiology 6:577, 1995

Sekar R, Stone PR: Trastuzumab use for metastatic breast cancer in pregnancy. Obstet Gynecol 110:507, 2007

Seligman NS, Almario CV, Hayes EJ, et al: Relationship between maternal methadone dose at delivery and neonatal abstinence syndrome. J Pediatr 157:428, 2010

Sheehan DM: Herbal medicines, phytoestrogens and toxicity: risk:benefit considerations. Proc Soc Exp Biol Med 217:379, 1998

Shepard TH: Annual commentary on human teratogens. Teratology 66:275, 2002a

Shepard TH: Letters: "proof" of human teratogenicity. Teratology 50:97, 1994

Shepard TH, Brent RL, Friedman JM, et al: Update on new developments in the study of human teratogens. Teratology 65:153, 2002b

Singer LT, Arendt R, Minnes S, et al: Cognitive and motor outcomes of cocaine-exposed infants. JAMA 287:1952, 2002

Stewart RD, Nelson DB, Adhikari EH, et al: The obstetrical and neonatal impact of maternal opioid detoxification in pregnancy. Am J Obstet Gynecol 209(3):267, 2013

Stiefel Laboratories Soriatane (acitretin) Medication Guide. 2011. Available at: http://www.fda.gov/downloads/Drugs/DrugSafety/ucm089133.pdf. Accessed April 10, 2013

Stillerman KP, Mattison DR, Giudice LC, et al: Environmental exposures and adverse pregnancy outcomes: a review of the science. Reprod Sci 15(7):631, 2008

Stillman RJ: In utero exposure to diethylstilbestrol: adverse effects on the reproductive tract and reproductive performance in male and female offspring. Am J Obstet Gynecol 142:905, 1982

Strandberg-Larsen K, Nielsen NR, Grønbaek M, et al: Binge drinking in pregnancy and risk of fetal death. Obstet Gynecol 111(3):602, 2008

Streissguth AP, Clarren SK, Jones KL: Natural history of fetal alcohol syndrome: a 10-year follow-up of eleven patients. Lancet 2:85, 1985

Texas Department of State Health Services: Birth defect risk factor series: hypoplastic left heart syndrome. 2012. Available at: http://www.dshs.state.tx.us/birthdefects/risk/risk-hlhs.shtm. Accessed April 10, 2013

van der Heijden BJ, Carlus C, Narcy F, et al: Persistent anuria, neonatal death, and renal microcystic lesions after prenatal exposure to indomethacin. Am J Obstet Gynecol 171:617, 1994

Van Gelder MM, Reefhuis J, Caton AR, et al: Maternal periconceptional illicit drug use and the risk of congenital malformations. Epidemiology 20:60, 2009

Vermillion ST, Scardo JA, Lashus AG, et al: The effect of indomethacin tocolysis on fetal ductus arteriosus constriction with advancing gestational age. Am J Obstet Gynecol 177:256, 1997

Vessey MP: Epidemiological studies of the effects of diethylstilbestrol. IARC Sci Publ 335, 1989

Vitale N, DeFeo M, De Santo LS, et al: Dose-dependent fetal complications of warfarin in pregnant women with mechanical heart valves. J Am Coll Cardiol 33:1637, 1999

Walker MPR, Moore TR, Brace RA: Indomethacin and arginine vasopressin interaction in the fetal kidney. A mechanism of oliguria. Am J Obstet Gynecol 171:1234, 1994

Warkany J: Warfarin embryopathy. Teratology 14:205, 1976

Watson WJ: Herceptin (trastuzumab) therapy during pregnancy: association with reversible anhydramnios. Obstet Gynecol 105:642, 2005

Weinstein MR: Recent advances in clinical psychopharmacology. I. Lithium carbonate. Hosp Form 12:759, 1977

Weiss CF, Glazko AJ, Weston JK: Chloramphenicol in the newborn infant: a physiologic explanation of its toxicity when given in excessive doses. N Engl J Med 262:787, 1960

Werler MM: Teratogen update: smoking and reproductive outcomes. Teratology 55:382, 1997

Wilkins-Haug L: Teratogen Update: toluene. Teratology 55:145, 1997

Wilson KL, Zelig CM, Harvey JP, et al: Persistent pulmonary hypertension of the newborn is associated with mode of delivery and not with maternal use of selective serotonin reuptake inhibitors. Am J Perinatol 28:19, 2011

Wlodarczyk BJ, Palacios AM, Chapa CJ, et al: Genetic basis of susceptibility to teratogen induced birth defects. Am J Med Genet C Semin Med Genet 157:215, 2011

Zelson C, Lee SJ, Casalino M: Neonatal narcotic addiction: comparative effects of maternal intake of heroin and methadone. N Engl J Med 289:1216, 1973

CHAPTER 13

Genetics

Genetics is the study of genes, heredity, and the variation of inherited characteristics. Medical genetics deals with the etiology and pathogenesis of human diseases that are at least partially genetic in origin, along with their prediction and prevention. Thus, it is closely linked to genomics, which is the study of how genes function and interact. In addition to chromosomal, mendelian, and nonmendelian genetic conditions reviewed in this chapter, medical genetics includes preimplantation and prenatal diagnosis, gene therapy, and newborn screening, which are discussed in Chapters 14, 16, and 32, respectively.

Genetic disease is common. Between 2 and 3 percent of newborns have a recognized structural defect. In another 3 percent of individuals, a defect is diagnosed by age 5, and another 8 to 10 percent are discovered by age 18 to have one or more functional or developmental abnormalities. An astonishing two thirds of the population will experience a disease with a genetic component during their lifetime. Advances in genomics are used increasingly to provide information regarding susceptibility to genetic diseases, and there is every indication that this field will reshape prenatal diagnosis (Bodurtha, 2012).

GENOMICS IN OBSTETRICS

Completed in 2003, the Human Genome Project identified nearly 25,000 human genes and led to rapid expansion of genomic research to better understand disease biology (Bodurtha, 2012; Feero, 2010; McKusick, 2003). One example is the International HapMap (Haplotype Map) Project, which studies the effects of genetic variation (National Human Genome Research Institute, 2012). HapMap investigates the nearly 10 million single nucleotide polymorphisms that comprise 0.5 percent of our DNA. Researchers look at how groups of common polymorphisms affect factors such as propensity to particular diseases and response to treatment. Another example is dbGaP, the database of Genotypes and Phenotypes, which is maintained by the National Center for Biotechnology Information (NCBI) (2013a). This database includes studies of genotype and phenotype interactions, such as genome-wide association studies and medical diagnostic assays. It is hoped that data from dbGaP will be used to develop tests or products that address public health needs.

The NCBI also maintains several genetic and genomic databases useful in obstetrics and maternal-fetal medicine practice. These include Online Mendelian Inheritance in Man (OMIM), GeneTests, and the Genetics Home Reference. Each is freely accessible to clinicians and researchers. Of these, OMIM is a comprehensive catalog of human genes and phenotypes originally created by the National Library of Medicine in collaboration with Johns Hopkins University. Clinicians can use OMIM to gain detailed information regarding particular syndromes and their genetic basis. Or, if a syndrome is suspected but the diagnosis is unclear, it may aid formulation a differential diagnosis by searching for syndromes that include particular traits or abnormalities. As of 2013, OMIM included more than 14,000 different genes with known sequences and nearly 4000 mendelian or mitochondrial conditions—phenotypes—with a known molecular basis (Johns Hopkins University, 2013).

TABLE 13-1. Examples of Karyotype Designations Using the International System for Human Cytogenetic Nomenclature (2009)

Karyotype	Description
46,XY	Normal male chromosome constitution
47,XX,+21	Female with trisomy 21
47,XY,+21/46,XY	Male who is a mosaic of trisomy 21 cells and cells with normal constitution
46,XY,del(4)(p14)	Male with terminal deletion of the short arm of chromosome 4 at band p14
46,XX,dup(5)(p14p15.3)	Female with duplication of the short arm of chromosome 5 from band p14 to band p15.3
45,XY,der(13;14)(q10;q10)	Male with a "balanced" robertsonian translocation of the long arms of chromosomes 13 and 14—the karyotype now has one normal 13, one normal 14, and the translocation chromosome, thereby reducing the normal 46 chromosome complement to 45
46,XY,t(11;22)(q23;q11.2)	Male with a balanced reciprocal translocation between chromosomes 11 and 22—breakpoints are at 11q23 and 22q11.2
46,XX,inv(3)(p21q13)	Female with inversion of chromosome 3 that extends from p21 to q13. This is a pericentric inversion because it includes the centromere
46,X,r(X)(p22.1q27)	Female with one normal X and one ring X chromosome. The breakpoints indicate that the regions distal to p22.1 and q27 are deleted from the ring
46,X,i(X)(q10)	Female with one normal X chromosome and an isochromosome of the long arm of the other X chromosome

Adapted from Jorde, 2006. Table contributed by Dr. Frederick Elder.

Another database, GeneTests, provides information on genetic conditions, the benefits and limitations of available tests for a given disorder, and how to send a specimen to a particular laboratory. As of 2013, the GeneTests website contained 575 clinical reviews and more than 3000 genetic tests, and it provided contact information for more than 600 laboratories. Additional information regarding laboratories that perform genetic tests is available from the NCBI's Genetic Testing Registry (2013c). The NCBI (2013b) has also established a database of genetic information intended for patients, the Genetics Home Reference. This database contains information on more than 2000 genetic conditions and genes.

CHROMOSOMAL ABNORMALITIES

Chromosomal abnormalities figure prominently in genetic disease. They are present in approximately 50 percent of spontaneous abortions, 5 percent of stillbirths, and 0.5 percent of liveborn infants (Parker, 2010; Schwartz, 2012). In the European Surveillance of Congenital Anomalies (EUROCAT) network of population-based registries, chromosomal abnormalities were recognized in 0.4 percent of pregnancies, with Down syndrome comprising more than half of cases (Dolk, 2010).

Standard Nomenclature

In humans, the 22 pairs of autosomes and one pair of sex chromosomes may be affected by various abnormalities. Karyotypes are described using the International System for Human Cytogenetic Nomenclature, a standardized format agreed upon by the genetics community (Shaffer, 2009). Abnormalities fall into two broad categories—those of chromosome number, such as trisomy, and those of chromosome structure, such as a deletion or translocation. Each chromosome has a short arm, termed the "p" or petit arm, and a long arm known as the "q" arm, selected because it is the next letter of the alphabet. The two arms are separated by the centromere.

When reporting a karyotype, the total number of chromosomes is listed first, corresponding to the number of centromeres. This is followed by the sex chromosomes, XX or XY, and then by a description of any structural variation. Specific abnormalities are indicated by standard abbreviations, such as del (deletion) and inv (inversion). The affected region or bands of the p or q arms are then designated, so that the reader will know both the exact abnormality location and the way in which the chromosomal complement is abnormal. Some examples of standard karyotype nomenclature are shown in Table 13-1.

Abnormalities of Chromosome Number

The most easily recognized chromosomal abnormalities are numerical. Aneuploidy is inheritance of either an extra chromosome—resulting in trisomy, or loss of a chromosome—monosomy. These differ from polyploidy, which is an abnormal number of haploid chromosome sets, such as triploidy. The estimated incidence of various numerical chromosomal abnormalities is shown in Table 13-2.

Autosomal Trisomies

Trisomy accounts for approximately half of all chromosomal abnormalities. In most cases, it results from nondisjunction, which is failure of normal chromosomal pairing and separation during meiosis. Nondisjunction may occur if the chromosomes:

TABLE 13-2. Frequency of Numerical Chromosomal Abnormalities

	Frequency (%)		
Abnormality	Abortus	Stillborn	Liveborn
Trisomy, any	25	4	—
Trisomy 21, 18, or 13	4.5	2.7	0.14–0.16
Trisomy 21	—	—	0.12–0.14
Trisomy 18	—	—	0.01–0.02
Trisomy 13	—	—	0.01
Monosomy X	8.7	0.1	0.01
Triploidy	6.4	0.2	0.0002
Tetraploidy	2.4	—	—

Data from Cragan, 2009; Parker, 2010; Schwartz, 2012.

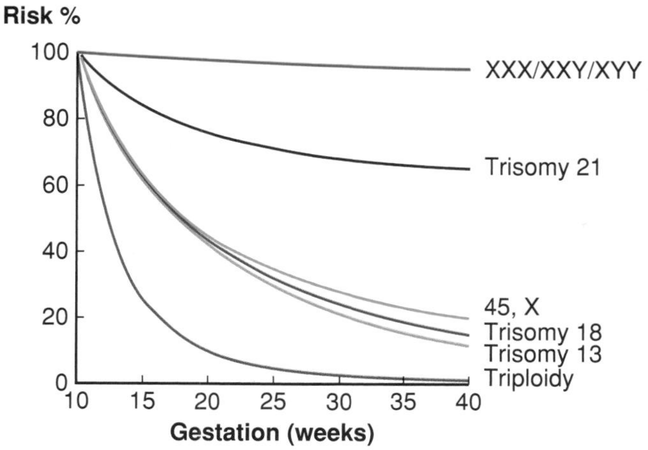

FIGURE 13-2 Gestational-age-related risk for selected chromosomal abnormalities, relative to the risk at 10 weeks' gestation. (Redrawn from Nicolaides, 2004, with permission.)

(1) fail to pair up, (2) pair up properly but separate prematurely, or (3) fail to separate.

The risk of any autosomal trisomy increases steeply with maternal age, particularly after age 35 (Fig. 13-1). Aging is thought to break down the chiasmata that keep the paired chromosomes aligned. Oocytes are held suspended in midprophase of meiosis I from birth until ovulation, in some cases for 50 years. Following completion of meiosis at the time of ovulation, nondisjunction will result in one gamete having two copies of the affected chromosome, leading to trisomy if fertilized. The other gamete, receiving no copy of the affected chromosome, will be monosomic if fertilized. Between 10 and 20 percent of oocytes are aneuploid secondary to meiotic errors, compared with 3 to 4 percent of sperm. Although each chromosome pair is equally likely to have a segregation error, it is rare for trisomies other than 21, 18, or 13 to result in a term pregnancy. As shown in Figure 13-2, many fetuses with autosomal trisomy will be lost before term.

Following a pregnancy with an autosomal trisomy, the risk for any autosomal trisomy in a future pregnancy is approximately 1 percent until the woman's age-related risk exceeds this. Accordingly, invasive prenatal diagnosis is offered in subsequent pregnancies (Chap. 14, p. 297). Parental chromosomal studies are not indicated unless Down syndrome was due to an unbalanced translocation.

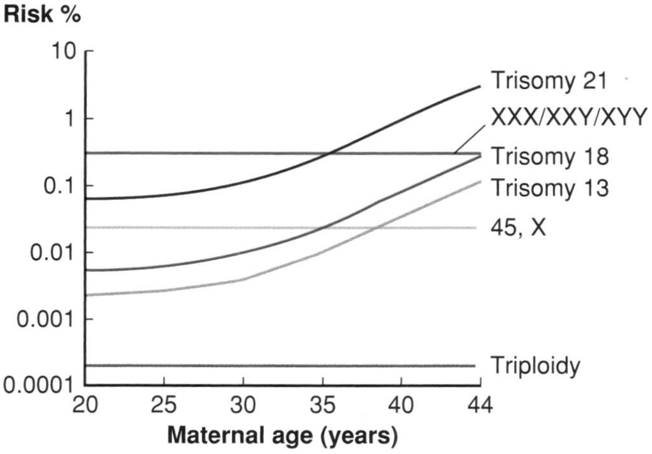

FIGURE 13-1 Maternal age-related risk for selected aneuploidies. (Redrawn from Nicolaides, 2004, with permission.)

Trisomy 21—Down Syndrome. In 1866, J. L. H. Down described a group of mentally retarded children with distinctive physical features. Nearly 100 years later, Lejeune (1959) demonstrated that Down syndrome is caused by an autosomal trisomy. The trisomy 21 karyotype is shown in Figure 13-3. Trisomy 21 is the etiology of 95 percent of Down syndrome cases, whereas 3 to 4 percent is due to a robertsonian translocation. The remaining 1 to 2 percent is secondary to an isochromosome or mosaicism. The nondisjunction that results in trisomy 21 occurs during meiosis I in almost 75 percent of cases. The remaining events occur during meiosis II.

Down syndrome is the most common nonlethal trisomy. Its prevalence is approximately 1 per 500 recognized pregnancies, including abortuses, stillbirths, and liveborn infants (Dolk, 2010). There is a significant fetal loss rate, as shown in Figure 13-2. Approximately 30 percent of fetuses with Down syndrome are lost between 12 and 40 weeks, and 20 percent between 16 and 40 weeks (Snijders, 1999). As a result, Down syndrome is found in 1 per 740 live births in the United States or 13.5 per 10,000. This represents an increase of approximately 33 percent compared with the rate in the late 1970s (Parker, 2010; Shin, 2009). The rise in prevalence is explained by the increase in maternal age distribution during this period.

Adult women with Down syndrome are fertile, and a third of their offspring will have Down syndrome (Scharrer, 1975). Contraceptive options are discussed in Chapter 38 (p. 695). Males with Down syndrome are almost always sterile because of markedly decreased spermatogenesis.

Clinical Findings. It is estimated that 25 to 30 percent of second-trimester fetuses with Down syndrome will have a major malformation that can be identified sonographically (Vintzileos, 1995). Approximately 40 percent of liveborn

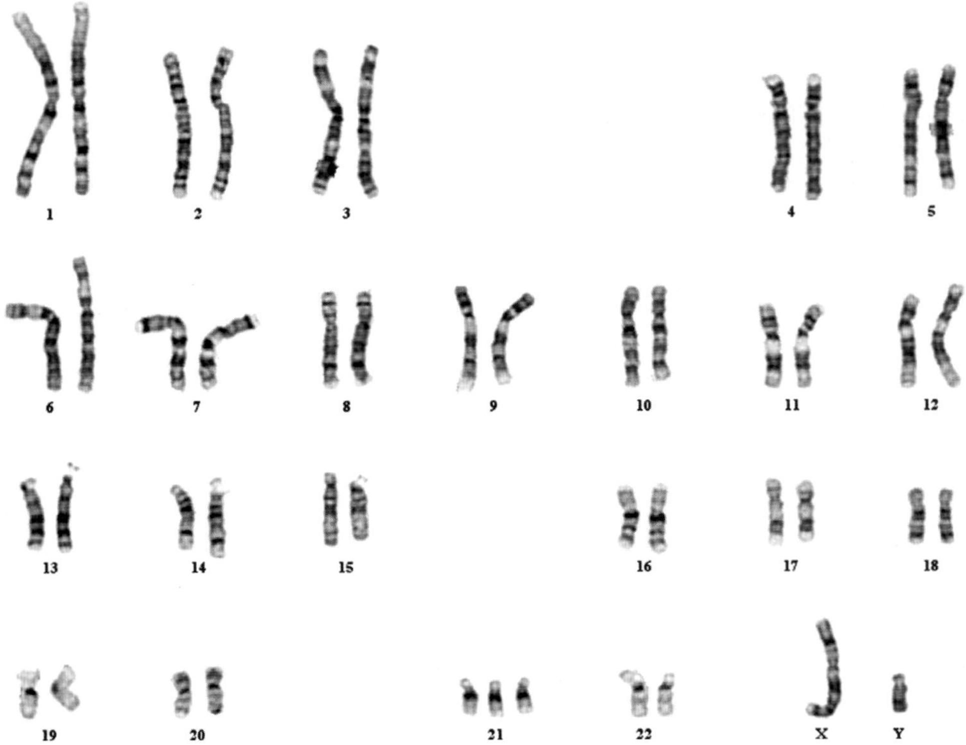

FIGURE 13-3 Abnormal male karyotype with trisomy 21, consistent with Down syndrome (47,XY,+21). (Photograph contributed by Dr. Frederick Elder.)

infants with Down syndrome are found to have cardiac defects, particularly endocardial cushion defects and ventricular septal defects (Figs. 10-22 and 10-23, p. 210). Gastrointestinal abnormalities develop in 7 percent and include duodenal atresia, esophageal atresia, and Hirschsprung disease (Fig. 10-28, p. 214) (Rankin, 2012).

Characteristic features of Down syndrome are shown in Figure 13-4. Typical findings include brachycephaly; epicanthal folds and up-slanting palpebral fissures; Brushfield spots, which are grayish spots on the periphery of the iris; a flat nasal bridge; and hypotonia. Infants often have loose skin at the nape of the neck, short fingers, a single palmar crease, hypoplasia of the middle phalanx of the fifth finger, and a prominent space or "sandal-toe gap" between the first and second toes. Some of these findings are sonographic markers for Down syndrome, which are reviewed in Chapter 14 (p. 292).

Health problems more common in children with Down syndrome include hearing loss in 75 percent, severe optical refractive errors in 50 percent, cataracts in 15 percent, thyroid disease in 15 percent, and an increased incidence of leukemia

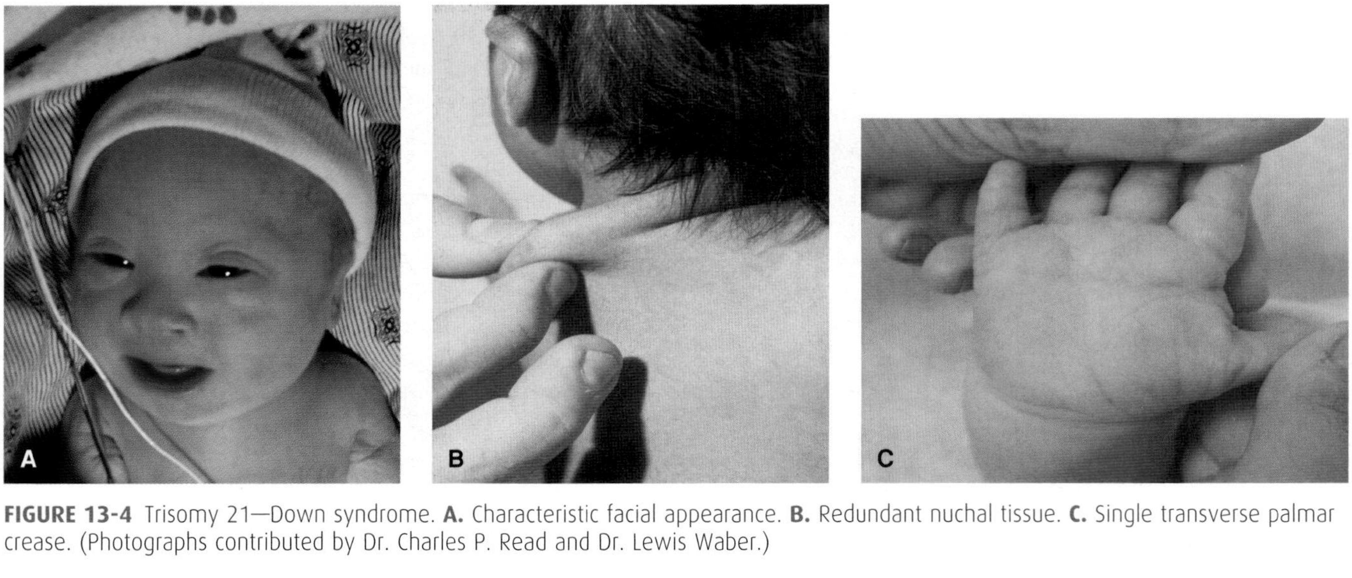

FIGURE 13-4 Trisomy 21—Down syndrome. **A.** Characteristic facial appearance. **B.** Redundant nuchal tissue. **C.** Single transverse palmar crease. (Photographs contributed by Dr. Charles P. Read and Dr. Lewis Waber.)

(American Academy of Pediatrics, 2001). The degree of mental impairment is usually mild to moderate, with an average intelligence quotient (IQ) score of 35 to 70. Social skills in affected children are often higher than predicted by their IQ scores.

Recent data suggest that approximately 95 percent of liveborn infants with Down syndrome survive the first year. The 10-year survival rate is at least 90 percent overall and is 99 percent if major malformations are absent (Rankin, 2012; Vendola, 2010). A number of organizations offer education and support for prospective parents faced with diagnosis of a Down syndrome fetus. These include the March of Dimes, National Down Syndrome Congress (www.ndsccenter.org), and National Down Syndrome Society (www.ndss.org).

Trisomy 18—Edwards Syndrome. This constellation of abnormalities and their association with another autosomal trisomy was first described by Edwards (1960). In population-based series, prevalence of trisomy 18 is approximately 1 per 2000 recognized pregnancies—including abortuses, stillbirths, and live births, and approximately 1 per 6600 liveborn infants (Dolk, 2010; Parker, 2010). The difference in prevalence is explained by the high in-utero lethality of the condition, as 85 percent of trisomy 18 fetuses are lost between 10 weeks' gestation and term (see Fig. 13-2). Perhaps not surprisingly, survival of liveborn infants is likewise bleak. More than half die within the first week, and the 1-year survival rate is only approximately 2 percent (Tennant, 2010; Vendola, 2010). The syndrome is three- to fourfold more common in females (Lin, 2006; Rosa, 2011). Unlike Down and Patau syndromes, which involve acrocentric chromosomes and thus may stem from a robertsonian translocation, it is uncommon for Edwards syndrome to result from a chromosomal rearrangement.

Clinical Findings. Virtually every organ system can be affected by trisomy 18. Common major anomalies include heart defects in almost 95 percent—particularly ventricular septal defects, as well as cerebellar vermian agenesis, enlarged cisterna magna, myelomeningocele, diaphragmatic hernia, omphalocele, imperforate anus, and renal anomalies such as horseshoe kidney (Lin, 2006; Rosa, 2011; Yeo, 2003). Sonographic images of several of these are shown in Chapter 10 (p. 200).

Cranial and extremity abnormalities are also particularly common and include a prominent occiput, posteriorly rotated and malformed ears, micrognathia, small mouth, clenched hands with overlapping digits, radial aplasia, hypoplastic nails, and rockerbottom or clubbed feet. Characteristic sonographic findings include a "strawberry-shaped" cranium and choroid plexus cysts (Fig. 13-5). In otherwise low-risk pregnancies, the risk for trisomy 18 is increased only when a choroid plexus cyst is associated with other abnormalities. Alone, this cyst may be considered a normal variant.

Pregnancies with trisomy 18 that reach the third trimester often develop fetal-growth restriction, and the mean birthweight is less than 2500 grams (Lin, 2006; Rosa, 2011). Mode of delivery should be discussed in advance, because abnormal fetal heart rate tracings are common during labor. In older reports, more than half of undiagnosed fetuses underwent cesarean delivery for "fetal distress" (Schneider, 1981).

Trisomy 13—Patau Syndrome. This constellation of fetal abnormalities and their association with yet another autosomal trisomy was described by Patau and colleagues (1960). The prevalence of trisomy 13 is approximately 1 per 12,000 live births and 1 per 5000 recognized pregnancies, which includes abortuses and stillbirths (Dolk, 2010; Parker, 2010). As with trisomy 18, trisomy 13 is highly lethal, and most affected fetuses are lost between 10 weeks and term (see Fig. 13-2).

Approximately 80 percent of pregnancies with Patau syndrome result from trisomy 13. The remainder are caused by a robertsonian translocation involving chromosomes 13 and 14, der(13;14)(q10;q10). This translocation is the most common structural chromosomal rearrangement. It is carried by approximately 1 in 1300 individuals, although the risk of an affected liveborn infant is less than 2 percent (Nussbaum, 2007).

Clinical Findings. Trisomy 13 is associated with abnormalities of virtually every organ system. One characteristic finding is holoprosencephaly. This is present in approximately two thirds of cases and may be accompanied by microcephaly, hypotelorism, and nasal abnormalities that range from a single nostril to a proboscis (Solomon, 2010). Cardiac defects are found in up to 90 percent of fetuses with trisomy 13 (Shipp, 2002).

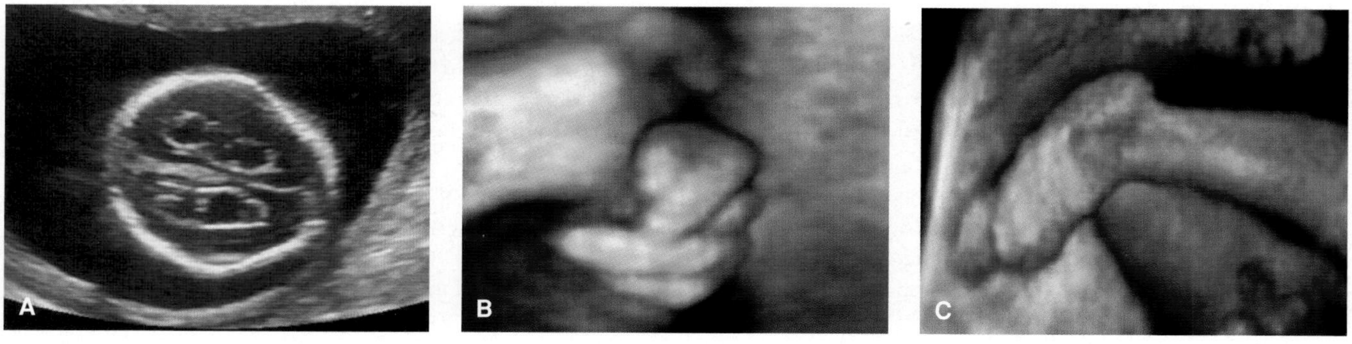

FIGURE 13-5 Trisomy 18–Edwards Syndrome. **A.** This transventricular sonographic view shows fetal choroid plexus cysts and a "strawberry-shaped" (unusually angulated) skull. Although not shown here, the fetal profile typically demonstrates micrognathia, with a very small, recessed mandible. **B.** This three-dimensional (3-D) sonographic image shows the characteristic hand position of clenched fists with overlapping digits. **C.** 3-D sonographic image displays a rockerbottom foot.

Other abnormalities that suggest trisomy 13 include neural-tube defects—particularly cephalocele, microphthalmia, cleft lip-palate, omphalocele, cystic renal dysplasia, polydactyly, rocker-bottom feet, and areas of skin aplasia (Lin, 2007). For the fetus or infant with a cephalocele, cystic kidneys, and polydactyly, the differential diagnosis includes trisomy 13 and the autosomal-recessive Meckel-Gruber syndrome, which is lethal. Sonographic images of several of these abnormalities are shown in Chapter 10 (p. 201).

Few trisomy 13 fetuses survive until birth. Of those that do, the 1-week survival is approximately 40 percent, and 1-year survival is only about 3 percent (Tennant, 2010; Vendola, 2010). Counseling regarding prenatal diagnosis and management options is similar to that described with trisomy 18.

For the mother, trisomy 13 is the only aneuploidy linked with an increased risk for preeclampsia. Hyperplacentosis and preeclampsia develop in up to half of pregnancies with trisomy 13 carried beyond the second trimester (Tuohy, 1992). Chromosome 13 contains the gene for soluble fms-like tyrosine kinase-1, called sFlt-1, which is an antiangiogenic protein associated with preeclampsia. Investigators have documented overexpression of the sflt-1 protein by trisomic 13 placentas and in serum of women with preeclampsia (Bdolah, 2006; Silasi, 2011). The role of antiangiogenic growth factors in the etiopathogenesis of preeclampsia is discussed in Chapter 40 (p. 735).

Other Trisomies. In the absence of mosaicism, which is discussed below, it is rare for other autosomal trisomies to result in a live birth. There are case reports of live births with trisomy 9 and with trisomy 22 (Kannan, 2009; Tinkle, 2003). Trisomy 16 is the most common trisomy found with first-trimester losses, accounting for 16 percent, but it is not identified later in gestation. Trisomy 1 has never been reported.

Monosomy

Nondisjunction creates an equal number of nullisomic and disomic gametes. As a rule, missing chromosomal material is more devastating than having extra chromosomal material, and almost all monosomic conceptuses are lost before implantation. The one exception is monosomy for the X chromosome, Turner syndrome, which is discussed subsequently. Despite the strong association between maternal age and trisomy, there is no association between maternal age and monosomy (see Fig. 13-1).

Polyploidy

This is an abnormal number of complete haploid chromosomal sets. Polyploidy accounts for approximately 20 percent of spontaneous abortions but is rarely encountered later in gestation.

Triploid pregnancies have three haploid sets or 69 chromosomes. To have three haploid chromosomal sets, one parent must contribute two sets, and the phenotypic presentation differs according to the parent of origin. In *diandric triploidy*, also known as type I triploidy, the extra chromosomal set is paternal, resulting from fertilization of one egg by two sperm or by a single diploid—and thus abnormal—sperm. Diandric triploidy produces a partial molar pregnancy, which is discussed in Chapter 20 (p. 396). Diandric triploidy accounts for most triploid conceptions, but the first-trimester loss rate is extremely high. As a result, two thirds of triploid pregnancies identified beyond the first trimester are caused instead by *digynic triploidy* (Jauniaux 1999). In a digynic triploid pregnancy, also known as type II triploidy, the extra chromosomal set is maternal, and the egg fails to undergo the first or second meiotic division before fertilization. Digynic triploid placentas do not develop molar changes. However, the fetus often displays asymmetric growth restriction (Jauniaux, 1999).

Triploidy is a lethal aneuploidy, and more than 90 percent of fetuses with either the diandric or digynic form have multiple structural anomalies. These include abnormalities of the central nervous system, heart, face, and extremities, as well as severe growth restriction (Jauniaux, 1999). Counseling, prenatal diagnosis, and delivery options are similar to those for trisomies 18 and 13. The recurrence risk for a woman whose triploid fetus survived past the first trimester is 1 to 1.5 percent, and thus prenatal diagnosis is offered in future pregnancies (Gardner, 1996).

Tetraploid pregnancies have 4 haploid sets or 92 chromosomes. Four sets of chromosomes results in either 92,XXXX or 92,XXYY. This suggests a postzygotic failure to complete an early cleavage division. The conceptus invariably succumbs, and the recurrence risk is minimal.

Sex Chromosome Abnormalities

45,X—Turner Syndrome. This is the only monosomy compatible with life. However, it is also the most common aneuploidy in abortuses and accounts for 20 percent of first-trimester losses. The prevalence of Turner syndrome is approximately 1 per 5000 live births or 1 per 2500 girls (Cragan, 2009; Dolk, 2010). The missing X chromosome is paternally derived in 80 percent of cases (Cockwell, 1991; Hassold, 1991).

Monosomy X encompasses three distinct phenotypes. Approximately 98 percent of these conceptuses are so abnormal that they abort early in the first trimester. In a second group, large cystic hygromas are identified in either the first or second trimester, frequently accompanied by hydrops (Fig. 10-16, p. 206 and Chap. 15, p. 315). In such cases, fetal demise almost invariably results. Only the third and least-common phenotype has the potential for postnatal survival. Affected fetuses may have small cystic hygromas visible in the first or second trimester, which do not result in hydrops, and they often have other major abnormalities. One reason for the wide range of Turner syndrome phenotype is that only half of liveborn infants actually have monosomy X. Approximately one fourth have mosaicism, such as 45,X/46,XX or 45,X/46,XY. Another 15 percent have isochromosome X, that is, 46,X,i(Xq)(Milunsky, 2004; Nussbaum, 2007).

Abnormalities associated with Turner syndrome include a major cardiac malformation—such as coarctation of the aorta or bicuspid aortic valve—in 30 to 50 percent; renal anomalies, particularly horseshoe kidney; and hypothyroidism. Other features include short stature, broad chest with widely spaced nipples, congenital lymphedema, webbed posterior neck (resulting from cystic hygromas), and minor bone and cartilage abnormalities. Intelligence is generally in the normal range, although affected individuals are more likely to have visual-spatial organization deficits and difficulties with nonverbal problem solving and interpretation of social cues (Jones, 2006). Growth hormone is typically administered in childhood to ameliorate short stature (Kappelgaard, 2011). More than 90 percent have ovarian dysgenesis and require estrogen repletion beginning just before adolescence. An exception is if a mosaicism involves a Y chromosome. Such cases are at risk for germ cell neoplasm—regardless of whether the child is phenotypically male or female, and eventual prophylactic bilateral gonadectomy is indicated (Cools, 2011; Schorge, 2012).

47,XXX. Approximately 1 in 1000 female infants has an additional X chromosome—47,XXX. The extra X is maternally derived in more than 90 percent of cases (Milunsky, 2004). Pubertal development and fertility are usually normal, although premature ovarian failure has been reported (Holland, 2001). Tall stature is common. The overall major malformation rate is not increased with 47,XXX. That said, atypical phenotypic features have been described in some individuals and include epicanthal folds, clinodactyly, hypotonia, genitourinary problems, and seizure disorders (Tartaglia, 2010). Attention deficit disorder and delays in language development and motor skills have also been reported (Linden, 2002). It is estimated that because of the variability in presentation and subtlety of abnormal findings, only 10 percent of affected children are ascertained clinically.

Females with two or more extra X chromosomes—48,XXXX or 49,XXXXX—are likely to have physical abnormalities apparent at birth. These abnormal X complements are associated with varying degrees of mental retardation. For both males and females, the IQ score is lower with each additional X chromosome.

47,XXY—Klinefelter Syndrome. This is the most common sex chromosome abnormality. It occurs in approximately 1 per 600 male infants. The additional X chromosome is maternally or paternally derived with equal propensity (Jacobs, 1995; Lowe, 2001). There is also a slight association with either advanced maternal age or advanced paternal age (Milunsky, 2004).

Infants with XXY appear phenotypically normal and usually do not have an increased incidence of anomalies. As children, boys are typically tall and have normal prepubertal development. However, they have gonadal dysgenesis, do not undergo normal virilization, and require testosterone supplementation beginning in adolescence. They may develop gynecomastia. In general, IQ scores are within the normal range but slightly below those of siblings, and delays in speech, reading, and motor skills are not uncommon (Girardin, 2011).

47,XYY. This aneuploidy occurs in approximately 1 in 1000 male infants. There is no association with paternal age, anomaly rates are not increased, and there are no unusual phenotypic features. These boys tend to be tall, they have normal puberty, and fertility is unimpaired. They are at increased risk for oral and written language impairments, but intelligence is generally normal (Ross, 2009). A commonly held misconception was that XYY karyotype was associated with criminal or violent behavior. However, these early reports have been refuted.

Males with more than two Y chromosomes—48,XYYY—or with both additional X and Y chromosomes—48,XXYY or 49,XXXYY—have obvious physical abnormalities and significant mental retardation.

Abnormalities of Chromosome Structure

Structural chromosomal abnormalities include deletions, duplications, translocations, isochromosomes, inversions, ring chromosomes, and mosaicism (see Table 13-1). Their overall birth prevalence is approximately 0.3 percent (Nussbaum, 2007). Identification of a structural chromosomal abnormality raises two primary questions. First, what phenotypic abnormalities or later developmental abnormalities are associated with this finding? Second, is evaluation of parental karyotype indicated—specifically, are the parents at increased risk to carry this abnormality? If so, what is their risk to have future affected offspring?

Deletions and Duplications

A chromosomal deletion indicates that a portion of a chromosome is missing, and a duplication means that a portion has been included twice. Deletions involving DNA segments large enough to be seen with standard cytogenetic karyotyping are identified in approximately 1 per 7000 births (Nussbaum, 2007). Common deletions may be referred to by eponyms—for example, del 5p is called cri du chat syndrome.

Most deletions and duplications occur during meiosis and result from malalignment or mismatching during the pairing of homologous chromosomes. When this happens, the misaligned segment may be deleted (Fig. 13-6). Or, if the mismatch remains when the two chromosomes recombine, it may result in a deletion in one chromosome and a duplication in the other. When a deletion or duplication is identified in a fetus or

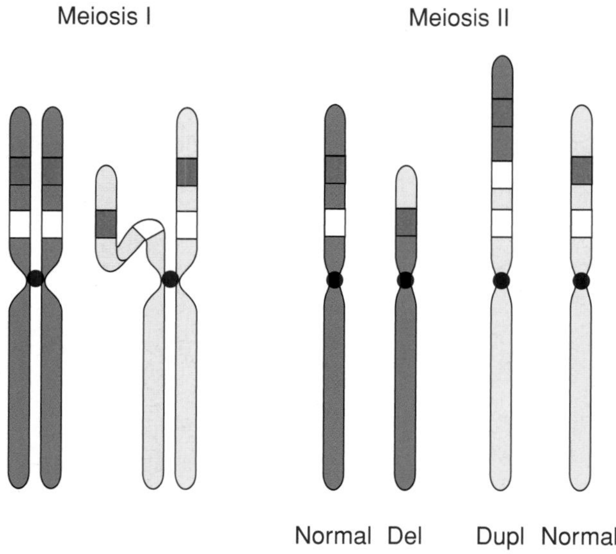

FIGURE 13-6 A mismatch during pairing of homologous chromosomes may lead to a deletion in one chromosome and a duplication in the other. del = deletion; dup = duplication.

infant, the parents should be offered karyotyping to determine if either carries a balanced translocation—as this would significantly increase the recurrence risk.

Microdeletion Syndromes. A chromosomal deletion smaller than 3 million base pairs may not be detectable with standard karyotyping. Termed microdeletions, these may require molecular cytogenetic techniques for identification. Despite the relatively small size, a microdeletion may involve a stretch of DNA that contains multiple genes—causing a contiguous gene syndrome, which can include serious but unrelated phenotypic abnormalities (Schmickel, 1986). When a specific microdeletion syndrome is suspected, it is usually confirmed using fluorescence in situ hybridization (p. 276). Examples of common microdeletion syndromes are listed in Table 13-3.

The region of DNA that is deleted in a microdeletion syndrome (or duplicated in a microduplication) is termed a *genomic copy number variant* when applied to chromosomal microarray analysis discussed on page 277. Use of array-based technology has identified copy number variants that result in previously uncharacterized microdeletion syndromes—including single gene and intragenic deletions (Mikhail, 2011; Schwartz, 2012). It is likely that continued expansion of this technology will dramatically advance our knowledge of the genetic basis of disease.

22q11 Microdeletion Syndrome. This syndrome is also known as DiGeorge syndrome, Shprintzen syndrome, and velocardiofacial syndrome. It is the most common microdeletion, with prevalence of 1 per 2000 to 7000 births (Shprintzen, 2008). Although it is inherited in an autosomal dominant fashion, most cases arise from de novo mutations. The full deletion includes 3 million base pairs, encompasses 40 genes, and may include 180 different features—thus posing some counseling challenges (Shprintzen, 2008). It was once thought that different constellations of features characterized the DiGeorge and Shprintzen phenotypes, but it is now accepted that they represent the same microdeletion (McDonald-McGinn, 2011).

Associated abnormalities include conotruncal cardiac anomalies in more than 75 percent of affected individuals, such as tetralogy of Fallot, pulmonary atresia, truncus arteriosus, interrupted aortic arch, and ventricular septal defects. Immune deficiency, such as T-cell lymphopenia, also develops in approximately 75 percent. More than 70 percent have velopharyngeal insufficiency or cleft palate. Other manifestations include learning disabilities and mental retardation, hypocalcemia, renal anomalies, esophageal dysmotility, hearing loss, behavioral disorders, and psychiatric illness. Short palpebral fissures, bulbous nose tip, micrognathia, short philtrum, and small or posteriorly rotated ears are characteristic facial features (McDonald-McGinn, 2011).

Microduplication Syndromes. These syndromes are caused by duplication of DNA regions smaller than 3 million base pairs. In some cases, a microduplication may involve the exact DNA region that causes a recognized microdeletion syndrome. Examples of these include the velocardiofacial, Smith-Magenis, and Williams-Beuren syndromes (Hassed, 2004; Potocki, 2000; Somerville, 2005).

Chromosomal Translocations

These are DNA rearrangements in which a segment of DNA breaks away from one chromosome and attaches to another. The rearranged chromosomes are called derivative (der)

TABLE 13-3. Some Microdeletion Syndromes Detectable by Fluorescence In Situ Hybridization (FISH)

Syndrome	Features	Location
Angelman	Dysmorphic facies—"happy puppet" appearance, mental retardation, ataxia, hypotonia, seizures	15q11.2–q13 (maternal genes)
Cri du chat	Abnormal laryngeal development with "cat-like" cry, hypotonia, mental retardation	5p15.2–15.3
Langer-Giedion	Trichorhinophalangeal syndrome, dysmorphic facies, sparse hair, redundant skin, mental retardation	8q24.1
Miller-Dieker	Neuronal migration abnormalities with lissencephaly, microcephaly, dysmorphic facies	17p13.3
Prader-Willi	Obesity, hypotonia, mental retardation, hypogonadotropic hypogonadism, small hands and feet	15q11.2–q13 (paternal genes)
Smith-Magenis	Dysmorphic facies, speech delay, hearing loss, sleep disturbances, self-destructive behaviors	17p11.2
Velocardiofacial/DiGeorge	May include conotruncal cardiac defects, cleft palate, velopharyngeal incompetence, thymic and parathyroid abnormalities, learning disability	22q11.2
WAGR	Wilms tumor, aniridia, genitourinary anomalies (including ambiguous genitalia), mental retardation	11p13
Wolf-Hirschhorn	Dysmorphic facies, mental retardation, polydactyly, cutis aplasia	4p16.3
X-linked ichthyosis/Kallmann syndrome	Ichthyosis: steroid sulfatase deficiency, corneal opacities. Kallmann: hypogonadotropic hypogonadism, anosmia	Xp22.3

Data from Online Mendelian Inheritance in Man (Johns Hopkins University, 2013).

chromosomes. There are two types—reciprocal and robertsonian translocations.

Reciprocal Translocations. A double-segment or reciprocal translocation develops when there are breaks in two different chromosomes and the broken fragments are exchanged, so that each affected chromosome contains a fragment of the other. If no chromosomal material is gained or lost in this process, the translocation is considered balanced. The prevalence of reciprocal translocations is approximately 1 per 600 births (Nussbaum, 2007). Although transposition of chromosomal segments can cause abnormalities—due to repositioning of specific genes—the balanced carrier is usually phenotypically normal. The risk of a major structural or developmental abnormality in an apparent balanced translocation carrier is approximately 6 percent. Interestingly, using microarray-based studies, as many as 20 percent of individuals who would otherwise appear to have a balanced translocation may have missing or redundant DNA segments that are below the resolution of a standard karyotype (Manning, 2010).

Balanced translocation carriers are at risk to produce unbalanced gametes that result in abnormal offspring. As shown in Figure 13-7, if an oocyte or sperm contains a translocated chromosome, fertilization results in an unbalanced translocation—monosomy for part of one affected chromosome and trisomy for part of the other. The observed risk of a specific translocation can often be estimated by a genetic counselor. In general, translocation carriers identified after the birth of an abnormal child have a 5- to 30-percent risk of having liveborn offspring with unbalanced chromosomes. Carriers identified for other reasons, for example, during an infertility evaluation, have only a 5-percent risk. This is probably because the gametes are so abnormal that conceptions are nonviable.

Robertsonian Translocations. These involve only *acrocentric* chromosomes, which are chromosomes 13, 14, 15, 21, and 22. In an acrocentric chromosome, the p arm is extremely short. In a robertsonian translocation, the q arms of two acrocentric chromosomes fuse at one centromere to form a derivative chromosome. Also, one centromere and the p arms of each chromosome are lost. The p arms contain the satellite regions, which contain only genes coding for ribosomal RNA. As these are present in multiple copies on other acrocentric chromosomes, the translocation carrier is usually phenotypically normal. Because the number of centromeres determines the chromosome count, a robertsonian translocation carrier has only 45 chromosomes.

Robertsonian translocations are found in approximately 1 per 1000 newborns. Balanced carriers have reproductive difficulties for a number of reasons. If the fused chromosomes are homologous, from the same chromosome pair, the carrier can produce only unbalanced gametes. Each egg or sperm contains either both copies of the translocated chromosome, which would result in trisomy if fertilized, or no copy, which would result in monosomy. If the fused chromosomes are nonhomologous, four of the six possible gametes would be abnormal.

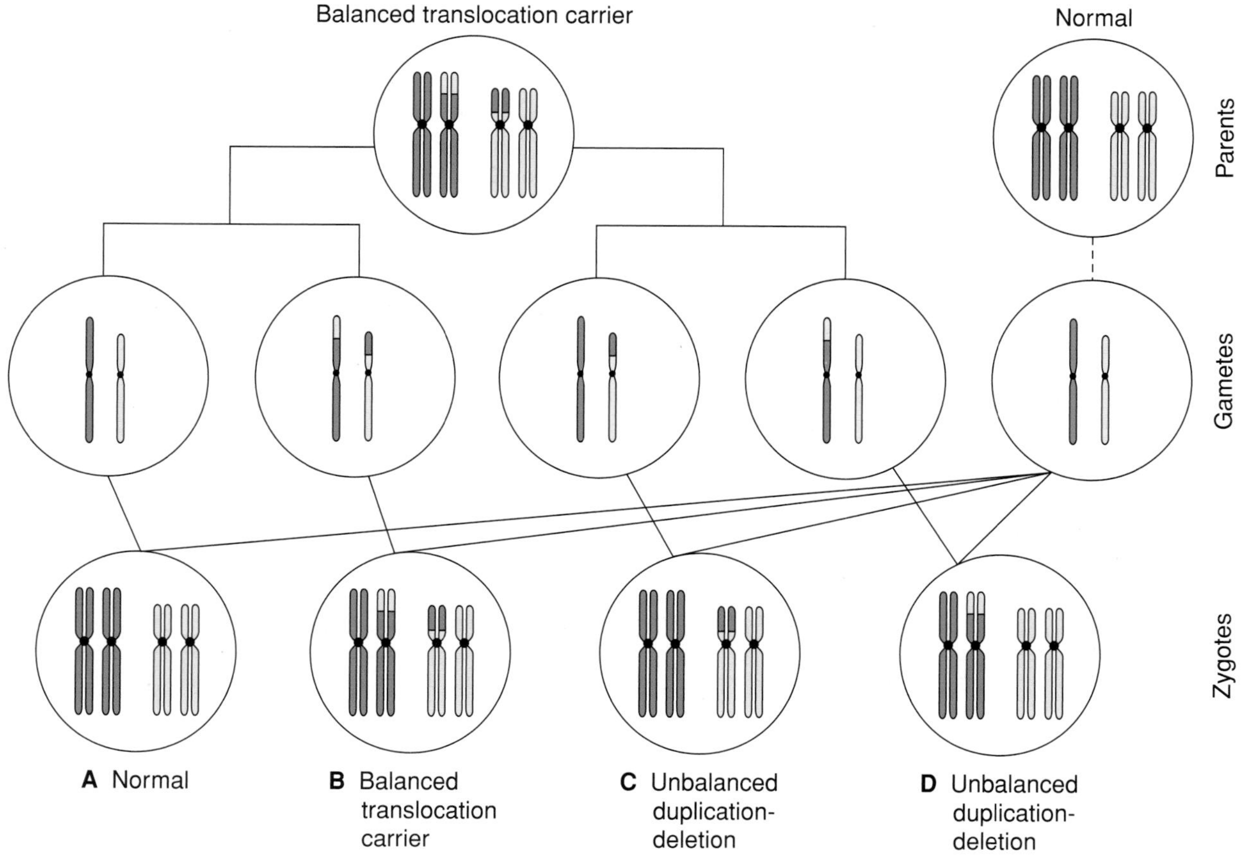

FIGURE 13-7 A carrier of a balanced translocation may produce offspring who are also carriers of the balanced rearrangement **(B)**, offspring with unbalanced translocations **(C, D)**, or offspring with normal chromosomal complements **(A)**.

The most common robertsonian translocation is der(13;14)(q10;q10), which may result in Patau syndrome, discussed on page 263. The observed incidence of abnormal offspring is approximately 15 percent if a robertsonian translocation is carried by the mother and 2 percent if carried by the father. Robertsonian translocations are not a major cause of miscarriage and are found in fewer than 5 percent of couples with recurrent pregnancy loss. When a fetus or child is found to have a translocation trisomy, both parents should be offered karyotype analysis. If neither parent is a carrier, the recurrence risk is extremely low.

Isochromosomes

These abnormal chromosomes are composed of either two q arms or two p arms of one chromosome fused together. Isochromosomes are thought to arise when the centromere breaks transversely instead of longitudinally during meiosis II or mitosis. They can also result from a meiotic error in a chromosome with a robertsonian translocation. An isochromosome containing the q arms of an acrocentric chromosome behaves like a homologous robertsonian translocation, and such a carrier can produce only abnormal unbalanced gametes. When an isochromosome involves nonacrocentric chromosomes, with p arms containing functional genetic material, the fusion and abnormal centromere break results in two isochromosomes. One is composed of both p arms, and one is composed of both q arms. It is likely that one of these isochromosomes would be lost during cell division, resulting in the deletion of all the genes located on the lost arm. Thus, a carrier is usually phenotypically abnormal and produces abnormal gametes. The most common isochromosome involves the long arm of the X chromosome, i(Xq), which is the etiology of 15 percent of Turner syndrome cases.

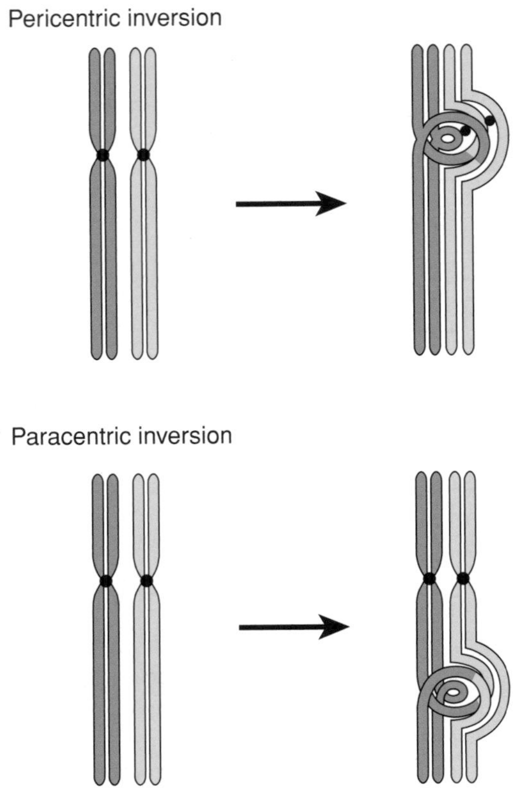

FIGURE 13-8 Mechanism of meiosis in the setting of either pericentric inversion (one involving the centromere) or paracentric inversion (not involving the centromere). Individuals with pericentric inversions are at increased risk to produce offspring with a duplication/deletion. Those with paracentric inversions are at increased risk for early pregnancy loss.

Chromosomal Inversions

When there are two breaks in the same chromosome, and the intervening genetic material is inverted before the breaks are repaired, the result is a chromosomal inversion. Although no genetic material is lost or duplicated, the rearrangement may alter gene function. There are two types—pericentric and paracentric.

Pericentric Inversion. If there are breaks in both the p and q arms of a chromosome, such that the inverted material includes the centromere, the inversion is pericentric (Fig. 13-8). This causes problems in chromosomal alignment during meiosis and confers significant risk for the carrier to produce abnormal gametes and abnormal offspring. In general, the observed risk of abnormal offspring in a pericentric inversion carrier is 5 to 10 percent if ascertainment was made after the birth of an abnormal child. However, the risk is only 1 to 3 percent if prompted by another indication. An important exception is a pericentric inversion on chromosome 9—inv(9)(p11q12), which is a normal variant present in approximately 1 percent of individuals.

Paracentric Inversion. If there are two breaks within one arm of a chromosome, and the inverted material does not include the centromere, the inversion is paracentric (see Fig. 13-8). The carrier makes either normal balanced gametes or gametes that are so abnormal as to preclude fertilization. Thus, although infertility may be a problem, the risk of having an abnormal offspring is extremely low.

Ring Chromosomes

If deletions occur at both ends of the same chromosome, the ends may come together to form a ring chromosome. The regions at the end of each chromosome are called telomeres and contain specialized nucleoprotein complexes that stabilize chromosomes. If only telomeres are lost, all necessary genetic material is retained, so the carrier is essentially balanced. With deletions extending more proximally than the telomeres, the carrier is likely to be phenotypically abnormal. An example of this is a ring X chromosome, which may result in Turner syndrome.

Ring chromosome carriers have reproductive difficulties. The ring prevents normal chromosome alignment during meiosis and thus produces abnormal gametes. It also disrupts cell division, which may cause abnormal tissue growth and lead to short stature, borderline to moderate mental deficiency, and minor dysmorphisms. A ring chromosome may form de novo or may be inherited from a carrier parent. Parent-to-child transmission is always maternal, possibly because of compromised spermatogenesis.

Chromosomal Mosaicism

A mosaic individual has two or more cytogenetically distinct cell lines that are derived from a single zygote. Phenotypic expression of mosaicism depends on several factors, including whether the cytogenetically abnormal cells involve the placenta, the fetus, part of the fetus, or some combination. For example, mosaicism found in cells from amnionic fluid culture does not always reflect the fetal chromosome complement. The different levels of mosaicism and their clinical significance are presented in Table 13-4. When the abnormal cells are present in only a single flask of amnionic fluid, the finding is likely pseudomosaicism, caused by cell-culture artifact (Bui, 1984; Hsu, 1984). When abnormal cells involve multiple cultures, however, true mosaicism is more likely, and further testing of fetal blood or skin fibroblasts may be warranted. A second cell line is verified in 60 to 70 percent of these fetuses (Hsu, 1984; Worton, 1984).

Confined Placental Mosaicism. According to studies of chorionic villus sampling (CVS), 2 percent of placentas are mosaic, even though the associated fetus is usually normal (Henderson, 1996). The mechanism underlying confined placental mosaicism may be either mitotic nondisjunction or partial correction of a meiotic error, and the mechanism appears to be chromosome-specific (Robinson, 1997). Fifteen to 20 percent of cases are associated with an adverse pregnancy outcome, such as miscarriage, fetal-growth restriction, or stillbirth (Reddy, 2009).

Fetal-growth restriction from placental mosaicism may arise in one of two ways. If the placenta has a population of aneuploid cells, impaired placental function may affect the growth of a cytogenetically normal fetus (Kalousek, 1983). Alternatively, if the fetus receives two otherwise normal copies of one chromosome, but both copies are from the same parent—uniparental disomy, then abnormal growth may result (p. 273).

In some cases, survival of cytogenetically abnormal fetuses may be due to placental mosaicism. Examples are trisomy 13 and 18 fetuses, who survive to term because of early "trisomic correction" in some cells that become trophoblasts (Kalousek, 1989).

Gonadal Mosaicism. Mosaicism confined to the gonads likely arises from a mitotic error in cells destined to become the gonad and results in a population of abnormal germ cells. Because spermatogonia and oogonia divide throughout fetal life, and spermatogonia continue to divide throughout adulthood, gonadal mosaicism may also follow a meiotic error in previously normal germ cells. Gonadal mosaicism may explain de novo autosomal dominant mutations in the offspring of normal parents. It may cause autosomal dominant diseases such as achondroplasia and osteogenesis imperfecta, as well as X-linked diseases such as Duchenne muscular dystrophy. Gonadal mosaicism may also explain the recurrence of such diseases in more than one child in a previously unaffected family. The potential for gonadal mosaicism explains the 6-percent recurrence risk after the birth of a child with a disease caused by a "new" mutation.

MODES OF INHERITANCE

Monogenic (Mendelian) Inheritance

A monogenic disorder is caused by a mutation or alteration in a single locus or gene in one or both members of a gene pair. Monogenic disorders are also called mendelian to signify that their transmission follows the laws of inheritance proposed by Gregor Mendel. Types of mendelian inheritance include autosomal dominant, autosomal recessive, X-linked, and Y-linked. Other monogenic patterns of inheritance are mitochondrial inheritance, uniparental disomy, imprinting, and trinucleotide repeat expansion, which is also termed anticipation. By age 25, approximately 0.4 percent of the population exhibits an abnormality attributed to a monogenic disorder, and 2 percent will have at least one such disorder during their lifetime. Some common single-gene disorders are listed in Table 13-5.

Relationship between Phenotype and Genotype

When considering inheritance, it is the phenotype that is dominant or recessive, not the genotype. With a dominant disease, the normal gene may direct the production of normal protein, but the phenotype is abnormal because it is determined by protein produced by the abnormal gene. With a recessive disease, a heterozygous carrier may produce detectable levels of an abnormal gene product but have no features of the condition because the phenotype is directed by the product of the normal co-gene. For example, erythrocytes from carriers of sickle-cell anemia contain approximately 30 percent hemoglobin S, but

TABLE 13-4. Types of Mosaicism Encountered in Amnionic Fluid Cultures

Type	Prevalence (%)	Description and Significance
Level I	2–3	Single cell with an abnormal karyotype in a single culture—confined to one of several flasks or to one of several colonies on a coverslip. This is usually a cell-culture artifact, that is, pseudomosaicism
Level II	1	Multiple cells with an abnormal karyotype in a single culture—confined to one of several flasks or to one of several colonies on a coverslip. This is usually a cell-culture artifact, that is, pseudomosaicism
Level III	0.1–0.3	Multiple cells in multiple cultures with an abnormal karyotype. Requires further evaluation as 60–70 percent of fetuses will have a second cell line, that is, true mosaicism

TABLE 13-5. Some Common Single-Gene Disorders

Autosomal Dominant
Achondroplasia
Acute intermittent porphyria
Adult polycystic kidney disease
Antithrombin III deficiency
BRCA1 and BRCA2 breast and/or ovarian cancer
Ehlers-Danlos syndrome
Familial adenomatous polyposis
Familial hypercholesterolemia
Hereditary hemorrhagic telangiectasia
Hereditary spherocytosis
Huntington disease
Hypertrophic obstructive cardiomyopathy
Long QT syndrome
Marfan syndrome
Myotonic dystrophy
Neurofibromatosis type 1 and 2
Tuberous sclerosis
von Willebrand disease
Autosomal Recessive
α_1-Antitrypsin deficiency
Congenital adrenal hyperplasia
Cystic fibrosis
Gaucher disease
Hemochromatosis
Homocystinuria
Phenylketonuria
Sickle-cell anemia
Tay-Sachs disease
Thalassemia syndromes
Wilson disease
X-Linked
Androgen insensitivity syndrome
Chronic granulomatous disease
Color blindness
Fabry disease
Fragile X syndrome
Glucose-6-phosphate deficiency
Hemophilia A and B
Hypophosphatemic rickets
Muscular dystrophy—Duchenne and Becker
Ocular albinism type 1 and 2

because the other 70 percent is hemoglobin A, these cells do not sickle in vitro.

Heterogeneity. Genetic heterogeneity explains how different genetic mechanisms can result in the same phenotype. Locus heterogeneity indicates that a specific disease phenotype can be caused by mutations in different genetic loci. It also explains why some diseases appear to follow more than one type of inheritance. An example is retinitis pigmentosa, which may develop following mutations in at least 35 different genes or loci and may result in autosomal dominant, autosomal recessive, or X-linked forms.

Allelic heterogeneity describes how different mutations of the same gene may affect presentation of a particular disease. For example, although only one gene has been associated with cystic fibrosis—the *cystic fibrosis conductance transmembrane regulator* gene (CFTR)—more than 1000 mutations in this gene have been described and result in varying disease severity. This is discussed in Chapter 14 (p. 295).

Phenotypic heterogeneity explains how different disease states can arise from different mutations in the same gene. For example, mutations in the *fibroblast growth factor receptor 3 (FGFR3)* gene may result in several different skeletal disorders, including achondroplasia and thanatophoric dysplasia, both of which are discussed in Chapter 10 (p. 217).

Autosomal Dominant Inheritance

If only one member of a gene pair determines the phenotype, that gene is considered to be dominant. Carriers have a 50-percent chance of passing on the affected gene with each conception. A gene with a dominant mutation generally specifies the phenotype in preference to the normal gene. That said, not all individuals will necessarily manifest an autosomal dominant condition the same way. Factors that affect the phenotype of an autosomal dominant condition include penetrance, expressivity, and occasionally, presence of codominant genes.

Penetrance. This term describes whether or not a dominant gene is expressed at all. A gene with recognizable phenotypic expression in all individuals has 100-percent penetrance. If some carriers express the gene but some do not, then penetrance is incomplete. This is quantitatively expressed by the ratio of those individuals with any phenotypic characteristics of the gene to the total number of gene carriers. For example, a gene that is expressed in some way in 80 percent of individuals who have that gene is 80-percent penetrant. Incomplete penetrance explains why some autosomal dominant diseases appear to "skip" generations.

Expressivity. Individuals with the same autosomal dominant trait—even within the same family—may manifest the condition differently. Genes with such variable expressivity can produce disease manifestations from mild to very severe. Examples include neurofibromatosis, tuberous sclerosis, and adult polycystic kidney disease.

Codominant Genes. If two different alleles in a gene pair are both expressed in the phenotype, they are considered to be codominant. Blood type, for example, is determined by expression of dominant A and B red-cell antigens that can be expressed simultaneously. Another example is the group of genes responsible for hemoglobin production. An individual with one gene directing production of hemoglobin S and the other directing production of hemoglobin C will produce both S and C hemoglobin.

Advanced Paternal Age. Paternal age older than 40 is associated with increased risk for spontaneous genetic mutations, particularly single base substitutions. This may result in offspring with new autosomal dominant disorders or X-linked carrier states. The risk is greater for some conditions than for others. In particular, advanced paternal age has been associated with mutations in the *fibroblast growth factor receptor 2 (FGFR2)* gene, which may cause craniosynostosis syndromes such as Apert, Crouzon, and Pfeiffer syndromes; mutations in the *FGFR3* gene, which may result in achondroplasia and thanatophoric dysplasia; and mutations in the *RET proto-oncogene,* which may cause multiple endocrine neoplasia syndromes (Jung, 2003; Toriello, 2008). Because these disorders are uncommon, the actual risk for any individual condition is low.

Advanced paternal age has also been associated with a slightly increased risk for Down syndrome and for isolated structural abnormalities (Grewal, 2011; Toriello, 2008; Yang, 2007). It is not generally considered to pose an increased risk for other aneuploidies, probably because the aneuploid sperm cannot fertilize an egg.

Autosomal Recessive Inheritance

A recessive trait is expressed only when both copies of the gene function in the same way. Thus, autosomal recessive diseases develop only when both gene copies are abnormal. Heterozygous carriers are usually undetectable clinically but may have biochemical test abnormalities. Many enzyme deficiency diseases display autosomal recessive inheritance, and enzyme activity in the carrier is approximately half of normal. Although this reduction usually does not cause clinical disease, it provides a phenotypic alteration that can be used for carrier screening. Other recessive conditions can be identified only by molecular genetic testing.

Unless carriers are screened for a specific disease, such as cystic fibrosis, they usually are recognized only after the birth of an affected child or the diagnosis of an affected family member (Chap. 14, p. 295). If a couple has a child with an autosomal recessive disease, the recurrence risk is 25 percent for each subsequent pregnancy. Thus, 1/4 of offspring will be homozygous normal, 2/4 will be heterozygous carriers, and 1/4 will be homozygous abnormal. In other words, three of four children will be phenotypically normal, and 2/3 of phenotypically normal siblings are actually carriers.

A heterozygous carrier of a recessive condition is only at risk to have affected children if his or her partner is heterozygous or homozygous for the disease. Genes for rare autosomal recessive conditions have low prevalence in the general population. Thus, the likelihood that a partner will be a gene carrier is low—unless there is consanguinity or the partner is a member of an at-risk group (American College of Obstetricians and Gynecologists, 2009b). This is discussed further in Chapter 14 (p. 294).

Inborn Errors of Metabolism. Most of these autosomal recessive diseases result from absence of a crucial enzyme, leading to incomplete metabolism of proteins, lipids, or carbohydrates. The metabolic intermediates that build up are toxic to a variety of tissues and may result in mental retardation or other abnormalities.

Phenylketonuria. This classic example of an autosomal recessive disease is caused by mutations in the *phenylalanine hydroxylase (PAH)* gene. PAH is needed to metabolize phenylalanine to tyrosine, and homozygotes have diminished or absent enzyme activity. This leads to abnormally high levels of phenylalanine, resulting in progressive intellectual impairment, autism, seizures, motor deficits, and neuropsychological abnormalities (Blau, 2010). Also, because phenylalanine competitively inhibits tyrosine hydroxylase—which is essential for melanin production, affected individuals have hair, eye, and skin hypopigmentation.

Approximately 3000 reproductive-aged women in the United States have phenylketonuria (PKU). The carrier frequency is approximately 1 in 60, and the disease affects 1 in 10,000 to 15,000 white newborns (American College of Obstetricians and Gynecologists, 2009a). PKU is one of the few metabolic disorders for which there is treatment. Early diagnosis and limitation of dietary phenylalanine beginning in infancy are essential to prevent neurological damage. Accordingly, all states and many countries now mandate newborn screening for PKU, and approximately 100 cases per million births are identified worldwide. The special diet should be continued indefinitely, as those who abandon the phenylalanine-restricted diet have a significantly lower IQ and neuropsychological impairments (Blau, 2010).

Affected women who do not adhere to a phenylalanine-free diet are at risk to have otherwise normal (heterozygous) offspring who sustain in utero damage as a result of being exposed to toxic phenylalanine concentrations. Phenylalanine is actively transported to the fetus, and hyperphenylalaninemia increases the risk for miscarriage and for PKU embryopathy. This is characterized by mental retardation, microcephaly, seizures, growth impairment, and cardiac anomalies. Among women on unrestricted diets, the risk to have a child with mental retardation may exceed 90 percent, and as many as 1 in 8 children have cardiac defects (Lenke, 1980). The Maternal Phenylketonuria Collaborative Study, which included 572 pregnancies followed more than 18 years, reported that maintenance of serum phenylalanine levels between 160 and 360 μmol/L (2 to 6 mg/dL) significantly reduced the fetal abnormality risk (Koch, 2003; Platt, 2000). Women who achieved optimal phenylalanine levels before 10 weeks' gestation had children with mean IQ scores in the normal range when assessed at age 6 to 7 years (Koch, 2003). Preconceptional counseling is recommended with a goal of maintaining an optimal phenylalanine concentration from 3 months before conception and continuing this throughout pregnancy (American College of Obstetricians and Gynecologists, 2009a).

Consanguinity. Two individuals are considered consanguineous if they have at least one recent ancestor in common. First-degree relatives share half of their genes, second-degree relatives share a fourth, and third-degree relatives—cousins—share one eighth. Because of the potential for shared deleterious genes, consanguinity confers an increased risk to have offspring with otherwise rare autosomal recessive diseases or multifactorial disorders. First cousins have a twofold increased risk—4 to 6 percent overall, in the absence of a family history of genetic disease.

Incest is defined as a sexual relationship between first-degree relatives such as parent-child or brother-sister and is universally illegal. Progeny of such unions carry the highest risk of abnormal outcomes, and up to 40 percent of offspring are abnormal as a result of recessive and multifactorial disorders (Freire-Maia, 1984; Nadiri, 1979).

X-Linked and Y-Linked Inheritance

Most X-linked diseases are recessive. Common examples include color blindness, hemophilia A and B, and Duchenne and Becker muscular dystrophy. When a woman carries a gene causing an X-linked recessive condition, each of her sons has a 50-percent risk of being affected, and each daughter has a 50-percent chance of being a carrier.

Males with an X-linked recessive gene are usually affected because they lack a second X chromosome to express the normal dominant gene. A male with an X-linked disease cannot have affected sons because they cannot receive his X chromosome. Women with an X-linked recessive gene are generally unaffected by the disease it causes. In some cases, however, the random inactivation of one X chromosome in each cell—termed lyonization—is skewed, and female carriers may have features of the condition. For example, approximately 10 percent of female carriers of hemophilia A display factor VIII levels less than 30 percent of normal, and a similar proportion of female hemophilia B carriers have factor IX levels less than 30 percent. With either type of hemophilia, the female carrier is at increased risk for abnormal bleeding at the time of delivery (Plug, 2006). Similarly, because female carriers of Duchenne or Becker muscular dystrophy are at increased risk for cardiomyopathy, periodic evaluation for cardiac dysfunction and neuromuscular disorders is recommended (American Academy of Pediatrics, 2005).

X-linked dominant disorders mainly affect females, because they tend to be lethal in males. Two examples are vitamin D-resistant rickets and incontinentia pigmenti. One exception is fragile X syndrome, which is discussed subsequently.

The prevalence of Y-linked chromosomal disorders is low. This chromosome carries genes important for sex determination and a variety of cellular functions related to spermatogenesis and bone development. Deletion of genes on the long arm of Y results in severe spermatogenic defects, whereas genes at the tip of the short arm are critical for chromosomal pairing during meiosis and for fertility.

Mitochondrial Inheritance

Human cells contain hundreds of mitochondria, each with its own genome and associated replication system. Oocytes contain approximately 100,000, but sperm contain only about 100, and these are destroyed after fertilization. Each mitochondrion has multiple copies of a 16.5-kb circular DNA molecule that contains 37 genes. Mitochondrial DNA encodes peptides required for oxidative phosphorylation, as well as ribosomal and transfer RNAs.

Mitochondria are inherited exclusively from the mother. Thus, although males and females both can be affected by a mitochondrial disorder, transmission is only through the mother. When a cell replicates, mitochondrial DNA sorts randomly into each of the daughter cells, a process termed replicative segregation. A consequence of replicative segregation is that any mitochondrial mutation will be propagated randomly into the daughter cells. Because there are multiple copies of mitochondrial DNA in each cell, the mitochondrion may contain only normal or only abnormal DNA—homoplasmy, or it may contain both normal and abnormally mutated DNA—heteroplasmy. If a heteroplasmic oocyte is fertilized, the relative proportion of abnormal DNA may affect whether the individual manifests a given mitochondrial disease. It is not possible to predict the potential degree of heteroplasmy among offspring, and this poses a challenge for genetic counseling.

As of 2013, 28 mitochondrial diseases or conditions with known molecular basis were described in OMIM (Johns Hopkins University, 2013). Examples include myoclonic epilepsy with ragged red fibers (MERRF), Leber optic atrophy, Kearns-Sayre syndrome, Leigh syndrome, several forms of mitochondrial myopathy and cardiomyopathy, and susceptibility to both aminoglycoside-induced deafness and chloramphenicol toxicity. Even aging is considered a mitochondrial disease!

DNA Triplet Repeat Expansion—Anticipation

Mendel's first law is that genes are passed unchanged from parent to progeny, and barring new mutations, this is true for many genes or traits. However, certain genes are unstable, and their size, and thus function, may be altered during parent-to-child transmission. This is manifested clinically by anticipation—a phenomenon in which disease symptoms seem to be more severe and to appear at an earlier age in each successive generation. Examples of some DNA triplet (trinucleotide) repeat diseases are shown in Table 13-6.

Fragile X Syndrome. This is the most common inherited form of mental retardation and affects approximately 1 in 3600 males and 1 in 4000 to 6000 females (American College of Obstetricians and Gynecologists, 2010). Fragile X syndrome is caused by expansion of a repeated trinucleotide DNA segment—cytosine-guanine-guanine (CGG)—at chromosome Xq27. When the CGG repeat number reaches a critical size—the full mutation—the *fragile X mental retardation 1 (FMR1)* gene becomes methylated. Methylation inactivates the gene, which halts expression of FMR1 protein.

Although transmission of the syndrome is X-linked, both the sex of the affected individual and the number of CGG repeats determine whether offspring are affected and to what degree. Intellectual disability is generally more severe in males, in whom

TABLE 13-6. Some Disorders Caused by DNA Triplet Repeat Expansion

Dentatorubral pallidoluysian atrophy
Fragile X syndrome
Friedreich ataxia
Huntington disease
Kennedy disease—spinal bulbar muscular atrophy
Myotonic dystrophy
Spinocerebellar ataxias

average IQ scores are 35 to 45 (Nelson, 1995). Affected individuals may have speech and language problems and attention deficit-hyperactivity disorder. Fragile X syndrome is also the most common known cause of autism. Associated phenotypic abnormalities become more prominent with age and include a narrow face with large jaw, prominent ears, connective tissue abnormalities, and macroorchidism in postpubertal males. Clinically, four groups have been described (American College of Obstetricians and Gynecologists, 2010):

- Full mutation—more than 200 repeats
- Premutation—55 to 200 repeats
- Intermediate—45 to 54 repeats
- Unaffected—fewer than 45 repeats

When a full mutation is present, males typically have significant cognitive and behavioral abnormalities and phenotypic features. In females, however, random X-inactivation results in variable expression, and the disability may be much less severe.

For individuals with a premutation, evaluation and counseling are more complex. A female with the fragile X premutation is at risk to have offspring with the full mutation. The likelihood of expansion to a critical full mutation depends on the current number of maternal repeats. The risk of a full mutation in an offspring is 5 percent or less if the CGG repeat number is below 70 but exceeds 95 percent with 100 to 200 CGG repeats (Nolin, 2003). Expansion is extremely unlikely in a male premutation carrier, but all of his daughters will carry the premutation. Among women with no risk factors, approximately 1 in 250 carries a fragile X premutation, and the risk is about 1 in 90 in those with a family history of mental retardation (Cronister, 2008). Premutation carriers may themselves experience significant health consequences. Males with the premutation are at increased risk for the fragile X tremor ataxia syndrome (FXTAS). Females are less likely to have FXTAS, although they have a 20-percent risk for fragile X-associated primary ovarian insufficiency.

The American College of Obstetricians and Gynecologists (2010) recommends testing for women with a family history of fragile X syndrome; individuals with unexplained mental retardation, developmental delay, or autism; and women with premature ovarian insufficiency. Prenatal diagnosis can be accomplished by amniocentesis or CVS (Chap. 14, p. 297). Specimens obtained by either can be used to accurately determine the CGG repeat number, although CVS may not accurately determine *FMR1* gene methylation status. Thus, DNA-based molecular testing with Southern blot and polymerase chain reaction are preferred.

Uniparental Disomy

This occurs when both members of a chromosome pair are inherited from the same parent. Often, uniparental disomy does not have clinical consequences. However, if chromosomes 6, 7, 11, 14, or 15 are involved, offspring are at increased risk for an abnormality because of parent-of-origin differences in gene expression (Shaffer, 2001). Although several genetic mechanisms may cause uniparental disomy, the most common is trisomic rescue, shown in Figure 13-9. After a nondisjunction event produces a trisomic conceptus, one of the three homologues may be lost. This will result in uniparental disomy for that chromosome in approximately one third of cases.

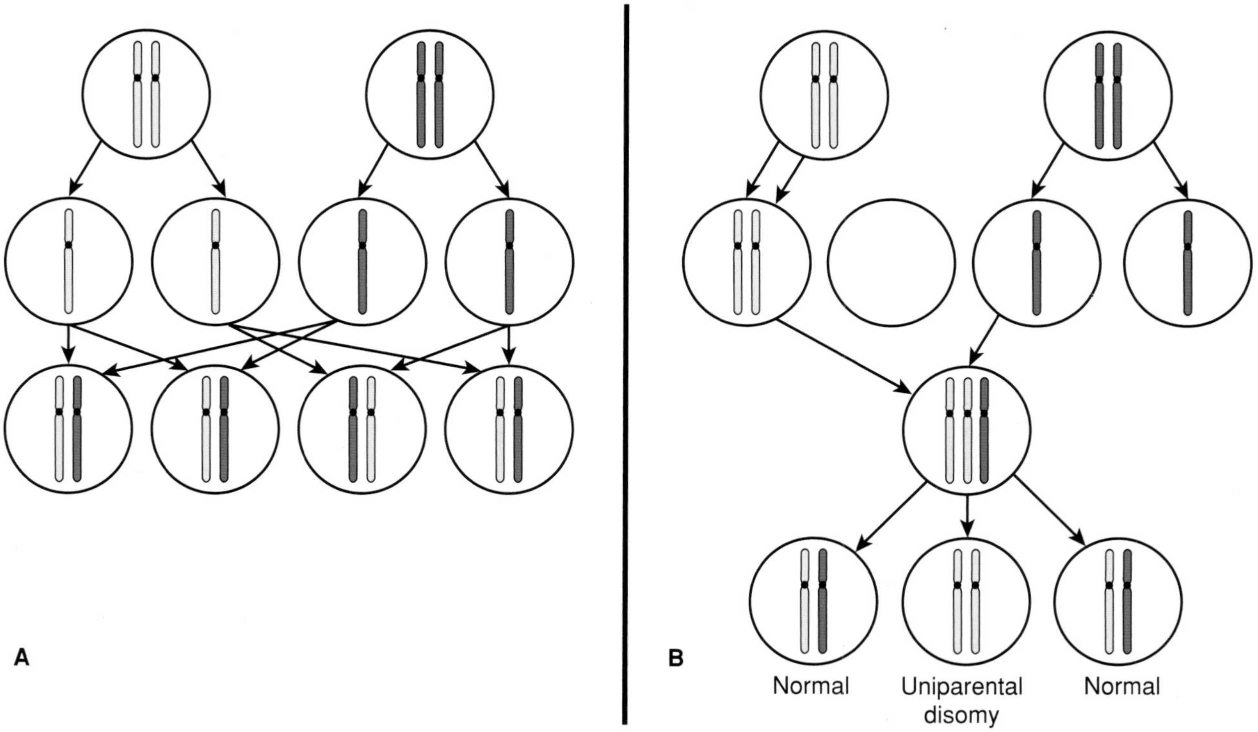

FIGURE 13-9 Mechanism of uniparental disomy arising from trisomic "rescue." **A.** In normal meiosis, one member of each pair of homologous chromosomes is inherited from each parent. **B.** If nondisjunction results in a trisomic conceptus, one homologue is sometimes lost. In a third of cases, loss of one homologue leads to uniparental disomy.

Isodisomy is the unique situation in which an individual receives two identical copies of one chromosome in a pair from one parent. This mechanism explains some cases of cystic fibrosis, in which only one parent is a carrier but the fetus inherits two copies of the same abnormal chromosome from that parent (Spence, 1988; Spotila, 1992). It also has been implicated in abnormal growth related to placental mosaicism.

Imprinting

A gene may be inherited in a transcriptionally silent state—inherited but not expressed—depending on whether it is inherited from the mother or father. The phenotype of the individual varies according to the parent of origin. Imprinting affects gene expression by epigenetic control, that is, gene activity regulation by modification of genetic structure other than alteration of the underlying nucleotide sequence. For example, methyl group addition may alter gene expression and thereby affect the phenotype without changing the genotype. Importantly, the effect may be reversed in a subsequent generation, because a female who inherits an imprinted gene from her father will pass it on in her oocytes with a maternal—rather than paternal—imprint, and vice versa.

Selected diseases that can involve imprinting are shown in Table 13-7. A useful example includes two very different diseases that may be caused by microdeletion, uniparental disomy, or imprinting for the 15q11-q13 DNA region. First, Prader–Willi syndrome is characterized by obesity and hyperphagia; short stature; small hands, feet, and external genitalia; and mild mental retardation. In more than 70 percent of cases, Prader-Willi syndrome is caused by microdeletion or disruption for the paternal 15q11.2-q13. The remaining cases are due to maternal uniparental disomy or due to maternal gene imprinting with the paternal gene inactivated.

In contrast, Angelman syndrome includes severe mental retardation; normal stature and weight; absent speech; seizure disorder; ataxia and jerky arm movements; and paroxysms of inappropriate laughter. In approximately 70 percent of cases, Angelman syndrome is caused by microdeletion for the maternal 15q11.2-q13. In 2 percent, the syndrome is caused by paternal uniparental disomy, and another 2 to 3 percent are due to paternal gene imprinting with the maternal genes inactivated.

TABLE 13-7. Some Disorders That Can Involve Imprinting

Disorder	Chromosomal Region	Parental Origin
Angelman	15q11.2-q13	Maternal
Beckwith-Wiedemann	11p15.5	Paternal
Myoclonic-dystonia	7q21	Maternal
Prader-Willi	15q11.2-q13	Paternal
Pseudohypoparathyroidism	20q13.2	Depends on type
Russell-Silver syndrome	7p11.2	Maternal

Data from Online Mendelian Inheritance in Man (Johns Hopkins University, 2013).

There are other examples of imprinting important to obstetrics. Complete hydatidiform mole, with a paternally derived diploid chromosomal complement, is characterized by abundant placental growth with no fetal structures (Chap. 20, p. 396). Conversely, an ovarian teratoma, with a maternally derived diploid chromosomal complement, is characterized by the growth of various fetal but no placental tissues (Porter, 1993). It thus appears that paternal genes are vital for placental development, maternal genes essential for fetal development, and that both are necessary for normal fetal development.

Multifactorial Inheritance

Traits or diseases are considered to have multifactorial inheritance if they are determined by the combination of multiple genes and environmental factors. Polygenic traits are determined by the combined effects of more than one gene. Most congenital and acquired conditions, as well as common traits, display multifactorial inheritance. Examples include malformations such as clefts and neural-tube defects, diseases such as diabetes and heart disease, and features or traits such as head size or height. Abnormalities that display multifactorial inheritance tend to recur in families, but not according to a mendelian pattern. If a couple has had a child with a multifactorial birth defect, their empiric risk to have another affected child is 3 to 5 percent. This risk declines exponentially with successively more distant relationships. Some characteristics of multifactorial conditions are shown in Table 13-8.

Multifactorial traits that have a normal distribution in the population are termed continuously variable. A measurement that is more than two standard deviations above or below the population mean is considered abnormal. Continuously variable traits tend to be less extreme in the offspring of affected individuals, because of the statistical principle of regression to the mean.

Threshold Traits. Some multifactorial traits do not appear until a threshold is exceeded. Genetic and environmental factors that create propensity or liability for the trait are themselves

TABLE 13-8. Characteristics of Multifactorial Diseases

There is a genetic contribution:
- No mendelian pattern of inheritance
- No evidence of single-gene disorder

Nongenetic factors are also involved in disease causation:
- Lack of penetrance despite predisposing genotype
- Monozygotic twins may be discordant

Familial aggregation may be present:
- Relatives are more likely to have disease-predisposing alleles

Expression more common among close relatives:
- Becomes less common in less closely related relatives—fewer predisposing alleles
- Greater concordance in monozygotic than dizygotic twins

Adapted from Nussbaum, 2007.

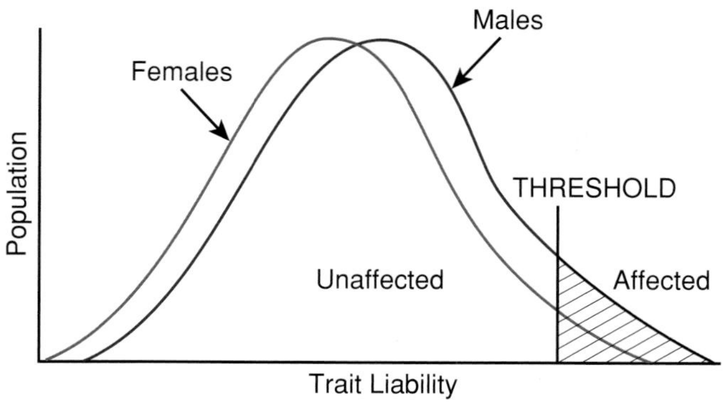

FIGURE 13-10 Schematic example of a threshold trait, such as pyloric stenosis, which has a predilection for males. Each gender is normally distributed, but at the same threshold, more males than females will develop the condition.

normally distributed, and only individuals at the extreme of the distribution exceed the threshold and exhibit the trait or defect. Phenotypic abnormality is thus an all-or-none phenomenon. Examples include cleft lip-palate and pyloric stenosis.

Certain threshold traits have a clear male or female predominance. If an individual of the less common gender has the characteristic or defect, the recurrence risk is greater in his or her offspring (Fig. 13-10). An example is pyloric stenosis, which is approximately four times more common in males (Krogh, 2012). A female with pyloric stenosis has likely inherited more predisposing genetic factors than are necessary to produce the defect in a male, and the recurrence risk for her children or siblings is thus higher than the expected 3 to 5 percent. Her male siblings or male offspring would have the highest liability because they not only will inherit more than the usual number of predisposing genes but also are the more susceptible gender.

The recurrence risk for threshold traits is also greater if the defect is severe. An example is that the recurrence risk after the birth of a child with bilateral cleft lip and palate is approximately 8 percent, but it is only about 4 percent following a child with unilateral cleft lip alone.

Cardiac Defects. Structural cardiac anomalies are the most common birth defects, with a birth prevalence of 8 per 1000. More than 100 genes believed to be involved in cardiovascular morphogenesis have been identified, including those directing production of various proteins, protein receptors, and transcription factors (Olson, 2006; Weismann, 2007).

The risk to have a child with a cardiac anomaly is approximately 5 to 6 percent if the mother has the defect and 2 to 3 percent if the father has the defect (Burn, 1998). Selected left-sided lesions, including hypoplastic left heart syndrome, coarctation of the aorta, and bicuspid aortic valve, may have recurrence risks four- to sixfold higher (Lin, 1988; Lupton, 2002; Nora, 1988). Observed recurrence risks for specific cardiac malformations are listed in Table 49-4 (p. 977).

Neural-Tube Defects. This is the second most common class of birth defects after cardiac anomalies. Their sonographic features and prenatal diagnosis are described in Chapters 10 (p. 201) and 14 (p. 283), respectively, and their prevention with folic acid is discussed in Chapter 9 (p. 181).

Neural-tube defects (NTDs) are classic examples of multifactorial inheritance. Their development may be influenced by hyperthermia, hyperglycemia, teratogen exposure, ethnicity, family history, fetal gender, and various genes. Selected risk factors are more strongly associated with specific NTD location. Hyperthermia has been associated with anencephaly risk; pregestational diabetes with cranial and cervical-thoracic defects; and valproic acid exposure with lumbosacral defects (Becerra, 1990; Hunter, 1984; Lindhout, 1992).

Almost 50 years ago, Hibbard and Smithells (1965) postulated that abnormal folate metabolism was responsible for many NTDs. For a woman with a prior affected child, the recurrence risk of 3 to 5 percent is decreased by at least 70 percent—and potentially by as much as 85 to 90 percent—with periconceptional folic acid supplementation at a dosage of 4 mg/day (Grosse, 2007; MRC Vitamin Study Research Group, 1991). However, most NTD cases do not occur in the setting of maternal folic acid deficiency, and it has become clear that the gene-nutrient interactions underlying folate-responsive NTDs are complex. The NTD risk may be affected by genetic variation in folate transport or accumulation, impaired folate utilization via secondary nutrient deficiencies such as vitamin B_{12} or choline deficiency, and genetic variation in activity of folate-dependent metabolic enzymes (Beaudin, 2009).

GENETIC TESTS

The two most common prenatal genetic tests, cytogenetic analysis and fluorescence in situ hybridization (FISH), are used primarily for aneuploidy detection. For the diagnosis of a specific disease in which the genetic basis is known, DNA-based tests are often employed, typically using polymerase chain reaction (PCR) for rapid amplification of DNA sequences. A new technology that has become clinically available is chromosomal microarray analysis (CMA), which allows the entire genome to be screened for differences in small DNA sequences that characterize genetic disease. Traditionally, each of the above tests has been performed on amnionic fluid or chorionic villi. Recently, however, attention has focused on use of cell-free fetal DNA found in the maternal circulation. A technique known as massively parallel sequencing has enabled researchers to identify trisomy 21 and other aneuploidies using cell-free fetal DNA from maternal blood, and there is potential for cell-free fetal DNA to be used to diagnose a wide range of genetic conditions in the future.

Cytogenetic Analysis

Any tissue containing dividing cells or cells that can be stimulated to divide is suitable for cytogenetic analysis. The dividing cells are arrested in metaphase, and their chromosomes are stained to reveal light and dark bands. The most commonly used technique is Giemsa staining, which yields the G-bands shown in Figure 13-3. Each chromosome has a unique banding pattern that permits its identification as well as detection of deleted, duplicated, or rearranged segments. The accuracy of cytogenetic analysis increases with the number of bands produced. High-resolution metaphase banding routinely yields

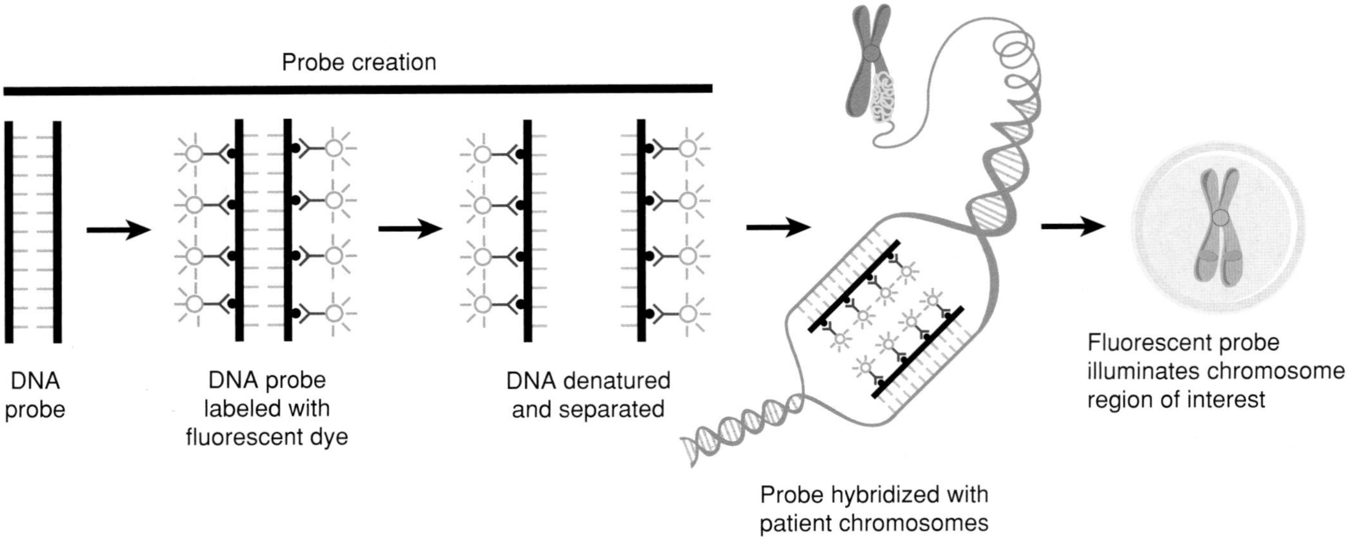

FIGURE 13-11 Steps in fluorescence in situ hybridization (FISH).

450 to 550 visible bands per haploid chromosome set. Banding of prophase chromosomes generally yields 850 bands.

Because only dividing cells can be evaluated, the rapidity with which results are obtained correlates with the rapidity of cell growth in culture. Fetal blood cells often produce results in 36 to 48 hours. Amnionic fluid, which contains epithelial cells, gastrointestinal mucosal cells, and amniocytes, usually yields results in 7 to 10 days. If fetal skin fibroblasts are evaluated postmortem, stimulation of cell growth can be more difficult, and cytogenetic analysis may take 2 to 3 weeks.

Fluorescence In Situ Hybridization

This tool provides a rapid method for determining numerical changes of selected chromosomes and confirming the presence or absence of a specific gene or DNA sequence. FISH is particularly useful for the rapid identification of a specific aneuploidy and for verification of suspected microdeletion or duplication syndromes. Speed is important in some instances because these findings may alter pregnancy management.

To perform FISH, cells are fixed onto a glass slide, and fluorescent-labeled chromosome or gene probes are hybridized to the fixed chromosomes, as shown in Figures 13-11 and 13-12. Each probe is a DNA sequence that is complementary to a unique region of the chromosome or gene being investigated. If the DNA sequence of interest is present, hybridization is detected as a bright signal, visible by microscopy. The number of signals indicates the number of chromosomes or genes of that type in the cell being analyzed. Findings are probe-specific. Thus, FISH does not provide information on the entire chromosomal complement but merely the chromosomal or gene region of interest.

The most common prenatal application of FISH involves testing interphase chromosomes with DNA sequences specific to chromosomes 21, 18, 13, X, and Y. Shown in Figure 13-12 is an example of interphase FISH using α-satellite probes for chromosomes 18, X, and Y to confirm trisomy 18. In a review of more than 45,000 cases, the concordance between FISH analysis and standard cytogenetic karyotyping was 99.8 percent (Tepperberg, 2001). The American College of Medical Genetics (2000) recommends that clinical decision making based on FISH also incorporate consistent clinical information or confirmatory chromosomal analysis.

Southern Blotting

This technique, named after Edward Southern, allows identification of one or several DNA fragments of interest from among the million or so typically obtained by enzyme digestion of the entire genome. As illustrated in Figure 13-13, a restriction endonuclease enzyme digests the DNA, resulting in fragments that are then separated using agarose gel electrophoresis. This is followed by transfer to a nitrocellulose membrane that binds DNA. Probes homologous for the DNA segment of interest are

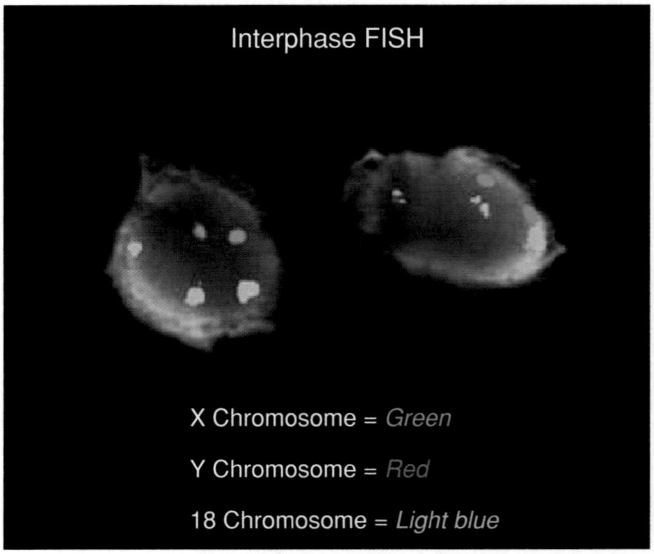

FIGURE 13-12 Interphase fluorescence in situ hybridization (FISH) using α-satellite probes for chromosomes 18, X, and Y. In this case, the three light blue signals, two green signals, and absence of red signals indicate that this is a female fetus with trisomy 18. (Image contributed by Dr. Frederick Elder.)

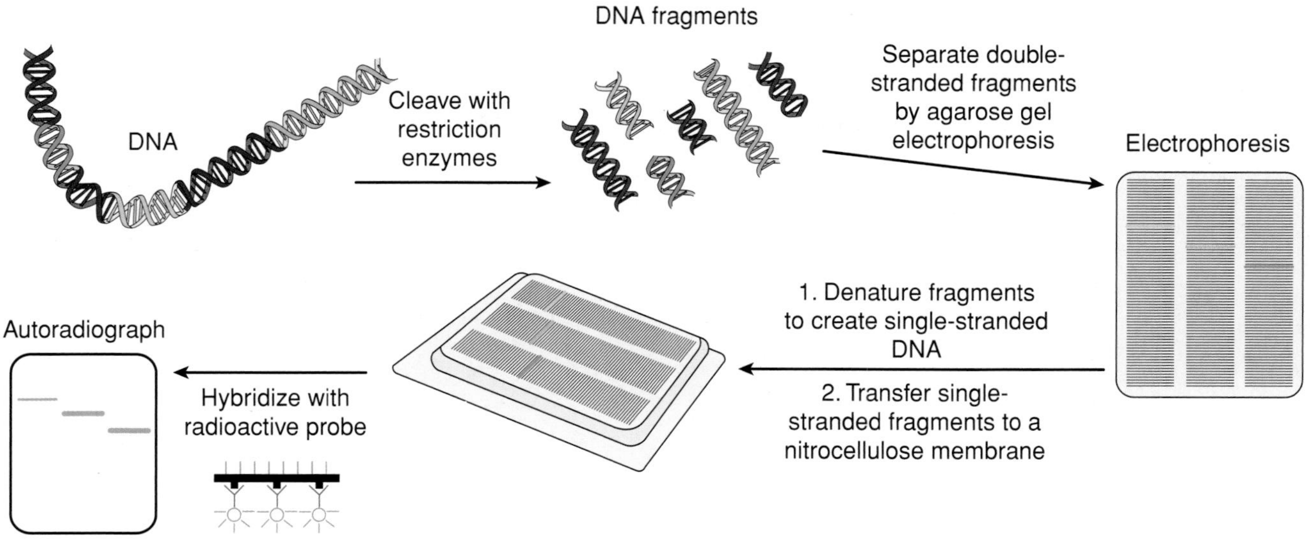

FIGURE 13-13 Southern blotting analysis. Genomic DNA is isolated from leukocytes or amniocytes and digested with a restriction enzyme. This procedure yields a series of reproducible fragments that are separated by agarose gel electrophoresis. The separated DNA fragments are then transferred ("blotted") to a nitrocellulose membrane that binds DNA. The membrane is treated with a solution containing a radioactive single-stranded nucleic acid probe, which forms a double-stranded nucleic acid complex at membrane sites when homologous DNA is present. These regions are then detected by autoradiography.

then hybridized to the DNA bound to the membrane, using a marker that permits their identification. Basic principles of the Southern blot technique also can be applied to RNA—known as Northern blotting—and to proteins—Western blotting.

Polymerase Chain Reaction

This tool enables the rapid synthesis of large amounts of a specific DNA sequence or gene. To do this, either the entire gene sequence must be known or the DNA sequences at the beginning and end of the gene must be known. PCR involves three steps that are repeated many times. First, double-stranded DNA is denatured by heating. Then, oligonucleotide primers corresponding to a target sequence on each separated DNA strand are added and become annealed to either end of the target sequence. Finally, a mixture of nucleotides and heat-stable DNA polymerase is added to elongate the primer sequence, and new complementary strands of DNA are synthesized. The procedure is repeated multiple times to permit exponential amplification of the DNA segment.

Real-time PCR is used to amplify a specific gene while simultaneously quantifying the target gene. This allows accurate quantification of gene expression. *Massively parallel genomic sequencing* or "shotgun sequencing" uses random small DNA fragments, which are amplified using millions of sequence tags. These small amplified sequences are computer-aligned, allowing the entire genome sequence to be ascertained. The number of unique sequences can then be counted and expressed as a percentage. This permits relative quantification of specific genes or, in the case of aneuploidy determination, chromosomes.

Linkage Analysis

If a specific disease-causing gene has not been identified, then linkage analysis may be used to estimate the likelihood that an individual or fetus has inherited the abnormal trait. This technique is used to estimate the location of different genes and their approximate distance from each other.

Specific scattered markers are selected for study based on the suspected location of the gene responsible for the condition. DNA from each family member is analyzed to determine whether any of the selected markers have been transmitted along with the disease gene. If individuals with the disease have the marker but individuals without the disease do not, the gene causing the disease is said to be linked to that marker. This suggests that they lie close to each other on the same chromosome. Limitations of this technique are that it is imprecise, that it depends on family size and availability of family members for testing, and that it relies on the presence of informative markers near the gene.

Chromosomal Microarray Analysis

This testing uses the principles of PCR and nucleic acid hybridization to screen DNA for many different genes or mutations simultaneously. Doing so can identify deletions and duplications as small as 1 kilobase—termed genomic copy number variants—whereas the resolution of standard karyotyping is approximately 3 megabases. Two types of arrays are used clinically: (1) comparative genomic hybridization (CGH) arrays, which detect microdeletions and microduplications in DNA and (2) single-nucleotide polymorphism (SNP) arrays, in which the variation may involve just one nucleotide. As shown in Figure 13-14, the CGH microarray platform contains DNA fragments of known sequence. DNA from the individual (or fetus) to be tested is labeled with a fluorescent dye and then exposed to the DNA fragments fixed on the chip. Normal control DNA is labeled with a different fluorescent probe. Finally, the intensity of fluorescent probe signals is determined with a laser scanner. Use of SNP arrays is similar, except that the

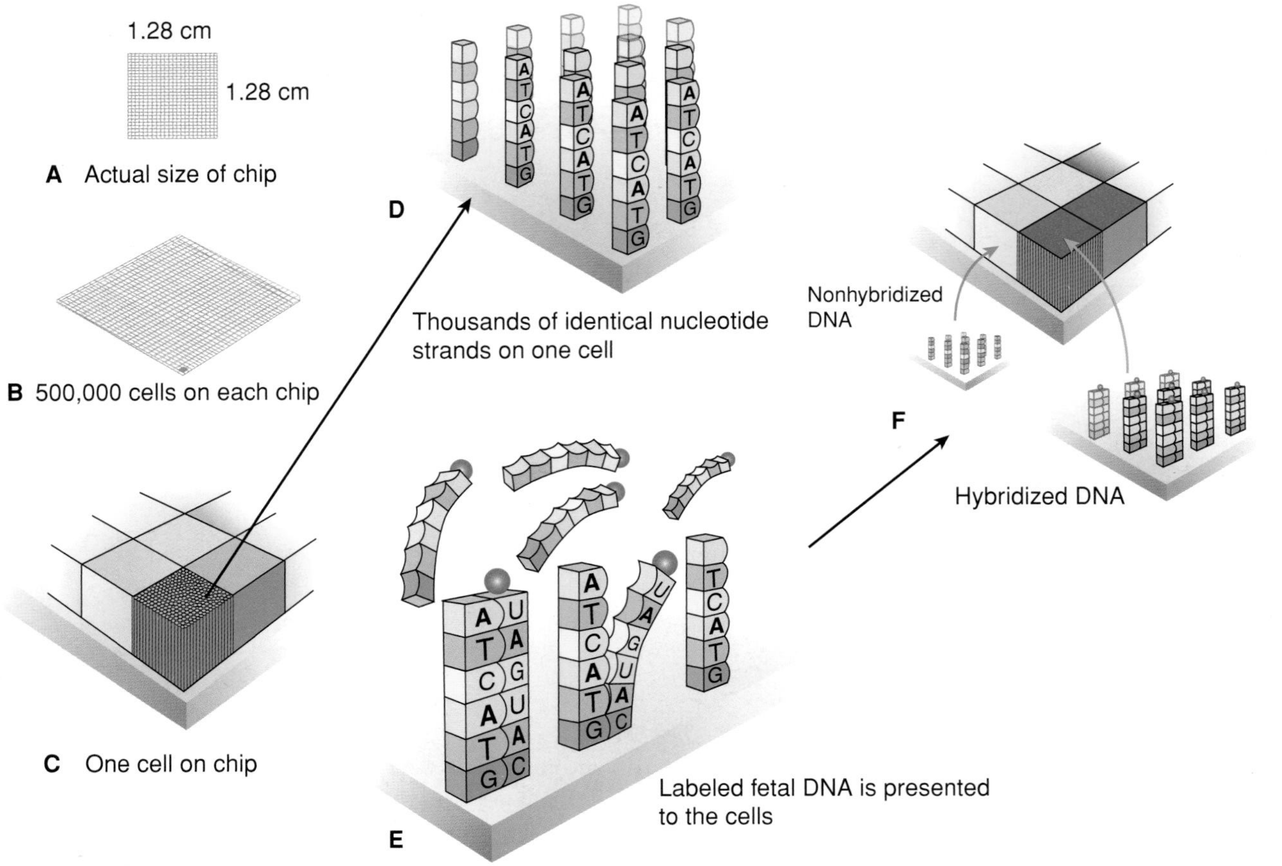

FIGURE 13-14 Chromosomal microarray analysis. **A.** Actual microarray chip size. **B.** Each chip contains thousands of cells (squares). **C & D.** Each cell contains thousands of identical oligonucleotides on its surface, and each cell is unique in its nucleotide content. **E.** During genetic analysis, a mixture containing tagged fetal DNA is presented to the chip. Complementary DNA sequences bind. **F.** If a laser is shined on the chip, DNA sequences that have bound will glow. This identifies a matching sequence. (From Doody, 2012, with permission.)

DNA is compared with known sequence variants, allowing determination of whether the fetus is heterozygous or homozygous for a mutation.

Arrays may be genome-wide or may be targeted to known genetic syndromes. Genome-wide arrays are used in research settings, for example, to identify novel microdeletion syndromes in individuals with intellectual disability (Slavotinek, 2008). In the prenatal setting, only targeted arrays are used. A major drawback of either type is the detection of *copy number variants of uncertain clinical significance* (Manning, 2010). When an abnormal pregnancy is found to have a variant that has not previously been associated with an abnormality, it may not be possible to determine whether the variant is benign or pathological.

Clinical Applications

CMA is used clinically for prenatal diagnosis and for stillbirth evaluation. The technique is expected to identify autosomal trisomies, sex chromosomal abnormalities, and other unbalanced chromosomal rearrangements visible with standard karyotype analysis. However, balanced chromosomal rearrangements such as translocations and inversions may *not* be identified. In addition, CGH arrays will not detect triploidy, mosaicism below 20 percent, or some marker chromosomes (Bui, 2011). A potential benefit of SNP arrays is the detection of triploidy. SNP arrays may also demonstrate *loss of heterozygosity* in a specimen, important for detection of uniparental disomy and consanguinity.

In pediatrics, CMA is considered a first-tier diagnostic test for children with mental retardation, congenital abnormalities, or dysmorphic features but with a normal karyotype. In such cases, CMA identifies an abnormality in up to 15 percent (Manning, 2010; Miller, 2010).

For stillbirth evaluation, CMA is more likely to provide a genetic diagnosis than standard karyotyping, in part because it does not require dividing cells. The Stillbirth Collaborative Research Network found that when karyotyping was uninformative, approximately 6 percent of cases had either aneuploidy or a pathogenic copy number variant identified with CMA (Reddy, 2012). Overall, CMA yielded results nearly 25 percent more often than standard karyotyping alone.

Targeted arrays are performed in the prenatal setting using chorionic villi or amnionic fluid. In a multicenter trial of more than 4000 pregnancies, Wapner and coworkers (2012) found that CMA identified all cases of common aneuploidies and unbalanced chromosomal rearrangements seen with standard karyotyping. When standard karyotyping results were normal, a microdeletion or microduplication of known or likely clinical significance was found in 6 percent if the indication was a fetal structural abnormality and in nearly 2 percent if performed for advanced maternal age or abnormal serum aneuploidy screening. Similar results have been reported by others (Hillman, 2011). Of concern is that variants of uncertain clinical significance are also identified in approximately 2 percent, which poses a challenge for counseling (Dugoff, 2012; Wapner, 2012). When copy number variants of uncertain clinical significance are encountered, parental testing is indicated.

Recently, the American College of Obstetricians and Gynecologists (2013) endorsed offering CMA testing when prenatal sonography identifies major fetal abnormalities. If the abnormalities suggest trisomy 21, 18, or 13, then karyotype analysis or FISH may be the initial test, and CMA can also be considered. Comprehensive genetic counseling is required before and after CMA testing. Also, depending on the platform used, it may need to include not only the potential to detect findings of uncertain clinical significance, but also adult-onset disease, consanguinity, and even non-paternity (American College of Obstetricians and Gynecologists, 2013).

Fetal DNA in the Maternal Circulation

Fetal cells are present in maternal blood at a very low concentration, only 2 to 6 cells per milliliter (Bianchi, 2006). And, some intact fetal cells may persist in the maternal circulation for decades following delivery. Persistent fetal cells may result in microchimerism, which has been implicated in maternal autoimmune diseases such as scleroderma, systemic lupus erythematosus, and Hashimoto thyroiditis. For prenatal diagnosis, the use of intact fetal cells is limited by their low concentration, persistence into successive pregnancies, and difficulties in distinguishing fetal from maternal cells. Cell-free fetal DNA overcomes these limitations.

Cell-Free Fetal DNA

This is released from apoptotic placental trophoblast—rather than actual fetal cells—and can be reliably detected in maternal blood after 7 weeks' gestation (Bodurtha, 2012). It comprises 3 to 6 percent of the circulating cell-free DNA in maternal plasma, with proportions increasing as gestation advances (Lo, 1998). Unlike intact fetal cells, cell-free fetal DNA is cleared within minutes from maternal blood (Lo, 1999). In the research setting, cell-free fetal DNA has been used to detect numerous single-gene disorders through paternally inherited alleles. These include myotonic dystrophy, achondroplasia, Huntington disease, congenital adrenal hyperplasia, cystic fibrosis, and β-thalassemia (Wright, 2009). Clinical applications of cell-free fetal DNA include determination of Rh (CDE) genotype, determination of fetal gender, and detection of autosomal trisomies (Fig. 13-15).

Rh D Genotype Evaluation. Fetal Rh D genotype assessment from maternal blood offers several potential benefits. Administration of anti-D immune globulin to an Rh D-negative pregnant woman carrying an Rh D-negative fetus can be eliminated. In the setting of Rh D alloimmunization, early identification of an Rh D-negative fetus can avoid unnecessary amniocentesis and/or serial fetal middle cerebral artery Doppler assessment. Rh D genotype evaluation using cell-free fetal DNA is done using real-time PCR to target multiple exons of the *RHD* gene. In a metaanalysis of more than 3000 pregnancies by Geifman-Holtzman and associates (2006), the average diagnostic accuracy approximated 95 percent, and only 3 percent of samples had inconclusive results. Subsequent studies have described accuracies of 99 to 100 percent (Minon, 2008; Tynan, 2011). Rh D genotyping using cell-free fetal DNA is used routinely in Europe. However, as of 2013, it has not been widely adopted in the United States. A theoretical concern is that women with false-negative test results would not receive anti-D immune globulin, leading to a potential increase in Rh D alloimmunization (Szczepura, 2011).

Fetal Sex Determination. From the standpoint of genetic disease, fetal sex determination may be clinically useful if the

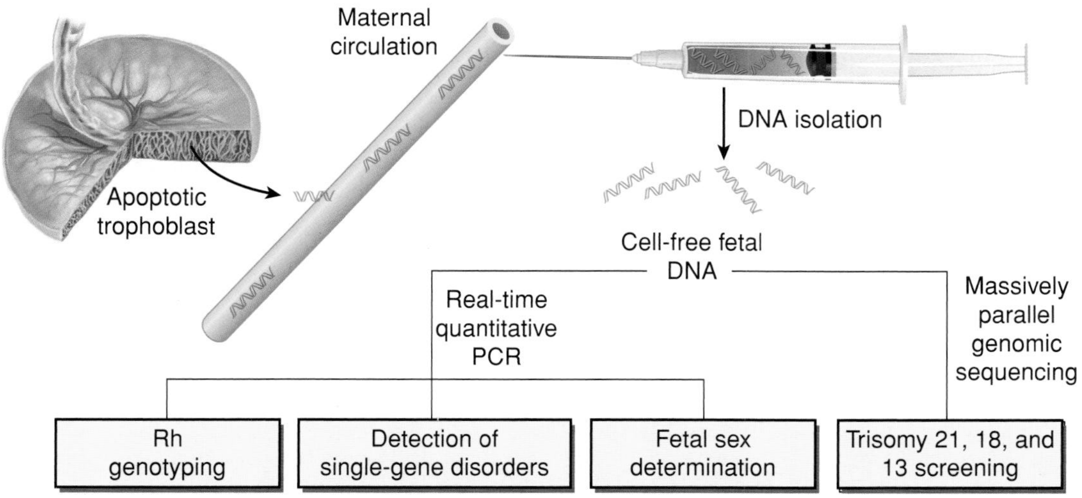

FIGURE 13-15 Cell-free fetal DNA is actually derived from apoptotic trophoblast. The DNA is isolated from maternal plasma, and real-time quantitative PCR may be used to target specific regions or sequences. This may be used for Rh D genotyping, identification of paternally inherited single-gene disorders, or fetal sex determination. Using a technique called massively parallel genomic sequencing, screening for trisomies 21, 18, and 13 may be performed.

fetus is at risk for an X-linked disorder. It may also be beneficial if the fetus is at risk for congenital adrenal hyperplasia because maternal corticosteroid therapy may be avoided if the fetus is male. In a metaanalysis of more than 6000 pregnancies by Devaney and colleagues (2011), the sensitivity of cell-free fetal DNA testing for fetal sex determination approximated 95 percent between 7 and 12 weeks' gestation, improving to 99 percent after 20 weeks. The test specificity was 99 percent at both time periods, suggesting that cell-free fetal DNA is a reasonable alternative to invasive testing in selected cases.

Aneuploidy Screening. Fetal Down syndrome and other autosomal trisomies can be detected from maternal plasma using massively parallel sequencing or by targeted (selective) sequencing of chromosome-specific regions (Chiu, 2008; Fan, 2008; Sparks, 2012). By simultaneously sequencing millions of DNA fragments, investigators can identify whether the proportion or ratio of fragments from one chromosome is higher than expected. Because sequences of fetal DNA are specific to individual chromosomes, samples from those with Down syndrome have a larger proportion of DNA sequences from chromosome 21. This technology has been termed noninvasive prenatal testing (NIPT).

Recent trials of NIPT in high-risk pregnancies have yielded detection rates for trisomies 21, 18, and 13 of approximately 98 percent, at a false-positive rate of 0.5 percent or less (American College of Obstetricians and Gynecologists, 2012; Bianchi, 2012; Palomaki, 2011, 2012). NIPT has recently become clinically available as a screening test, but it is not currently considered a replacement diagnostic test. Pretest counseling is recommended, with formal genetic counseling if an abnormal result is identified. Recommendations for its use are discussed in Chapter 14 (p. 292).

Limitations. There are several important limitations to using cell-free fetal DNA testing in its present form (Benn, 2012; Geifman-Holtzman, 2006). Because placental cells are being evaluated, confined placental mosaicism may yield abnormal results that do not reflect fetal karyotype. Similarly, results may not be as accurate in a multifetal gestation or with a vanishing twin (Chap. 45, p. 892). There may be false-negative results if fetal DNA levels are insufficient in the sample. This theoretically results in failure to detect an Rh-negative fetus. In the case of aneuploidy, there may be inability to differentiate trisomy from unbalanced translocation (Benn, 2012; Geifman-Holtzman, 2006). Finally, because the technology identifies differences in the relative proportion of chromosomal fragments, triploidy may not be identified.

REFERENCES

American Academy of Pediatrics: Health supervision for children with Down syndrome. Pediatrics 107(2):442, 2001

American Academy of Pediatrics Section on Cardiology and Cardiac Surgery: Clinical report: cardiovascular health supervision for individuals affected by Duchenne or Becker muscular dystrophy. Pediatrics 116(6):1569, 2005

American College of Medical Genetics: Technical and clinical assessment of fluorescence in situ hybridization: an ACMG/ASHG position statement. I. Technical considerations. Genet Med 2(6):356, 2000

American College of Obstetricians and Gynecologists: Maternal phenylketonuria. Committee Opinion No. 449, December 2009a

American College of Obstetricians and Gynecologists: Preconception and prenatal carrier screening for genetic diseases in individuals of Eastern European Jewish descent. Committee Opinion No. 442, October 2009b

American College of Obstetricians and Gynecologists: Carrier screening for fragile X syndrome. Committee Opinion No. 469, October 2010

American College of Obstetricians and Gynecologists, Society for Maternal-Fetal Medicine: Noninvasive testing for fetal aneuploidy. Committee Opinion No. 545, December 2012

American College of Obstetricians and Gynecologists: Array comparative genomic hybridization in prenatal diagnosis. Committee Opinion No. 581, December 2013

Bdolah Y, Palomaki GE, Yaron Y, et al: Circulating angiogenic proteins in trisomy 13. Am J Obstet Gynecol 194(1):239, 2006

Beaudin AE, Stover PJ: Insights into metabolic mechanisms underlying folate-responsive neural tube defects: a minireview. Birth Defects Res A Clin Mol Teratol 85(4):274, 2009

Becerra JE, Khoury MJ, Cordero JF, et al: Diabetes mellitus during pregnancy and the risks for specific birth defects: a population-based case-control study. Pediatrics 85(1):1, 1990

Benn P, Cuckle H, Pergament E: Non-invasive prenatal diagnosis for Down syndrome: the paradigm will shift, but slowly. Ultrasound Obstet Gynecol 39(2):127, 2012

Bianchi DW, Hanson J: Sharpening the tools: a summary of a National Institutes of Health workshop on new technologies for detection of fetal cells in maternal blood for early prenatal diagnosis. J Matern Fetal Neonatal Med 19(4):199, 2006

Bianchi DW, Platt LD, Goldberg JD, et al: Genome-wide fetal aneuploidy detection by maternal plasma DNA sequencing. Obstet Gynecol 119(5):890, 2012

Blau N, van Spronsen FJ, Levy HL: Phenylketonuria. Lancet 376(9750):1417, 2010

Bodurtha J, Strauss JF III: Genomics and perinatal care. N Engl J Med 366(1):64, 2012

Bradshaw: Anatomic disorders. In Hoffman BL, Schorge JO, Schaffer JI, et al (eds): Williams Gynecology, 2nd ed. New York, McGraw-Hill, 2012, p 490

Bui TH, Iselius L, Lindsten J: European collaborative study on prenatal diagnosis: mosaicism, pseudomosaicism and single abnormal cells in amniotic fluid cultures. Prenat Diagn 4(7):145, 1984

Bui TH, Vetro A, Zuffardi O, et al: Current controversies in prenatal diagnosis 3: is conventional chromosomal analysis necessary in the post-array CGH era? Prenat Diagn 31(3):235, 2011

Burn J, Brennan P, Little J, et al: Recurrence risks in offspring of adults with major heart defects: results from first cohort of British collaborative study. Lancet 351(9099):311, 1998

Chiu RW, Chan KC, Gao Y, et al: Noninvasive prenatal diagnosis of fetal chromosomal aneuploidy by massively parallel genomic sequencing of DNA in maternal plasma. Proc Natl Acad Sci USA 105(51):20458, 2008

Cockwell A, MacKenzie M, Youings S, et al: A cytogenetic and molecular study of a series of 45,X fetuses and their parents. J Med Genet 28(3):151, 1991

Cools M, Pleskacova J, Stoop H, et al: Gonadal pathology and tumor risk in relation to clinical characteristics in patients with 45,X/46,XY mosaicism. J Clin Endocrinol Metab 96(7):E1171, 2011

Cragan JD, Gilboa SM: Including prenatal diagnoses in birth defects monitoring: experience of the Metropolitan Atlanta Congenital Defects Program. Birth Defects Res A Clin Mol Teratol 85(1):20, 2009

Cronister A, Teicher J, Rohlfs EM, et al: Prevalence and instability of fragile X alleles: implications for offering fragile X premutation diagnosis. Obstet Gynecol 111(3):596, 2008

Devaney SA, Palomaki GE, Scott JA, et al: Noninvasive fetal sex determination using cell-free fetal DNA: a systematic review and meta-analysis. JAMA 306(6):627, 2011

Dolk H, Loane M, Garne E: The prevalence of congenital anomalies in Europe. Adv Exp Med Biol 686:349, 2010

Doody KJ: Treatment of the infertile couple. In Hoffman BL, Schorge JO, Schaffer JI (eds): Williams Gynecology, 2nd ed. New York, McGraw-Hill, 2012

Dugoff L: Application of genomic technology in prenatal diagnosis. N Engl J Med 367(23):2249, 2012

Edwards JH, Harnden DG, Cameron AH, et al: A new trisomic syndrome. Lancet 1(7128):787, 1960

Fan HC, Blumenfeld YJ, Chitkara U, et al: Noninvasive diagnosis of fetal aneuploidy by shotgun sequencing DNA from maternal blood. Proc Natl Acad Sci USA 105(42):16266, 2008

Feero WG, Guttmacher AE, Collins FS: Genomic medicine—an updated primer. N Engl J Med 362(21):2001, 2010

Freire-Maia N: Effects of consanguineous marriages on morbidity and precocious mortality: genetic counseling. Am J Med Genet 18(3):401, 1984

Gardner RJM, Sutherland GR: Chromosome Abnormalities and Genetic Counseling, 2nd ed. Oxford Monographs on Medical Genetics No. 29. Oxford, Oxford University Press, 1996

Geifman-Holtzman O, Grotegut CA, Gaughan JP: Diagnostic accuracy of noninvasive fetal Rh genotyping from maternal blood—a meta-analysis. Am J Obstet Gynecol 195(4):1163, 2006

Girardin CM, Vliet GV: Counselling of a couple faced with a prenatal diagnosis of Klinefelter syndrome. Acta Pediatr 100(6):917, 2011

Grewal J, Carmichael SL, Yang W, et al: Paternal age and congenital malformations in offspring in California, 1989–2002. Matern Child Health J 16(2):385, 2012

Grosse SD, Collins JS: Folic acid supplementation and neural tube defect recurrence prevention. Birth Defects Res A Clin Mol Teratol 79(11):737, 2007

Halvorson LM: Amenorrhea. In Hoffman BL, Schorge JO, Schaffer JI, et al (eds): Williams Gynecology, 2nd ed. New York, McGraw-Hill, 2012, p 445

Hassed SJ, Hopcus-Niccum D, Zhang L, et al: A new genomic duplication syndrome complementary to the velocardiofacial (22q11 deletion) syndrome. Clin Genet 65(5):400, 2004

Hassold T, Arnovitz K, Jacobs PA, et al: The parental origin of the missing or additional chromosome in 45,X and 47,XXX females. Birth Defects Orig Artic Ser 26(4):297, 1990

Henderson KG, Shaw TE, Barrett IJ, et al: Distribution of mosaicism in human placentae. Hum Genet 97(5):650, 1996

Hibbard ED, Smithells RW: Folic acid metabolism and human embryopathy. Lancet 1:1254, 1965

Hillman SC, Pretlove S, Coomarasamy A, et al: Additional information from array comparative genomic hybridization technology over conventional karyotyping in prenatal diagnosis: a systematic review and meta-analysis. Ultrasound Obstet Gynecol 37(1):6 2011

Holland CM: 47,XXX in an adolescent with premature ovarian failure and autoimmune disease. J Pediatr Adolesc Gynecol 14(2):77, 2001

Hsu LY, Perlis TE: United States survey on chromosome mosaicism and pseudomosaicism in prenatal diagnosis. Prenat Diagn 4(7):97, 1984

Hunter AGW: Neural tube defects in Eastern Ontario and Western Quebec: demography and family data. Am J Med Genet 19(1):45, 1984

Jacobs PA, Hassold TJ: The origin of numerical chromosomal abnormalities. Adv Genet 33:101, 1995

Jauniaux E: Partial moles: from postnatal to prenatal diagnosis. Placenta 20(5–6):379, 1999

Johns Hopkins University: Online Mendelian Inheritance in Man (OMIM): OMIM entry statistics. 2013. Available at: http://omim.org/statistics/entry. Accessed April 4, 2013

Jones KL: Smith's Recognizable Patterns of Human Malformation, 6th ed. Philadelphia, Elsevier Saunders, 2006

Jorde LB, Carey JC, Bamshad MJ, et al: Medical Genetics, 3rd ed. Philadelphia, Elsevier-Mosby-Saunders, 2006

Jung A, Schuppe HC, Schill WB: Are children of older fathers at risk for genetic disorders? Andrologia 35(4):191, 2003

Kalousek DK, Barrett IJ, McGillivray BC: Placental mosaicism and intrauterine survival of trisomies 13 and 18. Am J Hum Genet 44(3):338, 1989

Kalousek DK, Dill FJ: Chromosomal mosaicism confined to the placenta in human conceptions. Science 221(4611):665, 1983

Kannan TP, Hemlatha S, Ankathil R, et al: Clinical manifestations in trisomy 9. Indian J Pediatr 76(7):745, 2009

Kappelgaard A, Laursen T: The benefits of growth hormone therapy in patients with Turner syndrome, Noonan syndrome, and children born small for gestational age. Growth Horm IGF Res 21(6):305, 2011

Koch R, Hanley W, Levy H, et al: The Maternal Phenylketonuria International Study: 1984–2002. Pediatrics 112(6 Pt 2):1523, 2003

Krogh C, Gortz S, Wohlfahrt J, et al: Pre- and perinatal risk factors for pyloric stenosis and their influence on the male predominance. Am J Epidemiol 176(1):24, 2012

Lejeune J, Turpin R, Gautier M: Chromosomic diagnosis of mongolism. Arch Fr Pediatr 16:962, 1959

Lenke RR, Levy HL: Maternal phenylketonuria and hyperphenylalaninemia. An international survey of the outcome of untreated and treated pregnancies. N Engl J Med 303(21):1202, 1980

Lin AE, Garver KL: Genetic counseling for congenital heart defects. J Pediatr 113(6):1105, 1988

Lin HY, Chen YJ, Hung HY, et al: Clinical characteristics and survival of trisomy 18 in a medical center in Taipei, 1988–2004. Am J Med Genet 140(9):945, 2006

Lin HY, Lin SP, Chen YJ, et al: Clinical characteristics and survival of trisomy 13 in a medical center in Taiwan, 1985–2004. Pediatr Int 49(3):380, 2007

Linden MG, Bender BG: Fifty-one prenatally diagnosed children and adolescents with sex chromosome abnormalities. Am J Med Genet 110(1):11, 2002

Lindhout D, Omtzigt JGC, Cornel MC: Spectrum of neural tube defects in 34 infants prenatally exposed to antiepileptic drugs. Neurology 42(suppl 5):111, 1992

Lo YM, Tein MS, Lau TK, et al: Quantitative analysis of fetal DNA in maternal plasma and serum: implications for noninvasive prenatal diagnosis. Am J Hum Genet 62(4):768, 1998

Lo YM, Zhang J, Leung TN, et al: Rapid clearance of fetal DNA from maternal plasma. Am J Hum Genet 64(1):218, 1999

Lowe X, Eskenazi B, Nelson DO, et al: Frequency of XY sperm increases with age in fathers of boys with Klinefelter syndrome. Am J Hum Genet 69(5):1046, 2001

Lupton M, Oteng-Ntim E, Ayida G, et al: Cardiac disease in pregnancy. Curr Opin Obstet Gynecol 14(2):137, 2002

Manning M, Hudgins L, Professional Practice and Guidelines Committee: Array-based technology and recommendations for utilization in medical genetics practice for detection of chromosomal abnormalities. Genet Med 12(11):742, 2010

McDonald-McGinn DM, Sullivan KE: Chromosome 22q11.2 deletion syndrome (DiGeorge syndrome/velocardiofacial syndrome). Medicine 90(1):1, 2011

McKusick VA, Ruddle FH: A new discipline, a new name, a new journal. Genomics 1:1, 2003

Mikhail FM, Lose EJ, Robin NH, et al: Clinically relevant single gene or intragenic deletions encompassing critical neurodevelopmental genes in patients with developmental delay, mental retardation, and/or autism spectrum disorders. Am J Med Genet A 155A(10):2386, 2011

Miller DT, Adam MP, Aradhya S, et al: Consensus statement: chromosomal microarray is a first-tier clinical diagnostic test for individuals with developmental disabilities or congenital anomalies. Am J Hum Genet 86(5):749, 2010

Milunsky A, Milunsky JM: Genetic counseling: preconception, prenatal, and perinatal. In Milunsky A (ed): Genetic Disorders of the Fetus: Diagnosis, Prevention, and Treatment, 5th ed. Baltimore, Johns Hopkins University Press, 2004

Minon JM, Gerard C, Senterre JM, et al: Routine fetal RHD genotyping with maternal plasma: a four-year experience in Belgium. Transfusion 48(2):373, 2008

MRC Vitamin Study Research Group: Prevention of neural tube defects: results of the Medical Research Council Vitamin Study. Lancet 338(8760):131, 1991

Nadiri S: Congenital abnormalities in newborns of consanguineous and nonconsanguineous parents. Obstet Gynecol 53(2):195, 1979

National Center for Biotechnology Information: dbGaP: database of genotypes and phenotypes. 2013a. Available at: http://www.ncbi.nlm.nih.gov/projects/gap/cgi-bin/about.html#dac. Accessed April 4, 2013

National Center for Biotechnology Information: Genetics home reference. 2013b. Available at: http://ghr.nlm.nih.gov./ Accessed April 4, 2013

National Center for Biotechnology Information: Genetic Testing Registry. 2013c. Available at: http://www.ncbi.nlm.nih.gov/gtr./ Accessed April 4, 2013

National Human Genome Research Institute: International HapMap Project. 2012. Available at: http://www.genome.gov/10001688. Accessed April 4, 2013

Nelson DL: The fragile X syndromes. Semin Cell Biol 6(1):5, 1995

Nicolaides KH: The 11 to 13 +6 Weeks Scan. London, Fetal Medicine Foundation, 2004

Nolin SL, Brown WT, Glickspan A, et al: Expansion of the fragile X CGG repeat in females with premutation or intermediate alleles. Am J Hum Genet 72(2):454, 2003

Nora JJ, Nora AH: Updates on counseling the family with a first-degree relative with a congenital heart defect. Am J Med Genet 29(1):137, 1988

Nussbaum RL, McInnes RR, Willard HF (eds): Clinical cytogenetics: disorders of the autosomes and sex chromosomes. In Thompson & Thompson Genetics in Medicine, 7th ed. Elsevier-Saunders, 2007, p 89

Olson EN: Gene regulatory networks in the evolution and development of the heart. Science 313(5795):1922, 2006

Palomaki GE, Deciu C, Kloza EM, et al: DNA sequencing of maternal plasma reliably identifies trisomy 18 and trisomy 13 as well as Down syndrome: an international collaborative study. Genet Med 14(3):296, 2012

Palomaki GE, Kloza EM, Lambert-Messerlian GM, et al: DNA sequencing of maternal plasma to detect Down syndrome: an international clinical validation study. Genet Med 13(11):913, 2011

Parker SE, Mai CT, Canfield MA, et al: Updated national birth prevalence estimates for selected birth defects in the United States, 2004–2006. Birth Defects Res A Clin Mol Teratol 88(12):1008, 2010

Patau K, Smith DW, Therman E, et al: Multiple congenital anomaly caused by an extra autosome. Lancet 1(7128):790, 1960

Platt LD, Koch R, Hanley WB, et al: The international study of pregnancy outcome in women with maternal phenylketonuria: report of a 12-year study. Am J Obstet Gynecol 182(2):326, 2000

Plug I, Mauser-Bunschoten EP, Brocker-Vriends AH, et al: Bleeding in carriers of hemophilia. Blood 108(1):52, 2006
Porter S, Gilks CB: Genomic imprinting: a proposed explanation for the different behaviors of testicular and ovarian germ cell tumors. Med Hypotheses 41(1):37, 1993
Potocki L, Chen KS, Park SS, et al: Molecular mechanism for duplication 17p11.2—the homologous recombination reciprocal of the Smith-Magenis microdeletion. Nat Genet 24(1):84, 2000
Rankin J, Tennant PWG, Bythell M, et al: Predictors of survival in children born with Down syndrome: a registry-based study. Pediatrics 129(6):e1373, 2012
Reddy UM, Goldenber R, Silver R, et al: Stillbirth classification—developing an international consensus for research: executive summary of a National Institute of Child Health and Human Development workshop. Obstet Gynecol 114(4):901, 2009
Reddy UM, Grier PP, Saade GR, et al: Karyotype versus microarray testing for genetic abnormalities after stillbirth. N Engl J Med 367(23):2185, 2012
Robinson WP, Barrett IJ, Bernard L, et al: Meiotic origin of trisomy in confined placental mosaicism is correlated with presence of fetal uniparental disomy, high levels of trisomy in trophoblast, and increased risk of fetal intrauterine growth restriction. Am J Hum Genet 60(4):917, 1997
Rosa RFM, Rosa RCM, Lorenzen MB, et al: Trisomy 18: experience of a reference hospital from the south of Brazil. Am J Med Genet A 155A(7):1529, 2011
Ross JL, Zeger MP, Kushner H, et al: An extra X or Y chromosome: contrasting the cognitive and motor phenotypes in childhood in boys with 47,XYY syndrome or 47,XXY Klinefelter syndrome. Dev Disabil Res Rev 15(4):309, 2009
Scharrer S, Stengel-Rutkowski S, Rodewald-Rudescu A, et al: Reproduction in a female patient with Down's syndrome. Case report of a 46,XY child showing slight phenotypical anomalies born to a 47,XX, +21 mother. Humangenetik 26(3):207, 1975
Schmickel RD: Contiguous gene syndromes: a component of recognizable syndromes. J Pediatr 109(2):231, 1986
Schneider AS, Mennuti MT, Zackai EH: High cesarean section rate in trisomy 18 births: a potential indication for late prenatal diagnosis. Am J Obstet Gynecol 140(4):367, 1981
Schorge JO: Ovarian germ cell and sex cord-stromal tumors. In Hoffman BL, Schorge JO, Schaffer JI, et al (eds): Williams Gynecology, 2nd ed. New York, McGraw-Hill, 2012, p 882
Schwartz S, Hassold T: Chromosome disorders. In Longo DL, Kasper DL, Jameson JL, et al (eds): Harrison's Principles of Internal Medicine, 18th ed. New York, McGraw-Hill, 2012
Shaffer LG, Agan N, Goldberg JD, et al: American College of Medical Genetics Statement on diagnostic testing for uniparental disomy. Genet Med 3(3):206, 2001
Shaffer LG, Slovak ML, Campbell LJ (eds): ISCN 2009: International System for Human Cytogenetic Nomenclature (2009): Recommendations of the International Standing Committee on Human Cytogenetics Nomenclature. Basel, Karger, 2009
Shin M, Besser LM, Kucik JE, et al: Prevalence of Down syndrome in children and adolescents in 10 regions of the United States. Pediatrics 124(6):1565, 2009
Shipp TD, Benacerraf BR: Second trimester ultrasound screening for chromosomal abnormalities. Prenat Diagn 22(4):296, 2002
Shprintzen RJ: Velo-cardio-facial syndrome: 30 years of study. Dev Disabil Res Rev 14(1):3, 2008
Silasi M, Rana S, Powe C, et al: Placental expression of angiogenic factors in trisomy 13. Am J Obstet Gynecol 204(6):546.e1, 2011
Slavotinek AM: Novel microdeletion syndromes detected by chromosomal microarrays. Hum Genet 124(1):1, 2008
Snijders RJ, Sundberg K, Holzgreve W, et al: Maternal age- and gestation-specific risk for trisomy 21. Ultrasound Obstet Gynecol 13(3):167, 1999
Solomon BD, Rosenbaum KN, Meck JM, et al: Holoprosencephaly due to numeric chromosome abnormalities. Am J Med Genet C Semin Med Genet 154C(1):146, 2010
Somerville MJ, Mervis CB, Young EJ, et al: Severe expressive-language delay related to duplication of the Williams-Beuren locus. N Engl J Med 353(16):1694, 2005
Sparks AB, Wang ET, Struble CA, et al: Selective analysis of cell-free DNA in maternal blood for evaluation of fetal trisomy. Prenat Diagn 32(1):3, 2012
Spence JE, Perciaccante RG, Greig FM, et al: Uniparental disomy as a mechanism for human genetic disease. Am J Hum Genet 42(2):217, 1988
Spotila LD, Sereda L, Prockop DJ: Partial isodisomy for maternal chromosome 7 and short stature in an individual with a mutation at the COLIA2 locus. Am J Hum Genet 51(6):1396, 1992
Szczepura A, Osipenko L, Freeman K: A new fetal RHD genotyping test: costs and benefits of mass testing to target *antenatal* anti-D prophylaxis in England and Wales. BMC Pregnancy Childbirth 18(11):5.e1, 2011
Tartaglia NR, Howell S, Sutherland A, et al: A review of trisomy X (47,XXX). Orphanet J Rare Dis 5:8, 2010
Tennant PW, Pearce MS, Bythell M, et al: 20-year survival of children born with congenital anomalies: a population-based study. Lancet 375(9715):649, 2010
Tepperberg J, Pettenati MJ, Rao PN, et al: Prenatal diagnosis using interphase fluorescence in situ hybridization (FISH): 2-year multi-center retrospective study and review of the literature. Prenat Diagn 21(4):293, 2001
Tinkle BT, Walker ME, Blough-Pfau RI, et al: Unexpected survival in a case of prenatally diagnosed non-mosaic trisomy 22: clinical report and review of the natural history. Am J Med Genet A 118A(1):90, 2003
Toriello HV, Meck JM, Professional Practice and Guidelines Committee: Statement on guidance for genetic counseling in advanced paternal age. Genet Med 10(6):457, 2008
Tuohy JF, James DK: Pre-eclampsia and trisomy 13. Br J Obstet Gynaecol 99(11):891, 1992
Tynan JA, Angkachatchai V, Ehrich M, et al: Multiplexed analysis of circulating cell-free fetal nucleic acids for noninvasive prenatal diagnostic RHD testing. Am J Obstet Gynecol 204(3):251.e1, 2011
Vendola C, Canfield M, Daiger SP, et al: Survival of Texas infants born with trisomies 21, 18, and 13. Am J Med Genet A 152A(2):360, 2010
Vintzileos AM, Egan JF: Adjusting the risk for trisomy 21 on the basis of second-trimester ultrasonography. Am J Obstet Gynecol 172(3):837, 1995
Wapner RJ, Martin CL, Levy B: Chromosomal microarray versus karyotyping for prenatal diagnosis. N Engl J Med 367(23):2175, 2012
Weismann CG, Gelb BD: The genetics of congenital heart disease: a review of recent developments. Curr Opin Cardiol 22(3):200, 2007
Worton RG, Stern R: A Canadian collaborative study of mosaicism in amniotic fluid cell cultures. Prenat Diagn 4(7):131, 1984
Wright CF, Burton H: The use of cell-free fetal nucleic acids in maternal blood for non-invasive prenatal diagnosis. Hum Reprod Update 15(1):139, 2009
Yang Q, Wen SW, Leader A, et al: Paternal age and birth defects: how strong is the association? Human Reprod 22(3):696, 2007
Yeo L, Guzman ER, Day-Salvatore D, et al: Prenatal detection of fetal trisomy 18 through abnormal sonographic features. J Ultrasound Med 22(6):581, 2003

CHAPTER 14

Prenatal Diagnosis

Major congenital abnormalities are identified during pregnancy or shortly after birth in 2 to 3 percent of pregnancies. They account for 20 percent of infant deaths in the United States, surpassing preterm birth as the most common cause (Kochanek, 2011). Prenatal diagnosis is the science of identifying malformations, disruptions, chromosomal abnormalities, and other genetic syndromes in the fetus. It encompasses routine screening tests for aneuploidy and neural-tube defects, invasive diagnostic tests such as chorionic villus sampling and amniocentesis, additional screening and diagnostic tests offered to those at risk for specific genetic disorders, and the diagnosis of structural malformations with specialized sonography and other fetal imaging techniques discussed in Chapter 10. The goal of prenatal diagnosis is to provide accurate information regarding short- and long-term prognosis, recurrence risk, and potential therapy and to thereby improve counseling and optimize outcomes.

Structural fetal abnormalities may develop in at least three ways. The most common mechanism is *malformation*—an intrinsic abnormality "programmed" in development, regardless of whether a precise genetic etiology is known. Examples include spina bifida and omphalocele. A second mechanism is *deformation,* by which a fetus develops abnormally because of extrinsic mechanical forces imposed by the uterine environment. An example is limb contractures that develop with oligohydramnios from bilateral renal agenesis. A third type is *disruption,* which is a more severe change in form or function that occurs when genetically normal tissue is modified as the result of a specific insult. An example is damage from an amnionic band, which can cause a limb-reduction defect.

Multiple structural or developmental abnormalities may also present together as a syndrome, sequence, or association. A *syndrome* is a cluster of several anomalies or defects that have the same cause—for example, trisomy 18. A *sequence* describes anomalies that all developed sequentially from one initial insult. An example is the Pierre-Robin sequence in which micrognathia causes posterior displacement of the tongue—glossoptosis—which leads to a posterior rounded cleft in the palate. An *association* is a group of specific abnormalities that occur together frequently but do not seem to be linked etiologically. Diagnosis of the VACTERL association, for example, includes three or more of the following: vertebral defects, anal atresia, cardiac defects, tracheoesophageal fistula, renal anomalies, and limb abnormalities. Because of overlap of anomaly patterns, it is readily apparent that classification of fetal malformations is challenging, and reclassification is required periodically.

NEURAL-TUBE DEFECTS

These defects include anencephaly, spina bifida, cephalocele, and other rare spinal fusion (schisis) abnormalities. Features of these anomalies are detailed in Chapter 10 (p. 201), and fetal surgery for spina bifida is discussed in Chapter 16 (p. 325). Neural-tube defects (NTDs) are the second most common class of birth defect after cardiac anomalies, and their reported frequency is approximately 0.9 per 1000 births (Cragan, 2009; Dolk, 2010). More than 40 years ago, Brock and associates (1972, 1973) observed that pregnancies complicated by NTDs

TABLE 14-1. Risk Factors for Neural-Tube Defects

Genetic Cause	
Family history—multifactorial inheritance	
MTHFR mutation—677C→T	
Syndromes with autosomal recessive inheritance—Meckel Gruber, Roberts, Joubert, Jarcho-Levin, HARDE (hydrocephalus-agyria-retinal dysplasia-encephalocele)	
Aneuploidy—trisomy 13 and 18, triploidy	
Environmental Exposures	
Diabetes—hyperglycemia	
Hyperthermia—hot tub or sauna, fever (controversial)	
Medications—valproic acid, carbamazepine, coumadin, thalidomide, efavirenz	
Geographical—Ethnicity, Diet, and Other Factors	
United Kingdom, India, China, Egypt, Mexico, Southern Appalachian United States	

MTHFR = methylene tetrahydrofolate reductase.

had higher levels of alpha-fetoprotein (AFP) in both maternal serum and amnionic fluid. This formed the basis for the first maternal serum screening test for a fetal defect.

Risk Factors

Selected risk factors for NTDs are listed in Table 14-1, and genetic factors represent the largest category. Isolated NTDs display multifactorial inheritance. The recurrence risk is approximately 3 to 5 percent if a couple has previously had a child with either anencephaly or spina bifida, 5 percent if either parent was born with an NTD, and as high as 10 percent if a couple has two affected children. Importantly, almost 95 percent of NTDs develop in the absence of a family history. Polymorphisms in the methylene tetrahydrofolate reductase gene, which leads to impaired homocysteine and folate metabolism, have been associated with increased risk for anencephaly and spina bifida, as well as for cardiac malformations (Aneji, 2012; Harisha, 2010; Munoz, 2007; Yin, 2012). NTDs are a component of more than 80 genetic syndromes, many including other anomalies that may be amenable to prenatal diagnosis (Milunsky, 2004).

Other risk factors for NTDs include hyperthermia, medications that disturb folic acid metabolism, and hyperglycemia from insulin-dependent diabetes. Although the exact mechanism by which diabetes causes these anomalies is unknown, rodent studies have found that oxidative stress from embryonic hyperglycemia is associated with apoptosis in the developing neural tube (Li, 2012; Sugimura, 2009; Yang, 2008). The risk for these defects is also increased in certain racial or ethnic groups as well as in populations from selected geographical regions. For example, recent data from population-based registries indicate an NTD prevalence of 1.0 to 1.3 per 1000 births in the United Kingdom, which compares with 0.9 per 1000 in the United States (Cragan, 2009; Dolk, 2010). In the United States, the risk may be twice as high among Mexican-born women (Velie, 2006).

Prevention

Most women at increased risk for NTDs benefit from 4 mg folic acid taken daily before conception and through the first trimester. This is particularly important if a woman has one or more prior affected children or if either the pregnant woman or her partner has such a defect. Folic acid supplementation may not decrease the risk for NTDs in those with valproic acid exposure, pregestational diabetes, first-trimester fever or hot tub exposure, or defects associated with a genetic syndrome (American College of Obstetricians and Gynecologists, 2013b).

The policy of routine fortification of cereal grains with folic acid, which has been in place in the United States since 1998, provides approximately 200 additional micrograms of folic acid daily and may reduce the first occurrence of NTDs in *low-risk women* by approximately 20 percent (Honein, 2001). It is recommended that all women at low risk take 400 μg of folic acid orally every day before conception and through the first trimester, to reduce the NTD risk by as much as 80 percent (Chap. 8, p. 159).

Maternal Serum Alpha-Fetoprotein Screening (MSAFP)

Alpha-fetoprotein (AFP) is a glycoprotein synthesized by the fetal yolk sac and later by the fetal gastrointestinal tract and liver. It is the major serum protein in the embryo and fetus and is thus analogous to albumin. As shown in Figure 14-1, its concentration increases steadily in both fetal serum and amnionic fluid until 13 weeks' gestation, after which, levels rapidly decline. Conversely, AFP is found in steadily increasing quantities in maternal serum after 12 weeks. The normal concentration gradient between fetal plasma and maternal serum is

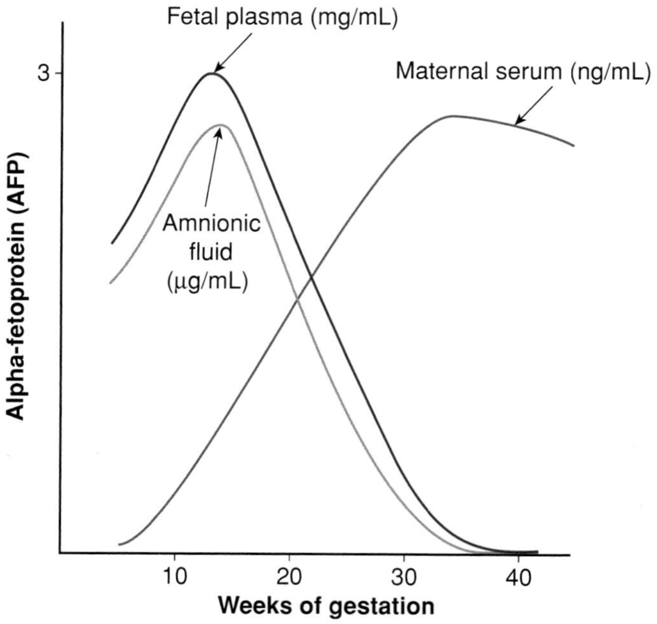

FIGURE 14-1 Diagram of alpha-fetoprotein (AFP) concentration across gestational age in fetal plasma, amnionic fluid, and maternal serum. The scale refers to the fetal plasma level, which is approximately 150 times greater than the amnionic fluid concentration and 50,000 times greater than the maternal serum concentration.

on the order of 50,000:1. Defects in fetal integument, such as neural-tube and ventral wall defects, permit AFP to leak into the amnionic fluid, resulting in dramatically increased maternal serum AFP levels.

It was shown more than 30 years ago that maternal serum AFP concentrations at 16 to 18 weeks exceeded 2.5 multiples of the median (MoM) in a large proportion of women carrying fetuses with either anencephaly or spina bifida (Wald, 1977). Since the mid-1980s, MSAFP concentration has been routinely measured as a screening test for NTDs.

Maternal serum AFP screening is generally performed from 15 through 20 weeks, within a protocol that includes quality control, counseling, and follow-up. AFP is measured in nanograms per milliliter and reported as multiples of the median (MoM) of the unaffected population. Using MoM normalizes the distribution of AFP levels and permits comparison of results from different laboratories and populations. Using a maternal serum AFP level of 2.0 or 2.5 MoM as the upper limit of normal, most laboratories report a detection rate—*test sensitivity*—of at least 90 percent for anencephaly and 80 percent for spina bifida at a screen-positive rate of 3 to 5 percent (Milunsky, 2004). The *positive predictive value*—the proportion with AFP elevation that have an affected fetus—is only 2 to 6 percent. This is explained by the overlap in AFP distributions in affected and unaffected pregnancies, as shown in Figure 14-2.

Several factors influence maternal serum AFP levels and are considered when calculating the AFP MoM:

1. Maternal weight—The AFP concentration is adjusted for the maternal volume of distribution.
2. Gestational age—The maternal serum concentration increases by approximately 15 percent per week during the second trimester (Knight, 1992). In general, the MoM should be recalculated if the biparietal diameter differs from the stated gestational age by more than 1 week.
3. Race/ethnicity—African American women have at least 10-percent higher serum AFP concentrations but are at lower risk for fetal NTDs.
4. Diabetes—Serum levels may be 10 to 20 percent lower in women with insulin-treated diabetes, despite a three- to fourfold increased risk for NTDs (Greene, 1988; Huttly, 2004). There is controversy whether such adjustment remains necessary or if results should apply to all types of diabetes (Evans, 2002; Sancken, 2001; Thornburg, 2008).
5. Multifetal gestation—Higher screening threshold values are used in twin pregnancies (Cuckle, 1990). At Parkland Hospital, an AFP level is considered elevated in a twin pregnancy if greater than 3.5 MoM, but other laboratories use 4.0 or even 5.0 MoM.

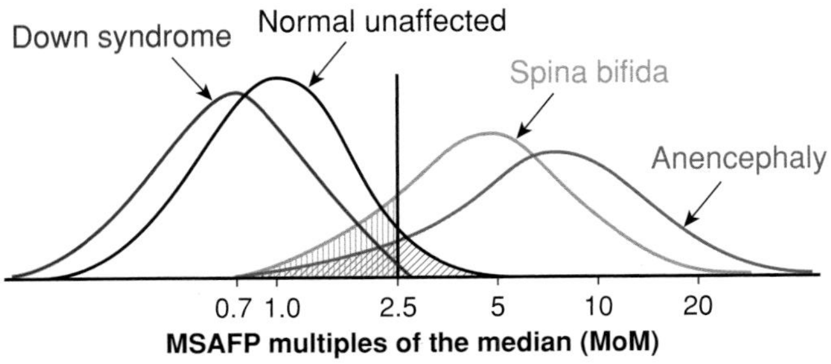

FIGURE 14-2 Maternal serum alpha-fetoprotein distribution for singleton pregnancies at 15 to 20 weeks. The screen cut-off value of 2.5 multiples of the median is expected to result in a false-positive rate of up to 5 percent (*black hatched area*) and false-negative rates of up to 20 percent for spina bifida (*tan hatched area*) and 10 percent for anencephaly (*red hatched area*).

According to the American College of Obstetricians and Gynecologists (2013b), all pregnant women should be offered screening for NTDs. Women who present for care early in pregnancy often have the option of several different screening tests for aneuploidy, as discussed subsequently. Those who elect second-trimester multiple marker serum screening will have a maternal serum AFP level measured as a component. Those who elect first-trimester screening or chorionic villus sampling may receive neural-tube defect screening either with serum AFP at 15 to 20 weeks or with sonography (American College of Obstetricians and Gynecologists, 2013c).

MSAFP Elevation

One algorithm for evaluating elevated maternal serum AFP levels is shown in Figure 14-3. The evaluation begins with a standard sonogram, if not already performed earlier in gestation, as this can reliably exclude three common causes of AFP level elevation: underestimation of gestational age, multifetal gestation, and fetal demise. Virtually all cases of anencephaly and many cases of spina bifida may be detected or suspected during a standard second-trimester sonographic examination (Dashe, 2006). Once the gestational age is verified and the screening test is confirmed to be abnormal, a patient is offered diagnostic evaluation.

Numerous fetal and placental abnormalities have been associated with AFP elevation (Table 14-2). The likelihood of one of these abnormalities or of an adverse pregnancy outcome in the absence of a recognized abnormality increases in proportion to the AFP level. More than 40 percent of pregnancies may be abnormal if the AFP level is greater than 7 MoM (Reichler, 1994).

For the foregoing reasons, women with a confirmed serum AFP level elevation should be referred for additional counseling and offered a diagnostic test, either specialized sonography or amniocentesis. Some women have risk factors that warrant referral for a diagnostic test even in the setting of a normal AFP level. These include personal history of or first-degree relative with an NTD, insulin-treated diabetes, and first-trimester exposure to a medication associated with increased risk.

Targeted Sonography

More than 25 years ago, Nicolaides and colleagues (1986) described frontal bone scalloping—the *lemon sign*, and anterior curvature of the cerebellum with effacement of the cisterna magna—the *banana sign*—in second-trimester fetuses with open spina bifida (Fig. 14-4). These investigators also frequently noted a small biparietal diameter and ventriculomegaly in such cases. Watson and coworkers (1991) reported that 99 percent of fetuses with open spina bifida had one or more of these findings. In addition to these cranial findings, transverse and sagittal images of the spine are increasingly used to characterize

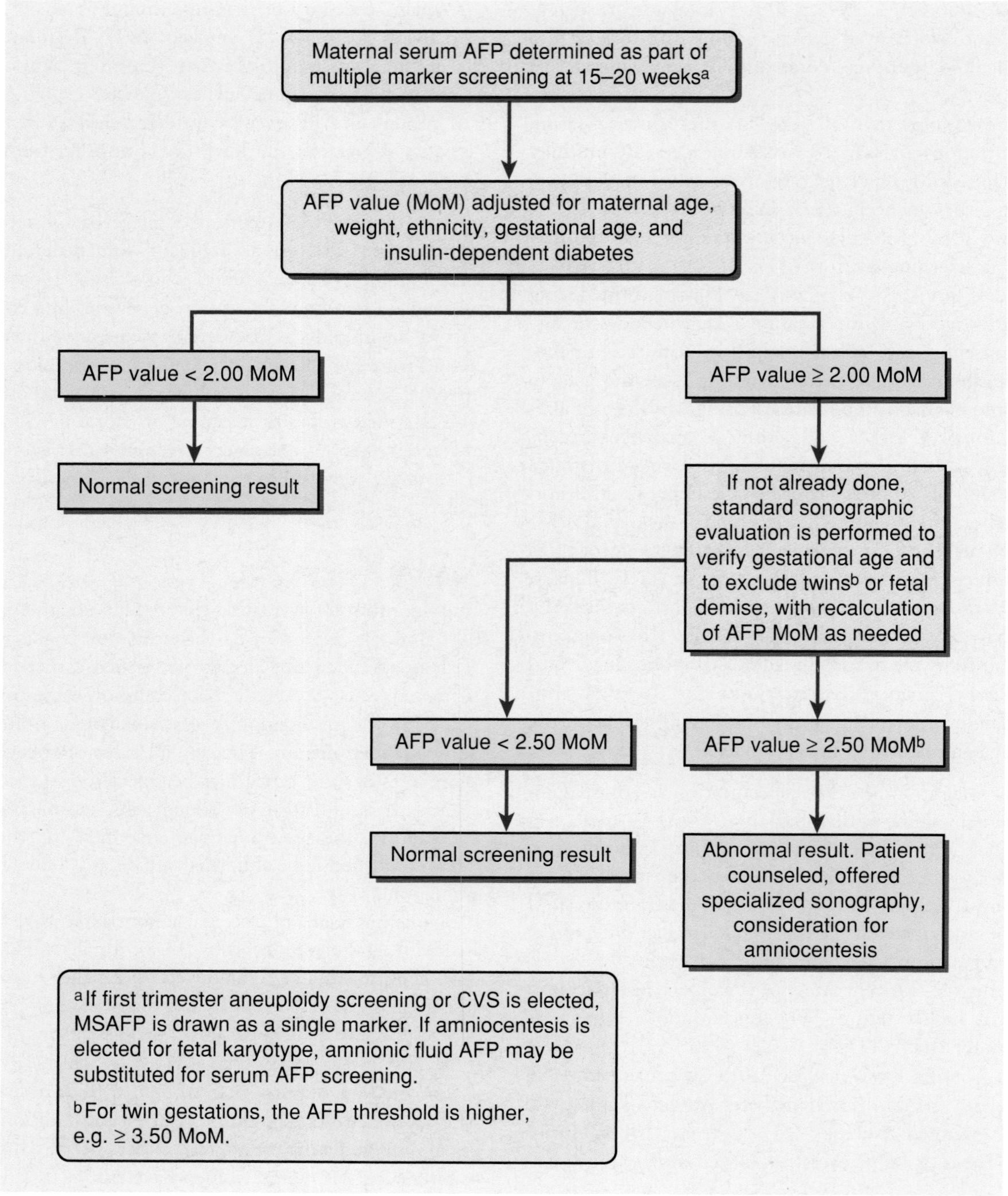

FIGURE 14-3 Example of an algorithm for evaluating maternal serum alpha-fetoprotein screening values (MSAFP). CVS = chorionic villus sampling; MoM = multiples of the median.

the size and location of spinal defects (Chap. 10, p. 202). Using these findings, experienced investigators have described nearly 100-percent detection of open NTDs (Norem, 2005; Sepulveda, 1995). Overall NTD risk may be reduced by at least 95 percent when no spine or cranial abnormality is observed (Morrow, 1991; Van den Hof, 1990).

Most centers use targeted sonography as the primary method of evaluating maternal serum AFP level elevation. The American College of Obstetricians and Gynecologists (2013b) recommends that women be counseled regarding the risks and benefits of targeted sonography and amniocentesis, the risk associated with the degree of AFP level elevation or other risk factors, and the quality and findings of the sonographic examination before making a decision.

Amniocentesis

Although amniocentesis for amnionic fluid AFP measurement was once considered the standard for open NTD diagnosis, it has been replaced in most centers by targeted sonography. If the amnionic fluid AFP level was elevated, an assay for acetylcholinesterase was performed, and if positive, was considered diagnostic of an NTD. Acetylcholinesterase leaks directly from exposed neural tissue into the amnionic fluid. The overall sensitivity of amniocentesis is approximately 98 percent for open

TABLE 14-2. Conditions Associated with Abnormal Maternal Serum Alpha-Fetoprotein Concentrations

Elevated Levels
Underestimated gestational age
Multifetal gestation[a]
Fetal death
Neural-tube defect
Gastroschisis
Omphalocele
Cystic hygroma
Esophageal or intestinal obstruction
Liver necrosis
Renal anomalies—polycystic kidneys, renal agenesis, congenital nephrosis, urinary tract obstruction
Cloacal exstrophy
Osteogenesis imperfecta
Sacrococcygeal teratoma
Congenital skin abnormality
Pilonidal cyst
Chorioangioma of placenta
Placenta intervillous thrombosis
Placental abruption
Oligohydramnios
Preeclampsia
Fetal-growth restriction
Maternal hepatoma or teratoma
Low Levels
Obesity[a]
Diabetes mellitus[a]
Trisomies 21 or 18
Gestational trophoblastic disease
Fetal death
Overestimated gestational age

[a]Alpha-fetoprotein is adjusted for these factors when multiples of the median are calculated.

NTDs, with a false-positive rate of 0.4 percent (Milunsky, 2004). Other fetal abnormalities associated with elevated amnionic fluid AFP levels and positive assay for acetylcholinesterase include ventral wall defects, esophageal atresia, fetal teratoma, cloacal exstrophy, and skin abnormalities such as epidermolysis bullosa.

Unexplained Maternal Serum AFP Level Elevation

If no fetal or placental abnormality is detected after a specialized sonographic evaluation, with or without amniocentesis, then an MSAFP elevation is considered unexplained. These pregnancies are at increased risk for various subsequent adverse pregnancy outcomes. These include fetal abnormalities or genetic syndromes not detectable sonographically, fetal-growth restriction, oligohydramnios, placental abruption, preterm membrane rupture, preterm birth, and fetal death. Many of these complications are assumed to result from placental damage or dysfunction. Importantly, AFP level elevation is *not* considered to be clinically useful as a screening tool for adverse pregnancy outcomes, due to its low sensitivity and positive predictive value. No specific program of maternal or fetal surveillance has been found to favorably affect pregnancy outcomes (Dugoff, 2010). At Parkland Hospital, prenatal care for these women is not altered unless a specific complication arises. Despite the extensive list of possible adverse outcomes, it is reassuring that most women with unexplained AFP level elevation have normal outcomes. Abnormally high or low values of other serum analytes used in aneuploidy screening protocols are reviewed on page 290.

Management of the Fetus with Spina Bifida

The optimal mode of delivery for a fetus with open spina bifida remains controversial. Some have recommended cesarean delivery before the onset of labor, positing that it may reduce the risk of mechanical trauma and spinal infection. Although some have found improved motor function in children delivered

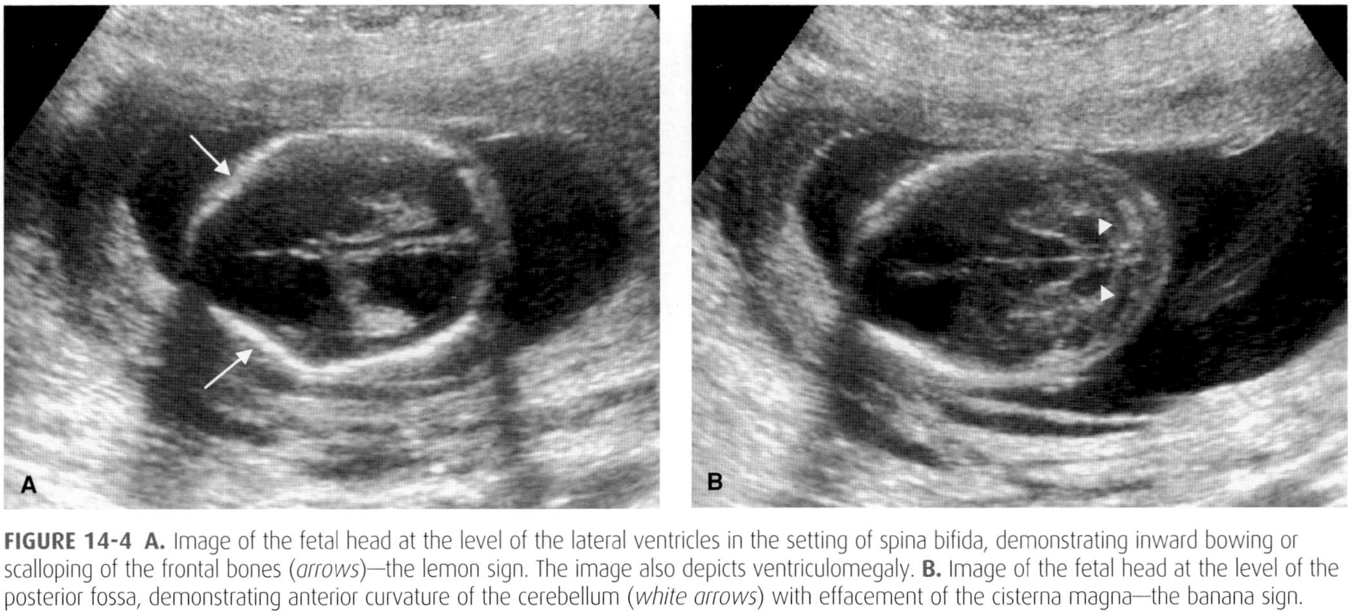

FIGURE 14-4 A. Image of the fetal head at the level of the lateral ventricles in the setting of spina bifida, demonstrating inward bowing or scalloping of the frontal bones (*arrows*)—the lemon sign. The image also depicts ventriculomegaly. **B.** Image of the fetal head at the level of the posterior fossa, demonstrating anterior curvature of the cerebellum (*white arrows*) with effacement of the cisterna magna—the banana sign.

operatively, others have not identified benefit in short- or long-term outcomes (Lewis, 2004; Luthy, 1991; Merrill, 1998). The American College of Obstetricians and Gynecologists (2013b) recommends that the route of delivery for the fetus with spina bifida should be individualized.

Open fetal surgery to repair NTDs has been the subject of several clinical studies. A landmark trial designed to compare open fetal surgery for spina bifida with standard postnatal care was described by Adzick and colleagues (2011). These authors of the Management of Myelomeningocele or MOMS trial found that in selected cases, fetal surgery resulted in improved motor outcomes and reduced need for ventriculoperitoneal shunt placement at age 2 to 3 years. They also reported, however, that the surgery itself was associated with significant maternal and fetal risks. This is discussed further in Chapter 16 (p. 325).

DOWN SYNDROME AND OTHER ANEUPLOIDIES

At least 8 percent of conceptuses are aneuploid, accounting for 50 percent of first-trimester abortions and 5 to 7 percent of all stillbirths and neonatal deaths. As discussed in Chapter 13 (p. 260), the risk of fetal trisomy increases with maternal age, particularly after age 35. Specific maternal age-related aneuploidy risks for singleton and twin pregnancies are shown in Tables 14-3 and 14-4. Other significant risk factors include a prior pregnancy with autosomal trisomy or triploidy or a woman or her partner with a numerical chromosomal abnormality or structural chromosomal rearrangement, such as a balanced translocation.

Types of Screening Tests

Until the mid-1980s, prenatal diagnostic testing for fetal aneuploidy was offered for "advanced maternal age." However, age alone is a poor screening test, because approximately 70 percent of Down syndrome pregnancies are in women younger than 35 years. Nearly 30 years ago, Merkatz and associates (1984) observed that pregnancies with Down syndrome were characterized by lower maternal serum AFP levels at 15 to 20 weeks, and screening became available for younger women. During the past two decades, there have been four major advances in the area of aneuploidy screening:

1. The addition of other serum analytes to second-trimester screening has improved Down syndrome detection rates to approximately 80 percent for the quadruple marker test (Table 14-5).
2. First-trimester screening at 11 to 14 weeks' gestation, using the fetal nuchal translucency measurement together with serum analytes, has achieved Down syndrome detection rates comparable to those for second-trimester screening in women younger than 35 years (American College of Obstetricians and Gynecologists, 2013c).
3. Combinations of first- and second-trimester screening yield Down syndrome detection rates as high as 90 to 95 percent (Malone, 2005b).
4. Maternal serum cell-free fetal DNA testing for trisomy 21, 18, and 13 has become available as a screening test for high-risk pregnancies, with a 98-percent detection rate and a false-positive rate of 0.5 percent (American College of Obstetricians and Gynecologists, 2012b; Bianchi, 2012; Palomaki, 2011, 2012).

With the exception of cell-free fetal DNA testing, each first- and/or second-trimester aneuploidy screening test is based on a composite likelihood ratio, and the maternal age-related risk is multiplied by this ratio. This principle also applies to modification of the Down syndrome risk by selected sonographic findings (p. 292). Each woman is provided with a specific risk,

TABLE 14-3. Maternal Age-Related Risk for Down Syndrome and Any Aneuploidy at Midtrimester and at Term in Singleton Pregnancies

	Down Syndrome		Any Aneuploidy	
Age	Midtrimester	Term	Midtrimester	Term
35	1/250	1/385	1/132	1/204
36	1/192	1/303	1/105	1/167
37	1/149	1/227	1/83	1/130
38	1/115	1/175	1/65	1/103
39	1/89	1/137	1/53	1/81
40	1/69	1/106	1/40	1/63
41	1/53	1/81	1/31	1/50
42	1/41	1/64	1/25	1/39
43	1/31	1/50	1/19	1/30
44	1/25	1/38	1/15	1/24
45	1/19	1/30	1/12	1/19

Adapted from Hook, 1983.

TABLE 14-4. Maternal Age-Related Risk for Down Syndrome and Any Aneuploidy at Midtrimester and at Term in Dizygotic Twin Pregnancies[a]

	Down Syndrome		Any Aneuploidy	
Age	Midtrimester	Term	Midtrimester	Term
32	1/256	1/409	1/149	1/171
33	1/206	1/319	1/116	1/151
34	1/160	1/257	1/91	1/126
35	1/125	1/199	1/71	1/101
36	1/98	1/153	1/56	1/82
37	1/77	1/118	1/44	1/67
38	1/60	1/92	1/35	1/54
39	1/47	1/72	1/27	1/44
40	1/37	1/56	1/21	1/35
41	1/29	1/44	1/17	1/28
42	1/23	1/33	1/13	1/22

[a]Risk applies to one or both fetuses.
Adapted from Meyers, 1997.

TABLE 14-5. Selected Down Syndrome Screening Strategies and Their Detection Rate

Strategy	Analytes	Detection Rate[a] (%)
First-trimester screen	NT, PAPP-A, and hCG or free β-hCG	79–87
NT	NT alone	64–70
Triple test	MSAFP, hCG or free β-hCG, uE3	61–70
Quadruple (Quad) test	MSAFP, hCG or free β-hCG, uE3, inh	74–81
Integrated screen	First-trimester screen and Quad test; results withheld until Quad test completed	94–96
Stepwise sequential screen	First-trimester screen and Quad test 1% offered diagnostic test after first-trimester screen 99% proceed to Quad test, results withheld until Quad test completed	90–95
Contingent sequential screen	First-trimester screen and Quad test 1% offered diagnostic test after first-trimester screen 15% proceed to Quad test; results withheld until Quad test completed 84% have no additional test after first-trimester screen	88–94
Cell-free fetal DNA testing (high-risk pregnancies)	No analytes—massively parallel genomic sequencing	98

[a]Based on a 5-percent positive screen rate.
Free β-hCG = free β-subunit hCG; hCG = human chorionic gonadotropin; inh = dimeric inhibin α; MSAFP = maternal serum alpha-fetoprotein; NT = nuchal translucency; PAPP-A = pregnancy-associated plasma protein-A; uE3 = unconjugated estriol.
Data from Alldred, 2012; American College of Obstetricians and Gynecologists, 2012b; Cuckle, 2005; Malone, 2005b; Wapner, 2003.

expressed as a ratio—1:X. However, each screening test has a predetermined value at which it is deemed "positive" or abnormal. For second-trimester tests, this threshold has traditionally been set at the risk for fetal Down syndrome in a woman aged 35 years—approximately 1 in 385 at term (see Table 14-3). Women with a positive screening test result should be offered a diagnostic test for fetal karyotype by either chorionic villus sampling or amniocentesis (American College of Obstetricians and Gynecologists, 2012a).

Counseling

Because technology advances have resulted in improved aneuploidy detection with available screening tests, the American College of Obstetricians and Gynecologists (2013c) recommends that all women who present for prenatal care before 20 weeks be offered screening. Available screening paradigms are shown in Table 14-5. A positive screening test result indicates increased risk, but it is not diagnostic of aneuploidy. Conversely, a negative screening test indicates that the risk is not increased, but it does not guarantee a normal fetus. Although Down syndrome is the focus of most aneuploidy screening protocols, it accounts for only half of all fetal chromosomal abnormality cases. Invasive diagnostic tests such as chorionic villus sampling and amniocentesis are safe and effective. Regardless of age, *all* women are counseled regarding the differences between screening and diagnostic tests, and they are given the option of invasive diagnostic testing.

First-Trimester Screening

The most commonly used protocol involves measurement of sonographic nuchal translucency and two maternal serum analytes. This is performed between 11 and 14 weeks' gestation.

Nuchal Translucency (NT)

This is the maximum thickness of the subcutaneous translucent area between the skin and soft tissue overlying the fetal spine at the back of the neck (Fig. 14-5). It is measured in the sagittal plane, when the crown-rump length measures between 38 and 84 mm. Specific criteria for NT measurement are listed in Table 10-3 (p. 196). The NT measurement is expressed as a multiple of the gestational age-specific median, similar to serum markers used for aneuploidy screening. An increased NT thickness itself is not a fetal abnormality, but rather is a marker that confers increased risk. Approximately one third of fetuses with increased nuchal translucency thickness will have a chromosome abnormality, nearly half of which are Down syndrome (Snijders, 1998).

As shown in Table 14-5, as an isolated marker, NT detects 64 to 70 percent of fetuses with Down syndrome at a false-positive rate of 5 percent, and it has maximal sensitivity at 11 weeks (Malone, 2005b). The risk conferred by an increased NT thickness is independent of that of serum analytes, and combining NT with serum analyte values results in greatly

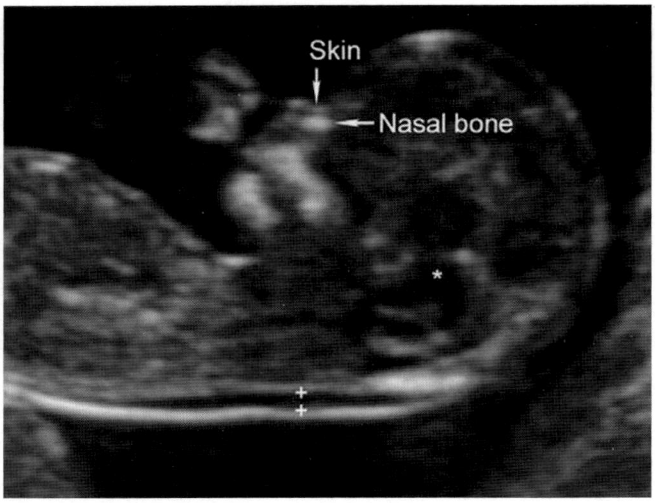

FIGURE 14-5 Sagittal image of a normal, 12-week fetus demonstrating correct caliper placement (+) for nuchal translucency measurement. The fetal nasal bone and overlying skin are indicated. The nasal tip and the 3rd and 4th ventricles (*asterisk*), which are other landmarks that should be visible in the nasal bone image, are also shown. (Image contributed by Dr. Michael Zaretsky.)

improved aneuploidy detection (Spencer, 1999). Thus, NT is generally used as an isolated marker only in screening for multifetal gestations, in which serum screening is not as accurate or may not be available (American College of Obstetricians and Gynecologists, 2013c). An exception is that if the NT measurement is increased to 3 to 4 mm, then the aneuploidy risk is unlikely to be normalized using serum analyte assessment, and invasive testing should be offered (Comstock, 2006).

Increased NT thickness is also associated with other aneuploidies, genetic syndromes, and various birth defects, especially fetal cardiac anomalies (Atzei, 2005; Simpson, 2007). Because of this, if the NT measurement is 3.5 mm or greater, the patient should be offered targeted sonography, with or without fetal echocardiography, in addition to fetal karyotyping (American College of Obstetricians and Gynecologists, 2013c).

The NT must be imaged and measured with a high degree of precision for aneuploidy detection to be accurate. This has led to standardized training, certification, and ongoing quality review programs. In the United States, training, credentialing, and monitoring are available through the Nuchal Translucency Quality Review (NTQR) program (www.ntqr.org). Training is also available through the Fetal Medicine Foundation (www.fetalmedicineusa.com). In addition to nuchal translucency, NTQR provides an educational process leading to certification in measurement of the fetal nasal bone, which is discussed on page 294 and shown in Figure 14-5.

Serum Analytes

Two analytes used for first-trimester aneuploidy screening are *human chorionic gonadotropin*—either intact or free β-hCG—and *pregnancy-associated plasma protein A (PAPP-A)*. In cases of fetal Down syndrome, the first-trimester serum free β-hCG level is higher, approximately 2.0 MoM, and the PAPP-A level is lower, approximately 0.5 MoM. With trisomy 18 and trisomy 13, levels of both analytes are lower (Cuckle, 2000; Malone, 2005b; Spencer, 1999, 2000; Tul, 1999). If gestational age is correct, the use of these serum markers—*without NT measurement*—results in detection rates for fetal Down syndrome up to 67 percent at a false-positive rate of 5 percent (Wapner, 2003). Aneuploidy detection is significantly greater if these first-trimester analytes are either: (1) combined with the sonographic NT measurement or (2) combined with second-trimester analytes, which is termed *serum integrated screening* (p. 291).

In twin pregnancies, serum free β-hCG and PAPP-A levels are approximately doubled compared with singleton values (Vink, 2012). Even with specific curves, a normal dichorionic cotwin will tend to normalize screening results, and thus, the aneuploidy detection rate is at least 15-percent lower (Bush, 2005).

Combined First-Trimester Screening

The most commonly used screening protocol combines the NT measurement with serum hCG and PAPP-A. Using this protocol, Down syndrome detection rates in large prospective trials range from 79 to 87 percent, at a false-positive rate of 5 percent (see Table 14-5). The detection rate is approximately 5-percent higher if performed at 11 compared with 13 weeks (Malone, 2005b). The detection rate for trisomies 18 and 13 is approximately 90 percent, at a 2-percent false-positive rate (Nicolaides, 2004; Wapner, 2003).

Maternal age does affect the performance of first-trimester aneuploidy screening tests. In prospective trials, combined first-trimester screening resulted in Down syndrome detection rates of 67 to 75 percent in women younger than 35 years at delivery, which are 10-percent lower than the overall detection rates in these studies (Malone, 2005b; Wapner, 2003). Among women older than 35 at delivery, however, Down syndrome detection rates were 90 to 95 percent, albeit at a higher false-positive rate of 15 to 22 percent.

Unexplained Abnormalities of First-Trimester Analytes

There is a significant association between serum PAPP-A levels below the 5th percentile and preterm birth, growth restriction, preeclampsia, and fetal demise (Dugoff, 2004). Similarly, low levels of free β-hCG have been associated with fetal demise (Goetzl, 2004). The sensitivity and positive-predictive values of these markers are considered too low to be clinically useful as screening tests. As with other serum analyte level abnormalities, no management strategies have been demonstrated to improve pregnancy outcomes when these marker levels are abnormally low (Dugoff, 2010).

Second-Trimester Screening

Pregnancies with fetal Down syndrome are characterized by lower maternal serum AFP levels—approximately 0.7 MoM, higher hCG levels—approximately 2.0 MoM, and lower unconjugated estriol levels—approximately 0.8 MoM (Merkatz, 1984; Wald, 1988). This *triple test* can detect 61 to 70 percent of Down syndrome cases as shown in Table 14-5

(Alldred, 2012). Levels of all three markers are decreased in the setting of trisomy 18, with a detection rate similar to that for Down syndrome at a false-positive rate of only 0.5 percent (Benn, 1999).

Levels of a fourth marker—*dimeric inhibin alpha*—are elevated in Down syndrome, with an average value of 1.8 MoM (Spencer, 1996). The addition of dimeric inhibin to the other three markers is the *quadruple* or *quad test,* which has a trisomy 21 detection rate of approximately 80 percent at a false-positive rate of 5 percent (see Table 14-5). As with first-trimester screening, aneuploidy detection rates will be slightly lower in younger women and higher in women older than 35 years at delivery. If second-trimester serum screening is used in twin pregnancies, aneuploidy detection rates are significantly lower (Vink, 2012).

The quad test is the most commonly used second-trimester serum screening test for aneuploidy. As a stand-alone test, it is generally used if women do not begin care until the second-trimester or if first-trimester screening is not available. As subsequently discussed, combining the quad test with first-trimester screening yields even greater aneuploidy detection rates.

Unexplained Abnormalities of Second-Trimester Analytes

There is a significant association between second-trimester elevation of either hCG or dimeric inhibin alpha levels and adverse pregnancy outcomes. The outcomes reported are similar to those associated with AFP level elevation and include fetal-growth restriction, preeclampsia, preterm birth, fetal demise, and stillbirth. Moreover, the likelihood of adverse outcome is increased when multiple marker levels are elevated (Dugoff, 2005). However, the sensitivity and positive predictive values of these markers are considered too low to be useful for screening or management (Dugoff, 2010).

Low Maternal Serum Estriol Levels. A maternal serum estriol level < 0.25 MoM has been associated with two uncommon but important conditions. The first, Smith-Lemli-Opitz syndrome, is an autosomal recessive condition characterized by mutations in the 7-dehydrocholesterol reductase gene. It may be associated with central nervous system, heart, kidney, and extremity abnormalities, with ambiguous genitalia, and with fetal-growth restriction. For this reason, the Society for Maternal-Fetal Medicine has recommended that sonographic evaluation be performed if an unconjugated estriol level is < 0.25 MoM (Dugoff, 2010). If abnormalities are identified, an elevated amnionic fluid 7-dehydrocholesterol level can confirm the diagnosis.

The second condition is steroid sulfatase deficiency, also known as X-linked ichthyosis. It is typically an isolated condition, but it may also occur in the setting of a contiguous gene deletion syndrome (Chap. 13, p. 266). In such cases, it may be associated with Kallmann syndrome, chondrodysplasia punctata, and/or mental retardation (Langlois, 2009). If the estriol level is < 0.25 MoM and the fetus appears to be male, fluorescence in situ hybridization to assess the steroid sulfatase locus on the X-chromosome may be considered (Dugoff, 2010).

Combined First- and Second-Trimester Screening

Combined screening strategies enhance aneuploidy detection. For this reason, the American College of Obstetricians and Gynecologists (2013c) recommends that a strategy incorporating both first- and second-trimester screening should be offered to women who seek prenatal care in the first trimester. Three types of screening strategies are available:

1. *Integrated screening* combines results of first- and second-trimester tests. This includes a combined measurement of fetal NT and serum analyte levels at 11 to 14 weeks' gestation plus quadruple markers at 15 to 20 weeks. An aneuploidy risk is then calculated from these seven parameters. As expected, integrated screening has the highest Down syndrome detection rate—94 to 96 percent at a false-positive rate of 5 percent (see Table 14-5). If NT measurement is not available, *serum integrated screening* includes all six serum markers to calculate risk. This screening, however, is less effective.
2. *Sequential screening* discloses the results of first-trimester screening to women at highest risk, who are then offered invasive testing with chorionic villus sampling or amniocentesis. There are two testing strategies in this category:
   - With *stepwise sequential screening,* women with first-trimester screen results that confer risk for Down syndrome above a particular threshold are offered invasive testing, and the remaining women receive second-trimester screening. The threshold is set at approximately 1 percent, because in a screened population, the 1 percent at highest risk includes approximately 70 percent of Down syndrome pregnancies (Cuckle, 2005). This method of screening may achieve up to a 95-percent detection rate (see Table 14-5).
   - With *contingent sequential screening,* women are divided into high-, moderate-, and low-risk groups. Those at highest risk, for example, the top 1 percent, are offered invasive testing. Women at moderate risk, who comprise 15 to 20 percent of the population, undergo second-trimester screening. The remaining 80 to 85 percent, who are at or below a 1:1000 risk, receive negative screening test results and have no further testing (Cuckle, 2005). Thus, most of those screened are provided with results almost immediately while still maintaining a high detection rate. This rate ranges from 88 to 94 percent (see Table 14-5). This option is also more cost-effective because a second-trimester test is obviated in up to 85 percent of patients.

Integrated and sequential screening strategies require coordination between the provider and laboratory to ensure that the second sample is obtained during the appropriate gestational age window, sent to the same laboratory, and linked to the first-trimester results.

Cell-Free Fetal DNA Screening

Using *massively parallel sequencing* or *chromosome selective sequencing* to isolate cell-free fetal DNA from maternal plasma, fetal Down syndrome and other autosomal trisomies may be detected as early as 10 weeks' gestation (Chap. 13, p. 279). Recent trials of these techniques in high-risk pregnancies have yielded detection rates for trisomies 21, 18, and 13 of approximately 98 percent at a false-positive rate of 0.5 percent or less (American College of Obstetricians and Gynecologists, 2012b; Bianchi, 2012; Palomaki, 2011, 2012; Sparks, 2012). This novel technology has recently become clinically available as a screening test, but it is not considered a replacement diagnostic test. Pretest counseling is recommended. If an abnormal result is identified, genetic counseling should be performed, and invasive prenatal diagnostic testing should be offered to confirm the results. The American College of Obstetricians and Gynecologists (2012b) currently recommends that the test may be offered to the following groups:

- Women 35 years or older at delivery
- Those with sonographic findings indicating increased risk for fetal aneuploidy
- Those with a prior pregnancy complicated by trisomy 21, 18, or 13
- Patient or partner carries a balanced robertsonian translocation indicating increased risk for fetal trisomy 21 or 13
- Those with an abnormal first-, second-, or combined first- and second-trimester screening test result for aneuploidy.

The College does not recommend offering the test to women with low-risk pregnancies or multifetal gestations (American College of Obstetricians and Gynecologists, 2012b).

Sonographic Screening

Major abnormalities and minor sonographic markers contribute significantly to aneuploidy detection. As shown in Table 14-6, with few exceptions, the aneuploidy risk associated with any major abnormality is high enough to warrant offering an invasive test for fetal karyotype and/or chromosomal microarray analysis (Chap. 13, p. 275). Importantly, a fetus with one abnormality may have others that are less likely to be detected sonographically or even undetectable sonographically but that greatly affect the prognosis nonetheless. Most fetuses with aneuploidy that is likely to be lethal in utero—such as trisomy 18 and 13 and triploidy—usually have sonographic abnormalities that can be seen by the second trimester. However, only 25 to 30 percent of second-trimester fetuses with Down syndrome will have a major malformation that can be identified sonographically (Vintzileos, 1995).

Second-Trimester Sonographic Markers—"Soft Signs"

For more than two decades, investigators have recognized that the sonographic detection of aneuploidy, particularly Down syndrome, may be improved by minor markers that are collectively referred to as "soft signs." Minor markers are normal variants rather than fetal abnormalities, and in the absence of aneuploidy or an associated abnormality, they do not significantly affect prognosis. Examples of these sonographic findings are listed in Table 14-7. Six of these markers have been the focus of genetic sonogram studies, in which likelihood ratios have been derived that allow a numerical risk to be calculated (Table 14-8). They are generally used only from 15 to 20 or 22 weeks' gestation. The aneuploidy risk increases steeply with the number of markers identified.

Unfortunately, at least 10 percent of unaffected pregnancies will have one of these soft signs, significantly limiting their utility for general population screening (Bromley, 2002; Nyberg, 2003). The incorporation of minor markers into second-trimester screening protocols has been studied primarily in high-risk populations. In this setting, detection rates of 50 to 75 percent for Down syndrome have been reported (American College of Obstetricians and Gynecologists, 2013c). With the exception of increased nuchal skinfold thickness, the identification of an isolated second-trimester marker in an otherwise low-risk pregnancy is not generally considered sufficient to warrant "high-risk" status. A metaanalysis concluded that if minor markers

TABLE 14-6. Aneuploidy Risk Associated with Selected Major Fetal Anomalies

Abnormality	Birth Prevalence	Aneuploidy Risk (%)	Common Aneuploidies[a]
Cystic hygroma	1/5000	50–70	45,X; 21; 18; 13; triploidy
Nonimmune hydrops	1/1500–4000	10–20	21, 18, 13, 45X, triploidy
Ventriculomegaly	1/1000–2000	5–25	13, 18, 21, triploidy
Holoprosencephaly	1/10,000–15,000	30–40	13, 18, 22, triploidy
Dandy-Walker malformation	1/12,000	40	18, 13, 21, triploidy
Cleft lip/palate	1/1000	5–15	18, 13
Cardiac defects	5–8/1000	10–30	21; 18; 13; 45,X; 22q11.2 microdeletion
Diaphragmatic hernia	1/3000–4000	5–15	18, 13, 21
Esophageal atresia	1/4000	10	18, 21
Duodenal atresia	1/10,000	30	21
Gastroschisis	1/2000–4000	No increase	
Omphalocele	1/4000	30–50	18, 13, 21, triploidy
Clubfoot	1/1000	5–30	18, 13

[a]Numbers indicate autosomal trisomies except where indicated; for example, 45,X indicates Turner syndrome.
Data from Best, 2012; Canfield, 2006; Colvin, 2005; Cragan, 2009; Dolk, 2010; Ecker, 2000; Gallot, 2007; Long, 2006; Orioli, 2010; Pedersen, 2012; Sharma, 2011; Solomon, 2010; Walker, 2001.

TABLE 14-7. Second-Trimester Sonographic Markers or "Soft Signs" Associated with Down Syndrome Fetuses

Sonographic Marker[a]
Brachycephaly or shortened frontal lobe
Clinodactyly (hypoplasia of the 5th digit middle phalanx)
Echogenic bowel
Flat facies
Echogenic intracardiac focus
Nasal bone absence or hypoplasia
Nuchal fold thickening
Renal pelvis dilation (mild)
"Sandal gap" between first and second toes
Shortened ear length
Single transverse palmar crease
Single umbilical artery
Short femur
Short humerus
Widened iliac angle

[a]Listed alphabetically.

TABLE 14-8. Likelihood Ratios and False-Positive Rates for Isolated Second-Trimester Markers Used in Down Syndrome Screening Protocols

Sonographic Marker	Likelihood Ratio	Prevalence in Unaffected Fetuses (%)
Nuchal skinfold thickening	11–17	0.5
Renal pelvis dilation	1.5–1.9	2.0–2.2
Echogenic intracardiac focus	1.4–2.8	3.8–3.9[a]
Echogenic bowel	6.1–6.7	0.5–0.7
Short femur	1.2–2.7	3.7–3.9
Short humerus	5.1–7.5	0.4
Any one marker	1.9–2.0	10.0–11.3
Two markers	6.2–9.7	1.6–2.0
Three or more	80–115	0.1–0.3

[a]Higher in Asian individuals.
Data from Bromley, 2002; Nyberg, 2001; Smith-Bindman, 2001.

were used as a basis to decide whether to offer amniocentesis, more fetal losses would result than cases of Down syndrome identified (Smith-Bindman, 2001). The American College of Obstetricians and Gynecologists (2013c) recommends that risk adjustment based on second-trimester sonographic markers be limited to specialized centers.

The *nuchal skinfold* is measured in the transcerebellar view of the fetal head, from the outer edge of the skull to the outer border of the skin (Fig. 14-6A). A measurement ≥ 6 mm is typically considered abnormal (Benacerraf, 1985). This finding is present in approximately 1 per 200 pregnancies and confers a more than tenfold risk for Down syndrome (Bromley,

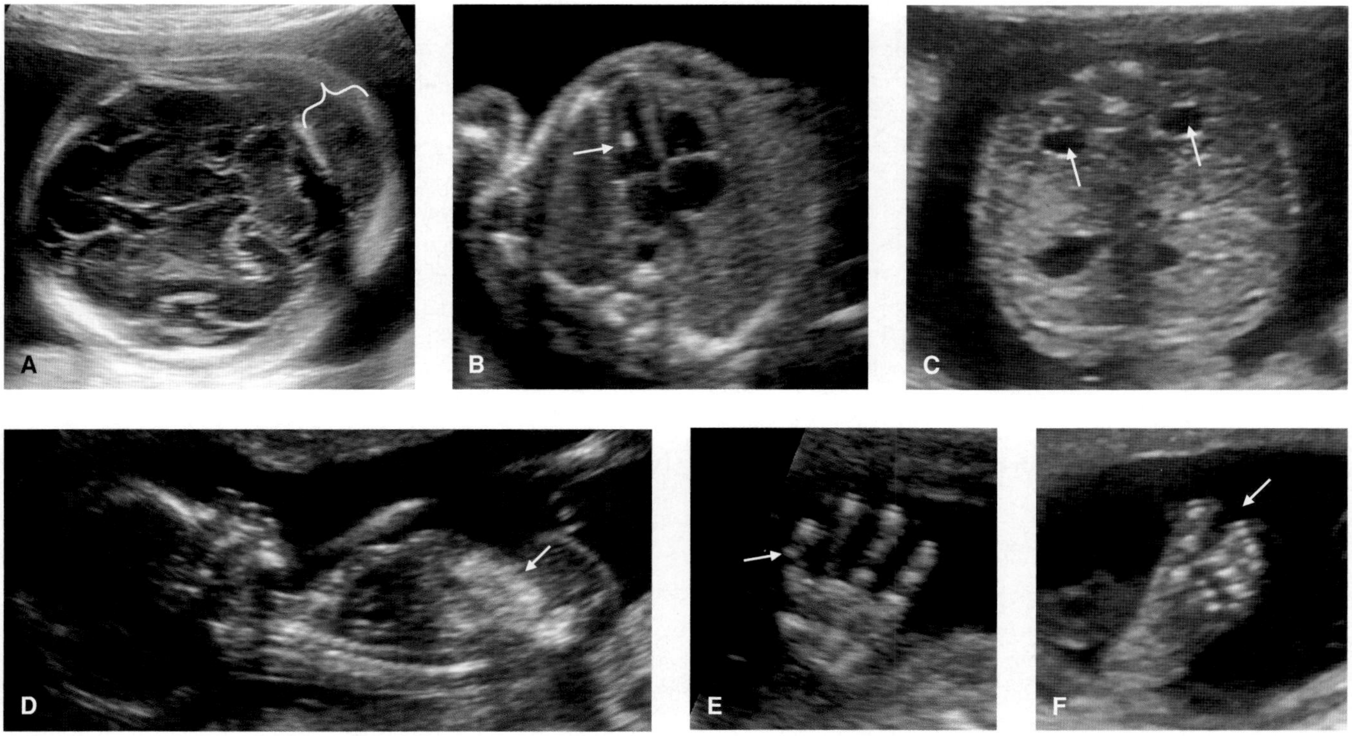

FIGURE 14-6 Minor sonographic markers that are associated with increased risk for fetal Down syndrome. **A.** Nuchal skinfold thickening (*bracket*). **B.** Echogenic intracardiac focus (*arrow*). **C.** Mild renal pelvis dilatation (pyelectasis) (*arrows*). **D.** Echogenic bowel (*arrow*). **E.** Clinodactyly—hypoplasia of the 5th finger middle phalanx creates an inward curvature (*arrow*). **F.** "Sandal-gap."

2002; Nyberg, 2001; Smith-Bindman, 2001). Unlike the other markers listed in Table 14-8, nuchal skinfold thickening should prompt targeted sonography and consideration of amniocentesis even as an isolated finding in an otherwise low-risk patient.

An *echogenic intracardiac focus (EIF)* is a focal papillary muscle calcification that is neither a structural nor functional cardiac abnormality. It is usually left-sided (Fig. 14-6B). An EIF is present in approximately 4 percent of fetuses, but it may be found in up to 30 percent of Asian individuals (Shipp, 2000). As an isolated finding, an EIF approximately doubles the risk for fetal Down syndrome (see Table 14-8). Particularly if bilateral, they are also common with trisomy 13 (Nyberg, 2001).

As discussed in Chapter 10 (p. 214), mild *renal pelvis dilatation* is usually transient or physiological and does not represent an underlying abnormality (Nguyen, 2010). The renal pelves are measured in a transverse image of the kidneys, anterior-to-posterior, with calipers placed at the inner borders of the fluid collection (Fig. 14-6C). A measurement 4 mm or greater is found in about 2 percent of fetuses and approximately doubles the risk for Down syndrome (see Table 14-8). The degree of pelvic dilatation beyond 4 mm correlates with the likelihood of an underlying renal abnormality, and additional evaluation is generally performed at approximately 34 weeks (Chap. 10, p. 215).

Echogenic fetal bowel appears as bright as bone and is seen in approximately 0.5 percent of pregnancies (Fig. 14-6D). Although typically associated with normal outcomes, it increases the risk for Down syndrome approximately sixfold (see Table 14-8). Echogenic bowel may represent small amounts of swallowed blood and may be seen in the setting of AFP level elevation (p. 287). It has also been associated with fetal cytomegalovirus infection and cystic fibrosis—representing inspissated meconium in the latter.

The femur and humerus are slightly shorter in Down syndrome fetuses, although the femur length to abdominal circumference (FL/AC) ratio is generally within the normal range in the second trimester. The femur is considered "short" for Down syndrome screening if it measures ≤ 90 percent of that expected. The expected femur length is that which correlates with the measured biparietal diameter (Benacerraf, 1987). Although this finding may be identified in approximately 4 percent of fetuses, its sensitivity may vary with ethnicity. As an isolated finding in an otherwise low-risk pregnancy, it is generally not considered to pose great enough risk to warrant counseling modification. Similarly, a humerus shortened to ≤ 89 percent of expected, based on a given biparietal diameter, has also been associated with an increased risk for Down syndrome (see Table 14-8).

First-Trimester Sonographic Findings

Unlike second-trimester soft signs, which may be readily visible during a standard sonogram, first-trimester findings associated with aneuploidy require specialized training. The fetal NT is unique in that it has become a component of aneuploidy screening offered to all women. Other first-trimester findings associated with an increased risk for fetal Down syndrome include an absent fetal nasal bone, wider frontomaxillary facial angle—indicating a flat facial profile, tricuspid regurgitation, and abnormal ductus venosus flow (Borenstein, 2008; Cicero, 2001; Faiola, 2005; Huggon, 2003; Matias, 1998; Sonek, 2007). Each has also been associated with an increased risk for trisomies 18 and 13 and other aneuploidies. However, these signs have not become widely adopted for routine use in the United States.

Fetal Nasal Bone. In approximately two thirds of fetuses with Down syndrome, the nasal bone is not visible at the 11- to 14-week examination (Cicero, 2004; Rosen, 2007; Sonek, 2006). Currently, this is the only first-trimester marker, other than NT, for which the Nuchal Translucency Quality Review Program has established a training program. Criteria for adequate assessment include that the fetus occupies most of the image; that there be a 45-degree angle of insonation with the fetal profile; that the profile be well defined in the midsagittal plane, with the tip of the nose and the third and fourth ventricles visible; and that the nasal bone brightness be greater than or equal to that of the overlying skin (Nuchal Translucency Quality Review Program, 2013). An example is shown in Figure 14-5. Initial optimism for this marker was somewhat dampened when the FASTER (First- and Second-Trimester Evaluation of Risk) trial concluded that difficulty in performing the assessment would limit its usefulness for aneuploidy screening (Malone, 2004, 2005a).

PREGNANCIES AT INCREASED RISK FOR GENETIC DISORDERS

Couples with a personal or family history of a heritable genetic disorder should be offered genetic counseling. They should be given an estimated risk of having an affected infant and provided information concerning benefits and limitations of available prenatal testing options. As discussed in Chapter 13 (p. 260), the publicly funded GeneTests website contains detailed information regarding hundreds of specific genetic conditions and laboratory testing information for more than 3000 genetic disorders (http://www.ncbi.nlm.nih.gov/sites/GeneTests). Prenatal diagnosis may be available if the disease-causing mutation or mutations are known. That said, many genetic disorders are characterized by a high degree of penetrance but variable expressivity, such that prediction of phenotype—even when family members are affected—is not currently possible. Common examples include neurofibromatosis, tuberous sclerosis, and Marfan syndrome. There are also conditions for which risk may be refined by detection of associated sonographic abnormalities or by gender determination if X-linked.

Ethnicity-based carrier screening is performed for certain autosomal recessive disorders that are found with increased frequency in specific racial or ethnic groups (Table 14-9). When an otherwise rare gene is found with increased frequency within a certain population and can be traced back to a single family member or small group of ancestors, it is called the *founder effect*. This phenomenon may occur when generations of individuals procreate only within their own groups because of religious or ethnic prohibitions or geographical isolation. Carrier screening should be offered to those at increased risk for selected autosomal recessive conditions, either prior to conception or early in pregnancy.

TABLE 14-9. Autosomal Recessive Diseases Found with Increased Frequency in Certain Ethnic Groups

Disease	Heritage of Groups at Increased Risk
Sickle hemoglobinopathies	African, Mediterranean, Middle Eastern, Indian
α-Thalassemia	African, Mediterranean, Middle Eastern, West Indian, Southeast Asian
β-Thalassemia	African, Mediterranean, Middle Eastern, Indian, Southeast Asian
Cystic fibrosis	Non-Hispanic white, Ashkenazi Jewish, Native American (Zuni, Pueblo)
Inborn errors of metabolism:	Ashkenazi Jewish
Tay-Sachs disease	Tay-Sachs is also more common among groups with French-Canadian and Cajun heritage
Canavan disease	
familial dysautonomia	
Fanconi anemia group C	
Niemann-Pick disease type A	
mucolipidosis IV	
Bloom syndrome	
Gaucher disease	

Cystic Fibrosis

This disorder is caused by a mutation in the *cystic fibrosis conductance transmembrane regulator (CFTR)* gene, which is located on the long arm of chromosome 7 and encodes a chloride-channel protein. Although the most common CFTR gene mutation associated with classic cystic fibrosis (CF) is the *ΔF508* mutation, more than 1900 mutations have been identified (Cystic Fibrosis Mutation Database, 2012). Cystic fibrosis may be caused by either *homozygosity* or *compound heterozygosity* for mutations in the CFTR gene. In other words, one mutation must be present in each copy of the gene, but they need not be the same mutation. As expected, this results in a tremendous range of clinical disease severity. Median survival is approximately 37 years, but approximately 15 percent have a milder disease form and can survive for decades longer (American College of Obstetricians and Gynecologists, 2011). Care for the pregnant woman with CF is discussed in Chapter 51 (p. 1022).

The current screening panel contains 23 panethnic CF gene mutations, selected because they are present in at least 0.1 percent of patients with classic CF (American College of Obstetricians and Gynecologists, 2011). The CF carrier frequency is approximately 1 in 25 in non-Hispanic white Americans and those of Ashkenazi Jewish descent, who are from Eastern Europe. Thus, the incidence of CF in a child born to a non-Hispanic white couple is approximately $\frac{1}{4} \times \frac{1}{25} \times \frac{1}{25}$, or 1:2500. As shown in Table 14-10, both CF incidence and the sensitivity of the screening test are lower for other ethnicities.

Current recommendations for CF carrier screening from the American College of Obstetricians and Gynecologists (2011) are as follows:

- Information regarding CF carrier screening should be made available to all couples presenting for preconceptional counseling or prenatal care.
- When both partners are from a high-risk ethnicity, carrier screening should be offered before conception or early in pregnancy.
- Acknowledging that it is becoming increasingly difficult to assign individuals a single ethnicity, it is reasonable to offer CF carrier screening to patients of all ethnicities.
- For individuals with a family or personal history of CF, screening with an expanded mutation panel or even complete CFTR gene sequencing may be necessary if not already obtained.

Although a negative screening test result does not preclude the possibility of carrying a less-common mutation, it reduces the risk substantively from the background rate (see Table 14-10). If both parents are carriers, the fetus can be tested using chorionic villus sampling or amniocentesis to determine whether he or she has inherited one or both of the parental mutations. Counseling following identification of two disease-causing mutations is challenging, because phenotype prediction is reasonably accurate only for pancreatic disease, and only then for well-characterized mutations. Prognosis depends most on degree of pulmonary disease, which varies considerably even among individuals with the most common genotype associated with classic disease, that is, those homozygous for the *ΔF508* mutation. This likely reflects the effect of genetic modifiers on protein function, which may further vary depending on CFTR mutation and on exposure and susceptibility to environmental factors (Cutting, 2005; Drumm, 2005).

TABLE 14-10. Cystic Fibrosis Detection and Carrier Rates before and after Testing

Racial or Ethnic Group	Detection (%)	Carrier Risk before Test	Carrier Risk after Negative Test
Ashkenazi Jewish	94.0	1/24	1 in 384
Caucasian	88.3	1/25	1 in 206
Hispanic American	71.7	1/58	1 in 203
African American	64.5	1/61	1 in 171
Asian American	48.9	1/94	1 in 183

Modified from the American College of Medical Genetics, 2006.

Sickle Hemoglobinopathies

This group includes sickle-cell anemia, sickle-cell hemoglobin C disease, and sickle-cell β-thalassemia. Sickle-cell anemia is the most common inherited life-shortening disease of childhood onset in the United States. Normal adult hemoglobin consists of two α-chains and two β-chains. As discussed in Chapter 56 (p. 1107), hemoglobin S results from a single point mutation in the gene that encodes the β-chain. A heterozygous individual has one copy each of hemoglobin A and S, that is, *hemoglobin AS* or sickle-cell trait. A homozygous individual inherits one copy of hemoglobin S from each parent to express *hemoglobin SS* or sickle-cell anemia. Hemoglobin C is inherited in a similar manner and SC disease results from one copy each of hemoglobin S and C.

African and African American patients are at increased risk to carry hemoglobin S and other hemoglobinopathies and should be offered preconceptional or prenatal screening. One in 12 African Americans has sickle-cell trait, one in 40 carries hemoglobin C, and one in 40 carries the trait for β-thalassemia. Hemoglobin S is also more common among individuals of Mediterranean, Middle Eastern, and Asian Indian descent (Davies, 2000). The American College of Obstetricians and Gynecologists (2013a) recommends that patients of African descent be offered hemoglobin electrophoresis. If a couple is at risk to have a child with a sickle hemoglobinopathy, genetic counseling should be offered. Prenatal diagnosis can be performed with either chorionic villus sampling or amniocentesis.

Thalassemias

These syndromes are the most common single-gene disorders worldwide, and up to 200 million people carry a gene for one of these hemoglobinopathies. Some individuals with thalassemia have microcytic anemia secondary to decreased synthesis of either α- or β-hemoglobin chains. In general, *deletions* of α-globin chains cause α-thalassemia, whereas *mutations* in β-globin chains cause β-thalassemia. Less commonly, an α-globin chain mutation also causes α-thalassemia. Care for the pregnant woman with thalassemia is discussed in Chapter 56 (p. 1112).

Alpha-Thalassemia

The number of α-globin genes that are deleted may range from one to all four. If two α-globin genes are deleted, both may be deleted from the same chromosome—*cis* configuration (αα/–), or one may be deleted from each chromosome—*trans* configuration (α-/α-). Alpha-thalassemia trait is common among individuals of African, Mediterranean, Middle Eastern, West Indian, and Southeast Asian descent and results in mild anemia. The *cis* configuration is more prevalent among Southeast Asians, whereas those of African descent are more likely to inherit the *trans* configuration. The clinical significance of this difference is that when both parents carry *cis* deletions, offspring are at risk for the absence of α-hemoglobin, called Hb Barts disease, which typically leads to hydrops and fetal loss (Chap. 15, p. 315).

Detection of α-thalassemia or α-thalassemia trait is based on molecular genetic testing and is not detectable using hemoglobin electrophoresis. Because of this, routine carrier screening is not offered. If there is microcytic anemia in the absence of iron deficiency, and the hemoglobin electrophoresis is normal, then testing for α-thalassemia should be considered, particularly among individuals of Southeast Asian descent (American College of Obstetricians and Gynecologists, 2013a).

Beta-Thalassemia

Mutations in β-globin genes may cause reduced or absent production of β-globin chains. If the mutation affects one gene, it results in β-thalassemia minor. If both copies are affected, the result is either β-thalassemia major—termed Cooley anemia—or β-thalassemia intermedia. Because of reduced production of hemoglobin A among carriers, electrophoresis demonstrates elevation of hemoglobins that do not contain β-chains, including hemoglobins F and A_2.

Beta-thalassemia minor is more common among individuals of African, Mediterranean, and Southeast Asian descent. The American College of Obstetricians and Gynecologists (2013a) recommends that they be offered carrier screening with hemoglobin electrophoresis, particularly if found to have microcytic anemia in the absence of iron deficiency. Hemoglobin A_2 levels exceeding 3.5 percent confirm the diagnosis. Other ethnicities at increased risk include those of Middle Eastern, West Indian, and Hispanic descent.

Tay-Sachs Disease

This autosomal recessive lysosomal-storage disease is characterized by absence of the hexosaminidase A enzyme. This leads to a buildup of GM2 gangliosides in the central nervous system, progressive neurodegeneration, and death in early childhood. Affected individuals have almost complete absence of the enzyme, whereas carriers are asymptomatic but have less than 55-percent hexosaminidase A activity. The carrier frequency of Tay-Sachs disease in Jewish individuals of Eastern European (Ashkenazi) descent is approximately 1 in 30, but it is much lower, only about 1 in 300, in the general population. Other groups at increased risk for Tay-Sachs disease include those of French-Canadian and Cajun descent. An international Tay-Sachs carrier-screening campaign was initiated in the 1970s and met with unprecedented success in the Ashkenazi Jewish population. The incidence of Tay-Sachs disease subsequently declined more than 90 percent (Kaback, 1993). Most cases of Tay-Sachs now occur in non-Jewish individuals.

The American College of Obstetricians and Gynecologists (2010) has the following screening recommendations for Tay-Sachs disease:

- Screening should be offered before pregnancy if both members of a couple are of Ashkenazi Jewish, French-Canadian, or Cajun descent, or if there is a family history of Tay-Sachs disease.
- When only one member of the couple is of one of the above ethnicities, the high-risk partner may be screened first, and if found to be a carrier, the other partner also should be offered screening. If the couple is already pregnant, then both partners may be screened simultaneously.

- Targeted mutation analysis of the *HEXA* gene has a sensitivity of 94 percent in Ashkenazi Jewish individuals but is not recommended for screening in low-risk groups because the detection rate may be below 50 percent.
- Biochemical analysis by determining the hexosaminidase A serum level has a sensitivity of 98 percent and is the test that should be performed in individuals from low-risk ethnicities. *Leukocyte testing* must be used if the woman is already pregnant or taking oral contraceptives.
- Ambiguous or positive screening test results should be confirmed by biochemical and DNA analysis for the most common mutation. This will detect patients who carry genes associated with mild disease or pseudodeficiency states. Referral to a genetics specialist may be helpful in such cases.
- If both partners are found to be carriers of Tay-Sachs disease, genetic counseling and prenatal diagnosis should be offered. Hexosaminidase activity may be measured from chorionic villus sampling or amniocentesis specimens.

Other Recessive Diseases in Ashkenazi Jewish Individuals

The carrier rate among individuals of Eastern European (Ashkenazi) Jewish descent is approximately 1 in 30 for Tay-Sachs disease, 1 in 40 for Canavan disease, and 1 in 32 for familial dysautonomia. Fortunately, the detection rate of screening tests for each is at least 98 percent in this population. Because of their relatively high prevalence and consistently severe and predictable phenotype, the American College of Obstetricians and Gynecologists (2009a) recommends that carrier screening for these three conditions be offered to Ashkenazi Jewish individuals, either before conception or during early pregnancy. In addition, other conditions for which carrier screening should be made available include mucolipidosis IV, Niemann-Pick disease type A, Fanconi anemia group C, Bloom syndrome, and Gaucher disease. Features of these conditions are shown in Table 14-11. Gaucher disease differs from the other conditions listed in that it is has a wide range in phenotype—from childhood illness to absence of symptoms throughout life. Also, there is effective treatment available in the form of enzyme therapy (Zuckerman, 2007).

The American College of Obstetricians and Gynecologists (2009a) has the following recommendations for carrier screening:

- When only one partner is of Ashkenazi Jewish descent, that individual should be screened first, and if found to be a carrier, the other partner is offered screening. With the exception of cystic fibrosis and Tay-Sachs disease, the carrier frequency and detection rate for each of the conditions listed in Table 14-11 is unknown.
- Individuals with a positive family history of one of these disorders should be offered carrier screening for it and may benefit from genetic counseling.
- When both partners are carriers of one of these disorders, they should be referred for genetic counseling and offered prenatal diagnosis.
- When a carrier is identified, they should be encouraged to inform relatives at risk for carrying the same mutation.

PRENATAL AND PREIMPLANTATION DIAGNOSTIC TESTING

Invasive procedures used in prenatal diagnosis—amniocentesis, chorionic villus sampling, and fetal blood sampling—enable a vast array of sophisticated genetic diagnoses to be made before birth. Preimplantation genetic diagnosis permits similar diagnoses to be made in oocytes or embryos before implantation.

Improvements in aneuploidy screening tests during the past decade as described in the preceding section have resulted in a significant decrease in the number of prenatal diagnostic procedures. In a study of more than 160,000 pregnant women 35 years and older, patient acceptance of amniocentesis procedures decreased from 56 to 36 percent between 2001 and 2008, while that of chorionic villus sampling decreased from 36 to 24 percent (Nakata, 2010). Fetal blood sampling procedures have also decreased, but for different reasons. Namely, amniocentesis with fluorescence in situ hybridization (FISH) has decreased the need for rapid karyotyping from fetal blood (Chap. 13, p. 276); the number of DNA-based tests performed on amnionic fluid has greatly expanded; and fetal middle cerebral artery Doppler studies have improved the accuracy of fetal anemia detection (Chap. 10, p. 221).

Amniocentesis

Transabdominal withdrawal of amnionic fluid remains the most common procedure used to diagnose fetal aneuploidy and other genetic conditions. It is generally performed between 15 and 20 weeks' gestation but may be performed later as well. The indication is usually to assess fetal karyotype, although use of FISH and array-based comparative genomic hybridization studies have increased considerably as discussed in Chapter 13 (p. 275). Because the amniocytes must be cultured before fetal karyotype can be assessed, the time needed for karyotyping is 7 to 10 days. Outside the context of prenatal genetic analysis, amnionic fluid occasionally may be removed in large amounts therapeutically to relieve symptomatic hydramnios (Chap. 11, p. 236). The same technique described next is also used for this indication.

Technique

Amniocentesis is performed using aseptic technique, under direct sonographic guidance, using a 20- to 22-gauge spinal needle (Fig. 14-7). A standard spinal needle is approximately 9 cm long, and depending on patient habitus, a longer needle may be required. The needle is directed into a clear pocket of amnionic fluid, while avoiding the fetus and umbilical cord and ideally without traversing the placenta. Efforts are made to puncture the chorioamnion rather than to "tent" it away from the underlying uterine wall. Discomfort from the procedure is considered minor, and local anesthetic is not typically used (Mujezinovic, 2011).

The volume of fluid generally needed for commonly performed analyses is shown in Table 14-12. Because the initial 1 to 2 mL of fluid aspirate may be contaminated with maternal cells, it is generally discarded. Approximately 20 mL of fluid is

TABLE 14-11. Autosomal Recessive Genetic Diseases More Common in Individuals of Eastern European Jewish Descent

Disorder	Disease Incidence	Carrier Frequency[a]	Percent Detection Rate	Description
Tay-Sachs disease	1/3000	1/30	94—molecular testing 98—biochemical testing	Hexosaminidase A deficiency; neurological motor and mental dysfunction with childhood death; no effective treatment
Canavan disease	1/6400	1/40	98	Aspartoacylase deficiency; neurological disorder with developmental delay, hypotonia, large head, seizures, blindness, gastrointestinal reflux, and childhood death; no effective treatment
Cystic fibrosis	1/2500–3000	1/24	94	Mutations in CFTR gene; classic form associated with progressive pulmonary impairment as well as pancreatic involvement; median survival 37 years; males often have congenital absence of vas deferens and infertility
Familial dysautonomia	1/3600	1/32	99	Mutations in IKBKAP gene; neurological disorder with poor feeding, abnormal sweating, pain and temperature insensitivity, labile blood pressure, and scoliosis; no cure, but some treatments lengthen and improve quality of life
Fanconi anemia group C	1/32,000	1.89	99	Recessive mutations; severe anemia, pancytopenia, developmental delay, failure to thrive, and later-childhood death; congenital anomalies, microcephaly, and mental retardation; bone-marrow transplantation may be successful
Niemann-Pick disease type A	1/32,000	1/90	95	Sphingomyelinase deficiency; neurodegenerative disorder with childhood death; no effective treatment
Mucolipidosis IV	1/62,500	1/127	95	Neurodegenerative lysosomal storage disorder with growth failure, marked psychomotor retardation, and retinal degeneration; life expectancy may be normal; no effective treatment
Bloom syndrome	1/40,000	1/100	95–97	Increased chromosome breakage; susceptibility to infections and malignancies, growth deficiency, skin findings, and mental retardation; death usually in 20s and related to cancer; no effective treatment
Gaucher disease (Type 1)	1/900	1/15	95	β-glucosidase deficiency; affects spleen, liver, and bones; develops at any age with a wide clinical spectrum including anemia, bruising and bleeding, hepatosplenomegaly, and osteoporosis; enzyme therapy improves quality of life

[a]Non-Jewish carrier frequency and detection rates are unknown except for Tay-Sachs disease and cystic fibrosis.
CFTR = cystic fibrosis transmembrane conductance regulator; IKBKAP = inhibitor of kappa light polypeptide gene enhancer in B-cells, kinase complex-associated protein.
Data from the American College of Obstetricians and Gynecologists, 2009a, 2010; National Institute of Neurological Disorders and Stroke, 2012a–d.

then collected for fetal chromosomal analysis before removing the needle. Sonography is used to observe the uterine puncture site for bleeding, and fetal cardiac motion is documented at the end of the procedure. If the patient is Rh D-negative and unsensitized, anti-D immune globulin is administered following the procedure (Chap. 15, p. 311).

The color and clarity of the fluid are documented. Amnionic fluid should be clear and colorless or pale yellow. Blood-tinged fluid is more frequent if there is transplacental passage of the needle, however, it generally clears with continued aspiration. The placenta is attached to the anterior uterine wall in approximately half of pregnancies, and if this is the case, it will be

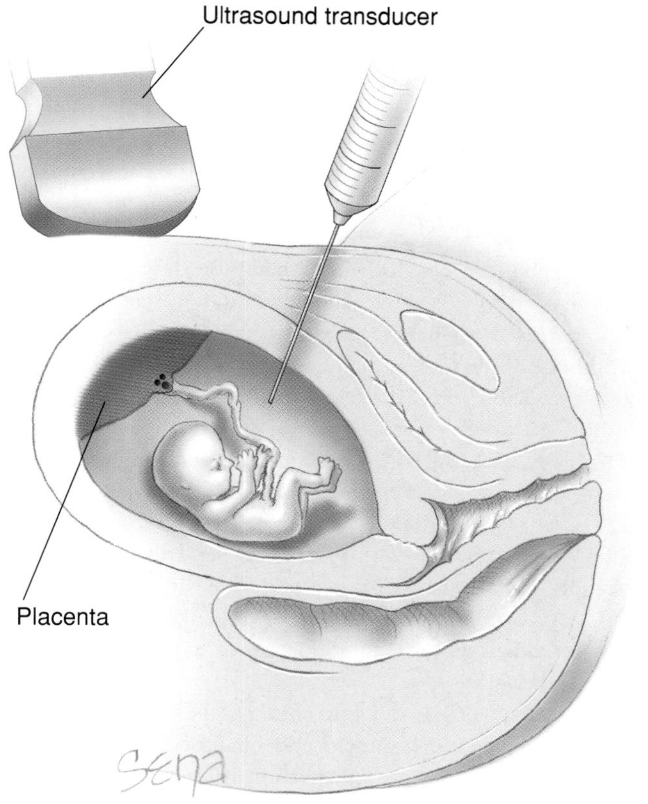

FIGURE 14-7 Amniocentesis.

traversed by the needle about 60 percent of the time (Bombard, 1995). Fortunately, this has not been associated with pregnancy loss (Marthin, 1997). Dark brown or greenish fluid may represent a past episode of intraamnionic bleeding.

Amniocentesis in Multifetal Pregnancy. For twin gestations, a small quantity of dilute indigo carmine dye is often injected before removing the needle from the first sac. This can be accomplished using 2 mL of a solution in which 1 mL of indigo carmine has been diluted in 10 mL of sterile saline. When the second sac is entered, the return of clear amnionic fluid verifies needle positioning within the second sac. Methylene blue dye is contraindicated because it has been associated with jejunal atresia and neonatal methemoglobinemia (Cowett, 1976; van der Pol, 1992). Because isolated cases of jejunal atresia have also been reported following use of indigo carmine dye, it has been suggested that sonographic visualization should be clear enough to avert the need for dye (Brandenburg, 1997).

TABLE 14-12. Selected Tests Performed on Amnionic Fluid and Typical Volume of Fluid Required

Test	Volume (mL)[a]
Fetal karyotype	20
Fluorescence in situ hybridization[b]	10
Alpha-fetoprotein	2
PCR tests for cytomegalovirus, toxoplasmosis, or parvovirus	1–2 each test
Cytomegalovirus culture	2–3
Delta OD 450 (bilirubin analysis)	2–3
Genotype studies (alloimmunization)	20
Fetal lung maturity tests	10

[a]The volume of fluid needed for each test may vary according to individual laboratory specifications.
[b]FISH: Fluorescence in situ hybridization is typically performed for chromosomes 21, 18, 13, X, and Y, or in the case of a fetal conotruncal cardiac abnormality, for the 22q.1.1 microdeletion.
PCR = polymerase chain reaction.

Complications

The procedure-related loss rate following midtrimester amniocentesis is considered to be 1 per 300 to 500 (American College of Obstetricians and Gynecologists, 2012a). The loss rate may be doubled in women with class 3 obesity–those with a body mass index (BMI) $\geq$ 40 kg/m^2 (Harper, 2012). In twin pregnancies, Cahill and coworkers (2009) reported an increased loss rate attributable to amniocentesis of 1.8 percent. Some losses are unrelated to the procedure and instead are due to abnormal placental implantation or abruption, uterine abnormalities, fetal anomalies, or infection. Wenstrom and colleagues (1990) analyzed 66 fetal deaths following nearly 12,000 second-trimester amniocenteses and found that 12 percent were caused by preexisting intrauterine infection.

Other complications of amniocentesis include amnionic fluid leakage in 1 to 2 percent and chorioamnionitis in less than 0.1 percent (American College of Obstetricians and Gynecologists, 2012a). Following leakage of amnionic fluid, which generally occurs within 48 hours of the procedure, fetal survival exceeds 90 percent (Borgida, 2000). Needle injuries to the fetus are rare. Amnionic fluid culture is successful in more than 99 percent of cases, although cells are less likely to grow if the fetus is abnormal (Persutte, 1995).

Early Amniocentesis

If performed between 11 and 14 weeks, amniocentesis is termed "early." The technique is the same as for traditional amniocentesis, although sac puncture may be more challenging due to lack of membrane fusion to the uterine wall. Also, less fluid is typically withdrawn—approximately 1 mL for each gestational week (Shulman, 1994; Sundberg, 1997).

Early amniocentesis is associated with significantly higher rates of procedure-related complications than other fetal procedures. In the Canadian Early and Mid-Trimester Amniocentesis Trial (1998) that involved more than 4000 women undergoing early amniocentesis, rates of amnionic fluid leakage, fetal loss, and talipes equinovarus (clubfoot) were all significantly higher following early amniocentesis than with traditional amniocentesis. Compared with chorionic villus sampling, early amniocentesis was similarly found to be associated with a fourfold increased rate of talipes equinovarus (Philip, 2004). Another problem with early amniocentesis is that the cell culture failure rate is higher, thus necessitating a second procedure. For all these reasons, the American College of Obstetricians and Gynecologists (2012a) recommends against the use of early amniocentesis.

Chorionic Villus Sampling (CVS)

Biopsy of chorionic villi is generally performed between 10 and 13 weeks' gestation. Although most procedures are performed to assess fetal karyotype, numerous specialized genetic tests can also be performed by chorionic villus sampling (CVS). Very few analyses specifically require either amnionic fluid or placental tissue. The primary advantage of villus biopsy is that results are available earlier in pregnancy, allowing safer pregnancy termination, if desired. A full karyotype is available in 7 to 10 days, and some laboratories provide preliminary results within 48 hours.

Technique

Chorionic villi may be obtained transcervically or transabdominally, using aseptic technique. Both approaches are considered equally safe and effective (American College of Obstetricians and Gynecologists, 2012a; Jackson, 1992). Transcervical villus sampling is performed using a specifically designed catheter made from flexible polyethylene that contains a blunt-tipped, malleable stylet. Transabdominal sampling is performed using an 18- or 20-gauge spinal needle. With either technique, transabdominal sonography is used to guide the catheter or needle into the early placenta—*chorion frondosum*, followed by aspiration of villi into a syringe containing tissue culture media (Fig. 14-8). Fetal cardiac motion is documented following the procedure.

Relative contraindications include vaginal bleeding or spotting, active genital tract infection, extreme uterine ante- or retroflexion, or body habitus precluding adequate visualization. If the patient is Rh D-negative and unsensitized, anti-D immune globulin is administered following the procedure as discussed in Chapter 15 (p. 311).

Complications

The overall loss rate following CVS is higher than that following midtrimester amniocentesis because of background spontaneous losses, that is, those that would have occurred between the first and second trimester in the absence of a fetal procedure. The procedure-related fetal loss rate is comparable to that with amniocentesis (American College of Obstetricians and Gynecologists, 2012a). Caughey and colleagues (2006) found that the overall loss rate following CVS was approximately 2 percent compared with less than 1 percent following amniocentesis. However, the adjusted procedure-related loss rate was about 1 per 400 for either procedure. The indication for CVS will also affect the loss rate. For example, fetuses with increased nuchal translucency thickness have a higher likelihood of demise. Finally, there is a "learning curve" effect associated with safe performance of CVS (Silver, 1990; Wijnberger, 2003).

An early problem with CVS was its association with *limb-reduction defects* and *oromandibular limb hypogenesis* (Burton, 1992; Firth, 1991, 1994; Hsieh, 1995). These were subsequently found to be associated with procedures performed at 7 weeks' gestation (Holmes, 1993). When performed at ≥ 10 weeks' gestation, as is commonly done today, the incidence of limb defects does not exceed the background rate of 1 per 1000 (Evans, 2005; Kuliev, 1996).

Vaginal spotting is not uncommon following transcervical sampling, but it is self-limited and not associated with pregnancy loss. The incidence of infection is less than 0.5 percent (American College of Obstetricians and Gynecologists, 2012a).

A limitation of CVS is that chromosomal mosaicism is identified in up to 2 percent of specimens. In most cases, the mosaicism reflects confined placental mosaicism rather than a true second cell line within the fetus. Amniocentesis should be offered, and if the result is normal, the mosaicism is presumed to be confined to the placenta. Confined placental mosaicism has been associated with fetal-growth impairment and stillbirth.

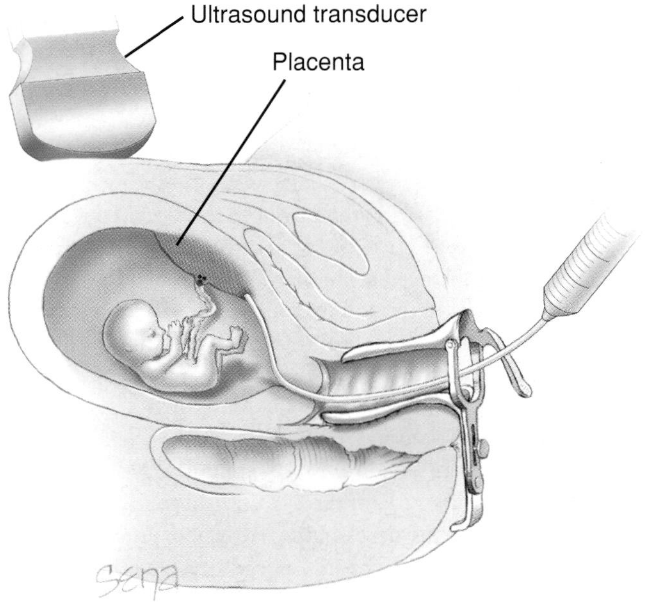

FIGURE 14-8 Transcervical chorionic villus sampling (CVS).

Fetal Blood Sampling

This procedure is also called cordocentesis or percutaneous umbilical blood sampling (PUBS). It was initially described for fetal transfusion of red blood cells in the setting of anemia from alloimmunization, as discussed in Chapter 15 (p. 310), and fetal anemia assessment remains the most common indication. Fetal blood sampling is also performed for assessment and treatment of platelet alloimmunization and for fetal karyotype determination, particularly in cases of mosaicism identified following amniocentesis or CVS. Fetal blood karyotyping can be accomplished within 24 to 48 hours. Thus, it is significantly quicker than the 7- to 10-day turnaround time with amniocentesis or CVS. Although fetal blood *can* be analyzed for virtually any test performed on neonatal blood, improvements in tests available with amniocentesis and CVS have eliminated the need for fetal venipuncture in most cases (Society for Maternal-Fetal Medicine, 2013).

Technique

Under direct sonographic guidance, using aseptic technique, the operator introduces a 22- or 23-gauge spinal needle into the umbilical vein, and blood is slowly withdrawn into a heparinized syringe. Adequate visualization of the needle is essential. As with

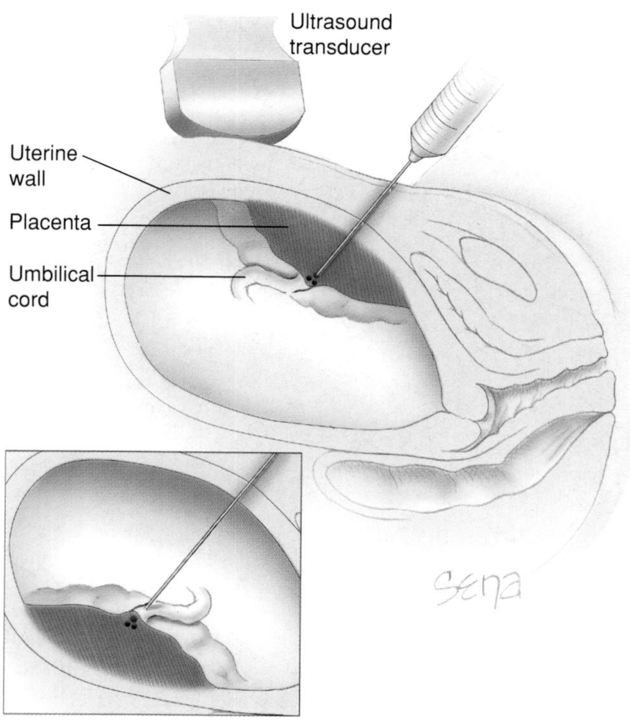

FIGURE 14-9 Fetal blood sampling. Access to the umbilical vein varies depending on placental location and cord position. With an anterior placenta, the needle may traverse the placenta. **Inset:** With posterior placentation, the needle passes through amnionic fluid before penetrating the umbilical vein. Alternatively, a free loop of cord may be accessed.

amniocentesis, a longer needle may be required depending on patient habitus. Fetal blood sampling is often performed near the placental cord insertion site, where it may be easier to enter the cord if the placenta is anterior (Fig. 14-9). Alternatively, a free loop of cord may be punctured. Because fetal blood sampling requires more time than other fetal procedures, a local anesthetic may be administered. Prophylactic antibiotics are used at some centers, although there are no trials to support this policy. Arterial puncture is avoided, because it may result in vasospasm and fetal bradycardia. After the needle is removed, fetal cardiac motion is documented, and the site is observed for bleeding.

Complications

The procedure-related fetal loss rate following fetal blood sampling is approximately 1.4 percent (Ghidini, 1993; Maxwell, 1991; Tongsong 2001). The actual loss rate varies according to the procedure indication and the fetal status. Other complications may include cord vessel bleeding in 20 to 30 percent of cases, fetal-maternal bleeding in approximately 40 percent of cases in which the placenta is traversed, and fetal bradycardia in 5 to 10 percent (Boupaijit, 2012; Ghidini, 1993; Society for Maternal-Fetal Medicine, 2013). Most complications are transitory, with complete recovery, but some result in fetal loss.

In a series of more than 2000 procedures comparing fetal blood sampling near the placental cord insertion site with puncture of a free loop, there were no differences in rates of procedure success, pregnancy loss, visible bleeding from the cord, or fetal bradycardia. Time to complete the procedure was significantly shorter if the cord was sampled at the placental insertion site rather than at a free loop—5 versus 7 minutes. However, sampling at the insertion site had a higher rate of maternal blood contamination (Tangshewinsirikul, 2011).

Preimplantation Genetic Testing

For couples undergoing in vitro fertilization (IVF), genetic testing performed on oocytes or embryos before implantation may provide valuable information regarding the chromosomal complement and single-gene disorders. There are two separate categories of testing—*preimplantation genetic diagnosis* and *preimplantation genetic screening*—each with different indications. Comprehensive genetic counseling is required before consideration of these procedures. There are three techniques that are used for both categories of preimplantation genetic testing:

1. *Polar body analysis* is a technique used to infer whether a developing oocyte is affected by a maternally inherited genetic disorder. The first and second polar bodies are normally extruded from the developing oocyte following meiosis I and II, and their sampling should not affect fetal development (Fig. 5-8, p. 89). In one recent series, this technique was used to diagnose 146 mendelian disorders, with reported accuracy exceeding 99 percent. The main disadvantages of polar body analysis are that the paternal genetic contribution is not evaluated and that an additional procedure may be required in complex cases (Kuliev, 2011).
2. *Blastomere biopsy* is done at the 6- to 8-cell (cleavage) stage when an embryo is 3 days old, and it is the technique most commonly used for preimplantation testing. One cell is typically removed through a hole made in the zona pellucida, as shown in Figure 14-10. The technique is associated with a 10-percent reduction in the pregnancy rate (Mastenbroek, 2007, 2011; Simpson, 2012). As discussed subsequently, a particular limitation of using this technique for aneuploidy assessment is that mosaicism of the blastomeres may not reflect the chromosomal complement of the developing embryo (American Society for Reproductive Medicine, 2008).
3. *Trophectoderm biopsy* involves removal of 5 to 7 cells from a 5- to 6-day blastocyst (Fig. 14-11). An advantage is that because the trophectoderm cells give rise to the trophoblast—the placenta—no cells are removed from the developing embryo. Disadvantageously, because the procedure is performed later in development, if genetic analysis cannot be performed rapidly, then cryopreservation and embryo transfer during a later IVF cycle may be required.

Preimplantation Genetic Diagnosis (PGD)

A genetic abnormality—rather than infertility—may be the reason why a couple has elected IVF. When either or both members of a couple are known carriers of a specific genetic disease or a balanced chromosomal rearrangement, preimplantation genetic diagnosis (PGD) may be performed to determine if an oocyte or embryo has the defect (American Society for Reproductive Medicine, 2008). Only embryos without the abnormality would be implanted.

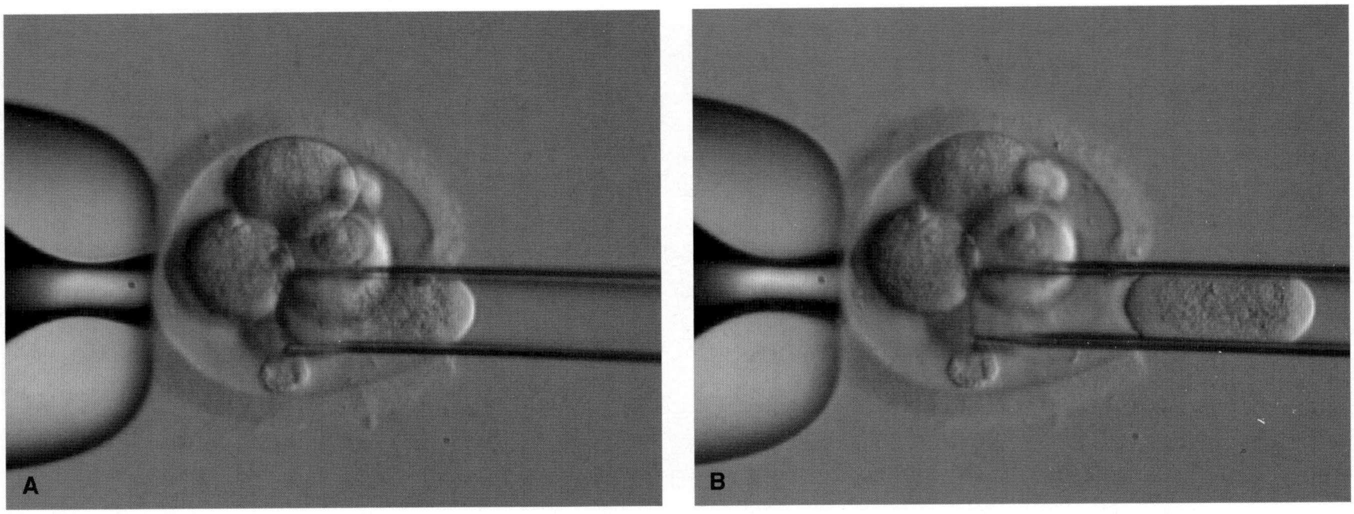

FIGURE 14-10 Blastomere biopsy. **A.** A blastomere is selected. **B.** This cell is then drawn into the pipette. (From Doody, 2012, with permission.)

This procedure has a vast number of applications. It is used to diagnose single-gene disorders such as cystic fibrosis, β-thalassemia, and hemophilia; to determine gender in X-linked diseases; to identify mutations such as BRCA-1 that do not cause disease but confer significantly increased risk; and to match human leukocyte antigens for umbilical cord stem cell transplantation for a sibling (de Wert, 2007; Flake, 2003; Fragouli, 2007; Grewal, 2004; Jiao, 2003; Rund, 2005; Xu, 2004).

To determine whether the known carrier has transmitted a specific genetic mutation, polymerase chain reaction (PCR) is used to amplify the genome region containing the segment of interest (Chap. 13, p. 277). If PGD is performed to identify a translocation or other structural chromosomal rearrangement carried by either parent, FISH is typically used. Because typically only one or two cells are available for analysis and because a rapid completion time is essential, this procedure is technically challenging. Risks include failure to amplify the genetic region of interest, selection of a cell that does not contain a nucleus, and maternal cell contamination. Infrequently, affected embryos thought to be normal are implanted, and unaffected embryos are misdiagnosed as abnormal and discarded. Because of this, the American Society for Reproductive Medicine (2008) encourages further prenatal diagnostic testing—either CVS or amniocentesis—to confirm PGD results.

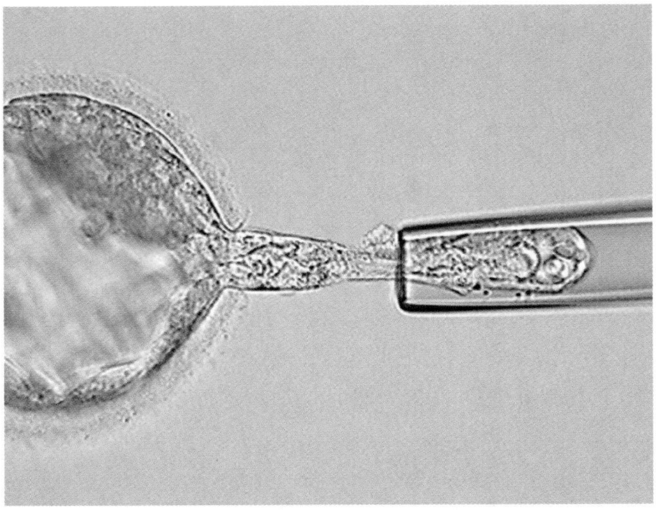

FIGURE 14-11 Photomicrograph of trophectoderm biopsy used in preimplantation genetic testing. The trophectoderm is distinct from the embryonic inner cell mass and gives rise to trophoblastic cells, which initiate placental development. (From Doody, 2012, with permission.)

Preimplantation Genetic Screening (PGS)

This term is used for aneuploidy screening that is performed on oocytes or embryos before IVF transfer. Such screening is used with couples who are not known to have or carry a genetic abnormality. Although preimplantation screening has obvious theoretical advantages, it has faced significant challenges in practice.

Most commonly, FISH is used to identify the copy number of selected chromosomes, and it is performed on a single blastomere (American Society for Reproductive Medicine, 2008). Because the number of chromosome pairs per cell nucleus that can be evaluated with FISH is limited, efforts have also focused on the use of chromosomal microarray analysis (Chap. 13, p. 277). Mosaicism is common in cleavage-stage embryo blastomeres, and it may not be clinically significant because it often does not reflect the actual embryonic chromosomal complement (American College of Obstetricians and Gynecologists, 2009b). In addition, among women 35 years or older, pregnancy rates following preimplantation screening are significantly lower than those observed following IVF without it (Mastenbroek, 2007, 2011). For these reasons, the American College of Obstetricians and Gynecologists (2009b) recommends against use of preimplantation screening with FISH for advanced maternal age screening. It also recommends against it for women with recurrent pregnancy loss or recurrent implantation failure outside the setting of a research trial.

REFERENCES

Adzick NS, Thom EA, Spong CY, et al: A randomized trial of prenatal versus postnatal repair of myelomeningocele. N Engl J Med 364(11):993, 2011

Alldred SK, Deeks JJ, Guo B, et al: Second trimester serum tests for Down's syndrome screening. Cochrane Database Syst Rev 6:CD009925, 2012

American College of Medical Genetics: Technical Standards and Guidelines for CFTR Mutation Testing, 2006. Available at: https://www.acmg.net/Pages/ACMG_Activities/stds-2002/cf.htm. Accessed March 3, 2014

American College of Obstetricians and Gynecologists: Preconception and prenatal carrier screening for genetic diseases in individuals of Eastern European Jewish descent. Committee Opinion No. 442, October 2009a

American College of Obstetricians and Gynecologists: Preimplantation genetic screening for aneuploidy. Committee Opinion No. 430, March 2009b

American College of Obstetricians and Gynecologists: Screening for Tay-Sachs disease. Committee Opinion No. 318, October 2005, Reaffirmed 2010

American College of Obstetricians and Gynecologists: Update on carrier screening for cystic fibrosis. Committee Opinion No. 486, April 2011

American College of Obstetricians and Gynecologists: Invasive prenatal testing for aneuploidy. Practice Bulletin No. 88, December 2007, Reaffirmed 2012a

American College of Obstetricians and Gynecologists: Noninvasive prenatal testing for fetal aneuploidy. Committee Opinion No. 545, December 2012b

American College of Obstetricians and Gynecologists: Hemoglobinopathies in pregnancy. Practice Bulletin No. 78, January 2007, Reaffirmed 2013a

American College of Obstetricians and Gynecologists: Neural tube defects. Practice Bulletin No. 44, July 2003, Reaffirmed 2013b

American College of Obstetricians and Gynecologists: Screening for fetal chromosomal abnormalities. Practice Bulletin No. 77, January 2007, Reaffirmed 2013c

American College of Obstetricians and Gynecologists: Genetics and molecular diagnostic testing. Technology Assessment No. 11, February 2014

American Society for Reproductive Medicine: Preimplantation genetic testing: a Practice Committee Opinion. Fertil Steril 90: S136, 2008

Aneji CN, Northrup H, Au KS: Deep sequencing study of the MTHFR gene to identify variants associated with myelomeningocele. Birth Defects Res A Clin Mol Teratol 94(2):84, 2012

Atzei A, Gajewska K, Huggon IC, et al: Relationship between nuchal translucency thickness and prevalence of major cardiac defects in fetuses with normal karyotype. Ultrasound Obstet Gynecol 26(2):154, 2005

Benacerraf BR, Barss VA, Laboda LA: A sonographic sign for the detection in the second trimester of the fetus with Down syndrome. Am J Obstet Gynecol 151(8):1078, 1985

Benacerraf BR, Gelman R, Frigoletto FD: Sonographic identification of second-trimester fetuses with Down's syndrome. N Engl J Med 317(22):1371, 1987

Benn PA, Leo MV, Rodis JF, et al: Maternal serum screening for fetal trisomy 18: a comparison of fixed cutoff and patient-specific risk protocols. Obstet Gynecol 93 (5 Pt 1):707, 1999

Best KE, Tennant PW, Addor MC, et al: Epidemiology of small intestinal atresia in Europe: a register-based study. Arch Dis Child Fetal Neonatal Ed 97(5):F353, 2012

Bianchi DW, Platt LD, Goldberg JD, et al: Genome-wide fetal aneuploidy detection by maternal plasma DNA sequencing. Obstet Gynecol 119(5):890, 2012

Bombard AT, Powers JF, Carter S, et al: Procedure-related fetal losses in transplacental versus nontransplacental genetic amniocentesis. Am J Obstet Gynecol 172(3):868, 1995

Borenstein M, Persico N, Kagan KO: Frontomaxillary facial angle in screening for trisomy 21 at 11+0 to 13+6 weeks. Ultrasound Obstet Gynecol 32(1):5, 2008

Borgida AF, Mills AA, Feldman DM, et al: Outcome of pregnancies complicated by ruptured membranes after genetic amniocentesis. Am J Obstet Gynecol 183(4):937, 2000

Boupaijit K, Wanapirak C, Piyamongkol W, et al: Effect of placental penetration during cordocentesis at mid-pregnancy on fetal outcomes. Prenat Diagn 32(1):83, 2012

Brandenburg H: The use of synthetic dyes for identification of the amniotic sacs in multiple pregnancies. Prenat Diagn 17(3):281, 1997

Brock DJ, Bolton AE, Monaghan JM: Prenatal diagnosis of anencephaly through maternal serum-alpha-fetoprotein measurement. Lancet 2(7835): 923, 1973

Brock DJ, Sutcliffe RG: Alpha-fetoprotein in the antenatal diagnosis of anencephaly and spina bifida. Lancet 2(7770):197, 1972

Bromley B, Lieberman E, Shipp TD, et al: The genetic sonogram, a method for risk assessment for Down syndrome in the mid trimester. J Ultrasound Med 21(10):1087, 2002

Burton BK, Schulz CJ, Burd LI: Limb anomalies associated with chorionic villus sampling. Obstet Gynecol 79 (5 Pt 1):726, 1992

Bush MC, Malone FD: Down syndrome screening in twins. Clin Perinatol 32(2):373, 2005

Cahill AG, Macones GA, Stamilio DM, et al: Pregnancy loss rate after mid-trimester amniocentesis in twin pregnancies. Am J Obstet Gynecol 200(3):257.e1, 2009

Canadian Early and Mid-Trimester Amniocentesis Trial (CEMAT) Group: Randomised trial to assess safety and fetal outcome of early and midtrimester amniocentesis. Lancet 351(9098):242, 1998

Canfield MA, Honein MA, Yuskiv N, et al: National estimates and race/ethnic-specific variation of selected birth defects in the United States, 1999–2001. Birth Defects Res A Clin Mol Teratol 76(11):747, 2006

Caughey AB, Hopkins LM, Norton ME. Chorionic villus sampling compared with amniocentesis and the difference in the rate of pregnancy loss. Obstet Gynecol 108(3):612, 2006

Cicero S, Curcio P, Papageorghiou A, et al: Absence of nasal bone in fetuses with trisomy 21 at 11–14 weeks of gestation: an observational study. Lancet 358(9294):1665, 2001

Cicero S, Rembouskos G, Vandecruys H, et al: Likelihood ratio for trisomy 21 in fetuses with absent nasal bone at the 11–14-week scan. Ultrasound Obstet Gynecol 23(3):218, 2004

Colvin J, Bower C, Dickinson JE, et al: Outcomes of congenital diaphragmatic hernia: a population-based study in Western Australia. Pediatrics 116(3):e356, 2005

Comstock CH, Malone FD, Robert H, et al: Is there a nuchal translucency millimeter measurement above which there is no added benefit from first trimester screening? Am J Obstet Gynecol 195(3):843, 2006

Cowett MR, Hakanson DO, Kocon RW, et al: Untoward neonatal effect of intraamniotic administration of methylene blue. Obstet Gynecol 48(1 Suppl): 74S, 1976

Cragan JD, Gilboa SM: Including prenatal diagnoses in birth defects monitoring: experience of the Metropolitan Atlanta Congenital Defects Program. Birth Defects Res A Clin Mol Teratol 85(1):20, 2009

Cuckle H: Biochemical screening for Down syndrome. Eur J Obstet Gynecol Reprod Biol 92(1):97, 2000

Cuckle H, Benn P, Wright D: Down syndrome screening in the first and/or second trimester: model predicted performance using meta-analysis parameters. Semin Perinatol 29(4):252, 2005

Cuckle H, Wald N, Stevenson JD, et al: Maternal serum alpha-fetoprotein screening for open neural tube defects in twin pregnancies. Prenat Diagn 10(2):71, 1990

Cutting GR: Modifier genetics: cystic fibrosis. Annu Rev Genomics Hum Genet 6:237, 2005

Cystic Fibrosis Mutation Database: CFMDB statistics. 2012 Available at: http://www.genet.sickkids.on.ca/StatisticsPage.html. Accessed February 25, 2013

Dashe JS, Twickler DM, Santos-Ramos R, et al: Alpha-fetoprotein detection of neural tube defects and the impact of standard ultrasound. Am J Obstet Gynecol 195(6):1623, 2006

Davies SC, Cronin E, Gill M, et al: Screening for sickle cell disease and thalassemia: a systematic review with supplementary research. Heath Technol Assess 4(3):1, 2000

de Wert G, Liebaers I, Van De Velde H: The future (r)evolution of preimplantation genetic diagnosis/human leukocyte antigen testing: ethical reflections. Stem Cells 25(9):2167, 2007

Dolk H, Loane M, Garne E: The prevalence of congenital anomalies in Europe. Adv Exp Med Biol 686:349, 2010

Doody KJ: Treatment of the infertile couple. In Hoffman BL, Schorge JO, Schaffer JI, et al (eds): Williams Gynecology, 2nd ed. New York, McGraw-Hill, 2012

Drumm ML, Konstan MW, Schluchter MD, et al: Genetic modifiers of lung disease in cystic fibrosis. N Engl J Med 353(14):1443, 2005

Dugoff L, Hobbins JC, Malone FD, et al: First-trimester maternal serum PAPP-A and free-beta subunit human chorionic gonadotropic concentrations and nuchal translucency are associated with obstetric complications: a population-based screening study (The FASTER Trial). Am J Obstet Gynecol 191(6):1446, 2004

Dugoff L, Hobbins JC, Malone FD, et al: Quad screen as a predictor of adverse pregnancy outcome. Obstet Gynecol 106(2):260, 2005

Dugoff L, Society for Maternal-Fetal Medicine: First- and second-trimester maternal serum markers for aneuploidy and adverse pregnancy outcomes. Obstet Gynecol 115(5):1052, 2010

Ecker JL, Shipp TD, Bromley B, et al: The sonographic diagnosis of Dandy-Walker and Dandy-Walker variant: associated findings and outcomes. Prenat Diagn 20(3):328, 2000

Evans MI, Harrison HH, O'Brien JE, et al: Correction for insulin-dependent diabetes in maternal serum alpha-fetoprotein testing has outlived its usefulness. Am J Obstet Gynecol 187(4):1084, 2002

SECTION 5

Evans MI, Wapner RJ: Invasive prenatal diagnostic procedures. Semin Perinatol 29(4):215, 2005

Faiola S, Tsoi E, Huggon C, et al: Likelihood ratio for trisomy 21 in fetuses with tricuspid regurgitation at the 11 to 13+6-week scan. Ultrasound Obstet Gynecol 26(1):22, 2005

Firth HV, Boyd PA, Chamberlain PF, et al: Analysis of limb reduction defects in babies exposed to chorionic villus sampling. Lancet 343(8905):1069, 1994

Firth HV, Boyd PA, Chamberlain P, et al: Severe limb abnormalities after chorion villus sampling at 56–66 days' gestation. Lancet 337(8744):762, 1991

Flake AW: Stem cell and genetic therapies for the fetus. Semin Pediatr Surg 12(3):202, 2003

Fragouli E: Preimplantation genetic diagnosis: present and future. J Assist Reprod Genet 24(6):201, 2007

Gallot D, Boda C, Ughetto S, et al: Prenatal detection and outcome of congenital diaphragmatic hernia: a French registry-based study. Ultrasound Obstet Gynecol 29(3):276, 2007

Ghidini A, Sepulveda W, Lockwood CJ, et al: Complications of fetal blood sampling. Am J Obstet Gynecol 168(5):1339, 1993

Goetzl L, Krantz D, Simpson JL, et al: Pregnancy-associated plasma protein A, free beta-hCG, nuchal translucency, and risk of pregnancy loss. Obstet Gynecol 104(1):30, 2004

Greene MF, Haddow JE, Palomaki GE, et al: Maternal serum alpha-fetoprotein levels in diabetic pregnancies. Lancet 2(8606):345, 1988

Grewal SS, Kahn JP, MacMillan ML, et al: Successful hematopoietic stem cell transplantation for Fanconi anemia from an unaffected HLA-genotype-identical sibling selected using preimplantation genetic diagnosis. Blood 103(3):1147, 2004

Harisha PN, Devi BI, Christopher R, et al: Impact of 5,10-methylenetetrohydrofolate reductase gene polymorphism on neural tube defects. J Neurosurg Pediatr 6(4):364, 2010

Harper LM, Cahill AG, Smith K, et al: Effect of maternal obesity on the risk of fetal loss after amniocentesis and chorionic villus sampling. Obstet Gynecol 119(4):745, 2012

Holmes LB: Report of National Institute of Child Health and Human Development Workshop on Chorionic Villus Sampling and Limb and Other Defects, October 20, 1992. Teratology 48(4):7, 1993

Honein MA, Paulozzi LJ, Mathews TJ, et al: Impact of folic acid fortification of the US food supply on the occurrence of neural tube defects. JAMA 285(23):2981, 2001

Hook EB, Cross PK, Schreinemachers DM: Chromosomal abnormality rates at amniocentesis and in live-born infants. JAMA 249(15):2034, 1983

Hsieh FJ, Shyu MK, Sheu BC, et al: Limb defects after chorionic villus sampling. Obstet Gynecol 85(1):84, 1995

Huggon IC, DeFigueiredo DB, Allan LD: Tricuspid regurgitation in the diagnosis of chromosomal anomalies in the fetus at 11–14 weeks of gestation. Heart 89(9):1071, 2003

Huttly W, Rudnicka A, Wald NJ: Second-trimester prenatal screening markers for Down syndrome in women with insulin-dependent diabetes mellitus. Prenat Diagn 24(10):804, 2004

Jackson LG, Zachary JM, Fowler SE, et al: A randomized comparison of transcervical and transabdominal chorionic-villus sampling. The U.S. National Institute of Child Health and Human Development Chorionic-Villus Sampling and Amniocentesis Study Group. N Engl J Med 327(9):636, 1992

Jiao Z, Zhou C, Li J, et al: Birth of healthy children after preimplantation diagnosis of beta-thalassemia by whole-genome amplification. Prenat Diagn 23(8):646, 2003

Kaback M, Lim-Steele J, Dabholkar D, et al: Tay Sachs disease: carrier screening, prenatal diagnosis, and the molecular era. JAMA 270:2307, 1993

Knight GK, Palomaki GE: Maternal serum alpha-fetoprotein and the detection of open neural tube defects. In Elias S, Simpson JL (eds): Maternal Serum Screening. New York, Churchill Livingstone, 1992, p 41

Kochanek KD, Jiaquan XU, Murphy SL, et al: Deaths: final data for 2009. Natl Vital Stat Rep Vol 60, 2011

Kuliev A, Jackson L, Froster U, et al: Chorionic villus sampling safety. Report of World Health Organization/EURO meeting in association with the Seventh International Conference on Early Prenatal Diagnosis of Genetic Diseases, Tel Aviv, Israel, May 21, 1994. Am J Obstet Gynecol 174(3):807, 1996

Kuliev A, Rechitsky S: Polar body-based preimplantation genetic diagnosis for Mendelian disorders. Mol Hum Reprod 17:275, 2011

Langlois S, Armstrong L, Gall K, et al: Steroid sulfatase deficiency and contiguous gene deletion syndrome amongst pregnant patients with low serum unconjugated estriols. Prenat Diagn 29(10):966, 2009

Lewis D, Tolosa JE, Kaufmann M, et al: Elective cesarean delivery and long-term motor function or ambulation status in infants with meningomyelocele. Obstet Gynecol 103(3):469, 2004

Li Z, Weng H, Xu C, et al: Oxidative stress-induced JNK1/2 activation triggers proapoptotic signaling and apoptosis that leads to diabetic embryopathy. Diabetes 61(8):2084, 2012

Long A, Moran P, Robson S: Outcome of fetal cerebral posterior fossa anomalies. Prenat Diagn 26(8):707, 2006

Luthy DA, Wardinsky T, Shurtleff DB, et al: Cesarean section before the onset of labor and subsequent motor function in infants with meningomyelocele diagnosed antenatally. N Engl J Med 324(10):662, 1991

Malone FD, Ball RH, Nyberg DA: First-trimester nasal bone evaluation for aneuploidy in the general population. Obstet Gynecol 104(6):1222, 2004

Malone FD, Ball RH, Nyberg DA, et al: First-trimester nasal bone evaluation for aneuploidy in the general population: reply. Obstet Gynecol 105(4):901, 2005a

Malone FD, Canick JA, Ball RH, et al: First-trimester or second-trimester screening, or both, for Down's syndrome. N Engl J Med 353(19):2001, 2005b

Marthin T, Liedgren S, Hammar M: Transplacental needle passage and other risk-factors associated with second trimester amniocentesis. Acta Obstet Gynecol Scand 76(8):728, 1997

Mastenbroek S, Twisk M, van der Veen F, et al: Preimplantation genetic screening: a systematic review and meta-analysis of RCTs. Hum Reprod Update 17(4):454, 2011

Mastenbroek S, Twisk M, van Echten-Arends J, et al: In vitro fertilization with preimplantation genetic screening. N Engl J Med 357(1):9, 2007

Matias A, Gomes C, Flack N: Screening for chromosomal abnormalities at 10–14 weeks: the role of ductus venous blood flow. Ultrasound Obstet Gynecol 12(6):380, 1998

Maxwell DJ, Johnson P, Hurley P, et al: Fetal blood sampling and pregnancy loss in relation to indication. Br J Obstet Gynaecol 98(9):892, 1991

Merkatz IR, Nitowsky HM, Macri JN, et al: An association between low maternal serum α-fetoprotein and fetal chromosomal abnormalities. Am J Obstet Gynecol 148(7):886, 1984

Merrill DC, Goodwin P, Burson JM, et al: The optimal route of delivery for fetal meningomyelocele. Am J Obstet Gynecol 179(1):235, 1998

Meyers C, Adam R, Dungan J, et al: Aneuploidy in twin gestations: when is maternal age advanced? Obstet Gynecol 89(2):248, 1997

Milunsky A, Canick JA: Maternal serum screening for neural tube and other defects. In Milunsky A (ed): Genetic Disorders and the Fetus. Diagnosis, Prevention, and Treatment, 5th ed. Baltimore, The Johns Hopkins University Press, 2004, p 719

Morrow RJ, McNay MB, Whittle MJ: Ultrasound detection of neural tube defects in patients with elevated maternal serum alpha-fetoprotein. Obstet Gynecol 78(6):1055, 1991

Mujezinovic F, Alfirevic Z: Analgesia for amniocentesis or chorionic villus sampling. Cochrane Database Syst Rev 11:CD008580, 2011

Munoz JB, Lacasana M, Cavazos RG, et al: Methylenetetrahydrofolate reductase gene polymorphisms and risk of anencephaly in Mexico. Mol Hum Reprod 13(6):419, 2007

Nakata N, Wang Y, Bhatt S: Trends in prenatal screening and diagnostic testing among women referred for advanced maternal age. Prenat Diagn 30(3):198, 2010

National Institute of Neurological Disorders and Stroke: NINDS Canavan disease information page. Available at: http://www.ninds.nih.gov/disorders/canavan/canavan.htm. Accessed December 20, 2012a

National Institute of Neurological Disorders and Stroke: NINDS Gaucher disease information page. , 2012b

National Institute of Neurological Disorders and Stroke: NINDS Niemann-Pick disease information page. http://www.ninds.nih.gov/disorders/niemann/niemann.htm. Accessed December 20, 2012c

National Institute of Neurological Disorders and Stroke: NINDS Tay-Sachs disease information page. Available at: http://www.ninds.nih.gov/disorders/taysachs/taysachs.htm. Accessed December 20, 2012d

Nguyen HT, Herndon CDA, Cooper C, et al: The Society for Fetal Urology consensus statement on the evaluation and management of antenatal hydronephrosis. J Pediatr Urol 6(3):212, 2010

Nicolaides KH: Nuchal translucency and other first-trimester sonographic markers of chromosomal abnormalities. Am J Obstet Gynecol 191(1):45, 2004

Nicolaides KH, Campbell S, Gabbe SG, et al: Ultrasound screening for spina bifida: cranial and cerebellar signs. Lancet 12(8498):72, 1986

Norem CT, Schoen EJ, Walton DL, et al: Routine ultrasonography compared with maternal serum alpha-fetoprotein for neural tube defect screening. Obstet Gynecol 106(4):747, 2005

Nuchal Translucency Quality Review Program: Nasal bone education. 2013. Available at: https://www.ntqr.org/SM/wfNasalBoneInfo.aspx. Accessed February 3, 2013

Nyberg DA, Souter VL: Use of genetic sonography for adjusting the risk for fetal Down syndrome. Semin Perinatol 27(2):130, 2003

Nyberg DA, Souter VL, El-Bastawissi A, et al: Isolated sonographic markers for detection of fetal Down syndrome in the second trimester of pregnancy. J Ultrasound Med 20(10):1053, 2001

Orioli IM, Catilla EE: Epidemiology of holoprosencephaly: prevalence and risk factors. Am J Med Genet Part C Semin Med Genet 154C:13 2010

Palomaki GE, Kloza EM, Lambert-Messerlian GM, et al: DNA sequencing of maternal plasma to detect Down syndrome: an international clinical validation study. Genet Med 13(11):913, 2011

Palomaki GE, Deciu C, Kloza EM, et al: DNA sequencing of maternal plasma reliably identifies trisomy 18 and trisomy 13 as well as Down syndrome: an international collaborative study. Genet Med 14(3):296, 2012

Pedersen RN, Calzolari E, Husby S, et al: Oesophageal atresia: prevalence, prenatal diagnosis, and associated anomalies in 23 European regions. Arch Dis Child 97(3):227, 2012

Persutte WH, Lenke RR: Failure of amniotic-fluid-cell growth: is it related to fetal aneuploidy? Lancet 345(8942):96, 1995

Philip J, Silver RK, Wilson RD, et al: Late first-trimester invasive prenatal diagnosis: results of an international randomized trial. Obstet Gynecol 103(6):1164, 2004

Reichler A, Hume RF Jr, Drugan A, et al: Risk of anomalies as a function of level of elevated maternal serum α-fetoprotein. Am J Obstet Gynecol 171(4):1052, 1994

Rosen T, D'Alton ME, Platt LD, et al: First-trimester ultrasound assessment of the nasal bone to screen for aneuploidy. Obstet Gynecol 110(2 Pt 1):339, 2007

Rund D, Rachmilewitz E: β-Thalassemia. N Engl J Med 353(11):1135, 2005

Sancken U, Bartels I: Biochemical screening for chromosomal disorders and neural tube defects (NTD): is adjustment of maternal alpha-fetoprotein (AFP) still appropriate in insulin-dependent diabetes mellitus (IDDM)? Prenat Diagn 21(5):383, 2001

Sepulveda W, Donaldson A, Johnson RD, et al: Are routine alpha-fetoprotein and acetylcholinesterase determinations still necessary at second-trimester amniocentesis? Impact of high-resolution ultrasonography. Obstet Gynecol 85:105, 1995

Sharma R, Stone S, Alzouebi A, et al: Perinatal outcome of prenatally diagnosed congenital talipes equinovarus. Prenat Diagn 31(2):142, 2011

Shipp TD, Bromley B, Lieberman E, et al: The frequency of the detection of fetal echogenic intracardiac foci with respect to maternal race. Ultrasound Obstet Gynecol 15(6):460, 2000

Shulman LP, Elias S, Phillips OP, et al: Amniocentesis performed at 14 weeks' gestation or earlier: Comparison with first-trimester transabdominal chorionic villus sampling. Obstet Gynecol 83(4):543, 1994

Silver RK, MacGregor SN, Sholl JS, et al: An evaluation of the chorionic villus sampling learning curve. Am J Obstet Gynecol 163(3):917, 1990

Simpson JL: Preimplantation genetic diagnosis to improve pregnancy outcomes in subfertility. Best Pract Res Clin Obstet Gynaecol 26(6):805, 2012

Simpson LL, Malone FD, Bianchi DW, et al: Nuchal translucency and the risk of congenital heart disease. Obstet Gynecol 109(2 Pt 1):376, 2007

Smith-Bindman R, Hosmer W, Feldstein VA, et al: Second-trimester ultrasound to detect fetuses with Down syndrome. A meta-analysis. JAMA 285(8):1044, 2001

Snijders RJ, Noble P, Sebire N, et al: UK multicentre project on assessment of risk of trisomy 21 by maternal age and fetal nuchal-translucency thickness at 10–14 weeks of gestation. Fetal Medicine Foundation First Trimester Screening Group. Lancet 352(9125):337, 1998

Society for Maternal-Fetal Medicine (SMFM), Berry SM, Stone J, et al: Fetal blood sampling. Am J Obstet Gynecol 209(3):170, 2013

Solomon BD, Rosenbaum KN, Meck JM, et al: Holoprosencephaly due to numeric chromosome abnormalities. Am J Med Genet C Semin Med Genet 154C:146, 2010

Sonek J, Borenstein M, Daklis T: Frontomaxillary facial angle in fetuses with trisomy 21 at 11–13(6) weeks. Am J Obstet Gynecol 196(3):271.e1, 2007

Sonek JD, Cicero S, Neiger R, et al: Nasal bone assessment in prenatal screening for trisomy 21. Am J Obstet Gynecol 195(5):1219, 2006

Sparks AB, Wang ET, Struble CA, et al: Selective analysis of cell-free DNA in maternal blood for evaluation of fetal trisomy. Prenat Diagn 32(1):3, 2012

Spencer K, Ong C, Skentou H, et al: Screening for trisomy 13 by fetal nuchal translucency and maternal serum free beta hCG and PAPP-A at 10–14 weeks of gestation. Prenat Diagn 20:411, 2000

Spencer K, Souter V, Tul N, et al: A screening program for trisomy 21 at 10–14 weeks using fetal nuchal translucency, maternal serum free beta-human chorionic gonadotropin and pregnancy-associated plasma protein-A. Ultrasound Obstet Gynecol 13(4):231, 1999

Spencer K, Wallace EM, Ritoe S: Second-trimester dimeric inhibin-A in Down's syndrome screening. Prenat Diagn 15(12):1101, 1996

Sugimura Y, Murase T, Oyama K, et al: Prevention of neural tube defects by loss of function of inducible nitric oxide synthase in fetuses of a mouse model of streptozocin-induced diabetes. Diabetologia 52(5):962, 2009

Sundberg K, Bang J, Smidt-Jensen S, et al: Randomised study of risk of fetal loss related to early amniocentesis versus chorionic villus sampling. Lancet 350(9079):697, 1997

Tangshewinsirikul C, Wanapirak C, Piyamongkol W, et al: Effect of cord puncture site on cordocentesis at mid-pregnancy on pregnancy outcome. Prenat Diagn 31;861, 2011

Thornburg LL, Knight KM, Peterson CJ, et al: Maternal serum alpha-fetoprotein values in type 1 and type 2 diabetic patients. Am J Obstet Gynecol 199(2):135.e1, 2008

Tongsong T, Wanapirak C, Kunavikatikul C, et al: Fetal loss rate associated with cordocentesis at midgestation. Am J Obstet Gynecol 184(4):719, 2001

Tul N, Spencer K, Noble P, et al: Screening for trisomy 18 by fetal nuchal translucency and maternal serum free beta hCG and PAPP-A at 10–14 weeks of gestation. Prenat Diagn 19(11):1035, 1999

Van den Hof MC, Nicolaides KH, Campbell J, et al: Evaluation of the lemon and banana signs in one hundred thirty fetuses with open spina bifida. Am J Obstet Gynecol 162(2):322, 1990

van der Pol JG, Wolf H, Boer K, et al: Jejunal atresia related to the use of methylene blue in genetic amniocentesis in twins. Br J Obstet Gynaecol 99(2):141, 1992

Velie EM, Shaw GM, Malcoe LH, et al: Understanding the increased risk of neural tube defect-affected pregnancies among Mexico-born women in California: immigration and anthropomorphic factors. Paediatr Perinat Epidemiol 20(3):219, 2006

Vintzileos AJ, Egan JF: Adjusting the risk for trisomy 21 on the basis of second-trimester ultrasonography. Am J Obstet Gynecol 172(3):837, 1995

Vink J, Wapner R, D'Alton ME: Prenatal diagnosis in twin gestations. Semin Perinatol 36(3):169, 2012

Wald NJ, Cuckle H, Brock JH, et al: Maternal serum-alpha-fetoprotein measurement in antenatal screening for anencephaly and spina bifida in early pregnancy. Report of UK Collaborative Study on Alpha-Fetoprotein in Relation to Neural-tube Defects. Lancet 1(8026):1323, 1977

Wald NJ, Cuckle HS, Densem JW, et al: Maternal serum unconjugated estriol as an antenatal screening test for Down's syndrome. Br J Obstet Gynaecol 95(4):334, 1988

Walker SJ, Ball RH, Babcook CJ, et al: Prevalence of aneuploidy and additional anatomic abnormalities in fetuses and neonates with cleft lip with or without cleft palate. A population-based study in Utah. J Ultrasound Med 20(11):1175, 2001.

Wapner R, Thom E, Simpson JL, et al: First-trimester screening for trisomies 21 and 18. N Engl J Med 349(15):1471, 2003

Watson WJ, Chescheir NC, Katz VL, et al: The role of ultrasound in evaluation of patients with elevated maternal serum alpha-fetoprotein: a review. Obstet Gynecol 78(1):123, 1991

Wenstrom KD, Weiner CP, Williamson RA, et al: Prenatal diagnosis of fetal hyperthyroidism using funipuncture. Obstet Gynecol 76(3 Pt 2):513, 1990

Wijnberger LD, van der Schouw YT, Christiaens GC: Learning in medicine: chorionic villus sampling. Prenat Diagn 20(3):241, 2003

Xu K, Rosenwaks Z, Beaverson K, et al: Preimplantation genetic diagnosis for retinoblastoma: the first reported liveborn. Am J Ophthalmol 137(1):18, 2004

Yang P, Zhao Z, Reece EA: Activation of oxidative stress signaling that is implicated in apoptosis with a mouse model of diabetic embryopathy. Am J Obstet Gynecol 198(1):130.e1, 2008

Yin M, Dong L, Zheng J, et al: Meta analysis of the association between MTHFR C677T polymorphism and the risk of congenital heart defects. Ann Hum Genet 76(1):9, 2012

Zuckerman A, Lahad A, Shmueli A, et al: Carrier screening for Gaucher disease: lessons for low-penetrance, treatable diseases. JAMA 298(11):1281, 2007

CHAPTER 15

Fetal Disorders

Fetal disorders may be acquired—such as *alloimmunization*, they may be genetic—*congenital adrenal hyperplasia* or *α4-thalassemia*, or they may be sporadic developmental abnormalities—like many structural malformations. Reviewed in this chapter are fetal anemia and thrombocytopenia, along with immune and nonimmune fetal hydrops. Hydrops is perhaps the quintessential fetal disorder, as it can be a manifestation of severe illness from a wide variety of etiologies. Fetal structural malformations are reviewed in Chapter 10; genetic abnormalities are reviewed in Chapters 13 and 14; and other conditions amenable to fetal medical and surgical treatment are reviewed in Chapter 16. Because congenital infections arise as a result of maternal infection or colonization, they are considered in Chapters 64 and 65.

FETAL ANEMIA

Of the many causes of fetal anemia, the most common is red cell alloimmunization, which results from transplacental passage of maternal antibodies that destroy fetal red cells. Alloimmunization leads to overproduction of immature fetal and neonatal red cells—*erythroblastosis fetalis*–a condition now referred to as *hemolytic disease of the fetus and newborn (HDFN)*. Several congenital infections are also associated with fetal anemia, particularly *parvovirus B19*, discussed in Chapter 64 (p. 1244). In Southeast Asian populations, α4-thalassemia is a common cause of severe anemia and nonimmune hydrops. Fetomaternal hemorrhage occasionally creates severe fetal anemia and is discussed on page 312. Rare causes of anemia include red cell production disorders—such as *Blackfan-Diamond anemia* and *Fanconi anemia*; red cell enzymopathies—*glucose-6-phosphate dehydrogenase deficiency* and *pyruvate kinase deficiency*; red cell structural abnormalities—*hereditary spherocytosis* and *elliptocytosis*; and myeloproliferative disorders—*leukemias*. Anemia may be identified through fetal blood sampling as described in Chapter 14 (p. 300) or by Doppler evaluation of the fetal middle cerebral artery (MCA) peak systolic velocity as described on page 310.

Progressive fetal anemia from any cause leads to heart failure, hydrops fetalis, and ultimately death. Fortunately, the prevention of Rh D alloimmunization with *anti-D immune globulin*, and the identification and treatment of fetal anemia with MCA Doppler studies and intrauterine transfusions, respectively, have dramatically changed the prevalence and course of this otherwise devastating disorder. Severely anemic fetuses transfused in utero have survival rates exceeding 90 percent, and even in cases of hydrops fetalis, survival rates approach 80 percent (Lindenburg, 2013; van Kamp, 2001).

Red Cell Alloimmunization

There are currently 30 different blood group systems and 328 red cell antigens recognized by the International Society of Blood Transfusion (Storry, 2011). Although some of these are immunologically and genetically important, many are so rare as to be of little clinical significance. Any individual who lacks a specific red cell antigen may produce an antibody when exposed to that antigen. Such antibodies can prove harmful to that individual if she receives an incompatible blood transfusion, and they may be harmful to her fetus during pregnancy.

Accordingly, blood banks routinely screen for erythrocyte antigens. These antibodies may also be harmful to a mother's fetus during pregnancy. As noted, maternal antibodies formed against fetal erythrocyte antigens may cross the placenta to cause fetal red cell lysis and anemia.

Typically, a fetus inherits at least one red cell antigen from the father that is lacking in the mother. Thus, the mother may become sensitized if enough fetal erythrocytes reach her circulation to elicit an immune response. Even so, alloimmunization is uncommon for the following reasons: (1) low prevalence of incompatible red cell antigens; (2) insufficient transplacental passage of fetal antigens or maternal antibodies; (3) maternal-fetal ABO incompatibility, which leads to rapid clearance of fetal erythrocytes before they elicit an immune response; (4) variable antigenicity; and (5) variable maternal immune response to the antigen.

In population-based screening studies, the prevalence of red cell alloimmunization in pregnancy is approximately 1 percent (Howard, 1998; Koelewijn, 2008). Most cases of severe fetal anemia requiring antenatal transfusion are attributable to anti-D, anti-Kell, or anti-c alloimmunization.

Alloimmunization Detection

A blood type and antibody screen are routinely assessed at the first prenatal visit, and unbound antibodies in maternal serum are detected by the *indirect Coombs test* (Chap. 9, p. 174). With positive results, specific antibodies are identified, their immunoglobulin subtype is determined as either IgG or IgM, and the titer is quantified. Only IgG antibodies are of concern because IgM antibodies do not cross the placenta. Selected antibodies and their potential to cause fetal hemolytic anemia are listed in Table 15-1. The *critical titer* is the level at which significant fetal anemia could potentially develop. This may be different for each antibody, is determined individually by each laboratory, and usually ranges between 1:8 and 1:32. If the critical titer for anti-D antibodies is 1:16, a titer ≥ 1:16 indicates the possibility of severe hemolytic disease. An important exception is Kell sensitization, which is discussed on page 308.

CDE (Rh) Blood Group Incompatibility

The rhesus system includes five red cell proteins or antigens: C, c, D, E, and e. No "d" antigen has been identified, and Rh D-negativity is defined as the absence of the D antigen. Although most people are Rh D positive or negative, more than 200 D antigen variants exist (Daniels, 2013).

CDE antigens are clinically important. Rh D-negative individuals may become sensitized after a single exposure to as little as 0.1 mL of fetal erythrocytes (Bowman, 1988). The two responsible genes—*RHD* and *RHCE*—are located on the short arm of chromosome 1 and are inherited together, independent of other blood group genes. Their incidence varies according to racial and ethnic origin. Nearly 85 percent of non-Hispanic white Americans are Rh D-positive, as are approximately 90 percent of Native Americans, 93 percent of African Americans and Hispanic Americans, and 99 percent of Asian individuals (Garratty, 2004).

The prevalence of Rh D alloimmunization complicating pregnancy ranges from 0.5 to 0.9 percent (Howard, 1998; Koelewijn, 2008; Martin, 2005). Without anti-D immune globulin prophylaxis, an Rh D-negative woman delivered of an Rh D-positive, *ABO-compatible* infant has a 16-percent likelihood of developing alloimmunization. Two percent will become sensitized by the time of delivery, 7 percent by 6 months postpartum, and the remaining 7 percent will be "*sensibilized*"—producing detectable antibodies only in a subsequent pregnancy (Bowman, 1985). If there is *ABO incompatibility*, the Rh D alloimmunization risk is approximately 2 percent without prophylaxis (Bowman, 2006). The reason for the differing rates relative to ABO blood type results from erythrocyte destruction of ABO-incompatible cells and thus limitation of sensitizing opportunities. Rh D sensitization also may occur following first-trimester pregnancy complications, prenatal diagnostic procedures, and maternal trauma (Table 15-2).

The Rh C, c, E, and e antigens have lower immunogenicity than the Rh D antigen, but they too can cause hemolytic disease. Sensitization to E, c, and C antigens complicates approximately 0.3 percent of pregnancies in screening studies and accounts for about 30 percent of red cell alloimmunization cases (Howard, 1998; Koelewijn, 2008). Anti-E alloimmunization is the most common, but the need for fetal or neonatal transfusions is significantly greater with anti-c alloimmunization than with anti-E or anti-C (Hackney, 2004; Koelewijn, 2008).

The Grandmother Effect. In virtually all pregnancies, small amounts of maternal blood enter the fetal circulation. Real-time polymerase chain reaction (PCR) has been used to identify maternal Rh D-positive DNA in peripheral blood from preterm and full-term Rh D-negative newborns (Lazar, 2006). Thus, it is possible for an Rh D-negative female fetus exposed to maternal Rh D-positive red cells to develop sensitization. When such an individual reaches adulthood, she may produce anti-D antibodies even before or early in her first pregnancy. This mechanism is called the *grandmother theory* because the fetus in the current pregnancy is jeopardized by maternal antibodies that were initially provoked by his or her *grandmother's* erythrocytes.

Alloimmunization to Minor Antigens

Because routine administration of anti-D immunoglobulin prevents anti-D alloimmunization, proportionately more cases of hemolytic disease are caused by red cell antigens other than D—also known as minor antigens (see Table 15-1). *Kell antibodies* are among the most frequent. *Duffy group A antibodies—anti-Fy^a*—are also fairly common, as are *anti-MNSs* and *anti-Jk^a—Kidd group* (Geifman-Holtzman, 1997). Most cases of sensitization to minor antigens result from incompatible blood transfusions (American College of Obstetricians and Gynecologists, 2012). If an IgG red cell antibody is detected and there is any doubt as to its significance, the clinician should err on the side of caution, and the pregnancy should be evaluated for hemolytic disease.

There are only a few blood group antigens that pose *no* fetal risk. Lewis antibodies—Le^a and Le^b, as well as I antibodies, are cold agglutinins. They are predominantly IgM and are not

TABLE 15-1. Minor Red Cell Antigens and Their Relationship to Fetal Hemolytic Disease

Blood Group System	Antigens Related to Hemolytic Disease	Hemolytic Disease Severity	Proposed Management
Lewis	*		
I	*		
Kell	K	Mild to severe[†]	Fetal assessment
	k, Ko, Kp^a Kp^b, Js^a, Js^b	Mild	Routine care
Rh (non-D)	E, C, c	Mild to severe[†]	Fetal assessment
Duffy	Fy^a	Mild to severe[†]	Fetal assessment
	Fy^b	None	Routine care
	By^3	Mild	Routine care
Kidd	Jk^a	Mild to severe	Fetal assessment
	Jk^b, Jk^3	Mild	Routine care
MNSs	M, S, s, U	Mild to severe	Fetal assessment
	N	Mild	Routine care
	Mi^a	Moderate	Fetal assessment
MSSSs	Mt^a	Moderate	Fetal assessment
	Vw, Mur, Hil, Hut	Mild	Routine care
Lutheran	Lu^a, Lu^b	Mild	Routine care
Diego	$D1^a$, Di^b	Mild to severe	Fetal assessment
Xg	Xg^a	Mild	Routine care
P	$PP_{1pk}(Tj^a)$	Mild to severe	Fetal assessment
Public antigens	Yt^a	Moderate to severe	Fetal assessment
	Yt^b, Lan, Ge, Jr^a, $CO^{1\text{-}b\text{-}}$	Mild	Routine care
	En^a	Moderate	Fetal assessment
	Co^a	Severe	Fetal assessment
Private antigens	Batty, Becker, Berrens, Evans, Gonzales, Hunt, Jobbins, Rm, Ven, $Wright^b$	Mild	Routine care
	Biles, Heibel, Radin, Zd	Moderate	Fetal assessment
	Good, $Wright^a$	Severe	Fetal assessment

*Not a proven cause of hemolytic disease of the fetus and newborn.
[†]With hydrops fetalis.
Modified from Weinstein, 1982.

expressed on fetal red cells. Another antibody that does not cause fetal hemolysis is *Duffy group B—Fy^b*.

Kell Alloimmunization. Approximately 90 percent of whites and up to 98 percent of African Americans are Kell negative. Kell type is not routinely determined, and approximately 90 percent of Kell sensitization cases result from transfusion with Kell-positive blood. Thus, transfusion history is important.

If Kell sensitization develops from maternal–fetal incompatibility, it may develop more rapidly and may be more severe than with sensitization to Rh D and other blood group antigens. This is because Kell antibodies attach to fetal bone marrow erythrocyte precursors and prevent a hemopoietic response to anemia. With fewer erythrocytes produced, there is less hemolysis. Because of these vicissitudes, severe anemia may not be predicted by either the maternal Kell antibody titer or the amnionic fluid bilirubin level (p. 310). One option is to use a lower critical titer—1:8—for Kell sensitization (Moise, 2012). The American College of Obstetricians and Gynecologists (2012) has recommended that antibody titers not be used to monitor Kell-sensitized pregnancies. Van Wamelen and colleagues (2007) have advocated MCA Doppler studies beginning at 16 to 17 weeks' gestation for pregnancies with anti-Kell titers ≥ 1:2.

ABO Blood Group Incompatibility

Incompatibility for the major blood group antigens A and B is the most common cause of hemolytic disease in newborn infants, but it does not cause appreciable hemolysis in the fetus. Approximately 20 percent of newborns have ABO blood group incompatibility, however, only 5 percent are clinically affected, and the resulting anemia is usually mild. The condition differs from Rh CDE incompatibility in several respects. First, ABO incompatibility is often seen in firstborn infants, whereas sensitization to other blood group antigens is *not*. This is because most group O women have developed anti-A and anti-B isoagglutinins before pregnancy from exposure to bacteria displaying similar antigens. Second, ABO alloimmunization can affect future pregnancies, but unlike CDE disease, it rarely becomes progressively more severe. Last, most anti-A and anti-B antibodies

TABLE 15-2. Causes of Fetomaternal Hemorrhage Associated with Red Cell Antigen Alloimmunization[a]

Pregnancy Loss
Ectopic pregnancy
Spontaneous abortion
Elective abortion
Fetal death (any trimester)
Procedures
Chorionic villus sampling
Amniocentesis
Fetal blood sampling
Other
Delivery
Trauma
Placental abruption
Unexplained vaginal bleeding during pregnancy
External cephalic version

[a]For each of the above, anti-D immune globulin is recommended.
Data from The American Academy of Pediatrics and American College of Obstetricians and Gynecologists, 2012.

are immunoglobulin M (IgM), which do not cross the placenta. Fetal red cells also have fewer A and B antigenic sites than adult cells and are thus less immunogenic. For these reasons, ABO alloimmunization is generally a pediatric disease rather than an obstetrical concern. There is no need to monitor for fetal hemolysis or to deliver the fetus early. Careful neonatal observation is essential, because hyperbilirubinemia may require treatment with phototherapy or occasionally transfusion (Chap. 33, p. 644).

Management of the Alloimmunized Pregnancy

An estimated 25 to 30 percent of fetuses from Rh D-alloimmunized pregnancies will have mild to moderate hemolytic anemia, and without treatment, up to 25 percent will develop hydrops (Tannirandorn, 1990). If alloimmunization is detected and the titer is below the critical value, the titer is generally repeated every 4 weeks for the duration of the pregnancy (American College of Obstetricians and Gynecologists, 2012). Importantly, however, if a woman has had a prior pregnancy complicated by alloimmunization, serial titer assessment is inadequate for surveillance of fetal anemia. In these instances, pregnancy is assumed to be at risk and is followed as discussed on page 310. Once a titer has reached a critical value, there is no benefit to repeating it. The pregnancy is at risk even if the titer decreases, and further evaluation is still required.

Determining Fetal Risk

The presence of maternal anti-D antibodies reflects her sensitization, but it does not necessarily indicate that the fetus will be affected or is even Rh D-positive. For example, in a non-Hispanic white couple in which the woman is Rh D-negative, there is an 85-percent chance that the man is Rh D-positive, but in 60 percent of these cases he will be heterozygous at the D-locus (American College of Obstetricians and Gynecologists, 2012). If he is heterozygous, then only half of his children will be at risk for hemolytic disease. Another consideration is that if a woman became sensitized in a prior pregnancy, her antibody titer might rise to high levels during the current pregnancy even if the current fetus is Rh D-negative. This is termed an *amnestic response.* Additionally, alloimmunization to a red cell antigen other than Rh D may have occurred following a blood transfusion in the past, and if that antigen is not present on paternal erythrocytes, the pregnancy is not at risk.

Initial evaluation of alloimmunization begins with determining the paternal erythrocyte antigen status. *Provided that paternity is certain*, if the father is negative for the red cell antigen to which the mother is sensitized, the pregnancy is not at risk. In an Rh D alloimmunized pregnancy in which the father is Rh D-positive, it is helpful to determine prenatal paternal zygosity for the Rh D antigen, and DNA-based analysis will establish this. If the father is heterozygous or if paternity is in question, the patient should be offered assessment of fetal antigen type. In the Unites States, this has traditionally been done with amniocentesis and PCR testing of uncultured amniocytes to assess fetal blood type (Chap. 13, p. 277) (American College of Obstetricians and Gynecologists, 2012). This test has a positive-predictive value of 100 percent and negative-predictive value of approximately 97 percent (Van den Veyver, 1996). Chorionic villus sampling is not generally performed because it is associated with greater risk for fetomaternal hemorrhage and may worsen alloimmunization. Fetal testing for other antigens is also available from reference laboratories using amniocentesis specimens. Examples include testing for E/e, C/c, Duffy, Kell, Kidd, and M/N.

More recently, noninvasive fetal Rh D blood typing has been performed using cell-free fetal DNA from maternal plasma (Chap. 13, p. 279). Accuracy is reported to be as high as 99 to 100 percent (Minon, 2008; Tynan, 2011). In a metaanalysis, only 3 percent of samples had inconclusive results (Geifman-Holtzman, 2006). Fetal Rh D blood typing with cell-free fetal DNA is routinely used in parts of Europe. There are two potential indications in Rh D negative pregnant women: (1) in women *with* Rh D alloimmunization, testing can identify fetuses who are also Rh D negative and do not require anemia surveillance, and (2) in women *without* Rh D alloimmunization, anti-D immune globulin might be withheld if the fetus is Rh D negative. However, concerns have been raised that use of the test to limit anti-D immune globulin administration could lead to an increased prevalence of Rh D alloimmunization (Goodspeed, 2013; Szczepura, 2011). As of 2013, cell-free fetal DNA testing for fetal Rh type has not been widely adopted in the United States.

Management of the alloimmunized pregnancy is individualized and may consist of maternal antibody titer surveillance, sonographic monitoring of the fetal MCA peak systolic velocity, amnionic fluid bilirubin studies, or fetal blood sampling. Accurate pregnancy dating is critical. The gestational age at which fetal anemia developed in prior pregnancies is important because anemia tends to occur earlier and be sequentially more severe.

Middle Cerebral Artery Doppler Velocimetry. In most specialized centers, serial measurement of the peak systolic velocity of the fetal middle cerebral artery has replaced amniocentesis for the detection of fetal anemia. The anemic fetus shunts blood preferentially to the brain to maintain adequate oxygenation. The velocity increases because of increased cardiac output and decreased blood viscosity (Moise, 2008a). The technique, which is discussed in Chapter 10 (p. 221), should be used only with adequate training and experience (American College of Obstetricians and Gynecologists, 2012).

In a landmark study, Mari and coworkers (2000) measured the MCA peak systolic velocity serially in 111 fetuses at risk for anemia and in 265 normal control fetuses. Threshold values > 1.5 multiples of the median (MoM) for given gestational ages correctly identified all fetuses with moderate or severe anemia. This provided a sensitivity of 100 percent, with a false-positive rate of 12 percent.

The MCA peak systolic velocity is followed serially, and values are plotted on a curve like the one shown in Figure 15-1. If the velocity is between 1.0 and 1.5 MoM and the slope is increasing—such that the value is approaching 1.5 MoM—surveillance is generally increased to weekly Doppler interrogation. If the MCA peak systolic velocity exceeds 1.5 MoM, further evaluation by fetal blood sampling is necessary to assess need for fetal transfusion. The false-positive rate increases significantly beyond 35 weeks, due to the normal increase in cardiac output that develops at this gestational age (Moise, 2008a; Zimmerman, 2002).

Amnionic Fluid Spectral Analysis. More than 50 years ago, Liley (1961) demonstrated the utility of amnionic fluid spectral analysis to measure bilirubin concentration. This permitted an estimate of hemolysis severity and indirect assessment of anemia. Amnionic fluid bilirubin is measured by a spectrophotometer and is demonstrable as a change in optical density absorbance at 450 nm—*ΔOD_{450}*. The likelihood of fetal anemia is determined by plotting the ΔOD_{450} value on a graph that is divided into several zones. The original Liley graph is valid from 27 to 42 weeks' gestation and contains three zones. Zone 1 indicates an Rh D-negative fetus or one with only mild disease. Zone 2 indicates fetal anemia, with hemoglobin concentrations of 11.0 to 13.9 g/dL for values in lower zone 2 and those of 8.0 to 10.9 g/dL for upper zone 2. Zone 3 indicates severe anemia, with hemoglobin concentration < 8.0 g/dL.

The Liley graph was subsequently modified by Queenan and associates (1993) to include gestational ages as early as 14 weeks (Fig. 15-2). The naturally high amnionic fluid bilirubin level at midpregnancy results in a large *indeterminate zone.* Here, bilirubin concentrations do not accurately predict fetal hemoglobin concentration. For this reason, if evaluation indicated that severe fetal anemia or hydrops before 25 weeks was likely, then fetal blood sampling was often performed.

Middle cerebral artery velocimetry is noninvasive and does not confer the risks for pregnancy loss or increased alloimmunization associated with amniocentesis. Importantly, it is also more accurate than ΔOD_{450} assessment, particularly early in pregnancy. Oepkes and coworkers (2006) compared MCA Doppler velocimetry and amnionic fluid bilirubin studies. They found that MCA Doppler had significantly greater sensitivity and accuracy. For these reasons, amnionic fluid spectral analysis is currently used only when Doppler velocimetry is not readily available. It also may be considered if the MCA peak systolic velocity exceeds 1.5 MoM after 35 weeks' gestation. In the latter situation, if ΔOD_{450} assessment indicates only mild hemolysis, delivery at 37 to 38 weeks has been recommended (American College of Obstetricians and Gynecologists, 2012; Moise, 2008b).

Fetal Blood Transfusion

If there is evidence of severe fetal anemia, either because of elevated MCA peak systolic velocity or development of fetal hydrops, management is strongly influenced by gestational age. The preterm fetus is usually evaluated with fetal blood sampling, as described in Chapter 14 (p. 300). Some recommend fetal transfusion until 30 to 32 weeks' gestation and delivery at

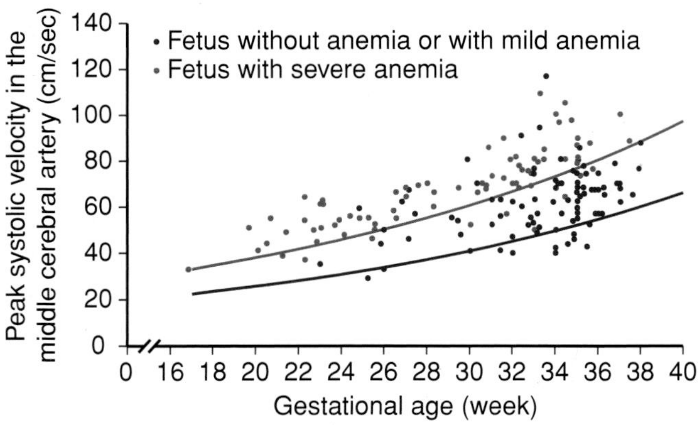

FIGURE 15-1 Doppler measurements of the peak systolic velocity in the middle cerebral artery in 165 fetuses at risk for severe anemia. The blue line indicates the median peak systolic velocity in normal pregnancies, and the red line shows 1.5 multiples of the median. (Redrawn from Oepkes, 2006, with permission.)

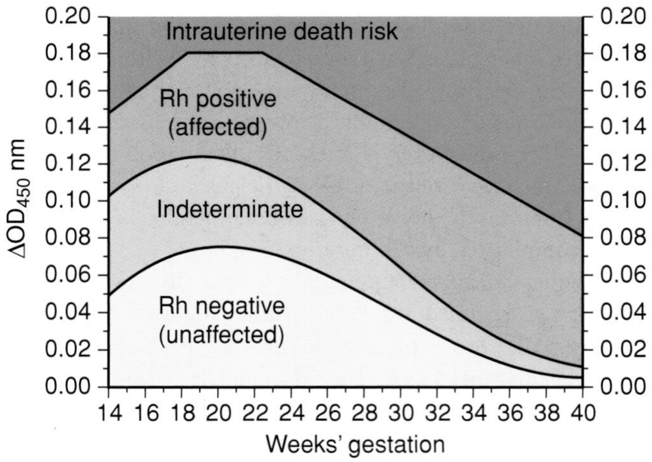

FIGURE 15-2 Proposed amnionic fluid ΔOD_{450} management zones in pregnancies from 14 to 40 weeks. (Redrawn from Queenan, 1993, with permission.)

32 to 34 weeks. To decrease neonatal morbidity from prematurity, others suggest intrauterine transfusion up to 36 weeks followed by delivery at 37 to 38 weeks (American College of Obstetricians and Gynecologists, 2012).

Intravascular transfusion into the umbilical vein under sonographic guidance is the preferred method of fetal transfusion. Peritoneal transfusion may be necessary with severe, early-onset hemolytic disease in the early second trimester, a time when the umbilical vein is too narrow to readily permit needle entry (Fox, 2008; Howe, 2007). With hydrops, although peritoneal absorption is impaired, some prefer to transfuse into both the peritoneal cavity and the umbilical vein.

Transfusion is generally recommended if the fetal hematocrit is < 30 percent. Once hydrops has developed, however, the hematocrit is generally 15 percent or lower. The red cells transfused are type O, Rh D negative, cytomegalovirus-negative, packed to a hematocrit of about 80 percent to prevent volume overload, irradiated to prevent fetal graft-versus-host reaction, and leukocyte-poor. The fetal-placental volume allows rapid infusion of a relatively large quantity of blood. Before transfusion, a paralytic agent such as vecuronium may be given to the fetus to minimize movements and potential needlestick trauma. In a nonhydropic fetus, the target hematocrit is generally 40 to 50 percent. The volume transfused may be estimated by multiplying the estimated fetal weight in grams by 0.02 for each 10-percent increase in hematocrit needed (Giannina, 1998). In the severely anemic fetus, less blood is transfused initially, and another transfusion is planned for about 2 days later.

Subsequent transfusions usually take place every 2 to 4 weeks, depending on the hematocrit. The sensitivity of the MCA peak systolic velocity to detect severe anemia appears to be lower following an initial transfusion, such that it may not be reliable (Scheier, 2006). One schedule is to perform a second transfusion in 10 days, the third 2 weeks later, and any additional transfusions 3 weeks later (Moise, 2012). Following transfusion, the fetal hematocrit generally decreases by approximately 1 volume percent per day. A more rapid initial decline may be seen with hydropic fetuses.

Outcomes. Procedure-related complications have been reported in up to 9 percent of transfused pregnancies (van Kamp, 2005). These include fetal death in approximately 3 percent, neonatal death in about 2 percent, need for emergent cesarean delivery in 6 percent, and infection in 1 percent. Considering that fetal transfusion is potentially lifesaving in severely compromised fetuses, these risks should not dissuade therapy.

The overall survival rate following fetal transfusion approximates 90 percent (Lindenberg, 2013; Van Kamp, 2005). If transfusion is required before 20 weeks, survival rates are lower but may reach 80 percent at experienced centers (Canlorde, 2011; Lindenberg, 2013). Van Kamp and colleagues (2001) reported that if hydrops had developed, the survival rate approached 75 to 80 percent. However, of the nearly two thirds with resolution of hydrops following transfusion, more than 95 percent survived. The survival rate was below 40 percent if hydrops persisted.

Lindenberg and associates (2012) recently reviewed long-term outcomes following intrauterine transfusion in a cohort of more than 450 alloimmunized pregnancies. Alloimmunization was secondary to Rh D in 80 percent, Kell in 12 percent, and Rh c in 5 percent. Approximately a fourth of affected fetuses had hydrops, and more than half also required exchange transfusion in the neonatal period. The overall survival rate approximated 90 percent. Among nearly 300 children aged 2 to 17 years who participated in neurodevelopmental testing, fewer than 5 percent had severe impairments. These included severe developmental delay in 3 percent, cerebral palsy in 2 percent, and deafness in 1 percent.

Prevention of Rh D Alloimmunization

Anti-D immune globulin has been used for more than four decades to prevent Rh D alloimmunization and is one of the success stories of modern obstetrics. In countries without access to anti-D immune globulin, nearly 10 percent of Rh D-negative pregnancies are complicated by hemolytic disease of the fetus and newborn (Zipursky, 2011). With immunoprophylaxis, however, the alloimmunization risk is reduced to < 0.2 percent. Despite longstanding and widespread use, its mechanism of action is not completely understood.

As many as 90 percent of alloimmunization cases occur from fetomaternal hemorrhage at delivery. Routine postpartum administration of anti-D immune globulin to at-risk pregnancies within 72 hours of delivery decreases the alloimmunization rate by 90 percent (Bowman, 1985). Additionally, provision of anti-D immune globulin at 28 weeks' gestation reduces the third-trimester alloimmunization rate from approximately 2 percent to 0.1 percent (Bowman, 1988).

Whenever there is doubt whether to give anti–D immunoglobulin, it should be given. Even if not needed, it will cause no harm, but failing to give it when needed can have severe consequences.

Current preparations of anti-D immune globulin are derived from human plasma donated by individuals with high-titer anti-D antibodies. Formulations prepared by cold ethanol fractionation and ultrafiltration can only be administered intramuscularly, because they contain plasma proteins that could result in anaphylaxis if given intravenously. However, newer formulations, prepared using ion exchange chromatography, may be administered either intramuscularly or intravenously. This is important for treatment of significant fetomaternal hemorrhage, which is discussed subsequently. Both preparation methods effectively remove viral particles, including hepatitis and human immunodeficiency viruses. Depending on the preparation, the half-life of anti-D immune globulin ranges from 16 to 24 days, which is why it is given both in the third trimester and following delivery. The standard intramuscular dose of anti-D immune globulin—300 μg or 1500 international units (IU)—will protect the average-sized mother from a fetal hemorrhage of up to 30 mL of fetal whole blood or 15 mL of fetal red cells.

In the United States, anti-D immune globulin is given prophylactically to all Rh D-negative, unsensitized women at approximately 28 weeks, and a second dose is given after delivery if the infant is Rh D-positive (American College of Obstetricians and Gynecologists, 2010). Before the 28-week dose of anti-D immune globulin, repeat antibody screening is recommended to identify individuals who have become alloimmunized (American Academy of Pediatrics and American College of Obstetricians and Gynecologists 2012). Following delivery, anti-D immune globulin should be given within 72 hours. Importantly, if immune globulin is inadvertently not administered following delivery, it should be given as soon as the omission is recognized, because there may be some protection up to 28 days postpartum (Bowman, 2006). Anti-D immune globulin is also administered after pregnancy-related events that could result in fetomaternal hemorrhage (see Table 15-2).

Anti-D immune globulin may produce a weakly positive—1:1 to 1:4—indirect Coombs titer in the mother. This is harmless and should not be confused with development of alloimmunization. Additionally, as the body mass index increases above 27 to 40 kg/m^2, serum antibody levels decrease by 30 to 60 percent and may be less protective (MacKenzie, 2006; Woelfer, 2004). Rh D-negative women who receive other types of blood products—including platelet transfusions and plasmapheresis—are also at risk of becoming sensitized, and this can be prevented with anti-D immune globulin. Rarely, a small amount of antibody crosses the placenta and results in a weakly positive direct Coombs test in cord and infant blood. Despite this, passive immunization does not cause significant fetal or neonatal hemolysis.

In approximately 1 percent of pregnancies, the volume of fetomaternal hemorrhage exceeds 30 mL of whole blood (Ness, 1987). A single dose of anti-D immune globulin would be insufficient in such situations. If additional anti-D immune globulin is considered only for women with risk factors—examples include abdominal trauma, placental abruption, placenta previa, intrauterine manipulation, multifetal gestation, or manual placenta removal—*half* of those who require more than the 1500-IU dose may be missed. Because of these observations, the American Association of Blood Banks recommends that all D-negative women be tested at delivery with a *rosette test* or *Kleihauer-Betke test* (Snyder, 1998).

The rosette test is used to identify whether fetal Rh D-positive cells are present in the circulation of an Rh D-negative woman. It is a qualitative test. A sample of maternal blood is mixed with anti-D antibodies that coat any Rh D-positive fetal cells present in the sample. Indicator red cells bearing the D-antigen are then added, and rosettes form around the fetal cells as the indicator cells attach to them by the antibodies. Thus, if rosettes are visualized, there are fetal Rh D-positive cells in that sample.

The Kleihauer-Betke test is a quantitative test used either in the setting of Rh D incompatibility or any time a large fetomaternal hemorrhage is suspected—regardless of antigen status. It is discussed on page 313.

The dosage of anti-D immune globulin is calculated from the estimated volume of the fetal-to-maternal hemorrhage, as described on page 311. One 1500-IU (300 μg) ampule is given for each 15 mL of fetal red cells or 30 mL of fetal whole blood to be neutralized. If using an intramuscular preparation of anti-D immune globulin, no more than five doses may be given in a 24-hour period. If using an intravenous preparation, two ampules—totaling 3000 IU (600 μg)—may be given every 8 hours. To determine if the administered dose was adequate, the indirect Coombs test may be performed. A positive result indicates that there is excess anti–D immunoglobulin in maternal serum, thus demonstrating that the dose was sufficient. Alternatively, a rosette test may be performed to assess whether circulating fetal cells remain.

Weak D Antigens

Women who are positive for *weak D antigens*, formerly called D^u, are not considered at risk for hemolytic disease and do not require anti-D immune globulin (American College of Obstetricians and Gynecologists, 2010). There are, however, D-antigen variants—termed *partial D antigens*—that can result in Rh D alloimmunization and cause hemolytic disease (Daniels, 2013). If a D-negative woman delivers a weak D-positive infant, she should be given anti-D immune globulin. It is worth emphasizing that if there is any doubt regarding D-antigen status, then immune globulin should be given.

Fetomaternal Hemorrhage

It is likely that all pregnant women experience a small fetomaternal hemorrhage, and in two-thirds, this may be sufficient to provoke an antigen-antibody reaction. As shown in Figure 15-3, the incidence increases with gestational age, as does the volume of fetal blood in the maternal circulation. Large volumes of blood loss—true fetomaternal hemorrhage—are fortunately rare. In a series of more than 30,000 pregnancies, de Almeida and Bowman (1994) found evidence of fetomaternal hemorrhage > 80 mL in approximately 1 per 1000 births, and hemorrhage > 150 mL in 1 per 5000 births.

Fetomaternal hemorrhage may follow maternal trauma, may occur with placenta previa or vasa previa, and may follow amniocentesis or external cephalic version (Giacoia, 1997; Rubod, 2007). In more than 80 percent of cases, however, no cause is identified. With significant hemorrhage, the most

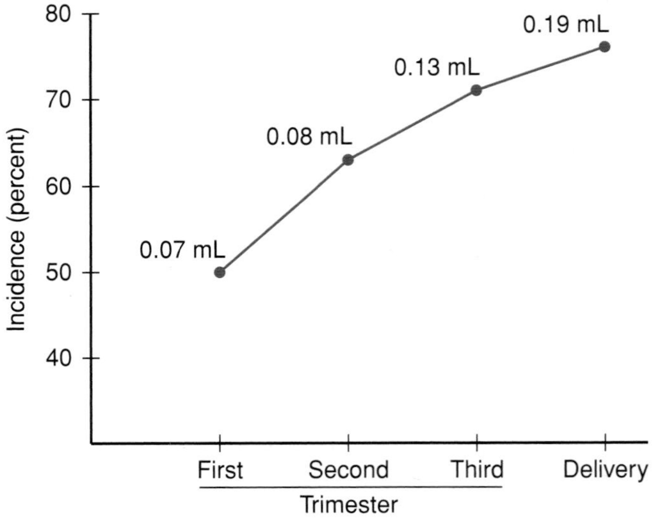

FIGURE 15-3 Incidence of fetal-to-maternal hemorrhage during pregnancy. The numbers at each data point represent total volume of fetal blood estimated to have been transferred into the maternal circulation. (Data from Choavaratana, 1997.)

common presenting complaint is decreased fetal movement (Eichbaum, 2006; Hartung, 2000; Wylie, 2010). A sinusoidal fetal heart rate pattern, although uncommon, is occasionally seen and warrants immediate evaluation (Chap. 24, p. 482). Sonography may demonstrate elevated MCA peak systolic velocity, and hydrops may be identified (Eichbaum, 2006; Giacoia, 1997; Hartung, 2000). If fetomaternal hemorrhage is suspected based on either a sinusoidal fetal heart rate pattern or positive Kleihauer-Betke test result, then the finding of an elevated MCA peak systolic velocity or hydrops should prompt consideration of either fetal transfusion or delivery.

One limitation of quantitative tests for fetal cells in the maternal circulation is that they do not provide information regarding hemorrhage timing or chronicity (Wylie, 2010). In general, anemia developing gradually or chronically, as in alloimmunization, is better tolerated by the fetus than acute anemia. Chronic anemia may not produce fetal heart rate abnormalities until the fetus is moribund. In contrast, significant acute hemorrhage is poorly tolerated by the fetus and may cause profound fetal neurological impairment from cerebral hypoperfusion, ischemia, and infarction. In some cases, fetomaternal hemorrhage is identified during stillbirth evaluation (Chap. 35, p. 664).

Tests for Fetomaternal Hemorrhage

Once fetomaternal hemorrhage is recognized, the volume of fetal blood loss can be estimated. The volume may influence obstetrical management and is essential to determining the appropriate dose of anti D-immune globulin if the woman is Rh D-negative.

The most commonly used quantitative test for fetal red cells in the maternal circulation is the acid elution or *Kleihauer-Betke (KB) test* (Kleihauer, 1957). Fetal erythrocytes contain hemoglobin F, which is more resistant to acid elution than hemoglobin A. After exposure to acid, only fetal hemoglobin remains, such that after staining, the fetal erythrocytes appear red and adult cells appear as "ghosts" (Fig. 15-4). Fetal cells are counted and expressed as a percentage of adult cells. The test is labor intensive. Moreover, it may be less accurate in two situations: (1) cases of maternal hemoglobinopathy in which maternal red cells carry excess fetal hemoglobin and (2) cases near or at term, at which time the fetus has already started to produce hemoglobin A.

The hemorrhaged fetal blood volume is calculated from the Kleihauer-Betke test result using the following formula:

$$\text{Fetal blood volume} = \frac{\text{MBV} \times \text{maternal Hct} \times \%\ \text{fetal cells in KB}}{\text{newborn Hct}}$$

One method is to estimate the maternal blood volume (MBV) as 5000 mL for a normal-size, normotensive women at term. Thus, for 1.7-percent positive KB-stained cells in a woman of average size with a hematocrit of 35 percent giving birth to a term infant weighing 3000 g and whose hematocrit is 50 percent:

$$\text{Fetal blood volume} = \frac{5000 \times 0.35 \times 0.017}{0.5} = 60 \text{ mL}$$

The fetal-placental blood volume at term approximates 125 mL/kg. For this 3000-g fetus, that would equate to 375 mL. Thus, this fetus has lost approximately 15 percent (60 ÷ 375 mL) of the fetal-placental volume. Because the hematocrit is 50 percent in a term fetus, this 60 mL of whole blood represents 30 mL of red cells lost over time into the maternal circulation. This loss should be well tolerated hemodynamically but would require two 300-μg doses of anti-D immunoglobulin to prevent alloimmunization. A more precise method to estimate the maternal blood volume includes a calculation based on the maternal height, weight, and anticipated blood volume increase due to gestational age (Chap. 41, p. 781).

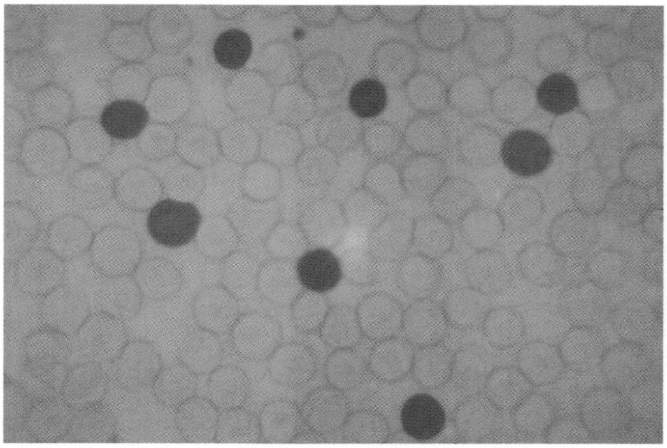

FIGURE 15-4 Kleihauer-Betke test demonstrating massive fetal-to-maternal hemorrhage. After acid-elution treatment, fetal red cells rich in hemoglobin F stain darkly, whereas maternal red cells with only very small amounts of hemoglobin F stain lightly.

Fetomaternal hemorrhage can also be quantified using flow cytometry to measure red cell size (Dziegiel, 2006). This is an automated test and is unaffected by maternal levels of fetal hemoglobin F or by fetal levels of hemoglobin A. In direct comparison studies with the Kleihauer-Betke test, flow cytometry has been reported to be more sensitive and accurate (Chambers, 2012; Fernandes, 2007).

FETAL THROMBOCYTOPENIA

Alloimmune Thrombocytopenia

This condition is also referred to as *neonatal alloimmune thrombocytopenia (NAIT)* or *fetal and neonatal alloimmune thrombocytopenia (FNAIT)*. Alloimmune thrombocytopenia (AIT) is the most common cause of severe thrombocytopenia among term newborns, with a frequency of 1 to 2 per 1000 (Kamphuis, 2010; Pacheco, 2013; Risson, 2012). AIT is caused by maternal alloimmunization to paternally inherited fetal platelet antigens. The resulting maternal antiplatelet antibodies cross the placenta in a manner similar to red cell alloimmunization (p. 306). Unlike *immune thrombocytopenia*, the maternal platelet count is normal. And unlike Rh-D alloimmunization, severe sequelae may affect the *first* at-risk pregnancy.

Maternal platelet alloimmunization is most commonly against human platelet antigen-1a (HPA-1a). This is followed by HPA-5b, HPA-1b, and HPA-3a, and alloimmunization to other antigens accounts for only 1 percent of reported cases. Alloimmunization to HPA-1a accounts for 80 to 90 percent of cases and is associated with the greatest severity (Bussel, 1997; Knight, 2011; Tiller, 2013).

Approximately 85 percent of white individuals are positive for HPA-1a. Two percent are homozygous for HPA-1b and thus are at risk for alloimmunization. But, only 10 percent of homozygous HPA-1b mothers carrying an HPA-1a fetus will produce anti-platelet antibodies. Approximately a third of affected fetuses or neonates will develop severe thrombocytopenia, and 10 to 20 percent with severe thrombocytopenia sustain an intracranial hemorrhage (ICH) (Kamphuis, 2010). As a result, population-based screening studies have identified FNAIT-associated ICH in 1 per 25,000 to 60,000 pregnancies (Kamphuis, 2010; Knight, 2011).

FNAIT has a broad spectrum of presentation. In some, neonatal thrombocytopenia may be an incidental finding or the infant may present with petechiae. Alternatively, the fetus or neonate may develop devastating ICH—often before birth. Of 600 pregnancies with alloimmune thrombocytopenia identified through a large international registry, fetal or neonatal ICH complicated 7 percent of cases (Tiller, 2013). Hemorrhage affected the firstborn child in 60 percent and occurred before 28 weeks' gestation in half. A third of affected children died soon after birth, and 50 percent of survivors had severe neurological disabilities. Bussel and coworkers (1997) evaluated fetal platelet counts before therapy in 107 fetuses with FNAIT. Thrombocytopenia severity was predicted by a prior sibling with perinatal ICH, and 98 percent of cases were identified this way. The initial platelet count was < 20,000/mL in 50 percent. In cases in which the platelet count was initially > 80,000/mL, they noted that it dropped by more than 10,000/mL each week without therapy.

Diagnosis and Management

The diagnosis of alloimmune thrombocytopenia is usually made after the first affected pregnancy in a woman with a normal platelet count whose neonate is found to have unexplained severe thrombocytopenia. Rarely, the diagnosis is ascertained after finding fetal ICH. The condition recurs in 70 to 90 percent of subsequent pregnancies, is often severe, and usually develops earlier with each successive pregnancy. Traditionally, fetal blood sampling was performed to detect fetal thrombocytopenia and tailor therapy, and platelets were transfused if the fetal platelet count was < 50,000/mL. But, concern with procedure-related complications has led experts to recommend abandoning routine fetal platelet sampling in favor of empiric treatment with intravenous immune globulin (IVIG) and prednisone (Berkowitz, 2006; Pacheco, 2011).

Therapy is stratified according to whether a prior affected pregnancy was complicated by perinatal ICH, and if so, at what gestational age (Table 15-3). Pioneering work by Bussel (1996) and Berkowitz (2006) and their colleagues demonstrated the efficacy of such treatment. In one series of 50 pregnancies with fetal thrombocytopenia secondary to FNAIT, IVIG resulted in an increased platelet count of approximately 50,000/mL, and no fetus developed ICH (Bussel, 1996). Among pregnancies at particularly high risk—based on platelet count < 20,000/mL or sibling with FNAIT-associated ICH—the addition of corticosteroids to IVIG increased the platelet count in 80 percent of cases (Berkowitz, 2006). Cesarean delivery has been recommended at or near term. A *noninstrumental* vaginal delivery may be considered only if fetal blood sampling has demonstrated a platelet count > 100,000/mL (Pacheco, 2011).

Additional considerations include risks and costs associated with therapy. Side effects of IVIG may include fever, headache, nausea/vomiting, myalgia, and rash. Maternal hemolysis also has been described (Rink, 2013). As of 2011, costs for various preparations of IVIG were approximately $70 per gram or nearly $10,000 for each weekly 2-g/kg infusion for an average-size pregnant woman (Pacheco, 2011).

TABLE 15-3. Fetal-Neonatal Alloimmune Thrombocytopenia (FNAIT) Treatment Recommendations

Risk Group	Criteria	Suggested Management
1	Prior fetus or newborn with ICH, but no maternal anti-HPA antibody identified	Maternal anti-HPA antibody screening and cross-matching with paternal platelets at 12, 24, and 32 weeks' gestation; no treatment for negative test results
2	Prior fetus or newborn with thrombocytopenia and maternal anti-HPA antibody, but no ICH	Beginning at 20 wks: IVIG 1g/kg/wk and prednisone 0.5 mg/kg/d ***or*** IVIG 2 g/kg/wk. Beginning at 32 weeks: IVIG 2 g/kg/wk and prednisone 0.5 mg/kg/d. Continue until delivery
3	Prior fetus with 3rd-trimester ICH or prior newborn with ICH, and maternal anti-HPA antibody	Beginning at 12 wks: IVIG 1 g/kg/wk. Beginning at 20 wks: either increase IVIG to 2 g/kg/wk ***or*** add prednisone 0.5 mg/kg/d. Beginning at 28 wks: IVIG 2 g/kg/wk ***and*** prednisone 0.5 mg/kg/d. Continue until delivery
4	Prior fetus with ICH before the 3rd trimester and maternal anti-HPA antibody	Beginning at 12 wks: IVIG 2 g/kg/wk. Beginning at 20 wks: add prednisone 1 mg/kg/d. Continue both until delivery

HPA = human platelet antigen; ICH = intracerebral hemorrhage; IVIG = intravenous immunoglobulin G.
Adapted from Pacheco, 2011.

Immune Thrombocytopenia

In pregnant women with immune thrombocytopenia (ITP), autoimmune antiplatelet IgG antibodies may cross the placenta and cause fetal thrombocytopenia. Maternal ITP is discussed in Chapter 56 (p. 1114). Fetal thrombocytopenia is usually mild. However, neonatal platelet levels may fall rapidly after birth and reach a nadir at 48 to 72 hours of life. Neither the maternal platelet count or identification of antiplatelet antibodies, nor treatment with corticosteroids is predictive of fetal or neonatal platelet counts. Importantly, fetal platelet counts are usually adequate to allow vaginal delivery without an increased risk of ICH. Fetal bleeding complications are considered rare, and fetal blood sampling is not recommended (Neunert, 2011). Delivery mode is based on standard obstetrical indications.

HYDROPS FETALIS

The term *hydrops* refers to excessive accumulation of serous fluid in the body, and strictly defined, *hydrops fetalis* is edema of the fetus. Traditionally, the diagnosis was made after delivery of a massively edematous neonate, often stillborn (Fig. 15-5). With sonography, hydrops has become a prenatal diagnosis. It is defined as two or more fetal effusions—pleural, pericardial, or ascites—or one effusion plus anasarca. With condition progression, edema is invariably a component, often accompanied by placentomegaly and hydramnios. Hydrops may result from a wide range of conditions with varying pathophysiologies, each with the potential to make the fetus severely ill. It is divided into two categories. If found in association with red cell alloimmunization, it is termed *immune*, otherwise, it is *nonimmune*.

Immune Hydrops

The incidence of immune hydrops has dramatically decreased with the advent of anti-D immune globulin, MCA Doppler studies for detection of severe anemia, and prompt fetal transfusion when needed. Only an estimated 10 percent of hydrops cases are caused by red cell alloimmunization (Bellini, 2009, 2012; Santolaya, 1992).

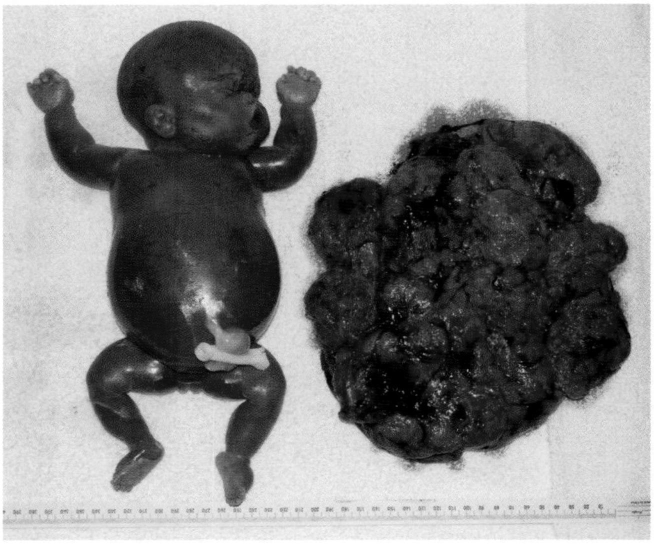

FIGURE 15-5 Hydropic, macerated stillborn infant and characteristically large placenta. The etiology was B19 parvovirus infection. (Photograph contributed by Dr. April Bleich.)

The pathophysiology underlying hydrops remains unknown. Immune hydrops is postulated to share several physiological abnormalities with nonimmune hydrops. As shown in Figure 15-6, these include decreased colloid oncotic pressure, increased hydrostatic (or central venous) pressure, and increased vascular permeability. Immune hydrops results from transplacental passage of maternal antibodies that destroy fetal red cells. Resultant anemia stimulates marrow erythroid hyperplasia and extramedullary hematopoiesis in the spleen and liver. The latter likely causes portal hypertension and impaired hepatic protein synthesis, which decreases plasma oncotic pressure (Nicolaides, 1985). Fetal anemia also may raise central venous pressure (Weiner, 1989). Finally, tissue hypoxia from anemia may increase capillary permeability, such that fluid collects in the fetal thorax, abdominal cavity, and/or subcutaneous tissue.

The degree of anemia in immune hydrops is typically severe. Nicolaides and associates (1988) reported that the hemoglobin concentration was 7 to 10 g/dL below the normal mean for gestational age in a cohort of 48 fetuses with immune hydrops. Similarly, in a series of 70 pregnancies with fetal anemia from red cell alloimmunization, Mari and coworkers (2000) found that all those with immune hydrops had hemoglobin values *below 5 g/dL*. As discussed on page 310, immune hydrops is treated with fetal blood transfusions (van Kamp, 2001).

Nonimmune Hydrops

Currently, nearly 90 percent of cases of hydrops are nonimmune (Bellini, 2009, 2012; Santolaya, 1992). The prevalence estimate is 1 per 1500 second-trimester pregnancies (Heinonen, 2000). The number of specific disorders that can lead to nonimmune hydrops is extensive. Etiologies and the proportion of births within each hydrops category from a review of more than 5400 affected pregnancies are summarized in Table 15-4. A cause is identified in at least 60 percent prenatally and in more than 80 percent postnatally (Bellini, 2009; Santo, 2011). As shown in Figure 15-6, there are several different pathophysiological processes proposed to account for the final common pathway of hydrops fetalis.

Importantly, the etiology of nonimmune hydrops varies according to when in gestation it is identified. Of those diagnosed prenatally, aneuploidy accounts for approximately 20 percent, cardiovascular abnormalities for 15 percent, and infections for 14 percent—the most common of these being parvovirus B19 (Santo, 2011). Overall, only 40 percent of pregnancies with nonimmune hydrops result in a liveborn neonate. For these, the neonatal survival rate is only about 50 percent. Sohan and colleagues (2001) reviewed 87 pregnancies with hydrops and found that 45 percent of those diagnosed before 24 weeks' gestation had a chromosomal abnormality. The most common was 45, X—*Turner syndrome* (Chap. 10, p. 205), and in such cases, the survival rate was < 5 percent. If hydrops is detected in the first trimester, the aneuploidy risk is nearly 50 percent, and most have cystic hygromas (Fig. 10-16, p. 206) (Has, 2001).

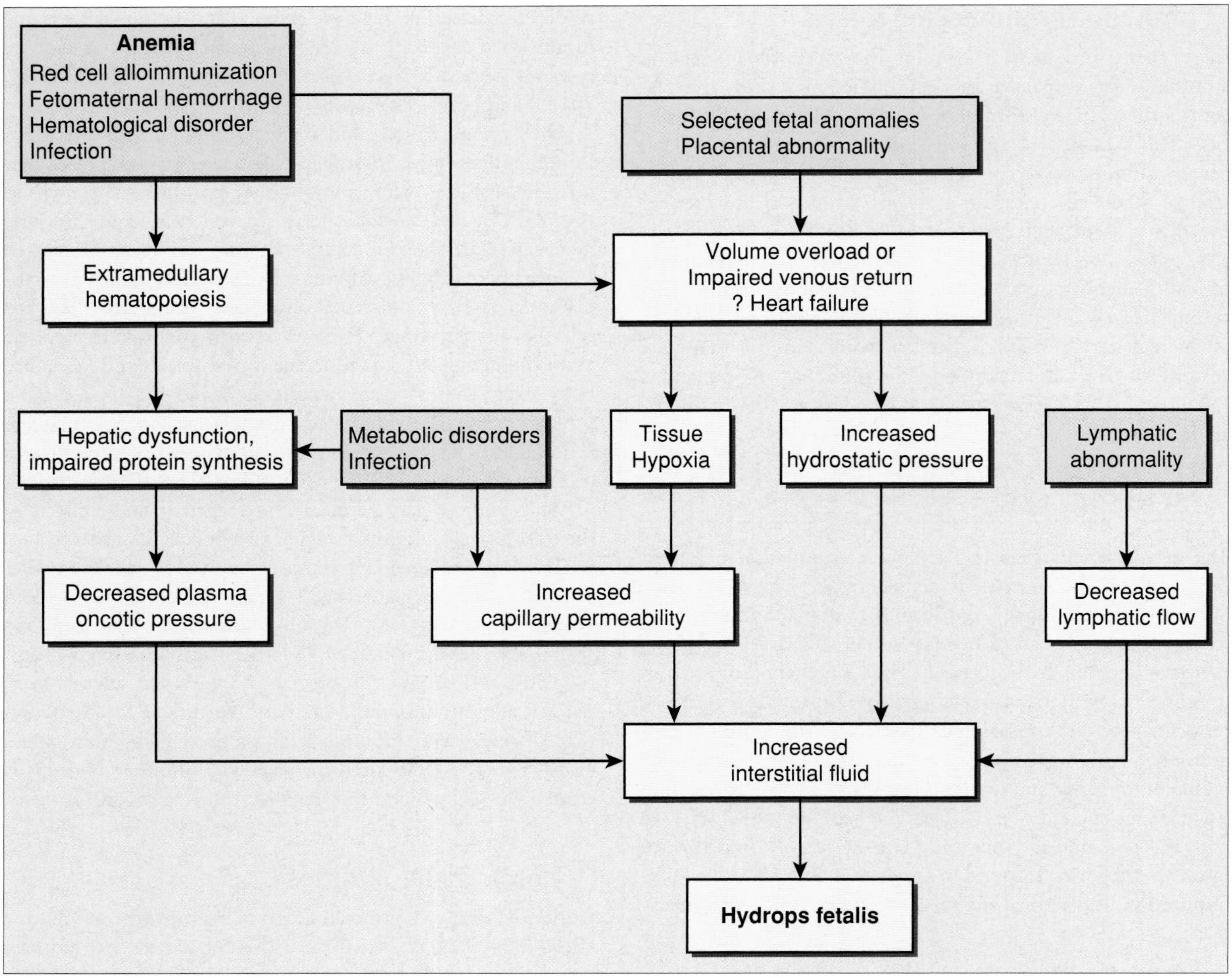

FIGURE 15-6 Proposed pathogenesis of immune and nonimmune hydrops fetalis. (Adapted from Bellini, 2009; Lockwood, 2009.)

Thus, the prognosis of nonimmune hydrops is guarded but is heavily dependent on etiology. In large series from Thailand and Southern China, α_4-thalassemia is the predominant cause of nonimmune hydrops, accounting for 30 to 50 percent of cases and conferring an extremely poor prognosis (Liao, 2007; Ratanasiri, 2009; Suwanrath-Kengpol, 2005). In contrast, Sohan and associates (2001) found that treatable causes of nonimmune hydrops—parvovirus, chylothorax, and tachyarrhythmias—each comprised about 10 percent of cases, and with fetal therapy, two thirds of fetuses with these etiologies survived.

Diagnostic Evaluation

Hydrops is readily detected sonographically. As noted, two effusions or one effusion plus anasarca are required for diagnosis. Edema may be particularly prominent around the scalp, or equally obvious around the trunk and extremities. Effusions are visible as fluid outlining the lungs, heart, or abdominal viscera (Fig. 15-7).

In many cases, targeted sonographic and laboratory evaluation will identify the underlying cause of fetal hydrops. These include cases due to fetal anemia, arrhythmia, structural abnormality, aneuploidy, placental abnormality, or complications of monochorionic twinning. Depending on the circumstances, initial evaluation includes the following:

1. Indirect Coombs test for alloimmunization
2. Targeted sonographic fetal and placental examination, including:
   - A detailed anatomic survey to assess for the structural abnormalities listed in Table 15-4
   - MCA Doppler velocimetry to assess for fetal anemia
   - Fetal echocardiography with M-mode evaluation
3. Amniocentesis for fetal karyotype and for B19 parvovirus, cytomegalovirus, and toxoplasmosis testing as discussed in Chapter 64. Consideration of chromosomal microarray analysis if fetal anomalies are present
4. Consideration of Kleihauer-Betke test for fetomaternal hemorrhage if anemia is suspected, depending on findings and test results
5. Consideration of testing for α-thalassemia and/or inborn errors of metabolism.

Isolated Effusion or Edema. Although one effusion or anasarca alone is not diagnostic for hydrops, the above evaluation

TABLE 15-4. Some Etiologies of Nonimmune Hydrops Fetalis

Category	Percent[a]
Cardiovascular	22
Structural defects: Ebstein anomaly, Fallot tetralogy with absent pulmonary valve, hypoplastic left or right heart, premature closure of ductus arteriosus, arteriovenous malformation (vein of Galen aneurysm)	
Cardiomyopathies	
Tachyarrhythmias	
Bradycardia, as may occur in heterotaxy syndrome with endocardial cushion defect or in maternal SLE with anti-Ro/La antibodies	
Chromosomal	13
Turner syndrome (45,X), triploidy, trisomies 21, 18, and 13	
Hematological	10
Hemoglobinopathies, such as α4-thalassemia	
Erythrocyte enzyme and membrane disorders	
Erythrocyte aplasia/dyserythropoiesis	
Decreased erythrocyte production (myeloproliferative disorders)	
Fetomaternal hemorrhage	
Infections	7
Parvovirus B19, syphilis, cytomegalovirus, toxoplasmosis, rubella, enterovirus, varicella, herpes simplex, coxsackievirus, listeriosis, leptospirosis, Chagas disease, Lyme disease	
Thoracic Abnormalities	6
Cystic adenomatoid malformation	
Pulmonary sequestration	
Diaphragmatic hernia	
Hydro/chylothorax	
Congenital high airway obstruction sequence	
Mediastinal tumors	
Skeletal dysplasia with very small thorax	
Lymphatic Abnormalities	6
Cystic hygroma, systemic lymphangiectasis, pulmonary lymphangiectasis	
Placental, Twin, and Cord Abnormalities	6
Placental chorioangioma, twin-twin transfusion syndrome, twin reversed arterial perfusion sequence, twin anemia polycythemia sequence, cord vessel thrombosis	
Kidney and Urinary Tract	2
Kidney malformations	
Bladder outlet obstructions	
Congenital (Finnish) nephrosis, Bartter syndrome, mesoblastic nephroma	
Syndromic	4
Arthrogryposis multiplex congenita, lethal multiple pterygium, congenital lymphedema, myotonic dystrophy type I, Neu-Laxova, Noonan, and Pena-Shokeir syndromes	
Other Rare Disorders	6
Inborn errors of metabolism: Gaucher disease, galactosialidosis, GM_1 gangliosidosis, sialidosis, mucopolysaccharidoses, mucolipidoses	
Tumors: sacrococcygeal teratoma, hemangioendothelioma with Kassabach-Merritt syndrome	
Idiopathic	18

[a]Percentages reflect the proportion within each category from a systematic review of more than 5400 pregnancies with nonimmune hydrops.
SLE = systemic lupus erythematosus.
Modified from Bellini, 2009.

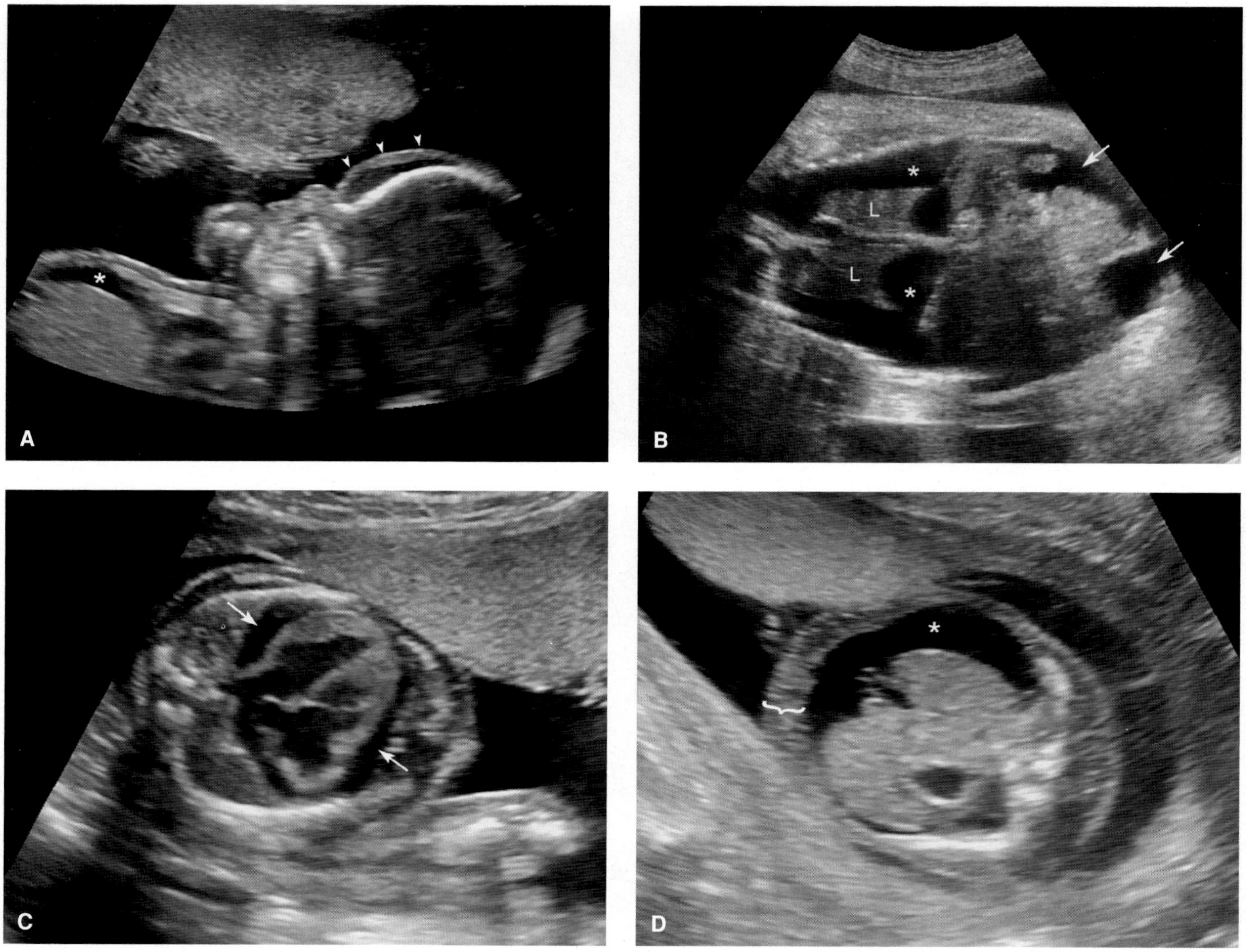

FIGURE 15-7 Hydropic features. **A.** This profile of a 23-week fetus with nonimmune hydrops secondary to B19 parvovirus infection depicts scalp edema (*arrowheads*) and ascites (*). **B.** In this coronal image, prominent pleural effusions (*) outline the lungs (*L*). This 34-week fetus had hydrops secondary to an arteriovenous malformation in the brain, known as a vein of Galen aneurysm. Fetal ascites is also present (*arrows*), as is anasarca. **C.** This axial (transverse) image depicts a pericardial effusion (*arrows*) in a 23-week fetus with hydrops from B19 parvovirus infection. The degree of cardiomegaly is impressive, and the ventricular hypertrophy raises concern for myocarditis, which can accompany parvovirus infection. **D.** This axial (transverse) image depicts fetal ascites (*) in a 15-week fetus with hydrops secondary to large cystic hygromas. Anasarca is also seen (*brackets*).

should be considered if these are encountered, as hydrops may develop. For example, an isolated pericardial effusion may be the initial finding in fetal B19 parvovirus infection (Chap. 64, p. 1244). An isolated pleural effusion may represent a chylothorax, which is amenable to prenatal diagnosis, and for which fetal therapy may be lifesaving if hydrops develops (Chap. 16, p. 329). Isolated ascites also may be the initial finding in fetal B19 parvovirus infection or it may result from a gastrointestinal abnormality such as meconium peritonitis. Finally, isolated edema, particularly involving the upper torso or the dorsum of the hands and feet, may be found in Turner or Noonan syndrome or may represent congenital lymphedema syndrome (Chap. 13, p. 264).

Mirror Syndrome

An association between fetal hydrops and development of maternal edema in which the fetus *mirrors* the mother is attributed to Ballantyne. He called the condition *triple edema* because the fetus, mother, and placenta all became edematous. The etiology of the hydrops is not related to development of mirror syndrome. It has been associated with hydrops from Rh D alloimmunization, twin-twin transfusion syndrome, placental chorioangioma, and with fetal cystic hygroma, Ebstein anomaly, sacrococcygeal teratoma, chylothorax, bladder outlet obstruction, supraventricular tachycardia, vein of Galen aneurysm, and various congenital infections (Braun, 2010).

In a review of more than 50 cases of mirror syndrome, Braun and coworkers (2010) found that approximately 90 percent of women had edema, 60 percent had hypertension, 40 percent had proteinuria, 20 percent had liver enzyme elevation, and nearly 15 percent had headache and visual disturbances. Based on these findings, it is reasonable to consider mirror syndrome a form of severe preeclampsia (Espinoza, 2006; Midgley, 2000). Others, however, have suggested that it is a separate disease process with hemodilution rather than hemoconcentration (Carbillon, 1997; Livingston, 2007). There have been recent reports describing the same imbalance of angiogenic and antiangiogenic factors observed with preeclampsia and thus supporting a common pathophysiology (Espinoza, 2006; Goa, 2013; Llurba, 2012). These findings, which include elevated concentrations of soluble fms-like tyrosine kinase-1 (sFlt-1), decreased placental growth factor (PlGF) levels, and elevation of soluble vascular endothelial growth factor receptor-1 (sVEGFR-1) concentrations, are discussed further Chapter 40 (p. 735).

In most cases with mirror syndrome, prompt delivery is indicated and followed by resolution of maternal edema and other findings in approximately 9 days (Braun, 2010). There are, however, isolated cases of fetal anemia, supraventricular tachycardia, hydrothorax, and bladder outlet obstruction in which successful fetal treatment resulted in resolution of both fetal hydrops and maternal mirror syndrome (Goa, 2013; Livingston, 2007; Llurba, 2012; Midgley, 2000). In two of these cases, normalization of the angiogenic imbalance also occurred following fetal transfusion for B19 parvovirus infection (Goa, 2013; Llurba, 2012). Fetal therapy for these conditions is reviewed in Chapter 16. Given the parallels to severe preeclampsia, delaying delivery to effect fetal therapy should be considered only with caution. If the maternal condition deteriorates, delivery is recommended.

REFERENCES

American Academy of Pediatrics and American College of Obstetricians and Gynecologists: Guidelines for Perinatal Care. 7th ed. Washington, 2012

American College of Obstetricians and Gynecologists: Carrier screening for fragile X syndrome. Committee Opinion No. 469, October 2010

American College of Obstetricians and Gynecologists: Management of alloimmunization during pregnancy. Practice Bulletin No. 75, August 2006, Reaffirmed 2012

Bellini C, Hennekam RCM: Non-immune hydrops fetalis: a short review of etiology and pathophysiology. Am J Med Genet 158A(3):597, 2012

Bellini C, Hennekam RC, Fulcheri E, et al: Etiology of nonimmune hydrops fetalis: a systematic review. Am J Med Genet A 149A(5):844, 2009

Berkowitz RL, Kolb EA, McFarland JG, et al: Parallel randomized trials of risk-based therapy for fetal alloimmune thrombocytopenia. Obstet Gynecol 107(1):91, 2006

Bowman J: Rh-immunoglobulin: Rh prophylaxis. Best Pract Res Clin Haematol 19(1):27, 2006

Bowman JM: Controversies in Rh prophylaxis: who needs Rh immune globulin and when should it be given? Am J Obstet Gynecol 151:289, 1985

Bowman JM: The prevention of Rh immunization. Transfus Med Rev 2:129, 1988

Braun T, Brauer M, Fuchs I, et al: Mirror syndrome: a systematic review of fetal associated conditions, maternal presentation, and perinatal outcome. Fetal Diagn Ther 27(4):191, 2010

Bussel JB, Berkowitz RL, Lynch L, et al: Antenatal management of alloimmune thrombocytopenia with intravenous gamma-globulin: a randomized trial of the addition of low-dose steroid to intravenous gamma-globulin. Am J Obstet Gynecol 174(5):1414, 1996

Bussel JB, Zabusky MR, Berkowitz RL, et al: Fetal alloimmune thrombocytopenia. N Engl J Med 337:22, 1997

Canlorde G, Mace G, Cortey A, et al: Management of very early fetal anemia resulting from red-cell alloimmunization before 20 weeks of gestation. Obstet Gynecol 118(6):1323, 2011

Carbillon L, Oury JF, Guerin JM, et al: Clinical biological features of Ballantyne syndrome and the role of placental hydrops. Obstet Gynecol Surv 52(5):310, 1997

Chambers E, Davies L, Evans S, et al: Comparison of haemoglobin F detection by the acid elution test, flow cytometry and high-performance liquid chromatography in maternal blood samples analysed for fetomaternal haemorrhage. Transfus Med 22(3):199, 2012

Choavaratana R, Uer-Areewong S, Makanantakocol S: Fetomaternal transfusion in normal pregnancy and during delivery. J Med Assoc Thai 80:96, 1997

Daniels G: Variants of RhD—current testing and clinical consequences. Br J Haematol 161(4):461, 2013

de Almeida V, Bowman JM: Massive fetomaternal hemorrhage: Manitoba experience. Obstet Gynecol 83:323, 1994

Dziegiel MH, Nielsen LK, Berkowicz A: Detecting fetomaternal hemorrhage by flow cytometry. Curr Opin Hematol 13(6):490, 2006

Eichbaum M, Gast AS, Sohn C: Doppler sonography of the fetal middle cerebral artery in the management of massive fetomaternal hemorrhage. Fetal Diagn Ther 21(4):334, 2006

Espinoza J, Romero R, Nien JK, et al: A role of the anti-angiogenic factor sVEGFR-1 in the "mirror syndrome" (Ballantyne's syndrome). J Matern Fetal Neonatal Med 19(10):607, 2006

Fernandes BJ, von Dadelszen P, Fazal I, et al: Flow cytometric assessment of feto-maternal hemorrhage; a comparison with Betke-Kleihauer. Prenat Diagn 27(7):641, 2007

Fox C, Martin W, Somerset DA, et al: Early intraperitoneal transfusion and adjuvant maternal immunoglobulin therapy in the treatment of severe red cell alloimmunization prior to fetal intravascular transfusion. Fetal Diagn Ther 23(2):159, 2008

Garratty G, Glynn SA, McEntire R, et al: ABO and Rh(D) phenotype frequencies of different racial/ethnic groups in the United States. Transfusion 44(5):703, 2004

Geifman-Holtzman O, Grotegut CA, Gaughan JP: Diagnostic accuracy of noninvasive fetal Rh genotyping from maternal blood—a meta-analysis. Am J Obstet Gynecol 195:1163, 2006

Geifman-Holtzman O, Wojtowycz M, Kosmas E, et al: Female alloimmunization with antibodies known to cause hemolytic disease. Obstet Gynecol 89:272, 1997

Giacoia GP. Severe fetomaternal hemorrhage: a review. Obstet Gynecol Surv 52:372, 1997

Giannina G, Moise KJ Jr, Dorman K: A simple method to estimate the volume for fetal intravascular transfusion. Fetal Diagn Ther 13:94, 1998

Goa S, Mimura K, Kakigano A, et al: Normalisation of angiogenic imbalance after intra-uterine transfusion for mirror syndrome caused by parvovirus B19. Fetal Diagn Ther 34(3):176, 2013

Goodspeed TA, Allyse M, Sayres LC, et al: Translating cell-free fetal DNA technology: structural lessons from non-invasive RhD blood typing. Trends Biotechnol 31(1):7, 2013

Hackney DN, Knudtson EJ, Rossi KQ, et al: Management of pregnancies complicated by anti-c isoimmunization. Obstet Gynecol 103:24, 2004

Hartung J, Chaoui R, Bollmann R: Nonimmune hydrops from fetomaternal hemorrhage treated with serial fetal intravascular transfusion. Obstet Gynecol 96(5 pt 2):844, 2000

Has R: Non-immune hydrops fetalis in the first trimester: a review of 30 cases. Clin Exp Obstet Gynecol 28(3):187, 2001

Heinonen S, Ruynamen M, Kirkinen P: Etiology and outcome of second trimester nonimmunological fetal hydrops. Scand J Obstet Gynecol 79:15, 2000

Howard H, Martlew V, McFadyen I, et al: Consequences for fetus and neonate of maternal red cell allo-immunization. Arch Dis Child Fetal Neonat Ed 78:F62, 1998

Howe DT, Michaitidis GD: Intraperitoneal transfusion in severe, early-onset Rh isoimmunization. Obstet Gynecol 110:880, 2007

Kamphuis MM, Paridaans N, Porcelijn L, et al: Screening in pregnancy for fetal or neonatal alloimmune thrombocytopenia: systematic review. BJOG 117(11):1335, 2010

Kleihauer B, Braun H, Betke K: Demonstration of fetal hemoglobin in erythrocytes of a blood smear. Klin Wochenschr 35(12):637, 1957

Knight M, Pierce M, Allen D, et al: The incidence and outcomes of fetomaternal alloimmune thrombocytopenia: a UK national study using three data sources. Br J Haematol 152(4):460, 2011

Koelewijn JM, Vrijkotte TGM, van der Schoot CE, et al: Effect of screening for red cell antibodies, other than anti-D, to detect hemolytic disease of the fetus and newborn: a population study in the Netherlands. Transfusion 48:941, 2008

Lazar L, Harmath AG, Ban Z, et al: Detection of maternal deoxyribonucleic acid in peripheral blood of premature and mature newborn infants. Prenat Diagn 26(2):168, 2006

Liao C, Wei J, Li Q, et al: Nonimmune hydrops fetalis diagnosed during the second half of pregnancy in Southern China. Fetal Diagn Ther 22(4):302, 2007

Liley AW: Liquor amnii analysis in management of pregnancy complicated by rhesus sensitization. Am J Obstet Gynecol 82:1359, 1961

Lindenburg I, van Kamp I, van Zwet E, et al: Increased perinatal loss after intrauterine transfusion for alloimmune anaemia before 20 weeks of gestation. BJOG 120:847, 2013

Lindenburg IT, Smits-Wintjens VE, van Klink JM, et al: Long-term neurodevelopmental outcome after intrauterine transfusion for hemolytic disease of the fetus/newborn: the LOTUS study. Am J Obstet Gynecol 206:141.e1, 2012
Livingston JC, Malik KM, Crombleholme TM, et al: Mirror syndrome: a novel approach to therapy with fetal peritoneal-amniotic shunt. Obstet Gynecol 110(2 pt 2):540, 2007
Llurba E, Marsal G, Sanchez O, et al: Angiogenic and antiangiogenic factors before and after resolution of maternal mirror syndrome. Ultrasound Obstet Gynecol 40(3):367, 2012
Lockwood CJ, Nadel AS, King ME, et al: A 32-year old pregnant woman with an abnormal fetal ultrasound study. Case 16-2009. N Engl J Med 360(21):2225, 2009
MacKenzie IZ, Roseman F, Findlay J, et al: The kinetics of routine antenatal prophylactic intramuscular injections of polyclonal anti-D immunoglobulin. BJOG 113:97, 2006
Mari G, Deter RL, Carpenter RL, et al: Noninvasive diagnosis by Doppler ultrasonography of fetal anemia due to maternal red-cell alloimmunization. N Engl J Med 342:9, 2000
Martin JA, Hamilton BE, Sutton PD, et al: Births: final data for 2003. Natl Vital Stat Rep 54(2):1, 2005
Midgley DY, Hardrug K: The Mirror syndrome. Eur J Obstet Gynecol Reprod Biol 8:201, 2000
Minon JM, Gerard C, Senterre JM, et al: Routine fetal RHD genotyping with maternal plasma: a four-year experience in Belgium. Transfusion 48(2):373, 2008
Moise KJ: Fetal anemia due to non-Rhesus-D red-cell alloimmunization. Semin Fetal Neonatal Med 13(4):207, 2008a
Moise KJ Jr: Management of rhesus alloimmunization in pregnancy. Obstet Gynecol 112:164, 2008b
Moise KJ, Argoti PS: Management and prevention of red cell alloimmunization in pregnancy. A systematic review. Obstet Gynecol 120(5):1132, 2012
Ness PM, Baldwin ML, Niebyl JR: Clinical high-risk designation does not predict excess fetal–maternal hemorrhage. Am J Obstet Gynecol 156:154, 1987
Neunert C, Lim W, Crowther M, et al: The American Society of Hematology 2011 evidence-based practice guideline for immune thrombocytopenia. Blood 117(16):4190, 2011
Nicolaides KH, Clewell WH, Mibashan RS, et al: Fetal haemoglobin measurement in the assessment of red cell isoimmunization. Lancet 1:1073, 1988
Nicolaides KH, Warenski JC, Rodeck CH: The relationship of fetal plasma protein concentration and hemoglobin level to the development of hydrops in rhesus isoimmunization. Am J Obstet Gynecol 152:341, 1985
Oepkes D, Seaward PG, Vandenbussche FP, et al: Doppler ultrasonography versus amniocentesis to predict fetal anemia. N Engl J Med 355: 156, 2006
Pacheco LD, Berkowitz RL, Moise KJ, et al: Fetal and neonatal alloimmune thrombocytopenia. A management algorithm based on risk stratification. Obstet Gynecol 118(5):1157, 2011
Queenan JT, Thomas PT, Tomai TP, et al: Deviation in amniotic fluid optical density at a wavelength of 450 nm in Rh isoimmunized pregnancies from 14 to 40 weeks' gestation: a proposal for clinical management. Am J Obstet Gynecol 168:1370, 1993
Ratanasiri T, Komwilaisak R, Sittivech A, et al: Incidence, causes, and pregnancy outcomes of hydrops fetalis at Srinagarind Hospital, 1996–2005: a 10-year review. J Med Assoc Thai 92(5):594, 2009
Rink BD, Gonik B, Chmait RH, et al: Maternal hemolysis after intravenous immunoglobulin treatment in fetal and neonatal alloimmune thrombocytopenia. Obstet Gynecol 121(2):471, 2013
Risson DC, Davies MW, Williams BA: Review of neonatal alloimmune thrombocytopenia. J Pediatr Child Health 48(9):816, 2012
Rubod C, Deruelle P, Le Goueff F, et al: Long-term prognosis for infants after massive fetomaternal hemorrhage. Obstet Gynecol 110(2 pt 1), 2007
Santo S, Mansour S, Thilaganathan B, et al: Prenatal diagnosis of non-immune hydrops fetalis: what do we tell the parents? Prenat Diagn 31:186, 2011
Santolaya J, Alley D, Jaffe R, et al: Antenatal classification of hydrops fetalis. Obstet Gynecol 79:256, 1992
Scheier M, Hernandez-Andrade E, Fonseca EB, et al: Prediction of severe fetal anemia in red blood cell alloimmunization after previous intrauterine transfusion. Am J Obstet Gynecol 195 (6):1550, 2006
Snyder EL: Prevention of hemolytic disease of the newborn due to anti-D. Prenatal/perinatal testing and Rh immune globulin administration. Am Assoc Blood Banks Assoc Bull 98:1 (Level III), 1998
Sohan K, Carroll SG, De La Fuente S, et al: Analysis of outcome in hydrops fetalis in relation to gestational age at diagnosis, cause, and treatment. Acta Obstet Gynecol Scand 80(8):726, 2001
Storry JR, Castilho L, Daniels G, et al: International Society of Blood Transfusion Working Party on red cell immunogenics and blood group terminology: Berlin Report. Vox Sanguinis 101:77, 2011
Suwanrath-Kengpol C, Kor-anantakul O, Suntharasaj T, et al: Etiology and outcome of non-immune hydrops fetalis in southern Thailand. Gynecol Obstet Invest 59(3):134, 2005
Szczepura A, Osipenko L, Freeman K. A new fetal RHD genotyping test: costs and benefits of mass testing to target antenatal anti-D prophylaxis in England and Wales. BMC Pregnancy Childbirth 11:5, 2011
Tannirandorn Y, Rodeck CH: New approaches in the treatment of haemolytic disease of the fetus. Ballieres Clin Haematol 3(2):289, 1990
Tiller H, Kamphuis MM, Flodmark O, et al: Fetal intracranial hemorrhages caused by fetal and neonatal alloimmune thrombocytopenia: an observational cohort study of 43 cases from an international multicentre registry. BMJ 3:e002490, 2013
Tynan JA, Angkachatchai V, Ehrich M, et al: Multiplexed analysis of circulating cell-free nucleic acids for noninvasive prenatal diagnostic RHD testing. Am J Obstet Gynecol 204(3):251.e1, 2011
Van den Veyver IB, Moise KJ: Fetal RhD typing by polymerase chain reaction in pregnancies complicated by rhesus alloimmunization. Obstet Gynecol 88:1061, 1996
Van Kamp IL, Klumper FJ, Bakkum RS, et al: The severity of immune fetal hydrops is predictive of fetal outcome after intrauterine treatment. Am J Obstet Gynecol 185:668, 2001
Van Kamp IL, Klumper FJ, Oepkes D, et al: Complications of intrauterine intravascular transfusion for fetal anemia due to maternal red-cell alloimmunization. Am J Obstet Gynecol 192:171, 2005
van Wamelen DJ, Klumper FJ, de Haas M, et al: Obstetric history and antibody titer in estimating severity of Kell alloimmunization in pregnancy. Obstet Gynecol 109:1093, 2007
Weiner CP, Pelzer GD, Heilskov J, et al: The effect of intravascular transfusion on umbilical venous pressure in anemic fetuses with and without hydrops. Am J Obstet Gynecol 161:1498, 1989
Weinstein L: Irregular antibodies causing hemolytic disease of the newborn: a continuing problem. Clin Obstet Gynecol 25(2):321, 1982
Woelfer B, Schuchter K, Janisiw M, et al: Postdelivery levels of anti-D IgG prophylaxis in mothers depend on maternal body weight. Transfusion 44:512, 2004
Wylie BJ, D'Alton ME: Fetomaternal hemorrhage. Obstet Gynecol 115(5): 1039, 2010
Zimmerman R, Carpenter RJ Jr, Durig P, et al: Longitudinal measurement of peak systolic velocity in the fetal middle cerebral artery for monitoring pregnancies complicated by red cell alloimmunization: a prospective multicenter trial with intention-to-treat. BJOG 109(7):746, 2002
Zipursky A: Prevention of vitamin K deficiency bleeding in newborns. Br J Haematol 104:430, 1999

CHAPTER 16

Fetal Therapy

Interventions developed during the past three decades have dramatically altered the course of selected fetal anomalies and conditions. Reviewed in this chapter are fetal disorders amenable to treatment with either maternal medication or surgical procedures. The treatment of fetal anemia and thrombocytopenia is reviewed in Chapter 15, and the treatment of some fetal infections is discussed in Chapters 64 and 65.

MEDICAL THERAPY

Fetal pharmacotherapy, administered to the mother and transported transplacentally, can be used to treat an array of serious conditions. Two well-described examples are *fetal tachyarrhythmia* treatment with medications such as digoxin, and corticosteroid therapy to prevent virilization of female fetuses with *congenital adrenal hyperplasia.* More recently, a course of corticosteroid therapy—the same used to promote lung maturity before preterm birth—has been used to stabilize the growth of large fetal lung masses and avoid fetal surgery.

Arrhythmias

Fetal cardiac rhythm disturbances may be broadly categorized as *tachyarrhythmias,* heart rates > 180 beats per minute (bpm); *bradyarrhythmia,* heart rate < 110 bpm; and ectopy, typically premature atrial contractions. Fetal M-mode sonography (p. 322) should be performed to determine the atrial and ventricular rate to clarify the relationship between atrial and ventricular beats, thereby diagnosing the rhythm disturbance type.

Premature Atrial Contractions

This is by far the most common arrhythmia. Premature atrial contractions are identified in 1 to 2 percent of pregnancies and are generally a benign finding (Hahurij, 2011; Strasburger, 2010). They represent immaturity of the cardiac conduction system and typically resolve either with advancing gestation or in the neonatal period. Although they may be conducted, they are more commonly blocked, and with handheld Doppler or fetoscope, they sound like a dropped beat. Premature atrial contractions are not associated with major structural cardiac abnormalities, but they sometimes occur with an atrial septal aneurysm. As shown in Figure 10-24 (p. 212), M-mode evaluation demonstrates that the dropped beat is a compensatory pause following the premature atrial contraction. They may occur as frequently as every other beat, known as *blocked atrial bigeminy.* This results in an auscultated fetal ventricular rate as low as 60 to 80 beats per minute. Unlike other causes of bradycardia, this carries a benign prognosis and does not require treatment (Strasburger, 2010).

Approximately 2 percent of fetuses with premature atrial contractions are later identified to develop *supraventricular tachycardia (SVT)* and require urgent treatment to prevent development of hydrops (Copel, 2000; Srinivasan, 2008). Given the importance of identifying such tachycardia, the fetus with premature atrial contractions is often monitored with heart rate assessment every 1 to 2 weeks until ectopy resolution.

Tachyarrhythmias

The two most common are *supraventricular tachycardia* and *atrial flutter.* SVT is characterized by an abrupt increase in the fetal heart rate to 180 to 300 bpm with 1:1 atrioventricular concordance. The typical range is 200 to 240 bpm. SVT may develop secondary to an ectopic focus or to an accessory atrioventricular pathway leading to a reentrant tachycardia. Atrial flutter is characterized by a much higher atrial rate—300 to 500 bpm. There are varying degrees of atrioventricular block, such that the ventricular rate may range from below normal to approximately 250 bpm (Fig. 16-1). In contrast, fetal *sinus tachycardia* typically presents with a gradual heart rate rise to a rate slightly above normal. There is often a readily discernible cause such as maternal fever or hyperthyroidism, or rarely, fetal anemia or infection.

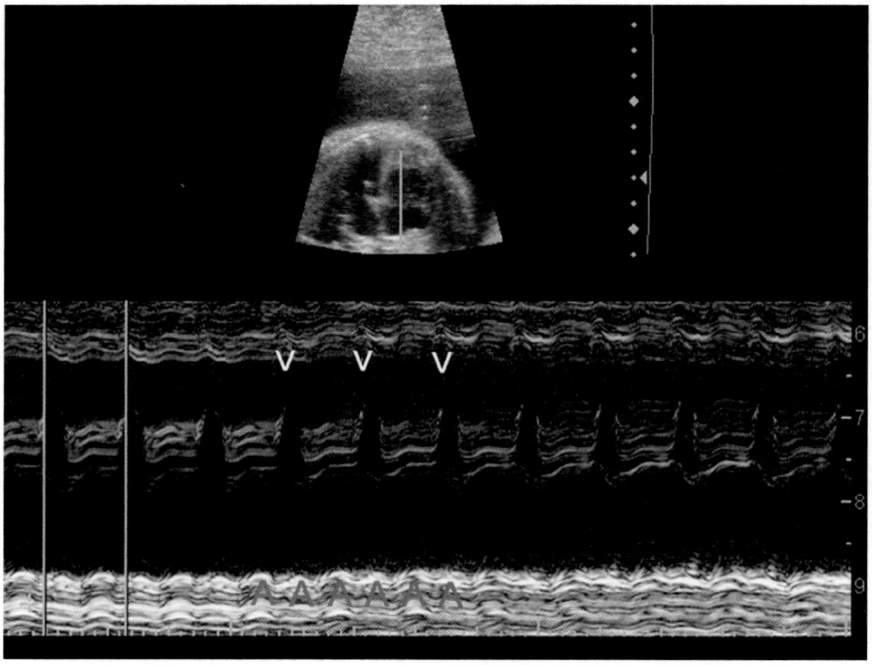

FIGURE 16-1 Atrial flutter. In this M-mode image at 28 weeks, calipers mark the ventricular rate, which is approximately 225 bpm. There are two atrial beats (*A*) for each ventricular beat (*V*), such that the atrial rate is approximately 450 bpm with 2:1 atrioventricular block.

If a tachyarrhythmia is identified, it is important to determine whether it is *sustained*—defined as present for at least 50 percent of the time. It may be necessary to monitor the fetal heart rate for 12 to 24 hours upon initial detection, and then periodically to reassess (Srinivasan, 2008). Nonsustained or intermittent tachyarrhythmias *generally* do not require treatment, provided that fetal surveillance is reassuring.

Sustained fetal tachyarrhythmia with ventricular rates exceeding 200 bpm impairs ventricular filling to such a degree that the risk of hydrops is significant. With atrial flutter, lack of coordinated atrioventricular contractions may further compound this risk. Maternal administration of antiarrhythmic agents that cross the placenta may convert the rhythm to normal or lower the baseline heart rate to forestall heart failure. Therapy may require dosages at the upper end of the therapeutic adult range. A maternal electrocardiogram should be performed before and during therapy. If the fetus has become hydropic, the drug may need to be administered directly via the umbilical vein (Mangione, 1999; Simpson, 2006).

Various antiarrhythmic medications have been used, most commonly digoxin, sotalol (Betapace), flecainide (Tambocor), and procainamide (Pronestyl). Their selection depends on the type of tachyarrhythmia as well as provider familiarity and experience with the drug. Digoxin is usually the first-line agent. Amiodarone (Cordarone) has been associated with fetal and neonatal hypothyroidism, which may be severe (Niinikoski, 2007; Simpson, 2006).

In a review of 485 cases of fetal tachyarrhythmia, hydrops was reported in approximately 40 percent of those with either SVT or atrial flutter (Krapp, 2003). Digoxin was the first-line agent selected in two thirds with either tachyarrhythmia. Treatment was more effective in nonhydropic fetuses than in those in whom hydrops had already developed. With therapy, the neonatal survival rate with either arrhythmia exceeded 90 percent (Krapp, 2003).

Bradyarrhythmia

The most common etiology of pronounced fetal bradycardia is *congenital heart block*. Approximately 50 percent of cases occur in the setting of a structural cardiac abnormality involving the conduction system. These include *heterotaxy*, in particular *left-atrial isomerism*; *endocardial cushion defect*; and *corrected transposition of the great vessels* (Srinivasan, 2008). The prognosis of heart block secondary to a structural cardiac anomaly is extremely poor, and fetal loss rates exceed 80 percent (Glatz, 2008; Strasburger, 2010). In a structurally normal heart, 85 percent of cases of atrioventricular block develop secondary to transplacental passage of maternal anti-SSA/Ro or anti-SSB/La antibodies (Buyon, 2009). Many of these women have, or subsequently develop, systemic lupus erythematosus or another connective-tissue disease (Chap. 59, p. 1172). The risk of third-degree heart block with these antibodies is only 2 to 5 percent, but it may be up to 20 percent if a prior infant has been affected. Immune-mediated congenital heart block confers a mortality rate of 20 to 30 percent, requires permanent pacing in two thirds of surviving children, and also poses a risk for cardiomyopathy (Buyon, 2009). If associated with effusions, bradyarrhythmias, or endocardial fibroelastosis, neonatal status may progressively worsen after birth (Cuneo, 2007).

Research efforts have focused on maternal corticosteroid therapy to reverse fetal heart block or forestall it. Friedman and colleagues (2008, 2009) conducted a prospective multicenter trial of pregnancies with anti-SSA/Ro antibodies—the PR Interval and Dexamethasone (PRIDE) study. Weekly sonography was used to monitor for fetal heart block. If identified, maternal treatment was dexamethasone 4 mg orally daily. There were several important findings. First-degree block was rare and did not generally precede to more advanced block; progression from second- to third-degree block was not prevented with maternal dexamethasone therapy; and third-degree atrioventricular block was *irreversible* (Friedman, 2008, 2009). In rare cases, there was a potential benefit in reversing first-degree atrioventricular block. However, the authors cautioned that there was a need to weigh this potential benefit against the risks of chronic antepartum corticosteroid treatment, including impaired fetal growth (Friedman, 2009).

Maternal terbutaline has also been administered to increase the fetal heart rate in cases with sustained bradycardia of any cause in which the fetal heart rate is ≤ 55 bpm. Cuneo and associates (2007) reported reversal of hydrops with this therapy in a few cases. However, outcomes in those with structural abnormalities remained poor.

Congenital Adrenal Hyperplasia

Several autosomal recessive enzyme deficiencies cause impaired fetal synthesis of cortisol from cholesterol by the adrenal cortex, resulting in congenital adrenal hyperplasia (CAH). This is the most common etiology of androgen excess in females with pseudohermaphroditism (Chap. 7, p. 148). Lack of cortisol stimulates adrenocorticotrophic hormone (ACTH) secretion by the anterior pituitary, and the resulting androstenedione and testosterone overproduction leads to virilization of female fetuses. Sequelae may include formation of labioscrotal folds, development of a urogenital sinus, or even creation of a penile urethra and scrotal sac (Fig. 7-18, p. 149).

More than 90 percent of CAH cases are caused by 21-hydroxylase deficiency, which is found in classic and nonclassic forms. The incidence of classic CAH is approximately 1:15,000 overall and is higher in selected populations. For example, it develops in approximately 1:300 Yupik Eskimos (Nimkarn, 2010). Among those with classic CAH, 75 percent are at risk for *salt-wasting adrenal crises* and require postnatal treatment with mineralocorticoids and glucocorticoids. The remaining 25 percent with classic CAH have the *simple virilizing type* and require glucocorticoid supplementation. Without prompt recognition and treatment, infants with the salt-wasting form can develop hyponatremia, dehydration, hypotension, and cardiovascular collapse. As discussed in Chapter 32 (p. 631), all states mandate newborn screening for CAH.

The efficacy of maternal dexamethasone treatment to suppress fetal androgen overproduction and either obviate or ameliorate virilization of female fetuses has been recognized for nearly 30 years (David, 1984; New, 2012). Prenatal corticosteroid therapy is considered successful in 80 to 85 percent of cases (Miller, 2013; Speiser, 2010). The alternative is consideration of postnatal genitoplasty, a complex and somewhat controversial surgical procedure, which may involve vaginoplasty, clitoroplasty, and labioplasty (Braga, 2009).

If treatment is elected, the typical regimen is oral dexamethasone given to the mother at a dosage of 20 μg/kg/d—up to 1.5 mg per day, divided in three doses. The critical period for external genitalia development is 7 to 12 weeks' gestation. To prevent virilization, treatment should be initiated by 9 weeks, *before it is known whether the fetus is at risk.* Because this is an autosomal recessive condition, affected females comprise only 1 in 8 at-risk conceptions.

Typically, carrier parents are identified after the birth of an affected child. Molecular genetic testing is clinically available for common mutations and deletions of the *CYP21A2* gene, which encodes the 21-hydroxylase enzyme. It is informative in 80 to 98 percent of cases, and for the remainder, gene sequencing may detect rarer alleles (Nimkarn, 2010). Women who elect treatment do so with a plan to undergo prenatal diagnosis and stop therapy if the fetus is male or an unaffected female. Prenatal diagnosis with molecular genetic testing may be performed on chorionic villi—at 10 to 12 weeks' gestation—or on amniocytes after 15 weeks. Ideally, the goal is to limit dexamethasone exposure in males and in unaffected females.

Recently, maternal treatment with dexamethasone has become a topic of significant controversy. The Endocrine Society has recommended that treatment be given only in the context of research protocols (Miller, 2013; Speiser, 2010). If therapy is initiated shortly before 9 weeks, the dosage of dexamethasone used is not considered to have significant teratogenic potential because organogenesis of major organs has already taken place (McCullough, 2010). There are ongoing concerns, however, about the potential effects of either excess *endogenous* androgens or excess *exogenous* dexamethasone on the developing brain. Although maternal dexamethasone has been used for many years to prevent virilization of female fetuses with CAH, long-term safety data are relatively limited.

Development of cell-free fetal DNA testing of maternal serum has potential to replace invasive tests such as chorionic villus sampling and amniocentesis for CAH (Chap. 13, p. 279). Determination of fetal gender using cell-free fetal DNA is reported to have at least 95-percent sensitivity when performed at or beyond 7 weeks' gestation (Devaney, 2011). Although not yet clinically available in 2013, DNA analysis of the *CYP21A2* gene has also been reported using cell-free fetal DNA testing.

Congenital Cystic Adenomatoid Malformation

Also called congenital pulmonary airway malformation (CPAM), this lung mass is a hamartomatous overgrowth of terminal bronchioles. Sonographically, congenital cystic adenomatoid malformation (CCAM) is a well-circumscribed mass that may appear solid and echogenic or may have one or multiple variably sized cysts (Fig. 10-18, p. 207). Lesions with cysts 5 mm or larger are generally termed macrocystic, whereas microcystic lesions have smaller cysts or appear solid (Adzick, 1985). Therapy for macrocystic CCAM is discussed on page 330.

Infrequently, a microcystic CCAM may demonstrate rapid growth between 18 and 26 weeks' gestation. The mass may become so large that it causes mediastinal shift, compromised cardiac output and venous return, and resultant hydrops (Cavoretto, 2008). A CCAM-volume ratio (CVR) has been used to quantify size and risk for hydrops in these severe cases (Crombleholme, 2002). The CVR is an estimate of the CCAM volume—length × width × height × 0.52—divided by the head circumference. In the absence of a dominant cyst, a

CVR exceeding 1.6 has been associated with a hydrops risk of approximately 75 percent, whereas the risk is < 5 percent with a smaller CVR.

If the CVR exceeds 1.4 or 1.6 or if signs of hydrops develop, corticosteroid treatment has been advocated to improve outcome. Regimens include dexamethasone—6.25 mg every 12 hours for four doses, or betamethasone—12.5 mg intramuscularly every 24 hours for two doses. In some reports, hydrops has resolved in nearly 80 percent of cases, and approximately 85 percent of these treated cases survived (Curran, 2010; Loh, 2012; Peranteau, 2007). However, others found that high-risk CCAMs displayed a variable response to corticosteroid treatment, and perinatal mortality rates were > 40 percent (Morris, 2009c).

Thyroid Disease

Identification of fetal thyroid disease is rare and usually prompted by sonographic detection of a fetal goiter. There are several possibilities to consider. If a woman has previously been treated for Graves disease with either thyroid ablation or surgical resection, she may continue to produce IgG thyroid-stimulating immunoglobulins. These cross the placenta to cause *fetal thyrotoxicosis*. In a woman receiving medication for Graves disease, transplacental passage of propylthiouracil or methimazole usually prevents this, as discussed in Chapter 58 (p. 1149). Occasionally, maternal treatment—or overtreatment—for thyrotoxicosis may cause *fetal hypothyroidism* (Bliddal, 2011a). Other potential causes of fetal hypothyroidism resulting in goiter include transplacental passage of thyroid peroxidase antibodies and fetal thyroid dyshormonogenesis (Agrawal, 2002).

If a goiter is identified, it is important to determine whether the fetus is hyper- or hypothyroid. Thyroid hormone levels may be measured in amnionic fluid, but *fetal blood sampling,* discussed in Chapter 14 (p. 300), is preferred for guiding treatment (Abuhamad, 1995; Ribault, 2009). A primary purpose of therapy—in addition to correcting the physiological abnormality—is to decrease goiter size. The goiter may compress the trachea and esophagus to such a degree that the fetus may develop severe hydramnios and the neonate may develop airway compromise. Hyperextension of the fetal neck by a goiter may result in labor dystocia.

Fetal Thyrotoxicosis

Untreated fetal thyrotoxicosis may present with goiter, tachycardia, growth restriction, hydramnios, accelerated bone maturation, and even heart failure and hydrops (Huel, 2009; Peleg, 2002). The cause is usually Graves disease with transplacental passage of thyroid-stimulating immunoglobulins. Most recommend fetal blood sampling to confirm the diagnosis (Duncombe, 2001; Heckel, 1997; Srisupundit, 2008). Confirmed fetal thyrotoxicosis is followed by maternal antithyroid treatment, and if the mother develops hypothyroidism, she is given supplemental levothyroxine (Hui, 2011).

Fetal Hypothyroidism

Goitrous hypothyroidism may lead to hydramnios, neck hyperextension, and delayed bone maturation. If the mother is receiving antithyroid medication, discontinuation is generally recommended, along with intraamnionic levothyroxine injection (Bliddal, 2011a; Ribault, 2009). There have been numerous case reports of intraamnionic levothyroxine treatment. However, optimal dosage and frequency have not been established, and reported dosages range from 50 to 800 mg every 1 to 4 weeks (Abuhamad, 1995; Bliddal, 2011b; Ribault, 2009).

Fetal Stem-Cell Transplantation

In theory, stem-cell transplantation could be used to treat various hematological, metabolic, and immunological diseases. It could also serve as a delivery vehicle for gene transfer to treat other genetic conditions. The fetal period is ideal for this because in the first and early second trimesters, the fetus lacks an adaptive immune response to foreign antigens—described as *preimmune* (Tiblad, 2008). Also, pretreatment chemotherapy or radiation is not necessary before transplantation, and graft-versus-host disease is less likely.

Fetal stem-cell transplantation has been most successful in the treatment of immunodeficiency syndromes. Engraftment has been achieved in fetuses with severe combined immunodeficiency and bare lymphocyte syndrome (Tiblad, 2008). Treatment of red blood cell and metabolic disorders, however, has not been successful (Mummery, 2011). Stem-cell transplantation has been attempted to treat hemoglobinopathies without success. Some children with α- and β-thalassemia have remained transfusion dependent despite achieving engraftment (Tiblad, 2008; Westgren, 1996). One fetus with osteogenesis imperfecta, type II, was transplanted with fetal mesenchymal stem cells and developed both engraftment and chimerism (Le Blanc, 2005; Mummery, 2011). Although long-term outcomes of such cases remain uncertain, the technology holds great promise.

SURGICAL THERAPY

Also called *maternal-fetal surgery*, these procedures are offered for selected congenital abnormalities in which the likelihood of fetal deterioration is so great that delaying treatment until after delivery would risk fetal death or substantially greater postnatal morbidity (Walsh, 2011). Open fetal surgery is a highly specialized, multidisciplinary intervention performed at relatively few centers in the United States and for only a few fetal conditions. It was pioneered more than three decades ago by Harrison and coworkers (1982) at the University of California, San Francisco. Criteria for consideration of fetal surgery are listed in Table 16-1. In many cases, data regarding the safety and efficacy of these procedures are lacking. The Agency for Healthcare Research and Quality has stressed that when considering fetal surgery, the overriding concern must be maternal and fetal safety. Accomplishing the fetal goals of the procedure are secondary (Walsh, 2011).

Some abnormalities amenable to fetal surgical treatment, antepartum or intrapartum, are shown in Table 16-2. Information regarding the procedures, their indications, and complications is provided to assist patient evaluation and

TABLE 16-1. Guiding Principles for Fetal Surgical Procedures

Accurate prenatal diagnosis for the defect is available, with staging if applicable
The defect appears isolated, with no evidence of other abnormality or underlying genetic syndrome that would significantly worsen survival or quality of life
The defect results in a high likelihood of death or irreversible organ destruction, and postnatal therapy is inadequate
The procedure is technically feasible, and a multidisciplinary team is in agreement regarding the treatment plan
Maternal risks from the procedure are well documented and considered acceptable
There is comprehensive parental counseling
It is recommended that there is an animal model for the defect and procedure

Modified from Deprest, 2010; Harrison, 1982; Vrecenak, 2013; Walsh, 2011.

counseling. It is beyond the scope of this text to provide technical information necessary to perform these procedures or address individual circumstances in which their benefits may outweigh potential risks.

TABLE 16-2. Selected Fetal Abnormalities Amenable to Fetal Surgery

Open Fetal Surgery
Myelomeningocele
Congenital cystic adenomatoid malformation (CCAM)
Extralobar pulmonary sequestration
Sacrococcygeal teratoma
Fetoscopic Surgery
Twin-twin transfusion: laser of placental anastomoses
Diaphragmatic hernia: fetal endoscopic tracheal occlusion (FETO)
Posterior urethral valves: cystoscopic laser
Congenital high airway obstruction: vocal cord laser
Amnionic band release
Percutaneous Procedures
Shunt therapy
Posterior-urethral valves/bladder outlet obstruction
Pleural effusion: chylothorax or sequestration
Dominant cyst in CCAM
Radiofrequency ablation
Twin-reversed arterial perfusion (TRAP) sequence
Monochorionic twins with severe anomaly(ies) of 1 twin
Chorioangioma
Fetal intracardiac catheter procedures
Aortic or pulmonic valvuloplasty for stenosis
Atrial septostomy for hypoplastic left heart with restrictive atrial septum
Ex-Utero Intrapartum Treatment (EXIT) Procedures
Congenital diaphragmatic hernia after FETO
Congenital high airway obstruction sequence (CHAOS)
Severe micrognathia
Tumors involving neck or airway
EXIT-to-resection: resection of fetal thoracic or mediastinal mass
EXIT-to-extracorporeal membrane oxygenation (ECMO): congenital diaphragmatic hernia

Open Fetal Surgery

These procedures require a highly-skilled multidisciplinary team and extensive preoperative counseling. The mother must undergo general endotracheal anesthesia to suppress both uterine contractions and fetal responses. Using sonographic guidance to avoid the placental edge, a hysterotomy incision is made with a stapling device that seals the edges for hemostasis. To replace amnionic fluid losses, warmed fluid is continuously infused into the uterus thorough a rapid infusion device. The fetus is gently manipulated to permit pulse oximetry monitoring and venous access, in case fluids or blood are emergently needed. The surgical procedure is then performed. After completion, the hysterotomy is closed and tocolysis begun. Tocolysis typically includes intravenous magnesium sulfate for 24 hours, oral indomethacin for 48 hours, and at some centers, oral nifedipine until delivery (Wu, 2009). Prophylactic antibiotics are also administered and generally continued for 24 hours following the procedure. Cesarean delivery will be needed later in gestation and for all future deliveries.

Risks

Morbidities associated with fetal surgery have been well characterized. In a review of 87 open procedures from the University of California, San Francisco, Golombeck and colleagues (2006) reported the following morbidities: pulmonary edema—28 percent, placental abruption—9 percent, blood transfusion—13 percent, premature rupture of membranes—52 percent, and preterm delivery—33 percent. Wilson and associates (2010) from Children's Hospital of Philadelphia reviewed subsequent pregnancy outcomes following open fetal surgery and reported that 14 percent experienced uterine rupture and 14 percent had uterine dehiscence. Morbidities identified in the recent *Management of Myelomeningocele Study—MOMS*—are shown in Table 16-3 (Adzick, 2011). Other potential risks include maternal sepsis and fetal death during or following the procedure.

Myelomeningocele Surgery

As depicted and described in Chapters 10 (p. 202) and 14 (p. 287), spina bifida, that is, a congenital open vertebral defect, may be associated with herniation of meninges alone (meningocele) or of meninges and spinal cord nerve roots (myelomeningocele). Despite postnatal repair, affected individuals may have varying degrees of paralysis, bladder and bowel

TABLE 16-3. Benefits and Risks of Fetal Myelomeningocele Surgery versus Postnatal Repair

	Fetal Surgery (n = 78)	Postnatal Surgery (n = 80)	*p* value
Benefits (primary outcomes)			
Perinatal death or shunt by 12 months[a]	68%	98%	< 0.001
Shunt placement by 12 months	40%	82%	< 0.001
Score derived from Bayley Mental Development Index and difference between functional and anatomical level of lesion (30 months)[a]	149 ± 58	123 ± 57	0.007
Hindbrain herniation (any)	64%	96%	< 0.001
Brainstem kinking (any)	20%	48%	< 0.001
Independent walking (30 months)	42%	21%	0.01
Risks			
Maternal pulmonary edema	6%	0	0.03
Placental abruption	6%	0	0.03
Maternal transfusion at delivery	9%	1%	0.03
Oligohydramnios	21%	4%	0.001
Gestational age at delivery	34 ± 3	37 ± 1	< 0.001
Preterm birth			
< 37 weeks	79%	15%	< 0.001
< 35 weeks	46%	5%	
< 30 weeks	13%	0	

[a]Each primary outcome had two components. The perinatal death components of the primary outcomes as well as the Bayley Mental Development Index at 30 months did not differ between the two study cohorts.
Data from Adzick, 2011.

dysfunction, developmental delays, and brainstem dysfunction from the Arnold-Chiari II malformation. Evidence from animal and human studies supports a two-hit hypothesis. Spinal cord damage results from both failure of neurulation during embryonic development and ongoing exposure throughout gestation of the neural elements to amnionic fluid (Adzick, 2010; Meuli, 1995, 1997).

Spina bifida is the first nonlethal birth defect for which fetal surgery has been offered. It meets all of the criteria listed in Table 16-1. Preliminary reports demonstrated that compared with historical controls, infants who had undergone fetal myelomeningocele surgery had reversal of the Arnold-Chiari II malformation and were less likely to require ventriculoperitoneal shunt placement (Bruner, 1999; Sutton, 1999).

Based on this evidence, the National Institutes of Health sponsored a randomized multicenter trial of prenatal versus postnatal myelomeningocele repair—the *Management of Myelomeningocele Study—MOMS* (Adzick, 2011). Criteria for participation in the MOMS trial included: (1) singleton fetus at 19.0 to 25.9 weeks' gestation; (2) upper myelomeningocele boundary between T1 and S1 as confirmed by fetal magnetic resonance (MR) imaging; (3) evidence of hindbrain herniation; and (4) normal karyotype and no evidence of a fetal anomaly unrelated to the myelomeningocele. Women at risk for preterm birth or placental abruption, those with a contraindication to fetal surgery, and women with body mass index ≥ 35 kg/m^2 were excluded. Using these criteria and following comprehensive multidisciplinary counseling, only 15 percent of screened patients underwent the procedure.

The MOMS trial demonstrated improved infant outcomes in the prenatal surgery cohort (see Table 16-3). Infants who had undergone prenatal surgery were *twice* as likely to walk independently by 30 months. They had significantly less hindbrain herniation and were only *half* as likely to undergo ventriculoperitoneal shunting by the age of 1 year. A primary outcome was a composite score that was derived from the Bayley Mental Development Index and from the difference between the functional and anatomical level of the lesion at 30 months. This outcome was also significantly better in the prenatal surgery group.

When counseling prospective families, however, it is essential to place these results into context. For example, despite improvements in the proportion with independent ambulation, *most* children who received fetal surgery were not able to ambulate independently, and nearly 30 percent were not able to ambulate at all. Prenatal surgery did not confer improvements in fetal or neonatal death rates or in the Bayley Mental Development Index score at age 30 months. And, as shown in Table 16-3, surgery was associated with a small but significant risk for placental abruption and maternal pulmonary edema. Moreover, nearly half were delivered ≤ 34 weeks, which significantly increased the risk for respiratory distress syndrome (Adzick, 2011). Long-term data from this trial are pending.

Since publication of the MOMS trial, fetal myelomeningocele has become the most common indication for open fetal surgery at the University of California, San Francisco (Vrecenak, 2013). This is not unexpected, as myelomeningocele is more common than other defects for which open fetal surgery is offered. Also, with other abnormalities, surgery is offered only in the most severe cases—usually prompted by development of hydrops. Rapid expansion of centers offering fetal myelomeningocele surgery has raised concerns about the importance of training and ongoing experience, adherence to the MOMS trial criteria, and need for a registry to ensure that future cases achieve the same success as in the MOMS trial (Cohen, 2014; Vrecenak, 2013).

Thoracic Masses

In the past, if hydrops developed in a fetus with a large extralobar pulmonary sequestration or cystic adenomatoid malformation without a dominant cyst, open fetal surgery with lobectomy was the only treatment available other than preterm delivery (Chap. 10, p. 207). Because most thoracic masses are small and have a benign prognosis, fetal surgery is rarely necessary for fetuses with such masses. Also, larger masses are generally treated with a trial of corticosteroids, and open fetal surgery is reserved for those cases prior to 32 weeks in which hydrops is developing. In fetuses with early hydrops and minimal placentomegaly, the survival rate following open lobectomy approximates 60 percent (Vrecenak, 2013). Use of the ex-utero intrapartum treatment procedure in the treatment of fetal lung masses is discussed on page 331.

Sacrococcygeal Teratoma

This germ cell tumor has a birth prevalence of about 1 per 28,000 (Derikx, 2006; Swamy, 2008). Sonographically, a sacrococcygeal teratoma (SCT) is a solid and/or cystic mass that arises from the anterior sacrum (Fig. 16-2). It may grow rapidly, usually extending inferiorly and externally (Fig. 10-12, p. 204). Hydramnios is common, and hydrops may develop from high-output cardiac failure, either as a consequence of tumor vascularity or secondary to bleeding within the tumor and resultant anemia. *Mirror syndrome*—maternal preeclampsia developing along with fetal hydrops—may occur in this setting (Chap. 15, p. 318). Fetal MR imaging may be helpful in evaluating the extent of the internal tumor component.

In 30 pregnancies with a prenatal diagnosis of SCT, the perinatal mortality rate exceeded 40 percent (Hedrick, 2004). Fetal loss approaches 100 percent if hydrops or placentomegaly develop (Vrecenak, 2013). The group at the Children's Hospital of Philadelphia has recommended consideration of open fetal surgery for SCT only in cases in which the tumor is completely external (Type I) and in which high cardiac output with early hydrops has developed in the second trimester (Vrecenak, 2013). As shown in Figure 16-2, hysterotomy is performed and the external component resected. The coccyx and any deep tumor are left in place for postnatal removal. Because tumor debulking interrupts the vascular steal, normal fetal physiology may be restored.

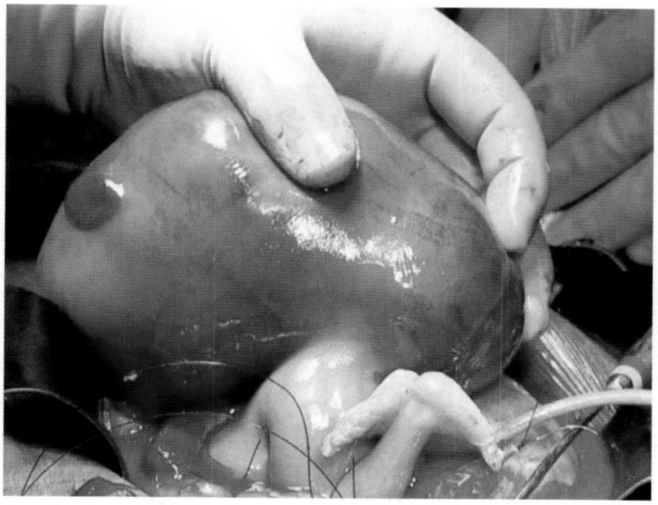

FIGURE 16-2 Photograph of open fetal surgery for resection of a sacrococcygeal teratoma. Hysterotomy has been completed, and the caudal portion of the fetus has been delivered onto the surgical field. The tumor is held by the surgeon's hand. (Photograph contributed by Dr. Timothy M. Crombleholme.)

Fetoscopic Surgery

These procedures use fiberoptic endoscopes only 1 to 2 mm in diameter to cross the maternal abdominal wall, the uterine wall, and membranes. Instruments such as lasers fit through 3- to 5-mm cannulae that surround the endoscope. Thus, fetoscopic surgeries are usually performed at highly specialized centers, and many are considered investigational. Morbidities are generally lower than with open fetal surgery, but they still may be formidable, particularly if maternal laparotomy is required for access (Golombeck, 2006). Examples of some conditions treated by fetoscopy are listed in Table 16-2.

Twin-Twin Transfusion Syndrome

As discussed in Chapter 45 (p. 907), fetoscopic laser ablation of placental anastomoses has become the preferred management for many cases of severe twin-twin transfusion syndrome (TTTS). It is generally performed between 16 and 26 weeks' gestation for monochorionic-diamnionic twin pregnancies with stage II to stage IV TTTS. These categories of the Quintero Staging System are described in Chapter 45 (Quintero, 1999; Society for Maternal-Fetal Medicine, 2013). In this country, pregnancies with stage I TTTS are not routinely offered laser ablation. However, following a consensus conference held by the North American Fetal Therapy Network (NAFTNet), as of 2013, a randomized trial that includes laser therapy for stage I TTTS is underway (Stamilio, 2010).

Technique. The procedure is typically performed under epidural analgesia with intravenous sedation. A fetoscope is used to view the vascular equator that separates the placental cotyledons supplying each twin to permit selective laser photocoagulation of arteriovenous anastomoses that cross this equator (Fig. 16-3).

The randomized trial of TTTS conducted in the United States and reported by Crombleholme and associates (2007) used the following methodology. First, a small skin incision

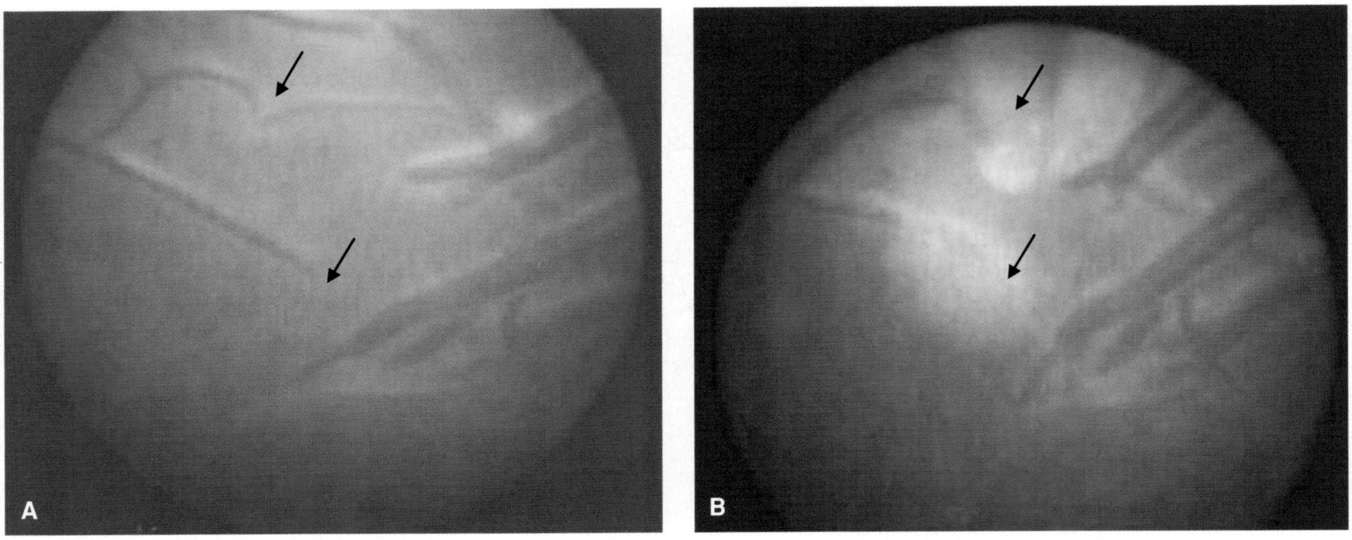

FIGURE 16-3 Laser therapy for twin-twin transfusion syndrome (TTTS). Fetoscopic photograph of the fetal surface of the placenta. **A.** Vascular anastomoses (*arrows*) are shown before selective laser ablation. **B.** Sites of ablation are seen as blanched yellow-white areas (*arrows*). (Photographs contributed by Dr. Timothy M. Crombleholme.)

allows ultrasound-guided placement of a 3.3-mm fetoscope containing separate ports for the lens, the laser, and rapid infusion of saline as needed. More recently, fetoscopes as small as 1.2 mm have been used (Chalouhi, 2011). Next, the chorionic plate of the placenta is mapped three times: first to identify all anastomoses at the vascular equator, then to mark and record the location of each connecting vessel, and after photocoagulation, to verify that no connecting vessels were missed or had recanalized. Vessels are photocoagulated with 60 watts of power using a 600-μm diameter diode laser with the endostat placed 1 cm from the vessel surface. A 400-μm neodymium:yttrium-aluminum-garnet (Nd:YAG) laser also may be used. At the end of the procedure, amnioreduction is performed to decrease the single deepest pocket of amnionic fluid to below 5 cm, and antibiotics are injected into the amnionic cavity.

If cardiomyopathy has been identified in the recipient twin, nifedipine, 20 mg every 6 hours, may be given to the mother 24 to 48 hours before photocoagulation and continued following the procedure, in an effort to improve recipient twin survival (Crombleholme, 2010).

Complications. Families should have reasonable expectations of procedural success and potential complications. Without treatment, the perinatal mortality rate for severe TTTS is 70 to 100 percent (Society for Maternal-Fetal Medicine, 2013). Following laser therapy, the anticipated perinatal mortality rate approximates 30 to 50 percent, with a 5- to 20-percent risk for long-term neurological handicap (Society for Maternal-Fetal Medicine, 2013). Cystic periventricular leukomalacia and grade III to IV interventricular hemorrhage are identified neonatally in up to 10 percent of laser-treated cases (Lopriore, 2006).

Procedure-related complications include preterm prematurely ruptured membranes in up to 25 percent, placental abruption in 8 percent, vascular laceration in 3 percent, amnionic band syndrome resulting from laser laceration of the membranes in 3 percent, and twin-anemia polycythemia sequence in 2 to 12 percent (Habli, 2009; Robyr, 2006). Finally, almost 85 percent of laser-treated TTTS pregnancies deliver before 34 weeks (Habli, 2009).

Twin anemia polycythemia sequence (TAPS) is a type of chronic fetofetal transfusion. It is characterized by large differences in hemoglobin concentrations between the twins of a monochorionic pair in the absence of amnionic fluid volume differences. It may occur spontaneously in 3 to 5 percent of monochorionic twins, although it has been recognized more frequently as a complication of laser-treated TTTS. Differences in middle cerebral artery peak systolic velocity, described in Chapter 10 (p. 221), between the twins may assist in identifying this complication (Robyr, 2006; Slaghekke, 2010).

Congenital Diaphragmatic Hernia

Fetal therapy for this anomaly is more controversial than for others. The prevalence of congenital diaphragmatic hernia (CDH) is approximately 1 in 3000 to 4000 births, and the overall survival rate is 50 to 60 percent (Chap. 10, p. 206). Associated anomalies occur in 40 percent of cases and confer a considerably lower survival rate. With isolated CDH, the major causes of mortality are pulmonary hypoplasia and pulmonary hypertension. The major risk factor is liver herniation, which complicates at least half of cases and is associated with a 30-percent reduction in the survival rate (Mullassery, 2010).

Because of maternal and fetal risks associated with fetal surgical intervention, efforts have focused on identifying those least likely to survive with postnatal therapy alone. Cases with associated anomalies are typically excluded, as are those without liver herniation. Prediction is further hampered because of improvements in neonatal care for infants with CDH. These include permissive hypercapnia, "gentle ventilation" to avoid barotrauma, and delayed surgery.

Lung-to-Head Ratio. This sonographic ratio was developed by investigators from the University of California, San Francisco to improve prediction of survival in fetuses with isolated left-sided CDH diagnosed before 25 weeks' gestation (Metkus, 1996). The lung-to-head ratio (LHR) is a measurement of the right lung area, taken at the level of the four-chamber view of the heart (Fig. 10-20, p. 209), divided by the head circumference. Investigators found that the survival rate was 100 percent if the LHR was above 1.35, and there were no survivors if it was below 0.6. Nearly three fourths of pregnancies had values between 0.6 and 1.35, and prediction was difficult in this large group because the overall survival rate was about 60 percent (Metkus, 1996).

Jani and coworkers (2006) evaluated the LHR in 184 cases from an international registry of isolated CDH between 22 and 28 weeks' gestation. The survival rate was 15 percent if the LHR was 0.8 to 1.0, 65 percent with LHRs 1.0 to 1.5, and 80 percent with LHRs 1.6 or more. There were no survivors with LHRs below 0.8. As of 2013, trials underway in the United States and Europe have selected a threshold LHR of 1.0 or lower for inclusion.

Magnetic Resonance Imaging. This has been used to estimate the volume of lung tissue ipsilateral and contralateral to the diaphragmatic hernia, which may then be compared with a gestational age-matched reference. Mayer and colleagues (2011) performed a metaanalysis of 19 studies involving more than 600 pregnancies in which isolated CDH was evaluated with fetal MR imaging. Factors significantly associated with neonatal survival included the side of the defect, total fetal lung volume, observed-to-expected lung volume, and fetal liver position.

Fetal MR imaging has also been used to quantify the volume of herniated liver (Fig. 10-44, p. 225). Two reasons underlie the rationale for assessing liver volume. The first is that liver herniation is perhaps the strongest predictor of outcome in fetuses with isolated CDH. Second, liver volume might be a more reliable predictor because lungs are inherently more compressible than liver. In preliminary reports, MR assessment of the degree of liver herniation has been found to correlate with postnatal survival rates and may even be more useful as a predictor than lung volume (Cannie, 2008; Walsh, 2000; Worley, 2009).

Tracheal Occlusion. Early attempts to treat severe diaphragmatic herniation used open fetal surgery. Unfortunately, repositioning of the liver into the abdomen resulted in kinking of the umbilical vein with subsequent fetal demise (Harrison, 1993).

Knowledge that fetal lungs normally produce fluid and that fetuses with upper airway obstruction develop hyperplastic lungs formed the rationale for tracheal occlusion (Hedrick, 1994). Initially, the trachea was occluded with an external clip (Harrison, 1993). Currently, a detachable silicone balloon is placed within the trachea endoscopically, using a 3-mm operating sheath and fetoscopes as small as 1 mm (Deprest, 2011; Ruano, 2012). The ex-utero intrapartum treatment procedure (p. 331) was developed in tandem with these procedures, and it is used at delivery during reversal of the tracheal occlusion.

A randomized trial of the *fetal endoscopic tracheal occlusion (FETO)* technique was conducted in pregnancies with isolated CDH, liver herniation, and LHR below 1.4 (Harrison, 2003). Pregnancies included had a predicted survival rate < 40 percent with conventional postnatal therapy based on historical data. The trial was stopped after only 24 women had been enrolled because no benefit was identified. Survival rates 90 days after birth were unexpectedly high in both groups and approximated 75 percent. Potential benefits of FETO may have been offset by the high rate of early preterm birth. The mean age at delivery was just older than 30 weeks, and fetuses were delivered an average of 6 weeks after the procedure. This left less time for catch-up growth (Wenstrom, 2003).

Following this study, there has been continued enthusiasm for the technique, particularly outside the United States. Using a lower lung-to-head ratio threshold of 1.0 for inclusion, significantly higher postnatal survival rates have been reported. Rates improved from < 25 percent with postnatal therapy to approximately 50 percent with FETO (Jani, 2009; Ruano, 2012).

Percutaneous Procedures

Sonographic guidance can be used to permit therapy with a shunt, radiofrequency ablation needle, or angioplasty catheter. With these procedures, desired instruments cross the maternal abdominal wall, uterine wall, and membranes to reach the amnionic cavity and fetus. Risks include maternal infection, preterm labor or prematurely ruptured membranes, and fetal injury or loss. Percutaneous shunts are used to drain fluid in cases of selected urinary and thoracic abnormalities. Radiofrequency ablation has become increasingly available for selected indications such as twin-reversed arterial perfusion sequence. Fetal cardiac catheterization procedures hold promise for pregnancies with severe hypoplastic left heart syndrome but currently remain investigational.

Thoracic Shunts

A shunt placed from the fetal pleural cavity into the amnionic cavity may be used to drain pleural fluid. A large effusion may cause a significant mediastinal shift, resulting in pulmonary hypoplasia or in heart failure and hydrops. The most common etiology of a primary effusion is *chylothorax*—caused by lymphatic obstruction. Pleural effusions may also be secondary to congenital viral infection or aneuploidy, or they may be associated with a malformation such as *extralobar pulmonary sequestration.* Yinon and associates (2010) reported aneuploidy in approximately 5 percent and associated anomalies in 10 percent of cases.

Typically, the effusion is first drained using a 22-gauge needle under sonographic guidance. Tests for aneuploidy and infection are performed, as well as a cell count. A pleural-fluid cell count with greater than 80-percent lymphocytes, in the absence of infection, is diagnostic of chylothorax. If the fluid reaccumulates, a trocar and cannula may be inserted through the fetal chest wall, and a double-pigtail shunt may be placed to drain the effusion (Fig. 16-4). If the effusion is right-sided, the shunt is placed in the lower third of the chest to permit maximum expansion of the lung. If left-sided, the shunt is placed along the upper axillary line to allow the heart to return to

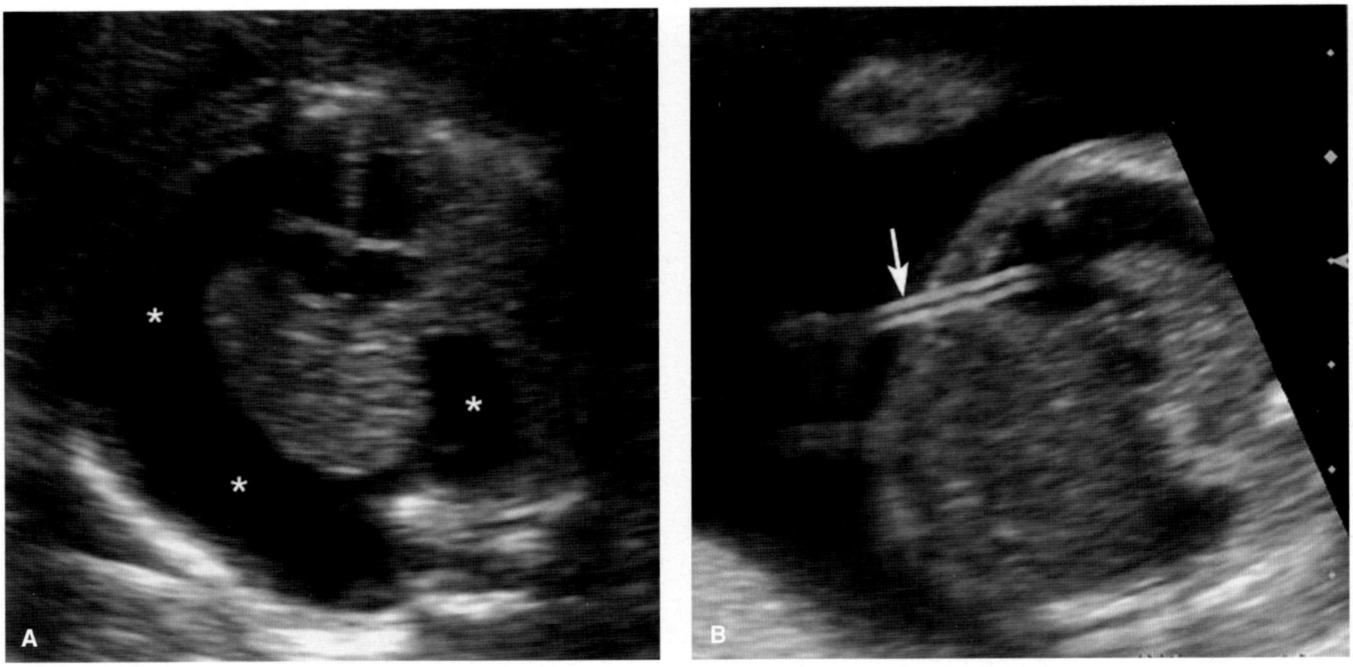

FIGURE 16-4 Thoraco-amnionic shunt placement. **A.** A large, right-sided fetal pleural effusion (*asterisks*) and ascites were identified at 18 weeks' gestation. The effusion was drained but rapidly reaccumulated. The xanthochromic fluid contained 95-percent lymphocytes, consistent with chylothorax. **B.** A double-pigtail shunt (*arrow*) was inserted under ultrasound guidance. Following shunt placement, the effusion and ascites resolved.

normal position (Mann, 2010). The overall survival rate is reported to be 70 percent, and that of hydropic fetuses approximates 50 percent (Mann, 2010; Yinon, 2010). Shunt displacement into the amnionic cavity is not uncommon. If the shunt remains in place, it must be clamped immediately upon delivery of the infant to avoid pneumothorax.

Shunts have also been used to drain a dominant cyst in fetuses with macrocystic *congenital cystic adenomatoid malformation*. Fortunately, cysts rarely are large enough to pose a risk for hydrops or pulmonary hypoplasia. Shunt placement may reduce the volume of the CCAM by as much as 70 percent and may reverse hydrops and improve survival rates (Knox, 2006; Mann, 2010). Survival rates following shunt placement for CCAM approximate 70 percent (Wilson, 2004).

Urinary Shunts

Vesicoamnionic shunts are used in fetuses with bladder-outlet obstruction that would otherwise have a grim prognosis. Distal obstruction of the urinary tract occurs more often in male fetuses, and the most common etiology is *posterior urethral valves,* followed by *urethral atresia* and by *prune belly syndrome*, which is also called *Eagle-Barrett syndrome*. Diagnosis is discussed in Chapter 10 (p. 216). Sonographic findings include dilatation of the bladder and proximal urethra, termed the "keyhole" sign, along with bladder wall thickening (Fig. 10-33, p. 217). Oligohydramnios before midpregnancy leads to pulmonary hypoplasia. Unfortunately, the outcome may be poor even when amnionic fluid volume is normal. Evaluation includes a careful search for associated anomalies, which may coexist in 40 percent of cases, and for aneuploidy, which has been reported in 5 to 8 percent of cases (Hayden, 1988; Hobbins, 1984; Mann, 2010; Manning, 1986).

Shunt placement allows urine to drain from the bladder into the amnionic cavity. This attempts to preserve renal function and improve oligohydramnios to prevent pulmonary hypoplasia. Potential candidates are fetuses without other severe anomalies or aneuploidy and without sonographic features that confer poor prognosis, for example, renal cortical cysts. Therapy is generally offered only if the fetus is male, because in females, the type of anomaly tends to be even more severe. Serial bladder drainage—vesicocentesis—is performed at 24- to 48-hour intervals under sonographic guidance to determine the urine electrolyte and protein content. This permits classification of the renal prognosis as good or poor (Table 16-4).

Amnioinfusion is usually performed before shunting to aid placement of the distant end of the catheter into the amnionic

TABLE 16-4. Fetal Urinary Analyte Values with Bladder Outlet Obstruction

Analyte	Good Prognosis	Poor Prognosis
Sodium	< 90 mmol/L	> 100 mmol/L
Chloride	< 80 mmol/L	> 90 mmol/L
Calcium	< 7 mg/dL	> 8 mg/dL
Osmolality	< 180 mmol/L	> 200 mmol/L
β_2-Microglobulin	< 6 mg/L	> 10 mg/L
Total protein	< 20 mg/dL	> 40 mg/dL

Good or poor prognosis is based on values from serial vesicocentesis performed between 18 and 22 weeks' gestation, using the last specimen obtained.
Data from Mann, 2010.

cavity. Amnioinfusion also assists sonographic fetal anatomical survey to ensure than no other abnormalities are present. A small trocar and cannula are then inserted into the fetal bladder under sonographic guidance. The shunt is placed as low as possible within the bladder to avoid dislodgement after bladder decompression. A double-pigtail catheter is used, with the distal end within the fetal bladder and the proximal end within the amnionic cavity.

Complications include displacement of the shunt out of the fetal bladder in up to 40 percent of cases, urinary ascites in about 20 percent, and development of gastroschisis in 10 percent (Freedman, 2000; Mann, 2010). Preterm delivery is common, and infant survival rates have ranged from 50 to 90 percent (Biard, 2005; Walsh, 2011). It is not known whether vesicoamnionic shunt placement confers a benefit in terms of long-term renal function (Holmes, 2001). A third of surviving children have required dialysis or renal transplantation, and almost half have respiratory problems (Biard, 2005).

Radiofrequency Ablation

With this procedure, high-frequency alternating current is used to coagulate and desiccate tissue. Radiofrequency ablation (RFA) has become a favored modality for the treatment of *twin-reversed arterial perfusion (TRAP) sequence,* also known as *acardiac twin* (Chap. 45, p. 908). Without treatment, the mortality rate for the normal or pump twin in TRAP sequence exceeds 50 percent. The procedure is also used for selective termination with other monochorionic twin complications (Bebbington, 2012).

The procedure is performed under sonographic guidance, and a 17- or 19-gauge RFA needle is placed into the base of the umbilical cord of the acardiac twin and into its abdomen. After a 2-cm area of coagulation is achieved, color Doppler sonography is used to verify absent flow into this twin. Several centers have reported a significantly improved rate of survival for the normal twin following RFA for TRAP sequence (Lee, 2007; Livingston, 2007). RFA was performed at approximately 20 weeks in 98 pregnancies with TRAP sequence reported by the North American Fetal Therapy Network (Lee, 2013). The median gestational age at delivery was 37 weeks, and the neonatal survival rate was 80 percent. The major complication was prematurely ruptured membranes and preterm birth—12 percent were delivered at about 26 weeks.

RFA has generally been offered to TRAP sequence pregnancies when the volume of the acardiac twin is large. In the NAFTNet series cited above, the median size of the acardius relative to the pump twin was 90 percent (Lee, 2013). Considering procedure-related risks, expectant management with close fetal surveillance is recommended if the estimated weight of the acardius is < 50 percent of the pump twin (Jelin, 2010).

Fetal Intracardiac Catheter Procedures

Selected fetal cardiac lesions may worsen during gestation, further complicating, or even obviating, options for postnatal repair. Severe narrowing of a cardiac outflow tract may result in progressive myocardial damage in utero, but intervention may permit muscle growth and preserve ventricular function (Walsh, 2011). Possible fetal procedures include *aortic valvuloplasty* for critical aortic stenosis; *atrial septostomy* for hypoplastic left heart syndrome with intact interatrial septum; and *pulmonary valvuloplasty* for pulmonary atresia with intact interventricular septum. There is a registry for these cases—the International Fetal Cardiac Intervention Registry (www.ifcir.org).

Of these, fetal aortic valvuloplasty is the most commonly performed. It is offered for selected cases of critical aortic stenosis in which the left ventricle is either normal sized or dilated. The goal is to prevent development of hypoplastic left heart and permit postnatal biventricular repair (McElhinney, 2010). Under sonographic guidance, an 18-gauge needle is inserted into the left ventricle with the tip positioned in front of the stenotic aortic valve. A 2.5- to 4.5-mm balloon catheter is then guided into the aortic annulus and inflated several times. Arzt and Tulzer (2011) reviewed the collective experience of two major centers that perform fetal cardiac procedures—one in Boston and the other in Linz, Austria. Technical procedural success was achieved in 75 percent of cases, and there was a 9-percent fetal loss rate. All required postnatal aortic valvuloplasty, two thirds needed early aortic valve replacement, and less than half achieved the goal of postnatal biventricular repair.

Fetal atrial septostomy, also using a percutaneous balloon catheter, has been offered in selected cases of hypoplastic left heart with an intact or highly restrictive interatrial septum. This condition has a postnatal mortality rate of approximately 80 percent (Glantz, 2007). In one report of 21 cases, the procedure-related loss was about 10 percent, and the short-term neonatal survival rate was 58 percent (Marshall, 2008).

Fetal pulmonary valvuloplasty has been offered in cases of pulmonary atresia with intact interventricular septum to prevent development of hypoplastic right heart syndrome. Success has been reported in approximately two thirds of cases. However, it is not yet clear whether outcomes are improved compared with standard postnatal repair (Artz, 2011; McElhinney, 2010).

Ex-Utero Intrapartum Treatment

This procedure is designed to allow the fetus to remain perfused by the placental circulation after being partially delivered, so that life-saving treatment can be performed before completing the delivery. The technique was first developed to obtain an airway with fetal tumors involving the oropharynx and neck (Catalano, 1992; Kelly, 1990; Langer, 1992). It was refined when tracheal occlusion was developed to treat congenital diaphragmatic hernia, because it was necessary to reestablish an airway after the trachea had been "plugged" or "clipped" (Mychaliska, 1997). Components of the procedure are shown in Table 16-5.

Some indications for the ex-utero intrapartum treatment (EXIT) procedure are listed in Table 16-2. It is the procedure of choice for intrapartum management of giant neck masses such as the one shown in Figure 16-5. Also, it is frequently used to remove the endotracheal balloon following fetal surgery for congenital diaphragmatic hernia (Laje, 2012; Ruano, 2012). Less common indications include treatment of *congenital high airway obstruction sequence (CHAOS)* and selected cases of severe fetal *micrognathia*, both discussed in Chapter 10 (Figs. 10-14 and 10-19, p. 205). Morris and coworkers (2009b) have proposed that in addition to a fetal jaw measurement below the 5th percentile, cases to be

SECTION 5

TABLE 16-5. Components of the Ex-Utero Intrapartum Treatment (EXIT) Procedure

Comprehensive preoperative evaluation: specialized sonography, fetal echocardiography, magnetic resonance imaging, fetal karyotype if possible
Uterine relaxation with deep general anesthesia and tocolysis
Intraoperative sonography to confirm placental margin and fetal position and to visualize vessels at uterine entry
Placement of stay-sutures followed by use of uterine stapling device to decrease uterine entry bleeding
Maintenance of uterine volume during the procedure via continuous amnioinfusion of warmed physiological solution to help prevent placental separation
Delivery of the fetal head, neck, and upper torso to permit access as needed
Fetal injection of intramuscular vecuronium, fentanyl, and atropine
Fetal peripheral intravenous access, pulse oximeter, and cardiac ultrasound
Following procedure, umbilical lines placed prior to cord clamping
Uterotonic agents administered as needed

Adapted from Moldenhauer, 2013.

considered for EXIT procedures are those with indirect evidence of obstruction, including hydramnios, an absent stomach bubble, or glossoptosis. Fetal MR imaging may be helpful in this setting (Chap. 10, p. 226).

This procedure can also be used as a bridge to other procedures. For example, during an EXIT procedure, resection of large thoracic masses may be accomplished by fetal thoracotomy performed with the placental circulation intact. In a series of 16 fetuses with CCAM volume ratios > 1.6 or hydrops, all of whom had mediastinal compression, Cass and colleagues (2013) reported that nine undergoing *EXIT-to-resection* survived. In contrast, there were no survivors with urgent postnatal surgery done alone. Similarly, Moldenhauer (2013) reported that 20 of 22 infants treated with EXIT-to-resection for lung masses survived. The EXIT procedure has also been used as a bridge to extracorporeal membrane oxygenation—*EXIT-to-ECMO*—in pregnancies with severe congenital diaphragmatic hernia. However, it has not been found to clearly confer survival benefit in such cases (Morris, 2009a; Stoffan, 2012).

An EXIT procedure is performed by a multidisciplinary team, which may include an obstetrician, maternal-fetal medicine specialist, pediatric surgeon(s), pediatric otolaryngologist, pediatric cardiologist, anesthesiologists for the mother and fetus, and neonatologists, as well as nursing personnel from many of these specialties. Counseling should include procedure-related risks such as hemorrhage from placental abruption or uterine atony, need for cesarean delivery in future pregnancies, increased risk for subsequent uterine rupture or dehiscence, possible need for hysterectomy, and fetal death or permanent neonatal disability. Compared with cesarean delivery, the EXIT procedure is also associated with a longer operating time—approximately 40 minutes longer depending on the procedure, increased blood loss, and a higher incidence of wound complications (Noah, 2002).

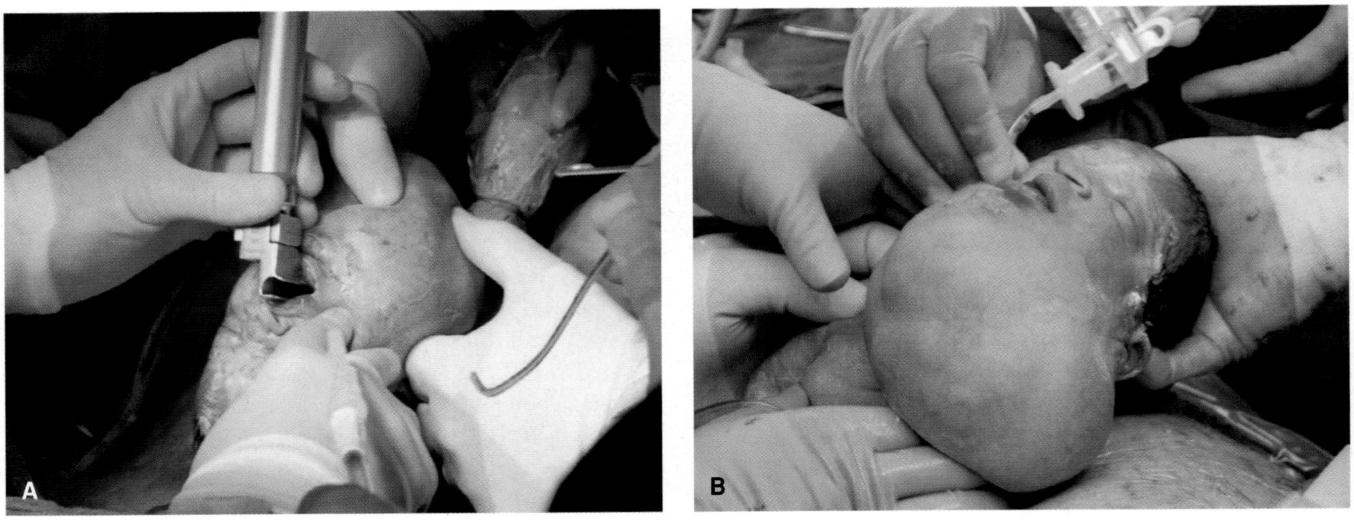

FIGURE 16-5 Ex-utero intrapartum treatment—EXIT procedure. **A.** This fetus was diagnosed prenatally with a large venolymphatic abnormality involving the face and neck. Involvement of the floor of the mouth, proximity to the anterior trachea, and mediastinal extension were evident on magnetic resonance imaging. Upon delivery of the head, placental circulation was maintained and an airway was established over the course of 20 minutes by a team of pediatric subspecialists that included a surgeon, anesthesiologist, and otolaryngologist. **B.** Following a controlled intubation, the fetus was ready for delivery and transfer to the neonatal intensive care unit team. (Photographs contributed by Drs. Stacey Thomas and Patricia Santiago-Muñoz.)

REFERENCES

Abuhamad AZ, Fisher DA, Warsof SL, et al: Antenatal diagnosis and treatment of fetal goitrous hypothyroidism: case report and review of the literature. Ultrasound Obstet Gynecol 6:368, 1995

Adzick NS: Fetal myelomeningocele: natural history, pathophysiology, and in utero intervention. Semin Fetal Neonatal Med. 15(1):9, 2010

Adzick NS, Harrison MR, Glick PL, et al: Fetal cystic adenomatoid malformation: prenatal diagnosis and natural history. J Pediatr Surg 20:483, 1985

Adzick NS, Thom EA, Spong CY, et al: A randomized trial of prenatal versus postnatal repair of myelomeningocele. N Engl J Med 364(11):993, 2011

Agrawal P, Ogilvy-Stuart A, Lees C: Intrauterine diagnosis and management of congenital goitrous hypothyroidism. Ultrasound Obstet Gynecol 19:501, 2002

Arzt W, Tulzer G: Fetal surgery for cardiac lesions. Prenat Diagn 31(7):695, 2011

Bebbington MW, Danzer E, Moldenhauer J, et al: Radiofrequency ablation vs bipolar umbilical cord coagulation in the management of complicated monochorionic pregnancies. Ultrasound Obstet Gynecol 40(3):319, 2012

Biard JM, Johnson MP, Carr MC, et al: Long-term outcomes in children treated by prenatal vesicoamniotic shunting for lower urinary tract obstruction. Obstet Gynecol 106:503, 2005

Bliddal S, Rasmussen AK, Sundberg K, et al: Antithyroid drug-induced fetal goitrous hypothyroidism. Nat Rev Endocrinol 7:396, 2011a

Bliddal S, Rasmussen ÅK, Sundberg K, et al: Graves' disease in two pregnancies complicated by fetal goitrous hypothyroidism: successful in utero treatment with levothyroxine. Thyroid 21(1):75, 2011b

Braga LH, Pippi Salle JL: Congenital adrenal hyperplasia: a critical reappraisal of the evolution of feminizing genitoplasty and the controversies surrounding gender reassignment. Eur J Pediatr Surg 19:203, 2009

Bruner JP, Tulipan N, Paschall RL, et al: Fetal surgery for myelomeningocele and the incidence of shunt-dependent hydrocephalus. JAMA 282(19):1819, 1999

Buyon JP, Clancy RM, Friedman DM: Autoimmune associated congenital heart block: integration of clinical and research clues in the management of the maternal/fetal dyad at risk. J Intern Med 265(6):653, 2009

Cannie M, Jani J, Chaffiotte C, et al: Quantification of intrathoracic liver herniation by magnetic resonance imaging and prediction of postnatal survival in fetuses with congenital diaphragmatic hernia. Ultrasound Obstet Gynecol 32:627, 2008

Cass DL, Olutoye OO, Cassady CI, et al: EXIT-to-resection for fetuses with large lung masses and persistent mediastinal compression near birth. J Pediatr Surg 48(1):138, 2013

Catalano PJ, Urken ML, Alvarez M, et al: New approach to the management of airway obstruction in "high risk" neonates. Arch Otolaryngol Head Neck Surg 118:306, 1992

Cavoretto P, Molina F, Poggi S, et al: Prenatal diagnosis and outcome of echogenic fetal lung lesions. Ultrasound Obstet Gynecol 32:769, 2008

Chalouhi GE, Essaoui M, Stirnemann J, et al: Laser therapy for twin-to-twin transfusion syndrome (TTTS). Prenat Diagn 31(7):637, 2011

Cohen AR, Couto J, Cummings JJ: Position statement on fetal myelomeningocele repair. Am J Obstet Gynecol 210(2):107, 2014

Copel JA, Liang RI, Demasio K, et al: The clinical significance of the irregular fetal heart rhythm. Am J Obstet Gynecol 182:813, 2000

Crombleholme TM, Coleman B, Hedrick H, et al: Cystic adenomatoid volume ratio predicts outcome in prenatally diagnosed cystic adenomatoid malformation of the lung. J Pediatr Surg 37(3):331, 2002

Crombleholme TM, Lim FY, Habli M, et al: Improved recipient twin survival with maternal nifedipine in twin-twin transfusion syndrome complicated by TTTS cardiomyopathy undergoing selective fetoscopic laser photocoagulation. Am J Obstet Gynecol 203(4):397.e1, 2010

Crombleholme TM, Shera D, Lee H, et al: A prospective, randomized, multicenter trial of amnioreduction vs selective fetoscopic laser photocoagulation for the treatment of twin-twin transfusion syndrome. Am J Obstet Gynecol 197:396, 2007

Cuneo BF, Zhao H, Strasburger JF, et al: Atrial and ventricular rate response and patterns of heart rate acceleration during maternal-fetal terbutaline treatment of fetal complete heart block. Am J Cardiol 100(4):661, 2007

Curran PF, Jelin EB, Rand L, et al: Prenatal steroids for microcystic congenital cystic adenomatoid malformations. J Pediatr Surg 45:145, 2010

David M, Forest MG: Prenatal treatment of congenital adrenal hyperplasia resulting from 21-hydroxylase deficiency. J Pediatr 105(5):799, 1984

Deprest J, Nicolaides K, Done E, et al: Technical aspects of fetal endoscopic tracheal occlusion for congenital diaphragmatic hernia. J Pediatr Surg 46(1): 22, 2011

Deprest JA, Flake AW, Gratacos E, et al: The making of fetal surgery. Prenat Diagn 30(7):653, 2010

Derikx JPM, De Backer A, Van De Schoot L, et al: Factors associated with recurrence and metastasis in sacrococcygeal teratoma. Brit J Surg 93:1543, 2006

Devaney SA, Palomaki GE, Scott JA, et al: Noninvasive fetal sex determination using cell-free fetal DNA: a systematic review and meta-analysis. JAMA 306(6):627, 2011

Duncombe GJ, Dickinson JE: Fetal thyrotoxicosis after maternal thyroidectomy. Aust N Z J Obstet Gynaecol 41(2):224, 2001

Freedman AL, Johnson MP, Gonzalez R: Fetal therapy for obstructive uropathy: past, present. . . future? Pediatr Nephrol 14:167, 2000

Friedman DM, Kim MY, Copel JA, et al: Prospective evaluation of fetuses with autoimmune associated congenital heart block followed in the PR interval and dexamethasone evaluation (PRIDE) study. Am J Cardiol 103(8):1102, 2009

Friedman DM, Kim MY, Copel JA: Utility of cardiac monitoring in fetuses at risk for congenital heart block: the PR Interval and Dexamethasone (PRIDE) Prospective Study. Circulation 117:485, 2008

Glantz JA, Tabbutt S, Gaynor JW, et al: Hypoplastic left heart syndrome with atrial level restriction in the era of prenatal diagnosis. Ann Thorac Surg 84:1633, 2007

Glatz AC, Gaynor JW, Rhodes LA, et al: Outcome of high-risk neonates with congenital complete heart block paced in the first 24 hours after birth. J Thorac Cardiovasc Surg 136(3):767, 2008

Golombeck K, Ball RH, Lee H, et al: Maternal morbidity after maternal-fetal surgery. Am J Obstet Gynecol 194:834, 2006

Habli M, Bombrys A, Lewis D, et al: Incidence of complications in twin-twin transfusion syndrome after selective fetoscopic laser photocoagulation: a single-center experience. Am J Obstet Gynecol 201(4):417.e1, 2009

Hahurij ND, Blom NA, Lopriore E, et al: Perinatal management and long-term cardiac outcome in fetal arrhythmia. Early Hum Dev 87:83, 2011

Harrison MR, Filly RA, Golbus MS, et al: Fetal treatment. N Engl J Med 307:1651, 1982

Harrison MR, Keller RL, Hawgood SB, et al: A randomized trial of fetal endoscopic tracheal occlusion for severe fetal congenital diaphragmatic hernia. N Engl J Med 349:1916, 2003

Harrison MR, Sydorak MR, Farrell JA, et al: Fetoscopic temporary tracheal occlusion for congenital diaphragmatic hernia: prelude to a randomized controlled trial. J Pediatr Surg 38:1012, 1993

Hayden SA, Russ PD, Pretorius DH, et al: Posterior urethral obstruction. Prenatal sonographic findings and clinical outcome in fourteen cases. J Ultrasound Med 7(7):371, 1988

Heckel S, Favre R, Schlienger JL, et al: Diagnosis and successful in utero treatment of a fetal goitrous hyperthyroidism caused by maternal Graves disease. A case report. Fetal Diagn Ther 12(1):54, 1997

Hedrick MH, Estes JM, Sullivan KM, et al: Plug the lung until it grows (PLUG): a new method to treat congenital diaphragmatic hernia in utero. J Pediatr Surg 29(5):612, 1994

Hedrick HL, Flake AW, Crombleholme TM, et al: Sacrococcygeal teratoma: prenatal assessment, fetal intervention, and outcome. J Pediatr Surg 39(3):430, 2004

Hobbins JC, Robero R, Grannum P, et al: Antenatal diagnosis of renal anomalies with ultrasound: I. Obstructive uropathy. Am J Obstet Gynecol 148:868, 1984

Holmes N, Harrison MR, Baskin LS, et al: Fetal surgery for posterior urethral valves: long-term postnatal outcomes. Pediatrics 108(1):E7, 2001

Huel C, Guibourdenche J, Vuillard E, et al: Use of ultrasound to distinguish between fetal hyperthyroidism and hypothyroidism on discovery of a goiter. Ultrasound Obstet Gynecol 33:412, 2009

Hui L, Bianchi DW: Prenatal pharmacotherapy for fetal anomalies: a 2011 update. Prenat Diagn 31:735, 2011

Jani JC, Keller RL, Benachi A, et al: Prenatal prediction of survival in isolated left-sided diaphragmatic hernia. Ultrasound Obstet Gynecol 27:18, 2006

Jani JC, Nicolaides KH, Gratacos E, et al: Severe diaphragmatic hernia treated by fetal endoscopic tracheal occlusion. Ultrasound Obstet Gynecol 34:304, 2009

Jelin E, Hirose S, Rand L, et al: Perinatal outcome of conservative management versus fetal intervention for twin reversed arterial perfusion sequence with a small acardiac twin. Fetal Diagn Ther 27:138, 2010

Kelly MF, Berenholz L, Rizzo KA, et al: Approach for oxygenation of the newborn with airway obstruction due to a cervical mass. Ann Oto Rhinol Laryngol 99(3 pt 1):179, 1990

Knox EM, Kilby MD, Martin WL, et al: In-utero pulmonary drainage in the management of primary hydrothorax and congenital cystic lung lesion: a systematic review. Ultrasound Obstet Gynecol 28:726, 2006

Krapp M, Kohl T, Simpson JM, et al: Review of diagnosis, treatment, and outcome of fetal atrial flutter compared with supraventricular tachycardia. Heart 89:913, 2003

Laje P, Johnson MP, Howell LJ, et al: Ex utero intrapartum treatment in the management of giant cervical teratomas. J Pediatr Surg 47(6):1208, 2012

Langer JC, Tabb T, Thompson P, et al: Management of prenatally diagnosed tracheal obstruction: access to the airway in utero prior to delivery. Fetal Diagn Ther 7(1):12, 1992

Le Blanc K, Götherström C, Ringdén O, et al: Fetal mesenchymal stem-cell engraftment in bone after in utero transplantation in a patient with severe osteogenesis imperfecta. Transplantation 79:1607, 2005

Lee H, Bebbington M, Crombleholme TM, et al: The North American Fetal Therapy Network Registry data on outcomes of radiofrequency ablation for twin-reversed arterial perfusion sequence. Fetal Diagn Ther 33(4):224, 2013

Lee H, Wagner AJ, Sy E, et al: Efficacy of radiofrequency ablation for twin-reversed arterial perfusion sequence. Am J Obstet Gynecol 196:459, 2007

Livingston JC, Lim FY, Polzin W, et al: Intrafetal radiofrequency ablation for twin reversed arterial perfusion (TRAP): a single-center experience. Am J Obstet Gynecol 197:399, 2007

Loh K, Jelin E, Hirose S, et al: Microcystic congenital pulmonary airway malformation with hydrops fetalis: steroids vs. open fetal resection. J Pediatr Surg 47(1):36, 2012

Lopriore E, van Wezel-Meijler G, Middlethorp JM, et al: Incidence, origin, and character of cerebral injury in twin-to-twin transfusion syndrome treated with fetoscopic laser surgery. Am J Obstet Gynecol 194(5):1215, 2006

Mangione R, Guyon F, Vergnaud A, et al: Successful treatment of refractory supraventricular tachycardia by repeat intravascular injection of amiodarone in a fetus with hydrops. Eur J Obstet Gynecol Reprod Biol 86:105, 1999

Mann S, Johnson MP, Wilson RD: Fetal thoracic and bladder shunts. Semin Fetal Neonatal Med 15:28, 2010

Manning FA, Harrison MR, Rodeck C: Catheter shunts for fetal hydronephrosis and hydrocephalus. Report of the International Fetal Surgery Registry. N Engl J Med 315:336, 1986

Marshall AC, Levine J, Morash D, et al: Results of in utero atrial septoplasty in fetuses with hypoplastic left heart syndrome. Prenat Diagn 28(11):1023, 2008

Mayer S, Klaritsch P, Petersen S, et al: The correlation between lung volume and liver herniation measurements by fetal MRI in isolated congenital diaphragmatic hernia: a systematic review and meta-analysis of observational studies. Prenat Diagn 31(11):1086, 2011

McCullough LB, Chervenak FA, Brent RL, et al: A case study in unethical transgressive bioethics: "Letter of Concern from Bioethicists" about the prenatal administration of dexamethasone. Am J Bioeth 10(9):35, 2010

McElhinney DB, Tworetsky W, Lock JE: Current status of fetal cardiac intervention. Circulation 121(10):1256, 2010

Metkus AP, Filly RA, Stringer MD, et al: Sonographic predictors of survival in fetal diaphragmatic hernia. J Pediatr Surg 31(1): 148, 1996

Meuli M, Meuli-Simmen C, Hutchins GM, et al: In utero surgery rescues neurological function at birth in sheep with spina bifida. Nat Med 1(4):342, 1995

Meuli M, Meuli-Simmen C, Hutchins GM, et al: The spinal cord lesion in human fetuses with myelomeningocele: implications for fetal surgery. J Pediatr Surg 32(3):448, 1997

Miller WL, Witchel SF: Prenatal treatment of congenital adrenal hyperplasia: risks outweigh benefits. Am J Obstet Gynecol 208(5):354, 2013

Moldenhauer JS: Ex utero intrapartum therapy. Semin Pediatr Surg 22(1):44, 2013

Morris LM, Lim FY, Crombleholme TM: Ex utero intrapartum treatment procedure: a peripartum management strategy in particularly challenging cases. J Pediatr 154(1):126, 2009a

Morris LM, Lim F-Y, Elluru RG, et al: Severe micrognathia: indications for EXIT-to-Airway. Fetal Diagn Ther 26:162, 2009b

Morris LM, Lim FY, Livingston JC, et al: High-risk fetal congenital pulmonary airway malformations have a variable response to steroids. J Pediatr Surg 44(1):60, 2009c

Mullassery D, Ba'ath ME, Jesudason EC, et al: Value of liver herniation in prediction of outcome in fetal congenital diaphragmatic hernia: a systematic review and meta-analysis. Ultrasound Obstet Gynecol 35(5):609, 2010

Mummery C, Westgren M, Sermon S: Current controversies in prenatal diagnosis 1: is stem cell therapy ready for human fetuses? Prenat Diagn 31:228, 2011

Mychaliska GB, Bealer JF, Graf JL, et al: Operating on placental support: the ex utero intrapartum treatment procedure. J Pediatr Surg 32(2):227, 1997

New MI, Abraham M, Yuen T, et al: An update on prenatal diagnosis and treatment of congenital adrenal hyperplasia. Semin Reprod Med 30(5):396, 2012

Niinikoski H, Mamalainen Am, Ekblad H, et al: Neonatal hypothyroidism after amiodarone therapy. Acta Paediatr 96:773, 2007

Nimkarn S, New MI: 21-Hydroxylase-deficient congenital adrenal hyperplasia. In Pagon RA, Bird TD, Dolan CR, et al (eds): GeneReviews™, Seattle, University of Washington, 2010. Available at: http://www.ncbi.nlm.nih.gov/books/NBK1171. Accessed June 10, 2013

Noah MM, Norton ME, Sandberg P, et al: Short-term maternal outcomes that are associated with the EXIT procedure, as compared with cesarean delivery. Am J Obstet Gynecol 186(4):773, 2002

Peleg D, Cada S, Peleg A, et al: The relationship between maternal serum thyroid-stimulating immunoglobulin and neonatal thyrotoxicosis. Obstet Gynecol 99(6):1040, 2002

Peranteau WH, Wilson RD, Liechty KW, et al: Effect of maternal betamethasone administration on prenatal congenital cystic adenomatoid malformation growth and fetal survival. Fetal Diagn Ther 22:365, 2007

Quintero RA, Morales WJ, Allen MH, et al: Staging of twin-twin transfusion syndrome. J Perinatol 19:550, 1999

Ribault V, Castanet M, Bertrand AM, et al: Experience with intraamniotic thyroxine treatment in nonimmune fetal goitrous hypothyroidism in 12 cases. J Clin Endocrinol Metab 94:3731, 2009

Robyr R, Lewi L, Salomon LJ, et al: Prevalence and management of late fetal complications following successful selective laser coagulation of chorionic plate anastomoses in twin-to-twin transfusion syndrome. Am J Obstet Gynecol 194(3):796, 2006

Ruano R, Yoshisaki CT, da Silva MM, et al: A randomized controlled trial of fetal endoscopic tracheal occlusion versus postnatal management of severe isolated congenital diaphragmatic hernia. Ultrasound Obstet Gynecol 39(1):20, 2012

Simpson JL: Fetal arrhythmias. Ultrasound Obstet Gynecol 27:599, 2006

Slaghekke F, Kist WJ, Oepkes D, et al: Twin anemia-polycythemia sequence: diagnostic criteria, classification, perinatal management, and outcome. Fetal Diagn Ther 27(4):181, 2010

Society for Maternal-Fetal Medicine, Simpson LL: Twin-twin transfusion syndrome. Am J Obstet Gynecol 208(1):3, 2013

Speiser PW, Azziz, Baskin LS, et al: Congenital adrenal hyperplasia due to steroid 21-hydroxylase deficiency: an Endocrine Society Clinical Practice Guideline. J Clin Endocrinol Metab 95(9):4133, 2010

Srinivasan S, Strasburger J: Overview of fetal arrhythmias. Curr Opin Pediatr 20:522, 2008

Srisupundit K, Sirichotiyakul S, Tongprasent F, et al: Fetal therapy in fetal thyrotoxicosis: a case report. Fetal Diagn Ther 23(2):114, 2008

Stamilio DM, Fraser WD, Moore TR: Twin-twin transfusion syndrome: an ethics-based and evidence-based argument for clinical research. Am J Obstet Gynecol 203(1):3, 2010

Stoffan AP, Wilson JM, Jennings RW, et al: Does the ex utero intrapartum treatment to extracorporeal membrane oxygenation procedure change outcomes for high-risk patients with congenital diaphragmatic hernia? J Pediatr Surg 47(6):1053, 2012

Strasburger JF, Wakai RT: Fetal cardiac arrhythmia detection and *in utero* therapy. Nat Rev Cardiol 7(5):277, 2010

Sutton LN, Adzick NS, Bilaniuk LT, et al: Improvement in hindbrain herniation demonstrated by serial fetal magnetic resonance imaging following fetal surgery for myelomeningocele. JAMA 282(19):1826, 1999

Swamy R, Embleton N, Hale J, et al: Sacrococcygeal teratoma over two decades: birth prevalence, prenatal diagnosis and clinical outcomes. Prenat Diagn 28:1048, 2008

Tiblad E, Westgren M: Fetal stem-cell transplantation. Best Pract Res Clin Obstet Gynaecol 22:189, 2008

Vrecenak JD, Flake AW: Fetal surgical intervention: progress and perspectives. Pediatr Surg Int 29(5):407, 2013

Walsh DS, Hubbard AM, Olutoye OO, et al: Assessment of fetal lung volumes and liver herniation with magnetic resonance imaging in congenital diaphragmatic hernia. Am J Obstet Gynecol 183:1067, 2000

Walsh WF, Chescheir NC, Gillam-Krakauer M, et al: Maternal-Fetal Surgical Procedures. Technical Brief No. 5. AHRQ Publication No. 10(11)-EHC059-EF, Rockville, Agency for Healthcare Research and Quality, 2011

Wenstrom KD: Perspective: fetal surgery for congenital diaphragmatic hernia. N Engl J Med 349(20):1887, 2003

Westgren M, Ringden O, Eik-Nes S, et al: Lack of evidence of permanent engraftment after in utero fetal stem cell transplantation in congenital hemoglobinopathies. Transplantation 61:1176, 1996

Wilson RD, Baxter JK, Johnson MP, et al: Thoracoamniotic shunts: fetal treatment of pleural effusions and congenital cystic adenomatoid malformations. Fetal Diagn Ther 19(5):413, 2004

Wilson RD, Lemerand K, Johnson MP, et al: Reproductive outcomes in subsequent pregnancies after a pregnancy complicated by open maternal-fetal surgery (1996–2007). Am J Obstet Gynecol 203(3):209.e1, 2010

Worley KC, Dashe JS, Barber RG, et al: Fetal magnetic resonance imaging in isolated diaphragmatic hernia: volume of herniated liver and neonatal outcome. Am J Obstet Gynecol 200;318.e1, 2009

Wu D, Ball RH: The maternal side of maternal-fetal surgery. Clin Perinatol 36(2):247, 2009

Yinon Y, Grisaru-Granovsky S, Chaddha V, et al: Perinatal outcome following fetal chest shunt insertion for pleural effusion. Ultrasound Obstet Gynecol 36:58, 2010

CHAPTER 17

Fetal Assessment

Available techniques employed to forecast fetal well-being focus on fetal biophysical findings that include heart rate, movement, breathing, and amnionic fluid production. These findings are used to perform antepartum fetal surveillance to accomplish the stated goals of the American College of Obstetricians and Gynecologists and the American Academy of Pediatrics (2012), which includes prevention of fetal death and avoidance of unnecessary interventions. In most cases, a negative, that is, normal test result is highly reassuring, because fetal deaths within 1 week of a normal test are rare. Indeed, negative-predictive values—a true negative test—for most of the tests described are 99.8 percent or higher. In contrast, estimates of the positive-predictive values—a true positive test—for abnormal test results are low and range between 10 and 40 percent. Importantly, the widespread use of antepartum fetal surveillance is primarily based on circumstantial evidence because there have been no definitive randomized clinical trials (Grivell, 2012; Hofmeyr, 2012).

FETAL MOVEMENTS

Passive unstimulated fetal activity commences as early as 7 weeks' gestation and becomes more sophisticated and coordinated by the end of pregnancy (Vindla, 1995). Indeed, beyond 8 menstrual weeks, fetal body movements are never absent for periods exceeding 13 minutes (DeVries, 1985). Between 20 and 30 weeks, general body movements become organized, and the fetus starts to show rest-activity cycles (Sorokin, 1982). Fetal movement maturation continues until approximately 36 weeks, when behavioral states are established in most normal fetuses. Nijhuis and colleagues (1982) described four fetal behavioral states:

- State 1F is a quiescent state—quiet sleep—with a narrow oscillatory bandwidth of the fetal heart rate.
- State 2F includes frequent gross body movements, continuous eye movements, and wider oscillation of the fetal heart rate. This state is analogous to rapid eye movement (REM) or active sleep in the neonate.
- State 3F includes continuous eye movements in the absence of body movements and no heart rate accelerations. The existence of this state is disputed (Pillai, 1990a).
- State 4F is one of vigorous body movement with continuous eye movements and heart rate accelerations. This state corresponds to the awake state in newborns.

Fetuses spend most of their time in states 1F and 2F. For example, at 38 weeks, 75 percent of time is spent in these two states. These behavioral states—particularly 1F and 2F, which correspond to quiet sleep and active sleep—have been used to develop an increasingly sophisticated understanding of fetal behavior. In a study of fetal urine production, as shown in Figure 17-1, bladder volumes increased during state 1F quiet sleep. During state 2F, the fetal heart rate baseline bandwidth increased appreciably, and bladder volume was significantly diminished due to fetal voiding as well as decreased

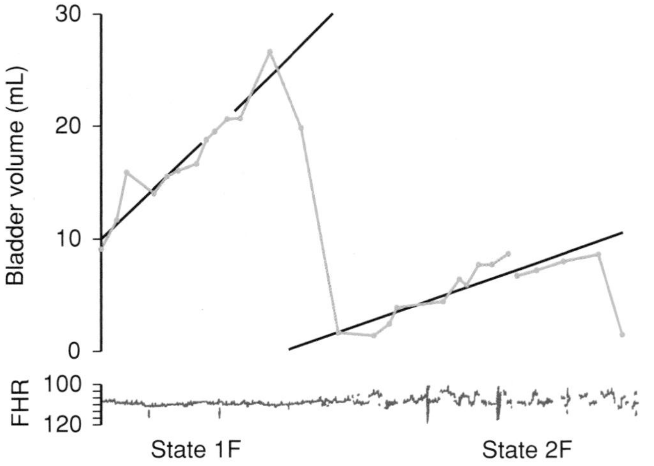

FIGURE 17-1 Fetal bladder volume measurements together with fetal heart rate (FHR) variation recorded in relation to 1F or 2F behavior states. State 1F fetal heart rate has a narrow bandwidth consistent with quiet sleep. State 2F heart rate shows wide oscillation of the baseline consistent with active sleep. (Modified from Oosterhof, 1993.)

urine production. These phenomena were interpreted to represent reduced renal blood flow during active sleep. Knight and coworkers (2012) studied 456 term pregnancies with the prenatal diagnosis of oligohydramnios and compared them with matched controls without oligohydramnios. Oligohydramnios was associated with lower birthweight and small-for-gestational age infants, as well as renal malformations, congenital torticollis, and congenitally dislocated hips.

An important determinant of fetal activity appears to be sleep-awake cycles, which are independent of the maternal sleep-awake state. Sleep cyclicity has been described as varying from approximately 20 minutes to as much as 75 minutes. Timor-Tritsch and associates (1978) reported that the mean length of the quiet or inactive state for term fetuses was 23 minutes. Patrick and associates (1982) measured gross fetal body movements with real-time sonography for 24-hour periods in 31 normal pregnancies and found the longest period of inactivity to be 75 minutes. *Amnionic fluid volume* is another important determinant of fetal activity. Sherer and colleagues (1996) assessed the number of fetal movements in 465 pregnancies during biophysical profile testing in relation to amnionic fluid volume. They observed decreased fetal activity with diminished amnionic volumes and suggested that a restricted uterine space might physically limit fetal movements.

Sadovsky and coworkers (1979b) studied fetal movements in 120 normal pregnancies and classified the movements into three categories according to both maternal perceptions and independent recordings using piezoelectric sensors. Weak, strong, and rolling movements were described, and their relative contributions to total weekly movements throughout the last half of pregnancy were quantified. As pregnancy advances, weak movements decrease and are superseded by more vigorous movements, which increase for several weeks and then subside at term. Presumably, declining amnionic fluid and space account for diminishing activity at term.

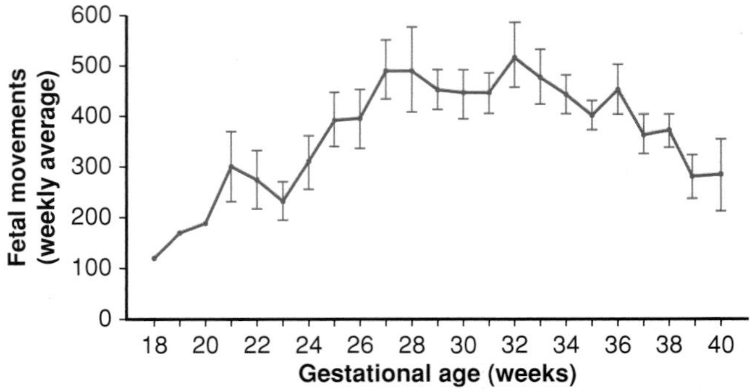

FIGURE 17-2 Graph depicts averages of fetal movements counted during 12-hour periods (mean ± SEM). (Data from Sadovsky, 1979a.)

Figure 17-2 shows fetal movements during the last half of gestation in 127 pregnancies with normal outcomes. The mean number of weekly movements calculated from 12-hour daily recording periods increased from approximately 200 at 20 weeks to a maximum of 575 movements at 32 weeks. Fetal movements then declined to an average of 282 at 40 weeks. Normal weekly maternal counts of fetal movements ranged between 50 and 950, with large daily variations that included counts as low as 4 to 10 per 12-hour period in normal pregnancies.

Clinical Application

Diminished fetal activity may be a harbinger of impending fetal death (Sadovsky, 1973). Because of this, various methods have been described to quantify movement of the fetus to forecast its well-being. Methods include use of a tocodynamometer, visualization with sonography, and maternal subjective perceptions. Most, but not all, investigators have reported excellent correlation between maternally perceived fetal motion and movements documented by instrumentation. For example, Rayburn (1980) found that 80 percent of all movements observed during sonographic monitoring were perceived by the mother. In contrast, however, Johnson and colleagues (1992) reported that beyond 36 weeks, mothers perceived only 16 percent of fetal body movements. Fetal motions lasting more than 20 seconds were more likely to be identified than shorter episodes. Although several fetal-movement counting protocols have been used, neither the optimal number of movements nor the ideal duration for counting them has been defined. For example, in one method, perception of 10 fetal movements in up to 2 hours is considered normal (Moore, 1989). In another, women are instructed to count fetal movements for 1 hour a day, and the count is accepted as reassuring if it equals or exceeds a previously established baseline count (Neldam, 1983).

Commonly, women may present in the third trimester complaining of subjectively reduced fetal movement. Harrington and associates (1998) reported that 7 percent of nearly 6800 women presented with a complaint of decreased fetal movement. Fetal heart rate monitoring tests were employed if sonographic scans for fetal growth or Doppler velocimetry were abnormal. Pregnancy outcomes for women who complained of decreased fetal movement were not significantly different from those for women without this complaint. Nonetheless, the authors recommended evaluation to reassure the mother.

Grant and coworkers (1989) performed an unparalleled investigation of maternally perceived fetal movements and pregnancy outcome. More than 68,000 pregnancies were randomly assigned between 28 and 32 weeks. Women in the fetal movement arm of the study were instructed by specially employed midwives to record the time needed to feel 10 movements each day. This required an average of 2.7 hours each day. Women in the control group were informally asked about movements during prenatal visits. Reports of decreased fetal motion were evaluated with tests of fetal well-being. Antepartum death rates for otherwise normal singleton fetuses were similar in the two study groups. Despite the counting policy, most stillborn fetuses were dead by the time the mothers reported for medical attention. Importantly, rather than concluding that maternal perceptions of fetal activity were meaningless, these investigators concluded that informal maternal perceptions were as valuable as formally recorded fetal movement.

The most recent randomized study of fetal movements was performed in Norway by Saastad and colleagues (2011). A total of 1076 women were randomly assigned to standardized fetal movement counting from gestational week 28 or to no counting. Growth-restricted fetuses were identified before birth significantly more often when fetal movement counting was used. There was also a significant reduction (0.4 versus 2.3 percent) in 1-minute Apgar scores ≤ 3 when counting was used. Also, Warrander and associates (2012) performed the first study of placental pathology in pregnancies complicated by decreased fetal movements. Decreased movement was associated with a variety of placental abnormalities including infarction.

FETAL BREATHING

After decades of uncertainty as to whether the fetus normally breathes, Dawes and coworkers (1972) showed small inward and outward flows of tracheal fluid in fetal sheep, indicating thoracic movement. These chest wall movements differed from those following birth in that they were discontinuous. Another interesting feature of fetal respiration was *paradoxical chest wall movement,* which is depicted in Figure 17-3. In the newborn or adult, the opposite occurs. One interpretation of the paradoxical respiratory motion might be coughing to clear amnionic fluid debris. Although the physiological basis for the breathing reflex is not completely understood, such exchange of amnionic fluid appears to be essential for normal lung development.

Dawes (1974) identified two types of respiratory movements. The first are *gasps* or *sighs,* which occurred at a frequency of 1 to 4 per minute. The second, *irregular bursts of breathing,* occurred at rates up to 240 cycles per minute. These latter rapid respiratory movements were associated with rapid eye movements–REM. Badalian and associates (1993) studied the maturation of normal fetal breathing using color flow and spectral Doppler analysis of nasal fluid flow as an index of lung function. They suggested that fetal respiratory rate decreased in conjunction with increased respiratory volume at 33 to 36 weeks and coincidental with lung maturation.

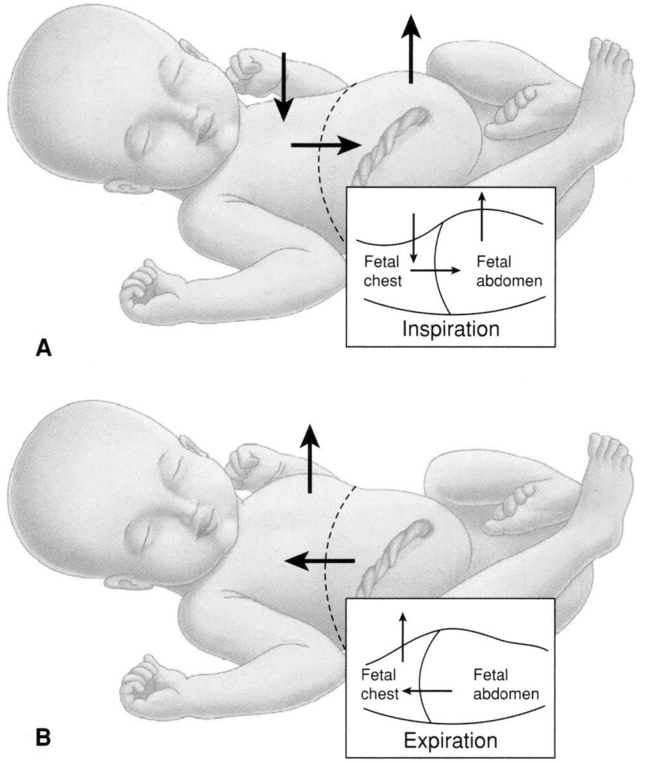

FIGURE 17-3 Paradoxical chest movement with fetal respiration. During inspiration **(A)**, the chest wall paradoxically *collapses* and the abdomen protrudes, whereas during expiration **(B)**, the chest wall *expands*. (Adapted from Johnson, 1988.)

Many investigators have examined fetal breathing movements using sonography to determine whether chest wall movements might reflect fetal health. Several variables in addition to hypoxia were found to affect fetal respiratory movements. These included hypoglycemia, sound stimuli, cigarette smoking, amniocentesis, impending preterm labor, gestational age, the fetal heart rate itself, and labor—during which it is normal for respiration to cease.

Because fetal breathing movements are episodic, interpretation of fetal health when respirations are absent may be tenuous. Patrick and associates (1980) performed continuous 24-hour observation using sonography to characterize fetal breathing patterns during the last 10 weeks of pregnancy. There was a total of 1224 hours of fetal observation in 51 pregnancies. Figure 17-4 displays the percentages of time spent breathing near term. Clearly, there is diurnal variation, because breathing substantively diminishes during the night. In addition, breathing activity increases somewhat following maternal meals. Total absence of breathing was observed in some of these normal fetuses for up to 122 minutes, indicating that fetal evaluation to diagnose absent respiratory motion may require long periods of observation.

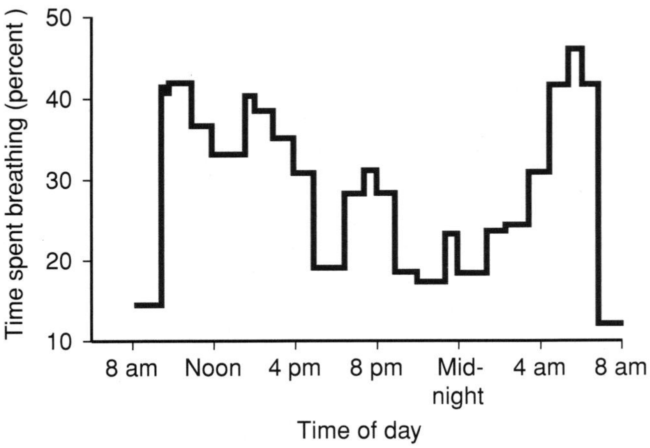

FIGURE 17-4 The percentage of time spent breathing by 11 fetuses at 38 to 39 weeks demonstrated a significant increase in fetal breathing activity after breakfast. Breathing activity diminished during the day and reached its minimum between 8 PM and midnight hours. There was a significant increase in the percentage of time spent breathing between 4 and 7 AM, when mothers were asleep. (Adapted from Patrick, 1980.)

The potential for breathing activity to be an important marker of fetal health is unfulfilled because of the multiplicity of factors that normally affect breathing. Most clinical applications have included assessment of other fetal biophysical indices, such as heart rate. As will be discussed, fetal breathing has become a component of the *biophysical profile.*

CONTRACTION STRESS TESTING

As amnionic fluid pressure increases with uterine contractions, myometrial pressure exceeds collapsing pressure for vessels coursing through uterine muscle. This ultimately decreases blood flow to the intervillous space. Brief periods of impaired oxygen exchange result, and if uteroplacental pathology is present, these elicit late fetal heart rate decelerations (Chap. 24, p. 483). Contractions also may produce a pattern of variable decelerations as a result of cord compression, suggesting oligohydramnios, which is often a concomitant of placental insufficiency.

Ray and colleagues (1972) used this concept in 66 complicated pregnancies and developed the *oxytocin challenge test,* which was later called the *contraction stress test.* Intravenous oxytocin was used to stimulate contractions, and the fetal heart rate response was recorded. The criterion for a positive test result, that is, an abnormal result, was uniform repetitive late fetal heart rate decelerations. These reflected the uterine contraction waveform and had an onset at or beyond the contraction acme. Such late decelerations could be the result of uteroplacental insufficiency. The tests were generally repeated on a weekly basis, and the investigators concluded that negative contraction stress test results, that is, normal results, forecasted fetal health. One disadvantage cited was that the average contraction stress test required 90 minutes to complete.

To perform the test, the fetal heart rate and uterine contractions are recorded simultaneously with an external monitor. If at least three spontaneous contractions of 40 seconds or longer are present in 10 minutes, no uterine stimulation is necessary (American College of Obstetricians and Gynecologists, 2012a). Contractions are induced with either oxytocin or nipple stimulation if there are fewer than three in 10 minutes. For oxytocin use, a dilute intravenous infusion is initiated at a rate of 0.5 mU/min and doubled every 20 minutes until a satisfactory contraction pattern is established (Freeman, 1975). The results of the contraction stress test are interpreted according to the criteria shown in Table 17-1.

TABLE 17-1. Criteria for Interpretation of the Contraction Stress Test

Negative: no late or significant variable decelerations
Positive: late decelerations following 50% or more of contractions (even if the contraction frequency is fewer than three in 10 minutes)
Equivocal-suspicious: intermittent late decelerations or significant variable decelerations
Equivocal-hyperstimulatory: fetal heart rate decelerations that occur in the presence of contractions more frequent than every 2 minutes or lasting longer than 90 seconds
Unsatisfactory: fewer than three contractions in 10 minutes or an uninterpretable tracing

Nipple stimulation to induce uterine contractions is usually successful for contraction stress testing (Huddleston, 1984). One method recommended by the American College of Obstetricians and Gynecologists (2012a) involves a woman rubbing one nipple through her clothing for 2 minutes or until a contraction begins. This 2-minute nipple stimulation ideally will induce a pattern of three contractions per 10 minutes. If not, after a 5-minute interval, she is instructed to retry nipple stimulation to achieve the desired pattern. If this is unsuccessful, then dilute oxytocin may be used. Advantages include reduced cost and shortened testing times. Some have reported unpredictable uterine hyperstimulation and fetal distress, whereas others did not find excessive activity to be harmful (Frager, 1987; Schellpfeffer, 1985).

NONSTRESS TESTS

Freeman (1975) and Lee and colleagues (1975) introduced the *nonstress test* to describe fetal heart rate acceleration in response to fetal movement as a sign of fetal health. This test involved the use of Doppler-detected fetal heart rate acceleration coincident with fetal movements perceived by the mother. By the end of the 1970s, the nonstress test had become the primary method of testing fetal health. The nonstress test was easier to perform, and normal results were used to further discriminate false-positive contraction stress tests. Simplistically, the nonstress test is primarily a test of *fetal condition,* and it differs from the contraction stress test, which is a test of *uteroplacental function.* Currently, nonstress testing is the most widely used primary testing method for assessment of fetal well-being and has also been incorporated into the biophysical profile testing system subsequently discussed.

Fetal Heart Rate Acceleration

There are autonomic influences mediated by sympathetic or parasympathetic impulses from brainstem centers that normally increase or decrease the fetal heart rate. *Beat-to-beat variability* is also under the control of the autonomic nervous system (Matsuura, 1996). Consequently, pathological loss of acceleration may be seen in conjunction with significantly decreased beat-to-beat variability of the fetal heart rate (Chap. 24, p. 479). Loss of such reactivity, however, is most commonly associated with sleep cycles as discussed on page 335. It also may be caused by central depression from medications or cigarette smoking (Jansson, 2005).

The nonstress test is based on the hypothesis that the heart rate of a fetus that is not acidemic as a result of hypoxia or neurological depression will temporarily accelerate in response to fetal movement. Fetal movements during testing are identified by maternal perception and recorded. As hypoxia develops, these fetal heart rate accelerations diminish (Smith, 1988).

Gestational age influences acceleration or reactivity of the fetal heart rate. Pillai and James (1990b) studied the development of fetal heart rate acceleration patterns during normal pregnancy. The percentage of body movements that is accompanied by accelerations and the amplitude of these accelerations increase with gestational age (Fig. 17-5). Guinn and colleagues (1998) studied nonstress test results between 25 and 28 weeks in 188 normal fetuses. Only 70 percent of these normal fetuses demonstrated the required 15 beats per minute (bpm) or more of heart rate acceleration. Lesser degrees of acceleration, that is, 10 bpm, occurred in 90 percent of the fetuses.

The National Institute of Child Health and Human Development Fetal Monitoring Workshop defined normal acceleration based on gestational age (Macones, 2008). In fetuses at or beyond 32 weeks, the acceleration acme is 15 bpm or more above the baseline rate, and the acceleration lasts 15 seconds or longer but less than 2 minutes. Before 32 weeks, accelerations are defined as having an acme that is 10 bpm or more above baseline for 10 seconds or longer. Cousins and associates (2012) compared the Workshop criteria recommended before 32 weeks, that is, 10 bpm/10 seconds, with standard 15 bpm/15 seconds criteria in a randomized trial of 143 women. They found no differences in perinatal outcomes.

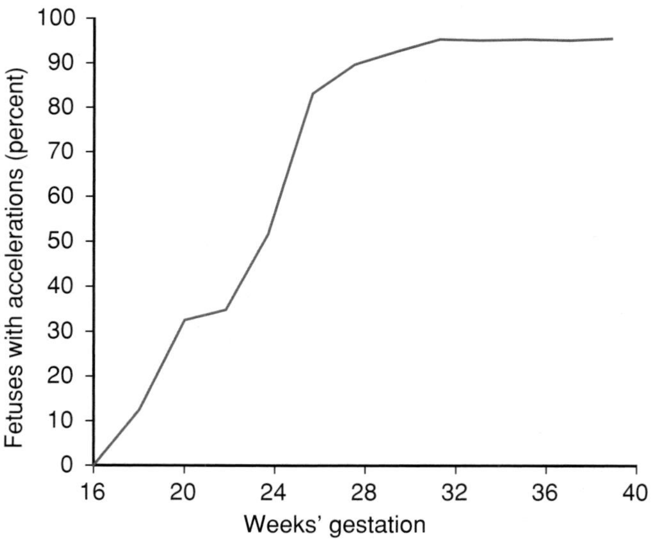

FIGURE 17-5 Percentage of fetuses with at least one acceleration of 15 bpm sustained for 15 seconds concurrent with fetal movement. (Adapted from Pillai, 1990b.)

Normal Nonstress Tests

There have been many different definitions of normal nonstress test results. They vary as to the number, amplitude, and duration of acceleration, as well as the test duration. The definition currently recommended by the American College of Obstetricians and Gynecologists and the American Academy of Pediatrics (2012) is two or more accelerations that peak at 15 bpm or more above baseline, each lasting 15 seconds or more, and all occurring within 20 minutes of beginning the test (Fig. 17-6). It was also recommended that accelerations with or without fetal movements be accepted, and that a 40-minute or longer tracing—to account for fetal sleep cycles—should be performed before concluding that there was insufficient fetal reactivity. Miller and coworkers (1996b) reviewed outcomes in fetuses with nonstress tests considered as nonreactive because there was only one acceleration. They concluded that one acceleration was just as reliable as two in predicting healthy fetal status.

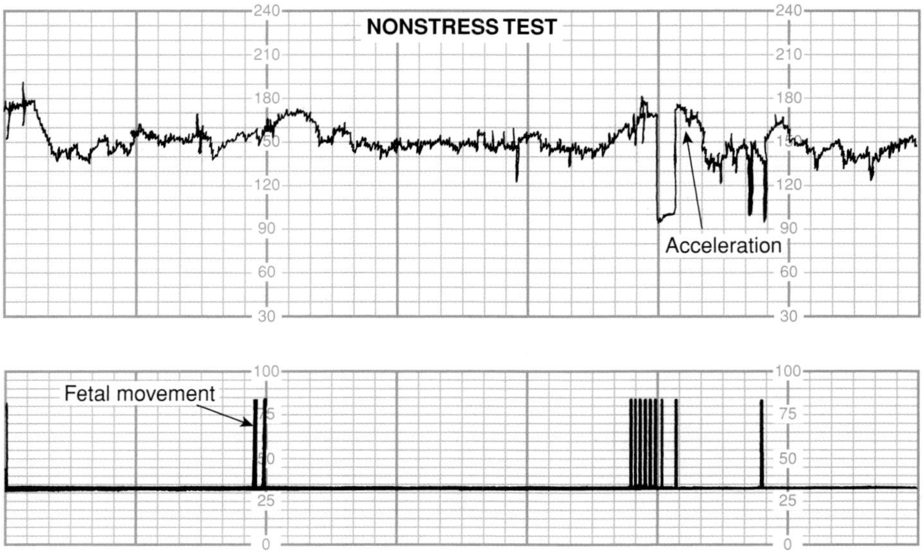

FIGURE 17-6 Reactive nonstress test. In the upper panel, notice the increase of fetal heart rate by more than 15 beats/min for longer than 15 seconds following fetal movements, which are indicated by the vertical marks (*lower panel*).

Although a normal number and amplitude of accelerations seems to reflect fetal well-being, their absence does not invariably predict fetal compromise. Indeed, some investigators have reported 90-percent or higher false-positive rates (Devoe, 1986). Because healthy fetuses may not move for periods of up to 75 minutes, some have considered that a longer duration of nonstress testing might increase the positive-predictive value of an abnormal, that is, nonreactive, test (Brown, 1981). In this scheme, either the test became reactive during a period up to 80 minutes or the test remained nonreactive for 120 minutes, which indicated that the fetus was very ill.

Not only are there many different definitions of normal nonstress test results, but the reproducibility of interpretations is problematic. For example, Hage (1985) mailed five nonstress tests, blinded to specific patient clinical data, to a national sample of obstetricians for their interpretations. He concluded that although nonstress testing is popular, the reliability of test interpretation needs improvement.

Abnormal Nonstress Tests

Based on the foregoing, an abnormal nonstress test is not always malignant. The example shown in Figure 17-7, however, was ominous. Such a pattern can also be seen with a sleeping fetus. Also, an abnormal test can revert to normal as the fetal condition changes, such as the example shown in Figure 17-8. Importantly, a normal nonstress test can become abnormal if the fetal condition deteriorates. There are abnormal patterns that reliably forecast severe fetal jeopardy. Devoe and coworkers (1985) concluded that nonstress tests that were nonreactive for 90 minutes were almost invariably—93 percent—associated with significant perinatal pathology. Hammacher and coworkers (1968) described tracings with what they termed a *silent oscillatory pattern* that he considered dangerous. This pattern consisted of a fetal heart rate baseline that oscillated less than 5 bpm and presumably indicated absent acceleration and beat-to-beat variability.

Visser and associates (1980) described a *terminal cardiotocogram,* which included: (1) baseline oscillation of less than 5 bpm, (2) absent accelerations, and (3) late decelerations with spontaneous uterine contractions. These results were similar to experiences from Parkland Hospital in which absence of accelerations during an 80-minute recording period in 27 fetuses was associated consistently with evidence of uteroplacental pathology (Leveno, 1983). The latter included fetal-growth restriction in 75 percent, oligohydramnios in 80 percent, fetal acidemia in 40 percent, meconium in 30 percent, and placental infarction in 93 percent.

Interval between Testing

Set originally rather arbitrarily at 7 days, the interval between tests appears to have been shortened as experience evolved with nonstress testing. According to the American College of Obstetricians and Gynecologists (2012a), more frequent testing is advocated by some investigators for women with postterm pregnancy, multifetal gestation, type 1 diabetes mellitus, fetal-growth restriction, or gestational hypertension. In these circumstances, some investigators perform twice-weekly tests, with additional testing completed for maternal or fetal deterioration regardless of the time elapsed since the last test. Others perform nonstress tests daily or even more frequently, such as with severe preeclampsia remote from term (Chap. 40, p. 755).

Decelerations During Nonstress Testing

Fetal movements commonly produce heart rate decelerations. Timor-Tritsch and associates (1978) reported this during nonstress testing in half to two thirds of tracings, depending on the

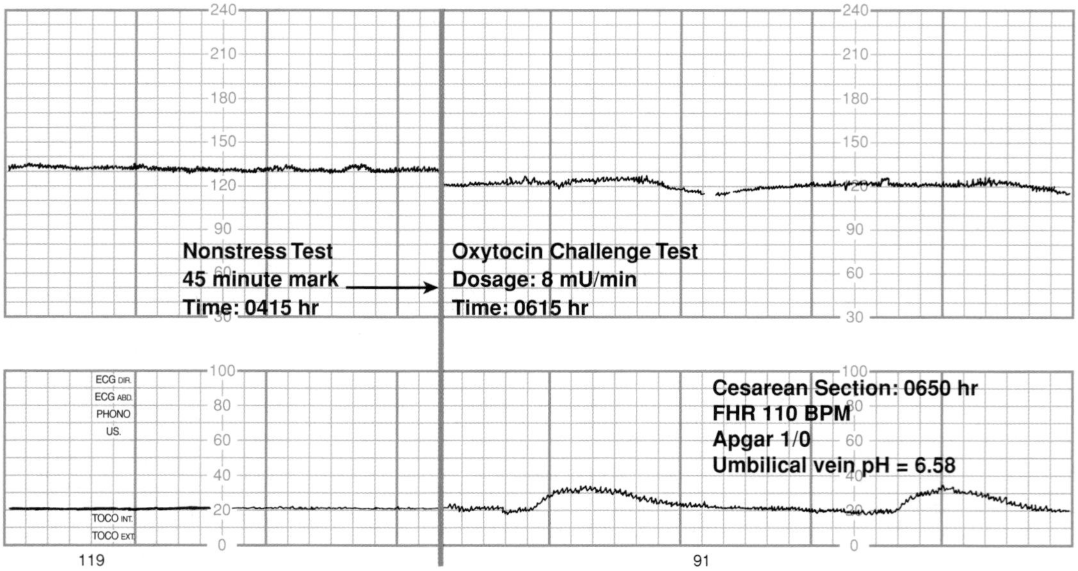

FIGURE 17-7 Nonreactive nonstress test (*left side of tracing*) followed by contraction stress test showing mild, late decelerations (*right side of tracing*). Cesarean delivery was performed, and the severely acidemic fetus could not be resuscitated.

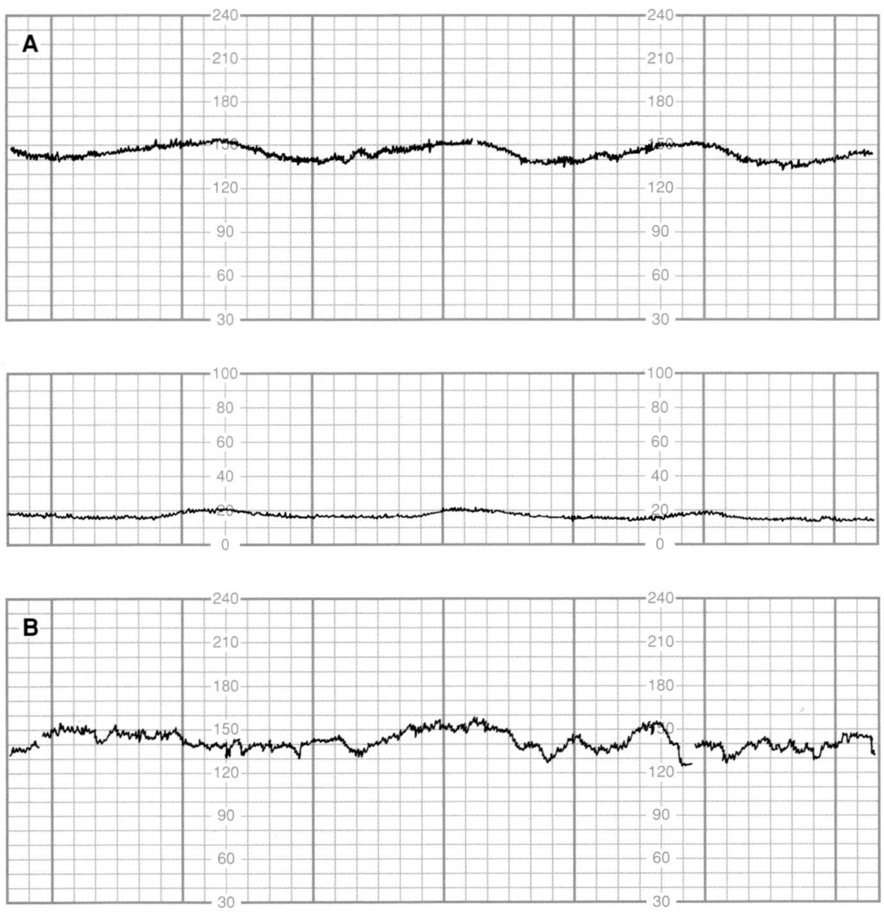

FIGURE 17-8 Two antepartum fetal heart rate (FHR) tracings in a 28-week pregnant woman with diabetic ketoacidosis. **A.** FHR tracing (*upper panel*) and accompanying contraction tracing (*second panel*). Tracing, obtained during maternal and fetal acidemia, shows absence of accelerations, diminished variability, and late decelerations with weak spontaneous contractions. **B.** FHR tracing shows return of normal accelerations and variability of the fetal heart rate following correction of maternal acidemia.

vigor of the fetal motion. This high incidence of decelerations inevitably makes interpretation of their significance problematic. Indeed, Meis and coworkers (1986) reported that variable fetal heart rate decelerations during nonstress tests were not a sign of fetal compromise. The American College of Obstetricians and Gynecologists (2012a) has concluded that variable decelerations, if nonrepetitive and brief—less than 30 seconds—do not indicate fetal compromise or the need for obstetrical intervention. In contrast, repetitive variable decelerations—at least three in 20 minutes—even if mild, have been associated with an increased risk of cesarean delivery for fetal distress. Decelerations lasting 1 minute or longer have been reported to have an even worse prognosis (Bourgeois, 1984; Druzin, 1981; Pazos, 1982).

Hoskins and associates (1991) attempted to refine interpretation of testing that shows variable decelerations by adding sonographic estimation of amnionic fluid volume. The incidence of cesarean delivery for intrapartum fetal distress progressively increased concurrently with the severity of variable decelerations and decline of amnionic fluid volume. Severe variable decelerations during a nonstress test plus an amnionic fluid index of ≤ 5 cm resulted in a 75-percent cesarean delivery rate. Fetal distress in labor, however, also frequently developed in those pregnancies with variable decelerations but with normal amounts of amnionic fluid. Similar results were reported by Grubb and Paul (1992).

False-Normal Nonstress Tests

Smith and associates (1987) performed a detailed analysis of the causes of fetal death within 7 days of normal nonstress tests. The most common indication for testing was postterm pregnancy. The mean interval between testing and death was 4 days, with a range of 1 to 7 days. The single most common autopsy finding was meconium aspiration, often associated with some type of umbilical cord abnormality. They concluded that an acute asphyxial insult had provoked fetal gasping. They also concluded that nonstress testing was inadequate to preclude such an acute asphyxial event and that other biophysical characteristics might be beneficial. Importantly, assessment of amnionic fluid volume was considered valuable. Other ascribed frequent causes of fetal death included intrauterine infection, abnormal cord position, malformations, and placental abruption.

ACOUSTIC STIMULATION TESTS

Loud external sounds have been used to startle the fetus and thereby provoke heart rate acceleration—an *acoustic stimulation nonstress test*. A commercially available acoustic stimulator is positioned on the maternal abdomen, and a stimulus of 1 to 2 seconds is applied (Eller, 1995). This may be repeated up to three times for up to 3 seconds (American College of Obstetricians and Gynecologists, 2012a). A positive response is defined as the rapid appearance of a qualifying acceleration following stimulation (Devoe, 2008). In a randomized trial of 113 women undergoing nonstress testing, vibroacoustic stimulation shortened the average time of testing from 24 to 15 minutes (Perez-Delboy, 2002). Similar results were reported by Turitz and coworkers (2012). Laventhal and colleagues (2003) reported that fetal tachyarrhythmia was provoked with vibroacoustic stimulation.

BIOPHYSICAL PROFILE

Manning and colleagues (1980) proposed the combined use of five fetal biophysical variables as a more accurate means of assessing fetal health than a single element. Typically, these

SECTION 5

TABLE 17-2. Components and Scores for the Biophysical Profile

Component	Score 2	Score 0
Nonstress test[a]	≥ 2 accelerations of ≥ 15 beats/min for ≥ 15 sec within 20–40 min	0 or 1 acceleration within 20–40 min
Fetal breathing	≥ 1 episode of rhythmic breathing lasting ≥ 30 sec within 30 min	< 30 sec of breathing within 30 min
Fetal movement	≥ 3 discrete body or limb movements within 30 min	< 3 discrete movements
Fetal tone	≥ 1 episode of extremity extension and subsequent return to flexion	0 extension/flexion events
Amnionic fluid volume[b]	A pocket of amnionic fluid that measures at least 2 cm in two planes perpendicular to each other (2 × 2 cm pocket)	Largest single vertical pocket ≤ 2 cm

[a]May be omitted if all four sonographic components are normal.
[b]Further evaluation warranted, regardless of biophysical composite score, if largest vertical amnionic fluid pocket ≤ 2 cm.

tests require 30 to 60 minutes of examiner time. Shown in Table 17-2 are the five fetal biophysical components assessed: (1) heart rate acceleration, (2) breathing, (3) movements, (4) tone, and (5) amnionic fluid volume. Normal variables were assigned a score of 2 each, and abnormal variables were given a score of 0. Thus, the highest score possible for a normal fetus is 10. Maternal medications such as morphine can significantly decrease the score (Kopecky, 2000). Ozkaya and associates (2012) found that biophysical test scores were higher if a test was performed in late evening (8 to 10 PM) compared with 8 to 10 AM.

Manning and colleagues (1987) tested more than 19,000 pregnancies using the biophysical profile interpretation and management shown in Table 17-3. More than 97 percent of the pregnancies tested had normal test results. They reported a false-normal test rate—defined by an antepartum death of a structurally normal fetus—of approximately 1 per 1000. The most common identifiable causes of fetal death after a normal biophysical profile include fetomaternal hemorrhage, umbilical cord accidents, and placental abruption (Dayal, 1999).

Manning and coworkers (1993) published a remarkable description of 493 fetuses in which biophysical scores were performed immediately before measurement of umbilical venous blood pH values obtained via cordocentesis. Approximately 20 percent of tested fetuses had growth restriction, and the remainder had alloimmune hemolytic anemia. As shown in Figure 17-9, a biophysical score of 0 was almost invariably associated with significant fetal acidemia, whereas a normal score of 8 or 10 was associated with normal pH. An equivocal test result—a score of 6—was a poor predictor of abnormal outcome. As the abnormal score decreased from 2 or 4 down to a very abnormal score of zero, this was a progressively more accurate predictor of abnormal fetal outcome.

In a similar study in 41 diabetic pregnancies, Salvesen and associates (1993) correlated the biophysical profile with umbilical venous blood pH obtained at cordocentesis. They too found that an abnormal pH was significantly associated with abnormal biophysical profile scores. They concluded, however, that the biophysical profile was of limited value in the prediction of fetal pH, because nine mildly acidemic fetuses had normal

TABLE 17-3. Interpretation of Biophysical Profile Score

Biophysical Profile Score	Interpretation	Recommended Management
10	Normal, nonasphyxiated fetus	No fetal indication for intervention; repeat test weekly except in diabetic patients and postterm pregnancy (twice weekly)
8/10 (Normal AFV) 8/8 (NST not done)	Normal, nonasphyxiated fetus	No fetal indication for intervention; repeat testing per protocol
8/10 (Decreased AFV)	Chronic fetal asphyxia suspected	Deliver
6	Possible fetal asphyxia	If amnionic fluid volume abnormal, deliver If normal fluid at > 36 weeks with favorable cervix, deliver If repeat test ≤ 6, deliver If repeat test > 6, observe and repeat per protocol
4	Probable fetal asphyxia	Repeat testing same day; if biophysical profile score ≤ 6, deliver
0 to 2	Almost certain fetal asphyxia	Deliver

AFV = amnionic fluid volume; NST = nonstress test.
From Manning, 1987, with permission.

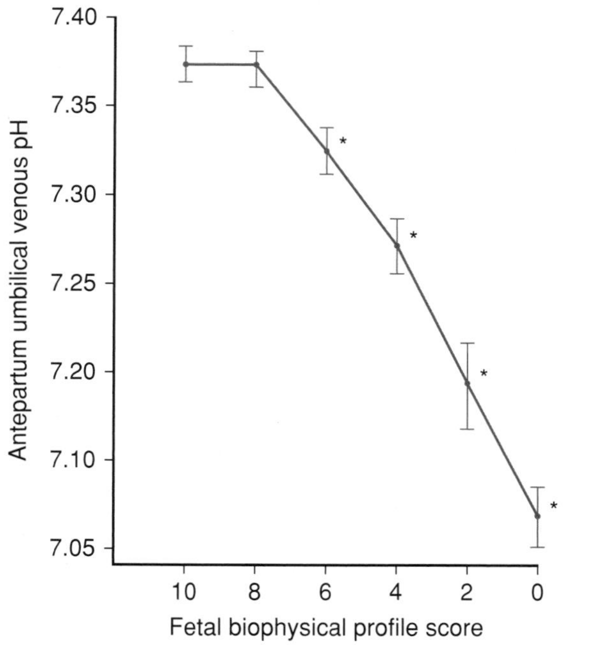

FIGURE 17-9 Mean umbilical vein pH (±2 SD) in relation to fetal biophysical profile score category. (Data from Manning, 1993.)

biophysical profile scores. Weiner and coworkers (1996) assessed 135 overtly growth-restricted fetuses and came to a similar conclusion. Morbidity and mortality in these latter fetuses were linked primarily to gestational age and birthweight and not to abnormal fetal test results. Lalor and associates (2008) performed a Cochrane review and concluded that there is insufficient evidence to support the use of the biophysical profile as a fetal well-being test in high-risk pregnancies. Kaur and colleagues (2008) performed daily biophysical profiles to ascertain the optimal delivery time in 48 growth-restricted preterm fetuses who weighed < 1000 g. Despite scores of 8 in 27 fetuses and 6 in 13, there were six deaths and 21 acidemic fetuses. These investigators concluded that a high incidence of false-positive and -negative results is seen in very preterm fetuses.

Modified Biophysical Profile

Because the biophysical profile is labor intensive and requires a person trained in sonography, Clark and coworkers (1989) used an abbreviated biophysical profile as a first-line screening test in 2628 singleton pregnancies. Specifically, a vibroacoustic nonstress test was performed twice weekly and combined with amnionic fluid index determination for which < 5 cm was considered abnormal (Chap. 11, p. 233). This abbreviated biophysical profile required approximately 10 minutes to perform, and they concluded that it was a superb antepartum surveillance method because there were no unexpected fetal deaths.

Nageotte and colleagues (1994) also combined biweekly nonstress tests with the amnionic fluid index and considered ≤ 5 cm to be abnormal. They performed 17,429 modified biophysical profiles in 2774 women and concluded that such testing was an excellent fetal surveillance tool. Miller and associates (1996a) reported results with more than 54,000 modified biophysical profiles performed in 15,400 high-risk pregnancies. They described a false-negative rate of 0.8 per 1000 and a false-positive rate of 1.5 percent.

The American College of Obstetricians and Gynecologists and the American Academy of Pediatrics (2012) have concluded that the modified biophysical profile test is as predictive of fetal well-being as other approaches to biophysical fetal surveillance.

AMNIONIC FLUID VOLUME

The importance of amnionic fluid volume estimation is indicated by its inclusion into virtually all schemes by which fetal health is assessed (Frøen, 2008). This is based on the rationale that decreased uteroplacental perfusion may lead to diminished fetal renal blood flow, decreased urine production, and ultimately, oligohydramnios. As discussed in Chapter 11 (p. 232), the *amnionic fluid index*, the *deepest vertical pocket*, and the *2 × 2-cm pocket* used in the biophysical profile are some sonographic techniques used to estimate amnionic fluid volume. The American College of Obstetricians and Gynecologists (2011) has concluded that either an amnionic fluid index < 5 cm or a maximum deepest vertical pocket < 2 cm are acceptable criteria for diagnosis of oligohydramnios.

In their review of 42 reports on the amnionic fluid index published between 1987 and 1997, Chauhan and coworkers (1999) concluded that an index ≤ 5.0 cm significantly increased the risk of either cesarean delivery for fetal distress or a low 5-minute Apgar score. Similarly, in a retrospective analysis of 6423 pregnancies managed at Parkland Hospital, Casey and colleagues (2000) found that an amnionic fluid index ≤ 5 cm was associated with significantly increased perinatal morbidity and mortality rates. Locatelli and associates (2004) also reported an increased rate of low-birthweight infants if there was oligohydramnios.

Not all investigators agree with the concept that an index of ≤ 5 cm portends adverse outcomes. Magann and colleagues (2011) recommend use of the single deepest pocket. They note that use of the amnionic fluid index leads to an increased diagnosis of oligohydramnios and results in more labor inductions and cesarean deliveries without neonatal outcome improvement. Driggers and coworkers (2004) and Zhang and associates (2004) did not find a correlation with poor outcomes in pregnancies in which the index was < 5 cm. In a randomized trial, Conway and colleagues (2000) concluded that nonintervention to permit spontaneous onset of labor was as effective as induction in term pregnancies with amnionic fluid index values ≤ 5 cm. Similar results were reported by Trudell and coworkers (2012). Patrelli and colleagues (2012) studied 68 women with amnionic fluid indices < 5 cm who were given 7 days of 1500-mL isotonic solution infusions plus daily oral hydration. The amnionic fluid index was significantly increased in hydrated women.

DOPPLER VELOCIMETRY

Blood flow velocity measured by Doppler ultrasound reflects downstream impedance (Chap. 10, p. 219). Three fetal vascular circuits—umbilical artery, middle cerebral artery, and ductus venosus—are currently assessed to determine fetal health and to aid in the decision to intervene for growth-restricted fetuses. Maternal uterine artery Doppler velocimetry has also been evaluated to predict placental dysfunction, with the goal to balance stillbirth against the risks of preterm delivery (Ghidini, 2007).

Doppler Blood Flow Velocity

Waveforms were first studied systematically in the umbilical arteries late in pregnancy, and abnormal waveforms correlated with placental villous hypovascularity, such as shown in Figure 17-10. Of the small placental arterial channels, 60 to 70 percent need to be obliterated before the umbilical artery Doppler waveform becomes abnormal. Such extensive placental vascular pathology has a major effect on fetal circulation.

According to Trudinger (2007), because more than 40 percent of the combined fetal ventricular output is directed to the placenta, obliteration of placental vascular channel increases afterload and leads to fetal hypoxemia. This in turn leads to dilatation and redistribution of middle cerebral artery blood flow. Ultimately, pressure rises in the ductus venosus due to afterload in the right side of the fetal heart. In this scheme, placental vascular dysfunction results in increased umbilical artery blood flow resistance, which progresses to decreased middle cerebral artery impedance followed ultimately by abnormal flow in the ductus venosus (Baschat, 2004). Clinically, abnormal Doppler waveforms in the ductus venosus are a late finding in the progression of fetal deterioration due to chronic hypoxemia.

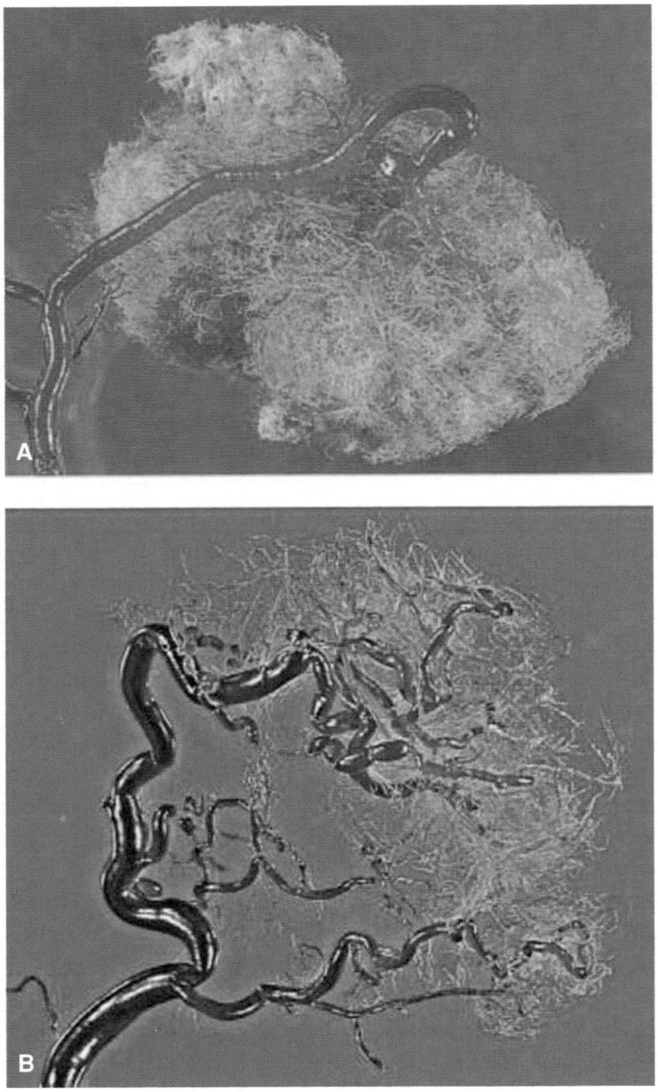

FIGURE 17-10 Acrylic casts of the umbilical arterial vascular tree within a placental lobule. They were prepared by injection of the umbilical artery at the site of cord insertion and later acid digestion of the tissue. **A.** Normal placenta. **B.** Placenta from a pregnancy with absent end-diastolic flow in the umbilical artery recorded before delivery. (From Trudinger, 2007, with permission.)

Umbilical Artery Velocimetry

The umbilical artery systolic-diastolic (S/D) ratio is considered abnormal if it is above the 95th percentile for gestational age or if diastolic flow is either absent or reversed (Chap. 10, p. 219). Absent or reversed end-diastolic flow signifies increased impedance to umbilical artery blood flow (Fig. 10-39, p. 220). It is reported to result from poorly vascularized placental villi and is seen in extreme cases of fetal-growth restriction (Todros, 1999). According to Zelop and colleagues (1996), the perinatal mortality rate for absent end-diastolic flow was approximately 10 percent, and for reversed end-diastolic flow, it approximated 33 percent. Spinillo and associates (2005) studied neurodevelopmental outcome at 2 years of age in 266 growth-restricted fetuses delivered between 24 and 35 weeks' gestation. Of infants with absent or reversed umbilical artery flow, 8 percent had evidence of cerebral palsy compared with 1 percent of those in whom Doppler flow was either normal or > 95th percentile but without reversed flow.

Doppler ultrasound of the umbilical artery has been subjected to more extensive assessment with randomized controlled trials than has any previous test of fetal health. Williams and colleagues (2003) randomized 1360 high-risk women to either nonstress testing or Doppler velocimetry. They found a significantly increased incidence of cesarean delivery for fetal distress in the nonstress test group compared with that for those tested with Doppler velocimetry—8.7 versus 4.6 percent, respectively. One interpretation of this finding is that the nonstress test more frequently identified fetuses in jeopardy. Conversely, Gonzalez and associates (2007) found that abnormal umbilical artery Doppler findings in a cohort of growth-restricted fetuses were the best predictors of perinatal outcomes.

The utility of umbilical artery Doppler velocimetry was reviewed by the American College of Obstetricians and Gynecologists (2013). It was concluded that no benefit has been demonstrated other than in pregnancies with suspected fetal-growth restriction. Specifically, no benefits have been demonstrated for velocimetry for other conditions such as postterm pregnancy, diabetes, systemic lupus erythematosus, or antiphospholipid antibody syndrome. Similarly, velocimetry has not proved valuable as a screening test for fetal compromise in the general obstetrical population.

Middle Cerebral Artery

Doppler velocimetry interrogation of the middle cerebral artery (MCA) has received particular attention because of observations that the hypoxic fetus attempts *brain sparing* by reducing cerebrovascular impedance and thus increasing blood flow. Such brain sparing in growth-restricted fetuses has been documented to undergo reversal (Konje, 2001). Investigators reported that 8 of 17 fetuses with this reversal died. Ott and coworkers (1998) randomized 665 women undergoing modified biophysical profile evaluation to either the profile alone or combined with middle cerebral and umbilical artery velocity flow assessment. There were no significant differences in pregnancy outcomes between these two study groups.

In a different application, Oepkes and colleagues (2006) used middle cerebral artery Doppler velocimetry to detect severe fetal anemia in 165 fetuses with D alloimmunization. They prospectively compared serial amniocentesis for measurement of bilirubin levels with Doppler measurement of peak systolic velocity in the middle cerebral artery. These investigators concluded that Doppler could safely replace amniocentesis in the management of alloimmunized pregnancies. And as discussed in Chapter 15 (p. 310), middle cerebral artery Doppler velocimetry is useful for detection and management of fetal anemia of any cause (Moise, 2008). The American College of Obstetricians and Gynecologists (2012b) also concluded that such use of Doppler is appropriate in centers with personnel trained in the procedure.

Ductus Venosus

The use of Doppler ultrasound to assess the fetal venous circulation is the most recent application of this technology. Bilardo and colleagues (2004) prospectively studied umbilical artery and ductus venosus Doppler velocimetry in 70 growth-restricted fetuses at 26 to 33 weeks' gestation. They concluded that ductus venosus velocimetry was the best predictor of perinatal outcome. Importantly, negative or reversed flow in the ductus venosus was a late finding because these fetuses had already sustained irreversible multiorgan damage due to hypoxemia. Also, gestational age at delivery was a major determinant of perinatal outcome independent of ductus venosus flow. Specifically, 36 percent of growth-restricted fetuses delivered between 26 and 29 weeks succumbed compared with only 5 percent delivered from 30 to 33 weeks.

Baschat and coworkers (2007) systemically studied 604 growth-restricted fetuses using umbilical artery, middle cerebral artery, and ductus venosus Doppler velocimetry and reached similar conclusions. Specifically, absent or reversed flow in the ductus venosus was associated with profound generalized fetal metabolic collapse. They too reported that gestational age was a powerful cofactor in ultimate perinatal outcome for growth-restricted fetuses delivered before 30 weeks. Put another way, by the time severely abnormal flow is seen in the ductus venosus, it is too late because the fetus is already near death. Conversely, earlier delivery puts the fetus at risk for death due to preterm delivery. Ghidini (2007) concluded that these reports do not support routine use of ductus venosus Doppler in the monitoring of growth-restricted fetuses and recommended further study.

Uterine Artery

Vascular resistance in the uterine circulation normally decreases in the first half of pregnancy due to invasion of maternal uterine vessels by trophoblastic tissue (Chap. 5, p. 93). This process can be detected using Doppler flow velocimetry, and uterine artery Doppler may be most helpful in assessing pregnancies at high risk of uteroplacental insufficiency (Abramowicz, 2008). Persistence or development of high-resistance patterns has been linked to a variety of pregnancy complications (Lees, 2001; Yu, 2005). In a study of 30,519 unselected British women, Smith and colleagues (2007) assessed uterine artery velocimetry at 22 to 24 weeks. The risk of fetal death before 32 weeks when associated with abruption, preeclampsia, or fetal-growth restriction was significantly linked to high-resistance flow. This has led to suggestions for continued research of uterine artery Doppler velocimetry as a screening tool to detect pregnancies at risk for stillbirth (Reddy, 2008). Sciscione and Hayes (2009) reviewed the use of uterine artery Doppler flow studies in obstetrical practice. Because standards for the study technique and criteria for an abnormal test are lacking, they noted that uterine artery Doppler studies should not be considered standard practice in either low- or high-risk populations.

CURRENT ANTENATAL TESTING RECOMMENDATIONS

According to the American College of Obstetricians and Gynecologists (2012a), there is no "best test" to evaluate fetal well-being. Three testing systems—contraction stress test, nonstress test, and biophysical profile—have different end points to consider depending on the clinical situation.

The most important consideration in deciding when to begin antepartum testing is the prognosis for neonatal survival. The severity of maternal disease is another important consideration. In general, with the majority of high-risk pregnancies, most authorities recommend that testing begin by 32 to 34 weeks. Pregnancies with severe complications might require testing as early as 26 to 28 weeks. The frequency for repeating tests has been arbitrarily set at 7 days, but more frequent testing is often done.

Significance of Fetal Testing

Does antenatal fetal testing really improve fetal outcome? Platt and coworkers (1987) reviewed its impact between 1971 and 1985 at Los Angeles County Hospital. During this 15-year period, more than 200,000 pregnancies were managed, and nearly 17,000 of these women underwent antepartum testing of various types. Fetal surveillance increased from less than 1 percent of pregnancies in the early 1970s to 15 percent in the mid-1980s. These authors concluded that such testing was clearly beneficial because the fetal death rate was significantly less in the tested high-risk pregnancies compared with the rate in those not tested. The study, however, did not consider other innovations incorporated into practice during those 15 years. Preliminary results from Ghana suggest that nonstress testing may be beneficial in low-resource countries (Anderson, 2012). In an observational study of 316 pregnancies complicated by gestational hypertension, women undergoing nonstress testing had a nonsignificant decreased risk for stillbirth compared with those not tested—3.6 versus 9.2 percent, respectively.

The benefits of antenatal fetal testing have not been sufficiently evaluated in randomized controlled trials according to Thacker and Berkelman (1986). This was concluded after reviewing 600 reports, which included only four randomized trials and all conducted with nonstress testing without a contraction stress test. The numbers in these four trials were considered too small to permit detection of important benefits and did not support a specific test. Enkin and colleagues (2000) reviewed evidence in the Cochrane Library database from controlled trials of antepartum fetal surveillance and concluded that "despite their widespread use, most tests of fetal well-being should be considered of experimental value only rather than validated clinical tools."

Another important and unanswered question is whether antepartum fetal surveillance identifies fetal asphyxia early enough to prevent brain damage. Todd and coworkers (1992) attempted to correlate cognitive development in infants up to age 2 years following either abnormal umbilical artery Doppler velocimetry or nonstress test results. Only abnormal nonstress tests were associated with marginally poorer cognitive outcomes. These investigators concluded that by the time fetal compromise is diagnosed with antenatal testing, fetal damage has already been sustained. Low and colleagues (2003) reached a similar conclusion in their study of 36 preterm infants delivered based on antepartum test results. Manning and coworkers (1998) studied the incidence of cerebral palsy in 26,290 high-risk pregnancies managed with serial biophysical profile testing. These outcomes were compared with those of 58,657 low-risk pregnancies in which antepartum testing was not performed. The rate of cerebral palsy was 1.3 per 1000 in tested pregnancies compared with 4.7 per 1000 in untested women.

Antenatal forecasts of fetal health have clearly been the focus of intense interest for four decades. When such testing is reviewed, several themes emerge:

1. Methods of fetal forecasting have evolved continually, a phenomenon that at least suggests dissatisfaction with the precision or efficacy of any given method.
2. The fetal biophysical performance is characterized by wide ranges of normal biological variation, resulting in difficulty determining when such performance should be considered abnormal. How many movements, respirations, or accelerations? In what time period? Unable to easily quantify normal fetal biophysical performance, most investigators have resorted to somewhat arbitrary answers to such questions.
3. Despite the invention of increasingly complex testing methods, abnormal results are seldom reliable, prompting many clinicians to use antenatal testing to forecast fetal *wellness* rather than *illness.*

REFERENCES

Abramowicz JS, Sheiner E: Ultrasound of the placenta: a systemic approach. Part II: Function assessment (Doppler). Placenta 29(11):921, 2008

American Academy of Pediatrics and American College of Obstetricians and Gynecologists: Guidelines for perinatal care, 7th ed. Washington, 2012

American College of Obstetricians and Gynecologists: Ultrasonography in pregnancy. Practice Bulletin No. 101, February 2009, Reaffirmed 2011

American College of Obstetricians and Gynecologists: Antepartum fetal surveillance. Practice Bulletin No. 9, October 1999, Reaffirmed 2012a

American College of Obstetricians and Gynecologists: Management of alloimmunization during pregnancy. Practice Bulletin No. 75, August 2006, Reaffirmed 2012b

American College of Obstetricians and Gynecologists: Intrauterine growth restriction. Practice Bulletin No. 134, May 2013

Anderson F, Seffah J, Owusu J, et al: Improved perinatal outcomes with fetal monitoring in Ghana. Abstract No. 692. Presented at the 32nd Annual Meeting of the Society for Maternal-Fetal Medicine. 6–11 February 2012

Badalian SS, Chao CR, Fox HE, et al: Fetal breathing-related nasal fluid flow velocity in uncomplicated pregnancies. Am J Obstet Gynecol 169:563, 1993

Baschat AA: Opinion and review: Doppler application in the delivery timing in the preterm growth-restricted fetus: another step in the right direction. Ultrasound Obstet Gynecol 23:118, 2004

Baschat AA, Cosmi E, Bilardo C, et al: Predictors of neonatal outcome in early-onset placental dysfunction. Obstet Gynecol 109:253, 2007

Bilardo CM, Wolf H, Stigter RH, et al: Relationship between monitoring parameters and perinatal outcome in severe, early intrauterine growth restriction. Ultrasound Obstet Gynecol 23:199, 2004

Bourgeois FJ, Thiagarajah S, Harbert GM Jr: The significance of fetal heart rate decelerations during nonstress testing. Am J Obstet Gynecol 150:213, 1984

Brown R, Patrick J: The nonstress test: how long is enough? Am J Obstet Gynecol 141:646, 1981

Casey BM, McIntire DD, Bloom SL, et al: Pregnancy outcomes after antepartum diagnosis of oligohydramnios at or beyond 34 weeks' gestation. Am J Obstet Gynecol 182:909, 2000

Chauhan SP, Sanderson M, Hendrix NW, et al: Perinatal outcomes and amniotic fluid index in the antepartum and intrapartum periods: a meta-analysis. Am J Obstet Gynecol 181:1473, 1999

Clark SL, Sabey P, Jolley K: Nonstress testing with acoustic stimulation and amnionic fluid volume assessment: 5973 tests without unexpected fetal death. Am J Obstet Gynecol 160:694, 1989

Conway DL, Groth S, Adkins WB, et al: Management of isolated oligohydramnios in the term pregnancy: a randomized clinical trial. Am J Obstet Gynecol 182:S21, 2000

Cousins L, Poeltler D, Faron S, et al: Nonstress testing at ≤32.0 weeks gestation: a randomized trial comparing different assessment criteria. Abstract No. 696. Presented at the 32nd Annual Meeting of the Society for Maternal-Fetal Medicine. 6–11 February 2012

Dawes GS: Breathing before birth in animals and man. An essay in medicine. Physiol Med 290:557, 1974

Dawes GS, Fox HE, Leduc BM, et al: Respiratory movements and rapid eye movement sleep in the foetal lamb. J Physiol 220:119, 1972

Dayal AK, Manning FA, Berck DJ, et al: Fetal death after normal biophysical profile score: an eighteen year experience. Am J Obstet Gynecol 181:1231, 1999

Devoe LD: Antenatal fetal assessment: contraction stress test, nonstress test, vibroacoustic stimulation, amniotic fluid volume, biophysical profile, and modified biophysical profile—an overview. Semin Perinatol 32(4):247, 2008

Devoe LD, Castillo RA, Sherline DM: The nonstress test as a diagnostic test: a critical reappraisal. Am J Obstet Gynecol 152:1047, 1986

Devoe LD, McKenzie J, Searle NS, et al: Clinical sequelae of the extended nonstress test. Am J Obstet Gynecol 151:1074, 1985

DeVries JIP, Visser GHA, Prechtl NFR: The emergence of fetal behavior. II. Quantitative aspects. Early Hum Dev 12:99, 1985

Driggers RW, Holcroft CJ, Blakemore KJ, et al: An amniotic fluid index ≤5 cm within 7 days of delivery in the third trimester is not associated with decreasing umbilical arterial pH and base excess. J Perinatol 24:72, 2004

Druzin ML, Gratacos J, Keegan KA, et al: Antepartum fetal heart rate testing, 7. The significance of fetal bradycardia. Am J Obstet Gynecol 139: 194, 1981

Eller DP, Scardo JA, Dillon AE, et al: Distance from an intrauterine hydrophone as a factor affecting intrauterine sound pressure levels produced by the vibroacoustic stimulation test. Am J Obstet Gynecol 173:523, 1995

Enkin M, Keirse MJNC, Renfrew M, et al: A Guide to Effective Care in Pregnancy and Childbirth, 3rd ed. New York, Oxford University Press, 2000, p 225

Frager NB, Miyazaki FS: Intrauterine monitoring of contractions during breast stimulation. Obstet Gynecol 69:767, 1987

Freeman RK: The use of the oxytocin challenge test for antepartum clinical evaluation of uteroplacental respiratory function. Am J Obstet Gynecol 121: 481, 1975

Frøen JF, Tviet JV, Saastad E, et al: Management of decreased fetal movements. Semin Perinatol 32(4):307, 2008

Ghidini A: Doppler of the ductus venosus in severe preterm fetal growth restriction. A test in search of a purpose? Obstet Gynecol 109:250, 2007
Gonzalez JM, Stamilio DM, Ural S, et al: Relationship between abnormal fetal testing and adverse perinatal outcomes in intrauterine growth restriction. Am J Obstet Gynecol 196:e48, 2007
Grant A, Elbourne D, Valentin L, et al: Routine formal fetal movement counting and risk of antepartum late death in normally formed singletons. Lancet 2:345, 1989
Grivell RM, Wong L, Ghatia V: Regimens of fetal surveillance for impaired fetal growth. Cochrane Database Syst Rev 6:CD007113, 2012
Grubb DK, Paul RH: Amnionic fluid index and prolonged antepartum fetal heart rate decelerations. Obstet Gynecol 79:558, 1992
Guinn DA, Kimberlin KF, Wigton TR, et al: Fetal heart rate characteristics at 25 to 28 weeks gestation. Am J Perinatol 15:507, 1998
Hage ML: Interpretation of nonstress tests. Am J Obstet Gynecol 153:490, 1985
Hammacher K, Hüter KA, Bokelmann J, et al: Foetal heart frequency and perinatal condition of the foetus and newborn. Gynaecologia 166:349, 1968
Harrington K, Thompson O, Jorden L, et al: Obstetric outcomes in women who present with a reduction in fetal movements in the third trimester of pregnancy. J Perinat Med 26:77, 1998
Hofmeyr GJ, Novikova N: Management of reported decreased fetal movements for improving pregnancy outcomes. Cochrane Database Syst Rev 4:CD009148, 2012
Hoskins IA, Frieden FJ, Young BK: Variable decelerations in reactive nonstress tests with decreased amnionic fluid index predict fetal compromise. Am J Obstet Gynecol 165:1094, 1991
Huddleston JF, Sutliff JG, Robinson D: Contraction stress test by intermittent nipple stimulation. Obstet Gynecol 63:669, 1984
Jansson LM, DiPietro J, Elko A: Fetal response to maternal methadone administration. Am J Obstet Gynecol 193:611, 2005
Johnson MJ, Paine LL, Mulder HH, et al: Population differences of fetal biophysical and behavioral characteristics. Am J Obstet Gynecol 166:138, 1992
Johnson T, Besigner R, Thomas R: New clues to fetal behavior and well-being. Contemp Ob/Gyn May 1988
Kaur S, Picconi JL, Chadha R, et al: Biophysical profile in the treatment of intrauterine growth-restricted fetuses who weigh <1000 g. Am J Obstet Gynecol 199:264.e1, 2008
Knight M, Berg C, Brocklehurst P, et al: Amniotic fluid embolism incidence, risk factors, and outcomes: a review and recommendations. BMC Pregnancy Childbirth 12:7, 2012
Konje JC, Bell SC, Taylor DT: Abnormal Doppler velocimetry and blood flow volume in the middle cerebral artery in very severe intrauterine growth restriction: is the occurrence of reversal of compensatory flow too late? Br J Obstet Gynaecol 108:973, 2001
Kopecky EA, Ryan ML, Barrett JFR, et al: Fetal response to maternally administered morphine. Am J Obstet Gynecol 183:424, 2000
Lalor JG, Fawole B, Alfirevic Z, et al: Biophysical profile for fetal assessment in high risk pregnancies. Cochrane Database Syst Rev 1:CD000038, 2008
Laventhal NT, Dildy GA III, Belfort MA: Fetal tachyarrhythmia associated with vibroacoustic stimulation. Obstet Gynecol 101:116, 2003
Lee CY, DiLoreto PC, O'Lane JM: A study of fetal heart rate acceleration patterns. Obstet Gynecol 45:142, 1975
Lees C, Parra M, Missfelder-Lobos H, et al: Individualized risk assessment for adverse pregnancy outcome by uterine artery Doppler at 23 weeks. Obstet Gynecol 98:369, 2001
Leveno KJ, Williams ML, DePalma RT, et al: Perinatal outcome in the absence of antepartum fetal heart rate acceleration. Obstet Gynecol 61:347, 1983
Locatelli A, Vergani P, Toso L, et al: Perinatal outcome associated with oligohydramnios in uncomplicated term pregnancies. Arch Gynecol Obstet 269:130, 2004
Low JA, Killen H, Derrick EJ: Antepartum fetal complexia in the preterm pregnancy. Am J Obstet Gynecol 188:461, 2003
Macones GA, Hankins GD, Spong CY, et al: The 2008 National Institute of Child Health and Human Development workshop report on electronic fetal monitoring: update on definitions, interpretation, and research guidelines. Obstet Gynecol 112:661, 2008
Magann EF, Sandlin AT, Ounpraseuth ST: Amniotic fluid and the clinical relevance of the sonographically estimated amniotic fluid volume: oligohydramnios. J Ultrasound Med 30(11):1573, 2011
Manning FA, Bondaji N, Harman CR, et al: Fetal assessment based on fetal biophysical profile scoring VIII: the incidence of cerebral palsy in tested and untested perinates. Am J Obstet Gynecol 178:696, 1998
Manning FA, Morrison I, Harman CR, et al: Fetal assessment based on fetal biophysical profile scoring: experience in 19,221 referred high-risk pregnancies, 2. An analysis of false-negative fetal deaths. Am J Obstet Gynecol 157:880, 1987
Manning FA, Platt LD, Sipos L: Antepartum fetal evaluation: development of a fetal biophysical profile. Am J Obstet Gynecol 136:787, 1980
Manning FA, Snijders R, Harman CR, et al: Fetal biophysical profile score, VI. Correlation with antepartum umbilical venous fetal pH. Am J Obstet Gynecol 169:755, 1993
Matsuura M, Murata Y, Hirano T, et al: The effects of developing autonomous nervous system on FHR variabilities determined by the power spectral analysis. Am J Obstet Gynecol 174:380, 1996
Meis PJ, Ureda JR, Swain M, et al: Variable decelerations during nonstress tests are not a sign of fetal compromise. Am J Obstet Gynecol 154:586, 1986
Miller DA, Rabello YA, Paul RH: The modified biophysical profile: antepartum testing in the 1990s. Am J Obstet Gynecol 174:812, 1996a
Miller F, Miller D, Paul R, et al: Is one fetal heart rate acceleration during a nonstress test as reliable as two in predicting fetal status? Am J Obstet Gynecol 174:337, 1996b
Moise KJ Jr: The usefulness of middle cerebral artery Doppler assessment in the treatment of the fetus at risk for anemia. Am J Obstet Gynecol 198:161.e1, 2008
Moore TR, Piaquadio K: A prospective evaluation of fetal movement screening to reduce the incidence of antepartum fetal death. Am J Obstet Gynecol 160:1075, 1989
Nageotte MP, Towers CV, Asrat T, et al: Perinatal outcome with the modified biophysical profile. Am J Obstet Gynecol 170:1672, 1994
Neldam S: Fetal movements as an indicator of fetal well being. Dan Med Bull 30:274, 1983
Nijhuis JG, Prechtl HFR, Martin CB Jr, et al: Are there behavioural states in the human fetus? Early Hum Dev 6:177, 1982
Oepkes D, Seaward PG, Vandenbussche FP, et al: Doppler ultrasonography versus amniocentesis to predict fetal anemia. N Engl J Med 355:156, 2006
Oosterhof H, vd Stege JG, Lander M, et al: Urine production rate is related to behavioural states in the near term human fetus. Br J Obstet Gynaecol 100:920, 1993
Ott WJ, Mora G, Arias F, et al: Comparison of the modified biophysical profile to a "new" biophysical profile incorporating the middle cerebral artery to umbilical artery velocity flow systolic/diastolic ratio. Am J Obstet Gynecol 178:1346, 1998
Ozkaya E, Baser E, Cinar M, et al: Does diurnal rhythm have an impact on fetal biophysical profile? J Matern Fetal Neonatal Med 25(4):335, 2012
Patrelli TS, Gizzo S, Cosmi E, et al: Maternal hydration therapy improves the quality of amniotic fluid and the pregnancy outcome in third-trimester isolated oligohydramnios: a controlled randomized institutional trial. J Ultrasound Med 31(2):239, 2012
Patrick J, Campbell K, Carmichael L, et al: Patterns of gross fetal body movements over 24-hour observation intervals during the last 10 weeks of pregnancy. Am J Obstet Gynecol 142:363, 1982
Patrick J, Campbell K, Carmichael L, et al: Patterns of human fetal breathing during the last 10 weeks of pregnancy. Obstet Gynecol 56:24, 1980
Pazos R, Vuolo K, Aladjem S, et al: Association of spontaneous fetal heart rate decelerations during antepartum nonstress testing and intrauterine growth retardation. Am J Obstet Gynecol 144:574, 1982
Perez-Delboy A, Weiss J, Michels A, et al: A randomized trial of vibroacoustic stimulation for antenatal fetal testing. Am J Obstet Gynecol 187:S146, 2002
Pillai M, James D: Behavioural states in normal mature human fetuses. Arch Dis Child 65:39, 1990a
Pillai M, James D: The development of fetal heart rate patterns during normal pregnancy. Obstet Gynecol 76:812, 1990b
Platt LD, Paul RH, Phelan J, et al: Fifteen years of experience with antepartum fetal testing. Am J Obstet Gynecol 156:1509, 1987
Ray M, Freeman R, Pine S, et al: Clinical experience with the oxytocin challenge test. Am J Obstet Gynecol 114:1, 1972
Rayburn WF: Clinical significance of perceptible fetal motion. Am J Obstet Gynecol 138:210, 1980
Reddy UM, Filly RA, Copel JA, et al: Prenatal imaging: ultrasonography and magnetic resonance imaging. Obstet Gynecol 112(1):145, 2008
Saastad E, Winje BA, Stray Penderson B, et al: Fetal movement counting improved identification of fetal growth restriction and perinatal outcomes—a multi-centre, randomized, controlled trial. PLoS One 6(12):e28482, 2011
Sadovsky E, Evron S, Weinstein D: Daily fetal movement recording in normal pregnancy. Riv Obstet Ginecol Practica Med Perinatal 59:395, 1979a
Sadovsky E, Laufer N, Allen JW: The incidence of different types of fetal movement during pregnancy. Br J Obstet Gynaecol 86:10, 1979b
Sadovsky E, Yaffe H: Daily fetal movement recording and fetal prognosis. Obstet Gynecol 41:845, 1973
Salvesen DR, Freeman J, Brudenell JM, et al: Prediction of fetal acidemia in pregnancies complicated by maternal diabetes by biophysical scoring and fetal heart rate monitoring. Br J Obstet Gynaecol 100:227, 1993

Schellpfeffer MA, Hoyle D, Johnson JWC: Antepartum uterine hypercontractility secondary to nipple stimulation. Obstet Gynecol 65:588, 1985
Sciscione AC, Hayes EJ: Uterine artery Doppler flow studies in obstetric practice. Am J Obstet Gynecol 201(2):121, 2009
Sherer DM, Spong CY, Ghidini A, et al: In preterm fetuses decreased amniotic fluid volume is associated with decreased fetal movements. Am J Obstet Gynecol 174:344, 1996
Smith CV, Nguyen HN, Kovacs B, et al: Fetal death following antepartum fetal heart rate testing: a review of 65 cases. Obstet Gynecol 70:18, 1987
Smith GCS, Yu CKH, Papageorghiou AT, et al: Maternal uterine artery Doppler flow velocimetry and the risk of stillbirth. Obstet Gynecol 109:144, 2007
Smith JH, Anand KJ, Cotes PM, et al: Antenatal fetal heart rate variation in relation to the respiratory and metabolic status of the compromised human fetus. Br J Obstet Gynaecol 95:980, 1988
Sorokin Y, Bottoms SF, Dierker CJ, et al: The clustering of fetal heart rate changes and fetal movements in pregnancies between 20 and 30 weeks gestation. Am J Obstet Gynecol 143:952, 1982
Spinillo A, Montanari L, Bergante C, et al: Prognostic value of umbilical artery Doppler studies in unselected preterm deliveries. Obstet Gynecol 105:613, 2005
Thacker SB, Berkelman RL: Assessing the diagnostic accuracy and efficacy of selected antepartum fetal surveillance techniques. Obstet Gynecol Surv 41:121, 1986
Timor-Tritsch IE, Dierker LJ, Hertz RH, et al: Studies of antepartum behavioral state in the human fetus at term. Am J Obstet Gynecol 132:524, 1978
Todd AL, Tridinger BJ, Cole MJ, et al: Antenatal tests of fetal welfare and development at age 2 years. Am J Obstet Gynecol 167:66, 1992
Todros T, Sciarrone A, Piccoli E, et al: Umbilical Doppler waveforms and placental villous angiogenesis in pregnancies complicated by fetal growth restriction. Obstet Gynecol 93:499, 1999
Trudell A, Ott W, Morris B: Isolated oligohydramnios after 34 weeks: obstetric and neonatal outcomes. Abstract No. 689. Presented at the 32nd Annual Meeting of the Society for Maternal-Fetal Medicine. 6–11 February 2012
Trudinger B: Doppler: more or less? Ultrasound Obstet Gynecol 29 (3):243, 2007
Turitz AL, Bastek JA, Sammel MD, et al: Vibroacoustic stimulation significantly reduces time that high risk patients spend in an urban antenatal testing unit. Abstract No. 690. Presented at the 32nd Annual Meeting of the Society for Maternal-Fetal medicine. 6–11 February 2012
Vindla S, James D: Fetal behavior as a test of fetal well-being. Br J Obstet Gynaecol 102:597, 1995
Visser GHA, Redman CWG, Huisjes HJ, et al: Nonstressed antepartum heart rate monitoring: implications of decelerations after spontaneous contractions. Am J Obstet Gynecol 138:429, 1980
Warrander LK, Batra G, Bernatavicius G, et al: Maternal perception of reduced fetal movements is associated with altered placental structure and function. PloS One 7(4):e34851, 2012
Weiner Z, Divon MY, Katz N, et al: Multi-variant analysis of antepartum fetal test in predicting neonatal outcome of growth retarded fetuses. Am J Obstet Gynecol 174:338, 1996
Williams KP, Farquharson DF, Bebbington M, et al: Screening for fetal well-being in a high-risk pregnant population comparing the nonstress test with umbilical artery Doppler velocimetry: a randomized controlled clinical trial. Am J Obstet Gynecol 188:1366, 2003
Yu CK, Smith GC, Papageorghiou AT, et al: An integrated model for the prediction of preeclampsia using maternal factors and uterine artery Doppler velocimetry in unselected low-risk women. Am J Obstet Gynecol 193:429, 2005
Zelop CM, Richardson DK, Heffner LJ: Outcomes of severely abnormal umbilical artery Doppler velocimetry in structurally normal singleton fetuses. Obstet Gynecol 87:434, 1996
Zhang J, Troendle J, Meikle S, et al: Isolated oligohydramnios is not associated with adverse perinatal outcomes. Br J Obstet Gynaecol 111:220, 2004

SECTION 6

EARLY PREGNANCY COMPLICATIONS

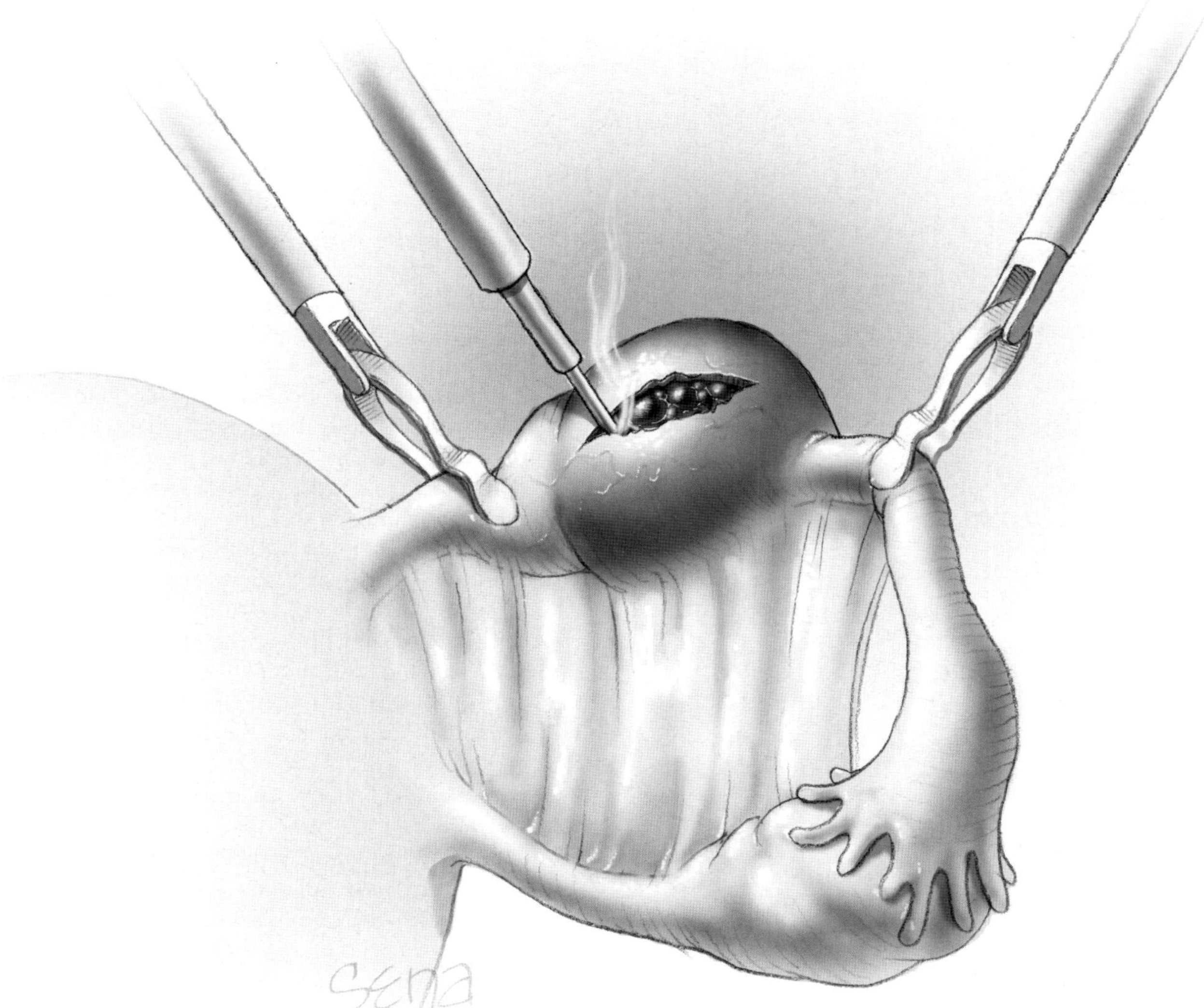

CHAPTER 18

Abortion

The word *abortion* derives from the Latin *aboriri*—to miscarry. Abortion is defined as the spontaneous or induced termination of pregnancy before fetal viability. It thus is appropriate that miscarriage and abortion are terms used interchangeably in a medical context. But because popular use of *abortion* by laypersons implies a deliberate intact pregnancy termination, many prefer *miscarriage* for spontaneous fetal loss. Newer terms made possible by widespread use of sonography and human chorionic gonadotropin measurements that identify extremely early pregnancies include *early pregnancy loss, wastage,* or *failure*. Throughout this book, these are all used at one time or another.

NOMENCLATURE

Terminology used to define fetal viability and thus an abortus has tremendous medical, legal, and social import. Viability lies between the lines that separate abortion from preterm birth. It is usually defined by pregnancy duration and fetal birthweight for statistical and legal purposes (Chap. 1, p. 2). This has led to incongruities in definitions from authoritative organizations. Importantly, the National Center for Health Statistics, the Centers for Disease Control and Prevention, and the World Health Organization all define *abortion* as pregnancy termination before 20 weeks' gestation or with a fetus born weighing < 500 g. These criteria, however, are somewhat contradictory because the mean birthweight of a 20-week fetus is 320 g, whereas 500 g is the mean for 22 to 23 weeks (Moore, 1977). Further confusion may derive from criteria set by state laws that define abortion even more widely.

As indicated above, technological developments have revolutionized current abortion terminology. Transvaginal sonography (TVS) and precise measurement of serum human chorionic gonadotropin (hCG) concentrations are used to identify extremely early pregnancies as well as those with an intrauterine versus ectopic location. Ubiquitous application of these practices makes it possible to distinguish between a *chemical* and a *clinical* pregnancy. An ad hoc international consensus group has proposed the term *pregnancy of unknown location—PUL*—with the goal of early identification and management of ectopic pregnancy (Barnhart, 2011; Doubilet, 2013). Management options for ectopic gestation are described in Chapter 19 (p. 384). Uterine pregnancies that eventuate in a spontaneous abortion are also termed *early pregnancy loss* or *early pregnancy failure.*

Terms that have been in clinical use for many decades are generally used to describe later pregnancy losses. These include:

1. Spontaneous abortion—this category includes threatened, inevitable, incomplete, complete, and missed abortion.

Septic abortion is used to further classify any of these that are complicated further by infection.

2. Recurrent abortion—this term is variably defined, but it is meant to identify women with repetitive spontaneous abortions so that an underlying factor(s) can be treated to achieve a viable newborn.
3. Induced abortion—this term is used to describe surgical or medical termination of a live fetus that has not reached viability.

FIRST-TRIMESTER SPONTANEOUS ABORTION

Pathogenesis

More than 80 percent of spontaneous abortions occur within the first 12 weeks of gestation. With first-trimester losses, death of the embryo or fetus nearly always precedes spontaneous expulsion. Death is usually accompanied by hemorrhage into the decidua basalis. This is followed by adjacent tissue necrosis that stimulates uterine contractions and expulsion. An intact gestational sac is usually filled with fluid and may or may not contain an embryo or fetus. Thus, the key to determining the cause of early miscarriage is to ascertain the cause of fetal death. In contradistinction, in later pregnancy losses, the fetus usually does not die before expulsion, and thus other explanations are sought.

Incidence

Statistics regarding the incidence of spontaneous abortion vary according to the diligence used for its recognition. Wilcox and colleagues (1988) studied 221 healthy women through 707 menstrual cycles and found that 31 percent of pregnancies were lost after implantation. They used highly specific assays for minute concentrations of maternal serum β-hCG and reported that two thirds of these early losses were *clinically silent*.

Currently, there are factors known to influence clinically apparent spontaneous abortion, however, it is unknown if these same factors affect clinically silent miscarriages. By way of example, the rate of clinical miscarriages is almost doubled when either parent is older than 40 years (Gracia, 2005; Kleinhaus, 2006). But, it is not known if clinically silent miscarriages are similarly affected by parental age.

Fetal Factors

As shown in Table 18-1, approximately half of miscarriages are *anembryonic*, that is, with no identifiable embryonic elements. Less accurately, the term *blighted ovum* may be used (Silver, 2011). The other 50 percent are *embryonic* miscarriages, which commonly display a developmental abnormality of the zygote, embryo, fetus, or at times, the placenta. Of embryonic miscarriage, half of these—25 percent of all abortuses—have chromosomal anomalies and thus are *aneuploid abortions*. The remaining cases are *euploid abortions*, that is, carrying a normal chromosomal complement.

TABLE 18-1. Chromosomal Findings in First-Trimester Abortuses

Chromosomal Studies	Incidence Range (%)
Embryonic	~50
Euploid	
46,XY and 46,XX	45 to 55
Aneuploid	
Autosomal trisomy	22 to 32
Monosomy X (45,X)	5 to 20
Triploidy	6 to 8
Tetraploidy	2 to 4
Structural anomaly	2
Anembryonic (blighted ovum)	~50

Data from Eiben, 1990; Kajii, 1980; Simpson, 1980, 2007.

Aneuploid Abortion

Both abortion rates and chromosomal anomalies decrease with advancing gestational age. As shown in Figure 18-1, 50 percent of embryonic abortions are aneuploid, but chromosomal abnormalities are found in just a third of second-trimester fetal losses and in only 5 percent of third-trimester stillbirths. Aneuploid abortion occurs at earlier gestational ages. Kajii and associates (1980) noted that 75 percent of aneuploid abortions occurred by 8 weeks. Of these, 95 percent of chromosomal abnormalities are caused by maternal gametogenesis errors, and 5 percent by paternal errors (Jacobs, 1980). Some found most common are listed in Table 18-1.

With first-trimester miscarriages, *autosomal trisomy* is the most frequently identified chromosomal anomaly. Although most trisomies result from *isolated nondisjunction*, balanced structural chromosomal rearrangements are found in one partner in 2 to 4 percent of couples with recurrent miscarriages. Trisomies have been identified in abortuses for all except chromosome number 1, and those with 13, 16, 18, 21,

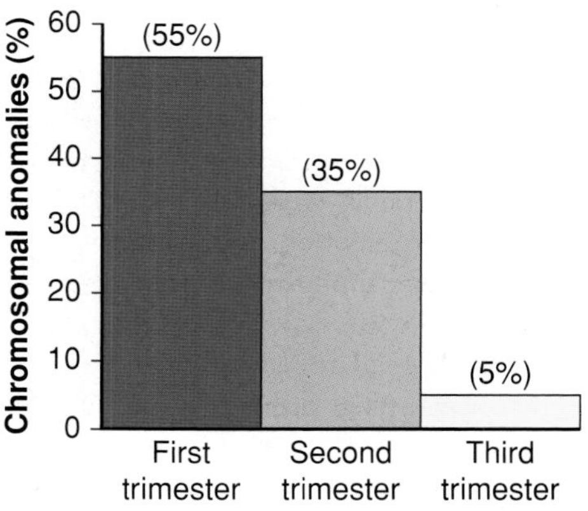

FIGURE 18-1 Frequency of chromosomal anomalies in abortuses and stillbirths during each trimester. Approximate percentages for each group are shown. (Data from Eiben, 1990; Fantel, 1980; Warburton, 1980.)

and 22 are most common. A previous miscarriage increases the baseline risk for aneuploidy in a subsequent fetus from 1.4 to 1.7 percent (Bianco, 2006). With two or three previous miscarriages, the risk increases to 1.8 and 2.2 percent, respectively.

Monosomy X (45,X) is the single most frequent specific chromosomal abnormality. This is *Turner syndrome*, which usually results in abortion, but liveborn females are described (Chap. 13, p. 264). Conversely, *autosomal monosomy* is rare and incompatible with life.

Triploidy is often associated with hydropic or molar placental degeneration (Chap. 20, p. 398). The fetus within a partial hydatidiform mole frequently aborts early, and the few carried longer are all grossly deformed. Advanced maternal and paternal age do not increase the incidence of triploidy. *Tetraploid* fetuses most often abort early in gestation, and they are rarely liveborn. Last, *chromosomal structural abnormalities* infrequently cause abortion.

Euploid Abortion

Chromosomally normal fetuses abort later than those that are aneuploid. Specifically, the rate of euploid abortions peaks at approximately 13 weeks (Kajii, 1980). In addition, the incidence of euploid abortions increases dramatically after maternal age exceeds 35 years (Stein, 1980).

Maternal Factors

The causes of euploid abortions are poorly understood, but various medical disorders, environmental conditions, and developmental abnormalities have been implicated. One example is the well-known influence of maternal age just described.

Infections

Some common viral, bacterial, and other infectious agents that invade the normal human can cause pregnancy loss. Many are systemic and infect the fetoplacental unit by bloodborne organisms. Others may infect locally through genitourinary infection or colonization. However, despite the numerous infections acquired in pregnancy, these uncommonly cause early abortion. *Brucella abortus, Campylobacter fetus,* and *Toxoplasma gondii* infections cause abortion in livestock, but their role in human pregnancy is less clear (Feldman, 2010; Hide, 2009; Mohammad, 2011; Vilchez, 2014). There appear to be no abortifacient effects of infections caused by *Listeria monocytogenes*, parvovirus, cytomegalovirus, or herpes simplex virus (Brown, 1997; Feldman, 2010). One possible exception is infection with *Chlamydia trachomatis,* which was found to be present in 4 percent of abortuses compared with < 1 percent of controls (Baud, 2011). Another is polymicrobial infection from periodontal disease that has been linked with a two- to fourfold increased risk (Holbrook, 2004; Moore, 2004; Xiong, 2007).

Data concerning a link between some other infections and increased abortion are conflicting. Examples are *Mycoplasma* and *Ureaplasma* (Quinn, 1983a,b; Temmerman, 1992). Another is an association with human immunodeficiency virus (HIV) (Quinn, 1983a,b; van Benthem, 2000). Oakeshott and coworkers (2002) reported an association between second-, but not first-, trimester miscarriage and *bacterial vaginosis.*

Medical Disorders

In general, early abortions are rarely due to chronic wasting diseases such as tuberculosis or carcinomatosis. There are a few specific disorders possibly linked with increased early pregnancy loss. Those associated with diabetes mellitus and thyroid disease are discussed subsequently. Another example is *celiac disease,* which has been reported to cause recurrent abortions as well as both male and female infertility (Sharshiner, 2013; Sher, 1994). Unrepaired cyanotic heart disease is likely a risk for abortion, and in some, this may persist after repair (Canobbio, 1996). Eating disorders—*anorexia nervosa* and *bulimia nervosa*—have been linked with subfertility, preterm delivery, and fetal-growth restriction. Their association with miscarriage, however, is less well studied (Andersen, 2009; Sollid, 2004). Inflammatory bowel disease and systemic lupus erythematosus may increase the risk (Al Arfaj, 2010; Khashan, 2012). *Chronic hypertension* does not appear to confer significant risk (Ankumah, 2013). Perhaps related, women with a history of recurrent miscarriages were reported to be at increased risk for fetal-growth restriction (Catov, 2008). Another possible link with vascular disease is that women with multiple miscarriages are more likely to later suffer a myocardial infarction (Kharazmi, 2011).

Medications. Only a few medications have been evaluated concerning a role with early pregnancy loss. Oral contraceptives or spermicidal agents used in contraceptive creams and jellies are not associated with an increased miscarriage rate. Similarly, nonsteroidal antiinflammatory drugs or ondansetron are not linked (Edwards, 2012; Pasternak, 2013). A pregnancy with an intrauterine device (IUD) in situ has an increased risk of abortion and specifically of septic abortion (Chap. 38, p. 700). With the newer IUDs, Moschos and Twickler (2011) reported that only 6 of 26 intact pregnancies aborted before 20 weeks. Finally, studies have shown no increase in pregnancy loss rates with meningococcal conjugate or trivalent inactivated influenza vaccines (Irving, 2013; Zheteyeva, 2013).

Cancer. Therapeutic doses of radiation are undeniably abortifacient, but doses that cause abortion are not precisely known (Chap. 46, p. 930). According to Brent (2009), exposure to < 5 rads does not increase the risk.

Cancer survivors who were previously treated with abdominopelvic radiotherapy may later be at increased risk for miscarriage. Wo and Viswanathan (2009) reported an associated two- to eightfold increased risk for miscarriages, low-birthweight and growth-restricted infants, preterm delivery, and perinatal mortality in women previously treated with radiotherapy. Hudson (2010) found an associated increased risk for miscarriage in those given radiotherapy and chemotherapy in the past for a childhood cancer.

The effects of chemotherapy in causing abortion are not well defined (Chap. 12, p. 248). Particularly worrisome are women with an early normal gestation erroneously treated with methotrexate for an ectopic pregnancy (Chap. 19, p. 384). In a report of eight such cases, two viable-size fetuses had multiple malformations. In the remaining six cases, three each had a spontaneous or induced abortion (Nurmohamed, 2011).

Diabetes Mellitus

The abortifacient effects of uncontrolled diabetes are well-known. Optimal glycemic control will mitigate much of this loss and is discussed in Chapters 8 (p. 157) and 57 (p. 1128). Spontaneous abortion and major congenital malformation rates are both increased in women with insulin-dependent diabetes. This is directly related to the degree of periconceptional glycemic and metabolic control.

Thyroid Disorders

These have long been suspected to cause early pregnancy loss and other adverse pregnancy outcomes. Severe iodine deficiency, which is infrequent in developed countries, has been associated with increased miscarriage rates (Castañeda, 2002). Varying degrees of thyroid hormone insufficiency are common in women. Although the worst—overt hypothyroidism—is infrequent in pregnancy, subclinical hypothyroidism has an incidence of 2 to 3 percent (Casey, 2005; Garber, 2012). Both are usually caused by autoimmune *Hashimoto thyroiditis,* in which both incidence and severity accrue with age. Despite this common prevalence, any increased risks for miscarriage due to hypothyroidism are still unclear (Krassas, 2010; Negro, 2010). That said, De Vivo (2010) reported that subclinical thyroid hormone deficiency may be associated with very early pregnancy loss.

The prevalence of abnormally high serum levels of antibodies to thyroid peroxidase or thyroglobulin is nearly 15 percent in pregnant women (Abbassi-Ghanavati, 2010; Haddow, 2011). Although most of these women are euthyroid, those with clinical hypothyroidism tend to have higher concentrations of antibodies. Even in euthyroid women, however, antibodies are a marker for increased miscarriage (Benhadi, 2009; Chen, 2011; Thangaratinam, 2011). This has been confirmed by two prospective studies, and preliminary data from one suggest that thyroxine supplementation decreases this risk (Männistö, 2009; Negro, 2006). Effects associated with thyroid disorders in women with *recurrent miscarriage* are considered further on page 359.

Surgical Procedures

The risk of miscarriage caused by surgery is not well studied. There is extensive interest in pregnancy outcomes following *bariatric surgery,* because as discussed on page 353, obesity is an uncontested risk factor for miscarriage. However, currently, it is not known if this risk is mitigated by weight-reduction surgery (Guelinckx, 2009).

It is likely that *uncomplicated* surgical procedures performed during early pregnancy do not increase the risk for abortion (Mazze, 1989). Ovarian tumors can generally be resected without causing miscarriage (Chap. 63, p. 1227). An important exception involves early removal of the corpus luteum or the ovary in which it resides. If performed before 10 weeks' gestation, supplemental progesterone should be given. Between 8 and 10 weeks, a single 150-mg intramuscular injection of 17-hydroxyprogesterone caproate is given at the time of surgery. If between 6 to 8 weeks, then two additional 150-mg injections should be given 1 and 2 weeks after the first. Other progesterone regimens include: (1) oral micronized progesterone (Prometrium), 200 or 300 mg orally once daily, or (2) 8-percent progesterone vaginal gel (Crinone) given intravaginally as one premeasured applicator daily *plus* micronized progesterone 100 or 200 mg orally once daily continued until 10 weeks' gestation.

Trauma seldom causes first-trimester miscarriage, and although Parkland Hospital is a busy trauma center, this is an infrequent association. Major trauma—especially abdominal—can cause fetal loss, but is more likely as pregnancy advances (Chap. 47, p. 950).

Nutrition

Extremes of nutrition—severe dietary deficiency and morbid obesity—are associated with increased miscarriage risks. Dietary quality may also be important, as this risk may be reduced in women who consume fresh fruit and vegetables daily (Maconochie, 2007).

Sole deficiency of one nutrient or moderate deficiency of all does not appear to increase risks for abortion. Even in extreme cases—for example, *hyperemesis gravidarum*—abortion is rare (Maconochie, 2007). Other examples discussed on page 352 are *anorexia* and *bulimia nervosa*. Importantly, Bulik and colleagues (2010) reported that half of pregnancies in women with anorexia nervosa were unplanned.

Obesity is associated with a litany of adverse pregnancy outcomes (Chap. 48, p. 965). These include subfertility and an increased risk of miscarriage and recurrent abortion (Jarvie, 2010; Lashen, 2004; Satpathy, 2008). In a study of 6500 women who conceived with in vitro fertilization (IVF), live birth rates were reduced progressively for each body mass index (BMI) unit increase (Bellver, 2010a). As noted earlier, although the risks for many adverse late-pregnancy outcomes are decreased after bariatric surgery, any salutary effects on the miscarriage rate are not clear (Guelinckx, 2009).

Social and Behavioral Factors

Lifestyle choices reputed to be associated with an increased miscarriage risk are most commonly related to chronic and especially heavy use of *legal* substances. The most common used is alcohol, with its potent teratogenic effects discussed in Chapter 12 (p. 245). That said, an increased miscarriage risk is only seen with regular or heavy use (Floyd, 1999; Maconochie, 2007). In fact, low-level alcohol consumption does not significantly increase the abortion risk (Cavallo, 1995; Kesmodel, 2002).

At least 15 percent of pregnant women admit to *cigarette smoking* (Centers for Disease Control and Prevention, 2013). It seems intuitive, but unproven, that cigarettes could cause early pregnancy loss by a number of mechanisms that cause adverse late-pregnancy outcomes (Catov, 2008).

Excessive caffeine consumption—not well defined—has been associated with an increased abortion risk. There are reports that heavy intake of approximately five cups of coffee per day—about 500 mg of caffeine—slightly increases the abortion risk (Armstrong, 1992; Cnattingus, 2000; Klebanoff, 1999). Studies of "moderate"—less than 200 mg daily—did not increase the risk (Savitz, 2008; Weng, 2008). Currently, the American College of Obstetricians and Gynecologists (2013b) has concluded that moderate consumption likely is not a major abortion risk and that any associated risk with higher intake is unsettled. Adverse effects of *illicit drugs* are discussed in Chapter 12 (p. 253).

Occupational and Environmental Factors

It is intuitive to limit exposure of pregnant women to any toxin. That said, although some environmental toxins such as benzene are implicated in fetal malformations, data with miscarriage risk is less clear (Lupo, 2011). The major reason is that it is not possible to accurately assess environmental exposures. Earlier reports that implicated some chemicals as increasing miscarriage risk include arsenic, lead, formaldehyde, benzene, and ethylene oxide (Barlow, 1982). More recently, there is evidence that DDT—dichlorodiphenyltrichloroethane—may cause excessive miscarriage rates (Eskenazi, 2009). In fact, use of DDT-containing insecticides had been suspended. But in 2006, it was again and is still endorsed by the World Health Organization (2011) for mosquito control for malaria prevention.

There are even fewer studies of occupational exposures and abortion risks. In a follow-up of the Nurses Health Study II, Lawson and associates (2012) reported slightly increased miscarriage risks in nurses exposed to antineoplastic drugs, sterilizing agents, and x-rays. Some of these found that exposure to *video display terminals* or to *ultrasound* did not increase miscarriage rates (Schnorr, 1991; Taskinen, 1990). Increased miscarriage risk was found for dental assistants exposed to more than 3 hours of nitrous oxide daily if there was no gas-scavenging equipment (Boivin, 1997; Rowland, 1995). Conclusions from a metaanalysis were that there is a small incremental risk for spontaneous abortion in women who worked with *cytotoxic antineoplastic chemotherapeutic agents* (Dranitsaris, 2005).

Immunological Factors

The immune tolerance of the mother to the paternal-haploid fetal combination remains enigmatic (Calleja-Agius, 2011; Williams, 2012). This is discussed in greater detail in Chapter 5 (p. 97). There is, however, an increased risk for early pregnancy loss with some immune-mediated disorders. The most potent of these are antiphospholipid antibodies directed against binding proteins in plasma (Erkan, 2011). These along with clinical and laboratory findings provide criteria for the *antiphospholipid antibody syndrome—APS* (American College of Obstetricians and Gynecologists, 2012). Because associated pregnancy loss can be repetitive, recurrent miscarriage due to APS is discussed on page 359.

Inherited Thrombophilias

Although thrombophilias were initially linked to various pregnancy outcomes, most putative associations have been refuted. Currently, the American College of Obstetricians and Gynecologists (2013a) is of the opinion that there is not a definitive causal link between these thrombophilias and adverse pregnancy outcomes in general, and abortion in particular.

Uterine Defects

Various inherited and acquired uterine defects are known to cause both early and late recurrent miscarriages, and they are considered on page 358.

Paternal Factors

These factors in the genesis of miscarriage are not well studied. Chromosomal abnormalities in sperm reportedly had an increased abortion risk (Carrell, 2003). Increasing paternal age was significantly associated with increased risk for abortion in the Jerusalem Perinatal Study (Kleinhaus, 2006). This risk was lowest before age 25 years, after which it progressively increased at 5-year intervals.

Clinical Classification of Spontaneous Abortion

Threatened Abortion

The clinical diagnosis of threatened abortion is presumed when bloody vaginal discharge or bleeding appears through a closed cervical os during the first 20 weeks (Hasan, 2009). Bleeding in early pregnancy must be differentiated from implantation bleeding, which some women have at the time of the expected menses (Chap. 5, p. 90). Almost a fourth of women develop clinically significant bleeding during early gestation that may persist for days or weeks. With miscarriage, bleeding usually begins first, and cramping abdominal pain follows hours to days later. There may be low-midline clearly rhythmic cramps; persistent low backache with pelvic pressure; or dull and midline suprapubic discomfort. Bleeding is by far the most predictive risk factor for pregnancy loss (Eddleman, 2006). Overall, approximately half will abort, but this risk is substantially less if there is fetal cardiac activity (Tongsong, 1995).

Even if miscarriage does not follow early bleeding, the risk for later adverse pregnancy outcomes is increased as shown in Table 18-2. In the study of almost 1.8 million pregnancies from the Danish National Patient Registry, there was a threefold risk for many of these pregnancy complications.

Threatened Abortion versus Ectopic Pregnancy. Every woman with an early pregnancy, vaginal bleeding, and pain should be evaluated. The primary goal is prompt diagnosis of an ectopic pregnancy. As discussed in Chapter 19

TABLE 18-2. Adverse Outcomes That are Increased in Women with Threatened Abortion

Maternal	Perinatal
Placenta previa	Preterm ruptured membranes
Placental abruption	Preterm birth
Manual removal of placenta	Low-birthweight infant
Cesarean delivery	Fetal-growth restriction
	Fetal and neonatal death

From Johns, 2006; Lykke, 2010; Saraswat, 2010; Wijesiriwardana, 2006.

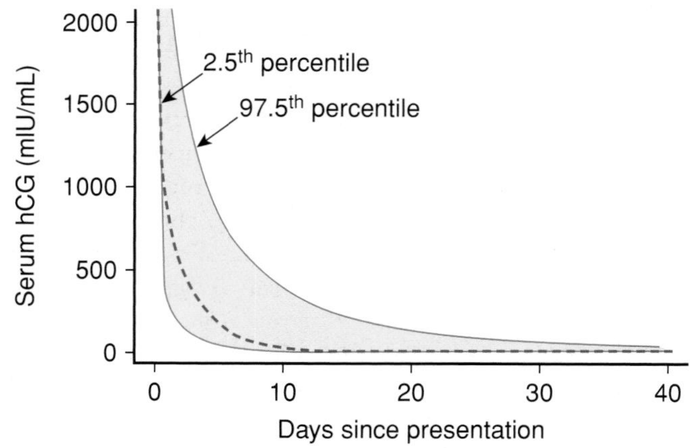

FIGURE 18-2 Composite curve describing decline in serial human chorionic gonadotropin (hCG) values starting at a level of 2000 mIU/mL following early spontaneous miscarriage. The dashed line is the predicted curve based on the summary of data from all women. The colored area within the dashed lines represents the 95-percent confidence intervals. (Data from Barnhart, 2004a.)

(p. 381), serial quantitative serum β-hCG and progesterone levels and transvaginal sonography are used to ascertain if there is an intrauterine live fetus. Because these are not 100-percent accurate to confirm early fetal death or location, repeat evaluations are often necessary. Serum hCG levels in women with bleeding who went on to have an early miscarriage are shown in Figure 18-2 and in Table 19-1 (p. 381). Values for women with early pregnancy bleeding who went on to have a normal pregnancy are shown in Figure 18-3. Several predictive models have been described (Barnhart, 2010; Condous, 2007; Connolly, 2013). With a robust uterine pregnancy, serum β-hCG levels should increase at least 53 to 66 percent every 48 hours (Barnhart, 2004a; Kadar, 1982). Serum progesterone concentrations < 5 ng/mL suggest a dying pregnancy, whereas values > 20 ng/mL support the diagnosis of a healthy pregnancy.

Transvaginal sonography is used to locate the pregnancy and determine if the fetus is alive. If this cannot be done, then *pregnancy of unknown location* is diagnosed (Chap. 19, p. 381).

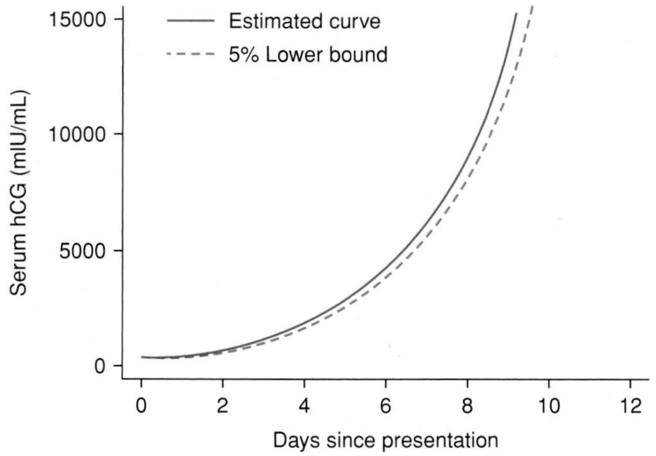

FIGURE 18-3 Composite curve of increasing serum levels of beta-human chorionic gonadotropin (β-hCG) in women with early bleeding and subsequent normal pregnancy. (Data from Barnhart, 2004b.)

The gestational sac—an anechoic fluid collection that represents the exocoelomic cavity—may be seen by 4.5 weeks (Fig. 9-3, p. 170). At this same time, β-hCG levels are generally considered to be 1500 to 2000 mIU/mL (Barnhart, 1994; Timor-Tritsch, 1988). Connolly and colleagues (2013) observed that this value could be as low as 390 mIU/mL, but also noted that a threshold as high as 3500 mIU/mL may be needed to identify the gestational sac in 99 percent of cases.

Another caveat is that a gestational sac may appear similar to other intrauterine fluid accumulations—the so-called *pseudogestational sac* (Fig. 19-5, p. 382). This pseudosac may be seen with ectopic pregnancy and is easier to exclude once a yolk sac is seen. Typically, the yolk sac is visible by 5.5 weeks and with a mean gestational-sac diameter of 10 mm. Thus, the diagnosis of a uterine pregnancy should be made cautiously if the yolk sac is not yet seen (American College of Obstetricians and Gynecologists, 2011e).

At 5 to 6 weeks, a 1- to 2-mm embryo adjacent to the yolk sac can be seen (Daya, 1993). Absence of an embryo in a sac with a mean sac diameter of 16 to 20 mm suggests a dead fetus (Levi, 1988; Nyberg, 1987). Finally, fetal cardiac activity can be detected at 6 to 6.5 weeks with an embryonic length of 1 to 5 mm and a mean sac diameter of 13 to 18 mm. A 5-mm embryo without cardiac activity is likely dead (Goldstein, 1992; Levi, 1990).

There are various management schemes derived from these findings. At Parkland Hospital, to ensure that live intrauterine pregnancies are not interrupted, we define the threshold of embryo fetal death based on values two standard deviations from the mean. Thus, an anembryonic gestation is diagnosed when the mean gestational sac diameter measures ≥ 20 mm and no embryo is seen. Embryonic death is also diagnosed if an embryo measuring ≥ 10 mm has no cardiac activity.

Management. Acetaminophen-based analgesia will help relieve discomfort from cramping. If uterine evacuation is not indicated, bed rest is often recommended but does not improve outcomes. Neither has treatment with a host of medications that include chorionic gonadotropin (Devaseelan, 2010). With persistent or heavy bleeding, the hematocrit is determined. If there is significant anemia or hypovolemia, then pregnancy evacuation is generally indicated. In these cases in which there is a live fetus, some choose transfusion and further observation.

Anti-D Immunoglobulin. With spontaneous miscarriage, 2 percent of Rh D-negative women will become alloimmunized if not provided passive isoimmunization. With an induced abortion, this rate may reach 5 percent. The American College of Obstetricians and Gynecologists (2013c) recommends anti-Rh_0 (D) immunoglobulin given as 300 μg intramuscularly (IM) for all gestational ages, or 50 μg IM for pregnancies ≤ 12 weeks and 300 μg for ≥ 13 weeks.

With threatened abortion, immunoglobulin prophylaxis is controversial because of sparse evidence-based data (American College of Obstetricians and Gynecologists, 2013c; Hannafin, 2006; Weiss, 2002). That said, some choose to administer anti-D immunoglobulin up to 12 weeks' gestation for a threatened abortion and a live fetus. At Parkland Hospital, we administer a 50-μg dose to all Rh D-negative women with first-trimester bleeding.

Inevitable Abortion

In the first trimester, gross rupture of the membranes along with cervical dilatation is nearly always followed by either uterine contractions or infection. A gush of vaginal fluid during the first half of pregnancy usually has serious consequences. In some cases not associated with pain, fever, or bleeding, fluid may have collected previously between the amnion and chorion. If this is documented, then diminished activity with observation is a reasonable course. After 48 hours, if no additional amnionic fluid has escaped and if there is no bleeding, cramping, or fever, then a woman may resume ambulation and pelvic rest. With bleeding, cramping, or fever, abortion is considered inevitable, and the uterus is evacuated.

Incomplete Abortion

Bleeding that follows partial or complete placental separation and dilation of the cervical os is termed incomplete abortion. The fetus and the placenta may remain entirely within the uterus or partially extrude through the dilated os. Before 10 weeks, they are frequently expelled together, but later, they deliver separately. Management options of incomplete abortion include curettage, medical abortion, or expectant management in clinically stable women as discussed on page 357. With surgical therapy, additional cervical dilatation may be necessary before suction curettage. In others, retained placental tissue simply lies loosely within the cervical canal and can be easily extracted with ring forceps.

Complete Abortion

At times, expulsion of the entire pregnancy may be completed before a woman presents to the hospital. A history of heavy bleeding, cramping, and passage of tissue or a fetus is common. Importantly, during examination, the cervical os is closed. Patients are encouraged to bring in passed tissue, which may be a complete gestation, blood clots, or a decidual cast. The last is a layer of endometrium in the shape of the uterine cavity that when sloughed can appear as a collapsed sac (Fig. 19-3, p. 379).

If an expelled complete gestational sac is not identified, sonography is performed to differentiate a complete abortion from threatened abortion or ectopic pregnancy. Characteristic findings of a complete abortion include a minimally thickened endometrium without a gestational sac. However, this does not guarantee a recent uterine pregnancy. Condous and associates (2005) described 152 women with heavy bleeding, an empty uterus with endometrial thickness < 15 mm, and a diagnosis of completed miscarriage. Six percent were subsequently proven to have an ectopic pregnancy. Thus, unless products of conception are seen or unless sonography confidently documents, at first an intrauterine pregnancy, and then later an empty cavity, a complete abortion cannot be surely diagnosed. In unclear settings, serial serum hCG measurements aid clarification. With complete abortion, these levels drop quickly (Connolly, 2013).

Missed Abortion

Also termed early pregnancy failure or loss, missed abortion, as originally defined, is contemporaneously misused compared with its meaning many decades ago. Historically, the term was used to describe dead products of conception that were retained for days, weeks, or even months in the uterus with a closed cervical os. Early pregnancy appeared to be normal with amenorrhea, nausea and vomiting, breast changes, and uterine growth. Because suspected fetal death could not be confirmed, expectant management was the sole option, and spontaneous miscarriage would eventually ensue. And because the time of fetal death could not be determined clinically, pregnancy duration—and thus fetal age—was erroneously calculated from the last menses. To elucidate these disparities, Streeter (1930) studied aborted fetuses and reported that the mean death-to-abortion interval was approximately 6 weeks.

This historical description of missed abortion is in contrast to that defined currently based on results of serial serum β-hCG assays and transvaginal sonography (Fig. 18-4). With rapid confirmation of fetal or embryonic death, many women choose uterine evacuation. Although many classify these as a missed abortion, the term is used interchangeably with early pregnancy loss or wastage (Silver, 2011).

Septic Abortion

Horrific infections and maternal deaths associated with criminal septic abortions have become rare with legalized abortion. Still, perhaps 1 to 2 percent of women with threatened or incomplete miscarriage develop a pelvic infection and sepsis syndrome. Elective abortion, either surgical or medical, is also occasionally complicated by severe and even fatal infections (Barrett, 2002; Ho, 2009). Bacteria gain uterine entry and colonize dead conception products. Organisms may invade myometrial tissues and extend to cause parametritis, peritonitis, septicemia, and, rarely, endocarditis (Vartian, 1991). Particularly worrisome are severe necrotizing infections and toxic shock syndrome caused by group A streptococcus—*S pyogenes* (Daif, 2009).

During the last few years, rare but severe infections with otherwise low-virulence organisms have complicated medical abortions. Deaths have been reported from toxic shock syndrome due to

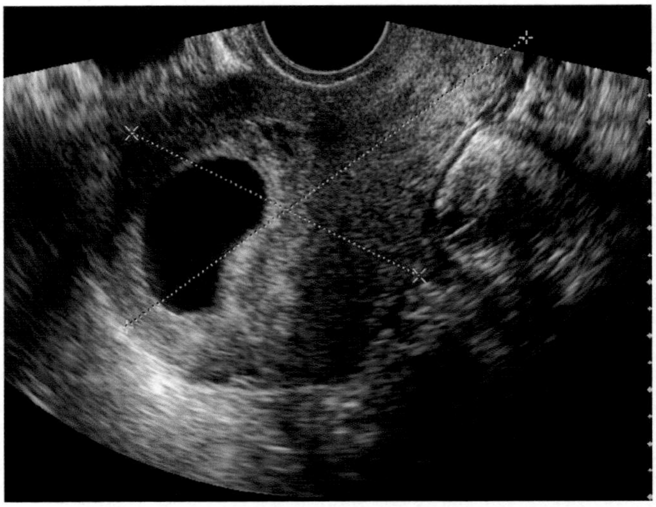

FIGURE 18-4 Transvaginal sonogram displays a large anechoic sac consistent with an anembryonic gestation. Calipers measure uterine length and anteroposterior thickness in a sagittal plane.

Clostridium perfringens (Centers for Disease Control and Prevention, 2005). Similar infections are caused by *Clostridium sordellii* and have clinical manifestations that begin within a few days after an abortion. Women may be afebrile when first seen with severe endothelial injury, capillary leakage, hemoconcentration, hypotension, and a profound leukocytosis (Cohen, 2007; Fischer, 2005; Ho, 2009). Maternal deaths from these clostridial species approximate 0.58 per 100,000 medical abortions (Meites, 2010).

Management of clinical infection includes prompt administration of broad-spectrum antibiotics as discussed in Chapter 37 (p. 685). If there are retained products or fragments, then suction curettage is also performed. Most women respond to this treatment within 1 to 2 days, and they are discharged when afebrile. Follow-up oral antibiotic treatment is likely unnecessary (Savaris, 2011). In a very few women, severe sepsis syndrome causes acute respiratory distress syndrome, acute kidney injury, or disseminated intravascular coagulopathy. In these cases, intensive supportive care is essential (Chap. 47, p. 940).

To prevent postabortal sepsis, prophylactic antibiotics are given at the time of induced abortion or spontaneous abortion that requires medical or surgical intervention. The American College of Obstetricians and Gynecologists (2011b) recommends doxycycline, 100 mg orally 1 hr before and then 200 mg orally after a surgical evacuation. At Planned Parenthood clinics, for medical abortion, doxycycline 100 mg is taken orally daily for 7 days and begins with abortifacient administration (Fjerstad, 2009b).

Management of Spontaneous Abortion

With embryofetal death now easy to verify with current sonographic technology, management can be more individualized. Unless there is serious bleeding or infection with an incomplete abortion, any of three options are reasonable—expectant, medical, or surgical management. Each has its own risks and benefits—for example, the first two are associated with unpredictable bleeding, and some women will undergo unscheduled curettage. Also, success of any method depends on whether the woman has an incomplete or missed abortion. Some of the risks and benefits are summarized as follows:

1. Expectant management of spontaneous incomplete abortion has failure rates as high as 50 percent.
2. Medical therapy with prostaglandin E_1 (PGE_1) has varying failure rates of 5 to 40 percent. In 1100 women with suspected first-trimester abortion, 81 percent had a spontaneous resolution (Luise, 2002).
3. Curettage usually results in a quick resolution that is 95- to 100-percent successful. It is invasive and not necessary for all women.

It is possible that patients and clinicians opt for surgical methods when there is not a strict protocol for medical treatment (Kollitz, 2011).

Several randomized studies that compared these management schemes were reviewed by Neilson (2010). A major drawback cited for between-study comparisons was varied inclusion criteria and techniques. For example, studies that included women with vaginal bleeding reported greater success for medical therapy than did studies that excluded such women (Creinin, 2006). With these caveats in mind, selected studies reported since 2005 are listed in Table 18-3. Importantly, Smith and coworkers (2009) reported that subsequent pregnancy rates did not differ among these management methods.

TABLE 18-3. Randomized Controlled Studies for Management of Various Types of First-Trimester Pregnancy Loss

Study	Inclusion Criteria	No.	Treatment Arms	Outcomes
Nguyen (2005)	Incomplete SAB	149	(1) PGE_1, 600 μg orally (2) PGE_1, 600 μg orally initially and at 4 hr	60% completed at 3 d 95% at 7 d; 3% curettage
Zhang (2005)	Pregnancy failure[b]	652	(1) PGE_1, 800 μg vaginally (2) Vacuum aspiration	71% completed at 3 d; 16% failure 97% successful
Trinder (2006) (MIST Trial)	Incomplete SAB; missed AB	1200	(1) Expectant (2) PGE_1, 800 μg vaginally + 200 mg mifepristone (3) Suction curettage	50% curettage 38% curettage 5% repeat curettage
Dao (2007)	Incomplete SAB	447	(1) PGE_1, 600 μg orally (2) Vacuum aspiration	95% completed 100% curettage
Torre (2012)	First-trimester miscarriage[b]	174	(1) Immediate—PGE_1, 200 μg orally now; 400 μg vaginally day 2 (2) Delayed—no Rx; TVS days 7 and 14	81% completed 19% curettage 57% completed 43% curettage

[a]Includes anembryonic gestation, embryonic or fetal death, without signs of incomplete SAB.
[b]Includes anembryonic gestation, embryonic or fetal death, or incomplete or inevitable SAB.
SAB = spontaneous abortion; PGE_1 = prostaglandin E_1; TVS = transvaginal sonography.

RECURRENT MISCARRIAGE

Other terms that have been used to describe repetitive early spontaneous pregnancy losses include *recurrent spontaneous abortion, recurrent pregnancy loss,* and *habitual abortion.* It is generally accepted that approximately 1 percent of fertile couples have recurrent miscarriages classically defined as three or more consecutive pregnancy losses at ≤ 20 weeks or with a fetal weight < 500 grams. Most of these are embryonic or early losses, and the remainder either are anembryonic or occur after 14 weeks. Studies are difficult to compare because of nonstandardized definitions. For example, some investigators include women with two instead of three consecutive losses, and yet others include women with three *nonconsecutive* losses. Documentation of pregnancy with β-hCG levels, sonography, and pathological examination also varies widely.

At minimum, recurrent miscarriage should be distinguished from sporadic pregnancy loss that implies intervening pregnancies that reached viability. Although women in the latter category were thought to have a much lower risk of yet another abortion, there are reports such as the one shown in Table 18-4 that question this assumption. In two studies, the risk for subsequent miscarriage is similar following either two or three pregnancy losses. Remarkably, the chances for a successful pregnancy are > 50 percent even after five losses (Brigham, 1999).

The American Society for Reproductive Medicine (2008) proposed that recurrent pregnancy loss be defined as two or more failed clinical pregnancies confirmed by either sonographic or histopathological examination. A thorough evaluation certainly is warranted after three losses, and treatment is initiated earlier in couples with concordant subfertility (Jaslow, 2010; Reddy, 2007). Treatment considerations are beyond the scope of this book. The reader is referred to Chapters 6 and 20 in the 2nd edition of *Williams Gynecology* (Cunningham, 2012; Doody, 2012).

Etiology

There are many putative causes of recurrent abortion, however, only three are widely accepted: parental chromosomal abnormalities, antiphospholipid antibody syndrome, and a subset of uterine abnormalities. Other suspected but not proven causes are alloimmunity, endocrinopathies, environmental toxins, and various infections. Infections seldom cause even sporadic loss. Thus, most are unlikely to cause recurrent miscarriage, especially since maternal antibodies usually have developed. For years, various inherited thrombophilia mutations that include factor V Leiden, prothrombin G20210A, protein C and S deficiency, and antithrombin deficiency were suspected. But, as discussed in Chapter 52 (p. 1029), large studies have refuted an association between increased pregnancy wastage and these thrombophilias (American College of Obstetricians and Gynecologists, 2013a).

There is some evidence to support a role for various polymorphisms of gene expression in miscarriages. Just a few examples include polymorphisms that alter VEGF-A expression, those that exaggerate platelet aggregation, and those with a specific maternal type of Th1 and Th2 immune response (Calleja-Agius, 2011; Corardetti, 2013; Eller, 2011; Flood, 2010).

The timing of recurrent loss may offer clues, and in some women, each miscarriage may occur near the same gestational age (Heuser, 2010). Genetic factors usually result in early embryonic losses, whereas autoimmune or uterine anatomical abnormalities more likely cause second-trimester losses (Schust, 2002). As mentioned, first-trimester losses in recurrent miscarriage have a significantly lower incidence of genetic abnormalities than sporadic losses—25 versus 50 percent (Sullivan, 2004). That said, routine chromosomal evaluation of abortuses is costly and may not accurately reflect the fetal karyotype.

TABLE 18-4. Predicted Miscarriage Rate in Scottish Women with Their Next Pregnancy According to Number of Prior Miscarriages[a]

	Number of Prior Pregnancy Losses			
	0	1	2	3
Initial pregnancy with miscarriage (n)	143,595	6577	700	115
Subsequent risk for miscarriage	7%	14%	26%	28%

[a]Nonconsecutive miscarriages showed the same pattern of risk as consecutive miscarriages.
Data from Bhattacharya, 2010.

Parental Chromosomal Abnormalities

Although these account for only 2 to 4 percent of recurrent losses, karyotypic evaluation of both parents is considered by many to be a critical part of evaluation. In an earlier study, balanced reciprocal translocations accounted for half of chromosomal abnormalities, robertsonian translocations for a fourth, and X chromosome mosaicism—47,XXY or *Klinefelter syndrome*—for 12 percent (Therapel, 1985). These chromosomal abnormalities are repetitive for consecutive losses (van den Boogaard, 2010). Inheritance of translocation syndromes and their sequelae are discussed in detail in Chapter 13 (p. 266).

After thorough genetic counseling, couples with an abnormal karyotype can usually be managed with IVF followed by preimplantation genetic diagnosis. These techniques are described in detail in Chapter 20 of *Williams Gynecology* (Doody, 2012).

Anatomical Factors

Several genital tract abnormalities have been implicated in recurrent miscarriage and other adverse pregnancy outcomes, but not infertility (Reichman, 2010). According to Devi Wold and colleagues (2006), 15 percent of women with three or more consecutive miscarriages will be found to have a congenital or acquired uterine anomaly.

Of acquired abnormalities, uterine synechiae—*Asherman syndrome*—usually result from destruction of large areas of endometrium. This can follow uterine curettage or ablative procedures. Characteristic multiple filling defects are seen with hysterosalpingography or saline-infusion sonography. Treatment is done using directed hysteroscopic lysis of adhesions. In many women, this lowers miscarriage rates and improves the "take home" pregnancy rate (Al-Inany, 2001; Goldenberg, 1995).

Uterine leiomyomas are found in a large proportion of adult women and can cause miscarriage, especially if located near the placental implantation site. That said, data indicating them to be a significant cause of recurrent pregnancy loss are not convincing (Saravelos, 2011). Uterine cavity distortion is apparently not requisite for bad outcomes (Sunkara, 2010). But in women undergoing IVF, pregnancy outcomes were adversely affected by submucous but not subserosal or intramural leiomyomas (Jun, 2001; Ramzy, 1998). As discussed in Chapter 63 (p. 1226), most agree that consideration be given to excision of submucosal and intracavitary leiomyomas in women with recurrent losses. Ironically, women undergoing uterine artery embolization of myomas had an increased risk for miscarriage in a subsequent pregnancy (Homer, 2010).

In contrast, congenital genital tract anomalies commonly originate from abnormal müllerian duct formation or abnormal fusion. These have an overall incidence of approximately 1 in 200 women (Nahum, 1998). The distribution of anomalies and associated loss rates are shown in Table 18-5. Depending on their anatomy, some may increase risks for early miscarriage, whereas others may cause midtrimester abortion or preterm delivery. Unicornuate, bicornuate, and septate uteri are associated with all three types of loss (Reichman, 2010). Looked at another way, developmental uterine anomalies were found in approximately 20 percent of women with recurrent pregnancy losses compared with about 7 percent of controls (Salim, 2003).

It has proven difficult to demonstrate that correction of uterine anomalies improves early pregnancy outcome. Additional discussion regarding the incidence, clinical impact, and treatment of anatomical abnormalities is found in Chapter 3 (p. 38), as well as in Chapter 18 of *Williams Gynecology* (Bradshaw, 2012).

TABLE 18-5. Estimated Prevalence and Pregnancy Loss Rate for Some Congenital Uterine Malformations

Uterine Anomaly[a]	Proportion of All Anomalies (%)	Pregnancy Loss Rate (%)[b]
Bicornuate	39	40–70
Septate or unicornuate	14–24	34–88
Didelphys	11	40
Arcuate	7	
Hypo- or aplastic	4	

[a]Estimated overall prevalence 1:200 women.
[b]Includes first- and second-trimester losses.
Data from Bradshaw, 2012; Buttram, 1979; Nahum, 1998; Reddy, 2007; Valli, 2001.

Immunological Factors

In their analysis of published studies, Yetman and Kutteh (1996) determined that 15 percent of more than 1000 women with recurrent miscarriage had recognized autoimmune factors. Two primary pathophysiological models are the *autoimmune theory*—immunity directed against self, and the *alloimmune theory*—immunity against another person.

As discussed on page 352, miscarriages are more common in women with systemic lupus erythematosus, an autoimmune disease (Clowse, 2008; Warren, 2004). Many of these women were found to have *antiphospholipid antibodies*, a family of autoantibodies that bind to phospholipid-binding plasma proteins (Erkan, 2011). Women with recurrent spontaneous pregnancy loss have a higher frequency of these antibodies compared with normal controls—5 to 15 versus 2 to 5 percent, respectively (Branch, 2010). The *antiphospholipid antibody syndrome (APS)* is defined by these antibodies found together with various forms of reproductive losses along with substantively increased risks for venous thromboembolism (American College of Obstetricians and Gynecologists, 2011d, 2013a). Mechanisms that cause pregnancy loss are discussed along with treatment in Chapter 59 (p. 1173).

With regard to alloimmunity, a provocative theory suggests that normal pregnancy requires formation of blocking factors that prevent maternal rejection of foreign fetal antigens that are paternally derived (Chap. 5, p. 98). Factors said to prevent this include *human leukocyte antigen (HLA)* similarity with the father, altered natural killer cell activity, regulatory T cell stimulation, and HLA-G gene mutations (Berger, 2010; Williams, 2012). Various tests and treatment options proposed to address this have not withstood rigorous scrutiny, and they are currently investigational (Reddy, 2007). Proposed therapies using paternal or third-party leukocyte immunization or intravenous immunoglobulin (IVIG) have not proved beneficial in women with idiopathic miscarriage (American Society for Reproductive Medicine, 2006; Stephenson, 2010).

Endocrine Factors

According to Arredondo and Noble (2006), 8 to 12 percent of recurrent miscarriages are caused by endocrine factors. Studies to evaluate these have been inconsistent and generally underpowered. Two examples, both controversial, are progesterone deficiency caused by a *luteal-phase defect* and *polycystic ovarian syndrome* (Bukulmez, 2004; Cocksedge, 2008; Nawaz, 2010).

In contrast, the well-known abortifacient effects of uncontrolled diabetes are detailed in Chapter 57. Optimal periconceptional glycemic control will mitigate much of this loss.

Likewise, the effects on early pregnancy loss of overt hypothyroidism and severe iodine deficiency are well known and discussed on page 353. Correction with supplementation reverses these effects. Also, the effects of subclinical hypothyroidism and antithyroid antibodies are sporadic, and thus any effects on recurrent miscarriage rates have been debated (Garber, 2012). That said, however, two recent metaanalyses reported convincingly positive associations between these antibodies and an increased risk for sporadic and recurrent miscarriages (Chen, 2011; Thangaratinam, 2011). Less convincing are preliminary data regarding thyroid hormone treatment for antibody-positive women.

MIDTRIMESTER ABORTION

The timespan that defines a midtrimester fetal loss extends from the end of the first trimester until the fetus weighs ≥ 500 g or gestational age reaches 20 weeks. For reasons discussed on page 350, a gestational age of 22 to 23 weeks is more accurate. Importantly, in many of these losses, an etiology can be found if a careful evaluation is completed.

Incidence and Etiology

Abortion becomes much less common by the end of the first trimester, and its incidence decreases successively thereafter. Overall, spontaneous loss in the second trimester is estimated at 1.5 to 3 percent, and after 16 weeks, it is only 1 percent (Simpson, 2007; Wyatt, 2005). First-trimester bleeding doubles the incidence of second-trimester loss (Hasan, 2009; Velez Edwards, 2012). Unlike earlier miscarriages that frequently are caused by chromosomal aneuploidies, these later fetal losses are due to a multitude of causes and more closely reflect those discussed in the section under Recurrent Miscarriage (p. 358). There are no data to accurately estimate the incidences of these various causes, but some of the more common etiologies are listed in Table 18-6. One frequently overlooked factor is that many second-trimester abortions are medically induced because of fetal abnormalities detected by prenatal screening programs for chromosome trisomies and structural defects.

Risk factors for second-trimester abortion include race, ethnicity, prior poor obstetrical outcomes, and extremes of maternal age. First-trimester bleeding was cited previously as a potent risk factor (Hasan, 2009). Edlow and colleagues (2007) observed that 27 percent of women with such a loss in the index pregnancy had a recurrent second-trimester loss in their next pregnancy. Moreover, a third of these women had a subsequent preterm birth.

TABLE 18-6. Some Causes of Midtrimester Spontaneous Pregnancy Losses

Fetal anomalies
Chromosomal
Structural
Uterine defects
Congenital
Leiomyomas
Incompetent cervix
Placental causes
Abruption, previa
Defective spiral artery transformation
Chorioamnionitis
Maternal disorders
Autoimmune
Infections
Metabolic

Data from Allanson, 2010; Dukhovny, 2009; Joo, 2009; Romero, 2011; Saravelos, 2011; Stout, 2010.

Fetal and Placental Evaluation

Because etiology is closely linked to recurrence risk, a thorough evaluation of obstetrical and perinatal findings is warranted. Pathological examination of the fetus and placenta is essential (Dukhovny, 2009). In women older than 35 years, chromosomal abnormalities explain 80 percent of recurrences (Marguard, 2010). In a study of 486 women of all ages with second-trimester miscarriages, fetal malformations were identified in 13 percent (Joo, 2009). In another, a third of otherwise normal fetuses had associated chorioamnionitis that was judged to have preceded labor (Allanson, 2010). Indeed, according to Srinivas and associates (2008), 95 percent of placentas in midtrimester abortions are abnormal. Other abnormalities are vascular thromboses and infarctions.

Management

Midtrimester abortions are classified similarly to first-trimester abortions. Management is also similar in many regards, and the schemes shown in Table 18-3 are frequently successful with a dead fetus or an incomplete midtrimester abortion. An exception is that at these later gestational ages, oxytocin in concentrated doses is highly effective for labor induction or augmentation. As subsequently discussed on page 366, surgical midtrimester abortion for fetal demise is technically more difficult. That said, there can be significant morbidity with either medical or surgical termination of these. Overall, however, for elective delivery, available data suggest that surgical termination by dilatation and evacuation has fewer complications than labor induction (Bryant, 2011; Edlow, 2011).

Cervical Insufficiency

Also known as incompetent cervix, this is a discrete obstetrical entity characterized classically by painless cervical dilatation in the second trimester. It can be followed by prolapse and ballooning of membranes into the vagina, and ultimately, expulsion of an immature fetus. Unless effectively treated, this sequence may repeat in future pregnancies. Many of these women have a history and clinical findings that make it difficult to verify *classic* cervical incompetence. For example, in a randomized trial of almost 1300 women with an atypical history, cerclage was found to be only marginally beneficial—13 versus 17 percent—to prolong pregnancy past 33 weeks (MacNaughton, 1993). It seems likely that many of these women with such a nonclassic history had preterm labor instead of classic cervical incompetence. In this study, for every 25 cerclage procedures, only one birth before 33 weeks was prevented. In a systematic review of similar women, however, indicated cerclages that were placed based on physical examination findings provided superior perinatal outcomes compared with expectant management (Ehsanipoor, 2013).

Because of these difficulties in identification of classic cervical insufficiency, interest has been focused on the predictive value of transvaginal sonography. Some findings assessed include cervical length as well as the presence of *funneling*, which is ballooning of the membranes into a dilated internal os, but with a closed external os (Owen, 2003). In women with these problems, early randomized trials were inconclusive in proving the clinical relevance of cerclage to prevent preterm birth (Rust, 2001; To, 2004). A multicenter randomized trial of 302 high-risk women with cervical length < 25 mm reported that cerclage prevented birth before viability but not birth before 34 weeks (Owen, 2009). Subsequently, however, Berghella and coworkers (2011) included five trials in a metaanalysis and showed that cerclage for these high-risk women significantly reduced preterm birth before 24, 28, 32, 35, and 37 weeks. One retrospective analysis found no improved outcomes with twin pregnancies in women with a cervical length ≤ 25 mm (Stoval, 2013).

Risk Factors

Although the cause of incompetence is obscure, previous cervical trauma such as dilatation and curettage, conization, cauterization, or amputation has been implicated. A Norwegian cohort study of more than 15,000 women with prior cervical conization found a fourfold risk of pregnancy loss before 24 weeks (Albrechtsen, 2008). Even though prior dilatation and evacuation (D&E) has an incidence of cervical injury of 5 percent, neither it nor dilatation and extraction (D&X) after 20 weeks increased the likelihood of an incompetent cervix (Chasen, 2005). In other instances, abnormal cervical development, including that following in utero exposure to diethylstilbestrol (DES), may play a role (Hoover, 2011). This is discussed further in Chapter 3 (p. 42).

Evaluation and Treatment

Sonography is performed to confirm a living fetus with no major anomalies. Cervical secretions are tested for gonorrhea and chlamydia infection. These and other obvious cervical infections are treated. For at least a week before and after surgery, sexual intercourse is prohibited.

Classic cervical incompetence is treated surgically with cerclage, which reinforces a weak cervix by a purse-string suture. Contraindications to cerclage usually include bleeding, uterine contractions, or ruptured membranes. With ruptured membranes and bleeding or contractions or both, the likelihood of failure is substantially increased. Thus, prophylactic cerclage before dilatation is preferable. At times, this may not be possible, and a *rescue cerclage* is performed emergently after the cervix is found to be dilated, effaced, or both. In some or even many of these women, cerclage is unknowingly being used incorrectly to treat preterm labor with cervical dilatation rather than an incompetent cervix.

The timing of surgery depends on clinical circumstances. In women who are diagnosed with cervical insufficiency based on their previous obstetrical outcomes, elective cerclage is usually done between 12 and 14 weeks' gestation. If the diagnosis is made in high-risk women using transvaginal sonography to document cervical shortening < 25 mm, then cerclage is done at that time. For the remainder who undergo emergent rescue cerclage, there is debate as to how late this should be performed. The conundrum is that the more advanced the pregnancy, the greater the risk that surgical intervention will stimulate preterm labor or membrane rupture. Although this practice is not evidence based, we usually do not perform cerclage after 23 weeks. Others, however, recommend placement later than this (Caruso, 2000; Terkildsen, 2003).

When outcomes of cerclage are evaluated, women with similar clinical presentations should be compared. For example, in the study of elective cerclage by Owen and associates (2009), approximately a third of women delivered before 35 weeks, and there were few complications with surgery. By contrast, in a 10-year review of 75 women undergoing emergency cerclage procedures, Chasen and Silverman (1998) reported that only half were delivered after 36 weeks. Importantly, only 44 percent of those with bulging membranes at the time of cerclage reached 28 weeks. Terkildsen and colleagues (2003) had similar experiences. Caruso and coworkers (2000) described emergency cerclage done in 23 women from 17 to 27 weeks who had a dilated cervix and protruding membranes. There were 11 liveborn infants, and these researchers concluded that success was unpredictable. Our experiences at Parkland Hospital are that rescue cerclages have a high failure rate, and women are counseled accordingly.

If the clinical indication for cerclage is questionable, these women may be advised to instead decrease physical activity and abstain from intercourse. Most undergo cervical examinations each week or every 2 weeks to assess effacement and dilatation. Unfortunately, rapid effacement and dilatation can develop despite such precautions (Witter, 1984).

Cerclage Procedures

Of the two vaginal cerclage operations, most use the simpler procedure developed by McDonald (1963) and shown in Figure 18-5. The more complicated operation is a modification of the procedure described by Shirodkar (1955) and shown in Figure 18-6. When either technique is performed prophylactically, women with a classic history of cervical incompetence have excellent outcomes (Caspi, 1990; Kuhn, 1977). As emphasized by Karl and Katz (2012), it is important to place the suture as high as possible and into the dense cervical stroma. There is some evidence that two cerclage sutures are not more effective than one (Giraldo-Isaza, 2013). For either vaginal or abdominal cerclage, there is insufficient evidence to recommend perioperative antibiotic prophylaxis (American College of Obstetricians and Gynecologist, 2011f, 2014).

Emergency or rescue cerclage is, of course, more difficult to perform. Replacement of the prolapsed amnionic sac back into the uterus will usually aid suture placement (Locatelli, 1999). This is sometimes made easier by tilting the operating table in the head-down position along with filling the bladder with 600 mL of saline through an indwelling Foley catheter. Although this may reduce the prolapsing membranes, it also may carry the cervix cephalad and away from the operating field. Some advocate placing a Foley catheter through the cervix and inflating the 30-mL balloon to deflect the amnionic sac cephalad. The balloon is deflated gradually as the cerclage suture is tightened around the catheter. In some

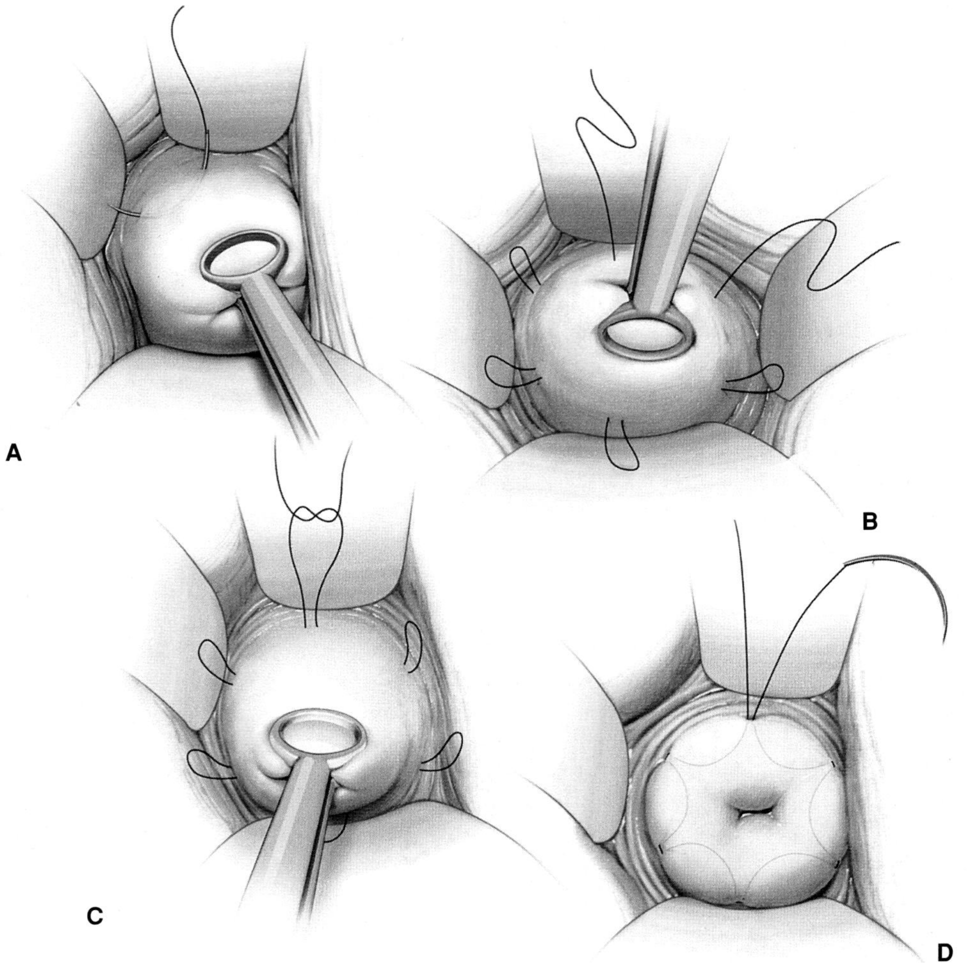

FIGURE 18-5 McDonald cerclage procedure for incompetent cervix. **A.** Start of the cerclage procedure with a No. 2 monofilament suture being placed in the body of the cervix very near the level of the internal os. **B.** Continuation of suture placement in the body of the cervix so as to encircle the os. **C.** Encirclement completed. **D.** The suture is tightened around the cervical canal sufficiently to reduce the diameter of the canal to 5 to 10 mm, and then the suture is tied. The effect of the suture placement on the cervical canal is apparent. A second suture placed somewhat higher may be of value if the first is not in close proximity to the internal os.

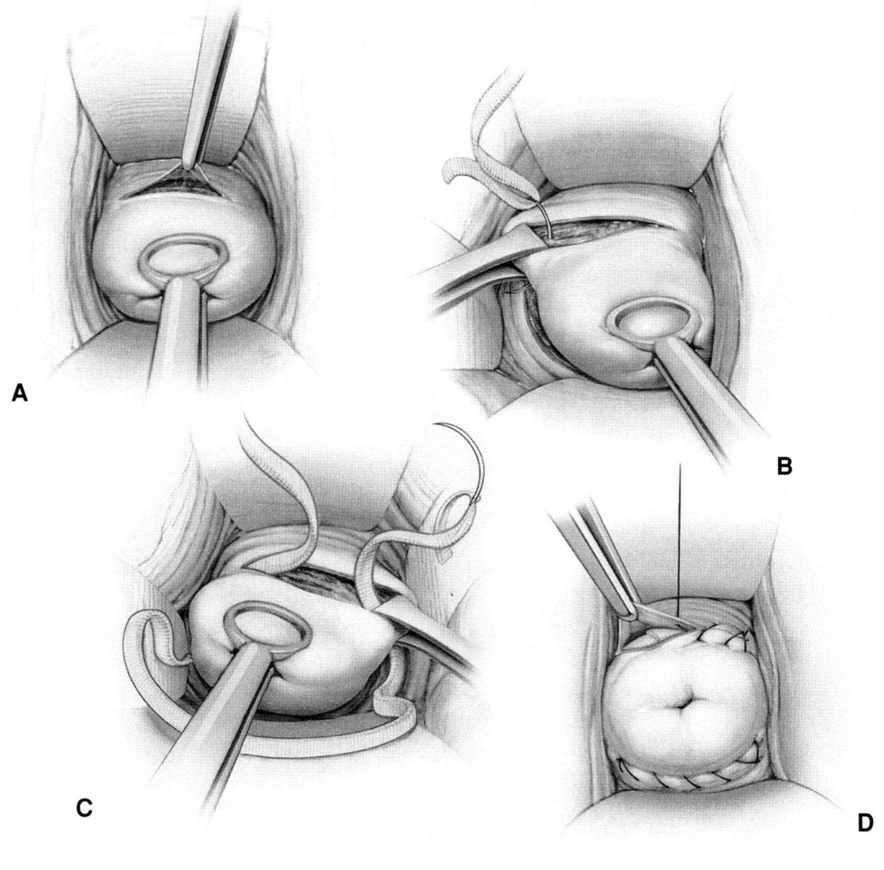

FIGURE 18-6 Modified Shirodkar cerclage for incompetent cervix. **A.** A transverse incision is made in the mucosa overlying the anterior cervix, and the bladder is pushed cephalad. **B.** A 5-mm Mersilene tape on a swaged-on or Mayo needle is passed anteriorly to posteriorly. **C.** The tape is then directed posteriorly to anteriorly on the other side of the cervix. Allis clamps are placed so as to bunch the cervical tissue. This diminishes the distance that the needle must travel submucosally and aids tape placement. **D.** The tape is snugly tied anteriorly, after ensuring that all slack has been taken up. The cervical mucosa is then closed with continuous stitches of chromic suture to bury the anterior knot.

women with bulging membranes, transabdominal amnionic fluid aspiration may be helpful. If this is done, bacterial cultures of the fluid should be obtained.

Transabdominal cerclage with the suture placed at the uterine isthmus can be used if there are severe cervical anatomical defects or if there have been prior transvaginal cerclage failures (Cammarano, 1995; Gibb, 1995). Zaveri and associates (2002) reviewed 14 observational studies in which a prior transvaginal cerclage had failed to prevent preterm delivery. The risk of perinatal death or delivery before 24 weeks was only slightly lower following transabdominal cerclage compared with the risk following repeat transvaginal cerclage—6 versus 13 percent, respectively. Importantly, 3 percent of women who underwent transabdominal cerclage had serious operative complications, whereas there were none in women in the transvaginal group. Whittle and coworkers (2009) described 31 women in whom transabdominal cervicoisthmic cerclage was done laparoscopically between 10 and 16 weeks. The procedure was converted to laparotomy in 25 percent, and there were four failures due to chorioamnionitis. Overall, fetal survival rate approximated 80 percent.

Complications. Principal complications of cerclage are membrane rupture, preterm labor, hemorrhage, infection, or combinations thereof. All are uncommon with prophylactic cerclage. In the multicenter study by Owen and colleagues (2009), of 138 procedures, there was one instance each of ruptured membranes and bleeding. In the trial by MacNaughton and associates (1993), membrane rupture complicated only 1 of more than 600 procedures done before 19 weeks. Thomason and coworkers (1982) found that perioperative antimicrobial prophylaxis failed to prevent most infection, and tocolytics failed to arrest most labor. In our view, clinical infection mandates immediate removal of the suture with labor induced or augmented. Similarly, with imminent abortion or delivery, the suture should be removed at once because uterine contractions can tear through the uterus or cervix.

Membrane rupture during suture placement or within the first 48 hours following surgery is considered by some to be an indication for cerclage removal because of the likelihood of serious fetal or maternal infection (Kuhn, 1977). That said, the range of management options includes observation, removal of the cerclage and observation, or removal of the cerclage and labor induction (Barth, 1995; O'Connor, 1999).

If subsequent cervical thinning is detected by sonographic assessment, then some consider a *reinforcement cerclage*. In one retrospective study, reinforcing cerclage sutures placed later did not significantly prolong pregnancy (Woo, 2013).

INDUCED ABORTION

The term induced abortion is defined as the medical or surgical termination of pregnancy before the time of fetal viability. Definitions to describe its frequency include: (1) *abortion ratio*—the number of abortions per 1000 live births, and (2) *abortion rate*—the number of abortions per 1000 women aged 15 to 44 years.

In the United States, abortion statistics most likely are underreported. This probably is because clinics inconsistently give statistics for medically induced abortions. For example, the Guttmacher Institute (2011) found that 1.2 million procedures were performed annually from 2005 through 2008. But for 2010, there were only about 765,650 elective abortions reported to the Centers for Disease Control and Prevention (Pazol, 2013). The abortion ratio was 227 per 1000 live births and the abortion rate was 15.1 per 1000 women aged 15 to 44 years. For the same year, women aged 20 to 29 years accounted for 58 percent of abortions and had the highest abortion rate. Black women had an abortion ratio of 477 per 1000 live births, white women had 140 per 1000, and Hispanic women had 195 per 1000. In 2009, 64 percent of abortions were done ≤ 8 weeks; 92 percent ≤ 13 weeks; 7 percent at 14 to 20 weeks; and only 1.3 percent were performed at ≥ 21 weeks. Global statistics for abortion rates are reported by the World Health Organization. According to its latest report, approximately 1 in 5 pregnancies were aborted worldwide in 2008 (Sedgh, 2012). Sadly, almost half of these abortions were considered unsafe.

Classification

Therapeutic Abortion

There are several diverse medical and surgical disorders that are indications for termination of pregnancy. Examples include persistent cardiac decompensation, especially with fixed pulmonary hypertension; advanced hypertensive vascular disease or diabetes; and malignancy. In cases of rape or incest, most consider termination reasonable. The most common indication currently is to prevent birth of a fetus with a significant anatomical, metabolic, or mental deformity. The seriousness of fetal deformities is wide ranging and usually defies social, legal, or political classification.

Elective or Voluntary Abortion

The interruption of pregnancy before viability at the request of the woman, but not for medical reasons, is usually termed *elective* or *voluntary abortion*. Regardless of terminology, these are stigmatized in this country (Harris, 2012). Most abortions done today are elective, and thus, it is one of the most commonly performed medical procedures. The pregnancy-associated mortality rate is 14-fold greater than the abortion-related mortality rate—8 versus 0.6 deaths per 100,000 (Raymond, 2012). From the Guttmacher Institute, Jones and Kavanaugh (2011) estimate that a third of American women will have at least one elective abortion by age 45. The Executive Board of the American College of Obstetricians and Gynecologists (2013d) supports the legal right of women to obtain an abortion prior to fetal viability and considers this a medical matter between a woman and her physician.

Abortion in the United States

The legality of elective abortion was established by the United States Supreme Court in the case of *Roe v. Wade*. The Court defined the extent to which states might regulate abortion and ruled that first-trimester procedures must be left to the medical judgment of the physician. After this, the State could regulate abortion procedures in ways reasonably related to maternal health. Finally, subsequent to viability, the State could promote its interest in the potential of human life and regulate and even proscribe abortion, except for the preservation of the life or health of the mother.

Other legislation soon followed. The 1976 Hyde Amendment forbids use of federal funds to provide abortion services except in case of rape, incest, or life-threatening circumstances. The Supreme Court in 1992 reviewed *Planned Parenthood v. Casey* and upheld the fundamental right to abortion, but established that regulations before viability are constitutional as long as they do not impose an "undue burden" on the woman. Subsequently, many states passed legislation that imposes counseling requirements, waiting periods, parental consent or notification for minors, facility requirements, and funding restrictions. One major choice-limiting decision was the 2007 Supreme Court decision that reviewed *Gonzales v. Carhart* and upheld the 2003 Partial-Birth Abortion Ban Act. This was problematic because there is no medically approved definition of partial-birth abortion according to the American College of Obstetricians and Gynecologists (2011a). According to the Guttmacher Institute, 41 states set new limits on abortion during 2011 and 2012 (Tanner, 2012).

Residency Training in Abortion Techniques

Because of its inherent controversial aspects, abortion training for residents has been both championed and assailed. The American College of Obstetricians and Gynecologists (2009a) supports abortion training, and the Accreditation Council for Graduate Medical Education mandated in 1996 that Obstetrics and Gynecology residency education must include access to experience with induced abortion. The Kenneth J. Ryan Residency Training Program was established in 1999 at the University of California at San Francisco to work with residency programs to improve training in abortion and family planning. By 2013, 59 Ryan programs had been started in the United States and in Canada (Heartwell, 2013). These programs provide comprehensive didactics and evidence-based, opt-out clinical training in all pregnancy-termination methods and contraceptive methodology.

Other programs are less codified, but teach residents technical aspects through their management of early incomplete and missed abortions as well as pregnancy interruption for fetal death, severe fetal anomalies, and life-threatening medical or surgical disorders. Freedman and colleagues (2010) rightfully emphasize that considerations for abortion training should include social, moral, and ethical aspects.

Programs have been designed for postresidency training in abortion and contraceptive techniques. Formal fellowships in Family Planning are 2-year postgraduate programs that, by 2010, were located in 22 departments of obstetrics and gynecology at academic centers across the country. Training includes experience with high-level research and with all methods of pregnancy prevention and termination.

Abortion Providers

The American College of Obstetricians and Gynecologists (2013d) respects the need and responsibility of health-care providers to determine their individual positions on induced abortion. It also emphasizes the need to provide standard-of-care counseling and timely referral if providers have individual beliefs that preclude pregnancy termination. From a mail survey of 1800 obstetrician-gynecologists, 97 percent had encountered women seeking an abortion, but only 14 percent performed them (Stulberg, 2011). Still, most practitioners help women find an abortion provider (Harris, 2011). And at least for midtrimester procedures, maternal-fetal medicine specialists provide some services (Kerns, 2012). In any event, it is imperative that any physician who cares for women must be familiar with various abortion techniques so that complications can be managed or referrals made for suitable care (Steinauer, 2005a,b).

Counseling before Elective Abortion

There are three basic choices available to a woman considering an abortion: (1) continued pregnancy with its risks and parental responsibilities; (2) continued pregnancy with arranged adoption; or (3) termination of pregnancy with its risks. Knowledgeable and compassionate counselors should objectively describe and provide information regarding these choices so that a woman or couple can make an informed decision (Baker, 2009; Templeton, 2011).

TECHNIQUES FOR ABORTION

In the absence of serious maternal medical disorders, abortion procedures do not require hospitalization. With outpatient abortion, capabilities for cardiopulmonary resuscitation and for immediate transfer to a hospital must be available.

First-trimester abortions can be performed either medically or surgically by several methods that are listed in Table 18-7. Results

TABLE 18-7. Some Techniques Used for First-Trimester Abortion[a]

Surgical
Dilatation and curettage
Vacuum aspiration
Menstrual aspiration
Medical
Prostaglandins E_2, $F_{2\alpha}$, E_1, and analogues
Vaginal insertion
Parenteral injection
Oral ingestion
Sublingual
Antiprogesterones—RU-486 (mifepristone) and epostane
Methotrexate—intramuscular and oral
Various combinations of the above

[a]All procedures are aided by pretreatment using hygroscopic cervical dilators.

TABLE 18-8. Comparisons of Some Advantages and Drawbacks to Medical versus Surgical Abortion

Factor	Medical	Surgical
Invasive	Usually no	Yes
Pain	More	Less
Vaginal bleeding	Prolonged, unpredictable	Light, predictable
Incomplete abortion	More common	Uncommon
Failure rate	2–5%	1%
Severe bleeding	0.1%	0.1%
Infection rate	Low	Low
Anesthesia	Usually none	Yes
Time involved	Multiple visits, follow-up exam	Usually one visit, no follow-up exam

are comparable with methods for spontaneous miscarriages discussed previously on page 357 and shown in Table 18-3. They have a high success rate—95 percent with medical and 99 percent with surgical techniques. Further comparison of medical and surgical methods is shown in Table 18-8. Medical therapy has more drawbacks in that it is more time consuming; it has an unpredictable outcome—extending for days up to a few weeks; and bleeding is usually heavier and unpredictable (Niinimäki, 2009; Robson, 2009). Likely for these reasons, only 10 percent of abortions in the United States are managed using medical methods (Templeton, 2011).

Cervical Preparation

There are several methods that will soften and slowly dilate the cervix to minimize trauma from mechanical dilatation (Newmann, 2014). A Cochrane review confirmed that hygroscopic dilators and cervical ripening medications had similar efficacy in decreasing the length of first-trimester procedures (Kapp, 2010).

Of these, hygroscopic dilators are devices that draw water from cervical tissues and expand to gradually dilate the cervix. One type is derived from various species of *Laminaria* algae that are harvested from the ocean floor (Figs. 18-7 and 18-8). Another is *Dilapan-S,* which is composed of an acrylic-based gel.

Schneider and associates (1991) described 21 cases in which women who had a hygroscopic dilator placed changed their minds. Of 17 women who chose to continue their pregnancy, there were 14 term deliveries, two preterm deliveries, and one miscarriage 2 weeks later. None suffered infection-related morbidity, including three untreated women with cervical cultures positive for *Chlamydia trachomatis.*

In contrast to these devices, there are medications used for cervical preparations. The most common is misoprostol (Cytotec), which is used off-label, and patients are counseled accordingly (Tang, 2013). The dose is 400 to 600 μg administered orally, sublingually, or placed into the posterior vaginal fornix. In a multicenter randomized trial, Meirik and coworkers (2012) enrolled nearly 4900 women undergoing an elective first-trimester abortion. Half were given two 200-μg tablets orally 3 hours preprocedure, and the other group was given placebo. Marginal benefits ascribed to misoprostol included easier cervical dilatation and a lower composite complication rate. Another effective cervical-ripening agent is the progesterone antagonist *mifepristone* (Mifeprex). With this, 200 to 600 μg is given orally. Other options include formulations of *prostaglandins* E_2 and F_{2a}, which have unpleasant side effects and are usually reserved as second-line drugs (Kapp, 2010).

Surgical Abortion

Surgical pregnancy termination includes a transvaginal approach through an appropriately dilated cervix or, rarely, laparotomy with either hysterotomy or hysterectomy. With transvaginal

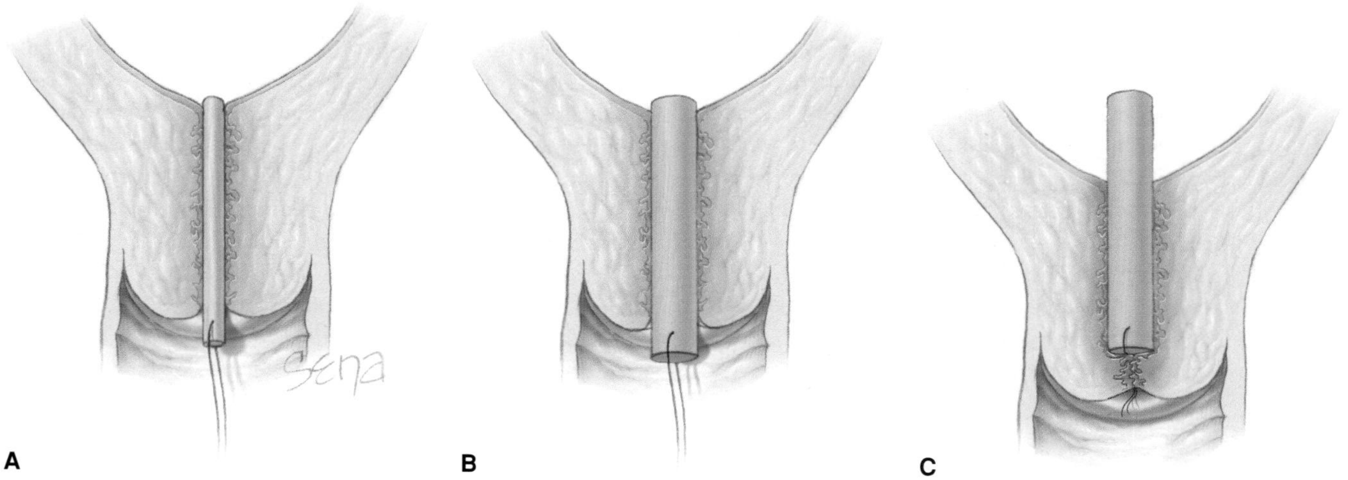

FIGURE 18-7 Insertion of laminaria before dilatation and curettage. **A.** Laminaria immediately after being appropriately placed with its upper end just through the internal os. **B.** Several hours later the laminaria is now swollen, and the cervix is dilated and softened. **C.** Laminaria inserted too far through the internal os; the laminaria may rupture the membranes.

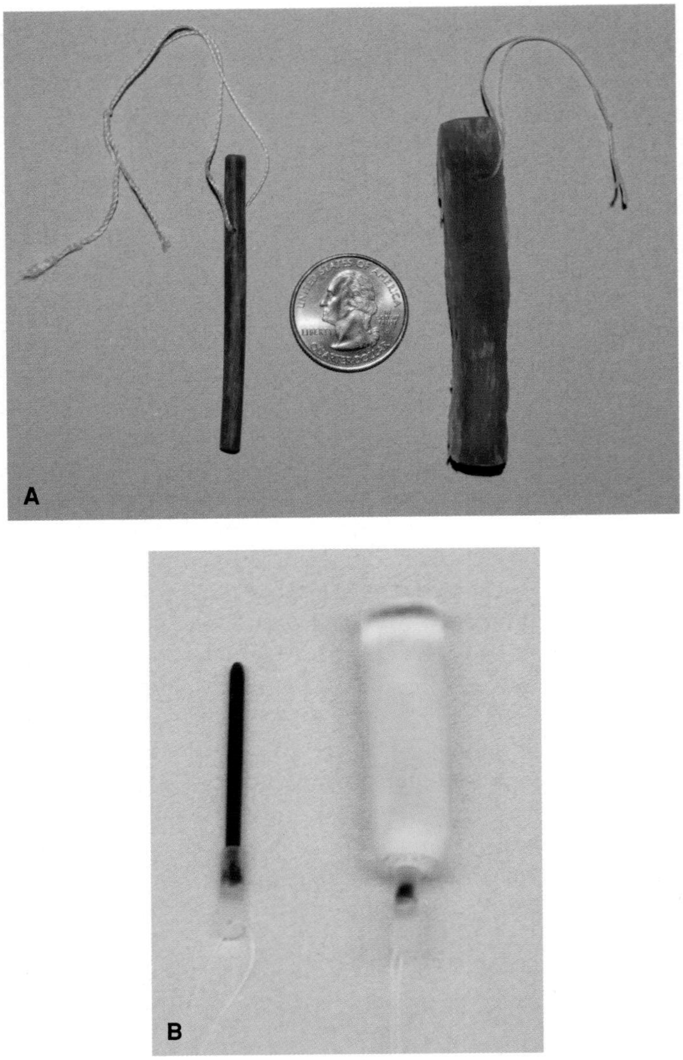

FIGURE 18-8 Hygroscopic dilators. With each type, the dry unit (*left*) expands exponentially when exposed to water (*right*) as in the endocervical canal. **A.** Laminaria. **B.** Dilapan-S.

evacuation, preoperative cervical ripening is favored and is typically associated with less pain, a technically easier procedure, and shorter operating times (Kapp, 2010). Curettage usually requires intravenously or orally administered sedatives or analgesics, and some also use paracervical blockade with lidocaine (Allen, 2009; Cansino, 2009; Renner, 2012). Perioperative antibiotic prophylaxis is described on page 357. No recommendations specifically address venous thromboembolism (VTE) prophylaxis for curettage in low-risk pregnant patients. The American College of Chest Physicians (Bates, 2012) recommends only early ambulation for cesarean delivery in those without risk factors, and at our hospital, we apply this also to less invasive curettage.

Dilatation and Curettage (D&C)

Transcervical approaches to surgical abortion require first dilating the cervix and then evacuating the pregnancy by mechanically scraping out the contents—sharp curettage, by suctioning out the contents—suction curettage, or both. Vacuum aspiration, the most common form of suction curettage, requires a rigid cannula attached to an electric-powered vacuum source or to a handheld syringe for its vacuum source (Goldberg, 2004; MacIsaac, 2000; Masch, 2005).

Curettage—either sharp or suction—is recommended for gestations ≤ 15 weeks. Complication rates increase after the first trimester. Perforation, cervical laceration, hemorrhage, incomplete removal of the fetus or placenta, and postoperative infections are among these. Niinimäki and associates (2009) reported results from more than 20,000 Finnish women undergoing surgical termination before 63 days. The 5.6-percent complication rate was made up equally of hemorrhage, incomplete abortion, and infection. A second curettage procedure was necessary in 2 percent. As further discussed on page 368, there was a 20-percent complication rate in the more than 22,000 women undergoing a medical termination.

Technique. After bimanual examination is performed to determine uterine size and orientation, a speculum is inserted, and the cervix is swabbed with povidone-iodine or equivalent solution. The anterior cervical lip is grasped with a toothed tenaculum. The cervix, vagina, and uterus are richly supplied by nerves of Frankenhäuser plexus, which lies within connective tissue lateral to the uterosacral and cardinal ligaments. Thus, a paracervical block is effective to relieve pain (Renner, 2012). A local anesthetic, such as 5 mL of 1- or 2-percent lidocaine, is most effective if placed immediately lateral to the insertion of the uterosacral ligaments into the uterus at 4 and 8 o'clock. An intracervical block with 5-mL aliquots of 1-percent lidocaine injected at 12, 3, 6, and 9 o'clock was reported to be equally effective (Mankowski, 2009). Dilute vasopressin may be added to the local anesthetic to decrease blood loss (Keder, 2003).

Uterine sounding measures the depth and inclination of the cavity before other instrument insertion. If required, the cervix is further dilated with Hegar, Hank, or Pratt dilators until a suction cannula of the appropriate diameter can be inserted. Small cannulas carry the risk of leaving retained intrauterine tissue postoperatively, whereas large cannulas risk cervical injury and more discomfort. The fourth and fifth fingers of the hand introducing the dilator should rest on the perineum and buttocks as the dilator is pushed through the internal os (Fig. 18-9). This technique minimizes forceful dilatation and provides a safeguard against uterine perforation. The suction cannula is moved toward the fundus and then back toward the os and is turned circumferentially to cover the entire surface of the uterine cavity (Fig. 18-10). When no more tissue is aspirated, a gentle sharp curettage should follow to remove any remaining placental or fetal fragments (Fig. 18-11).

Because uterine perforation usually occurs with insertion of any of these instruments, manipulations should be carried out with the thumb and forefinger only (see Fig. 18-9). For pregnancies beyond 16 weeks, the fetus is extracted, usually in parts, using Sopher forceps and other destructive instruments. Inherent risks include uterine perforation, cervical laceration, and uterine bleeding due to the larger fetus and placenta and to the thinner uterine walls. Morbidity can be minimized if careful attention is paid to performing the steps outlined above.

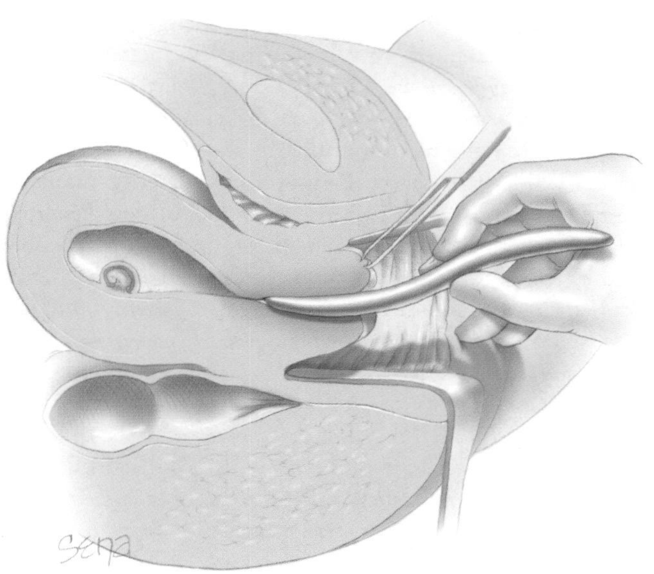

FIGURE 18-9 Dilatation of cervix with a Hegar dilator. Note that the fourth and fifth fingers rest against the perineum and buttocks, lateral to the vagina. This maneuver is an important safety measure because if the cervix relaxes abruptly, these fingers prevent a sudden and uncontrolled thrust of the dilator, a common cause of uterine perforation.

Complications. The incidence of uterine perforation with elective abortion is variable, and determinants include clinician skill and uterine position. Perforation is more common with a retroverted uterus and is usually recognized when the instrument passes without resistance deep into the pelvis. Observation is usually sufficient if the uterine perforation is small, as when produced by a uterine sound or narrow dilator. Although perforations through old cesarean incision or myomectomy scars are potentially possible, Chen and colleagues (2008) reported no perforations through such scars in 78 women undergoing medical or surgical abortion.

If some instruments—especially suction and sharp curettes—pass through a uterine defect and into the peritoneal cavity, considerable intraabdominal damage can ensue (Keegan, 1982). In these women, laparotomy or laparoscopy to examine the abdominal contents is often the safest course of action. Bowel injury can cause severe peritonitis and sepsis (Kambiss, 2000). A rare complication of curettage with more advanced pregnancies is sudden, severe consumptive coagulopathy.

If prophylactic antimicrobials are given, pelvic sepsis is decreased by 40 to 90 percent and depends on whether the procedure is surgical or medical. Most infections that do develop respond readily to appropriate antimicrobial treatment (Chap. 37, p. 685). Rarely, infections such as bacterial endocarditis will develop, but they can be fatal (Jeppson, 2008). Uncommon long-term complications of curettage include cervical insufficiency or uterine synechiae.

Dilatation and Evacuation (D&E)

Beginning at 16 weeks, fetal size and structure dictate use of this technique. Wide mechanical cervical dilatation, achieved with metal or hygroscopic dilators, precedes mechanical destruction

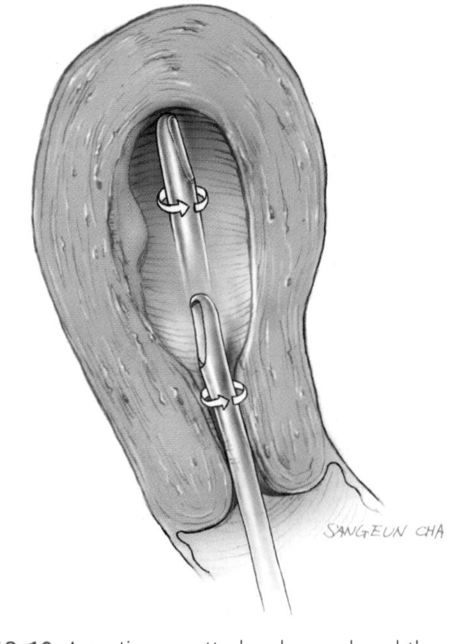

FIGURE 18-10 A suction curette has been placed through the cervix into the uterus. The figure shows the rotary motion used to aspirate the contents. (From Word, 2012, with permission.)

and evacuation of fetal parts. With complete removal of the fetus, a large-bore vacuum curette is used to remove the placenta and remaining tissue. This is better accomplished using intraoperative sonographic imaging.

Dilatation and Extraction (D&X)

This is similar to dilatation and evacuation except that a suction cannula is used to evacuate the intracranial contents after

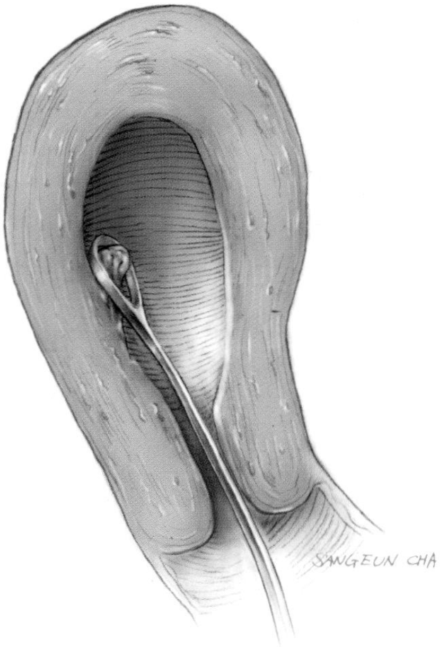

FIGURE 18-11 A sharp curette is advanced into the uterine cavity while the instrument is held with the thumb and forefinger as shown in Figure 18-9. In the movement of the curette, only the strength of these two fingers should be used. (From Word, 2012, with permission.)

delivery of the fetal body through the dilated cervix. This aids extraction and minimizes uterine or cervical injury from instruments or fetal bones. In political parlance, this procedure has been termed *partial birth abortion*.

Menstrual Aspiration

This is done within 1 to 3 weeks after a missed menstrual period and with a positive serum or urine pregnancy test result. It is performed with a flexible 5- or 6-mm Karman cannula that is attached to a syringe. This procedure has been referred to as *menstrual extraction, menstrual induction, instant period, traumatic abortion, and mini-abortion*. A distinct drawback is that because the pregnancy is so small, an implanted zygote can be missed by the curette, or an ectopic pregnancy can be unrecognized. To identify placenta in the aspirate, MacIsaac and Darney (2000) recommend that the syringe contents be rinsed in a strainer to remove blood, then placed in a clear plastic container with saline and examined with back lighting. Placental tissue macroscopically appears soft, fluffy, and feathery. A magnifying lens, colposcope, or microscope also can improve visualization. Despite the possibility of missing the products, Paul and coworkers (2002) reported a 98-percent success rate with more than 1000 such procedures.

Manual Vacuum Aspiration

This procedure is similar to menstrual aspiration but is used for early pregnancy failures or elective termination up to 12 weeks. Some recommend that pregnancy terminations done in the office with this method be limited to ≤ 10 weeks because blood loss rises sharply between 10 and 12 weeks (Masch, 2005; Westfall, 1998). For pregnancies ≤ 8 weeks, preprocedure cervical ripening is usually not necessary. After this time, some recommend that osmotic dilators be placed the day prior or misoprostol given 2 to 4 hours before the procedure. Paracervical blockade with or without sedation is used. The technique employs a hand-operated 60-mL syringe and cannula. A vacuum is created in the syringe attached to the cannula, which is inserted transcervically into the uterus. The vacuum produces up to 60 mm Hg suction. Complications are similar to other surgical methods (Goldberg, 2004).

Hysterotomy or Hysterectomy

In some women with second-trimester pregnancies who desire sterilization, hysterotomy with tubal ligation is reasonable. If there is significant uterine disease, then hysterectomy may provide ideal treatment. In some cases of a failed second-trimester medical induction, either of these may be considered.

Medical Abortion

According to the American College of Obstetricians and Gynecologists (2011c), outpatient medical abortion is an acceptable alternative to surgical pregnancy termination in appropriately selected pregnant women less than 49 days' menstrual age. After this time, available data—albeit less robust—support surgical abortion as preferable. Throughout history, many natural substances have been given for alleged abortifacient effects. In many of these, serious illness and even death have resulted. Currently, there are only three medications for early medical abortion that have been widely studied. These are used either alone or in combination and include: (1) the antiprogestin *mifepristone,* (2) the antimetabolite *methotrexate,* and (3) the prostaglandin *misoprostol*. Mifepristone and methotrexate increase uterine contractility by reversing progesterone-induced inhibition, whereas misoprostol directly stimulates the myometrium. Clark and associates (2006) have reported that mifepristone causes cervical collagen degradation, possibly from increased expression of matrix metalloprotease-2 (MMP-2). *Methotrexate and misoprostol are both teratogens. Thus there must be a commitment to completing the abortion once these drugs have been given.*

With these three agents, a number of dosing schemes have been proven effective, and some are shown in Table 18-9. *For all three, misoprostol is given initially*. This is either used alone or given with methotrexate or mifepristone. In each instance, it is followed by further but variable misoprostol doses. As shown in Table 18-3, any regimen used for "early pregnancy loss" is likely to be successful for elective pregnancy interruption. For elective termination at ≤ 63 days' gestation, randomized trials by von Hertzen (2009, 2010) and Winikoff (2008) and their colleagues showed 92- to 96-percent efficacy when one of the mifepristone/misoprostol regimens was used. Similar results were reported from 10 large urban Planned Parenthood clinics (Fjerstad, 2009a). In this latter study, buccal misoprostol-oral mifepristone regimens were 87-to 98-percent successful for abortion induction with pregnancies < 10 weeks' gestation, and this rate diminished with advancing gestations. In another study of 122 women at 9 to 12 weeks' gestation, the success rate was approximately 80 percent (Dalenda, 2010).

Contraindications

In many cases, contraindications to medical abortion evolved from exclusion criteria that were used in initial clinical trials. Thus, some are relative contraindications: in situ intrauterine device; severe anemia, coagulopathy, or anticoagulant use; and significant medical conditions such as active liver disease, cardiovascular disease, or uncontrolled seizure disorders. Because misoprostol diminishes glucocorticoid activity, women with disorders requiring glucocorticoid therapy are usually excluded (American College of Obstetricians and Gynecologists, 2009b). In women with renal insufficiency, the methotrexate dose should be modified and given with caution, or preferably, another regimen should be chosen (Kelly, 2006).

Administration

With the mifepristone/misoprostol regimen, mifepristone treatment is followed by misoprostol given at that same time or up to 72 hours later as shown in Table 18-9. Some prefer that misoprostol be administered on site, after which the woman typically remains for 4 hours. Symptoms are common within 3 hours and include lower abdominal pain, vomiting, diarrhea, fever, and chills or shivering. In the first few hours after misoprostol is given, if the pregnancy appears to have been expelled, a pelvic examination is done to confirm this. If not and if the pregnancy is still intact, the woman is discharged and appointed to return in 1 to 2 weeks. Some choose to repeat a prostaglandin dose (Dickinson, 2014). Conversely, if there

TABLE 18-9. Regimens for Medical Termination of Early Pregnancy

Mifepristone/Misoprostol
[a]Mifepristone, 100–600 mg orally followed by:
[b]Misoprostol, 200–600 μg orally or 400–800 μg vaginally, buccally, or sublingually given immediately or up to 72 hours
Methotrexate/Misoprostol
[c]Methotrexate, 50 mg/m^2 BSA intramuscularly or orally followed by:
[d]Misoprostol, 800 μg vaginally in 3–7 days. Repeat if needed 1 week after methotrexate initially given
Misoprostol alone
[e]800 μg vaginally or sublingually, repeated for up to three doses

[a]Doses of 200 versus 600 mg similarly effective.
[b]Oral route may be less effective and have more nausea and diarrhea. Sublingual route has more side effects than vaginal route. Shorter intervals (6 hours) with misoprostol may be less effective when given > 36 hours.
[c]Efficacy similar for routes of administration.
[d]Similar efficacy when given on day 3 versus day 5.
[e]Intervals 3–12 hours given vaginally; 3–4 hours given sublingually.
BSA = body surface area.
Data from the American College of Obstetricians and Gynecologists, 2011c, 2013e; Borgatta, 2001; Coyaji, 2007; Creinin, 2001, 2007; Fekih, 2010; Fjerstad, 2009a; Guest, 2007; Hamoda, 2005; Honkanen, 2004; Jain, 2002; Pymar, 2001; Raghavan, 2009; Schaff, 2000; Shannon, 2006; von Hertzen, 2003, 2007, 2009, 2010; Winikoff, 2008.

is an incomplete abortion on clinical or sonographic evaluation, then suction curettage usually is recommended. Other complications are hemorrhage and infection (Niinimäki, 2009; von Hertzen, 2010).

With the methotrexate regimens, misoprostol is given 3 to 7 days later, and women are seen again at least 24 hours after misoprostol administration. They are next seen approximately 7 days after methotrexate is given, and sonographic examination is performed. If an intact pregnancy is seen, then another dose of misoprostol is given. Afterward, the woman is seen again in 1 week if fetal cardiac activity is present or in 4 weeks if there is no heart motion. If abortion has not occurred by the second visit, it is usually completed by suction curettage.

Complications

In a 2-year review of more than 233,000 medical abortions performed at Planned Parenthood affiliates, there were 1530 (0.65 percent) significant adverse events. Most of these were ongoing pregnancy (Cleland, 2013). Bleeding and cramping with medical termination can be significantly worse than menstrual cramps. Thus adequate analgesia, usually including a narcotic, is provided. The American College of Obstetricians and Gynecologists (2011c) recommends that if there is enough blood to soak two or more pads per hour for at least 2 hours, the woman is instructed to contact her provider to determine whether she needs to be seen.

Unnecessary surgical intervention in women undergoing medical abortion can be avoided if properly indicated follow-up sonographic results are interpreted appropriately. Specifically, if no gestational sac is seen and there is no heavy bleeding, then intervention is unnecessary. This is true even when, as is common, the uterus contains sonographically evident debris. Another study reported that a multilayered sonographic pattern indicated a successful abortion (Tzeng, 2013). Clark and coworkers (2010) provided data that routine postabortal sonographic examination is unnecessary. They instead recommend assessment of the clinical course along with bimanual pelvic examination. Follow-up serum β-hCG levels have shown promise in preliminary investigations (Dayananda, 2013).

Midtrimester Abortion

There have long been invasive means of midtrimester surgical abortion as shown in Table 18-10 and discussed on page 367.

TABLE 18-10. Some Techniques Used for Midtrimester Abortion[a]

Surgical
Dilatation and curettage (D&C)
Dilatation and evacuation (D&E)
Dilatation and extraction (D&X)
Laparotomy
Hysterotomy
Hysterectomy
Medical
Intravenous oxytocin
Intraamnionic hyperosmotic fluid
20-percent saline
30-percent urea
Prostaglandins E_2, $F_{2\alpha}$, E_1
Intraamnionic injection
Extraovular injection
Vaginal insertion
Parenteral injection
Oral ingestion

[a]All procedures are aided by pretreatment using hygroscopic cervical dilators.

TABLE 18-11. Concentrated Oxytocin Protocol for Midtrimester Abortion

50 units oxytocin in 500 mL of normal saline infused over 3 hr; then 1-hr diuresis (no oxytocin)
100 units oxytocin in 500 mL of normal saline infused over 3 hr; then 1-hr diuresis (no oxytocin)
150 units oxytocin in 500 mL of normal saline infused over 3 hr; then 1-hr diuresis (no oxytocin)
200 units oxytocin in 500 mL of normal saline infused over 3 hr; then 1-hr diuresis (no oxytocin)
250 units oxytocin in 500 mL of normal saline infused over 3 hr; then 1-hr diuresis (no oxytocin)
300 units oxytocin in 500 mL of normal saline infused over 3 hr; then 1-hr diuresis (no oxytocin)

Modified from Ramsey, 2000.

In the past 25 years, medical methods that safely and effectively accomplish midtrimester abortion have also evolved considerably. Risks versus benefits of medical versus surgical midtrimester termination are similar to those shown in Table 18-8 (Bryant, 2011; Edlow, 2011; Kelly, 2010; Mentula, 2011). Principal among noninvasive methods is high-dose intravenous oxytocin. Others include a number of prostaglandin analogues that can be given orally, vaginally, or parenterally. Regardless of method, hygroscopic dilators as shown in Figure 18-7 and 18-8 shorten the duration (Goldberg, 2005).

Oxytocin

Given alone in high doses, oxytocin will result in second-trimester abortion in 80 to 90 percent of cases. Oxytocin is delivered in an isotonic solution. Thus, by avoiding excessive administration of dilute intravenous solutions, hyponatremia or water intoxication is rare. One regimen is shown in Table 18-11.

Prostaglandins E_2 (PGE_2) and E_1 (PGE_1)

A 20-mg prostaglandin E_2 suppository placed in the posterior vaginal fornix is an effective means of inducing a second-trimester abortion. It is not more effective than high-dose oxytocin, and it causes more frequent side effects such as nausea, vomiting, fever, and diarrhea (Owen, 1992). If PGE_2 is used, simultaneous administration of an antiemetic such as metoclopramide, an antipyretic such as acetaminophen, and an antidiarrheal such as diphenoxylate/atropine will help prevent or treat symptoms.

Misoprostol (Cytotec) used alone is also a simple and effective method for second-trimester pregnancy termination. In one randomized trial, a 600-μg misoprostol dose given vaginally was followed by 400 μg every 4 hours (Ramsey, 2004). This regimen effected abortion significantly faster than concentrated oxytocin plus PGE_2—median time to abortion 12 versus 17 hours, respectively. By 24 hours, 95 percent of women given misoprostol had aborted compared with 85 percent in the oxytocin-PGE_2 cohort. Two percent of women in the misoprostol group required curettage for retained placenta compared with 15 percent in the oxytocin-PGE_2 group. In another study, 200 mg mifepristone given orally 1 day before misoprostol reduced the median time-to-expulsion from 10.6 to 8.1 hours (Ngoc, 2011).

Outcomes of medically induced second-trimester abortion in women with a prior cesarean delivery were at first discouraging, but recent evidence is less pessimistic. In two systematic reviews, the risk of uterine rupture in such women given misoprostol was reported to be 0.3 to 0.4 percent (Berghella, 2009; Goyal, 2009).

CONSEQUENCES OF ELECTIVE ABORTION

Maternal Mortality

Because they are common, regulated, and reportable, most abortion statistics are for elective procedures. Even so, abortion-related deaths are likely underreported (Horon, 2005). With this caveat in mind, legally induced abortion, performed by trained gynecologists during the first 2 months of pregnancy, has a mortality rate of less than 1 per 100,000 procedures (Pazol, 2011). In a report from Finland comprising nearly 43,000 abortions performed before 63 days, only one procedure-related death was documented (Niinimaki, 2009). Early abortions are even safer, and the relative mortality risk of abortion approximately doubles for each 2 weeks after 8 weeks' gestation. The Centers for Disease Control and Prevention identified 12 abortion-related deaths in the United States in 2008 (Pazol, 2012). As emphasized by Raymond and Grimes (2012), mortality rates are 14-fold greater for pregnancies that are continued.

Health and Future Pregnancies

Data relating abortion to overall maternal health and to subsequent pregnancy outcome are limited. From studies, there is no evidence for excessive mental disorders (Munk-Olsen, 2011; Steinberg, 2014). There are few data regarding subsequent reproductive health, although the rates of infertility or ectopic pregnancy are not increased. There may be exceptions if there are postabortal infections, especially those caused by chlamydiae. Also, other data suggest that some adverse pregnancy outcomes are more common in women who have had an induced abortion (Maconochie, 2007). Specifically, several studies note an approximate 1.5-fold increased incidence of preterm delivery—22 to 32 weeks (Hardy, 2013; Moreau, 2005; Swingle, 2009). Multiple sharp curettage procedures may increase the subsequent risk of placenta previa, whereas vacuum aspiration procedures likely do not (Johnson, 2003).

It appears that subsequent pregnancy outcomes are similar regardless of whether a prior induced abortion was completed medically or surgically. In a report of 30,349 procedures from the Danish Abortion Registry, there were 16,883 women who had a subsequent pregnancy (Virk, 2007). Rates of ectopic pregnancy, miscarriage, and preterm delivery were not significantly different in those with prior surgical abortion or previous medical termination.

CONTRACEPTION FOLLOWING MISCARRIAGE OR ABORTION

Ovulation may resume as early as 2 weeks after an early pregnancy termination. Lahteenmaki and Luukkainen (1978) detected surges of luteinizing hormone (LH) 16 to 22 days after abortion in 15 of 18 women studied. Plasma progesterone levels, which had plummeted after the abortion, increased soon after LH surges. These hormonal events agree with histological changes observed in endometrial biopsies by Boyd and Holmstrom (1972).

Thus, it is important that unless another pregnancy is desired right away, effective contraception should be initiated very soon after abortion. There is no reason to delay this, and an intrauterine device can be inserted after the procedure is completed (Bednarek, 2011; Shimoni, 2011). Alternatively, any of the various forms of hormonal contraception can be initiated at this time (Madden, 2009; Reeves, 2007). For women who desire another pregnancy, sooner may be preferable to later. Specifically, Love and colleagues (2010) analyzed the next pregnancy outcomes in nearly 31,000 women following miscarriage and found that conceptions within 6 months after miscarriage had better pregnancy outcomes compared with pregnancies conceived after 6 months.

REFERENCES

Abbassi-Ghanavati M, Casey BM, Spong CY, et al: Pregnancy outcomes in women with thyroid peroxidase antibodies. Obstet Gynecol 116:381, 2010

Albrechtsen S, Rasmussen S, Thoresen S, et al: Pregnancy outcome in women before and after cervical conization: population based cohort study. BMJ 18:337, 2008

Al Arfaj AS, Khalil N: Pregnancy outcome in 396 pregnancies in patients with SLE in Saudi Arabia. Lupus 19:1665, 2010

Al-Inany H: Intrauterine adhesions. An update. Acta Obstet Gynecol Scand 80:986, 2001

Allanson B, Jennings B, Jacques A, et al: Infection and fetal loss in the mid-second trimester of pregnancy. Aust N Z J Obstet Gynaecol 50(3):221, 2010

Allen RH, Fitzmaurice G, Lifford KL, et al: Oral compared with intravenous sedation for first-trimester surgical abortion: a randomized controlled trial. Obstet Gynecol 113(2 pt 1):276, 2009

American College of Obstetricians and Gynecologists: Abortion access and training. Committee Opinion No. 424, January 2009a

American College of Obstetricians and Gynecologists: Misoprostol for postabortion care. Committee Opinion No. 427, February 2009b

American College of Obstetricians and Gynecologists: Abortion policy. College Statement of Policy. January 1993, Reaffirmed 2011a

American College of Obstetricians and Gynecologists: Antibiotic prophylaxis for gynecologic procedures. Practice Bulletin No. 104, May 2009, Reaffirmed 2011b

American College of Obstetricians and Gynecologists: Medical management of abortion. Practice Bulletin No. 67, October 2005, Reaffirmed 2011c

American College of Obstetricians and Gynecologists: Thromboembolism in pregnancy. Practice Bulletin No. 123, September 2011d

American College of Obstetricians and Gynecologists: Ultrasonography in pregnancy. Practice Bulletin No. 101, February 2009, Reaffirmed 2011e

American College of Obstetricians and Gynecologists: Use of prophylactic antibiotics in labor and delivery. Practice Bulletin No. 120, June 2011f

American College of Obstetricians and Gynecologists: Antiphospholipid syndrome. Practice Bulletin No. 132, December 2012

American College of Obstetricians and Gynecologists: Inherited thrombophilias in pregnancy. Practice Bulletin No. 138, September 2013a

American College of Obstetricians and Gynecologists: Moderate caffeine consumption during pregnancy. Committee Opinion No. 462, August 2010, Reaffirmed 2013b

American College of Obstetricians and Gynecologists: Prevention of Rh D alloimmunization. Practice Bulletin No. 4, May 1999, Reaffirmed 2013c

American College of Obstetricians and Gynecologists: The limits of conscientious refusal in reproductive medicine. Committee Opinion No. 385, November 2007, Reaffirmed 2013d

American College of Obstetricians and Gynecologists: Second-trimester abortion. Practice Bulletin No. 135, June 2013e

American College of Obstetricians and Gynecologists: Cerclage for management of cervical insufficiency. Practice Bulletin No. 142, February 2014

American Society for Reproductive Medicine: Definitions of infertility and recurrent pregnancy loss. Fertil Steril 90(Suppl 3):S60, 2008

American Society for Reproductive Medicine: Intravenous immunoglobulin and recurrent spontaneous pregnancy loss. Fertil Steril 86(5 Suppl 1):S22b, 2006

Andersen AE, Ryan GL: Eating disorders in the obstetric and gynecologic patient population. Obstet Gynecol 114(6):1353, 2009

Ankumah NA, Tita A, Cantu J, et al: Pregnancy outcome vary by blood pressure level in women with mild-range chronic hypertension. Abstract No. 614, Am J Obstet Gynecol 208(1):S261, 2013

Armstrong BG, McDonald AD, Sloan M: Cigarette, alcohol, and coffee consumption and spontaneous abortion. Am J Public Health 82:85, 1992

Arredondo F, Noble LS: Endocrinology of recurrent pregnancy loss. Semin Reprod Med 1:33, 2006

Baker A, Beresford T: Informed consent, patient education, and counseling. In Paul M, Lichtenberg ES, Borgatta L, et al (eds): Management of Unintended and Abnormal Pregnancy. West Sussex, Wiley-Blackwell, 2009, p 48

Barlow S, Sullivan FM: Reproductive Hazards of Industrial Chemicals: An Evaluation of Animal and Human Data. New York, Academic Press, 1982

Barnhart K, Mennuti MT, Benjamin I, et al: Prompt diagnosis of ectopic pregnancy in an emergency department setting. Obstet Gynecol 84(6):1010, 1994

Barnhart K, van Mello NM, Bourne T, et al: Pregnancy of unknown location: a consensus statement of nomenclature, definitions, and outcome. Fertil Steril 95(3):857, 2011

Barnhart K, Sammel MD, Chung K, et al: Decline of serum human chorionic gonadotropin and spontaneous complete abortion: defining the normal curve. Obstet Gynecol 104:975, 2004a

Barnhart KT, Sammel MD, Appleby D, et al: Does a prediction model for pregnancy of unknown location developed in the UK validate on a US population? Hum Reprod 25(10):2434, 2010

Barnhart KT, Sammel MD, Rinaudo PF: Symptomatic patients with an early viable intrauterine pregnancy: hCG curves redefined. Obstet Gynecol 104:50, 2004b

Barrett JP, Whiteside JL, Boardman LA: Fatal clostridial sepsis after spontaneous abortion. Obstet Gynecol 99:899, 2002

Barth WH: Operative procedures of the cervix. In Hankins GDV, Clark SL, Cunningham FG, et al (eds): Operative Obstetrics. Norwalk, Appleton & Lange, 1995, p 753

Bates SM, Greer IA, Middledorp S, et al: VTE, thrombophilia, antithrombotic therapy, and pregnancy: Antithrombotic Therapy and Prevention of Thrombosis, 9th ed: American College of Chest Physicians Evidence-Based Clinical Practice Guidelines. Chest 141:e691S, 2012

Baud D, Goy G, Jaton K, et al: Role of *Chlamydia trachomatis* in miscarriage. Emerg Infect Dis 17(9):1630, 2011

Bednarek PH, Creinin MD, Reeves MF, et al: Immediate versus delayed IUD insertion after uterine aspiration. N Engl J Med 364(21):2208, 2011

Bellver J, Ayllón Y, Ferrando M, et al: Female obesity impairs in vitro fertilization outcome without affecting embryo quality. Fertil Steril 93(2):447, 2010a

Benhadi N, Wiersinga WM, Reitsma JB, et al: Higher maternal TSH levels in pregnancy are associated with increased risk for miscarriage, fetal or neonatal death. Eur J Endocrinol 160:985, 2009

Berger DS, Hogge WA, Barmada MM, et al: Comprehensive analysis of HLA-G: implications for recurrent spontaneous abortion. Reprod Sci 17(4):331, 2010

Berghella V, Airoldi J, O'Neill AM, et al: Misoprostol for second trimester pregnancy termination in women with prior caesarean: a systematic review. BJOG 116(9):1151, 2009

Berghella V, Mackeen D: Cervical length screening with ultrasound-indicated cerclage compared with history-indicated cerclage for prevention of preterm birth: a meta-analysis. Obstet Gynecol 118(1):148, 2011

Bhattacharya S, Townend J, Bhattacharya S: Recurrent miscarriage: are three miscarriages one too many? Analysis of a Scottish population-based database of 151,021 pregnancies. Eur J Obstet Gynecol Reprod Biol 150:24, 2010

Bianco K, Caughey AB, Shaffer BL, et al: History of miscarriage and increased incidence of fetal aneuploidy in subsequent pregnancy. Obstet Gynecol 107:1098, 2006

Boivin JF: Risk of spontaneous abortion in women occupationally exposed to anaesthetic gases: a meta-analysis. Occup Environ Med 54:541, 1997

Borgatta L, Burnhill MS, Tyson J, et al: Early medical abortion with methotrexate and misoprostol. Obstet Gynecol 97:11, 2001

Boyd EF Jr, Holmstrom EG: Ovulation following therapeutic abortion. Am J Obstet Gynecol 113:469, 1972

Bradshaw KD: Anatomic disorders. In Hoffman BL, Schorge JO, Schaffer JI, et al: Williams Gynecology, 2nd ed. McGraw-Hill, New York, 2012

Branch DW, Gibson M, Silver RM: Recurrent miscarriage. N Engl J Med 363:18, 2010

Brent RL: Saving lives and changing family histories: appropriate counseling of pregnant women and men and women of reproductive age, concerning the risk of diagnostic radiation exposures during and before pregnancy. Am J Obstet Gynecol 200(1):4, 2009

Brigham SA, Conlon C, Farquhason RG: A longitudinal study of pregnancy outcome following idiopathic recurrent miscarriage. Hum Reprod 14(11):2868, 1999

Brown ZA, Selke S, Zeh J, et al: The acquisition of herpes simplex virus during pregnancy. N Engl J Med 337:509, 1997

Bryant AG, Grimes DA, Garrett JM: Second-trimester abortion for fetal anomalies or fetal death. Labor induction compared with dilation and evacuation. Obstet Gynecol 117(4):788, 2011

Bukulmez O, Arici A: Luteal phase defect: myth or reality. Obstet Gynecol Clin North Am 31:727, 2004

Bulik CM, Hoffman ER, Von Holle A, et al: Unplanned pregnancy in women with anorexia nervosa. Obstet Gynecol 116:1136, 2010

Buttram VC Jr, Gibbons WE: Mullerian anomalies: a proposed classification (an analysis of 144 cases). Fertil Steril 32(1):40, 1979

Calleja-Agius J, Muttukrishna S, Pizzey AR, et al: Pro- and anti-inflammatory cytokines in threatened miscarriages. Am J Obstet Gynecol 205:83.e8–16, 2011

Cammarano CL, Herron MA, Parer JT: Validity of indications for transabdominal cervicoisthmic cerclage for cervical incompetence. Am J Obstet Gynecol 172:1871, 1995

Canobbio MM, Mair DD, van der Velde M, et al: Pregnancy outcomes after the Fontan repair. J Am Coll Cardiol 28(3):763, 1996

Cansino C, Edelman A, Burke A, et al: Paracervical block with combined ketorolac and lidocaine in first-trimester surgical abortion: a randomized controlled trial. Obstet Gynecol 114(6):1220, 2009

Carrell DT, Wilcox AL, Lowy L, et al: Male chromosomal factors of unexplained recurrent pregnancy loss. Obstet Gynecol 101:1229, 2003

Caruso A, Trivellini C, De Carolis S, et al: Emergency cerclage in the presence of protruding membranes: is pregnancy outcome predictable? Acta Obstet Gynecol Scand 79:265, 2000

Casey BM, Dashe JS, Wells CE, et al: Subclinical hypothyroidism and pregnancy outcomes. Obstet Gynecol 105(2):239, 2005

Caspi E, Schneider DF, Mor Z, et al: Cervical internal os cerclage: description of a new technique and comparison with Shirodkar operation. Am J Perinatol 7:347, 1990

Castañeda R, Lechuga D, Ramos RI, et al: Endemic goiter in pregnant women: utility of the simplified classification of thyroid size by palpation and urinary iodine as screening tests. BJOG 109:1366, 2002

Catov JM, Nohr EA, Olsen J, et al: Chronic hypertension related to risk for preterm and term small for gestational age births. Obstet Gynecol 112(2 pt 1):290, 2008

Cavallo F, Russo R, Zotti C, et al: Moderate alcohol consumption and spontaneous abortion. Alcohol 30:195, 1995

Centers for Disease Control and Prevention: *Clostridium sordellii* toxic shock syndrome after medical abortion with mifepristone and intravaginal misoprostol—United States and Canada, 2001–2005. MMWR 54(29):724, 2005

Centers for Disease Control and Prevention: Tobacco use and pregnancy. 2013. Available at: http://www.cdc.gov/reproductivehealth/TobaccoUsePregnancy/index.htm. Accessed May 22, 2013

Chasen ST, Kalish RB, Gupta M, et al: Obstetric outcomes after surgical abortion at > or = 20 weeks' gestation. Am J Obstet Gynecol 193:1161, 2005

Chasen ST, Silverman NS: Mid-trimester emergent cerclage: a ten year single institution review. J Perinatol 18:338, 1998

Chen BA, Reeves MF, Creinin MD, et al: Misoprostol for treatment of early pregnancy failure in women with previous uterine surgery. Am J Obstet Gynecol 198:626.e1, 2008

Chen L, Hu R: Thyroid autoimmunity and miscarriage: a meta-analysis. Clin Endocrinol 74:513, 2011

Clark K, Ji H, Feltovich H, et al: Mifepristone-induced cervical ripening: structural, biomechanical, and molecular events. Am J Obstet Gynecol 194:1391, 2006

Clark W, Bracken H, Tanenhaus J, et al: Alternatives to a routine follow-up visit for early medical abortion. Obstet Gynecol 115(2 Pt 1):264, 2010

Cleland K, Creinin M, Nucatola D, et al: Significant adverse events and outcomes after medical abortion. Obstet Gynecol 121(1):166, 2013

Clowse ME, Jamison M, Myers E, et al: A national study of the complications of lupus in pregnancy. Am J Obstet Gynecol 199:127.e1, 2008

Cnattingius S, Signorello LB, Anneren G, et al: Caffeine intake and the risk of first-trimester spontaneous abortion. N Engl J Med 343:1839, 2000

Cocksedge KA, Li TC, Saravelos SH, et al: A reappraisal of the role of polycystic ovary syndrome in recurrent miscarriage. Reprod Biomed Online 17:151, 2008

Cohen AL, Bhatnagar J, Reagan S, et al: Toxic shock associated with *Clostridium sordellii* and *Clostridium perfringens* after medical and spontaneous abortion. Obstet Gynecol 110:1027, 2007

Condous G, Okaro E, Khalid A, et al: Do we need to follow up complete miscarriages with serum human chorionic gonadotrophin levels? BJOG 112:827, 2005

Condous G, Van Calster B, Kirk E, et al: Clinical information does not improve the performance of mathematical models in predicting the outcome of pregnancies of unknown location. Fertil Steril 88(3):572, 2007

Connolly A, Ryan DH, Stuebe AM, et al: Reevaluation of discriminatory and threshold levels for serum β-hCG in early pregnancy. Obstet Gynecol 121(1):65, 2013

Corardetti A, Cecati M, Sartini D, et al: Deregulated cytokine and chemokine expression in endometrium from women with recurrent pregnancy loss. Abstract No. 88, Am J Obstet Gynecol 208(1 Suppl):S52, 2013

Coyaji K, Krishna U, Ambardekar S, et al: Are two doses of misoprostol after mifepristone for early abortion better than one? BJOG 114(3):271, 2007

Creinin MD, Huang X, Westhoff C: et al: Factors related to successful misoprostol treatment for early pregnancy failure. Obstet Gynecol 107:901, 2006

Creinin MD, Pymar HC, Schwartz JL: Mifepristone 100 mg in abortion regimens. Obstet Gynecol 98:434, 2001

Creinin MD, Schreiber CA, Bednarek P: Mifepristone and misoprostol administered simultaneously versus 24 hours apart for abortion. Obstet Gynecol 109(4):885, 2007

Cunningham FG, Halvorson LM: First-trimester abortion. In Hoffman BL, Schorge JO, Schaffer JI, et al (eds): Williams Gynecology, 2nd ed. McGraw-Hill, New York, 2012

Daif JL, Levie M, Chudnoff S, et al: Group A streptococcus causing necrotizing fasciitis and toxic shock syndrome after medical termination of pregnancy. Obstet Gynecol 113(2 Pt 2):504, 2009

Dalenda C, Ines N, Fathia B, et al: Two medical abortion regimens for late first-trimester termination of pregnancy: a prospective randomized trial. Contraception 81(4):323, 2010

Dao B, Blum J, Thieba B, et al: Is misoprostol a safe, effective and acceptable alternative to manual vacuum aspiration for postabortion care? Results from a randomized trial in Burkina Faso, West Africa. BJOG 114(11):1368, 2007

Daya S: Accuracy of gestational age estimation by means of fetal crown-rump length measurement. Am J Obstet Gynecol 168(3 Pt 1):903, 1993

Dayananda I, Maurer R, Fortin J, et al: Medical abortion follow-up serum human chorionic gonadotropin compared with ultrasonography. Obstet Gynecol 121(3):607, 2013

Devaseelan P, Fogarty PP, Regan L: Human chorionic gonadotropin for threatened abortion. Cochrane Database Syst Rev 5:DC007422, 2010

Devi Wold AS, Pham N, Arici A: Anatomic factors in recurrent pregnancy loss. Semin Reprod Med 1:25, 2006

De Vivo A, Mancuso A, Giacobbe A, et al: Thyroid function in women found to have early pregnancy loss. Thyroid 20(6):633, 2010

Dickinson J, Jennings B, Doherty D: Comparison of three regimens using mifepristone and misoprostol for second trimester pregnancy termination. Am J Obstet Gynecol 210:S36, 2014

Doody KJ: Treatment of the infertile couple. In Hoffman BL, Schorge JO, Schaffer JI, et al (eds): Williams Gynecology, 2nd ed. McGraw-Hill, New York, 2012

Doubilet PM, Benson CB, Bourne T, et al: Diagnostic criteria for nonviable pregnancy early in the first trimester. N Engl J Med 369:1443, 2013

Dranitsaris G, Johnston M, Poirier S, et al: Are health care providers who work with cancer drugs at an increased risk for toxic events? A systematic review and meta-analysis of the literature. J Oncol Pharm Pract 2:69, 2005

Dukhovny S, Zutshi P, Abbott JF: Recurrent second trimester pregnancy loss: evaluation and management. Curr Opin Endocrinol Diabetes Obes 16:451, 2009

Eddleman K, Sullivan L, Stone J, et al: An individualized risk for spontaneous pregnancy loss: a risk function model. J Soc Gynecol Investig 13:197A, 2006

Edlow AG, Hou MY, Maurer R, et al: Uterine evacuation for second-trimester fetal death and maternal morbidity. Obstet Gynecol 117(2, part 1):307, 2011

Edlow AG, Srinivas SK, Elovitz MA: Second-trimester loss and subsequent pregnancy outcomes: what is the real risk? Am J Obstet Gynecol 197:581.e1, 2007

Edwards DRV, Aldridge T, Baird DD, et al: Periconceptional over-the-counter nonsteroidal anti-inflammatory drug exposure and risk for spontaneous abortion. Obstet Gynecol 120(1):113, 2012

Ehsanipoor R, Selligman N, Szymanski L, et al: Physical exam indicated cerclage versus expectant management: a systematic review and meta-analysis. Abstract No. 152, Am J Obstet Gynecol 208(1 Suppl):S76, 2013
Eiben B, Bartels I, Bahr-Prosch S, et al: Cytogenetic analysis of 750 spontaneous abortions with the direct-preparation method of chorionic villi and its implications for studying genetic causes of pregnancy wastage. Am J Hum Genet 47:656, 1990
Eller AG, Branch DW, Nelson L, et al: Vascular endothelial growth factor-A gene polymorphisms in women with recurrent pregnancy loss. J Reprod Immunol 88(1):48, 2011
Erkan D, Kozora E, Lockshin MD: Cognitive dysfunction and white matter abnormalities in antiphospholipid syndrome. Pathophysiology 18(1):93, 2011
Eskenazi B, Chevrier J, Rosas LG, et al: The Pine River statement: human health consequences of DDT use. Environ Health Perspect 117(9):1359, 2009
Fantel AG, Shepard TH, Vadheim-Roth C, et al: Embryonic and fetal phenotypes: prevalence and other associated factors in a large study of spontaneous abortion. In Porter IH, Hook EM (eds): Human Embryonic and Fetal Death. New York, Academic Press, 1980, p 71
Fekih M, Fathallah K, Ben Regaya L, et al: Sublingual misoprostol for first trimester termination of pregnancy. Int J Gynaecol Obstet 109(1):67, 2010
Feldman DM, Timms D, Borgida AF: Toxoplasmosis, parvovirus, and cytomegalovirus in pregnancy. Clin Lab Med 30(3):709, 2010
Fischer M, Bhatnagar J, Guarner J, et al: Fatal toxic shock syndrome associated with *Clostridium sordellii* after medical abortion. N Engl J Med 353:2352, 2005
Fjerstad M, Sivin I, Lichtenberg ES, et al: Effectiveness of medical abortion with mifepristone and buccal misoprostol through 59 gestational days. Contraception 80(3):282, 2009a
Fjerstad M, Trussell J, Sivin I, et al: Rates of serious infection after changes in regimens for medical abortion. N Engl J Med 361:145, 2009b
Flood K, Peace A, Kent E, et al: Platelet reactivity and pregnancy loss. Am J Obstet Gynecol 203:281.e1, 2010
Floyd RL, Decoufle P, Hungerford DW: Alcohol use prior to pregnancy recognition. Am J Prev Med 17:101, 1999
Freedman L, Landy U, Steinauer J: Obstetrician-gynecologist experiences with abortion training: physician insights from a qualitative study. Contraception 81(6):525, 2010
Garber J, Cobin R, Gharib H, et al: Clinical practice guidelines for hypothyroidism in adults: cosponsored by the American Association of Clinical Endocrinologists and the American Thyroid Association. Thyroid 22(12):1200, 2012
Gibb DM, Salaria DA: Transabdominal cervicoisthmic cerclage in the management of recurrent second trimester miscarriage and preterm delivery. Br J Obstet Gynaecol 102:802, 1995
Giraldo-Isaza MA, Fried GP, Hegarty SE, et al: Comparison of 2 stitches vs 1 stitch for transvaginal cervical cerclage for preterm birth prevention. Am J Obstet Gynecol 208:209.e1, 2013
Goldberg AB, Dean G, Kang MS, et al: Manual versus electric vacuum aspiration for early first-trimester abortion: a controlled study of complication rates. Obstet Gynecol 103:101, 2004
Goldberg AB, Drey EA, Whitaker AK: Misoprostol compared with laminaria before early second-trimester surgical abortion: a randomized trial. Obstet Gynecol 106:234, 2005
Goldenberg M, Sivan E, Sharabi Z, et al: Reproductive outcome following hysteroscopic management of intrauterine septum and adhesions. Human Reprod 10:2663, 1995
Goldstein SR: Significance of cardiac activity on endovaginal ultrasound in very early embryos. Obstet Gynecol 80(4):670, 1992
Goyal V: Uterine rupture in second-trimester misoprostol-induced abortion of cesarean delivery: a systematic review. Obstet Gynecol 112:1117, 2009
Gracia CR, Sammel MD, Chittams J, et al: Risk factors for spontaneous abortion in early symptomatic first-trimester pregnancies. Obstet Gynecol 106:993, 2005
Guelinckx I, Devlieger R, Vansant G: Reproductive outcome after bariatric surgery: a critical review. Hum Reprod Update 15(2):189, 2009
Guest J, Chien PF, Thomson MA, et al: Randomised controlled trial comparing the efficacy of same-day administration of mifepristone and misoprostol for termination of pregnancy with the standard 36 to 48 hour protocol. BJOG 114(2):207, 2007
Guttmacher Institute: US abortion rate levels off after 30-year decline. Reuters Health Information, January 12, 2011
Haddow JE, McClain MR, Palomaki GE, et al: Thyroperoxidase and thyroglobulin antibodies in early pregnancy and placental abruption. Obstet Gynecol 117:287, 2011
Hamoda H, Ashok PW, Flett GMM, et al: A randomised controlled trial of mifepristone in combination with misoprostol administered sublingually or vaginally for medical abortion up to 13 weeks of gestation. BJOG 112(8):1102, 2005
Hannafin B, Lovecchio F, Blackburn P: Do Rh-negative women with first trimester spontaneous abortions need Rh immune globulin? Am J Obstet Gynecol 24:487, 2006
Hardy G, Benjamin A, Abenhaim HA: Effect of induced abortions on early preterm births and adverse perinatal outcomes. J Obstet Gynaecol Can 35(2):138, 2013
Harris LH: Stigma and abortion complications in the United States. Obstet Gynecol 120(6):1472, 2012
Harris LH, Cooper A, Rasinski KA, et al: Obstetrician-gynecologists' objections to and willingness to help patients obtain an abortion. Obstet Gynecol 118(4):905, 2011
Hasan R, Baird DD, Herring AH, et al: Association between first-trimester vaginal bleeding and miscarriage. Obstet Gynecol 114:860, 2009
Heartwell SF, Deputy Director, Domestic Programs, Susan Thompson Buffett Foundation, March 2013
Heuser C, Dalton J, Macpherson C, et al: Idiopathic recurrent pregnancy loss recurs at similar gestational ages. Am J Obstet Gynecol 203(4):343.e1, 2010
Hide G, Morley EK, Hughes JM, et al: Evidence for high levels of vertical transmission in *Toxoplasma gondii*. Parasitology 136(14):1877, 2009
Ho CS, Bhatnagar J, Cohen AL, et al: Undiagnosed cases of fatal *Clostridium*-associated toxic shock in Californian women of childbearing age. Am J Obstet Gynecol 201:459.e1–7, 2009
Holbrook WJ, Oskarsdottir A, Fridjonsson T, et al: No link between low-grade periodontal disease and preterm birth: a pilot study in a health Caucasian population. Acta Odontol Scand 62:177, 2004
Homer H, Saridogan E: Uterine artery embolization for fibroids is associated with an increased risk of miscarriage. Fertil Steril 94(1):324, 2010
Honkanen H, Piaggio G, Hertzen H, et al: WHO multinational study of three misoprostol regimens after mifepristone for early medical abortion. BJOG 111(7):715, 2004
Hoover RN, Hyer M, Pheiffer RM, et al: Adverse health outcomes in women exposed in utero to diethylstilbestrol. N Engl J Med 365(14):1304, 2011
Horon IL: Underreporting of maternal deaths on death certificates and the magnitude of the problem of maternal mortality. Am J Public Health 95:478, 2005
Hudson MM: Reproductive outcomes for survivors of childhood cancer. Obstet Gynecol 116:1171, 2010
Irving A, Kieke B, Donahue J, et al: Trivalent inactivated influenza vaccine and spontaneous abortion. Obstet Gynecol 121(1):159, 2013
Jacobs PA, Hassold TJ: The origin of chromosomal abnormalities in spontaneous abortion. In Porter IH, Hook EB (eds): Human Embryonic and Fetal Death. New York, Academic Press, 1980, p 289
Jain JK, Harwood B, Meckstroth KR, et al: A prospective randomized, double-blinded, placebo-controlled trial comparing mifepristone and vaginal misoprostol to vaginal misoprostol alone for elective termination of early pregnancy. Hum Reprod 17:1477, 2002
Jarvie E, Ramsay JE: Obstetric management of obesity in pregnancy. Semin Fetal Neonatal Med 15(2):83, 2010
Jaslow CR, Carney JL, Kutteh WH: Diagnostic factors identified in 1020 women with two versus three or more recurrent pregnancy losses. Fertil Steril 93(4):1234, 2010
Jeppson PC, Park A, Chen CC: Multivalvular bacterial endocarditis after suction curettage abortion. Obstet Gynecol 112:452, 2008
Johns J, Jauniaux E: Threatened miscarriage as a predictor of obstetric outcome. Obstet Gynecol 107:845, 2006
Johnson LG, Mueller BA, Daling JR: The relationship of placenta previa and history of induced abortion. Int J Gynaecol Obstet 81:191, 2003
Jones RK, Kavanaugh ML: Changes in abortion rates between 2000 and 2008 and lifetime incidence of abortion. Obstet Gynecol 117(6):1358, 2011
Joo JG, Beke A, Berkes E, et al: Fetal pathology in second-trimester miscarriages. Fetal Diagn Ther 25(2):186, 2009
Jun SH, Ginsburg ES, Racowsky C, et al: Uterine leiomyomas and their effect on in vitro fertilization outcome: a retrospective study. J Assist Reprod Genet 18:139, 2001
Kadar N, DeCherney AH, Romero R: Receiver operating characteristic (ROC) curve analysis of the relative efficacy of single and serial chorionic gonadotropin determinations in the early diagnosis of ectopic pregnancy. Fertil Steril 37:542, 1982
Kajii T, Ferrier A, Niikawa N, et al: Anatomic and chromosomal anomalies in 639 spontaneous abortions. Hum Genet 55:87, 1980
Kambiss SM, Hibbert ML, Macedonia C, et al: Uterine perforation resulting in bowel infarction: sharp traumatic bowel and mesenteric injury at the time of pregnancy termination. Milit Med 165:81, 2000
Kapp N, Lohr PA, Ngo TD, et al: Cervical preparation for first trimester surgical abortion. Cochrane Database Syst Rev 2:CD007207, 2010
Karl K, Katz M: A stepwise approach to cervical cerclage. OBG Management 24:31, 2012
Keder LM: Best practices in surgical abortion. Am J Obstet Gynecol 189:418, 2003

Keegan GT, Forkowitz MJ: A case report: uretero-uterine fistula as a complication of elective abortion. J Urol 128:137, 1982
Kelly H, Harvey D, Moll S: A cautionary tale. Fatal outcome of methotrexate therapy given for management of ectopic pregnancy. Obstet Gynecol 107:439, 2006
Kerns JL, Steinauer JE, Rosenstein MG, et al: Maternal-fetal medicine subspecialists' provision of second-trimester termination services. Am J Perinatol 29:709, 2012
Kesmodel U, Wisborg K, Olsen SF, et al: Moderate alcohol intake in pregnancy and the risk of spontaneous abortion. Alcohol 37:87, 2002
Kharazmi E, Dossus L, Rohrmann S, et al: Pregnancy loss and risk of cardiovascular disease: a prospective population-based cohort study (EPIC-Heidelberg). Heart 97(1):49, 2011
Khashan AS, Quigley EMM, McNamee R, et al: Increased risk of miscarriage and ectopic pregnancy among women with irritable bowel syndrome. Clin Gastroenterol Hepatol 10(8):902, 2012
Klebanoff MA, Levine RJ, DerSimonian R, et al: Maternal serum paraxanthine, a caffeine metabolite, and the risk of spontaneous abortion. N Engl J Med 341:1639, 1999
Kleinhaus K, Perrin M, Friedlander Y, et al: Paternal age and spontaneous abortion. Obstet Gynecol 108:369, 2006
Kollitz K, Meyn, Lohr P, Creinin M: Mifepristone and misoprostol for early pregnancy failure: a cohort analysis. Am J Obstet Gynecol 204:386.e1–6, 2011
Krassas GE, Poppe K, Glinoer D: Thyroid function and human reproductive health. Endo Rev 31:702, 2010
Kuhn RPJ, Pepperell RJ: Cervical ligation: a review of 242 pregnancies. Aust N Z J Obstet Gynaecol 17:79, 1977
Lahteenmaki P, Luukkainen T: Return of ovarian function after abortion. Clin Endocrinol 2:123, 1978
Lashen H, Fears K, Sturdee D: Obesity is associated with increased risk of early and recurrent miscarriage: matched case control study. Hum Reprod 19:1644, 2004
Lawson CC, Rocheleau CM, Whelan EA, et al: Occupational exposures among nurses and risk of spontaneous abortion. Am J Obstet Gynecol 206:327.e1, 2012
Levi CS, Lyons EA, Lindsay DJ: Early diagnosis of nonviable pregnancy with endovaginal US. Radiology 167(2):383, 1988
Levi CS, Lyons EA, Zheng XH, et al: Endovaginal US: demonstration of cardiac activity in embryos of less than 5.0 mm in crown-rump length. Radiology 176(1):71, 1990
Locatelli A, Vergani P, Bellini P, et al: Amnioreduction in emergency cerclage with prolapsed membranes: comparison of two methods for reducing the membranes. Am J Perinatol 16:73, 1999
Love ER, Bhattacharya S, Smith NC, et al: Effect of interpregnancy interval on outcomes of pregnancy after miscarriage: retrospective analysis of hospital episode statistics in Scotland. BMJ 341:c3967, 2010
Luise C, Jermy K, May C, et al: Outcome of expectant management of spontaneous first trimester miscarriage: observational study. BMJ 324:873, 2002
Lupo PJ, Symanski E, Waller DK, et al: Maternal exposure to ambient levels of benzene and neural tube defects among offspring, Texas, 1999–2004. Environ Health Perspect 119:397, 2011
Lykke JA, Dideriksen KL, Lidegaard Ø, et al: First-trimester vaginal bleeding and complications later in pregnancy. Obstet Gynecol 115:935, 2010
MacIsaac L, Darney P: Early surgical abortion: an alternative to and backup for medical abortion. Am J Obstet Gynecol 183:S76, 2000
MacNaughton MC, Chalmers IG, Dubowitz V, et al: Final report of the Medical Research Council/Royal College of Obstetricians and Gynaecologists Multicentre Randomized Trial of Cervical Cerclage. Br J Obstet Gynaecol 100:516, 1993
Maconochie N, Doyle P, Prior S, et al: Risk factors for first trimester miscarriage—results from a UK-population-based case-control study. BJOG 114:170, 2007
Madden T, Westhoff C: Rates of follow-up and repeat pregnancy in the 12 months after first-trimester induced abortion. Obstet Gynecol 113:663, 2009
Mankowski JL, Kingston J, Moran T, et al: Paracervical compared with intracervical lidocaine for suction curettage: a randomized controlled trial. Obstet Gynecol 113:1052, 2009
Männistö T, Vääräsmäki M, Pouta A, et al: Perinatal outcome of children born to mothers with thyroid dysfunction or antibodies: a prospective population-based cohort study. J Clin Endocrinol Metab 94:772, 2009
Marguard K, Westphal LM, Milki AA, et al: Etiology of recurrent pregnancy loss in women over the age of 35 years. Fertil Steril 94(4):1473, 2010
Masch RJ, Roman AS: Uterine evacuation in the office. Contemp Ob Gyn 51:66, 2005
Mazze RI, Källén B: Reproductive outcome after anesthesia and operation during pregnancy: a registry study of 5405 cases. Am J Obstet Gynecol 161:1178, 1989
McDonald IA: Incompetent cervix as a cause of recurrent abortion. J Obstet Gynaecol Br Commonw 70:105, 1963
Meirik O, Huang NTM, Piaggio G, et al: Complications of first-trimester abortion by vacuum aspiration after cervical preparation with and without misoprostol: a multicentre randomized trial. Lancet 379:1817, 2012
Meites E, Zane S, Gould C: Fatal *Clostridium sordellii* infections after medical abortions. N Engl J Med 363(14):1382, 2010
Mentula M, Suhonen S, Heikinheimo O: One- and two-day intervals between mifepristone and misoprostol in second trimester medical termination of pregnancy. Hum Reprod 26(10):2690, 2011
Mohammad KL, Ghazaly MM, Zaalouk TK, et al: Maternal brucellosis and human pregnancy. J Egypt Soc Parasitol 41(2):485, 2011
Moore S, Ide M, Coward PY, et al: A prospective study to investigate the relationship between periodontal disease and adverse pregnancy outcome. Br Dent J 197:251, 2004
Moreau C, Kaminski M, Ancel PY, et al: Previous induced abortions and the risk of very preterm delivery: results of the EPIPAGE study. BJOG 112:430, 2005
Moschos E, Twickler DM: Intrauterine devices in early pregnancy: findings on ultrasound and clinical outcomes. Am J Obstet Gynecol 204:427.e1–6, 2011
Munk-Olsen T, Laursen T, Pedersen, C, et al: Induced first-trimester abortion and risk of mental disorder. N Engl J Med 364(4):332, 2011
Nahum GG: Uterine anomalies. How common are they, and what is their distribution among subtypes? J Reprod Med 43(10):877, 1998
Nawaz FH, Rizvi J: Continuation of metformin reduces early pregnancy loss in obese Pakistani women with polycystic ovarian syndrome. Gynecol Obstet Invest 69(3):184, 2010
Negro R, Formoso G, Mangieri T, et al: Levothyroxine treatment in euthyroid pregnant women with autoimmune thyroid disease: effects on obstetrical complications. J Clin Endocrinol Metab 91(7):2587, 2006
Negro R, Schwartz A, Gismondi R, et al: Universal screening versus case finding for detection and treatment of thyroid hormonal dysfunction during pregnancy. J Clin Endocrinol Metab 95(4):1699, 2010
Neilson JP, Gyte GM, Hickey M, et al: Medical treatments for incomplete miscarriage (less than 24 weeks). Cochrane Database Syst Rev 1:CD007223, 2010
Newmann SJ, Sokoloff A, Tharyil M, et al: Same-day synthetic osmotic dilators compared with overnight laminaria before abortion at 14-18 weeks of gestation: a randomized controlled trial. Obstet Gynecol 123:271, 2014
Ngoc NT, Shochet T, Raghavan S, et al: Mifepristone and misoprostol compared with misoprostol alone for second-trimester abortion. Obstet Gynecol 118(3):601, 2011
Nguyen NT, Blum J, Durocher J, et al: A randomized controlled study comparing 600 versus 1200 μg oral misoprostol for medical management of incomplete abortion. Contraception 72:438, 2005
Niinimäki M, Pouta A, Bloigu A, et al: Immediate complications after medical compared with surgical termination of pregnancy. Obstet Gynecol 114:795, 2009
Nurmohamed L, Moretti ME, Schechter T, et al: Outcome following high-dose methotrexate in pregnancies misdiagnosed as ectopic. Am J Obstet Gynecol 205:533.e1, 2011
Nyberg DA, Mack LA, Laing FC, et al: Distinguishing normal from abnormal gestational sac growth in early pregnancy. J Ultrasound Med 6(1):23, 1987
Oakeshott P, Hay P, Hay S, et al: Association between bacterial vaginosis or chlamydial infection and miscarriage before 16 weeks' gestation: prospective, community based cohort study. BMJ 325:1334, 2002
O'Connor S, Kuller JA, McMahon MJ: Management of cervical cerclage after preterm premature rupture of membranes. Obstet Gynecol Surv 54:391, 1999
Owen J, Hankins G, Iams J, et al: Multicenter randomized trial of cerclage for preterm birth prevention in high-risk women with shortened midtrimester cervical length. Am J Obstet Gynecol 201(4):375, 2009
Owen J, Hauth JC, Winkler CL, et al: Midtrimester pregnancy termination: a randomized trial of prostaglandin E2 versus concentrated oxytocin. Am J Obstet Gynecol 167:1112, 1992
Owen J, Iams JD, Hauth JC: Vaginal sonography and cervical incompetence. Am J Obstet Gynecol 188:586, 2003
Pasternak B, Svanström H, Hviid A: Ondansetron in pregnancy and risk of adverse fetal outcomes. N Engl J Med 368(9):814, 2013
Paul ME, Mitchell CM, Rogers AJ, et al: Early surgical abortion: efficacy and safety. Am J Obstet Gynecol 187:407, 2002
Pazol K, Creanga AA, Burley KD, et al: Abortion surveillance—United States 2010. MMWR 62(ss08):1, 2013
Pazol K, Creanga AA, Zane S, et al: Abortion surveillance—United States, 2009. MMWR 61(8):1, 2012
Pazol K, Zane SB, Parker WY, et al: Abortion surveillance—United States, 2008. MMWR 60(15):1, 2011

Pymar HC, Creinin MD, Schwartz JL: Mifepristone followed on the same day by vaginal misoprostol for early abortion. Contraception 64:87, 2001
Quinn PA, Shewchuck AB, Shuber J, et al: Efficacy of antibiotic therapy in preventing spontaneous pregnancy loss among couples colonized with genital mycoplasmas. Am J Obstet Gynecol 145:239, 1983a
Quinn PA, Shewchuck AB, Shuber J, et al: Serologic evidence of *Ureaplasma urealyticum* infection in women with spontaneous pregnancy loss. Am J Obstet Gynecol 145:245, 1983b
Raghavan S, Comendant R, Digol I, et al: Two-pill regimens of misoprostol after mifepristone medical abortion through 63 days' gestational age: a randomized controlled trial of sublingual and oral misoprostol. Contraception 79(2):84, 2009
Ramsey PS, Owen J: Midtrimester cervical ripening and labor induction. Clin Obstet Gynecol 43(3):495, 2000
Ramsey PS, Savage K, Lincoln T, Owen J: Vaginal misoprostol versus concentrated oxytocin and vaginal PGE2 for second-trimester labor induction. Obstet Gynecol 104:138, 2004
Ramzy AM, Sattar M, Amin Y, et al: Uterine myomata and outcome of assisted reproduction. Hum Reprod 13:198, 1998
Raymond E, Grimes D: The comparative safety of legal induced abortion and childbirth in the United States. Obstet Gynecol 119(2, Part 1):215, 2012
Reddy UM: Recurrent pregnancy loss: nongenetic causes. Contemp Ob Gyn 52:63, 2007
Reeves MF, Smith KJ, Creinin MD: Contraceptive effectiveness of immediate compared with delayed insertion of intrauterine devices after abortion. Obstet Gynecol 109:1286, 2007
Reichman DE, Laufer MR: Congenital uterine anomalies affecting reproduction. Best Pract Res Clin Obstet Gynecol 24(2):193, 2010
Renner RM, Nichols MD, Jensen JT, et al: Paracervical block for pain control in first-trimester surgical abortion. Obstet Gynecol 119:1030, 2012
Robson SC, Kelly T, Howel D, et al: Randomised preference trial of medical versus surgical termination of pregnancy less than 14 weeks' gestation (TOPS). Health Technol Assess 13(53):1, 2009
Romero R, Kusanovic JP, Chaiworapongsa T, et al: Placental bed disorders in preterm labor, preterm PROM, spontaneous abortion and abruptio placentae. Best Pract Res Clin Obstet Gynaecol 25(3):313, 2011
Rowland AS, Baird DD, Shore DL, et al: Nitrous oxide and spontaneous abortion in female dental assistants. Am J Epidemiol 141:531, 1995
Rust OA, Atlas RO, Reed J, et al: Revisiting the short cervix detected by transvaginal ultrasound in the second trimester: why cerclage may not help. Am J Obstet Gynecol 185:1098, 2001
Salim R, Regan L, Woelfer B, et al: A comparative study of the morphology of congenital uterine anomalies in women with and without a history of recurrent first trimester miscarriage. Hum Reprod 18:162, 2003
Saraswat L, Bhattacharya S, Maheshwari A, et al: Maternal and perinatal outcome in women with threatened miscarriage in the first trimester: a systematic review. BJOG 117:245, 2010
Saravelos SH, Yan J, Rehmani H, et al: The prevalence and impact of fibroids and their treatment on the outcome of pregnancy in women with recurrent miscarriage. Hum Reprod 26:3274, 2011
Satpathy HK, Fleming A, Frey D, et al: Maternal obesity and pregnancy. Postgrad Med 120(3):E01, 2008
Savaris RF, Silva de Moraes G, Cristovam RA, et al: Are antibiotics necessary after 48 hours of improvement in infected/septic abortions? A randomized controlled trial followed by a cohort study. Am J Obstet Gynecol 204:301.e1, 2011
Savitz DA, Chan RL, Herring AH, et al: Caffeine and miscarriage risk. Epidemiology 19:55, 2008
Schaff EA, Fielding SL, Westhoff C, et al: Vaginal misoprostol administered 1, 2, or 3 days after mifepristone for early medical abortion. A randomized trial. JAMA 284:1948, 2000
Schneider D, Golan A, Langer R, et al: Outcome of continued pregnancies after first and second trimester cervical dilatation by laminaria tents. Obstet Gynecol 78:1121, 1991
Schnorr TM, Grajewski BA, Hornung RW, et al: Video display terminals and the risk of spontaneous abortion. N Engl J Med 324:727, 1991
Schust D, Hill J: Recurrent pregnancy loss. In Berek J (ed): Novak's Gynecology, 13th ed. Philadelphia, Lippincott Williams & Wilkins, 2002
Sedgh G, Singh S, Shah I, et al: Induced abortion: incidence and trends worldwide from 1995 to 2008. Lancet 379:625, 2012
Shannon C, Wiebe E, Jacot F: Regimens of misoprostol with mifepristone for early medical abortion: a randomized trial. BJOG 113:621, 2006
Sharshiner R, Romero S, Silver R, et al: Celiac disease serum markers and recurrent pregnancy loss. Abstract No. 151, Am J Obstet Gynecol 208(1 Suppl):S76, 2013
Sher KS, Jayanthi V, Probert CS, et al: Infertility, obstetric and gynaecological problems in coeliac sprue. Digest Dis 12:186, 1994
Shimoni N, Davis A, Ramos M, et al: Timing of copper intrauterine device insertion after medical abortion. Obstet Gynecol 118(3):623, 2011
Shirodkar VN: A new method of operative treatment for habitual abortions in the second trimester of pregnancy. Antiseptic 52:299, 1955
Silver RM, Branch DW, Goldenberg R, et al: Nomenclature for pregnancy outcomes. Obstet Gynecol 118(6):1402, 2011
Simpson JL: Causes of fetal wastage. Clin Obstet Gynecol 50(1):10, 2007
Simpson JL: Genes, chromosomes, and reproductive failure. Fertil Steril 33(2):107, 1980
Smith LF, Ewings PD, Guinlan C: Incidence of pregnancy after expectant, medical, or surgical management of spontaneous first trimester miscarriage: long term follow-up of miscarriage treatment (MIST) randomized controlled trial. BMJ 339:b3827, 2009
Sollid CP, Wisborg K, Hjort JH, et al: Eating disorder that was diagnosed before pregnancy and pregnancy outcome. Am J Obstet Gynecol 190:206, 2004
Srinivas SK, Ernst LM, Edlow AG, et al: Can placental pathology explain second-trimester pregnancy loss and subsequent pregnancy outcomes? Am J Obstet Gynecol 199:402.e1, 2008
Stein Z, Kline J, Susser E, et al: Maternal age and spontaneous abortion. In Porter IH, Hook EB (eds): Human Embryonic and Fetal Death. New York, Academic Press, 1980, p 107
Steinauer J, Darney P, Auerbach RD: Should all residents be trained to do abortions? Contemp Ob Gyn 51:56, 2005a
Steinauer J, Drey EA, Lewis R, et al: Obstetrics and gynecology resident satisfaction with an integrated, comprehensive abortion rotation. Obstet Gynecol 105:1335, 2005b
Steinberg JR, McCulloch CE, Adler NE: Abortion and mental health. Obstet Gynecol 123:263, 2014
Stephenson MD, Kutteh WH, Purkiss S, et al: Intravenous immunoglobulin and idiopathic secondary recurrent miscarriage: a multicentered randomized placebo-controlled trial. Hum Reprod 25(9):2203, 2010
Stout MJ, Odibo AO, Graseck AS, et al: Leiomyomas at routine second-trimester ultrasound examination and adverse obstetric outcomes. Obstet Gynecol 116:1056, 2010
Stoval N, Sibai B, Habli M: Is there a role for cerclage in twin gestation with short cervical length (CL)? Single center experience. Abstract No. 143, Am J Obstet Gynecol 208(1 Suppl):S73, 2013
Streeter GL: Focal deficiencies in fetal tissues and their relation to intra-uterine amputation. Carnegie Institute of Washington 1930, Publication No. 414, p 5
Stulberg DB, Dude AM, Dahlguist I, et al: Abortion provision among practicing obstetrician-gynecologists. Obstet Gynecol 1189):609, 2011
Sullivan AE, Silver RM, LaCoursiere DY, et al: Recurrent fetal aneuploidy and recurrent miscarriage. Obstet Gynecol 104:784, 2004
Sunkara SK, Khairy M, El-Toukhy T, et al: The effect of intramural fibroids without uterine cavity involvement on the outcome of IVF treatment: a systematic review and meta-analysis. Hum Reprod 25(2):418, 2010
Swingle HM, Colaizy TT, Zimmerman MB, et al: Abortion and the risk of subsequent preterm birth. J Reprod Med 54:95, 2009
Tang J, Kapp N, Dragoman M, et al: WHO recommendations for misoprostol use for obstetric and gynecologic indications. Int J Gynaecol Obstet 121(2):186, 2013
Tanner L: Abortion in America: restrictions on the rise. The Associated Press, October 12, 2012
Taskinen H, Kyyrönen P, Hemminki K: Effects of ultrasound, shortwaves, and physical exertion on pregnancy outcome in physiotherapists. J Epidemiol Community Health 44:196, 1990
Temmerman M, Lopita MI, Sanghvi HC, et al: The role of maternal syphilis, gonorrhea and HIV-1 infections in spontaneous abortion. Int J STD AIDS 3:418, 1992
Templeton A, Grimes D: A request for abortion. N Engl J Med 365(23):2198, 2011
Terkildsen MFC, Parilla BV, Kumar P, et al: Factors associated with success of emergent second-trimester cerclage. Obstet Gynecol 101:565, 2003
Thangaratinam S, Tan A, Knox E, et al: Association between thyroid autoantibodies and miscarriage and preterm birth: meta-analysis of evidence. BMJ 342:d2616, 2011
Therapel AT, Tharapel SA, Bannerman RM: Recurrent pregnancy losses and parental chromosome abnormalities: a review. Br J Obstet Gynecol 92:899, 1985
Thomason JL, Sampson MB, Beckman CR, et al: The incompetent cervix: a 1982 update. J Reprod Med 27:187, 1982
Timor-Tritsch IE, Farine D, Rosen MG: A close look at early embryonic development with the high-frequency transvaginal transducer. Am J Obstet Gynecol 159(3):676, 1988
To MS, Alfirevic Z, Heath VCF, et al: Cervical cerclage for prevention of preterm delivery in women with short cervix: randomised controlled trial. Lancet 363:1849, 2004
Tongsong T, Srisomboon J, Wanapirak C, et al: Pregnancy outcome of threatened abortion with demonstrable fetal cardiac activity: a cohort study. J Obstet Gynaecol 21:331, 1995

Torre A, Huchon C, Bussieres L, et al: Immediate versus delayed medical treatment for first-trimester miscarriage: a randomized trial. Am J Obstet Gynecol 206:215.e1, 2012

Trinder J, Brocklehurst P, Porter R, et al: Management of miscarriage: expectant, medical, or surgical? Results of randomized controlled trial (miscarriage treatment (MIST) trial). BMJ 332(7552):1235, 2006

Tzeng CR, Hwang JL, Au HK, et al: Sonographic patterns of the endometrium in assessment of medical abortion outcomes. Contraception 88(1):153, 2013

Valli E, Zupi E, Marconi D, et al: Hysteroscopic findings in 344 women with recurrent spontaneous abortion. J Am Assoc Gynecol Laparosc 8(3):398, 2001

van Benthem BH, de Vincenzi I, Delmas MD, et al: Pregnancies before and after HIV diagnosis in a European cohort of HIV-infected women. European study on the natural history of HIV infection in women. AIDS 14:2171, 2000

van den Boogaard E, Kaandorp SP, Franssen MT, et al: Consecutive or non-consecutive recurrent miscarriage: is there any difference in carrier status? Hum Reprod 25(6):1411, 2010

Vartian CV, Septimus EJ: Tricuspid valve group B streptococcal endocarditis following elective abortion. Rev Infect Dis 13:997, 1991

Velez Edwards DR, Baird DD, Hasan R, et al: First-trimester bleeding characteristics associate with increased risk of preterm birth: data from a prospective pregnancy cohort. Hum Reprod 27(1):54, 2012

Vilchez G, Saona P, Bahado-Singh R, et al: Adverse obstetrical outcomes of brucellosis in pregnancy: a 42-year experience in Peru. Am J Obstet Gynecol 210:S216, 2014

Virk J, Zhang J, Olsen J: Medical abortion and the risk of subsequent adverse pregnancy outcomes. N Engl J Med 357:648, 2007

von Hertzen H, Honkanen H, Piaggio G, et al: WHO multinational study of three misoprostol regimens after mifepristone for early medical abortion. I: efficacy. BJOG 110:808, 2003

von Hertzen H, Huong NTM, Piaggio G, et al: Misoprostol dose and route after mifepristone for early medical abortion: a randomized controlled non-inferiority trial. BJOG 117(10):1186, 2010

von Hertzen H, Piaggio G, Huong NT, et al: Efficacy of two intervals and two routes of administration of misoprostol for termination of early pregnancy: a randomized controlled equivalence trial. Lancet 369:1938, 2007

von Hertzen H, Piaggio G, Wojdyla D, et al: Two mifepristone doses and two intervals of misoprostol administration for termination of early pregnancy: a randomized factorial controlled equivalence trial. BJOG 116(3):381, 2009

Warburton D, Stein Z, Kline J, et al: Chromosome abnormalities in spontaneous abortion: data from the New York City study. In Porter IH, Hook EB (eds): Human Embryonic and Fetal Death. New York, Academic Press, 1980, p 261

Warren JB, Silver RM: Autoimmune disease in pregnancy: systemic lupus erythematosus and antiphospholipid syndrome. Obstet Gynecol Clin North Am 31:345, 2004

Weiss J, Malone F, Vidaver J, et al: Threatened abortion: a risk factor for poor pregnancy outcome—a population based screening study (the FASTER Trial). Am J Obstet Gynecol 187:S70, 2002

Weng X, Odouki R, Li DK: Maternal caffeine consumption during pregnancy and the risk of miscarriage: a prospective cohort study. Am J Obstet Gynecol 198:279.e1, 2008

Westfall JM, Sophocles A, Burggraf H, et al: Manual vacuum aspiration for first-trimester abortion. Arch Fam Med 7:559, 1998

Whittle WL, Singh SS, Allen L, et al: Laparoscopic cervico-isthmic cerclage: surgical technique and obstetric outcomes. Am J Obstet Gynecol 201:364.e1, 2009

Wijesiriwardana A, Bhattacharya S, Shetty A, et al: Obstetric outcome in women with threatened miscarriage in the first trimester. Obstet Gynecol 107:557, 2006

Wilcox AF, Weinberg CR, O'Connor JF, et al: Incidence of early loss of pregnancy. N Engl J Med 319:189, 1988

Williams Z: Inducing tolerance to pregnancy. N Engl J Med 367(12):1159, 2012

Winikoff B, Dzuba IG, Creinin MD, et al: Two distinct oral routes of misoprostol in mifepristone medical abortion: a randomized controlled trial. Obstet Gynecol 112(6):1303, 2008

Witter FR: Negative sonographic findings followed by rapid cervical dilatation due to cervical incompetence. Obstet Gynecol 64:136, 1984

Wo JY, Viswanathan AN: Impact of radiotherapy on fertility, pregnancy, and neonatal outcomes in female cancer patients. Int J Radiat Oncol Biol Phys 73(5):1304, 2009

Woo J, Arrabal P, O'Reilly G: Pregnancy outcome after placement of reinforcement cerclage. Abstract No. 798, Am J Obstet Gynecol 208(1 Suppl):S335, 2013

Word L, Hoffman BL: Surgeries for benign gynecologic conditions. In Hoffman BL, Schorge JO, Schaffer JI, et al: Williams Gynecology, 2nd ed. McGraw-Hill, New York, 2012

World Health Organization: The use of DDT in malaria vector control: WHO position statement. 2011. Available at: http://whqlibdoc.who.int/hq/2011/WHO_HTM_GMP_2011_eng.pdf. Accessed May 21, 2013

Wyatt PR, Owolabi T, Meier C, et al: Age-specific risk of fetal loss observed in a second trimester serum screening population. Am J Obstet Gynecol 192:240, 2005

Xiong X, Buekens P, Vastardis S, et al: Periodontal disease and pregnancy outcomes: state-of-the-science. Obstet Gynecol Surv 62(9):605, 2007

Yetman DL, Kutteh WH: Antiphospholipid antibody panels and recurrent pregnancy loss: prevalence of anticardiolipin antibodies compared with other antiphospholipid antibodies. Fertil Steril 66:540, 1996

Zaveri V, Aghajafari F, Amankwah K, et al: Abdominal versus vaginal cerclage after a failed transvaginal cerclage: a systematic review. Am J Obstet Gynecol 187:868, 2002

Zhang J, Gilles JM, Barnhart K, et al: A comparison of medical management with misoprostol and surgical management for early pregnancy failure. N Engl J Med 353:761, 2005

Zheteyeva Y, Moro PL, Xue X, et al: Safety of meningococcal polysaccharide-protein conjugate vaccine in pregnancy: a review of the Vaccine Adverse Event Reporting System. Am J Obstet Gynecol 208(6):478.e1, 2013

CHAPTER 19

Ectopic Pregnancy

Following fertilization and fallopian tube transit, the blastocyst normally implants in the endometrial lining of the uterine cavity. Implantation elsewhere is considered ectopic and comprises 1 to 2 percent of all first-trimester pregnancies in the United States. This small proportion disparately accounts for 6 percent of all pregnancy-related deaths (Berg, 2010; Stulberg, 2013). In addition, the chance for a subsequent successful pregnancy is reduced after an ectopic pregnancy. Fortunately, urine and serum beta-human chorionic gonadotropin (β-hCG) assays and transvaginal sonography have made earlier diagnosis possible. And as a result, both maternal survival rates and conservation of reproductive capacity are improved.

TUBAL PREGNANCY

Classification

Nearly 95 percent of ectopic pregnancies are implanted in the various segments of the fallopian tube and give rise to fimbrial, ampullary, isthmic, or interstitial tubal pregnancies (Fig. 19-1). As shown, the ampulla is the most frequent site, followed by the isthmus. The remaining 5 percent of nontubal ectopic pregnancies implant in the ovary, peritoneal cavity, cervix, or prior cesarean scar. Occasionally, a multifetal pregnancy is composed of one conceptus with normal uterine implantation coexisting with one implanted ectopically. The natural incidence of these *heterotopic pregnancies* approximates 1 per 30,000 pregnancies. However, because of assisted reproductive technologies (ART), their incidence has increased to 1 in 7000 overall, and following ovulation induction, it may be as high as 0.5 to 1 percent (Mukul, 2007). Rarely, twin tubal pregnancy with both embryos in the same tube or with one in each tube has been reported (Eze, 2012; Svirsky, 2010).

Regardless of location, D-negative women with an ectopic pregnancy who are not sensitized to D-antigen should be given IgG anti-D immunoglobulin (American College of Obstetricians and Gynecologists, 2013). In first-trimester pregnancies, a 50-μg or a 300-μg dose is appropriate, whereas a standard 300-μg dose is used for later gestations.

Risks

Abnormal fallopian tube anatomy underlies many cases of tubal ectopic pregnancy. Surgeries for a prior tubal pregnancy, for fertility restoration, or for sterilization confer the highest risk of tubal implantation. After one previous ectopic pregnancy, the chance of another approximates 10 percent (Ankum, 1996; Skjeldestad, 1998). Prior sexually transmitted disease or other tubal infection, which can distort normal tubal anatomy, is another common risk factor. Specifically, one episode of salpingitis can be followed by a subsequent ectopic pregnancy in up to 9 percent of women (Westrom, 1992). Similarly, peritubal adhesions subsequent to salpingitis, appendicitis, or endometriosis may increase the risk for tubal pregnancy. Salpingitis isthmica nodosa, which is a condition in which epithelium-lined diverticula extend into a hypertrophied muscularis layer,

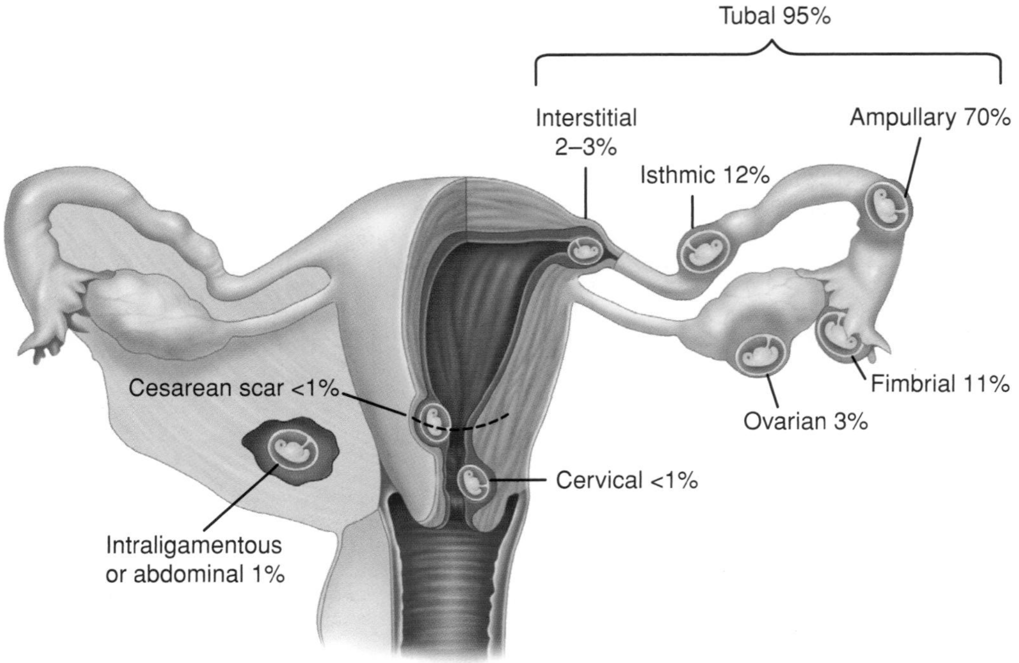

FIGURE 19-1 Sites of implantation of 1800 ectopic pregnancies from a 10-year population-based study. (Data from Callen, 2000; Bouyer, 2003.)

also poses an increased risk (Schippert, 2012). Congenital fallopian tube anomalies, especially those secondary to in utero diethylstilbestrol exposure, can also lead to malformed tubes and higher ectopic rates (Hoover, 2011).

Infertility, per se, as well as the use of ART to overcome it, is linked to substantively increased risks for ectopic pregnancy (Clayton, 2006). And "atypical" implantations—cornual, abdominal, cervical, ovarian, and heterotopic pregnancy—are more common following ART procedures. Smoking is also a known association, although the underlying mechanism is unclear (Waylen, 2009). Last, with any form of contraception, the absolute number of ectopic pregnancies is decreased because pregnancy occurs less often. However, with some contraceptive method failures, the relative number of ectopic pregnancies is increased. Examples include tubal sterilization, copper and progestin-releasing intrauterine devices (IUDs), and progestin-only contraceptives (Furlong, 2002).

Evolution and Potential Outcomes

With tubal pregnancy, because the fallopian tube lacks a submucosal layer, the fertilized ovum promptly burrows through the epithelium. The zygote comes to lie near or within the muscularis, which is invaded in most cases by rapidly proliferating trophoblast. The embryo or fetus in an ectopic pregnancy is often absent or stunted.

Outcomes of ectopic pregnancy include tubal rupture, tubal abortion, or pregnancy failure with resolution. With rupture, the invading expanding products of conception and associated hemorrhage may tear rents in the fallopian tube at any of several sites. As a rule, if the tube ruptures in the first few weeks, the pregnancy is most likely located in the isthmic portion, whereas the ampulla is slightly more distensible (Fig. 19-2). However, if the fertilized ovum implants within the interstitial portion, rupture usually occurs later. Tubal ectopic pregnancies usually burst spontaneously but may occasionally rupture following coitus or bimanual examination.

Alternatively, the pregnancy may abort out the distal fallopian tube, and the frequency of this depends in part on the initial implantation site. Abortion is common in fimbrial and ampullary pregnancies, whereas rupture is the usual outcome with those in the tubal isthmus. With tubal abortion, hemorrhage disrupts the connection between the placenta and membranes and the tubal wall. If placental separation is complete,

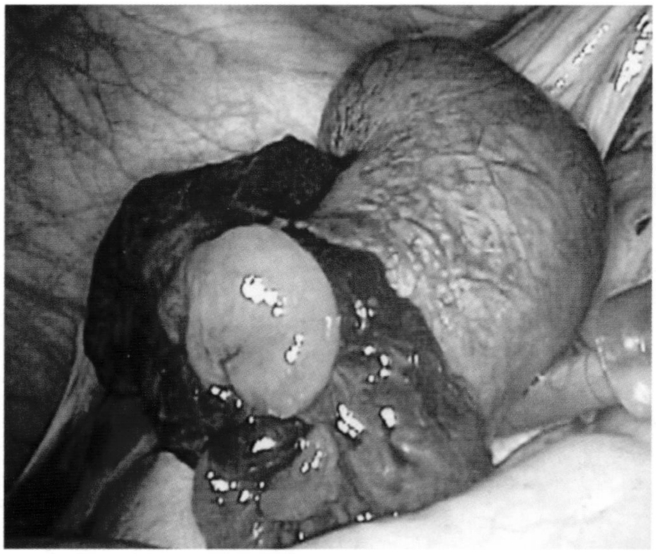

FIGURE 19-2 Ruptured ampullary early tubal pregnancy. (Photograph contributed by Dr. Togas Tulandi.)

the entire conceptus may be extruded through the fimbriated end into the peritoneal cavity. At this point, hemorrhage may cease and symptoms eventually disappear. Some bleeding usually persists as long as products remain in the tube. Blood slowly trickles from the tubal fimbria into the peritoneal cavity and typically pools in the rectouterine cul-de-sac. If the fimbriated extremity is occluded, the fallopian tube may gradually become distended by blood, forming a hematosalpinx.

Last, an unknown number of ectopic pregnancies spontaneously fail and are reabsorbed. This may be documented now more regularly with the advent of sensitive β-hCG assays.

There are differences between "acute" ectopic pregnancy just described and "chronic" ectopic pregnancy. The more common acute ectopic pregnancies are those with a high serum β-hCG level and rapid growth, leading to an immediate diagnosis. These carry a higher risk of tubal rupture (Barnhart, 2003c). With chronic ectopic pregnancy, abnormal trophoblast die early, and thus negative or lower, static serum β-hCG levels are found (Brennan, 2000). Chronic ectopic pregnancies typically rupture late, if at all, but commonly form a complex pelvic mass, which often is the reason prompting diagnostic surgery (Cole, 1982; Grynberg, 2009; Uğur, 1996).

Clinical Manifestations

Earlier patient presentation and more precise diagnostic technology typically allow identification before rupture. In these cases, symptoms and signs of ectopic pregnancy are often subtle or even absent. The woman does not suspect tubal pregnancy and assumes that she has a normal early pregnancy or is having a miscarriage.

With later diagnosis, a "classic" presentation is characterized by the triad of delayed menstruation, pain, and vaginal bleeding or spotting. With tubal rupture, there is usually severe lower abdominal and pelvic pain that is frequently described as sharp, stabbing, or tearing. There is tenderness during abdominal palpation. Bimanual pelvic examination, especially cervical motion, causes exquisite pain. The posterior vaginal fornix may bulge from blood in the rectouterine cul-de-sac, or a tender, boggy mass may be felt to one side of the uterus. Although minimal early, later the uterus may be pushed to one side by an ectopic mass. The uterus may also be slightly enlarged due to hormonal stimulation. Symptoms of diaphragmatic irritation, characterized by pain in the neck or shoulder, especially on inspiration, develop in perhaps half of women with sizable hemoperitoneum.

Some degree of vaginal spotting or bleeding is reported by 60 to 80 percent of women with tubal pregnancy. Although profuse vaginal bleeding is suggestive of an incomplete abortion, such bleeding occasionally is seen with tubal gestations. Moreover, tubal pregnancy can lead to significant intraabdominal hemorrhage. Responses to moderate bleeding include no change in vital signs, a slight rise in blood pressure, or a vasovagal response with bradycardia and hypotension. Birkhahn and colleagues (2003) noted that in 25 women with ruptured ectopic pregnancy, most at presentation had a heart rate < 100 beats per minute and a systolic blood pressure > 100 mm Hg. Blood pressure will fall and pulse will rise only if bleeding continues and hypovolemia becomes significant. Vasomotor disturbances develop, ranging from vertigo to syncope.

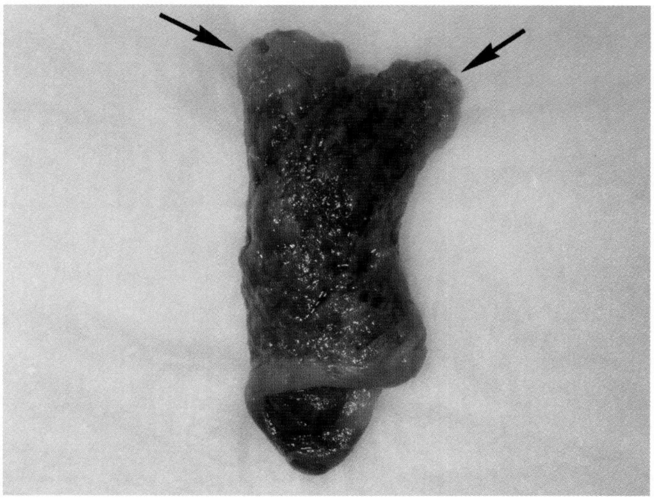

FIGURE 19-3 This decidual cast was passed by a patient with a tubal ectopic pregnancy. The cast mirrors the shape of the endometrial cavity, and each arrow marks the portion of decidua that lined the cornua.

Even after substantive hemorrhage, hemoglobin or hematocrit readings may at first show only a slight reduction. Hence, after an acute hemorrhage, a decline in hemoglobin or hematocrit level over several hours is a more valuable index of blood loss than is the initial level. In approximately half of women with a ruptured ectopic pregnancy, varying degrees of leukocytosis up to 30,000/μL may be documented.

Decidua is endometrium that is hormonally prepared for pregnancy, and the degree to which the endometrium is converted with ectopic pregnancy is variable. Thus, in addition to bleeding, women with ectopic tubal pregnancy may pass a *decidual cast*, which is the entire sloughed endometrium that takes the form of the endometrial cavity (Fig. 19-3). Importantly, decidual sloughing may also occur with uterine abortion. Thus, tissue should be carefully evaluated visually and then histologically for evidence of a conceptus. If no clear gestational sac is visually seen or if no villi are identified histologically within the cast, then the possibility of ectopic pregnancy must still be considered.

Multimodality Diagnosis

The differential diagnosis for abdominal pain coexistent with pregnancy is extensive. Pain may derive from uterine conditions such as miscarriage, infection, degenerating or enlarging leiomyomas, molar pregnancy, or round-ligament pain. Adnexal disease may include ectopic pregnancy; hemorrhagic, ruptured, or torsed ovarian masses; salpingitis; or tuboovarian abscess. Last, appendicitis, cystitis, renal stone, or gastroenteritis may be nongynecological sources of lower abdominal pain in early pregnancy.

A number of algorithms have been proposed to identify ectopic pregnancy. Most include these key components: physical findings, transvaginal sonography (TVS), serum β-hCG level measurement—both the initial and the subsequent pattern of rise or decline, and diagnostic surgery, which includes uterine curettage, laparoscopy, and occasionally, laparotomy (Fig. 19-4). Algorithm use applies only to hemodynamically stable women—those with presumed rupture should undergo

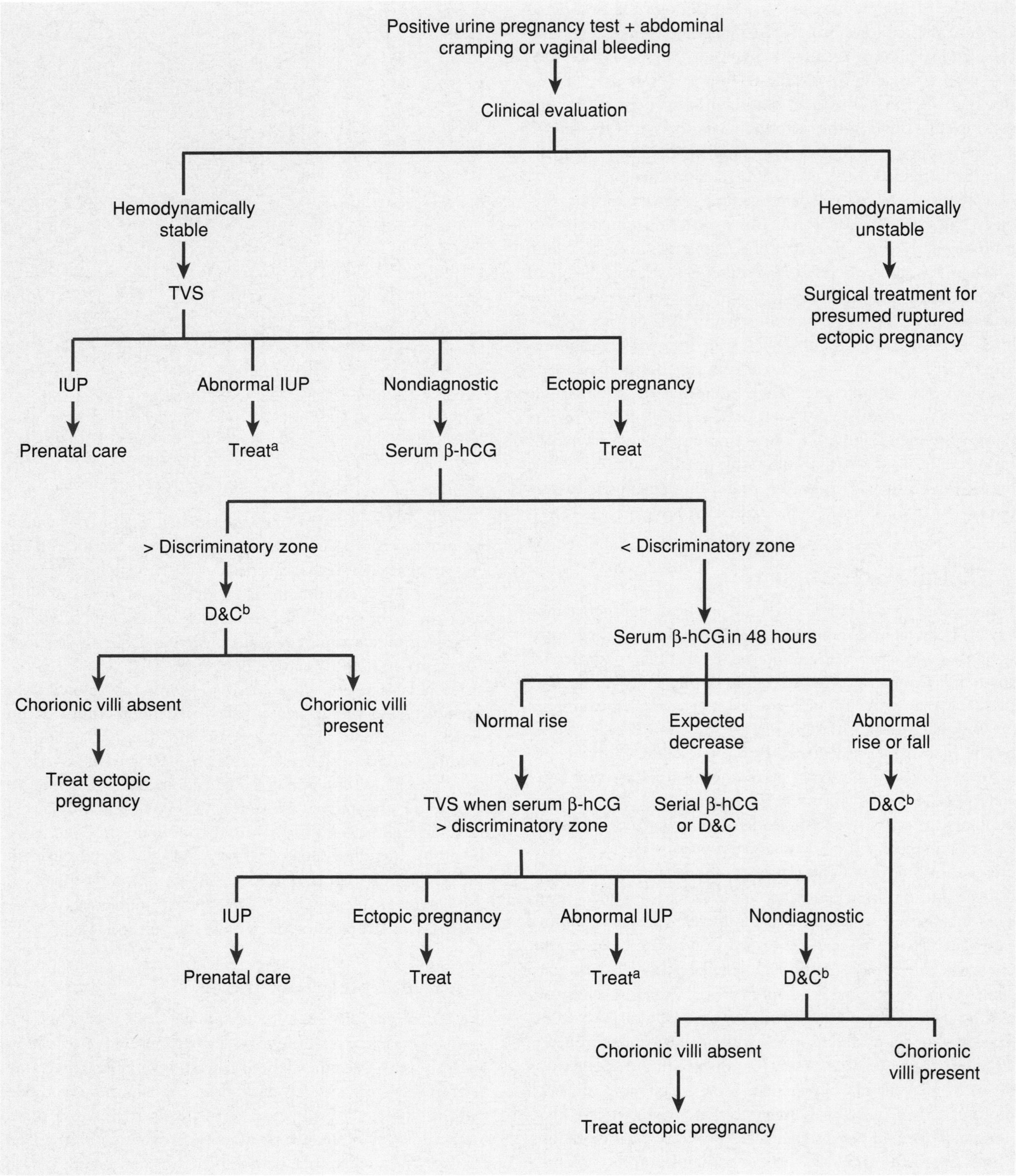

FIGURE 19-4 One suggested algorithm for evaluation of a woman with a suspected ectopic pregnancy. [a]Expectant management, D&C, or medical regimens are suitable options. [b]Serial serum β-hCG levels may be appropriate if a normal uterine pregnancy or if completed abortion is suspected clinically. β-hCG = beta human chorionic gonadotropin; D&C = dilatation and curettage; IUP = intrauterine pregnancy; TVS = transvaginal sonography. (Modified from Gala, 2012.)

prompt surgical therapy. For a suspected unruptured ectopic pregnancy, all diagnostic strategies involve trade-offs. Strategies that maximize detection of ectopic pregnancy may result in termination of a normal pregnancy. Conversely, those that reduce the potential for normal pregnancy interruption will delay ectopic pregnancy diagnosis. Patient desires for the index pregnancy are also discussed and may influence these trade-offs.

Beta Human Chorionic Gonadotropin

Rapid and accurate determination of pregnancy is essential to identify an ectopic pregnancy. Current serum and urine pregnancy tests that use enzyme-linked immunosorbent assays (ELISAs) for β-hCG are sensitive to levels of 10 to 20 mIU/mL and are positive in > 99 percent of ectopic pregnancies (Kalinski, 2002). Rare cases of chronic ectopic pregnancy, described earlier, with negative serum β-hCG assay results have been reported.

With bleeding or pain and a positive pregnancy test result, an initial TVS is typically performed to identify gestation location. If a yolk sac, embryo, or fetus is identified within the uterus or the adnexa, then a diagnosis can be made. In many cases however, TVS is nondiagnostic, and tubal pregnancy is still a possibility. In these cases in which neither intrauterine nor extrauterine pregnancy is identified, the term *pregnancy of unknown location (PUL)* is used until additional clinical information allows determination of pregnancy location.

Levels above the Discriminatory Zone. A number of investigators have described discriminatory β-hCG levels above which failure to visualize an intrauterine pregnancy (IUP) indicates that the pregnancy either is not alive or is ectopic. Barnhart and colleagues (1994) reported that an empty uterus with a serum β-hCG concentration ≥ 1500 mIU/mL was 100-percent accurate in excluding a live uterine pregnancy. Some institutions set their discriminatory threshold higher at ≥ 2000 mIU/mL. Moreover, Connolly and associates (2013) reported evidence to suggest an even higher threshold. They noted that with live uterine pregnancies, a gestational sac was seen 99 percent of the time with a discriminatory level of 3510 mIU/mL.

If the initial β-hCG level exceeds the set discriminatory level and no evidence for a uterine pregnancy is seen with TVS, then the diagnosis is narrowed in most cases to a failed uterine pregnancy, completed abortion, or an ectopic pregnancy. Early multifetal gestation also remains a possibility. If there is a suspicion in a stable patient that a PUL could be a normal pregnancy, it is prudent to continue expectant management with serial β-hCG level assessment to avoid harming an early normal pregnancy. If patient history or extruded uterine tissue suggests a completed abortion, then serial β-hCG levels will drop rapidly. Otherwise, curettage will distinguish an ectopic from a nonliving uterine pregnancy. Some do not recommend diagnostic curettage because it results in unnecessary surgical therapy (Barnhart, 2002). This is countered by concern for methotrexate toxicity if this drug is given erroneously to women with a presumed ectopic pregnancy.

Levels below the Discriminatory Zone. If the initial β-hCG level is below the set discriminatory value, pregnancy location is often not technically discernible with TVS. With these PULs, serial β-hCG level assays are done to identify patterns that indicate either a growing or failing uterine pregnancy. Levels that rise or fall outside these expected parameters increase the concern for ectopic pregnancy. Thus, appropriately selected women with a possible ectopic pregnancy, but whose initial β-hCG level is below the discriminatory threshold, are seen 2 days later for further evaluation. First, with early normal progressing uterine pregnancies, Kadar and Romero (1987) reported that mean doubling time for serum β-hCG levels was approximately 48 hours. The lowest normal value for this increase was 66 percent. Barnhart and coworkers (2004) reported a 53-percent 48-hour minimum rise with a 24-hour minimum rise of 24 percent. Seeber and associates (2006) used an even more conservative 35-percent 48-hour rise. Importantly, Silva and colleagues (2006) caution that a third of women with an ectopic pregnancy will have a 53-percent rise at 48 hours. They further reported that no single pattern characterizes ectopic pregnancy and that approximately half of ectopic pregnancies will show decreasing β-hCG levels, whereas the other half will have increasing levels.

With a failing intrauterine pregnancy, patterned rates of β-hCG level decline can also be anticipated. Rates of decline ranging between 21 and 35 percent are commonly used. As seen in Table 19-1, the percentage drop is greater if the initial β-hCG level is higher.

In pregnancies without these expected rises or falls in β-hCG levels, distinction between a nonliving intrauterine and an ectopic pregnancy may be aided by repeat β-hCG level evaluation (Zee, 2013). Also, uterine curettage is an option. Barnhart and associates (2003b) reported that endometrial biopsy was less sensitive than curettage. Before curettage, a second TVS examination may be indicated and may display new informative findings.

Serum Progesterone

A single serum progesterone measurement may clarify the diagnosis in a few cases (Stovall, 1989, 1992b). A value exceeding 25 ng/mL excludes ectopic pregnancy with 92.5-percent

TABLE 19-1. Expected Minimum Percentage Decline of Initial Serum β-hCG Levels to Subsequently Drawn Values for Nonliving Pregnancies

Initial hCG (mIU/mL)	By day 2: (% decline)	By day 4: (% decline)	By day 7: (% decline)
50	12	26	34
100	16	35	47
300	22	45	62
500	24	50	68
1000	28	55	74
2000	31	60	79
3000	33	63	81
4000	34	64	83
5000	35	66	84

Data from Barnhart, 2004; Chung, 2006.

sensitivity (Lipscomb, 1999a; Pisarska, 1998). Conversely, values below 5 ng/mL are found in only 0.3 percent of normal pregnancies (Mol, 1998). Thus, values < 5 ng/mL suggest either a nonliving uterine pregnancy or an ectopic pregnancy. Because in most ectopic pregnancies, progesterone levels range between 10 and 25 ng/mL, the clinical utility is limited (American College of Obstetricians and Gynecologists, 2012). One caveat is that pregnancy achieved with ART may be associated with higher than usual progesterone levels (Perkins, 2000).

A number of preliminary studies have been done to evaluate novel markers to detect ectopic pregnancy (Rausch, 2012; Senapati, 2013). However, none of these are in current clinical use.

Transvaginal Sonography

Endometrial Findings. In a woman in whom ectopic pregnancy is suspected, TVS is performed to look for findings indicative of intrauterine or ectopic pregnancy. During endometrial cavity evaluation, an intrauterine gestational sac is usually visible between 4½ and 5 weeks. The yolk sac appears between 5 and 6 weeks, and a fetal pole with cardiac activity is first detected at 5½ to 6 weeks (Fig. 9-3, p. 170). With transabdominal sonography, these structures are visualized slightly later.

In contrast, with ectopic pregnancy, a trilaminar endometrial pattern can be diagnostic (Fig. 19-5). Its specificity is 94 percent, but with a sensitivity of only 38 percent (Hammoud, 2005). In addition, Moschos and Twickler (2008b) determined that in women with PUL at presentation, no normal pregnancies had a stripe thickness < 8 mm.

Anechoic fluid collections, which might normally suggest an early intrauterine gestational sac, may also be seen with ectopic pregnancy. These include pseudogestational sac and decidual cyst. First, a pseudosac is a fluid collection between the endometrial layers and conforms to the cavity shape (see Fig. 19-5). If a pseudosac is noted, the risk of ectopic pregnancy is increased (Hill, 1990; Nyberg, 1987). Second, a decidual cyst is identified as an anechoic area lying within the endometrium

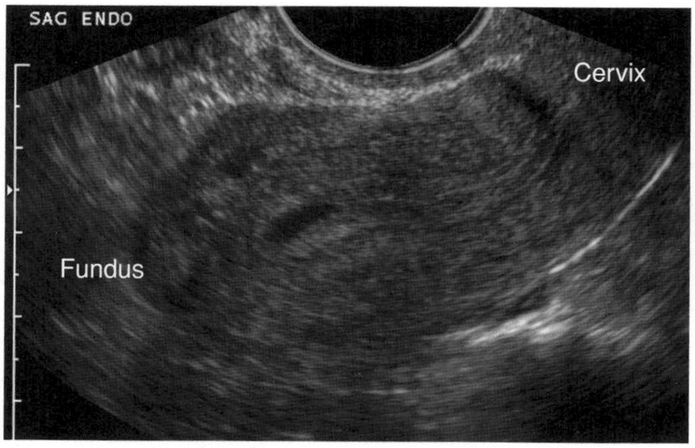

FIGURE 19-5 Transvaginal sonography of a pseudogestational sac within the endometrial cavity. Its cavity-conforming shape and central location are characteristic of these anechoic fluid collections. Distal to this fluid, the endometrial stripe has a trilaminar pattern, which is a common finding with ectopic pregnancy. (Image contributed by Dr. Elysia Moschos.)

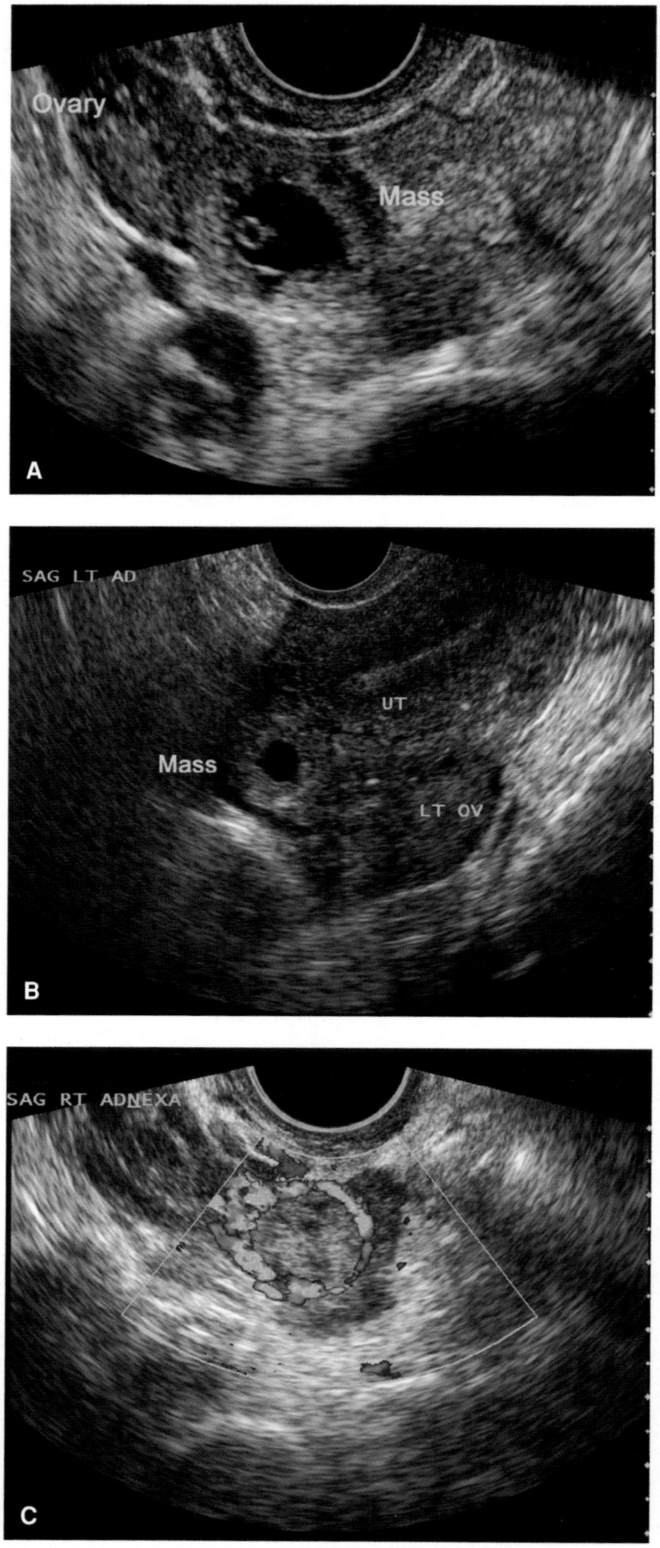

FIGURE 19-6 Various transvaginal sonographic findings with ectopic tubal pregnancies. For sonographic diagnosis, an ectopic mass should be seen in the adnexa separate from the ovary and may be seen as: **(A)** a yolk sac (shown here) and/or fetal pole with or without cardiac activity within an extrauterine sac, **(B)** an empty extrauterine sac with a hyperechoic ring, or **(C)** an inhomogeneous adnexal mass. In this last image, color Doppler shows a classic "ring of fire," which reflects increased vascularity typical of ectopic pregnancies. LT OV = left ovary; SAG LT AD = sagittal left adnexal; UT = uterus.

but remote from the canal and often at the endometrial-myometrial border. Ackerman and colleagues (1993b) suggested that this finding represents early decidual breakdown and precedes decidual cast formation.

These two findings contrast with the intradecidual sign seen with intrauterine pregnancy. This is an early gestational sac and is eccentrically located within one of the endometrial stripe layers (Dashefsky, 1988). The American College of Obstetricians and Gynecologists (2011) advises caution in diagnosing a uterine pregnancy in the absence of a definite yolk sac or embryo.

Adnexal Findings. The sonographic diagnosis of ectopic pregnancy rests on visualization of an adnexal mass separate from the ovary (Fig. 19-6). If fallopian tubes and ovaries are visualized and an extrauterine yolk sac, embryo, or fetus is identified, then an ectopic pregnancy is clearly confirmed. In other cases, a hyperechoic halo or tubal ring surrounding an anechoic sac can be seen. Alternatively, an inhomogeneous complex adnexal mass is usually caused by hemorrhage within the ectopic sac or by an ectopic pregnancy that has ruptured into the tube. Overall, approximately 60 percent of ectopic pregnancies are seen as an inhomogeneous mass adjacent to the ovary; 20 percent appear as a hyperechoic ring; and 13 percent have an obvious gestational sac with a fetal pole (Condous, 2005). Importantly, not all adnexal masses represent an ectopic pregnancy, and integration of sonographic findings with other clinical information is necessary.

Placental blood flow within the periphery of the complex adnexal mass—the *ring of fire*—can be seen with transvaginal color Doppler imaging. Although this can aid in the diagnosis, this finding can also be seen with a corpus luteum of pregnancy, and differentiation can be challenging.

Hemoperitoneum. In women with suspected ectopic pregnancy, evaluation for hemoperitoneum can add valuable clinical information. More commonly, this is completed using sonography, but assessment can also be made by culdocentesis. Sonographically, hemoperitoneum is anechoic or hypoechoic fluid. Blood initially collects in the dependent retrouterine cul-de-sac, and then additionally surrounds the uterus as it fills the pelvis (Fig. 19-7). As little as 50 mL can be seen in the cul-de-sac using TVS, and transabdominal imaging helps to assess the hemoperitoneum extent. For example, with significant intraabdominal hemorrhage, blood will track up the pericolic gutters to fill Morison pouch near the liver. Free fluid in this pouch typically is not seen until accumulated blood reaches 400 to 700 mL (Branney, 1995; Rodgerson, 2001; Rose, 2004). Diagnostically, peritoneal fluid in conjunction with an adnexal mass is highly predictive of ectopic pregnancy (Nyberg, 1991). Importantly, however, a small amount of peritoneal fluid is physiologically normal.

Culdocentesis is a simple technique used commonly in the past to identify hemoperitoneum. The cervix is pulled outward and upward toward the symphysis with a tenaculum, and a long 18-gauge needle is inserted through the posterior vaginal fornix into the retrouterine cul-de-sac. If present, fluid can be aspirated. However, a failure to do so is interpreted only as unsatisfactory entry into the cul-de-sac and does not exclude ectopic pregnancy. Fluid containing fragments of old clots or bloody fluid that does not clot is compatible with the diagnosis of hemoperitoneum. In contrast, if the blood sample clots, it may have been obtained from an adjacent blood vessel or from a briskly bleeding ectopic pregnancy. A number of studies have challenged its usefulness, and culdocentesis has been largely replaced by TVS (Glezerman, 1992; Vermesh, 1990).

Laparoscopy

Direct visualization of the fallopian tubes and pelvis by laparoscopy offers a reliable diagnosis in most cases of suspected

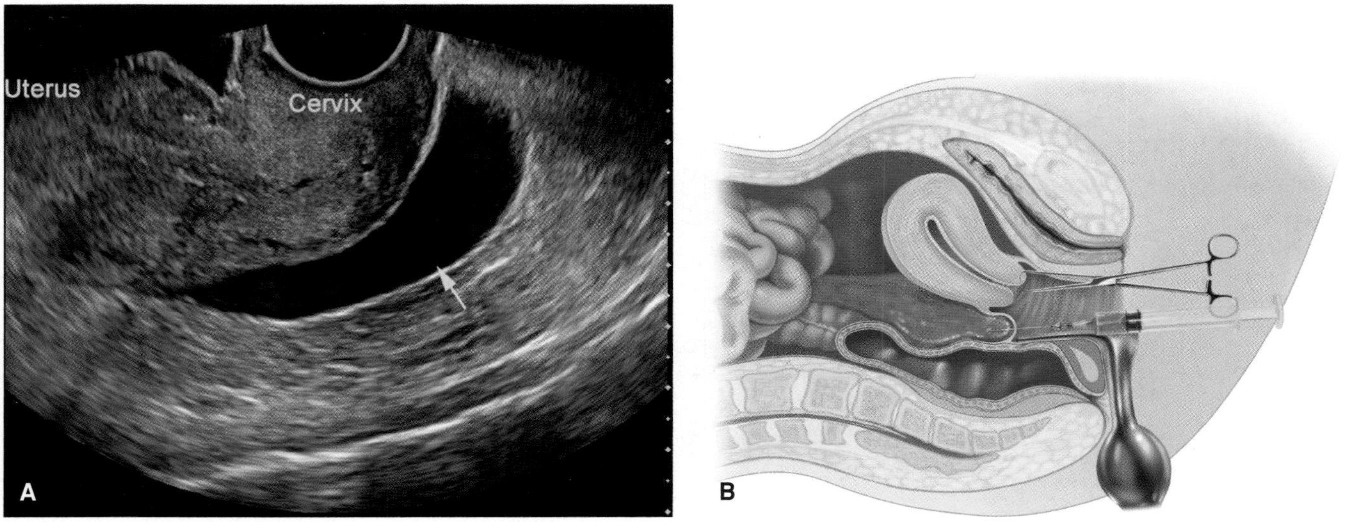

FIGURE 19-7 Techniques to identify hemoperitoneum. **A.** Transvaginal sonography of an anechoic fluid collection (*arrow*) in the retrouterine cul-de-sac. **B.** Culdocentesis: with a 16- to 18-gauge spinal needle attached to a syringe, the cul-de-sac is entered through the posterior vaginal fornix as upward traction is applied to the cervix with a tenaculum.

ectopic pregnancy. There is also a ready transition to definitive operative therapy, which is discussed subsequently.

Treatment Options

Options for ectopic tubal pregnancy treatment include medical and surgical approaches, and their comparison is discussed on page 387. Medical therapy traditionally involves the antimetabolite methotrexate. Surgical choices include mainly salpingostomy or salpingectomy.

Medical Management

Regimen Options

Methotrexate is a folic acid antagonist. It tightly binds to dihydrofolate reductase, blocking the reduction of dihydrofolate to tetrahydrofolate, which is the active form of folic acid. As a result, de novo purine and pyrimidine synthesis is halted, which leads to arrested DNA, RNA, and protein synthesis. Thus, methotrexate is highly effective against rapidly proliferating tissue such as trophoblast, and overall ectopic tubal pregnancy resolution rates approximate 90 percent with its use. However, bone marrow, gastrointestinal mucosa, and respiratory epithelium can also be harmed. It is directly toxic to hepatocytes and is renally excreted. Importantly, methotrexate is a potent teratogen, and methotrexate embryopathy is notable for craniofacial and skeletal abnormalities and fetal-growth restriction (Chap. 12, p. 248) (Nurmohamed, 2011). In addition, methotrexate is excreted into breast milk and may accumulate in neonatal tissues and interfere with neonatal cellular metabolism (American Academy of Pediatrics, 2001; Briggs, 2011). Based on all these findings, a list of contraindications and pretherapy laboratory testing is found in Table 19-2. Methotrexate is bound primarily to albumin, and its displacement by other medications such as phenytoin, tetracyclines, salicylates, and sulfonamides can increase methotrexate serum drug levels. Moreover, renal clearance of methotrexate may be impaired by nonsteroidal antiinflammatory drugs, probenecid, aspirin, or penicillins (Stika, 2012). Last, vitamins containing folic acid may lower methotrexate efficacy.

For ease and efficacy, intramuscular methotrexate administration is used most frequently for ectopic pregnancy resolution, and single-dose and multidose methotrexate protocols are available (see Table 19-2). As noted, methotrexate can lead to bone marrow depression. This toxicity can be blunted by early administration of leucovorin, which is folinic acid and has activity equivalent to folic acid. Thus, leucovorin, which is given within the multidose protocol, allows for some purine and pyrimidine synthesis to buffer side effects.

In comparing these two protocols, trade-offs are recognized. For example, single-dose therapy offers simplicity, less expense, and less intensive posttherapy monitoring and does not require leucovorin rescue. However, some but not all studies report a higher success rate for the multidose regimen (Alleyassin, 2006; Barnhart, 2003a; Lipscomb, 2005). At our institution, we use single-dose methotrexate.

A third hybrid "two dose" protocol has been proposed in an effort to balance the efficacy and convenience of the two most commonly used protocols (Barnhart, 2007). The regimen involves administering 50 mg/m^2 of methotrexate on days 0 and 4 without leucovorin rescue. Data are limited on its comparative efficacy with the two standard regimens, but one study showed single-dose to be as effective as the two-dose regimen (Gungorduk, 2011).

TABLE 19-2. Medical Treatment Protocols for Ectopic Pregnancy

	Single Dose	Multidose
Dosing	One dose; repeat if necessary	Up to four doses of both drugs until serum β-hCG declines by 15%
Medication Dosage		
Methotrexate	50 mg/m^2 BSA (day 1)	1 mg/kg, days 1, 3, 5, and 7
Leucovorin	NA	0.1 mg/kg days 2, 4, 6, and 8
Serum β-hCG level	Days 1 (baseline), 4, and 7	Days 1, 3, 5, and 7
Indication for additional dose	If serum β-hCG level does not decline by 15% from day 4 to day 7 Less than 15% decline during weekly surveillance	If serum β-hCG declines < 15%, give additional dose; repeat serum β-hCG in 48 hours and compare with previous value; maximum four doses
Posttherapy surveillance	Weekly until serum β-hCG undetectable	
	Methotrexate Contraindications	
Sensitivity to MTX Evidence of tubal rupture Breast feeding	Intrauterine pregnancy Hepatic, renal, or hematological dysfunction	Peptic ulcer disease Active pulmonary disease Evidence of immunodeficiency

BSA = body surface area; β-hCG = β-human chorionic gonadotropin; MTX = methotrexate; NA = not applicable.
From American College of Obstetricians and Gynecologists, 2012; Practice Committee of American Society for Reproductive Medicine, 2013.

Patient Selection

The best candidate for medical therapy is the woman who is asymptomatic, motivated, and compliant. With medical therapy, some classic predictors of success include a low initial serum β-hCG level, small ectopic pregnancy size, and absent fetal cardiac activity. Of these, initial serum β-hCG level is the single best prognostic indicator of successful treatment with single-dose methotrexate. Specifically, reported failure rates are 1.5 percent if the initial serum β-hCG concentration is < 1000 mIU/mL; 5.6 percent with 1000 to 2000 mIU/mL; 3.8 percent with 2000 to 5000 mIU/mL; and 14.3 percent when levels are between 5000 and 10,000 mIU/mL (Menon, 2007). Interestingly, the initial serum β-hCG value is not a valid indicator of the number of doses needed for successful resolution (Nowak-Markwitz, 2009).

Many early trials also used "large size" as an exclusion criterion, although these data are less precise. Lipscomb and colleagues (1998) reported a 93-percent success rate with single-dose methotrexate when the ectopic mass was < 3.5 cm. This compared with success rates between 87 and 90 percent when the mass was > 3.5 cm. Last, most studies report increased failure rates if there is cardiac activity. Lipscomb and colleagues (1998) reported an 87-percent success rate in such cases.

Treatment Side Effects

These regimens are associated with minimal laboratory changes and symptoms, although occasional toxicity may be severe. Kooi and Kock (1992) reviewed 16 studies and reported that adverse effects were resolved by 3 to 4 days after methotrexate was discontinued. The most common were liver involvement—12 percent, stomatitis—6 percent, and gastroenteritis—1 percent. One woman had bone marrow depression. Regarding long-term effects, Oriol and coworkers (2008), using antimüllerian hormone assays, concluded that ovarian reserve was not compromised by single-dose methotrexate therapy.

Importantly, 65 to 75 percent of women initially given methotrexate will have increasing pain beginning several days after therapy. This separation pain generally is mild and relieved by analgesics. In a series of 258 methotrexate-treated women by Lipscomb and colleagues (1999b), 20 percent had pain severe enough to require evaluation in the clinic or emergency room. Ultimately, 10 of these 53 underwent surgical exploration. Said another way, 20 percent of women given single-dose methotrexate will have significant pain, and 20 percent of these will require laparoscopy.

Overall, the failure rate is similar for either medical or surgical management. In three randomized trials, 5 to 14 percent of women treated initially with methotrexate ultimately required surgery, whereas 4 to 20 percent of those undergoing laparoscopic resection eventually received methotrexate for persistent trophoblast (Fernandez, 1998; Hajenius, 1997, 2007; Saraj, 1998). Rupture of persistent ectopic pregnancy is the worst form of primary therapy failure and occurs in 5 to 10 percent of women treated medically. Lipscomb and associates (1998) described a 14-day mean time to rupture, but one woman had tubal rupture 32 days after single-dose methotrexate.

Monitoring Therapy Efficacy

Serum β-hCG levels are used to monitor response to both medical and surgical therapy. After linear salpingostomy, serum β-hCG levels decline rapidly over days and then more gradually, with a mean resolution time of approximately 20 days. In contrast, after single-dose methotrexate, mean serum β-hCG levels increase for the first 4 days, and then gradually decline, with a mean resolution time of 27 days. Lipscomb and colleagues (1998) used single-dose methotrexate to successfully treat 287 women and reported that the average time to resolution—defined as a serum β-hCG level < 15 mIU/mL, was 34 days. Importantly, the longest time was 109 days.

As shown in Table 19-2, monitoring single-dose therapy calls for serum β-hCG determinations at days 4 and 7 following initial injection on day 1. If the level fails to drop more than 15 percent between days 4 and 7, then a second dose of methotrexate is required. This is necessary in 15 to 20 percent of women treated with single-dose therapy. With multidose methotrexate, levels are measured at 48-hour intervals until they fall more than 15 percent. Once appropriately dropping levels are achieved in either regimen, serum β-hCG determinations are then measured weekly until undetectable. Outpatient surveillance is preferred, but if there is any question of safety or compliance, the woman is hospitalized. Failure is judged when the β-hCG level plateaus or rises or tubal rupture occurs. Importantly, tubal rupture can occur in the face of declining β-hCG levels.

Surgical Management

Laparoscopy is the preferred surgical treatment for ectopic pregnancy unless a woman is hemodynamically unstable. There have been only a few prospective studies that compare laparotomy with laparoscopic surgery. Hajenius and associates (2007) performed a Cochrane Database review and found that subsequent uterine pregnancy rates and tubal patency rates in those treated with salpingostomy were comparable with either abdominal entry route. Subsequent ectopic pregnancies were fewer in women treated laparoscopically, although this was not statistically significant. As experience has accrued, cases previously managed by laparotomy—for example, ruptured tubal pregnancies or interstitial pregnancies—can safely be managed laparoscopically by those with suitable expertise. Before surgery, future fertility desires of the patient should be discussed. In those desiring permanent sterilization, the unaffected tube can be ligated concurrently with salpingectomy for the affected fallopian tube.

Tubal surgery is considered conservative when there is tubal salvage, such as with salpingostomy. Radical surgery is defined by salpingectomy. Some have shown conservative surgery may increase the rate of subsequent uterine pregnancy but is associated with higher rates of persistently functioning trophoblast (Bangsgaard, 2003; de Bennetot, 2012). This may not be the case, however. In a randomized controlled trial, Fernandez and associates (2013) evaluated 2-year rates of attaining an intrauterine pregnancy following either salpingostomy or salpingectomy. Although pregnancy rates with salpingectomy were 64 percent compared with 71 percent following salpingostomy, these differences were not statistically significant.

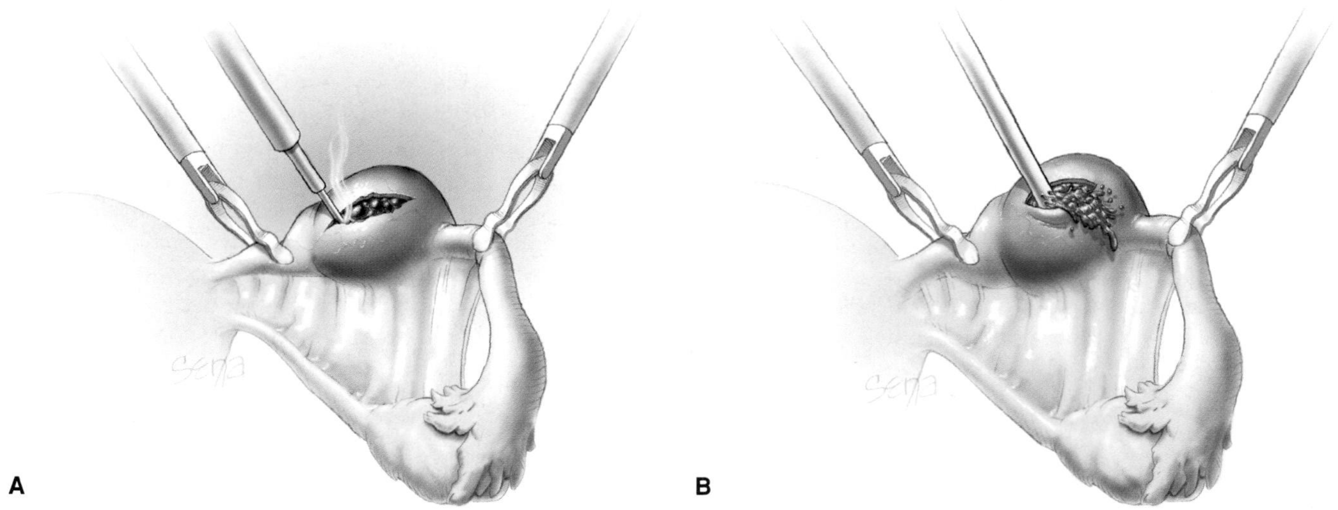

FIGURE 19-8 Linear salpingostomy for ectopic pregnancy. **A.** A linear incision for removal of a small tubal pregnancy is created on the antimesenteric border of the tube. **B.** Products of conception may be flushed from the tube using an irrigation probe. Alternatively, products may be removed with grasping forceps. Following evacuation of the tube, bleeding sites are treated with electrosurgical coagulation. The incision is not sutured. (From Thompson, 2012, with permission.)

Salpingostomy

This procedure is typically used to remove a small unruptured pregnancy that is usually < 2 cm in length and located in the distal third of the fallopian tube (Fig. 19-8). Natale and associates (2003) reported that serum β-hCG levels > 6000 mIU/mL are associated with a higher risk of implantation into the muscularis and thus with more tubal damage.

With surgery, a 10- to 15-mm linear incision is made on the antimesenteric border over the pregnancy. The products usually will extrude from the incision. These can be carefully removed or flushed out using high-pressure irrigation that more thoroughly removes the trophoblastic tissue (Al-Sunaidi, 2007). Small bleeding sites are controlled with needlepoint electrocoagulation, and the incision is left unsutured to heal by secondary intention.

Seldom performed today, salpingotomy is essentially the same procedure as salpingostomy except that the incision is closed with delayed-absorbable suture. According to Tulandi and Guralnick (1991), there is no difference in prognosis with or without suturing.

Salpingectomy

Tubal resection may be used for both ruptured and unruptured ectopic pregnancies. To minimize the rare recurrence of pregnancy in the tubal stump, complete excision of the fallopian tube is advised. With one laparoscopic technique, the affected fallopian tube is lifted and held with atraumatic grasping forceps (Thompson, 2012). One of several suitable bipolar grasping devices is placed across the fallopian tube at the uterotubal junction. Once desiccated, the tube is cut. The bipolar device is then advanced across the most proximal portion of mesosalpinx. Similarly, current is applied, and the desiccated tissue cut. This process moves serially from the proximal mesosalpinx to its distal extent under the tubal ampulla. Alternatively, an endoscopic suture loop can be used to encircle and ligate the knuckle of fallopian tube that contains the ectopic pregnancy and its underlying vascular supply within the mesosalpinx. Two consecutive suture loops are placed, and the tube distal to these ligatures is then cut free with scissors.

Most tubal ectopic pregnancies are small and pliant. Accordingly, they can be held firmly by grasping forceps and drawn up into one of the accessory site cannulas. Larger tubal ectopic pregnancies may be placed in an endoscopic sac to prevent fragmentation as they are removed through the laparoscopic port site. Importantly, to remove all trophoblastic tissue, the pelvis and abdomen should be irrigated and suctioned free of blood and tissue debris. Slow and systematic movement of the patient from Trendelenburg to reverse Trendelenburg positioning during irrigation can also assist in dislodging stray tissue and fluid. These should be suctioned and removed from the peritoneal cavity.

Persistent Trophoblast

Incomplete removal of trophoblast may result in persistent trophoblastic tissue. This complicates 5 to 20 percent of salpingostomies and can be identified by stable or rising β-hCG levels. Usually, β-hCG levels fall quickly and are at approximately 10 percent of preoperative values by day 12 (Hajenius, 1995; Vermesh, 1988). Also, if the postoperative day 1 serum β-hCG value is less than 50 percent of the preoperative value, then persistent trophoblast rarely is a problem (Spandorfer, 1997). According to Seifer (1997), factors that increase the risk of persisting trophoblast include: pregnancies less than 2 cm, early pregnancy less than 42 menstrual days, serum β-hCG level > 3000 mIU/mL, or implantation medial to the salpingostomy site. With stable or increasing β-hCG levels, additional surgical or medical therapy is necessary. Currently, standard therapy for this is single-dose methotrexate, 50 mg/m^2 × body surface area (BSA). To prevent persistent trophoblastic tissue, some advocate postoperative administration of "prophylactic" methotrexate with a dose of 1 mg/m^2 BSA (Akira, 2008; Graczykowski, 1997).

Medical versus Surgical Therapy

Several randomized trials have compared methotrexate treatment with laparoscopic surgery. One multicenter trial compared a multidose methotrexate protocol with laparoscopic salpingostomy and found no differences for tubal preservation and primary treatment success (Hajenius, 1997). However, in this same study group, health-related quality of life factors such as pain, posttherapy depression, and decreased perception of health were significantly impaired after systemic methotrexate compared with laparoscopic salpingostomy (Nieuwkerk, 1998). In their randomized controlled trial, Fernandez and coworkers (2013) compared multidose medical therapy against salpingostomy and found that medical and conservative surgery provided similar 2-year rates of attaining an intrauterine pregnancy.

There is conflicting evidence when single-dose methotrexate is compared with surgical intervention. In two separate studies, single-dose methotrexate was overall less successful in resolving pregnancy than laparoscopic salpingostomy, although tubal patency and subsequent uterine pregnancy rates were similar between both groups (Fernandez, 1998; Sowter, 2001). Women treated with methotrexate had significantly better physical functioning immediately following therapy, but there were no differences in psychological functioning. Krag Moeller and associates (2009) reported the results from their randomized trial that had a median surveillance period of 8.6 years during which future pregnancy rates were evaluated. Ectopic-resolution success rates were not significantly different between those managed surgically and those treated with methotrexate. Moreover, cumulative spontaneous intrauterine pregnancy rates were not different between the methotrexate group (73 percent) and the surgical group (62 percent). Based on these studies, we conclude that women who are hemodynamically stable and in whom there is a small tubal diameter, no fetal cardiac activity, and serum β-hCG concentrations < 5000 mIU/mL have similar outcomes with medical or surgical management. Despite lower success rates with medical therapy for women with larger tubal size, higher serum β-hCG levels, and fetal cardiac activity, medical management can be offered to the motivated woman who understands the risks.

Expectant Management

In select cases, it is reasonable to observe very early tubal pregnancies that are associated with stable or falling serum β-hCG levels. As many as a third of such women will present with declining β-hCG levels (Shalev, 1995). Stovall and Ling (1992a) restrict expectant management to women with tubal ectopic pregnancies only, decreasing serial β-hCG levels, diameter of the ectopic mass ≤ 3.5 cm, and no evidence of intraabdominal bleeding or rupture by transvaginal sonography. Mavrelos and coworkers (2013) noted that almost one third of 333 tubal ectopic pregnancies measuring < 3 cm and with β-hCG levels < 1500 mIU/mL resolved without intervention. Noted by the American College of Obstetricians and Gynecologists (2012), 88 percent of ectopic pregnancies will resolve if the β-hCG is < 200 mIU/mL.

With expectant management, subsequent rates of tubal patency and intrauterine pregnancy are comparable with surgery and medical management. The potentially grave consequences of tubal rupture, coupled with the established safety of medical and surgical therapy, require that expectant therapy be undertaken only in appropriately selected and counseled women.

INTERSTITIAL PREGNANCY

Diagnosis

These pregnancies implant within the proximal tubal segment that lies within the muscular uterine wall (Fig. 19-9). Incorrectly, they may be called cornual pregnancies, but this term describes a conception that develops in the rudimentary horn of a uterus with a müllerian anomaly. Risk factors are similar to others

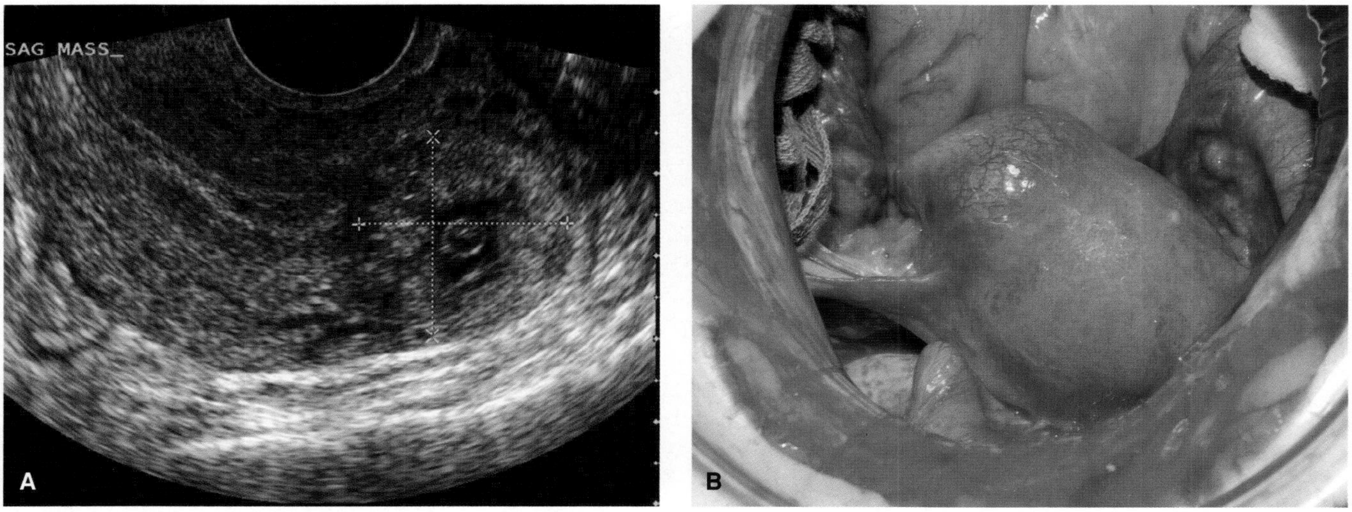

FIGURE 19-9 Interstitial ectopic pregnancy. **A.** This parasagittal view using transvaginal sonography shows an empty uterine cavity and a mass that is cephalad and lateral to the uterine fundus (*calipers*). **B.** Intraoperative photograph during laparotomy and before cornual resection of the same ectopic pregnancy. In this frontal view, the bulging right-sided interstitial ectopic pregnancy is lateral to the round ligament insertion and medial to the isthmic portion of the fallopian tube. (Photograph contributed by Drs. David Rogers and Elaine Duryea.)

discussed for tubal ectopic pregnancy, although previous ipsilateral salpingectomy is a specific risk factor for interstitial pregnancy (Lau, 1999). Undiagnosed interstitial pregnancies usually rupture following 8 to 16 weeks of amenorrhea, which is later than for more distal tubal ectopic pregnancies. This is due to greater distensibility of the myometrium covering the interstitial fallopian tube segment. Because of the proximity of these pregnancies to the uterine and ovarian arteries, there is a risk of severe hemorrhage, which is associated with mortality rates as high as 2.5 percent (Tulandi, 2004).

With TVS and serum β-hCG assays, interstitial pregnancy can now be diagnosed early in many cases, but diagnosis can be challenging. These pregnancies sonographically can appear similar to an eccentrically implanted intrauterine pregnancy, especially in a uterus with a müllerian anomaly. Criteria that may aid differentiation include: an empty uterus, a gestational sac seen separate from the endometrium and > 1 cm away from the most lateral edge of the uterine cavity, and a thin, < 5-mm myometrial mantle surrounding the sac (Timor-Tritsch, 1992). Moreover, an echogenic line, known as the "interstitial line sign," extending from the gestational sac to the endometrial cavity most likely represents the interstitial portion of the fallopian tube and is highly sensitive and specific (Ackerman, 1993a). In unclear cases, three-dimensional sonography, magnetic resonance (MR) imaging, or diagnostic laparoscopy may also provide clarification (Izquierdo, 2003; Parker, 2012). Laparoscopically, an enlarged protuberance lying outside the round ligament coexistent with normal distal fallopian tubes and ovaries is found.

Management

Surgical management with either cornual resection or cornuostomy may be performed via laparotomy or laparoscopy, depending on patient hemodynamic stability and surgeon expertise (Word, 2012; Zuo, 2012). With either approach, intraoperative intramyometrial vasopressin injection may limit surgical blood loss, and β-hCG levels should be monitored postoperatively to exclude remnant trophoblast. Cornual resection removes the gestational sac and surrounding cornual myometrium by means of a wedge excision (Fig. 19-10). Alternatively, cornuostomy involves incision of the cornua and suction or instrument extraction of the pregnancy.

With early diagnosis, conservative medical management may be considered. However, because of the low incidence, consensus regarding methotrexate route or regimen is lacking. In their small series, Jermy and associates (2004) reported a 94-percent success with systemic methotrexate using a dose of 50 mg/m^2 BSA. Others have described direct methotrexate injection into the gestational sac (Timor-Tritsch, 1996). Importantly, because these women typically have higher initial serum β-hCG levels at diagnosis, longer surveillance is usually needed.

The risk of uterine rupture with subsequent pregnancies following either medical or conservative surgical management is unclear. Thus, careful observation of these women during pregnancy, along with strong consideration of elective cesarean delivery, is warranted.

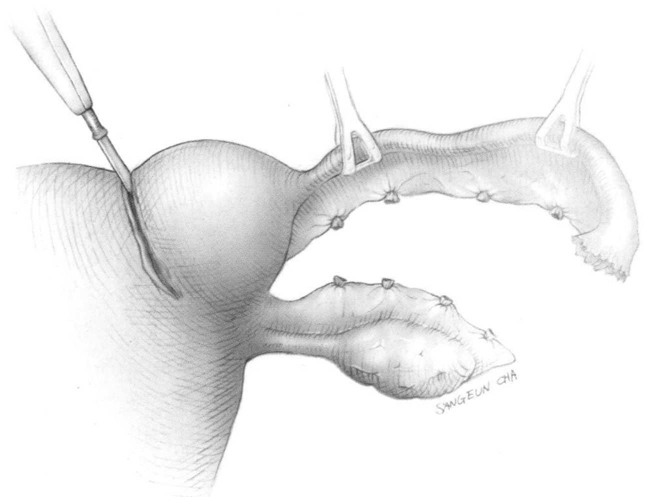

FIGURE 19-10 During cornual resection, the pregnancy, surrounding myometrium, and ipsilateral fallopian tube are excised en bloc. The incision is angled inward as it is deepened. This creates a characteristic wedge shape into the myometrium, which is then closed in layers with delayed-absorbable suture. The serosa is closed with subcuticular style suturing. (From Word, 2012, with permission.)

Distinct from interstitial pregnancy, the term *angular pregnancy* describes intrauterine implantation in one of the lateral angles of the uterus and medial to the uterotubal junction and round ligament. This distinction is important because angular pregnancies can sometimes be carried to term but with increased risk of abnormal placentation and its consequences (Jansen, 1981).

ABDOMINAL PREGNANCY

Diagnosis

Strictly defined, abdominal pregnancy is an implantation in the peritoneal cavity exclusive of tubal, ovarian, or intraligamentous implantations. These are rare ectopic pregnancies with an estimated incidence of 1 in 10,000 to 25,000 live births (Atrash, 1987; Worley, 2008). Although a zygote can traverse the tube and implant primarily in the peritoneal cavity, most abdominal pregnancies are thought to follow early tubal rupture or abortion with reimplantation. In cases of advanced extrauterine pregnancy, it is not unusual that the placenta is still at least partially attached to the uterus or adnexa (Fig. 19-11).

Diagnosis may be difficult. First, symptoms may be absent or vague. Laboratory tests are typically uninformative, although maternal serum alpha-fetoprotein levels may be elevated. Clinically, abnormal fetal positions may be palpated, or the cervix is displaced (Zeck, 2007). Sonographically, findings with an abdominal pregnancy may not be recognized, and the diagnosis is often missed (Costa, 1991). Oligohydramnios is common but nonspecific. Other clues include a fetus seen separate from the uterus or eccentrically positioned within the pelvis; lack of myometrium between the fetus and the maternal anterior abdominal wall or bladder; and extrauterine placental tissue

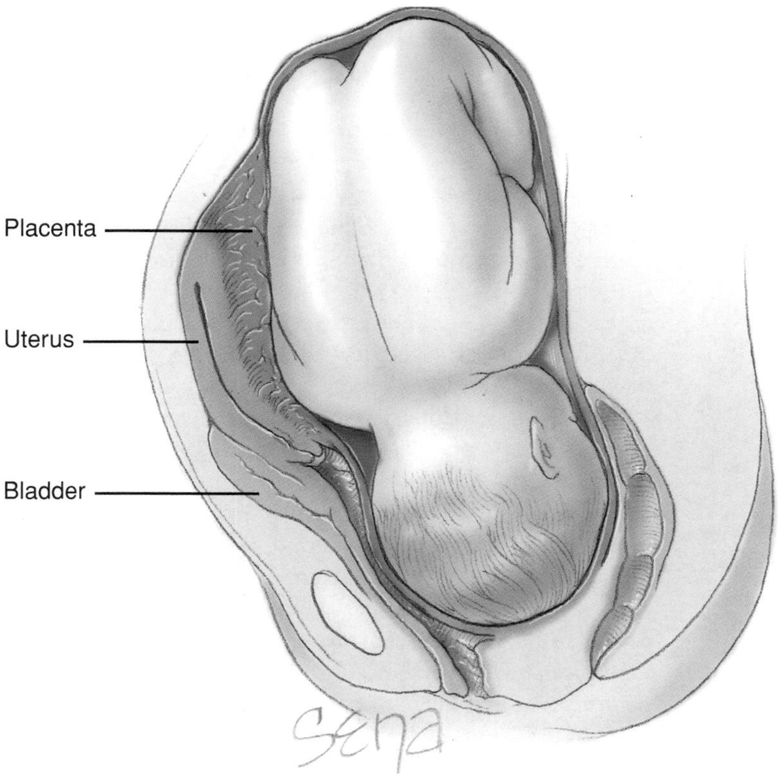

FIGURE 19-11 Sagittal view of an abdominal pregnancy at term. The placenta is implanted on the posterior surface of the uterus and broad ligament. The enlarged, flattened uterus is located just beneath the anterior abdominal wall and to the level of the umbilicus. The cervix and vagina are pulled up and are dislodged anteriorly and superiorly by the large fetal head in the cul-de-sac.

(Sherer, 2007). If additional anatomical information is needed, MR imaging can be used to confirm the diagnosis and provide maximal information concerning placental implantation (Bertrand, 2009; Mittal, 2012).

Management

An abdominal pregnancy can be life-threatening, and management depends on the gestational age at diagnosis. Some describe waiting until fetal viability with close surveillance (Gomez, 2008; Varma, 2003). Of note, Stevens (1993) reported fetal malformations and deformations in 20 percent. The most common malformations were limb deficiency and central nervous system anomalies. The most common deformations were facial and/or cranial asymmetry and various joint abnormalities. Conservative management also carries a maternal risk for sudden and dangerous hemorrhage. We are of the opinion that termination generally is indicated when the diagnosis is made. Certainly, before 24 weeks, conservative treatment rarely is justified.

Once placental implantation has been assessed, several options are available. Preoperative angiographic embolization has been used successfully in some women with advanced abdominal pregnancy. Alternatively, catheters placed in the uterine arteries may be inflated to decrease intraoperative blood loss. In either case, vascularization of ectopic placental implantation may be difficult to occlude. Other preoperative considerations include insertion of ureteral catheters, bowel preparation, assurance of sufficient blood products, and availability of a multidisciplinary surgical team or elective transfer to a tertiary care facility. In many ways, surgical management is similar to that for placenta percreta, which is detailed in Chapter 41 (p. 807).

The principal surgical objectives involve delivery of the fetus and careful assessment of placental implantation without provoking hemorrhage. Unnecessary exploration is avoided because the anatomy is commonly distorted and surrounding areas will be extremely vascular. Importantly, placental removal may precipitate torrential hemorrhage because the normal hemostatic mechanism of myometrial contraction to constrict hypertrophied blood vessels is lacking. If it is obvious that the placenta can be safely removed or if there is already hemorrhage from its implantation site, then removal begins immediately. When possible, blood vessels supplying the placenta should be ligated first.

Some advocate leaving the placenta in place as the lesser of two evils. It decreases the chance of immediate life-threatening hemorrhage, but at the expense of long-term sequelae. If left in the abdominal cavity, the placenta commonly becomes infected, with subsequent formation of abscesses, adhesions, intestinal or ureteral obstruction, and wound dehiscence (Bergstrom, 1998; Martin, 1988). In many of these cases, surgical removal becomes inevitable. If the placenta is left, its involution may be monitored using sonography and serum β-hCG levels (France, 1980; Martin, 1990). Color Doppler sonography can be used to assess changes in blood flow. In some cases, and usually depending on its size, placental function rapidly declines, and the placenta is resorbed. However, placental resorption may take years (Roberts, 2005; Valenzano, 2003).

If the placenta is left in place, postoperative methotrexate use is controversial. It has been recommended to hasten involution but has been reported to cause accelerated placental destruction with accumulation of necrotic tissue and infection with abscess formation (Rahman, 1982). It is difficult to envision a supporting role for the use of an antimetabolite for a senescent organ (Worley, 2008).

INTRALIGAMENTOUS PREGNANCY

In zygotes implanted toward the mesosalpinx, rupture may occur at the portion of the tube not immediately covered by peritoneum. The gestational contents may then be extruded into a space formed between the broad ligament leaves and become an intraligamentous or broad ligament pregnancy. These are rare, and information accrues from case reports (Seckin, 2011). Clinical findings and management mirror those for abdominal pregnancy. Although laparotomy is required in most instances, a few case reports describe laparoscopic excision of early small pregnancies (Apantaku, 2006; Cormio, 2006).

OVARIAN PREGNANCY

Ectopic implantation of the fertilized egg in the ovary is rare and is diagnosed if four clinical criteria are met. These were outlined by Spiegelberg (1878): (1) the ipsilateral tube is intact and distinct from the ovary; (2) the ectopic pregnancy occupies the ovary; (3) the ectopic pregnancy is connected by the uteroovarian ligament to the uterus; and (4) ovarian tissue can be demonstrated histologically amid the placental tissue (Fig. 19-12). Risk factors are similar to those for tubal pregnancies, but ART or IUD failure seems to be disproportionately associated (Ko, 2012). Presenting complaints and findings mirror tubal ectopic pregnancy. Although the ovary can accommodate the expanding pregnancy more easily than the fallopian tube, rupture at an early stage is the usual consequence.

TVS use has resulted in a more frequent diagnosis of unruptured ovarian pregnancies. Sonographically, an internal anechoic area is surrounded by a wide echogenic ring, which in turn is surrounded by ovarian cortex (Comstock, 2005). In their review of 49 cases, Choi and associates (2011) noted that the diagnosis may not be made until surgery as many cases are presumed tubal ectopic pregnancy. Moreover, at surgery, an early ovarian pregnancy may be considered to be a hemorrhagic corpus luteum cyst or a bleeding corpus luteum.

Evidence-based management accrues mainly from case reports (Hassan, 2012; Scutiero, 2012). Classically, management for ovarian pregnancies has been surgical. Small lesions have been managed by ovarian wedge resection or cystectomy, whereas larger lesions require oophorectomy. Finally, systemic or locally injected methotrexate has been used successfully to treat small unruptured ovarian pregnancies (Pagidas, 2013). With conservative surgery or medical management, β-hCG levels should be monitored to exclude remnant trophoblast.

CERVICAL PREGNANCY

Diagnosis

This ectopic pregnancy is defined by cervical glands noted histologically opposite the placental attachment site and by part or all of the placenta found below the entrance of the uterine vessels or below the peritoneal reflection on the anterior uterus. In a typical case, the endocervix is eroded by trophoblast, and the pregnancy develops in the fibrous cervical wall. The more cephalad that the trophoblast is implanted along the cervical canal, the greater is its capacity to grow and hemorrhage. The incidence of cervical pregnancy lies between 1 in 8600 and 1 in 12,400 pregnancies, but the incidence is increasing as a result of ART (Ginsburg, 1994). Another risk according to Jeng and colleagues (2007) is previous dilation and curettage.

Painless vaginal bleeding is reported by 90 percent of women with a cervical pregnancy—a third of these have massive hemorrhage (Ushakov, 1997). As pregnancy progresses, a distended, thin-walled cervix with a partially dilated external os may be evident. Above the cervical mass, a slightly enlarged uterine fundus can be felt. Identification of cervical pregnancy is based on speculum examination, palpation, and TVS. Sonographic findings typical of cervical pregnancy are shown and described in Figure 19-13. MR imaging and 3-D sonography have also been used to confirm the diagnosis (Jung, 2001; Sherer, 2008).

Management

Cervical pregnancy may be treated medically or surgically. In many centers, including ours, methotrexate has become the first-line therapy in stable women, and administration follows protocols listed in Table 19-2 (Verma, 2011; Zakaria, 2011). The drug has also been injected directly into the gestational sac, alone or with systemic doses (Jeng, 2007; Kirk, 2006). Others describe methotrexate infusion combined

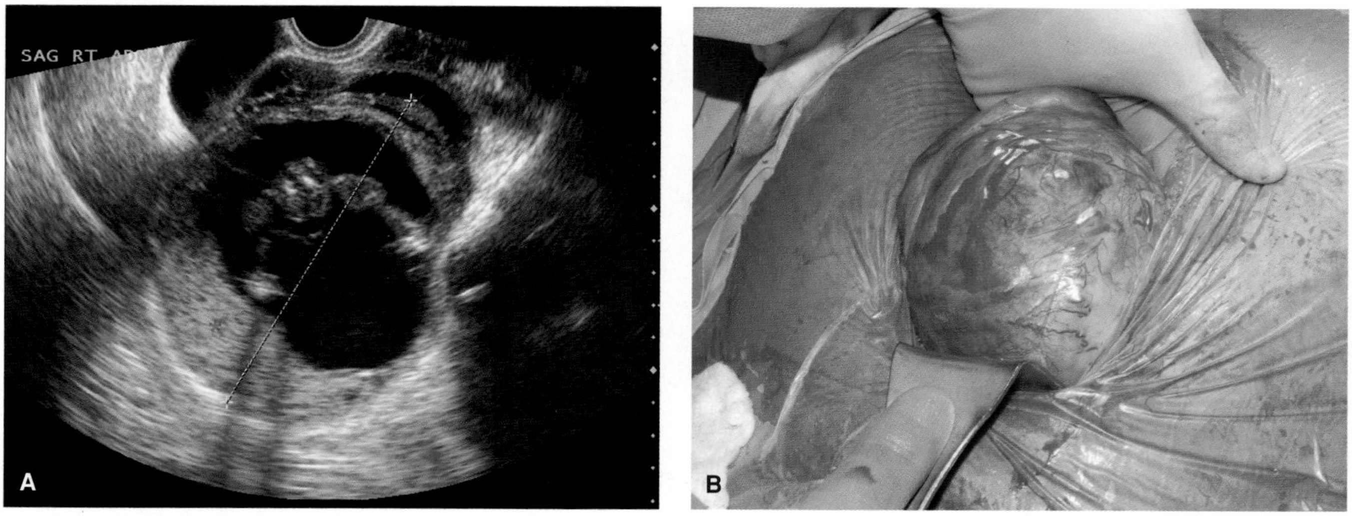

FIGURE 19-12 Ovarian pregnancy. **A.** Transvaginal sonogram shows a gestational sac containing fetal parts of a 16-week gestation. The placenta is marked by a red asterisk. **B.** Due to concern for extensive parasitic blood supply to the pregnancy, exploratory laparotomy was performed. Here, the right ovary is lifted by the surgeon, and the fallopian tube is the cordlike structure stretched across the top of the mass. Due to mass size and vascularity and scant normal ovarian stroma, this patient was treated by right salpingo-oophorectomy. (Photograph contributed by Dr. Kyler Elwell.)

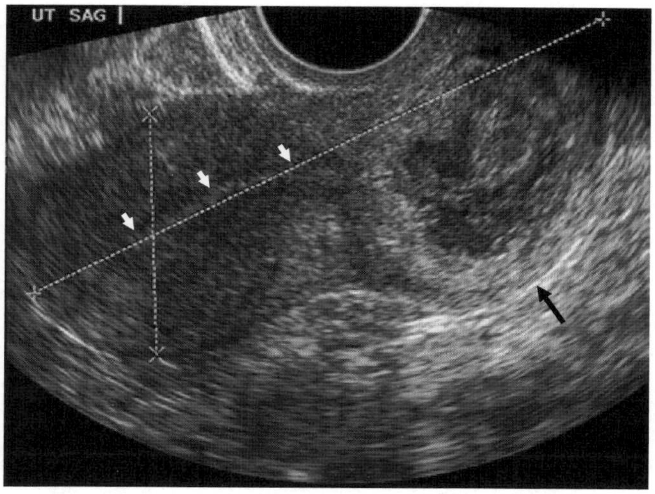

FIGURE 19-13 Cervical pregnancy. Transvaginal sonographic findings may include: (1) an hourglass uterine shape and ballooned cervical canal; (2) gestational tissue at the level of the cervix (*black arrow*); (3) absent intrauterine gestational tissue (*white arrows*); and (4) a portion of the endocervical canal seen interposed between the gestation and the endometrial canal. (Image contributed by Dr. Elysia Moschos.)

with uterine artery embolization (Xiaolin, 2010). With methotrexate regimens, resolution and uterine preservation are achieved for gestations < 12 weeks in 91 percent of cases (Kung, 1997). In selecting appropriate candidates, Hung and colleagues (1996) noted higher risks of systemic methotrexate treatment failure in those with a gestational age > 9 weeks, β-hCG levels > 10,000 mIU/mL, crown-rump length > 10 mm, and fetal cardiac activity. For this reason, many induce fetal death with intracardiac or intrathoracic injection of potassium chloride. With a single-dose intramuscular methotrexate protocol, a dose between 50 and 75 mg/m^2 BSA is typical. For women in whom fetal cardiac activity is detectable, a sonographically guided fetal intracardiac injection of 2 mL (2 mEq/mL) potassium chloride solution can be given (Verma, 2009). If β-hCG levels do not decline more than 15 percent after 1 week, a second dose of methotrexate can be given. Song and associates (2009) described management of 50 cases and observed that sonographic resolution lagged far behind serum β-hCG regression.

As an adjunct to medical or surgical therapy, uterine artery embolization has been described either as a response to bleeding or as a preprocedural preventive tool (Hirakawa, 2009; Nakao, 2008; Zakaria, 2011). The specifics of this interventional radiological technique are detailed in Chapter 41 (p. 820). Also in the event of hemorrhage, a 26F Foley catheter with a 30-mL balloon can be placed intracervically and inflated to effect hemostasis by vessel tamponade and to monitor uterine drainage. The balloon remains inflated for 24 to 48 hours and is gradually decompressed over a few days (Ushakov, 1997).

Although conservative management is feasible for many women with cervical pregnancies, suction curettage or hysterectomy may be selected. Moreover, hysterectomy may be required with bleeding uncontrolled by conservative methods. Unfortunately, due to the close proximity of the ureters to the ballooned cervix, urinary tract injury rates are of concern with hysterectomy.

Suction curettage may be especially favored in rare cases of a heterotopic pregnancy composed of a cervical and a desired uterine pregnancy (Moragianni, 2012). If cervical curettage is planned, intraoperative bleeding may be lessened by preoperative uterine artery embolization, by ligation of the descending branches of the uterine arteries, by vasopressin injection, or by a cerclage placed at the internal cervical os to compress feeding vessels (Davis, 2008; De La Vega, 2007; Trojano, 2009; Wang, 2011). Of these, cervical branches of the uterine artery can effectively be ligated with placement of hemostatic cervical sutures on the lateral aspects of the cervix at 3 and 9 o'clock. Cerclage placement is described in Chapter 18 (p. 361). Following curettage, a Foley balloon is placed to tamponade bleeding and is managed as described earlier.

CESAREAN SCAR PREGNANCY

This term describes implantation within the myometrium of a prior cesarean delivery scar. Its incidence approximates 1 in 2000 normal pregnancies and has increased alongside the cesarean delivery rate (Ash, 2007; Rotas, 2006). The pathogenesis of cesarean scar pregnancy (CSP) has been likened to that for placenta accreta and carries similar risk for serious hemorrhage (Timor-Tritsch, 2012a). It is unknown if the incidence increases with multiple cesarean deliveries or if it is affected by either one- or two-layer uterine incision closure.

Women with CSP usually present early, and pain and bleeding are common. However, up to 40 percent of women are asymptomatic, and the diagnosis is made during routine sonographic examination (Rotas, 2006). Rarely, early rupture can lead to an abdominal pregnancy (Teng, 2007).

Sonographically, differentiating between a cervicoisthmic intrauterine pregnancy and CSP can be difficult, and several investigators have described sonographic findings (Jurkovic, 2003; Moschos, 2008a). According to Godin (1997), there are four sonographic criteria that should be satisfied for the diagnosis, which are shown and described in Figure 19-14. Although TVS is the typical first-line imaging tool, MR imaging is useful when sonography is equivocal or inconclusive before intervention (Osborn, 2012).

Treatment standards are lacking, and several options are available. Hysterectomy is an acceptable initial choice in those desiring sterilization. It is sometimes a necessary option with heavy uncontrolled bleeding. Fertility-preserving options include systemic or locally injected methotrexate, either alone or combined with conservative surgery (Shen, 2012; Timor-Tritsch, 2012b; Yang, 2010). Surgeries include visually guided suction curettage or transvaginal aspiration, hysteroscopic removal, or isthmic excision. These are completed solely or more typically with adjunctive methotrexate (Michener, 2009; Seow, 2004, 2013; Timor-Tritsch, 2012a; Wang, 2009, 2012; Yang, 2009). Often uterine artery embolization is used preoperatively to minimize hemorrhage risk (Zhang, 2012; Zhuang, 2009).

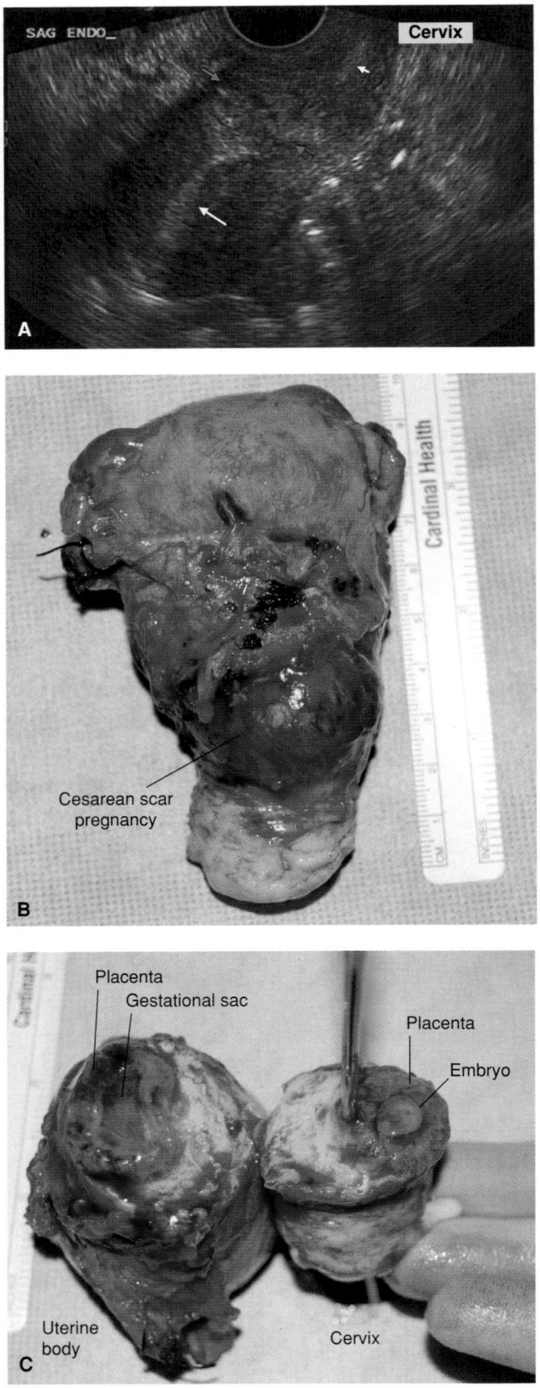

FIGURE 19-14 Cesarean scar pregnancy. **A.** Transvaginal sonogram of a uterus with a cesarean scar pregnancy (CSP) in a sagittal plane. An empty uterine cavity is identified by a bright hyperechoic endometrial stripe (*long, white arrow*). An empty cervical canal is similarly identified (*short, white arrow*). Last, an intrauterine mass is seen in the anterior part of the uterine isthmus (*red arrows*). Healthy myometrium between the bladder and gestational sac is absent. (Image contributed by Dr. Elysia Moschos.) **B.** Hysterectomy specimen containing a cesarean scar pregnancy. **C.** This same hysterectomy specimen is transversely sectioned at the level of the uterine isthmus and through the gestational sac. The uterine body lies to the left, and the cervix is on the right. A metal probe is placed through the endocervical canal to show the eccentric development of this gestation. Only a thin layer of myometrium overlies this pregnancy, which pushes anteriorly through the uterine wall. (Photographs contributed by Drs. Sunil Balgobin, Manisha Sharma, Rebecca Stone.)

OTHER SITES OF ECTOPIC PREGNANCY

Ectopic placental implantations in less expected sites have been described in case reports and include the omentum, spleen, liver, and retroperitoneum, among others (Chin, 2010; Chopra, 2009; Gang, 2010; Martínez-Varea, 2011). Also, intramural uterine implantations at sites other than a cesarean scar have been noted in women with prior uterine surgeries, ART, or adenomyosis (Memtsa, 2013; Wu, 2013). Although laparotomy is preferred by many for these ectopic sites, laparoscopic excision in hemodynamically stable patients by those with suitable skills is gaining acceptance.

REFERENCES

Ackerman TE, Levi CS, Dashefsky SM, et al: Interstitial line: sonographic finding in interstitial (cornual) ectopic pregnancy. Radiology 189(1):83, 1993a

Ackerman TE, Levi CS, Lyons EA, et al: Decidual cyst: endovaginal sonographic sign of ectopic pregnancy. Radiology 189(3):727, 1993b

Akira S, Negishi Y, Abe T, et al: Prophylactic intratubal injection of methotrexate after linear salpingostomy for prevention of persistent ectopic pregnancy. J Obstet Gynaecol Res 34:885, 2008

Alleyassin A, Khademi A, Aghahosseini M, et al: Comparison of success rates in the medical management of ectopic pregnancy with single-dose and multiple-dose administration of methotrexate: a prospective, randomized clinical trial. Fertil Steril 85(6):1661, 2006

Al-Sunaidi M, Tulandi T: Surgical treatment of ectopic pregnancy. Semin Reprod Med 25(2):117, 2007

American Academy of Pediatrics Committee on Drugs: Transfer of drugs and other chemicals into human milk. Pediatrics 108(3):776, 2001

American College of Obstetricians and Gynecologists: Ultrasonography in pregnancy. Practice Bulletin No. 101, February 2009, Reaffirmed 2011

American College of Obstetricians and Gynecologists: Medical management of ectopic pregnancy. Practice Bulletin No. 94, June 2008, Reaffirmed 2012

American College of Obstetricians and Gynecologists: Prevention of Rh D alloimmunization. Practice Bulletin No. 4, May 1999, Reaffirmed 2013

Ankum WM, Mol BWJ, Van der Veen F, et al: Risk factors for ectopic pregnancy: a meta-analysis. Fertil Steril 65:1093, 1996

Apantaku O, Rana P, Inglis T: Broad ligament ectopic pregnancy following in-vitro fertilisation in a patient with previous bilateral salpingectomy. J Obstet Gynaecol 26(5):474, 2006

Ash A, Smith A, Maxwell D: Caesarean scar pregnancy. BJOG 114:253, 2007

Atrash HK, Friede A, Hogue CJ: Abdominal pregnancy in the United States: Frequency and maternal mortality. Obstet Gynecol 69:333, 1987

Bakken IJ, Skjeldestad FE, Lydersen S, et al: Births and ectopic pregnancies in a large cohort of women tested for *Chlamydia trachomatis*. Sex Transm Dis 34:739, 2007a

Bakken IJ, Skjeldestad FE, Nordbo SA: *Chlamydia trachomatis* infections increase the risk for ectopic pregnancy: a population-based, nested case-control study. Sex Transm Dis 34:166, 2007b

Bangsgaard N, Lund CO, Ottesen B, et al: Improved fertility following conservative surgical treatment of ectopic pregnancy. Br J Obstet Gynaecol 110:765, 2003

Barnhart K, Hummel AC, Sammel MD, et al: Use of "2-dose" regimen of methotrexate to treat ectopic pregnancy. Fertil Steril 87(2):250, 2007

Barnhart K, Mennuti MT, Benjamin I, et al: Prompt diagnosis of ectopic pregnancy in an emergency department setting. Obstet Gynecol 84:1010, 1994

Barnhart KT, Gosman G, Ashby R, et al: The medical management of ectopic pregnancy: a meta-analysis comparing "single dose" and "multidose" regimens. Obstet Gynecol 101:778, 2003a

Barnhart KT, Gracia CR, Reindl B, et al: Usefulness of Pipelle endometrial biopsy in the diagnosis of women at risk for ectopic pregnancy. Am J Obstet Gynecol 188:906, 2003b

Barnhart KT, Katz I, Hummel A, et al: Presumed diagnosis of ectopic pregnancy. Obstet Gynecol 100:505, 2002

Barnhart KT, Rinaudo P, Hummel A, et al: Acute and chronic presentation of ectopic pregnancy may be two clinical entities. Fertil Steril 80:1345, 2003c

Barnhart KT, Sammel MD, Gracia CR, et al: Risk factors for ectopic pregnancy in women with symptomatic first-trimester pregnancies. Fertil Steril 86:36, 2006

Barnhart KT, Sammel MD, Rinaudo PF, et al: Symptomatic patients with an early viable intrauterine pregnancy: hCG curves redefined. Obstet Gynecol 104:50, 2004
Berg CJ, Callaghan WM, Syverson C, et al: Pregnancy-related mortality in the United States, 1998–2005. Obstet Gynecol 116:1302, 2010
Bergstrom R, Mueller G, Yankowitz J: A case illustrating the continued dilemmas in treating abdominal pregnancy and a potential explanation for the high rate of postsurgical febrile morbidity. Gynecol Obstet Invest 46:268, 1998
Bertrand G, Le Ray C, Simard-Émond L, et al: Imaging in the management of abdominal pregnancy: a case report and review of the literature. J Obstet Gynaecol Can 31(1):57, 2009
Birkhahn RH, Gaieta TJ, Van Deusen SK, et al: The ability of traditional vital signs and shock index to identify ruptured ectopic pregnancy. Am J Obstet Gynecol 189:1293, 2003
Bouyer J, Coste J, Shojaei T, et al: Risk factors for ectopic pregnancy: a comprehensive analysis based on a large case-control, population-based study in France. Am J Epidemiol 157:185, 2003
Branney SW, Wolfe RE, Moore EE, et al: Quantitative sensitivity of ultrasound in detecting free intraperitoneal fluid. J Trauma 40(6):1052, 1995
Brennan DF, Kwatra S, Kelly M, et al: Chronic ectopic pregnancy—two cases of acute rupture despite negative beta hCG. J Emerg Med 19(3):249, 2000
Briggs GG, Freeman RK, Yaffe SJ: Drugs in Pregnancy and Lactation, 9th ed. Philadelphia, Lippincott Williams & Wilkins, 2011, pp 928, 932
Callen PW (ed): Ultrasonography in Obstetrics and Gynecology, 4th ed. Philadelphia, WB Saunders, 2000, p 919
Chin PS, Wee HY, Chern BS: Laparoscopic management of primary hepatic pregnancy. Aust N Z J Obstet Gynaecol 50(1):95, 2010
Choi HJ, Im KS, Jung HJ, et al: Clinical analysis of ovarian pregnancy: a report of 49 cases. Eur J Obstet Gynecol Reprod Biol 158(1):87, 2011
Chopra S, Keepanasseril A, Suri V, et al: Primary omental pregnancy: case report and review of literature. Arch Gynecol Obstet 279(4):441, 2009
Chung K, Sammel M, Zhou L, et al: Defining the curve when initial levels of human chorionic gonadotropin in patients with spontaneous abortions are low. Fertil Steril 85:508, 2006
Clayton HB, Schieve LA, Peterson HB, et al: Ectopic pregnancy risk with assisted reproductive technology procedures. Obstet Gynecol 107(3):595, 2006
Cole T, Corlett RC Jr: Chronic ectopic pregnancy. Obstet Gynecol 59(1):63, 1982
Comstock C, Huston K, Lee W: The ultrasonographic appearance of ovarian ectopic pregnancies. Obstet Gynecol 105:42, 2005
Condous G, Okaro E, Khalid A, et al: The accuracy of transvaginal ultrasonography for the diagnosis of ectopic pregnancy prior to surgery. Hum Reprod 20(5):1404, 2005
Connolly A, Ryan DH, Stuebe AM, et al: Reevaluation of discriminatory and threshold levels for serum β-hCG in early pregnancy. Obstet Gynecol 121(1):65, 2013
Cormio G, Ceci O, Loverro G, et al: Spontaneous left broad ligament pregnancy after ipsilateral salpingo-oophorectomy. J Minim Invasive Gynecol 13(2):84, 2006
Costa SD, Presley J, Bastert G: Advanced abdominal pregnancy. Obstet Gynecol Surv 46:515, 1991
Davis LB, Lathi RB, Milki AA, et al: Transvaginal ligation of the cervical branches of the uterine artery and injection of vasopressin in a cervical pregnancy as an initial step to controlling hemorrhage: a case report. J Reprod Med 53(5):365, 2008
Dashefsky SM, Lyons EA, Levi CS, et al: Suspected ectopic pregnancy: endovaginal and transvesical US. Radiology 169:181, 1988
de Bennetot M, Rabischong B, Aublet-Cuvelier B, et al: Fertility following tubal ectopic pregnancy: results of a population-based study. Fertil Steril 98(5):1271, 2012
De La Vega GA, Avery C, Nemiroff R, et al: Treatment of early cervical pregnancy with cerclage, carboprost, curettage, and balloon tamponade. Obstet Gynecol 109(2 Pt 2):505, 2007
Eze JN, Obuna JA, Ejikeme BN: Bilateral tubal ectopic pregnancies: a report of two cases. Ann Afr Med 11(2):112, 2012
Fernandez H, Capmas P, Lucot JP, et al: Fertility after ectopic pregnancy: the DEMETER randomized trial. Hum Reprod 28(5):1247, 2013
Fernandez H, Yves Vincent SCA, Pauthier S, et al: Randomized trial of conservative laparoscopic treatment and methotrexate administration in ectopic pregnancy and subsequent fertility. Hum Reprod 13:3239, 1998
France JT, Jackson P: Maternal plasma and urinary hormone levels during and after a successful abdominal pregnancy. Br J Obstet Gynaecol 87:356, 1980
Furlong LA: Ectopic pregnancy risk when contraception fails. A review. J Reprod Med 47(11):881, 2002
Gala RB: Ectopic pregnancy. In Hoffman BL, Schorge JO, Schaffer JI, et al (eds): Williams Gynecology, 2nd ed. New York, McGraw-Hill, 2012, p 198
Gang G, Yudong Y, Zhang G: Successful laparoscopic management of early splenic pregnancy: case report and review of literature. J Minim Invasive Gynecol 17(6):794, 2010
Ginsburg ES, Frates MC, Rein MS, et al: Early diagnosis and treatment of cervical pregnancy in an in vitro fertilization program. Fertil Steril 61:966, 1994
Glezerman M, Press F, Carpman M: Culdocentesis is an obsolete diagnostic tool in suspected ectopic pregnancy. Arch Gynecol Obstet 252:5, 1992
Godin PA, Bassil S, Donnez J: An ectopic pregnancy developing in a previous caesarian section scar. Fertil Steril 67:398, 1997
Gomez E, Vergara L, Weber C, et al: Successful expectant management of an abdominal pregnancy diagnosed at 14 weeks. J Matern Fetal Neonatal Med 21(12):917, 2008
Graczykowski JW, Mishell DR Jr: Methotrexate prophylaxis for persistent ectopic pregnancy after conservative treatment by salpingostomy. Obstet Gynecol 89:118, 1997
Grynberg M, Teyssedre J, Andre C, et al: Rupture of ectopic pregnancy with negative serum beta-hCG leading to hemorrhagic shock. Obstet Gynecol 113:537, 2009
Gungorduk K, Asicioglu O, Yildirim G, et al: Comparison of single-dose and two-dose methotrexate protocols for the treatment of unruptured ectopic pregnancy. J Obstet Gynaecol 31(4):330, 2011
Hajenius PJ, Engelsbel S, Mol BW, et al: Randomised trial of systemic methotrexate versus laparoscopic salpingostomy in tubal pregnancy. Lancet 350:774, 1997
Hajenius PJ, Mol BWJ, Ankum WM, et al: Clearance curves of serum human chorionic gonadotropin for the diagnosis of persistent trophoblast. Hum Reprod 10:683, 1995
Hajenius PJ, Mol F, Mol BW, et al: Intervention for tubal ectopic pregnancy. Cochrane Database Syst Rev 1:CD000324, 2007
Hammoud AO, Hammoud I, Bujold E, et al: The role of sonographic endometrial patterns and endometrial thickness in the differential diagnosis of ectopic pregnancy. Am J Obstet Gynecol 192:1370, 2005
Hassan S, Arora R, Bhatia K: Primary ovarian pregnancy: case report and review of literature. BMJ Case Rep Nov 21, 2012
Hill LM, Kislak S, Martin JG: Transvaginal sonographic detection of the pseudogestational sac associated with ectopic pregnancy. Obstet Gynecol 75(6):986, 1990
Hirakawa M, Tajima T, Yoshimitsu K, et al: Uterine artery embolization along with the administration of methotrexate for cervical ectopic pregnancy: technical and clinical outcomes. AJR Am J Roentgenol 192(6):1601, 2009
Hoover RN, Hyer M, Pfeiffer RM, et al: Adverse health outcomes in women exposed in utero to diethylstilbestrol. N Engl J Med 365(14):1304, 2011
Hung TH, Jeng CJ, Yang YC, et al: Treatment of cervical pregnancy with methotrexate. Int J Gynaecol Obstet 53:243, 1996
Izquierdo LA, Nicholas MC: Three-dimensional transvaginal sonography of interstitial pregnancy. J Clin Ultrasound 31(9):484, 2003
Jansen RP, Elliott PM: Angular intrauterine pregnancy. Obstet Gynecol 58(2):167, 1981
Jeng CJ, Ko ML, Shen J: Transvaginal ultrasound-guided treatment of cervical pregnancy. Obstet Gynecol 109:1076, 2007
Jermy K, Thomas J, Doo A, et al: The conservative management of interstitial pregnancy. BJOG 111:1283, 2004
Jung SE, Byun JY, Lee JM, et al: Characteristic MR findings of cervical pregnancy. J Magn Reson Imaging 13(6):918, 2001
Jurkovic D, Hillaby K, Woelfer B, et al: First-trimester diagnosis and management of pregnancies implanted into the lower uterine segment cesarean section scar. Ultrasound Obstet Gynecol 21(3):220, 2003
Kadar N, Romero R: Observations on the log human chorionic gonadotropin–time relationship in early pregnancy and its practical implications. Am J Obstet Gynecol 157:73, 1987
Kalinski MA, Guss DA: Hemorrhagic shock from a ruptured ectopic pregnancy in a patient with a negative urine pregnancy test result. Ann Emerg Med 40:102, 2002
Karaer A, Avsar FA, Batioglu S: Risk factors for ectopic pregnancy: a case-control study. Aust N Z J Obstet Gynaecol 46:521, 2006
Kirk E, Condous G, Haider Z, et al: The conservative management of cervical ectopic pregnancies. Ultrasound Obstet Gynecol 27(4):430, 2006
Ko PC, Lo LM, Hsieh TT, et al: Twenty-one years of experience with ovarian ectopic pregnancy at one institution in Taiwan. Int J Gynaecol Obstet 119(2):154, 2012
Kooi S, Kock HC: A review of the literature on nonsurgical treatment in tubal pregnancy. Obstet Gynecol Surv 47:739, 1992
Krag Moeller LB, Moeller C, Thomsen SG, et al: Success and spontaneous pregnancy rates following systemic methotrexate versus laparoscopic surgery for tubal pregnancies: a randomized trial. Acta Obstet Gynecol Scand 88(12):1331, 2009
Kung FT, Chang SY, Tsai YC, et al: Subsequent reproduction and obstetric outcome after methotrexate treatment of cervical pregnancy: a review of

original literature and international collaborative follow-up. Hum Reprod 12:591, 1997
Lau S, Tulandi T: Conservative medical and surgical management of interstitial ectopic pregnancy. Fertil Steril 72:207, 1999
Lipscomb GH, Bran D, McCord ML, et al: Analysis of three hundred fifteen ectopic pregnancies treated with single-dose methotrexate. Am J Obstet Gynecol 178:1354, 1998
Lipscomb GH, Givens VM, Meyer NL, et al: Comparison of multidose and single-dose methotrexate protocols for the treatment of ectopic pregnancy. Am J Obstet Gynecol 192:1844, 2005
Lipscomb GH, McCord ML, Stovall TG, et al: Predictors of success of methotrexate treatment in women with tubal ectopic pregnancies. N Engl J Med 341:1974, 1999a
Lipscomb GH, Puckett KJ, Bran D, et al: Management of separation pain after single-dose methotrexate therapy for ectopic pregnancy. Obstet Gynecol 93:590, 1999b
Martin JN Jr, McCaul JF IV: Emergent management of abdominal pregnancy. Clin Obstet Gynecol 33:438, 1990
Martin JN Jr, Sessums JK, Martin RW, et al: Abdominal pregnancy: current concepts of management. Obstet Gynecol 71:549, 1988
Martínez-Varea A, Hidalgo-Mora JJ, Payá V, et al: Retroperitoneal ectopic pregnancy after intrauterine insemination. Fertil Steril 95(7):2433.e1, 2011
Mavrelos D, Nicks H, Jamil A, et al: Efficacy and safety of a clinical protocol for expectant management of selected women diagnosed with a tubal ectopic pregnancy. Ultrasound Obstet Gynecol 42(1):102, 2013
Memtsa M, Jamil A, Sebire N, et al: Rarity revisited: diagnosis and management of intramural ectopic pregnancy. Ultrasound Obstet Gynecol 42(3):359, 2013
Menon S, Colins J, Barnhart KT: Establishing a human chorionic gonadotropin cutoff to guide methotrexate treatment of ectopic pregnancy: a systematic review. Fertil Steril 87(3):481, 2007
Michener C, Dickinson JE: Caesarean scar ectopic pregnancy: a single centre case series. Aust N Z J Obstet Gynaecol 49(5):451, 2009
Mittal SK, Singh N, Verma AK, et al: Fetal MRI in the pre-operative diagnosis and assessment of secondary abdominal pregnancy: a rare sequela of a previous caesarean section. Diagn Interv Radiol 18(5):496, 2012
Mol BWJ, Lijmer JG, Ankum WM, et al: The accuracy of single serum progesterone measurement in the diagnosis of ectopic pregnancy: a meta-analysis. Hum Reprod 13:3220, 1998
Moragianni VA, Hamar BD, McArdle C, et al: Management of a cervical heterotopic pregnancy presenting with first-trimester bleeding: case report and review of the literature. Fertil Steril 98(1):89, 2012
Moschos E, Sreenarasimhaiah S, Twickler DM: First-trimester diagnosis of cesarean scar ectopic pregnancy. J Clin Ultrasound 36(8):504, 2008a
Moschos E, Twickler DM: Endometrial thickness predicts intrauterine pregnancy in patients with pregnancy of unknown location. Ultrasound Obstet Gynecol 32(7):929, 2008b
Mukul LV, Teal SB: Current management of ectopic pregnancy. Obstet Gynecol Clin North Am 34:403, 2007
Nakao Y, Yokoyama, Iwasaka T: Uterine artery embolization followed by dilation and curettage for cervical pregnancy. Obstet Gynecol 111:505, 2008
Natale AM, Candiani M, Merlo D, et al: Human chorionic gonadotropin level as a predictor of trophoblastic infiltration into the tubal wall in ectopic pregnancy: a blinded study. Fertil Steril 79:981, 2003
Nieuwkerk PT, Hajenius PJ, Ankum WM, et al: Systemic methotrexate therapy versus laparoscopic salpingostomy in patients with tubal pregnancy. Part I. Impact on patients' health-related quality of life. Fertil Steril 70:511, 1998
Nowak-Markwitz E, Michalak M, Olejnik M, et al: Cutoff value of human chorionic gonadotropin in relation to the number of methotrexate cycles in the successful treatment of ectopic pregnancy. Fertil Steril 92(4):1203, 2009
Nurmohamed L, Moretti ME, Schechter T, et al: Outcome following high-dose methotrexate in pregnancies misdiagnosed as ectopic. Am J Obstet Gynecol 205(6):533.e1, 2011
Nyberg DA, Hughes MP, Mack LA, et al: Extrauterine findings of ectopic pregnancy of transvaginal US: importance of echogenic fluid. Radiology 178:823, 1991
Nyberg DA, Mack LA, Laing FC, et al: Distinguishing normal from abnormal gestational sac growth in early pregnancy. J Ultrasound Med 6(1):23, 1987
Oriol B, Barrio A, Pacheco A, et al: Systemic methotrexate to treat ectopic pregnancy does not affect ovarian reserve. Fertil Steril 90(5):1579, 2008
Osborn DA, Williams TR, Craig BM: Cesarean scar pregnancy: sonographic and magnetic resonance imaging findings, complications, and treatment. J Ultrasound Med 31(9):1449, 2012
Pagidas K, Frishman GN: Nonsurgical management of primary ovarian pregnancy with transvaginal ultrasound-guided local administration of methotrexate. J Minim Invasive Gynecol 20(2):252, 2013
Parker RA 3rd, Yano M, Tai AW, et al: MR imaging findings of ectopic pregnancy: a pictorial review. Radiographics 32(5):1445, 2012
Perkins SL, Al-Ramahi M, Claman P: Comparison of serum progesterone as an indicator of pregnancy nonviability in spontaneously pregnant emergency room and infertility clinic patient populations. Fertil Steril 73:499, 2000
Pisarska MD, Carson SA, Buster JE: Ectopic pregnancy. Lancet 351:1115, 1998
Practice Committee of American Society for Reproductive Medicine: Medical treatment of ectopic pregnancy: a committee opinion. Fertil Steril 100(3):638, 2013
Rahman MS, Al-Suleiman SA, Rahman J, et al: Advanced abdominal pregnancy—observations in 10 cases. Obstet Gynecol 59:366, 1982
Rausch ME, Barnhart KT: Serum biomarkers for detecting ectopic pregnancy. Clin Obstet Gynecol 55(2):418, 2012
Roberts RV, Dickinson JE, Leung Y, et al: Advanced abdominal pregnancy: still an occurrence in modern medicine. Aust N Z J Obstet Gynaecol 45(6):518, 2005
Rodgerson JD, Heegaard WG, Plummer D, et al: Emergency department right upper quadrant ultrasound is associated with a reduced time to diagnosis and treatment of ruptured ectopic pregnancies. Acad Emerg Med 8(4):331, 2001
Rose JS: Ultrasound in abdominal trauma. Emerg Med Clin North Am 22(3):581, 2004
Rotas MA, Haberman S, Levgur M: Cesarean scar ectopic pregnancies. Obstet Gynecol 107:1373, 2006
Saraj AJ, Wilcox JG, Najmabadi S, et al: Resolution of hormonal markers of ectopic gestation: a randomized trial comparing single-dose intramuscular methotrexate with salpingostomy. Obstet Gynecol 92:989, 1998
Schippert C, Soergel P, Staboulidou I, et al: The risk of ectopic pregnancy following tubal reconstructive microsurgery and assisted reproductive technology procedures. Arch Gynecol Obstet 285(3):863, 2012
Scutiero G, Di Gioia P, Spada A, et al: Primary ovarian pregnancy and its management. JSLS 16(3):492, 2012
Seckin B, Turkcapar FA, Tarhan I, et al: Advanced intraligamentary pregnancy resulting in a live birth. J Obstet Gynaecol 31(3):260, 2011
Seeber BE, Sammel MD, Guo W, et al: Application of redefined human chorionic gonadotropin curves for the diagnosis of women at risk for ectopic pregnancy. Fertil Steril 86(2):454, 2006
Seifer DB: Persistent ectopic pregnancy: an argument for heightened vigilance and patient compliance. Fertil Steril 68:402, 1997
Senapati S, Barnhart KT: Biomarkers for ectopic pregnancy and pregnancy of unknown location. Fertil Steril 99(4):1107, 2013
Seow KM, Huang LW, Lin YH: Cesarean scar pregnancy: issues in management. Ultrasound Obstet Gynecol 23(3):247, 2004
Seow KM, Wang PH, Huang LW, et al: Transvaginal sono-guided aspiration of gestational sac concurrent with a local methotrexate injection for the treatment of unruptured cesarean scar pregnancy. Arch Gynecol Obstet 288(2):361, 2013
Shalev E, Peleg D, Tsabari A, et al: Spontaneous resolution of ectopic tubal pregnancy: natural history. Fertil Steril 63:15, 1995
Shen L, Tan A, Zhu H: Bilateral uterine artery chemoembolization with methotrexate for cesarean scar pregnancy. Am J Obstet Gynecol 207(5):386.e1, 2012
Sherer DM, Dalloul M, Gorelick C, et al: Unusual maternal vasculature in the placental periphery leading to the diagnosis of abdominal pregnancy at 25 weeks' gestation. J Clin Ultrasound 35(5):268, 2007
Sherer DM, Gorelick C, Dalloul M, et al: Three-dimensional sonographic findings of a cervical pregnancy. J Ultrasound Med 27(1):155, 2008
Silva C, Sammel MD, Zhou L, et al: Human chorionic gonadotropin profile for women with ectopic pregnancy. Obstet Gynecol 107:605, 2006
Skjeldestad FE, Hadgu A, Eriksson N: Epidemiology of repeat ectopic pregnancy: a population-based prospective cohort study. Obstet Gynecol 91:129, 1998
Song MJ, Moon MH, Kim JA, et al: Serial transvaginal sonographic findings of cervical ectopic pregnancy treated with high-dose methotrexate. J Ultrasound Med 28:55, 2009
Sowter MC, Farquhar CM, Petrie KJ, et al: A randomised trial comparing single dose systemic methotrexate and laparoscopic surgery for the treatment of unruptured tubal pregnancy. BJOG 108(2):192, 2001
Spandorfer SD, Sawin SW, Benjamin I, et al: Postoperative day 1 serum human chorionic gonadotropin level as a predictor of persistent ectopic pregnancy after conservative surgical management. Fertil Steril 68:430, 1997
Spiegelberg O: Zur Casuistic der Ovarialschwangerschaft. Arch Gynaekol 13:73, 1878
Stevens CA: Malformations and deformations in abdominal pregnancy. Am J Med Genet 47:1189, 1993
Stika CS: Methotrexate: the pharmacology behind medical treatment for ectopic pregnancy. Clin Obstet Gynecol 55(2):433, 2012
Stovall TG, Ling FW: Some new approaches to ectopic pregnancy management. Contemp Obstet Gynecol 37:35, 1992a

Stovall TG, Ling FW, Carson SA, et al: Serum progesterone and uterine curettage in differential diagnosis of ectopic pregnancy. Fertil Steril 57:456, 1992b

Stovall TG, Ling FW, Cope BJ, et al: Preventing ruptured ectopic pregnancy with a single serum progesterone. Am J Obstet Gynecol 160:1425, 1989

Stulberg DB, Cain LR, Dahlquist I, et al: Ectopic pregnancy rates in the Medicaid population. Am J Obstet Gynecol 208(4):274.e1, 2013

Svirsky R, Maymon R, Vaknin Z, et al: Twin tubal pregnancy: a rising complication? Fertil Steril 94(5):1910.e13, 2010

Teng HC, Kumar G, Ramli NM: A viable secondary intra-abdominal pregnancy resulting from rupture of uterine scar: role of MRI. Br J Radiol 80:e134, 2007

Thompson M, Kho K: Minimally invasive surgery. In Hoffman BL, Schorge JO, Schaffer JI, et al (eds): Williams Gynecology, 2nd ed. New York, McGraw-Hill, 2012, p 1132

Timor-Tritsch IE, Monteagudo A: Unforeseen consequences of the increasing rate of cesarean deliveries: early placenta accreta and cesarean scar pregnancy. A review. Am J Obstet Gynecol 207(1):14, 2012a

Timor-Tritsch IE, Monteagudo A, Lerner JP: A "potentially safer" route for puncture and injection of cornual ectopic pregnancies. Ultrasound Obstet Gynecol 7(5):353, 1996

Timor-Tritsch IE, Monteagudo A, Matera C, et al: Sonographic evolution of cornual pregnancies treated without surgery. Obstet Gynecol 79(6):1044, 1992

Timor-Tritsch IE, Monteagudo A, Santos R, et al: The diagnosis, treatment, and follow-up of cesarean scar pregnancy. Am J Obstet Gynecol 207(1):44.e1, 2012b

Trojano G, Colafiglio G, Saliani N, et al: Successful management of a cervical twin pregnancy: neoadjuvant systematic methotrexate and prophylactic high cervical cerclage before curettage. Fertil Steril 91:935.e17, 2009

Tulandi T, Al-Jaroudi D: Interstitial pregnancy: results generated from the Society of Reproductive Surgeons. Obstet Gynecol 103:47, 2004

Tulandi T, Guralnick M: Treatment of tubal ectopic pregnancy by salpingotomy with or without tubal suturing and salpingectomy. Fertil Steril 55:53, 1991

Uğur M, Turan C, Vicdan K, et al: Chronic ectopic pregnancy: a clinical analysis of 62 cases. Aust N Z J Obstet Gynaecol 36(2):186, 1996

Ushakov FB, Elchalal U, Aceman PJ, et al: Cervical pregnancy: past and future. Obstet Gynecol Surv 52:45, 1997

Valenzano M, Nicoletti L, Odicino F, et al: Five-year follow-up of placental involution after abdominal pregnancy. J Clin Ultrasound 31(1):39, 2003

Varma R, Mascarenhas L, James D: Successful outcome of advanced abdominal pregnancy with exclusive omental insertion. Ultrasound Obstet Gynecol 12:192, 2003

Verma U, English D, Brookfield K: Conservative management of nontubal ectopic pregnancies. Fertil Steril 96(6):1391, 2011

Verma U, Goharkhay N: Conservative management of cervical ectopic pregnancy. Fertil Steril 91(3):671, 2009

Vermesh M, Graczykowski JW, Sauer MV: Reevaluation of the role of culdocentesis in the management of ectopic pregnancy. Am J Obstet Gynecol 162:411, 1990

Vermesh M, Silva PD, Sauer MV, et al: Persistent tubal ectopic gestation: patterns of circulating beta-human chorionic gonadotropin and progesterone and management options. Fertil Steril 50:584, 1988

Virk J, Zhang J, Olsen J: Medical abortion and the risk of subsequent adverse pregnancy outcomes. N Engl J Med 357:648, 2007

Wang JH, Xu KH, Lin J, et al: Methotrexate therapy for cesarean section scar pregnancy with and without suction curettage. Fertil Steril 92(4):1208, 2009

Wang Y, Xu B, Dai S, et al: An efficient conservative treatment modality for cervical pregnancy: angiographic uterine artery embolization followed by immediate curettage. Am J Obstet Gynecol 204(1):31.e1, 2011

Wang Z, Le A, Shan L, et al: Assessment of transvaginal hysterotomy combined with medication for cesarean scar ectopic pregnancy. J Minim Invasive Gynecol 19(5):639, 2012

Waylen AL, Metwally M, Jones GL, et al: Effects of cigarette smoking upon clinical outcomes of assisted reproduction: a meta-analysis. Hum Reprod Update 15:31, 2009

Westrom L, Joesoef R, Reynolds G, et al: Pelvic inflammatory disease and fertility: a cohort study of 1,844 women with laparoscopically verified disease and 657 control women with normal laparoscopic results. Sex Transm Dis 19(4):185, 1992

Word L, Hoffman BL: Surgeries for benign gynecologic conditions. In Hoffman BL, Schorge JO, Schaffer JI, et al (eds): Williams Gynecology, 2nd ed. New York, McGraw-Hill, 2012, p 1037

Worley KC, Hnat MD, Cunningham FG: Advanced extrauterine pregnancy: diagnostic and therapeutic challenges. Am J Obstet Gynecol 198:297e1, 2008

Wu PJ, Han CM, Wang CJ, et al: Early detection and minimally invasive management of intramural pregnancy. J Minim Invasive Gynecol 20(1):123, 2013

Xiaolin Z, Ling L, Chengxin Y, et al: Transcatheter intraarterial methotrexate infusion combined with selective uterine artery embolization as a treatment option for cervical pregnancy. J Vasc Interv Radiol 21(6):836, 2010

Yang Q, Piao S, Wang G, et al: Hysteroscopic surgery of ectopic pregnancy in the cesarean section scar. J Minim Invasive Gynecol 16(4):432, 2009

Yang XY, Yu H, Li KM, et al: Uterine artery embolisation combined with local methotrexate for treatment of caesarean scar pregnancy. BJOG 117(8):990, 2010

Zakaria MA, Abdallah ME, Shavell VI, et al: Conservative management of cervical ectopic pregnancy: utility of uterine artery embolization. Fertil Steril 95(3):872, 2011

Zeck W, Kelters I, Winter R, et al: Lessons learned from four advanced abdominal pregnancies at an East African Health Center. J Perinat Med 35(4):278, 2007

Zee J, Sammel MD, Chung K, et al: Ectopic pregnancy prediction in women with a pregnancy of unknown location: data beyond 48 h are necessary. Hum Reprod December 18, 2013 [Epub ahead of print]

Zhang B, Jiang ZB, Huang MS, et al: Uterine artery embolization combined with methotrexate in the treatment of cesarean scar pregnancy: results of a case series and review of the literature. J Vasc Interv Radiol 23(12):1582, 2012

Zhuang Y, Huang L: Uterine artery embolization compared with methotrexate for the management of pregnancy implanted within a cesarean scar. Am J Obstet Gynecol 201(2):152.e1, 2009

Zuo X, Shen A, Chen M: Successful management of unruptured interstitial pregnancy in 17 consecutive cases by using laparoscopic surgery. Aust N Z J Obstet Gynaecol 52(4):387, 2012

CHAPTER 20

Gestational Trophoblastic Disease

Gestational trophoblastic disease (GTD) is the term used to encompass a group of tumors typified by abnormal trophoblast proliferation. Trophoblast produce human chorionic gonadotropin (hCG), thus the measurement of this peptide hormone in serum is essential for GTD diagnosis, management, and surveillance. GTD histologically is divided into *hydatidiform moles,* which are characterized by the presence of villi, and nonmolar trophoblastic neoplasms, which lack villi.

Hydatidiform moles are excessively edematous immature placentas (Benirschke, 2012). These include the benign *complete hydatidiform mole* and *partial hydatidiform mole* and the malignant *invasive mole.* Invasive mole is deemed malignant due to its marked penetration into and destruction of the myometrium as well as its ability to metastasize.

Nonmolar trophoblastic neoplasms include choriocarcinoma, placental site trophoblastic tumor, and epithelioid trophoblastic tumor. These three are differentiated by the type of trophoblast they contain.

The malignant forms of gestational trophoblastic disease are termed *gestational trophoblastic neoplasia (GTN).* These include invasive mole, choriocarcinoma, placental site trophoblastic tumor, and epithelioid trophoblastic tumor. Other terms applied to GTN are *malignant gestational trophoblastic disease* and *persistent gestational trophoblastic disease.* These malignancies develop weeks or years following any type of pregnancy, but frequently occur after a hydatidiform mole.

Each of the GTN tumor types is histologically distinct and varies in its propensity to invade and metastasize. However, histological confirmation is typically not available. Instead, measurement of serum hCG levels combined with clinical findings—rather than a histological specimen—is used to diagnose and treat this malignancy. Accordingly, GTN is often identified and effectively treated as a group.

In the past, these metastatic tumors had a prohibitively high mortality rate. However, with chemotherapy, currently most tumors are highly curable (Goldstein, 2010). Early-stage GTN is typically cured with single-agent chemotherapy, whereas later-stage disease usually responds to combination chemotherapy.

HYDATIDIFORM MOLE—MOLAR PREGNANCY

The classic histological findings of molar pregnancy include villous stromal edema and trophoblast proliferation (Fig. 20-1). The degree of histological changes, karyotypic differences, and the absence or presence of embryonic elements are used to classify them as either *complete* or *partial moles.* These two also vary in associated risks for developing medical comorbidities and postevacuation GTN. Of the two, GTN more frequently follows complete hydatidiform mole.

A complete mole has abnormal chorionic villi that grossly appear as a mass of clear vesicles. These vary in size and often hang in clusters from thin pedicles. In contrast, a partial molar pregnancy has focal and less advanced hydatidiform changes and contains some fetal tissue. Although both forms of moles usually fill the uterine cavity, they rarely may be tubal or other forms of ectopic pregnancy (Sebire, 2005).

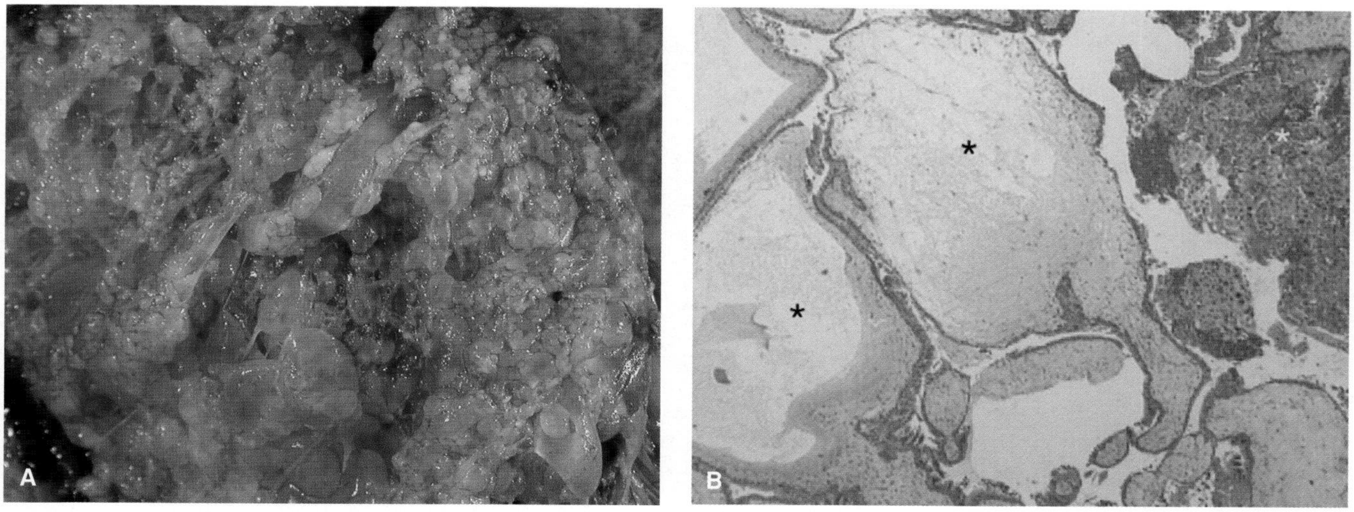

FIGURE 20-1 Complete hydatidiform mole. **A.** Gross specimen with characteristic vesicles of variable size. (Image contributed by Dr. Brian Levenson.) **B.** Low-magnification photomicrograph shows generalized edema and cistern formation (*black asterisks*) within avascular villi. Haphazard trophoblastic hyperplasia is marked by a yellow asterisk on the right. (Image contributed by Dr. Erika Fong.)

Epidemiology and Risk Factors

There is an ethnic predisposition to hydatidiform mole, which has increased prevalence in Asians, Hispanics, and American Indians (Drake, 2006; Lee, 2011; Smith, 2006). The incidence in the United States and Europe has been relatively constant at 1 to 2 per 1000 deliveries (Lee, 2011; Lybol, 2011; Salehi, 2011).

The strongest risk factors are age and a history of prior hydatidiform mole. Women at both extremes of reproductive age are most vulnerable. Specifically, adolescents and women aged 36 to 40 years have a twofold risk, but those older than 40 have an almost tenfold risk (Altman, 2008; Sebire, 2002a). For those with a prior complete mole, the risk of another mole is 1.5 percent. With a previous partial mole, the rate is 2.7 percent (Garrett, 2008). After two prior molar pregnancies, Berkowitz and associates (1998) reported that 23 percent of women had a third mole.

Pathogenesis

With rare exceptions, molar pregnancies arise from chromosomally abnormal fertilizations. Complete moles most often have a diploid chromosomal composition (Table 20-1). These usually are 46,XX and result from *androgenesis,* meaning both sets of chromosomes are paternal in origin. As shown in Figure 20-2A, an ovum is fertilized by a haploid sperm, which

TABLE 20-1. Features of Partial and Complete Hydatidiform Moles

Feature	Partial Mole	Complete Mole
Karyotype[a]	69,XXX or 69,XXY	46,XX
Clinical Presentation		
Diagnosis	Missed abortion	Molar gestation
Uterine size	Small for dates	Large for dates
Theca-lutein cysts	Rare	25–30% of cases
Initial hCG levels	< 100,000 mIU/mL	> 100,000 mIU/mL
Medical complications[b]	Rare	Uncommon
Rate of subsequent GTN	1–5% of cases	15–20% of cases
Pathology		
Embryo-fetus	Often present	Absent
Amnion, fetal erythrocytes	Often present	Absent
Villous edema	Focal	Widespread
Trophoblastic proliferation	Focal, slight to moderate	Slight to severe
Trophoblast atypia	Mild	Marked
$p57^{KIP2}$ immunostaining	Positive	Negative

[a]Typical karyotypes.
[b]These include anemia, hyperthyroidism, hyperemesis gravidarum, preeclampsia, and infection.
GTN = gestational trophoblastic neoplasia; hCG = human chorionic gonadotropin.

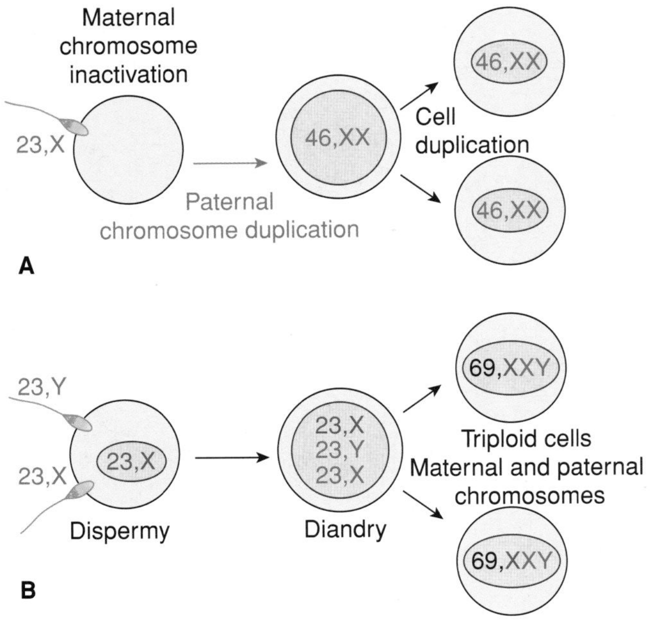

FIGURE 20-2 Typical pathogenesis of complete and partial moles. **A.** A 46,XX complete mole may be formed if a 23,X-bearing haploid sperm penetrates a 23,X-containing haploid egg whose genes have been "inactivated." Paternal chromosomes then duplicate to create a 46,XX diploid complement solely of paternal origin. **B.** A partial mole may be formed if two sperm—either 23,X- or 23,Y-bearing—both fertilize (*dispermy*) a 23,X-containing haploid egg whose genes have not been inactivated. The resulting fertilized egg is triploid with two chromosome sets being donated by the father (*diandry*).

then duplicates its own chromosomes after meiosis. The chromosomes of the ovum are either absent or inactivated. Less commonly, the chromosomal pattern may be 46,XY or 46,XX and due to fertilization by two sperm, that is, *dispermic fertilization* or *dispermy* (Lawler, 1991; Lipata, 2010).

Partial moles usually have a triploid karyotype—69,XXX, 69,XXY—or much less commonly, 69,XYY. These are each composed of two paternal haploid sets of chromosomes contributed by dispermy and one maternal haploid set (see Fig. 20-2B). Less frequently, a similar haploid egg may be fertilized by an unreduced diploid 46,XY sperm. These triploid zygotes result in some embryonic development, however, it ultimately is a lethal fetal condition. Fetuses that reach advanced ages have severe growth restriction, multiple congenital anomalies, or both.

Twin Pregnancy Comprised of a Normal Fetus and Coexistent Complete Mole

Rarely, in some twin pregnancies, one chromosomally normal fetus is paired with a complete diploid molar pregnancy. These are recognized in only 1 in 22,000 to 100,000 pregnancies (Steller, 1994). It is important that these cases be distinguished from a single partial molar pregnancy with its abnormal associated fetus. Amniocentesis done for fetal karyotyping is used to confirm the diagnosis.

There are a number of unique pregnancy complications with this twin pregnancy. And, many women may choose to terminate the pregnancy, if diagnosed early. In those with continuing pregnancy, survival of the normal fetus is variable and dependent on complications that commonly develop from the molar component. The most worrisome are preeclampsia or hemorrhage, which frequently necessitate preterm delivery. Wee and Jauniaux (2005) reviewed outcomes in 174 women of whom 82 chose termination. Of the remaining 92 pregnancies, 42 percent either miscarried or had a perinatal death; approximately 60 percent delivered preterm; and only 40 percent delivered at term.

Another concern for those continuing their pregnancy is the possible risk for developing subsequent GTN. Sebire and colleagues (2002b) reviewed such twin pregnancies and reported that in those not terminated, 21 percent of mothers subsequently required chemotherapy. But, this was not significantly different from a rate of 16 percent among women who chose termination. Others have reported rates up to 50 percent following continuation (Massardier, 2009). At this time, most data indicate that women with these twin pregnancies are not at greater risk for subsequent neoplasia than those with a singleton complete mole (Niemann, 2007b). Postdelivery surveillance is conducted as for any molar pregnancy and is discussed on page 401.

Clinical Findings

The clinical presentation of women with a molar pregnancy has changed remarkably over the past several decades because prenatal care is sought much earlier and because sonography is virtually universal. As a result, most molar pregnancies are detected when they are small and before complications ensue (Kerkmeijer, 2009; Mangili, 2008).

Typically, there are usually 1 to 2 months of amenorrhea before discovery. In 41 women with a complete mole diagnosed at a mean of 10 weeks, Gemer and colleagues (2000) reported that 41 percent were asymptomatic and 58 percent had vaginal bleeding. Moreover, only 2 percent had anemia or hyperemesis, and none had other manifestations that in the past were common in these women.

As gestation advances, symptoms generally tend to be more pronounced with complete compared with partial moles (Niemann, 2007a). Untreated molar pregnancies will almost always cause uterine bleeding that varies from spotting to profuse hemorrhage. Bleeding may presage spontaneous molar abortion, but more often, it follows an intermittent course for weeks to months. In more advanced moles with considerable concealed uterine hemorrhage, moderate iron-deficiency anemia develops. Many women have uterine growth that is more rapid than expected. The enlarged uterus has a soft consistency, but typically no fetal heart motion is detected. Nausea and vomiting may become significant. The ovaries contain multiple theca-lutein cysts in 25 to 60 percent of women with a complete mole (Fig. 20-3). These likely result from overstimulation of lutein elements by sometimes massive amounts of hCG. Because theca-lutein cysts regress following pregnancy evacuation, expectant management is preferred. Occasionally a larger cyst may undergo torsion, infarction, and hemorrhage. However, oophorectomy is not performed unless there is extensive infarction that persists after untwisting.

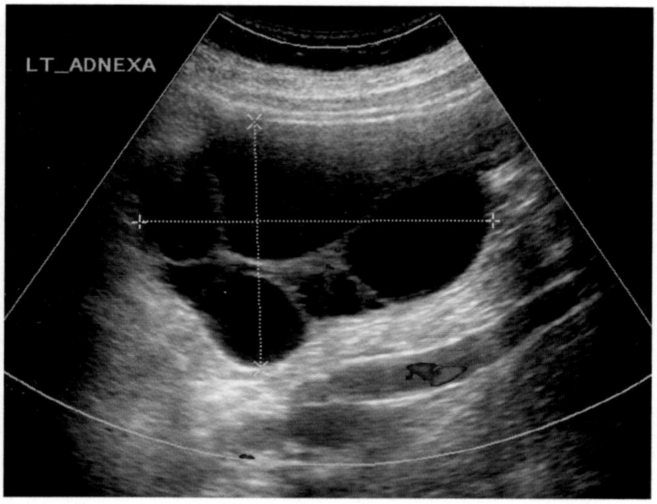

FIGURE 20-3 Sonographic image of an ovary with theca-lutein cysts in a woman with a hydatidiform mole.

The thyrotropin-like effects of hCG frequently cause serum free thyroxine (fT_4) levels to be elevated and thyroid-stimulating hormone (TSH) levels to be decreased. Despite this, clinically apparent thyrotoxicosis is unusual and, in our experience, can be mimicked by bleeding and sepsis from infected products. Moreover, the serum free T_4 levels rapidly normalize after uterine evacuation. Despite this, a case of presumed "thyroid storm" has been reported (Moskovitz, 2010).

Severe preeclampsia and eclampsia are relatively common with large molar pregnancies. However, these are seldom seen today because of early diagnosis and evacuation. An exception is in the case of a normal fetus coexisting with a complete mole, described earlier. In those cases in which pregnancy is not terminated, severe preeclampsia frequently mandates preterm delivery. The predilection for preeclampsia is explained by the hypoxic trophoblastic mass, which releases antiangiogenic factors that activate endothelial damage (Chap. 40, p. 733).

Diagnosis

Most women initially have amenorrhea that is followed by irregular bleeding that almost always prompts pregnancy testing and sonography. Some women will present with spontaneous passage of molar tissue.

Serum β-HCG Measurements

With a complete molar pregnancy, serum β-hCG levels are commonly elevated above those expected for gestational age. With more advanced moles, values in the millions are not unusual. Importantly, these high values can lead to erroneous false-negative *urine* pregnancy test results because of oversaturation of the test assay by excessive β-hCG hormone (Chap. 9, p. 169). In these cases, *serum* β-hCG determinations with or without sample dilution will clarify the conundrum. With a partial mole, β-hCG levels may also be significantly elevated, but more commonly concentrations fall into ranges expected for gestational age.

Sonography

Although sonographic imaging is the mainstay of trophoblastic disease diagnosis, not all cases are confirmed initially. Sonographically, a complete mole appears as an echogenic uterine mass with numerous anechoic cystic spaces but without a fetus or amnionic sac. The appearance is often described as a "snowstorm" (Figure 20-4). A partial mole has features that include a thickened, multicystic placenta along with a fetus or at least fetal tissue. In early pregnancy, however, these sonographic characteristics are seen in fewer than half of hydatidiform moles (Fowler, 2006). The most common misdiagnosis is incomplete or missed abortion. Occasionally, molar pregnancy may be confused for a multifetal pregnancy or a uterine leiomyoma with cystic degeneration.

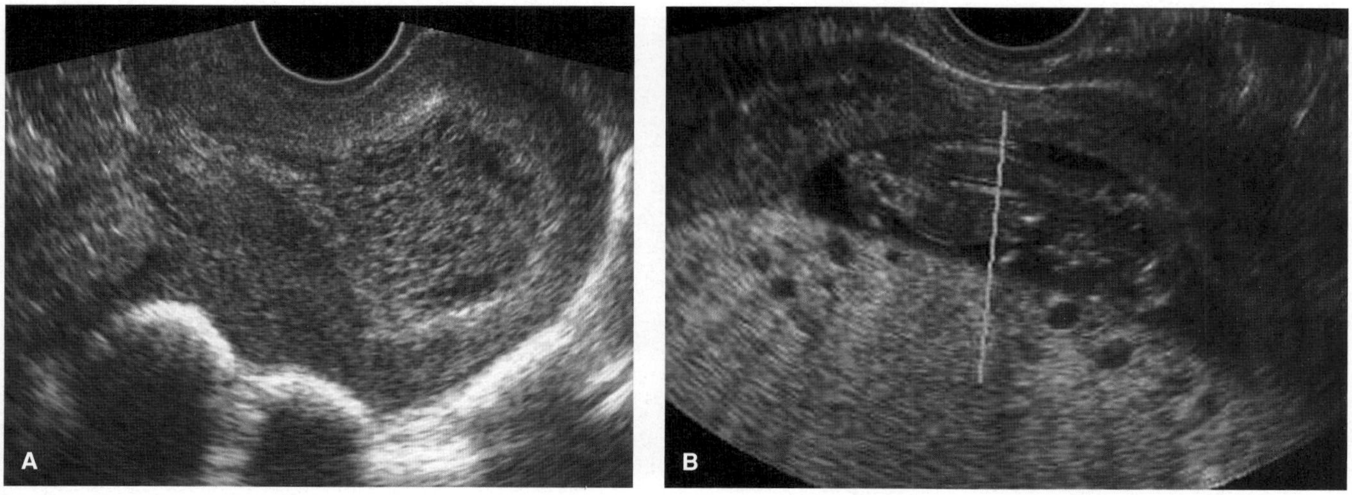

FIGURE 20-4 Sonograms of hydatidiform moles. **A.** Sagittal view of a uterus with a complete hydatidiform mole. The characteristic "snowstorm" appearance is due to an echogenic uterine mass that has numerous anechoic cystic spaces. Notably, a fetus and amnionic sac are absent. **B.** In this image of a partial hydatidiform mole, the fetus is seen above a multicystic placenta. (Image contributed by Dr. Elysia Moschos.)

Pathological Diagnosis

Surveillance for subsequent neoplasia following molar pregnancy is crucial. Thus, moles must be histologically distinguished from other types of pregnancy failure that have hydropic placental degeneration, which can mimic molar villous changes. Some distinguishing histological characteristics are shown in Table 20-1.

In pregnancies before 10 weeks, classic molar changes may not be apparent because villi may not be enlarged and molar stroma may not yet be edematous and avascular (Paradinas, 1996). In such situations, other techniques are used to differentiate. One takes advantage of the differing ploidy to distinguish partial (triploid) moles from diploid entities. Complete moles and nonmolar pregnancies with hydropic placental degeneration are both diploid.

Another technique involves histological immunostaining to identify the $p57^{KIP2}$ nuclear protein. Because the gene that expresses $p57^{KIP2}$ is paternally imprinted, only maternally donated genes are expressed. Because complete moles contain only paternal genetic material, they cannot express this gene; do not produce $p57^{KIP2}$; and thus, do not pick up this immunostain. In contrast, this nuclear protein is strongly expressed in partial moles and in nonmolar pregnancies with hydropic change (Castrillon, 2001). As a result, the combined use of ploidy analysis and $p57^{KIP2}$ immunostaining can be used to differentiate: (1) a complete mole (diploid/$p57^{KIP2}$-negative), (2) a partial mole (triploid/$p57^{KIP2}$-positive), and spontaneous abortion with hydropic placental degeneration (diploid/$p57^{KIP2}$-positive) (Merchant, 2005).

Management

Maternal deaths from molar pregnancies are rare because of early diagnosis, timely evacuation, and vigilant postevacuation surveillance for GTN. Preoperative evaluation attempts to identify known potential complications such as preeclampsia, hyperthyroidism, anemia, electrolyte depletions from hyperemesis, and metastatic disease (Table 20-2) (Lurain, 2010). Most recommend chest x-ray, whereas computed tomography (CT) and magnetic resonance (MR) imaging are not routinely done unless the chest radiograph shows lung lesions or unless there is evidence of other extrauterine disease such as in the brain or liver.

Termination of Molar Pregnancy

Regardless of uterine size, molar evacuation by suction curettage is usually the preferred treatment. Preoperative cervical dilatation with an osmotic agent is recommended if the cervix is minimally dilated. Intraoperative bleeding can be greater with molar pregnancy than with a comparably sized uterus containing nonmolar products. Thus with large moles, adequate anesthesia, sufficient intravenous access, and blood-banking support is imperative. The cervix is mechanically dilated to allow insertion of a 10- to 14-mm suction curette. As evacuation is begun, oxytocin is infused to limit bleeding. Intraoperative sonography is recommended to

TABLE 20-2. Some Considerations for Management of Hydatidiform Mole

Preoperative
Laboratory
Hemogram; serum β-hCG, creatinine, and hepatic aminotransferase levels
TSH, free T_4 levels
Type and Rh; group and screen or crossmatch
Chest radiograph
Consider hygroscopic dilators
Intraoperative
Large-bore intravenous catheter(s)
Regional or general anesthesia
Oxytocin (Pitocin): 20 units in 1000 mL RL for continuous infusion
One or more other uterotonic agents may be added as needed:
Methylergonovine (Methergine): 0.2 mg = 1 mL = 1 ampule IM every 2 hr prn
Carboprost tromethamine ($PGF_{2\alpha}$) (Hemabate): 250 μg = 1 mL = 1 ampule IM every 15–90 min prn
Misoprostol (PGE_1) (Cytotec): 200 mg tablets for rectal administration, 800–1000 mg once
Karman cannula—size 10 or 12
Consider sonography machine
Postevacuation
Anti-D immune globulin (Rhogam) if Rh D-negative
Initiate effective contraception[a]
Review pathology report
Serum hCG levels: within 48 hours of evacuation, weekly until undetectable, then monthly for 6 months

[a]Intrauterine devices are not suitable during surveillance.
GTN = gestational trophoblastic neoplasia; hCG = human chorionic gonadotropin; IM = intramuscular; PG = prostaglandin; RL = Ringer lactate; T_4 = thyroxine; TSH = thyroid-stimulating hormone.

help ensure that the uterine cavity has been emptied. When the myometrium has contracted, thorough but gentle curettage with a sharp large-loop Sims curette is performed. If bleeding continues despite uterine evacuation and oxytocin infusion, other uterotonic agents shown in Table 20-2 are given. In some cases, pelvic arterial embolization or hysterectomy may be necessary (Tse, 2007). Profuse hemorrhage and surgical methods that may be useful for its management are discussed in Chapter 41 (p. 818).

It is invariable that some degree of trophoblastic deportation into the pelvic venous system takes place during molar evacuation (Hankins, 1987). With large molar pregnancies, the volume of tissue may be sufficient to produce clinically apparent respiratory insufficiency, pulmonary edema, or even embolism. In our earlier experiences with very large moles, these and their chest x-ray manifestations clear rapidly without specific treatment. However, fatalities have been described (Delmis, 2000). Because of deportation, there is concern that trophoblastic tissue will thrive within the lung parenchyma to cause persistent disease or even overt malignancy. Fortunately, there is no evidence that this is a major problem.

Following curettage, anti-D immunoglobulin (Rhogam) is given to Rh D-negative women because fetal tissues with a partial mole may include red cells with D-antigen (Chap. 15, p. 311). Those with suspected complete mole are similarly treated because a definitive diagnosis of complete versus partial mole may not be confirmed until pathological evaluation of the evacuated products.

Following evacuation, the long-term prognosis for women with a hydatidiform mole is not improved with prophylactic chemotherapy (Goldstein, 1995). Moreover, chemotherapy toxicity—including death—may be significant, and thus it is not recommended routinely by the American College of Obstetricians and Gynecologists (2012).

Methods other than suction curettage may be considered for select cases. Hysterectomy with ovarian preservation may be preferable for women who have completed childbearing. Of women aged 40 and older, approximately a third will subsequently develop GTN, and hysterectomy markedly reduces this likelihood (Hanna, 2010). Theca-lutein cysts seen at the time of hysterectomy do not require removal, and they spontaneously regress following molar termination. Some recommend aspiration of larger cysts to minimize pain and torsion risk. In contrast, labor induction or hysterotomy is seldom used for molar evacuation in the United States. Both will likely increase blood loss and theoretically may increase the incidence of persistent trophoblastic disease (American College of Obstetricians and Gynecologists, 2012).

Postevacuation Surveillance

Close biochemical surveillance for persistent gestational neoplasia should follow hydatidiform mole evacuation. Concurrently, reliable contraception is imperative to avoid confusion caused by rising β-hCG levels from a new pregnancy. Most recommend either combination hormonal contraception or injectable medroxyprogesterone acetate. The latter is particularly useful if there is poor compliance. Intrauterine devices are not used until β-hCG levels are undetectable because of the risk of uterine perforation if there is an invasive mole. Finally, barrier and other methods are not recommended because of their relatively high failure rates.

Biochemical surveillance is by serial measurements of serum β-hCG to detect persistent or renewed trophoblastic proliferation. The initial β-hCG level is obtained within 48 hours after evacuation. This serves as the baseline, which is compared with β-hCG quantification done thereafter every 1 to 2 weeks until levels progressively decline to become undetectable.

The median time for such resolution is 7 weeks for partial moles and 9 weeks for complete moles. Once β-hCG is undetectable, this is confirmed with monthly determinations for another 6 months. After this, surveillance is discontinued and pregnancy allowed. Because such intensive monitoring has a high noncompliance rate, a truncated approach has been studied, and it may be unnecessary to verify undetectable β-hCG levels for 6 months. Specifically, it was shown that no woman with a partial or complete mole whose serum β-hCG level became undetectable subsequently developed neoplasia (Lavie, 2005; Wolfberg, 2004). Importantly, during the time during which β-hCG levels are monitored, either increasing or persistently plateaued levels mandate evaluation for trophoblastic neoplasia. If the woman has not become pregnant, then these levels signify increasing trophoblastic proliferation that is most likely malignant.

There are a number of risk factors for developing trophoblastic neoplasia following molar evacuation. Most important, complete moles have a 15 to 20 percent incidence of malignant sequelae, compared with 1 to 5 percent following partial moles. Surprisingly, with much earlier recognition and evacuation of molar pregnancies, the risk for neoplasia has not been lowered (Schorge, 2000). Other risk factors are older age, β-hCG levels > 100,000 mIU/mL, uterine size that is large-for-gestational age, theca-lutein cysts > 6 cm, and slow decline in β-hCG levels (Berkowitz, 2009; Kang, 2012; Wolfberg, 2005). Although not routine, postevacuation uterine sonographic surveillance showing myometrial nodules or hypervascularity may be a predictor of subsequent neoplasia (Garavaglia, 2009).

GESTATIONAL TROPHOBLASTIC NEOPLASIA

This group includes invasive mole, choriocarcinoma, placental site trophoblastic tumor, and epithelioid trophoblastic tumor. These tumors almost always develop with or follow some form of recognized pregnancy. Half follow hydatidiform mole, a fourth follow miscarriage or tubal pregnancy, and another fourth develop after a preterm or term pregnancy (Goldstein, 2012). Although these four tumor types are histologically distinct, they are usually diagnosed solely by persistently elevated serum β-hCG levels because tissue is frequently not available for pathological study. Criteria for the diagnosis of postmolar gestational trophoblastic neoplasia are shown in Table 20-3.

Clinical Findings

These placental tumors are characterized clinically by their aggressive invasion into the myometrium and propensity to metastasize. The most common finding with gestational trophoblastic neoplasms is irregular bleeding associated with uterine subinvolution. The bleeding may be continuous or

TABLE 20-3. Criteria for Diagnosis of Gestational Trophoblastic Neoplasia

1. Plateau of serum β-hCG level (± 10 percent) for four measurements during a period of 3 weeks or longer—days 1, 7, 14, 21
2. Rise of serum β-hCG level > 10 percent during three weekly consecutive measurements or longer, during a period of 2 weeks or more—days 1, 7, 14
3. Serum β-hCG level remains detectable for 6 months or more
4. Histological criteria for choriocarcinoma

intermittent, with sudden and sometimes massive hemorrhage. Myometrial perforation from trophoblastic growth may cause intraperitoneal hemorrhage. In some women, lower genital tract metastases are evident, whereas in others there are only distant metastases with no trace of a uterine tumor.

Diagnosis, Staging, and Prognostic Scoring

Consideration for the possibility of gestational trophoblastic neoplasia is the most important factor in its recognition. Unusually persistent bleeding after any type of pregnancy should prompt measurement of serum β-hCG levels and consideration for diagnostic curettage. Uterine size is assessed along with careful examination for lower genital tract metastases, which usually appear as bluish vascular masses (Cagayan, 2010). Tissue diagnosis is unnecessary, thus biopsy is not required and may cause significant bleeding.

Once the diagnosis is verified, in addition to a baseline serum β-hCG level and hemogram, a search for local disease and metastases includes tests of liver and renal function, transvaginal sonography, chest CT scan or radiograph, and brain and abdominopelvic CT scan or MR imaging. Less commonly, positron-emission tomographic (PET) scanning and cerebrospinal fluid β-hCG level determination are used to identify metastases (Lurain, 2011).

Gestational trophoblastic neoplasia is staged clinically using the system of the International Federation of Gynecology and Obstetrics (FIGO) (2009). This includes a modification of the World Health Organization (1983) prognostic index score, with which scores of 0 to 4 are given for each of the categories shown in Table 20-4. Women with WHO scores of 0 to 6 are considered to have low-risk disease, whereas those with a score ≥ 7 are considered in the high-risk group.

Histological Classification

Again, it is stressed that the diagnosis of trophoblastic neoplasias is usually made by persistently elevated serum β-hCG levels without confirmation by pathological tissue study. Clinical staging is arrived at without regard for histological findings, even if available. Still, there are distinct histological types that are described next.

Invasive Mole

These are the most common trophoblastic neoplasms that follow hydatidiform moles, and almost all invasive moles arise

TABLE 20-4. International Federation of Gynecology and Obstetrics (FIGO) Staging and Diagnostic Scoring System for Gestational Trophoblastic Neoplasia

Anatomical Staging	
Stage I	Disease confined to the uterus
Stage II	GTN extends outside of the uterus but is limited to the genital structures (adnexa, vagina, broad ligament)
Stage III	GTN extends to the lungs, with or without known genital tract involvement
Stage IV	All other metastatic sites

Modified World Health Organization (WHO) Prognostic Scoring System[a]

Scores[b]	0	1	2	4
Age (years)	< 40	≥ 40	—	—
Antecedent pregnancy	Mole	Abortion	Term	—
Interval after index pregnancy (mo)	< 4	4–6	7–12	> 12
Pretreatment serum β-hCG (mIU/mL)	$< 10^3$	10^3 to 10^4	10^4 to 10^5	$\geq 10^5$
Largest tumor size (including uterus)	< 3 cm	3–4 cm	≥ 5 cm	—
Site of metastases		Spleen, kidney	GI	Liver, brain
Number of metastases	—	1–4	5–8	> 8
Previous failed chemotherapy drugs	—	—	1	≥ 2

[a]Adapted by FIGO.
[b]Low risk = WHO score of 0 to 6; high risk = WHO score of ≥ 7.
β-hCG = beta human chorionic gonadotropin; GI = gastrointestinal; GTN = gestational trophoblastic neoplasia.
Adapted from FIGO Committee on Gynecologic Oncology, 2009.

from partial or complete moles (Sebire, 2005). Previously known as *chorioadenoma destruens*, invasive mole is characterized by extensive tissue invasion by trophoblast and whole villi. There is penetration deep into the myometrium, sometimes with involvement of the peritoneum, adjacent parametrium, or vaginal vault. Although locally aggressive, invasive moles are less prone to metastasize such as with choriocarcinoma.

Gestational Choriocarcinoma

This is the most common type of trophoblastic neoplasm to follow a term pregnancy or a miscarriage, and only a third of cases follow a molar gestation (Soper, 2006). Choriocarcinoma is composed of cells reminiscent of early cytotrophoblast and syncytiotrophoblast, however, it contains no villi. This rapidly growing tumor invades both myometrium and blood vessels to create hemorrhage and necrosis. Myometrial tumor may spread outward and become visible on the uterine surface as dark, irregular nodules. Metastases often develop early and are generally blood-borne (Fig. 20-5). The most common sites are the lungs and vagina, but tumor may be metastatic to the vulva, kidneys, liver, ovaries, brain, and bowel. Choriocarcinomas are commonly accompanied by ovarian theca-lutein cysts.

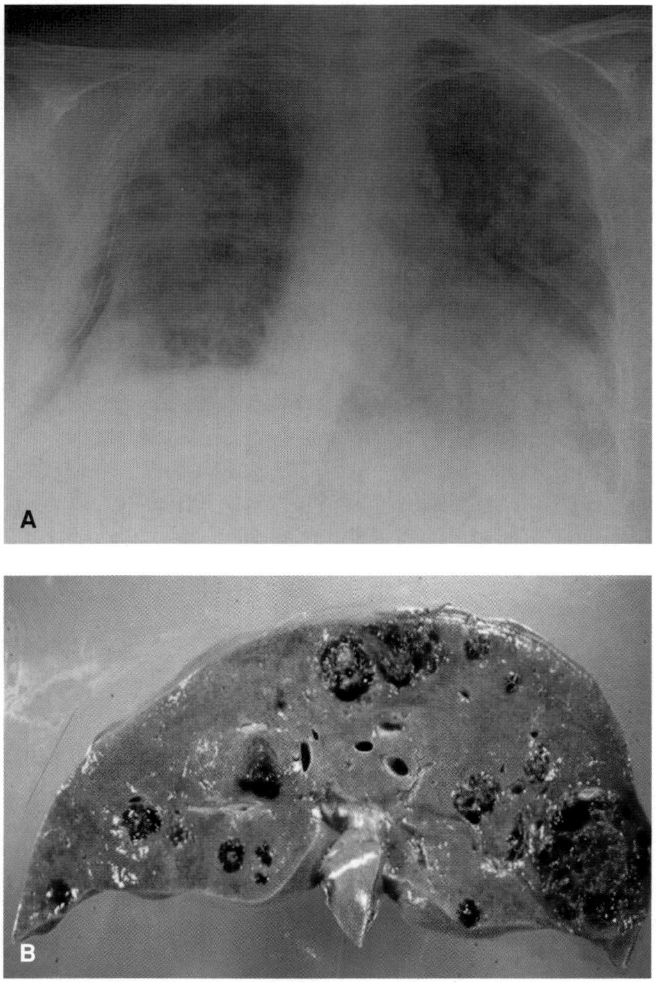

FIGURE 20-5 Metastatic choriocarcinoma. **A.** Chest radiograph demonstrates widespread metastatic lesions. **B.** Autopsy specimen with multiple hemorrhagic hepatic metastases. (Images contributed by Dr. Michael Conner.)

Placental Site Trophoblastic Tumor (PSST)

This uncommon tumor arises from implantation site-intermediate trophoblast. These tumors have associated serum β-hCG levels that may be only modestly elevated, but they produce variant forms of hCG, and identification of a high proportion of free β-hCG (> 30 percent) is considered diagnostic. Treatment of placental site trophoblastic tumor by hysterectomy is preferred because these locally invasive tumors are usually resistant to chemotherapy (Baergen, 2006). For higher-risk stage I and for later stages, adjuvant multidrug chemotherapy is also given (Schmid, 2009).

Epithelioid Trophoblastic Tumor

This rare tumor develops from chorionic-type intermediate trophoblast. Grossly, the tumor grows in a nodular fashion. Primary treatment is hysterectomy because this tumor is relatively resistant to chemotherapy. Approximately a fourth of women with this neoplasm will have metastatic disease, and they are given combination chemotherapy (Morgan, 2008).

Treatment

Women with gestational trophoblastic neoplasia are best managed by oncologists. Chemotherapy is usually the primary treatment, and repeat evacuation is not recommended by most because of risks for uterine perforation, bleeding, infection, or intrauterine adhesion formation. In a few, suction curettage may be necessary if there is bleeding or a substantial amount of retained molar tissue. Although controversial, some also consider a second uterine evacuation to be an initial therapeutic option in some cases of GTN following molar evacuation in an effort to avoid or minimize chemotherapy (Pezeshki, 2004; van Trommel, 2005). Moreover, in specific cases, hysterectomy may be primary or adjuvant treatment (Clark, 2010).

Single-agent chemotherapy protocols are usually sufficient for nonmetastatic or low-risk metastatic neoplasia (Horowitz, 2009). In their review of 108 women with low-risk disease, Abrão and colleagues (2008) reported that monotherapy protocols with either methotrexate or actinomycin D were equally effective compared with a regimen containing both. In general, methotrexate is less toxic than actinomycin D (Chan, 2006; Seckl, 2010). Regimens are repeated until serum β-hCG levels are undetectable.

Combination chemotherapy is given for high-risk disease, and reported cure rates approximate 90 percent (Lurain, 2010). A number of regimens have been used with success. One is *EMA-CO,* which includes *e*toposide, *m*ethotrexate, *a*ctinomycin D, *c*yclophosphamide, and *o*ncovin (vincristine). Adjuvant surgical and radiotherapy may also be employed (Hanna, 2010).

With either low- or high-risk disease, once serum β-hCG levels are undetectable, serosurveillance is continued for 1 year. During this time, effective contraception is crucial to avoid any teratogenic effects of chemotherapy to the fetus as well as to mitigate confusion from rising β-hCG levels caused by superimposed pregnancy.

A small number of women during surveillance, despite no evidence of metastases, will be found to have very low β-hCG levels that plateau. This phenomenon is referred to as quiescent hCG and presumably is caused by dormant trophoblast. Close observation without therapy is recommended, and 20 percent will eventually have recurrent active and progressive trophoblastic neoplasia (Khanlian, 2003).

SUBSEQUENT PREGNANCY

Women with prior gestational trophoblastic disease or successfully treated neoplasia usually do not have impaired fertility, and their pregnancy outcomes are usually normal (Tse, 2012). The primary concern in these women is their 2-percent risk for developing trophoblastic disease in a subsequent pregnancy (Garrett, 2008). Sonographic evaluation is recommended in early pregnancy, and subsequently if indicated. At delivery, the placenta or products of conception are sent for pathological evaluation, and a serum β-hCG level is measured 6 weeks postpartum.

REFERENCES

Abrão RA, de Andrade JM, Tiezzi DG, et al: Treatment for low-risk gestational trophoblastic disease: comparison of single-agent methotrexate, dactinomycin and combination regimens. Gynecol Oncol 108:149, 2008

Altman AD, Bently B, Murray S, et al: Maternal age-related rate of gestational trophoblastic disease. Obstet Gynecol 112:244, 2008

American College of Obstetricians and Gynecologists: Diagnosis and treatment of gestational trophoblastic disease. Practice Bulletin No. 53, June 2004, Reaffirmed 2012

Baergen RN, Rutgers JL, Young RH, et al: Placental site trophoblastic tumor: a study of 55 cases and review of the literature emphasizing factors of prognostic significance. Gynecol Oncol 100:511, 2006

Benirschke K, Burton GJ, Baergen RN (eds): Molar pregnancies. In Pathology of the Human Placenta, 6th ed. New York, Springer, 2012, p 687

Berkowitz RS, Goldstein DP: Current management of gestational trophoblastic diseases. Gynecol Oncol 112(3):654, 2009

Berkowitz RS, Im SS, Bernstein MR, et al: Gestational trophoblastic disease. Subsequent pregnancy outcome, including repeat molar pregnancy. J Reprod Med 43:81, 1998

Cagayan MS: Vaginal metastases complicating gestational trophoblastic neoplasia. J Reprod Med 55(5–6):229, 2010

Castrillon DH, Sun D, Weremowicz S, et al: Discrimination of complete hydatidiform mole from its mimics by immunohistochemistry of the paternally imprinted gene product p57KIP2. Am J Surg Pathol 25(10):1225, 2001

Chan KK, Huang Y, Tam KF, et al: Single-dose methotrexate regimen in the treatment of low-risk gestational trophoblastic neoplasia. Am J Obstet Gynecol 195:1282, 2006

Clark RM, Nevadunsky NS, Ghosh S, et al: The evolving role of hysterectomy in gestational trophoblastic neoplasia at the New England Trophoblastic Disease Center. J Reprod Med 55(5–6):194, 2010

Delmis J, Pfeifer D, Ivanisecvic M, et al: Sudden death from trophoblastic embolism in pregnancy. Eur J Obstet Gynecol Reprod Biol 92:225, 2000

Drake RD, Rao GG, McIntire DD, et al: Gestational trophoblastic disease among Hispanic women: a 21-year hospital-based study. Gynecol Oncol 103:81, 2006

FIGO Committee on Gynecologic Oncology: Current FIGO staging for cancer of the vagina, fallopian tube, ovary, and gestational trophoblastic neoplasia. Int J Gynaecol Obstet 105:3, 2009

Fowler DJ, Lindsay I, Seckl MJ, et al: Routine pre-evacuation ultrasound diagnosis of hydatidiform mole: experience of more than 1000 cases from a regional referral center. Ultrasound Obstet Gynecol 27(1):56, 2006

Garavaglia E, Gentile C, Cavoretto P, et al: Ultrasound imaging after evacuation as an adjunct to beta-hCG monitoring in posthydatidiform molar gestational trophoblastic neoplasia. Am J Obstet Gynecol 200(4):417.e1, 2009

Garrett LA, Garner EIO, Feltmate CM, et al: Subsequent pregnancy outcomes in patients with molar pregnancy and persistent gestational trophoblastic neoplasia. J Reprod Med 53:481, 2008

Gemer O, Segal S, Kopmar A, et al: The current clinical presentation of complete molar pregnancy. Arch Gynecol Obstet 264(1):33, 2000

Goldstein DP: Gestational trophoblastic neoplasia: where we came from, where we stand today, where we are heading. Keynote address. J Reprod Med 55(5–6):184, 2010

Goldstein DP, Berkowitz RS: Current management of gestational trophoblastic neoplasia. Hematol Oncol Clin North Am 26(1):111, 2012

Goldstein DP, Berkowitz RS: Prophylactic chemotherapy of complete molar pregnancy. Semin Oncol 22:157, 1995

Hankins GD, Wendel GD, Snyder RR, et al: Trophoblastic embolization during molar evacuation: central hemodynamic observations. Obstet Gynecol 63:368, 1987

Hanna RK, Soper JT: The role of surgery and radiation therapy in the management of gestational trophoblastic disease. Oncologist 15(6):593, 2010

Horowitz NS, Goldstein DP, Berkowitz RS: Management of gestational trophoblastic neoplasia. Semin Oncol 36(2):181, 2009

Kang WD, Choi HS, Kim SM: Prediction of persistent gestational trophoblastic neoplasia: the role of hCG level and ratio in 2 weeks after evacuation of complete mole. Gynecol Oncol 124(2):250, 2012

Kerkmeijer LG, Massuger LF, Ten Kate-Booij MJ, et al: Earlier diagnosis and serum human chorionic gonadotropin regression in complete hydatidiform moles. Obstet Gynecol 113:326, 2009

Khanlian SA, Smith HO, Cole LA: Persistent low levels of human chorionic gonadotropin: a premalignant gestational trophoblastic disease. Am J Obstet Gynecol 188(5):1254, 2003

Lavie I, Rao GG, Castrillon DH, et al: Duration of human chorionic gonadotropin surveillance for partial hydatidiform moles. Am J Obstet Gynecol 192:1362, 2005

Lawler SD, Fisher RA, Dent J: A prospective genetic study of complete and partial hydatidiform moles. Am J Obstet Gynecol 164:1270, 1991

Lee C, Smith HO, Kim SJ: Epidemiology. In Hancock BW, Seckl MJ, Berkowitz RS, et al (eds): Gestational trophoblastic disease, 3rd ed. London, International Society for the Study of Trophoblastic Disease, 2011, p 57. Available at: http://www.isstd.org/index.html. Accessed January 17, 2012

Lipata F, Parkash V, Talmor M, et al: Precise DNA genotyping diagnosis of hydatidiform mole. Obstet Gynecol 115(4):784, 2010

Lurain JR: Gestational trophoblastic disease I: epidemiology, pathology, clinical presentation and diagnosis of gestational trophoblastic disease, and management of hydatidiform mole. Am J Obstet Gynecol 203(6):531, 2010

Lurain JR: Gestational trophoblastic disease II: classification and management of gestational trophoblastic neoplasia. Am J Obstet Gynecol 204(1):11, 2011

Lybol C, Thomas CM, Bulten J: et al: Increase in the incidence of gestational trophoblastic disease in The Netherlands. Gynecol Oncol 121(2):334, 2011

Mangili G, Garavaglia E, Cavoretto P, et al: Clinical presentation of hydatidiform mole in northern Italy: has it changed in the last 20 years? Am J Obstet Gynecol 198(3):302.e1, 2008

Massardier J, Golfner F, Journet D, et al: Twin pregnancy with complete hydatidiform mole and coexistent fetus obstetrical and oncological outcomes in a series of 14 cases. Eur J Obstet Gynecol Reprod Biol 143:84, 2009

Merchant SH, Amin MB, Viswanatha DS, et al: p57KIP2 immunohistochemistry in early molar pregnancies: emphasis on its complementary role in the differential diagnosis of hydropic abortuses. Hum Pathol 36:180, 2005

Morgan JM, Lurain JR: Gestational trophoblastic neoplasia: an update. Curr Oncol Rep 10(6):497, 2008

Moskovitz JB, Bond MC: Molar pregnancy-induced thyroid storm. J Emerg Med 38(5):e71, 2010

Niemann I, Petersen LK, Hansen ES, et al: Differences in current clinical features of diploid and triploid hydatidiform mole. BJOG 114:1273, 2007a

Niemann I, Sunde L, Petersen LK: Evaluation of the risk of persistent trophoblastic disease after twin pregnancy with diploid hydatidiform mole and coexisting normal fetus. Am J Obstet Gynecol 197:45.e1, 2007b

Paradinas FJ, Browne P, Fisher RA, et al: A clinical, histopathological and flow cytometric study of 149 complete moles, 146 partial moles and 107 non-molar hydropic abortions. Histopathology 28(2):101, 1996

Pezeshki M, Hancock BW, Silcocks P: The role of repeat uterine evacuation in the management of persistent gestational trophoblastic disease. Gynecol Oncol 95(3):423, 2004

Salehi S, Eloranta S, Johansson AL: Reporting and incidence trends of hydatidiform mole in Sweden 1973–2004. Acta Oncol 50(3):367, 2011

Schmid P, Nagai Y, Agarwal R: Prognostic markers and long-term outcome of placental-site trophoblastic tumours: a retrospective observational study. Lancet 374(9683):48, 2009

Schorge JO, Goldstein DP, Bernstein MR, et al: Recent advances in gestational trophoblastic disease. J Reprod Med 45:692, 2000

Sebire NJ, Foskett M, Fisher RA, et al: Risk of partial and complete hydatidiform molar pregnancy in relation to maternal age. Br J Obstet Gynaecol 109:99, 2002a

Sebire NJ, Foskett M, Parainas FJ, et al: Outcome of twin pregnancies with complete hydatidiform mole and healthy co-twin. Lancet 359:2165, 2002b

Sebire NJ, Lindsay I, Fisher RA: Overdiagnosis of complete and partial hydatidiform mole in tubal ectopic pregnancies. Int J Gynecol Pathol 24(3):260, 2005

Seckl MJ, Sebire NJ, Berkowitz RS: Gestational trophoblastic disease. Lancet 376(9742):717, 2010

Smith HO, Wiggins C, Verschraegen CF, et al: Changing trends in gestational trophoblastic disease. J Reprod Med 51:777, 2006

Soper JT: Gestational trophoblastic disease. Obstet Gynecol 108:176, 2006

Steller MA, Genest DR, Bernstein MR, et al: Clinical features of multiple conception with partial or complete molar pregnancy and coexisting fetuses. J Reprod Med 39(3):147, 1994

Tse KY, Chan KK, Tam KF: 20-year experience of managing profuse bleeding in gestational trophoblastic disease. J Reprod Med (5):397, 2007

Tse KY, Ngan HY: Gestational trophoblastic disease. Best Pract Res Clin Obstet Gynaecol 26(3):357, 2012

van Trommel NE, Massuger LF, Verheijen RH, et al: The curative effect of a second curettage in persistent trophoblastic disease: a retrospective cohort survey. Gynecol Oncol 99:6, 2005

Wee L, Jauniaux E: Prenatal diagnosis and management of twin pregnancies complicated by a co-existing molar pregnancy. Prenat Diagn 25(9):772, 2005

Wolfberg AJ, Berkowitz RS, Goldstein DP: Postevacuation hCG levels and risk of gestational trophoblastic neoplasia in women with complete molar pregnancy. Obstet Gynecol 106(3):548, 2005

Wolfberg AJ, Feltmate C, Goldstein DP, et al: Low risk of relapse after achieving undetectable hCG levels in women with complete molar pregnancy. Obstet Gynecol 104:551, 2004

World Health Organization Scientific Group: Gestational trophoblastic disease. WHO Tech Rep Ser 692:1, 1983

SECTION 7

LABOR

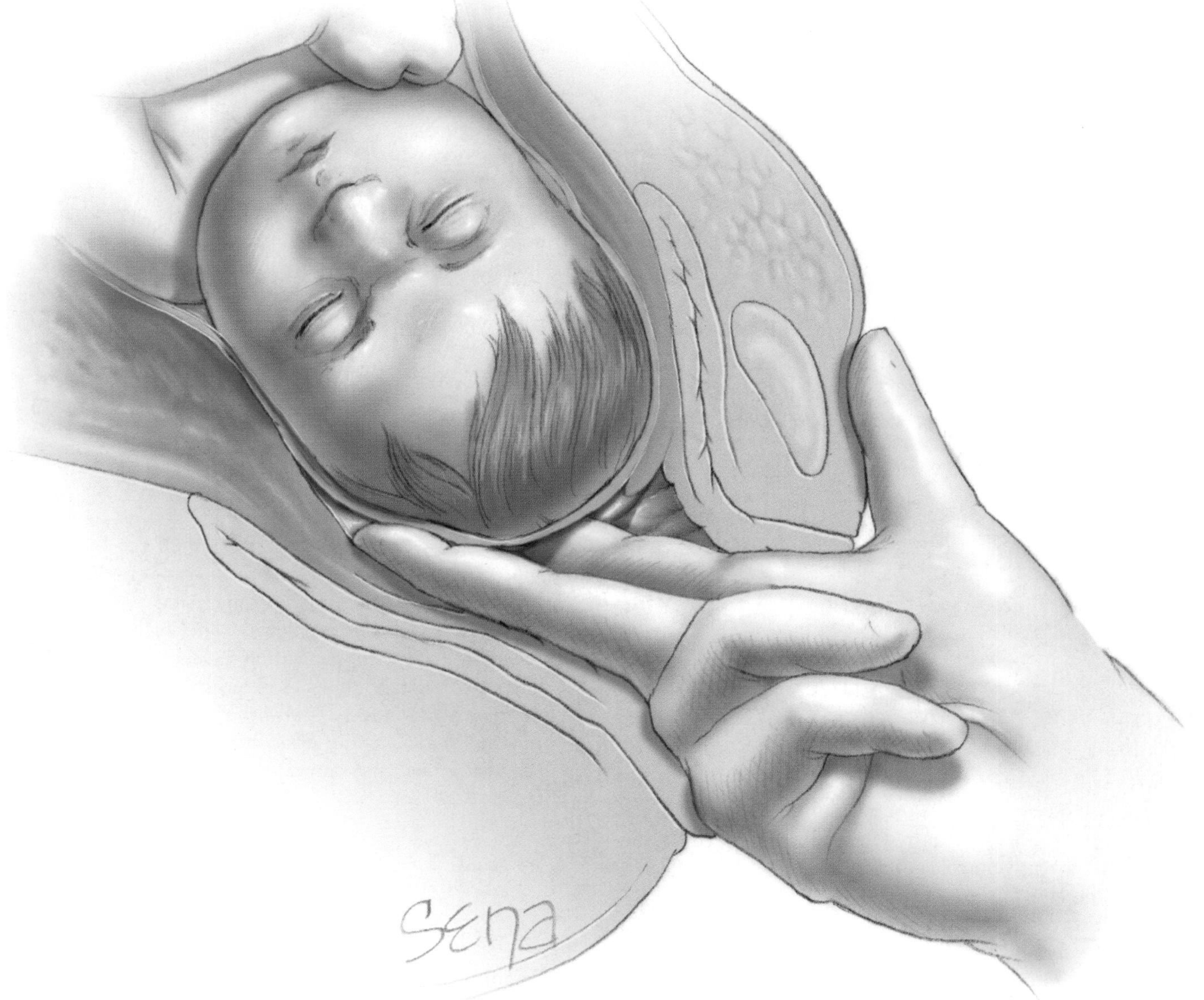

CHAPTER 21

Physiology of Labor

The last few hours of human pregnancy are characterized by forceful and painful uterine contractions that effect cervical dilatation and cause the fetus to descend through the birth canal. There are extensive preparations in both the uterus and cervix long before this. During the first 36 to 38 weeks of normal gestation, the myometrium is in a preparatory yet unresponsive state. Concurrently, the cervix begins an early stage of remodeling—termed *softening*—yet maintains structural integrity. Following this prolonged uterine quiescence, there is a transitional phase during which myometrial unresponsiveness is suspended, and the cervix undergoes ripening, effacement, and loss of structural integrity.

The physiological processes that regulate parturition and the onset of labor continue to be defined. It is clear, however, that labor onset represents the culmination of a series of biochemical changes in the uterus and cervix. These result from endocrine and paracrine signals emanating from both mother and fetus. Their relative contributions vary between species, and it is these differences that complicate elucidation of the exact factors that regulate human parturition. When parturition is abnormal, then preterm labor, dystocia, or postterm pregnancy may result. Of these, preterm labor remains the major contributor to neonatal mortality and morbidity in developed countries.

PHASES OF PARTURITION

The bringing forth of young—*parturition*—requires well-orchestrated transformations in both uterine and cervical function. As shown in Figure 21-1, parturition can be arbitrarily divided into four overlapping phases that correspond to the major physiological transitions of the myometrium and cervix during pregnancy (Casey, 1993, 1997; Challis, 2000; Word, 2007). These phases of parturition include: (1) a prelude to it, (2) the preparation for it, (3) the process itself, and (4) recovery. Importantly, the *phases of parturition* should not be confused with the *clinical stages of labor,* that is, the first, second, and third stages—which comprise the third phase of parturition (Fig. 21-2).

Phase 1 of Parturition: Uterine Quiescence and Cervical Softening

Uterine Quiescence

Beginning even before implantation, a remarkably effective period of myometrial quiescence is imposed. This phase normally comprises 95 percent of pregnancy and is characterized by uterine smooth muscle tranquility with maintenance of cervical structural integrity. The inherent propensity of the myometrium to contract is held in abeyance, and uterine muscle is rendered unresponsive to natural stimuli. Concurrently, the uterus must initiate extensive changes in its size and vascularity to accommodate the pregnancy and

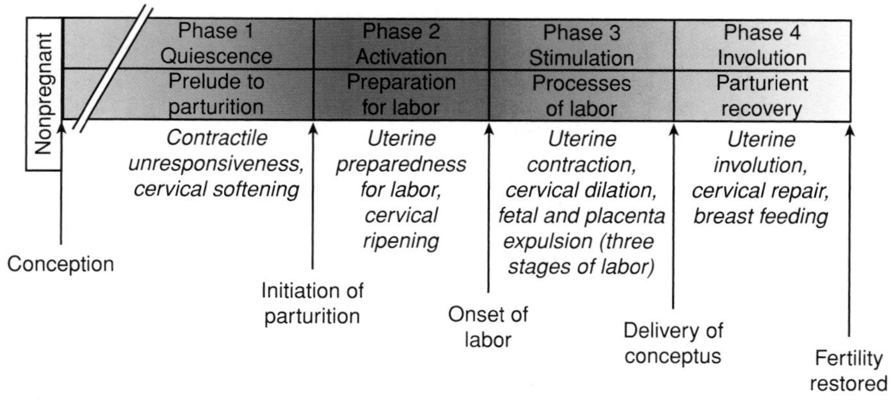

FIGURE 21-1 The phases of parturition.

prepare for uterine contractions. The myometrial unresponsiveness of phase 1 continues until near the end of pregnancy. Some low-intensity myometrial contractions are felt during the quiescent phase, but they do not normally cause cervical dilatation. Contractions of this type become more common toward the end of pregnancy, especially in multiparous women, and are referred to as *Braxton Hicks contractions* or *false labor* (Chap. 4, p. 47).

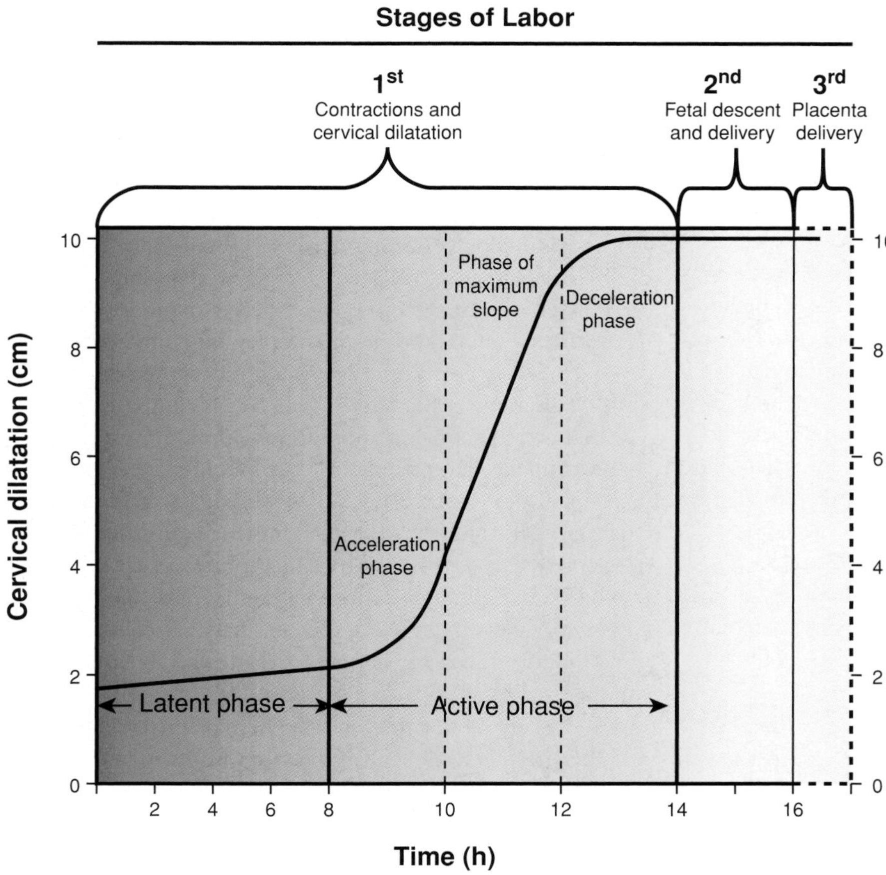

FIGURE 21-2 Composite of the average dilatation curve for labor in nulliparous women. The curve is based on analysis of data derived from a large, nearly consecutive series of women. The first stage is divided into a relatively flat latent phase and a rapidly progressive active phase. In the active phase, there are three identifiable component parts: an acceleration phase, a linear phase of maximum slope, and a deceleration phase. (Redrawn from Friedman, 1978.)

Cervical Softening

The cervix has multiple functions during pregnancy that include: (1) maintenance of barrier function to protect the reproductive tract from infection, (2) maintenance of cervical competence despite increasing gravitational forces, and (3) orchestration of extracellular matrix changes that allow progressive increases in tissue compliance.

In nonpregnant women, the cervix is closed and firm, and its consistency is similar to nasal cartilage. By the end of pregnancy, the cervix is easily distensible, and its consistency is similar to the lips of the oral cavity. Thus, the first stage of this remodeling—termed *softening*—is characterized by an increase in tissue compliance, yet the cervix remains firm and unyielding. Hegar (1895) first described palpable softening of the lower uterine segment at 4 to 6 weeks' gestation, and this sign was once used to diagnose pregnancy.

Clinically, the maintenance of cervical anatomical and structural integrity is essential for continuation of pregnancy to term. Preterm cervical dilatation, structural incompetence, or both may forecast delivery (Iams, 1996).

Structural Changes with Softening. Cervical softening results from increased vascularity, stromal hypertrophy, glandular hypertrophy and hyperplasia, and slow, progressive compositional or structural changes of the extracellular matrix (House, 2009; Leppert, 1995; Mahendroo, 2012; Word, 2007). During matrix changes, collagen, the main structural protein in the cervix, undergoes conformational changes that alter tissue strength and flexibility. Specifically, collagen processing and the number or type of covalent cross-links between collagen triple helices are altered. These cross-links are normally required for stable collagen fibril formation (Canty, 2005). A reduction in cross-links between newly synthesized collagen monomers results from reduced expression and activity of the cross-link forming enzymes, lysyl hydroxylase and lysyl oxidase, beginning in early pregnancy (Akins, 2011; Drewes, 2007; Ozasa, 1981). Concurrently there is reduced expression of the matricellular proteins thrombospondin 2 and tenascin C. These proteins also influence collagen fibril structure and strength. Together, these early pregnancy changes contribute to the gradual increase in tissue compliance during pregnancy.

The clinical importance of these matrix changes is supported by the greater prevalence of cervical insufficiency in those with inherited defects in collagen and elastin synthesis or assembly (Anum, 2009; Hermanns-Lê, 2005; Paternoster, 1998; Rahman, 2003; Wang, 2006). Examples are Ehlers-Danlos and Marfan syndromes, discussed in Chapter 59 (p. 1181). Additionally, human cervical stromal cells express a transcription factor, microphthalmia-associated transcription factor (MiTF-Cx). During pregnancy, this factor maintains cervical competency by repressing the expression of genes involved in cervical dilation and parturition (Hari Kishore, 2012).

Phase 2 of Parturition: Preparation for Labor

To prepare for labor, the myometrial tranquility of phase 1 of parturition must be suspended—so-called *uterine awakening* or *activation.* This phase 2 is a progression of uterine changes during the last 6 to 8 weeks of pregnancy. Importantly, shifting events associated with phase 2 can cause either preterm or delayed labor.

Myometrial Changes

Phase 2 myometrial changes prepare it for labor contractions. This shift probably results from alterations in the expression of key proteins that control contractility. These *contraction-associated proteins (CAPs)* include the oxytocin receptor, prostaglandin F receptor, and connexin 43 (Smith, 2007). Thus, myometrial oxytocin receptors markedly increase along with increased numbers and surface areas of gap junction proteins such as connexin 43. Together, these lead to increased uterine irritability and responsiveness to *uterotonins*—agents that stimulate contractions.

Another critical change in phase 2 is formation of the lower uterine segment from the isthmus. With this development, the fetal head often descends to or even through the pelvic inlet—so-called *lightening.* The abdomen commonly undergoes a shape change, sometimes described by women as "the baby dropped." It is also likely that the lower segment myometrium is unique from that in the upper uterine segment, resulting in distinct roles for each during labor. This is supported by baboon studies that demonstrate differential expression of prostaglandin receptors within myometrial regions. There are also human studies that report an expression gradient of oxytocin receptors, with greater expression in fundal myometrial cells (Fuchs, 1984; Havelock, 2005; Smith, 2001).

Cervical Ripening During Phase 2

Before contractions begin, the cervix must undergo more extensive remodeling. This eventually results in cervical yielding and dilatation upon initiation of forceful uterine contractions. Cervical modifications during this second phase principally involve connective tissue changes—so-called *cervical ripening.* The transition from the softening to the ripening phase begins weeks or days before onset of contractions. During this transformation, the total amount and composition of proteoglycans and glycosaminoglycans within the matrix are altered. Many of the processes that aid cervical remodeling are controlled by the same hormones regulating uterine function. That said, the molecular events of each are varied because of differences in cellular composition and physiological requirements. The uterine corpus is predominantly smooth muscle, whereas the cervix is primarily connective tissue. Cellular components of the cervix include fibroblasts, epithelia, and few smooth muscle cells.

Endocervical Epithelia

During pregnancy, endocervical epithelial cells proliferate such that endocervical glands occupy a significant percentage of cervical mass. The endocervical canal is lined with mucus-secreting columnar and stratified squamous epithelia, which protect against microbial invasion. Mucosal epithelia function as sentinels for antigens by expressing Toll-like receptors that recognize pathogens. In addition, epithelia respond in ways that lead to bacterial and viral killing. For this, the epithelia express antimicrobial peptides and protease inhibitors and signal to underlying immune cells when a pathogenic challenge exceeds their protective capacity (Wira, 2005).

In mice, studies suggest that cervical epithelia may also aid cervical remodeling by regulating tissue hydration and maintenance of barrier function. Hydration may be regulated by expression of *aquaporins*—water channel proteins. Maintenance of barrier function and paracellular transport of ion and solutes is regulated by tight junction proteins, such as claudins 1 and 2 (Anderson, 2006; Timmons, 2007). In the human cervical and vaginal mucosal epithelia, junctional proteins are also reported to be expressed (Blaskewicz, 2011).

Cervical Connective Tissue

Collagen. The cervix is an extracellular matrix-rich tissue. Constituents of the matrix include type I, III, and IV collagen, glycosaminoglycans, matricellular proteins, proteoglycans, and elastin. Of these, collagen is largely responsible for structural disposition of the cervix. Collagen is the most abundant mammalian protein and has a complex biosynthesis pathway that includes at least six enzymes and chaperones to accomplish maturation. Each collagen molecule is composed of three alpha chains, which wind around each other to form procollagen. Multiple collagen triple-helical molecules are cross-linked to one another by the actions of lysyl oxidase to form fibrils. Collagen fibrils interact with small proteoglycans such as decorin or biglycan, as well as matricellular proteins such as thrombospondin 2. These interactions determine fibril size, packing, and organization (Fig. 21-3). This ensures that collagen fibrils are of uniform diameter and are packed together in a regular and highly organized pattern (Canty, 2005).

During cervical ripening, collagen fibril diameter is increased, and there is increased spacing between fibrils. These changes may result in part from accumulation of poorly cross-linked collagen and reduced expression of matricellular proteins. Dispersion of collagen fibrils leads to a loss of tissue integrity and increased tissue compliance. Matrix metalloproteases (MMPs) are proteases capable of degrading extracellular matrix proteins. Of these, collagenase members of the MMP family degrade collagen. Some studies support a role of MMPs in cervical ripening. But, others suggest that the biomechanical changes are not consistent solely with collagenase activation and

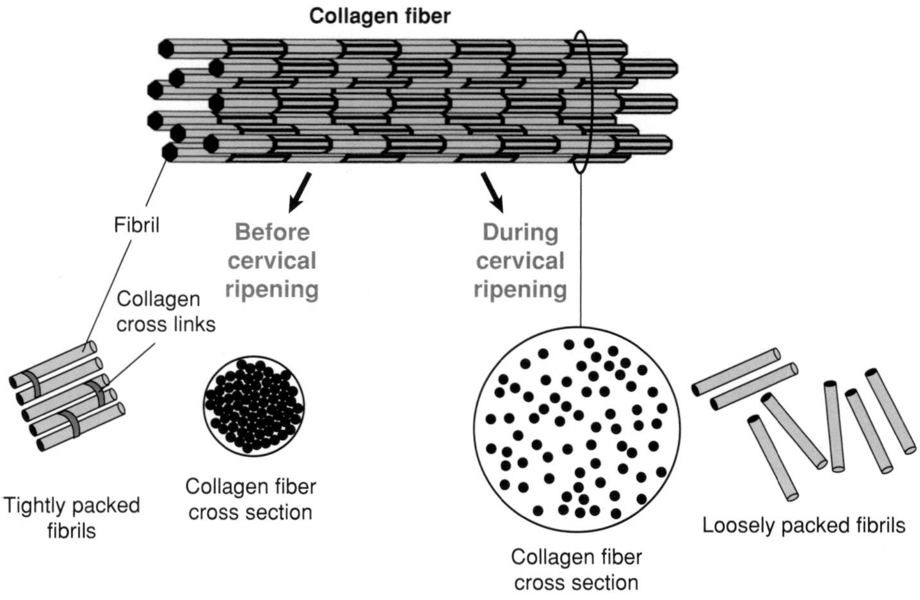

FIGURE 21-3 Fibrillar collagen synthesis and organization. Collagen fibrils are assembled into collagen fibers. Fibril size and packing are regulated in part by small proteoglycans such as decorin that bind collagen. Before cervical ripening, fibril size is uniform, and fibrils are well packed and organized. During cervical ripening, fibril size is less uniform, and spacing between collagen fibrils and fibers is increased and disorganized.

loss of collagen. For example, Buhmschi and colleagues (2004) performed tissue biomechanical studies in the rat and suggest that ripening correlates with changes in the three-dimensional structure of collagen rather than its degradation by collagenases. Moreover, mouse and human studies document no changes in collagen content between nonpregnancy and term pregnancy (Akins, 2011; Myers, 2008; Read, 2007).

Thus, it is likely that dynamic changes in collagen structure rather than collagen content may regulate remodeling. This point is well illustrated in specialized microscopy images of mouse and human cervical collagen (Zhang, 2012). In further support, polymorphisms or mutations in genes required for collagen assembly are associated with an increased incidence of cervical insufficiency (Anum, 2009; Paternoster, 1998; Rahman, 2003; Warren, 2007).

Glycosaminoglycans (GAGs). These are high-molecular-weight polysaccharides that complex with proteins to form proteoglycans. One glycosaminoglycan is hyaluronan (HA), a carbohydrate polymer whose synthesis is carried out by hyaluronan synthase isoenzymes. Expression of these enzymes is increased in the cervix during ripening (Akgul, 2012; Osmers, 1993; Straach, 2005). The functions of hyaluronans are dependent on size, and the breakdown of large- to small-molecular-weight molecules is carried out by a family of hyaluronidase enzymes. Hyaluronidase genes are expressed in both the mouse and human cervix, and increased hyaluronidase activity is reported in the mouse cervix at term (Akgul, 2012). Large-molecular-weight HA predominates in the mouse cervix during ripening and has a dynamic role to increase viscoelasticity and matrix disorganization. Low-molecular-weight HA has proinflammatory properties, and studies in mice and women reveal increased concentrations during labor and in the puerperium (Akgul, 2012; Ruscheinsky, 2008). The importance of regulated changes in HA size during cervical ripening and dilatation is supported by a study reporting hyaluronidase administration to the cervix for ripening in term pregnant women (Spallicci, 2007). Activation of intracellular signaling cascades and other biological functions requires interactions with cell-associated HA-binding proteins such as *versican* (Ruscheinsky, 2008).

Proteoglycans. These glycoproteins are composed of a protein core and GAG chains. Changes in the amount of core protein or in the number, length, or degree of sulfation of GAG chains can influence proteoglycan function. Although not well-defined, changes in proteoglycan composition are thought to accompany cervical ripening. At least three small leucine-rich proteoglycans are expressed in the cervix—decorin, biglycan, and fibromodulin (Westergren-Thorsson, 1998). In other connective tissues, decorin and other family members interact with collagen and influence the packing and order of collagen fibrils (Ameye, 2002). Collagen fibrils are rearranged in the skin of decorin-deficient mice and result in collagen fibers that are weakened, shortened, and disorganized (see Fig. 21-3). In addition to the cervix, these proteoglycans are expressed in the fetal membranes and uterus. Changes in expression levels may regulate fetal membrane tensile strength and uterine function (Meiner, 2007; Wu, 2012).

Inflammatory Changes. The marked changes within the extracellular matrix during cervical ripening in phase 2 are accompanied by stromal invasion with inflammatory cells. This has led to a model in which cervical ripening is considered an inflammatory process. As such, cervical chemoattractants attract inflammatory cells, which in turn release proteases that may aid degradation of collagen and other matrix components. In phase 3 or 4 of parturition, there is increased cervical expression of chemokines and collagenase/protease activity. It was assumed that processes regulating phases 3 and 4 of dilation and postpartum recovery of the cervix were similar to those in phase 2 of cervical ripening (Bokström, 1997; Osman, 2003; Sennström, 2000; Young, 2002). This has been challenged by observations from both human and animal studies. Sakamoto and associates (2004, 2005) found no correlation between the degree of clinical cervical ripening and the tissue concentrations of cervical neutrophil-chemoattractant interleukin 8 (IL-8). Microarray studies comparing gene expression patterns at term before and after cervical ripening report little increase in expression of proinflammatory genes. In contrast, there is a robust increase in proinflammatory and immunosuppressive genes in the cervix after delivery compared with during cervical ripening (Bollapragada, 2009; Hassan, 2006, 2009).

In mouse models, monocyte migration, but not activation, takes place before labor (Timmons, 2006, 2007, 2009). Mice deficient in the chemokine receptor CCR2, important in monocyte homing to tissues, have normally timed labor. This further supports the suggestion that labor is not initiated by an inflammatory response (Menzies, 2012). Furthermore, tissue depletion of neutrophils before birth has no effect on the timing or success of parturition. Finally, activation of neutrophils, proinflammatory M1 macrophages, and alternatively of activated M2 macrophages is increased within 2 hours after birth. This suggests a role for inflammatory cells in postpartum cervical remodeling and repair.

Induction and Prevention of Cervical Ripening

There are no therapies to prevent premature cervical ripening. Cervical cerclage is used to circumvent cervical insufficiency, although success appears limited (Owen, 2012). In contrast, treatment to promote cervical ripening for labor induction includes direct application of prostaglandins E_2 (PGE_2) and $F_{2\alpha}$ ($PGF_{2\alpha}$). Prostaglandins likely modify extracellular matrix structure to aid ripening. Although the role of prostaglandins in the normal physiology of cervical ripening remains unclear, this property is useful clinically to assist labor induction (Chap. 26, p. 526). In some nonhuman species, the cascades of events that allow cervical ripening are induced by decreasing serum progesterone concentrations. And in humans, administration of progesterone antagonists causes cervical ripening. As discussed later, humans may have developed unique mechanisms to localize decreases in progesterone action in the cervix and myometrium.

Phase 3 of Parturition: Labor

This phase is synonymous with active labor, which is customarily divided into three stages. These compose the commonly used labor graph shown in Figure 21-2. The clinical stages of labor may be summarized as follows. The first stage begins when spaced uterine contractions of sufficient frequency, intensity, and duration are attained to bring about cervical thinning, or *effacement*. This labor stage ends when the cervix is fully dilated—about 10 cm—to allow passage of the term-sized fetus. The first stage of labor, therefore, is the *stage of cervical effacement and dilatation.*

The second stage begins when cervical dilatation is complete and ends with delivery. Thus, the second stage of labor is the *stage of fetal expulsion.* Last, the third stage begins immediately after delivery of the fetus and ends with the delivery of the placenta. Thus, the third stage of labor is the *stage of placental separation and expulsion.*

First Stage of Labor: Clinical Onset of Labor

In some women, forceful uterine contractions that effect delivery begin suddenly. In others, labor initiation is heralded by spontaneous release of a small amount of blood-tinged mucus from the vagina. This extrusion of the mucus plug that had previously filled the cervical canal during pregnancy is referred to as "show" or "bloody show." There is very little blood with the mucous plug, and its passage indicates that labor is already in progress or likely will ensue in hours to days.

Uterine Labor Contractions

Unique among physiological muscular contractions, those of uterine smooth muscle during labor are painful. The cause of this is not known definitely, but several possibilities have been suggested: (1) hypoxia of the contracted myometrium—such as that with angina pectoris; (2) compression of nerve ganglia in the cervix and lower uterus by contracted interlocking muscle bundles; (3) cervical stretching during dilatation; and (4) stretching of the peritoneum overlying the fundus.

Of these, compression of nerve ganglia in the cervix and lower uterine segment by the contracting myometrium is an especially attractive hypothesis. Paracervical infiltration with local anesthetic usually produces appreciable pain relief with contractions (Chap. 25, p. 509). Uterine contractions are involuntary and, for the most part, independent of extrauterine control. Neural blockade from epidural analgesia does not diminish their frequency or intensity. In other examples, myometrial contractions in paraplegic women and in women after bilateral lumbar sympathectomy are normal but painless.

Mechanical stretching of the cervix enhances uterine activity in several species, including humans. This phenomenon has been referred to as the *Ferguson reflex* (Ferguson, 1941). Its exact mechanism is not clear, and release of oxytocin has been suggested but not proven. Manipulation of the cervix and "stripping" the fetal membranes is associated with an increase in blood levels of prostaglandin $F_{2\alpha}$ metabolite (PGFM).

The interval between contractions diminishes gradually from approximately 10 minutes at the onset of first-stage labor to as little as 1 minute or less in the second stage. Periods of relaxation between contractions, however, are essential for fetal welfare. Unremitting contractions compromise uteroplacental blood flow sufficiently to cause fetal hypoxemia. In active-phase labor, the duration of each contraction ranges from 30 to 90 seconds, averaging about 1 minute. There is appreciable variability in contraction intensity during normal labor. Specifically, amnionic fluid pressures generated by contractions during spontaneous labor average 40 mm Hg, but vary from 20 to 60 mm Hg (Chap. 24, p. 498).

Distinct Lower and Upper Uterine Segments. During active labor, the anatomical uterine divisions that were initiated in phase 2 of parturition become increasingly evident (Figs. 21-4 and 21-5). By abdominal palpation, even before membrane rupture, the two segments can sometimes be differentiated. The upper segment is firm during contractions, whereas the lower segment is softer, distended, and more passive. This mechanism is imperative because if the entire myometrium, including the lower uterine segment and cervix, were to contract simultaneously and with equal intensity, the net expulsive force would be markedly decreased. Thus, the upper segment contracts, retracts, and expels the fetus. In response to these contractions, the softened lower uterine segment and cervix dilate and thereby form a greatly expanded, thinned-out tube through which the fetus can pass.

The myometrium of the upper segment does not relax to its original length after contractions. Instead, it becomes relatively fixed at a shorter length. The upper active uterine segment

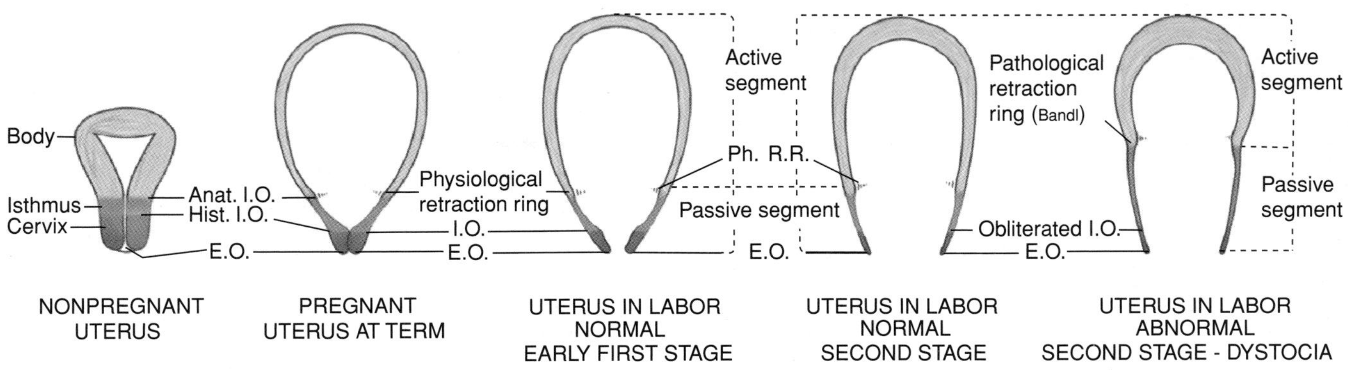

FIGURE 21-4 Sequence of development of the segments and rings in the uterus at term and in labor. Note comparison between the uterus of a nonpregnant woman, the uterus at term, and the uterus during labor. The passive lower uterine segment is derived from the isthmus, and the physiological retraction ring develops at the junction of the upper and lower uterine segments. The pathological retraction ring develops from the physiological ring. Anat. I.O. = anatomical internal os; E.O. = external os; Hist. I.O. = histological internal os; Ph. R.R. = physiological retraction ring.

contracts down on its diminishing contents, but myometrial tension remains constant. The net effect is to take up slack, thus maintaining the advantage gained in expulsion of the fetus. Concurrently, the uterine musculature is kept in firm contact with the uterine contents. As the consequence of retraction, each successive contraction commences where its predecessor left off. Thus, the upper part of the uterine cavity becomes slightly smaller with each successive contraction. Because of the successive shortening of the muscular fibers, the upper active segment becomes progressively thickened throughout first- and second-stage labor (see Fig. 21-4). This process continues and results in a tremendously thickened upper uterine segment immediately after delivery.

Clinically, it is important to understand that the phenomenon of upper segment retraction is contingent on a decrease in the volume of its contents. For this to happen, particularly early in labor when the entire uterus is virtually a closed sac with only minimal cervical dilatation, the musculature of the lower segment must stretch. This permits an increasing portion of the uterine contents to occupy the lower segment. The upper segment retracts only to the extent that the lower segment distends and the cervix dilates.

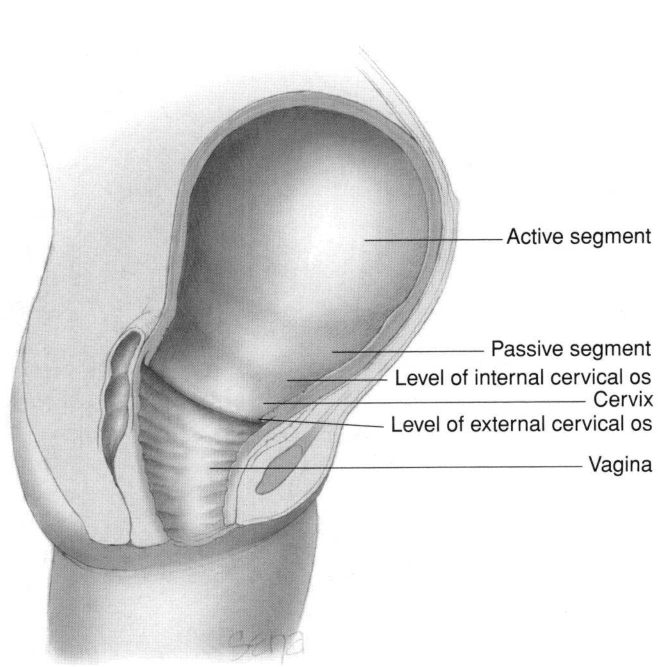

FIGURE 21-5 The uterus at the time of vaginal delivery. The active upper segment retracts around the presenting part as the fetus descends through the birth canal. In the passive lower segment, there is considerably less myometrial tone.

Relaxation of the lower uterine segment mirrors the same gradual progression of retraction. Recall that after each contraction of the upper segment, the muscles do not return to their previous length, but tension remains essentially the same. By comparison, in the lower segment, successive lengthening of the fibers with labor is accompanied by thinning, normally to only a few millimeters in the thinnest part. As a result of the lower segment thinning and concomitant upper segment thickening, a boundary between the two is marked by a ridge on the inner uterine surface—the *physiological retraction ring.* When the thinning of the lower uterine segment is extreme, as in obstructed labor, the ring is prominent and forms a *pathological retraction ring.* This abnormal condition is also known as the *Bandl ring,* which is discussed further and illustrated in Chapter 23 (p. 470).

Changes in Uterine Shape During Labor. Each contraction produces an elongation of the ovoid uterine shape with a concomitant decrease in horizontal diameter. This change in shape has important effects on the labor process. First, there is increased *fetal axis pressure,* that is, the decreased horizontal diameter serves to straighten the fetal vertebral column. This presses the upper pole of the fetus firmly against the fundus, whereas the lower pole is thrust farther downward. The lengthening of the ovoid shape has been estimated at 5 and 10 cm. Second, with lengthening of the uterus, the longitudinal muscle fibers are drawn taut. As a result, the lower segment and cervix are the only parts of the uterus that are flexible, and these are pulled upward and around the lower pole of the fetus.

Ancillary Forces in Labor

After the cervix is dilated fully, the most important force in fetal expulsion is that produced by maternal intraabdominal pressure. Contraction of the abdominal muscles simultaneously with forced respiratory efforts with the glottis closed is referred to as *pushing.* The force is similar to that with defecation, but the intensity usually is much greater. The importance of intraabdominal pressure is shown by the prolonged descent during labor in paraplegic women and in those with a dense epidural block. And, although increased intraabdominal pressure is necessary to complete second-stage labor, pushing accomplishes little in the first stage. It exhausts the mother, and its associated increased intrauterine pressures may be harmful to the fetus.

Cervical Changes

As the result of contraction forces, two fundamental changes—effacement and dilatation—occur in the already-ripened cervix. For an average-sized fetal head to pass through the cervix, its canal must dilate to a diameter of approximately 10 cm. At this time, the cervix is said to be completely or fully dilated. Although there may be no fetal descent during cervical effacement, most commonly the presenting fetal part descends somewhat as the cervix dilates. During second-stage labor in nulliparas, the presenting part typically descends slowly and steadily. In multiparas, however, particularly those of high parity, descent may be rapid.

Cervical effacement is "obliteration" or "taking up" of the cervix. It is manifest clinically by shortening of the cervical

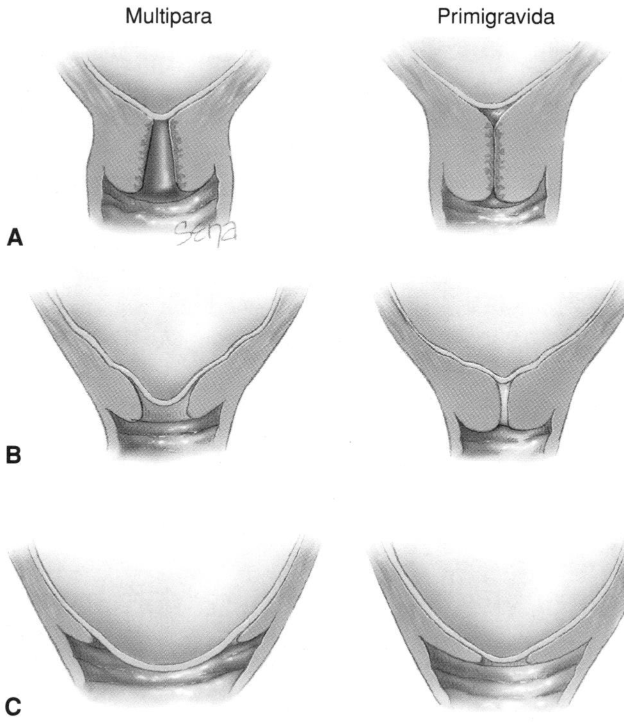

FIGURE 21-6 Schematic showing effacement and dilatation. **A.** Before labor, the primigravid cervix is long and undilated in contrast to that of the multipara, which has dilatation of the internal and external os. **B.** As effacement begins, the multiparous cervix shows dilatation and funneling of the internal os. This is less apparent in the primigravid cervix. **C.** As complete effacement is achieved in the primigravid cervix, dilation is minimal. The reverse is true in the multipara.

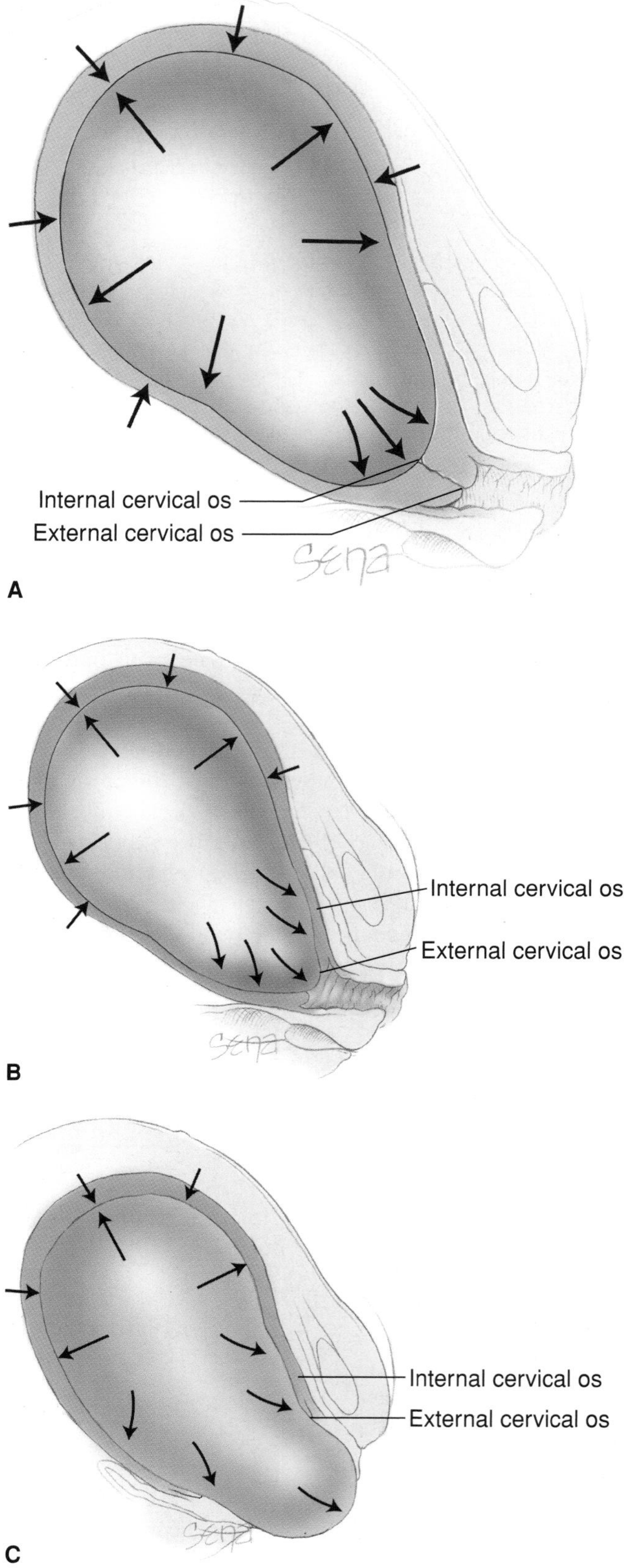

FIGURE 21-7 Hydrostatic action of membranes in effecting cervical effacement and dilatation. With labor progression, note the changing relations of the internal and external os in **(A)**, **(B)**, and **(C)**. Although not shown in this diagram, with membrane rupture, the presenting part, applied to the cervix and the forming lower uterine segment, acts similarly.

canal from a length of approximately 2 cm to a mere circular orifice with almost paper-thin edges. The muscular fibers at the level of the internal cervical os are pulled upward, or "taken up," into the lower uterine segment. The condition of the external os remains temporarily unchanged (Fig. 21-6).

Effacement may be compared to a funneling process in which the whole length of a narrow cylinder is converted into a very obtuse, flaring funnel with a small circular opening. Because of increased myometrial activity during uterine preparedness for labor, appreciable effacement of a softened cervix sometimes is accomplished before active labor begins. Effacement causes expulsion of the mucous plug as the cervical canal is shortened.

Because the lower segment and cervix have lesser resistance during a contraction, a centrifugal pull is exerted on the cervix and creates *cervical dilatation* (Fig. 21-7). As uterine contractions cause pressure on the membranes, the hydrostatic action of the amnionic sac in turn dilates the cervical canal like a wedge. In the absence of intact membranes, the pressure of the presenting fetal part against the cervix and lower uterine segment is similarly effective. Early rupture of the membranes does not retard cervical dilatation so long as the presenting fetal part is positioned to exert pressure against the cervix and lower segment. The process of cervical effacement and dilatation causes formation of the *forebag* of amnionic fluid. This is the leading portion of fluid and amnionic sac located in front of the presenting part.

Referring back to Figure 21-2, recall that cervical dilatation is divided into latent and active phases. The active phase is subdivided further into the acceleration phase, the phase of maximum slope, and the deceleration phase (Friedman, 1978). The duration of the latent phase is more variable and sensitive to changes by extraneous factors. For example, sedation may prolong the latent phase, and myometrial stimulation shortens it. The latent phase duration has little bearing on the subsequent course of labor, whereas the characteristics of the accelerated phase are usually predictive of labor outcome. Completion of cervical dilatation during the active phase is accomplished by cervical retraction about the presenting part. The first stage ends when cervical dilatation is complete. Once the second stage commences, only progressive descent of the presenting part will foretell further progress.

Second Stage of Labor: Fetal Descent

In many nulliparas, engagement of the head is accomplished before labor begins. That said, the head may not descend further until late in labor. In the descent pattern of normal labor, a typical hyperbolic curve is formed when the station of the fetal head is plotted as a function of labor duration. *Station* describes descent of the fetal biparietal diameter in relation to a line drawn between maternal ischial spines (Chap. 22, p. 449). Active descent usually takes place after dilatation has progressed for some time (Fig. 21-8). In nulliparas, increased rates of descent are observed ordinarily during cervical dilatation phase of maximum slope. At this time, the speed of descent is also maximal and is maintained until the presenting part reaches the perineal floor (Friedman, 1978).

Pelvic Floor Changes During Labor

The birth canal is supported and is functionally closed by several layers of tissues that together form the pelvic floor. These anatomical structures are shown in detail in Chapter 2 (p. 22). The most important are the levator ani muscle and the fibromuscular connective tissue covering its upper and lower surfaces. There are marked changes in the biomechanical properties of these structures and of the vaginal wall during parturition. These result from altered extracellular matrix structure or composition (Lowder, 2007; Rahn, 2008). The levator ani consists of the pubovisceral, puborectalis, and iliococcygeus muscles, which close the lower end of the pelvic cavity as a diaphragm. Thereby, a concave upper and a convex lower surface are presented. The posterior and lateral portions of the pelvic floor, which are not spanned by the levator ani, are occupied bilaterally by the piriformis and coccygeus muscles.

The levator ani muscle varies in thickness from 3 to 5 mm, although its margins encircling the rectum and vagina are somewhat thicker. During pregnancy, the levator ani usually undergoes hypertrophy, forming a thick band that extends backward from the pubis and encircles the vagina about 2 cm above the plane of the hymen. On contraction, the levator ani draws both the rectum and the vagina forward and upward in the direction of the symphysis pubis and thereby acts to close the vagina.

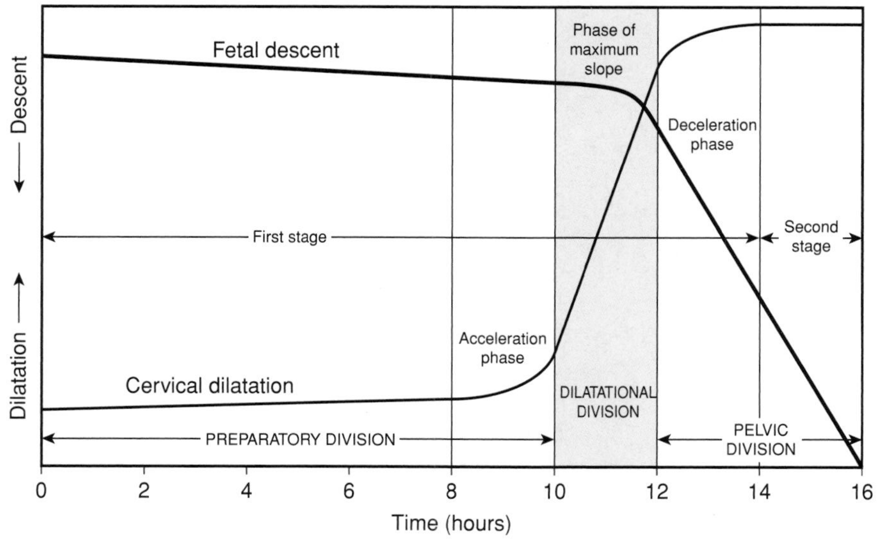

FIGURE 21-8 Labor course divided on the basis of expected evolution of the dilatation and descent curves into three functional divisions. The preparatory division includes the latent and acceleration phases. The dilatational division is the phase of maximum slope of dilatation. The pelvic division encompasses both the deceleration phase and the second stage, which is concurrent with the phase of maximum slope of fetal descent. (Redrawn from Friedman, 1978.)

In the first stage of labor, the membranes, when intact, and the fetal presenting part serve to dilate the upper vagina. The most marked change consists of stretching of the levator ani muscle fibers. This is accompanied by thinning of the central portion of the perineum, which becomes transformed from a wedge-shaped, 5-cm-thick tissue mass to a thin, almost transparent membranous structure less than 1 cm thick. When the perineum is distended maximally, the anus becomes markedly dilated and presents an opening that varies from 2 to 3 cm in diameter and through which the anterior wall of the rectum bulges.

Third Stage of Labor: Delivery of Placenta and Membranes

This stage begins immediately after fetal delivery and involves separation and expulsion of the placenta and membranes. As the neonate is born, the uterus spontaneously contracts around its diminishing contents. Normally, by the time the newborn is completely delivered, the uterine cavity is nearly obliterated. The organ consists of an almost solid mass of muscle, several centimeters thick, above the thinner lower segment. The uterine fundus now lies just below the level of the umbilicus.

This sudden diminution in uterine size is inevitably accompanied by a decrease in the area of the placental implantation site (Fig. 21-9). For the placenta to accommodate itself to this reduced area, it increases in thickness, but because of limited placental elasticity, it is forced to buckle. The resulting tension pulls the weakest layer—decidua spongiosa—from that site. Thus, placental separation follows the disproportion created between the relatively unchanged placental size and the reduced size of the implantation site.

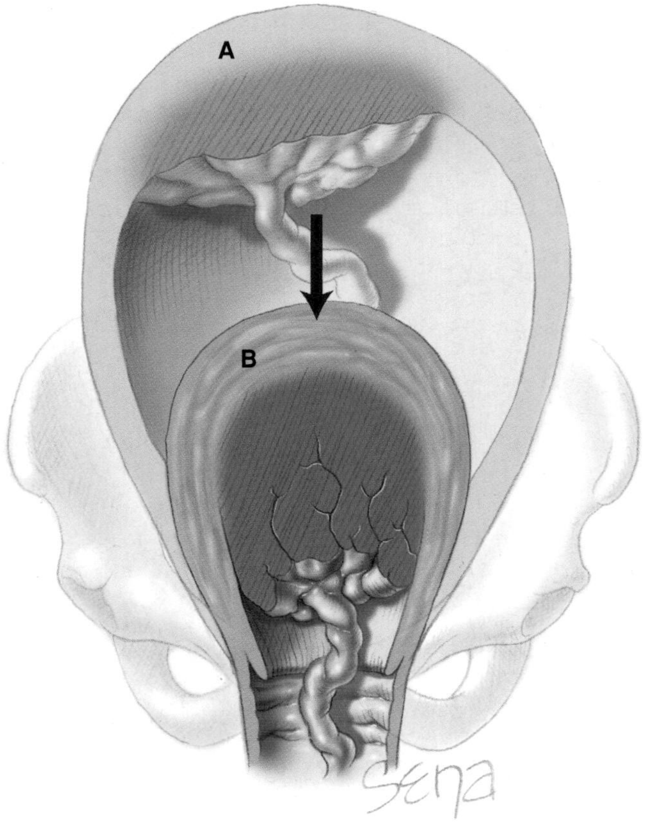

FIGURE 21-9 Diminution in size of the placental site after birth of the infant. **A.** Spatial relations before birth. **B.** Placental spatial relations after birth.

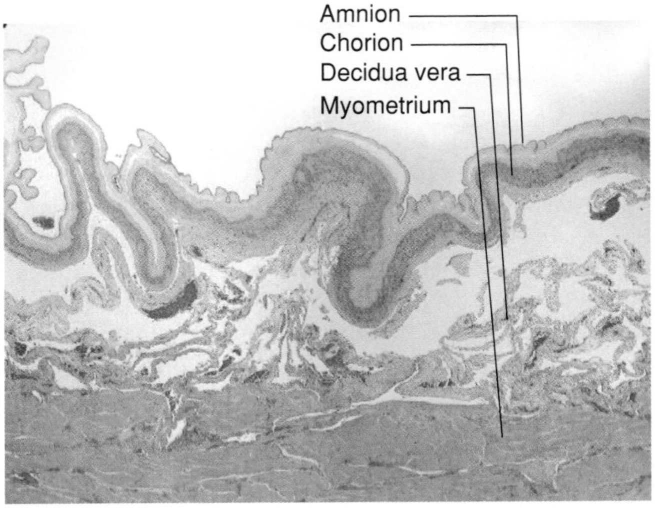

FIGURE 21-10 Postpartum, membranes are thrown up into folds as the uterine cavity decreases in size. (Photograph contributed by Dr. Kelley S. Carrick.)

Cleavage of the placenta is aided greatly by the loose structure of the spongy decidua, which may be likened to the row of perforations between postage stamps. As separation proceeds, a hematoma forms between the separating placenta/decidua and the decidua that remains attached to the myometrium. The hematoma is usually the result rather than the cause of the separation, because in some cases bleeding is negligible.

Fetal Membrane Separation and Placental Extrusion. The great decrease in uterine cavity surface area simultaneously throws the fetal membranes—the amniochorion and the parietal decidua—into innumerable folds (Fig. 21-10). Membranes usually remain in situ until placental separation is nearly completed. These are then peeled off the uterine wall, partly by further contraction of the myometrium and partly by traction that is exerted by the separated placenta.

After the placenta has separated, it may be expelled by increased abdominal pressure. Completion of the third stage is also accomplished by alternately compressing and elevating the fundus, while exerting minimal traction on the umbilical cord (Fig. 27-12, p. 546). The retroplacental hematoma either follows the placenta or is found within the inverted sac formed by the membranes. In this process, known as the *Schultze mechanism* of placental expulsion, blood from the placental site pours into the membrane sac and does not escape externally until after extrusion of the placenta. In the other form of placental extrusion, known as the *Duncan mechanism,* the placenta separates first at the periphery and blood collects between the membranes and the uterine wall and escapes from the vagina. In this circumstance, the placenta descends sideways, and its maternal surface appears first.

Phase 4 of Parturition: The Puerperium

Immediately and for about an hour or so after delivery, the myometrium remains in a state of rigid and persistent contraction and retraction. This directly compresses large uterine vessels and allows thrombosis of their lumens to prevent hemorrhage (Fig. 2-11, p. 27). This is typically augmented by uterotonics (Chap. 27, p. 547).

Uterine involution and cervical repair, both remodeling processes that restore these organs to the nonpregnant state, follow in a timely fashion. These protect the reproductive tract from invasion by commensal microorganisms and restore endometrial responsiveness to normal hormonal cyclicity.

During the early puerperium, there is onset of lactogenesis and milk let-down in mammary glands, as described in Chapter 36 (p. 672). Reinstitution of ovulation signals preparation for the next pregnancy. This generally occurs within 4 to 6 weeks after birth, but it is dependent on the duration of breast feeding and lactation-induced, prolactin-mediated anovulation and amenorrhea.

PHYSIOLOGICAL AND BIOCHEMICAL PROCESSES REGULATING PARTURITION

There are two general contemporaneous theorems concerning labor initiation. Viewed simplistically, the first is the *functional loss of pregnancy maintenance factors,* whereas the second focuses on *synthesis of factors that induce parturition.* Some investigators also speculate that the mature fetus is the source of the initial signal for parturition commencement. Others suggest that one or more uterotonins, produced in increased amounts, or an increased population of myometrial uterotonin receptors is the proximate cause. Indeed, an obligatory role for one or more uterotonins is included in most parturition theories, as either a primary or a secondary phenomenon in the final events of childbirth. Both rely on careful regulation of smooth muscle contraction.

Myometrial Action

Anatomical and Physiological Considerations

There are unique characteristics of smooth muscle, including myometrium, compared with those of skeletal muscle that may confer advantages for uterine contraction efficiency and fetal delivery. First, the degree of smooth-muscle cell shortening with contractions may be one order of magnitude greater than that attained in striated muscle cells. Second, forces can be exerted in smooth muscle cells in multiple directions. In contrast, the contraction force generated by skeletal muscle is always aligned with the axis of the muscle fibers. Third, smooth muscle is not organized in the same manner as skeletal muscle. In myometrium, the thick and thin filaments are found in long, random bundles throughout the cells. This plexiform arrangement aids greater shortening and force-generating capacity. Last, greater multidirectional force generation in the uterine fundus compared with that of the lower uterine segment permits versatility in expulsive force directionality. These forces thus can be brought to bear irrespective of the fetal lie or presentation.

Regulation of Myometrial Contraction and Relaxation

Myometrial contraction is controlled by transcription of key genes, which produce proteins that repress or enhance cellular contractility. These proteins function to: (1) enhance the interactions between the actin and myosin proteins that cause muscle contraction, (2) increase excitability of individual myometrial cells, and (3) promote intracellular cross talk that allows development of synchronous contractions.

Actin-Myosin Interactions. The interaction of myosin and actin is essential to muscle contraction. This interaction requires that actin be converted from a globular to a filamentous form. Moreover, actin must be attached to the cytoskeleton at focal points in the cell membrane to allow development of tension (Fig. 21-11). Actin must partner with myosin, which is composed of multiple light and heavy chains. The interaction of myosin and actin activates adenosine triphosphatase (ATPase), hydrolyzes adenosine triphosphate, and generates force. This interaction is brought about by enzymatic phosphorylation of the 20-kDa light chain of myosin (Stull, 1988, 1998). This is catalyzed by the enzyme *myosin light-chain kinase,* which is activated by calcium. Calcium binds to *calmodulin,* a calcium-binding regulatory protein, which in turn binds to and activates myosin light-chain kinase.

Intracellular Calcium. Agents that promote contraction act on myometrial cells to increase intracellular cytosolic calcium concentration—$[Ca^{2+}]_i$. Or, they allow an influx of extracellular calcium through ligand- or voltage-regulated calcium channels (see Fig. 21-11). For example, prostaglandin $F_{2\alpha}$ and oxytocin bind their respective receptors during labor to open ligand-activated calcium channels. Activation of these receptors also releases calcium from the sarcoplasmic reticulum to cause decreased electronegativity within the cell. Voltage-gated ion channels open, additional calcium ions move into the cell, and cellular depolarization follows. The increase in $[Ca^{2+}]_i$ is often transient, but contractions can be prolonged through the inhibition of myosin phosphatase activity (Woodcock, 2004).

Conditions that decrease $[Ca^{2+}]_i$ and increase intracellular concentrations of cyclic adenosine monophosphate (cAMP) or cyclic guanosine monophosphate (cGMP) ordinarily promote uterine relaxation. Corticotropin-releasing hormone is one of several factors reported to regulate $[Ca^{2+}]_i$ and subsequently modulate expression of the large-conductance potassium channels (BKCa) in the human myometrium (Xu, 2011; You, 2012). Genetic studies in humans and transgenic overexpression in mice reveal that small-conductance calcium-activated K^+ isoform 3 (SK3) channels may also be important in maintenance of uterine relaxation (Day, 2011; Rada, 2012). SK3 channel expression declines at the end of term pregnancy as contractility is increased and overexpression of SK3 in transgenic mice dampens uterine contraction force to prevent delivery. Yet another potential mechanism for maintenance of relaxation shown in Figure 21-11 is the promotion of actin in a globular form rather than in fibrils required for contraction (Macphee, 2000; Yu, 1998).

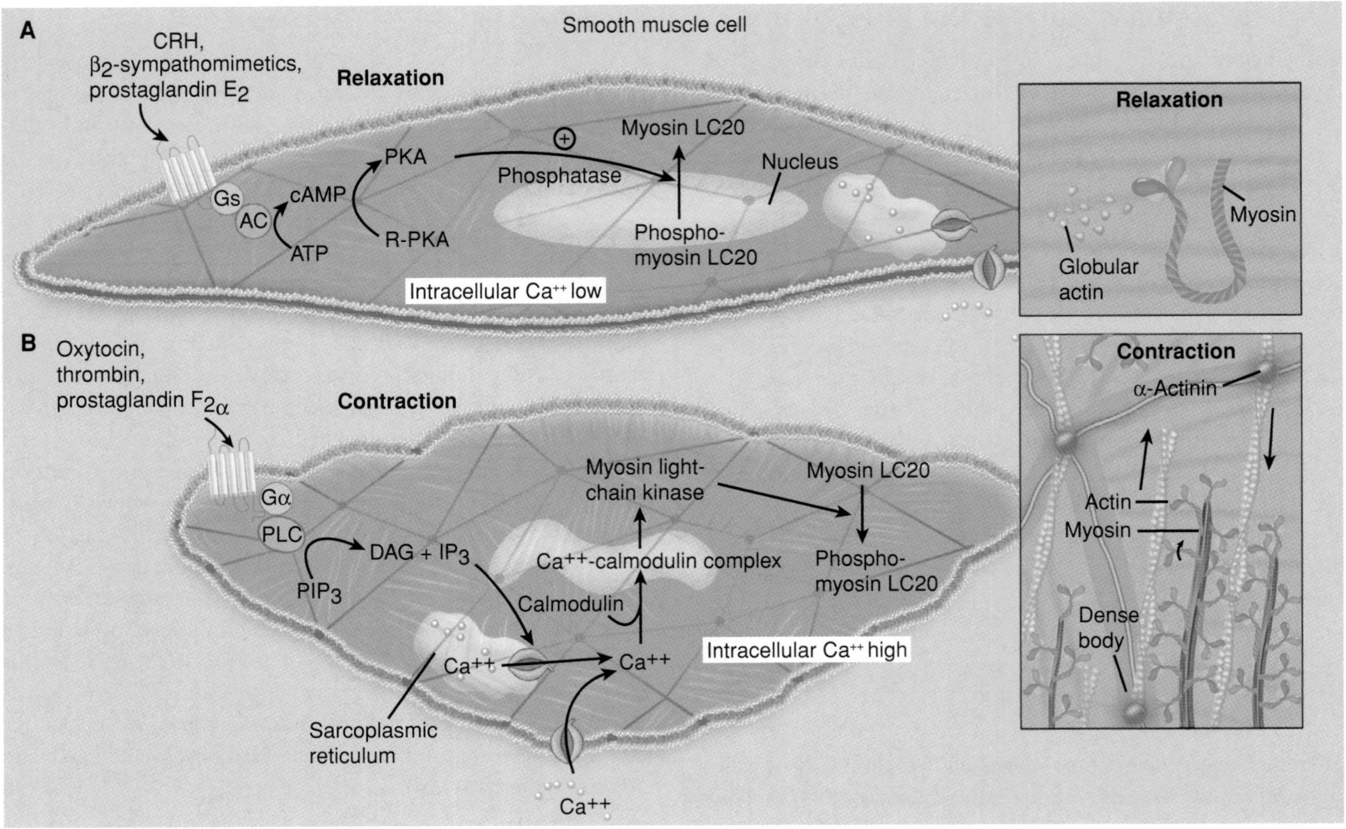

FIGURE 21-11 Uterine myocyte relaxation and contraction. **A.** Uterine relaxation is maintained by factors that increase myocyte cyclic adenosine monophosphate (cAMP). This activates protein kinase A (PKA) to promote phosphodiesterase activity with dephosphorylation of myosin light-chain kinase (MLCK). There are also processes that serve to maintain actin in a globular form, and thus to prevent fibril formation necessary for contractions. **B.** Uterine contractions result from reversal of these sequences. Actin now assumes a fibrillar form, and calcium enters the cell to combine with calmodulin to form complexes. These complexes activate MLCK to bring about phosphorylation of the myosin light chains. This generates ATPase activity to cause sliding of myosin over the actin fibrils, which is a uterine contractor. AC = adenylyl cyclase; Ca^{++} = calcium; DAG = diacylglycerol; Gs and Gα = G-receptor proteins; IP_3 = inositol triphosphate; LC20 = light chain 20; PIP_3 = phosphatidylinositol 3,4,5-triphosphate; PLC = phospholipase C; R-PKA = inactive protein kinase. (Redrawn from Smith, 2007.)

In addition to myocyte contractility, myocyte excitability is also regulated by changes in the electrochemical potential gradient across the plasma membrane. Before labor, myocytes maintain a relatively high interior electronegativity. This state is maintained by the combined actions of the ATPase-driven sodium-potassium pump and the large conductance voltage- and Ca^{2+}-sensitive K channel—*maxi-K channel* (Parkington, 2001). During uterine quiescence, the maxi-K channel is open and allows potassium to leave the cell to maintain interior electronegativity. At the time of labor, changes in electronegativity lead to depolarization and contraction (Brainard, 2005; Chanrachakul, 2003). And, as parturition progresses, there is increased synchronization of electrical uterine activity.

Myometrial Gap Junctions. Cellular signals that control myometrial contraction and relaxation can be effectively transferred between cells through intercellular junctional channels. Communication is established between myocytes by gap junctions, which aid the passage of electrical or ionic coupling currents as well as metabolite coupling. The transmembrane channels that make up the gap junctions consist of two protein "hemi-channels" (Sáez, 2005). These *connexons* are each composed of six *connexin* subunit proteins (Fig. 21-12). These pairs of connexons establish a conduit between coupled cells for the exchange of small molecules that can be nutrients, waste, metabolites, second messengers, or ions.

Optimal numbers of gap junctions are believed to be important for electrical myometrial synchrony. Four described in the uterus are connexins 26, 40, 43, and 45. Connexin 43 junctions are scarce in the nonpregnant uterus, and they increase in size and abundance during human parturition (Chow, 1994). Also, mouse models deficient in connexin 43-enriched gap junctions exhibit delayed parturition, further supporting their role (Döring, 2006; Tong, 2009).

Cell Surface Receptors. There are various cell surface receptors that can directly regulate myocyte contractile state. Three major classes are G-protein-linked, ion channel-linked, and enzyme-linked. Multiple examples of each have been identified in human myometrium. These further appear to be modified during the phases of parturition. Most G-protein-coupled receptors are associated with adenylyl cyclase activation. Examples are the CRHR1α and the LH

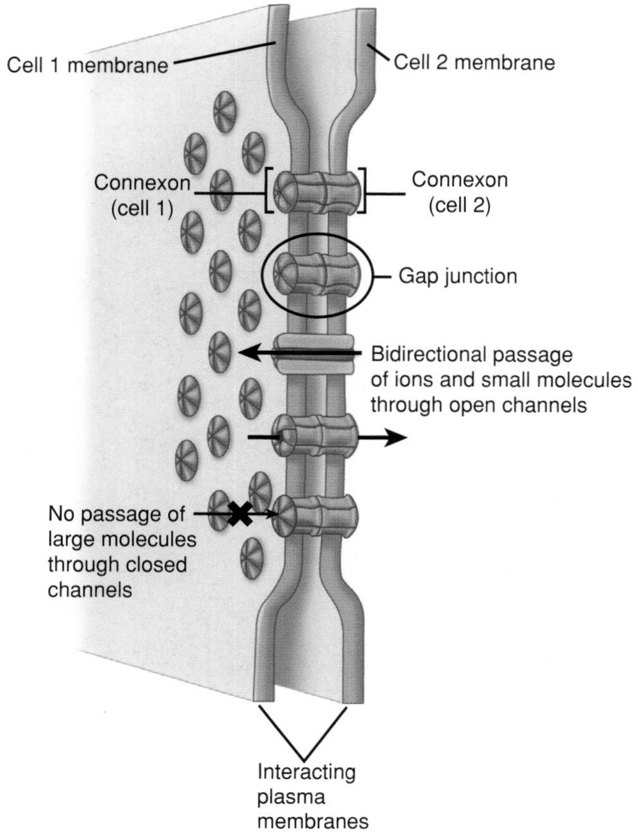

FIGURE 21-12 The protein subunits of gap junction channels are called connexins. Six connexins form a hemichannel (connexon), and two connexons (one from each cell) form a gap junction channel. Connexons and gap junction channels can be formed from one or more connexin proteins. The composition of the gap junction channel is important for their selectivity with regard to passage of molecules and communication between cells.

receptors (Fig. 21-13). Other G-protein-coupled myometrial receptors, however, are associated with G-protein-mediated activation of phospholipase C. Ligands for the G-protein-coupled receptors include numerous neuropeptides, hormones, and autacoids. Many of these are available to the myometrium during pregnancy in high concentration via *endocrine* or *autocrine* mechanisms (Fig. 21-14).

Cervical Dilatation During Labor

There is a large influx of leukocytes into the cervical stroma with cervical dilatation (Sakamoto, 2004, 2005). Cervical tissue levels of leukocyte chemoattractants such as IL-8 are increased just after delivery, as are IL-8 receptor levels. Identification of genes upregulated just after vaginal delivery further suggests that dilatation and early stages of postpartum repair are aided by inflammatory responses, apoptosis, and activation of proteases that degrade extracellular matrix components (Hassan, 2006; Havelock, 2005). The composition of glycosaminoglycans, proteoglycans, and poorly formed collagen fibrils that were necessary during ripening and dilatation must be rapidly removed to allow reorganization and recovery of cervical structure. In the days that follow parturition, recovery of cervical structure involves processes that resolve inflammation, promote tissue repair, and regenerate dense cervical connective tissue with structural integrity and mechanical strength.

Phase 1: Uterine Quiescence and Cervical Competence

Myometrial quiescence is so remarkable and successful that it probably is induced by multiple independent and cooperative biomolecular processes. Individually, some of these processes may be redundant to ensure pregnancy continuance. It is likely that all manners of molecular systems—neural, endocrine, paracrine, and autocrine—are called on to implement and coordinate a state of relative uterine unresponsiveness. Moreover, a complementary "fail-safe" system that protects the uterus against agents that could perturb the tranquility of phase 1 also must be in place (see Fig. 21-14).

As shown in Figure 21-15, phase 1 of human parturition and its quiescence are likely the result of many factors that include: (1) actions of estrogen and progesterone via intracellular receptors, (2) myometrial cell plasma membrane receptor-mediated increases in cAMP, (3) generation of cGMP, and (4) other systems, including modification of myometrial-cell ion channels.

Progesterone and Estrogen Contributions

In many species, the role of the sex steroid hormones is clear—progesterone inhibits and estrogen promotes the events leading to parturition. In humans, however, it seems most likely that both estrogen and progesterone are components of a broader-based molecular system that implements and maintains uterine quiescence. In many species, the removal of progesterone, that is, *progesterone withdrawal,* directly precedes progression of phase 1 into phase 2 of parturition. In addition, providing progesterone to some species will delay parturition via a decrease in myometrial activity and continued cervical competency (Challis, 1994). Studies in these species have led to a better understanding of why the progesterone-replete myometrium of phase 1 is relatively noncontractile.

Plasma levels of estrogen and progesterone in normal pregnancy are enormous and in great excess of the affinity constants for their receptors. For this reason, it is difficult to comprehend how relatively subtle changes in the ratio of their concentrations could modulate physiological processes during pregnancy. The teleological evidence, however, for an increased progesterone-to-estrogen ratio in the maintenance of pregnancy and a decline in the progesterone-to-estrogen ratio for parturition is overwhelming. In all species studied to date, including humans, administration of the progesterone-receptor antagonists *mifepristone (RU-486)* or *onapristone* will promote some or all key features of parturition. These include cervical ripening, increased cervical distensibility, and increased uterine sensitivity to uterotonins (Bygdeman, 1994; Chwalisz, 1994a; Wolf, 1993).

The exact role of estrogen in regulating human uterine activity and cervical competency is less well understood. That said, it appears that estrogen can act to promote progesterone

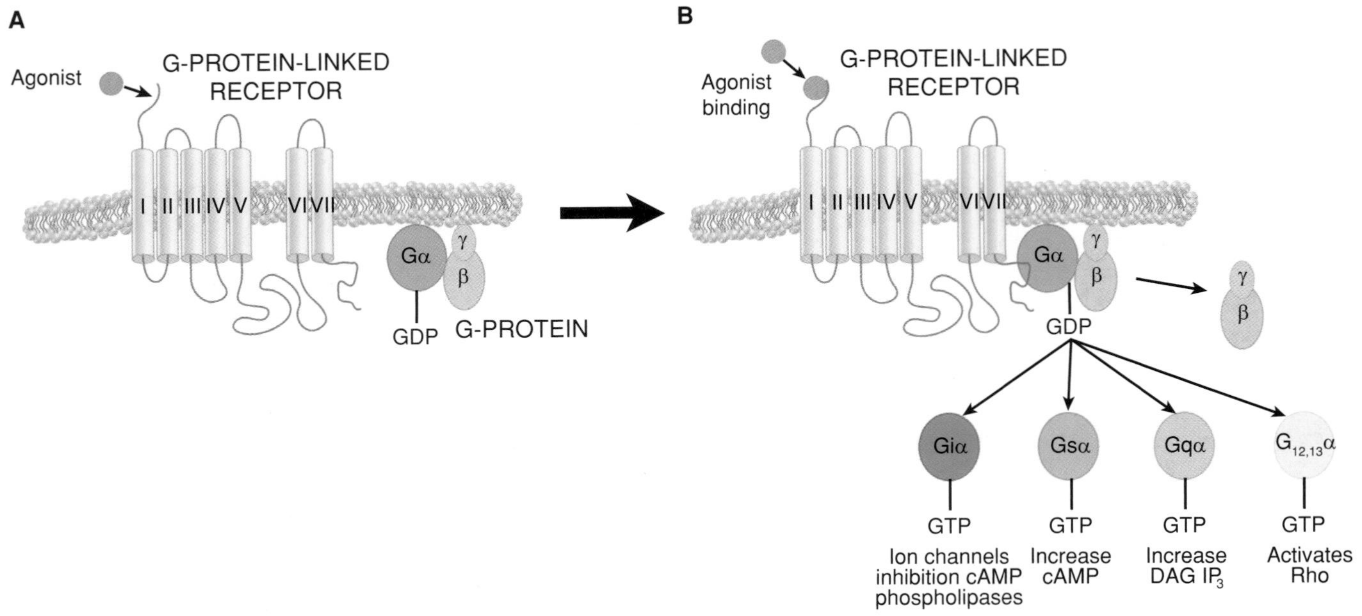

FIGURE 21-13 G-protein-coupled receptor signal transduction pathways. **A.** Receptors coupled to heterotrimeric guanosine-triphosphate (GTP)-binding proteins (G proteins) are integral transmembrane proteins that transduce extracellular signals to the cell interior. G-protein-coupled receptors exhibit a common structural motif consisting of seven membrane-spanning regions. **B.** Receptor occupation promotes interaction between the receptor and the G protein on the interior surface of the membrane. This induces an exchange of guanosine diphosphate (GDP) for GTP on the G protein α subunit and dissociation of the α subunit from the βγ heterodimer. Depending on its isoform, the GTP-α subunit complex mediates intracellular signaling either indirectly by acting on effector molecules such as adenylyl cyclase (AC) or phospholipase C (PLC), or directly by regulating ion channel or kinase function. cAMP = cyclic adenosine monophosphate; DAG = diacylglycerol; IP_3 = inositol triphosphate.

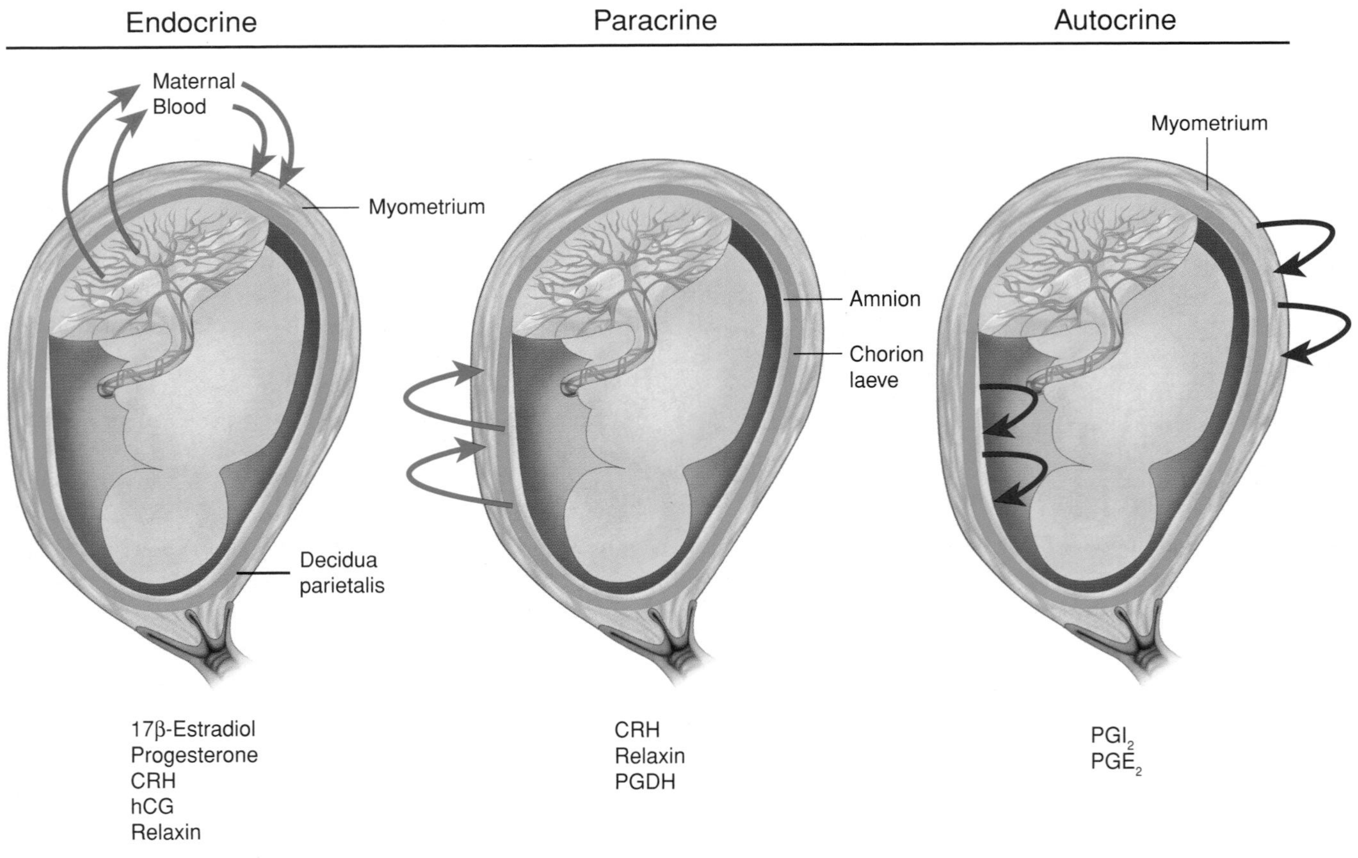

FIGURE 21-14 Theoretical fail-safe system involving endocrine, paracrine, and autocrine mechanisms for the maintenance of phase 1 of parturition, uterine quiescence. CRH = corticotropin-releasing hormone; hCG = human chorionic gonadotropin; PGE_2 = prostaglandin E_2; PGI_2 = prostaglandin I_2; PGDH = 15-hydroxyprostaglandin dehydrogenase.

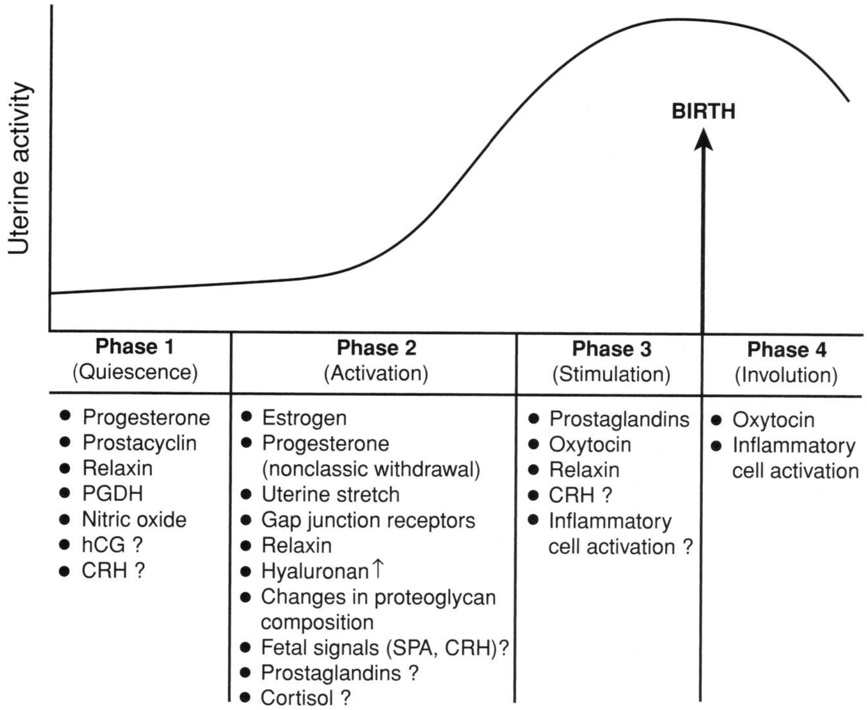

FIGURE 21-15 The key factors thought to regulate the phases of parturition. CRH = corticotropin-releasing hormone; hCG = human chorionic gonadotropin; SPA = surfactant protein A. (Adapted from Challis, 2002.)

responsiveness and, in doing so, promote uterine quiescence. The estrogen receptor, acting via the estrogen-response element of the progesterone-receptor gene, induces progesterone-receptor synthesis, which allows increased progesterone-mediated function.

Myometrial Cell-to-Cell Communication. Progesterone maintains uterine quiescence by various mechanisms that cause decreased expression of the contraction-associated proteins (CAPs)(p. 410). Progesterone can promote expression of the inhibitory transcription factor ZEB1—zinc finger E-box binding homeobox protein 1—which can inhibit expression of the CAP genes, connexin 43, and oxytocin receptor (Renthal, 2010). As another mechanism, progesterone bound to the progesterone receptor (PR) can recruit coregulatory factors. These include PSF—polypyrimidine tract binding protein-associated splicing factor—and Sin3A/HDACs—yeast switch-dependent3 homologue A/histone deacetylase corepressor complex—which inhibit expression of the gene encoding the gap junctional protein connexin 43 in rat and human myocytes (Xie, 2012).

At the end of pregnancy, increased stretch along with increased estrogen dominance results in a decline in PSF and Sin/HDAC levels, thus abrogating the suppression of connexin 43 expression by progesterone. Additionally, with loss of progesterone function at term, ZEB1 levels decline due to increased production of small regulatory RNAs termed microRNAs. This releases inhibition of connexin 43 and oxytocin receptor levels to promote increased uterine contractility (Renthal, 2010; Williams, 2012b).

G-Protein–Coupled Receptors

A number of G-protein-coupled receptors that normally are associated with $G\alpha_s$-mediated activation of adenylyl cyclase and increased levels of cAMP are present in myometrium. These receptors together with appropriate ligands may act in concert with sex steroid hormones as part of a fail-safe system to maintain uterine quiescence (Price, 2000; Sanborn, 1998).

Beta-Adrenoreceptors. These receptors are prototypical examples of cAMP signaling causing myometrium relaxation. Agents binding to these receptors have been used for tocolysis with preterm labor and include ritodrine and terbutaline (Chap. 42, p. 852). β-Adrenergic receptors mediate $G\alpha_s$-stimulated increases in adenylyl cyclase, increased levels of cAMP, and myometrial cell relaxation. The rate-limiting factor is likely the number of receptors expressed and the level of adenylyl cyclase expression.

Luteinizing Hormone (LH) and Human Chorionic Gonadotropin (hCG) Receptors. These hormones share the same receptor, and this G-protein-coupled receptor has been demonstrated in myometrial smooth muscle and blood vessels (Lei, 1992; Ziecik, 1992). Levels of myometrial LH-hCG receptors during pregnancy are greater before than during labor (Zuo, 1994). Chorionic gonadotropin acts to activate adenylyl cyclase by way of a plasma membrane receptor–$G_{\alpha s}$-linked system. This decreases contraction frequency and force and decreases the number of tissue-specific myometrial cell gap junctions (Ambrus, 1994; Eta, 1994). Thus, high circulating levels of hCG may be one mechanism causing uterine quiescence.

Relaxin. This peptide hormone consists of an A and B chain and is structurally similar to the insulin family of proteins (Bogic, 1995; Weiss, 1995). Relaxin mediates lengthening of the pubic ligament, cervical softening, vaginal relaxation, and inhibition of myometrial contractions. There are two separate human relaxin genes, designated *H1* and *H2*. The *H1* gene is primarily expressed in the decidua, trophoblast, and prostate, whereas the *H2* gene is primarily expressed in the corpus luteum.

Relaxin in plasma of pregnant women is believed to originate exclusively from corpus luteum secretion. Plasma levels peak at approximately 1 ng/mL between 8 and 12 weeks' gestation. Thereafter, they decline to lower levels that persist until term. Its plasma membrane receptor—*relaxin family peptide receptor 1 (RXFP1)*—mediates activation of adenylyl cyclase. Relaxin inhibits contractions of nonpregnant myometrial strips, but not those of uterine tissue taken from pregnant women. It also effects cervical remodeling through cell proliferation and modulation of extracellular matrix components such as collagen and hyaluronan (Park, 2005; Soh, 2012).

Corticotropin-Releasing Hormone (CRH). This hormone is synthesized in the placenta and hypothalamus. As discussed later, CRH plasma levels increase dramatically during the final 6 to 8 weeks of normal pregnancy and have been implicated in the mechanisms controlling the timing of human parturition (Smith, 2007; Wadhwa, 1998). CRH appears to promote myometrial quiescence during most of pregnancy and aids myometrial contractions with onset of parturition. Recent studies suggest that these opposing actions are achieved by differential actions of CRH via its receptor CRHR1. In the term nonlaboring myometrium, the interaction of CRH with its CRHR1 receptor results in activation of the Gs-adenylate cyclase-cAMP signaling pathway. This results in inhibition of inositol triphosphate (IP_3) production and a stabilization of $[Ca^{2+}]_i$ (You, 2012). In term laboring myometrium, $[Ca^{2+}]_i$ is increased by CRH activation of G proteins Gq and Gi and leads to stimulation of IP_3 production and increased contractility. Another aspect of CRH regulation is union of CRH to its binding protein, which can limit bioavailability. CRH-binding protein levels are high during pregnancy and are reported to decline at the time of labor.

Prostaglandins. These interact with a family of eight different G-protein-coupled receptors, several of which are expressed in myometrium (Myatt, 2004). Prostaglandins usually are considered as uterotonins. However, their effects are diverse, and some act as smooth muscle relaxants.

The major synthetic pathways involved in prostaglandin biosynthesis are shown in Figure 21-16. Prostaglandins are produced using plasma membrane-derived arachidonic acid, which usually is released by the action of the phospholipases A_2 or C. Arachidonic acid can then act as substrate for both type 1 and type 2 prostaglandin H synthase (PGHS-1 and -2), which are also called cyclooxygenase-1 and -2 (COX-1 and -2). Both PGHS isoforms convert arachidonic acid to the unstable endoperoxide prostaglandin G_2 and then to prostaglandin H_2. These enzymes are the target of many nonsteroidal antiinflammatory drugs (NSAIDs). Indeed, the tocolytic actions of specific NSAIDs, as discussed in Chapter 42 (p. 852), were considered promising until they were shown to have adverse fetal effects (Loudon, 2003; Olson, 2003, 2007).

Through prostaglandin isomerases, prostaglandin H_2 is converted to active prostaglandins, including PGE_2, $PGF_{2\alpha}$, and PGI_2. Isomerase expression is tissue-specific and thereby controls the relative production of various prostaglandins. Another important control point for prostaglandin activity is its metabolism, which most often is through the action of 15-hydroxyprostaglandin dehydrogenase (PGDH). Expression of this enzyme can be regulated in the uterus, which is important because of its ability to rapidly inactivate prostaglandins.

The effect of prostaglandins on tissue targets is complicated in that there are a number of G-protein-coupled prostaglandin receptors (Coleman, 1994). This family of receptors is classified according to the binding specificity of a given receptor to a particular prostaglandin. Both PGE_2 and PGI_2 could potentially act to maintain uterine quiescence by increasing cAMP signaling, yet PGE_2 can promote uterine contractility through binding to prostaglandin E receptors 1 and 3 (EP_1 and EP_3). Also, PGE_2, PGD_2, and PGI_2 have been shown to cause vascular smooth muscle relaxation and vasodilatation in many circumstances. Thus, either the generation of specific prostaglandins or the relative expression of the various prostaglandin receptors may determine myometrial responses to prostaglandins (Lyall, 2002; Olson, 2003, 2007; Smith, 2001; Smith, 1998).

In addition to gestational changes, other studies show that there may be regional changes in the upper and lower uterine segments. COX-2 expression is spatially regulated in the myometrium and cervix in pregnancy and labor, with an increasing concentration gradient from the fundus to the cervix (Havelock, 2005). Thus, it is entirely possible that prostanoids contribute to myometrial relaxation at one stage of pregnancy and to regional fundal myometrial contractions after parturition initiation (Myatt, 2004).

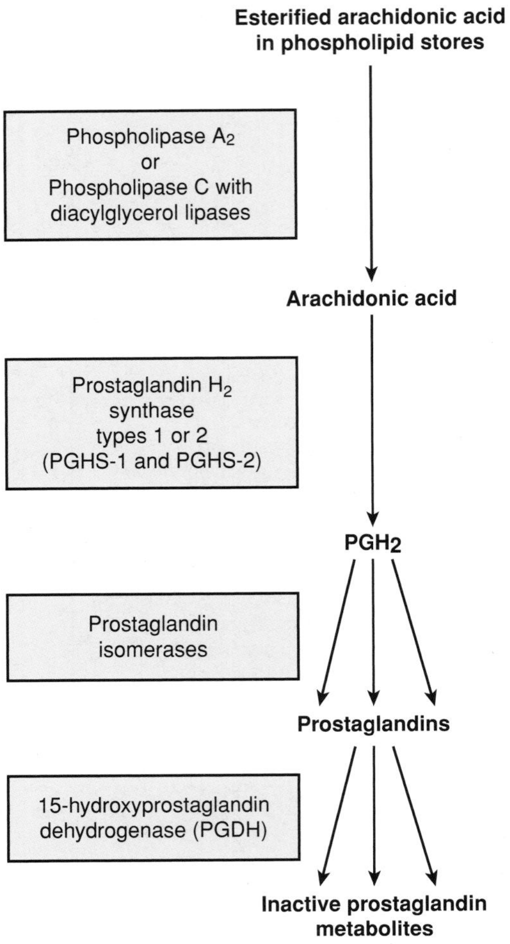

FIGURE 21-16 Overview of the prostaglandin biosynthetic pathway.

Atrial and Brain Natriuretic Peptides and Cyclic Guanosine Monophosphate (cGMP)

Activation of guanylyl cyclase increases intracellular cGMP levels, which promotes smooth muscle relaxation (Word, 1993). Intracellular cGMP levels are increased in the pregnant myometrium and can be stimulated by atrial natriuretic peptide (ANP), brain natriuretic peptide (BNP) receptors, and nitric oxide (Telfer, 2001). All of these factors and their receptors are expressed in the pregnant uterus. However, it remains unclear if these factors and intracellular cGMP play a role in uterine quiescence in normal pregnancy physiology (Itoh, 1994; Yallampalli, 1994a,b).

Accelerated Uterotonin Degradation

In addition to pregnancy-induced compounds that promote myometrial cell refractoriness, there are striking increases in the activity of enzymes that degrade or inactivate endogenously produced uterotonins. Some of these and their degradative enzymes include: PGDH and prostaglandins; enkephalinase and endothelins; oxytocinase and oxytocin; diamine oxidase and histamine; catechol *O*-methyltransferase and catecholamines; angiotensinases and angiotensin-II; and platelet-activating factor (PAF) acetylhydrolase and PAF. Activities of several of these enzymes are increased by progesterone, and many decrease late in gestation (Bates, 1979; Casey, 1980; Germain, 1994).

Phase 2: Uterine Activation and Cervical Ripening

Classic Progesterone Withdrawal and Parturition

Key factors in uterine activation are depicted in Figure 21-15. In species that exhibit progesterone withdrawal, parturition progression to labor can be blocked by administering progesterone to the mother. However, there are conflicting reports as to whether progesterone administration in pregnant women can delay the timely onset of parturition or prevent preterm labor. The possibility that progesterone-containing injections or vaginal suppositories may be used to prevent preterm labor has been studied in a number of randomized trials conducted during the past 15 years. These are discussed in Chapter 42 (p. 844), but in general, their use has marginal clinical benefits in preventing recurrent preterm birth and its associated perinatal morbidity.

Progesterone Receptor Antagonists and Human Parturition

When the steroidal antiprogestin mifepristone (RU-486) is administered during the latter phase of the ovarian cycle, it induces menstruation prematurely. It is also an effective abortifacient during early pregnancy (Chap. 18, p. 368). Mifepristone is a classic steroid antagonist, acting at the level of the progesterone receptor. Although less effective in inducing abortion or labor in women later in pregnancy, mifepristone appears to have some effect on cervical ripening and on increasing myometrial sensitivity to uterotonins (Berkane, 2005; Chwalisz, 1994a,b). These data suggest that humans have a mechanism for progesterone inactivation, whereby the myometrium and cervix become refractory to the inhibitory actions of progesterone.

Functional Progesterone Withdrawal in Human Parturition

As an alternative to classic progesterone withdrawal resulting from decreased secretion, research has focused on mechanisms that inhibit progesterone action in human pregnancy. Functional progesterone withdrawal or antagonism is possibly mediated through several mechanisms: (1) changes in the relative expression of the nuclear progesterone-receptor isoforms, PR-A, PR-B, and PR-C; (2) changes in the relative expression of membrane-bound progesterone receptors; (3) posttranslational modifications of the progesterone receptor; (4) alterations in PR activity through changes in the expression of coactivators or corepressors that directly influence receptor function; (5) local inactivation of progesterone by steroid-metabolizing enzymes or synthesis of a natural antagonist; and (6) microRNA regulation of progesterone-metabolizing enzymes and transcription factors that modulate uterine quiescence.

There is evidence that progesterone-receptor activity is decreased late in gestation. A series of studies have shown that the relative ratio of PR-A to PR-B within the myometrium, decidua, and chorion shifts late in gestation (Madsen, 2004; Mesiano, 2002; Pieber, 2001). Specifically, increased PR-A levels during parturition depress the antiinflammatory actions of PR-B and thereby promote proinflammatory gene expression at term (Tan, 2012). Moreover, these activities have been shown to be specific for the upper and lower uterine segments (Condon, 2003, 2006). Similarly, studies of cervical stroma suggest changes in receptor isoform concentrations (Stjernholm-Vladic, 2004). In addition, membrane PR isoforms are also expressed in the myometrium and placenta. However, it remains to be determined if they play a role to promote the transition from myometrial quiescence to activation (Chapman, 2006; Karteris, 2006; Zachariades, 2012). There is evidence in rodent models that local action of enzymes such as steroid 5α-reductase type 1 or 20α-hydroxysteroid dehydrogenase (20α-HSD) catabolize progesterone to metabolites that have a weak affinity for the progesterone receptor (Mahendroo, 1999; Piekorz, 2005). In the human cervix, decreased activity of 17β-hydroxysteroid dehydrogenase type 2 at term results in a net increase in estrogen and decline in progesterone levels (Andersson, 2008). Recent studies provide new insights into the regulatory role of small noncoding RNAs (microRNAs) in regulating expression of the steroid metabolizing enzyme 20α-HSD (Williams, 2012a). Increased expression of microRNA200a in the term myometrium blunts the expression of STAT5b, an inhibitor of 20α-HSD. Reduced STAT5b function allows increased 20α-HSD levels that result in increased progesterone metabolism and reduced progesterone function.

Taken together, all of these observations support the concept that multiple pathways exist for a functional progesterone withdrawal that includes changes in PR isoform and receptor coactivator levels, microRNA regulation, and increased local hormone metabolism to less active products.

Oxytocin Receptors

Because of its longstanding application for labor induction, it seemed logical that oxytocin must play a central role in spontaneous human labor. But this venerable hormone may have only a minor supporting role. Currently, it still is controversial whether oxytocin plays a role in the early phases of uterine activation or whether its sole function is in the expulsive phase of labor. Most studies of regulation of myometrial oxytocin-receptor synthesis have been performed in rodents. Disruption of the oxytocin receptor gene in the mouse does not affect parturition. This suggests that, at least in this species, multiple systems likely ensure that parturition occurs. There is little doubt, however, that there is an increase in myometrial oxytocin receptors during phase 2 of parturition. Moreover, their activation results in increased phospholipase C activity and subsequent increases in cytosolic calcium levels and uterine contractility.

Progesterone and estradiol appear to be the primary regulators of oxytocin receptor expression. Estradiol treatment in vivo or in myometrial explants increases myometrial oxytocin receptor concentrations. This action, however, is prevented by simultaneous treatment with progesterone (Fuchs, 1983). Progesterone also may act within the myometrial cell to increase oxytocin-receptor degradation and inhibit oxytocin activation of its receptor at the cell surface (Bogacki, 2002). These data indicate that one of the mechanisms whereby progesterone maintains uterine quiescence is through the inhibition of myometrial oxytocin response.

The increase in oxytocin receptor levels in nonhuman species appears to be mainly regulated either directly or indirectly by estradiol. Treatment of several species with estrogen leads to increased uterine oxytocin receptor levels (Blanks, 2003; Challis, 1994). Moreover, the level of oxytocin receptor mRNA in human myometrium at term is greater than that found in preterm myometrium (Wathes, 1999). Thus, increased receptors at term may be attributable to increased gene transcription. An estrogen response element, however, is not present in the oxytocin receptor gene, suggesting that the stimulatory effects of estrogen may be indirect.

Human studies suggest that inflammatory-related rapid-response genes may regulate oxytocin receptors (Bethin, 2003; Kimura, 1999; Massrieh, 2006). These receptors also are present in human endometrium and in decidua at term and stimulate prostaglandin production. In addition, these receptors are found in the myometrium and at lower levels in amniochorion-decidual tissues (Benedetto, 1990; Wathes, 1999).

Relaxin

Although relaxin may contribute to uterine quiescence, it also has roles in phase 2 of parturition. These include remodeling of the extracellular matrix of the uterus, cervix, vagina, breast, and pubic symphysis as well as promoting cell proliferation and inhibiting apoptosis. Its actions on cell proliferation and apoptosis are mediated through the G-protein-coupled receptor, RXFP1, whereas some but not all actions of relaxin on matrix remodeling are mediated through this receptor (Samuel, 2009; Yao, 2008). The precise mechanisms for modulation of matrix turnover have not been fully elucidated. However, relaxin appears to mediate glycosaminoglycan and proteoglycan synthesis and degrade matrix macromolecules such as collagen by induction of matrix metalloproteases. Relaxin promotes growth of the cervix, vagina, and pubic symphysis and is necessary for breast remodeling for lactation. Consistent with its proposed roles, mice deficient in relaxin or the RXFP1 receptor have protracted labor; show reduced growth of the cervix, vagina, and symphysis; and are unable to nurse because of incomplete nipple development (Feng, 2005; Park, 2005; Rosa, 2012; Soh, 2012; Yao, 2008).

Fetal Contributions to Initiation of Parturition

It is intellectually intriguing to envision that the mature human fetus provides the signal to initiate parturition. Teleologically, this seems most logical because such a signal could be transmitted in several ways to suspend uterine quiescence. The fetus may provide a signal through a blood-borne agent that acts on the placenta. Research is ongoing to better understand the fetal signals that contribute to parturition initiation (Mendelson, 2009). Although signals may arise from the fetus, the uterus and cervix likely first must be prepared for labor before a uterotonin produced by or one whose release is stimulated by the fetus can be optimally effective (Casey, 1994).

Uterine Stretch and Parturition

There is now considerable evidence that fetal growth is an important component in uterine activation in phase 1 of parturition. In association with fetal growth, significant increases in myometrial tensile stress and amnionic fluid pressure follow (Fisk, 1992). With uterine activation, stretch is required for induction of specific contraction-associated proteins (CAPs). Specifically, stretch increases expression of the gap junction protein—connexin 43 and of oxytocin receptors. Gastrin-releasing peptide, a stimulatory agonist for smooth muscle, is increased by stretch in the myometrium (Tattersall, 2012). Others have hypothesized that stretch plays an integrated role with fetal-maternal endocrine cascades of uterine activation (Lyall, 2002; Ou, 1997, 1998).

Clinical support for a role of stretch comes from the observation that multifetal pregnancies are at a much greater risk for preterm labor than singletons. And preterm labor is also significantly more common in pregnancies complicated by hydramnios. Although the mechanisms causing preterm birth in these two examples are debated, a role for uterine stretch must be considered.

Cell signaling systems used by stretch to regulate the myometrial cell continue to be defined. This process—*mechanotransduction*—may include activation of cell-surface receptors or ion channels, transmission of signals through extracellular matrix, or release of autocrine molecules that act directly on myometrium (Shynlova, 2009; Young, 2011). For example, the extracellular matrix protein fibronectin and its cell-surface receptor, alpha 5 integrin receptor, are induced in the rodent by stretch (Shynlova, 2007). This interaction may aid force transduction during labor contraction by anchoring hypertrophied myocytes to the uterine extracellular matrix.

Fetal Endocrine Cascades Leading to Parturition

The ability of the fetus to provide endocrine signals that initiate parturition has been demonstrated in several species. Liggins and associates (1967, 1973) demonstrated that the fetus provides the signal for the timely onset of parturition in sheep. This signal was shown to come from the fetal hypothalamic-pituitary-adrenal axis (Whittle, 2001).

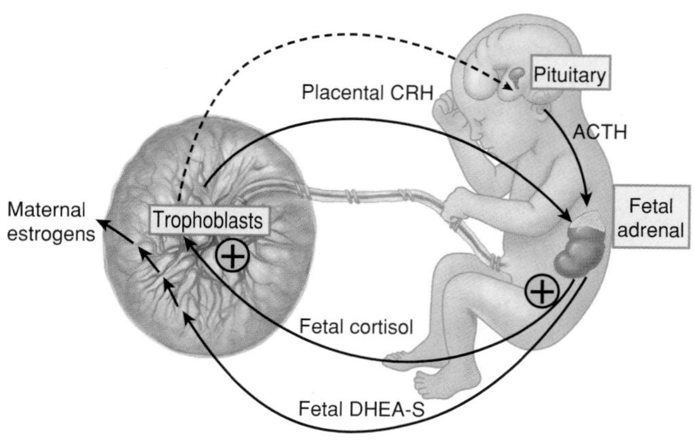

FIGURE 21-17 The placental–fetal adrenal endocrine cascade. In late gestation, placental corticotropin-releasing hormone (CRH) stimulates fetal adrenal production of dehydroepiandrosterone sulfate (DHEA-S) and cortisol. The latter stimulates production of placental CRH, which leads to a feed-forward cascade that enhances adrenal steroid hormone production. ACTH = adrenocorticotropic hormone.

Defining the exact mechanisms regulating human parturition has proven more difficult, and all evidence suggests that it is not regulated in the exact manner seen in the sheep. Even so, activation of the human fetal hypothalamic-pituitary-adrenal-placental axis is considered a critical component of normal parturition. Moreover, premature activation of this axis is considered to prompt many cases of preterm labor (Challis, 2000, 2001). As in the sheep, steroid products of the human fetal adrenal gland are believed to have effects on the placenta and membranes that eventually transform myometrium from a quiescent to contractile state. A key component in the human may be the unique ability of the placenta to produce large amounts of CRH, as shown in Figure 21-17.

Placental Corticotropin-Releasing Hormone Production. A CRH hormone identical to maternal and fetal hypothalamic CRH is synthesized by the placenta in relatively large amounts (Grino, 1987; Saijonmaa, 1988). One important difference is that, unlike hypothalamic CRH, which is under glucocorticoid negative feedback, cortisol has been shown to *stimulate* placental CRH production. This is by activation of the transcription factor, nuclear factor kappa B (NF-κB) (Jones, 1989; Marinoni, 1998; Thomson, 2013). This ability makes it possible to create a feed-forward endocrine cascade that does not end until delivery.

Maternal plasma CRH levels are low in the first trimester and rise from midgestation to term. In the last 12 weeks, CRH plasma levels rise exponentially, peaking during labor and then falling precipitously after delivery (Frim, 1988; Sasaki, 1987). Amnionic fluid CRH levels similarly increase in late gestation. CRH is the only trophic hormone-releasing factor to have a specific serum binding protein. During most of pregnancy, it appears that CRH-binding protein (CRH-BP) binds most maternal circulating CRH, and this inactivates it (Lowry, 1993). During later pregnancy, however, CRH-BP levels in both maternal plasma and amnionic fluid decline, leading to markedly increased levels of bioavailable CRH (Perkins, 1995; Petraglia, 1997).

In pregnancies in which the fetus can be considered to be "stressed" from various complications, concentrations of CRH in fetal plasma, amnionic fluid, and maternal plasma are increased compared with those seen in normal gestation (Berkowitz, 1996; Goland, 1993; McGrath, 2002; Perkins, 1995). The placenta is likely the source for this increased CRH concentration (Torricelli, 2011). For example, placental CRH content was fourfold higher in placentas from women with preeclampsia than in those from normal pregnancies (Perkins, 1995). Such increases in placental CRH production during normal gestation and the excessive secretion of placental CRH in complicated pregnancies may play a role in fetal adrenal cortisol synthesis (Murphy, 1982). They also may result in the supranormal levels of umbilical cord blood cortisol noted in stressed neonates (Falkenberg, 1999; Goland, 1994).

Corticotropin-Releasing Hormones and Parturition Timing

Placental CRH has been proposed to play several roles in parturition regulation. Placental CRH may enhance fetal cortisol production to provide positive feedback so that the placenta produces more CRH. Late in pregnancy—phase 2 or 3 of parturition—modification in the CRH receptor favors a switch from cAMP formation to increased myometrial cell calcium levels via protein kinase C activation (You, 2012). Oxytocin acts to attenuate CRH-stimulated accumulation of cAMP in myometrial tissue. And, CRH augments the contraction-inducing potency of a given dose of oxytocin in human myometrial strips (Quartero, 1991, 1992). CRH acts to increase myometrial contractile force in response to $PGF_{2\alpha}$ (Benedetto, 1994). Finally, CRH has been shown to stimulate fetal adrenal C_{19}-steroid synthesis, thereby increasing substrate for placental aromatization. Increased production of estrogens would shift the estrogen-to-progesterone ratio and promote the expression of a series of myometrial contractile proteins.

Some have proposed that the rising level of CRH at the end of gestation reflects a *fetal-placental clock* (McLean, 1995). CRH levels vary greatly among women, and it appears that the rate of increase in maternal CRH levels is a more accurate predictor of pregnancy outcome than is a single measurement (Leung, 2001; McGrath, 2002). In this regard, the placenta and fetus, through endocrinological events, influence the timing of parturition at the end of normal gestation.

Fetal Lung Surfactant and Parturition

Surfactant protein A (SP-A) produced by the fetal lung is required for lung maturation. Its levels are increased in amnionic fluid at term in mice. Studies in the mouse suggest that the increasing SP-A concentrations in amnionic fluid activate fluid macrophages to migrate into the myometrium and induce NF-κB (Condon, 2004). This factor activates inflammatory response genes in the myometrium, which in turn promote uterine contractility. This model supports the supposition that fetal signals play a role in parturition initiation. SP-A is expressed by the human amnion and decidua, is present in the amnionic fluid, and prompts signaling pathways in human myometrial cells (Garcia-Verdugo, 2008; Lee, 2010; Snegovskikh, 2011). The exact mechanisms by which SP-A activates myometrial contractility in women, however, remains to be clarified (Leong, 2008). SP-A selectively inhibits prostaglandin $F_{2\alpha}$ in the term decidua, and amnionic fluid concentration of SP-A declines at term (Chaiworapongsa, 2008).

Fetal Anomalies and Delayed Parturition

There is fragmentary evidence that pregnancies with markedly diminished estrogen production may be associated with prolonged gestation. These "natural experiments" include fetal anencephaly with adrenal hypoplasia and those with inherited placental sulfatase deficiency. The broad range of gestational length seen with these disorders calls into question the exact role of estrogen in human parturition initiation.

Other fetal abnormalities that prevent or severely reduce the entry of fetal urine into amnionic fluid—renal agenesis, or into lung secretions—pulmonary hypoplasia, do not prolong human pregnancy. Thus, a fetal signal through the paracrine arm of the fetal-maternal communication system does not appear to be mandated for parturition initiation.

Some brain anomalies of the fetal calf, fetal lamb, and sometimes the human fetus delay the normal timing of parturition. More than a century ago, Rea (1898) observed an association between fetal anencephaly and prolonged human gestation. Malpas (1933) extended these observations and described a pregnancy with an anencephalic fetus that was prolonged to 374 days—53 weeks. He concluded that the association between anencephaly and prolonged gestation was attributable to anomalous fetal brain-pituitary-adrenal function. The adrenal glands of the anencephalic fetus are very small and, at term, may be only 5 to 10 percent as large as those of a normal fetus. This is caused by developmental failure of the fetal zone that normally accounts for most of fetal adrenal mass and production of C_{19}-steroid hormones (Chap. 5, p. 108). Such pregnancies are associated with delayed labor and suggest that the fetal adrenal glands are important for the timely onset of parturition (Anderson, 1973).

Phase 3: Uterine Stimulation

This parturition phase is synonymous with uterine contractions that bring about progressive cervical dilatation and delivery. Current data favor the *uterotonin theory of labor initiation.* Increased uterotonin production would follow once phase 1 is suspended and uterine phase 2 processes are implemented. A number of uterotonins may be important to the success of phase 3, that is, active labor (see Fig. 21-15). Just as multiple processes likely contribute to myometrial unresponsiveness of phase 1 of parturition, other processes may contribute jointly to a system that ensures labor success.

Uterotonins that are candidates for labor induction include oxytocin, prostaglandins, serotonin, histamine, PAF, angiotensin II, and many others. All have been shown to stimulate smooth muscle contraction through G-protein coupling.

Oxytocin and Phase 3 of Parturition

Late in pregnancy, during phase 2 of parturition, there is a 50-fold or more increase in the number of myometrial oxytocin receptors (Fuchs, 1982; Kimura, 1996). This increase coincides with an increase in uterine contractile responsiveness to oxytocin. Moreover, prolonged gestation is associated with a delay in the increase of these receptors (Fuchs, 1984).

Oxytocin—literally, *quick birth*—was the first uterotonin to be implicated in parturition initiation. This nanopeptide is synthesized in the magnocellular neurons of the supraoptic and paraventricular neurons. The prohormone is transported with its carrier protein, *neurophysin*, along the axons to the neural lobe of the posterior pituitary gland in membrane-bound vesicles for storage and later release. The prohormone is converted enzymatically to oxytocin during transport (Gainer, 1988; Leake, 1990).

Role of Oxytocin in Phases 3 and 4 of Parturition. Because of successful labor induction with oxytocin, it was logically suspected in parturition initiation. First, in addition to its effectiveness in inducing labor at term, oxytocin is a potent uterotonin and occurs naturally in humans. Subsequent observations provide additional support for this theory: (1) the number of oxytocin receptors strikingly increases in myometrial and decidual tissues near the end of gestation; (2) oxytocin acts on decidual tissue to promote prostaglandin release; and (3) oxytocin is synthesized directly in decidual and extraembryonic fetal tissues and in the placenta (Chibbar, 1993; Zingg, 1995).

Although little evidence suggests a role for oxytocin in phase 2 of parturition, abundant data support its important role during second-stage labor and in the puerperium—phase 4 of parturition. Specifically, there are increased maternal serum oxytocin levels: (1) during second-stage labor, which is the end of phase 3 of parturition; (2) in the early puerperium; and (3) during breast feeding (Nissen, 1995). Immediately after delivery of the fetus, placenta, and membranes, which completes parturition phase 3, firm and persistent uterine contractions and myometrial retraction are essential to prevent postpartum hemorrhage. Oxytocin likely causes persistent contractions.

Oxytocin infusion in women promotes increased levels of mRNAs from myometrial genes that encode proteins essential for uterine involution. These include interstitial collagenase, monocyte chemoattractant protein-1, interleukin-8, and urokinase plasminogen activator receptor. Therefore, oxytocin action at the end of labor may be involved in uterine involution.

Prostaglandins and Phase 3 of Parturition

Although their role in parturition phase 2 of noncomplicated pregnancies is less well defined, a critical role for prostaglandins in phase 3 of parturition is clear (MacDonald, 1993). First, levels of prostaglandins—or their metabolites—in amnionic fluid, maternal plasma, and maternal urine are increased during labor (Fig. 21-18. Second, treatment of pregnant women with

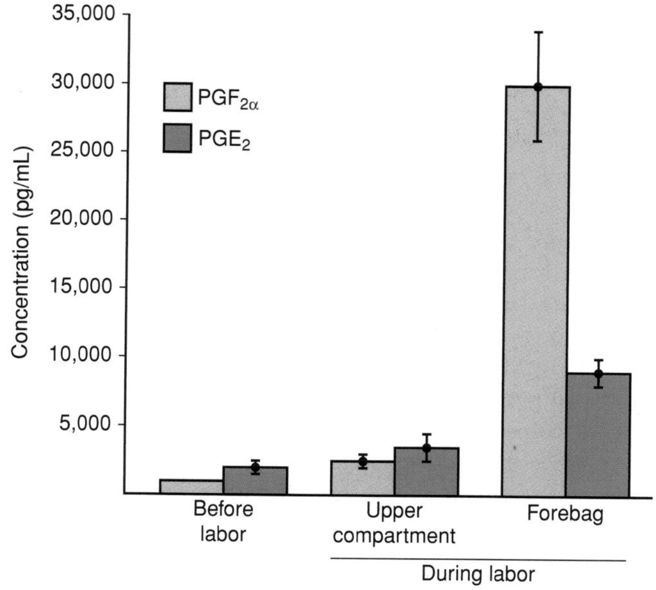

FIGURE 21-18 Mean (±SD) concentrations of prostaglandin $F_{2\alpha}$ ($PGF_{2\alpha}$) and prostaglandin E_2 (PGE_2) in amnionic fluid at term before labor and in the upper and forebag compartments during labor at all stages of cervical dilatation. (Data from MacDonald, 1993.)

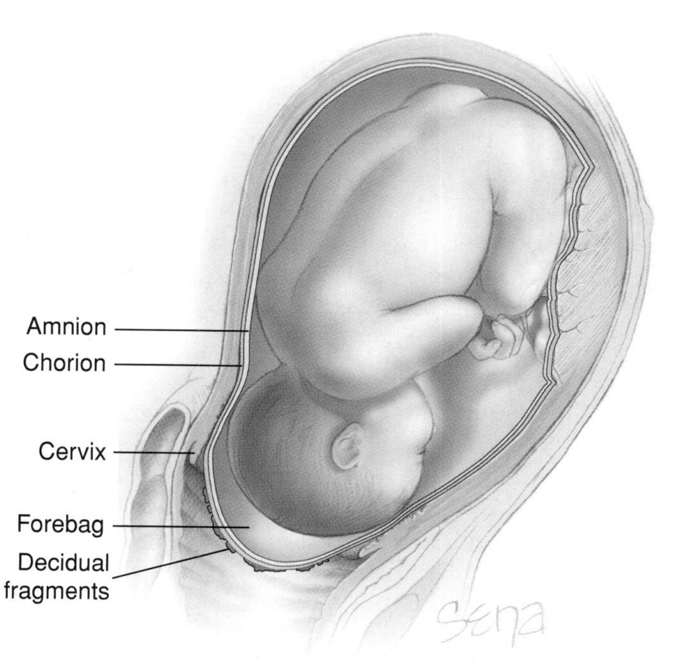

FIGURE 21-19 Sagittal view of the exposed forebag and attached decidual fragments after cervical dilatation during labor. (Redrawn from MacDonald, 1996.)

prostaglandins, by any of several administration routes, causes abortion or labor at all gestational stages. Moreover, administration of prostaglandin H synthase type 2 (PGHS-2) inhibitors to pregnant women will delay spontaneous labor onset and sometimes arrest preterm labor (Loudon, 2003). Last, prostaglandin treatment of myometrial tissue in vitro sometimes causes contraction, dependent on the prostanoid tested and the physiological status of the tissue treated.

Uterine Events Regulating Prostaglandin Production. During labor, prostaglandin production within the myometrium and decidua is an efficient mechanism of activating contractions. For example, prostaglandin synthesis is high and unchanging in the decidua during phase 2 and 3 of parturition. Moreover, the receptor level for $PGF_{2\alpha}$ is increased in the decidua at term, and this increase most likely is the regulatory step in prostaglandin action in the uterus. The myometrium synthesizes PGHS-2 with labor onset, but most prostaglandins likely come from the decidua.

The fetal membranes and placenta also produce prostaglandins. Primarily PGE_2, but also $PGF_{2\alpha}$, are detected in amnionic fluid at all gestational stages. As the fetus grows, prostaglandins levels in the amnionic fluid increase gradually. Their major increases in concentration within amnionic fluid, however, are demonstrable after labor begins (see Fig. 21-18). These higher levels likely result as the cervix dilates and exposes decidual tissue (Fig. 21-19). These increased levels in the forebag compared with those in the upper compartment are believed to follow an inflammatory response that signals the events leading to active labor. Together, the increases in cytokines and prostaglandins further degrade the extracellular matrix, thus weakening fetal membranes.

Findings of Kemp and coworkers (2002) and Kelly (2002) support a possibility that inflammatory mediators aid cervical dilatation and alterations to the lower uterine segment. It can be envisioned that they, along with the increased prostaglandin levels measured in vaginal fluid during labor, add to the relatively rapid cervical changes that are characteristic of parturition.

Endothelin-1

The endothelins are a family of 21-amino acid peptides that powerfully induce myometrial contraction (Word, 1990). The endothelin A receptor is preferentially expressed in smooth muscle and effects an increase in intracellular calcium. Endothelin-1 is produced in myometrium of term gestations and is able to induce synthesis of other contractile mediators such as prostaglandins and inflammatory mediators (Momohara, 2004; Sutcliffe, 2009). The requirement of endothelin-1 in normal parturition physiology remains to be established. However, there is evidence of pathologies associated with aberrant endothelin-1 expression, such as premature birth and uterine leiomyomas (Tanfin, 2011, 2012).

Angiotensin II

There are two G-protein-linked angiotensin II receptors expressed in the uterus—AT1 and AT2. In nonpregnant women, the AT2 receptor is predominant, but the AT1 receptor is preferentially expressed in pregnant women (Cox, 1993). Angiotensin II binding to the plasma-membrane receptor evokes contraction. During pregnancy, the vascular smooth muscle that expresses the AT2 receptor is refractory to the pressor effects of infused angiotensin II (Chap. 4, p. 61). In myometrium near term, however, angiotensin II may be another component of the uterotonin system of parturition phase 3 (Anton, 2009).

Contribution of Intrauterine Tissues to Parturition

Although they have a potential role in parturition initiation, the amnion, chorion laeve, and decidua parietalis more likely have an alternative role. The membranes and decidua make up an important tissue shell around the fetus that serves as a physical, immunological, and metabolic shield to protect against untimely initiation of parturition. Late in gestation, however, the fetal membranes may indeed act to prepare for labor.

Amnion

Virtually all of the tensile strength—resistance to tearing and rupture—of the fetal membranes is provided by the amnion (Chap. 5, p. 98). This avascular tissue is highly resistant to penetration by leukocytes, microorganisms, and neoplastic cells. It also constitutes a selective filter to prevent fetal particulate-bound lung and skin secretions from reaching the maternal compartment. In this manner, maternal tissues are protected from amnionic fluid constituents that could worsen decidual or myometrial function or could promote adverse events such as amnionic-fluid embolism (Chap. 41, p. 812).

Several bioactive peptides and prostaglandins that cause myometrial relaxation or contraction are synthesized in amnion (Fig. 21-20). Late in pregnancy, amnionic prostaglandin biosynthesis is increased, and phospholipase A_2 and PGHS-2 show increased activity (Johnson, 2002). Accordingly, many hypothesize that prostaglandins regulate events leading to parturition. It is likely that amnion is the major source for amnionic fluid prostaglandins, and their role in activation of cascades that promote membrane rupture is clear. The influence of amnion-derived prostaglandins on uterine quiescence and activation, however, is less clear. This is because prostaglandin transport from the amnion through the chorion to access maternal tissues is limited by expression of the inactivating enzyme, prostaglandin dehydrogenase.

Chorion Laeve

This tissue layer also is primarily protective and provides immunological acceptance. The chorion laeve is also enriched with enzymes that inactivate uterotonins. Enzymes include prostaglandin dehydrogenase (PGDH), oxytocinase, and enkephalinase (Cheung, 1990; Germain, 1994). As noted, PGDH inactivates amnion-derived prostaglandins. With chorionic rupture, this barrier would be lost, and prostaglandins could readily influence adjacent decidua and myometrium.

There is also evidence that PGDH levels found in the chorion decline during labor. This would allow increased prostaglandin-stimulated matrix metalloproteinase activity associated with membrane rupture. It would further allow prostaglandin entry into the maternal compartment to promote myometrial contractility (Patel, 1999; Van Meir, 1996; Wu, 2000). It is likely that progesterone maintains chorion PGDH expression, whereas cortisol decreases its expression. Thus, PGDH levels would decrease late in gestation as fetal cortisol production increases and as part of progesterone withdrawal.

Decidua

A metabolic contribution of decidual activation to parturition initiation is an appealing possibility for both anatomical and functional reasons. The generation of decidual uterotonins that act in a paracrine manner on contiguous myometrium is intuitive. In addition, decidua expresses steroid metabolizing enzymes such as 20α-HSD and steroid 5αR1 that may regulate local progesterone withdrawal. Decidual activation is characterized by increased proinflammatory cells and increased expression of proinflammatory cytokines, prostaglandins, and uterotonins such as oxytocin receptors and connexin 43.

Cytokines produced in the decidua can either increase uterotonin production—principally prostaglandins. Or they can act directly on myometrium to cause contraction. Examples are tumor necrosis factor-α (TNF-α) and interleukins 1, 6, 8, and 12. These molecules also can act as chemokines that recruit to the myometrium neutrophils and eosinophils, which further increase contractions and labor (Keelan, 2003).

There is uncertainty whether prostaglandin concentration or output from the decidua increases with term labor onset. Olson and Ammann (2007) suggest that the major regulation

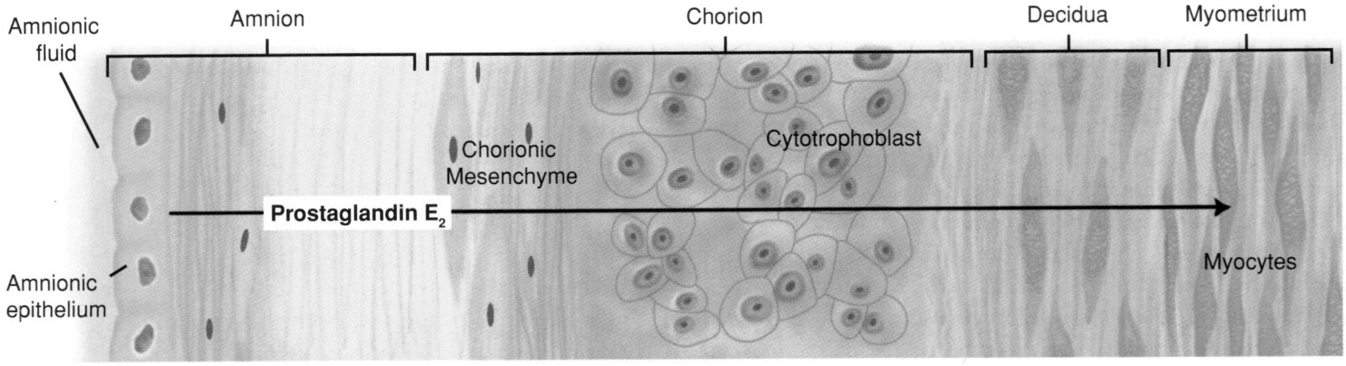

FIGURE 21-20 The amnion synthesizes prostaglandins, and late in pregnancy, synthesis is increased by increased phospholipase A_2 and prostaglandin H synthase, type 2 (PGHS-2) activity. During pregnancy, the transport of prostaglandins from the amnion to maternal tissues is limited by expression of the inactivating enzymes, prostaglandin dehydrogenase (PGDH), in the chorion. During labor, PGDH levels decline, and amnion-derived prostaglandins can influence membrane rupture and uterine contractility. The role of decidual activation in parturition is unclear but may involve local progesterone metabolism and increased prostaglandin receptor concentrations, thus enhancing uterine prostaglandin actions and cytokine production. (Adapted from Smith, 2007.)

of decidual prostaglandin action is not their synthesis but rather increased $PGF_{2\alpha}$ receptor expression.

Summary: Regulation of Phase 3 and 4 of Parturition

It is likely that multiple and possibly redundant processes contribute to the success of the three active labor phases once phase 1 of parturition is suspended and phase 2 is initiated. Phase 3 is highlighted by increased activation of G-protein-coupled receptors that inhibit cAMP formation, increase intracellular calcium stores, and promote interaction of actin and myosin and subsequent force generation. Simultaneously, cervical proteoglycan composition and collagen structure are altered to a form that promotes tissue distensibility and increased compliance. The net result is initiation of coordinated myometrial contractions of sufficient amplitude and frequency to dilate the prepared cervix and push the fetus through the birth canal. Multiple regulatory ligands orchestrate these processes and vary from endocrine hormones such as oxytocin to locally produced prostaglandins.

In phase 4 of parturition, a complicated series of repair processes are initiated to resolve inflammatory responses and remove glycosaminoglycans, proteoglycans, and structurally compromised collagen. Simultaneously, matrix and cellular components required for complete uterine involution are synthesized, and the dense connective tissue and structural integrity of the cervix is reformed.

REFERENCES

Akins ML, Luby-Phelps, K, Bank RA, et al: Cervical softening during pregnancy: regulated changes in collagen cross-linking and composition of matricellular proteins in the mouse. Biol Reprod 84(5):1053, 2011

Akgul Y, Holt R, Mummert M, et al: Dynamic changes in cervical glycosaminoglycan composition during normal pregnancy and preterm birth. Endocrinology 153(7):3493, 2012

Ambrus G, Rao CV: Novel regulation of pregnant human myometrial smooth muscle cell gap junctions by human chorionic gonadotropin. Endocrinology 135:2772, 1994

Ameye L, Young MF: Mice deficient in small leucine-rich proteoglycans: novel *in vivo* models for osteoporosis, osteoarthritis, Ehlers-Danlos syndrome, muscular dystrophy, and corneal diseases. Glycobiology 12(9): 107R, 2002

Anderson ABM, Turnbull AC: Comparative aspects of factors involved in the onset of labor in ovine and human pregnancy. In Klopper A, Gardner J (eds): Endocrine Factors in Labour. London, Cambridge University Press, 1973, p 141

Anderson J, Brown N, Mahendroo MS, et al: Utilization of different aquaporin water channels in the mouse cervix during pregnancy and parturition and in the models of preterm and delayed cervical ripening. Endocrinology 147: 130, 2006

Andersson S, Minjarez D, Yost NP, et al: Estrogen and progesterone metabolism in the cervix during pregnancy and parturition. J Clin Endocrinol Metab 93(6):2366, 2008

Anton L, Merrill DC, Neves LA, et al: The uterine placental bed renin-angiotensin system in normal and preeclamptic pregnancy. Endocrinology 150(9):4316, 2009

Anum EA, Hill LD, Pandya A, et al: Connective tissue and related disorders and preterm birth: clues to genes contributing to prematurity. Placenta 30(3):207, 2009

Bates GW, Edman CD, Porter JC, et al: Catechol-*O*-methyltransferase activity in erythrocytes of women taking oral contraceptive steroids. Am J Obstet Gynecol 133:691, 1979

Benedetto C, Petraglia F, Marozio L, et al: Corticotropin-releasing hormone increases prostaglandin-$F_{2\alpha}$ activity on human myometrium in vitro. Am J Obstet Gynecol 171:126, 1994

Benedetto MT, DeCicco F, Rossiello F, et al: Oxytocin receptor in human fetal membranes at term and during delivery. J Steroid Biochem 35:205, 1990

Berkane N, Verstraete L, Uzan S, et al: Use of mifepristone to ripen the cervix and induce labor in term pregnancies. Am J Obstet Gynecol 192:114, 2005

Berkowitz GS, Lapinski RH, Lockwood CJ, et al: Corticotropin-releasing factor and its binding protein: maternal serum levels in term and preterm deliveries. Am J Obstet Gynecol 174:1477, 1996

Bethin KE, Nagai Y, Sladek R, et al: Microarray analysis of uterine gene expression in mouse and human pregnancy. Mol Endocrinol 17:1454, 2003

Blanks AM, Vatish M, Allen MJ, et al: Paracrine oxytocin and estradiol demonstrate a spatial increase in human intrauterine tissues with labor. J Clin Endocrinol Metab 88:3392, 2003

Blaskewicz CD, Pudney J, Anderson DJ: Structure and function of intercellular junctions in human cervical and vaginal mucosal epithelia. Biol Reprod 85(1):97, 2011

Bogacki M, Silvia WJ, Rekawiecki R, et al: Direct inhibitory effect of progesterone on oxytocin-induced secretion of prostaglandin F (2alpha) from bovine endometrial tissue. Biol Reprod 67:184, 2002

Bogic LV, Mandel M, Bryant-Greenwood GD: Relaxin gene expression in human reproductive tissues by in situ hybridization. J Clin Endocrinol Metab 80:130, 1995

Bokström H, Brännström M, Alexandersson M, et al: Leukocyte subpopulations in the human uterine cervical stroma at early and term pregnancy. Hum Reprod 12:586, 1997

Bollapragada S, Youssef R, Jordan F, et al: Term labor is associated with a core inflammatory response in human fetal membranes, myometrium, and cervix. Am J Obstet Gynecol 200(1):104.e1, 2009

Brainard AM, Miller AJ, Martens JR, et al: Maxi-K channels localize to caveolae in human myometrium: a role for an actin–channel–caveolin complex in the regulation of myometrial smooth muscle K^+ current. Am J Physiol Cell Physiol 289:C49, 2005

Buhimschi IA, Dussably L, Buhimschi CS, et al: Physical and biomechanical characteristics of rat cervical ripening are not consistent with increased collagenase activity. Am J Obstet Gynecol 191:1695, 2004

Bygdeman M, Swahn ML, Gemzell-Danielsson K, et al: The use of progesterone antagonists in combination with prostaglandin for termination of pregnancy. Hum Reprod 9:121, 1994

Canty EG, Kadler KE: Procollagen trafficking, processing and fibrillogenesis. Cell Sci 118:1341, 2005

Casey ML, Hemsell DL, MacDonald PC, et al: NAD^+-dependent 15-hydroxyprostaglandin dehydrogenase activity in human endometrium. Prostaglandins 19:115, 1980

Casey ML, MacDonald PC: Human parturition. In Bruner JP (ed): Infertility and Reproductive Medicine Clinics of North America. Philadelphia, Saunders, 1994, p 765

Casey ML, MacDonald PC: Human parturition: distinction between the initiation of parturition and the onset of labor. In Ducsay CA (ed): Seminars in Reproductive Endocrinology. New York, Thieme, 1993, p 272

Casey ML, MacDonald PC: The endocrinology of human parturition. Ann N Y Acad Sci 828:273, 1997

Chaiworapongsa T, Hong JS, Hull WM, et al: The concentration of surfactant protein-A in amniotic fluid decreases in spontaneous human parturition at term. J Matern Fetal Neonatal Med 21(9):652, 2008

Challis JR, Sloboda DM, Alfaidy N, et al: Prostaglandins and mechanisms of preterm birth. Reproduction 124:1, 2002

Challis JR, Smith SK: Fetal endocrine signals and preterm labor. Biol Neonate 79:163, 2001

Challis JRG, Lye SJ: Parturition. In Knobil E, Neill JD (eds): The Physiology of Reproduction, 2nd ed, Vol II. New York, Raven, 1994, p 985

Challis JRG, Matthews SG, Gibb W, et al: Endocrine and paracrine regulation of birth at term and preterm. Endocr Rev 21:514, 2000

Chanrachakul B, Matharoo-Ball B, Turner A, et al: Immunolocalization and protein expression of the alpha subunit of the large-conductance calcium-activated potassium channel in human myometrium. Reproduction 126:43, 2003

Chapman NR, Kennelly MM, Harper KA, et al: Examining the spatio-temporal expression of mRNA encoding the membrane G protein-coupled receptor-alpha isoform in human cervix and myometrium during pregnancy and labour. Mol Hum Reprod 12(1):19, 2006

Cheung PY, Walton JC, Tai HH, et al: Immunocytochemical distribution and localization of 15-hydroxyprostaglandin dehydrogenase in human fetal membranes, decidua, and placenta. Am J Obstet Gynecol 163:1445, 1990

Chibbar R, Miller FD, Mitchell BF: Synthesis of oxytocin in amnion, chorion, and decidua may influence the timing of human parturition. J Clin Invest 91:185, 1993

Chow L, Lye SJ: Expression of the gap junction protein connexin-43 is increased in the human myometrium toward term and with the onset of labor. Am J Obstet Gynecol 170:788, 1994

Chwalisz K: The use of progesterone antagonists for cervical ripening and as an adjunct to labour and delivery. Hum Reprod Suppl 1:131, 1994a

Chwalisz K, Garfield RE: Antiprogestins in the induction of labor. Ann N Y Acad Sci 734:387, 1994b

Coleman RA, Smith WL, Narumiya S: Eighth International Union of Pharmacology. Classification of prostanoid receptors: properties, distribution, and structure of the receptor and their subtypes. Pharmacol Rev 46:205, 1994

Condon JC, Hardy DB, Kovaric K, et al: Up-regulation of the progesterone receptor (PR)-C isoform in laboring myometrium by activation of nuclear factor-kappaB may contribute to the onset of labor through inhibition of PR function. Mol Endocrinol 20:764, 2006

Condon JC, Jeyasuria P, Faust JM, et al: A decline in the levels of progesterone receptor coactivators in the pregnant uterus at term may antagonize progesterone receptor function and contribute to the initiation of parturition. Proc Natl Acad Sci USA 100:9518, 2003

Condon JC, Jeyasuria P, Faust JM, et al: Surfactant protein secreted by the maturing mouse fetal lung acts as a hormone that signals the initiation of parturition. Proc Natl Acad Sci USA 101:4978, 2004

Cox BE, Ipson MA, Shaul PW, et al: Myometrial angiotensin II receptor subtypes change during ovine pregnancy. J Clin Invest 92:2240, 1993

Day LJ, Schaa KL, Ryckman KK, et al: Single-nucleotide polymorphisms in the KCNN3 gene associate with preterm birth. Reprod Sci 18(3):286, 2011

Döring B, Shynlova O, Tsui P, et al: Ablation of connexin43 in uterine smooth muscle cells of the mouse causes delayed parturition. J Cell Sci 119:1715, 2006

Drewes PG, Yanagisawa H, Starcher B, et al: Pelvic organ prolapse in fibulin-5 knockout mice: pregnancy-induced changes in elastic fiber homeostasis in mouse vagina. Am J Pathol 170:578, 2007

Eta E, Ambrus G, Rao CV: Direct regulation of human myometrial contractions by human chorionic gonadotropin. J Clin Endocrinol Metab 79:1582, 1994

Falkenberg ER, Davis RO, DuBard M, et al: Effects of maternal infections on fetal adrenal steroid production. Endocr Res 25:239, 1999

Feng S, Bogatcheva NV, Kamat AA, et al: Genetic targeting of relaxin and Insl3 signaling in mice. Ann N Y Acad Sci 1041:82, 2005

Ferguson JKW: A study of the motility of the intact uterus at term. Surg Gynecol Obstet 73:359, 1941

Fisk NM, Ronderos-Dumit D, Tannirandorn Y, et al: Normal amniotic pressure throughout gestation. Br J Obstet Gynaecol 99:18, 1992

Friedman EA: Labor: Clinical Evaluation and Management, 2nd ed. New York, Appleton-Century-Crofts, 1978

Frim DM, Emanuel RL, Robinson BG, et al: Characterization and gestational regulation of corticotropin-releasing hormone messenger RNA in human placenta. J Clin Invest 82:287, 1988

Fuchs AR, Fuchs F, Husslein P, et al: Oxytocin receptors and human parturition. A dual role for oxytocin in the initiation of labor. Science 215:1396, 1982

Fuchs AR, Fuchs F, Husslein P, et al: Oxytocin receptors in the human uterus during pregnancy and parturition. Am J Obstet Gynecol 150:734, 1984

Fuchs AR, Periyasamy S, Alexandrova M, et al: Correlation between oxytocin receptor concentration and responsiveness to oxytocin in pregnant rat myometrium: effect of ovarian steroids. Endocrinology 113:742, 1983

Gainer H, Alstein M, Whitnall MH, et al: The biosynthesis and secretion of oxytocin and vasopressin. In Knobil E, Neill J (eds): The Physiology of Reproduction, Vol II. New York, Raven, 1988, p 2265

Garcia-Verdugo I, Tanfin Z, Dallot E, et al: Surfactant protein A signaling pathways in human uterine smooth muscle cells. Biol Reprod 79(2):348, 2008

Germain A, Smith J, MacDonald PC, et al: Human fetal membrane contribution to the prevention of parturition: uterotonin degradation. J Clin Endocrinol Metab 78:463, 1994

Goland RS, Jozak S, Conwell I: Placental corticotropin-releasing hormone and the hypercortisolism of pregnancy. Am J Obstet Gynecol 171:1287, 1994

Goland RS, Jozak S, Warren WB, et al: Elevated levels of umbilical cord plasma corticotropin-releasing hormone in growth-retarded fetuses. J Clin Endocrinol Metab 77:1174, 1993

Grino M, Chrousos GP, Margioris AN: The corticotropin releasing hormone gene is expressed in human placenta. Biochem Biophys Res Commun 148:1208, 1987

Hari Kishore A, Li XH, Word RA: Hypoxia and PGE_2 regulate MiTF-CX during cervical ripening. Mol Endocrinol 26(12):2031, 2012

Hassan SS, Romero R, Haddad R, et al: The transcriptome of the uterine cervix before and after spontaneous term parturition. Am J Obstet Gynecol 195(3):778, 2006

Hassan SS, Romero R, Tarca AL, et al: The transcriptome of cervical ripening in human pregnancy before the onset of labor at term: identification of novel molecular functions involved in this process. J Matern Fetal Neonatal Med 33(12):1183, 2009

Havelock J, Keller P, Muleba N, et al: Human myometrial gene expression before and during parturition. Biol Reprod 72:707, 2005

Hegar A: Diagnose der frühesten Schwangerschaftsperiode. Dtsch Med Wochenschr 21:565, 1895

Hermanns-Lê T, Piérard G, Quatresooz P: Ehlers-Danlos-like dermal abnormalities in women with recurrent preterm premature rupture of fetal membranes. Am J Dermatopathol 27(5), 407, 2005

House M, Kaplan DL, Socrate S: Relationships between mechanical properties and extracellular matrix constituents of the cervical stroma during pregnancy. Semin Perinatol 33(5):300, 2009

Iams JD, Goldenberg RL, Meis PJ, et al: The length of the cervix and the risk of spontaneous premature delivery. N Engl J Med 334:567, 1996

Itoh H, Sagawa N, Hasegawa M, et al: Expression of biologically active receptors for natriuretic peptides in the human uterus during pregnancy. Biochem Biophys Res Commun 203:602, 1994

Johnson RF, Mitchell CM, Giles WB, et al: The in vivo control of prostaglandin H synthase-2 messenger ribonucleic acid expression in the human amnion at parturition. J Clin Endocrinol Metab 87:2816, 2002

Jones SA, Brooks AN, Challis JR: Steroids modulate corticotropin-releasing hormone production in human fetal membranes and placenta. J Clin Endocrinol Metab 68:825, 1989

Karteris E, Zervou S, Pang Y, et al: Progesterone signaling in human myometrium through two novel membrane G protein-coupled receptors: potential role in functional progesterone withdrawal at term. Mol Endocrinol 20:1519, 2006

Keelan JA, Blumenstein M, Helliwell RJ, et al: Cytokines, prostaglandins and parturition—a review. Placenta 24:S33, 2003

Kelly RW: Inflammatory mediators and cervical ripening. J Reprod Immunol 57:217, 2002

Kemp B, Menon R, Fortunato SJ, et al: Quantitation and localization of inflammatory cytokines interleukin-6 and interleukin-8 in the lower uterine segment during cervical dilatation. J Asst Reprod Genet 19:215, 2002

Kimura T, Ivell R, Rust W, et al: Molecular cloning of a human MafF homologue, which specifically binds to the oxytocin receptor gene in term myometrium. Biochem Biophys Res Commun 264:86, 1999

Kimura T, Takemura M, Nomura S, et al: Expression of oxytocin receptor in human pregnant myometrium. Endocrinology 137:780, 1996

Leake RD: Oxytocin in the initiation of labor. In Carsten ME, Miller JD (eds): Uterine Function. Molecular and Cellular Aspects. New York, Plenum, 1990, p 361

Lee DC, Romero R, Kim CJ, et al: Surfactant protein-A as an anti-inflammatory component in the amnion: implications for human pregnancy. J Immunol 184(11):6479, 2010

Lei ZM, Reshef E, Rao CV: The expression of human chorionic gonadotropin/luteinizing hormone receptors in human endometrial and myometrial blood vessels. J Clin Endocrinol Metab 75:651, 1992

Leong AS, Norman JE, Smith R: Vascular and myometrial changes in the human uterus at term. Reprod Sci 15:59, 2008

Leppert PC: Anatomy and physiology of cervical ripening. Clin Obstet Gynecol 38:267, 1995

Leung TN, Chung TK, Madsen G, et al: Rate of rise in maternal plasma corticotrophin-releasing hormone and its relation to gestational length. BJOG 108:527, 2001

Liggins GC, Fairclough RJ, Grieves SA, et al: The mechanism of initiation of parturition in the ewe. Recent Prog Horm Res 29:111, 1973

Liggins GC, Kennedy PC, Holm LW: Failure of initiation of parturition after electrocoagulation of the pituitary of the fetal lamb. Am J Obstet Gynecol 98:1080, 1967

Loudon JA, Groom KM, Bennett PR: Prostaglandin inhibitors in preterm labour. Best Pract Res Clin Obstet Gynaecol 17:731, 2003

Lowder JL, Debes KM, Moon DK, et al: Biomechanical adaptations of the rat vagina and supportive tissues in pregnancy to accommodate delivery. Obstet Gynecol 109:136, 2007

Lowry PJ: Corticotropin-releasing factor and its binding protein in human plasma. Ciba Found Symp 172:108, 1993

Lyall F, Lye S, Teoh T, et al: Expression of Gsalpha, connexin-43, connexin-26, and EP1, 3, and 4 receptors in myometrium of prelabor singleton versus multiple gestations and the effects of mechanical stretch and steroids on Gsalpha. J Soc Gynecol Invest 9:299, 2002

MacDonald PC, Casey ML: Preterm birth. Sci Am 3:42, 1996

MacDonald PC, Casey ML: The accumulation of prostaglandins (PG) in amniotic fluid is an aftereffect of labor and not indicative of a role for PGE2 and PGE2 alpha in the initiation of human parturition. J Clin Endocrinol Metab 76:1332, 1993

Macphee DJ, Lye SJ: Focal adhesion signaling in the rat myometrium is abruptly terminated with the onset of labor. Endocrinology 141:274, 2000

Madsen G, Zakar T, Ku CY, et al: Prostaglandins differentially modulate progesterone receptor-A and -B expression in human myometrial cells: evidence for prostaglandin-induced functional progesterone withdrawal. J Clin Endocrinol Metab 89:1010, 2004

Mahendroo M: Cervical remodeling in term and preterm birth: insights from an animal model. Reproduction 143(4):429, 2012

Mahendroo MS, Porter A, Russell DW, et al: The parturition defect in steroid 5alpha-reductase type 1 knockout mice is due to impaired cervical ripening. Mol Endocrinol 13:981, 1999

Malpas P: Postmaturity and malformation of the fetus. J Obstet Gynaecol Br Emp 40:1046, 1933

Marinoni E, Korebrits C, Di Iorio R, et al: Effect of betamethasone in vivo on placental corticotropin-releasing hormone in human pregnancy. Am J Obstet Gynecol 178:770, 1998

Massrieh W, Derjuga A, Doualla-Bell F, et al: Regulation of the MAFF transcription factor by proinflammatory cytokines in myometrial cells. Biol Reprod 74:699, 2006

McGrath S, McLean M, Smith D, et al: Maternal plasma corticotropin-releasing hormone trajectories vary depending on the cause of preterm delivery. Am J Obstet Gynecol 186:257, 2002

McLean M, Bisits A, Davies J, et al: A placental clock controlling the length of human pregnancy. Nat Med 1:460, 1995

Meinert M, Malmström A, Tufvesson E, et al: Labour induces increased concentrations of biglycan and hyaluronan in human fetal membranes. Placenta 28(5–6)482, 2007

Mendelson CR: Minireview: fetal-maternal hormonal signaling in pregnancy and labor. Mol Endocrinol 23(7):947, 2009

Menzies FM, Khan AH, Higgins CA, et al: The chemokine receptor CCR2 is not required for successful initiation of labor in mice. Biol Reprod 86(4):118, 2012

Mesiano S, Chan EC, Fitter JT, et al: Progesterone withdrawal and estrogen activation in human parturition are coordinated by progesterone receptor A expression in the myometrium. J Clin Endocrinol Metab 87:2924, 2002

Momohara Y, Sakamoto S, Obayashi S, et al: Roles of endogenous nitric oxide synthase inhibitors and endothelin-1 for regulating myometrial contractions during gestation in the rat. Mol Hum Reprod 10(7):505, 2004

Murphy BE: Human fetal serum cortisol levels related to gestational age: evidence of a midgestational fall and a steep late gestational rise independent of sex or mode of delivery. Am J Obstet Gynecol 144:276, 1982

Myatt L, Lye SJ: Expression, localization and function of prostaglandin receptors in myometrium. Prostaglandins Leukot Essent Fatty Acids 70:137, 2004

Myers KM, Paskaleva AP, House M, et al: Mechanical and biochemical properties of human cervical tissue. Acta Biomater 4:104, 2008

Nissen E, Lilja G, Widstrom AM, et al: Elevation of oxytocin levels early post partum in women. Acta Obstet Gynecol Scand 74:530, 1995

Olson DM, Ammann C: Role of the prostaglandins in labour and prostaglandin receptor inhibitors in the prevention of preterm labour. Front Biosci 12:1329, 2007

Olson DM, Zaragoza DB, Shallow MC: Myometrial activation and preterm labour: evidence supporting a role for the prostaglandin F receptor—a review. Placenta 24:S47, 2003

Osman I, Young A, Ledingham MA, et al: Leukocyte density and pro-inflammatory cytokine expression in human fetal membranes, decidua, cervix and myometrium before and during labour at term. Mol Hum Reprod 9:41, 2003

Osmers R, Rath W, Pflanz MA, et al: Glycosaminoglycans in cervical connective tissue during pregnancy and parturition. Obstet Gynecol 81:88, 1993

Ou CW, Chen ZQ, Qi S, et al: Increased expression of the rat myometrial oxytocin receptor messenger ribonucleic acid during labor requires both mechanical and hormonal signals. Biol Reprod 59:1055, 1998

Ou CW, Orsino A, Lye SJ: Expression of connexin-43 and connexin-26 in the rat myometrium during pregnancy and labor is differentially regulated by mechanical and hormonal signals. Endocrinology 138:5398, 1997

Owen J, Mancuso M: Cervical cerclage for the prevention of preterm birth. Obstet Gynecol Clin North Am 39(1):25, 2012

Ozasa H, Tominaga T, Nishimura T, et al: Lysyl oxidase activity in the mouse uterine cervix is physiologically regulated by estrogen. Endocrinology 109:618, 1981

Park JI, Chang CL, Hsu SY: New insights into biological roles of relaxin and relaxin-related peptides. Rev Endocr Metab Disord 6:291, 2005

Parkington HC, Coleman HA: Excitability in uterine smooth muscle. Front Horm Res 27:179, 2001

Patel FA, Clifton VL, Chwalisz K, et al: Steroid regulation of prostaglandin dehydrogenase activity and expression in human term placenta and choriodecidua in relation to labor. J Clin Endocrinol Metab 84:291, 1999

Paternoster DM, Santarossa C, Vettore N, et al: Obstetric complications in Marfan's syndrome pregnancy. Minerva Ginecol 50:441, 1998

Perkins AV, Wolfe CD, Eben F, et al: Corticotrophin-releasing hormone-binding protein in human fetal plasma. J Endocrinol 146:395, 1995

Petraglia F, Florio P, Simoncini T, et al: Cord plasma corticotropin-releasing factor-binding protein (CRF-BP) in term and preterm labour. Placenta 18:115, 1997

Pieber D, Allport VC, Hills F, et al: Interactions between progesterone receptor isoforms in myometrial cells in human labour. Mol Hum Reprod 7:875, 2001

Piekorz RP, Gingras S, Hoffmeyer A, et al: Regulation of progesterone levels during pregnancy and parturition by signal transducer and activator of transcription 5 and 20α-hydroxysteroid dehydrogenase. Mol Endocrinol 19:431, 2005

Price SA, Pochun I, Phaneuf S, et al: Adenylyl cyclase isoforms in pregnant and nonpregnant human myometrium. J Endocrinol 164:21, 2000

Quartero HWP, Noort WA, Fry CH, et al: Role of prostaglandins and leukotrienes in the synergistic effect of oxytocin and corticotropin-releasing hormone (CRH) on the contraction force in human gestational myometrium. Prostaglandins 42:137, 1991

Quartero HWP, Strivatsa G, Gillham B: Role for cyclic adenosine monophosphate in the synergistic interaction between oxytocin and corticotrophin-releasing factor in isolated human gestational myometrium. Clin Endocrinol 36:141, 1992

Rada CC, Pierce SL, Nuno DW, et al: Overexpression of the SK3 channel alters vascular remodeling during pregnancy leading to fetal demise. Am J Physiol Endocrinol Metab 303(7):E825, 2012

Rahman J, Rahman FZ, Rahman W, et al: Obstetric and gynecologic complications in women with Marfan syndrome. J Reprod Med 48:723, 2003

Rahn DD, Ruff MD, Brown SA, et al: Biomechanical properties of the vaginal wall: effect of pregnancy, elastic fiber deficiency, and pelvic organ prolapse. Am J Obstet Gynecol 198:590.e1, 2008

Rea C: Prolonged gestation, acrania, monstrosity and apparent placenta praevia in one obstetrical case. JAMA 30:1166, 1898

Read CP, Word RA, Ruscheinsky MA, et al: Cervical remodeling during pregnancy and parturition: molecular characterization of the softening phase in mice. Reproduction 134:327, 2007

Renthal NE, Chen CC, Williams KC, et al: MiR-200 family and targets, ZEB1 and ZEB2, modulate uterine quiescence and contractility during pregnancy and labor. Proc Natl Acad Sci U S A 107(48):20828, 2010

Rosa RG, Akgul Y, Joazeiro PP, et al: Changes of large molecular weight hyaluronan and versican in the mouse pubic symphysis through pregnancy. Biol Reprod 82(2):44, 2012

Ruscheinsky M, De la Motte C, Mahendroo M: Hyaluronan and its binding proteins during cervical ripening and parturition: dynamic changes in size, distribution and temporal sequence. Matrix Biol, March 17, 2008

Sáez JC, Retamal MA, Basilio D, et al: Connexin-based gap junction hemichannels: gating mechanisms. Biochim Biophys Acta 1711:215, 2005

Saijonmaa O, Laatikainen T, Wahlstrom T: Corticotrophin-releasing factor in human placenta: localization, concentration and release in vitro. Placenta 9:373, 1988

Sakamoto Y, Moran P, Bulmer JN, et al: Macrophages and not granulocytes are involved in cervical ripening. J Reprod Immunol 66(2):161, 2005

Sakamoto Y, Moran P, Searle RF, et al: Interleukin-8 is involved in cervical dilatation but not in prelabour cervical ripening. Clin Exp Immunol 138:151, 2004

Samuel CS, Royce SG, Chen B, et al: Relaxin family peptide receptor-1 protects against airway fibrosis during homeostasis but not against fibrosis associated with chronic allergic airways disease. Endocrinology 150(3):1495, 2009

Sanborn BM, Yue C, Wang W, et al: G-protein signaling pathways in myometrium: affecting the balance between contraction and relaxation. Rev Reprod 3:196, 1998

Sasaki A, Shinkawa O, Margioris AN, et al: Immunoreactive corticotropin-releasing hormone in human plasma during pregnancy, labor, and delivery. J Clin Endocrinol Metab 64:224, 1987

Sennström MB, Ekman G, Westergren-Thorsson G, et al: Human cervical ripening, an inflammatory process mediated by cytokines. Mol Hum Reprod 6:375, 2000

Shynlova O, Tsui P, Jaffer S, et al: Integration of endocrine and mechanical signals in the regulation of myometrial functions during pregnancy and labour. Eur J Obstet Gynecol Reprod Biol 144(Suppl 1):S2, 2009

Shynlova O, Williams SJ, Draper H, et al: Uterine stretch regulates temporal and spatial expression of fibronectin protein and its alpha 5 integrin receptor in myometrium of unilaterally pregnant rats. Biol Reprod 77:880, 2007

Smith GC, Wu WX, Nathanielsz PW: Effects of gestational age and labor on expression of prostanoid receptor genes in baboon uterus. Biol Reprod 64:1131, 2001

Smith R: Parturition. N Engl J Med 356:271, 2007
Smith R, Mesiano S, Chan EC, et al: Corticotropin-releasing hormone directly and preferentially stimulates dehydroepiandrosterone sulfate secretion by human fetal adrenal cortical cells. J Clin Endocrinol Metab 83:2916, 1998
Snegovskikh VV, Bhandari V, Wright JR, et al: Surfactant protein-A (SP-A) selectively inhibits prostaglandin F2alpha (PGF2alpha) production in term decidua: implications for the onset of labor. J Clin Endocrinol Metab 96(4):E624, 2011
Soh YM, Tiwari A, Mahendroo M, et al: Relaxin regulates hyaluronan synthesis and aquaporins in the cervix of late pregnant mice. Endocrinology 153(12):6054, 2012
Spallicci MD, Chiea MA, Singer JM, et al: Use of hyaluronidase for cervical ripening: a randomized trial. Eur J Obstet Gynecol 130(1):46, 2007
Stjernholm-Vladic Y, Wang H, Stygar D, et al: Differential regulation of the progesterone receptor A and B in the human uterine cervix at parturition. Gynecol Endocrinol 18:41, 2004
Straach KJ, Shelton JM, Richardson JA, et al: Regulation of hyaluronan expression during cervical ripening. Glycobiology 15:55, 2005
Stull JT, Lin PJ, Krueger JK, et al: Myosin light chain kinase: functional domains and structural motifs. Acta Physiol Scand 164:471, 1998
Stull JT, Taylor DA, MacKenzie LW, et al: Biochemistry and physiology of smooth muscle contractility. In McNellis D, Challis JRG, MacDonald PC, et al (eds): Cellular and Integrative Mechanisms in the Onset of Labor. An NICHD Workshop. Ithaca, Perinatology, 1988, p 17
Sutcliffe AM, Clarke DL, Bradbury DA, et al: Transcriptional regulation of monocyte chemotactic protein-1 release by endothelin-1 in human airway smooth muscle cells involves NF-kappaB and AP-1. Br J Pharmacol 157(3):436, 2009
Tan H, Yi L, Rose NS, et al: Progesterone receptor-A and –B have opposite effects on proinflammatory gene expression in human myometrial cells: implications of progesterone actions in human pregnancy and parturition. J Clin Endocrinol Metab 97(5):E719, 2012
Tanfin Z, Breuiller-Fouché M: The endothelin axis in uterine leiomyomas: new insights. Biol Reprod 87(1):5, 2012
Tanfin Z, Leibe D, Robin P, et al: Endothelin-1: physiological and pathological role in myometrium. Int J Biochem Cell Biol 43(3):299, 2011
Tattersall M, Cordeaux Y, Charnock-Jones DS, et al: Expression of gastrin-releasing peptide is increased by prolonged stretchy of human myometrium, and antagonists of its receptor inhibit contractility. J Physiol 590(Pt 9):2081, 2012
Telfer JF, Itoh H, Thomson AJ, et al: Activity and expression of soluble and particulate guanylate cyclases in myometrium from nonpregnant and pregnant women: down-regulation of soluble guanylate cyclase at term. J Clin Endocrinol Metab 86(12):5934, 2001
Thomson M: The physiological roles of placental corticotropin releasing hormone in pregnancy and childbirth. J Physiol Biochem 69(3):559, 2013
Timmons BC, Fairhurst AM, Mahendroo MS: Temporal changes in myeloid cells in the cervix during pregnancy and parturition. J Immunol 182(5):2700, 2009
Timmons BC, Mahendroo M: Processes regulating cervical ripening differ from cervical dilation and postpartum repair: insights from gene expression studies. Reprod Sci 14:53, 2007
Timmons BC, Mahendroo MS: Timing of neutrophil activation and expression of proinflammatory markers do not support a role for neutrophils in cervical ripening in the mouse. Biol Reprod 74:236, 2006
Tong D, Lu X, Wang HS, et al: A dominant loss-of-function GJA1(Cx43) mutant impairs parturition in the mouse. Biol Reprod 80(6):1099, 2009
Torricelli M, Novembri R, Bloise E, et al: Changes in placental CRH, urocortins, and CRH-receptor mRNA expression associated with preterm delivery and chorioamnionitis. J Clin Endocrinol Metab 96(2):534, 2011
Van Meir CA, Sangha RK, Walton JC, et al: Immunoreactive 15-hydroxyprostaglandin dehydrogenase (PGDH) is reduced in fetal membranes from patients at preterm delivery in the presence of infection. Placenta 17:291, 1996
Wadhwa PD, Porto M, Garite TJ, et al: Maternal corticotropin-releasing hormone levels in the early third trimester predict length of gestation in human pregnancy. Am J Obstet Gynecol 179:1079, 1998
Wang H, Parry S, Macones G, et al: A functional SNP in the promoter of the SERPINH1 gene increases risk of preterm premature rupture of membranes in African Americans. Proc Natl Acad Sci USA 103:13463, 2006
Warren JE, Silver RM, Dalton J, et al: Collagen 1A1 and transforming growth factor-β polymorphisms in women with cervical insufficiency. Obstet Gynecol 110:619, 2007
Wathes DC, Borwick SC, Timmons PM, et al: Oxytocin receptor expression in human term and preterm gestational tissues prior to and following the onset of labour. J Endocrinol 161:143, 1999
Weiss G: Relaxin used to produce the cervical ripening of labor. Clin Obstet Gynecol 38:293, 1995
Westergren-Thorsson G, Norman M, Björnsson S, et al: Differential expressions of mRNA for proteoglycans, collagens and transforming growth factor-beta in the human cervix during pregnancy and involution. Biochim Biophys Acta 1406:203, 1998
Whittle WL, Patel FA, Alfaidy N, et al: Glucocorticoid regulation of human and ovine parturition: the relationship between fetal hypothalamic-pituitary-adrenal axis activation and intrauterine prostaglandin production. Biol Reprod 64:1019, 2001
Williams KC, Renthal NE, Condon JC, et al: MicroRNA-200a serves a key role in the decline of progesterone receptor function leading to term and preterm labor. Proc Natl Acad Sci U S A 109(19)7529, 2012a
Williams KC, Renthal NE, Gerard RD, et al: The microRNA (miR)-199a/214 cluster mediates opposing effects of progesterone and estrogen on uterine contractility during pregnancy and labor. Mol Endocrinol 26(11):1857, 2012b
Wira CR, Grant-Tschudy KS, Crane-Godreau MA: Epithelial cells in the female reproductive tract: a central role as sentinels of immune protection. Am J Reprod Immunol 53:65, 2005
Wolf JP, Simon J, Itskovitz J, et al: Progesterone antagonist RU 486 accommodates but does not induce labour and delivery in primates. Hum Reprod 8:759, 1993
Woodcock NA, Taylor CW, Thornton S: Effect of an oxytocin receptor antagonist and rho kinase inhibitor on the $[Ca^{++}]_i$ sensitivity of human myometrium. Am J Obstet Gynecol 190:222, 2004
Word RA, Kamm KE, Stull JT, et al: Endothelin increases cytoplasmic calcium and myosin phosphorylation in human myometrium. Am J Obstet Gynecol 162:1103, 1990
Word RA, Li XH, Hnat M, et al: Dynamics of cervical remodeling during pregnancy and parturition: mechanisms and current concepts. Semin Reprod Med, 25(1):69, 2007
Word RA, Stull JT, Casey ML, et al: Contractile elements and myosin light chain phosphorylation in myometrial tissue from nonpregnant and pregnant women. J Clin Invest 92:29, 1993
Wu WX, Ma XH, Smith GC, et al: Prostaglandin dehydrogenase mRNA in baboon intrauterine tissues in late gestation and spontaneous labor. Am J Physiol Regul Integr Comp Physiol 279:R1082, 2000
Wu Z, Aron AW, Macksoud EE, et al: Uterine dysfunction in biglycan and decorin deficient mice leads to dystocia during parturition. PLoS ONE 7(1):e2927, 2012
Xie N, Liu L, Li Y, et al: Expression and function of myometrial PSF suggest a role in progesterone withdrawal and the initiation of labor. Mol Endocrinol 26(8):1370, 2012
Xu C, Gao L, You X, et al: CRH acts on CRH-1 and –R2 to differentially modulate the expression of large-conductance calcium-activated potassium channels in human pregnant myometrium. Endocrinology 152(11):4406, 2011
Yallampalli C, Byam-Smith M, Nelson SO, et al: Steroid hormones modulate the production of nitric oxide and cGMP in the rat uterus. Endocrinology 134:1971, 1994a
Yallampalli C, Izumi H, Byam-Smith M, et al: An L-arginine-nitric oxide-cyclic guanosine monophosphate system exists in the uterus and inhibits contractility during pregnancy. Am J Obstet Gynecol 170:175, 1994b
Yao L, Agoulnik AI, Cooke S, et al: Relaxin acts on stromal cells to promote epithelial and stromal proliferation and inhibit apoptosis in the mouse cervix and vagina. Endocrinology 149(5):2072, 2008
You X, Gao L, Liu J, et al: CRH activation of different signaling pathways results in differential calcium signaling in human pregnant myometrium before and during labor. J Clin Endocrinol Metab 97(10):1851, 2012
Young A, Thomson AJ, Ledingham M, et al: Immunolocalization of proinflammatory cytokines in myometrium, cervix, and fetal membranes during human parturition at term. Biol Reprod 66:445, 2002
Young RC, Goloman G: Mechanotransduction in rat myometrium: coordination of contractions of electrically and chemically isolated tissues. Reprod Sci 18(1):64, 2011
Yu JT, López Bernal A: The cytoskeleton of human myometrial cells. J Reprod Fertil 112:185, 1998
Zachariades E, Mparmpakas D, Pang Y, et al: Changes in placental progesterone receptors in term and preterm labour. Placenta 33(5):367, 2012
Zhang Y, Akins ML, Murari K, et al: A compact fiber-optic SHG scanning endomicroscope and its application to visualize cervical remodeling during pregnancy. Proc Natl Acad Sci USA 109(32):12878, 2012
Ziecik AJ, Derecka-Reszka K, Rzucidlo SJ: Extragonadal gonadotropin receptors, their distribution and function. J Physiol Pharmacol 43:33, 1992
Zingg HH, Rozen F, Chu K, et al: Oxytocin and oxytocin receptor gene expression in the uterus. Recent Prog Horm Res 50:255, 1995
Zuo J, Lei ZM, Rao CV: Human myometrial chorionic gonadotropin/luteinizing hormone receptors in preterm and term deliveries. J Clin Endocrinol Metab 79:907, 1994

CHAPTER 22

Normal Labor

Labor is the process that leads to childbirth. It begins with the onset of regular uterine contractions and ends with delivery of the newborn and expulsion of the placenta. The term *labor* in the obstetrical context takes on several connotations from the English language. It is undoubtedly true that pregnancy and birth are physiological processes, and as such, labor and delivery should be considered to be normal for most women (Lawrence, 2012). This understanding of normal labor and delivery as a physiological process has come under some scrutiny in the past decade because pelvic floor disorders have been observed to be more prevalent among women who have delivered at least one child (Handa, 2011; Nygaard, 2008). Determining which aspects of childbirth contribute most to this risk has become an area of intense investigation and discussed further in Chapter 30 (p. 588).

MECHANISMS OF LABOR

At the onset of labor, the position of the fetus with respect to the birth canal is critical to the route of delivery and thus should be determined in early labor. Important relationships include fetal lie, presentation, attitude, and position.

Fetal Lie

The relation of the fetal long axis to that of the mother is termed *fetal lie* and is either *longitudinal* or *transverse.* Occasionally, the fetal and the maternal axes may cross at a 45-degree angle, forming an *oblique lie.* This lie is unstable and becomes longitudinal or transverse during labor. A longitudinal lie is present in more than 99 percent of labors at term. Predisposing factors for transverse fetal position include multiparity, placenta previa, hydramnios, and uterine anomalies (Chap. 23, p. 468).

Fetal Presentation

The *presenting part* is that portion of the fetal body that is either foremost within the birth canal or in closest proximity to it. It typically can be felt through the cervix on vaginal examination. Accordingly, in longitudinal lies, the presenting part is either the fetal head or breech, creating *cephalic* and *breech presentations*, respectively. When the fetus lies with the long axis transversely, the *shoulder* is the presenting part. Table 22-1 describes the incidences of the various fetal presentations.

Cephalic Presentation

Such presentations are classified according to the relationship between the head and body of the fetus (Fig. 22-1). Ordinarily, the head is flexed sharply so that the chin is in contact with the thorax. The occipital fontanel is the presenting part, and this presentation is referred to as a *vertex* or *occiput presentation.* Much

TABLE 22-1. Fetal Presentation in 68,097 Singleton Pregnancies at Parkland Hospital

Presentation	Percent	Incidence
Cephalic	96.8	—
Breech	2.7	1:36
Transverse lie	0.3	1:335
Compound	0.1	1:1000
Face	0.05	1:2000
Brow	0.01	1:10,000

less commonly, the fetal neck may be sharply extended so that the occiput and back come in contact, and the face is foremost in the birth canal—*face presentation* (Fig. 23-6, p. 466). The fetal head may assume a position between these extremes, partially flexed in some cases, with the anterior (large) fontanel, or bregma, presenting—*sinciput presentation*—or partially extended in other cases, to have a *brow presentation* (Fig. 23-8, p. 468). These latter two presentations are usually transient. As labor progresses, sinciput and brow presentations almost always convert into vertex or face presentations by neck flexion or extension, respectively. Failure to do so can lead to dystocia, as discussed in Chapter 23 (p. 455).

The term fetus usually presents with the vertex, most logically because the uterus is piriform or pear shaped. Although the fetal head at term is slightly larger than the breech, the entire *podalic pole* of the fetus—that is, the breech and its flexed extremities—is bulkier and more mobile than the cephalic pole. The *cephalic pole* is composed of the fetal head only. Until approximately 32 weeks, the amnionic cavity is large compared with the fetal mass, and the fetus is not crowded by the uterine walls. Subsequently, however, the ratio of amnionic fluid volume decreases relative to the increasing fetal mass. As a result, the uterine walls are apposed more closely to the fetal parts.

If presenting by the breech, the fetus often changes polarity to make use of the roomier fundus for its bulkier and more mobile podalic pole. As discussed in Chapter 28 (p. 559), the incidence of breech presentation decreases with gestational age. It approximates 25 percent at 28 weeks, 17 percent at 30 weeks, 11 percent at 32 weeks, and then decreases to approximately 3 percent at term. The high incidence of breech presentation in hydrocephalic fetuses is in accord with this theory, as the larger fetal cephalic pole requires more room than its podalic pole.

Breech Presentation

When the fetus presents as a breech, the three general configurations are *frank, complete,* and *footling presentations* and are described in Chapter 28 (p. 559). Breech presentation may result from circumstances that prevent normal version from taking place. One example is a septum that protrudes into the uterine cavity (Chap. 3, p. 42). A peculiarity of fetal attitude, particularly extension of the vertebral column as seen in frank breeches, also may prevent the fetus from turning. If the placenta is implanted in the lower uterine segment, it may distort normal intrauterine anatomy and result in a breech presentation.

Fetal Attitude or Posture

In the later months of pregnancy, the fetus assumes a characteristic posture described as attitude or habitus as shown in Figure 22-1. As a rule, the fetus forms an ovoid mass that corresponds roughly to the shape of the uterine cavity. The fetus becomes folded or bent upon itself in such a manner that the back becomes markedly convex; the head is sharply flexed so that the chin is almost in contact with the chest; the thighs are flexed over the abdomen; and the legs are bent at the knees. In all cephalic presentations, the arms are usually crossed over the thorax or become parallel to the sides. The umbilical cord lies in the space between them and the lower extremities. This characteristic posture results from the mode of fetal growth and its accommodation to the uterine cavity.

Abnormal exceptions to this attitude occur as the fetal head becomes progressively more extended from the vertex to the face presentation (see Fig. 22-1). This results in a progressive change in fetal attitude from a convex (flexed) to a concave (extended) contour of the vertebral column.

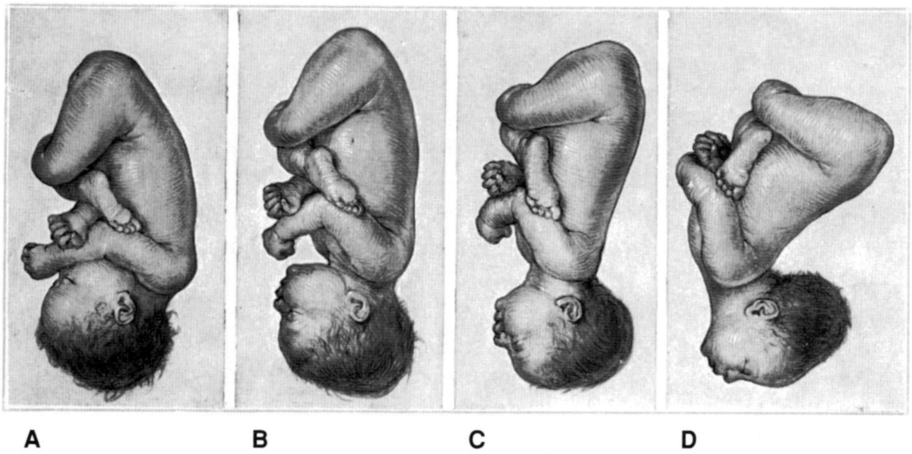

FIGURE 22-1 Longitudinal lie. Cephalic presentation. Differences in attitude of the fetal body in **(A)** vertex, **(B)** sinciput, **(C)** brow, and **(D)** face presentations. Note changes in fetal attitude in relation to fetal vertex as the fetal head becomes less flexed.

Fetal Position

Position refers to the relationship of an arbitrarily chosen portion of the fetal presenting part to the right or left side of the birth canal. Accordingly, with each presentation there may be two positions—right or left. The fetal occiput, chin (mentum), and sacrum are the determining points in vertex, face, and breech presentations, respectively (Figs. 22-2 to 22-6). Because the presenting part may be in either the left or right position, there are left and right occipital, left and right mental, and left and right sacral presentations. These are abbreviated as LO and RO, LM and RM, and LS and RS, respectively.

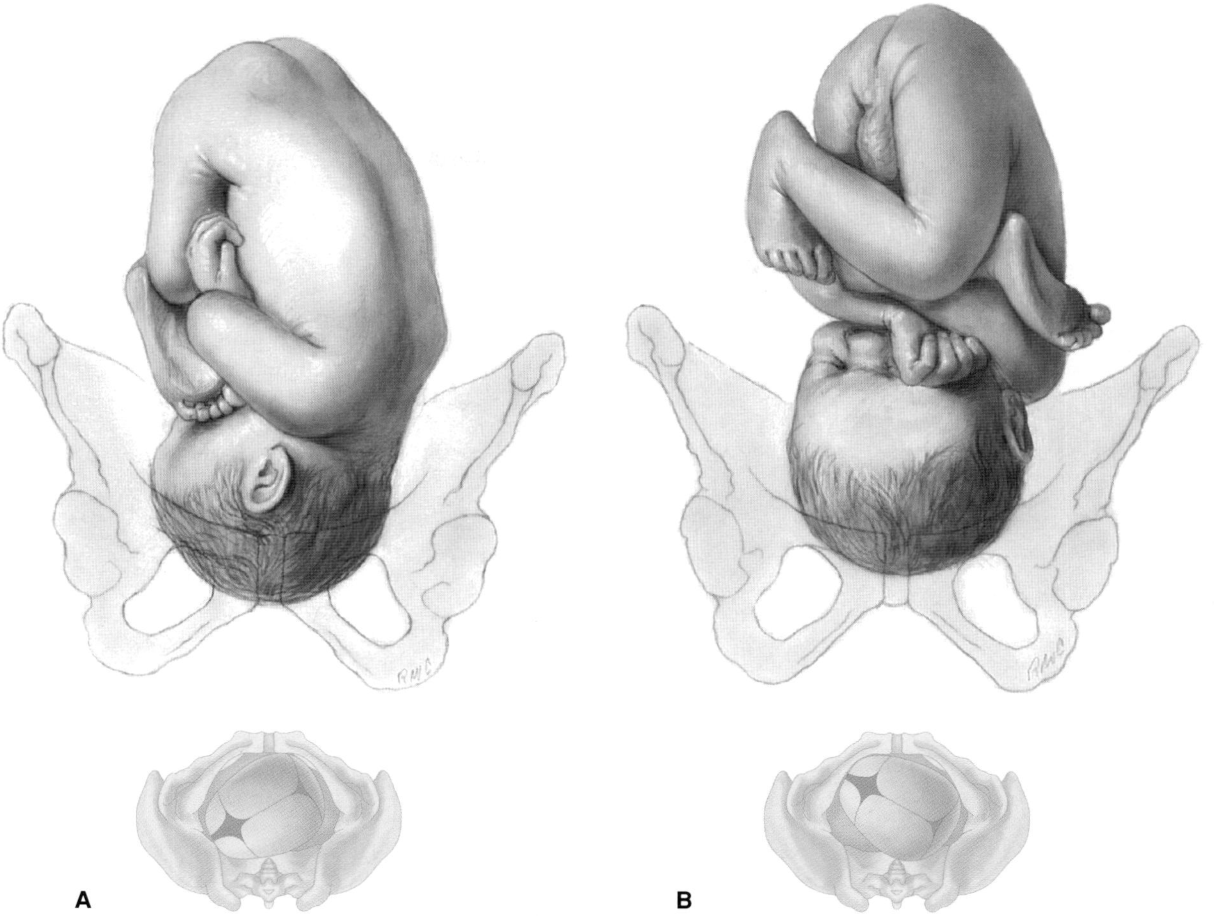

FIGURE 22-2 Longitudinal lie. Vertex presentation. **A.** Left occiput anterior (LOA). **B.** Left occiput posterior (LOP).

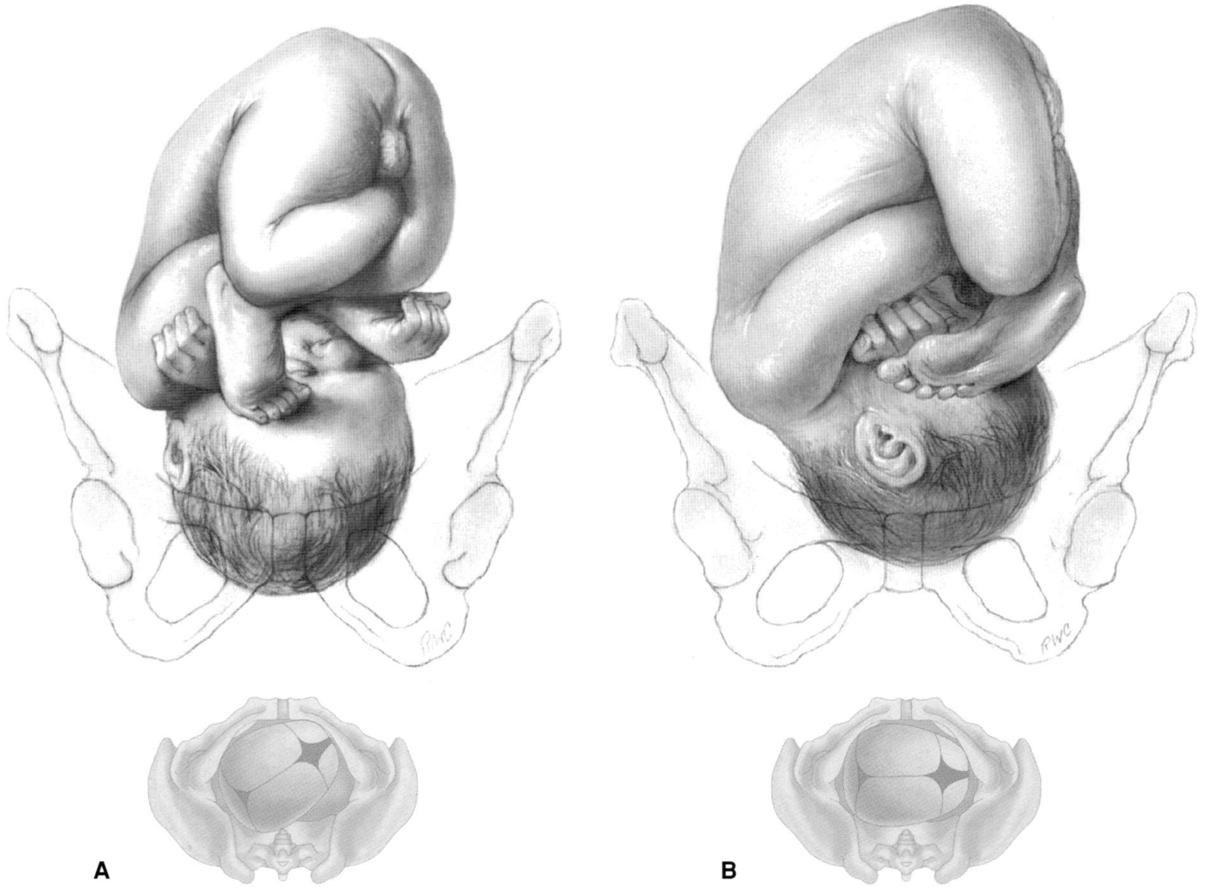

FIGURE 22-3 Longitudinal lie. Vertex presentation. **A**. Right occiput posterior (ROP). **B**. Right occiput transverse (ROT).

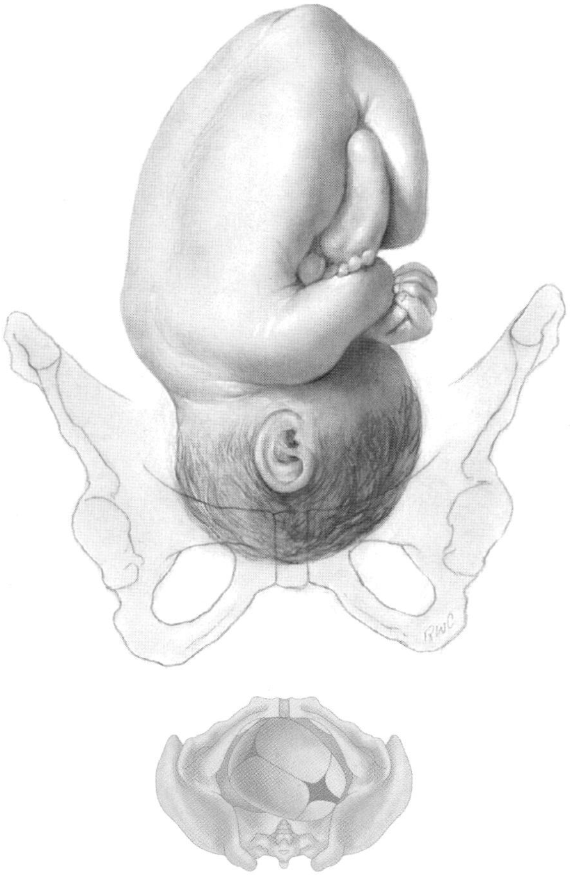

FIGURE 22-4 Longitudinal lie. Vertex presentation. Right occiput anterior (ROA).

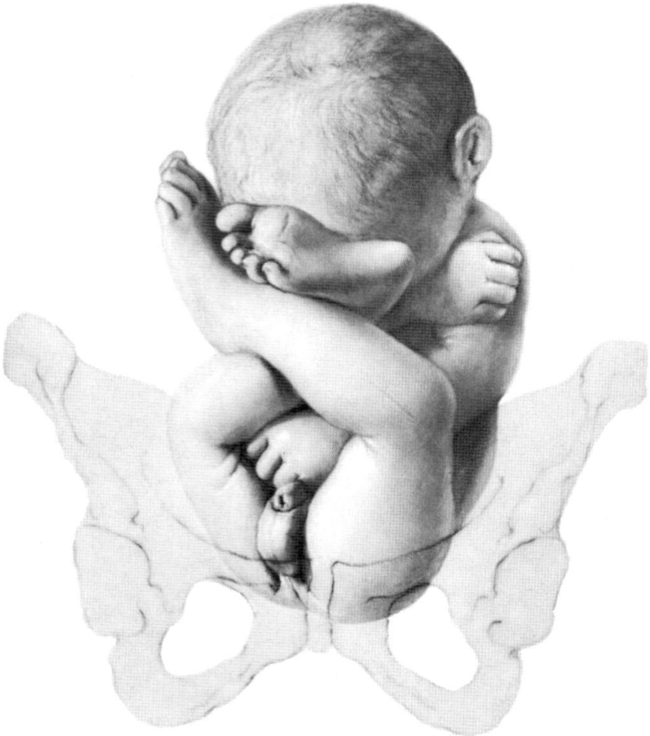

FIGURE 22-6 Longitudinal lie. Breech presentation. Left sacrum posterior (LSP).

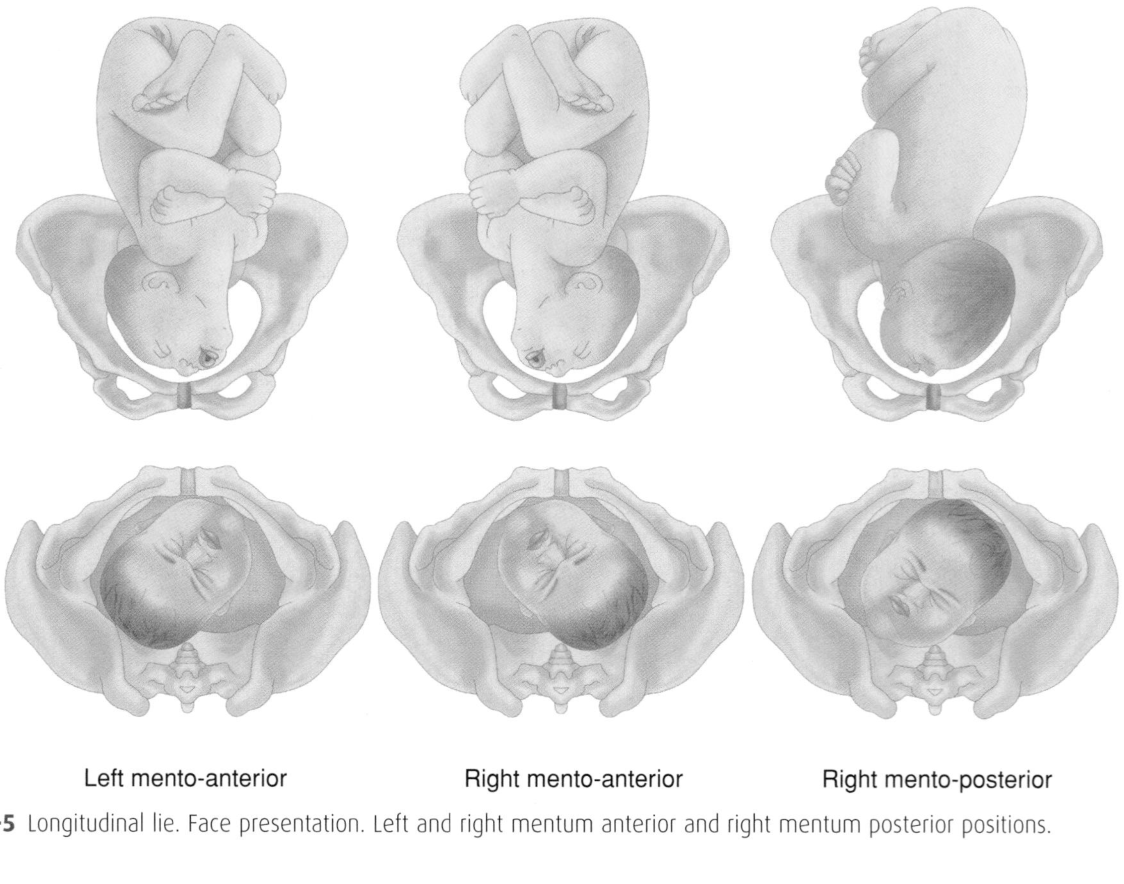

FIGURE 22-5 Longitudinal lie. Face presentation. Left and right mentum anterior and right mentum posterior positions.

Varieties of Presentations and Positions

For still more accurate orientation, the relationship of a given portion of the presenting part to the anterior, transverse, or posterior portion of the maternal pelvis is considered. Because the presenting part in right or left positions may be directed anteriorly (A), transversely (T), or posteriorly (P), there are six varieties of each of the three presentations as shown in Figures 22-2 to 22-6. Thus, in an occiput presentation, the presentation, position, and variety may be abbreviated in clockwise fashion as:

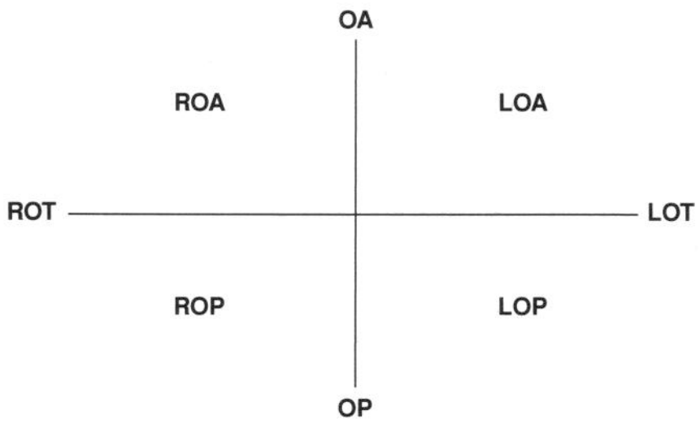

Approximately two thirds of all vertex presentations are in the left occiput position, and one third in the right.

In shoulder presentations, the acromion (scapula) is the portion of the fetus arbitrarily chosen for orientation with the maternal pelvis. One example of the terminology sometimes employed for this purpose is illustrated in Figure 22-7. The acromion or back of the fetus may be directed either posteriorly or anteriorly and superiorly or inferiorly. Because it is impossible to differentiate exactly the several varieties of shoulder presentation by clinical examination and because such specific differentiation serves no practical purpose, it is customary to refer to all transverse lies simply as *shoulder presentations.* Another term used is *transverse lie,* with *back up* or *back down,* which is clinically important when deciding incision type for cesarean delivery (Chap. 23, p. 468).

Diagnosis of Fetal Presentation and Position

Several methods can be used to diagnose fetal presentation and position. These include abdominal palpation, vaginal examination, auscultation, and, in certain doubtful cases, sonography. Rarely, plain radiographs, computed tomography, or magnetic resonance imaging may be used.

Abdominal Palpation—Leopold Maneuvers

Abdominal examination can be conducted systematically employing the four maneuvers described by Leopold in 1894 and shown in Figure 22-8. The mother lies supine and comfortably positioned with her abdomen bared. These maneuvers may be difficult if not impossible to perform and interpret if the patient is obese, if there is excessive amnionic fluid, or if the placenta is anteriorly implanted.

The first maneuver permits identification of which fetal pole—that is, cephalic or podalic—occupies the uterine fundus. The breech gives the sensation of a large, nodular mass, whereas the head feels hard and round and is more mobile and ballottable.

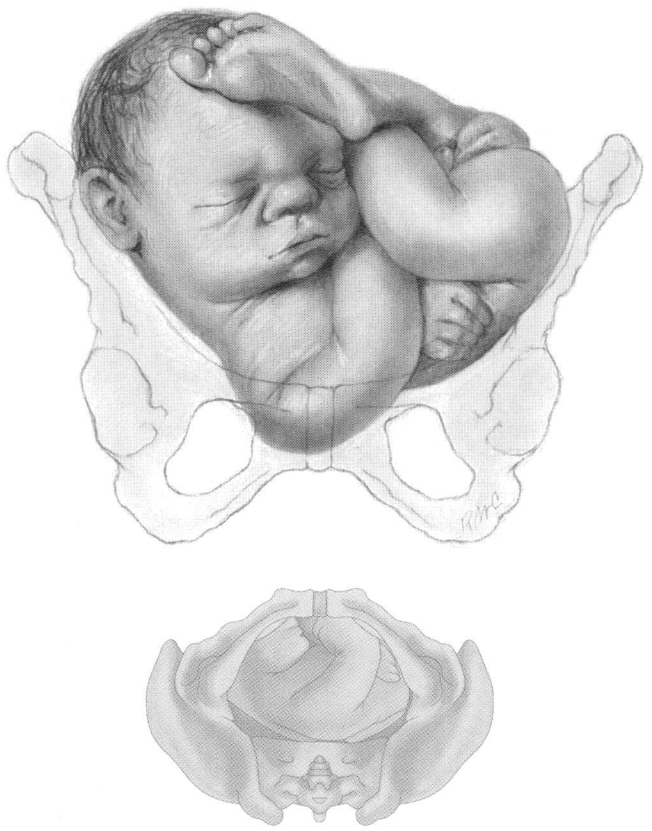

FIGURE 22-7 Transverse lie. Right acromiodorsoposterior (RADP). The shoulder of the fetus is to the mother's right, and the back is posterior.

Performed after determination of fetal lie, the second maneuver is accomplished as the palms are placed on either side of the maternal abdomen, and gentle but deep pressure is exerted. On one side, a hard, resistant structure is felt—the back. On the other, numerous small, irregular, mobile parts are felt—the fetal extremities. By noting whether the back is directed anteriorly, transversely, or posteriorly, fetal orientation can be determined.

The third maneuver is performed by grasping with the thumb and fingers of one hand the lower portion of the maternal abdomen just above the symphysis pubis. If the presenting part is not engaged, a movable mass will be felt, usually the head. The differentiation between head and breech is made as in the first maneuver. If the presenting part is deeply engaged, however, the findings from this maneuver are simply indicative that the lower fetal pole is in the pelvis, and details are then defined by the fourth maneuver.

To perform the fourth maneuver, the examiner faces the mother's feet and, with the tips of the first three fingers of each hand, exerts deep pressure in the direction of the axis of the pelvic inlet. In many instances, when the head has descended into the pelvis, the anterior shoulder may be differentiated readily by the third maneuver.

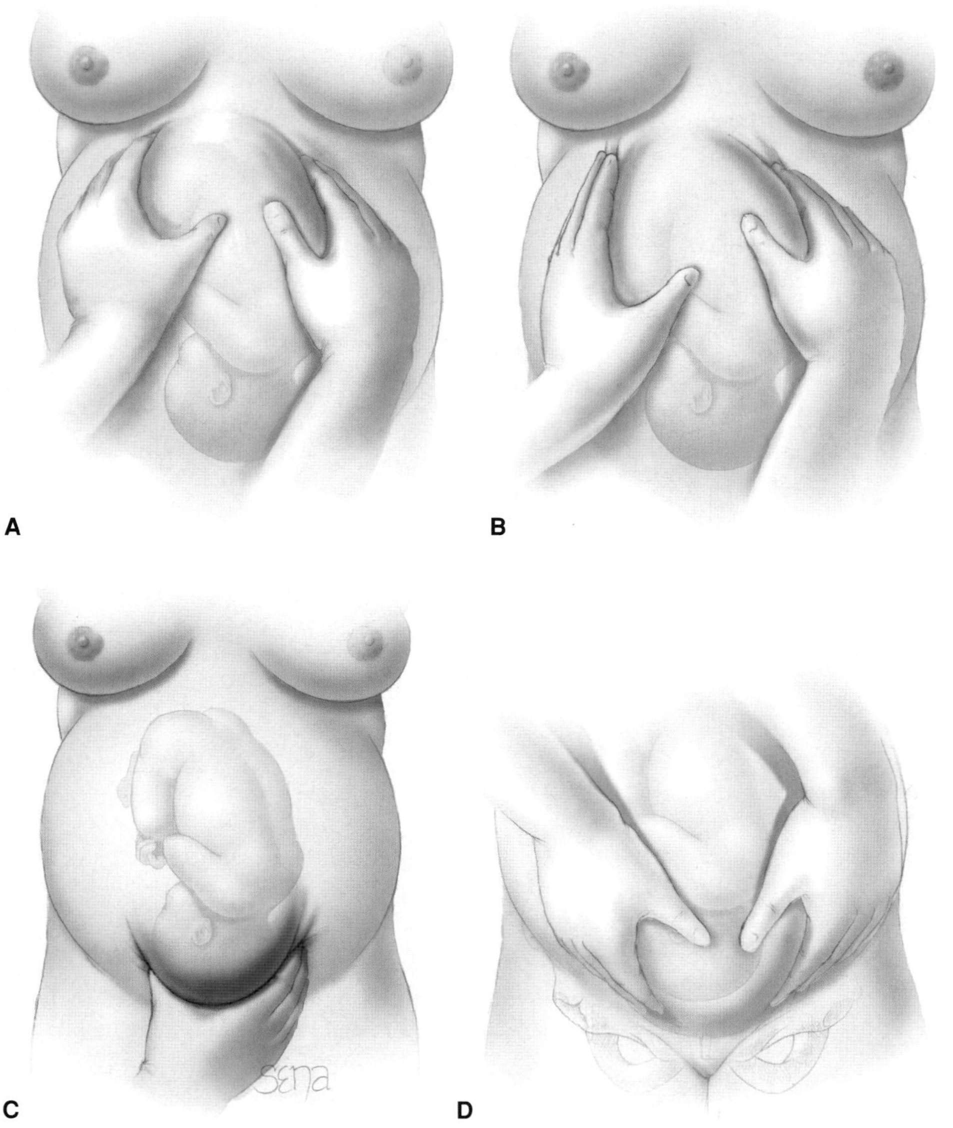

FIGURE 22-8 Leopold maneuvers **(A–D)** performed in a fetus with a longitudinal lie in the left occiput anterior position (LOA).

Abdominal palpation can be performed throughout the latter months of pregnancy and during and between the contractions of labor. With experience, it is possible to estimate the size of the fetus. According to Lydon-Rochelle and colleagues (1993), experienced clinicians accurately identify fetal malpresentation using Leopold maneuvers with a high sensitivity—88 percent, specificity—94 percent, positive-predictive value—74 percent, and negative-predictive value—97 percent.

Vaginal Examination

Before labor, the diagnosis of fetal presentation and position by vaginal examination is often inconclusive because the presenting part must be palpated through a closed cervix and lower uterine segment. With the onset of labor and after cervical dilatation, vertex presentations and their positions are recognized by palpation of the various fetal sutures and fontanels. Face and breech presentations are identified by palpation of facial features and fetal sacrum, respectively.

In attempting to determine presentation and position by vaginal examination, it is advisable to pursue a definite routine, comprising four movements. First, the examiner inserts two fingers into the vagina and the presenting part is found. Differentiation of vertex, face, and breech is then accomplished readily. Second, if the vertex is presenting, the fingers are directed posteriorly and then swept forward over the fetal head toward the maternal symphysis (Fig. 22-9). During this movement, the fingers necessarily cross the sagittal suture and its linear course is delineated. Next, the positions of the two fontanels are ascertained. For this, fingers are passed to the most anterior extension of the sagittal suture, and the fontanel encountered there is examined and identified. Then, with a sweeping motion, the fingers pass along the suture to the other end of the head until the other fontanel is felt and differentiated (Fig. 22-10). Last, the station, or extent to which the presenting part has descended into the pelvis, can also be established at this time (p. 449). Using these maneuvers, the various sutures and fontanels are located readily (Fig. 7-11, p. 139).

Sonography and Radiography

Sonographic techniques can aid fetal position identification, especially in obese women or in women with rigid abdominal walls. Zahalka and associates (2005) compared digital examinations with transvaginal and transabdominal sonography for fetal head position determination during second-stage labor and reported that transvaginal sonography was superior.

Occiput Anterior Presentation

In most cases, the vertex enters the pelvis with the sagittal suture lying in the transverse pelvic diameter. The fetus enters the pelvis in the *left occiput transverse (LOT)* position in 40 percent of labors and in the *right occiput transverse (ROT)* position in 20 percent (Caldwell, 1934). In *occiput anterior positions—LOA* or *ROA*—the head either enters the pelvis with the occiput rotated 45 degrees anteriorly from the transverse position, or this rotation occurs subsequently. The mechanism of labor in all these presentations is usually similar.

The positional changes of the presenting part required to navigate the pelvic canal constitute the *mechanisms of labor.*

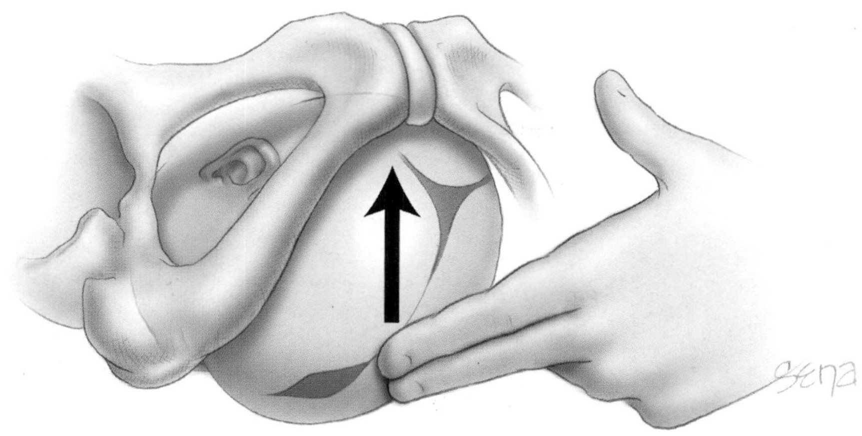

FIGURE 22-9 Locating the sagittal suture by vaginal examination.

The *cardinal movements of labor* are engagement, descent, flexion, internal rotation, extension, external rotation, and expulsion (Fig. 22-11). During labor, these movements not only are sequential but also show great temporal overlap. For example, as part of engagement, there is both flexion and descent of the head. It is impossible for the movements to be completed unless the presenting part descends simultaneously. Concomitantly, uterine contractions effect important modifications in fetal attitude, or habitus, especially after the head has descended into the pelvis. These changes consist principally of fetal straightening, with loss of dorsal convexity and closer application of the extremities to the body. As a result, the fetal ovoid is transformed into a cylinder, with the smallest possible cross section typically passing through the birth canal.

Engagement

The mechanism by which the biparietal diameter—the greatest transverse diameter in an occiput presentation—passes through the pelvic inlet is designated *engagement*. The fetal head may engage during the last few weeks of pregnancy or not until after labor commencement. In many multiparous and some nulliparous women, the fetal head is freely movable above the pelvic inlet at labor onset. In this circumstance, the head is sometimes referred to as "floating." A normal-sized head usually does not engage with its sagittal suture directed anteroposteriorly. Instead, the fetal head usually enters the pelvic inlet either transversely or obliquely. Segel and coworkers (2012) analyzed labor in 5341 nulliparous women and found that fetal head engagement before labor onset did not affect vaginal delivery rates in either spontaneous or induced labor.

Asynclitism. The fetal head tends to accommodate to the transverse axis of the pelvic inlet, whereas the sagittal suture, while remaining parallel to that axis, may not lie exactly midway between the symphysis and the sacral promontory. The sagittal suture frequently is deflected either posteriorly toward the promontory or anteriorly toward the symphysis (Fig. 22-12). Such lateral deflection to a more anterior or posterior position in the pelvis is called *asynclitism*. If the sagittal suture approaches the sacral promontory, more of the anterior parietal bone presents itself to the examining fingers, and the condition is called *anterior asynclitism*. If, however, the sagittal suture lies close to the symphysis, more of the posterior parietal bone will present, and the condition is called *posterior asynclitism*. With extreme posterior asynclitism, the posterior ear may be easily palpated.

Moderate degrees of asynclitism are the rule in normal labor. However, if severe, the condition is a common reason for cephalopelvic disproportion even with an otherwise normal-sized pelvis. Successive shifting from posterior to anterior asynclitism aids descent.

Descent

This movement is the first requisite for birth of the newborn. In nulliparas, engagement may take place before the onset of labor, and further descent may not follow until the onset of the second stage. In multiparas, descent usually begins with engagement. Descent is brought about by one or more of four forces: (1) pressure of the amnionic fluid, (2) direct pressure of the fundus upon the breech with contractions, (3) bearing-down efforts of maternal abdominal muscles, and (4) extension and straightening of the fetal body.

Flexion

As soon as the descending head meets resistance, whether from the cervix, pelvic walls, or pelvic floor, it normally flexes. With this movement, the chin is brought into more intimate contact with the fetal thorax, and the appreciably shorter suboccipitobregmatic diameter is substituted for the longer occipitofrontal diameter (Figs. 22-13 and 22-14).

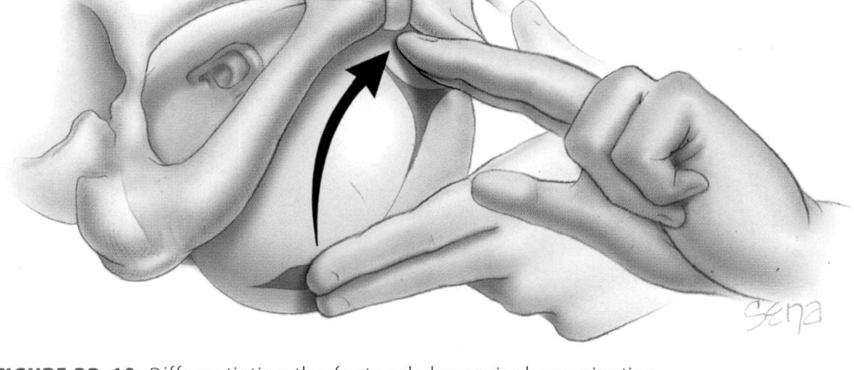

FIGURE 22-10 Differentiating the fontanels by vaginal examination.

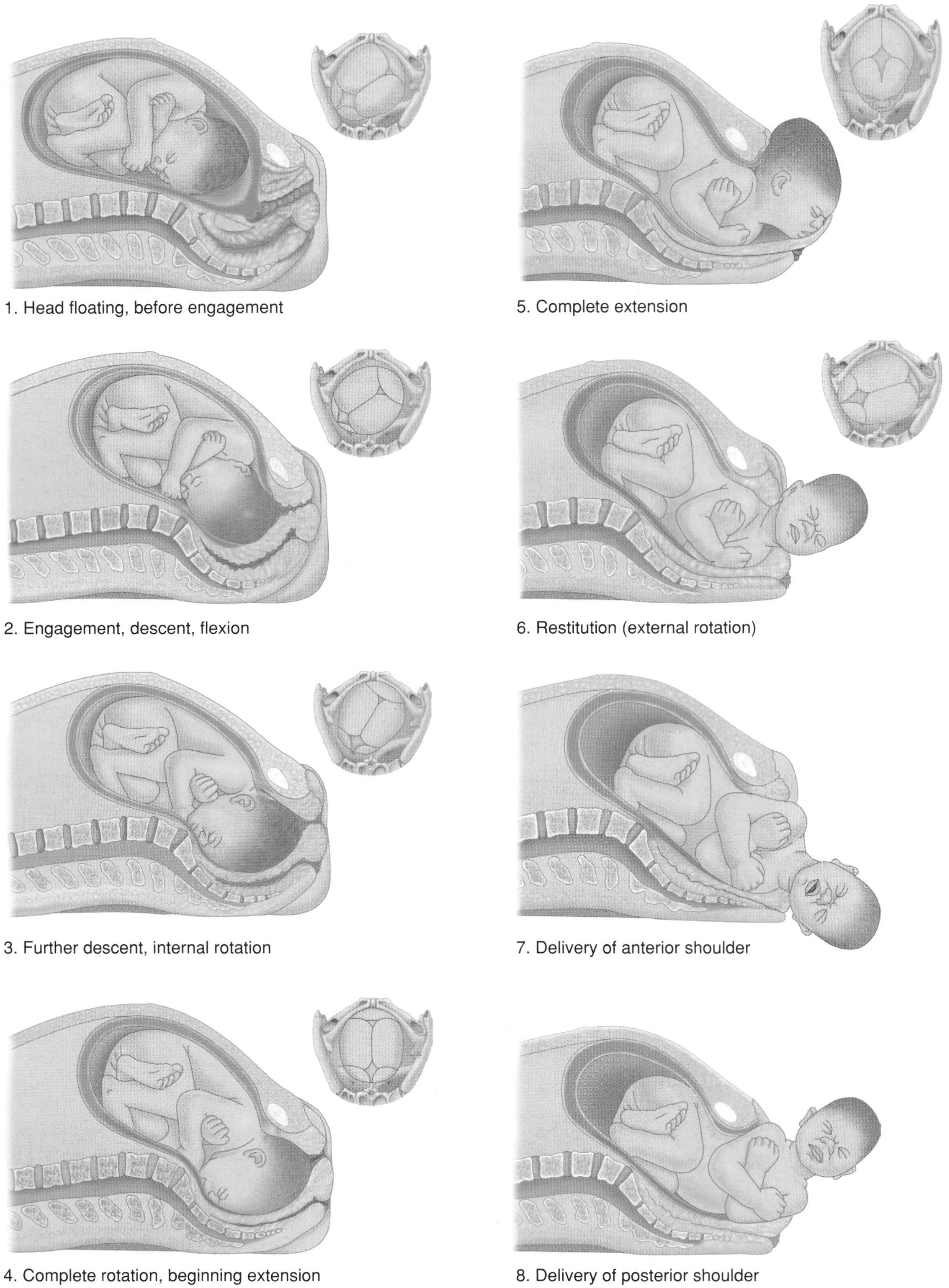

FIGURE 22-11 Cardinal movements of labor and delivery from a left occiput anterior position.

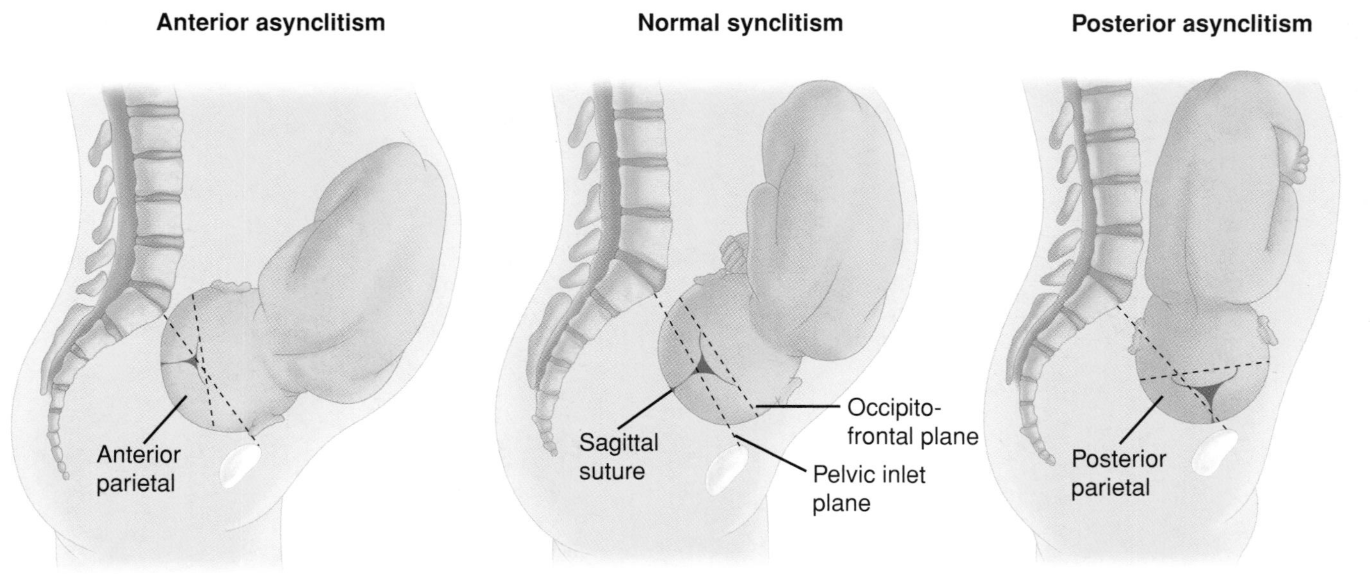

FIGURE 22-12 Synclitism and asynclitism.

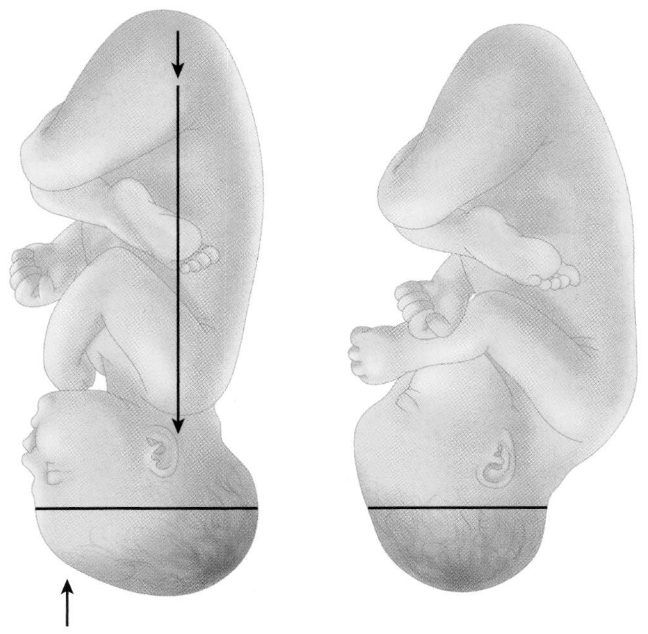

FIGURE 22-13 Lever action produces flexion of the head. Conversion from occipitofrontal to suboccipitobregmatic diameter typically reduces the anteroposterior diameter from nearly 12 to 9.5 cm.

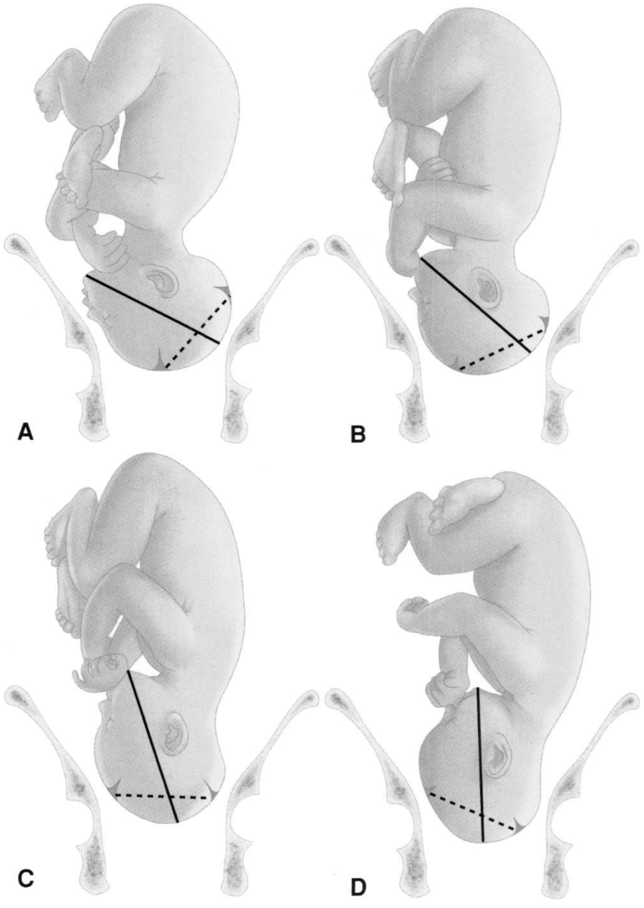

FIGURE 22-14 Four degrees of head flexion. The solid line represents the occipitomental diameter, whereas the broken line connects the center of the anterior fontanel with the posterior fontanel. **A.** Flexion poor. **B.** Flexion moderate. **C.** Flexion advanced. **D.** Flexion complete. Note that with complete flexion, the chin is on the chest. The suboccipitobregmatic diameter, the shortest anteroposterior diameter of the fetal head, is passing through the pelvic inlet.

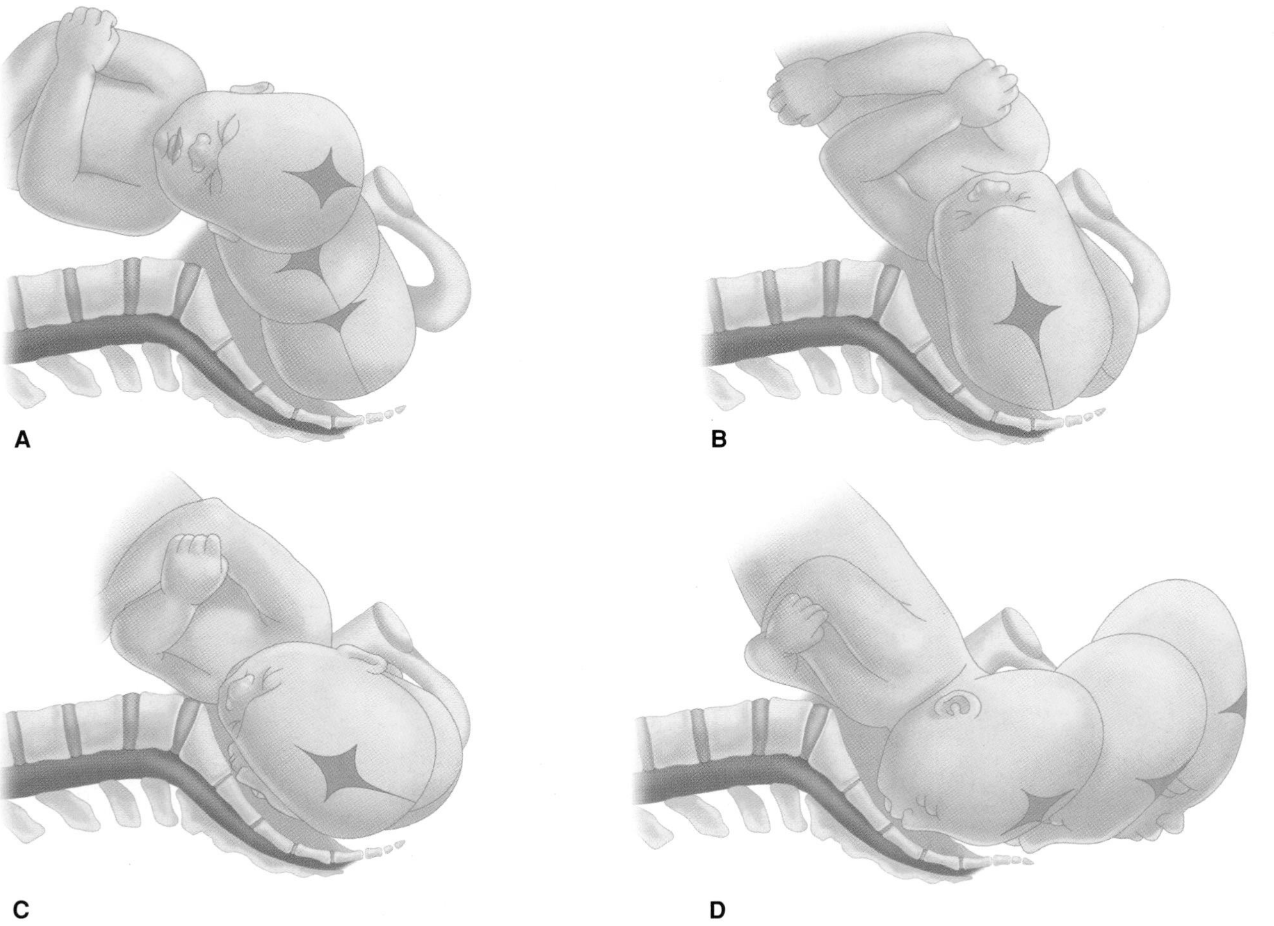

FIGURE 22-15 Mechanism of labor for the left occiput transverse position, lateral view. **A.** Engagement. **B.** After engagement, further descent. **C.** Descent and initial internal rotation. **D.** Rotation and extension.

Internal Rotation

This movement consists of a turning of the head in such a manner that the occiput gradually moves toward the symphysis pubis anteriorly from its original position or, less commonly, posteriorly toward the hollow of the sacrum (Figs. 22-15 to 22-17). Internal rotation is essential for completion of labor, except when the fetus is unusually small.

Calkins (1939) studied more than 5000 women in labor to ascertain the time of internal rotation. He concluded that in approximately two thirds, internal rotation is completed by the time the head reaches the pelvic floor; in about another fourth, internal rotation is completed shortly after the head reaches the pelvic floor; and in the remaining 5 percent, rotation does not take place. When the head fails to turn until reaching the pelvic floor, it typically rotates during the next one or two contractions in multiparas. In nulliparas, rotation usually occurs during the next three to five contractions.

Extension

After internal rotation, the sharply flexed head reaches the vulva and undergoes extension. If the sharply flexed head, on reaching the pelvic floor, did not extend but was driven farther downward, it would impinge on the posterior portion of the perineum and would eventually be forced through the perineal tissues. When the head presses on the pelvic floor, however, two forces come into play. The first force, exerted by the uterus, acts more posteriorly, and the second, supplied by the resistant pelvic floor and the symphysis, acts more anteriorly. The resultant vector is in the direction of the vulvar opening, thereby causing head extension. This brings the base of the occiput into direct contact with the inferior margin of the symphysis pubis (see Fig. 22-16).

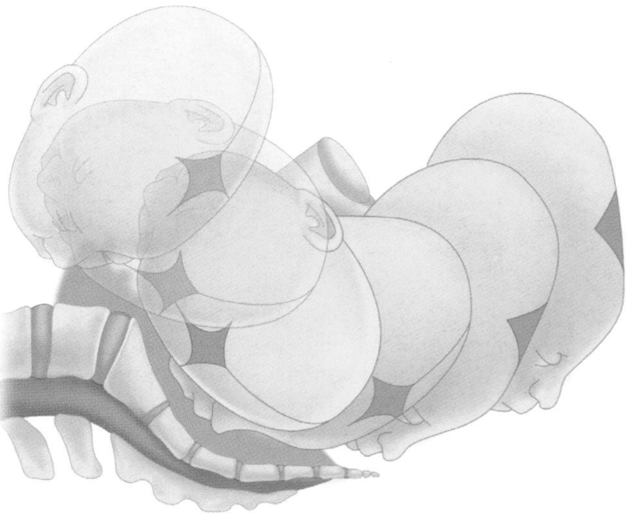

FIGURE 22-16 Mechanism of labor for left occiput anterior position.

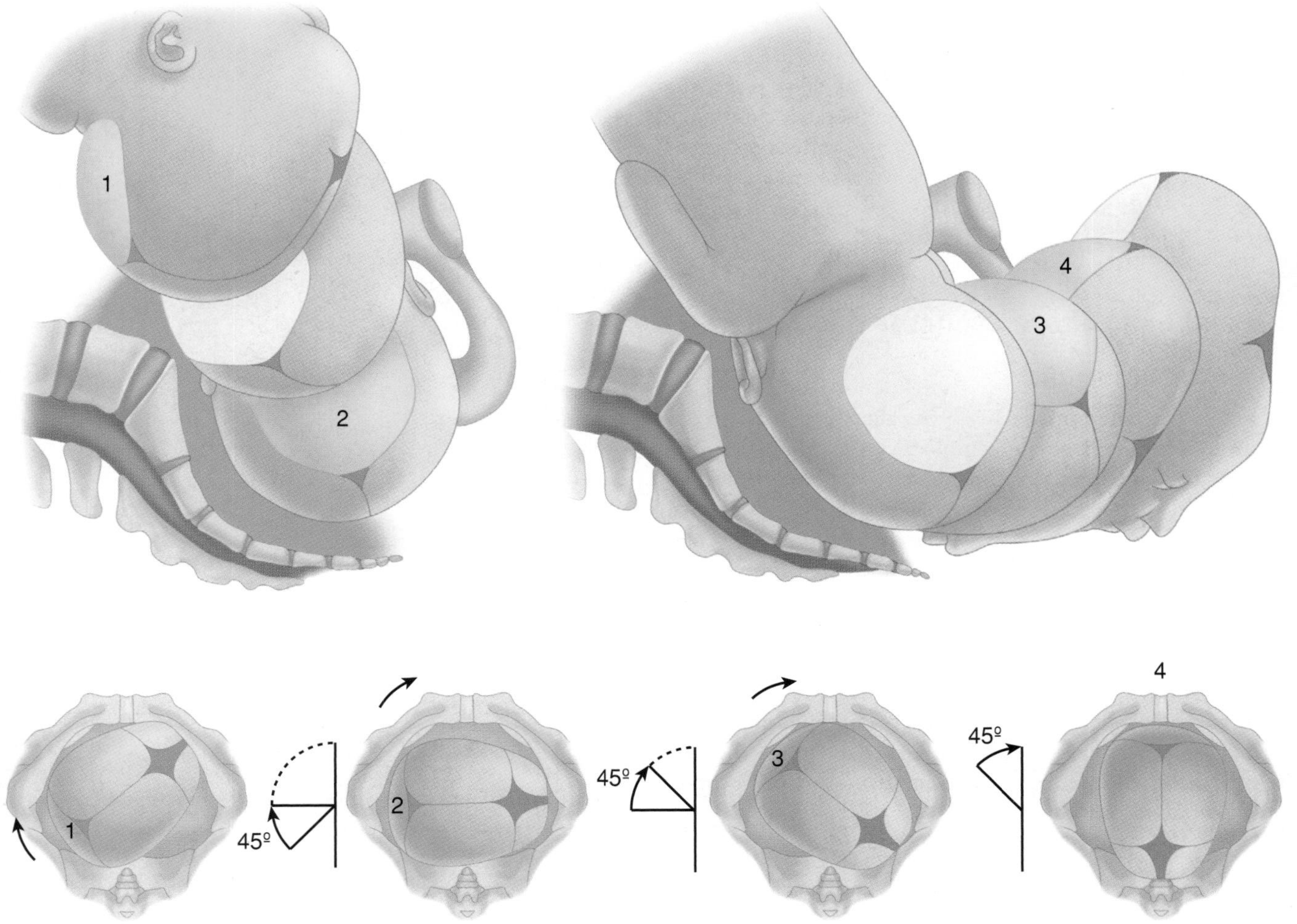

FIGURE 22-17 Mechanism of labor for right occiput posterior position showing anterior rotation.

With progressive distention of the perineum and vaginal opening, an increasingly larger portion of the occiput gradually appears. The head is born as the occiput, bregma, forehead, nose, mouth, and finally the chin pass successively over the anterior margin of the perineum (see Fig. 22-17). Immediately after its delivery, the head drops downward so that the chin lies over the maternal anus.

External Rotation

The delivered head next undergoes *restitution* (see Fig. 22-11). If the occiput was originally directed toward the left, it rotates toward the left ischial tuberosity. If it was originally directed toward the right, the occiput rotates to the right. Restitution of the head to the oblique position is followed by external rotation completion to the transverse position. This movement corresponds to rotation of the fetal body and serves to bring its bisacromial diameter into relation with the anteroposterior diameter of the pelvic outlet. Thus, one shoulder is anterior behind the symphysis and the other is posterior. This movement apparently is brought about by the same pelvic factors that produced internal rotation of the head.

Expulsion

Almost immediately after external rotation, the anterior shoulder appears under the symphysis pubis, and the perineum soon becomes distended by the posterior shoulder. After delivery of the shoulders, the rest of the body quickly passes.

Occiput Posterior Presentation

In approximately 20 percent of labors, the fetus enters the pelvis in an *occiput posterior (OP)* position (Caldwell, 1934). The right occiput posterior (ROP) is slightly more common than the left (LOP). It appears likely from radiographic evidence that posterior positions are more often associated with a narrow forepelvis. They also are more commonly seen in association with anterior placentation (Gardberg, 1994a).

In most occiput posterior presentations, the mechanism of labor is identical to that observed in the transverse and anterior varieties, except that the occiput has to internally rotate to the symphysis pubis through 135 degrees, instead of 90 and 45 degrees, respectively (see Fig. 22-17).

Effective contractions, adequate head flexion, and average fetal size together permit most posteriorly positioned occiputs to rotate promptly as soon as they reach the pelvic floor, and labor is not lengthened appreciably. In perhaps 5 to 10 percent of cases, however, rotation may be incomplete or may not take place at all, especially if the fetus is large (Gardberg, 1994b). Poor contractions, faulty head flexion, or epidural analgesia, which diminishes abdominal muscular pushing and relaxes pelvic floor muscles, may predispose to incomplete rotation. If rotation is incomplete, transverse arrest may result. If no rotation toward the symphysis takes place, the occiput may remain in the direct occiput posterior position, a condition known as *persistent occiput posterior.* Both persistent occiput posterior and transverse arrest represent deviations from the normal mechanisms of labor and are considered further in Chapter 23.

Fetal Head Shape Changes

Caput Succedaneum

In vertex presentations, labor forces alter fetal head shape. In prolonged labors before complete cervical dilatation, the portion of the fetal scalp immediately over the cervical os becomes edematous (Fig. 33-1, p. 647). This swelling, known as the *caput succedaneum,* is shown in Figures 22-18 and 22-19. It usually attains a thickness of only a few millimeters, but in prolonged labors it may be sufficiently extensive to prevent differentiation of the various sutures and fontanels. More commonly, the caput is formed when the head is in the lower portion of the birth canal and frequently only after the resistance of a rigid vaginal outlet is encountered. Because it develops over the most dependent area of the head, one may deduce the original fetal head position by noting the location of the caput succedaneum.

Molding

In addition to soft tissue changes, the bony fetal head shape is also altered by external compressive forces and is referred to as *molding* (see Fig. 22-19). Possibly related to Braxton Hicks contractions, some molding develops before labor. Most studies indicate that there is seldom overlapping of the parietal bones. A "locking" mechanism at the coronal and lambdoidal connections actually prevents such overlapping (Carlan, 1991). Molding results in a shortened suboccipitobregmatic diameter and a lengthened mentovertical diameter. These changes are of greatest importance in women with contracted pelves or asynclitic presentations. In these circumstances, the degree to which the head is capable of molding may make the difference between spontaneous vaginal delivery and an operative delivery. Some older literature cited severe head molding as a cause for possible cerebral trauma. Because of the multitude of associated factors, for example, prolonged labor with fetal sepsis and acidosis, it is impossible to link molding to any alleged fetal or neonatal neurological sequelae. Most cases of molding resolve within the week following delivery, although persistent cases have been described (Graham, 2006).

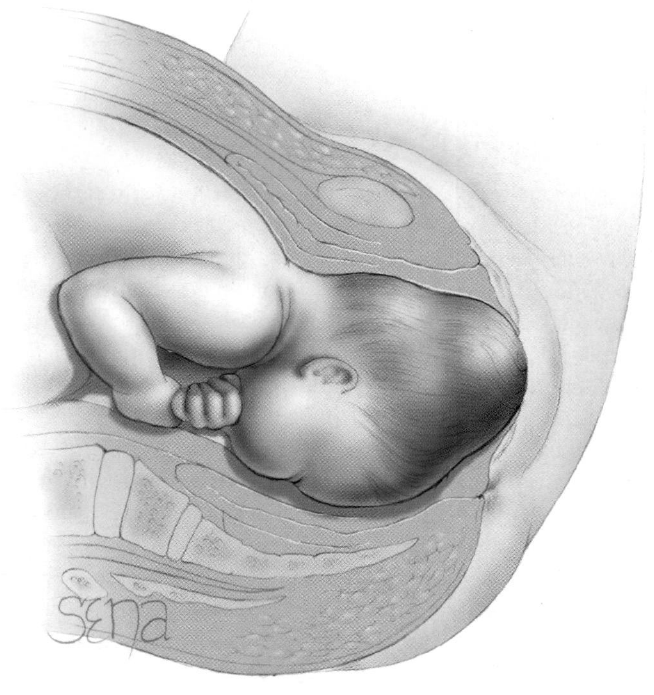

FIGURE 22-18 Formation of caput succedaneum and head molding.

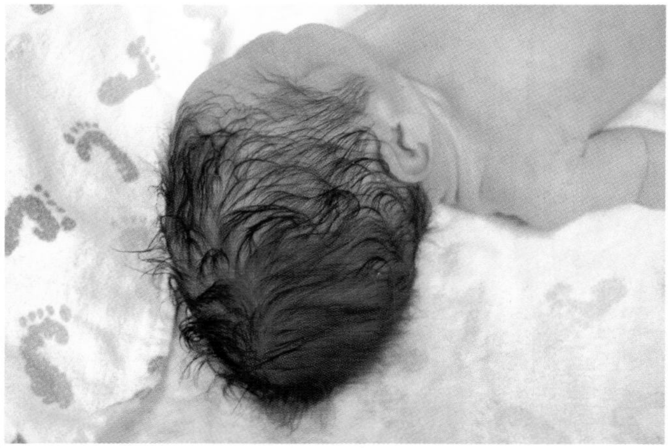

FIGURE 22-19 Considerable molding of the head and caput succedaneum formation in a recently delivered newborn.

CHARACTERISTICS OF NORMAL LABOR

The greatest impediment to understanding normal labor is recognizing its start. The strict definition of labor—*uterine contractions that bring about demonstrable effacement and dilatation of the cervix*—does not easily aid the clinician in determining when labor has actually begun, because this diagnosis is confirmed only retrospectively. Several methods may be used to define its start. One defines onset as the clock time when painful contractions become regular. Unfortunately, uterine activity that causes discomfort, but that does not represent true labor, may develop at any time during pregnancy. False labor often stops spontaneously, or it may proceed rapidly into effective contractions.

A second method defines the onset of labor as beginning at the time of admission to the labor unit. In the United States, admission for labor is frequently based on the extent of cervical dilatation accompanied by painful contractions. If a woman has intact membranes, then a cervical dilatation of 3 to 4 cm or greater is presumed to be a reasonably reliable threshold for the diagnosis of labor. In this case, labor onset commences

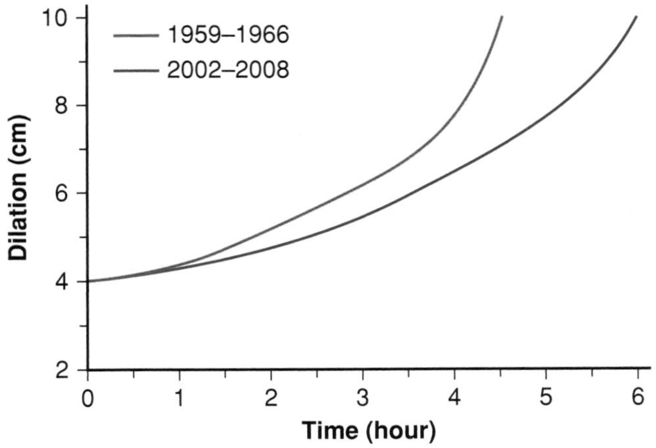

FIGURE 22-20 Average labor curves for women with singleton term pregnancies presenting in spontaneous labor with vaginal delivery for nulliparas for 1959–1966 compared with 2002–2008. (From Zhang, 2002.)

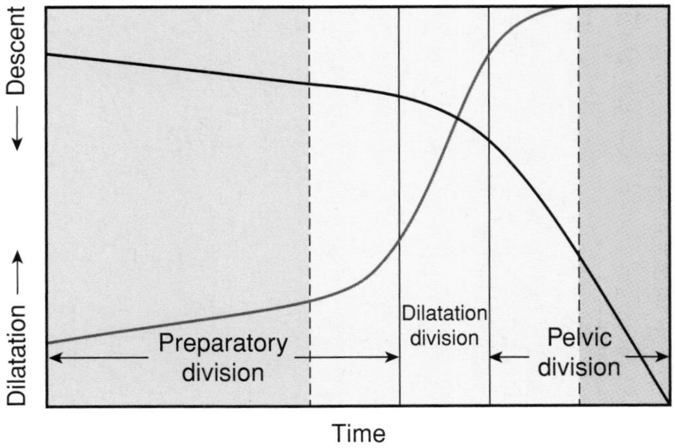

FIGURE 22-21 Labor course divided functionally on the basis of dilatation and descent curves into: (1) a preparatory division, including latent and acceleration phases; (2) a dilatational division, occupying the phase of maximum slope; and (3) a pelvic division, encompassing both deceleration phase and second stage concurrent with the phase of maximum slope of descent. (Redrawn from Friedman, 1978.)

with the time of admission. This presumptive method obviates many of the uncertainties in diagnosing labor during earlier stages of cervical dilatation. Laughon and colleagues (2012) compared the duration of spontaneous labor at term in nulliparas delivered in the United States between 1959 and 1966 to that of those delivered from 2002 to 2008. As shown in Figure 22-20, the length of labor increased by approximately 2 hours during those 50 years.

First Stage of Labor

Assuming that the diagnosis has been confirmed, what then are the expectations for the progress of normal labor? A scientific approach was begun by Friedman (1954), who described a characteristic sigmoid pattern for labor by graphing cervical dilatation against time. This graphical approach, based on statistical observations, changed labor management. Friedman developed the concept of three functional labor divisions to describe the physiological objectives of each division as shown in Figure 22-21. First, during the *preparatory division,* although the cervix dilates little, its connective tissue components change considerably (Chap. 21, p. 410). Sedation and conduction analgesia are capable of arresting this labor division. The *dilatational division,* during which dilatation proceeds at its most rapid rate, is unaffected by sedation. Last, the *pelvic division* commences with the deceleration phase of cervical dilatation. The classic labor mechanisms that involve the cardinal fetal movements of the cephalic presentation take place principally during this pelvic division. In actual practice, however, the onset of the pelvic division is seldom clearly identifiable.

As shown in Figure 22-21, the pattern of cervical dilatation during the preparatory and dilatational divisions of normal labor is a sigmoid curve. Two phases of cervical dilatation are defined. The *latent phase* corresponds to the preparatory division, and the *active phase* to the dilatational division. And as shown in Figure 22-22, Friedman subdivided the active phase into the *acceleration phase,* the *phase of maximum slope,* and the *deceleration phase.*

Latent Phase

The onset of latent labor, as defined by Friedman (1972), is the point at which the mother perceives regular contractions. The latent phase for most women ends once dilatation of 3 to 5 cm is achieved. This threshold may be clinically useful, for it defines dilatation limits beyond which active labor can be expected.

This concept of a latent phase has great significance in understanding normal human labor, because labor is considerably longer when a latent phase is included. To better illustrate

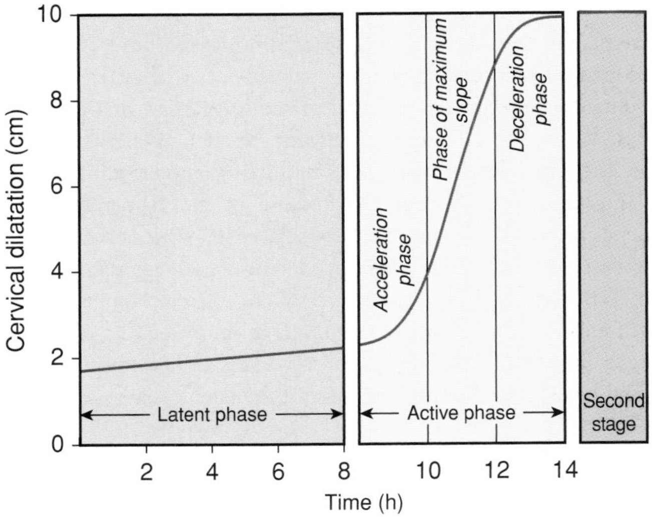

FIGURE 22-22 Composite of the average dilatation curve for nulliparous labor. The first stage is divided into a relatively flat latent phase and a rapidly progressive active phase. In the active phase, there are three identifiable component parts that include an acceleration phase, a phase of maximum slope, and a deceleration phase. (Redrawn from Friedman, 1978.)

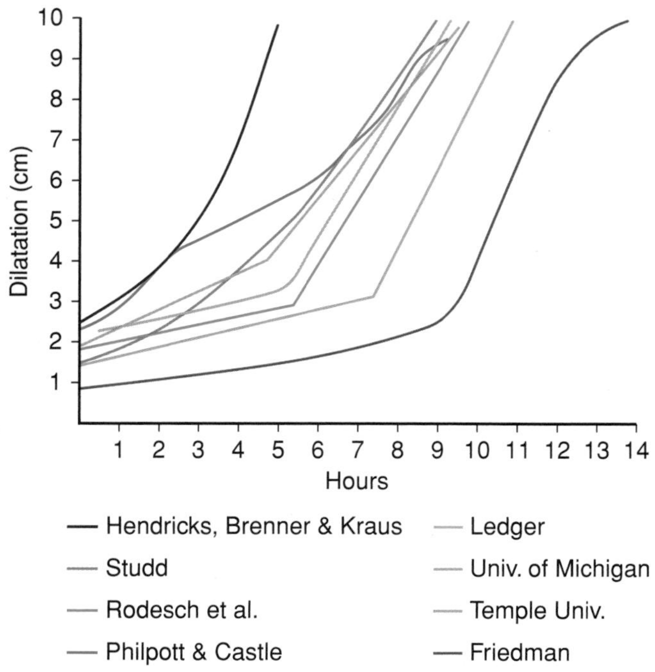

FIGURE 22-23 Progress of labor in primigravid women from the time of admission. When the starting point on the abscissa begins with admission to the hospital, a latent phase is not observed.

this, Figure 22-23 shows eight labor curves from nulliparas in whom labor was diagnosed beginning with their admission, rather than with the onset of regular contractions. When labor is defined similarly, there is remarkable similarity of individual labor curves.

Prolonged Latent Phase. Friedman and Sachtleben (1963) defined this by a latent phase exceeding 20 hours in the nullipara and 14 hours in the multipara. These times corresponded to the 95th percentiles. Factors that affected latent phase duration include excessive sedation or epidural analgesia; unfavorable cervical condition, that is, thick, uneffaced, or undilated; and false labor. In those who had been administered heavy sedation, 85 percent of women eventually entered active labor. In another 10 percent, uterine contractions ceased, suggesting that they had false labor. The remaining 5 percent experienced persistence of an abnormal latent phase and required oxytocin stimulation. Amniotomy was discouraged because of the 10-percent incidence of false labor. Sokol and associates (1977) reported a 3- to 4- percent incidence of prolonged latent phase, regardless of parity. Friedman (1972) reported that latent phase prolongation did not adversely influence fetal or maternal morbidity or mortality rates. However, Chelmow and coworkers (1993) disputed the long-held belief that prolongation of the latent phase is benign.

Active Labor

The progress of labor in nulliparas has particular significance because these curves all reveal a rapid change in the slope of cervical dilatation rates between 3 and 5 cm (see Fig. 22-23). *Thus, cervical dilatation of 3 to 5 cm or more, in the presence of uterine contractions, can be taken to reliably represent the threshold for active labor.* Similarly, these curves provide useful guideposts for labor management.

Turning again to Friedman (1955), the mean duration of active-phase labor in nulliparas was 4.9 hours. But the standard deviation of 3.4 hours is large, hence, the active phase was reported to have a statistical maximum of 11.7 hours. Indeed, rates of cervical dilatation ranged from a minimum of 1.2 up to 6.8 cm/hr. Friedman (1972) also found that multiparas progress somewhat faster in active-phase labor, with a *minimum* normal rate of 1.5 cm/hr. His analysis of active-phase labor concomitantly describes rates of fetal descent and cervical dilatation (see Fig. 22-21). Descent begins in the later stage of active dilatation, commencing at 7 to 8 cm in nulliparas and becoming most rapid after 8 cm.

Active-Phase Abnormalities. These have bee reported to occur in 25 percent of nulliparous and 15 percent of multiparous labors (Sokol, 1977). Friedman (1972) subdivided active-phase problems into *protraction* and *arrest disorders*. Protraction is defined as a *slow rate* of cervical dilatation or descent, which for nulliparas was < 1.2 cm dilatation per hour or < 1 cm descent per hour. For multiparas, protraction was defined as < 1.5 cm dilatation per hour or < 2 cm descent per hour. Friedman defined arrest as a *complete cessation* of dilatation or descent. *Arrest of dilatation* was defined as 2 hours with no cervical change, and *arrest of descent* as 1 hour without fetal descent. The prognosis for protraction and arrest disorders differs considerably. Friedman found that approximately 30 percent of women with protraction disorders had cephalopelvic disproportion (CPD). This compared with a 45-percent CPD rate for women in whom an arrest disorder developed. Abnormal labor patterns, diagnostic criteria, and treatment methods are summarized in Chapter 23 (p. 456).

Hendricks and colleagues (1970) challenged Friedman's conclusions about the course of normal human labor. Their principal differences included: (1) absence of a latent phase, (2) no deceleration phase, (3) brevity of labor, and (4) dilatation at similar rates for nulliparas and multiparas after 4 cm. They disputed the concept of a latent phase because they observed that the cervix dilated and effaced slowly during the 4 weeks preceding labor. They contended that the *latent phase* actually progressed over several weeks. They also reported that labor was relatively rapid. Specifically, the average time from admission to complete dilatation was 4.8 hours for nulliparas and 3.2 hours for multiparas.

There have been other reports in which investigators have reassessed the Friedman labor curves. Zhang and associates (2010) studied electronic labor records from 62,415 parturients with spontaneous labor at term and vaginal birth. They found that normal labor may take more than 6 hours to progress from 4 to 5 cm and more than 3 hours to progress from 5 to 6 cm dilation. Thereafter, labor accelerated much faster in multiparas. In a study performed at Parkland Hospital, epidural analgesia was found to lengthen the active phase of the Friedman labor curve by 1 hour (Alexander, 2002). This increase was the result of a slight but significant decrease in the rate of cervical dilatation—1.4 cm/hr in women given epidural analgesia compared with 1.6 cm/hr in those without such analgesia. There are now several reports that maternal obesity lengthens the first stages of labor by 30 to 60 minutes (Chin, 2012; Kominiarek, 2011). Finally, Adams and coworkers (2012) found that maternal fear increased labor by approximately 45 minutes.

Second Stage of Labor

This stage begins with complete cervical dilatation and ends with fetal delivery. The median duration is approximately 50 minutes for nulliparas and about 20 minutes for multiparas, but it is highly variable (Kilpatrick, 1989). In a woman of higher parity with a previously dilated vagina and perineum, two or three expulsive efforts after full cervical dilatation may suffice to complete delivery. Conversely, in a woman with a contracted pelvis, with a large fetus, or with impaired expulsive efforts from conduction analgesia or sedation, the second stage may become abnormally long. Robinson and colleagues (2011) found that increasing maternal body mass index did not interfere with the second stage of labor. Abnormalities of this labor stage are described in Chapter 23 (p. 456).

Duration of Labor

Our understanding of the normal duration of labor may be clouded by the many clinical variables that affect conduct of labor in modern obstetrical units. Kilpatrick and Laros (1989) reported that the mean length of first- and second-stage labor was approximately 9 hours in nulliparous women without regional analgesia, and that the 95th percentile upper limit was 18.5 hours. Corresponding times for multiparous women were a mean of 6 hours with a 95th percentile maximum of 13.5 hours. These authors defined labor onset as the time when a woman recalled regular, painful contractions every 3 to 5 minutes that led to cervical change.

Spontaneous labor was analyzed in nearly 25,000 women delivered at term at Parkland Hospital in the early 1990s. Almost 80 percent of women were admitted with a cervical dilatation of 5 cm or less. Parity—nulliparous versus multiparous—and cervical dilatation at admission were significant determinants of the length of spontaneous labor. The median time from admission to spontaneous delivery for all parturients was 3.5 hours, and 95 percent of all women delivered within 10.1 hours. These results suggest that normal human labor is relatively short. Zhang and associates (2009a,b) described similar findings in their study of 126,887 deliveries from 12 United States institutions.

Summary of Normal Labor

Labor is characterized by brevity and considerable biological variation. Active labor can be reliably diagnosed when cervical dilatation is 3 cm or more in the presence of uterine contractions. Once this cervical dilatation threshold is reached, normal progression to delivery can be expected, depending on parity, in the ensuing 4 to 6 hours. Anticipated progress during a 1- to 2-hour second stage is monitored to ensure fetal safety. Finally, most women in spontaneous labor, regardless of parity, if left unaided, will deliver within approximately 10 hours after admission for spontaneous labor. Insufficient uterine activity is a common and correctable cause of abnormal labor progress. *Therefore, when the length of otherwise normal labor exceeds the expected norm, interventions other than cesarean delivery—for example, oxytocin administration—must be first considered.*

TABLE 22-2. Recommended Nurse/Patient Ratios for Labor and Delivery

Ratio	Clinical Setting
1:2	Patients in labor
1:1	Patients in second-stage labor
1:1	Patients with medical/obstetrical complications
1:2	Oxytocin induction/augmentation
1:1	During epidural analgesia initiation
1:1	Circulation for cesarean delivery

MANAGEMENT OF NORMAL LABOR

The ideal management of labor and delivery requires two potentially opposing viewpoints on the part of clinicians. First, birthing should be recognized as a normal physiological process that most women experience without complications. Second, intrapartum complications, often arising quickly and unexpectedly, should be anticipated. Thus, clinicians must simultaneously make every woman and her supporters feel comfortable, yet ensure safety for the mother and newborn should complications suddenly develop. Principles such as these are the basis for a recent *"Call to Action"* by seven national organizations intended to emphasize quality patient care in labor and delivery (Lawrence, 2012). The American Academy of Pediatrics and the American College of Obstetricians and Gynecologists (2012) have collaborated in the development of *Guidelines for Perinatal Care.* These provide detailed information on the appropriate content of intrapartum care, including both personnel and facility requirements. Shown in Table 22-2 are the recommended nurse-to-patient ratios recommended for labor and delivery. Shown in Table 22-3 are the recommended room dimensions for these functions.

TABLE 22-3. Recommended Minimum Room Dimensions for Labor and Delivery

Function	Net Floor Space (square feet)
LDR	340
Intensive care	200
Vaginal delivery	340
Cesarean delivery	440

LDR = labor, delivery, and recovery.
Data from American Academy of Pediatrics and American College of Obstetricians and Gynecologists, 2012.

Admission Procedures

Pregnant women should be urged to report early in labor rather than to procrastinate until delivery is imminent for fear that they might be experiencing false labor. Early admittance to the labor and delivery unit is important, especially if during antepartum care the woman, her fetus, or both have been identified as being at risk.

Identification of Labor

Although the differentiation between false and true labor is difficult at times, the diagnosis usually can be clarified by contraction frequency and intensity and by cervical dilatation. In those instances when a diagnosis of labor cannot be established with certainty, observation for a longer period is often wise.

Pates and associates (2007) studied the commonly used recommendations given to pregnant women that, in the absence of ruptured membranes or bleeding, uterine contractions 5 minutes apart for 1 hour—that is, ≥ 12 contractions in 1 hour—may signify labor onset. Among 768 women studied at Parkland Hospital, active labor defined as cervical dilatation ≥ 4 cm was diagnosed within 24 hours in three fourths of women with ≥ 12 contractions per hour. Bailit and coworkers (2005) compared labor outcomes of 6121 women who presented in active labor defined as uterine contractions plus cervical dilatation ≥ 4 cm with those of 2697 women who presented in the latent phase. Women admitted during latent-phase labor had more active-phase arrest, more frequent need for oxytocin labor stimulation, and higher rates of chorioamnionitis. It was concluded that physician interventions in women presenting in the latent phase may have been the cause of subsequent labor abnormalities.

Emergency Medical Treatment and Labor Act—EMTALA

Congress enacted EMTALA in 1986 to ensure public access to emergency services regardless of the ability to pay. All Medicare-participating hospitals with emergency services must provide an appropriate screening examination for any pregnant woman experiencing contractions and presenting to the emergency department for evaluation.

The definition of an emergency condition makes specific reference to a pregnant woman who is having contractions. Labor is defined as "the process of childbirth beginning with the latent phase of labor continuing through delivery of the placenta. A woman experiencing contractions is in true labor unless a physician certifies that after a reasonable time of observation the woman is in false labor." A woman in true labor is considered "unstable" for interhospital transfer purposes until the newborn and placenta are delivered. An unstable woman may, however, be transferred at the direction of the patient or by a physician who certifies that the benefits of treatment at another facility outweigh the transfer risks. Physicians and hospitals violating these federal requirements are subject to civil penalties up to $50,000 and termination from the Medicare program.

Electronic Fetal Heart Rate Monitoring

As discussed in Chapter 24 (p. 473), electronic fetal heart rate monitoring is routinely used for high-risk pregnancies commencing at admission. Some investigators recommend monitoring women with low-risk pregnancies upon admission as a test of fetal well-being—the so-called *fetal admission test.* If no fetal heart rate abnormalities are detected, continuous electronic monitoring is replaced by intermittent assessment for the remainder of labor. We are of the view that electronic fetal heart rate monitoring is reasonable in the preadmission evaluation of women, including those who subsequently are discharged. At Parkland Hospital, external electronic monitoring is performed for at least 1 hour before discharging the woman who was ascertained to have false labor.

Home Births

A major emphasis of obstetrical care during the 20th century was the movement to birthing in hospitals rather than in homes. In 2006, 98.9 percent of births in the United States took place in hospitals (Martin, 2011). Of the other 1.1 percent, 67.2 percent were in homes, and 27.6 percent were in birthing centers. Between 2004 and 2008, more than half of all states had an increase in home births (MacDorman, 2011). As discussed in Chapter 1 (p. 11) most studies suggest increased risks with home deliveries (Berghella, 2008; Cheng, 2013; de Jonge, 2013; Grunebaum, 2013). Indeed, Chervenak and colleagues (2013) have questioned the ethics of physicians voluntarily involved in home births.

Initial Evaluation

Maternal blood pressure, temperature, pulse, and respiratory rate are recorded. The pregnancy record is promptly reviewed to identify complications. Problems identified or anticipated during prenatal care should be displayed prominently in the pregnancy record. Most often, *unless there has been bleeding in excess of bloody show,* a vaginal examination is performed. The gloved index and second fingers are then introduced into the vagina while avoiding the anal region (Fig. 22-24). The number of vaginal examinations correlates with infection-related morbidity, especially in cases of early membrane rupture.

Ruptured Membranes

The woman should be instructed during the antepartum period to be aware of fluid leakage from the vagina and to report such an event promptly. Rupture of the membranes is significant for three reasons. First, if the presenting part is not fixed in the pelvis, the possibility of umbilical cord prolapse and compression is greatly increased. Second, labor is likely to begin soon if the pregnancy is at or near term. Third, if delivery is delayed after membrane rupture, intrauterine infection is more likely as the time interval increases (Herbst, 2007).

Upon sterile speculum examination, ruptured membranes are diagnosed if amnionic fluid pools in the posterior fornix or clear fluid flows from the cervical canal. Although several

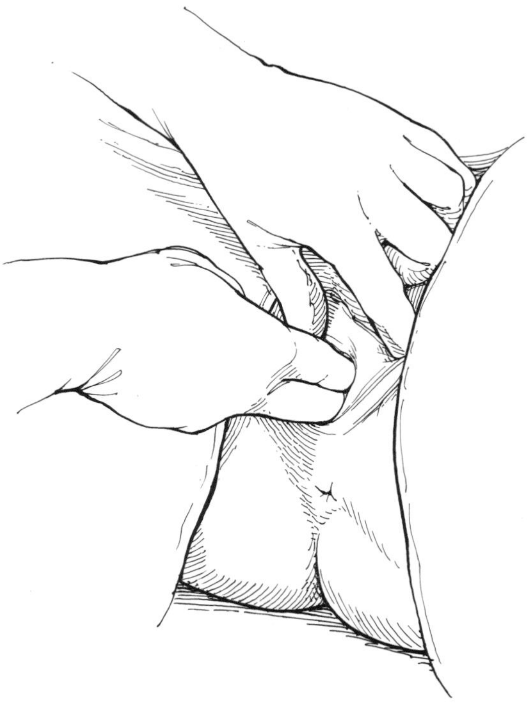

FIGURE 22-24 To perform vaginal examination, the labia have been separated with one hand, and the first and second fingers of the other hand are carefully inserted into the introitus.

diagnostic tests for the detection of ruptured membranes have been recommended, none is completely reliable. If the diagnosis remains uncertain, another method involves pH determination of vaginal fluid. The pH of vaginal secretions normally ranges from 4.5 to 5.5, whereas that of amnionic fluid is usually 7.0 to 7.5. The use of the indicator *nitrazine* to identify ruptured membranes is a simple and fairly reliable method. Test papers are impregnated with the dye, and the color of the reaction between these paper strips and vaginal fluids is interpreted by comparison with a standard color chart. A pH above 6.5 is consistent with ruptured membranes. False-positive test results may occur with coexistent blood, semen, or bacterial vaginosis, whereas false-negative tests may result with scant fluid.

Other tests include arborization or ferning of vaginal fluid, which suggests amnionic rather than cervical fluid. Amnionic fluid crystallizes to form a fernlike pattern due to its relative concentrations of sodium chloride, proteins, and carbohydrates (Fig. 4-2, p. 49). Detection of alpha-fetoprotein in the vaginal vault has been used to identify amnionic fluid (Yamada, 1998). Although rarely required, identification may also follow injection of indigo carmine into the amnionic sac via abdominal amniocentesis.

Cervical Assessment

The degree of *cervical effacement* usually is expressed in terms of the length of the cervical canal compared with that of an uneffaced cervix. When the length of the cervix is reduced by one half, it is 50-percent effaced. When the cervix becomes as thin as the adjacent lower uterine segment, it is completely, or 100-percent, effaced.

Cervical dilatation is determined by estimating the average diameter of the cervical opening by sweeping the examining finger from the margin of the cervical opening on one side to that on the opposite side. The diameter traversed is estimated in centimeters. The cervix is said to be dilated fully when the diameter measures 10 cm, because the presenting part of a term-size newborn usually can pass through a cervix this widely dilated.

The *position* of the cervix is determined by the relationship of the cervical os to the fetal head and is categorized as posterior, mid-position, or anterior. Along with position, the *consistency* of cervix is determined to be soft, firm, or intermediate between these two.

The level—or *station*—of the presenting fetal part in the birth canal is described in relationship to the ischial spines, which are halfway between the pelvic inlet and the pelvic outlet. When the lowermost portion of the presenting fetal part is at the level of the spines, it is designated as being at zero (0) station. In the past, the long axis of the birth canal above and below the ischial spines was arbitrarily divided into thirds by some and into fifths (approximately 1 cm) by other groups. In 1989, the American College of Obstetricians and Gynecologists adopted the classification of station that divides the pelvis above and below the spines into fifths. Each fifth represents 1 cm above or below the spines. Thus, as the presenting fetal part descends from the inlet *toward* the ischial spines, the designation is –5, –4, –3, –2, –1, then 0 station. Below the spines, as the presenting fetal part descends, it passes +1, +2, +3, +4, and +5 stations to delivery. Station +5 cm corresponds to the fetal head being visible at the introitus.

If the leading part of the fetal head is at 0 station or below, most often the fetal head has engaged—thus, the biparietal plane has passed through the pelvic inlet. *If the head is unusually molded or if there is an extensive caput formation or both, engagement might not have taken place although the head appears to be at 0 station.*

In a study done at five teaching centers in Denver, residents, nurses, and faculty were surveyed to determine what definitions were being used to describe fetal station (Carollo, 2004). Four different definitions were in use. Disturbingly, these investigators found that few caregivers were aware that others were using different definitions of station! Dupuis and colleagues (2005) tested the reliability of clinical estimations of station using the position of the leading part in centimeters above or below the spines as recommended by the American Academy of Pediatrics and the American College of Obstetricians and Gynecologists (2012). A birth simulator was used in which station could be precisely measured and compared with the vaginal examination done by clinicians. They reported that the clinical examiners were incorrect a third of the time.

These five characteristics: cervical dilatation, effacement, consistency, position, and fetal station are assessed when tabulating the Bishop score. This score is commonly used to predict labor induction outcome and is discussed in Chapter 26 (p. 526).

Laboratory Studies

When a woman is admitted in labor, most often the hematocrit or hemoglobin concentration should be rechecked. The hematocrit can be measured easily and quickly. At Parkland Hospital, blood is collected in a standard collection tube with anticoagulant. From this, a heparinized capillary tube is filled to spin in a microhematocrit centrifuge in the labor and delivery unit. This provides a hematocrit value within 3 minutes. The initial collection tube is also sent to the hematology laboratory for evaluation. Another labeled tube of blood is allowed to clot and sent to the blood bank for blood type and antibody screen, if needed. A final sample is collected for syphilis and human immunodeficiency virus (HIV) serology. We obtain a urine specimen for protein determination in hypertensive women only (Chap. 40, p. 729). In some labor units, however, a clean-catch voided specimen is examined in all women for protein and glucose.

Women who have had no prenatal care should be considered to be at risk for syphilis, hepatitis B, and HIV (Chap. 65, p. 1265). In those with no prior prenatal care, these laboratory studies, as well as a blood type and antibody screen, should be performed (American Academy of Pediatrics and American College of Obstetricians and Gynecologists, 2012). Some states, for example, Texas, require routine testing for syphilis, hepatitis B, and HIV in all women admitted to labor and delivery units, even if these were done during prenatal care.

Management of the First Stage of Labor

As soon as possible after admittance, the remainder of a general examination is completed. Whether a pregnancy is normal can best be determined when all examinations, including record and laboratory review, are completed. A rational plan for monitoring labor can then be established based on the needs of the fetus and the mother. Because there are marked individual variations in labor lengths, precise statements as to its anticipated duration are unwise.

Intrapartum Fetal Monitoring

This is discussed in detail in Chapter 24. Briefly, the American Academy of Pediatrics and American College of Obstetricians and Gynecologists (2012) recommend that during first-stage labor, in the absence of any abnormalities, the fetal heart rate should be checked immediately after a contraction at least every 30 minutes and then every 15 minutes during the second stage. If continuous electronic monitoring is used, the tracing is evaluated at least every 30 minutes during the first stage and at least every 15 minutes during second-stage labor. For women with pregnancies at risk, fetal heart auscultation is performed at least every 15 minutes during first-stage labor and every 5 minutes during the second stage. Continuous electronic monitoring may be used with evaluation of the tracing every 15 minutes during the first stage of labor, and every 5 minutes during the second stage.

Uterine Contractions

Although usually assessed by electronic monitoring as also discussed in Chapter 24, contractions can be both quantitatively and qualitatively evaluated manually. With the palm of the hand resting lightly on the uterus, the time of contraction onset is determined. Its intensity is gauged from the degree of firmness the uterus achieves. At the acme of effective contractions, the finger or thumb cannot readily indent the uterus during a "firm" contraction. The time at which the contraction disappears is noted next. This sequence is repeated to evaluate the frequency, duration, and intensity of uterine contractions.

Maternal Vital Signs

Temperature, pulse, and blood pressure are evaluated at least every 4 hours. If membranes have been ruptured for many hours before labor onset or if there is a borderline temperature elevation, the temperature is checked hourly. Moreover, with prolonged membrane rupture, defined as greater than 18 hours, antimicrobial administration for prevention of group B streptococcal infections is recommended. This is discussed in Chapter 64 (p. 1249).

Subsequent Cervical Examinations

During the first stage of labor, the need for subsequent vaginal examinations to monitor cervical change and presenting part position will vary considerably. When the membranes rupture, an examination to exclude cord prolapse should be performed expeditiously if the fetal head was not definitely engaged at the previous examination. The fetal heart rate should also be checked immediately and during the next uterine contraction to help detect occult umbilical cord compression. At Parkland Hospital, periodic pelvic examinations are typically performed at 2- to 3-hour intervals to evaluate labor progress.

Oral Intake

Food should be withheld during active labor and delivery. Gastric emptying time is remarkably prolonged once labor is established and analgesics are administered. As a consequence, ingested food and most medications remain in the stomach and are not absorbed. Instead, they may be vomited and aspirated (Chap. 25, p. 519). According to the American Academy of Pediatrics and the American College of Obstetricians and Gynecologists (2007), sips of clear liquids, occasional ice chips, and lip moisturizers are permitted.

Intravenous Fluids

Although it has become customary in many hospitals to establish an intravenous infusion system routinely early in labor, there is seldom any real need for this in the normal pregnant woman, at least until analgesia is administered. An intravenous infusion system is advantageous during the immediate puerperium to administer oxytocin prophylactically and at times therapeutically when uterine atony persists. Moreover, with longer labors, the administration of glucose, sodium, and water to the otherwise fasting woman at the rate of 60 to 120 mL/hr prevents dehydration and acidosis. Shrivastava and associates (2009) noted shorter labors in nulliparas delivering vaginally who were provided an intravenous normal saline with dextrose solution compared with those given saline solution only. Garite and coworkers (2000) randomly assigned 195 women in labor to receive either 125 or 250 mL/hr of lactated Ringer or isotonic sodium chloride solution. The mean volume of total intravenous fluid was 2008 mL in the 125 mL/hr group and 2487 mL in the 250 mL/hr group. Labor lasted > 12 hours in significantly more (26 versus 13 percent) of the women given a 125 mL/hr infusion compared with those given 250 mL/hr—26 versus 13 percent, respectively.

Maternal Position

The normal laboring woman need not be confined to bed early in labor. A comfortable chair may be beneficial psychologically and perhaps physiologically. In bed, the laboring woman should be allowed to assume the position she finds most comfortable—this will be lateral recumbency most of the time. She must not be restricted to lying supine because of resultant aortocaval compression and its potential to lower uterine perfusion (Chap. 4, p. 60). Bloom and colleagues (1998) conducted a randomized trial of walking during labor in more than 1000 women with low-risk pregnancies. They found that walking neither enhanced nor impaired active labor and that it was not harmful. Lawrence and associates (2009) reached similar findings in their Cochrane database review.

Analgesia

This is discussed in detail in Chapter 25. In general, pain relief should depend on the needs and desires of the woman. The American College of Obstetricians and Gynecologists (2009) has specified optimal goals for anesthesia care in obstetrics.

Amniotomy

If the membranes are intact, there is a great temptation, even during normal labor, to perform amniotomy. The presumed benefits are more rapid labor, earlier detection of meconium-stained amnionic fluid, and the opportunity to apply an electrode to the fetus or insert a pressure catheter into the uterine cavity for monitoring. The advantages and disadvantages of amniotomy are discussed in Chapter 26 (p. 531). Importantly, the fetal head must be well applied to the cervix and not be dislodged from the pelvis during the procedure to avert umbilical cord prolapse.

Urinary Bladder Function

Distention of the bladder should be avoided because it can hinder descent of the fetal presenting part and lead to subsequent bladder hypotonia and infection. During each abdominal examination, the suprapubic region should be inspected and palpated to detect distention. If the bladder is readily seen or palpated above the symphysis, the woman should be encouraged to void. At times, those who may be unable to void on a bedpan may be able to ambulate with assistance to a toilet and successfully void. If the bladder is distended and voiding is not possible, catheterization is indicated. Carley and coworkers (2002) found that 51 of 11,332 vaginal deliveries (1 in 200) were complicated by urinary retention. Most women resumed normal voiding before discharge from the hospital. Musselwhite and associates (2007) reported retention in 4.7 percent of women who had labor epidural analgesia. Risk factors for retention were primiparity, oxytocin-induced or -augmented labor, perineal lacerations, operative vaginal delivery, catheterization during labor, and labor duration > 10 hours.

Management of the Second Stage of Labor

With full cervical dilatation, which signifies the onset of the second stage, a woman typically begins to bear down. With descent of the presenting part, she develops the urge to defecate. Uterine contractions and the accompanying expulsive forces may now last 1 minutes and recur at an interval no longer than 1½ minute. As discussed on page 447, the median duration of the second stage is 50 minutes in nulliparas and 20 minutes in multiparas, although the interval can be highly variable. Monitoring of the fetal heart rate is discussed on page 450, and interpretation of second-stage electronic fetal heart rate patterns is discussed in Chapter 24 (p. 487).

Expulsive Efforts

In most cases, bearing down is reflexive and spontaneous during second-stage labor. Occasionally, a woman may not employ her expulsive forces to good advantage and coaching is desirable. Her legs should be half-flexed so that she can push with them against the mattress. When the next uterine contraction begins, she is instructed to exert downward pressure as though she were straining at stool. A woman is not encouraged to push beyond the completion of each contraction. Instead, she and her fetus should be allowed to rest and recover. During this period of actively bearing down, the fetal heart rate auscultated immediately after the contraction is likely to be slow but should recover to normal range before the next expulsive effort.

Several positions during the second stage have been recommended to augment pushing efforts. Eason and colleagues (2000) performed an extensive review of various positions and their effect on the incidence of perineal trauma. They found that the supported upright position had no advantages over the recumbent one. Upright positions include sitting, kneeling, squatting, or resting with the back at a 30-degree elevation. Conversely, in their systematic review, Berghella and coworkers (2008) reported good-quality data that supported the upright position. Fetal and obstetrical outcomes appear to be unaffected whether pushing is coached or uncoached during second-stage labor (Bloom, 2006; Tuuli, 2012). The maternal effects of coached pushing were reported by Schaffer and colleagues (2005), who performed urodynamic testing in primigravidas 3 months following delivery. Women coached to push during second-stage labor had decreased bladder capacity and decreased first urge to void compared with women encouraged to push or rest as desired. The long-term effects of this practice are yet to be defined.

As the head descends through the pelvis, the perineum begins to bulge and the overlying skin becomes stretched. Now the scalp of the fetus may be visible through the vulvar opening. At this time, the woman and her fetus are prepared for delivery, which is described in Chapter 27 (p. 537).

LABOR MANAGEMENT PROTOCOLS

An orderly and systematic approach to labor management results in reproducible maternal and perinatal outcomes. This was proven by Althabe and coworkers (2008), who randomized implementation of evidence-based care in 19 hospitals in Argentina and Uruguay. Several labor management protocols are subsequently presented. These include those from the National Maternity Hospital in Dublin, the World Health Organization, and from Parkland Hospital.

Active Management of Labor

More than 30 years ago, O'Driscoll and associates (1984) pioneered the concept that a disciplined, standardized labor management protocol reduced the number of cesarean deliveries for dystocia. Their overall cesarean delivery rate was 5 percent in the 1970s and 1980s with such management. The approach is now referred to as *active management of labor*. Two of its components—amniotomy and oxytocin—have been widely used, especially in English-speaking countries outside the United States. With this protocol, labor is diagnosed when painful contractions are accompanied by complete cervical effacement, bloody "show," or ruptured membranes. Women with such findings are committed to delivery within 12 hours. Pelvic examination is performed each hour for the next 3 hours, and thereafter at 2-hour intervals. When dilatation has not increased by at least 1 cm/hr, amniotomy is performed. Progress is again assessed at 2 hours and high-dose oxytocin infusion, described in Chapter 26 (p. 530), is started unless dilatation of at least 1 cm/hr is documented. Women are constantly attended by midwives. If membranes rupture before admission, oxytocin is begun for no progress at the 1-hour mark.

López-Zeno and colleagues (1992) prospectively compared such active management with their "traditional" approach to labor management at Northwestern Memorial Hospital in Chicago. They randomly assigned 705 nulliparas with uncomplicated pregnancies in spontaneous labor at term. The cesarean delivery rate was significantly lower with active versus traditional management—10.5 versus 14.1 percent, respectively. Subsequent studies did not show this. Wei and associates (2009) in a Cochrane database review found a modest reduction in cesarean delivery rates when active management of labor was compared with standard care. Frigoletto and coworkers (1995) reported another randomized trial with 1934 nulliparous women at Brigham and Women's Hospital in Boston. Although they found that such management somewhat shortened labor, it did not affect the cesarean delivery rate. These observations have since been reported by many others (Brown, 2008).

World Health Organization Partograph

A *partograph* was designed by the World Health Organization (WHO) for use in developing countries (Dujardin, 1992). According to Orji (2008), the partograph is similar for nulliparas and multiparas. Labor is divided into a latent phase, which should last no longer than 8 hours, and an active phase. The active phase starts at 3 cm dilatation, and progress should be no slower than 1 cm/hr. A 4-hour wait is recommended before intervention when the active phase is slow. Labor is graphed, and analysis includes use of alert and action lines. Lavender and colleagues (2006) randomized 3000 nulliparous women to labor interventions at 2 hours versus 4 hours as recommended by WHO. Their cesarean delivery rate was unaffected, and they concluded that interventions such as amniotomy and oxytocin were needlessly increased using the 2-hour time interval. After their Cochrane Database review, Lavender and associates (2008) do not recommend use of the partograph for standard labor management.

Parkland Hospital Labor Management Protocol

Women are admitted if active labor—defined as cervical dilatation of 3 to 4 cm or more in the presence of uterine contractions—is diagnosed or if ruptured membranes are confirmed. Management guidelines summarized in Figure 22-25 stipulate that a pelvic examination be performed approximately every 2 hours. Ineffective labor is suspected when the cervix does not dilate within approximately 2 hours of admission. Amniotomy is then performed, and labor progress determined at the next 2-hour evaluation. In women whose labors do not progress, an intrauterine pressure catheter is placed to assess uterine function. Hypotonic contractions and no cervical dilatation after an additional 2 to 3 hours result in stimulation of labor using the high-dose oxytocin regimen described in Chapter 26 (p. 530). The goal is uterine activity of 200 to 250 Montevideo units for 2 to 4 hours before dystocia can be diagnosed.

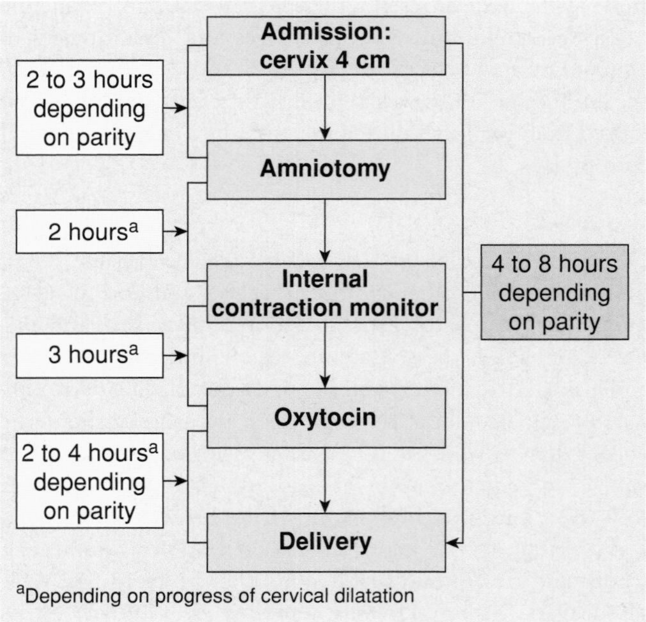

FIGURE 22-25 Schematic of labor management protocol in use at Parkland Hospital. The total admission-to-delivery times are shorter than the potential sum of the intervention intervals because not every woman requires every intervention.

Dilatation rates of 1 to 2 cm/hr are accepted as evidence of progress after satisfactory uterine activity has been established with oxytocin. This can require up to 8 hours or more before cesarean delivery is performed for dystocia. The cumulative time required to effect this stepwise management approach permits many women to establish effective labor. This management protocol has been evaluated in more than 20,000 women with uncomplicated pregnancies. Importantly, these labor interventions and the relatively infrequent use of cesarean delivery did not jeopardize the fetus-newborn.

REFERENCES

Adams SS, Eberhard-Gran M, Eskild A: Fear of childbirth and duration of labour: a study of 2206 women with intended vaginal delivery. BJOG 119(10):1238, 2012

Alexander JM, Sharma SK, McIntire DD, et al: Epidural analgesia lengthens the Friedman active phase of labor. Obstet Gynecol 100:46, 2002

Althabe F, Buekens P, Bergel E, et al: A behavioral intervention to improve obstetrical care. N Engl J Med 358:1929, 2008

American Academy of Pediatrics and the American College of Obstetricians and Gynecologists: Guidelines for Perinatal Care, 6th ed. Washington, 2007

American Academy of Pediatrics and the American College of Obstetricians and Gynecologists: Guidelines for Perinatal Care, 7th ed. Washington, 2012

American College of Obstetricians and Gynecologists: Obstetric forceps. Committee Opinion 71, August 1989

American College of Obstetricians and Gynecologists: Optimal goals for anesthesia care in obstetrics. Committee Opinion No. 433, May 2009

Bailit JL, Dierker L, Blanchard MH, et al: Outcomes of women presenting in active versus latent phase of spontaneous labor. Obstet Gynecol 105:77, 2005

Berghella V, Baxter JK, Chauhan SP: Evidence-based labor and delivery management. Am J Obstet Gynecol 199:445, 2008

Bloom SL, Casey BM, Schaffer JI, et al: A randomized trial of coached versus uncoached maternal pushing during the second stage of labor. Am J Obstet Gynecol 194:10, 2006

Bloom SL, McIntire DD, Kelly MA, et al: Lack of effect of walking on labor and delivery. N Engl J Med 339:76, 1998

Brown HC, Paranjothy S, Dowswell T, et al: Package of care for active management in labour for reducing caesarean section rates in low-risk women. Cochrane Database Syst Rev 8:CD004907, 2008

Caldwell WE, Moloy HC, D'Esopo DA: A roentgenologic study of the mechanism of engagement of the fetal head. Am J Obstet Gynecol 28:824, 1934

Calkins LA: The etiology of occiput presentations. Am J Obstet Gynecol 37:618, 1939

Carlan SJ, Wyble L, Lense J, et al: Fetal head molding: diagnosis by ultrasound and a review of the literature. J Perinatol 11:105, 1991

Carley ME, Carley JM, Vasdev G, et al: Factors that are associated with clinically overt postpartum urinary retention after vaginal delivery. Am J Obstet Gynecol 187:430, 2002

Carollo TC, Reuter JM, Galan HL, et al: Defining fetal station. Am J Obstet Gynecol 191:1793, 2004

Chelmow D, Kilpatrick SJ, Laros RK Jr: Maternal and neonatal outcomes after prolonged latent phase. Obstet Gynecol 81:486, 1993

Cheng YW, Snowden JM, King TL, et al: Selected perinatal outcomes associated with planned home births in the United States. Am J Obstet Gynecol 209(4):325.e1, 2013

Chervenak FA, McCullough LB, Brent RL, et al: Planned home birth: the professional responsibility response. Am J Obstet Gynecol 208(1):31, 2013

Chin JR, Henry E, Holmgren CM, et al: Maternal obesity and contraction strength in the first stage of labor. Am J Obstet Gynecol 207:129.e1, 2012

de Jonge A, Mesman JAJM, Manniën J, et al: Severe adverse maternal outcomes among low risk women with planned home versus hospital births in the Netherlands: nationwide cohort study. BMJ 346:f3263, 2013

Dujardin B, De Schampheleire I, Sene H, et al: Value of the alert and action lines on the partogram. Lancet 339:1336, 1992

Dupuis O, Silveira R, Zentner A, et al: Birth simulator: Reliability of transvaginal assessment of fetal head station as defined by the American College of Obstetricians and Gynecologists classification. Am J Obstet Gynecol 192:868, 2005

Eason E, Labrecque M, Wells G, et al: Preventing perineal trauma during childbirth: a systematic review. Obstet Gynecol 95:464, 2000

Friedman E: The graphic analysis of labor. Am J Obstet Gynecol 68:1568, 1954

Friedman EA: An objective approach to the diagnosis and management of abnormal labor. Bull N Y Acad Med 48:842, 1972

Friedman EA: Labor: Clinical Evaluation and Management, 2nd ed. New York, Appleton-Century-Crofts, 1978

Friedman EA: Primigravid labor: a graphicostatistical analysis. Obstet Gynecol 6:567, 1955

Friedman EA, Sachtleben MR: Amniotomy and the course of labor. Obstet Gynecol 22:755, 1963

Frigoletto FD Jr, Lieberman E, Lang JM, et al: A clinical trial of active management of labor. N Engl J Med 333:745, 1995

Gardberg M, Tuppurainen M: Anterior placental location predisposes for occiput posterior presentation near term. Acta Obstet Gynecol Scand 73:151, 1994a

Gardberg M, Tuppurainen M: Persistent occiput posterior presentation—a clinical problem. Acta Obstet Gynecol Scand 73:45, 1994b

Garite TJ, Weeks J, Peters-Phair K, et al: A randomized controlled trial of the effect of increased intravenous hydration on the course of labor in nulliparous women. Am J Obstet Gynecol 183:1544, 2000

Graham JM Jr, Kumar A: Diagnosis and management of extensive vertex birth molding. Clin Pediatr (Phila) 45(7):672, 2006

Grunebaum A, McCullough LB, Sapra KJ, et al: Apgar scores of 0 at 5 minutes and neonatal outcomes or serious neurologic dysfunction in relation to birth setting. Am J Obstet Gynecol 209:323.e1, 2013

Handa VL, Blomquist JL, Knoepp LR, et al: Pelvic floor disorder 5–10 years after vaginal or cesarean childbirth. Obstet Gynecol 118:777, 2011

Hendricks CH, Brenner WE: Cardiovascular effects of oxytocic drugs used postpartum. Am J Obstet Gynecol 108:751, 1970

Herbst A, Källén K: Time between membrane rupture and delivery and septicemia in term neonates. Obstet Gynecol 110:612, 2007

Kilpatrick SJ, Laros RK Jr: Characteristics of normal labor. Obstet Gynecol 74:85, 1989

Kominiarek MA, Zhang J, VanVeldhuisen P, et al: Contemporary labor patterns: the impact of maternal body mass index. Am J Obstet Gynecol 205:244.e1, 2011

Laughon SK, Branch W, Beaver J, et al: Changes in labor patterns over 50 years. Am J Obstet Gynecol 206:419.e1.9, 2012

Lavender T, Alfirevic A, Walkinshaw S: Effect of different partogram action lines on birth outcomes. Obstet Gynecol 108:295, 2006

Lavender T, Hart A, Smyth RM: Effect of partogram use on outcomes for women in spontaneous labour at term. Cochrane Database Syst Rev 8:CD005461, 2008

Lawrence A, Lewis L, Hofmeyr GJ, et al: Maternal positions and mobility during first stage labour. Cochrane Database Syst Rev 2:CD003934, 2009

Lawrence HC, Copel JA, O'Keeffe DF, et al: Quality patient care in labor and delivery: a call to action. Am J Obstet Gynecol 207(3):147, 2012

Leopold J: Conduct of normal births through external examination alone. Arch Gynaekol 45:337, 1894

López-Zeno JA, Peaceman AM, Adashek JA, et al: A controlled trial of a program for the active management of labor. N Engl J Med 326:450, 1992

Lydon-Rochelle M, Albers L, Gorwoda J, et al: Accuracy of Leopold maneuvers in screening for malpresentation: a prospective study. Birth 20:132, 1993

MacDorman MF, Declerq E, Mathews TJ: United States home births increase 20 percent from 2004 to 2008. Birth 38(3):185, 2011

Martin JA, Hamilton BE, Ventura SJ, et al: Births: final data for 2009. Natl Vital Stat Rep 60(1):1, 2011

Musselwhite KL, Faris P, Moore K, et al: Use of epidural anesthesia and the risk of acute postpartum urinary retention. Am J Obstet Gynecol 196:472, 2007

Nygaard I, Barber MD, Burgio KL, et al: Prevalence of symptomatic pelvic floor disorders in US women. JAMA 300:1311, 2008

O'Driscoll K, Foley M, MacDonald D: Active management of labor as an alternative to cesarean section for dystocia. Obstet Gynecol 63:485, 1984

Orji E: Evaluating progress of labor in nulliparas and multiparas using the modified WHO partograph. Int J Gynaecol Obstet 102:249, 2008

Pates JA, McIntire DD, Leveno KJ: Uterine contractions preceding labor. Obstet Gynecol 110:566, 2007

Robinson BK, Mapp DC, Bloom SL, et al: Increasing maternal body mass index and characteristics of the second stage of labor. Obstet Gynecol 118:1309, 2011

Schaffer JI, Bloom SL, Casey BM, et al: A randomized trial of the effects of coached vs uncoached maternal pushing during the second stage of labor on postpartum pelvic floor structure and function. Am J Obstet Gynecol 192:1692, 2005

Segel SY, Carreño CA, Weiner MS, et al: Relationship between fetal station and successful vaginal delivery in nulliparous women. Am J Perinatol 29:723, 2012

Shrivastava VK, Garite TJ, Jenkins SM, et al: A randomized, double-blinded, controlled trial comparing parenteral normal saline with and without dextrose on the course of labor in nulliparas. Am J Obstet Gynecol 200(4):379.e1, 2009

Sokol RJ, Stojkov J, Chik L, et al: Normal and abnormal labor progress: I. A quantitative assessment and survey of the literature. J Reprod Med 18:47, 1977

Tuuli MG, Frey HA, Odibo AO, et al: Immediate compared with delayed pushing in the second stage of labor. Obstet Gynecol 120:660, 2012

Wei S, Wo BL, Xu H, et al: Early amniotomy and early oxytocin for prevention of, or therapy for, delay in first stage spontaneous labour compared with routine care. Cochrane Database Syst Rev 2:CD006794, 2009

Yamada H, Kishida T, Negishi H, et al: Silent premature rupture of membranes, detected and monitored serially by an AFP kit. J Obstet Gynaecol Res 24:103, 1998

Zahalka N, Sadan O, Malinger G, et al: Comparison of transvaginal sonography with digital examination and transabdominal sonography for the determination of fetal head position in the second stage of labor. Am J Obstet Gynecol 193:381, 2005

Zhang J, Landy HJ, Branch DW, et al: Contemporary patterns of spontaneous labor with normal neonatal outcomes. Obstet Gynecol 116:1281, 2010

Zhang J, Troendle J, Mikolajczyk R, et al: Natural history of labor progression [Abstract 134]. Presented at the 29th Annual Meeting of the Society for Maternal-Fetal Medicine in San Diego, CA, January 26–31, 2009a

Zhang J, Troendle JF, Yancey MK: Reassessing the labor curve in nulliparous women. Am J Obstet Gynecol 187:824, 2002

Zhang J, Vanveldhuisen P, Troendle J, et al: Normal labor patterns in U.S. women [Abstract 80]. Presented at the 29th Annual Meeting of the Society for Maternal–Fetal Medicine in San Diego, CA, January 26–31, 2009b

CHAPTER 23

Abnormal Labor

DYSTOCIA

There are several labor abnormalities that may interfere with the orderly progression to spontaneous delivery. Generally, these are referred to as *dystocia*. Dystocia literally means *difficult labor* and is characterized by abnormally slow labor progress. It arises from four distinct abnormalities that may exist singly or in combination. First, expulsive forces may be abnormal. For example, uterine contractions may be insufficiently strong or inappropriately coordinated to efface and dilate the cervix—uterine dysfunction. Also, there may be inadequate voluntary maternal muscle effort during second-stage labor. Second, fetal abnormalities of presentation, position, or development may slow labor. Also, abnormalities of the maternal bony pelvis may create a contracted pelvis. And last, soft tissue abnormalities of the reproductive tract may form an obstacle to fetal descent. More simply, these abnormalities can be mechanistically simplified into three categories that include abnormalities of the *powers*—uterine contractility and maternal expulsive effort; the *passenger*—the fetus; and the *passage*—the pelvis. Common clinical findings in women with these labor abnormalities are summarized in Table 23-1.

Dystocia Descriptors

Abnormalities that are shown in Table 23-1 often interact in concert to produce dysfunctional labor. Commonly used expressions today such as *cephalopelvic disproportion* and *failure to progress* are used to describe ineffective labors. Of these, *cephalopelvic disproportion* is a term that came into use before the 20th century to describe obstructed labor resulting from disparity between the fetal head size and maternal pelvis. But the term originated at a time when the main indication for cesarean delivery was overt pelvic contracture due to rickets (Olah, 1994). Such absolute disproportion is now rare, and most cases result from malposition of the fetal head within the pelvis (asynclitism) or from ineffective uterine contractions. True disproportion is a tenuous diagnosis because two thirds or more of women

TABLE 23-1. Common Clinical Findings in Women with Ineffective Labor

Inadequate cervical dilation or fetal descent:
Protracted labor—slow progress
Arrested labor—no progress
Inadequate expulsive effort—ineffective pushing
Fetopelvic disproportion:
Excessive fetal size
Inadequate pelvic capacity
Malpresentation or position of the fetus
Ruptured membranes without labor

TABLE 23-2. Abnormal Labor Patterns, Diagnostic Criteria, and Methods of Treatment

Labor Pattern	Diagnostic Criteria: Nulliparas	Diagnostic Criteria: Multiparas	Preferred Treatment	Exceptional Treatment
Prolongation Disorder				
Prolonged latent phase	> 20 hr	> 14 hr	Bed rest	Oxytocin or cesarean delivery for urgent problems
Protraction Disorders				
Protracted active-phase dilatation	< 1.2 cm/hr	1.5 cm/hr	Expectant and support	Cesarean delivery for CPD
Protracted descent	< 1 cm/hr	< 2 cm/hr		
Arrest Disorders				
Prolonged deceleration phase	> 3 hr	> 1 hr	Evaluate for CPD: CPD: cesarean; No CPD: oxytocin	Rest if exhausted; Cesarean delivery
Secondary arrest of dilatation	> 2 hr	> 2 hr		
Arrest of descent	> 1 hr	> 1 hr		
Failure of descent	No descent in deceleration phase or second stage			

CPD = cephalopelvic disproportion.
Modified from Cohen, 1983.

undergoing cesarean delivery for this reason subsequently deliver even larger newborns vaginally. A second phrase, *failure to progress* in either spontaneous or stimulated labor, has become an increasingly popular description of ineffectual labor. This term reflects lack of progressive cervical dilatation or lack of fetal descent. Neither of these two expressions is specific. Terms presented in Table 23-2 and their diagnostic criteria more precisely describe abnormal labor.

Mechanisms of Dystocia

Dystocia as described by Williams (1903) in the first edition of this text is still true today. Figure 23-1 demonstrates the mechanical process of labor and potential obstacles. The cervix and lower uterus are shown at the end of pregnancy and at the end of labor. At the end of pregnancy, the fetal head, to traverse the birth canal, must encounter a relatively thick lower uterine segment and undilated cervix. The uterine fundus muscle is less developed and presumably less powerful. Uterine contractions, cervical resistance, and the forward pressure exerted by the leading fetal part are the factors influencing the progress of first-stage labor.

As also shown in Figure 23-1B, after complete cervical dilatation, the mechanical relationship between the fetal head size and position and the pelvic capacity, namely *fetopelvic proportion*, becomes clearer as the fetus descends. Because of this, abnormalities in fetopelvic proportions become more apparent once the second stage is reached.

Uterine muscle malfunction can result from uterine overdistention or obstructed labor or both. *Thus, ineffective labor is generally accepted as a possible warning sign of fetopelvic disproportion.*

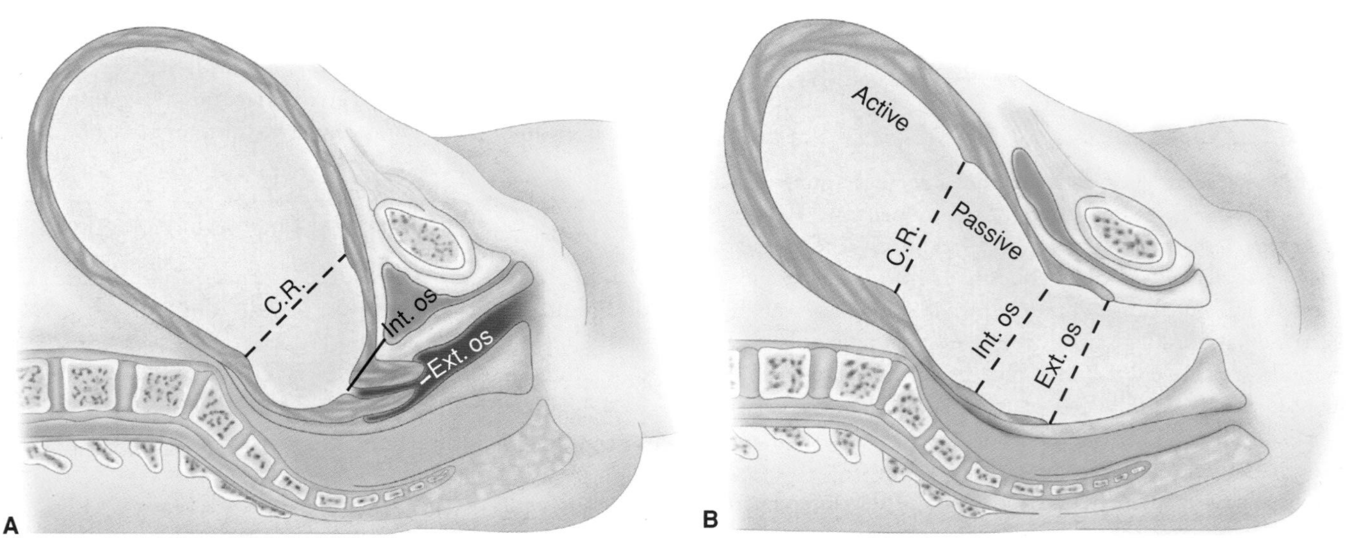

FIGURE 23-1 Diagrams of the birth canal. **A.** At the end of pregnancy. **B.** During the second-stage of labor, showing formation of the birth canal. C.R. = contraction ring; Int. = internal; Ext = external. (Adapted from Williams, 1903.)

Although artificial separation of labor abnormalities into pure *uterine dysfunction* and *fetopelvic disproportion* simplifies classification, it is an incomplete characterization because these two abnormalities are so closely interlinked. Indeed, according to the American College of Obstetricians and Gynecologists (2013), the bony pelvis rarely limits vaginal delivery. In the absence of objective means of precisely distinguishing these two causes of labor failure, clinicians must rely on a *trial of labor* to determine if labor can be successful in effecting vaginal delivery.

Revised Dystocia Diagnosis

In 2009, the total cesarean delivery rate for all births in the United States reached a record high of 32.9 percent (Martin, 2011). This was the 13th consecutive year in which the cesarean rate increased, and it represented a nearly 60-percent increase compared with 20.7 percent in 1996. The 2010 rate of 32.8 percent could suggest that this long trend of increasing cesarean rates may now be moderating (Martin, 2012). Given that many repeat cesarean deliveries are performed after primary operations for dystocia, it is estimated that 60 percent of all cesarean deliveries in the United States are ultimately attributable to the diagnosis of abnormal labor (American College of Obstetricians and Gynecologists, 2013).

To address this increasing cesarean delivery rate, a workshop was convened by the National Institute of Child Health and Human Development (NICHD) and the American College of Obstetricians and Gynecologists (Spong, 2012). The workshop recommended new definitions for arrest of labor progress to prevent unnecessary first cesarean deliveries. Specifically, it concluded that "adequate time for normal latent and active phases of the first stage and for the second stage should be allowed as long as the maternal and fetal conditions permit. The adequate time for each of these stages appears to be longer than traditionally estimated." The implication of this viewpoint is that changing the diagnostic criteria of abnormal labor will reduce the excessive cesarean birth rate. Shown in Table 23-3 is a synopsis of some of these workshop recommendations for revised labor management criteria. According to the workshop, these definitions "vary somewhat from published criteria and are recommended in recognition of more recent findings regarding labor progress that challenge our long-held practices based on the Friedman curve."

These proposed new criteria listed in Table 23-3 for normal, and therefore also abnormal labor, were heavily dependent on results of the NICHD-sponsored *Safe Labor Consortium* and on an NICHD-sponsored report on second-stage labor duration (Rouse, 2009; Zhang, 2010). Shown in Table 23-4 is a comparison of active labor phase duration in the *Safe Labor Consortium* compared with other contemporary reports. It is important to note that almost half of the *Consortium* cohort received oxytocin and 84 percent had received epidural analgesia—both factors associated with longer active-phase labor. Indeed, cases using oxytocin and epidural analgesia in the studies of Graseck (2012) and Alexander (2002) had similar active-labor phase durations to those from the *Consortium*. Importantly, all these reports were based on contemporary obstetrical practices.

The *Safe Labor Consortium* report by Zhang and associates (2010) was a multicenter retrospective study using abstracted 2002 to 2008 data from electronic medical records in 19 hospitals across the United States. One purpose of this study was to analyze labor patterns and develop contemporary criteria for labor progress in nulliparas. Shown in Figure 23-2 is a synopsis of the study cohort, which formed the basis of the proposed new criteria for labor progress. Importantly, all women with cesarean delivery were excluded as were all of those with compromised newborn infants. Because of these major exclusions, the pattern of labor now defined as normal is problematic given that only women who achieved vaginal birth with a *normal* infant outcome were included. It is also problematic to conclude that these revised labor criteria will reduce the cesarean rate when the overall rate in the *Safe Labor Consortium* was 30.5 percent using the newly proposed first-stage labor intervals. The authors of a report from the Maternal Fetal Medicine Units Network of the NICHD analyzed labor management practices

TABLE 23-4. Duration of Active Phase Labor: Comparison in Contemporary Reports[a]

Investigator	Oxytocin (%)	Epidural (%)	Active Phase, 4–10 cm Dilation
Zhang (2010)[b]	47	84	6 hr
Graseck (2012)	0	70	5 hr
Alexander (2002)	44	100	7.4 hr

[a]Includes nulliparous women at term with spontaneous labor and cervical dilatation 4 cm.
[b]*Safe Labor Consortium.*

TABLE 23-3. Evidence for Adequate and Arrested Labor

Arrest of labor: *". . . the diagnosis of arrest of labor should not be made until adequate time has elapsed."*
Adequate labor: *". . . includes greater than 6 cm dilation with membrane rupture and 4 or more hours of adequate contractions (e.g., greater than 200 Montevideo units) or 6 hours or more if contractions inadequate with no cervical change. . . ."*
Second-stage labor: *". . . no progress for more than 4 hours in nulliparous women with an epidural, more than 3 hours in nulliparous women without an epidural. . . ."*
"No cesarean before these time limits . . . in the presence of reassuring maternal and fetal status."

From Spong, 2012.

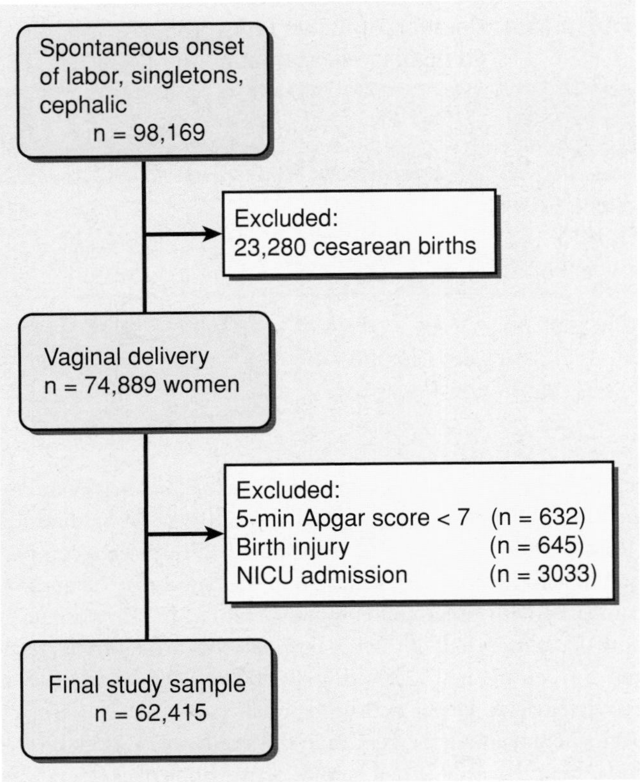

FIGURE 23-2 Study cohort for the analysis of spontaneous labor in the *Safe Labor Consortium*. NICU = neonatal intensive care unit. (Data from Zhang, 2010.)

in 8546 women undergoing primary cesarean delivery for dystocia in a wide cross section of hospitals in the United States (Alexander, 2003). Approximately 92 percent of the cesareans for dystocia were performed in the active phase of labor defined as ≥ 4 cm cervical dilatation. The median admission to delivery interval was 17 hours, and the median cervical dilation was 6 cm before the dystocia diagnosis in women in active-phase labor. Oxytocin was used in 90 percent of women diagnosed with dystocia. It was concluded that bona-fide efforts were being made in contemporary practice to achieve active labor before diagnosing dystocia leading to cesarean delivery.

The report by Rouse and colleagues (2009) on second-stage labor was a secondary analysis of 4126 nulliparous women who reached the second stage during a randomized trial to study fetal pulse oximetry. Of the 360 women—9 percent—whose second stage was > 3 hours, 95 percent had received epidural analgesia. A third of these 360 women—3.5 percent of the whole cohort—had a second stage > 4 hours. The results of this study were interpreted as support for extending the duration of the second stage in nulliparas to beyond the current recommended 3 hours when epidural analgesia is used (American College of Obstetricians and Gynecologists, 2013). The investigators concluded that a fetus born after a > 3-hour second stage had a higher—albeit still low—neonatal intensive care unit (NICU) admission rate and a low risk for brachial plexus injury (Rouse, 2009).

These latter results are in contrast to those associated with prolonged second-stage labors at Parkland Hospital (Bleich, 2012). This study included 21,991 women of whom 7 percent had a second-stage labor > 3 hours. Most of the 2 percent of women reaching 4 hours in the second stage had been given epidural analgesia and were awaiting cesarean delivery that was decided on at the 3-hour time point. Typically, oxytocin had been discontinued, and they also had reassuring fetal heart rate tracings that permitted temporization awaiting operative space. Thus, such prolonged second stages were *unintentional* in that further efforts to effect vaginal delivery were not made. Despite these caveats, virtually every adverse infant outcome analyzed increased significantly when the second stage exceeded 3 hours in women with labor epidural analgesia (Table 23-5).

We conclude that at this time, an improved definition of the adequacy of a trial of labor before diagnosing dystocia remains an elusive goal. The newly proposed criteria for first-stage labor are already in use in contemporary practice, and thus they are unlikely to have much impact on the cesarean delivery rate for abnormal labor. Importantly, the purported safety of the proposed new criteria for second-stage labor management should be viewed with caution until more published experiences accrue.

ABNORMALITIES OF THE EXPULSIVE FORCES

Cervical dilatation and propulsion and expulsion of the fetus are brought about by contractions of the uterus, which are reinforced during the second stage by voluntary or involuntary muscular action of the abdominal wall—"pushing." The diagnosis of uterine dysfunction in the latent phase is difficult and sometimes can be made only in retrospect (Chap. 22, p. 446). Women who are not yet in active labor commonly are erroneously treated for uterine dysfunction.

Beginning in the 1960s, there have been at least three significant advances in the treatment of uterine dysfunction. First is the realization that undue labor prolongation may contribute to maternal and perinatal morbidity and mortality rates. Second, dilute intravenous infusion of oxytocin is used for treatment of certain types of uterine dysfunction. Last, cesarean delivery is selected rather than difficult midforceps delivery when oxytocin fails or its use is inappropriate.

Types of Uterine Dysfunction

Reynolds and coworkers (1948) emphasized that uterine contractions of normal labor are characterized by a gradient of myometrial activity. These forces are greatest and last longest at the fundus—considered *fundal dominance*—and they diminish toward the cervix. Caldeyro-Barcia and colleagues (1950) from Montevideo, Uruguay, inserted small balloons into the myometrium at various levels (Chap. 24, p. 498). They reported that in addition to a gradient of activity, there was a time differential in the onset of the contractions in the fundus, midzone, and lower uterine segments. Larks (1960) described the stimulus as starting in one cornu and then several milliseconds later in the other. The excitation waves then join and sweep over the fundus and down the uterus. Normal spontaneous contractions often exert pressures approximating 60 mm Hg (Hendricks, 1959). Even so, the Montevideo group ascertained that the lower limit of contraction pressure required to dilate the cervix is 15 mm Hg.

TABLE 23-5. Neonatal Outcomes in Relation to Second-Stage Labor Duration

	Second-Stage Duration			
Outcome	< 3 hours n = 20,502	3–4 hours n = 1062	≥ 4 hours n = 427	p value
Birthweight ≥ 4000 g	962 (5)	150 (14)[a]	71 (17)[a]	< 0.001
Apgar scores ≤ 3 at 5 minutes	14 (0.1)	3 (0.3)[a]	2 (0.5)[a]	0.002
Umbilical artery blood pH < 7.0	75 (0.4)	8 (0.8)[a]	4 (1)[d]	0.024
Resuscitation at delivery	120 (0.6)	18 (2)[a]	13 (3)[a]	< 0.001
Admission to intensive care	150 (0.7)	22 (2)[a]	8 (2)[a]	< 0.001
Seizures[b]	23 (0.1)	18 (1.7)[a]	13 (3)[a]	< 0.001
Sepsis[c]	32 (0.2)	7 (0.7)[a]	0	< 0.001
Erb palsy	67 (0.3)	15 (1.4)[a]	2 (0.5)	< 0.001
Neonatal death	3 (0.02)	0	0	0.897

All data shown as n (%).
[a]Significantly different compared to < 3 hours.
[b]Seizure within the first 24 hours of life.
[c]Sepsis defined as positive blood culture.
[d]Significant compared to < 3 hours after adjustment for age, race, body mass index, and epidural analgesia.
Data from Bleich, 2012.

From these observations, it is possible to define two types of uterine dysfunction. In the more common *hypotonic uterine dysfunction,* there is no basal hypertonus and uterine contractions have a normal gradient pattern (synchronous), but pressure during a contraction is insufficient to dilate the cervix. In the second type, *hypertonic uterine dysfunction* or *incoordinate uterine dysfunction,* either basal tone is elevated appreciably or the pressure gradient is distorted. Gradient distortion may result from more forceful contraction of the uterine midsegment than the fundus or from complete asynchrony of the impulses originating in each cornu or a combination of these two.

Active-Phase Disorders

Labor abnormalities are divided into either a slower-than-normal progress—*protraction disorder*—or a complete cessation of progress—*arrest disorder*. A woman must be in the active phase of labor with cervical dilatation to at least 3 to 4 cm to be diagnosed with either of these. Handa and Laros (1993) diagnosed active-phase arrest, defined as no dilatation for 2 hours or more, in 5 percent of term nulliparas. This incidence has not changed since the 1950s (Friedman, 1978). Inadequate uterine contractions, defined as less than 180 Montevideo units, calculated as shown in Figure 23-3, were diagnosed in 80 percent of women with active-phase arrest.

Protraction disorders are less well described, and the time necessary before diagnosing slow progress is undefined. The World Health Organization (1994) has proposed a labor management *partograph* in which protraction is defined as less than 1 cm/hr cervical dilatation for a minimum of 4 hours. Criteria for the diagnosis of protraction and arrest disorders have been recommended by the American College of Obstetricians and Gynecologists (2013). These criteria were adapted from those of Cohen and Friedman (1983), shown in Table 23-2.

Hauth and coworkers (1986, 1991) reported that when labor is effectively induced or augmented with oxytocin, 90 percent of women achieve 200 to 225 Montevideo units, and 40 percent achieve at least 300 Montevideo units. These results suggest that there are certain minimums of uterine activity that should be achieved before performing cesarean delivery for dystocia. Accordingly, the American College of Obstetricians and Gynecologists (2013) has suggested that before the diagnosis of first-stage labor arrest is made, specific criteria should be met. First, the latent phase has been completed, and the cervix is dilated 4 cm or more. Also, a uterine contraction pattern of 200 Montevideo units or more in a 10-minute period has been present for 2 hours without cervical change. Rouse and associates (1999) have challenged the "2-hour rule" on the grounds that a longer time, that is, at least 4 hours, is necessary before concluding that the active phase of labor has failed. We agree.

Second-Stage Disorders

As discussed in Chapter 21 (p. 415), fetal descent largely follows complete dilatation. Moreover, the second stage incorporates many of the cardinal movements necessary for the fetus to negotiate the birth canal. Accordingly, disproportion of the fetus and pelvis frequently becomes apparent during second-stage labor.

Until recently, there have been largely unquestioned second-stage rules that limited its duration. These rules were established in American obstetrics by the beginning of the 20th century. They stemmed from concerns about maternal and fetal health, likely regarding infection, and led to difficult forceps operations. The second stage in nulliparas was limited to 2 hours and extended to 3 hours when regional analgesia was used. For multiparas, 1 hour was the limit, extended to 2 hours with regional analgesia.

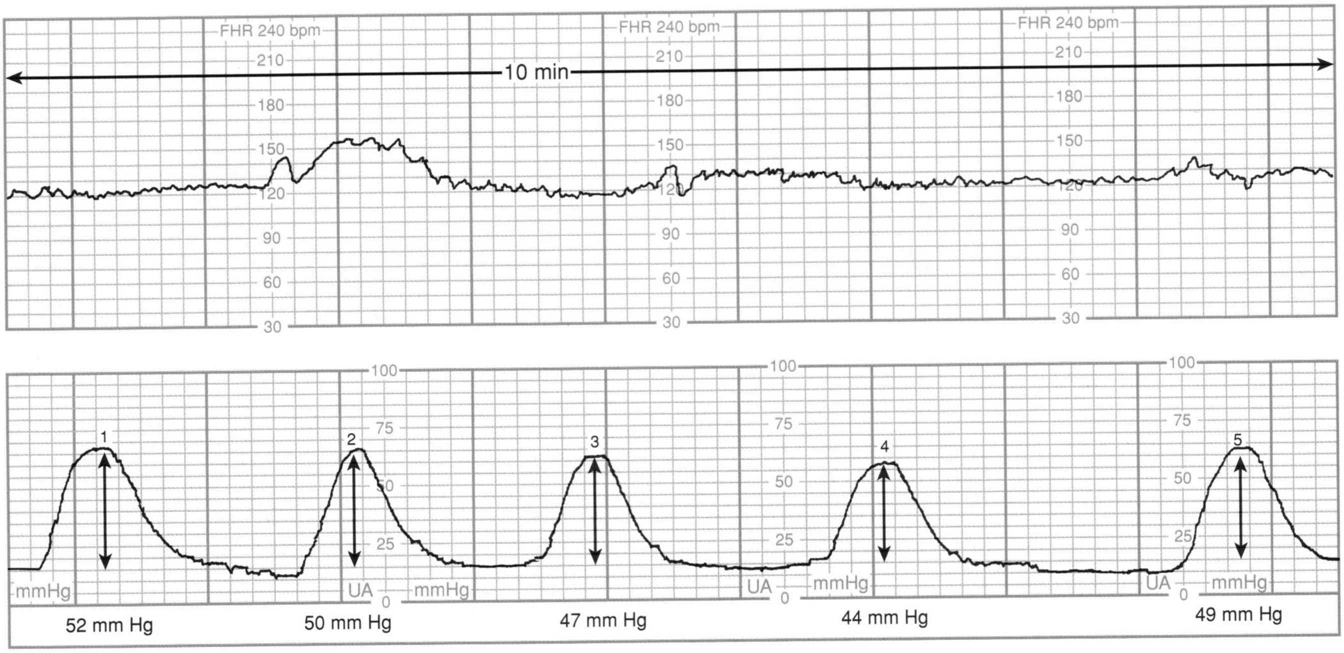

FIGURE 23-3 Montevideo units are calculated by subtracting the baseline uterine pressure from the peak contraction pressure for each contraction in a 10-minute window and adding the pressures generated by each contraction. In the example shown, there were five contractions, producing pressure changes of 52, 50, 47, 44, and 49 mm Hg, respectively. The sum of these five contractions is 242 Montevideo units.

Cohen (1977) investigated the fetal effects of second-stage labor length at Beth Israel Hospital. He included 4403 term nulliparas in whom electronic fetal heart rate monitoring was performed. The neonatal mortality rate was not increased in women whose second-stage labor exceeded 2 hours. Epidural analgesia was used commonly, and this likely accounted for the large number of pregnancies with a prolonged second stage. These data influenced decisions to permit an additional hour for the second stage when regional analgesia is used.

Menticoglou and coworkers (1995a,b) challenged the prevailing dictums on second-stage duration. These arose because of grave neonatal injuries associated with forceps rotations to shorten second-stage labor. As a result, they allowed a longer second stage to decrease the operative vaginal delivery rate. Between 1988 and 1992, second-stage labor exceeded 2 hours in a fourth of 6041 nulliparas at term. Labor epidural analgesia was used in 55 percent. The length of the second stage, even in those lasting up to 6 hours or more, was not related to neonatal outcome. These results were attributed to careful use of electronic monitoring and scalp pH measurements. These investigators concluded that there is no compelling reason to intervene with a possibly difficult forceps or vacuum extraction because a certain number of hours have elapsed. They observed, however, that after 3 hours in the second stage, delivery by cesarean or other operative method increased progressively. By 5 hours, the prospects for spontaneous delivery in the subsequent hour are only 10 to 15 percent.

Adverse maternal outcomes, however, are increased with prolonged second-stage labor. Myles and Santolaya (2003) analyzed both the maternal and neonatal consequences of this in 7818 women in Chicago between 1996 and 1999. Adverse maternal outcomes in relation to the duration of second-stage labor were increased as shown in Table 23-6. Neonatal mortality and morbidity rates were not related to the length of the second stage.

Relationship between First- and Second-Stage Labor Duration

It is possible that prolonged first-stage labor presages that with the second stage. Nelson and associates (2013) studied the relationships between the lengths of the first and second stages of labor in 12,523 nulliparous women at term delivered at Parkland Hospital. The length of the second stage significantly increased concomitantly with increasing length of the first stage. The 95th percentile was 15.6 and 2.9 hours for the first and second stages, respectively. Women with first stages lasting longer than 15.6 hr (> 95th percentile) had a 16.3 percent rate of a second-stage labor lasting 3 hr (95th percentile) compared with a 4.5-percent rate in women with first-stages labors lasting less than the 95th percentile.

TABLE 23-6. Clinical Outcomes in Relation to the Duration of Second-Stage Labor

Clinical Outcome (%)	Duration of Second Stage < 2 hr n = 6529	2–4 hr n = 384	> 4 hr n = 148
Cesarean delivery	1.2	9.2	34.5
Instrumented delivery	3.4	16.0	35.1
Perineal trauma	3.6	13.4	26.7
Postpartum hemorrhage	2.3	5.0	9.1
Chorioamnionitis	2.3	8.9	14.2

Adapted from Myles, 2003.

Maternal Pushing Efforts

With full cervical dilatation, most women cannot resist the urge to "bear down" or "push" each time the uterus contracts (Chap. 22, p. 451). The combined force created by contractions of the uterus and abdominal musculature propels the fetus downward. Bloom and colleagues (2006) studied effects of actively coaching expulsive efforts. They reported that although the second stage was slightly shorter in coached women, there were no other maternal advantages.

At times, force created by abdominal musculature is compromised sufficiently to slow or even prevent spontaneous vaginal delivery. Heavy sedation or regional analgesia may reduce the reflex urge to push and may impair the ability to contract abdominal muscles sufficiently. In other instances, the inherent urge to push is overridden by the intense pain created by bearing down. Two approaches to second-stage pushing in women with epidural analgesia have yielded contradictory results. The first advocates pushing forcefully with contractions after complete dilation, regardless of the urge to push. With the second, analgesia infusion is stopped and pushing begun only after the woman regains the sensory urge to bear down. Fraser and coworkers (2000) found that delayed pushing reduced difficult operative deliveries, whereas Manyonda and associates (1990) reported the opposite. Hansen and colleagues (2002) randomly assigned 252 women with epidural analgesia to one of the two approaches. There were no adverse maternal or neonatal outcomes linked to delayed pushing despite significantly prolonging second-stage labor. Plunkett and coworkers (2003), in a similar study, confirmed these findings.

Fetal Station at Onset of Labor

Descent of the leading edge of the presenting part to the level of the ischial spines (0 station) is defined as engagement. Friedman and Sachtleben (1965, 1976) reported a significant association between higher station at the onset of labor and subsequent dystocia. Handa and Laros (1993) found that fetal station at the time of arrested labor was also a risk factor for dystocia. Roshanfekr and associates (1999) analyzed fetal station in 803 nulliparous women at term in active labor. At admission, the third with the fetal head at or below 0 station had a 5-percent cesarean delivery rate. This is compared with a 14-percent rate for those with higher stations. The prognosis for dystocia, however, was not related to incrementally higher fetal head stations above the pelvic midplane (0 station). Importantly, 86 percent of nulliparous women without fetal head engagement at diagnosis of active labor delivered vaginally. These observations apply especially for parous women because the head typically descends later in labor.

Reported Causes of Uterine Dysfunction

Epidural Analgesia

Various labor factors have been implicated as causes of uterine dysfunction. Of these, epidural analgesia can slow labor (Sharma, 2000). As shown in Table 23-7, epidural analgesia has been associated with lengthening of both first- and second-stage labor and with slowing of the rate of fetal descent. This is documented further in Chapter 25 (p. 515).

TABLE 23-7. Effect of Epidural Analgesia on the Progress of Labor in 199 Nulliparous Women Delivered Spontaneously at Parkland Hospital

Factor[a]	Epidural Analgesia	Meperidine Analgesia	*p* value
Cervical dilatation at analgesia	4.1 cm	4.2 cm	NS
Active phase	7.9 hr	6.3 hr	.005
Second stage	60 min	48 min	.03
Fetal descent	4.2 cm/hr	7.9 cm/hr	.003

[a]Mean values are listed.
NS = not stated.
Data from Alexander, 1998.

Chorioamnionitis

Because of the association of prolonged labor with maternal intrapartum infection, some clinicians have suggested that infection itself contributes to abnormal uterine activity. Satin and coworkers (1992) studied the effects of chorioamnionitis on oxytocin stimulation in 266 pregnancies. Infection diagnosed late in labor was found to be a marker of cesarean delivery performed for dystocia, whereas this was not a marker in women diagnosed as having chorioamnionitis early in labor. Specifically, 40 percent of women developing chorioamnionitis after requiring oxytocin for dysfunctional labor later required cesarean delivery for dystocia. It is likely that uterine infection in this clinical setting is a consequence of dysfunctional, prolonged labor rather than a cause of dystocia.

Maternal Position During Labor

Advocacy for recumbency or ambulation during labor has vacillated. Proponents of walking report it to shorten labor, decrease rates of oxytocin augmentation, decrease the need for analgesia, and lower the frequency of operative vaginal delivery (Flynn, 1978; Read, 1981). But other observations do not support this. According to Miller (1983), the uterus contracts more frequently but with less intensity with the mother lying on her back rather than on her side. Conversely, contraction frequency and intensity have been reported to increase with sitting or standing. Lupe and Gross (1986) concluded, however, that there is no conclusive evidence that upright maternal posture or ambulation improves labor. They reported that women preferred to lie on their side or sit in bed. Few chose to walk, fewer to squat, and none wanted the knee-chest position. They tended to assume fetal positions in later labor. Most women enthusiastic about ambulation returned to bed when active labor began (Carlson, 1986; Williams, 1980).

Bloom and colleagues (1998) conducted a randomized trial to study the effects of walking during first-stage labor. In 1067 women with uncomplicated term pregnancies delivered at Parkland Hospital, these investigators reported that ambulation did not affect labor duration. Ambulation did not reduce the need for analgesia, nor was it harmful to the perinate. Because of these observations, we give women without complications the option to select either recumbency or supervised ambulation during labor. This policy is in agreement with the American College of Obstetricians and Gynecologists (2013), which has concluded that ambulation in labor is not harmful, and mobility may result in greater comfort.

Birthing Position in Second-Stage Labor

Considerable interest has been shown in alternative second-stage labor birth positions and their effect on labor. Gupta and Hofmeyr (2004) in their Cochrane database review compared upright positions with supine or lithotomy positions. Upright positions included sitting in a "birthing chair," kneeling, squatting, or resting with the back at a 30-degree elevation. With these positions, they found a 4-minute shorter interval to delivery, less pain, and a lower incidence both of nonreassuring fetal heart rate patterns and of operative vaginal delivery. There was, however, an increased rate of blood loss > 500 mL with the upright positions. Berghella and colleagues (2008) hypothesized that parity, less intense aortocaval compression, improved fetal alignment, and larger pelvic outlet diameters might explain these findings. In an earlier study, Russell (1969) described a 20- to 30-percent increase in the area of the pelvic outlet with squatting compared with that in the supine position. Finally, Babayer and associates (1998) cautioned that prolonged sitting or squatting during the second stage may cause common fibular nerve neuropathy.

Water Immersion

A birthing tub or bath has been advocated as a means of relaxation that may contribute to more efficient labor. Cluett and coworkers (2004) randomly assigned 99 laboring women at term in first-stage labor identified to have dystocia to immersion in a birthing pool or to oxytocin augmentation. Water immersion lowered the rate of epidural analgesia use but did not alter the rate of operative delivery. More infants of women in the immersion group were admitted to the NICU. These findings were similar to their subsequent Cochrane database review, except that NICU admission rates were not increased (Cluett, 2009).

Robertson and associates (1998) reported that immersion was not associated with chorioamnionitis or uterine infection. Moreover, Kwee and coworkers (2000) studied the effects of immersion in 20 women and reported that blood pressure decreased, whereas fetal heart rate was unaffected. Neonatal complications unique to underwater birth that have been described include drowning, hyponatremia, waterborne infection, cord rupture, and polycythemia (Austin, 1997; Pinette, 2004).

PREMATURELY RUPTURED MEMBRANES AT TERM

Membrane rupture at term without spontaneous uterine contractions complicates approximately 8 percent of pregnancies. Until recently, management generally included labor stimulation if contractions did not begin after 6 to 12 hours. This intervention evolved more than 50 years ago because of maternal and fetal complications due to chorioamnionitis (Calkins, 1952). Such routine intervention was the accepted practice until challenged by Kappy and colleagues (1979). These investigators reported excessive cesarean delivery in term pregnancies with ruptured membranes managed with labor stimulation compared with those expectantly managed.

Subsequent research included that of Hannah (1996) and Peleg (1999) and their associates, who enrolled a total of 5042 pregnancies with ruptured membranes in a randomized investigation. They measured the effects of induction versus expectant management and also compared induction using intravenous oxytocin with that using prostaglandin E_2 gel. There were approximately 1200 pregnancies in each of the four study arms. They concluded that labor induction with intravenous oxytocin was the preferred management. This determination was based on significantly fewer intrapartum and postpartum infections in women whose labor was induced. There were no significant differences in cesarean delivery rates. Subsequent analysis by Hannah and coworkers (2000) indicated increased adverse outcomes when expectant management at home was compared with in-hospital observation. Mozurkewich and associates (2009) reported lower rates of chorioamnionitis, metritis, and NICU admissions for women with term ruptured membranes whose labors were induced compared with those managed expectantly. At Parkland Hospital, labor is induced soon after admission when ruptured membranes are confirmed at term. The benefit of prophylactic antibiotics in women with ruptured membranes before labor at term is unclear (Passos, 2012).

PRECIPITOUS LABOR AND DELIVERY

Labor can be too slow, but it also can be abnormally rapid. *Precipitous labor and delivery* is extremely rapid labor and delivery. It may result from an abnormally low resistance of the soft parts of the birth canal, from abnormally strong uterine and abdominal contractions, or rarely from the absence of painful sensations and thus a lack of awareness of vigorous labor.

According to Hughes (1972), precipitous labor terminates in expulsion of the fetus in < 3 hours. Using this definition, 89,047 live births—2 percent—were complicated by precipitous labor in the United States during 2006 (Martin, 2009). Despite this incidence, there is little published information concerning adverse effects.

Maternal Effects

Precipitous labor and delivery seldom are accompanied by serious maternal complications if the cervix is effaced appreciably and compliant, if the vagina has been stretched previously, and if the perineum is relaxed. Conversely, vigorous uterine contractions combined with a long, firm cervix and a noncompliant birth canal may lead to uterine rupture or extensive lacerations of the cervix, vagina, vulva, or perineum. It is in these latter circumstances that the rare condition of *amnionic-fluid embolism* most likely develops (Chap. 41, p. 812).

Precipitous labor is frequently followed by uterine atony. *The uterus that contracts with unusual vigor before delivery is likely to be hypotonic after delivery.* Postpartum hemorrhage from uterine atony is discussed in Chapter 41 (p. 784).

Mahon and colleagues (1994) described 99 pregnancies delivered within 3 hours of labor onset. *Short labors* were defined as a rate of cervical dilatation of 5 cm/hr or faster for nulliparas and 10 cm/hr for multiparas. Such short labors were more common in multiparas who typically had contractions at intervals less than 2 minutes and were associated with placental abruption, meconium, postpartum hemorrhage, cocaine abuse, and low Apgar scores.

Fetal and Neonatal Effects

Adverse perinatal outcomes from precipitous labor may be increased considerably for several reasons. The tumultuous uterine contractions, often with negligible intervals of relaxation, prevent appropriate uterine blood flow and fetal oxygenation. Resistance of the birth canal may rarely cause intracranial trauma. Acker and coworkers (1988) reported that Erb or Duchenne brachial palsy was associated with such labors in a third of cases (Chap. 33, p. 648). Finally, during an unattended birth, the newborn may fall to the floor and be injured, or it may need resuscitation that is not immediately available.

Treatment

Unusually forceful spontaneous uterine contractions are not likely to be modified to a significant degree by analgesia. The use of tocolytic agents such as magnesium sulfate is unproven in these circumstances. Use of general anesthesia with agents that impair uterine contractibility, such as isoflurane, is often excessively heroic. Certainly, any oxytocin agents being administered should be stopped immediately.

FETOPELVIC DISPROPORTION

Pelvic Capacity

Fetopelvic disproportion arises from diminished pelvic capacity, excessive fetal size, or more usually both. Any contraction of the pelvic diameters that diminishes its capacity can create dystocia during labor. There may be a contraction of the pelvic inlet, the midpelvis, or the pelvic outlet, or a generally contracted pelvis may be caused by combinations of these. Normal pelvic dimension are additionally discussed in Chapter 2 (p. 32).

Contracted Inlet

The pelvic inlet usually is considered to be contracted if its shortest anteroposterior diameter is < 10 cm or if the greatest transverse diameter is < 12 cm. The anteroposterior diameter of the inlet is commonly approximated by manually measuring the diagonal conjugate, which is approximately 1.5 cm greater (Chap. 2, p. 33). Therefore, inlet contraction usually is defined as a diagonal conjugate < 11.5 cm.

Using clinical and at times, imaging pelvimetry, it is important to identify the shortest anteroposterior diameter through which the fetal head must pass. Occasionally, the body of the first sacral vertebra is displaced forward so that the shortest distance may actually be between this abnormal sacral promontory and the symphysis pubis.

Before labor, the fetal biparietal diameter has been shown to *average* from 9.5 to as much as 9.8 cm. Therefore, it might prove difficult or even impossible for some fetuses to pass through an inlet that has an anteroposterior diameter of less than 10 cm. Mengert (1948) and Kaltreider (1952), employing x-ray pelvimetry, demonstrated that the incidence of difficult deliveries is increased to a similar degree when either the anteroposterior diameter of the inlet is < 10 cm or the transverse diameter is < 12 cm. As expected, when both diameters are contracted, dystocia is much greater than when only one is contracted.

A small woman is likely to have a small pelvis, but she is also likely to have a small neonate. Thoms (1937) studied 362 nulliparas and found that the mean birthweight of their offspring was significantly lower—280 g—in women with a small pelvis than in those with a medium or large pelvis. In veterinary obstetrics, in most species, maternal size rather than paternal size is the important determinant of fetal size.

Normally, cervical dilatation is aided by hydrostatic action of the unruptured membranes or after their rupture, by direct application of the presenting part against the cervix (Fig. 21-7, p. 414). In contracted pelves, however, because the head is arrested in the pelvic inlet, the entire force exerted by the uterus acts directly on the portion of membranes that contact the dilating cervix. Consequently, early spontaneous rupture of the membranes is more likely.

After membrane rupture, absent pressure by the head against the cervix and lower uterine segment predisposes to less effective contractions. Hence, further dilatation may proceed very slowly or not at all. Cibils and Hendricks (1965) reported that the mechanical adaptation of the fetal passenger to the bony passage plays an important part in determining the efficiency of contractions. The better the adaptation, the more efficient the contractions. Thus, cervical response to labor provides a prognostic view of labor outcome in women with inlet contraction.

A contracted inlet also plays an important part in the production of abnormal presentations. In normal nulliparas, the presenting part at term commonly descends into the pelvic cavity before labor onset. When the inlet is contracted considerably or there is marked asynclitism, descent usually does not take place until after labor onset, if at all. Cephalic presentations still predominate, but the head floats freely over the pelvic inlet or rests more laterally in one of the iliac fossae. Accordingly, very slight influences may cause the fetus to assume other presentations. In women with contracted pelves, face and shoulder presentations are encountered three times more frequently, and the cord prolapses four to six times more often.

Contracted Midpelvis

This finding is more common than inlet contraction. It frequently causes transverse arrest of the fetal head, which potentially can lead to a difficult midforceps operation or to cesarean delivery.

The obstetrical plane of the midpelvis extends from the inferior margin of the symphysis pubis through the ischial spines and touches the sacrum near the junction of the fourth and fifth vertebrae (Chap. 2, p. 33). A transverse line theoretically connecting the ischial spines divides the midpelvis into anterior and posterior portions. The former is bounded anteriorly by the lower border of the symphysis pubis and laterally by the ischiopubic rami. The posterior portion is bounded dorsally by the sacrum and laterally by the sacrospinous ligaments, forming the lower limits of the sacrosciatic notch.

Average midpelvis measurements are as follows: *transverse,* or interischial spinous, 10.5 cm; *anteroposterior,* from the lower border of the symphysis pubis to the junction of S_{4-5}, 11.5 cm; and *posterior sagittal,* from the midpoint of the interspinous line to the same point on the sacrum, 5 cm. The definition of midpelvic contractions has not been established with the same precision possible for inlet contractions. Even so, the midpelvis is likely contracted when the sum of the interspinous and posterior sagittal diameters of the midpelvis—normally, 10.5 plus 5 cm, or 15.5 cm—falls to 13.5 cm or less. This concept was emphasized by Chen and Huang (1982) in evaluating possible midpelvic contraction. There is reason to suspect midpelvic contraction whenever the interspinous diameter is < 10 cm. When it measures < 8 cm, the midpelvis is contracted.

Although there is no precise manual method of measuring midpelvic dimensions, a suggestion of contraction sometimes can be inferred if the spines are prominent, the pelvic sidewalls converge, or the sacrosciatic notch is narrow. Moreover, Eller and Mengert (1947) noted that the relationship between the intertuberous and interspinous diameters of the ischium is sufficiently constant that narrowing of the interspinous diameter can be anticipated when the intertuberous diameter is narrow. A normal intertuberous diameter, however, does not always exclude a narrow interspinous diameter.

Contracted Outlet

This finding usually is defined as an interischial tuberous diameter of 8 cm or less. The pelvic outlet may be roughly likened to two triangles, with the interischial tuberous diameter constituting the base of both. The sides of the anterior triangle are the pubic rami, and its apex is the inferoposterior surface of the symphysis pubis. The posterior triangle has no bony sides but is limited at its apex by the tip of the last sacral vertebra—not the tip of the coccyx. Diminution of the intertuberous diameter with consequent narrowing of the anterior triangle must inevitably force the fetal head posteriorly. Floberg and associates (1987) reported that outlet contractions were found in almost 1 percent of more than 1400 unselected nulliparas with term pregnancies. A contracted outlet may cause dystocia not so much by itself but by an often-associated midpelvic contraction. *Outlet contraction without concomitant midplane contraction is rare.*

Although the disproportion between the fetal head and the pelvic outlet is not sufficiently great to give rise to severe dystocia, it may play an important part in perineal tears. With increased narrowing of the pubic arch, the occiput cannot emerge directly beneath the symphysis pubis but is forced farther down upon the ischiopubic rami. The perineum, consequently, becomes increasingly distended and thus exposed to risk of laceration.

Pelvic Fractures

Vallier (2012) reviewed experiences with pelvic fractures and pregnancy. Trauma from automobile collisions was the most common cause. Moreover, they note that fracture pattern, minor malalignment, and retained hardware are not absolute indications for cesarean delivery. A history of pelvic fracture warrants careful review of previous radiographs and possibly pelvimetry later in pregnancy.

Estimation of Pelvic Capacity

The techniques for clinical evaluation using digital examination of the bony pelvis during labor are described in detail in Chapter 2 (p. 32). Briefly, the examiner attempts to judge the anteroposterior diameter of the inlet—the diagonal conjugate, the interspinous diameter of the midpelvis, and the intertuberous distances of the pelvic outlet. A narrow pelvic arch of less than 90 degrees can signify a narrow pelvis. An unengaged fetal head can indicate either excessive fetal head size or reduced pelvic inlet capacity.

The value of radiologic imaging to assess pelvic capacity has also been examined. First, with x-ray pelvimetry alone, the prognosis for successful vaginal delivery in any given pregnancy cannot be established (Mengert, 1948). Thus, the American College of Obstetricians and Gynecologists (2009) considers x-ray pelvimetry to be of limited value in the management of labor with a cephalic presentation.

Advantages of pelvimetry with computed tomography (CT), such as that shown in Figure 23-4, compared with those of conventional x-ray pelvimetry include reduced radiation exposure, greater accuracy, and easier performance. With either method, costs are comparable, and x-ray exposure is small (Chap. 46, p. 934). Depending on the machine and technique employed, fetal doses with CT pelvimetry may range from 250 to 1500 mrad (Moore, 1989).

Advantages of magnetic resonance (MR) pelvimetry include lack of ionizing radiation, accurate measurements, complete fetal imaging, and the potential for evaluating soft tissue dystocia (McCarthy, 1986; Stark, 1985). Zaretsky and colleagues (2005) used MR imaging to measure pelvic and fetal head volume to identify those women at greatest risk of undergoing cesarean delivery for dystocia. Although significant associations were found with some of the measures and cesarean delivery for dystocia, these researchers could not with accuracy predict which individual women would require cesarean delivery. Others have reported similar findings (Sporri, 1997).

Fetal Dimensions in Fetopelvic Disproportion

Fetal size alone is seldom a suitable explanation for failed labor. Even with the evolution of current technology, a fetal size threshold to predict fetopelvic disproportion is still elusive. Most cases of disproportion arise in fetuses whose weight is well within the range of the general obstetrical population. As shown in Figure 23-5, two thirds of neonates who required cesarean delivery after failed forceps delivery weighed less than 3700 g. Thus, other factors—for example, malposition of the head—obstruct fetal passage through the birth canal. These include asynclitism, occiput posterior position, and face and brow presentations.

Estimation of Fetal Head Size

Efforts to clinically and radiographically predict fetopelvic disproportion based on fetal head size have proved disappointing.

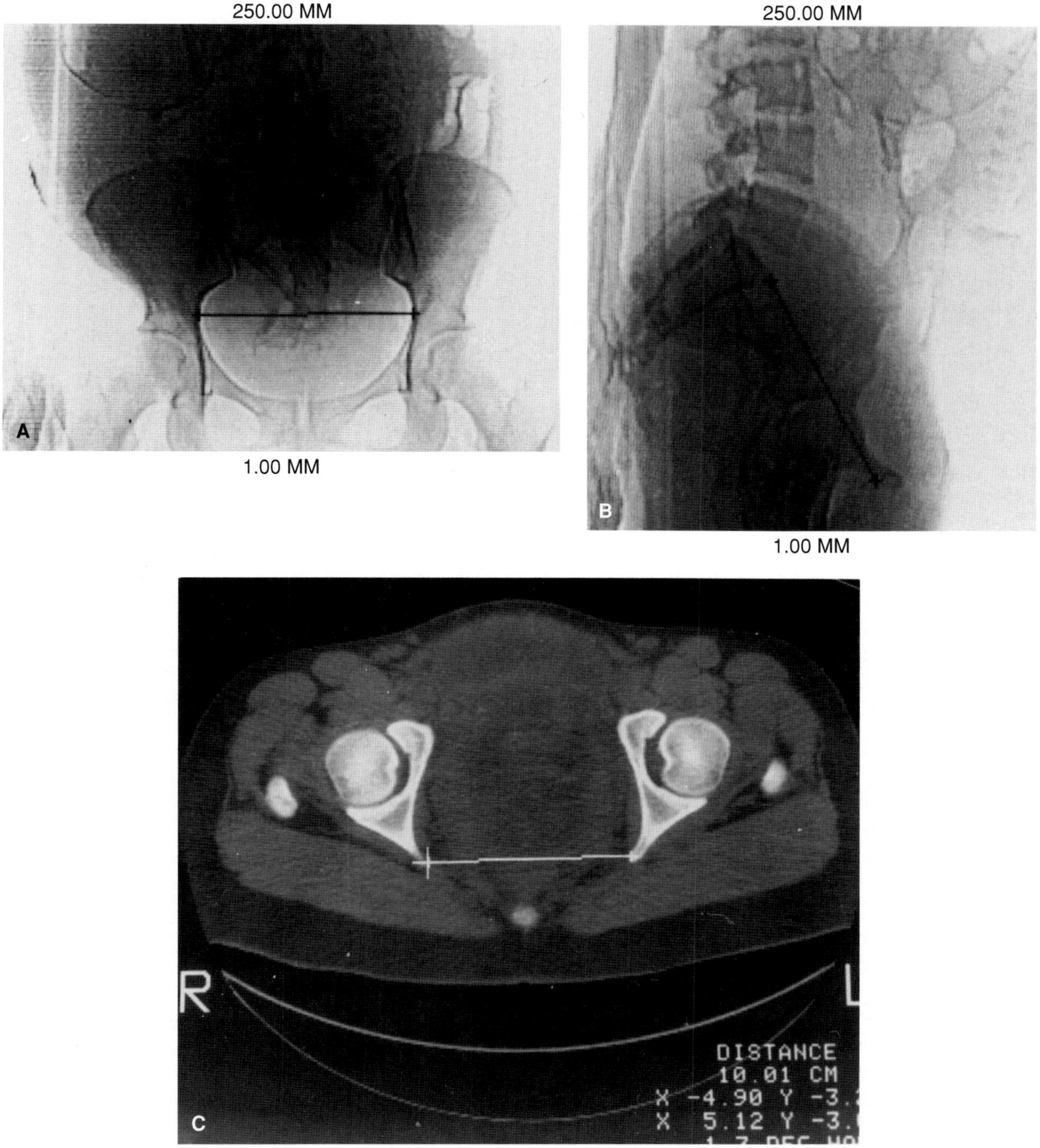

FIGURE 23-4 **A.** Anteroposterior view of a digital radiograph. Illustrated is the measurement of the transverse diameter of the pelvic inlet using an electronic cursor. The fetal body is clearly outlined. **B.** Lateral view of a digital radiograph. Illustrated are measurements of the anteroposterior diameters of the inlet using the electronic cursor. **C.** An axial computed tomographic section through the midpelvis. The level of the fovea of the femoral heads was ascertained from the anteroposterior digital radiograph because it corresponds to the level of the ischial spines. The interspinous diameter is measured using the electronic cursor. The total fetal radiation dose using these three exposures is approximately 250 mrad.

Mueller (1885) and Hillis (1930) described a clinical maneuver to predict disproportion. The fetal brow and the suboccipital region are grasped through the abdominal wall with the fingers, and firm pressure is directed downward in the axis of the inlet. If no disproportion exists, the head readily enters the pelvis, and vaginal delivery can be predicted. Thorp and coworkers (1993) performed a prospective evaluation of the *Mueller-Hillis maneuver* and concluded that there was no relationship between dystocia and failed descent during the maneuver.

Measurements of fetal head diameters using plain radiographic techniques are not used because of parallax distortions. The biparietal diameter and head circumference can be measured sonographically, and there have been attempts to use this information in the management of dystocia. Thurnau and

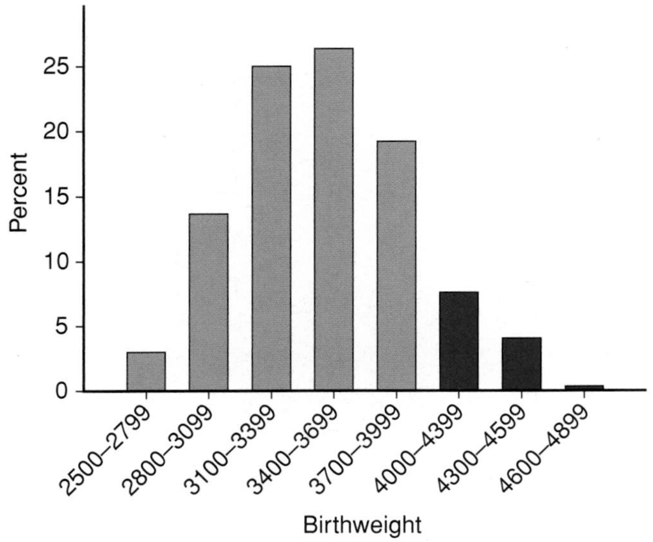

FIGURE 23-5 Birthweight distribution of 362 newborns born by cesarean delivery at Parkland Hospital (1989–1999) after a failed forceps attempt. Only 12 percent (n = 44) of the newborns weighed > 4000 g (*dark bars*).

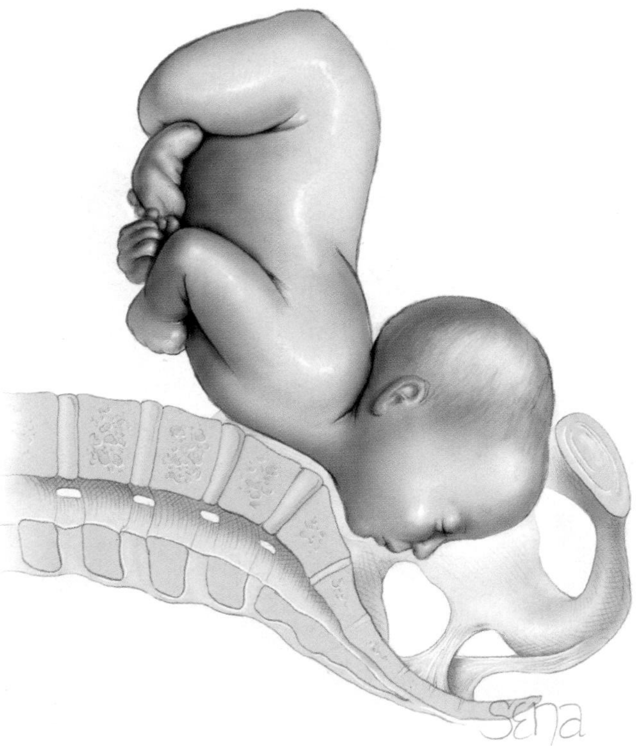

FIGURE 23-6 Face presentation. The occiput is the longer end of the head lever. The chin is directly posterior. Vaginal delivery is impossible unless the chin rotates anteriorly.

colleagues (1991) used the *fetal-pelvic index* to identify labor complications. Unfortunately, the sensitivity of such measurements to predict cephalopelvic disproportion is poor (Ferguson, 1998). We are of the view that there is no currently satisfactory method for accurate prediction of fetopelvic disproportion based on head size.

Face Presentation

With this presentation, the head is hyperextended so that the occiput is in contact with the fetal back, and the chin (mentum) is presenting (Fig. 23-6). The fetal face may present with the chin (mentum) anteriorly or posteriorly, relative to the maternal symphysis pubis (Chap. 22, p. 436). Although some mentum posterior presentations persist, most convert spontaneously to anterior even in late labor (Duff, 1981). If not, the fetal brow (bregma) is pressed against the maternal symphysis pubis. This position precludes flexion of the fetal head necessary to negotiate the birth canal. Thus, a mentum posterior presentation is undeliverable except with a very preterm fetus.

Face presentations rarely deliver as such vaginally. Cruikshank and White (1973) reported an incidence of 1 in 600, or 0.17 percent. As shown in Table 22-1 (p. 434), among more than 70,000 singleton newborns delivered at Parkland Hospital, approximately 1 in 2000 had a face presentation at delivery.

Etiology

Causes of face presentations are numerous and include conditions that favor extension or prevent head flexion. Preterm infants, with their smaller head dimensions, can engage before conversion to vertex position (Shaffer, 2006). In exceptional instances, marked enlargement of the neck or coils of cord around the neck may cause extension. Bashiri and associates (2008) reported that fetal malformations and hydramnios were risk factors for face or brow presentations. Anencephalic fetuses naturally present by the face.

Extended positions develop more frequently when the pelvis is contracted or the fetus is very large. In a series of 141 face presentations studied by Hellman and coworkers (1950), the incidence of inlet contraction was 40 percent. This high incidence of pelvic contraction should be kept in mind when considering management.

High parity is a predisposing factor to face presentation (Fuchs, 1985). In these cases, a pendulous abdomen permits the back of the fetus to sag forward or laterally, often in the same direction in which the occiput points. This promotes extension of the cervical and thoracic spine.

Diagnosis

Face presentation is diagnosed by vaginal examination and palpation of facial features. As discussed in Chapter 28 (p. 560), it is possible to mistake a breech for a face presentation because the anus may be mistaken for the mouth and the ischial tuberosities for the malar prominences. The radiographic demonstration of the hyperextended head with the facial bones at or below the pelvic inlet is characteristic.

Mechanism of Labor

Face presentations rarely are observed above the pelvic inlet. Instead, the brow generally presents early and is usually converted to present the face after further extension of the head during descent. The mechanism of labor in these cases consists of the cardinal movements of descent, internal rotation, and flexion, and the accessory movements of extension and external rotation (Fig. 23-7). Descent is brought about by the same

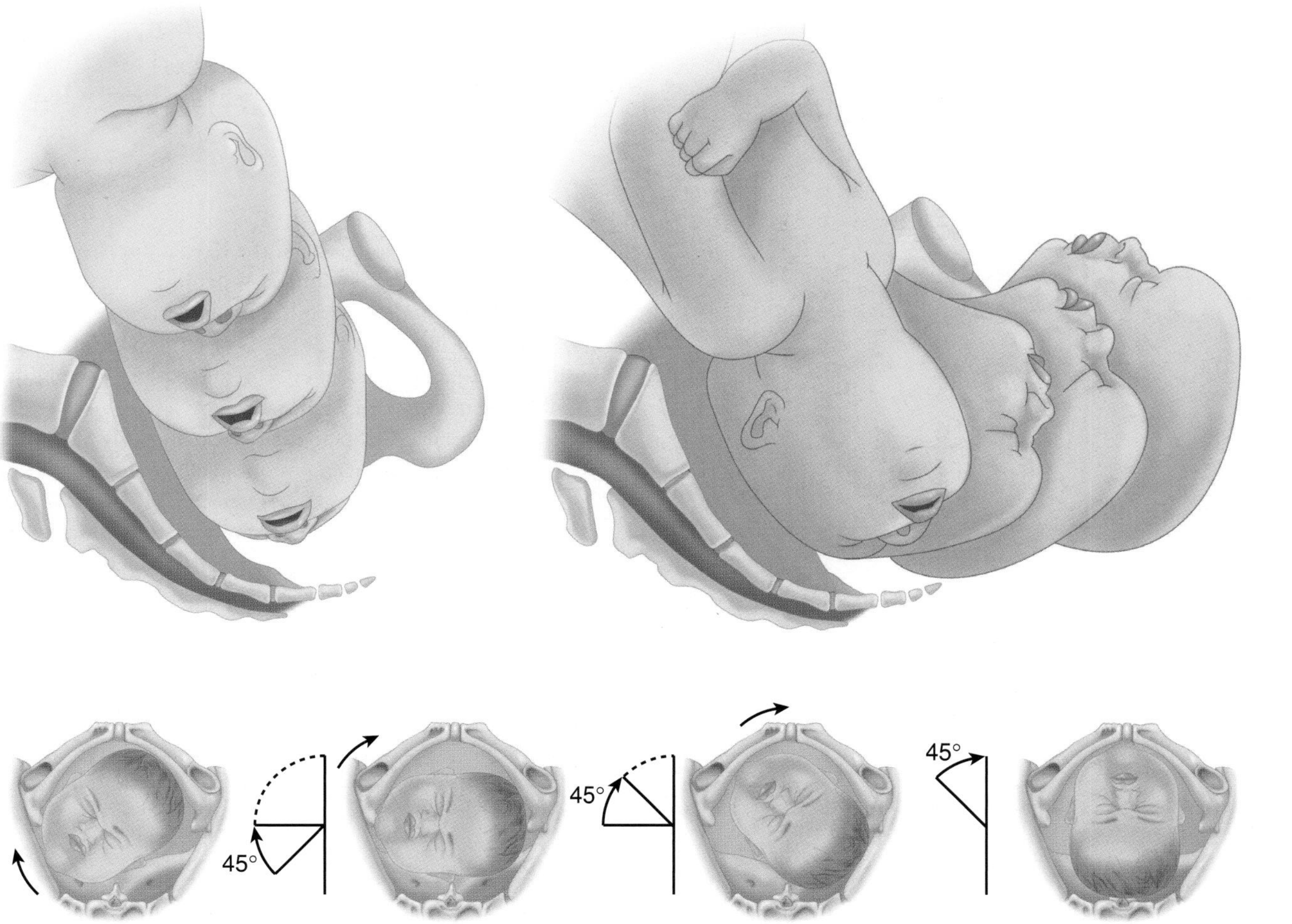

FIGURE 23-7 Mechanism of labor for right mentoposterior position with subsequent rotation of the mentum anteriorly and delivery.

factors as in cephalic presentations. Extension results from the relation of the fetal body to the deflected head, which is converted into a two-armed lever, the longer arm of which extends from the occipital condyles to the occiput. When resistance is encountered, the occiput must be pushed toward the back of the fetus while the chin descends.

The objective of internal rotation of the face is to bring the chin under the symphysis pubis. Only in this way can the neck traverse the posterior surface of the symphysis pubis. If the chin rotates directly posteriorly, the relatively short neck cannot span the anterior surface of the sacrum, which measures about 12 cm in length. Moreover, the fetal brow (bregma) is pressed against the maternal symphysis pubis. This position precludes flexion necessary to negotiate the birth canal. Hence, birth of the head from a mentum posterior position is impossible unless the shoulders enter the pelvis at the same time, an event that is impossible except when the fetus is extremely small or macerated. Internal rotation results from the same factors as in vertex presentations.

After anterior rotation and descent, the chin and mouth appear at the vulva, the undersurface of the chin presses against the symphysis, and the head is delivered by flexion. The nose, eyes, brow (bregma), and occiput then appear in succession over the anterior margin of the perineum. After birth of the head, the occiput sags backward toward the anus. Next, the chin rotates externally to the side toward which it was originally directed, and the shoulders are born as in cephalic presentations.

Edema may sometimes significantly distort the face. At the same time, the skull undergoes considerable molding, manifested by an increase in length of the occipitomental diameter of the head.

Management

In the absence of a contracted pelvis, and with effective labor, successful vaginal delivery usually will follow. Fetal heart rate monitoring is probably better done with external devices to avoid damage to the face and eyes. Because face presentations among term-size fetuses are more common when there is some degree of pelvic inlet contraction, cesarean delivery frequently is indicated. Attempts to convert a face presentation manually into a vertex presentation, manual or forceps rotation of a persistently posterior chin to a mentum anterior position, and internal podalic version and extraction are dangerous and should not be attempted.

Brow Presentation

This rare presentation is diagnosed when that portion of the fetal head between the orbital ridge and the anterior fontanel

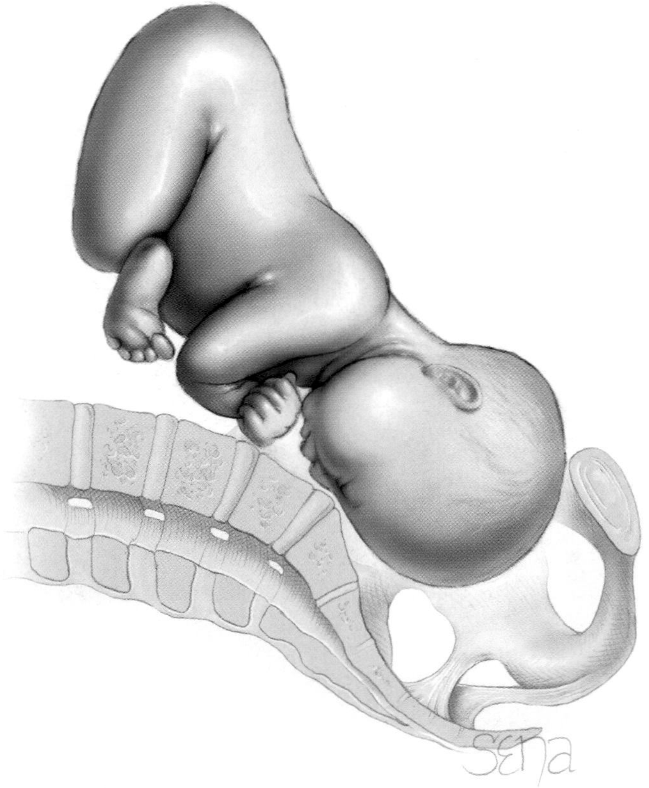

FIGURE 23-8 Brow posterior presentation.

presents at the pelvic inlet. As shown in Figure 23-8, the fetal head thus occupies a position midway between full flexion (occiput) and extension (face). Except when the fetal head is small or the pelvis is unusually large, engagement of the fetal head and subsequent delivery cannot take place as long as the brow presentation persists.

Etiology and Diagnosis

The causes of persistent brow presentation are the same as those for face presentation. A brow presentation is commonly unstable and often converts to a face or an occiput presentation (Cruikshank, 1973). The presentation may be recognized by abdominal palpation when both the occiput and chin can be palpated easily, but vaginal examination is usually necessary. The frontal sutures, large anterior fontanel, orbital ridges, eyes, and root of the nose are felt on vaginal examination, but neither the mouth nor the chin is palpable.

Mechanism of Labor

With a very small fetus and a large pelvis, labor is generally easy, but with a larger fetus, it is usually difficult. This is because engagement is impossible until there is marked molding that shortens the occipitomental diameter or more commonly, until there is either flexion to an occiput presentation or extension to a face presentation. The considerable molding essential for vaginal delivery of a persistent brow characteristically deforms the head. The caput succedaneum is over the forehead, and it may be so extensive that identification of the brow by palpation is impossible. In these instances, the forehead is prominent and squared, and the occipitomental diameter is diminished.

In transient brow presentations, the prognosis depends on the ultimate presentation. If the brow persists, prognosis is poor for vaginal delivery unless the fetus is small or the birth canal is large. Principles of management are the same as those for a face presentation.

Transverse Lie

In this position, the long axis of the fetus is approximately perpendicular to that of the mother. When the long axis forms an acute angle, an *oblique lie* results. The latter is usually only transitory, because either a longitudinal or transverse lie commonly results when labor supervenes. For this reason, the oblique lie is called an *unstable lie* in Great Britain.

In a transverse lie, the shoulder is usually positioned over the pelvic inlet. The head occupies one iliac fossa, and the breech the other. This creates a *shoulder presentation* in which the side of the mother on which the acromion rests determines the designation of the lie as right or left acromial. And because in either position the back may be directed anteriorly or posteriorly, superiorly or inferiorly, it is customary to distinguish varieties as dorsoanterior and dorsoposterior (Fig. 23-9).

Transverse lie was found once in 322 singleton deliveries (0.3 percent) at both the Mayo Clinic and the University of Iowa Hospital (Cruikshank, 1973; Johnson, 1964). This is remarkably similar to the incidence at Parkland Hospital of approximately 1 in 335 singleton fetuses.

Etiology

Some of the more common causes of transverse lie include: (1) abdominal wall relaxation from high parity, (2) preterm fetus, (3) placenta previa, (4) abnormal uterine anatomy, (5) hydramnios, and (6) contracted pelvis.

Women with four or more deliveries have a tenfold incidence of transverse lie compared with nulliparas. A relaxed and pendulous abdomen allows the uterus to fall forward, deflecting the long axis of the fetus away from the axis of the birth canal and into an oblique or transverse position. Placenta previa and pelvic contraction act similarly. A transverse or oblique lie occasionally develops in labor from an initial longitudinal position.

Diagnosis

A transverse lie is usually recognized easily, often by inspection alone. The abdomen is unusually wide, whereas the uterine fundus extends to only slightly above the umbilicus. No fetal pole is detected in the fundus, and the ballottable head is found in one iliac fossa and the breech in the other. The position of the back is readily identifiable. When the back is anterior (Fig. 23-9, p. 469), a hard resistance plane extends across the front of the abdomen. When it is posterior, irregular nodulations representing fetal small parts are felt through the abdominal wall.

On vaginal examination, in the early stages of labor, if the side of the thorax can be reached, it may be recognized by the "gridiron" feel of the ribs. With further dilatation, the scapula and the clavicle are distinguished on opposite sides of the thorax. The position of the axilla indicates the side of the mother toward which the shoulder is directed.

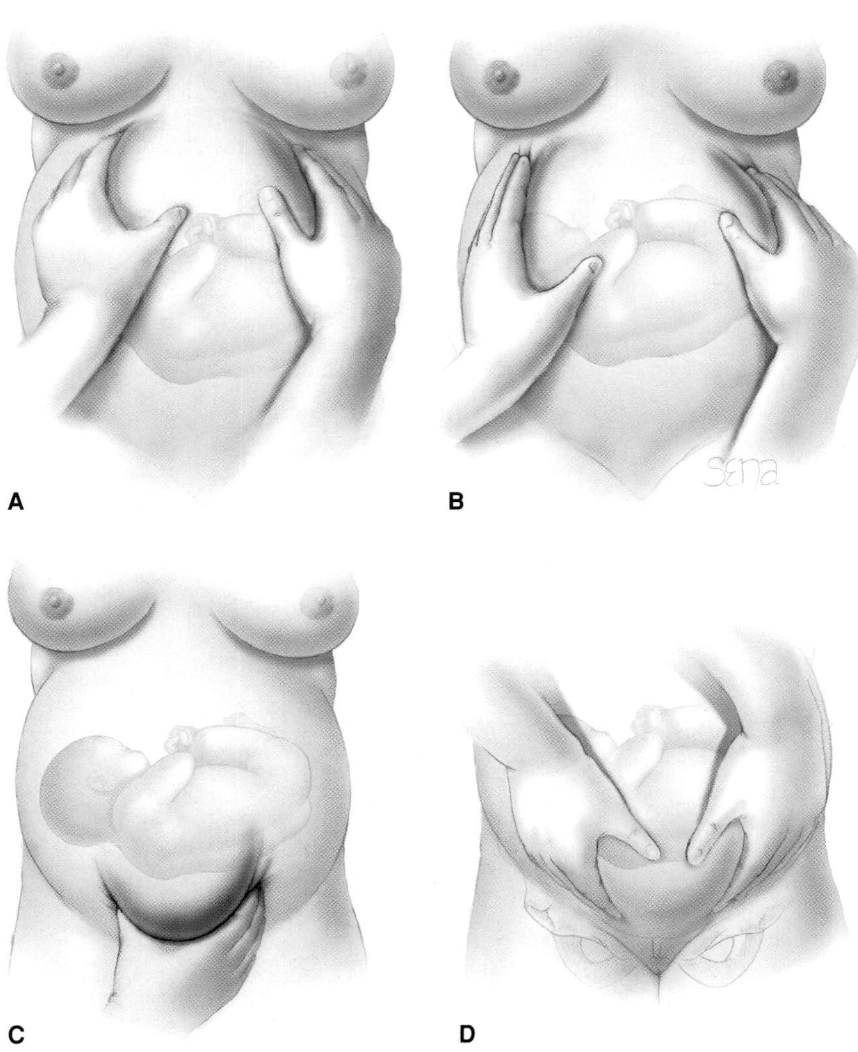

FIGURE 23-9 Leopold maneuver performed on a woman with a fetal transverse lie, right acromiodorsoanterior position. **A.** First maneuver. **B.** Second maneuver. **C.** Third maneuver. **D.** Fourth maneuver.

Mechanism of Labor

Spontaneous delivery of a fully developed newborn is impossible with a persistent transverse lie. After rupture of the membranes, if labor continues, the fetal shoulder is forced into the pelvis, and the corresponding arm frequently prolapses (Fig. 23-10). After some descent, the shoulder is arrested by the margins of the pelvic inlet, with the head in one iliac fossa and the breech in the other. As labor continues, the shoulder is impacted firmly in the upper part of the pelvis. The uterus then contracts vigorously in an unsuccessful attempt to overcome the obstacle. With time, a retraction ring rises increasingly higher and becomes more marked. With this *neglected transverse lie,* the uterus will eventually rupture. Even without this complication, morbidity is increased because of the frequent association with placenta previa, the increased likelihood of cord prolapse, and the necessity for major operative efforts.

If the fetus is small—usually < 800 g—and the pelvis is large, spontaneous delivery is possible despite persistence of the abnormal lie. The fetus is compressed with the head forced against its abdomen. A portion of the thoracic wall below the shoulder thus becomes the most dependent part, appearing at the vulva. The head and thorax then pass through the pelvic cavity at the same time. The fetus, which is doubled upon itself and thus sometimes referred to as *conduplicato corpore*, is expelled.

Management

Active labor in a woman with a transverse lie is usually an indication for cesarean delivery. Before labor or early in labor, with the membranes intact, attempts at external version are worthwhile in the absence of other complications. If the fetal head can be maneuvered by abdominal manipulation into the pelvis, it should be held there during the next several contractions in an attempt to fix the head in the pelvis.

With cesarean delivery, because neither the feet nor the head of the fetus occupies the lower uterine segment, a low transverse incision into the uterus may lead to difficult fetal extraction. This is especially true of dorsoanterior presentations. Therefore, a vertical incision is typically indicated (Chap. 30, p. 598).

Compound Presentation

Incidence and Etiology

In a compound presentation, an extremity prolapses alongside the presenting part, and both present simultaneously in the pelvis (Fig. 23-11). Goplerud and Eastman (1953) identified a hand or arm prolapsed alongside the head once in every 700 deliveries. Much less common was prolapse of one or both lower extremities alongside a cephalic presentation or a hand alongside a breech. At Parkland Hospital, compound presentations were identified in only 68 of more than 70,000 singleton fetuses—an incidence of approximately 1 in 1000. Causes of compound presentations are conditions that prevent complete occlusion of the pelvic inlet by the fetal head, including preterm labor.

Management and Prognosis

In most cases, the prolapsed part should be left alone, because most often it will not interfere with labor. If the arm is prolapsed alongside the head, the condition should be observed closely to ascertain whether the arm retracts out of the way with descent of the presenting part. If it fails to retract and if it appears to prevent descent of the head, the prolapsed arm should be pushed gently upward and the head simultaneously downward by fundal pressure. Tebes and coworkers (1999) described a tragic outcome in a newborn delivered spontaneously with the hand alongside the head. The infant developed

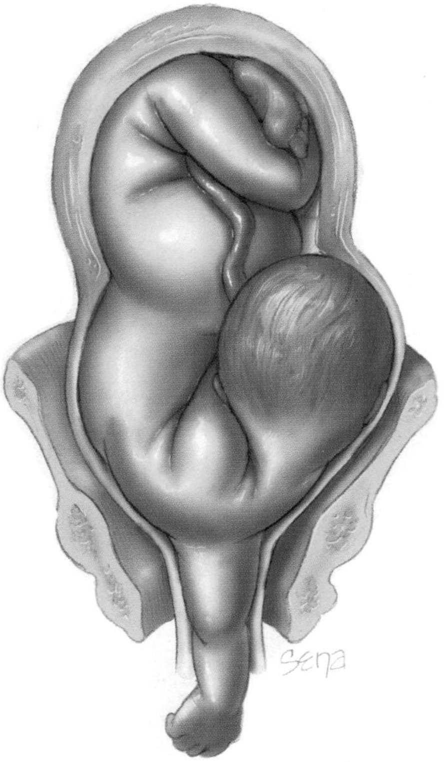

FIGURE 23-10 Neglected shoulder presentation. A thick muscular band forming a pathological retraction ring has developed just above the thin lower uterine segment. The force generated during a uterine contraction is directed centripetally at and above the level of the pathological retraction ring. This serves to stretch further and possibly to rupture the thin lower segment below the retraction ring.

ischemic necrosis of the presenting forearm, which required amputation. In general, rates of perinatal mortality and morbidity are increased as a result of concomitant preterm delivery, prolapsed cord, and traumatic obstetrical procedures.

COMPLICATIONS WITH DYSTOCIA

Maternal Complications

Dystocia, especially if labor is prolonged, is associated with an increased incidence of several common obstetrical and neonatal complications. Intrapartum chorioamnionitis and postpartum pelvic infection are more common with desultory and prolonged labors. Postpartum hemorrhage from atony is increased with prolonged and augmented labors. There is also a higher incidence of uterine tears with hysterotomy if the fetal head is impacted in the pelvis.

Uterine Rupture

Abnormal thinning of the lower uterine segment creates a serious danger during prolonged labor, particularly in women of high parity and in those with a prior cesarean delivery (Chap. 41, p. 790). When disproportion is so pronounced that there is no engagement or descent, the lower uterine segment becomes increasingly stretched, and rupture may follow. In such cases, there is usually an exaggeration of the normal *contraction ring* shown in Figure 23-1.

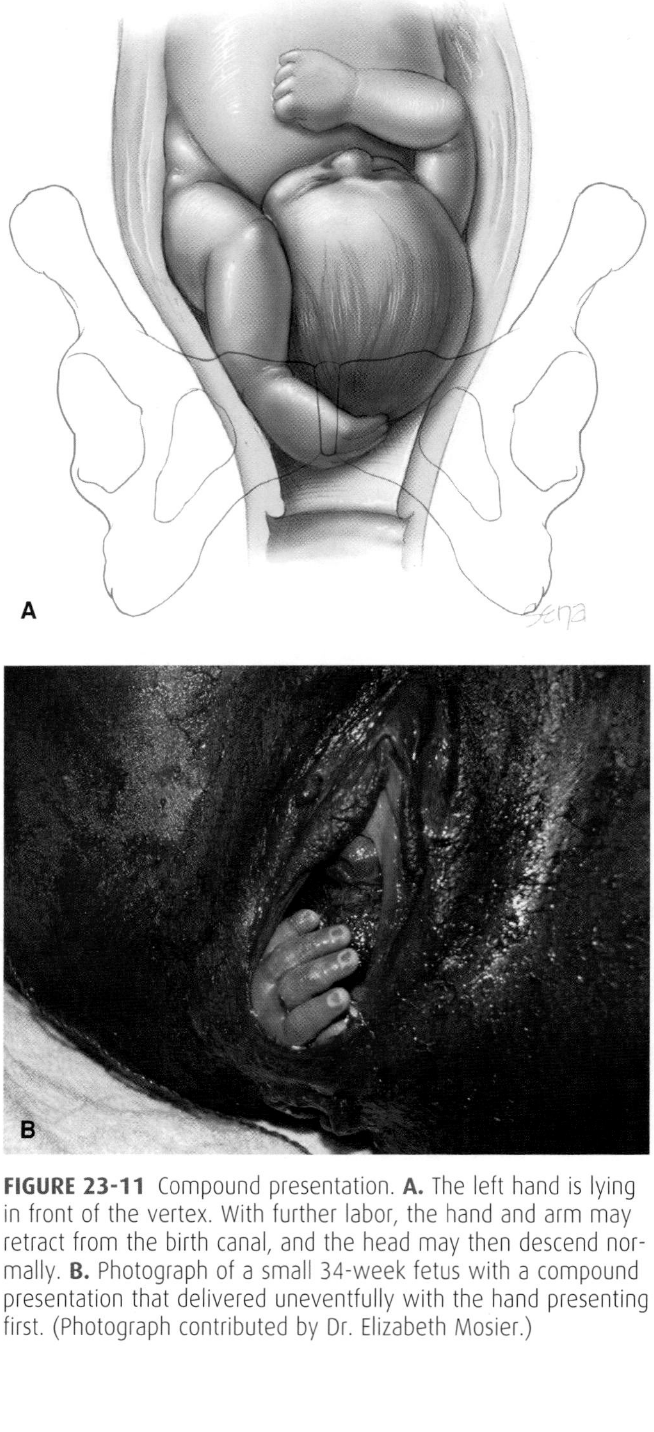

FIGURE 23-11 Compound presentation. **A.** The left hand is lying in front of the vertex. With further labor, the hand and arm may retract from the birth canal, and the head may then descend normally. **B.** Photograph of a small 34-week fetus with a compound presentation that delivered uneventfully with the hand presenting first. (Photograph contributed by Dr. Elizabeth Mosier.)

Pathological Retraction Ring. Localized rings or constrictions of the uterus develop in association with prolonged obstructed labors that are seldom encountered today. The *pathological retraction ring of Bandl* is associated with marked stretching and thinning of the lower uterine segment. The ring may be seen clearly as a uterine indentation and signifies impending rupture of the lower uterine segment.

Following birth of a first twin, a pathological ring may still develop occasionally as hourglass constrictions of the uterus. The ring can sometimes be relaxed and delivery effected with appropriate general anesthesia, but occasionally prompt cesarean delivery offers a better prognosis for the second twin (Chap. 45, p. 917).

Fistula Formation

With dystocia, the presenting part is firmly wedged into the pelvic inlet and does not advance for a considerable time. Tissues of the birth canal lying between the leading part and the pelvic wall may be subjected to excessive pressure. Because of impaired circulation, necrosis may result and become evident several days after delivery as vesicovaginal, vesicocervical, or rectovaginal fistulas. Most often, pressure necrosis follows a very prolonged second stage. They are rarely seen today except in undeveloped countries.

Pelvic Floor Injury

During childbirth, the pelvic floor is exposed to direct compression from the fetal head and to downward pressure from maternal expulsive efforts. These forces stretch and distend the pelvic floor, resulting in functional and anatomical alterations in the muscles, nerves, and connective tissues. There is accumulating evidence that such effects on the pelvic floor during childbirth lead to urinary incontinence and to pelvic organ prolapse (Handa, 2011). As discussed in Chapter 27 (p. 548), the anal sphincter is torn in 3 to 6 percent of deliveries, and many of these women report subsequent fecal or gas incontinence. Many of these long-term sequelae have contributed to the current trend of *cesarean delivery on maternal request* discussed in Chapter 30 (p. 589).

Postpartum Lower Extremity Nerve Injury

Wong and colleagues (2003) reviewed neurological injury involving the lower extremities in association with labor and delivery. The most common mechanism is external compression of the common fibular (fomerly common peroneal) nerve. This is usually caused by inappropriate leg positioning in stirrups, especially during prolonged second-stage labor. These and other injuries are discussed in Chapter 36 (p. 676). Fortunately, symptoms resolve within 6 months of delivery in most women.

Perinatal Complications

Similar to the mother, the incidence of peripartum fetal sepsis is increased with longer labors. *Caput succedaneum* and *molding* develop commonly and may be impressive (Fig. 22-19, p. 444) (Buchmann, 2008). Mechanical trauma such as nerve injury, fractures, and cephalohematoma are also more frequent and discussed fully in Chapter 33 (p. 645).

REFERENCES

Acker DB, Gregory KD, Sachs BP, et al: Risk factors for Erb-Duchenne palsy. Obstet Gynecol 71:389, 1988

Alexander J: MFMU Cesarean Registry: Labor characteristics of women undergoing cesarean delivery for dystocia. Am J Obstet Gynecol 189(6):S138, 2003

Alexander JM, Lucas MJ, Ramin SM, et al: The course of labor with and without epidural analgesia. Am J Obstet Gynecol 178:516, 1998

Alexander JM, Sharma SK, McIntire DD, at el: Epidural analgesia lengthens the Friedman active phase of labor. Obstet Gynecol 100:46, 2002

American College of Obstetricians and Gynecologists: Guidelines for diagnostic imaging during pregnancy. Committee Opinion No. 299, September 2004, Reaffirmed 2009

American College of Obstetricians and Gynecologists: Dystocia and augmentation of labor. Practice Bulletin No. 49, December 2003, Reaffirmed 2013

Austin T, Bridges N, Markiewicz M, et al: Severe neonatal polycythaemia after third stage of labour underwater. Lancet 350 (9089):1445, 1997

Babayer M, Bodack MP, Creatura C: Common peroneal neuropathy secondary to squatting during childbirth. Obstet Gynecol 91:830, 1998

Bashiri A, Burstein E, Bar-David J, et al: Face and brow presentation: independent risk factors. J Matern Fetal Neonatal Med 21(6):357, 2008

Berghella V, Baxter JK, Chauhan SP: Evidence-based labor and delivery management. Am J Obstet Gynecol 199(5):445, 2008

Bleich AT, Alexander JM, McIntire DD, et al: An analysis of second-stage labor beyond 3 hours in nulliparous women. Am J Perinatol 29:717, 2012

Bloom SL, Casey BM, Schaffer JI, et al: A randomized trial of coached versus uncoached maternal pushing during the second stage of labor. Am J Obstet Gynecol 194; 10, 2006

Bloom SL, McIntire DD, Kelly MA, et al: Lack of effect of walking on labor and delivery. N Engl J Med 339:76, 1998

Buchmann EJ, Libhaber E: Sagittal suture overlap in cephalopelvic disproportion: blinded and non-participant assessment. Acta Obstet Gynecol Scand 87(7):731, 2008

Caldeyro-Barcia R, Alvarez H, Reynolds SRM: A better understanding of uterine contractility through simultaneous recording with an internal and a seven channel external method. Surg Obstet Gynecol 91:641, 1950

Calkins LA: Premature spontaneous rupture of the membranes. Am J Obstet Gynecol 64:871, 1952

Carlson JM, Diehl JA, Murray MS, et al: Maternal position during parturition in normal labor. Obstet Gynecol 68:443, 1986

Chen HY, Huang SC: Evaluation of midpelvic contraction. Int Surg 67:516, 1982

Cibils LA, Hendricks CH: Normal labor in vertex presentation. Am J Obstet Gynecol 91:385, 1965

Cluett ER, Burns E: Immersion in water in labour and birth. Cochrane Database Syst Rev 2:CD000111, 2009

Cluett ER, Pickering RM, Getliffe K, et al: Randomised controlled trial of labouring in water compared with standard augmentation for management of dystocia in first stage of labour. BMJ 328:314, 2004

Cohen W: Influence of the duration of second stage labor on perinatal outcome and puerperal morbidity. Obstet Gynecol 49:266, 1977

Cohen W, Friedman EA (eds): Management of Labor. Baltimore, University Park Press, 1983

Cruikshank DP, White CA: Obstetric malpresentations: twenty years' experience. Am J Obstet Gynecol 116:1097, 1973

Duff P: Diagnosis and management of face presentation. Obstet Gynecol 57:105, 1981

Eller WC, Mengert WF: Recognition of mid-pelvic contraction. Am J Obstet Gynecol 53:252, 1947

Ferguson JE, Newberry YG, DeAngelis GA, et al: The fetal-pelvic index has minimal utility in predicting fetal-pelvic disproportion. Am J Obstet Gynecol 179:1186, 1998

Floberg J, Belfrage P, Ohlsén H: Influence of pelvic outlet capacity on labor: a prospective pelvimetry study of 1429 unselected primi-paras. Acta Obstet Gynecol Scand 66:121, 1987

Flynn AM, Kelly J, Hollins G, et al: Ambulation in labour. BMJ 2:591, 1978

Fraser WD, Marcoux S, Krauss I, et al: Multicenter, randomized, controlled trial of delayed pushing for nulliparous women in the second stage of labor with continuous epidural analgesia. Am J Obstet Gynecol 182:1165, 2000

Friedman EA: Labor. Clinical Evaluation and Management, 2nd ed. New York, Appleton-Century-Crofts, 1978

Friedman EA, Sachtleben MR: Station of the fetal presenting part II: effect on the course of labor. Am J Obstet Gynecol 93:530, 1965

Friedman EA, Sachtleben MR: Station of the fetal presenting part IV: arrest of descent in nulliparas. Obstet Gynecol 47:129, 1976

Fuchs K, Peretz BA, Marcovici R, et al: The grand multipara—is it a problem? Int J Gynaecol Obstet 73:321, 1985

Goplerud J, Eastman NJ: Compound presentation: survey of 65 cases. Obstet Gynecol 1:59, 1953

Graseck A, Odibo AO, Tuuli M, et al: Normal first stage of labor in women undergoing trial of labor after cesarean delivery. Obstet Gynecol 119:732, 2012

Gupta JK, Hofmeyr GJ: Position for women during second stage of labour. Cochrane Database Syst Rev 1:CD002006, 2004

Handa VL, Blomquist JL, Knoepp LR, et al: Pelvic floor disorders 5–10 years after vaginal or cesarean childbirth. Obstet Gynecol 118(4):777, 2011

Handa VL, Laros RK: Active-phase arrest in labor: predictors of cesarean delivery in a nulliparous population. Obstet Gynecol 81:758, 1993

Hannah ME, Hodnett ED, Willan A, et al: Prelabor rupture of the membranes at term: expectant management at home or in hospital? Obstet Gynecol 96:533, 2000

Hannah M, Ohlsson A, Farine D, et al: International Term PROM Trial: a RCT of induction of labor for prelabor rupture of membranes at term. Am J Obstet Gynecol 174:303, 1996

Hansen SL, Clark SL, Foster JC: Active pushing versus passive fetal descent in the second stage of labor: a randomized controlled trial. Obstet Gynecol 99:29, 2002

Hauth JC, Hankins GD, Gilstrap LC III: Uterine contraction pressures achieved in parturients with active phase arrest. Obstet Gynecol 78:344, 1991

Hauth JC, Hankins GD, Gilstrap LC III, et al: Uterine contraction pressures with oxytocin induction/augmentation. Obstet Gynecol 68:305, 1986

Hellman LM, Epperson JWW, Connally F: Face and brow presentation: the experience of the Johns Hopkins Hospital, 1896 to 1948. Am J Obstet Gynecol 59:831, 1950

Hendricks CH, Quilligan EJ, Tyler AB, et al: Pressure relationships between intervillous space and amniotic fluid in human term pregnancy. Am J Obstet Gynecol 77:1028, 1959

Hillis DS: Diagnosis of contracted pelvis by the impression method. Surg Gynecol Obstet 51:857, 1930

Hughes EC: Obstetric-Gynecologic Terminology. Philadelphia, Davis, 1972, p 390

Johnson CE: Transverse presentation of the fetus. JAMA 187:642, 1964

Kaltreider DF: Criteria of midplane contraction. Am J Obstet Gynecol 63:392, 1952

Kappy KA, Cetrulo C, Knuppel RA: Premature rupture of membranes: conservative approach. Am J Obstet Gynecol 134:655, 1979

Kwee A, Graziosi GCM, van Leeuwen JHS, et al: The effect of immersion on haemodynamic and fetal measures in uncomplicated pregnancies of nulliparous women. Br J Obstet Gynaecol 107:663, 2000

Larks SD: Electrohysterography. Springfield, Thomas, 1960

Lupe PJ, Gross TL: Maternal upright posture and mobility in labor: a review. Obstet Gynecol 67:727, 1986

Mahon TR, Chazotte C, Cohen WR: Short labor: characteristics and outcome. Obstet Gynecol 84:47, 1994

Manyonda IT, Shaw DE, Drife JO: The effect of delayed pushing in the second stage of labor with continuous lumbar epidural analgesia. Acta Obstet Gynecol Scand 69:291, 1990

Martin JA, Hamilton BE, Sutton PD, et al: Births: final data for 2006. Natl Vital Stat Rep 57(7):1, 2009

Martin JA, Hamilton BE, Ventura SJ, et al: Births: final data for 2009. Natl Vital Stat Rep 60(1):1, 2011

Martin JA, Hamilton BE, Ventura SJ, et al: Births: final data for 2010. Natl Vital Stat Rep 61(1):1, 2012

McCarthy S: Magnetic resonance imaging in obstetrics and gynecology. Magn Reson Imaging 4:59, 1986

Mengert WF: Estimation of pelvic capacity. JAMA 138:169, 1948

Menticoglou SM, Manning F, Harman C, et al: Perinatal outcomes in relation to second-stage duration. Am J Obstet Gynecol 173:906, 1995a

Menticoglou SM, Perlman M, Manning FA: High cervical spinal cord injury in neonates delivered with forceps: report of 15 cases. Obstet Gynecol 86:589, 1995b

Miller FC: Uterine motility in spontaneous labor. Clin Obstet Gynecol 26:78, 1983

Moore MM, Shearer DR: Fetal dose estimates for CT pelvimetry. Radiology 171:265, 1989

Mozurkewich E, Chilimigras J, Koepke E, et al: Indications for induction of labour: a best-evidence review. BJOG 116(5):626, 2009

Mueller P: About the prognosis for delivery with a narrow pelvis. Arch Gynaekol 27:311, 1885

Myles TD, Santolaya J: Maternal and neonatal outcomes in patients with a prolonged second stage of labor. Obstet Gynecol 102(1):52, 2003

Nelson DB, McIntire DD, Leveno KJ: Relationship of the length of the first stage of labor to the length of the second stage. Obstet Gynecol 122:27, 2013

Olah KSJ, Neilson J: Failure to progress in the management of labour. Br J Obstet Gynaecol 101:1, 1994

Passos F, Cardose K, Coelho AM, et al: Antibiotic prophylaxis in premature rupture of membranes at term. Obstet Gynecol 120:1045, 2012

Peleg D, Hannah ME, Hodnett ED, et al: Predictors of cesarean delivery after prelabor rupture of membranes at term. Obstet Gynecol 93:1031, 1999

Pinette MG, Wax J, Wilson E: The risks of underwater birth. Am J Obstet Gynecol 190(5):1211, 2004

Plunkett BA, Lin A, Wong CA, et al: Management of the second stage of labor in nulliparas with continuous epidural analgesia. Obstet Gynecol 102:109, 2003

Read JA, Miller FC, Paul RH: Randomized trial of ambulation versus oxytocin for labor enhancement: a preliminary report. Am J Obstet Gynecol 139:669, 1981

Reynolds SRM, Heard OO, Bruns P, et al: A multichannel strain-gauge tocodynamometer: an instrument for studying patterns of uterine contractions in pregnant women. Bull Johns Hopkins Hosp 82:446, 1948

Robertson PA, Huang LJ, Croughan-Minihane MS, et al: Is there an association between water baths during labor and the development of chorioamnionitis or endometritis? Am J Obstet Gynecol 178:1215, 1998

Roshanfekr D, Blakemore KJ, Lee J, et al: Station at onset of active labor in nulliparous patients and risk of cesarean delivery. Obstet Gynecol 93:329, 1999

Rouse DJ, Owen J, Hauth JC: Active-phase labor arrest: oxytocin augmentation for at least 4 hours. Obstet Gynecol 93:323, 1999

Rouse DJ, Weiner SJ, Bloom SL, et al: Second-stage labor duration in nulliparous women: relationship to maternal and perinatal outcomes. Am J Obstet Gynecol 201:357.e1, 2009

Russell JG: Moulding of the pelvic outlet. J Obstet Gynaecol Br Commonw 76:817, 1969

Satin AJ, Maberry MC, Leveno KJ, et al: Chorioamnionitis: a harbinger of dystocia. Obstet Gynecol 79:913, 1992

Shaffer BL, Cheng YW, Vargas JE, et al: Face presentation: predictors and delivery route. Am J Obstet Gynecol 194(5):e10, 2006

Sharma SK, Leveno KJ: Update: epidural analgesia during labor does not increase cesarean births. Curr Anesth Rep 2:18, 2000

Spong CY, Berghella V, Wenstrom KD, et al: Preventing the first cesarean delivery: summary of a joint Eunice Kennedy Shriver National Institute of Child Health and Human Development, Society of Maternal-Fetal Medicine, and American College of Obstetricians and Gynecologists workshop. Obstet Gynecol 120:1181, 2012

Sporri S, Hanggi W, Brahetti A, et al: Pelvimetry by magnetic resonance imaging as a diagnostic tool to evaluate dystocia. Obstet Gynecol 89:902, 1997

Stark DD, McCarthy SM, Filly RA, et al: Pelvimetry by magnetic resonance imaging. Am J Radiol 144:947, 1985

Tebes CC, Mehta P, Calhoun DA, et al: Congenital ischemic forearm necrosis associated with a compound presentation. J Matern Fetal Med 8:281, 1999

Thoms H: The obstetrical significance of pelvic variations: a study of 450 primiparous women. BMJ 2:210, 1937

Thorp JM Jr, Pahel-Short L, Bowes WA Jr: The Mueller-Hillis maneuver: can it be used to predict dystocia? Obstet Gynecol 82:519, 1993

Thurnau GR, Scates DH, Morgan MA: The fetal-pelvic index: a method of identifying fetal-pelvic disproportion in women attempting vaginal birth after previous cesarean delivery. Am J Obstet Gynecol 165:353, 1991

Vallier HA, Cureton BA, Schubeck D: Pregnancy outcomes after pelvic ring injury. J Orthop Trauma 26(5):302, 2012

Williams JW: Obstetrics: A Textbook for the Use of Students and Practitioners, 1st ed. New York, Appleton, 1903, p 282

Williams RM, Thom MH, Studd JW: A study of the benefits and acceptability of ambulation in spontaneous labor. Br J Obstet Gynaecol 87:122, 1980

Wong CA, Scavone BM, Dugan S, et al: Incidence of postpartum lumbosacral spine and lower extremity nerve injuries. Obstet Gynecol 101:279, 2003

World Health Organization: Partographic management of labour. Lancet 343:1399, 1994

Zaretsky MV, Alexander JM, McIntire DD, et al: Magnetic resonance imaging pelvimetry and the prediction of labor dystocia. Obstet Gynecol 106:919, 2005

Zhang J, Landy HJ, Branch DW, et al: Contemporary patterns of spontaneous labor with normal neonatal outcomes. Obstet Gynecol 116:1281, 2010

CHAPTER 24

Intrapartum Assessment

Following earlier work by Hon (1958), continuous electronic fetal monitoring (EFM) was introduced into obstetrical practice in the late 1960s. No longer were intrapartum fetal surveillance and the suspicion of fetal distress based on periodic auscultation with a fetoscope. Instead, the continuous graph-paper portrayal of the fetal heart rate was potentially diagnostic in assessing pathophysiological events affecting the fetus. Indeed, there were great expectations: (1) that electronic fetal heart rate monitoring provided accurate information, (2) that the information was of value in diagnosing fetal distress, (3) that it would direct intervention to prevent fetal death or morbidity, and (4) that continuous electronic fetal heart rate monitoring was superior to intermittent methods.

When first introduced, electronic fetal heart rate monitoring was used primarily in complicated pregnancies, but gradually became used in most pregnancies. By 1978, it was estimated that nearly two thirds of American women were being monitored electronically during labor (Banta, 1979). Currently, more than 85 percent of all live births in the United States undergo electronic fetal monitoring (Ananth, 2013). Indeed, fetal monitoring has become the most prevalent obstetrical procedure in this country.

ELECTRONIC FETAL MONITORING

Internal (Direct) Electronic Monitoring

The fetus can be monitored electronically by direct or indirect methods. Direct fetal heart measurement is accomplished by attaching a bipolar spiral electrode directly to the fetus (Fig. 24-1). The wire electrode penetrates the fetal scalp, and the second pole is a metal wing on the electrode. Vaginal body fluids create a saline electrical bridge that completes the circuit and permits measurement of the voltage differences between the two poles. The two wires of the bipolar electrode are attached to a reference electrode on the maternal thigh to eliminate electrical interference. The electrical fetal cardiac signal—P wave, QRS complex, and T wave—is amplified and fed into a cardiotachometer for heart rate calculation. The peak R-wave voltage is the portion of the fetal electrocardiogram most reliably detected.

An example of the method of fetal heart rate processing employed when a scalp electrode is used is shown in Figure 24-2. Time (t) in milliseconds between fetal R waves is fed into a cardiotachometer, where a new fetal heart rate is set with the arrival of each new R wave. As also shown in Figure 24-2, a premature atrial contraction is computed as a heart rate acceleration because the interval (t_2) is shorter than the preceding one (t_1). The phenomenon of continuous R-to-R wave fetal heart rate computation is known as *beat-to-beat variability.* The physiological event being counted, however, is not a mechanical event corresponding to a heartbeat but rather an electrical event.

Electrical cardiac complexes detected by the electrode include those generated by the mother. Although the maternal

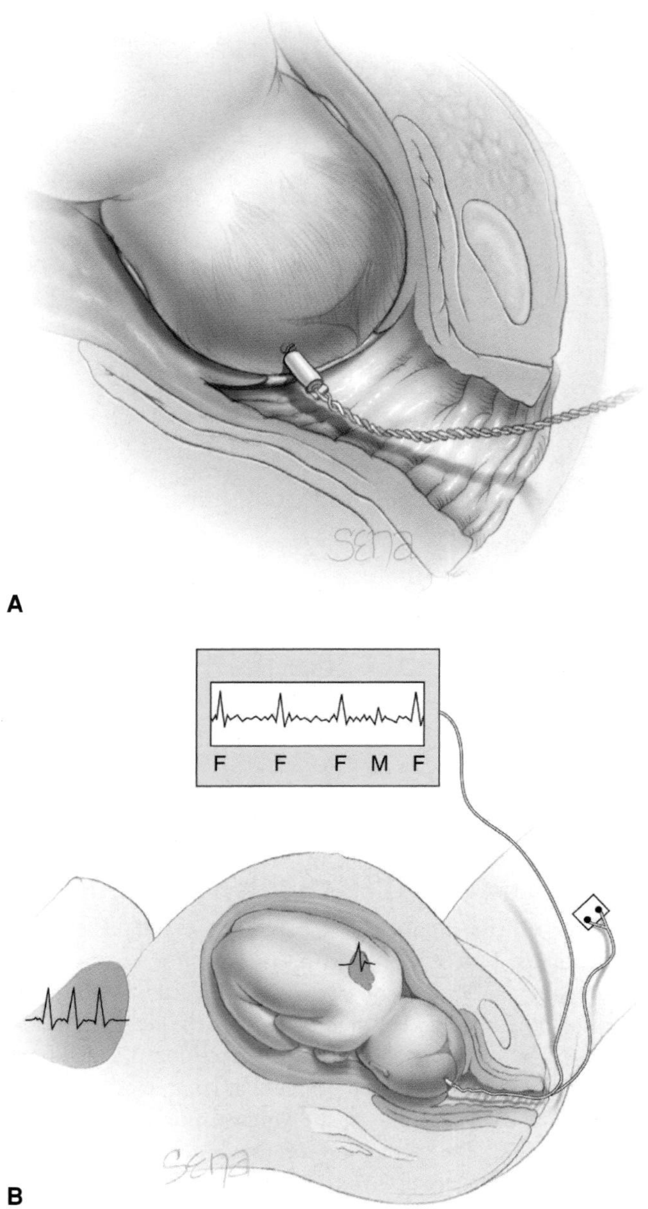

FIGURE 24-1 Internal electronic fetal monitoring. **A.** Scalp electrode penetrates the fetal scalp by means of a coiled electrode. **B.** Schematic representation of a bipolar electrode attached to the fetal scalp for detection of fetal QRS complexes (F). Also shown is the maternal heart and corresponding electrical complex (M) that is detected.

electrocardiogram (ECG) signal is approximately five times stronger than the fetal ECG, its amplitude is diminished when it is recorded through the fetal scalp electrode. In a live fetus, this low maternal ECG signal is detected but masked by the fetal ECG. If the fetus is dead, the weaker maternal signal will be amplified and displayed as the "fetal" heart rate (Freeman, 2003). Shown in Figure 24-3 are simultaneous recordings of maternal chest wall ECG signals and fetal scalp electrode ECG signals. This fetus is experiencing premature atrial contractions, which cause the cardiotachometer to rapidly and erratically seek new heart rates, resulting in the "spiking" shown in the standard fetal monitor tracing. Importantly, when the fetus

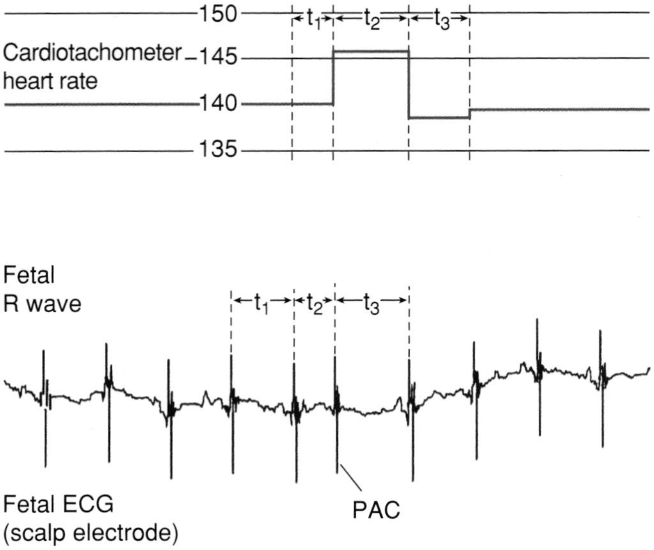

FIGURE 24-2 Schematic representation of fetal electrocardiographic signals used to compute continuing beat-to-beat heart rate with scalp electrodes. Time intervals (t_1, t_2, t_3) in milliseconds between successive fetal R waves are used by a cardiotachometer to compute instantaneous fetal heart rate. ECG = electrocardiogram; PAC = premature atrial contraction.

is dead, the maternal R waves are still detected by the scalp electrode as the next best signal and are counted by the cardiotachometer (Fig. 24-4).

External (Indirect) Electronic Monitoring

Membrane rupture may be avoided by use of external detectors to monitor fetal heart action. External monitoring, however, does not provide the precision of fetal heart rate measurement afforded by internal monitoring (Nunes, 2014).

The fetal heart rate is detected through the maternal abdominal wall using the *ultrasound Doppler principle* (Fig. 24-5). Ultrasound waves undergo a shift in frequency as they are reflected from moving fetal heart valves and from pulsatile blood ejected during systole (Chap. 10, p. 209). The unit consists of a transducer that emits ultrasound and a sensor to detect a shift in frequency of the reflected sound. The transducer is placed on the maternal abdomen at a site where fetal heart action is best detected. A coupling gel must be applied because air conducts ultrasound waves poorly. The device is held in position by a belt. Care should be taken that maternal arterial pulsations are not confused with fetal cardiac motion (Neilson, 2008).

Ultrasound Doppler signals are edited electronically before fetal heart rate data are printed onto monitor paper. Reflected ultrasound signals from moving fetal heart valves are analyzed through a microprocessor that compares incoming signals with the most recent previous signal. This process, called *autocorrelation*, is based on the premise that the fetal heart rate has regularity whereas "noise" is random and without regularity. Several fetal heart motions must be deemed electronically acceptable by the microprocessor before the fetal heart rate is printed. Such electronic editing has greatly improved the tracing quality of the externally recorded fetal heart rate.

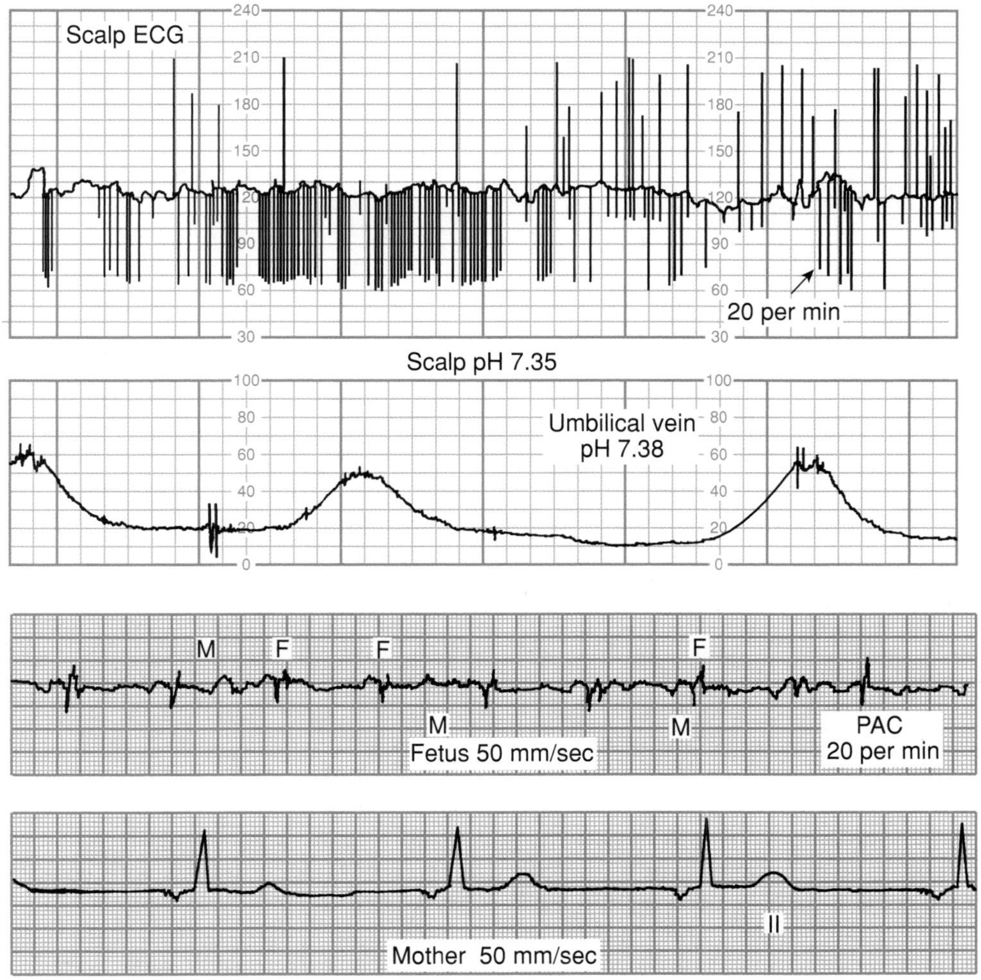

FIGURE 24-3 The top tracing shows standard fetal monitor tracing of heart rate using a fetal scalp electrode. Spiking of the fetal rate in the monitor tracing is due to premature atrial contractions. The second panel displays accompanying contractions. The bottom two tracings represent cardiac electrical complexes detected from fetal scalp and maternal chest wall electrodes. ECG = electrocardiogram; F = fetus; M = mother; PAC = fetal premature atrial contraction.

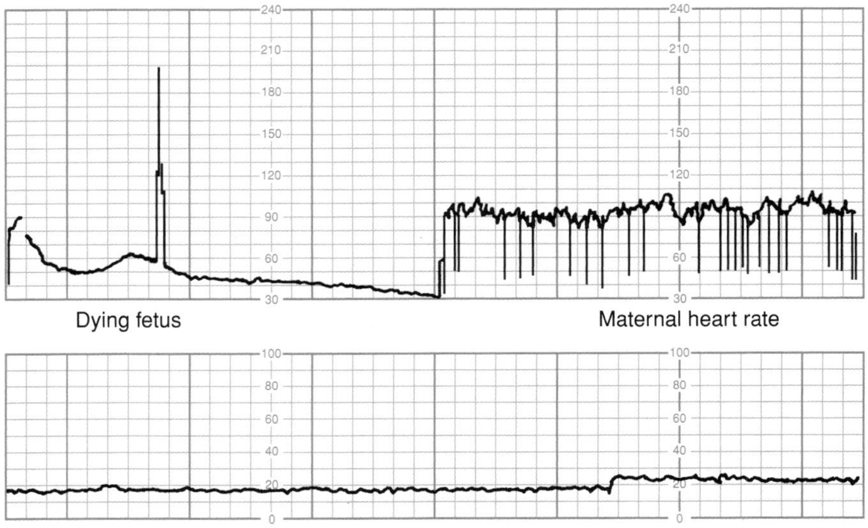

FIGURE 24-4 Placental abruption. In the upper panel, the fetal scalp electrode first detected the heart rate of the dying fetus. After fetal death, the maternal electrocardiogram complex is detected and recorded. The second panel displays an absence of uterine contractions.

Fetal Heart Rate Patterns

It is now generally accepted that interpretation of fetal heart rate patterns can be problematic because of the lack of agreement on definitions and nomenclature (American College of Obstetricians and Gynecologists, 2013b). In one example, Blackwell and colleagues (2011) asked three maternal-fetal medicine specialists to independently interpret 154 fetal heart rate tracings. Interobserver agreement was poor for the most ominous tracings and "moderate" for less severe patterns. The authors cautioned that their results represented idealized circumstances that should not be considered reflective of routine clinical practice.

The National Institute of Child Health and Human Development (NICHD) Research Planning Workshop

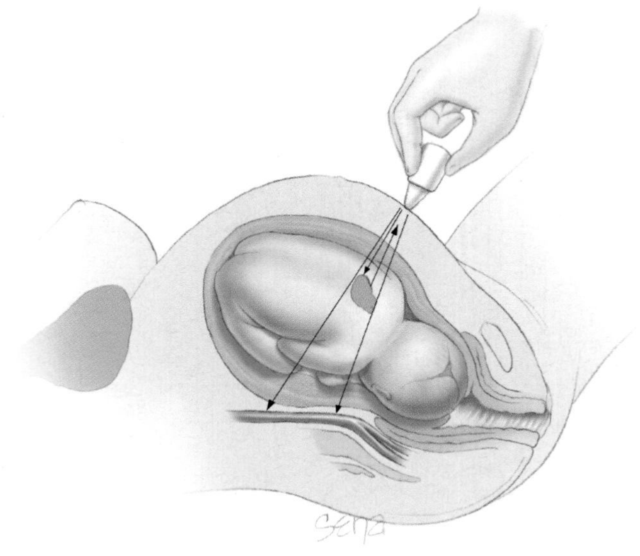

FIGURE 24-5 Ultrasound Doppler principle used externally to measure fetal heart motions. Pulsations of the maternal aorta also may be detected and erroneously counted. (Adapted from Klavan, 1977.)

(1997) brought together investigators with expertise in the field to propose standardized, unambiguous definitions for interpretation of fetal heart rate patterns during labor. This workshop was repeated in 2008. The definitions proposed and shown in Table 24-1 as a result of this second workshop are used in this chapter. First, it is important to recognize that interpretation of electronic fetal heart rate data is based on the visual pattern of the heart rate as portrayed on chart recorder graph paper. Thus, the choice of vertical and horizontal scaling greatly affects the appearance of the fetal heart rate. Scaling factors recommended by the workshop are 30 beats per minute (beats/min or bpm) per vertical cm (range, 30 to 240 bpm) and 3 cm/min chart recorder paper speed. Fetal heart rate variation is falsely displayed at the slower 1 cm/min paper speed compared with that of the smoother baseline recorded at 3 cm/min (Fig. 24-6). Thus, pattern recognition can be considerably distorted depending on the scaling factors used.

Baseline Fetal Heart Activity

This refers to the modal characteristics that prevail apart from periodic accelerations or decelerations associated with uterine contractions. Descriptive characteristics of baseline fetal heart activity include *rate, beat-to-beat variability, fetal arrhythmia*, and distinct patterns such as *sinusoidal* or *saltatory* fetal heart rates.

Rate

With increasing fetal maturation, the heart rate decreases. This continues postnatally such that the average rate is 90 bpm by age 8 (Behrman, 1992). Pillai and James (1990) longitudinally studied fetal heart rate characteristics in 43 normal pregnancies. The baseline fetal heart rate decreased an average of 24 bpm between 16 weeks and term, or approximately 1 beat/min per week. This normal gradual slowing of the fetal heart rate is thought to correspond to maturation of parasympathetic (vagal) heart control (Renou, 1969).

The baseline fetal heart rate is the approximate mean rate rounded to increments of 5 bpm during a 10-minute tracing

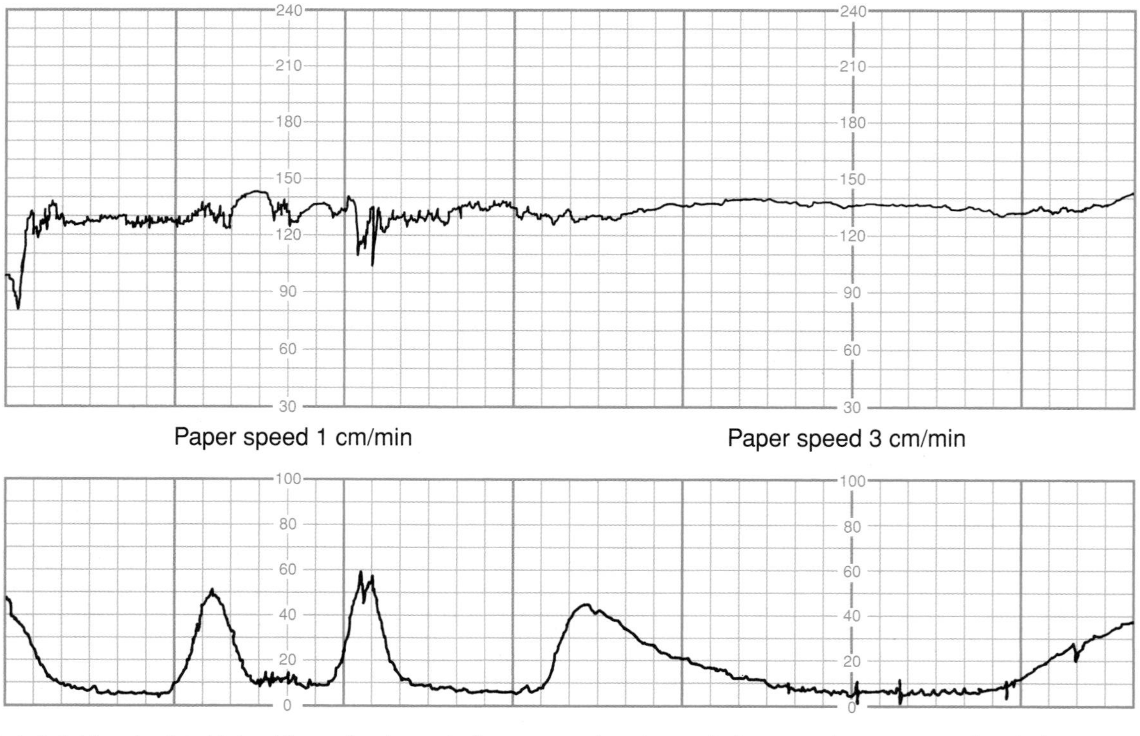

FIGURE 24-6 Fetal heart rate obtained by scalp electrode (*upper panel*) and recorded at 1 cm/min compared with that at 3 cm/min chart recorder paper speed. Concurrent uterine contractions are shown (*lower panel*).

TABLE 24-1. Electronic Fetal Monitoring Definitions

Pattern	Definition
Baseline	• The mean FHR rounded to increments of 5 bpm during a 10-min segment, excluding: —Periodic or episodic changes —Segments of baseline that differ by more than 25 bpm • The baseline must be for a minimum of 2 min in any 10-min segment or the baseline for that time period is indeterminate. In this case, one may refer to the prior 10-min window for determination of baseline. • Normal FHR baseline: 110–160 bpm • Tachycardia: FHR baselines > 160 bpm • Bradycardia: FHR baseline < 110 bpm
Baseline variability	• Fluctuations in the baseline FHR that are irregular in amplitude and frequency • Variability is visually quantified as the amplitude of peak-to-trough in bpm —Absent: amplitude range undetectable —Minimal: amplitude range detectable but ≤ 5 bpm or fewer —Moderate (normal): amplitude range 6–25 bpm —Marked: amplitude range > 25 bpm
Acceleration	• A visually apparent abrupt increase (onset to peak in < 30 sec) in the FHR • At 32 weeks and beyond, an acceleration has a peak of 15 bpm or more above baseline, with a duration of 15 sec or more but less than 2 min from onset to return • Before 32 weeks, an acceleration has a peak of 10 bpm or more above baseline, with a duration of ≥ 10 sec but < 2 min from onset to return • Prolonged acceleration lasts ≥ 2 min, but < 10 min • If an acceleration lasts 10 min, it is a baseline change
Early deceleration	• Visually apparent usually symmetrical gradual decrease and return of the FHR associated with a uterine contraction • A gradual FHR decrease is defined as from the onset to the FHR nadir of ≥ 30 sec • The decrease in FHR is calculated from the onset to the nadir of the deceleration • The nadir of the deceleration occurs at the same time as the peak of the contraction • In most cases the onset, nadir, and recovery of the deceleration are coincident with the beginning, peak, and ending of the contraction, respectively
Late deceleration	• Visually apparent usually symmetrical gradual decrease and return of the FHR associated with a uterine contraction • A gradual FHR decrease is defined as from the onset to the FHR nadir of ≥ 30 sec • The decrease in FHR is calculated from the onset to the nadir of the deceleration • The deceleration is delayed in timing, with the nadir of the deceleration occurring after the peak of the contraction • In most cases the onset, nadir, and recovery of the deceleration occur after the beginning, peak, and ending of the contraction, respectively
Variable deceleration	• Visually apparent abrupt decrease in FHR • An abrupt FHR decrease is defined as from the onset to the FHR nadir of < 30 sec • The decrease in FHR is calculated from the onset to the nadir of the deceleration • The decrease in FHR is ≥ 15 bpm, lasting ≥ 15 sec, and < 2 min in duration • When variable decelerations are associated with uterine contraction, their onset, depth, and duration commonly vary with successive uterine contractions
Prolonged deceleration	• Visually apparent decrease in the FHR below the baseline • Decrease in FHR from the baseline that is ≥ 15 bpm, lasting ≥ 2 min but < 10 min in duration • If a deceleration lasts ≥ 10 min, it is a baseline change
Sinusoidal pattern	• Visually apparent, smooth, sine wave-line undulating pattern in FHR baseline with a cycle frequency of 3–5 per minute which persists for 20 min or more

bpm = beats per minute; FHR = fetal heart rate.
Summarized from the National Institute of Child Health and Human Development Research Planning Workshop, 1997.

segment. In any 10-minute window, the minimum interpretable baseline duration must be at least 2 minutes. If the baseline fetal heart rate is less than 110 bpm, it is termed *bradycardia.* If the baseline rate is greater than 160 bpm, it is termed *tachycardia.* The average fetal heart rate is considered the result of tonic balance between *accelerator* and *decelerator* influences on pacemaker cells. In this concept, the sympathetic system is the accelerator influence, and the parasympathetic system is the decelerator factor mediated via vagal slowing of heart rate (Dawes, 1985). Heart rate also is under the control of arterial chemoreceptors such that both hypoxia and hypercapnia can modulate rate. More severe and prolonged hypoxia, with a rising blood lactate level and severe metabolic acidemia, induces a prolonged fall in heart rate (Thakor, 2009).

Bradycardia. In the third trimester, the normal mean baseline fetal heart rate has generally been accepted to range between 120 and 160 bpm. The lower normal limit is disputed internationally, with some investigators recommending 110 bpm (Manassiev, 1996). Pragmatically, a rate between 100 and 119 bpm, in the absence of other changes, usually is not considered to represent fetal compromise. Such low but potentially normal baseline heart rates also have been attributed to head compression from occiput posterior or transverse positions, particularly during second-stage labor (Young, 1976). Such mild bradycardias were observed in 2 percent of monitored pregnancies and averaged approximately 50 minutes in duration. Freeman and associates (2003) have concluded that bradycardia within the range of 80 to 120 bpm with good variability is reassuring. Interpretation of rates less than 80 bpm is problematic, and such rates generally are considered nonreassuring.

Some causes of fetal bradycardia include congenital heart block and serious fetal compromise (Jaeggi, 2008; Larma, 2007). Figure 24-7 shows bradycardia in a fetus dying from placental abruption. Maternal hypothermia under general anesthesia for repair of a cerebral aneurysm or during maternal cardiopulmonary bypass for open-heart surgery also can cause fetal bradycardia. Sustained fetal bradycardia in the setting of severe pyelonephritis and maternal hypothermia also has been reported (Hankins, 1997). These infants apparently are not harmed by several hours of such bradycardia.

Tachycardia. Fetal tachycardia is defined as a baseline heart rate greater than 160 bpm. The most common explanation for fetal tachycardia is maternal fever from chorioamnionitis, although fever from any source can increase baseline fetal heart rate. Such infections also have been observed to induce fetal tachycardia before overt maternal fever is diagnosed (Gilstrap, 1987). Fetal tachycardia caused by maternal infection typically is not associated with fetal compromise unless there are associated periodic heart rate changes or fetal sepsis.

Other causes of fetal tachycardia include fetal compromise, cardiac arrhythmias, and maternal administration of parasympathetic (atropine) or sympathomimetic (terbutaline) drugs. The key feature to distinguish fetal compromise in association

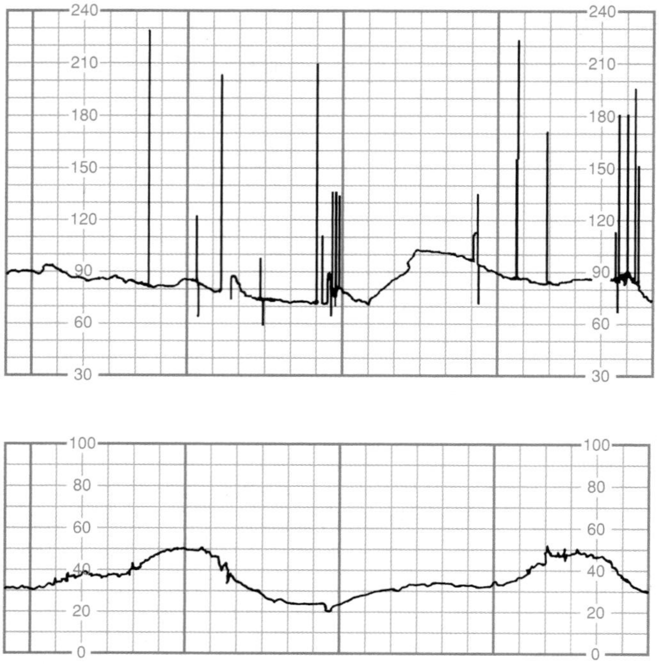

FIGURE 24-7 Fetal bradycardia measured with a scalp electrode (*upper panel*) in a pregnancy complicated by placental abruption and subsequent fetal death. Concurrent uterine contractions are shown in the lower panel.

with tachycardia seems to be concomitant heart rate decelerations. Prompt relief of the compromising event, such as correction of maternal hypotension caused by epidural analgesia, can result in fetal recovery.

Wandering Baseline. This baseline rate is unsteady and "wanders" between 120 and 160 bpm (Freeman, 2003). This rare finding is suggestive of a neurologically abnormal fetus and may occur as a preterminal event.

Beat-to-Beat Variability

Baseline variability is an important index of cardiovascular function and appears to be regulated largely by the autonomic nervous system (Kozuma, 1997). That is, a sympathetic and parasympathetic "push and pull" mediated via the sinoatrial node produces moment-to-moment or beat-to-beat oscillation of the baseline heart rate. Such heart rate change is defined as baseline variability. Variability can be further divided into short term and long term, although these terms have fallen out of use. *Short-term variability* reflects the instantaneous change in fetal heart rate from one beat—or R wave—to the next. This variability is a measure of the time interval between cardiac systoles (Fig. 24-8). Short-term variability can most reliably be determined to be normally present only when electrocardiac cycles are measured directly with a scalp electrode. *Long-term variability* is used to describe the oscillatory changes during 1 minute and result in the waviness of the baseline (Fig. 24-9). The normal frequency of such waves is three to five cycles per minute (Freeman, 2003).

It should be recognized that precise quantitative analysis of both short- and long-term variability presents a number

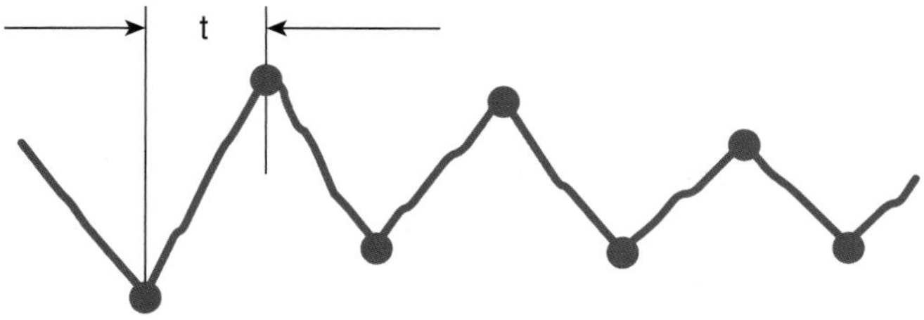

FIGURE 24-8 Schematic representation of short-term beat-to-beat variability measured by a fetal scalp electrode. t = time interval between successive fetal R waves. (Adapted from Klavan, 1977.)

of frustrating problems due to technical and scaling factors. For example, Parer and coworkers (1985) evaluated 22 mathematical formulas designed to quantify heart rate variability and found most to be unsatisfactory. Consequently, most clinical interpretation is based on visual analysis with subjective judgment of the smoothness or flatness of the baseline. According to Freeman and colleagues (2003), there is no current evidence that the distinction between short- and long-term variability has any clinical relevance. Similarly, the NICHD Workshop (1997) did not recommend differentiating short- and long-term variability because in actual practice they are visually determined as a unit. The workshop panel defined baseline variability as those baseline fluctuations of two cycles per minute or greater. They recommended the criteria shown in Figure 24-10 for quantification of variability. Normal beat-to-beat variability was accepted to be 6 to 25 bpm.

Increased Variability. Several physiological and pathological processes can affect or interfere with beat-to-beat variability. Dawes and associates (1981) described increased variability during *fetal breathing.* In healthy infants, short-term variability is attributable to respiratory sinus arrhythmia (Divon, 1986). *Fetal body movements* also affect variability (Van Geijn, 1980). Pillai and James (1990) reported increased baseline variability with *advancing gestation.* Up to 30 weeks, baseline characteristics were similar during both fetal rest and activity. After 30 weeks, fetal inactivity was associated with diminished baseline variability and conversely, variability was increased during fetal activity. Fetal gender does not affect heart rate variability (Ogueh, 1998).

The baseline fetal heart rate becomes more physiologically fixed (less variable) as the rate increases. Conversely, there is more instability or variability of the baseline at lower heart

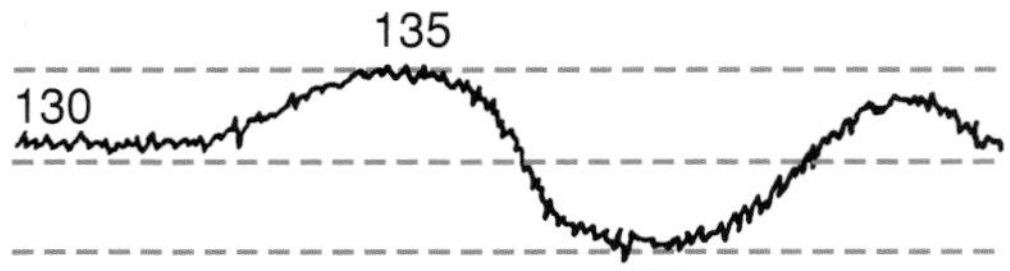

FIGURE 24-9 Schematic representation of long-term beat-to-beat variability of the fetal heart rate ranging between 125 and 135 bpm. (Adapted from Klavan, 1977.)

rates. This phenomenon presumably reflects less cardiovascular physiological wandering as beat-to-beat intervals shorten due to increasing heart rate.

Decreased Variability. Diminished beat-to-beat variability can be an ominous sign indicating a seriously compromised fetus. Paul and coworkers (1975) reported that loss of variability in combination with decelerations was associated with *fetal acidemia.* They analyzed variability in the 20 minutes preceding delivery in 194 pregnancies. Decreased variability was defined as 5 or fewer bpm excursion of the baseline (see Fig. 24-10), whereas acceptable variability exceeded this range. Fetal scalp pH was measured 1119 times in these pregnancies, and mean values were found to be increasingly acidemic when decreased variability was added to progressively intense heart rate decelerations. For example, mean fetal scalp pH of approximately 7.10 was found when severe decelerations were combined with 5 bpm or less variability, compared with a pH of approximately 7.20 when greater variability was associated with similarly severe decelerations. Severe *maternal acidemia* also can cause decreased fetal beat-to-beat variability, as shown in Figure 24-11 in a mother with diabetic ketoacidosis.

The precise pathological mechanisms by which fetal hypoxemia results in diminished beat-to-beat variability are not totally understood. Interestingly, mild degrees of fetal hypoxemia have been reported actually to *increase* variability, at least at the outset of the hypoxic episode (Murotsuki, 1997). According to Dawes (1985), it seems probable that the loss of variability is a result of metabolic acidemia that causes depression of the fetal brainstem or the heart itself. Thus, diminished beat-to-beat variability, when it reflects fetal compromise, likely reflects acidemia rather than hypoxia.

A common cause of diminished beat-to-beat variability is administration of *analgesic drugs* during labor (Chap. 25, p. 506). Various central nervous system depressant drugs can cause transient diminished beat-to-beat variability. Included are narcotics, barbiturates, phenothiazines, tranquilizers, and general anesthetics. Variability regularly diminishes within 5 to 10 minutes following intravenous meperidine administration, and the effects may last up to 60 minutes or longer depending on the dosage given (Petrie, 1993). Butorphanol given intravenously diminishes fetal heart rate reactivity (Schucker, 1996). In a study performed at Parkland Hospital, Hill and colleagues (2003) found that 5 bpm or less variability occurred in 30 percent of women given continuous intravenous meperidine compared with 7 percent in those given continuous labor epidural analgesia.

Magnesium sulfate, widely used in the United States for tocolysis as well as management of hypertensive women, has been arguably associated with diminished beat-to-beat variability. Hallak and associates (1999) randomly assigned 34 normal, nonlaboring women to standard magnesium sulfate infusion versus isotonic saline. Magnesium sulfate was associated with statistically decreased variability only in the third hour of the infusion. The average decrease in variability was deemed clinically insignificant, however, because the mean variability was

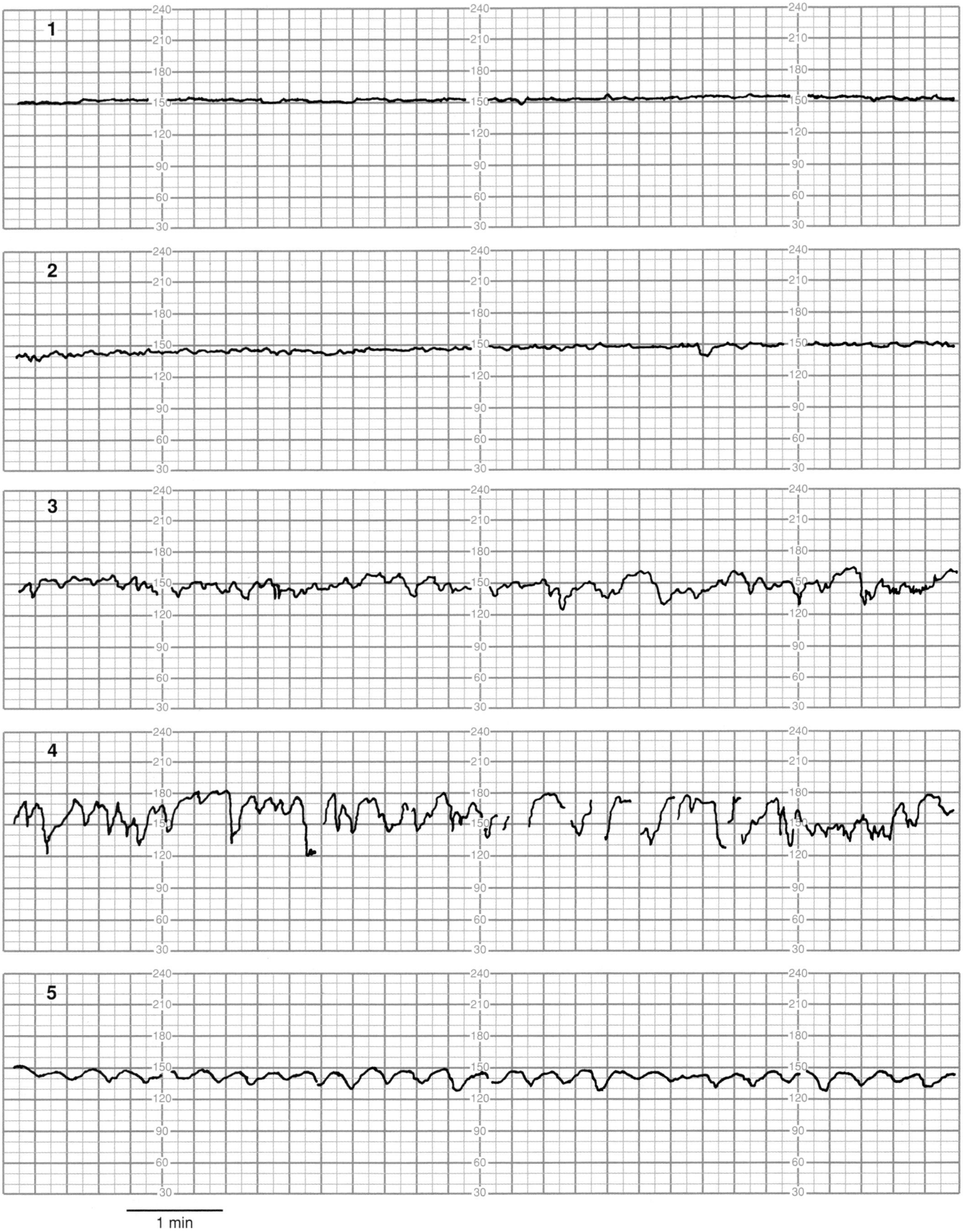

FIGURE 24-10 Grades of baseline fetal heart rate variability shown in the following five panels. **1.** Undetectable, absent variability. **2.** Minimal variability, ≤ 5 bpm. **3.** Moderate (normal) variability, 6 to 25 bpm. **4.** Marked variability, > 25 bpm. **5.** Sinusoidal pattern. This differs from variability in that it has a smooth, sinelike pattern of regular fluctuation and is excluded in the definition of fetal heart rate variability. (Adapted from National Institute of Child Health and Human Development Research Planning Workshop, 1997.)

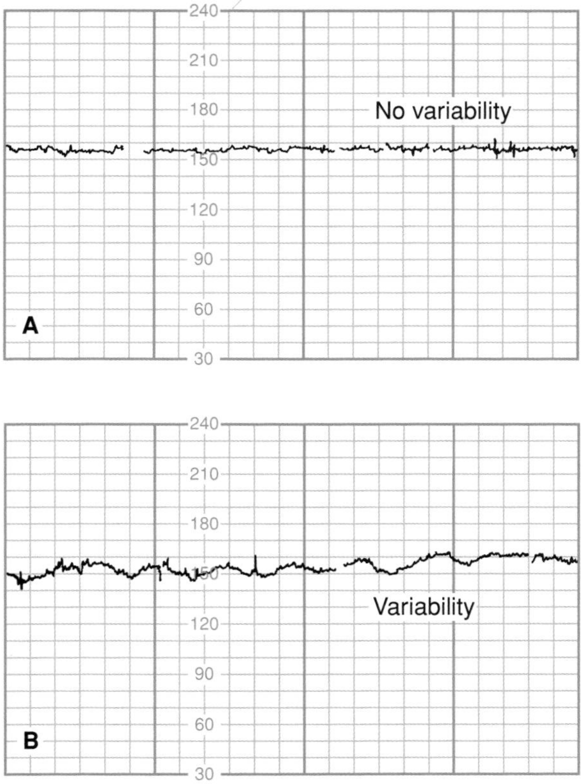

FIGURE 24-11 **A.** External fetal heart recording showing lack of long-term variability at 31 weeks during maternal diabetic keto-acidosis (pH 7.09). **B.** Recovery of fetal long-term variability after correction of maternal acidemia.

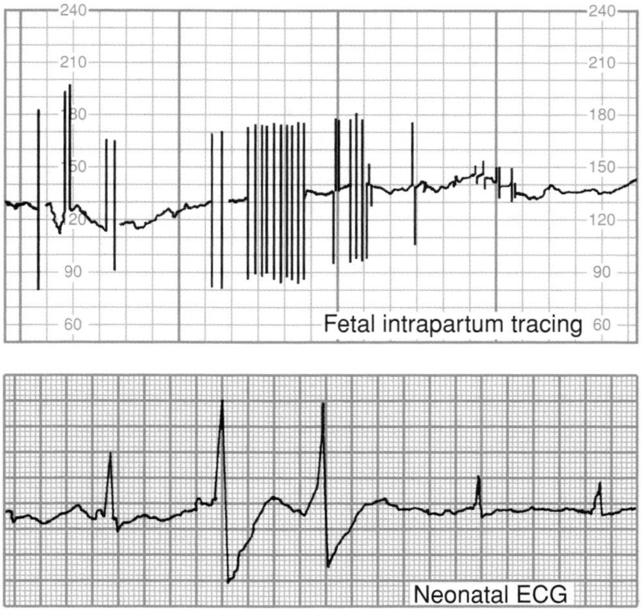

FIGURE 24-12 Internal fetal monitoring at term demonstrated occasional abrupt beat-to-beat fetal heart rate spiking due to erratic extrasystoles shown in the corresponding fetal electrocardiogram. The normal infant was delivered spontaneously and had normal cardiac rhythm in the nursery.

2.7 bpm in the third hour of magnesium infusion compared with 2.8 bpm at baseline. Magnesium sulfate also blunted the frequency of accelerations.

It is generally believed that reduced baseline heart rate variability is the single most reliable sign of fetal compromise. Smith and coworkers (1988) performed a computerized analysis of beat-to-beat variability in growth-restricted fetuses before labor. They observed that diminished variability (4.2 bpm or less) that was maintained for 1 hour was diagnostic of developing acidemia and imminent fetal death. By contrast, Samueloff and associates (1994) evaluated variability as a predictor of fetal outcome during labor in 2200 consecutive deliveries. They concluded that variability by itself could not be used as the only indicator of fetal well-being. Conversely, they also concluded that good variability should not be interpreted as necessarily reassuring. Blackwell and associates (2011) found that even experts often disagreed as to whether variability was absent or minimal (< 5 beats per minute).

In summary, beat-to-beat variability is affected by various pathological and physiological mechanisms. Variability has considerably different meaning depending on the clinical setting. The development of decreased variability in the absence of decelerations is unlikely to be due to fetal hypoxia (Davidson, 1992). A persistently flat fetal heart rate baseline—absent variability—within the normal baseline rate range and without decelerations may reflect a previous insult to the fetus that has resulted in neurological damage (Freeman, 2003).

Cardiac Arrhythmia

When fetal cardiac arrhythmias are first suspected using electronic monitoring, findings can include baseline bradycardia, tachycardia, or most commonly in our experience, *abrupt baseline spiking* (Fig. 24-12). Intermittent baseline bradycardia is frequently due to congenital heart block. As discussed in Chapter 59 (p. 1172), conduction defects, most commonly complete atrioventricular (AV) block, usually are found in association with maternal connective-tissue diseases. An arrhythmia can only be documented, practically speaking, when scalp electrodes are used. Some fetal monitors can be adapted to output the scalp electrode signals into an electrocardiographic recorder. Because only a single lead is obtained, analysis and interpretation of rhythm and rate disturbances are severely limited.

Southall and associates (1980) studied antepartum fetal cardiac rate and rhythm disturbances in 934 normal pregnancies between 30 and 40 weeks. Arrhythmias, episodes of bradycardia < 100 bpm, or tachycardia > 180 bpm were encountered in 3 percent. Most supraventricular arrhythmias are of little significance during labor unless there is coexistent heart failure as evidenced by fetal hydrops. Many supraventricular arrhythmias disappear in the immediate neonatal period, although some are associated with structural cardiac defects (Api, 2008). Copel and coworkers (2000) used echocardiography to evaluate 614 fetuses referred for auscultated irregular heart rate without hydrops. Only 10 fetuses (2 percent) were found to have significant arrhythmias, and all but one of these infants survived.

Boldt and colleagues (2003) followed 292 consecutive fetuses diagnosed with a cardiac arrhythmia through birth and into childhood. Atrial extrasystoles were the most common arrhythmia (68 percent), followed by atrial tachycardias (12 percent), atrioventricular block (12 percent), sinus bradycardia (5 percent), and ventricular extrasystoles (2.5 percent). Chromosomal anomalies were found in 1.7 percent of the fetuses. Fetal hydrops developed in 11 percent, and 2 percent had intrauterine death. Fetal hydrops was a bad prognostic finding. Overall, 93 percent of the study population was alive at a median follow-up period of 5 years, and 3 percent—seven infants—had neurological handicaps. Of the infants with atrial extrasystoles, 97 percent lived, and none suffered neurological injury. Only 6 percent required postnatal cardiac medications. Lopriore and associates (2009) found low rates of death and long-term neurological impairment in fetuses with supraventricular tachycardia or atrial flutter. In contrast, higher mortality rates were noted in those with atrioventricular block.

Although most fetal arrhythmias are of little consequence during labor when there is no evidence of fetal hydrops, such arrhythmias impair interpretation of intrapartum heart rate tracings. Sonographic evaluation of fetal anatomy and echocardiography may be useful. Some clinicians use fetal scalp sampling as an adjunct. Generally, in the absence of fetal hydrops, neonatal outcome is not measurably improved by pregnancy intervention. At Parkland Hospital, intrapartum fetal cardiac arrhythmias, especially those associate with clear amnionic fluid, are managed conservatively. Freeman and colleagues (2003) have extensively reviewed interpretation of the fetal electrocardiogram during labor.

Sinusoidal Heart Rate

A true sinusoidal pattern such as that shown in panel 5 of Figure 24-10 may be observed with fetal intracranial hemorrhage, with severe fetal asphyxia, and with severe fetal anemia from Rh alloimmunization, fetomaternal hemorrhage, twin-twin transfusion syndrome, or vasa previa with bleeding (Modanlou, 2004). Insignificant sinusoidal patterns have been reported following administration of meperidine, morphine, alphaprodine, and butorphanol (Angel, 1984; Egley, 1991; Epstein, 1982). Shown in Figure 24-13 is a sinusoidal pattern seen with maternal meperidine administration. An important characteristic of this pattern when due to narcotics is the sine frequency of 6 cycles per minute. A sinusoidal pattern also has been described with chorioamnionitis, fetal distress, and umbilical cord occlusion (Murphy, 1991). Young (1980a) and Johnson (1981) with their coworkers concluded that intrapartum sinusoidal fetal heart patterns were not generally associated with fetal compromise.

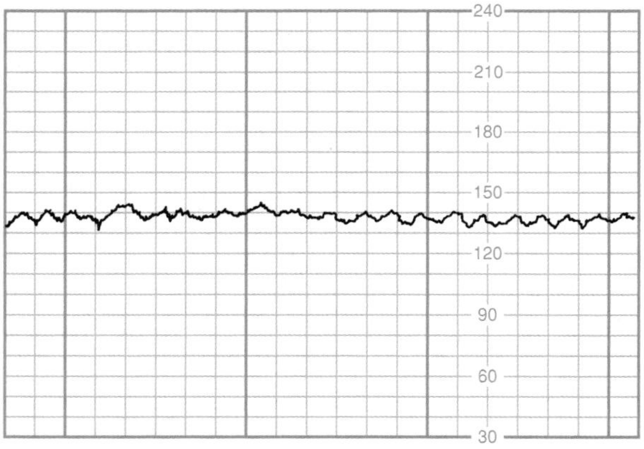

FIGURE 24-13 Sinusoidal fetal heart rate pattern associated with maternal intravenous meperidine administration. Sine waves are occurring at a rate of 6 cycles per minute.

Modanlou and Freeman (1982), based on their extensive review, proposed adoption of a strict definition:

1. Stable baseline heart rate of 120 to 160 bpm with regular oscillations,
2. Amplitude of 5 to 15 bpm (rarely greater),
3. Long-term variability frequency of 2 to 5 cycles per minute,
4. Fixed or flat short-term variability,
5. Oscillation of the sinusoidal waveform above or below a baseline, and
6. Absent accelerations.

Although these criteria were selected to define a sinusoidal pattern that is most likely ominous, they observed that the pattern associated with alphaprodine is indistinguishable. Other investigators have proposed a classification of sinusoidal heart rate patterns into mild—amplitude 5 to 15 bpm, intermediate—16 to 24 bpm, and major—25 or more bpm to quantify fetal risk (Murphy, 1991; Neesham, 1993).

Some investigators have defined intrapartum sine wavelike baseline variation with periods of acceleration as *pseudosinusoidal.* Murphy and colleagues (1991) reported that pseudosinusoidal patterns were seen in 15 percent of monitored labors. Mild pseudosinusoidal patterns were associated with use of meperidine and epidural analgesia. Intermediate pseudosinusoidal patterns were linked to fetal sucking or transient episodes of fetal hypoxia caused by umbilical cord compression. Egley and associates (1991) reported that 4 percent of fetuses demonstrated sinusoidal patterns transiently during normal labor. These authors observed patterns for up to 90 minutes in some cases and also in association with oxytocin or alphaprodine usage, or both.

The pathophysiology of sinusoidal patterns is unclear, in part due to various definitions. There seems to be general agreement that *antepartum* sine wave baseline undulation portends severe fetal anemia. Still, few D-alloimmunized fetuses develop this pattern (Nicolaides, 1989). The sinusoidal pattern has been reported to develop or disappear after fetal transfusion (Del Valle, 1992; Lowe, 1984). Ikeda and associates (1999) have proposed, based on studies in fetal lambs, that the sinusoidal fetal heart rate pattern is related to waves of arterial blood pressure, reflecting oscillations in the baroreceptor-chemoreceptor feedback mechanism for control of the circulation.

Periodic Fetal Heart Rate Changes

The periodic fetal heart rate refers to deviations from baseline that are temporally related to uterine contractions. *Acceleration* refers to an increase in fetal heart rate above baseline and *deceleration* to a decrease below the baseline rate. The nomenclature most commonly used in the United States is based on the *timing* of the deceleration in relation to contractions—thus, *early, late,* or *variable* in onset related to the corresponding uterine contraction. The waveform of these decelerations is also significant for pattern recognition. In early and late decelerations, the slope of fetal heart rate change is gradual, resulting in a curvilinear and uniform or symmetrical waveform. With variable decelerations, the slope of fetal heart rate change is abrupt and erratic, giving the waveform a jagged appearance. The 1997 workshop proposed that decelerations be defined as *recurrent* if they occur with 50 percent or more of contractions in any 20-minute period.

Another system now used less often to describe decelerations is based on the pathophysiological events considered most likely to cause the pattern. In this system, early decelerations are termed *head compression,* late decelerations are termed *uteroplacental insufficiency,* and variable decelerations become *cord compression patterns.*

Accelerations

These are visually apparent abrupt increases—defined as onset of acceleration to a peak in less than 30 seconds—in the fetal heart rate baseline (American College of Obstetricians and Gynecologists, 2013b). At 32 weeks' gestation and beyond, the acceleration has a peak of 15 bpm with a duration of 15 seconds or more but less than 2 minutes (see Table 24-1). Before 32 weeks, a peak of 10 bpm for 15 seconds to 2 minutes is considered normal. Prolonged acceleration was defined as 2 minutes or more but less than 10 minutes.

According to Freeman and coworkers (2003), accelerations most often occur antepartum, in early labor, and in association with variable decelerations. Proposed mechanisms for intrapartum accelerations include fetal movement, stimulation by uterine contractions, umbilical cord occlusion, and fetal stimulation during pelvic examination. Fetal scalp blood sampling and acoustic stimulation also incite fetal heart rate acceleration (Clark, 1982). Finally, accelerations can occur during labor without any apparent stimulus. Indeed, they are common in labor and are nearly always associated with fetal movement. These accelerations are virtually always reassuring and almost always confirm that the fetus is not acidemic at that time.

Accelerations seem to have the same physiological explanations as beat-to-beat variability in that they represent intact neurohormonal cardiovascular control mechanisms linked to fetal behavioral states. Krebs and colleagues (1982) analyzed electronic heart rate tracings in nearly 2000 fetuses and found sporadic accelerations during labor in 99.8 percent. Fetal heart accelerations during the first or last 30 minutes during labor, or both, was a favorable sign for fetal well-being. The absence of such accelerations during labor, however, is not necessarily an unfavorable sign unless coincidental with other nonreassuring changes. There is an approximately 50-percent chance of acidemia in the fetus who fails to respond to stimulation in the presence of an otherwise nonreassuring pattern (Clark, 1984; Smith, 1986).

Early Deceleration

This consists of a gradual decrease and return to baseline associated with a contraction (Fig. 24-14). Such early deceleration was first described by Hon (1958), who observed that there was a heart rate drop with contractions and that this was related to cervical dilatation. He considered these findings to be physiological.

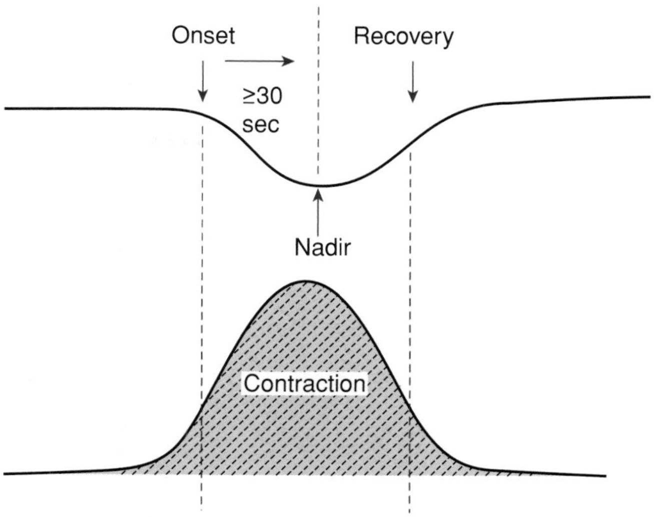

FIGURE 24-14 Features of early fetal heart rate deceleration. Characteristics include a gradual decline in the heart rate with both onset and recovery coincident with the onset and recovery of the contraction. The nadir of the deceleration is 30 seconds or more after the deceleration onset.

Freeman and associates (2003) defined early decelerations as those generally seen in active labor between 4 and 7 cm dilatation. In their definition, the degree of deceleration is generally proportional to the contraction strength and rarely falls below 100 to 110 bpm or 20 to 30 bpm below baseline. Such decelerations are common during active labor and not associated with tachycardia, loss of variability, or other fetal heart rate changes. Importantly, early decelerations are not associated with fetal hypoxia, acidemia, or low Apgar scores.

Head compression probably causes vagal nerve activation as a result of dural stimulation, and this mediates the heart rate deceleration (Paul, 1964). Ball and Parer (1992) concluded that fetal head compression is a likely cause not only of the deceleration shown in Figure 24-14 but also of those shown in Figure 24-15, which typically occur during second-stage labor. Indeed, they observed that head compression is the likely cause of many variable decelerations classically attributed to cord compression.

Late Deceleration

The fetal heart rate response to uterine contractions can be an index of either uterine perfusion or placental function. A late deceleration is a smooth, gradual, symmetrical decrease in fetal heart rate beginning at or after the contraction peak and returning to baseline only after the contraction has ended. A gradual decrease is defined as 30 seconds or more from the onset of the deceleration to the nadir. In most cases, the onset, nadir, and recovery of the deceleration occur after the beginning, peak, and ending of the contraction, respectively (Fig. 24-16). The magnitude of late decelerations is seldom more than 30 to 40 bpm below baseline and typically not more

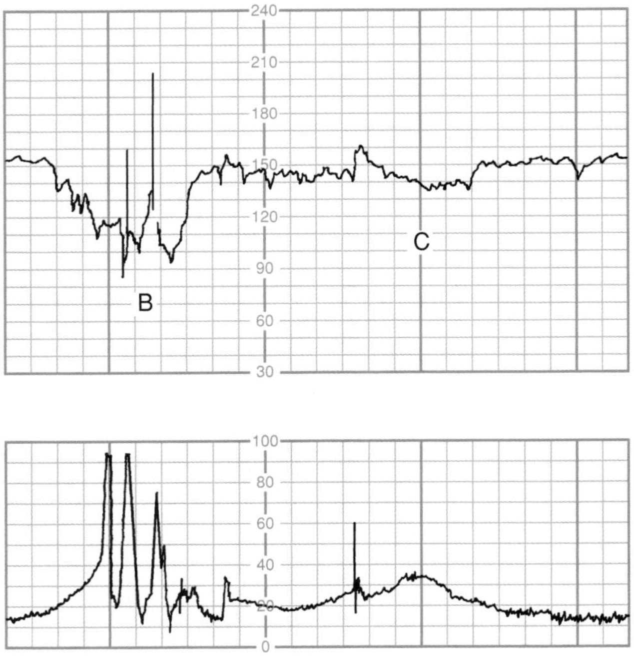

FIGURE 24-15 Two different fetal heart rate patterns during second-stage labor that are likely both due to head compression (*upper panel*). Maternal pushing efforts (*lower panel*) correspond to the spikes with uterine contractions. Fetal heart rate deceleration (*C*) is consistent with the pattern of head compression shown in Figure 24-14. Deceleration (*B*), however, is "variable" in appearance because of its jagged configuration and may alternatively represent cord occlusion.

than 10 to 20 bpm. Late decelerations usually are not accompanied by accelerations.

Myers and associates (1973) studied monkeys in which they compromised uteroplacental perfusion by lowering maternal aortic blood pressure. The interval or lag from the contraction onset until the late deceleration onset was directly related to basal fetal oxygenation. They demonstrated that the length of the lag phase was predictive of the fetal Po_2 but not fetal pH.

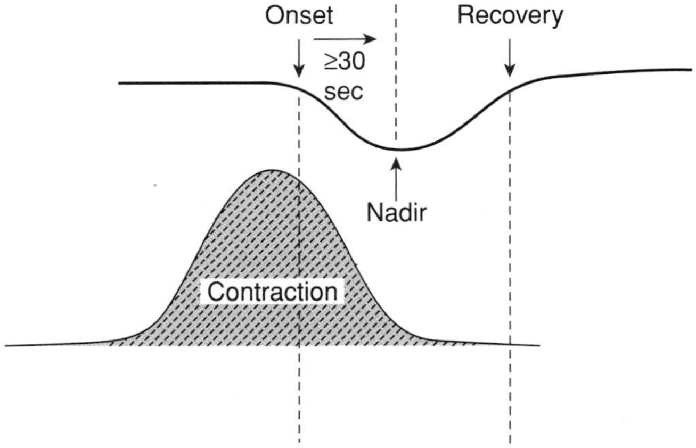

FIGURE 24-16 Features of late fetal heart rate deceleration. Characteristics include gradual decline in the heart rate with the contraction nadir, and recovery occurring after the end of the contraction. The nadir of the deceleration occurs 30 seconds or more after the onset of the deceleration.

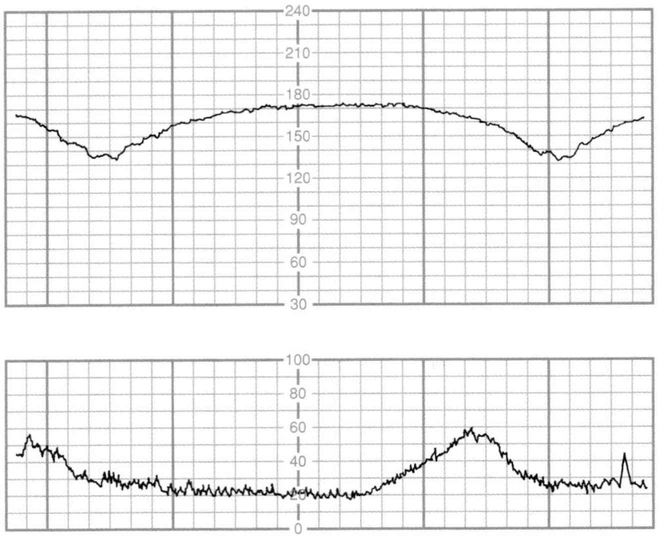

FIGURE 24-17 Late decelerations due to uteroplacental insufficiency resulting from placental abruption. Immediate cesarean delivery was performed. Umbilical artery pH was 7.05 and the Po_2 was 11 mm Hg.

The lower the fetal Po_2 before contractions, the shorter the lag phase to onset of late decelerations. This lag period reflected the time necessary for the fetal Po_2 to fall below a critical level necessary to stimulate arterial chemoreceptors, which mediated decelerations.

Murata and coworkers (1982) also showed that a late deceleration was the first fetal heart rate consequence of uteroplacental-induced hypoxia. During the course of progressive hypoxia that led to death over 2 to 13 days, monkey fetuses invariably exhibited late decelerations before development of acidemia. Variability of the baseline heart rate disappeared as acidemia developed.

Numerous clinical circumstances can result in late decelerations. Generally, any process that causes maternal hypotension, excessive uterine activity, or placental dysfunction can induce late decelerations. The two most common causes are hypotension from epidural analgesia and uterine hyperactivity caused by oxytocin stimulation. Maternal diseases such as hypertension, diabetes, and collagen-vascular disorders can cause chronic placental dysfunction. Placental abruption can cause acute late decelerations (Fig. 24-17).

Variable Deceleration

The most common deceleration patterns encountered during labor are variable decelerations attributed to umbilical cord occlusion. Melchior and Bernard (1985) identified variable decelerations in 40 percent of more than 7000 monitor tracings when labor had progressed to 5 cm dilatation and in 83 percent by the end of the first stage of labor. Variable deceleration is defined as an abrupt decrease in the fetal heart rate beginning with the onset of the contraction and reaching a nadir in less than 30 seconds. The decrease must last between ≥ 15 seconds and 2 minutes and must be ≥ 15 bpm in amplitude. The onset of deceleration typically varies with successive contractions (Fig. 24-18).

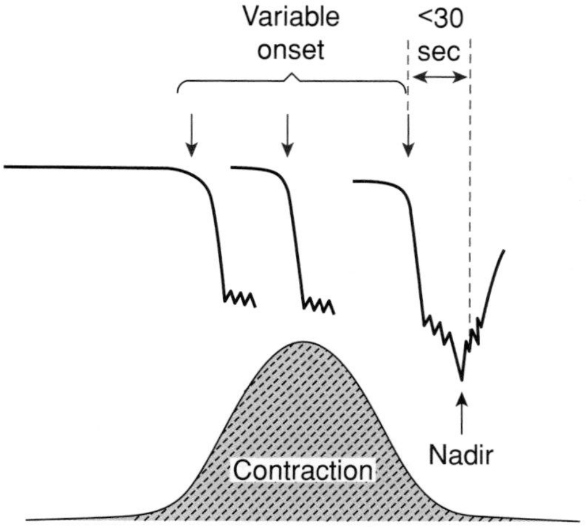

FIGURE 24-18 Features of variable fetal heart rate decelerations. Characteristics include an abrupt decline in the heart rate, and onset that commonly varies with successive contractions. The decelerations measure ≥ 15 bpm for ≥ 15 seconds and have an onset-to-nadir phase of < 30 seconds. Total duration is < 2 minutes.

Very early in the development of electronic monitoring, Hon (1959) tested the effects of umbilical cord compression on fetal heart rate (Fig. 24-19). Similar complete occlusion of the umbilical cord in experimental animals produces abrupt, jagged-appearing deceleration of the fetal heart rate (Fig. 24-20). Concomitantly, fetal aortic pressure increases. Itskovitz and colleagues (1983) observed that variable decelerations in fetal lambs occurred only after umbilical blood flow was reduced by at least 50 percent.

Two types of variable decelerations are shown in Figure 24-21. The deceleration denoted by "A" is very much like that

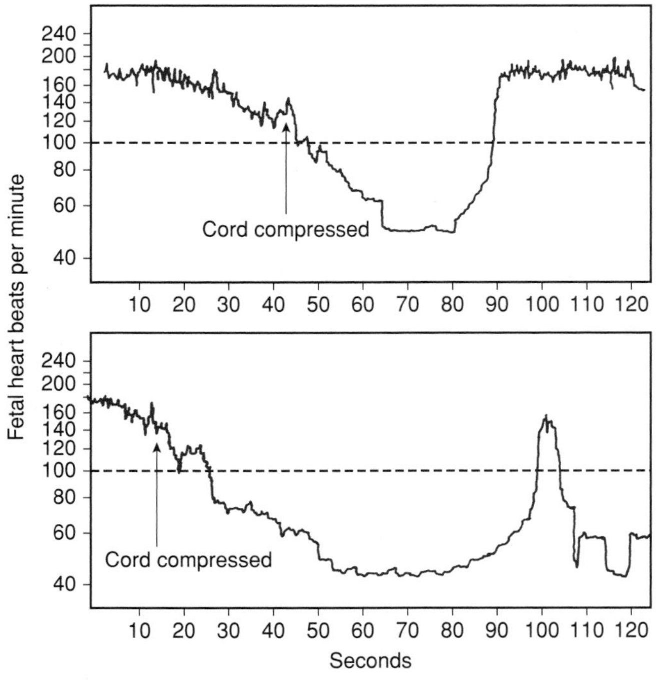

FIGURE 24-19 A. The effects of 25-second cord compression compared with those of 40 seconds in panel **(B)**. (Redrawn from Hon, 1959, with permission.)

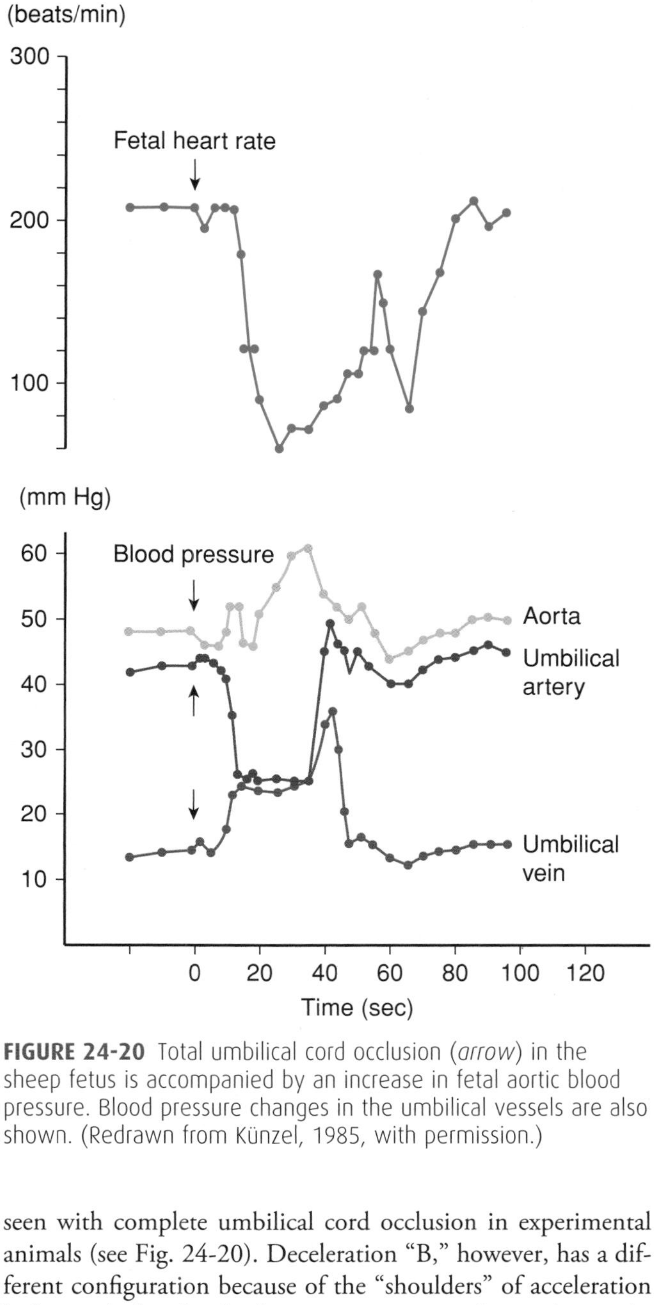

FIGURE 24-20 Total umbilical cord occlusion (*arrow*) in the sheep fetus is accompanied by an increase in fetal aortic blood pressure. Blood pressure changes in the umbilical vessels are also shown. (Redrawn from Künzel, 1985, with permission.)

seen with complete umbilical cord occlusion in experimental animals (see Fig. 24-20). Deceleration "B," however, has a different configuration because of the "shoulders" of acceleration before and after the deceleration component. Lee and coworkers (1975) proposed that this form of variable deceleration was caused by differing degrees of partial cord occlusion. In this physiological scheme, occlusion of only the vein reduces fetal blood return, thereby triggering a baroreceptor-mediated acceleration. With increasing intrauterine pressure and subsequent complete cord occlusion, fetal systemic hypertension develops due to obstruction of umbilical artery flow. This stimulates a baroreceptor-mediated deceleration. Presumably, the aftercoming shoulder of acceleration represents the same events occurring in reverse (Fig. 24-22).

Ball and Parer (1992) concluded that variable decelerations are mediated vagally and that the vagal response may be due to chemoreceptor or baroreceptor activity or both. Partial or complete cord occlusion produces an increase in afterload (baroreceptor) and a decrease in fetal arterial oxygen content (chemoreceptor). These both result in vagal activity leading to deceleration. In fetal monkeys, the baroreceptor reflexes appear to operate during the first 15 to 20 seconds of umbilical cord occlusion followed by decline in Po_2 at approximately 30 seconds, which then serves as a chemoreceptor stimulus (Mueller-Heubach, 1982).

Thus, variable decelerations represent fetal heart rate reflexes that reflect either blood pressure changes due to interruption of umbilical flow or changes in oxygenation. It is likely that most fetuses have experienced brief but recurrent periods of hypoxia due to umbilical cord compression during gestation. The frequency and inevitability of cord occlusion undoubtedly have provided the fetus with these physiological mechanisms as a means of coping. The great dilemma for the obstetrician in managing variable fetal heart rate decelerations is determining when variable decelerations are pathological. According to the American College of Obstetricians and Gynecologists (2013a), recurrent variable decelerations with minimal to moderate variability are *indeterminate,* whereas those with absent variability are *abnormal.*

Other fetal heart rate patterns have been associated with umbilical cord compression. *Saltatory* baseline heart rate (Fig. 24-23) was first described by Hammacher and colleagues (1968) and linked to umbilical cord complications during labor. The pattern consists of rapidly recurring couplets of acceleration and deceleration causing relatively large oscillations of the baseline fetal heart rate. We also observed a relationship between cord occlusion and the saltatory pattern (Leveno, 1984). In the absence of other fetal heart rate findings, these do not signal fetal compromise. *Lambda* is a pattern involving an acceleration followed by a variable deceleration with no acceleration at the end of the deceleration. This pattern typically is seen in early labor and is not ominous (Freeman, 2003). This lambda pattern may result from mild cord compression or

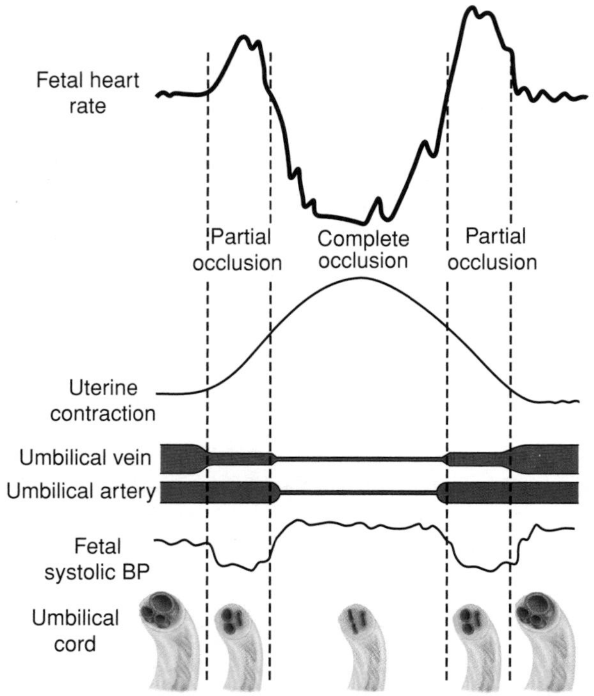

FIGURE 24-22 Schematic representation of the fetal heart rate effects with partial and complete umbilical cord occlusion. Uterine pressures generated early in a contraction cause cord compression predominantly of the thin-walled umbilical vein. The resulting decrease in fetal cardiac output leads to an initial compensatory rise in fetal heart rate. As cord compression intensifies, umbilical arteries are then also compressed. The resulting rise in fetal systolic blood pressure leads to a vagal-mediated fetal heart rate deceleration. As the contraction abates and compression is relieved first on the umbilical arteries, elevated fetal systolic blood pressures drop and the deceleration resolves. A final increase in fetal heart rate is seen as a result of persistent umbilical vein occlusion. With completion of the uterine contraction and cord compression, the fetal heart rate returns to baseline. BP = blood pressure. (Adapted from Lee, 1975.)

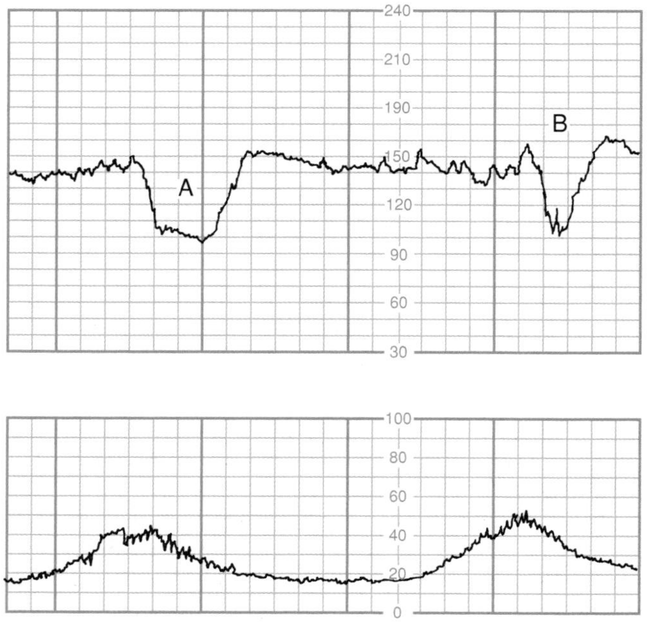

FIGURE 24-21 Varying (variable) fetal heart rate decelerations. Deceleration (*B*) exhibits "shoulders" of acceleration compared with deceleration (*A*). (Adapted from Künzel, 1985, with permission.)

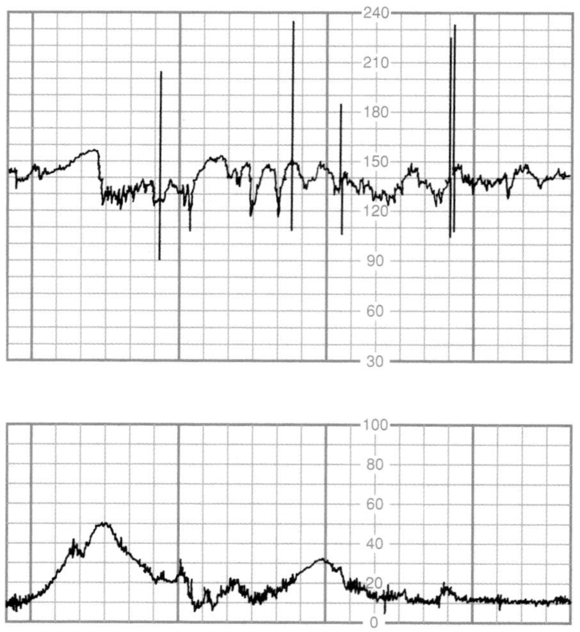

FIGURE 24-23 Saltatory baseline fetal heart rate showing rapidly recurring couplets of acceleration combined with deceleration.

stretch. *Overshoot* is a variable deceleration followed by acceleration. The clinical significance of this pattern is controversial (Westgate, 2001).

Prolonged Deceleration

This pattern, which is shown in Figure 24-24, is defined as an isolated deceleration greater than 15 bpm lasting 2 minutes or longer but < 10 minutes from onset to return to baseline. Prolonged decelerations are difficult to interpret because they are seen in many different clinical situations. Some of the more common causes include cervical examination, uterine hyperactivity, cord entanglement, and maternal supine hypotension.

Epidural, spinal, or paracervical analgesia may induce prolonged deceleration of the fetal heart rate. For example, Eberle and coworkers (1998) reported that prolonged decelerations occurred in 4 percent of normal parturients given either epidural or intrathecal labor analgesia. Hill and associates (2003) observed prolonged deceleration in 1 percent of women given epidural analgesia during labor at Parkland Hospital. Other causes of prolonged deceleration include maternal hypoperfusion or hypoxia from any cause, placental abruption, umbilical cord knots or prolapse, maternal seizures including eclampsia and epilepsy, application of a fetal scalp electrode, impending birth, or even maternal Valsalva maneuver.

The placenta is very effective in resuscitating the fetus if the original insult does not recur immediately. Occasionally, such self-limited prolonged decelerations are followed by loss of beat-to-beat variability, baseline tachycardia, and even a period of late decelerations, all of which resolve as the fetus recovers. Freeman and colleagues (2003) emphasize rightfully that the fetus may die during prolonged decelerations. Thus, management of prolonged decelerations can be extremely tenuous. Management of isolated prolonged decelerations is based on bedside clinical judgment, which inevitably will sometimes be imperfect given the unpredictability of these decelerations.

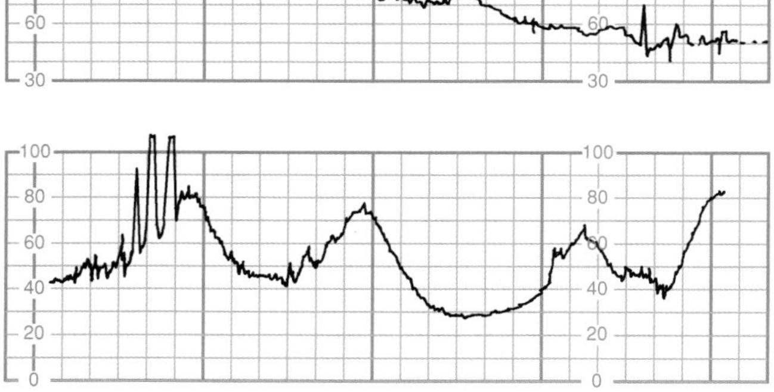

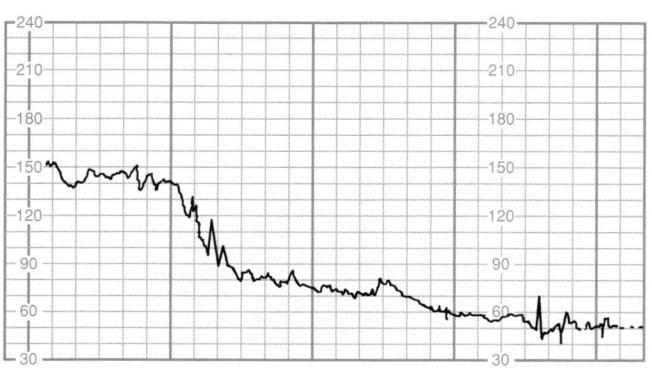

FIGURE 24-24 Prolonged fetal heart rate deceleration due to uterine hyperactivity. Approximately 3 minutes of the tracing are shown, but the fetal heart rate returned to normal after uterine hypertonus resolved. Vaginal delivery later ensued.

Fetal Heart Rate Patterns During Second-Stage Labor

Decelerations are virtually ubiquitous during the second stage. Melchior and Bernard (1985) reported that only 1.4 percent of more than 7000 deliveries lacked decelerations during second-stage labor. Both cord compression and fetal head compression have been implicated as causes of decelerations and baseline bradycardia during second-stage labor. The high incidence of such patterns minimized their potential significance during the early development and interpretation of electronic monitoring. For example, Boehm (1975) described profound, prolonged fetal heart rate deceleration in the 10 minutes preceding vaginal delivery of 18 healthy infants. However, Herbert and Boehm (1981) later reported another 18 pregnancies with similar prolonged second-stage decelerations. There was one stillbirth and one neonatal death. These experiences attest to the unpredictability of the fetal heart rate during second-stage labor.

Spong and associates (1998) analyzed the characteristics of second-stage variable fetal heart rate decelerations in 250 deliveries and found that as the total number of decelerations to < 70 bpm increased, the 5-minute Apgar score decreased. Put another way, the longer a fetus was exposed to variable decelerations, the lower the Apgar score was at 5 minutes.

Picquard and coworkers (1988) analyzed heart rate patterns during second-stage labor in 234 women in an attempt to identify specific patterns to diagnose fetal compromise. Loss of beat-to-beat variability and baseline fetal heart rate < 90 bpm were predictive of fetal acidemia. Krebs and associates (1981) also found that persistent or progressive baseline bradycardia and baseline tachycardia were associated with low Apgar scores. Gull and colleagues (1996) observed that abrupt fetal heart rate deceleration to < 100 bpm associated with loss of beat-to-beat variability for 4 minutes or longer was predictive of fetal acidemia. Thus, abnormal baseline heart rate—either bradycardia or tachycardia, absent beat-to-beat variability, or both—in the presence of second-stage decelerations, is associated with increased but not inevitable fetal compromise (Fig. 24-25).

Admission Fetal Monitoring in Low-Risk Pregnancies

With this approach, women with low-risk pregnancies are monitored for a short time on admission for labor, and continuous monitoring is used only if fetal heart rate abnormalities are subsequently identified. Mires and coworkers (2001) randomly assigned 3752 low-risk women in spontaneous labor at admission either to auscultation of the fetal heart or to 20 minutes of electronic fetal monitoring. Use of admission electronic fetal monitoring did not improve infant outcome. Moreover, its use

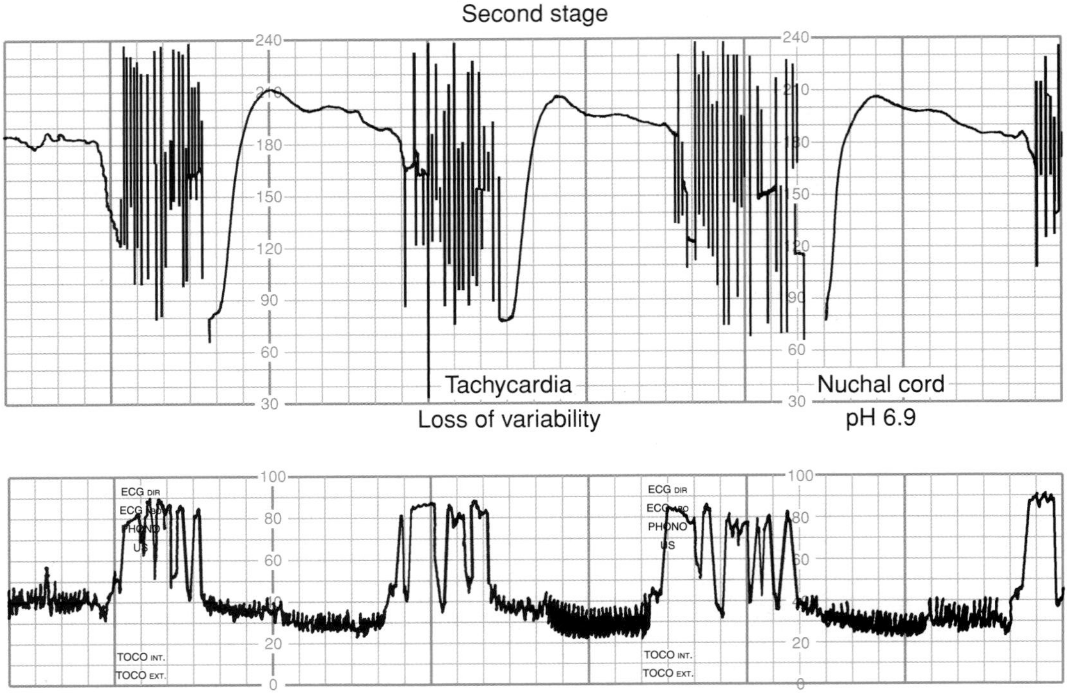

FIGURE 24-25 Cord-compression fetal heart rate decelerations in second-stage labor associated with tachycardia and loss of variability. The umbilical cord arterial pH was 6.9.

resulted in increased interventions, including operative delivery. Impey and associates (2003) performed a similar study in 8588 low-risk women and also found no improvement in infant outcome. More than half of the women enrolled in these studies, whether they received admission electronic monitoring or auscultation, eventually required continuous monitoring for diagnosed abnormalities in the fetal heart rate.

With the increasing rate of scheduled cesarean deliveries in the United States, clinicians and hospitals must decide whether fetal monitoring is required before the procedure in low-risk women. The American College of Obstetricians and Gynecologists (2010) has concluded that data are insufficient to determine the value of fetal monitoring under these circumstances.

Centralized Monitoring

Technological advances have made it possible to observe fetal heart rate monitors from a remote, centralized location. Such intrapartum monitoring equipment has become common in American labor and delivery units. The rationale behind centralized monitoring is that the ability to monitor several patients simultaneously would lead to better outcomes. What is the evidence that this rationale is correct? To our knowledge, only one study on centralized fetal monitoring has been reported. Anderson and colleagues (2011) measured the ability of 12 individuals to detect critical signals in fetal heart rate tracings on one, two, or four monitors. The results showed that detection accuracy declined as the number of displays increased.

OTHER INTRAPARTUM ASSESSMENT TECHNIQUES

Fetal Scalp Blood Sampling

According to the American College of Obstetricians and Gynecologists (2009), measurements of the pH in capillary scalp blood may help to identify the fetus in serious distress. That said, it also emphasized that neither normal nor abnormal scalp pH results have been shown to be predictive of infant outcome. The College also indicated that the procedure is now used uncommonly and is not even available at some hospitals.

For completion, an illuminated endoscope is inserted through the dilated cervix after membrane rupture so as to press firmly against the fetal scalp (Fig. 24-26). The skin is wiped clean with a cotton swab and coated with a silicone gel to cause the blood to accumulate as discrete globules. An incision is made through the skin to a depth of 2 mm with a special blade on a long handle. As a drop of blood forms on the surface, it is immediately collected into a heparinized glass capillary tube. The pH of the blood is measured promptly.

The pH of fetal capillary scalp blood is usually lower than that of umbilical venous blood and approaches that of umbilical arterial blood. Zalar and Quilligan (1979) recommended a protocol to try to confirm fetal distress. If the pH is > 7.25, labor is observed, and if between 7.20 and 7.25, the pH measurement is repeated within 30 minutes. If the pH is < 7.20, another scalp blood sample is collected immediately, and the mother is taken to an operating room and prepared for surgery. Delivery is performed promptly if the low pH is confirmed. Otherwise, labor is allowed to continue, and scalp blood samples are repeated periodically.

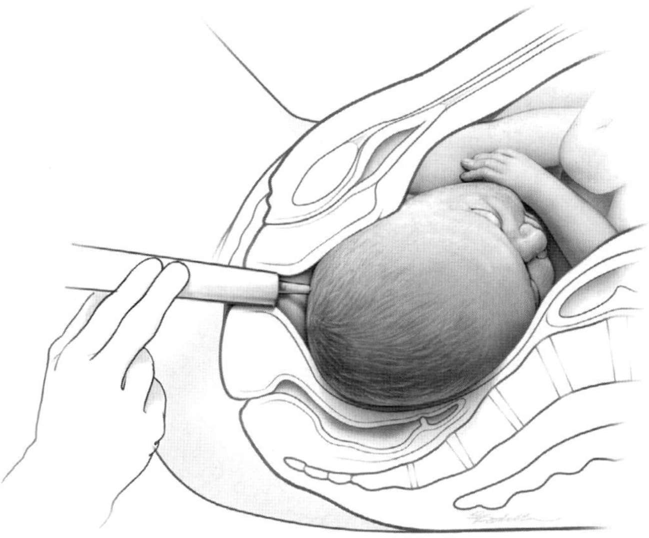

FIGURE 24-26 The technique of fetal scalp sampling using an amnioscope. The end of the endoscope is displaced from the fetal vertex approximately 2 cm to show the disposable blade against the fetal scalp before incision. (Adapted from Hamilton, 1974.)

The only benefits reported for scalp pH testing are fewer cesarean deliveries for fetal distress (Young, 1980b). Goodwin and coworkers (1994), however, in a study of 112,000 deliveries, showed a decrease in the scalp pH sampling rate. The rate dropped from approximately 1.8 percent in the mid-1980s to 0.03 percent by 1992 but with no increased delivery rate for fetal distress. They concluded that scalp pH sampling was unnecessary. Kruger and colleagues (1999) have advocated the use of fetal scalp blood lactate concentration as an adjunct to pH. Wiberg-Itzel and associates (2008) randomized 1496 fetuses to scalp blood pH analysis and 1496 to scalp blood lactate analysis. They found either to be equivalent in predicting fetal acidemia. The advantage of lactate measurement was that a smaller amount of blood was needed, which led to a lower procedural failure rate compared with scalp sampling for pH.

Scalp Stimulation

Clark and coworkers (1984) have suggested that scalp stimulation is an alternative to scalp blood sampling. This proposal was based on the observation that heart rate acceleration in response to pinching of the scalp with an Allis clamp just before obtaining blood was invariably associated with a normal pH. Conversely, failure to provoke acceleration was not uniformly predictive of fetal acidemia. Later, Elimian and associates (1997) reported that of 58 cases in which the fetal heart rate accelerated ≥ 10 bpm after 15 seconds of gentle digital stroking of the scalp, 100 percent had a scalp pH of ≥ 7.20. Without an acceleration, however, only 30 percent had a scalp pH < 7.20.

Vibroacoustic Stimulation

Fetal heart rate acceleration in response to vibroacoustic stimulation has been recommended as a substitute for scalp sampling (Edersheim, 1987). The technique uses an electronic artificial larynx placed approximately 1 cm from or directly onto the maternal abdomen (Chap. 17, p. 341). Response to vibroacoustic stimulation is considered normal if a fetal heart rate acceleration of at least 15 bpm for at least 15 seconds occurs within 15 seconds after the stimulation and with prolonged fetal movements (Sherer, 1994). Lin and colleagues (2001) prospectively studied vibroacoustic stimulation in 113 women in labor with either moderate to severe variable or late fetal heart rate decelerations. They concluded that this technique is an effective predictor of fetal acidosis in the setting of variable decelerations. The predictability for fetal acidosis, however, is limited in the setting of late decelerations. Other investigators have reported that although vibroacoustic stimulation in second-stage labor is associated with fetal heart rate reactivity, the quality of the response did not predict neonatal outcome or enhance labor management (Anyaegbunam, 1994).

Skupski and coworkers (2002) performed a metaanalysis of reports on intrapartum fetal stimulation tests published between 1966 and 2000. Four types of fetal stimulation were analyzed and included scalp puncture for pH testing, Allis clamp pinching of the fetal scalp, vibroacoustic stimulation, and digital stroking of the scalp. Results were similar for all four methods. These investigators concluded that intrapartum stimulation tests were useful to exclude fetal acidemia. They cautioned, however, that these tests are "less than perfect."

Fetal Pulse Oximetry

Using technology similar to that of adult pulse oximetry, instrumentation has been developed that may allow assessment of fetal oxyhemoglobin saturation once membranes are ruptured. A unique padlike sensor such as shown in Figure 24-27 is inserted through the cervix and positioned against the fetal face, where it is held in place by the uterine wall. A transabdominal fetal pulse oximeter has also been described in

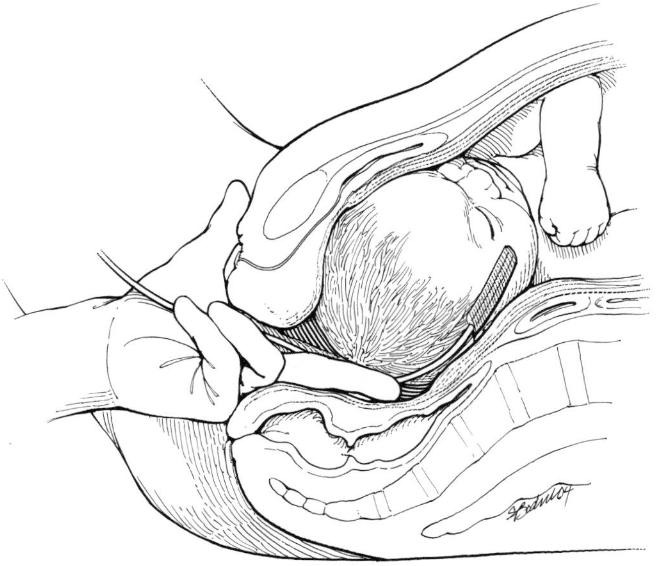

FIGURE 24-27 Schematic diagram of fetal pulse oximeter sensor placement.

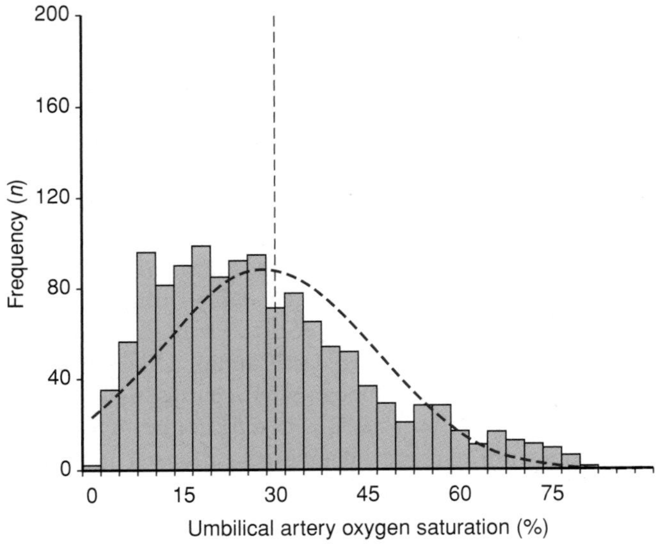

FIGURE 24-28 Frequency distribution of umbilical artery oxygen saturation values in 1281 vigorous newborn infants. Dotted line indicates normal distribution. (Redrawn from Arikan, 2000, with permission.)

a preliminary study (Vintzileos, 2005). As reviewed by Yam and coworkers (2000), the transcervical device has been used extensively by many investigators. It has been reported to reliably register fetal oxygen saturation in 70 to 95 percent of women throughout 50 to 88 percent of their labors. The lower limit for normal fetal oxygen saturation is generally considered to be 30 percent by investigators (Gorenberg, 2003; Stiller, 2002). As shown in Figure 24-28, however, fetal oxygen saturation normally varies greatly when measured in umbilical artery blood (Arikan, 2000). Bloom and associates (1999) reported that brief, transient fetal oxygen saturations below 30 percent were common during labor because such values were observed in 53 percent of fetuses with normal outcomes. Saturation values below 30 percent, however, when persistent for 2 minutes or longer, were associated with an increased risk of potential fetal compromise.

Garite and colleagues (2000) randomly assigned 1010 women with term pregnancies and in whom predefined abnormal fetal heart rate patterns developed. Patients received either conventional fetal monitoring alone or fetal monitoring plus continuous fetal pulse oximetry. Cesarean delivery for fetal distress was performed when pulse oximetry values remained < 30 percent for the entire interval between two contractions or when the fetal heart rate patterns met predefined guidelines. The use of fetal pulse oximetry significantly reduced the cesarean delivery rate for nonreassuring fetal status from 10.2 to 4.5 percent. Alternatively, the cesarean delivery rate for dystocia increased significantly from 9 to 19 percent when pulse oximetry was used. There were no neonatal benefits or adverse effects associated with fetal pulse oximetry. Based on these observations, in 2000, the Obstetrics and Gynecology Devices Panel of the Medical Devices Advisory Committee of the Food and Drug Administration (FDA) (2012) approved marketing of the Nellcor N-400 Fetal Oxygen Monitoring System.

Since then, another three randomized trials of fetal pulse oximetry have been reported. Of these, Klauser and colleagues (2005) randomly assigned 360 women with nonreassuring fetal heart rate patterns to standard fetal monitoring plus fetal pulse oximetry or to standard monitoring alone and found no benefits for oximetry. East and coworkers (2006) randomized 600 women with nonreassuring fetal heart rate patterns to standard monitoring either alone or with added fetal pulse oximetry. These investigators reported that addition of oximetry significantly reduced cesarean delivery rates for a nonreassuring fetal heart rate pattern. They further reported, however, that neonatal outcomes were not different between the study groups. Also, Bloom and associates (2006) reported the largest trial, which was performed by the Maternal-Fetal Units Network. A total of 5341 women in labor at term underwent placement of the fetal oximetry sensor, but the information was randomly withheld from care providers. Unlike the earlier studies, participants were not required to have nonreassuring fetal heart rate patterns. Sensor application was generally successful and fetal oxygen saturation values were registered 75 percent of the time. Knowledge of fetal oxygen saturation did not change the cesarean delivery rates in the overall population or in the subgroup of 2168 women who had nonreassuring fetal heart rate patterns. Moreover, neonatal outcomes were not improved by knowledge of fetal oxygen saturation status. Because of these findings, in 2005, the manufacturer discontinued sale of the fetal oximeter system in the United States.

Fetal Electrocardiography

As fetal hypoxia worsens, there are changes in the T-wave and in the ST segment of the fetal ECG. Because of this, several investigators have assessed the value of analyzing these parameters as an adjunct to conventional fetal monitoring. The technique requires internal fetal heart monitoring and special equipment to process the fetal ECG. The rationale behind this technology is based on the observation that the mature fetus exposed to hypoxemia develops an elevated ST segment with a progressive rise in T-wave height that can be expressed as a T:QRS ratio (Fig. 24-29). It is postulated that increasing T:QRS ratios reflect fetal cardiac ability to adapt to hypoxia and appears before neurological damage. Worsening hypoxia results in an increasingly negative ST-segment deflection such that it appears as a biphasic waveform (Fig. 24-30). In 2005, the manufacturer—Neoventa Medical—received FDA (2012) approval for their ST analysis program—the STAN system.

There have been a few studies of ST-segment changes with fetal monitoring. Westgate and coworkers (1993) conducted a randomized trial of 2400 pregnancies. Infant outcomes were not improved compared with those in whom conventional fetal monitoring alone was used. There was, however, a reduction in the cesarean delivery rate for fetal distress. In another randomized trial of 4966 Swedish women, Amer-Wåhlin and colleagues (2001, 2007) found that the addition of ST-segment analysis to conventional fetal monitoring significantly reduced cesarean delivery rates for fetal distress and metabolic acidemia

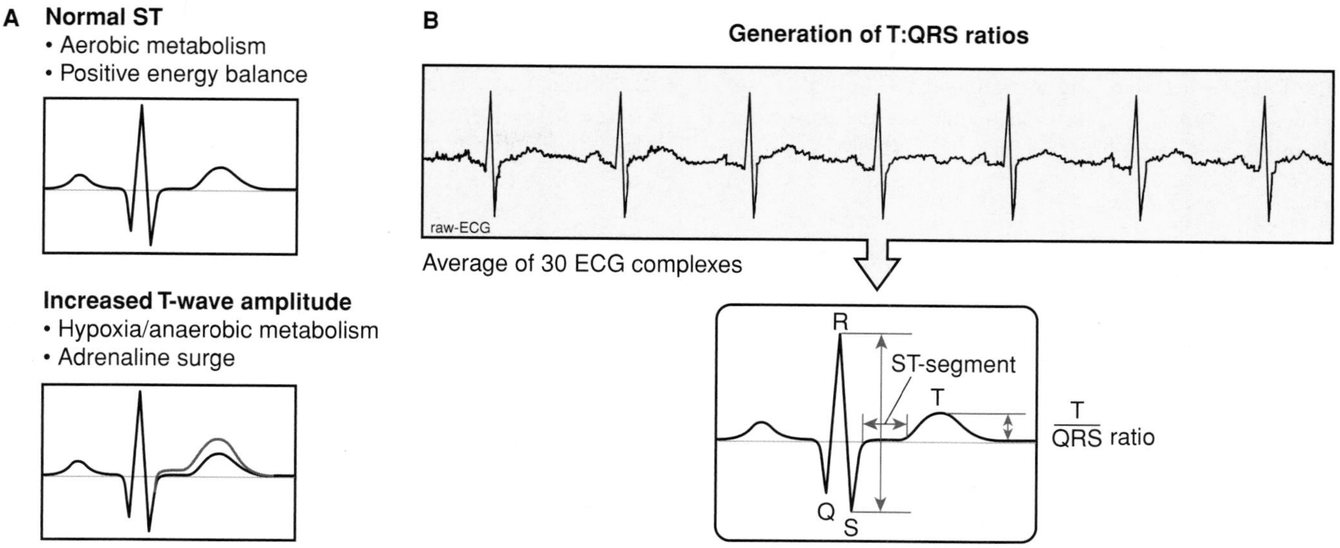

FIGURE 24-29 A. ST segment changes in normal and hypoxic conditions. **B.** Generation of T:QRS ratios. (Redrawn from Devoe, 2006, with permission.)

in umbilical artery blood. Subsequently, Doria and associates (2007) introduced STAN as a clinical practice in a London hospital and reported no changes in the incidence of operative delivery or neonatal encephalopathy. Most recently, Becker and colleagues (2012) performed a metaanalysis of five randomized trials comprising 15,352 patients and found that use of ST-segment analysis did not reduce the rates of cesarean delivery or fetal metabolic acidemia at birth.

It must be considered that ST-segment abnormalities might occur late in the course of fetal compromise. Neilson (2013) reviewed the Cochrane Database to assess fetal ECG analysis during labor. There were 16,295 women in which such monitoring was performed. He concluded that fetal ST-segment waveform analysis was perhaps useful in preventing fetal acidosis and neonatal encephalopathy when standard fetal heart rate monitoring suggested abnormal patterns. Although no randomized trials have yet been performed in the United States, the Maternal-Fetal Medicine Units Network has one in progress.

Intrapartum Doppler Velocimetry

Doppler analysis of the umbilical artery has been studied as another potential adjunct to conventional fetal monitoring. Further described in Chapter 10 (p. 219), abnormal Doppler waveforms may signify pathological umbilical-placental vessel resistance. From their review, Farrell and associates (1999) concluded that this technique was a poor predictor of adverse perinatal outcomes. They concluded that Doppler velocimetry had little if any role in fetal surveillance during labor.

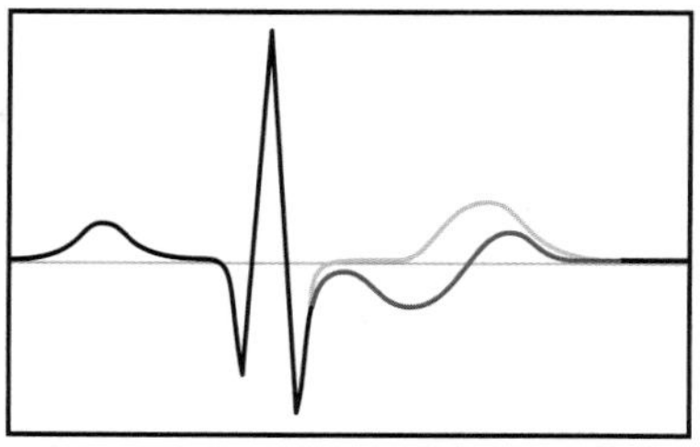

FIGURE 24-30 Biphasic ST-segment waveform with progressive fetal hypoxia. (Adapted from Devoe, 2006.)

FETAL DISTRESS

The terms *fetal distress* and *birth asphyxia* are too broad and vague to be applied with any precision to clinical situations (American College of Obstetricians and Gynecologists, 2005). Uncertainty regarding the diagnosis based on interpretation of fetal heart rate patterns has given rise to descriptions such as *reassuring* or *nonreassuring*. The term "reassuring" suggests a restoration of confidence by a particular pattern, whereas "nonreassuring" suggests inability to remove doubt. These patterns during labor are dynamic—they can rapidly change from reassuring to nonreassuring and vice versa. In this situation, obstetricians experience surges of both confidence and doubt. Put another way, most diagnoses of fetal distress using heart rate patterns occur when obstetricians lose confidence or cannot assuage doubts about fetal condition. *These assessments are subjective clinical judgments that are inevitably subject to imperfection and must be recognized as such.*

Pathophysiology

Why is the diagnosis of fetal distress based on heart rate patterns so tenuous? One explanation is that these patterns are more a reflection of fetal physiology than of pathology. Physiological control of heart rate includes various interconnected mechanisms that depend on blood flow and oxygenation. Moreover, the activity of these control mechanisms is influenced by the preexisting state of fetal oxygenation, for example, as seen with chronic placental insufficiency. Importantly, the fetus is tethered by an umbilical cord, whereby blood flow is constantly in jeopardy. Moreover, normal labor is a process of increasing acidemia (Rogers, 1998). Thus, normal labor is a process of repeated fetal hypoxic events resulting inevitably in acidemia. Put another way, and assuming that "asphyxia" can be defined as hypoxia leading to acidemia, normal parturition is an asphyxiating event for the fetus.

Diagnosis

Because of the above uncertainties, it follows that identification of "fetal distress" based on fetal heart rate patterns is imprecise and controversial. It is well known that experts in interpretation of these patterns often disagree with each other. In fact, Parer (1997), a strong advocate of electronic fetal heart rate monitoring and an organizer of the 1997 NICHD fetal monitoring workshop, lightheartedly compared the experts in attendance to marine iguanas of the Galapagos Islands, to wit: "all on the same beach but facing different directions and spitting at one another constantly!"

Ayres-de-Campos and colleagues (1999) investigated interobserver agreement of fetal heart rate pattern interpretation and found that agreement—or conversely, disagreement—was related to whether the pattern was normal, suspicious, or pathological. Specifically, experts agreed on 62 percent of normal patterns, 42 percent of suspicious patterns, and only 25 percent of pathological patterns. Keith and coworkers (1995) asked each of 17 experts to review 50 tracings on two occasions, at least 1 month apart. Approximately 20 percent changed their own interpretations, and approximately 25 percent did not agree with the interpretations of their colleagues. And although Murphy and associates (2003) concluded that at least part of the interpretation problem is due to a lack of formalized education in American training programs, this is obviously only a small modifier. Put another way, how can the teacher enlighten the student if the teacher is uncertain?

National Institutes of Health Workshops Three-Tier Classification System

The NICHD (1997) held a succession of workshops in 1995 and 1996 to develop standardized and unambiguous definitions of fetal heart rate (FHR) tracings and published recommendations for interpreting these patterns. In 2008, a second workshop was convened to reevaluate the 1997 recommendations and to clarify terminology (see Table 24-1)(Macones, 2008). A major result was the recommendation of a three-tier system for classification of FHR patterns (Table 24-2). The American College of Obstetricians and Gynecologists (2013b) subsequently recommended use of this tiered system.

TABLE 24-2. Three-Tier Fetal Heart Rate Interpretation System

Category I—Normal
Include all of the following:
- Baseline rate: 110–160 bpm
- Baseline FHR variability: moderate
- Late or variable decelerations: absent
- Early decelerations: present or absent
- Accelerations: present or absent

Category II—Indeterminate
Include all FHR tracings not categorized as Category I or III. Category II tracings may represent an appreciable fraction of those encountered in clinical care. Examples include any of the following:

Baseline rate
- Bradycardia not accompanied by absent baseline variability
- Tachycardia

Baseline FHR variability
- Minimal baseline variability
- Absent baseline variability not accompanied by recurrent decelerations
- Marked baseline variability

Accelerations
- Absence of induced accelerations after fetal stimulation

Periodic or episodic decelerations
- Recurrent variable decelerations accompanied by minimal or moderate baseline variability
- Prolonged deceleration ≥ 2 min but < 10 min
- Recurrent late decelerations with moderate baseline variability
- Variable decelerations with other characteristics, such as slow return to baseline, "overshoots," or "shoulders"

Category III—Abnormal
Include either:
- Absent baseline FHR variability and any of the following:
  Recurrent late decelerations
  Recurrent variable decelerations
  Bradycardia
- Sinusoidal pattern

bpm = beats per minute; FHR = fetal heart rate.
From Macones, 2008, with permission.

A few studies have been done to assess the three-tiered system. Jackson and coworkers (2011) studied 48,444 women in labor and found that category I (normal FHR) patterns were observed during labor in 99.5 percent of tracings. Category II (indeterminate FHR) patterns were found in 84.1 percent of tracings, and category III (abnormal FHR) patterns were seen in 0.1 percent (54 women). Most—84 percent of women—had a mix of categories during labor. Cahill and colleagues (2012) retrospectively studied the incidence of umbilical cord acidemia (pH ≤ 7.10) correlated with fetal heart rate characteristics during the 30 minutes preceding delivery. None of the three categories demonstrated a significant association with cord blood acidemia. The American College of Obstetricians and Gynecologists and the American Academy of Pediatrics (2014) concluded that a category I or II tracing with a 5-minute Apgar score > 7 or normal arterial blood acid-base values was not consistent with an acute hypoxic-ischemic event.

Sholapurkar (2012) also challenged the validity of the three-tier system because most abnormal fetal heart rate patterns fall into the indeterminate category II, that is, one for which no definite management recommendations can be made. It was further suggested that this resulted from most fetal heart rate decelerations being inappropriately classified as *variable* decelerations due to cord compression.

Parer and King (2010) compared the current situation in the United States with that of other countries in which a consensus on classification and management has been reached by a number of professional societies. Some of these include the Royal College of Obstetricians and Gynecologists, the Society of Obstetricians and Gynecologists of Canada, the Royal Australian and New Zealand College of Obstetricians and Gynecologists, and the Japan Society of Obstetrics and Gynecology. Parer and King (2010) further comment that the NICHD three-tier system is inadequate because category II—indeterminate FHR—consists of a "vast heterogenous mixture of patterns" that prevents development of a management strategy. Parer and Ikeda (2007) had previously proposed a color-coded five-tier system for both FHR interpretation *and management.* There have been two reports comparing the five-tier and three-tier systems. Bannerman and associates (2011) found that the two systems were similar in fetal heart rate interpretations for tracings that were either very normal or very abnormal. Coletta and coworkers (2012) found that the five-tier system had better sensitivity than the three-tier system. It is apparent that, after 50 years of continuous electronic fetal heart rate monitoring use, there is not a consensus on interpretation and management recommendations for FHR patterns (Parer, 2011).

Meconium in the Amnionic Fluid

Obstetrical teaching throughout the past century has included the concept that meconium passage is a potential warning of fetal asphyxia. In 1903, J. Whitridge Williams observed and attributed meconium passage to "relaxation of the sphincter ani muscle induced by faulty aeration of the (fetal) blood." Even so, obstetricians have also long realized that the detection of meconium during labor is problematic in the prediction of fetal distress or asphyxia. In their review, Katz and Bowes (1992) emphasized the prognostic uncertainty of meconium by referring to the topic as a "murky subject." Indeed, although 12 to 22 percent of labors are complicated by meconium, only a few are linked to infant mortality. In an investigation from Parkland Hospital, meconium was found to be a "low-risk" obstetrical hazard because the perinatal mortality rate attributable to meconium was 1 death per 1000 live births (Nathan, 1994).

Three theories have been suggested to explain fetal passage of meconium and in part may explain the tenuous connection between its detection and infant mortality. First, the pathological explanation proposes that fetuses pass meconium in response to hypoxia and that meconium therefore signals fetal compromise (Walker, 1953). Second, the physiological explanation is that in utero passage of meconium represents normal gastrointestinal tract maturation under neural control (Mathews, 1979). A final theory posits that meconium passage follows vagal stimulation from common but transient umbilical cord entrapment with resultant increased bowel peristalsis (Hon, 1961). Thus, meconium release may represent physiological processes.

Ramin and associates (1996) studied almost 8000 pregnancies with meconium-stained amnionic fluid delivered at Parkland Hospital. Meconium aspiration syndrome was significantly associated with fetal acidemia at birth. Other significant correlates of aspiration included cesarean delivery, forceps to expedite delivery, intrapartum heart rate abnormalities, depressed Apgar scores, and need for assisted ventilation at delivery. Analysis of the type of fetal acidemia based on umbilical blood gases suggested that the fetal compromise associated with meconium aspiration syndrome was an acute event. This is because most acidemic fetuses had abnormally increased P_{CO_2} values rather than a pure metabolic acidemia.

Dawes and coworkers (1972) observed that such hypercarbia in fetal lambs induces gasping and resultant increased amnionic fluid inhalation. Jovanovic and Nguyen (1989) observed that meconium gasped into the fetal lungs caused aspiration syndrome only in asphyxiated animals. Ramin and colleagues (1996) hypothesized that the pathophysiology of meconium aspiration syndrome includes, but is not limited to, fetal hypercarbia, which stimulates fetal respiration leading to aspiration of meconium into the alveoli. Lung parenchymal injury is secondary to acidemia-induced alveolar cell damage. In this pathophysiological scenario, meconium in amnionic fluid is a fetal environmental hazard rather than a marker of preexistent compromise. This proposed pathophysiological sequence is not all-inclusive, because it does not account for approximately half of the cases of meconium aspiration syndrome in which the fetus was not acidemic at birth.

Thus, it was concluded that the high incidence of meconium observed in the amnionic fluid during labor often represents fetal passage of gastrointestinal contents in conjunction with normal physiological processes. Although normal, such meconium becomes an environmental hazard when fetal acidemia supervenes. Importantly, such acidemia occurs acutely, and therefore meconium aspiration is unpredictable and likely unpreventable. Moreover, Greenwood and colleagues (2003) showed that clear amnionic fluid was also a poor predictor. In a prospective study of 8394 women with clear amnionic fluid, they found that clear fluid was an unreliable sign of fetal well-being.

Growing evidence indicates that many infants with meconium aspiration syndrome have suffered chronic hypoxia before birth (Ghidini, 2001). Blackwell and associates (2001) found that 60 percent of infants diagnosed with meconium aspiration syndrome had umbilical artery blood pH ≥ 7.20, implying that the syndrome was unrelated to the neonatal condition at delivery. Similarly, markers of chronic hypoxia, such as fetal erythropoietin levels and nucleated red blood cell counts in newborn infants, suggest that chronic hypoxia is involved in many meconium aspiration syndrome cases (Dollberg, 2001; Jazayeri, 2000).

In the recent past, routine obstetrical management of a newborn with meconium-stained amnionic fluid included intrapartum suctioning of the oropharynx and nasopharynx. Guidelines from the American Academy of Pediatrics and the American College of Obstetricians and Gynecologists, however, recommend that such infants no longer routinely receive intrapartum suctioning because it does not prevent meconium aspiration syndrome (Perlman, 2010). As discussed in Chapter 32

(p. 626), if the infant is depressed, the trachea is intubated, and meconium suctioned from beneath the glottis. If the newborn is vigorous, defined as having strong respiratory efforts, good muscle tone, and a heart rate > 100 bpm, then tracheal suction is not necessary and may injure the vocal cords.

Management Options

The principal management options for significantly variable fetal heart rate patterns consist of correcting any fetal insult, if possible. Measures suggested by the American College of Obstetricians and Gynecologists (2013b,c) are listed in Table 24-3. Moving the mother to the lateral position, correcting maternal hypotension caused by regional analgesia, and discontinuing oxytocin serve to improve uteroplacental perfusion. Examination is done to exclude prolapsed cord or impending delivery. Simpson and James (2005) assessed benefits of three maneuvers in 52 women with fetal oxygen saturation sensors already in place. They used intravenous hydration—500 to 1000 mL of lactated Ringer solution given over 20 minutes; lateral versus supine position; and using a nonrebreathing mask that administered supplemental oxygen at 10 L/min. Each of these maneuvers significantly increased fetal oxygen saturation levels, although the increments were small.

Tocolysis

A single intravenous or subcutaneous injection of 0.25 mg of terbutaline sulfate given to relax the uterus has been described as a temporizing maneuver in the management of nonreassuring fetal heart rate patterns during labor. The rationale is that inhibition of uterine contractions might improve fetal oxygenation, thus achieving in utero resuscitation. Cook and Spinnato (1994) described their experience during 10 years with terbutaline tocolysis for fetal resuscitation in 368 pregnancies. Such resuscitation improved fetal scalp blood pH values, although all fetuses underwent cesarean delivery. These investigators concluded that although the studies were small and rarely randomized, most reported favorable results with terbutaline tocolysis for nonreassuring patterns. Small intravenous doses of nitroglycerin—60 to 180 μg—also have been reported to be beneficial (Mercier, 1997). The American College of Obstetricians and Gynecologists (2013b) has concluded that there is insufficient evidence to recommend tocolysis for nonreassuring fetal heart rate patterns.

Amnioinfusion

Gabbe and coworkers (1976) showed in monkeys that removal of amnionic fluid produced variable decelerations and that replenishment of fluid with saline relieved the decelerations. Miyazaki and Taylor (1983) infused saline through an intrauterine pressure catheter in laboring women who had either variable decelerations or prolonged decelerations attributed to cord entrapment. Such therapy improved the heart rate pattern in half of the women studied. Later, Miyazaki and Nevarez (1985) randomly assigned 96 nulliparous women in labor with cord compression patterns and found that those who were treated with amnioinfusion required cesarean delivery for fetal distress less often.

Based on many of these early reports, transvaginal amnioinfusion has been extended into three clinical areas. These include: (1) treatment of variable or prolonged decelerations, (2) prophylaxis for women with oligohydramnios, as with prolonged ruptured membranes, and (3) attempts to dilute or wash out thick meconium (Chap. 33, p. 638).

Many different amnioinfusion protocols have been reported, but most include a 500- to 800-mL bolus of warmed normal

TABLE 24-3. Some Resuscitative Measures for Category II or Category III Tracings

Goal	Associated Fetal Heart Rate Abnormality[a]	Potential Intervention(s)[b]
Improve fetal oxygenation and uteroplacental blood flow	Recurrent late decelerations Prolonged decelerations or bradycardia Minimal or absent FHR variability	Initial lateral decubitus positioning Administer maternal oxygen Administer intravenous fluid bolus Reduce uterine contraction frequency
Take steps to diminish uterine activity	Tachysystole with category II or III tracing	Discontinue oxytocin or prostaglandins Tocolytics, e.g., terbutaline, magnesium sulfate
Relieve umbilical cord compression	Recurrent variable decelerations Prolonged decelerations or bradycardia	Reposition mother Amnioinfusion With prolapse of cord, manually elevate the presenting part while preparing for immediate delivery

[a]Simultaneous evaluation of the suspected cause(s) is also an important step in management of abnormal FHR tracings.
[b]The combination of multiple interventions simultaneously may be appropriate and potentially more effective than doing them individually or serially.
FHR = fetal heart rate.

TABLE 24-4. Complications Associated with Amnioinfusion from a Survey of 186 Obstetrical Units

Complication	Centers No. (%)
Uterine hypertonus	27 (14)
Abnormal fetal heart rate tracing	17 (9)
Chorioamnionitis	7 (4)
Cord prolapse	5 (2)
Uterine rupture	4 (2)
Maternal cardiac or respiratory compromise	3 (2)
Placental abruption	2 (1)
Maternal death	2 (1)

Adapted from Wenstrom, 1995.

saline followed by a continuous infusion of approximately 3 mL per minute (Owen, 1990; Pressman, 1996). In another study, Rinehart and colleagues (2000) randomly gave a 500-mL bolus of normal saline at room temperature alone or 500-mL bolus plus continuous infusion of 3 mL per minute. Their study included 65 women with variable decelerations, and the investigators found neither method to be superior. Wenstrom and associates (1995) surveyed use of amnioinfusion in teaching hospitals in the United States. The procedure was used in 96 percent of the 186 centers surveyed, and it was estimated that 3 to 4 percent of all women delivered at these centers received such infusion. Potential complications of amnioinfusion are summarized in Table 24-4.

Prophylactic Amnioinfusion for Variable Decelerations. Hofmeyr and Lawrie (2012) used the Cochrane Database to specifically analyze the effects of amnioinfusion in the management of fetal heart rate patterns associated with umbilical cord compression. Nineteen suitable studies were identified, most with fewer than 200 participants. It was concluded that amnioinfusion appeared to be useful in reducing the occurrence of variable decelerations, improving neonatal outcome, and reducing cesarean delivery rates. The American College of Obstetricians and Gynecologists (2013a) recommends consideration of amnioinfusion with persistent variable decelerations.

Prophylactic Amnioinfusion for Oligohydramnios. Amnioinfusion in women with oligohydramnios has been used prophylactically to avoid intrapartum fetal heart rate patterns from cord occlusion. Nageotte and coworkers (1991) found that this resulted in significantly decreased frequency and severity of variable decelerations in labor. However, the cesarean delivery rate or condition of term infants was not improved. In a randomized investigation, Macri and colleagues (1992) studied prophylactic amnioinfusion in 170 term and postterm pregnancies complicated by both thick meconium and oligohydramnios. Amnioinfusion significantly reduced cesarean delivery rates for fetal distress and meconium aspiration syndrome. In contrast, Ogundipe and associates (1994) randomly assigned 116 term pregnancies with an amnionic fluid index < 5 cm to receive prophylactic amnioinfusion or standard obstetrical care. There were no significant differences in overall cesarean delivery rates, delivery rates for fetal distress, or umbilical cord acid-base studies.

Amnioinfusion for Meconium-Stained Amnionic Fluid. Pierce and associates (2000) summarized the results of 13 prospective trials of intrapartum amnioinfusion in 1924 women with moderate to thick meconium-stained fluid. Infants born to women treated by amnioinfusion were significantly less likely to have meconium below the vocal cords and were less likely to develop meconium aspiration syndrome than infants born to women not undergoing amnioinfusion. The cesarean delivery rate was also lower in the amnioinfusion group. Similar results were reported by Rathore and coworkers (2002). In contrast, several investigators were not supportive of amnioinfusion for meconium staining. For example, Usta and associates (1995) reported that amnioinfusion was not feasible in half of women with moderate or thick meconium who were randomized to this treatment. These investigators were unable to demonstrate any improvement in neonatal outcomes. Spong and coworkers (1994) also concluded that although prophylactic amnioinfusion did dilute meconium, it did not improve perinatal outcome. Last, Fraser and colleagues (2005) randomized amnioinfusion in 1998 women with thick meconium staining of the amnionic fluid in labor and found no benefits. Because of these findings, the American College of Obstetricians and Gynecologists (2012a, 2013c) does not recommend amnioinfusion to dilute meconium-stained amnionic fluid. According to Xu and coworkers (2007), in areas lacking continuous monitoring, amnioinfusion may be used to lower the incidence of meconium aspiration syndrome.

Fetal Heart Rate Patterns and Brain Damage

Attempts to correlate fetal heart rate patterns with brain damage have been based primarily on studies of infants identified as a result of medicolegal actions. Phelan and Ahn (1994) reported that among 48 fetuses later found to be neurologically impaired, a persistent nonreactive fetal heart rate tracing was already present at the time of admission in 70 percent. They concluded that fetal neurological injury occurred predominately before arrival to the hospital. When they looked retrospectively at heart rate patterns in 209 brain-damaged infants, they concluded that there was not a single unique pattern associated with fetal neurological injury (Ahn, 1996). Graham and associates (2006) reviewed the world literature published between 1966 and 2006 on the effect of fetal heart rate monitoring to prevent perinatal brain injury and found no benefit.

Experimental Evidence

Fetal heart rate patterns necessary for perinatal brain damage have been studied in experimental animals. Myers (1972) described the effects of complete and partial asphyxia in rhesus monkeys in studies of brain damage due to perinatal asphyxia. Complete asphyxia was produced by total occlusion of umbilical blood flow that led to prolonged deceleration (Fig. 24-31). Fetal arterial pH did not drop to 7.0 until approximately

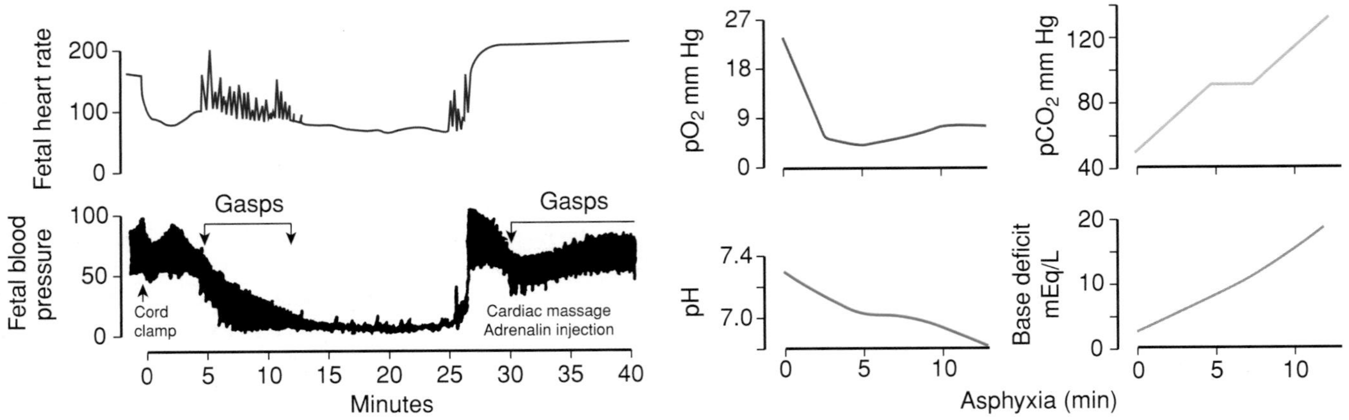

FIGURE 24-31 Prolonged deceleration in a rhesus monkey shown with blood pressure and biochemical changes during total occlusion of umbilical cord blood flow. (Adapted from Myers, 1972.)

8 minutes after complete cessation of oxygenation and umbilical flow. At least 10 minutes of such prolonged deceleration was required before there was evidence of brain damage in surviving fetuses.

Myers (1972) also produced partial asphyxia in rhesus monkeys by impeding maternal aortic blood flow. This resulted in late decelerations due to uterine and placental hypoperfusion. He observed that several hours of these late decelerations did not damage the fetal brain unless the pH fell below 7.0. Indeed, Adamsons and Myers (1977) reported subsequently that late decelerations were a marker of partial asphyxia long before brain damage occurred.

The most common fetal heart rate pattern during labor—due to umbilical cord occlusion—requires considerable time to significantly affect the fetus in experimental animals. Clapp and colleagues (1988) partially occluded the umbilical cord for 1 minute every 3 minutes in fetal sheep. Rocha and associates (2004) totally occluded the umbilical cord for 90 seconds every 30 minutes for 3 to 5 hours a day for 4 days without producing necrotic brain cell injury. Results from such studies suggest that the effects of umbilical cord entrapment depend on the degree of occlusion—partial versus total, the duration of individual occlusions, and the frequency of such occlusions.

Human Evidence

The contribution of intrapartum events to subsequent neurological handicaps has been greatly overestimated, as discussed in further detail in Chapter 33 (p. 638). It is clear that for brain damage to occur, the fetus must be exposed to much more than a brief period of hypoxia. Moreover, the hypoxia must cause profound, just barely sublethal metabolic acidemia. Because of this, the American College of Obstetricians and Gynecologists (2012b) recommends umbilical cord blood gases be obtained whenever there is cesarean delivery for fetal compromise, a low 5-minute Apgar score, severe fetal-growth restriction, an abnormal fetal heart rate tracing, maternal thyroid disease, or multifetal gestation (Chap. 32, p. 628). Fetal heart rate patterns consistent with these sublethal conditions are fortunately rare.

Benefits of Electronic Fetal Heart Rate Monitoring

There are several fallacious assumptions behind expectations of improved perinatal outcome with electronic monitoring. One assumption is that fetal distress is a slowly developing phenomenon and that electronic monitoring permits early detection of the compromised fetus. This assumption is illogical—that is, how can all fetuses die slowly? Another presumption is that all fetal damage develops in the hospital. Within the past 20 years, attention has been focused on the reality that most damaged fetuses suffered insults before arrival at labor units. The very term *fetal monitor* implies that this inanimate technology in some fashion "monitors." The assumption is made that if a dead or damaged infant is delivered, the tracing strip must provide some clue, because this device was monitoring fetal condition. All of these assumptions led to great expectations and fostered the belief that all neonatal deaths or injuries were preventable.

By the end of the 1970s, questions regarding the efficacy, safety, and costs of electronic monitoring were being voiced from the Office of Technology Assessment, the United States Congress, and the Centers for Disease Control and Prevention. Banta and Thacker (2002) reviewed 25 years of the controversy on the benefits, or lack thereof, of electronic fetal monitoring. Using the Cochrane Database, Alfirevic and colleagues (2013) reviewed 13 randomized trials involving more than 37,000 women. They concluded that electronic fetal monitoring increased the rate of cesarean and operative vaginal deliveries but produced no declines in rates of perinatal mortality, neonatal seizures, or cerebral palsy. Grimes and Peipert (2010) wrote a *Current Commentary* on electronic fetal monitoring in *Obstetrics & Gynecology.* They summarized that such monitoring, although it has been used in 85 percent of the almost 4 million annual births in the United States, has failed as a public health screening program. They noted that the positive predictive value of electronic fetal monitoring for fetal death in labor or cerebral palsy is near zero—meaning that "almost every positive test result is wrong."

There have been two recent attempts to study the epidemiological effects of electronic fetal monitoring in the United States, each using national vital statistics of births linked to infant deaths. Chen and coworkers (2011) used 2004 data on 1,732,211 singleton live births, 89 percent of which underwent electronic fetal monitoring. They reported that monitoring increased operative delivery rates but decreased early neonatal mortality rates. This benefit was gestational age dependent, however, and the highest impact was seen in preterm fetuses. Most recently, Ananth and colleagues (2013) reported a similar but larger epidemiological study using United States birth certificate data linked with infant death certificate data. They studied 57,983,286 nonanomalous singleton livebirths born between 1990 and 2004. The temporal increase in fetal monitoring use between 1990 and 2004 was associated with a decline in neonatal mortality rates, especially in preterm gestations. In an accompanying editorial, Resnik (2013) cautioned that an epidemiological association between fetal monitoring and reduced neonatal death does not establish causation. He suggested that the limitations of the study by Ananth "should make the reader skeptical of the findings." He opined that the electronic fetal monitoring debate "goes on . . . and on . . . and on." And it does indeed.

TABLE 24-5. Guidelines for Methods of Intrapartum Fetal Heart Rate Monitoring

Surveillance	Low-Risk Pregnancies	High-Risk Pregnancies
Acceptable methods		
Intermittent auscultation	Yes	Yes[a]
Continuous electronic monitoring (internal or external)	Yes	Yes[b]
Evaluation intervals		
First-stage labor (active)	30 min	15 min[a,b]
Second-stage labor	15 min	5 min[a,c]

[a]Preferably before, during, and after a uterine contraction.
[b]Includes tracing evaluation and charting at least every 15 min.
[c]Tracing should be evaluated at least every 5 min.
From the American Academy of Pediatrics and the American College of Obstetricians and Gynecologists, 2012.

Parkland Hospital Experience: Selective versus Universal Monitoring

In July 1982, an investigation began at Parkland Hospital to ascertain whether all women in labor should undergo electronic monitoring (Leveno, 1986). In alternating months, universal electronic monitoring was rotated with selective heart rate monitoring, which was the prevailing practice. During the 3-year investigation, 17,410 labors were managed using universal electronic monitoring, and these outcomes were compared with a similar-sized cohort of women selectively monitored electronically. No significant differences were found in any perinatal outcomes. There was a small but significant increase in the cesarean delivery rate for fetal distress associated with universal monitoring. Thus, increased application of electronic monitoring at Parkland Hospital did not improve perinatal results, but it slightly increased the frequency of cesarean delivery for fetal distress.

Current Recommendations

The methods most commonly used for intrapartum fetal heart rate monitoring include auscultation with a fetal stethoscope or a Doppler ultrasound device, or continuous electronic monitoring of the heart rate and uterine contractions. No scientific evidence has identified the most effective method, including the frequency or duration of fetal surveillance that ensures optimum results. Summarized in Table 24-5 are the recommendations of the American Academy of Pediatrics and the American College of Obstetricians and Gynecologists (2012). Intermittent auscultation or continuous electronic monitoring is considered an acceptable method of intrapartum surveillance in both low- and high-risk pregnancies. The recommended interval between checking the heart rate, however, is longer in the uncomplicated pregnancy. When auscultation is used, it is recommended that it be performed after a contraction and for 60 seconds. It also is recommended that a 1-to-1 nurse–patient ratio be used if auscultation is employed. The position taken by the American College of Obstetricians and Gynecologists (2013b) in their *Practice Bulletin,* however, is somewhat different. While acknowledging that the available data do not show a clear benefit for the use of electronic monitoring over intermittent auscultation, the committee recommends limiting use of auscultation to low-risk pregnancies and further recommends recording the fetal heart rate every 15 minutes in active first stage labor and every 5 minutes in the second stage.

INTRAPARTUM SURVEILLANCE OF UTERINE ACTIVITY

Analysis of electronically measured uterine activity permits some generalities concerning the relationship of certain contraction patterns to labor outcome. There is considerable normal variation, however, and caution must be exercised before judging true labor or its absence solely from a monitor tracing. Uterine muscle efficiency to effect delivery varies greatly. To use an analogy, 100-meter sprinters all have the same muscle groups yet cross the finish line at different times.

Internal Uterine Pressure Monitoring

Amnionic fluid pressure is measured between and during contractions by a fluid-filled plastic catheter with its distal tip located above the presenting part (Fig. 24-32). The catheter is connected to a strain-gauge pressure sensor adjusted to the same level as the catheter tip in the uterus. The amplified electrical signal produced in the strain gauge by variation in pressure within the fluid system is recorded on a calibrated moving paper strip simultaneously with the fetal heart rate recording (see Fig. 24-6). Intrauterine pressure catheters are now available that have the pressure sensor in the catheter tip, which obviates the need for the fluid column.

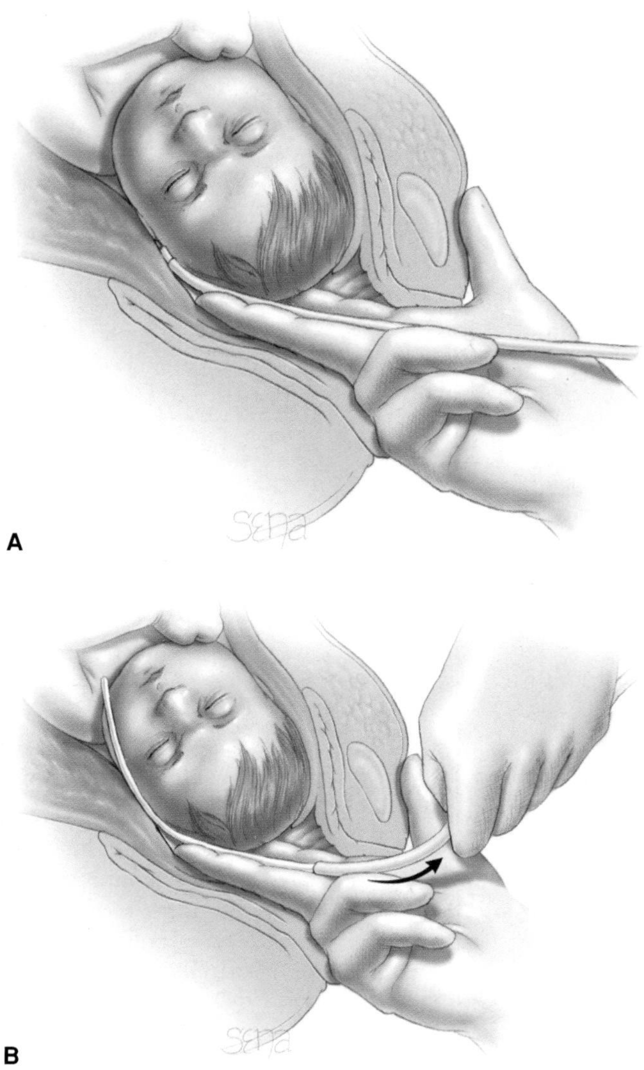

FIGURE 24-32 Placement of an intrauterine pressure catheter to monitor contractions and their pressures. **A.** The white catheter, contained within the blue introducer, is inserted into the birth canal and placed along one side of the fetal head. **B.** The catheter is then gently advanced into the uterus, and the introducer is withdrawn.

External Monitoring

Uterine contractions can be measured by a displacement transducer in which the transducer button, or "plunger," is held against the abdominal wall. As the uterus contracts, the button moves in proportion to the strength of the contraction. This movement is converted into a measurable electrical signal that indicates the *relative* intensity of the contraction. It has generally been accepted to not give an accurate measure of intensity. Bakker and associates (2010) performed a randomized trial comparing internal versus external monitoring of uterine contractions in 1456 women. The two methods were equivalent in terms of operative deliveries and neonatal outcomes.

Patterns of Uterine Activity

Caldeyro-Barcia and Poseiro (1960), from Montevideo, Uruguay, were pioneers who have done much to elucidate the patterns of spontaneous uterine activity throughout pregnancy. Contractile waves of uterine activity were usually measured using intraamnionic pressure catheters. But early in their studies, as many as four simultaneous intramyometrial microballoons were also used to record uterine pressure. These investigators also introduced the concept of *Montevideo units* to define uterine activity (Chap. 23, p. 458). By this definition, uterine performance is the product of the intensity—increased uterine pressure above baseline tone—of a contraction in mm Hg multiplied by contraction frequency per 10 minutes. For example, three contractions in 10 minutes, each of 50 mm Hg intensity, would equal 150 Montevideo units.

During the first 30 weeks of pregnancy, uterine activity is comparatively quiescent. Contractions are seldom greater than 20 mm Hg, and these have been equated with those first described in 1872 by John Braxton Hicks. Uterine activity increases gradually after 30 weeks, and it is noteworthy that these *Braxton Hicks contractions* also increase in intensity and frequency. Further increases in uterine activity are typical of the last weeks of pregnancy, termed *prelabor.* During this phase, the cervix ripens (Chap. 21, p. 410).

According to Caldeyro-Barcia and Poseiro (1960), clinical labor usually commences when uterine activity reaches values between 80 and 120 Montevideo units. This translates into approximately three contractions of 40 mm Hg every 10 minutes. Importantly, there is no clear-cut division between prelabor and labor, but rather a gradual and progressive transition.

During first-stage labor, uterine contractions increase progressively in intensity from approximately 25 mm Hg at commencement of labor to 50 mm Hg at the end. At the same time, frequency increases from three to five contractions per 10 minutes, and uterine baseline tone from 8 to 12 mm Hg. Uterine activity further increases during second-stage labor, aided by maternal pushing. Indeed, contractions of 80 to 100 mm Hg are typical and occur as frequently as five to six per 10 minutes. Interestingly, the duration of uterine contractions—60 to 80 seconds—does not increase appreciably from early active labor through the second stage (Bakker, 2007; Pontonnier, 1975). Presumably, this duration constancy serves fetal respiratory gas exchange. During a uterine contraction, as the intrauterine pressure exceeds that of the intervillous space, respiratory gas exchange is halted. This leads to functional fetal "breath holding," which has a 60- to 80-second limit that remains relatively constant.

Caldeyro-Barcia and Poseiro (1960) also observed empirically that uterine contractions are clinically palpable only after their intensity exceeds 10 mm Hg. Moreover, until the intensity of contractions reaches 40 mm Hg, the uterine wall can readily be depressed by the finger. At greater intensity, the uterine wall then becomes so hard that it resists easy depression. Uterine contractions usually are not associated with pain until their intensity exceeds 15 mm Hg, presumably because this is the minimum pressure required for distending the lower uterine segment and cervix. It follows that Braxton Hicks contractions exceeding 15 mm Hg may be perceived as uncomfortable because distention of the uterus, cervix, and birth canal is generally thought to produce discomfort.

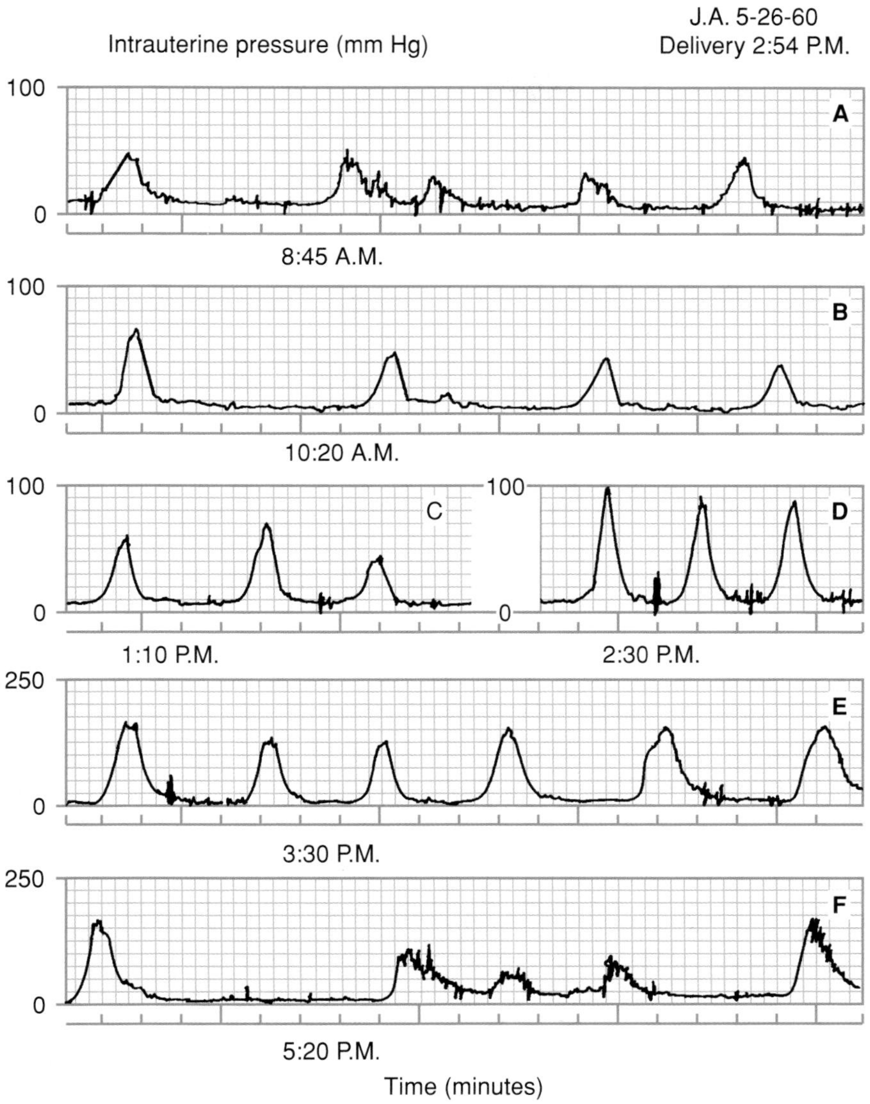

FIGURE 24-33 Intrauterine pressure recorded through a single catheter. **A.** Prelabor. **B.** Early labor. **C.** Active labor. **D.** Late labor. **E.** Spontaneous activity ½ hour postpartum. **F.** Spontaneous activity 2½ hours postpartum. (Redrawn from Hendricks, 1968, with permission.)

Hendricks (1968) observed that "the clinician makes great demands upon the uterus." The uterus is expected to remain well relaxed during pregnancy, to contract effectively but intermittently during labor, and then to remain in a state of almost constant contraction for several hours postpartum. Figure 24-33 demonstrates an example of normal uterine activity during labor. Uterine activity progressively and gradually increases from prelabor through late labor. Interestingly, as shown in Figure 24-33, uterine contractions after birth are identical to those resulting in delivery of the infant. It is therefore not surprising that the uterus that performs poorly before delivery is also prone to atony and puerperal hemorrhage.

Origin and Propagation of Contractions

The uterus has not been studied extensively in terms of its nonhormonal physiological mechanisms of function. The normal contractile wave of labor originates near the uterine end of one of the fallopian tubes. Thus, these areas act as "pacemakers" (Fig. 24-34). The right pacemaker usually predominates over the left and starts most contractile waves. Contractions spread from the pacemaker area throughout the uterus at 2 cm/sec, depolarizing the whole organ within 15 seconds. This depolarization wave propagates downward toward the cervix. Intensity is greatest in the fundus, and it diminishes in the lower uterus. This phenomenon is thought to reflect reductions in myometrial thickness from the fundus to the cervix. Presumably, this descending gradient of pressure serves to direct fetal descent toward the cervix and to efface the cervix. Importantly, all parts of the uterus are synchronized and reach their peak pressure almost simultaneously, giving rise to the curvilinear waveform shown in Figure 24-34. Young and Zhang (2004) have shown that the initiation of each contraction is triggered by a tissue-level bioelectric event.

The pacemaker theory also serves to explain the varying intensity of adjacent coupled contractions shown in panels A and B of Figure 24-33. Such coupling was termed *incoordination* by Caldeyro-Barcia and Poseiro (1960). A contractile wave begins in one cornual-region pacemaker, but does not synchronously depolarize the entire uterus. As a result, another contraction begins in the contralateral pacemaker and produces the second contractile wave of the couplet. These small contractions alternating with larger ones appear to be typical of early labor. Indeed, labor may progress with such uterine activity, albeit at a slower pace. These authors also observed that labor would progress slowly if regular contractions were hypotonic—that is, contractions with intensity less than 25 mm Hg or frequency less than 2 per 10 minutes.

Hauth and coworkers (1986) quantified uterine contraction pressures in 109 women at term who received oxytocin for labor induction or augmentation. Most of these women achieved 200 to 225 Montevideo units, and 40 percent had up to 300 units to effect delivery. The authors suggested that these levels of uterine activity should be sought before consideration of cesarean delivery for presumed dystocia.

New Terminology for Uterine Contractions

This has been recommended by the American College of Obstetricians and Gynecologists (2013b), for the description and quantification of uterine contractions. *Normal uterine activity* is defined as five or fewer contractions in 10 minutes, averaged over a 30-minute window. *Tachysystole* was defined

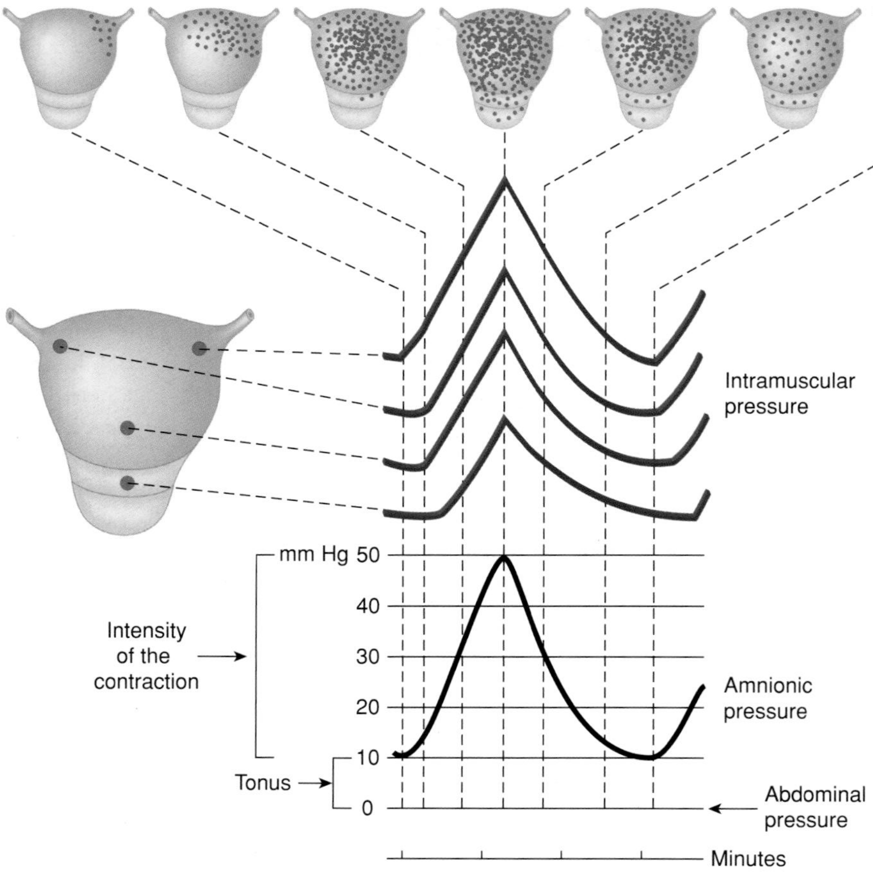

FIGURE 24-34 Schematic representation of the normal contractile wave of labor. Large uterus on the left shows the four points at which intramyometrial pressure was recorded with microballoons. Four corresponding pressure tracings are shown in relation to each other by shading on the small uteri at top. (Adapted from Caldeyro-Barcia, 1960.)

as more than five contractions in 10 minutes, averaged over 30 minutes. Tachysystole can be applied to spontaneous or induced labor (Chap. 26, p. 527). The term *hyperstimulation* was abandoned. Stewart and associates (2012) prospectively studied uterine tachysystole in 584 women undergoing labor induction with misoprostol at Parkland Hospital. There was no association of adverse infant outcomes with increasing number of contractions per 10 minutes or per 30 minutes. Six or more contractions in 10 minutes, however, were significantly associated with fetal heart rate decelerations.

Complications of Electronic Fetal Monitoring

Electrodes for fetal heart rate evaluation and catheters for uterine contraction measurement are both associated with infrequent but potentially serious complications. Rarely, an intrauterine pressure catheter during placement may lacerate a fetal vessel in the placenta. Also with insertion, placental and possibly uterine perforation can cause hemorrhage, serious morbidity, and spurious recordings that have resulted in inappropriate management. Severe cord compression has been described from entanglement with the pressure catheter. Injury to the fetal scalp or breech by a heart rate electrode is rarely severe. However, application at some other site—such as the eye in face presentations—can be serious.

Both the fetus and the mother may be at increased risk of *infection* from internal monitoring (Faro, 1990). Scalp wounds from the electrode may become infected, and subsequent cranial osteomyelitis has been reported (Brook, 2005; Eggink, 2004; McGregor, 1989). The American Academy of Pediatrics and the American College of Obstetricians and Gynecologists (2012) have recommended that certain maternal infections, including human immunodeficiency virus (HIV), herpes simplex virus, and hepatitis B and C virus, are relative contraindications to internal fetal monitoring.

REFERENCES

Adamsons K, Myers RE: Late decelerations and brain tolerance of the fetal monkey to intrapartum asphyxia. Am J Obstet Gynecol 128:893, 1977

Ahn MO, Korst L, Phelan JP: Intrapartum fetal heart rate patterns in 209 brain damaged infants. Am J Obstet Gynecol 174:492, 1996

Alfirevic Z, Devane D, Gyte GM: Continuous cardiotocography (CTG) as a form of electronic fetal monitoring (EFM) for fetal assessment during labour. Cochrane Database Syst Rev 5:CD006066, 2013

Amer-Wåhlin I, Arulkumaran S, Hagberg H, et al: Fetal electrocardiogram: ST waveform analysis in intrapartum surveillance. BJOG 114:1191, 2007

Amer-Wåhlin I, Hellsten C, Norén H, et al: Cardiotocography only versus cardiotocography plus ST analysis of fetal electrocardiogram for intrapartum fetal monitoring: a Swedish randomized controlled trial. Lancet 358:534, 2001

American Academy of Pediatrics and the American College of Obstetricians and Gynecologists: Intrapartum and postpartum care of the mother. In Guidelines for Perinatal Care, 7th ed. Washington, 2012

American College of Obstetricians and Gynecologists and American Academy of Pediatrics: Neonatal encephalopathy and neurologic outcome. Washington, March 2014, In press

American College of Obstetricians and Gynecologists: Inappropriate use of the terms fetal distress and birth asphyxia. Committee Opinion No. 326, December 2005

American College of Obstetricians and Gynecologists: Fetal monitoring prior to scheduled cesarean delivery. Committee Opinion No. 382, October 2007, Reaffirmed 2010

American College of Obstetricians and Gynecologists: Amnioinfusion does not prevent meconium aspiration syndrome. Committee Opinion No. 346, October 2006, Reaffirmed 2012a

American College of Obstetricians and Gynecologists: Umbilical cord blood gas and acid-base analysis. Committee Opinion No. 348, November 2006, Reaffirmed 2012b

American College of Obstetricians and Gynecologists: Intrapartum fetal heart rate monitoring: nomenclature, interpretation, and general management principles. Practice Bulletin No. 106, July 2009, Reaffirmed 2013a

American College of Obstetricians and Gynecologists: Management of intrapartum fetal heart rate tracings. Practice Bulletin No. 116, November 2010, Reaffirmed 2013b

American College of Obstetricians and Gynecologists: Management of delivery of a newborn with meconium stained amniotic fluid. Committee Opinion No. 379, September 2007, Reaffirmed 2013c

Ananth CV, Chauhan SP, Chen HY, et al: Electronic fetal monitoring in the United States. Obstet Gynecol 121(5):927, 2013

Anderson BL, Scerbo MW, Belfore LA, et al: Time and number of displays impact critical signal detection in fetal heart rate tracings. Am J Perinatol 28(6):435, 2011

Angel J, Knuppel R, Lake M: Sinusoidal fetal heart rate patterns associated with intravenous butorphanol administration. Am J Obstet Gynecol 149:465, 1984

Anyaegbunam AM, Ditchik A, Stoessel R, et al: Vibroacoustic stimulation of the fetus entering the second stage of labor. Obstet Gynecol 83:963, 1994

Api O, Carvalho JS: Fetal dysrhythmias. Best Pract Res Clin Obstet Gynaecol 22(1):31, 2008

Arikan GM, Scholz HS, Petru E, et al: Cord blood oxygen saturation in vigorous infants at birth: what is normal? BJOG 107:987, 2000

Ayres-de-Campos D, Bernardes J, Costa-Pereira A, et al: Inconsistencies in classification by experts of cardiotocograms and subsequent clinical decision. BJOG 106:1307, 1999

Bakker JJH, Verhoeven CJM, Janssen PF, et al: Outcomes after internal versus external tocodynamometry for monitoring labor. N Engl J Med 362:306, 2010

Bakker PC, Kurver PH, Duik DJ, et al: Elevated uterine activity increases the risk of fetal acidosis at birth. Am J Obstet Gynecol 196:313, 2007

Ball RH, Parer JT: The physiologic mechanisms of variable decelerations. Am J Obstet Gynecol 166:1683, 1992

Bannerman CG, Grobman WA, Antoniewicz L: Assessment of the concordance among 2-tier, 3-tier, and 5-tier fetal heart rate classification systems. Am J Obstet Gynecol 205(3):288.e1, 2011

Banta HD, Thacker SB: Assessing the costs and benefits of electronic fetal monitoring. Obstet Gynecol Surv 34:627, 1979

Banta HD, Thacker SB: Electronic fetal monitoring: lessons from a formative case of health technology assessment. Int J Technol Assess Health Care 18:762, 2002

Becker JH, Bax L, Amer-Wåhlin I, et al: ST analysis of the fetal electrocardiogram in intrapartum fetal monitoring. Obstet Gynecol 119:145, 2012

Behrman RE: The cardiovascular system. In Behrman RE, Kliegman RM, Nelson WE, et al (eds): Nelson Textbook of Pediatrics, 14th ed. Philadelphia, Saunders, 1992, p 1127

Blackwell SC, Groman WA, Antoniewicz L, et al: Interobserver and intraobserver reliability of the NICHD 3-tier fetal heart rate interpretation system. Am J Obstet Gynecol 205:378.e1, 2011

Blackwell SC, Moldenhauer J, Hassan SS, et al: Meconium aspiration syndrome in term neonates with normal acid-base status at delivery: is it different? Am J Obstet Gynecol 184:1422, 2001

Bloom SL, Spong CY, Thom E, et al: Fetal pulse oximetry and cesarean delivery. N Engl J Med 335:21, 2006

Bloom SL, Swindle RG, McIntire DD, et al: Fetal pulse oximetry: duration of desaturation and intrapartum outcome. Obstet Gynecol 93:1036, 1999

Boehm FH: Prolonged end stage fetal heart rate deceleration. Obstet Gynecol 45:579, 1975

Boldt T, Eronen M, Andersson S: Long-term outcome in fetuses with cardiac arrhythmias. Obstet Gynecol 102:1372, 2003

Brook I: Infected neonatal cephalohematomas caused by anaerobic bacteria. J Perinat Med 33(3):255, 2005

Cahill AG, Roehl KA, Odibo AO, et al: Association and prediction of neonatal acidemia. Am J Obstet Gynecol 207:206.e1, 2012

Caldeyro-Barcia R, Poseiro JJ: Physiology of the uterine contraction. Clin Obstet Gynecol 3:386, 1960

Chen HY, Chauhan SP, Ananth C: Electronic fetal heart monitoring and its relationship to neonatal and infant mortality in the United States. Am J Obstet Gynecol 204(6):491.e1, 2011

Clapp JF, Peress NS, Wesley M, et al: Brain damage after intermittent partial cord occlusion in the chronically instrumented fetal lamb. Am J Obstet Gynecol 159:504, 1988

Clark SL, Gimovsky ML, Miller FC: Fetal heart rate response to scalp blood sampling. Am J Obstet Gynecol 14:706, 1982

Clark SL, Gimovsky ML, Miller FC: The scalp stimulation test: a clinical alternative to fetal scalp blood sampling. Am J Obstet Gynecol 148:274, 1984

Coletta J, Murphy E, Rubeo Z, et al: The 5-tier system of assessing fetal heart rate tracings is superior to the 3-tier system in identifying fetal acidemia. Am J Obstet Gynecol 206:226.e1, 2012

Cook VD, Spinnato JA: Terbutaline tocolysis prior to cesarean section for fetal distress. J Matern Fetal Med 3:219, 1994

Copel JA, Liang RI, Demasio K, et al: The clinical significance of the irregular fetal heart rhythm. Am J Obstet Gynecol 182:813, 2000

Davidson SR, Rankin JH, Martin CB Jr, et al: Fetal heart rate variability and behavioral state: analysis by power spectrum. Am J Obstet Gynecol 167:717, 1992

Dawes GS: The control of fetal heart rate and its variability in counts. In Kunzel W (ed): Fetal Heart Rate Monitoring. Berlin, Springer, 1985, p 188

Dawes GS, Fox HE, Leduc BM, et al: Respiratory movements and rapid eye movement sleep in the foetal lamb. J Physiol 220:119, 1972

Dawes GS, Visser GHA, Goodman JDS, et al: Numerical analysis of the human fetal heart rate: modulation by breathing and movement. Am J Obstet Gynecol 140:535, 1981

Del Valle GO, Joffe GM, Izquierdo LA, et al: Acute posttraumatic fetal anemia treated with fetal intravascular transfusion. Am J Obstet Gynecol 166:127, 1992

Devoe L: ECG analysis: the next generation in electronic fetal monitoring? Contemporary Ob/Gyn, September 15, 2006, p 6

Divon MY, Winkler H, Yeh SY, et al: Diminished respiratory sinus arrhythmia in asphyxiated term infants. Am J Obstet Gynecol 155:1263, 1986

Dollberg S, Livny S, Mordecheyev N, et al: Nucleated red blood cells in meconium aspiration syndrome. Obstet Gynecol 97:593, 2001

Doria V, Papageorghiou AT, Gustafsson A, et al: Review of the first 1502 cases of ECG-ST waveform analysis during labour in a teaching hospital. BJOG 114:1202, 2007

East CE, Brennecke SP, King JF, et al: The effect of intrapartum fetal pulse oximetry, in the presence of a nonreassuring fetal heart rate pattern, on operative delivery rates: a multicenter, randomized, controlled trial (the FOREMOST trial). Am J Obstet Gynecol 194:606, 2006

Eberle RL, Norris MC, Eberle AM, et al: The effect of maternal position on fetal heart rate during epidural or intrathecal labor analgesia. Am J Obstet Gynecol 179:150, 1998

Edersheim TG, Hutson JM, Druzin ML, et al: Fetal heart rate response to vibratory acoustic stimulation predicts fetal pH in labor. Am J Obstet Gynecol 157:1557, 1987

Eggink BH, Richardson CJ, Rowen JL: *Gardnerella vaginalis*–infected scalp hematoma associated with electronic fetal monitoring. Pediatr Infect Dis J 23:276, 2004

Egley CC, Bowes WA, Wagner D: Sinusoidal fetal heart rate pattern during labor. Am J Perinatol 8:197, 1991

Elimian A, Figueroa R, Tejani N: Intrapartum assessment of fetal well-being: a comparison of scalp stimulation with scalp pH sampling. Obstet Gynecol 89:373, 1997

Epstein H, Waxman A, Gleicher N, et al: Meperidine induced sinusoidal fetal heart rate pattern and reversal with naloxone. Obstet Gynecol 59:225, 1982

Faro S, Martens MG, Hammill HA, et al: Antibiotic prophylaxis: is there a difference? Am J Obstet Gynecol 162:900, 1990

Farrell T, Chien PFW, Gordon A: Intrapartum umbilical artery Doppler velocimetry as a predictor of adverse perinatal outcome: a systematic review. BJOG 106:783, 1999

Food and Drug Administration: OxiFirst Fetal Oxygen Saturation Monitoring System. 2012. Available at: http://www.fda.gov/MedicalDevices/ProductsandMedicalProcedures/DeviceApprovalsandClearances/Recently-ApprovedDevices/ucm089789.htm. Accessed August 21, 2013

Food and Drug Administration: STAN S31 Fetal Heart Monitor—P020001. 2012. Available at: http://www.fda.gov/MedicalDevices/ProductsandMedicalProcedures/DeviceApprovalsandClearances/Recently-ApprovedDevices/ucm078446.htm. Accessed August 21, 2013

Fraser WD, Hofmeyer J, Lede R, et al: Amnioinfusion for the prevention of the meconium aspiration syndrome. N Engl J Med 353:9, 2005

Freeman RK, Garite TH, Nageotte MP: Fetal Heart Rate Monitoring, 3rd ed. Philadelphia, Lippincott Williams & Wilkins, 2003

Gabbe SG, Ettinger BB, Freeman RK, et al: Umbilical cord compression associated with amniotomy: laboratory observations. Am J Obstet Gynecol 126:353, 1976

Garite TJ, Dildy GA, McNamara H, et al: A multicenter controlled trial of fetal pulse oximetry in the intrapartum management of nonreassuring fetal heart rate patterns. Am J Obstet Gynecol 183:1049, 2000

Ghidini A, Spong CY: Severe meconium aspiration syndrome is not caused by aspiration of meconium. Am J Obstet Gynecol 185:931, 2001

Gilstrap LC III, Hauth JC, Hankins GDV, et al: Second stage fetal heart rate abnormalities and type of neonatal acidemia. Obstet Gynecol 70:191, 1987

Goodwin TM, Milner-Masterson L, Paul RH: Elimination of fetal scalp blood sampling on a large clinical service. Obstet Gynecol 83:971, 1994

Gorenberg DM, Pattillo C, Hendi P, et al: Fetal pulse oximetry: correlation between oxygen desaturation, duration, and frequency and neonatal outcomes. Am J Obstet Gynecol 189:136, 2003

Graham EM, Petersen SM, Christo DK, et al: Intrapartum electronic fetal heart rate monitoring and the prevention of perinatal brain injury. Obstet Gynecol 108:656, 2006

Greenwood C, Lalchandani S, MacQuillan K, et al: Meconium passed in labor: how reassuring is clear amniotic fluid? Obstet Gynecol 102:89, 2003

Grimes DA, Peipert JF: Electronic fetal monitoring as a public health screening program. Obstet Gynecol 116:1397, 2010

Gull I, Jaffa AJ, Oren M, et al: Acid accumulation during end-stage bradycardia in term fetuses: how long is too long? BJOG 103:1096, 1996

Hallak M, Martinez-Poyer J, Kruger ML, et al: The effect of magnesium sulfate on fetal heart rate parameters: a randomized, placebo-controlled trial. Am J Obstet Gynecol 181:1122, 1999

Hamilton LA Jr, McKeown MJ: Biochemical and electronic monitoring of the fetus. In Wynn RM (ed): Obstetrics and Gynecology Annual, 1973. New York, Appleton-Century-Crofts, 1974

Hammacher K, Huter K, Bokelmann J, et al: Foetal heart frequency and perinatal conditions of the fetus and newborn. Gynaecologia 166:349, 1968

Hankins GDV, Leicht TL, Van Houk JW: Prolonged fetal bradycardia secondary to maternal hypothermia in response to urosepsis. Am J Perinatol 14:217, 1997

Hauth JC, Hankins GV, Gilstrap LC, et al: Uterine contraction pressures with oxytocin induction/augmentation. Obstet Gynecol 68:305, 1986

Hendricks CH: Uterine contractility changes in the early puerperium. Clin Obstet Gynecol 11(1):125, 1968

Herbert CM, Boehm FH: Prolonged end-stage fetal heart deceleration: a reanalysis. Obstet Gynecol 57:589, 1981

Hill JB, Alexander JM, Sharma SK, et al: A comparison of the effects of epidural and meperidine analgesia during labor on fetal heart rate. Obstet Gynecol 102:333, 2003

Hofmeyr GJ, Lawrie TA: Amnioinfusion for potential or suspected umbilical cord compression in labour. Cochrane Database Syst Rev 1:CD000013, 2012

Hon EH: The electronic evaluation of the fetal heart rate. Am J Obstet Gynecol 75:1215, 1958

Hon EH: The fetal heart rate patterns preceding death in utero. Am J Obstet Gynecol 78:47, 1959

Hon EH, Bradfield AM, Hess OW: The electronic evaluation of the fetal heart rate. Am J Obstet Gynecol 82:291, 1961

Ikeda T, Murata Y, Quilligan EJ, et al: Two sinusoidal heart rate patterns in fetal lambs undergoing extracorporeal membrane oxygenation. Am J Obstet Gynecol 180:462, 1999

Impey L, Raymonds M, MacQuillan K, et al: Admission cardiotocography: a randomised controlled trial. Lancet 361:465, 2003

Itskovitz J, LaGamma EF, Rudoloph AM: Heart rate and blood pressure response to umbilical cord compression in fetal lambs with special reference to the mechanisms of variable deceleration. Am J Obstet Gynecol 147:451, 1983

Jackson M, Holmgren CM, Esplin MS, et al: Frequency of fetal heart rate categories and short-term neonatal outcome. Obstet Gynecol 118:803, 2011

Jaeggi ET, Friedberg MK: Diagnosis and management of fetal bradyarrhythmias. Pacing Clin Electrophysiol 31 Suppl 1:S50, 2008

Jazayeri A, Politz L, Tsibris JCM, et al: Fetal erythropoietin levels in pregnancies complicated by meconium passage: does meconium suggest fetal hypoxia? Am J Obstet Gynecol 183:188, 2000

Johnson TR Jr, Compton AA, Rotmeusch J, et al: Significance of the sinusoidal fetal heart rate pattern. Am J Obstet Gynecol 139:446, 1981

Jovanovic R, Nguyen HT: Experimental meconium aspiration in guinea pigs. Obstet Gynecol 73:652, 1989

Katz VL, Bowes WA: Meconium aspiration syndrome: reflections on a murky subject. Am J Obstet Gynecol 166:171, 1992

Keith RDF, Beckley S, Garibaldi JM, et al: A multicentre comparative study of 17 experts and an intelligent computer system for managing labour using the cardiotocogram. BJOG 102:688, 1995

Klauser CK, Christensen EE, Chauhan SP, et al: Use of fetal pulse oximetry among high-risk women in labor: a randomized clinical trial. Am J Obstet Gynecol 192:1810, 2005

Klavan M, Laver AT, Boscola MA: Clinical concepts of fetal heart rate monitoring. Waltham, Hewlett-Packard, 1977

Kozuma S, Watanabe T, Bennet L, et al: The effect of carotid sinus denervation on fetal heart rate variation in normoxia, hypoxia and post-hypoxia in fetal sleep. BJOG 104:460, 1997

Krebs HB, Petres RE, Dunn LJ: Intrapartum fetal heart rate monitoring, 5. Fetal heart rate patterns in the second stage of labor. Am J Obstet Gynecol 140:435, 1981

Krebs HB, Petres RE, Dunn LJ, et al: Intrapartum fetal heart rate monitoring, 6. Prognostic significance of accelerations. Am J Obstet Gynecol 142:297, 1982

Kruger K, Hallberg B, Blennow M, et al: Predictive value of fetal scalp blood lactate concentration and pH as markers of neurologic disability. Am J Obstet Gynecol 181:1072, 1999

Künzel W: Fetal heart rate alterations in partial and total cord occlusion. In Künzel W (ed): Fetal Heart Rate Monitoring: Clinical Practice and Pathophysiology. Berlin, Springer, 1985, p 114

Larma JD, Silva AM, Holcroft CJ, et al: Intrapartum electronic fetal heart rate monitoring and the identification of metabolic acidosis and hypoxic-ischemic encephalopathy. Am J Obstet Gynecol 197(3):301.e1, 2007

Lee CV, DiLaretto PC, Lane JM: A study of fetal heart rate acceleration patterns. Obstet Gynecol 45:142, 1975

Leveno KJ, Cunningham FG, Nelson S: Prospective comparison of selective and universal electronic fetal monitoring in 34,995 pregnancies. N Engl J Med 315:615, 1986

Leveno KJ, Quirk JG, Cunningham FG, et al: Prolonged pregnancy: observations concerning the causes of fetal distress. Am J Obstet Gynecol 150:465, 1984

Lin CC, Vassallo B, Mittendorf R: Is intrapartum vibroacoustic stimulation an effective predictor of fetal acidosis? J Perinat Med 29:506, 2001

Lopriore E, Aziz MI, Nagel HT, et al: Long-term neurodevelopmental outcome after fetal arrhythmia. Am J Obstet Gynecol 87(2):83, 2009

Lowe TW, Leveno KJ, Quirk JG, et al: Sinusoidal fetal heart rate patterns after intrauterine transfusion. Obstet Gynecol 64:215, 1984

Macri CJ, Schrimmer DB, Leung A, et al: Prophylactic amnioinfusion improves outcome of pregnancy complicated by thick meconium and oligohydramnios. Am J Obstet Gynecol 167:117, 1992

Macones GA, Hankins GD, Spong CY, et al: The 2008 National Institute of Child Health and Human Development workshop report on electronic fetal monitoring: update on definitions, interpretation, and research guidelines. Obstet Gynecol 112(3):661, 2008

Manassiev N: What is the normal heart rate of a term fetus? BJOG 103:1272, 1996

Mathews TG, Warshaw JB: Relevance of the gestational age distribution of meconium passage in utero. Pediatrics 64:30, 1979

McGregor JA, McFarren T: Neonatal cranial osteomyelitis: a complication of fetal monitoring. Obstet Gynecol 73(2):490, 1989

Melchior J, Bernard N: Incidence and pattern of fetal heart rate alterations during labor. In Kunzel W (ed): Fetal Heart Rate Monitoring: Clinical Practice and Pathophysiology. Berlin, Springer, 1985, p 73

Mercier FJ, Dounas M, Bouaziz H, et al: Intravenous nitroglycerin to relieve intrapartum fetal distress related to uterine hyperactivity: a prospective observation study. Anesth Analg 84:1117, 1997

Mires G, Williams F, Howie P: Randomised controlled trial of cardiotocography versus Doppler auscultation of fetal heart at admission in labour in low risk obstetric population. BMJ 322:1457, 2001

Miyazaki FS, Nevarez F: Saline amnioinfusion for relief of repetitive variable decelerations: a prospective randomized study. Am J Obstet Gynecol 153:301, 1985

Miyazaki FS, Taylor NA: Saline amnioinfusion for relief of variable or prolonged decelerations. Am J Obstet Gynecol 146:670, 1983

Modanlou H, Freeman RK: Sinusoidal fetal heart rate pattern: its definition and clinical significance. Am J Obstet Gynecol 142:1033, 1982

Modanlou HD, Murata Y: Sinusoidal heart rate pattern: reappraisal of its definition and clinical significance. J Obstet Gynaecol Res 30(3):169, 2004

Mueller-Heubach E, Battelli AF: Variable heart rate decelerations and transcutaneous PO_2 (tc PO_2) during umbilical cord occlusion in the fetal monkey. Am J Obstet Gynecol 144:796, 1982

Murata Y, Martin CB, Ikenoue T, et al: Fetal heart rate accelerations and late decelerations during the course of intrauterine death in chronically catheterized rhesus monkeys. Am J Obstet Gynecol 144:218, 1982

Murotsuki J, Bocking AD, Gagnon R: Fetal heart rate patterns in growth-restricted fetal sleep induced by chronic fetal placental embolization. Am J Obstet Gynecol 176:282, 1997

Murphy AA, Halamek LP, Lyell DJ, et al: Training and competency assessment in electronic fetal monitoring: a national survey. Obstet Gynecol 101:1243, 2003

Murphy KW, Russell V, Collins A, et al: The prevalence, aetiology and clinical significance of pseudo-sinusoidal fetal heart rate patterns in labour. BJOG 98:1093, 1991

Myers RE: Two patterns of perinatal brain damage and their conditions of occurrence. Am J Obstet Gynecol 112:246, 1972
Myers RE, Mueller-Heubach E, Adamsons K: Predictability of the state of fetal oxygenation from a quantitative analysis of the components of late deceleration. Am J Obstet Gynecol 115:1083, 1973
Nageotte MP, Bertucci L, Towers CV, et al: Prophylactic amnioinfusion in pregnancies complicated by oligohydramnios: a prospective study. Obstet Gynecol 77:677, 1991
Nathan L, Leveno KJ, Carmody TJ, et al: Meconium: a 1990s perspective on an old obstetric hazard. Obstet Gynecol 83:328, 1994
National Institute of Child Health and Human Development Research Planning Workshop: Electronic fetal heart rate monitoring: research guidelines for integration. Am J Obstet Gynecol 177:1385, 1997
Neesham DE, Umstad MP, Cincotta RB, et al: Pseudo-sinusoidal fetal heart rate pattern and fetal anemia: case report and review. Aust N Z J Obstet Gynaecol 33:386, 1993
Neilson DR Jr, Freeman RK, Mangan S: Signal ambiguity resulting in unexpected outcome with external fetal heart rate monitoring. Am J Obstet Gynecol 198:717, 2008
Neilson JP: Fetal electrocardiogram (ECG) for fetal monitoring during labour. Cochrane Database System Rev 5:CD000116, 2013
Nicolaides KH, Sadovsky G, Cetin E: Fetal heart rate patterns in red blood cell isoimmunized pregnancies. Am J Obstet Gynecol 161:351, 1989
Nunes I, Ayres-de-Campos D, Costa-Santos C, et al: Differences between external and internal fetal heart rate monitoring during the second stage of labor: a prospective observational study. J Perinat Med January 16, 2014 [Epub ahead of print]
Ogueh O, Steer P: Gender does not affect fetal heart rate variation. BJOG 105:1312, 1998
Ogundipe OA, Spong CY, Ross MG: Prophylactic amnioinfusion for oligohydramnios: a re-evaluation. Obstet Gynecol 84:544, 1994
Owen J, Henson BV, Hauth JC: A prospective randomized study of saline solution amnioinfusion. Am J Obstet Gynecol 162:1146, 1990
Parer J: NIH sets the terms for fetal heart rate pattern interpretation. OB/Gyn News, September 1, 1997
Parer JT: Personalities, politics and territorial tiffs: a half century of fetal heart rate monitoring. Am J Obstet Gynecol 204(6):548, 2011
Parer JT, Ikeda T: A framework for standardized management of intrapartum fetal heart rate pattern. Am J Obstet Gynecol 197:26, 2007
Parer JT, King TL: Fetal heart rate monitoring: the next step? Am J Obstet Gynecol 203(6):520, 2010
Parer WJ, Parer JT, Holbrook RH, et al: Validity of mathematical models of quantitating fetal heart rate variability. Am J Obstet Gynecol 153:402, 1985
Paul RH, Snidon AK, Yeh SY: Clinical fetal monitoring, 7. The evaluation and significance of intrapartum baseline FHR variability. Am J Obstet Gynecol 123:206, 1975
Paul WM, Quilligan EJ, MacLachlan T: Cardiovascular phenomena associated with fetal head compression. Am J Obstet Gynecol 90:824, 1964
Perlman JM, Wylie J, Kattwinkel J: Part 11: Neonatal resuscitation: 2010 International consensus on cardiopulmonary resuscitation and emergency cardiovascular care science with treatment recommendations. Circulation 122(16 Suppl 2):S516, 2010
Petrie RH: Dose/response effects of intravenous meperidine in fetal heart rate variability. J Matern Fetal Med 2:215, 1993
Phelan JP, Ahn MO: Perinatal observations in forty-eight neurologically impaired term infants. Am J Obstet Gynecol 171:424, 1994
Picquard F, Hsiung R, Mattauer M, et al: The validity of fetal heart rate monitoring during the second stage of labor. Obstet Gynecol 72:746, 1988
Pierce J, Gaudier FL, Sanchez-Ramos L: Intrapartum amnioinfusion for meconium-stained fluid: meta-analysis of prospective clinical trials. Obstet Gynecol 95:1051, 2000
Pillai M, James D: The development of fetal heart rate patterns during normal pregnancy. Obstet Gynecol 76:812, 1990
Pontonnier G, Puech F, Grandjean H, et al: Some physical and biochemical parameters during normal labour. Fetal and maternal study. Biol Neonate 26:159, 1975
Pressman EK, Blakemore KJ: A prospective randomized trial of two solutions for intrapartum amnioinfusion: effects on fetal electrolytes, osmolality, and acid-base status. Am J Obstet Gynecol 175:945, 1996
Ramin KD, Leveno KJ, Kelly MS, et al: Amnionic fluid meconium: a fetal environmental hazard. Obstet Gynecol 87:181, 1996
Rathore AM, Singh R, Ramji S, et al: Randomised trial of amnioinfusion during labour with meconium stained amniotic fluid. BJOG 109:17, 2002
Renou P, Warwick N, Wood C: Autonomic control of fetal heart rate. Am J Obstet Gynecol 105:949, 1969
Resnik R: Electronic fetal monitoring: the debate goes on . . . and on . . . and on. Obstet Gynecol 121(5):917, 2013
Rinehart BK, Terrone DA, Barrow JH, et al: Randomized trial of intermittent or continuous amnioinfusion for variable decelerations. Obstet Gynecol 96:571, 2000
Rocha E, Hammond R, Richardson B: Necrotic cell injury in the preterm and near-term ovine fetal brain after intermittent umbilical cord occlusion. Am J Obstet Gynecol 191:488, 2004
Rogers MS, Mongelli M, Tsang KH, et al: Lipid peroxidation in cord blood at birth: the effect of labour. BJOG 105:739, 1998
Samueloff A, Langer O, Berkus M, et al: Is fetal heart rate variability a good predictor of fetal outcome? Acta Obstet Gynecol Scand 73:39, 1994
Schucker JL, Sarno AP, Egerman RS, et al: The effect of butorphanol on the fetal heart rate reactivity during labor. Am J Obstet Gynecol 174:491, 1996
Sherer DM: Blunted fetal response to vibroacoustic stimulation associated with maternal intravenous magnesium sulfate therapy. Am J Perinatol 11:401, 1994
Sholapurkar SL: The conundrum of vanishing early decelerations in British obstetrics, a step backwards? Detailed appraisal of British and American classifications of fetal heart rate decelerations—fallacies of emphasis on waveform and putative aetiology. J Obstet Gynaecol 32(6):505, 2012
Simpson KR, James DC: Efficacy of intrauterine resuscitation techniques in improving fetal oxygen status during labor. Obstet Gynecol 105:1362, 2005
Skupski DW, Rosenberg CR, Eglinton GS: Intrapartum fetal stimulation tests: a meta-analysis. Obstet Gynecol 99:129, 2002
Smith CV, Nguyen HN, Phelan JP, et al: Intrapartum assessment of fetal well-being: a comparison of fetal acoustic stimulation with acid–base determinations. Am J Obstet Gynecol 155:726, 1986
Smith JH, Anand KJ, Cotes PM, et al: Antenatal fetal heart rate variation in relation to the respiratory and metabolic status of the compromised human fetus. BJOG 95:980, 1988
Southall DP, Richards J, Hardwick RA, et al: Prospective study of fetal heart rate and rhythm patterns. Arch Dis Child 55:506, 1980
Spong CY, Ogundipe OA, Ross MG: Prophylactic amnioinfusion for meconium-stained amniotic fluid. Am J Obstet Gynecol 171:931, 1994
Spong CY, Rasul C, Collea JV, et al: Characterization and prognostic significance of variable decelerations in the second stage of labor. Am J Perinatol 15:369, 1998
Stewart RD, Bleich AT, Lo JY, et al: Defining uterine tachysystole: how much is too much? Am J Obstet Gynecol 207:290.e1–6, 2012
Stiller R, von Mering R, König V, et al: How well does reflectance pulse oximetry reflect intrapartum fetal acidosis? Am J Obstet Gynecol 186:1351, 2002
Thakor AS, Giussani DA: Effects of acute acidemia on the fetal cardiovascular defense to acute hypoxemia. Am J Physiol Regul Integr Comp Physiol 296(1):R90, 2009
Usta IM, Mercer BM, Aswad NK, et al: The impact of a policy of amnioinfusion for meconium-stained amniotic fluid. Obstet Gynecol 85:237, 1995
Van Geijn HP, Jongsma HN, deHaan J, et al: Heart rate as an indicator of the behavioral state. Am J Obstet Gynecol 136:1061, 1980
Vintzileos AM, Nioka S, Lake M, et al: Transabdominal fetal pulse oximetry with near-infrared spectroscopy. Am J Obstet Gynecol 192(1):129, 2005
Walker J: Foetal anoxia. J Obstet Gynaecol Br Commonw 61:162, 1953
Wenstrom K, Andrews WW, Maher JE: Amnioinfusion survey: prevalence protocols and complications. Obstet Gynecol 86:572, 1995
Westgate J, Harris M, Curnow JSH, et al: Plymouth randomized trial of cardiotocogram only versus ST waveform plus cardiotocogram for intrapartum monitoring in 2400 cases. Am J Obstet Gynecol 169:1151, 1993
Westgate JA, Bennet L, De Haan HH, et al: Fetal heart rate overshoot during repeated umbilical cord occlusion in sheep. Obstet Gynecol 97:454, 2001
Wiberg-Itzel E, Lipponer C, Norman M, et al: Determination of pH or lactate in fetal scalp blood in management of intrapartum fetal distress: randomised controlled multicenter trial. BMJ 336:1284, 2008
Williams JW: Williams Obstetrics, 1st ed. New York, Appleton, 1903
Xu H, Hofmeyr J, Roy C, et al: Intrapartum amnioinfusion for meconium-stained amniotic fluid: a systematic review of randomised controlled trials. BJOG 114:383, 2007
Yam J, Chua S, Arulkumaran S: Intrapartum fetal pulse oximetry. Part I: principles and technical issues. Obstet Gynecol Surv 55:163, 2000
Young BK, Katz M, Wilson SJ: Sinusoidal fetal heart rate, 1. Clinical significance. Am J Obstet Gynecol 136:587, 1980a
Young BK, Weinstein HM: Moderate fetal bradycardia. Am J Obstet Gynecol 126:271, 1976
Young DC, Gray JH, Luther ER, et al: Fetal scalp blood pH sampling: its value in an active obstetric unit. Am J Obstet Gynecol 136:276, 1980b
Young RC, Zhang P: Functional separation of deep cytoplasmic calcium from subplasmalemmal space calcium in cultured human uterine smooth muscle cells. Cell Calcium 36(1):11, 2004
Zalar RW, Quilligan EJ: The influence of scalp sampling on the cesarean section rate for fetal distress. Am J Obstet Gynecol 135:239, 1979

CHAPTER 25

Obstetrical Analgesia and Anesthesia

Obstetrical anesthesia presents unique challenges. Labor begins without warning, and anesthesia may be required within minutes of a full meal. Vomiting with aspiration of gastric contents is a constant threat. The usual physiological adaptations of pregnancy require special consideration, especially with disorders such as preeclampsia, placental abruption, or sepsis syndrome.

Of all anesthesia-related deaths in the United States from 1995 to 2005, 3.6 percent were in pregnant women (Li, 2009). Berg and colleagues (2010) analyzed deaths of women during or within 1 year of pregnancy in the United States from 1998 through 2005. They found that 54 of 4693—1.2 percent—such deaths were attributable to anesthesia complications. Hawkins and associates (2011) analyzed anesthesia-related maternal mortality in this country between 1979 and 2002. As shown in Table 25-1, anesthetic-related maternal mortality rates decreased nearly 60 percent during this time, and there currently is approximately one anesthetic death per million live births. About two thirds of deaths associated with general anesthesia were caused by intubation failure or induction problems during cesarean delivery. Deaths associated with regional analgesia were caused by high spinal or epidural blocks—26 percent; respiratory failure—19 percent; and drug reaction—19 percent. The improved case-fatality rate for general anesthesia was especially notable considering that such anesthesia is now used for the highest-risk patients and the most hurried emergencies, that is, decision-incision intervals < 15 minutes (Bloom, 2005).

Several factors have contributed to improved obstetrical anesthesia safety (Hawkins, 2011). The most significant is the increased use of regional analgesia. Increased availability of in-house anesthesia coverage almost certainly is another important reason. Despite these encouraging results suggesting the safety of general anesthesia, there are now reports of increasing complications with regional analgesia techniques.

GENERAL PRINCIPLES

Obstetrical Anesthesia Services

The American College of Obstetricians and Gynecologists (2008) reaffirmed its joint position with the American Society of Anesthesiologists that a woman's request for labor pain relief is sufficient medical indication for its provision. Identification of any of the risk factors shown in Table 25-2 should prompt consultation with anesthesia personnel to permit a joint management plan. This plan should include strategies to minimize the need for emergency anesthesia in women for whom such anesthesia would be especially hazardous.

Goals for optimizing obstetrical anesthesia services have been jointly established by the American College of Obstetricians and Gynecologists and the American Society of Anesthesiologists (2009) and include:

1. Availability of a licensed practitioner who is credentialed to administer an appropriate anesthetic whenever necessary and to maintain support of vital functions in an obstetrical emergency
2. Availability of anesthesia personnel to permit the start of a cesarean delivery within 30 minutes of the decision to perform the procedure

TABLE 25-1. Case-Fatality Rates and Rate Ratios of Anesthesia-Related Deaths During Cesarean Delivery by Type of Anesthesia in the United States, 1979–2002

	Case-Fatality Rates[a]		
Year of Death	General Anesthesia	Regional Analgesia	Rate Ratios
1979–1984	20.0	8.6	2.3 (95% CI 1.9–2.9)
1985–1990	32.3	1.9	16.7 (95% CI 12.9–21.8)
1991–1996	16.8	2.5	6.7 (95% CI 3.0–14.9)
1997–2002	6.5	3.8	1.7 (95% CI 0–4.6)

[a]Deaths per million general or regional anesthetics.
CI = confidence interval.
Data from Hawkins, 2011.

3. Anesthesia personnel immediately available to perform an emergency cesarean delivery during the active labor of a woman attempting vaginal birth after cesarean (Chap. 31, p. 615)
4. Appointment of a qualified anesthesiologist to be responsible for all anesthetics administered
5. Availability of a qualified physician with obstetrical privileges to perform operative vaginal or cesarean delivery during administration of anesthesia
6. Availability of equipment, facilities, and support personnel equal to that provided in the surgical suite

TABLE 25-2. Maternal Factors That May Prompt Anesthetic Consultation

Morbid obesity
Severe edema or anatomical abnormalities of the face, neck, or spine, including trauma or surgery
Abnormal dentition, small mandible, or difficulty opening the mouth
Extremely short stature, short neck, or neck arthritis
Goiter
Serious maternal medical problems, such as cardiac, pulmonary, or neurological disease
Bleeding disorders
Severe preeclampsia
Prior anesthetic complications
Obstetrical complications likely to lead to operative delivery—examples include placenta previa, preterm breech presentation, or higher-order multifetal gestation

Adapted from the American Academy of Pediatrics and American College of Obstetricians and Gynecologists: Guidelines for Perinatal Care, 7th ed. Washington, 2012.

7. Immediate availability of personnel, other than the surgical team, to assume responsibility for resuscitation of a depressed newborn (Chap. 32, p. 625).

To meet these goals, 24-hour in-house anesthesia coverage is usually necessary. Providing such service in smaller facilities is more challenging—a problem underscored by the fact that approximately a third of all hospitals providing obstetrical care have fewer than 500 deliveries per year (American College of Obstetricians and Gynecologists, 2009).

Bell and coworkers (2000) calculated the financial burden that may be incurred to provide 24/7 obstetrical anesthesia coverage. Given the average indemnity and Medicaid reimbursement for labor epidural analgesia, they concluded that such coverage could not operate profitably at their tertiary referral institution. Compounding this burden, some third-party payers have denied reimbursement for epidural analgesia in the absence of a specific medical indication—an approach repudiated by the American College of Obstetricians and Gynecologists and the American Society of Anesthesiologists (2008).

Role of an Obstetrician

Every obstetrician should be proficient in local and pudendal analgesia that may be administered in appropriately selected circumstances. In general, however, it is preferable for an anesthesiologist or anesthetist to provide pain relief so that the obstetrician can focus attention on the laboring woman and her fetus.

Principles of Pain Relief

In a scholarly review, Hawkins (2010) emphasized that labor pain is a highly individual response to variable stimuli that are uniquely received and interpreted (Fig. 25-1). These stimuli are modified by emotional, motivational, cognitive, social, and cultural circumstances. Labor pain caused by uterine contractions and cervical dilation is transmitted through visceral afferent sympathetic nerves entering the spinal cord from T_{10} through L_1. Later in labor, perineal stretching transmits painful stimuli through the pudendal nerve and sacral nerves S_2 through S_4. Cortical responses to pain and anxiety during labor are complex and may be influenced by maternal expectations for childbirth, her age and preparation through education, the presence of emotional support, and other factors. Pain perception is heightened by fear and the need to move into various positions. A woman may be motivated to have a certain type of birthing experience, and these opinions will influence her judgment regarding pain management and other choices during labor and delivery.

Maternal physiological responses to labor pain may influence maternal and fetal well-being and labor progress. For example, hyperventilation may induce hypocarbia. An increased metabolic rate increases oxygen consumption. Increases in cardiac output and vascular resistance may increase maternal blood pressure. Pain, stress, and anxiety cause release of stress hormones such as cortisol and β-endorphins. The sympathetic nervous system response to pain leads to a marked increase

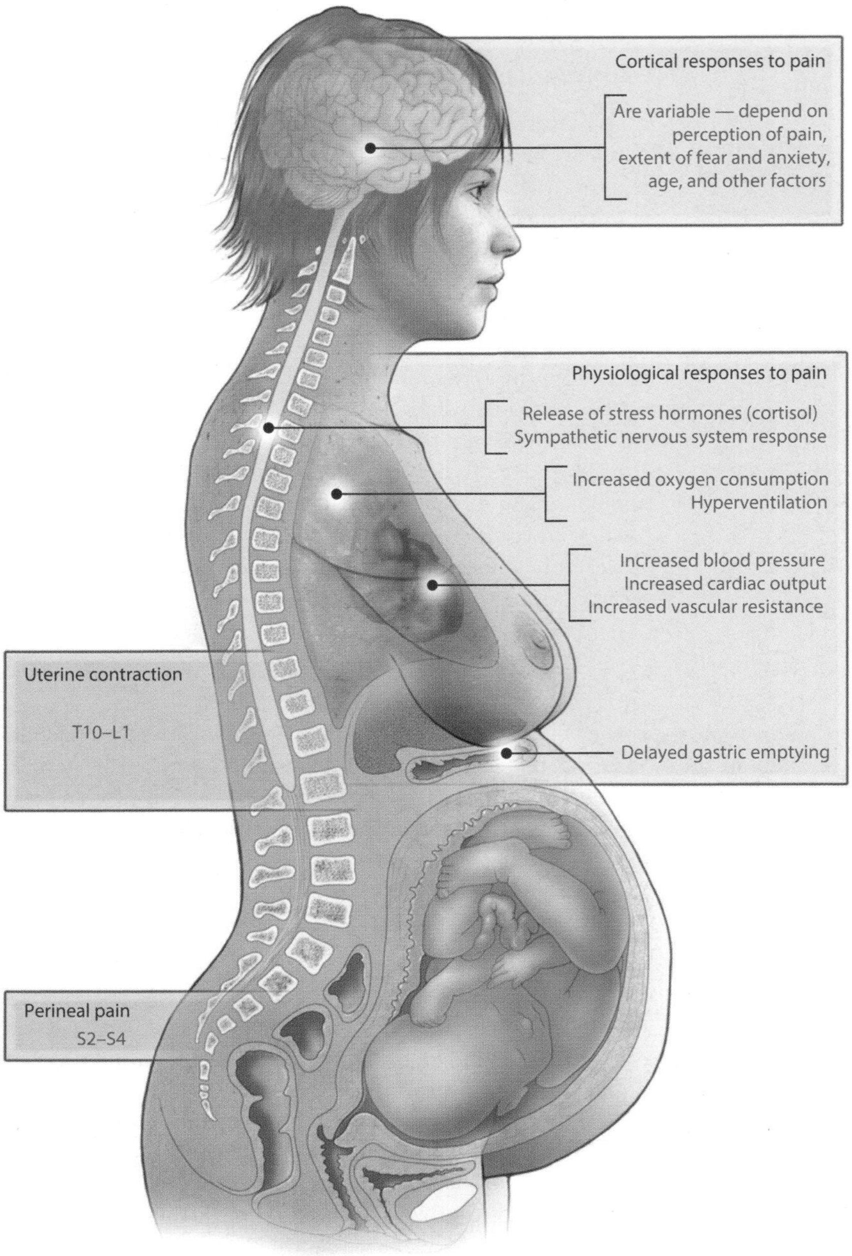

FIGURE 25-1 Sources of pain during labor and maternal physiological responses. (From Hawkins, 2010, with permission.)

in circulating catecholamines that can adversely affect uterine activity and uteroplacental blood flow. Effective analgesia attenuates or eliminates these responses.

ANALGESIA AND SEDATION DURING LABOR

If uterine contractions and cervical dilatation cause discomfort, pain relief with a narcotic such as meperidine (Demerol), plus one of the tranquilizer drugs such as promethazine (Phenergan), is usually appropriate. With a successful program of analgesia and sedation, the mother should rest quietly between contractions. In this circumstance, discomfort usually is felt at the acme of an effective uterine contraction. Appropriate drug selection and administration of the medications shown in Table 25-3 should safely accomplish these objectives.

Parenteral Agents

Meperidine and Promethazine

Meperidine, 50 to 100 mg, with promethazine, 25 mg, may be administered intramuscularly at intervals of 2 to 4 hours. A more rapid effect is achieved by giving meperidine intravenously in doses of 25 to 50 mg every 1 to 2 hours. Whereas analgesia is maximal 30 to 45 minutes after an intramuscular injection, it develops almost immediately following intravenous administration. Meperidine readily crosses the placenta, and its half-life in the newborn is approximately 13 hours or longer (American College of Obstetricians and Gynecologists, 2013b). Its depressant effect in the fetus follows closely behind the peak maternal analgesic effect.

According to Bricker and Lavender (2002), meperidine is the most common opioid used worldwide for pain relief from labor. Tsui and associates (2004) found meperidine to be superior to placebo for pain relief in the first stage of labor. In a randomized investigation of epidural analgesia conducted at Parkland Hospital, patient-controlled intravenous analgesia with meperidine was found to be an inexpensive and reasonably effective method for labor analgesia (Sharma, 1997). Women randomized to self-administered analgesia were given 50-mg meperidine with 25-mg promethazine intravenously as an initial bolus. Thereafter, an infusion pump was set to deliver 15 mg of meperidine every 10 minutes as needed until delivery. Neonatal sedation, as measured by need for naloxone treatment in the delivery room, was identified in 3 percent of newborns.

Butorphanol (Stadol)

This synthetic narcotic, given in 1- to 2-mg doses, compares favorably with 40 to 60 mg of meperidine (Quilligan, 1980). Its major side effects are somnolence, dizziness, and dysphoria. Neonatal respiratory depression is reported to be less than with meperidine. Importantly, the two drugs are not given contiguously because butorphanol antagonizes the narcotic effects of meperidine. Hatjis and Meis (1986) described a transient sinusoidal fetal heart rate pattern

TABLE 25-3. Some Parenteral Analgesic Agents for Labor Pain

Agent	Usual Dose	Frequency	Onset	Neonatal Half-Life
Meperidine	25–50 mg (IV)	Q 1–2 hr	5 min (IV)	~18–20 hr
	50–100 mg (IM)	Q 2–4 hr	30–45 min (IM)	~60 hr
Fentanyl	50–100 μg (IV)	Q 1 hr	1 min	~5 hr
Nalbuphine	10 mg (IV or IM)	Q 3 hr	2–3 min (IV) 15 min (IM)	~4 hr
Butorphanol	1–2 mg (IV or IM)	Q 4 hr	1–2 min (IV) 10–30 min (IM)	Unknown
Morphine	2–5 mg (IV) 10 mg (IM)	Q 4 hr	5 min (IV) 30–40 min (IM)	~7 hr

IV = intravenously; IM = intramuscularly; Q = every.

following butorphanol administration but with no short-term maternal or neonatal adverse sequelae (Chap. 24, p. 482).

Fentanyl

This short-acting and potent synthetic opioid may be given in doses of 50 to 100 μg intravenously every hour. Its main disadvantage is a short duration of action, which requires frequent dosing or use of a patient-controlled intravenous pump. Moreover, Atkinson and coworkers (1994) reported that butorphanol provided better initial analgesia than fentanyl and was associated with fewer requests for additional medication or for epidural analgesia.

Efficacy and Safety of Parenteral Agents

Parenteral sedation is not without risks. Hawkins and colleagues (1997) reported that 4 of 129 maternal anesthetic-related deaths were from such sedation—one from aspiration, two from inadequate ventilation, and one from overdosage.

Narcotics used during labor may cause newborn respiratory depression. Naloxone is a narcotic antagonist capable of reversing respiratory depression induced by opioid narcotics. It acts by displacing the narcotic from specific receptors in the central nervous system. Withdrawal symptoms may be precipitated in recipients who are physically dependent on narcotics. For this reason, naloxone is contraindicated in a newborn of a narcotic-addicted mother (American Academy of Pediatrics and American College of Obstetricians and Gynecologists, 2012). After adequate ventilation has been established, naloxone may be given to reverse respiratory depression in a newborn infant whose mother received narcotics (Chap. 32, p. 626).

Nitrous Oxide

A self-administered mixture of 50-percent nitrous oxide (N_2O) and oxygen may provide satisfactory analgesia during labor (Rosen, 2002a). Some preparations are premixed in a single cylinder (Entonox), and in others, a blender mixes the two gases from separate tanks (Nitronox). The gases are connected to a breathing circuit through a valve that opens only when the patient inspires. The use of intermittent nitrous oxide for labor pain has been reviewed by Rosen (2002a).

NERVE BLOCKS

Various nerve blocks have been developed over the years to provide pain relief during labor and/or delivery. These include pudendal, paracervical, and neuraxial blocks such as spinal, epidural, and combined spinal-epidural techniques.

Anesthetic Agents

Some of the more commonly used nerve block anesthetics, along with their usual concentrations, doses, and durations of action, are summarized in Table 25-4. The dose of each agent varies widely and is dependent on the particular nerve block and physical status of the woman. The onset, duration, and quality of analgesia can be enhanced by increasing the dose. This can be done safely only by incrementally administering small-volume boluses of the agent and by carefully monitoring early warning signs of toxicity. Administration of these agents must be followed by appropriate monitoring for adverse reactions. Equipment and personnel to manage these reactions must be immediately available.

Most often, serious toxicity follows inadvertent intravenous injection. Systemic toxicity from local anesthetics typically manifests in the central nervous and cardiovascular systems. For this reason, when epidural analgesia is initiated, dilute epinephrine is sometimes added and given as a test dose. A sudden significant rise in the maternal heart rate or blood pressure immediately after administration suggests intravenous catheter placement. Local analgesic agents are manufactured in more than one concentration and ampule size, which increases the potential for dosing errors.

Central Nervous System Toxicity

Early symptoms are those of *stimulation* but, as serum levels increase, *depression* follows. Symptoms may include lightheadedness, dizziness, tinnitus, metallic taste, and numbness of the tongue and mouth. Patients may show bizarre behavior, slurred speech, muscle fasciculation and excitation, and ultimately, generalized convulsions, followed by loss of consciousness.

For management, the convulsions should be controlled, an airway established, and oxygen delivered. Succinylcholine

TABLE 25-4. Local Anesthetic Agents Commonly Used in Obstetrics

Anesthetic Agent[a]	Usual Concentration (%)	Usual Volume (mL)	Onset	Average Duration (min)	Maximum Dose (mg)	Clinical Use
Aminoesters[b]						
2-Chloroprocaine	2	10–20	Rapid	30–60	800	Local infiltration or pudendal block
	3	10–20		30–60		Epidural *only* for cesarean
Aminoamides[b]						
Bupivacaine	0.25	5–10	Slow	60–90	175	Epidural for labor
	0.5	10–20		90–150		Epidural for cesarean
	0.75	1.5–2		60–120		Spinal for cesarean
Lidocaine	1–1.5	10–20	Rapid	30–60	300	Local infiltration or pudendal block
	1.5–2	5–20		60–90		Epidural for labor or cesarean
	5	1.5–2		45–60		Spinal for D&C or puerperal tubal
Ropivacaine	0.2–0.5	5–10	Slow	60–90	200	Epidural for labor
	0.5–1	10–30		90–150	250	Epidural for cesarean

[a]Without epinephrine.
[b]Esters are hydrolyzed by plasma cholinesterases and amides by hepatic clearance.
D&C = dilatation and curettage.
Adapted from Liu, 2009. Courtesy of Drs. Shiv Sharma and Erica Grant.

abolishes the peripheral manifestations of the convulsions and allows tracheal intubation. Diazepam (Valium) can be used to inhibit convulsions. Magnesium sulfate, administered according to the regimen for eclampsia, also controls convulsions (Chap. 40, p. 758). Abnormal fetal heart rate patterns such as late decelerations or persistent bradycardia may develop from maternal hypoxia and lactic acidosis induced by convulsions. With arrest of convulsions, administration of oxygen, and application of other supportive measures, the fetus usually recovers more quickly in utero than following immediate cesarean delivery. Moreover, the mother is better served if delivery is forestalled until the intensity of hypoxia and metabolic acidosis has diminished.

Cardiovascular Toxicity

These manifestations generally develop later than those from cerebral toxicity, and they may not develop at all because they are induced by higher serum drug levels. The notable exception is bupivacaine, which is associated with the development of neurotoxicity and cardiotoxicity at virtually identical levels (Mulroy, 2002). Because of this risk of systemic toxicity, use of 0.75-percent solution of bupivacaine for epidural injection has been proscribed by the Food and Drug Administration. Similar to neurotoxicity, cardiovascular toxicity is characterized first by stimulation and then by depression. Accordingly, there is hypertension and tachycardia, which soon is followed by hypotension, cardiac arrhythmias, and impaired uteroplacental perfusion.

Hypotension is managed initially by turning the woman onto either side to avoid aortocaval compression. A crystalloid solution is infused rapidly along with intravenously administered ephedrine. Emergency cesarean delivery is considered if maternal vital signs have not been restored within 5 minutes of cardiac arrest (Chap. 47, p. 956). As with convulsions, however, the fetus is likely to recover more quickly in utero once maternal cardiac output is reestablished.

Pudendal Block

Pain with vaginal delivery arises from stimuli from the lower genital tract. These are transmitted primarily through the pudendal nerve, the peripheral branches of which provide sensory innervation to the perineum, anus, vulva, and clitoris. The pudendal nerve passes beneath the posterior surface of the sacrospinous ligament just as the ligament attaches to the ischial spine. Sensory nerve fibers of the pudendal nerve are derived from ventral branches of the S_2 through S_4 nerves.

The pudendal nerve block is a relatively safe and simple method of providing analgesia for spontaneous delivery. As shown in Figure 25-2, a tubular introducer is used to sheath and guide a 15-cm 22-gauge needle into position over the pudendal nerve. The end of the introducer is placed against the vaginal mucosa just beneath the tip of the ischial spine.

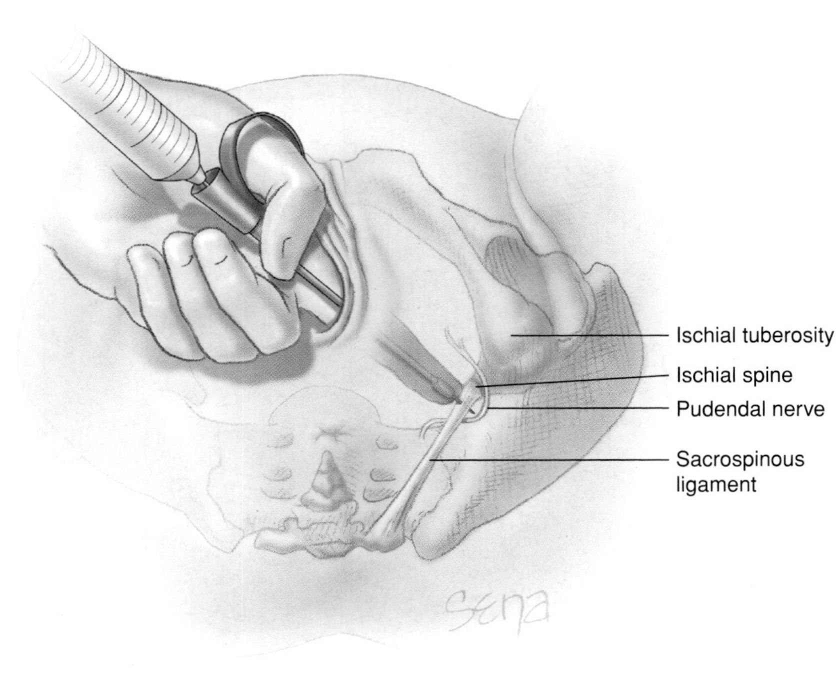

FIGURE 25-2 Local infiltration of the pudendal nerve. Transvaginal technique showing the needle extended beyond the needle guard and passing through the sacrospinous ligament to reach the pudendal nerve.

The introducer allows 1.0 to 1.5 cm of needle to protrude beyond its tip, and the needle is pushed beyond the introducer tip into the mucosa. A mucosal wheal is made with 1 mL of 1-percent lidocaine solution or an equivalent dose of another local anesthetic (see Table 25-3). To guard against intravascular infusion, aspiration is attempted before this and all subsequent injections. The needle is then advanced until it touches the sacrospinous ligament, which is infiltrated with 3 mL of lidocaine. The needle is advanced farther through the ligament. As it pierces the loose areolar tissue behind the ligament, the resistance of the plunger decreases. Another 3 mL of solution is injected into this region. Next, the needle is withdrawn into the introducer, which is moved to just above the ischial spine. The needle is inserted through the mucosa and 3 more mL is deposited. The procedure is then repeated on the other side.

Within 3 to 4 minutes of injection, the successful pudendal block will allow pinching of the lower vagina and posterior vulva bilaterally without pain. If delivery occurs before the pudendal block becomes effective and an episiotomy is indicated, then the fourchette, perineum, and adjacent vagina can be infiltrated with 5 to 10 mL of 1-percent lidocaine solution directly at the planned episiotomy site. By the time of repair, the pudendal block usually has become effective.

Pudendal block usually does not provide adequate analgesia when delivery requires extensive obstetrical manipulation. Moreover, such analgesia is usually inadequate for women in whom complete visualization of the cervix and upper vagina or manual exploration of the uterine cavity is indicated.

Infrequently, complications may follow this block. As previously described, intravascular injection of a local anesthetic agent may cause serious systemic toxicity. Hematoma formation from perforation of a blood vessel is most likely when there is a coagulopathy (Lee, 2004). Rarely, severe infection may originate at the injection site. The infection may spread posteriorly to the hip joint, into the gluteal musculature, or into the retropsoas space (Svancarek, 1977).

Paracervical Block

This block usually provides satisfactory pain relief during first-stage labor. However, because the pudendal nerves are not blocked, additional analgesia is required for delivery. For paracervical blockade, usually lidocaine or chloroprocaine, 5 to 10 mL of a 1-percent solution, is injected into the cervix laterally at 3 and 9 o'clock. Because these anesthetics are relatively short acting, paracervical block may have to be repeated during labor. We do not use it at Parkland Hospital.

Fetal bradycardia is a worrisome complication that occurs in approximately 15 percent of paracervical blocks (Rosen, 2002b). Bradycardia usually develops within 10 minutes and may last up to 30 minutes. Doppler studies have shown an increase in the pulsatility index of the uterine arteries following paracervical blockade (Chap. 10, p. 219). These observations support the hypothesis of drug-induced arterial vasospasm as a cause of fetal bradycardia (Manninen, 2000). For these reasons, paracervical block should not be used in situations of potential fetal compromise.

Neuraxial Regional Blocks

Epidural, spinal, or combined spinal-epidural techniques were the more common methods used for relief of pain during labor and/or delivery in the United States in 2008 (Osterman, 2011b). Nearly two out of three mothers receive neuraxial anesthesia for relief of pain either during labor or during vaginal or cesarean delivery. Neuraxial techniques were more common in vaginal deliveries assisted by forceps—84 percent or vacuum extraction—77 percent than spontaneous vaginal deliveries—60 percent (Osterman, 2011a). Among first births, 68 percent of women delivered vaginally received neuraxial pain relief compared with 57 percent of women delivering their second or higher number child.

Epidural *analgesia* via a catheter as shown in Figure 25-3 is typically used for relief of labor pain, although it can also be used for *anesthesia* during operative vaginal and cesarean delivery. Spinal analgesia is typically given as a single intrathecal injection of a local anesthetic at the time of operative vaginal delivery or cesarean. Continuous spinal analgesia during labor via an indwelling spinal catheter is also under investigation. Combined spinal-epidural analgesia/anesthesia also illustrated in Figure 25-3 consists of a single intrathecal injection followed by a catheter placed into the epidural space

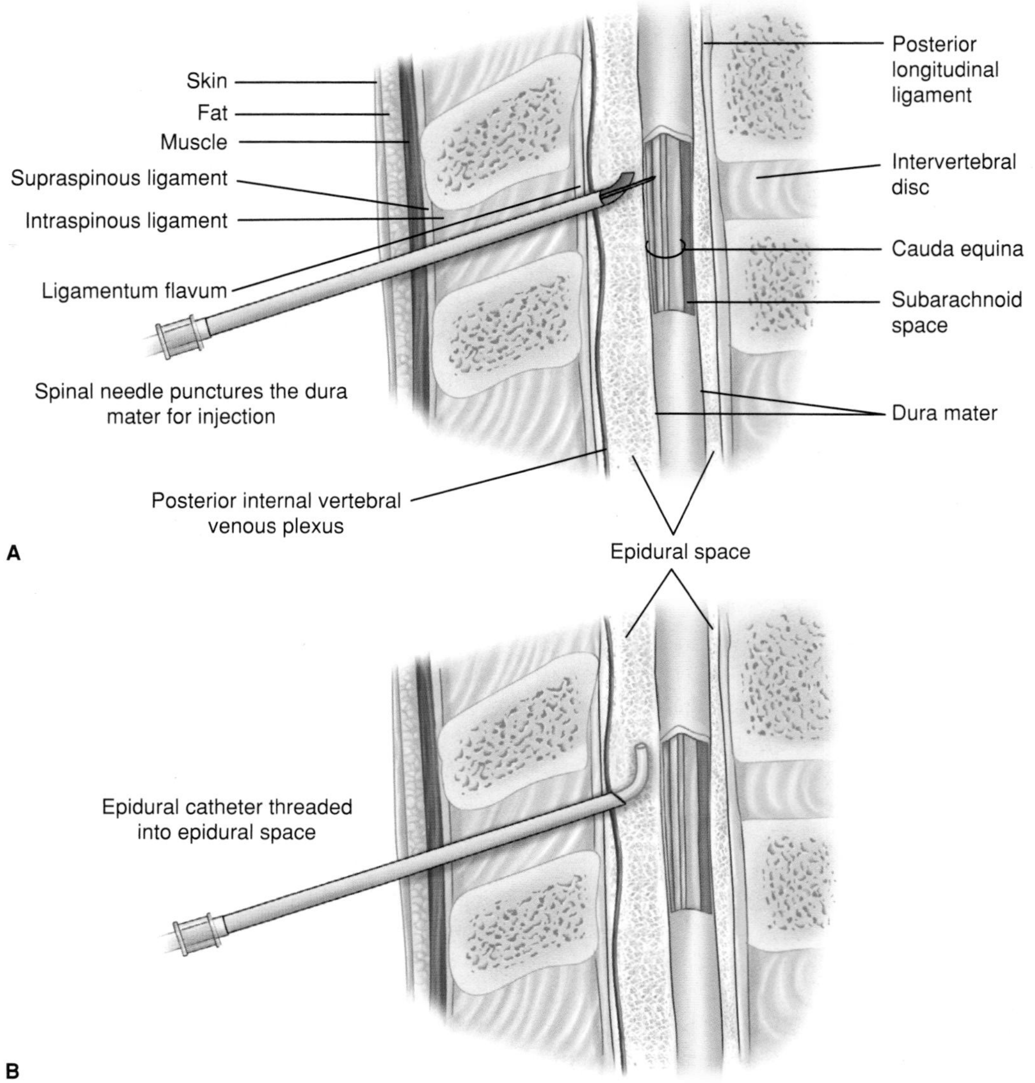

FIGURE 25-3 Neuraxial analgesia. **A.** Combined spinal-epidural analgesia. **B.** Epidural analgesia.

for either patient- or provider-controlled infusion of a local anesthetic and/or an opioid such as fentanyl. The combined spinal-epidural technique has the advantages of immediate pain relief from the spinal injection coupled with a portal for continuous analgesia via the epidural catheter. Unlike the spinal injection, the relief provided by the epidural catheter takes approximately 30 minutes to become effective. Perhaps as many as a third of epidural catheter tips will migrate during labor, resulting in ineffective pain control should cesarean be necessary.

Spinal (Subarachnoid) Block

Introduction of a local anesthetic into the subarachnoid space to effect analgesia has long been used for delivery. Advantages include a short procedure time, rapid blockade onset, and high success rate. Because of the smaller subarachnoid space during pregnancy, likely the consequence of internal vertebral venous plexus engorgement, the same amount of anesthetic agent in the same volume of solution produces a much higher blockade in parturients than in nonpregnant women.

Vaginal Delivery

Low spinal block can be used for operative vaginal delivery. The level of analgesia should extend to the T_{10} dermatome, which corresponds to the level of the umbilicus. Blockade to this level provides excellent relief from the pain of uterine contractions (Fig. 25-4).

Several local anesthetic agents have been used for spinal analgesia (see Table 25-4). Addition of glucose to any of these agents creates a hyperbaric solution, which is heavier and denser than cerebrospinal fluid. A sitting position causes a hyperbaric solution to settle caudally, whereas a lateral position will have a greater effect on the dependent side. Lidocaine given in a hyperbaric solution produces excellent analgesia and has the advantage of a rapid onset and relatively short duration. Bupivacaine in an 8.25-percent dextrose solution provides satisfactory anesthesia to the lower

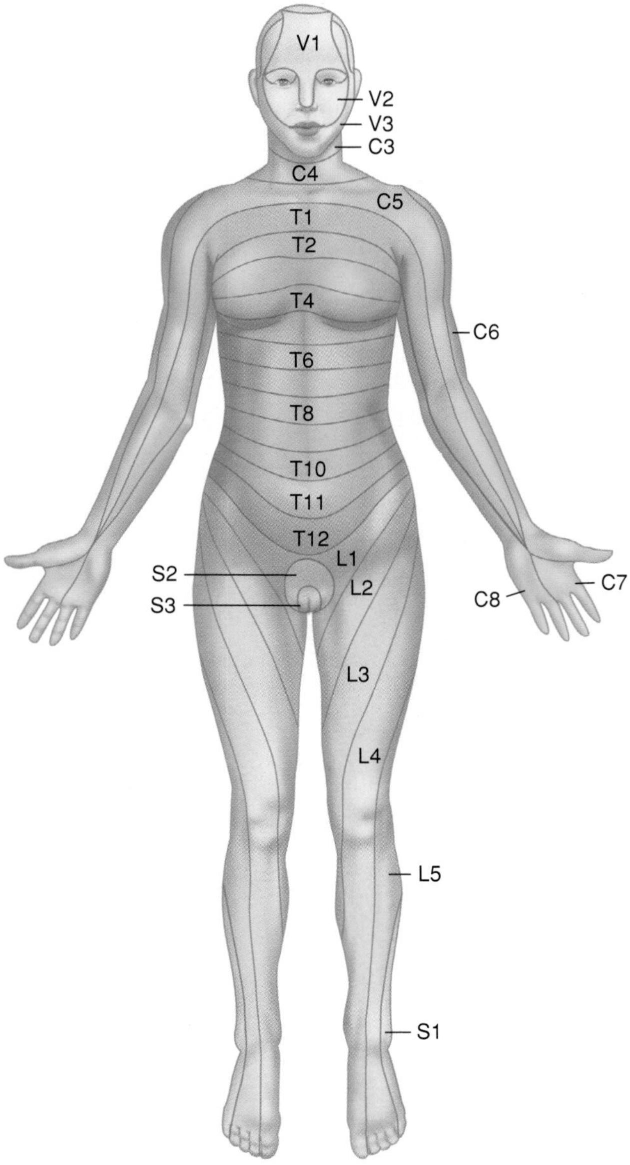

FIGURE 25-4 Dermatome distribution.

vagina and the perineum for more than 1 hour. Neither is administered until the cervix is fully dilated, and all other criteria for safe forceps delivery have been fulfilled (Chap. 29, p. 575). Preanalgesic intravenous hydration with 1 L of crystalloid solution will prevent or minimize hypotension in many cases.

Cesarean Delivery

A level of sensory blockade extending to the T_4 dermatome is desired for cesarean delivery (see Fig. 25-4). Depending on maternal size, 10 to 12 mg of bupivacaine in a hyperbaric solution or 50 to 75 mg of lidocaine hyperbaric solution are administered. The addition of 20 to 25 μg of fentanyl increases the rapidity of blockade onset and reduces shivering. The addition of 0.2 mg of morphine improves pain control during delivery and postoperatively.

TABLE 25-5. Complications of Regional Analgesia

Complication	Incidence (%)
Hypotension (in prehydrated women undergoing cesarean delivery)	
Spinal	25–67
Epidural (in prehydrated women in labor)	28–31
Epidural	8.5–9
Fever > 100.4°F (excess rate over women treated with narcotics)	
Nulliparous women	19
Multiparous women	1
Postdural puncture headache	
Spinal	1.5–3
Epidural	2
Combined spinal epidural	1–2.8
Transient fetal heart decelerations	8
Pruritus (with added opioid only)	
Epidural	1.3–26
Spinal	41–85
Inadequate pain relief: epidural	9–15

Adapted from the American College of Obstetricians and Gynecologists, 2013b.

Complications

Shown in Table 25-5 are some of the more common complications associated with neuraxial analgesia. Importantly, obese women have significantly impaired ventilation and thus close clinical monitoring is imperative (Vricella, 2011).

Hypotension. This common complication may develop soon after injection of the local anesthetic agent. It is the consequence of vasodilatation from sympathetic blockade and is compounded by obstructed venous return due to uterine compression of the great vessels. In the supine position, even in the absence of maternal hypotension measured in the brachial artery, placental blood flow may still be significantly reduced. Treatment includes uterine displacement by left lateral patient positioning, intravenous crystalloid hydration, and intravenous bolus injections of ephedrine or phenylephrine.

Ephedrine is a sympathomimetic drug that binds to alpha- and beta-receptors but also indirectly enhances norepinephrine release. It raises blood pressure by increasing heart rate and cardiac output and by variably elevating peripheral vascular resistance. In animal studies, ephedrine preserves uteroplacental blood flow during pregnancy compared with $alpha_1$-receptor agonists. Accordingly, it is a preferred vasopressor for obstetrical use. Phenylephrine is a pure alpha agonist and raises blood pressure solely through vasoconstriction. A metaanalysis of seven randomized trials by Lee (2002a) suggests that the safety profiles of ephedrine and phenylephrine are comparable. Following their systematic review of 14 reports, Lee (2002b) questioned whether routine prophylactic ephedrine is needed for elective cesarean delivery. But although fetal acidemia has been reported with prophylactic ephedrine use, this was not observed with prophylactic phenylephrine use (Ngan Kee, 2004).

Hypotension is the more common blood pressure perturbation. However, paradoxically, hypertension from ergonovine or methylergonovine injections following delivery is more common in women who have received a spinal or epidural block.

High Spinal Blockade. Most often, complete spinal blockade follows administration of an excessive dose of local anesthetic. This is certainly not always the case, because accidental total spinal block has even occurred following an epidural test dose. With complete spinal blockade, hypotension and apnea promptly develop and must be immediately treated to prevent cardiac arrest. In the undelivered woman: (1) the uterus is immediately displaced laterally to minimize aortocaval compression, (2) effective ventilation is established, preferably with tracheal intubation, and (3) intravenous fluids and ephedrine are given to correct hypotension.

Postdural Puncture Headache. Leakage of cerebrospinal fluid (CSF) from the meningeal puncture site can lead to postdural puncture or "spinal headache." Presumably, when the woman sits or stands, the diminished CSF volume creates traction on pain-sensitive central nervous system structures.

Rates of this complication can be reduced by using a small-gauge spinal needle and avoiding multiple punctures. In a prospective, randomized study of five different spinal needles, Vallejo and associates (2000) concluded that Sprotte and Whitacre needles had the lowest risks of postdural puncture headaches. Sprigge and Harper (2008) reported that the incidence of postdural puncture headache was 1 percent in more than 5000 women undergoing spinal analgesia. Postdural puncture headaches are much less frequent with epidural blockade because the dura is not intentionally punctured. The incidence of inadvertent dural puncture with epidural analgesia approximates 0.2 percent (Introna, 2012; Katircioglu, 2008). There is no good evidence that placing a woman absolutely flat on her back for several hours is effective in preventing headache. Vigorous hydration may be of value, but compelling evidence to support its use is also lacking.

If a headache develops, the administration of *caffeine,* a cerebral vasoconstrictor, has been shown in randomized studies to afford temporary relief (Camann, 1990). With severe headache, an *epidural blood patch* is most effective. Ten to 20 mL of autologous blood are obtained aseptically by venipuncture into a tube *without anticoagulant.* This blood is then injected into the epidural space at the site of dural puncture. Further CSF leakage is halted by either mass effect or coagulation. Relief is immediate, and complications are uncommon. In a randomized trial of 64 women, Scavone and coworkers (2004) found that prophylactic blood patch did not decrease either the incidence of postdural puncture headache or the need for a subsequent therapeutic blood patch.

If a headache does not have the pathognomonic postural characteristics or persists despite treatment with a blood patch, other diagnoses should be considered. For example, Chisholm and Campbell (2001) described a case of superior sagittal sinus thrombosis that manifested as a postural headache. Chan and Paech (2004) have described persistent CSF leak in three women. Smarkusky and colleagues (2006) described pneumocephalus, which caused immediate cephalgia. Finally, intracranial and intraspinal subarachnoid hematomas have developed after spinal analgesia (Dawley, 2009; Liu, 2008).

Convulsions. In rare instances, postdural puncture cephalgia is associated with temporary blindness and convulsions. Shearer and associates (1995) described eight such cases associated with 19,000 regional analgesic procedures done at Parkland Hospital. It is presumed that these too are caused by CSF hypotension. Immediate treatment of seizures and blood patch was usually effective in these cases.

Bladder Dysfunction. With spinal analgesia, bladder sensation is likely to be obtunded and bladder emptying impaired for several hours after delivery. As a consequence, bladder distention is a frequent postpartum complication, especially if appreciable volumes of intravenous fluid are given. Millet (2012) randomized 146 women with neuraxial analgesia to either intermittent or continuous bladder catheterizations and found that the intermittent method was associated with significantly higher rates of bacteriuria.

Arachnoiditis and Meningitis. Local anesthetics are no longer preserved in alcohol, formalin, or other toxic solutes, and disposable equipment is used by most. These practices, coupled with aseptic technique, have made meningitis and arachnoiditis rare but have not eliminated them (Centers for Disease Control and Prevention, 2010).

Contraindications to Spinal Analgesia

Shown in Table 25-6 are the absolute contraindications to regional analgesia according to the American College of Obstetricians and Gynecologists (2013b). Obstetrical complications that are associated with maternal hypovolemia and hypotension—for example, severe hemorrhage—are contraindications to spinal blockade. The additive cardiovascular effects of spinal blockade in the presence of acute blood loss in nonpregnant patients were documented by Kennedy and coworkers (1968).

Disorders of coagulation and defective hemostasis also preclude spinal analgesia use. Although there are no randomized studies to guide the management of anticoagulation at the time of delivery, consensus opinion suggests that women given

TABLE 25-6. Absolute Contraindications to Neuraxial Analgesia

Refractory maternal hypotension
Maternal coagulopathy
Thrombocytopenia (variously defined)
Low-molecular-weight heparin within 12 hours
Untreated maternal bacteremia
Skin infection over site of needle placement
Increased intracranial pressure caused by a mass lesion

subcutaneous unfractionated heparin or low-molecular-weight heparin should be instructed to stop therapy when labor begins (Krivak, 2007). Subarachnoid puncture is also contraindicated if there is cellulitis at the needle entry site. Neurological disorders are considered by many to be a contraindication, if for no other reason than that exacerbation of the neurological disease might be attributed without cause to the anesthetic agent. Other maternal conditions, such as significant aortic stenosis or pulmonary hypertension, are also relative contraindications to spinal analgesia (Chap. 49, p. 983).

As with significant hemorrhage, severe preeclampsia is another complication in which markedly decreased blood pressure can be predicted when neuraxial analgesia is used. Wallace and associates (1995) randomly assigned 80 women with severe preeclampsia undergoing cesarean delivery at Parkland Hospital to receive general anesthesia or either epidural or combined spinal-epidural analgesia. There were no differences in maternal or neonatal outcomes. Still, 30 percent of women given epidural analgesia and 22 percent of those given spinal-epidural blockade developed hypotension—the average reduction in mean arterial pressure was between 15 and 25 percent.

Epidural Analgesia

Relief of labor and childbirth pain, including cesarean delivery, can be accomplished by injection of a local anesthetic agent into the epidural or peridural space (see Fig. 25-3). This potential space contains areolar tissue, fat, lymphatics, and the internal vertebral venous plexus. This plexus becomes engorged during pregnancy such that the volume of the epidural space is appreciably reduced. Entry for obstetrical analgesia is usually through a lumbar intervertebral space. Although only one injection may be given, usually an indwelling catheter is placed for subsequent agent administration or continuous infusion. Infusions use a volumetric pump controlled either by the patient or by a caregiver. The American College of Obstetricians and Gynecologists and the American Society of Anesthesiologists (2008) believe that under appropriate physician supervision, labor and delivery nursing personnel who have been specifically trained in the management of epidural infusions should be able to adjust dosage and also discontinue infusions.

Continuous Lumbar Epidural Block

Complete analgesia for the pain of labor and vaginal delivery necessitates a block from the T_{10} to the S_5 dermatomes (Figs. 25-1 and 25-4). For cesarean delivery, a block extending from the T_4 to the S_1 dermatomes is desired. The effective spread of anesthetic depends upon the catheter tip location; the dose, concentration, and volume of anesthetic agent used; and whether the mother is head-down, horizontal, or head-up (Setayesh, 2001). Individual variations in anatomy or presence of synechiae may preclude a completely satisfactory block. Finally, the catheter tip may migrate from its original location during labor.

Technique. One example of the sequential steps and techniques for performance of epidural analgesia is detailed in Table 25-7. Before injection of the local anesthetic therapeutic dose, a test dose is given. The woman is observed for features of toxicity from intravascular injection and for signs of spinal

TABLE 25-7. Technique for Labor Epidural Analgesia

Informed consent is obtained, and the obstetrician consulted
Monitoring includes the following:
- Blood pressure every 1 to 2 minutes for 15 minutes after giving a bolus of local anesthetic
- Continuous maternal heart rate monitoring during analgesia induction
- Continuous fetal heart rate monitoring
- Continual verbal communication

Hydration with 500 to 1000 mL of lactated Ringer solution
The woman assumes a lateral decubitus or sitting position
The epidural space is identified with a loss-of-resistance technique
The epidural catheter is threaded 3 to 5 cm into the epidural space
A test dose of 3 mL of 1.5% lidocaine with 1:200,000 epinephrine or 3 mL of 0.25% bupivacaine with 1:200,000 epinephrine is injected after careful aspiration to avert intravascular injection and after a uterine contraction. This minimizes the chance of confusing tachycardia that results from labor pain with that of tachycardia from intravenous injection of the test dose
If the test dose is negative, one or two 5-mL doses of 0.25% bupivacaine are injected to achieve a sensory T_{10} level
After 15 to 20 minutes, the block is assessed using loss of sensation to cold or pinprick. If no block is evident, the catheter is replaced. If the block is asymmetrical, the epidural catheter is withdrawn 0.5 to 1.0 cm and an additional 3 to 5 mL of 0.25% bupivacaine is injected. If the block remains inadequate, the catheter is replaced
The woman is positioned in the lateral or semilateral position to avoid aortocaval compression
Subsequently, maternal blood pressure is recorded every 5 to 15 minutes. The fetal heart rate is monitored continuously
The level of analgesia and intensity of motor blockade are assessed at least hourly

From Glosten, 1999, with permission.

blockade from subarachnoid injection. If these are absent, only then is a full dose given. Analgesia is maintained by intermittent boluses of similar volume, or small volumes of the drug are delivered continuously by infusion pump (Halpern, 2009). The addition of small doses of a short-acting narcotic—fentanyl or sufentanil—has been shown to improve analgesic efficacy while avoiding motor blockade (Chestnut, 1988). As with spinal blockade, it is imperative that close monitoring, including the level of analgesia, be performed by trained personnel. Appropriate resuscitation equipment and drugs must be available during administration of epidural analgesia.

Complications

Total Spinal Blockade. As shown in Table 25-5, there are certain problems inherent in epidural analgesia use. Dural puncture with inadvertent subarachnoid injection may cause total spinal blockade. Sprigge and Harper (2008) cited an incidence of 0.91 percent recognized accidental dural punctures at the time of epidural analgesia in more than 18,000 women. Personnel and facilities must be immediately available to manage this complication as described on page 504.

Ineffective Analgesia. Using currently popular continuous epidural infusion regimens such as 0.125-percent bupivacaine with 2-mg/mL fentanyl, 90 percent of women rate their pain relief as good to excellent (Sharma, 1997). Alternatively, a few women find epidural analgesia to be inadequate for labor. In a study of almost 2000 parturients, Hess and associates (2001) found that approximately 12 percent complained of three or more episodes of pain or pressure. Risk factors for such breakthrough pain included nulliparity, heavier fetal weights, and epidural catheter placement at an earlier cervical dilatation. Dresner and colleagues (2006) reported that epidural analgesia was more likely to fail as body mass index increased. If epidural analgesia is allowed to dissipate before another injection of anesthetic drug, subsequent pain relief may be delayed, incomplete, or both.

In some women, epidural analgesia is not sufficient for cesarean delivery. For example, in a Maternal Fetal Medicine Units (MFMU) Network study, 4 percent of women initially given epidural analgesia required a general anesthetic for cesarean delivery (Bloom, 2005). Also at times, perineal analgesia for delivery is difficult to obtain, especially with the lumbar epidural technique. When this situation is encountered, pudendal block or systemic analgesia or rarely general anesthesia may be added.

Hypotension. Sympathetic blockade from epidurally injected analgesic agents may cause hypotension and decreased cardiac output. According to Miller and coworkers (2013), hypotension is more common—20 percent—in women with an admission pulse pressure < 45 mm Hg compared with 6 percent in those whose pulse pressure is > 45 mm Hg. In normal pregnant women, hypotension induced by epidural analgesia usually can be prevented by rapid infusion of 500 to 1000 mL of crystalloid solution as described for spinal analgesia. Danilenko-Dixon and associates (1996) showed that maintaining a lateral position compared with the supine position minimized hypotension. Despite these precautions, hypotension is the most frequent side effect and is severe enough to require treatment in a third of women (Sharma, 1997).

Central Nervous Stimulation. Convulsions are an uncommon but serious complication, the immediate management of which was described previously (p. 507). Also cited was the case described by Smarkusky and coworkers (2006) of acute onset of intrapartum headache due to a postdural pneumocephalus.

Maternal Fever. Fusi and colleagues (1989) observed that the mean temperature increased in laboring women given epidural analgesia. Subsequently, several randomized and retrospective cohort studies have confirmed that some women develop intrapartum fever following this procedure. Many studies are limited by inability to control for other risk factors, such as labor length, duration of ruptured membranes, and number of vaginal examinations. With this in mind, the frequency of intrapartum fever associated with epidural analgesia was found by Lieberman and O'Donoghue (2002) to be 10 to 15 percent above the baseline rate.

The two general theories concerning the etiology of maternal hyperthermia are *maternal-fetal infection* or *dysregulation of body temperature.* Dashe and coworkers (1999) studied placental histopathology in laboring women given epidural analgesia and identified intrapartum fever only when there was placental inflammation. This suggests that fever is due to infection. The other proposed mechanisms include alteration of the hypothalamic thermoregulatory set point, impairment of peripheral thermoreceptor input to the central nervous system with selective blockage of warm stimuli, or imbalance between heat production and heat loss. Sharma (2014) randomized 400 nulliparas with labor epidural analgesia to receive cefoxitin 2 g prophylactically versus placebo. It was hypothesized that epidural-related fever was due to infection and that prophylactic antimicrobial use should significantly reduce the rate of fever. Approximately equal proportions—about 40 percent—of women developed fever $\geq 38°C$ during labor. This result suggested that infection was unlikely to be the cause of fever associated with epidural analgesia during labor. Whatever the mechanism, women with persistent fever are usually treated with antimicrobials for presumed chorioamnionitis.

Back Pain. An association between epidural analgesia and back pain has been reported by some but not all. In a prospective cohort study, Butler and Fuller (1998) reported that back pain after delivery was common with epidural analgesia, however, persistent pain was uncommon. Based on their systematic review, Lieberman and O'Donoghue (2002) concluded that available data do not support an association between epidural analgesia and development of de novo, long-term backache.

Miscellaneous Complications. A spinal or epidural hematoma is a rare complication of an epidural catheter (Grant, 2007). Epidural abscesses are equally rare (Darouiche, 2006). Uncommonly, the plastic epidural catheter is sheared off (Noblett, 2007).

Effect on Labor

Most studies, including the combined five randomized trials from Parkland Hospital shown in Table 25-8, report that epidural analgesia prolongs labor and increases the use of oxytocin stimulation. Alexander and associates (2002) examined the effects of epidural analgesia on the Friedman (1955) labor curve described in Chapter 22 (p. 445). There were 459 nulliparas randomly assigned to patient-controlled epidural analgesia or patient-controlled intravenous meperidine. Compared with original Friedman criteria, epidural analgesia prolonged the active phase of labor by 1 hour. As further shown in Table 25-8, epidural analgesia also increased the need for operative vaginal delivery because of prolonged second-stage labor, but importantly, without adverse neonatal effects (Chestnut, 1999). This association between epidural analgesia and prolonged second-stage labor as well as operative vaginal delivery has been attributed to local-anesthetic induced motor blockade and resultant impaired maternal expulsive efforts. Craig and colleagues (2014) randomized 310 nulliparous women with labor epidural analgesia to bupivacaine plus fentanyl or fentanyl alone during second-stage labor. Epidural bupivacaine analgesia did cause motor blockade during the second stage, however, the duration of the second stage was not increased. Neither obstetrical nor neonatal outcomes were different between the two study groups. Patient satisfaction was high, irrespective of the method.

TABLE 25-8. Selected Labor Events in 2703 Nulliparous Women Randomized to Epidural Analgesia or Intravenous Meperidine Analgesia

Event[a]	Epidural Analgesia n = 1339	Intravenous Meperidine n = 1364	*p* value
Labor outcomes			
First-stage duration (hr)[b]	8.1 ± 5	7.5 ± 5	0.011
Second-stage duration (min)	60 ± 56	47 ± 57	< 0.001
Oxytocin after analgesia	641 (48)	546 (40)	< 0.001
Type of delivery			
Spontaneous vaginal	1027 (77)	1122 (82)	< 0.001
Forceps	172 (13)	101 (7)	< 0.001
Cesarean	140 (10.5)	141 (10.3)	0.92

[a]Data are presented as n (%) or mean ± SD.
[b]First stage = initiation of analgesia to complete cervical dilatation.
Adapted from Sharma, 2004.

Fetal Heart Rate. Hill and associates (2003) examined the effects of epidural analgesia with 0.25-percent bupivacaine on fetal heart rate patterns. Compared with intravenous meperidine, no deleterious effects were identified. Reduced beat-to-beat variability and fewer accelerations were more common in fetuses whose mothers received meperidine (Chap. 24, p. 479). Based on their systematic review, Reynolds and coworkers (2002) reported that epidural analgesia was associated with improved neonatal acid-base status compared with meperidine.

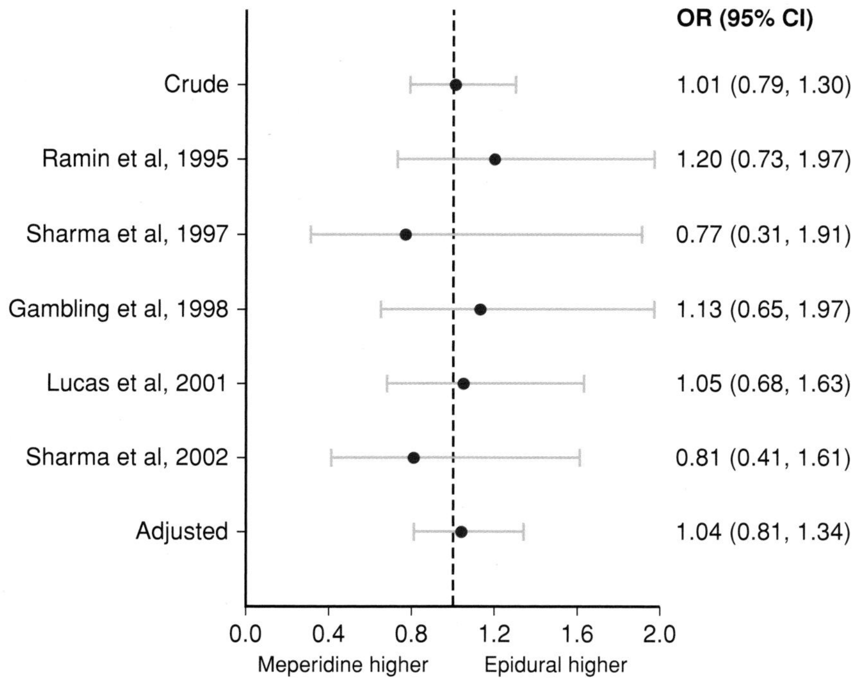

FIGURE 25-5 Results of five studies comparing the incidence of cesarean delivery in women given either epidural analgesia or intravenous meperidine. The individual odds ratios (ORs) with 95-percent confidence intervals (CIs) for each randomized study, as well as overall crude and adjusted ORs with 95-percent CIs, are shown. An OR of less than 1.0 favored epidural over meperidine analgesia. From Sharma, 2004, with permission.

Cesarean Delivery Rates. A contentious issue in the past was whether epidural analgesia increased the risk for cesarean delivery. Evidence that it did was from the era when dense blocks of local anesthetic agents were used that impaired motor function and therefore likely did contribute to increased rates of cesarean delivery. As techniques were refined, however, many investigators believed that epidural administration of *dilute* anesthetic solutions did not increase cesarean delivery rates. Some observational studies have suggested a decreased risk for cesarean delivery with oxytocin induction (Hants, 2013).

Several studies conducted at Parkland Hospital were designed to answer this and related questions. From 1995 to 2002, a total of 2703 nulliparas at term and in spontaneous labor were enrolled in five trials to evaluate epidural analgesia techniques compared with methods of intravenous meperidine administration. The results from these are summarized in Figure 25-5 and show that epidural analgesia does not significantly increase cesarean delivery rates.

Yancey and colleagues (1999) described the effects of an on-demand labor epidural analgesia service at Tripler Army Hospital in Hawaii. This followed a policy change in military medical centers. As a result, the incidence of labor epidural analgesia increased from 1 percent before the policy to 60 percent within 2 years. The primary cesarean delivery rate was 13.4 percent before and 13.2 percent after this dramatic change. In a follow-up study, Yancey and coworkers (2001) reported that fetal malpresentations at vaginal delivery were not more common after epidural usage increased. The only significant difference that they found was an increased duration of second-stage labor of approximately 25 minutes (Zhang, 2001).

Based on these randomized studies and a metaanalysis of 14 such trials, Sharma and Leveno (2003) and Leighton and Halpern (2002) concluded that epidural analgesia is not associated with an increased cesarean delivery rate.

Timing of Epidural Placement

In several retrospective studies, epidural placement in early labor was linked to an increased risk of cesarean delivery (Lieberman, 1996; Rogers, 1999; Seyb, 1999). These observations prompted at least five randomized trials, which showed that timing of epidural placement has no effect on the risk of cesarean birth, forceps delivery, or fetal malposition (Chestnut, 1994a,b; Luxman, 1998; Ohel, 2006; Wong, 2005, 2009). Thus, withholding epidural placement until some arbitrary cervical dilation has been attained is unsupportable and serves only to deny women maximal labor pain relief. The American College of Obstetricians and Gynecologists (2013b) recommends that the decision for epidural analgesia should be made individually with each patient and that women should not be required to reach 4 to 5 cm cervical dilation before receiving epidural analgesia.

Safety

The relative safety of epidural analgesia is reflected by the extraordinary experiences reported by Crawford (1985) from the Birmingham Maternity Hospital in England. From 1968 through 1985, more than 26,000 women were given epidural analgesia for labor, and there were no maternal deaths. The nine potentially life-threatening complications followed either inadvertent intravenous or intrathecal injection of lidocaine, bupivacaine, or both. Similarly, according to the Confidential Enquiries into Maternal Deaths in the United Kingdom between 2003 and 2005, there were few anesthesia-related deaths associated with epidural use (Lewis, 2007).

There were no anesthesia-related maternal deaths among nearly 20,000 women who received epidural analgesia in the MFMU Network study cited earlier (Bloom, 2005). And finally, Ruppen and associates (2006) reviewed data from 27 studies involving 1.4 million pregnant women who received epidural analgesia. They calculated risks of 1:145,000 for deep epidural infection, 1:168,000 for epidural hematoma, and 1:240,000 for persistent neurological injury.

Contraindications

As with spinal analgesia, contraindications to epidural analgesia include actual or anticipated serious maternal hemorrhage, infection at or near the puncture site, and suspicion of neurological disease (see Table 25-6).

Thrombocytopenia. Although low platelet counts are intuitively worrisome, the level at which epidural bleeding *might* develop is unknown according to the American Society of Anesthesiologists Task Force on Obstetrical Anesthesia (2007). Epidural hematomas are rare, and incidence of nerve damage from a hematoma is estimated to be 1 in 150,000 (Grant, 2007). The American College of Obstetricians and Gynecologists (2013b) has concluded that women with a platelet count of 50,000 to 100,000/μL may be candidates for regional analgesia.

Anticoagulation. Women receiving anticoagulation therapy who are given regional analgesia are at increased risk for spinal cord hematoma and compression (Chap. 52, p. 1039). The American College of Obstetricians and Gynecologists (2013b) has concluded the following:

1. Women receiving unfractionated heparin therapy should be able to receive regional analgesia if they have a normal activated partial thromboplastin time (aPTT)
2. Women receiving prophylactic doses of unfractionated heparin or low-dose aspirin are not at increased risk and can be offered regional analgesia
3. For women receiving once-daily low-dose low-molecular-weight heparin, regional analgesia should not be placed until 12 hours after the last injection
4. Low-molecular-weight heparin should be withheld for at least 2 hours after epidural catheter removal
5. The safety of regional analgesia in women receiving twice-daily low-molecular-weight heparin has not been studied sufficiently. It is not known whether delaying regional analgesia for 24 hours after the last injection is adequate.

Severe Preeclampsia-Eclampsia. Potential concerns with epidural analgesia in those with severe preeclampsia include hypotension as well as hypertension from pressor agents given to correct hypotension. Additionally, there is the potential for pulmonary edema following infusion of large volumes of crystalloid. These are outweighed by disadvantages of general anesthesia. Tracheal intubation may be difficult because of upper airway edema. Moreover, general anesthesia can lead to severe, sudden hypertension that can cause pulmonary or cerebral edema or intracranial hemorrhage.

With improved techniques for infusion of dilute local anesthetics into the epidural space, most obstetricians and obstetrical anesthesiologists have come to favor epidural blockade for labor and delivery in women with severe preeclampsia. There seems to be no argument that epidural analgesia for women with severe preeclampsia-eclampsia can be safely used when trained anesthesiologists and obstetricians are responsible for the woman and her fetus. In a study from Parkland Hospital, Lucas and colleagues (2001) randomly assigned 738 women with hypertension to epidural analgesia or patient-controlled intravenous analgesia during labor. A standardized protocol for prehydration, incremental epidural administration, and ephedrine use was employed. They concluded that labor epidural analgesia was safe in women with hypertensive disorders.

Women with severe preeclampsia have remarkably diminished intravascular volume compared with normal pregnancy

(Zeeman, 2009). Conversely, total body water is increased because of the capillary leak caused by endothelial cell activation (Chap. 40, p. 734). This imbalance is manifested as pathological peripheral edema, proteinuria, ascites, and total lung water. For all of these reasons, aggressive volume replacement increases the risk for pulmonary edema, especially in the first 72 hours postpartum. In one study, Hogg and associates (1999) reported that 3.5 percent of women with severe preeclampsia developed pulmonary edema when preloaded without a protocol limitation to volume. Importantly, this risk can be reduced or obviated with judicious prehydration—usually with 500 to 1000 mL of crystalloid solution. Specifically, in the study by Lucas and colleagues (2001) cited earlier, there were no instances of pulmonary edema among the women in whom the crystalloid preload was limited to 500 mL. Moreover, vasodilation produced by epidural blockade is less abrupt if the analgesia level is achieved slowly with dilute solutions of local anesthetic agents. This allows maintenance of blood pressure while simultaneously avoiding infusion of large crystalloid volumes.

With vigorous intravenous crystalloid therapy, there is also concern about development of cerebral edema (Chap. 40, p. 745). Finally, Heller and coworkers (1983) demonstrated that most cases of pharyngolaryngeal edema were related to aggressive volume therapy.

Epidural Opiate Analgesia

Injection of opiates into the epidural space to relieve pain from labor has become popular. Their mechanism of action derives from interaction with specific receptors in the dorsal horn and dorsal roots. Opiates alone usually will not provide adequate analgesia, and they most often are given with a local anesthetic agent such as bupivacaine. The major advantages of using such a combination are the rapid onset of pain relief, a decrease in shivering, and less dense motor blockade. Side effects are common and include pruritus and urinary retention. Naloxone, given intravenously, will abolish these symptoms without affecting the analgesic action.

Combined Spinal-Epidural Techniques

The combination of spinal and epidural techniques has increased in popularity and may provide rapid and effective analgesia for labor and for cesarean delivery. An introducer needle is first placed in the epidural space. A small-gauge spinal needle is then introduced through the epidural needle into the subarachnoid space—this is called the *needle-through-needle technique* (see Figure 25-3). A single bolus of an opioid, sometimes in combination with a local anesthetic, is injected into the subarachnoid space. The spinal needle is withdrawn, and an epidural catheter is then placed through the introducer needle. A subarachnoid opioid bolus results in the rapid onset of profound pain relief with virtually no motor blockade. The epidural catheter permits repeated analgesia dosing. Miro (2008) compared epidural analgesia with combined spinal-epidural analgesia for labor in 6497 women and found the overall outcomes and complications to be similar for the two techniques. In a randomized comparison, however, Abrão and colleagues (2009) reported that combined spinal-epidural analgesia was associated with a greater incidence of fetal heart rate abnormalities related to uterine hypertonus than was epidural analgesia alone. Beamon and coworkers (2014) reported similar results.

Continuous Spinal Analgesia During Labor

There is emerging interest in continuous spinal analgesia for relief of labor pain. This neuraxial technique was first used more than 60 years ago (Hinebaugh, 1944). Frequent severe postdural puncture headaches led to its abandonment. With redesigned needles and catheters, Arkoosh (2008) subsequently randomized 429 women to either continuous spinal or conventional epidural analgesia during labor. There were no differences in complications between these two neuraxial techniques. However, the technique remains investigational.

Local Infiltration for Cesarean Delivery

A local block is occasionally useful to augment an inadequate or "patchy" regional block that was given emergently. Rarely, local infiltration may be needed to perform an emergency cesarean delivery to save the life of a fetus in the absence of anesthesia support. Young (2012) reviewed regional analgesia techniques used for cesarean delivery that provide analgesia to the parietal peritoneum as well as skin and muscles of the anterior abdominal wall.

In one technique, the skin is infiltrated along the proposed incision, and the subcutaneous, muscle, and rectus sheath layers are injected as the abdomen is opened. A dilute solution of lidocaine—30 mL of 2-percent with 1:200,000 epinephrine diluted with 60 mL of normal saline—is prepared, and a total of 100 to 120 mL is infiltrated. Injection of large volumes into the fatty layers, which are relatively devoid of nerve supply, is avoided to limit the total dose of local anesthetic needed.

A second technique involves a field block of the major branches supplying the abdominal wall, to include the 10th, 11th, and 12th intercostal nerves and the ilioinguinal and genitofemoral nerves. As shown in Figure 25-6, the former group of nerves is located at a point midway between the costal margin and iliac crest in the midaxillary line. The latter group is found at the level of the external inguinal ring. Only one skin puncture is made at each of the four sites (right and left sides). At the intercostal block site, the needle is directed medially, and injection is carried down to the transversalis fascia, avoiding injection of the subcutaneous fat. Approximately 5 to 8 mL of 0.5-percent lidocaine is injected. The procedure is repeated at a 45-degree angle cephalad and caudad to this line. The other side is then injected. At the ilioinguinal and genitofemoral sites, the injection is started at a site 2 to 3 cm lateral from the pubic tubercle at a 45-degree angle. Finally, the skin overlying the planned incision is injected.

GENERAL ANESTHESIA

Trained personnel and specialized equipment—including fiberoptic intubation—are mandatory for the safe use of general anesthesia. This is because a common cause of death cited for

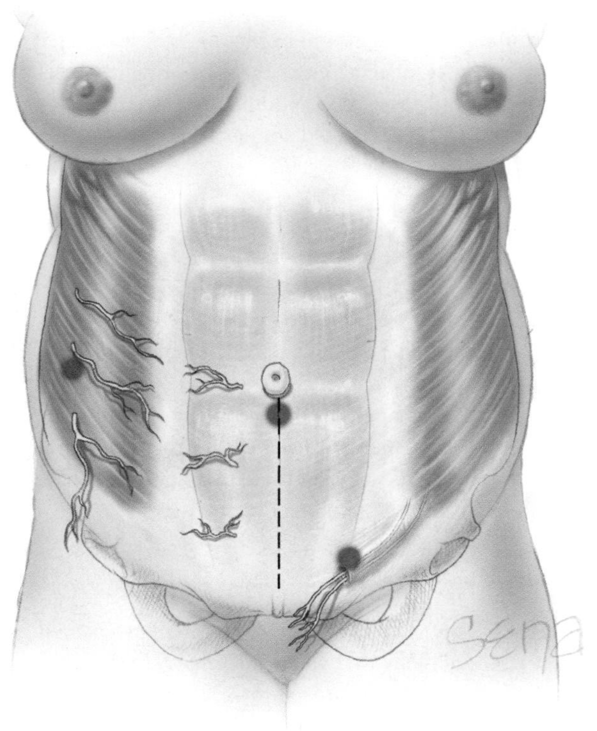

FIGURE 25-6 Local anesthetic block for cesarean delivery. The first injection site is halfway between the costal margin and iliac crest in the midaxillary line to block the 10th, 11th, and 12th intercostal nerves. A second injection at the external inguinal ring blocks branches of the genitofemoral and ilioinguinal nerves. These sites are infiltrated bilaterally. A final site is along the line of proposed skin incision.

general anesthesia is failed intubation. This occurs in approximately 1 of every 250 general anesthetics administered to pregnant women—a tenfold higher rate than in nonpregnant patients (Hawkins, 2011; Quinn, 2013). The American College of Obstetricians and Gynecologists (2013b) has concluded that this relative increase in morbidity and mortality rates suggests that neuraxial analgesia is the preferred method of pain control and should be used unless contraindicated (see Table 25-6). Indeed, in two reports from the MFMU Network, 93 percent of more than 54,000 cesarean deliveries were performed using neuraxial analgesia (Bloom, 2005; Brookfield, 2013). Butwick and coworkers (2014) cited a higher incidence of general anesthesia use among non-white women.

Patient Preparation

Before anesthesia induction, several steps should be taken to help minimize the complication risks. These include antacid use, lateral uterine displacement, and preoxygenation.

Antacid administration shortly before anesthesia induction has probably decreased mortality rates from general anesthesia more than any other single practice. The American Society of Anesthesiologists Task Force on Obstetrical Anesthesia (2007) recommends timely administration of a nonparticulate antacid, an H_2-receptor antagonist, or metoclopramide. For many years, we have recommended administration of 30 mL of Bicitra—sodium citrate with citric acid—a few minutes before anesthesia induction by either general or major neuraxial block. If more than 1 hour has passed after the first dose was given and anesthesia has not yet been induced, then a second dose is given.

Lateral uterine displacement is also provided as the uterus may compress the inferior vena cava and aorta when the mother is supine. With uterine displacement, the duration of general anesthesia has less effect on neonatal condition than if the woman remains supine (Crawford, 1972).

Last, because functional reserve lung capacity is reduced, the pregnant woman becomes hypoxemic more rapidly during periods of apnea than do nonpregnant patients. Obesity exacerbates this tendency (McClelland, 2009). To minimize hypoxia between the time of muscle relaxant injection and intubation, it is important first to replace nitrogen in the lungs with oxygen. This preoxygenation is accomplished by administering 100-percent oxygen via face mask for 2 to 3 minutes before anesthesia induction. In an emergency, four vital capacity breaths of 100-percent oxygen via a tight breathing circuit will provide similar benefit (Norris, 1985).

Induction of Anesthesia

Thiopental given intravenously was widely used and offered easy and rapid induction, prompt recovery, and minimal risk of vomiting. Unfortunately, this thiobarbiturate is no longer available in the United States because the sole European manufacturer stopped production on the basis that the drug was also being used for capital punishment (American Society of Anesthesiologists, 2011). It was deemed "an unfortunate irony that many more lives will be lost or put in jeopardy as a result of not having thiopental available for its legitimate medical use." Drugs now being used in lieu of thiopental include propofol or etomidate. Propofol has the undesirable side effect of hypotension.

Ketamine also may be used to render a patient unconscious. Doses of 1 mg/kg induce general anesthesia. Alternatively, given intravenously in low doses of 0.2 to 0.3 mg/kg, ketamine may be used to produce analgesia and sedation just before vaginal delivery. Ketamine may also prove useful in women with acute hemorrhage because it is not associated with hypotension. Conversely, it usually causes a rise in blood pressure, and thus it generally should be avoided in women who are already hypertensive. Unpleasant delirium and hallucinations are commonly induced by this agent.

Intubation

Immediately after a patient is rendered unconscious, a muscle relaxant is given to aid intubation. *Succinylcholine,* a rapid-onset and short-acting agent, frequently is used. Cricoid pressure—the *Sellick maneuver*—is applied by a trained assistant to occlude the esophagus from the onset of induction until intubation is completed. Before the operation begins, proper placement of the endotracheal tube must be confirmed.

Failed Intubation

Although uncommon, failed intubation is a major cause of anesthesia-related maternal mortality. A history of prior difficult intubation and a careful anatomical assessment of the neck and the maxillofacial, pharyngeal, and laryngeal structures may help predict intubation complications. Even in cases in which the initial airway assessment was unremarkable, edema may develop intrapartum and present considerable challenges. Morbid obesity is also a major risk factor for failed or difficult intubation. The American Society of Anesthesiologists Task Force on Obstetrical Anesthesia (2007) stresses the importance of appropriate preoperative preparation. This includes the immediate availability of specialized equipment such as different-shaped laryngoscopes, laryngeal mask airways, fiberoptic bronchoscope, and transtracheal ventilation set, as well as liberal use of awake oral intubation techniques.

Management. An important principle is to start the operative procedure only after it has been ascertained that tracheal intubation has been successful and that adequate ventilation can be accomplished. Even with an abnormal fetal heart rate pattern, cesarean delivery initiation will only serve to complicate matters if there is difficult or failed intubation. Frequently, the woman must be allowed to awaken and a different technique used, such as an awake intubation or regional analgesia.

Following failed intubation, the woman is ventilated by mask and cricoid pressure is applied to reduce the aspiration risk. Surgery may proceed with mask ventilation, or the woman may be allowed to awaken. In those cases in which the woman has been paralyzed and in which ventilation cannot be reestablished by insertion of an oral airway, by laryngeal mask airway, or by use of a fiberoptic laryngoscope to intubate the trachea, then a life-threatening emergency exists. To restore ventilation, percutaneous or even open cricothyrotomy is performed, and jet ventilation begun. Failed intubation drills have been recommended to optimize response to such an emergency.

Gas Anesthetics

Once the endotracheal tube is secured, a 50:50 mixture of nitrous oxide and oxygen is administered to provide analgesia. Usually, a volatile halogenated agent is added to provide amnesia and additional analgesia. The mechanisms of action of inhaled anesthetics have been reviewed by Campagna and associates (2003).

The most commonly used volatile anesthetics in the United States include *isoflurane* and two of its derivatives, *desflurane* and *sevoflurane.* They are usually added in low concentrations to the nitrous oxide-oxygen mixture to provide amnesia. They are potent, nonexplosive agents that produce remarkable uterine relaxation when given in high concentrations. These are used when relaxation is a requisite, such as for internal podalic version of the second twin, breech decomposition, and replacement of the acutely inverted uterus.

Extubation

The endotracheal tube may be safely removed only if the woman is conscious to a degree that enables her to follow commands and is capable of maintaining oxygen saturation with spontaneous respiration. Consideration should be given to emptying the stomach via a nasogastric tube before extubation. As induction has become safer, extubation may now be more perilous. Of 15 anesthesia-related deaths of pregnant women from 1985 to 2003 in Michigan, none occurred during induction, whereas five resulted from hypoventilation or airway obstruction during emergence, extubation, or recovery (Mhyre, 2007).

Aspiration

Massive gastric acidic inhalation may cause pulmonary insufficiency from aspiration pneumonitis. Such pneumonitis has in the past been the most common cause of anesthetic deaths in obstetrics and therefore deserves special attention. To minimize this risk, antacids should be given routinely, intubation should be accompanied by cricoid pressure, and regional analgesia should be employed when possible.

Fasting

According to the American Society of Anesthesiologists Task Force on Obstetrical Anesthesia (2007) and the American College of Obstetricians and Gynecologists (2013a), there are insufficient data regarding fasting times for clear liquids and the risk of pulmonary aspiration during labor. Recommendations are that modest amounts of clear liquids such as water, clear tea, black coffee, carbonated beverages, and pulp-free fruit juices be allowed in uncomplicated laboring women. Obvious solid foods should be avoided. A fasting period of 6 to 8 hours, depending on the type of food ingested, is recommended for uncomplicated parturients undergoing elective cesarean delivery or puerperal tubal ligation.

O'Sullivan (2009) randomized 2426 low-risk nulliparas to consume either water and ice chips alone or small amounts of bread, biscuits, vegetables, fruits, yogurt, soup, and fruit juice. Approximately 30 percent of women in each arm of the study underwent cesarean delivery. No cases of aspiration occurred during the study, although approximately a third of women in each study arm vomited during labor or delivery. Epidural analgesia during labor was used in this study, although the authors did not report the type of anesthesia used for cesarean deliveries. Presumably neuraxial analgesia was used for cesarean deliveries, and this greatly minimized the pulmonary aspiration risk associated with general anesthesia. Given the low prevalence of aspiration, this trial, albeit large, was not powered to measure whether feeding during labor was safe. Our policy at Parkland Hospital is to prohibit oral intake during labor and delivery.

Pathophysiology

In 1952, Teabeaut demonstrated experimentally that if the pH of aspirated fluid was below 2.5, severe chemical pneumonitis developed. It was later demonstrated that the gastric juice pH of nearly half of women tested intrapartum was < 2.5 (Taylor, 1966). The right mainstem bronchus usually offers the simplest pathway for aspirated material to reach the lung parenchyma, and therefore, the right lower lobe is most often involved. In severe cases, there is bilateral widespread involvement.

The woman who aspirates may develop evidence of respiratory distress immediately or several hours after aspiration, depending in part on the material aspirated and the severity of the response. Aspiration of a large amount of solid material causes obvious airway obstruction signs. Smaller particles without acidic liquid may lead to patchy atelectasis and later to bronchopneumonia.

When highly acidic liquid is inspired, decreased oxygen saturation along with tachypnea, bronchospasm, rhonchi, rales, atelectasis, cyanosis, tachycardia, and hypotension are likely to develop. At the injury sites, there is pulmonary capillary leakage and exudation of protein-rich fluid containing numerous erythrocytes into the lung interstitium and alveoli. This causes decreased pulmonary compliance, shunting of blood, and severe hypoxemia. Radiographic changes may not appear immediately, and these may be variable, although the right lung most often is affected. Therefore, chest radiographs alone should not be used to exclude aspiration.

Treatment

The methods recommended for treatment of aspiration have changed appreciably in recent years, indicating that previous therapy was not very successful. Suspicion of aspiration of gastric contents demands close monitoring for evidence of pulmonary damage. Respiratory rate and oxygen saturation as measured by pulse oximetry are the most sensitive and earliest indicators of injury.

Inhaled fluid should be immediately and thoroughly wiped from the mouth and removed from the pharynx and trachea by suction. Saline lavage may further disseminate the acid throughout the lung and is not recommended. If large particulate matter is inspired, bronchoscopy may be indicated to relieve airway obstruction. There is no convincing clinical or experimental evidence that corticosteroid therapy or prophylactic antimicrobial administration is beneficial (Marik, 2001). If clinical evidence of infection develops, however, then vigorous treatment is given. If acute respiratory distress syndrome develops, mechanical ventilation with positive end-expiratory pressure may prove lifesaving (Chap. 47, p. 944).

REFERENCES

Abrão KC, Francisco RP, Miyadahira S, et al: Elevation of uterine basal tone and fetal heart rate abnormalities after labor analgesia: a randomized controlled trial. Obstet Gynecol 113(10):41, 2009

Alexander JM, Sharma SK, McIntire DD, et al: Epidural analgesia lengthens the Friedman active phase of labor. Obstet Gynecol 100:46, 2002

American Academy of Pediatrics and American College of Obstetricians and Gynecologists: Guidelines for Perinatal Care, 7th ed. Washington, 2012

American College of Obstetricians and Gynecologists: Oral intake during labor. Committee Opinion No. 441, September 2009, Reaffirmed 2013a

American College of Obstetricians and Gynecologists: Obstetric analgesia and anesthesia. Practice Bulletin 36, July 2002, Reaffirmed 2013b

American College of Obstetricians and Gynecologists and the American Society of Anesthesiologists: Pain relief during labor. Committee Opinion No. 295, July 2004, Reaffirmed 2008

American College of Obstetricians and Gynecologists and the American Society of Anesthesiologists: Optimal goals for anesthesia care in obstetrics. Committee Opinion No.433, May 2009

American Society of Anesthesiologists: ASA Statement on Sodium thiopental's removal from the market, January 21, 2011. Available at: http://www.asahq.org/For-the-Public-and-Media/Press-Room/ASA-News/ASA-Statement-on-Thiopental-Removal-from-the-Market.aspx. Accessed August 1, 2013

American Society of Anesthesiologists Task Force on Obstetrical Anesthesia: Practice guidelines for obstetrical anesthesia. Anesthesiology 106:843, 2007

Arkoosh V, Palmer C, Yun E, et al: A randomized, double-masked, multicenter comparison of the safety of continuous intrathecal labor analgesia using a 28-gauge catheter versus continuous epidural labor analgesia. Anesthesiology 108(2):286, 2008

Atkinson BD, Truitt LJ, Rayburn WF, et al: Double-blind comparison of intravenous butorphanol (Stadol) and fentanyl (Sublimaze) for analgesia during labor. Am J Obstet Gynecol 171:993, 1994

Beamon C, Stuebe A, Edwards L, et al: Effect of mode of regional anesthesia on neonatal outcomes in preeclamptic patients. Am J Obstet Gynecol 210:S173, 2014

Bell ED, Penning DH, Cousineau EF, et al: How much labor is in a labor epidural? Manpower cost and reimbursement for an obstetric analgesia service in a teaching institution. Anesthesiology 92:851, 2000

Berg CJ, Callaghan WM, Syverson C, et al: Pregnancy-related mortality in the United States, 1998 to 2005. Obstet Gynecol 116:1302, 2010

Bloom SL, Spong CY, Weiner SJ, et al: Complications of anesthesia for cesarean delivery. Obstet Gynecol 106:281, 2005

Bricker L, Lavender T: Parenteral opioids for labor pain relief: A systematic review. Am J Obstet Gynecol 186:S94, 2002

Brookfield K, Osmundson S, Jaqvi M, et al: General anesthesia at cesarean delivery portends worse maternal and neonatal outcomes. Abstract No. 672. Am J Obstet Gynecol 208(1 Suppl):S28, 2013

Butler R, Fuller J: Back pain following epidural anaesthesia in labour. Can J Anaesth 45:724, 1998

Butwick A, Blumenfeld Y, Brookfeld K, et al: Ethnic disparities among patients undergoing general anesthesia for cesarean delivery. Am J Obstet Gynecol 210:S259, 2014

Camann WR, Murray RS, Mushlin PS, et al: Effects of oral caffeine on postdural puncture headache: a double-blinded, placebo-controlled trial. Anesth Analg 70:181, 1990

Campagna JA, Miller KW, Forman SA: Mechanisms of actions of inhaled anesthetics. N Engl J Med 348:2110, 2003

Centers for Disease Control and Prevention: Bacterial meningitis after intrapartum anesthesia—New York and Ohio, 2008–2009. MMWR 59(3):65, 2010

Chan BO, Paech MJ: Persistent cerebrospinal fluid leak: a complication of the combined spinal-epidural technique. Anesth Analg 98:828, 2004

Chestnut DH: Effect on the progress of labor and method of delivery. In Chestnut DH (ed): Obstetric Anesthesia: Principles and Practice, 2nd ed. St Louis: Mosby-Year Book, 1999, p 408

Chestnut DH, McGrath JM, Vincent RD Jr, et al: Does early administration of epidural analgesia affect obstetric outcome in nulliparous women who are in spontaneous labor? Anesthesiology 80:1201, 1994a

Chestnut DH, Owen CL, Bates JN, et al: Continuous infusion epidural analgesia during labor: a randomized, double-blind comparison of 0.625% bupivacaine/0.0002% fentanyl versus 0.125% bupivacaine. Anesthesiology 68:754, 1988

Chestnut DH, Vincent RD Jr, McGrather JM, et al: Does early administration of epidural analgesia affect obstetric outcome in nulliparous women who are receiving intravenous oxytocin? Anesthesiology 80:1193, 1994b

Chisholm ME, Campbell DC: Postpartum postural headache due to superior sagittal sinus thrombosis mistaken for spontaneous intracranial hypotension. Can J Anaesth 48:302, 2001

Craig MG, Tao W, McIntire DD, et al: A randomized trial of bupivacaine plus fentanyl versus only fentanyl for epidural analgesia during the second stage of labor. Anesth Analg 2014 In press

Crawford JS: Some maternal complications of epidural analgesia for labour. Anaesthesia 40:1219, 1985

Crawford JS, Burton M, Davies P: Time and lateral tilt at caesarean section. Br J Anaesth 44:477, 1972

Danilenko-Dixon DR, Tefft L, Haydon B, et al: The effect of maternal position on cardiac output with epidural analgesia in labor [Abstract]. Am J Obstet Gynecol 174:332, 1996

Darouiche RO: Spinal epidural abscess. N Engl J Med 355:2012, 2006

Dashe JS, Rogers BB, McIntire DD, et al: Epidural analgesia and intrapartum fever: placental findings. Obstet Gynecol 93:341, 1999

Dawley B, Hendrix A: Intracranial subdural hematoma after spinal anesthesia in a parturient. Obstet Gynecol 113(2):570, 2009

Dresner M, Brocklesby J, Bamber J: Audit of the influence of body mass index on the performance of epidural analgesia in labour and the subsequent mode of delivery. Br J Obstet Gynaecol 113:1178, 2006

Friedman EA: Primigravid labor: a graphicostatistical analysis. Obstet Gynecol 6:567, 1955

Fusi L, Steer PJ, Maresh MJA, et al: Maternal pyrexia associated with the use of epidural analgesia in labour. Lancet 1:1250, 1989

Gambling DR, Sharma SK, Ramin SM, et al: A randomized study of combined spinal-epidural analgesia versus intravenous meperidine during labor: impact on cesarean delivery rate. Anesthesiology 89(6):1336, 1998

Glosten B: Local anesthetic techniques. In Chestnut DH (ed): Obstetric Anesthesia: Principles and Practice, 2nd ed. St Louis, Mosby-Year Book, 1999, p 363

Grant GJ: Safely giving regional anesthesia to gravidas with clotting disorders. Contemp OB Gyn August, 2007
Halpern SH, Carvalho B: Patient-controlled epidural analgesia for labor. Anesth Analg 108(3):921, 2009
Hants Y, Kabiri D, Gat R, et al: Neuraxial analgesia may reduce the risk for cesarean delivery during induced labor. Abstract No. 339. Am J Obstet Gynecol 208(1 Suppl):S151, 2013
Hatjis CG, Meis PJ: Sinusoidal fetal heart rate pattern associated with butorphanol administration. Obstet Gynecol 67:377, 1986
Hawkins JL: Epidural analgesia for labor and delivery. N Engl J Med 362:1503, 2010
Hawkins JL, Chang J, Palmer SK, et al: Anesthesia-related maternal mortality in the United States: 1979–2002. Obstet Gynecol 117:69, 2011
Hawkins JL, Koonin LM, Palmer SK, et al: Anesthesia-related deaths during obstetric delivery in the United States, 1979–1990. Anesthesiology 86:277, 1997
Heller PJ, Scheider EP, Marx GF: Pharyngolaryngeal edema as a presenting symptom in preeclampsia. Obstet Gynecol 62:523, 1983
Hess PE, Pratt SD, Lucas TP, et al: Predictors of breakthrough pain during labor epidural analgesia. Anesth Analg 93:414, 2001
Hill JB, Alexander JM, Sharma SK, et al: A comparison of the effects of epidural and meperidine analgesia during labor on fetal heart rate. Obstet Gynecol 102:333, 2003
Hinebaugh M, Lang W: Continuous spinal anesthesia for labor and delivery: a preliminary report. Ann Surg 120(2):143, 1944
Hogg B, Hauth JC, Caritis SN, et al: Safety of labor epidural anesthesia for women with severe hypertensive disease. Am J Obstet Gynecol 181:1096, 1999
Introna RPS, Blair JR, Neeld JB: What is the incidence of inadvertent dural puncture during epidural anesthesia in obstetrics? Anesthesiology 117(3):686, 2012
Katircioglu K, Hasegeli L, Ibrahimhakkioglu HF, et al: A retrospective review of 34,109 epidural anesthetics for obstetric and gynecologic procedures at a single private hospital in Turkey. Anesth Analg 107:1742, 2008
Kennedy WF Jr, Bonica JJ, Akamatsu TJ, et al: Cardiovascular and respiratory effects of subarachnoid block in the presence of acute blood loss. Anesthesiology 29:29, 1968
Krivak TC, Zorn KK: Venous thromboembolism in obstetrics and gynecology. Obstet Gynecol 109(3):761, 2007
Lee A, Ngan Kee WD, Gin T: A quantitative, systematic review of randomized controlled trials of ephedrine versus phenylephrine for the management of hypotension during spinal anesthesia for cesarean delivery. Anesth Analg 94:920, 2002a
Lee A, Ngan Kee WD, Gin T: Prophylactic ephedrine prevents hypotension during spinal anesthesia for cesarean delivery but does not improve neonatal outcome: a quantitative systematic review. Can J Anaesth 49:588, 2002b
Lee LA, Posner KL, Domino KB, et al: Injuries associated with regional anesthesia in the 1980s and 1990s: a closed claims analysis. Anesthesiology 101:143, 2004
Leighton BL, Halpern SH: The effects of epidural analgesia on labor, maternal, and neonatal outcomes: a systematic review. Am J Obstet Gynecol 186:569, 2002
Lewis G (ed): The Confidential Enquiry into Maternal and Child Health (CEMACH). Saving Mothers' Lives. London, CEMACH, 2007
Li G, Warner M, Lang BH et al: Epidemiology of anesthesia-related mortality in the United States, 1999–2005. Anesthesiology 110(4):759, 2009
Lieberman E, Lang JM, Cohen A, et al: Association of epidural analgesia with cesarean delivery in nulliparas. Obstet Gynecol 88:993, 1996
Lieberman E, O'Donoghue C: Unintended effects of epidural analgesia during labor: a systematic review. Am J Obstet Gynecol 186:531, 2002
Liu SS, Lin Y: Local anesthetics. In Barash P, Cullen B, Stoeling R, et al (eds): Clinical Anesthesia, 6th ed. Philadelphia, Lippincott Williams & Wilkins, 2009, p 541
Liu WH, Lin JH, Lin JC, et al: Severe intracranial and intraspinal subarachnoid hemorrhage after lumbar puncture: a rare case report. Am J Emerg Med 26:633, 2008
Lucas MJ, Sharma SK, McIntire DD, et al: A randomized trial of labor analgesia in women with pregnancy-induced hypertension. Am J Obstet Gynecol 185:970, 2001
Luxman D, Wholman I, Groutz A, et al: The effect of early epidural block administration on the progression and outcome of labor. Int J Obstet Anesth 7:161, 1998
Manninen T, Aantaa R, Salonen M, et al: A comparison of the hemodynamic effects of paracervical block and epidural anesthesia for labor analgesia. Acta Anaesthesiol Scand 44:441, 2000
Marik PE: Aspiration pneumonitis and aspiration pneumonia. N Engl J Med 344:665, 2001
McClelland SH, Bogod DG, Hardman JG: Pre-oxygenation and apnoea in pregnancy: changes during labour and with obstetric morbidity in a computational simulation. Anaesthesia 64(4):371, 2009
Mhyre JM, Riesner MN, Polley LS, et al: A series of anesthesia-related maternal deaths in Michigan, 1985–2003. Anesthesiology 106:1096, 2007
Miller N, Cypher R, Thomas S, et al: Admission pulse pressure is a novel predictor of fetal heart rate abnormalities following initial dosing of a labour epidural: a retrospective cohort study. Abstract No. 333. Am J Obstet Gynecol 208(1 Suppl):S149, 2013
Millet L, Shaha S, Bartholomew ML: Rates of bacteriuria in laboring with epidural analgesia: continuous vs intermittent bladder catheterization. Am J Obstet Gynecol 206:316, 2012
Miro M, Guasch E, Gilsanz F: Comparison of epidural analgesia with combined spinal-epidural for labor: a retrospective study of 6497 cases. Int J Obstet Anesth 17:15, 2008
Mulroy MF: Systemic toxicity and cardiotoxicity from local anesthetics: incidence and preventive measures. Reg Anesth Pain Med 27:556, 2002
Ngan Kee WD, Khaw KS, Ng FF, et al: Prophylactic phenylephrine infusion for preventing hypotension during spinal anesthesia for cesarean delivery. Anesth Analg 98:815, 2004
Noblett K, McKinney A, Kim R: Sheared epidural catheter during an elective procedure. Obstet Gynecol 109:566, 2007
Norris MC, Dewan DM: Preoxygenation for cesarean section: A comparison of two techniques. Anesthesiology 62:827, 1985
Ohel G, Gonen R, Vaida S, et al: Early versus late initiation of epidural analgesia in labor: does it increase the risk of cesarean section? A randomized trial. Am J Obstet Gynecol 194:600, 2006
Osterman MJK, Martin JA: Epidural and spinal anesthesia use during labor, 2008. Natl Vital Stat Rep 59(5):1, 2011a
Osterman MJK, Martin JA, Mathews TJ, et al: Expanded data from the new birth certificate, 2008. Natl Vital Stat Rep 59(7):1, 2011b
O'Sullivan G, Liu B, Hart D, et al: Effect of food intake during labour on obstetric outcome: randomised controlled trial. BMJ 338:b784, 2009
Quilligan EJ, Keegan KA, Donahue MJ: Double-blind comparison of intravenously injected butorphanol and meperidine in parturients. Int J Gynaecol Obstet 18:363, 1980
Quinn AC, Milne D, Columb M, et al: Failed tracheal intubation in obstetric anaesthesia: 2 yr national case-control study in the UK. Br J Anaesth 110(1):74, 2013
Ramin SM, Gambling DR, Lucas MJ, et al: Randomized trial of epidural versus intravenous analgesia during labor. Obstet Gynecol 86(5):783, 1995
Reynolds F, Sharma SK, Seed PT: Analgesia in labour and fetal acid-base balance: a meta-analysis comparing epidural with systemic opioid analgesia. Br J Obstet Gynaecol 109:1344, 2002
Rogers R, Gilson G, Kammerer-Doak D: Epidural analgesia and active management of labor: effects on length of labor and mode of delivery. Obstet Gynecol 93:995, 1999
Rosen MA: Nitrous oxide for relief of labor pain: a systematic review. Am J Obstet Gynecol 186:S110, 2002a
Rosen MA: Paracervical block for labor analgesia: a brief historic review. Am J Obstet Gynecol 186:S127, 2002b
Ruppen W, Derry S, McQuay H, et al: Incidence of epidural hematoma, infection, and neurologic injury in obstetric patients with epidural analgesia/anesthesia. Anesthesiology 105:394, 2006
Scavone BM, Wong CA, Sullivan JT, et al: Efficacy of a prophylactic epidural blood patch in preventing post dural puncture headache in parturients after inadvertent dural puncture. Anesthesiology 101:1422, 2004
Setayesh AR, Kholdebarin AR, Moghadam MS, et al: The Trendelenburg position increases the spread and accelerates the onset of epidural anesthesia for cesarean section. Can J Anaesth 48:890, 2001
Seyb ST, Berka RJ, Socol ML, et al: Risk of cesarean delivery with elective induction of labor at term in nulliparous women. Obstet Gynecol 94:600, 1999
Sharma SK, Alexander JM, Messick G, et al: Cesarean delivery: a randomized trial of epidural analgesia versus intravenous meperidine analgesia during labor in nulliparous women. Anesthesiology 96(3):546, 2002
Sharma SK, Leveno KJ: Regional analgesia and progress of labor. Clin Obstet Gynecol 46:633, 2003
Sharma SK, McIntire DD, Wiley J, et al: Labor analgesia and cesarean delivery. An individual patient meta-analysis of nulliparous women. Anesthesiology 100:142, 2004
Sharma SK, Rogers BB, Alexander JM, et al: A randomized trial of the effects of antibiotic prophylaxis on epidural related fever in labor. Anesth Analg 2014 In press
Sharma SK, Sidawi JE, Ramin SM, et al: Cesarean delivery: a randomized trial of epidural versus patient-controlled meperidine analgesia during labor. Anesthesiology 87:487, 1997
Shearer VE, Jhaveri HS, Cunningham FG: Puerperal seizures after post-dural puncture headache. Obstet Gynecol 85:255, 1995

Smarkusky L, DeCarvalho H, Bermudez A, et al: Acute onset headache complicating labor epidural caused by intrapartum pneumocephalus. Obstet Gynecol 108:795, 2006

Sprigge JS, Harper SJ: Accidental dural puncture and post dural puncture headache in obstetric anaesthesia: presentation and management: a 23-year survey in a district general hospital. Anaesthesia 63:36, 2008

Svancarek W, Chirino O, Schaefer G Jr, et al: Retropsoas and subgluteal abscesses following paracervical and pudendal anesthesia. JAMA 237:892, 1977

Taylor G, Pryse-Davies J: The prophylactic use of antacids in the prevention of the acid pulmonary aspiration syndrome (Mendelson's syndrome). Lancet 1:288, 1966

Teabeaut JR II: Aspiration of gastric contents: an experimental study. Am J Pathol 28:51, 1952

Tsui MHY, Kee WDN, Ng FF, et al: A double blinded randomized placebo controlled study of intramuscular pethidine for pain relief in the first stage of labour. Br J Obstet Gynaecol 111:648, 2004

Vallejo MC, Mandell GL, Sabo DP, et al: Postdural puncture headache: a randomized comparison of five spinal needles in obstetric patients. Anesth Analg 91:916, 2000

Vricella LK, Louis JM, Mercer BM, et al: Impact of morbid obesity on epidural anesthesia complications in labor. Am J Obstet Gynecol 205:307, 2011

Wallace DH, Leveno KJ, Cunningham FG, et al: Randomized comparison of general and regional anesthesia for cesarean delivery in pregnancies complicated by severe preeclampsia. Obstet Gynecol 86:193, 1995

Wong CA, McCarthy RJ, Sullivan JT, et al: Early compared with late neuraxial analgesia in nulliparous labor induction. Obstet Gynecol 113(5):1066, 2009

Wong CA, Scavone BM, Peaceman AM, et al: The risk of cesarean delivery with neuraxial analgesia given early versus late in labor. N Engl J Med 352:655, 2005

Yancey MK, Pierce B, Schweitzer D, et al: Observations on labor epidural analgesia and operative delivery rates. Am J Obstet Gynecol 180:353, 1999

Yancey MK, Zhang J, Schweitzer DL, et al: Epidural analgesia and fetal head malposition at vaginal delivery. Obstet Gynecol 97:608, 2001

Young MJ, Gorlin AW, Modes VE, et al: Clinical implications of the transversus abdominis plane block in adults. Anesthesiol Res Pract 2012:731645, 2012

Zeeman GG, Cunningham FG, Pritchard JA: The magnitude of hemoconcentration with eclampsia. Hypertens Preg 28(2):127, 2009

Zhang J, Yancey MK, Klebanoff MA, et al: Does epidural analgesia prolong labor and increase risk of cesarean delivery? A natural experiment. Am J Obstet Gynecol 185:128, 2001

CHAPTER 26

Induction and Augmentation of Labor

Induction implies stimulation of contractions before the spontaneous onset of labor, with or without ruptured membranes. When the cervix is closed and uneffaced, labor induction will often commence with *cervical ripening*, a process that generally employs prostaglandins to soften and open the cervix.

Augmentation refers to enhancement of spontaneous contractions that are considered inadequate because of failed cervical dilation and fetal descent. In the United States, the incidence of labor induction more than doubled from 9.5 percent in 1991 to 23.2 percent in 2011 (Martin, 2013). The incidence is variable between practices. At Parkland Hospital approximately 35 percent of labors are induced or augmented. By comparison, at the University of Alabama at Birmingham Hospital, labor is induced in approximately 20 percent of women, and another 35 percent are given oxytocin for augmentation—a total of 55 percent. This chapter includes an overview of indications for labor induction and augmentation and a description of various techniques to effect preinduction cervical ripening.

LABOR INDUCTION

Indications

Induction is indicated when the benefits to either mother or fetus outweigh those of pregnancy continuation. The more common indications include membrane rupture without labor, gestational hypertension, oligohydramnios, nonreassuring fetal status, postterm pregnancy, and various maternal medical conditions such as chronic hypertension and diabetes (American College of Obstetricians and Gynecologists, 2013b).

Contraindications

Methods to induce or augment labor are contraindicated by most conditions that preclude spontaneous labor or delivery. The few maternal contraindications are related to prior uterine incision type, contracted or distorted pelvic anatomy, abnormally implanted placentas, and uncommon conditions such as active genital herpes infection or cervical cancer. Fetal factors include appreciable macrosomia, severe hydrocephalus, malpresentation, or nonreassuring fetal status.

Techniques

Oxytocin has been used for decades to induce or augment labor. Other effective methods include prostaglandins, such as misoprostol and dinoprostone, and mechanical methods that encompass stripping of membranes, artificial rupture of membranes, extraamnionic saline infusion, transcervical balloons, and hygroscopic cervical dilators. Importantly, and as recommended in *Guidelines for Perinatal Care*, each obstetrical department should have its own written protocols that describe administration of these methods for labor induction and augmentation (American Academy of Pediatrics and American College of Obstetricians and Gynecologists, 2012).

Risks

Maternal complications associated with labor induction consist of cesarean delivery, chorioamnionitis, uterine scar rupture, and postpartum hemorrhage from uterine atony.

Cesarean Delivery Rate

This is especially increased in nulliparas undergoing induction (Luthy, 2004; Yeast, 1999). Indeed, several investigators have reported a two- to threefold increased risk (Hoffman, 2003; Maslow, 2000; Smith, 2003). Moreover, these rates are inversely related with cervical favorability at induction, that is, the *Bishop score* (Vahratian, 2005; Vrouenraets, 2005). The increased risk for cesarean delivery with labor induction does not appear to be lowered with preinduction cervical ripening in the nullipara with an unfavorable cervix (Mercer, 2005). In fact, the cesarean delivery rate following elective induction was significantly increased even in women with a Bishop score of 7 or greater compared with that in those with spontaneous labor (Hamar, 2001). Station and position of the fetal vertex may also affect success rates. For example, in nulliparas at > 41 weeks' gestation and with an unengaged vertex, the cesarean delivery rate was increased 12-fold compared with that in women with an engaged fetal vertex (Shin, 2004).

The premise that elective labor induction increases the risk of cesarean delivery has been questioned (Macones, 2009). Many studies have compared women undergoing labor induction to those laboring spontaneously. However, using women undergoing expectant management, Osmundson and colleagues (2010, 2011) reported similar cesarean delivery rates in more than 4000 women undergoing elective induction between 39 and nearly 41 weeks with or without a favorable cervix. Currently, this subject remains unresolved.

Chorioamnionitis

Amniotomy is often selected to augment labor (p. 531). Women whose labor is managed with amniotomy have an increased incidence of chorioamnionitis compared with those in spontaneous labor (American College of Obstetricians and Gynecologists, 2013a).

Rupture of a Prior Uterine Incision

Uterine rupture during labor in women with a history of prior uterine surgery can be catastrophic (Chap. 31, p. 613). Some of these risks were quantified by Lydon-Rochelle and associates (2001), who reported that the uterine rupture risk is increased threefold for women in spontaneous labor with a uterine scar. With oxytocin labor induction without prostaglandins, the risk was fivefold increased, and with prostaglandins, it was strikingly increased 15.6-fold. The Maternal-Fetal Medicine Units Network also reported a threefold increased risk of uterine scar rupture with oxytocin, and this was even higher when prostaglandins were also used (Landon, 2004). The American College of Obstetricians and Gynecologists (2013d) recommends against the use of misoprostol for preinduction cervical ripening or labor induction in women with a prior uterine scar (Chap. 31, p. 615).

Uterine Atony

Postpartum hemorrhage from uterine atony is more common in women undergoing induction or augmentation. And, atony with intractable hemorrhage, especially during cesarean delivery, is a frequent indication for peripartum hysterectomy (Shellhaas, 2009). In a study from Parkland Hospital, labor induction was associated with 17 percent of 553 emergency peripartum hysterectomies (Hernandez, 2013). In the United States, Bateman and coworkers (2012) reported that the postpartum hysterectomy rate increased 15 percent between 1994 and 2007. This was largely attributable to increased rates of atony associated with more medical labor inductions and more primary and repeat cesarean deliveries. Finally, elective induction was associated with more than a threefold increased rate of hysterectomy in the analysis by Bailit and colleagues (2010).

Elective Labor Induction

There can be no doubt that elective induction for convenience has become more prevalent. In the United States between 1991 and 2006, rates of early term labor induction increased significantly for all race and ethnicity groups (Murthy, 2011). This was highest for non-Hispanic white women in 2006. In this group, the rate was 20.5 percent if there was either diabetes or hypertension and was 9 percent for women without these indications. Clark and coworkers (2009) reported data from 14,955 deliveries at 37 weeks or greater. They noted that 32 percent were elective deliveries, and 19 percent were elective labor inductions.

The American College of Obstetricians and Gynecologists (2013b) does not endorse this widespread practice. Occasional exceptions might include logistical and other reasons such as a risk of rapid labor, a woman who lives a long distance from the hospital, or psychosocial indications. We are also of the opinion that routine elective induction at term is not justified because of the increased risks for adverse maternal outcomes. Elective delivery before 39 completed weeks is also associated with significant and appreciable adverse neonatal morbidity (Chiossi, 2013; Clark, 2009; Tita, 2009). If elective induction is considered at term, inherent risks must be discussed, informed consent obtained, and guidelines followed as promulgated by the American College of Obstetricians and Gynecologists (2013b), which are detailed in Chapter 31 (p. 610).

Guidelines to discourage elective inductions have been described by Fisch (2009) and Oshiro (2013) and their associates. Both groups reported significant decreases in elective delivery rates following guideline initiation. Tanne (2013) surveyed more than 800 United States hospitals and reported that efforts to reduce early term deliveries are succeeding.

Factors Affecting Successful Induction

Several factors increase or decrease the ability of labor induction to achieve vaginal delivery. Favorable factors include multiparity, body mass index (BMI) < 30, favorable cervix, and birthweight < 3500 g (Peregrine, 2006; Pevzner, 2009). For both nulliparas and multiparas, Kominiarek and colleagues (2011) found that labor duration to reach the active phase and to complete dilatation was adversely affected by a higher BMI.

In many cases, the uterus is simply poorly prepared for labor. One example is an "unripe cervix." Indeed, investigators with the *Consortium on Safe Labor* reported that elective induction resulted in vaginal delivery in 97 percent of multiparas and 76 percent of nulliparas, but that induction was more often successful with a ripe cervix (Laughon, 2012a). The increased cesarean delivery risk associated with induction is likely also strongly influenced by the induction attempt duration, especially with an unfavorable cervix (Spong, 2012). Simon and Grobman (2005) concluded that a latent phase as long as 18 hours during induction allowed most of these women to achieve a vaginal delivery without a significantly increased risk of maternal or neonatal morbidity. Rouse and associates (2000) recommend a minimum of 12 hours of uterine stimulation with oxytocin after membrane rupture.

PREINDUCTION CERVICAL RIPENING

As noted, the condition of the cervix—described as cervical "ripeness" or "favorability"—is important to successful labor induction. That said, at least some estimates of favorability are highly subjective. In either case, there are pharmacological and mechanical methods that can enhance cervical favorability—also termed *preinduction cervical ripening*.

Some of the techniques described may have benefits when compared with oxytocin induction alone (Table 26-1). Some are also quite successful for initiating labor. That said, few data support the premise that any of these techniques results in a reduced cesarean delivery rate or in less maternal or neonatal morbidity compared with that in women in whom these methods are not used.

Cervical "Favorability"

One quantifiable method used to predict labor induction outcomes is the score described by Bishop (1964) and presented in Table 26-2. As favorability or Bishop score decreases, the rate of induction to effect vaginal delivery also declines. A *Bishop score* of 9 conveys a high likelihood for a successful induction. Put another way, most practitioners would consider that a woman whose cervix is 2-cm dilated, 80-percent effaced, soft, and midposition and with the fetal occiput at –1 station would have a successful labor induction. For research purposes, a Bishop score of 4 or less identifies an unfavorable cervix and may be an indication for cervical ripening.

TABLE 26-1. Some Commonly Used Regimens for Preinduction Cervical Ripening and/or Labor Induction

Techniques	Agent	Route/Dose	Comments
Pharmacological			
Prostaglandin E_2	Dinoprostone gel, 0.5 mg (Prepidil)	Cervical 0.5 mg; repeat in 6 hr; permit 3 doses total	1. Shorter I-D times with oxytocin infusion than oxytocin alone
	Dinoprostone insert, 10 mg (Cervidil)	Posterior fornix, 10 mg	1. Insert has shorter I-D times than gel 2. 6–12 hr interval from last insert to oxytocin infusion
Prostaglandin E_1[a]	Misoprostol tablet, 100 or 200 μg (Cytotec)[b]	Vaginal, 25 μg; repeat 3–6 hr prn Oral, 50–100 μg; repeat 3–6 hr prn	1. Contractions within 30–60 min 2. Comparable success with oxytocin for ruptured membranes at term and/or favorable cervix 3. Tachysystole common with vaginal doses > 25 μg
Mechanical			
Transcervical 36F Foley catheter	30-mL balloon		1. Improves Bishop scores rapidly 2. 80-mL balloon more effective 3. Combined with oxytocin infusion is superior to PGE_1 vaginally 4. Results improved with EASI with possible decreased infection rate
Hygroscopic dilators		Laminaria, magnesium sulfate	1. Rapidly improves Bishop score 2. May not shorten I-D times with oxytocin 3. Uncomfortable, requires speculum and placement on an examination table

[a]Off-label use.
[b]Tablets must be divided for 25- and 50-μg dose, but drug is evenly dispersed.
EASI = extraamnionic saline infusion at 30–40 mL/hr; I-D = induction-to-delivery.

TABLE 26-2. Bishop Scoring System Used for Assessment of Inducibility

	Cervical Factor				
Score	Dilatation (cm)	Effacement (%)	Station (−3 to +2)	Consistency	Position
0	Closed	0–30	−3	Firm	Posterior
1	1–2	40–50	−2	Medium	Midposition
2	3–4	60–70	−1	Soft	Anterior
3	≥ 5	≥ 80	+1, +2	—	—

From Bishop, 1964.

Laughon and coworkers (2011) attempted to simplify the Bishop score by performing a regression analysis on 5610 singleton, uncomplicated deliveries by nulliparas between $37^{0/7}$ and $41^{6/7}$ weeks. Only cervical dilation, station, and effacement were significantly associated with successful vaginal delivery. Thus, a simplified Bishop score, which incorporated only these three parameters, had a similar or improved positive- or negative-predictive value compared with that of the original Bishop score.

Transvaginal sonographic measurement of cervical length has been evaluated as a Bishop score alternative. Hatfield and associates (2007) performed a metaanalysis of 20 trials in which cervical length was used to predict successful induction. Because of study criteria heterogeneity—including the definition of "successful induction"—the authors concluded that the question remains unanswered. Both this study and the one by Uzun and colleagues (2013) found that sonographically determined cervical length was not superior to the Bishop score for predicting induction success.

Pharmacological Techniques

Unfortunately, women frequently have an indication for induction but also have an unfavorable cervix. Thus, considerable research has been directed toward techniques to "ripen" the cervix before uterine contraction stimulation. Importantly, more often than not, techniques used to improve cervical favorability also stimulate contractions and thereby aid subsequent labor induction or augmentation. Techniques most commonly used for preinduction cervical ripening and induction include several prostaglandin analogues.

Prostaglandin E_2

Dinoprostone is a synthetic analogue of prostaglandin E_2. It is commercially available in three forms: a gel, a time-release vaginal insert, and a 10-mg suppository. The gel and time-release vaginal insert formulations are indicated only for cervical ripening before labor induction. However, the 10-mg suppository is indicated for pregnancy termination between 12 and 20 weeks and for evacuation of the uterus after fetal demise up to 28 weeks.

Local application of dinoprostone is commonly used for cervical ripening (American College of Obstetricians and Gynecologists, 2013b). Its gel form—*Prepidil*—is available in a 2.5-mL syringe for an intracervical application of 0.5 mg of dinoprostone. With the woman supine, the tip of a prefilled syringe is placed intracervically, and the gel is deposited just below the internal cervical os. After application, the woman remains reclined for at least 30 minutes. Doses may be repeated every 6 hours, with a maximum of three doses recommended in 24 hours.

A 10-mg dinoprostone vaginal insert—*Cervidil*—is also approved for cervical ripening. This is a thin, flat, rectangular polymeric wafer held within a small, white, mesh polyester sac (Fig. 26-1). The sac has a long attached tail to allow easy removal from the vagina. The insert provides slower release of medication—0.3 mg/hr—than the gel form. Cervidil is used as a single dose placed transversely in the posterior vaginal fornix. Lubricant should be used sparingly, if at all, because it can coat the device and hinder dinoprostone release. Following insertion, the woman should remain recumbent for at least 2 hours. The insert is removed after 12 hours or with labor onset and at least 30 minutes before the administration of oxytocin.

Most metaanalyses of dinoprostone efficacy report a reduced time to delivery within 24 hours. However, they do not consistently show a reduction in the cesarean delivery rate. Kelly and coworkers (2009) provided a Cochrane review of 63 trials and 10,441 women given vaginal prostaglandins or either placebo or no treatment. These investigators reported a higher vaginal delivery rate within 24 hours when prostaglandins were used. They also found that cesarean delivery rates were unchanged. Similar results were reported after another Cochrane review of intracervical dinoprostone gel by Boulvain and associates (2008). Compared with placebo or no treatment, a reduced risk of cesarean delivery was found only in a subgroup of women

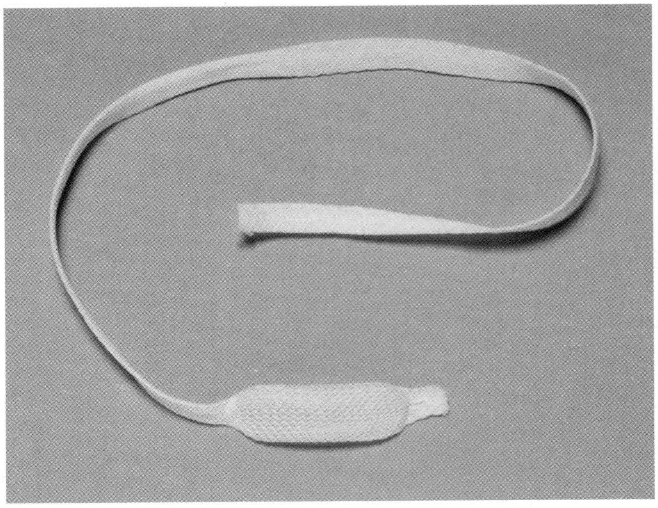

FIGURE 26-1 Cervidil vaginal insert contains 10 mg of dinoprostone designed to release approximately 0.3 mg/hr during a 10-hour period.

with an unfavorable cervix and intact membranes. Finally, the Foley catheter versus vaginal prostaglandin E_2 gel for induction of labor at term (PROBAAT trials) were unblinded, randomized trials comparing these two options (Jozwiak, 2011, 2013a, 2014). There was no difference in cesarean delivery rate, a finding consistent with accompanying metaanalyses.

Side Effects. Uterine tachysystole has been reported to follow vaginally administered prostaglandin E_2 in 1 to 5 percent of women (Hawkins, 2012). Although definitions of uterine activity vary among studies, most use the definition recommended by the American College of Obstetricians and Gynecologists (2013c):

1. *Uterine tachysystole* is defined as > 5 contractions in a 10-minute period. It should always be qualified by the presence or absence of fetal heart rate abnormalities.
2. *Uterine hypertonus, hyperstimulation, and hypercontractility are terms no longer defined, and their use is not recommended.*

Because uterine tachysystole associated with fetal compromise may develop when prostaglandins are used with preexisting spontaneous labor, such use is not recommended. If tachysystole follows the 10-mg insert, its removal by pulling on the tail of the surrounding net sac will usually reverse this effect. Irrigation to remove the gel preparation has not been shown to be helpful.

The manufacturers recommend caution when these preparations are used in women with ruptured membranes. Caution is also recommended when they are used in women with glaucoma or asthma. In a review of 189 women with asthma, however, dinoprostone was not associated with asthma worsening or exacerbation (Towers, 2004). Other contraindications listed by the manufacturers include a history of dinoprostone hypersensitivity, suspicion of fetal compromise or cephalopelvic disproportion, unexplained vaginal bleeding, women already receiving oxytocin, those with six or more previous term pregnancies, those with a contraindication to vaginal delivery, or women with a contraindication to oxytocin or who may be endangered by prolonged uterine contractions, for example, those with a history of cesarean delivery or uterine surgery.

Administration. Prostaglandin E_2 preparations should only be administered in or near the delivery suite. Moreover, uterine activity and fetal heart rate should be monitored (American College of Obstetricians and Gynecologists, 2013b). These guidelines stem from the risk of uterine tachysystole. When contractions begin, they are usually apparent in the first hour and show peak activity in the first 4 hours. According to manufacturer guidelines, oxytocin induction that follows prostaglandin use for cervical ripening should be delayed for 6 to 12 hours following prostaglandin E_2 gel administration or for at least 30 minutes after removal of the vaginal insert.

Prostaglandin E_1

Misoprostol—*Cytotec*—is a synthetic prostaglandin E_1 that is approved as a 100- or 200-μg tablet for peptic ulcer prevention. It has been used "off label" for preinduction cervical ripening and may be administered orally or vaginally. The tablets are stable at room temperature. Although widespread, the off-label use of misoprostol has been controversial (Wagner, 2005; Weeks, 2005). Specifically, G. D. Searle & Company (Cullen, 2000) notified physicians that misoprostol is not approved for labor induction or abortion. At the same time, however, the American College of Obstetricians and Gynecologists (2013b) reaffirmed its recommendation for use of the drug because of proven safety and efficacy. It currently is the preferred prostaglandin for cervical ripening at Parkland Hospital.

Vaginal Administration. Numerous studies have reported equivalent or superior efficacy for cervical ripening or labor induction with vaginally administered misoprostol tablets compared with intracervical or intravaginal prostaglandin E_2. A metaanalysis of 121 trials also confirmed these findings (Hofmeyr, 2010). Compared with oxytocin or with intravaginal or intracervical dinoprostone, misoprostol increased the vaginal delivery rate within 24 hours. Moreover, although the uterine tachysystole rate increased, this did not affect cesarean delivery rates. Compared with dinoprostone, misoprostol decreased the need for oxytocin induction, but it increased the frequency of meconium-stained amnionic fluid. Higher doses of misoprostol are associated with a decreased need for oxytocin but more uterine tachysystole with and without fetal heart rate changes. The American College of Obstetricians and Gynecologists (2013b) recommends the 25-μg vaginal dose—a fourth of a 100-μg tablet. The drug is evenly distributed among these quartered tablets.

Wing and colleagues (2013) recently described use of a vaginal polymer insert containing 200 μg of PGE_1. They compared its efficacy with 10-mg dinoprostone inserts, and preliminary observations are favorable.

Oral Administration. Prostaglandin E_1 tablets are also effective when given orally. Ho and coworkers (2010) performed a randomized controlled trial comparing titrated oral misoprostol with oxytocin. They found similar rates of vaginal delivery and side effects. In a metaanalysis of nine trials including nearly 3000 women, however, there were reported improvements in various outcomes with oral misoprostol (Kundodyiwa, 2009). In particular, there was a significantly lower cesarean delivery rate for the five trials comparing oral misoprostol with dinoprostone—relative risk 0.82. For the two trials comparing oral with vaginal misoprostol, oral misoprostol was associated with a lower rate of uterine tachysystole with fetal heart rate changes, but there were no significant differences with respect to rates of cesarean delivery or other outcomes.

Nitric Oxide Donors

Several findings have led to a search for clinical agents that stimulate nitric oxide (NO) production locally (Chanrachakul, 2000a). This is because nitric oxide is likely a mediator of cervical ripening (Chap. 21, p. 423). Also, cervical nitric oxide metabolite concentrations are increased at the beginning of uterine contractions. Last, cervical nitric oxide production is very low in postterm pregnancy (Väisänen-Tommiska, 2003, 2004).

Bullarbo and colleagues (2007) reviewed rationale and use of two nitric oxide donors, *isosorbide mononitrate* and *glyceryl trinitrate*. Isosorbide mononitrate induces cervical cyclooxygenase 2 (COX-2), and it also brings about cervical ultrastructure rearrangement similar to that seen with spontaneous cervical ripening (Ekerhovd, 2002, 2003). Despite this, clinical trials have not shown nitric oxide donors to be as effective as prostaglandin E_2 for cervical ripening (Chanrachakul, 2000b; Osman, 2006). Moreover, the addition of isosorbide mononitrate to either dinoprostone or misoprostol did not enhance cervical ripening either in early or term pregnancy nor did it shorten time to vaginal delivery (Collingham, 2010; Ledingham, 2001; Wölfler, 2006). A metaanalysis of 10 trials including 1889 women concluded that nitric oxide donors do not appear to be useful for cervical ripening during labor induction (Kelly, 2011).

Mechanical Techniques

These include transcervical placement of a Foley catheter with or without extraamnionic saline infusion, hygroscopic cervical dilators, and membrane stripping. In a recent metaanalysis of 71 randomized trials including 9722 women, Jozwiak and associates (2012) reported that mechanical techniques reduced the risk of uterine tachysystole compared with prostaglandins, although cesarean delivery rates were unchanged. Trials comparing mechanical techniques with oxytocin found a lower rate of cesarean delivery with mechanical methods. Trials comparing mechanical techniques with dinoprostone found a higher rate of multiparous women undelivered at 24 hours with mechanical techniques. Another metaanalysis done to compare Foley catheter placement with intravaginal dinoprostone inserts also found similar rates of cesarean delivery and less frequent uterine tachysystole (Jozwiak, 2013a).

Transcervical Catheter

Generally, these techniques are only used when the cervix is unfavorable because the catheter tends to come out as the cervix opens. In most cases, a Foley catheter is placed through the internal cervical os, and downward tension is created by taping the catheter to the thigh (Mei-Dan, 2014). A modification of this—*extraamnionic saline infusion (EASI)*—consists of a constant saline infusion through the catheter into the space between the internal os and placental membranes (Fig. 26-2). Karjane and coworkers (2006) reported that chorioamnionitis was significantly less frequent when infusion was done compared with no infusion—6 versus 16 percent. A systematic review and metaanalysis of 30 trials found that Foley catheter induction alone compared with prostaglandins resulted in higher infection rates unless saline was infused (Heinemann, 2008).

Most studies of transcervical catheters do not show a reduction in the cesarean delivery rate compared with prostaglandins. Cromi and colleagues (2012) compared a double-tipped Foley catheter and the dinoprostone vaginal insert. They found higher rates of delivery within 24 hours with the mechanical technique, but no differences in the cesarean delivery rates. The PROBAAT trials, in which cervical ripening with a Foley catheter was compared with

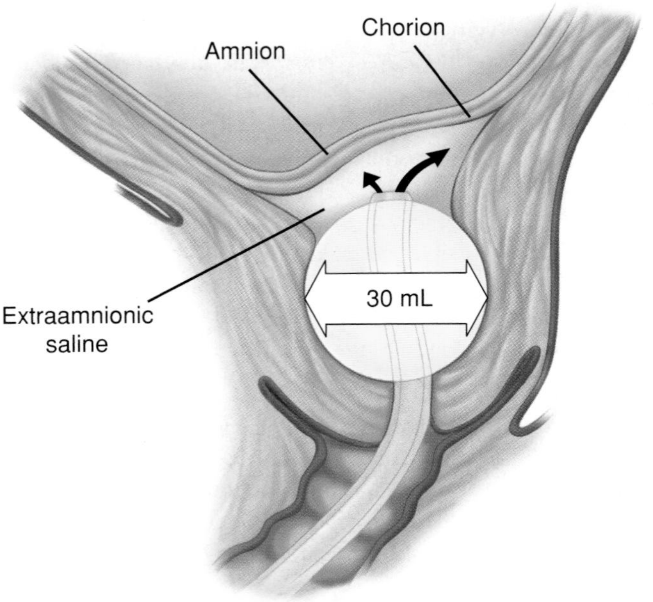

FIGURE 26-2 Extraamnionic saline infusion (EASI) through a 26F Foley catheter that is placed through the cervix. The 30-mL balloon is inflated with saline and pulled snugly against the internal os, and the catheter is taped to the thigh. Room-temperature normal saline is infused through the catheter port of the Foley at 30 or 40 mL/hour by intravenous infusion pump.

vaginal dinoprostone gel, dinoprostone vaginal inserts, and vaginal misoprostol, reported similar outcomes between the mechanical technique and the prostaglandin agents. Also, fewer overall cases of cardiotocographic changes were seen in the mechanical technique group (Jozwiak, 2011, 2013a, 2014; Wang, 2014).

Hygroscopic Cervical Dilators

Cervical dilatation can be accomplished using hygroscopic osmotic cervical dilators, as described for early pregnancy termination (Chap. 18, p. 365). These mechanical dilators have been successfully used for more than 40 years when inserted before pregnancy termination. They have also been used for cervical ripening before labor induction. Intuitive concerns of ascending infection have not been verified. Thus, their use appears to be safe, although anaphylaxis has rarely followed laminaria insertion (Lichtenberg, 2004). Dilators are attractive because of their low cost. However, placement generally requires a speculum and positioning of the woman on an examination table, which can be cumbersome and uncomfortable. A handful of studies performed in the 1990s compared hygroscopic cervical dilators and prostaglandins. There were few benefits of this mechanical technique other than cost.

METHODS OF INDUCTION AND AUGMENTATION

Labor induction has primarily been effected with the use of amniotomy, prostaglandins, and oxytocin, alone or in combination. Because preinduction cervical ripening frequently eventuates in labor, studies to determine induction efficacy for some of these agents have produced sometimes confusing results. The use of prostaglandins for labor augmentation has generally been considered experimental.

Prostaglandin E_1

As discussed on page 527, both vaginal and oral misoprostol are used for either cervical ripening or labor induction. Hofmeyr and associates (2010) performed a Cochrane systematic review of agents for labor induction. They reported that vaginal misoprostol, followed by oxytocin if needed, compared with oxytocin alone resulted in fewer failures within 24 hours. As expected, prostaglandin use led to a higher incidence of uterine tachysystole, but cesarean delivery rates were similar.

It appears that 100 μg of oral or 25 μg of vaginal misoprostol are similar in efficacy compared with intravenous oxytocin for labor induction in women at or near term with either prematurely ruptured membranes or a favorable cervix (Lin, 2005; Lo, 2003). Misoprostol may be associated with an increased rate of uterine tachysystole, particularly at higher doses. Also, induction with prostaglandin E_1 may prove ineffective and require subsequent induction or augmentation with oxytocin. Thus, although there are trade-offs regarding the risks, costs, and ease of administration of each drug, either is suitable for labor induction.

For *labor augmentation*, results of a randomized controlled trial showed oral misoprostol, 75 μg given at 4-hour intervals for a maximum of two doses, to be safe and effective (Bleich, 2011). The 75-μg dose was based on a previous dose-finding study (Villano, 2011). Although there was more uterine tachysystole among women with labor augmented with misoprostol, there were no significant differences in the frequency of nonreassuring fetal status or cesarean delivery.

Oxytocin

As discussed, in most instances, preinduction cervical ripening and labor induction are simply a continuum. Thus, "ripening" will also stimulate labor. If not, induction or augmentation may be continued with solutions of oxytocin given by infusion pump. Synthetic oxytocin is one of the most frequently used medications in the United States. It was the first polypeptide hormone synthesized, an achievement for which the 1955 Nobel Prize in chemistry was awarded (du Vigneaud, 1953). Oxytocin may be used for labor induction or for augmentation. With oxytocin use, the American College of Obstetricians and Gynecologists (2013b) recommends fetal heart rate and contraction monitoring similar to that for any high-risk pregnancy. Contractions can be monitored either by palpation or by electronic means (Chap. 24, p. 497).

Intravenous Oxytocin Administration

The goal of induction or augmentation is to effect uterine activity sufficient to produce cervical change and fetal descent, while avoiding development of a nonreassuring fetal status. In general, oxytocin should be discontinued if the number of contractions persists with a frequency of more than five in a 10-minute period or more than seven in a 15-minute period or with a persistent nonreassuring fetal heart rate pattern. Oxytocin discontinuation nearly always rapidly decreases contraction frequency. When oxytocin is stopped, its concentration in plasma rapidly falls because the half-life is approximately 3 to 5 minutes. Seitchik and coworkers (1984) found that the uterus contracts within 3 to 5 minutes of beginning an oxytocin infusion and that a plasma steady state is reached in 40 minutes. Response is highly variable and depends on preexisting uterine activity, cervical status, pregnancy duration, and individual biological differences. Caldeyro-Barcia and Poseiro (1960) reported that the uterine response to oxytocin increases from 20 to 30 weeks' gestation and increases rapidly at term (Chap. 24, p. 498).

Oxytocin Dosage. A 1-mL ampule containing 10 units usually is diluted into 1000 mL of a crystalloid solution and administered by infusion pump. A typical infusate consists of 10 or 20 units, which is 10,000 or 20,000 mU or one or two 1-mL vials, mixed into 1000 mL of lactated Ringer solution. This mixture results in an oxytocin concentration of 10 or 20 mU/mL, respectively. To avoid bolus administration, the infusion should be inserted into the main intravenous line close to the venipuncture site.

Oxytocin is generally very successful when used to stimulate labor. A Cochrane metaanalysis of 12 trials involving 12,819 women comparing oxytocin with expectant management reported that fewer women—8 versus 54 percent—failed to deliver vaginally within 24 hours when oxytocin was used (Alfirevic, 2009). This metaanalysis studied different oxytocin dosing regimens. A smaller metaanalysis of four trials involving 660 women and comparing high-dose and low-dose oxytocin regimens reported that high-dose regimens were associated with reduced length of labor and cesarean delivery rate and with a concomitant increased spontaneous vaginal delivery rate (Mori, 2011).

Oxytocin Regimens

As a result of numerous studies, several regimens for labor stimulation are now recommended by the American College of Obstetricians and Gynecologists (2013a). These and others are shown in Table 26-3. Initially, only variations of low-dose protocols were used in the United States. Then O'Driscoll and colleagues (1984) described their Dublin protocol for the active management of labor that called for oxytocin at a starting dosage of 6 mU/min and advanced in 6-mU/min increments. Subsequent comparative trials during the 1990s studied high-dose—4 to 6 mU/min—versus conventional low-dose—0.5 to 1.5 mU/min—regimens, both for labor induction and for augmentation.

From Parkland Hospital, Satin and associates (1992) evaluated an oxytocin regimen using an initial and incremental dosage of 6 mU/min compared with one using 1 mU/min. Increases at 20-minute intervals were provided as needed. Among 1112 women undergoing induction, the 6-mU/min regimen resulted in a shorter mean admission-to-delivery time, fewer failed inductions, and no cases of neonatal sepsis. Among 1676 women who had labor augmentation, those who received the 6-mU/min regimen had a shorter duration-to-delivery

TABLE 26-3. Various Low- and High-Dose Oxytocin Regimens Used for Labor Induction

Regimen	Starting Dose (mU/min)	Incremental Increase (mU/min)	Interval (min)
Low-dose	0.5–1.5	1	15–40
	2	4, 8, 12, 16, 20, 25, 30	15
High-dose	4	4	15
	4.5	4.5	15–30
	6	6[a]	20–40[b]

[a]With uterine tachysystole and after oxytocin infusion is discontinued, it is restarted at the previous dose and increased at 3 mU/min incremental doses.
[b]Uterine tachysystole is more common with shorter intervals.
Data from Merrill, 1999; Satin, 1992, 1994; Xenakis, 1995.

time, fewer forceps deliveries, fewer cesarean deliveries for dystocia, and decreased rates of intrapartum chorioamnionitis or neonatal sepsis. With this protocol, uterine tachysystole is managed by oxytocin discontinuation followed by resumption when indicated and at half the stopping dosage. Thereafter, the dosage is increased at 3 mU/min when appropriate, instead of the usual 6-mU/min increase used for women without tachysystole. No adverse neonatal effects were observed.

Xenakis and coworkers (1995) reported benefits using an incremental oxytocin regimen starting at 4 mU/min. In a comparative study of 1307 women by Merrill and Zlatnik (1999), 816 women were randomized for labor induction and 816 for augmentation with incremental oxytocin given at either 1.5 or 4.5 mU/min. Women randomized to the 4.5 mU/min dosage had significantly decreased mean durations of induction-to-second-stage labor and induction-to-delivery. Nulliparas randomized to the 4.5 mU/min dosage had a significantly lower cesarean delivery rate for dystocia compared with those given 1.5 mU/min dosage—5.9 versus 11.9 percent.

Thus, benefits favor higher-dose regimens of 4.5 to 6 mU/min compared with lower dosages of 0.5 to 1.5 mU/min. In 1990 at Parkland Hospital, routine use of the 6-mU/min oxytocin beginning and incremental dosage was incorporated and continues through today. In other labor units, a 2-mU/min beginning and incremental oxytocin regimen is preferred and administered. With either regimen, these dosages are employed for either labor induction or augmentation.

Interval between Incremental Dosing

Intervals to increase oxytocin doses vary from 15 to 40 minutes as shown in Table 26-3. Satin and colleagues (1994) addressed this aspect with a 6-mU/min regimen providing increases at either 20- or 40-minute intervals. Women assigned to the 20-minute interval regimen for labor augmentation had a significantly reduced cesarean delivery rate for dystocia compared with that for the 40-minute interval regimen—8 versus 12 percent. As perhaps expected, uterine tachysystole was significantly more frequent with the 20-minute escalation regimen.

Other investigators reported even more frequent incremental increases. Frigoletto (1995) and Xenakis (1995) and their coworkers gave oxytocin at 4 mU/min with increases as needed every 15 minutes. Merrill and Zlatnik (1999) started with 4.5 mU/min, with increases every 30 minutes. López-Zeno and associates (1992) began at 6 mU/min with increases every 15 minutes. Thus, there are several acceptable oxytocin protocols that at least appear dissimilar. But a comparison of protocols from two institutions indicates that this is not so:

1. The Parkland Hospital protocol calls for a starting dose of oxytocin at 6 mU/min and with 6-mU/min increases every 40 minutes, but it employs flexible dosing based on uterine tachysystole.
2. The University of Alabama at Birmingham Hospital protocol begins oxytocin at 2 mU/min and increases it as needed every 15 minutes to 4, 8, 12, 16, 20, 25, and 30 mU/min.

Thus, although the regimens at first appear disparate, if there is no uterine activity, either regimen is delivering 12 mU/min by 45 minutes into the infusion.

Maximal Dosage

The *maximal* effective dose of oxytocin to achieve adequate contractions in all women is different. Wen and colleagues (2001) studied 1151 consecutive nulliparas and found that the likelihood of progression to vaginal delivery decreased at and beyond an oxytocin dosage of 36 mU/min. Still, at a dosage of 72 mU/min, half of the nulliparas were delivered vaginally. Thus, if contractions are not adequate—less than 200 Montevideo units—and if the fetal status is reassuring and labor has arrested, an oxytocin infusion dose greater than 48 mU/min has no apparent risks.

Risks versus Benefits

Unless the uterus is scarred, uterine rupture associated with oxytocin infusion is rare, even in parous women (Chap. 41, p. 790). Flannelly and associates (1993) reported no uterine ruptures, with or without oxytocin, in 27,829 nulliparas. There were eight instances of overt uterine rupture during labor in 48,718 parous women. Only one of these was associated with oxytocin use.

Oxytocin has amino-acid homology similar to arginine vasopressin. Because of this, it has significant antidiuretic action, and when infused at doses of 20 mU/min or more, renal free water clearance decreases markedly. If aqueous fluids are infused in appreciable amounts along with oxytocin, *water intoxication* can lead to convulsions, coma, and even death. In general, if oxytocin is to be administered in high doses for a considerable period of time, its concentration should be increased rather than increasing the flow rate of a more dilute solution. Consideration also should be given to use of crystalloids—either normal saline or lactated Ringer solution.

Uterine Contraction Pressures

Contraction forces in spontaneously laboring women range from 90 to 390 Montevideo units. As described in Chapter 24

(p. 498), the latter are calculated by subtracting the baseline uterine pressure from the peak contraction pressure for each contraction in a 10-minute window. The pressures generated by each contraction are then summed. Caldeyro-Barcia (1950) and Seitchik (1984) with their coworkers found that the mean or median spontaneous uterine contraction pattern resulting in a progression to a vaginal delivery was between 140 and 150 Montevideo units.

In the management of active-phase arrest, and with no contraindication to intravenous oxytocin, decisions must be made with knowledge of the safe upper range of uterine activity. Hauth and colleagues (1986) described an effective and safe protocol for oxytocin augmentation for active-phase arrest. With it, more than 90 percent of women achieved an average of at least 200 to 225 Montevideo units. Hauth and associates (1991) later reported that nearly all women in whom active-phase arrest persisted despite oxytocin generated more than 200 Montevideo units. Importantly, despite no labor progression, there were no adverse maternal or perinatal effects in those undergoing cesarean delivery. There are no data regarding safety and efficacy of contraction patterns in women with a prior cesarean delivery, with twins, or with an overdistended uterus.

Active-Phase Arrest

First-stage arrest of labor is defined by the American College of Obstetricians and Gynecologists (2013a) as a completed latent phase along with contractions exceeding 200 Montevideo units for more than 2 hours without cervical change. Some investigators have attempted to define a more accurate duration for active-phase arrest (Spong, 2012). Arulkumaran and coworkers (1987) extended the 2-hour limit to 4 hours and reported a 1.3-percent cesarean delivery rate in women who continued to have adequate contractions and progressive cervical dilatation of at least 1 cm/hr. In women without progressive cervical dilatation who were allowed another 4 hours of labor, half required cesarean delivery.

Rouse and colleagues (1999) prospectively managed 542 women at term with active-phase arrest and no other complications. Their protocol was to achieve a sustained pattern of at least 200 Montevideo units for a *minimum* of 4 hours. This time frame was extended to 6 hours if activity of 200 Montevideo units or greater could not be sustained. Almost 92 percent of these women were delivered vaginally. As discussed in Chapter 23 (p. 459), these and other studies support the practice of allowing an active-phase arrest of 4 hours (Rouse, 2001; Solheim, 2009).

Zhang and coworkers (2002) analyzed labor duration from 4 cm to complete dilatation in 1329 nulliparas at term. They found that before dilatation of 7 cm was reached, lack of progress for more than 2 hours was not uncommon in those who delivered vaginally. Alexander and associates (2002) reported that epidural analgesia prolonged active labor by 1 hour compared with duration of the active phase as defined by Friedman (1955). Consideration of these changes in the management of labor, especially in nulliparas, may safely reduce the cesarean delivery rate.

As data have accrued, investigators have increasingly questioned the thresholds for labor arrest disorders established by Friedman and others in the 1960s. In particular, investigators with the *Consortium on Safe Labor* reported that half of cases of dystocia after labor induction occurred before 6 cm of cervical dilation (Boyle, 2013; Zhang, 2010c). Even for women with spontaneous labor, these researchers found that active-phase labor was more likely to occur at 6 cm, and after slow progress between 4 and 6 cm (Zhang, 2010a). Additionally, they reported that a 2-hour threshold for diagnosing arrest disorders may be too brief when cervical dilation is < 6 cm (Zhang, 2010b). It was also shown that the duration of first-stage labor was more than 2 hours longer than had been reported using data from the Collaborative Perinatal Project (Laughon, 2012b).

Amniotomy for Induction and Augmentation

A common indication for artificial rupture of the membranes—*surgical amniotomy*—includes the need for direct monitoring of the fetal heart rate or uterine contractions or both. During amniotomy, to minimize cord prolapse risk, dislodgement of the fetal head is avoided. For this, fundal or suprapubic pressure or both may be helpful. Some clinicians prefer to rupture membranes during a contraction. If the vertex is not well applied to the lower uterine segment, a gradual egress of amnionic fluid can sometimes be accomplished by several membrane punctures with a 26-gauge needle held with a ring forceps and with direct visualization using a vaginal speculum. In many of these, however, membranes tear and fluid is lost rapidly. Because of the risk of cord prolapse or rarely abruption, the fetal heart rate is assessed before and immediately after amniotomy.

Elective Amniotomy

Membrane rupture with the intention of accelerating labor is often performed. In the investigations presented in Table 26-4, amniotomy at approximately 5-cm dilation accelerated spontaneous labor by 1 to 1½ hours. Importantly, neither the need for oxytocin stimulation nor the overall cesarean delivery rate was increased. Although mild and moderate cord compression patterns were increased following amniotomy, cesarean delivery rates for fetal distress were not increased. Most importantly, there were no adverse perinatal effects.

Amniotomy Induction

Artificial rupture of the membranes—sometimes called *surgical induction*—can be used to induce labor, and it always implies a commitment to delivery. The main disadvantage of amniotomy used alone for labor induction is the unpredictable and occasionally long interval until labor onset. That said, in a randomized trial, Bakos and Bäckström (1987) found that amniotomy alone or combined with oxytocin was superior to oxytocin alone. Mercer and colleagues (1995) randomized 209 women undergoing oxytocin induction to either early amniotomy at 1 to 2 cm or late amniotomy at 5 cm. Early amniotomy was associated with a significant 4-hour reduction in labor duration. With early amniotomy, however, there was an increased incidence of chorioamnionitis.

Amniotomy Augmentation

It is common practice to perform amniotomy when labor is abnormally slow. Rouse and associates (1994) found that amniotomy

TABLE 26-4. Randomized Clinical Trials of Elective Amniotomy in Early Spontaneous Labor at Term

		Effects of Amniotomy					
Study	Number	Mean Dilatation at Amniotomy	Mean Shortening of Labor	Need for Oxytocin	Cesarean Delivery Rate	Abnormal Tracing	Neonatal Effects
Fraser (1993)	925	< 5 cm	125 min	None	None[a]	None	None
Garite (1993)	459	5.5 cm	81 min	Decreased	None	Increased[b]	None
UK Amniotomy Group (1994)	1463	5.1 cm	60 min	None	None	NA	None

[a]No effect on overall rate; cesarean delivery for fetal distress significantly increased.
[b]Increased mild and moderate umbilical cord compression patterns.
NA = not assessed.

with oxytocin augmentation for arrested active-phase labor shortened the time to delivery by 44 minutes compared with that of oxytocin alone. Although amniotomy did not alter the delivery route, one drawback was that it significantly increased the incidence of chorioamnionitis. The American College of Obstetricians and Gynecologists (2013a) recommends the use of amniotomy to enhance progress in active labor, but cautions that this may increase the risks of infection and maternal fever.

Membrane Stripping for Labor Induction

Labor induction by membrane "stripping" is a frequent practice. Several studies have suggested that membrane stripping is safe and decreases the incidence of postterm pregnancy without consistently increasing the incidence of ruptured membranes, infection, or bleeding. Authors of a metaanalysis of 22 trials including 2797 women reported that membrane stripping reduced the number of women remaining undelivered after 41 weeks without increasing the infection risk. They concluded that eight women would need to undergo membrane stripping to avoid one labor induction. Downsides are discomfort and associated bleeding (Boulvain, 2005).

ACTIVE MANAGEMENT OF LABOR

This term describes a codified approach to the management of labor, which is discussed in detail in Chapter 22 (p. 452).

REFERENCES

Alexander JM, Sharma SK, McIntire D, et al: Epidural analgesia lengthens the Friedman active phase of labor. Obstet Gynecol 100:46, 2002

Alfirevic Z, Kelly AJ, Dowswell T: Intravenous oxytocin alone for cervical ripening and induction of labour. Cochrane Database Syst Rev 4:CD003246, 2009

American Academy of Pediatrics and American College of Obstetricians and Gynecologists: Guidelines for Perinatal Care, 7th ed. 2012

American College of Obstetricians and Gynecologists: Dystocia and augmentation of labor. Practice Bulletin No. 49, December 2003, Reaffirmed 2013a

American College of Obstetricians and Gynecologists: Induction of labor. Practice Bulletin No. 107, August 2009, Reaffirmed 2013b

American College of Obstetricians and Gynecologists: Intrapartum fetal heart rate monitoring: nomenclature, interpretation, and general management principles. Practice Bulletin No. 106, July 2009, Reaffirmed 2013c

American College of Obstetricians and Gynecologists: Vaginal birth after previous cesarean delivery. Practice Bulletin 115, August 2010, Reaffirmed 2013d

Arulkumaran S, Koh CH, Ingemarsson I, et al: Augmentation of labour—mode of delivery related to cervimetric progress. Aust NZ J Obstet Gynaecol 27:304, 1987

Bakos O, Bäckström T: Induction of labor: a prospective, randomized study into amniotomy and oxytocin as induction methods in a total unselected population. Acta Obstet Gynecol Scand 66:537, 1987

Bailit JL, Gregory KD, Reddy UM, et al: Maternal and neonatal outcomes by labor onset type and gestational age. Am J Obstet Gynecol 202(3):245.e1, 2010

Bateman BT, Mhyre JM, Callaghan WM, et al: Peripartum hysterectomy in the United States: nationwide 14 year experience. Am J Obstet Gynecol 206(1):63.e1, 2012

Bishop EH: Pelvic scoring for elective induction. Obstet Gynecol 24:266, 1964

Bleich AT, Villano KS, Lo JY, et al: Oral misoprostol for labor augmentation: a randomized controlled trial. Obstet Gynecol 118(6):1255, 2011

Boulvain M, Kelly A, Irion O: Intracervical prostaglandins for induction of labour. Cochrane Database Syst Rev 1:CD006971, 2008

Boulvain M, Stan C, Irion O: Membrane sweeping for induction of labour. Cochrane Database Syst Rev 1:CD000451, 2005

Boyle A, Reddy UM, Landy HJ, et al: Primary cesarean delivery in the United States. Obstet Gynecol 122(1):33, 2013

Bullarbo M, Orrskog ME, Andersch B, et al: Outpatient vaginal administration of the nitric oxide donor isosorbide mononitrate for cervical ripening and labor induction postterm: a randomized controlled study. Am J Obstet Gynecol 196:50.e1, 2007

Caldeyro-Barcia R, Alvarez H, Reynolds SRM: A better understanding of uterine contractility through simultaneous recording with an internal and a seven channel external method. Surg Obstet Gynecol 91:641, 1950

Caldeyro-Barcia R, Poseiro JJ: Physiology of the uterine contraction. Clin Obstet Gynecol 3:386, 1960

Chanrachakul B, Herabutya Y, Punyavachira P: Potential efficacy of nitric oxide for cervical ripening in pregnancy at term. Int J Gynaecol Obstet 71(3):217, 2000a

Chanrachakul B, Herabutya Y, Punyavachira P: Randomized comparison of glyceryl trinitrate and prostaglandin E_2 for cervical ripening at term. Obstet Gynecol 96:549, 2000b

Chiossi G, Lai Y, Landon MB, et al: Timing of delivery and adverse outcomes in term singleton repeat cesarean deliveries. Obstet Gynecol 121(3):561, 2013

Clark SL, Miller DD, Belfort MA, et al: Neonatal and maternal outcomes associated with elective term delivery. Am J Obstet Gynecol 200(2):156.e1, 2009

Collingham J, Fuh K, Caughey A, et al: Oral misoprostol and vaginal isosorbide mononitrate for labor induction: a randomized controlled trial. Obstet Gynecol 116(1):121, 2010

Cromi A, Ghezzi F, Uccella S, et al: A randomized trial of preinduction cervical ripening: dinoprostone vaginal insert versus double-balloon catheter. Am J Obstet Gynecol 207(2):125.e1, 2012

Cullen M: Important drug warning concerning unapproved use of intravaginal or oral misoprostol in pregnant women for induction of labor or abortion. August 23, 2000. Available at: http://www.fda.gov/ohrms/dockets/dailys/00/Nov00/111500/cp0001.pdf. Accessed September 14, 2013

du Vigneaud V, Ressler C, Swan JM, et al: The synthesis of oxytocin. J Am Chem Soc 75:4879, 1953

Ekerhovd E, Bullarbo M, Andersch B, et al: Vaginal administration of the nitric oxide donor isosorbide mononitrate for cervical ripening at term: a randomized controlled study. Am J Obstet Gynecol 189:1692, 2003

Ekerhovd E, Weijdegärd B, Brännström I, et al: Nitric oxide induced cervical ripening in the human: involvement of cyclic guanosine monophosphate, prostaglandin $F_2\alpha$, and prostaglandin E_2. Am J Obstet Gynecol 186:745, 2002
Fisch JM, English D, Pedaline S, et al: Labor induction process improvement: a patient quality-of-care initiative. Obstet Gynecol 113(4):797, 2009
Flannelly GM, Turner MJ, Rassmussen MJ, et al: Rupture of the uterus in Dublin: an update. J Obstet Gynaecol 13:440, 1993
Fraser W, Marcoux S, Moutquin JM, et al: Effect of early amniotomy on the risk of dystocia in nulliparous women. N Engl J Med 328:1145, 1993
Friedman EA: Primigravid labor: a graphicostatistical analysis. Obstet Gynecol 6:567, 1955
Frigoletto FD, Lieberman E, Lang JM, et al: A clinical trial of active management of labor. N Engl J Med 333:745, 1995
Garite TJ, Porto M, Carlson NJ, et al: The influence of elective amniotomy on fetal heart rate patterns and the course of labor in term patients: a randomized study. Am J Obstet Gynecol 168:1827, 1993
Hamar B, Mann S, Greenberg P, et al: Low-risk inductions of labor and cesarean delivery for nulliparous and parous women at term. Am J Obstet Gynecol 185:S215, 2001
Hatfield AS, Sanchez-Ramos L, Kaunitz AM: Sonographic cervical assessment to predict the success of labor induction: a systematic review with meta-analysis. Am J Obstet Gynecol 197:186, 2007
Hauth JC, Hankins GD, Gilstrap LC III: Uterine contraction pressures achieved in parturients with active phase arrest. Obstet Gynecol 78:344, 1991
Hauth JC, Hankins GD, Gilstrap LC III: Uterine contraction pressures with oxytocin induction/augmentation. Obstet Gynecol 68:305, 1986
Hawkins JS, Wing DA: Current pharmacotherapy options for labor induction. Expert Opin Pharmacother 13(14):2005, 2012
Heinemann J, Gillen G, Sanchez-Ramos L, et al: Do mechanical methods of cervical ripening increase infectious morbidity? A systematic review. Am J Obstet Gynecol 199(2):177, 2008
Hernandez JS, Wendel GD Jr, Sheffield JS: Trends in emergency peripartum hysterectomy at a single institution: 1988–2009. Am J Perinatol 30(5):365, 2013
Ho M, Cheng SY, Li TC: Titrated oral misoprostol solution compared with intravenous oxytocin for labor augmentation: a randomized controlled trial. Obstet Gynecol 116(3):612, 2010
Hoffman MK, Sciscione AC: Elective induction with cervical ripening increases the risk of cesarean delivery in multiparous women. Obstet Gynecol 101:7S, 2003
Hofmeyr GJ, Gülmezoglu AM, Pileggi C: Vaginal misoprostol for cervical ripening and induction of labour. Cochrane Database Syst Rev 10:CD000941, 2010
Jozwiak M, Bloemenkamp KW, Kelly AJ, et al: Mechanical methods for induction of labour. Cochrane Database Syst Rev 3:CD001233, 2012
Jozwiak M, Oude Rengerink K, Benthem M, et al: Foley catheter versus vaginal prostaglandin E2 gel for induction of labour at term (PROBAAT trial): an open-label, randomised controlled trial. Lancet 378(9809):2095, 2011
Jozwiak M, Oude Rengerink K, Ten Eikelder ML, et al: Foley catheter or prostaglandin E2 inserts for induction of labour at term: an open-label randomized controlled trial (PROBAAT-P trial) and systematic review of literature. Eur J Obstet Gynecol Reprod Biol 170(1):137, 2013a
Jozwiak M, Ten Eikelder M, Rengerink KO, et al: Foley catheter versus vaginal misoprostol: randomized controlled trial (PROBAAT-M Study) and systematic review and meta-analysis of literature. Am J Perinatol 31:145, 2014
Karjane NW, Brock EL, Walsh SW: Induction of labor using a Foley balloon, with and without extra-amniotic saline infusion. Obstet Gynecol 107:234, 2006
Kelly AJ, Alfirevic Z, Dowswell T: Outpatient versus inpatient induction of labour for improving birth outcomes. Cochrane Database Syst Rev 2: CD007372, 2009
Kelly AJ, Munson C, Minden L: Nitric oxide donors for cervical ripening and induction of labour. Cochrane Database Syst Rev 6:CD006901, 2011
Kominiarek MA, Zhang J, Vanveldhuisen P, et al: Contemporary labor patterns: the impact of maternal body mass index. Am J Obstet Gynecol 205(3):244.e1, 2011
Kundodyiwa TW, Alfirevic Z, Weeks AD: Low-dose oral misoprostol for induction of labor: a systematic review. Obstet Gynecol 113(2 Pt 1):374, 2009
Landon MB, Hauth JC, Leveno KJ, et al: Maternal and perinatal outcomes associated with a trial of labor after prior cesarean delivery. N Engl J Med 351(25):2581, 2004
Laughon SK, Branch DW, Beaver J, et al: Changes in labor patterns over 50 years. Am J Obstet Gynecol 206(5):419.e1, 2012a
Laughon SK, Zhang J, Grewal J, et al: Induction of labor in a contemporary obstetric cohort. Am J Obstet Gynecol 206(6):486.e1, 2012b
Laughon SK, Zhang J, Troendle J, et al: Using a simplified Bishop score to predict vaginal delivery. Obstet Gynecol 117(4):805, 2011
Ledingham MA, Thomson AJ, Lunan CB, et al: A comparison of isosorbide mononitrate, misoprostol and combination therapy for first trimester pre-operative cervical ripening: a randomised controlled trial. Br J Obstet Gynecol 108:276, 2001
Lichtenberg ES: Complications of osmotic dilators. Obstet Gynecol Surv 59(7):528, 2004
Lin MG, Nuthalapaty FS, Carver AR, et al: Misoprostol for labor induction in women with term premature rupture of membranes: a meta-analysis. Obstet Gynecol 106:593, 2005
Lo JY, Alexander JM, McIntire DD, et al: Ruptured membranes at term: randomized, double-blind trial of oral misoprostol for labor induction. Obstet Gynecol 101:685, 2003
López-Zeno JA, Peaceman AM, Adashek JA, et al: A controlled trial of a program for the active management of labor. N Engl J Med 326:450, 1992
Luthy DA, Malmgren JA, Zingheim RW: Cesarean delivery after elective induction in nulliparous women: the physician effect. Am J Obstet Gynecol 191:1511, 2004
Lydon-Rochelle M, Holt VL, Easterling TR, et al: Risk of uterine rupture during labor among women with a prior cesarean delivery. N Engl J Med 345(1):3, 2001
Macones GA: Elective induction of labor: waking the sleeping dogma? Ann Intern Med 151(4):281, 2009
Martin JA, Hamilton BE, Ventura SJ, et al: Births: final data for 2011. Natl Vital Stat Rep 62(1), 1, 2013
Maslow AS, Sweeny AL: Elective induction of labor as a risk factor for cesarean delivery among low-risk women at term. Obstet Gynecol 95:917, 2000
Mei-Dan E, Walfisch A, Valencia C, et al: Making cervical ripening EASI: a prospective controlled comparison of single versus double balloon catheters. J Matern Fetal Neonatal Med January 8, 2014 [Epub ahead of print]
Mercer BM: Induction of labor in the nulliparous gravida with an unfavorable cervix. Obstet Gynecol 105:688, 2005
Mercer BM, McNanley T, O'Brien JM, et al: Early versus late amniotomy for labor induction: a randomized trial. Am J Obstet Gynecol 173:1371, 1995
Merrill DC, Zlatnik FJ: Randomized, double-masked comparison of oxytocin dosage in induction and augmentation of labor. Obstet Gynecol 94:455, 1999
Mori R, Tokumasu H, Pledge D, et al: High dose versus low dose oxytocin for augmentation of delayed labour. Cochrane Database Syst Rev 10:CD007201, 2011
Murthy K, Grobman WA, Lee TA, et al: Trends in induction of labor at early-term gestation. Am J Obstet Gynecol 204(5):435.e1, 2011
O'Driscoll K, Foley M, MacDonald D: Active management of labor as an alternative to cesarean section for dystocia. Obstet Gynecol 63:485, 1984
Oshiro BT, Kowalewski L, Sappenfield W, et al: A multistate quality improvement program to decrease elective deliveries before 39 weeks of gestation. Obstet Gynecol 121(5):1025, 2013
Osman I, MacKenzie F, Norrie J, et al: The "PRIM" study: a randomized comparison of prostaglandin E_2 gel with the nitric oxide donor isosorbide mononitrate for cervical ripening before the induction of labor at term. Am J Obstet Gynecol 194:1012, 2006
Osmundson S, Ou-Yang RJ, Grobman WA: Elective induction compared with expectant management in nulliparous women with an unfavorable cervix. Obstet Gynecol 117(3):583, 2011
Osmundson SS, Ou-Yang RJ, Grobman WA: Elective induction compared with expectant management in nulliparous women with a favorable cervix. Obstet Gynecol 116(3):601, 2010
Peregrine E, O'Brien P, Omar R, et al: Clinical and ultrasound parameters to predict the risk of cesarean delivery after induction of labor. Obstet Gynecol 107(2 Pt 1):227, 2006
Pevzner L, Rayburn WF, Rumney P, et al: Factors predicting successful labor induction with dinoprostone and misoprostol vaginal inserts. Obstet Gynecol 114(2 Pt 1):261, 2009
Rouse DJ, McCullough C, Wren AL, et al: Active-phase labor arrest: a randomized trial of chorioamnion management. Obstet Gynecol 83:937, 1994
Rouse DJ, Owen J, Hauth JC: Active-phase labor arrest: oxytocin augmentation for at least 4 hours. Obstet Gynecol 93:323, 1999
Rouse DJ, Owen J, Hauth JC: Criteria for failed labor induction: prospective evaluation of a standardized protocol. Obstet Gynecol 96:671, 2000
Rouse DJ, Owen J, Savage KG, et al: Active phase labor arrest: revisiting the 2-hour minimum. Obstet Gynecol 98:550, 2001
Satin AJ, Leveno KJ, Sherman ML, et al: High- versus low-dose oxytocin for labor stimulation. Obstet Gynecol 80:111, 1992
Satin AJ, Leveno KJ, Sherman ML, et al: High-dose oxytocin: 20- versus 40-minute dosage interval. Obstet Gynecol 83:234, 1994

Seitchik J, Amico J, Robinson AG, et al: Oxytocin augmentation of dysfunctional labor. IV. Oxytocin pharmacokinetics. Am J Obstet Gynecol 150:225, 1984

Shellhaas CS, Gilbert S, Landon MB, et al: The frequency and complication rates of hysterectomy accompanying cesarean delivery. Obstet Gynecol 114(2 Pt 1):224, 2009

Shin KS, Brubaker KL, Ackerson LM: Risk of cesarean delivery in nulliparous women at greater than 41 weeks' gestational age with an unengaged vertex. Am J Obstet Gynecol 190:129, 2004

Simon CE, Grobman WA: When has an induction failed? Obstet Gynecol 105: 705, 2005

Smith KM, Hoffman MK, Sciscione A: Elective induction of labor in nulliparous women increases the risk of cesarean delivery. Obstet Gynecol 101:45S, 2003

Solheim K, Myers D, Sparks T, et al: Continuing a trial of labor after 2 hours of active-phase labor arrest: a cost-effectiveness analysis. Abstract No 205. Presented at the 29th Annual Meeting of the Society for Maternal-Fetal Medicine. 26–31 January 2009

Spong CY, Berghella V, Wenstrom KD, et al: Preventing the first cesarean delivery. Summary of a Joint Eunice Kennedy Shriver National Institute of Child Health and Human Development, Society for Maternal-Fetal Medicine, and American College of Obstetricians and Gynecologists Workshop. Obstet Gynecol 120(5):1181, 2012

Tanne JH: US hospitals are reducing early elective deliveries. BMJ 346:f1417, 2013

Tita AT, Landon MB, Spong CY, et al: Timing of elective repeat cesarean delivery at term and neonatal outcomes. N Engl J Med 360(2):111, 2009

Towers CV, Briggs GG, Rojas JA: The use of prostaglandin E2 in pregnant patients with asthma. Am J Obstet Gynecol 190(6):1777, 2004

UK Amniotomy Group: A multicentre randomised trial of amniotomy in spontaneous first labour at term. Br J Obstet Gynaecol 101:307, 1994

Uzun I, Sik A, Sevket O, et al: Bishop score versus ultrasound of the cervix before induction of labor for prolonged pregnancy: which one is better for prediction of cesarean delivery. J Matern Fetal Neonatal Med 26(14):1450, 2013

Vahratian A, Zhang J, Troendle JF, et al: Labor progression and risk of cesarean delivery in electively induced nulliparas. Obstet Gynecol 105: 698, 2005

Väisänen-Tommiska M, Nuutila M, Aittomäki K, et al: Nitric oxide metabolites in cervical fluid during pregnancy: further evidence for the role of cervical nitric oxide in cervical ripening. Am J Obstet Gynecol 188:779, 2003

Väisänen-Tommiska M, Nuutila M, Ylikorkala O: Cervical nitric oxide release in women postterm. Obstet Gynecol 103:657, 2004

Villano KS, Lo JY, Alexander JM: A dose-finding study of oral misoprostol for labor augmentation. Am J Obstet Gynecol 204(6):560.e1, 2011

Vrouenraets FPJM, Roumen FJME, Dehing CJG, et al: Bishop score and risk of cesarean delivery after induction of labor in nulliparous women. Am J Obstet Gynecol 105: 690, 2005

Wagner M: Off-label use of misoprostol in obstetrics: a cautionary tale. BJOG 112: 266, 2005

Wang W, Zheng J, Fu J, et al: Which is the safer method of labor induction for oligohydramnios women? Transcervical double balloon catheter or dinoprostone vaginal insert. J Matern Fetal Neonatal Med January 8, 2014 [Epub ahead of print]

Weeks AD, Fiala C, Safar P: Misoprostol and the debate over off-label drug use. BJOG 112: 269, 2005

Wen T, Beceir A, Xenakis E, et al: Is there a maximum effective dose of Pitocin? Am J Obstet Gynecol 185:S212, 2001

Wing DA, Brown R, Plante LA, et al: Misoprostol vaginal insert and time to vaginal delivery. A randomized controlled trial. Obstet Gynecol 122(2 pt 1): 201, 2013

Wölfler MM, Facchinetti F, Venturini P, et al: Induction of labor at term using isosorbide mononitrate simultaneously with dinoprostone compared to dinoprostone treatment alone: a randomized, controlled trial. Am J Obstet Gynecol 195:1617, 2006

Xenakis EMJ, Langer O, Piper JM, et al: Low-dose versus high-dose oxytocin augmentation of labor—a randomized trial. Am J Obstet Gynecol 173: 1874, 1995

Yeast JD, Jones A, Poskin M: Induction of labor and the relationship to cesarean delivery: a review of 7001 consecutive inductions. Am J Obstet Gynecol 180:628, 1999

Zhang J, Landy HJ, Branch DW, et al: Contemporary patterns of spontaneous labor with normal neonatal outcomes. Obstet Gynecol 116(6):1281, 2010a

Zhang J, Troendle J, Mikolajczyk R, et al: The natural history of the normal first stage of labor. Obstet Gynecol 115(4):705, 2010b

Zhang J, Troendle J, Reddy UM, et al: Contemporary cesarean delivery practice in the United States. Am J Obstet Gynecol 203(4):326.e1, 2010c

Zhang J, Troendle JF, Yancey MK: Reassessing the labor curve in nulliparous women. Am J Obstet Gynecol 187:824, 2002

SECTION 8

DELIVERY

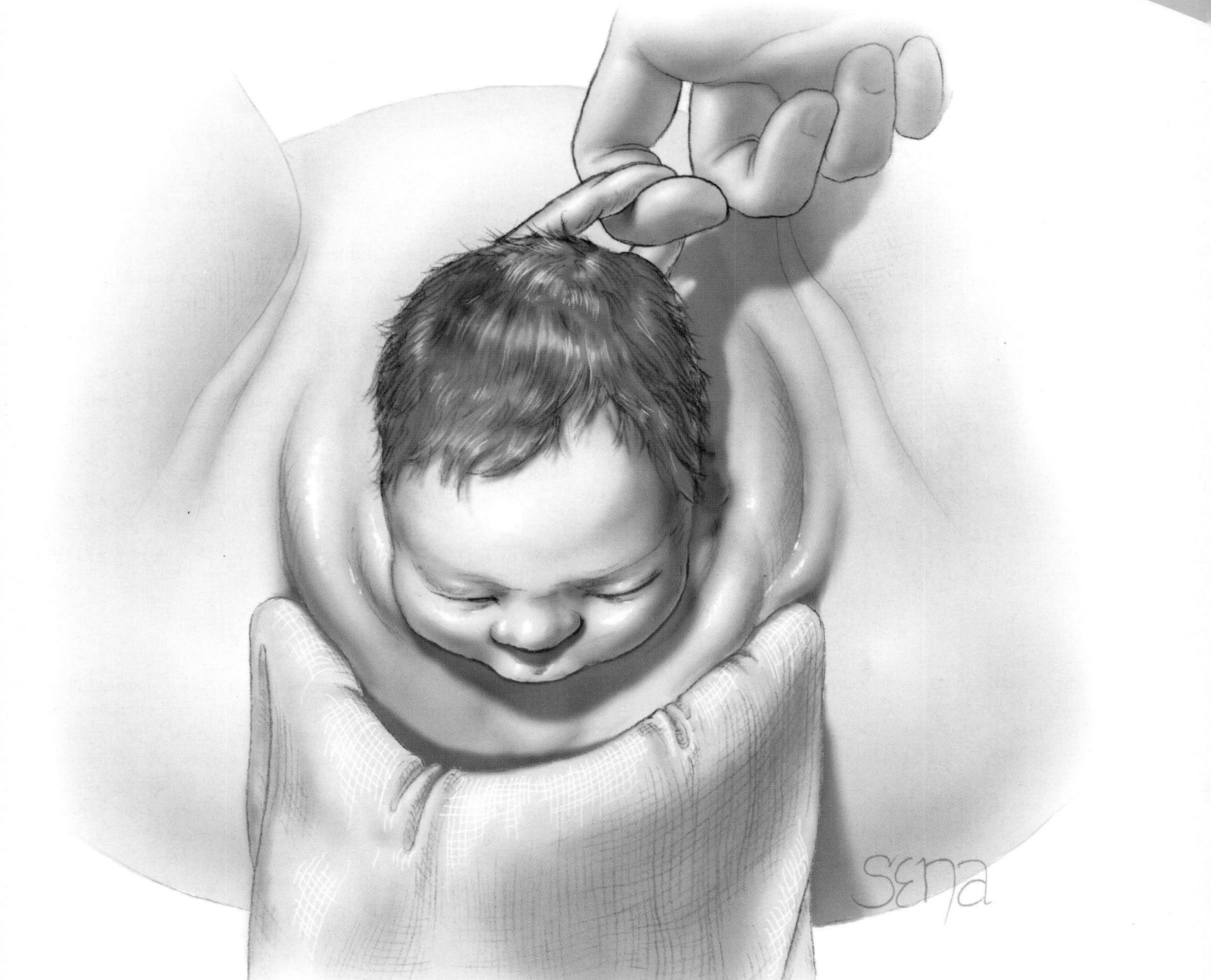

CHAPTER 27

Vaginal Delivery

The natural culmination of second-stage labor is controlled vaginal delivery of a healthy neonate with minimal trauma to the mother. Vaginal delivery is the preferred route of delivery for most fetuses, although certain clinical settings may favor cesarean delivery. Spontaneous vaginal delivery is typical, however, maternal or fetal complications may warrant operative vaginal delivery as described in Chapter 29. Last, a malpresenting fetus or multifetal gestation in many cases may be delivered vaginally but requires special techniques. These are described in Chapters 28—Breech Delivery and 45—Multifetal Pregnancy.

ROUTE OF DELIVERY

In general, spontaneous vaginal vertex delivery poses the lowest risk of most maternal and fetal comorbidity. Compared with cesarean delivery, spontaneous vaginal delivery has lower associated rates of maternal infection, hemorrhage, anesthesia complications, and peripartum hysterectomy, among others. In contrast, for women undergoing spontaneous vaginal delivery compared with cesarean delivery, pelvic floor disorders may be increased (Handa, 2011; Rortveit, 2003). Longitudinal studies, however, suggest that initial pelvic floor protection advantages gained from cesarean delivery are lost as women age (Dolan, 2010; Glazener, 2013; Rortveit, 2001). During their State-of-the-Science Conference, the National Institutes of Health panel (2006) summarized that stress urinary incontinence rates after elective cesarean delivery are lower than those following vaginal delivery. However, the duration of this protection is unclear, particularly in older and multiparous populations. This same conference considered the evidence implicating vaginal delivery in other pelvic floor disorders to be weak and not favoring either delivery route.

PREPARATION FOR DELIVERY

The end of second-stage labor is heralded as the perineum begins to distend, the overlying skin becomes stretched, and the fetal scalp is seen through the separating labia. Increased perineal pressure from the fetal head creates reflexive bearing-down efforts, which are encouraged when appropriate. At this time, preparations are made for delivery. Some considerations that arise during labor and which are also discussed in Chapter 22 (p. 451) are reiterated. For example, the bladder is palpated, and if it is distended, catheterization may be necessary. Continued attention is also given to fetal heart rate monitoring. As one example, a nuchal cord often tightens with descent and may lead to deepening variable decelerations. Antibiotic prophylaxis against infective endocarditis is not recommended for vaginal delivery in most women with cardiac conditions. Exceptions are in women with cyanotic heart disease or prosthetic valves or both. For these women, prophylaxis as outlined in Table 49-10 (p. 991) is indicated

30 to 60 minutes before the anticipated procedure (American College of Obstetricians and Gynecologists, 2011).

During second-stage labor, pushing positions may vary. But for delivery, dorsal lithotomy position is the most widely used and often the most satisfactory. For better exposure, leg holders or stirrups are used. Corton and associates (2012) found no increased rates of perineal lacerations with stirrup use compared to without their use. With positioning, legs are not separated too widely or placed one higher than the other. Within the leg holder, the popliteal region should rest comfortably in the proximal portion and the heel in the distal portion. The legs are not strapped into the stirrups, thereby allowing quick flexion of the thighs backward onto the abdomen should shoulder dystocia develop (p. 541). Legs may cramp during the second stage, in part, because of pressure by the fetal head on pelvic nerves. Cramping may be relieved by repositioning the affected leg or by brief massage.

Preparation for delivery includes vulvar and perineal cleansing. If desired, sterile drapes may be placed in such a way that only the immediate area around the vulva is exposed. In the past, scrubbing, gowning, gloving, and donning protective mask and eyewear was done to protect the laboring woman from infectious agents. Although these considerations remain valid, infectious disease exposure concerns today must also be extended to health-care providers.

OCCIPUT ANTERIOR POSITION

By the time of perineal distention, the position of the presenting occiput is usually known. In some cases, however, molding and caput formation have precluded accurate identification. At this time, careful assessment is again performed as described in Chapter 22 (p. 438). In most cases, presentation is directly occiput anterior or is rotated slightly oblique. But, in perhaps 5 percent, persistent occiput posterior is identified. Rarely, the vertex will be presenting in the occiput transverse position when the head bulges the perineum.

Delivery of the Head

With each contraction, the vulvovaginal opening is dilated by the fetal head to gradually form an ovoid and finally, an almost circular opening (Fig. 27-1). This encirclement of the largest head diameter by the vulvar ring is termed *crowning*. Unless an episiotomy has been made as described later, the perineum thins and especially in nulliparous women, may undergo spontaneous laceration. The anus becomes greatly stretched, and the anterior wall of the rectum may be easily seen through it.

There once was considerable controversy concerning routine episiotomy use. It is now clear that episiotomy increases the risk of a tear into the external anal sphincter, the rectum, or both. Conversely, anterior tears involving the urethra and labia are more common in women in whom an episiotomy is avoided. Most, including us, advocate individualization and do not routinely perform episiotomy.

To limit spontaneous vaginal laceration, some perform intrapartum perineal massage to widen the introitus for head passage. With this, the perineum is grasped in the midline by

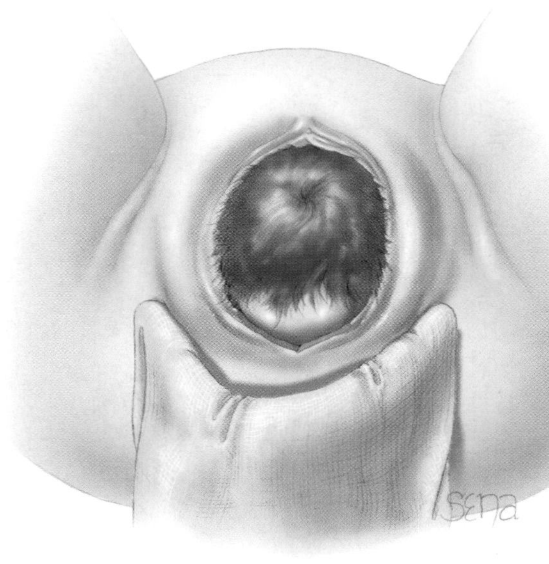

FIGURE 27-1 Delivery of the head. The occiput is being kept close to the symphysis by moderate pressure on the fetal chin at the tip of the maternal coccyx.

both hands using the thumb and opposing fingers. Outward and lateral stretch against the perineum is then repeatedly applied. Evidence for this technique is limited and mixed regarding efficacy for perineal protection when applied either antepartum or intrapartum (Geranmayeh, 2012; Mei-dan, 2008; Stamp, 2001).

When the head distends the vulva and perineum enough to open the vaginal introitus to a diameter of 5 cm or more, a gloved hand may be used to support the perineum (Fig. 27-2). The other hand is used to guide and control the fetal head to avoid expulsive delivery. Slow delivery of the head may decrease

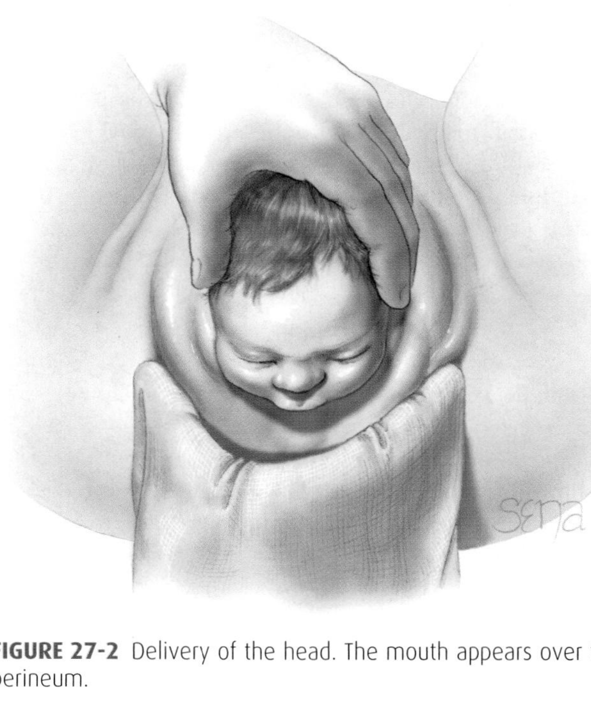

FIGURE 27-2 Delivery of the head. The mouth appears over the perineum.

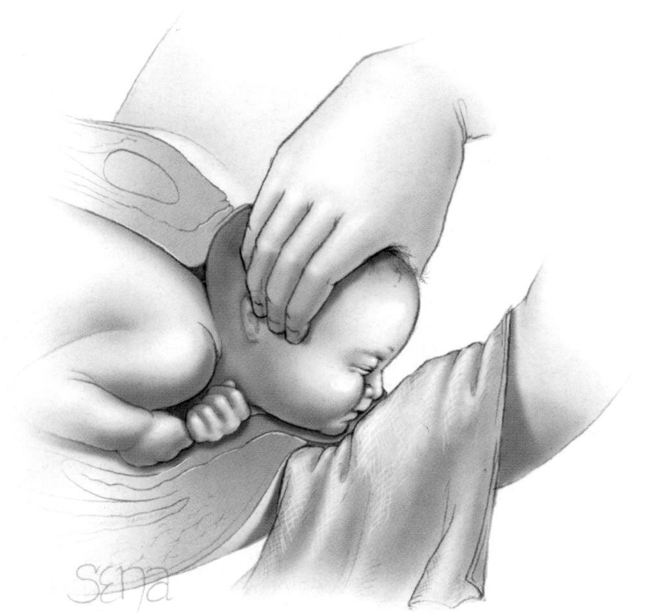

FIGURE 27-3 Modified Ritgen maneuver. Moderate upward pressure is applied to the fetal chin by the posterior hand covered with a sterile towel, while the suboccipital region of the fetal head is held against the symphysis.

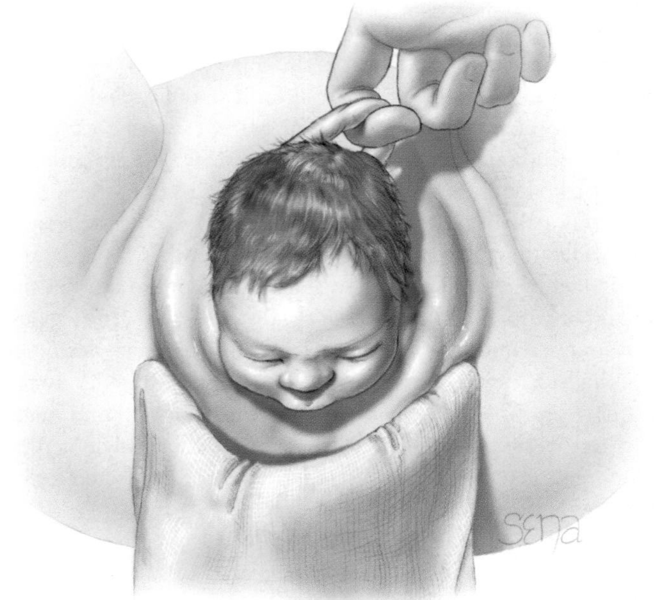

FIGURE 27-4 The umbilical cord, if identified around the neck, is readily slipped over the head.

lacerations (Laine, 2008). Alternatively, if expulsive efforts are inadequate or expeditious delivery is needed, the modified *Ritgen maneuver* may be employed. With this, gloved fingers beneath a draped towel exert forward pressure on the fetal chin through the perineum just in front of the coccyx. Concurrently, the other hand presses superiorly against the occiput (Fig. 27-3). Originally described in 1855, the Ritgen maneuver allows controlled fetal head delivery (Cunningham, 2008). It also favors neck extension so that the head passes through the introitus and over the perineum with its smallest diameters. Comparing the Ritgen maneuver with simple perineal support in 1623 women, Jönsson and colleagues (2008) found a similar incidence of third- and fourth-degree tears—5.5 percent with the maneuver and 4.4 percent with simple support. Last, some espouse a "hands-poised" method, in which the attendant does not touch the perineum during delivery of the head (Mayerhofer, 2002; McCandlish, 1998). Compared with traditional perineal support, this expectant method does not appear to offer greater third-degree laceration protection (Aasheim, 2011).

Delivery of the Shoulders

Following delivery of the fetal head, a finger should be passed across the fetal neck to determine whether it is encircled by one or more umbilical cord loops (Fig. 27-4). A nuchal cord is found in approximately 25 percent of deliveries and ordinarily causes no harm. If an umbilical cord coil is felt, it should be slipped over the head if loose enough. If applied too tightly, the loop should be cut between two clamps. Such tight nuchal cords complicate approximately 6 percent of all deliveries but are not associated with worse neonatal outcome than those without a cord loop (Henry, 2013).

Following its delivery, the fetal head falls posteriorly, bringing the face almost into contact with the maternal anus. The occiput promptly turns toward one of the maternal thighs, and the head assumes a transverse position (Fig. 27-5). This external rotation indicates that the bisacromial diameter, which is the transverse diameter of the thorax, has rotated into the anteroposterior diameter of the pelvis.

Most often, the shoulders appear at the vulva just after external rotation and are born spontaneously. If delayed, extraction aids controlled delivery. The sides of the head are grasped with two hands, and gentle downward traction is applied until the anterior shoulder appears under the pubic arch. Next, by an upward movement, the posterior shoulder is delivered. During delivery, abrupt or powerful force is avoided to avert brachial plexus injury.

The rest of the body almost always follows the shoulders without difficulty. With prolonged delay, however, its birth may be hastened by moderate traction on the head and moderate pressure on the uterine fundus. Hooking the fingers in the axillae is avoided. This can injure upper extremity nerves and produce a transient or possibly permanent paralysis. Traction, furthermore, should be exerted only in the direction of the long axis of the neonate. If applied obliquely, it causes neck bending and excessive brachial plexus stretching. Immediately after delivery of the newborn, there is usually a gush of amnionic fluid, often blood-tinged but not grossly bloody.

Previously, immediate nasopharyngeal bulb suctioning of the newborn was routine to remove secretions. It was found, however, that suctioning of the nasopharynx may lead to neonatal bradycardia (Gungor, 2006). The American Heart Association neonatal resuscitation recommendations currently

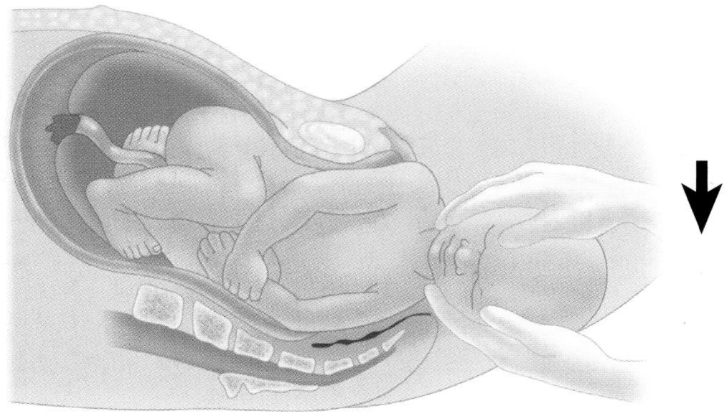

A

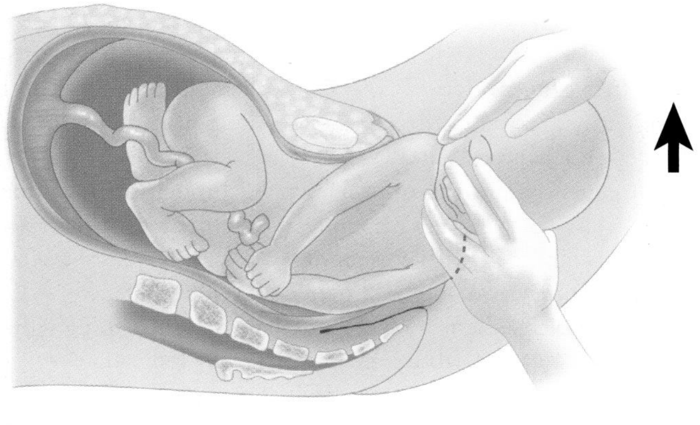

B

FIGURE 27-5 Delivery of the shoulders. **A.** Gentle downward traction to effect descent of the anterior shoulder. **B.** Delivery of the anterior shoulder completed. Gentle upward traction to deliver the posterior shoulder.

eschew most suctioning immediately following birth—even with meconium present. This includes bulb syringe aspiration. Suctioning should be reserved for neonates who have obvious obstruction to spontaneous breathing or who require positive-pressure ventilation (Kattwinkel, 2010). Similarly, if meconium is present and the newborn is depressed, then intubation and tracheal suctioning is recommended (American College of Obstetricians and Gynecologists, 2013b). These aspects are discussed in further detail in Chapter 33 (p. 638).

Clamping the Cord

The umbilical cord is cut between two clamps placed 6 to 8 cm from the fetal abdomen, and later an umbilical cord clamp is applied 2 to 3 cm from its insertion into the fetal abdomen. A plastic clamp that is safe, efficient, and fairly inexpensive, such as the Double Grip Umbilical Clamp (Hollister), is used at Parkland Hospital.

For term neonates, the timing of umbilical cord clamping remains debatable. A delay in umbilical cord clamping for up to 60 seconds may increase total body iron stores, expand blood volume, and decrease anemia incidence in the neonate (Andersson, 2011; Yao, 1974). This may be particularly valuable in populations in which iron deficiency is prevalent (Abalos, 2009). Conversely, and as discussed in Chapter 33 (p. 643), higher hemoglobin concentration increases risks for hyperbilirubinemia and extended hospitalization for neonatal phototherapy (McDonald, 2008). Delayed cord clamping may also hinder timely and needed neonatal resuscitation. Fortunately, in general, delayed umbilical cord clamping compared with early clamping does not worsen Apgar scores, umbilical cord pH, or respiratory distress caused by polycythemia. Regarding maternal outcomes, rates of postpartum hemorrhage are similar between early and delayed clamping groups (Andersson, 2013). Fewer data are available regarding cord "milking," in which the operator pushes blood through the cord toward the newborn. This maneuver appears safe and may be advantageous if rapid cord clamping is clinically indicated (Upadhyay, 2013).

For the preterm neonate, delayed cord clamping has several benefits. These include higher red cell volume, decreased need for blood transfusion, better circulatory stability, and lower rates of intraventricular hemorrhage and of necrotizing enterocolitis (Rabe, 2012; Raju, 2013; Sommers, 2012).

The American College of Obstetricians and Gynecologists (2012c) has concluded that there is insufficient evidence to support or refute benefits from delayed umbilical cord clamping for term neonates in resource-rich settings. For preterm newborns, however, evidence supports delaying umbilical cord clamping to 30 to 60 seconds after birth. This opinion is also endorsed by the American Academy of Pediatrics (2013). Our policy is to clamp the cord after assessing the need to clear the airway, all of which usually requires approximately 30 seconds. The newborn is not elevated above the introitus at vaginal delivery or much above the maternal abdominal wall at the time of cesarean delivery.

PERSISTENT OCCIPUT POSTERIOR POSITION

Approximately 2 to 10 percent of singleton term cephalic fetuses deliver in an occiput posterior (OP) position (Cheng, 2010). As shown in Figure 27-6, many fetuses delivering OP were occiput anterior (OA) in early labor and reflect malrotation during labor. Predisposing risks include epidural analgesia, nulliparity, greater fetal weight, and prior OP position delivery (Cheng, 2006a; Gardberg, 2004; Lieberman, 2005).

Morbidity

Women with a persistent OP position have higher associated rates of prolonged second-stage labor, cesarean delivery, and operative vaginal delivery. For women who deliver vaginally, rates of blood loss and of third- and fourth-degree laceration, so-called higher-order vaginal lacerations, are increased (Senécal, 2005).

Infants delivered from an OP position have many more complications then those born positioned OA. Cheng and coworkers (2006b) compared outcomes of 2591 women undergoing delivery with a persistent OP position with those of 28,801 women whose newborns were delivered OA. Virtually every possible delivery complication was found more frequently with persistent OP position. Only 46 percent of these women

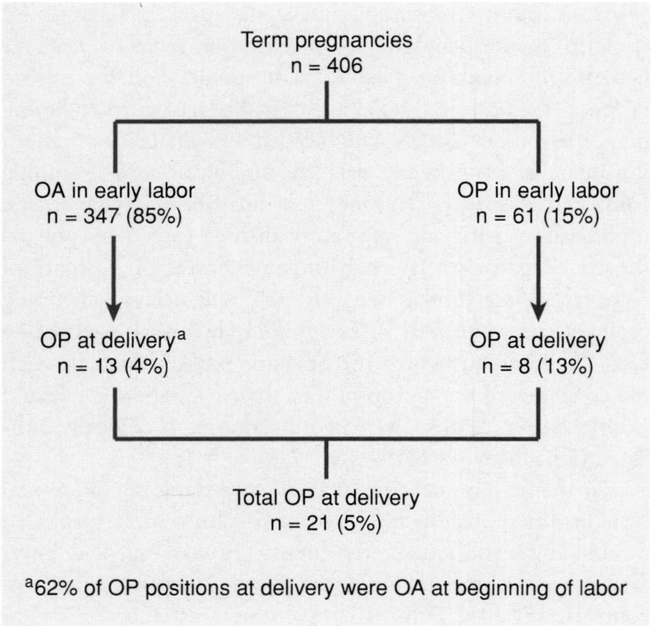

FIGURE 27-6 Occiput posterior (OP) presentation in early labor compared with presentation at delivery. Sonography was used to determine position of the fetal head in early labor. OA = occiput anterior. (Data from Gardberg, 1998.)

delivered spontaneously, and the remainder accounted for 9 percent of cesarean deliveries performed. These investigators also found that an OP position at delivery was associated with increased adverse short-term neonatal outcomes that included acidemic umbilical cord gases, birth trauma, Apgar scores < 7, and intensive care nursery admission, among others. Similar results were reported by Ponkey (2003) and Fitzpatrick (2001) and their associates.

Methods to prevent persistent OP position and its associated morbidity have been investigated. First, digital examination for identification of fetal head position can be inaccurate, and sonography can be used to increase accuracy (Dupuis, 2005; Souka, 2003; Zahalka, 2005). Such information may provide an explanation for prolonged second-stage labor or may identify suitable candidates for manual rotation. In contrast, varying maternal position either before or during labor does not appear to lower rates of persistent OP position (Desbriere, 2013; Kariminia, 2004).

Delivery of Persistent Occiput Posterior Position

Delivery of a fetus with an OP position may be completed by spontaneous or operative vaginal delivery. First, if the pelvic outlet is roomy and the vaginal outlet and perineum are somewhat relaxed from prior deliveries, rapid spontaneous OP delivery will often take place. Conversely, if the vaginal outlet is resistant to stretch and the perineum is firm, second-stage labor may be appreciably prolonged. During each expulsive effort, the head is driven against the perineum to a much greater degree than when the head position is OA. This leads to greater rates of higher-order perineal lacerations (Groutz, 2011; Melamed, 2013).

In some cases, spontaneous vaginal delivery from an OP position does not appear feasible or expedited delivery is needed. Here, manual rotation with spontaneous delivery from an OA position may be preferred. This technique is described fully in Chapter 29 (p. 580). Successful rotation rates range from 47 to 90 percent. And, as would be expected, lower rates of cesarean delivery, vaginal laceration, and maternal blood loss follow rotation to OA position and vaginal delivery (Le Ray, 2005; Sen, 2013; Shaffer, 2006, 2011). Disadvantageously, manual rotation is linked with higher cervical laceration rates. Thus, careful inspection of the cervix following rotation is prudent.

For exigent delivery, forceps or vacuum device can be applied to a persistent OP position. This is often performed in conjunction with an episiotomy. Also, if the head is engaged, the cervix fully dilated, and the pelvis adequate, forceps rotation may be attempted. These circumstances most likely prevail when expulsive efforts of the mother during the second stage are ineffective. Both these operative vaginal techniques are detailed in Chapter 29 (p. 582).

Infrequently, protrusion of fetal scalp through the introitus is the consequence of marked elongation of the fetal head from molding combined with formation of a large caput succedaneum. In some cases, the head may not even be engaged—that is, the biparietal diameter may not have passed through the pelvic inlet. In these, labor is characteristically long and descent of the head is slow. Careful palpation above the symphysis may disclose the fetal head to be above the pelvic inlet. Prompt cesarean delivery is appropriate.

At Parkland Hospital, spontaneous delivery or manual rotation is preferred for management of persistent OP position. In other cases, either manual rotation to OA position followed by forceps delivery or forceps delivery from the OP position is used. If neither can be completed with relative ease, cesarean delivery is performed.

OCCIPUT TRANSVERSE POSITION

In the absence of a pelvic architecture abnormality or asynclitism, the occiput transverse position is usually transitory. Thus, unless contractions are hypotonic, the head usually spontaneously rotates to an OA position. If hypotonic uterine contractions are suspected and cephalopelvic disproportion is absent, then an oxytocin infusion can be used to stimulate labor.

If rotation ceases because of poor expulsive forces, vaginal delivery usually can be accomplished readily in a number of ways. The easiest is manual rotation of the occiput either anteriorly to OA or less commonly, posteriorly to OP. If either is successful, Le Ray and coworkers (2007) reported a 4-percent cesarean delivery rate compared with a 60-percent rate in women in whom manual rotation was not successful. Some recommend rotation with Kielland forceps for the persistent occiput transverse position as outlined in Chapter 29 (p. 582). These forceps are used to rotate the occiput to the anterior position, and delivery is accomplished with the same forceps or by substitution with either Simpson or Tucker–McLane forceps.

In some cases, there may be an underlying cause leading to the persistent occiput transverse position that is not easily overcome. For example, a platypelloid pelvis is flattened anteroposteriorly and an android pelvis is heart shaped. With these, there may be inadequate space for occipital rotation to either an OA or OP position (Fig. 2-20, p. 34). Because of these concerns, undue force should be avoided if forceps delivery is attempted.

SHOULDER DYSTOCIA

Following complete emergence of the fetal head during vaginal delivery, the remainder of the body may not rapidly follow. The anterior fetal shoulder can become wedged behind the symphysis pubis and fail to deliver using normally exerted downward traction and maternal pushing. Because the umbilical cord is compressed within the birth canal, such dystocia is an emergency. Several maneuvers, in addition to downward traction on the fetal head, may be performed to free the shoulder. This requires a team approach, in which effective communication and leadership are critical.

Consensus regarding a specific definition of shoulder dystocia is lacking. Some investigators focus on whether maneuvers to free the shoulder are needed, whereas others use the head-to-body delivery time interval as defining (Beall, 1998). Spong and coworkers (1995) reported that the mean head-to-body delivery time in normal births was 24 seconds compared with 79 seconds in those with shoulder dystocia. These investigators proposed that a head-to-body delivery time > 60 seconds be used to define shoulder dystocia. Currently, however, the diagnosis continues to rely on the clinical perception that the normal downward traction needed for fetal shoulder delivery is ineffective.

Because of these differing definitions, the incidence of shoulder dystocia varies. Current reports cite an incidence between 0.6 percent and 1.4 percent (American College of Obstetricians and Gynecologists, 2012b). There is evidence that the incidence has increased in recent decades, likely due to increasing fetal birthweight (MacKenzie, 2007). Alternatively, this increase may be due to more attention given to appropriate documentation of dystocia (Nocon, 1993).

Maternal and Neonatal Consequences

In general, shoulder dystocia poses greater risk to the fetus than the mother. Postpartum hemorrhage, usually from uterine atony but also from vaginal lacerations, is the main maternal risk (Jangö, 2012; Rahman, 2009). In contrast, significant neonatal neuromusculoskeletal injury and even mortality are concerns. MacKenzie and associates (2007) reviewed 514 cases of shoulder dystocia and found that 11 percent were associated with serious neonatal trauma. Brachial plexus injury was diagnosed in 8 percent, and 2 percent suffered a clavicle, humeral, or rib fracture. Seven percent showed evidence of acidosis at delivery, and 1.5 percent required cardiac resuscitation or developed hypoxic ischemic encephalopathy. Mehta and colleagues (2007) found a similar number of injuries in a study of 205 shoulder dystocia cases, in which 17 percent had injury. Again, most involved the brachial plexus. These specific injuries are described more fully in Chapter 33 (p. 648). Of predictors, increasing fetal weight, maternal body mass index, and second-stage duration and a prior shoulder dystocia appear to raise the neonatal injury risk with shoulder dystocia (Bingham, 2010; Mehta, 2006).

Prediction and Prevention

There has been considerable evolution in obstetrical thinking regarding the preventability of shoulder dystocia. Although there are clearly several risk factors associated with this complication, identification of individual instances before the fact has proved to be impossible. The American College of Obstetricians and Gynecologists (2012b) reviewed studies and concluded that:

1. Most cases of shoulder dystocia cannot be accurately predicted or prevented.
2. Elective induction of labor or elective cesarean delivery for all women suspected of having a macrosomic fetus is not appropriate.
3. Planned cesarean delivery may be considered for the nondiabetic woman with a fetus whose estimated fetal weight is > 5000 g or for the diabetic woman whose fetus is estimated to weigh > 4500 g.

Birthweight

Commonly cited maternal characteristics associated with increased fetal birthweight are obesity, postterm pregnancy, multiparity, diabetes, and gestational diabetes. There is universal agreement that increasing birthweight is associated with an increasing incidence of shoulder dystocia. In one study of nearly 2 million vaginal deliveries, Overland and coworkers (2012) noted that in 75 percent of shoulder dystocia cases, newborns weighed > 4000 g. That said, the concept that cesarean delivery is indicated for large fetuses, even those estimated to weigh 4500 g, should be tempered. Rouse and Owen (1999) concluded that a prophylactic cesarean delivery policy for macrosomic fetuses would require more than 1000 cesarean deliveries with attendant morbidity as well as millions of dollars to avert a single permanent brachial plexus injury.

Intrapartum Factors

Some labor characteristics have been associated with an increased shoulder dystocia risk and include prolonged second-stage labor, operative vaginal delivery, and prior shoulder dystocia (Mehta, 2004; Moragianni, 2012; Overland, 2009). Of these, the risk of recurrent shoulder dystocia ranges from 1 to 13 percent (Bingham, 2010; Moore, 2008; Ouzounian, 2013). For many women with prior shoulder dystocia, a trial of labor may be reasonable. The American College of Obstetricians and Gynecologists (2012b) recommends that estimated fetal weight, gestational age, maternal glucose intolerance, and severity of prior neonatal injury be evaluated and risks and benefits of cesarean delivery discussed with any woman with a history of shoulder dystocia. After discussion, either mode of delivery is appropriate.

Management

Because shoulder dystocia cannot be accurately predicted, clinicians should be well versed in its management principles. Because of ongoing cord compression with this dystocia, one goal is to reduce the head-to-body delivery time. This is balanced against the second goal, which is avoidance of fetal and maternal injury from aggressive manipulations. Accordingly, an initial gentle attempt at traction, assisted by maternal expulsive efforts, is recommended. Adequate analgesia is certainly ideal. Some clinicians advocate performing a large episiotomy to provide room for manipulations. Of note, Paris (2011) and Gurewitsch (2004) and their colleagues reported no change in the brachial plexus injury rate for groups in which episiotomy was not performed during shoulder dystocia management.

After gentle traction, various techniques can be used to free the anterior shoulder from its impacted position behind the symphysis pubis. Of these, moderate *suprapubic pressure* can be applied by an assistant, while downward traction is applied to the fetal head. Pressure is applied with the heel of the hand to the anterior shoulder wedged above and behind the symphysis. The anterior shoulder is thus either depressed or rotated, or both, so the shoulders occupy the oblique plane of the pelvis and the anterior shoulder can be freed.

The *McRoberts maneuver* was described by Gonik and associates (1983) and named for William A. McRoberts, Jr., who popularized its use at the University of Texas at Houston. The maneuver consists of removing the legs from the stirrups and sharply flexing them up onto the abdomen (Fig. 27-7). Gherman and associates (2000) analyzed the McRoberts maneuver using x-ray pelvimetry. They found that the procedure caused straightening of the sacrum relative to the lumbar vertebrae, rotation of the symphysis pubis toward the maternal head, and a decrease in the angle of pelvic inclination. Although this does not increase pelvic dimensions, pelvic rotation cephalad tends to free the impacted anterior shoulder. Gonik and coworkers (1989) tested the McRoberts position objectively with laboratory models and found that the maneuver reduced the forces needed to free the fetal shoulder.

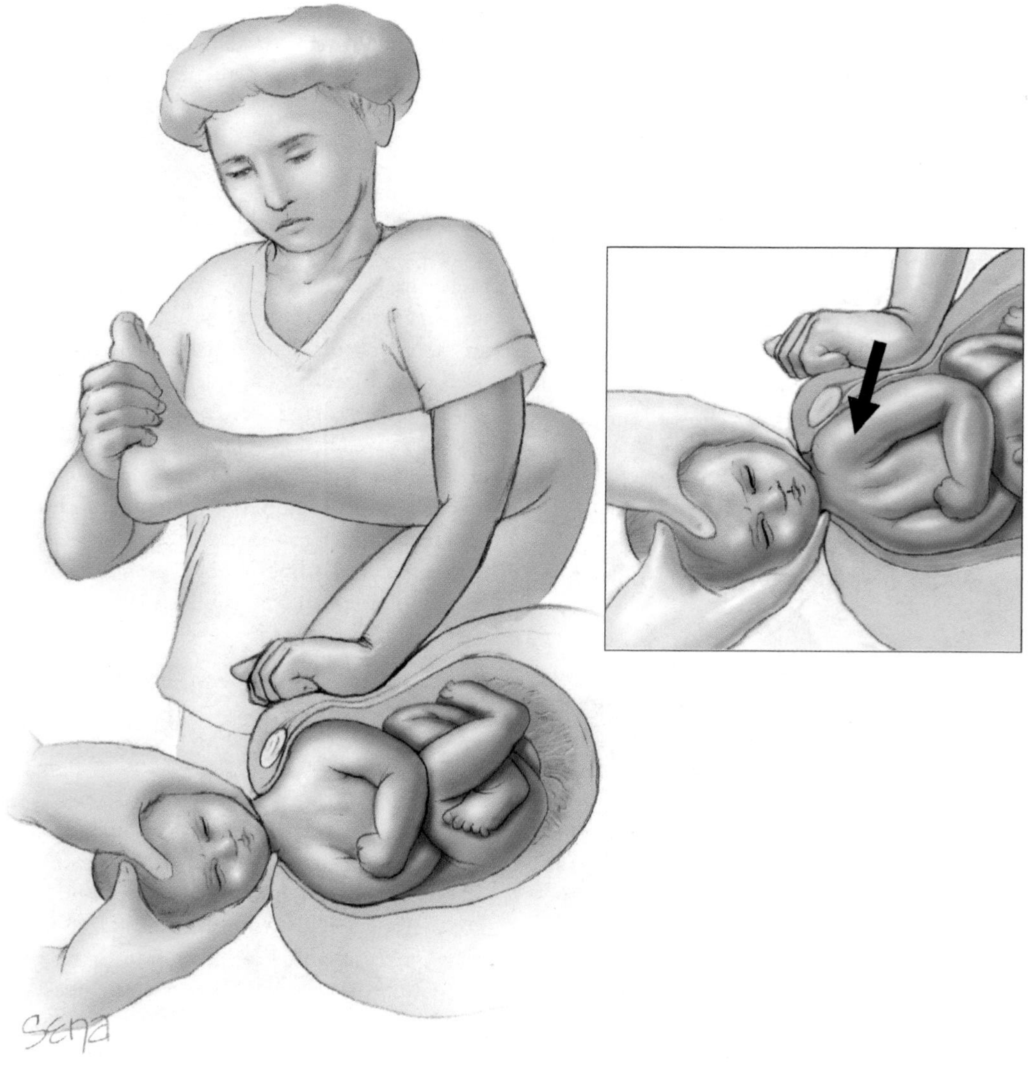

FIGURE 27-7 The McRoberts maneuver. The maneuver consists of removing the legs from the stirrups and sharply flexing the thighs up onto the abdomen. The assistant is also providing suprapubic pressure simultaneously (*arrow*).

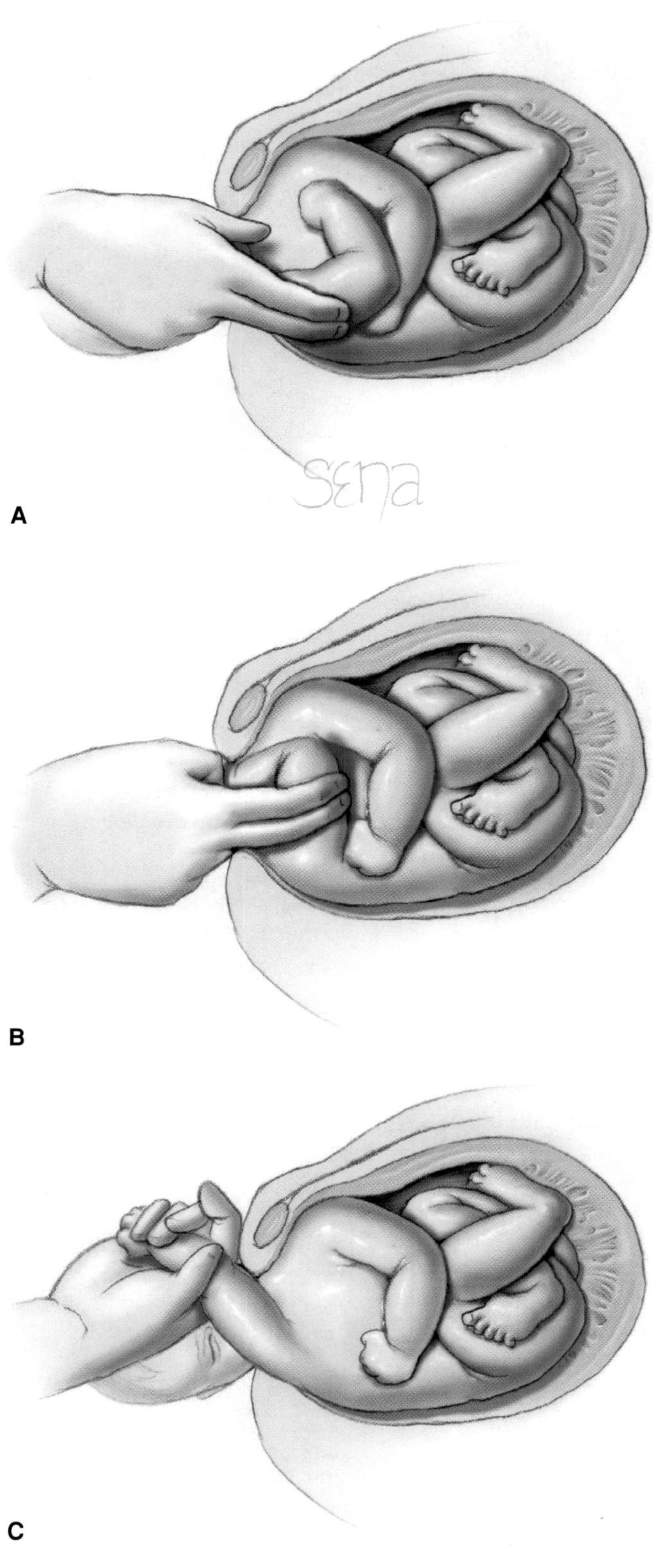

FIGURE 27-8 Delivery of the posterior shoulder for relief of shoulder dystocia. **A.** The operator's hand is introduced into the vagina along the fetal posterior humerus. **B.** The arm is splinted and swept across the chest, keeping the arm flexed at the elbow. **C.** The fetal hand is grasped and the arm extended along the side of the face. The posterior arm is delivered from the vagina.

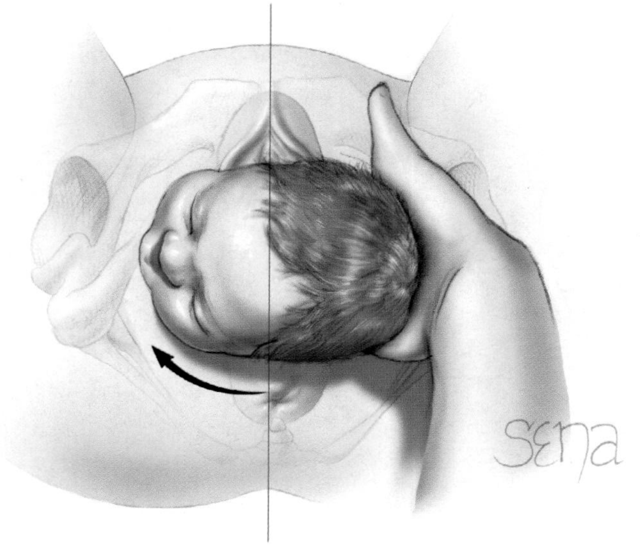

FIGURE 27-9 Woods maneuver. The hand is placed behind the posterior shoulder of the fetus. The shoulder is then rotated progressively 180 degrees in a corkscrew manner so that the impacted anterior shoulder is released.

Another maneuver, *delivery of the posterior shoulder,* consists of carefully sweeping the posterior arm of the fetus across its chest, followed by delivery of the arm. The shoulder girdle is then rotated into one of the oblique diameters of the pelvis with subsequent delivery of the anterior shoulder (Fig. 27-8).

Woods (1943) reported that by progressively rotating the posterior shoulder 180 degrees in a corkscrew fashion, the impacted anterior shoulder could be released. This is frequently referred to as the *Woods corkscrew maneuver* (Fig. 27-9). Rubin (1964) recommended two maneuvers. First, the fetal shoulders are rocked from side to side by applying force to the maternal abdomen. If this is not successful, the pelvic hand reaches the most easily accessible fetal shoulder, which is then pushed toward the anterior surface of the chest. This maneuver most often abducts both shoulders, which in turn produces a smaller shoulder-to-shoulder diameter. This permits displacement of the anterior shoulder from behind the symphysis (Fig. 27-10).

Importantly, progression from one maneuver to the next should be organized and methodical. As noted, the urgency to relieve the dystocia should be balanced against potentially injurious traction forces and manipulations. Lerner and coworkers (2011) in their evaluation of 127 shoulder dystocia cases reported that all neonates without sequelae from shoulder dystocia were born by 4 minutes. Conversely, most depressed neonates—57 percent—had head-to-body delivery intervals > 4 minutes. The percentage of depressed neonates rose sharply after 3 minutes.

Deliberate *fracture of the anterior clavicle* by using the thumb to press it toward and against the pubic ramus can be attempted to free the shoulder impaction. In practice, however, deliberate fracture of a large neonate clavicle is difficult. If successful, the fracture will heal rapidly and is usually trivial compared with brachial nerve injury, asphyxia, or death.

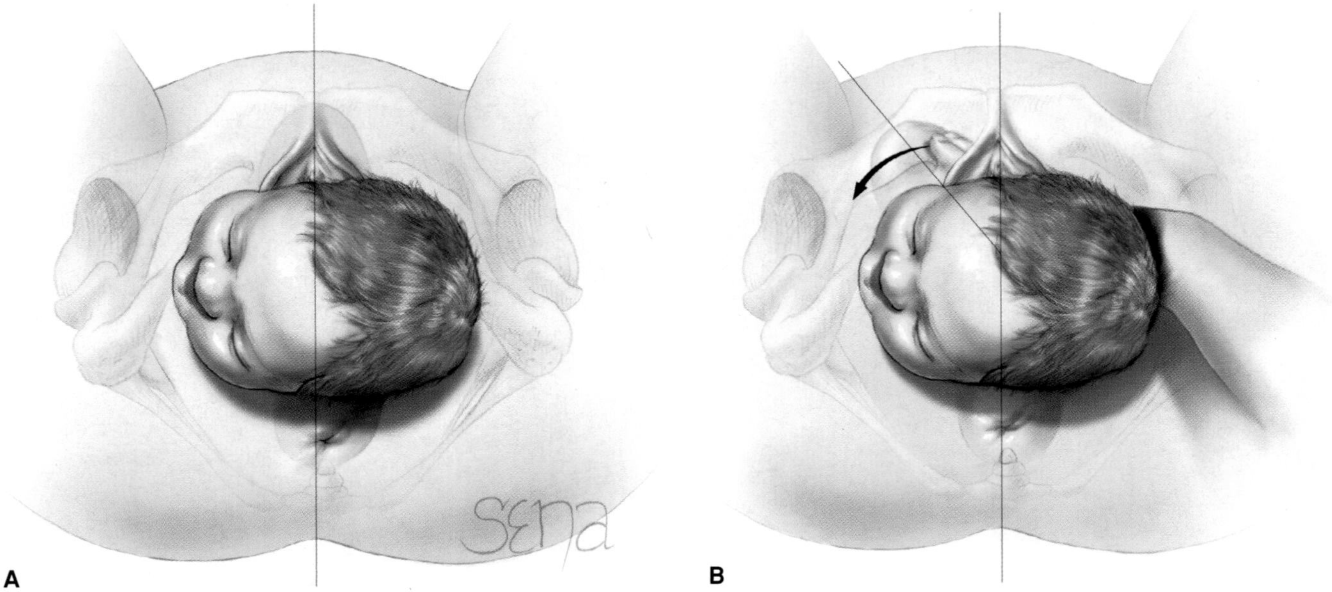

FIGURE 27-10 The second Rubin maneuver. **A.** The shoulder-to-shoulder diameter is aligned vertically. **B.** The more easily accessible fetal shoulder (the anterior is shown here) is pushed toward the anterior chest wall of the fetus (*arrow*). Most often, this results in abduction of both shoulders, which reduces the shoulder-to-shoulder diameter and frees the impacted anterior shoulder.

Hibbard (1982) recommended that pressure be applied to the fetal jaw and neck in the direction of the maternal rectum, with strong fundal pressure applied by an assistant as the anterior shoulder is freed. Strong fundal pressure, however, applied at the wrong time may result in even further impaction of the anterior shoulder. Gross and associates (1987) reported that fundal pressure in the absence of other maneuvers "resulted in a 77-percent complication rate and was strongly associated with (fetal) orthopedic and neurologic damage."

Sandberg (1985) reported the *Zavanelli maneuver* for cephalic replacement into the pelvis followed by cesarean delivery. The first part of the maneuver consists of returning the head to the occiput anterior or posterior position. Terbutaline, 0.25 mg, is given subcutaneously to produce uterine relaxation. The operator flexes the head and slowly pushes it back into the vagina. Cesarean delivery is then performed. Sandberg (1999) reviewed 103 reported cases in which the Zavanelli maneuver was used. It was successful in 91 percent of cephalic cases and in all cases of breech head entrapments. Despite successful replacement, fetal injuries were common but may have resulted from the multiple manipulations used before the Zavanelli maneuver (Sandberg, 2007). Six stillbirths, eight neonatal deaths, and 10 neonates who suffered brain damage were described. Uterine rupture also was reported.

Symphysiotomy, in which the intervening symphyseal cartilage and much of its ligamentous support is cut to widen the symphysis pubis, is described in Chapter 28 (p. 567). It has been used successfully for shoulder dystocia (Hartfield, 1986). Goodwin and colleagues (1997) reported three cases in which symphysiotomy was performed after the Zavanelli maneuver had failed. All three neonates died, and maternal morbidity was significant due to urinary tract injury. *Cleidotomy* consists of cutting the clavicle with scissors or other sharp instruments and is usually done for a dead fetus (Schramm, 1983).

Hernandez and Wendel (1990) suggested use of a *shoulder dystocia drill* to better organize emergency management:

1. Call for help—mobilize assistants and anesthesia and pediatric personnel. Initially, a gentle attempt at traction is made. Drain the bladder if it is distended.
2. A generous episiotomy may be desired to afford room posteriorly.
3. Suprapubic pressure is used initially by most practitioners because it has the advantage of simplicity. Only one assistant is needed to provide suprapubic pressure, while normal downward traction is applied to the fetal head.
4. The McRoberts maneuver requires two assistants. Each assistant grasps a leg and sharply flexes the maternal thigh against the abdomen.

These maneuvers will resolve most cases of shoulder dystocia.

If the above listed steps fail, the following steps may be attempted, and any of the maneuvers may be repeated:

5. Delivery of the posterior arm is attempted. With a fully extended arm, however, this is usually difficult to accomplish.
6. Woods screw maneuver is applied.
7. Rubin maneuver is attempted.

Other techniques generally should be reserved for cases in which all other maneuvers have failed. These include intentional fracture of the anterior clavicle and the Zavanelli maneuver. The American College of Obstetricians and Gynecologists (2012b) has concluded that no one maneuver is superior to another in releasing an impacted shoulder or reducing the chance of injury. Performance of the McRoberts maneuver, however, was deemed a reasonable initial approach. The College (2012a) also has created a Patient Safety Checklist to guide the documentation process with shoulder dystocia.

Shoulder dystocia training and protocols using simulation-based education and drills has evidence-based support. These tools improve performance and retention of drill steps (Buerkle, 2012; Crofts, 2008; Grobman, 2011). Their use has translated into improved neonatal outcome in some, but not all, investigations (Draycott, 2008; Inglis, 2011; Walsh, 2011).

SPECIAL POPULATIONS

Typical vaginal delivery may be challenging in women with perineal limitations or with a large anomalous fetus. Delivery in women with prior pelvic reconstructive surgeries and in those with scarring from female genital mutilation is described here. The special needs of women with congenital vaginal septa, giant condyloma, Crohn disease, or connective-tissue disorders are discussed in chapters covering those topics.

Female Genital Mutilation

Inaccurately called female circumcision, mutilation refers to medically unnecessary vulvar and perineal modification. In the United States it is a federal crime to perform unnecessary genital surgery on a girl younger than 18 years. That said, forms of female genital mutilation are practiced in countries throughout Africa, the Middle East, and Asia. As many as 130 million women worldwide have undergone one of these procedures, and approximately 230,000 live in the United States (Nour, 2006). Cultural sensitivity is imperative, because many women may be offended by the suggestion that they have been assaulted or mutilated (American College of Obstetricians and Gynecologists, 2007).

The World Health Organization (1997) classifies genital mutilations into four types (Table 27-1). Complications include infertility, dysmenorrhea, diminished sexual quality of life, and propensity for vulvovaginal infection (Almroth, 2005; Andersson, 2012; Nour, 2006). In general, women with significant symptoms following type III procedures are candidates for corrective surgery. Specifically, division of midline scar tissue to reopen the vulva is termed defibulation or deinfibulation.

Female genital mutilation has been associated with some adverse maternal and neonatal complications. The World Health Organization (2006) estimated that these procedures increased perinatal morbidity rates by 10 to 20 per 1000. Small increased risks for prolonged labor, cesarean delivery, postpartum hemorrhage, and early neonatal death are found by some but not all (Chibber, 2011; Rouzi, 2012; Wuest, 2009). Importantly, the psychiatric consequences can be profound.

TABLE 27-1. World Health Organization Classification of Female Genital Mutilation

Type I	Prepuce excision with or without clitoral excision
Type II	Clitoral excision with or without partial or total labia minora excision
Type III	Partial or complete labial minora and/or majora excision with or without clitoridectomy and then fusion of the wound, termed infibulation.
Type IV	Unclassified and includes pricking, piercing, incision, stretching, and introduction of corrosive substances into the vagina

Adapted from the World Health Organization, 1997.

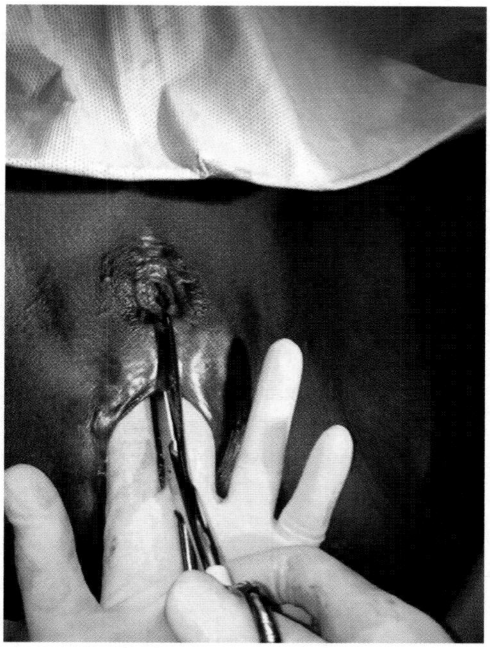

FIGURE 27-11 Process of defibulation. Although not shown here, lidocaine is first infiltrated along the planned incision. As protection, two fingers of one hand are insinuated behind the shelf created by fused labia but in front of the urethra and crowning head. The shelf is then incised in the midline. After delivery, the raw edges are sutured with rapidly absorbable material to secure hemostasis. (From Rouzi, 2012, with permission.)

For those women who do not desire defibulation until they become pregnant, the procedure can be done at midpregnancy using spinal analgesia (Nour, 2006). Or, as shown in Figure 27-11, another option is to wait until delivery. In women not undergoing defibulation, anal sphincter tear rates with vaginal delivery may be increased (Berggren, 2013; Wuest, 2009). In our experiences, intrapartum defibulation in many cases allows successful vaginal delivery without major complications.

Prior Pelvic Reconstructive Surgery

These surgeries are performed with increasing frequency in reproductive-aged women, and thus pregnancy following these procedures is not uncommon. Logically, there are concerns for symptom recurrence following vaginal delivery, and high-quality data to aid evidenced-based decisions are limited. For women with prior stress urinary incontinence surgery, slightly greater protection against postpartum incontinence is gained by elective cesarean delivery (Pollard, 2012; Pradhan, 2013). Stated another way, most women with prior anti-incontinence surgery can be delivered vaginally without symptom recurrence. Also, cesarean delivery is not always protective.

Obviously, symptom recurrence and the need for additional vaginal surgery should be weighed against the surgical risk of cesarean delivery (Groenen, 2008). In those with prior surgeries for anal incontinence or pelvic organ prolapse, only scant information regarding outcomes is available. Such cases require individualization.

Anomalous Fetuses

Rarely, delivery can be obstructed by extreme macrocephaly secondary to hydrocephaly or by massive fetal abdomen enlargement from a greatly distended bladder, ascites, or large kidneys or liver. With milder forms of hydrocephaly, if the biparietal diameter is < 10 cm or if the head circumference is < 36 cm, then vaginal delivery may be permitted (Anteby, 2003).

In rare cases in which neonatal death has occurred or is certain due to associated anomalies, vaginal delivery may be reasonable, but the head or abdomen must be reduced in size for delivery. Removal of fluid by cephalocentesis or paracentesis with sonographic guidance can be performed intrapartum. For hydrocephalic fetuses that are breech, cephalocentesis can be accomplished suprapubically when the aftercoming head enters the pelvis. For those that require cesarean delivery, fluid removal before hysterotomy circumvents extending a low transverse or lengthening a vertical incision.

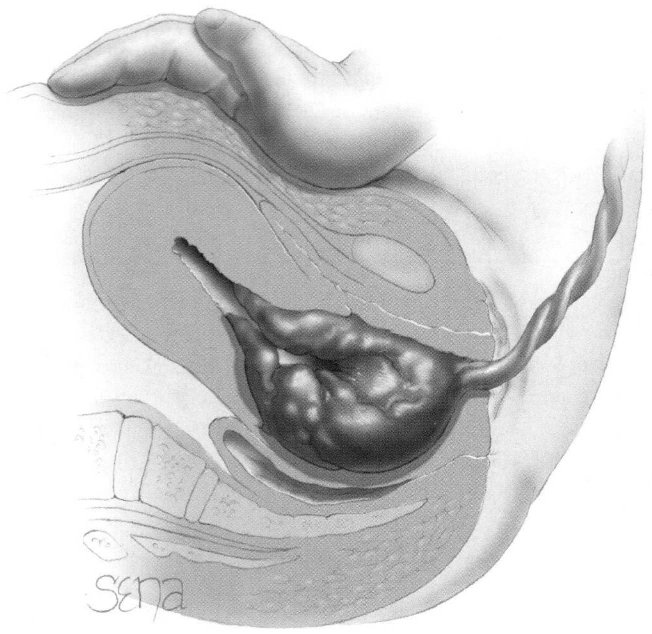

FIGURE 27-12 Expression of placenta. Note that the hand is *not* trying to push the fundus of the uterus through the birth canal! As the placenta leaves the uterus and enters the vagina, the uterus is elevated by the hand on the abdomen while the cord is held in position. The mother can aid in the delivery of the placenta by bearing down. As the placenta reaches the perineum, the cord is lifted, which in turn lifts the placenta out of the vagina.

THIRD STAGE OF LABOR

Delivery of the Placenta

Third-stage labor begins immediately after fetal birth and ends with placental delivery. Goals include delivery of an intact placenta and avoidance of uterine inversion or postpartum hemorrhage. The latter two are grave intrapartum complications and constitute emergencies, as described in Chapter 41 (p. 783).

Immediately after newborn birth, uterine fundal size and consistency are examined. If the uterus remains firm and there is no unusual bleeding, watchful waiting until the placenta separates is the usual practice. Massage is not employed, but the fundus is frequently palpated to ensure that it does not become atonic and filled with blood from placental separation. To prevent uterine inversion, umbilical cord traction must not be used to pull the placenta from the uterus. Moreover, placental expression is not forced before placental separation. Signs of separation include a sudden gush of blood into the vagina, a globular and firmer fundus, a lengthening of the umbilical cord as the placenta descends into the vagina, and a rise of the uterus into the abdomen. With the last, the placenta, having separated, passes down into the lower uterine segment and vagina. Here, its bulk pushes the uterus upward.

These signs sometimes appear within 1 minute after newborn delivery and usually within 5 minutes. Once the placenta has detached from the uterine wall, it should be determined that the uterus is firmly contracted. The mother may be asked to bear down, and the intraabdominal pressure often expels the placenta into the vagina. These efforts may fail or may not be possible because of analgesia. After ensuring that the uterus is contracted firmly, pressure is exerted by a hand wrapped around the fundus to propel the detached placenta into the vagina (Fig. 27-12). The umbilical cord is kept slightly taut but is not pulled. Concurrently, the heel of the hand exerts downward pressure between the symphysis pubis and the uterine fundus. This also aids inversion prevention. Once the placenta passes through the introitus, pressure on the uterus is relieved. The placenta is then gently lifted away (Fig. 27-13). Care is taken to prevent placental membranes from being torn off and left behind. If the membranes begin to tear, they are grasped with a clamp and removed by gentle teasing (Fig. 27-14).

Manual Removal of Placenta

Occasionally, the placenta will not separate promptly. This is especially common with preterm delivery (Dombrowski, 1995). If there is brisk bleeding and the placenta cannot be delivered by the above technique, manual removal of the placenta is indicated, using the safeguards described in Chapter 41 (p. 784). It is unclear how much time should elapse in the absence of bleeding before the placenta is manually removed (Deneux-Tharaux, 2009). If labor analgesia is still intact, some obstetricians practice routine manual removal of any placenta that has not separated spontaneously by the time they have completed

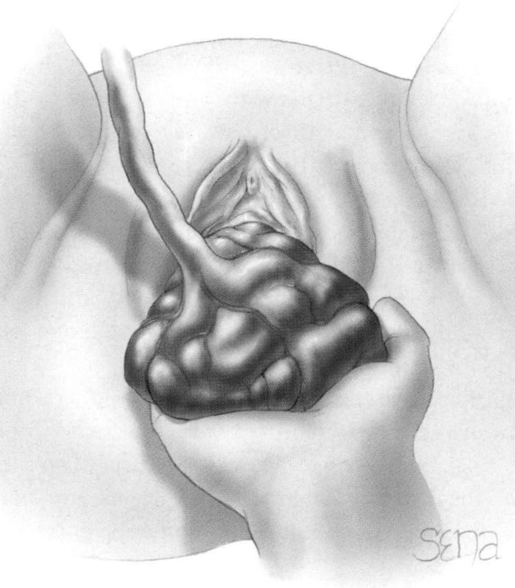

FIGURE 27-13 The placenta is removed from the vagina by lifting the cord.

delivery of the newborn and care of the cord. The benefits of this practice, however, have not been proven, and most obstetricians await spontaneous placental detachment unless bleeding is excessive. When manual removal is performed, some administer a single dose of intravenous antibiotics similar to that used for cesarean infection prophylaxis (Chap. 30, p. 590). The American College of Obstetricians and Gynecologists (2011) has concluded that there are no data to either support or refute this practice.

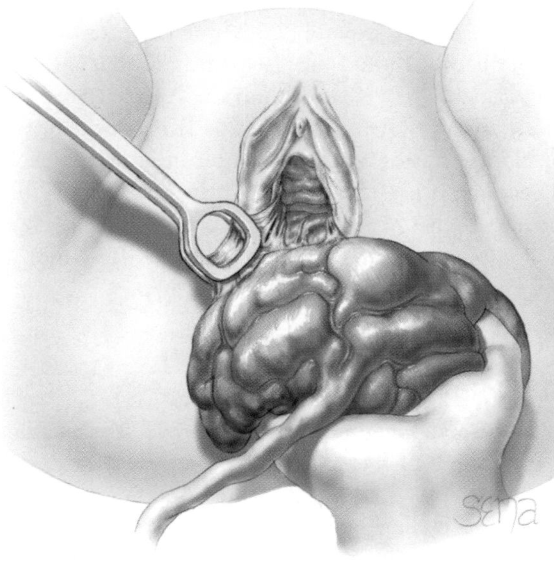

FIGURE 27-14 Membranes that were somewhat adhered to the uterine lining are separated by gentle traction with a ring forceps.

Management of the Third Stage

Practices within the third stage of labor may be broadly considered as either physiological or active management. Physiological or expectant management involves waiting for placental separation signs and allowing the placenta to deliver either spontaneously or aided by nipple stimulation or gravity (World Health Organization, 2012). In contrast, active management of third-stage labor consists of early cord clamping, controlled cord traction during placental delivery, and immediate administration of prophylactic uterotonics. The goal of this triad is to limit postpartum hemorrhage (Begley, 2011; Jangsten, 2011; Prendiville, 1988). In addition, uterine massage following placental delivery is recommended by many but not all to prevent postpartum hemorrhage. We support this with the caveat that evidence for this practice is not strong (Abdel-Aleem, 2010). As noted earlier (p. 539), immediate cord clamping does not increase postpartum hemorrhage rates and thus is a less important component of this trio. Similarly, cord traction may also be less critical (Gülmezoglu, 2012).

Therefore, uterotonics appear to be the most important factor to decrease postpartum blood loss. Choices include oxytocin (Pitocin), misoprostol (Cytotec), carboprost (Hemabate), and the ergots, namely ergonovine (Ergotrate) and methylergonovine (Methergine). In addition, a combination agent of oxytocin and ergonovine (Syntometrine) is used outside the United States. Also in other countries, carbetocin (Duratocin), a long-acting oxytocin analogue, is available and effective for hemorrhage prevention during cesarean delivery (Attilakos, 2010; Su, 2012). Of these, the World Health Organization (2012) recommends oxytocin as a first-line agent. Ergot-based drugs and misoprostol are alternatives in settings that lack oxytocin.

Uterotonics may be given before or after placental expulsion without increasing rates of postpartum hemorrhage, placental retention, or third-stage labor length (Soltani, 2010). If they are given before delivery of the placenta, however, they may entrap an undiagnosed, undelivered second twin. Thus, abdominal palpation should confirm no additional fetuses.

High-Dose Oxytocin

Synthetic oxytocin is identical to that produced by the posterior pituitary. Its action is noted at approximately 1 minute, and it has a mean half-life of 3 to 5 minutes. When given as a bolus, oxytocin can cause profound hypotension. Secher and coworkers (1978) reported that an intravenous bolus of 10 units of oxytocin caused a marked transient fall in blood pressure with an abrupt increase in cardiac output. Svanström and associates (2008) confirmed those findings in 10 healthy women following cesarean delivery. Mean pulse rate increased 28 bpm, mean arterial pressure decreased 33 mm Hg, and electrocardiogram changes of myocardial ischemia as well as chest pain and subjective discomfort were noted. These hemodynamic changes could be dangerous for women hypovolemic from hemorrhage or those with cardiac disease. Thus, oxytocin should not be given intravenously as a large bolus. Rather, it should be given as a dilute solution by continuous intravenous infusion or as an intramuscular injection.

Water intoxication can result from the antidiuretic action of high-dose oxytocin if administered in a large volume of electrolyte-free dextrose solution (Whalley, 1963). In a case report, Schwartz and Jones (1978) described convulsions in both a mother and her newborn following administration of 6.5 liters of 5-percent dextrose solution and 36 units of oxytocin before delivery. The cord plasma sodium concentration was 114 mEq/L. Accordingly, if oxytocin is to be administered in high doses for a considerable period of time, its concentration should be increased rather than increasing the infusion flow rate (Chap. 26, p. 530).

Despite the routine use of oxytocin, no standard prophylactic dose has been established for its use following either vaginal or cesarean delivery. In an analysis of studies that compared oxytocin dosage, investigators found higher infusion doses to be more effective than lower doses or protracted fixed-dose administration (Roach, 2013; Tita, 2012). Our standard practice, if an intravenous infusion is established, is to add 20 units (2 mL) of oxytocin per liter of infusate. This solution is administered after delivery of the placenta at a rate of 10 to 20 mL/min (200 to 400 mU/min) for a few minutes until the uterus remains firmly contracted and bleeding is controlled. The infusion rate then is reduced to 1 to 2 mL/min until the mother is ready for transfer from the recovery suite to the postpartum unit. The infusion is usually then discontinued. For women without intravenous access, 10 units of intramuscular oxytocin are provided.

Ergonovine and Methylergonovine

These ergot alkaloids have similar activity levels in myometrium, and only methylergonovine is currently manufactured in the United States. These agents require very specific storage conditions, as they deteriorate rapidly with exposure to light, heat, and humidity.

Whether given intramuscularly or orally, both are powerful stimulants of myometrial contraction, exerting an effect that may persist for hours. In pregnant women, an intramuscular or oral dose of 0.2 mg results in tetanic uterine contractions. Effects develop within a few minutes after intramuscular or oral administration. Moreover, the response is sustained with little tendency toward relaxation. *Ergots are dangerous for the fetus and mother when given before delivery*. Moreover, cases of serious injury and death have been reported when methylergonovine was administered accidentally to newborns in the labor and delivery room instead of vitamin K, hepatitis B vaccine, or naloxone (Aeby, 2003; American Regent, 2012a; Bangh, 2005). The Food and Drug Administration (2012) has added a warning to the package insert recommending a 12-hour delay between the last methylergonovine dose and breast feeding. Despite this, no adverse effects attributable to this drug in breast milk have been reported (Briggs, 2011).

In addition to neonatal concerns, parenteral administration of ergot alkaloids, especially by the intravenous route, may induce transient maternal hypertension. Other reported side effects include nausea, vomiting, tinnitus, headache, and painful uterine contractions. Hypertension is more likely to be severe in women with gestational hypertension. These drugs are contraindicated in patients with hypertension, cardiac disease or occlusive vascular disorders, severe hepatic or renal disease, and sepsis (Novartis, 2012; Sanders-Bush, 2011). Moreover, this drug is not routinely given intravenously to avoid inducing sudden hypertensive and cerebrovascular accidents. If considered a lifesaving measure, however, intravenous methylergonovine should be given slowly during no less than 60 seconds with careful monitoring of blood pressure (American Reagent, 2012b).

Ergot alkaloid agents do not provide superior protection against postpartum hemorrhage compared with oxytocin. Moreover, safety and tolerability are greater with oxytocin (Liabsuetrakul, 2007). For these reasons, ergot alkaloid agents are considered second-line for third-stage labor prevention of hemorrhage.

Misoprostol

This prostaglandin E_1 analogue has proved inferior to oxytocin for postpartum hemorrhage prevention (Tunçalp, 2012). Although oxytocin is preferred, in resource-poor settings that lack oxytocin, misoprostol is suitable for hemorrhage prophylaxis and is given as a single oral 600-μg dose (Mobeen, 2011; World Health Organization, 2012). Side effects include shivering in 30 percent and fever in 5 percent. Unlike some other prostaglandins, nausea or diarrhea is infrequent (Derman, 2006; Lumbiganon, 1999; Walraven, 2005).

"FOURTH STAGE" OF LABOR

The hour immediately following delivery of the placenta is critical, and it has been designated by some as the fourth stage of labor. During this time, lacerations are repaired. Although uterotonics are administered, postpartum hemorrhage as the result of uterine atony is most likely at this time. Hematomas may expand. Consequently, uterine tone and the perineum should be frequently evaluated. The American Academy of Pediatrics and the American College of Obstetricians and Gynecologists (2012) recommend that maternal blood pressure and pulse be recorded immediately after delivery and every 15 minutes for the first 2 hours. The placenta, membranes, and umbilical cord should be examined for completeness and for anomalies, as described in Chapter 6 (p. 117).

Birth Canal Lacerations

Lower genital tract lacerations may involve the cervix, vagina, or perineum. Those of the cervix and vagina are described in Chapter 41 (p. 788). Perineal tears may follow any vaginal delivery and are classified by their depth. Complete definitions and visual examples are given in Figure 27-15. As noted, third- and fourth-degree lacerations are considered higher-order lacerations. Short-term, these are associated with greater blood loss, puerperal pain, and wound disruption or infection risk.

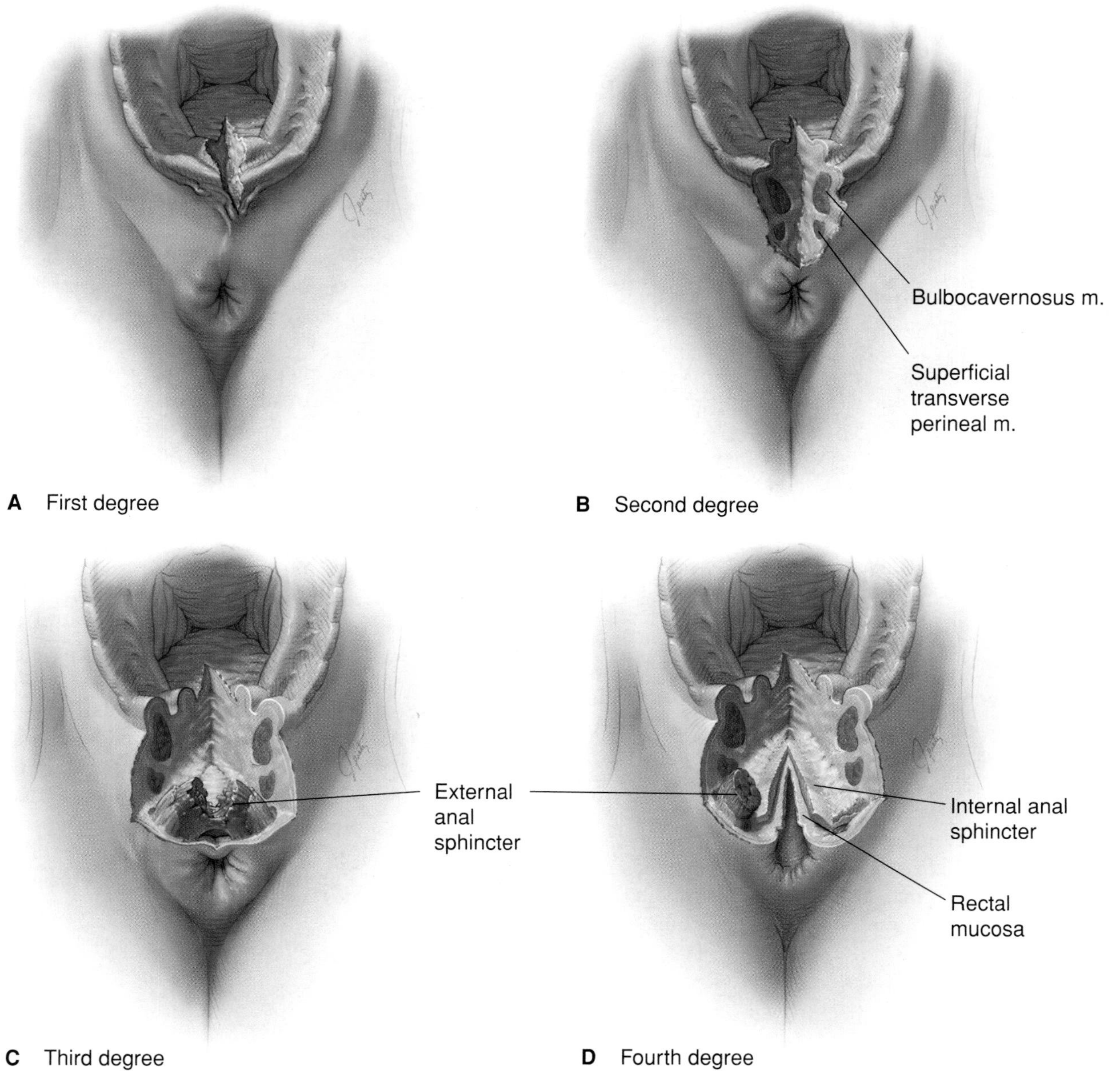

FIGURE 27-15 Classification of perineal lacerations. **A.** First-degree lacerations involve the fourchette, perineal skin, and vaginal mucous membrane but not the underlying fascia and muscle. These included periurethral lacerations, which may bleed profusely. **B.** Second-degree lacerations involve, in addition, the fascia and muscles of the perineal body but not the anal sphincter. These tears may be midline, but often extend upward on one or both sides of the vagina, forming an irregular triangle. **C.** Third-degree lacerations extend farther to involve the external anal sphincter. **D.** Fourth-degree lacerations extend completely through the rectal mucosa to expose its lumen and thus involves disruption of both the external and internal anal sphincters. (Used with permission from Drs. Shayzreen Roshanravan and Marlene Corton.)

Long-term, they are linked with higher rates of anal incontinence and dyspareunia. The incidence of higher-order lacerations varies from 0.25 to 6 percent (Garrett, 2014; Groutz, 2011; Melamed, 2013; Stock, 2013). Risk factors for these more complex lacerations include midline episiotomy, nulliparity, longer second-stage labor, precipitous delivery, persistent occiput posterior position, operative vaginal delivery, Asian race, and increasing fetal birthweight (Landy, 2011; Melamed, 2013). Epidural analgesia was found to be protective (Jango, 2014).

Morbidity rates rise as laceration severity increases. Stock and coworkers (2013) reported that approximately 7 percent of 909 higher-order lacerations had complications. Williams and Chames (2006) found that mediolateral episiotomy was the most powerful predictor of wound disruption. Goldaber and associates (1993) found that 21 of 390 or 5.4 percent of women with fourth-degree lacerations experienced significant morbidity. There were 1.8 percent dehiscences, 2.8 percent infections plus a dehiscence, and 0.8 percent with isolated infections.

The repair of perineal lacerations is virtually the same as that of episiotomy incisions, albeit sometimes less satisfactory because of tear irregularities. Thus, laceration repair technique is discussed with episiotomy repair.

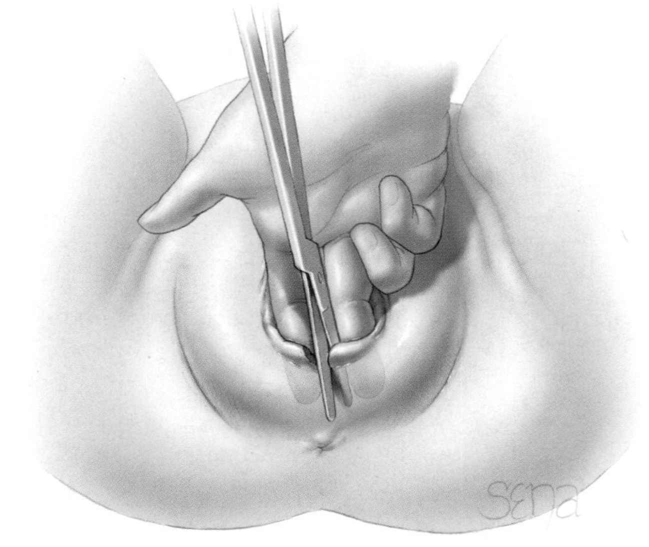

FIGURE 27-16 Midline episiotomy. Two fingers are insinuated between the perineum and fetal head, and the episiotomy is then cut vertically downward.

Episiotomy

The word episiotomy derives from the Greek *episton*—pubic region—plus *-tomy*—to cut. In a strict sense, episiotomy is incision of the pudendum—the external genital organs. Perineotomy is incision of the perineum. In common parlance, however, the term episiotomy often is used synonymously with perineotomy, a practice that we follow here. The incision may be made in the midline, creating a median or midline episiotomy (Fig. 27-16). It may also begin off the midline and directed laterally and downward away from the rectum, termed a mediolateral episiotomy.

Episiotomy Indications and Consequences

Although episiotomy is still a common obstetrical procedure, its use has decreased remarkably over the past 30 years. Oliphant and coworkers (2010) used the National Hospital Discharge Survey to analyze episiotomy rates between 1979 and 2006 in the United States. They noted a 75-percent decline in the episiotomy age-adjusted rate. Through the 1970s, however, it was common practice to cut an episiotomy for almost all women having their first delivery. The reasons for its popularity included substitution of a straight surgical incision, which was easier to repair, for the ragged laceration that otherwise might result. The long-held beliefs that postoperative pain is less and healing improved with an episiotomy compared with a tear, however, appeared to be incorrect (Larsson, 1991).

Another commonly cited but unproven benefit of routine episiotomy was that it prevented pelvic floor disorders. A number of observational studies and randomized trials, however, showed that routine episiotomy is associated with an *increased* incidence of anal sphincter and rectal tears (Angioli, 2000; Nager, 2001; Rodriguez, 2008).

Carroli and Mignini (2009) reviewed the Cochrane Pregnancy and Childbirth Group trials registry. There were lower rates of posterior perineal trauma, surgical repair, and healing complications in women managed with a restrictive use of episiotomy. Alternatively, the incidence of anterior perineal trauma was lower in the group managed with routine use of episiotomy.

With these findings came the realization that episiotomy did not protect the perineal body but contributed to anal sphincter incontinence by increasing the risk of higher-order lacerations. Signorello and associates (2000) reported that fecal and flatal incontinence was increased four- to sixfold in women with an episiotomy compared with a group of women delivered with an intact perineum. Even compared with spontaneous lacerations, episiotomy tripled the risk of fecal incontinence and doubled it for flatal incontinence. Episiotomy without extension did not lower this risk. Despite repair of a third-degree extension, 30 to 40 percent of women have long-term anal incontinence (Gjessing, 1998; Poen, 1998). Finally, Alperin and associates (2008) reported that episiotomy performed for the first delivery conferred a fivefold risk for second-degree or higher-order laceration with the second delivery.

The American College of Obstetricians and Gynecologists (2013a) has concluded that restricted use of episiotomy is preferred to routine use. We are of the view that the procedure should be applied selectively for appropriate indications. Thus, episiotomy should be *considered* for indications such as shoulder dystocia, breech delivery, macrosomic fetuses, operative vaginal deliveries, persistent occiput posterior positions, and other instances in which failure to perform an episiotomy will result in significant perineal rupture. The final rule is that there is no substitute for surgical judgment and common sense.

Episiotomy Type and Timing

Before episiotomy, analgesia may be provided by existing labor epidural analgesia, by bilateral pudendal nerve blockade, or by infiltration of 1-percent lidocaine. If performed unnecessarily early, bleeding from the episiotomy may be considerable during the interval between incision and delivery. If it is performed too late, lacerations will not be prevented. Typically, episiotomy is completed when the head is visible during a contraction to a diameter of approximately 4 cm, that is, crowning. When used in conjunction with forceps delivery, most perform an episiotomy after application of the blades (Chap. 29, p. 580).

Technique

For midline episiotomy, fingers are insinuated between the crowning head and the perineum. The scissors are positioned at 6 o'clock on the vaginal opening and directed posteriorly (see Fig. 27-16). The incision length varies from 2 to 3 cm depending on perineal length and degree of tissue thinning. The incision is customized for specific delivery needs but should stop well before reaching the external anal sphincter. With mediolateral

TABLE 27-2. Midline versus Mediolateral Episiotomy

	Type of Episiotomy	
Characteristic	Midline	Mediolateral
Surgical repair	Easy	More difficult
Faulty healing	Rare	More common
Postoperative pain	Minimal	Common
Anatomical results	Excellent	Occasionally faulty
Blood loss	Less	More
Dyspareunia	Rare	Occasional
Extensions	Common	Uncommon

episiotomy, scissors are positioned at 7 o'clock or at 5 o'clock, and the incision is extended 3 to 4 cm toward the ipsilateral ischial tuberosity.

Differences between the two types of episiotomies are summarized in Table 27-2. Except for the important issue of third- and fourth-degree extensions, midline episiotomy is superior. Anthony and colleagues (1994) presented data from the Dutch National Obstetric Database of more than 43,000 deliveries. They found a more than fourfold decrease in severe perineal lacerations following mediolateral episiotomy compared with rates after midline incision. Proper selection of cases can minimize this one disadvantage. For example, if episiotomy is required during operative vaginal delivery, several studies have reported a protective effect from mediolateral episiotomy against higher-order perineal lacerations (de Leeuw, 2008; de Vogel, 2012; Hirsch, 2008).

Repair of Episiotomy or Perineal Laceration

Typically, episiotomy repair is deferred until the placenta has been delivered. This policy permits undivided attention to the signs of placental separation and delivery. A further advantage is that episiotomy repair is not interrupted or disrupted by the obvious necessity of delivering the placenta, especially if manual removal must be performed that may disrupt a newly repaired episiotomy. The major disadvantage is continuing blood loss until the repair is completed. Direct pressure from an applied gauze sponge will help to limit this loss.

For suitable repair, an understanding of perineal support and anatomy is necessary and is discussed in Chapter 2 (p. 21). Adequate analgesia is imperative, and Sanders and coworkers (2002) emphasized that women without regional analgesia can experience high levels of pain during perineal suturing. Again, local lidocaine can be used solely or as a supplement to bilateral pudendal nerve blockade. In those with epidural analgesia, additional dosing may be necessary.

There are many ways to repair an episiotomy incision, but hemostasis and anatomical restoration without excessive suturing are essential. A technique that commonly is employed for midline repair is shown in Figure 27-17. Some

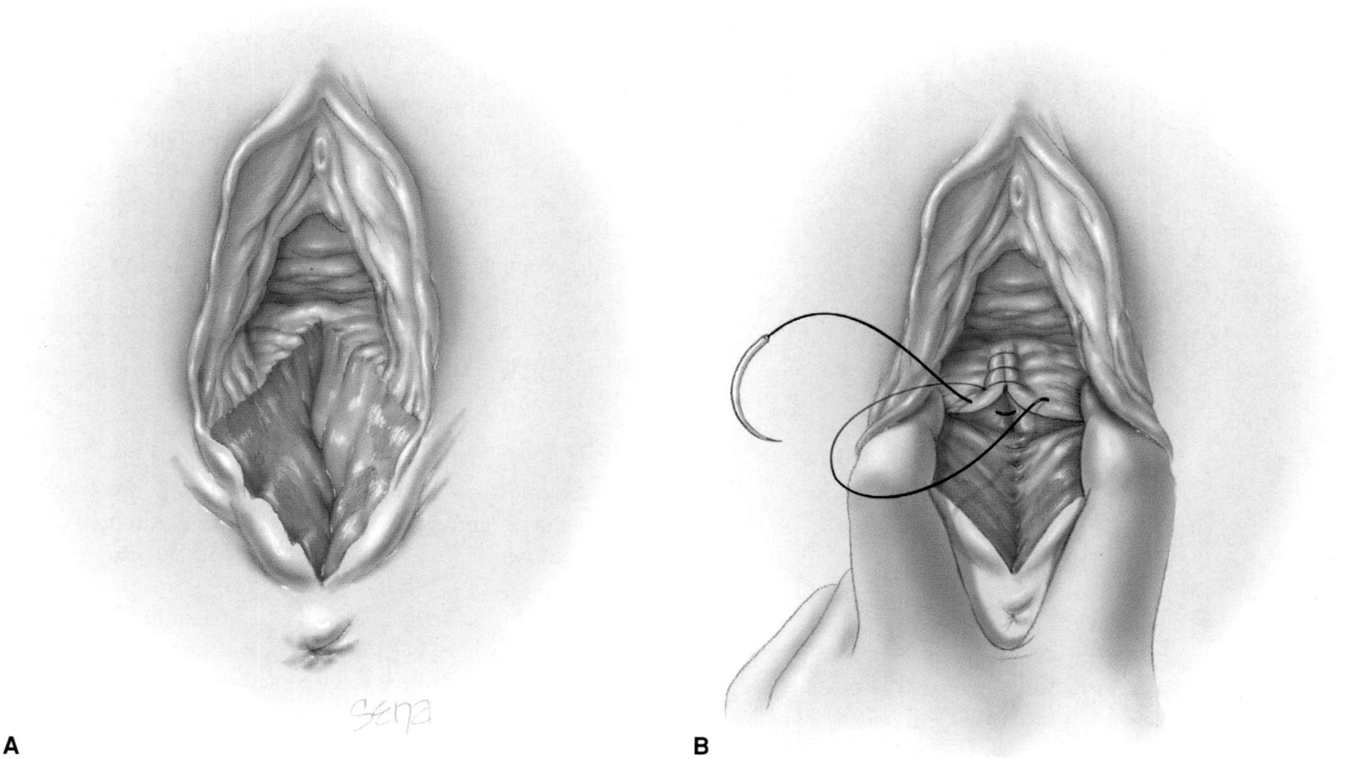

A B

FIGURE 27-17 Repair of midline episiotomy. **A.** Disruption of the hymenal ring and bulbocavernosus and superficial transverse perineal muscles are seen within the diamond-shaped episiotomy incision. **B.** An anchor stitch is placed above the wound apex to begin a running closure. Absorbable 2–0 or 3–0 suture is used for continuous closure of the vaginal mucosa and submucosa with interlocking stitches. (*continued*)

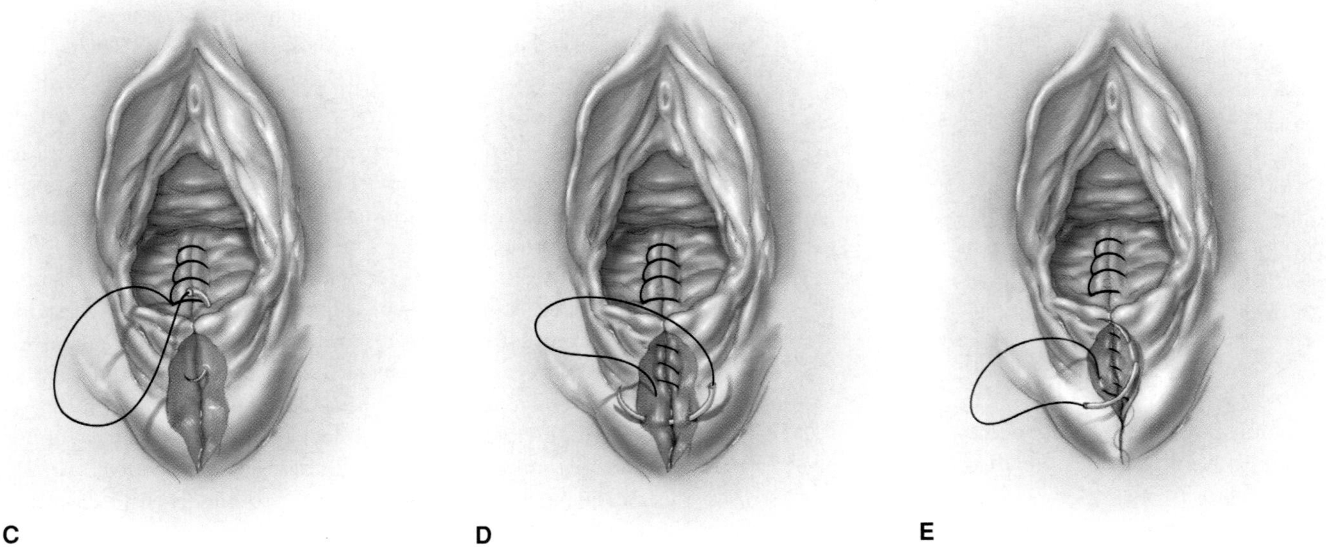

FIGURE 27-17 (*Continued*) **C.** After closing the vaginal incision and reapproximating the cut margins of the hymenal ring, the needle and suture are positioned to close the perineal incision. **D.** A continuous closure with absorbable 2–0 or 3–0 suture is used to close the fascia and muscles of the incised perineum. This aids restoration of the perineal body for long-term support. **E.** The continuous suture is then carried upward as a subcuticular stitch. The final knot is tied proximal to the hymenal ring.

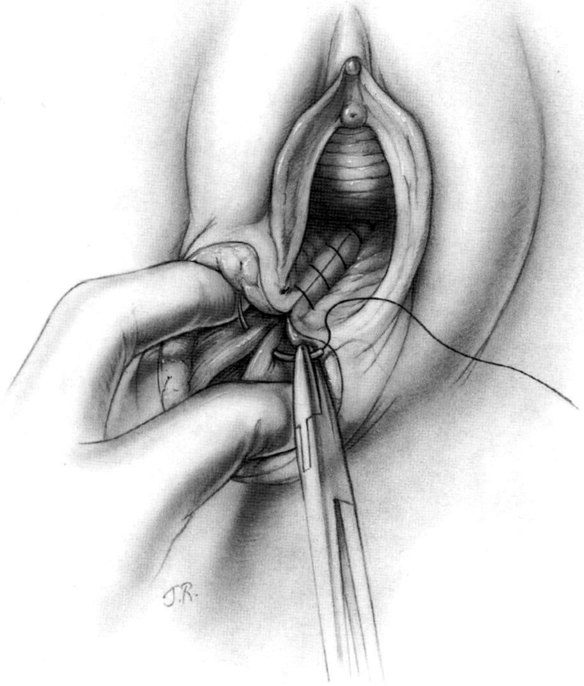

FIGURE 27-18 Mediolateral episiotomy repair. The vaginal mucosa is shown as already closed using 2–0 absorbable suture in a running interlocking stitch similar to that for midline repair. As illustrated, perineal reapproximation begins with reunion of bulbocavernosus and transverse perineal muscles. These will assist reestablishment of perineal body support. Distal to these muscles, abundant fat in the ischiorectal fossa is incorporated in the same running closure. A second layer atop this first perineal layer may be required to adequately close dead space. The skin is then closed with a subcuticular stitch as used for midline closure.

studies have found similar postoperative pain scores using either continuous or interrupted closure (Kindberg, 2008; Valenzuela, 2009). Others note less pain with continuous suturing (Kettle, 2012). Moreover, continuous suturing is faster and uses less suture material. Mornar and Perlow (2008) have shown that blunt needles are suitable and likely decrease the incidence of needlestick injuries. The suture material commonly used is 2–0 chromic catgut. Sutures made of polyglycolic acid derivatives are also frequently used. A decrease in postsurgical pain is cited as the major advantage of synthetic materials. Closures with these materials, however, occasionally require suture removal from the repair site because of pain or dyspareunia. According to Kettle and associates (2002), this disadvantage may be reduced using a rapidly absorbed polyglactin 910 (Vicryl Rapide).

Repair of a mediolateral episiotomy is similar to a midline repair. The technique is shown in Figure 27-18.

Fourth-Degree Laceration Repair

Two methods are used to repair a laceration involving the anal sphincter and rectal mucosa. The first is the end-to-end technique, which we prefer, and the second is the overlapping technique.

The *end-to-end technique* is shown in Figure 27-19. In all techniques that have been described, it is essential to approximate the torn edges of the rectal mucosa with sutures placed in the rectal muscularis approximately 0.5 cm apart. One suitable choice is 2–0 or 3–0 chromic gut. This muscular layer then is covered by reapproximation of the internal anal sphincter. Finally, the cut ends of the external anal sphincter are isolated, approximated, and sutured together end-to-end with three or four interrupted stitches. The remainder of the repair is the same as for a midline episiotomy.

The *overlapping technique* is an alternative method to approximate the external anal sphincter. Data based on randomized controlled trials do not support that this method yields superior anatomical or functional results compared with those of the traditional end-to-end method (Farrell, 2012; Fitzpatrick, 2000).

We, as well as others, recommend perioperative antimicrobial prophylaxis for the reduction of infectious morbidity associated with higher-order perineal injury repair (Goldaber, 1993; Stock, 2013). A single dose of a second-generation cephalosporin is suitable, or clindamycin for penicillin-allergic women. Although such prophylaxis has some evidence-based support, the American College of Obstetricians and Gynecologists (2011) has concluded that this practice has not been extensively studied (Duggal, 2008; Stock, 2013). Postoperatively, stool softeners should be prescribed for a week, and enemas and suppositories should be avoided.

Unfortunately, normal function is not always ensured even with correct and complete surgical repair. Some women may experience continuing fecal incontinence caused by injury to the innervation of the pelvic floor musculature (Roberts, 1990).

Postepisiotomy Pain

Pudendal nerve blockade can aid relief of perineal pain postoperatively (Aissaoui, 2008). Locally applied ice packs help reduce swelling and allay discomfort. Topical application of 5-percent lidocaine ointment was not effective in relieving episiotomy or perineal laceration discomfort in one randomized trial (Minassian, 2002). Analgesics such as codeine give considerable relief. Because pain may be a signal of a large vulvar, paravaginal, or ischiorectal fossa hematoma or perineal cellulitis, these sites should be examined carefully if pain is severe or persistent. Management of these complications is discussed in Chapters 37 and 41 (p. 689 and p. 790). In addition to pain, urinary retention may complicate episiotomy recovery (Mulder, 2012). Its management is described in Chapter 36 (p. 676).

For those with second-degree or greater lacerations, intercourse is usually proscribed until after the first puerperal visit at 4 to 6 weeks. Signorello and coworkers (2001) surveyed 615 women 6 months postpartum and reported that those delivered with an intact perineum reported better sexual function compared with those who had perineal trauma. In another

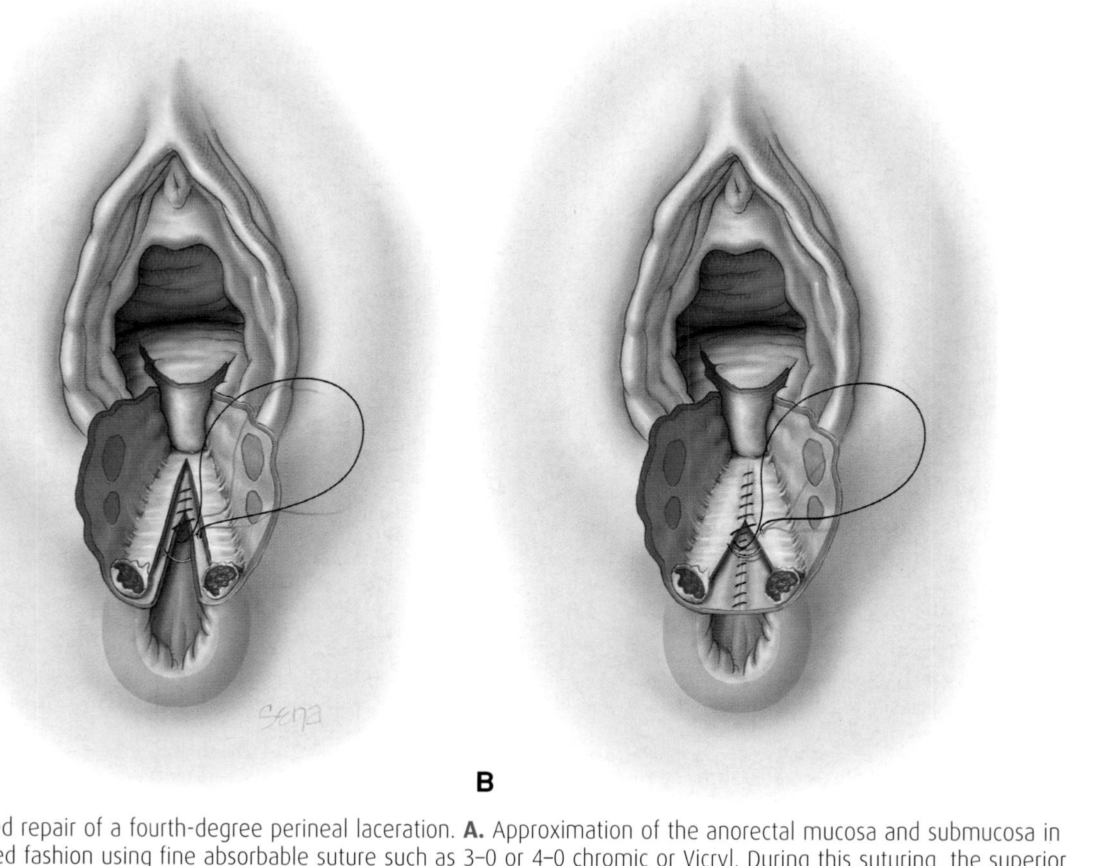
A B

FIGURE 27-19 Layered repair of a fourth-degree perineal laceration. **A.** Approximation of the anorectal mucosa and submucosa in a running or interrupted fashion using fine absorbable suture such as 3–0 or 4–0 chromic or Vicryl. During this suturing, the superior extent of the anterior anal laceration is identified, and the sutures are placed through the submucosa of the anorectum approximately 0.5 cm apart down to the anal verge. **B.** A second layer is placed through the rectal muscularis using 3–0 Vicryl suture in a running or interrupted fashion. This "reinforcing layer" should incorporate the torn ends of the internal anal sphincter, which is identified as the thickening of the circular smooth muscle layer at the distal 2 to 3 cm of the anal canal. It can be identified as the glistening white fibrous structure lying between the anal canal submucosa and the fibers of the external anal sphincter (EAS). In many cases, the internal sphincter retracts laterally and must be sought and retrieved for repair. (*continued*)

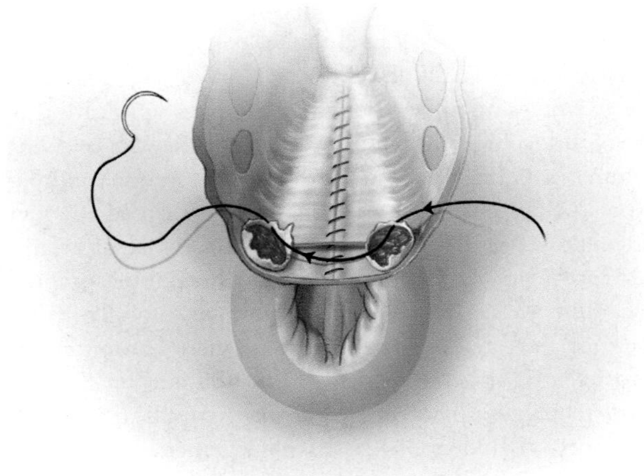

C

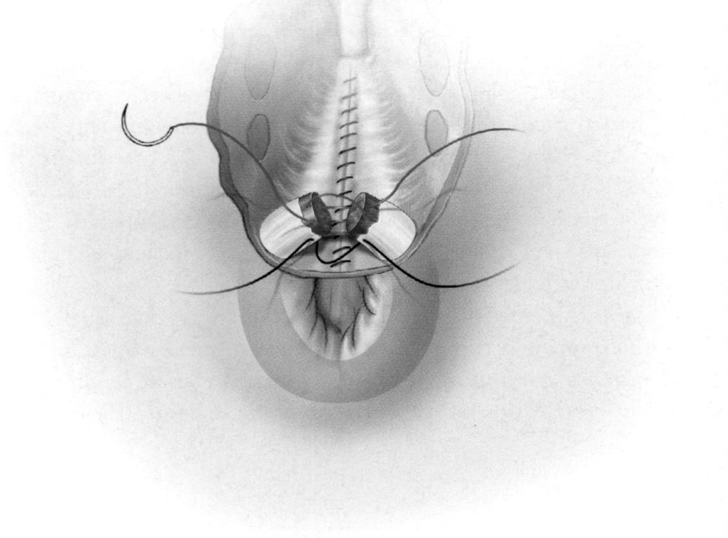

D

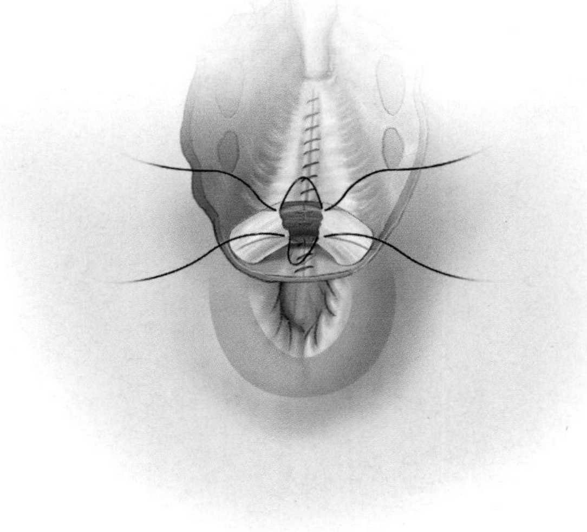

E

FIGURE 27-19 (*Continued*) **C.** In overview, with traditional end-to-end approximation of the EAS, a suture is placed through the EAS muscle, and four to six simple interrupted 2–0 or 3–0 Vicryl sutures are placed at the 3, 6, 9, and 12 o'clock positions through the connective tissue capsule of the sphincter. The sutures through the inferior and posterior portions of the sphincter should be placed first to aid this part of the repair. To begin this portion of the closure, the disrupted ends of the striated EAS muscle and capsule are identified and grasped with Allis clamps. Suture is placed through the posterior wall of the EAS capsule. **D.** Sutures through the EAS (*blue suture*) and inferior capsule wall. **E.** Sutures to reapproximate the anterior and superior walls of the EAS capsule. The remainder of the repair is similar to that described for a midline episiotomy in Figure 27-17.

follow-up of 2490 women, Rådestad and associates (2008) reported delayed intercourse at 3 and 6 months, but not at 1 year, in women with and without perineal trauma.

REFERENCES

Aasheim V, Nilsen AB, Lukasse M, et al: Perineal techniques during the second stage of labour for reducing perineal trauma. Cochrane Database Syst Rev 12:CD006672, 2011

Abalos E: Effect of timing of umbilical cord clamping of term infants on maternal and neonatal outcomes: RHL commentary. World Health Organization. 2009. Available at: http://apps.who.int/rhl/pregnancy_childbirth/childbirth/3rd_stage/cd004074_abalose_com/en./ Accessed April 25, 2013

Abdel-Aleem H, Singata M, Abdel-Aleem M, et al: Uterine massage to reduce postpartum hemorrhage after vaginal delivery. Int J Gynaecol Obstet 111(1):32, 2010

Aeby A, Johansson AB, De Schuiteneer B, Blum D: Methylergometrine poisoning in children: review of 34 cases. J Toxicol Clin Toxicol 41(3):249, 2003

Aissaoui Y, Bruyère R, Mustapha H, et al: A randomized controlled trial of pudendal nerve block for pain relief after episiotomy. Anesth Analg 107:625, 2008

Almroth L, Elmusharaf S, El Hadi N, et al: Primary infertility after genital mutilation in girlhood in Sudan: a case-control study. Lancet 366:385, 2005

Alperin M, Krohn MA, Parviainen K: Episiotomy and increase in the risk of obstetric laceration in a subsequent vaginal delivery. Obstet Gynecol 111:1274, 2008

American Academy of Pediatrics: Timing of umbilical cord clamping after birth. Pediatrics 131(4):e1323, 2013

American Academy of Pediatrics and the American College of Obstetricians and Gynecologists: Guidelines for Perinatal Care, 7th ed. Washington, AAP and ACOG, 2012, p 195

American College of Obstetricians and Gynecologists: Guidelines for Women's Health Care, 3rd ed. Washington, 2007, p 243

American College of Obstetricians and Gynecologists: Prophylactic antibiotics in labor and delivery. Practice Bulletin No. 120, June 2011

American College of Obstetricians and Gynecologists: Documenting shoulder dystocia. Patient Safety Checklist No. 6, August 2012a

American College of Obstetricians and Gynecologists: Shoulder dystocia. Practice Bulletin No. 40, November 2002, Reaffirmed 2012b

American College of Obstetricians and Gynecologists: Timing of umbilical cord clamping after birth. Committee Opinion No. 543, December 2012c

American College of Obstetricians and Gynecologists: Episiotomy. Practice Bulletin No. 71, April 2006, Reaffirmed 2013a

American College of Obstetricians and Gynecologists: Management of delivery of a newborn with meconium-stained amniotic fluid. Committee Opinion No. 379, September 2007, Reaffirmed 2013b

American Regent: Methylergonovine maleate injection, USP. 2012a. Healthcare Professional Correspondence. Available at: http://www.americanregent.com/documents/news/6tuNxatD2c = .pdf. Accessed April 29, 2013

American Regent: Methylergonovine maleate injection, USP. Prescribing Information. 2012b. Available at: http://www.americanregent.com/documents/Product77PrescribingInformation.pdf. Accessed May 13, 2013

Andersson O, Hellström-Westas L, Andersson D, et al: Effects of delayed compared with early umbilical cord clamping on maternal postpartum hemorrhage and cord blood gas sampling: a randomized trial. Acta Obstet Gynecol Scand 92(5):567, 2013

Andersson O, Hellström-Westas L, Andersson D, et al: Effect of delayed versus early umbilical cord clamping on neonatal outcomes and iron status at 4 months: a randomised controlled trial. BMJ 343:d7157, 2011

Andersson SH, Rymer J, Joyce DW, et al: Sexual quality of life in women who have undergone female genital mutilation: a case-control study. BJOG 119(13):1606, 2012

Angioli R, Gomez-Marin O, Cantuaria G, et al: Severe perineal lacerations during vaginal delivery: the University of Miami experience. Am J Obstet Gynecol 182:1083, 2000

Anteby EY, Yagel S: Route of delivery of fetuses with structural anomalies. Eur J Obstet Gynecol Reprod Biol 106(1):5, 2003

Anthony S, Buitendijk SE, Zondervan KT, et al: Episiotomies and the occurrence of severe perineal lacerations. Br J Obstet Gynaecol 101:1064, 1994

Attilakos G, Psaroudakis D, Ash J, et al: Carbetocin versus oxytocin for the prevention of postpartum haemorrhage following caesarean section: the results of a double-blind randomised trial. BJOG 117(8):929, 2010

Bangh SA, Hughes KA, Roberts DJ, et al: Neonatal ergot poisoning: a persistent iatrogenic illness. Am J Perinatol 22(5):239, 2005

Beall MH, Spong C, McKay J, et al: Objective definition of shoulder dystocia: a prospective evaluation. Am J Obstet Gynecol 179:934, 1998

Begley CM, Gyte GM, Devane D, et al: Active versus expectant management for women in the third stage of labour. Cochrane Database Syst Rev 11:CD007412, 2011

Berggren V, Gottvall K, Isman E, et al: Infibulated women have an increased risk of anal sphincter tears at delivery: a population-based Swedish register study of 250 000 births. Acta Obstet Gynecol Scand 92(1):101, 2013

Bingham J, Chauhan SP, Hayes E, et al: Recurrent shoulder dystocia: a review. Obstet Gynecol Surv 65(3):183, 2010

Briggs GG, Freeman RK, Yaffe SJ (eds): Drugs in Pregnancy and Lactation, 9th ed. Philadelphia, Lippincott Williams & Wilkins, 2011, p 939

Buerkle B, Pueth J, Hefler LA, et al: Objective structured assessment of technical skills evaluation of theoretical compared with hands-on training of shoulder dystocia management: a randomized controlled trial. Obstet Gynecol 120(4):809, 2012

Carroli G, Mignini L: Episiotomy for vaginal birth. Cochrane Database Syst Rev 1:CD000081, 2009

Cheng YW, Hubbard A, Caughey AB, et al: The association between persistent fetal occiput posterior position and perinatal outcomes: an example of propensity score and covariate distance matching. Am J Epidemiol 171(6):656, 2010

Cheng YW, Shaffer BL, Caughey AB: Associated factors and outcomes of persistent occiput posterior position: a retrospective cohort study from 1976 to 2001. J Matern Fetal Neonatal Med 19(9):563, 2006a

Cheng YW, Shaffer BL, Caughey AB: The association between persistent occiput posterior position and neonatal outcomes. Obstet Gynecol 107(4):837, 2006b

Chibber R, El-Saleh E, El Harmi J: Female circumcision: obstetrical and psychological sequelae continues unabated in the 21st century. J Matern Fetal Neonatal Med 24(6):833, 2011

Corton MM, Lankford JC, Ames R, et al: A randomized trial of birthing with and without stirrups. Am J Obstet Gynecol 207(2):133.e1, 2012

Crofts JF, Fox R, Ellis D, et al: Observations from 450 shoulder dystocia simulations: lessons for skills training. Obstet Gynecol 112(4):906, 2008

Cunningham FG: The Ritgen maneuver: another sacred cow questioned. Obstet Gynecol 112:210, 2008

de Leeuw JW, de Wit C, Kuijken JP, et al: Mediolateral episiotomy reduces the risk for anal sphincter injury during operative vaginal delivery. BJOG 115:104, 2008

Deneux-Tharaux C, Macfarlane A, Winter C, et al: Policies for manual removal of placenta at vaginal delivery: variations in timing within Europe. BJOG 116(1):119, 2009

Derman RJ, Kodkany BS, Goudar SS, et al: Oral misoprostol in preventing postpartum haemorrhage in resource poor communities: a randomised controlled trial. Lancet 368:1248, 2006

Desbriere R, Blanc J, Le Dû R, et al: Is maternal posturing during labor efficient in preventing persistent occiput posterior position? A randomized controlled trial. Am J Obstet Gynecol 208(1):60.e1, 2013

de Vogel J, van der Leeuw-van Beek A, Gietelink D, et al: The effect of a mediolateral episiotomy during operative vaginal delivery on the risk of developing obstetrical anal sphincter injuries. Am J Obstet Gynecol 206(5):404, 2012

Dolan LM, Hilton P: Obstetric risk factors and pelvic floor dysfunction 20 years after first delivery. Int Urogynecol 21(5):535, 2010

Dombrowski MP, Bottoms SF, Saleh AAA, et al: Third stage of labor: analysis of duration and clinical practice. Am J Obstet Gynecol 172:1279, 1995

Draycott TJ, Crofts JF, Ash JP, et al: Improving neonatal outcome through practical shoulder dystocia training. Obstet Gynecol 112:12, 2008

Duggal N, Mercado C, Daniels K, et al: Antibiotic prophylaxis for prevention of postpartum perineal wound complications: a randomized controlled trial. Obstet Gynecol 111(6):1268, 2008

Dupuis O, Ruimark S, Corinne D, et al: Fetal head position during the second stage of labor: comparison of digital vaginal examination and transabdominal ultrasonographic examination. Eur J Obstet Gynecol Reprod Biol 123(2):193, 2005

Farrell SA, Flowerdew G, Gilmour D, et al: Overlapping compared with end-to-end repair of complete third-degree or fourth-degree obstetric tears: three-year follow-up of a randomized controlled trial. Obstet Gynecol 120(4):803, 2012

Fitzpatrick M, Behan M, O'Connell PR, et al: A randomized clinical trial comparing primary overlap with approximation repair of third-degree obstetric tears. Am J Obstet Gynecol 183:1220, 2000

Fitzpatrick M, McQuillan K, O'Herlihy C: Influence of persistent occiput posterior position on delivery outcome. Obstet Gynecol 98(6):1027, 2001

Food and Drug Administration: Methergine (methylergonovine maleate) tablet and injection. 2012. Available at: http://www.fda.gov/Safety/MedWatch/SafetyInformation/ucm310728.htm. Accessed April 29, 2013

Gardberg M, Laakkonen E, Sälevaara M: Intrapartum sonography and persistent occiput posterior position: a study of 408 deliveries. Obstet Gynecol 91(5 Pt 1):746, 1998

Gardberg M, Stenwall O, Laakkonen E: Recurrent persistent occipito-posterior position in subsequent deliveries. BJOG 111(2):170, 2004

Garrett A, El-Nashar S, Famuyide A: Prediction of third and fourth degree perineal lacerations in primiparas: a case control study. Am J Obstet Gynecol 210:S271, 2014

Geranmayeh M, Rezaei Habibabadi Z, et al: Reducing perineal trauma through perineal massage with Vaseline in second stage of labor. Arch Gynecol Obstet 285(1):77, 2012

Gherman RB, Tramont J, Muffley P, et al: Analysis of McRoberts' maneuver by x-ray pelvimetry. Obstet Gynecol 95:43, 2000

Gjessing H, Backe B, Sahlin Y: Third degree obstetric tears; outcome after primary repair. Acta Obstet Gynecol Scand 77:736, 1998

Glazener C, Elders A, Macarthur C, et al: Childbirth and prolapse: long-term associations with the symptoms and objective measurement of pelvic organ prolapse. BJOG 120(2):161, 2013

Goldaber KG, Wendel PJ, McIntire DD, et al: Postpartum perineal morbidity after fourth-degree perineal repair. Am J Obstet Gynecol 168:489, 1993

Gonik B, Allen R, Sorab J: Objective evaluation of the shoulder dystocia phenomenon: effect of maternal pelvic orientation on force reduction. Obstet Gynecol 74:44, 1989

Gonik B, Stringer CA, Held B: An alternate maneuver for management of shoulder dystocia. Am J Obstet Gynecol 145(7):882, 1983

Goodwin TM, Banks E, Millar LK, et al: Catastrophic shoulder dystocia and emergency symphysiotomy. Am J Obstet Gynecol 177:463, 1997

Grobman WA, Miller D, Burke C, et al: Outcomes associated with introduction of a shoulder dystocia protocol. Am J Obstet Gynecol 205(6):513, 2011

Groenen R, Vos MC, Willekes C, et al: Pregnancy and delivery after mid-urethral sling procedures for stress urinary incontinence: case reports and a review of literature. Int Urogynecol J Pelvic Floor Dysfunct 19(3):441, 2008

Gross SJ, Shime J, Farine D: Shoulder dystocia: predictors and outcome: a five-year review. Am J Obstet Gynecol 156:334, 1987

Groutz A, Hasson J, Wengier A, et al: Third- and fourth-degree perineal tears: prevalence and risk factors in the third millennium. Am J Obstet Gynecol 204(4):347.e1, 2011

Gülmezoglu AM, Lumbiganon P, Landoulsi S, et al: Active management of the third stage of labour with and without controlled cord traction: a randomised, controlled, non-inferiority trial. Lancet 379(9827):1721, 2012

Gungor S, Kurt E, Teksoz E, et al: Oronasopharyngeal suction versus no suction in normal and term infants delivered by elective cesarean section: a prospective randomized controlled trial. Gynecol Obstet Invest 61(1):9, 2006

Gurewitsch ED, Donithan M, Stallings SP, et al: Episiotomy versus fetal manipulation in managing severe shoulder dystocia: a comparison of outcomes. Am J Obstet Gynecol 191(3):911, 2004

Handa VL, Blomquist JL, Knoepp LR, et al: Pelvic floor disorders 5–10 years after vaginal or cesarean childbirth. Obstet Gynecol 118(4):777, 2011

Hartfield VJ: Symphysiotomy for shoulder dystocia. Am J Obstet Gynecol 155:228, 1986

Henry E, Andres RL, Christensen RD: Neonatal outcomes following a tight nuchal cord. J Perinatol 33(3):231, 2013

Hernandez C, Wendel GD: Shoulder dystocia. In Pitkin RM (ed): Clinical Obstetrics and Gynecology, Vol XXXIII. Hagerstown, Lippincott, 1990, p 526

Hibbard LT: Coping with shoulder dystocia. Contemp Ob/Gyn 20:229, 1982

Hirsch E, Haney EI, Gordon TE, et al: Reducing high-order perineal laceration during operative vaginal delivery. Am J Obstet Gynecol 198(6):668.e1, 2008

Inglis SR, Feier N, Chetiyaar JB, et al: Effects of shoulder dystocia training on the incidence of brachial plexus injury. Am J Obstet Gynecol 204(4):322.e1, 2011

Jangö H, Langhoff-Roos J, Rosthoj S, et al: Modifiable risk factors of obstetric anal sphincter injury in primiparous women: a population-based cohort study. Am J Obstet Gynecol 210:59, 2014

Jangö H, Langhoff-Roos J, Rosthøj S, et al: Risk factors of recurrent anal sphincter ruptures: a population-based cohort study. BJOG 119(13):1640, 2012

Jangsten E, Mattsson LÅ, Lyckestam I, et al: A comparison of active management and expectant management of the third stage of labour: a Swedish randomised controlled trial. BJOG 118(3):362, 2011

Jönsson ER, Elfaghi I, Rydhström, et al: Modified Ritgen's maneuver for anal sphincter injury at delivery: a randomized controlled trial. Obstet Gynecol 112:212, 2008

Kariminia A, Chamberlain ME, Keogh J, et al: Randomised controlled trial of effect of hands and knees posturing on incidence of occiput posterior position at birth. 328(7438):490, 2004

Kattwinkel J, Perlman JM, Aziz K, et al: Part 15: neonatal resuscitation: 2010 American Heart Association Guidelines for Cardiopulmonary Resuscitation and Emergency Cardiovascular Care. Circulation 122(18 Suppl 3):S909, 2010

Kettle C, Dowswell T, Ismail KM: Continuous and interrupted suturing techniques for repair of episiotomy or second-degree tears. Cochrane Database Syst Rev 11:CD000947, 2012

Kettle C, Hills RK, Jones P, et al: Continuous versus interrupted perineal repair with standard or rapidly absorbed sutures after spontaneous vaginal birth: a randomized controlled trial. Lancet 359:2217, 2002

Kindberg S, Stehouwer M, Hvidman L, et al: Postpartum perineal repair performed by midwives: a randomized trial comparing two suture techniques leaving the skin unsutured. BJOG 115:472, 2008

Laine K, Pirhonen T, Rolland R, et al: Decreasing the incidence of anal sphincter tears during delivery. Obstet Gynecol 111:1053, 2008

Landy HJ, Laughon SK, Bailit JL, et al: Characteristics associated with severe perineal and cervical lacerations during vaginal delivery. Obstet Gynecol 117(3):627, 2011

Larsson P, Platz-Christensen J, Bergman B, et al: Advantage or disadvantage of episiotomy compared with spontaneous perineal laceration. Gynecol Obstet Invest 31:213, 1991

Le Ray C, Carayol M, Jaquemin S, et al: Is epidural analgesia a risk factor for occiput posterior or transverse positions during labour? Eur J Obstet Gynecol Reprod Biol 123(1):22, 2005

Le Ray C, Serres P, Schmitz T, et al: Manual rotation in occiput posterior or transverse positions: risk factors and consequences on the cesarean delivery rate. Obstet Gynecol 110(4):873, 2007

Lerner H, Durlacher K, Smith S, et al: Relationship between head-to-body delivery interval in shoulder dystocia and neonatal depression. Obstet Gynecol 118(2 Pt 1):318, 2011

Liabsuetrakul T, Choobun T, Peeyananjarassri K, et al: Prophylactic use of ergot alkaloids in the third stage of labour. Cochrane Database Syst Rev 2:CD005456, 2007

Lieberman E, Davidson K, Lee-Parritz A, et al: Changes in fetal position during labor and their association with epidural analgesia. Obstet Gynecol 105 (5 Pt 1):974, 2005

Lumbiganon P, Hofmeyr J, Gülmezoglu AM, et al: Misoprostol dose-related shivering and pyrexia in the third stage of labour. WHO Collaborative Trial of Misoprostol in the Management of the Third Stage of Labour. Br J Obstet Gynaecol 106(4):304, 1999

MacKenzie IZ, Shah M, Lean K, et al: Management of shoulder dystocia: trends in incidence and maternal and neonatal morbidity. Obstet Gynecol 110:1059, 2007

Mayerhofer K, Bodner-Adler B, Bodner K, et al: Traditional care of the perineum during birth: a prospective, randomized, multicenter study of 1,076 women. J Reprod Med 47:477, 2002

McCandlish R, Bowler U, Van Asten H, et al: A randomised controlled trial of care of the perineum during second stage of normal labour. Br J Obstet Gynaecol 105(12):1262, 1998

McDonald SJ, Middleton P: Effect of timing of umbilical cord clamping of term infants on maternal and neonatal outcomes. Cochrane Database Syst Rev 16:CD004074, 2008

Mehta SH, Blackwell SC, Bujold E, et al: What factors are associated with neonatal injury following shoulder dystocia? J Perinatol 26(2):85, 2006

Mehta SH, Blackwell SC, Chadha R, et al: Shoulder dystocia and the next delivery: outcomes and management. J Matern Fetal Neonatal Med 20(10):729, 2007

Mehta SH, Bujold E, Blackwell SC, et al: Is abnormal labor associated with shoulder dystocia in nulliparous women? Am J Obstet Gynecol 190(6):1604, 2004

Mei-dan E, Walfisch A, Raz I, et al: Perineal massage during pregnancy: a prospective controlled trial. Isr Med Assoc J 10(7):499, 2008

Melamed N, Gavish O, Eisner M, et al: Third- and fourth-degree perineal tears—incidence and risk factors. J Matern Fetal Neonatal Med 26(7):660, 2013

Minassian VA, Jazayeri A, Prien SD, et al: Randomized trial of lidocaine ointment versus placebo for the treatment of postpartum perineal pain. Obstet Gynecol 100:1239, 2002

Mobeen N, Durocher J, Zuberi N, et al: Administration of misoprostol by trained traditional birth attendants to prevent postpartum haemorrhage in homebirths in Pakistan: a randomised placebo-controlled trial. BJOG 118(3):353, 2011

Moore HM, Reed SD, Batra M, et al: Risk factors for recurrent shoulder dystocia, Washington state, 1987–2004. Am J Obstet Gynecol 198:e16, 2008

Moragianni VA, Hacker MR, Craparo FJ: The impact of length of second stage of labor on shoulder dystocia outcomes: a retrospective cohort study. J Perinat Med 40(4):463, 2012

Mornar SJ, Perlow JH: Blunt suture needle use in laceration and episiotomy repair at vaginal delivery. Am J Obstet Gynecol 198:e14, 2008

Mulder FE, Schoffelmeer MA, Hakvoort RA, et al: Risk factors for postpartum urinary retention: a systematic review and meta-analysis. BJOG 119(12):1440, 2012

Nager CW, Helliwell JP: Episiotomy increases perineal laceration length in primiparous women. Am J Obstet Gynecol 185:444, 2001

National Institutes of Health: NIH state-of-the-science conference: cesarean delivery on maternal request. 2006. Available at: http://consensus.nih.gov/2006/cesareanstatement.htm. Accessed April 23, 2013

Nocon JJ, McKenzie DK, Thomas LJ, et al: Shoulder dystocia: an analysis of risks and obstetric maneuvers. Am J Obstet Gynecol 168:1732, 1993

Nour NM, Michels KB, Bryant AE: Defibulation to treat female genital cutting: effect on symptoms and sexual function. Obstet Gynecol 108:55, 2006

Novartis: Syntometrime (synthetic oxytocin/ergometrine maleate). 2012. Available at: http://www.google.com/search?q=novartis+syntometrine+prescribing+information&rls=com.microsoft:en-us:IE-SearchBox&ie=UTF-8&oe=UTF-8&sourceid = ie7&rlz=1I7ADRA_enUS425. Accessed April 29, 2013

Oliphant SS, Jones KA, Wang L, et al: Trends over time with commonly performed obstetric and gynecologic inpatient procedures. Obstet Gynecol 116(4):926, 2010

Ouzounian JG, Korst LM, Miller DA, et al: Brachial plexus palsy and shoulder dystocia: obstetric risk factors remain elusive. Am J Perinatol 30(4):303, 2013

Overland EA, Spydslaug A, Nielsen CS, et al: Risk of shoulder dystocia in second delivery: does a history of shoulder dystocia matter? Am J Obstet Gynecol 200(5):506.e1, 2009

Overland EA, Vatten LJ, Eskild A: Risk of shoulder dystocia: associations with parity and offspring birthweight. A population study of 1 914 544 deliveries. Acta Obstet Gynecol Scand 91(4):483, 2012

Paris AE, Greenberg JA, Ecker JL, et al: Is an episiotomy necessary with a shoulder dystocia? Am J Obstet Gynecol 205(3):217.e1, 2011

Poen AC, Felt-Bersma RJ, Strijers RL, et al: Third-degree obstetric perineal tear: long-term clinical and functional results after primary repair. Br J Surg 85:1433, 1998

Pollard ME, Morrisroe S, Anger JT: Outcomes of pregnancy following surgery for stress urinary incontinence: a systematic review. J Urol 187(6):1966, 2012

Ponkey SE, Cohen AP, Heffner LJ, et al: Persistent fetal occiput posterior position: obstetric outcomes. Obstet Gynecol 101(5 Pt 1):915, 2003

Pradhan A, Tincello DG, Kearney R: Childbirth after pelvic floor surgery: analysis of Hospital Episode Statistics in England, 2002–2008. BJOG 120(2):200, 2013

Prendiville WJ, Harding JE, Elbourne DR, et al: The Bristol third stage trial: active versus physiological management of third stage of labour. Br Med J 297:1295, 1988

Rabe H, Diaz-Rossello JL, Duley L, et al: Effect of timing of umbilical cord clamping and other strategies to influence placental transfusion at preterm birth on maternal and infant outcomes. Cochrane Database Syst Rev 8:CD003248, 2012

Rådestad I, Olsson A, Nissen E, et al: Tears in the vagina, perineum, sphincter ani, and rectum and first sexual intercourse after childbirth: a nationwide follow-up. Birth 35:98, 2008

Rahman J, Bhattee G, Rahman MS: Shoulder dystocia in a 16-year experience in a teaching hospital. J Reprod Med 54(6):378, 2009

Raju TN: Timing of umbilical cord clamping after birth for optimizing placental transfusion. Curr Opin Pediatr 25(2):180, 2013

Ritgen G: Concerning his method for protection of the perineum. Monatschrift für Geburtskunde 6:21, 1855. See English translation, Wynn RM: Am J Obstet Gynecol 93:421, 1965

Roach MK, Abramovici A, Tita AT: Dose and duration of oxytocin to prevent postpartum hemorrhage: a review. Am J Perinatol 30(7):523, 2013

Roberts PL, Coller JA, Schoetz DJ, et al: Manometric assessment of patients with obstetric injuries and fecal incontinence. Dis Colon Rectum 33:16, 1990

Rodriguez A, Arenas EA, Osorio AL, et al: Selective vs routine midline episiotomy for the prevention of third- or fourth-degree lacerations in nulliparous women. Am J Obstet Gynecol 198:285.e1, 2008

Rortveit G, Daltveit AK, Hannestad YS, et al: Urinary incontinence after vaginal delivery or cesarean section. N Engl J Med 348:9000, 2003

Rortveit G, Hannestad YS, Daltveit AK, et al: Age- and type-dependent effects of parity on urinary incontinence: the Norwegian EPINCONT study. Obstet Gynecol 98(6):1004, 2001

Rouse DJ, Owen J: Prophylactic cesarean delivery for fetal macrosomia diagnosed by means of ultrasonography—a Faustian bargain? Am J Obstet Gynecol 181:332, 1999

Rouzi AA, Al-Sibiani SA, Al-Mansouri NM, et al: Defibulation during vaginal delivery for women with type III female genital mutilation. Obstet Gynecol 120(1):98, 2012

Rubin A: Management of shoulder dystocia. JAMA 189:835, 1964

Sandberg EC: Shoulder dystocia: associated with versus caused by the Zavanelli maneuver. Am J Obstet Gynecol 197(1):115, 2007

Sandberg EC: The Zavanelli maneuver: 12 years of recorded experience. Obstet Gynecol 93:312, 1999

Sandberg EC: The Zavanelli maneuver: a potentially revolutionary method for the resolution of shoulder dystocia. Am J Obstet Gynecol 152:479, 1985

Sanders J, Campbell R, Peters TJ: Effectiveness of pain relief during perineal suturing. Br J Obstet Gynaecol 109:1066, 2002

Sanders-Bush E, Hazelwood L: 5-Hydroxytryptamine (serotonin) and dopamine. In Brunton LL, Chabner BA, Knollmann BC (eds): Goodman and Gilman's The Pharmacological Basis of Therapeutics, 12th ed. New York, McGraw-Hill, 2011

Schramm M: Impacted shoulders—a personal experience. Aust N Z J Obstet Gynaecol 23:28, 1983

Schwartz RH, Jones RWA: Transplacental hyponatremia due to oxytocin. Br Med J 1:152, 1978

Secher NJ, Arnso P, Wallin L: Haemodynamic effects of oxytocin (Syntocinon) and methylergometrine (Methergin) on the systemic and pulmonary circulations of pregnant anaesthetized women. Acta Obstet Gynecol Scand 57:97, 1978

Sen K, Sakamoto H, Nakabayashi Y, et al: Management of the occiput posterior presentation: a single institute experience. J Obstet Gynaecol Res 39(1):160, 2013

Senécal J, Xiong X, Fraser WD, et al: Effect of fetal position on second-stage duration and labor outcome. Obstet Gynecol 105(4):763, 2005

Shaffer BL, Cheng YW, Vargas JE, et al: Manual rotation of the fetal occiput: predictors of success and delivery. Am J Obstet Gynecol 194(5):e7, 2006

Shaffer BL, Cheng YW, Vargas JE, et al: Manual rotation to reduce caesarean delivery in persistent occiput posterior or transverse position. J Matern Fetal Neonatal Med 24(1):65, 2011

Signorello LB, Harlow BL, Chekos AK, et al: Midline episiotomy and anal incontinence: retrospective cohort study. Br Med J 320:86, 2000

Signorello LB, Harlow BL, Chekos AK, et al: Postpartum sexual functioning and its relationship to perineal trauma: a retrospective cohort study of primiparous women. Am J Obstet Gynecol 184:881, 2001

Soltani H, Hutchon DR, Poulose TA: Timing of prophylactic uterotonics for the third stage of labour after vaginal birth. Cochrane Database Syst Rev 8:CD006173, 2010

Sommers R, Stonestreet BS, Oh W, et al: Hemodynamic effects of delayed cord clamping in premature infants. Pediatrics 129(3):e667, 2012

Souka AP, Haritos T, Basayiannis K, et al: Intrapartum ultrasound for the examination of the fetal head position in normal and obstructed labor. J Matern Fetal Neonatal Med 13(1):59, 2003

Spong CY, Beall M, Rodrigues D, et al: An objective definition of shoulder dystocia: prolonged head-to-body delivery intervals and/or the use of ancillary obstetric maneuvers. Obstet Gynecol 86:433, 1995

Stamp G, Kruzins G, Crowther C: Perineal massage in labour and prevention of perineal trauma: randomised controlled trial. BMJ 322(7297):1277, 2001

Stock L, Basham E, Gossett DR, et al: Factors associated with wound complications in women with obstetric anal sphincter injuries (OASIS). Am J Obstet Gynecol 208(4):327.e1, 2013

Su LL, Chong YS, Samuel M: Carbetocin for preventing postpartum haemorrhage. Cochrane Database Syst Rev 4:CD005457, 2012

Svanström MC, Biber B, Hanes M, et al: Signs of myocardial ischaemia after injection of oxytocin: a randomized double-blind comparison of oxytocin and methylergometrine during caesarean section. Br J Anaesth 100:683, 2008

Tita AT, Szychowski JM, Rouse DJ, et al: Higher-dose oxytocin and hemorrhage after vaginal delivery: a randomized controlled trial. Obstet Gynecol 119(2 Pt 1):293, 2012

Tunçalp Ö, Hofmeyr GJ, Gülmezoglu AM: Prostaglandins for preventing postpartum haemorrhage. Cochrane Database Syst Rev 8:CD000494, 2012

Upadhyay A, Gothwal S, Parihar R, et al: Effect of umbilical cord milking in term and near term infants: randomized control trial. Am J Obstet Gynecol 208(2):120.e1, 2013

Valenzuela P, Saiz Puente MS, Valero JL, et al: Continuous versus interrupted sutures for repair of episiotomy or second-degree perineal tears: a randomised controlled trial. BJOG 116(3):436, 2009

Walraven G, Blum J, Dampha Y, et al: Misoprostol in the management of the third stage of labour in the home delivery setting in rural Gambia: a randomised controlled trial. BJOG 112:1277, 2005

Walsh JM, Kandamany N, Ni Shuibhne N, et al: Neonatal brachial plexus injury: comparison of incidence and antecedents between 2 decades. Am J Obstet Gynecol 204(4):324.e1, 2011

Whalley PJ, Pritchard JA: Oxytocin and water intoxication. JAMA 186:601, 1963

Williams MK, Chames MC: Risk factors for the breakdown of perineal laceration repair after vaginal delivery. Am J Obstet Gynecol 195:755, 2006

Woods CE: A principle of physics is applicable to shoulder delivery. Am J Obstet Gynecol 45:796, 1943

World Health Organization: Female genital mutilation: a joint WHO/UNICEF/UNFPA statement. Geneva: World Health Organization, 1997

World Health Organization: Female genital mutilation and obstetric outcome: WHO collaborative prospective study in six African countries. Lancet 367:1835, 2006

World Health Organization: WHO Recommendations for the Prevention and Treatment of Postpartum Haemorrhage. Geneva, World Health Organization, 2012, p 4

Wuest S, Raio L, Wyssmueller D, et al: Effects of female genital mutilation on birth outcomes in Switzerland. BJOG 116(9):1204, 2009

Yao AC, Lind J: Placental transfusion. Am J Dis Child 127:128, 1974

Zahalka N, Sadan O, Malinger G, et al: Comparison of transvaginal sonography with digital examination and transabdominal sonography for the determination of fetal head position in the second stage of labor. Am J Obstet Gynecol 193:381, 2005

CHAPTER 28

Breech Delivery

Near term, the fetus typically turns spontaneously to a cephalic presentation as the increasing bulk of the buttocks seeks the more spacious fundus. However, if the fetal buttocks or legs enter the pelvis before the head, the presentation is breech. This fetal lie is more common remote from term as each fetal pole is of similar bulk earlier in pregnancy (Fig. 28-1). That said, breech presentation persists at term in 3 to 4 percent of singleton deliveries. The annual rate of breech presentation at delivery in nearly 270,000 singleton newborns at Parkland Hospital has varied from only 3.3 to 3.9 percent during the past 30 years.

Current obstetrical thinking regarding vaginal delivery of the breech fetus has been tremendously influenced by results reported from the Term Breech Trial Collaborative Group (Hannah, 2000). This trial included 1041 women randomly assigned to planned cesarean and 1042 to planned vaginal delivery. In the planned vaginal delivery group, 57 percent were actually delivered vaginally. Planned cesarean delivery was associated with a lower risk of perinatal mortality compared with planned vaginal delivery—3 per 1000 versus 13 per 1000. Cesarean delivery was also associated with a lower risk of "serious" neonatal morbidity—1.4 versus 3.8 percent.

The reaction to these findings by the American College of Obstetricians and Gynecologists (2001) resulted in an abrupt decline in the rate of attempted vaginal breech deliveries. Since those times, however, a more moderate plan was reached for management of breech delivery.

Critics of the Term Breech Trial emphasized that most of the outcomes included in the "serious" neonatal morbidity composite did not actually portend long-term disability. Moreover, as data from countries with low perinatal mortality rates became available, they showed infrequent perinatal deaths, and rates did not differ significantly between mode-of-delivery groups. Also, only nulliparas were included in the Term Breech Trial, and fewer than 10 percent underwent radiological pelvimetry. And last, the 2-year outcomes for children born during the original multicenter trial showed that planned cesarean delivery was not associated with a reduction in the rate of death or developmental delay (Whyte, 2004). Some of the large studies reporting the safety and risks of vaginal delivery for the term breech singleton are discussed further on page 561.

These findings prompted the American College of Obstetricians and Gynecologists (2012b) to modify its stance on breech presentation, and it currently recommends that "the decision regarding the mode of delivery should depend on the experience of the health care provider" and that "planned vaginal delivery of a term singleton breech fetus may be reasonable under hospital-specific protocol guidelines." This has been echoed by

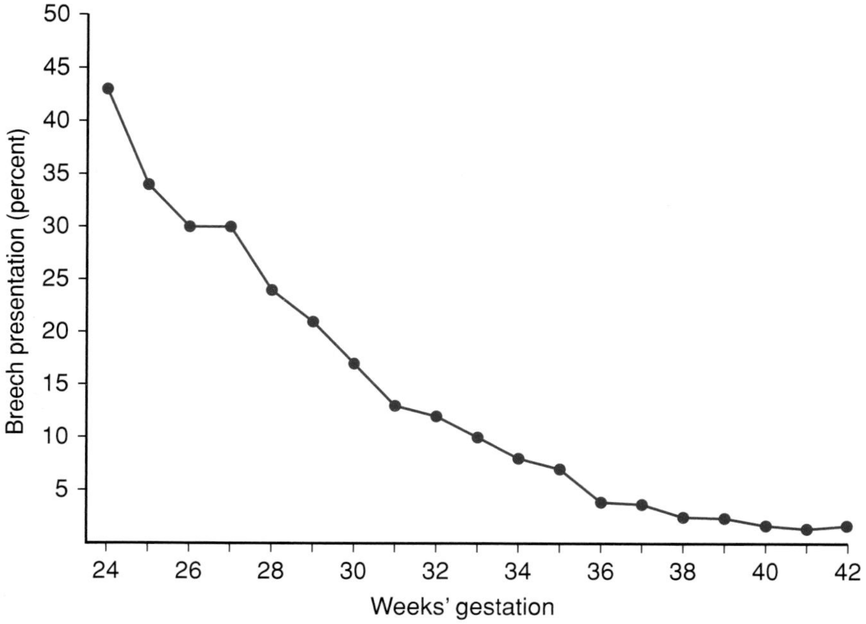

FIGURE 28-1 Prevalence of breech presentation by gestational age at delivery in 58,842 singleton pregnancies at the University of Alabama at Birmingham Hospitals 1991 to 2006. (Data courtesy of Dr. John Hauth and Ms. Sue Cliver.)

other obstetrical organizations (Carbonne, 2001; Kotaska, 2009; Royal College of Obstetricians and Gynaecologists, 2009).

CLASSIFICATION OF BREECH PRESENTATIONS

The varying relations between the lower extremities and buttocks of breech fetuses form the categories of frank, complete, and incomplete breech presentations. With a frank breech presentation, the lower extremities are flexed at the hips and extended at the knees, and thus the feet lie in close proximity to the head (Fig. 28-2). A complete breech differs in that one or both knees are flexed (Fig. 28-3). With incomplete breech presentation, one or both hips are not flexed, and one or both feet or knees lie below the breech, such that a foot or knee is lowermost in the birth canal (Fig. 28-4). A footling breech is an incomplete breech with one or both feet below the breech.

In perhaps 5 percent of term breech fetuses, the head may be in extreme hyperextension. These presentations have been referred to as the *stargazer fetus*, and in Britain as the *flying foetus*. With such hyperextension, vaginal delivery may result in injury to the cervical spinal cord. Thus, if present after labor has begun, this is an indication for cesarean delivery (Svenningsen, 1985).

DIAGNOSIS

Risk Factors

Understanding the clinical settings that predispose to breech presentation can aid early recognition. Other than early gestational age, risk factors include abnormal amnionic fluid

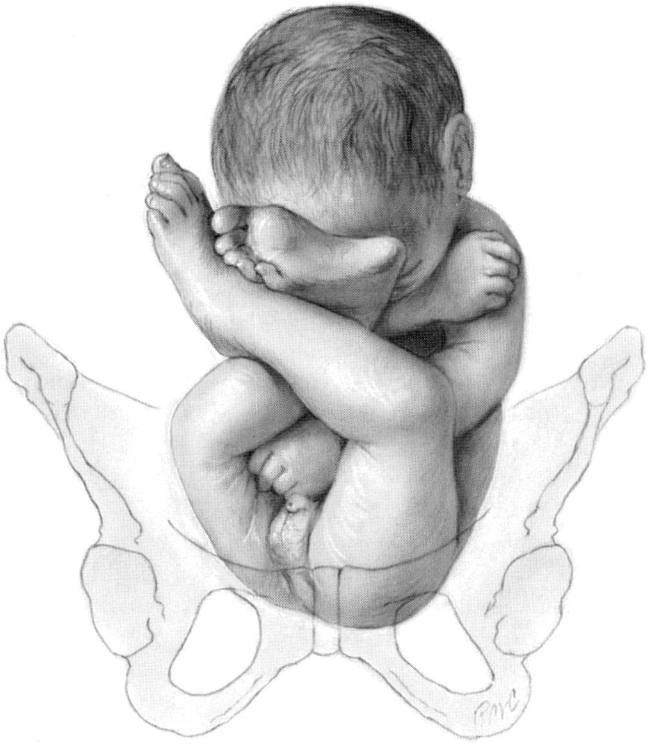

FIGURE 28-2 Frank breech presentation.

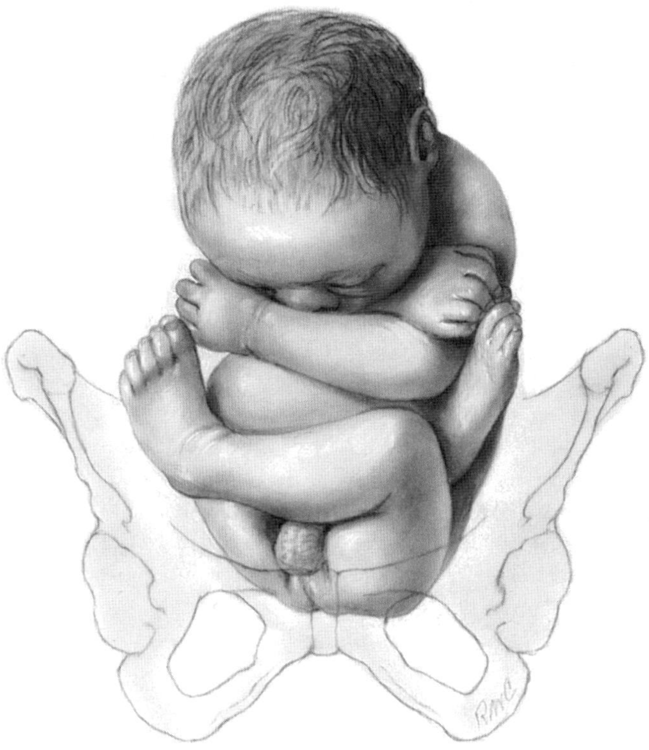

FIGURE 28-3 Complete breech presentation.

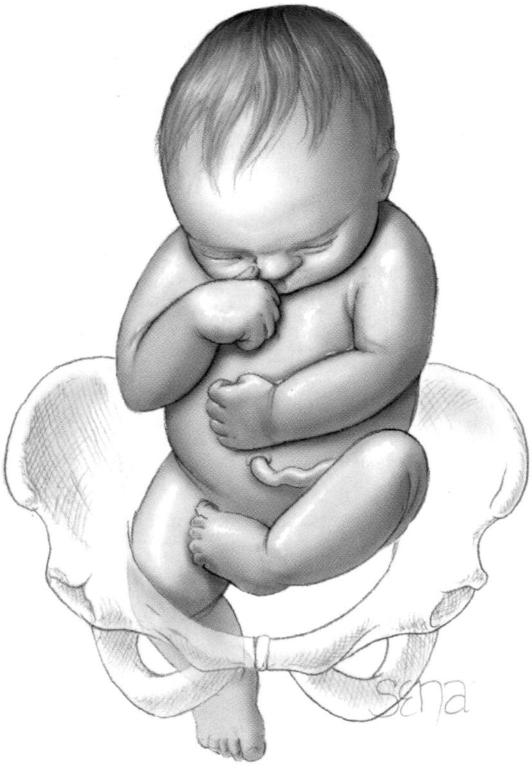

FIGURE 28-4 Incomplete breech presentation.

volume, multifetal gestation, hydrocephaly, anencephaly, uterine anomalies, placenta previa, fundal placental implantation, pelvic tumors, high parity with uterine relaxation, and prior breech delivery. Specifically, following one breech delivery, the recurrence rate for a second pregnancy with breech presentation was nearly 10 percent, and that for a subsequent third pregnancy was 27 percent (Ford, 2010). Prior cesarean delivery has also been described by some to increase twofold the incidence of breech presentation (Kalogiannidis, 2010; Vendittelli, 2008). Last, smoking may be a modifiable cause of this presentation (Rayl, 1996; Witkop, 2008).

Examination

Leopold maneuvers to ascertain fetal presentation are discussed in Chapter 22 (p. 438). With the first maneuver, the hard, round, ballottable fetal head may be found to occupy the fundus. The second maneuver indicates the back to be on one side of the abdomen and the small parts on the other. With the third maneuver, if not engaged, the breech is movable above the pelvic inlet. After engagement, the fourth maneuver shows the firm breech to be beneath the symphysis. The accuracy of this palpation varies (Lydon-Rochelle, 1993; Nassar, 2006). Thus, with suspected breech presentation—or any presentation other than cephalic—sonographic evaluation is indicated.

With a frank breech during vaginal examination, no feet are appreciated, but the fetal ischial tuberosities, sacrum, and anus are usually palpable. After further fetal descent, the external genitalia may also be distinguished. Especially when labor is prolonged, the fetal buttocks may become markedly swollen, rendering differentiation of a face and breech difficult. In some cases, the anus may be mistaken for the mouth and the ischial tuberosities for the malar eminences. With careful examination, however, the finger encounters muscular resistance with the anus, whereas the firmer, less yielding jaws are felt through the mouth. The finger, upon removal from the anus, may be stained with meconium. The mouth and malar eminences form a triangular shape, whereas the ischial tuberosities and anus lie in a straight line. With a complete breech, the feet may be felt alongside the buttocks. In footling presentations, one or both feet are inferior to the buttocks.

The fetal sacrum and its spinous processes are palpated also to establish position. As with cephalic presentations described in Chapter 22 (p. 434), fetal positions are designated as left sacrum anterior (LSA), right sacrum anterior (RSA), left sacrum posterior (LSP), right sacrum posterior (RSP), or sacrum transverse (ST) to reflect the relations of the fetal sacrum to the maternal pelvis.

ROUTE OF DELIVERY

Multiple factors aid determination of the best delivery route for a given mother-fetus pair. These include fetal characteristics, pelvic dimensions, coexistent pregnancy complications, operator experience, patient preference, and hospital capabilities.

Term and Preterm Breech Fetus

Although sharing the similarity of presentation, preterm breech fetuses have distinct risks related to immaturity compared with their term breech counterparts. Accordingly, separation of term and preterm breech fetuses for discussion allows a more accurate evaluation of information.

Term Breech Fetus

Data regarding superior perinatal outcomes for planned cesarean delivery of a singleton term breech are conflicting. As described earlier (p. 558), the Term Breech Trial reported lower neonatal morbidity and mortality rates with planned cesarean delivery for breech presentation. Additional data favoring cesarean delivery comes from the World Health Organization (Lumbiganon, 2010). From their evaluation of more than 100,000 deliveries from nine participating Asian countries, they reported improved perinatal outcomes associated with planned cesarean compared with planned vaginal delivery of the term breech fetus. Other studies have evaluated neonatal outcome with cesarean delivery and also found lowered neonatal morbidity and mortality rates (Hartnack Tharin, 2011; Mailàth-Pokorny, 2009; Rietberg, 2005; Swedish Collaborative Breech Study Group, 2005).

In contrast, the *Presentation et Mode d'Accouchement*—which translates as presentation and mode of delivery (PREMODA)—study showed no differences in corrected neonatal mortality rates and neonatal outcomes according to delivery mode (Goffinet, 2006). This French prospective observational study involved more than 8000 women with term breech singletons. Strict criteria were used to select 2526 of these for planned vaginal delivery, and 71 percent of that group were delivered vaginally. Similarly, data from the Lille Breech Study Group in France showed no excessive morbidity in term breech singletons delivered vaginally provided strict fetal biometric and maternal pelvimetry parameters were applied (Michel, 2011). Other smaller studies also support these findings as long as guidelines are part of the selection process (Alarab, 2004; Albrechtsen, 1997; Giuliani, 2002; Toivonen, 2012). Long-term evidence in support of vaginal breech delivery comes from Eide and associates (2005). These researchers analyzed intelligence testing scores of more than 8000 men delivered breech and found no differences in intellectual performance in those delivered vaginally or by cesarean.

Despite evidence on both sides of the debate, at least in this country, rates of planned vaginal delivery attempts continue to decline (Hehir, 2012). And as predicted, the number of skilled operators able to safely select and vaginally deliver breech fetuses continues to dwindle (Chinnock, 2007). Moreover, obvious medicolegal concerns makes physician training in such deliveries difficult. In response, some institutions have developed birth simulators to improve resident competence in vaginal breech delivery (Deering, 2006; Maslovitz, 2007).

Preterm Breech Fetus

Although there are no randomized studies regarding delivery of the preterm breech fetus, planned cesarean delivery appears to confer a survival advantage. Reddy and associates (2012) reported data from an National Institutes of Health retrospective multicenter cohort study involving 208,695 deliveries between 24 and 32 weeks' gestation. For breech fetuses within these gestational ages, attempting vaginal delivery yielded a low completion rate, and those completed were associated with higher neonatal mortality rates compared with planned cesarean delivery. Other studies have reported similar findings (Demirci, 2012; Lee, 1998; Muhuri, 2006). There are, however, a few smaller studies that describe no improved survival rate in fetuses at earlier gestational ages—24 to 29 weeks—delivered by planned cesarean (Kayem, 2008; Stohl, 2011).

There are limited data regarding any preferable delivery route for preterm breech fetuses between 32 and 37 weeks. In these cases, fetal weight rather than gestational age is likely most important. The Maternal Fetal Medicine Committee of the Society of Obstetricians and Gynaecologists of Canada (SOGC) recommend that vaginal breech delivery is reasonable when the estimated fetal weight is > 2500 g (Kotaska, 2009).

Delivery Complications

Maternal Morbidity and Mortality

Increased rates of maternal and perinatal morbidity can be anticipated with breech presentations. For the mother, with either cesarean or vaginal delivery, genital tract laceration can be problematic. With cesarean delivery, added stretching of the lower uterine segment by forceps or by a poorly molded fetal head can extend hysterotomy incisions. With vaginal delivery, especially with a thinned lower uterine segment, delivery of the aftercoming head through an incompletely dilated cervix or application of forceps may cause vaginal wall or cervical lacerations. Manipulations may also extend an episiotomy, create deep perineal tears, and increase infection risks. Anesthesia sufficient to induce appreciable uterine relaxation during vaginal delivery may cause uterine atony and in turn, postpartum hemorrhage. Death is a rare complication, but rates appear higher in those with planned cesarean delivery for breech presentation—a case fatality rate of 0.47 maternal deaths per 1000 births (Schutte, 2007). Last, as described in Chapter 30 (p. 588), the risks associated with vaginal breech delivery are balanced against general cesarean delivery risks, which include those associated with vaginal birth after cesarean (VBAC) or those with repeated cesarean hysterotomy.

Perinatal Morbidity and Mortality

Preterm delivery is a common association, and there is an increased rate of congenital anomalies. In addition, birth trauma, although uncommon, can contribute to death of the breech fetus. Importantly, these are seen both with vaginal as well as cesarean delivery. Some of the more common injuries are fractures of the humerus, clavicle, and femur (Canpolat, 2010; Matsubara, 2008). In some cases, traction may separate scapular, humeral, or femoral epiphyses.

Rare traumatic injuries may involve bony or soft tissues. Neonatal perineal tears have been reported from fetal scalp electrodes (Freud, 1993). Upper extremity paralysis—Erb or Duchenne—may follow brachial plexus stretching (Al-Qattan, 2010). When the fetus is extracted through a contracted pelvis, spoon-shaped depressions or actual fractures of the skull may result. The spinal cord may be injured or vertebra fractured if great force is employed (Vialle, 2007). Hematomas of the sternocleidomastoid muscles occasionally develop after delivery, although they usually disappear spontaneously. Last, testicular injury may follow breech delivery (Mathews, 1999). These are discussed in further detail in Chapter 33 (p. 645).

Compared with cephalic presentation, umbilical cord prolapse is more frequent with breech fetuses. Huang and coworkers (2012) analyzed 40 cases of prolapse and reported that half were associated with malpresentation or vaginal delivery of a second twin.

Some perinatal outcomes may be inherent to the breech position rather than delivery. For example, development of hip dysplasia is more common in breech compared with cephalic presentation and is unaffected by delivery mode (de Hundt, 2012; Fox, 2010; Ortiz-Neira, 2012).

Imaging Techniques

In many fetuses—especially those that are preterm—the breech is smaller than the aftercoming head. Moreover, unlike cephalic presentations, the head of a breech-presenting fetus does not undergo appreciable molding during labor. Thus, to avoid head entrapment following delivery of the breech, pelvic dimensions should be assessed before vaginal delivery. In addition, fetal size, type of breech, and degree of neck flexion or extension should be identified. To evaluate these, several imaging techniques can be used.

Sonography

In most cases, sonographic fetal evaluation will have been performed as part of prenatal care. If not, gross fetal abnormalities, such as hydrocephaly or anencephaly, can be rapidly ascertained with sonography. This will identify many fetuses not suitable for vaginal delivery and will help to ensure that a cesarean delivery is not performed under emergency conditions for an anomalous fetus with no chance of survival.

Head flexion can usually also be determined sonographically, and for vaginal delivery, the fetal head should not be extended (Fontenot, 1997; Rojansky, 1994). If imaging is uncertain, then simple two-view radiography of the abdomen is useful to define head inclination. The sonographic accuracy of fetal weight estimation does not appear limited by breech presentation (McNamara, 2012). Although variable, many protocols use fetal weights < 2500 g and > 3800 to 4000 g or evidence of growth restriction as exclusion criteria for planned vaginal delivery (Azria, 2012; Kotaska, 2009). Similarly, a biparietal diameter (BPD) > 90 to 100 mm is often considered exclusionary (Giuliani, 2002; Roman, 2008).

TABLE 28-1. Factors Favoring Cesarean Delivery of the Breech Fetus

Lack of operator experience
Patient request for cesarean delivery
Large fetus: > 3800 to 4000 g
Apparently healthy and viable preterm fetus either with active labor or with indicated delivery
Severe fetal-growth restriction
Fetal anomaly incompatible with vaginal delivery
Prior perinatal death or neonatal birth trauma
Incomplete or footling breech presentation
Hyperextended head
Pelvic contraction or unfavorable pelvic shape determined clinically or with pelvimetry
Prior cesarean delivery

Pelvimetry

This assessment of the bony pelvis before vaginal delivery may be completed with one-view computed tomography (CT), magnetic resonance imaging, or plain film radiographs. Although there are no comparative data among these modalities for pelvimetry, computed tomography is favored due to its accuracy, low radiation dose, and widespread availability (Thomas, 1998). At Parkland Hospital, we use CT pelvimetry when possible to assess the critical dimensions of the pelvis (Chap. 2, p. 32). Although variable, some suggest specific measurements to permit a planned vaginal delivery: inlet anteroposterior diameter ≥ 105 mm; inlet transverse diameter ≥ 120 mm; and midpelvic interspinous diameter ≥ 100 mm (Azria, 2012; Vendittelli, 2006). Others use maternal-fetal biometry correlation. Appropriate values include: the sum of the inlet obstetrical conjugate minus the fetal BPD is ≥ 15 mm; the inlet transverse diameter minus the BPD is ≥ 25 mm; and the midpelvis interspinous diameter minus the BPD is ≥ 0 mm (Michel, 2011).

Decision-Making Summary

As outlined by the American College of Obstetricians and Gynecologists (2012b), risks versus benefits are weighed and discussed with the patient. If possible, this is preferably done before admission. A diligent search is made for any other complications, actual or anticipated, that might warrant cesarean delivery. Common circumstances are listed in Table 28-1. For a favorable outcome with any breech delivery, at the very minimum, the birth canal must be sufficiently large to allow passage of the fetus without trauma. The cervix must be fully dilated, and if not, then a cesarean delivery nearly always is the more appropriate method of delivery if suspected fetal compromise develops.

MANAGEMENT OF LABOR AND DELIVERY

Methods of Vaginal Delivery

There are important fundamental differences between labor and delivery in cephalic and breech presentations. With a cephalic presentation, once the head is delivered, the rest of the body typically follows without difficulty. With a breech, however, successively larger and less compressible parts are born. Spontaneous complete expulsion of the fetus that presents as a breech, as subsequently described, is seldom accomplished successfully. Therefore, as a rule, vaginal delivery requires skilled participation for a favorable outcome.

There are three general methods of breech delivery through the vagina:

1. Spontaneous breech delivery. The fetus is expelled entirely spontaneously without any traction or manipulation other than support of the newborn.
2. Partial breech extraction. The fetus is delivered spontaneously as far as the umbilicus, but the remainder of the body is extracted or delivered with operator traction and assisted maneuvers, with or without maternal expulsive efforts.
3. Total breech extraction. The entire body of the fetus is extracted by the obstetrician.

Labor Induction and Augmentation

Induction or augmentation of labor in women with a breech presentation is controversial, and data are limited. Marzouk and associates (2011) found similar perinatal neonatal outcomes with spontaneous labor or with cervical preparation and induced labor. In many studies, improved rates of successful vaginal delivery and neonatal outcome are associated with orderly labor progression. Thus, some protocols avoid augmentation, whereas others recommend it only for hypotonic contractions (Alarab, 2004; Kotaska, 2009). In women with a viable fetus, at Parkland Hospital, we attempt amniotomy induction but prefer cesarean delivery instead of oxytocin induction or augmentation.

Management of Labor

On arrival, rapid assessment should be made to establish the status of the membranes, labor, and fetal condition. Surveillance of fetal heart rate and uterine contractions begins at admission, and immediate recruitment of necessary staff should include:

(1) an obstetrician skilled in the art of breech extraction, (2) an associate to assist with the delivery, (3) anesthesia personnel who can ensure adequate analgesia or anesthesia when needed, and (4) an individual trained in newborn resuscitation.

For the mother, an intravenous catheter is inserted, and crystalloid infusion begun. Emergency induction of anesthesia or maternal resuscitation following hemorrhage from lacerations or from uterine atony are but two of many reasons that may require immediate intravenous access.

Assessment of cervical dilatation and effacement and the station of the presenting part is essential for planning the route of delivery. If labor is too far advanced, there may not be sufficient time to obtain pelvimetry. This alone, however, should not force the decision for cesarean delivery. Commonly, satisfactory progress in labor is the best indicator of pelvic adequacy (Biswas, 1993; Nwosu, 1993). Sonographic fetal biometry and assessment of head flexion are completed. And if not performed as part of earlier prenatal care, fetal anatomy is evaluated. Ultimately, the choice of abdominal or vaginal delivery is based on factors discussed earlier and listed in Table 28-1.

For managing labor and delivery of a breech fetus, additional help is required. One-on-one nursing is ideal during labor because of the risk of cord prolapse or occlusion, and physicians must be readily available for such emergencies. Guidelines for monitoring the high-risk fetus are applied as discussed in Chapter 24 (p. 497). During the first stage of labor, the fetal heart rate is recorded at least every 15 minutes. Most clinicians prefer continuous electronic monitoring. If a nonreassuring fetal heart rate pattern develops, then a decision must be made regarding the necessity of cesarean delivery.

When membranes are ruptured, either spontaneously or artificially, the cord prolapse risk is appreciable and is increased when the fetus is small or when the breech is not frank (Dilbaz, 2006; Erdemoglu, 2010). Therefore, a vaginal examination should be performed following rupture to exclude prolapse, and special attention should be directed to the fetal heart rate for the first 5 to 10 minutes following membrane rupture.

Cardinal Movements with Breech Delivery

Engagement and descent of the breech usually take place with the bitrochanteric diameter in one of the oblique pelvic diameters. The anterior hip usually descends more rapidly than the posterior hip, and when the resistance of the pelvic floor is met, internal rotation of 45 degrees usually follows, bringing the anterior hip toward the pubic arch and allowing the bitrochanteric diameter to occupy the anteroposterior diameter of the pelvic outlet. If the posterior extremity is prolapsed, however, it, rather than the anterior hip, rotates to the symphysis pubis.

After rotation, descent continues until the perineum is distended by the advancing breech, and the anterior hip appears at the vulva. By lateral flexion of the fetal body, the posterior hip then is forced over the perineum, which retracts over the fetal buttocks, thus allowing the infant to straighten out when the anterior hip is born. The legs and feet follow the breech and may be born spontaneously or require aid.

After the birth of the breech, there is slight external rotation, with the back turning anteriorly as the shoulders are brought into relation with one of the oblique diameters of the pelvis. The shoulders then descend rapidly and undergo internal rotation, with the bisacromial diameter occupying the anteroposterior plane. Immediately following the shoulders, the head, which is normally sharply flexed on the thorax, enters the pelvis in one of the oblique diameters and then rotates in such a manner as to bring the posterior portion of the neck under the symphysis pubis. The head is then born in flexion.

The breech may engage in the transverse diameter of the pelvis, with the sacrum directed anteriorly or posteriorly. The mechanism of labor in the transverse position differs only in that internal rotation is through an arc of 90 rather than 45 degrees. Infrequently, rotation occurs in such a manner that the back of the fetus is directed posteriorly instead of anteriorly. Such rotation should be prevented if possible. Although the head may be delivered by allowing the chin and face to pass beneath the symphysis, the slightest traction on the body may cause extension of the head, which increases the diameter of the head that must pass through the pelvis.

Partial Breech Extraction

With all breech deliveries, unless there is considerable relaxation of the perineum, an episiotomy should be made and is an important adjunct to delivery. Ideally, the breech is allowed to deliver spontaneously to the umbilicus. Delivery is easier, and in turn, morbidity and mortality rates are, at least intuitively, lower. Delivery of the breech draws the umbilicus and attached cord into the pelvis, which stretches and compresses the cord. Therefore, once the breech has passed beyond the vaginal introitus, the abdomen, thorax, arms, and head must be delivered promptly either spontaneously or assisted, as described here.

The posterior hip will deliver, usually from the 6 o'clock position, and often with sufficient pressure to evoke passage of thick meconium (Fig. 28-5). The anterior hip then delivers, followed by external rotation to a sacrum anterior position. The mother should be encouraged to continue to push.

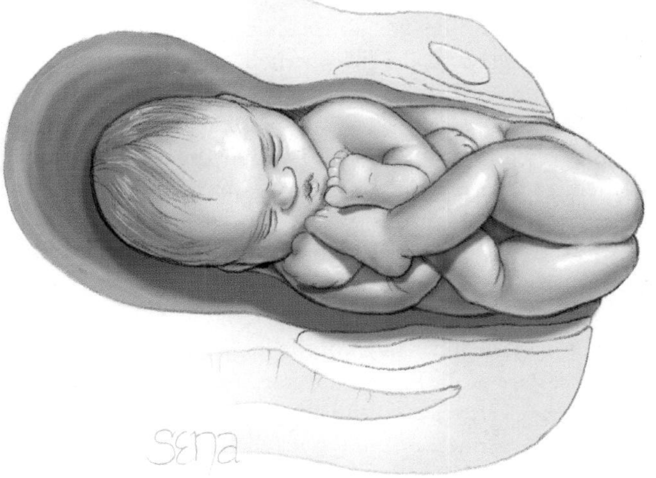

FIGURE 28-5 The hips of the frank breech are delivering over the perineum. The anterior hip usually is delivered first.

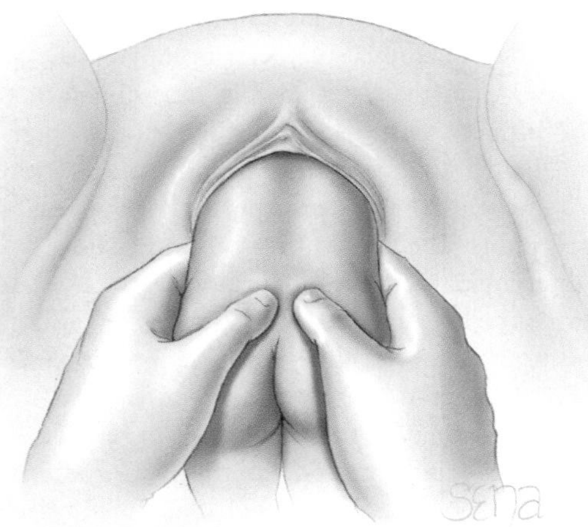

FIGURE 28-6 Delivery of the body. The hands are applied, but not above the pelvic girdle. With thumbs over the sacrum, gentle downward traction is accomplished until the scapulas are clearly visible.

As the fetus continues to descend, the legs are sequentially delivered by splinting the medial aspect of each femur with the operator's fingers positioned parallel to each femur, and by exerting pressure laterally to sweep each leg away from the midline.

Following delivery of the legs, the fetal bony pelvis is grasped with both hands, using a cloth towel moistened with warm water. The fingers should rest on the anterior superior iliac crests and the thumbs on the sacrum, minimizing the chance of fetal abdominal soft tissue injury (Fig. 28-6). Maternal expulsive efforts are used in conjunction with downward traction to effect delivery.

A cardinal rule in successful breech extraction is to employ steady, gentle, downward traction until the lower halves of the scapulas are delivered, making no attempt at delivery of the shoulders and arms until one axilla becomes visible. As the scapulas become visible, the fetal back tends to turn spontaneously toward the side of the mother to which it was originally directed. The appearance of one axilla indicates that the time has arrived for shoulder delivery. It makes little difference which shoulder is delivered first, and there are two methods for their delivery. In the first method, with the scapulas visible, the trunk is rotated in such a way that the anterior shoulder and arm appear at the vulva and can easily be released and delivered first (Fig. 28-7). The body of the fetus is then rotated 180 degrees in the reverse direction to deliver the other shoulder and arm (Fig. 28-8).

The second method is employed if trunk rotation is unsuccessful. With this maneuver, the posterior shoulder is delivered first. For this, the feet are grasped in one hand and drawn upward over the inner thigh of the mother, toward which the ventral surface of the fetus is directed (Fig. 28-9). In this manner, leverage is exerted on the posterior shoulder, which slides out over the perineal margin, usually followed by the arm and hand. Then, by depressing the body of the fetus, the anterior shoulder emerges beneath the pubic arch, and the arm and hand usually follow spontaneously.

These rotational and downward traction maneuvers will decrease the persistence of nuchal arms, which can prevent descent and may result in a traumatic delivery. These maneuvers are frequently most easily effected with the operator at the level of the maternal pelvis and with one knee on the floor.

After both shoulders are delivered, the back of the fetus tends to rotate spontaneously in the direction of the symphysis. If upward rotation fails to occur, it is completed by manual rotation of the body. Delivery of the head may then be accomplished.

Unfortunately, the process is not always so simple, and it is sometimes necessary to assist delivery of the arms. There is more space available in the posterior and lateral segments of the normal pelvis than elsewhere. Therefore, in difficult cases, the posterior arm should be freed first. Because the corresponding axilla is already visible, upward traction on the feet is continued, and two fingers of the other hand are passed along the humerus until the elbow is reached (see Fig. 28-9). The fingers are placed parallel to the humerus and used to splint the arm, which is swept downward and delivered through the vulva. To deliver the anterior arm, depression of the fetal body is sometimes all that is required to allow the anterior arm to slip out spontaneously. In other instances, the anterior arm can be swept down over the thorax using two of the operator's fingers as a splint.

In some cases, the body must be held with the thumbs over the scapulas and rotated to bring the undelivered shoulder near the closest sacrosciatic notch. The legs then are carried upward to bring the ventral surface of the fetus to the opposite inner thigh of the mother. Subsequently, the arm can be delivered posteriorly as described previously. If the arms have become extended over the head, their delivery, although more difficult, usually can be accomplished by the maneuvers just described. In so doing, particular care must be taken by the operator to carry his or her fingers up to the elbow and to use them as a splint to prevent fracture of the fetal humerus.

Nuchal Arm

As just mentioned, one or both fetal arms occasionally may be found around the back of the neck—the nuchal arm—and impacted at the pelvic inlet. In this situation, delivery is more difficult. If the nuchal arm cannot be freed in the manner just described, extraction may be aided, especially with a single nuchal arm, by rotating the fetus through a half circle in such a direction that the friction exerted by the birth canal will serve to draw the elbow toward the face (Fig. 28-10). Should rotation of the fetus fail to free the nuchal arm(s), it may be necessary to push the fetus upward in an attempt to release it. If the rotation is still unsuccessful, the nuchal arm often is extracted by hooking a finger(s) over it and forcing the arm over the shoulder, and down the ventral surface for delivery of the arm. In this event, fracture of the humerus or clavicle is common.

Modified Prague Maneuver

Rarely, the back of the fetus fails to rotate to the anterior. In this situation, rotation of the back to the anterior may be achieved

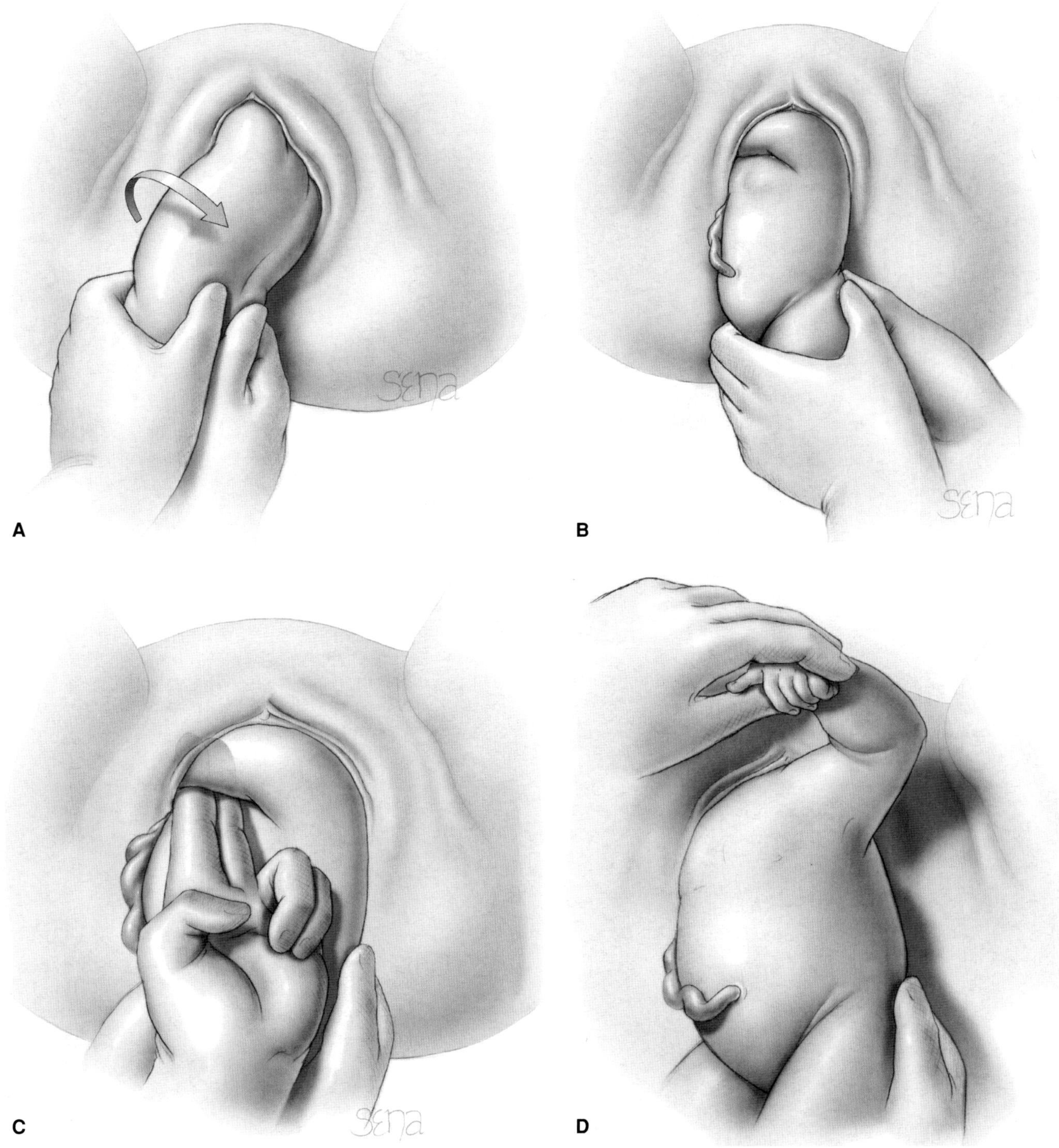

FIGURE 28-7 Clockwise rotation of the fetal pelvis and abdomen 90 degrees brings the sacrum from anterior to left sacrum transverse (LST). Simultaneously, the application of gentle downward traction effects delivery of the scapula **(A)** and arm **(B–D)**.

by using stronger traction on the fetal legs or bony pelvis. If the back still remains oriented posteriorly, extraction may be accomplished using the Mauriceau maneuver, described next, and delivering the fetus back down. If this is impossible, the fetus still may be delivered using the modified Prague maneuver, which, as practiced today, consists of two fingers of one hand grasping the shoulders of the back-down fetus from below while the other hand draws the feet up and over the maternal abdomen (Fig. 28-11).

Delivery of the Aftercoming Head

Mauriceau Maneuver. Normally, the fetal head may be extracted with forceps or by one of several maneuvers. With the Mauriceau maneuver, the index and middle finger of one hand

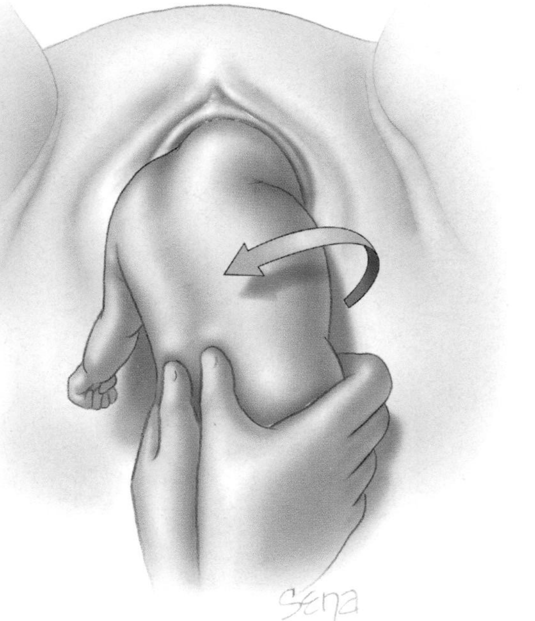

FIGURE 28-8 Counterclockwise rotation from right sacrum anterior (RSA) to right sacrum transverse (RST) along with gentle downward traction effects delivery of the right scapula.

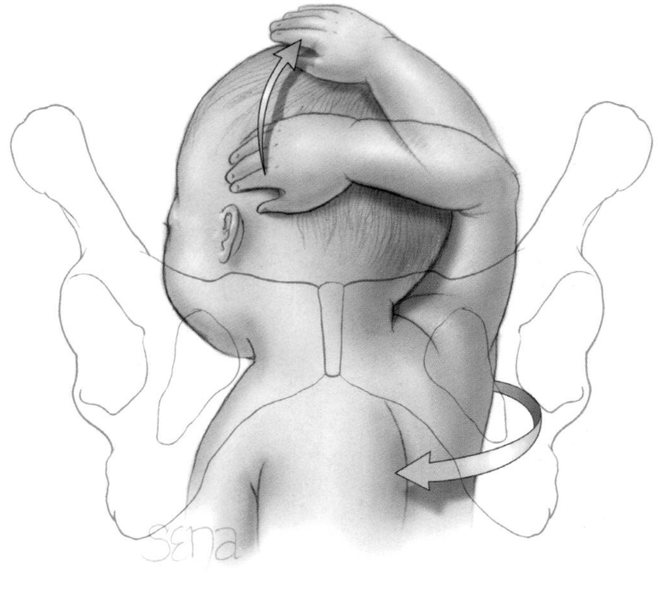

FIGURE 28-10 Reduction of nuchal arm being accomplished by rotating the fetus through half a circle counterclockwise so that the friction exerted by the birth canal will draw the elbow toward the face.

are applied over the maxilla, to flex the head, while the fetal body rests on the palm of the hand and forearm (Fig. 28-12). The operator's forearm is straddled by the fetal legs. Two fingers of the other hand then are hooked over the fetal neck, and grasping the shoulders, downward traction is concurrently applied until the suboccipital region appears under the symphysis. Gentle suprapubic pressure simultaneously applied by an assistant helps keep the head flexed. The body then is elevated toward the maternal abdomen, and the mouth, nose, brow, and eventually the occiput emerge successively over the

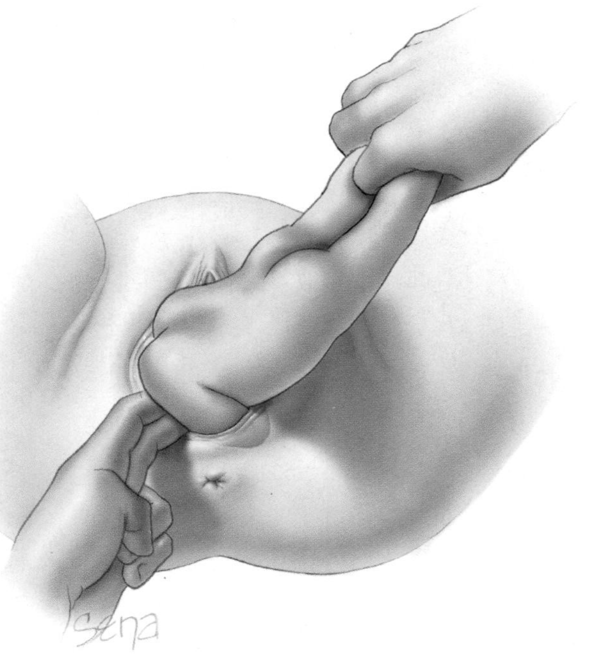

FIGURE 28-9 As breech extraction continues, upward traction is employed with the fetus drawn to the mother's left inner thigh, thus effecting delivery of the posterior shoulder. This is followed by delivery of the posterior arm. The fetal body is then depressed and delivery of the anterior shoulder follows.

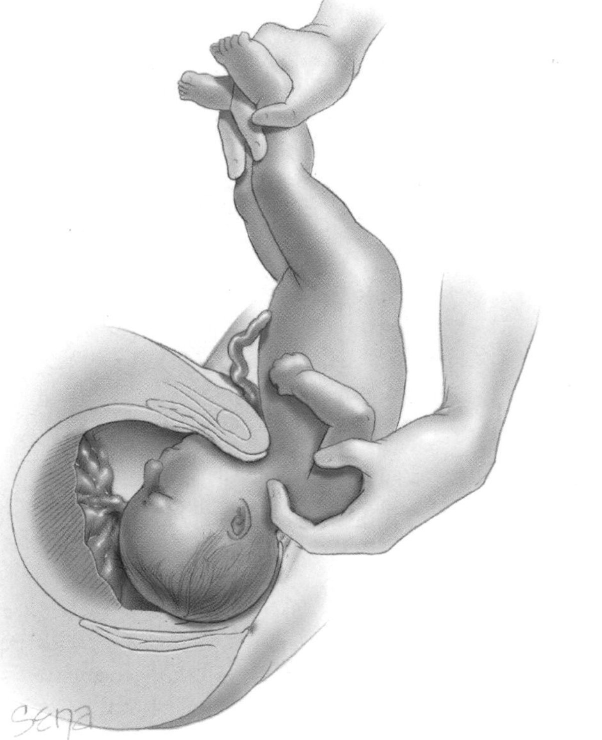

FIGURE 28-11 Delivery of the aftercoming head using the modified Prague maneuver necessitated by failure of the fetal trunk to rotate anteriorly.

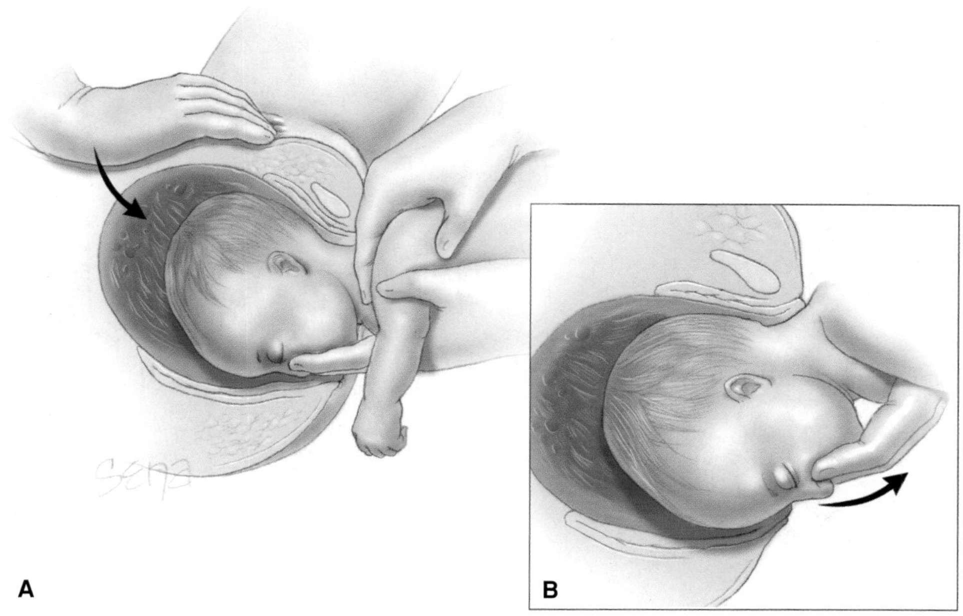

FIGURE 28-12 **A.** Delivery of the aftercoming head using the Mauriceau maneuver. Note that as the fetal head is being delivered, flexion of the head is maintained by suprapubic pressure provided by an assistant. **B.** Pressure on the maxilla is applied simultaneously by the operator as upward and outward traction is exerted.

perineum. With this maneuver, the operator uses both hands simultaneously and in tandem to exert continuous downward gentle traction simultaneously on the fetal neck and on the maxilla. At the same time, appropriate suprapubic pressure is applied by an assistant (see Fig. 28-12).

Forceps to Aftercoming Head. Specialized forceps can also be used to deliver the aftercoming head. Piper forceps, shown in Figure 28-13, or divergent Laufe forceps may be applied electively or when the Mauriceau maneuver cannot be accomplished easily. The blades of the forceps should not be applied to the aftercoming head until it has been brought into the pelvis by gentle traction, combined with suprapubic pressure, and is engaged. Suspension of the body of the fetus in a towel effectively holds the fetus up and helps keep the arms and cord out of the way as the forceps blades are applied.

Because the forceps blades are directed upward from the level of the perineum, some choose to apply them from a one-knee kneeling position. Piper forceps have a downward arch in the shank to accommodate the fetal body and lack a pelvic curve. This shape permits a direct application of the cephalic curve of the blade along the length of the maternal vagina and fetal parietal bone. The blade to be placed on the maternal left is held in the operator's left hand. The right hand slides between the fetal head and left maternal vaginal sidewall to guide the blade inward and around the parietal bone. The opposite blade mirrors this application. Once in place, the blades are articulated, and the fetal body rests across the shanks. The head is delivered by pulling gently outward and raising the handle simultaneously. This rolls the face over the perineum, while the occiput remains beneath the symphysis until after the brow delivers. Ideally, the head and body move in unison to minimize trauma.

Entrapment of the Aftercoming Head. Occasionally—especially with a small preterm fetus—the incompletely dilated cervix will constrict around the neck and impede delivery of the aftercoming head. At this point, it must be assumed that there is significant and even total cord compression, and thus time management is essential. With gentle traction on the fetal body, the cervix, at times, may be manually slipped over the occiput. If this is not successful, then Dührssen incisions as shown in Figure 28-14 may be necessary. Other alternatives include intravenous nitroglycerin—typically 100 μg—to provide cervical relaxation (Dufour, 1997; Wessen, 1995). There is, however, no compelling evidence of its efficacy for this purpose. General anesthesia with halogenated agents is another option.

As a last resort, replacement of the fetus higher into the vagina and uterus, followed by cesarean delivery, can be used to rescue an entrapped breech fetus that cannot be delivered vaginally. This maneuver was described for the protruding head with intractable shoulder dystocia and is termed the *Zavanelli maneuver* as described by Sandberg (1988). It was subsequently reported by Steyn and Pieper (1994) to be used to deliver the entrapped aftercoming head in a 2590-g breech fetus. Sandberg (1999) reviewed 11 breech deliveries in which this maneuver was used.

Symphysiotomy is also used to aid delivery of an entrapped aftercoming head. Using local analgesic, this operation surgically divides the intervening symphyseal cartilage and much of its ligamentous support to widen the symphysis pubis up to 2.5 cm (Basak, 2011). Lack of operator training and potentially serious maternal pelvic or urinary tract injury explain its rare use in the United States. That said, if cesarean section is not available or unsafe for the mother, symphysiotomy may be lifesaving for both mother and baby (Hofmeyr, 2012).

Total Breech Extraction

Complete or Incomplete Breech

At times, total extraction of a complete or incomplete breech may be required. A hand is introduced through the vagina, and both fetal feet are grasped. The ankles are held with the second finger lying between them. With gentle traction, the feet are brought through the introitus. If difficulty is experienced in grasping both feet, first one foot should be drawn into the vagina but not through the introitus, and then the other foot is advanced in a similar fashion. Now both feet are grasped and pulled through the vulva simultaneously (Fig. 28-15).

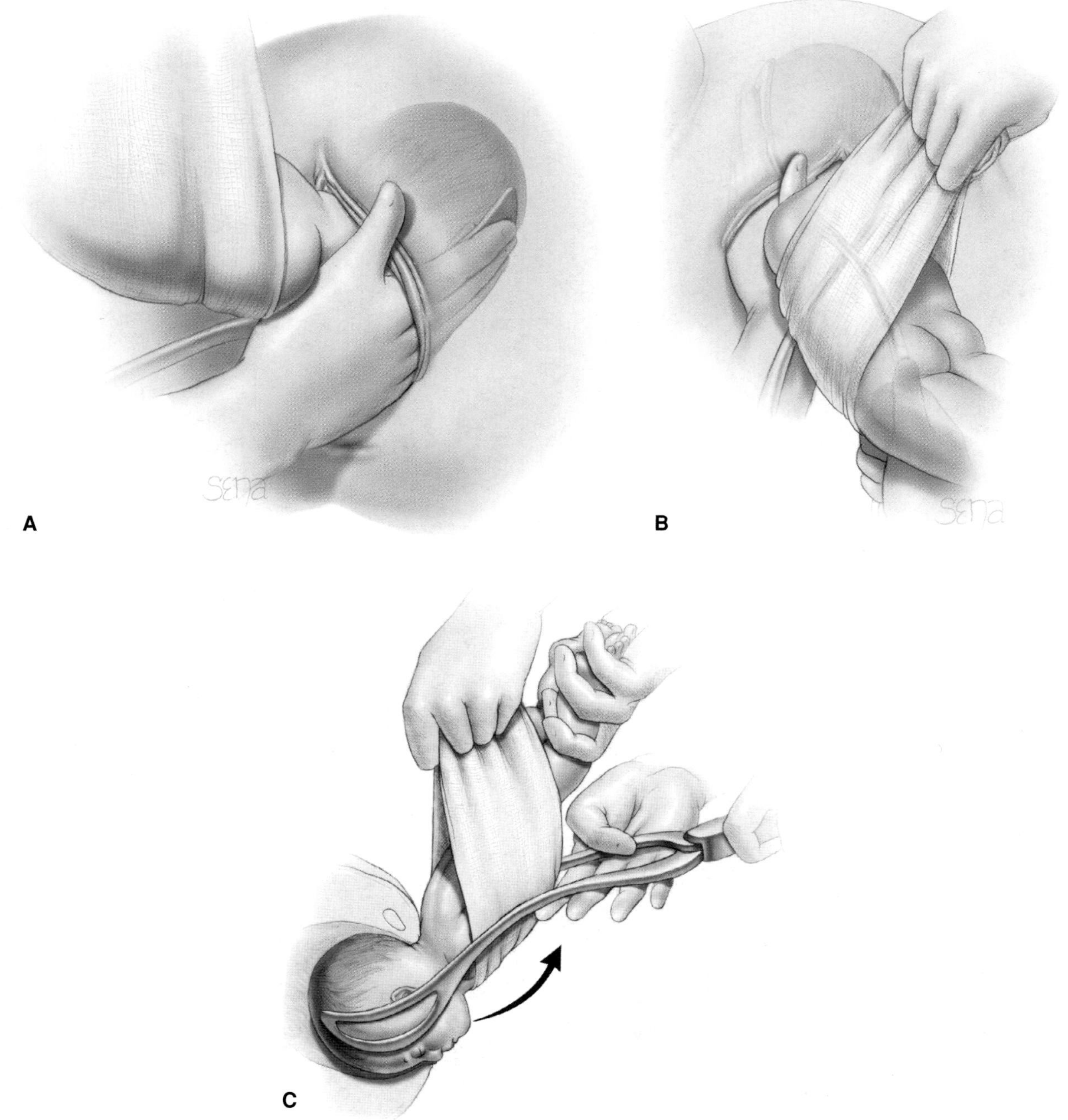

FIGURE 28-13 Piper forceps for delivery of the aftercoming head. **A.** The fetal body is held elevated using a warm towel and the left blade of forceps is applied to the aftercoming head. **B.** The right blade is applied with the body still elevated. **C.** Forceps delivery of the aftercoming head. Note the direction of movement shown by the arrow.

As the legs begin to emerge through the vulva, downward gentle traction is continued. As the legs emerge, successively higher portions are grasped, first the calves and then the thighs. When the breech appears at the vaginal outlet, gentle traction is applied until the hips are delivered. As the buttocks emerge, the back of the fetus usually rotates to the anterior. The thumbs are then placed over the sacrum and the fingers over the hips, and breech extraction is completed, as described for partial breech extraction (p. 564). During cesarean delivery, these maneuvers are also used during delivery of a complete, incomplete, or footling breech through the hysterotomy incision.

Frank Breech

During complete extraction of a frank breech, moderate traction is exerted by a finger in each groin and aided by a generous episiotomy (Fig. 28-16). Once the breech is pulled through the introitus, the steps described for partial breech extraction are then completed (p. 564). These maneuvers are also used during cesarean delivery of the frank breech through the hysterotomy incision.

If moderate traction does not effect delivery, then vaginal delivery can be accomplished only by breech decomposition. This procedure involves manipulation within the birth canal

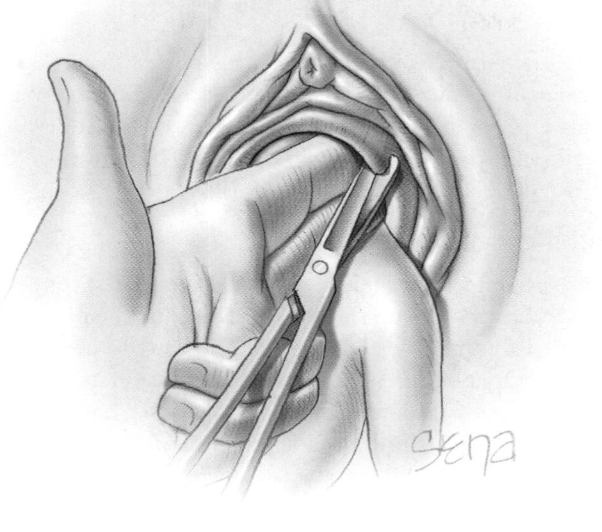

FIGURE 28-14 Dührssen incision being cut at 2 o'clock, which is followed by a second incision at 10 o'clock. Infrequently, an additional incision is required at 6 o'clock. The incisions are so placed as to minimize bleeding from the laterally located cervical branches of the uterine artery. After delivery, the incisions are repaired as described in Chapter 41 (p. 790).

to convert the frank breech into a footling breech. It is accomplished more readily if the membranes have ruptured only recently, and it becomes extremely difficult if there is minimal amnionic fluid. In such cases, the uterus may have become tightly contracted around the fetus. Pharmacological relaxation by general anesthesia, intravenous magnesium sulfate, or a betamimetic agent such as terbutaline, 250 μg subcutaneously, may be required.

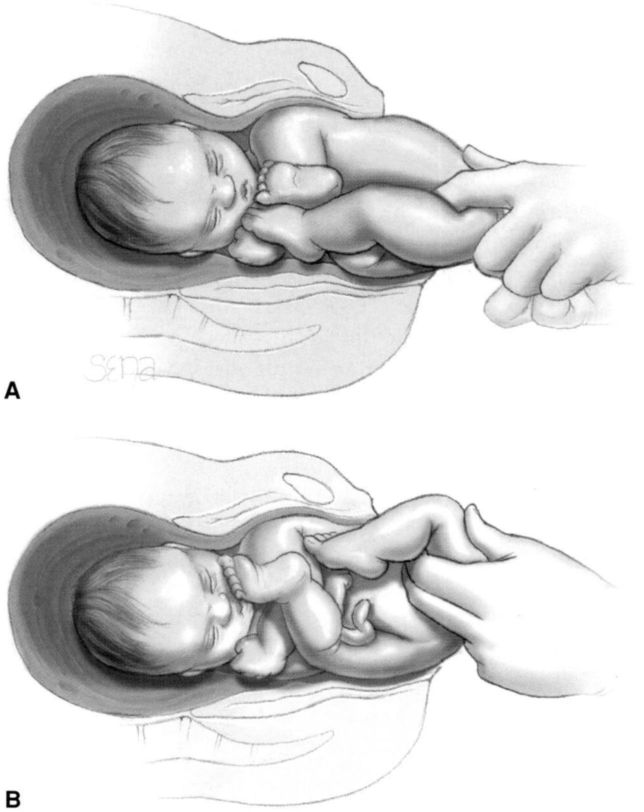

FIGURE 28-16 **A.** Extraction of frank breech using fingers in groins. **B.** Once the hips are delivered, each hip and knee is flexed to deliver them from the vagina.

Breech decomposition is accomplished by the maneuver attributed to Pinard (1889). It aids in bringing the fetal feet within reach of the operator. As shown in Figure 28-17, two fingers are carried up along one extremity to the knee to push it away from the midline. Spontaneous flexion usually follows,

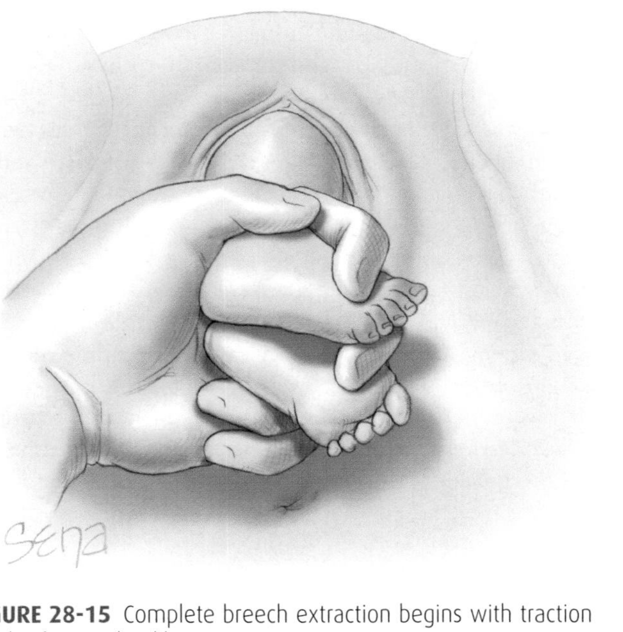

FIGURE 28-15 Complete breech extraction begins with traction on the feet and ankles.

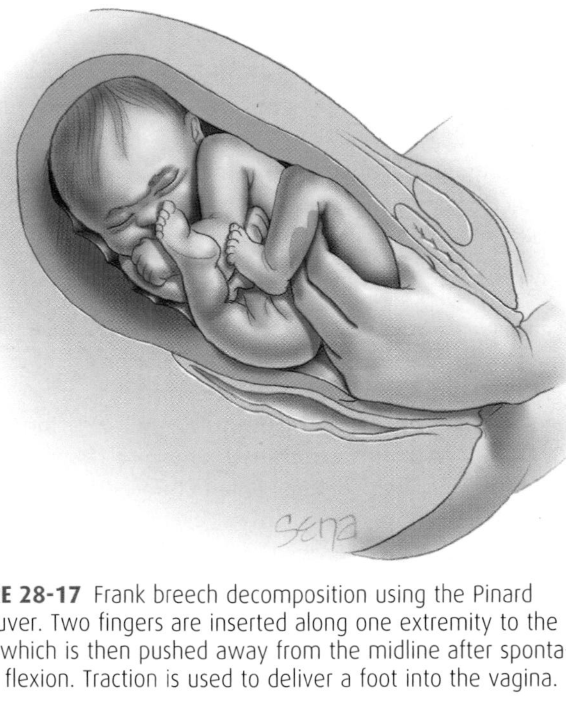

FIGURE 28-17 Frank breech decomposition using the Pinard maneuver. Two fingers are inserted along one extremity to the knee, which is then pushed away from the midline after spontaneous flexion. Traction is used to deliver a foot into the vagina.

and the foot of the fetus is felt to impinge on the back of the hand. The fetal foot then may be grasped and brought down.

ANALGESIA AND ANESTHESIA

Continuous epidural analgesia, as described in Chapter 25 (p. 509), is advocated by some as ideal for women in labor with a breech presentation. This may increase the need for labor augmentation and may prolong second-stage labor (Chadha, 1992; Confino, 1985). These potential disadvantages must be weighed against the advantages of better pain relief and increased pelvic relaxation should extensive manipulation be required. Analgesia must be sufficient for episiotomy, for breech extraction, and for Piper forceps application. Nitrous oxide plus oxygen inhalation provides further relief from pain. If general anesthesia is required, it must be induced quickly.

Anesthesia for breech decomposition and extraction must provide sufficient relaxation to allow intrauterine manipulations. Although successful decomposition has been accomplished using epidural or spinal analgesia, increased uterine tone may render the operation more difficult. Under such conditions, general anesthesia with a halogenated agent may be required.

VERSION

With this procedure, fetal presentation is altered by physical manipulation, either substituting one pole of a longitudinal presentation for the other, or converting an oblique or transverse lie into a longitudinal presentation. According to whether the head or breech is made the presenting part, the operation is designated cephalic or podalic version, respectively. With external version, the manipulations are performed exclusively through the abdominal wall. With internal version, they are accomplished inside the uterine cavity.

External Cephalic Version

For breech fetuses near term, the American College of Obstetricians and Gynecologists (2012a,b) recommends that version should be offered and attempted whenever possible. Its success rate ranges from 35 to 86 percent, with an average of 58 percent. For women with a transverse lie, the overall success rate is significantly higher.

Indications

In general, external version is attempted before labor in a woman who has reached 36 weeks' gestation with a breech fetus. Before this time, a breech presentation still has a high likelihood of correcting spontaneously. And, if performed too early, time may allow a return back to breech (Bogner, 2012). Last, if version causes a need for immediate delivery, complications of iatrogenic preterm delivery generally are not severe.

Version is contraindicated if vaginal delivery is not an option. Examples include placenta previa or nonreassuring fetal status. Other contraindications include rupture of membranes, known uterine malformation, multifetal gestation, and recent uterine bleeding. As discussed in Chapter 31 (p. 616), prior uterine incision is a relative contraindication. In a few small studies, external version was not associated with uterine rupture (Abenhaim, 2009; Sela, 2009). At Parkland Hospital, external version is not attempted in these women, but larger studies are needed.

Several factors can improve the chances of a successful version attempt. These include multiparity, abundant amnionic fluid, unengaged presenting part, fetal size 2500 to 3000 g, posterior placenta, and nonobese patient (Buhimschi, 2011; de Hundt, 2012; Kok, 2008, 2009, 2011).

Complications

Patient counseling includes projected success rates, conversion back to breech, and risks of the procedure itself. Risks include placental abruption, uterine rupture, fetomaternal hemorrhage, alloimmunization, preterm labor, fetal compromise, and even death. Most worrisome is the report by Stine and coworkers (1985) of a maternal death due to amnionic fluid embolism. That said, fetal deaths are rare, serious complication rates are typically very low, and emergent cesarean rates are 0.5 percent or less (Collaris, 2004; Collins, 2007; Grootscholten, 2008).

Importantly, even after successful version, several reports suggest that the cesarean delivery rate does not completely revert to the baseline for vertex presentations. Specifically, dystocia, malpresentation, and nonreassuring fetal heart patterns may be more common in these fetuses despite successful version (Chan, 2004; Vézina, 2004).

Technique

External cephalic version should be carried out in an area that has ready access to a facility equipped to perform an emergency cesarean delivery (American College of Obstetricians and Gynecologists, 2012a). Sonographic examination is performed to confirm nonvertex presentation, document amnionic fluid volume adequacy, exclude obvious fetal anomalies if not done previously, and identify placental location. External monitoring is performed to assess fetal heart rate reactivity. Anti-D immune globulin is given to Rh-D negative women.

A forward roll of the fetus usually is attempted first. Each hand grasps one fetal pole, and the fetal buttocks are elevated from the maternal pelvis and displaced laterally (Fig. 28-18). The buttocks are then gently guided toward the fundus, while the head is directed toward the pelvis. If the forward roll is unsuccessful, then a backward flip is attempted. Version attempts are discontinued for excessive discomfort, persistently abnormal fetal heart rate, or after multiple failed attempts. Failure is not always absolute. Ben-Meir and colleagues (2007) reported a spontaneous version rate of 7 percent among 226 failed versions—2 percent among nulliparas and 13 percent among parous women.

If version is successful, the nonstress test is repeated until a normal test result is obtained. If version is completed before 39 weeks' gestation, then awaiting spontaneous labor and fetal maturity is preferred.

Tocolysis

Existing evidence may support the use of tocolytic agents during external version attempts (American College of Obstetricians

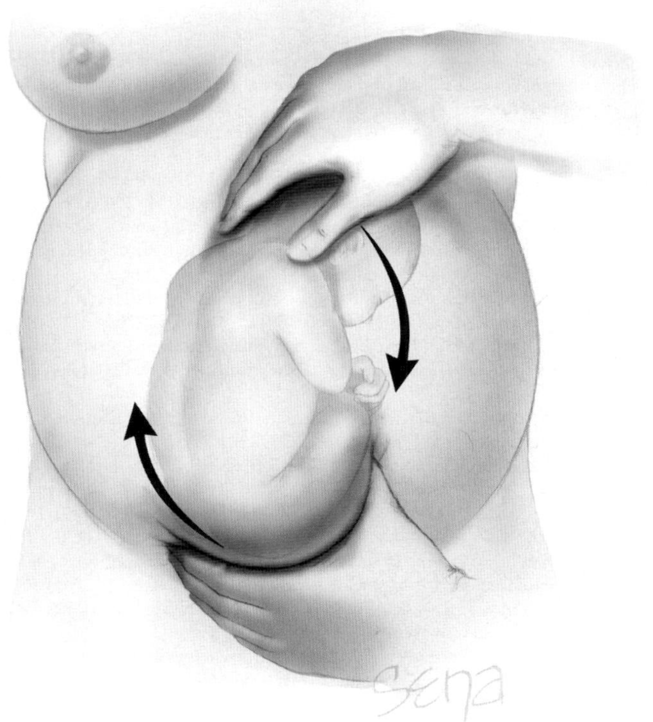

FIGURE 28-18 External cephalic version. With an attempted forward roll, clockwise pressure is exerted against the fetal poles.

and Gynecologists, 2012a). Agents investigated include betamimetics, such as terbutaline, ritodrine, or salbutamol; calcium-channel blockers, such as nifedipine; and nitric oxide donors, such as nitroglycerin. Most randomized investigations have evaluated betamimetics. In one such trial, Fernandez and coworkers (1996) reported that the success rate with subcutaneous terbutaline—52 percent—was significantly higher than without—27 percent. Other studies of betamimetics support their efficacy, although not universally (Marquette, 1996; Robertson, 1987; Vani, 2009). There is less evidence to support the use of nifedipine and nitroglycerin (Cluver, 2012; Wilcox, 2011). Our policy at Parkland Hospital is to administer 250 μg of terbutaline subcutaneously to most women before attempted version. When maternal tachycardia—a known side effect of terbutaline—is noted, then the version attempt is begun.

Conduction Analgesia

Epidural analgesia has been reported to increase version success rates (Mancuso, 2000; Schorr, 1997). But Sullivan and associates (2009) noted no improvement with combined spinal-epidural analgesia. In two small randomized trials, Weiniger and associates (2007, 2010) reported that spinal analgesia increased version success rate. In the trials by Dugoff (1999) and Delisle (2003) and their colleagues, spinal analgesia was not of benefit. According to the American College of Obstetricians and Gynecologists (2012a), there is not enough consistent evidence to recommend conduction analgesia routinely for external version.

With the exception of rare severe complications, Collaris and Oei (2004) concluded that external cephalic version is safe. One caveat was that complications were more common when conduction analgesia was used. Use of nitrous oxide or conduction analgesia was associated with twice as many abnormal fetal heart rate tracings. Moreover, vaginal bleeding and procedure-related emergency cesarean deliveries were increased tenfold. These reviewers concluded that diminished pain in these women likely encouraged overzealous application of force during the version attempts. In another small study, however, Suen and associates (2012) showed that the force applied during version under spinal analgesia was actually less.

Other Methods

There are some unconventional interventions that have been used to help effect version. Moxibustion is a traditional Chinese medicine technique that burns a cigarette-shaped stick of ground *Artemisia vulgaris*—which is also known as mugwort or in Japanese as *moxa.* At the BL 67 acupuncture point, the stick is directly placed against the skin or indirectly heats an acupuncture needle at the site to increase fetal movement and promote spontaneous breech version. It is performed usually between 33 and 36 weeks' gestation to permit a trial of external cephalic version if not successful. Results from randomized controlled studies are conflicting. However, a Cochrane Database review found some evidence to support moxibustion use when combined with acupuncture (Cardini, 1998, 2005; Coyle, 2012; Guittier, 2009; Neri, 2004).

Internal Podalic Version

This maneuver is used only for delivery of a second twin. With the membranes preferably still intact, a hand is inserted into the uterine cavity to turn the fetus manually. The operator seizes one or both feet and draws them through the fully dilated cervix, while using the other hand transabdominally to push the upper portion of the fetal body in the opposite direction as shown in Chapter 45 (p. 918). This is then followed by breech extraction.

REFERENCES

Abenhaim HA, Varin J, Boucher M: External cephalic version among women with a previous cesarean delivery: report on 36 cases and review of the literature. J Perinat Med 37(2):156, 2009

Alarab M, Regan C, O'Connell MP, et al: Singleton vaginal breech delivery at term: still a safe option. Obstet Gynecol 103:407, 2004

Albrechtsen S, Rasmussen S, Reigstad H, et al: Evaluation of a protocol for selecting fetuses in breech presentation for vaginal delivery or cesarean section. Am J Obstet Gynecol 177:586, 1997

Al-Qattan MM, El-Sayed AA, Al-Zahrani AY, et al: Obstetric brachial plexus palsy: a comparison of affected infants delivered vaginally by breech or cephalic presentation. Hand Surg Eur 35(5):366, 2010

American College of Obstetricians and Gynecologists: Mode of term singleton breech delivery. Committee Opinion No. 265, December 2001

American College of Obstetricians and Gynecologists: External cephalic version. Practice Bulletin No. 13, February 2000, Reaffirmed 2012a

American College of Obstetricians and Gynecologists: Mode of term in singleton breech delivery. Committee Opinion No. 340, July 2006, Reaffirmed 2012b

Azria E, Le Meaux JP, Khoshnood B, et al: Factors associated with adverse perinatal outcomes for term breech fetuses with planned vaginal delivery. Am J Obstet Gynecol 207(4):285.e1, 2012

Basak S, Kanungo S, Majhi C: Symphysiotomy: is it obsolete? J Obstet Gynaecol Res 37(7):770, 2011

Ben-Meir A, Elram T, Tsafrir A, et al: The incidence of spontaneous version after failed external cephalic version. Am J Obstet Gynecol 196(2):157, 2007

Biswas A, Johnstone MJ: Term breech delivery: does x-ray pelvimetry help? Aust N Z J Obstet Gynaecol 33:150, 1993
Bogner G, Xu F, Simbrunner C, et al: Single-institute experience, management, success rate, and outcome after external cephalic version at term. Int J Gynaecol Obstet 116(2):134, 2012
Buhimschi CS, Buhimschi IA, Wehrum MJ, et al: Ultrasonographic evaluation of myometrial thickness and prediction of a successful external cephalic version. Obstet Gynecol 118(4):913, 2011
Canpolat FE, Köse A, Yurdakök M: Bilateral humerus fracture in a neonate after cesarean delivery. Arch Gynecol Obstet 281(5):967, 2010
Carbonne B, Goffinet F, Breart G, et al: The debate on breach presentation: delivery of breach presentations: the position of the National College of French Gynecologists. [French] J Gynecol Obstet Biol Reprod (Paris) 30:191, 2001
Cardini F, Lombardo P, Regalia AL, et al: A randomized controlled trial of moxibustion for breech presentation. Br J Obstet Gynaecol 112(6):743, 2005
Cardini F, Weixin H: Moxibustion for correction of breech presentation: a randomized controlled trial. JAMA 280:1580, 1998
Chadha YC, Mahmood TA, Dick MJ, et al: Breech delivery and epidural analgesia. Br J Obstet Gynaecol 99:96, 1992
Chan LY, Tang JL, Tsoi KF, et al: Intrapartum cesarean delivery after successful external cephalic version: a meta-analysis. Obstet Gynecol 104:155, 2004
Chinnock M, Robson S: Obstetric trainees' experience in vaginal breech delivery. Obstet Gynecol 110:900, 2007
Cluver C, Hofmeyr GJ, Gyte GM, et al: Interventions for helping to turn term breech babies to head first presentation when using external cephalic version. Cochrane Database Syst Rev 1:CD000184, 2012
Collaris RJ, Oei SG: External cephalic version: a safe procedure? A systematic review of version-related risks. Acta Obstet Gynecol Scand 83:511, 2004
Collins S, Ellaway P, Harrington D, et al: The complications of external cephalic version: results from 805 consecutive attempts. Br J Obstet Gynaecol 114(5):636, 2007
Confino E, Ismajovich B, Rudick V, et al: Extradural analgesia in the management of singleton breech delivery. Br J Anaesth 57:892, 1985
Coyle ME, Smith CA, Peat B: Cephalic version by moxibustion for breech presentation. Cochrane Database Syst Rev 5:CD003928, 2012
Deering S, Brown J, Hodor J, et al: Simulation training and resident performance of singleton vaginal breech delivery. Obstet Gynecol 107(1): 86, 2006
de Hundt M, Vlemmix F, Bais JM, et al: Risk factors for developmental dysplasia of the hip: a meta-analysis. Eur J Obstet Gynecol Reprod Biol 165(1):8, 2012
Delisle MF, Kamani AA, Douglas MJ, et al: Antepartum external cephalic version under spinal anesthesia: a randomized controlled study [Abstract]. J Obstet Gynaecol Can 25:S13, 2003
Demirci O, Tuğrul AS, Turgut A, et al: Pregnancy outcomes by mode of delivery among breech births. Arch Gynecol Obstet 285(2):297, 2012
Dilbaz B, Ozturkoglu E, Dilbaz S, et al: Risk factors and perinatal outcomes associated with umbilical cord prolapse. Arch Gynecol Obstet 274(2):104, 2006
Dufour PH, Vinatier D, Orazi G, et al: The use of intravenous nitroglycerin for emergency cervico-uterine relaxation. Acta Obstet Gynecol Scand 76:287, 1997
Dugoff L, Stamm CA, Jones OW III, et al: The effect of spinal anesthesia on the success rate of external cephalic version: a randomized trial. Obstet Gynecol 93:345, 1999
Eide MG, Øyen N, Skjaerven R, et al: Breech delivery and intelligence: a population-based study of 8,738 breech infants. Obstet Gynecol 105(1):4, 2005
Erdemoglu M, Kale A, Kuyumcuoglu U, et al: Umbilical cord prolapse in the southeast region of Turkey: evaluation of 79 cases. Clin Exp Obstet Gynecol 37(2):141, 2010
Fernandez CO, Bloom S, Wendel G: A prospective, randomized, blinded comparison of terbutaline versus placebo for singleton, term external cephalic version. Am J Obstet Gynecol 174:326, 1996
Fontenot T, Campbell B, Mitchell-Tutt E, et al: Radiographic evaluation of breech presentation: is it necessary? Ultrasound Obstet Gynecol 10:338, 1997
Ford JB, Roberts CL, Nassar N, et al: Recurrence of breech presentation in consecutive pregnancies. BJOG 117(7):830, 2010
Fox AE, Paton RW: The relationship between mode of delivery and developmental dysplasia of the hip in breech infants: a four-year prospective cohort study. J Bone Joint Surg Br 92(12):1695, 2010
Freud E, Orvieto R, Merlob P: Neonatal labioperineal tear from fetal scalp electrode insertion, a case report. J Reprod Med 38:647, 1993
Giuliani A, Scholl WMJ, Basver A, et al: Mode of delivery and outcome of 699 term singleton breech deliveries at a single center. Am J Obstet Gynecol 187:1694, 2002
Goffinet F, Carayol M, Foidart JM, et al: Is planned vaginal delivery for breech presentation at term still an option? Results of an observational prospective survey in France and Belgium. Am J Obstet Gynecol 194(4):1002, 2006
Grootscholten K, Kok M, Oei SG, et al: External cephalic version-related risks: a meta-analysis. Obstet Gynecol 112(5):1143, 2008
Guittier MJ, Pichon M, Dong H, et al: Moxibustion for breech version: a randomized controlled trial. Obstet Gynecol 114(5):1034, 2009
Hannah ME, Hannah WJ, Hewson SA, et al: Planned caesarean section versus planned vaginal birth for breech presentation at term: a randomised multicentre trial. Lancet 356:1375, 2000
Hartnack Tharin JE, Rasmussen S, Krebs L: Consequences of the Term Breech Trial in Denmark. Acta Obstet Gynecol Scand 90(7):767, 2011
Hehir MP, O'Connor HD, Kent EM, et al: Changes in vaginal breech delivery rates in a single large metropolitan area. Am J Obstet Gynecol 206(6):498.e1, 2012
Hofmeyr GJ, Shweni PM: Symphysiotomy for feto-pelvic disproportion. Cochrane Database Syst Rev 10:CD005299, 2012
Huang JP, Chen CP, Chen CP, et al: Term pregnancy with umbilical cord prolapse. Taiwan J Obstet Gynecol 51(3):375, 2012
Kalogiannidis I, Masouridou N, Dagklis T, et al: Previous cesarean section increases the risk for breech presentation at term pregnancy. Clin Exp Obstet Gynecol 37(1):29, 2010
Kayem G, Baumann R, Goffinet F, et al: Early preterm breech delivery: is a policy of planned vaginal delivery associated with increased risk of neonatal death? Am J Obstet Gynecol 198(3):289.e1, 2008
Kok M, Cnossen J, Gravendeel L, et al: Clinical factors to predict the outcome of external cephalic version: a metaanalysis. Am J Obstet Gynecol 199(6):630.e1, 2008
Kok M, Cnossen J, Gravendeel L, et al: Ultrasound factors to predict the outcome of external cephalic version: a meta-analysis. Ultrasound Obstet Gynecol 33(1):76, 2009
Kok M, van der Steeg JW, van der Post JA, et al: Prediction of success of external cephalic version after 36 weeks. Am J Perinatol 28(2):103, 2011
Kotaska A, Menticoglou S, Gagnon R: SOGC clinical practice guideline: vaginal delivery of breech presentation: no. 226, June 2009. Int J Gynaecol Obstet 107(2):169, 2009
Lee KS, Khoshnood B, Sriram S, et al: Relationship of cesarean delivery to lower birth weight-specific neonatal mortality in singleton breech infants in the United States. Obstet Gynecol 92(5):769, 1998
Lumbiganon P, Laopaiboon M, Gülmezoglu AM, et al: Method of delivery and pregnancy outcomes in Asia: the WHO global survey on maternal and perinatal health 2007–08. Lancet 375(9713):490, 2010
Lydon-Rochelle M, Albers L, Gorwoda J, et al: Accuracy of Leopold maneuvers in screening for malpresentation: a prospective study. Birth 20:132, 1993
Mailàth-Pokorny M, Preyer O, Dadak C, et al: Breech presentation: a retrospective analysis of 12-years' experience at a single center. Wien Klin Wochenschr 121(5–6):209, 2009
Mancuso KM, Yancey MK, Murphy JA, et al: Epidural analgesia for cephalic version: a randomized trial. Obstet Gynecol 95:648, 2000
Marquette GP, Boucher M, Theriault D, et al: Does the use of a tocolytic agent affect the success rate of external cephalic version? Am J Obstet Gynecology 175:859, 1996
Marzouk P, Arnaud E, Oury JF, et al: Induction of labour and breech presentation: experience of a French maternity ward. [French] J Gynecol Obstet Biol Reprod (Paris) 40(7):668, 2011
Maslovitz S, Barkai G, Lessing JB, et al: Recurrent obstetric management mistakes identified by simulation. Obstet Gynecol 109(6):1295, 2007
Mathews R, Sheridan ME, Patil U: Neonatal testicular loss secondary to perinatal trauma in breech presentation. BJU Int 83(9):1069, 1999
Matsubara S, Izumi A, Nagai T, et al: Femur fracture during abdominal breech delivery. Arch Gynecol Obstet 278(2):195, 2008
McNamara JM, Odibo AO, Macones GA, et al: The effect of breech presentation on the accuracy of estimated fetal weight. Am J Perinatol 29(5):353, 2012
Michel S, Drain A, Closset E, et al: Evaluation of a decision protocol for type of delivery of infants in breech presentation at term. Eur J Obstet Gynecol Reprod Biol 158(2):194, 2011
Muhuri PK, Macdorman MF, Menacker F: Method of delivery and neonatal mortality among very low birth weight infants in the United States. Matern Child Health J 10:47, 2006
Nassar N, Roberts CL, Cameron CA, et al: Diagnostic accuracy of clinical examination for detection of non-cephalic presentation in late pregnancy: cross sectional analytic study. BMJ 333:578, 2006

Neri I, Airola G, Contu G, et al: Acupuncture plus moxibustion to resolve breech presentation: a randomized controlled study. J Matern Fetal Neonatal Med 15(4):247, 2004
Nwosu EC, Walkinshaw S, Chia P: Undiagnosed breech. Br J Obstet Gynaecol 100:531, 1993
Ortiz-Neira CL, Paolucci EO, Donnon T: A meta-analysis of common risk factors associated with the diagnosis of developmental dysplasia of the hip in newborns. Eur J Radiol 81(3):e344, 2012
Pinard A: On version by external maneuvers. In: Traite du Palper Abdominal. Paris, Lauwereyns, 1889
Rayl J, Gibson PJ, Hickok DE: A population-based case-control study of risk factors for breech presentation. Am J Obstet Gynecol 174(1 Pt 1):28, 1996
Reddy UM, Zhang J, Sun L, et al: Neonatal mortality by attempted route of delivery in early preterm birth. Am J Obstet Gynecol 207(2):117.e1, 2012
Rietberg CC, Elferink-Stinkens PM, Visser GH: The effect of the Term Breech Trial on medical intervention behaviour and neonatal outcome in The Netherlands: an analysis of 35,453 term breech infants. Br J Obstet Gynaecol 112(2):205, 2005
Robertson AW, Kopelman JN, Read JA, et al: External cephalic version at term: is a tocolytic necessary? Obstet Gynecol 70:896, 1987
Rojansky N, Tanos V, Lewin A, et al: Sonographic evaluation of fetal head extension and maternal pelvis in cases of breech presentation. Acta Obstet Gynecol Scand 73:607, 1994
Roman H, Carayol M, Watier L, et al: Planned vaginal delivery of fetuses in breech presentation at term: prenatal determinants predictive of elevated risk of cesarean delivery during labor. Eur J Obstet Gynecol Reprod Biol 138(1):14, 2008
Royal College of Obstetricians and Gynaecologists: The management of breech presentation. RCOG Green Top Guidelines, No. 20b. London, 2006
Sandberg EC: The Zavanelli maneuver: 12 years of recorded experience. Obstet Gynecol 93:312, 1999
Sandberg EC: The Zavanelli maneuver extended: progression of a revolutionary concept. Am J Obstet Gynecol 158(6 Pt 1):1347, 1988
Schorr SJ, Speights SE, Ross EL, et al: A randomized trial of epidural anesthesia to improve external cephalic version success. Am J Obstet Gynecol 177:1133, 1997
Schutte JM, Steegers EA, Santema JG, et al: Maternal deaths after elective cesarean section for breech presentation in the Netherlands. Acta Obstet Gynecol Scand 86(2):240, 2007
Sela HY, Fiegenberg T, Ben-Meir A, et al: Safety and efficacy of external cephalic version for women with a previous cesarean delivery. Eur J Obstet Gynecol Reprod Biol 142(2):111, 2009
Steyn W, Pieper C: Favorable neonatal outcome after fetal entrapment and partially successful Zavanelli maneuver in a case of breech presentation. Am J Perinatol 11:348, 1994
Stine LE, Phelan JP, Wallace R, et al: Update on external cephalic version performed at term. Obstet Gynecol 65:642, 1985
Stohl HE, Szymanski LM, Althaus JJ: Vaginal breech delivery in very low birth weight (VLBW) neonates: experience of a single center. J Perinat Med 39(4):379, 2011
Suen SS, Khaw KS, Law LW, et al: The force applied to successfully turn a foetus during reattempts of external cephalic version is substantially reduced when performed under spinal analgesia. J Matern Fetal Neonatal Med 25(6):719, 2012
Sullivan JT, Grobman WA, Bauchat JR, et al: A randomized controlled trial of the effect of combined spinal-epidural analgesia on the success of external cephalic version for breech presentation. Int J Obstet Anesth 18(4):328, 2009
Svenningsen NW, Westgren M, Ingemarsson I: Modern strategy for the term breech delivery—a study with a 4-year follow-up of the infants. J Perinat Med 13:117, 1985
Swedish Collaborative Breech Study Group: Term breech delivery in Sweden: mortality relative to fetal presentation and planned mode of delivery. Acta Obstet Gynecol Scand 84(6):593, 2005
Thomas SM, Bees NR, Adam EJ: Trends in the use of pelvimetry techniques. Clin Radiol 53(4):293, 1998
Toivonen E, Palomäki O, Huhtala H, et al: Selective vaginal breech delivery at term—still an option. Acta Obstet Gynecol Scand 91(10):1177, 2012
Vani S, Lau SY, Lim BK, et al: Intravenous salbutamol for external cephalic version. Int J Gynecol Obstet 104(1):28, 2009
Vendittelli F, Pons JC, Lemery D, et al: The term breech presentation: neonatal results and obstetric practices in France. Eur J Obstet Gynecol Reprod Biol 125(2):176, 2006
Vendittelli F, Rivière O, Creen-Hébert C, et al: Is a breech presentation at term more frequent in women with a history of cesarean delivery? Am J Obstet Gynecol 198(5):521.e1, 2008
Vézina Y, Bujold E, Varin J, et al: Cesarean delivery after successful external cephalic version of breech presentation at term: a comparative study. Am J Obstet Gynecol 190:763, 2004
Vialle R, Piétin-Vialle C, Ilharreborde B, et al: Spinal cord injuries at birth: a multicenter review of nine cases. J Matern Fetal Neonatal Med 20(6):435, 2007
Weiniger CF, Ginosar Y, Elchalal U, et al: External cephalic version for breech presentation with or without spinal analgesia in nulliparous women at term. Obstet Gynecol 110:1343, 2007
Weiniger CF, Ginosar Y, Elchalal U, et al: Randomized controlled trial of external cephalic version in term multiparae with or without spinal analgesia. Br J Anaesth 104(5):613, 2010
Wessen A, Elowsson P, Axemo P, et al: The use of intravenous nitroglycerin for emergency cervico-uterine relaxation. Acta Anaesthesiol Scand 39:847, 1995
Wilcox CB, Nassar N, Roberts CL: Effectiveness of nifedipine tocolysis to facilitate external cephalic version: a systematic review. BJOG 118(4):423, 2011
Witkop CT, Zhang J, Sun W, et al: Natural history of fetal position during pregnancy and risk of nonvertex delivery. Obstet Gynecol 111(4):875, 2008
Whyte H, Hannah ME, Saigal S, et al: Outcomes of children at 2 years after planned cesarean birth versus planned vaginal birth for breech presentation at term: the International Randomized Term Breech Trial. Am J Obstet Gynecol 191(3):864, 2004

CHAPTER 29

Operative Vaginal Delivery

Operative deliveries are vaginal deliveries accomplished with the use of a vacuum device or forceps. Once either is applied to the fetal head, outward traction generates forces that augment maternal pushing to deliver the fetus vaginally. The most important function of both devices is traction. In addition, however, forceps may also be used for rotation, particularly from occiput transverse and posterior positions.

The precise frequency of operative vaginal delivery in the United States is unknown. According to the birth certificate data from the National Vital Statistics Report, forceps- or vacuum-assisted vaginal delivery was used for 3.6 percent of births in the United States in 2010. According to Yeomans (2010), the vacuum-to-forceps delivery ratio is 4:1. Figure 29-1 depicts the decline in the rates of this type of delivery since 1990. In general, operative vaginal delivery attempts are successful. In the United States in 2006, only 0.4 percent of forceps trials and 0.8 percent of vacuum extraction attempts failed to result in vaginal delivery (Osterman, 2009).

INDICATIONS

If it is technically feasible and can be safely accomplished, termination of second-stage labor by operative vaginal delivery is indicated in any condition threatening the mother or fetus that is likely to be relieved by delivery. Some fetal indications for operative vaginal delivery include nonreassuring fetal heart rate pattern and premature placental separation. In the past, forceps delivery was believed to be somewhat protective of the fragile preterm infant head. Subsequent studies, however, reported no significant differences in outcomes for neonates who weighed 500 to 1500 g between those delivered spontaneously and those delivered by outlet forceps (Fairweather, 1981; Schwartz, 1983).

Some maternal indications include heart disease, pulmonary injury or compromise, intrapartum infection, and certain neurological conditions. The most common are exhaustion and prolonged second-stage labor. For nulliparas, the latter is defined as > 3 hours with or > 2 hours without regional analgesia (American College of Obstetricians and Gynecologists, 2012). In parous women, it is defined as > 2 hours with and > 1 hour without regional analgesia.

Operative vaginal delivery should generally be performed from either a low or outlet station. Additionally, forceps or vacuum delivery generally should not be used *electively* until the criteria for an outlet delivery have been met. In these circumstances, operative vaginal delivery is a simple and safe operation, although with some risk of maternal lower reproductive tract injury (Yancey, 1991). Moreover, there is no evidence that use of prophylactic operative delivery is beneficial in the otherwise normal delivery.

CLASSIFICATION AND PREREQUISITES

The American College of Obstetricians and Gynecologists (2012) classifies operative vaginal deliveries as summarized in Table 29-1. It emphasizes that the two most important discriminators of risk for both mother and infant are station and rotation. Station is measured in centimeters, –5 to 0 to +5. Zero station reflects a line drawn between the

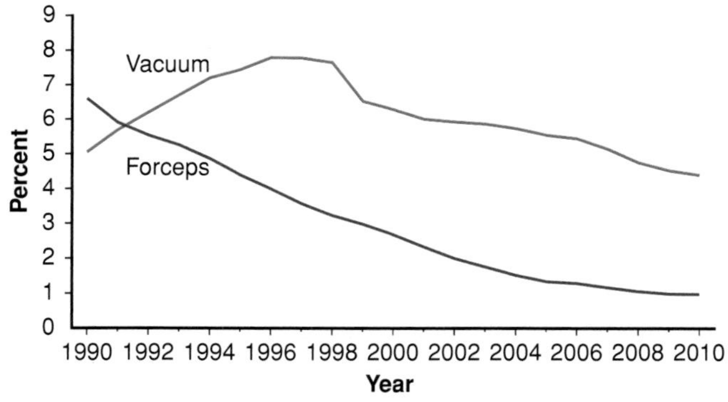

FIGURE 29-1 Decline in operative vaginal delivery rates, 1990–2010. (From Martin, 2012.)

ischial spines. Deliveries are categorized as outlet, low, and midpelvic procedures. High forceps, in which instruments are applied above 0 station, have no place in contemporary obstetrics.

TABLE 29-1. Operative Vaginal Delivery Prerequisites and Classification According to Station and Rotation[a]

Procedure	Criteria
Outlet forceps	• Scalp is visible at the introitus without separating the labia • Fetal skull has reached pelvic floor • Fetal head is at or on perineum • Sagittal suture is in anteroposterior diameter or right or left occiput anterior or posterior position, and • Rotation does not exceed 45 degrees
Low forceps (2 types)	Leading point of fetal skull is at station ≥ +2 cm, and not on the pelvic floor, and: a) Rotation is 45 degrees or less, *or* b) Rotation is greater than 45 degrees
Midforceps	Station is between 0 and +2 cm
High	Not included in classification
Prerequisites	
Experienced operator	
Engaged head	
Ruptured membranes	
Vertex presentation[b]	
Completely dilated cervix	
Precisely assessed fetal head position	
Cephalopelvic disproportion not suspected	
No fetal coagulopathy or bone demineralization disorder	

[a]Classification for the vacuum delivery system is the same as for forceps except that vacuum is used for traction but not rotation.
[b]Forceps, but not vacuum extractor, may be used for delivery of a face presentation with mentum anterior.

Once station and rotation are assessed, there are several prerequisites for operative vaginal delivery (see Table 29-1). In addition and specific to vacuum extraction, fetuses should be at least 34 weeks gestational age, and although infrequently used in the United States, fetal scalp blood sampling should not have been recently performed.

Regional analgesia or general anesthesia is preferable for low forceps or midpelvic procedures, although pudendal blockade may prove adequate for outlet forceps. Before operative vaginal delivery, the bladder should also be emptied to provide additional pelvic space and minimize bladder trauma.

MORBIDITY

In general, a higher station and/or greater degrees of rotation increase the chance of maternal or fetal injury. In the discussion of operative vaginal delivery, morbidity is most properly compared with morbidity from cesarean delivery, and not with that from spontaneous vaginal delivery. This is because the alternative to indicated operative vaginal delivery is cesarean delivery. As examples, postpartum uterine infection and pelvic cellulitis are more frequent, and often more severe, in women following cesarean delivery compared with that following operative vaginal delivery (Robertson, 1990). Moreover, in a study of more than 1 million births, Spiliopoulos and associates (2011) reported cesarean delivery, but not operative vaginal delivery, as a risk for peripartum hysterectomy.

Maternal Morbidity

Lacerations

The very conditions that lead to indications for operative vaginal delivery also increase the need for episiotomy and the likelihood of lacerations (de Leeuw, 2008). That said, operative vaginal delivery is associated with higher rates of third- and fourth-degree lacerations as well as vaginal wall and cervical lacerations (Hamilton, 2011; Hirayama, 2012; Landy, 2011). These appear to occur more frequently with forceps compared with vacuum extraction, and especially if there is a midline episiotomy (Kudish, 2006; O'Mahony, 2010). Hagadorn-Freathy and coworkers (1991) reported a 13-percent rate of third- and fourth-degree episiotomy extensions and vaginal lacerations for outlet forceps, 22 percent for low forceps with less than 45-degree rotation, 44 percent for low forceps with more than 45-degree rotation, and 37 percent for midforceps deliveries.

In an effort to lower rates of third- and fourth-degree lacerations, and coincident with overall efforts to reduce routine episiotomy use, many advocate only indicated episiotomy with operative vaginal delivery. For example, Ecker and colleagues (1997) reported a significant decrease in the episiotomy rate with both forceps—96 to 30 percent—as well as vacuum—89 to 39 percent—deliveries from 1984 to 1994. During this time, there was a decrease in fourth-degree but no change in third-degree lacerations. If episiotomy is required, several studies have reported a protective effect from mediolateral episiotomy against these more extensive perineal lacerations (de Leeuw, 2008; de Vogel, 2012; Hirsch, 2008). But as discussed in Chapter 27 (p. 551), this is balanced against the additional potential morbidity compared with a midline episiotomy. Early disarticulation of forceps and cessation of maternal pushing during disarticulation can also be protective. Last, these injuries are more common with operative vaginal delivery from an occiput posterior position (Damron, 2004). Thus, manual or forceps rotation from occiput posterior to occiput anterior position and then subsequent operative vaginal delivery may decrease lower-reproductive-tract injury.

Pelvic Floor Disorders

This term encompasses urinary incontinence, anal incontinence, and pelvic organ prolapse. Operative vaginal delivery has been suggested as a possible risk for each of these. Proposed mechanisms include structural compromise and/or pelvic floor denervation secondary to forces exerted during delivery.

Urinary retention and bladder dysfunction are often short-term effects of forceps and vacuum deliveries (Mulder, 2012). Importantly, episiotomy and epidural analgesia, both common associates of operative vaginal delivery, are also identified risks for urinary retention. Symptoms are brief and typically resolve with 24 to 48 hours of passive catheter bladder drainage.

Regarding more sustained urinary dysfunction, parity and specifically vaginal delivery are known risk factors for urinary incontinence (Gyhagen, 2013; Rortveit, 2003). And, a few studies show a greater attributable risk with operative vaginal delivery (Baydock, 2009; Handa, 2011). But, many studies do not support an increased risk compared with vaginal delivery alone (Handa, 2012; Leijonhufvud, 2011; MacArthur, 2006; Thom, 2011).

Evidence linking anal incontinence with operative vaginal delivery is conflicting. Some studies show that anal sphincter disruption caused by higher-order episiotomy, but not delivery mode, is the main etiological factor strongly associated with anal incontinence (Baud, 2011; Bols, 2010; Evers, 2012; Nygaard, 1997). In contrast, others directly link operative vaginal delivery with this complication (MacArthur, 2005; Pretlove, 2008). But, these studies may not be incongruous as operative vaginal delivery, as previously discussed, is associated with increased rates of higher-order episiotomy. Importantly, several studies and reviews have not found cesarean delivery to be protective for anal incontinence (Nelson, 2010).

Last, evidence linking pelvic organ prolapse with operative vaginal delivery also shows mixed results (Gyhagen, 2013; Handa, 2011). Interestingly, Glazener and associates (2013) evaluated women 12 years after delivery by means of a symptom questionnaire and physical examination. Complaints of prolapse *symptoms* were linked to operative vaginal delivery, but true *objective measurement of prolapse* showed a protective effect from this delivery mode compared with vaginal delivery alone.

Perinatal Morbidity

Acute Perinatal Injuries

These are more frequent with operative vaginal deliveries than with cesarean delivery or spontaneous vaginal delivery alone. Although these may be seen with either method, they are more commonly seen with vacuum extraction. Some injuries include cephalohematoma, subgaleal hemorrhage, retinal hemorrhage, neonatal jaundice secondary to these hemorrhages, shoulder dystocia, clavicular fracture, and scalp lacerations. Cephalohematoma and subgaleal hemorrhage are both extracranial lesions described in Chapter 33 (p. 646).

In 1998, the Food and Drug Administration issued a Public Health Advisory regarding the possible association of vacuum-assisted delivery with serious fetal complications, including death. In response, the American College of Obstetricians and Gynecologists (1998) issued a Committee Opinion recommending the continued use of vacuum-assisted delivery devices when appropriate. At that time, they estimated that there was approximately one adverse event per 45,455 vacuum extractions per year.

In contrast, forceps-assisted vaginal delivery has higher rates of facial nerve injury, brachial plexus injury, depressed skull fracture, and corneal abrasion (Demissie, 2004; Dupuis, 2005; American College of Obstetricians and Gynecologists, 2012). And while some studies have associated vacuum extraction with higher rates of intracranial hemorrhage, others show similar rates with either of the two methods (Towner, 1999; Wen, 2001; Werner, 2011).

As a group, if operative vaginal delivery is compared with cesarean delivery, rates of extracranial hematoma, skull fracture, facial nerve or brachial plexus injury, retinal hemorrhage, and facial or scalp laceration are lower with cesarean delivery, and shoulder dystocia is eliminated. Importantly, however, fetal acidemia rates are not increased with operative vaginal delivery (Contag, 2010; Walsh, 2013). Intracranial hemorrhage rates are similar among infants delivered by vacuum extraction, forceps, or cesarean delivery during labor (Towner, 1999). But, these rates are higher than among those delivered spontaneously or by cesarean delivery before labor. These authors suggest that the common risk factor for intracranial hemorrhage is abnormal labor. Werner and associates (2011), in their evaluation of more than 150,000 singleton deliveries, reported that forceps-assisted delivery was associated with fewer total neurological complications compared with vacuum-assisted or cesarean delivery. However, as a subset, subdural hemorrhage was significantly more frequent in both operative vaginal delivery cohorts compared with infants in the cesarean delivery group.

Reports of neonatal morbidity rates compared between midforceps and cesarean delivery are conflicting. In the study by Towner and colleagues (1999), similar risks were reported for intracranial hemorrhage. Bashore and associates (1990) observed comparable Apgar scores, cord blood acid-base values, neonatal intensive care unit admission, and birth trauma between these two. In another study, however, Robertson and coworkers (1990) reported significantly higher rates of these adverse outcomes in the midforceps group. And Hagadorn-Freathy and colleagues (1991) reported an increased risk for facial nerve palsy—9 percent—with midforceps delivery.

Mechanisms of Acute Injury

In general, with operative vaginal delivery, the types of fetal injury can usually be explained by the forces exerted. In cases of cephalohematoma or subgaleal hemorrhage, suction and perhaps rotation during vacuum extraction may lead to a primary vessel laceration (Fig. 33-1, p. 647). Intracranial hemorrhage may result from skull fracture and vessel laceration or from vessel laceration alone due to exerted forces. With facial nerve palsy, one of the forceps blades may compress the nerve against the facial bones (Duval, 2009; Falco, 1990). The higher rates of shoulder dystocia seen with vacuum extraction may result from the angle of traction. With the vacuum, this angle creates vector forces that actually pull the anterior shoulder into the symphysis pubis (Caughey, 2005). To explain brachial plexus injury, Towner and Ciotti (2007) proposed that as the fetal head descends down the birth canal, the shoulders may stay above the pelvic inlet. Thus, similar to shoulder dystocia at the symphysis, this "shoulder dystocia at the pelvic inlet" is overcome by traction forces but with concomitant stretch on the brachial plexus.

Long-Term Infant Morbidity

Evidence regarding long-term neurodevelopmental outcomes in children delivered by operative vaginal delivery is reassuring. Seidman and colleagues (1991) evaluated more than 52,000 Israeli Defense Forces draftees at age 17 years and found that regardless of delivery mode, there were similar rates of physical or cognitive impairments. Wesley and associates (1992) noted similar intelligence scores among 5-year-olds following spontaneous, forceps, or vacuum deliveries. Murphy and coworkers (2004) found no association between forceps delivery and epilepsy in a cohort of 21,441 adults. In their epidemiological review, O'Callaghan and colleagues (2011) found no association between cerebral palsy and operative vaginal delivery. A prospective study by Bahl and associates (2007) included children of 264 women who underwent operative delivery. Their incidence of neurodevelopmental morbidity was similar in those undergoing successful forceps delivery, failed forceps with cesarean delivery, or cesarean delivery without forceps.

Data regarding midforceps deliveries are for the most part reassuring. Broman and coworkers (1975) reported that infants delivered by midforceps had slightly higher intelligence scores at age 4 years compared with those of children delivered spontaneously. Using the same database, however, Friedman and associates (1977, 1984) analyzed intelligence assessments at or after age 7 years. They concluded that children delivered by midforceps had lower mean intelligence quotients compared with children delivered by outlet forceps. In yet another report from this same database, Dierker and colleagues (1986) compared long-term outcomes of children delivered by midforceps with those of children delivered by cesarean after dystocia. The strength of this study is the appropriateness of the control group. These investigators reported that delivery by midforceps was not associated with neurodevelopmental disability. Last, Nilsen (1984) evaluated 18-year-old men and found that those delivered by Kielland forceps had higher intelligence scores than those delivered spontaneously, by vacuum extraction, or by cesarean. As discussed on page 582, Burke and coworkers (2012) reported 144 cases of attempted Kielland forceps rotation and described minimal morbidity.

TRIAL OF OPERATIVE VAGINAL DELIVERY

If an attempt to perform an operative vaginal delivery is expected to be difficult, then it should be considered a trial. Delivery is conducted preferably in an operating room equipped and staffed for immediate cesarean delivery. If forceps cannot be satisfactorily applied, then the procedure is stopped and either vacuum extraction or cesarean delivery is performed. With the former, if there is no descent with traction, the trial should be abandoned and cesarean delivery performed.

With such caveats, cesarean delivery after an attempt at operative vaginal delivery was not associated with adverse neonatal outcomes if there was a reassuring fetal heart rate tracing (Alexander, 2009). A similar study evaluated 122 women who had a trial of midcavity forceps or vacuum extraction in a setting with full preparations for cesarean delivery (Lowe, 1987). Investigators found no significant difference in immediate neonatal or maternal morbidity compared with that of 42 women delivered for similar indications by cesarean but without such a trial. Conversely, in 61 women who had "unexpected" vacuum or forceps failure in which there was no prior preparation for immediate cesarean delivery, neonatal morbidity was higher.

Factors associated with operative delivery failure are persistent occiput posterior position, absence of regional or general anesthesia, and birthweight > 4000 g (Ben-Haroush, 2007). In general, to avert morbidity with failed forceps or vacuum delivery, the American College of Obstetricians and Gynecologists (2012) cautions that these trials should be attempted only if the clinical assessment is highly suggestive of a successful outcome. We also emphasize proper training.

Sequential instrumentation most frequently involves an attempt at vacuum extraction followed by one with forceps. This most likely stems from the higher completion rate with forceps compared with vacuum extraction noted earlier (p. 574). There is no evidence to justify this practice, as it significantly increases risks for fetal trauma (Dupuis, 2005; Murphy, 2001; Gardella, 2001). Because of these adverse outcomes, the American College of Obstetricians and Gynecologists (2012) recommends against the sequential use of instruments unless there is a "compelling and justifiable reason."

TRAINING

As the rate of operative vaginal delivery has declined, so have opportunities for training. Fifteen years ago, Hankins and colleagues (1999) reported that fewer than half of residency directors expected proficiency with midforceps delivery. From the data shown in Figure 29-1, we, and others, would expect that number to be much lower today (Miller, 2014). In many programs, training in even low and outlet forceps procedures has reached critically low levels. For residents completing training in 2012, the Accreditation Council for Graduate Medical Education (2012) lists a median of only six forceps deliveries, and that for vacuum deliveries was 16.

Because traditional hands-on training has evolved, residency programs should have readily available skilled operators to teach these procedures by simulation as well as through actual cases (Spong, 2012). And, the effectiveness of simulation training has been reported (Bahl, 2009; Dupuis, 2006, 2009; Leslie, 2005). In one program, there were lowered rates of maternal and neonatal morbidity associated with operative vaginal delivery after the implementation of a formal education

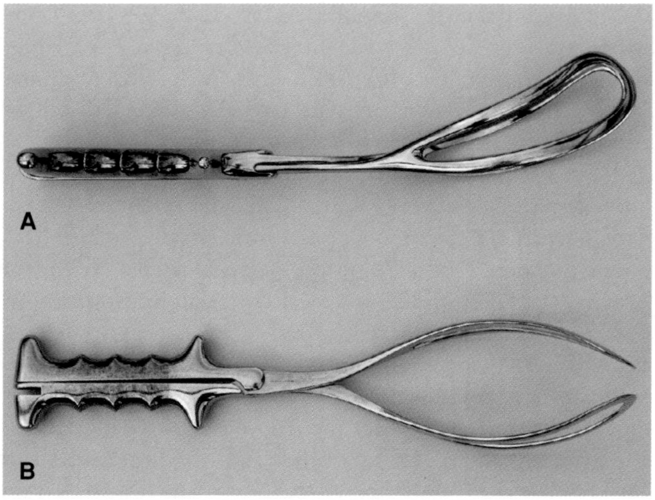

FIGURE 29-2 Elliot forceps. **A.** Note the ample pelvic curve in the blades. **B.** The cephalic curve, which accommodates the fetal head, is evident in the articulated blades. The fenestrated blade and the overlapping shank in front of the English-style lock characterize these forceps.

program that included a manikin and pelvic model (Cheong, 2004). In another, assignment of a labor and delivery attending with the specific goal to increase forceps delivery education led to a 59-percent increase in forceps-assisted vaginal delivery rates.

FORCEPS DELIVERY

Forceps Design

These instruments consist basically of two crossing branches. Each branch has four components: blade, shank, lock, and handle. Each blade has two curves: the outward cephalic curve conforms to the round fetal head, and the upward pelvic curve corresponds more or less to the axis of the birth canal. Some varieties have an opening within or a depression along the blade surface and are termed *fenestrated* or *pseudofenestrated*, respectively (Fig. 29-2). These blade modifications permit a firmer grasp of the fetal head, but at the expense of increased blade thickness, which may increase vaginal trauma. In general, Simpson or Elliot forceps, with their fenestrated blades, are used to deliver a fetus with a molded head, as is common in nulliparous women. The Tucker-McLane forceps have thin smooth blades and are often used for a fetus with a rounded head, which is more characteristic in multiparas (Fig. 29-3). In most situations, however, any of these are appropriate.

The blades are connected to the handles by shanks. The common method of articulation, the English lock, consists of a socket located on the shank at the junction with the handle, into which fits a socket similarly located on the opposite shank (see Fig. 29-3). A sliding lock is used in some forceps, such as Kielland forceps (Fig. 29-4).

Forceps Blade Application and Delivery

Forceps blades grasp the head and are applied according to fetal head position. If the head is in an occiput anterior position, two or more fingers of the right hand are introduced inside the left posterior portion of the vulva and then into the vagina beside the fetal head. The handle of the left branch is grasped between the thumb and two fingers of the left hand (Fig. 29-5). The blade tip is then gently passed into the vagina between the fetal head and the palmar surface of the fingers of the right hand (Fig. 29-6). For application of the right blade, two or more fingers of the left hand are introduced into the right posterior portion of the vagina to serve as a guide for the right blade. This blade is held in the right hand and introduced into the vagina as described for the left blade. After positioning, the branches are articulated (Fig. 29-7). If the head is positioned in a left occiput anterior or right occiput anterior position, then the lower of the two blades is typically placed first.

The blades are constructed so that their cephalic curve is closely adapted to the sides of the fetal head. The biparietal

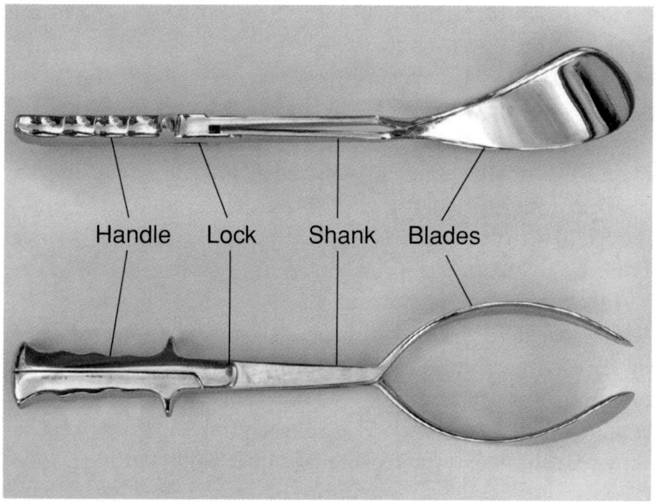

FIGURE 29-3 Tucker-McLane forceps. The blade is solid, and the shank is narrow.

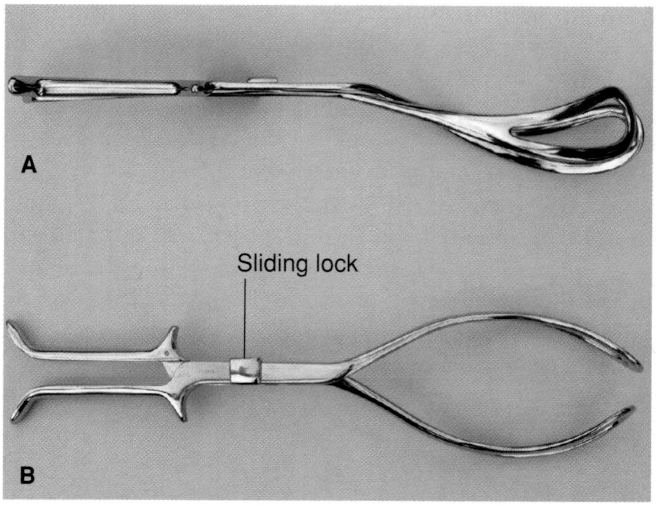

FIGURE 29-4 Kielland forceps. The characteristic features are minimal pelvic curvature **(A)**, sliding lock **(B)**, and light weight.

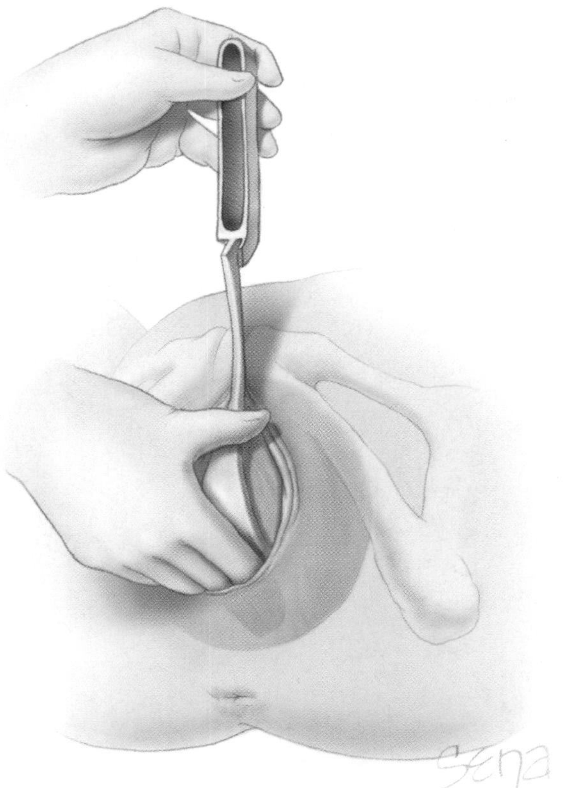

FIGURE 29-5 The left handle of the forceps is held in the left hand. The blade is introduced into the left side of the pelvis between the fetal head and the fingers of the operator's right hand.

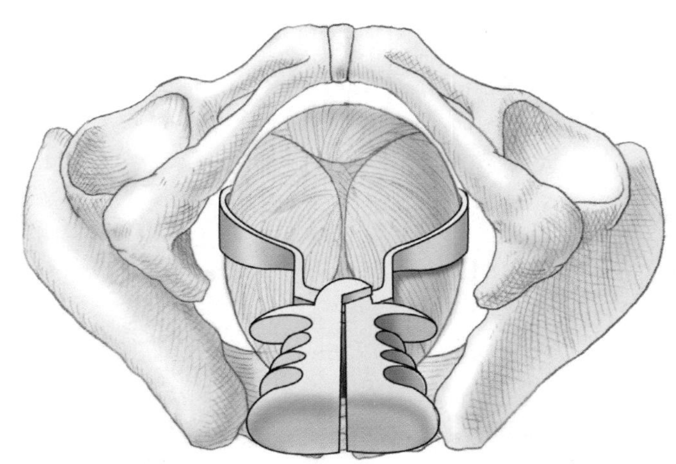

FIGURE 29-7 The vertex is now occiput anterior, and the forceps are symmetrically placed and articulated.

diameter of the fetal head corresponds to the greatest distance between appropriately applied blades. Consequently, the fetal head is perfectly grasped only when the long axis of the blades corresponds to the occipitomental diameter. These diameters are depicted in Figure 7-12 (p. 140). As a result, most of the blade lies over the face. If the fetus is in an occiput anterior position, then the concave arch of the blades is directed toward the sagittal suture. If the fetus is in an occiput posterior position, then the concave arch is directed toward the fetal face.

For the occiput anterior position, appropriately applied blades are equidistant from the sagittal suture, and each blade is equidistant from its adjacent lambdoidal suture. In the occiput posterior position, the blades are equidistant from the midline of the face and brow. Also for occiput posterior position, blades are symmetrically placed relative to the sagittal suture and each coronal suture. Applied in this way, the forceps should not slip, and traction may be applied most advantageously. With most forceps, if one blade is applied over the brow and the other over the occiput, the instrument cannot be locked, or if locked, the blades will slip off when traction is applied (Fig. 29-8). For these reasons, the forceps must be applied directly to the sides of the fetal head along the occipitomental diameter.

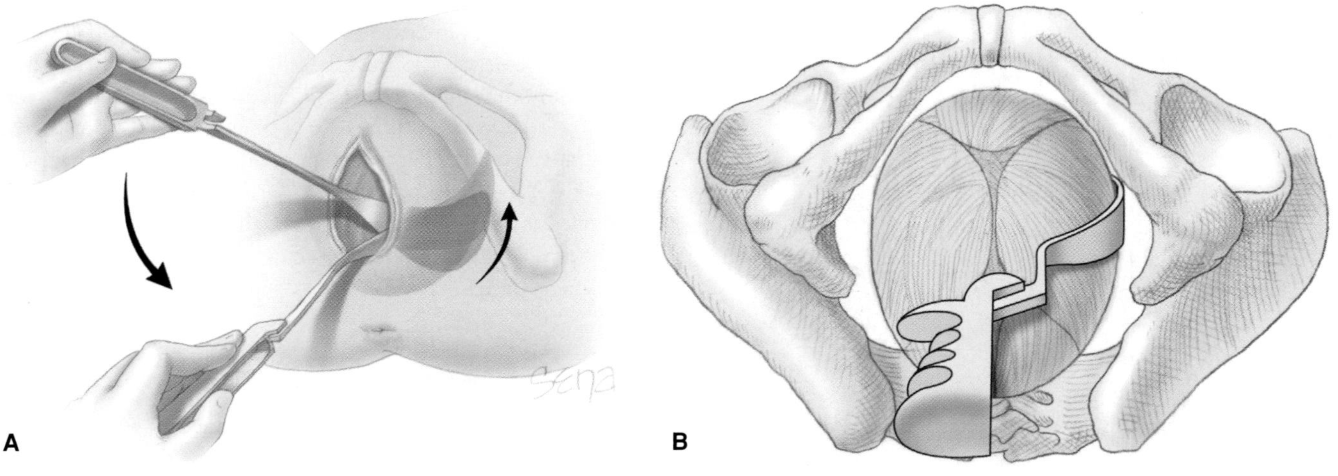

A B

FIGURE 29-6 A. Continued insertion of the left blade. The right hand, not shown here, guides the blade during placement. Note the arc of the handles as they rotate to be applied to the mother's left. **B.** First blade in place. An assistant's hand can hold this handle in place as the second blade is applied.

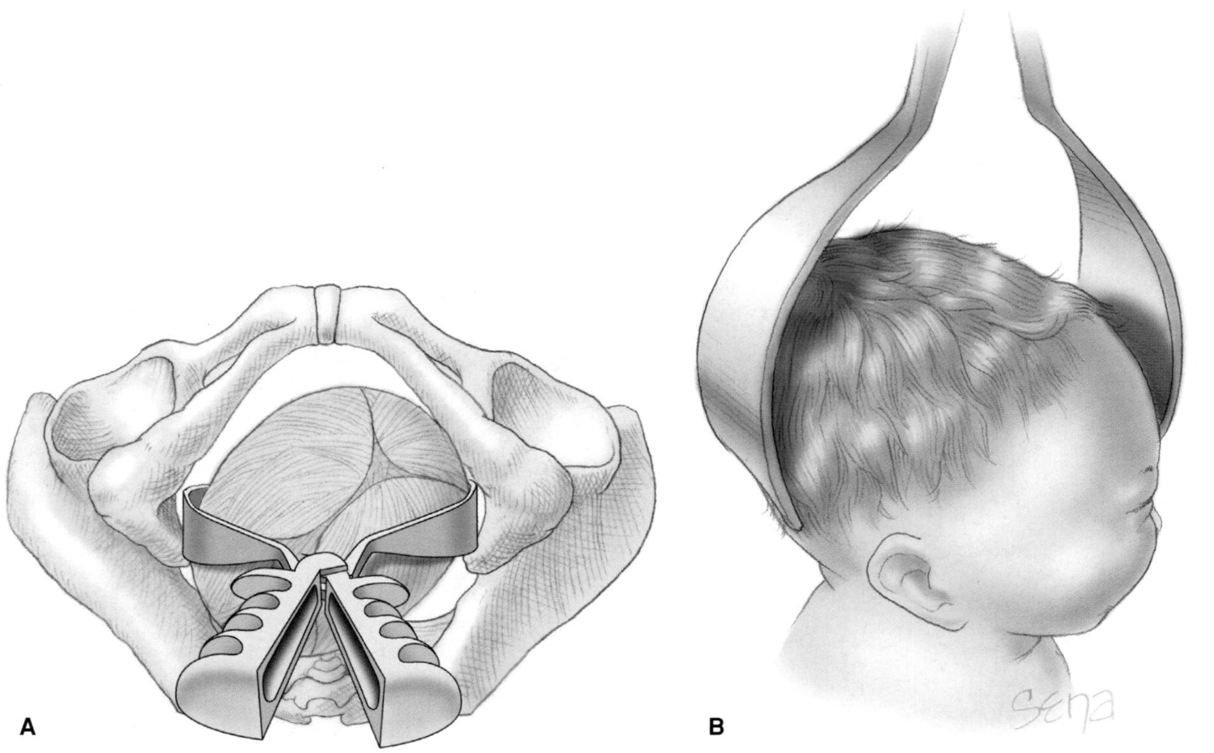

FIGURE 29-8 Incorrect application of forceps. **A.** One blade over the occiput and the other over the brow. Forceps cannot be locked. **B.** With incorrect placement, blades tend to slip off with traction.

If necessary, rotation to occiput anterior is performed before traction is applied (Fig. 29-9). When it is certain that the blades are placed satisfactorily, then gentle, intermittent, horizontal traction is exerted concurrent with maternal efforts until the perineum begins to bulge (Fig. 29-10). With traction, as the vulva is distended by the occiput, an episiotomy may be performed if indicated. Additional horizontal traction is applied, and the handles are gradually elevated, eventually pointing almost directly upward as the parietal bones emerge (Figs. 29-11 and 29-12). As the handles are raised, the head is extended. During the birth of the head, spontaneous delivery should be simulated as closely as possible.

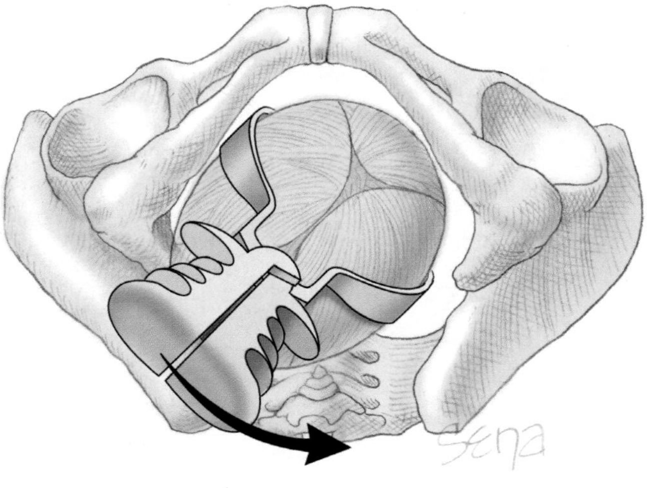

FIGURE 29-9 Forceps have been locked. Vertex is rotated from left occiput anterior to occiput anterior (*arrow*).

The force produced by the forceps on the fetal skull is a complex function of both traction and compression by the forceps, as well as friction produced by maternal tissues. It is impossible to ascertain the amount of force exerted by forceps for an individual patient. Traction should therefore be intermittent, and the head should be allowed to recede between contractions, as in spontaneous labor. Except when urgently indicated, as in severe fetal bradycardia, delivery should be sufficiently slow, deliberate, and gentle to prevent undue head compression. It is preferable to apply traction only with each uterine contraction. Maternal pushing will augment these efforts.

After the vulva has been well distended by the head, the delivery may be completed in several ways. Some clinicians keep the forceps in place to control the advance of the head. If done, however, the thickness of the blades adds to vulvar distention, thus increasing the likelihood of laceration or necessitating a large episiotomy. To prevent this, the forceps may be removed, and delivery is then completed by maternal pushing (Fig. 29-13). Importantly, if blades are disarticulated and removed too early, the head may recede and lead to a prolonged delivery. Pushing in some cases may be aided by addition of the modified Ritgen maneuver.

Delivery of Occiput Posterior Positions

Prompt delivery may at times become necessary when the small occipital fontanel is directed toward one of the sacroiliac synchondroses, that is, in right occiput or left occiput posterior positions. When delivery is required in either instance, the head is often imperfectly flexed. In some cases, when the hand is introduced into the vagina to locate the posterior ear, the occiput rotates spontaneously toward the anterior, indicating that manual rotation of the fetal head might easily be accomplished.

With manual rotation, an open hand is inserted into the vagina. The palm straddles the sagittal suture of the fetal head. The operator's fingers wrap around one side of the fetal face and thumb extends along the other side. If the occiput is in a right posterior position, rotation is clockwise to bring it to a right occiput anterior or to a straight occiput anterior position. With left occiput posterior position, rotation is counterclockwise. If resistance is met during rotation, the head may be slightly elevated but should not be disengaged, as this risks cord prolapse. After the occiput has reached the anterior position, labor may be allowed to continue, or forceps can be applied. Le Ray and colleagues (2007, 2013) reported a success rate of greater than 90 percent with manual rotation.

Manual rotations are most easily completed in multiparas. If manual rotation cannot be easily accomplished, application of forceps blades to the head in the posterior position and delivery from the

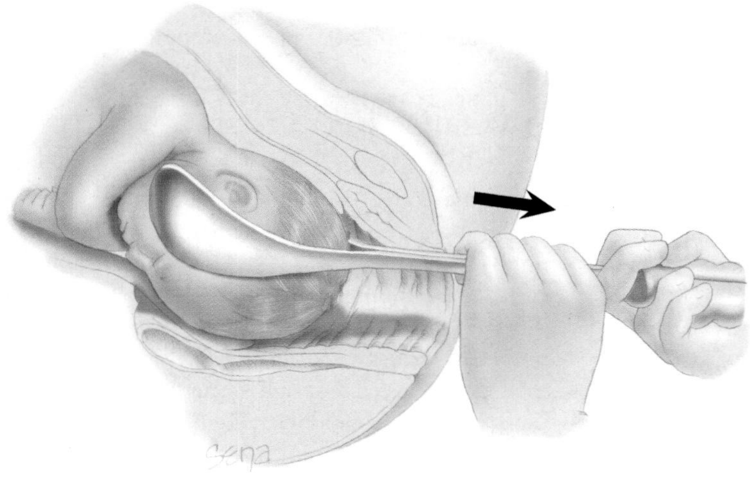

FIGURE 29-10 Occiput anterior. Delivery by low forceps. The direction of gentle traction for delivery of the head is indicated (*arrow*).

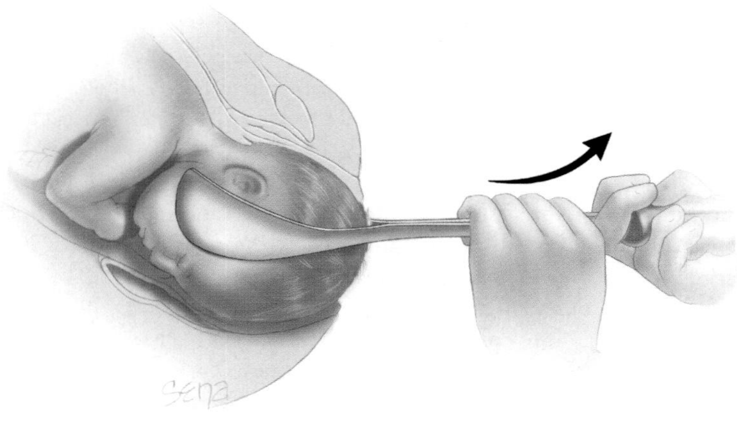

FIGURE 29-11 Upward arching traction (*arrow*) is used as the head is delivered.

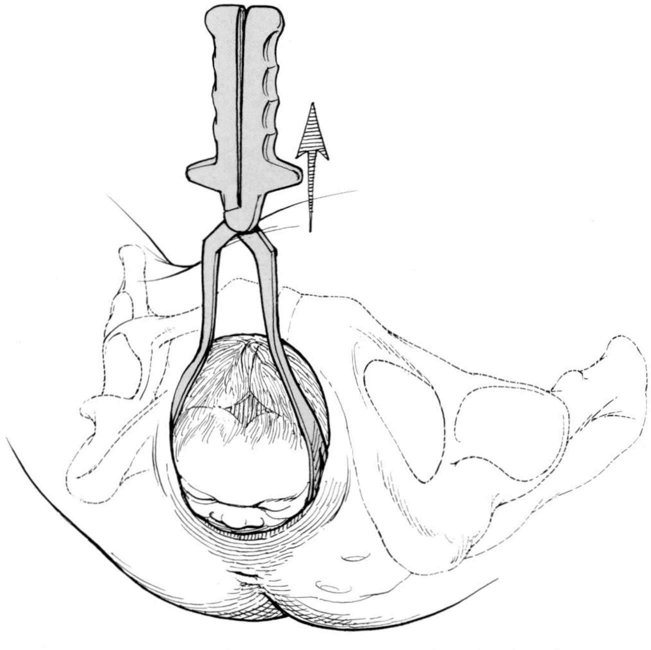

FIGURE 29-12 Upward traction is continued as the head is delivered.

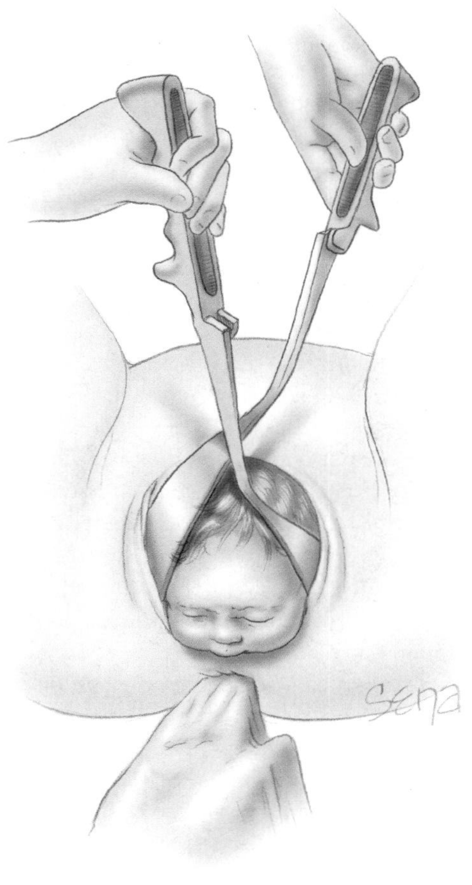

FIGURE 29-13 Forceps may be disarticulated as the head is delivered. Modified Ritgen maneuver may be used to complete delivery of the head.

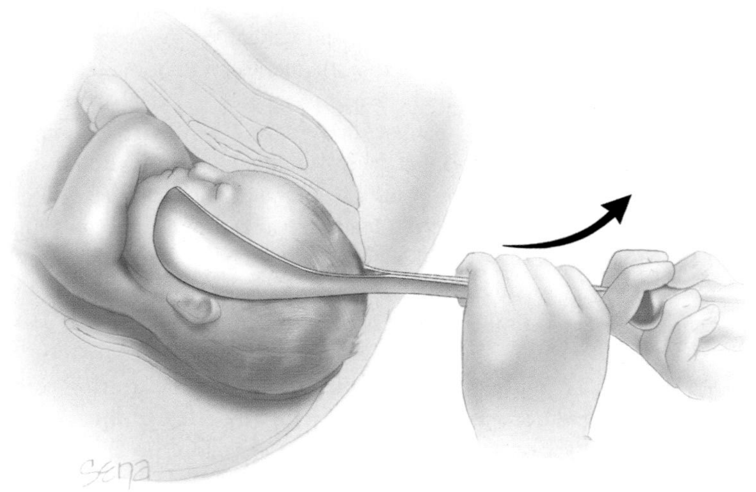

FIGURE 29-14 Outlet forceps delivery from an occiput posterior position. The head should be flexed after the bregma passes under the symphysis.

occiput posterior position may be the safest procedure (Fig. 29-14). In many cases, the cause of the persistent occiput posterior position and of the difficulty in accomplishing rotation is an anthropoid pelvis. This architecture opposes rotation and predisposes to posterior delivery (Fig. 2-20, p. 34).

With forceps delivery from an occiput posterior position, horizontal traction should be applied until the base of the nose is under the symphysis. The handles should then be slowly elevated until the occiput gradually emerges over the anterior margin of the perineum. Then, the forceps are directed in a downward motion, and the nose, mouth, and chin successively emerge from the vulva.

Occiput posterior delivery causes greater distention of the vulva, and a large episiotomy may be needed. Pearl and associates (1993) reviewed 564 occiput posterior deliveries and compared them with 1068 occiput anterior deliveries as controls. The occiput posterior group had a higher incidence of severe perineal lacerations and extensive episiotomy compared with the occiput anterior group. From The Netherlands, de Leeuw and associates (2008) studied more than 28,500 operative vaginal deliveries and reported similar findings. Consequences of these perineal tears are discussed in Chapter 27 (p. 536). Also, infants delivered from the occiput posterior position had a higher incidence of Erb and facial nerve palsies, 1 and 2 percent, respectively, than did those delivered from the occiput anterior position. As expected, rotations to occiput anterior ultimately decrease perineal delivery trauma (Bradley, 2013).

For rotations from the occiput posterior position, Tucker-McLane, Simpson, or Kielland forceps may be used. The oblique occiput may be rotated 45 degrees to the posterior position, or 135 degrees to the anterior position. If rotation is performed with Tucker-McLane or Simpson forceps, the head must be flexed, but this is not necessary with Kielland forceps because they have a less pronounced pelvic curve. In rotating the occiput anteriorly with Tucker-McLane or Simpson forceps, the pelvic curvature, originally directed upward, is, at the completion of rotation, inverted and directed posteriorly. Attempted delivery with the instrument in this position is likely to cause vaginal sulcus tears and sidewall lacerations. To avoid such trauma, it is essential to remove and reapply the instrument as previously described for occiput anterior delivery.

Rotation from Occiput Transverse Positions

When the occiput is obliquely anterior, it gradually rotates spontaneously to the symphysis pubis as traction is exerted. When it is directly transverse, however, a rotary motion of the forceps is required. When the occiput is directed toward the patient's left, rotation counterclockwise from the left side toward the midline is required. For right occiput transverse positions, clockwise rotation is required.

With experienced operators, high success rates with minimal maternal morbidity can be achieved (Burke, 2012; Stock, 2013). Either standard forceps, such as Simpson, or specialized forceps, such as Kielland, are employed. The latter have a sliding lock and almost no pelvic curve (see Fig. 29-4). On each handle is a small knob that indicates the direction of the occiput. The station of the fetal head must be accurately ascertained to be at, or preferably below, the level of the ischial spines, especially in the presence of extreme molding.

Kielland described two methods of applying the anterior blade. The first is the wandering or gliding method in which the anterior blade is introduced at the side of the pelvis over the brow or face. The blade is then arched around the brow or face to an anterior position, with the handle of the blade held close to the opposite maternal buttock throughout the maneuver. The second blade is introduced posteriorly and the branches are locked.

The second is the classic application in which the anterior blade is introduced first with its cephalic curve directed upward, curving under the symphysis. After it has been advanced far enough toward the upper vagina, it is turned on its axis through 180 degrees to adapt the cephalic curvature to the head. For a more detailed description of Kielland forceps procedures, see the second edition of *Operative Obstetrics* (Gilstrap, 2002).

Application of forceps to an occiput transverse positioned fetus in these women with a platypelloid pelvis should not be attempted until the fetal head has reached or approached the pelvic floor. Regardless of the original position of the head, after rotation, delivery eventually is accomplished by exerting traction downward until the occiput appears at the vulva. After this, the rest of the operation is completed as previously described for occiput anterior delivery.

Face Presentation Forceps Delivery

With a mentum anterior face presentation, forceps can be used to effect vaginal delivery. The blades are applied to the sides of the head along the occipitomental diameter, with the pelvic curve directed toward the neck. Downward traction is exerted until the chin appears under the symphysis. Then, by an upward movement, the face is slowly extracted, with the nose, eyes, brow, and occiput appearing in succession over the anterior margin of the perineum. Forceps should not be applied to the mentum posterior presentation because vaginal delivery is impossible except in very small fetuses.

VACUUM EXTRACTION

Vacuum Extractor Design

With vacuum delivery technique, suction is created within a cup placed on the fetal scalp such that traction on the cup aids fetal expulsion. In the United States, *vacuum extractor* is the preferred term for the devices shown in Figure 29-15, whereas in Europe it is commonly called a *ventouse*—from French, literally, "soft cup." Theoretical advantages of this tool compared with forceps include simpler requirements for precise positioning on the fetal head and avoidance of space-occupying blades within the vagina, thereby lowering maternal trauma rates.

As noted, vacuum devices contain a cup, shaft, handle, and vacuum generator. Vacuum cups may be metal, hard plastic, or soft plastic and may also differ in their shape, size, and reusability. In the United States, nonmetal cups are generally preferred, and there are two main types. The soft cup is a pliable funnel- or bell-shaped dome, whereas the rigid type has a firm flattened mushroom-shaped cup and circular ridge around the cup rim (Table 29-2). When compared, rigid mushroom cups generate significantly more traction force (Hofmeyr, 1990; Muise, 1993). With occiput posteriorly positioned heads or with asynclitism, the flatter cup also permits improved placement at the flexion point, which is typically less accessible with these head positions. The trade-off is that the flatter cups have higher scalp laceration rates. Thus, many manufacturers recommend soft bell cups for more straightforward occiput anterior deliveries. Rigid mushroom cups may be preferred for occiput posterior or transverse presentation or for asynclitism.

Several investigators have compared outcomes with various rigid and soft cups. Metal cups provide higher success rates

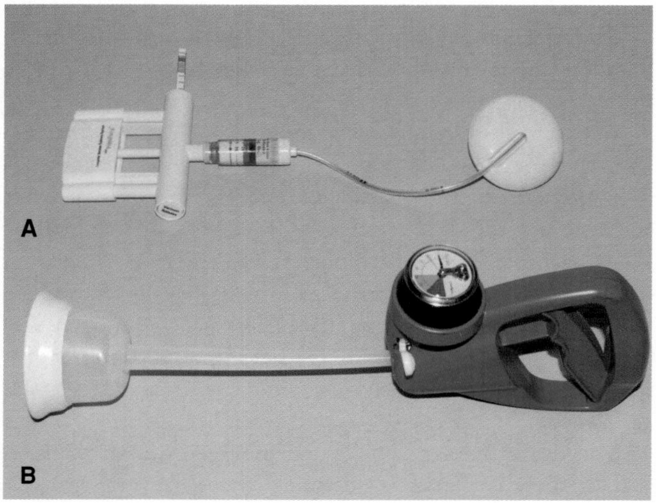

FIGURE 29-15 Vacuum delivery systems. **A.** The *Kiwi OmniCup* contains a handheld vacuum-generating pump, which is attached via flexible tubing to a rigid plastic mushroom cup. **B.** The *Mityvac Mystic II MitySoft Bell Cup* has a soft bell cup attached by a semirigid shaft to a handheld pump.

TABLE 29-2. Vacuum Cups for Operative Vaginal Delivery

Cup Style	Manufacturer
Soft Bell Cup	
GentleVac	OB Scientific
Kiwi ProCup	Clinical Innovations
Mityvac MitySoft Bell	CooperSurgical
Pearl Edge Bell Cup	CooperSurgical
Secure Cup	Utah Medical Products
Soft Touch	Utah Medical Products
Tender Touch	Utah Medical Products
Tender Touch Ultra	Utah Medical Products
Velvet Touch[a]	Utah Medical Products
Reusable vacuum delivery cup[a]	CooperSurgical
Rigid Mushroom Cup	
Flex Cup	Utah Medical Products
Mityvac M-Style	CooperSurgical
Super M-Style	CooperSurgical
Mityvac M-Select[b]	CooperSurgical
Kiwi OmniCup[b]	Clinical Innovations
Kiwi Omni-C Cup[c]	Clinical Innovations

[a]Reusable cups.
[b]Suitable for occiput posterior positions or asynclitism.
[c]For extractions through a hysterotomy incision during cesarean delivery.

but greater rates of scalp injuries, including cephalohematomas (O'Mahony, 2010). In another study, Kuit and coworkers (1993) found that the only advantage of the soft cups was a lower incidence of scalp injury. They reported a 14-percent episiotomy extension rate with both rigid and pliable cups. Associated perineal lacerations occurred with 16 percent of rigid cup extractions and 10 percent with the pliable cup. In a review, Vacca (2002) concluded that there were fewer scalp lacerations with the soft cup, but that the rate of cephalohematomas and subgaleal hemorrhage was similar between soft and rigid cups. Importantly, high-pressure vacuum generates large amounts of force regardless of the cup used (Duchon, 1998).

Aside from the cup, the shaft that connects the cup and handle may be flexible or semiflexible. Tubing-like flexible shafts may be preferred for occiput posterior or asynclitic presentation to permit better seating of the cup (see Fig. 29-15A). Last, the vacuum generator may be handheld and actuated by the operator or may be held and operated by an assistant.

Technique

An important step in vacuum extraction is proper cup placement over the *flexion point*. This pivot point maximizes traction, minimizes cup detachment, flexes but averts twisting of the fetal head, and delivers the smallest head diameter through the pelvic outlet. This improves success rates, lowers fetal scalp injury rates, and lessens perineal trauma because the smallest fetal head diameter distends the vulva (Baskett, 2008).

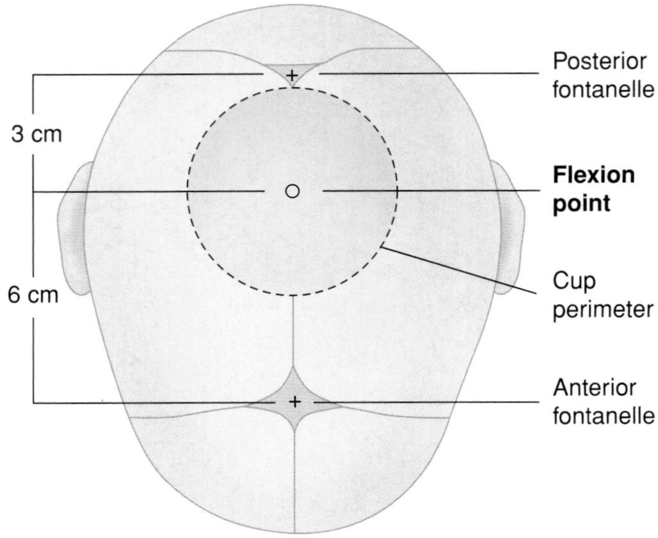

FIGURE 29-16 Drawing demonstrates correct cup placement at the flexion point. Along the sagittal suture, this spot lies 3 cm from the posterior fontanel and 6 cm from the anterior fontanel.

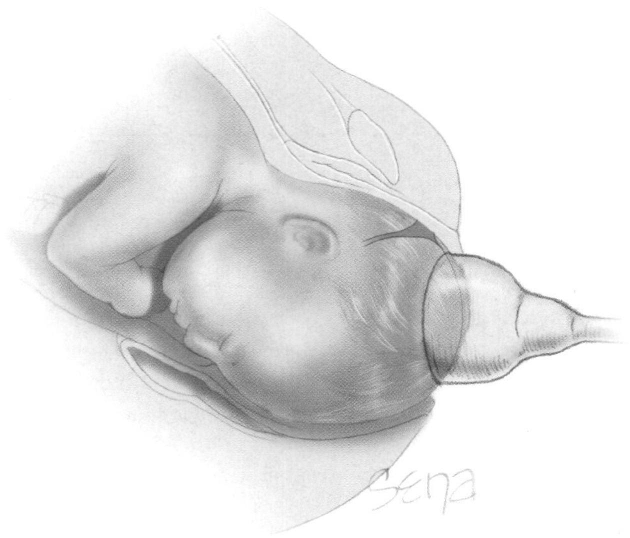

FIGURE 29-17 Cup placed before application of traction.

The flexion point is found along the sagittal suture, approximately 3 cm in front of the posterior fontanel and approximately 6 cm from the anterior fontanel. Because cup diameters range from 5 to 6 cm, when properly placed, the cup rim lies 3 cm from the anterior fontanel (Fig. 29-16). Placement of the cup more anteriorly on the fetal cranium—near the anterior fontanel—should be avoided as it leads to cervical spine extension during traction unless the fetus is small. Such placement also delivers a wider fetal head diameter through the vaginal opening. Last, asymmetrical placement relative to the sagittal suture may worsen asynclitism. For elective use, cup placement in occiput anterior positions is seldom difficult. In contrast, when the indication for delivery is failure to descend caused by occipital malposition—with or without asynclitism or deflexion—cup positioning can be difficult.

During cup placement, maternal soft tissue entrapment predisposes the mother to lacerations and virtually ensures cup dislodgement. Thus, the entire cup circumference should be palpated both before and after the vacuum has been created as well as prior to traction to exclude such entrapment. Gradual vacuum creation is advocated by some and is generated by increasing the suction in increments of 0.2 kg/cm^2 every 2 minutes until a total negative pressure of 0.8 kg/cm^2 is reached (Table 29-3). That said, other studies have shown that negative pressure can be increased to 0.8 kg/cm^2 in < 2 minutes without a significant difference in efficacy or in maternal and fetal outcomes (Suwannachat, 2011, 2012).

TABLE 29-3. Vacuum Pressure Conversions

mm Hg	cm Hg	inches Hg	lb/in^2	kg/cm^2
100	10	3.9	1.9	0.13
200	20	7.9	3.9	0.27
300	30	11.8	5.8	0.41
400	40	15.7	7.7	0.54
500	50	19.7	9.7	0.68
600	60	23.6	11.6	0.82

Once suction is created, the instrument handle is grasped, and traction is initiated (Fig. 29-17). Effort should be intermittent and coordinated with maternal expulsive efforts. Similar to forceps delivery, traction is usually directed initially downward, then progressively extended upward as the head emerges. Manual torque to the cup is avoided as it may cause cup displacement or cephalohematomas and with metal cups, "cookie-cutter"–type scalp lacerations. Thus, occiput anterior oblique positions are corrected not by rotation, but solely by downward outward traction. During pulls, the operator should place the nondominant hand within the vagina, with the thumb on the extractor cup and one or more fingers on the fetal scalp. So positioned, descent of the presenting part can be judged and the traction angle can be adjusted with head descent. In addition, the relationship of the cup edge to the scalp can be assessed to help detect cup separation.

Between contractions, some physicians will lower the suction levels to decrease rates of scalp injury, whereas others will maintain suction in cases of nonreassuring fetal heart tones to aid rapid delivery. No differences in maternal or fetal outcome could be demonstrated if the level of vacuum was decreased between contractions or if an effort was made to prevent fetal loss of station (Bofill, 1997). Once the head is extracted, the vacuum pressure is relieved, the cup removed, and the usual techniques to complete vaginal delivery are followed.

Vacuum extraction should be considered a trial. Without early and clear evidence of descent toward delivery, an alternative delivery approach should be considered. As a general guideline, progressive descent should accompany each traction attempt. Neither data nor consensus are available regarding the number of pulls required to effect delivery, the maximum number of cup "pop-offs" that can be tolerated, or optimal total duration of the procedure. Some manufacturers have recommendations regarding these in their instructional literature (Clinical Innovations, LLC, 2013; CooperSurgical, 2011).

During a vacuum extraction trial, cup dislodgement due to technical failure or less than optimal placement should not be equated with dislodgement under ideal conditions of exact cup placement and optimal vacuum maintenance. These cases may merit either additional attempts at placement or alternatively, a trial of forceps (Ezenagu, 1999; Williams, 1991). The least desirable cases are those in which traction without progress or multiple disengagements occur following correct cup application and appropriate traction. As with forceps procedures, there should be a willingness to abandon attempts at vacuum extraction if satisfactory progress is not made (American College of Obstetricians and Gynecologists, 2012).

REFERENCES

Accreditation Council for Graduate Medical Education: Obstetrics and Gynecology Case Logs. 2012. Available at: http://www.acgme.org/acgmeweb/Portals/0/ObGynNatData1112.pdf. Accessed April 13, 2013

Alexander JM, Leveno KJ, Hauth JC, et al: Failed operative vaginal delivery. Obstet Gynecol 114(5):1017, 2009

American College of Obstetricians and Gynecologists: Delivery by vacuum extraction. Committee Opinion No. 208, September 1998

American College of Obstetricians and Gynecologists: Operative vaginal delivery. Practice Bulletin No. 17, June 2000, Reaffirmed 2012

Bahl R, Murphy DJ, Strachan B: Qualitative analysis by interviews and video recordings to establish the components of a skilled low-cavity non-rotational vacuum delivery. BJOG 116(2):319, 2009

Bahl R, Patel RR, Swingler R, et al: Neurodevelopmental outcome at 5 years after operative delivery in the second stage of labor: a cohort study. Am J Obstet Gynecol 197:147, 2007

Bashore RA, Phillips WH Jr, Brinkman CR III: A comparison of the morbidity of midforceps and cesarean delivery. Am J Obstet Gynecol 162(6):1428, 1990

Baskett TF, Fanning CA, Young DC: et al: A prospective observational study of 1000 vacuum assisted deliveries with the OmniCup device. J Obstet Gynaecol Can 30(7):573, 2008

Baud D, Meyer S, Vial Y, et al: Pelvic floor dysfunction 6 years post-anal sphincter tear at the time of vaginal delivery. Int Urogynecol J 22(9):1127, 2011

Baydock SA, Flood C, Schulz JA, et al: Prevalence and risk factors for urinary and fecal incontinence four months after vaginal delivery. J Obstet Gynaecol Can 31(1):36, 2009

Ben-Haroush A, Melamed N, Kaplan B, et al: Predictors of failed operative vaginal delivery: a single-center experience. Am J Obstet Gynecol 197:308.e1, 2007

Bofill JA, Rust OA, Schorr SJ, et al: A randomized trial of two vacuum extraction techniques. Obstet Gynecol 89(5 Pt 1):758, 1997

Bols EM, Hendriks EJ, Berghmans BC, et al: A systematic review of etiological factors for postpartum fecal incontinence. Acta Obstet Gynecol Scand 89(3):302, 2010

Bradley MS, Kaminski RJ, Streitman DC, et al: Effect of rotation on perineal lacerations in forceps-assisted vaginal deliveries. Obstet Gynecol 122(1):132, 2013

Broman SH, Nichols PL, Kennedy WA: Preschool IQ: prenatal and early developmental correlates. Hillside, Lawrence Erlbaum Associates, 1975

Burke N, Field K, Mujahid F, et al: Use and safety of Kielland's forceps in current obstetric practice. Obstet Gynecol 120(4):766, 2012

Caughey AB, Sandberg PL, Zlatnik MG, et al: Forceps compared with vacuum. Rates of neonatal and maternal morbidity. Obstet Gynecol 106:908, 2005

Cheong YC, Abdullahi H, Lashen H, et al: Can formal education and training improve the outcome of instrumental delivery? Eur J Obstet Gynecol 113:139, 2004

Clinical Innovations, LLC: Kiwi complete vacuum delivery system instructions for use. Available at: http://www.clinicalinnovations.com/site_files/files/Kiwi%20IFU%20Rev%20F.pdf. Accessed November 19, 2013

Contag SA, Clifton RG, Bloom SL, et al: Neonatal outcomes and operative vaginal delivery versus cesarean delivery. Am J Perinatol 27(6):493, 2010

CooperSurgical: Mityvac vacuum assist delivery system directions for use. Trumbull, CooperSurgical, 2011

Damron DP, Capeless EL: Operative vaginal delivery: a comparison of forceps and vacuum for success rate and risk of rectal sphincter injury. Am J Obstet Gynecol 191:907, 2004

de Leeuw JW, de Wit C, Kuijken JP, et al: Mediolateral episiotomy reduces the risk for anal sphincter injury during operative vaginal delivery. BJOG 115:104, 2008

Demissie K, Rhoads GG, Smulian JC, et al: Operative vaginal delivery and neonatal and infant adverse outcomes: population based retrospective analysis. BMJ 329(7456):24, 2004

de Vogel J, van der Leeuw-van Beek A, Gietelink D, et al: The effect of a mediolateral episiotomy during operative vaginal delivery on the risk of developing obstetrical anal sphincter injuries. Am J Obstet Gynecol 206(5):404, 2012

Dierker LJ, Rosen MG, Thompson K, et al: Midforceps deliveries: long-term outcome of infants. Am J Obstet Gynecol 154:764, 1986

Duchon MA, DeMund MA, Brown RH: Laboratory comparison of modern vacuum extractors. Obstet Gynecol 72:155, 1998

Dupuis O, Moreau R, Pham MT: Assessment of forceps blade orientations during their placement using an instrumented childbirth simulator. BJOG 116(2):327, 2009

Dupuis O, Moreau R, Silveira R, et al: A new obstetric forceps for the training of junior doctors: a comparison of the spatial dispersion of forceps blade trajectories between junior and senior obstetricians. Am J Obstet Gynecol 194:1524, 2006

Dupuis O, Silveira R, Dupont C, et al: Comparison of "instrument-associated" and "spontaneous" obstetric depressed skull fractures in a cohort of 68 neonates. Am J Obstet Gynecol 192(1):165, 2005

Duval M, Daniel SJ: Facial nerve palsy in neonates secondary to forceps use. Arch Otolaryngol Head Neck Surg 123(7):634, 2009

Ecker JL, Tan WM, Bansal RK, et al: Is there a benefit to episiotomy at operative vaginal delivery? Observations over ten years in a stable population. Am J Obstet Gynecol 176:411, 1997

Evers EC, Blomquist JL, McDermott KC, et al: Obstetrical anal sphincter laceration and anal incontinence 5–10 years after childbirth. Am J Obstet Gynecol 207(5):425.e1, 2012

Ezenagu LC, Kakaria R, Bofill JA: Sequential use of instruments at operative vaginal delivery: is it safe? Am J Obstet Gynecol 180:1446, 1999

Fairweather D: Obstetric management and follow-up of the very low-birth-weight infant. J Reprod Med 26:387, 1981

Falco NA, Eriksson E: Facial nerve palsy in the newborn: incidence and outcome. Plast Reconstr Surg 85:1, 1990

Food and Drug Administration Public Health Advisory: Need for CAUTION When Using Vacuum Assisted Delivery Devices. 1998. Available at: http://www.fda.gov/MedicalDevices/Safety/AlertsandNotices/PublicHealthNotifications/ucm062295.htm. Accessed December 20, 2012

Friedman EA, Sachtleben MR, Bresky PA: Dysfunctional labor, 12. Long-term effects on the fetus. Am J Obstet Gynecol 127:779, 1977

Friedman EA, Sachtleben-Murray MR, Dahrouge D, et al: Long-term effects of labor and delivery on offspring: a matched-pair analysis. Am J Obstet Gynecol 150:941, 1984

Gardella C, Taylor M, Benedetti T, et al: The effect of sequential use of vacuum and forceps for assisted vaginal delivery on neonatal and maternal outcomes. Am J Obstet Gynecol 185(4): 896, 2001

Gilstrap LC III: Forceps delivery. In Gilstrap LC III, Cunningham FG, VanDorsten JP (eds): Operative Obstetrics, 2nd ed. New York, McGraw-Hill, 2002

Glazener C, Elders A, Macarthur C, et al: Childbirth and prolapse: long-term associations with the symptoms and objective measurement of pelvic organ prolapse. BJOG 120(2):161, 2013

Gyhagen M, Bullarbo M, Nielsen T, et al: The prevalence of urinary incontinence 20 years after childbirth: a national cohort study in singleton primiparae after vaginal or caesarean delivery. BJOG 120:144, 2013

Hagadorn-Freathy AS, Yeomans ER, Hankins GDV: Validation of the 1988 ACOG forceps classification system. Obstet Gynecol 77:356, 1991

Hamilton EF, Smith S, Yang L, et al: Third- and fourth-degree perineal lacerations: defining high-risk clinical clusters. Am J Obstet Gynecol 204(4):309.e1, 2011

Handa VL, Blomquist JL, Knoepp LR, et al: Pelvic floor disorders 5–10 years after vaginal or cesarean childbirth. Obstet Gynecol 118(4):777, 2011

Handa VL, Blomquist JL, McDermott KC, et al: Pelvic floor disorders after vaginal birth: effect of episiotomy, perineal laceration, and operative birth. Obstet Gynecol 119(2 Pt 1):233, 2012

Hankins GD, Uckan E, Rowe TF, et al: Forceps and vacuum delivery: expectations of residency and fellowship training program directors. Am J Perinatol 16:23, 1999

Hirayama F, Koyanagi A, Mori R, et al: Prevalence and risk factors for third- and fourth-degree perineal lacerations during vaginal delivery: a multi-country study. BJOG 119(3):340, 2012

Hirsch E, Haney EI, Gordon TE, et al: Reducing high-order perineal laceration during operative vaginal delivery. Am J Obstet Gynecol 198(6):668.e1, 2008

Hofmeyr GJ, Gobetz L, Sonnendecker EW, et al: New design rigid and soft vacuum extractor cups: a preliminary comparison of traction forces. Br J Obstet Gynaecol 97(8):681, 1990

Kudish B, Blackwell S, Mcneeley SG, et al: Operative vaginal delivery and midline episiotomy: a bad combination for the perineum. Am J Obstet Gynecol 195(3):749, 2006

Kuit JA, Eppinga HG, Wallenburg HCS, et al: A randomized comparison of vacuum extraction delivery with a rigid and a pliable cup. Obstet Gynecol 82:280, 1993

Landy HJ, Laughon SK, Bailit JL, et al: Characteristics associated with severe perineal and cervical lacerations during vaginal delivery. Obstet Gynecol 117(3):627, 2011

Leijonhufvud A, Lundholm C, Cnattingius S, et al: Risks of stress urinary incontinence and pelvic organ prolapse surgery in relation to mode of childbirth. Am J Obstet Gynecol 204(1):70.e1, 2011

Le Ray C, Deneux-Tharaux C, Khireddine I, et al: Manual rotation to decrease operative delivery in posterior or transverse positions. Obstet Gynecol 122(3):634, 2013

Le Ray C, Serres P, Schmitz T, et al: Manual rotation in occiput posterior or transverse positions. Obstet Gynecol 110:873, 2007

Leslie KK, Dipasquale-Lehnerz P, Smith M: Obstetric forceps training using visual feedback and the isometric strength testing unit. Obstet Gynecol 105:377, 2005

Lowe B: Fear of failure: a place for the trial of instrumental delivery. Br J Obstet Gynaecol 94:60, 1987

MacArthur C, Glazener C, Lancashire R, et al: Faecal incontinence and mode of first and subsequent delivery: a six-year longitudinal study. Br J Obstet Gynaecol 112:1075, 2005

MacArthur C, Glazener CM, Wilson PD, et al: Persistent urinary incontinence and delivery mode history: a six-year longitudinal study. BJOG 113:218, 2006

Martin JA, Hamilton BE, Ventura SJ, et al: Births: final data for 2010. Natl Vital Stat Rep 61(1):1, 2012

Miller ES, Barber EL, McDonald KD, et al: Association between obstetrician forceps volume and maternal and fetal outcomes. Obstet Gynecol 123:248, 2014

Muise KL, Duchon MA, Brown RH: The effect of artificial caput on performance of vacuum extractors. Obstet Gynecol 81(2):170, 1993

Mulder F, Schoffelmeer M, Hakvoort R, et al: Risk factors for postpartum urinary retention: a systematic review and meta-analysis. BJOG 119(12):1440, 2012

Murphy DJ, Libby G, Chien P, et al: Cohort study of forceps delivery and the risk of epilepsy in adulthood. Am J Obstet Gynecol 191:392, 2004

Murphy DJ, Liebling RE, Verity L, et al: Early maternal and neonatal morbidity associated with operative delivery in second stage of labour: a cohort study. Lancet 358:1203, 2001

Nelson RL, Furner SE, Westercamp M, et al: Cesarean delivery for the prevention of anal incontinence. Cochrane Database Syst Rev 2:CD006756, 2010

Nilsen ST: Boys born by forceps and vacuum extraction examined at 18 years of age. Acta Obstet Gynecol Scand 63:549, 1984

Nygaard IE, Rao SS, Dawson JD: Anal incontinence after anal sphincter disruption: a 30 year retrospective cohort study. Obstet Gynecol 89:896, 1997

O'Callaghan ME, MacLennan AH, Gibson CS, et al: Epidemiologic associations with cerebral palsy. Obstet Gynecol 118(3):576, 2011

O'Mahony F, Hofmeyr GJ, Menon V: Choice of instruments for assisted vaginal delivery. Cochrane Database Syst Rev 11:CD005455, 2010

Osterman MJ, Martin JA, Menacker F: Expanded health data from the new birth certificate, 2006. Natl Vital Stat Rep 58(5):1, 2009

Pearl ML, Roberts JM, Laros RK, et al: Vaginal delivery from the persistent occiput posterior position: influence on maternal and neonatal morbidity. J Reprod Med 38:955, 1993

Pretlove SJ, Thompson PJ, Toozs-Hobson PM, et al: Does the mode of delivery predispose women to anal incontinence in the first year postpartum? A comparative systematic review. BJOG 115:421, 2008

Robertson PA, Laros RK, Zhao RL: Neonatal and maternal outcome in low-pelvic and mid-pelvic operative deliveries. Am J Obstet Gynecol 162:1436, 1990

Rortveit G, Daltveit AK, Hannestad YS, et al: Urinary incontinence after vaginal delivery or cesarean section. N Engl J Med 348:9000, 2003

Schwartz DB, Miodovnik M, Lavin JP Jr: Neonatal outcome among low birth weight infants delivered spontaneously or by low forceps. Obstet Gynecol 62:283, 1983

Seidman DS, Laor A, Gale R, et al: Long-term effects of vacuum and forceps deliveries. Lancet 337:1583, 1991

Solt I, Jackson S, Moore T, et al: Teaching forceps: the impact of proactive faculty. Am J Obstet Gynecol 204(5):448.e1, 2011

Spiliopoulos M, Kareti A, Jain NJ, et al: Risk of peripartum hysterectomy by mode of delivery and prior obstetric history: data from a population-based study. Arch Gynecol Obstet 283(6):1261, 2011

Spong CY, Berghella V, Wenstrom KD, et al: Preventing the First Cesarean Delivery: summary of a Joint Eunice Kennedy Shriver National Institute of Child Health and Human Development, Society for Maternal-Fetal Medicine, and American College of Obstetricians and Gynecologists Workshop. Obstet Gynecol 120(5):1181, 2012

Stock SJ, Josephs K, Farquharson S, et al: Maternal and neonatal outcomes of successful Kielland's rotational forceps delivery. Obstet Gynecol 121(5):1032, 2013

Suwannachat B, Laopaiboon M, Tonmat S, et al: Rapid versus stepwise application of negative pressure in vacuum extraction-assisted vaginal delivery: a multicentre randomised controlled non-inferiority trial. BJOG 118(10):1247, 2011

Suwannachat B, Lumbiganon P, Laopaiboon M: Rapid versus stepwise negative pressure application for vacuum extraction assisted vaginal delivery. Cochrane Database Syst Rev 8:CD006636, 2012

Thom DH, Brown JS, Schembri M, et al: Parturition events and risk of urinary incontinence in later life. Neurourol Urodyn 30:1456, 2011

Towner D, Castro MA, Eby-Wilkens E, et al: Effect of mode of delivery in nulliparous women on neonatal intracranial injury. N Engl J Med 341:1709, 1999

Towner DR, Ciotti MC: Operative vaginal delivery: a cause of birth injury or is it? Clin Obstet Gynecol 50(3):563, 2007

Vacca A: Vacuum-assisted delivery. Best Pract Res Clin Obstet Gynaecol 16:17, 2002

Walsh CA, Robson M, McAuliffe FM: Mode of delivery at term and adverse neonatal outcomes. Obstet Gynecol 121(1):122, 2013

Wen SW, Liu S, Kramer MS, et al: Comparison of maternal and infant outcomes between vacuum extraction and forceps deliveries. Am J Epidemiol 153(2):103, 2001

Werner EF, Janevic TM, Illuzzi J, et al: Mode of delivery in nulliparous women and neonatal intracranial injury. Obstet Gynecol 118(6):1239, 2011

Wesley B, Van den Berg B, Reece EA: The effect of operative vaginal delivery on cognitive development. Am J Obstet Gynecol 166:288, 1992

Williams MC, Knuppel RA, O'Brien WF, et al: A randomized comparison of assisted vaginal delivery by obstetric forceps and polyethylene vacuum cup. Obstet Gynecol 78:789, 1991

Yancey MK, Pierce B, Schweitzer D, et al: Observations on labor epidural analgesia and operative delivery rates. Am J Obstet Gynecol 180(2 Pt 1):353, 1999

Yeomans ER: Operative vaginal delivery. Obstet Gynecol 115(3):645, 2010

CHAPTER 30

Cesarean Delivery and Peripartum Hysterectomy

Cesarean delivery defines the birth of a fetus via laparotomy and then hysterotomy. The origin of *caesarean* is uncertain and was reviewed in the 23rd edition of *Williams Obstetrics* (Cunningham, 2010). There are two general types of cesarean delivery—*primary* refers to a first-time hysterotomy and *secondary* denotes a uterus with one or more prior hysterotomy incisions. Neither definition includes removal of the fetus from the abdominal cavity in the case of uterine rupture or with abdominal pregnancy. Rarely, hysterotomy is performed in a woman who has just died or in whom death is expected soon—postmortem or perimortem cesarean delivery (Chap. 47, p. 956).

In some instances, and most often because of emergent complications such as intractable hemorrhage, abdominal hysterectomy is indicated following delivery. When performed at the time of cesarean delivery, the operation is termed *cesarean hysterectomy*. If done within a short time after delivery, it is termed *postpartum hysterectomy*. *Peripartum hysterectomy* is a broader term that combines these two. In most cases, hysterectomy is total, but supracervical hysterectomy is also an option. The adnexa are not typically removed.

CESAREAN DELIVERY IN THE UNITED STATES

From 1970 to 2010, the cesarean delivery rate in the United States rose from 4.5 percent of all deliveries to 32.8 percent. In 2010, this rate actually declined from a peak of 32.9 percent in 2009 (Martin, 2012). The other, albeit brief, decline was between 1989 and 1996 (Fig. 31-1, p. 610). This more profound decrease was largely due to a significantly increased rate of *vaginal birth after cesarean (VBAC)* and to a closely mirrored decrease in the primary rate. These trends were short lived, and in 2007, the primary cesarean delivery rate was above 30 percent, whereas VBAC rates had dropped to 8 percent (MacDorman, 2011).

The reasons for the continued increase in the cesarean rates are not completely understood, but some explanations include the following:

1. Women are having fewer children, thus, a greater percentage of births are among *nulliparas*, who are at increased risk for cesarean delivery.
2. The average *maternal age* is rising, and older women, especially nulliparas, are at increased risk of cesarean delivery.
3. The use of *electronic fetal monitoring* is widespread. This technique is associated with an increased cesarean delivery rate compared with intermittent fetal heart rate auscultation (Chap. 24, p. 496). Cesarean delivery performed primarily for "fetal distress" comprises only a minority of all such procedures. In many more cases, concern for an abnormal or "nonreassuring" fetal heart rate tracing lowers the threshold for cesarean delivery.
4. Most fetuses presenting as *breech* are now delivered by cesarean. As discussed in Chapter 28 (p. 561), concern for fetal injury, as well as the infrequency with which a breech presentation meets criteria for a labor trial, almost guarantee that most will be delivered by cesarean.
5. The frequency of *forceps* and *vacuum deliveries* has decreased (Chap. 29, p. 574).

6. Rates of *labor induction* continue to rise, and induced labor, especially among nulliparas, increases the cesarean delivery rate (Chap. 26, p. 523).
7. The prevalence of *obesity* has risen dramatically, and obesity increases the cesarean delivery risk (Chap. 48, p. 965).
8. Rates of cesarean delivery for women with preeclampsia have increased, whereas labor induction rates for these patients have declined.
9. *Vaginal birth after cesarean—VBAC*—has decreased from a high of 28 percent in 1996 to 8 percent in 2007 (Chap. 31, p. 610).
10. Elective cesarean deliveries are increasingly being performed for a variety of indications including concern for *pelvic floor injury* associated with vaginal birth, medically indicated *preterm birth*, reduction of *fetal injury risk*, and for *maternal request*.
11. *Malpractice litigation* related to fetal injury during spontaneous or operative vaginal delivery continues to contribute significantly to the present cesarean delivery rate.

CESAREAN DELIVERY INDICATIONS AND RISKS

Some indications for performing cesarean delivery are shown in Table 30-1. More than 85 percent of these operations are performed for four reasons—prior cesarean delivery, dystocia, fetal jeopardy, or abnormal fetal presentation.

TABLE 30-1. Some Indications for Cesarean Delivery

Maternal
Prior cesarean delivery
Abnormal placentation
Maternal request
Prior classical hysterotomy
Unknown uterine scar type
Uterine incision dehiscence
Prior full-thickness myomectomy
Genital tract obstructive mass
Invasive cervical cancer
Prior trachelectomy
Permanent cerclage
Prior pelvic reconstructive surgery
Pelvic deformity
HSV or HIV infection
Cardiac or pulmonary disease
Cerebral aneurysm or arteriovenous malformation
Pathology requiring concurrent intraabdominal surgery
Perimortem cesarean delivery
Maternal-Fetal
Cephalopelvic disproportion
Failed operative vaginal delivery
Placenta previa or placental abruption
Fetal
Nonreassuring fetal status
Malpresentation
Macrosomia
Congenital anomaly
Abnormal umbilical cord Doppler study
Thrombocytopenia
Prior neonatal birth trauma

HIV = human immunodeficiency virus; HSV = herpes simplex virus.

Maternal Mortality and Morbidity

To provide accurate informed consent, understanding both maternal and neonatal risks and benefits with surgery is essential. As a broad overview, cesarean delivery has higher maternal surgical risks for the current and subsequent pregnancies. This is balanced against lower rates of perineal injury and short-term pelvic floor disorders, described in Chapter 27 (p. 536). For the neonate, cesarean delivery offers lower rates of birth trauma and stillbirth. Conversely, rates of initial respiratory difficulties are greater with cesarean delivery.

For the mother, death attributable solely to cesarean delivery is rare in the United States. Even so, numerous studies attest to increased mortality risks. Clark and colleagues (2008), in a review of nearly 1.5 million pregnancies, found maternal mortality rates of 2.2 per 100,000 cesarean deliveries compared with 0.2 per 100,000 vaginal births. In a metaanalysis of 203 studies, Guise and coworkers (2010) reported a maternal mortality rate of 13 per 100,000 with elective repeat cesarean delivery compared with 4 per 100,000 women undergoing a trial of labor during VBAC attempt.

Similar to mortality rates, the frequency of some maternal complications is increased with all cesarean compared with vaginal deliveries (Table 30-2). Villar and associates (2007) reported that maternal morbidity rates increased twofold with cesarean compared with vaginal delivery. Principal among these are infection, hemorrhage, and thromboembolism. In addition, anesthetic complications, which also rarely include death, have a greater incidence with cesarean compared with vaginal delivery (Cheesman, 2009; Hawkins, 2011). Adjacent organs may be injured. The bladder laceration rate is 1 to 3 per 1000 cesarean deliveries, whereas that for ureteral injury approximates 0.3 per 1000 cases (Güngördük, 2010; Phipps, 2005; Rajasekar, 1997). Bowel damage occurs in approximately 1 in 1000 cesarean deliveries (Silver, 2006).

Women expressing a desire for elective primary cesarean delivery may be counseled that surgery offers decreased risks for hemorrhage and chorioamnionitis compared with planned primary vaginal birth. But this is again balanced against higher maternal rates of thromboembolism, hysterectomy, and rehospitalization for infection or wound complications; longer initial hospital stays; and greater rates of uterine rupture or abnormal placental implantation in subsequent pregnancies (Declercq, 2007; Geller, 2010; Liu, 2007).

Women who undergo a cesarean delivery are much more likely to be delivered by a repeat operation in subsequent pregnancies. For women undergoing subsequent cesarean, the maternal risks just described are even greater (Cahill, 2006; Marshall, 2011; Silver, 2006).

As an advantage, there is evidence that cesarean delivery is associated with lower rates of urinary incontinence and pelvic

TABLE 30-2. Complications Associated with Low-Risk Planned Cesarean Delivery[a] Compared with Planned Vaginal Delivery among Healthy Women in Canada, 1991–2005

Complication	Type of Planned Delivery[b] Cesarean n = 46,766	Vaginal n = 2,292,420
Overall morbidity	1279 (2.73)	20,639 (0.9)
Hysterectomy	39 (0.09)	254 (0.01)
Transfusion	11 (0.02)	1500 (0.07)
Anesthetic complications	247 (0.53)	4793 (0.21)
Hypovolemic shock	3 (0.01)	435 (0.02)[c]
Cardiac arrest	89 (0.19)	887 (0.04)
Venous thromboembolism	28 (0.06)	623 (0.03)
Puerperal infection	281 (0.60)	4833 (0.21)
Wound disruption	41 (0.09)	1151 (0.05)
Wound hematoma	607 (1.3)	6263 (0.27)
In-hospital deaths	0	41 (0.002)

[a]Healthy women with a singleton gestation and no previous cesarean delivery who underwent cesarean delivery for breech presentation were used as a surrogate for a low-risk planned cesarean delivery group.
[b]Data are shown as number (%).
[c]Nonsignificant comparison. For all other comparisons $p < 0.05$.
Modified from Liu, 2007.

organ prolapse (Glazener, 2013; Gyhagen, 2013; Handa, 2011; Leijonhufvud, 2011; Rortveit, 2003). This protective advantage may persist to some degree over time, but cesarean delivery is not wholly protective (Dolan, 2010; MacArthur, 2011; Rortveit, 2001). Finally, cesarean delivery is not protective long-term for fecal incontinence (MacArthur, 2011, 2013; Nelson, 2010).

Neonatal Morbidity

Cesarean delivery is associated with less risk of fetal trauma. And this in many instances influences the choice of cesarean delivery despite the associated maternal risks. Alexander and colleagues (2006) found that fetal injury complicated 1 percent of cesarean deliveries. Skin laceration was most common, but others included cephalohematoma, clavicular fracture, brachial plexopathy, skull fracture, and facial nerve palsy. Cesarean deliveries following a failed operative vaginal delivery attempt had the highest injury rate, whereas the lowest rate—0.5 percent—occurred in the elective cesarean delivery group. That said, Worley and colleagues (2009) found that approximately a third of pregnant women who were delivered at Parkland Hospital entered spontaneous labor at term, and 96 percent of these delivered vaginally without adverse neonatal outcomes.

Although physical injury risks are lower, cesarean delivery per se may have no bearing on the neurodevelopmental prognosis of the infant. Scheller and Nelson (1994) in a report from the National Institutes of Health and Lien and associates (1995) presented data specifically refuting any association between cesarean delivery and lower rates of either cerebral palsy or seizures. Moreover, as discussed in Chapter 33 (p. 638), the incidences of neonatal seizures or cerebral palsy have not diminished as the rate of cesarean delivery has increased (Miller, 2008; Miller, 2013).

Patient Choice in Cesarean Delivery

As women have taken a more active role in their obstetrical care, some request elective cesarean delivery. Data regarding the true incidence of *cesarean delivery on maternal request (CDMR)* are limited, however, estimates are a 1- to 7-percent rate in the United States in 2003 (Gossman, 2006; Menacker, 2006).

Reasons for requested cesarean delivery include reduced risk of fetal injury, avoidance of the uncertainty and pain of labor, protection of pelvic floor support, and convenience. Thus, the debate surrounding CDMR includes its medical rationale from both a maternal and fetal-neonatal standpoint, the concept of informed free choice by the woman, and the autonomy of the physician in offering this choice.

To address this, the National Institutes of Health (2006) held a State-of-the-Science Conference on Cesarean Delivery on Maternal Request. A panel of experts critically reviewed available literature to form recommendations based on identified risks and benefits. It is noteworthy that most of the maternal and neonatal outcomes examined had insufficient data to permit such recommendations. Indeed, one of the main conclusions of the conference was that more high-quality research is needed to fully evaluate the issues. The American College of Obstetricians and Gynecologists (2013) concluded that data comparing planned cesarean and planned vaginal delivery were minimal and thus should be interpreted cautiously.

The panel was able to draw a few conclusions from existing information. Cesarean delivery on maternal request should not be performed before 39 weeks' gestation unless there is evidence of fetal lung maturity. It should be avoided in women desiring several children because of the risk of placental implantation abnormalities and cesarean hysterectomy. Finally, it should not be motivated by the unavailability of effective pain management.

PATIENT PREPARATION

Delivery Availability

There is no nationally recognized standard of care that codifies an acceptable time interval to begin performance of a cesarean delivery. Previously, a 30-minute decision-to-incision interval was recommended. In most instances, however, operative delivery is not necessary within this 30-minute time frame. Bloom and coworkers (2001) reported for the Maternal-Fetal Medicine Units Network that 69 percent of 7450 cesareans performed in labor commenced more than 30 minutes after the decision to operate. In a second study, Bloom and colleagues (2006) evaluated cesarean deliveries performed for emergency indications. They reported that failure to achieve a cesarean delivery decision-to-incision time of less than 30 minutes was not associated with a negative neonatal outcome. On the other hand, when faced with an acute, catastrophic deterioration in fetal condition, cesarean delivery usually is indicated as rapidly as possible, and thus purposeful delays are inappropriate. The American Academy of Pediatrics and the American College of Obstetricians and Gynecologists (2012) recommend that facilities giving obstetrical care should have the ability to initiate cesarean delivery in a time frame that best incorporates maternal and fetal risks and benefits.

Informed Consent

Obtaining informed consent is a process and not merely a medical record document (American College of Obstetricians and Gynecologists, 2012a). This conversation between a clinician and patient should enhance a woman's awareness of her diagnosis and contain a discussion of medical and surgical care alternatives, procedure goals and limitations, and surgical risks. For women with a prior cesarean delivery, the option of a trial of labor should be included for suitable candidates. Also, in those desiring permanent sterilization, consenting for tubal ligation, as described in Chapter 39 (p. 720), can be completed at this time.

Timing of Scheduled Cesarean Delivery

Adverse neonatal sequelae from neonatal immaturity with elective delivery before 39 completed weeks are appreciable (Clark, 2009; Tita, 2009a). To avoid these, assurance of fetal maturity before scheduled elective surgery is essential as outlined by the American Academy of Pediatrics and the American College of Obstetricians and Gynecologists (2012) and discussed in Chapter 31 (p. 615). To assist with this and other components of cesarean delivery planning, the American College of Obstetricians and Gynecologists (2011a,c) has created Patient Safety Checklists to be completed before the planned surgery.

Perioperative Care

If cesarean delivery is scheduled, a sedative may be given at bedtime the night before surgery. In general, no other sedatives, narcotics, or tranquilizers are administered until after the fetus is born. Oral intake is stopped at least 8 hours before the procedure. The woman scheduled for repeat cesarean delivery typically is admitted the day of surgery and evaluated by the obstetrical and anesthesia teams. Recently performed hematocrit and indirect Coombs test are reviewed, and if the latter is positive, then availability of compatible blood must be ensured.

As discussed in Chapter 25 (p. 509), regional analgesia is preferred for cesarean delivery. An antacid is given shortly before regional analgesia or induction with general anesthesia. One example is Bicitra, 30 mL orally in a single dose. This minimizes the lung injury risk from gastric acid aspiration. Once the woman is supine, a wedge beneath the right hip creates a left lateral tilt to aid venous return and avoid hypotension. According to the American College of Obstetricians and Gynecologists (2010), there are insufficient data to determine the value of fetal monitoring before scheduled cesarean delivery in women without risk factors. That said, fetal heart sounds should be documented in the operating room prior to surgery.

For further preparation, if hair obscures the operative field it should be removed the day of surgery by clipping. This is associated with fewer surgical site infections compared with shaving (Tanner, 2011). An indwelling bladder catheter is typically placed at Parkland Hospital to collapse the bladder away from the hysterotomy incision, to avert urinary retention secondary to regional analgesia, and to allow accurate postoperative urine measurement. Small studies support the nonuse of catheterization in hemodynamically stable women to minimize urinary infections (Li, 2011; Nasr, 2009).

The risk of thromboembolism is increased with pregnancy and almost doubled in those undergoing cesarean delivery (James, 2006). For this reason, for all women not already receiving thromboprophylaxis, the American College of Obstetricians and Gynecologists (2011d) recommends initiation of pneumatic compression hose before cesarean delivery. These are usually discontinued once the woman ambulates. In contrast, we favor the recommendations of American College of Chest Physicians for early ambulation for women without risk factors who are undergoing cesarean delivery (Bates, 2012). For women already receiving prophylaxis or those with increasing risk factors, prophylaxis is escalated as discussed in Chapter 52 and shown in Table 52-8 (p. 1046).

Some women scheduled for cesarean delivery have concurrent comorbidity that requires specific management in anticipation of surgery. Among others, these include insulin-requiring or gestational diabetes, coagulopathy or thrombophilia, chronic corticosteroid use, and significant reactive airway disease. Preparations for surgery in these women are discussed in the respective chapters covering these topics.

Infection Prevention

Febrile morbidity is frequent after cesarean delivery. Numerous good-quality trials have proved that that a single dose of an antimicrobial agent given at the time of cesarean delivery significantly decreases infection morbidity. Although more obvious for women undergoing unscheduled cesarean delivery, this practice also significantly lowers the postoperative infection rate in women undergoing elective surgery (American College of Obstetricians and Gynecologists, 2011b). Depending on drug allergies, most recommend a single intravenous dose of a β-lactam antimicrobial—either a cephalosporin or extended-spectrum penicillin derivative. A 1-g dose of cefazolin is an efficacious and cost-effective choice. For obese women, a 2-g dose usually provides adequate coverage, although Pevzner and associates (2011) showed this dose may be inadequate for those with body mass index > 40. In women with significant penicillin or cephalosporin allergy, a single 600-mg intravenous dose of clindamycin combined with a weight-based dose of aminoglycoside is an alternative. A 900-mg clindamycin dose is used for obese patients.

Antimicrobial administration before surgical incision has been shown to lower postoperative infection rates without adverse neonatal effects compared with drug administration after umbilical cord clamping (Sullivan, 2007; Tita, 2009b; Witt, 2011). For this reason, the American College of Obstetricians and Gynecologists (2011b) recommends that prophylaxis be administered within the 60 minutes prior to the start of planned cesarean delivery. For emergent delivery, prophylaxis should be given as soon as feasible.

Preoperative preparation of the abdominal wall skin is effective to prevent wound infection. Either chlorhexidine or povidone-iodine solutions can be used. In addition, to prevent postoperative metritis following cesarean delivery, preoperative vaginal cleansing with a povidone-iodine scrub has been evaluated in small randomized trials (Haas, 2013). Some show benefit, whereas others do not (Reid, 2001; Starr, 2005; Yildirim, 2012). Vaginal cleansing is not a part of preoperative preparation at Parkland Hospital.

Antibiotic prophylaxis against infective endocarditis is not recommended for most with cardiac conditions—exceptions are women with cyanotic heart disease, prosthetic valves, or both (American College of Obstetricians and Gynecologists, 2011b). Regimens selected for routine cesarean infection prophylaxis will also serve as appropriate endocarditis coverage (Chap. 49, p. 991).

Surgical Safety

The Joint Commission (2013) established a protocol to prevent surgical errors that encompasses three components: (1) preprocedure verification of all relevant documents, (2) marking the operative site, and (3) completion of a "time out" before procedure initiation. The "time out" requires attention of the entire team to confirm that the patient, site, and procedure are correct. Important discussions also include introduction of the patient-care team members, verification of prophylactic antibiotics, estimation of procedure length, and communication of anticipated complications. Additionally, requests for special instrumentation should be addressed preoperatively to prevent potential patient compromise and intraoperative delays.

An instrument, sponge, and needle count before and after surgery and vaginal delivery is crucial to surgical safety. If counts are not reconciled following abdominal or vaginal examination, then radiographic imaging for retained foreign objects is obtained (American College of Obstetricians and Gynecologists, 2012b).

TECHNIQUE FOR CESAREAN DELIVERY

With minor variations, surgical performance of cesarean delivery is comparable worldwide. Most steps are founded on evidence-based data, and these have been reviewed by Dahlke (2013) and Hofmeyr (2009) and their associates. As with all surgery, a clear understanding of relevant anatomy is essential, and this is described and illustrated in Chapter 2 (p. 16).

Abdominal Incision

In obstetrics, usually a midline vertical or a suprapubic transverse incision is chosen for laparotomy. Transverse abdominal entry is by either Pfannenstiel or Maylard incisions. Of these, the Pfannenstiel incision is selected most frequently for cesarean delivery. Transverse incisions follow Langer lines of skin tension, and superior cosmetic results compared with vertical incisions can be achieved. Additionally, decreased rates of postoperative pain, fascial wound dehiscence, and incisional hernia compared with vertical entry are benefits. Use of the Pfannenstiel incision, however, is often discouraged for cases in which a large operating space is essential or in which access to the upper abdomen may be needed. Because of the layers created during incision of the internal and external oblique aponeuroses with transverse incisions, purulent fluid can collect between these. Therefore, cases with high infection risks may favor a midline incision. Last, neurovascular structures, which include the ilioinguinal and iliohypogastric nerves and superficial and inferior epigastric vessels, are often encountered with transverse incisions. Logically, bleeding, wound hematoma, and neurological disruption may more frequently complicate these incisions compared with vertical incision. With repeat cesarean delivery, reentry through a Pfannenstiel incision usually is more time consuming and difficult because of scarring.

The Maylard incision differs mainly from the Pfannenstiel in that the bellies of the rectus abdominis muscles are transected horizontally to widen the operating space. It is technically more difficult due to its required isolation and ligation of the inferior epigastric arteries, which lie lateral to these muscle bellies.

Vertical infraumbilical incisions provide quick entry to shorten incision-to-delivery time (Wylie, 2010). Moreover, this incision has minimal blood loss, superior access to the upper abdomen, generous operating room, and the flexibility for easy wound extension if greater space or access is needed. No important neurovascular structures traverse this incision, and aponeuroses at the linea alba are fused. Main disadvantages are poorer cosmetic results, higher fascial dehiscence or incisional hernia rates, and greater postoperative pain. For morbidly obese patients, a vertical incision that extends up and around the umbilicus may be preferable to avoid cutting through a large pannus (Fig. 48-7, p. 968).

Transverse Incisions

With the Pfannenstiel incision, the skin and subcutaneous tissue are incised using a low, transverse, slightly curvilinear incision. This is made at the level of the pubic hairline, which is typically 3 cm above the superior border of the symphysis pubis. The incision is extended somewhat beyond the lateral borders of the rectus abdominis muscles. It should be of adequate width to accommodate delivery—12 to 15 cm is typical.

Sharp dissection is continued through the subcutaneous layer to the fascia. The superficial epigastric vessels can usually be identified halfway between the skin and fascia, several centimeters from the midline, and coagulated. If lacerated, these may be suture ligated with 3-0 plain gut suture or coagulated with an electrosurgical blade.

The fascia is then incised sharply at the midline. The anterior abdominal fascia is typically composed of two visible layers, the aponeurosis from the external oblique muscle and a fused layer containing aponeuroses of the internal oblique and transverse abdominis muscles. Ideally, the two layers are individually incised during lateral extension of the fascial incision. The inferior epigastric vessels typically lie outside the lateral border of the rectus abdominis muscle and beneath the fused aponeuroses of the internal oblique and transverse abdominis muscles. Thus, although infrequently required, extension of the fascial incision further laterally may cut these vessels. Therefore, if lateral extension is needed, these vessels should be identified and coagulated or ligated to prevent bleeding and vessel retraction.

Once the fascia is incised, the inferior fascial edge is grasped with suitable clamps and elevated by the assistant as the operator separates the fascial sheath from the underlying rectus muscles either bluntly or sharply until the superior border of the symphysis pubis is reached. Any blood vessels coursing between the sheath and muscles are clamped, cut, and ligated, or they are coagulated with an electrosurgery blade. Next, the superior fascial edge is grasped and again, separation of fascia from the rectus muscles is completed. Meticulous hemostasis is imperative to lower rates of infection and bleeding. The fascial separation is carried near enough to the umbilicus to permit an adequate midline longitudinal incision of the peritoneum. The rectus abdominis and pyramidalis muscles are then separated in the midline by sharp and blunt dissection to expose the transversalis fascia and peritoneum.

The transversalis fascia and preperitoneal fat are dissected carefully to reach the underlying peritoneum. The peritoneum near the upper end of the incision is opened carefully, either bluntly or by elevating it with two hemostats placed approximately 2 cm apart. The tented fold of peritoneum between the clamps is examined and palpated to ensure that omentum, bowel, or bladder is not adjacent. The peritoneum is then incised. The incision is extended superiorly to the upper pole of the incision and downward to just above the peritoneal reflection over the bladder. Importantly, in women who have had previous intraabdominal surgery, including cesarean delivery, omentum or bowel may be adhered to the undersurface of the peritoneum. Moreover, in women with obstructed labor, the bladder may be pushed cephalad almost to the level of the umbilicus.

Vertical Incision

An infraumbilical midline vertical incision begins 2 to 3 cm above the superior margin of the symphysis and should be of sufficient length to allow fetal delivery without difficulty. Therefore, its length should correspond with the estimated fetal size, and 12 to 15 cm is typical. Sharp or electrosurgical dissection is performed to the level of the anterior rectus sheath. A small opening is made sharply with scalpel in the upper half of the linea alba. Placement here avoids potential cystotomy. Index and middle fingers are placed beneath the fascia, and the fascial incision is extended superiorly and inferiorly with scissors or scalpel. Midline separation of the rectus muscles and pyramidalis muscles and peritoneal entry are then similar to those with the Pfannenstiel incision.

Hysterotomy

Most often, the lower uterine segment is incised transversely as described by Kerr in 1921. Occasionally, a low-segment vertical incision as described by Krönig in 1912 may be used. The classical incision is a vertical incision into the body of the uterus above the lower uterine segment and reaches the uterine fundus. In practice, however, the classical incision is similar to the low-vertical incision, which is typically extended cephalad only to the extent required for fetal delivery. For most cesarean deliveries, the transverse incision is preferred. Compared with a classical incision, it is easier to repair, is located in the inactive segment and thus least likely to rupture during a subsequent pregnancy, causes less incision-site bleeding, and promotes less bowel or omentum adherence to the myometrial incision.

Low Transverse Cesarean Incision

Before any hysterotomy, the surgeon should palpate the fundus and adnexa to identify degrees of uterine rotation. The uterus may be dextrorotated so that the left round ligament is more anterior and closer to the midline. In such cases, hysterotomy placement is modified to keep the incision centered within the lower segment. This avoids extension into and laceration of the left uterine artery. With thick meconium or infected amnionic fluid, some surgeons prefer to put a moistened laparotomy sponge in each lateral peritoneal gutter to absorb fluid and blood that escape from the opened uterus. A moist sponge may also be used to pack protruding bowel away from the operative field.

The reflection of peritoneum above the upper margin of the bladder and overlying the anterior lower uterine segment—termed the bladder flap—is grasped in the midline with forceps and incised transversely with scissors (Fig. 30-1). Bladder flap creation effectively moves the bladder away from

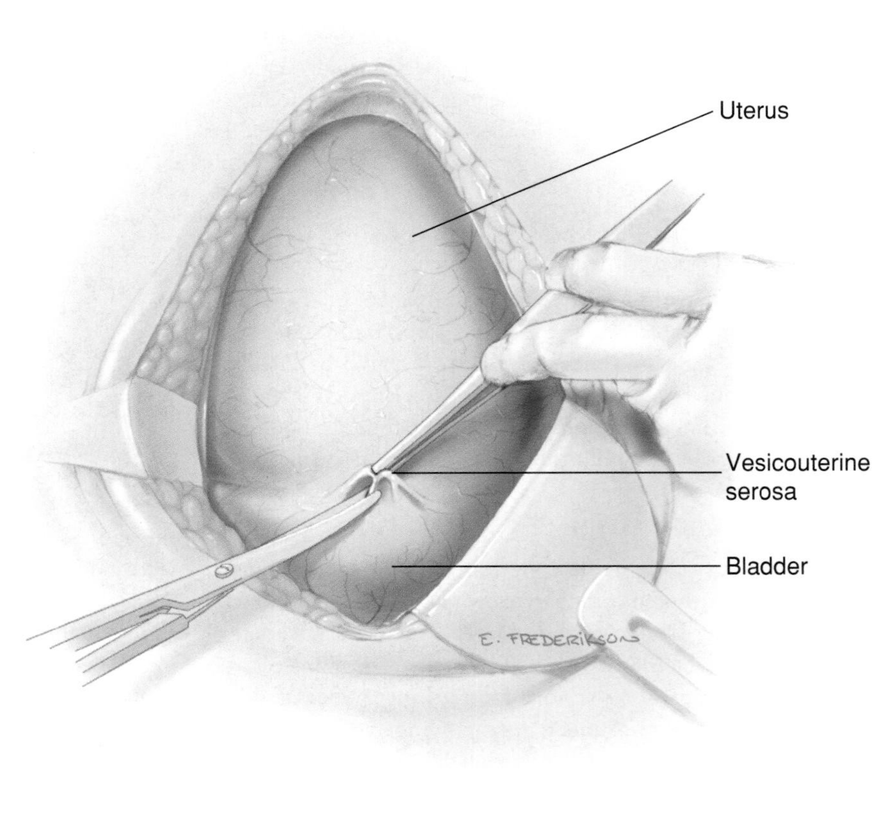

FIGURE 30-1 The loose vesicouterine serosa above the bladder reflection is grasped with forceps and incised with Metzenbaum scissors.

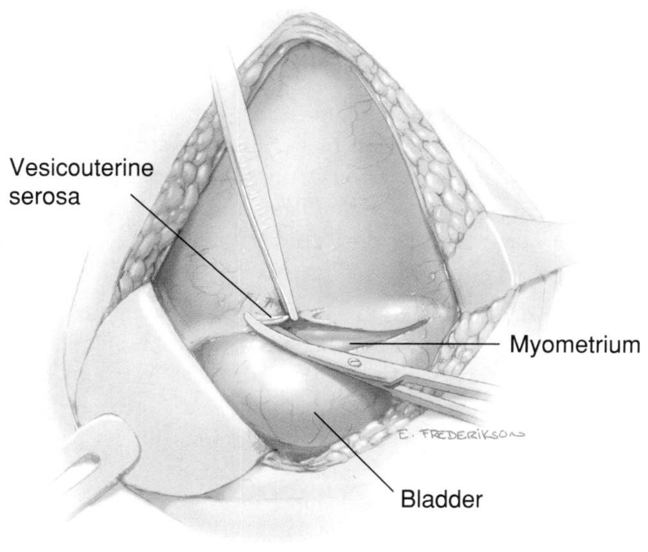

FIGURE 30-2 The loose serosa above the upper margin of the bladder is elevated and incised laterally.

the planned hysterotomy site and prevents bladder laceration if an unintended inferior hysterotomy extension occurs during fetal delivery.

Following this initial incision, scissors are inserted between the vesicouterine serosa and myometrium of the lower uterine segment. The scissors are pushed laterally from the midline on each side to further open the visceral peritoneum and expose the myometrium. This transverse peritoneal incision extends almost the full length of the lower uterine segment. As the lateral margin on each side is approached, the scissors are directed somewhat more cephalad (Fig. 30-2). The lower edge of peritoneum is elevated, and the bladder is gently separated from the underlying myometrium with blunt or sharp dissection within this vesicouterine space (Fig. 30-3).

In general, this caudad separation of bladder does not exceed 5 cm and usually is less. It is possible, especially with an effaced, dilated cervix, to dissect downward so caudally as to inadvertently expose and then enter the underlying vagina rather than the lower uterine segment. However, in instances in which cesarean hysterectomy is planned or anticipated, extended caudad bladder dissection is recommended to aid total hysterectomy and decrease the risk of cystotomy.

Some surgeons do not create a bladder flap. The main advantage is a shorter skin incision-to-delivery time, however, data supporting this practice are limited (Hohlagschwandtner, 2001; Tuuli, 2012).

The uterus is entered through the lower uterine segment approximately 1 cm below the upper margin of the peritoneal reflection. It is important to place the uterine incision relatively higher in women with advanced or complete cervical dilatation. Failure to adjust increases the risk of lateral extension of the incision into the uterine arteries. It may also lead to incision of the cervix or vagina rather than the lower uterine segment. Such incisions into the cervix can create significant postoperative distortion of cervical anatomy. Correct placement uses the vesicouterine serosal reflection as a guide.

Uterine Incision. The uterus can be incised by a variety of techniques. Each is initiated by using a scalpel to transversely incise the exposed lower uterine segment for 1 to 2 cm in the midline (Fig. 30-4). This must be done carefully to avoid fetal laceration. Careful blunt entry using hemostats or fingertip to split the muscle may be helpful. Once the uterus is opened, the incision can be extended by simply spreading the incision, using lateral and slightly upward pressure applied with each index finger (Fig. 30-5). Alternatively, if the lower uterine segment is thick, then cutting laterally and then slightly upward with bandage scissors will extend the incision. Importantly, when scissors are used, the index and midline fingers of the nondominant hand should be insinuated beneath the myometrium and above fetal parts to prevent fetal laceration. Comparing blunt and sharp extensions of the initial uterine incision, sharp extension is associated with an increased estimated blood loss, but postoperative hematocrit changes, need for transfusion, and infection rates are not different (Xu, 2013).

The uterine incision should be made large enough to allow delivery of the head and trunk of the fetus without either tearing into or having to cut into the uterine vessels that course along the lateral uterine margins. If the placenta is encountered in the incision line, it must be either detached or incised. *When*

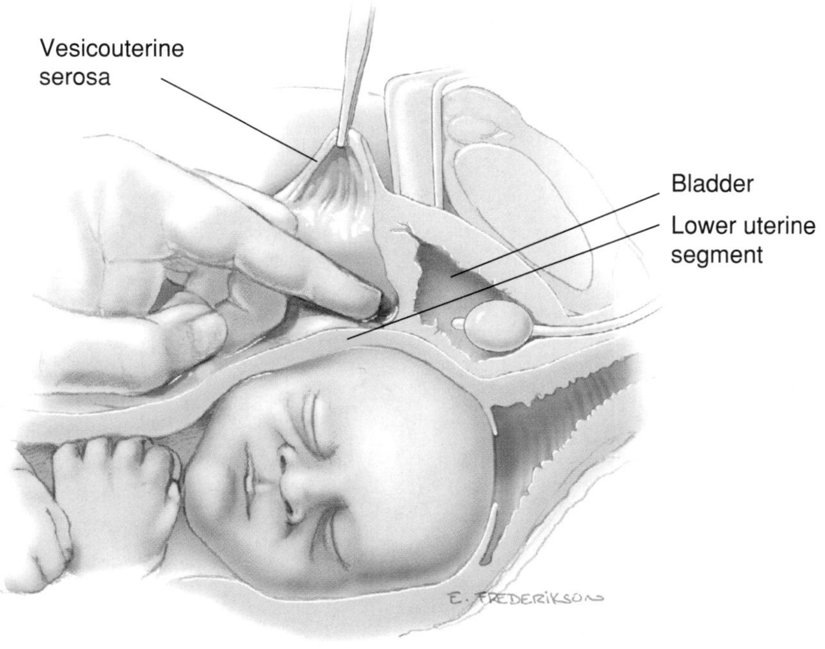

FIGURE 30-3 Cross section shows blunt dissection of the bladder off the uterus to expose the lower uterine segment.

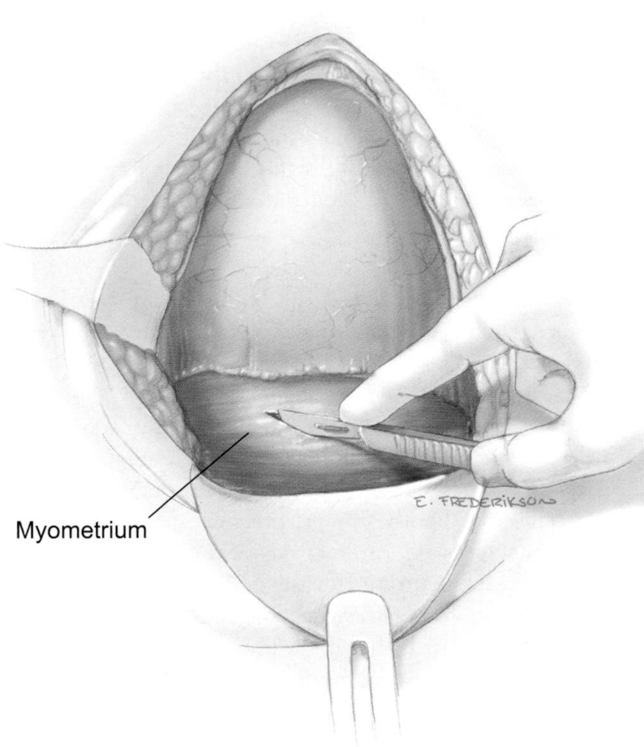

FIGURE 30-4 The myometrium is carefully incised to avoid cutting the fetal head.

the placenta is incised, fetal hemorrhage may be severe. Thus, delivery and cord clamping should be performed as soon as possible.

At times, a low-transverse hysterotomy is selected but provides inadequate room for delivery. In such instances, one corner of the hysterotomy incision is extended cephalad into the contractile portion of the myometrium—a *J incision*. If this is completed bilaterally, a *U incision* is formed. Last, some prefer to extend in the midline—a *T incision*. As expected, these have been linked with higher intraoperative blood loss (Boyle, 1996; Patterson, 2002). Moreover, as these extend into the contractile portion, a trial of labor and vaginal delivery are more likely contraindicated in future pregnancies.

Delivery of the Fetus. In a cephalic presentation, a hand is slipped into the uterine cavity between the symphysis and fetal head. The head is elevated gently with the fingers and palm through the incision. Once the head enters the incision, delivery may be aided by modest transabdominal fundal pressure (Fig. 30-6).

After a long labor with cephalopelvic disproportion, the fetal head may be tightly wedged in the birth canal. This situation can have disastrous results, and there are three considerations for delivery. First, a "push" method may be used. With this, upward pressure exerted by a hand in the vagina by an assistant will help to dislodge the head and allow its delivery above the symphysis. Relief of such head impaction increases the risk of hysterotomy extension and associated blood loss as well as fetal skull fracture. As an alternative, a "pull" method is used in which the fetal legs are grasped and delivered through the hysterotomy opening. The fetus is then delivered by traction as one would complete a breech extraction. Support for this latter approach comes only from small randomized trials and case series (Bastani, 2012; Shazly, 2013; Veisi, 2012). Last, a low vertical hysterotomy incision, which will give more room for the "pull" technique, may be selected. If a low transverse

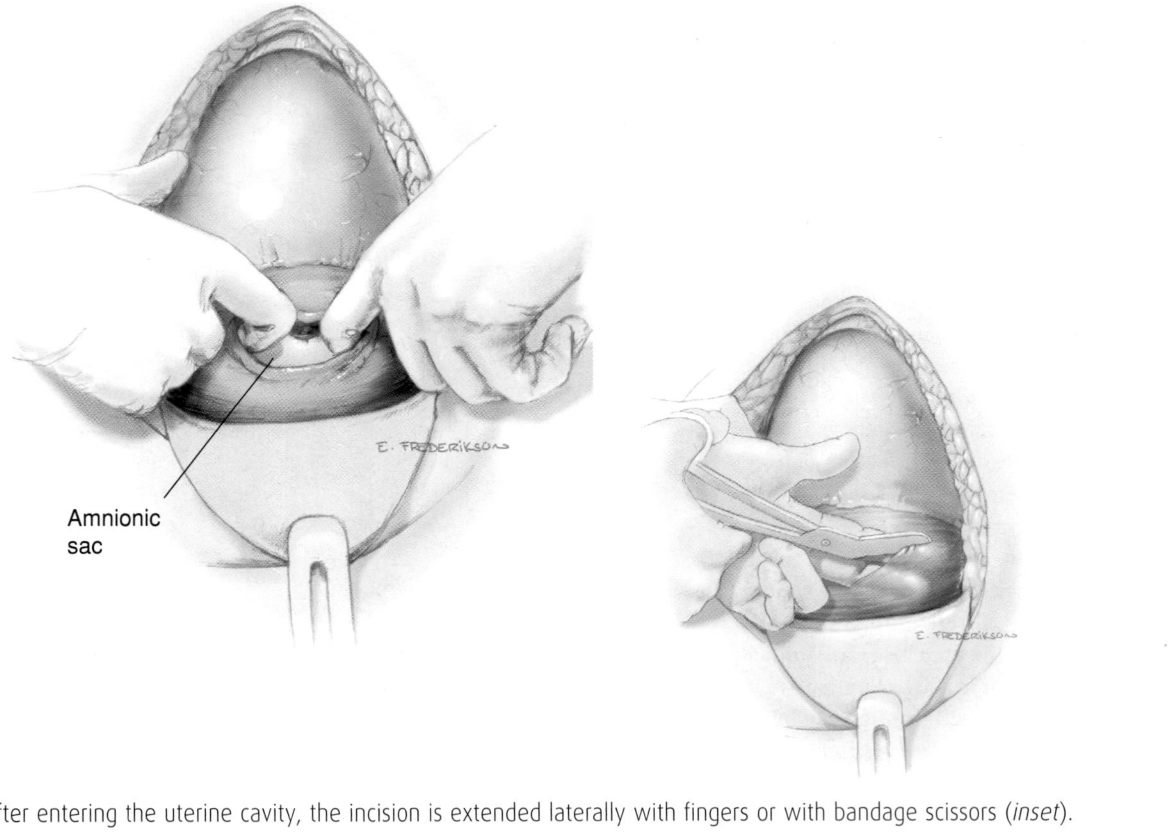

FIGURE 30-5 After entering the uterine cavity, the incision is extended laterally with fingers or with bandage scissors (*inset*).

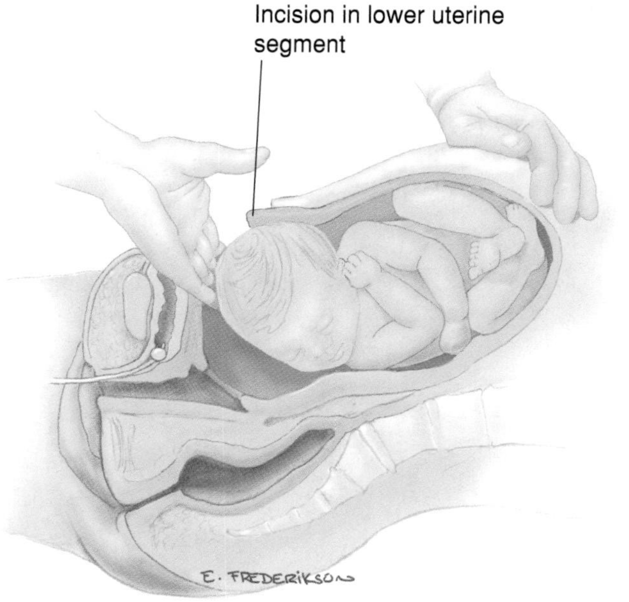

FIGURE 30-6 Delivery of the fetal head.

incision has already been made, then this can be extended to a J-, U-, or T-incision for room.

Conversely, in women without labor, the fetal head may be unmolded and without a leading cephalic point. The round head may be difficult to lift through the uterine incision in a relatively thick lower segment that is unattenuated by labor. In such instances, either forceps or a vacuum device may be used to deliver the fetal head as shown in Figure 30-7.

After head delivery, a finger should be passed across the fetal neck to determine whether it is encircled by one or more umbilical cord loops. If an umbilical cord coil is felt, it should be slipped over the head. The head is rotated to an occiput transverse position, which aligns the fetal bisacromial diameter vertically. The sides of the head are grasped with two hands, and gentle downward traction is applied until the anterior shoulder enters the hysterotomy incision (Fig. 30-8). Next, by upward movement, the posterior shoulder is delivered. During delivery, abrupt or powerful force is avoided to avert brachial plexus injury. With steady outward traction, the rest of the body then readily follows. Gentle fundal pressure may aid this.

With some exceptions, current American Heart Association neonatal resuscitation recommendations eschew suctioning immediately following birth, even with meconium present (Kattwinkel, 2010). A fuller discussion of this and the timing of umbilical cord clamping as it relates to neonatal outcome are found in Chapter 27 (p. 539). The umbilical cord is clamped, and the newborn is given to the team member who will conduct resuscitative efforts as needed (Chap. 32, p. 625).

The American Academy of Pediatrics and the American College of Obstetricians and Gynecologists (2012) recommend that "a qualified person who is skilled in neonatal resuscitation should be in the delivery room, with all equipment needed for neonatal resuscitation, to care for the neonate." Jacob and Phenninger (1997) compared 834 cesarean deliveries with 834 low-risk vaginal deliveries. They found that with regional analgesia, there is rarely a need for infant resuscitation after elective repeat cesarean delivery or cesarean delivery for dystocia without fetal heart rate abnormalities and that a pediatrician may not be necessary at such deliveries. At Parkland Hospital, pediatric nurse practitioners attend uncomplicated, scheduled cesarean deliveries.

After birth, an intravenous infusion containing two ampules or 20 units of oxytocin per liter of crystalloid is infused at 10 mL/min. Some prefer higher infusion dosages, however, bolus doses are avoided because of associated hypotension (Roach, 2013). Once the uterus contracts satisfactorily, the rate can be reduced. An alternative is carbetocin—a longer-acting oxytocin derivative that is not available in the United States—that provides suitable, albeit more expensive, hemorrhage

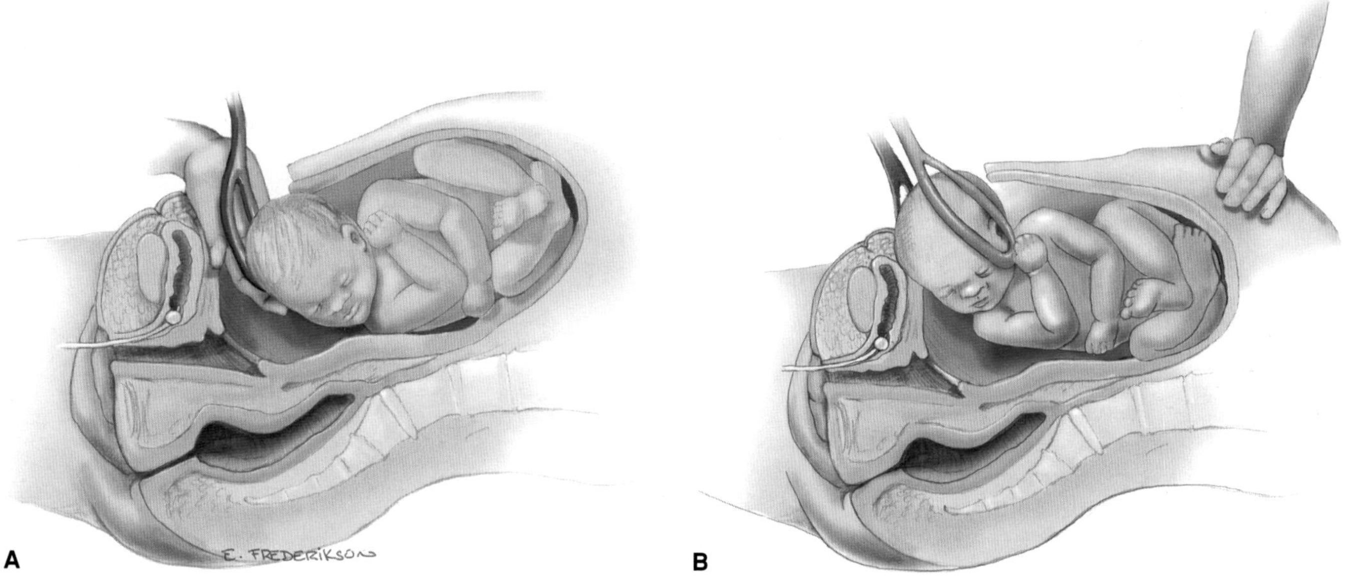

FIGURE 30-7 **A.** The first cesarean forceps blade is placed. **B.** Slight upward and outward traction is used to lift the head through the incision.

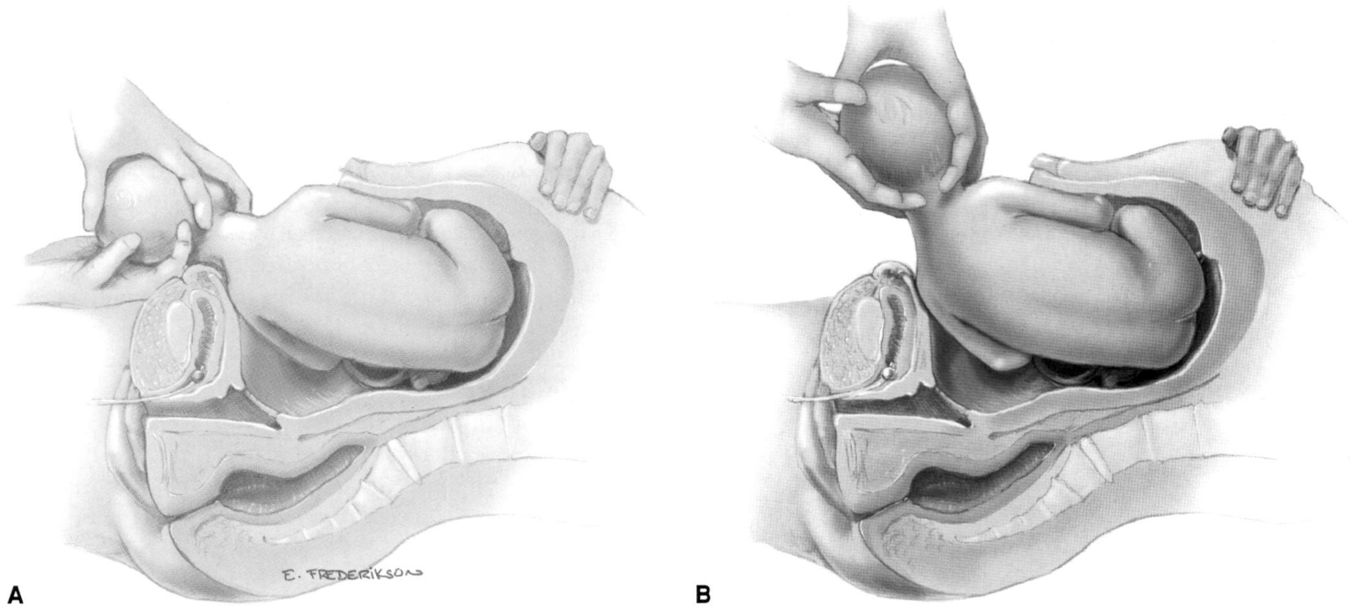

FIGURE 30-8 The anterior **(A)** and then the posterior **(B)** shoulder are delivered.

prophylaxis (Su, 2012). Second-tier agents are ergot-alkaloids, which carry hypertensive side effects, and misoprostol, which provides inferior postpartum hemorrhage protection compared with oxytocin. Last, the use of tranexamic acid (Cyklokapron) has recently been described in a few small studies to lower blood loss during cesarean delivery (Abdel-Aleem, 2013; Güngördük, 2011). Its antifibrinolytic action and effects on thromboembolism rates in pregnant surgical patients are unclear, and larger trials are needed before widespread use. Additional discussions of all these agents are found in Chapters 27 (p. 547) and 41 (p. 785).

Placental Delivery. The uterine incision is observed for any vigorously bleeding sites. These should be promptly clamped with Pennington or ring forceps. The placenta is then delivered unless it has already done so spontaneously. Many surgeons prefer manual removal, but spontaneous delivery, as shown in Fig. 30-9, along with some cord traction may reduce the risk of operative blood loss and infection (Anorlu, 2008; Baksu, 2005). Fundal massage may begin as soon as the fetus is delivered to hasten placental separation and delivery.

Immediately after delivery and gross inspection of the placenta, the uterine cavity is suctioned and wiped out with a gauze sponge to remove avulsed membranes, vernix, and clots. Previously, double-gloved fingers or ring forceps placed through the hysterotomy incision were used to dilate an ostensibly closed cervix. This practice does not improve infection rates from potential hematometra and is not recommended (Güngördük, 2009; Liabsuetrakul, 2011).

Uterine Repair. After placental delivery, the uterus is lifted through the incision onto the draped abdominal wall, and the fundus is covered with a moistened laparotomy sponge. Although some clinicians prefer to avoid such uterine exteriorization, it often has benefits that outweigh its disadvantages. For example, the relaxed, atonic uterus can be recognized quickly and massage applied. The incision and bleeding points are more easily visualized and repaired, especially if there have been extensions. Adnexal exposure is superior, and thus, tubal sterilization is easier. The principal disadvantage is discomfort

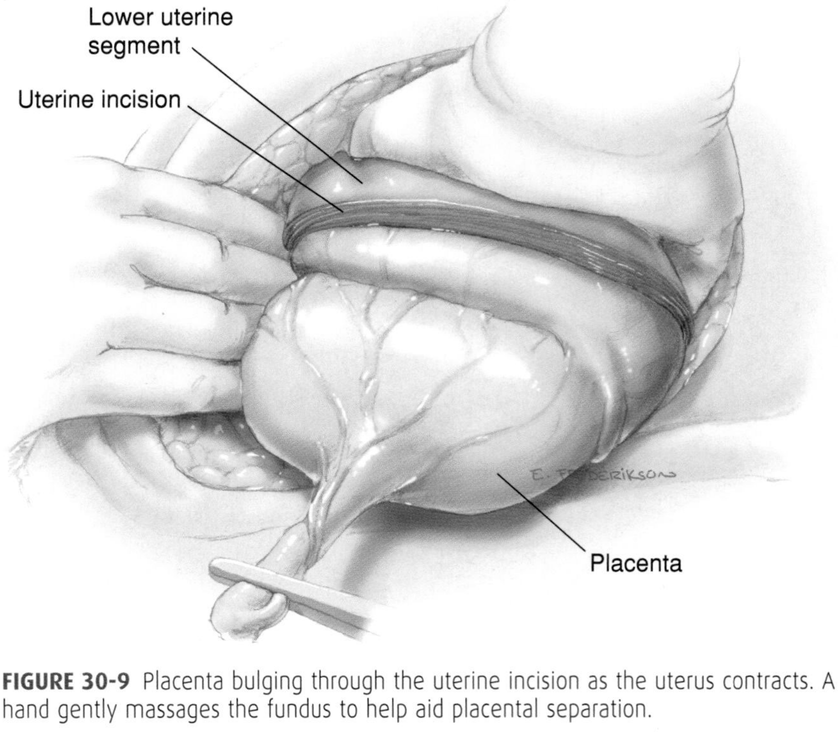

FIGURE 30-9 Placenta bulging through the uterine incision as the uterus contracts. A hand gently massages the fundus to help aid placental separation.

and vomiting caused by traction in cesarean deliveries performed under regional analgesia. Importantly, rates of febrile morbidity or blood loss do not appear to be increased with uterine exteriorization (Coutinho, 2008; Walsh, 2009).

Before hysterotomy closure, previously clamped large vessels may be ligated separately or incorporated within the running incision closure. One angle of the uterine incision is grasped to stabilize and maneuver the incision. The uterine incision is then closed with one or two layers of continuous 0- or No. 1 absorbable suture (Fig. 30-10). Chromic suture is used by many, but some prefer synthetic delayed-absorbable sutures. Single-layer closure is typically faster and is not associated with higher rates of infection or transfusion (CAESAR study collaborative group, 2010; Dodd, 2008; Hauth, 1992). Moreover, most studies observed that the type of uterine closure does not significantly affect complications in the next pregnancy (Chapman, 1997; Durnwald, 2003; Roberge, 2011).

At Parkland Hospital, we favor the one-layer uterine closure. The initial suture is placed just beyond one angle of the uterine incision. A running-lock suture for hemostasis is then performed, with each suture penetrating the full thickness of the myometrium. Concern has been expressed by some clinicians that sutures through the decidua may lead to endometriosis or adenomyosis in the hysterotomy scar, but this is rare. It is important to carefully select the site of each stitch and to avoid withdrawing the needle once it penetrates the myometrium. This minimizes perforation of unligated vessels and subsequent bleeding. The running-lock suture is continued just beyond the opposite incision angle. If approximation is not satisfactory after a single-layer continuous closure or if bleeding sites persist, then more sutures are required. Either another layer of running suture is placed to achieve approximation and hemostasis, or individual bleeding sites can be secured with figure-of-eight or mattress sutures.

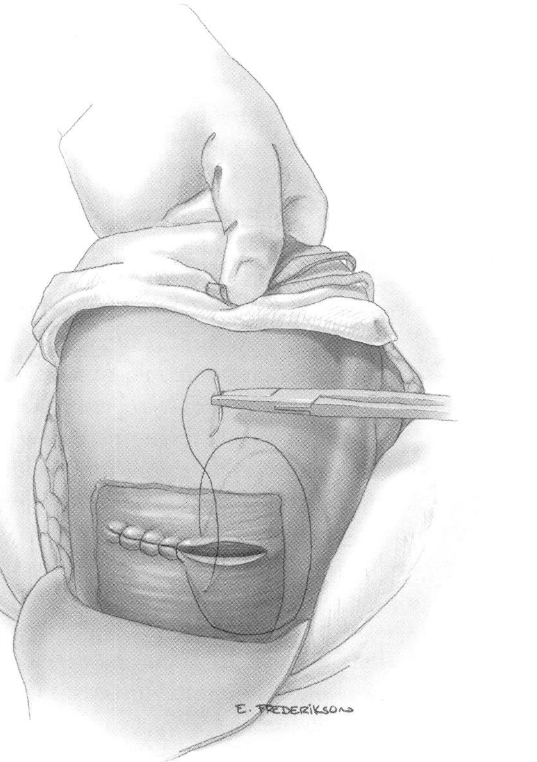

FIGURE 30-10 The cut edges of the uterine incision are approximated with a running-lock suture anchored at either angle of the incision.

Traditionally, serosal edges overlying the uterus and bladder have been approximated with a continuous 2-0 chromic catgut suture. Multiple randomized trials suggest that omission of this step causes no postoperative complications (Grundsell, 1998; Irion, 1996; Nagele, 1996). If tubal sterilization is to be performed, it is now done as described in Chapter 39 (p. 720).

Adhesions

Following cesarean delivery, adhesions commonly form within the vesicouterine space or between the anterior abdominal wall and uterus. And with each successive pregnancy, the percentage of affected women and adhesion severity increases (Morales, 2007; Tulandi, 2009). Adhesions can significantly lengthen incision-to-delivery times and total operative time (Rossouw, 2013; Sikirica, 2012). Although occurring infrequently, rates of cystotomy and bowel injury are also increased (Rahman, 2009; Silver, 2006).

Intuitively, scarring can be reduced by handling tissues delicately, achieving hemostasis, and minimizing tissue ischemia, infection, and foreign-body reaction. Data are conflicting regarding closure of the bladder flap (visceral peritoneum) or of the abdominal cavity (parietal peritoneum) and its effect on subsequent adhesions. Some note benefit from closure of one, but not the other, or neither (CAESAR study collaborative group, 2010; Cheong, 2009; Kapustian, 2012; Lyell, 2005, 2012).

Benefit from placement of an adhesion barrier at the repaired hysterotomy site is limited to only two nonrandomized studies (Chapa, 2011; Fushiki, 2005). Currently, there is an ongoing multicenter randomized trial to evaluate use of the barrier *Seprafilm* at the time of cesarean delivery (National Institutes of Health, 2012).

Abdominal Closure

Any laparotomy sponges are removed, and the paracolic gutters and cul-de-sac are gently suctioned of blood and amnionic fluid. Some surgeons irrigate the gutters and cul-de-sac, especially in the presence of infection or meconium. Routine irrigation in low-risk women, however, leads to greater intraoperative nausea and without lower postoperative infection rates (Harrigill, 2003; Viney, 2012).

After sponge and instrument counts are found to be correct, the abdominal incision is closed in layers. Many surgeons omit the parietal peritoneal closure. In addition to ambiguity regarding adhesion prevention, data are also conflicting as to whether nonclosure of parietal peritoneum decreases postoperative discomfort and analgesia requirements (Chanrachakul, 2002; Lyell, 2005; Rafique, 2002). However, if there is distended bowel in the incision site, we find that peritoneal closure may help to protect the bowel when fascial sutures are placed.

As each layer is closed, bleeding sites are located, clamped, and ligated or coagulated with an electrosurgical blade. The rectus abdominis muscles are allowed to fall into place. With significant diastasis, the rectus muscles may be approximated with one or two figure-of-eight sutures of 0 or No. 1 chromic gut suture. The overlying rectus fascia is closed by a continuous, nonlocking technique with a delayed-absorbable suture. In patients with a higher risk for infection, there may be theoretical value in selecting a monofilament suture here rather than braided material.

The subcutaneous tissue usually need not be closed if it is less than 2 cm thick. With thicker layers, however, closure is recommended to minimize seroma and hematoma formation, which can lead to wound infection and/or disruption (Bohman, 1992; Chelmow, 2004). Addition of a subcutaneous drain does not prevent significant wound complications (Hellums, 2007; Ramsey, 2005). Skin is closed with a running subcuticular stitch using 4-0 delayed-absorbable suture or with staples. In comparison, final cosmetic results and infection rates appear similar, skin suturing takes longer, but wound separation rates are higher with staples (Basha, 2010; Figueroa, 2013; Mackeen, 2012; Tuuli, 2011).

Joel-Cohen and Misgav-Ladach Techniques

The Pfannenstiel-Kerr technique just described has been used for decades. More recently, the Joel-Cohen and Misgav-Ladach modifications have been described. These differ from traditional Pfannenstiel-Kerr entry mainly by their initial incision placement and greater use of blunt dissection.

The Joel-Cohen technique creates a straight 10-cm transverse skin incision 3 cm below the level of the anterior superior iliac spines. The subcutaneous tissue layer is opened sharply 2 to 3 cm in the midline. This is carried down, without lateral extension, to the fascia. A small transverse incision is made in the fascia, and a finger from each hand is hooked into the lateral angles of this fascial incision. The incision is then stretched transversely. Once the fascia is opened and rectus abdominis muscle bellies identified, an index finger from each hand is inserted between the bellies. One is moved cranially and the other caudally, in opposition, to further separate the bellies. Index finger dissection is used to enter the peritoneum, and again, cranial and caudad opposing stretch with index fingers will open this layer. All the layers of the abdominal wall are then manually stretched laterally in opposition to further open the incision. The visceral peritoneum is incised in the midline above the bladder, and the bladder is bluntly reflected inferiorly to separate it from the underlying lower uterine segment. The myometrium is incised transversely in the midline and then opened and extended laterally with one finger hooked into each corner of the hysterotomy incision. Interrupted sutures are used for hysterotomy closure. Neither visceral nor parietal peritoneum is closed. The Misgav-Ladach technique is similar and differs mainly in that myometrial incision closure is completed with a single-layer locking continuous suture (Hofmeyr, 2009; Holmgren, 1999).

These techniques have been associated with shorter operative times and with lower rates of intraoperative blood loss and postoperative pain (Hofmeyr, 2008). They may, however, prove difficult for women with anterior rectus fibrosis and peritoneal adhesions (Bolze, 2013). Moreover, long-term outcomes with these techniques, such as subsequent uterine rupture, are unknown.

Classical Cesarean Incision

This incision is usually avoided because it encompasses the active upper uterine segment and thus is prone to rupture with subsequent pregnancies.

Indications. A classical incision is occasionally preferred for delivery. Some indications stem from difficulty in exposing or safely entering the lower uterine segment. For example, a *densely adhered bladder* from previous surgery is encountered; a *leiomyoma* occupies the lower uterine segment; the cervix has been *invaded by cancer*; or *massive maternal obesity* precludes safe access to the lower uterine segment. A classical incision is also preferred in some cases of *placenta previa with anterior implantation*, especially those complicated by placenta accrete syndromes.

In other instances, fetal indications dictate the need. *Transverse lie of a large fetus*, especially if the membranes are ruptured and the shoulder is impacted in the birth canal, usually necessitates a classical incision. A fetus presenting as a back-down transverse lie is particularly difficult to deliver through a transverse uterine incision. In instances when the fetus is very small, especially if breech, a classical incision may be preferable (Osmundson, 2013). In such cases, the poorly developed lower uterine segment provides inadequate space for the manipulations required for breech delivery. Or, less commonly, the small fetal head may become entrapped by a contracting uterine fundus following membrane rupture. Last, with multiple fetuses, a classical incision again may be needed to provide suitable room for extraction of fetuses that may be malpositioned or preterm.

Uterine Incision and Repair. A vertical uterine incision is initiated with a scalpel beginning as low as possible and preferably within the lower uterine segment (Fig. 30-11). If adhesions, insufficient exposure, a tumor, or placenta percreta preclude development of a bladder flap, then the incision is made above the level of the bladder. Once the uterus is entered with a scalpel, the incision is extended cephalad with bandage scissors until it is long enough to permit delivery of the fetus. With scissor use, the fingers of the nondominant hand are insinuated between the myometrium and fetus to prevent fetal laceration. As the incision is opened, numerous large vessels that bleed profusely are commonly encountered within the myometrium. The remainder of fetal and placental delivery mirrors that with a low transverse hysterotomy.

For incision closure, one method employs a layer of 0- or No. 1 chromic catgut with a continuous stitch to approximate the deeper halves of the incision (Fig. 30-12). The outer depth of myometrium is then closed with similar suture and with a running stitch or figure-of-eight sutures. No unnecessary needle tracks should be made lest myometrial vessels be perforated, leading to subsequent hemorrhage or hematomas. To achieve good approximation and to prevent the suture from tearing through the myometrium, it is helpful to have an assistant compress the uterus on each side of the wound toward the midline as each stitch is placed.

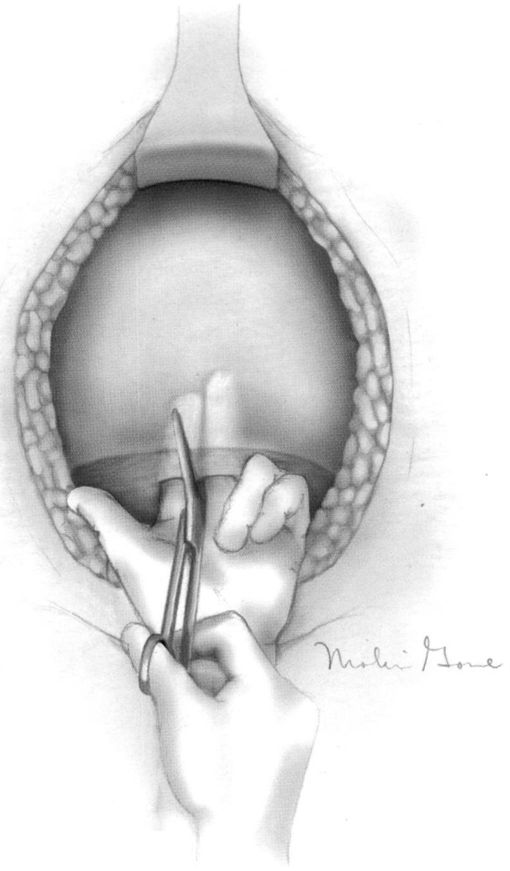

FIGURE 30-11 An initial small vertical hysterotomy incision is made in the lower uterine segment. Fingers are insinuated between the myometrium and fetus to avoid fetal laceration. Scissors extend the incision cephalad as needed for delivery.

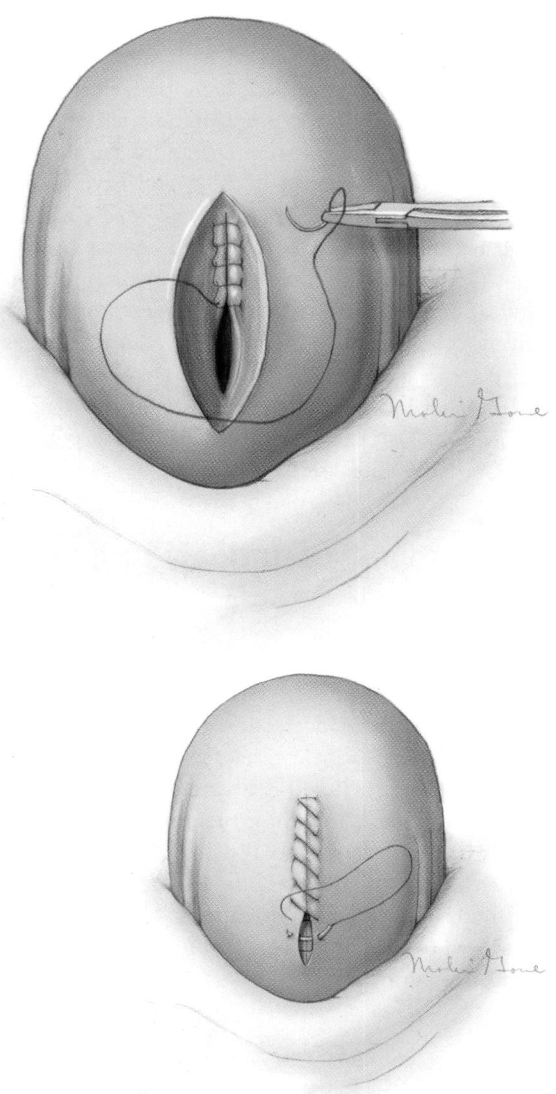

A

B

FIGURE 30-12 Classical incision closure. The deeper half **(A)** and superficial half **(B)** of the incision are closed in a running fashion.

PERIPARTUM HYSTERECTOMY

Indications

Hysterectomy is more commonly performed during or after cesarean delivery but may be needed following vaginal birth. If all deliveries are considered, the rate ranges from 0.4 to 2.5 per 1000 births and has risen significantly during the past few decades. During a 25-year period, the rate of peripartum hysterectomy at Parkland Hospital was 1.7 per 1000 births (Hernandez, 2012). Most of this increase is attributed to the increasing rates of cesarean delivery and its associated complications in subsequent pregnancy (Bateman, 2012; Bodelon, 2009; Flood, 2009; Orbach, 2011). Of hysterectomies, approximately one half to two thirds are total, whereas the remaining cases are supracervical (Rossi, 2010; Shellhaas, 2009).

Cesarean hysterectomies are most commonly performed to arrest or prevent hemorrhage from intractable uterine atony or abnormal placentation (Bateman, 2012; Hernandez, 2012; Owolabi, 2013). These as well as other less frequent indications are found in Table 30-3. For example, large leiomyomas may preclude satisfactory hysterotomy closure and necessitate hysterectomy. Or, postpartum infectious morbidity from an infected, necrotic uterus will prompt uterine removal for recovery (Fig. 37-4, p. 688). Logically, risk factors for peripartum hysterectomy mirror the risks of these indicated complications, which are described throughout the text.

Major complications of peripartum hysterectomy include increased blood loss and greater risk of urinary tract damage. Blood loss is usually appreciable because hysterectomy is being

TABLE 30-3. Some Indications for Peripartum Hysterectomy
Uterine atony
Abnormal placentation
Bleeding
Accrete syndromes
Uterine extension
Uterine rupture
Cervical laceration
Postpartum uterine infection
Leiomyoma
Invasive cervical cancer
Ovarian neoplasia

performed for hemorrhage that frequently is torrential, and the procedure itself is associated with substantial blood loss. Although many cases with such hemorrhage cannot be anticipated, those with abnormal implantation can often be identified antepartum. Preoperative preparations for placenta accreta are discussed in Chapter 41 (p. 807) and have also been outlined by the Society for Maternal-Fetal Medicine (2010) and American College of Obstetricians and Gynecologists (2012c).

An important factor affecting the cesarean hysterectomy complication rate is whether the operation is performed electively or emergently (Briery, 2007). After anticipated or planned cesarean hysterectomy, there are lower rates of blood loss, less need for blood transfusions, and fewer urinary tract complications compared with emergent procedures (Briery, 2007; Glaze, 2008; Sakse, 2007).

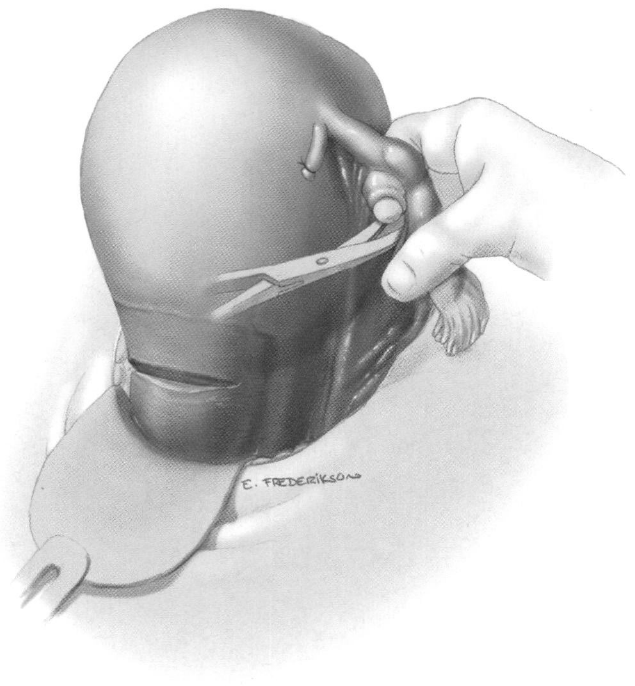

FIGURE 30-14 The posterior leaf of the broad ligament adjacent to the uterus is perforated just beneath the fallopian tube, utero-ovarian ligaments, and ovarian vessels.

Peripartum Hysterectomy Technique

Supracervical or total hysterectomy is performed using standard operative techniques. For this, adequate exposure is essential. Initially, placement of a self-retaining retractor such as a Balfour is not necessary. Rather, satisfactory exposure is obtained with cephalad traction on the uterus by an assistant, along with handheld retractors such as a Richardson or Deaver. The bladder flap is deflected downward to the level of the cervix if possible to permit total hysterectomy. In cases in which cesarean hysterectomy is planned or strongly suspected, extended bladder flap dissection is ideally completed before initial hysterotomy. Later attempts at bladder dissection may be obscured by bleeding, or excess blood may be lost while this dissection is performed.

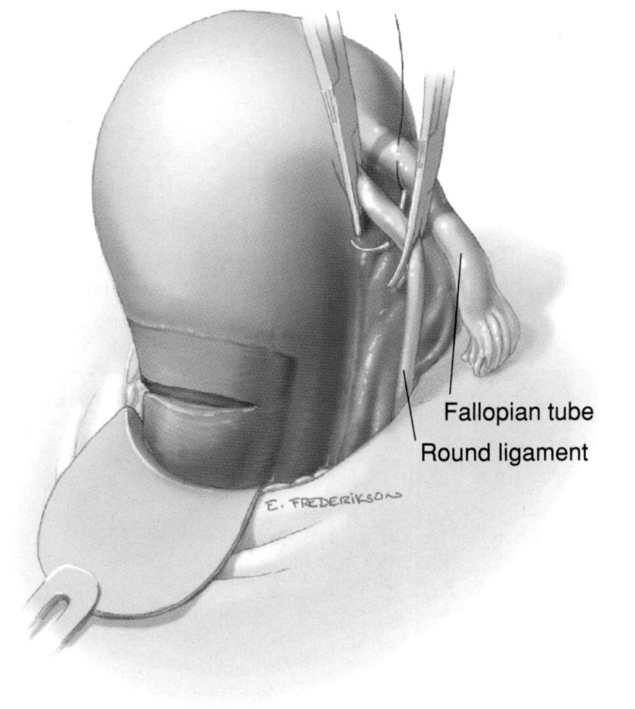

FIGURE 30-13 The round ligaments are clamped, doubly ligated, and transected bilaterally.

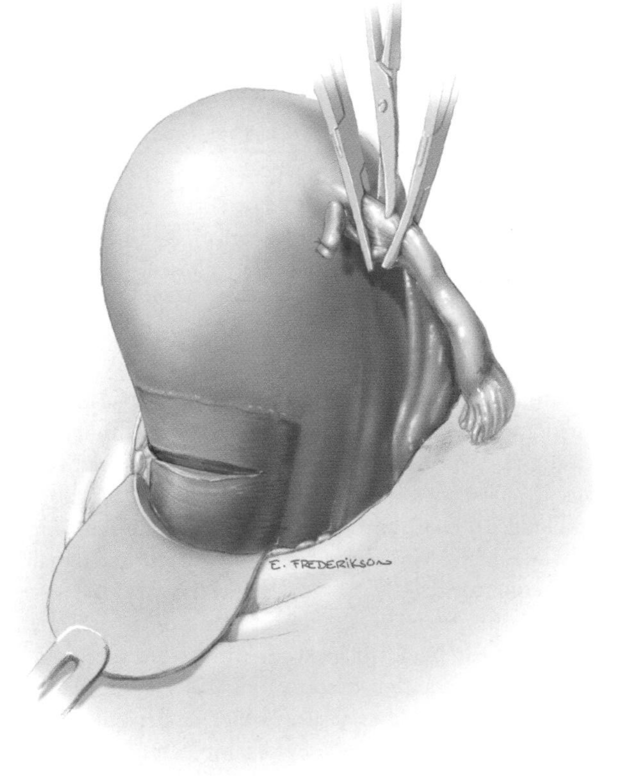

FIGURE 30-15 The uteroovarian ligament and fallopian tube are doubly clamped and cut bilaterally. The lateral pedicle is doubly ligated.

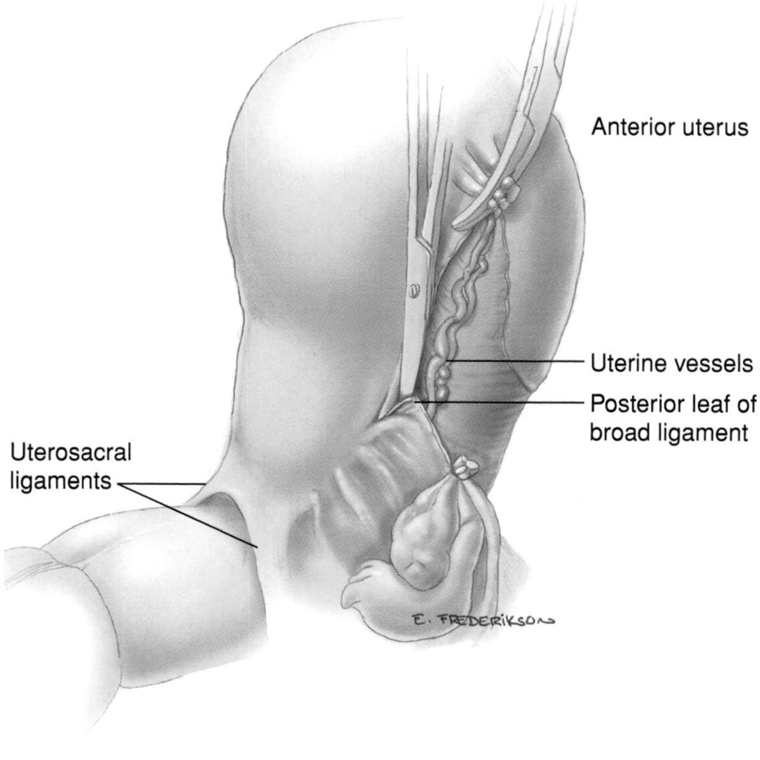

FIGURE 30-16 The posterior leaf of the broad ligament is divided inferiorly toward the uterosacral ligament.

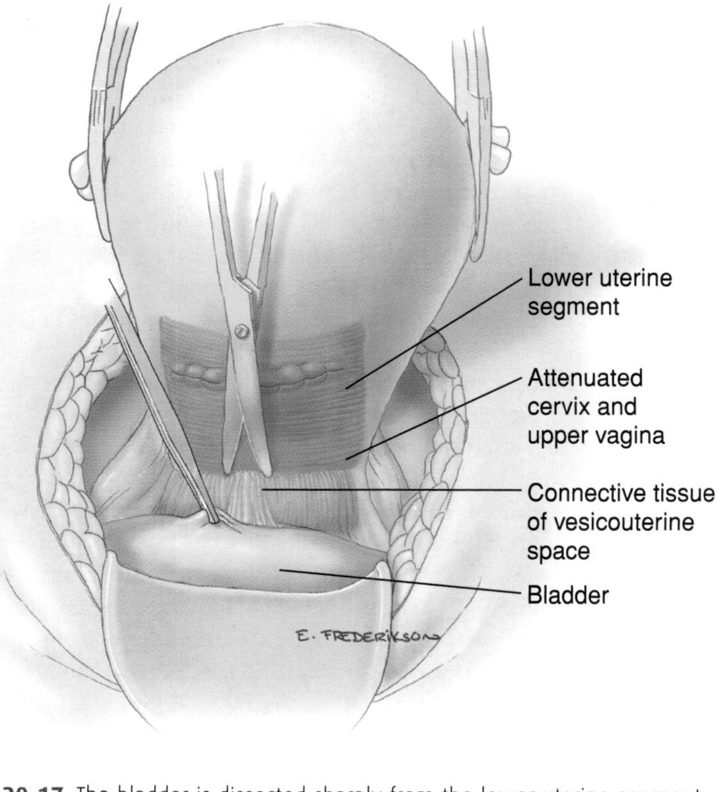

FIGURE 30-17 The bladder is dissected sharply from the lower uterine segment.

After cesarean delivery, the placenta is typically removed. In cases of placenta accrete syndromes, in which hysterectomy is already planned, the placenta is usually left undisturbed in situ. In either situation, if the hysterotomy incision is bleeding appreciably, it can be sutured or Pennington or sponge forceps can be applied for hemostasis. If bleeding is minimal, neither maneuver is necessary.

The round ligaments are divided close to the uterus between Kocher clamps and doubly ligated (Fig. 30-13). Either 0 or No. 1 suture can be used in either chromic gut or delayed-absorbable material. The incision in the vesicouterine serosa that was made to mobilize the bladder is extended laterally and upward through the anterior leaf of the broad ligament to reach the incised round ligaments. The posterior leaf of the broad ligament adjacent to the uterus is perforated just beneath the fallopian tubes, uteroovarian ligaments, and ovarian vessels (Fig. 30-14). These structures together are then doubly clamped close to the uterus and divided, and the lateral pedicle is doubly ligated (Fig. 30-15). The posterior leaf of the broad ligament is divided toward the uterosacral ligaments (Fig. 30-16). Next, the bladder and attached peritoneal flap are further deflected and dissected as needed from the lower uterine segment and retracted out of the operative field. If the bladder flap is unusually adhered, as it may be after previous hysterotomy incisions, careful sharp dissection may be necessary (Fig. 30-17).

Special care is required from this point on to avoid injury to the ureters, which pass beneath the uterine arteries. To help accomplish this, an assistant places constant traction to pull the uterus in the direction away from the side on which the uterine vessels are being ligated. The ascending uterine artery and veins on either side are identified near their origin. These pedicles are then doubly clamped immediately adjacent to the uterus, divided, and doubly suture ligated. As shown in Figure 30-18, we prefer to use three heavy clamps—Heaney or Ballantine—to incise the tissue between the most medial clamps, and then ligate the pedicle in the clamps lateral to the uterus.

With cesarean hysterectomy, it may be more advantageous in cases of profuse hemorrhage to rapidly double clamp and divide all of the vascular pedicles between clamps to gain hemostasis. The operator can then return to ligate all of the pedicles.

Total Hysterectomy

Even if total hysterectomy is planned, we find it in many cases technically easier to finish the operation after amputating the uterine fundus and placing Ochsner or Kocher clamps on the cervical stump for traction and hemostasis.

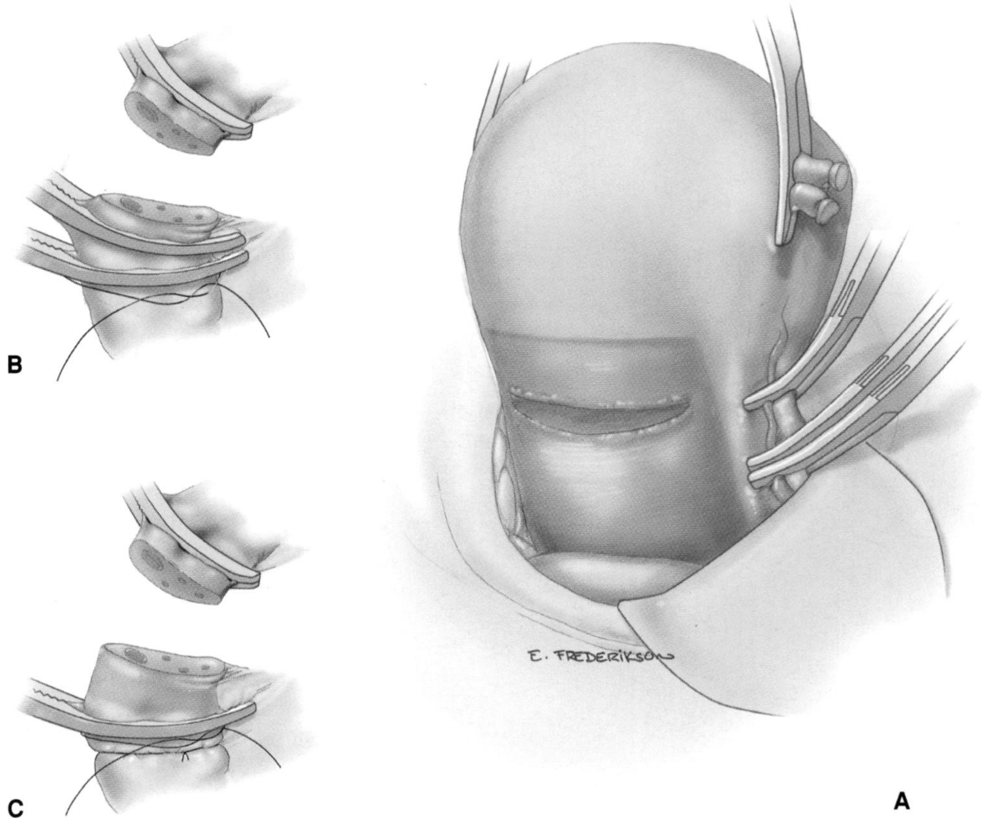

FIGURE 30-18 A. The uterine artery and veins on either side are doubly clamped immediately adjacent to the uterus and divided. A third medial clamp will prevent "back bleeding." **B & C.** The vascular pedicle is doubly suture ligated.

Self-retaining retractors also may be placed at this time. To remove the cervix, the bladder is mobilized further if needed. This carries the ureters caudad as the bladder is retracted beneath the symphysis and will prevent laceration or suturing of the bladder during cervical excision and vaginal cuff closure.

If the cervix is effaced and dilated considerably, its softness may obscure palpable identification of the cervicovaginal junction. The junction location can be ascertained through a vertical uterine incision made anteriorly in the midline, either through the open hysterotomy incision or through an incision created at the level of the ligated uterine vessels. A finger is directed inferiorly through the incision to identify the free margin of the dilated, effaced cervix and the anterior vaginal fornix. The contaminated glove is replaced. Another useful method to identify the cervical margins is to transvaginally place four metal skin clips or brightly colored sutures at 12, 3, 6, and 9 o'clock positions on the cervical edges in cases of planned hysterectomy.

The cardinal ligaments, the uterosacral ligaments, and the many large vessels these ligaments contain are clamped systematically with Heaney-type curved or straight clamps (Fig. 30-19). The clamps are placed as close to the cervix as possible, taking care not to include excessive tissue in each clamp. The tissue between the pair of clamps is incised, and the lateral pedicle is suture ligated. These steps are repeated caudally until the level of the lateral vaginal fornix is reached. In this way, the descending branches of the uterine vessels are clamped, cut, and ligated as the cervix is dissected from the cardinal ligaments.

Immediately below the level of the cervix, a curved clamp is placed across the lateral vaginal fornix, and the tissue is incised above the clamp (Fig. 30-20). The excised lateral vaginal fornix can be simultaneously doubly ligated and sutured to the stump of the cardinal ligament. The cervix is inspected to ensure that it has been completely removed, and the vagina is then repaired. Each of the angles of the lateral vaginal fornix is secured to the cardinal and uterosacral ligaments to mitigate later vaginal prolapse (Fig. 30-21). Following this step, some surgeons prefer to close the vagina using figure-of-eight sutures. Others achieve hemostasis by using a running-lock stitch placed through the mucosa and adjacent endopelvic fascia around the circumference of the vaginal cuff (Fig. 30-22).

If a self-retaining retractor has not already been placed, some clinicians choose to insert one at this point. The bowel is then packed out of the field, and all sites are examined carefully for bleeding. One technique is to perform a systematic bilateral survey from the fallopian tube and ovarian ligament pedicles to the vaginal vault and bladder flap. Bleeding sites are ligated with care to avoid the ureters. The abdominal wall normally is closed in layers, as previously described for cesarean delivery (p. 597).

Supracervical Hysterectomy

To perform a subtotal hysterectomy, the uterine body is amputated immediately above the level of uterine artery ligation. The

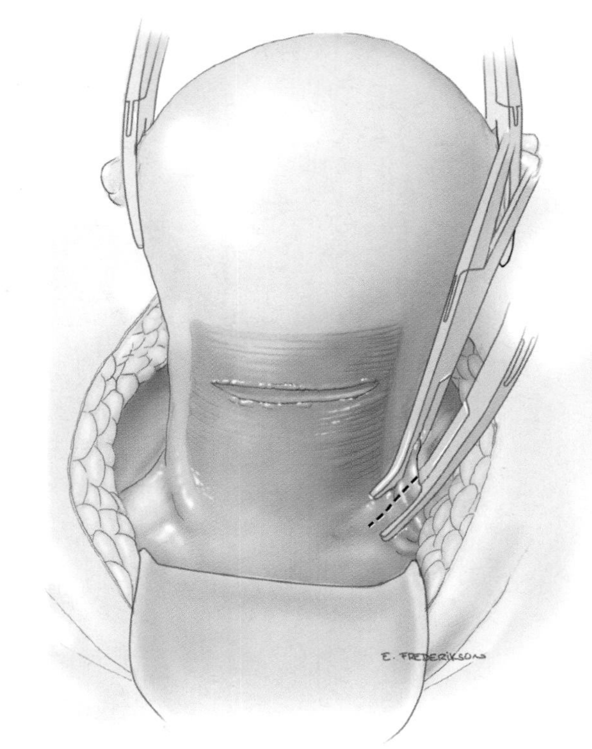

FIGURE 30-19 The cardinal ligaments are clamped, incised, and ligated.

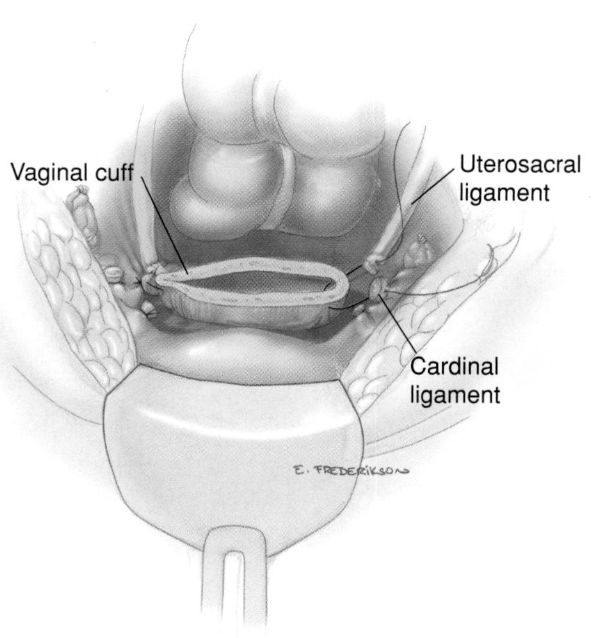

FIGURE 30-21 The lateral angles of the vaginal cuff are secured to the cardinal and uterosacral ligaments.

cervical stump may be closed with continuous or interrupted chromic catgut sutures of 0 or No. 1 gauge. Subtotal hysterectomy is often all that is necessary to stop hemorrhage. It may be preferred for women who would benefit from a shorter surgery or for those with extensive adhesions that threaten significant urinary tract injury.

Salpingo-Oophorectomy

Because of the large adnexal vessels and their close proximity to the uterus, it may be necessary to remove one or both adnexa to obtain hemostasis. Briery and colleagues (2007) reported unilateral or bilateral oophorectomy in a fourth of cases. Preoperative counseling should include this possibility.

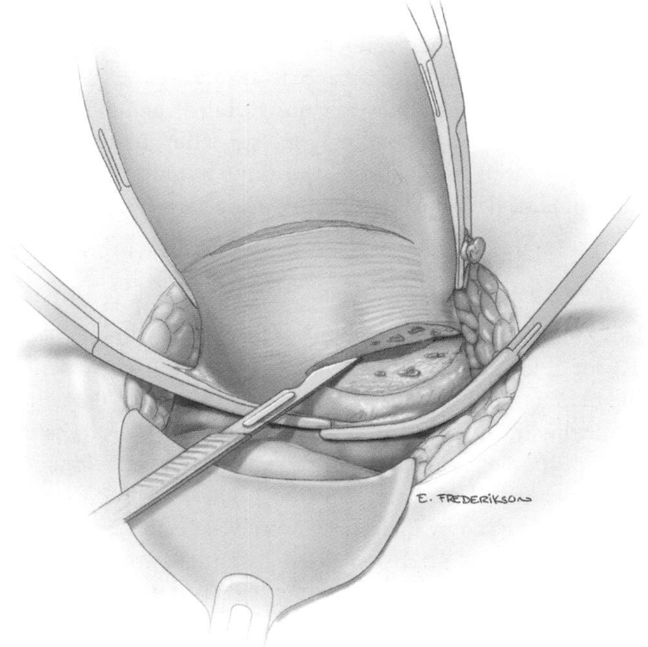

FIGURE 30-20 A curved clamp is placed across the lateral vaginal fornix below the level of the cervix, and the tissue incised medially to the point of the clamp.

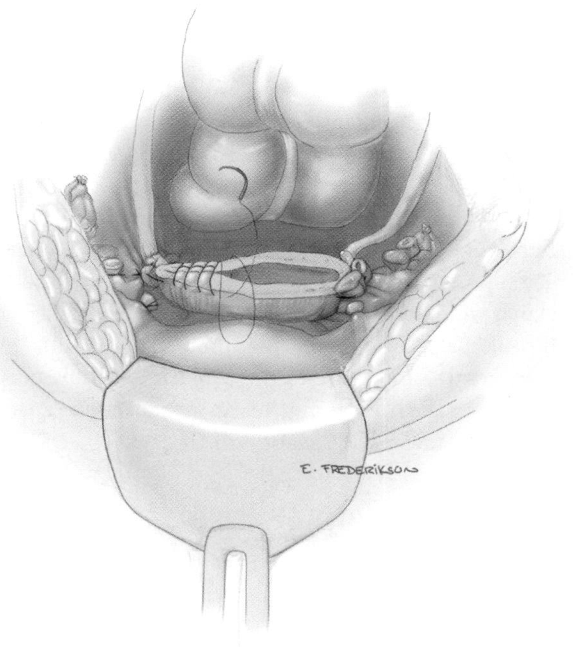

FIGURE 30-22 A running-lock suture approximates the vaginal wall edges.

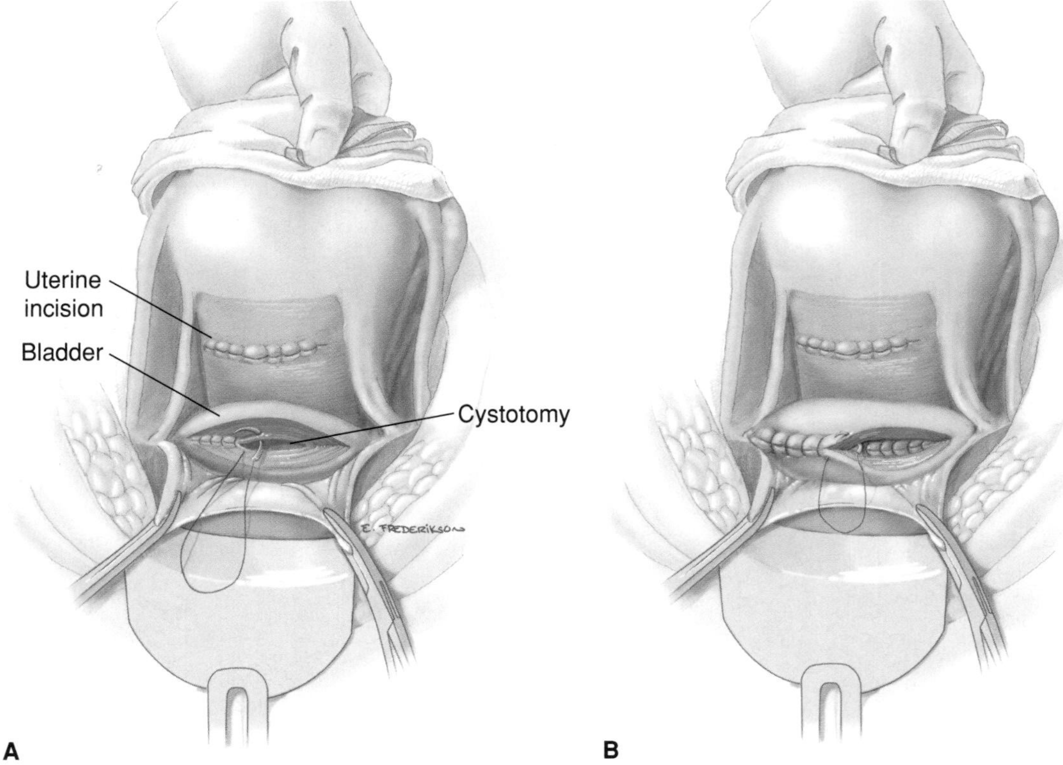

FIGURE 30-23 Cystotomy repair. **A.** The primary layer inverts the bladder mucosa with running or interrupted sutures of 3-0 delayed-absorbable or absorbable suture. **B.** Second and possibly a third layer approximate the bladder muscularis to reinforce the incision closure.

Cystotomy

Rarely, and usually in women who have had a previous cesarean delivery, the bladder may be lacerated. This complication may occur during cesarean delivery, but it is more common with cesarean hysterectomy, especially if there is abnormal placental implantation.

Bladder injury is typically identified at the time of surgery, and initially, a gush of clear fluid into the operating field may be seen. If cystotomy is suspected, it may be confirmed with retrograde instillation of sterile infant formula through a Foley catheter into the bladder. Leakage of opaque milk aids in laceration identification and delineation of its borders. In some cases, cystoscopy may be indicated to further define bladder injury. Primary repair is preferred and lowers the risk of postoperative vesicovaginal fistula formation. Once ureteral patency is confirmed, the bladder may be closed with a two- or three-layer running closure using a 3-0 absorbable or delayed-absorbable suture (Fig. 30-23). The first layer inverts the mucosa into the bladder, and subsequent layers reapproximate bladder muscularis. Postoperative care requires continuous bladder drainage for 7 to 10 days.

PERIPARTUM MANAGEMENT

Intravenous Fluids

During and after cesarean delivery, requirements for intravenous fluids can vary considerably. Intravenously administered fluids consist of either lactated Ringer solution or a similar crystalloid solution with 5-percent dextrose. Typically, at least 2 to 3 L is infused during surgery. Blood loss with uncomplicated cesarean delivery approximates 1000 mL. The average-sized woman with a hematocrit of 30 percent or more and with a normally expanded blood and extracellular fluid volume most often will tolerate blood loss up to 2000 mL without difficulty. Unappreciated bleeding through the vagina during the procedure, bleeding concealed in the uterus after its closure, or both commonly lead to underestimation.

Blood loss averages 1500 mL with elective cesarean hysterectomy, although this is variable (Pritchard, 1965). Most peripartum hysterectomies are unscheduled, and blood loss in these cases is correspondingly greater. Thus, in addition to close monitoring of vital signs and urine output, the hematocrit should be determined intra- or postoperatively as indicated (Chap. 41, p. 781).

Recovery Suite

Close monitoring of the amount of vaginal bleeding is necessary for at least an hour in the immediate postoperative period. The uterine fundus is also identified frequently by palpation to ensure that the uterus remains firmly contracted. Unfortunately, as conduction analgesia fades or the woman awakens from general anesthesia, abdominal palpation is likely to produce pain. An analgesic given by intermittent intravenous injection can be effective (Table 30-4). A sterile thin abdominal wound dressing is sufficient, and indeed, a thick, heavily taped padded dressing will interfere with fundal palpation and massage. Deep breathing and coughing are encouraged. Once regional analgesia begins to fade or the woman becomes fully awake following general anesthesia, criteria for transfer to the postpartum ward include minimal bleeding, stable vital signs, and adequate urine output.

TABLE 30-4. Typical Settings for Administration of Intravenous Opioids via a Patient-Controlled Analgesia Pump

Recovery room:
IV meperidine, 25 mg every 5 min up to 100 mg
or
IV morphine, 2 mg every 5 min up to 10 mg

Postpartum ward (first 24 hr after surgery)[a]:
IM meperidine, 50–75 mg every 3–4 hr as needed
or
PCA intravenous meperidine, 10 mg with a 6 min lockout interval and maximum dose of 200 mg in 4 hr as needed. An additional 25-mg booster dose is permitted for a maximum of 2 doses
or
IM morphine, 10–15 mg every 3–4 hr as needed
or
PCA intravenous morphine, 1 mg with a 6-min lockout interval and maximum dose of 30 mg in 4 hr as needed. An additional 2-mg booster dose is permitted for a maximum of 2 doses

[a]Each postpartum ward regimen also included promethazine, 25 mg intravenously every 6 hr as needed for nausea.
IM = intramuscular; IV = intravenous; PCA = patient-controlled analgesia.
From Yost, 2004, with permission.

Hospital Care until Discharge

Analgesia, Vital Signs, Intravenous Fluids

A number of schemes are suitable for postoperative pain control. Some basic regimens are shown in Table 30-4. In a trial at Parkland Hospital, Yost and associates (2004) found that morphine provided superior pain relief to meperidine and was associated with significantly higher rates of breast feeding and continuation of infant rooming in. Breast feeding can be initiated the day of surgery. If the mother elects not to breast feed, a binder that supports the breasts without marked compression usually will minimize discomfort (Chap. 36, p. 675).

After transfer to her room, the woman is assessed at least hourly for 4 hours, and thereafter at intervals of 4 hours. Vital signs, uterine tone, urine output, and bleeding are evaluated. The hematocrit is routinely measured the morning after surgery. It is checked sooner if there was unusual blood loss or if there is hypotension, tachycardia, oliguria, or other evidence to suggest hypovolemia. If the hematocrit is decreased significantly from the preoperative level, the measurement is repeated and a search is instituted to identify the cause. If the hematocrit stabilizes, the mother can be allowed to ambulate, and if there is little likelihood of further blood loss, iron therapy is preferred to transfusion.

As described in Chapter 36 (p. 671), the puerperium is characterized by excretion of fluid that was retained during pregnancy. At least with elective cesarean delivery, significant extracellular fluid sequestration in the bowel wall and lumen does not occur, unless perhaps it was necessary to pack the bowel away from the operative field. Thus, the woman who undergoes routine cesarean delivery rarely develops fluid sequestration in the extracellular space. On the contrary, she normally begins surgery with a physiologically enlarged extravascular volume acquired during pregnancy that she mobilizes and excretes after delivery. As a generalization, 3 L of fluid should prove adequate during the first 24 hours after surgery. If urine output falls below 30 mL/hr, however, the woman should be reevaluated promptly. The cause of the oliguria may range from unrecognized blood loss to an antidiuretic effect from infused oxytocin.

Women undergoing unscheduled cesarean delivery may have pathological retention or constriction of the extracellular fluid compartment caused by severe preeclampsia, sepsis syndrome, vomiting, prolonged labor without adequate fluid intake, and increased blood loss.

Bladder and Bowel Function

The Foley catheter most often can be removed by 12 hours postoperatively, or more conveniently, the morning after surgery. The prevalence of urinary retention following cesarean delivery approximates 3 to 7 percent. Regional analgesia and failure to progress in labor are identified risks (Chai, 2008; Liang, 2007). Thus, surveillance for bladder overdistention should be implemented as with vaginal delivery.

In uncomplicated cases, solid food may be offered within 8 hours of surgery (Bar, 2008; Orji, 2009). Although some degree of adynamic ileus follows virtually every abdominal operation, in most cases of cesarean delivery, it is negligible. Symptoms include abdominal distention, gas pains, and an inability to pass flatus or stool. The pathophysiology of postoperative ileus is complex and involves inflammatory and neural factors that are incompletely understood (van Bree, 2012). If associated with otherwise unexplained fever, an unrecognized bowel injury may be responsible. Treatment for ileus has changed little during the past several decades and involves intravenous fluid and electrolyte supplementation. If severe, nasogastric decompression is necessary.

Ambulation and Wound Care

As discussed on page 590, women undergoing cesarean delivery have an increased risk of venous thromboembolism compared with those delivering vaginally. Additional risks include age > 35; obesity; parity > 3; emergency cesarean; cesarean hysterectomy; concurrent infection, major illness, preeclampsia, or gross varicosities; recent immobility; and prior deep-vein thrombosis or thrombophilia (Marik, 2008). Postoperative thromboprophylaxis is discussed in Chapter 52 (p. 1045). Early ambulation lowers the risk of venous thromboembolism. In most instances, by the day after surgery, a woman should get briefly out of bed with assistance at least twice to walk. Ambulation can be timed so that a recently administered analgesic will minimize discomfort. By the second day, she may walk without assistance.

The incision is inspected each day, and skin sutures or clips often can be removed on the fourth postoperative day. If there is concern, however, for superficial wound separation—for example, in obese patients—the suture or clips should remain in place for 7 to 10 days. By the third postpartum day, showering is not harmful to the incision.

Hospital Discharge

Unless there are complications during the puerperium, the mother generally is discharged on the third or fourth postpartum day (Buie, 2010). Data from small studies suggest that earlier discharge may be feasible for properly selected and motivated women (Strong, 1993; Tan, 2012). Activities during the first week should be restricted to self-care and newborn care with assistance. Driving can be resumed when pain does not limit the ability to brake quickly and when narcotic medications are not in use. Return to work is variable. Six weeks is commonly cited, although many women use the Family and Medical Leave Act to allow up to 12 weeks for recovery and newborn bonding.

REFERENCES

Abdel-Aleem H, Alhusaini T, Abdel-Aleem M, et al: Effectiveness of tranexamic acid on blood loss in patients undergoing elective cesarean section: randomized clinical trial. J Matern Fetal Neonatal Med 26(17):1705, 2013

Alexander JM, Leveno KJ, Hauth J, et al: Fetal injury associated with cesarean delivery. Obstet Gynecol 108(4):885, 2006

American Academy of Pediatrics and American College of Obstetricians and Gynecologists: Guidelines for Perinatal Care, 7th ed. Elk Grove, American Academy of Pediatrics, 2012

American College of Obstetricians and Gynecologists: Fetal monitoring prior to scheduled cesarean delivery. Committee Opinion No. 382, October 2007, Reaffirmed 2010

American College of Obstetricians and Gynecologists: Preoperative planned cesarean delivery. Patient Safety Checklist No. 4, December 2011a

American College of Obstetricians and Gynecologists: Prophylactic antibiotics in labor and delivery. Practice Bulletin No. 120, June 2011b

American College of Obstetricians and Gynecologists: Scheduling planned cesarean delivery. Patient Safety Checklist No. 3, December 2011c

American College of Obstetricians and Gynecologists: Thromboembolism in pregnancy. Practice Bulletin No. 123, September 2011d

American College of Obstetricians and Gynecologists: Informed consent. Committee Opinion No. 439, August 2009, Reaffirmed 2012a

American College of Obstetricians and Gynecologists: Patient safety in the surgical environment. Committee Opinion No. 464, September 2010, Reaffirmed 2012b

American College of Obstetricians and Gynecologists: Placenta accreta. Committee Opinion No. 529, July 2012c

American College of Obstetricians and Gynecologists: Cesarean delivery on maternal request. Committee Opinion No. 559, April 2013

Anorlu RI, Maholwana B, Hofmeyr GJ: Methods of delivering the placenta at caesarean section. Cochrane Database Syst Rev 3:CD004737, 2008

Baksu A, Kalan A, Ozkan A, et al: The effect of placental removal method and site of uterine repair on postcesarean endometritis and operative blood loss. Acta Obstet Gynecol Scand 84(3):266, 2005

Bar G, Scheiner E, Lezerovizt A, et al: Early maternal feeding following caesarean delivery: a prospective randomized study. Acta Obstet Gynecol Scand 87(1):68, 2008

Basha SL, Rochon ML, Quiñones JN, et al: Randomized controlled trial of wound complication rates of subcuticular suture vs staples for skin closure at cesarean delivery. Am J Obstet Gynecol 203(3):285.e1, 2010

Bastani P, Pourabolghasem S, Abbasalizadeh F, et al: Comparison of neonatal and maternal outcomes associated with head-pushing and head-pulling methods for impacted fetal head extraction during cesarean delivery. Int J Gynaecol Obstet 118(1):1, 2012

Bateman BT, Mhyre JM, Callaghan WM, et al: Peripartum hysterectomy in the United States: nationwide 14 year experience. Am J Obstet Gynecol 206(1):63.e1, 2012

Bates SM, Greer IA, Middeldorp S, et al: VTE, thrombophilia, antithrombotic therapy, and pregnancy: Antithrombotic Therapy and Prevention of Thrombosis, 9th ed: American College of Chest Physicians Evidence-Based Clinical Practice Guidelines. Chest 141(2 Suppl):e691S, 2012

Bloom SL, for the National Institute of Child Health and Human Development Maternal–Fetal Medicine Units Cesarean Registry: Decision to incision times and infant outcome. Am J Obstet Gynecol 185:S121, 2001

Bloom SL, Leveno KJ, Spong CY, et al: Decision-to-incision times and maternal and fetal outcomes. Obstet Gynecol 108(1):6, 2006

Bodelon C, Bernabe-Ortiz A, Schiff MA, et al: Factors associated with peripartum hysterectomy. Obstet Gynecol 114(1):115, 2009

Bohman VR, Gilstrap L, Leveno K, et al: Subcutaneous tissue: to close or not to close at cesarean section. Am J Obstet Gynecol 166:407, 1992

Bolze PA, Massoud M, Gaucherand P, et al: What about the Misgav-Ladach surgical technique in patients with previous cesarean Sections? Am J Perinatol 30(3):197, 2013

Boyle JG, Gabbe SG: T and J vertical extensions in low transverse cesarean births. Obstet Gynecol 87(2):238, 1996

Briery CM, Rose CH, Hudson WT, et al: Planned vs emergent cesarean hysterectomy. Am J Obstet Gynecol 197(2):154.e1, 2007

Buie VC, Owings MF, DeFrances CJ, et al: National Hospital Discharge Survey: 2006 summary. National Center for Health Statistics. Vital Health Stat 13(168):1, 2010

CAESAR study collaborative group: Caesarean section surgical techniques: a randomised factorial trial (CAESAR). BJOG 117(11):1366, 2010

Cahill AG, Stamilio DM, Odibo AO, et al: Is vaginal birth after cesarean (VBAC) or elective repeat cesarean safer in women with a prior vaginal delivery? Am J Obstet Gynecol 195(4):1143, 2006

Chai AH, Wong T, Mak HL, et al: Prevalence and associated risk factors of retention of urine after caesarean section. Int Urogynecol J Pelvic Floor Dysfunct 194(4):537, 2008

Chanrachakul B, Hamontri S, Herabutya Y: A randomized comparison of postcesarean pain between closure and nonclosure of peritoneum. Eur J Obstet Gynecol Reprod Biol 101:31, 2002

Chapa HO, Venegas G, Vanduyne CP, et al: Peritoneal adhesion prevention at cesarean section: an analysis of the effectiveness of an absorbable adhesion barrier. J Reprod Med 56(3–4):103, 2011

Chapman SJ, Owen J, Hauth JC: One versus two-layer closure of a low transverse cesarean: the next pregnancy. Obstet Gynecol 89:16, 1997

Cheesman K, Brady JE, Flood P, et al: Epidemiology of anesthesia-related complications in labor and delivery, New York State, 2002–2005. Anesth Analg 109:1174, 2009

Chelmow D, Rodriguez EJ, Sabatini MM: Suture closure of subcutaneous fat and wound disruption after cesarean delivery: a meta-analysis. Obstet Gynecol 103:974, 2004

Cheong Y, Premkumar G, Metwally M, et al: To close or not to close? A systematic review and a meta-analysis of peritoneal non-closure and adhesion formation after caesarean section. Eur J Obstet Gynecol Reprod Biol 147(1):3, 2009

Clark SL, Belfort MA, Dildy GA, et al: Maternal death in the 21st century: causes, prevention, and relationship to cesarean delivery. Am J Obstet Gynecol 199(1):36.e1, 2008

Clark SL, Miller DD, Belfort MA, et al: Neonatal and maternal outcomes associated with elective term delivery. Am J Obstet Gynecol 200(2):156.e1, 2009

Coutinho IC, Ramos de Morim MM, Katz L, et al: Uterine exteriorization compared with in situ repair at cesarean delivery. Obstet Gynecol 111:639, 2008

Cunningham FG, Leveno KJ, Bloom SL, et al (eds): Cesarean delivery and peripartum hysterectomy. In Williams Obstetrics, 23rd ed. New York, McGraw-Hill, 2010

Dahlke JD, Mendez-Figueroa H, Rouse DJ, et al: Evidence-based surgery for cesarean delivery: an updated systematic review. Am J Obstet Gynecol 209(4):294, 2013

Declercq E, Barger M, Cabral HJ, et al: Maternal outcomes associated with planned primary cesarean births compared with planned vaginal births. Obstet Gynecol 109(3):669, 2007

Dodd JM, Anderson ER, Gates S: Surgical techniques for uterine incision and uterine closure at the time of caesarean section. Cochrane Database Syst Rev 3:CD004732, 2008

Dolan LM, Hilton P: Obstetric risk factors and pelvic floor dysfunction 20 years after first delivery. Int Urogynecol J 21(5):535, 2010

Durnwald C, Mercer B: Uterine rupture, perioperative and perinatal morbidity after single-layer and double-layer closure at cesarean delivery. Am J Obstet Gynecol 189:925, 2003

Figueroa D, Jauk VC, Szychowski JM, et al: Surgical staples compared with subcuticular suture for skin closure after cesarean delivery: a randomized controlled trial. Obstet Gynecol 121(1):33, 2013

Flood KM, Said S, Geary M, et al: Changing trends in peripartum hysterectomy over the last 4 decades. Am J Obstet Gynecol 200(6):632.e1, 2009
Fushiki H, Ikoma T, Kobayashi H, et al: Efficacy of Seprafilm as an adhesion prevention barrier in cesarean sections. Obstet Gynecol Treat 91:557, 2005
Geller EJ, Wu JM, Jannelli ML, et al: Maternal outcomes associated with planned vaginal versus planned primary cesarean delivery. Am J Perinatol 27(9):675, 2010
Glaze S, Ekwalanga P, Roberts G, et al: Peripartum hysterectomy: 1999 to 2006. Obstet Gynecol 111(3):732, 2008
Glazener C, Elders A, Macarthur C, et al: Childbirth and prolapse: long-term associations with the symptoms and objective measurement of pelvic organ prolapse. BJOG 120(2):161, 2013
Gossman GL, Joesch JM, Tanfer K: Trends in maternal request cesarean delivery from 1991 to 2004. Obstet Gynecol 108: 1506, 2006
Grundsell HS, Rizk DE, Kumar RM: Randomized study of non-closure of peritoneum in lower segment cesarean section. Acta Obstet Gynecol Scand 77:110, 1998
Guise JM, Denman MA, Emeis C, et al: Vaginal birth after cesarean: new insights on maternal and neonatal outcomes. Obstet Gynecol 115(6):1267, 2010
Güngördük K, Asicioglu O, Celikkol O, et al: Iatrogenic bladder injuries during caesarean delivery: a case control study. J Obstet Gynaecol 30(7):667, 2010
Güngördük K, Yildirim G, Ark C: Is routine cervical dilatation necessary during elective caesarean section? A randomised controlled trial. Aust N Z J Obstet Gynaecol 49(3):263, 2009
Güngördük K, Yıldırım G, Asıcıoğlu O, et al: Efficacy of intravenous tranexamic acid in reducing blood loss after elective cesarean section: a prospective, randomized, double-blind, placebo-controlled study. Am J Perinatol 28(3):233, 2011
Gyhagen M, Bullarbo M, Nielsen TF, et al: The prevalence of urinary incontinence 20 years after childbirth: a national cohort study in singleton primiparae after vaginal or caesarean delivery. BJOG 120(2):144, 2013
Haas DM, Morgan S, Contreras K: Vaginal preparation with antiseptic solution before cesarean section for preventing postoperative infections. Cochrane Database Syst Rev 1:CD007892, 2013
Handa VL, Blomquist JL, Knoepp LR, et al: Pelvic floor disorders 5–10 years after vaginal or cesarean childbirth. Obstet Gynecol 118(4):777, 2011
Harrigill KM, Miller HS, Haynes DE: The effect of intraabdominal irrigation at cesarean delivery on maternal morbidity: a randomized trial. Obstet Gynecol 101:80, 2003
Hauth JC, Owen J, Davis RO, et al: Transverse uterine incision closure: one versus two layers. Am J Obstet Gynecol 167:1108, 1992
Hawkins JL, Chang J, Palmer SK, et al: Anesthesia-related maternal mortality in the United States: 1979–2002. Obstet Gynecol 117(1):69, 2011
Hellums EK, Lin MG, Ramsey PS: Prophylactic subcutaneous drainage for prevention of wound complications after cesarean delivery—a metaanalysis. Am J Obstet Gynecol 197(3):229, 2007
Hernandez JS, Nuangchamnong N, Ziadie M, et al: Placental and uterine pathology in women undergoing peripartum hysterectomy. Obstet Gynecol 119(6):1137, 2012
Hofmeyr GJ, Mathai M, Shah A, et al: Techniques for caesarean section. Cochrane Database Syst Rev 1:CD004662, 2008
Hofmeyr JG, Novikova N, Mathai M, et al: Techniques for cesarean section. Am J Obstet Gynecol 201(5):431, 2009
Hohlagschwandtner M, Ruecklinger E, Husslein P, et al: Is the formation of a bladder flap at cesarean necessary? A randomized trial. Obstet Gynecol 98(6):1089, 2001
Holmgren G, Sjöholm L, Stark M: The Misgav Ladach method for cesarean section: method description. Acta Obstet Gynecol Scand 78(7):615, 1999
Irion O, Luzuy F, Beguin F: Nonclosure of the visceral and parietal peritoneum at caesarean section: a randomised controlled trial. Br J Obstet Gynaecol 103:690, 1996
Jacob J, Phenninger J: Cesarean deliveries: When is a pediatrician necessary? Obstet Gynecol 89:217, 1997
James AH, Jamison MG, Brancazio LR, et al: Venous thromboembolism during pregnancy and the postpartum period: incidence, risk factors, and mortality. Am J Obstet Gynecol 194:1311, 2006
Kapustian V, Anteby EY, Gdalevich M, et al: Effect of closure versus nonclosure of peritoneum at cesarean section on adhesions: a prospective randomized study. Am J Obstet Gynecol 206(1):56.e1, 2012
Kattwinkel J, Perlman JM, Aziz K, et al: Part 15: neonatal resuscitation: 2010 American Heart Association Guidelines for Cardiopulmonary Resuscitation and Emergency Cardiovascular Care. Circulation 122(18 Suppl 3):S909, 2010
Kerr JMM: The lower uterine segment incision in conservative caesarean section. J Obstet Gynaecol Br Emp 28:475, 1921
Krönig B: Transperitonealer cervikaler Kaiserschnitt. In: Doderlein A, Krönig B (eds): Operative Gynäkologie, 3rd ed. Leipzig, Thieme, 1912, p 879
Leijonhufvud A, Lundholm C, Cnattingius S, et al: Risks of stress urinary incontinence and pelvic organ prolapse surgery in relation to mode of childbirth. Am J Obstet Gynecol 204(1):70.e1, 2011
Li L, Wen J, Wang L, et al: Is routine indwelling catheterisation of the bladder for caesarean section necessary? A systematic review. BJOG 118(4):400, 2011
Liabsuetrakul T, Peeyananjarassri K: Mechanical dilatation of the cervix at non-labour caesarean section for reducing postoperative morbidity. Cochrane Database Syst Rev 11:CD008019, 2011
Liang CC, Chang SD, Chang YL, et al: Postpartum urinary retention after cesarean delivery. Int J Gynaecol Obstet 99(3):229, 2007
Lien JM, Towers CV, Quilligan EJ, et al: Term early-onset neonatal seizures: obstetric characteristics, etiologic classifications, and perinatal care. Obstet Gynecol 85:163, 1995
Liu SL, Liston RM, Joseph KS, et al: Maternal mortality and severe morbidity associated with low-risk planned cesarean delivery versus planned vaginal delivery at term. CMAJ 176(4):455, 2007
Lyell DJ, Caughey AB, Hu E, et al: Peritoneal closure at primary cesarean delivery and adhesions. Obstet Gynecol 106(2):275, 2005
Lyell DJ, Caughey AB, Hu E, et al: Rectus muscle and visceral peritoneum closure at cesarean delivery and intraabdominal adhesions. Am J Obstet Gynecol 206(6):515.e1, 2012
MacArthur C, Glazener C, Lancashire R, et al: Exclusive caesarean section delivery and subsequent urinary and faecal incontinence: a 12-year longitudinal study. BJOG 118(8):1001, 2011
MacArthur C, Wilson D, Herbison P, et al: Faecal incontinence persisting after childbirth: a 12 year longitudinal study. BJOG 120(2):169, 2013
MacDorman M, Declercq E, Menacker F: Recent trends and patterns in cesarean and vaginal birth after cesarean (VBAC) deliveries in the United States. Clin Perinatol 38(2):179, 2011
Mackeen AD, Berghella V, Larsen ML: Techniques and materials for skin closure in caesarean section. Cochrane Database Syst Rev 11:CD003577, 2012
Marik PE, Plante LA: Venous thromboembolic disease and pregnancy. N Engl J Med 359(19):2025, 2008
Marshall NE, Fu R, Guise JM: Impact of multiple cesarean deliveries on maternal morbidity: a systematic review. Am J Obstet Gynecol 205(3):262.e1, 2011
Martin JA, Hamilton BE, Ventura SJ, et al: Births: final data for 2010. Natl Vital Stat Rep 61(1):1, 2012
Menacker F, Declercq E, Macdorman MF: Cesarean delivery: background, trends, and epidemiology. Semin Perinatol 30(5):235, 2006
Miller ES, Hahn K, Grobman WA, et al: Consequences of a primary elective cesarean delivery across the reproductive life. Obstet Gynecol 121(4):789, 2013
Miller R, Depp R: Minimizing perinatal neurologic injury at term: is cesarean section the answer? Clin Perinatol 35(3):549, 2008
Morales KJ, Gordon MC, Bates GW Jr: Postcesarean delivery adhesions associated with delayed delivery of infant. Am J Obstet Gynecol 196(5):461.e1, 2007
Nagele F, Karas H, Spitzer D, et al: Closure or nonclosure of the visceral peritoneum at cesarean delivery. Am J Obstet Gynecol 174:1366, 1996
Nasr AM, ElBigawy AF, Abdelamid AE, et al: Evaluation of the use vs nonuse of urinary catheterization during cesarean delivery: a prospective, multicenter, randomized controlled trial. J Perinatol 29(6):416, 2009
National Institutes of Health: ClinicalTrials.gov: Seprafilm adhesion barrier and cesarean delivery. 2012. Available at: http://clinicaltrials.gov/ct2/show/NCT00565643. Accessed May 6, 2013
National Institutes of Health: State-of-the-Science Conference Statement on Cesarean Delivery on Maternal Request. NIH Consens Sci Statements. 2006. Mar 27–29; 23(1):1, 2006
Nelson RL, Furner SE, Westercamp M, et al: Cesarean delivery for the prevention of anal incontinence. Cochrane Database Syst Rev 2:CD006756, 2010
Orbach A, Levy A, Wiznitzer A, et al: Peripartum cesarean hysterectomy: critical analysis of risk factors and trends over the years. J Matern Fetal Neonatal Med 24(3):480, 2011
Orji EO, Olabode TO, Kuti O, et al: A randomised controlled trial of early initiation of oral feeding after cesarean section. J Matern Fetal Neonatal Med 22(1):65, 2009
Osmundson SS, Garabedian MJ, Lyell DJ: Risk factors for classical hysterotomy by gestational age. Obstet Gynecol 122:845, 2013
Owolabi MS, Blake RE, Mayor MT, et al: Incidence and determinants of peripartum hysterectomy in the metropolitan area of the District of Columbia. J Reprod Med 58(3–4):167, 2013
Patterson LS, O'Connell CM, Baskett TF: Maternal and perinatal morbidity associated with classic and inverted T cesarean incisions. Obstet Gynecol 100(4):633, 2002

Pevzner L, Swank M, Krepel C, et al: Effects of maternal obesity on tissue concentrations of prophylactic cefazolin during cesarean delivery. Obstet Gynecol 117(4):877, 2011

Phipps MG, Watabe B, Clemons JL, et al: Risk factors for bladder injury during cesarean delivery. Obstet Gynecol 105(1):156, 2005

Pritchard JA: Changes in the blood volume during pregnancy and delivery. Anesthesiology 26:393, 1965

Rafique Z, Shibli KU, Russell IF, et al: A randomised controlled trial of the closure or non-closure of peritoneum at caesarean section: effect on postoperative pain. Br J Obstet Gynaecol 109:694, 2002

Rahman MS, Gasem T, Al Suleiman SA, et al: Bladder injuries during cesarean section in a university hospital: a 25-year review. Arch Gynecol Obstet 279(3):349, 2009

Rajasekar D, Hall M: Urinary tract injuries during obstetric intervention. Br J Obstet Gynaecol 104:731, 1997

Ramsey PS, White AM, Guinn DA, et al: Subcutaneous tissue reapproximation, alone or in combination with drain, in obese women undergoing cesarean delivery. Obstet Gynecol 105(5 Pt 1):967, 2005

Reid VC, Hartmann KE, McMahon M, et al: Vaginal preparation with povidone iodine and postcesarean infectious morbidity: a randomized controlled trial. Obstet Gynecol 97(1):147, 2001

Roach MK, Abramovici A, Tita AT: Dose and duration of oxytocin to prevent postpartum hemorrhage: a review. Am J Perinatol 30(7):523, 2013

Roberge S, Chaillet N, Boutin A, et al: Single- versus double-layer closure of the hysterotomy incision during cesarean delivery and risk of uterine rupture. Int J Gynaecol Obstet 115(1):5, 2011

Rortveit G, Daltveit AK, Hannestad YS, et al: Urinary incontinence after vaginal delivery or cesarean section. N Engl J Med 348(10):900, 2003

Rortveit G, Hannestad YS, Daltveit AK, et al: Age- and type-dependent effects of parity on urinary incontinence: the Norwegian EPINCONT study. Obstet Gynecol 98(6):1004, 2001

Rossi AC, Lee RH, Chmait RH. Emergency postpartum hysterectomy for uncontrolled postpartum bleeding: a systematic review. Obstet Gynecol 115(3):637, 2010

Rossouw JN, Hall D, Harvey J: Time between skin incision and delivery during cesarean. Int J Gynaecol Obstet 121(1):82, 2013

Sakse A, Weber T, Nickelsen C, et al: Peripartum hysterectomy in Denmark 1995–2004. Acta Obstet Gynecol Scand 86(12):1472, 2007

Scheller JM, Nelson KB: Does cesarean delivery prevent cerebral palsy or other neurologic problems of childhood? Obstet Gynecol 83:624, 1994

Shazly SA, Elsayed AH, Badran SM, et al: Abdominal disimpaction with lower uterine segment support as a novel technique to minimize fetal and maternal morbidities during cesarean section for obstructed labor: a case series. Am J Perinatol 30(8):695, 2013

Shellhaas CS, Gilbert S, Landon MB, et al: The frequency and complication rates of hysterectomy accompanying cesarean delivery. Obstet Gynecol 114(2 Pt 1):224, 2009

Sikirica V, Broder MS, Chang E, et al: Clinical and economic impact of adhesiolysis during repeat cesarean delivery. Acta Obstet Gynecol Scand 91(6):719, 2012

Silver RM, Landon MB, Rouse DJ, et al: Maternal morbidity associated with multiple repeat cesarean deliveries. Obstet Gynecol 107:1226, 2006

Society for Maternal-Fetal Medicine, Belfort MA: Placenta accreta. Am J Obstet Gynecol 203(5):430, 2010

Starr RV, Zurawski J, Ismail M: Preoperative vaginal preparation with povidone-iodine and the risk of postcesarean endometritis. Obstet Gynecol 105(5 Pt 1):1024, 2005

Strong TH, Brown WL Jr, Brown WL, et al: Experience with early postcesarean hospital dismissal. Am J Obstet Gynecol 169:116, 1993

Su LL, Chong YS, Samuel M: Carbetocin for preventing postpartum haemorrhage. Cochrane Database Syst Rev 2:CD005457, 2012

Sullivan SA, Smith T, Chang E, et al: Administration of cefazolin prior to skin incision is superior to cefazolin at cord clamping in preventing postcesarean infectious morbidity: a randomized controlled trial. Am J Obstet Gynecol 196:455, 2007

Tan PG, Norazilah MJ, Omar SZ: Hospital discharge on the first compared with the second day after a planned cesarean delivery: a randomized controlled trial. Obstet Gynecol 120(6):1273, 2012

Tanner J, Norrie P, Melen K: Preoperative hair removal to reduce surgical site infection. Cochrane Database Syst Rev 11:CD004122, 2011

The Joint Commission: Facts about the Universal Protocol. 2013. Available at: http://www.jointcommission.org/standards_information/up.aspx. Accessed May 12, 2013

Tita AT, Landon MB, Spong CY, et al: Timing of elective repeat cesarean delivery at term and neonatal outcomes. N Engl J Med 360(2):111, 2009a

Tita AT, Rouse DJ, Blackwell S, et al: Emerging concepts in antibiotic prophylaxis for cesarean delivery: a systematic review. Obstet Gynecol 113(3):675, 2009b

Tulandi T, Agdi M, Zarei A, Miner L, et al: Adhesion development and morbidity after repeat cesarean delivery. Am J Obstet Gynecol 201(1):56.e1, 2009

Tuuli MG, Odibo AO, Fogertey P, et al: Utility of the bladder flap at cesarean delivery: a randomized controlled trial. Obstet Gynecol 119(4):815, 2012

Tuuli MG, Rampersad RM, Carbone JF, et al: Staples compared with subcuticular suture for skin closure after cesarean delivery: a systematic review and meta-analysis. Obstet Gynecol 117(3):682, 2011

van Bree SH, Nemethova A, Cailotto C, et al: New therapeutic strategies for postoperative ileus. Nat Rev Gastroenterol Hepatol 9(11):675, 2012

Veisi F, Zangeneh M, Malekkhosravi S, et al: Comparison of "push" and "pull" methods for impacted fetal head extraction during cesarean delivery. Int J Gynaecol Obstet 118(1):4, 2012

Villar J, Carroli G, Zavaleta N, et al: Maternal and neonatal individual risks and benefits associated with caesarean delivery: multicentre prospective study. BJM 335:1025, 2007

Viney R, Isaacs C, Chelmow D: Intra-abdominal irrigation at cesarean delivery: a randomized controlled trial. Obstet Gynecol 119(6):1106, 2012

Walsh CA, Walsh SR: Extraabdominal vs intraabdominal uterine repair at cesarean delivery: a metaanalysis. Am J Obstet Gynecol 200(6):625.e1, 2009

Worley KC, McIntire DD, Leveno KJ: The prognosis for spontaneous labor in women with uncomplicated term pregnancies: implications for cesarean delivery on maternal request. Obstet Gynecol 113(4):812, 2009

Witt A, Döner M, Petricevic L, et al: Antibiotic prophylaxis before surgery vs after cord clamping in elective cesarean delivery: a double-blind, prospective, randomized, placebo-controlled trial. Arch Surg 146(12):1404, 2011

Wylie BJ, Gilbert S, Landon MB, et al: Comparison of transverse and vertical skin incision for emergency cesarean delivery. Obstet Gynecol 115(6):1134, 2010

Xu LL, Chau AM, Zuschmann A: Blunt vs. sharp uterine expansion at lower segment cesarean section delivery: a systematic review with metaanalysis. Am J Obstet Gynecol 208(1):62.e1, 2013

Yildirim G, Güngördük K, Asicioğlu O, et al: Does vaginal preparation with povidone-iodine prior to caesarean delivery reduce the risk of endometritis? A randomized controlled trial. J Matern Fetal Neonatal Med 25(11):2316, 2012

Yost NP, Bloom SL, Sibley MK, et al: A hospital-sponsored quality improvement study of pain management after cesarean delivery. Am J Obstet Gynecol 190:1341, 2004

CHAPTER 31

Prior Cesarean Delivery

Once a cesarean, always a cesarean.
Cragin, 1916

Once a cesarean, always a trial of labor?
Pauerstein, 1966

Once a cesarean, always a controversy.
Flamm, 1997

Few issues in modern obstetrics have been as controversial as the management of the woman who has undergone a prior cesarean delivery. As we approach the 100th anniversary of the oft-quoted remark by Cragin, the issue remains unsettled.

100 YEARS OF CONTROVERSY

Management of the woman who has undergone a previous cesarean delivery has been—for good reasons—a controversial topic for more than 100 years. By the beginning of the 20th century, cesarean delivery had become relatively safe. But, as women survived the first operation and conceived again, they were now at risk for uterine rupture. This was because of the prevailing use of vertical hysterotomy—and especially the classical incision (Williams, 1903). The inherent dangers of uterine rupture led to the dictum above by Edwin B. Cragin (1916). It was not until later that Kerr (1921) described use of a transverse low-segment uterine incision that was predicted to be less likely to rupture with subsequent labor.

Perhaps contrary to popular belief, these events did not result in strict adherence to repeat cesarean delivery. In the 10th edition of *Williams Obstetrics*, Eastman (1950) stated a preference for vaginal delivery in these women and described a 30-percent vaginal delivery rate at Johns Hopkins Hospital. But while only 2 percent of women who labored had a uterine rupture, they had a 10-percent maternal mortality rate. Subsequent observational studies from the 1960s also suggested that vaginal delivery was a reasonable option (Pauerstein 1966, 1969). Germane to this is that through the 1960s, the overall cesarean delivery rate was only approximately 5 percent. Beginning then, however, well-intentioned efforts to improve perinatal outcomes were accompanied by a rapidly escalating cesarean delivery rate that exceeded 20 percent by 1985 (Chap. 30, p. 587). In addition, the concept of *cesarean delivery on maternal request* has increased the primary operation rate (American College of Obstetricians and Gynecologists, 2013b). And as expected, as the primary cesarean rate increased, the rate for repeat operations followed (Rosenstein, 2013).

To address this, a National Institutes of Health (NIH) Consensus Development Conference (1981) was convened, and it questioned the necessity of routine repeat cesarean delivery. With support and encouragement from the American College of Obstetricians and Gynecologists (1988, 1994), enthusiastic attempts were begun to increase the use of *vaginal birth after cesarean—VBAC*. These attempts were highly successful, and VBAC rates increased from 3.4 percent in 1980 to a peak of 28.3 percent in 1996. These rates, along with a concomitant

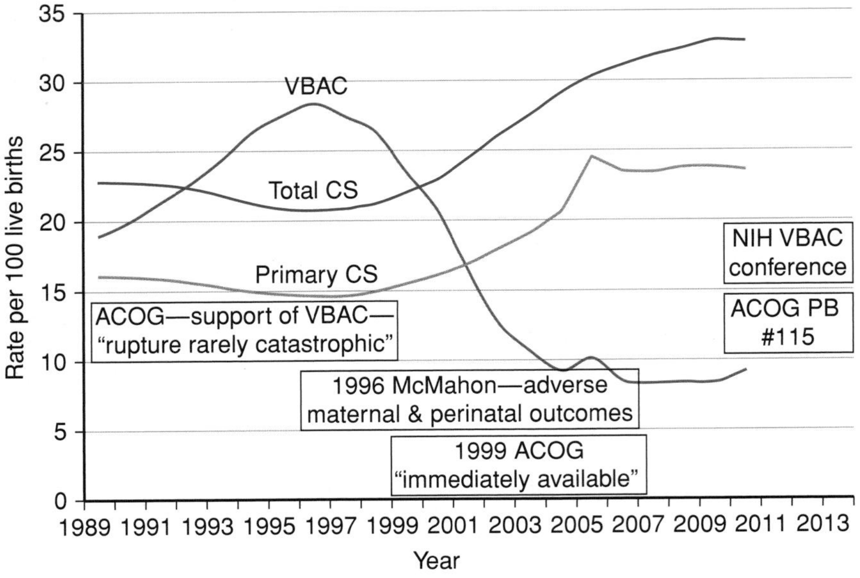

FIGURE 31-1 Total and primary cesarean delivery (CS) rates and vaginal birth after previous cesarean (VBAC) rate: United States, 1989–2010. Epochs denoted within rectangles represent contemporaneous ongoing events related to these rates. (Data from National Institutes of Health: NIH Consensus Development Conference, 2010; Martin, 2012a,b).

decline in total cesarean delivery rates for the United States, are shown in Figure 31-1.

As the vaginal delivery rate increased, so did reports of uterine rupture-related maternal and perinatal morbidity and mortality (McMahon, 1996; Sachs, 1999). These dampened prevailing enthusiasm for a *trial of labor* and stimulated the American College of Obstetricians and Gynecologists (1998) to caution that such trials should be attempted only in appropriately equipped institutions with physicians *readily available* to provide emergency care. Less than a year later, the College (1999) recommended that physicians should be *immediately available*. Many believe that this one-word change—from *readily* to *immediately* available—was in large part responsible for the decade-long decline in national VBAC rates illustrated in Figure 31-1 (Cheng, 2014; Leeman, 2013). The VBAC rate leveled at approximately 8 percent by 2009 and 2010, while the total cesarean delivery rate increased to 32.8 percent in 2011 (Martin, 2011, 2012a,b). Because the success rate of a trial of labor resulting in a VBAC is not 100 percent, another way of examining these changes was described by Uddin and colleagues (2013). These investigators reported the proportion of women with a prior cesarean delivery who underwent a trial of labor. This number peaked in 1997, when slightly more than half of all of these women chose a trial of labor. Thereafter, this percentage plummeted and reached a nadir of about 16 percent in 2005. Since that time, the proportion has increased and averaged 20 to 25 percent through 2009. Ironically, during this same decade, there were continuing reports that described the success and safety of VBAC in selected clinical settings.

In reality, there are several other interrelated factors—both medical and nonmedical—that have undoubtedly contributed to declining VBAC rates. Because of their complexity and importance, the *Eunice Kennedy Shriver* National Institute of Child Health and Human Development (NICHD) and the Office of Medical Applications of Research (OMAR) convened a National Institutes of Health Consensus Development Conference Panel (2010) to study these issues. The Panel report included a contemporaneous summary concerning the risks and benefits of repeat cesarean versus vaginal delivery. These findings are subsequently described along with summaries of current recommendations by various professional organizations. However, data from California indicate that VBAC rates have not perceptibly increased since the 2010 NIH Consensus Conference that encouraged greater access to a trial of labor after cesarean delivery (Barger, 2013).

FACTORS THAT INFLUENCE A TRIAL OF LABOR

Delivery planning for the woman who has had a previous cesarean delivery can begin with preconceptional counseling, but should definitely be addressed early in prenatal care. Importantly, any decision arrived at is subject to continuing revisions as dictated by exigencies that arise during the course of pregnancy. Assuming no mitigating circumstances, there are two basic choices. First is a *trial of labor after cesarean (TOLAC)* with the goal of achieving *VBAC*. If cesarean delivery becomes necessary during the trial, then it is termed a "failed trial of labor." A second choice is *elective repeat cesarean delivery (ERCD)*. This includes scheduled cesarean delivery as well as unscheduled but planned cesarean delivery for spontaneous labor or another indication.

Selection should consider factors known to influence a successful trial of labor as well as benefits and risks. In general, appropriately selected women who attempt VBAC have success rates that approximate 75 percent. These rates vary between institutions and providers and are affected by prepregnancy, antepartum, intrapartum, and nonmedical factors.

Some medical variables that influence a successful trial of labor are listed in Table 31-1. As for economical and medicolegal factors, professional liability concerns and insufficient resources to provide adequate staffing for hospitals to accommodate a trial of labor weigh heavily.

TRIAL OF LABOR VERSUS REPEAT CESAREAN DELIVERY

As evidence mounted that the risk of uterine rupture and perinatal morbidity and mortality might be greater than expected, the American College of Obstetricians and Gynecologists (1988, 1998, 1999, 2013a) issued updated Practice Bulletins supporting labor trials but also urging a more cautious approach. It is problematic that both options have risks and benefits to mother and fetus but that these are not always congruent.

Maternal Risks

Uterine rupture and its associated complications clearly are increased with a trial of labor. It is this increased risk that

TABLE 31-1. Some Factors That Influence a Successful Trial of Labor in a Woman with Prior Cesarean Delivery

Low-Risk	Favors Success	Increased Failure Rate	High-Risk[a]
Transverse incision Prior vaginal delivery Appropriate counseling Sufficient personnel and equipment	Teaching hospital White race Spontaneous labor Prior fetal malpresentation 1 or 2 prior transverse incisions Nonrecurrent indication Current preterm pregnancy	Single mother Increased maternal age Macrosomic fetus Obesity Breech Multifetal pregnancy Preeclampsia EGA > 40 weeks Low-vertical incision Unknown incision Labor induction Medical disease Multiple prior cesarean deliveries Education < 12 years Short interdelivery interval Liability concerns	Classical or T incision Prior rupture Patient refusal Transfundal surgery Obstetrical contraindication, e.g., previa Inadequate facilities

[a]Most consider these absolute contraindications.
EGA = estimated gestational age.

underpins most of the angst in attempting a trial of labor. Despite this, some have argued that these factors should weigh only minimally in the decision to attempt a trial because their absolute risk is low. One of the largest and most comprehensive studies designed to examine risks associated with vaginal birth in women with a prior cesarean delivery was conducted by the Maternal-Fetal Medicine Units (MFMU) Network (Landon, 2004). In this prospective study conducted at 19 academic medical centers, the outcomes of nearly 18,000 women who attempted a trial of labor were compared with those of more than 15,000 women who underwent elective repeat cesarean delivery. As shown in Table 31-2, although the risk of uterine rupture was higher among women undergoing a trial of labor, the absolute risk was small—only 7 per 1000. To the contrary, however, there were no uterine ruptures in the elective cesarean delivery group. Not surprisingly, rates of stillbirth

TABLE 31-2. Complications in Women with a Prior Cesarean Delivery Enrolled in the NICHD Maternal-Fetal Medicine Units Network, 1999–2002

Complication	Trial of Labor Group n = 17,898 No. (%)	Elective Repeat Cesarean Group n = 15,801 No. (%)	Odds Ratio (95% CI)	*p* value
Uterine rupture	124 (0.7)	0	NA	< .001
Uterine dehiscence	119 (0.7)	76 (0.5)	1.38 (1.04–1.85)	.03
Hysterectomy	41 (0.2)	47 (0.3)	0.77 (0.51–1.17)	.22
Thromboembolic disease	7 (0.04)	10 (0.1)	0.62 (0.24–1.62)	.32
Transfusion	304 (1.7)	158 (1.0)	1.71 (1.41–2.08)	< .001
Uterine infection	517 (2.9)	285 (1.8)	1.62 (1.40–1.87)	< .001
Maternal death	3 (0.02)	7 (0.04)	0.38 (0.10–1.46)	.21
Antepartum stillbirth[a]				
37–38 weeks	18 (0.4)	8 (0.1)	2.93 (1.27–6.75)	.008
≥ 39 weeks	16 (0.2)	5 (0.1)	2.70 (0.99–7.38)	.07
Intrapartum stillbirth[a]	2	0	NA	NS
Term HIE[a]	12 (0.08)	0	NA	< .001
Term neonatal death[a]	13 (0.08)	7 (0.05)	1.82 (0.73–4.57)	.19

[a]Denominator is 15,338 for the trial of labor group and 15,014 for the elective repeat cesarean delivery group.
CI = confidence interval; HIE = hypoxic ischemic encephalopathy; NA = not applicable; NICHD = National Institute of Child Health and Human Development; NS = not significant.
Adapted from Landon, 2004.

and hypoxic ischemic encephalopathy were significantly greater in the trial of labor arm. Others have reported similar results (Chauhan, 2003; Mozurkewich, 2000). In one study of nearly 25,000 women with a prior cesarean delivery, perinatal death risk was 1.3 per 1000 among the 15,515 women who had a trial of labor (Smith, 2002). Although the absolute risk is small, it is *11 times greater* than the risk found in 9014 women with a planned repeat cesarean delivery.

Most studies suggest that the maternal *mortality* rate does not differ significantly between women undergoing a trial of labor compared with those undergoing an elective repeat cesarean delivery (Landon, 2004; Mozurkewich, 2000). One outlier was a retrospective cohort study of more than 300,000 Canadian women with a prior cesarean delivery (Wen, 2005). In this study, the maternal death rate for women undergoing an elective repeat cesarean delivery was 5.6 per 100,000 compared with 1.6 per 100,000 for those having a trial of labor.

Estimates of maternal *morbidity* have also produced conflicting results. In the metaanalysis by Mozurkewich and Hutton (2000), women undergoing a trial of labor were approximately half as likely to require a blood transfusion or hysterectomy compared with those undergoing repeat cesarean delivery. Conversely, in the MFMU Network study, Landon and coworkers (2004) observed that the risks of transfusion and infection were significantly greater for women attempting a trial of labor (see Table 31-2). Rossi and D'Addario (2008) reported similar findings in their metaanalysis. McMahon and associates (1996), in a population-based study of 6138 women, found that major complications—hysterectomy, uterine rupture, or operative injury—were almost twice as common in women undergoing a trial of labor compared with those undergoing an elective cesarean delivery. *Importantly, compared with a successful trial of labor, the risk of these major complications was fivefold greater in women whose attempted vaginal delivery failed.* The metaanalysis cited above also reported an increased incidence of overall maternal complications when women with a failed vaginal delivery were compared with those undergoing successful vaginal delivery—17 versus 3 percent, respectively (Rossi, 2008). Similar findings have been reported from the Network Cesarean Registry (Babbar, 2013).

Fetal and Neonatal Risks

The Panel found little or no evidence regarding short- and long-term neonatal outcomes after TOLAC versus ERCD. Most of the available evidence documents differences comparing *actual* rather than *intended* mode of delivery and is of low quality. A trial of labor is associated with significantly higher *perinatal mortality* rates compared with ERCD—perinatal mortality rate 0.13 versus 0.05 percent; neonatal mortality rate 0.11 versus 0.06 (Guise, 2010). A trial of labor also appears to be associated with a higher risk of *hypoxic ischemic encephalopathy (HIE)* than ERCD. The Maternal-Fetal Medicine Networks Unit study reported the incidence of HIE at term to be 46 per 100,000 trials of labor compared with zero cases in women undergoing ERCD (Landon, 2004).

Analysis of pooled data suggests that the absolute risk of *transient tachypnea of the newborn* is slightly higher with ERCD compared with TOLAC—4.2 versus 3.6 percent (Guise, 2010). But, neonatal bag and mask ventilation was used more often in infants delivered following TOLAC than in those delivered by ERCD—5.4 versus 2.5 percent. Finally, there are no significant differences in *5-minute Apgar scores* or *neonatal intensive care unit admissions* for infants delivered by TOLAC compared with those delivered by ERCD. *Birth trauma* from lacerations is more commonly seen in infants born by ERCD.

Maternal versus Fetal Risks

Relative risks for mother and baby differ between modes of delivery. Regarding overall risks, the Panel (2010) concluded that in a hypothetical group of 100,000 women of *any* gestational age who undergo TOLAC, there will be 4 maternal deaths, 468 cases of uterine rupture, and 133 perinatal deaths. In comparison, in a hypothetical group of 100,000 women of *any* gestational age who undergo ERCD, there will be 13 maternal deaths, 26 uterine ruptures, and 50 perinatal deaths.

Despite potential concerns of increased complications, an elective repeat cesarean delivery is considered by many women to be preferable to a trial of labor. Frequent reasons include the convenience of a scheduled delivery and the fear of a prolonged and potentially dangerous labor. In an earlier study, Abitbol and colleagues (1993) found that these preferences persisted despite extensive antepartum counseling.

CANDIDATES FOR A TRIAL OF LABOR

There are few high-quality data available to guide selection of trial of labor candidates (Guise, 2004; Hashima, 2004). That said, having fewer complicating risk factors increases the likelihood of success (Gregory, 2008). Several algorithms and nomograms have been developed to aid prediction, but none has demonstrated reasonable prognostic value (Grobman, 2007b, 2008, 2009; Macones, 2006; Metz, 2013; Srinivas, 2007). Use of a predictive model for failed trial of labor, however, was found to be somewhat predictive of uterine rupture or dehiscence (Stanhope, 2013). Despite these limitations for precision, several points are pertinent to the evaluation of these women and are described in the next sections. Current recommendations of the American College of Obstetricians and Gynecologists (2013a) are that most women with one previous cesarean delivery with a low-transverse hysterotomy are candidates, and if appropriate, they should be counseled regarding a trial of labor versus elective repeat cesarean delivery.

Prior Uterine Incision

Prior Incision Type

The type and number of prior cesarean deliveries are overriding factors in recommending a trial of labor. Women with one prior low-transverse hysterotomy have the lowest risk of symptomatic scar separation (Table 31-3). The highest risks are with prior vertical incisions extending into the fundus, such as the classical incision shown in Figure 31-2 (Society for Maternal Fetal Medicine, 2013). Importantly, in some women, the classical scar will rupture before the onset of labor, and this can happen several weeks before term. In a review of 157 women

TABLE 31-3. Types of Prior Uterine Incisions and Estimated Risks for Uterine Rupture

Prior Incision	Estimated Rupture Rate (%)
Classical	2–9
T-shaped	4–9
Low-vertical[a]	1–7
One low-transverse	0.2–0.9
Multiple low-transverse	0.9–1.8
Prior preterm cesarean delivery	"increased"
Prior uterine rupture	
Lower segment	2–6
Upper uterus	9–32

[a]See text for definition.
Data from the American College of Obstetricians and Gynecologists, 2013a; Cahill, 2010b; Chauhan, 2002; Landon, 2006; Macones, 2005; Martin, 1997; Miller, 1994; Sciscione, 2008; Society for Maternal-Fetal Medicine, 2012; Tahseen, 2010.

with a prior classical cesarean delivery, one woman had a complete uterine rupture before the onset of labor, whereas 9 percent had a uterine dehiscence (Chauhan, 2002).

The risk of uterine rupture in women with a prior vertical incision that did not extend into the fundus is unclear. Martin (1997) and Shipp (1999) and their coworkers reported that these low-vertical uterine incisions did not have an increased risk for rupture compared with low-transverse incisions. The American College of Obstetricians and Gynecologists (2013a) concluded that although there is limited evidence, women with a prior vertical incision in the lower uterine segment without fundal extension may be candidates for a trial of labor. This is in contrast to prior classical or T-shaped uterine incisions, which are considered by most as contraindications to labor.

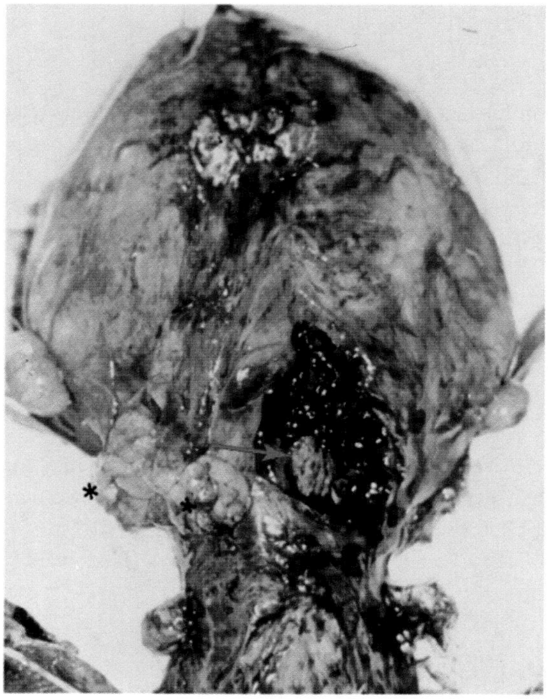

FIGURE 31-2 Ruptured vertical cesarean section scar (*arrow*) identified at time of repeat cesarean delivery early in labor. The two black asterisks to the left indicate some sites of densely adhered omentum.

Currently, there are few indications for a primary vertical incision (Osmundson, 2013). In those instances—for example, preterm breech fetus with an undeveloped lower segment—the "low vertical" incision almost invariably extends into the active segment. It is not known, however, how far upward the incision has to extend before risks become those of a true classical incision. It is helpful in the operative report to document its exact extent.

Prior preterm cesarean delivery may have an increased risk for rupture. Although the type of prior incision was not known, Sciscione and associates (2008) reported that women who had a prior preterm cesarean delivery were twice as likely to suffer a uterine rupture compared with those with a prior term cesarean delivery. This may be in part explained by the increased likelihood with a preterm fetus of extension of the uterine incision into the contractile portion. Conversely, Harper and colleagues (2009) did not find a significantly increased rate of rupture during subsequent VBAC in women with a prior cesarean delivery performed at or before 34 weeks.

There are special considerations for women with uterine malformations who have undergone cesarean delivery. Earlier reports suggested that the uterine rupture risk in a subsequent pregnancy was increased compared with the risk in those with a prior low-transverse hysterotomy and normally formed uterus (Ravasia, 1999). But, in a study of 103 women with müllerian duct anomalies who had one prior cesarean delivery and who attempted a trial of labor, there were no cases of uterine rupture (Erez, 2007). Given the wide range of risk for uterine rupture associated with the various uterine incision types, it is not surprising that most fellows of the American College of Obstetricians and Gynecologists consider the type of prior incision to be the most important factor when considering a trial of labor (Coleman, 2005).

Prior Incision Closure

As discussed in Chapter 30 (p. 596), the low-transverse hysterotomy incision can be sutured in either one or two layers. Whether the risk of subsequent uterine rupture is affected by these is unclear. Chapman (1997) and Tucker (1993) and their associates found no relationship between a one- and two-layer closure and the risk of subsequent uterine rupture. And although Durnwald and Mercer (2003) also found no increased risk of rupture, they reported that uterine dehiscence was more common after single-layer closure. In contrast, Bujold and coworkers (2002) found that a single-layer closure was associated with nearly a fourfold increased risk of rupture compared with a double-layer closure. In response, Vidaeff and Lucas (2003) argued that experimental models have not demonstrated advantages of a double-layer closure and that the evidence is insufficient to routinely recommend a double-layer closure. At Parkland Hospital we routinely suture the low-segment incision with one running locking suture.

Number of Prior Cesarean Incisions

There are at least three studies that reported a doubling of the rupture rate—from approximately 0.6 to 1.85 percent—in women with two versus one prior transverse hysterotomy incision (Macones, 2005a; Miller, 1994; Tahseen, 2010). In contrast, analysis of the MFMU Network database by Landon and colleagues (2006) did not confirm this. Instead, they reported an insignificant difference in the uterine rupture rate in 975 women with multiple prior cesarean deliveries compared with 16,915 women with a single prior operation—0.9 versus 0.7 percent, respectively. As discussed subsequently, other serious maternal morbidity increases along with the number of prior cesarean deliveries (Marshall, 2011).

Imaging of Prior Incision

Sonographic measurement of a prior hysterotomy incision has been used to predict the likelihood of rupture with a trial of labor. Large defects in the hysterotomy scar in a nonpregnant uterus forecast a greater risk for rupture (Osser, 2011). Naji and associates (2013a,b) found that the *residual myometrial thickness* decreased as pregnancy progressed and that rupture correlates with a thinner scar. From their review, however, Jastrow and coworkers (2010) found no ideal thickness to be suitably predictive. The optimal safe threshold value for the lower uterine segment—smallest measurement from amnionic fluid to bladder—ranged from 2.0 to 3.5 mm. For the myometrial layer—smallest measurement of the hypoechoic portion of the lower segment, it was 1.4 to 2.0 mm. With a lower segment < 2.0 mm, the risk of uterine rupture was increased 11-fold. With myometrial thickness < 1.4 mm, uterine rupture was increased fivefold. The measurements, however, are not predictive for an individual woman (Bergeron, 2009).

Prior Uterine Rupture

Women who have previously sustained a uterine rupture are at increased risk for recurrence during a subsequent attempted VBAC. As shown in Table 31-3, those with a previous low-segment rupture have a 2- to 6-percent recurrence risk, whereas prior upper segment uterine rupture confers a 9- to 32-percent risk (Reyes-Ceja, 1969; Ritchie, 1971). We believe that women with a prior uterine rupture or classical or T-shaped incision ideally should undergo repeat cesarean delivery when fetal pulmonary maturity is assured, and preferably before the onset of labor. They should also be counseled regarding the hazards of unattended labor and signs of possible uterine rupture.

Interdelivery Interval

Magnetic resonance imaging studies of myometrial healing suggest that complete uterine involution and restoration of anatomy may require at least 6 months (Dicle, 1997). To explore this further, Shipp and colleagues (2001) examined the relationship between interdelivery interval and uterine rupture in 2409 women who had one prior cesarean delivery. There were 29 women with a uterine rupture—1.4 percent. Interdelivery intervals of ≤ 18 months were associated with a threefold increased risk of symptomatic rupture during a subsequent trial of labor compared with intervals > 18 months. Similarly, Stamilio and coworkers (2007) noted a threefold increased risk of uterine rupture in women with an interpregnancy interval of < 6 months compared with one ≥ 6 months. But they also reported that interpregnancy intervals of 6 to 18 months did not significantly increase the risk.

Prior Vaginal Delivery

Prior vaginal delivery, either before or after a cesarean birth, significantly improves the prognosis for a subsequent vaginal delivery with either spontaneous or induced labor (Grinstead, 2004; Hendler, 2004; Mercer, 2008). Prior vaginal delivery also lowers the risk of subsequent uterine rupture and other morbidities (Cahill, 2006; Hochler, 2014; Zelop, 2000). Indeed, the most favorable prognostic factor is prior vaginal delivery.

Indication for Prior Cesarean Delivery

Considering all women who elect trial of labor, 60 to 80 percent will have a successful vaginal delivery (American College of Obstetricians and Gynecologists, 2013a). Women with a nonrecurring indication—for example, breech presentation—have the highest success rate of nearly 90 percent (Wing, 1999). Those with a prior cesarean delivery for fetal compromise have an approximately 80-percent success rate, and for those done for labor arrest, success rates approximate 60 percent (Bujold, 2001; Peaceman, 2006). Prior second-stage cesarean delivery can be associated with second-stage uterine rupture in a subsequent pregnancy (Jastrow, 2013).

Fetal Size

Most studies show that increasing fetal size is inversely related to successful trial of labor. The risk for uterine rupture is less robust. Zelop and associates (2001) compared the outcomes of almost 2750 women undergoing a trial of labor, and 1.1 percent had a uterine rupture. The rate increased—albeit not significantly—with increasing fetal weight. The rate was 1.0 percent for fetal weight < 4000 g, 1.6 percent for > 4000 g, and 2.4 percent for > 4250 g. Similarly, Elkousy and colleagues (2003) reported that the relative risk of rupture doubled if birthweight was > 4000 g. Conversely, Baron and coworkers (2013a) did not find increased uterine rupture with birthweights > 4000 g.

Fetal size at the opposite end of the spectrum may increase the chances of a successful VBAC. Specifically, women who attempt a trial of labor with a preterm fetus have higher successful VBAC rates and lower rupture rates (Durnwald, 2006; Quiñones, 2005).

Multifetal Gestation

Perhaps surprisingly, twin pregnancy does not appear to increase the uterine rupture risk with trial of labor. Ford and associates (2006) analyzed the outcomes of 1850 such women and reported a 45-percent successful vaginal delivery rate and a rupture rate of 0.9 percent. Similar studies by Cahill (2005) and Varner (2007) and their colleagues reported rupture rates of 0.7 to 1.1 percent and vaginal delivery rates of 75 to 85 percent. According to the American College of Obstetricians and Gynecologists (2013a), women with twins and a prior low-transverse hysterotomy who are otherwise candidates for vaginal delivery can safely undergo a trial of labor.

Maternal Obesity

Obesity decreases the success rate of trial of labor. Hibbard and coworkers (2006) reported the following vaginal delivery rates: 85 percent with a normal body mass index (BMI), 78 percent with a BMI between 25 and 30, 70 percent with a BMI between 30 and 40, and 61 percent with a BMI of 40 or greater. Similar findings were reported by Juhasz and associates (2005).

Fetal Death

Most women with a prior cesarean delivery and fetal death in the current pregnancy would prefer a VBAC. Although fetal concerns are obviated, available data suggest that maternal risks are increased. Nearly 46,000 women with a prior cesarean delivery in the Network database had a total of 209 fetal deaths (Ramirez, 2010). There were 76 percent who had a trial of labor with a success rate of 87 percent. Overall, the rupture rate was 2.4 percent. Four of five ruptures were during induction in 116 women with one prior transverse incision—3.4 percent.

LABOR AND DELIVERY CONSIDERATIONS

If elective repeat cesarean delivery is planned, it is essential that the fetus be mature. As shown in Figure 31-3, significant and appreciable adverse neonatal morbidity has been reported

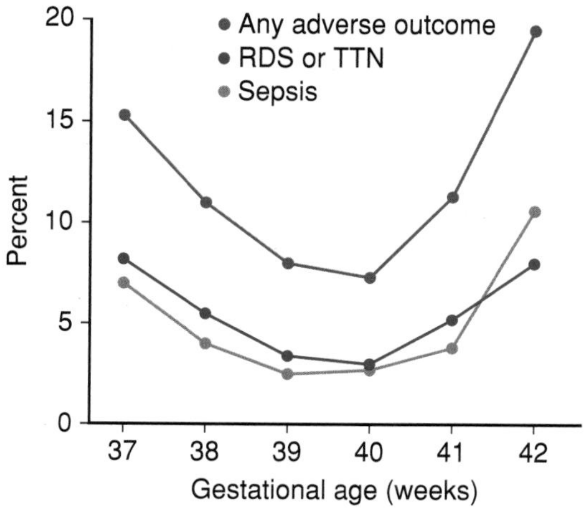

FIGURE 31-3 Neonatal morbidity and mortality rates seen with 13,258 elective repeat cesarean deliveries. Any adverse outcome includes death. Sepsis includes suspected and proven. RDS = respiratory distress syndrome; TTN = transient tachypnea of the newborn. (From Tita, 2009.)

with elective delivery before 39 completed weeks (Chiossi, 2013; Clark, 2009; Tita, 2009). The American Academy of Pediatrics and the American College of Obstetricians and Gynecologists (2012) have established the following guidelines for timing an elective operation, and at least one of these three must be documented:

1. Ultrasound measurement < 20 weeks supports a gestational age of ≥ 39 weeks.
2. Fetal heart sounds have been documented for 30 weeks by Doppler ultrasound.
3. A positive serum or urine β-hCG test result has been documented for ≥ 36 weeks.

Accurate gestational dating is suitable using any of the above criteria. Other options are to await spontaneous labor or to document fetal pulmonary maturation by amnionic-fluid analysis (Chap. 34, p. 655).

Informed Consent

The risks and benefits of a trial of labor versus a repeat cesarean delivery should be thoroughly discussed, and the decision to attempt a trial of labor is made by the informed woman in conjunction with her health-care provider (American Academy of Pediatrics and the American College of Obstetricians and Gynecologists, 2012). As previously emphasized, no woman with a prior uterine incision should be forced to undergo a trial of labor.

Intrapartum Care

Because of the risks of uterine rupture for women undergoing a trial of labor, the American Academy of Pediatricians and the American College of Obstetricians and Gynecologists (2012) recommend that such trials be undertaken only in facilities with staff immediately available to provide emergency care. Moreover, these centers should have a plan for managing uterine rupture.

Some argue that these provisions deny women full access to choices. For example in an earlier survey of Ohio hospitals, 15 percent of Level I, 63 percent of Level II, and 100 percent of Level III institutions met these requirements (Lavin, 2002). Moreover, an obstetrical anesthesia workforce survey reported that these rules were in place in 86 percent of hospitals with ≥ 1500 annual deliveries, in 45 percent of those with 500 to 1499 deliveries, and in 33 percent of those with < 500 deliveries.

Cervical Ripening and Labor Stimulation

As discussed, labor induction is associated with a higher failure rate for a trial of labor. The risks for uterine rupture, however, are less clear with induction or augmentation, with the exception of prostaglandin E_1—misoprostol—which is contraindicated (American College of Obstetricians and Gynecologists, 2013a; Ophir, 2012). While most institutions are not so conservative, we do not induce or augment labor pharmacologically in these women at Parkland Hospital. Instead, we attempt induction by amniotomy. Other considerations are to avoid induction or augmentation in women with an unknown prior incision type, an unfavorable cervix, or pregnancy > 40 weeks.

Oxytocin

Induction or augmentation of labor with oxytocin has been *implicated* in increased rates of uterine rupture in some studies (Zelop, 1999). In the Network study reported by Landon and colleagues (2004), uterine rupture was more frequent in women induced—1.1 percent—than in those in spontaneous labor—0.4 percent. Among women in this trial who had never had a prior vaginal delivery, the uterine rupture risk associated with an oxytocin induction was 1.8 percent—a fourfold increased risk compared with spontaneous labor (Grobman, 2007a). In contrast, in one case-control study, induction was not associated with a higher risk for rupture (Harper, 2012a). In an observational study, the success rate of induction was 67 percent (Shatz, 2012).

Cahill and coworkers (2008) reported a dose-related risk of rupture with oxytocin. At an infusion dose of 21 to 30 mU/min, the uterine rupture risk was fourfold greater than that in women not given oxytocin. Goetzl and associates (2001) described similar findings. They concluded, however, that differences in the dose or patterns of oxytocin use associated with uterine rupture were not substantive enough to require development of different induction protocols.

Prostaglandins

Various prostaglandin preparations that are commonly employed for cervical ripening or labor induction are discussed in Chapter 26 (p. 526). Safety with their use in women with a prior cesarean delivery is not clear because of conflicting data. For example, Wing and colleagues (1998) described a comparative study of PGE_1—*misoprostol*—versus oxytocin for labor induction in women with a prior cesarean delivery. They terminated their trial after two of the first 17 women assigned to misoprostol developed a uterine rupture. Other studies confirmed this, and most consider misoprostol to be contraindicated (American College of Obstetricians and Gynecologists, 2013a).

Studies to evaluate other prostaglandins for induction have mixed results. Ravasia and coworkers (2000) compared uterine rupture in 172 women given PGE_2 gel with 1544 women in spontaneous labor. The rupture rate was significantly greater in women treated with PGE_2 gel—2.9 percent—compared with 0.9 percent in those with spontaneous labor. Lydon-Rochelle and associates (2001) also reported that induction with prostaglandins for a trial of labor increased the uterine rupture risk.

Not all studies report an increased risk of uterine rupture with prostaglandins. In the Network study cited previously, there was a uterine rupture rate of 1.4 percent when any prostaglandin was used in combination with oxytocin (Landon, 2004). But in the subgroup of 227 women in whom labor was induced with a prostaglandin only, there were no ruptures. Similar findings were reported in that intravaginal prostaglandins were not found to be associated with an increased uterine rupture risk (Macones, 2005b). These latter investigators, along with Kayani and colleagues (2005), found that sequential use of a prostaglandin followed by oxytocin was associated with a threefold-increased risk of rupture compared with spontaneous labor.

After reviewing these more contemporaneous reports, the American College of Obstetricians and Gynecologists (2013a) concluded that labor induction for some women who attempt a trial of labor is a reasonable option. The College also concluded that it is reasonable to (1) avoid misoprostol, (2) select women most likely to have a successful trial of labor, and (3) avoid sequential use of prostaglandins and oxytocin.

Epidural Analgesia

Concerns that epidural analgesia for labor might mask the pain of uterine rupture have not been verified. Fewer than 10 percent of women with scar separation experience pain and bleeding, and fetal heart rate decelerations are the most likely sign of rupture (Kieser, 2002). That said, Cahill and coworkers (2010a) documented that more frequent episodes of epidural dosing were associated with increasing uterine rupture rates. Successful VBAC rates are similar, and in some cases higher, among women with labor epidural analgesia compared with those using other forms of analgesia (Landon, 2005). Perhaps related, almost a fourth of successful VBAC deliveries were completed with either forceps or vacuum (Inbar, 2013). The American Academy of Pediatrics and the American College of Obstetricians and Gynecologists (2012) have concluded that epidural analgesia may safely be used during a trial of labor.

Uterine Scar Exploration

Some clinicians routinely document the integrity of a prior scar by placing a hand through the dilated cervix and along the inner surface of the lower uterine segment following successful vaginal delivery. However, routine uterine exploration is considered by others to be unnecessary. Currently, the benefits of scar evaluation in the asymptomatic woman are unclear. There is general agreement, however, that surgical correction of a scar dehiscence is necessary only if significant bleeding is encountered. Our practice is to routinely examine these prior incision sites. Any decision for laparotomy and repair takes into consideration the extent of the tear, whether the peritoneal cavity has been entered, and the presence of active bleeding.

External Cephalic Version

External cephalic version for breech presentation is acceptable in women with a prior cesarean delivery who are contemplating a trial of labor (American College of Obstetricians and Gynecologists, 2013a). This procedure is addressed in Chapter 28 (p. 570).

UTERINE RUPTURE

Classification

Uterine rupture typically is classified as either (1) *complete* when all layers of the uterine wall are separated, or (2) *incomplete* when the uterine muscle is separated but the visceral peritoneum is intact. Incomplete rupture is also commonly referred to as *uterine dehiscence*. As expected, morbidity and mortality rates are appreciably greater when rupture is complete. The greatest risk factor for either form of rupture is prior cesarean delivery. In a review of all uterine rupture cases in Nova Scotia between 1988 and 1997, Kieser and Baskett (2002) reported that 92 percent were in women with a prior cesarean birth. Holmgren and associates (2012) described 42 cases of rupture in women with a prior hysterotomy. Of these, 36 were in labor at the time of rupture.

Diagnosis

Progress of labor in women attempting VBAC is similar to regular labor, and there is no specific pattern that presages uterine rupture (Graseck, 2012; Harper, 2012b). Before hypovolemic shock develops, symptoms and physical findings in women with uterine rupture may appear bizarre unless the possibility is kept in mind. For example, hemoperitoneum from a ruptured uterus may result in diaphragmatic irritation with pain referred to the chest—directing one to a diagnosis of pulmonary or amnionic fluid embolism instead of uterine rupture. The most common sign of uterine rupture is a nonreassuring fetal heart rate pattern with variable heart rate decelerations that may evolve into late decelerations and bradycardia as shown in Figure 31-4 (American Academy of Pediatrics and American College of Obstetricians and Gynecologists, 2012). In 36 cases of such rupture during a trial of labor, there were fetal signs in 24, maternal in eight, and both in three (Holmgren, 2012). Few women experience cessation of contractions following uterine rupture, and the use of intrauterine pressure catheters has not been shown to assist reliably in the diagnosis (Rodriguez, 1989).

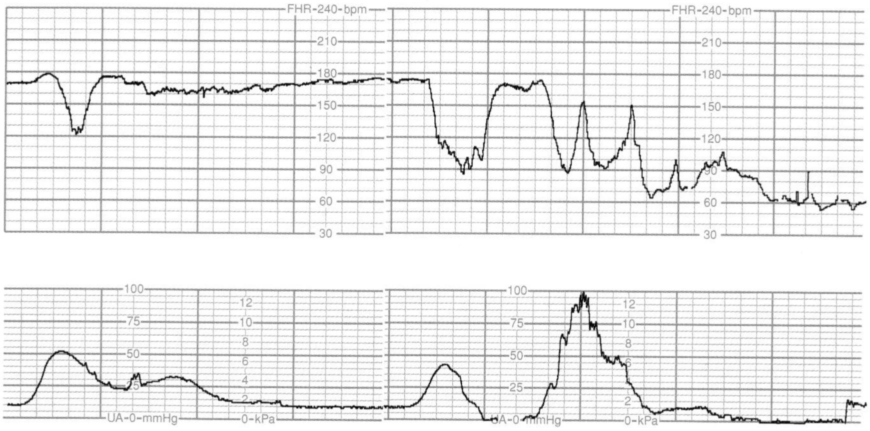

FIGURE 31-4 Fetal heart rate tracing in a woman whose uterus ruptured during labor while pushing. The rupture apparently stimulated a reflex push, after which uterine tone diminished and fetal bradycardia worsened.

In some women, the appearance of uterine rupture is identical to that of placental abruption. In most, however, there is remarkably little appreciable pain or tenderness. Also, because most women in labor are treated for discomfort with either narcotics or epidural analgesia, pain and tenderness may not be readily apparent. The condition usually becomes evident because of fetal distress signs and occasionally because of maternal hypovolemia from concealed hemorrhage.

If the fetal presenting part has entered the pelvis with labor, loss of station may be detected by pelvic examination. If the fetus is partly or totally extruded from the uterine rupture site, abdominal palpation or vaginal examination may be helpful to identify the presenting part, which will have moved away from the pelvic inlet. A firm contracted uterus may at times be felt alongside the fetus.

Decision-to-Delivery Time

With rupture and expulsion of the fetus into the peritoneal cavity, the chances for intact fetal survival are dismal, and reported mortality rates range from 50 to 75 percent. *Fetal condition depends on the degree to which the placental implantation remains intact, although this can change within minutes.* With rupture, the only chance of fetal survival is afforded by immediate delivery—most often by laparotomy—otherwise, hypoxia is inevitable. If rupture is followed by immediate total placental separation, then very few intact fetuses will be salvaged. *Thus, even in the best of circumstances, fetal salvage will be impaired.* The Utah experiences are instructive here (Holmgren, 2012). Of the 35 laboring patients with a uterine rupture, the decision-to-delivery time was < 18 minutes in 17, and none of these infants had an adverse neurological outcome. Of the 18 born > 18 minutes from decision time, the three infants with long-term neurological impairments were delivered at 31, 40, and 42 minutes. There were no deaths, thus severe neonatal neurological morbidity developed in 8 percent of these 35 women with uterine rupture.

In a study using the Swedish Birth Registry, Kaczmarczyk and colleagues (2007) found that the risk of neonatal death following uterine rupture was 5 percent—a 60-fold increase in risk compared with pregnancies not complicated by uterine rupture. In the Network study, seven of the 114 uterine ruptures—6 percent—associated with a trial of labor were complicated by the development of neonatal hypoxic ischemic encephalopathy (Spong, 2007).

Maternal deaths from rupture are uncommon. For example, of 2.5 million women who gave birth in Canada between 1991 and 2001, there were 1898 cases of uterine rupture, and four of these—0.2 percent—resulted in maternal death (Wen, 2005). In other regions of the world, however, maternal mortality rates associated with uterine rupture are much higher. In a report from rural India, for example, the maternal mortality rate associated with uterine rupture was 30 percent (Chatterjee, 2007).

Hysterectomy versus Repair

With complete rupture during a trial of labor, hysterectomy may be required. In the reports by McMahon (1996) and Miller (1997) and their coworkers, 10 to 20 percent of such women required hysterectomy for hemostasis. In selected cases, however, suture repair with uterine preservation may be performed. Sheth (1968) described outcomes from a series of 66 women in whom repair of a uterine rupture was elected rather than hysterectomy. In 25 instances, the repair was accompanied by tubal sterilization. Thirteen of the 41 mothers who did not have tubal sterilization had a total of 21 subsequent pregnancies. Uterine rupture recurred in four of these—approximately 25 percent. Usta and associates (2007) identified 37 women with a prior complete uterine rupture delivered during a 25-year period in Lebanon. Hysterectomy was performed in 11, and in the remaining 26 women, the rupture was repaired. Twelve of these women had 24 subsequent pregnancies, one third of which were complicated by recurrent uterine rupture. In another study, however, women with a uterine dehiscence were not more likely to have uterine rupture with a subsequent pregnancy (Baron, 2013b).

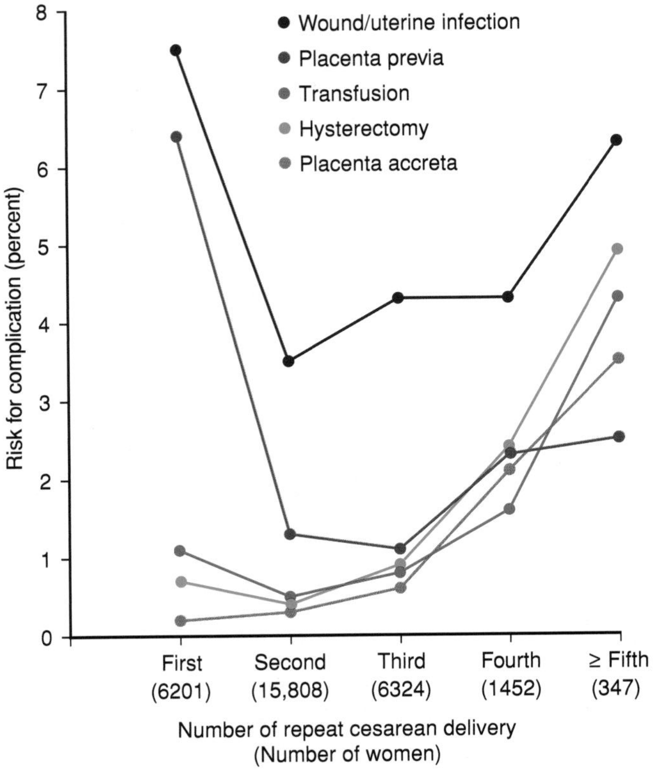

FIGURE 31-5 Maternal-Fetal Medicine Units Network: rates of some complications with increasing number of repeat cesarean deliveries. (Data from Silver, 2006.)

COMPLICATIONS WITH MULTIPLE REPEAT CESAREAN DELIVERIES

Because of the concerns with attempting a trial of labor—even in the woman with excellent criteria that forecast successful VBAC—most women in the United States undergo elective repeat cesarean delivery. This choice is not without several significant maternal complications, and rates of these increase in women who have multiple repeat operations. The incidences of some common complications for women with one prior transverse cesarean delivery who undergo an elective repeat cesarean delivery were shown in Table 31-2. Finally, half of cesarean hysterectomies done at Parkland Hospital are in women with one or more prior cesarean deliveries (Hernandez, 2013).

The Network addressed issues of increased morbidity in a cohort of 30,132 women who had from one to six repeat cesarean deliveries (Silver, 2006). This report addressed a list of morbidities, most of which increased as a trend with increasing number of repeat operations. The rates of some of the more common or serious complications are depicted in Figure 31-5. In addition to the ones shown, rates of bowel or bladder injury, admission to an intensive care unit or ventilator therapy, and maternal mortality, as well as operative and hospitalization length, showed significantly increasing trends. Similar results have been reported by others (Nisenblat, 2006; Usta, 2005). More difficult to quantify are risks for bowel obstructions and pelvic pain from peritoneal adhesive disease, both of which increase with each successive cesarean delivery (Andolf, 2010; Mankuta, 2013).

Cook and colleagues (2013) from the United Kingdom Obstetric Surveillance System (UKOSS) described adverse sequelae of women with multiple cesarean deliveries. Outcomes of those undergoing a fifth or greater operation were compared with those from women having a second through fourth procedure. Those having five or more cesarean deliveries had significantly increased rates of morbidity compared with rates in women having fewer than five procedures. Specifically, the major hemorrhage rate increased 18-fold; visceral damage, 17-fold; critical care admissions, 15-fold; and delivery < 37 weeks, sixfold. Much of this morbidity was in the 18 percent who had placenta previa or accrete syndromes (Chap. 41, p. 799). A percreta may invade the bladder or other adjacent structures. With this, difficult resection carries an inordinately high risk of hysterectomy, massive hemorrhage with transfusion, and maternal mortality.

STATE OF VAGINAL BIRTH AFTER CESAREAN—2014

The "best answer" for a given woman with a prior cesarean delivery is unknown. We agree with Scott (2011) regarding a "common-sense" approach. Thus, the woman—and her partner if she wishes—are encouraged to actively participate with her health-care provider in the final decision after appropriate counseling. For women who wish TOLAC despite a factor that increases their specific risk, additions to the consent form are recommended (American College of Obstetricians and Gynecologists, 2013a). Bonanno and colleagues (2011) have provided such an example.

TABLE 31-4. Some Recommendations of Professional Societies Concerning a Trial of Labor to Attempt VBAC

	Counseling	Facilities	Other
American College of Obstetricians and Gynecologists (2013a)	Offer to most women with one prior low-transverse incision; consider for two prior low-transverse incisions	Safest with ability for immediate cesarean delivery; patients should be allowed to accept increased risk when not available	Not precluded: twins, macrosomia, prior low-vertical or unknown type of incision
Society of Obstetricians and Gynaecologists of Canada (2005)	Offer to women with one prior transverse low-segment cesarean delivery; with > 1 prior CD then VBAC likely successful but increased risks	Should deliver in hospital in which timely cesarean delivery is available; approximate timeframe of 30 minutes	Oxytocin or Foley catheter induction safe, but prostaglandins should not be used; macrosomia, diabetes, postterm pregnancy, twins are not contraindications
Royal College of Obstetricians and Gynaecologists (2007)	Discuss VBAC option with women with prior low-segment cesarean delivery; decision between obstetrician and patient	Suitable delivery suite with continuous care and monitoring; immediate cesarean delivery capability	Caution with twins and macrosomia

CD = cesarean delivery; VBAC = vaginal birth after cesarean.

Brief synopses of professional society guidelines are shown in Table 31-4. Guidelines that tend to be more conservative are shown in Table 31-5.

TABLE 31-5. Conservative Guidelines to Approach a Trial of Labor Following Cesarean Delivery

Follow ACOG practice guidelines
Education and counseling
Preconceptionally
Provide ACOG patient pamphlet
Early during prenatal care
Develop preliminary plan
Revisit at least each trimester
Be willing to alter decision
Have facilities availability
Risk assessment
Review previous operative note(s)
Review relative and absolute contraindications
Reconsider risks as pregnancy progresses
Tread carefully: > 1 prior transverse CD, unknown incision, twins, macrosomia
Labor and delivery
Cautions for induction—unfavorable cervix, high station
Consider AROM
Avoid prostaglandins
Respect oxytocin—know when to quit
Beware of abnormal labor progress
Respect EFM pattern abnormalities
Know when to abandon a trial of labor

ACOG = American College of Obstetricians and Gynecologists; AROM = artificial rupture of membranes; CD = cesarean delivery; EFM = electronic fetal monitoring.

REFERENCES

Abitbol MM, Castillo I, Taylor UB, et al: Vaginal birth after cesarean section: the patient's point of view. Am Fam Physician 47:129, 1993

American Academy of Pediatrics and the American College of Obstetricians and Gynecologists: Guidelines for Perinatal Care, 7th ed., 2012

American College of Obstetricians and Gynecologists: Guidelines for vaginal delivery after a previous cesarean birth. Committee Opinion No. 64, October 1988

American College of Obstetricians and Gynecologists: Vaginal delivery after previous cesarean birth. Committee Opinion No. 143, October 1994

American College of Obstetricians and Gynecologists: Vaginal birth after previous cesarean delivery. Practice Bulletin No. 2, October 1998

American College of Obstetricians and Gynecologists: Vaginal birth after previous cesarean delivery. Practice Bulletin No. 5, July 1999

American College of Obstetricians and Gynecologists: Vaginal birth after previous cesarean delivery. Practice Bulletin No. 115, Reaffirmed 2013a

American College of Obstetricians and Gynecologists: Cesarean delivery on maternal request. Committee Opinion No. 559, April 2013b

Andolf E, Thorsell M, Källén K: Cesarean delivery and risk for postoperative adhesions and intestinal obstruction: a nested case-control study of the Swedish Medical Birth Registry. Am J Obstet Gynecol 203:406.e1, 2010

Babbar S, Chauhan S, Hammas I, et al: Failed trial of labor after cesarean delivery: indications for failure and peripartum complications. Abstract No. 818, Am J Obstet Gynecol 208 (1 Suppl):S342, 2013

Barger MK, Dunn JT, Bearman S, et al: A survey of access to trial of labor in California hospitals in 2012. BMC Pregnancy Childbirth 13:83, 2013

Baron J, Weintraub A, Sergienko R, et al: Is vaginal delivery of a macrosomic infant after cesarean section really so dangerous? Abstract No. 799, Am J Obstet Gynecol 208(1 Suppl):S335, 2013a

Baron J, Weintraub A, Eshcoli T, et al: The significance of a previous uterine scar dehiscence on subsequent births. Abstract No. 800. Am J Obstet Gynecol 208(1 Suppl):S336, 2013b

Bergeron M-E, Jastrow N, Brassard N, et al: Sonography of lower uterine segment thickness and prediction of uterine rupture. Obstet Gynecol 113(2):520, 2009

Bonanno C, Clausing M, Berkowitz R: VBAC: a medicolegal perspective. Clin Perinatol 38:217, 2011

Bujold E, Bujold C, Hamilton EF, et al: The impact of a single-layer or double-layer closure on uterine rupture. Am J Obstet Gynecol 186:1326, 2002

Bujold E, Gauthier RJ: Should we allow a trial of labor after a previous cesarean for dystocia in the second stage of labor? Obstet Gynecol 98:652, 2001

Cahill A, Stamilio DM, Paré E, et al: Vaginal birth after cesarean (VBAC) attempt in twin pregnancies: is it safe? Am J Obstet Gynecol 193:1050, 2005

Cahill AG, Odibo AO, Allsworth JE, et al: Frequent epidural dosing as a marker for impending uterine rupture in patients who attempt vaginal birth after cesarean delivery. Am J Obstet Gynecol 202:355.e1, 2010a

Cahill AG, Stamilio DM, Odibo A, et al: Is vaginal birth after cesarean (VBAC) or elective repeat cesarean safer in women with a prior vaginal delivery? Am J Obstet Gynecol 195:1143, 2006

Cahill AG, Tuuli M, Odibo AO, et al: Vaginal birth after caesarean for women with three or more prior caesareans: assessing safety and success. BJOG 117:422, 2010b

Cahill AG, Waterman BM, Stamilio DM, et al: Higher maximum doses of oxytocin are associated with an unacceptably high risk for uterine rupture in patients attempting vaginal birth after cesarean delivery. Am J Obstet Gynecol 199:32.e1, 2008

Chapman SJ, Owen J, Hauth JC: One- versus two-layer closure of a low transverse cesarean: the next pregnancy. Obstet Gynecol 89:16, 1997

Chatterjee SR, Bhaduri S: Clinical analysis of 40 cases of uterine rupture at Durgapur Subdivisional Hospital: an observational study. J Indian Med Assoc 105:510, 2007

Chauhan SP, Magann EF, Wiggs CD, et al: Pregnancy after classic cesarean delivery. Obstet Gynecol 100:946, 2002

Chauhan SP, Martin JN Jr, Henrichs CE, et al: Maternal and perinatal complications with uterine rupture in 142,075 patients who attempted vaginal birth after cesarean delivery: a review of the literature. Am J Obstet Gynecol 189:408, 2003

Cheng Y, Snowden J, Cottrell E, et al: Trends in proportions of hospitals with VBAC: impact of ACOG guidelines. Am J Obstet Gynecol 210:S241, 2014

Chiossi G, Lai Y, Landon MB, et al: Timing of delivery and adverse outcomes in term singleton repeat cesarean deliveries. Obstet Gynecol 121:561, 2013

Clark SL, Miller DD, Belfort MA, et al: Neonatal and maternal outcomes associated with elective term delivery. Am J Obstet Gynecol 200(2):156.e1, 2009

Coleman VH, Erickson K, Schulkin J, et al: Vaginal birth after cesarean delivery. J Reprod Med 50:261, 2005

Cook J, Javis S, Knight M, et al: Multiple repeat caesarean section in the UK: incidence and consequences to mother and child. A national, prospective, cohort study. BJOG 120(1):85, 2013

Cragin E: Conservatism in obstetrics. N Y Med J 104:1, 1916

Dicle O, Kücükler C, Pirnar T: Magnetic resonance imaging evaluation of incision healing after cesarean sections. Eur Radiol 7:31, 1997

Durnwald C, Mercer B: Uterine rupture, perioperative and perinatal morbidity after single-layer and double-layer closure at cesarean delivery. Am J Obstet Gynecol 189:925, 2003

Durnwald CP, Rouse DJ, Leveno KJ, et al: The Maternal-Fetal Medicine Units Cesarean Registry: safety and efficacy of a trial of labor in preterm pregnancy after a prior cesarean delivery. Am J Obstet Gynecol 195:1119, 2006

Eastman NJ: Williams Obstetrics, 10th ed. Appleton-Century-Crofts, New York, 1950

Elkousy MA, Sammel M, Stevens E, et al: The effect of birth weight on vaginal birth after cesarean delivery success rates. Am J Obstet Gynecol 188:824, 2003

Erez O, Dulder D, Novack L, et al: Trial of labor and vaginal birth after cesarean section in patients with uterine Müllerian anomalies: a population-based study. Am J Obstet Gynecol 196:537.e1, 2007

Flamm BL: Once a cesarean, always a controversy. Obstet Gynecol 90:312, 1997

Ford AA, Bateman BT, Simpson LL: Vaginal birth after cesarean delivery in twin gestations: a large, nationwide sample of deliveries. Am J Obstet Gynecol 195:1138, 2006

Goetzl L, Shipp TD, Cohen A, et al: Oxytocin dose and the risk of uterine rupture in trial of labor after cesarean. Obstet Gynecol 97:381, 2001

Graseck AS, Odibo AO, Tuuli M, et al: Normal first stage of labor in women undergoing trial of labor after cesarean delivery. Obstet Gynecol 119(4):732, 2012

Gregory KD, Korst LM, Fridman M, et al: Vaginal birth after cesarean: clinical risk factors associated with adverse outcome. Am J Obstet Gynecol 198:452.e1, 2008

Grinstead J, Grobman WA: Induction of labor after one prior cesarean: predictors of vaginal delivery. Obstet Gynecol 103:534, 2004

Grobman WA, Gilbert S, Landon MB, et al: Outcomes of induction of labor after one prior cesarean. Obstet Gynecol 109:262, 2007a

Grobman WA, Lai Y, Landon MB, et al: Can a prediction model for vaginal birth after cesarean also predict the probability of morbidity related to a trial of labor? Am J Obstet Gynecol 200(1):56.e1, 2009

Grobman WA, Lai Y, Landon MB, et al: Development of a nomogram for prediction of vaginal birth after cesarean delivery. Obstet Gynecol 109:806, 2007b

Grobman WA, Lai Y, Landon MB, et al: Prediction of uterine rupture associated with attempted vaginal birth after cesarean delivery. Am J Obstet Gynecol 199:30.e1, 2008

Guise JM, Berlin M, McDonagh M, et al: Safety of vaginal birth after cesarean: a systematic review. Obstet Gynecol 103:420, 2004

Guise JM, Denman MA, Emeis C, et al: Vaginal birth after cesarean: new insights on maternal and neonatal outcomes. Obstet Gynecol 115:1267, 2010

Harper LM, Cahill AG, Boslaugh S, et al: Association of induction of labor and uterine rupture in women attempting vaginal birth after cesarean: a survival analysis. Am J Obstet Gynecol 206:51.e1, 2012a

Harper LM, Cahill AG, Roehl KA, et al: The pattern of labor preceding uterine rupture. Am J Obstet Gynecol 207(3):210.e1, 2012b

Harper LM, Cahill AG, Stamilio DM, et al: Effect of gestational age at the prior cesarean delivery on maternal morbidity in subsequent VBAC attempt. Am J Obstet Gynecol 200(3):276.e1, 2009

Hashima JN, Eden KB, Osterweil P, et al: Predicting vaginal birth after cesarean delivery: a review of prognostic factors and screening tools. Am J Obstet Gynecol 190:547, 2004

Hendler I, Gauthier RJ, Bujold E: The effects of prior vaginal delivery compared to prior VBAC on the outcomes of current trial of VBAC. Abstract No. 384. J Soc Gynecol Investig 11:202A, 2004

Hernandez JS, Wendel GD, Sheffield JS: Trends in emergency peripartum hysterectomy at a single institution: 1988–2009. Am J Perinatol 30:365, 2013

Hibbard JU, Gilbert S, Landon MB, et al: Trial of labor or repeat cesarean delivery in women with morbid obesity and previous cesarean delivery. Obstet Gynecol 108:125, 2006

Hochler H, Yaffe H, Schwed P, et al: Safety of a trial of labor after cesarean delivery in grandmultiparous women. Obstet Gynecol 123:304, 2014

Holmgren C, Scott JR, Porter TF, et al: Uterine rupture with attempted vaginal birth after cesarean delivery. Obstet Gynecol 119:725, 2012

Inbar R, Mazaaki S, Kalter A, et al: Vaginal birth after cesarean (VBAC) is associated with an increased risk of instrumental delivery. Abstract No. 812, Am J Obstet Gynecol 208 (1 Suppl):S340, 2013

Jastrow N, Chailet N, Roberge S, et al: Sonographic lower uterine segment thickness and risk of uterine scar defect: a systematic review. J Obstet Gynaecol Can 32(4):321, 2010

Jastrow N, Demers S, Gauthier RI, et al: Adverse obstetric outcomes in women with previous cesarean for dystocia in second stage labor. Am J Perinatol 30:173, 2013

Juhasz G, Gyamfi C, Gyamfi P, et al: Effect of body mass index and excessive weight gain on success of vaginal birth after cesarean delivery. Obstet Gynecol 106:741, 2005

Kaczmarczyk M, Sparén P, Terry P, et al: Risk factors for uterine rupture and neonatal consequences of uterine rupture: a population-based study of successive pregnancies in Sweden. BJOG 114:1208, 2007

Kayani SI, Alfirevic Z: Uterine rupture after induction of labour in women with previous caesarean section. BJOG 112:451, 2005

Kerr JN: The lower uterine segment incision in conservative cesarean section. J Obstet Gynaecol Br Emp 28:475, 1921

Kieser KE, Baskett TF: A 10-year population-based study of uterine rupture. Obstet Gynecol 100:749, 2002

Landon MB, Hauth JC, Leveno KJ, et al: Maternal and perinatal outcomes associated with a trial of labor after prior cesarean delivery. N Engl J Med 351:2581, 2004

Landon MB, Leindecker S, Spong CY, et al: The MFMU Cesarean Registry: factors affecting the success of trial of labor after previous cesarean delivery. Am J Obstet Gynecol 193:1016, 2005

Landon MB, Spong CY, Thom E, et al: Risk of uterine rupture with a trial of labor in women with multiple and single prior cesarean delivery. Obstet Gynecol 108:12, 2006

Lavin JP, DiPasquale L, Crane S, et al: A state-wide assessment of the obstetric, anesthesia, and operative team personnel who are available to manage the labors and deliveries and to treat the complications of women who attempt vaginal birth after cesarean delivery. Am J Obstet Gynecol 187:611, 2002

Leeman LM, Beagle M, Espey E, et al: Diminishing availability of trial of labor after cesarean delivery in New Mexico hospitals. Obstet Gynecol 122:242, 2013

Lydon-Rochelle M, Holt VL, Easterling TR, et al: Risk of uterine rupture during labor among women with a prior cesarean delivery. N Engl J Med 345:3, 2001

Macones GA, Cahill A, Pare E, et al: Obstetric outcomes in women with two prior cesarean deliveries: is vaginal birth after cesarean delivery a viable option? Am J Obstet Gynecol 192:1223, 2005a

Macones GA, Cahill AG, Stamilio DM, et al: Can uterine rupture in patients attempting vaginal birth after cesarean delivery be predicted? Am J Obstet Gynecol 195:1148, 2006

Macones GA, Peipert J, Nelson DB, et al: Maternal complications with vaginal birth after cesarean delivery: a multicenter study. Am J Obstet Gynecol 193:1656, 2005b

Mankuta D, Mansour M, Alon SA: Maternal and fetal morbidity due to abdominal adhesions after repeated cesarean section. Abstract No. 792, Am J Obstet Gynecol 208(1 Suppl):S332, 2013

Marshall NE, Fu R, Guise JM: Impact of multiple cesarean deliveries on maternal morbidity: a systematic review. Am J Obstet Gynecol 205:262.e1, 2011
Martin JA, Hamilton BE, Ventura SJ, et al: Births: final data for 2009. Natl Vital Stat Rep 60(1):1, 2011
Martin JA, Hamilton BE, Ventura SJ, et al: Births: final data for 2010. Natl Vital Stat Rep 61(1):1, 2012a
Martin JA, Hamilton BE, Ventura SJ, et al: Births: preliminary data for 2011. Natl Vital Stat Rep 61(5):1, 2012b
Martin JN, Perry KG, Roberts WE, et al: The care for trial of labor in the patients with a prior low-segment vertical cesarean incision. Am J Obstet Gynecol 177:144, 1997
McMahon MJ, Luther ER, Bowes WA Jr, et al: Comparison of a trial of labor with an elective second cesarean section. N Engl J Med 335:689, 1996
Mercer BM, Gilbert S, Landon MB, et al: Labor outcomes with increasing number of prior vaginal births after cesarean delivery. Obstet Gynecol 111:285, 2008
Metz TD, Stoddard GJ, Henry E, et al: Simple, validated vaginal birth after cesarean delivery prediction model for use at the time of admission. Obstet Gynecol 122:571, 2013
Miller DA, Diaz FG, Paul RH: Vaginal birth after cesarean: a 10-year experience. Obstet Gynecol 84(2):255, 1994
Miller DA, Goodwin TM, Gherman RB, et al: Intrapartum rupture of the unscarred uterus. Obstet Gynecol 89:671, 1997
Mozurkewich EL, Hutton EK: Elective repeat cesarean delivery versus trial of labor: a meta-analysis of the literature from 1989 to 1999. Am J Obstet Gynecol 183(5):1187, 2000
Naji O, Daemen A, Smith A, et al: Changes in cesarean section scar dimensions during pregnancy: a prospective longitudinal study. Ultrasound Obstet Gynecol 41(5):556, 2013a
Naji O, Wynants L, Smith A, et al: Predicting successful vaginal birth after cesarean section using a model based on cesarean scar features examined using transvaginal sonography. Ultrasound Obstet Gynecol 41(6):672, 2013
National Institutes of Health: Consensus Development Conference of Cesarean Childbirth, September 1980. NIH Pub No. 82–2067, Bethesda, NIH, 1981
National Institutes of Health Consensus Development Conference Panel: National Institutes of Health Consensus Development conference statement: vaginal birth after cesarean: new insights. March 8–10, 2010. Obstet Gynecol 115:1279, 2010
Nisenblat V, Barak S, Griness OB, et al: Maternal complications associated with multiple cesarean deliveries. Obstet Gynecol 108:21, 2006
Ophir E, Odeh M, Hirsch Y, et al: Uterine rupture during trial of labor: controversy of induction's methods. Obstet Gynecol Surv 67(11):734, 2012
Osmundson SS, Garabedian MJ, Lyell DJ: Risk factors for classical hysterotomy by gestational age. Obstet Gynecol 122:845, 2013
Osser OV, Valentin L: Clinical importance of appearance of cesarean hysterotomy scar at transvaginal ultrasonography in nonpregnant women. Obstet Gynecol 117:525, 2011
Pauerstein CJ: Once a section, always a trial of labor? Obstet Gynecol 28:273, 1966
Pauerstein CJ, Karp L, Muher S: Trial of labor after low segment cesarean section. S Med J 62:925, 1969
Peaceman AM, Gersnoviez R, Landon MB, et al: The MFMU cesarean registry: impact of fetal size on trial of labor success for patients with previous cesarean for dystocia. Am J Obstet Gynecol 195:1127, 2006
Quiñones JN, Stamilio DM, Paré E, et al: The effect of prematurity on vaginal birth after cesarean delivery: success and maternal morbidity. Obstet Gynecol 105:519, 2005
Ramirez MM, Gilbert S, Landon MB, et al: Mode of delivery in women with antepartum fetal death and prior cesarean delivery. Am J Perinatol 27:825, 2010
Ravasia DJ, Brain PH, Pollard JK: Incidence of uterine rupture among women with müllerian duct anomalies who attempt vaginal birth after cesarean delivery. Am J Obstet Gynecol 181:877, 1999
Ravasia DJ, Wood SL, Pollard JK: Uterine rupture during induced trial of labor among women with previous cesarean delivery. Am J Obstet Gynecol 183:1176, 2000
Reyes-Ceja L, Cabrera R, Insfran E, et al: Pregnancy following previous uterine rupture: study of 19 patients. Obstet Gynecol 34:387, 1969
Ritchie EH: Pregnancy after rupture of the pregnant uterus: a report of 36 pregnancies and a study of cases reported since 1932. J Obstet Gynaecol Br Commonw 78:642, 1971
Rodriguez MH, Masaki DI, Phelan JP, et al: Uterine rupture: are intrauterine pressure catheters useful in the diagnosis? Am J Obstet Gynecol 161:666, 1989
Rosenstein MG, Kuppermann M, Gregorich SE, et al: Association between vaginal birth after cesarean delivery and primary cesarean delivery rates. 122:1010, 2013
Rossi AC, D'Addario V: Maternal morbidity following a trial of labor after cesarean section vs elective repeat cesarean delivery: a systematic review with metaanalysis. Am J Obstet Gynecol 199(3):224, 2008
Royal College of Obstetricians and Gynaecologists: Birth after previous caesarean birth. Green-top Guideline No. 45, February 2007
Sachs BP, Koblin C, Castro MA, et al: The risk of lowering the cesarean-delivery rate. N Engl J Med 340:5, 1999
Sciscione AC, Landon MB, Leveno KJ, et al: Previous preterm cesarean delivery and risk of subsequent uterine rupture. Obstet Gynecol 111:648, 2008
Scott JR: Vaginal birth after cesarean delivery: a common-sense approach. Obstet Gynecol 118:342, 2011
Shatz L, Novack L, Mazor M, et al: Induction of labor after a prior cesarean delivery: lessons from a population-based study. J Perinat Med 41:171, 2013
Sheth SS: Results of treatment of rupture of the uterus by suturing. J Obstet Gynaecol Br Commonw 75:55, 1968
Shipp TD, Zelop CM, Repke JT, et al: Interdelivery interval and risk of symptomatic uterine rupture. Obstet Gynecol 97:175, 2001
Shipp TD, Zelop CM, Repke JT, et al: Intrapartum uterine rupture and dehiscence in patients with prior lower uterine segment vertical and transverse incisions. Obstet Gynecol 94:735, 1999
Silver RM, Landon MB, Rouse DJ, et al: Maternal morbidity associated with multiple repeat cesarean deliveries. Obstet Gynecol 207:1226, 2006
Smith GC, Pell JP, Cameron AD, et al: Risk of perinatal death associated with labor after previous cesarean delivery in uncomplicated term pregnancies. JAMA 287:2684, 2002
Society for Maternal-Fetal Medicine: Counseling and management of women with prior classical cesarean delivery. Contemp OB/GYN 57(6):26, 2012
Society for Maternal-Fetal Medicine: Prior non-lower segment uterine scar: when to plan for cesarean delivery. Contemp OB/GYN 58(12):50, 2013
Society of Obstetricians and Gynaecologists of Canada: SOGC clinical practice guidelines. Guidelines for vaginal birth after previous caesarean birth. Number 155 (replaces guideline Number 147), February 2005. Int J Gynaecol Obstet 89(3):319, 2005
Spong CY, Landon MB, Gilbert S, et al: Risk of uterine rupture and adverse perinatal outcome at term after cesarean delivery. Obstet Gynecol 110:801, 2007
Srinivas SK, Stamilio DM, Stevens EJ, et al: Predicting failure of a vaginal birth attempt after cesarean delivery. Obstet Gynecol 109:800, 2007
Stamilio DM, DeFranco E, Paré E, et al: Short interpregnancy interval. Risk of uterine rupture and complications of vaginal birth after cesarean delivery. Obstet Gynecol 110, 1075, 2007
Stanhope T, El-Nasher S, Garrett A, et al: Prediction of uterine rupture or dehiscence during trial of labor after cesarean delivery: a cohort study. Abstract No. 821, Am J Obstet Gynecol 208(1 Suppl):S343, 2013
Tahseen S, Griffiths M: Vaginal birth after two caesarean sections (VBAC-2)—a systematic review with meta-analysis of success rate and adverse outcomes of VBAC-2 versus VBAC-1 and repeat (third) caesarean sections. BJOG 117:5, 2010
Tita AT, Landon MB, Spong CY, et al: Timing of elective repeat cesarean delivery at term and neonatal outcomes. N Engl J Med 360(2):111, 2009
Tucker JM, Hauth JC, Hodgkins P, et al: Trial of labor after a one- or two-layer closure of a low transverse uterine incision. Am J Obstet Gynecol 168:545, 1993
Uddin SFG, Simon AE: Rates and success rates of trial of labor after cesarean delivery in the United States, 1990–2009. Matern Child Health J 17:1309, 2013
Usta IM, Hamdi MA, Abu Musa AA, et al: Pregnancy outcome in patients with previous uterine rupture. Acta Obstet Gynecol 86:172, 2007
Usta IM, Hobeika EM, Abu-Musa AA, et al: Placenta previa-accreta: risk factors and complications. Am J Obstet Gynecol 193:1045, 2005
Varner MW, Thom E, Spong CY, et al: Trial of labor after one previous cesarean delivery for multifetal gestation. Obstet Gynecol 110:814, 2007
Vidaeff AC, Lucas MJ: Impact of single- or double-layer closure on uterine rupture. Am J Obstet Gynecol 188:602, 2003
Wen SW, Huang L, Liston R, et al: Severe maternal morbidity in Canada, 1991–2001. CMAJ 173:759, 2005
Williams JW: Obstetrics: A Textbook for the Use of Students and Practitioners, 1st ed. Appleton & Co, New York, 1903
Wing DA, Lovett K, Paul RH: Disruption of prior uterine incision following misoprostol for labor induction in women with previous cesarean delivery. Obstet Gynecol 91:828, 1998
Wing DA, Paul RH: Vaginal birth after cesarean section: selection and management. Clin Obstet Gynecol 42:836, 1999
Zelop CM, Shipp TD, Repke JT, et al: Effect of previous vaginal delivery on the risk of uterine rupture during a subsequent trial of labor. Am J Obstet Gynecol 183:1184, 2000
Zelop CM, Shipp TD, Repke JT, et al: Outcomes of trial of labor following previous cesarean delivery among women with fetuses weighing > 4000 g. Am J Obstet Gynecol 185:903, 2001
Zelop CM, Shipp TD, Repke JT, et al: Uterine rupture during induced or augmented labor in gravid women with one prior cesarean delivery. Am J Obstet Gynecol 181:882, 1999

SECTION 9

THE NEWBORN

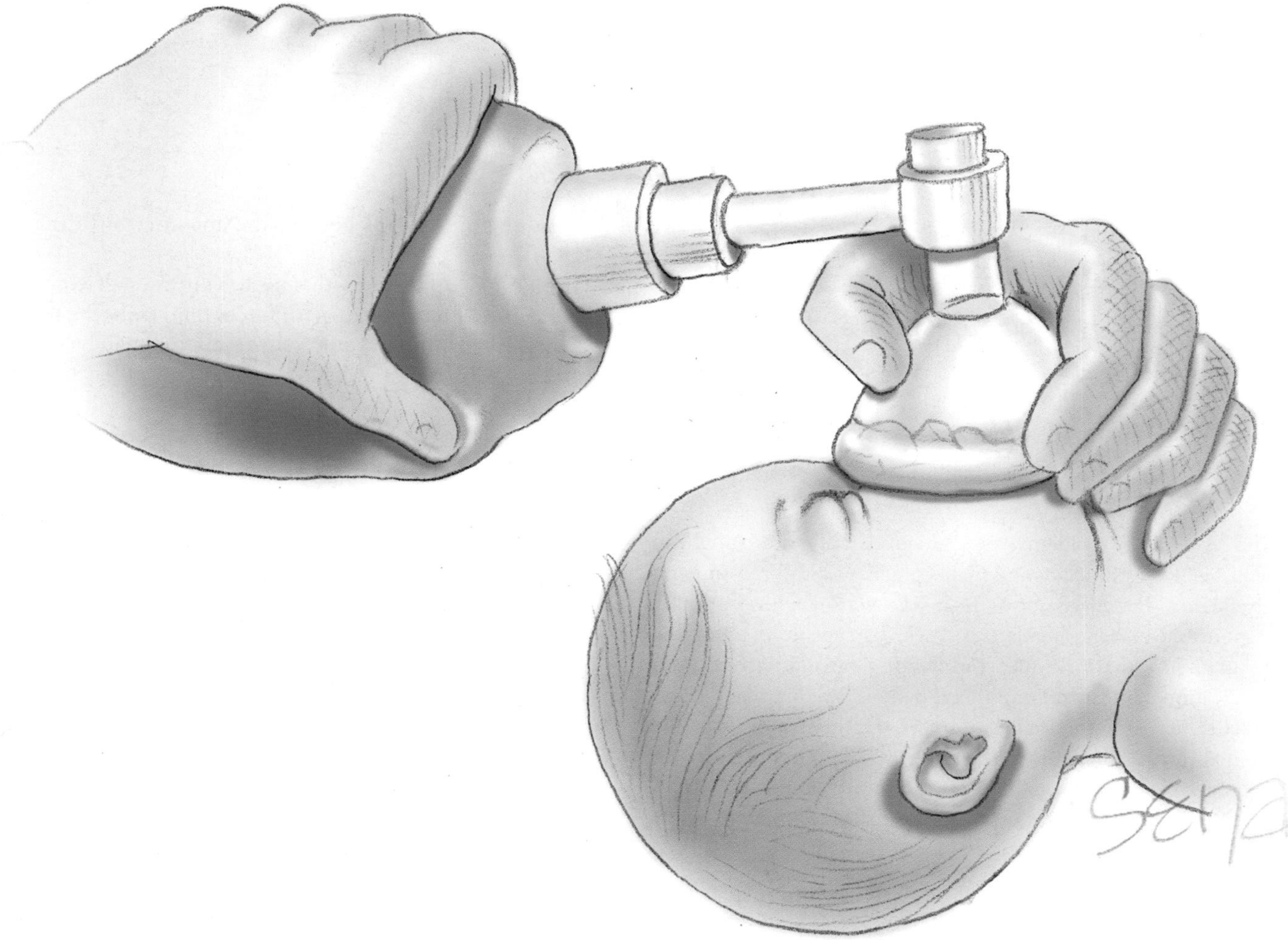

CHAPTER 32

The Newborn

The American Academy of Pediatrics and the American College of Obstetricians and Gynecologists (2012) recommend attendance at delivery of at least one person whose primary responsibility is the neonate and who is capable of initiating resuscitation that includes intubation, vascular access, and medication administration. This usually is a pediatrician, nurse practitioner, anesthesiologist, nurse anesthetist, or specially trained nurse. However, in their absence, the responsibility for neonatal resuscitation falls to the obstetrical attendant. Thus, obstetricians should be well versed in measures for immediate care of the newborn.

INITIATION OF AIR BREATHING

Immediately following birth, the infant must promptly convert to air breathing as the fluid-filled alveoli expand with air and pulmonary perfusion is established. The newborn begins to breathe and cry almost immediately after birth, which indicates establishment of active respiration. Some factors that appear to influence the first breath include:

- Physical stimulation—examples include handling the neonate during delivery.
- Oxygen deprivation and carbon dioxide accumulation—these serve to increase the frequency and magnitude of breathing movements both before and after birth (Dawes, 1974).
- Thoracic compression—this occurs during pelvic descent, following which vaginal birth forces fluid from the respiratory tract in volume equivalent to approximately a fourth of the ultimate functional residual capacity (Saunders, 1978).
- Aeration of the newborn lung does not involve the inflation of a collapsed structure, but instead, the rapid replacement of bronchial and alveolar fluid by air. After delivery, the residual alveolar fluid is cleared through the pulmonary circulation and to a lesser degree, through the pulmonary lymphatics (Chernick, 1978). Delay in fluid removal from the alveoli probably contributes to the syndrome of transient tachypnea of the newborn (TTN) (Guglani, 2008). As fluid is replaced by air, compression of the pulmonary vasculature is reduced considerably, and in turn, resistance to blood flow is lowered. With the fall in pulmonary arterial blood pressure, the ductus arteriosus normally closes (Fig. 7-8, p. 136).

High negative intrathoracic pressures are required to bring about the initial entry of air into the fluid-filled alveoli. Normally, from the first breath after birth, progressively more residual air accumulates in the lung, and with each successive breath, lower pulmonary opening pressure is required. In the normal mature newborn, by approximately the fifth breath, pressure-volume changes achieved with each respiration are very similar to those of the adult. Thus, the breathing pattern shifts from the shallow episodic inspirations characteristic of the fetus to regular, deeper inhalations (Chap. 17, p. 337). Surfactant, which is synthesized by type II pneumocytes and already present in the alveoli, lowers alveolar surface tension and thereby prevents lung collapse. Insufficient surfactant, common in preterm infants, leads promptly to respiratory distress syndrome, which is described in Chapter 34 (p. 653).

CARE IN THE DELIVERY ROOM

Personnel designated for infant support are responsible for immediate care and for acute resuscitation initiation if needed.

Immediate Care

Before and during delivery, careful consideration must be given to several determinants of neonatal well-being including: (1) maternal health status; (2) prenatal complications, including any suspected fetal malformations; (3) gestational age; (4) labor complications; (5) duration of labor and ruptured membranes; (6) type and duration of anesthesia; (7) difficulty with delivery; and (8) medications given during labor and their dosages, administration routes, and timing relative to delivery.

Newborn Resuscitation

The International Liaison Committee on Resuscitation (ILCOR) updated its guidelines for neonatal resuscitation that are sanctioned by the American Academy of Pediatrics and the American Heart Association (Biban, 2011; Perlman, 2010). These substantially revised guidelines are incorporated into the following sections.

Approximately 10 percent of newborns require some degree of active resuscitation to stimulate breathing, and 1 percent require extensive resuscitation. It is perhaps not coincidental that there is a two- to threefold risk of death for newborns delivered at home compared with those delivered in hospitals (American College of Obstetricians and Gynecologists, 2013b). When deprived of oxygen, either before or after birth, neonates demonstrate a well-defined sequence of events leading to apnea (Fig. 32-1). With oxygen deprivation, there is a transient period of rapid breathing, and if it persists, breathing stops, which is termed *primary apnea.* This stage is accompanied by a fall in heart rate and loss of neuromuscular tone. Simple stimulation and exposure to oxygen will usually reverse primary apnea. If oxygen deprivation and asphyxia persist, however, the newborn will develop deep gasping respirations, followed by secondary apnea. This latter stage is associated with a further decline in heart rate, falling blood pressure, and loss of neuromuscular tone. Neonates in secondary apnea will not respond to stimulation and will not spontaneously resume respiratory efforts. Unless ventilation is assisted, death follows. Clinically, primary and secondary apneas are indistinguishable. Thus, secondary apnea must be assumed and resuscitation of the apneic newborn must be started immediately.

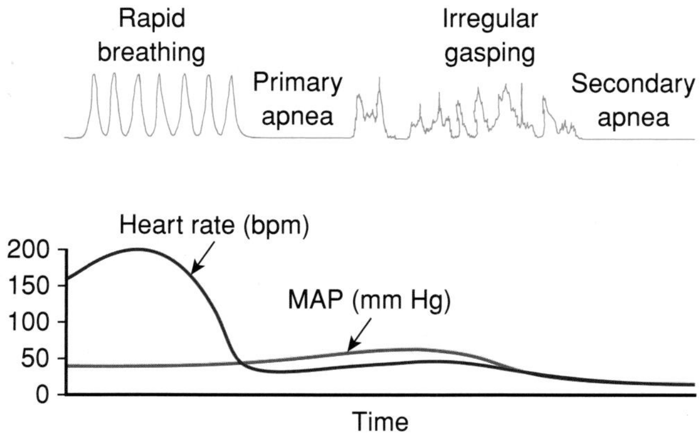

FIGURE 32-1 Physiological changes associated with primary and secondary apnea in the newborn. bpm = beats per minute; HR = heart rate; MAP = mean arterial pressure. (Adapted from Kattwinkel, 2006.)

Resuscitation Protocol

The updated algorithm for newborn resuscitation recommended by ILCOR and the International Consensus on Cardiopulmonary Resuscitation is shown in Figure 32-2. Many of its tenets follow below.

Basic Measures

The vigorous newborn is first placed in a warm environment to minimize heat loss, the airway is cleared, and the infant dried. Routine gastric aspiration has been shown to be nonbeneficial and even harmful (Kiremitci, 2011). And although previously recommended, there is no evidence that bulb suctioning for clear or meconium-stained fluid is beneficial, even if the newborn is depressed (Chap. 33, p. 638). With stimulation, the healthy newborn will take a breath within a few seconds of birth and cry within half a minute, after which routine supportive care is provided.

Assessment at 30 Seconds of Life. Apnea, gasping respirations, or heart rate < 100 bpm beyond 30 seconds after delivery should prompt administration of positive-pressure ventilation with *room air* (Fig. 32-3). Assisted ventilation rates of 30 to 60 breaths per minute are commonly employed, and the percent of oxygen saturation is monitored by pulse oximetry. At this point, supplemental oxygen can be given in graduated increasing percentages to maintain oxygen saturation (Spo_2) values within a normal range (Vento, 2011). Adequate ventilation is indicated by improved heart rate.

Assessment at 60 Seconds of Life. If the heart rate remains < 100 bpm, then ventilation is inadequate. The head position should be checked as shown in Figure 32-3, secretions cleared, and if necessary, inflation pressure increased. If the heart rate persists below 100 bpm beyond 60 seconds, tracheal intubation is considered. A number of conditions may be the cause of inadequate response, including the following:

- Hypoxemia or acidosis from any cause
- Drugs administered to the mother before delivery
- Immaturity
- Upper airway obstruction
- Pneumothorax
- Lung abnormalities
- Meconium aspiration
- Central nervous system developmental abnormality
- Sepsis syndrome.

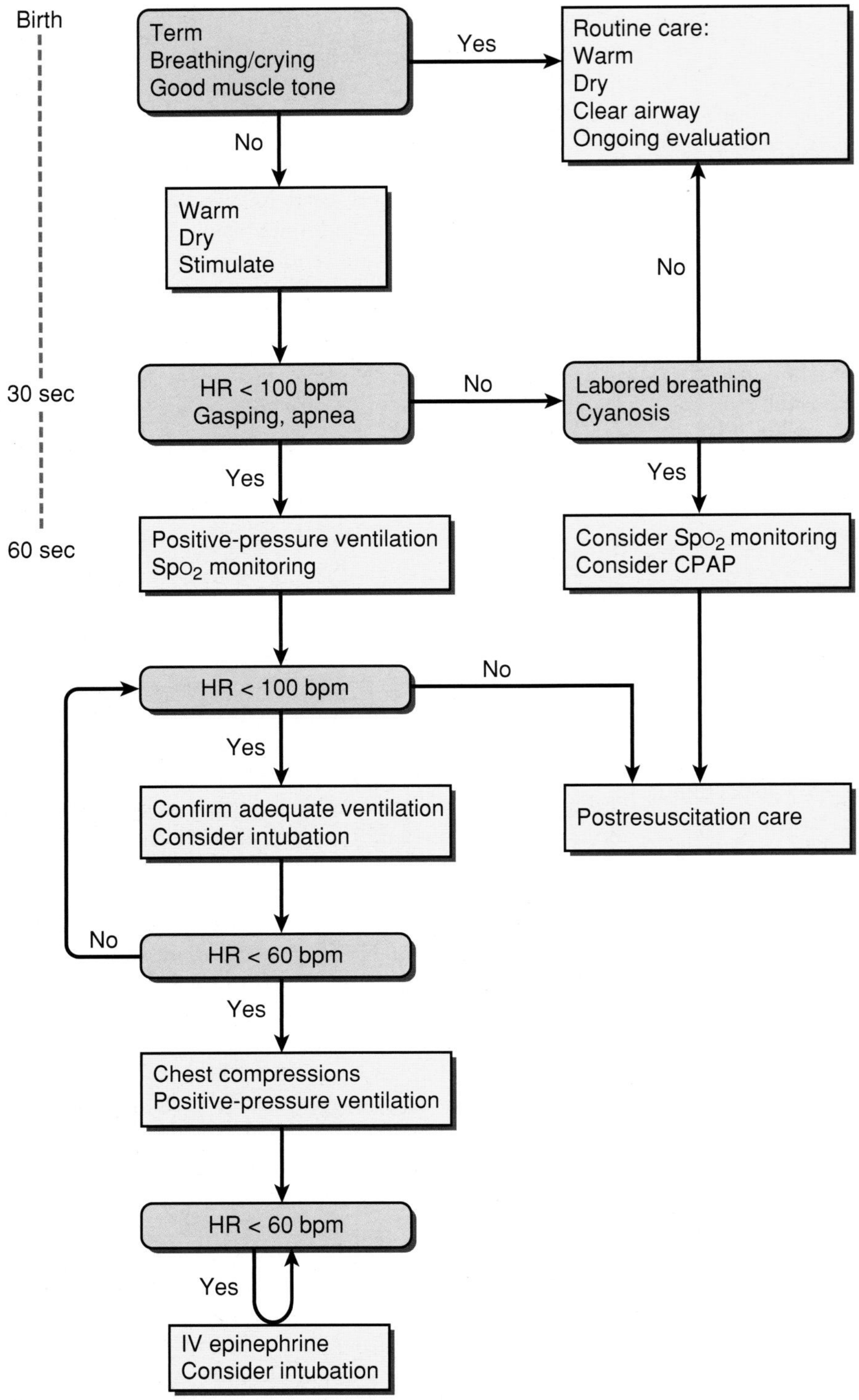

FIGURE 32-2 Algorithm for resuscitation of the newborn. CPAP = continuous positive airway pressure; HR = heart rate; IV = intravenous. (Adapted from Perlman, 2010.)

Tracheal Intubation

If bag-and-mask ventilation is ineffective or prolonged, tracheal intubation is then performed. Other indications include the need for chest compressions or tracheal administration of medications, or special circumstances such as extremely low birthweight or a congenital diaphragmatic hernia. A laryngoscope with a straight blade—size 0 for a preterm infant and size 1 for a term neonate—is introduced at the side of the mouth and then directed posteriorly toward the oropharynx as shown in Figure 32-4. The laryngoscope is next moved gently into the vallecula—the space between the base of the tongue and the epiglottis. Gentle elevation of the laryngoscope tip will raise the epiglottis and expose the glottis and the vocal cords. The tube is then introduced through the vocal cords. Gentle cricoid pressure may be useful. Tube sizes vary from 3.5 to 4.0 mm for term infants down to 2.5 mm for those < 28 weeks or < 1000 g.

Several steps are taken to ensure that the tube is positioned in the trachea and not the esophagus: observation for symmetrical chest wall motion; auscultation for equal breath sounds, especially in the axillae; and auscultation for the absence of breath sounds or gurgling over the stomach. Tracheal suctioning is no longer recommended or discouraged. Using an appropriate ventilation bag attached to the tracheal tube, puffs of air are delivered into the tube at 1- to 2-second intervals with a force adequate to gently lift the chest wall. In term infants, pressures of 30 to 40 cm H_2O typically will expand the alveoli without causing barotrauma. For preterm infants, pressures are 20 to 25 cm H_2O. An increase in heart rate and Spo_2 levels within acceptable ranges reflect a positive response.

Chest Compressions

If the heart rate remains < 60 bpm despite adequate ventilation for 30 seconds, chest compressions are initiated. These are delivered on the lower third of the sternum at a depth sufficient to generate a palpable pulse. A 3:1 compressions-to-ventilation ratio is recommended, with 90 compressions and 30 breaths to achieve approximately 120 events each minute. The heart rate is reassessed every 30 seconds, and chest compressions are continued until the spontaneous heart rate is at least 60 bpm.

Epinephrine and Volume Expansion

Intravenously administered epinephrine is indicated when the heart rate remains < 60 bpm after adequate ventilation and chest compressions. Epinephrine may be given through the endotracheal tube if venous access has not been established. The recommended intravenous dose is 0.01 to 0.03 mg/kg. If given through the tracheal tube, higher doses are employed—0.05 to 0.1 mg/kg.

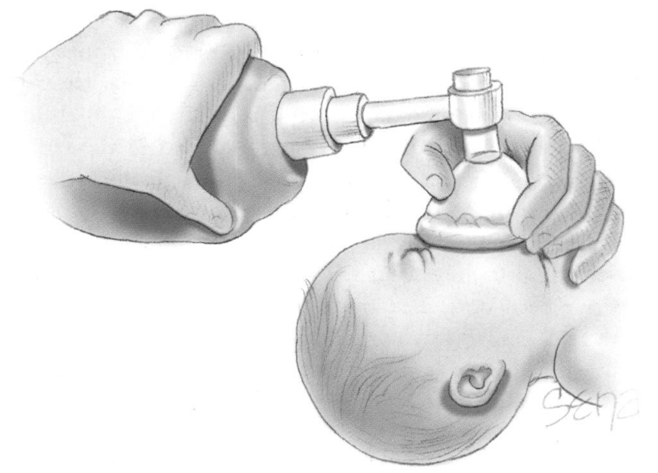

FIGURE 32-3 Correct use of bag-and-mask ventilation. The head should be in a sniffing position with the tip of the nose pointing to the ceiling. The neck should not be hyperextended.

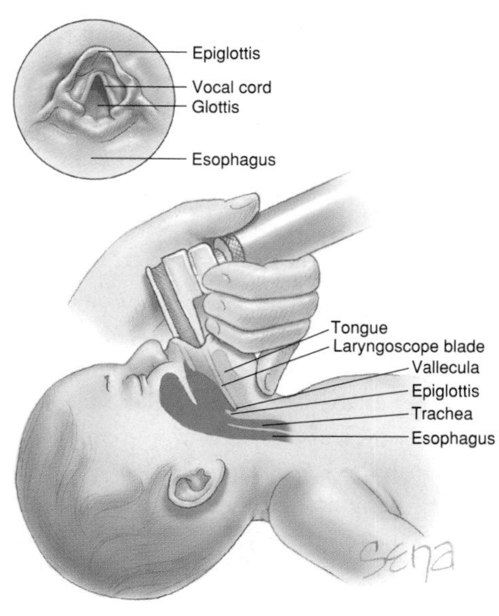

FIGURE 32-4 Sagittal view of laryngoscope positioning during intubation. The laryngoscope blade is inserted between the tongue base and epiglottis. Upward tilting of the tongue also lifts the epiglottis. The endotracheal tube is then threaded below the epiglottis and between the vocal cords (*inset*) to enter the trachea.

For infants with blood loss, early volume replacement with crystalloid or packed red cells is indicated if they do not respond to resuscitation.

Discontinuation of Resuscitation

As expected, newborns with cardiopulmonary arrest who do not respond promptly to resuscitation are at great risk for death, and if they survive, for severe morbidity (Haddad, 2000). The International Consensus Committee concluded that discontinuation of resuscitative efforts may be appropriate in a neonate without a heartbeat for 10 minutes of continuous and adequate resuscitative efforts (Perlman, 2010). This committee cites lack of data for more specific recommendations regarding the infant whose heart rate remains < 60 bpm.

EVALUATION OF NEWBORN CONDITION

Apgar Score

The scoring system described in 1953 by Dr. Virginia Apgar remains a useful clinical tool to identify those neonates who require resuscitation and to assess the effectiveness of any resuscitative measures. As shown in Table 32-1, each of the five easily identifiable characteristics—heart rate, respiratory effort, muscle tone, reflex irritability, and color—is assessed and assigned a value of 0 to 2. The total score, based on the sum of the five components, is determined in all neonates at 1 and 5 minutes after delivery. In depressed infants, the score may be calculated at further 5-minute intervals until a 20-minute Apgar score is assessed.

The 1-minute Apgar score reflects the need for immediate resuscitation. The 5-minute score, and particularly the change in score between 1 and 5 minutes, is a useful index of the effectiveness of resuscitative efforts. The 5-minute Apgar score also has prognostic significance for neonatal survival because survival is related closely to the condition of the neonate in the delivery room (Apgar, 1958). In an analysis of more than 150,000 infants delivered at Parkland Hospital, Casey and associates (2001b) assessed the significance of the 5-minute score for predicting survival during the first 28 days of life. They found that in term neonates, the risk of neonatal death was approximately 1 in 5000 for those with Apgar scores of 7 to 10. This risk compares with a mortality rate of 1 in 4 for term infants with 5-minute scores of 3 or less. Low 5-minute scores were comparably predictive of neonatal death in preterm infants. These investigators concluded that the Apgar scoring system

TABLE 32-1. Apgar Scoring System

Sign	0 Points	1 Point	2 Points
Heart rate	Absent	< 100 bpm	≥ 100 bpm
Respiratory effort	Absent	Slow, irregular	Good, crying
Muscle tone	Flaccid	Some extremity flexion	Active motion
Reflex irritability	No response	Grimace	Vigorous cry
Color	Blue, pale	Body pink, extremities blue	Completely pink

bpm = beats per minute.
Data from Apgar, 1953.

is as relevant for the prediction of neonatal survival today as it was more than 50 years ago.

There have been attempts to use Apgar scores to define asphyxial injury and to predict subsequent neurological outcome—uses for which the Apgar score was never intended. Such associations are difficult to measure with reliability given that both asphyxial injury and low Apgar scores are infrequent outcomes. For example, according to United States birth certificate records for 2010, only 1.8 percent of newborns had a 5-minute score below 7 (Martin, 2012). Similarly, in a population-based study of more than 1 million term infants born in Sweden between 1988 and 1997, the incidence of 5-minute Apgar scores of 3 or less was approximately 2 per 1000 (Thorngren-Jerneck, 2001).

Despite the methodological challenges, erroneous definitions of asphyxia by many groups were established based solely on low Apgar scores. These prompted the American College of Obstetricians and Gynecologists and the American Academy of Pediatrics (2010) to issue a series of joint opinions with important caveats regarding limitations of use of the Apgar score. One is that because certain elements of the Apgar score are partially dependent on the physiological maturity of the newborn, a healthy preterm infant may receive a low score only because of immaturity (Catlin, 1986). Apgar scores may be influenced by a variety of factors including, but not limited to, fetal malformations, maternal medications, and infection. Therefore, it is inappropriate to use an Apgar score alone to diagnose asphyxia. A 5-minute Apgar score of 3 correlates poorly with adverse future neurological outcomes, and thus scores are measured also at 10, 15, and 20 minutes when the score remains 3 or less (Freeman, 1988; Nelson, 1981).

Importantly, the Apgar score alone cannot establish hypoxia as the cause of cerebral palsy. As discussed in Chapter 33 (p. 638), a neonate who has had an asphyxial insult proximate to delivery that is severe enough to result in acute neurological injury will demonstrate most of the following: (1) profound acidemia with cord artery blood pH < 7 and acid-base deficit ≥ 12 mmol/L; (2) Apgar score of 0–3 persisting for 10 minutes or longer; (3) neurological manifestations such as seizures, coma, or hypotonia; and (4) multisystem organ dysfunction—cardiovascular, gastrointestinal, hematological, pulmonary, or renal (American College of Obstetricians and Gynecologists and the American Academy of Pediatrics, 2003).

Umbilical Cord Blood Acid–Base Studies

Blood taken from umbilical vessels may be used for acid-base studies to assess the metabolic status of the neonate. Blood collection is performed following delivery by immediately isolating a 10- to 20-cm segment of cord with two clamps placed near the neonate and another two clamps nearer the placenta. The importance of clamping the cord is underscored by the fact that delays of 20 to 30 seconds can alter both the PCO_2 and pH (Valero, 2012; White, 2012). The cord is then cut between the two proximal clamps and then the two distal clamps.

Arterial blood is drawn from the isolated cord segment into a 1- to 2-mL commercially prepared plastic syringe containing lyophilized heparin or a similar syringe that has been flushed with a heparin solution containing 1000 U/mL. Once sampling is completed, the needle is capped and the syringe transported, on ice, to the laboratory. Although efforts should be made for prompt transport, neither the pH nor PCO_2 values change significantly in blood kept at room temperature for up to 60 minutes (Duerbeck, 1992). Mathematical models have been developed that allow reasonable prediction of birth acid–base status in properly collected cord blood samples analyzed as late as 60 hours after delivery (Chauhan, 1994). Also, Swedish investigators reported significant variances in acid-base measurements with the use of different analyzers (Mokarami, 2012).

Fetal Acid-Base Physiology

The fetus produces both carbonic and organic acids. Carbonic acid (H_2CO_3) is formed by oxidative metabolism of CO_2. The fetus usually rapidly clears CO_2 through the placental circulation. If CO_2 clearance is lowered, then carbonic acid levels rise. When H_2CO_3 accumulates in fetal blood and there is no concurrent increase in organic acids, the result is termed respiratory acidemia. This often follows impaired placental exchange.

In contrast, organic acids primarily include lactic and β-hydroxybutyric acids. Levels of these increase with persistent placental exchange impairment and result from anaerobic glycolysis. These organic acids are cleared slowly from fetal blood, and when they accumulate without a concurrent increase in H_2CO_3, the result is termed metabolic acidemia. With the development of metabolic acidemia, bicarbonate (HCO_3^-) decreases because it is used to buffer the organic acid. An increase in H_2CO_3 accompanied by an increase in organic acid reflected by decreased HCO_3^- causes mixed respiratory-metabolic acidemia.

In the fetus, respiratory and metabolic acidemia and ultimately tissue acidosis are most likely part of a progressively worsening continuum. This is different from the adult pathophysiology, in which distinct conditions result in either respiratory acidosis—for example, pulmonary disease, or metabolic acidosis—for example, diabetes. In the fetus, the placenta serves as both the lungs and to a certain degree, the kidneys. One principal cause of fetal acidemia is a decrease in uteroplacental perfusion. This results in the retention of CO_2, that is, respiratory acidemia, and if protracted and severe enough, a mixed or metabolic acidemia.

Assuming that maternal pH and blood gases are normal, the actual pH of fetal blood is dependent on the proportion of carbonic and organic acids and the amount of bicarbonate, which is the major buffer in blood. This can best be illustrated by the Henderson–Hasselbalch equation:

$$pH = pK + \log \frac{[base]}{[acid]} \text{ or, } pH = pK + \log \frac{HCO_3^-}{H_2CO_3}$$

For clinical purposes, HCO_3^- represents the metabolic component and is reported in mEq/L. The H_2CO_3 concentration represents the respiratory component and is reported as the Pco_2 in mm Hg. Thus:

$$pH = pK + \log \frac{\text{metabolic } (HCO_3^- \text{ mEq/L})}{\text{respiratory } (Pco_2 \text{ mm Hg})}$$

The result of this equation is a pH value. Because pH is a logarithmic term, it does not give a linear measure of acid accumulation. For example, a change in hydrogen ion concentration associated with a fall in pH from 7.0 to 6.9 is almost twice that which is associated with a fall in pH from 7.3 to 7.2. For this reason, the change in base, termed delta base, offers a more linear measure of the degree of accumulation of metabolic acid (Armstrong, 2007). The delta base is a calculated number used as a measure of the change in buffering capacity of bicarbonate (HCO_3^-). The formula for calculating the base excess (BE) is as follows:

$$BE = 0.02786 \times Pco_2 \times 10^{(pH - 6.1)} \times 13.77 \times pH - 124.58$$

Shown in Figure 32-5 is a nomogram developed from which these can be calculated if only two parameters are known. For example, HCO_3^- concentration will be decreased with a metabolic acidemia as it is consumed to maintain a normal pH. A base deficit occurs when HCO_3^- concentration decreases to below normal levels, and a base excess occurs when HCO_3^- values are above normal. Importantly, a mixed respiratory–metabolic acidemia with a large base deficit and a low HCO_3^-, for example 12 mmol/L, is more often associated with a depressed neonate than is a mixed acidemia with a minimal base deficit and a more nearly normal HCO_3^- level.

Clinical Significance of Acidemia

Fetal oxygenation and pH generally decline during the course of normal labor. Normal umbilical cord blood pH and blood gas values at delivery in term newborns are summarized in Table 32-2. Similar values have been reported for preterm infants (Dickinson, 1992; Ramin, 1989; Riley, 1993). The lower limits of normal pH in the newborn have been found to range from 7.04 to 7.10 (Boylan, 1994). Thus, these values should be considered to define neonatal acidemia. Even so, most fetuses will tolerate intrapartum acidemia with a pH as low as 7.00 without incurring neurological impairment (Freeman, 1988; Gilstrap, 1989). However, in a study of newborns with a pH < 7.0 from Parkland Hospital, there were inordinate proportions of neonatal deaths—8 percent, intensive-care admission—39 percent, intubations—14 percent, and seizures—13 percent (Goldaber, 1991). And in a study from Oxford of more than 51,000 term infants, the incidence of neonatal encephalopathy with the pH < 7.0 was 3 percent (Yeh, 2012).

Another important prognostic consideration is the direction of pH change from birth to the immediate neonatal period. For example, the risk of seizures during the first 24 hours of life was reduced fivefold if an umbilical artery cord pH below 7.2 normalized within 2 hours after delivery (Casey, 2001a).

Respiratory Acidemia

Acute interruption in placental gas exchange is accompanied by subsequent CO_2 retention and respiratory acidemia. The most common antecedent factor is transient umbilical cord compression. Generally, respiratory acidemia is not harmful to the fetus (Low, 1994).

The degree to which pH is affected by Pco_2—the respiratory component of the acidosis—can be calculated. First, the upper normal neonatal Pco_2 of 49 mm Hg is subtracted from the cord blood gas Pco_2 value.

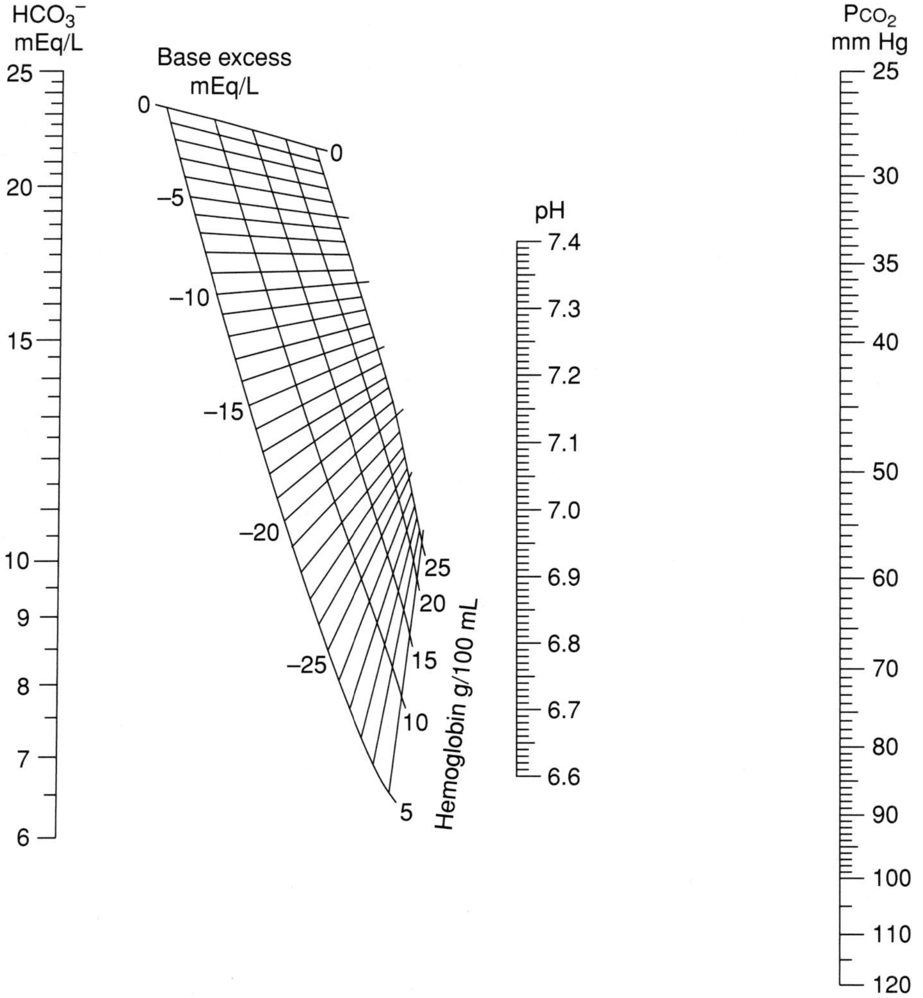

FIGURE 32-5 Nomogram for determining the delta base. (Adapted from Siggaard-Andersen, 1963).

SECTION 9

TABLE 32-2. Umbilical Cord Blood pH and Blood Gas Values in Normal Term Newborns

Values	Ramin, 1989[a] Spontaneous Delivery n = 1292[c]	Riley, 1993[b] Spontaneous Delivery n = 3522[c]	Kotaska, 2010[b] Spontaneous Delivery n = 303[d]	Kotaska, 2010[e] Cesarean Delivery n = 189[d]
Arterial Blood				
pH	7.28 (0.07)	7.27 (0.069)	7.26 (7.01–7.39)	7.3 (7.05–7.39)
P_{CO_2} (mm Hg)	49.9 (14.2)	50.3 (11.1)	51 (30.9–85.8)	54 (37.5–79.5)
HCO_3^- (mEq/L)	23.1 (2.8)	22.0 (3.6)	—	—
Base excess (mEq/L)	−3.6 (2.8)	−2.7 (2.8)	—	—
Venous Blood				
pH	—	7.34 (0.063)	7.31 (7.06–7.44)	7.34 (7.10–7.42)
P_{CO_2} (mm Hg)	—	40.7 (7.9)	41 (24.9–70.9)	44 (29.1–70.2)
HCO_3^- (mEq/L)	—	21.4 (2.5)	—	—
Base excess (mEq/L)	—	−2.4 (2)	—	—

[a]Infants of selected women with uncomplicated vaginal deliveries.
[b]Infants of unselected women with vaginal deliveries.
[c]Data shown as mean (SD).
[d]Data shown as range with 2.5 or 97.5 percentile.
[e]Cesarean delivery—labor not stated.

Each additional 10 mm Hg P_{CO_2} increment will lower the pH by 0.08 units (Eisenberg, 1987). Thus, in a mixed respiratory–metabolic acidemia, the benign respiratory component can be calculated. As an example, acute cord prolapse during labor prompts cesarean delivery of an infant 20 minutes later. The umbilical artery blood gas pH was 6.95 and the P_{CO_2} was 89 mm Hg. To calculate the degree to which the cord compression and subsequent impairment of CO_2 exchange affected the pH, the relationship given earlier is applied: 89 mm Hg minus 49 mm Hg = 40 mm Hg excess CO_2. To correct pH: $(40 \div 10) \times 0.08 = 0.32$; $6.95 + 0.32 = 7.27$. Therefore, the pH before cord prolapse was approximately 7.27, well within normal limits, and thus the low pH resulted from respiratory acidosis.

Metabolic Acidemia

The fetus begins to develop metabolic acidemia when oxygen deprivation is of sufficient duration and magnitude to require anaerobic metabolism for cellular energy needs. Low and associates (1997) defined fetal acidosis as a base deficit ≥ 12 mmol/L and severe fetal acidosis as a base deficit ≥ 16 mmol/L. In the Parkland study of more than 150,000 newborns cited earlier, metabolic acidemia was defined using umbilical cord blood gas cutoffs that were 2 standard deviations below the mean (Casey, 2001b). Thus, metabolic acidemia was an umbilical artery blood pH < 7.00 accompanied by a P_{CO_2} of ≤ 76.3 mm Hg, with higher values indicating a respiratory component; HCO_3^- concentration ≤ 17.7 mmol/L; and base deficit ≥ 10.3 mEq/L. From the standpoint of *possible* cerebral palsy causation, the American College of Obstetricians and Gynecologists and the American Academy of Pediatrics (2003), in their widely endorsed monograph, defined metabolic acidosis as umbilical arterial pH < 7.0 and a base deficit ≥ 12 mmol/L.

Metabolic acidemia is associated with a high rate of multiorgan dysfunction. In rare cases, such hypoxia-induced metabolic acidemia may be so severe that it causes subsequent neurological impairment—*hypoxic-ischemic encephalopathy* (Chap. 33, p. 639). In fact, a fetus without such acidemia cannot by definition have suffered recent hypoxic-induced injury. That said, severe metabolic acidosis is poorly predictive of subsequent neurological impairment in the term neonate. Although metabolic acidosis was associated with an increase in immediate neonatal complications in a group of infants with depressed 5-minute Apgar scores, there were no differences in umbilical artery blood gas measurements among infants who subsequently developed cerebral palsy compared with those with normal neurological outcomes (Socol, 1994).

In very-low-birthweight infants, that is, those < 1000 g, newborn acid-base status may be more closely linked to long-term neurological outcome (Gaudier, 1994; Low, 1995). In the study cited above, Casey and coworkers (2001b) described the association between metabolic acidemia, low Apgar scores, and neonatal death in term and preterm infants. Regarding term neonates, as shown in Figure 32-6, relative to newborns with a 5-minute Apgar score of at least 7, the risk of neonatal death was more than 3200-fold greater in term infants with metabolic acidemia and 5-minute scores of 3 or less.

Recommendations for Cord Blood Gas Determinations

A cost-effectiveness analysis for universal cord blood gas measurements has not been conducted. In some centers, such as ours at Parkland Hospital, cord gas analysis is performed in all neonates at birth. The American College of Obstetricians and

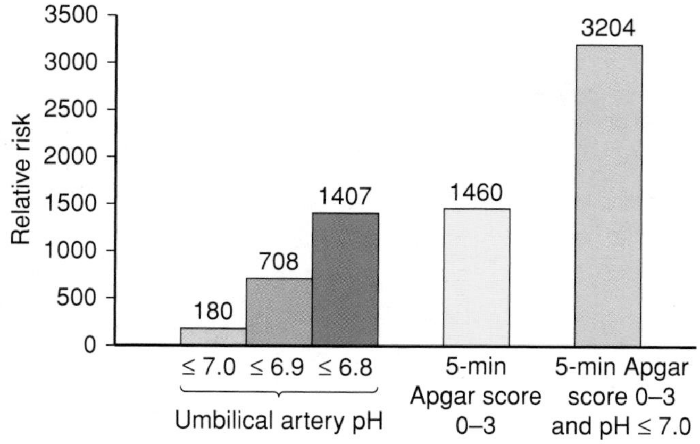

FIGURE 32-6 Relative risk for neonatal death in term infants with low Apgar score or umbilical artery acidemia—or both. The relative risk is cited above each bar. (Data from Casey, 2001b.)

Gynecologists (2012) recommends that cord blood gas and pH analyses be obtained in the following circumstances:

- Cesarean delivery for fetal compromise
- Low 5-minute Apgar score
- Severe fetal-growth restriction
- Abnormal fetal heart rate tracing
- Maternal thyroid disease
- Intrapartum fever
- Multifetal gestation.

Although umbilical cord acid-base blood determinations are poorly predictive of either immediate or long-term adverse neurological outcome, they provide the most objective evidence of the fetal metabolic status at birth.

PREVENTIVE CARE

Eye Infection Prophylaxis

Gonococcal Infection

Ophthalmia neonatorum is mucopurulent conjunctivitis of newborns. Some form of conjunctivitis affects 1 to 12 percent of all neonates, and gonococcal and chlamydial infections are some of the most common causes (Zuppa, 2011). Blindness was previously common in children who developed *Neisseria gonorrhoeae* infection. However, in 1884, Credé, a German obstetrician, introduced a 1-percent ophthalmic solution of silver nitrate that largely eliminated this. Various other antimicrobial agents have also proven to be effective, and gonococcal prophylaxis is now mandatory for all neonates (American Academy of Pediatrics and American College of Obstetricians and Gynecologists, 2012). Recommendations for gonococcal eye prophylaxis include a single application of either 1-percent silver nitrate solution or 0.5-percent erythromycin or 1-percent tetracycline ophthalmic ointment soon after delivery. Treatment of presumptive gonococcal ophthalmia, that is, conjunctivitis in a neonate born to a mother with untreated gonorrhea, is given with single-dose ceftriaxone, 100 mg/kg, either intramuscularly or intravenously. Testing for both gonococcus and chlamydia should be obtained before treatment.

Chlamydial Infection

Adequate neonatal prophylaxis against chlamydial conjunctivitis is complex. Ideally, prenatal screening and treatment for *Chlamydia trachomatis* obviates conjunctival infection (Hammerschlag, 2011). Of neonates delivered vaginally of mothers with an active chlamydial infection, from 12 to 25 percent will develop conjunctivitis for up to 20 weeks (Teoh, 2003). Prophylactic topical eye treatments do not reliably reduce the incidence of chlamydial conjunctivitis. In a study from Kenya, 2.5-percent povidone-iodine solution was reported to be superior to either 1-percent silver nitrate solution or 0.5-percent erythromycin ointment in preventing chlamydial conjunctivitis (Isenberg, 1995). In another study from Iran, povidone-iodine eye drops were twice as effective in preventing clinical conjunctivitis as erythromycin drops—9 versus 18 percent failure rate, respectively (Ali, 2007). In an Israeli study, tetracycline ointment was marginally superior to povidone-iodine (David, 2011). For all of these reasons, conjunctivitis in a newborn up to 3 months old should prompt consideration for chlamydial infection. Treatment for chlamydial infection is with oral azithromycin for 5 days or erythromycin for 14 days.

Hepatitis B Immunization

Routine immunization of all newborns with thimerosal-free vaccine against hepatitis B before hospital discharge is standard practice (American Academy of Pediatrics and American College of Obstetricians and Gynecologists, 2012). This vaccine does not appear to increase the number of febrile episodes, sepsis evaluations, or adverse neurological sequelae (Lewis, 2001). Some advocate treatment of high-risk or even all seropositive women with antiviral nucleoside or nucleotide analogues during pregnancy to minimize transmission to the fetus (Dusheiko, 2012; Tran, 2012). Certainly, if the mother is seropositive for hepatitis B surface antigen, then the neonate should also be passively immunized with hepatitis B immune globulin as discussed in Chapter 55 (p. 1090).

Vitamin K

This injection is provided to prevent vitamin K-dependent hemorrhagic disease of the newborn, which is discussed in Chapter 33 (p. 644). A single dose of 0.5- to 1-mg intramuscular vitamin K is given within 1 hour of birth (American Academy of Pediatrics and American College of Obstetricians and Gynecologists, 2012).

Newborn Screening

State-based public-health newborn screening programs were solidified when, in response to calls for a uniform national policy, the Maternal and Child Health Bureau appointed a committee of the American College of Medical Genetics to recommend a panel of tests (Watson, 2006). Technical advances have made a large number of relatively simply performed mass

SECTION 9

TABLE 32-3. Newborn Screening Core Panel—Estimated Number of Children Shown in Parentheses Identified in the United States in 2006

Acylcarnitine Disorders[a]				
Organic Acid Metabolism	**Fatty Acid Metabolism**	**Amino Acid Metabolism[a]**	**Hemoglobin Disorders**	**Others**
Isovaleric (32)	Medium-chain acyl-CoA dehydrogenase (239)	Phenylketonuria (215)	SS disease (1128)	Congenital hypothyroidism (2156)
Glutaric type I (38)	Very long-chain acyl-CoA dehydrogenase (69)	Maple syrup (urine) (26)	S-β-thalassemia (163)	Biotinidase (62)
3-Hydroxy-3-methyl glutaric (3)	Long-chain 3-OH acyl-CoA dehydrogenase (13)	Homocystinuria (11)	SC disease (484)	Congenital adrenal hyperplasia (202)
Multiple carboxylase (3)	Trifunctional protein (2)	Citrullinemia (24)		Galactosemia (224)
Methylmalonic mutase (50)	Carnitine uptake (85)	Arginosuccinic (7)		Hearing loss (5073)
3-Methylcrotonyl-CoA carboxylase (100)		Tyrosinemia I		Cystic fibrosis (1248)
Methylmalonic acid (cobalamine A, B) (12)				Critical congenital heart disease[b]
Propionic (15)				Severe combined immunodeficiency[b]
β-Ketothiolase (7)				

[a]Determined by tandem mass spectrometry.
[b]Added after 2006.
From Centers for Disease Control and Prevention, 2012b; Watson, 2006.

screening tests available for newborn conditions, and many are mandated by various state laws (American College of Obstetricians and Gynecologists, 2011b). Since then, two have been added to the original core panel of 29 congenital conditions, and all are shown in Table 32-3.

According to the Centers for Disease Control and Prevention (2012b), the programs have been successful and cost effective. For example, neonatal screening for hearing loss was shown in a Dutch study to diagnose problems a mean of 6 months earlier and improve long-term outcomes (Durieux-Smith, 2008). A successful screening program for medium chain acyl-CoA dehydrogenase deficiency was described in a Danish study (Anderson, 2012). The use of pulse oximetry to screen for severe congenital heart disease was reviewed by Thangaratinam (2012).

Most states require that all tests in the core panel be performed. Supplemental conditions—*secondary targets*—are also listed on the Maternal and Child Health Bureau website. Some states require some of these 24 in addition to their mandated core panel. Each practitioner should be familiar with their individual state requirements, which are available at http://genes-r-us.uthscsa.edu/resources/consumer/statemap.htm and http://www.hrsa.gov/advisorycommittee/mchbadvisory/heritabledisorders/recommendedpanel/index/html.

ROUTINE NEWBORN CARE

Gestational Age Estimation

Newborn gestational age can be estimated very soon after delivery. The relationship between gestational age and birthweight should be used to identify neonates at risk for complications (McIntire, 1999). For example, neonates who are either small or large for gestational age are at increased risk for hypoglycemia and polycythemia, and measurements of blood glucose and hematocrit are indicated (American Academy of Pediatrics and American College of Obstetricians and Gynecologists, 2012).

Care of Skin and Umbilical Cord

All excess vernix, blood, and meconium should be gently wiped off at the time of delivery while keeping the infant warm. Any remaining vernix is readily absorbed and disappears within 24 hours. The first bath should be postponed until the neonate's temperature has stabilized.

Aseptic precautions should be observed in the immediate care of the cord. The American Academy of Pediatrics and the American College of Obstetrics and Gynecologists (2012) have concluded that keeping the cord dry is sufficient care. The umbilical cord begins to lose water from Wharton jelly shortly after birth. Within 24 hours, the cord stump loses its characteristic bluish-white, moist appearance and soon becomes dry and black. Within several days to weeks, the stump sloughs and leaves a small, granulating wound, which after healing forms the umbilicus. Separation usually takes place within the first 2 weeks, with a range of 3 to 45 days (Novack, 1988). The umbilical cord dries more quickly and separates more readily when exposed to air. Thus, a dressing is not recommended.

In resource-poor countries, prophylaxis is reasonable. Triple-dye applied to the cord was reported superior to soap and water care in preventing colonization and exudate formation

(Janssen, 2003). In a Nepalese study, cleansing the cord stump with 4-percent chlorhexidine reduced severe omphalitis by 75 percent compared with soap and water cleansing (Mullany, 2006). Likewise, 0.1-percent chlorhexidine powder was superior to dry cord care (Kapellen, 2009).

Despite precautions, a serious umbilical infection—omphalitis—is sometimes encountered. In a German study of more than 750 newborns with aseptic cord care, 1.3 percent developed omphalitis (Kapellen, 2009). The most likely offending organisms are *Staphylococcus aureus, Escherichia coli,* and group B streptococcus. Typical signs of cellulitis and stump discharge usually aid diagnosis. However, mild erythema and some bleeding at the stump site with cord detachment is common, and some cases may present no outward signs. Thus, the diagnosis can be elusive.

Feeding and Weight Loss

According to the American College of Obstetricians and Gynecologists (2013a), exclusive breast feeding is preferred until 6 months. In many hospitals, infants begin breast feeding in the delivery room. Most term newborns thrive best when fed 8 to 12 times daily for approximately 15 minutes per episode. Preterm or growth-restricted newborns require feedings at shorter intervals.

One goal of *Healthy People 2020* of the United States Department of Health and Human Services (2010) is to increase the proportion of mothers who breast feed their infants. Substantial progress toward this goal has been made. In 2009, 77 percent of infants were initially breast fed, and 47 percent were still breast fed at 6 months and 26 percent at 1 year (Centers for Disease Control and Prevention, 2012a). Breast feeding is discussed further in Chapter 36 (p. 673). Because most neonates actually receive little nutriment for the first 3 or 4 days of life, they progressively lose weight until the flow of maternal milk has been established or other feeding is instituted. Preterm infants lose relatively more weight and regain their birthweight more slowly. Conversely, growth-restricted but otherwise healthy infants regain their initial weight more quickly than those born preterm. With proper nourishment, birthweight of term infants usually is regained by the end of the 10th day.

Stools and Urine

For the first 2 or 3 days after birth, the colon contains soft, brownish-green meconium. This consists of desquamated epithelial cells from the intestinal tract, mucus, epidermal cells, and lanugo (fetal hair) that have been swallowed along with amnionic fluid. The characteristic color results from bile pigments. During fetal life and for a few hours after birth, the intestinal contents are sterile, but bacteria quickly colonize the bowel.

Meconium stooling is seen in 90 percent of newborns within the first 24 hours, and most of the rest within 36 hours. Usually, newborns first void shortly after birth, but may not until the second day. Meconium and urine passage indicates patency of the gastrointestinal and urinary tracts, respectively. Failure of the newborn to stool or urinate after these times suggests a congenital defect, such as imperforate anus or a urethral valve. After the third or fourth day, as a result of milk ingestion, meconium is replaced by light-yellow homogenous feces with a consistency similar to peanut butter.

Icterus Neonatorum

Between the second and fifth day of life approximately one third of all neonates develop so-called physiological jaundice of the newborn. It has special significance considering most hospitals have policies for early discharge. Correspondingly, it has been the subject of several recent reviews and is discussed further in Chapter 33 (p. 644) (Dijk, 2012; Gazzin, 2011; Hansen, 2011; Lauer, 2011).

Newborn Male Circumcision

Neonatal circumcision has been a controversial topic in the United States for at least 25 years. For centuries, newborn male circumcision has been performed as a religious ritual. Even so, scientific evidence supports several medical benefits that include prevention of phimosis, paraphimosis, and balanoposthitis. Circumcision also decreases the incidence of penile cancer and of cervical cancer among their sexual partners. In 1999, the American Academy of Pediatrics concluded that existing evidence was insufficient to recommend *routine* neonatal circumcision. It seems that this policy has had only a negligible effect on practices in this country. Specifically, the Centers for Disease Control and Prevention (2011) estimated that the newborn male circumcision rate decreased during a 12-year period from approximately 60 percent in 2009 to only 55 percent in 2010.

Subsequent studies have again endorsed health benefits of circumcision. In two large randomized trials from regions of Africa with a high prevalence of human immunodeficiency virus (HIV), adult male circumcision was found to lower the risk of HIV acquisition by half (Bailey, 2007; Gray, 2007). And adult male circumcision was reported to decrease incidences of HIV, HPV, and herpes infections (Tobian, 2009). These and other studies were considered by the American Academy of Pediatrics Task Force on Circumcision (2012). In its policy statement, the Task Force concluded that health benefits of newborn male circumcision outweigh the risks, and thus, access to the procedure is justified for families who choose it. Benefits cited include prevention of urinary infections, penile cancer, and transmission of some sexually transmitted infections, including HIV infection. The Task Force stopped short of recommending circumcision for *all* newborns. The American College of Obstetricians and Gynecologists (2011a) endorses these views.

Anesthesia for Circumcision

The American Academy of Pediatrics Task Force (2012) recommends that if circumcision is performed, procedural analgesia should be provided. Various pain relief techniques have been described, including lidocaine-prilocaine topical cream, local analgesia infiltration, dorsal penile nerve block, or ring block. Several studies attest to the efficacy of the dorsal penile nerve block (Arnett, 1990; Stang, 1988). Studies show that the dorsal penile nerve block or the ring block techniques are both superior to topical analgesia (Hardwick-Smith, 1998; Lander, 1997; Taddio, 1997). The use of a pacifier dipped in sucrose is a useful adjunct to these methods (Kaufman, 2002).

After appropriate penile cleansing, the ring block technique consists of placing a wheal of 1-percent lidocaine at the base of the penis and advancing the needle in a 180-degree arc around the base of the penis first to one side and then the other to achieve a circumferential ring of analgesia. The maximum dose of lidocaine is 1.0 mL. *No vasoactive compounds such as epinephrine should ever be added to the local analgesic agent.*

Surgical Technique

Newborn circumcision should be performed only on a healthy neonate. Other contraindications include any genital abnormalities such as hypospadias and a family history of a bleeding disorder unless excluded in the infant. The most commonly used instruments are shown in Figure 32-7 and include Gomco and Mogen clamps and the Plastibell device. Compared with the Gomco procedure, Kaufman and colleagues (2002) reported that the Mogen technique required less time to perform and was associated with less apparent discomfort for the newborn. Regardless of the method used, the goal is to remove enough shaft skin and inner preputial epithelium so that the glans is exposed sufficiently to prevent phimosis. In all techniques: (1) the amount of external skin to be removed must be accurately estimated, (2) the preputial orifice must be dilated to visualize the glans and ensure that it is normal, (3) the inner preputial epithelium must be freed from the glans epithelium, and (4) the circumcision device must be left in place long enough to produce hemostasis before amputating the prepuce (Lerman, 2001). For a detailed description of surgical techniques, see the second edition of *Operative Obstetrics* (Mastrobattista, 2002).

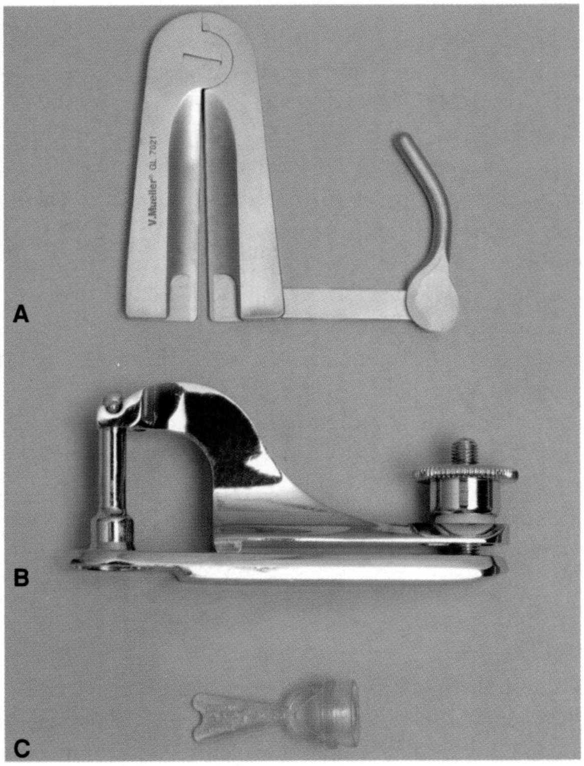

FIGURE 32-7 Three different tools used for circumcision. **A.** Mogen clamp. The arms of the clamp open to a 3-mm maximum width. **B.** Gomco clamp, assembled. **C.** Plastibell device.

Circumcision Complications

As with any surgical procedure, there is a risk of bleeding, infection, and hematoma formation. These risks, however, are low (Christakis, 2000). Unusual complications reported as isolated cases include distal glans amputation, acquisition of human immunodeficiency virus-1 (HIV-1) infection or other sexually transmitted diseases, meatal stenosis, penile denudation, penile destruction with electrosurgical coagulation, subsequent epidermal inclusion cyst and urethrocutaneous fistula, and ischemia following the inappropriate use of lidocaine with epinephrine (Amukele, 2003; Berens, 1990; Gearhart, 1989; Neulander, 1996; Nicoll, 1997; Pippi-Salle, 2013; Upadhyay, 1998).

Rooming-In

This model of maternity care place newborns in their mothers' rooms instead of central nurseries. Termed rooming-in, this approach first appeared in United States hospitals in the early 1940s (Temkin, 2002). In part, rooming-in stems from a trend to make all phases of childbearing as natural as possible and to foster early mother-child relationships. By 24 hours, the mother is generally fully ambulatory. Thereafter, with rooming-in, she can usually provide routine care for herself and her newborn. An obvious advantage is her increased ability to assume full care of the infant when she arrives home.

Hospital Discharge

Traditionally, the newborn is discharged with its mother, and in most cases, maternal stay has determined that of the neonate. Safe discharge for late preterm infants has special concerns (Whyte, 2012). From 1970 to the mid-1990s, average maternal postpartum length of stay declined steadily, and many mothers were discharged in under 48 hours. Although it is clear that most newborns can be safely discharged within 48 hours, this is not uniformly true. For example, using data from the Canadian Institute for Health Information, Liu and colleagues (2000) examined readmission rates in more than 2.1 million neonatal discharges. As the length of hospital stay decreased from 4.2 days in 1990 to 2.7 days in 1997, the readmission rate increased from 27 to 38 per 1000 births. Dehydration and jaundice accounted for most of these readmissions, and brain damage from icterus neonatorum is discussed in Chapter 33 (p. 644). Using Washington state neonatal discharge data, Malkin and coworkers (2000) found that the 28-day mortality rate was increased fourfold and the 1-year mortality rate increased twofold in newborns discharged within 30 hours of birth.

Because of the increased scrutiny regarding short hospital stays, federal legislation—*The Newborns' and Mothers' Health Protection Act of 1996*—was enacted to prohibit insurers from restricting hospital stays for mothers and newborns to less than 2 days for vaginal delivery or 4 days for cesarean delivery. As a result, the average length of hospital stay for childbirth increased from 2.1 days in 1995 to 2.5 days in 2000. This increase reflected the reduced number of very short hospital stays following childbirth (Hall, 2002). Although Mosen and associates (2002) found that implementation of the new legislation was associated with a 6-percent increase in cost, readmission rates within 7 days of discharge decreased by nearly half. In an analysis of more than 662,000 births in California, Datar and Sood (2006) found decreased rates of readmission of 9, 12, and 20 percent, respectively, at 1, 2, and 3 years after the legislation was implemented.

REFERENCES

Ali A, Khadije D, Elahe A, et al: Prophylaxis of ophthalmia neonatorum comparison of Betadine, erythromycin and no prophylaxis. J Trop Pediatr 53(6):388, 2007

American Academy of Pediatrics and the American College of Obstetricians and Gynecologists: Care of the newborn. In: Guidelines for Perinatal Care, 7th ed. Washington, 2012, p 265

American Academy of Pediatrics, Task Force on Circumcision: Circumcision Policy Statement. Pediatrics 103:686, 1999

American Academy of Pediatrics, Task Force on Circumcision: Circumcision Policy Statement. Pediatrics 130(3):585, 2012

American College of Obstetricians and Gynecologists: Breastfeeding: maternal and infant aspects. Committee Opinion No. 361, Reaffirmed 2013a

American College of Obstetricians and Gynecologists: Circumcision. Committee Opinion No. 260, October 2001, Reaffirmed 2011a

American College of Obstetricians and Gynecologists: Newborn screening. Committee Opinion No. 481, March 2011b

American College of Obstetricians and Gynecologists: Planned home birth. Committee Opinion No. 476, February 2011, Reaffirmed 2013b

American College of Obstetricians and Gynecologists: Umbilical cord blood gas and acid–base analysis. Committee Opinion No. 348, November 2006, Reaffirmed 2012

American College of Obstetricians and Gynecologists and the American Academy of Pediatrics: Neonatal encephalopathy and cerebral palsy: defining the pathogenesis and pathophysiology. January 2003

American College of Obstetricians and Gynecologists and the American Academy of Pediatrics: The Apgar score. Committee Opinion No. 333, May 2006, Reaffirmed 2010

Amukele SA, Lee GW, Stock JA, et al: 20-year experience with iatrogenic penile injury. J Urol 170:1691, 2003

Anderson S, Botti C, Li B, et al: Medium chain acyl-CoA dehydrogenase deficiency detected among Hispanics by New Jersey newborn screening. Am J Med Genet A 158A(9):2100, 2012

Apgar V: A proposal for a new method of evaluation of the newborn infant. Curr Res Anesth Analg 32:260, 1953

Apgar V, Holaday DA, James LS, et al: Evaluation of the newborn infant—second report. JAMA 168:1985, 1958

Armstrong L, Stenson BJ: Use of umbilical cord blood gas analysis in the assessment of the newborn. Arch Dis Child Fetal Neonatal Ed 92:430, 2007

Arnett RM, Jones JS, Horger EO III: Effectiveness of 1% lidocaine dorsal penile nerve block in infant circumcision. Am J Obstet Gynecol 163:1074, 1990

Bailey RC, Moses S, Parker CB, et al: Male circumcision for HIV prevention in young men in Kismu, Kenya: a randomized controlled trial. Lancet 369:643, 2007

Berens R, Pontus SP Jr: A complication associated with dorsal penile nerve block. Reg Anesth 15:309, 1990

Biban P, Filipovic-Grcic B, Biarent D, et al: New cardiopulmonary resuscitation guidelines 2010: managing the newly born in delivery room. Early Hum Dev 87 Suppl 1:S9, 2011

Boylan PC, Parisi VM: Fetal acid–base balance. In Creasy RK, Resnik R (eds): Maternal–Fetal Medicine, 3rd ed. Philadelphia, Saunders, 1994

Casey BM, Goldaber KG, McIntire DD, et al: Outcomes among term infants when two-hour postnatal pH is compared with pH at delivery. Am J Obstet Gynecol 184:447, 2001a

Casey BM, McIntire DD, Leveno KJ: The continuing value of the Apgar score for the assessment of newborn infants. N Engl J Med 344:467, 2001b

Catlin EA, Carpenter MW, Brann BS, et al: The Apgar score revisited: influence of gestational age. J Pediatr 109:865, 1986

Centers for Disease Control and Prevention: Breastfeeding report card—United States, 2012. Available at: http://www.cdc.gov/breastfeeding/data/reportcard2.htm. Accessed October 10, 2012a

Centers for Disease Control and Prevention: CDC grand rounds: newborn screening and improved outcomes. MMWR 61(21)390, 2012b

Centers for Disease Control and Prevention: Trends in in-hospital newborn male circumcision—United States, 1999—2010. MMWR 60(34):1167, 2011

Chauhan SP, Cowan BD, Meydrech EF, et al: Determination of fetal acidemia at birth from a remote umbilical arterial blood gas analysis. Am J Obstet Gynecol 170:1705, 1994

Chernick V: Fetal breathing movements and the onset of breathing at birth. Clin Perinatol 5:257, 1978

Christakis DA, Harvey E, Zerr DM, et al: A trade-off analysis of routine newborn circumcision. Pediatrics 105:246, 2000

Credé CSF: Die Verhütung der Augenenzündung der Neugeborenen. Berlin, Hirschwald, 1884

Datar A, Sood N: Impact of postpartum hospital-stay legislation on newborn length of stay, readmission, and mortality in California. Pediatrics 118:63, 2006

David M, Rumelt S, Weintraub Z: Efficacy comparison between povidone iodine 2.5% and tetracycline 1% in prevention of ophthalmia neonatorum. Ophthalmology 118(7):1454, 2011

Dawes GS: Breathing before birth in animals or man. N Engl J Med 290:557, 1974

Dickinson JE, Eriksen NL, Meyer BA, et al: The effect of preterm birth on umbilical cord blood gases. Obstet Gynecol 79:575, 1992

Dijk PH, Hulzebos CV: An evidence-based view on hyperbilirubinemia. Acta Paediatr Suppl 101(464):3, 2012

Duerbeck NB, Chaffin DG, Seeds JW: A practical approach to umbilical artery pH and blood gas determinations. Obstet Gynecol 79:959, 1992

Durieux-Smith A, Fitzpatrick E, Whittingham J: Universal newborn hearing screening: a question of evidence. Int J Audiol 47(1):12, 2008

Dusheiko G: Interruption of mother-to-infant transmission of hepatitis B: time to include selective antiviral prophylaxis? Lancet 379(9830):2019, 2012

Eisenberg MS, Cummins RO, Ho MT: Code Blue: Cardiac Arrest and Resuscitation. Philadelphia, Saunders, 1987, p 146

Freeman JM, Nelson KB: Intrapartum asphyxia and cerebral palsy. Pediatrics 82:240, 1988

Gaudier FL, Goldenberg RL, Nelson KG, et al: Acid–base status at birth and subsequent neurosensory impairment in surviving 500 to 1000 gm infants. Am J Obstet Gynecol 170:48, 1994

Gazzin S, Tiribelli C: Bilirubin-induced neurological damage. J Matern Fetal Neonatal Med 24(Suppl 1):154, 2011

Gearhart JP, Rock JA: Total ablation of the penis after circumcision with electrocautery: a method of management and long-term follow-up. J Urol 142:799, 1989

Gilstrap LC III, Leveno KJ, Burris J, et al: Diagnosis of birth asphyxia on the basis of fetal pH, Apgar score, and newborn cerebral dysfunction. Am J Obstet Gynecol 161:825, 1989

Goldaber KG, Gilstrap LC III, Leveno KJ, et al: Pathologic fetal acidemia. Obstet Gynecol 78:1103, 1991

Gray RH, Kigozi G, Serwadda D, et al: Male circumcision for HIV prevention in Rakai, Uganda: a randomized trial. Lancet 369:657, 2007

Guglani L, Lakshminrusimha S, Ryan RM: Transient tachypnea of the newborn. Pediatr Rev 29(11):e59, 2008

Haddad B, Mercer BM, Livingston JC, et al: Outcome after successful resuscitation of babies born with Apgar scores of 0 at both 1 and 5 minutes. Am J Obstet Gynecol 182:1210, 2000

Hall MJ, Owings MF: 2000 National hospital discharge survey. Adv Data 329:1, 2002

Hammerschlag MR: Chylamydial and gonococcal infections in infants and children. Clin Infect Dis 53(3):S99, 2011

Hansen TW: Prevention of neurodevelopmental sequelae of jaundice in the newborn. Dev Med Child Neurol 53(Suppl 4): 24, 2011

Hardwick-Smith S, Mastrobattista JM, Wallace PA, et al: Ring block for neonatal circumcision. Obstet Gynecol 91:930, 1998

Isenberg SJ, Apt L, Wood M: A controlled trial of povidone-iodine as prophylaxis against ophthalmia neonatorum. N Engl J Med 332:562, 1995

Janssen PA, Selwood BL, Dobson SR, et al: To dye or not to dye: a randomized clinical trial of a triple dye/alcohol regime versus dry cord care. Pediatrics 111:15, 2003

Kapellen TM, Gebauer CM, Brosteanu O, et al: Higher rate of cord-related adverse events in neonates with dry umbilical cord care compared to chlorhexidine powder. Results of a randomized controlled study to compare efficacy and safely of chlorhexidine powder versus dry care in umbilical cord care of the newborn. Neonatology 96(1):13, 2009

Kattwinkel J: Textbook of Neonatal Resuscitation, 5th ed. American Academy of Pediatrics and American Heart Association, 2006, p 1–8

Kaufman GE, Cimo S, Miller LW, et al: An evaluation of the effects of sucrose on neonatal pain with 2 commonly used circumcision methods. Am J Obstet Gynecol 186:564, 2002

Kiremitci S, Tuzun F, Yesilirmak DC, et al: Is gastric aspiration needed for newborn management in delivery room? Resuscitation 82(1):40–4, 2011

Kotaska K, Urinovska R, Klapkova E, et al: Re-evaluation of cord blood arterial and venous reference ranges for pH, pO_2, pCO_2, according to spontaneous or cesarean delivery. J Clin Lab Anal 24(5):300, 2010

Lander J, Brady-Fryer B, Metcalfe JB, et al: Comparison of ring block, dorsal penile nerve block, and topical anesthesia for neonatal circumcision: a randomized controlled trial. JAMA 278:2157, 1997

Lauer BJ, Spector ND: Hyperbilirubinemia in the newborn. Pediatr Rev 32(8):341, 2011

Lerman SE, Liao JC: Neonatal circumcision. Pediatr Clin North Am 48:1539, 2001

Lewis E, Shinefield HR, Woodruff BA, et al: Safety of neonatal hepatitis B vaccine administration. Pediatr Infect Dis J 20:1049, 2001

Liu S, Wen SW, McMillan D, et al: Increased neonatal readmission rate associated with decreased length of hospital stay at birth in Canada. Can J Public Health 91:46, 2000

Low JA, Lindsay BG, Derrick EJ: Threshold of metabolic acidosis associated with newborn complications. Am J Obstet Gynecol 177:1391, 1997

Low JA, Panagiotopoulos C, Derrick EJ: Newborn complications after intrapartum asphyxia with metabolic acidosis in the preterm fetus. Am J Obstet Gynecol 172:805, 1995

Low JA, Panagiotopoulos C, Derrick EJ: Newborn complications after intrapartum asphyxia with metabolic acidosis in the term fetus. Am J Obstet Gynecol 170:1081, 1994

Malkin JD, Garber S, Broder MS, et al: Infant mortality and early postpartum discharge. Obstet Gynecol 96:183, 2000

Martin JA, Hamilton BE, Ventura SJ, et al: Births: Final Data for 2010. Natl Vital Stat Rep 61(1), 2012

Mastrobattista JM, Swaim LS: Circumcision. In Gilstrap LC III, Cunningham FG, VanDorsten JP (eds): Operative Obstetrics, 2nd ed. New York, McGraw-Hill, 2002, p 657

McIntire DD, Bloom SL, Casey BM, Leveno KJ: Birth weight in relation to morbidity and mortality among newborn infants. N Engl J Med 340:1234, 1999

Mokarami P, Wiberg N, Olofsson P: An overlooked aspect on metabolic acidosis at birth: blood gas analyzers calculate base deficit differently. Acta Obstet Gynecol Scand 91(5):574, 2012

Mosen DM, Clark SL, Mundorff MB, et al: The medical and economic impact of the Newborns' and Mothers' Health Protection Act. Obstet Gynecol 99:116, 2002

Mullany LC, Darmstadt GL, Khatry SK, et al: Topical applications of chlorhexidine to the umbilical cord for prevention of omphalitis and neonatal mortality in southern Nepal: a community-based, cluster randomized trial. Lancet 367:910, 2006

Nelson KB, Ellenberg JH: Apgar scores as predictors of chronic neurologic disability. Pediatrics 68:36, 1981

Neulander E, Walfisch S, Kaneti J: Amputation of distal penile glans during neonatal ritual circumcision—a rare complication. Br J Urol 77:924, 1996

Nicoll A: Routine male neonatal circumcision and risk of infection with HIV-1 and other sexually transmitted diseases. Arch Dis Child 77:194, 1997

Novack AH, Mueller B, Ochs H: Umbilical cord separation in the normal newborn. Am J Dis Child 142:220, 1988

Perlman JM, Wyllie J, Kattwinkel J, et al: Part 11: Neonatal resuscitation: 2010 international consensus on cardiopulmonary resuscitation and emergency cardiovascular care science with treatment recommendations. Circulation 122(16 Suppl 2):S516, 2010

Pippi-Salle JL, Jesus LE, Lorenzo AJ, et al: Glans amputation during routine neonatal circumcision: mechanism of injury and strategy for prevention. J Pediatr Urol 9:763, 2013

Ramin SM, Gilstrap LC, Leveno KJ, et al: Umbilical artery acid–base status in the preterm infant. Obstet Gynecol 74:256, 1989

Riley RJ, Johnson JWC: Collecting and analyzing cord blood gases. Clin Obstet Gynecol 36:13, 1993

Saunders RA, Milner AD: Pulmonary pressure/volume relationships during the last phase of delivery and the first postnatal breaths in human subjects. J Pediatr 93:667, 1978

Siggaard-Anderson O: Blood acid–base alignment nomogram. Scand J Clin Laborat Invest 15:211, 1963

Socol ML, Garcia PM, Riter S: Depressed Apgar scores, acid–base status, and neurologic outcome. Am J Obstet Gynecol 170:991, 1994

Stang HJ, Gunnar MR, Snellman L, et al: Local anesthesia for neonatal circumcision: effects on distress and cortisol response. JAMA 259:1507, 1988

Taddio A, Stevens B, Craig K, et al: Efficacy and safety of lidocaine-prilocaine cream for pain during circumcision. N Engl J Med 336:1197, 1997

Temkin E: Rooming-in: redesigning hospitals and motherhood in Cold War America. Bull Hist Med 76:271, 2002

Teoh D, Reynolds S: Diagnosis and management of pediatric conjunctivitis. Pediatr Emerg Care 19:48, 2003

Thangaratinam S, Brown K, Zamora J, et al: Pulse oximetry screening for critical congenital hear defects in asymptomatic newborn babies: a systemic review and meta-analysis. Lancet 379:2459, 2012

Thorngren-Jerneck K, Herbst A: Low 5-minute Apgar score: a population-based register study of 1 million term births. Obstet Gynecol 98:65, 2001

Tobian AA, Serwadda D, Quinn TC, et al: Male circumcision for the prevention of HSV-2 and HPV infections and syphilis. N Engl J Med 360(13): 1298, 2009

Tran TT: Hepatitis B: treatment to prevent perinatal transmission. Clin Obstet Gynecol 55(2):541, 2012

United States Department of Health and Human Services: Healthy People 2020: Maternal, Infant, and Child Health. 2010. Available at: http://www.healthypeople.gov/2020/topicsobjectives2020/objectiveslist.aspx?topicId=26. Accessed December 27, 2012

Upadhyay V, Hammodat HM, Pease PWB: Post circumcision meatal stenosis: 12 years' experience. N Z Med J 111:57, 1998

Valero J, Desantes D, Perales-Puchalt A, et al: Effect of delayed umbilical cord clamping on blood gas analysis. Eur J Obstet Gynecol Reprod Biol 162(1):21, 2012

Vento M, Saugstad OD: Oxygen supplementation in the delivery room: updated information. J Pediatr 158(2 Suppl):e5, 2011

Watson MS, Mann MY, Lloyd-Puryear MA, et al: Newborn screening: towards a uniform screening panel and system. Executive summary. Genet Med 8(Suppl 5):1S, 2006

White CR, Mok T, Doherty DA, et al: The effect of time, temperature and storage device on umbilical cord blood gas and lactate measurement: a randomized controlled trial. J Matern Fetal Neonatal Med 25(6):587–94, 2012

Whyte RK: Neonatal management and safe discharge of late and moderate preterm infants. Semin Fetal neonatal Med 17(3):153, 2012

Yeh P, Emary K, Impey L: The relationship between umbilical cord arterial pH and serious adverse neonatal outcome: analysis of 51,519 consecutive validated samples. BJOG 119(7):824, 2012

Zuppa AA, D'Andrea V, Catenazzi P, et al: Ophthalmia neonatorum: what time of prophylaxis? J Matern Fetal Neonatal Med 24(6):769, 2011

CHAPTER 33

Diseases and Injuries of the Term Newborn

Term newborns are susceptible to a wide spectrum of illnesses. In many instances, clinical manifestations of these disorders are extensions of pathological effects already incurred by the fetus. A common example is the newborn who is depressed and acidotic because of intrapartum septicemia. Because many of these disorders are differently manifested, those more common in term newborns are considered here, whereas those more frequent in preterm neonates are discussed in Chapter 34. Specific disorders that are the direct consequence of maternal diseases are discussed in pertinent chapters.

RESPIRATORY DISTRESS SYNDROME

At the time of delivery, the newborn must convert rapidly to air breathing as described in Chapter 7 (p. 142). With inspiration, there is alveolar expansion, fluid clearance, and surfactant secretion by type II pneumocytes to prevent lung collapse. Interference with these functions can create respiratory insufficiency with hypoxemia and compensatory tachypnea, which is generally referred to as neonatal *respiratory distress syndrome* or simply *RDS*. In preterm infants, this is caused by lung immaturity and insufficient surfactant, and variants may be seen in severely ill older children and adults (Chap. 47, p. 943). All of these have some element of surfactant deficiency because the inciting agent damages alveolar epithelium. As fetuses approach term, surfactant deficiency as a cause of RDS diminishes. In a report from Beijing that described 125 term infants with RDS, the most frequent causes were perinatal infection with sepsis syndrome in 50 percent, elective cesarean delivery in 27 percent, severe asphyxia in 10 percent, and meconium aspiration in 7 percent (Liu, 2010).

Surfactant Deficiency

Inadequate surfactant secretion that leads to respiratory distress syndrome becomes less frequent with increasing gestational age. That said, even with a low incidence in term infants, RDS from surfactant deficiency is not rare (Berthelot-Ricou, 2012). Male gender and white race are independent risk factors (Anadkat, 2012). Also, mutations of genes that encode for surfactant protein synthesis may augment the deficiency (Garmany, 2008; Wambach, 2012). Regardless of etiology, when surfactant secretion is diminished, the pulmonary pathophysiology, clinical course, and management are similar to that for preterm infants. Treatment includes mechanical ventilation and replacement of surfactant by insufflation (Chap. 34, p. 654). There is no evidence that antenatal maternal corticosteroid treatment will enhance surfactant synthesis in late preterm fetuses (Gyamfi-Bannerman, 2012). The prognosis in term newborns largely depends on the cause, severity, and response to treatment.

Meconium Aspiration Syndrome

The physiology of meconium passage and amnionic fluid contamination is considered in detail in Chapter 24 (p. 493). In some instances, inhalation of meconium-stained fluid at or near delivery causes acute airway obstruction, chemical pneumonitis, surfactant dysfunction or inactivation, and pulmonary hypertension (Swarnam, 2012). If severe, hypoxemia may lead to neonatal death or long-term neurological sequelae in survivors.

Given the high frequency—10 to 20 percent—of meconium-stained amnionic fluid in laboring women at term, it is reasonable to assume that meconium aspiration must be relatively common. Fortunately, severe aspiration leading to overt respiratory failure is much less frequent. And although the exact incidence of meconium aspiration is not known, Singh and associates (2009) reported it to be 1.8 percent for all deliveries. In a French study of nearly 133,000 term newborns, the prevalence of severe aspiration syndrome was 0.07 percent, and this increased progressively from 37 to 43 weeks' gestation (Fischer, 2012). Mortality rates depend on severity. In an earlier report from Parkland Hospital, for all patients, meconium aspiration caused 1 death per 1000 live births (Nathan, 1994).

Fetal morbidity is more often associated with thicker meconium content. It is presumed that in most cases, amnionic fluid is ample to dilute the meconium to permit prompt clearance by normal fetal physiological mechanisms. Meconium aspiration syndrome occasionally develops with light staining. Many newborns are affected after a normal labor and uncomplicated delivery. However, some associated obstetrical factors include postterm pregnancy and fetal-growth restriction. These fetuses are at highest risk because there frequently is diminished amnionic fluid and labor with cord compression or uteroplacental insufficiency. These may increase the likelihood of meconium passage that is thick and undiluted (Leveno, 1984).

Prevention

It was once widely held that aspiration was stimulated by fetal hypoxic episodes, and fetal heart rate tracing abnormalities were used to identify fetuses at greatest risk during labor. Unfortunately, this was found to be an unreliable predictor (Dooley, 1985). Preliminary studies reported that the incidence and severity of the syndrome could be mitigated by *oropharyngeal suctioning* after delivery of the fetal head, but before the chest. For a while, this was standard care, but it was abandoned when shown that strict adherence to this protocol did not reduce syndrome incidence or severity (Davis, 1985; Wiswell, 1990). At the same time, reports described that pulmonary hypertension caused by aspirated meconium was characterized by abnormal arterial muscularization beginning well before birth. These findings led some to conclude that only chronically asphyxiated fetuses developed meconium aspiration syndrome (Katz, 1992). Proof of this never materialized, and Richey (1995) and Bloom (1996) and their colleagues found no correlation between meconium aspiration and markers of *acute* asphyxia—for example, umbilical artery acidosis. Conversely, others have reported that thick meconium is an independent risk factor for neonatal acidosis (Maisonneuve, 2011).

Conflicted findings regarding suctioning stimulated performance of an 11-center randomized trial designed to compare suctioning with no suctioning (Vain, 2004). There was an identical 4-percent incidence of meconium aspiration syndrome in both groups. Subsequently, a committee that represented the American Heart Association and American Academy of Pediatrics (Perlman, 2010), as well as the American College of Obstetricians and Gynecologists (2013b), has recommended *against* routine intrapartum oro- and nasopharyngeal suctioning at delivery. Instead, for depressed newborns, management includes intubation and suctioning to remove meconium and other aspirated material from beneath the glottis (Chap. 32, p. 626).

Intrapartum amnioinfusion has been used successfully in laboring women with decreased amnionic fluid volume and frequent variable fetal heart rate decelerations (Chap. 24, p. 494). It has also been studied as a preventive measure in labors complicated by meconium staining (Spong, 1994). Although amnioinfusion apparently posed little or no increased risk, it was found to be of no benefit because fetuses usually inhaled meconium before labor (Bryne, 1987; Wenstrom, 1995). To further settle this issue, a trial was conducted with almost 2000 women at 36 weeks' gestation or later and in whom labor was complicated by thick meconium (Fraser, 2005). The perinatal death rate with and without amnioinfusion was 0.05 percent in both groups. Rates of moderate or severe meconium aspiration were also not significantly different—4.4 percent with and 3.1 percent without amnioinfusion. Finally, cesarean delivery rates were similar—32 versus 29 percent, respectively. Currently, the American College of Obstetrics and Gynecologists (2012c) does not recommend amnioinfusion to reduce meconium aspiration syndrome.

Treatment

Ventilatory support is given as needed. Because some aspects of meconium aspiration syndrome are caused by surfactant deficiency, replacement therapy has been given in some studies. *Extracorporeal membrane oxygenation—ECMO*—therapy is reserved for neonates who remain poorly oxygenated despite maximal ventilatory assistance. In their Cochrane review of randomized trials, El Shahed and colleagues (2007) found that surfactant replacement significantly decreased need for extracorporeal membrane oxygenation. Although they found that surfactant administration did not lower the mortality rate, a subsequent trial suggested that it was reduced (Dargaville, 2011). The proportion that requires ECMO treatment varies. In the report by Singh and coworkers (2009), 1.4 percent of 7518 term newborns with the syndrome required such treatment, and these had a 5-percent mortality rate. Ramachandrappa and colleagues (2011) reported a higher mortality rate in late-preterm infants compared with term infants. Finally, pulmonary lavage with surfactant is being evaluated (Choi, 2012).

NEONATAL ENCEPHALOPATHY AND CEREBRAL PALSY

Few events evoke more fear and apprehension in parents and obstetricians than the specter of "brain damage," which immediately conjures visions of disabling cerebral palsy and hopeless intellectual disability. Although most brain disorders or injuries are less horrific, history has helped to perpetuate the more dismal outlook. In the first edition of this textbook, J. Whitridge Williams (1903) limited discussions of brain injury to that sustained from birth trauma. When later editions introduced the concept that *asphyxia neonatorum* was another cause of cerebral palsy, this too was linked to traumatic birth. Even as brain damage caused by traumatic delivery became uncommon during the ensuing decades, the belief—albeit erroneous—was that intrapartum events caused most neurological disability. This was a major reason for the escalating cesarean delivery rate beginning in the 1970s. Unfortunately, because in most cases the genesis of cerebral palsy occurred long before labor, this did little to mitigate risks for cerebral palsy (O'Callaghan, 2013).

These realizations stimulated scientific investigations to determine the etiopathogenesis of fetal brain disorders to include those leading to cerebral palsy. Seminal observations include those of Nelson and Ellenberg (1984, 1985, 1986a), discussed subsequently. These investigators are appropriately credited with proving that these neurological disorders are due to complex multifactorial processes caused by a combination of genetic, physiological, environmental, and obstetrical factors. Importantly, these studies showed that few neurological disorders were associated with peripartum events. Continuing international interest was garnered to codify the potential role of intrapartum events. In 2000, President Frank Miller of the American College of Obstetricians and Gynecologists appointed a task force to study the vicissitudes of neonatal encephalopathy and cerebral palsy. From this, the 2003 Task Force findings were promulgated by the American College of Obstetricians and Gynecologists and the American Academy of Pediatrics (2003). The multispecialty coalition reviewed contemporaneous data and provided criteria to define various neonatal brain disorders.

In 2010, 10 years later, President Richard Waldman of the American College of Obstetricians and Gynecologists appointed a second task force to update these findings. The 2014 Task Force has now published its findings (American College of Obstetricians and Gynecologists and the American Academy of Pediatrics, 2014). The 2014 Task Force findings are more circumspect in contrast to the earlier ones. Specifically, more limitations are cited in identifying cause(s) of peripartum *hypoxic-ischemic encephalopathy* compared with other etiologies of neonatal encephalopathy. The 2014 Task Force recommends multidimensional assessment of each affected infant. They add the caveat that no one strategy is infallible, and thus, no single strategy will achieve 100-percent certainty in attributing a cause to neonatal encephalopathy.

Neonatal Encephalopathy

The 2014 Task Force defined neonatal encephalopathy as a syndrome of neurological dysfunction identified in the earliest days of life in neonates born at ≥ 35 weeks' gestation. It is manifested by subnormal levels of consciousness or seizures and often accompanied by difficulty with initiating and maintaining respiration and by depressed tone and reflexes. The incidence of encephalopathy has been cited to be 0.27 to 1.1 per 1000 term liveborn neonates, and it is much more frequent in preterm infants (Ensing, 2013; Plevani, 2013; Takenouchi, 2012; Wu, 2011). Although the 2014 Task Force concluded that there are many causes of encephalopathy and cerebral palsy, it focused on those termed *hypoxic-ischemic encephalopathy (HIE)* and thought to be incurred intrapartum. To identify affected infants, a thorough evaluation is necessary, including maternal history, obstetrical antecedents, intrapartum factors, placental pathology, and newborn course, along with laboratory and neuroimaging findings.

There are three clinically defined levels. *Mild encephalopathy* is characterized by hyperalertness, irritability, jitteriness, and hypertonia and hypotonia. *Moderate encephalopathy* is manifest by lethargy, severe hypertonia, and occasional seizures. *Severe encephalopathy* is manifest by coma, multiple seizures, and recurrent apnea.

The 2014 Task Force also concluded that of the several forms of cerebral palsy, only the *spastic quadriplegic* type can result from acute peripartum ischemia. Other forms—*hemiparetic* or *hemiplegic cerebral palsy, spastic diplegia,* and *ataxia*—are unlikely to result from an intrapartum event. Purely dyskinetic or ataxic cerebral palsy, especially when accompanied by a learning disorder, usually has a genetic origin (Nelson, 1998).

Criteria for Hypoxic-Ischemic Encephalopathy

The 2014 Task Force radically revised its 2003 criteria used to define an acute peripartum event that is consistent with a hypoxic-ischemic episode and neonatal encephalopathy. These are outlined in Table 33-1 and are considered with the following caveats.

Apgar Scores. Low 5- and 10-minute Apgar scores are associated with increased risks for neurological impairment. There are many causes of low Apgar scores, and most of these infants will not develop cerebral palsy. If the 5-minute Apgar is ≥ 7, it is unlikely that peripartum HIE caused cerebral palsy.

Acid-Base Studies. Low pH and base deficit levels increase the likelihood that neonatal encephalopathy was caused by HIE. Decreasing levels form a continuum of increasing risk, but most acidemic neonates will be neurologically normal (Wayock, 2013). A cord artery pH > 7.2 is very unlikely to be associated with HIE.

Neuroimaging Studies. Magnetic resonance (MR) imaging or spectroscopy (MRS) is the best modality with which to

TABLE 33-1. Findings Consistent with an Acute Peripartum or Intrapartum Event Leading to Hypoxic-Ischemic Encephalopathy

Neonatal Findings
Apgar score: < 5 at 5 and 10 minutes
Umbilical arterial acidemia: pH < 7.0 and/or base deficit ≥ 12 mmol/L
Neuroimaging evidence of acute brain injury: MRI or MRS consistent with HIE
Multisystem involvement consistent with HIE
Type and Timing of Contributing Factors
Sentinel hypoxic or ischemic event occurring immediately before or during delivery
Fetal heart rate monitor patterns consistent with an acute peripartum or intrapartum event

HIE = hypoxic ischemic encephalopathy; MRI = magnetic resonance imaging; MRS = magnetic resonance spectroscopy.

From the American College of Obstetricians and Gynecologists and the American Academy of Pediatrics, 2014.

visualize findings consistent with HIE. The 2014 Task Force concludes that cranial sonography and computed tomography (CT) lack sensitivity in the term newborn. Normal MR imaging/MRS findings after the first 24 hours of life, however, effectively exclude a hypoxic-ischemic cause of encephalopathy. MR imaging between 24 and 96 hours may be more sensitive for the timing of peripartum cerebral injury, and MR imaging at 7 to 21 days following birth is the best technique to delineate the full extent of cerebral injury.

Multisystem Involvement. Neonatal manifestations of multisystem injury are consistent with HIE. These include renal, gastrointestinal, hepatic, or cardiac injury; hematological abnormalities; or combinations of these. The severity of neurological injury does not necessarily correlate with injuries to these other systems.

Contributing Factors

The 2014 Task Force also found that certain contributing factors may be consistent with an acute peripartum event.

Sentinel Event. Adverse obstetrical events that may lead to catastrophic clinical outcomes are designated sentinel events. Examples given by the 2014 Task Force include ruptured uterus, severe placental abruption, cord prolapse, and amnionic-fluid embolism. Martinez-Biarge and associates (2012) studied almost 58,000 deliveries and identified 192 cases with one of these sentinel events. Of these 192 infants, 6 percent died intrapartum or in the early neonatal period, and 10 percent developed neonatal encephalopathy. In a study of 307 cases of cord prolapse, the fetal death rate was 6.8 percent (Hartigan, 2013). Besides these sentinel events, other risk factors for neonatal acidosis include prior cesarean delivery, maternal age ≥ 35 years, thick meconium, chorioamnionitis, and general anesthesia (Johnson, 2014; Maisonneuve, 2011).

Fetal Heart Rate Patterns. The 2014 Task Force emphasized the importance of differentiating an abnormal fetal heart rate (FHR) tracing on presentation versus one that develops subsequently. A category 1 or 2 FHR tracing associated with Apgar scores ≥ 7 at 5 minutes, normal cord gases (±1 SD), or both, is not consistent with an acute HIE event (Anderson, 2013). An FHR pattern at the time of presentation with persistently minimal or absent variability and lacking accelerations, with duration ≥ 60 minutes, and even without decelerations is suggestive of an already compromised fetus. The Task Force further recommended that if fetal well-being cannot be established with these findings present, the woman should be evaluated for the method and timing of delivery.

Application of 2003 Task Force Criteria

It seemed likely that strict adherence to all of the criteria set forth by the 2003 Task Force would exclude some infants who go on to develop cerebral palsy as a result of neonatal encephalopathy (Strijbis, 2006). To test these criteria, Phelan and coworkers (2011) retrospectively applied the 2003 Task Force criteria to 39 term infants with permanent central nervous system impairment. They found that the Task Force criteria and these 39 cases correlated in varying degrees. Of the essential criteria, pH < 7.0 and base deficit ≥ 12 mmol/L showed a 97- and 100-percent correlation, respectively; moderate to severe encephalopathy—97 percent correlation; spastic quadriplegia or dyskinetic form—92 percent; and no other identifiable cause—100 percent. Of the nonspecific criteria, a sentinel hypoxic event had an 80-percent correlation; fetal heart rate requirements—100 percent; Apgar score ≤ 3 beyond 5 minutes—29 percent; and multisystem involvement—100 percent. As discussed subsequently, a sentinel event alone had only a 10-percent predictive value for newborn encephalopathy (Martinez-Biarge, 2012).

Prevention

Most prophylactic measures for neonatal encephalopathy have been evaluated in preterm infants (Chap. 42, p. 854). One of these—hypothermia—may prevent death and mitigate moderate to severe neurological disability in term infants (Nelson, 2014; Pfister, 2010; Shankaran, 2005, 2012). MR imaging studies have demonstrated a slowing of diffusional abnormalities and fewer infarctions with hypothermia (Bednarek, 2012; Shankaran, 2012). Most randomized trials have shown improved outcomes with hypothermia in infants born at 36 weeks or older (Azzopardi, 2009; Guillet, 2012; Jacobs, 2011). In a metaanalysis of more than 1200 newborns, Tagin and colleagues (2012) concluded that hypothermia improves survival rates and neurodevelopment. More recently, clinical trials to evaluate concomitant erythropoietin therapy for neuroprophylaxis are being conducted (Wu, 2012). Preliminary data from a Dutch multicenter trial of maternal allopurinol therapy indicate some mitigation of cerebral damage from hypoxia and ischemia (Kaandorp, 2013).

Cerebral Palsy

This term refers to a group of nonprogressive disorders of movement or posture caused by abnormal development or damage to brain centers for motor control. Cerebral palsy is further classified by the type of neurological dysfunction—spastic, dyskinetic, or ataxic—as well as the number and distribution of limbs involved—quadriplegia, diplegia, hemiplegia, or monoplegia. Together, the major types are *spastic quadriplegia*—the most common—which has a strong association with mental retardation and seizure disorders; *diplegia,* which is common in preterm or low-birthweight infants; *hemiplegia; choreoathetoid types;* and *mixed varieties.* Although epilepsy and mental retardation frequently accompany cerebral palsy, these two disorders seldom are associated with perinatal asphyxia in the absence of cerebral palsy.

Incidence and Epidemiological Correlates

According to the Centers for Disease Control and Prevention (2011), the prevalence of cerebral palsy is variably reported in the United States. In one multisite surveillance program in 2006, the average prevalence was 2.9 per 1000 8-year-old children. *It is crucial to emphasize that this rate is derived from all children—including preterm infants.* Because of the remarkably increased survival rates of the latter, the overall rate of cerebral palsy and other developmental disabilities reported in the 1950s has remained essentially unchanged (Boyle, 2011).

Long-term follow-up studies of more than 900,000 Norwegian nonanomalous term infants cite an incidence of 1 per 1000 (Moster, 2008). By contrast, the incidence was 91 per 1000 for infants born at 23 to 27 weeks. In absolute numbers, term infants comprise half of cerebral palsy cases because there are proportionately far fewer preterm births. It is again emphasized that most studies have not made distinctions between term and preterm infants.

As noted earlier, Nelson and Ellenberg (1984, 1985, 1986a) made many foundational observations concerning cerebral palsy. Their initial studies emanated from data from the Collaborative Perinatal Project. This included children from almost 54,000 pregnancies who were followed until age 7. They found that the most frequently associated risk factors for cerebral palsy were: (1) evidence of genetic abnormalities such as maternal mental retardation or fetal congenital malformations; (2) birthweight < 2000 g; (3) birth before 32 weeks; and (4) perinatal infection. They also found that obstetrical complications were not strongly predictive, and only a fifth of affected children had markers of perinatal asphyxia. *For the first time, there was solid evidence that the cause of most cases of cerebral palsy was unknown, and importantly, only a small proportion was caused by neonatal hypoxic-ischemic encephalopathy.* Equally importantly, there was no foreseeable single intervention that would likely prevent a large proportion of cases.

Numerous studies have since confirmed many of these findings and identified an imposing list of other risk factors that are shown in Table 33-2. As expected, preterm birth continues to be the single most important risk factor (Goepfert, 1996; Thorngren-Jerneck, 2006). Small-for-gestational-age infants are also at increased risk. Stoknes and associates (2012) showed that in more than 90 percent of growth-restricted infants, cerebral palsy was due to antepartum factors. A myriad other placental and neonatal risk factors has been correlated with neurodevelopmental abnormalities (Ahlin, 2013; Avagliano, 2010; Blair, 2011; Redline, 2005, 2008). Some placental factors are discussed further in Chapter 6, and in just one example, there is a substantively increased risk with chorioamnionitis (Gilbert, 2010; Shatrov, 2010). An example of a neonatal cause is arterial ischemic stroke, which may be associated with inherited fetal thrombophilias (Gibson, 2005; Harteman, 2013; Kirton, 2011). Also, neonates with isolated congenital heart lesions have an increased risk for microcephaly, possibly due to chronic fetal hypoxemia (Barbu, 2009). Other miscellaneous causes of cerebral palsy include fetal anemia, twin-twin transfusion syndrome, intrauterine transfusions, and fetal alcohol syndrome (DeJong, 2012; Lindenburg, 2013; O'Leary, 2012; Rossi, 2011; Spruijt, 2012).

TABLE 33-2. Perinatal Risk Factors Reported to Be Increased in Children with Cerebral Palsy

Risk Factors	Risk Ratio	95% CI
Hydramnios	6.9	1.0–49.3
Placental abruption	7.6	2.7–21.1
Interval between pregnancies < 3 months or > 3 years	3.7	1.0–4.4
Spontaneous preterm labor	3.4	1.7–6.7
Preterm delivery at 23–27 weeks	78.9	56.5–110
Breech or face presentation, transverse lie	3.8	1.6–9.1
Severe birth defect	5.6	8.1–30.0
Nonsevere birth defect	6.1	3.1–11.8
Time to cry > 5 minutes	9.0	4.3–18.8
Low placental weight	3.6	1.5–8.4
Placental infarction	2.5	1.2–5.3
Chorioamnionitis		
Clinical	2.4	1.5–3.8
Histological	1.8	1.2–2.9
Others[a]	—	—

[a]Includes respiratory distress syndrome, meconium aspiration, emergent cesarean or operative vaginal delivery, hypoglycemia, gestational hypertension, hypotension, advanced maternal age, nighttime delivery, seizures, fetal-growth restriction, male gender, and nulliparity.
From Ahlin, 2013; Blair, 2011; Livinec, 2005; McIntyre, 2013; Moster, 2008; Nelson, 1985; 1986a, 2012; O'Callaghan, 2011; Redline, 2005; Shatrov, 2010; Takenouchi, 2012; Torfs, 1990; Wu, 2012.

Intrapartum Events. The National Collaborative Perinatal Project found that intrapartum hypoxemia was linked to a minority of cerebral palsy cases. However, because the study was carried out in the 1960s, there were inconsistent criteria to accurately assign cause. The contribution of hypoxic-ischemic encephalopathy to subsequent neurological disorders is discussed in detail on page 639. Thus, the 2003 Task Force applied these criteria to more contemporaneous outcomes and determined that only 1.6 cases of cerebral palsy per 10,000 deliveries are attributable solely to intrapartum hypoxia. This finding is supported by a study from Western Australia that spanned from 1975 to 1980 (Stanley, 1991). These latter investigators concluded that intrapartum injury as the cause of cerebral palsy was unlikely in 92 percent of cases; in 3 percent, it was possible; and in only 5 percent was it likely. In another review of 209 infants with neurological impairment, 75 percent were classified as nonpreventable (Phelan, 1996). In yet another study of 213 such children, only 2 percent of cases could be attributed to intrapartum hypoxia (Strijbis, 2006).

Intrapartum Fetal Heart Rate Monitoring

Despite persistent attempts to validate continuous intrapartum electronic fetal monitoring as effective to prevent adverse perinatal outcomes, evidence does not support its ability to predict or reduce cerebral palsy risk (Clark, 2003; Devoe, 2011; MacDonald, 1985; Thacker, 1995). Importantly, there are no specific fetal heart rate patterns predictive of cerebral palsy, and no relationship has been found between the clinical response to abnormal patterns and neurological outcome (Melone, 1991; Nelson, 1996). Indeed, an abnormal heart rate pattern in fetuses that ultimately develop cerebral palsy may reflect a preexisting neurological abnormality (Phelan, 1994). Because of these studies, the American College of Obstetricians and Gynecologists (2013a) has concluded that electronic fetal monitoring does not reduce the incidence of long-term neurological impairment.

Apgar Scores

In general, 1- and 5-minute Apgar scores are poor predictors of long-term neurological impairment. When the 5-minute Apgar score is 3 or less, however, neonatal death or the risk of neurological sequelae is increased substantially (Dijxhoorn, 1986; Nelson, 1984). In a Swedish study, 5 percent of such children subsequently required special schooling (Stuart, 2011). In a Norwegian study, the incidence of these low Apgar scores was 0.1 percent in more than 235,000 newborns. Almost a fourth died, and 10 percent of survivors developed cerebral palsy (Moster, 2001).

Persistence past 5 minutes of these extremely low scores correlates strongly with an increased risk for neurological morbidity and death (Grünebaum, 2013). This of course is not absolute, and the 2003 Task Force cited a 10-percent risk for cerebral palsy for infants with 10-minute scores of 0 to 3. For 15-minute scores ≤ 2, there is a 53-percent mortality rate and a 36-percent cerebral palsy rate, and for 20-minute scores ≤ 2, there is a 60-percent mortality rate and a 57-percent rate of cerebral palsy. Some outcomes in the Norwegian Study of infants with these low 5-minute Apgar scores are shown in Table 33-3. Survivors with Apgar scores of 0 at 10 minutes have even worse outcomes. In a review of 94 such infants, 78 died, and *all* survivors assessed had long-term disabilities (Harrington, 2007).

Umbilical Cord Blood Gas Studies

As outlined on page 639, objective evidence for metabolic acidosis—cord arterial blood pH < 7.0 and base deficit ≥ 12 mmol/L—is a risk factor for encephalopathy as well as for cerebral palsy. The risk increases as acidosis worsens. From their review of 51 studies, Malin and coworkers (2010) found that low cord arterial pH correlates with increased risk for neonatal encephalopathy and cerebral palsy. When used alone, however, these determinations are not accurate in predicting long-term neurological sequelae (Dijxhoorn, 1986; Yeh, 2012).

TABLE 33-3. Comparison of Mortality and Morbidity in Norwegian Infants Weighing > 2500 g According to 5-Minute Apgar Scores

Outcome	Apgar 0–3	Apgar 7–10	Relative Risk (95% CI)
Number	292	233, 500	
Mortality rates			
Neonatal	16.5%	0.05%	386 (270–552)
Infant	19.2%	0.3%	76 (56–103)
1–8 years	3%	0.2%	18 (8–39)
Morbidity rates			
Cerebral palsy	6.8%	0.09%	81 (48–128)
Mental retardation	1.3%	0.1%	9 (3–29)
Other neurological	4.2%	0.5%	9 (5–17)
Non-neurological	3.4%	2.0%	2 (0.8–5.5)

Data from Moster, 2001.

Data from several studies corroborate that a pH < 7.0 is the threshold for clinically significant acidemia (Gilstrap, 1989; Goldaber, 1991). The likelihood of neonatal death increases as the cord artery pH falls to 7.0 or less. Casey and colleagues (2001) reported that when the pH was 6.8 or lower, the neonatal mortality rate was increased 1400-fold. When the cord pH was ≤ 7.0 *and* the 5-minute Apgar score was 0 to 3, there was a 3200-fold increased risk of neonatal death.

In the study from Oxford, adverse neurological outcomes were 0.36 percent with pH < 7.1 and 3 percent with pH < 7.0 (Yeh, 2012). As mentioned, newborn complications increase coincident with increasing severity of acidemia at birth. According to the American College of Obstetricians and Gynecologists (2012d), encephalopathy develops in 10 percent of newborns whose umbilical arterial base deficit is 12 to 16 mmol/L, and in 40 percent of those whose deficit is > 16 mmol/L. In a Swedish study, researchers observed that cord blood lactate levels may prove to be superior to base deficit for prognostication of neurological disorders (Wiberg, 2010).

Nucleated Red Blood Cells and Lymphocytes

Both immature red cells and lymphocytes enter the circulation of term infants in response to hypoxia or hemorrhage. During the past two decades, quantification of these cells has been proposed as a measure of hypoxia, but most studies do not support this premise (Hankins, 2002; Silva, 2006; Walsh, 2011, 2013). The 2003 Task Force concluded that their use was investigational.

Neuroimaging Studies in Encephalopathy and Cerebral Palsy

Various neuroimaging techniques have provided important insight into the etiology and evolution of perinatal hypoxic-ischemic encephalopathy and later cerebral palsy (p. 639). Importantly, findings are highly dependent on fetal age. The preterm neonatal brain responds quite differently to an ischemic episode compared with that of a term infant. Other factors include insult severity and duration as well as restoration of cerebrovascular hypoperfusion. *Thus, precise timing of an injury with neuroimaging studies is not a realistic goal.* Reports are of two types—those in which neuroimaging was done during the neonatal period and those done when older children are diagnosed with cerebral palsy.

Neuroimaging in Neonatal Period

Regarding early use, the 2014 Task Force concluded that these imaging techniques provide the following information:

1. Sonographic studies are generally normal on the day of birth. Increasing echogenicity in the thalami and basal ganglia is seen beginning at approximately 24 hours. This progresses over 2 to 3 days and persists for 5 to 7 days.
2. Computed tomography scans are usually normal the first day in term infants. Decreased density in the thalami or basal ganglia is seen beginning at about 24 hours and persists for 5 to 7 days.
3. Magnetic resonance imaging will detect some abnormalities on the first day. Within 24 hours, MR imaging may

show restricted water diffusion that peaks at about 5 days and disappears within 2 weeks. Acquisitions with T1- and T2-weighted images show variable abnormalities, which have an onset from less than 24 hours to several days. In a study of 175 term infants with acute encephalopathy, it was reported that MR imaging showing basal ganglia lesions accurately predicted motor impairment at 2 years of age (Martinez-Biarge, 2012).

The 2014 Task Force concluded that for term infants, imaging studies are helpful in timing an injury, but they provide only a window in time that is imprecise. Findings in preterm infants are considered in Chapter 34 (p. 656).

Neuroimaging in Older Children with Cerebral Palsy

Imaging studies performed in children diagnosed with cerebral palsy frequently show abnormal findings. Wu and associates (2006) used CT or MR imaging to study 273 children who were born after 36 weeks and who were diagnosed later in childhood with cerebral palsy. Although a third of these studies were normal, focal arterial infarction was seen in 22 percent; brain malformations in 14 percent; and periventricular white-matter injuries in 12 percent. In another study of 351 children with cerebral palsy—about half were born near term—MR imaging findings were abnormal in 88 percent (Bax, 2006). Similar findings were reported in an Australian study (Robinson, 2008).

CT and MR imaging techniques have also been used in older children in an attempt to define the timing of fetal or perinatal cerebral injury. Wiklund and coworkers (1991a,b) studied 83 children between ages 5 and 16 years who were born at term and who developed hemiplegic cerebral palsy. Nearly 75 percent had abnormal CT findings, and these investigators concluded that more than half had CT findings that suggested a *prenatal injury*. Approximately 20 percent was attributed to a *perinatal injury*. In a similar study, Robinson and colleagues (2008) used MR imaging. They reported pathological findings in 84 percent of children with spastic quadriplegia, which is the neurological lesion that the 2014 Task Force reported to correlate with neonatal encephalopathy.

Intellectual Disability and Seizure Disorders

The term *intellectual disability* is the preferred substitute term for the older culturally insensitive term *mental retardation* (Centers for Disease Control and Prevention, 2012). It describes a spectrum of disabilities and seizure disorders that frequently accompany cerebral palsy. But when either of these manifests alone, they are seldom caused by perinatal hypoxia (Nelson, 1984, 1986a,b). Severe mental retardation has a prevalence of 3 per 1000 children, and its most frequent causes are chromosomal, gene mutations, and other congenital malformations. Finally, preterm birth is a common association for these (Moster, 2008).

The major predictors of seizure disorders are fetal malformations—cerebral and noncerebral; family history of seizures; and neonatal seizures (Nelson, 1986b). Neonatal encephalopathy causes a small proportion of seizure disorders. Reports from the Neonatal Research Network and other studies concluded that increasing severity of encephalopathy correlates best with seizures (Glass, 2011; Kwon, 2011).

Autism Spectrum Disorders

According to the Centers for Disease Control and Prevention (2012), the frequency of autism is almost 0.5 percent, and for attention deficit hyperactivity disorders, it is 6.7 percent. Although these may be associated with maternal metabolic conditions, none has been linked convincingly to peripartum events (Krakowiak, 2012).

HEMATOLOGICAL DISORDERS

There are a few neonatal disorders of erythrocytes, platelets, and coagulation with which the obstetrician should be familiar. As is the case for most other conditions manifest by the newborn shortly after birth, many of these hematological problems were acquired by the fetus and persist in the newborn.

Anemia

After 35 weeks' gestation, the mean cord hemoglobin concentration is approximately 17 g/dL, and values below 14 g/dL are considered abnormal. A review of nearly 3000 deliveries found that late cord clamping was associated with a mean hemoglobin increase of 2.2 g/dL (McDonald, 2008). Unfortunately, this practice almost doubled the incidence of hyperbilirubinemia requiring phototherapy. The American College of Obstetricians and Gynecologists (2012b) has concluded that optimal timing of cord clamping for term infants is unknown. Conversely, cord blood hemoglobin concentration may be abnormally low, or it may fall after delivery. Fetal anemia results from many causes and is discussed in Chapter 15 (p. 306).

Acute anemia with hypovolemia is seen with deliveries in which the placenta is cut or torn, if a fetal vessel is perforated or lacerated, or if the infant is held well above the level of the placenta for some time before cord clamping. Intracranial or extracranial injury or trauma to fetal intraabdominal organs can also cause hemorrhage with acute anemia (Akin, 2011).

Polycythemia and Hyperviscosity

Neonatal polycythemia with hyperviscosity can be associated with chronic hypoxia in utero, twin-twin transfusion syndrome, placental- and fetal-growth restriction, fetal macrosomia from maternal diabetes, and transfusion at delivery. Current recommendations by the International Liaison Committee on Resuscitation (ILCOR) are to delay cord clamping for at least 1 minute after delivery (Davis, 2012). When the hematocrit rises above 65, blood viscosity markedly increases and may cause neonatal plethora, cyanosis, or neurological aberrations. Because of the shorter lifespan of macrocytic fetal erythrocytes, hyperbilirubinemia commonly accompanies polycythemia as subsequently discussed. Other findings include thrombocytopenia, fragmented erythrocytes, and hypoglycemia. Partial exchange transfusion may be necessary in some neonates.

Hyperbilirubinemia

Even in term fetuses, hepatic maturation is not complete, and thus some unconjugated bilirubin—either albumin bound or free—is cleared by placental transfer to be conjugated in the maternal liver (Chap. 7, p. 141). Fetal protection from unconjugated bilirubin is lost after delivery if it is not cleared rapidly. Because clearance is totally dependent on neonatal hepatic function, varying degrees of neonatal hyperbilirubinemia result. Even in the mature newborn, serum bilirubin usually increases for 3 to 4 days to reach levels up to 10 mg/dL. After this, concentrations usually fall rapidly. In one large study, 1 to 2 percent of neonates delivered at 35 weeks' gestation or later had a maximum serum bilirubin level > 20 mg/dL (Eggert, 2006). In approximately 15 percent of term newborns, bilirubin levels cause clinically visible skin color changes termed *physiological jaundice* (Burke, 2009). As expected, in preterm infants, the bilirubin increase is greater and more prolonged.

Acute Bilirubin Encephalopathy and Kernicterus

Excessive serum bilirubin levels can be neurotoxic for newborns (Dijk, 2012; Watchako, 2013). The pathogenesis is complex, and toxicity has two forms. *Acute bilirubin encephalopathy* is encountered in the first days of life and is characterized by hypotonia, poor feeding, lethargy, and abnormal auditory-evoked responses (Kaplan, 2011). Immediate recognition and treatment will usually mitigate progressive neurotoxicity. The chronic form is termed *kernicterus*—from Greek *jaundice of the nuclei*. Neurotoxicity follows bilirubin deposition and staining of the basal ganglia and hippocampus and is further characterized by profound neuronal degeneration. Survivors have spasticity, muscular incoordination, and varying degrees of mental retardation. Although there is a positive correlation between kernicterus and unconjugated bilirubin levels above 18 to 20 mg/dL, it can develop at much lower concentrations, especially in very preterm neonates (Sgro, 2011). Continuing hemolysis is a risk factor for kernicterus, and experiences from the Collaborative Perinatal Project were that bilirubin levels ≥ 25 mg/dL correlated with kernicterus only with ongoing Coombs-positive hemolysis (Kuzniewicz, 2009). This was recently verified in a study by Vandborg and associates (2012).

Prevention and Treatment

Various forms of phototherapy are used to prevent as well as treat neonatal hyperbilirubinemia (Hansen, 2011). These "bili-lights" emit a spectrum of 460 to 490 nm, which increases bilirubin oxidation to enhance its renal clearance and lower serum levels. Light that penetrates the skin also increases peripheral blood flow, which further enhances photo-oxidation. It is problematic that available devices are not standardized (Bhutani, 2011). Another advantage is that exchange transfusions are seldom required with phototherapy. There are studies in both preterm and term newborns that attest to phototherapy efficacy (Watchko, 2013). A Neonatal Research Network study reported that aggressive phototherapy in low-birthweight neonates reduced rates of neurodevelopmental impairment (Newman, 2006).

For term infants, the American Academy of Pediatrics and the American College of Obstetricians and Gynecologists (2012b) stress early detection and prompt phototherapy to prevent bilirubin encephalopathy. Despite these measures, bilirubin encephalopathy persists, and this is somewhat related to early hospital discharges (Gazzin, 2011; Kaplan, 2011; Sgro, 2011). According to Burke and coworkers (2009), hospitalizations for kernicterus in term infants were 5.1 per 100,000 in 1988. Since then, however, this rate has decreased to 0.4 to 2.7 cases per 100,000 births (Watchko, 2013).

Hemorrhagic Disease of the Newborn

This disorder is characterized by spontaneous internal or external bleeding beginning any time after birth. Most hemorrhagic disease results from abnormally low levels of the vitamin K-dependent clotting factors—V, VII, IX, X, prothrombin, and proteins C and S (Zipursky, 1999). Infants whose mothers took anticonvulsant drugs are at higher risk because these suppress maternal hepatic synthesis of some of these factors (Chap. 60, p. 1190). Classic hemorrhagic disease is usually apparent 2 to 5 days after birth in infants not given vitamin K prophylaxis at delivery (Busfield, 2013). Delayed hemorrhage may occur at 2 to 12 weeks in exclusively breast-fed infants because breast milk contains little vitamin K. Other causes of neonatal hemorrhage include hemophilia, congenital syphilis, sepsis, thrombocytopenia purpura, erythroblastosis, and intracranial hemorrhage.

The American Academy of Pediatrics and the American College of Obstetricians and Gynecologists (2012) recommends routine prophylaxis for hemorrhagic disease with a 0.5 to 1 mg dose of vitamin K_1 (phytonadione) given intramuscularly. Oral administration is not effective, and maternal vitamin K administration results in very little transport to the fetus. For treatment of active bleeding, vitamin K is injected intravenously.

Thrombocytopenia

Abnormally low platelet concentrations in term newborns may be due to various etiologies such as immune disorders, infections, drugs, or inherited platelet defects, or they may be part of a congenital syndrome. In many, thrombocytopenia is an extension of a fetal disorder such as infection with B19 parvovirus, cytomegalovirus, toxoplasmosis, and others discussed in Chapters 64 and 65. Term infants admitted to neonatal intensive care units, especially those with sepsis, have accelerated platelet consumption (Eissa, 2013). In these, transfusions are occasionally indicated (Sallmon, 2012).

Immune Thrombocytopenia

In women with an autoimmune disorder such as systemic lupus erythematosus or immunological thrombocytopenia, maternal antiplatelet IgG is transferred to the fetus and can cause accelerated platelet destruction. Most cases are mild, and platelet levels usually reach a nadir at 48 to 72 hours. Maternal corticosteroid therapy generally has no effect on fetal platelets. Fetal blood sampling for platelet determination is seldom necessary, and platelets are usually adequate to prevent fetal hemorrhage during delivery (Chap. 56, p. 1115).

Alloimmune Thrombocytopenia

Alloimmune thrombocytopenia (AIT) or neonatal alloimmune thrombocytopenia (NAIT) is caused by maternal-fetal platelet antigen disparity. If maternal alloimmunization is stimulated, then transplacental antiplatelet IgG antibodies cause severe fetal thrombocytopenia, which is considered in detail in Chapter 15 (p. 313).

Preeclampsia Syndrome

Maternal platelet function and destruction can be severely affected in women with severe preeclampsia. That said, fetal or neonatal thrombocytopenia is rarely caused by the preeclampsia syndrome even when the mother has severe thrombocytopenia. The large study of mother-infant pairs delivered at Parkland Hospital dispelled earlier reports of an association of neonatal thrombocytopenia with preeclampsia (Pritchard, 1987). Instead, neonatal thrombocytopenia was found to be associated with preterm delivery and its myriad complications (Chap. 34, p. 653).

INJURIES OF THE NEWBORN

Birth injuries can potentially complicate any delivery. Thus, although some are more likely associated with "traumatic" delivery by forceps or vacuum, others are seen with otherwise uncomplicated vaginal or cesarean delivery. In this section, some injuries are discussed in general, but specific injuries are described elsewhere in connection with their associated obstetrical complications, for example, breech delivery in Chapter 28 or multifetal gestation in Chapter 45.

Incidence

In three population studies that included more than 8 million term infants, the overall incidence of birth trauma was 20 to 26 per 1000 deliveries (Baskett, 2007; Linder, 2012; Moczygemba, 2010). Of these studies, data from Nova Scotia are shown in Table 33-4 with an overall trauma risk of 19.5 per 1000 deliveries. Only 1.6 per 1000 were due to major trauma, and these rates were highest with failed instrumented delivery and lowest with cesarean delivery without labor. Thus, most traumatic injuries were minor and had an incidence of 18 per 1000 deliveries.

Injuries associated with cesarean delivery from a Maternal-Fetal Medicine Units Network study were described by Alexander and coworkers (2006). Four hundred injuries were identified from a total of 37,100 operations—a rate of 11 per 1000 cesarean deliveries. Although skin lacerations predominated—7 per 1000—more serious injuries in these 400 infants included 88 cephalohematomas, 11 clavicular fractures, 11 facial nerve palsies, nine brachial plexopathies, and six skull fractures.

TABLE 33-4. Incidence of Major and Minor Birth Trauma—Nova Scotia, 1988–2001

Type of Delivery (Trauma Rate per 1000)	Number	Birth Trauma (Rate per 1000) Major[a]	Minor[b]
Spontaneous (14)	88,324	1.2	13
Assisted			
Vacuum (71)	3175	3.7	67
Forceps (58)	10,478	5.2	53
Failed assisted			
Vacuum (105)	609	8.3	100
Forceps (56)	714	7.0	50
Cesarean (8.6)	16,132	0.3	8.3
Labor (12)	10,731	0.4	11.9
No labor (1.2)	5401	0.2	1.1
All (19.5)	119,432	1.6	18

[a]Major trauma = depressed skull fracture, intracranial hemorrhage, brachial plexopathy, or combination.
[b]Minor trauma = linear skull fracture, other fractures, facial palsy, cephalohematoma, or combination.
Data from Baskett, 2007.

Cranial Injuries

Traumatic head injuries that are associated with labor or delivery can be *external* and obvious, such as a skull or mandibular fracture; they can be *intracranial*; and in some, they are *covert*. The fetal head has considerable plasticity and can undergo appreciable molding. Rarely, severe molding can result in tearing of bridging cortical veins that empty into the sagittal sinus, internal cerebral veins, the vein of Galen, or of the tentorium itself. As a result, intracranial, subdural, and even epidural hemorrhage can be seen after an apparently uneventful vaginal delivery (Scheibl, 2012). Bleeding may also be asymptomatic. Conversely, subgaleal hemorrhages associated with instrumented delivery can be life threatening (Doumouchtsis, 2008; Swanson, 2012). In rare severe head trauma cases, there is embolization of fetal brain tissue to the heart or lungs (Cox, 2009).

Intracranial Hemorrhage

Most aspects of neonatal intracranial hemorrhage are related to gestational age. Specifically, most hemorrhage in preterm neonates results from hypoxia and ischemia, whereas in term newborns, trauma is the most frequent cause. Some varieties are shown in Table 33-5. *Importantly, in some infants, a putative cause is not found.* In many cases, intracranial hemorrhage is asymptomatic. The reported incidence varies, but it is highest with operative deliveries—both vaginal and cesarean deliveries. In the study by Moczygemba and colleagues (2010), for more than 8 million singleton deliveries, the overall intracranial hemorrhage rate was approximately 0.2 per 1000 births—1 per 5000. In a study from New York City, Werner and associates (2011) cited a combined incidence in more than 120,000 nulliparous singleton operative deliveries of 0.12 percent, or about 1 in

TABLE 33-5. Major Types of Neonatal Intracranial Hemorrhage

Type	Etiology and Neuropathogenesis	Clinical Outcomes
Subdural	Trauma—tentorial, falx, or venous (sinus) laceration causing hematoma	Uncommon but potentially serious; symptom onset is variable depending on hematoma expansion, but usually < 24 hours: irritability, lethargy, and brainstem compression
Primary subarachnoid	Possibly due to trauma or hypoxia—excludes SAH associated with subdural, intraventricular, intracerebral (AVM, aneurysm), or intracerebellar hemorrhage	Common but almost always benign
Intracerebellar	Trauma and perhaps hypoxia—most cases in preterm infants	Uncommon but serious
Intraventricular	Trauma and hypoxia (no discernible cause in 25 percent)—hemorrhage usually from choroid plexus	Uncommon but serious; symptoms as for subdural hemorrhage
Miscellaneous	Trauma with epidural or intracerebral hemorrhage Hemorrhagic infarction—embolism or thrombosis in artery or vein Coagulopathies—thrombocytopenia or inherited factor deficiencies Vascular defect—aneurysm or AVM	Depends on cause

AVM = arteriovenous malformation; SAH = subarachnoid hemorrhage.
Data from Volpe, 1995.

750 procedures. The rates of intracranial hemorrhage were 1:385 with vacuum delivery; 1:515 with forceps, and 1:1210 with cesarean delivery. In another study, its incidence was nearly 1 percent following vacuum-assisted deliveries (Simonson, 2007). According to the American College of Obstetricians and Gynecologists (2012a), the incidence of intracranial hemorrhage from birth trauma has been substantively decreased by elimination of difficult operative vaginal deliveries. This was verified in a recent report of carefully conducted Kielland forceps deliveries (Burke, 2012).

The prognosis after hemorrhage depends on its location and extent, as shown in Table 33-5. For example, subdural and subarachnoid hemorrhage seldom results in neurological abnormalities, whereas large hematomas are serious. Any bleeding into the parenchyma from intraventricular or intracerebellar hemorrhage often causes serious permanent damage or death. Periventricular hemorrhage rarely causes the type of sequelae that are common in those born preterm (Chap. 34, p. 656).

Infants who have traumatic subdural or infratentorial hemorrhage tears will have neurological abnormalities from the time of birth (Volpe, 1995). Those most severely affected have stupor or coma, nuchal rigidity, and opisthotonos that worsen over minutes to hours. Some newborns who are born depressed appear to improve until about 12 hours of age, when drowsiness, apathy, feeble cry, pallor, failure to nurse, dyspnea, cyanosis, vomiting, and convulsions become evident.

Spontaneous intracranial hemorrhage has also been documented in healthy term neonates (Huang, 2004; Rutherford, 2012). In a prospective MR imaging study, Whitby and coworkers (2004) found that 6 percent of those delivered spontaneously and 28 percent of those delivered by forceps had a subdural hemorrhage. None of these had clinical findings, and hematomas resolved by 4 weeks in all infants.

Extracranial Hematomas

These blood collections accumulate outside the calvarium and are categorized as a *cephalohematoma* or *subgaleal hemorrhage* (Fig. 33-1). From its most superficial inward, the scalp is composed of skin, subcutaneous tissue, galea aponeurotica, subgaleal space, and calvarium periosteum. The galea aponeurotica is dense fibrous tissue, whereas the subgaleal space contains loose, fibroareolar tissue. Traversing across the subgaleal space are large, valveless *emissary veins*, which connect the dural sinuses inside the skull with the superficial scalp veins. Both the galea aponeurotica and subgaleal space span across the occipital, parietal, and frontal bones. In contrast, periosteum invests each individual skull bone and does not cross suture lines.

Cephalohematomas are cranial subperiosteal hematomas. These develop from shearing forces during labor and delivery that lacerate the emissary or diploic veins. Fortunately, the densely adhered periosteum impedes rapid enlargement and limits final hematoma size. Hemorrhage can be over one or both parietal bones, but palpable edges can be appreciated as the blood reaches the limits of the periosteum. These hematomas must be differentiated from *caput succedaneum*, also shown in Figure 33-1. A cephalohematoma may not be apparent until hours after delivery, when bleeding sufficient to raise the periosteum has occurred. After it is identified, it often grows larger and persists for weeks or even months, and bleeding may be

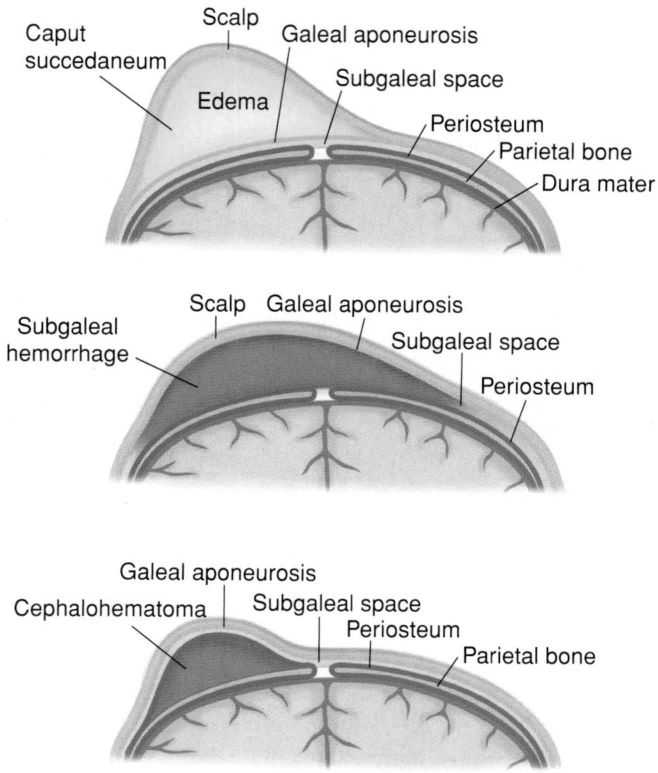

FIGURE 33-1 Schematic of extracranial lesions in the neonate.

sufficient to cause anemia. By contrast, with caput succedaneum, swelling of the scalp causes edema that overlies the periosteum. The caput is maximal at birth, rapidly grows smaller, and usually disappears within hours or a few days. Occasionally, it becomes infected, and abscess may form (Kersten, 2008).

Cephalohematomas are common, and in the study from Nova Scotia shown in Table 33-3, these accounted for 80 percent of traumatic injuries with an incidence of 16 per 1000 (Baskett, 2007). They rarely develop in the absence of birth trauma, and an 11-percent incidence was reported in 913 term infants delivered by vacuum extraction (Simonson, 2007). In the Network study of cesarean delivery outcomes cited above, the incidence of cephalohematoma was 2.4 per 1000 operations (Alexander, 2006). Others have reported lower incidences, although cephalohematoma is more common with vacuum compared with forceps deliveries—0.8 versus 2.7 per 1000 operative deliveries (Werner, 2011).

Subgaleal hemorrhage results from laceration of one of the emissary veins, with bleeding between the galea aponeurotica and the skull periosteum. Because of its loose areolar tissue and large surface area, significant blood volumes can collect in this potential space and can extend from the neck to the orbits and laterally to the temporal fascia above the ears. Resulting hypotension can lead to significant morbidity, and cited mortality rates range from 12 to 18 percent (Chang, 2007; Kilani, 2006).

Skull Fractures

These are rare but are especially worrisome because of their association with serious intracranial hemorrhages as discussed above. Volpe (1995) considers three types of skull injuries to be fractures—linear and depressed fractures and occipital osteodiastasis. In a French study of nearly 2 million deliveries from 1990 to 2000, the incidence of skull fractures was reported to be 3.7 per 100,000 births, and 75 percent were associated with operative vaginal deliveries (Dupuis, 2005). These are occasionally seen with spontaneous or cesarean delivery such as the depressed skull fracture shown in Figure 33-2. These latter fractures are more common when the head is tightly wedged in the pelvis. In such cases, there are at least three possible causes. A fracture may result from skull compression against the sacral promontory, by hand pressure used to lift the head at cesarean delivery, or from transvaginally applied upward hand pressure by an assistant. Fractures are managed with surgical decompression, although spontaneous resolution can follow (Basaldella, 2011).

Spinal Cord Injury

Overstretching of the spinal cord and associated hemorrhage and edema are rare injuries. They are usually caused by excessive longitudinal or lateral traction of the spine or by torsion during delivery. In some cases, there is fracture or dislocation of the vertebrae. Menticoglou and associates (1995) described 15 neonates with this type of high cervical spinal cord injury and found that all of the injuries were associated with forceps rotations. Spinal cord injury also can occur during breech delivery. Ross and coworkers (2006) described C_{5-6} vertebral dislocation associated with a Zavanelli maneuver done because of shoulder dystocia (Chap. 27, p. 544).

Peripheral Nerve Injuries

Traumatic injuries to nerves can be serious and distressing, especially if permanent. Injury can involve a single nerve, or it can affect a nerve root, plexus, or trunk (Volpe, 1995).

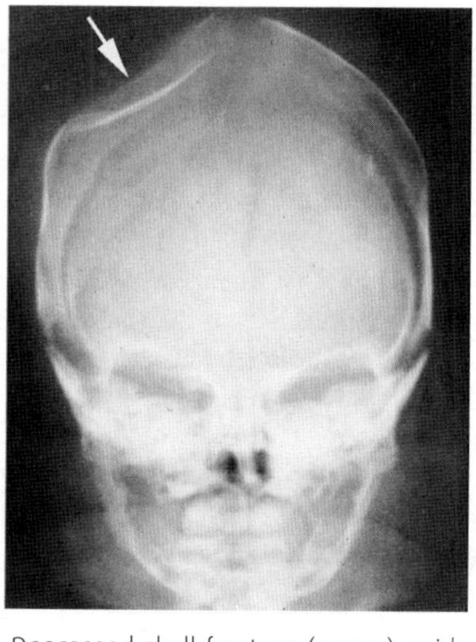

FIGURE 33-2 Depressed skull fracture (*arrow*) evident immediately after cesarean delivery. Labor had progressed, and the head was deep in the pelvis. Dislodgment of the head from the birth canal was performed by an assistant using manual pressure upward through the vagina.

Brachial Plexopathy

Injuries to the brachial plexus are relatively common. They are identified in 1 to 3 per 1000 term births (Baskett, 2007; Joyner, 2006; Lindqvist, 2012). In the study of more than 8 million singleton births reported by Moczygemba and colleagues (2010), the incidence of brachial nerve injury was 1.5 per 1000 vaginal deliveries and 0.17 per 1000 cesarean deliveries. Breech delivery and shoulder dystocia are risks for this trauma. However, severe plexopathy may also occur without risk factors or shoulder dystocia (Torki, 2012).

The injury with plexopathy is actually to the nerve roots that supply the brachial plexus—C_{5-8} and T_1. With hemorrhage and edema, axonal function may be temporarily impaired, but the recovery chances are good. However, with avulsion, the prognosis is poor. In 90 percent of cases, there is damage to the C_{5-6} nerve roots causing *Erb* or *Duchenne paralysis* (Volpe, 1995). Injuries with breech delivery are normally of this type, whereas the more extensive lesions follow difficult cephalic deliveries (Ubachs, 1995). The C_{5-6} roots join to form the upper trunk of the plexus, and injury leads to paralysis of the deltoid, infraspinatus, and flexor muscles of the forearm. The affected arm is held straight and internally rotated, the elbow is extended, and the wrist and fingers flexed. Finger function usually is retained. Because lateral head traction is frequently employed to effect delivery of the shoulders in normal vertex presentations, most cases of Erb paralysis follow deliveries that do not appear difficult. Damage to the C_8-T_1 roots supplying the lower plexus results in *Klumpke paralysis,* in which the hand is flaccid. Total involvement of all brachial plexus nerve roots results in flaccidity of the arm and hand, and with severe damage, there may also be *Horner syndrome.*

Unfortunately, as discussed in Chapter 27 (p. 541), shoulder dystocia cannot be accurately predicted. In most cases, axonal death does not occur and the prognosis is good. Lindqvist and associates (2012) reported complete recovery in 86 percent of children with C_{5-6} trauma, which was the most common injury, and in 38 percent of those with C_{5-7} damage. However, those with global C_{5-8}-T_1 injuries always had permanent disability. Surgical exploration and possible repair may improve function if there is persistent paralysis (Malessy, 2009).

Facial Paralysis

Trauma to the facial nerve commonly occurs as it emerges from the stylomastoid foramen, and this can cause facial paralysis (Fig. 33-3). The incidence, which ranges from 0.2 to 7.5 per 1000 term births, is likely influenced by the vigor with which the diagnosis is sought (Al Tawil, 2010; Moczygemba, 2010). Facial paralysis may be apparent at delivery or may develop shortly after birth. It most frequently is associated with uncomplicated vaginal delivery. However, in one series, a fourth of cases followed cesarean delivery (Alexander, 2006; Al Tawil, 2010; Moczygemba, 2010). Facial nerve damage is likely more common with low forceps (Hagadorn-Freathy, 1991; Levine, 1984). It is possible that damage is caused by pressure exerted by the posterior blade when forceps have been placed obliquely on the fetal head. In these cases, forceps marks indicate the cause of injury. Spontaneous recovery within a few days is the rule, however, permanent paralysis has been described (Al Tawil, 2010; Duval, 2009).

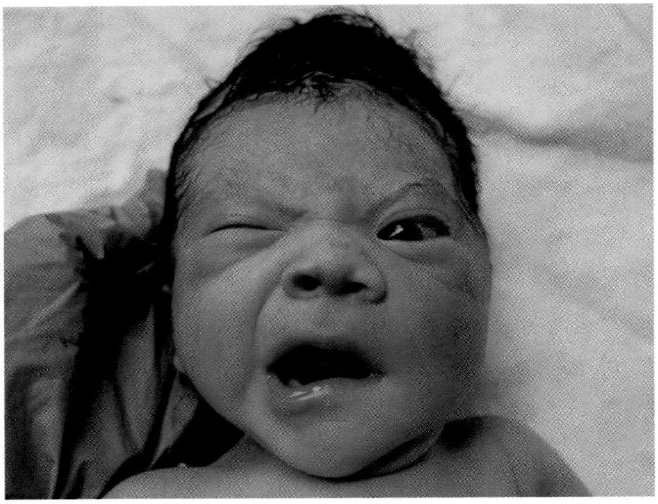

FIGURE 33-3 Left facial nerve injury. This was almost completely resolved two days after delivery.

Fractures

Most long-bone fractures follow difficult deliveries, however, this is not always the case. At minimum, palpation of the clavicles and long bones is indicated for all newborns after a difficult delivery. Crepitation or unusual irregularity should prompt radiographic examination.

Clavicular fractures are common, unpredictable, and unavoidable complications of normal birth. Their incidence averages 5 to 10 per 1000 live births (Linder, 2012; Moczygemba, 2010). Other than female gender, no specific risk factors—including birthweight and mode of delivery—have been identified.

Humeral fractures are infrequent, and 70 percent follow an uneventful birth (Turpenny, 1993). Others are associated with difficult delivery of the shoulders in cephalic deliveries and of an extended arm in breech deliveries. Radiographically, they are often of the greenstick type, although complete fracture with overriding bones can be seen. Sonography has also been used to confirm diagnosis (Sherr-Lurie, 2011).

Femoral fractures are relatively rare and usually are associated with vaginal breech delivery. They occasionally follow cesarean delivery, and in one report, they were bilateral (Cebesoy, 2009). Because most breech-presenting fetuses now undergo cesarean delivery, most of these fractures are associated with this mode (Alexander, 2006; Cebesoy, 2009).

Mandibular fractures have been reported, are rare, and have been reviewed by Vasconcelos and coworkers (2009). The rare cases of cervical vertebral dislocation in fetuses delivered as breech or after the Zavanelli maneuver are discussed above (Ross, 2006).

Muscle Injuries

Sternocleidomastoid muscle injury was usually seen with vaginal breech delivery (Roemer, 1954). Hematomas of the muscle or the fascial sheath may resolve slowly with cicatricial contraction. With normal neck growth, the less-elastic damaged muscle does not elongate appropriately. As a result, the head is gradually turned toward the side of the injury—*torticollis.*

Soft Tissue Injuries

Conceivably, any fetal organ or part could be injured with either vaginal or cesarean delivery. Some of these include subcapsular hepatic hematomas that presented as inguinal and scrotal hematoma. In such cases, ecchymoses of the inguinal region are termed *Stabler sign,* and those of the scrotum are termed *Bryant sign* (Heyman, 2011; Lee, 2011). Thymic gland traumatic hemorrhage in those with underlying hyperplasia or cyst has been described before, during, and after delivery (Eifinger, 2007; Saksenberg, 2001). Injuries to the sixth cranial nerve with resultant lateral rectus ocular muscle paralysis have also been reported following operative vaginal delivery (Galbraith, 1994).

Congenital Deformity Injuries

There are several injuries creating morphological defects that the fetus can sustain long before delivery. One is the amnionic band syndrome caused when a free strip of amnion forms a focal ring around an extremity or digit. Eventually, deformation or amputation may result. Occasionally, the amputated part may be found within the uterus. The genesis of such bands is debated and discussed in Chapter 6 (p. 121). A similar anomaly is a *limb-reduction defect* associated with chorionic villus sampling performed before 9 weeks' gestation as discussed in Chapter 14 (p. 300).

Various congenital postural anomalies form when a normally developed fetal structure becomes deformed by intrauterine mechanical factors. Examples of the latter include chronic oligohydramnios, restricted fetal movement imposed by an abnormally shaped or small uterine cavity, or by the presence of additional fetuses. Some mechanical deformations include talipes equinovarus (clubfoot), scoliosis, and hip dislocation (Miller, 1981). Talipes and other positional foot abnormalities are associated with membrane rupture from early amniocentesis between 11 and 13 weeks' gestation (Chap. 14, p. 299). Finally, somewhat related, hypoplastic lungs also can result from oligohydramnios (Chap. 11, p. 237).

REFERENCES

Ahlin K, Himmelmann K, Hagberg G, et al: Cerebral palsy and perinatal infection in children born at term. Obstet Gynecol 122:41, 2013

Akin MA, Coban D, Doganay S, et al: Intrahepatic and adrenal hemorrhage as a rare cause of neonatal anemia. J Perinat Med 39(3):353, 2011

Alexander JM, Leveno KJ, Hauth J, et al: Fetal injury associated with cesarean delivery. Obstet Gynecol 108:885, 2006

Al Tawil K, Saleem N, Kadri H, et al: Traumatic facial nerve palsy in newborns: is it always iatrogenic? Am J Perinatol 27:711, 2010

American Academy of Pediatrics and American College of Obstetricians and Gynecologists: Guidelines for perinatal care. 7th ed. Washington, 2012, p 301

American College of Obstetricians and Gynecologists: Intrapartum fetal heart rate monitoring: nomenclature, interpretation, and general management principles. Practice Bulletin No. 106, July 2009, Reaffirmed 2013a

American College of Obstetricians and Gynecologists: Management of delivery of a newborn with meconium-stained amnionic fluid. Committee Opinion No. 379, 2007, Reaffirmed 2013b

American College of Obstetricians and Gynecologists: Amnioinfusion does not prevent meconium aspiration syndrome. Committee Opinion No. 346, 2006, Reaffirmed 2012c

American College of Obstetricians and Gynecologists: Umbilical cord blood gas and acid-base analysis. Committee Opinion No. 348, November 2006, Reaffirmed 2012d

American College of Obstetricians and Gynecologists: Operative vaginal delivery. Practice Bulletin No. 17, June 2000, Reaffirmed 2012a

American College of Obstetricians and Gynecologists: Timing of cord clamping after birth. Committee Opinion No. 543. December 2012b

American College of Obstetricians and Gynecologists and American Academy of Pediatrics: Neonatal encephalopathy and cerebral palsy. Defining the pathogenesis and pathophysiology. Washington, January 2003

American College of Obstetricians and Gynecologists and American Academy of Pediatrics: Neonatal encephalopathy and neurologic outcome, 2nd ed. Washington, March 2014

Anadkat KS, Kuzniewicz MW, Chaudhari BP, et al: Increased risk for respiratory distress among white, male, late preterm and term infants. J Perinatol 32(10):750, 2012

Anderson C, Witter F, Graham E: Identification of neonates with hypoxic-ischemic encephalopathy (HIE) using debt-time, a measure of intrapartum electronic fetal heart rate (FHR). Abstract No. 749, Am J Obstet Gynecol 208(1 Suppl):S315, 2013

Avagliano L, Marconi AM, Candiani M, et al: Thrombosis of the umbilical vessels revisited. An observational study of 317 consecutive autopsies at a single institution. Hum Pathol 41:971, 2010

Azzopardi DV, Strohm B, Edwards AD, et al: Moderate hypothermia to treat perinatal asphyxial encephalopathy. N Engl J Med 361:1349, 2009

Barbu D, Mert I, Kruger M, et al: Evidence of fetal central nervous system injury in isolated congenital heart defects: microcephaly at birth. Am J Obstet Gynecol 201(1):43.e1, 2009

Basaldella L, Marton E, Bekelis K, et al: Spontaneous resolution of atraumatic intrauterine ping-pong fractures in newborns delivered by cesarean section. J Child Neurol 26:1149, 2011

Baskett TF, Allen VM, O'Connell CM, et al: Fetal trauma in term pregnancy. Am J Obstet Gynecol 197:499.e1, 2007

Bax M, Tydeman C, Flodmark O: Clinical and MRI correlates of cerebral palsy: the European cerebral palsy study. JAMA 296:1602, 2006

Bednarek N, Mathur A, Inder T, et al: Impact of therapeutic hypothermia on MRI diffusion changes in neonatal encephalopathy. Neurology 78:1420, 2012

Berthelot-Ricou A, Lacroze V, Courbiere B, et al: Respiratory distress syndrome after elective caesarean section in near term infants: a 5-year cohort study. J Matern Fetal Neonatal Med 26(2):176, 2012

Bhutani VK, Committee on Fetus and Newborn, American Academy of Pediatrics: Phototherapy to prevent severe neonatal hyperbilirubinemia in the newborn infant 35 or more weeks of gestation. Pediatrics 128(4):e1046, 2011

Blair E, de Groot JH, Nelson KD: Placental infarction identified by macroscopic examination and risk of cerebral palsy in infants at 35 weeks of gestational age and over. Am J Obstet Gynecol 205(2):124.e1, 2011

Bloom S, Ramin S, Neyman S, et al: Meconium stained amniotic fluid: is it associated with elevated erythropoietin levels? Am J Obstet Gynecol 174:360, 1996

Boyle CA, Boulet S, Schieve LA, et al: Trends in the prevalence of developmental disabilities in US children, 1997–2008. Pediatrics 127:1034, 2011

Bryne DL, Gau G: In utero meconium aspiration: an unpreventable cause of neonatal death. BJOG 94:813, 1987

Burke BL, Robbins JM, Bird TM, et al: Trends in hospitalizations for neonatal jaundice and kernicterus in the United States, 1988–2005. Pediatrics 123(2):524, 2009

Burke N, Field K, Mujahid F, et al: Use and safety of Kielland's forceps in current obstetric practice. Obstet Gynecol 120(4):766, 2012

Busfield A, Samuel R, McNinch A, et al: Vitamin K deficiency bleeding after NICE guidance and withdrawal of Konakion Neonatal: British Paediatric Surveillance Unit study, 2006–2008. Arch Dis Child 98:41, 2013

Casey BM, McIntire DD, Leveno KJ: The continuing value of the Apgar score for the assessment of newborn infants. N Engl J Med 344:467, 2001

Cebesoy FB, Cebesoy O, Incebiyik A: Bilateral femur fracture in a newborn: an extreme complication of cesarean delivery. Arch Gynecol Obstet 279:73, 2009

Centers for Disease Control and Prevention: Cerebral palsy occurrence in the US. National Center on Birth Defects and Developmental Disabilities, Health Communication Science Office. 2011. Available at: http://www.cdc.gov/Features/dsCerebralPalsy. Accessed June 6, 2013

Centers for Disease Control and Prevention: Key findings: trends in the prevalence of developmental disabilities in U.S. children 1997–2008. 2012. Available at: http://www.cdc.gov/ncbddd/features/birthdefects-dd-keyfindings.html. Accessed June 6, 2013

Chang HY, Peng CC, Kao HA, et al: Neonatal subgaleal hemorrhage: clinical presentation, treatment, and predictors of poor prognosis. Pediatr Int 49(6):903, 2007

Choi HJ, Hahn S, Lee J, et al: Surfactant lavage therapy for meconium aspiration syndrome: a systematic review and meta-analysis. Neonatology 101:183, 2012

Clark SL, Hankins GD: Temporal and demographic trends in cerebral palsy—fact and fiction. Am J Obstet Gynecol 188:628, 2003
Cox P, Silvestri E, Lazda E, et al: Embolism of brain tissue in intrapartum and early neonatal deaths: report of 9 cases. Pediatr Dev Pathol 12(6):464, 2009
Dargaville PA, Copnell B, Mills JF, et al: Randomized controlled trial of lunch lavage with dilute surfactant for meconium aspiration syndrome. J Pediatr 158(3):383, 2011
Davis PG, Dawson JA: New concepts in neonatal resuscitation. Curr Opin Pediatr 24(2):147, 2012
Davis RO, Phillips JB III, Harris BA Jr, et al: Fatal meconium aspiration syndrome occurring despite airway management considered appropriate. Am J Obstet Gynecol 141:731, 1985
DeJong EP Lindenburg IT, van Klink JM, et al: Intrauterine transfusion for parvovirus B19 infection: long term neurodevelopmental outcome. Am J Obstet Gynecol 206(3):204.e1, 2012
Devoe LD: Electronic fetal monitoring: does it really lead to better outcomes? Am J Obstet Gynecol 204(6):455, 2011
Dijk PH, Hulzebos C: An evidence-based view on hyperbilirubinaemia. Acta Paediatr Suppl 101(464):3, 2012
Dijxhoorn MJ, Visser GHA, Fidler VJ, et al: Apgar score, meconium and acidemia at birth in relation to neonatal neurological morbidity in term infants. Br J Obstet Gynaecol 86:217, 1986
Dooley SL, Pesavento DJ, Depp R, et al: Meconium below the vocal cords at delivery: correlation with intrapartum events. Am J Obstet Gynecol 153:767, 1985
Doumouchtsis SK, Arulkumaran S: Head trauma after instrumental births. Clin Perinatol 35:69, 2008
Dupuis O, Silveira R, Dupont C, et al: Comparison of "instrument-associated" and "spontaneous" obstetric depressed skull fractures in a cohort of 68 neonates. Am J Obstet Gynecol 192:165, 2005
Duval M, Daniel SJ: Facial nerve palsy in neonates secondary to forceps use. Arch Otolaryngol Head Neck Surg 135:634, 2009
Eggert LD, Wiedmeier SE, Wilson J, et al: The effect of instituting a prehospital-discharge newborn bilirubin screening program in an 18-hospital health system. Pediatrics 117:e855, 2006
Eifinger F, Ernestus K, Benz-Bohm G, et al: True thymic hyperplasia associated with severe thymic cyst bleeding in a newborn: a case report and review of the literature. Ann Diagn Pathol 11:358, 2007
Eissa DS, El-Farrash RA: New insights into thrombopoiesis in neonatal sepsis. Platelets 24(2):122, 2013
El Shahed AI, Dargaville P, Ohisson A, et al: Surfactant for meconium aspiration syndrome in full term/near term infants. Cochrane Database Syst Rev 3:CD002054, 2007
Ensing S, Abu-Hanna A, Schaaf J, et al: Trends in birth asphyxia among live born term singletons. Abstract No. 453, Am J Obstet Gynecol 208 (1 Suppl):S197, 2013
Fischer C, Rybakowski C, Ferdynus C, et al: A population-based study of meconium aspiration syndrome in neonates born between 37 and 43 weeks of gestation. Int J Pediatr 2012:321545, 2012
Fraser WD, Hofmeyr J, Lede R, et al: Amnioinfusion for the prevention of the meconium aspiration syndrome. Amnioinfusion Trial Group. N Engl J Med 353:909, 2005
Galbraith RS: Incidence of sixth nerve palsy in relation to mode of delivery. Am J Obstet Gynecol 170:1158, 1994
Garmany TH, Wambach JA, Heins HB, et al: Population and disease-based prevalence of the common mutations associated with surfactant deficiency. Pediatr Res 63(6):645, 2008
Gazzin S, Tiribelli C: Bilirubin-induced neurological damage. J Matern Fetal Neonatal Med 24:154, 2011
Gibson CS, MacLennan AH, Hague WM, et al: Associations between inherited thrombophilias, gestational age, and cerebral palsy. Am J Obstet Gynecol 193:1437, 2005
Gilbert WM, Jacoby BN, Xing G: Adverse obstetric events are associated with significant risk of cerebral palsy. Am J Obstet Gynecol 203:328, 2010
Gilstrap LC III, Leveno KJ, Burris J, et al: Diagnosis of asphyxia on the basis of fetal pH, Apgar score, and newborn cerebral dysfunction. Am J Obstet Gynecol 161:825, 1989
Glass HG, Hong KJ, Rogers EE, et al: Risk factors for epilepsy in children with neonatal encephalopathy. Pediatr Res 70(5):535, 2011
Goepfert AR, Goldenberg RL, Hauth JC, et al: Obstetrical determinants of neonatal neurological morbidity. Am J Obstet Gynecol 174:470, 1996
Goldaber KG, Gilstrap LC III, Leveno KJ, et al: Pathologic fetal acidemia. Obstet Gynecol 78:1103, 1991
Grünebaum A, McCullough LB, Sapra KJ, et al: Apgar score of 0 at 5 minutes and neonatal seizures or serious neurologic dysfunction in relation to birth setting. Am J Obstet Gynecol 200:323.e1, 2013
Guillet R, Edwards AD, Thoresen M, et al: Seven-to-eight year follow-up of the CoolCap trial of head cooling for neonatal encephalopathy. Pediatr Res 71(12):205, 2012
Gyamfi-Bannerman C, Gilbert S, Landon MB, et al: Effect of antenatal corticosteroids on respiratory morbidity in singletons after late-preterm birth. Obstet Gynecol 119:555, 2012
Hagadorn-Freathy AS, Yeomans ER, Hankins GD: Validation of the 1988 ACOG forceps classification system. Obstet Gynecol 77(3):356, 1991
Hankins GD, Koen S, Gei AF, et al: Neonatal organ system injury in acute birth asphyxia sufficient to result in neonatal encephalopathy. Obstet Gynecol 99:688, 2002
Hansen TWR: Prevention of neurodevelopmental sequelae of jaundice in the newborn. Dev Med Child Neurol 53(Suppl 4):24, 2011
Harrington DJ, Redman CW, Moulden M, et al: Long-term outcome in surviving infants with Apgar zero at 10 minutes: a systematic review of the literature and hospital-based cohort. Am J Obstet Gynecol 196:463, 2007
Harteman J, Groenendaal F, Benders M, et al: Role of thrombophilic factors in full-term infants with neonatal encephalopathy. Pediatr Res 73(1):80, 2013
Hartigan L, Hehir M, McHugh A, et al: Analysis of incidence and outcomes of umbilical cord prolapse over 20 years at a large tertiary referral center. Abstract No. 431, Am J Obstet Gynecol 208(1 Suppl):S188, 2013
Heyman S, Vervloessem D: Bryant's and Stabler's signs after a difficult delivery. N Engl J Med 365:1824, 2011
Huang AH, Robertson RL: Spontaneous superficial parenchymal and leptomeningeal hemorrhage in term neonates. AJNR Am J Neuroadiol 25(3): 469, 2004
Jacobs SE, Morley CJ, Inder TE, et al: Whole-body hypothermia for term and near-term newborns with hypoxic-ischemic encephalopathy: a randomized controlled trial. Arch Pediatr Adolesc Med 165(8):692, 2011
Johnson C, Burd I, Northington F, et al: Clinical chorioamnionitis is associated with a more severe metabolic acidosis in neonates with suspected hypoxic-ischemic encephalopathy. Am J Obstet Gynecol 210:S205, 2014
Joyner B, Soto MA, Adam HM: Brachial plexus injury. Pediatr Rev 27:238, 2006
Kaandorp J, Benders M, Schuit E, et al: Maternal allopurinol administration during term labor for neuroprotection in case of fetal asphyxia: a multicenter randomized controlled trial. Abstract No. 20, Am J Obstet Gynecol 208 (1 Suppl):S14, 2013
Kaplan M, Bromiker R, Hammerman C: Severe neonatal hyperbilirubinemia and kernicterus: are these still problems in the third millennium? Neonatology 100(4):354, 2011
Katz VL, Bowes WA Jr: Meconium aspiration syndrome: reflections on a murky subject. Am J Obstet Gynecol 166(1 Pt 1):171, 1992
Kersten CM, Moellering CM, Mato S: Spontaneous drainage of neonatal cephalohematoma: a delayed complication of scalp abscess. Clin Pediatr 47(2):183, 2008
Kilani RA, Wetmore J: Neonatal subgaleal hematoma: presentation and outcome—radiological findings and factors associated with mortality. Am J Perinatol 23(1):41, 2006
Kirton A, Armstrong-Wells J, Chang T, et al: Symptomatic neonatal arterial ischemic stroke: the International Pediatric Stroke Study. Pediatrics 128(6):e1402, 2011
Krakowiak P, Walker CK, Bremer AA, et al: Maternal metabolic conditions and risk for autism and other neurodevelopmental disorders. Pediatrics 129(5):1, 2012
Kuzniewicz M, Newman TB: Interaction of hemolysis and hyperbilirubinemia on neurodevelopmental outcomes in the collaborative perinatal project. Pediatrics 123(3):1045, 2009
Kwon JM, Guillet R, Shankaran S, et al: Clinical seizures in neonatal hypoxic-ischemic encephalopathy have no independent impact on neurodevelopmental outcome: secondary analyses of data from the neonatal research network hypothermia trial. J Child Neurol 26:322, 2011
Lee JH, Im SA: Neonatal subcapsular hepatic hematomas presenting as a scrotal wall hematoma. Pediatr Int 53:777, 2011
Leveno KJ, Quirk JG Jr, Cunningham FG, et al: Prolonged pregnancy. I. Observations concerning the causes of fetal distress. Am J Obstet Gynecol 150:465, 1984
Levine MG, Holroyde J, Woods JR, et al: Birth trauma: incidence and predisposing factors. Obstet Gynecol 63:792, 1984
Lindenburg IT, van Klink JM, Smits-Wintjens EHJ, et al: Long-term neurodevelopmental and cardiovascular outcome after intrauterine transfusions for fetal anaemia: a review. Prenat Diagn 33:815, 2013
Linder I, Melamed N, Kogan A, et al: Gender and birth trauma in full-term infants. J Matern Fetal Neonatal Med 25(9):1603, 2012
Lindqvist PG, Erichs K, Molnar C, et al: Characteristics and outcome of brachial plexus birth palsy in neonates. Acta Paediatr 101(6):579, 2012

Liu J, Shi Y, Dong JY, et al: Clinical characteristics, diagnosis and management of respiratory distress syndrome in full-term neonates. Clin Med J (Engl) 123:2640, 2010

Livinec F, Ancel PY, Marret S, et al: Prenatal risk factors for cerebral palsy in very preterm singletons and twins. Obstet Gynecol 105:1341, 2005

MacDonald D, Grant A, Sheridan-Pereira M, et al: The Dublin randomized controlled trial of intrapartum fetal heart rate monitoring. Am J Obstet Gynecol 152:524, 1985

Maisonneuve E, Audibert F, Guilbaud L, et al: Risk factors for severe neonatal acidosis. Obstet Gynecol 118(4):818, 2011

Malessy MJ, Pondaag W: Obstetric brachial plexus injuries. Neurosurg Clin North Am 20(1):1, 2009

Malin GL, Morris RK, Khan KS: Strength of association between umbilical cord pH and perinatal and long term outcomes: systematic review and meta-analysis. BMJ 340:c1471, 2010

Martinez-Biarge M, Madero R, Gonzalez A, et al: Perinatal morbidity and risk of hypoxic-ischemic encephalopathy associated with intrapartum sentinel events. Am J Obstet Gynecol 206(2):148, 2012

McDonald SJ, Middleton P: Effect of timing of umbilical cord clamping of term infants on maternal and neonatal outcomes. Cochrane Database Syst Rev 2:CD004074, 2008

McIntyre S, Blair E, Badawi N, et al: Antecedents of cerebral palsy and perinatal death in term and late pretem singletons. Obstet Gynecol 122:869, 2013

Melone PJ, Ernest JM, O'Shea MD Jr, et al: Appropriateness of intrapartum fetal heart rate management and risk of cerebral palsy. Am J Obstet Gynecol 165:272, 1991

Menticoglou SM, Perlman M, Manning FA: High cervical spinal cord injury in neonates delivered with forceps: report of 15 cases. Obstet Gynecol 86:589, 1995

Miller ME, Graham JM Jr, Higginbottom MC, et al: Compression-related defects from early amnion rupture: evidence for mechanical teratogenesis. J Pediatr 98:292, 1981

Moczygemba CK, Paramsothy P, Meikle S, et al: Route of delivery and neonatal birth trauma. Am J Obstet Gynecol 202(4):361.e1, 2010

Moster D, Lie RT, Irgens LM: The association of the Apgar score with subsequent death and cerebral palsy: a population-based study in term infants. J Pediatr 138(6):798, 2001

Moster D, Lie RT, Markestad T: Long-term medical and social consequences of preterm birth. N Engl J Med 359:262, 2008

Nathan L, Leveno KJ, Carmody TJ III, et al: Meconium: a 1990s perspective on an old obstetric hazard. Obstet Gynecol 83(3):329, 1994

Nelson DB, Lucke AM, McIntire DD, et al: Obstetric antecedents to body cooling treatment of the newborn infant. Am J Obstet Gynecol, In press, 2014

Nelson KB, Bingham P, Edwards EM, et al: Antecedents of neonatal encephalopathy in the Vermont Oxford network encephalopathy registry. Pediatrics 130(5):878, 2012

Nelson KB, Dambrosia JM, Ting TY, et al: Uncertain value of electronic fetal monitoring in predicting cerebral palsy. N Engl J Med 334:613, 1996

Nelson KB, Ellenberg JH: Antecedents of cerebral palsy: multivariate analysis of risk. N Engl J Med 315:81, 1986a

Nelson KB, Ellenberg JH: Antecedents of cerebral palsy: univariate analysis of risks. Am J Dis Child 139:1031, 1985

Nelson KB, Ellenberg JH: Antecedents of seizure disorders in early childhood. Am J Dis Child 140:1053, 1986b

Nelson KB, Ellenberg JH: Obstetric complications as risk factors for cerebral palsy or seizure disorders. JAMA 251:1843, 1984

Nelson KB, Grether JK: Potentially asphyxiating conditions and spastic cerebral palsy in infants of normal birth weight. Am J Obstet Gynecol 179:507, 1998

Newman TB, Liljestrand P, Jeremy RJ, et al: Outcomes among newborns with total serum bilirubin levels of 25 mg per deciliter or more. N Engl J Med 354:1889, 2006

O'Callaghan M, MacLennan A: Cesarean delivery and cerebral palsy: a systematic review and meta-analysis. Obstet Gynecol 122:1169, 2013

O'Callaghan ME, MacLennan AH, Gibson CS, et al: Epidemiologic associations with cerebral palsy. Obstet Gynecol 118(3):576, 2011

O'Leary CM, Watson L, D'Antoine H, et al: Heavy maternal alcohol consumption and cerebral palsy in the offspring. Dec Med Child Neurol 54: 224, 2012

Perlman JM, Wyllie J, Kattwinkel J, et al: Part 11: Neonatal resuscitation. 2010 International Consensus on Cardiopulmonary Resuscitation and Emergency Cardiovascular Care Science with Treatment Recommendations. Circulation 122:S516, 2010

Pfister RH, Soll RF: Hypothermia for the treatment of infants with hypoxic-ischemic encephalopathy. J Perinatol 30(Suppl):S82, 2010

Phelan JP, Ahn MO: Perinatal observations in forty-eight neurologically impaired term infants. Am J Obstet Gynecol 171:424, 1994

Phelan JP, Ahn MO, Korst L, et al: Is intrapartum fetal brain injury in the term fetus preventable? Am J Obstet Gynecol 174:318, 1996

Phelan JP, Korst LM, Martin GI: Application of criteria developed by the Task Force on Neonatal Encephalopathy and Cerebral Palsy to acutely asphyxiated neonates. Obstet Gynecol 118(4):824, 2011

Plevani C, Pozzi I, Locatelli A, et al: Risk factors of neurological damage in infants with asphyxia. Abstract No. 414, Am J Obstet Gynecol 208(1 Suppl):S182, 2013

Pritchard JA, Cunningham FG, Pritchard SA, et al: How often does maternal preeclampsia–eclampsia incite thrombocytopenia in the fetus? Obstet Gynecol 69:292, 1987

Redline RW: Placental pathology: a systematic approach with clinical correlations. Placenta 22:S86, 2008

Redline RW: Severe fetal placental vascular lesions in term infants with neurologic impairment. Am J Obstet Gynecol 192:452, 2005

Ramachandrappa A, Rosenberg ES, Wagoner S, et al: Morbidity and mortality in late preterm infants with severe hypoxic respiratory failure on extracorporeal membrane oxygenation. J Pediatr 159(2):192, 2011

Richey S, Ramin SM, Bawdon RE, et al: Markers of acute and chronic asphyxia in infants with meconium-stained amniotic fluid. Am J Obstet Gynecol 172:1212, 1995

Robinson MN, Peake LJ, Ditchfield MR, et al: Magnetic resonance imaging findings in a population-based cohort of children with cerebral palsy. Dev Med Child Neurol 51(1):39, 2008

Roemer RJ: Relation of torticollis to breech delivery. Am J Obstet Gynecol 67:1146, 1954

Ross MG, Beall MH: Cervical neck dislocation associated with the Zavanelli maneuver. Obstet Gynecol 108:737, 2006

Rossi AC, Vanderbilt D, Chmait RH: Neurodevelopmental outcomes after laser therapy for twin-twin transfusion syndrome: a systematic review and meta-analysis. Obstet Gynecol 118(5):1145, 2011

Rutherford MA, Ramenghi LA, Cowan FM: Neonatal stroke. Arch Dis Child Fetal Neonatal Ed 97(5):F377, 2012

Saksenberg V, Bauch B, Reznik S: Massive acute thymic haemorrhage and cerebral haemorrhage in an intrauterine fetal death. J Clin Pathol 54:796, 2001

Sallmon H, Sola-Visner M: Clinical and research issues in neonatal anemia and thrombocytopenia. Curr Opin Pediatr 24(1):16, 2012

Scheibl A, Calderon EM, Borau MJ, et al: Epidural hematoma. J Pediatr Surg 47(2):e19, 2012

Sgro M, Campbell D, Barozzino T, et al: Acute neurological findings in a national cohort of neonates with severe neonatal hyperbilirubinemia. J Perinatol 31(6):392, 2011

Shankaran S, Branes PD, Hintz SR. et al: Brain injury following trial of hypothermia for neonatal hypoxic-ischaemic encephalopathy. Arch Dis Child Fetal Neonatal Ed 97(6):F398, 2012

Shankaran S, Laptook AR, Ehrenkranz RA, et al: Whole-body hypothermia for neonates with hypoxic-ischemic encephalopathy. N Engl J Med 353:1574, 2005

Shatrov JG, Birch SC, Lam FT, et al: Chorioamnionitis and cerebral palsy: a meta-analysis. Obstet Gynecol 116:387, 2010

Sherr-Lurie N, Bialik GM, Ganel A, et al: Fractures of the humerus in the neonatal period. Isr Med Assoc J 13(6):363, 2011

Silva AM, Smith RN, Lehmann CU, et al: Neonatal nucleated red blood cells and the prediction of cerebral white matter injury in preterm infants. Obstet Gynecol 107:550, 2006

Simonson C, Barlow P, Dehennin N, et al: Neonatal complications of vacuum-assisted delivery. Obstet Gynecol 110:189, 2007

Singh BS, Clark RH, Powers RJ, et al: Meconium aspiration syndrome remains a significant problem in the NICU: outcomes and treatment patterns in term neonates admitted for intensive care during a ten-year period. J Perinatol 29(7):497, 2009

Spong CY, Ogundipe OA, Ross MG: Prophylactic amnioinfusion for meconium stained amniotic fluid. Am J Obstet Gynecol 171:931, 1994

Spruijt M, Steggerda S, Rath M, et al: Cerebral injury in twin-twin transfusion syndrome treated with fetoscopic laser surgery. Obstet Gynecol 120(1):15, 2012

Stanley FJ, Blair E: Why have we failed to reduce the frequency of cerebral palsy? Med J Aust 154:623, 1991

Stoknes M, Andersen GL, Dahlseng MO, et al: Cerebral palsy and neonatal death in term singletons born small for gestational age. Pediatrics 130(6):e1629, 2012

Strijbis EM, Oudman I, van Essen P, et al: Cerebral palsy and the application of the international criteria for acute intrapartum hypoxia. Obstet Gynecol 107:1357, 2006

Stuart A, Olausson PO, Kallen K: Apgar scores at 5 minutes after birth in relation to school performance at 16 years of age. Obstet Gynecol 118 (2 Pt 1):201, 2011

Swanson AE, Veldman A, Wallace EM, et al: Subgaleal hemorrhage: risk factors and outcomes. Acta Obstet Gynecol Scand 91(2):260, 2012

Swarnam K, Soraisham AS, Sivanandan S: Advances in the management of meconium aspiration syndrome. Int J Pediatr 2012:359571, 2012

Tagin MA, Woolcott CG, Vincer MJ, et al: Hypothermia for neonatal hypoxic ischemic encephalopathy: an updated systematic review and meta-analysis. Arch Pediatr Adolesc Med 166(6):558, 2012

Takenouchi T, Kasdorf E, Engel M, et al: Changing pattern of perinatal brain injury in term infants in recent years. Pediatr Neurol 46(2):106, 2012

Thacker SB, Stroup DF, Peterson HB: Efficacy and safety of intrapartum electronic fetal monitoring: an update. Obstet Gynecol 86:613, 1995

Thorngren-Jerneck K, Herbst A: Perinatal factors associated with cerebral palsy in children born in Sweden. Obstet Gynecol 108:1499, 2006

Torfs CP, van den Berg B, Oechsli FW, et al: Prenatal and perinatal factors in the etiology of cerebral palsy. J Pediatr 116:615, 1990

Torki M, Barton L, Miller D, et al: Severe brachial plexus palsy in women without shoulder dystocia. Obstet Gynecol 120(3):539, 2012

Turpenny PD, Nimmo A: Fractured clavicle of the newborn in a population with a high prevalence of grand-multiparity: analysis of 78 consecutive cases. Br J Obstet Gynaecol 100:338, 1993

Ubachs JMH, Slooff ACJ, Peeters LLH: Obstetric antecedents of surgically treated obstetric brachial plexus injuries. Br J Obstet Gynaecol 102:813, 1995

Vain NE, Szyld EG, Prudent LM, et al: Oropharyngeal and nasopharyngeal suctioning of meconium-stained neonates before delivery of their shoulders: multicentre, randomized controlled trial. Lancet 364:597, 2004

Vandborg PK, Hansen BM, Greisen G, et al: Follow-up of neonates with total serum bilirubin levels ≥ 25 mg/dL: a Danish population-based study. Pediatrics 130(1):61, 2012

Vasconcelos BC, Lago CA, Nogueira RV, et al: Mandibular fracture in a premature infant: a case report and review of the literature. J Oral Maxillofac Surg 67(1):218, 2009

Volpe JJ: Neurology of the Newborn, 3rd ed. Philadelphia, Saunders, 1995, p 373

Walsh B, Boylan G, Dempsey E, et al: Association of nucleated red blood cells and severity of encephalopathy in normothermic and hypothermic infants. Acta Paediatr 102(2):e64, 2013

Walsh BH, Bovian GB, Murray DM: Nucleated red blood cells and early EEG: predicting Sarnat stage and two year outcome. Early Hum Dev 87(5):335, 2011

Wambach JA, Wegner DJ, Depass K, et al: Single ABCA3 mutations increase risk for neonatal respiratory distress syndrome. Pediatrics 130(6):e1575, 2012

Watchko JF, Tiribelli C: Bilirubin-induced neurologic damage--mechanisms and management approaches. N Engl J Med 369:21, 2013

Wayock C, Greenberg B, Jennings J, et al: Perinatal risk factors for severe hypoxic-ischemic encephalopathy in neonates treated with whole body hypothermia. Abstract No. 176, Am J Obstet Gynecol 208(1 Suppl):S76, 2013

Wenstrom KD, Andrews WW, Maher JE: Amnioinfusion survey: prevalence, protocols, and complications. Obstet Gynecol 86:572, 1995

Werner EF, Janevic TM, Illuzzi J, et al: Mode of delivery in nulliparous women and neonatal intracranial injury. Obstet Gynecol 118(6):1239, 2011

Whitby EH, Griffiths PD, Rutter S, et al: Frequency and natural history of subdural haemorrhages in babies and relation to obstetrical factors. Lancet 363:846, 2004

Wiberg N, Kallen K, Herbst A, et al: Relation between umbilical cord blood pH, base deficit, lactate, 5-minute Apgar score and development of hypoxic ischemic encephalopathy. Acta Obstet Gynecol Scand 89:1263, 2010

Wiklund LM, Uvebrant P, Flodmark O: Computed tomography as an adjunct in etiological analysis of hemiplegic cerebral palsy, 1. Children born preterm. Neuropediatrics 22:50, 1991a

Wiklund LM, Uvebrant P, Flodmark O: Computed tomography as an adjunct in etiological analysis of hemiplegic cerebral palsy, 2. Children born at term. Neuropediatrics 22:121, 1991b

Williams, JW: Obstetrics: a Text-book for the Use of Students and Practitioners. New York, Appleton, 1903

Wiswell TE, Tuggle JM, Turner BS: Meconium aspiration syndrome: have we made a difference? Pediatrics 85:715, 1990

Wu YW, Bauer LA, Ballard RA, et al: Erythropoietin for neuroprotection in neonatal encephalopathy: safety and pharmacokinetics. Pediatrics 130(4):683, 2012

Wu YW, Croen LA, Shah SJ, et al: Cerebral palsy in a term population: risk factors and neuroimaging findings. Pediatrics 118:691, 2006

Wu YW, Pham TN, Danielsen B, et al: Nighttime delivery and risk of neonatal encephalopathy. Am J Obstet Gynecol 204(1):37.e1, 2011

Yeh P, Emary K, Impey L: The relationship between umbilical cord arterial pH and serious adverse neonatal outcome: analysis of 51,519 consecutive validated samples. BJOG 119(7):824, 2012

Zipursky A: Prevention of vitamin K deficiency bleeding in newborns. Br J Haematol 104:430, 1999

CHAPTER 34

The Preterm Newborn

The preterm infant is susceptible to various serious medical complications during the newborn period as well as morbidities extending later into life (Table 34-1). These complications are primarily the consequence of immature organs that result from abbreviated gestation. A less commonly cited cause of morbidity and mortality is congenital malformations, which are much more prevalent in preterm births. For example, between 2010 and 2013 at Parkland Hospital, major malformations were diagnosed in 67 per 1000 singleton births < 37 weeks' gestation. This compared with 15 per 1000 in those ≥ 38 weeks—an almost fivefold excess. The pivotal complication, however, is *respiratory distress syndrome (RDS)*. This results from immature lungs that are unable to sustain necessary oxygenation. Resulting hypoxia is an underlying associated cause of neurological damage such as cerebral palsy. In addition, hyperoxia, a side effect of RDS treatment, causes bronchopulmonary dysplasia and retinopathy of prematurity. These complications of prematurity can be placed in perspective in terms of the *human consequences.* In 2009, two thirds of all infant deaths in the United States were in the 12 percent of infants who were born < 37 weeks (Mathews, 2013).

RESPIRATORY DISTRESS SYNDROME

To provide blood gas exchange immediately following delivery, the lungs must rapidly fill with air while being cleared of fluid. Concurrently, pulmonary arterial blood flow must increase remarkably. Some of the fluid is expressed as the chest is compressed during vaginal delivery, and the remainder is absorbed through the pulmonary lymphatics. Sufficient surfactant, synthesized by type II pneumocytes, is essential to stabilize the air-expanded alveoli. It lowers surface tension and thereby prevents lung collapse during expiration (Chap. 7, p. 142). If surfactant is inadequate, hyaline membranes form in the distal bronchioles and alveoli, and RDS develops. Although respiratory insufficiency is generally a disease of preterm neonates, it does develop in term newborns, especially with sepsis or meconium aspiration.

Clinical Course

In typical RDS, tachypnea develops, the chest wall retracts, and expiration is accompanied by *grunting* and *nostril flaring.* Shunting of blood through nonventilated lung contributes to hypoxemia and metabolic and respiratory acidosis. Poor peripheral circulation and systemic hypotension may be evident. The chest radiograph shows a diffuse reticulogranular infiltrate and an air-filled tracheobronchial tree—*air bronchogram.*

As discussed further in Chapter 33 (p. 637), respiratory insufficiency can also be caused by sepsis, pneumonia, meconium aspiration, pneumothorax, persistent fetal circulation, heart failure, and malformations involving thoracic structures, such as diaphragmatic hernia. Evidence is also accruing that common mutations in surfactant protein production may cause RDS (Garmany, 2008; Shulenin, 2004).

TABLE 34-1. Complications of Prematurity

Respiratory distress syndrome (RDS, HMD)
Bronchopulmonary dysplasia (BPD)
Pneumothorax
Pneumonia/sepsis
Patent ductus arteriosus (PDA)
Necrotizing enterocolitis (NEC)
Retinopathy of prematurity (ROP)
Intraventricular hemorrhage (IVH)
Periventricular leukomalacia (PVL)
Cerebral palsy (CP)

HMD = hyaline membrane disease.

Pathology

With inadequate surfactant, alveoli are unstable, and low pressures cause collapse at end expiration. Pneumocyte nutrition is compromised by hypoxia and systemic hypotension. Partial persistence of the fetal circulation may lead to pulmonary hypertension and a relative right-to-left shunt. Eventually, alveolar cells undergo ischemic necrosis. When oxygen therapy is initiated, the pulmonary vascular bed dilates, and the shunt reverses. Protein-filled fluid leaks into the alveolar ducts, and the cells lining the ducts slough. Hyaline membranes composed of fibrin-rich protein and cellular debris line the dilated alveoli and terminal bronchioles. The epithelium underlying the membrane becomes necrotic. With hematoxylin-eosin staining, these membranes appear amorphous and eosinophilic, like hyaline cartilage. Because of this, respiratory distress in the newborn is also termed *hyaline membrane disease.*

Treatment

The most important factor influencing survival is neonatal intensive care. Although hypoxemia prompts supplemental oxygen, excess oxygen can damage the pulmonary epithelium and the retina. However, advances in mechanical ventilation technology have improved neonatal survival rates. For example, *continuous positive airway pressure (CPAP)* prevents the collapse of unstable alveoli. This allows high inspired-oxygen concentrations to be reduced, thereby minimizing its toxicity. Disadvantages include overstretch of the endothelium and epithelium, which results in barotrauma and impaired venous return (Verbrugge, 1999). *High-frequency oscillatory ventilation* may reduce the barotrauma risk by using a constant, low-distending pressure and small oscillations to promote alveolar patency. This technique allows optimal lung volume to be maintained and carbon dioxide to be cleared without damaging alveoli. Although mechanical ventilation has undoubtedly improved survival rates, it is also an important factor in the genesis of chronic lung disease—*bronchopulmonary dysplasia.*

Treatment of the ventilator-dependent neonate with *glucocorticoids* was used previously to prevent chronic lung disease. The American Academy of Pediatrics now recommends against their use because of limited benefits and increased adverse neuropsychological effects (Watterberg, 2010). Yeh and colleagues (2004) described significantly impaired motor and cognitive function and school performance in exposed neonates. A review by Halliday and associates (2009) supports late postnatal corticosteroid treatment only for infants who could not be weaned from mechanical ventilation. In some studies, *inhaled nitric oxide* was shown to be associated with improved outcomes for neonates undergoing mechanical ventilation (Ballard, 2006; Kinsella, 2006; Mestan, 2005). Other studies showed no benefits (van Meurs, 2005). Currently, such treatment is considered investigational (Chock, 2009; Stark, 2006).

Surfactant Prophylaxis

Exogenous surfactant products can prevent RDS. They contain biological or animal surfactants such as bovine—*Survanta,* calf—*Infasurf,* porcine—*Curosurf,* or synthetic—*Exosurf.* Lucinactant—*Surfaxin R*—is a synthetic form that contains sinulpeptide KL4 to diminish lung inflammation (Zhu, 2008). In a Cochrane review, Pfister and coworkers (2007) found that animal-derived and synthetic surfactants were comparable.

Surfactant therapy has been credited with the largest drop in infant mortality rates observed in 25 years (Jobe, 1993). It has been used for *prophylaxis* of preterm, at-risk newborns and for *rescue* of those with established disease. Given together, antenatal corticosteroids and surfactant result in an even greater reduction in the overall death rate. In their review, Seger and Soll (2009) found that infants who received prophylactic surfactant had decreased risks of pneumothorax, pulmonary interstitial emphysema, bronchopulmonary dysplasia, and mortality.

Complications

Persistent hyperoxia injures the lung, especially the alveoli and capillaries. High oxygen concentrations given at high pressures can cause *bronchopulmonary dysplasia.* With this, alveolar and bronchiolar epithelial damage leads to hypoxia, hypercarbia, and chronic oxygen dependence from peribronchial and interstitial fibrosis. According to Baraldi and Filippone (2007), most cases are now seen in infants born before 30 weeks' gestation and represent a developmental disorder secondary to alveolarization injury. Severe disease and death rates are decreasing, however, long-term pulmonary dysfunction is encountered later. *Pulmonary hypertension* is another frequent complication. If hyperoxemia is sustained, the infant also is at risk of developing *retinopathy of prematurity,* formerly called *retrolental fibroplasia* (p. 656). When any of these develop, the likelihood of subsequent neurosensory impairment is substantively increased (Schmidt, 2003).

Prevention

Antenatal Corticosteroids

The National Institutes of Health (1994, 2000) concluded that a single course of antenatal corticosteroid therapy reduced respiratory distress and intraventricular hemorrhage in preterm infants born between 24 and 34 weeks (p. 657). The

American College of Obstetricians and Gynecologists and American Academy of Pediatrics (2012) considers all women at risk for preterm birth in this gestational-age range to be potential candidates for therapy. This is discussed further is Chapter 42 (p. 850). After 34 weeks, approximately 4 percent of infants develop respiratory distress syndrome (Consortium on Safe Labor, 2010).

Amniocentesis for Fetal Lung Maturity

Delivery for fetal indications is necessary when the risks to the fetus from a hostile intrauterine environment are greater than the risk of severe neonatal problems, even if the fetus is preterm. If this degree of risk is absent and the criteria for elective delivery at term are not met, then amniocentesis and amnionic fluid analysis can be used to confirm fetal lung maturity. To accomplish this, there are several methods to determine the relative concentration of surfactant-active phospholipids in amnionic fluid. Fluid acquisition is similar to that described for second-trimester amniocentesis (Chap. 16, p. 297). With this sampling, complications requiring urgent delivery arise in up to 1 percent of procedures (American College of Obstetricians and Gynecologists, 2008). Following analysis, the probability of respiratory distress developing in a given infant depends on the test used and fetal gestational age. Importantly, administration of corticosteroids to induce pulmonary maturation has variable effects on some of these tests.

Lecithin–Sphingomyelin (L/S) Ratio. Although not used nearly as much as in the past, the labor-intensive *L/S ratio* for many years was the gold-standard test. Dipalmitoylphosphatidylcholine (DPPC), that is, lecithin—along with phosphatidylinositol and especially phosphatidylglycerol (PG)—is an important component of the surface-active layer that prevents alveolar collapse (Chap. 32, p. 624). Before 34 weeks, lecithin and sphingomyelin are present in amnionic fluid in similar concentrations. At 32 to 34 weeks, the concentration of lecithin relative to sphingomyelin begins to rise (Fig. 34-1).

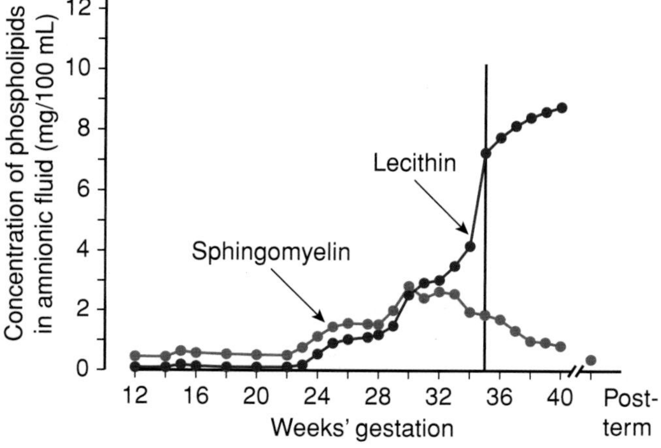

FIGURE 34-1 Changes in mean concentrations of lecithin and sphingomyelin in amnionic fluid during gestation in normal pregnancy. (Redrawn from Gluck, 1973, with permission.)

Gluck (1971) reported that the risk of neonatal respiratory distress is slight whenever the concentration of lecithin is at least twice that of sphingomyelin—the L/S ratio. Conversely, there is increased risk of respiratory distress when this ratio is < 2. Because lecithin and sphingomyelin are found in blood and meconium, contamination with these substances may falsely lower a mature L/S ratio.

Phosphatidylglycerol. Previously, respiratory distress was thought to develop despite an L/S ratio > 2 in infants of women with diabetes. Some recommend that phosphatidylglycerol be documented in amnionic fluid of these women. Based on current evidence, it is unclear if either diabetes, per se, or its level of control causes false-positive phospholipid test results for fetal lung maturity (American College of Obstetricians and Gynecologists, 2008).

Fluorescence Polarization. This automated assay measures the surfactant-to-albumin ratio in uncentrifuged amnionic fluid and gives results in approximately 30 minutes. A ratio of ≥ 50 with the commercially available *TDx-FLM* test predicted fetal lung maturity in 100 percent of cases (Steinfeld, 1992). Subsequent investigators found the TDx-FLM to be equal or superior to the L/S ratio, foam stability index, or phosphatidylglycerol assessment, including testing in diabetic pregnancies (Eriksen, 1996; Karcher, 2005). The recently modified *TDx-FLM II* is used by many hospitals as their primary test of pulmonary maturity, with a threshold ratio of 55 mg/g.

Other Tests. The *foam stability* or *shake test* depends on the ability of surfactant in amnionic fluid, when mixed appropriately with ethanol, to generate stable foam at the air–liquid interface (Clements, 1972). Problems include errors caused by slight contamination and frequent false-negative test results. Alternatively, the *Lumadex-FSI test, fluorescent polarization (microviscometry),* and *amnionic fluid absorbance at 650-nm wavelength* have all been used with variable success. The *lamellar body count* is a rapid, simple, and accurate method of assessing fetal lung maturity and is comparable to TDx-FLM and L/S ratio (Karcher, 2005).

NECROTIZING ENTEROCOLITIS

This newborn bowel disorder has clinical findings of abdominal distention, ileus, and bloody stools. There is usually radiological evidence of *pneumatosis intestinalis*—bowel wall gas derived from invading bacteria. Bowel perforation may prompt resection. Necrotizing enterocolitis is seen primarily in low-birthweight newborns but occasionally is encountered in mature neonates. Various hypothesized causes include perinatal hypotension, hypoxia, sepsis, umbilical catheterization, exchange transfusions, and the feeding of cow milk and hypertonic solutions (Kliegman, 1984). All of these can ultimately lead to intestinal ischemia, and reperfusion injury likely also has a role (Czyrko, 1991). The unifying hypothesis for these pathological processes is the uncontrolled inflammatory response to bacterial colonization of the preterm intestine (Grave, 2007).

Treatment for necrotizing enterocolitis is controversial (van Vliet, 2013). A randomized trial of laparotomy versus peritoneal drainage found no difference in survival rates in preterm infants (Moss, 2006). In an observational study, however, Blakely (2006) found that death rates and neurodevelopmental outcomes assessed at 18 to 22 months were more favorable with laparotomy compared with drainage.

RETINOPATHY OF PREMATURITY

Formerly known as *retrolental fibroplasia,* by 1950, retinopathy of prematurity had become the largest single cause of blindness in this country. After the discovery that the disease resulted from hyperoxemia, its frequency decreased remarkably. The fetal retina vascularizes centrifugally from the optic nerve starting at approximately the fourth month and continues until shortly after birth. During vascularization, excessive oxygen induces severe retinal vasoconstriction with endothelial damage and vessel obliteration, especially in the temporal portion. Neovascularization results, and the new vessels penetrate the retina and extend into the vitreous. Here, they are prone to leak proteins or burst with subsequent hemorrhage. Adhesions then form, which detach the retina.

Precise levels of hyperoxemia that can be sustained without causing retinopathy are not known. Preterm birth results in a "relative" hyperoxia compared with in utero oxygen content even in infants not exposed to higher FiO_2. To better understand the oxygen saturation threshold necessary to minimize retinopathy without increasing other adverse outcomes, the National Institute of Child Health and Human Development (NICHD) Neonatal Network performed a randomized trial of oxygenation in 1316 infants born between 24 and 27 weeks (SUPPORT Study Group, 2010). The target range of oxygen saturation was 85 to 89 percent in one arm of this trial and 91 to 95 percent in the other arm. Death before discharge occurred significantly more frequently in the lower-oxygen saturation group—20 versus 16 percent. However, severe retinopathy among survivors developed significantly less often in the lower-oxygen saturation group—8.6 versus 17.9 percent. This study generated considerable controversy as to whether the consent process was adequate for a trial with such end points (Drazen, 2013).

BRAIN DISORDERS

Central nervous system injury in preterm infants usually creates different neuroanatomical sequelae compared with that in term infants (Chap. 33, p. 639). In preterm infants, cerebral lesions detected by neuroimaging include intraventricular hemorrhage, periventricular hemorrhagic infarction, cystic periventricular leukomalacia, and diffuse white matter injury. All of these are strongly associated with adverse neurodevelopmental outcome. Locatelli and colleagues (2010) found a significantly increased incidence of neurological damage in preterm infants who had periventricular hemorrhage, periventricular leukomalacia, or both.

Cranial sonography remains the preferred approach for detecting frequently occurring brain abnormalities and acute events. It is readily available and reliable for detecting common abnormalities and monitoring brain growth. Because cystic injuries may take 2 to 5 weeks to evolve, serial scans are obtained during this time. In infants whose findings are transient and resolve in the neonatal period, prognosis is improved compared with those whose lesions remain and evolve. At the same time, however, between 4 and 10 percent of prematurely born children may develop cerebral palsy in the absence of lesions. Put another way, 90 to 96 percent of preterm infants with cerebral palsy have cerebral lesions that are detectable using cranial sonography.

Intracranial Hemorrhage

There are four major categories of intracranial hemorrhage in the neonate (Volpe, 1995). *Subdural hemorrhage* is usually the result of trauma. *Subarachnoid hemorrhage* and *intracerebellar hemorrhage* usually result from trauma in term infants and hypoxia in preterm infants. *Periventricular-intraventricular hemorrhage* results from either trauma or asphyxia in half of term infants and has no discernible cause in a fourth. In preterm neonates, the pathogenesis of periventricular hemorrhage is multifactorial and includes hypoxic-ischemic events, anatomical factors, coagulopathy, and many others. The prognosis after hemorrhage depends on its location and extent. For example, subdural and subarachnoid hemorrhage often result in minimal, if any, neurological abnormalities. Bleeding into the parenchyma, however, can cause serious permanent damage.

Periventricular-Intraventricular Hemorrhage

When the fragile capillaries in the germinal matrix rupture, there is bleeding into surrounding tissues that may extend into the ventricular system and brain parenchyma. This type of hemorrhage is common in preterm neonates, especially those born before 32 weeks. However, it can also develop at later gestational ages and even in term neonates. Most hemorrhages develop within 72 hours of birth, but they have been observed as late as 24 days (Perlman, 1986). Because intraventricular hemorrhage usually is recognized within 3 days of delivery, its genesis is often erroneously attributed to birth events. It is important to realize that *prelabor* intraventricular hemorrhage also can occur (Achiron, 1993; Nores, 1996).

Almost half of hemorrhages are clinically silent, and most small germinal matrix hemorrhages and those confined to the cerebral ventricles resolve without impairment (Weindling, 1995). Large lesions can result in hydrocephalus or in degenerated cystic areas termed *periventricular leukomalacia* (p. 657). Importantly, the extent of periventricular leukomalacia correlates with cerebral palsy risk.

Pathology. Damage to the germinal matrix capillary network predisposes to subsequent extravasation of blood into the surrounding tissue. In preterm infants, this capillary network is especially fragile for several reasons. First, the subependymal germinal matrix provides poor support for the vessels coursing through it. Second, venous anatomy in this region causes stasis and congestion, which makes vessels susceptible to bursting with increased intravascular pressure. Third, vascular autoregulation is impaired before 32 weeks (Matsuda, 2006; Volpe, 1987). Even if extensive hemorrhage or other complications of preterm birth do not cause death, survivors can have major neurodevelopmental handicaps. DeVries and associates (1985) attribute most long-term sequelae of intraventricular-periventricular hemorrhage to *periventricular leukomalacia*. These degenerated cystic areas develop *most* commonly as a result of ischemia and *least* commonly in direct response to hemorrhage.

Incidence and Severity. The incidence of ventricular hemorrhage depends on gestational age at birth. Approximately half of all neonates born before 34 weeks, but only 4 percent of those born at term, will have some evidence of hemorrhage (Hayden, 1985). Very-low-birthweight infants have the earliest onset of hemorrhage, the greatest likelihood of parenchymal tissue involvement, and thus the highest mortality rate (Perlman, 1986). Preterm black infants are at disparate risk for intraventricular hemorrhage (Reddick, 2008).

The severity of intraventricular hemorrhage can be assessed by neuroimaging studies. Papile and coworkers (1978) devised the most widely used grading scheme to quantify the extent of a lesion and estimate prognosis.

Grade I—hemorrhage limited to the germinal matrix
Grade II—intraventricular hemorrhage
Grade III—hemorrhage with ventricular dilatation
Grade IV—parenchymal extension of hemorrhage

Data from the Neonatal Research Network indicate that 30 percent of infants born weighing 501 to 1500 g develop intracranial hemorrhage, and 12 percent are grade III or IV (Fanaroff, 2007). Jakobi and associates (1992) showed that infants with grade I or II intraventricular hemorrhage had a greater than 90-percent survival rate and a 3-percent rate of handicap—similar to control infants without hemorrhage of the same age. The survival rate for infants with grade III or IV hemorrhage, however, was only 50 percent. Extremely-low-birthweight infants with grade I or II hemorrhage have poorer neurodevelopmental outcomes at 20 months than controls (Patra, 2006).

Contributing Factors. Events that predispose to germinal matrix hemorrhage and subsequent periventricular leukomalacia are multifactorial and complex. As noted, the preterm fetus has fragile intracranial blood vessels that make it particularly susceptible. Moreover, preterm birth is frequently associated with infection, which further predisposes to endothelial activation, platelet adherence, and thrombi (Redline, 2008). RDS and mechanical ventilation are commonly associated factors (Sarkar, 2009).

Prevention with Antenatal Corticosteroids. These agents, given at least 24 hours before delivery, appear to prevent or reduce intraventricular hemorrhage incidence and severity. A Consensus Development Conference of the National Institutes of Health (1994) concluded that such therapy reduced rates of mortality, respiratory distress, and intraventricular hemorrhage in preterm infants born between 24 and 32 weeks and that the benefits were additive with those from surfactant therapy. The consensus panel also concluded that benefits of antenatal corticosteroid therapy probably extend to women with preterm premature membrane rupture. A second consensus statement by the National Institutes of Health (2000) recommended that repeated courses of corticosteroids should not be given. They noted that there were insufficient data to prove benefit or to document the safety of multiple courses (Chap. 42, p. 850).

Subsequently, the Maternal-Fetal Medicine Units Network reported that repeated corticosteroid courses were associated with some improved preterm neonatal outcomes, but also with reduced birthweight and increased risk for fetal-growth restriction (Wapner, 2006). Surveillance of this cohort through age 2 to 3 years found that children exposed to repeated—versus single-dose—steroid courses did not differ significantly in physical or neurocognitive measures (Wapner, 2007). It was worrisome, however, that there was a nonsignificant 5.7-fold relative risk of cerebral palsy in infants exposed to multiple steroid courses. At the same time, the 2-year follow-up of the Australasian Collaborative Trial was reported by Crowther (2007). In more than 1100 infants, the incidence of cerebral palsy was almost identical—4.2 versus 4.8 percent—in those given repeated versus single-course steroids, respectively.

Other Preventative Methods. The efficacy of *phenobarbital, vitamin K, vitamin E*, or *indomethacin* in diminishing the frequency and severity of intracranial hemorrhage, when administered either to the neonate or to the mother during labor, remains controversial (Chiswick, 1991; Hanigan, 1988; Thorp, 1995). Data from various sources suggest that *magnesium sulfate* may prevent the sequelae of periventricular hemorrhage, as discussed on page 659.

It is generally agreed that avoiding significant hypoxia both before and after preterm delivery is paramount (Low, 1995). There is presently no convincing evidence, however, that routine cesarean delivery for the preterm fetus presenting cephalic will decrease the incidence of periventricular hemorrhage. Anderson and colleagues (1992) found no significant difference in the overall frequency of hemorrhage in infants whose birthweights were below 1750 g and who were delivered without labor compared with those delivered during latent or active labor. Infants delivered of mothers in active labor, however, tended to have more grade III or IV hemorrhages.

Periventricular Leukomalacia

This pathological description refers to cystic areas deep in brain white matter that develop after hemorrhagic or ischemic infarction. Tissue ischemia leads to regional necrosis. Because brain tissue does not regenerate and the preterm neonate has minimal gliosis, these irreversibly damaged areas appear as echolucent cysts on neuroimaging studies. Generally, they require at least 2 weeks to form but may develop as long as 4 months after the initial insult. Thus, their presence at birth may help to determine the timing of a hemorrhagic event.

Cerebral Palsy

This term refers to a group of conditions that are characterized by chronic movement or posture abnormalities that are cerebral in origin, arise early in life, and are nonprogressive (Nelson, 2003).

Epilepsy and mental retardation frequently accompany cerebral palsy. The cause(s) of cerebral palsy are different in preterm and term infants (Chap. 33, p. 640).

Cerebral palsy is commonly classified by the type of neurological dysfunction—spastic, dyskinetic, or ataxic—as well as the number and distribution of limbs involved—quadriplegia, diplegia, hemiplegia, or monoplegia. The major types and their frequencies are:

1. *Spastic quadriplegia,* which has a strong association with mental retardation and seizure disorders—20 percent
2. *Diplegia,* which is common in preterm or low-birthweight infants—30 percent
3. *Hemiplegia*—30 percent
4. *Choreoathetoid types*—15 percent
5. *Mixed varieties* (Freeman, 1988; Rosen, 1992).

Incidence and Epidemiological Correlates

According to the Centers for Disease Control and Prevention, the prevalence of cerebral palsy in the United States was 3.1 per 1000 children in 2000 (Bhasin, 2006). Importantly, this rate either has remained essentially unchanged or has increased since the 1950s (Torfs, 1990; Winter, 2002). In some countries, the incidence has risen because advances in the care of very preterm infants have improved their survival, but not their neurological prognosis. For example, Moster and associates (2008) presented long-term follow-up of more than 900,000 births in Norway. Of nonanomalous term infants, the cerebral palsy rate was 0.1 percent compared with 9.1 percent in those born at 23 to 27 weeks. Similarly, O'Callaghan and coworkers (2011) studied the epidemiological associations of cerebral palsy and found preterm birth to be the greatest risk factor.

Intraventricular Hemorrhage

Various clinical and pathological data link severe intraventricular hemorrhage—grade III or IV—and resulting periventricular leukomalacia to cerebral palsy. As described earlier, grade I or II hemorrhages usually resolve without extensive tissue injury. Luthy (1987) reported a 16-fold increased risk of cerebral palsy for low-birthweight infants who had grade III or IV hemorrhage compared with the risk in infants who had either no or grade I or II hemorrhage.

Ischemia

Preterm infants are most susceptible to brain ischemia and periventricular leukomalacia. Before 32 weeks, the vascular anatomy of the brain is composed of two systems. One penetrates into the cortex—the *ventriculopedal system.* The other reaches down to the ventricles, but then curves to flow outward—the *ventriculofugal system* (Weindling, 1995). There are no vascular anastomoses connecting these two systems. As a result, the area between these systems, through which the pyramidal tracts pass near the lateral cerebral ventricles, is a watershed area vulnerable to ischemia. Vascular insufficiency before 32 weeks leading to ischemia would affect this watershed area first. Resulting damage of the pyramidal tracts may cause spastic diplegia. After 32 weeks, vascular flow shifts toward the cortex. Thus, hypoxic injury after this time primarily damages the cortical region.

Perinatal Infection

Periventricular leukomalacia is more strongly linked to infection and inflammation than to intraventricular hemorrhage. Zupan and colleagues (1996) studied 753 infants born between 24 and 32 weeks, 9 percent of whom developed periventricular leukomalacia. Those born before 28 weeks, those who had inflammatory events during the last days to weeks before delivery, or those who had both were at highest risk. Perlman and associates (1996) found that periventricular leukomalacia was strongly associated with prolonged membrane rupture, chorioamnionitis, and neonatal hypotension. Bailis and coworkers (2008) reported that chronic—and not acute—placental inflammation was associated with leukomalacia.

Fetal infection may be the key element in the pathway between preterm birth and cerebral palsy (Burd, 2012; Leviton, 2010). In the pathway proposed in Figure 34-2, antenatal reproductive tract infection evokes the production of cytokines such as tumor necrosis factor and interleukins-1, -6, and -8. These in turn stimulate prostaglandin production and preterm labor (Chap. 42, p. 838). Preterm intracranial blood vessels are susceptible to rupture and damage, and the cytokines that stimulate preterm labor also have direct toxic effects on oligodendrocytes and myelin. Vessel rupture, tissue hypoxia, and cytokine-mediated damage result in massive neuronal cell death. Glutamate is released, stimulating membrane receptors to allow excess calcium to enter the neurons. High intracellular calcium levels are toxic to white matter, and glutamate may be directly toxic to oligodendrocytes (Oka, 1993).

Many studies have shown that infection and cytokines can directly damage the immature brain. Inoculation of rabbit embryos with *Escherichia coli* causes histological damage in white matter (Yoon, 1997a). Moreover, tumor necrosis factor

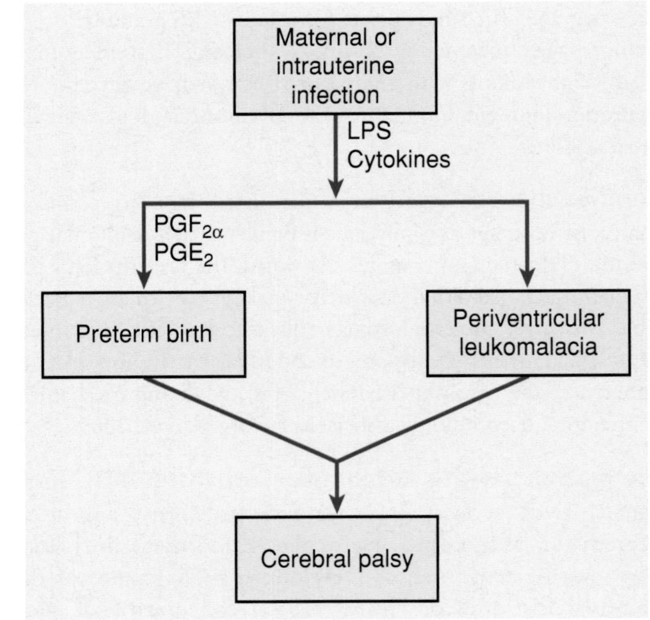

FIGURE 34-2 Schematic representation of the hypothesized pathway between maternal or intrauterine infection and preterm birth or periventricular leukomalacia. Both potentially lead to cerebral palsy. LPS = lipopolysaccharide; PG = prostaglandin.

and interleukin-6 were more frequently found in the brains of infants who died with periventricular leukomalacia (Yoon, 1997b). Cytokines are strongly linked to white matter lesions even when organisms cannot be demonstrated (Yoon, 2000).

Andrews and colleagues (2008) provided data that raise questions regarding an increased incidence of adverse neurodevelopmental outcomes related to chorioamnionitis. In a cohort of infants born between 23 and 32 weeks, they studied several surrogate indicators and direct markers of in utero inflammation. These included clinical findings, cytokine levels, histological findings, and microbial culture results. Infants undergoing comprehensive psychoneurological testing had similar incidences of intelligence quotient (IQ) scores < 70, cerebral palsy, or both, regardless of these markers. The researchers interpreted their findings to support current practices that employ efforts to delay delivery with preterm pregnancies in the absence of overt intrauterine infection. This does not apply to preterm pregnancy in which clinical chorioamnionitis is diagnosed (Soraisham, 2009). Of 3094 singletons born < 33 weeks, 15 percent had evidence of clinical chorioamnionitis, which included foul-smelling amnionic fluid, maternal fever, uterine tenderness, fetal tachycardia, and maternal leukocytosis. Compared with noninfected infants, cases complicated by chorioamnionitis had significantly increased rates of early-onset sepsis—4.8 versus 0.9 percent—and intraventricular hemorrhage—22 versus 12 percent.

Prevention—Neuroprotection

Because epidemiological evidence suggested that maternal magnesium sulfate therapy had a fetal neuroprotective effect, three large randomized trials have been performed to investigate this hypothesis. These studies are discussed in detail in Chapter 42 (p. 854), as well as other evidence that magnesium sulfate is effective in reducing cerebral palsy in preterm infants.

REFERENCES

Achiron R, Pinchas OH, Reichman B, et al: Fetal intracranial haemorrhage: clinical significance of in-utero ultrasonic diagnosis. Br J Obstet Gynaecol 100:995, 1993

American College of Obstetricians and Gynecologists: Fetal lung maturity. Practice Bulletin No. 97, September 2008

American College of Obstetricians and Gynecologists and American Academy of Pediatrics: Guidelines for perinatal care. 7th ed. Washington, 2012

Anderson GD, Bada HS, Shaver DC, et al: The effect of cesarean section on intraventricular hemorrhage in the preterm infant. Am J Obstet Gynecol 166:1091, 1992

Andrews WW, Cliver SP, Biasini F, et al: Early preterm birth: association between in utero exposure to acute inflammation and severe neurodevelopmental disability at 6 years of age. Am J Obstet Gynecol 198:466, 2008

Bailis A, Maleki Z, Askin F, et al: Histopathological placental features associated with development of periventricular leukomalacia in preterm infants. Am J Obstet Gynecol 199(6):S43, 2008

Ballard RA, Truog WE, Cnaan A, et al: Inhaled nitric oxide in preterm infants undergoing mechanical ventilation. N Engl J Med 355:343, 2006

Baraldi E, Filippone M: Chronic lung disease after premature birth. N Engl J Med 357:1946, 2007

Bhasin TK, Brocksen S, Avchen RN, et al: Prevalence of four developmental disabilities among children aged 8 years—metropolitan Atlanta developmental disabilities surveillance program, 1996 and 2000. MMWR 55:22, 2006

Blakely ML, Tyson JE, Lally KP, et al: Laparotomy versus peritoneal drainage for necrotizing enterocolitis or isolated intestinal perforation in extremely low birth weight infants: outcomes through 18 months adjusted age. Pediatrics 117:e680, 2006

Burd I, Balakrishnan B, Kannan S: Models of fetal brain injury, intrauterine inflammation, and preterm birth. Am J Reprod Immunol 67(4):287, 2012

Chiswick M, Gladman G, Sinha S, et al: Vitamin E supplementation and periventricular hemorrhage in the newborn. Am J Clin Nutr 53:370S, 1991

Chock VY, Van Meurs KP, Hintz SR, et al: Inhaled nitric oxide for preterm premature rupture of membranes, oligohydramnios, and pulmonary hypoplasia. Am J Perinatol 26(4):317, 2009

Clements JA, Platzker ACG, Tierney DF, et al: Assessment of the risk of respiratory distress syndrome by a rapid test for surfactant in amniotic fluid. N Engl J Med 286:1077, 1972

Consortium on Safe Labor: Respiratory morbidity in late preterm births. JAMA 304(4):419, 2010

Crowther CA, Doyle LW, Haslam RR, et al: Outcomes at 2 years of age after repeat doses of antenatal corticosteroids. N Engl J Med 357:1179, 2007

Czyrko C, Steigman C, Turley DL, et al: The role of reperfusion injury in occlusive intestinal ischemia of the neonate: malonaldehyde-derived fluorescent products and correlation of histology. J Surg Res 51:1, 1991

DeVries LS, Dubowitz V, Lary S, et al: Predictive value of cranial ultrasound in the newborn baby: a reappraisal. Lancet 2:137, 1985

Drazen JM, Solomon CG, Greene MF: Informed consent and SUPPORT. N Engl J Med 368(20):1929, 2013

Eriksen N, Tey A, Prieto J, et al: Fetal lung maturity in diabetic patients using the TDx FLM assay. Am J Obstet Gynecol 174:348, 1996

Fanaroff AA, Stoll BJ, Wright LL, et al: Trends in neonatal morbidity and mortality for very low birthweight infants. Am J Obstet Gynecol 196:147.e1, 2007

Freeman JM, Nelson KB: Intrapartum asphyxia and cerebral palsy. Pediatrics 82:240, 1988

Garmany TH, Wambach JA, Heins HB, et al: Population and disease-based prevalence of the common mutations associated with surfactant deficiency. Pediatr Res 63(6):645, 2008

Gluck L, Kulovich MV: Lecithin-sphingomyelin ratios in amniotic fluid in normal and abnormal pregnancy. Am J Obstet Gynecol 115:539, 1973

Gluck L, Kulovich MV, Borer RC Jr, et al: Diagnosis of the respiratory distress syndrome by amniocentesis. Am J Obstet Gynecol 109:440, 1971

Grave G, Nelson SA, Walker A, et al: New therapies and preventive approaches for necrotizing enterocolitis: report of a research planning workshop. Pediatr Res 62:1, 2007

Halliday HL, Ehrenkranz RA, Doyle LW: Late (> 7 days) postnatal corticosteroids for chronic lung disease in preterm infants. Cochrane Database Syst Rev 1:CD001145, 2009

Hanigan WC, Kennedy G, Roemisch F, et al: Administration of indomethacin for the prevention of periventricular–intraventricular hemorrhage in high-risk neonates. J Pediatr 112:941, 1988

Hayden CK, Shattuck KE, Richardson CJ, et al: Subependymal germinal matrix hemorrhage in full-term neonates. Pediatrics 75:714, 1985

Jakobi P, Weissman A, Zimmer EZ, et al: Survival and long-term morbidity in preterm infants with and without a clinical diagnosis of periventricular, intraventricular hemorrhage. Eur J Obstet Gynecol Reprod Biol 46:73, 1992

Jobe AH: Pulmonary surfactant therapy. N Engl J Med 328:861, 1993

Karcher R, Sykes E, Batton D, et al: Gestational age-specific predicted risk of neonatal respiratory distress syndrome using lamellar body count and surfactant-to-albumin ratio in amniotic fluid. Am J Obstet Gynecol 193:1680, 2005

Kinsella JP, Cutter GR, Walsh WF, et al: Early inhaled nitric oxide therapy in premature newborns with respiratory failure. N Engl J Med 355:354, 2006

Kliegman RM, Fanaroff AA: Necrotizing enterocolitis. N Engl J Med 310:1093, 1984

Leviton A, Allred EN, Kuban KCK, et al: Microbiologic and histologic characteristics of the extremely preterm infant's placenta predict white matter damage and later cerebral palsy. The ELGAN study. Pediatr Res 67:95, 2010

Locatelli A, Andreani M, Pizzardi A, et al: Antenatal variables associated with severe adverse neurodevelopmental outcome among neonates born at less than 32 weeks. Eur J Obstet Gynecol Reprod Biol 152(2):143, 2010

Low JA, Panagiotopoulos C, Derrick EJ: Newborn complications after intrapartum asphyxia with metabolic acidosis in the preterm fetus. Am J Obstet Gynecol 172:805, 1995

Luthy DA, Shy KK, Strickland D, et al: Status of infants at birth and risk for adverse neonatal events and long-term sequelae: a study in low birthweight infants. Am J Obstet Gynecol 157:676, 1987

Mathews TJ, MacDorman MF: Infant mortality statistics from the 2009 period linked birth/infant death data set. Natl Vital Stat Rep 61(8):1, 2013

Matsuda T, Okuyama K, Cho K, et al: Cerebral hemodynamics during the induction of antenatal periventricular leukomalacia by hemorrhagic hypotension in chronically instrumented fetal sheep. Am J Obstet Gynecol 194:1057, 2006

Mestan KK, Marks JD, Hecox K, et al: Neurodevelopmental outcomes of premature infants treated with inhaled nitric oxide. N Engl J Med 353:23, 2005

Moss RL, Dimmitt RA, Barnhart DC, et al: Laparotomy versus peritoneal drainage for necrotizing enterocolitis and perforation. N Engl J Med 354:2225, 2006

Moster D, Lie RT, Markestad T: Long-term medical and social consequences of preterm birth. N Engl J Med 359:262, 2008

National Institutes of Health: Antenatal corticosteroids revisited: repeat courses. NIH Consens Statement 17(2):1, 2000

National Institutes of Health: The effects of corticosteroids for fetal maturation on perinatal outcomes. NIH Consens Statement 12(2):1, 1994

Nelson KB: Can we prevent cerebral palsy? N Engl J Med 349:1765, 2003

Nores J, Roberts A, Carr S: Prenatal diagnosis and management of fetuses with intracranial hemorrhage. Am J Obstet Gynecol 174:424, 1996

O'Callaghan ME, MacLennan AH, Gibson, CS, et al: Epidemiologic associations with cerebral palsy. Obstet Gynecol 118:576, 2011

Oka A, Belliveau MJ, Rosenberg PA, et al: Vulnerability of oligodendroglia to glutamate: pharmacology, mechanisms, and prevention. J Neurosci 13:1441, 1993

Papile LA, Burstein J, Burstein R, et al: Incidence and evolution of subependymal and intraventricular hemorrhage: a study of infants with birth weights less than 1500 gm. J Pediatr 92:529, 1978

Patra K, Wilson-Costello D, Taylor HG, et al: Grades I-II intraventricular hemorrhage in extremely low birth weight infants: effects on neurodevelopment. J Pediatr 149:169, 2006

Perlman JM, Risser R, Broyles RS: Bilateral cystic periventricular leukomalacia in the premature infant: associated risk factors. Pediatrics 97:822, 1996

Perlman JM, Volpe JJ: Intraventricular hemorrhage in extremely small premature infants. Am J Dis Child 140:1122, 1986

Pfister RH, Soll RF, Wiswell T: Protein containing synthetic surfactant versus animal derived surfactant extract for the prevention and treatment of respiratory distress syndrome. Cochrane Database Syst Rev 4:CD006069, 2007

Reddick K, Canzoneri B, Roeder H, et al: Racial disparities and neonatal outcomes in preterm infants with intraventricular hemorrhage. Am J Obstet Gynecol 199(6):S71, 2008

Redline RW: Placental pathology: a systematic approach with clinical correlations. Placenta 22:S86, 2008

Rosen MG, Dickinson JC: The incidence of cerebral palsy. Am J Obstet Gynecol 167:417, 1992

Sarkar S, Bhagat I, Dechert R, et al: Severe intraventricular hemorrhage in preterm infants: comparison of risk factors and short-term neonatal morbidities between grade 3 and grade 4 intraventricular hemorrhage. Am J Perinatol 26:419, 2009

Schmidt B, Asztalos EV, Roberts RS, et al: Impact of bronchopulmonary dysplasia, brain injury, and severe retinopathy on the outcome of extremely low-birth-weight infants at 18 months. JAMA 289:1124, 2003

Seger N, Soll R: Animal derived surfactant extract for treatment of respiratory distress syndrome. Cochrane Database Syst Rev 2:CD007836, 2009

Shulenin S, Nogee LM, Annilo T, et al: ABCA3 gene mutations in newborns with fatal surfactant deficiency. N Engl J Med 350:1296, 2004

Soraisham AS, Singhal Nalini, McMillan DD, et al: A multicenter study on the clinical outcome of chorioamnionitis in preterm infants. Am J Obstet Gynecol 200:372.e1, 2009

Stark AR: Inhaled NO for preterm infants—getting to yes? N Engl J Med 355:404, 2006

Steinfeld JD, Samuels P, Bulley MA, et al: The utility of the TDx test in the assessment of fetal lung maturity. Obstet Gynecol 79:460, 1992

SUPPORT Study Group of the Eunice Kennedy Shriver NICHD Neonatal Research Network: Target ranges of oxygen saturation in extremely preterm infants. N Engl J Med 362(21):1959, 2010

Thorp JA, Ferette-Smith D, Gaston L, et al: Antenatal vitamin K and phenobarbital for preventing intracranial hemorrhage in the premature newborn: a randomized double-blind placebo-controlled trial. Am J Obstet Gynecol 172:253, 1995

Torfs CP, van den Berg B, Oechsli FW, et al: Prenatal and perinatal factors in the etiology of cerebral palsy. J Pediatr 116:615, 1990

van Meurs KP, Wright LL, Ehrenkranz RA, et al: Inhaled nitric oxide for premature infants with severe respiratory failure. N Engl J Med 353:13, 2005

van Vliet EO, de Kleviet JF, Oosterlaan J, et al: Perinatal infections and neurodevelopmental outcome in very preterm and very low-birth-weight infants: a meta-analysis. JAMA Pediatr 167(7):662, 2013

Verbrugge SJ, Lachmann B: Mechanisms of ventilation-induced lung injury: physiological rationale to prevent it. Monaldi Arch Chest Dis 54:22, 1999

Volpe JJ: Neurology of the Newborn, 3rd ed. Philadelphia, Saunders, 1995, p 373

Volpe JJ, Hill A: Neurologic disorders. In Avery GB (ed): Neonatology, 3rd ed. Philadelphia, JB Lippincott, 1987, p 1073

Wapner RJ, Sorokin Y, Mele L, et al: Long-term outcomes after repeated doses of antenatal corticosteroids. N Engl J Med 357:1190, 2007

Wapner RJ, Sorokin Y, Thom EA, et al: Single versus weekly courses of antenatal corticosteroids: evaluation of safety and efficacy. Am J Obstet Gynecol 195:633, 2006

Watterberg KL; American Academy of Pediatrics Committee on Fetus and Newborn: Policy statement–postnatal corticosteroids to prevent or treat bronchopulmonary dysplasia. Pediatrics 126(4):800, 2010

Weindling M: Periventricular haemorrhage and periventricular leukomalacia. Br J Obstet Gynaecol 102:278, 1995

Winter S, Autry A, Boyle C, et al: Trends in the prevalence of cerebral palsy in a population-based study. Pediatrics 110:1220, 2002

Yeh TF, Lin YJ, Lin HC, et al: Outcomes at school age after postnatal dexamethasone therapy for lung disease of prematurity. N Engl J Med 350:1304, 2004

Yoon BH, Kim CJ, Romero R, et al: Experimentally induced intrauterine infection causes fetal brain white matter lesions in rabbits. Am J Obstet Gynecol 177:797, 1997a

Yoon BH, Romero R, Kim CJ, et al: High expression of tumor necrosis factor-alpha and interleukin-6 in periventricular leukomalacia. Am J Obstet Gynecol 177:406, 1997b

Yoon BH, Romero R, Park JS, et al: Fetal exposure to an intra-amniotic inflammation and the development of cerebral palsy at the age of three years. Am J Obstet Gynecol 182:675, 2000

Zhu Y, Miller TL, Chidekel A, et al: KL4-surfactant (lucinactant) protects human airway epithelium from hyperoxia. Pediatr Res 64(2):154, 2008

Zupan V, Gonzalez P, Lacaze-Masmonteil T, et al: Periventricular leukomalacia: risk factors revisited. Dev Med Child Neurol 38:1061, 1996

CHAPTER 35

Stillbirth

Fetal mortality—the intrauterine death of a fetus at any gestational age—is considered a major but often overlooked public health issue. It is estimated that there are more than 1 million fetal losses each year in the United States, and most occur before 20 weeks' gestation. Fetal mortality data from the National Vital Statistics system are usually presented for fetal deaths at 20 weeks' gestation or older (MacDorman, 2012). Using this definition, there are nearly as many fetal deaths as infant deaths (Fig. 35-1). As shown in Figure 35-2, fetal deaths rates at 20 weeks or more are gestational-age related, reaching a nadir that plateaus between approximately 27 and 33 weeks. Following this, there is a progressive rate increase.

DEFINITION OF FETAL MORTALITY

The definition of fetal death adopted by the Centers for Disease Control and Prevention National Center for Health Statistics is based on the definitions recommended by the World Health Organization (MacDorman, 2012). This definition is as follows:

> *Fetal death means death prior to complete expulsion or extraction from the mother of a product of human conception irrespective of the duration of pregnancy and which is not an induced termination of pregnancy. The death is indicated by the fact that after such expulsion or extraction, the fetus does not breathe or show any other evidence of life such as beating of the heart, pulsation of the umbilical cord, or definite movement of voluntary muscles. Heartbeats are to be distinguished from transient cardiac contractions; respirations are to be distinguished from fleeting respiratory efforts or gasps.*

Reporting requirements for fetal deaths are determined by each state, and thus, requirements differ significantly (Chap. 1, p. 2). Most states require reporting of fetal deaths at 20 weeks' gestation or older or a minimum 350-g birthweight—roughly equivalent to 20 weeks—or some combination of these two. Seven states require fetal deaths before 20 weeks to be reported, and one state sets the threshold at 16 weeks. Three states require reporting of fetal deaths with birthweights 500 g or more—roughly equivalent to 22 weeks. There is substantial evidence that not all fetal deaths for which reporting is required are actually recorded (MacDorman, 2012). This is most likely at the earlier gestations of various state requirements.

The overall fetal mortality rate at 20 weeks or more for the United States has steadily declined since 1985 from 7.8 to 6.1 per 1000 total births in 2006 (MacDorman, 2012). Before this, declines were even more impressive and likely due to elimination of deaths of anomalous fetuses at later gestational ages that were "prevented" by early pregnancy terminations (Fretts, 1992).

Fetal mortality is generally divided into three periods: early, or < 20 completed weeks; intermediate, 20–27 weeks; and late, 28 weeks or more. The fetal death rate after 28 weeks has declined since 1990, whereas deaths from 20 to 27 weeks are largely unchanged (Fig. 35-3).

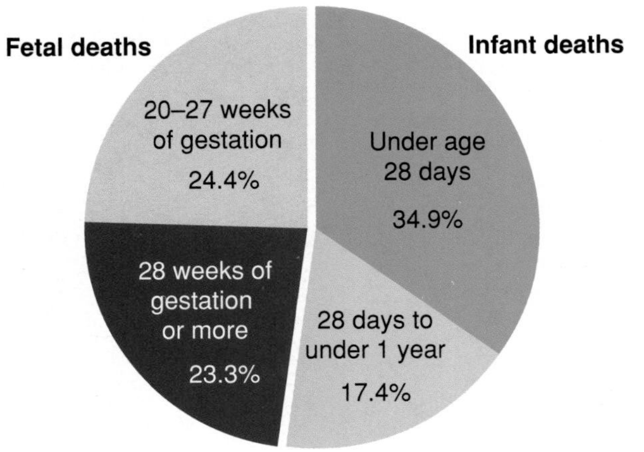

FIGURE 35-1 Percent distribution of fetal deaths at 20 weeks' gestation or more, and infant deaths: United States 2006. (From MacDorman, 2012.)

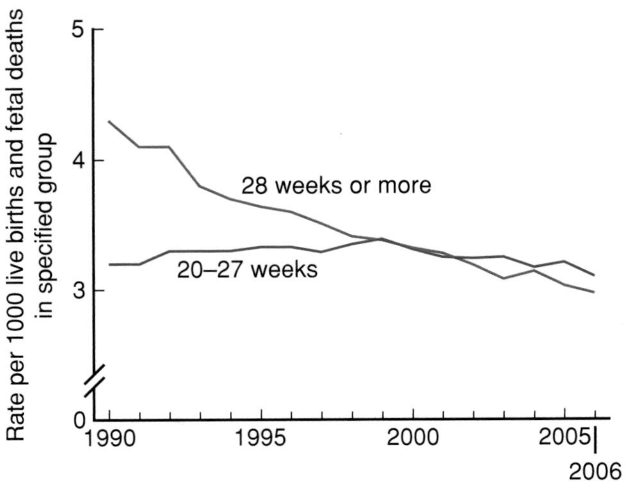

FIGURE 35-3 Fetal mortality rates by period of gestation: United States, 1990–2006. (From MacDorman, 2012.)

CAUSES OF FETAL DEATH

The *Eunice Kennedy Shriver* National Institute of Child Health and Human Development (NICHD) created the Stillbirth Collaborative Research Network to ascertain stillbirth causes in a racially and geographically diverse population in the United States. From this, the Stillbirth Collaborative Research Writing Group (2011b) ascertained stillbirths at 20 weeks or later between 2006 and 2008 in 59 tertiary care and community hospitals in five states. Standardized evaluations that included autopsy, placental histology, and testing of maternal or fetal blood/tissues—including fetal karyotyping—were performed in 500 women with 512 stillbirths. Of these, 83 percent were before labor and were considered antepartum stillbirths. Causes of stillbirth were divided into eight categories shown in Table 35-1. These categories were then classified as probable, possible, or unknown. As an example, diabetes was considered a *probable cause* if the fetus had diabetic embryopathy with lethal anomalies or the mother had diabetic ketoacidosis, but it was a *possible cause* if the mother had poor glycemic control and the fetus had abnormal growth. Overall, a probable or possible source was identified in 76 percent of cases.

This Network study of stillbirths is unprecedented in the United States for several reasons. It was a population-based cohort of stillbirths, all of which underwent systematic and thorough evaluation. Each cause of fetal death assigned is reasonably straightforward and comprehensible except for "placental abnormalities," which includes "uteroplacental insufficiency" as well as a few other entities less clearly defined. This aside, the leading reasons for fetal death were obstetrical complications that primarily included abruption, multifetal gestation, and spontaneous labor or ruptured membranes before viability. The major contribution of this study was that systematic evaluation led to a likely cause in approximately three fourths of stillbirths. This rate is considerably higher then most analyses of stillbirth etiologies and serves to emphasize the importance of careful evaluations.

RISK FACTORS FOR FETAL DEATH

Factors that have been associated with an increased risk of antepartum stillbirth include advanced maternal age; African-American race; smoking; illicit drug use; maternal medical

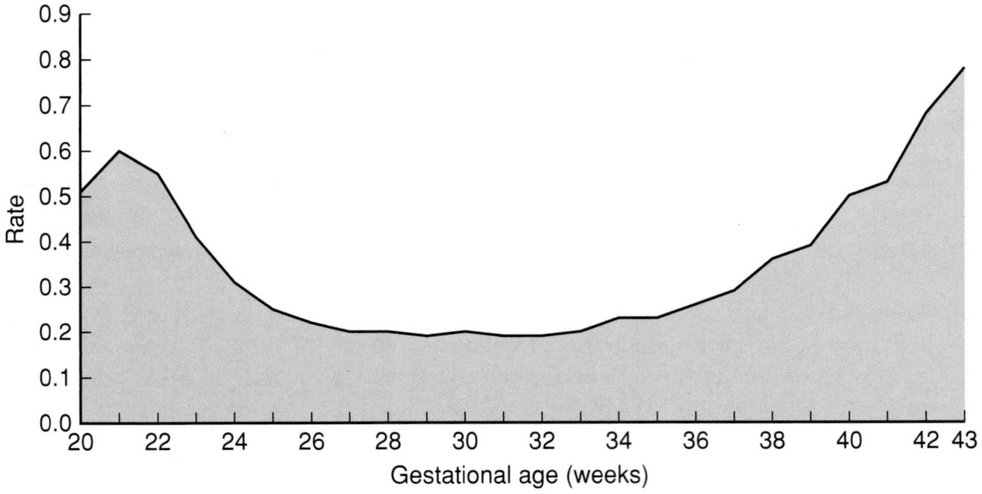

FIGURE 35-2 Fetal mortality rate per 1000 births by single weeks of gestation: United States, 2006. (From MacDorman, 2012.)

TABLE 35-1. Causes of 512 Stillbirths in the Stillbirth Collaborative Research Network Study

Cause	Examples	Percent
Obstetrical complications	Abruption; multifetal gestation; ruptured preterm membranes at 20–24 weeks	29
Placental abnormalities	Uteroplacental insufficiency; maternal vascular disorders	24
Fetal malformations	Major structural abnormalities and/or genetic abnormalities	14
Infection	Involving the fetus or placenta	13
Umbilical cord abnormalities	Prolapse; stricture; thrombosis	10
Hypertensive disorders	Preeclampsia; chronic hypertension	9
Medical complications	Diabetes; antiphospholipid antibody syndrome	8
Undetermined	NA	24

NA = not applicable.
Percentages are rounded and total more than 100 percent because some stillbirths had more than one cause. Overall, a cause was identified in 76 percent of stillbirths.
Adapted from the Stillbirth Collaborative Research Network Writing Group, 2011b.

diseases—such as overt diabetes or chronic hypertension; assisted reproductive technology; nulliparity; obesity; and previous adverse pregnancy outcomes—such as prior preterm birth or growth-restricted newborn (Reddy, 2010; Varner, 2014). There have been two major recent studies in which the investigators assessed whether it was possible to identify stillbirth risk factors either before or shortly after confirmation of pregnancy. Reddy and colleagues (2010) analyzed data from the NICHD Consortium on Safe Labor. Briefly, the pregnancy outcomes of 206,969 women delivered between 2002 and 2008 at 19 hospitals in the United States were analyzed. Shown in Figure 35-4 is the distribution of stillbirths according to gestational age. Clearly, the tragedy of stillbirth occurs primarily in term pregnancies. Reddy and colleagues (2010) found individual risk factors that included race, parity, advanced maternal age, and obesity performed poorly as predictors of stillbirth at term. They concluded that these results did not support routine antenatal surveillance for any of these demographic risk factors. This is discussed further subsequently.

The second recent analysis of stillbirth risk factors was included in the Stillbirth Collaborative Research Network study described earlier. Investigators studied stillbirth prediction based on risks identified in early pregnancy. They found that pregnancy factors known at the start of pregnancy accounted for a small proportion of stillbirth risk. Except for prior stillbirth or pregnancy loss such as preterm birth or fetal-growth restriction, other risks had limited predictive value (Stillbirth Collaborative Research Network Writing Group, 2011a). The importance of prior stillbirth as a risk for recurrence has been emphasized by Sharma and associates (2006). Specifically, stillbirth risk was fivefold higher in women with a prior stillbirth, and this recurrence risk was almost tripled in African-American women. Rasmussen (2009) analyzed 864,531 births in Norway between 1967 and 2005 and reported that prior preterm birth, fetal-growth restriction, preeclampsia, and placental abruption were strongly associated with subsequent stillbirth. Shown in Table 35-2 are estimates of stillbirth risk according to maternal factors including prior loss.

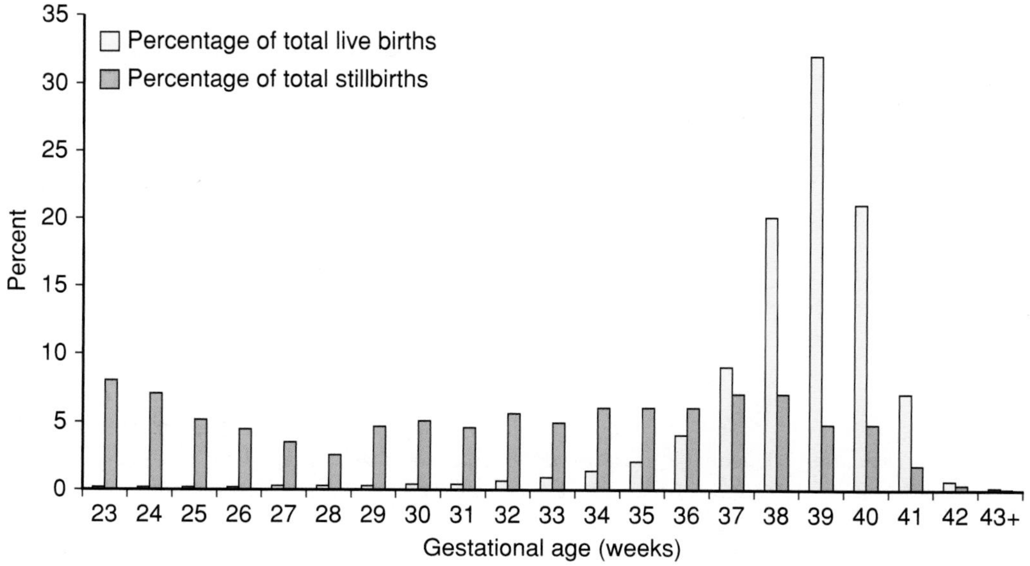

FIGURE 35-4 Distribution of livebirths and stillbirths in the National Institute of Child Health and Development Safe Labor Consortium according to gestational age. (From Reddy, 2010.)

TABLE 35-2. Estimated Maternal Risk Factors and Risk of Stillbirth

Condition	Prevalence (%)	Estimated Rate of Stillbirth (per 1000 births)	OR[a]
All pregnancies		6.4	1.0
Low-risk pregnancies	80	4.0–5.5	0.86
Hypertensive disorders			
Chronic hypertension	6–10	6–25	1.5–2.7
Pregnancy-induced hypertension			
Mild	5.8–7.7	9–51	1.2–4.0
Severe	1.3–3.3	12–29	1.8–4.4
Diabetes			
Diet alone	2.5–5	6–10	1.2–2.2
Insulin + diet	2.4	6–35	1.7–7.0
Systemic lupus erythematosus	< 1	40–150	6–20
Renal disease	< 1	15–200	2.2–30
Thyroid disease	0.2–2	12–20	2.2–3.0
Thrombophilia	1–5	18–40	2.8–5.0
Cholestasis of pregnancy	< 0.1	12–30	1.8–4.4
Smoking > 10 cigarettes	10–20	10–15	1.7–3.0
Obesity			
BMI 25–29.9 kg/m^2	21	12–15	1.9–2.7
BMI > 30	20	13–18	2.1–2.8
Education (< 12 y vs ≥ 12 y)	30	10–13	1.6–2.0
Prior growth-restricted infant (< 10%)	6.7	12–30	2–4.6
Prior stillbirth	0.5–1	9–20	1.4–3.2
Multifetal gestation			
Twins	2.7	12	1.0–2.8
Triplets	0.14	34	2.8–3.7
Maternal age (reference < 35 y)			
35–39 y	15–18	11–14	1.8–2.2
≥ 40 y	2	11–21	1.8–3.3
Black women compared with white women	15	12–14	2.0–2.2

[a]Odds ratio of the factor present compared with the risk factor absent.
From Fretts, 2005, with permission.

EVALUATION OF THE STILLBORN

Determining the cause of fetal death aids maternal psychological adaptation to a significant loss, helps assuage the guilt that is part of grieving, permits more accurate counseling regarding recurrence risk, and may prompt therapy or intervention to prevent a similar outcome in the next pregnancy (American College of Obstetricians and Gynecologists, 2012). Identification of inherited syndromes also provides useful information for other family members.

Clinical Examination

Important tests in stillbirth evaluation are neonatal autopsy and karyotyping and examination of the placenta, cord, and membranes (Pinar, 2014). An algorithm provided by the American College of Obstetricians and Gynecologists (2012) is shown in Figure 35-5. A thorough examination of the fetus, placenta, and membranes is recommended at delivery, with careful documentation in the medical record. The details of relevant prenatal events should be provided. Photographs should be taken whenever possible, and a full radiograph of the fetus—a *fetogram*—may be performed. Magnetic resonance (MR) imaging and sonography may be especially important in providing anatomical information if parents decline a full autopsy.

Laboratory Evaluation

If autopsy and chromosomal studies are performed, up to 35 percent of stillborns are discovered to have major structural anomalies (Faye-Petersen, 1999). Approximately 20 percent have dysmorphic features or skeletal abnormalities, and 8 percent have chromosomal abnormalities (Pauli, 1994; Saller, 1995). The American College of Obstetricians and Gynecologists (2012) recommends karyotyping all stillborns. Reddy and coworkers (2012) have recently reported that microarray analysis is more likely than karyotype analysis to provide a genetic diagnosis, primarily because of its success with nonviable tissue. In the absence

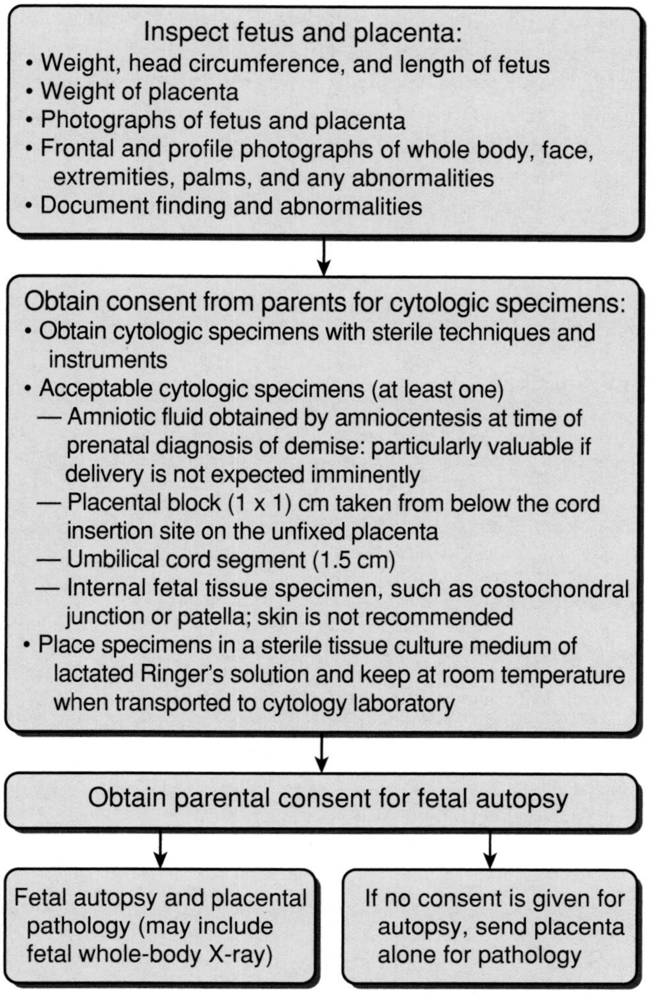
Inspect fetus and placenta:
• Weight, head circumference, and length of fetus
• Weight of placenta
• Photographs of fetus and placenta
• Frontal and profile photographs of whole body, face, extremities, palms, and any abnormalities
• Document finding and abnormalities
Obtain consent from parents for cytologic specimens:
• Obtain cytologic specimens with sterile techniques and instruments
• Acceptable cytologic specimens (at least one)
— Amniotic fluid obtained by amniocentesis at time of prenatal diagnosis of demise: particularly valuable if delivery is not expected imminently
— Placental block (1 x 1) cm taken from below the cord insertion site on the unfixed placenta
— Umbilical cord segment (1.5 cm)
— Internal fetal tissue specimen, such as costochondral junction or patella; skin is not recommended
• Place specimens in a sterile tissue culture medium of lactated Ringer's solution and keep at room temperature when transported to cytology laboratory
Obtain parental consent for fetal autopsy
Fetal autopsy and placental pathology (may include fetal whole-body X-ray)
If no consent is given for autopsy, send placenta alone for pathology

FIGURE 35-5 Flow chart for fetal and placental evaluation. (From Management of stillbirth. ACOG Practice Bulletin No. 102. American College of Obstetricians and Gynecologists. Obstet Gynecol 2009;113:748–61.

of morphological anomalies, up to 5 percent of stillborns will have a chromosomal abnormality (Korteweg, 2008).

Appropriate consent must be obtained to take fetal tissue samples, including fluid obtained postmortem by needle aspiration. A total of 3 mL of fetal blood, obtained from the umbilical cord or by cardiac puncture, is placed into a sterile, heparinized tube for cytogenetic studies. If blood cannot be obtained, the American College of Obstetricians and Gynecologists (2012) recommends at least one of the following samples: (1) a placental block measuring about 1 × 1 cm taken below the cord insertion site in the unfixed specimen; (2) umbilical cord segment approximately 1.5 cm long; or (3) internal fetal tissue specimen such as costochondral junction or patella. *Importantly, skin is no longer recommended for a tissue sample.* Tissue is washed with sterile saline before being placed in lactated Ringer solution or sterile cytogenetic medium. Placement in formalin or alcohol kills remaining viable cells and prevents cytogenetic analysis.

A full karyotype may not be possible in cases with prolonged fetal death. For example, Korteweg and associates (2008) reported that they successfully performed cytogenetic analysis in only a third of macerated fetuses. Fluorescence in situ hybridization might be used to exclude numerical abnormalities or to document certain common deletions such as that causing DiGeorge syndrome. Maternal blood should be obtained for Kleihauer-Betke staining; for antiphospholipid antibody and lupus anticoagulant testing if indicated; and for serum glucose measurement to exclude overt diabetes (Silver, 2013).

Autopsy

Parents should be offered and encouraged to allow a full autopsy. However, valuable information can still be obtained from limited studies. Pinar and colleagues (2012) described the autopsy protocol used by the Stillbirth Collaborative Research Network. In the absence of an autopsy, a gross external examination combined with photography, radiography, MR imaging, bacterial cultures, and selective use of chromosomal and histopathological studies often can aid determination of the cause of death.

A complete autopsy is more likely to yield valuable information. An analysis of 400 consecutive fetal deaths in Wales found that autopsy altered the presumed cause of death in 13 percent and provided new information in another 26 percent (Cartlidge, 1995). Other investigators have shown that autopsy results changed the recurrence risk estimates and parental counseling in 25 to 50 percent of cases (Faye-Petersen, 1999; Silver, 2007).

According to the survey by Goldenberg and coworkers (2013), most hospitals do not audit stillbirths. In other centers, however, maternal records and autopsy findings are reviewed on a monthly basis by a stillbirth committee composed of obstetricians, maternal-fetal medicine specialists, neonatologists, clinical geneticists, and perinatal pathologists. If possible, the cause of death is assigned based on available evidence. Most importantly, parents should then be contacted and offered counseling regarding the reason for death, the recurrence risk if any, and possible strategies to avoid recurrence in future pregnancies.

PSYCHOLOGICAL ASPECTS

Fetal death is psychologically traumatic for the woman and her family. Further stress results from an interval of more than 24 hours between the diagnosis of fetal death and the induction of labor, not seeing her infant for as long as she desires, and having no tokens of remembrance (Radestad, 1996). As discussed in Chapter 61 (p. 1205), the woman experiencing a stillbirth or even an early miscarriage is at increased risk for postpartum depression and should be closely monitored (Nelson, 2013). This and other significant life events increase the risks for another subsequent stillborn (Hogue, 2013).

MANAGEMENT OF WOMEN WITH PRIOR STILLBIRTH

The American College of Obstetricians and Gynecologists (2012) has provided a management outline for women with prior stillbirth (Table 35-3). Importantly, these recommendations are based primarily on limited or inconsistent scientific evidence or on expert opinions. Unfortunately, few studies

TABLE 35-3. Management of Subsequent Pregnancy after Stillbirth

Preconceptional or Initial Prenatal Visit
Detailed medical and obstetrical history
Evaluation and workup of previous stillbirth
Determination of recurrence risk
Smoking cessation
Weight loss in obese women (preconceptional only)
Genetic counseling if family genetic condition exists
Diabetes screen
Thrombophilia workup: antiphospholipid antibodies (only if specifically indicated)
Support and reassurance
First Trimester
Dating ultrasonography
First-trimester screen: pregnancy-associated plasma protein A, human chorionic gonadotropin, and nuchal translucency[a]
Support and reassurance
Second Trimester
Fetal ultrasonographic anatomic survey at 18–20 weeks of gestation
Maternal serum screening (quadruple) or single-marker alpha fetoprotein if first trimester screening[a]
Support and reassurance
Third Trimester
Ultrasonographic screening for fetal-growth restriction after 28 weeks
Kick counts starting at 28 weeks
Antepartum fetal surveillance starting at 32 weeks or 1–2 weeks earlier than prior stillbirth
Support and reassurance
Delivery
Elective induction at 39 weeks
Delivery before 39 weeks only with documented fetal lung maturity by amniocentesis

[a]Provides risk modification but does not alter management.
Adapted from American College of Obstetricians and Gynecologists, 2012; Reddy, 2007.

address management of such women. Those with modifiable risk factors for stillbirth such as hypertension or diabetes control require specific management strategies. According to Reddy (2007), because almost half of fetal deaths are associated with growth restriction, fetal sonographic anatomical assessment beginning at midpregnancy is recommended. This is followed by serial growth studies beginning at 28 weeks.

Weeks and associates (1995) evaluated fetal biophysical testing in 300 women whose only indication was prior stillbirth. There was only one recurrent stillbirth, and only three fetuses had abnormal testing results before 32 weeks. There was no relationship between the gestational age of the previous stillborn and the incidence or timing of abnormal test results or fetal jeopardy in the subsequent pregnancy. These investigators concluded that antepartum surveillance should begin at 32 weeks or later in the otherwise healthy woman with a history of stillbirth. This recommendation is supported by the American College of Obstetricians and Gynecologists (2012) with the caveat that it increases the iatrogenic preterm delivery rate.

Delivery at 39 weeks is recommended by induction or by cesarean delivery for those with a contraindication to induction. This minimizes fetal mortality rates, although the degree of risk reduction may be greater for older women (Page, 2013).

REFERENCES

American College of Obstetricians and Gynecologists: Management of stillbirth. Practice Bulletin No.102, March 2009, Reaffirmed 2012

Cartlidge PHT, Stewart JH: Effect of changing the stillbirth definition on evaluation of perinatal mortality rates. Lancet 346:486, 1995

Faye-Petersen OM, Guinn DA, Wenstrom KD: Value of perinatal autopsy. Obstet Gynecol 94(6):915, 1999

Fretts RC: Etiology and prevention of stillbirth. Am J Obstet Gynecol 193(6):1923, 2005

Fretts RC, Boyd ME, Usher RH, et al: The changing pattern of fetal death, 1961–1988. Obstet Gynecol 79:35, 1992

Goldenberg RL, Farrow V, McClure EM, et al: Stillbirth: knowledge and practice among U.S. obstetrician-gynecologists. Am J Perinatol 30(10):813, 2013

Hogue CJR, Parker CB, Willinger M, et al: A population-based case-control study of stillbirth: the relationship of significant life events to the racial disparity for African Americans. Am J Epidemiol 177(8):755, 2013

Korteweg FJ, Bouman K, Erwich JJ, et al: Cytogenetic analysis after evaluation of 750 fetal deaths. Obstet Gynecol 111:865, 2008

MacDorman MF, Kirmeyer SE, Wilson EC: Fetal and perinatal mortality, United States, 2006. Natl Vital Stat Rep 60(8):1, 2012

Nelson DB, Freeman MP, Johnson, NL, et al: A prospective study of postpartum depression in 17,648 parturients. J Matern Fetal Neonatal Med 26(12):1155, 2013

Page JM, Snowden JM, Cheng YW, et al: The risk of stillbirth and infant death by each additional week of expectant management stratified by maternal age. Am J Obstet Gynecol 209(4):375.e1, 2013

Pauli RM, Reiser CA: Wisconsin Stillbirth Service Program: II. Analysis of diagnoses and diagnostic categories in the first 1,000 referrals. Am J Med Genet 50:135, 1994

Pinar H, Goldenberg RL, Koch MA, et al: Placental findings in singleton stillbirths. Obstet Gynecol 123:325, 2014

Pinar H, Koch MA, Hawkins H, et al: The Stillbirth Collaborative Research Network Postmortem Examination protocol. Am J Perinatol 29:187, 2012

Radestad I, Steineck G, Nordin C, et al: Psychological complications after stillbirth—influence of memories and immediate management: population based study. BMJ 312:1505, 1996

Rasmussen S, Irgens LM, Skjaerven R, et al: Prior adverse pregnancy outcome and the risk of stillbirth. Obstet Gynecol 114(6):1259, 2009

Reddy UM: Prediction and prevention of recurrent stillbirth. Obstet Gynecol 110:1151, 2007

Reddy UM, Laughon SK, Sun L, et al: Prepregnancy risk factors for antepartum stillbirth in the United States. Obstet Gynecol 116:1119, 2010

Reddy UM, Page GP, Saade GR, et al: Karyotype versus microarray testing for genetic abnormalities after stillbirth. N Engl J Med 367(23):2185, 2012

Saller DN Jr, Lesser KB, Harrel U, et al: The clinical utility of the perinatal autopsy. JAMA 273:663, 1995

Sharma PP, Salihu HM, Oyelese Y, et al: Is race a determinant of stillbirth recurrence? Obstet Gynecol 107(2 Pt 1):391, 2006

Silver RM: Fetal death. Obstet Gynecol 109:153, 2007

Silver RM, Parker CB, Reddy UM, et al: Antiphospholipid antibodies in stillbirth. Obstet Gynecol 122(3):641, 2013

Stillbirth Collaborative Research Network Writing Group: Association between stillbirth and risk factors known at pregnancy confirmation. JAMA 306(22):2469, 2011a

Stillbirth Collaborative Research Network Writing Group: Causes of death among stillbirths. JAMA 306(22):2459, 2011b

Varner JW, Silver RM, Rowland Hogue CJ, et al: Association between stillbirth and illicit drug use and smoking during pregnancy. Obstet Gynecol 123:113, 2014

Weeks JW, Asrat T, Morgan MA, et al: Antepartum surveillance for a history of stillbirth: when to begin? Am J Obstet Gynecol 172:486, 1995

SECTION 10

THE PUERPERIUM

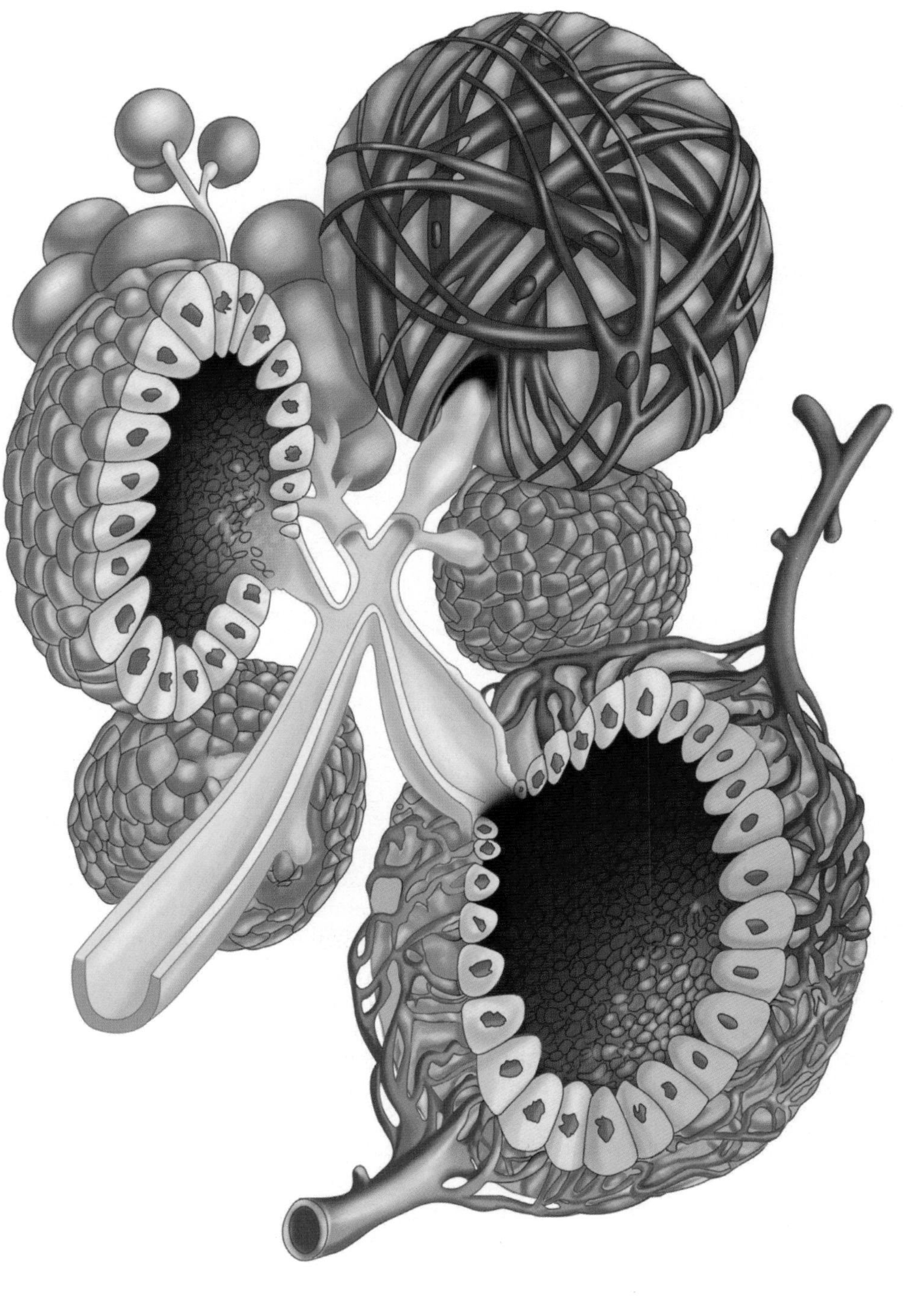

CHAPTER 36

The Puerperium

The word *puerperium* is derived from Latin—*puer,* child + *parus,* bringing forth. Currently, it defines the time following delivery during which pregnancy-induced maternal anatomical and physiological changes return to the nonpregnant state. Its duration is understandably inexact, but is considered to be between 4 and 6 weeks. Although much less complex compared with pregnancy, the puerperium has appreciable changes, some of which may be either bothersome or worrisome for the new mother. Importantly, several complications can develop, and some are serious.

The puerperium may be a time of intense anxiety for many women. Some mothers have feelings of abandonment following delivery because of a newly aimed focus on the infant. Kanotra and colleagues (2007) analyzed challenges that women faced from 2 to 9 months following delivery. A third of these new mothers felt the need for social support, and 25 percent had concerns with breast feeding (Table 36-1).

INVOLUTION OF THE REPRODUCTIVE TRACT

Birth Canal

Return to the nonpregnant state begins soon after delivery. The vagina and its outlet gradually diminish in size but rarely regain their nulliparous dimensions. Rugae begin to reappear by the third week but are less prominent than before. The hymen is represented by several small tags of tissue, which scar to form the *myrtiform caruncles.* Vaginal epithelium begins to proliferate by 4 to 6 weeks, usually coincidental with resumed ovarian estrogen production. Lacerations or stretching of the perineum during delivery may result in vaginal outlet relaxation. Some damage to the pelvic floor may be inevitable, and parturition predisposes to urinary incontinence and pelvic organ prolapse. This is discussed in detail in Chapter 27 (p. 536).

Uterus

The massively increased uterine blood flow necessary to maintain pregnancy is made possible by significant hypertrophy and remodeling of pelvic vessels. After delivery, their caliber gradually diminishes to approximately that of of the prepregnant state. Within the puerperal uterus, larger blood vessels become obliterated by hyaline changes, are gradually resorbed, and are replaced by smaller ones. Minor vestiges of the larger vessels, however, may persist for years.

During labor, the margin of the dilated cervix, which corresponds to the external os, may be lacerated. The cervical opening contracts slowly and for a few days immediately after labor, readily admits two fingers. By the end of the first week, this opening narrows, the cervix thickens, and the endocervical canal reforms. The external os does not completely resume its pregravid appearance. It remains somewhat wider, and typically, ectocervical depressions at the site of lacerations become permanent. These changes are characteristic of a parous cervix (Fig. 36-1). The markedly attenuated lower uterine segment

TABLE 36-1. Pregnancy Risk Assessment Surveillance System—PRAMS.[a] Concerns Raised by Women in the First 2–9 Months Postpartum

Concerns	Percent
Need for social support	32
Breast-feeding issues	24
Inadequate education about newborn care	21
Help with postpartum depression	10
Perceived need for extended hospital stay	8
Need for maternal insurance coverage postpartum	6

[a]Centers for Disease Control and Prevention, 2012b.
Data from Kanotra, 2007.

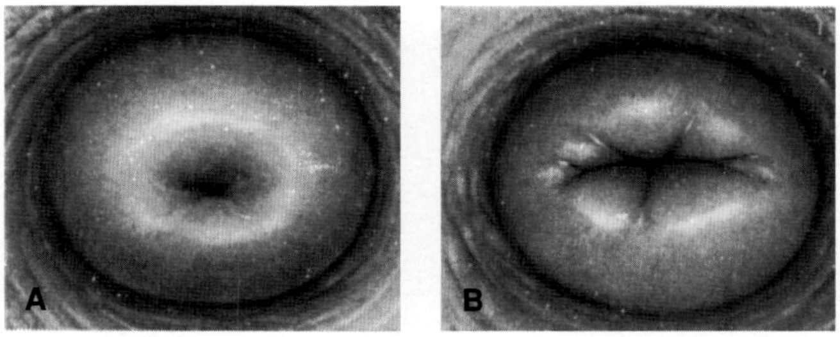

FIGURE 36-1 Common appearance of nulliparous **(A)** and parous **(B)** cervices.

contracts and retracts, but not as forcefully as the uterine corpus. During the next few weeks, the lower segment is converted from a clearly distinct substructure large enough to accommodate the fetal head to a barely discernible uterine isthmus located between the corpus and internal os.

Cervical epithelium also undergoes considerable remodeling, and this actually may be salutary. Ahdoot and associates (1998) found that approximately half of women showed regression of high-grade dysplasia following vaginal delivery. Kaneshiro and coworkers (2005) found similar regression—about 60 percent overall—regardless of delivery mode.

Postpartum, the fundus of the contracted uterus lies slightly below the umbilicus. It consists mostly of myometrium covered by serosa and internally lined by basal decidua. The anterior and posterior walls, which lie in close apposition, are each 4 to 5 cm thick (Buhimschi, 2003). At this time, the uterus weighs approximately 1000 g. Because blood vessels are compressed by the contracted myometrium, the uterus on section appears ischemic compared with the reddish-purple hyperemic pregnant organ.

Myometrial involution is a truly remarkable *tour de force* of destruction or deconstruction that begins as soon as 2 days after delivery as shown in Figure 36-2. As emphasized by Hytten (1995), studies that describe the degree of decreasing uterine weight postpartum are poor quality. Best estimates are that by 1 week, the uterus weighs approximately 500 g; by 2 weeks, about 300 g; and at 4 weeks, involution is complete and the uterus weighs approximately 100 g. After each successive delivery, the uterus is usually slightly larger than before the most recent pregnancy. The total number of myocytes does not decrease appreciably—rather, their size decreases markedly.

Sonographic Findings

Uterine size dissipates rapidly in the first week (Fig. 36-3). And the uterus and endometrium return to pregravid size by 8 weeks after delivery (Belachew, 2012; Steinkeler, 2012). In a study of 42 normal women postpartum, Tekay and Jouppila (1993) identified fluid in the endometrial cavity in 78 percent at 2 weeks, 52 percent at 3 weeks, 30 percent at 4 weeks, and 10 percent at 5 weeks. Demonstrable uterine cavity contents are seen for up to 2 months following delivery. Belachew and colleagues (2012) used 3-dimensional sonography and visualized

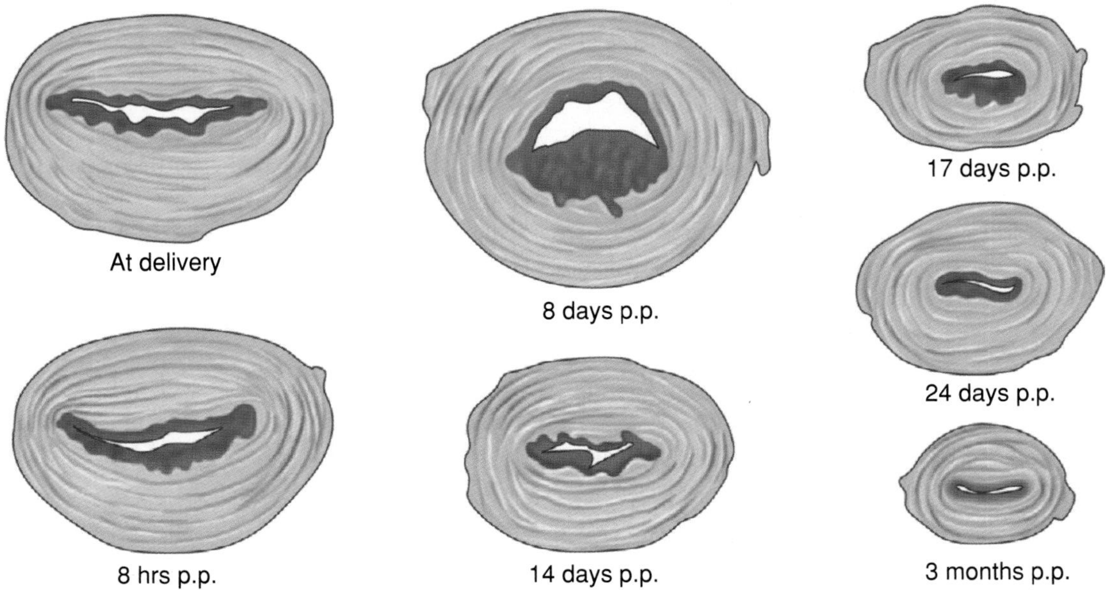

FIGURE 36-2 Cross sections of uteri made at the level of the involuting placental site at varying times after delivery. p.p. = postpartum. (Redrawn from Williams, 1931.)

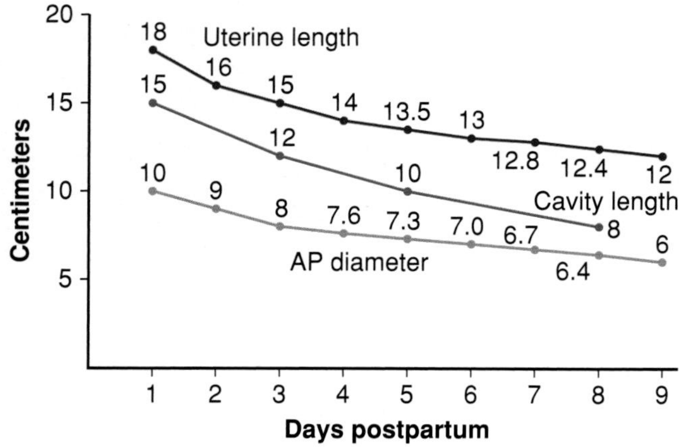

FIGURE 36-3 Sonographic measurements of uterine involution during the first 9 days postpartum. AP = anteroposterior. (Data from Hytten, 1995.)

intracavitary tissue matter in a third on day 1, 95 percent on day 7, 87 percent on day 14, and 28 percent on day 28. By day 56, the small cavity was empty. Sohn and associates (1988) described Doppler ultrasound results showing continuously increasing uterine artery vascular resistance during the first 5 days postpartum.

Decidua and Endometrial Regeneration

Because separation of the placenta and membranes involves the spongy layer, the decidua basalis is not sloughed. The remaining decidua has striking variations in thickness, it has an irregular jagged appearance, and it is infiltrated with blood, especially at the placental site (see Fig. 36-2).

Within 2 or 3 days after delivery, the remaining decidua becomes differentiated into two layers. The superficial layer becomes necrotic and is sloughed in the lochia. The basal layer adjacent to the myometrium remains intact and is the source of new endometrium. This arises from proliferation of the endometrial glandular remnants and the stroma of the interglandular connective tissue.

Endometrial regeneration is rapid, except at the placental site. Within a week or so, the free surface becomes covered by epithelium, and Sharman (1953) identified fully restored endometrium in all biopsy specimens obtained from the 16th day onward. Histological endometritis is part of the normal reparative process. Moreover, microscopic inflammatory changes characteristic of acute salpingitis are seen in almost half of women between 5 and 15 days, but these findings do not reflect infection (Andrews, 1951).

Clinical Aspects

Afterpains. In primiparous women, the uterus tends to remain tonically contracted following delivery. In multiparas, however, it often contracts vigorously at intervals and gives rise to *afterpains,* which are similar to but milder than labor contractions. These are more pronounced as parity increases and worsen when the infant suckles, likely because of oxytocin release (Holdcroft, 2003). Usually, afterpains decrease in intensity and become mild by the third day. We have encountered unusually severe and persistent afterpains in women with postpartum uterine infections.

Lochia. Early in the puerperium, sloughing of decidual tissue results in a vaginal discharge of variable quantity. The discharge is termed *lochia* and contains erythrocytes, shredded decidua, epithelial cells, and bacteria. For the first few days after delivery, there is blood sufficient to color it red—*lochia rubra.* After 3 or 4 days, lochia becomes progressively pale in color—*lochia serosa.* After approximately the 10th day, because of an admixture of leukocytes and reduced fluid content, lochia assumes a white or yellow-white color—*lochia alba.* The average duration of lochial discharge ranges from 24 to 36 days (Fletcher, 2012).

Placental Site Involution

Complete extrusion of the placental site takes up to 6 weeks (Williams, 1931). Immediately after delivery, the placental site is approximately palm-sized. Within hours of delivery, it normally consists of many thrombosed vessels that ultimately undergo organization (see Fig. 36-2). By the end of the second week, it is 3 to 4 cm in diameter.

Placental site involution is an exfoliation process, which is prompted in great part by undermining of the implantation site by new endometrial proliferation (Williams, 1931). Thus, involution is not simply absorption in situ. Exfoliation consists of both extension and "downgrowth" of endometrium from the margins of the placental site, as well as development of endometrial tissue from the glands and stroma left deep in the decidua basalis after placental separation. Anderson and Davis (1968) concluded that placental site exfoliation results from sloughing of infarcted and necrotic superficial tissues followed by a remodeling process.

Subinvolution

In some cases, uterine involution is hindered because of infection, retained placental fragments, or other causes. Such subinvolution is accompanied by varied intervals of prolonged lochia as well as irregular or excessive uterine bleeding. On bimanual examination, the uterus is larger and softer than would be expected. Ergonovine (Ergotrate) or methylergonovine (Methergine), 0.2 mg orally every 3 to 4 hours for 24 to 48 hours, is recommended by many, but its efficacy is questionable. Of these, only methylergonovine is currently available in the United States. If there is infection, antimicrobial therapy usually leads to a good response. In an earlier study, Wager and coworkers (1980) reported that a third of these late cases of postpartum metritis are caused by *Chlamydia trachomatis.* Empirical therapy with azithromycin or doxycycline usually prompts resolution regardless of bacterial etiology.

Another cause of subinvolution is incompletely remodeled uteroplacental arteries (Andrew, 1989; Kavalar, 2012). These noninvoluted vessels are filled with thromboses and lack an endothelial lining. Perivascular trophoblasts are also identified in the vessel walls, suggesting an aberrant interaction between uterine cells and trophoblasts.

Late Postpartum Hemorrhage

The American College of Obstetricians and Gynecologists (2013b) defines *secondary postpartum hemorrhage* as bleeding 24 hours to 12 weeks after delivery. Clinically worrisome uterine hemorrhage develops within 1 to 2 weeks in perhaps 1 percent of women. Such bleeding most often is the result of abnormal involution of the placental site. It occasionally is caused by retention of a placental fragment or by a uterine artery pseudoaneurysm. Usually, retained products undergo necrosis with fibrin deposition and may eventually form a so-called *placental polyp*. As the eschar of the polyp detaches from the myometrium, hemorrhage may be brisk. As discussed in Chapter 56 (p. 1118), delayed postpartum hemorrhage may also be caused by von Willebrand disease or other inherited coagulopathies (Lipe, 2011).

In our experiences, few women with delayed hemorrhage are found to have retained placental fragments. Thus, we and others do not routinely perform curettage (Lee, 1981). Another concern is that curettage may worsen bleeding by avulsing part of the implantation site. Thus, in a stable patient, if sonographic examination shows an empty cavity, then oxytocin, methylergonovine, or a prostaglandin analogue is given. Antimicrobials are added if uterine infection is suspected. If large clots are seen in the uterine cavity with sonography, then *gentle* suction curettage is considered. Otherwise curettage is carried out only if appreciable bleeding persists or recurs after medical management.

URINARY TRACT

Normal pregnancy-induced glomerular hyperfiltration persists on the first postpartum day but returns to prepregnancy baseline by 2 weeks (Hladunewich, 2004). Also, dilated ureters and renal pelves return to their prepregnant state during the course of 2 to 8 weeks postpartum. Because of this dilated collecting system, coupled with residual urine and bacteriuria in a traumatized bladder, urinary tract infection is a concern in the puerperium.

Bladder trauma is associated most closely with labor length and thus to some degree is a normal accompaniment of vaginal delivery. Funnell and colleagues (1954) used cystoscopy immediately postpartum and described varying degrees of submucosal hemorrhage and edema. Postpartum, the bladder has an increased capacity and a relative insensitivity to intravesical pressure. Thus, overdistention, incomplete emptying, and excessive residual urine are common. Their management is discussed on page 676.

It is unusual for urinary incontinence to manifest during the puerperium. That said, much attention has been given to the potential for subsequent development of urinary incontinence and other pelvic floor disorders in the years following delivery. A fuller discussion is found in Chapter 30 (p. 588).

PERITONEUM AND ABDOMINAL WALL

The broad and round ligaments require considerable time to recover from stretching and loosening during pregnancy. As a result of ruptured elastic fibers in the skin and prolonged distention by the pregnant uterus, the abdominal wall remains soft and flaccid. If the abdomen is unusually flabby or pendulous, an ordinary girdle is often satisfactory. An abdominal binder is at best a temporary measure. Several weeks are required for these structures to return to normal, and recovery is aided by exercise. These may be started anytime following vaginal delivery and as soon as abdominal soreness diminishes after cesarean delivery. Silvery abdominal striae commonly develop as *striae gravidarum* (Chap. 4, p. 51). Except for these, the abdominal wall usually resumes its prepregnancy appearance. When muscles remain atonic, however, the abdominal wall also remains lax. Marked separation of the rectus abdominis muscles—*diastasis recti*—may result.

HEMATOLOGICAL PARAMETERS AND PREGNANCY HYPERVOLEMIA

Hematological and Coagulation Changes

Marked leukocytosis and thrombocytosis may occur during and after labor. The white blood cell count sometimes reaches 30,000/μL, with the increase predominantly due to granulocytes. There is a relative lymphopenia and an absolute eosinopenia. Normally, during the first few postpartum days, hemoglobin concentration and hematocrit fluctuate moderately. If they fall much below the levels present just before labor, a considerable amount of blood has been lost (Chap. 41, p. 781).

By the end of pregnancy, there are many changes in laboratory findings that assess coagulation (Kenny, 2014). These are discussed in Chapter 4 (p. 57) and listed in the Appendix (p. 1288). Many persist in the puerperium. One example is that the markedly increased levels of plasma fibrinogen are maintained at least through the first week, and hence, so is the increase in sedimentation rate.

Pregnancy-Induced Hypervolemia

When the amount of blood attained by normal pregnancy hypervolemia is lost as postpartum hemorrhage, the woman almost immediately regains her nonpregnant blood volume (Chap. 41, p. 781). If less has been lost at delivery, it appears that in most women, blood volume has nearly returned to its nonpregnant level by 1 week after delivery. Cardiac output usually remains elevated for 24 to 48 hours postpartum and declines to nonpregnant values by 10 days (Robson, 1987). Heart rate changes follow this pattern. Systemic vascular resistance and blood pressure rise (Fig. 36-4). Systemic vascular resistance remains in the lower range characteristic of pregnancy for 2 days postpartum and then begins to steadily increase to normal nonpregnant values (Hibbard, 2014).

Normal pregnancy is associated with an appreciable increase in extracellular sodium and water, and postpartum diuresis is a physiological reversal of this process. Chesley and coworkers (1959) demonstrated a decrease in sodium space of approximately 2 L during the first week postpartum. This also corresponds with loss of residual pregnancy hypervolemia. In preeclampsia, pathological retention of fluid antepartum and its diuresis postpartum may be prodigious (Chap. 40, p. 768).

Postpartum diuresis results in relatively rapid weight loss of 2 to 3 kg, which is added to the 5 to 6 kg incurred by delivery and normal blood loss. Weight loss from pregnancy itself is likely to be maximal by the end of the second week postpartum.

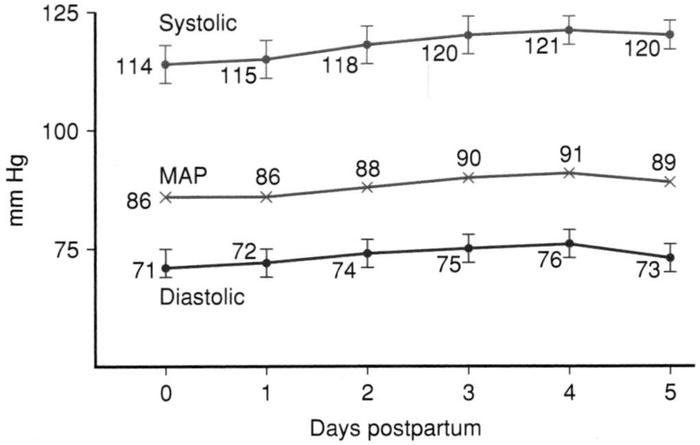

FIGURE 36-4 During the early puerperium, blood pressure normally rises toward nonpregnant values. MAP = mean arterial pressure.

It follows that any residual increased weight compared with prepregnancy values probably represents fat stores that will persist. According to Schauberger and associates (1992), women approach their self-reported prepregnancy weight 6 months after delivery but still retain an average surplus of 1.4 kg (3 lb).

BREASTS AND LACTATION

Breast Anatomy and Products

Each mature mammary gland or breast is composed of 15 to 25 lobes. They are arranged radially and are separated from one another by varying amounts of fat. Each lobe consists of several lobules, which in turn are composed of numerous alveoli. Each alveolus is provided with a small duct that joins others to form a single larger duct for each lobe as shown in Figure 36-5. These *lactiferous ducts* open separately on the nipple, where they may be distinguished as minute but distinct orifices. The alveolar secretory epithelium synthesizes the various milk constituents, described next.

After delivery, the breasts begin to secrete *colostrum*, which is a deep lemon-yellow liquid. It usually can be expressed from the nipples by the second postpartum day. Compared with mature milk, colostrum is rich in immunological components and contains more minerals and amino acids (Ballard, 2013). It also has more protein, much of which is globulin, but less sugar and fat. Secretion persists for 5 days to 2 weeks, with gradual conversion to mature milk by 4 to 6 weeks. The colostrum content of immunoglobulin A (IgA) offers the newborn protection against enteric pathogens. Other host resistance factors found in colostrum and milk include complement, macrophages, lymphocytes, lactoferrin, lactoperoxidase, and lysozymes.

Mature milk is a complex and dynamic biological fluid that includes fat, proteins, carbohydrates, bioactive factors, minerals, vitamins, hormones, and many cellular products. The concentrations and contents of human milk change even during a single feed and are influenced by maternal diet, as well as infant age, health, and needs. A nursing mother easily produces 600 mL of milk daily, and maternal gestational weight gain has little impact on its quantity or quality (Institute of Medicine, 1990). Milk is isotonic with plasma, and lactose accounts for half of the osmotic pressure. Essential amino acids are derived from blood, and nonessential amino acids are derived in part from blood or synthesized in the mammary gland. Most milk proteins are unique and include α-lactalbumin, β-lactoglobulin, and casein. Fatty acids are synthesized in the alveoli from glucose and are secreted by an apocrine-like process. Most vitamins are found in human milk, but in variable amounts. Vitamin K is virtually absent, and thus, an intramuscular dose is given to the newborn (Chap. 33, p. 644). Vitamin D content is low—22 IU/mL. Thus, newborn supplementation is also recommended by the American Academy of Pediatrics (Wagner, 2008).

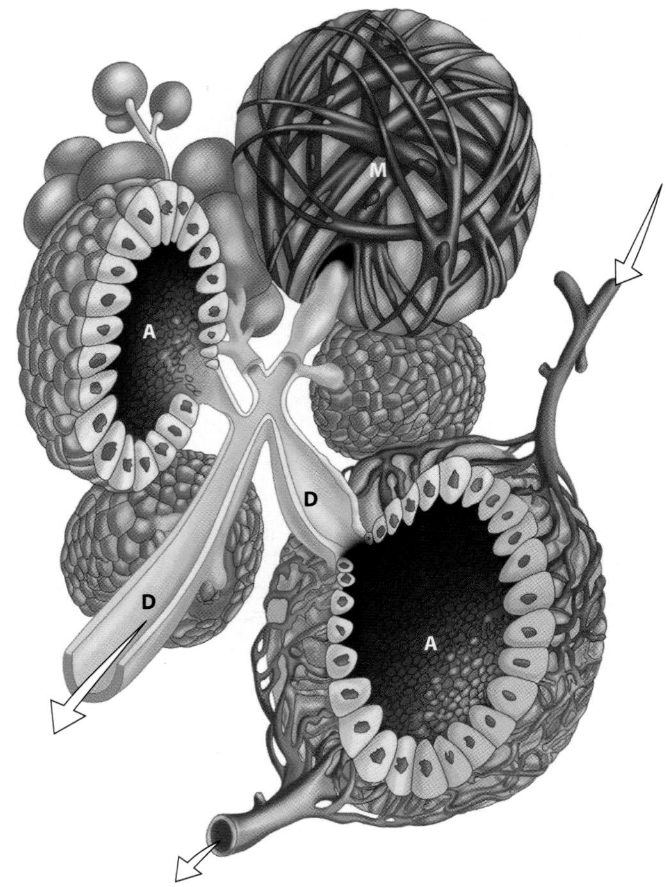

FIGURE 36-5 Schematic of the alveolar and ductal system during lactation. Note the myoepithelial fibers (*M*) that surround the outside of the uppermost alveolus. The secretions from the glandular elements are extruded into the lumen of the alveoli (*A*) and ejected by the myoepithelial cells into the ductal system (*D*), which empties through the nipple. Arterial blood supply to the alveolus is identified by the upper right arrow and venous drainage by the arrow beneath.

Whey is milk serum and has been shown to contain large amounts of interleukin-6 (Saito, 1991). Human milk has a whey-to-casein ratio of 60:40, considered ideal for absorption. *Prolactin* appears to be actively secreted into breast milk (Yuen, 1988). *Epidermal growth factor (EGF)* has been identified in human milk. And because it is not destroyed by gastric proteolytic enzymes, it may be absorbed to promote growth and maturation of newborn intestinal mucosa (McCleary, 1991).

Other critical components in human milk include lactoferrin, melatonin, oligosaccharides, and essential fatty acids.

Endocrinology of Lactation

The precise humoral and neural mechanisms involved in lactation are complex. Progesterone, estrogen, and placental lactogen, as well as prolactin, cortisol, and insulin, appear to act in concert to stimulate the growth and development of the milk-secreting apparatus (Porter, 1974). With delivery, there is an abrupt and profound decrease in the levels of progesterone and estrogen. This decrease removes the inhibitory influence of progesterone on α-lactalbumin production and stimulates lactose synthase to increase milk lactose. Progesterone withdrawal also allows prolactin to act unopposed in its stimulation of α-lactalbumin production. Serotonin is produced in mammary epithelial cells and has a role in maintaining milk production. This may explain the decreased milk production in women taking selective serotonin-reuptake inhibitors—SSRIs (Collier, 2012).

The intensity and duration of subsequent lactation are controlled, in large part, by the repetitive stimulus of nursing and emptying of milk from the breast. Prolactin is essential for lactation, and women with extensive pituitary necrosis—*Sheehan syndrome*—do not lactate (Chap. 58, p. 1163). Although plasma prolactin levels fall after delivery to levels lower than during pregnancy, each act of suckling triggers a rise in levels (McNeilly, 1983). Presumably a stimulus from the breast curtails the release of dopamine, also known as prolactin-inhibiting factor, from the hypothalamus. This in turn transiently induces increased prolactin secretion.

The posterior pituitary secretes oxytocin in pulsatile fashion. This stimulates milk expression from a lactating breast by causing contraction of myoepithelial cells in the alveoli and small milk ducts (see Fig. 36-4). Milk ejection, or *letting down*, is a reflex initiated especially by suckling, which stimulates the posterior pituitary to liberate oxytocin. The reflex may even be provoked by an infant cry and can be inhibited by maternal fright or stress.

Immunological Consequences of Breast Feeding

Human milk contains several protective immunological substances, including secretory IgA and growth factors. The antibodies in human milk are specifically directed against maternal environmental antigens such as against *Escherichia coli* (Iyengar, 2012). As a result, breast-fed infants are less prone to enteric infections than bottle-fed ones (Cravioto, 1991). Human milk also provides protection against rotavirus infections, a major cause of infant gastroenteritis (Newburg, 1998). Moreover, the risks of atopic dermatitis and respiratory infections are reduced (Ip, 2009). Bartick and Reinhold (2010) calculated that significant economic burdens from pediatric disease could be lessened by improved breast-feeding rates.

Much attention has been directed to the role of maternal breast-milk lymphocytes in neonatal immunological processes. Milk contains both T and B lymphocytes, but the T lymphocytes appear to differ from those found in blood. Specifically, milk T lymphocytes are almost exclusively composed of cells that exhibit specific membrane antigens. These memory T cells appear to be an avenue for the neonate to benefit from the maternal immunological experience (Bertotto, 1990).

Nursing

Human milk is ideal food for neonates. It provides age-specific nutrients as well as immunological factors and antibacterial substances (American College of Obstetricians and Gynecologists, 2013a). Milk also contains factors that act as biological signals for promoting cellular growth and differentiation. The American Academy of Pediatrics (2012) has provided a list of dose-response benefits of nursing (Table 36-2). For both mother and infant, the benefits of breast feeding are long-term. For example, women who breast feed have a lower risk of breast and reproductive cancer, and their children have increased adult intelligence independent of a wide range of possible confounding factors (Jong, 2012; Kramer, 2008). Breast feeding is associated with decreased postpartum weight retention (Baker, 2008). In addition, rates of sudden-infant-death syndrome are significantly lower among breast-fed infants. Last, in the Nurses' Health Study, women who reported breast feeding for at least 2 cumulative years had a 23-percent lower risk of coronary heart disease (Stuebe, 2009). For all these reasons, the American Academy of Pediatrics (2012) supports the World Health Organization (2011) recommendations of exclusive breast feeding for up to 6 months, with avoidance of exposure to cow milk proteins.

The Surgeon General of the U.S. Department of Health and Human Services (2011) lists some barriers for breast feeding and suggests practical means of overcoming them. Educational initiatives that include father and peer counseling may improve these rates (Pisacane, 2005; Wolfberg, 2004). The *Baby Friendly Hospital Initiative* is an international program to increase rates of exclusive breast feeding and to extend its duration. It is based on the World Health Organization (1989) *Ten Steps to Successful Breastfeeding* (Table 36-3). Worldwide, almost 20,000 hospitals are designated as "baby-friendly." Forrester-Knauss and coworkers (2013) described successful trends toward exclusive breast feeding in Switzerland during 9 years

TABLE 36-2. Advantages of Breast Feeding

Nutritional
Immunological
Developmental
Psychological
Social
Economical
Environmental
Optimal growth and development
Decrease risks for acute and chronic diseases

Summarized from the American Academy of Pediatrics and the American College of Obstetricians and Gynecologists, 2012.

TABLE 36-3. Ten Steps to Successful Breast Feeding

1. Have a written breast-feeding policy that is regularly communicated to all health-care staff
2. Train all staff in skills necessary to implement this policy
3. Inform all pregnant women about the benefits and management of breast feeding
4. Help mothers initiate breast feeding within an hour of birth
5. Show mothers how to breast feed and how to sustain lactation, even if they should be separated from their infants
6. Feed newborn infants nothing but breast milk, unless medically indicated, and under no circumstances provide breast milk substitutes, feeding bottles, or pacifiers free of charge or at low cost
7. Practice rooming-in, which allows mothers and infants to remain together 24 hours a day
8. Encourage breast feeding on demand
9. Give no artificial pacifiers to breast-feeding infants
10. Help start breast-feeding support groups and refer mothers to them

Adapted from the World Health Organization, 1989.

in which a Baby-Friendly Hospital Initiative was implemented. However, in 2011 in the United States, fewer than 10 percent of births in 43 states and the District of Columbia occurred in "baby friendly" hospitals (Centers for Disease Control and Prevention, 2012a). In a large population-based study, fewer than two thirds of term neonates were exclusively breast fed at the time of discharge (McDonald, 2012).

There are a variety of individual resources available for breast-feeding mothers that include online information from the American Academy of Pediatrics (http://www.aap.org) and La Leche League International (http://www.lalecheleague.org).

Care of Breasts

The nipples require little attention other than cleanliness and attention to skin fissures. Fissured nipples render nursing painful, and they may have a deleterious influence on milk production. These cracks also provide a portal of entry for pyogenic bacteria. Because dried milk is likely to accumulate and irritate the nipples, washing the areola with water and mild soap is helpful before and after nursing. When the nipples are irritated or fissured, it may be necessary to use topical lanolin and a nipple shield for 24 hours or longer. If fissuring is severe, the infant should not be permitted to nurse on the affected side. Instead, the breast should be emptied regularly with a pump until the lesions are healed. Poor latching of the neonate to the breast can create such fissures. Proper technique for positioning the mother and infant during *latch-on* and nursing has been reviewed by the American College of Obstetricians and Gynecologists (2013a).

Contraindications to Breast Feeding

Nursing is contraindicated in women who take street drugs or do not control their alcohol use; have an infant with galactosemia; have human immunodeficiency virus (HIV) infection; have active, untreated tuberculosis; take certain medications; or are undergoing breast cancer treatment (American Academy of Pediatrics and American College of Obstetricians and Gynecologists, 2012; Faupel-Badger, 2013). Breast feeding has been recognized for some time as a mode of HIV transmission and is proscribed in developed countries in which adequate nutrition is otherwise available (Chap. 65, p. 1282). Other viral infections do not contraindicate breast feeding. For example, with maternal cytomegalovirus infection, both virus and antibodies are present in breast milk. And although hepatitis B virus is excreted in milk, breast feeding is not contraindicated if hepatitis B immune globulin is given to the newborns of affected mothers. Maternal hepatitis C infection is not a contraindication because breast feeding has not been shown to transmit infection. Women with active herpes simplex virus may suckle their infants if there are no breast lesions and if particular care is directed to hand washing before nursing.

Drugs Secreted in Milk

Most drugs given to the mother are secreted in breast milk, although the amount ingested by the infant typically is small. Many factors influence drug excretion and include plasma concentration, degree of protein binding, plasma and milk pH, degree of ionization, lipid solubility, and molecular weight (Rowe, 2013). The ratio of drug concentration in breast milk to that in maternal plasma is the *milk-to-plasma drug-concentration ratio*. Most drugs have a ratio of ≤ 1, approximately 25 percent have a ratio > 1, and about 15 percent have a ratio > 2 (Ito, 2000). Ideally, to minimize infant exposure, medication selection should favor drugs with a shorter half-life, poorer oral absorption, and lower lipid solubility. If multiple daily drug doses are required, then each is taken by the mother *after* the closest feed. Single daily-dosed drugs may be taken just before the longest infant sleep interval—usually at bedtime (Spencer, 2002).

There are only a few drugs that are absolutely contraindicated while breast feeding (Berlin, 2013; Bertino, 2012). Cytotoxic drugs may interfere with cellular metabolism and potentially cause immune suppression or neutropenia, affect growth, and, at least theoretically, increase the risk of childhood cancer. Examples include cyclophosphamide, cyclosporine, doxorubicin, methotrexate, and mycophenolate. If a medication presents a concern, then the importance of therapy should be ascertained. It should be determined whether there is a safer alternative or whether neonatal exposure can be minimized if the medication dose is taken immediately after each breast feeding (American Academy of Pediatrics and the American College of Obstetricians and Gynecologists, 2012). Data on individual drugs are available through the National Institutes of Health website, LactMed, which can be found at: toxnet.nlm.nih.gov/cgi-bin/sis/htmlgen?LACT.

Radioactive isotopes of copper, gallium, indium, iodine, sodium, and technetium rapidly appear in breast milk.

Consultation with a nuclear medicine specialist is recommended before performing a diagnostic study with these isotopes (Chap. 46, p. 934). The goal is to use a radionuclide with the shortest excretion time in breast milk. The mother should pump her breasts before the study and store enough milk in a freezer for feeding the infant. After the study, she should pump her breasts to maintain milk production but discard all milk produced during the time that radioactivity is present. This ranges from 15 hours up to 2 weeks, depending on the isotope used. Importantly, radioactive iodine concentrates and persists in the thyroid. Its special considerations are discussed in Chapter 63 (p. 1231).

Breast Engorgement

This is common in women who do not breast feed and is typified by milk leakage and breast pain. These peak 3 to 5 days after delivery (Spitz, 1998). Up to half of affected women require analgesia for breast-pain relief, and as many as 10 percent report severe pain for up to 14 days.

Evidence is insufficient to firmly support any specific treatment (Mangesi, 2010). That said, breasts can be supported with a well-fitting brassiere, breast binder, or "sports bra." Cool packs and oral analgesics for 12 to 24 hours aid discomfort. Pharmacological or hormonal agents are not recommended to suppress lactation.

Fever caused by breast engorgement was common before the renaissance of breast feeding. In one study, Almeida and Kitay (1986) reported that 13 percent of postpartum women had fever from engorgement that ranged from 37.8 to 39°C. Fever seldom persists for longer than 4 to 16 hours. The incidence and severity of engorgement, and fever associated with it, are much lower if women breast feed. Other causes of fever, especially those due to infection, must be excluded. Of these, *mastitis* is infection of the mammary parenchyma. It is relatively common in lactating women and is discussed in Chapter 37 (p. 691).

Other Issues with Lactation

With *inverted nipples*, lactiferous ducts open directly into a depression at the center of the areola. With these depressed nipples, nursing is difficult. If the depression is not deep, milk sometimes can be made available by use of a breast pump. If instead the nipple is greatly inverted, daily attempts should be made during the last few months of pregnancy to draw or "tease" the nipple out with the fingers.

Extra breasts—*polymastia*, or extra nipples—*polythelia*, may develop along the former embryonic mammary ridge. Also termed the *milk line*, this line extends from the axilla to the groin bilaterally. In some women, there may be vulvar breast tissue (Wagner, 2013). The incidence of accessory breast tissue ranges from 0.22 to 6 percent in the general population (Loukas, 2007). These breasts may be so small as to be mistaken for pigmented moles, or if without a nipple, for lymphadenopathy or lipoma. Polymastia has no obstetrical significance, although occasionally enlargement of these accessory breasts during pregnancy or engorgement postpartum may result in discomfort and anxiety.

Galactocele is a milk duct that becomes obstructed by inspissated secretions. The amount is ordinarily limited, but an excess may form a fluctuant mass—a galactocele—that may cause pressure symptoms and have the appearance of an abscess. It may resolve spontaneously or require aspiration.

There are marked individual variations in the amount of milk secreted. Many of these are dependent not on general maternal health but on breast glandular development. Rarely, there is complete lack of mammary secretion—*agalactia*. Occasionally, mammary secretion is excessive—*polygalactia*.

MATERNAL CARE DURING THE PUERPERIUM

Hospital Care

For 2 hours after delivery, blood pressure and pulse should be taken every 15 minutes, or more frequently if indicated. Temperature is assessed every 4 hours for the first 8 hours and then at least every 8 hours subsequently (American Academy of Pediatrics and American College of Obstetricians and Gynecologists, 2012). The amount of vaginal bleeding is monitored, and the fundus palpated to ensure that it is well contracted. If relaxation is detected, the uterus should be massaged through the abdominal wall until it remains contracted. Uterotonics are also sometimes required. Blood may accumulate within the uterus without external bleeding. This may be detected early by uterine enlargement during fundal palpation in the first postdelivery hours. Because the likelihood of significant hemorrhage is greatest immediately postpartum, even in normal births, the uterus is closely monitored for at least 1 hour after delivery. Postpartum hemorrhage is discussed in Chapter 41 (p. 783). If regional analgesia or general anesthesia was used for labor or delivery, the mother should be observed in an appropriately equipped and staffed recovery area.

Women are out of bed within a few hours after delivery. An attendant should be present for at least the first time, in case the woman becomes syncopal. The many confirmed advantages of early ambulation include fewer bladder complications, less frequent constipation, and reduced rates of puerperal venous thromboembolism. Almost half of thromboembolic events associated with pregnancy develop in the puerperium. Jacobsen and colleagues (2008) reported that pulmonary embolism is most common in the first 6 weeks postpartum. In a recent audit of puerperal women at Parkland Hospital, the frequency of venous thromboembolism was found to be 0.008 percent after a vaginal birth and 0.04 percent following cesarean delivery. We attribute this low incidence to early ambulation. Risk factors and other measures to diminish the frequency of thromboembolism are discussed in Chapter 52 (p. 1029).

There are no dietary restrictions for women who have been delivered vaginally. Two hours after normal vaginal delivery, if there are no complications, a woman should be allowed to eat. With breast feeding, the level of calories and protein consumed during pregnancy should be increased slightly as recommended by the Food and Nutrition Board of the National Research Council (Chap. 9, p. 178). If the mother does not breast feed, dietary requirements are the same as for a nonpregnant woman. It is standard practice in our hospital to continue oral iron supplementation for at least 3 months after delivery and to check the hematocrit at a first postpartum visit.

Perineal Care

The woman is instructed to cleanse the vulva from anterior to posterior—the vulva toward the anus. A cool pack applied to the perineum may help reduce edema and discomfort during the first 24 hours if there is a laceration or an episiotomy. Most women also appear to obtain a measure of relief from the periodic application of a local anesthetic spray. Severe discomfort usually indicates a problem, such as a hematoma within the first day or so and infection after the third or fourth day (Chap. 37, p. 689 and Chap. 41, p 790). *Severe perineal, vaginal, or rectal pain always warrants careful inspection and palpation.* Beginning approximately 24 hours after delivery, moist heat as provided by warm sitz baths can be used to reduce local discomfort. Tub bathing after uncomplicated delivery is allowed. The episiotomy incision normally is firmly healed and nearly asymptomatic by the third week.

Rarely, the cervix, and occasionally a portion of the uterine body, may protrude from the vulva following delivery. This is accompanied by variable degrees of anterior and posterior vaginal wall prolapse. Symptoms include a palpable mass at or past the introitus, voiding difficulties, or pressure. Puerperal procidentia typically improves with time as the weight of the uterus lessens with involution. As a temporizing measure in those with pronounced prolapse, the uterus can be replaced and held in position with a suitable pessary.

Bladder Function

In most delivery units, intravenous fluids are infused during labor and for an hour or so after delivery. Oxytocin, in doses that have an antidiuretic effect, is typically infused postpartum, and rapid bladder filling is common. Moreover, both bladder sensation and capability to empty spontaneously may be diminished by local or conduction analgesia, by trauma to the bladder, by episiotomy or lacerations, or by operative vaginal delivery. Thus, urinary retention and bladder overdistention is common in the early puerperium. Ching-Chung and associates (2002) reported retention in 4 percent of women delivered vaginally. Musselwhite and coworkers (2007) reported retention in 4.7 percent of women who had labor epidural analgesia. Risk factors that increased likelihood of retention were primiparity, perineal lacerations, oxytocin-induced or -augmented labor, operative vaginal delivery, catheterization during labor, and labor duration > 10 hours.

Prevention of bladder overdistention demands observation after delivery to ensure that the bladder does not overfill and that it empties adequately with each voiding. The enlarged bladder can be palpated suprapubically, or it is evident abdominally indirectly as it elevates the fundus above the umbilicus. Van Os and Van der Linden (2006) have investigated the use of an automated sonography system to detect high bladder volumes and thus postpartum urinary retention.

If a woman has not voided within 4 hours after delivery, it is likely that she cannot. If she has trouble voiding initially, she also is likely to have further trouble. An examination for perineal and genital-tract hematomas is made. With an overdistended bladder, an indwelling catheter should be left in place until the factors causing retention have abated. Even without a demonstrable cause, it usually is best to leave the catheter in place for at least 24 hours. This prevents recurrence and allows recovery of normal bladder tone and sensation.

When the catheter is removed, it is necessary subsequently to demonstrate ability to void appropriately. If a woman cannot void after 4 hours, she should be catheterized and the urine volume measured. If more than 200 mL, the bladder is not functioning appropriately, and the catheter is left for another 24 hours. If less than 200 mL of urine is obtained, the catheter can be removed and the bladder rechecked subsequently as just described. Harris and coworkers (1977) reported that 40 percent of such women develop bacteriuria, and thus a single dose or short course of antimicrobial therapy is reasonable after the catheter is removed.

Pain, Mood, and Cognition

Discomfort and its causes following cesarean delivery are considered in Chapter 30 (p. 605). During the first few days after vaginal delivery, the mother may be uncomfortable because of afterpains, episiotomy and lacerations, breast engorgement, and at times, postdural puncture headache. Mild analgesics containing codeine, aspirin, or acetaminophen, preferably in combinations, are given as frequently as every 3 hours during the first few days.

It is fairly common for a mother to exhibit some degree of depressed mood a few days after delivery. Termed *postpartum blues,* this likely is the consequence of several factors that include emotional letdown that follows the excitement and fears experienced during pregnancy and delivery, discomforts of the early puerperium, fatigue from sleep deprivation, anxiety over the ability to provide appropriate infant care, and body image concerns.

In most women, effective treatment includes anticipation, recognition, and reassurance. This disorder is usually mild and self-limited to 2 to 3 days, although it sometimes lasts for up to 10 days. Should these moods persist or worsen, an evaluation for symptoms of major depression is done (Chap. 61, p. 1205). Suicidal or infanticidal ideation is dealt with emergently. Because major postpartum depression recurs in at least a fourth of women in subsequent pregnancies, some recommend pharmacological prophylaxis beginning in late pregnancy or immediately postpartum.

Last, postpartum hormonal changes in some women may affect brain function. Bannbers and colleagues (2013) compared a measure of executive function in postpartum women and controls and observed a decrease in postpartum subjects.

Neuromusculoskeletal Problems

Obstetrical Neuropathies

Pressure on branches of the lumbosacral nerve plexus during labor may manifest as complaints of intense neuralgia or cramplike pains extending down one or both legs as soon as the head descends into the pelvis. If the nerve is injured, pain may continue after delivery, and there also may be variable degrees of sensory loss or muscle paralysis. In some cases, there is footdrop, which can be secondary to injury at the level of the lumbosacral plexus, sciatic nerve, or common fibular (peroneal) nerve. Components of the lumbosacral plexus cross the pelvic brim and can be compressed by the fetal head or by forceps. The common fibular nerves may be externally compressed when the legs are positioned in stirrups, especially during prolonged second-stage labor.

Obstetrical neuropathy is relatively infrequent. Wong and associates (2003) evaluated more than 6000 delivered women and found that approximately 1 percent had a confirmed nerve injury. Lateral femoral cutaneous neuropathies were the most common (24), followed by femoral neuropathies (14). A motor deficit accompanied a third of injuries. Nulliparity, prolonged second-stage labor, and pushing for a long duration in the semi-Fowler position were risk factors. The median duration of symptoms was 2 months, and the range was 2 weeks to 18 months.

Nerve injuries with cesarean delivery include the iliohypogastric and ilioinguinal nerves (Rahn, 2010). These are discussed further in Chapter 2 (p. 17).

Musculoskeletal Injuries

Pain in the pelvic girdle, hips, or lower extremities may follow stretching or tearing injuries sustained at normal or difficult delivery. Magnetic resonance (MR) imaging is often informative. One example is the piriformis muscle hematoma shown in Figure 36-6. Most injuries resolve with antiinflammatory agents and physical therapy. Rarely, there may be septic pyomyositis such as with iliopsoas muscle abscess (Nelson, 2010; Young, 2010).

Separation of the symphysis pubis or one of the sacroiliac synchondroses during labor leads to pain and marked interference with locomotion. Estimates of the frequency of this event vary widely from 1 in 600 to 1 in 30,000 deliveries (Reis, 1932; Taylor, 1986). In our experiences, symptomatic separations are uncommon. Their onset of pain is often acute during delivery, but symptoms may manifest either antepartum or up to 48 hours postpartum (Snow, 1997). Treatment is generally conservative, with rest in a lateral decubitus position and an appropriately fitted pelvic binder. Surgery is occasionally necessary in some symphyseal separations of more than 4 cm (Kharrazi, 1997). The recurrence risk is > 50 percent in subsequent pregnancy, and Culligan and associates (2002) recommend consideration for cesarean delivery. In rare cases, fractures of the sacrum or pubic ramus are caused by even uncomplicated deliveries (Alonso-Burgos, 2007). As discussed in Chapter 58 (p. 1159), the latter are more likely with osteoporosis associated with heparin or corticosteroid therapy (Cunningham, 2005). In rare but serious cases, bacterial osteomyelitis—*osteitis pubis*—can be devastating (Fig. 36-7). Lawford and coworkers (2010) reported such a case that caused massive vulvar edema.

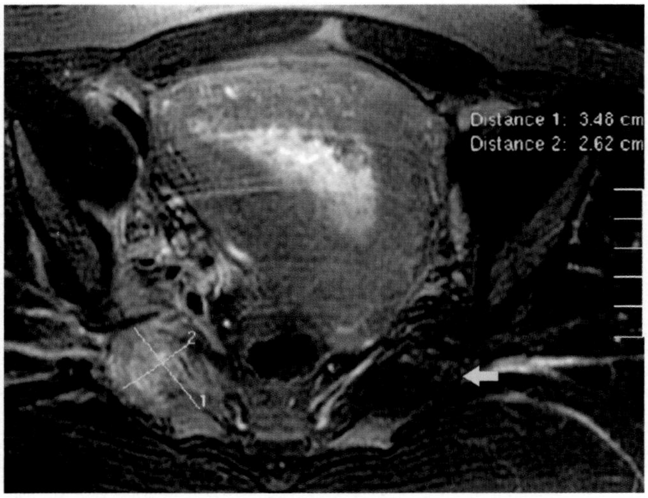

FIGURE 36-6 Magnetic resonance image of a piriformis hematoma. A large inhomogeneous mass of the right piriformis muscle consistent with a hematoma (*yellow cursor measurements*) is compared with the normal-appearing left piriformis muscle (*yellow arrow*).

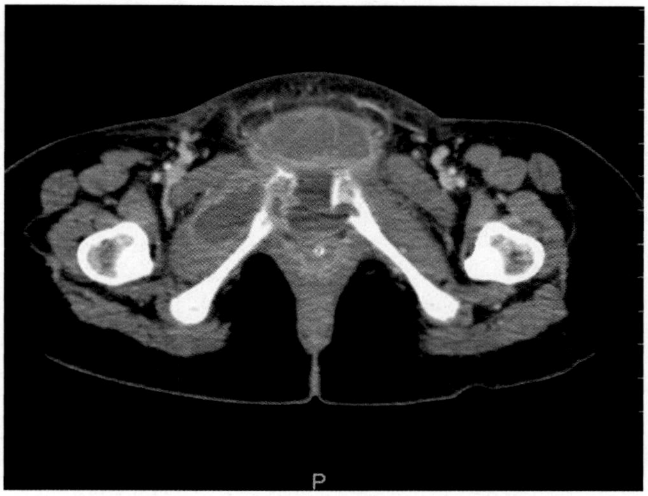

FIGURE 36-7 Bacterial osteitis pubis–osteomyelitis caused by *Streptococcus milleri* in a woman with symptomatic symphyseal separation.

Immunizations

The D-negative woman who is not isoimmunized and whose infant is D-positive is given 300 μg of anti-D immune globulin shortly after delivery (Chap. 15, p. 311). Women who are not already immune to rubella or rubeola measles are excellent candidates for combined measles-mumps-rubella vaccination before discharge (Chap. 9, p. 184). Unless contraindicated, at Parkland Hospital a diphtheria-tetanus toxoid booster injection is also given to postpartum women.

Hospital Discharge

Following uncomplicated vaginal delivery, hospitalization is seldom warranted for more than 48 hours. A woman should receive instructions concerning anticipated normal physiological puerperal changes, including lochia patterns, weight loss from diuresis, and milk let-down. She also should receive instructions concerning fever, excessive vaginal bleeding, or leg pain, swelling, or tenderness. Persistent headaches, shortness of breath, or chest pain warrant immediate concern.

Hospital stay length following labor and delivery is now regulated by federal law (Chap. 32, p. 634). Currently, the norms are hospital stays up to 48 hours following uncomplicated vaginal delivery and up to 96 hours following uncomplicated cesarean delivery (American Academy of Pediatrics and the American College of Obstetricians and Gynecologists, 2012). Earlier hospital discharge is acceptable for appropriately selected women if they desire it.

Contraception

During the hospital stay, a concerted effort should be made to provide family planning education. Various forms of contraception are discussed throughout Chapter 38 and sterilization procedures in Chapter 39.

Women not breast feeding have return of menses usually within 6 to 8 weeks. At times, however, it is difficult clinically to assign a specific date to the first menstrual period after delivery. A minority of women bleed small to moderate amounts intermittently, starting soon after delivery. Ovulation occurs at a mean of 7 weeks, but ranges from 5 to 11 weeks (Perez, 1972). That said, ovulation before 28 days has been described (Hytten, 1995). Thus, conception is possible during the artificially defined 6-week puerperium. *Women who become sexually active during the puerperium, and who do not desire to conceive, should initiate contraception.* Kelly and associates (2005) reported that by the third month postpartum, 58 percent of adolescents had resumed sexual intercourse, but only 80 percent of these were using contraception. Because of this, many recommend long-acting reversible contraceptives—LARC (Baldwin, 2013).

Women who breast feed ovulate much less frequently compared with those who do not, but there are great variations. Timing of ovulation depends on individual biological variation as well as the intensity of breast feeding. Lactating women may first menstruate as early as the second or as late as the 18th month after delivery. Campbell and Gray (1993) analyzed daily urine specimens to determine the time of ovulation in 92 lactating women. As shown in Figure 36-8, breast feeding in general delays resumption of ovulation, although as already emphasized, it does not invariably forestall it. Other findings in their study included the following:

1. Resumption of ovulation was frequently marked by return of normal menstrual bleeding.
2. Breast-feeding episodes lasting 15 minutes seven times daily delayed ovulation resumption.
3. Ovulation can occur without bleeding.
4. Bleeding can be anovulatory.
5. The risk of pregnancy in breast-feeding women was approximately 4 percent per year.

For the breast-feeding woman, progestin-only contraceptives—mini-pills, depot medroxyprogesterone, or progestin implants—do not affect the quality or quantity of milk. These may be initiated any time during the puerperium. Estrogen-progestin contraceptives likely reduce the quantity of breast milk, but under the proper circumstances, they too can be used by breast-feeding women. However, these are withheld until after the first 4 weeks because of their higher thromboembolic risk in puerperal patients. These hormonal methods are summarized in Table 36-4 and are discussed in Chapter 38 (p. 695).

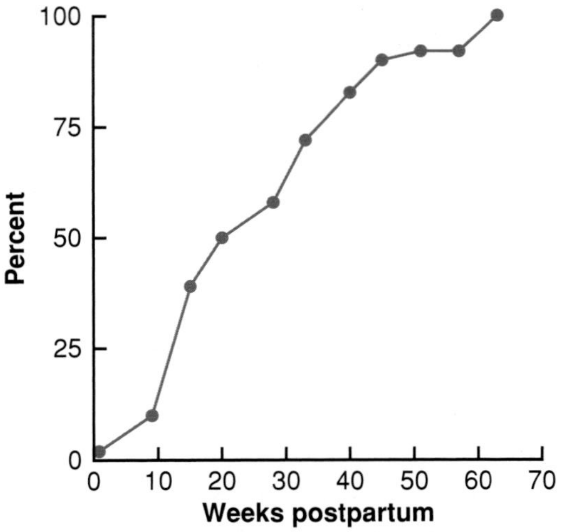

FIGURE 36-8 Cumulative proportion of breast-feeding women who ovulated during the first 70 weeks following delivery. (Data from Campbell, 1993.)

HOME CARE

Coitus

There are no evidence-based data concerning resumption of coitus after delivery. It seems best to use common sense (Minig, 2009). After 2 weeks, coitus may be resumed *based on desire and comfort.* Barrett and colleagues (2000) reported that almost 90 percent of 484 primiparous women resumed sexual activity by 6 months. And although 65 percent of these reported problems, only 15 percent discussed them with a health-care provider.

Intercourse too soon may be unpleasant, if not frankly painful, due to incomplete healing of the episiotomy or lacerations. Moreover, the vaginal epithelium is thin, and very little lubrication follows sexual stimulation. This is due to the hypoestrogenic state following delivery, which lasts until ovulation resumes. It may be particularly problematic in breast-feeding women who are hypoestrogenic for many months postpartum (Palmer, 2003; Wisniewski, 1991). For treatment, small amounts of topical estrogen cream can be applied daily for

TABLE 36-4. Some Hormonal Contraceptive Regimens for Breast-Feeding Women[a]

Progestin-only "mini pill"
Intramuscular depot medroxyprogesterone acetate
Progesterone-releasing implants
Progesterone-releasing intrauterine systems
Combination oral contraceptives—low-dose estrogen

[a]See also Chapter 38 (p. 695).

several weeks to vulvar tissues. Additionally, vaginal lubricants may be used with coitus.

Late Maternal Morbidity

Taken together, major and minor maternal morbidity are surprisingly common in the months following childbirth (MacArthur, 1991). In a survey of 1249 British mothers followed for up to 18 months, 3 percent required hospital readmission within 8 weeks (Glazener, 1995; Thompson, 2002). Milder health problems during the first 8 weeks were reported by 87 percent (Table 36-5). Moreover, almost three fourths continued to have various problems for up to 18 months. Practitioners should be aware of these potential issues in their patients convalescing from birthing.

Follow-Up Care

By discharge, women who had an uncomplicated course can resume most activities, including bathing, driving, and household functions. Jimenez and Newton (1979) tabulated cross-cultural information on 202 societies from various international geographical regions. Following childbirth, most societies did not restrict work activity, and approximately half expected a return to full duties within 2 weeks. Wallace and coworkers (2013) reported that 80 percent of women who worked during pregnancy resume work by 1 year after delivery. Despite this, Tulman and Fawcett (1988) reported that only half of mothers regained their usual level of energy by 6 weeks. Women who delivered vaginally were twice as likely to have normal energy levels at this time compared with those with a cesarean delivery. Ideally, the care and nurturing of the infant should be provided by the mother with ample help from the father.

The American Academy of Pediatrics and the American College of Obstetricians and Gynecologists (2012) recommend a postpartum visit between 4 and 6 weeks. This has proven quite satisfactory to identify abnormalities beyond the immediate puerperium and to initiate contraceptive practices.

TABLE 36-5. Puerperal Morbidity Reported by 8 Weeks

Morbidity	Percent[a]
Fatigue	59
Breast problems	36
Anemia	25
Backache	24
Hemorrhoids	23
Headache	22
"Blues"	21
Constipation	20
Suture breakdown	16
Vaginal discharge	15

[a]At least one symptom was reported by 87 percent of all women.
Data from Glazener, 1995.

REFERENCES

Ahdoot D, Van Nostrand KM, Nguyen NJ, et al: The effect of route of delivery on regression of abnormal cervical cytologic findings in the postpartum period. Am J Obstet Gynecol 178:1116, 1998

Almeida OD Jr, Kitay DZ: Lactation suppression and puerperal fever. Am J Obstet Gynecol 154:940, 1986

Alonso-Burgos A, Royo P, Diaz L, et al: Labor-related sacral and pubic fractures. J Bone Joint Surg 89:396, 2007

American Academy of Pediatrics: Breastfeeding and the use of human milk. Pediatrics 129(3):e827, 2012

American Academy of Pediatrics and the American College of Obstetricians and Gynecologists: Guidelines for Perinatal Care, 7th ed. Washington, AAP and ACOG, 2012

American College of Obstetricians and Gynecologists: Breastfeeding: maternal and infant aspects. Committee Opinion No. 361, February 2007, Reaffirmed 2013a

American College of Obstetricians and Gynecologists: Postpartum hemorrhage. Practice Bulletin No. 76, October 2006, Reaffirmed 2013b

Anderson WR, Davis J: Placental site involution. Am J Obstet Gynecol 102:23, 1968

Andrew AC, Bulmer JN, Wells M, et al: Subinvolution of the uteroplacental arteries in the human placental bed. Histopathology 15:395, 1989

Andrews MC: Epithelial changes in the puerperal fallopian tube. Am J Obstet Gynecol 62:28, 1951

Baker JL, Gamborg M, Heitmann BL, et al: Breastfeeding reduces postpartum weight retention. Am J Clin Nutr 88(6):1543, 2008

Baldwin MK, Edelman AB: The effect of long-acting reversible contraception on rapid repeat pregnancy in adolescents: a review. J Adolesc Health 52 (4 Suppl):S47, 2013

Ballard O, Morrow AL: Human milk composition: nutrients and bioactive factors. Pediatr Clin North Am 60(1):49, 2013

Bannbers E, Gingnell M, Engman J, et al: Prefrontal activity during response inhibition decreases over time in the postpartum period. Behav Brain Res 241:132, 2013

Barrett G, Pendry E, Peacock J, et al: Women's sexual health after childbirth. BJOG 107:186, 2000

Bartick M, Reinhold A: The burden of suboptimal breastfeeding in the United States: a pediatric cost analysis. Pediatrics 125(5):e1048, 2010

Belachew J, Axelsson O, Mulic-Lutvica A, et al: Longitudinal study of the uterine body and cavity with three-dimensional ultrasonography in the puerperium. Acta Obstet Gynecol Scand 91(10):1184, 2012

Berlin CM Jr, van den Anker, JN: Safety during breastfeeding: drugs, foods, environmental chemicals, and maternal infections. Semin Fetal Neonatal Med 18(1):13, 2013

Bertino E, Varalda A, Di Nicola P, et al: Drugs and breastfeeding: instructions for use. J Matern Fetal Neonatal Med 25(Suppl 4):78, 2012

Bertotto A, Gerli R, Fabietti G, et al: Human breast milk T lymphocytes display the phenotype and functional characteristics of memory T cells. Eur J Immunol 20:1877, 1990

Buhimschi CS, Buhimschi IA, Manlinow AM, et al: Myometrial thickness during human labor and immediately post partum. Am J Obstet Gynecol 188:553, 2003

Campbell OMR, Gray RH: Characteristics and determinants of postpartum ovarian function in women in the United States. Am J Obstet Gynecol 169:55, 1993

Centers for Disease Control and Prevention: Breastfeeding Report Card—United States, 2012a. Available at: http://www.cdc.gov/breastfeeding/data/reportcard.htm. Accessed May 18, 2013

Centers for Disease Control and Prevention: PRAMS, the Pregnancy Risk Assessment Monitoring System. 2012b. Available at: http://www.cdc.gov/prams/index.htm. Accessed May 18, 2013

Chesley LC, Valenti C, Uichano L: Alterations in body fluid compartments and exchangeable sodium in early puerperium. Am J Obstet Gynecol 77:1054, 1959

Ching-Chung L, Shuenn-Dhy C, Ling-Hong T, et al: Postpartum urinary retention: assessment of contributing factors and long-term clinical impact. Aust N Z J Obstet Gynaecol 42:365, 2002

Collier RJ, Hernandez LL, Horseman ND: Serotonin as a homeostatic regulator of lactation. Domest Anim Endocrinol 43(2):161, 2012

Cravioto A, Tello A, Villafan H, et al: Inhibition of localized adhesion of enteropathogenic *Escherichia coli* to HEp-2 cells by immunoglobulin and oligosaccharide fractions of human colostrum and breast milk. J Infect Dis 163:1247, 1991

Culligan P, Hill S, Heit M: Rupture of the symphysis pubis during vaginal delivery followed by two subsequent uneventful pregnancies. Obstet Gynecol 100:1114, 2002

Cunningham FG: Screening for osteoporosis. N Engl J Med 353(18):1975, 2005
Faupel-Badger JM, Arcaro KF, Balkam JJ, et al: Postpartum remodeling, lactation, and breast cancer risk: summary of a National Cancer Institute-sponsored workshop. J Natl Cancer Inst 105(3):166, 2013
Fletcher S, Grotegut CA, James AH: Lochia patterns among normal women: a systematic review. J Womens Health (Larchmt) 21(12):1290, 2012
Forrester-Knauss C, Merten S, Weiss C, et al: The Baby-Friendly Hospital Initiative in Switzerland: trends over a 9-year period. J Hum Lact 29(4):510, 2013
Funnell JW, Klawans AH, Cottrell TLC: The postpartum bladder. Am J Obstet Gynecol 67:1249, 1954
Glazener CM, Abdalla M, Stroud P, et al: Postnatal maternal morbidity: extent, causes, prevention and treatment. Br J Obstet Gynaecol 102: 282,1995
Harris RE, Thomas VL, Hui GW: Postpartum surveillance for urinary tract infection: patients at risk of developing pyelonephritis after catheterization. South Med J 70:1273, 1977
Hibbard JU, Schroff SG, Cunningham FG: Cardiovascular alterations in normal and preeclamptic pregnancy. In Taylor RN, Roberts JM, Cunningham FG (eds): Chesley's Hypertensive Disorders in Pregnancy, 4th ed. Amsterdam, Academic Press, 2014
Hladunewich MA, Lafayette RA, Derby GC, et al: The dynamics of glomerular filtration in the puerperium. Am J Physiol Renal Physiol 286:F496, 2004
Holdcroft A, Snidvongs S, Cason A, et al: Pain and uterine contractions during breast feeding in the immediate post-partum period increase with parity. Pain 104:589, 2003
Hytten F: The Clinical Physiology of the Puerperium. London, Farrand Press, 1995
Institute of Medicine: Nutrition During Pregnancy. Washington, National Academy of Science, 1990, p 202
Ip S, Chung M, Raman G, et al: A summary of the Agency for Healthcare Research and Quality's evidence report on breastfeeding in developed countries. Breastfeed Med 4(Suppl 1):S17, 2009
Ito S: Drug therapy for breast-feeding women. N Engl J Med 343:118, 2000
Iyengar SR, Walker WA: Immune factors in breast milk and the development of atopic disease. J Pediatr Gastroenterol Nutr 55(6):641, 2012
Jacobsen AF, Skjeldestad FE, Sandset PM: Incidence and risk patterns of venous thromboembolism in pregnancy and puerperium—a register-based case-control study. Am J Obstet Gynecol 198:233, 2008
Jimenez MH, Newton N: Activity and work during pregnancy and the postpartum period: a cross-cultural study of 202 societies. Am J Obstet Gynecol 135:171, 1979
Jong DE, Kikkert HR, Fidler V, et al: Effects of long-chain polyunsaturated fatty acid supplementation of infant formula on cognition and behavior at 9 years of age. Dev Med Child Neurol 54(12):1102, 2012
Kaneshiro BE, Acoba JD, Holzman J, et al: Effect of delivery route on natural history of cervical dysplasia. Am J Obstet Gynecol 192(5):1452, 2005
Kanotra S, D'Angelo D, Phares TM, et al: Challenges faced by new mothers in the early postpartum period: an analysis of comment data from the 2000 Pregnancy Risk Assessment Monitoring System (PRAMS) survey. Matern Child Health J 11(6):549, 2007
Kavalar R, Arko D, Fokter Dovnik N, et al: Subinvolution of placental bed vessels: case report and review of the literature. Wien Klin Wochenschr 124(19–20):725, 2012
Kelly LS, Sheeder J, Stevens-Simon C: Why lightning strikes twice: postpartum resumption of sexual activity during adolescence. J Pediatr Adolesc Gynecol 18:327, 2005
Kenny LC, McCrae KR, Cunningham FG: Platelets, coagulation, and the liver. In Taylor RN, Roberts JM, Cunningham FG (eds): Chesley's Hypertensive Disorders in Pregnancy, 4th ed. Amsterdam, Academic Press, 2014
Kharrazi FD, Rodgers WB, Kennedy JG, et al: Parturition-induced pelvic dislocation: a report of four cases. J Orthop Trauma 11:277, 1997
Kramer MS, Aboud F, Mironova E, et al: Breastfeeding and child cognitive development: new evidence from a large randomized trial. Arch Gen Psychiatry 65(5):578, 2008
Lawford AM, Scott K, Lust K: A case of massive vulvar oedema due to septic pubic symphysitis complicating pregnancy. Aust N Z J Obstet Gynaecol 50(6):576, 2010
Lee CY, Madrazo B, Drukker BH: Ultrasonic evaluation of the postpartum uterus in the management of postpartum bleeding. Obstet Gynecol 58:227, 1981
Lipe BC, Dumas MA, Ornstein DL: Von Willebrand disease in pregnancy. Hematol Oncol Clin North Am 25(2):335, 2011
Loukas M, Clarke P, Tubbs RS: Accessory breasts: a historical and current perspective. Am Surg 73(5):525, 2007
MacArthur C, Lewis M, Knox EG: Health after childbirth. Br J Obstet Gynaecol 98:1193, 1991
Mangesi L, Dowswell T: Treatments for breast engorgement during lactation. Cochrane Database Syst Rev 9:CD006946, 2010
McCleary MJ: Epidermal growth factor: an important constituent of human milk. J Hum Lact 7:123, 1991
McDonald SD, Pullenayegum E, Chapman B, et al: Prevalence and predictors of exclusive breastfeeding at hospital discharge. Obstet Gynecol 119(6):1171, 2012
McNeilly AS, Robinson ICA, Houston MJ, et al: Release of oxytocin and prolactin in response to suckling. BMJ (Clin Res Ed) 286:257, 1983
Minig L, Trimble EL, Sarsotti C, et al: Building the evidence base for postoperative and postpartum advice. Obstet Gynecol 114(4):892, 2009
Musselwhite KL, Faris P, Moore K, et al: Use of epidural anesthesia and the risk of acute postpartum urinary retention. Am J Obstet Gynecol 196:472, 2007
Nelson DB, Manders DB, Shivvers SA: Primary iliopsoas abscess and pregnancy. Obstet Gynecol 116(2 Pt 2):479, 2010
Newburg DS, Peterson JA, Ruiz-Palacias GM, et al: Role of human-milk lactadherin in protection against symptomatic rotavirus infection. Lancet 351(9110):1160, 1998
Palmer AR, Likis FE: Lactational atrophic vaginitis. J Midwifery Womens Health 48:282, 2003
Perez A, Vela P, Masnick GS, et al: First ovulation after childbirth: the effect of breastfeeding. Am J Obstet Gynecol 114:1041, 1972
Pisacane A, Continisio GI, Aldinucci M, et al: A controlled trial of the father's role in breastfeeding promotion. Pediatrics 116:e494, 2005
Porter JC: Proceedings: Hormonal regulation of breast development and activity. J Invest Dermatol 63:85, 1974
Rahn DD, Phelan JN, Roshanravan SM, et al: Anterior abdominal wall nerve and vessel anatomy: clinical implications for gynecologic surgery. Am J Obstet Gynecol 202(3):234.e1, 2010
Reis RA, Baer JL, Arens RA, et al: Traumatic separation of the symphysis pubis during spontaneous labor: with a clinical and x-ray study of the normal symphysis pubis during pregnancy and the puerperium. Surg Gynecol Obstet 55:336, 1932
Robson SC, Dunlop W, Hunter S: Haemodynamic changes during the early puerperium. BMJ (Clin Res Ed) 294:1065, 1987
Rowe H, Baker T, Hale TW: Maternal medication, drug use and breastfeeding. Pediatr Clin North Am 6(1); 275, 2013
Saito S, Maruyama M, Kato Y, et al: Detection of IL-6 in human milk and its involvement in IgA production. J Reprod Immunol 20:267, 1991
Schauberger CW, Rooney BL, Brimer LM: Factors that influence weight loss in the puerperium. Obstet Gynecol 79:424, 1992
Sharman A: Postpartum regeneration of the human endometrium. J Anat 87:1, 1953
Snow RE, Neubert AG: Peripartum pubic symphysis separation: a case series and review of the literature. Obstet Gynecol Surv 52:438, 1997
Sohn C, Fendel H, Kesternich P: Involution-induced changes in arterial uterine blood flow [German]. Z Geburtshilfe Perinatol 192:203, 1988
Spencer JP, Gonzalez LS III, Barnhart DJ: Medications in the breast-feeding mother. Am Fam Physician 65(2):170, 2002
Spitz AM, Lee NC, Peterson HB: Treatment for lactation suppression: little progress in one hundred years. Am J Obstet Gynecol 179:1485, 1998
Steinkeler J, Coldwell BJ, Warner MA: Ultrasound of the postpartum uterus. Ultrasound Q 28(2):97, 2012
Stuebe AM, Michels KB, Willett WC, et al: Duration of lactation and incidence of myocardial infarction in middle to late adulthood. Am J Obstet Gynecol 200(2):138.e1, 2009
Taylor RN, Sonson RD: Separation of the pubic symphysis. An underrecognized peripartum complication. J Reprod Med 31:203, 1986
Tekay A, Jouppila P: A longitudinal Doppler ultrasonographic assessment of the alterations in peripheral vascular resistance of uterine arteries and ultrasonographic findings of the involuting uterus during the puerperium. Am J Obstet Gynecol 168(1 Pt 1):190, 1993
Thompson JF, Roberts CL, Currie M, et al: Prevalence and persistence of health problems after childbirth: associations with parity and method of birth. Birth 29:83, 2002
Tulman L, Fawcett J: Return of functional ability after childbirth. Nurs Res 37:77, 1988
U.S. Department of Health and Human Services. Executive summary: the Surgeon General's call to action to support breastfeeding. 2011. Available at: http://www.surgeongeneral.gov/library/calls/breastfeeding/executivesummary.pdf. Accessed May 18, 2013
Van Os AFM, Van der Linden PJQ: Reliability of an automatic ultrasound system in the post partum period in measuring urinary retention. Acta Obstet Gynecol Scand 85:604, 2006

Wager GP, Martin DH, Koutsky L, et al: Puerperal infectious morbidity: relationship to route of delivery and to antepartum *Chlamydia trachomatis* infection. Am J Obstet Gynecol 138:1028, 1980
Wagner CL, Greer FR, American Academy of Pediatrics Section on Breastfeeding: Prevention of rickets and vitamin D deficiency in infants, children, and adolescents. Pediatrics 122(5):1142, 2008
Wagner IJ, Damitz LA, Carey E, et al: Bilateral accessory breast tissue of the vulva: a case report introducing a novel labiaplasty technique. Ann Plast Surg 70(5):549, 2013
Wallace M, Saurel-Cubizolles MJ, EDEN mother–child cohort study group: Returning to work one year after childbirth: data from the mother-child cohort EDEN. Matern Child Health J 17(8):1432, 2013
Williams JW: Regeneration of the uterine mucosa after delivery with especial reference to the placental site. Am J Obstet Gynecol 22:664, 1931
Wisniewski PM, Wilkinson EJ: Postpartum vaginal atrophy. Am J Obstet Gynecol 165(4 Pt 2):1249, 1991
Wolfberg AJ, Michels KB, Shields W, et al: Dads as breastfeeding advocates: results from a randomized controlled trial of an educational intervention. Am J Obstet Gynecol 191:708, 2004
Wong CA, Scavone BM, Dugan S, et al: Incidence of postpartum lumbosacral spine and lower extremity nerve injuries. Obstet Gynecol 101:279, 2003
World Health Organization: Exclusive breastfeeding for six months best for babies everywhere. 2011. Available at: http://www.who.int/mediacentre/news/statements/2011/breastfeeding_20110115/en/. Accessed May 17, 2013
World Health Organization: Protecting, promoting and supporting breastfeeding: the special role of maternity services. Geneva, World Health Organization, 1989, p iv
Young OM, Werner E, Sfakianaki AK: Primary psoas muscle abscess after an uncomplicated spontaneous vaginal delivery. Obstet Gynecol 116(2 Pt 2):477, 2010
Yuen BH: Prolactin in human milk: the influence of nursing and the duration of postpartum lactation. Am J Obstet Gynecol 158:583, 1988

CHAPTER 37

Puerperal Complications

Puerperal complications include many of those encountered during pregnancy, but there are some that are more common at this time. Typical of these is puerperal pelvic infection—a well-known killer of postpartum women. Other infections include mastitis and breast abscesses. Thromboembolism during the short 6-week puerperium is as frequent as during all 40 antepartum weeks.

PUERPERAL INFECTIONS

Traditionally, the term *puerperal infection* describes any bacterial infection of the genital tract after delivery. These infections as well as preeclampsia and obstetrical hemorrhage form the lethal triad of maternal death causes before and during the 20th century. Fortunately, because of effective antimicrobials, maternal mortality from infection has become uncommon. Berg and associates (2010) reported results from the Pregnancy Mortality Surveillance System, which contained 4693 pregnancy-related maternal deaths in the United States from 1998 through 2005. Infection caused 10.7 percent of pregnancy-related deaths and was the fifth leading cause. In a similar analysis of the North Carolina population from 1991 through 1999, Berg and colleagues (2005) reported that 40 percent of infection-related maternal deaths were preventable.

Puerperal Fever

A number of factors can cause fever—a temperature of 38.0°C (100.4°F) or higher—in the puerperium. *Most persistent fevers after childbirth are caused by genital tract infection.* Using this conservative definition of fever, Filker and Monif (1979) reported that only about 20 percent of women febrile within the first 24 hours after giving birth vaginally were subsequently diagnosed with pelvic infection. This was in contrast to 70 percent of those undergoing cesarean delivery. It must be emphasized that spiking fevers of 39°C or higher that develop within the first 24 hours postpartum may be associated with virulent pelvic infection caused by group A streptococcus and is discussed on page 683.

Other causes of puerperal fever include breast engorgement, urinary infections, episiotomy and abdominal incisions, perineal lacerations, and respiratory complications after cesarean delivery (Maharaj, 2007). Approximately 15 percent of women who do not breast feed develop postpartum fever from *breast engorgement.* As discussed in Chapter 36 (p. 675), the incidence of fever is lower in breast-feeding women. "Breast fever" rarely exceeds 39°C in the first few postpartum days and usually lasts < 24 hours. *Urinary infections* are uncommon postpartum because of the normal diuresis encountered then. That said, *acute pyelonephritis* has a variable clinical picture. The first sign of renal infection may be fever, followed later by costovertebral angle tenderness, nausea, and vomiting. *Atelectasis* following abdominal delivery is caused by hypoventilation and is best prevented by coughing and deep breathing on a fixed schedule following surgery. Fever associated with atelectasis is thought to follow infection by normal flora that proliferate distal to obstructing mucus plugs.

Uterine Infection

Postpartum uterine infection or puerperal sepsis has been called variously *endometritis, endomyometritis,* and *endoparametritis.* Because infection involves not only the decidua but also the myometrium and parametrial tissues, we prefer the inclusive term *metritis with pelvic cellulitis.*

Predisposing Factors

The route of delivery is the single most significant risk factor for the development of uterine infection (Burrows, 2004; Conroy, 2012; Koroukian, 2004). In the French Confidential Enquiry on Maternal Deaths, Deneux-Tharaux and coworkers (2006) cited a nearly 25-fold increased infection-related mortality rate with cesarean versus vaginal delivery. Rehospitalization rates for wound complications and endometritis were increased significantly in women undergoing a planned primary cesarean delivery compared with those having a planned vaginal birth (Declercq, 2007).

Vaginal Delivery. Compared with cesarean delivery, metritis following vaginal delivery is relatively infrequent. Women delivered vaginally at Parkland Hospital have a 1- to 2-percent incidence of metritis. Women at high risk for infection because of membrane rupture, prolonged labor, and multiple cervical examinations have a 5-to 6-percent frequency of metritis after vaginal delivery. If there is intrapartum chorioamnionitis, the risk of persistent uterine infection increases to 13 percent (Maberry, 1991). Finally, in one study, manual removal of the placenta, discussed in Chapter 41 (p. 784), increased the puerperal metritis rate threefold (Baksu, 2005).

Cesarean Delivery. Single-dose perioperative antimicrobial prophylaxis is recommended for all women undergoing cesarean delivery (American College of Obstetricians and Gynecologists, 2011). Such single-dose antimicrobial prophylaxis has done more to decrease the incidence and severity of postcesarean delivery infections than any other intervention in the past 30 years. Such practices decrease the puerperal pelvic infection risk by 65 to 75 percent (Smaill, 2010).

The magnitude of the risk is exemplified from reports that predate antimicrobial prophylaxis. Cunningham and associates (1978) described an overall incidence of 50 percent in women undergoing cesarean delivery at Parkland Hospital. Important risk factors for infection following surgery included prolonged labor, membrane rupture, multiple cervical examinations, and internal fetal monitoring. Women with all these factors who were not given perioperative prophylaxis had a 90-percent serious postcesarean delivery pelvic infection rate (DePalma, 1982).

Other Risk Factors. It is generally accepted that pelvic infection is more frequent in women of lower socioeconomic status (Maharaj, 2007). Except in extreme cases usually not seen in this country, it is unlikely that anemia or poor nutrition predispose to infection. *Bacterial colonization* of the lower genital tract with certain microorganisms—for example, group B streptococcus, *Chlamydia trachomatis, Mycoplasma hominis, Ureaplasma urealyticum,* and *Gardnerella vaginalis*—has been associated with an increased postpartum infection risk (Andrews, 1995; Jacobsson, 2002; Watts, 1990). Other factors associated with an increased infection risk include general anesthesia, cesarean delivery for multifetal gestation, young maternal age and nulliparity, prolonged labor induction, obesity, and meconium-stained amnionic fluid (Acosta, 2012; Jazayeri, 2002; Kabiru, 2004; Leth, 2011; Siriwachirachai, 2010; Tsai, 2011).

Microbiology

Most female pelvic infections are caused by bacteria indigenous to the genital tract. Over the past 20 years, there have been reports of group A β-hemolytic streptococcus causing toxic shock-like syndrome and life-threatening infection (Aronoff, 2008; Castagnola, 2008; Nathan, 1994; Palep-Singh, 2007). Prematurely ruptured membranes are a prominent risk factor in these infections (Anteby, 1999). In reviews by Crum (2002) and Udagawa (1999) and their colleagues, women in whom group A streptococcal infection was manifested before, during, or within 12 hours of delivery had a maternal mortality rate of almost 90 percent and fetal mortality rate > 50 percent. In the past 10 years, skin and soft-tissue infections due to community-acquired methicillin-resistant *Staphylococcus aureus*—*CA-MRSA*—have become common (Chap. 64, p. 1251). Although this variant is not a frequent cause of puerperal metritis, it is commonly implicated in abdominal incisional infections (Anderson, 2007; Patel, 2007). Rotas and coworkers (2007) reported a woman with episiotomy cellulitis from CA-MRSA and hematogenously spread necrotizing pneumonia.

Common Pathogens. Bacteria commonly responsible for female genital tract infections are listed in Table 37-1. Generally, infections are polymicrobial, which enhances bacterial synergy. Other factors that promote virulence are hematomas and devitalized tissue. Although the cervix and vagina routinely harbor such bacteria, the uterine cavity is usually sterile before rupture of the amnionic sac. As the consequence of labor and delivery and associated manipulations, the amnionic

TABLE 37-1. Bacteria Commonly Responsible for Female Genital Infections

Aerobes
Gram-positive cocci—group A, B, and D streptococci, enterococcus, *Staphylococcus aureus, Staphylococcus epidermidis*
Gram-negative bacteria—*Escherichia coli, Klebsiella, Proteus* species
Gram-variable—*Gardnerella vaginalis*
Others
Mycoplasma and *Chlamydia* species, *Neisseria gonorrhoeae*
Anaerobes
Cocci—*Peptostreptococcus* and *Peptococcus* species
Others—*Clostridium, Bacteroides,* and *Fusobacterium* species, *Mobiluncus* species

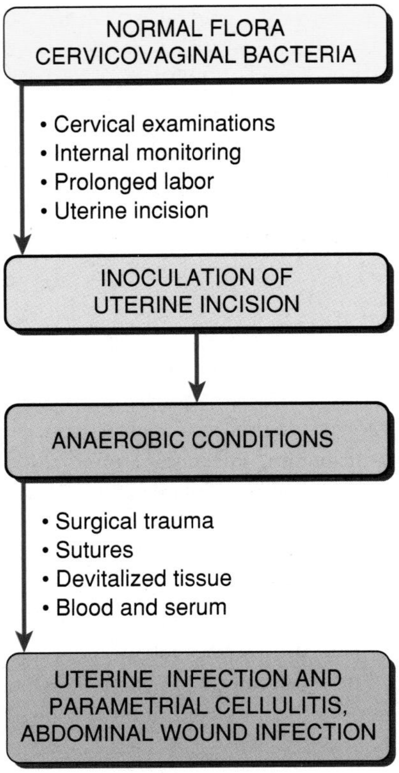

FIGURE 37-1 Pathogenesis of metritis following cesarean delivery. (Adapted from Gilstrap, 1979.)

fluid and uterus become contaminated with anaerobic and aerobic bacteria (Fig. 37-1). Intraamnionic cytokines and C-reactive protein are also markers of infection (Combs, 2013; Marchocki, 2013). In studies done before the use of antimicrobial prophylaxis, Gilstrap and Cunningham (1979) cultured amnionic fluid obtained at cesarean delivery in women in labor with membranes ruptured more than 6 hours. All had bacterial growth, and an average of 2.5 organisms was identified from each specimen. Anaerobic and aerobic organisms were identified in 63 percent, anaerobes alone in 30 percent, and aerobes alone in only 7 percent. Anaerobes included *Peptostreptococcus* and *Peptococcus* species in 45 percent, *Bacteroides* species in 9 percent, and *Clostridium* species in 3 percent. Aerobes included *Enterococcus* in 14 percent, group B streptococcus in 8 percent, and *Escherichia coli* in 9 percent of isolates. Sherman and coworkers (1999) later showed that bacterial isolates at cesarean delivery correlated with those taken from women with metritis at 3 days postpartum.

The role of other organisms in the etiology of these infections is unclear. Chlamydial infections have been implicated in late-onset, indolent metritis (Ismail, 1985). Observations of Chaim and colleagues (2003) suggest that when cervical colonization of *U urealyticum* is heavy, it may contribute to the development of metritis. Finally, Jacobsson and associates (2002) reported a threefold risk of puerperal infection in a group of Swedish women in whom bacterial vaginosis was identified in early pregnancy (Chap. 65, p. 1276).

Bacterial Cultures. Routine pretreatment genital tract cultures are of little clinical use and add significant costs. Similarly, routine blood cultures seldom modify care. In two earlier studies done before perioperative prophylaxis was used, blood cultures were positive in 13 percent of women with postcesarean metritis at Parkland Hospital and 24 percent in those at Los Angeles County Hospital (Cunningham, 1978; DiZerega, 1979). In a later Finnish study, Kankuri and associates (2003) confirmed bacteremia in only 5 percent of almost 800 women with puerperal sepsis.

Pathogenesis and Clinical Course

Puerperal infection following vaginal delivery primarily involves the placental implantation site, decidua and adjacent myometrium, or cervicovaginal lacerations. The pathogenesis of uterine infection following cesarean delivery is that of an infected surgical incision (see Fig. 37-1). Bacteria that colonize the cervix and vagina gain access to amnionic fluid during labor. Postpartum, they invade devitalized uterine tissue. Parametrial cellulitis next follows with infection of the pelvic retroperitoneal fibroareolar connective tissue. With early treatment, infection is contained within the parametrial and paravaginal tissue, but it may extend deeply into the pelvis.

Fever is the most important criterion for the diagnosis of postpartum metritis. Intuitively, the degree of fever is believed proportional to the extent of infection and sepsis syndrome. Temperatures commonly are 38 to 39°C. Chills that accompany fever suggest bacteremia or endotoxemia. Women usually complain of abdominal pain, and parametrial tenderness is elicited on abdominal and bimanual examination. Leukocytosis may range from 15,000 to 30,000 cells/μL, but recall that cesarean delivery itself increases the leukocyte count (Hartmann, 2000). Although an offensive odor may develop, many women have foul-smelling lochia without evidence for infection, and vice versa. Some other infections, notably those caused by group A β-hemolytic streptococci, may be associated with scant, odorless lochia.

Treatment

If nonsevere metritis develops following vaginal delivery, then treatment with an oral antimicrobial agent is usually sufficient. For moderate to severe infections, however, intravenous therapy with a broad-spectrum antimicrobial regimen is indicated. Improvement follows in 48 to 72 hours in nearly 90 percent of women treated with one of several regimens. Persistent fever after this interval mandates a careful search for causes of refractory pelvic infection. These include a parametrial phlegmon—an area of intense cellulitis; an abdominal incisional or pelvic abscess or infected hematoma; and septic pelvic thrombophlebitis. In our experience, persistent fever is seldom due to antimicrobial-resistant bacteria or due to drug side effects. The woman may be discharged home after she has been afebrile for at least 24 hours, and further oral antimicrobial therapy is not needed (Dinsmoor, 1991; French, 2004).

Choice of Antimicrobials. Although therapy is empirical, initial treatment following cesarean delivery is directed against elements of the mixed flora shown in Table 37-1. For infections following vaginal delivery, as many as 90 percent of women respond to regimens such as ampicillin plus gentamicin. In contrast, anaerobic coverage is included for infections following cesarean delivery (Table 37-2).

TABLE 37-2. Antimicrobial Regimens for Intravenous Treatment of Pelvic Infection Following Cesarean Delivery

Regimen	Comments
Clindamycin + gentamicin	"Gold standard," 90–97% efficacy, once-daily gentamicin dosing acceptable ***plus*** Ampicillin added to regimen with sepsis syndrome or suspected enterococcal infection
Clindamycin + aztreonam	Gentamicin substitute for renal insufficiency
Extended-spectrum penicillins	Piperacillin, piperacillin tazobactam, ampicillin/sulbactam, ticarcillin/clavulanate
Cephalosporins	Cefotetan, cefoxitin, cefotaxime
Vancomycin	Added to other regimens for suspected *S aureus* infections
Metronidazole + ampicillin + gentamicin	Metronidazole has excellent anaerobic coverage
Carbapenems	Imipenem/cilastatin, meropenem, ertapenem reserved for special indications

In 1979, DiZerega and colleagues compared the effectiveness of clindamycin plus gentamicin with that of penicillin G plus gentamicin for treatment of pelvic infections following cesarean delivery. Women given the clindamycin-gentamicin regimen had a 95-percent response rate, and this regimen is still considered by most to be the standard by which others are measured (French, 2004). Because enterococcal cultures may be persistently positive despite this standard therapy, some add ampicillin to the clindamycin-gentamicin regimen, either initially or if there is no response by 48 to 72 hours (Brumfield, 2000).

Many authorities recommend that serum gentamicin levels be periodically monitored. At Parkland Hospital, we do not routinely do so if the woman has normal renal function. Once-daily dosing versus multiple-dosing with gentamicin provides adequate serum levels, and either method has similar cure rates (Livingston, 2003).

Because of potential nephrotoxicity and ototoxicity with gentamicin in the event of diminished glomerular filtration, some have recommended a combination of clindamycin and a second-generation cephalosporin to treat such women. Others recommend a combination of clindamycin and aztreonam, which is a monobactam compound with activity similar to the aminoglycosides.

The spectra of *β-lactam antimicrobials* include activity against many anaerobic pathogens. Some examples include cephalosporins such as cefoxitin, cefotetan, cefotaxime, and ceftriaxone, as well as extended-spectrum penicillins such as piperacillin, ticarcillin, and mezlocillin. β-Lactam antimicrobials are inherently safe and except for allergic reactions, are free of major toxicity. The *β-lactamase inhibitors*, clavulanic acid, sulbactam, and tazobactam, have been combined with ampicillin, amoxicillin, ticarcillin, and piperacillin to extend their spectra. *Metronidazole* has superior in vitro activity against most anaerobes. This agent given with ampicillin and an aminoglycoside provides coverage against most organisms encountered in serious pelvic infections. It is also used to treat *Clostridium difficile* colitis.

Imipenem and similar antimicrobials are in the carbapenem family. These offer broad-spectrum coverage against most organisms associated with metritis. Imipenem is used in combination with *cilastatin*, which inhibits its renal metabolism. Preliminary findings with *ertapenem* indicated suboptimal outcomes (Brown, 2012). It seems reasonable from both a medical and an economic standpoint to reserve these drugs for serious nonobstetrical infections.

Vancomycin is a glycopeptide antimicrobial active against gram-positive bacteria. It is used in lieu of β-lactam therapy for a patient with a type 1 allergic reaction and given for suspected infections due to *Staphylococcus aureus* and to treat *C difficile* colitis (Chap. 54, p. 1074).

Perioperative Prophylaxis

As discussed, administration of antimicrobial prophylaxis at the time of cesarean delivery has remarkably reduced the postoperative pelvic and wound infection rates. Numerous studies have shown that prophylactic antimicrobials reduce the pelvic infection rate by 70 to 80 percent (Chelmow, 2001; Dinsmoor, 2009; Smaill, 2010; Witt, 2011). The observed benefit applies to both elective and nonelective cesarean delivery and also includes a reduction in abdominal incisional infection rates.

Single-dose prophylaxis with ampicillin or a first-generation cephalosporin is ideal, and both are as effective as broad-spectrum agents or a multiple-dose regimen (American College of Obstetricians and Gynecologists, 2011). Extended-spectrum prophylaxis with azithromycin added to standard single-dose prophylaxis has shown a further reduction in postcesarean metritis rates (Tita, 2008). These findings need to be verified. Women known to be colonized with methicillin-resistant *Staphylococcus aureus*—MRSA—are given vancomycin in addition to a cephalosporin (Chap. 64, p. 1251). Finally, it is controversial whether the infection rate is lowered more if the selected antimicrobial is given before the skin incision compared with after umbilical cord clamping (Baaqeel, 2012; Macones, 2012; Sun, 2013). The American College of Obstetricians and Gynecologists (2011) has concluded that the evidence favors predelivery administration. There may be additive salutary effects of preoperative vaginal cleansing with povidone-iodine rinse or application of metronidazole gel (Haas, 2013; Reid, 2011; Yildirim, 2012).

Other Methods of Prophylaxis. Several studies have evaluated the value of prenatal cervicovaginal cultures. These are obtained in the hope of identifying pathogens that might be eradicated to decrease incidences of preterm labor, chorioamnionitis, and puerperal infections. Unfortunately, treatment of asymptomatic vaginal infections has not been shown to prevent these complications. Carey and coworkers (2000) reported no beneficial effects for women treated for asymptomatic bacterial vaginosis. Klebanoff and colleagues (2001) reported a similar postpartum infection rate in women treated for second-trimester asymptomatic *Trichomonas vaginalis* infection compared with that of placebo-treated women.

Technical maneuvers done to alter the postpartum infection rate have been studied with cesarean delivery. For example, allowing the placenta to separate spontaneously compared with removing it manually lowers the infection risk. However, changing gloves by the surgical team after placental delivery does not (Atkinson, 1996). Exteriorizing the uterus to close the hysterotomy may decrease febrile morbidity (Jacobs-Jokhan, 2004). Postdelivery mechanical lower segment and cervical dilatation have not been shown to be effective (Liabsuetrakul, 2011). No differences were found in postoperative infection rates when single- versus two-layer uterine closure was compared (Hauth, 1992). Similarly, infection rates are not appreciatively affected by closure versus nonclosure of the peritoneum (Bamigboye, 2003; Tulandi, 2003). Importantly, although closure of subcutaneous tissue in obese women does not lower the wound infection rate, it does decrease the wound separation incidence (Chelmow, 2004; Magann, 2002; Naumann, 1995). Similarly, skin closure with staples versus suture has a higher incidence of noninfectious skin separation (Mackeen, 2012; Tuuli, 2011).

Complications of Uterine and Pelvic Infections

In more than 90 percent of women, metritis responds to treatment within 48 to 72 hours. In some of the remainder, any of several complications may arise. These include wound infections, complex pelvic infections such as phlegmons or abscesses, and septic pelvic thrombophlebitis (Jaiyeoba, 2012). As with other aspects of puerperal infections, the incidence and severity of these complications are remarkably decreased by perioperative antimicrobial prophylaxis.

Abdominal Incisional Infections

Wound infection is a common cause of persistent fever in women treated for metritis. Other wound infection risk factors include obesity, diabetes, corticosteroid therapy, immunosuppression, anemia, hypertension, and inadequate hemostasis with hematoma formation. If prophylactic antimicrobials are given as described above, the incidence of abdominal wound infection following cesarean delivery ranges from 2 to 10 percent depending on risk factors (Andrews, 2003; Chaim, 2000).

Incisional abscesses that develop following cesarean delivery usually cause persistent fever or fever beginning about the fourth day. In many cases, antimicrobials had been given to treat pelvic infection, yet fever persisted. There is wound erythema and drainage. Although organisms that cause wound infections are generally the same as those isolated from amnionic fluid at cesarean delivery, hospital-acquired pathogens may also be causative (Emmons, 1988; Owen, 1994). Treatment includes antimicrobials, surgical drainage, and debridement of devitalized tissue. The fascia is carefully inspected to document integrity.

Local wound care is typically completed twice daily. Before each dressing change, procedural analgesia is tailored to wound size and location, and oral, intramuscular, or intravenous dosage routes are suitable. Topical lidocaine may also be added. Necrotic tissue is removed, and the wound is repacked with moist gauze. At 4 to 6 days, healthy granulation tissue is typically present, and secondary en bloc closure of the open layers can usually be accomplished (Wechter, 2005). With this closure, a polypropylene or nylon suture of appropriate gauge enters 3 cm from one wound edge. It crosses the wound to incorporate the full wound thickness and emerges 3 cm from the other wound edge. These are placed in series to close the opening. In most cases, sutures may be removed on postprocedural day 10. Wound vacuum device use is gaining popularity. However, its efficacy remains unproven in randomized trials.

Wound Dehiscence

Wound disruption or dehiscence refers to separation of the fascial layer. This is a serious complication and requires secondary closure of the incision in the operating room. McNeeley and associates (1998) reported a fascial dehiscence rate of approximately 1 per 300 operations in almost 9000 women undergoing cesarean delivery. Most disruptions manifested on about the fifth postoperative day and were accompanied by a serosanguineous discharge. Two thirds of 27 fascial dehiscences identified in this study were associated with concurrent fascial infection and tissue necrosis.

Necrotizing Fasciitis

This uncommon, severe wound infection is associated with high mortality rates. In obstetrics, necrotizing fasciitis may involve abdominal incisions, or it may complicate episiotomy or other perineal lacerations. As the name implies, there is significant tissue necrosis. Of the risk factors for fasciitis summarized by Owen and Andrews (1994), three of these—*diabetes, obesity,* and *hypertension*—are relatively common in pregnant women. Like pelvic infections, these wound complications usually are polymicrobial and are caused by organisms that make up the normal vaginal flora. *In some cases, however, infection is caused by a single virulent bacterial species such as group A β-hemolytic streptococcus.* Occasionally, necrotizing infections are caused by rarely encountered pathogens (Swartz, 2004).

Goepfert and coworkers (1997) reviewed their experiences with necrotizing fasciitis at the University of Alabama Birmingham Hospital. Nine cases complicated more than 5000 cesarean deliveries—frequency of 1.8 per 1000. In two women, the infection was fatal. In a report from Brigham and Women's and Massachusetts General Hospitals, Schorge and colleagues (1998) described five women with fasciitis following cesarean delivery. None of these women had predisposing risk factors, and none died.

Infection may involve skin, superficial and deep subcutaneous tissues, and any of the abdominopelvic fascial layers (Fig. 37-2). In some cases, muscle is also involved—myofasciitis. Although some virulent infections, for example, from group A β-hemolytic streptococci, develop early postpartum, most of these necrotizing infections do not cause symptoms

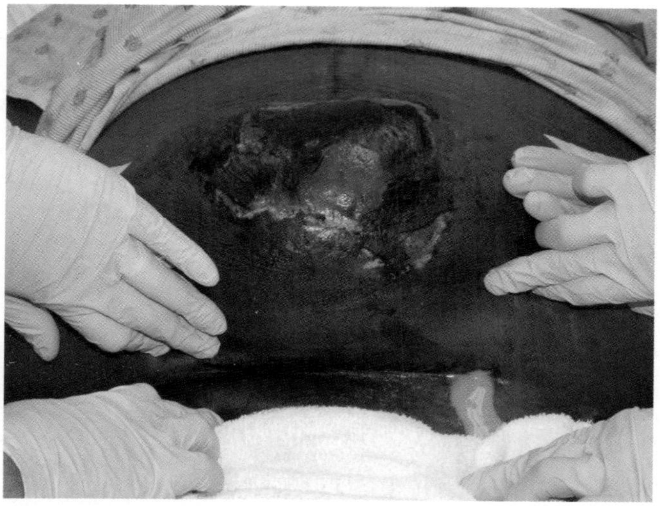

FIGURE 37-2 Necrotizing fasciitis involving the abdominal wall and Pfannenstiel incision. The skin rapidly became dusky and gangrenous, and pus is seen exuding from the left angle of the incision. Extensive debridement and supportive therapy were lifesaving.

until 3 to 5 days after delivery. Clinical findings vary, and it is frequently difficult to differentiate more innocuous superficial wound infections from an ominous deep fascial one. A high index of suspicion, with surgical exploration if the diagnosis is uncertain, may be lifesaving. We aggressively pursue early exploration. Certainly, if myofasciitis progresses, the woman may become ill from septicemia. Profound hemoconcentration from capillary leakage with circulatory failure commonly occurs, and death may soon follow as described in Chapter 47 (p. 947).

Early diagnosis, surgical debridement, antimicrobials, and intensive care are paramount to successfully treat necrotizing soft-tissue infections (Gallup, 2004; Urschel, 1999). Surgery includes extensive debridement of all infected tissue, leaving wide margins of healthy bleeding tissue. This may include extensive abdominal or vulvar debridement with unroofing and excision of abdominal, thigh, or buttock fascia. Death is virtually universal without surgical treatment, and rates approach 50 percent even if extensive debridement is performed. With extensive resection, synthetic mesh may ultimately be required later to close the fascial incision (Gallup, 2004; McNeeley, 1998).

Adnexal Abscesses and Peritonitis

An *ovarian abscess* rarely develops in the puerperium. These are presumably caused by bacterial invasion through a rent in the ovarian capsule (Wetchler, 1985). The abscess is usually unilateral, and women typically present 1 to 2 weeks after delivery. Rupture is common, and peritonitis may be severe.

Peritonitis is infrequent following cesarean delivery. It is almost invariably preceded by metritis. It most often is caused by uterine incisional necrosis and dehiscence, but it may be due to a ruptured adnexal abscess or an inadvertent bowel injury at cesarean delivery. Peritonitis is rarely encountered after vaginal delivery, and many such cases are due to virulent strains of group A β-hemocyte streptococci or similar organisms.

Importantly in postpartum women, abdominal rigidity may not be prominent with puerperal peritonitis because of abdominal wall laxity from pregnancy. Pain may be severe, but frequently, the first symptoms of peritonitis are those of *adynamic ileus.* Marked bowel distention may develop, and these findings are unusual after uncomplicated cesarean delivery. If the infection begins in an intact uterus and extends into the peritoneum, antimicrobial treatment alone usually suffices. Conversely, peritonitis caused by uterine incisional necrosis as discussed subsequently, or from bowel perforation, must be treated promptly with surgical intervention.

Parametrial Phlegmon

For some women in whom metritis develops following cesarean delivery, parametrial cellulitis is intensive and forms an area of induration—a *phlegmon*—within the leaves of the broad ligament (Fig. 37-3). These infections should be considered when fever persists longer than 72 hours despite intravenous antimicrobial therapy (Brown, 1999; DePalma, 1982).

Phlegmons are usually unilateral, and they frequently are limited to the parametrium at the base of the broad ligament. If the inflammatory reaction is more intense, cellulitis extends along natural lines of cleavage. The most common form of

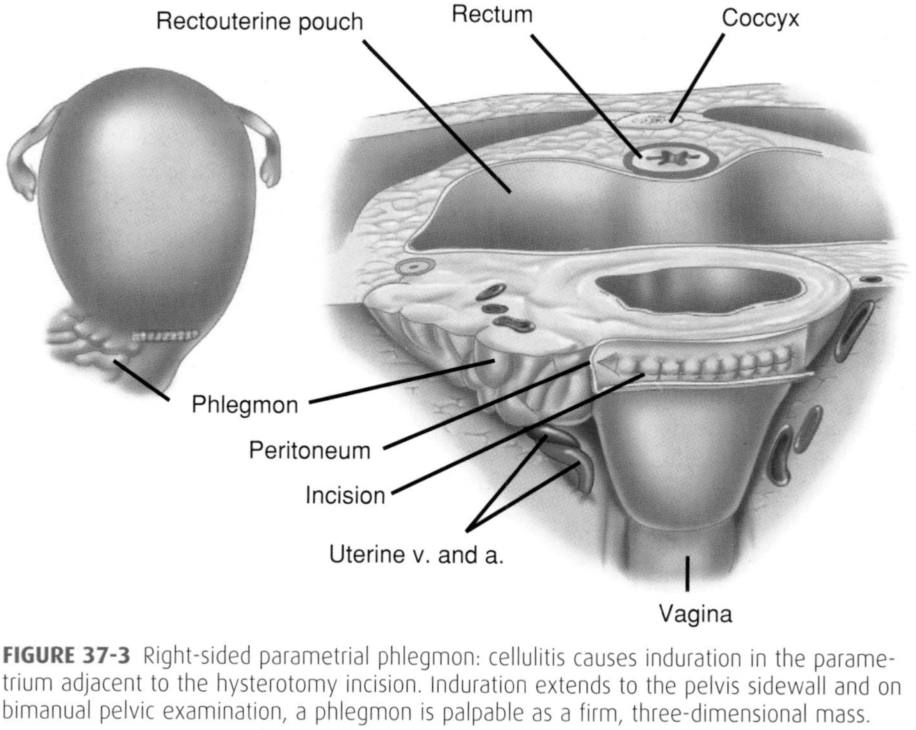

FIGURE 37-3 Right-sided parametrial phlegmon: cellulitis causes induration in the parametrium adjacent to the hysterotomy incision. Induration extends to the pelvis sidewall and on bimanual pelvic examination, a phlegmon is palpable as a firm, three-dimensional mass.

CHAPTER 37

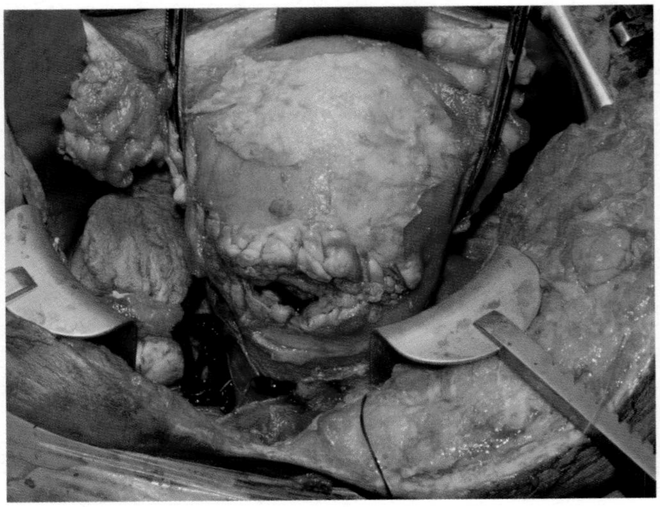

FIGURE 37-4 Necrotic hysterotomy infection. Severe cellulitis of the uterine incision resulted in dehiscence with subsequent leakage into the peritoneal cavity. Hysterectomy was required for sufficient debridement of necrotic tissue.

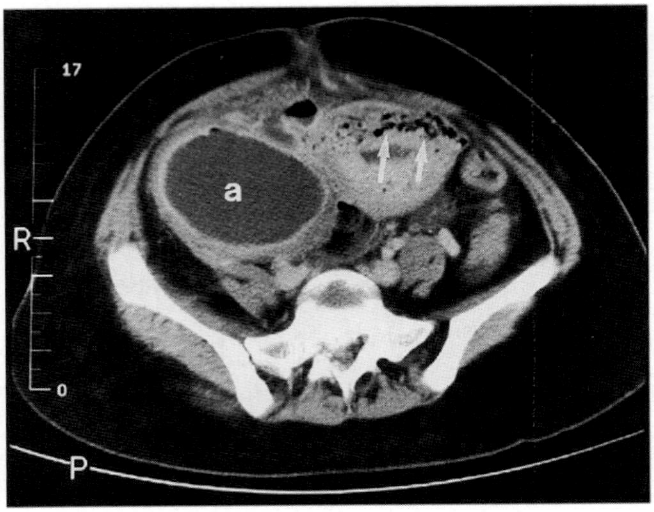

FIGURE 37-5 Pelvic computed tomography scan showing necrosis of the uterine incision with gas in the myometrium (*arrows*). There is also a large right-sided parametrial abscess (*a*).

extension is laterally along the broad ligament, with a tendency to extend to the pelvic sidewall. Occasionally, posterior extension may involve the rectovaginal septum, producing a firm mass posterior to the cervix. In most women with a phlegmon, clinical improvement follows continued treatment with a broad-spectrum antimicrobial regimen. Typically, fever resolves in 5 to 7 days, but in some cases, it persists longer. Absorption of the induration may require several days to weeks.

In some women, severe cellulitis of the uterine incision may lead to necrosis and separation (Treszezamsky, 2011). Extrusion of purulent material as shown in Figure 37-4 leads to intraabdominal abscess formation and peritonitis as described above. Surgery is reserved for women in whom uterine incisional necrosis is suspected because of ileus and peritonitis. For most, hysterectomy and surgical debridement are needed and are predictably difficult because the cervix and lower uterine segment are involved with an intense inflammatory process that extends to the pelvic sidewall. The adnexa are seldom involved, and one or both ovaries can usually be conserved. There is often appreciable blood loss, and transfusion may be necessary.

Imaging Studies

Persistent puerperal infections can be evaluated using computed tomography (CT) or magnetic resonance (MR) imaging. Brown and associates (1991) used CT imaging in 74 women in whom pelvic infection was refractory to 5 days of antimicrobial therapy. They found at least one abnormal radiological finding in 75 percent of these women, and in most, these were nonsurgical. Maldjian and coworkers (1999) used MR imaging in 50 women with persistent fever and found a bladder flap hematoma in two thirds. In three women, parametrial edema was seen, and another two had a pelvic hematoma. In most cases, imaging can be used to dissuade surgical exploration.

Uterine incisional dehiscence such as shown in Figure 37-4 is sometimes suspected based on CT scanning images. Another example is shown in Figure 37-5. These findings must be interpreted within the clinical context because apparent uterine incisional defects thought to represent edema can be seen even after uncomplicated cesarean delivery (Twickler, 1991).

Occasionally, a parametrial phlegmon suppurates, forming a fluctuant broad ligament mass that may point above the inguinal ligament. These abscesses may dissect anteriorly as shown in Figure 37-5 and be amenable to CT-directed needle drainage. Occasionally they dissect posteriorly to the rectovaginal septum, where surgical drainage is easily effected by colpotomy incision. A *psoas abscess* is rare, and despite antimicrobial therapy, percutaneous drainage may be required (Shahabi, 2002; Swanson, 2008).

Septic Pelvic Thrombophlebitis

This was a frequent complication in the preantibotic era. Collins and colleagues (1951) described suppurative thrombophlebitis in 70 women cared for from 1937 through 1946 at Charity Hospital in New Orleans. Septic embolization was common and caused a third of maternal deaths during that period. With the advent of antimicrobial therapy, the mortality rate and need for surgical therapy for these infections diminished.

Septic phlebitis arises as an extension along venous routes and may cause thrombosis as shown in Figure 37-6. Lymphangitis often coexists. The ovarian veins may then become involved because they drain the upper uterus and therefore the placental implantation site. The experiences of Witlin and Sibai (1995) and Brown and coworkers (1999) suggest that puerperal septic thrombophlebitis is likely to involve one or both ovarian venous plexuses (Fig. 37-7). In a fourth of women, the clot extends into the inferior vena cava and occasionally to the renal vein.

The incidence of septic phlebitis has varied in several reports. In a 5-year survey of 45,000 women who were delivered at Parkland Hospital, Brown and associates (1999) found an incidence of septic pelvic thrombophlebitis of 1 per 9000 following

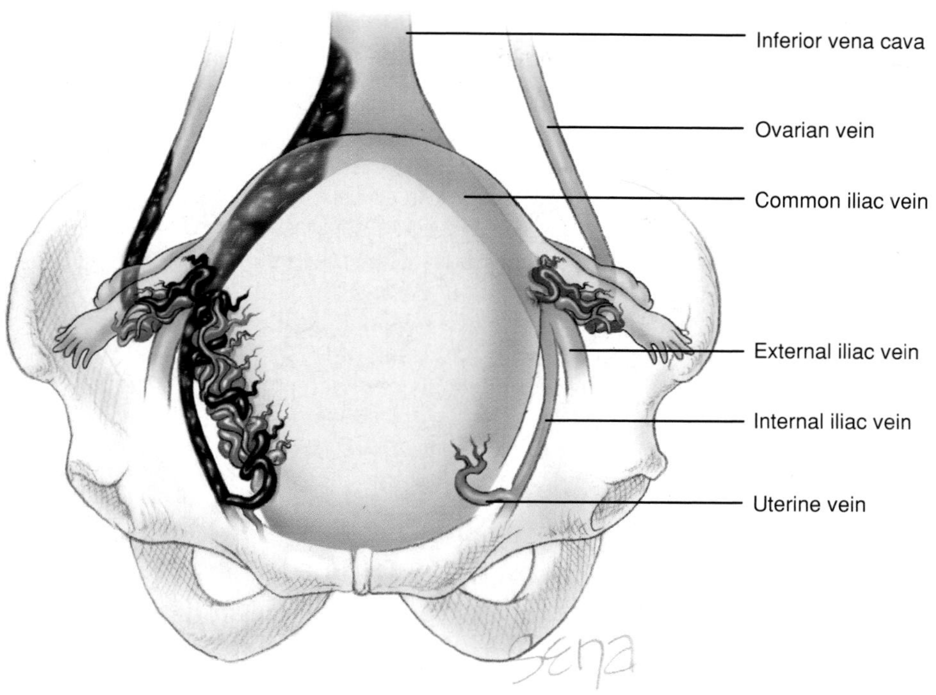

FIGURE 37-6 Septic pelvic thrombophlebitis: uterine and parametrial infection may extend to any pelvic vessel as well as the inferior vena cava. The clot in the right common iliac vein extends from the uterine and internal iliac veins and into the inferior vena cava. The ovarian vein septic thrombosis extends halfway to the vena cava.

vaginal delivery and 1 per 800 with cesarean delivery. The overall incidence of 1 per 3000 deliveries was similar to the 1 per 2000 reported by Dunnihoo and colleagues (1991). In a cohort of 16,650 women undergoing primary cesarean delivery, Rouse and coworkers (2004) reported an incidence of 1 per 400 cesarean deliveries. Incidences approximated 1 per 175 surgeries if there was antecedent chorioamnionitis but only 1 per 500 if there was no intrapartum infection.

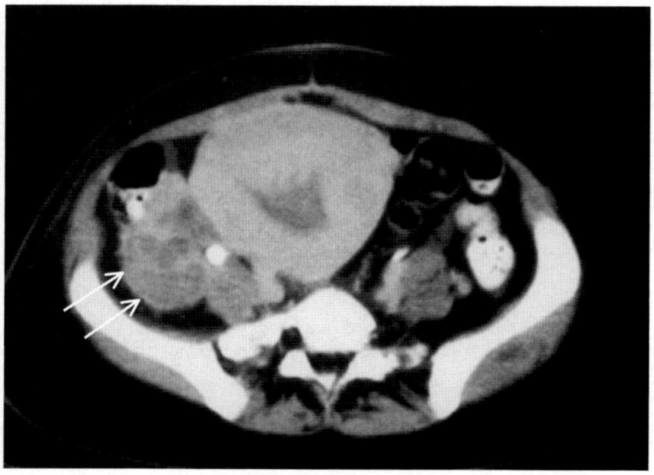

FIGURE 37-7 Ovarian vein thrombosis. Pelvic computed tomography scan shows enlargement of the right ovarian venous plexus with low density of the various lumens (*arrows*). The clotted vessels were easily palpable in this thin woman who had delivered vaginally 3 days earlier and was being treated with antimicrobials for metritis.

Women with septic thrombophlebitis usually have symptomatic improvement with antimicrobial treatment, however, they continue to have fever. Although there occasionally is pain in one or both lower quadrants, patients are usually asymptomatic except for chills. Diagnosis can be confirmed by either pelvic CT or MR imaging (Klima, 2008; Sheffield, 2001). Using either, Brown and colleagues (1999) found that 20 percent of 69 women with metritis who had fever despite ≥ 5 days of appropriate antimicrobial therapy had septic pelvic thrombophlebitis.

It has been disproven that intravenous heparin causes fever to dissipate with septic phlebitis (Brown, 1986; Witlin, 1995). And although Garcia and coworkers (2006) and Klima and Snyder (2008) advocate heparin therapy, we do not recommend anticoagulation. In a randomized study of 14 women by Brown and associates (1999), the addition of heparin to antimicrobial therapy for septic pelvic thrombophlebitis did not hasten recovery or improve outcome. Certainly, there is no evidence for long-term anticoagulation as given for non-infection-related venous thromboembolism.

Perineal Infections

Episiotomy infections are not common because the operation is performed much less frequently now than in the past (American College of Obstetricians and Gynecologists, 2013). Reasons for this are discussed further in Chapter 27 (p. 550). In an older study, Owen and Hauth (1990) described only 10 episiotomy infections in 20,000 women delivered at the University of Alabama at Birmingham. With infection, dehiscence is a concern. Ramin and colleagues (1992) reported an episiotomy dehiscence rate of 0.5 percent at Parkland Hospital—80 percent of these were infected. In a more recent study, Uygur and associates (2004) reported a 1-percent dehiscence rate and attributed two thirds to infection. There are no data to suggest that dehiscence is related to faulty repair.

Infection of a fourth-degree laceration can be more serious. Goldaber and coworkers (1993) described 390 women with a fourth-degree laceration, of whom 5.4 percent had morbidity. In these women, 2.8 percent had infection and dehiscence, 1.8 percent had only dehiscence, and 0.8 percent only infection. Stock and associates (2013) reported wound complications in 7.3 percent of women with anal sphincter injuries. They further observed that intrapartum antimicrobials were protective against infection. Although life-threatening septic shock is rare, it may still occur as a result of an infected episiotomy (Soltesz,

1999). Occasionally also, necrotizing fasciitis develops as discussed on page 686.

Pathogenesis and Clinical Course

Episiotomy dehiscence is most commonly associated with infection as discussed above. Other factors include coagulation disorders, smoking, and human papillomavirus infection (Ramin, 1994). Local pain and dysuria, with or without urinary retention, are common symptoms. Ramin and colleagues (1992), evaluating a series of 34 women with episiotomy dehiscence, reported that the most common findings were pain in 65 percent, purulent discharge in 65 percent, and fever in 44 percent. In extreme cases, the entire vulva may become edematous, ulcerated, and covered with exudate.

Vaginal lacerations may become infected directly or by extension from the perineum. The mucosa becomes red and swollen and may then become necrotic and slough. Parametrial extension may result in lymphangitis.

Cervical lacerations are common but seldom are noticeably infected, which may manifest as metritis. Deep lacerations which extend directly into the tissue at the base of the broad ligament may become infected and cause lymphangitis, parametritis, and bacteremia.

Treatment

Infected episiotomies are managed like other infected surgical wounds. Drainage is established, and in many cases, sutures are removed and the infected wound debrided. In women with obvious cellulitis but no purulence, close observation and broad-spectrum antimicrobial therapy alone may be appropriate. With dehiscence, local wound care is continued along with intravenous antimicrobials. Hauth and colleagues (1986) were the first to advocate early repair after infection subsided, and other studies have confirmed the efficacy of this approach. Hankins and coworkers (1990) described early repair of episiotomy dehiscence in 31 women with an average duration of 6 days from dehiscence to episiotomy repair. All but two had a successful repair. Each of the two women with failures developed a pinpoint rectovaginal fistula that was treated successfully with a small rectal flap. With episiotomy dehiscence due to infection, Ramin and coworkers (1992) reported successful early repair in 32 of 34 women (94 percent), and Uygur and colleagues (2004) noted a similarly high percentage. Rarely, intestinal diversion may be required to allow healing (Rose, 2005).

Early Repair of Infected Episiotomy

Before performing early repair, diligent preparation is essential as outlined in Table 37-3. The surgical wound must be properly cleaned and cleared of infection. Once the surface of the episiotomy wound is free of infection and exudate and covered by pink granulation tissue, secondary repair can be accomplished. The tissue must be adequately mobilized, with special attention to identify and mobilize the anal sphincter muscle. Secondary closure of the episiotomy is accomplished in layers, as described for primary episiotomy closure (Chap. 27, p. 551). Postoperative care includes local wound care, low-residue diet, stool softeners, and nothing per vagina or rectum until healed.

TABLE 37-3. Preoperative Protocol for Early Repair of Episiotomy Dehiscence

Open wound, remove sutures, begin intravenous antimicrobials
Wound care
Sitz bath several times daily or hydrotherapy
Adequate analgesia or anesthesia—regional analgesia or general anesthesia may be necessary for the first few debridements
Scrub wound twice daily with a povidone-iodine solution
Debride necrotic tissue
Closure when afebrile and with pink, healthy granulation tissue
Bowel preparation for fourth-degree repairs

Toxic Shock Syndrome

This acute febrile illness with severe multisystem derangement has a case-fatality rate of 10 to 15 percent. There is usually fever, headache, mental confusion, diffuse macular erythematous rash, subcutaneous edema, nausea, vomiting, watery diarrhea, and marked hemoconcentration. Renal failure followed by hepatic failure, disseminated intravascular coagulation, and circulatory collapse may follow in rapid sequence. During recovery, the rash-covered areas undergo desquamation. For some time, *Staphylococcus aureus* was recovered from almost all afflicted persons. Specifically, a staphylococcal exotoxin, termed *toxic shock syndrome toxin-1* (TSST-1) was found to cause the clinical manifestations by provoking profound endothelial injury. A very small amount of TSST-1 has been shown to activate 5 to 30 percent of T cells to create a "cytokine storm" as described by Que (2005) and Heying (2007) and their coworkers.

During the 1990s, sporadic reports of virulent group A β-hemolytic streptococcal infection began to appear. Heavy colonization or infection is complicated in some cases by *streptococcal toxic shock syndrome,* which is produced when pyrogenic exotoxin is elaborated. Serotypes M1 and M3 are particularly virulent (Beres, 2004; Okumura, 2004). Finally almost identical findings of toxic shock were reported by Robbie and associates (2000) in women with *Clostridium sordellii* colonization.

Thus, in some cases of toxic shock syndrome, infection is not apparent and colonization of a mucosal surface is the presumed source. Ten to 20 percent of pregnant women have vaginal colonization with *S aureus*. Thus, it is not surprising that the disease develops in postpartum women when there is luxuriant bacterial growth vaginally (Chen, 2006; Guerinot, 1982).

Delayed diagnosis and treatment may be associated with maternal mortality (Schummer, 2002). Crum and colleagues (2002) described a neonatal death following antenatal toxic shock syndrome. Principal therapy is supportive, while allowing reversal of capillary endothelial injury (Chap. 47, p. 947). Antimicrobial therapy that includes staphylococcal and streptococcal coverage is given. With evidence of pelvic infection, antimicrobial therapy must also include agents used for polymicrobial infections. Women with these infections may require extensive wound debridement and possibly hysterectomy. Because the toxin is so potent, the mortality rate is correspondingly high (Hotchkiss, 2003).

BREAST INFECTIONS

Parenchymal infection of the mammary glands is a rare antepartum complication but is estimated to develop in up to a third of breast-feeding women (Barbosa-Cesnik, 2003). Excluding breast engorgement, in our experiences, as well as that of Lee and associates (2010), the incidence of mastitis is much lower and probably approximates 1 percent. There is no evidence that any of several prophylactic measures prevent breast infection (Crepinsek, 2012). Risk factors include difficulties in nursing and mothers with outside employment (Branch-Elliman, 2012). Symptoms of suppurative mastitis seldom appear before the end of the first week postpartum and as a rule, not until the third or fourth week. Infection almost invariably is unilateral, and marked engorgement usually precedes inflammation. Symptoms include chills or actual rigors, which are soon followed by fever and tachycardia. There is severe pain, and the breast(s) becomes hard and red (Fig. 37-8). Approximately 10 percent of women with mastitis develop an abscess. Detection of fluctuation may be difficult, and sonography is usually diagnostic as also shown in Figure 37-8.

Etiology

Staphylococcus aureus, especially its methicillin-resistant strain, is the most commonly isolated organism. Matheson and coworkers (1988) reported it in 40 percent of women with mastitis. Other commonly isolated organisms are coagulase-negative staphylococci and viridans streptococci. The immediate source of organisms that cause mastitis is almost always the infant's nose and throat. Bacteria enter the breast through the nipple at the site of a fissure or small abrasion. The infecting organism can usually be cultured from milk. Toxic shock syndrome from mastitis caused by *S aureus* has been reported (Demey, 1989; Fujiwara, 2001).

At times, suppurative mastitis reaches epidemic levels among nursing mothers. Such outbreaks most often coincide with the appearance of a new strain of antibiotic-resistant staphylococcus. A contemporaneous example is community-acquired methicillin-resistant *S aureus* (CA-MRSA), which has rapidly become the most commonly isolated staphylococcal species in some areas (Klevens, 2007; Pallin, 2008). At Parkland Hospital from 2000 to 2004, Laibl and associates (2005) reported that a fourth of CA-MRSA isolates were from pregnant or postpartum women with puerperal mastitis. Hospital-acquired MRSA may cause mastitis when the infant becomes colonized after contact with nursery personnel who are colonized (Centers for Disease Control and Prevention, 2006). Stafford and colleagues (2008) found a higher incidence of subsequent abscess in those with CA-MRSA-associated mastitis. In one study of puerperal breast abscesses, 63 percent were due to methicillin-resistant strains (Berens, 2010).

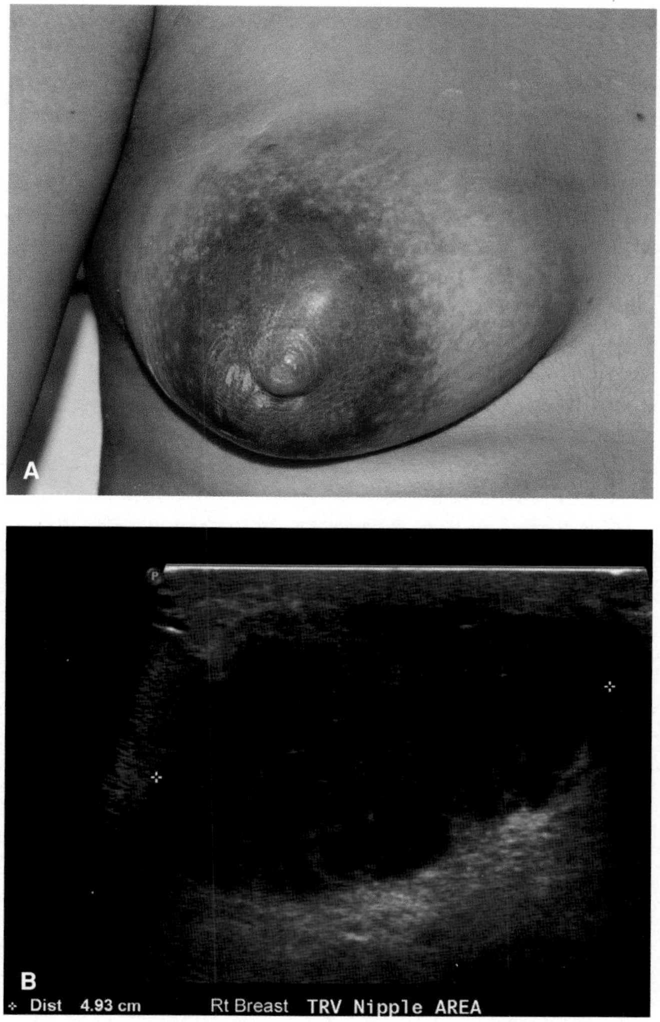

FIGURE 37-8 Puerperal mastitis with breast abscess. **A.** Photograph shows indurated, erythematous skin overlying area of right-sided breast infection. **B.** Sonographic picture of this 5-cm abscess. (Images contributed by Dr. Emily Adhikari.)

Management

Provided that appropriate therapy for mastitis is started before suppuration begins, the infection usually resolves within 48 hours. As discussed, abscess formation is more common with *S aureus* infection (Matheson, 1988). Most recommend that milk be expressed from the affected breast onto a swab and cultured before therapy is begun. Bacterial identification and antimicrobial sensitivities provide information mandatory for a successful program of nosocomial infection surveillance (Lee, 2010).

The initial antimicrobial choice is influenced by the current experience with staphylococcal infections at the institution. Although most are community-acquired organisms, as discussed above, these frequently include CA-MRSA. Dicloxacillin, 500 mg orally four times daily, may be started empirically. Erythromycin is given to women who are penicillin sensitive. If the infection is caused by resistant, penicillinase-producing staphylococci or if resistant organisms are suspected while awaiting the culture results, then vancomycin or another anti-MRSA antimicrobial should be given. Even though clinical response may be prompt, treatment should be continued for 10 to 14 days.

Marshall and coworkers (1975) demonstrated the importance of continued breast feeding. They reported that of 65 women with mastitis, the only three who developed abscesses were among the 15 women who quit breast feeding. Vigorous milk expression may be sufficient treatment alone (Thomsen, 1984). Sometimes the infant will not nurse on the inflamed breast. This probably is not related to any changes in the milk taste but is secondary to engorgement and edema, which can make the areola harder to grip. Pumping can alleviate this. When nursing bilaterally, it is best to begin suckling on the uninvolved breast. This allows let-down to commence before moving to the tender breast.

In resource-poor countries, breast feeding in women infected with the human immunodeficiency virus (HIV) is not contraindicated. In the setting of mastitis or breast abscess, it is recommended to stop feeding from the infected breast. This is because HIV RNA levels increase in affected breast milk. These levels return to baseline after symptoms resolve (Semrau, 2013).

Breast Abscess

In a population-based study of nearly 1.5 million Swedish women, the incidence of breast abscess was 0.1 percent (Kvist, 2005). An abscess should be suspected when defervescence does not follow within 48 to 72 hours of mastitis treatment or when a mass is palpable. Again, sonographic imaging is valuable (see Fig. 37-8). Breast abscesses can be quite large, and in one case report, 2 liters of pus was drained (Martic, 2012). Traditional therapy is surgical drainage, which usually requires general anesthesia. The incision should be made corresponding to Langer skin lines for a cosmetic result (Stehman, 1990). In early cases, a single incision over the most dependent portion of fluctuation is usually sufficient. Multiple abscesses, however, require several incisions and disruption of loculations. The resulting cavity is loosely packed with gauze, which should be replaced at the end of 24 hours by a smaller pack.

A more recently used technique that is less invasive is sonographically guided needle aspiration using local analgesia. This has an 80- to 90-percent success rate (O'Hara, 1996; Schwarz, 2001). In a randomized trial, Naeem and colleagues (2012) compared surgical drainage and aspiration. They found aspiration resulted in quicker healing at 8 weeks, 77 versus 93 percent, respectively.

REFERENCES

Acosta CD, Bhattacharya S, Tuffnell D, et al: Maternal sepsis: a Scottish population-based case-control study. BJOG 119(4):474, 2012

American College of Obstetricians and Gynecologists: Episiotomy. Practice Bulletin No. 71, April 2006, Reaffirmed 2013

American College of Obstetricians and Gynecologists: Use of prophylactic antibiotics in labor and delivery. Practice Bulletin No. 120, June 2011

Anderson DJ, Sexton DJ, Kanafani ZA, et al: Severe surgical site infection in community hospitals: epidemiology, key procedures, and the changing prevalence of methicillin-resistant *Staphylococcus aureus*. Infect Control Hosp Epidemiol 28 (9):1047, 2007

Andrews WW, Hauth JC, Cliver SP, et al: Randomized clinical trial of extended spectrum antibiotic prophylaxis with coverage for *Ureaplasma urealyticum* to reduce post-cesarean delivery endometritis. Obstet Gynecol 101:1183, 2003

Andrews WW, Shah SR, Goldenberg RL, et al: Association of post-cesarean delivery endometritis with colonization of the chorioamnion by *Ureaplasma urealyticum*. Obstet Gynecol 85:509, 1995

Anteby EY, Yagel S, Hanoch J, et al: Puerperal and intrapartum group A streptococcal infection. Infect Dis Obstet Gynecol 7:276, 1999

Aronoff DM, Mulla ZD: Postpartum invasive group A streptococcal disease in the modern era. Infect Dis Obstet Gynecol 796892:1, 2008

Atkinson MW, Owen J, Wren A, et al: The effect of manual removal of the placenta on post-cesarean endometritis. Obstet Gynecol 87:99, 1996

Baaqeel H, Baaqeel R: Timing of administration of prophylactic antibiotics for caesarean section: a systematic review and meta-analysis. BJOG 120(6):661, 2013

Baksu A, Kalan A, Ozkan A, et al: The effect of placental removal method and site of uterine repair on postcesarean endometritis and operative blood loss. Acta Obstet Gynecol Scand 84(3):266, 2005

Bamigboye AA, Hofmeyr GJ: Closure versus non-closure of the peritoneum at caesarean section. Cochrane Database Syst Rev 4:CD000163, 2003

Barbosa-Cesnik C, Schwartz K, et al: Lactation mastitis. JAMA 289:1609, 2003

Berens P, Swaim L, Peterson B: Incidence of methicillin-resistant *Staphylococcus aureus* in postpartum breast abscesses. Breastfeed Med 5(3):113, 2010

Beres SB, Sylva GL, Sturdevant DE, et al: Genome-wide molecular dissection of serotype M3 group A *Streptococcus* strains causing two epidemics of invasive infections. Proc Natl Acad Sci U S A 101:11833, 2004

Berg CJ, Callaghan WM, Syverson C, et al: Pregnancy-related mortality in the United States, 1998 to 2005. Obstet Gynecol 116(6):1302, 2010

Berg CJ, Harper MA, Atkinson SM, et al: Preventability of pregnancy-related deaths: results of a state-wide review. Obstet Gynecol 106:1228, 2005

Branch-Elliman W, Golen TH, Gold HS, et al: Risk factors for *Staphylococcus aureus* postpartum breast abscess. Clin Infect Dis 54(1):71, 2012

Brown CEL, Dunn DH, Harrell R, et al: Computed tomography for evaluation of puerperal infection. Surg Gynecol Obstet 172:2, 1991

Brown CEL, Lowe TW, Cunningham FG, et al: Puerperal pelvic thrombophlebitis: impact on diagnosis and treatment using x-ray computed tomography and magnetic resonance imaging. Obstet Gynecol 68:789, 1986

Brown CEL, Stettler RW, Twickler D, et al: Puerperal septic pelvic thrombophlebitis: incidence and response to heparin therapy. Am J Obstet Gynecol 181:143, 1999

Brown KR, Williams SF, Apuzzio JJ: Ertapenem compared to combination drug therapy for the treatment of postpartum endometritis after cesarean delivery. J Matern Fetal Neonatal Med 25(6):743, 2012

Brumfield, CG, Hauth JC, Andrews WW: Puerperal infection after cesarean delivery: evaluation of a standardized protocol. Am J Obstet Gynecol 182:1147, 2000

Burrows LJ, Meyn LA, Weber AM: Maternal morbidity associated with vaginal versus cesarean delivery. Obstet Gynecol 103:907, 2004

Carey JC, Klebanoff MA, Hauth JC, et al: Metronidazole to prevent preterm delivery in pregnant women with asymptomatic bacterial vaginosis. N Engl J Med 342:534, 2000

Castagnola DE, Hoffman MK, Carlson J, et al: Necrotizing cervical and uterine infection in the postpartum period caused by Group A *Streptococcus*. Obstet Gynecol 111:533, 2008

Centers for Disease Control and Prevention: Community-associated methicillin-resistant *Staphylococcus aureus* infection among healthy newborns—Chicago and Los Angeles County, 2004. MMWR 55(12):329, 2006

Chaim W, Bashiri A, Bar-David J, et al: Prevalence and clinical significance of postpartum endometritis and wound infection. Infect Dis Obstet Gynecol 8:77, 2000

Chaim W, Horowitz S, David JB, et al: *Ureaplasma urealyticum* in the development of postpartum endometritis. Eur J Obstet Reprod Biol 15:145, 2003

Chelmow D, Rodriguez EJ, Sabatini MM: Suture closure of subcutaneous fat and wound disruption after cesarean delivery: a meta-analysis. Obstet Gynecol 103:974, 2004

Chelmow D, Ruehli MS, Huang E: Prophylactic use of antibiotics for nonlaboring patients undergoing cesarean delivery with intact membranes: a meta-analysis. Am J Obstet Gynecol 184:656, 2001

Chen KT, Huard RC, Della-Latta P, et al: Prevalence of methicillin-sensitive and methicillin-resistant *Staphylococcus aureus* in pregnant women. Obstet Gynecol 108:482, 2006

Collins CG, McCallum EA, Nelson EW, et al: Suppurative pelvic thrombophlebitis: 1. Incidence, pathology, etiology; 2. Symptomatology and diagnosis; 3. Surgical techniques: a study of 70 patients treated by ligation of the inferior vena cava and ovarian veins. Surgery 30:298, 1951

Combs CA, Gravett M, Garite T, et al: Intramniotic inflammation may be more important than the presence of microbes as a determinant of perinatal outcome in preterm labor. Am J Obstet Gynecol 208(1):S44, 2013

Conroy K, Koenig AF, Yu YH, et al: Infectious morbidity after cesarean delivery: 10 strategies to reduce risk. Rev Obstet Gynecol 5 (2):69, 2012

Crepinsek MA, Crowe L, Michener K, et al: Interventions for preventing mastitis after childbirth. Cochrane Database Syst Rev 10:CD007239, 2012
Crum NF, Chun HM, Gaylord TG, et al: Group A streptococcal toxic shock syndrome developing in the third trimester of pregnancy. Infect Dis Obstet Gynecol 10:209, 2002
Cunningham FG, Hauth JC, Strong JD, et al: Infectious morbidity following cesarean: comparison of two treatment regimens. Obstet Gynecol 52:656, 1978
Declercq E, Barger M, Cabral HJ, et al: Maternal outcomes associated with planned primary cesarean births compared with planned vaginal births. Obstet Gynecol 109:669, 2007
Demey HE, Hautekeete MI, Buytaert P, et al: Mastitis and toxic shock syndrome. A case report. Acta Obstet Gynecol Scand 68:87, 1989
Deneux-Tharaux C, Carmona E, Bouvier-Colle MH, et al: Postpartum maternal mortality and cesarean delivery. Obstet Gynecol 108:541, 2006
DePalma RT, Cunningham FG, Leveno KJ, et al: Continuing investigation of women at high risk for infection following cesarean delivery. Obstet Gynecol 60:53, 1982
Dinsmoor MJ, Gilbert S, Landon MB, et al: Perioperative antibiotic prophylaxis for nonlaboring cesarean delivery. Obstet Gynecol 114(4):752, 2009
Dinsmoor MJ, Newton ER, Gibbs RS: A randomized, double-blind placebo-controlled trial of oral antibiotic therapy following intravenous antibiotic therapy for postpartum endometritis. Obstet Gynecol 77:60, 1991
DiZerega G, Yonekura L, Roy S, et al: A comparison of clindamycin-gentamicin and penicillin gentamicin in the treatment of post-cesarean section endomyometritis. Am J Obstet Gynecol 134:238, 1979
Dunnihoo DR, Gallaspy JW, Wise RB, et al: Postpartum ovarian vein thrombophlebitis: a review. Obstet Gynecol Surv 46:415, 1991
Emmons SL, Krohn M, Jackson M, et al: Development of wound infections among women undergoing cesarean section. Obstet Gynecol 72:559, 1988
Filker RS, Monif GRG: Postpartum septicemia due to group G streptococci. Obstet Gynecol 53;28S, 1979
French LM, Smaill FM: Antibiotic regimens for endometritis after delivery. Cochrane Database Syst Rev 4:CD001067, 2004
Fujiwara Y, Endo S: A case of toxic shock syndrome secondary to mastitis caused by methicillin-resistant *Staphylococcus aureus*. Kansenshogaku Zasshi 75:898, 2001
Gallup DG, Meguiar RV: Coping with necrotizing fasciitis. Contemp Ob/Gyn 49:38, 2004
Garcia J, Aboujaoude R, Apuzzio J, et al: Septic pelvic thrombophlebitis: diagnosis and management. Infect Dis Obstet Gynecol 2006(15614):1, 2006
Gilstrap LC III, Cunningham FG: The bacterial pathogenesis of infection following cesarean section. Obstet Gynecol 53:545, 1979
Goepfert AR, Guinn DA, Andrews WW, et al: Necrotizing fasciitis after cesarean section. Obstet Gynecol 89:409, 1997
Goldaber KG, Wendel PJ, McIntire DD, et al: Postpartum perineal morbidity after fourth degree perineal repair. Am J Obstet Gynecol 168:489, 1993
Guerinot GT, Gitomer SD, Sanko SR: Postpartum patient with toxic shock syndrome. Obstet Gynecol 59:43S, 1982
Haas DM, Morgan S, Contreras K: Vaginal preparation with antiseptic solution before cesarean section for preventing postoperative infections. Cochrane Database Syst Rev 1:CD007892, 2013
Hankins GDV, Hauth JC, Gilstrap LC, et al: Early repair of episiotomy dehiscence. Obstet Gynecol 75:48, 1990
Hartmann KE, Barrett KE, Reid VC, et al: Clinical usefulness of white blood cell count after cesarean delivery. Obstet Gynecol 96:295, 2000
Hauth JC, Gilstrap LC III, Ward SC, et al: Early repair of an external sphincter ani muscle and rectal mucosal dehiscence. Obstet Gynecol 67:806, 1986
Hauth JC, Owen J, Davis RO: Transverse uterine incision closure: one versus two layers. Am J Obstet Gynecol 167:1108, 1992
Heying R, van de Gevel J, Que YA, et al: Fibronectin-binding proteins and clumping factor A in *Staphylococcus aureus* experimental endocarditis: FnBPA is sufficient to activate human endothelial cells. Thromb Haemost 97:617, 2007
Hotchkiss RS, Karl IE: The pathophysiology and treatment of sepsis. N Engl J Med 348:2, 2003
Ismail MA, Chandler AE, Beem ME: Chlamydial colonization of the cervix in pregnant adolescents. J Reprod Med 30:549, 1985
Jacobs-Jokhan D, Hofmeyr G: Extra-abdominal versus intra-abdominal repair of the uterine incision at caesarean section. Cochrane Database Syst Rev 4:CD000085, 2004
Jacobsson B, Pernevi P, Chidekel L, et al: Bacterial vaginosis in early pregnancy may predispose for preterm birth and postpartum endometritis. Acta Obstet Gynecol Scand 81:1006, 2002
Jaiyeoba O: Postoperative infections in obstetrics and gynecology. Clin Obstet Gynecol 55(4):904, 2012
Jazayeri A, Jazayeri MK, Sahinler M, et al: Is meconium passage a risk factor for maternal infection in term pregnancies? Obstet Gynecol 99(4):548, 2002
Kabiru W, Raynor BD: Obstetric outcomes associated with increase in BMI category during pregnancy. Am J Obstet Gynecol 191:928, 2004
Kankuri E, Kurki T, Carlson P, et al: Incidence, treatment and outcome of peripartum sepsis. Acta Obstet Gynecol Scand 82:730, 2003
Klebanoff MA, Carey JC, Hauth JC, et al: Failure of metronidazole to prevent preterm delivery among pregnant women with asymptomatic *Trichomonas vaginalis* infection. N Engl J Med 345:487, 2001
Klevens RM, Morrison MA, Nadle J, et al: Invasive methicillin-resistant *Staphylococcus aureus* infections in the United States. JAMA 298:1763, 2007
Klima DA, Snyder TE: Postpartum ovarian vein thrombosis. Obstet Gynecol 111:431, 2008
Koroukian SM: Relative risk of postpartum complications in the Ohio Medicaid population: vaginal versus cesarean delivery. Med Care Res Rev 61:203, 2004
Kvist LJ, Rydhstroem H: Factors related to breast abscess after delivery: a population-based study. BJOG 112:1070, 2005
Laibl VR, Sheffield JS, Roberts S, et al: Clinical presentation of community-acquired methicillin-resistant *Staphylococcus aureus* in pregnancy. Obstet Gynecol 106:461, 2005
Lee IW, Kang L, Hsu HP, et al: Puerperal mastitis requiring hospitalization during a nine-year period. Am J Obstet Gynecol 203(4):332, 2010
Leth RA, Uldbjerg N, Norgaard M, et al: Obesity, diabetes, and the risk of infections diagnosed in hospital and post-discharge infections after cesarean section: a prospective cohort study. Acta Obstet Gynecol Scand 90(5):501, 2011
Liabsuetrakul T, Peeyananjarassri K: Mechanical dilatation of the cervix at non-labour caesarean section for reducing postoperative morbidity. Cochrane Database Syst Rev 11:CD008019, 2011
Livingston JC, Llata E, Rinehart E, et al: Gentamicin and clindamycin therapy in postpartum endometritis: the efficacy of daily dosing versus dosing every 8 hours. Am J Obstet Gynecol 188:149, 2003
Maberry MC, Gilstrap LC, Bawdon RE, et al: Anaerobic coverage for intra-amnionic infection: maternal and perinatal impact. Am J Perinatol 8:338, 1991
Mackeen AD, Berghella V, Larsen ML: Techniques and materials for skin closure in caesarean section. Cochrane Database Syst Rev 11:CD003577, 2012
Macones GA, Cleary KL, Parry S, et al: The timing of antibiotics at cesarean: a randomized controlled trial. Am J Perinatol 29(4):273, 2012
Magann EF, Chauhan SP, Rodts-Palenik S, et al: Subcutaneous stitch closure versus subcutaneous drain to prevent wound disruption after cesarean delivery: a randomized clinical trial. Am J Obstet Gynecol 186:1119, 2002
Maharaj D: Puerperal pyrexia: a review. Part II: Obstet Gynecol Surv 62:400, 2007
Maldjian C, Adam R, Maldjian J, et al: MRI appearance of the pelvis in the post cesarean-section patient. Magn Reson Imaging 17:223, 1999
Marchocki Z, O'Donoghue M, Collins K, et al: Clinical significance of elevated high-sensitivity C-reactive protein in amniotic fluid obtained at emergency caesarean section. Am J Obstet Gynecol 208(1)S314, 2013
Marshall BR, Hepper JK, Zirbel CC: Sporadic puerperal mastitis—an infection that need not interrupt lactation. JAMA 344:1377, 1975
Martic K, Vasilj O. Extremely large breast abscess in a breastfeeding mother. J Hum Lact 28(4):460, 2012
Matheson I, Aursnes I, Horgen M, et al: Bacteriological findings and clinical symptoms in relation to clinical outcome in puerperal mastitis. Acta Obstet Gynecol Scand 67:723, 1988
McNeeley SG Jr, Hendrix SL, Bennett SM, et al: Synthetic graft placement in the treatment of fascial dehiscence with necrosis and infection. Am J Obstet Gynecol 179:1430, 1998
Naeem M, Rahimnajjad MK, Rahimnajjad NA, et al: Comparison of incision and drainage against needle aspiration for the treatment of breast abscess. Am Surg 78(11):1224, 2012
Nathan L, Leveno KJ: Group A streptococcal puerperal sepsis: historical review and 1990s resurgence. Infect Dis Obstet Gynecol 1:252, 1994
Naumann RW, Hauth JC, Owen J, et al: Subcutaneous tissue approximation in relation to wound disruption after cesarean delivery in obese women. Obstet Gynecol 85:412, 1995
O'Hara RJ, Dexter SPL, Fox JN: Conservative management of infective mastitis and breast abscesses after ultrasonographic assessment. Br J Surg 83:1413, 1996
Okumura K, Schroff R, Campbell R, et al: Group A streptococcal puerperal sepsis with retroperitoneal involvement developing in a late postpartum woman: case report. Am Surg 70:730, 2004
Owen J, Andrews WW: Wound complications after cesarean section. Clin Obstet Gynecol 27:842, 1994
Owen J, Hauth JC: Episiotomy infection and dehiscence. In Gilstrap LC III, Faro S (eds): Infections in Pregnancy. New York, Liss, 1990, p 61
Palep-Singh M, Jayaprakasan J, Hopkisson JF: Peripartum group A streptococcal sepsis: a case report. J Reprod Med 52 (10):977, 2007

Pallin DJ, Egan DJ, Pelletier AJ, et al: Increased U.S. emergency department visits for skin and soft tissue infections, and changes in antibiotic choices, during the emergence of community-associated methicillin-resistant *Staphylococcus aureus*. Ann Emerg Med 51:291, 2008

Patel M, Kumar RA, Stamm AM, et al: USA300 genotype community-associated methicillin-resistant *Staphylococcus aureus* as a cause of surgical site infection. J Clin Microbiol 45 (10):3431, 2007

Que YA, Haefliger JA, Piroth L, et al: Fibrinogen and fibronectin binding cooperative for valve infection and invasion in *Staphylococcus aureus* experimental endocarditis. J Exp Med 201:1627, 2005

Ramin SM, Gilstrap LC: Episiotomy and early repair of dehiscence. Clin Obstet Gynecol 37:816, 1994

Ramin SM, Ramus R, Little B, et al: Early repair of episiotomy dehiscence associated with infection. Am J Obstet Gynecol 167:1104, 1992

Reid VC, Hartmann KE, McMahon M, et al: Vaginal preparation with povidone iodine and postcesarean infections morbidity: a randomized controlled trial. Obstet Gynecol 97:147, 2001

Robbie LA, Dummer S, Booth NA, et al: Plasminogen activator inhibitor 2 and urokinase-type plasminogen activator in plasma and leucocytes in patients with severe sepsis. Br J Haematol 109:342, 2000

Rose CH, Blessitt KL, Araghizadeh F: Episiotomy dehiscence that required intestinal diversion. Am J Obstet Gynecol 193:1759, 2005

Rotas M, McCalla S, Liu C, et al: Methicillin-resistant *Staphylococcus aureus* necrotizing pneumonia arising from an infected episiotomy site. Obstet Gynecol 109:533, 2007

Rouse DJ, Landon M, Leveno KJ, et al: The Maternal-Fetal Medicine Units cesarean registry: chorioamnionitis at term and its duration—relationship to outcomes. Am J Obstet Gynecol 191:211, 2004

Schorge JO, Granter SR, Lerner LH, et al: Postpartum and vulvar necrotizing fasciitis: early clinical diagnosis and histopathologic correlation. J Reprod Med 43:586, 1998

Schummer W, Schummer C: Two cases of delayed diagnosis of postpartal streptococcal toxic shock syndrome. Infect Dis Obstet Gynecol 10:217, 2002

Schwarz RJ, Shrestha R: Needle aspiration of breast abscesses. Am J Surg 182:117, 2001

Semrau K, Kuhn L, Brooks DR, et al: Dynamics of breast milk HIV-1 RNA with unilateral mastitis or abscess. J Acquir Immune Defic Syndr 62(3):348, 2013

Shahabi S, Klein JP, Rinaudo PF: Primary psoas abscess complicating a normal vaginal delivery. Obstet Gynecol 99:906, 2002

Sheffield JS, Cunningham FG: Detecting and treating septic pelvic thrombophlebitis. Contemp Ob/Gyn 3:15, 2001

Sherman D, Lurie S, Betzer M, et al: Uterine flora at cesarean and its relationship to postpartum endometritis. Obstet Gynecol 94:787, 1999

Siriwachirachai T, Sangkomkamhang US, Lumbiganon P, et al: Antibiotics for meconium-stained amniotic fluid in labour for preventing maternal and neonatal infections. Cochrane Database Syst Rev 12:CD007772, 2010

Smaill F, Gyte GM: Antibiotic prophylaxis versus no prophylaxis for preventing infection after cesarean section. Cochrane Database Syst Rev 1:CD007482, 2010

Soltesz S, Biedler A, Ohlmann P, et al: Puerperal sepsis due to infected episiotomy wound [German]. Zentralbl Gynakol 121:441, 1999

Stafford I, Hernandez J, Laibl V, et al: Community-acquired methicillin-resistant *Staphylococcus aureus* among patients with puerperal mastitis requiring hospitalization. Obstet Gynecol 112(3):533, 2008

Stehman FB: Infections and inflammations of the breast. In Hindle WH (ed): Breast Disease for Gynecologists. Norwalk, CT, Appleton & Lange, 1990, p 151

Stock L, Basham E, Gossett DR, et al: Factors associated with wound complications in women with obstetric and sphincter injuries (OASIS). Am J Obstet Gynecol 208(4):327.e1, 2013

Sun J, Ding M, Liu J, et al: Prophylactic administration of cefazolin prior to skin incision versus antibiotics at cord clamping in preventing postcesarean infectious morbidity: a systematic review and meta-analysis of randomized controlled trials. Gynecol Obstet Invest 75(3):175, 2013

Swanson A, Lau KK, Kornman T, et al: Primary psoas muscle abscess in pregnancy. Aust N Z J Obstet Gynaecol 48(6):607, 2008

Swartz MN: Cellulitis. N Engl J Med 350:904, 2004

Thomsen AC, Espersen T, Maigaard S: Course and treatment of milk stasis, noninfectious inflammation of the breast, and infectious mastitis in nursing women. Am J Obstet Gynecol 149:492, 1984

Tita ATN, Hauth JC, Grimes A, et al: Decreasing incidence of postcesarean endometritis with extended-spectrum antibiotic prophylaxis. Obstet Gynecol 111:51, 2008

Treszezamsky AD, Feldman D, Sarabanchong VO: Concurrent postpartum uterine and abdominal wall dehiscence and *Streptococcus anginosus* infection. Obstet Gynecol 118(2):449, 2011

Tsai PS, Hsu CS, Fan YC: General anaesthesia is associated with increased risk of surgical site infection after cesarean delivery compared with neuraxial anaesthesia: a population-based study. Br J Anaesth 107(5):757, 2011

Tulandi T, Al-Jaroudi D: Nonclosure of peritoneum: a reappraisal. Am J Obstet Gynecol 189:609, 2003

Tuuli MG, Rampersad RM, Carbone JF, et al: Staples compared with subcuticular suture for skin closure after cesarean delivery: a systematic review and meta-analysis. Obstet Gynecol 117(3):682, 2011

Twickler DM, Setiawan AT, Harrell RS, et al: CT appearance of the pelvis after cesarean section. AJR Am J Roentgenol 156:523, 1991

Udagawa H, Oshio Y, Shimizu Y: Serious group A streptococcal infection around delivery. Obstet Gynecol 94:153, 1999

Urschel JD: Necrotizing soft tissue infections. Postgrad Med J 75:645, 1999

Uygur D, Yesildaglar N, Kis S, et al: Early repair of episiotomy dehiscence. Aust N Z J Obstet Gynaecol 44:244, 2004

Watts DH, Krohn MA, Hillier SL, et al: Bacterial vaginosis as a risk factor for post-cesarean endometritis. Obstet Gynecol 75:52, 1990

Wechter ME, Pearlman MD, Hartmann KE: Reclosure of the disrupted laparotomy wound. A systematic review. Obstet Gynecol 106:376, 2005

Wetchler SJ, Dunn LJ: Ovarian abscess. Report of a case and a review of the literature. Obstet Gynecol Surv 40:476, 1985

Witlin AG, Sibai BM: Postpartum ovarian vein thrombosis after vaginal delivery: a report of 11 cases. Obstet Gynecol 85:775, 1995

Witt A, Doner M, Petricevic L, et al: Antibiotic prophylaxis before surgery vs after cord clamping in elective cesarean delivery: a double-blind, prospective, randomized placebo-controlled trial. Arch Surg 146(12):1404, 2011

Yildirim G, Gungorduk K, Asicioglu O, et al: Does vaginal preparation with povidone-iodine prior to cesarean delivery reduce the risk of endometritis? A randomized controlled trial. J Matern Fetal Neonatal Med 25(11):2316, 2012

CHAPTER 38

Contraception

Half of all pregnancies each year in the United States are unintended (Finer, 2011). These may follow contraceptive method failure or stem from lack of contraceptive use. Specifically, 10 percent of sexually active American women not pursuing pregnancy did not use any birth control method (Jones, 2012). And, for sexually active fertile women not using contraception, pregnancy rates approach 90 percent at 1 year.

For those seeking contraception, various effective contraceptive methods are available. Preferences of United States women are shown in Table 38-1. With these methods, wide variations are seen between estimated failure rates of perfect and typical use during the first year. Similarly, the World Health Organization (WHO) has grouped methods according to effectiveness tiers that reflect these failure rates (Table 38-2). Implants and intrauterine devices are found in the top tier. They are effective in lowering unintended pregnancy rates and are considered long-acting reversible contraception (LARC) (Winner, 2012). The American College of Obstetricians and Gynecologists (2013c) recognizes these efficacy tiers and the high unintended pregnancy rate. Thus, the College recommends that clinicians provide counseling on *all* options and encourages highly effective LARC for all appropriate candidates.

Unfortunately, no contraceptive method is completely without side effects. That said, an important tenet is that contraception usually poses less risk than pregnancy. During appropriate method selection, underlying patient health conditions should be known. Some disorders or the medications used for their treatment can increase the risk of some contraceptives. The WHO (2010) has provided evidence-based guidelines, termed *Medical Eligibility Criteria*, for the use of all highly effective reversible contraceptive methods by women with various health conditions. Individual countries have subsequently modified these. The *United States Medical Eligibility Criteria (US MEC)* was published in the United States by the Centers for Disease Control and Prevention (CDC) (2010b), and its use is encouraged by the American College of Obstetricians and Gynecologists (2011b). Shown on page 698, the CDC (2011, 2012) has since added updates to reflect changes for women at high risk for human immunodeficiency virus (HIV) infection and for women in the puerperium. The US MEC guidelines and these updates, as well as a free smart-phone application of the guidelines, are available at the CDC website: http://www.cdc.gov/reproductivehealth/UnintendedPregnancy/USMEC.htm.

In the US MEC, reversible contraceptive methods are organized into six groups by their similarity: combination hormonal contraceptives (CHCs), progestin-only pills (POPs), depot medroxyprogesterone acetate (DMPA), implants, levonorgestrel-releasing intrauterine system (LNG-IUS), and copper intrauterine devices (Cu-IUDs). For a given health condition, each method is categorized 1 through 4. The score describes a method's safety profile for a typical woman with that condition:

TABLE 38-1. Method Use among Women in the United States

Method	Percentage
Female sterilization	16.5
Male sterilization	6.2
Combination pill	17.1
Progestin-only pill	0.4
Implants or patch	0.9
DMPA	2.3
Vaginal ring	1.3
Intrauterine devices	3.5
Male condom	10.2
Periodic abstinence	
Calendar method	0.6
Natural family planning[a]	0.1
Withdrawal	3.2
Other methods[b]	0.3
Not using contraception[c]	37.8

[a]Methods using physiological changes to signal ovulation.
[b]Includes diaphragm, female condom, cervical cap, contraceptive sponge, spermicides, and emergency contraception.
[c]Includes those seeking pregnancy, surgically sterilized for noncontraceptive reasons, sexually inactive, pregnant or puerperal, and those who are sexually active but not using contraception.
DMPA = depot medroxyprogesterone acetate.
Data from Jones, 2012.

TABLE 38-2. Contraceptive Failure Rates During the First Year of Method Use in Women in the United States

Method[a]	Perfect Use	Typical Use
Top Tier: Most Effective		
Intrauterine devices		
Levonorgestrel system	0.2	0.2
T 380A copper	0.6	0.8
Levonorgestrel implants	0.05	0.05
Female sterilization	0.5	0.5
Male sterilization	0.1	0.15
Second Tier: Very Effective		
Combination pill	0.3	9
Vaginal ring	0.3	9
Patch	0.3	9
DMPA	0.2	6
Progestin-only pill	0.3	9
Third Tier: Effective		
Condom		
Male	2	18
Female	5	21
Diaphragm with spermicides	6	12
Fertility-awareness		24
Standard days	5	
Two day	4	
Ovulation	3	
Symptothermal	0.4	
Fourth Tier: Least Effective		
Spermicides	18	28
Sponge		
Parous women	20	24
Nulliparous women	9	12
No WHO Category		
Withdrawal	4	22
No contraception	85	85

[a]Methods organized according to tiers of efficacy by World Health Organization (WHO), Johns Hopkins Bloomberg School of Public Health, 2007.
DMPA = depot medroxyprogesterone acetate.
Data from Trussell, 2011a.

(1) no restriction of method use, (2) method advantages outweigh risks, (3) method risks outweigh advantages, and (4) method poses an unacceptably high health risk.

Alternatively, depending on the underlying disorder or patient desire, male or female sterilization may be a preferred or recommended permanent contraceptive method. These options are fully discussed in Chapter 39 (p. 720).

LONG-ACTING REVERSIBLE CONTRACEPTION: INTRAUTERINE DEVICES

These are the most commonly used method of reversible contraception worldwide, and in the United States, nearly 4 percent of women select this method (d'Arcanques, 2007; Jones, 2012). Fortunately, contraindications to IUD use are few.

Intrauterine devices (IUDs) that are *chemically inert* are composed of nonabsorbable materials. The three IUDs currently approved for use in the United States are *chemically active* and have continuous elution of copper or a progestin. Of these, there are two different levonorgestrel-releasing intrauterine systems—*Mirena* and *Skyla* (Fig. 38-1). Each releases the progestin into the uterus at a relatively constant rate, which reduces systemic effects. Their T-shaped radiopaque frames have a stem wrapped with a cylinder reservoir that contains the levonorgestrel. There are two trailing brown strings attached to the stem (Bayer Healthcare Pharmaceuticals, 2013a,b). Mirena is currently approved for 5 years of use following insertion, however, some evidence supports its efficacy for 7 years (Thonneau, 2008). Skyla is approved for 3 years of use. It has slightly smaller overall dimensions than its counterpart and was sized to more appropriately fit a nulliparous uterus (Gemzell-Danielsson, 2012). It can also be differentiated from *Mirena* visually and sonographically by a silver ring near the junction of the device's stem and arms.

The third device is the T 380A IUD, named *ParaGard*. It has a polyethylene and barium sulfate T-shaped frame wound with copper, and two strings extend from the stem base. Originally

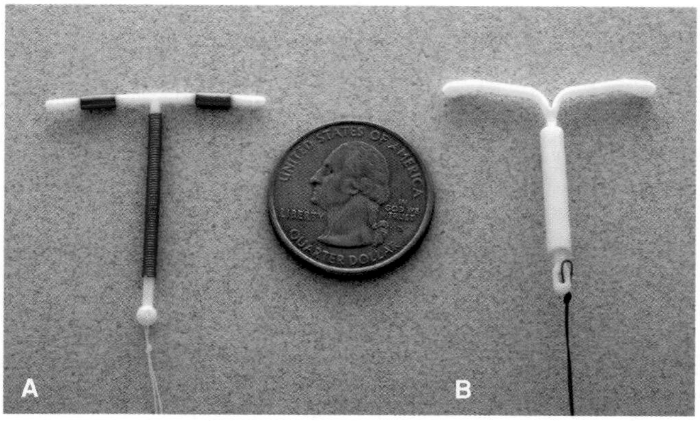

FIGURE 38-1 Intrauterine devices (IUDs). **A.** *ParaGard T 380A* copper IUD. **B.** *Mirena* levonorgestrel-releasing intrauterine system.

blue, the strings are now white. It is currently approved for 10 years of use following insertion (Teva Women's Health, 2011).

In addition to these three currently marketed, women may retain discontinued brands of IUD. A *Lippes Loop* has two "S" shapes stacked one on the other. The *Dalkon Shield* has a crab form, whereas a *Copper 7* mirrors that number. *Progestasert* is an early T-shaped progestin-releasing IUD. Last, various metal-eluting ring-shaped devices are common in Asia.

Contraceptive Action

All these IUDs are effective. Failure rates are well below 1 percent and similar overall to those of tubal sterilization (American College of Obstetricians and Gynecologists, 2013a; Thonneau, 2008; Trussell, 2011b). Their mechanisms have not been precisely defined, but prevention of fertilization is now favored. Within the uterus, an intense local endometrial inflammatory response is induced, especially by copper-containing devices. Cellular and humoral components of this inflammation are expressed in endometrial tissue and in fluid filling the uterine cavity and fallopian tubes. These lead to decreased sperm and egg viability (Ortiz, 2007). Also, in the unlikely event that fertilization does occur, the same inflammatory actions are directed against the blastocyst. The endometrium is transformed into a hostile site for implantation. With the copper IUD specifically, copper levels increase in the cervical mucus of users and decrease sperm motility and viability (Jecht, 1973). With the LNG-IUS, in addition to an inflammatory reaction, long-term progestin release leads to endometrial atrophy, which hinders normal implantation. Moreover, progestins create scant viscous cervical mucus that obstructs sperm motility. The LNG-IUS may also inconsistently release sufficient progestin to inhibit ovulation, although this is a lesser effect than its local actions.

Method-Specific Adverse Effects

Several method-specific complications may follow IUD insertion and include uterine perforation, device expulsion, menstrual changes, infection, and miscarriage if pregnancy occurs. Also, in the past, IUDs were perceived to increase the risk of ectopic pregnancy. However, this has been clarified. Specifically, IUDs are so effective as contraceptives that they lower the absolute number of ectopic pregnancies by half compared with the rate in noncontracepting women (World Health Organization, 1985, 1987). But, the IUD mechanisms of action are more effective in preventing *intrauterine* implantation. Thus, if an IUD fails, a higher proportion of pregnancies are likely to be ectopic (Backman, 2004; Furlong, 2002).

Perforation

During uterine sounding or IUD insertion, the uterus may be perforated, which is identified by the tool traveling further than the expected uterine length based on initial bimanual examination. Rates approximate 1 per 1000 insertions, and risks include puerperal insertion, lactation, provider inexperience, and extremes of uterine flexion (Harrison-Woolrych, 2003). Although devices may migrate spontaneously into and through the uterine wall, most perforations occur, or at least begin, at the time of insertion.

With the more common fundal perforation, bleeding typically is minimal due to myometrial contraction around the site. If no brisk or persistent bleeding is noted from the os following instrument removal, then patient observation alone is reasonable. Rarely, lateral perforations may lead to uterine artery laceration and brisk bleeding, which may prompt laparoscopy or laparotomy for control. Following any perforation, although this is not firmly evidence-based, a single dose of broad-spectrum antibiotic may mitigate infection.

Lost Device

Expulsion of an IUD from the uterus is most common during the first month. Thus, women should be examined approximately 1 month following IUD insertion, usually after menses, to identify the tails trailing from the cervix. Following this, a woman should be instructed to palpate the strings each month after menses.

If the tail of an IUD cannot be visualized, the device may have been expelled, may have perforated the uterus, or may be malpositioned. Some have found that IUD perforation, rotation, or embedding may cause pain or bleeding (Benacerraf, 2009; Moschos, 2011). Alternatively, the device may be normally positioned with its tail folded within the endocervical canal or uterine cavity. To investigate, after excluding pregnancy, a cytological brush can be twirled within the endocervical canal to entangle the strings and bring them gently into the vagina. If unsuccessful, the uterine cavity is probed gently with a Randall stone clamp or with a specialized rod with a terminal hook to retrieve the strings.

It should never be assumed that the device has been expelled unless it was seen. Thus, if tails are not visible and the device is not felt by gentle probing of the uterine cavity, transvaginal sonography can be used to ascertain if the device is within the uterus. Although traditional sonography will document IUD position adequately in most cases, three-dimensional sonography offers improved visualization, especially with the levonorgestrel-releasing IUD (Moschos, 2011). If sonography is inconclusive or if no device is seen, then a plain radiograph of the abdominopelvis is taken. Computed tomography (CT) scanning or less commonly, magnetic resonance (MR) imaging is an alternative (Boortz, 2012). It is safe to perform MR imaging at 1.5 and 3 Tesla (T) with an IUD in place (Pasquale, 1997; Zieman, 2007).

TABLE 38-3. Contraindications and Cautions with Specific Contraceptive Methods

Condition	CHC[a]	POP	DMPA	Implants	LNG-IUS	Cu-IUD
	1 = no method restrictions **2 = method benefits outweigh risks** **3 = method risks outweigh benefits** **4 = method poses an unacceptably high health risk** **Blank space indicates method is category 1 or 2**					
Pregnancy	4	4	4	4	4	4
Component allergy	4	4	4	4	4	4
Postpartum < 21 days	4					
21–42 days	2/3[b]					
Postpregnancy infection					4	4
Smoking & age ≥ 35 yr	3/4[c]					
Active breast cancer	4	4	4	4	4	
Breast cancer disease free ≥ 5 yr	3	3	3	3	3	
Multiple cardiovascular risks	3/4[d]		3			
Well-controlled or mild CHTN	3					
Systolic BP ≥ 160 or	4		3			
Diastolic BP ≥ 100	4		3			
Vascular disease	4		3			
Complicated heart valve disease	4					
Peripartum cardiomyopathy	3/4[d]					
Acute or prior VTE	3/4[d]					
Thrombophilia	4					
Surgery with long immobilization	4					
DM > 20 yr	3/4[d]		3			
DM & end-organ disease	3/4[d]		3			
Bariatric surgery & malabsorption	3[e]	3				
Inflammatory bowel disease	2/3[d]					
Cirrhosis (severe, decompensated)	4	3	3	3	3	
Liver tumors[f]	4	3	3	3	3	
Symptomatic gallbladder disease	3					
At risk for GC/CT					3	3
Distorted uterine cavity					4	4
GTD surveillance					4	4
Ritonavir-boosted PIs	3	3				
Enzyme-inducing anticonvulsants[g]	3	3				
Lamotrigine	3					
Rifampin/rifabutin	3	3				
			Start/Continue (S/C)[h]			
Condition	**S/C**	**S/C**	**S/C**	**S/C**	**S/C**	**S/C**
Current or history of ISHD	4	2/3	3/3	2/3	2/3	
Stroke	4	2/3	3/3	2/3		
Migraine with aura	4	2/3	2/3	2/3	2/3	
Migraine, no aura, < 35 yr	2/3					
≥ 35 yr	3/4					
Unexplained vaginal bleeding[i]			3	3	4/2	4/2
Cervical cancer before treatment					4/2	4/2
Endometrial cancer					4/2	4/2
Current PID or cervicitis					4/2	4/2
Rheumatoid arthritis			2/3[j]			
Acute viral hepatitis	4/2					
AIDS not controlled on ARV					3/2	3/2
Pelvic tuberculosis					4/3	4/3

TABLE 38-3. Continued

	Start/Continue (S/C)[h]					
Condition	S/C	S/C	S/C	S/C	S/C	S/C
SLE & positive or unknown APAs	4	3	3	3	3	
SLE & severe thrombocytopenia			3			3/2
Complicated solid-organ transplantation	4				3/2	3/2

[a]Combination hormone contraception (CHC) group includes pills, vaginal ring, and patch.
[b]Associated risks that increase category score include: age ≥ 35, transfusion at delivery, BMI ≥ 30, postpartum hemorrhage, cesarean delivery, smoking, preeclampsia.
[c]Smoking ≥ 15 cigarettes/day increases risk category to 4 in this age group.
[d]Risk category score is modified by associated risk factors and disease severity.
[e]Oral agents only. Ring and patch are category 1.
[f]Benign hepatic adenoma or hepatocellular cancer.
[g]These include phenytoin, barbiturates, carbamazepine, oxcarbazepine, primidone, topiramate.
[h]In those methods under Start/Continue columns, the first US MEC number refers to whether a method may be initiated in an affected patient. For patients who initially develop the condition while using a specific method, the second number refers to risks for continuing that method.
[i]Prior to evaluation.
[j]Those on chronic corticosteroids and at risk for bone fracture.
AIDS = acquired immunodeficiency syndrome; APA = antiphospholipid antibodies; ARV = antiretroviral; BP = blood pressure; CHTN = chronic hypertension; Cu-IUD = copper intrauterine device; DM = diabetes mellitus; DMPA = depot medroxyprogesterone acetate; GC/CT = gonorrhea/chlamydial infection; GTD = gestational trophoblastic disease; ISHD = ischemic heart disease; LNG-IUS = levonorgestrel-releasing intrauterine system; PI = protease inhibitor; PID = pelvic inflammatory disease; POP = progestin-only pills; SLE = system lupus erythematosus.
Adapted from Centers for Disease Control and Prevention, 2010b, 2011, 2013.

A device may penetrate the muscular uterine wall to varying degrees. Those with a predominantly intrauterine location are typically managed by hysteroscopic IUD removal. In contrast, devices that have nearly or completely perforated through the uterine wall are more easily removed laparoscopically. Chemically inert devices usually are removed easily from the peritoneal cavity. An extrauterine copper-bearing device, however, frequently induces an intense local inflammatory reaction and adhesions. Thus, copper IUDs may be more firmly adhered. Laparotomy may be necessary, and bowel preparation is considered. Perforations of large and small bowel and bladder and bowel fistulas have been reported remote from insertion (Lyon, 2012; Mascarenhas, 2012; Zeino, 2011).

Menstrual Changes

Women who choose the copper IUD should be informed that dysmenorrhea and menorrhagia may develop. These are often treated with nonsteroidal antiinflammatory drugs (NSAIDs) (Grimes, 2006). Heavy bleeding may cause iron deficiency anemia, for which oral iron salts are given (Hassan, 1999).

With the LNG-IUS, women are counseled to expect irregular spotting for up to 6 months after placement, and thereafter to expect monthly menses to be lighter or even absent (Bayer HealthCare Pharmaceuticals, 2013a). Specifically, the Mirena device is associated with progressive amenorrhea, which is reported by 30 percent of women after 2 years and by 60 percent after 12 years (Ronnerdag, 1999). This is often associated with improved dysmenorrhea.

Infection

The device-related infection risk is increased only during the first 20 days following insertion (Farley, 1992). Of those who develop an infection during this time, most usually have an unrecognized coexistent cervical infection. Accordingly, women at risk for sexually transmitted diseases (STDs) should be screened either before or at the time of IUD insertion (Centers for Disease Control and Prevention, 2010a; Sufrin, 2012). That said, device insertion need not be delayed while awaiting *Neisseria gonorrhoeae, Chlamydia trachomatis,* or PAP screening results in asymptomatic women. If these bacteria are found and the patient is without symptoms, then the IUD may remain and treatment prescribed as detailed in Chapter 65 (p. 1269). Importantly, *routine* antimicrobial prophylaxis before insertion is not recommended (Grimes, 2001; Walsh, 1998). Moreover, the American Heart Association does not recommend infective endocarditis prophylaxis with insertion (Wilson, 2007).

After these first 3 weeks, infection risk is not increased in IUD users who would otherwise be at low risk of STDs. Correspondingly, IUDs appear to cause little, if any, increase in the risk of infertility in these low-risk patients (Hubacher, 2001). For these reasons, the American College of Obstetricians and Gynecologists (2011a, 2012a) recommends that women at low risk for STDs, including adolescents, are good candidates for IUDs (Table 38-3). The IUD is also safe and effective in HIV-infected women and may be used in others who are immunosuppressed (Centers for Disease Control and Prevention, 2012).

If infection does develop, it may take several forms and typically requires broad-spectrum antimicrobials. *Septic abortion* mandates immediate uterine evacuation in addition to antimicrobials. Pelvic inflammatory disease (PID) without abscess is treated with systemic antibiotics. There are theoretical concerns that a coexistent IUD might worsen the infection or delay resolution. Although a provider may choose to remove an IUD in this setting, some evidence also supports allowing a device to remain during treatment in those hospitalized with mild or moderate PID (Centers for Disease Control and Prevention, 2010b; Tepper, 2013). Last, *tuboovarian abscess* may develop with PID and is treated aggressively with intravenous broad-spectrum antibiotics and IUD removal.

In addition to these infections, *Actinomyces israelii* is a gram-positive, slow-growing, anaerobic indigenous vaginal bacterium that rarely causes infection with abscess formation (Persson, 1984). Some have found it more frequently in the vaginal flora or on the Pap smears of IUD users (Curtis, 1981; Fiorino, 1996). Current recommendations advise that an asymptomatic woman may retain her IUD and does not require antibiotic treatment (American College of Obstetricians and Gynecologists, 2013c; Lippes, 1999; Westhoff, 2007a). However, if signs or symptoms of infection develop in women who harbor *Actinomyces* species, then the device should be removed and antimicrobial therapy instituted. Early findings with infection include fever, weight loss, abdominal pain, and abnormal vaginal bleeding or discharge. *Actinomyces* species are sensitive to antimicrobials with gram-positive coverage, notably the penicillins.

Pregnancy with an IUD

For women who become pregnant while using an IUD, ectopic pregnancy should be excluded (Chap. 19, p. 379). With intrauterine pregnancy, until approximately 14 weeks' gestation, the tail may be visible through the cervix, and if seen, it should be grasped and the IUD removed by gentle outward traction. This action reduces complications such as subsequent abortion, chorioamnionitis, and preterm birth (Brahmi, 2012; Kim, 2010). Tatum and coworkers (1976) reported an abortion rate of 54 percent with the device left in place compared with a rate of 25 percent if it was promptly removed.

If the tail is not visible, attempts to locate and remove the device may result in abortion. However, some practitioners have successfully used sonography to assist in device removal in cases without visible strings (Schiesser, 2004). After fetal viability is reached, it is unclear whether it is better to remove an IUD whose string is visible and accessible or to leave it in place. There is no evidence that fetal malformations are increased with a device in place (Tatum, 1976).

Second-trimester miscarriage with an IUD in place is more likely to be infected (Vessey, 1974). Sepsis may be fulminant and fatal. Pregnant women with a device in utero who demonstrate any evidence of pelvic infection are treated with intensive antimicrobial therapy and prompt uterine evacuation. Because of these risks, a woman should be given the option of early pregnancy termination if the device cannot be removed early in pregnancy. Last, in women who give birth with a device in place, appropriate steps should be taken at delivery to identify and remove the IUD.

Insertion

Timing

Immediately following miscarriage, surgical abortion, or delivery, an IUD may be inserted in the absence of infection. Also, Shimoni and colleagues (2011) describe "immediate" insertion 1 week after medical abortion. The risk of IUD expulsion is slightly higher if it is placed immediately following any of these recent pregnancies. That said, the advantages of preventing future unplanned pregnancies appear to outweigh this (Bednarek, 2011; Chen, 2010; Grimes, 2010a; Steenland, 2011).

Insertion techniques depend on uterine size. After first-trimester evacuation, the IUD can be placed using the manufacturer's standard instructions. If the uterine cavity is larger, the IUD can be placed using ring forceps with sonographic guidance (Stuart, 2012). Immediately following vaginal or cesarean delivery, an IUD can be placed by hand or with an instrument (Grimes, 2010b). To reduce expulsion rates and to minimize the perforation risk, some may choose to wait for complete involution—at least 6 weeks after delivery. Women delivered at Parkland Hospital are seen 3 weeks postpartum, and IUDs are inserted 6 weeks postpartum or sooner if involution is complete.

For placement not related to pregnancy, insertion near the end of normal menstruation, when the cervix is usually softer and somewhat more dilated, may be easier and at the same time may exclude early pregnancy. But, insertion is not limited to this time. For the woman who is sure she is not pregnant and does not want to be pregnant, insertion is done at any time.

Technique

Before insertion, several procedural steps are carried out. Any contraindications are identified. If there are none, the woman is counseled and written consent obtained. An oral NSAID, with or without codeine, can be used to allay cramps (Karabayirli, 2012). Strong evidence does not support an advantage to supplemental misoprostol, intrauterine or cervical canal instillation of lidocaine, or paracervical blockade to lessen insertional pain (McNicholas, 2012; Nelson, 2013; Swenson, 2012). Bimanual pelvic examination is performed to identify uterine position and size. Abnormalities are evaluated, as they may contraindicate insertion. Mucopurulent cervicitis or significant vaginitis should be appropriately treated and resolved before IUD insertion.

The cervical surface is cleansed with an antiseptic solution, and sterile instruments and a sterile IUD should be used. A tenaculum is placed on the cervical lip, and the canal and uterine cavity are straightened by applying gentle traction. The uterus is then sounded to identify the direction and depth of the uterine cavity. Specific steps of ParaGard and Mirena insertion are shown in Figures 38-2 and 38-3 and outlined in their respective package inserts.

Following insertion, only the threads should be visible trailing from the cervix. These are trimmed to allow 3 to 4 cm to protrude into the vagina, and their length is recorded. If there is suspicion that the device is not positioned correctly, then placement should be confirmed, using sonography if necessary.

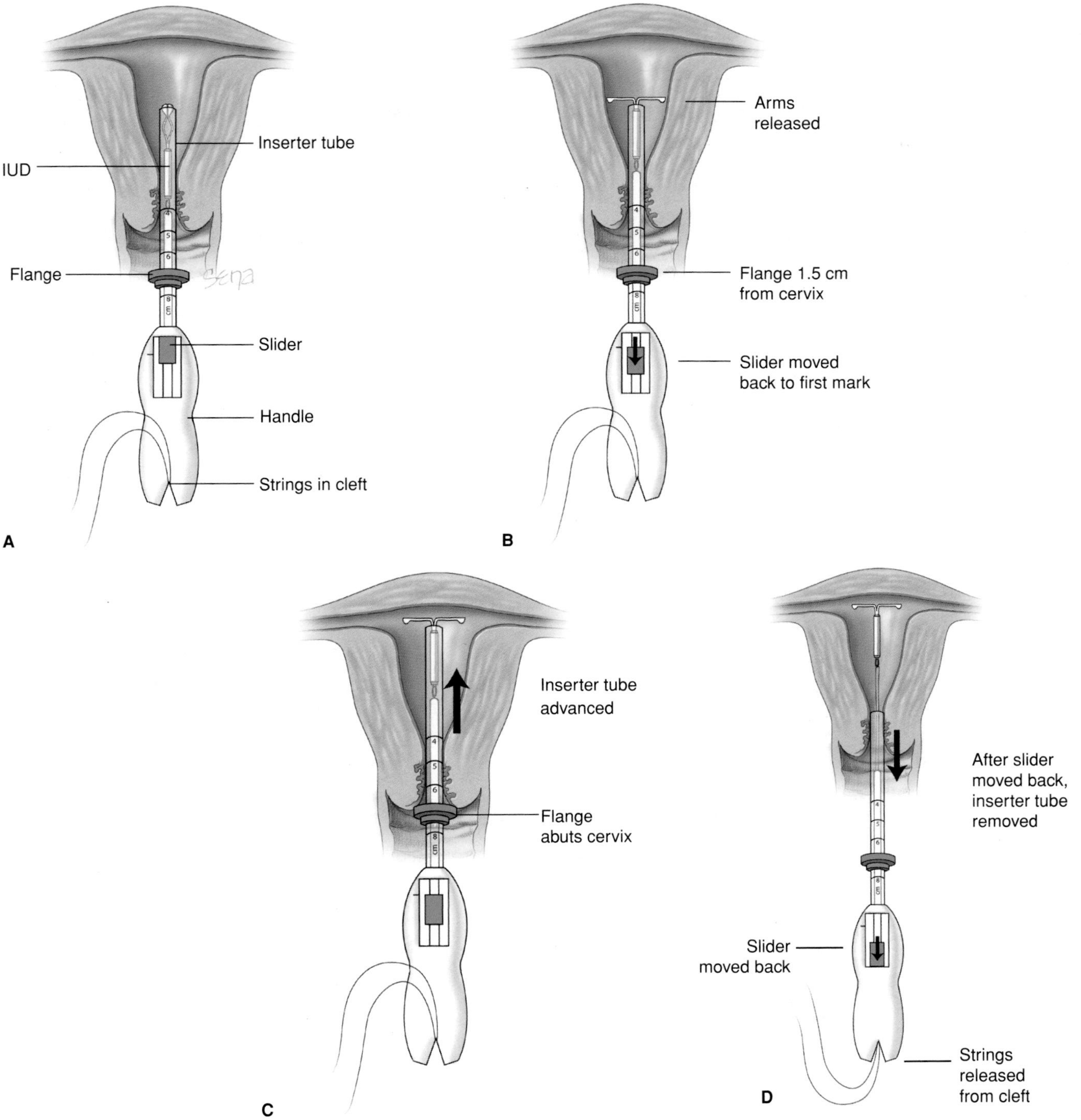

FIGURE 38-2 Insertion of the *Mirena* intrauterine system. Initially, threads from behind the slider are first released to hang freely. The slider found on the handle should be positioned at the top of the handle nearest the device. The IUD arms are oriented horizontally. A flange on the outside of the inserter tube is positioned from the IUD tip to reflect the depth found with uterine sounding. **A.** As both free threads are pulled, the *Mirena* IUD is drawn into the inserter tube. The threads are then tightly fixed from below into the handle's cleft. In these depictions, the inserter tube has been foreshortened. The inserter tube is gently inserted into the uterus until the flange lies 1.5 to 2 cm from the external cervical os to allow the arms to open. **B.** While holding the inserter steady, the IUD arms are released by pulling the slider back to reach the raised horizontal mark on the handle, but no further. **C.** The inserter is then gently guided into the uterine cavity until its flange touches the cervix. **D.** The device is released by holding the inserter firmly in position and pulling the slider down all the way. The threads will be released automatically from the cleft. The inserter may then be removed, and IUD strings trimmed.

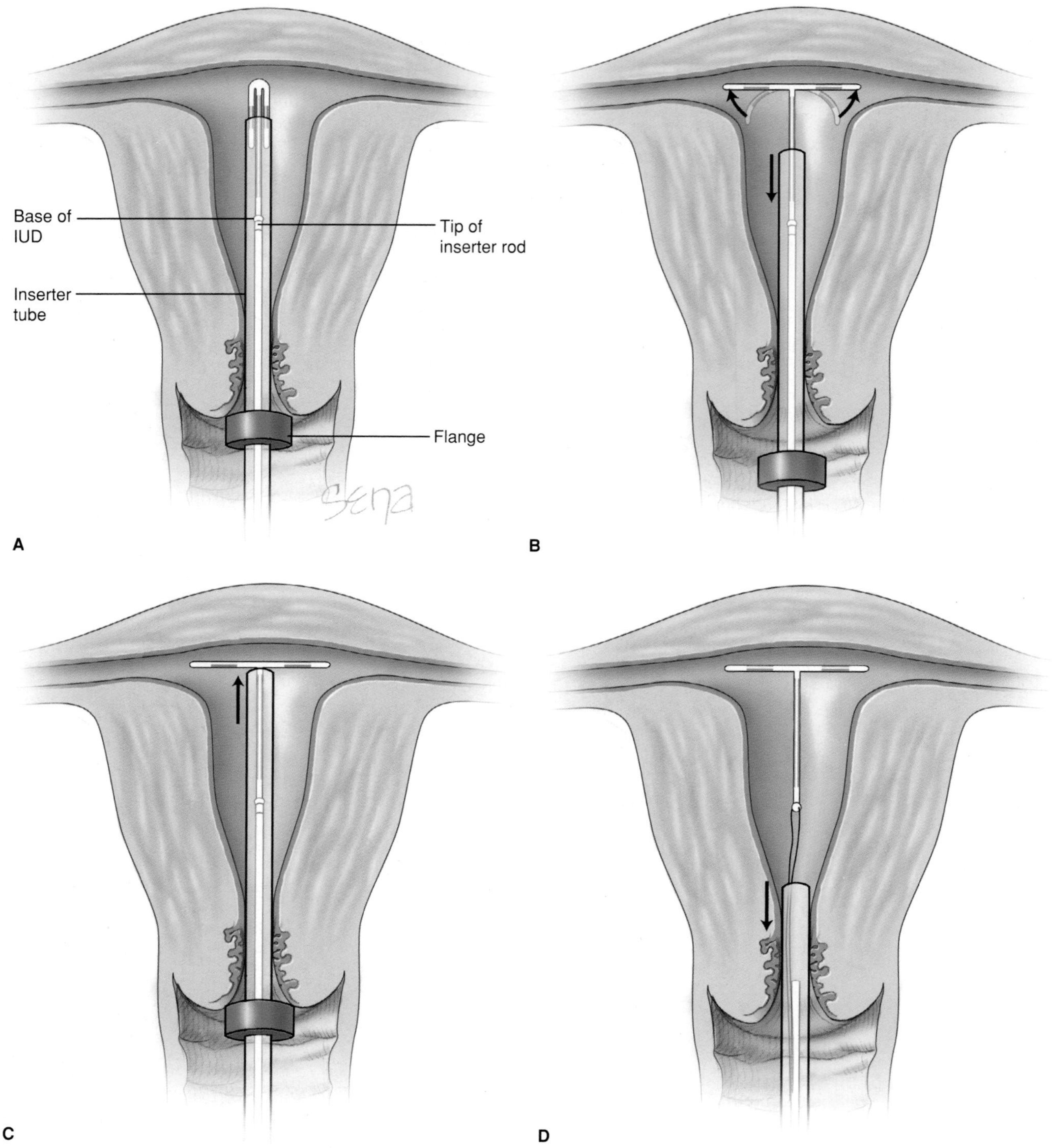

FIGURE 38-3 Insertion of *ParaGard T 380A*. The uterus is sounded, and the IUD is loaded into its inserter tube not more than 5 minutes before insertion. A blue plastic flange on the outside of the inserter tube is positioned from the IUD tip to reflect uterine depth. The IUD arms should lie in the same plane as the flat portion of the oblong blue flange. **A.** The inserter tube, with the IUD loaded, is passed into the endometrial cavity. A long, solid, white inserter rod abuts the base of the IUD. When the blue flange contacts the cervix, insertion stops. **B.** To release the IUD arms, the solid white rod within the inserter tube is held steady, while the inserter tube is withdrawn no more than 1 cm. **C.** The inserter tube, not the inserter rod, is then carefully moved upward toward the top of the uterus until slight resistance is felt. At no time during insertion is the inserter rod advanced forward. **D.** First, the solid white rod and then the inserter tube are withdrawn individually. At completion, only the threads should be visible protruding from the cervix. These are trimmed to allow 3 to 4 cm to extend into the vagina.

If the IUD is not positioned completely within the uterus, it is removed and replaced with a new device. An expelled or partially expelled device should not be reinserted.

LONG-ACTING REVERSIBLE CONTRACEPTION: PROGESTIN IMPLANTS

Etonogestrel Implant

Contraception can be provided by thin, pliable progestin-containing cylinders that are implanted subdermally and release hormone over many years. One of these, *Implanon* is a single-rod implant with 68 mg of etonogestrel covered by an ethylene vinyl acetate copolymer cover. The implant is placed subdermally on the medial surface of the upper arm 8 to 10 cm from the elbow in the biceps groove and is aligned with the long axis of the arm. It may be used as contraception for 3 years and then replaced at the same site or in the opposite arm (Merck, 2012a).

Implanon is not radiopaque, and a misplaced implant may be identified with sonography using a 10- to 15-MHz linear array transducer (Shulman, 2006). In some cases, MR imaging may be required if supplemental information is needed despite sonography (Correia, 2012). To improve radiologic detection, the manufacturer developed *Nexplanon*, which is similarly shaped and pharmacologically identical to *Implanon* but is radiopaque. Additionally, the *Nexplanon* inserter device is designed to assist with subdermal placement and avert deeper insertions. Both implants are highly effective, and the mechanism of action for progestin-only products is described on page 704 (Croxatto, 1998; Mommers, 2012). Although still approved by the Food and Drug Administration (FDA), *Implanon* is no longer distributed by the manufacturer.

Levonorgestrel Implants

The first progestin implants contained levonorgestrel, and systems are still available outside the United States. *Jadelle*, originally named *Norplant-2*, provides levonorgestrel and contraception for 5 years through two subdermally implanted Silastic rods. After this time, rods may be removed and if desired, new rods inserted at the same site (Bayer Schering Pharma Oy, 2010). *Jadelle* is approved by the FDA, however, it is not marketed or distributed in the United States (Population Council, 2013). Sino-implant II is a two-rod implant with the same amount (150 mg) of levonorgestrel and same mechanism of action as *Jadelle* but provides 4 years of contraception (Shanghai Dahua Pharmaceutical, 2012). Sino-implant II is manufactured in China and approved for use by several countries in Asia and Africa.

Both implant systems are highly effective, and the mechanism of action for progestin-only products is described on page 704. Like the etonogestrel implant, these systems are placed subdermally on the inner arm approximately 8 cm from the elbow and have similar removal steps. Implants vary regarding their insertion technique, and manufacturer instructions should be consulted.

The forerunner of these implants was the *Norplant System*, which provided levonorgestrel in six Silastic rods implanted subdermally. The manufacturer stopped distributing the system in 2002.

Method-Specific Adverse Effects

Risks that are specific to implants stem mainly from malpositioning. First, branches of the medial antebrachial cutaneous nerve can be injured if the implant or insertion needle is placed too deeply or if exploration for a lost implant is aggressive. Clinically, numbness and paresthesia over the anteromedial aspect of the forearm are noted (Brown, 2012; Wechselberger, 2006). Second, nonpalpable devices are not uncommon and may require radiological imaging for localization as described earlier. If imaging fails to locate an *Implanon* or *Nexplanon* implant, etonogestrel blood level determination can be used to verify that the implant is in situ.

Insertion

Timing

For those not currently using hormonal contraception, the etonogestrel implant is ideally inserted within 5 days of menses onset. If inserted later in the cycle, then alternative contraception is recommended for 7 days following placement. With levonorgestrel-releasing implants, contraception is established within 24 hours if inserted within the first 7 days of the menstrual cycle (Sivin, 1997; Steiner, 2010). For transitioning methods, an implant is placed on the day of the first placebo COC pill; on the day that the next DMPA injection would be due; or within 24 hours of taking the last POP (Merck, 2012a). Related to pregnancy, an implant may be inserted before discharge following delivery, miscarriage, or abortion.

Nexplanon Insertion Technique

With the patient lying down, her nondominant arm, forearm, and hand are outstretched on the bed with the inner aspects of each exposed upward, and the elbow is flexed. The insertion site is marked with a sterile pen 8 to 10 cm proximal to the medial condyle of the humerus. A second mark is placed 4 centimeters proximally and delineates the final path of the implant. The Nexplanon is inserted using sterile technique. The area is cleaned aseptically, and a 1-percent lidocaine anesthetic track is injected beneath the skin along the planned insertion path. The implant is then placed as shown in Figure 38-4. After placement, both patient and provider should palpate and identify both ends of the 4-cm implant. To minimize bruising at the site, a pressure bandage is created around the arm and is removed the following day.

With sterile implant removal, the proximal end of the implant is depressed with a finger to allow the distal end to bulge toward the skin. After anesthetizing the skin over this bulge, the skin is incised 2 mm toward the elbow along the long axis of the arm. The proximal butt of the implant is then pushed toward this incision. Once visible, the distal implant is grasped with a hemostat and removed. If present, superficial

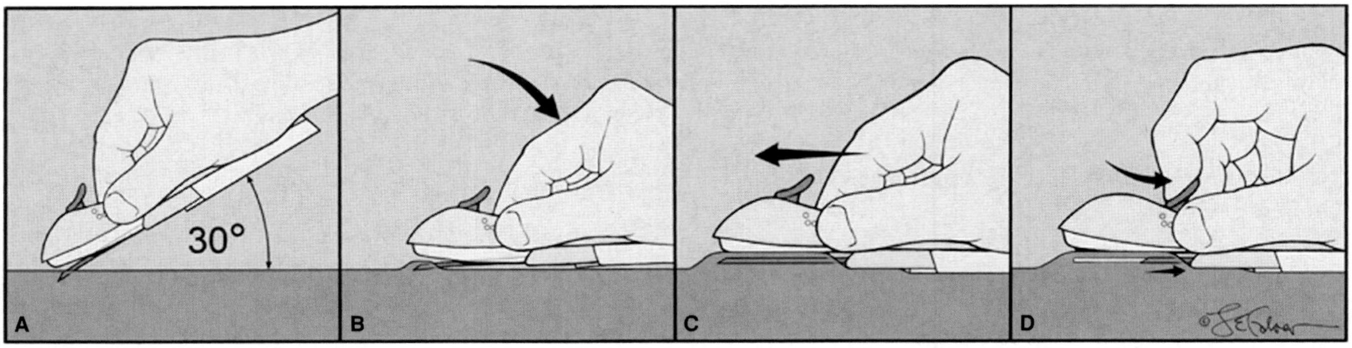

FIGURE 38-4 Nexplanon insertion. A sterile pen marks the insertion site, which is 8 to 10 cm proximal to the medial humeral condyle. A second mark is placed 4 cm proximally along the arm's long axis. The area is cleaned aseptically, and a 1-percent lidocaine anesthetic track is injected along the planned insertion path. **A.** The insertion device is grasped at its gripper bubbles found on either side, and the needle cap is removed outward. The device can be seen within the needle bore. The needle bevel then pierces the skin at a 30-degree angle. **B.** Once the complete bevel is subcutaneous, the needle is quickly angled downward to lie horizontally. **C.** Importantly, the skin is tented upward by the needle as the needle is slowly advanced horizontally and subdermally. **D.** Once the needle is completely inserted, the lever on the top of the device is pulled backward toward the operator. This retracts the needle and thereby deposits the implant. The device is then lifted away from the skin. After placement, both patient and operator should palpate the 4-cm implant.

adhesions surrounding an implant may be dissected away with hemostat tips placed into the incision.

PROGESTIN-ONLY CONTRACEPTIVE GROUP

Actions and Side Effects

Progestin-only contraceptives include the implants just described, pills, and injectables. As their primary contraceptive action, these progestins suppress luteinizing hormone (LH) and in turn block ovulation. As other effects, cervical mucus is thickened to retard sperm passage, and atrophy renders the endometrium unfavorable for implantation. Fertility is restored rapidly following cessation of progestin-only contraception, with the exception of DMPA as described on page 711 (Mansour, 2011).

For all progestin-only methods, irregular uterine bleeding is a distinct disadvantage. It may manifest as metrorrhagia or menorrhagia and is the most frequently reported adverse event leading to method discontinuation. Often, counseling and reassurance regarding this effect is sufficient. Particularly troublesome bleeding may be improved by one to two cycles of COCs, by a 1- to 3-week course of estrogen alone, or by a short course of NSAIDs combined with the established method. Fortunately, with prolonged use, progestins induce endometrial atrophy, which leads to sustained amenorrhea. And, for the well-counseled patient, this is often an advantage.

Most progestin-only contraceptive methods do not significantly affect lipid metabolism, glucose levels, hemostatic factors, liver function, thyroid function, and blood pressure (Dorflinger, 2002). Moreover, these have not been shown to increase the risk for thromboembolism, stroke, or cardiovascular disease (Mantha, 2012; World Health Organization, 1998). However, as described on page 711, the increased low-density lipoprotein (LDL) cholesterol and decreased high-density lipoprotein (HDL) cholesterol levels seen with DMPA may be less desirable if there are cardiac or vascular risks.

Progestin-only methods do not impair milk production and are an excellent choice for lactating women. There are no increased risks of genital tract or breast neoplasia (Wilailak, 2012; World Health Organization, 1991a,b, 1992). Weight gain and bone mineral density loss are not prominent side effects of this contraceptive group, except for DMPA, as noted on page 711 (Funk, 2005; Lopez, 2011). Functional ovarian cysts develop with a greater frequency in women using progestin-only agents, although they do not usually necessitate intervention (Brache, 2002; European Society of Human Reproduction and Embryology, 2001). Last, an association between depression and DMPA or POPs is unclear (Civic, 2000; Svendal, 2012; Westhoff, 1995). Women with depression may be prescribed these methods, but surveillance following initiation is reasonable.

Contraindications to Progestin-Only Contraceptives

These methods are ideal for most women, but contraindications and cautions are associated with a few conditions. Current breast cancer and pregnancy are the only two absolute contraindications. However, conditions for which limited and cautious use should be considered are listed in Table 38-3.

There are a few instances in which manufacturer restrictions differ from the US MEC. First, manufacturer prescribing information lists thrombosis or thromboembolic disorders as contraindications (Merck, 2012a; Pfizer, 2012). However, for individuals with these disorders, US MEC considers progestin-containing methods category 2. Second, for many progestin products, manufacturers note prior ectopic pregnancy as a contraindication. This is secondary to progesterone's effect to slow fallopian tube motility and thereby delay fertilized egg transport to the endometrial cavity. But again, US MEC considers progestin injectables and implants category 1, and progestin-only pills are category 2 for those with prior ectopic pregnancy.

VERY EFFECTIVE CONTRACEPTION: HORMONAL CONTRACEPTIVES

These currently are available in forms that contain both estrogen and progestin or contain only progestin. Progestin-only injectables and pills are considered very effective, yet second-tier agents, due to the need for increased patient compliance. Similarly, products containing both estrogen and progestin, often termed combination hormonal contraception (CHC), are considered in this tier. These may be supplied as pills, transvaginal rings, or transdermal patches.

Combination Hormonal Contraceptives Mechanism of Action

The contraceptive actions of CHCs are multiple, but the most important effect is suppression of hypothalamic gonadotropin-releasing factors. This in turn blocks pituitary secretion of follicle-stimulating hormone (FSH) and LH to inhibit ovulation. The progestin component provides ovulation prevention by suppressing LH; they thicken cervical mucus and thereby retard sperm passage; and they render the endometrium unfavorable for implantation. Estrogen blocks ovulation by suppressing FSH release. It also stabilizes the endometrium, which prevents intermenstrual bleeding—also known as *breakthrough bleeding*. The net effect is an extremely effective yet highly reversible method (Mansour, 2011).

Combination Oral Contraceptive Pills

Composition

Combination oral contraceptive pills are the most frequently used birth control method in the United States. In a 2006 to 2010 survey, 17 percent of US women were using these (Jones, 2012). COCs are marketed in an almost bewildering variety (Table 38-4). Most are also available as generics, and the FDA (2013) confirms the bioequivalence of COC generics. The American College of Obstetricians and Gynecologists (2013b) supports the use of either branded or generic preparations.

Pharmacologically, ethinyl estradiol is the most common estrogen present in COC formulations in the United States. Less frequently, mestranol or estradiol valerate is used. Unwanted effects most often attributed to the estrogen component include breast tenderness, fluid retention, weight gain, nausea, and headache.

COCs also contain one of several progestins that are structurally related to progesterone, testosterone, or spironolactone. Thus, these progestins bind variably to progesterone, androgen, estrogen, glucocorticoid, and mineralocorticoid receptors. These affinities explain many pill-related side effects and are often used to compare one progestin with another.

Most progestins used in COCs are related to testosterone and may impart androgenic side affects such as acne and adverse HDL and LDL levels. To avoid these effects, progestins more structurally similar to the progestone molecule have been developed. Medroxyprogesterone acetate is one example, but it is mainly used in a progestin-only injectable form. Another, nomegestrol acetate, is used in a COC approved outside the United States. Despite these pharmacological differences, the true advantage of one progestin over another is less apparent clinically (Lawrie, 2011; Moreau, 2007).

Another progestin, drospirenone, is structurally similar to spironolactone. The doses used in currently marketed COCs have effects similar to 25 mg of this diuretic hormone (Seeger, 2007). Drospirenone displays antiandrogenic activity, provides an antialdosterone action to minimize water retention, and has antimineralocorticoid properties that may, in theory, cause potassium retention and hyperkalemia (Krattenmacher, 2000). Thus, it is avoided in women with renal or adrenal insufficiency or with hepatic dysfunction. Moreover, serum potassium level monitoring is recommended in the first month for patients chronically treated concomitantly with any drug associated with potassium retention. These include NSAIDs, angiotensin-converting enzyme (ACE) inhibitors, angiotensin II antagonists, heparin, aldosterone antagonists, and potassium-sparing diuretics (Bayer HealthCare Pharmaceuticals, 2012).

Since the development of COCs, their estrogen and progestin content has dropped remarkably to minimize adverse effects. Currently, the lowest acceptable dose is limited by the ability to prevent pregnancy and to avoid unacceptable breakthrough bleeding. Thus, the daily estrogen content varies from 10 to 50 μg of ethinyl estradiol, and most contain 35 μg or less.

With COCs termed *monophasic pills*, the progestin dose remains constant throughout the cycle. In others, the dose frequently is varied, and terms *biphasic, triphasic,* or *quadriphasic pill* are used depending on the number of dose changes within the cycle. In some formulations, the estrogen dose also varies. In general, phasic pills were developed to reduce the total progestin content per cycle without sacrificing contraceptive efficacy or cycle control. The theoretical advantage of a lower total progesterone dose per cycle has not been borne out clinically (Moreau, 2007). Cycle control also appears to be comparable among mono- through triphasic pills (van Vliet, 2006, 2011a,b).

Administration

Hormones are taken daily for a specified time (21 to 81 days) and then replaced by placebo for a specified time (4 to 7 days), which is called the "pill-free interval." During these pill-free days, withdrawal bleeding is expected.

With the trend to lower estrogen doses to minimize side effects, there is concern for follicular development and ovulation. To counter this, the active-pill duration in some formulations is extended to 24 days. And, these 24/4 regimens do appear to reduce ovulation and breakthrough bleeding rates (Fels, 2013).

Alternatively, longer durations of active hormone, designed to minimize the number of withdrawal episodes, have been introduced (Edelman, 2006). These extended-cycle products produce a 13-week cycle, that is, 12 weeks of hormone use, followed by a week for withdrawal menses. The product *Amethyst* provides continuous active hormone pills for 365 days each year. Such extended or continuous regimens may be especially suited for women with significant menstrual symptoms.

TABLE 38-4. Combination Oral Contraceptives Formulations

Product Name	Estrogen	µg (days)[a]	Progestin	mg (days)
Monophasic Preparations				
20–25 µg estrogen				
Yaz, Loryna	EE	20 (24)	Drospirenone	3.00 (24)
Beyaz[b]	EE	20 (24)	Drospirenone	3.00 (24)
Aviane, Falmina, Lessina, Orsythia	EE	20	Levonorgestrel	0.10
Loestrin 1/20, Junel 1/20, Microgestin 1/20	EE	20	Norethindrone acetate	1.00
Loestrin Fe 1/20[c], Gildess Fe 1/20[c], Junel Fe 1/20[c], Microgestin Fe 1/20[c]	EE	20	Norethindrone acetate	1.00
Loestrin 24 Fe[c]	EE	20 (24)	Norethindrone acetate	1.00 (24)
30–35 µg estrogen				
Desogen, Ortho-Cept, Emoquette	EE	30	Desogestrel	0.15
Yasmin, Syeda	EE	30	Drospirenone	3.00
Safyral[b]	EE	30	Drospirenone	3.00
Kelnor, Zovia 1/35	EE	35	Ethynodiol diacetate	1.00
Nordette, Altavera, Introvale, Kurvelo, Levora, Marlissa, Portia	EE	30	Levonorgestrel	0.15
Lo/Ovral, Cryselle, Low-Ogestrel, Elinest	EE	30	Norgestrel	0.30
Ovcon-35, Balziva, Briellyn, Philith, Gildagia	EE	35	Norethindrone	0.40
Femcon Fe[c]	EE	35	Norethindrone	0.40
Brevicon, Modicon, Nortrel 0.5/35, Wera	EE	35	Norethindrone	0.50
Ortho-Novum 1/35, Norinyl 1+35, Nortrel 1/35, Norethin 1/35, Cyclafem 1/35, Alyacen 1/35, Dasetta 1/35	EE	35	Norethindrone	1.00
Loestrin 1.5/30, Junel 1.5/30, Microgestin 1.5/30	EE	30	Norethindrone acetate	1.50
Loestrin Fe 1.5/30[c], Junel Fe 1.5/30[c], Microgestin Fe 1.5/30[c] Gildess Fe 1.5/30[c]	EE	30	Norethindrone acetate	1.50
Ortho-Cyclen, Sprintec, Previfem, Estarylla, Mono-Linyah	EE	35	Norgestimate	0.25
50 µg estrogen				
Ogestrel	EE	50	Norgestrel	0.50
Zovia 1/50	EE	50	Ethynodiol diacetate	1.00
Norinyl 1+50	Mes	50	Norethindrone	1.00
Ovcon 50	EE	50	Norethindrone	1.00
Multiphasic Preparations				
10 µg estrogen				
Lo Loestrin Fe[c]	EE	10 (24) 10 (2)	Norethindrone acetate	1.00 (24)
20 µg estrogen				
Mircette, Kariva, Viorele	EE	20 (21) 0 (2) 10 (5)	Desogestrel	0.15
25 µg estrogen				
Ortho Tri-Cyclen Lo, Tri Lo Sprintec	EE	25	Norgestimate	0.18 (7) 0.215 (7) 0.25 (7)
Cyclessa, Velivet	EE	25	Desogestrel	0.1 (7) 0.125 (7) 0.15 (7)
30–35 µg estrogen				
Ortho Tri-Cyclen, Tri-Sprintec, Tri-Previfem, Tri-Linyah, Tri-Estarylla	EE	35	Norgestimate	0.18 (7) 0.215 (7) 0.25 (7)
Trivora, Enpresse, Levonest, Myzilra	EE	30 (6) 40 (5) 30 (10)	Levonorgestrel	0.05 (6) 0.075 (5) 0.125 (10)

TABLE 38-4. Continued

Product Name	Estrogen	µg (days)[a]	Progestin	mg (days)
Estrostep[c], Tri-Legest[c]	EE	20 (5) 30 (7) 35 (9)	Norethindrone acetate	1.00
Ortho-Novum 7/7/7, Alyacen 7/7/7, Cyclafem 7/7/7, Dasetta 7/7/7, Nortrel 7/7/7	EE	35	Norethindrone	0.50 (7) 0.75 (7) 1.0 (7)
Tri-Norinyl, Aranelle	EE	35	Norethindrone	0.50 (7) 1.00 (9) 0.50 (5)
Natazia	EV	3 (2) 2 (5) 2 (17) 1 (2)	Dienogest	– 2.00 (5) 3.00 (17) –
Progestin-Only Preparations				
Micronor, Nor-QD, Errin, Camila, Heather	None		Norethindrone	0.35 (c)
Extended-Cycle Preparations				
20 µg estrogen				
LoSeasonique[d]	EE	20 (84) 10 (7)	Levonorgestrel	0.10 (84)
30 µg estrogen				
Seasonale[d], Quasense[d]	EE	30 (84)	Levonorgestrel	0.15 (84)
Seasonique[e]	EE	30 (84) 10 (7)	Levonorgestrel	0.15 (84)
Continuous Preparation				
Amethyst[f]	EE	20 (28)	Levonorgestrel	0.09

EE = ethinyl estradiol; EV = estradiol valerate; LC = levomefolate calcium; Mes = mestranol.
[a]Administered for 21 days, variations listed in parentheses.
[b]0.451 mg of levomefolate calcium, which is a form of folic acid, is found in each pill.
[c]Contains or is available in formulas that contain 75-mg doses of ferrous fumarate within the placebo pills.
[d]12 weeks of active pills, 1 week of inert pills.
[e]12 weeks of active pills, 1 week of ethinyl estradiol only.
[f]One pill every day, 365 days each year.
Compiled from US Food and Drug Administration, 2013.

For general initiation, women should ideally begin COCs on the first day of a menstrual cycle. In such cases, a supplementary contraceptive method is unnecessary. With the more traditional "Sunday start," women begin pills on the first Sunday that follows menses onset, and an additional method is needed for 1 week to prevent conception. If menses begin on a Sunday, then pills are begun that day and no supplementary method is required. Alternatively, with the "Quick Start" method, COCs are started on any day, commonly the day prescribed, regardless of cycle timing. An additional method is used during the first week. This latter approach improves short-term compliance (Westhoff, 2002, 2007b). If the woman is already pregnant during Quick Start initiation, COCs are not teratogenic (Lammer, 1986; Rothman, 1978; Savolainen, 1981). Similarly, same-day initiation can be implemented with the contraceptive vaginal ring or patch (Murthy, 2005; Schafer, 2006).

For maximum efficiency, pills should be taken at the same time each day. If one dose is missed, contraception is likely not diminished with higher-dose monophasic COCs. Doubling the next dose will minimize breakthrough bleeding and maintain the pill schedule. If several doses are missed or if lower-dose pills are used, the pill may be stopped, and an effective barrier technique used until menses. The pill may then be restarted. Alternatively, a new pack can be started immediately following identification of missed pills, and a barrier method used for 1 week. If there is no withdrawal bleeding, the woman should continue her pills but seek attention to exclude pregnancy.

With initiation of COCs, spotting or bleeding is common. It does not reflect contraceptive failure and typically resolves within one to three cycles. If unscheduled bleeding persists, those with bleeding during the first part of a pill pack may benefit from an increase in the pill's estrogen dose, whereas those with bleeding during the second part may improve with a higher progestin dose (Nelson, 2011).

Method-Specific Effects

Altered Drug Efficacy

Combination oral contraceptives interfere with the actions of some drugs. In such cases, doses can be adjusted as shown in Table 38-5. Conversely, some drugs decrease the COC effectiveness. Three groups are notable: the antitubercular drugs rifampin and rifabutin; efavirenz and ritonavir-boosted protease inhibitors, which are used to treat HIV infection; and enzyme-inducing anticonvulsants, which include phenytoin (Dilantin), carbamazepine (Tegretol), oxcarbazepine (Trileptal), barbiturates, primidone (Mysoline), and topiramate (Topamax) (Gaffield, 2011; Panel on Antiretroviral Guidelines for Adults and Adolescents, 2013). With these, a method other than COCs is preferable. However, if a COC is selected for concurrent use with an agent from these three groups, then a preparation containing a minimum of 30 μg ethinyl estradiol should be chosen.

In obese women, COCs are highly effective (Lopez, 2010). That said, some but not all studies point to a potential increased pregnancy risk with COC use due to lowered hormone bioavailability (Brunner, 2005; Holt, 2002, 2005; Westhoff, 2010). With the transdermal patch method, however, there is stronger evidence that obesity may alter pharmacokinetics and lower efficacy (p. 701).

Metabolic Changes

Although their effects on carbohydrate metabolism are considered clinically insignificant, COCs do have notable effects on lipid and protein synthesis. In general, COCs increase serum levels of triglycerides and total cholesterol. Estrogen decreases LDL cholesterol concentrations but increases HDL and very-low density (VLDL) cholesterol levels. Some progestins cause the reverse. Despite this, the clinical consequences of these perturbations have almost certainly been overstated. Oral contraceptives are not atherogenic, and their impact on lipids is inconsequential for most women (Wallach, 2000). But in women with dyslipidemias, the American College of Obstetricians and Gynecologists

TABLE 38-5. Drugs Whose Effectiveness Is Influenced by Combination Oral Contraceptives

Interacting Drug	Documentation	Management
Analgesics		
Acetaminophen	Adequate	Larger doses of analgesic may be required
Aspirin	Probable	Larger doses of analgesic may be required
Meperidine	Suspected	Smaller doses of analgesic may be required
Morphine	Probable	Larger doses of analgesic may be required
Anticoagulants		
Dicumarol, warfarin	Controversial	
Anticonvulsant		
Lamotrigine monotherapy	Adequate	Avoid
Antidepressants		
Imipramine	Suspected	Decrease dosage about a third
Tranquilizers		
Diazepam, alprazolam	Suspected	Decrease dose
Temazepam	Possible	May need to increase dose
Other benzodiazepines	Suspected	Observe for increased effect
Anti-inflammatories		
Corticosteroids	Adequate	Watch for potentiation of effects, decrease dose accordingly
Bronchodilators		
Aminophylline, caffeine, theophylline	Adequate	Reduce starting dose by a third
Antihypertensives		
Cyclopenthiazide	Adequate	Increase dose
Metoprolol	Suspected	May need to lower dose
Antibiotics		
Troleandomycin	Suspected liver damage	Avoid
Cyclosporine	Possible	May use smaller dose

Modified from Gaffield, 2011; Wallach, 2000.

(2013e) recommends assessment of lipid levels following COC initiation. Moreover, for women with LDL cholesterol levels > 160 mg/dL or for those with multiple additional risk factors for cardiovascular disease, alternative contraceptive methods are recommended.

With COCs, protein metabolism is affected, and estrogens prompt increased hepatic production of various globulins. First, fibrinogen and many of the clotting factor levels are increased in direct proportion to estrogen dose and may lead to thrombosis (Comp, 1996). Angiotensinogen production is also augmented by COCs, and its conversion by renin to angiotensin I may be associated with "pill-induced hypertension" discussed subsequently. Last, COCs increase sex-hormone binding globulin (SHBG) levels, which decrease bioavailable testosterone concentrations and improve androgenic side effects.

Regarding carbohydrate metabolism, there are fortunately limited effects with current low-dose formulations in women who do not have diabetes (Lopez, 2012a). And, the risk of developing diabetes is not increased (Kim, 2002). Moreover, COCs may be used in nonsmoking, diabetic women younger than 35 years who have no associated vascular disease (American College of Obstetricians and Gynecologists, 2013e). Last, studies have not supported a connection between COCs and weight gain (Gallo, 2011).

Other metabolic changes, often qualitatively similar to those of pregnancy, have been identified in women taking oral contraceptives. For example, total plasma thyroxine (T_4) and thyroid-binding proteins are elevated. These pregnancy-like effects should be considered when evaluating laboratory tests in women using COCs.

Cardiovascular Effects

Despite increased plasma angiotensinogen (renin substrate) levels, most women using low-dose COCs formulations rarely develop clinically significant hypertension (Chasan-Taber, 1996). However, it is common practice for patients to return 8 to 12 weeks after COC initiation for evaluation of blood pressure and other symptoms.

During initial contraception selection, a history of gestational hypertension does not preclude subsequent COC use. Also, COCs are permissible in women with well-controlled uncomplicated hypertension who are nonsmokers, otherwise healthy, and younger than 35 (American College of Obstetricians and Gynecologists, 2013e). In contrast, severe forms of hypertension, especially those with end-organ involvement, usually preclude COC use.

For women with prior stroke, COCs should not be considered due to risks for repeat events. The risk for a first stroke is substantially increased in women who have hypertension, who smoke, or who have migraine headaches with visual aura or other focal neurological changes *and* use oral contraceptives (MacClellan, 2007). However, for nonsmoking women younger than 35, the risk of ischemic and hemorrhagic strokes is extremely low, and method benefits considerably outweigh risks (World Health Organization, 1996, 1998). Moreover, because of this low risk, the American College of Obstetricians and Gynecologists (2013e) notes that COCs may be considered for women with migraines that lack focal neurological signs if they are otherwise healthy, normotensive nonsmokers younger than 35 years.

For women with prior myocardial infarction, COCs should not be considered. Also, in women with multiple cardiovascular risk factors, which include smoking, hypertension, older age, and diabetes, the risk for myocardial infarction outweighs the benefits of this method. However, for those without these risks, low-dose oral contraceptives are not associated with an increased risk of myocardial infarction (Margolis, 2007; World Health Organization, 1997).

It has long been known that the risk of deep-vein thrombosis and pulmonary embolism is increased in women who use COCs (Stadel, 1981). These clearly are estrogen-dose related, and rates have substantively decreased with lower-dose formulations containing 10 to 35 μg of ethinyl estradiol. The incidence of venous thromboembolism (VTE) with COC use is only 3 to 4 per 10,000 woman-years and is lower than the incidence of 5 to 6 per 10,000 woman-years estimated for pregnancy (Chap. 52, p. 1028) (Mishell, 2000). The enhanced risk of VTE appears to decrease rapidly once COCs are stopped. And because these complications are increased in women smokers older than 35 years, COCs are not recommended for this population (Craft, 1989).

Those most at risk for VTE include women with thrombophilias (Comp, 1996). Other clinical factors that increase the risk of VTE with COC use are hypertension, obesity, diabetes, smoking, and a sedentary lifestyle (Pomp, 2007, 2008). Moreover, COC use during the month before a major operative procedure appears to double the risk for postoperative VTE (Robinson, 1991). Thus, the American College of Obstetricians and Gynecologists (2013d) recommends balancing the risks of VTE with those of unintended pregnancy during the 4 to 6 weeks required to reverse the thrombogenic effects of COCs before surgery. In the early puerperium, VTE risks are also increased, and COCs are not recommended for women within the first 4 weeks after delivery. For all women, an increased VTE risk with drospirenone-containing COCs has been shown in two studies. Accordingly, the FDA has encouraged an assessment of benefits and VTE risks in users of these pills (Food and Drug Administration, 2011; Jick, 2011; Parkin, 2011).

Neoplasia

Fortunately, most studies indicate that overall, COCs are not associated with an increased risk of cancer (Hannaford, 2007). In fact, a protective effect against ovarian and endometrial cancer has been shown (Collaborative Group on Epidemiological Studies of Ovarian Cancer, 2008; Tsilidis, 2011). Protection from these cancers decreases, however, as time from pill use lengthens (Tworoger, 2007). In contrast, the relative risk of cervical dysplasia and cervical cancer is increased in current COC users, but this declines after use is discontinued. Following 10 or more years, risk returns to that of never users (International Collaboration of Epidemiological Studies of Cervical Cancer, 2007).

Although COC use in the past was linked to development of hepatic *focal nodular hyperplasia* and *benign hepatic adenoma*, large studies do not support this (Heinemann, 1998). Moreover, there is also no evidence for increased risk of hepatocellular cancer (Maheshwari, 2007). For women with known tumors, COCs may be used in those with focal nodular hyperplasia, but avoided in those with benign hepatic adenoma and hepatocellular carcinoma (Kapp, 2009b). Rates of colorectal cancer appear to be reduced in ever users (Bosetti, 2009; Kabat, 2008).

It is unclear whether COCs contribute to the development of breast cancer, and major studies show no risk or a small risk among current users, which drops with time following cessation (Collaborative Group on Hormonal Factors in Breast Cancer, 1996; Marchbanks, 2002). In women who are carriers of the *BRCA1* or *BRCA2* gene mutation, risks for breast cancer are not increased by COC use (Brohet, 2007; Iodice, 2010). With regard to benign breast disease, COCs appear to lower rates (Vessey, 2007).

Other Effects

As summarized in Table 38-6, many noncontraceptive benefits are associated with COC use (American College of Obstetricians and Gynecologists, 2012c). And indeed, COCs may be used for these effects, even in those without contraceptive needs.

Low-dose estrogen formulations are not associated with depression or premenstrual mood changes and may actually improve the latter (Joffe, 2007). This is especially true with the drospirenone-containing COCs. Several studies have shown symptom improvement in women with premenstrual dysphoric disorder (PMDD) who use the drospirenone-containing COC *Yaz* (Lopez, 2012b; Pearlstein, 2005; Yonkers, 2005). And, the FDA has approved indications for this pill to include treatment of PMDD and moderate acne vulgaris for women requesting oral contraception.

Cholestasis and cholestatic jaundice are uncommon, but they resolve when COCs are discontinued. For women who have active hepatitis, COCs should not be initiated, but these may be continued in women who experience a flare of their liver disease while already taking COCs. Use of progestin-only contraception in these women is not restricted. Moreover, there is no reason to withhold COCs from women who have recovered. With cirrhosis, mild compensated disease does not limit the use of COCs or progestin-only methods. However, in those with severe decompensated disease, all hormonal methods should be avoided (Kapp, 2009a).

TABLE 38-6. Some Benefits of Combined Estrogen Plus Progestin Oral Contraceptives

Increased bone density
Reduced menstrual blood loss and anemia
Decreased risk of ectopic pregnancy
Improved dysmenorrhea from endometriosis
Fewer premenstrual complaints
Decreased risk of endometrial and ovarian cancer
Reduction in various benign breast diseases
Inhibition of hirsutism progression
Improvement of acne
Prevention of atherogenesis
Decreased incidence and severity of acute salpingitis
Decreased activity of rheumatoid arthritis

The progestin component of COCs reduces serum free testosterone levels and inhibits 5α-reductase to limit conversion of testosterone to its active metabolite, dihydrotestosterone. The estrogen component increases SHBG production and also lowers circulating androgen levels. The expected results of these actions are to improve androgenic conditions such as acne and hirsutism.

Hyperpigmentation of the face and forehead—chloasma—is more likely in women who demonstrated such a change during pregnancy. This is less common with low-dose estrogen formulations. Cervical mucorrhea, likely due to cervical ectopy, is common in response to the estrogen component of COCs (Critchlow, 1995). Although previously used for treating functional ovarian cysts, low-dose COC formulations have no effects related to cyst resolution or prevention (European Society of Human Reproduction and Embryology, 2001; Grimes, 2011).

Transdermal Patch

The *Ortho Evra* patch is another combination hormonal contraceptive formulation. It has an inner layer containing an adhesive and hormone matrix, and a water-resistant outer layer. Thus, women can wear the patch in bathtubs, showers, swimming pools, saunas, and whirlpools without decreased efficacy. The patch may be applied to buttocks, upper outer arm, lower abdomen, or upper torso, but the breasts are avoided. Because the hormones are combined with the adhesive, improper skin adherence will lower hormone absorption and efficacy. Therefore, if a patch is so poorly adhered that it requires reinforcement with tape, it should be replaced.

Initiation of the patch is the same as for COCs, and a new patch is applied weekly for 3 weeks, followed by a patch-free week to allow withdrawal bleeding. Although a patch is ideally worn no longer than 7 days, hormone levels remain in an effective range for up to 9 days. This affords a 2-day window for patch change delays (Abrams, 2001).

In general, the transdermal patch and vaginal ring produce metabolic changes, side effects, and efficacy rates comparable to those with COC pills. However, the patch has been associated with a higher VTE risk in some but not other studies (Cole, 2007; Jick, 2010; Lidegaard, 2012). And despite this lack of convincing association, the FDA (2008) ordered labeling for the patch to state that users *may* be at increased risk for developing VTE. Obesity—90 kg or greater—may be associated with an increased risk for patch contraceptive failure (Zieman, 2002). Last, application-site reaction and breast tenderness are more frequent during initial cycles in patch wearers (Urdl, 2005).

Transvaginal Ring

The *NuvaRing* is yet another form of combination hormonal contraception and is a flexible intravaginal ring. Constructed of ethinyl vinyl acetate, the ring measures 54 mm in diameter and 4 mm in cross section (Fig. 38-5). During insertion, the ring is compressed and threaded into the vagina, but no specific final intravaginal position is required. Its core releases ethinyl estradiol and the progestin etonogestrel, which are absorbed across the vaginal epithelium. Before being dispensed, the

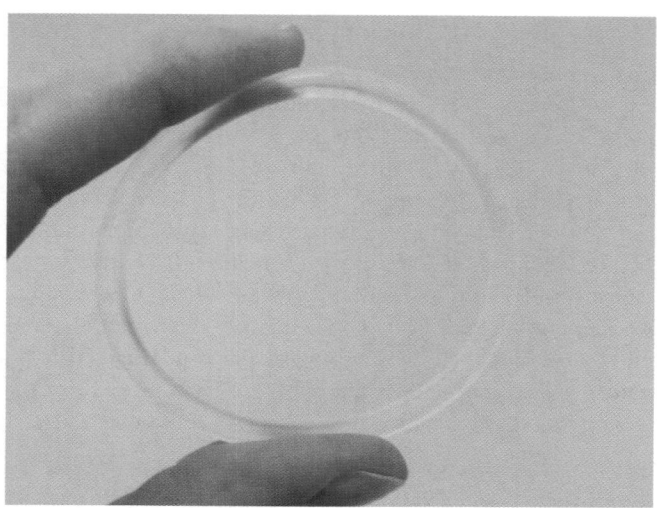

FIGURE 38-5 *NuvaRing*: estrogen-progestin—releasing vaginal contraceptive ring.

rings are refrigerated, and once dispensed, their shelf life is 4 months. The ring is placed within 5 days of menses onset and after 3 weeks of use, is removed for 1 week to allow withdrawal bleeding. Contraception will still be afforded if a ring is left in place for a fourth week (Merck, 2012b).

Patient satisfaction is high with this method, although vaginitis, ring-related events, and leukorrhea are more common (Oddsson, 2005). Despite this, no deleterious affect on vaginal flora or on lower reproductive-tract or endometrial epithelia has been found (Bulten, 2005; Veres, 2004). Approximately 70 percent of partners feel the ring during intercourse (Dieben, 2002). If this is bothersome, the ring may be removed for intercourse but should be replaced within 3 hours to maintain efficacy.

Injectable Progestin Contraceptives

Both intramuscular depot medroxyprogesterone acetate (Depo-Provera), 150 mg every 3 months, and norethisterone enanthate, 200 mg every 2 months, are injectable progestin contraceptives that have been effectively used worldwide for years. Available in the United States, DMPA is injected into the deltoid or gluteus muscle, but massage is avoided to ensure that the drug is released slowly. Alternatively, a subcutaneous version, *depo-subQ provera 104*, is also available and is injected into the subcutaneous tissue of the anterior thigh or abdomen every 3 months.

DMPA is an effective method, and as with other progestin-only methods, contraception is provided by ovulation inhibition, increased cervical mucus viscosity, and creation of an endometrium unfavorable for ovum implantation. Initial injection is given within the first 5 days following menses onset. Therapeutic serum levels sufficient to exert a consistent contraceptive effect are observed by 24 hours. Thus, no additional contraceptive method is required with initiation within this window. Alternatively, limited data support a "Quick Start" or initiation of DMPA regardless of cycle day. If so implemented, investigators recommend an initial negative pregnancy test result before injection, a supplemental contraceptive method during the 7 days following injection, and a second pregnancy test after 3 to 6 weeks to identify an early pregnancy (Rickert, 2007; Sneed, 2005). Fortunately, pregnancies conceived during DMPA use are not associated with an increased risk of fetal malformation (Katz, 1985). For women who present for intramuscular DMPA reinjection more than 13 weeks or subcutaneous DMPA reinjection more than 14 weeks after the prior dose, the manufacturer recommends exclusion of pregnancy before reinjection (Pfizer, 2010, 2012).

Actions and Side Effects

Injected progestins offer the convenience of a 3-month dosing schedule, contraceptive effectiveness comparable with or better than COCs, and minimal to no lactation impairment. Iron deficiency anemia is less likely in long-term users because of amenorrhea, which develops in up to 50 percent after 1 year and in 80 percent after 5 years.

Similar to other progestin-only contraceptive, irregular menstrual bleeding is common, and a fourth of women discontinued DMPA in the first year because of this (Cromer, 1994). Unique to DMPA, prolonged anovulation can follow discontinuation, which results in delayed fertility resumption. After injections are stopped, one fourth of patients do not resume regular menses for up to 1 year (Gardner, 1970). Accordingly, DMPA may not be ideal for women who plan to use birth control only briefly before attempting conception.

As with other progestins, DMPA has not been associated with cardiovascular events or stroke in otherwise healthy women. However, in those with severe hypertension, an increased risk of stroke has been found in DMPA users (World Health Organization, 1998). Moreover, the US MEC expresses concerns regarding hypoestrogenic effects and reduced HDL levels from DMPA in women with vascular disease or multiple risks for cardiovascular disease.

Weight gain is generally attributed to DMPA, and these increases are comparable between the two depot forms (Bahamondes, 2001; Nault, 2013; Westhoff, 2007c). In long-term users, loss of bone mineral density is also a potential problem (Petitti, 2000; Scholes, 1999). In 2004, the FDA added a black box warning to DMPA labeling, which notes that this concern is probably most relevant for adolescents, who are building bone mass, and perimenopausal women, who will soon have increased bone loss during menopause. That said, it is the opinion of the World Health Organization (1998) and American College of Obstetricians and Gynecologists (2008) that DMPA should not be restricted in those high-risk groups. And, it seems prudent to reevaluate overall risks and benefits during extended use (d'Arcangues, 2006).

It is somewhat reassuring that bone loss appears to be reversible after discontinuation of therapy but is still not complete after 18 to 24 months (Clark, 2006; Gai, 2011; Scholes, 2002).

Progestin-Only Pills

So-called *mini-pills* are progestin-only contraceptives that are taken daily. These contraceptives have not achieved widespread popularity and are used by only 0.4 percent of American women (Hall, 2012). Unlike COCs, they do not reliably inhibit ovulation. Rather, their effectiveness depends more on cervical mucus thickening and endometrial atrophy. Because mucus changes are not sustained longer than 24 hours, minipills should be taken at the same time every day to be maximally effective. If a progestin-only pill is taken even 4 hours late, a supplemental form of contraception must be used for the next 48 hours. Progestin-only pills are contraindicated in women with known breast cancer or pregnancy. Other cautions are listed in Table 38-3.

EFFECTIVE CONTRACEPTION: BARRIER METHODS

Male Condom

For many years, male and female condoms, vaginal diaphragms, and periodic abstinence have been used for contraception with variable success (see Table 38-2). The contraceptive efficacy of the male condom is enhanced appreciably by a reservoir tip and probably by the addition of a spermicide. Such agents, as well as those used for lubrication, should be water-based because oil-based products destroy latex condoms and diaphragms.

When used properly, condoms provide considerable but not absolute protection against a broad range of STDs. These include gonorrhea, syphilis, trichomoniasis, and HIV, herpetic, and chlamydial infections.

For individuals sensitive to latex, condoms made from lamb intestines are effective, but they do not provide infection protection. Fortunately, nonallergenic condoms have been developed that are made of polyurethane or of synthetic elastomers. Polyurethane condoms are effective against STDs but have a higher breakage and slippage rate than latex condoms (Gallo, 2006).

Female Condom

The only female condom available is marketed as the *FC2 Female Condom*. It is a synthetic nitrile sheath with one flexible polyurethane ring at each end. Its open ring remains outside the vagina, whereas its closed internal ring is fitted under the symphysis like a diaphragm (Fig. 38-6). The female condom can be used with both water-based and oil-based lubricants. Male condoms should not be used concurrently because simultaneous use may cause friction that leads to condom slipping, tearing, and displacement. Following use, the female condom outer ring should be twisted to seal the condom so that no semen spills. As an added value, in vitro tests have shown the female condom to be impermeable to HIV and other STDs.

Diaphragm Plus Spermicide

The diaphragm consists of a circular latex dome of various diameters supported by a circumferential latex-covered metal spring. It is effective when used in combination with spermicidal jelly or cream. The spermicide is applied into the dome cup and along the rim. The device is then positioned so that the cup faces the cervix and so that the cervix, vaginal fornices, and anterior vaginal wall are partitioned effectively from the remainder of the vagina and the penis. In this fashion, the centrally placed spermicide is held against the cervix. When appropriately positioned, one rim is lodged deep in the posterior vaginal fornix, and the opposite rim fits behind the inner surface of the symphysis and immediately below the urethra (Fig. 38-7). If a diaphragm is too small, it will not remain in place. If it is too large, it is uncomfortable when forced into position. A coexistent cystocele or uterine prolapse typically leads to instability and expulsion. Because size and spring flexibility must be individualized, the diaphragm is available only by prescription.

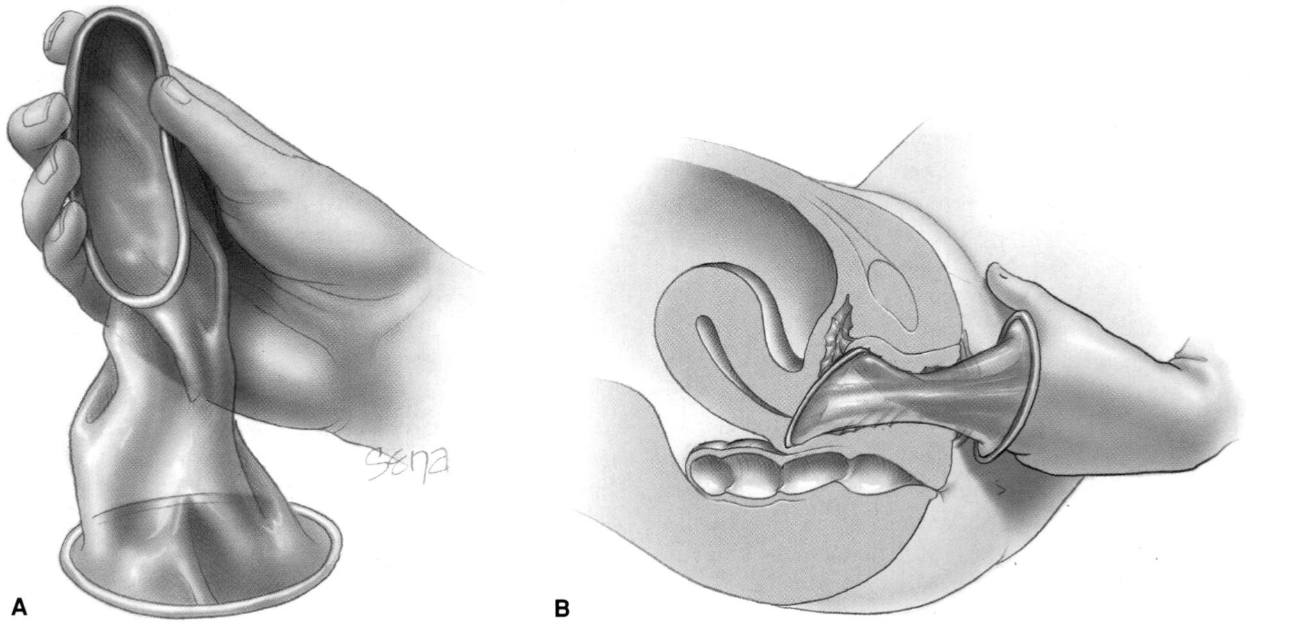

FIGURE 38-6 *FC2 Female Condom* insertion and positioning. **A.** The inner ring is squeezed for insertion. The sheath is inserted similarly to a diaphragm. **B.** The inner ring is pushed inward with an index finger.

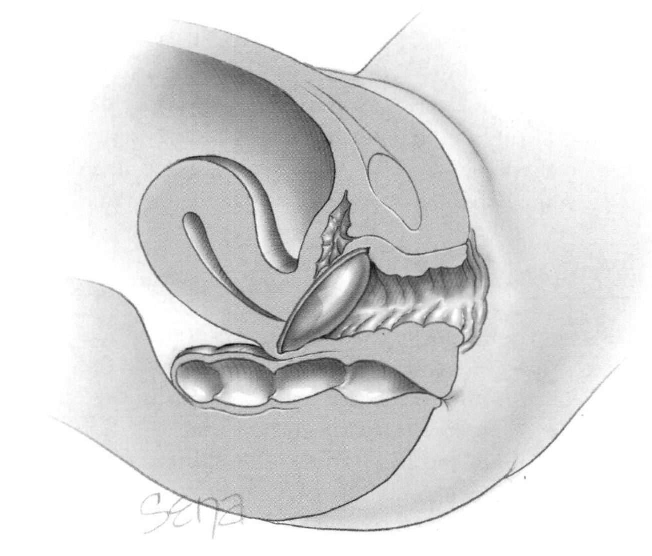

FIGURE 38-7 A diaphragm in place creates a physical barrier between the vagina and cervix.

With use, the diaphragm and spermicide can be inserted hours before intercourse, but if more than 6 hours elapse, additional spermicide should be placed in the upper vagina for maximum protection and be reapplied before each coital episode. The diaphragm should not be removed for at least 6 hours after intercourse. Because toxic shock syndrome has been described following its use, it may be worthwhile to remove the diaphragm at 6 hours, or at least the next morning, to minimize this rare event. Diaphragm use is associated with a slightly increased rate of urinary infections, presumably from urethral irritation by the ring under the symphysis.

Cervical Cap

FemCap is currently the only available cervical cap in the United States. Made of silicone rubber, it has a sailor-cap shape with a dome that covers the cervix and a flared brim, which allows the cap to be held in place by the muscular walls of the upper vagina. Available in 22-, 26-, and 30-mm sizes, it should be used with a spermicide applied once at insertion to both sides of the dome cup. For contraception, it should remain in place for 6 hours following coitus and may remain for up to 48 hours. Even with proper fitting and correct use, pregnancy rates with this method are higher that with the diaphragm (Gallo, 2002; Mauck, 1999).

Fertility Awareness-Based Methods

All of these family planning methods attempt to identify the fertile days each cycle and advise sexual abstinence during these days. However, their limited efficacy is shown in Table 38-2. Common forms of these fertility awareness-based (FAB) methods include Standard Days, Calendar Rhythm, Temperature Rhythm, Cervical Mucus, and Symptothermal Methods.

The *Standard Days Method* counsels women to avoid unprotected intercourse during cycle days 8 through 19. For successful use, women must have regular monthly cycles of 26 to 32 days. Those who use this method can mark a calendar or can use *Cycle-Beads*, which is a ring of counting beads, to keep track of their days.

The *Calendar Rhythm Method* requires counting the number of days in the shortest and longest menstrual cycle during a 6- to 12-month span. From the shortest cycle, 18 days are subtracted to calculate the first fertile day. From the longest cycle, 11 days are subtracted to identify the last fertile day. This is problematic because ovulation most often occurs 14 days before the onset of the next menses. Because this is not necessarily 14 days after the onset of the last menses, the calendar rhythm method is not reliable.

The *Temperature Rhythm Method* relies on slight changes—sustained 0.4°F increases—in the basal body temperature that usually occur just before ovulation. This method is much more likely to be successful if during each menstrual cycle, intercourse is avoided until well after the ovulatory temperature rise. For this method to be most effective, the woman must abstain from intercourse from the first day of menses through the third day after the temperature increase.

The *Cervical Mucus Method*, also called the Two-Day Method or Billings Method, relies on awareness of vaginal "dryness" and "wetness." These reflect changes in the amount and quality of cervical mucus at different times in the menstrual cycle. With the Billings Method, abstinence is required from the beginning of menses until 4 days after slippery mucus is identified. With the Two-Day method, intercourse is considered safe if a woman did not note mucus on the day of planned intercourse or the day prior.

The *Symptothermal Method* combines changes in cervical mucus—onset of fertile period; changes in basal body temperature—end of fertile period; and calculations to estimate the time of ovulation. This method is more complex to learn and apply, but it does not appreciably improve efficacy.

LESS EFFECTIVE CONTRACEPTION: SPERMICIDES

These contraceptives are marketed variously as creams, jellies, suppositories, films, and aerosol foam. They are especially useful for women who need temporary protection, for example, during the first week after starting COCs. Most can be purchased without a prescription.

Typically, spermicides function by providing a physical barrier to sperm penetration and a chemical spermicidal action. The active ingredient is nonoxynol-9 or octoxynol-9. Although these are spermicidal, they do not provide STD protection. Ideally, spermicides must be deposited high in the vagina in contact with the cervix shortly before intercourse. Their duration of maximal effectiveness is usually no more than 1 hour, and thereafter, they must be reinserted before repeat intercourse. Douching should be avoided for at least 6 hours after coitus.

High pregnancy rates are primarily attributable to inconsistent use rather than to method failure. Even if inserted regularly and correctly, however, they are considered a less effective method (see Table 38-2). Fortunately, if pregnancy does occur, they are not considered teratogenic (Briggs, 2011).

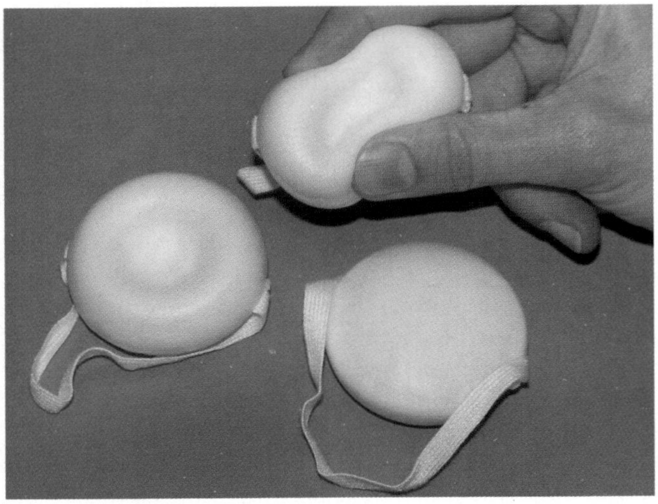

FIGURE 38-8 *Today* sponges. The sponge is moistened with tap water and gently squeezed to create light suds. It is then positioned with the dimple directly against the cervix. The fabric loop trails within the vagina and can be hooked with a finger to later extract the sponge.

Contraceptive Sponge

The *Today* contraceptive sponge is an over-the-counter, one-size-fits-all device. The nonoxynol-9–impregnated polyurethane disc is 2.5 cm thick and 5.5 cm wide and has a dimple on one side and satin loop on the other (Fig. 38-8). The sponge can be inserted up to 24 hours prior to intercourse, and while in place, it provides contraception regardless of coital frequency. It should remain in place for 6 hours after intercourse. Pregnancy is prevented primarily by the spermicide nonoxynol-9 and to a lesser extent, by covering the cervix and absorbing semen.

Although the sponge is possibly more convenient than the diaphragm or condom, it is less effective than either (Kuyoh, 2003). Most common causes for discontinuance are pregnancy, irritation, discomfort, or vaginitis (Beckman, 1989). Although toxic shock syndrome (TSS) has been reported with the contraceptive sponge, it is rare, and evidence suggests that the sponge may actually limit production of the responsible staphylococcal exotoxin (Remington, 1987). Still, it is recommended that the sponge not be used during menses or the puerperium.

EMERGENCY CONTRACEPTION

Many women present for contraceptive care following unprotected sexual intercourse. In this situation, several emergency contraception (EC) regimens substantially decrease the likelihood of an unwanted pregnancy when used correctly. Current methods include COCs, POPs, progesterone antagonists, and copper-containing IUDs (Table 38-7). Patients can obtain information regarding emergency contraception by calling 1-888-NOT-2-LATE or accessing The Emergency Contraception Website: http://not-2-late.com.

Hormonal Emergency Contraception

Also known as the *Yuzpe method*, one EC method provides a minimum of 100 μg of ethinyl estradiol and 0.5 mg of levonorgestrel in each of two doses. As shown in Table 38-7, a sufficient dose may be achieved by two or more pills. The first dose is taken ideally within 72 hours of intercourse but may be given up to 120 hours. The initial dose is followed 12 hours later by a second equivalent dose.

With progestin-only regimens, 1.5 mg of levonorgestrel is taken, either as a single, one-time 1.5-mg dose or as two tablets, each containing 0.75 mg levonorgestrel. With these regimens, the first dose is ideally taken within 72 hours of unprotected coitus but may be given up to 120 hours. With the two-pill

TABLE 38-7. Methods Available for Use as Emergency Contraception

Method	Formulation	Pills per Dose	Number of Doses[a]
Progestin-Only Pill			
Plan B, Next Choice	0.75 mg levonorgestrel	1	2
Plan B One-Step, Next Choice One Dose	150 mg levonorgestrel	1	1
PRM Pill			
Ella	30 mg ulipristal acetate	1	1
COC Pills[b,c]			
Ogestrel	0.05 mg EE + 0.5 mg norgestrel	2	2
Lo/Ovral, Low-Ogestrel	0.03 mg EE + 0.3 mg norgestrel	4	2
Enpresse (orange), Trivora (pink)	0.03 mg EE + 0.125 mg levonorgestrel	4	2
Nordette, Seasonale	0.03 mg EE + 0.15 mg levonorgestrel	4	2
Aviane, LoSeasonique (orange)	0.02 mg EE + 0.1 mg levonorgestrel	5	2
Copper-Containing IUD			
Paragard T 380A			

[a]Doses taken 12 hours apart.
[b]Other COC brands with formulations identical to those above may also be used (see Table 38-4).
[c]Use of an antiemetic agent before taking the medication will lessen the risk of nausea, which is a common side effect.
COC = combination oral contraceptive; EE = ethinyl estradiol; PRM = progesterone-receptor modulator.

regimen, the second dose follows 12 hours later, although a 24-hour interval between the doses is also effective (Ngai, 2005).

One progesterone-receptor modulator currently available for EC is ulipristal acetate and is marketed as *Ella*. It is taken as a single 30-mg tablet up to 120 hours after unprotected intercourse (Brache, 2010; Watson, 2010).

The major mechanism with all hormonal regimens is inhibition or delay of ovulation. Emergency hormonal contraceptive regimens are more effective the sooner they are taken and decrease the risk of pregnancy by up to 94 percent (American College of Obstetricians and Gynecologists, 2012b). Although highly effective, if EC fails to prevent pregnancy or is mistimed, no associations with major congenital malformation or pregnancy complications have been noted with estrogen- or progestin-containing regimens. Data regarding ulipristal acetate in this setting are limited.

With EC administration, nausea and vomiting can be a significant side effect (Gemzell-Danielsson, 2013). Accordingly, an oral antiemetic may be prescribed at least 1 hour before each dose. If a woman vomits within 2 hours of a dose, the dose must be repeated.

Copper-Containing Intrauterine Devices

For women who are candidates, copper IUD insertion is an effective EC method and provides an effective 10-year method of contraception (Cheng, 2012). If an IUD is placed up to 5 days after unprotected coitus, the failure rate approximates only 0.1 percent (Fasoli, 1989; Wu, 2010).

PUERPERAL CONTRACEPTION

For mothers who are nursing exclusively, ovulation during the first 10 weeks after delivery is unlikely. Nursing, however, is not a reliable method of family planning for women whose infants are on a daytime-only feeding schedule. Moreover, waiting for first menses involves a risk of pregnancy, because ovulation usually antedates menstruation. Certainly, after the first menses, contraception is essential unless the woman desires pregnancy.

For nursing mothers, progestin-only contraceptives are the preferred choice in most cases. In addition, IUDs have been recommended for the lactating sexually active woman. Estrogen-progestin contraceptives may reduce both the rate and the duration of milk production, although data are limited (Truitt, 2010). Moreover, very small quantities of the hormones are excreted in breast milk, but no adverse effects on infants have been reported (World Health Organization, 1988). Thus, in many cases, the benefits from pregnancy prevention by the use of COCs after the first 4 puerperal weeks would appear to outweigh the risks in selected patients. Immediate postpartum COC initiation is avoided due to VTE risks (Centers for Disease Control and Prevention, 2011).

REFERENCES

Abrams LS, Skee DM, Wong FA, et al: Pharmacokinetics of norelgestromin and ethinyl estradiol from two consecutive contraceptive patches. J Clin Pharmacol 41:1232, 2001

American College of Obstetricians and Gynecologists: Depot medroxyprogesterone acetate and bone effects. Practice Bulletin No. 415, September 2008

American College of Obstetricians and Gynecologists: Increasing use of contraceptive implants and intrauterine devices to reduce unintended pregnancy. Committee Opinion No. 450, December 2009, Reaffirmed 2011a

American College of Obstetricians and Gynecologists: Understanding and using the U.S. Medical Eligibility Criteria for Contraceptive Use, 2010. Committee Opinion No. 505, September 2011b

American College of Obstetricians and Gynecologists: Adolescents and long-acting reversible contraception: implants and intrauterine devices. Committee Opinion No. 539, October 2012a

American College of Obstetricians and Gynecologists: Emergency contraception. Practice Bulletin No. 112, May 2010, Reaffirmed 2012b

American College of Obstetricians and Gynecologists: Noncontraceptive use of hormonal contraceptives. Practice Bulletin No. 110, January 2010, Reaffirmed 2012c

American College of Obstetricians and Gynecologists: Benefits and risks of sterilization. Practice Bulletin No. 133, February 2013a

American College of Obstetricians and Gynecologists: Brand versus generic oral contraceptives. Committee Opinion No. 375, August 2007, Reaffirmed 2013b

American College of Obstetricians and Gynecologists: Long-acting reversible contraception: implants and intrauterine devices. Practice Bulletin No. 121, July 2011, Reaffirmed 2013c

American College of Obstetricians and Gynecologists: Prevention of deep vein thrombosis and pulmonary embolism. Practice Bulletin No. 84, August 2007, Reaffirmed 2013d

American College of Obstetricians and Gynecologists: Use of hormonal contraception in women with coexisting medical conditions. Practice Bulletin No. 73, June 2006, Reaffirmed 2013e

Backman T, Rauramo I, Huhtala S, et al: Pregnancy during the use of levonorgestrel intrauterine system. Am J Obstet Gynecol 190(1):50, 2004

Bahamondes L, Del Castillo S, Tabares G: Comparison of weight increase in users of depot medroxyprogesterone acetate and copper IUD up to 5 years. Contraception 64(4):223, 2001

Bayer HealthCare Pharmaceuticals: Mirena (levonorgestrel-releasing intrauterine system): highlights of prescribing information. 2013a. Available at: http://labeling.bayerhealthcare.com/html/products/pi/Mirena_PI.pdf. Accessed February 17, 2013

Bayer HealthCare Pharmaceuticals: Skyla (levonorgestrel-releasing intrauterine system): highlights of prescribing information. 2013b. Available at: http://labeling.bayerhealthcare.com/html/products/pi/Skyla_PI.pdf. Accessed March 2, 2013

Bayer HealthCare Pharmaceuticals: Yaz (drospirenone and ethinyl estradiol tablets): highlights of prescribing information. 2012. Available at: http://labeling.bayerhealthcare.com/html/products/pi/fhc/YAZ_PI.pdf?WT.mc_id=www.berlex.com. Accessed March 7, 2013

Bayer Shering Pharma Oy: Jadelle: data sheet. 2010. Available at: http://www.bayerresources.com.au/resources/uploads/DataSheet/file9537.pdf. Accessed February 16, 2013

Beckman LJ, Murray J, Harvey SM: The contraceptive sponge: factors in initiation and discontinuation of use. Contraception 40:481, 1989

Bednarek PH, Creinin MD, Reeves MF, et al: Immediate versus delayed IUD insertion after uterine aspiration. N Engl J Med 364(23):2208, 2011

Benacerraf BR, Shipp TD, Bromley B: Three-dimensional ultrasound detection of abnormally located intrauterine contraceptive devices which are a source of pelvic pain and abnormal bleeding. Ultrasound Obstet Gynecol 34(1):110, 2009

Boortz HE, Margolis DJ, Ragavendra N, et al: Migration of intrauterine devices: radiologic findings and implications for patient care. Radiographics 32(2):335, 2012

Bosetti C, Bravi F, Negri E, et al: Oral contraceptives and colorectal cancer risk: a systematic review and meta-analysis. Hum Reprod Update 15(5):489, 2009

Brache V, Cochon L, Jesam C, et al: Immediate pre-ovulatory administration of 30 mg ulipristal acetate significantly delays follicular rupture. Hum Reprod 25(9):2256, 2010

Brache V, Faundes A, Alvarez F, et al: Nonmenstrual adverse events during use of implantable contraceptives for women: data from clinical trials. Contraception 65(1):63, 2002

Brahmi D, Steenland MW, Renner RM, et al: Pregnancy outcomes with an IUD in situ: a systematic review. Contraception 85(2):131, 2012

Briggs GG, Freeman RK, Yaffe SJ: Drugs in Pregnancy and Lactation, 9th ed. Philadelphia, Lippincott Williams & Wilkins, 2011, p 1049

Brohet RM, Goldgar DE, Easton DF, et al: Oral contraceptives and breast cancer risk in the International BRCA 1/2 Carrier Cohort Study: a report from EMBRACE, GENEPSO, GEO-HEBON, and the IBCCS Collaborating Group. J Clin Oncol 25:5327, 2007

Brown M, Britton J: Neuropathy associated with etonogestrel implant insertion. Contraception 86(5):591, 2012

Brunner LR, Hogue CJ: The role of body weight in oral contraceptive failure: results from the 1995 national survey of family growth. Ann Epidemiol 15:492, 2005
Bulten J, Grefte J, Siebers B, et al: The combined contraceptive vaginal ring (NuvaRing) and endometrial histology. Contraception 72:362, 2005
Centers for Disease Control and Prevention: Sexually transmitted diseases treatment guidelines, 2010. MMWR 59 (12):1, 2010a
Centers for Disease Control and Prevention: Update to CDC's *U.S. Medical Eligibility Criteria for Contraceptive Use, 2010*: revised recommendations for the use of contraceptive methods during the postpartum period. MMWR 60(26):878, 2011
Centers for Disease Control and Prevention: Update to CDC's *U.S. Medical Eligibility Criteria for Contraceptive Use, 2010*: revised recommendations for the use of hormonal contraception among women at high risk for HIV infection or infected with HIV. MMWR 61(24):449, 2012
Centers for Disease Control and Prevention: U.S. medical eligibility criteria for contraceptive use, 2010. MMWR 59(4):1, 2010b
Centers for Disease Control and Prevention: U.S. selected practice recommendations for contraceptive use, 2013. MMWR 62 (5):1, 2013
Chasan-Taber L, Willett WC, Manson JE, et al: Prospective study of oral contraceptives and hypertension among women in the United States. Circulation 94:483, 1996
Chen BA, Reeves MF, Hayes JL, et al: Postplacental or delayed insertion of the levonorgestrel intrauterine device after vaginal delivery: a randomized controlled trial. Obstet Gynecol 116(5):1079, 2010
Cheng L, Che Y, Gulmezoglu AM: Interventions for emergency contraception. Cochrane Database Syst Rev 2:CD001324, 2012
Civic D, Scholes D, Ichikawa L, et al: Depressive symptoms in users and non-users of depot medroxyprogesterone acetate. Contraception 61(6):385, 2000
Clark MK, Sowers M, Levy B, et al: Bone mineral density loss and recovery during 48 months in first-time users of depot medroxyprogesterone acetate. Fertil Steril 86:1466, 2006
Cole JA, Norman H, Doherty M, et al: Venous thromboembolism, myocardial infarction, and stroke among transdermal contraceptive system users. Obstet Gynecol 109:339, 2007
Collaborative Group on Epidemiological Studies of Ovarian Cancer, Beral V, Doll R, et al: Ovarian cancer and oral contraceptives: collaborative reanalysis of data of 45 epidemiological studies including 23,257 women with ovarian cancer and 87,303 controls. Lancet 371:303, 2008
Collaborative Group on Hormonal Factors in Breast Cancer: Breast cancer and hormonal contraceptives: collaborative reanalysis of individual data on 53,297 women with breast cancer and 100,239 women without breast cancer from 54 epidemiological studies. Lancet 347:1713, 1996
Comp PC: Coagulation and thrombosis with OC use: physiology and clinical relevance. Dialogues Contracept 5:1, 1996
Correia L, Ramos AB, Machado AI, et al: Magnetic resonance imaging and gynecological devices. Contraception 85(6):538, 2012
Craft P, Hannaford PC: Risk factors for acute myocardial infarction in women: evidence from the Royal College of General Practitioners' Oral Contraceptive Study. BMJ 298:165, 1989
Critchlow CW, Wölner-Hanssen P, Eschenback DA, et al: Determinants of cervical ectopia and of cervicitis: age, oral contraception, specific cervical infection, smoking, and douching. Am J Obstet Gynecol 173:534, 1995
Cromer BA, Smith RD, Blair JM, et al: A prospective study of adolescents who choose among levonorgestrel implant (Norplant), medroxyprogesterone acetate (Depo-Provera), or the combined oral contraceptive pill as contraception. Pediatrics 94:687, 1994
Croxatto HB, Mäkäräinen L: The pharmacodynamics and efficacy of Implanon. An overview of the data. Contraception 58:91S, 1998
Curtis EM, Pine L: *Actinomyces* in the vaginas of women with and without intrauterine contraceptive devices. Am J Obstet Gynecol 140:880, 1981
d'Arcangues C: WHO statement on hormonal contraception and bone health. Contraception 73(5):443, 2006
d'Arcangues C: Worldwide use of intrauterine devices for contraception. Contraception 75:S2, 2007
Dieben TO, Roumen FJ, Apter D: Efficacy, cycle control, and user acceptability of a novel combined contraceptive vaginal ring. Obstet Gynecol 100:585, 2002
Dorflinger LJ: Metabolic effects of implantable steroid contraceptives for women. Contraception 65(1):47, 2002
Edelman A, Gallo MF, Nichols MD, et al: Continuous versus cyclic use of combined oral contraceptives for contraception: systematic Cochrane review of randomized controlled trials. Hum Reprod 21:573, 2006
European Society of Human Reproduction and Embryology—ESHRE Capri Workshop Group: Ovarian and endometrial function during hormonal contraception. Hum Reprod 16(7):1527, 2001
Farley TMM, Rosenberg MJ, Rowe PJ, et al: Intrauterine devices and pelvic inflammatory disease: an international perspective. Lancet 339:785, 1992
Fasoli M, Parazzini F, Cecchetti G, et al: Post-coital contraception: an overview of published studies. Contraception 39:459, 1989
Fels H, Steward R, Melamed A, et al: Comparison of serum and cervical mucus hormone levels during hormone-free interval of 24/4 vs. 21/7 combined oral contraceptives. Contraception 87(6):732, 2013
Finer LB, Zolna MR: Unintended pregnancy in the United States: incidence and disparities, 2006. Contraception 84(5):478, 2011
Fiorino AS: Intrauterine contraceptive device–associated actinomycotic abscess and *Actinomyces* detection on cervical smear. Obstet Gynecol 87:142, 1996
Food and Drug Administration: Drug safety communication: safety review update on the possible increased risk of blood clots with birth control pills containing drospirenone. 2011. Available at: http://www.fda.gov/Drugs/DrugSafety/ucm273021.htm. Accessed March 7, 2013
Food and Drug Administration: Orange book: approved drug products with therapeutic equivalence evaluations. 2013. Available at: http://www.accessdata.fda.gov/scripts/cder/ob/default.cfm. Accessed February 20, 2013
Funk S, Miller MM, Mishell DR Jr, et al: Safety and efficacy of Implanon, a single-rod implantable contraceptive containing etonogestrel. Contraception 71:319, 2005
Furlong LA: Ectopic pregnancy risk when contraception fails. J Reprod Med 47:881, 2002
Gaffield ME, Culwell KR, Lee CR: The use of hormonal contraception among women taking anticonvulsant therapy. Contraception 83(1):16, 2011
Gai L, Zhang J, Zhang H, et al: The effect of depot medroxyprogesterone acetate (DMPA) on bone mineral density (BMD) and evaluating changes in BMD after discontinuation of DMPA in Chinese women of reproductive age. Contraception 83(3):218, 2011
Gallo MF, Grimes DA, Lopez LM, et al: Non-latex versus latex male condoms for contraception. Cochrane Database Syst Rev 1:CD003550, 2006
Gallo MF, Grimes DA, Schulz KF: Cervical cap versus diaphragm for contraception. Cochrane Database Syst Rev 4:CD003551, 2002
Gallo MF, Lopez LM, Grimes DA, et al: Combination contraceptives: effects on weight. Cochrane Database Syst Rev 9:CD003987, 2011
Gardner JM, Mishell DR Jr: Analysis of bleeding patterns and resumption of fertility following discontinuation of a long-acting injectable contraceptive. Fertil Steril 21:286, 1970
Gemzell-Danielsson K, Berger C, Lalitkumar PG: Emergency contraception—mechanisms of action. Contraception 87(3):300, 2013
Gemzell-Danielsson K, Schellschmidt I, Apter D: A randomized, phase II study describing the efficacy, bleeding profile, and safety of two low-dose levonorgestrel-releasing intrauterine contraceptive systems and Mirena. Fertil Steril 97(3):616, 2012
Grimes DA, Hubacher D, Lopez LM, et al: Non-steroidal anti-inflammatory drugs for heavy bleeding or pain associated with intrauterine-device use. Cochrane Database Syst Rev 4:CD006034, 2006
Grimes DA, Jones LB, Lopez LM, et al: Oral contraceptives for functional ovarian cysts. Cochrane Database Syst Rev 9:CD006134, 2011
Grimes DA, Lopez LM, Schulz KF, et al: Immediate postabortal insertion of intrauterine devices. Cochrane Database Syst Rev 6:CD001777, 2010a
Grimes DA, Lopez LM, Schulz KF, et al: Immediate post-partum insertion of intrauterine devices. Cochrane Database Syst Rev 5:CD003036, 2010b
Grimes DA, Schulz KF: Antibiotic prophylaxis for intrauterine contraceptive device insertion. Cochrane Database Syst Rev 2:CD001327, 2001
Hall KS, Trussell J, Schwarz EB: Progestin-only contraceptive pill use among women in the United States. Contraception 86(6):653, 2012
Hannaford PC, Selvaraj S, Elliott AM, et al: Cancer risk among users of oral contraceptives: cohort data from the Royal College of General Practitioners' oral contraception study. BMJ 335:651, 2007
Harrison-Woolrych M, Ashton J, Coulter D: Uterine perforation on intrauterine device insertion: is the incidence higher than previously reported? Contraception 67:53, 2003
Hassan EO, el-Husseini M, el-Nahal N: The effect of 1-year use of the CuT 380A and oral contraceptive pills on hemoglobin and ferritin levels. Contraception 60(2):101, 1999
Heinemann LA, Weimann A, Gerken G, et al: Modern oral contraceptive use and benign liver tumors: the German Benign Liver Tumor Case-Control Study. Eur J Contracept Reprod Health Care 3:194, 1998
Holt VL, Cushing-Haugen KL, Daling JR: Body weight and risk of oral contraceptive failure. Obstet Gynecol 99:820, 2002
Holt VL, Scholes D, Wicklund KG, et al: Body mass index, weight, and oral contraceptive failure risk. Obstet Gynecol 105:46, 2005
Hubacher D, Lara-Ricalde R, Taylor DJ, et al: Use of copper intrauterine devices and the risk of tubal infertility among nulligravid women. N Engl J Med 345:561, 2001

International Collaboration of Epidemiological Studies of Cervical Cancer: Cervical cancer and hormonal contraceptives: collaborative reanalysis of individual data for 16,573 women with cervical cancer and 35,509 women without cervical cancer from 24 epidemiological studies. Lancet 370:1609, 2007
Iodice S, Barile M, Rotmensz N, et al: Oral contraceptive use and breast or ovarian cancer risk in BRCA1/2 carriers: a meta-analysis. Eur J Cancer 46(12):2275, 2010
Jecht EW, Bernstein GS: The influence of copper on the motility of human spermatozoa. Contraception 7:381, 1973
Jick SS, Hagberg KW, Kaye JA: ORTHO EVRA and venous thromboembolism: an update. Contraception 81(5):452, 2010
Jick SS, Hernandez RK: Risk of non-fatal venous thromboembolism in women using oral contraceptives containing drospirenone compared with women using oral contraceptives containing levonorgestrel: case-control study using United States claims data. BMJ 340:d2151, 2011
Joffe J, Petrillo LF, Viguera AC, et al: Treatment of premenstrual worsening depression with adjunctive oral contraceptive pills: a preliminary report. J Clin Psychiatry 68:1954, 2007
Jones J, Mosher W, Daniels K: Current contraceptive use in the United States, 2006–2010, and changes in patterns of use since 1995. Natl Health Stat Report 60:1, 2012
Kabat GC, Miller AB, Rohan TE: Oral contraceptive use, hormone replacement therapy, reproductive history and risk of colorectal cancer in women. Int J Cancer 122:643, 2008
Kapp N, Curtis KM: Hormonal contraceptive use among women with liver tumors: a systematic review. Contraception 80(4):387, 2009a
Kapp N, Tilley IB, Curtis KM: The effects of hormonal contraceptive use among women with viral hepatitis or cirrhosis of the liver: a systematic review. Contraception 80(4):381, 2009b
Karabayirli S, Ayrim AA, Muslu B: Comparison of the analgesic effects of oral tramadol and naproxen sodium on pain relief during IUD insertion. J Minim Invasive Gynecol 19(5):581, 2012
Katz Z, Lancet M, Skornik J, et al: Teratogenicity of progestogens given during the first trimester of pregnancy. Obstet Gynecol 65(6):775, 1985
Kim C, Siscovick DS, Sidney S, et al: Oral contraceptive use and association with glucose, insulin, and diabetes in young adult women: the CARDIA Study. Coronary Artery Risk Development in Young Adults. Diabetes Care 25:1027, 2002
Kim SK, Romero R, Kusanovic JP, et al: The prognosis of pregnancy conceived despite the presence of an intrauterine device (IUD). J Perinat Med 38(1):45, 2010
Krattenmacher R: Drospirenone: pharmacology and pharmacokinetics of a unique progestogen. Contraception 62:29, 2000
Kuyoh MA, Toroitich-Ruto C, Grimes DA, et al: Sponge versus diaphragm for contraception: a Cochrane review. Contraception 67:15, 2003
Lammer EJ, Cordero JF: Exogenous sex hormone exposure and the risk for major malformations. JAMA 255:3128, 1986
Lawrie TA, Helmerhorst FM, Maitra NK, et al: Types of progestogens in combined oral contraception: effectiveness and side-effects. Cochrane Database Syst Rev 5:CD004861, 2011
Lidegaard Ø, Nielsen LH, Skovlund CW, et al: Risk of venous thromboembolism from use of oral contraceptives containing different progestogens and oestrogen doses: Danish cohort study, 2001–9. BMJ 343:d6423, 2011
Lippes J: Pelvic actinomycosis: a review and preliminary look at prevalence. Am J Obstet Gynecol 180:265, 1999
Lopez LM, Edelman A, Chen-Mok M, et al: Progestin-only contraceptives: effects on weight. Cochrane Database Syst Rev 4:CD008815, 2011
Lopez LM, Grimes DA, Chen-Mok M, et al: Hormonal contraceptives for contraception in overweight or obese women. Cochrane Database Syst Rev 7:CD008452, 2010
Lopez LM, Grimes DA, Schulz KF: Steroidal contraceptives: effect on carbohydrate metabolism in women without diabetes mellitus. Cochrane Database Syst 2:CD006133, 2012a
Lopez LM, Kaptein AA, Helmerhorst FM: Oral contraceptives containing drospirenone for premenstrual syndrome. Cochrane Database Syst Rev 2:CD006586, 2012b
Lyon A, Pandravada A, Leung E, et al: Emergency laparoscopic sigmoid colectomy for perforation secondary to intrauterine contraceptive device. J Obstet Gynaecol 32(4):402, 2012
MacClellan LR, Giles W, Cole J, et al: Probable migraine with visual aura and risk of ischemic stroke: the Stroke Prevention in Young Women Study. Stroke 38:2438, 2007
Maheshwari S, Sarraj A, Kramer J, et al: Oral contraception and the risk of hepatocellular carcinoma. J Hepatol 47:506, 2007
Mansour D, Gemzell-Danielsson K, Inki P, et al: Fertility after discontinuation of contraception: a comprehensive review of the literature. Contraception 84(5):465, 2011
Mantha S, Karp R, Raghavan V, et al: Assessing the risk of venous thromboembolic events in women taking progestin-only contraception: a meta-analysis. BMJ 345:e4944, 2012
Marchbanks PA, McDonald JA, Wilson HG, et al: Oral contraceptives and the risk of breast cancer. N Engl J Med 346(26):2025, 2002
Margolis KL, Adami HO, Luo J, et al: A prospective study of oral contraceptive use and risk of myocardial infarction among Swedish women. Fertil Steril 88:310, 2007
Mascarenhas MP, Tiraboschi RB, Paschoalin VP, et al: Exercise-induced hematuria as the main manifestation of migration of intrauterine contraceptive device into the bladder. Case Rep Urol 2012:736426, 2012
Mauck C, Callahan M, Weiner DH, et al: A comparative study of the safety and efficacy of FemCap, a new vaginal barrier contraceptive, and the Ortho All-Flex diaphragm. The FemCap Investigators' Group. Contraception 60(2):71, 1999
McNicholas CP, Madden T, Zhao Q, et al: Cervical lidocaine for IUD insertional pain: a randomized controlled trial. Am J Obstet Gynecol 207(5): 384.e1, 2012
Merck: Nexplanon: highlights of prescribing information. 2012a. Available at: http://www.nexplanon-usa.com/en/hcp/main/prescribing-information.asp. Accessed February 16, 2013
Merck: Nuvaring: prescribing information. 2012b. Available at: http://www.merck.com/product/usa/pi_circulars/n/nuvaring/nuvaring_pi.pdf. Accessed March 7, 2013
Mishell DR Jr: Oral contraceptives and cardiovascular events: summary and application of data. Int J Fertil 45:121, 2000
Mommers E, Blum GF, Gent TG, et al: Nexplanon, a radiopaque etonogestrel implant in combination with a next-generation applicator: 3-year results of a noncomparative multicenter trial. Am J Obstet Gynecol 207(5):388.e1, 2012
Moreau C, Trussell J, Gilbert F, et al: Oral contraceptive tolerance: does the type of pill matter? Obstet Gynecol 109:1277, 2007
Moschos E, Twickler DM: Does the type of intrauterine device affect conspicuity on 2D and 3D ultrasound? AJR Am J Roentgenol 196(6):1439, 2011
Murthy AS, Creinin MD, Harwood B, et al: Same-day initiation of the transdermal hormonal delivery system (contraceptive patch) versus traditional initiation methods. Contraception 72(5):333, 2005
Nault AM, Peipert JF, Zhao Q, et al: Validity of perceived weight gain in women using long-acting reversible contraception and depot medroxyprogesterone acetate. Am J Obstet Gynecol 208(1):48.e1, 2013
Nelson AL, Cwiak C: Combined oral contraceptives (COCs). In Hatcher RA, Trussell J, Nelson AL, et al (eds): Contraceptive Technology, 20th ed. New York, Ardent Media, 2011, p 313
Nelson AL, Fong JK: Intrauterine infusion of lidocaine does not reduce pain scores during IUD insertion. Contraception 88(1):37, 2013
Ngai SW, Fan S, Li S, et al: A randomized trial to compare 24 h versus 12 h double dose regimen of levonorgestrel for emergency contraception. Hum Reprod 20:307, 2005
Oddsson K, Leifels-Fischer B, Wiel-Masson D, et al: Superior cycle control with a contraceptive vaginal ring compared with an oral contraceptive containing 30 microg ethinylestradiol and 150 microg levonorgestrel: a randomized trial. Hum Reprod 20:557, 2005
Ortiz ME, Croxatto HB: Copper-T intrauterine device and levonorgestrel intrauterine system: biological bases of their mechanism of action. Contraception 75:S16, 2007
Panel on Antiretroviral Guidelines for Adults and Adolescents. Guidelines for the use of antiretroviral agents in HIV-1-infected adults and adolescents. 2013. Available at http://aidsinfo.nih.gov/ContentFiles/AdultandAdolescentGL.pdf. Accessed March 3, 2013
Parkin L, Sharples K, Hernandez RK, et al: Risk of venous thromboembolism in users of oral contraceptives containing drospirenone or levonorgestrel: nested case-control study based on UK General Practice Research Database. BMJ 340:d2139, 2011
Pasquale SA, Russer TJ, Foldes R, et al: Lack of interaction between magnetic resonance imaging and the copper-T380A IUD. Contraception 55(3):169, 1997
Pearlstein TB, Bachmann GA, Zacur HA, et al: Treatment of premenstrual dysphoric disorder with a new drospirenone-containing oral contraceptive formulation. Contraception 72:414, 2005
Persson E, Holmberg K: A longitudinal study of *Actinomyces israelii* in the female genital tract. Acta Obstet Gynecol Scand 63:207, 1984
Petitti DB, Piaggio G, Mehta S, et al: Steroid hormone contraception and bone mineral density: a cross-sectional study in an international population. The WHO Study of Hormonal Contraception and Bone Health. Obstet Gynecol 95(5):736, 2000
Pfizer: Depo-Provera (medroxyprogesterone acetate) injectable suspension: highlights of prescribing information. 2012. Available at: http://labeling.pfizer.com/ShowLabeling.aspx?id=522. Accessed February 19, 2013

Pfizer: Depo-subQ Provera 104: physician information. 2010. Available at: http://labeling.pfizer.com/ShowLabeling.aspx?id=549. Accessed February 19, 2013

Pomp ER, le Cessie S, Rosendaal FR, et al: Risk of venous thrombosis: obesity and its joint effect with oral contraceptive use and prothrombotic mutations. Br J Haematol 139(2):289, 2007

Pomp ER, Rosendaal FR, Doggen CJ: Smoking increases the risk of venous thrombosis and acts synergistically with oral contraceptive use. Am J Hematol 83:97, 2008

Population Council: Jadelle. 2013. Available at: http://www.popcouncil.org/what/jadelle.asp. Accessed February 16, 2013

Remington KM, Buller RS, Kelly JR: Effect of the Today contraceptive sponge on growth and toxic shock syndrome toxin-1 production by *Staphylococcus aureus*. Obstet Gynecol 69:563, 1987

Rickert VI, Tiezzi L, Lipshutz J, et al: Depo Now: preventing unintended pregnancies among adolescents and young adults. J Adolesc Health 40(1):22, 2007

Robinson GE, Burren T, Mackie IJ, et al: Changes in haemostasis after stopping the combined contraceptive pill: implications for major surgery. BMJ 302:269, 1991

Ronnerdag M, Odlind V: Health effects of long-term use of the intrauterine levonorgestrel-releasing system. Acta Obstet Gynecol Scand 78:716, 1999

Rothman KJ, Louik C: Oral contraceptives and birth defects. N Engl J Med 299:522, 1978

Savolainen E, Saksela E, Saxen L: Teratogenic hazards of oral contraceptives analyzed in a national malformation register. Am J Obstet Gynecol 140:521, 1981

Schafer JE, Osborne LM, Davis AR, et al: Acceptability and satisfaction using Quick Start with the contraceptive vaginal ring versus an oral contraceptive. Contraception 73(5):488, 2006

Schiesser M, Lapaire O, Tercanli S, et al: Lost intrauterine devices during pregnancy: maternal and fetal outcome after ultrasound-guided extraction. An analysis of 82 cases. Ultrasound Obstet Gynecol 23:486, 2004

Scholes D, LaCroix AS, Ichikawa LE, et al: Injectable hormone contraception and bone density: results from a prospective study. Epidemiology 13:581, 2002

Scholes D, LaCroix AS, Ott SM, et al: Bone mineral density in women using depot medroxyprogesterone acetate for contraception. Obstet Gynecol 93:233, 1999

Seeger JD, Loughlin J, Eng PM, et al: Risk of thromboembolism in women taking ethinylestradiol/drospirenone and other oral contraceptives. Obstet Gynecol 110:587, 2007

Shanghai Dahua Pharmaceutical: Sino-implant (II): questions and answers for clients. 2012. Available at: http://www.k4health.org/toolkits/implants/sino-implant-ii%C2%AE-implants. Accessed February 16, 2013

Shimoni N, Davis A, Ramos ME, et al: Timing of copper intrauterine device insertion after medical abortion: a randomized controlled trial. Obstet Gynecol 118(3):623, 2011

Shulman LP, Gabriel H: Management and localization strategies for the nonpalpable Implanon rod. Contraception 73:325, 2006

Sivin I, Viegas O, Campodonico I, et al: Clinical performance of a new two-rod levonorgestrel contraceptive implant: a three-year randomized study with Norplant implants as controls. Contraception 55(2):73, 1997

Sneed R, Westhoff C, Morroni C, et al: A prospective study of immediate initiation of depot medroxyprogesterone acetate contraceptive injection. Contraception 71(2):99, 2005

Stadel BV: Oral contraceptives and cardiovascular disease. N Engl J Med 305:612, 1981

Steenland MW, Tepper NK, Curtis KM, et al: Intrauterine contraceptive insertion postabortion: a systematic review. Contraception 84(5):447, 2011

Steiner M, Lopez M, Grimes D, et al: Sino-implant (II)—a levonorgestrel releasing two-rod implant: systematic review of the randomized controlled trials. Contraception 81(3)197, 2010

Stuart GS, Cunningham FG: Contraception and sterilization. In Hoffman BL, Schorge JO, Schaffer JI, et al: Williams Gynecology, 2nd ed. New York, McGraw-Hill, 2012, p 139

Sufrin CB, Postlethwaite D, Armstrong MA, et al: *Neisseria gonorrhea* and *Chlamydia trachomatis* screening at intrauterine device insertion and pelvic inflammatory disease. Obstet Gynecol 120(6):1314, 2012

Svendal G, Berk M, Pasco JA, et al: The use of hormonal contraceptive agents and mood disorders in women. J Affect Disord 140(1):92, 2012

Swenson C, Turok DK, Ward K, et al: Self-administered misoprostol or placebo before intrauterine device insertion in nulliparous women: a randomized controlled trial. Obstet Gynecol 120(2 Pt 1):341, 2012

Tatum HJ, Schmidt FH, Jain AK: Management and outcome of pregnancies associated with Copper-T intrauterine contraceptive device. Am J Obstet Gynecol 126:869, 1976

Tepper NK, Steenland MW, Gaffield ME, et al: Retention of intrauterine devices in women who acquire pelvic inflammatory disease: a systematic review. Contraception 87(5):655, 2013

Teva Women's Health: ParaGard T 380A intrauterine copper contraceptive: prescribing information, 2011. Available at: http://hcp.paragard.com/images/ParaGard_info.pdf. Accessed February 17, 2013

Thonneau PF, Almont TE: Contraceptive efficacy of intrauterine devices. Am J Obstet Gynecol 198:248, 2008

Truitt ST, Fraser AB, Gallo MF, et al: Combined hormonal versus nonhormonal versus progestin-only contraception in lactation. Cochrane Database Syst Rev 2:CD003988, 2010

Trussell J: Contraceptive efficacy. In Hatcher RA, Trussell J, Nelson AL, et al (eds): Contraceptive Technology, 20th ed. New York, Ardent Media, 2011a, p 791

Trussell J: Contraceptive failure in the United States. Contraception 70:89, 2011b

Tsilidis KK, Allen NE, Key TJ, et al: Oral contraceptive use and reproductive factors and risk of ovarian cancer in the European Prospective Investigation into Cancer and Nutrition. Br J Cancer 105(9):1436, 2011

Tworoger SS, Fairfield KM, Colditz GA, et al: Association of oral contraceptive use, other contraceptive methods, and infertility with ovarian cancer risk. Am J Epidemiol 166(8):894, 2007

Urdl W, Apter D, Alperstein A, et al: Contraceptive efficacy, compliance and beyond: factors related to satisfaction with once-weekly transdermal compared with oral contraception. Eur J Obstet Gynecol Reprod Biol 121:202, 2005

Van Vliet HA, Grimes DA, Helmerhorst FM, et al: Biphasic versus monophasic oral contraceptives for contraception. Cochrane Database Syst Rev 3:CD002032, 2006

Van Vliet HA, Grimes DA, Lopez LM, et al: Triphasic versus monophasic oral contraceptives for contraception. Cochrane Database Syst Rev 11: CD003553, 2011a

Van Vliet HA, Raps M, Lopez LM, et al: Quadriphasic versus monophasic oral contraceptives for contraception. Cochrane Database Syst Rev 11: CD009038, 2011b

Veres S, Miller L, Burington B: A comparison between the vaginal ring and oral contraceptives. Obstet Gynecol 104:555, 2004

Vessey M, Yeates D: Oral contraceptives and benign breast disease: an update of findings in a large cohort study. Contraception 76:418, 2007

Vessey MP, Johnson B, Doll R, et al: Outcome of pregnancy in women using intrauterine devices. Lancet 1:495, 1974

Wallach M, Grimes DA (eds): Modern Oral Contraception. Updates from The Contraception Report. Totowa, Emron, 2000, pp 26, 90, 194

Walsh T, Grimes D, Frezieres R, et al: Randomised controlled trial of prophylactic antibiotics before insertion of intrauterine devices. IUD Study Group. Lancet 351:1005, 1998

Watson: Ella prescribing information. 2010. Available at: http://www.accessdata.fda.gov/drugsatfda_docs/label/2010/022474s000lbl.pdf. Accessed March 5, 2013

Wechselberger G, Wolfram D, Pülzl P, et al: Nerve injury caused by removal of an implantable hormonal contraceptive. Am J Obstet Gynecol 195(1):323, 2006

Westhoff C: IUDs and colonization or infection with *Actinomyces*. Contraception 75:S48, 2007a

Westhoff C, Heartwell S, Edwards S, et al: Initiation of oral contraceptive using a quick start compared with a conventional start: a randomized controlled trial. Obstet Gynecol 109:1270, 2007b

Westhoff C, Jain JK, Milson, et al: Changes in weight with depot medroxyprogesterone acetate subcutaneous injection 104 mg/0.65 mL. Contraception 75:261, 2007c

Westhoff C, Kerns J, Morroni C, et al: Quick start: novel oral contraceptive initiation method. Contraception 66:141, 2002

Westhoff C, Wieland D, Tiezzi L: Depression in users of depo-medroxyprogesterone acetate. Contraception 51(6):351, 1995

Westhoff CL, Torgal AH, Mayeda ER, et al: Pharmacokinetics of a combined oral contraceptive in obese and normal-weight women. Contraception 81(6):474, 2010

Wilailak S, Vipupinyo C, Suraseranivong V, et al: Depot medroxyprogesterone acetate and epithelial ovarian cancer: a multicentre case-control study. BJOG 119(6):672, 2012

Wilson W, Taubert KA, Gewitz M, et al: Prevention of infective endocarditis: Guidelines from the American Heart Association: a guideline from the American Heart Association Rheumatic Fever, Endocarditis, and Kawasaki Disease Committee, Council on Cardiovascular Surgery and Anesthesia, and the Quality of Care and Outcomes Research Interdisciplinary Working Group. Circulation 116:1736, 2007

Winner B, Peipert JF, Zhao Q, et al: Effectiveness of long-acting reversible contraception. N Engl J Med 366(21):1998, 2012

World Health Organization: A multinational case-control study of ectopic pregnancy. Clin Reprod Fertil 3:131, 1985
World Health Organization: Acute myocardial infarction and combined oral contraceptives: results of an international multi-center case-control study. Lancet 349:1202, 1997
World Health Organization: Cardiovascular disease and use of oral and injectable progestogen-only contraceptives and combined injectable contraceptives. Results of an international, multicenter, case-control study. Contraception 57:315, 1998
World Health Organization: Depot-medroxyprogesterone acetate (DMPA) and risk of endometrial cancer. Int J Cancer 49:186, 1991a
World Health Organization: Depot-medroxyprogesterone acetate (DMPA) and risk of invasive squamous cell cervical cancer. Contraception 45(4): 299, 1992
World Health Organization: Depot-medroxyprogesterone acetate (DMPA) and risk of liver cancer. Int J Cancer 49(2):182, 1991b
World Health Organization: Effects of hormonal contraceptives on breast milk composition and infant growth. Stud Fam Plann 19/361, 1988
World Health Organization: Ischaemic stroke and combined oral contraceptives: results of an international, multi-center case-control study. Lancet 348:498, 1996
World Health Organization: Mechanism of action, safety and efficacy of intrauterine devices. Technical Report No. 753, Geneva, Switzerland, WHO, 1987
World Health Organization: Medical Eligibility for Contraceptive Use, 4th ed. 2009. Geneva, World Health Organization, 2010
World Health Organization/Department of Reproductive Health and Research (WHO/RHR), Johns Hopkins Bloomberg School of Public Health (SHSPH): Family Planning Handbook for Providers, Baltimore and Geneva, 2007
Wu S, Godfrey EM, Wojdyla D, et al: Copper T380A intrauterine device for emergency contraception: a prospective, multicentre, cohort clinical trial. BJOG 117(10):1205, 2010
Yonkers KA, Brown C, Pearlstein TB, et al: Efficacy of a new low-dose oral contraceptive with drospirenone in premenstrual dysphoric disorder. Obstet Gynecol 106:492, 2005
Zeino MY, Wietfeldt ED, Advani V, et al: Laparoscopic removal of a copper intrauterine device from the sigmoid colon. JSLS 15(4):568, 2011
Zieman M, Guillebaud J, Weisberg E, et al: Contraceptive efficacy and cycle control with the Ortho Evra/Evra transdermal system: the analysis of pooled data. Fertil Steril 77:S13, 2002
Zieman M, Kanal E: Copper T 380A IUD and magnetic resonance imaging. Contraception 75:93, 2007

CHAPTER 39
Sterilization

Sterilization is a popular choice of contraception for millions of men and women. This procedure is indicated in those requesting sterilization and who clearly understand its permanence as well as its difficult and often unsuccessful reversal. The American College of Obstetricians and Gynecologists (2009, 2013) recommends that all persons considering sterilization should also be counseled regarding alternative contraceptive choices.

FEMALE STERILIZATION

Almost a fourth of all women using contraception in the United States from 2006 through 2008 chose a form of sterilization (Mosher, 2010). And, for women aged 35 to 44 years, surgical sterilization was their most commonly reported form of birth control (Brunner Huber, 2009).

Female sterilization is usually accomplished by occlusion or division of the fallopian tubes. *Puerperal sterilization* procedures performed in conjunction with cesarean or vaginal delivery follow approximately 8 percent of all live births in the United States (Chan, 2010). *Nonpuerperal tubal sterilization* is done at a time unrelated to recent pregnancy and is also termed interval sterilization. These latter procedures are usually accomplished via laparoscopy as outpatient surgery. Hysteroscopic or minilaparotomy approaches to occlusion are also available.

Puerperal Tubal Sterilization

For several days after delivery, the uterine fundus lies at the level of the umbilicus, and fallopian tubes are accessible directly beneath the abdominal wall. Moreover, abdominal laxity allows easy repositioning of the incision over each uterine cornu. Thus, puerperal sterilization is technically simple, and hospitalization need not be prolonged.

Some prefer to perform sterilization immediately following delivery, although others wait for 12 to 24 hours. At Parkland Hospital, puerperal tubal ligation is performed in the obstetrical surgical suite the morning after delivery. This minimizes hospital stay but lowers the likelihood that postpartum hemorrhage would complicate recovery following surgery. In addition, the status of the newborn can be better ascertained before surgery.

Various techniques are now used to disrupt tubal patency. In general, a midtubal segment of fallopian tube is excised, and the severed ends seal by fibrosis and peritoneal regrowth. Commonly used methods of interval sterilization include the Parkland, Pomeroy, and modified Pomeroy techniques (American College of Obstetricians and Gynecologists, 2013). Irving and Uchida techniques or Kroener fimbriectomy are rarely used because they involve increased dissection, operative time, and chance of mesosalpingeal injury. With fimbriectomy, unfavorably high failure rates stem from recanalization of the proximal tubal segment (Pati, 2000).

Surgical Technique

If scheduled for the first postpartum day, puerperal sterilization is typically completed using spinal analgesia. If done more proximate to delivery, the same epidural catheter used for labor analgesia can be used for sterilization analgesia. General anesthesia may be less desirable due to residual pregnancy-related airway changes (Bucklin, 2003).

The bladder is emptied before surgery. A small infraumbilical incision is made. Adequate exposure is critical, and Army-Navy or appendiceal retractors are usually suitable. For obese women, a slightly larger incision and narrow Deaver retractors may be required. If bowel or omentum is obstructing, then Trendelenburg position may be helpful. Digitally packing with a single, moist, fanned-out piece of surgical gauze may also be used, but a hemostat should always be attached to the distal end to avert its retention. It is sometimes helpful to tilt the entire table to the opposite side of the tube being exposed.

The fallopian tube is identified and grasped at its midportion with a Babcock clamp, and the distal fimbria confirmed. This prevents confusing the round ligament with the midportion of the tube. A common reason for sterilization failure is ligation of the wrong structure, typically the round ligament. Therefore, identification and isolation of the distal tube prior to ligation is necessary. Whenever the tube is inadvertently dropped, it is mandatory to repeat this identification procedure. Surgical steps for ligation are outlined in Figures 39-1 and 39-2.

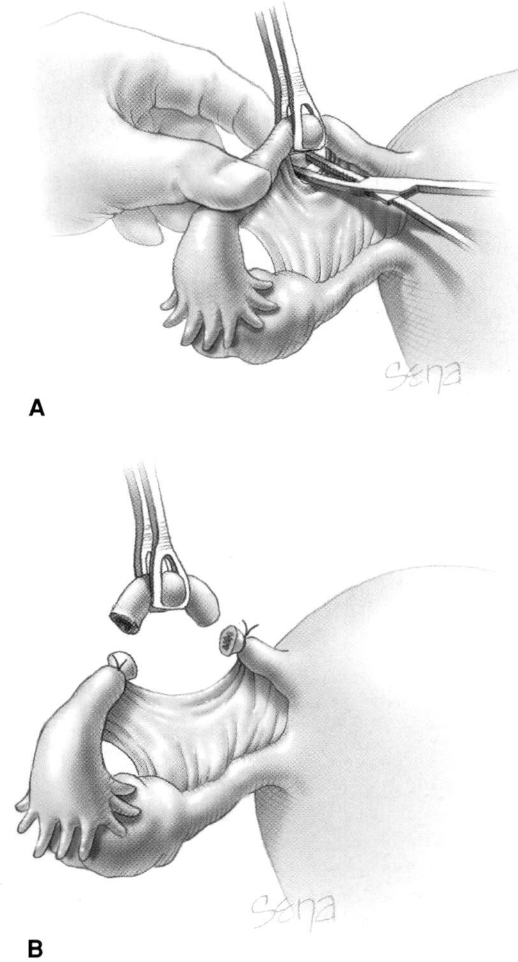

A

B

FIGURE 39-1 Parkland method. **A.** An avascular site in the mesosalpinx adjacent to the fallopian tube is perforated with a small hemostat. The jaws are opened to separate the fallopian tube from the adjacent mesosalpinx for approximately 2.5 cm. **B.** The freed fallopian tube is ligated proximally and distally with 0-chromic suture. The intervening segment of approximately 2 cm is excised, and the excision site is inspected for hemostasis. This method was designed to avoid the initial intimate proximity of the cut ends of the fallopian tube inherent with the Pomeroy procedure. (From Word, 2012, with permission.)

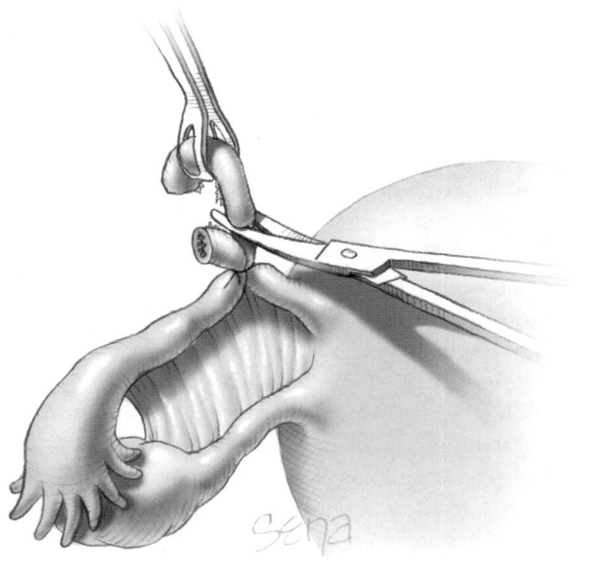

FIGURE 39-2 Pomeroy method. During ligation of a midsegment tubal loop, plain catgut is used to ensure prompt absorption of the ligature and subsequent separation of the severed tubal ends. (From Word, 2012, with permission.)

After surgery, diet is given as tolerated. Ileus is infrequent and should prompt concern for bowel injury, albeit rare. Most women have an uncomplicated course and are discharged on the first postoperative day.

Nonpuerperal (Interval) Surgical Tubal Sterilization

These techniques and other modifications basically consist of (1) ligation and resection at laparotomy as described earlier for puerperal sterilization; (2) application of permanent rings, clips, or inserts to the fallopian tubes by laparoscopy or hysteroscopy; or (3) electrocoagulation of a tubal segment, usually through a laparoscope. A detailed description and illustration of these can be found in *Williams Gynecology, 2nd edition* (Thompson, 2012).

In the United States, a laparoscopic approach to interval tubal sterilization is the most common. The procedure is frequently performed in an ambulatory surgical setting under general anesthesia. In almost all cases, the woman can be discharged within several hours. Minilaparotomy using a 3-cm suprapubic incision is also popular, especially in resource-poor countries (Kulier, 2004). Although not commonly used, the peritoneal cavity can be entered through the posterior vaginal fornix—colpotomy or culdotomy—to perform tubal interruption. Major morbidity is rare with either minilaparotomy or laparoscopy.

Long-Term Complications

Contraceptive Failure

Pregnancy following sterilization is uncommon. The Collaborative Review of Sterilization (CREST) study followed 10,863 women who had undergone tubal sterilization from 1978 through 1986

(Peterson, 1996). The cumulative failure rate for the various tubal procedures was 18.5 per 1000 or approximately 0.5 percent. The study found puerperal sterilization to be highly effective. The 5-year failure rate was 5 per 1000, and for 12 years, it was 7 per 1000.

Puerperal sterilization fails for two major reasons. First, surgical errors occur and include transection of the round ligament or only partial transection of the tube. For this reason, both tubal segments are submitted for pathological confirmation. Second, a fistulous tract or spontaneous reanastomosis may form between the severed tubal stumps.

Interval tubal sterilization may fail for several reasons. First, it may be due to equipment failure such as a defective current for electrosurgery or an insufficiently occlusive clip (Belot, 2008). Second, failure may result from fistula formation, especially with electrosurgical procedures, or the fallopian tube may undergo spontaneous reanastomosis. A third possibility is that the woman may have been already pregnant at the time of surgery—a so-called luteal phase pregnancy. To limit this possibility, surgery may ideally be performed during the follicular phase, and an effective contraceptive method used before surgery. Last, in some cases, no reason is found. Importantly, Soderstrom (1985) found that most sterilization failures were not preventable.

Approximately 30 percent of pregnancies that follow a failed tubal sterilization procedure are ectopic. This rate rises to 50 percent for those following a bipolar coagulation procedure (McCausland, 1980; Peterson, 1997). Thus, any symptoms of pregnancy in a woman after tubal sterilization must be investigated, and an ectopic pregnancy excluded.

Other Effects

Ovarian and breast cancer risks are either decreased or unaffected following sterilization (Ness, 2011; Press, 2011). Women who have undergone tubal sterilization are highly unlikely to subsequently have salpingitis (Levgur, 2000). An almost twofold increased incidence of functional ovarian cysts follows tubal sterilization (Holt, 2003). Several investigators have evaluated the risk of menorrhagia and intermenstrual bleeding following tubal sterilization, and most have found no association (DeStefano, 1985; Peterson, 2000; Shy, 1992).

Less objective but important psychological sequelae of sterilization have also been evaluated. In the CREST study, Costello (2002) found that tubal ligation did not change sexual interest or pleasure in 80 percent of women. In most of the 20 percent of women who did report a change, positive effects were 10 to 15 times more likely.

Invariably, a number of women express regrets regarding sterilization, and this is especially true if performed at a younger age (Curtis, 2006; Kelekçi, 2005). In the CREST study, Jamieson (2002) reported that 7 percent of women who had undergone tubal ligation had regrets by 5 years. This is not limited to their own sterilization, because 6.1 percent of women whose husbands had undergone vasectomy had similar regrets.

Reversal of Tubal Sterilization

No woman should undergo tubal sterilization believing that subsequent fertility is guaranteed by either surgery or by assisted reproductive techniques. Both approaches are technically difficult, expensive, and not always successful. Pregnancy rates following surgical reanastomosis are higher in younger women, in those with significant tubal length remaining, and in those with isthmic-to-isthmic repairs (American Society for Reproductive Medicine, 2012). With surgical reversals, pregnancy rates vary from 45 to 85 percent (Trussell, 2003; Van Voorhis, 2000). Almost 10 percent of women who became pregnant following reversal of tubal sterilization have an ectopic pregnancy.

Salpingectomy and Hysterectomy

Newer evidence suggests that the fallopian tube may be the origin of pelvic serous carcinomas, especially those of the ovary. With this knowledge, the Society of Gynecologic Oncologists (2013) has issued a practice statement recommending salpingectomy to lower cancer risks. Specifically, for women at average risk of ovarian cancer, risk-reducing salpingectomy should be discussed and considered with patients at the time of abdominal or pelvic surgery, with hysterectomy, or in lieu of tubal ligation. Initial steps of salpingectomy are shown in Figure 39–3. Further illustration and discussion of surgical steps are outlined in *Williams Gynecology, 2nd edition* (Word, 2012).

In the absence of uterine or other pelvic disease, hysterectomy solely for sterilization at the time of cesarean delivery, early in the puerperium, or even remote from pregnancy is difficult to justify. It carries significantly increased surgical morbidity compared with tubal sterilization (Jamieson, 2000; Nieboer, 2009).

Transcervical Sterilization

Intratubal Devices

There are several devices that are inserted via hysteroscopy to occlude the proximal fallopian tubes. These interval sterilization options include *Essure*, a microinsert that has a fine stainless-steel inner coil enclosed in polyester fibers and an

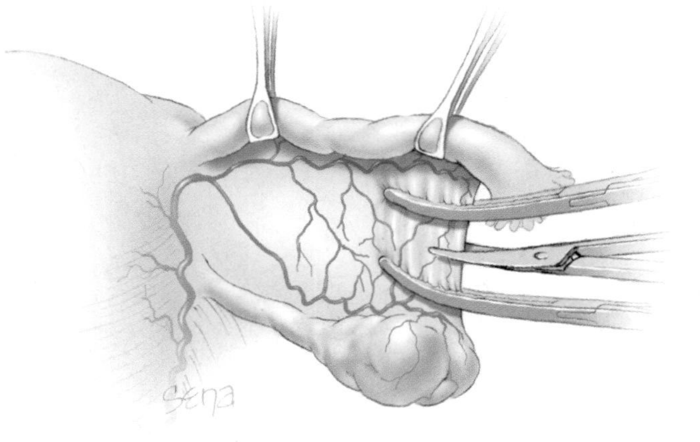

FIGURE 39-3 With salpingectomy, the mesosalpinx is sequentially clamped, cut, and ligated. (From Word, 2012, with permission.)

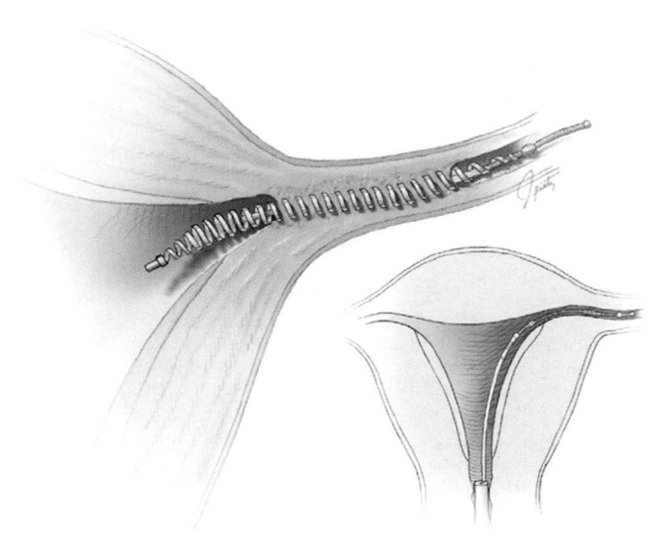

FIGURE 39-4 Essure microinsert placement hysteroscopically and ingrowth of tissue. (From Thompson, 2012, with permission.)

expandable outer coil of Nitinol—a nickel and titanium alloy (Fig. 39-4). The outer coil expands after placement, allowing the inner fibers also to expand. These synthetic fibers incite a chronic inflammatory response to prompt local tissue ingrowth that leads to complete tubal lumen occlusion (Valle, 2000).

For hysteroscopic placement, sedation, paracervical block, or both may be used, and in-office insertion is often selected. Devices cannot be placed in all women, and some do not tolerate the procedure awake (Duffy, 2005). Bilateral placement is achieved in 95 to 98 percent of cases (Anderson, 2011; Cooper, 2003; Miño, 2007). Rarely, intractable pelvic pain following insertion may require Essure removal (Beckwith, 2008; Lannon, 2007).

Because complete tubal blockage is not 100 percent, it must be confirmed by hysterosalpingography (HSG) 3 months following surgery (American College of Obstetricians and Gynecologists, 2012). With such confirmation, efficacy rates for these devices reach 98 to 99 percent (Anderson, 2011; Smith, 2010). Failures following transcervical sterilization include noncompliance with HSG or its misinterpretation, conception before insertion, insert expulsion, migration of one or both of the inserts, uterine perforation, and method failure (Levy, 2007; Veersema, 2010). Although data are limited to small case series, pregnancies conceived with Essure in place do not appear to be at increased risk from the device (Galen, 2011; Mijatovic, 2012; Veersema, 2013).

The other insert, *Adiana,* also stimulates tissue ingrowth for tubal occlusion using a cylindrical, 1.5 × 3.5 mm, nonabsorbent silicone elastomer matrix. However, for financial reasons, production of this device has now been discontinued by the manufacturer (Hologic, 2012).

Intratubal Chemical Methods

Although none is currently available in the United States, several chemical substances are used to cause sclerosis or obstruction of the tubal ostia (Abbott, 2007; Ogburn, 2007). Placement of quinacrine pellets into the uterine fundus with an IUD-type inserter method has been used worldwide in more than 100,000 women. The World Health Organization has lifted its ban on quinacrine use because studies have shown no evidence of carcinogenesis (Lippes, 2002). The major drawbacks are 1-, 5-, and 10-year cumulative pregnancy rates of 3, 10, and 12 percent, respectively (Sokal, 2008a,b, 2010).

MALE STERILIZATION

Currently, up to a half million men in the United States undergo vasectomy each year (Barone, 2006; Magnani, 1999). Through a small incision, the vas deferens lumen is disrupted to block the passage of sperm from the testes (Fig. 39-5). Alternatively, the no-scalpel method accomplishes this through a needle puncture in the scrotum. The latter method is associated with fewer minor surgical complications than the traditional incision technique, but each is equally effective (Cook, 2007).

Vasectomy is safer than tubal sterilization because it is less invasive and is performed with local analgesia (American College of Obstetricians and Gynecologists, 2013). In a review to compare the two, Hendrix and associates (1999) found that, compared with vasectomy, female tubal sterilization has a 20-fold increased complication rate, a 10- to 37-fold failure rate, and costs three times as much.

One disadvantage is that sterilization following vasectomy is not immediate. Complete release of sperm stored in the reproductive tract beyond the interrupted vas deferens takes approximately 3 months or 20 ejaculations. Although guidelines vary regarding the number and timing of postprocedural semen analyses, many investigators suggest that collection of only one azoospermic semen analysis at 3 months is sufficient evidence of sterility (Bodiwala, 2007; Griffin, 2005). During the period before azoospermia is documented, another form of contraception should be used.

The failure rate for vasectomy during the first year is 9.4 per 1000 procedures but only 11.4 per 1000 at 2, 3, and 5 years (Jamieson, 2004). Failures result from unprotected intercourse too soon after ligation, incomplete occlusion of the vas deferens, or recanalization (Awsare, 2005; Deneux-Tharaux, 2004).

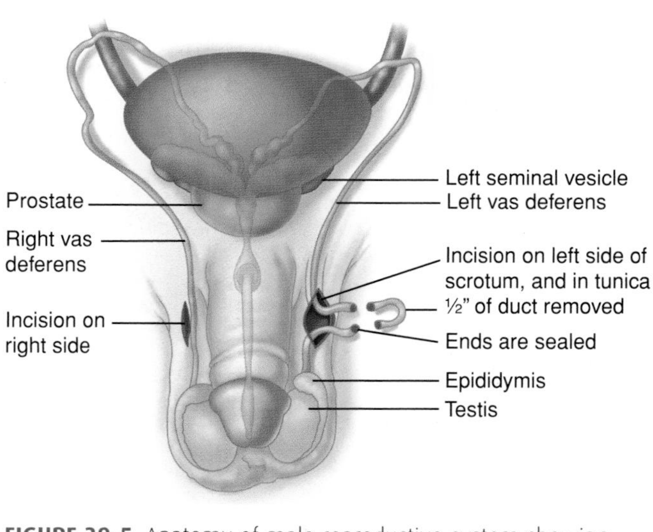

FIGURE 39-5 Anatomy of male reproductive system showing procedure for vasectomy.

Long-Term Effects

Other than regrets, long-term consequences are rare. A major one is troublesome chronic scrotal pain, which develops in up to 15 percent of men (Leslie, 2007; Manikandan, 2004). Previous concerns for atherogenesis, immune-complex mediated disease, testicular cancer, and prostate cancer have been allayed (Bernal-Delgado, 1998; Giovannucci, 1992; Goldacre, 1983; Møller, 1994).

Restoration of Fertility

Reanastomosis of the vas deferens can be completed most effectively using microsurgical techniques. Conception rates following reversal are adversely affected by longer duration from vasectomy, poor sperm quality found at reversal, and type of reversal procedure required (American Society for Reproductive Medicine, 2008).

REFERENCES

Abbott J: Transcervical sterilization. Curr Opin Obstet Gynecol 19:325, 2007

American College of Obstetricians and Gynecologists: Sterilization of women, including those with mental disabilities. Committee Opinion No. 371, July 2007, Reaffirmed 2009

American College of Obstetricians and Gynecologists: Use of hysterosalpingography after tubal sterilization. Committee Opinion No. 458, June 2010, Reaffirmed 2012

American College of Obstetricians and Gynecologists: Benefits and risks of sterilization. Practice Bulletin No. 133, February 2013

American Society for Reproductive Medicine: Committee Opinion: role of tubal surgery in the era of assisted reproductive technology. Fertil Steril 97(3):539, 2012

American Society for Reproductive Medicine: Vasectomy reversal. Fertil Steril 90:S78, 2008

Anderson TL, Vancaillie TG: The Adiana System for permanent contraception: safety and efficacy at 3 years. J Minim Invasive Gynecol 18(5):612, 2011

Awsare N, Krishnan J, Boustead GB, et al: Complications of vasectomy. Ann R Coll Surg Engl 87:406, 2005

Barone MA, Hutchison PL, Johnson CH, et al: Vasectomy in the Unites States, 2002. J Urol 176:232, 2006

Beckwith AW: Persistent pain after hysteroscopic sterilization with microinserts. Obstet Gynecol 111:511, 2008

Belot F, Louboutin A, Fauconnier A: Failure of sterilization after clip placement. Obstet Gynecol 111:515, 2008

Bernal-Delgado E, Latour-Pérez J, Pradas-Arnal F, et al: The association between vasectomy and prostate cancer: a systematic review of the literature. Fertil Steril 70:201, 1998

Bodiwala D, Jeyarajah S, Terry TR, et al: The first semen analysis after vasectomy: timing and definition of success. BJU Int 99:727, 2007

Brunner Huber LR, Huber KR: Contraceptive choices of women 35–44 years of age: findings from the Behavioral Risk Factor Surveillance System. Ann Epidemiol 19(11):823, 2009

Bucklin BA: Postpartum tubal ligation: timing and other anesthetic considerations. Clin Obstet Gynecol 46(3):657, 2003

Chan LM, Westhoff CL: Tubal sterilization trends in the United States. Fertil Steril 94(1):1, 2010

Cook LA, Pun A, van Vliet H, et al: Scalpel versus no-scalpel incision for vasectomy. Cochrane Database Syst Rev 18:CD004112, 2007

Cooper JM, Carignan CS, Cher D, et al: Microinsert nonincisional hysteroscopic sterilization. Obstet Gynecol 102(1):59, 2003

Costello C, Hillis S, Marchbanks P, et al: The effect of interval tubal sterilization on sexual interest and pleasure. Obstet Gynecol 100:3, 2002

Curtis KM, Mohllajee AP, Peterson HB: Regret following female sterilization at a young age: a systematic review. Contraception 73:205, 2006

Deneux-Tharaux C, Kahn E, Nazerali H, et al: Pregnancy rates after vasectomy: a survey of U.S. urologists. Contraception 69:401, 2004

DeStefano F, Perlman JA, Peterson HB, et al: Long term risk of menstrual disturbances after tubal sterilization. Am J Obstet Gynecol 152:835, 1985

Duffy S, Marsh F, Rogerson L, et al: Female sterilization: a cohort controlled comparative study of Essure versus laparoscopic sterilization. BJOG 112:1522, 2005

Galen DI, Khan N, Richter KS: Essure multicenter off-label treatment for hydrosalpinx before in vitro fertilization. J Minim Invasive Gynecol 18(3):338, 2011

Giovannucci E, Tosteson TD, Speizer FE, et al: A long-term study of mortality in men who have undergone vasectomy. N Engl J Med 326:1392, 1992

Goldacre JM, Holford TR, Vessey MP: Cardiovascular disease and vasectomy. N Engl J Med 308:805, 1983

Griffin T, Tooher R, Nowakowski K, et al: How little is enough? The evidence for post-vasectomy testing. J Urol 174:29, 2005

Hendrix NW, Chauhan SP, Morrison JC: Sterilization and its consequences. Obstet Gynecol Surv 54:766, 1999

Hologic: Hologic Announces Second Quarter Fiscal 2012 Operating Results. Available online at: http://investors.hologic.com/index.php?s=43&item=447. Accessed April 30, 2012

Holt VL, Cushing-Haugen KL, Daling JR: Oral contraceptives, tubal sterilization, and functional ovarian cyst risk. Obstet Gynecol 102:252, 2003

Jamieson DJ, Costello C, Trussell J, et al: The risk of pregnancy after vasectomy. Obstet Gynecol 103:848, 2004

Jamieson DJ, Hillis SD, Duerr A, et al: Complications of interval laparoscopic tubal sterilization: findings from the United States Collaborative Review of Sterilization. Obstet Gynecol 96:997, 2000

Jamieson DJ, Kaufman SC, Costello C, et al: A comparison of women's regret after vasectomy versus tubal sterilization. Obstet Gynecol 99:1073, 2002

Kelekçi S, Erdemoglu E, Kutluk S, et al: Risk factors for tubal ligation: regret and psychological effects. Impact of Beck Depression Inventory. Contraception 71:417, 2005

Kulier R, Boulvain M, Walker D, et al: Minilaparotomy and endoscopic techniques for tubal sterilization. Cochrane Database Syst Rev 3: CD0013282002, 2004

Lannon BM, Lee SY: Techniques for removal of the Essure hysteroscopic tubal occlusion device. Fertil Steril 88(2):497.e13, 2007

Leslie TA, Illing RO, Cranston DW, et al: The incidence of chronic scrotal pain after vasectomy: a prospective audit. BJU Int 100:1330, 2007

Levgur M, Duvivier R: Pelvic inflammatory disease after tubal sterilization: a review. Obstet Gynecol Surv 55:41, 2000

Levy B, Levie MD, Childers ME: A summary of reported pregnancies after hysteroscopic sterilization. J Minim Invasive Gynecol 14:271, 2007

Lippes J: Quinacrine sterilization: the imperative need for clinical trials. Fertil Steril 77:1106, 2002

Magnani RJ, Haws JM, Morgan GT, et al: Vasectomy in the United States, 1991 and 1995. Am J Public Health 89:92, 1999

Manikandan R, Srirangam SJ, Pearson E, et al: Early and late morbidity after vasectomy: a comparison of chronic scrotal pain at 1 and 10 years. BJU Int 93:571, 2004

McCausland A: High rate of ectopic pregnancy following laparoscopic tubal coagulation failures. Am J Obstet Gynecol 136:97, 1980

Mijatovic V, Dreyer K, Emanuel MH, et al: Essure hydrosalpinx occlusion prior to IVF-ET as an alternative to laparoscopic salpingectomy. Eur J Obstet Gynecol Reprod Biol 161(1):42, 2012

Miño M, Arjona JE, Cordón J, et al: Success rate and patient satisfaction with the Essure sterilisation in an outpatient setting: a prospective study of 857 women. BJOG 114:763, 2007

Møller H, Knudsen LB, Lynge E: Risk of testicular cancer after vasectomy: cohort study of over 73,000 men. BMJ 309:295, 1994

Moschos E, Twickler DM: Techniques used for imaging in gynecology. In Hoffman BL, Schorge JO, Schaffer JI, et al: Williams Gynecology, 2nd ed. New York, McGraw-Hill, 2012, p 48

Mosher WD, Jones J: Use of contraception in the United States: 1982–2008. National Center for Health Statistics. Vital Health Stat 23(29), 2010

Ness RB, Dodge RC, Edwards RP, et al: Contraception methods, beyond oral contraceptives and tubal ligation, and risk of ovarian cancer. Ann Epidemiol 21(3):188, 2011

Nieboer TE, Johnson N, Lethaby A, et al: Surgical approach to hysterectomy for benign gynaecological disease. Cochrane Database Syst Rev 3:CD003677, 2009

Ogburn T, Espey E: Transcervical sterilization: past, present and future. Obstet Gynecol Clin North Am 34:57, 2007

Pati S, Cullins V: Female sterilization: evidence. Obstet Gynecol Clin North Am 27:859, 2000

Peterson HB, Jeng G, Folger SG, et al: The risk of menstrual abnormalities after tubal sterilization. N Engl J Med 343:1681, 2000

Peterson HB, Xia Z, Hughes JM, et al: The risk of ectopic pregnancy after tubal sterilization. U.S. Collaborative Review of Sterilization Working Group. N Engl J Med 336(11):762, 1997

Peterson HB, Xia Z, Hughes JM, et al: The risk of pregnancy after tubal sterilization: findings from the U.S. Collaborative Review of Sterilization. Am J Obstet Gynecol 174:1161, 1996

Press DJ, Sullivan-Halley J, Ursin G, et al: Breast cancer risk and ovariectomy, hysterectomy, and tubal sterilization in the women's contraceptive and reproductive experiences study. Am J Epidemiol 173(1):38, 2011

Shy KK, Stergachis A, Grothaus LG, et al: Tubal sterilization and risk of subsequent hospital admission for menstrual disorders. Am J Obstet Gynecol 166:1698, 1992

Smith RD: Contemporary hysteroscopic methods for female sterilization. Int J Gynaecol Obstet 108(1):79, 2010

Society of Gynecologic Oncologists: SGO Clinical Practice Statement: Salpingectomy for Ovarian Cancer Prevention. Available at: https://www.sgo.org/clinical-practice/guidelines/sgo-clinical-practice-statement-salpingectomy-for-ovarian-cancer-prevention/. Accessed December 13, 2013

Soderstrom RM: Sterilization failures and their causes. Am J Obstet Gynecol 152:395, 1985

Sokal DC, Hieu do T, Loan ND, et al: Contraceptive effectiveness of two insertions of quinacrine: results from 10-year follow-up in Vietnam. Contraception 78:61, 2008a

Sokal DC, Hieu do T, Loan ND, et al: Safety of quinacrine contraceptive pellets: results from 10-year follow-up in Vietnam. Contraception 78:66, 2008b

Sokal DC, Trujillo V, Guzmán SC, et al: Cancer risk after sterilization with transcervical quinacrine: updated findings from a Chilean cohort. Contraception 81(1):75, 2010

Thompson M, Kho K: Minimally invasive surgery. In Hoffman BL, Schorge JO, Schaffer JI, et al: Williams Gynecology, 2nd ed. New York, McGraw-Hill, 2012, p 1172

Trussell J, Guilbert E, Hedley A: Sterilization failure, sterilization reversal, and pregnancy after sterilization reversal in Quebec. Obstet Gynecol 101: 677, 2003

Valle RF, Carignan CS, Wright TC, et al: Tissue response to the STOP microcoil transcervical permanent contraceptive device: results from a prehysterectomy study. Fertil Steril 76:974, 2001

Van Voorhis BJ: Comparison of tubal ligation reversal procedures. Clin Obstet Gynecol 43:641, 2000

Veersema S, Mijatovic V, Dreyer K, et al: Outcomes of Pregnancies in Women With Hysteroscopically Placed Micro-Inserts In Situ. J Minim Invasive Gynecol October 30, 2013 [Epub ahead of print]

Veersema S, Vleugels MP, Moolenaar LM, et al: Unintended pregnancies after Essure sterilization in the Netherlands. Fertil Steril 93(1):35, 2010

Word L, Hoffman BL: Surgeries for benign gynecologic conditions. In Hoffman BL, Schorge JO, Schaffer JI, et al: Williams Gynecology, 2nd ed. New York, McGraw-Hill, 2012, pp 1124, 1030, 1031

SECTION 11

OBSTETRICAL COMPLICATIONS

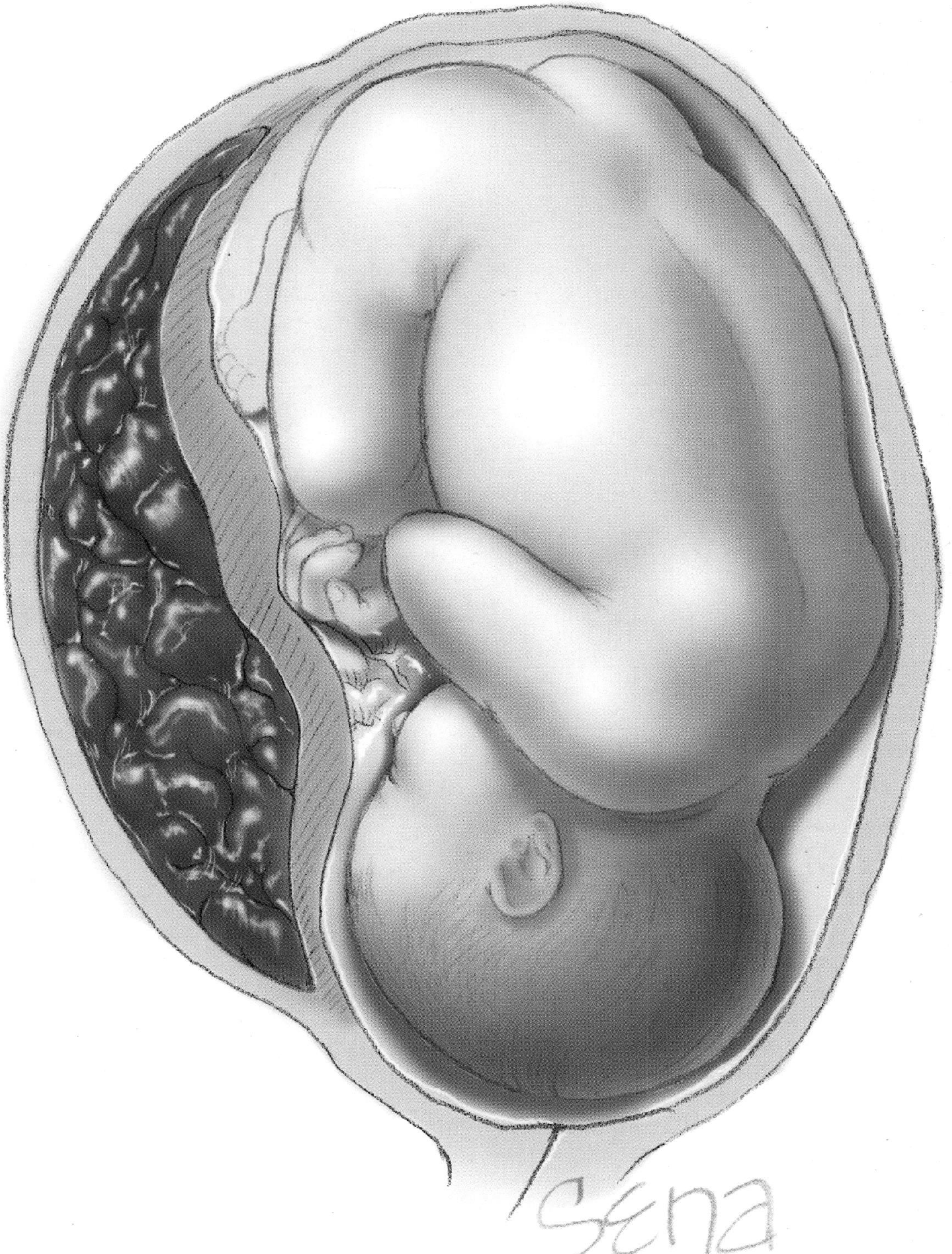

CHAPTER 40

Hypertensive Disorders

How pregnancy incites or aggravates hypertension remains unsolved despite decades of intensive research. Indeed, hypertensive disorders remain among the most significant and intriguing unsolved problems in obstetrics.

Hypertensive disorders complicate 5 to 10 percent of all pregnancies, and together they are one member of the deadly triad—along with hemorrhage and infection—that contributes greatly to maternal morbidity and mortality. Of these disorders, the *preeclampsia syndrome*, either alone or superimposed on chronic hypertension, is the most dangerous. As subsequently discussed, new-onset hypertension during pregnancy—termed *gestational hypertension*—is followed by signs and symptoms of preeclampsia almost half the time, and preeclampsia is identified in 3.9 percent of all pregnancies (Martin, 2012).

The World Health Organization (WHO) systematically reviews maternal mortality worldwide, and in developed countries, 16 percent of maternal deaths were reported to be due to hypertensive disorders (Khan, 2006). This proportion is greater than three other leading causes that include hemorrhage—13 percent, abortion—8 percent, and sepsis—2 percent. In the United States from 1998 to 2005, Berg and colleagues (2010) reported that 12.3 percent of 4693 pregnancy-related maternal deaths were caused by preeclampsia or eclampsia. The rate was similar to that of 10 percent for maternal deaths in France from 2003 through 2007 (Saucedo, 2013). Importantly, more than half of these hypertension-related deaths were preventable (Berg, 2005).

TERMINOLOGY AND DIAGNOSIS

In this country for the past two decades, pregnancy hypertension was considered using the terminology and classification promulgated by the Working Group of the National High Blood Pressure Education Program—NHBPEP (2000). To update these, a Task Force was appointed by President James Martin for the American College of Obstetricians and Gynecologists (2013b) to provide evidence-based recommendations for clinical practice. The basic classification was retained, as it describes four types of hypertensive disease:

1. Gestational hypertension—evidence for the preeclampsia syndrome does not develop and hypertension resolves by 12 weeks postpartum
2. Preeclampsia and eclampsia syndrome
3. Chronic hypertension of any etiology
4. Preeclampsia superimposed on chronic hypertension.

Importantly, this classification differentiates the preeclampsia syndrome from other hypertensive disorders because it is potentially more ominous. This concept aids interpretation of studies that address the etiology, pathogenesis, and clinical management of pregnancy-related hypertensive disorders.

Diagnosis of Hypertensive Disorders

Hypertension is diagnosed empirically when appropriately taken blood pressure exceeds 140 mm Hg systolic or 90 mm Hg diastolic. Korotkoff phase V is used to define diastolic pressure. Previously, incremental increases of 30 mm Hg systolic or 15 mm Hg diastolic from midpregnancy blood pressure values had

TABLE 40-1. Diagnostic Criteria for Pregnancy-Associated Hypertension

Condition	Criteria Required
Gestational hypertension	BP > 140/90 mmHg after 20 weeks in previously normotensive women
Preeclampsia—Hypertension and:	
Proteinuria	• ≥ 300 mg/24h, or • Protein: creatinine ratio ≥ 0.3 or • Dipstick 1+ persistent[a] *or*
Thrombocytopenia	• Platelets < 100,000/μL
Renal insufficiency	• Creatinine > 1.1 mg/dL or doubling of baseline[b]
Liver involvement	• Serum transaminase levels[c] twice normal
Cerebral symptoms	• Headache, visual disturbances, convulsions
Pulmonary edema	—

[a]Recommended only if sole available test.
[b]No prior renal disease.
[c]AST (aspartate aminotransferase) or ALT (alanine aminotransferase).
Modified from the American College of Obstetricians and Gynecologists, 2013b.

also been used as diagnostic criteria, even when absolute values were < 140/90 mm Hg. These incremental changes are no longer recommended criteria because evidence shows that such women are not likely to experience increased adverse pregnancy outcomes (Levine, 2000; North, 1999). That said, women who have a rise in pressure of 30 mm Hg systolic or 15 mm Hg diastolic should be observed more closely because eclamptic seizures develop in some of these women whose blood pressures have stayed < 140/90 mm Hg (Alexander, 2006). A sudden rise in mean arterial pressure later in pregnancy—also known as "delta hypertension"—may also signify preeclampsia even if blood pressure is < 140/90 mm Hg (Macdonald-Wallis, 2012; Vollaard, 2007).

Concept of "Delta Hypertension"

The systolic and diastolic blood pressure levels of 140/90 mm Hg have been arbitrarily used since the 1950s to define "hypertension" in nonpregnant individuals. As discussed in detail in Chapter 50 (p. 1000), these levels were selected by insurance companies for a group of middle-aged men. It seems more realistic to define normal-range blood pressures that fall between an upper and lower limit for blood pressure measurements for a particular population—such as young, healthy, pregnant women. A schematic example is shown in Figure 40-1 using arbitrary blood pressure readings. Data curves for both women show blood pressure measurements near the 25th percentile until 32 weeks. These begin to rise in patient B, who by term has substantively increased blood pressures. However, her pressures are still < 140/90 mm Hg, and thus she is considered to be "normotensive." We termed this rather acute increase in blood pressure as "delta hypertension." As discussed later, some of these women will develop eclamptic seizures or HELLP (hemolysis, elevated liver enzyme levels, low platelet count) syndrome while still normotensive.

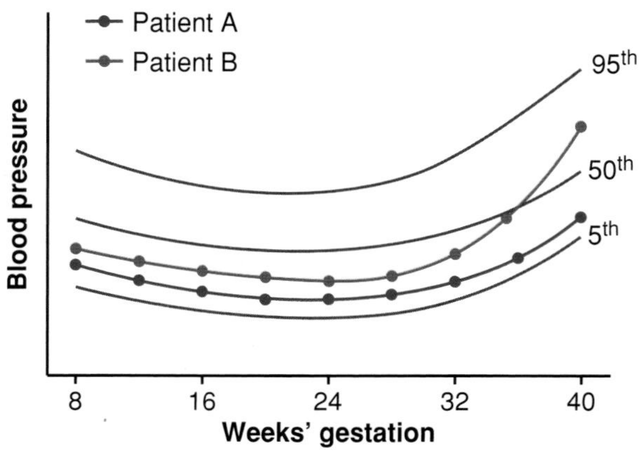

FIGURE 40-1 Schematic shows normal reference ranges for blood pressure changes across pregnancy. Patient A (*blue*) has blood pressures near the 20th percentile throughout pregnancy. Patient B (*red*) has a similar pattern with pressures at about the 25th percentile until about 36 weeks when blood pressure begins to increase. By term, it is substantively higher and in the 75th percentile, but she is still considered "normotensive."

Gestational Hypertension

This diagnosis is made in women whose blood pressures reach 140/90 mm Hg or greater for the first time after midpregnancy, but in whom *proteinuria is not identified* (Table 40-1). Almost half of these women subsequently develop preeclampsia syndrome, which includes findings such as headaches or epigastric pain, proteinuria, and thrombocytopenia. Even so, when blood pressure increases appreciably, it is dangerous to both mother and fetus to ignore this rise only because proteinuria has not yet developed. As Chesley (1985) emphasized, 10 percent of eclamptic seizures develop before overt proteinuria can be detected. Finally, gestational hypertension is reclassified by some as *transient hypertension* if evidence for preeclampsia does not develop and the blood pressure returns to normal by 12 weeks postpartum.

Preeclampsia Syndrome

As emphasized throughout this chapter, *preeclampsia is best described as a pregnancy-specific syndrome that can affect virtually every organ system.* And, although preeclampsia is much more than simply gestational hypertension with proteinuria, appearance of proteinuria remains an important diagnostic criterion. Thus, proteinuria is an *objective* marker and reflects the system-wide endothelial leak, which characterizes the preeclampsia syndrome.

Abnormal protein excretion is arbitrarily defined by 24-hour urinary excretion exceeding 300 mg; a urine protein:creatinine ratio ≥ 0.3; or persistent 30 mg/dL (1+ dipstick) protein in random urine samples (Lindheimer, 2008a). None of these values is sacrosanct, and urine concentrations vary widely during the day, as do dipstick readings. Thus, assessment may show a dipstick value of 1+ to 2+ from concentrated urine specimens from women who excrete < 300 mg/day. As discussed on page 740, it is likely that determination of a spot urine:creatinine ratio is a suitable replacement for a 24-hour urine measurement (Chap. 4, p. 65).

It is now appreciated that overt proteinuria may not be a feature in some women with the preeclampsia syndrome (Sibai, 2009). Because of this, the Task Force (2013) suggested other diagnostic criteria, which are shown in Table 40-1. Evidence of multiorgan involvement may include thrombocytopenia, renal dysfunction, hepatocellular necrosis ("liver dysfunction"), central nervous system perturbations, or pulmonary edema.

Indicators of Preeclampsia Severity

The markers listed in Table 40-1 are also used to classify preeclampsia syndrome severity. Although many use a dichotomous "mild" and "severe" classification, the Task Force (2013) discourages the use of "mild preeclampsia." It is problematic that there are criteria for the diagnosis of "severe" preeclampsia, but the default classification is either implied or specifically termed as "mild," "less severe," or "nonsevere" (Alexander, 2003; Lindheimer, 2008b). There are no generally agreed-on criteria for "moderate" preeclampsia—an elusive third category. We use the criteria listed in Table 40-2, which are categorized as "severe" versus "nonsevere." Importantly, while it is pragmatic that nonsevere classifications include "moderate" and "mild," these have not been specifically defined.

TABLE 40-2. Indicators of Severity of Gestational Hypertensive Disorders[a]

Abnormality	Nonsevere[b]	Severe
Diastolic BP	< 110 mm Hg	≥ 110 mm Hg
Systolic BP	< 160 mm Hg	≥ 160 mm Hg
Proteinuria[c]	None to positive	None to positive
Headache	Absent	Present
Visual disturbances	Absent	Present
Upper abdominal pain	Absent	Present
Oliguria	Absent	Present
Convulsion (eclampsia)	Absent	Present
Serum creatinine	Normal	Elevated
Thrombocytopenia (< 100,000/μL)	Absent	Present
Serum transaminase elevation	Minimal	Marked
Fetal-growth restriction	Absent	Obvious
Pulmonary edema	Absent	Present

[a]Compare with criteria in Table 40-1.
[b]Includes "mild" and "moderate" hypertension not specifically defined.
[c]Most disregard degrees of proteinuria as being nonsevere or severe.
BP = blood pressure.

Some symptoms are considered to be ominous. *Headaches* or *visual disturbances* such as *scotomata* can be premonitory symptoms of eclampsia. *Epigastric or right upper quadrant pain* frequently accompanies hepatocellular necrosis, ischemia, and edema that ostensibly stretches Glisson capsule. This characteristic pain is frequently accompanied by elevated serum hepatic transaminase levels. Finally, *thrombocytopenia* is also characteristic of worsening preeclampsia as it signifies platelet activation and aggregation as well as microangiopathic hemolysis. Other factors indicative of severe preeclampsia include renal or cardiac involvement and obvious fetal-growth restriction, which also attests to its duration.

As will be discussed, the more profound these signs and symptoms, the less likely they can be temporized, and the more likely delivery will be required. *A caveat is that differentiation between nonsevere and severe gestational hypertension or preeclampsia can be misleading because what might be apparently mild disease may progress rapidly to severe disease.*

Eclampsia

In a woman with preeclampsia, a convulsion that cannot be attributed to another cause is termed *eclampsia*. The seizures are generalized and may appear before, during, or after labor. The proportion who do not develop seizures until after 48 hours postpartum approximates 10 percent (Sibai, 2005). In some reports, up to a fourth of eclamptic seizures develop beyond 48 hours postpartum (Chames, 2002). Our experiences from Parkland Hospital, however, are that delayed postpartum eclampsia continues to occur in about 10 percent of cases—similar to what we first reported more than 20 years ago (Alexander, 2006; Brown, 1987). This lower percentage was also found in 222 women with eclampsia from The Netherlands (Zwart, 2008).

Preeclampsia Superimposed on Chronic Hypertension

Regardless of its cause, any chronic hypertensive disorder predisposes a woman to develop superimposed preeclampsia syndrome. Chronic underlying hypertension is diagnosed in women with documented blood pressures ≥ 140/90 mm Hg before pregnancy or before 20 weeks' gestation, or both. Hypertensive disorders can create difficult problems with diagnosis and management in women who are not first seen until after midpregnancy. This is because blood pressure normally decreases during the second and early third trimesters in both normotensive and chronically hypertensive women (Chap. 50, p. 1003). Thus, a woman with previously undiagnosed chronic vascular disease who is seen before 20 weeks frequently has blood pressures within the normal range. During the third trimester, however, as blood pressures return to their originally hypertensive levels, it may be difficult to determine whether hypertension is chronic or induced by pregnancy. Even a careful search for evidence of preexisting end-organ damage may be futile, as many of these women have mild disease and no evidence of ventricular hypertrophy, retinal vascular changes, or renal dysfunction.

In some women with chronic hypertension, their blood pressure increases to obviously abnormal levels, and this is typically after 24 weeks. If new-onset or worsening baseline hypertension is accompanied by new-onset proteinuria or other findings listed in Table 40-1, then superimposed preeclampsia is diagnosed. Compared with "pure" preeclampsia, superimposed preeclampsia commonly develops earlier in pregnancy. It also tends to be more severe and often is accompanied by fetal-growth restriction. The same criteria shown in Table 40-2 are also used to further characterize severity of superimposed preeclampsia.

INCIDENCE AND RISK FACTORS

Preeclampsia Syndrome

Young and nulliparous women are particularly vulnerable to developing preeclampsia, whereas older women are at greater risk for chronic hypertension with superimposed preeclampsia. The incidence is markedly influenced by race and ethnicity—and thus by genetic predisposition. By way of example, in nearly 2400 nulliparas enrolled in a Maternal-Fetal Medicine Units (MFMU) Network study, the incidence of preeclampsia was 5 percent in white, 9 percent in Hispanic, and 11 percent in African-American women (Myatt, 2012a,b).

Other factors include environmental, socioeconomic, and even seasonal influences (Lawlor, 2005; Palmer, 1999; Spencer, 2009). With consideration for these vicissitudes, in several worldwide studies reviewed by Staff and coworkers (2014), the incidence of preeclampsia in nulliparous populations ranged from 3 to 10 percent. The incidence of preeclampsia in multiparas is also variable but is less than that for nulliparas. Specifically, population studies from Australia, Canada, Denmark, Norway, Scotland, Sweden, and Massachusetts indicate an incidence of 1.4 to 4 percent (Roberts, 2011).

There are several other risk factors associated with preeclampsia. These include obesity, multifetal gestation, maternal age, hyperhomocysteinemia, and metabolic syndrome (Conde-Agudelo, 2000; Scholten, 2013; Walker, 2000). The relationship between maternal weight and the risk of preeclampsia is progressive. It increases from 4.3 percent for women with a body mass index (BMI) < 20 kg/m^2 to 13.3 percent in those with a BMI > 35 kg/m^2 (Fig. 48-5, p. 966). In women with a twin gestation compared with those with singletons, the incidence of gestational hypertension—13 versus 6 percent, and the incidence of preeclampsia—13 versus 5 percent, are both significantly increased (Sibai, 2000). It is interesting that this latter incidence is unrelated to zygosity (Maxwell, 2001).

Although smoking during pregnancy causes various adverse pregnancy outcomes, ironically, it has consistently been associated with a *reduced risk* for hypertension during pregnancy (Bainbridge, 2005; Zhang, 1999). Kraus and associates (2013) posit that this is because smoking upregulates placental adrenomedullin expression, which regulates volume homeostasis.

Women with preeclampsia in the first pregnancy are at greater risk in a second pregnancy compared with women normotensive during their first pregnancy (McDonald, 2009). And conversely, in the woman who was normotensive during her first pregnancy, the incidence of preeclampsia in a subsequent pregnancy is much lower than for a first pregnancy. In a population-based retrospective cohort analysis, Getahun and colleagues (2007) studied almost 137,000 second pregnancies in such women. The incidence for preeclampsia in secundigravida white women was 1.8 percent compared with 3 percent in African-American women.

Eclampsia

Presumably because it is somewhat preventable by adequate prenatal care, the incidence of eclampsia has decreased over the years in areas where health care is more readily available. In countries with adequate resources, its incidence averages 1 in 2000 deliveries. Ventura and associates (2000) estimated that the incidence in the United States in 1998 was 1 in 3250 births. According to the Royal College of Obstetricians and Gynaecologists (2006), it approximates 1 in 2000 in the United Kingdom. Akkawi and coworkers (2009) reported it to be 1 in 2500 in Dublin, Andersgaard and associates (2006) as 1 per 2000 for Scandinavia, and Zwart and colleagues (2008) as 1 per 1600 for The Netherlands.

ETIOPATHOGENESIS

Any satisfactory theory concerning the etiology and pathogenesis of preeclampsia must account for the observation that gestational hypertensive disorders are more likely to develop in women with the following characteristics:

- Are exposed to chorionic villi for the first time
- Are exposed to a superabundance of chorionic villi, as with twins or hydatidiform mole
- Have preexisting conditions of endothelial cell activation or inflammation such as diabetes or renal or cardiovascular disease
- Are genetically predisposed to hypertension developing during pregnancy.

A fetus is not a requisite for preeclampsia to develop. And, although chorionic villi are essential, they need not be intrauterine. For example, Worley and associates (2008) reported a 30-percent incidence in women with an extrauterine pregnancy exceeding 18 weeks' gestation. Regardless of precipitating etiology, the cascade of events leading to the preeclampsia syndrome is characterized by abnormalities that result in vascular endothelial damage with resultant vasospasm, transudation of plasma, and ischemic and thrombotic sequelae.

Phenotypic Expression of Preeclampsia Syndrome

The preeclampsia syndrome is widely variable in its clinical phenotypic expression. There are at least two major subtypes differentiated by whether or not remodeling of uterine spiral arterioles by endovascular trophoblastic invasion is defective. This concept has given rise to the "two-stage disorder" theory of preeclampsia etiopathogenesis. Ness and Roberts (1996) consider that the two-stage disorder includes "maternal and placental preeclampsia." According to Redman and coworkers (2014), stage 1 is caused by faulty endovascular trophoblastic remodeling that downstream causes the stage 2 clinical syndrome. Importantly, stage 2 is susceptible to modification by preexisting maternal conditions that are manifest by endothelial cell activation or inflammation. Such conditions include cardiovascular or renal disease, diabetes, obesity, immunological disorders, or hereditary influences.

Such compartmentalization is artificial, and it seems logical to us that preeclampsia syndrome presents clinically as a spectrum of worsening disease. Moreover, evidence is accruing that many "isoforms" exist as discussed below. Examples include differences in maternal and fetal characteristics, placental findings, and hemodynamic findings (Phillips, 2010; Valensise, 2008; van der Merwe, 2010).

Etiology

Writings describing eclampsia have been traced as far back as 2200 BC (Lindheimer, 2014). And, an imposing number of mechanisms have been proposed to explain its cause. Those currently considered important include:

1. Placental implantation with abnormal trophoblastic invasion of uterine vessels
2. Immunological maladaptive tolerance between maternal, paternal (placental), and fetal tissues
3. Maternal maladaptation to cardiovascular or inflammatory changes of normal pregnancy
4. Genetic factors including inherited predisposing genes and epigenetic influences.

Abnormal Trophoblastic Invasion

Normal implantation is characterized by extensive remodeling of the spiral arterioles within the decidua basalis as shown schematically in Figure 40-2 (Chap. 5, p. 93). Endovascular trophoblasts replace the vascular endothelial and muscular linings to enlarge the vessel diameter. The veins are invaded only superficially. In some cases of preeclampsia, however, there may be *incomplete trophoblastic invasion.* With this, decidual vessels, but not myometrial vessels, become lined with endovascular trophoblasts. The deeper myometrial arterioles do not lose their endothelial lining and musculoelastic tissue, and their mean external diameter is only half that of corresponding vessels in normal placentas (Fisher, 2014). In general, the magnitude of defective trophoblastic invasion is thought to correlate with severity of the hypertensive disorder (Madazli, 2000).

Using electron microscopy, De Wolf and coworkers (1980) examined arteries taken from the implantation site. They reported that early preeclamptic changes included endothelial damage, insudation of plasma constituents into vessel walls, proliferation of myointimal cells, and medial necrosis. Lipid accumulated first in myointimal cells and then within macrophages. These lipid-laden cell changes, shown in Figure 40-3, were referred to as *atherosis* by Hertig (1945). Nelson and colleagues (2014) completed placental examination in more than 1200 women with preeclampsia. These investigators reported that vascular lesions including spiral arteriole narrowing, atherosis, and infarcts were more common in placentas from women diagnosed with preeclampsia before 34 weeks.

Thus, the abnormally narrow spiral arteriolar lumen likely impairs placental blood flow. McMahon and colleagues (2014) have provided evidence that decreased soluble anti-angiogenic growth factors may be involved in faulty endovascular remodeling. Diminished perfusion and a hypoxic environment eventually lead to release of *placental debris* or *microparticles* that incite a systemic inflammatory response (Lee, 2012; Redman, 2012). Fisher and Roberts (2014) have provided an elegant review of the molecular mechanisms involved in these interactions.

Defective placentation is posited to further cause the susceptible (pregnant) woman to develop gestational hypertension, the preeclampsia syndrome, preterm delivery, a growth-restricted fetus, and/or placental abruption (Brosens, 2011; Kovo, 2010; McElrath, 2008; Nelson, 2014). In addition, Staff and coworkers (2013) have hypothesized that acute atherosis identifies a group of women at increased risk for later atherosclerosis and cardiovascular disease.

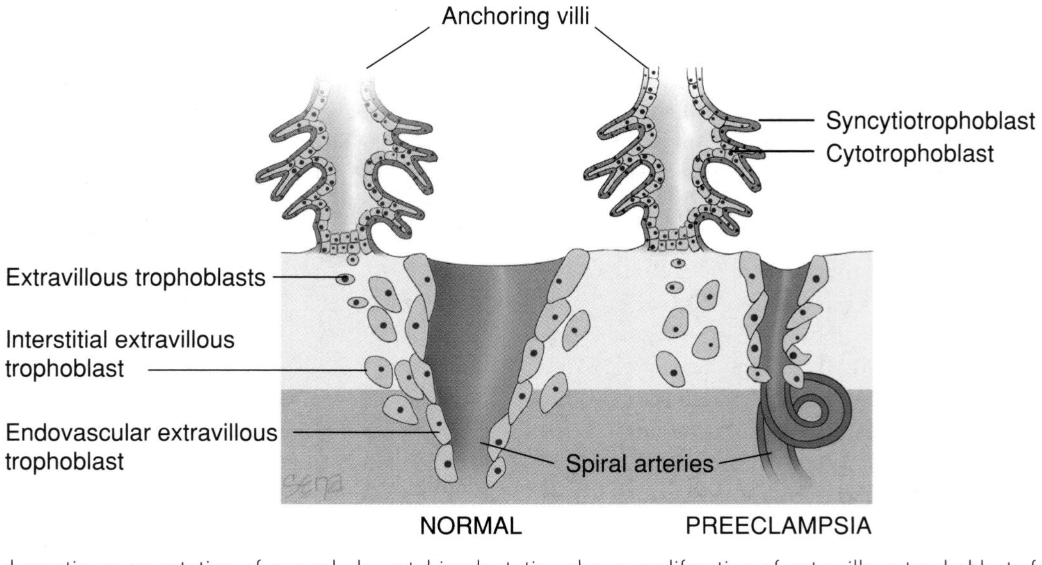

FIGURE 40-2 Schematic representation of normal placental implantation shows proliferation of extravillous trophoblasts from an anchoring villus. These trophoblasts invade the decidua and extend into the walls of the spiral arteriole to replace the endothelium and muscular wall to create a dilated low-resistance vessel. With preeclampsia, there is defective implantation characterized by incomplete invasion of the spiral arteriolar wall by extravillous trophoblasts. This results in a small-caliber vessel with high resistance to flow.

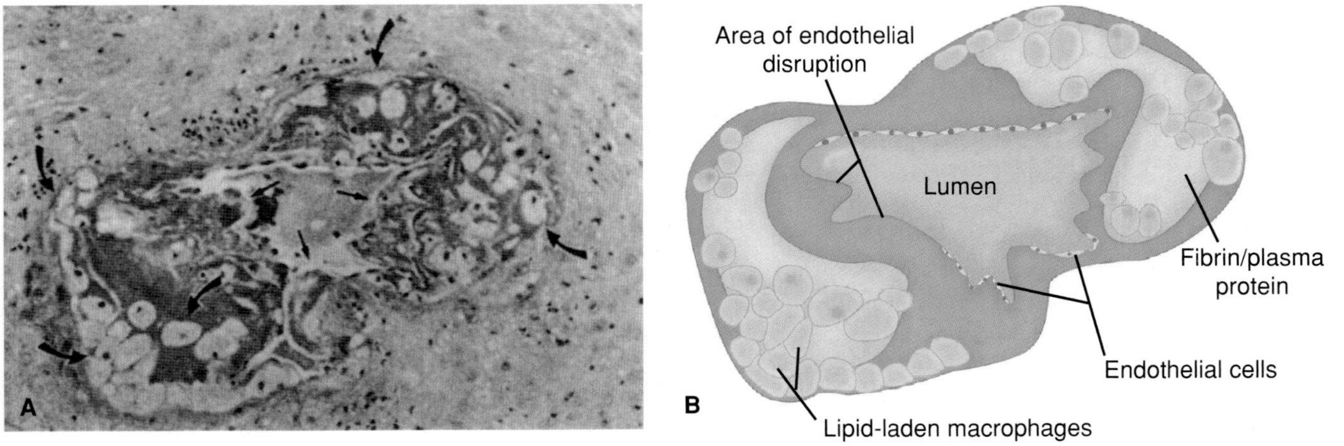

FIGURE 40-3 Atherosis in a blood vessel from a placental bed. **A.** Photomicrograph shows disruption of the endothelium that results in a narrowed lumen because of subendothelial accumulation of plasma proteins and foamy macrophages. Some of the foamy macrophages are shown by curved arrows, and straight arrows highlight areas of endothelial disruption. **B.** Schematic diagram of the photomicrograph. (Modified from Rogers, 1999, with permission.)

Immunological Factors

Maternal immune tolerance to paternally derived placental and fetal antigens is discussed in Chapter 5 (p. 97). Loss of this tolerance, or perhaps its *dysregulation*, is another theory cited to account for preeclampsia syndrome (Erlebacher, 2013). Certainly, the histological changes at the maternal-placental interface are suggestive of acute graft rejection. Some of the factors possibly associated with dysregulation include "immunization" from a previous pregnancy, some inherited human leukocyte antigen (HLA) and natural killer (NK)-cell receptor haplotypes, and possibly shared susceptibility genes with diabetes and hypertension (Fukui, 2012; Ward, 2014).

Inferential data also suggest preeclampsia to be an immune-mediated disorder. For example, the risk of preeclampsia is appreciably enhanced in circumstances in which formation of blocking antibodies to placental antigenic sites *might* be impaired. In this scenario, the first pregnancy would carry a higher risk. Tolerance dysregulation might also explain an increased risk when the paternal antigenic load is increased, that is, with two sets of paternal chromosomes—a "double dose." Namely, women with molar pregnancies have a high incidence of early-onset preeclampsia. Women with a trisomy 13 fetus also have a 30- to 40-percent incidence of preeclampsia. These women have elevated serum levels of antiangiogenic factors, and the gene for one of these factors, sFlt-1, is on chromosome 13 (Bdolah, 2006). Conversely, women previously exposed to paternal antigens, such as a prior pregnancy with the *same* partner, are "immunized" against preeclampsia. This phenomenon is not as apparent in women with a prior abortion. Strickland and associates (1986) studied more than 29,000 pregnancies at Parkland Hospital. These investigators reported that hypertensive disorder rates were decreased in women who previously had miscarried compared with nulligravidas. However, the difference, although statistically significant, was not great—22 versus 25 percent. Other studies have shown that multiparas impregnated by a new consort have an increased risk of preeclampsia (Mostello, 2002).

Redman and colleagues (2014) reviewed the possible role of *immune maladaptation* in preeclampsia pathophysiology. In women destined to be preeclamptic, extravillous trophoblasts early in pregnancy express reduced amounts of immunosuppressive nonclassic HLA G. Black women more commonly have the 1597ΔC allele that further predisposes to preeclampsia (Loisel, 2013). Zhou and coworkers (2012b) have shown this to be associated with high levels of placental oxidative products. These changes may contribute to defective placental vascularization in stage 1 of the preeclampsia syndrome (p. 732). Recall that as discussed in Chapter 4 (p. 56), during normal pregnancy, T-helper (Th) lymphocytes are produced so that type 2 activity is increased in relation to type 1—termed *type 2 bias* (Redman, 2012, 2014). Th2 cells promote humoral immunity, whereas Th1 cells stimulate inflammatory cytokine secretion. Beginning in the early second trimester in women who develop preeclampsia, Th1 action is increased and the Th1/Th2 ratio changes. Contributors to an enhanced immunologically mediated inflammatory reaction are stimulated by placental *microparticles* and by adipocytes (Redman, 2012, 2014).

Endothelial Cell Activation

In many ways, inflammatory changes are believed to be a continuation of the stage 1 changes caused by defective placentation as discussed above. In response to placental factors released by ischemic changes or by any other inciting cause, a cascade of events begins (Davidge, 2014). Thus, antiangiogenic and metabolic factors and other inflammatory mediators are thought to provoke endothelial cell injury.

Endothelial cell dysfunction may result from an extreme activated state of leukocytes in the maternal circulation (Faas, 2000; Gervasi, 2001). Briefly, cytokines such as tumor necrosis factor-α (TNF-α) and the interleukins (IL) may contribute to the oxidative stress associated with preeclampsia. This is characterized by reactive oxygen species and free radicals that lead to formation of self-propagating lipid peroxides (Manten, 2005). These in turn generate highly toxic radicals that injure endothelial cells, modify their nitric oxide production, and interfere with prostaglandin balance. Other consequences of oxidative stress include production of the lipid-laden macrophage foam cells seen in atherosis and shown in Figure 40-3; activation of microvascular coagulation manifest by thrombocytopenia; and increased capillary permeability manifest by edema and proteinuria.

These observations on the effects of oxidative stress in preeclampsia have given rise to increased interest in the potential benefit of antioxidants to prevent preeclampsia. Unfortunately, dietary supplementation with vitamins E (α-tocopherol) and C (ascorbic acid) to prevent preeclampsia has thus far proven unsuccessful (Task Force, 2013). This is discussed subsequently.

Nutritional Factors

John and colleagues (2002) showed that in the general population, a diet high in fruits and vegetables with antioxidant activity is associated with decreased blood pressure. Zhang and associates (2002) reported that the incidence of preeclampsia was doubled in women whose daily intake of ascorbic acid was less than 85 mg. These studies were followed by randomized trials to study dietary supplementation. Villar and coworkers (2006) showed that calcium supplementation in populations with a *low dietary calcium intake* had a small effect to lower perinatal mortality rates but no effect on preeclampsia incidence (p. 748). According to the 2013 Task Force, in several trials, supplementation with the antioxidant vitamins C or E showed no benefits.

Genetic Factors

From a hereditary viewpoint, preeclampsia is a multifactorial, polygenic disorder. In their comprehensive review, Ward and Taylor (2014) cite an incident risk for preeclampsia of 20 to 40 percent for daughters of preeclamptic mothers; 11 to 37 percent for sisters of preeclamptic women; and 22 to 47 percent for twins. In a study by Nilsson and colleagues (2004) that included almost 1.2 million Swedish births, there was a genetic component for gestational hypertension and for preeclampsia. They also reported 60-percent concordance in monozygotic female twin pairs.

The hereditary predisposition for preeclampsia likely is the result of interactions of literally hundreds of inherited genes—both maternal and paternal—that control myriad enzymatic and metabolic functions throughout every organ system. Plasma-derived factors may induce some of these genes in preeclampsia (Mackenzie, 2012). Thus, the clinical manifestation in any given woman with the preeclampsia syndrome will occupy a spectrum as previously discussed. In this regard, phenotypic expression will differ among similar genotypes depending on interactions with environmental factors (Yang, 2013).

Candidate Genes

Hundreds of genes have been studied for their possible association with preeclampsia (Buurma, 2013; Ward, 2014). Several of those that may have positive significant association with preeclampsia are listed in Table 40-3. Polymorphisms of the genes for Fas receptor, hypoxia-inducible factor-1α protein (HIF-1α), IL-1β, lymphotoxin-α, transforming growth factor beta 3 (TGF-β3), apolipoprotein E (ApoE), and TNF-α have also been studied with varying results (Borowski, 2009; Hefler, 2001; Jamalzei, 2013; Lachmeijer, 2001; Livingston, 2001; Wilson, 2009). Because of the heterogeneity of the preeclampsia syndrome and especially of the other genetic and environmental factors that interact with its complex phenotypic expression, it is doubtful that any *one* candidate gene will be found responsible. Indeed, Majander and associates (2013) have linked preeclampsia predisposition to *fetal* genes on chromosome 18.

TABLE 40-3. Genes with Possible Associations with Preeclampsia Syndrome

Gene (Polymorphism)	Function Affected
MTHFR (C677T)	Methylene tetrahydrofolate reductase
F5 (Leiden)	Factor V_{Leiden}
AGT (M235T)	Angiotensinogen
HLA (Various)	Human leukocyte antigens
NOS3 (Glu 298 Asp)	Endothelial nitric oxide
F2 (G20210A)	Prothrombin (factor II)
ACE (I/D^{at}Intron 16)	Angiotensin-converting enzyme
CTLA4	Cytotoxic T-lymphocyte-associated protein
LPL	Lipoprotein lipase
SERPINE1	Serine peptidase inhibitor

Data from Buurma, 2013; Staines-Urias, 2012; Ward, 2014.

Other Genetic Variables

An extensive list of other variables affect genotypic and phenotypic expression of the preeclampsia syndrome. Some include maternal and paternal genotypes, associated disorders, genomic ethnicity, gene-gene interactions, epigenetic phenomena, and gene-environmental interactions. Combinations of these are infinite. Ethnoracial factors are important as discussed regarding the high incidence of preeclampsia in African-American women. It may be that Latina women have a lower prevalence because of interactions of American Indian and white race genes (Shahabi, 2013).

Pathogenesis

Vasospasm

The concept of vasospasm with preeclampsia was advanced by Volhard (1918) based on his direct observations of small blood vessels in the nail beds, ocular fundi, and bulbar conjunctivae. It was also surmised from histological changes seen in various affected organs (Hinselmann, 1924; Landesman, 1954). Endothelial activation causes vascular constriction with increased resistance and subsequent hypertension. At the same time, endothelial cell damage causes interstitial leakage through which blood constituents, including platelets and fibrinogen, are deposited subendothelially. Wang and associates (2002) have also demonstrated disruption of endothelial junctional proteins. Suzuki and coworkers (2003) described ultrastructural changes in the subendothelial region of resistance arteries in preeclamptic women. The much larger venous circuit is similarly involved, and with diminished blood flow because of maldistribution, ischemia of the surrounding tissues can lead to necrosis, hemorrhage, and other end-organ disturbances characteristic of the syndrome. One important clinical correlate is the markedly attenuated blood volume seen in women with severe preeclampsia (Zeeman, 2009).

Endothelial Cell Injury

As discussed on page 733, during the past two decades, endothelial cell injury has become the centerpiece in the contemporary understanding of preeclampsia pathogenesis (Davidge, 2014). In this scheme, protein factor(s)—likely placental—are secreted into the maternal circulation and provoke activation and dysfunction of the vascular endothelium. Many of the facets of the clinical syndrome of preeclampsia are thought to result from these widespread endothelial cell changes. Grundmann and associates (2008) have reported that *circulating endothelial cell—CEC*—levels are elevated fourfold in the peripheral blood of preeclamptic women. Similarly, Petrozella and colleagues (2012) demonstrated increased levels of circulating endothelial microparticles—EMPs—in preeclamptic women.

Intact endothelium has anticoagulant properties, and endothelial cells blunt the response of vascular smooth muscle to agonists by releasing nitric oxide. Damaged or activated endothelial cells may produce less nitric oxide and secrete substances that promote coagulation and increase sensitivity to vasopressors (Gant, 1974). Further evidence of endothelial activation includes the characteristic changes in glomerular capillary endothelial morphology, increased capillary permeability, and elevated blood concentrations of substances associated with endothelial activation. These latter substances are transferable, and serum from women with preeclampsia stimulates some of these substances in greater amounts. It seems likely that multiple factors in plasma of preeclamptic women combine to have these vasoactive effects (Myers, 2007; Walsh, 2009).

Increased Pressor Responses

As discussed in Chapter 4 (p. 61), pregnant women normally develop refractoriness to infused vasopressors (Abdul-Karim, 1961). Women with early preeclampsia, however, have increased vascular reactivity to infused norepinephrine and angiotensin II (Raab, 1956; Talledo, 1968). Moreover, increased sensitivity to angiotensin II clearly precedes the onset of gestational hypertension (Gant, 1974).

Prostaglandins

Several prostanoids are thought to be central to preeclampsia syndrome pathophysiology. Specifically, the blunted pressor response seen in normal pregnancy is at least partially due to decreased vascular responsiveness mediated by endothelial prostaglandin synthesis. For example, compared with normal pregnancy, endothelial prostacyclin (PGI_2) production is decreased in preeclampsia. This action appears to be mediated by phospholipase A_2 (Davidge, 2014). At the same time, thromboxane A_2 secretion by platelets is increased, and the prostacyclin:thromboxane A_2 ratio decreases. The net result favors increased sensitivity to infused angiotensin II and, ultimately, vasoconstriction (Spitz, 1988). These changes are apparent as early as 22 weeks in women who later develop preeclampsia (Chavarria, 2003).

Nitric Oxide

This potent vasodilator is synthesized from L-arginine by endothelial cells. Withdrawal of nitric oxide results in a clinical picture similar to preeclampsia in a pregnant animal model (Conrad, 1989). Inhibition of nitric oxide synthesis increases mean arterial pressure, decreases heart rate, and reverses the pregnancy-induced refractoriness to vasopressors. In humans, nitric oxide likely is the compound that maintains the normal low-pressure vasodilated state characteristic of fetoplacental perfusion (Myatt, 1992; Weiner, 1992). It also is produced by fetal endothelium, and here it is increased in response to preeclampsia, diabetes, and sepsis (Parra, 2001; von Mandach, 2003).

The effects of nitric oxide production in preeclampsia are unclear (Davidge, 2014). It appears that the syndrome is associated with decreased endothelial nitric oxide synthase expression, thus increasing nitric oxide inactivation. These responses may be race related, with African-American women producing more nitric oxide (Wallace, 2009).

Endothelins

These 21-amino acid peptides are potent vasoconstrictors, and endothelin-1 (ET-1) is the primary isoform produced by human endothelium (George, 2011). Plasma ET-1 levels are increased in normotensive pregnant women, but women with preeclampsia have even higher levels (Ajne, 2003; Clark, 1992). According to Taylor and Roberts (1999), the placenta is not the source of increased ET-1 concentrations, and they likely arise from systemic endothelial activation. Interestingly, treatment of preeclamptic women with magnesium sulfate lowers ET-1 concentrations (Sagsoz, 2003).

Angiogenic and Antiangiogenic Proteins

Placental vasculogenesis is evident by 21 days after conception. There is an ever-expanding list of pro- and antiangiogenic substances involved in placental vascular development. The families of vascular endothelial growth factor (VEGF) and angiopoietin (Ang) are most extensively studied. *Angiogenic imbalance* is used to describe excessive amounts of antiangiogenic factors that are hypothesized to be stimulated by worsening hypoxia at the uteroplacental interface. Trophoblast of women destined to develop preeclampsia overproduces at least two antiangiogenic peptides that enter the maternal circulation (Karumanchi, 2014):

1. *Soluble Fms-like tyrosine kinase 1 (sFlt-1)* is a variant of the Flt-1 receptor for placental growth factor (PlGF) and for VEGF. Increased maternal sFlt-1 levels inactivate and decrease circulating free PlGF and VEGF concentrations,

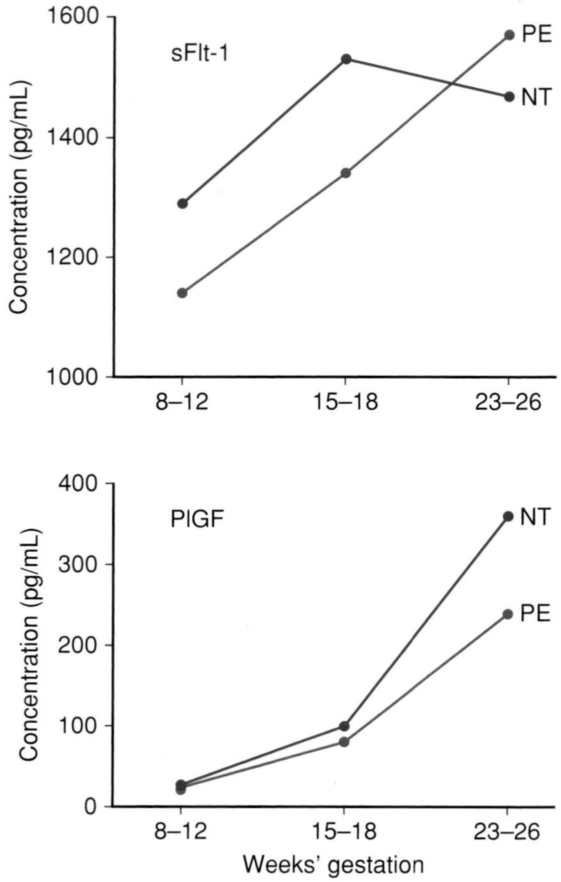

FIGURE 40-4 Angiogenic and antiangiogenic factors in normotensive (NT) and preeclamptic (PE) women across pregnancy. Both pairs of factors are significantly divergent by 23 to 26 weeks. sFlt = soluble Fms-like tyrosine kinase 1; PlGF = placental growth factor. (Data from Myatt, 2013.)

leading to endothelial dysfunction (Maynard, 2003). As shown in Figure 40-4, sFlt-1 levels begin to increase in maternal serum months before preeclampsia is evident. Haggerty and colleagues (2012) observed that these high levels in the second trimester were associated with a doubling of the risk for preeclampsia. This divergence from normal levels appears to occur even sooner with early-onset preeclampsia (Vatten, 2012).

2. *Soluble endoglin (sEng)* is a placenta-derived 65-kDa molecule that blocks endoglin, which is a surface coreceptor for the TGFβ family. Also called CD105, this soluble form of endoglin inhibits various TGFβ isoforms from binding to endothelial receptors and results in decreased endothelial nitric oxide-dependent vasodilatation (Levine, 2006; Venkatesha, 2006). Serum levels of sEng also begin to increase months before clinical preeclampsia develops (Haggerty, 2012).

The cause of placental overproduction of antiangiogenic proteins remains an enigma. Concentrations of the soluble forms are not increased in the fetal circulation or amnionic fluid, and their levels in maternal blood dissipate after delivery (Staff, 2007). Research currently is focused on immunological mechanisms, oxidative stress, mitochondrial pathology, and hypoxia genes (Karumanchi, 2014). Clinical research is directed at use of antiangiogenic proteins in the prediction and diagnosis of preeclampsia. In a systematic review, Widmer and associates (2007) concluded that third-trimester elevation of sFlt-1 levels and decreased PlGF concentrations correlate with preeclampsia development after 25 weeks. These results require verification in prospective studies. Subsequently, Haggerty and coworkers (2012) reported that doubling of expressions of sFlt-1 and sEng increased the preeclampsia risk 39 and 74 percent, respectively.

PATHOPHYSIOLOGY

Although the cause of preeclampsia remains unknown, evidence for its manifestation begins early in pregnancy with covert pathophysiological changes that gain momentum across gestation and eventually become clinically apparent. Unless delivery supervenes, these changes ultimately result in multiorgan involvement with a clinical spectrum ranging from an attenuated manifestation to one of cataclysmic deterioration that is life threatening for both mother and fetus. As discussed, these are thought to be a consequence of endothelial dysfunction, vasospasm, and ischemia. Although the many maternal consequences of the preeclampsia syndrome are usually described in terms of individual organ systems, they frequently are multiple, and they overlap clinically.

Cardiovascular System

Severe disturbances of normal cardiovascular function are common with preeclampsia syndrome. These are related to: (1) increased cardiac afterload caused by hypertension; (2) cardiac preload, which is affected negatively by pathologically diminished hypervolemia of pregnancy and is increased by intravenous crystalloid or oncotic solutions; and (3) endothelial activation with interendothelial extravasation of intravascular fluid into the extracellular space and importantly, into the lungs.

Hemodynamic Changes and Cardiac Function

The cardiovascular aberrations of pregnancy-related hypertensive disorders vary depending on several modifiers. These factors include hypertension severity, underlying chronic disease, preeclampsia severity, and in which part of the clinical spectrum these are studied. In some women, these cardiovascular changes may precede hypertension onset (De Paco, 2008; Easterling, 1990; Khalil, 2012; Melchiorre, 2013). Nevertheless, with the clinical onset of preeclampsia, cardiac output declines, due at least in part to increased peripheral resistance. When assessing cardiac function in preeclampsia, consideration is given to echocardiographic measures of *myocardial function* and to clinically relevant *ventricular function*.

Myocardial Function. Serial echocardiographic studies have documented in preeclampsia evidence for ventricular remodeling that is accompanied by diastolic dysfunction in 40 percent of women (Melchiorre, 2012). In some of these women, functional differences persisted up to 16 months after delivery (Evans, 2011). Ventricular remodeling was judged to be an

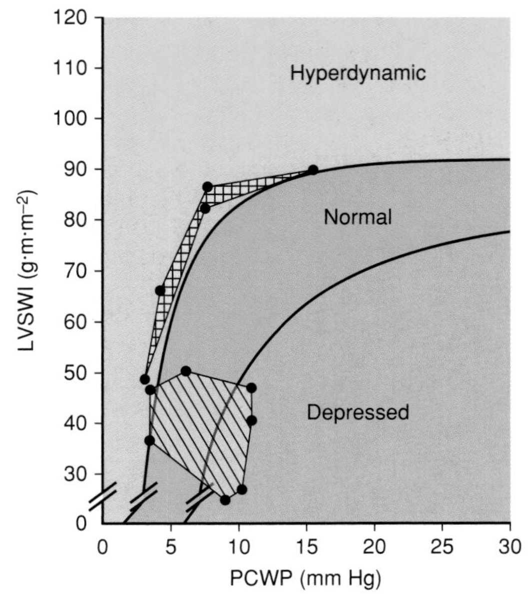

FIGURE 40-5 Ventricular function in normally pregnant women (*striped area*) and in women with eclampsia (*boxed area*) is plotted on a Braunwald ventricular function curve. Normal values are from Clark, 1989, and those for eclampsia are from Hankins, 1984. LVSWI = left ventricular stroke work index; PCWP = pulmonary capillary wedge pressure.

adaptive response to maintain normal contractility with the increased afterload of preeclampsia. In the otherwise healthy pregnant woman, these changes are usually clinically inconsequential. But when combined with underlying ventricular dysfunction—for example, concentric ventricular hypertrophy from chronic hypertension—further diastolic dysfunction may cause cardiogenic pulmonary edema as discussed in Chapters 47 (p. 943) and 49 (p. 990).

Ventricular Function. Despite the relatively high frequency of diastolic dysfunction with preeclampsia, in most women clinical cardiac function is appropriate. This has been shown by several studies in which ventricular function was assessed using invasive hemodynamic methods (Hibbard, 2014). Importantly, both normally pregnant women and those with preeclampsia syndrome can have normal or slightly hyperdynamic ventricular function (Fig. 40-5). Thus, both have a cardiac output that is appropriate for left-sided filling pressures. Data from preeclamptic women obtained by invasive hemodynamic studies are confounded because of the heterogeneity of populations and interventions that also may significantly alter these measurements. Some of these are crystalloid infusions, antihypertensive agents, and magnesium sulfate.

Ventricular function studies of preeclamptic women from several investigations are shown in Figure 40-6. Although cardiac function was hyperdynamic in all women, filling pressures were dependent on the volume of intravenous fluids. Specifically, aggressive hydration resulted in overtly hyperdynamic ventricular function in most women. However, this was accompanied by elevated pulmonary capillary wedge pressures. In some of these women, pulmonary edema may develop despite normal ventricular function because of an alveolar endothelial-epithelial leak. This is compounded by decreased oncotic pressure from a low serum albumin concentration (American College of Obstetricians and Gynecologists, 2012b).

Thus, increased cardiac output and hyperdynamic ventricular function is largely a result of low wedge pressures and not a result of augmented myocardial contractility. By comparison, women given appreciably larger volumes of fluid commonly had filling pressures that exceeded normal, but their ventricular function remained hyperdynamic because of concomitantly increased cardiac output.

From these studies, it is reasonable to conclude that aggressive fluid administration to otherwise normal women with severe preeclampsia substantially elevates normal left-sided filling pressures and increases a physiologically normal cardiac output to hyperdynamic levels.

Blood Volume

For nearly 100 years, *hemoconcentration* has been a hallmark of eclampsia. This was not precisely quantified until Zeeman and colleagues (2009) expanded the previous observations

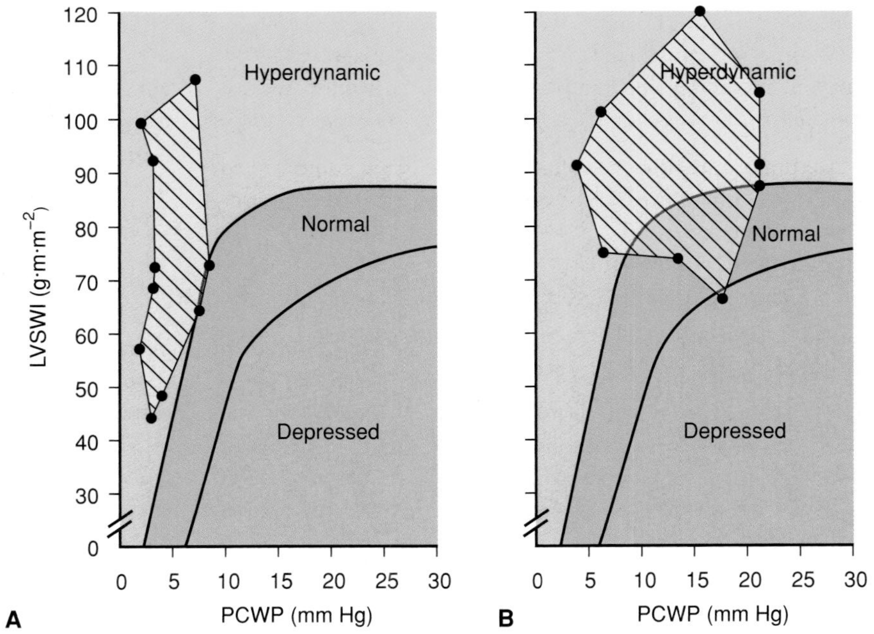

FIGURE 40-6 Ventricular function in women with severe preeclampsia–eclampsia plotted on the Braunwald ventricular function curve. The pulmonary capillary wedge pressures (PCWP) are lower in those managed with restricted fluid administration (*striped area in* **A**) compared with women managed with aggressive fluid therapy (*striped area in* **B**). In those managed with aggressive fluid infusions, eight developed pulmonary edema despite normal to hyperdynamic ventricular function in all but one. LVSWI = left ventricular stroke work index. (Data for **A** from Benedetti, 1980; Hankins, 1984; data for **B** from Rafferty, 1980; Phelan, 1982.)

of Pritchard and associates (1984) and showed in *eclamptic* women that the normally expected hypervolemia is severely curtailed (Fig. 40-7). Women of average size should have a blood volume of nearly 4500 mL during the last several weeks of a normal pregnancy. In nonpregnant women, this volume approximates only 3000 mL. With eclampsia, however, much or all of the anticipated normal excess 1500 mL is lost. Such hemoconcentration results from generalized vasoconstriction that follows endothelial activation and leakage of plasma into the interstitial space because of increased permeability. In women with *preeclampsia*, and depending on its severity, hemoconcentration is usually not as marked. Women with gestational hypertension, but without preeclampsia, usually have a normal blood volume (Silver, 1998).

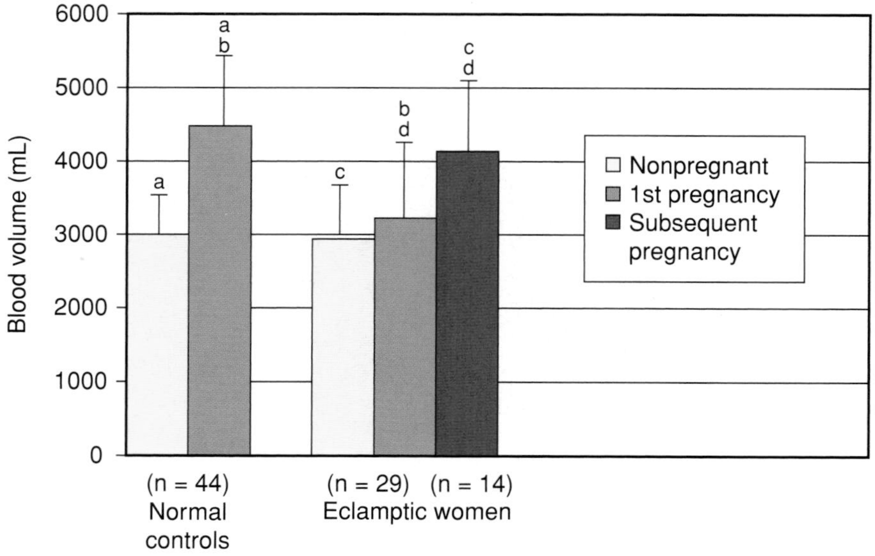

FIGURE 40-7 The two bar graphs on the left compare mean blood volumes in nonpregnant and term normally pregnant women. On the right, graphs display values for a group of 29 women with eclampsia and their nonpregnant values. The red bar reflects values for a subset of 14 who had a subsequent normotensive pregnancy. Extensions above bars represent one standard deviation. Comparison between values with identical lowercase letters, that is, a-a, b-b, c-c, d-d, are significant $p < .001$. (Data from Zeeman, 2009, with permission.)

For women with severe hemoconcentration, it was once taught that an acute fall in hematocrit suggested resolution of preeclampsia. In this scenario, hemodilution follows endothelial healing with return of interstitial fluid into the intravascular space. *Although this is somewhat correct, it is important to recognize that a substantive cause of this fall in hematocrit is usually the consequence of blood loss at delivery* (Chap. 41, p. 783). It may also partially result from increased erythrocyte destruction as subsequently described. Vasospasm and endothelial leakage of plasma may persist for a variable time after delivery as the endothelium is restored to normalcy. As this takes place, vasoconstriction reverses, and as the blood volume increases, the hematocrit usually falls. Thus, women with eclampsia:

- Are unduly sensitive to vigorous fluid therapy administered in an attempt to expand the contracted blood volume to normal pregnancy levels
- Are sensitive to amounts of blood loss at delivery that are considered normal for a normotensive woman.

Hematological Changes

Several hematological abnormalities are associated with the preeclampsia syndrome. Among those commonly identified is thrombocytopenia, which at times may become severe enough to be life threatening. Occasionally, the levels of some plasma clotting factors may be decreased, and erythrocytes display abnormal morphology and undergo rapid hemolysis.

Thrombocytopenia

Decreased platelet concentrations with eclampsia were described as early as 1922 by Stancke. The platelet count is routinely measured in women with any form of gestational hypertension. The frequency and intensity of thrombocytopenia vary and are dependent on the severity and duration of the preeclampsia syndrome and the frequency with which platelet counts are performed (Heilmann, 2007; Hupuczi, 2007). Overt thrombocytopenia—defined by a platelet count < 100,000/μL—indicates severe disease (see Table 40-2). In general, the lower the platelet count, the higher the rates of maternal and fetal morbidity and mortality (Leduc, 1992). In most cases, delivery is advisable because thrombocytopenia usually continues to worsen. After delivery, the platelet count may continue to decline for the first day or so. It then usually increases progressively to reach a normal level within 3 to 5 days. As discussed on page 768, in some instances with HELLP syndrome, the platelet count continues to fall after delivery. If these do not reach a nadir until 48 to 72 hours, then preeclampsia syndrome may be incorrectly attributed to one of the thrombotic microangiopathies (George, 2013). These syndromes are discussed in Chapter 56 (p. 1116).

Other Platelet Abnormalities

In addition to thrombocytopenia, there are myriad other platelet alterations described with the preeclampsia syndrome. These were reviewed by Kenny and coworkers (2014) and include platelet activation with increased α-degranulation producing β-thromboglobulin, factor 4, and increased clearance. Paradoxically, in most studies, in vitro platelet aggregation is decreased compared with the normal increase characteristic of pregnancy. This likely is due to platelet "exhaustion" following in vivo activation. Although the cause is unknown, immunological processes or simply platelet deposition at sites of endothelial damage may be implicated. Platelet-bound and circulating platelet-bindable immunoglobulins are increased, which suggest platelet surface alterations.

Neonatal Thrombocytopenia

Severe thrombocytopenia does not develop in the fetus or infant born to preeclamptic women despite severe maternal thrombocytopenia (Kenny, 2014; Pritchard, 1987). *Importantly, maternal thrombocytopenia in hypertensive women is not a fetal indication for cesarean delivery.*

Hemolysis

Severe preeclampsia is frequently accompanied by evidence of hemolysis as manifest by elevated serum lactate dehydrogenase levels and decreased haptoglobin levels. Other evidence comes from schizocytosis, spherocytosis, and reticulocytosis in peripheral blood (Cunningham, 1985; Pritchard, 1954, 1976). These derangements result in part from *microangiopathic hemolysis* caused by endothelial disruption with platelet adherence and fibrin deposition. Sanchez-Ramos and colleagues (1994) described increased erythrocyte membrane fluidity with HELLP syndrome. Cunningham and coworkers (1995) postulated that these changes were due to serum lipid alterations, and Mackay and associates (2012) found substantively decreased long-chain fatty acid content in erythrocytes of preeclamptic women. Erythrocytic membrane changes, increased adhesiveness, and aggregation may also promote a hypercoagulable state (Gamzu, 2001).

HELLP Syndrome. Subsequent to reports of hemolysis and thrombocytopenia with severe preeclampsia, descriptions followed that abnormally elevated serum liver transaminase levels were commonly found and were indicative of hepatocellular necrosis (Chesley, 1978). Weinstein (1982) referred to this combination of events as the *HELLP syndrome*—and this moniker now is used worldwide. Also, and as shown in Table 40-2, facets of the HELLP syndrome are included in criteria that differentiate severe from nonsevere preeclampsia. The HELLP syndrome is discussed in further detail on page 742.

Coagulation Changes

Subtle changes consistent with intravascular coagulation, and less often erythrocyte destruction, commonly are found with preeclampsia and especially eclampsia (Kenny, 2014). Some of these changes include increased factor VIII consumption, increased levels of fibrinopeptides A and B and of D-dimers, and decreased levels of regulatory proteins—antithrombin III and protein C and S. Except for thrombocytopenia discussed above, coagulation aberrations generally are mild and are seldom clinically significant (Kenny, 2014; Pritchard, 1984). Unless there is associated placental abruption, plasma fibrinogen levels do not differ remarkably from levels found in normal pregnancy. Fibrin degradation products such as D-dimers are elevated only occasionally. *Fibronectin*, a glycoprotein associated with vascular endothelial cell basement membrane, is elevated in women with preeclampsia (Brubaker, 1992). As preeclampsia worsens, so do abnormal findings with *thromboelastography* (Pisani-Conway, 2013). Despite these changes, routine laboratory assessments of coagulation, including prothrombin time, activated partial thromboplastin time, and plasma fibrinogen level, were found to be unnecessary in the management of pregnancy-associated hypertensive disorders (Barron, 1999).

Volume Homeostasis

The normal pregnancy-induced extra- and intracellular volume increases that are accompanied by vasodilatation undergo further complex shifts with the preeclampsia syndrome. In addition to blood volume changes shown in Figure 40-7, there are many hormonal, fluid, and electrolyte aberrations.

Endocrine Changes

Plasma levels of *renin, angiotensin II, angiotensin 1–7, aldosterone,* and *atrial natriuretic peptide* are substantively increased during normal pregnancy. *Deoxycorticosterone (DOC)* is a potent mineralocorticoid that is also increased remarkably in normal pregnancy (Chap. 4, p. 71). This compound results from conversion of plasma progesterone to DOC rather than increased maternal adrenal secretion. Because of this, DOC secretion is not reduced by sodium retention or hypertension. This may explain why women with preeclampsia retain sodium (Winkel, 1980). In pregnancy, the mineralocorticoid receptor becomes less sensitive to aldosterone (Armanini, 2012).

Vasopressin levels are similar in nonpregnant, normally pregnant, and preeclamptic women even though the metabolic clearance is increased in the latter two (Dürr, 1999).

Atrial natriuretic peptide is released during atrial wall stretching from blood volume expansion, and it responds to cardiac contractility (Chap. 4, p. 61). Serum levels rise in pregnancy, and its secretion is further increased in women with preeclampsia (Borghi, 2000; Luft, 2009). Levels of its precursor—proatrial natriuretic peptide—are also increased in preeclampsia (Sugulle, 2012).

Fluid and Electrolyte Changes

In women with severe preeclampsia, the volume of *extracellular fluid,* manifest as edema, is usually much greater than that in normal pregnant women. The mechanism responsible for pathological fluid retention is thought to be endothelial injury (Davidge, 2014). In addition to generalized edema and proteinuria, these women have reduced plasma oncotic pressure. This reduction creates a filtration imbalance and further displaces intravascular fluid into the surrounding interstitium.

Electrolyte concentrations do not differ appreciably in women with preeclampsia compared with those of normal pregnant women. This may not be the case if there has been vigorous diuretic therapy, sodium restriction, or administration of free water with sufficient oxytocin to produce antidiuresis.

Following an eclamptic convulsion, the *serum pH* and *bicarbonate* concentration are lowered due to lactic acidosis and compensatory respiratory loss of carbon dioxide. The intensity of acidosis relates to the amount of lactic acid produced—metabolic acidosis—and the rate at which carbon dioxide is exhaled—respiratory acidosis.

Kidney

During normal pregnancy, renal blood flow and glomerular filtration rate are increased appreciably (Chap. 4, p. 63). With development of preeclampsia, there may be a number of reversible anatomical and pathophysiological changes. Of clinical importance, renal perfusion and glomerular filtration are reduced. Levels that are much less than normal nonpregnant values are infrequent and are the consequence of severe disease.

A small degree of decreased glomerular filtration may result from reduced plasma volume. Most of the decrement, however, is from increased renal afferent arteriolar resistance that may be elevated up to fivefold (Conrad, 2014; Cornelis, 2011). There are also morphological changes characterized by *glomerular endotheliosis* blocking the filtration barrier. This is discussed further subsequently. Diminished filtration causes serum creatinine levels to rise to values seen in nonpregnant individuals, that is, 1 mg/mL, and sometimes even higher (Lindheimer, 2008a). Abnormal values usually begin to normalize 10 days or later after delivery (Spaan, 2012a).

In most preeclamptic women, urine sodium concentration is elevated. Urine osmolality, urine:plasma creatinine ratio, and fractional excretion of sodium also indicate that a prerenal mechanism is involved. Kirshon and coworkers (1988) infused dopamine intravenously into oliguric women with preeclampsia, and this renal vasodilator stimulated increased urine output, fractional sodium excretion, and free water clearance. As was shown in Figure 40-6, sodium-containing crystalloid infusion increases left ventricular filling pressure, and although oliguria temporarily improves, rapid infusions may cause clinically apparent pulmonary edema. *Intensive intravenous fluid therapy is not indicated as "treatment" for preeclamptic women with oliguria. Exceptions are diminished urine output from hemorrhage or fluid loss from vomiting or fever.*

Plasma uric acid concentration is typically elevated in preeclampsia. The elevation exceeds the reduction in glomerular filtration rate and likely is also due to enhanced tubular reabsorption (Chesley, 1945). At the same time, preeclampsia is associated with diminished urinary excretion of calcium, perhaps because of increased tubular reabsorption (Taufield, 1987). Another possibility is from increased placental urate production compensatory to increased oxidative stress.

Proteinuria

As shown in Table 40-1, some degree of proteinuria will establish the diagnosis of preeclampsia syndrome. Proteinuria may develop late, and some women may already be delivered or have had an eclamptic convulsion before it appears. For example, 10 to 15 percent of women with HELLP syndrome did not have proteinuria at presentation (Sibai, 2004). In another report, 17 percent of eclamptic women did not have proteinuria by the time of seizures (Zwart, 2008).

Problematically, the optimal method of establishing abnormal levels of either urine protein or albumin remains to be defined. Chen and associates (2008) have shown that clean-catch and catheterized urine specimens correlate well. But dipstick qualitative determinations depend on urinary concentration and are notorious for false-positive and -negative results. For a 24-hour quantitative specimen, the "consensus" threshold value used is > 300 mg/24 h (Task Force, 2013). Tun and colleagues (2012) have shown equivalent efficacy using protein excretion of 165 mg in a 12-hour sample. Importantly, these values have not been irrefutably established.

Determination of urinary protein:creatinine ratio may supplant the cumbersome 24-hour quantification (Ethridge, 2013; Kyle, 2008; Morris, 2012). In a systematic review, Papanna and associates (2008) concluded that random urine protein:creatinine ratios that are below 130 to 150 mg/g, that is, 0.13 to 0.15, indicate a low likelihood of proteinuria exceeding 300 mg/day. Midrange ratios, that is, 300 mg/g or 0.3 have poor sensitivity and specificity. Stout and colleagues (2013) found that values < 0.08 or > 1.19 had negative- or positive-predictive values of 86 and 96 percent, respectively. At this time, most recommend that with midrange ratio values, 24-hour protein excretion should be quantified.

There are several methods used to measure proteinuria, and none detect all of the various proteins normally excreted (Nayeri, 2013). A more accurate method involves measurement of albumin excretion. Albumin filtration exceeds that of larger globulins, and with glomerular disease such as preeclampsia, most of the protein in urine is albumin. There are test kits that permit rapid measurement of urinary albumin:creatinine ratios in an outpatient setting (Kyle, 2008).

Although worsening or nephrotic-range proteinuria has been considered by most to be a sign of severe disease, this does not appear to be the case (Airoldi, 2007). Certainly, this concept was not accepted by the 2013 Task Force. Finally, increasing proteinuria is more common in multifetal pregnancy complicated by preeclampsia (Zilberberg, 2013).

Anatomical Changes

Sheehan and Lynch (1973) commonly found changes identifiable at autopsy by light and electron microscopy in the kidneys of eclamptic women. Glomeruli are enlarged by approximately 20 percent, they are "bloodless," and capillary loops variably are dilated and contracted. Endothelial cells are swollen—termed *glomerular capillary endotheliosis* by Spargo and associates (1959). Endothelial cells are often so swollen that they block or partially block the capillary lumens (Fig. 40-8). Homogeneous subendothelial deposits of proteins and fibrin-like material are seen.

Endothelial swelling may result from angiogenic factor "withdrawal" caused by free angiogenic proteins complexing with the circulating antiangiogenic protein receptor discussed on page 735 (Conrad, 2014; Eremina, 2007; Karumanchi, 2009). The angiogenic proteins are crucial for podocyte health, and their inactivation leads to podocyte dysfunction and endothelial swelling. One marker of this is excretion of podocyte proteins such as nephrin, podocalyxin, and βig-h3 (transforming growth factor, β-induced) (Wang, 2012b). Also, eclampsia is characterized by increased excretion of urinary podocytes, a phenomenon shared by other proteinuric disorders (Garrett, 2013; Wagner, 2012). Of interest, podocytes are epithelia, and thus renal pathology involves both endothelial and epithelial cells (see Fig. 40-8).

Acute Kidney Injury

Rarely is *acute tubular necrosis* caused by preeclampsia alone. Although mild degrees are encountered in neglected cases, clinically apparent renal failure is invariably induced by coexistent hemorrhage with hypovolemia and hypotension (Chap. 41, p. 814). This is usually caused by severe obstetrical hemorrhage for which adequate blood replacement is not given. Drakeley and coworkers (2002) described 72 women with preeclampsia and renal failure. Half had HELLP syndrome, and a third had placental abruption. As discussed on page 742, Haddad and colleagues (2000) reported that 5 percent of 183 women

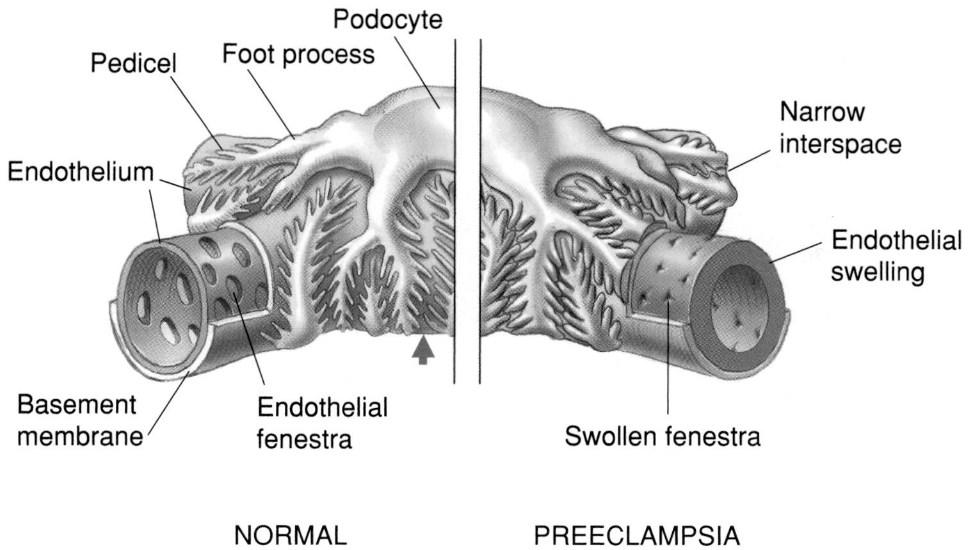

FIGURE 40-8 Schematic showing glomerular capillary endotheliosis. The capillary of the normal glomerulus shown on the left has wide endothelial fenestrations, and the pedicels emanating from the podocytes are widely spaced (*arrow*). The illustration on the right is of a glomerulus with changes induced by the preeclampsia syndrome. The endothelial cells are swollen and their fenestrae narrowed, as are the pedicels that now abut each other.

with HELLP syndrome had kidney injury. Half of these, however, also had a placental abruption, and most had postpartum hemorrhage. Rarely, irreversible *renal cortical necrosis* develops (Chap. 53, p. 1064).

Liver

Hepatic changes in women with fatal eclampsia were described in 1856 by Virchow. The characteristic lesions were regions of periportal hemorrhage in the liver periphery. In their elegant autopsy studies, Sheehan and Lynch (1973) described that some degree of hepatic infarction accompanied hemorrhage in almost half of women who died with eclampsia. These corresponded with reports that had appeared during the 1960s describing elevated serum hepatic transaminase levels. Along with the earlier observations by Pritchard and associates (1954), who described hemolysis and thrombocytopenia with eclampsia, this constellation of hemolysis, hepatocellular necrosis, and thrombocytopenia was later termed *HELLP syndrome* by Weinstein (1985) to call attention to its seriousness (p. 742).

Lesions as extensive as those shown in Figure 40-9 are unusual, even in the autopsy series by Sheehan and Lynch (1973). From a pragmatic point, liver involvement with preeclampsia may be clinically significant in several circumstances.

First, symptomatic involvement is considered a sign of severe disease. It typically manifests by moderate to severe right-upper quadrant or midepigastric pain and tenderness. In many cases, such women also have elevated levels of serum aminotransferase, namely, aspartate aminotransferase (AST) or alanine aminotransferase (ALT). In some cases, however, the amount of hepatic tissue involved with infarction may be surprisingly extensive yet still clinically insignificant. In our experiences, infarction may be worsened by hypotension from obstetrical hemorrhage, and it occasionally causes hepatic failure—so-called shock liver (Alexander, 2009).

Second, asymptomatic elevations of serum hepatic transaminase levels—AST and ALT—are also considered markers for severe preeclampsia. Values seldom exceed 500 U/L, but have been reported to be greater than 2000 U/L in some women (Chap. 55, p. 1085). In general, serum levels inversely follow platelet levels, and they both usually normalize within 3 days following delivery as previously discussed on page 738.

In a third example of liver involvement, hemorrhagic infarction may extend to form a hepatic hematoma. These in turn may extend to form a subcapsular hematoma that may rupture. They can be identified using computed tomography (CT) scanning or magnetic resonance (MR) imaging as shown in Figure 40-10. Unruptured hematomas are probably more common than clinically suspected and are more likely to be found with HELLP syndrome (Carlson, 2004; Vigil-De Gracia, 2012). Although once considered a surgical condition, contemporaneous management usually consists of observation and conservative treatment of hematomas unless hemorrhage is ongoing. In some cases, however, prompt surgical intervention may be lifesaving. Vigil-De Gracia and coworkers (2012) reviewed 180 cases of hepatic hematoma or rupture. More than 90 percent had HELLP syndrome, and in 90 percent, the capsule had ruptured. The maternal mortality rate was 22 percent, and the perinatal mortality rate was 31 percent. In rare cases, liver transplant is necessary (Hunter, 1995; Wicke, 2004).

Last, acute fatty liver of pregnancy is sometimes confused with preeclampsia (Nelson, 2013; Sibai, 2007a). It too has an onset in late pregnancy, and often there is accompanying

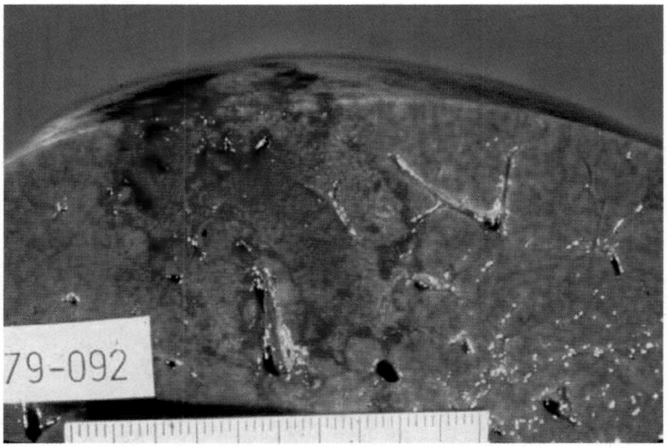

FIGURE 40-9 Gross liver specimen from a woman with preeclampsia who died from aspiration pneumonitis. Periportal hemorrhagic necrosis was seen microscopically. (From Cunningham, 1993.)

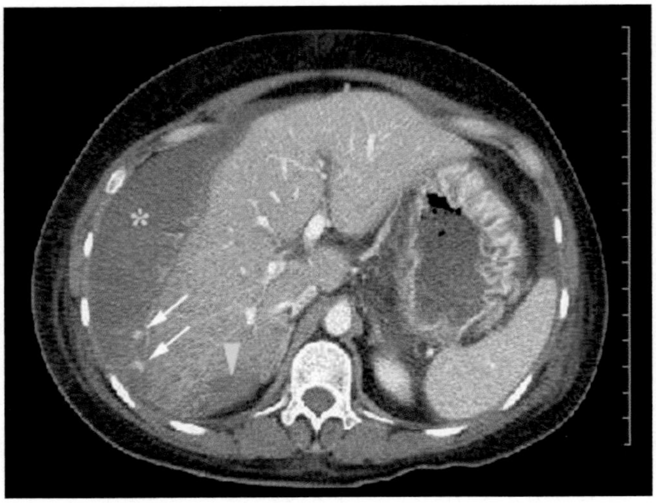

FIGURE 40-10 Abdominal CT imaging performed postpartum in a woman with severe HELLP syndrome and right-upper quadrant pain. A large subcapsular hematoma (*asterisk*) is seen confluent with intrahepatic infarction and hematoma (*arrowhead*). Numerous flame-shaped hemorrhages are seen at the hematoma interface (*arrows*).

hypertension, elevated serum transaminase and creatinine levels, and thrombocytopenia (Chap. 55, p. 1086).

HELLP Syndrome

There is no universally accepted strict definition of this syndrome, and thus its incidence varies by investigator. When it is identified, the likelihood of hepatic hematoma and rupture is substantially increased. In a multicenter study, Haddad and colleagues (2000) described 183 women with HELLP syndrome of whom 40 percent had adverse outcomes including two maternal deaths. The incidence of subcapsular liver hematoma was 1.6 percent. Other complications included eclampsia—6 percent, placental abruption—10 percent, acute kidney injury—5 percent, and pulmonary edema—10 percent. Other serious complications included stroke, coagulopathy, acute respiratory distress syndrome, and sepsis.

Women with preeclampsia complicated by the HELLP syndrome typically have worse outcomes than those without these findings (Kozic, 2011; Martin, 2012, 2013). In their review of 693 women with HELLP syndrome, Keiser and coworkers (2009) reported that 10 percent had concurrent eclampsia. Sep and associates (2009) also described a significantly increased risk for complications in women with HELLP syndrome compared with those with "isolated preeclampsia." These included eclampsia—15 versus 4 percent; preterm birth—93 versus 78 percent; and perinatal mortality rate—9 versus 4 percent, respectively. Because of these marked clinical differences, these investigators postulate that HELLP syndrome has a distinct pathogenesis. Others have shown a difference in the ratio of antiangiogenic and inflammatory acute-phase proteins in these two conditions and have reached similar conclusions (Reimer, 2013). Given all of the variables contributing to the incidence and pathophysiology of preeclampsia as discussed on page 736, this is a reasonable conclusion. Sibai and Stella (2009) have discussed some of these aspects under the rubric of "atypical preeclampsia-eclampsia."

Pancreas

According to Sheehan and Lynch (1973), there are no convincing data that the pancreas has special involvement with preeclampsia syndrome. If so, the occasional case reports of concurrent hemorrhagic pancreatitis are likely unrelated (Swank, 2012). That said, severe hemoconcentration may predispose to pancreatic inflammation.

Brain

Headaches and visual symptoms are common with severe preeclampsia, and associated convulsions define eclampsia. The earliest anatomical descriptions of brain involvement came from autopsy specimens, but CT- and MR-imaging and Doppler studies have added many important insights into cerebrovascular involvement.

Neuroanatomical Lesions

Most gross anatomical descriptions of the brain in eclamptic women are taken from eras when mortality rates were high. One consistent finding was that brain pathology accounted for only about a third of fatal cases such as the one shown in Figure 40-11. In fact, most deaths were from pulmonary edema, and brain lesions were coincidental. Thus, although gross intracerebral hemorrhage was seen in up to 60 percent of eclamptic women, it was fatal in only half of these (Melrose, 1984; Richards, 1988; Sheehan, 1973). As shown in Figure 40-12, other principal lesions found at autopsy of eclamptic women were cortical and subcortical petechial hemorrhages. The classic microscopic vascular lesions consist of fibrinoid necrosis of the arterial wall and perivascular microinfarcts and hemorrhages. Other frequently described major lesions include subcortical edema, multiple nonhemorrhagic areas of "softening" throughout the brain, and hemorrhagic areas in the white matter. There also may be hemorrhage in the basal ganglia or pons, often with rupture into the ventricles.

Cerebrovascular Pathophysiology

Clinical, pathological, and neuroimaging findings have led to two general theories to explain cerebral abnormalities with

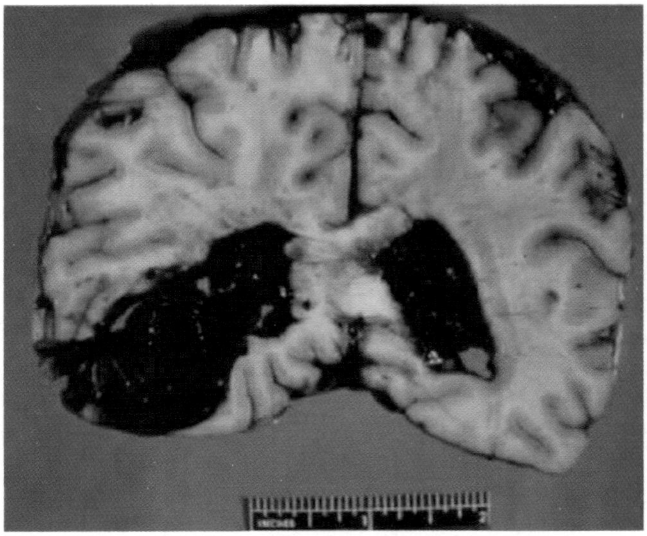

FIGURE 40-11 This autopsy brain slice shows a fatal hypertensive hemorrhage in a primigravida with eclampsia.

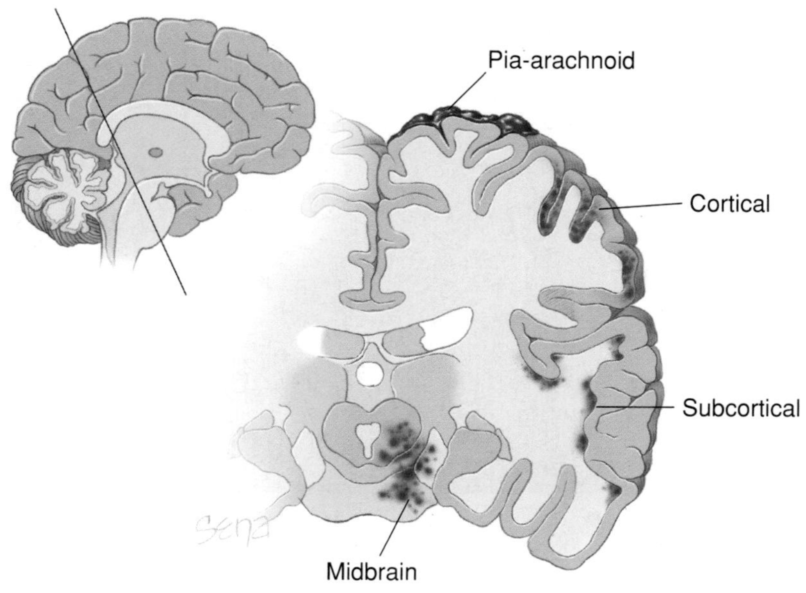

FIGURE 40-12 Composite illustration showing location of cerebral hemorrhages and petechiae in women with eclampsia. Insert shows the level of the brain from which the main image was constructed. (Data from Sheehan, 1973.)

eclampsia. Importantly, endothelial cell dysfunction that characterizes the preeclampsia syndrome likely plays a key role in both. The first theory suggests that in response to acute and severe hypertension, cerebrovascular overregulation leads to vasospasm (Trommer, 1988). This presumption is based on the angiographic appearance of diffuse or multifocal segmental narrowings suggestive of vasospasm (Ito, 1995). In this scheme, diminished cerebral blood flow is hypothesized to result in ischemia, cytotoxic edema, and eventually tissue infarction. Although this theory was widely embraced for many years, there is little objective evidence to support it.

The second theory is that sudden elevations in systemic blood pressure exceed the normal cerebrovascular autoregulatory capacity (Hauser, 1988; Schwartz, 2000). Regions of forced vasodilation and vasoconstriction develop, especially in arterial boundary zones. At the capillary level, disruption of end-capillary pressure causes increased hydrostatic pressure, hyperperfusion, and extravasation of plasma and red cells through endothelial tight-junction openings. This leads to *vasogenic edema*. This theory is incomplete because very few eclamptic women have mean arterial pressures that exceed limits of autoregulation—approximately 160 mm Hg.

It seems reasonable to conclude that the most likely mechanism is a combination of the two. Thus, a preeclampsia-associated interendothelial cell leak develops at blood pressure (hydraulic) levels much lower than those usually causing vasogenic edema and is coupled with a loss of upper-limit autoregulation (Zeeman, 2009). With imaging studies, these changes manifest as facets of the *reversible posterior leukoencephalopathy syndrome* (Hinchey, 1996). This subsequently became referred to as the *posterior reversible encephalopathy syndrome—PRES*. This term is misleading because although PRES lesions principally involve the posterior brain—the occipital and parietal cortices—in at least a third of cases, they also involve other brain areas (Edlow, 2013; Zeeman, 2004a). The most frequently affected region is the parietooccipital cortex—the boundary zone of the anterior, middle, and posterior cerebral arteries. Also, in most cases, these lesions are reversible (Cipolla, 2014).

Cerebral Blood Flow

Autoregulation is the mechanism by which cerebral blood flow remains relatively constant despite alterations in cerebral perfusion pressure. In nonpregnant individuals, this mechanism protects the brain from hyperperfusion when mean arterial pressures increase to as high as 160 mm Hg. These are pressures far greater than those seen in all but a very few women with eclampsia. Thus, to explain eclamptic seizures, it was theorized that autoregulation must be altered by pregnancy. Although species differences must be considered, studies by Cipolla and colleagues (2007, 2009, 2014) have convincingly shown that autoregulation is unchanged across pregnancy in rodents. That said, some, but not others, have provided evidence of impaired autoregulation in women with preeclampsia (Janzarik, 2014; van Veen, 2013).

Zeeman and associates (2003) showed that cerebral blood flow during the first two trimesters of normal pregnancy is similar to nonpregnant values, but thereafter, it significantly decreases by 20 percent during the last trimester. These investigators also documented significantly increased cerebral blood flow in women with severe preeclampsia compared with that of normotensive pregnant women (Zeeman, 2004b). Taken together, these findings suggest that eclampsia occurs when cerebral hyperperfusion forces capillary fluid interstitially because of endothelial damage, which leads to perivascular edema characteristic of the preeclampsia syndrome. In this regard, eclampsia is an example of the posterior reversible encephalopathy syndrome as previously discussed.

Neurological Manifestations

There are several neurological manifestations of the preeclampsia syndrome. Each signifies severe involvement and requires immediate attention. First, *headache and scotomata* are thought to arise from cerebrovascular hyperperfusion that has a predilection for the occipital lobes. According to Sibai (2005) and Zwart and coworkers (2008), 50 to 75 percent of women have headaches and 20 to 30 percent have visual changes preceding eclamptic convulsions. The headaches may be mild to severe and intermittent to constant. In our experiences, they are unique in that they do not usually respond to traditional analgesia, but they do improve after magnesium sulfate infusion is initiated.

Convulsions are a second potential manifestation and are diagnostic for eclampsia. These are caused by excessive release of excitatory neurotransmitters—especially glutamate; massive depolarization of network neurons; and bursts of action potentials (Meldrum, 2002). Clinical and experimental evidence suggest that extended seizures can cause significant brain injury and later brain dysfunction.

As a third manifestation, *blindness* is rare with preeclampsia alone, but it complicates eclamptic convulsions in up to 15 percent of women (Cunningham, 1995). Blindness has been reported to develop up to a week or more following delivery (Chambers, 2004). There are at least two types of blindness as discussed subsequently.

Last, *generalized cerebral edema* may develop and is usually manifest by mental status changes that vary from confusion to coma. This situation is particularly dangerous because fatal transtentorial herniation may result.

Neuroimaging Studies

With CT imaging, localized hypodense lesions at the gray- and white-matter junction, primarily in the parietooccipital lobes, are typically found in eclampsia. Such lesions may also be seen in the frontal and inferior temporal lobes, the basal ganglia, and thalamus (Brown, 1988). The spectrum of brain involvement is wide, and increasing involvement can be identified with CT imaging. Edema of the occipital lobes or diffuse cerebral edema may cause symptoms such as blindness, lethargy, and confusion (Cunningham, 2000). In the latter cases, widespread edema shows as a marked compression or even obliteration of the cerebral ventricles. Such women may develop signs of impending life-threatening transtentorial herniation.

Several MR imaging acquisitions are used to study eclamptic women. Common findings are hyperintense T2 lesions—posterior reversible encephalopathy syndrome (PRES)—in the subcortical and cortical regions of the parietal and occipital lobes (Fig. 40-13). There is also relatively common involvement of the basal ganglia, brainstem, and cerebellum (Brewer, 2013; Zeeman, 2004a). Although these PRES lesions are almost universal in women with eclampsia, their incidence in women with preeclampsia is less frequent. They are more likely to be found in women who have severe disease and who have neurological symptoms (Schwartz, 2000). And although usually reversible, a fourth of these hyperintense lesions represent cerebral infarctions that have persistent findings (Loureiro, 2003; Zeeman, 2004a).

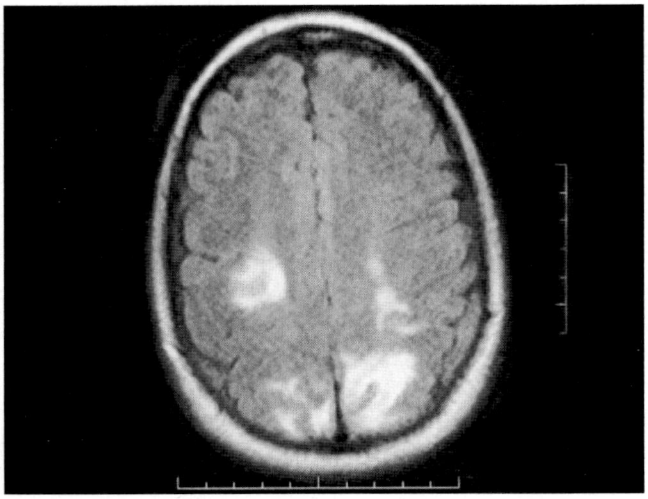

FIGURE 40-13 Cranial magnetic resonance imaging in a nullipara with eclampsia. Multilobe T2-FLAIR high-signal lesions are apparent. FLAIR = fluid-attenuated inversion recovery. (Image contributed by Dr. Gerda Zeeman.)

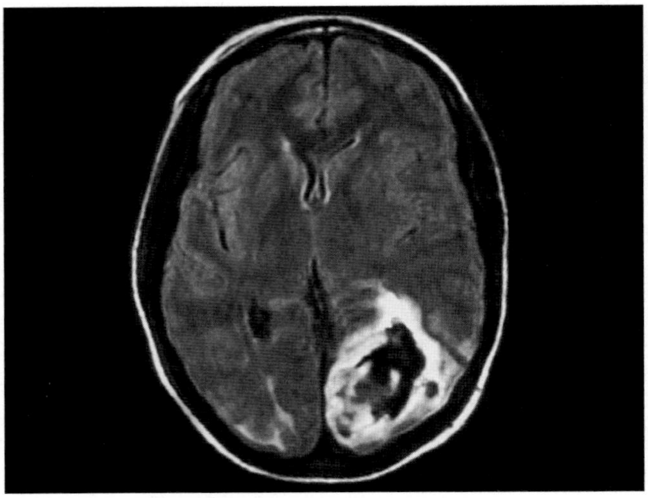

FIGURE 40-14 Cranial magnetic resonance imaging performed 3 days postpartum in a woman with eclampsia and HELLP syndrome. Neurovisual defects persisted at 1 year, causing job disability. (From Murphy, 2005, with permission.)

Visual Changes and Blindness

Scotomata, blurred vision, or diplopia are common with severe preeclampsia and eclampsia. These usually improve with magnesium sulfate therapy and/or lowered blood pressure. Blindness is less common, is usually reversible, and may arise from three potential areas. These are the visual cortex of the occipital lobe, the lateral geniculate nuclei, and the retina. In the retina, pathological lesions may be ischemia, infarction, or detachment (Roos, 2012).

Occipital blindness is also called *amaurosis*—from the Greek *dimming*. Affected women usually have evidence of extensive occipital lobe vasogenic edema on imaging studies. Of 15 women cared for at Parkland Hospital, occipital blindness lasted from 4 hours to 8 days, but it resolved completely in all cases (Cunningham, 1995). Rarely, extensive cerebral infarctions may result in total or partial visual defects (Fig. 40-14).

Blindness from retinal lesions is caused either by serous retinal detachment or rarely by retinal infarction, which is termed *Purtscher retinopathy* (Fig. 40-15). *Serous retinal detachment* is usually unilateral and seldom causes total visual loss. In fact, asymptomatic serous retinal detachment is relatively common (Saito, 1998). In most cases of eclampsia-associated blindness, visual acuity subsequently improves, but if caused by retinal artery occlusion, vision may be permanently impaired (Lara-Torre, 2002; Roos, 2012). In some women, these findings are additive. Moseman and Shelton (2002) described a woman with permanent blindness due to a combination of retinal infarctions and bilateral lesions in the lateral geniculate nuclei.

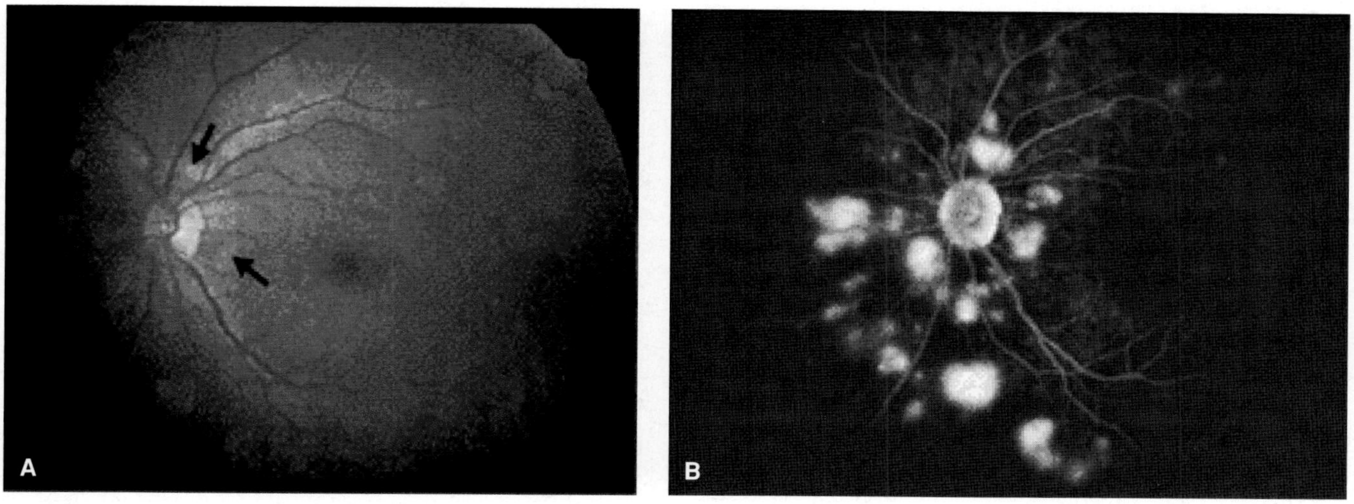

FIGURE 40-15 Purtscher retinopathy caused by choroidal ischemia and infarction in preeclampsia syndrome. **A.** Ophthalmoscopy shows scattered yellowish, opaque lesions of the retina (*arrows*). **B.** The late phase of fluorescein angiography shows areas of intense hyperfluorescence representing pooling of extravasated dye. (From Lam, 2001, with permission.)

Cerebral Edema

Clinical manifestations suggesting widespread cerebral edema are worrisome. During 13 years at Parkland Hospital, 10 of 175 women with eclampsia were diagnosed with symptomatic cerebral edema (Cunningham, 2000). Symptoms ranged from lethargy, confusion, and blurred vision to obtundation and coma. In most cases, symptoms waxed and waned. Mental status changes generally correlated with the degree of involvement seen with CT and MR imaging studies. *These women are very susceptible to sudden and severe blood pressure elevations, which can acutely worsen the already widespread vasogenic edema.* Thus, careful blood pressure control is essential. In the 10 women with generalized edema, three became comatose and had imaging findings of impending transtentorial herniation. One of these three died from herniation. Consideration is given for treatment with mannitol or dexamethasone.

Long-Term Neurocognitive Sequelae

Women with eclampsia have been shown to have some cognitive decline when studied 5 to 10 years following an eclamptic pregnancy. This is discussed further on page 770.

Uteroplacental Perfusion

Defects in endovascular trophoblastic invasion and placentation germane to development of the preeclampsia syndrome and fetal-growth restriction were discussed on page 732. Of immense clinical importance, compromised uteroplacental perfusion is almost certainly a major culprit in the increased perinatal morbidity and mortality rates. Thus, measurement of uterine, intervillous, and placental blood flow would likely be informative. Attempts to assess these in humans have been hampered by several obstacles that include inaccessibility of the placenta, the complexity of its venous effluent, and the need for radioisotopes or invasive techniques.

Measurement of uterine artery blood flow velocity has been used to estimate resistance to uteroplacental blood flow (Chap. 17, p. 345). Vascular resistance is estimated by comparing arterial systolic and diastolic velocity waveforms. By the completion of placentation, impedance to uterine artery blood flow is markedly decreased, but with abnormal placentation, abnormally high resistance persists (Everett, 2012; Ghidini, 2008; Napolitano, 2012). Earlier studies were done to assess this by measuring peak systolic:diastolic velocity ratios from uterine and umbilical arteries in preeclamptic pregnancies. The results were interpreted as showing that in some cases, but certainly not all, there was increased resistance (Fleischer, 1986; Trudinger, 1990).

Another Doppler waveform—uterine artery "notching"—has been reported to be associated with increased risks for preeclampsia or fetal-growth restriction (Groom, 2009). In the MFMU Network study reported by Myatt and colleagues (2012a), however, notching had a low predictive value except for early-onset severe disease.

Matijevic and Johnson (1999) measured resistance in *uterine spiral arteries*. Impedance was higher in peripheral than in central vessels—a so-called ring-like distribution. Mean resistance was higher in all women with preeclampsia compared with that in normotensive controls. Ong and associates (2003) used MR imaging and other techniques to assess placental perfusion ex vivo in the myometrial arteries removed from women with preeclampsia or fetal-growth restriction. These investigators confirmed that in both conditions myometrial arteries exhibited endothelium-dependent vasodilatory response. Moreover, other pregnancy conditions are also associated with increased resistance (Urban, 2007). One major adverse effect, fetal-growth restriction, is discussed in Chapter 44 (p. 874).

Pimenta and colleagues (2013) assessed placental vascularity using a three-dimensional power Doppler histogram. These researchers described the *placental vascularity index*, which was decreased in women with any pregnancy-associated hypertensive disorders—11.1 percent compared with 15.2 percent in normal controls.

Despite these findings, evidence for compromised uteroplacental circulation is found in only a few women who go on to develop preeclampsia. Indeed, when preeclampsia develops during the third trimester, only a third of women with severe disease have abnormal uterine artery velocimetry (Li, 2005). In a study of 50 women with HELLP syndrome, only a third had abnormal uterine artery waveforms (Bush, 2001). In general, the extent of abnormal waveforms correlates with severity of fetal involvement (Ghidini, 2008; Groom, 2009).

PREDICTION AND PREVENTION

Prediction

Measurement during early pregnancy—or across pregnancy—of various biological, biochemical, and biophysical markers implicated in preeclampsia syndrome pathophysiology has been proposed to predict its development. Attempts have been made to identify early markers of faulty placentation, impaired placental perfusion, endothelial cell activation and dysfunction, and activation of coagulation. For the most, these have resulted in testing strategies with poor sensitivity and with poor positive-predictive value for preeclampsia (Conde-Agudelo, 2014; Lindheimer, 2008b; Odibo, 2013). Currently, no screening tests are predictably reliable, valid, and economical (Kleinrouweler, 2012). There are, however, combinations of tests, some yet to be adequately evaluated, that may be promising (Dugoff, 2013; Kuc, 2011; Navaratnam, 2013; Olsen, 2012).

The list of predictive factors evaluated during the past three decades is legion. Although most have been evaluated in the first half of pregnancy, some have been tested as predictors of severity in the third trimester (Chaiworapongsa, 2013; Mosimann, 2013; Rana, 2012). Others have been used to forecast recurrent preeclampsia (Demers, 2014). Some of these tests are listed in Table 40-4, which is by no means all inclusive. Conde-Agudelo and coworkers (2014) have recently provided a thorough review of many of these testing strategies.

Vascular Resistance Testing and Placental Perfusion

Most of these are cumbersome, time consuming, and overall inaccurate.

Provocative Pressor Tests. Three tests have been extensively evaluated to assess the blood pressure rise in response to a stimulus. The *roll-over test* measures the hypertensive response in women at 28 to 32 weeks who are resting in the left lateral decubitus position and then roll over to the supine position. Increased blood pressure signifies a positive test. The *isometric exercise test* employs the same principle by squeezing a handball. The *angiotensin II infusion test* is performed by giving incrementally increasing doses intravenously, and the hypertensive response is quantified. In their updated metaanalysis, Conde-Agudelo and associates (2014) found sensitivities of all three tests to range from 55 to 70 percent, and specificities approximated 85 percent.

Uterine Artery Doppler Velocimetry. Faulty trophoblastic invasion of the spiral arteries, which is depicted in Figure 40-2, results in diminished placental perfusion and upstream increased uterine artery resistance. Increased uterine artery velocimetry determined by Doppler ultrasound in the first two trimesters should provide indirect evidence of this process and thus serve as a predictive test for preeclampsia (Gebb, 2009a,b; Groom, 2009). As described on page 745 and in Chapter 10 (p. 220), increased flow resistance results in an abnormal waveform represented by an exaggerated *diastolic notch*. These have value for fetal-growth restriction but not preeclampsia (American College of Obstetricians and Gynecologists, 2013a). Several flow velocity waveforms—alone or in combination—have been investigated for preeclampsia prediction. In some of these, predictive values for early-onset preeclampsia were promising (Herraiz, 2012).

TABLE 40-4. Predictive Tests for Development of the Preeclampsia Syndrome

Testing Related To:	Examples
Placental perfusion/ vascular resistance	Roll-over test, isometric handgrip or cold pressor test, pressor response to aerobic exercise, angiotensin-II infusion, midtrimester mean arterial pressure, platelet angiotensin-II binding, renin, 24-hour ambulatory blood pressure monitoring, uterine artery or fetal transcranial Doppler velocimetry
Fetal-placental unit endocrine dysfunction	Human chorionic gonadotropin (hCG), alpha-fetoprotein (AFP), estriol, pregnancy-associated protein A (PAPP A), inhibin A, activin A, placental protein 13, corticotropin-releasing hormone, A disintegrin, ADAM-12, kisspeptin
Renal dysfunction	Serum uric acid, microalbuminuria, urinary calcium or kallikrein, microtransferrinuria, *N*-acetyl-β-glucosaminidase, cystatin C, podocyturia
Endothelial dysfunction/ oxidant stress	Platelet count and activation, fibronectin, endothelial adhesion molecules, prostaglandins, prostacyclin, MMP-9, thromboxane, C-reactive protein, cytokines, endothelin, neurokinin B, homocysteine, lipids, insulin resistance, antiphospholipid antibodies, plasminogen activator-inhibitor (PAI), leptin, p-selectin, angiogenic factors such as placental growth factor (PlGF), vascular endothelial growth factor (VEGF), fms-like tyrosine kinase receptor-1 (sFlt-1), endoglin
Others	Antithrombin-III(AT-3), atrial natriuretic peptide (ANP), β_2-microglobulin, haptoglobin, transferrin, ferritin, 25-hydroxyvitamin D, genetic markers, cell-free fetal DNA, serum and urine proteomics and metabolomic markers, hepatic aminotransferases

ADAM12 = ADAM metallopeptidase domain 12; MMP = matrix metalloproteinase.
Adapted from Conde-Agudelo, 2014.

At this time, however, none is suitable for clinical use (Conde-Agudelo, 2014; Kleinrouweler, 2012; Myatt, 2012a).

Pulse Wave Analysis. Like the uterine artery, finger arterial pulse "stiffness" is an indicator of cardiovascular risk. Investigators have preliminarily evaluated its usefulness in preeclampsia prediction (Vollebregt, 2009).

Fetal-Placental Unit Endocrine Function

Several serum analytes that have been proposed to help predict preeclampsia are shown in Table 40-4. Newer ones are continuously added (Jeyabalan, 2009; Kanasaki, 2008; Kenny, 2009). Many of these gained widespread use in the 1980s to identify fetal malformations and were also found to be associated with other pregnancy abnormalities such as neural-tube defects and aneuploidy (Chap. 14, p. 289). Although touted for hypertension prediction, in general, none of these tests has been shown to be clinically beneficial for that purpose.

Tests of Renal Function

Serum Uric Acid. One of the earliest laboratory manifestations of preeclampsia is hyperuricemia (Powers, 2006). It likely results from reduced uric acid clearance from diminished glomerular filtration, increased tubular reabsorption, and decreased secretion (Lindheimer, 2008a). It is used by some to define preeclampsia, but Cnossen and coworkers (2006) reported that its sensitivity ranged from 0 to 55 percent, and specificity was 77 to 95 percent.

Microalbuminuria. As a predictive test for preeclampsia, microalbuminuria has sensitivities ranging from 7 to 90 percent and specificities between 29 and 97 percent (Conde-Agudelo, 2014). Poon and colleagues (2008) likewise found unacceptable sensitivity and specificity for urine albumin:creatinine ratios.

Endothelial Dysfunction and Oxidant Stress

As discussed on page 733, endothelial activation and inflammation are major participants in the pathophysiology of the preeclampsia syndrome. As a result, compounds such as those listed in Table 40-4 are found in circulating blood of affected women, and some have been assessed for their predictive value.

Fibronectins. These high-molecular-weight glycoproteins are released from endothelial cells and extracellular matrix following endothelial injury (Chavarria, 2002). More than 30 years ago, plasma concentrations were reported to be elevated in women with preeclampsia (Stubbs, 1984). Following their systematic review, however, Leeflang and associates (2007) concluded that neither cellular nor total fibronectin levels were clinically useful to predict preeclampsia.

Coagulation Activation. Thrombocytopenia and platelet dysfunction are integral features of preeclampsia as discussed on page 738. Platelet activation causes increased destruction and decreased concentrations, and mean platelet volume rises because of platelet immaturity (Kenny, 2014). Although markers of coagulation activation are increased, the substantive overlap with levels in normotensive pregnant women stultifies their predictive value.

Oxidative Stress. Increased levels of lipid peroxides coupled with decreased antioxidant activity have raised the possibility that markers of oxidative stress might predict preeclampsia. For example, malondialdehyde is a marker of lipid peroxidation. Other markers are various prooxidants or their potentiators. These include iron, transferrin, and ferritin; blood lipids, including triglycerides, free fatty acids, and lipoproteins; and antioxidants such as ascorbic acid and vitamin E (Bainbridge, 2005; Conde-Agudelo, 2014; Mackay, 2012; Powers, 2000). These have not been found to be predictive, and treatment to prevent preeclampsia with some of them has been studied as discussed on page 748.

Hyperhomocysteinemia causes oxidative stress and endothelial cell dysfunction and is characteristic of preeclampsia. Although women with elevated serum homocysteine levels at midpregnancy had a three- to fourfold risk of preeclampsia, these tests have not been shown to be clinically useful predictors (D'Anna, 2004; Mignini, 2005; Zeeman, 2003).

Angiogenic Factors. As discussed on page 735, evidence has accrued that an imbalance between proangiogenic and antiangiogenic factors is related to preeclampsia pathogenesis. Serum levels of some proangiogenic factors—vascular endothelial growth factor (VEGF) and placental growth factor (PlGF)—begin to decrease before clinical preeclampsia develops. And, recall as shown in Figure 40-4 that at the same time levels of some antiangiogenic factors such as sFlt-1 and sEng become increased (Maynard, 2008). In one study, these abnormalities were identified coincidentally with rising uterine artery Doppler resistance (Coolman, 2012).

Conde-Agudelo and colleagues (2014) reviewed the predictive accuracy of some of these factors for severe preeclampsia. Sensitivities for all cases of preeclampsia ranged from 30 to 50 percent, and specificity was about 90 percent. Their predictive accuracy was higher for early-onset preeclampsia. These preliminary results suggest a clinical role for preeclampsia prediction. However, until this role is better substantiated, their general clinical use is not currently recommended (Boucoiran, 2013; Kleinrouweler, 2012; Widmer, 2007). Automated assays are being studied, and the World Health Organization (WHO) began a multicenter trial in 2008 to evaluate these factors (Sunderji, 2009).

Cell-Free Fetal DNA

As discussed in Chapter 13 (p. 279), cell-free fetal DNA can be detected in maternal plasma. It has been reported that fetal-maternal cell trafficking is increased in pregnancies complicated by preeclampsia (Holzgreve, 1998). It is hypothesized that cell-free DNA is released by accelerated apoptosis of cytotrophoblasts (DiFederico, 1999). From their review, Conde-Agudelo and associates (2014) concluded that cell-free fetal DNA quantification is not yet useful for prediction purposes.

Proteomic, Metabolomic, and Transcriptomic Markers

Methods to study serum and urinary proteins and cellular metabolites have opened a new vista for preeclampsia prediction. Preliminary studies indicate that these may become useful (Bahado-Singh, 2013; Carty, 2011; Liu, 2013; Myers, 2013).

TABLE 40-5. Some Methods to Prevent Preeclampsia That Have Been Evaluated in Randomized Trials

Dietary manipulation—low-salt diet, calcium or fish oil supplementation
Exercise—physical activity, stretching
Cardiovascular drugs—diuretics, antihypertensive drugs
Antioxidants—ascorbic acid (vitamin C), α-tocopherol (vitamin E), vitamin D
Antithrombotic drugs—low-dose aspirin, aspirin/dipyridamole, aspirin + heparin, aspirin + ketanserin

Modified from Staff, 2014.

Prevention

Various strategies used to prevent or modify preeclampsia severity have been evaluated. Some are listed in Table 40-5. In general, none of these has been found to be convincingly and reproducibly effective.

Dietary and Lifestyle Modifications

A favorite of many theorists and faddists for centuries, dietary "treatment" for preeclampsia has produced some interesting abuses as chronicled by Chesley (1978).

Low-Salt Diet. One of the earliest research efforts to prevent preeclampsia was salt restriction (De Snoo, 1937). This interdiction was followed by years of inappropriate diuretic therapy. Although these practices were discarded, it ironically was not until relatively recently that the first randomized trial was done and showed that a sodium-restricted diet was ineffective in preventing preeclampsia in 361 women (Knuist, 1998). Guidelines from the United Kingdom National Institute for Health and Clinical Excellence (2010) recommend against salt restrictions.

Calcium Supplementation. Studies performed in the 1980s outside the United States showed that women with low dietary calcium intake were at significantly increased risk for gestational hypertension (Belizan, 1980; López-Jaramillo, 1989; Marya, 1987). Calcium supplementation has been studied in several trials, including one by the National Institute of Child Health and Human Development (NICHD) that included more than 4500 nulliparous women (Levine, 1997). In one recent metaanalysis, Patrelli and coworkers (2012) reported that increased calcium intake lowered the risk for preeclampsia in high-risk women. In aggregate, most of these trials have shown that unless women are calcium deficient, supplementation has no salutary effects (Staff, 2014).

Fish Oil Supplementation. Cardioprotective fatty acids found in some fatty fishes are plentiful in diets of Scandinavians and American Eskimos. The most common dietary sources are EPA—eicosapentaenoic acid, ALA—alpha-linoleic acid, and DHA—docosahexaenoic acid. With proclamations that supplementation with these fatty acids would prevent inflammatory-mediated atherogenesis, it was not a quantum leap to posit that they might also prevent preeclampsia. Unfortunately, randomized trials conducted thus far have shown no such benefits (Makrides, 2006; Olafsdottir, 2006; Olsen, 2000; Zhou, 2012a).

Exercise. There are a few studies done to assess the protective effects of physical activity on preeclampsia. In their systematic review, Kasawara and associates (2012) reported a trend toward risk reduction with exercise. More research is needed in this area (Staff, 2014).

Antihypertensive Drugs

Because of the putative effects of sodium restriction, diuretic therapy became popular with the introduction of chlorothiazide in 1957 (Finnerty, 1958; Flowers, 1962). In their metaanalysis, Churchill and colleagues (2007) summarized nine randomized trials that included more than 7000 pregnancies. They found that women given diuretics had a decreased incidence of edema and hypertension but not of preeclampsia.

Because women with chronic hypertension are at high risk for preeclampsia, several randomized trials—only a few placebo-controlled—have been done to evaluate various antihypertensive drugs to reduce the incidence of superimposed preeclampsia. A critical analysis of these trials by Staff and coworkers (2014) failed to demonstrate salutary effects.

Antioxidants

There are inferential data that an imbalance between oxidant and antioxidant activity may play an important role in the pathogenesis of preeclampsia (p. 747). Thus, naturally occurring antioxidants—vitamins C, D, and E—might decrease such oxidation. Indeed, women who developed preeclampsia were found to have reduced plasma levels of these antioxidants (De-Regil, 2012; Raijmakers, 2004). There have now been several randomized studies to evaluate vitamin supplementation for women at high risk for preeclampsia (Poston, 2006; Rumbold, 2006; Villar, 2007). The one by the MFMU Network included almost 10,000 low-risk nulliparas (Roberts, 2009). None of these studies showed reduced preeclampsia rates in women given vitamins C and E compared with those given placebo. The recent metaanalysis by De-Regil and colleagues (2012) likewise showed no benefits of vitamin D supplementation.

The rationale for the use of *statins* to prevent preeclampsia is that they stimulate hemoxygenase-1 expression that inhibits sFlt-1 release. There are preliminary animal data that statins may prevent hypertensive disorders of pregnancy. The MFMU Network plans a randomized trial to test pravastatin for this purpose (Costantine, 2013).

Antithrombotic Agents

There are sound theoretical reasons that antithrombotic agents might reduce the incidence of preeclampsia. As discussed on page 734, the syndrome is characterized by vasospasm, endothelial cell dysfunction, and inflammation, as well as activation of platelets and the coagulation-hemostasis system. Moreover, prostaglandin imbalance(s) may be operative, and other sequelae include placental infarction and spiral artery thrombosis (Nelson, 2014).

TABLE 40-6. Maternal-Fetal Medicine Units Network Trial of Low-Dose Aspirin in Women at High Risk for Preeclampsia

Risk Factors	No.	Preeclampsia (%)[a] Aspirin	Placebo
Normotensive, no proteinuria	1613	14.5	17.7
Proteinuria plus hypertension	119	31.7	22.0
Proteinuria only	48	25.0	33.3
Hypertension only	723	24.8	25.0
Insulin-dependent diabetes	462	18.3	21.6
Chronic hypertension	763	26.0	24.6
Multifetal gestation	678	11.5	15.9
Previous preeclampsia	600	16.7	19.0

[a]No statistically significant difference for any comparison between groups.
Data from Caritis, 1998.

Low-Dose Aspirin. In oral doses of 50 to 150 mg daily, aspirin effectively inhibits platelet thromboxane A2 biosynthesis but has minimal effects on vascular prostacyclin production (Wallenburg, 1986). However, clinical trials have shown limited benefits. For example, results in Table 40-6 are from the MFMU Network, and none of the outcomes shown were significantly improved. Some reports are more favorable. For example, the Paris Collaborative Group performed a metaanalysis that included 31 randomized trials involving 32,217 women (Askie, 2007). For women assigned to receive antiplatelet agents, the relative risk for development of preeclampsia, superimposed preeclampsia, preterm delivery, or any adverse pregnancy outcome was significantly decreased by 10 percent. Another review and metaanalysis reported marginal benefits for low-dose aspirin and severe preeclampsia (Roberge, 2012). A recent small Finnish multicenter trial included 152 women at high risk for preeclampsia (Villa, 2013). Although there were no benefits to low-dose aspirin, the accompanying metaanalysis reported a lowering of risk. The 2013 Task Force recommended the use of low-dose aspirin in some high-risk women to prevent preeclampsia.

Low-Dose Aspirin plus Heparin. In women with lupus anticoagulant, treatment with low-dose aspirin and heparin mitigates thrombotic sequelae (Chap. 59, p. 1175). Because of the high prevalence of placental thrombotic lesions found with severe preeclampsia, observational trials have been done to evaluate such treatments for affected women. Sergis and associates (2006) reviewed effects of prophylaxis with low-molecular-weight heparin plus low-dose aspirin on pregnancy outcomes in women with a history of severe early-onset preeclampsia and low-birthweight neonates. They reported better pregnancy outcomes in women given low-molecular-weight heparin plus low-dose aspirin compared with those given low-dose aspirin alone. Similar findings were reported in a trial that included 139 women with thrombophilia and a history of early-onset preeclampsia (de Vries, 2012). Despite these small trials, evidence is insufficient to recommend these regimens to prevent preeclampsia (National Institute for Health and Clinical Excellence, 2010; Staff, 2014).

MANAGEMENT

Pregnancy complicated by gestational hypertension is managed based on severity, gestational age, and presence of preeclampsia. With preeclampsia, management varies with the severity of endothelial cell injury and multiorgan dysfunction.

Preeclampsia cannot always be diagnosed definitively (p. 728). Thus, the Task Force of the American College of Obstetricians and Gynecologists (2013b) recommends more frequent prenatal visits if preeclampsia is "suspected." *Increases in systolic and diastolic blood pressure can be either normal physiological changes or signs of developing pathology.* Increased surveillance permits more prompt recognition of ominous changes in blood pressure, critical laboratory findings, and clinical signs and symptoms (Macdonald-Wallis, 2012).

The basic management objectives for any pregnancy complicated by preeclampsia are: (1) termination of pregnancy with the least possible trauma to mother and fetus, (2) birth of an infant who subsequently thrives, and (3) complete restoration of health to the mother. In many women with preeclampsia, especially those at or near term, all three objectives are served equally well by induction of labor. *One of the most important clinical questions for successful management is precise knowledge of fetal age.*

Early Diagnosis of Preeclampsia

Traditionally, the frequency of prenatal visits is increased during the third trimester, and this aids early detection of preeclampsia. *Women without overt hypertension, but in whom early developing preeclampsia is suspected during routine prenatal visits, are seen more frequently.* The protocol used successfully for many years at Parkland Hospital for women with new-onset diastolic blood pressures > 80 mm Hg but < 90 mm Hg or with sudden abnormal weight gain of more than 2 pounds per week includes, at minimum, return visits at 7-day intervals. Outpatient surveillance is continued unless overt hypertension, proteinuria, headache, visual disturbances, or epigastric discomfort supervene. Women with overt new-onset hypertension—either diastolic pressures ≥ 90 mm Hg or systolic pressures ≥ 140 mm Hg—are admitted to determine if the increase is due to preeclampsia, and if so, to evaluate its severity. Women with persistent severe disease are generally delivered, as discussed subsequently. Conversely, women with apparently mild disease can often be managed as outpatients, although there should be a low threshold for continued hospitalization for the nullipara, especially if there is proteinuria.

Evaluation

Hospitalization is considered at least initially for women with new-onset hypertension, especially if there is persistent or worsening hypertension or development of proteinuria. A systematic evaluation is instituted to include the following:

- Detailed examination, which is followed by daily scrutiny for clinical findings such as headache, visual disturbances, epigastric pain, and rapid weight gain
- Weight determined daily
- Analysis for proteinuria or urine protein:creatinine ratio on admittance and at least every 2 days thereafter
- Blood pressure readings in the sitting position with an appropriate-size cuff every 4 hours, except between 2400 and 0600 unless previous readings had become elevated
- Measurements of plasma or serum creatinine and hepatic aminotransferase levels and a hemogram that includes platelet quantification. The frequency of testing is determined by hypertension severity. Some recommend measurement of serum uric acid and lactic acid dehydrogenase levels and coagulation studies. However, the value of these tests has been called into question (Cnossen, 2006; Conde-Agudelo, 2014; Thangaratinam, 2006).
- Evaluation of fetal size and well-being and amnionic fluid volume, with either physical examination or sonography.

Goals of management include early identification of worsening preeclampsia and development of a management plan for timely delivery. If any of these observations lead to a diagnosis of severe preeclampsia as previously defined by the criteria in Table 40-2, further management is subsequently described.

Reduced physical activity throughout much of the day is likely beneficial, but as the 2013 Task Force concluded, absolute bed rest is not desirable. Ample protein and calories should be included in the diet, and sodium and fluid intake should not be limited or forced. Further management depends on: (1) preeclampsia severity, (2) gestational age, and (3) condition of the cervix.

Fortunately, many cases are sufficiently mild and near enough to term that they can be managed conservatively until labor commences spontaneously or until the cervix becomes favorable for labor induction. Complete abatement of all signs and symptoms, however, is uncommon until after delivery. *Almost certainly, the underlying disease persists until delivery is accomplished.*

Consideration for Delivery

Termination of pregnancy is the only cure for preeclampsia. Headache, visual disturbances, or epigastric pain are indicative that convulsions may be imminent, and oliguria is another ominous sign. Severe preeclampsia demands anticonvulsant and frequently antihypertensive therapy, followed by delivery. Treatment is identical to that described subsequently for eclampsia. The prime objectives are to forestall convulsions, to prevent intracranial hemorrhage and serious damage to other vital organs, and to deliver a healthy newborn.

When the fetus is preterm, the tendency is to temporize in the hope that a few more weeks in utero will reduce the risk of neonatal death or serious morbidity from prematurity. As discussed, such a policy certainly is justified in milder cases. Assessments of fetal well-being and placental function are performed, especially when the fetus is immature. Most recommend frequent performance of various tests to assess fetal well-being as described by the American College of Obstetricians and Gynecologists (2012a). These include the *nonstress test* or the *biophysical profile* (Chap. 17, pp. 338 and 341). Measurement of the lecithin-sphingomyelin (L/S) ratio in amnionic fluid may provide evidence of lung maturity (Chap. 34, p. 655).

With moderate or severe preeclampsia that does not improve after hospitalization, delivery is usually advisable for the welfare of both mother and fetus. This is true even when the cervix is unfavorable (Tajik, 2012). Labor induction is carried out, usually with preinduction cervical ripening from a prostaglandin or osmotic dilator (Chap. 26, p. 525). Whenever it appears that induction almost certainly will not succeed or attempts have failed, then cesarean delivery is indicated.

For a woman near term, with a soft, partially effaced cervix, even milder degrees of preeclampsia probably carry more risk to the mother and her fetus-infant than does induction of labor (Tajik, 2012). The decision to deliver late-preterm fetuses is not clear. Barton and coworkers (2009) reported excessive neonatal morbidity in women delivered before 38 weeks despite having stable, mild, nonproteinuric hypertension. The Netherlands study of 4316 newborns delivered between $34^{0/7}$ and $36^{6/7}$ weeks also described substantive neonatal morbidity in these cases (Langenveld, 2011). Most of these deliveries were before 36 weeks, and the higher cesarean delivery rates were associated with more respiratory complications. Conversely, one randomized trial of 756 women with mild preeclampsia supported delivery after 37 weeks (Koopmans, 2009).

Elective Cesarean Delivery

Once severe preeclampsia is diagnosed, labor induction and vaginal delivery have traditionally been considered ideal. Temporization with an immature fetus is considered subsequently. Several concerns, including an unfavorable cervix, a perceived sense of urgency because of preeclampsia severity, and a need to coordinate neonatal intensive care, have led some to advocate cesarean delivery. Alexander and colleagues (1999) reviewed 278 singleton liveborn neonates weighing 750 to 1500 g delivered of women with severe preeclampsia at Parkland Hospital. In half of the women, labor was induced, and the remainder underwent cesarean delivery without labor. Induction was successful in accomplishing vaginal delivery in a third, and it was not harmful to the very-low-birthweight infants. Alanis and associates (2008) reported similar observations. The results of a systematic review also confirmed these conclusions (Le Ray, 2009).

Hospitalization versus Outpatient Management

For women with mild to moderate stable hypertension—whether or not preeclampsia has been confirmed—surveillance is continued in the hospital, at home for some reliable patients, or in a day-care unit. At least intuitively, reduced physical activity throughout much of the day seems beneficial. Several observational studies and randomized trials have addressed the benefits of inpatient care and outpatient management.

Somewhat related, Abenhaim and coworkers (2008) reported a retrospective cohort study of 677 nonhypertensive women hospitalized for bed rest because of threatened preterm delivery. When outcomes of these women were compared with those of the general obstetrical population, bed rest was associated with a significantly reduced relative risk—RR 0.27—of developing preeclampsia. In a review of two small randomized trials totaling 106 women at high risk for preeclampsia, prophylactic bed rest for 4 to 6 hours daily at home was successful in significantly lowering the incidence of preeclampsia but not gestational hypertension (Meher, 2006).

These and other observations support the claim that restricted activity alters the underlying pathophysiology of the preeclampsia syndrome. That said, complete bed rest is not recommended by the 2013 Task Force. First, this is pragmatically unachievable because of the severe restrictions it places on otherwise well women. Also, as discussed in Chapter 52 (p. 1029), it likely also predisposes to thromboembolism (Knight, 2007).

High-Risk Pregnancy Unit

The concept of prolonged hospitalization for women with hypertension arose during the 1970s. At Parkland Hospital, an inpatient antepartum unit was established in 1973 by Dr. Peggy Whalley in large part to provide care for such women. Initial results from this unit were reported by Hauth (1976) and Gilstrap (1978) and their colleagues. Most hospitalized women have a beneficial response characterized by amelioration or improvement of hypertension. *These women are not "cured," and nearly 90 percent have recurrent hypertension before or during labor.* By 2013, more than 10,000 nulliparas with mild to moderate early-onset hypertension during pregnancy had been managed successfully in this unit. Provider costs—*not charges*—for this relatively simple physical facility, modest nursing care, no drugs other than iron and folate supplements, and few essential laboratory tests are minimal compared with the cost of neonatal intensive care for a preterm infant. None of these women have suffered thromboembolic disease.

Home Health Care

Many clinicians believe that further hospitalization is not warranted if hypertension abates within a few days, and this has legitimized third-party payers to deny hospitalization reimbursement. Consequently, many women with mild to moderate hypertension are managed at home. Outpatient management may continue as long as preeclampsia syndrome does not worsen and fetal jeopardy is not suspected. Sedentary activity throughout the greater part of the day is recommended. These women are instructed in detail to report symptoms. Home blood pressure and urine protein monitoring or frequent evaluations by a visiting nurse may prove beneficial. Caution is exercised regarding use of certain automated home blood pressure monitors (Lo, 2002; Ostchega, 2012).

In an observational study by Barton and associates (2002), 1182 nulliparas with mild gestational hypertension—20 percent had proteinuria—were managed with home health care. Their mean gestational ages were 32 to 33 weeks at enrollment and 36 to 37 weeks at delivery. Severe preeclampsia developed in approximately 20 percent, about 3 percent developed HELLP syndrome, and two women had eclampsia. Perinatal outcomes were generally good. In approximately 20 percent, there was fetal-growth restriction, and the perinatal mortality rate was 4.2 per 1000.

Several prospective studies have been designed to compare continued hospitalization with either home health care or a day-care unit. In a pilot study from Parkland Hospital, Horsager and colleagues (1995) randomly assigned 72 nulliparas with new-onset hypertension from 27 to 37 weeks either to continued hospitalization or to outpatient care. In all of these women, proteinuria had receded to less than 500 mg per day when they were randomized. Outpatient management included daily blood pressure monitoring by the patient or her family. Weight and dipstick spot urine protein determinations were evaluated three times weekly. A home health nurse visited twice weekly, and the women were seen weekly in the clinic. Perinatal outcomes were similar in each group. The only significant difference was that women in the home care group developed severe preeclampsia significantly more frequently than hospitalized women—42 versus 25 percent.

A larger randomized trial reported by Crowther and coworkers (1992) included 218 women with mild gestational nonproteinuric hypertension. After evaluation, half remained hospitalized, whereas the other half was managed as outpatients. As shown in Table 40-7, the mean duration of hospitalization was 22.2 days for women with inpatient management compared with only 6.5 days in the home-care group. Preterm delivery before 34 and before 37 weeks was increased twofold in the outpatient group, but maternal and infant outcomes otherwise were similar.

Day-Care Unit

Another approach, popular in European countries, is day care (Milne, 2009). This approach has been evaluated by several investigators. In the study by Tuffnell and associates (1992), 54 women with hypertension after 26 weeks' gestation were assigned to either day care or routine outpatient management (see Table 40-7). Progression to overt preeclampsia and labor inductions were significantly increased in the routine management group. Turnbull and coworkers (2004) enrolled 395 women who were randomly assigned to either day care or inpatient management (see Table 40-7). Almost 95 percent had mild to moderate hypertension. Of enrolled women, 288 were without proteinuria, and 86 had ≥ 1+ proteinuria. There were no perinatal deaths, and none of the women developed eclampsia or HELLP syndrome. Surprisingly, costs for either scheme were not significantly different. Perhaps not surprisingly, general satisfaction favored day care.

Summary of Hospitalization versus Outpatient Management

From the above, either inpatient or close outpatient management is appropriate for a woman with mild de novo hypertension, including those with nonsevere preeclampsia. Most of these studies were carried out in academic centers with dedicated management teams. That said, the key to success is close follow-up and a conscientious patient with good home support.

TABLE 40-7. Randomized Clinical Trials Comparing Hospitalization versus Routine Care for Women with Mild Gestational Hypertension or Preeclampsia

	Maternal Characteristics—Admission					Maternal Characteristics—Delivery				Perinatal Outcomes		
Study Groups	No.	$Para_0$ (%)	Chronic HTN (%)	EGA (wk)	Prot (%)	EGA (wk)	< 37 wk (%)	< 34 wk (%)	Mean Hosp (d)	Mean BW (g)	SGA (%)	PMR (%)
Crowther (1992)	218[a]											
Hospitalization	110	13	14	35.3	0	38.3	12	1.8	22.2	3080	14	0
Outpatient	108	13	17	34.6	0	38.2	22	3.7	6.5	3060	14	0
Tuffnell (1992)	54											
Day Unit	24	57	23	36	0	39.8	—	—	1.1	3320	—	0
Usual Care	30	54	21	36.5	21	39	—	—	5.1	3340	—	0
Turnbull (2004)	374[b]											
Hospitalization	125	63	0	35.9	22	39	—	—	8.5	3330	3.8	0
Day Unit	249	62	0	36.2	22	39.7	—	—	7.2	3300	2.3	0

[a]Excluded women with proteinuria at study entry.
[b]Included women with ≤ 1+ proteinuria.
BW = birthweight; EGA = estimated gestational age; HTN = hypertension; $Para_0$ = nulliparas; PMR = perinatal mortality rate; Prot = proteinuria; SGA = small for gestational age.

Antihypertensive Therapy for Mild to Moderate Hypertension

The use of antihypertensive drugs in attempts to prolong pregnancy or modify perinatal outcomes in pregnancies complicated by various types and severities of hypertensive disorders has been of considerable interest. Treatment for women with chronic hypertension complicating pregnancy is discussed in detail in Chapter 50 (p. 1005).

Drug treatment for early mild preeclampsia has been disappointing as shown in representative randomized trials listed in Table 40-8. Sibai and colleagues (1987a) evaluated the effectiveness of labetalol and hospitalization compared with hospitalization alone in 200 nulliparas with gestational hypertension from 26 to 35 weeks' gestation. Although women given labetalol had significantly lower mean blood pressures, there were no differences between the groups in terms of mean pregnancy prolongation, gestational age at delivery, or birthweight. The cesarean delivery rates were similar, as were the number of infants admitted to special-care nurseries. *The frequency of growth-restricted infants was doubled in women given labetalol—19 versus 9 percent.* The three other studies listed in Table 40-8 were performed to compare labetalol or the calcium-channel blockers, nifedipine and isradipine, with placebo. Except for fewer episodes of severe hypertension, none of these studies showed any benefits of antihypertensive treatment. Moreover, there may have been treatment-induced adverse fetal growth (Von Dadelszen, 2002).

Abalos and associates (2007) reviewed 46 randomized trials of active antihypertensive therapy compared with either no treatment or placebo given to women with mild to moderate gestational hypertension. Except for a halving of the risk for developing severe hypertension, active antihypertensive therapy had no beneficial effects. They further reported that fetal-growth restriction *was not increased* in treated women. In this vein, it is also controversial whether β-blocking agents cause fetal-growth restriction if given for chronic hypertension (August, 2014; Umans, 2014). Thus, any salutary or adverse effects of antihypertensive therapy seem minimal at most.

Delayed Delivery

Up through the early 1990s, it was the practice that all women with severe preeclampsia were delivered without delay. During the past 25 years, however, another approach for women with preterm severe preeclampsia has been advocated. This approach calls for "conservative" or "expectant" management with the aim of improving neonatal outcome without compromising maternal safety. Aspects of such management always include careful daily—and usually more frequent—inpatient monitoring of the mother and her fetus.

Expectant Management of Preterm Severe Preeclampsia

Theoretically, antihypertensive therapy has potential application when severe preeclampsia develops before intact neonatal survival is likely. Such management is controversial, and it may be dangerous. In one of the first studies, Sibai and the Memphis group (1985) attempted to prolong pregnancy because of fetal immaturity in 60 women with severe preeclampsia between 18 and 27 weeks. The results were disastrous. *The perinatal mortality rate was 87 percent. Although no mothers died, 13 suffered placental abruption, 10 had eclampsia, three developed renal failure, two had hypertensive encephalopathy, and one each had an intracerebral hemorrhage and a ruptured hepatic hematoma.*

Because of these catastrophic outcomes, the Memphis group redefined their study criteria and performed a randomized trial of expectant versus aggressive management for 95 women who had severe preeclampsia but with more advanced gestations of 28 to 32 weeks (Sibai, 1994). *Women with HELLP syndrome were excluded from this trial.* Aggressive management included glucocorticoid administration for fetal lung maturation followed by

TABLE 40-8. Randomized Placebo-Controlled Trials of Antihypertensive Therapy for Early Mild Gestational Hypertension

Study	Study Drug (No.)	Pregnancy Prolonged (d)	Severe HTN[a] (%)	Cesarean Delivery (%)	Placental Abruption (%)	Mean Birthweight (g)	Growth Restriction (%)	Neonatal Deaths (No.)
Sibai (1987a)[a] 200 inpatients	Labetalol (100)	21.3	5	36	2	2205	19[c]	1
	Placebo (100)	20.1	15[c]	32	0	2260	9	0
Sibai (1992)[b] 200 outpatients	Nifedipine (100)	22.3	9	43	3	2405	8	0
	Placebo (100)	22.5	18[c]	35	2	2510	4	0
Pickles (1992) 144 outpatients	Labetalol (70)	26.6	9	24	NS	NS	NS	NS
	Placebo (74)	23.1	10	26	NS	NS	NS	NS
Wide-Swensson (1995) 111 outpatients	Isradipine (54)	23.1	22	26	NS	NS	NS	0
	Placebo (57)	29.8	29	19	NS	NS	NS	0

[a]All women had preeclampsia.
[b]Includes postpartum hypertension.
[c]$p < .05$ when study drug compared with placebo.
HTN = hypertension; NS = not stated.

delivery in 48 hours. Expectantly managed women were observed at bed rest and given either labetalol or nifedipine orally if there was severe hypertension. In this study, pregnancy was prolonged for a mean of 15.4 days in the expectant management group. An overall improvement in neonatal outcomes was also reported.

Following these experiences, expectant management became more commonly practiced, but with the caveat that women with HELLP syndrome or growth-restricted fetuses were usually excluded. But in a subsequent follow-up observational study, the Memphis group compared outcomes in 133 preeclamptic women with and 136 without HELLP syndrome who presented between 24 and 36 weeks (Abramovici, 1999). Women were subdivided into three study groups. The first group included those with *complete HELLP syndrome*. The second group included women with *partial HELLP syndrome*—defined as either one or two but not all three of the defining laboratory findings. The third group included women who had severe preeclampsia without HELLP syndrome laboratory findings. Perinatal outcomes were similar in each group, and importantly, outcomes were not improved with procrastination. Despite this, the investigators concluded that women with partial HELLP syndrome and those with severe preeclampsia alone could be managed expectantly.

Sibai and Barton (2007b) reviewed expectant management of severe preeclampsia from 24 to 34 weeks. More than 1200 women were included, and although the average time gained ranged from 5 to 10 days, the maternal morbidity rates were formidable. As shown in Table 40-9, serious complications in some of these and in later studies included placental abruption, HELLP syndrome, pulmonary edema, renal failure, and eclampsia. Moreover, perinatal mortality rates averaged 90 per 1000. Fetal-growth restriction was common, and in the study from The Netherlands by Ganzevoort and associates (2005a,b), it was an astounding 94 percent. Perinatal mortality rates are disproportionately high in these growth-restricted infants, but maternal outcomes were not appreciably different from pregnancies in women without growth-restricted fetuses (Haddad, 2007; Shear, 2005).

The MEXPRE Latin Study was a multicenter trial that randomly assigned 267 women with severe preeclampsia at 28 to 32 weeks to prompt delivery or to expectant management (Vigil-De Gracia, 2013). The perinatal mortality rate approximated 9 percent in each group, and these investigators found no improvements in composite neonatal morbidity with expectant management. On the other hand, fetal-growth restriction—22 versus 9 percent—and placental abruption—7.6 versus 1.5 percent—were significantly higher in the group managed expectantly.

Barber and associates (2009) conducted a 10-year review of 3408 women with severe preeclampsia from 24 to 32 weeks. They found that increasing lengths of antepartum hospital stays were associated with slight but significantly increased rates of maternal and neonatal morbidity.

Expectant Management of Midtrimester Severe Preeclampsia

Several small studies have focused on expectant management of severe preeclampsia syndrome *before 28 weeks*. In their review, Bombrys and coworkers (2008) found eight such studies that included nearly 200 women with severe preeclampsia with an onset < 26 completed weeks. Maternal complications were common. Because there were no neonatal survivors in women presenting before 23 weeks, the Task Force of the American College of Obstetricians and Gynecologists (2013b) recommends

TABLE 40-9. Maternal and Perinatal Outcomes Reported Since 2005 with Expectant Management of Severe Preeclampsia from 24 to 34 Weeks

			Maternal Outcomes (%)					Perinatal Outcomes (%)	
Study	No.	Days Gained	Placental Abruption	HELLP	Pulm. Edema	ARF	Eclampsia	FGR	PMR
Oettle (2005)	131[a]	11.6	23	4.6	0.8	2.3	2.3	NS	13.8
Shear (2005)	155	5.3	5.8	27	3.9	NS	1.9	62	3.9
Ganzevoort (2005a, b)	216	11	1.8	18	3.6	NS	1.8	94	18
Sarsam (2008)	35	9.2	5.7	11	2.9	2.9	18	31	2.8
Bombrys (2009)	66	5	11	8	9	3	0	27	1.5
Abdel-Hady (2010)	211	12	3.3	7.6	0.9	6.6	0.9	NS	48
Vigil-De Gracia (2013)	131	10.3	7.6	14	1.5	4.5	0.8	22	8.7
Range	945	5–12	1.8–23	4.6–27	0.9–3.9	2.3–6.6	0.9–18	27–94	1.5–48

[a]Includes one maternal death.
ARF = acute renal failure; EGA = estimated gestational age; FGR = fetal-growth restriction; HELLP = hemolysis, elevated liver enzyme levels, low platelet count syndrome; NS = not stated; PMR = perinatal mortality rate; Pulm. = pulmonary.

pregnancy termination. For women with slightly more advanced pregnancies, however, the decision is less clear. For example, at 23 weeks' gestation, the perinatal survival rate was 18 percent, but long-term perinatal morbidity is yet unknown. For women with pregnancies at 24 to 26 weeks, perinatal survival approached 60 percent, and it averaged almost 90 percent for those at 26 weeks.

There have been at least five studies published since 2005 of women with severe midtrimester preeclampsia who were managed expectantly (Abdel-Hady, 2010; Belghiti, 2011; Bombrys, 2008; Budden, 2006; Gaugler-Senden, 2006). Maternal complications developed in 60 percent, and there was one death. Perinatal mortality was 65 percent. At this time, there are no comparative studies attesting to the perinatal benefits of such expectant treatment versus early delivery in the face of serious maternal complications that approach 50 percent.

Glucocorticoids for Lung Maturation

In attempts to enhance fetal lung maturation, glucocorticoids have been administered to women with severe hypertension who are remote from term. Treatment does not seem to worsen maternal hypertension, and a decrease in the incidence of respiratory distress and improved fetal survival has been cited. That said, there is only one randomized trial of corticosteroids given to hypertensive women for fetal lung maturation. This trial, by Amorim and colleagues (1999), included 218 women with severe preeclampsia between 26 and 34 weeks who were randomly assigned to betamethasone or placebo administration. Neonatal complications, including respiratory distress, intraventricular hemorrhage, and death, were decreased significantly when betamethasone was given compared with placebo. *On the heavily weighted negative side, there were two maternal deaths and 18 stillbirths.* We add these findings to buttress our unenthusiastic acceptance of attempts to prolong gestation in many of these women (Alexander, 2014; Bloom, 2003).

Corticosteroids to Ameliorate HELLP Syndrome

Almost 30 years ago, Thiagarajah and associates (1984) suggested that glucocorticoids might aid treatment of the laboratory abnormalities associated with HELLP syndrome. Subsequently, Tompkins (1999) and O'Brien (2002) and their colleagues reported less than salutary effects. Martin and coworkers (2003) reviewed observational outcomes of almost 500 such women treated at their institution and reported salutary results with treatment. Unfortunately, their subsequent randomized trial compared two corticosteroids and did not include a nontreated group (Isler, 2001).

Since these observational studies, at least two prospective randomized trials have addressed this question. Fonseca and associates (2005) randomly assigned 132 women with HELLP syndrome to either dexamethasone or placebo administration. Outcomes assessed included duration of hospitalization, recovery time of abnormal laboratory test results, resolution of clinical parameters, and complications that included acute renal failure, pulmonary edema, eclampsia, and death. None of these was significantly different between the two groups. In another randomized study, Katz and coworkers (2008) assigned 105 postpartum women with HELLP syndrome to treatment with dexamethasone or placebo. They analyzed outcomes similar to the Fonseca study and found no advantage to dexamethasone. Shown in Figure 40-16 are recovery times for platelet counts and serum aspartate aminotransferase (AST) levels. These times were almost identical in the two groups. For these reasons, the 2013 Task Force does not recommend corticosteroid treatment for thrombocytopenia with HELLP syndrome. A caveat is that in women with dangerously low platelet counts, corticosteroids *might* serve to increase platelets.

Expectant Managment—Risks versus Benefits—Recommendations

Taken in toto, these studies do not show overwhelming benefits compared with risks for expectant management of severe preeclampsia in those with gestations from 24 to 32 weeks. The Society for Maternal-Fetal Medicine (2011) has determined that such management is a reasonable alternative in selected women with severe preeclampsia before 34 weeks. The Task Force of the American College of Obstetricians and Gynecologists (2013b) supports this recommendation. As shown in Figure 40-17, such management calls for in-hospital maternal and fetal surveillance with delivery prompted by evidence for worsening severe preeclampsia or maternal or fetal compromise. Although attempts are made for vaginal delivery in most cases, the likelihood of cesarean delivery increases with decreasing gestational age.

Our view is more conservative. Undoubtedly, the overriding reason to terminate pregnancies with severe preeclampsia is maternal safety. There are no data to suggest that expectant management is beneficial for the mother. Indeed, it seems obvious that a delay to prolong gestation in women with severe preeclampsia may have serious maternal consequences such as those shown in Table 40-9. Notably, placental abruption develops in up to 20 percent, and pulmonary edema in as many as 4 percent. Moreover, there are substantive risks for eclampsia, cerebrovascular hemorrhage, and especially maternal death. These observations are even more pertinent when considered with the absence of convincing evidence that perinatal outcomes are markedly improved by the average prolongation of pregnancy of about 1 week. If undertaken, the caveats that mandate delivery shown in Table 40-10 should be strictly heeded.

Eclampsia

Preeclampsia complicated by generalized tonic-clonic convulsions appreciably increases the risk to both mother and fetus. Mattar and Sibai (2000) described outcomes in 399 consecutive women with eclampsia from 1977 through 1998. Major maternal complications included placental abruption—10 percent, neurological deficits—7 percent, aspiration pneumonia—7 percent, pulmonary edema—5 percent, cardiopulmonary arrest—4 percent, and acute renal failure—4 percent. Moreover, 1 percent of these women died.

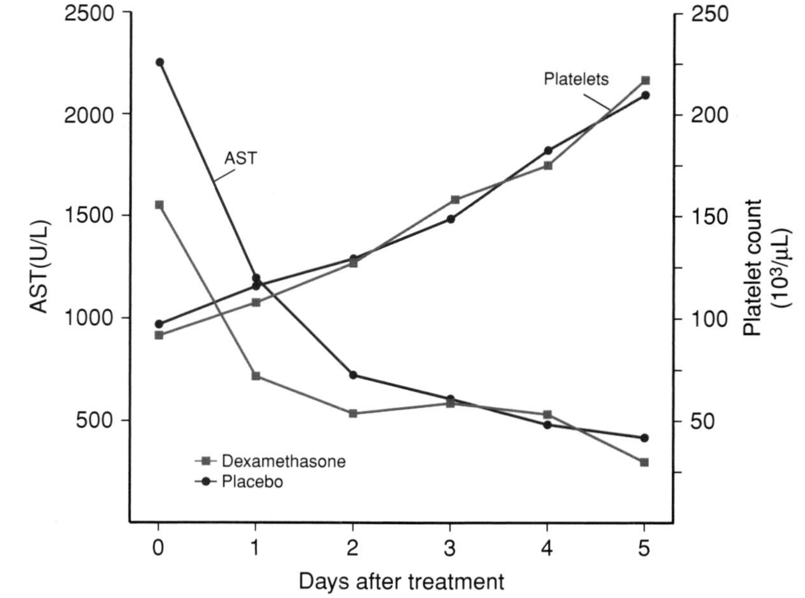

FIGURE 40-16 Recovery times for platelet counts and serum aspartate aminotransferase (AST) levels in women with HELLP syndrome assigned to receive treatment with dexamethasone or placebo. (Data from Katz, 2008.)

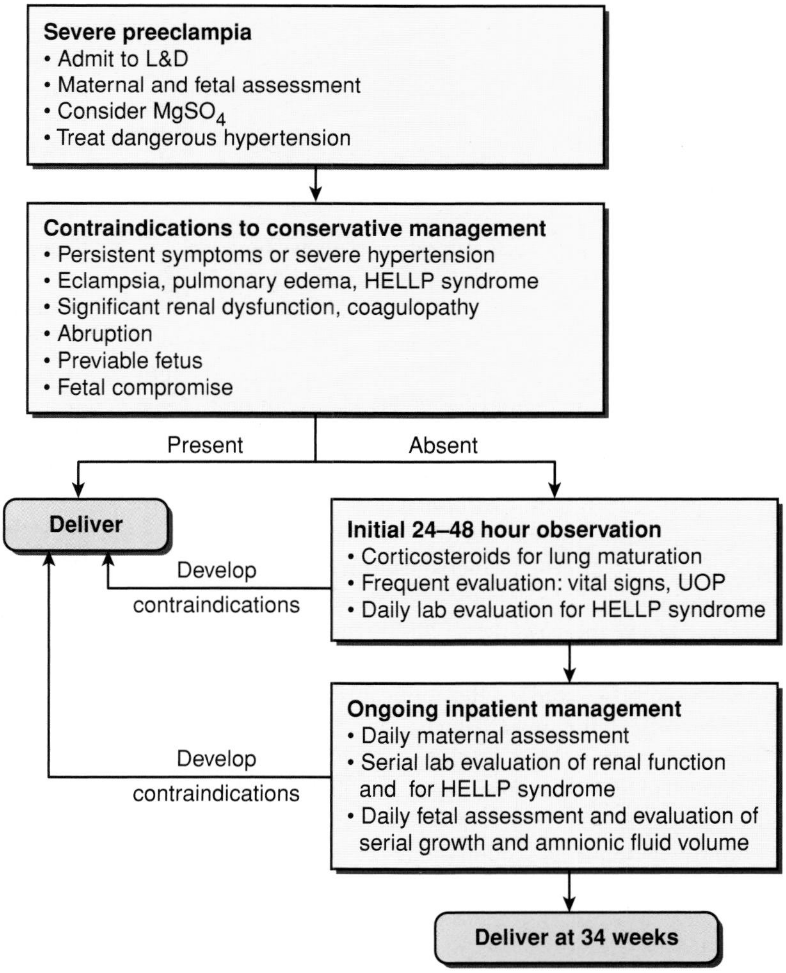

FIGURE 40-17 Schematic clinical management algorithm for suspected severe preeclampsia at < 34 weeks. HELLP = hemolysis, elevated liver enzyme levels, low platelet count; L&D = labor and delivery; $MgSO_4$ = magnesium sulfate; UOP = urine output. (Adapted from the Society for Maternal-Fetal Medicine, 2011.)

TABLE 40-10. Indications for Delivery in Women < 34 Weeks' Gestation Managed Expectantly

Corticosteroid Therapy for Lung Maturation[a] and Delivery after Maternal Stabilization:
Uncontrolled severe hypertension
Eclampsia
Pulmonary edema
Placental abruption
Disseminated intravascular coagulation
Nonreassuring fetal status
Fetal demise
Corticosteroid Therapy for Lung Maturation—Delay Delivery 48 hr If Possible:
Preterm ruptured membranes or labor
Thrombocytopenia < 100,000/μL
Hepatic transaminase levels twice upper limit of normal
Fetal-growth restriction
Oligohydramnios
Reversed end-diastolic Doppler flow in umbilical artery
Worsening renal dysfunction

[a]Initial dose only, do not delay delivery.
From the Society for Maternal-Fetal Medicine, 2011, and the Task Force of the American College of Obstetricians and Gynecologists, 2013b.

European maternity units also report excessive maternal and perinatal morbidity and mortality rates with eclampsia. In a report from Scandinavia, Andersgaard and associates (2006) described 232 women with eclampsia. Although there was but a single maternal death, a third of the women experienced major complications that included HELLP syndrome, renal failure, pulmonary edema, pulmonary embolism, and stroke. The United Kingdom Obstetric Surveillance System (UKOSS) audit reported by Knight (2007) described no maternal deaths in 214 eclamptic women, but five women experienced cerebral hemorrhage. In The Netherlands, there were three maternal deaths among 222 eclamptic women (Zwart, 2008). From Dublin, Akkawi and coworkers (2009) reported four maternal deaths among 247 eclamptic women (Akkawi, 2009). Data from Australia are similar (Thornton, 2013). Thus, in developed countries, the maternal mortality rate approximates 1 percent in women with eclampsia. In perspective, this is a thousand-fold increase above the overall maternal death rates for these countries.

Almost without exception—but at times unnoticed—preeclampsia precedes the onset of eclamptic convulsions. Depending on whether convulsions appear before, during, or after labor, eclampsia is designated as antepartum, intrapartum, or postpartum. Eclampsia is most common in the last trimester and becomes increasingly frequent as term approaches. In more recent years, the incidence of postpartum eclampsia has risen. This is presumably related to improved access to prenatal care, earlier detection of preeclampsia, and prophylactic use of magnesium sulfate (Chames, 2002). Importantly, other diagnoses should be considered in women with convulsions more than 48 hours postpartum or in women with focal neurological deficits, prolonged coma, or atypical eclampsia (Sibai, 2009, 2012).

Immediate Management of Seizure

Eclamptic seizures may be violent, and the woman must be protected, especially her airway. So forceful are the muscular movements that the woman may throw herself out of her bed, and if not protected, her tongue is bitten by the violent action of the jaws (Fig. 40-18). This phase, in which the muscles alternately contract and relax, may last approximately a minute. Gradually, the muscular movements become smaller and less frequent, and finally the woman lies motionless. After a seizure, the woman is postictal, but in some, a coma of variable duration ensues. When the convulsions are infrequent, the woman usually recovers some degree of consciousness after each attack. As the woman arouses, a semiconscious combative state may ensue. In severe cases, coma persists from one convulsion to another, and death may result. In rare instances, a single convulsion may be followed by coma from which the woman may never emerge. As a rule, however, death does not occur until after frequent convulsions. Finally and also rarely, convulsions continue unabated—*status epilepticus*—and require deep sedation and even general anesthesia to obviate anoxic encephalopathy.

Respirations after an eclamptic convulsion are usually increased in rate and may reach 50 or more per minute in response to hypercarbia, lactic acidemia, and transient hypoxia. Cyanosis may be observed in severe cases. High fever is a grave sign as it likely emanates from cerebrovascular hemorrhage.

Proteinuria is usually, but not always, present as discussed on page 730. Urine output may be diminished appreciably, and occasionally anuria develops. There may be hemoglobinuria, but hemoglobinemia is observed rarely. Often, as shown in

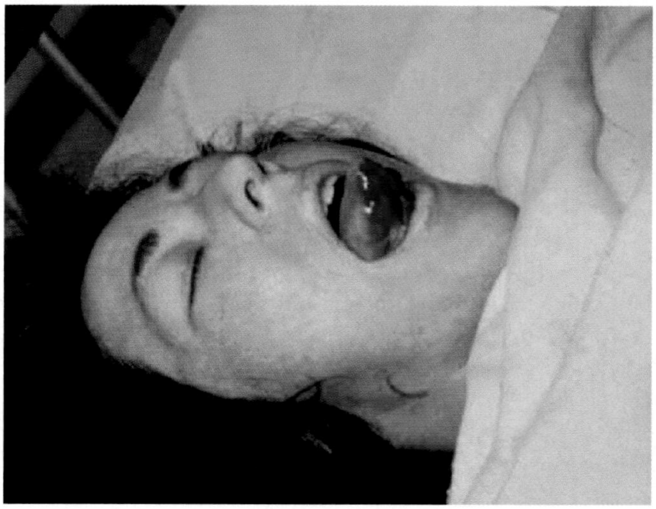

FIGURE 40-18 Hematoma of tongue from laceration during an eclamptic convulsion. Thrombocytopenia may have contributed to the bleeding.

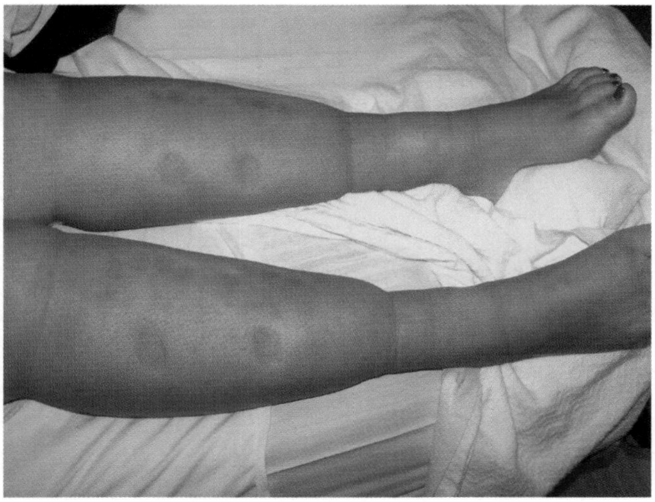

FIGURE 40-19 Severe edema in a young nullipara with antepartum preeclampsia. (Photograph contributed by Dr. Nidhi Shah.)

Figure 40-19, peripheral and facial edema is pronounced, but it may also be absent.

As with severe preeclampsia, an increase in urinary output after delivery is usually an early sign of improvement. If there is renal dysfunction, serum creatinine levels should be monitored. Proteinuria and edema ordinarily disappear within a week postpartum. In most cases, blood pressure returns to normal within a few days to 2 weeks after delivery (Berks, 2009). As subsequently discussed, the longer hypertension persists postpartum and the more severe it is, the more likely it is that the woman also has chronic vascular disease (Podymow, 2010).

In antepartum eclampsia, labor may begin spontaneously shortly after convulsions ensue and may progress rapidly. If the convulsions occur during labor, contractions may increase in frequency and intensity, and the duration of labor may be shortened. Because of maternal hypoxemia and lactic acidemia caused by convulsions, it is not unusual for fetal bradycardia to follow a seizure (Fig. 40-20). Bradycardia usually recovers within 3 to 5 minutes. If it persists more than about 10 minutes, however, then another cause such as placental abruption or imminent delivery must be considered.

Pulmonary edema may follow shortly after eclamptic convulsions or up to several hours later. This usually is caused by aspiration pneumonitis from gastric-content inhalation during vomiting that frequently accompanies convulsions. In some women, pulmonary edema may be caused by ventricular failure from increased afterload that may result from severe hypertension and further aggravated by vigorous intravenous fluid administration (Dennis, 2012b). Such pulmonary edema from ventricular failure is more common in morbidly obese women and in those with previously unappreciated chronic hypertension.

Occasionally, sudden death occurs synchronously with an eclamptic convulsion, or it follows shortly thereafter. Most often in these cases, death results from a massive cerebral hemorrhage (see Fig. 40-11). Hemiplegia may result from sublethal hemorrhage. Cerebral hemorrhages are more likely in older women with underlying chronic hypertension as discussed on page 761. Rarely, they may be due to a ruptured cerebral berry aneurysm or arteriovenous malformation (Witlin, 1997a).

In approximately 10 percent of women, some degree of blindness follows a seizure. The causes of blindness or impaired vision are discussed on page 744. Blindness with severe preeclampsia without convulsions is usually due to retinal detachment (Vigil-De Gracia, 2011). Conversely, blindness with eclampsia is almost always due to occipital lobe edema (Cunningham, 1995). In both instances, however, the prognosis for return to normal function is good and is usually complete within 1 to 2 weeks postpartum.

Up to 5 percent of women with eclampsia have substantively altered consciousness, including persistent coma, following a seizure. This is due to extensive cerebral edema, and transtentorial herniation may cause death as discussed on page 744 (Cunningham, 2000).

Rarely, eclampsia is followed by psychosis, and the woman becomes violent. This may last for several days to 2 weeks, but the prognosis for return to normal function is good, provided there was no preexisting mental illness. It is presumed to be similar to postpartum psychosis discussed in detail in Chapter 61 (p. 1210). Antipsychotic medications have proved effective in the few cases of posteclampsia psychosis treated at Parkland Hospital.

Differential Diagnosis

Generally, eclampsia is more likely to be diagnosed too frequently rather than overlooked. Epilepsy, encephalitis, meningitis, brain tumor, neurocysticercosis, amnionic fluid embolism, postdural puncture cephalgia, and ruptured cerebral

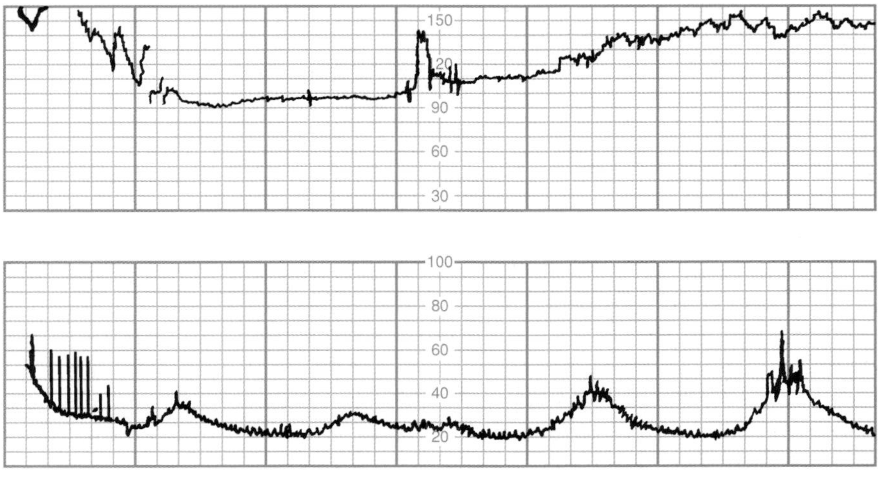

FIGURE 40-20 Fetal heart rate tracing shows fetal bradycardia following an intrapartum eclamptic convulsion. Bradycardia resolved and beat-to-beat variability returned approximately 5 minutes following the seizure.

TABLE 40-11. Magnesium Sulfate Dosage Schedule for Severe Preeclampsia and Eclampsia

Continuous Intravenous (IV) Infusion
Give 4- to 6-g loading dose of magnesium sulfate diluted in 100 mL of IV fluid administered over 15–20 min
Begin 2 g/hr in 100 mL of IV maintenance infusion. Some recommend 1 g/hr
Monitor for magnesium toxicity:
Assess deep tendon reflexes periodically
Some measure serum magnesium level at 4–6 hr and adjust infusion to maintain levels between 4 and 7 mEq/L (4.8 to 8.4 mg/dL)
Measure serum magnesium levels if serum creatinine ≥ 1.0 mg/dL
Magnesium sulfate is discontinued 24 hr after delivery
Intermittent Intramuscular Injections
Give 4 g of magnesium sulfate ($MgSO_4 \cdot 7H_2O$ USP) as a 20% solution intravenously at a rate not to exceed 1 g/min
Follow promptly with 10 g of 50% magnesium sulfate solution, one half (5 g) injected deeply in the upper outer quadrant of each buttock through a 3-inch-long 20-gauge needle. (Addition of 1.0 mL of 2% lidocaine minimizes discomfort.) If convulsions persist after 15 min, give up to 2 g more intravenously as a 20% solution at a rate not to exceed 1 g/min. If the woman is large, up to 4 g may be given slowly
Every 4 hr thereafter, give 5 g of a 50% solution of magnesium sulfate injected deeply in the upper outer quadrant of alternate buttocks, but only after ensuring that:
The patellar reflex is present,
Respirations are not depressed, and
Urine output the previous 4 hr exceeded 100 mL
Magnesium sulfate is discontinued 24 hr after delivery

aneurysm during late pregnancy and the puerperium may simulate eclampsia. Until other such causes are excluded, however, all pregnant women with convulsions should be considered to have eclampsia.

Management of Eclampsia

It has been long recognized that magnesium sulfate is highly effective in preventing convulsions in women with preeclampsia and in stopping them in those with eclampsia. In his review, Chesley (1978) cited observational data by Pritchard and colleagues (1955, 1975) from Parkland Hospital and from his own institution, Kings County Hospital in Brooklyn. At that time, most eclampsia regimens used in the United States adhered to a similar philosophy still in use today, the tenets of which include the following:

1. Control of convulsions using an intravenously administered loading dose of magnesium sulfate that is followed by a maintenance dose, usually intravenous, of magnesium sulfate
2. Intermittent administration of an antihypertensive medication to lower blood pressure whenever it is considered dangerously high
3. Avoidance of diuretics unless there is obvious pulmonary edema, limitation of intravenous fluid administration unless fluid loss is excessive, and avoidance of hyperosmotic agents
4. Delivery of the fetus to achieve a remission of preeclampsia.

Magnesium Sulfate to Control Convulsions

In more severe cases of preeclampsia and in eclampsia, magnesium sulfate administered parenterally is an effective anticonvulsant that avoids producing central nervous system depression in either the mother or the infant. It may be given intravenously by continuous infusion or intramuscularly by intermittent injection (Table 40-11). The dosages for severe preeclampsia are the same as for eclampsia. Because labor and delivery is a more likely time for convulsions to develop, women with preeclampsia-eclampsia usually are given magnesium sulfate during labor and for 24 hours postpartum.

Magnesium sulfate is almost universally administered intravenously. In most units, the intramuscular route has been abandoned. Of concern, magnesium sulfate solutions, although inexpensive to prepare, are not readily available in all parts of the developing world. And even when the solutions are available, the technology to infuse them may not be. Therefore, it should not be overlooked that the drug can be administered intramuscularly and that this route is as effective as intravenous administration (Salinger, 2013). In two reports from India, intramuscular regimens were nearly equivalent in preventing recurrent convulsions and maternal deaths in women with eclampsia (Chowdhury, 2009; Jana, 2013). These observations comport with earlier ones from Parkland Hospital as described by Pritchard and colleagues (1975, 1984).

Magnesium sulfate is not given to treat hypertension. Based on several studies cited subsequently and extensive clinical observations, magnesium most likely exerts a specific anticonvulsant action on the cerebral cortex. Typically, the mother stops convulsing after the initial 4-g loading dose. By an hour or two, she regains consciousness sufficiently to be oriented to place and time.

The magnesium sulfate dosages presented in Table 40-11 usually result in plasma magnesium levels illustrated in Figure 40-21. When magnesium sulfate is given to arrest eclamptic seizures, 10 to 15 percent of women will have a subsequent convulsion. If so, an additional 2-g dose of magnesium

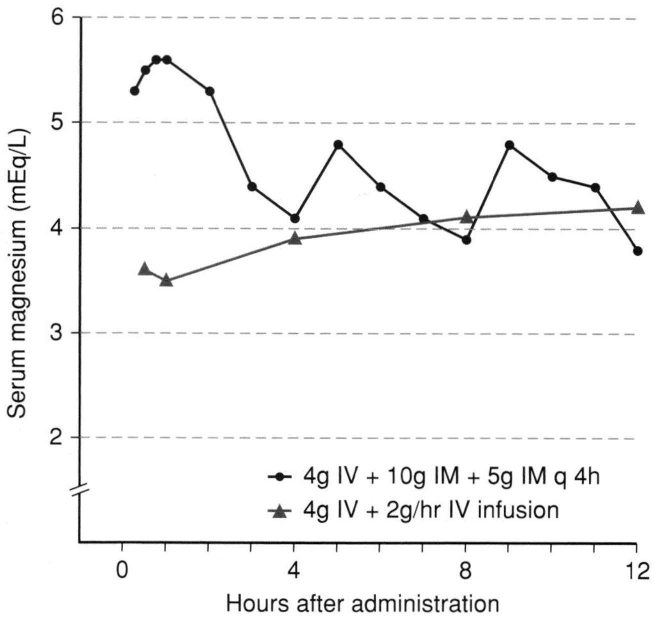

FIGURE 40-21 Comparison of serum magnesium levels in mEq/L following a 4-g intravenous loading dose of magnesium sulfate and then maintained by either an intramuscular or continuing infusion. Multiply by 1.2 to convert mEq/L to mg/dL. (Data from Sibai, 1984.)

sulfate in a 20-percent solution is slowly administered intravenously. In a small woman, this additional 2-g dose may be used once, but it can be given twice if needed in a larger woman. In only 5 of 245 women with eclampsia at Parkland Hospital was it necessary to use supplementary anticonvulsant medication to control convulsions (Pritchard, 1984). For these, an intravenous barbiturate is given slowly. Midazolam or lorazepam may be given in a small single dose, but prolonged use is avoided because it is associated with a higher mortality rate (Royal College of Obstetricians and Gynaecologists, 2006).

Maintenance magnesium sulfate therapy is continued for 24 hours after delivery. For eclampsia that develops postpartum, magnesium sulfate is administered for 24 hours after the onset of convulsions. Ehrenberg and Mercer (2006) studied abbreviated postpartum magnesium administration in 200 women with *mild* preeclampsia. Of 101 women randomized to 12-hour treatment, seven had worsening preeclampsia, and treatment was extended to 24 hours. None of these 101 women and none of the other cohort of 95 given the 24-hour magnesium infusion developed eclampsia. This abbreviated regimen needs further study before being routinely administered for severe preeclampsia or eclampsia.

Pharmacology and Toxicology. Magnesium sulfate USP is $MgSO_4 \cdot 7H_2O$ and not simple $MgSO_4$. It contains 8.12 mEq per 1 g. Parenterally administered magnesium is cleared almost totally by renal excretion, and magnesium intoxication is unusual when the glomerular filtration rate is normal or only slightly decreased. Adequate urine output usually correlates with preserved glomerular filtration rates. That said, magnesium excretion is not urine flow dependent, and urinary volume per unit time does not, per se, predict renal function. *Thus, serum creatinine levels must be measured to detect a decreased glomerular filtration rate.*

Eclamptic convulsions are almost always prevented or arrested by plasma magnesium levels maintained at 4 to 7 mEq/L, 4.8 to 8.4 mg/dL, or 2.0 to 3.5 mmol/L. Although laboratories typically report *total* magnesium levels, free or *ionized* magnesium is the active moiety for suppressing neuronal excitability. Taber and associates (2002) found poor correlation between total and ionized levels. Further studies are necessary to determine if either measurement provides a superior method for surveillance.

After a 4-g intravenous loading dose in nonobese women, magnesium levels observed with the intramuscular regimen and those observed with the maintenance infusion of 2 g/hr are similar (see Fig. 40-21). The obesity epidemic has affected these observations. Tudela and colleagues (2013) reported our observations from Parkland Hospital with magnesium administration to obese women. More than 60 percent of women whose body mass index (BMI) exceeded 30 kg/m^2 and who were receiving the 2-g/hr dose had subtherapeutic levels at 4 hours. Thus, 40 percent of obese women would require 3 g/hr to maintain effective plasma levels. That said, currently most do not recommend routine magnesium level measurements (American College of Obstetricians and Gynecologists, 2013b; Royal College of Obstetricians and Gynaecologists, 2006).

Patellar reflexes disappear when the plasma magnesium level reaches 10 mEq/L—about 12 mg/dL—presumably because of a curariform action. This sign serves to warn of impending magnesium toxicity. When plasma levels rise above 10 mEq/L, breathing becomes weakened. At 12 mEq/L or higher levels, respiratory paralysis and respiratory arrest follow. Somjen and coworkers (1966) induced marked hypermagnesemia in themselves by intravenous infusion and achieved plasma levels up to 15 mEq/L. Predictably, at such high plasma levels, respiratory depression developed that necessitated mechanical ventilation, but depression of the sensorium was not dramatic as long as hypoxia was prevented.

Treatment with calcium gluconate or calcium chloride, 1 g intravenously, along with withholding further magnesium sulfate, usually reverses mild to moderate respiratory depression. One of these agents should be readily available whenever magnesium is being infused. Unfortunately, the effects of intravenously administered calcium may be short-lived if there is a steady-state toxic level. For severe respiratory depression and arrest, prompt tracheal intubation and mechanical ventilation are lifesaving. Direct toxic effects on the myocardium from high levels of magnesium are uncommon. It appears that cardiac dysfunction associated with magnesium is due to respiratory arrest and hypoxia. With appropriate ventilation, cardiac action is satisfactory even when plasma magnesium levels are exceedingly high (McCubbin, 1981; Morisaki, 2000).

Because magnesium is cleared almost exclusively by renal excretion, the dosages described will become excessive if glomerular filtration is substantially decreased. The initial 4-g loading dose of magnesium sulfate can be safely administered regardless of renal function. It is important to administer the standard loading dose and not to reduce it under the mistaken conception that diminished renal function requires it. This is because after distribution, a loading dose achieves the desired therapeutic level, and the infusion maintains the steady-state level. *Thus, only the maintenance infusion rate should be altered with diminished glomerular filtration rate.* Renal function is estimated by measuring plasma creatinine. Whenever plasma creatinine levels are > 1.0 mg/mL, serum magnesium levels are measured to guide the infusion rate. With severe renal dysfunction, only the loading dose of magnesium sulfate is required to produce a steady-state therapeutic level.

Acute cardiovascular effects of parenteral magnesium in women with severe preeclampsia have been studied using data obtained by pulmonary and radial artery catheterization. After a 4-g intravenous dose administered over 15 minutes, mean arterial pressure fell slightly, accompanied by a 13-percent increase in cardiac index (Cotton, 1986b). Thus, magnesium decreased systemic vascular resistance and mean arterial pressure. At the same time, it increased cardiac output without evidence of myocardial depression. These findings were coincidental with transient nausea and flushing, and the cardiovascular effects persisted for only 15 minutes despite continued magnesium infusion.

Thurnau and associates (1987) showed that there was a small but highly significant increase in total magnesium concentration in the cerebrospinal fluid with magnesium therapy. The magnitude of the increase was directly proportional to the corresponding serum concentration.

Magnesium is anticonvulsant and neuroprotective in several animal models. Some proposed mechanisms of action include: (1) reduced presynaptic release of the neurotransmitter glutamate, (2) blockade of glutamatergic *N*-methyl-D-aspartate (NMDA) receptors, (3) potentiation of adenosine action, (4) improved calcium buffering by mitochondria, and (5) blockage of calcium entry via voltage-gated channels (Arango, 2006; Wang, 2012a).

Uterine Effects. Relatively high serum magnesium concentrations depress myometrial contractility both in vivo and in vitro. With the regimen described and the plasma levels that result, no evidence of myometrial depression has been observed beyond a transient decrease in activity during and immediately after the initial intravenous loading dose. Leveno and associates (1998) compared outcomes in 480 nulliparous women given phenytoin for preeclampsia with outcomes in 425 preeclamptic women given magnesium sulfate. Magnesium did not significantly alter the need for oxytocin stimulation of labor, admission-to-delivery intervals, or route of delivery. Similar results have been reported by others (Atkinson, 1995; Szal, 1999; Witlin, 1997b).

The mechanisms by which magnesium might inhibit uterine contractility are not established. It is generally assumed, however, that these depend on its effects on intracellular calcium as discussed in detail in Chapter 21 (p. 417). Inhibition of uterine contractility is magnesium dose dependent, and serum levels of at least 8 to 10 mEq/L are necessary to inhibit uterine contractions (Watt-Morse, 1995). This likely explains why there are few if any uterine effects seen clinically when magnesium sulfate is given for preeclampsia. And as discussed in Chapter 42 (p. 852), magnesium is also not considered to be an effective tocolytic agent.

Fetal and Neonatal Effects. Magnesium administered parenterally promptly crosses the placenta to achieve equilibrium in fetal serum and less so in amnionic fluid (Hallak, 1993). Levels in amnionic fluid increase with duration of maternal infusion (Gortzak-Uzen, 2005). Current evidence supports the view that magnesium sulfate has small but significant effects on the fetal heart rate pattern—specifically beat-to-beat variability. Hallak and coworkers (1999) compared an infusion of magnesium sulfate with a saline infusion. These investigators reported that magnesium was associated with a small and clinically insignificant decrease in variability. Similarly, in a retrospective study, Duffy and associates (2012) reported a lower heart rate baseline that was within the normal range; decreased variability; and fewer prolonged decelerations. They noted no adverse outcomes.

Overall, maternal magnesium therapy appears safe for perinates. For example, a recent MFMU Network study of more than 1500 exposed preterm neonates found no association between the need for neonatal resuscitation and cord blood magnesium levels (Johnson, 2012). Still, there are a few neonatal adverse events associated with its use. In a Parkland Hospital study of 6654 mostly term exposed newborns, 6 percent had hypotonia (Abbassi-Ghanavati, 2012). In addition, exposed neonates had lower 1- and 5-minute Apgar scores, a higher intubation rate, and more admissions to the special care nursery. The study showed that neonatal depression occurs only if there is *severe* hypermagnesemia at delivery.

Observational studies have suggested a protective effect of magnesium against the development of cerebral palsy in very-low-birthweight infants (Nelson, 1995; Schendel, 1996). At least five randomized trials have also assessed neuroprotective effects in preterm newborns. These findings are discussed in detail in Chapter 42 (p. 854). Nguyen and colleagues (2013) expanded this possibility to include term newborn neuroprotection. They performed a Cochrane Database review to compare term neonatal outcomes with and without exposure to peripartum magnesium therapy and reported that there were insufficient data to draw conclusions.

Finally, as discussed in Chapter 42 (p. 852), long-term use of magnesium, given for several days for tocolysis, has been associated with neonatal osteopenia (American College of Obstetricians and Gynecologists, 2013c).

Maternal Safety and Efficacy of Magnesium Sulfate. The multinational Eclampsia Trial Collaborative Group study (1995) involved 1687 women with eclampsia randomly allocated to different anticonvulsant regimens. In one cohort, 453 women were randomly assigned to be given magnesium sulfate and compared with 452 given diazepam. In a second cohort, 388 eclamptic women were randomly assigned to be given magnesium sulfate and compared with

TABLE 40-12. Randomized Comparative Trials of Magnesium Sulfate with Another Anticonvulsant to Prevent Recurrent Eclamptic Convulsions

		Recurrent Seizures			Maternal Deaths		
Study	Comparison Drug	$MgSO_4$ (%)	Other Drug (%)	RR (95% CI)	$MgSO_4$ (%)	Other Drug (%)	RR (95% CI)
Crowther (1990)	Diazepam	5/24	7/27	0.80 (0.29–2.2)	1/24	0/27	
Bhalla (1994)	Lytic cocktail	1/45	11/45	0.09 (0.1–0.68)	0/45	2/45	
Eclampsia Trial Collaborative Group (1995)	Phenytoin	60/453	126/452	0.48 (0.36–0.63)	10/388	20/387	0.5 (0.24–1.00)
	Diazepam	22/388	66/387	0.33 (0.21–0.53)	17/453	24/452	0.74 (0.40–1.36)
Totals		88/910 (9.7)	210/911 (23)	0.41 (0.32–0.51)	28/910 (3.1)	45/911 (4.9)	0.62 (0.39–0.99)

Data adapted from Alexander, 2014.

387 women given phenytoin. The results of these and other comparative studies that each enrolled at least 50 women are summarized in Table 40-12. In aggregate, magnesium sulfate therapy was associated with a significantly lower incidence of recurrent seizures compared with women given an alternative anticonvulsant—9.7 versus 23 percent. Importantly, the maternal death rate of 3.1 percent with magnesium sulfate was significantly lower than that of 4.9 percent for the other regimens.

Magnesium safety and toxicity was recently reviewed by Smith and coworkers (2013). In more than 9500 treated women, the overall rate of absent patellar tendon reflexes was 1.6 percent; respiratory depression 1.3 percent; and calcium gluconate administration 0.2 percent. They reported only one maternal death due to magnesium toxicity. Our anecdotal experiences are similar—in the estimated 50 years of its use in more than 40,000 women, there has been only one maternal death from an overdose (Pritchard, 1984).

Management of Severe Hypertension

Dangerous hypertension can cause cerebrovascular hemorrhage and hypertensive encephalopathy, and it can trigger eclamptic convulsions in women with preeclampsia. Other complications include hypertensive afterload congestive heart failure and placental abruption (Clark, 2012).

Because of these sequelae, the National High Blood Pressure Education Program Working Group (2000) and the 2013 Task Force recommend treatment to lower systolic pressures to or below 160 mm Hg and diastolic pressures to or below 110 mm Hg. Martin and associates (2005) reported provocative observations that highlight the importance of treating systolic hypertension. They described 28 selected women with severe preeclampsia who suffered an associated stroke. Most of these were hemorrhagic strokes—93 percent—and all women had systolic pressures > 160 mm Hg before suffering their stroke. By contrast, only 20 percent of these same women had diastolic pressures > 110 mm Hg. It seems likely that at least half of serious hemorrhagic strokes associated with preeclampsia are in women with chronic hypertension (Cunningham, 2005). Long-standing hypertension results in development of *Charcot-Bouchard aneurysms* in the deep penetrating arteries of the lenticulostriate branch of the middle cerebral arteries. These vessels supply the basal ganglia, putamen, thalamus, and adjacent deep white matter, as well as the pons and deep cerebellum. These unique aneurysmal weakenings predispose these small arteries to rupture during sudden hypertensive episodes (Chap. 50, p. 1007).

Antihypertensive Agents

Several drugs are available to rapidly lower dangerously elevated blood pressure in women with the gestational hypertensive disorders. The three most commonly employed are hydralazine, labetalol, and nifedipine. For years, parenteral hydralazine was the only one of these three available. But when parenteral labetalol was later introduced, it was considered to be equally effective for obstetrical use. Orally administered nifedipine has since then gained some popularity as first-line treatment for severe gestational hypertension.

Hydralazine

This is probably still the most commonly used antihypertensive agent in the United States for treatment of women with severe gestational hypertension. Hydralazine is administered intravenously with a 5-mg initial dose, and this is followed by 5- to 10-mg doses at 15- to 20-minute intervals until a satisfactory response is achieved (American College of Obstetricians and Gynecologists, 2012b). Some limit the total dose to 30 mg per treatment cycle (Sibai, 2003). The target response antepartum or intrapartum is a decrease in diastolic blood pressure to 90 to 110 mm Hg. Lower diastolic pressures risk compromised placental perfusion. Hydralazine has proven remarkably effective to prevent cerebral hemorrhage. Its onset of action can be as rapid as 10 minutes. Although repeated administration every 15 to 20 minutes may theoretically lead to undesirable hypotension, this has not been our experience when given in these 5- to 10-mg increments.

At Parkland Hospital, between 5 and 10 percent of all women with intrapartum hypertensive disorders are given a parenteral antihypertensive agent. Most often, we use hydralazine as described. We do not limit the total dose, and seldom has a second antihypertensive agent been needed. We estimate that nearly 6000 women have been so treated at Parkland during the past 50 years. Although less popular in Europe, hydralazine is used in some centers, according to the Royal College of Obstetricians and Gynaecologists (2006). A dissenting opinion for first-line intrapartum use of hydralazine was voiced by the Vancouver group after a systematic review (Magee, 2009). At the same time, however, Umans and coworkers (2014) concluded that objective outcome data did not support the use of one drug over another.

As with any antihypertensive agent, the tendency to give a larger initial dose of hydralazine if the blood pressure is higher must be avoided. The response to even 5- to 10-mg doses cannot be predicted by hypertension severity. Thus, our protocol is to always administer 5 mg as the initial dose. An adverse response to exceeding this initial dose is shown in Figure 40-22. This woman had chronic hypertension complicated by severe superimposed preeclampsia, and hydralazine was injected more frequently than recommended. Her blood pressure decreased in less than 1 hour from 240–270/130–150 mm Hg to 110/80 mm Hg, and fetal heart rate decelerations characteristic of uteroplacental insufficiency became evident. Decelerations persisted until her blood pressure was increased with rapid crystalloid infusion. In some cases, this fetal response to diminished uterine perfusion may be confused with placental abruption and may result in unnecessary and potentially dangerous emergent cesarean delivery.

Labetalol

This effective intravenous antihypertensive agent is an α_1- and nonselective β-blocker. Some prefer its use over hydralazine because of fewer side effects (Sibai, 2003). At Parkland Hospital, we give 10 mg intravenously initially. If the blood pressure has not decreased to the desirable level in 10 minutes, then 20 mg is given. The next 10-minute incremental dose is 40 mg and is followed by another 40 mg if needed. If a salutary response is not achieved, then an 80-mg dose is given. Sibai (2003) recommends 20 to 40 mg every 10 to 15 minutes as needed and a maximum dose of 220 mg per treatment cycle. The American College of Obstetricians and Gynecologists (2012b) recommends starting with a 20-mg intravenous bolus. If not effective within 10 minutes, this is followed by 40 mg, then 80 mg every 10 minutes. Administration should not exceed a 220-mg total dose per treatment cycle.

Hydralazine versus Labetalol

Comparative studies of these two antihypertensive agents show equivalent results (Umans, 2014). In an older trial, Mabie and colleagues (1987) compared intravenous hydralazine with labetalol for blood pressure control in 60 peripartum women. Labetalol lowered blood pressure more rapidly, and associated tachycardia was minimal. However, hydralazine lowered mean arterial pressures to safe levels more effectively. In a later trial, Vigil-De Gracia and associates (2007) randomly assigned 200 severely hypertensive women intrapartum to be given either: (1) intravenous hydralazine—5 mg, which could be given every 20 minutes and repeated to a maximum of five doses, or (2) intravenous labetalol—20 mg initially, followed by 40 mg in 20 minutes and then 80 mg every 20 minutes if needed up to a maximum 300-mg dose. Maternal and neonatal outcomes were similar. Hydralazine caused significantly more maternal tachycardia and palpitations, whereas labetalol more frequently caused maternal hypotension and bradycardia. Both drugs have been associated with a reduced frequency of fetal heart rate accelerations (Cahill, 2013).

Nifedipine

This calcium-channel blocking agent has become popular because of its efficacy for control of acute pregnancy-related hypertension. The NHBPEP Working Group (2000) and the Royal College of Obstetricians and Gynaecologists (2006) recommend a 10-mg initial oral dose to be repeated in 30 minutes if necessary. *Nifedipine given sublingually is no longer recommended.* Randomized trials that compared nifedipine with labetalol found neither drug definitively superior to the other. However, nifedipine lowered blood pressure more quickly (Scardo, 1999; Shekhar, 2013; Vermillion, 1999).

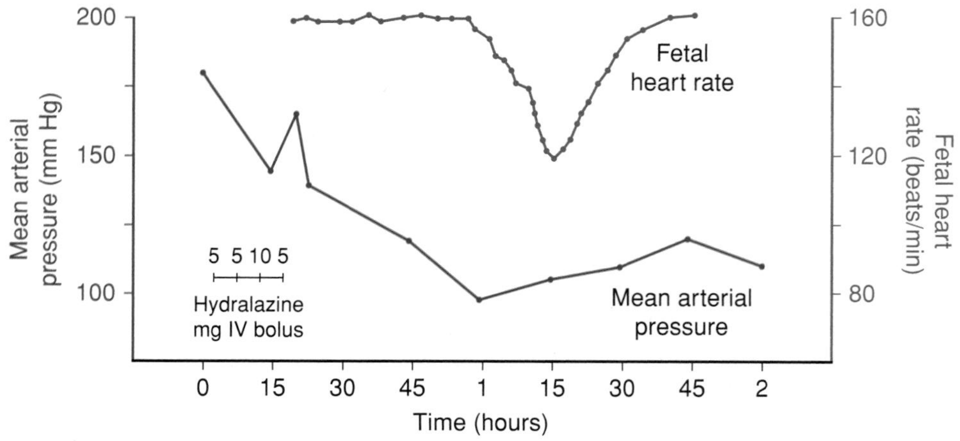

FIGURE 40-22 Hydralazine was given at 5-minute intervals instead of 15-minute intervals. The mean arterial pressure decreased from 180 to 90 mm Hg within 1 hour and was associated with fetal bradycardia. Rapid crystalloid infusion raised the mean pressure to 115 mm Hg, and the fetus recovered.

Other Antihypertensive Agents

A few other generally available antihypertensive agents have been tested in clinical trials but are not widely used (Umans, 2014). Belfort and associates (1990) administered the calcium antagonist *verapamil* by intravenous infusion at 5 to 10 mg per hour. Mean arterial pressure was lowered by 20 percent. Belfort and coworkers (1996, 2003) reported that *nimodipine* given either by continuous infusion or orally was effective to lower blood pressure in women with severe preeclampsia. Bolte and colleagues (1998, 2001) reported good results in preeclamptic women given intravenous *ketanserin*, a selective serotonergic ($5HT_{2A}$) receptor blocker. *Nitroprusside* or *nitroglycerine* is recommended by some if there is not optimal response to first-line agents. With these latter two agents, fetal cyanide toxicity may develop after 4 hours. We have not had the need for either due to our consistent success with first-line treatment using hydralazine, labetalol, or a combination of the two given in succession, but never simultaneously.

There are experimental antihypertensive drugs that may become useful for preeclampsia treatment. One is *calcitonin gene related peptide (CGRP),* a 37-amino acid potent vasodilator. Another is *antidigoxin antibody Fab (DIF)* directed against *endogenous digitalis-like factors*, also called *cardiotonic steroids* (Bagrov, 2008; Lam, 2013).

Diuretics

Potent loop diuretics can further compromise placental perfusion. Immediate effects include depletion of intravascular volume, which most often is already reduced compared with that of normal pregnancy (p. 737). Therefore, before delivery, diuretics are not used to lower blood pressure (Zeeman, 2009; Zondervan, 1988). We limit *antepartum* use of furosemide or similar drugs solely to treatment of pulmonary edema.

Fluid Therapy

Lactated Ringer solution is administered routinely at the rate of 60 mL to no more than 125 mL per hour unless there is unusual fluid loss from vomiting, diarrhea, or diaphoresis, or, more likely, excessive blood loss with delivery. Oliguria is common with severe preeclampsia. Thus, coupled with the knowledge that maternal blood volume is likely constricted compared with that of normal pregnancy, it is tempting to administer intravenous fluids more vigorously. But controlled, conservative fluid administration is preferred for the typical woman with severe preeclampsia who already has excessive extracellular fluid that is inappropriately distributed between intravascular and extravascular spaces. As discussed on page 737, infusion of large fluid volumes enhances the maldistribution of extravascular fluid and thereby appreciably increases the risk of pulmonary and cerebral edema (Dennis, 2012a; Sciscione, 2003; Zinaman, 1985). For labor analgesia with neuraxial analgesia, crystalloid solutions are infused slowly in graded amounts (Chap. 25, p. 516).

Pulmonary Edema

Women with severe preeclampsia-eclampsia who develop pulmonary edema most often do so postpartum (Cunningham, 1986, 2012; Zinaman, 1985). With pulmonary edema in the eclamptic woman, aspiration of gastric contents, which may be the result of convulsions, anesthesia, or oversedation, should be excluded. As discussed in Chapter 47 (p. 942), there are three common causes of pulmonary edema in women with severe preeclampsia syndrome—pulmonary capillary permeability edema, cardiogenic edema, or a combination of the two.

Some women with severe preeclampsia—especially if given vigorous fluid replacement—will have mild pulmonary congestion from permeability edema (see Fig. 40-6). This is caused by normal pregnancy changes magnified by the preeclampsia syndrome as discussed in Chapter 4 (p. 58). Importantly, plasma oncotic pressure decreases appreciably in normal term pregnancy because of decreased serum albumin concentration, and oncotic pressure falls even more with preeclampsia (Zinaman, 1985). And both increased extravascular fluid oncotic pressure and increased capillary permeability have been described in women with preeclampsia (Brown, 1989; Øian, 1986).

Invasive Hemodynamic Monitoring

Knowledge concerning cardiovascular and hemodynamic pathophysiological alterations associated with severe preeclampsia-eclampsia has accrued from studies done using invasive monitoring and a flow-directed pulmonary artery catheter (see Figs. 40-5 and 40-6). Clark and Dildy (2010) have reviewed such monitoring in obstetrics. Two conditions frequently cited as indications are preeclampsia associated with either oliguria or pulmonary edema. Somewhat ironically, it is usually vigorous treatment of the former that results in most cases of the latter. The American College of Obstetricians and Gynecologists (2013a) recommends against routine invasive monitoring. The College notes that such monitoring should be reserved for severely preeclamptic women with accompanying severe cardiac disease, renal disease, or both or in cases of refractory hypertension, oliguria, and pulmonary edema. An alternative noninvasive hemodynamic monitoring strategy has been evaluated in preliminary studies (Moroz, 2013).

Plasma Volume Expansion

Because the preeclampsia syndrome is associated with hemoconcentration, attempts to expand blood volume seem intuitively reasonable (Ganzevoort, 2004). This has led some to infuse various fluids, starch polymers, albumin concentrates, or combinations thereof to expand blood volume. There are, however, older observational studies that describe serious complications—especially pulmonary edema—with volume expansion (Benedetti, 1985; López-Llera, 1982; Sibai, 1987b). In general, these studies were not controlled or even comparative (Habek, 2006).

The Amsterdam randomized study reported by Ganzevoort and coworkers (2005a,b) was a well-designed investigation done to evaluate volume expansion. A total of 216 women with severe preeclampsia were enrolled between 24 and 34 weeks' gestation. The study included women whose preeclampsia was complicated by HELLP syndrome, eclampsia, or fetal-growth restriction. All women were given magnesium sulfate to prevent eclampsia, betamethasone to promote fetal pulmonary

TABLE 40-13. Maternal and Perinatal Outcomes in a Randomized Trial of Plasma Volume Expansion versus Saline Infusion in 216 Women with Severe Preeclampsia between 24 and 34 Weeks

Outcomes	Control Group[a] (n = 105)	Treatment Group[a] (n = 111)
Maternal Outcomes (%)		
Eclampsia (after enrollment)	1.9	1.8
HELLP (after enrollment)	19.0	17.0
Pulmonary edema	2.9	4.5
Placental abruption	3.8	1.0
Perinatal Outcomes		
Fetal deaths (%)	7	12
Prolongation of pregnancy (mean)	11.6 d	6.7 d
EGA at death (mean)	26.7 wk	26.3 wk
Birthweight (mean)	625 g	640 g
Live births (%)	93	88
Prolongation of pregnancy (mean)	10.5 d	7.4 d
EGA at delivery (mean)	31.6 wk	31.4 wk
RDS (%)	30	35
Neonatal death (%)	7.6	8.1
Perinatal mortality rate (n per 1000)	142/1000	207/1000

[a]All comparisons $p > 0.05$.
EGA = estimated gestational age; HELLP = hemolysis, elevated liver enzyme levels, low platelet count; RDS = respiratory distress syndrome.
Data from Ganzevoort, 2005a, b.

maturity, ketanserine to control dangerous hypertension, and normal saline infusions restricted only to deliver medications. In the group randomly assigned to volume expansion, each woman was given 250 mL of 6-percent hydroxyethyl starch infused over 4 hours twice daily. Their maternal and perinatal outcomes were compared with a control group and are shown in Table 40-13. None of these outcomes was significantly different between the two groups. Importantly, serious maternal morbidity and a substantive perinatal mortality rate accompanied their "expectant" management (see Table 40-9).

Neuroprophylaxis—Prevention of Seizures

There have been several randomized trials designed to test the efficacy of seizure prophylaxis for women with gestational hypertension, with or without proteinuria. In most of these, magnesium sulfate was compared with another anticonvulsant or with a placebo. *In all studies, magnesium sulfate was reported to be superior to the comparator agent to prevent eclampsia.* Four of the larger studies are summarized in Table 40-14. In the study from Parkland Hospital, Lucas and colleagues (1995) reported that magnesium sulfate therapy was superior to phenytoin to prevent eclamptic seizures in women with gestational hypertension and preeclampsia. Belfort and coworkers (2003) compared magnesium sulfate and nimodipine—a calcium-channel blocker with specific cerebral vasodilator activity—for eclampsia prevention. In this unblinded randomized trial involving 1650 women with severe preeclampsia, the rate of eclampsia was more than threefold higher for women allocated to the nimodipine group—2.6 versus 0.8 percent.

The largest comparative study was the entitled *MAGnesium Sulfate for Prevention of Eclampsia* and reported by the Magpie Trial Collaboration Group (2002). More than 10,000 women with severe preeclampsia from 33 countries were randomly allocated to treatment with magnesium sulfate or placebo. Women given magnesium had a 58-percent significantly lower risk of eclampsia than those given placebo. Smyth and associates (2009) provided follow-up data of infants born to these mothers given magnesium sulfate. At approximately 18 months, child behavior did not differ in those exposed compared with those not exposed to magnesium sulfate.

Who Should Be Given Magnesium Sulfate?

Magnesium will prevent proportionately more seizures in women with correspondingly worse disease. As previously discussed, however, severity is difficult to quantify, and thus it is difficult to decide which individual woman might benefit most from neuroprophylaxis. *The 2013 Task Force recommends that women with either eclampsia or severe preeclampsia should be given magnesium sulfate prophylaxis.* Again, criteria that establish "severity" are not totally uniform (see Table 40-2). At the same time, however, the 2013 Task Force suggests that all women with "mild" preeclampsia do not need magnesium sulfate neuroprophylaxis. The conundrum is whether or not to give neuroprophylaxis to any of these women with "nonsevere" gestational hypertension or preeclampsia (Alexander, 2006).

TABLE 40-14. Randomized Comparative Trials of Prophylaxis with Magnesium Sulfate and Placebo or Another Anticonvulsant in Women with Gestational Hypertension

	No. with Seizures/Total No. Treated (%)		
Study/Inclusions	Magnesium Sulfate	Control	Comparison[a]
Lucas et al (1995)		Phenytoin	
Gestational hypertension[b]	0/1049 (0)	10/1089 (0.9)	$p < 0.001$
Coetzee et al (1998)		Placebo	
Severe preeclampsia	1/345 (0.3)	11/340 (3.2)	RR = 0.09 (0.1–0.69)
Magpie Trial (2002)[c]		Placebo	
Severe preeclampsia	40/5055 (0.8)	96/5055 (1.9)	RR = 0.42 (0.26–0.60)
Belfort et al (2003)		Nimodipine	
Severe preeclampsia	7/831 (0.8)	21/819 (2.6)	RR = 0.33 (0.14–0.77)

[a]All comparisons significant $p < 0.05$.
[b]Included women with and without proteinuria and those with all severities of preeclampsia.
[c]Magpie Trial Collaboration Group, 2002.

In many other countries, and principally following dissemination of the Magpie Trial Collaboration Group (2002) study results, magnesium sulfate is now recommended for women with severe preeclampsia. In some, however, debate continues concerning whether therapy should be reserved for women who have an eclamptic seizure. We are of the opinion that eclamptic seizures are dangerous for reasons discussed on page 742. Maternal mortality rates of up to 5 percent have been reported even in recent studies (Andersgaard, 2006; Benhamou, 2009; Moodley, 2010; Schutte, 2008; Zwart, 2008). Moreover, there are substantially increased perinatal mortality rates in both industrialized countries and underdeveloped ones (Abd El Aal, 2012; Knight, 2007; Ndaboine, 2012; Schutte, 2008; von Dadelszen, 2012). Finally, the possibility of adverse long-term neuropsychological and vision-related sequelae of eclampsia described by Aukes (2009, 2012), Postma (2009), Wiegman (2012), and their coworkers, which are discussed on page 770, have raised additional concerns that eclamptic seizures are not "benign."

Selective versus Universal Magnesium Sulfate Prophylaxis

There is uncertainty around which women with nonsevere gestational hypertension should be given magnesium sulfate neuroprophylaxis. An opportunity to address these questions was afforded by a change in our prophylaxis protocol for women delivering at Parkland Hospital. Before this time, Lucas and associates (1995) had found that the risk of eclampsia without magnesium prophylaxis was approximately 1 in 100 for women with *mild preeclampsia*. Up until 2000, all women with gestational hypertension were given magnesium prophylaxis intramuscularly as first described by Pritchard in 1955. After 2000, we instituted a standardized protocol for intravenously administered magnesium sulfate (Alexander, 2006). At the same time, we also changed our practice of universal seizure prophylaxis for all women with gestational hypertension to one of selective prophylaxis given only to women who met our criteria for severe gestational hypertension. These criteria, shown in Table 40-15, included women with ≥ 2+ proteinuria measured by dipstick in a catheterized urine specimen.

Following this protocol change, 60 percent of 6518 women with gestational hypertension during a 4½-year period were

TABLE 40-15. Selective versus Universal Magnesium Sulfate Prophylaxis: Parkland Hospital Criteria to Define Severity of Gestational Hypertension

In a woman with new-onset proteinuric hypertension, at least one of the following criteria is required:
Systolic BP ≥ 160 or diastolic BP ≥ 110 mm Hg
Proteinuria ≥ 2+ by dipstick in a catheterized urine specimen
Serum creatinine > 1.2 mg/dL
Platelet count < 100,000/μL
Aspartate aminotransferase (AST) elevated two times above upper limit of normal range
Persistent headache or scotomata
Persistent midepigastric or right-upper quadrant pain

BP = blood pressure.
Criteria based on those from National High Blood Pressure Education Program Working Group, 2000; American College of Obstetricians and Gynecologists, 2012b; cited by Alexander, 2006.

TABLE 40-16. Selected Pregnancy Outcomes in 6518 Women with Gestational Hypertension According to Whether They Developed Eclampsia

Pregnancy Outcomes	Eclampsia No. (%)	Gest. HTN[a] No. (%)	*p* value
Number	87	6431	
Maternal			
Cesarean delivery	32 (37)	2423 (38)	0.86
Placental abruption	1 (1)	72 (1)	0.98
General anesthesia[b]	20 (23)	270 (4)	< 0.001
Neonatal			
Composite morbidity[c]	10 (12)	240 (1)	0.04

[a]Includes women who had preeclampsia.
[b]Emergent cesarean delivery.
[c]One or more: cord artery pH < 7.0; 5-minute Apgar score < 4; perinatal death; or unanticipated admission of term infant to an intensive care nursery.
Gest. HTN = gestational hypertension.
Data from Alexander, 2006.

given magnesium sulfate neuroprophylaxis (Table 40-16). The remaining 40 percent with nonsevere hypertension were not treated, and of these, 27 women developed eclamptic seizures—1 in 92. The seizure rate was only 1 in 358 for 3935 women with criteria for severe disease who were given magnesium sulfate, and thus these cases were treatment failures. To assess morbidity, outcomes in 87 eclamptic women were compared with outcomes in all 6431 noneclamptic hypertensive women. Although most maternal outcomes were similar, almost a fourth of women with eclampsia who underwent emergent cesarean delivery required general anesthesia. This is a great concern because eclamptic women have laryngotracheal edema and are at a higher risk for failed intubation, gastric acid aspiration, and death (American College of Obstetricians and Gynecologists, 2013d). Neonatal outcomes were also a concern because the composite morbidity defined in Table 40-16 was significantly increased tenfold in eclamptic compared with noneclamptic women—12 versus 1 percent, respectively.

Thus, if one uses the Parkland criteria for nonsevere gestational hypertension, about 1 of 100 such women who are not given magnesium sulfate prophylaxis can be expected to have an eclamptic seizure. A fourth of these women likely will require emergent cesarean delivery with attendant maternal and perinatal morbidity and mortality from general anesthesia. From this, the major question regarding management of nonsevere gestational hypertension remains—whether it is acceptable to avoid unnecessary treatment of 99 women to risk eclampsia in one? The answer appears to be yes as suggested by the 2013 Task Force.

Delivery

To avoid maternal risks from cesarean delivery, steps to effect vaginal delivery are used initially in women with eclampsia. Following a seizure, labor often ensues spontaneously or can be induced successfully even in women remote from term (Alanis, 2008). An immediate cure does not promptly follow delivery by any route, but serious morbidity is less common during the puerperium in women delivered vaginally.

Blood Loss at Delivery

Hemoconcentration or lack of normal pregnancy-induced hypervolemia is an almost predictable feature of severe preeclampsia-eclampsia as quantified by Zeeman and associates (2009) and shown in Figure 40-7. *These women, who consequently lack normal pregnancy hypervolemia, are much less tolerant of even normal blood loss than are normotensive pregnant women.* It is of great importance to recognize that an appreciable fall in blood pressure soon after delivery most often means excessive blood loss and not sudden resolution of vasospasm and endothelial damage. When oliguria follows delivery, the hematocrit should be evaluated frequently to help detect excessive blood loss. If identified, hemorrhage should be treated appropriately by careful crystalloid and blood transfusion.

Analgesia and Anesthesia

During the past 20 years, the use of conduction analgesia for women with preeclampsia syndrome has proven ideal. Initial problems with this method included hypotension and diminished uterine perfusion caused by sympathetic blockade in these women with attenuated hypervolemia. But pulmonary edema was mitigated by techniques that used slow induction of epidural analgesia with dilute solutions of anesthetic agents to counter the need for rapid infusion of large volumes of crystalloid or colloid to correct maternal hypotension (Hogg, 1999; Wallace, 1995). Moreover, epidural blockade avoids general anesthesia, in which the stimulation of tracheal intubation may cause sudden severe hypertension. Such blood pressure increases, in turn, can cause pulmonary edema, cerebral edema, or intracranial hemorrhage. Finally, tracheal intubation may be particularly difficult and thus hazardous in women with airway edema due to preeclampsia (American College of Obstetricians and Gynecologists, 2013d).

At least three randomized studies have been performed to evaluate these methods of analgesia and anesthesia. Wallace and colleagues (1995) studied 80 women at Parkland Hospital with severe preeclampsia who were to undergo cesarean delivery. They had not been given labor epidural analgesia and were randomized to receive general anesthesia, epidural analgesia, or combined spinal-epidural analgesia. Their average preoperative blood pressures approximated 170/110 mm Hg, and all had proteinuria. Anesthetic and obstetrical management included antihypertensive drug therapy and limited intravenous fluids as previously described. Perinatal outcomes in each group were similar. Maternal hypotension resulting from regional analgesia was managed with judicious intravenous fluid administration. In women undergoing general anesthesia, maternal blood pressure was managed to avoid severe hypertension (Fig. 40-23). There were no serious maternal or fetal complications attributable to any of the three anesthetic methods. It was concluded that all three are

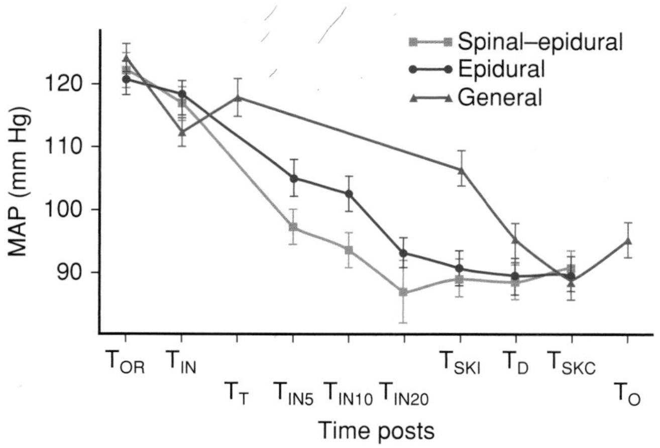

FIGURE 40-23 Blood pressure effects of general anesthesia versus epidural or spinal-epidural analgesia for cesarean delivery in 80 women with severe preeclampsia. MAP = mean arterial pressure. Time posts (T): OR = operating room; IN = induction of anesthesia; T = tracheal intubation; IN5 = induction + 5 min; IN10 = induction + 10 min; IN20 = induction + 20 min; SKI = skin incision; D = delivery; SKC = skin closure; O = extubation. (From Wallace, 1995, with permission.)

acceptable for use in women with pregnancies complicated by severe preeclampsia if steps are taken to ensure a careful approach to the selected method.

Another randomized study included 70 women with severe preeclampsia receiving spinal analgesia versus general anesthesia (Dyer, 2003). All had a nonreassuring fetal heart rate tracing as the indication for cesarean delivery, and outcomes were equivalent. Dyer and coworkers (2008) later showed that decreased mean arterial blood pressure induced by epidural blockade could be effectively counteracted by phenylephrine infusion to maintain cardiac output.

In a study from the University of Alabama at Birmingham, Head and colleagues (2002) randomly assigned 116 women with severe preeclampsia to receive either epidural or patient-controlled intravenous meperidine analgesia during labor. A standardized protocol limited intravenous fluids to 100 mL/hr. More women—9 percent—from the group assigned to epidural analgesia required ephedrine for hypotension. As expected, pain relief was superior in the epidural group, but maternal and neonatal complications were similar between groups. One woman in each group developed pulmonary edema.

It is important to emphasize that epidural analgesia is not to be considered *treatment* of preeclampsia. Lucas and associates (2001) studied 738 laboring women at Parkland Hospital who were 36 weeks or more and who had gestational hypertension of varying severity. Patients were randomly assigned to receive either epidural analgesia or patient-controlled intravenous meperidine analgesia. Maternal and neonatal outcomes were similar in the two study groups. However, as shown in Table 40-17, epidural analgesia resulted in a greater decrement of mean maternal arterial pressure compared with meperidine, but it was not superior in preventing recurrent severe hypertension later in labor.

For these reasons, judicious fluid administration is essential in severely preeclamptic women who receive regional analgesia. Newsome and coworkers (1986) showed that vigorous crystalloid infusion with epidural blockade in women with severe preeclampsia caused elevation of pulmonary capillary wedge pressures (see Fig. 40-6). Aggressive volume replacement in these women increases their risk for pulmonary edema, especially in the first 72 hours postpartum (Clark, 1985; Cotton, 1986a). When pulmonary edema develops, there is also concern for development of cerebral edema. Finally, Heller and associates (1983) demonstrated that most cases of pharyngolaryngeal edema were related to aggressive volume therapy.

Persistent Severe Postpartum Hypertension

The potential problem of antihypertensive agents causing serious compromise of uteroplacental perfusion and thus of fetal well-being is obviated by delivery. Postpartum, if difficulty arises in controlling severe hypertension or if intravenous hydralazine or labetalol are being used repeatedly, then oral regimens can be given. Examples include labetalol or another β-blocker, nifedipine or another calcium-channel blocker, and possible addition of a thiazide diuretic. Persistent or refractory hypertension is likely due to mobilization of pathological interstitial fluid and redistribution into the intravenous compartment, underlying chronic hypertension, or usually both (Sibai, 2012; Tan, 2002). In women with chronic hypertension and left-ventricular hypertrophy, severe postpartum hypertension can cause

TABLE 40-17. Comparison of Cardiovascular Effects of Epidural versus Patient-Controlled Meperidine Analgesia During Labor in Women with Gestational Hypertension

	Labor Analgesia		
Hemodynamic Change	Epidural (n = 372)	Meperidine (n = 366)	*p* value
Mean arterial pressure change (mean)	−25 mm Hg	−15 mm Hg	< 0.001
Ephedrine for hypotension (%)	11%	0	< 0.001
Severe hypertension after analgesia (%) (BP ≥ 160/110 mm Hg)	< 1%	1%	NS

NS = not significant.
Data from Lucas, 2001.

CHAPTER 40

pulmonary edema from cardiac failure (Cunningham, 1986, 2012; Sibai, 1987a).

Furosemide

Because persistence of severe hypertension corresponds to the onset and length of diuresis and extracellular fluid mobilization, it seems logical that furosemide-augmented diuresis might serve to hasten blood pressure control. To study this, Ascarelli and coworkers (2005) designed a randomized trial that included 264 postpartum preeclamptic women. After onset of spontaneous diuresis, patients were assigned to 20-mg oral furosemide given daily or no therapy. Women with mild disease had similar blood pressure control regardless of whether they received treatment or placebo. However, women with severe preeclampsia who were treated, compared with those receiving placebo, had a lower mean systolic blood pressure at 2 days—142 versus 153 mm Hg. They also required less frequently administered antihypertensive therapy during the remainder of hospitalization—14 versus 26 percent, respectively.

We have used a simple method to estimate excessive extracellular/interstitial fluid. The *postpartum weight* is compared with the most recent *prenatal weight*, either from the last clinic visit or on admission for delivery. On average, soon after delivery, maternal weight should be reduced by at least 10 to 15 pounds depending on infant and placental weight, amnionic fluid volume, and blood loss. Because of various interventions, especially intravenous crystalloid infusions given during operative vaginal or cesarean delivery, women with severe preeclampsia often have an immediate postpartum weight *in excess of their last prenatal weight*. If this weight increase is associated with severe persistent postpartum hypertension, then diuresis with intravenous furosemide is usually helpful in controlling blood pressure.

Plasma Exchange

Martin and colleagues (1995) have described an atypical syndrome in which severe preeclampsia-eclampsia persists despite delivery. These investigators described 18 such women whom they encountered during a 10-year period. They advocate single or multiple plasma exchange for these women. In some cases, 3 L of plasma was exchanged three times—a 36- to 45-donor unit exposure for each patient—before a response was forthcoming. Others have described plasma exchange performed in postpartum women with HELLP syndrome (Förster, 2002; Obeidat, 2002). In all of these cases, however, the distinction between HELLP syndrome and thrombotic thrombocytopenic purpura or hemolytic uremic syndrome was not clear. As further discussed in Chapter 56 (p. 1116), in our experiences with more than 50,000 women with gestational hypertension among nearly 450,000 pregnancies cared for at Parkland Hospital through 2012, we have encountered very few women with persistent postpartum hypertension, thrombocytopenia, and renal dysfunction who were diagnosed as having a thrombotic microangiopathy (Dashe, 1998). These latter syndromes complicating pregnancy were reviewed by Martin (2008) and George (2013) and their colleagues, who conclude that a rapid diagnostic test for ADAMTS-13 enzyme activity might be helpful to differentiate most of these syndromes.

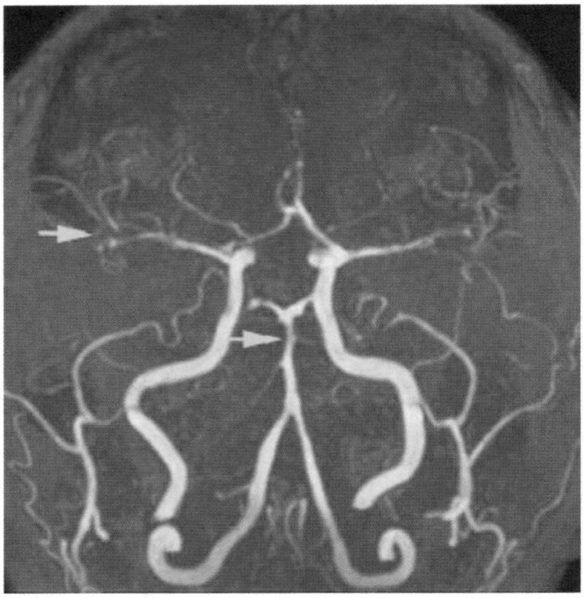

FIGURE 40-24 Reversible cerebral vasoconstriction syndrome. Magnetic resonance angiography shows generalized vasoconstriction of the anterior and posterior cerebral circulation (*arrows*). (From Garcia-Reitboeck, 2013, with permission.)

Reversible Cerebral Vasoconstriction Syndrome

This is another cause of persistent hypertension, "thunderclap" headaches, seizures, and central nervous system findings. It is a form of *postpartum angiopathy*. As shown in Figure 40-24, it is characterized by diffuse segmental constriction of cerebral arteries and may be associated with ischemic and hemorrhagic strokes. The reversible cerebral vasoconstriction syndrome has several inciting causes that include pregnancy, and particularly preeclampsia (Ducros, 2012). It is more common in women, and in some cases, vasoconstriction may be so severe as to cause cerebral ischemia and infarction. The appropriate management is not known at this time (Edlow, 2013).

COUNSELING FOR FUTURE PREGNANCIES

As discussed on page 732, defective remodeling of the spiral arteries in some placentations has been posited as the cause of at least one preeclampsia phenotype. Lack of deep placentation has been associated with preeclampsia, placental abruption, fetal-growth restriction, and preterm birth (Wikström, 2011). With this type of "overlap syndrome," hypertensive disorders may serve as markers for subsequent preterm labor and fetal-growth restriction. For example, even in subsequent nonhypertensive pregnancies, women who had preterm preeclampsia are at increased risk for preterm birth (Connealy, 2013.)

In addition, women who have had either gestational hypertension or preeclampsia are at higher risk to develop hypertension in future pregnancies. Generally, the earlier preeclampsia is diagnosed during the index pregnancy, the greater the likelihood of recurrence. Sibai and colleagues (1986, 1991) found that nulliparas diagnosed with preeclampsia before 30 weeks have a recurrence risk as high as 40 percent during a subsequent pregnancy. In a prospective study of 500 women previously delivered for preeclampsia at 37 weeks, the recurrence rate in a subsequent gestation was 23 percent (Bramham, 2011). These investigators also found an increased risk during subsequent pregnancies for preterm delivery and fetal-growth restriction even if these women remained normotensive.

In a study from the Denmark Birth Registry, Lykke and coworkers (2009b) analyzed singleton births in more than 535,000 women who had a first and second delivery. Women whose first pregnancy was complicated by preeclampsia between 32 and 36 weeks had a significant twofold increased incidence of preeclampsia in their second pregnancy—25 versus 14 percent—compared with women who were normotensive during the first pregnancy. Analyzed from another view, they also found that preterm delivery and fetal-growth restriction in the first pregnancy significantly increased the risk for preeclampsia in the second pregnancy.

As probably expected, women with HELLP syndrome have a substantive risk for recurrence in subsequent pregnancies. In two studies the risk ranged from 5 to 26 percent, but the true recurrence risk likely lies between these two extremes (Habli, 2009; Sibai, 1995). Even if HELLP syndrome does not recur with subsequent pregnancies, there is a high incidence of preterm delivery, fetal-growth restriction, placental abruption, and cesarean delivery (Habli, 2009; Hnat, 2002).

LONG-TERM CONSEQUENCES

Over the past 20 years, evidence has accrued that preeclampsia, like fetal-growth disorders and preterm birth, is a marker for subsequent cardiovascular morbidity and mortality. Thus, women with hypertension identified during pregnancy should be evaluated during the first several months postpartum and counseled regarding long-term risks. The Working Group concluded that hypertension attributable to pregnancy should resolve within 12 weeks of delivery (National High Blood Pressure Education Program, 2000). Persistence beyond this time is considered to be chronic hypertension (Chap. 50, p. 1000). The Magpie Trial Follow-Up Collaborative Group (2007) reported that 20 percent of 3375 preeclamptic women seen at a median of 26 months postpartum had hypertension. Importantly, even if hypertension does not persist in the short term, convincing evidence suggests that the risk for long-term cardiovascular morbidity is significantly increased in preeclamptic women.

Cardiovascular and Neurovascular Morbidity

With the advent of national databases, several studies confirm that any hypertension during pregnancy is a marker for an increased risk for morbidity and mortality in later life (American College of Obstetricians and Gynecologists, 2013c). In a case-control study from Iceland, Arnadottir and associates (2005) analyzed outcomes for 325 women who had hypertension complicating pregnancy and who were delivered from 1931 through 1947. At a median follow-up of 50 years, 60 percent of women with pregnancy-related hypertension compared with only 53 percent of controls had died. Compared with 629 normotensive pregnant controls, the prevalences of *ischemic heart disease*—24 versus 15 percent, and *stroke*—9.5 versus 6.5 percent, were significantly increased in the women who had gestational hypertension. In a Swedish population study of more than 400,000 nulliparas delivered between 1973 and 1982, Wikström and coworkers (2005) also found an increased incidence of ischemic heart disease in women with prior pregnancy-associated hypertension.

Lykke and associates (2009a) cited findings from a Danish registry of more than 780,000 nulliparous women. After a mean follow-up of almost 15 years, the incidence of *chronic hypertension* was significantly increased 5.2-fold in those who had gestational hypertension, 3.5-fold after mild preeclampsia, and 6.4-fold after severe preeclampsia. After two hypertensive pregnancies, there was a 5.9-fold increase in the incidence. Importantly, these investigators also reported a significant 3.5-fold increased risk for *type 2 diabetes*.

Bellamy and coworkers (2007) performed a systematic review and metaanalysis of long-term risks for cardiovascular disease in women with preeclampsia. As shown in Figure 40-25, the risks in later life were increased for hypertension, ischemic heart disease, stroke, venous thromboembolism, and all-cause mortality. As emphasized by several investigators, other cofactors or comorbidities are related to acquisition of these long-term adverse outcomes (Gastrich, 2012; Harskamp, 2007; Hermes, 2012; Spaan, 2012b). These include but are not limited to the metabolic syndrome, diabetes, obesity, dyslipidemia, and atherosclerosis. These conclusions are underscored by the findings of Berends and colleagues (2008), who confirmed shared constitutional risks for long-term vascular-related disorders in preeclamptic women and in their parents. Similar preliminary observations were reported by Smith (2009, 2012) and Stekkinger (2013) and their associates.

At least in some of these women, their hypertensive cardiovascular pathologies appear to have begun near the time of

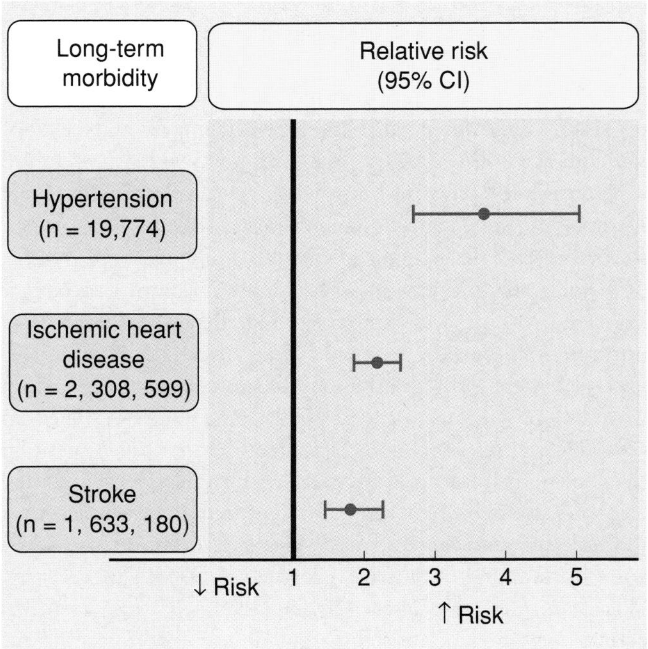

FIGURE 40-25 Long-term cardiovascular consequences of preeclampsia. All differences $p \leq .001$. (Data from Bellamy, 2007.)

their own births. For example, individuals who are born preterm have increased ventricular mass later in life (Lewandowski, 2013). Women who have preeclampsia and who develop chronic hypertension later in life have an increased ventricular mass index before they become hypertensive (Ghossein-Doha, 2013). A similar phenomenon is associated with preterm birth and with fetal-growth disorders.

Renal Sequelae

Preeclampsia appears to also be a marker for subsequent renal disease. In a preliminary study, the possibility was raised that persistent podocyturia might be a marker for such disease (Garrett, 2013). In a 40-year study of Norwegian birth and end-stage renal disease linked registries, although the absolute risk of renal failure was small, preeclampsia was associated with a fourfold increased risk (Vikse, 2008). Women with recurrent preeclampsia had an even greater risk. These data need to be considered in light of the findings that 15 to 20 percent of women with preeclampsia who undergo renal biopsy have evidence of chronic renal disease (Chesley, 1978). In another long-term follow-up study, Spaan and coworkers (2009) compared formerly preeclamptic women with a cohort of women who were normotensive at delivery. At 20 years following delivery, preeclamptic women were significantly more likely to be chronically hypertensive—55 versus 7 percent—compared with control women. They also had higher peripheral vascular and renovascular resistance and decreased renal blood flow. These data do not permit conclusions as to cause versus effect.

Neurological Sequelae

Until recently, eclamptic seizures were believed to have no significant long-term sequelae. Findings have now accrued, however, that this is not always the case. Recall that almost all eclamptic women have multifocal areas of perivascular edema, and about a fourth also have areas of cerebral infarction (Zeeman, 2004a).

A Dutch group has reported several long-term follow-up studies in women with severe preeclampsia and eclampsia (Aukes, 2007, 2009, 2012). These investigators found long-term persistence of brain white-matter lesions that were incurred during eclamptic convulsions (Aukes, 2009). When studied with MR imaging at a mean of 7 years, 40 percent of formerly eclamptic women had more numerous and larger aggregate white matter lesions compared with 17 percent of normotensive control women. These investigators later also observed these white-matter lesions in preeclamptic women without convulsions (Aukes, 2012). In studies designed to assess clinical relevance, Aukes and colleagues (2007) reported that formerly eclamptic women had subjectively impaired cognitive functioning. They also reported that women with multiple seizures had impaired sustained attention compared with normotensive controls (Postma, 2009). And recently, Wiegman and associates (2012) described that formerly eclamptic women at approximately 10 years had lower vision-related quality of life compared with control subjects. Because there were no studies done before these women suffered from preeclampsia or eclampsia, the investigators appropriately concluded that cause versus effect of these white-matter lesions remains unknown.

REFERENCES

Abalos E, Duley L, Steyn DW, et al: Antihypertensive drug therapy for mild to moderate hypertension during pregnancy. Cochrane Database Syst Rev 1:CD002252, 2007

Abbassi-Ghanavati M, Alexander JM, McIntire DD: Neonatal effects of magnesium sulfate given to the mother. Am J Perinatol 29(10):795, 2012

Abd El Aal DE, Shahin AY: Management of eclampsia at Assiut University Hospital, Egypt. Int J Gynaecol Obstet 116(3):232, 2012

Abdel-Hady ES, Fawzy M, El-Negri M, et al: Is expectant management of early-onset severe preeclampsia worthwhile in low-resource settings? Arch Gynecol Obstet 282(1):23, 2010

Abdul-Karim R, Assali NS: Pressor response to angiotonin in pregnant and nonpregnant women. Am J Obstet Gynecol 82:246, 1961

Abenhaim HA, Bujold E, Benjamin A, et al: Evaluating the role of bedrest on the prevention of hypertensive disease of pregnancy and growth restriction. Hypertens Pregnancy 27(2):197, 2008

Abramovici D, Friedman SA, Mercer BM, et al: Neonatal outcome in severe preeclampsia at 24 to 36 weeks' gestation: does the HELLP (hemolysis, elevated liver enzyme, and low platelet count) syndrome matter? Am J Obstet Gynecol 180:221, 1999

Airoldi J, Weinstein L: Clinical significance of proteinuria in pregnancy. Obstet Gynecol Surv 62:117, 2007

Ajne G, Wolff K, Fyhrquist F, et al: Endothelin converting enzyme (ECE) activity in normal pregnancy and preeclampsia. Hypertens Pregnancy 22:215, 2003

Akkawi C, Kent E, Geary M, et al: The incidence of eclampsia in a single defined population with a selective use of magnesium sulfate. Abstract No 798. Presented at the 29th Annual Meeting of the Society for Maternal-Fetal Medicine, January 26–31, 2009

Alanis MC, Robinson CJ, Hulsey TC, et al: Early-onset severe preeclampsia: induction of labor vs elective cesarean delivery and neonatal outcomes. Am J Obstet Gynecol 199:262.e1, 2008

Alexander JM, Bloom SL, McIntire DD, et al: Severe preeclampsia and the very low-birthweight infant: is induction of labor harmful? Obstet Gynecol 93:485, 1999

Alexander JM, Cunningham FG: Management. In Taylor RN, Roberts JM, Cunningham FG (eds): Chesley's Hypertensive Disorders in Pregnancy, 4th ed. Amsterdam, Academic Press, 2014

Alexander JM, McIntire DD, Leveno KJ, et al: Magnesium sulfate for the prevention of eclampsia in women with mild hypertension. Am J Obstet Gynecol 189:S89, 2003

Alexander JM, McIntire DD, Leveno KJ, et al: Selective magnesium sulfate prophylaxis for the prevention of eclampsia in women with gestational hypertension. Obstet Gynecol 108:826, 2006

Alexander JM, Sarode R, McIntire DD, et al: Use of whole blood in the management of hypovolemia due to obstetric hemorrhage. Obstet Gynecol 113(6):1320, 2009

American College of Obstetricians and Gynecologists: Antepartum fetal surveillance. Practice Bulletin No. 9, October 1999, Reaffirmed 2012a

American College of Obstetricians and Gynecologists: Diagnosis and management of preeclampsia and eclampsia. Practice Bulletin No. 33, January 2002, Reaffirmed 2012b

American College of Obstetricians and Gynecologists: Fetal growth restriction. Practice Bulletin No. 134, May 2013a

American College of Obstetricians and Gynecologists: Hypertension in pregnancy. Report of the American College of Obstetricians and Gynecologists' Task Force on Hypertension in pregnancy. Obstet Gynecol 122:1122, 2013b

American College of Obstetricians and Gynecologists: Magnesium sulfate use in obstetrics. Committee Opinion No. 573, September 2013c

American College of Obstetricians and Gynecologists: Obstetric analgesia and anesthesia. Practice Bulletin No. 36, July 2002, Reaffirmed 2013d

Amorim MMR, Santos LC, Faúndes A: Corticosteroid therapy for prevention of respiratory distress syndrome in severe preeclampsia. Am J Obstet Gynecol 180:1283, 1999

Andersgaard AB, Herbst A, Johansen M, et al: Eclampsia in Scandinavia: incidence, substandard care, and potentially preventable cases. Acta Obstet Gynecol 85:929, 2006

Arango MF, Mejia-Mantilla JH: Magnesium for acute traumatic brain injury. Cochrane Database Syst Rev 4:CD005400, 2006

Armanini D: Preeclampsia. The role of aldosterone in hypertension and inflammation. Hypertension 59(6):1099, 2012

Arnadottir GA, Geirsson RT, Arngrimsson Reynir, et al: Cardiovascular death in women who had hypertension in pregnancy: a case-control study. BJOG 112:286, 2005

Ascarelli MH, Johnson V, McCreary H, et al: Postpartum preeclampsia management with furosemide: a randomized clinical trial. Obstet Gynecol 105:29, 2005

Askie LM, Henderson-Smart DJ, Stewart LA: Antiplatelet agents for the prevention of preeclampsia: a meta-analysis of individual data. Lancet 369:179, 2007

Atkinson MW, Guinn D, Owen J, et al: Does magnesium sulfate affect the length of labor induction in women with pregnancy-associated hypertension? Am J Obstet Gynecol 173:1219, 1995

August P, Jeyabalan A, Roberts JM: Chronic hypertension. In Taylor RN, Roberts JM, Cunningham FG (eds): Chesley's Hypertensive Disorders in Pregnancy, 4th ed. Amsterdam, Academic Press, 2014

Aukes AM, de Groot JC, Aarnoudse JG, et al: Brain lesions several years after eclampsia. Am J Obstet Gynecol 200(5):504.e1, 2009

Aukes AM, de Groot JC, Wiegman MJ, et al: Long-term cerebral imaging after pre-eclampsia. BJOG 119(9):1117, 2012

Aukes AM, Wessel I, Dubois AM, et al: Self-reported cognitive functioning in formerly eclamptic women. Am J Obstet Gynecol 197(4):365.e1, 2007

Bagrov AY, Shapiro JI: Endogenous digitalis: Pathophysiologic roles and therapeutic applications. Nat Clin Pract Nephrol 4(7):378, 2008

Bahado-Singh RO, Akolekar R, Mandal R, et al: First-trimester metabolomic detection of late-onset preeclampsia. Am J Obstet Gynecol 208(1):58.e1, 2013

Bainbridge SA, Sidle EH, Smith GN: Direct placental effects of cigarette smoke protect women from pre-eclampsia: the specific roles of carbon monoxide and antioxidant systems in the placenta. Med Hypotheses 64:17, 2005

Barber D, Xing G, Towner D: Expectant management of severe eclampsia between 24–32 weeks gestation: a ten-year review. Abstract No 742. Presented at the 29th Annual Meeting of the Society for Maternal-Fetal Medicine, January 26–31, 2009

Barron WM, Heckerling P, Hibbard JU, et al: Reducing unnecessary coagulation testing in hypertensive disorders of pregnancy. Obstet Gynecol 94:364, 1999

Barton CR, Barton JR, O'Brien JM, et al: Mild gestational hypertension: differences in ethnicity are associated with altered outcomes in women who undergo outpatient treatment. Am J Obstet Gynecol 186:896, 2002

Barton J, Barton L, Istwan N, et al: The frequency of elective delivery at 34.0–36.9 weeks' gestation and its impact on neonatal outcomes in women with stable mild gestational hypertension (MGHTN). Abstract No 252. Presented at the 29th Annual Meeting of the Society for Maternal-Fetal Medicine, January 26–31, 2009

Bdolah Y, Palomaki GE, Yaron Y, et al: Circulating angiogenic proteins in trisomy 13. Am J Obstet Gynecol 194(1):239, 2006

Belfort M, Anthony J, Saade G, et al: A comparison of magnesium sulfate and nimodipine for the prevention of eclampsia. N Engl J Med 348:304, 2003

Belfort MA, Anthony J, Buccimazza A, et al: Hemodynamic changes associated with intravenous infusion of the calcium antagonist verapamil in the treatment of severe gestational proteinuric hypertension. Obstet Gynecol 75:970, 1990

Belfort MA, Taskin O, Buhur A, et al: Intravenous nimodipine in the management of severe preeclampsia: double blind, randomized, controlled clinical trial. Am J Obstet Gynecol 174:451, 1996

Belghiti J, Kayem G, Tsatsaris V, et al: Benefits and risks of expectant management of severe preeclampsia at less than 26 weeks gestation: the impact of gestational age and severe fetal growth restriction. Am J Obstet Gynecol 205(5):465.e1, 2011

Belizan JM, Villar J: The relationship between calcium intake and edema-, proteinuria-, and hypertension-getosis: an hypothesis. Am J Clin Nutr 33: 2202, 1980

Bellamy L, Casas JP, Hingorani AD, et al: Pre-eclampsia and risk of cardiovascular disease and cancer in later life: systematic review and meta-analysis. BMJ 335:974, 2007

Benedetti TJ, Cotton DB, Read JC, et al: Hemodynamic observations in severe preeclampsia with a flow-directed pulmonary artery catheter. Am J Obstet Gynecol 136:465, 1980

Benedetti TJ, Kates R, Williams V: Hemodynamic observations in severe preeclampsia complicated by pulmonary edema. Am J Obstet Gynecol 152:330, 1985

Benhamou D, Chassard D, Mercier FJ, et al: The seventh report of the confidential enquiries into maternal deaths in the United Kingdom: comparison with French data. Ann Fr Anesth Reanim 28:38, 2009

Berends AL, de Groot CJ, Sijbrands EJ, et al: Shared constitutional risks for maternal vascular-related pregnancy complications and future cardiovascular disease. Hypertension 51:1034, 2008

Berg CJ, Callaghan WM, Swerson C, et al: Pregnancy-related mortality in the United States, 1998 to 2006. Obstet Gynecol 116(6):1302, 2010

Berg CJ, Harper MA, Atkinson SM, et al: Preventability of pregnancy-related deaths. Obstet Gynecol 106:1228, 2005

Berks D, Steegers EAP, Molas M, et al: Resolution of hypertension and proteinuria after preeclampsia. Obstet Gynecol 114(6):1307, 2009

Bhalla AK, Dhall GI, Dhall K: A safer and more effective treatment regimen for eclampsia. Aust N Z J Obstet Gynecol 34:14, 1994

Bloom SL, Leveno KJ: Corticosteroid use in special circumstances: preterm ruptured membranes, hypertension, fetal growth restriction, multiple fetuses. Clin Obstet Gynecol 46:150, 2003

Bolte AC, Gafar S, van Eyck J, et al: Ketanserin, a better option in the treatment of preeclampsia? Am J Obstet Gynecol 178:S118, 1998

Bolte AC, van Eyck J, Gaffar SF, et al: Ketanserin for the treatment of preeclampsia. J Perinat Med 29:14, 2001

Bombrys AE, Barton JR, Habli M, Sibai BM: Expectant management of severe preeclampsia at 27 $^{0}/_{7}$ to 33 $^{6}/_{7}$ weeks' gestation: maternal and perinatal outcomes according to gestational age by weeks at onset of expectant management. Am J Perinatol 26:441, 2009

Bombrys AE, Barton JR, Nowacki EA, et al: Expectant management of severe preeclampsia at less than 27 weeks' gestation: maternal and perinatal outcomes according to gestational age by weeks at onset of expectant management. Am J Obstet Gynecol 199:247.e1, 2008

Borghi C, Esposti DD, Immordino V, et al: Relationship of systemic hemodynamics, left ventricular structure and function, and plasma natriuretic peptide concentrations during pregnancy complicated by preeclampsia. Am J Obstet Gynecol 183:140, 2000

Borowski K, Kair L, Zeng S, et al: Lack of association of FAS gene and preeclampsia. Abstract No 706. Presented at the 29th Annual Meeting of the Society for Maternal-Fetal Medicine, January 26–31, 2009

Boucoiran I, Thissier-Levy S, Wu Y, et al: Risks for preeclampsia and small for gestational age: predictive values of placental growth factor, soluble fms-like tyrosine kinase-1, and inhibin A in singleton and multiple-gestation pregnancies. Am J Perinatol 30(7):607, 2013

Bramham K, Briley AL, Seed P, et al: Adverse maternal and perinatal outcomes in women with previous preeclampsia: a prospective study. Am J Obstet Gynecol 204(6):512.e1, 2011

Brewer J, Owens MY, Wallace K, et al: Posterior reversible encephalopathy syndrome in 46 of 47 patients with eclampsia. Am J Obstet Gynecol 208(6):468.e1, 2013

Brosens I, Pijnenborg R, Vercruysse L, et al: The "Great Obstetrical Syndromes" are associated with disorders of deep placentation. Am J Obstet Gynecol 204(3):193, 2011

Brown CEL, Cunningham FG, Pritchard JA: Convulsions in hypertensive, proteinuric primiparas more than 24 hours after delivery: eclampsia or some other cause? J Reprod Med 32:499, 1987

Brown MA, Gallery EDM, Ross MR, et al: Sodium excretion in normal and hypertensive pregnancy: a prospective study. Am J Obstet Gynecol 159:297, 1988

Brown MA, Zammit VC, Lowe SA: Capillary permeability and extracellular fluid volumes in pregnancy-induced hypertension. Clin Sci 77:599, 1989

Brubaker DB, Ross MG, Marinoff D: The function of elevated plasma fibronectin in preeclampsia. Am J Obstet Gynecol 166:526, 1992

Budden A, Wilkinson L, Buksh MJ, et al: Pregnancy outcomes in women presenting with pre-eclampsia at less than 25 weeks gestation. Aust N Z J Obstet Gynaecol 46(5):407, 2006

Bush KD, O'Brien JM, Barton JR: The utility of umbilical artery Doppler investigation in women with HELLP (hemolysis, elevated liver enzymes, and low platelet count) syndrome. Am J Obstet Gynecol 184:1087, 2001

Buurma AJ, Turner RJ, Driessen JH, et al: Genetic variants in pre-eclampsia: a meta-analysis. Hum Reprod Update 19(3):289, 2013

Cahill A, Odibo A, Roehl K, et al: Impact of intrapartum antihypertensives on electronic fetal heart rate (EFM) patterns in labor. Abstract No. 615, Am J Obstet Gynecol 208(1 Suppl):S262, 2013

Caritis S, Sibai B, Hauth J, et al: Low-dose aspirin to prevent preeclampsia in women at high risk. National Institute of Child Health and Human Development Network of Maternal–Fetal Medicine Units. N Engl J Med 338:701, 1998

Carlson KL, Bader CL: Ruptured subcapsular liver hematoma in pregnancy: a case report of nonsurgical management. Am J Obstet Gynecol 190:558, 2004

Carty DM, Siwy J, Brennand JE, et al: Urinary proteomics for prediction of preeclampsia. Hypertension 57(3):561, 2011

Chaiworapongsa T, Robero R, Korzeniewski SJ, et al: Maternal plasma concentrations of angiogenic/antiangiogenic factors in the third trimester of pregnancy to identify the patient at risk for stillbirth at or near term and severe late preeclampsia. Am J Obstet Gynecol 208(4):287.e1, 2013

Chambers KA, Cain TW: Postpartum blindness: two cases. Ann Emerg Med 43:243, 2004

Chames MC, Livingston JC, Ivester TS, et al: Late postpartum eclampsia: a preventable disease? Am J Obstet Gynecol 186:1174, 2002
Chavarria ME, Lara-Gonzalez L, Gonzalez-Gleason A, et al: Maternal plasma cellular fibronectin concentrations in normal and preeclamptic pregnancies: a longitudinal study for early prediction of preeclampsia. Am J Obstet Gynecol 187:595, 2002
Chavarria ME, Lara-González L, González-Gleason A, et al: Prostacyclin/thromboxane early changes in pregnancies that are complicated by preeclampsia. Am J Obstet Gynecol 188:986, 2003
Chen BA, Parviainen K, Jeyabalan A: Correlation of catheterized and clean catch urine protein/creatinine ratios in preeclampsia evaluation. Obstet Gynecol 112:606, 2008
Chesley LC: Diagnosis of preeclampsia. Obstet Gynecol 65:423, 1985
Chesley LC (ed): Hypertensive Disorders in Pregnancy. Appleton-Century-Crofts, New York, 1978
Chesley LC, Williams LO: Renal glomerular and tubular function in relation to the hyperuricemia of preeclampsia and eclampsia. Am J Obstet Gynecol 50:367, 1945
Chowdhury JR, Chaudhuri S, Bhattacharyya N, et al: Comparison of intramuscular magnesium sulfate with low dose intravenous magnesium sulfate regimen for treatment of eclampsia. J Obstet Gynaecol Res 35:119, 2009
Churchill D, Beever GD, Meher S, et al: Diuretics for preventing preeclampsia. Cochrane Database Syst Rev 1:CD004451, 2007
Cipolla MJ: Brief review: cerebrovascular function during pregnancy and eclampsia. Hypertension 50:14, 2007
Cipolla MJ, Smith J, Kohlmeyer MM, et al: SKCa and IKCa channels, myogenic tone, and vasodilator responses in middle cerebral arteries and parenchymal arterioles: effect of ischemia and reperfusion. Stroke 40(4):1451, 2009
Cipolla MJ, Zeeman GG, Cunningham FG: Cerebrovascular (patho)physiology in preeclampsia/eclampsia. In Taylor RN, Roberts JM, Cunningham FG (eds): Chesley's Hypertensive Disorders in Pregnancy, 4th ed. Amsterdam, Academic Press, 2014
Clark BA, Halvorson L, Sachs B, et al: Plasma endothelin levels in preeclampsia: elevation and correlation with uric acid levels and renal impairment. Am J Obstet Gynecol 166:962, 1992
Clark SL, Cotton DB, Wesley L, et al: Central hemodynamic assessment of normal term pregnancy. Am J Obstet Gynecol 161:1439, 1989
Clark SL, Dildy GA III: Pulmonary artery catheterization. In Belfort M, Saade GR, Foley MR, et al (eds): Critical Care Obstetrics, 5th ed. West Sussex, Wiley-Blackwell, 2010, p 215
Clark SL, Divon MY, Phelan JP: Preeclampsia/eclampsia: hemodynamic and neurologic correlations. Obstet Gynecol 66:337, 1985
Clark SL, Hankins GD: Preventing maternal deaths: 10 clinical diamonds. Obstet Gynecol 119(2 Pt 1):360, 2012
Cnossen JS, de Ruyter-Hanhijarvi H, van der Post JA, et al: Accuracy of serum uric acid determination in predicting pre-eclampsia: a systematic review. Acta Obstet Gynecol Scand 85(5):519, 2006
Coetzee EJ, Dommisse J, Anthony J: A randomised controlled trial of intravenous magnesium sulphate versus placebo in the management of women with severe pre-eclampsia. Br J Obstet Gynaecol 105(3):300, 1998
Conde-Agudelo A, Belizan JM: Risk factors for pre-eclampsia in a large cohort of Latin American and Caribbean women. Br J Obstet Gynaecol 107:75, 2000
Conde-Agudelo A, Romero R, Roberts JM: Tests to predict preeclampsia. In Taylor RN, Roberts JM, Cunningham FG (eds): Chesley's Hypertensive Disorders in Pregnancy, 4th ed. Amsterdam, Academic Press, 2014
Connealy B, Carreno C, Kase B, et al: A history of prior preeclampsia is a major risk factor for preterm birth. Abstract No. 619, Am J Obstet Gynecol 208(1 Suppl):S264, 2013
Conrad KP, Stillman I, Lindheimer MD: The kidney in normal pregnancy and preeclampsia. In Taylor RN, Roberts JM, Cunningham FG (eds): Chesley's Hypertensive Disorders in Pregnancy, 4th ed. Amsterdam, Academic Press, 2014
Conrad KP, Vernier KA: Plasma level, urinary excretion and metabolic production of cGMP during gestation in rats. Am J Physiol 257:R847, 1989
Coolman M, Timmermans S, de Groot CJ, et al: Angiogenic and fibrinolytic factors in blood during the first half of pregnancy and adverse pregnancy outcomes. Obstet Gynecol 119(6):1190, 2012
Cornelis T, Adutayo A, Keunen J, et al: The kidney in normal pregnancy and preeclampsia. Semin Nephrol 31:4, 2011
Costantine MM, Cleary K, Eunice Kennedy Shriver National Institute of Child Health and Human Development Obstetric-Fetal Pharmacology Research Units Network: Pravastatin for the prevention of preeclampsia in high-risk pregnant women. Obstet Gynecol 121(2 Pt 1):349, 2013
Cotton DB, Jones MM, Longmire S, et al: Role of intravenous nitroglycerine in the treatment of severe pregnancy-induced hypertension complicated by pulmonary edema. Am J Obstet Gynecol 154:91, 1986a
Cotton DB, Longmire S, Jones MM, et al: Cardiovascular alterations in severe pregnancy-induced hypertension: effects of intravenous nitroglycerin coupled with blood volume expansion. Am J Obstet Gynecol 154:1053, 1986b
Crowther C: Magnesium sulphate versus diazepam in the management of eclampsia: a randomized controlled trial. Br J Obstet Gynaecol 97(2):110, 1990
Crowther CA, Bouwmeester AM, Ashurst HM: Does admission to hospital for bed rest prevent disease progression or improve fetal outcome in pregnancy complicated by non-proteinuric hypertension? Br J Obstet Gynaecol 99:13, 1992
Cunningham FG: Liver disease complicating pregnancy. Williams Obstetrics, 19th ed. (Suppl 1). Norwalk, Appleton & Lange, 1993
Cunningham FG: Peripartum cardiomyopathy: we've come a long way, but.... Obstet Gynecol 120(5):992, 2012
Cunningham FG: Severe preeclampsia and eclampsia: systolic hypertension is also important. Obstet Gynecol 105(2):237, 2005
Cunningham FG, Fernandez CO, Hernandez C: Blindness associated with preeclampsia and eclampsia. Am J Obstet Gynecol 172:1291, 1995
Cunningham FG, Lowe T, Guss S, et al: Erythrocyte morphology in women with severe preeclampsia and eclampsia. Am J Obstet Gynecol 153:358, 1985
Cunningham FG, Pritchard JA, Hankins GDV, et al: Peripartum heart failure: idiopathic cardiomyopathy or compounding cardiovascular events? Obstet Gynecol 67:157, 1986
Cunningham FG, Twickler D: Cerebral edema complicating eclampsia. Am J Obstet Gynecol 182:94, 2000
D'Anna R, Baviera G, Corrado F, et al: Plasma homocysteine in early and late pregnancy complicated with preeclampsia and isolated intrauterine growth restriction. Acta Obstet Gynecol Scand 83:155, 2004
Dashe JS, Ramin SM, Cunningham FG: The long-term consequences of thrombotic microangiopathy (thrombotic thrombocytopenic purpura and hemolytic uremic syndrome) in pregnancy. Obstet Gynecol 91:662, 1998
Davidge S, de Groot C, Taylor RN: Endothelial cell dysfunction and oxidative stress. In Taylor RN, Roberts JM, Cunningham FG (eds): Chesley's Hypertensive Disorders in Pregnancy, 4th ed. Amsterdam, Academic Press, 2014
Demers S, Bujold E, Arenas E, et al: Prediction of recurrent preeclampsia using first-trimester uterine artery Doppler. Am J Perinatol 31(2):99, 2014
Dennis AT, Castro J, Carr C, et al: Haemodynamics in women with untreated pre-eclampsia. Anaesthesia 67(10):1105, 2012a
Dennis AT, Solnordal CB: Acute pulmonary oedema in pregnant women. Anaesthesia 67(6):646, 2012b
De Paco C, Kametas N, Rencoret G, et al: Maternal cardiac output between 11 and 13 weeks of gestation in the prediction of preeclampsia and small for gestational age. Obstet Gynecol 111:292, 2008
De-Regil LM, Palacios C, Ansary A, et al: Vitamin D supplementation for women during pregnancy. Cochrane Database Syst Rev 2:CD008873, 2012
De Snoo K: The prevention of eclampsia. Am J Obstet Gynecol 34:911, 1937
de Vries JI, van Pampus MG, Hague WM: Low-molecular-weight heparin added to aspirin in the prevention of recurrent early-onset pre-eclampsia in women with inheritable thrombophilia: the FRUIT-RCT. J Thromb Haemost 10(1):64, 2012
De Wolf F, De Wolf-Peeters C, Brosens I, et al: The human placental bed: electron microscopic study of trophoblastic invasion of spiral arteries. Am J Obstet Gynecol 137:58, 1980
DiFederico E, Genbacev O, Fisher SJ: Preeclampsia is associated with widespread apoptosis of placental cytotrophoblasts within the uterine wall. Am J Pathol 155:293, 1999
Drakeley AJ, Le Roux PA, Anthony J, et al: Acute renal failure complicating severe preeclampsia requiring admission to an obstetric intensive care unit. Am J Obstet Gynecol 186:253, 2002
Ducros A: Reversible cerebral vasoconstriction syndrome. Lancet Neurol 11(10):906, 2012
Duffy CR, Odibo AO, Roehl KA, et al: Effect of magnesium sulfate on fetal heart rate patterns in the second stage of labor. Obstet Gynecol 119(6):1129, 2012
Dugoff L, Cuckle H, Behrendt N, et al: First-trimester prediction of preeclampsia using soluble P-selectin, follistatin-related protein 3, complement 3a, soluble TNF receptor type 1, PAPP-A, AFP, inhibin A, placental growth factor, uterine artery Doppler and maternal characteristics. Abstract No. 589, Am J Obstet Gynecol 208(1 Suppl):S252, 2013
Dürr JA, Lindheimer MD: Control of volume and body tonicity. In Lindheimer MD, Roberts JM, Cunningham FG (eds): Chesley's Hypertensive Disorders in Pregnancy, 2nd ed. Stamford, Appleton & Lange, 1999, p 103
Dyer RA, Els I, Farbas J, et al: Prospective, randomized trial comparing general with spinal anesthesia for cesarean delivery in preeclamptic patients with a nonreassuring fetal heart trace. Anesthesiology 99:561, 2003

Dyer RA, Piercy JL, Reed AR, et al: Hemodynamic changes associated with spinal anesthesia for cesarean delivery in severe preeclampsia. Anesthesiology 108(5):802, 2008

Easterling TR, Benedetti TJ, Schmucker BC, et al: Maternal hemodynamics in normal and preeclamptic pregnancies: a longitudinal study. Obstet Gynecol 76:1061, 1990

Eclampsia Trial Collaborative Group: Which anticonvulsant for women with eclampsia? Evidence from the collaborative eclampsia trial. Lancet 345:1455, 1995

Edlow JA, Caplan LR, O'Brien K, et al: Diagnosis of acute neurological emergencies in pregnant and post-partum women. Lancet Neurol 12(2):175, 2013

Ehrenberg HM, Mercer BM: Abbreviated postpartum magnesium sulphate therapy for women with mild preeclampsia: a randomized controlled trial. Obstet Gynecol 108(4):833, 2006

Eremina V, Baelde HJ, Quaggin SE: Role of the VEGF-A signaling pathway in the glomerulus: evidence for crosstalk between components of the glomerular filtration barrier. Nephron Physiol 106(2):32, 2007

Erlebacher A: Immunology of the maternal-fetal interface. Annu Rev Immunol 31:387, 2013

Ethridge J, Mercer B: Can preeclampsia be preliminarily diagnosed or excluded when the urine protein: creatinine ratio (TPCR) is < 300mg/g? Abstract No. 629, Am J Obstet Gynecol 208(1 Suppl):S267, 2013

Evans CS, Gooch L, Flotta D, et al: Cardiovascular system during the postpartum state in women with a history of preeclampsia. Hypertension 58:57, 2011

Everett TR, Mahendru AA, McEniery CM, et al: Raised uterine artery impedance is associated with increased maternal arterial stiffness in the late second trimester. Placenta 33(7):572, 2012

Faas MM, Schuiling GA, Linton EA, et al: Activation of peripheral leukocytes in rat pregnancy and experimental preeclampsia. Am J Obstet Gynecol 182:351, 2000

Finnerty FA, Buchholz JH, Tuckman J: Evaluation of chlorothiazide (Diuril) in the toxemias of pregnancy. JAMA 166:141, 1958

Fisher S, Roberts JM: The placenta in normal pregnancy and preeclampsia. In Taylor RN, Roberts JM, Cunningham FG (eds): Chesley's Hypertensive Disorders in Pregnancy, 4th ed. Amsterdam, Academic Press, 2014

Fleischer A, Schulman H, Farmakides G, et al: Uterine artery Doppler velocimetry in pregnant women with hypertension. Am J Obstet Gynecol 154:806, 1986

Flowers CE, Grizzle JE, Easterling WE, et al: Chlorothiazide as a prophylaxis against toxemia of pregnancy. A double-blind study. Am J Obstet Gynecol 84:919, 1962

Fonseca JE, Méndez F, Cataño C, et al: Dexamethasone treatment does not improve the outcome of women with HELLP syndrome: a double-blind, placebo-controlled, randomized clinical trial. Am J Obstet Gynecol 193:1591, 2005

Förster JG, Peltonen S, Kaaja R, et al: Plasma exchange in severe postpartum HELLP syndrome. Acta Anaesthesiol Scand 46:955, 2002

Fukui A, Yokota M, Funamiz A, et al: Changes in NK cells in preeclampsia. Am J Reprod Immunol 67(4):278, 2012

Gamzu R, Rotstein R, Fusman R, et al: Increased erythrocyte adhesiveness and aggregation in peripheral venous blood of women with pregnancy-induced hypertension. Obstet Gynecol 98:307, 2001

Gant NF, Chand S, Worley RJ, et al: A clinical test useful for predicting the development of acute hypertension in pregnancy. Am J Obstet Gynecol 120:1, 1974

Ganzevoort W, Rep A, Bonsel GJ, et al: A randomized trial of plasma volume expansion in hypertensive disorders of pregnancy: influence on the pulsatile indices of the fetal umbilical artery and middle cerebral artery. Am J Obstet Gynecol 192:233, 2005a

Ganzevoort W, Rep A, Bonsel GJ, et al: Plasma volume and blood pressure regulation in hypertensive pregnancy. J Hypertens 22:1235, 2004

Ganzevoort W, Rep A, PERTA investigators, et al: A randomized controlled trial comparing two temporizing management strategies, one with and one without plasma volume expansion, for severe and early onset pre-eclampsia. BJOG 112:1337, 2005b

Garcia-Reitboeck P, Al-Memar A: Images in clinical medicine: reversible cerebral vasoconstriction after preeclampsia. N Engl J Med 369(3):e4, 2013

Garrett A, Craici I, White W, et al: Persistent urinary podocyte loss after preeclamptic pregnancies may be a possible mechanism of chronic renal injury. Abstract No. 618, Am J Obstet Gynecol 208(1 Suppl):S263, 2013

Gastrich MD, Gandhi SK, Pantazopoulos J, et al: Cardiovascular outcomes after preeclampsia or eclampsia complicated by myocardial infarction or stroke. Obstet Gynecol 120(4), 823, 2012

Gaugler-Senden IP, Huijssoon AG, Visser W, et al: Maternal and perinatal outcome of preeclampsia with an onset before 24 weeks' gestation. Audit in a tertiary referral center. Eur J Obstet Gynecol Reprod Biol 128:216, 2006

Gebb J, Einstein F, Merkatz IR, et al: First trimester 3D power Doppler of the intervillous space in patients with decreased PAPP-A levels and increased uterine artery pulsatility index. Abstract No 279. Presented at the 29th Annual Meeting of the Society for Maternal-Fetal Medicine, January 26–31, 2009a

Gebb J, Landsberger E, Merkatz I, et al: First trimester uterine artery Doppler, PAPP-A and 3D power Doppler of the intervillous space in patients at risk for preeclampsia. Abstract No 251. Presented at the 29th Annual Meeting of the Society for Maternal-Fetal Medicine, January 26–31, 2009b

George EM, Granger JP: Endothelin: key mediator of hypertension in preeclampsia. Am J Hypertens 24(9):964, 2011

George JN, Charania RS: Evaluation of patients with microangiopathic hemolytic anemia and thrombocytopenia. Semin Thromb Hemost 39(2):153, 2013

Gervasi MT, Chaiworapongsa T, Pacora P, et al: Phenotypic and metabolic characteristics of monocytes and granulocytes in preeclampsia. Am J Obstet Gynecol 185:792, 2001

Getahun D, Ananth CV, Oyeese Y, et al: Primary preeclampsia in the second pregnancy. Obstet Gynecol 110:1319, 2007

Ghidini A, Locatelli A: Monitoring of fetal well-being: role of uterine artery Doppler. Semin Perinatol 32:258, 2008

Ghossein-Doha C, Peeters L, van Jeijster S, et al: Hypertension after preeclampsia is preceded by changes in cardiac structures and function. Hypertension 62(2):382, 2013

Gilstrap LC, Cunningham FG, Whalley PJ: Management of pregnancy-induced hypertension in the nulliparous patient remote from term. Semin Perinatol 2:73, 1978

Gortzak-Uzan L, Mezad D, Smolin A: Increasing amniotic fluid magnesium concentrations with stable maternal serum levels. A prospective clinical trial. J Reprod Med 50:817, 2005

Groom KM, North RA, Stone PR, et al: Patterns of change in uterine artery Doppler studies between 20 and 24 weeks of gestation and pregnancy outcomes. Obstet Gynecol 113(2):332, 2009

Grundmann M, Woywodt A, Kirsch T, et al: Circulating endothelial cells: a marker of vascular damage in patients with preeclampsia. Am J Obstet Gynecol 198:317.e1, 2008

Habek D, Bobic MV, Habek JC: Oncotic therapy in management of preeclampsia. Arch Med Res 37:619, 2006

Habli M, Eftekhari N, Wiebrach E, et al: Long term outcome of HELLP syndrome. Abstract No 763. Presented at the 29th Annual Meeting of the Society for Maternal-Fetal Medicine, January 26–31, 2009

Haddad B, Barton JR, Livingston JC, et al: Risk factors for adverse maternal outcomes among women with HELLP (hemolysis, elevated liver enzymes, and low platelet count) syndrome. Am J Obstet Gynecol 183:444, 2000

Haddad B, Kayem G, Deis S, et al: Are perinatal and maternal outcomes different during expectant management of severe preeclampsia in the presence of intrauterine growth restriction? Am J Obstet Gynecol 196:237.e1, 2007

Haggerty CL, Seifert ME, Tang G: Second trimester anti-angiogenic proteins and preeclampsia. Pregnancy Hypertens 2(2):158, 2012

Hallak M, Berry SM, Madincea F, et al: Fetal serum and amniotic fluid magnesium concentrations with maternal treatment. Obstet Gynecol 81:185, 1993

Hallak M, Martinez-Poyer J, Kruger ML, et al: The effect of magnesium sulfate on fetal heart rate parameters: a randomized, placebo-controlled trial. Am J Obstet Gynecol 181:1122, 1999

Hankins GDV, Wendel GW Jr, Cunningham FG, et al: Longitudinal evaluation of hemodynamic changes in eclampsia. Am J Obstet Gynecol 150:506, 1984

Harskamp RE, Zeeman GG: Preeclampsia: at risk for remote cardiovascular disease. Am J Med Sci 334(4):291, 2007

Hauser RA, Lacey DM, Knight MR: Hypertensive encephalopathy. Arch Neurol 45:1078, 1988

Hauth JC, Cunningham FG, Whalley PJ: Management of pregnancy-induced hypertension in the nullipara. Obstet Gynecol 48:253, 1976

Head BB, Owen J, Vincent RD Jr, et al: A randomized trial of intrapartum analgesia in women with severe preeclampsia. Obstet Gynecol 99:452, 2002

Hefler LA, Tempfer CB, Gregg AR: Polymorphisms within the interleukin-1β gene cluster and preeclampsia. Obstet Gynecol 97:664, 2001

Heilmann L, Rath W, Pollow K: Hemostatic abnormalities in patients with severe preeclampsia. Clin Appl Thromb Hemost 13: 285, 2007

Heller PJ, Scheider EP, Marx GF: Pharyngo-laryngeal edema as a presenting symptom in preeclampsia. Obstet Gynecol 62:523, 1983

Hermes W, Ket JC, van Pampus MG, et al: Biochemical cardiovascular risk factors after hypertensive pregnancy disorders: a systematic review and meta-analysis. Obstet Gynecol Surv 67(12):793, 2012

Herraiz I, Escribano D, Gómez-Arriaga PI, et al: Predictive value of sequential models of uterine artery Doppler in pregnancies at high risk for pre-eclampsia. Ultrasound Obstet Gynecol 40(1):68, 2012

Hertig AT: Vascular pathology in the hypertensive albuminuric toxemias of pregnancy. Clinics 4:602, 1945

Hibbard JU, Shroff SG, Cunningham FG: Cardiovascular alterations in normal and preeclamptic pregnancy. In Taylor RN, Roberts JM, Cunningham FG (eds): Chesley's Hypertensive Disorders in Pregnancy, 4th ed. Amsterdam, Academic Press, 2014

Hinchey J, Chaves C, Appignani B, et al: A reversible posterior leukoencephalopathy syndrome. N Engl J Med 334(8):494, 1996

Hinselmann H: Die Eklampsie. Bonn, F Cohen, 1924

Hnat MD, Sibai BM, Caritis S, et al: Perinatal outcome in women with recurrent preeclampsia compared with women who develop preeclampsia as nulliparas. Am J Obstet Gynecol 186:422, 2002

Hogg B, Hauth JC, Caritis SN, et al: Safety of labor epidural anesthesia for women with severe hypertensive disease. Am J Obstet Gynecol 181:1096, 1999

Holzgreve W, Ghezzi F, Di Naro E, et al: Disturbed fetomaternal cell traffic in preeclampsia. Obstet Gynecol 91:669, 1998

Horsager R, Adams M, Richey S, et al: Outpatient management of mild pregnancy induced hypertension. Am J Obstet Gynecol 172:383, 1995

Hubel CA, McLaughlin MK, Evans RW, et al: Fasting serum triglycerides, free fatty acids, and malondialdehyde are increased in preeclampsia, are positively correlated, and decrease within 48 hours postpartum. Am J Obstet Gynecol 174:975, 1996

Hunter SK, Martin M, Benda JA, et al: Liver transplant after massive spontaneous hepatic rupture in pregnancy complicated by preeclampsia. Obstet Gynecol 85:819, 1995

Hupuczi P, Nagy B, Sziller I, et al: Characteristic laboratory changes in pregnancies complicated by HELLP syndrome. Hypertens Pregnancy 26: 389, 2007

Isler CM, Barrilleaux PS, Magann EF, et al: A prospective, randomized trial comparing the efficacy of dexamethasone and betamethasone for the treatment of antepartum HELLP (hemolysis, elevated liver enzymes, and low platelet count) syndrome. Am J Obstet Gynecol 184:1332, 2001

Ito T, Sakai T, Inagawa S, et al: MR angiography of cerebral vasospasm in preeclampsia. AJNR Am J Neuroradiol 16(6):1344, 1995

Jamalzei B, Fallah S, Kashanian M, et al: Association of the apolipoprotein E variants with susceptibility to pregnancy with preeclampsia. Clin Lab 59(5–6):563, 2013

Jana N, Dasgupta S, Das DK, et al: Experience of a low-dose magnesium sulfate regimen for the management of eclampsia over a decade. Int J Gynaecol Obstet 122(1):13, 2013

Janzarik WG, Ehlers E, Ehmann R, et al: Dynamic cerebral autoregulation in pregnancy and the risk of preeclampsia. Hypertension 63:161, 2014

Jeyabalan A, Stewart DR, McGonigal SC, et al: Low relaxin concentrations in the first trimester are associated with increased risk of developing preeclampsia. Reprod Sci 16:101A, 2009

John JH, Ziebland S, Yudkin P, et al: Effects of fruit and vegetable consumption on plasma antioxidant concentrations and blood pressure: a randomized controlled trial. Lancet 359:1969, 2002

Johnson LH, Mapp DC, Rouse DJ: Association of cord blood magnesium concentration and neonatal resuscitation. J Pediatr 160(4):573, 2012

Kanasaki K, Palmsten K, Sugimoto H, et al: Deficiency in catechol-O-methyltransferase and 2-methoxyoestradiol is associated with pre-eclampsia. Nature 453:1117, 2008

Karumanchi A, Rana S, Taylor RN: Angiogenesis and preeclampsia. In Taylor RN, Roberts JM, Cunningham FG (eds): Chesley's Hypertensive Disorders in Pregnancy, 4th ed. Amsterdam, Academic Press, 2014

Karumanchi SA, Stillman IE, Lindheimer MD: Angiogenesis and preeclampsia. In Lindheimer MD, Roberts JM, Cunningham FG (eds): Chesley's Hypertensive Disorders of Pregnancy, 3rd ed. New York, Elsevier, 2009, p 87

Kasawara KT, do Nascimento SL, Costa ML, et al: Exercise and physical activity in the prevention of pre-eclampsia: systematic review. Acta Obstet Gynecol Scand 91(10):1147, 2012

Katz L, de Amorim MMR, Figueroa JN, et al: Postpartum dexamethasone for women with hemolysis, elevated liver enzymes, and low platelets (HELLP) syndrome: a double-blind, placebo-controlled, randomized clinical trial. Am J Obstet Gynecol 198:283.e1, 2008

Keiser S, Owens M, Parrish M, et al: HELLP syndrome II. Concurrent eclampsia in 70 cases. Abstract No 781. Presented at the 29th Annual Meeting of the Society for Maternal-Fetal Medicine, January 26–31, 2009

Kenny L, McCrae K, Cunningham FG: Platelets, coagulation, and the liver. In Taylor RN, Roberts JM, Cunningham FG (eds): Chesley's Hypertensive Disorders in Pregnancy, 4th ed. Amsterdam, Academic Press, 2014

Kenny LC, Broadhurst DI, Dunn W, et al: Early pregnancy prediction of preeclampsia using metabolomic biomarkers. Reprod Sci 16:102A, 2009

Khalil A, Akolekar R, Syngelaki A, et al: Maternal hemodynamics at 11–13 weeks' gestation and risk of pre-eclampsia. Ultrasound Obstet Gynecol 40(1):28, 2012

Khan KS, Wojdyla D, Say L, et al: WHO analysis of causes of maternal death: a systematic review. Lancet 367:1066, 2006

Kirshon B, Lee W, Mauer MB, et al: Effects of low-dose dopamine therapy in the oliguric patient with preeclampsia. Am J Obstet Gynecol 159:604, 1988

Kleinrouweler CE, Wiegerinck MM, Ris-Stalpers C, et al: Accuracy of circulating placental growth factor, vascular endothelial growth factor, soluble fms-like tyrosine kinase 1 and soluble endoglin in the prediction of preeclampsia: a systematic review and meta-analysis. BJOG 119(7):778, 2012

Knight M, UK Obstetric Surveillance System (UKOSS): Eclampsia in the United Kingdom 2005. BJOG 114:1072, 2007

Knuist M, Bonsel GJ, Zondervan HA, et al: Low sodium diet and pregnancy-induced hypertension: a multicentre randomized controlled trial. Br J Obstet Gynaecol 105:430, 1998

Koopmans CM, Bijlenga D, Groen H, et al: Induction of labour versus expectant monitoring for gestational hypertension or mild pre-eclampsia after 36 weeks' gestation (HYPITAT): a multicentre, open-label randomized controlled trial. Lancet 374(9694):979, 2009

Kovo M, Schreiber L, Ben-Haroush A, et al: Placental vascular lesion differences in pregnancy-induced hypertension and normotensive fetal growth restriction. Am J Obstet Gynecol 202(6):561,e1, 2010

Kozic JR, Benton SJ, Hutcheon JA, et al: Abnormal liver function tests as predictors of adverse maternal outcomes in women with preeclampsia. J Obstet Gynaecol Can 33(10:995, 2011

Kraus D, Fent L, Heine RP, et al: Smoking and preeclampsia protection: cigarette smoke increases placental adrenomedullin expression and improves trophoblast invasion via the adrenomedullin pathway. Abstract No. 43, Am J Obstet Gynecol 208(1):S26, 2013

Kuc S, Wortelboer EJ, van Rijn BB, et al: Evaluation of 7 serum biomarkers and uterine artery Doppler ultrasound for first-trimester prediction of preeclampsia: a systematic review. Obstet Gynecol Surv 66(4):225, 2011

Kyle PM, Fielder JN, Pullar B, et al: Comparison of methods to identify significant proteinuria in pregnancy in the outpatient setting. BJOG 115:523, 2008

Lachmeijer AMA, Crusius JBA, Pals G, et al: Polymorphisms in the tumor necrosis factor and lymphotoxin-α gene region and preeclampsia. Obstet Gynecol 98:612, 2001

Lam DS, Chan W: Images in clinical medicine. Choroidal ischemia in preeclampsia. N Engl J Med 344(10):739, 2001

Lam GK, Hopoate-Sitake M, Adair CD, et al: Digoxin antibody fragment, antigen binding (Fab), treatment of preeclampsia in women with endogenous digitalis-like factor: a secondary analysis of the DEEP trial. Am J Obstet Gynecol 209(2):119.e1, 2013

Landesman R, Douglas RG, Holze E: The bulbar conjunctival vascular bed in the toxemias of pregnancy. Am J Obstet Gynecol 68:170, 1954

Langenveld J, Ravelli ACJ, van Kaam AH, et al: Neonatal outcome of pregnancies complicated by hypertensive disorders between 34 and 37 weeks of gestation: a 7 year retrospective analysis of national registry. Am J Obstet Gynecol 205(6):540.e.1, 2011

Lara-Torre E, Lee MS, Wolf MA, et al: Bilateral retinal occlusion progressing to long-lasting blindness in severe preeclampsia. Obstet Gynecol 100:940, 2002

Lawlor DA, Morton SM, Nitsch D, Leon DA: Association between childhood and adulthood socioeconomic position and pregnancy induced hypertension: results from the Aberdeen children of the 1950s cohort study. J Epidemiol Community Health 59:49, 2005

Leduc L, Wheeler JM, Kirshon B, et al: Coagulation profile in severe preeclampsia. Obstet Gynecol 79:14, 1992

Lee SM, Romero R, Lee YJ, et al: Systemic inflammatory stimulation by microparticles derived from hypoxic trophoblast as a model for inflammatory response in preeclampsia. Am J Obstet Gynecol 207(4):337.e1, 2012

Leeflang MM, Cnossen JS, van der Post JA, et al: Accuracy of fibronectin tests for the prediction of pre-eclampsia: a systematic review. Eur J Obstet Gynecol Reprod Biol 133(1):12, 2007

Le Ray C, Wavrant S, Rey E, et al: Induction or elective caesarean in severe early-onset preeclampsia: a meta-analysis of observational studies. Abstract No 724. Presented at the 29th Annual Meeting of the Society for Maternal-Fetal Medicine, January 26–31, 2009

Leveno KJ, Alexander JM, McIntire DD, et al: Does magnesium sulfate given for prevention of eclampsia affect the outcome of labor? Am J Obstet Gynecol 178:707, 1998

Levine RJ, Ewell MG, Hauth JC, et al: Should the definition of preeclampsia include a rise in diastolic blood pressure of >/ = 15 mm Hg to a level < 90 mm Hg in association with proteinuria? Am J Obstet Gynecol 183:787, 2000

Levine RJ, Hauth JC, Curet LB, et al: Trial of calcium to prevent preeclampsia. N Engl J Med 337:69, 1997

Levine RJ, Lam C, Qian C et al: Soluble endoglin and other circulating antiangiogenic factors in preeclampsia. N Engl J Med 355:992, 2006

Lewandowski AJ, Augustine D, Lamata P, et al: Preterm heart in adult life. Cardiovascular magnetic resonance reveals distinct differences in left ventricular mass, geometry, and function. Circulation 127(2):197, 2013

Li H, Gudnason H, Olofsson P, et al: Increased uterine artery vascular impedance is related to adverse outcome of pregnancy but is present in only one-third of late third-trimester pre-eclampsia women. Ultrasound Obstet Gynecol 25:459, 2005

Lindheimer MD, Conrad K, Karumanchi SA: Renal physiology and disease in pregnancy. In Alpern RJ, Hebert SC (eds): Seldin and Giebisch's The Kidney: Physiology and Pathophysiology, 4th ed. New York, Elsevier, 2008a, p 2339

Lindheimer MD, Taler SJ, Cunningham FG: Hypertension in pregnancy [Invited Am Soc Hypertension position paper]. J Am Soc Hypertens 2:484, 2008b

Lindheimer MD, Taylor RN, Cunningham FG, et al: Introduction, history, controversies, and definitions. In Taylor RN, Roberts JM, Cunningham FG (eds): Chesley's Hypertensive Disorders in Pregnancy, 4th ed, Amsterdam, Academic Press, 2014

Liu L, Cooper M, Yang T, et al: Transcriptomics and proteomics ensemble analyses reveal serological protein panel for preeclampsia diagnosis. Abstract No. 642, Am J Obstet Gynecol 208(1 Suppl):S272, 2013

Livingston JC, Park V, Barton JR, et al: Lack of association of severe preeclampsia with maternal and fetal mutant alleles for tumor necrosis factor α and lymphotoxin α genes and plasma tumor necrosis α levels. Am J Obstet Gynecol 184:1273, 2001

Lo C, Taylor RS, Gamble G, et al: Use of automated home blood pressure monitoring in pregnancy: is it safe? Am J Obstet Gynecol 187:1321, 2002

Loisel DA, Billstrand C, Murray K, et al: The maternal HLA-G 1597 DC null mutation is associated with increased risk of pre-eclampsia and reduced HLA-G expression during pregnancy in African-American women. Mol Hum Reprod 19(3):144, 2013

López-Jaramillo P, Narváez M, Weigel RM, et al: Calcium supplementation reduces the risk of pregnancy-induced hypertension in an Andes population. Br J Obstet Gynaecol 96:648, 1989

López-Llera M: Complicated eclampsia: Fifteen years' experience in a referral medical center. Am J Obstet Gynecol 142:28, 1982

Loureiro R, Leite CC, Kahhale S, et al: Diffusion imaging may predict reversible brain lesions in eclampsia and severe preeclampsia: initial experience. Am J Obstet Gynecol 189:1350, 2003

Lucas MJ, Leveno KJ, Cunningham FG: A comparison of magnesium sulfate with phenytoin for the prevention of eclampsia. N Engl J Med 333:201, 1995

Lucas MJ, Sharma S, McIntire DD, et al: A randomized trial of the effects of epidural analgesia on pregnancy-induced hypertension. Am J Obstet Gynecol 185:970, 2001

Luft FC, Gallery EDM, Lindheimer MD: Normal and abnormal volume homeostasis. In Lindheimer MD, Roberts JM, Cunningham FG (eds): Chesley's Hypertensive Disorders of Pregnancy, 3rd ed. New York, Elsevier, 2009, p 271

Lykke JA, Langhoff-Roos J, Sibai BM, et al: Hypertensive pregnancy disorders and subsequent cardiovascular morbidity and type 2 diabetes mellitus in the mother. Hypertension 53:944, 2009a

Lykke JA, Paidas MJ, Langhoff-Roos J: Recurring complications in second pregnancy. Obstet Gynecol 113:1217, 2009b

Mabie WC, Gonzalez AR, Sibai BM, et al: A comparative trial of labetalol and hydralazine in the acute management of severe hypertension complicating pregnancy. Obstet Gynecol 70:328, 1987

Macdonald-Wallis C, Lawlor DA, Fraser A, et al: Blood pressure change in normotensive, gestational hypertensive, preeclamptic, and essential hypertensive pregnancies. Hypertension 59(6):1241, 2012

Mackay VA, Huda SS, Stewart FM, et al: Preeclampsia is associated with compromised maternal synthesis of long-chain polyunsaturated fatty acids, leading to offspring deficiency. Hypertension 60(4):1078, 2012

Mackenzie RM, Sandrim VC, Carty DM, et al: Endothelial FOS expression and preeclampsia. BJOG 119(13):1564, 2012

Madazli R, Budak E, Calay Z, et al: Correlation between placental bed biopsy findings, vascular cell adhesion molecule and fibronectin levels in pre-eclampsia. Br J Obstet Gynaecol 107:514, 2000

Magee LA, Yong PJ, Espinosa V, et al: Expectant management of severe preeclampsia remote from term: a structured systematic review. Hypertens Pregnancy 25:1, 2009

Magpie Trial Collaboration Group: Do women with pre-eclampsia, and their babies, benefit from magnesium sulphate? The Magpie Trial: a randomised placebo-controlled trial. Lancet 359:1877, 2002

Magpie Trial Follow-Up Collaborative Group: The Magpie Trial: a randomized trial comparing magnesium sulphate with placebo for pre-eclampsia. Outcome for women at 2 years. BJOG 114:300, 2007

Majander KK, Villa PM, Kivinen K, et al: A follow-up linkage study of Finnish pre-eclampsia families identifies a new fetal susceptibility locus on chromosome 18. Eur J Hum Genet 21(9):1024, 2013

Makrides M, Duley L, Olsen SF: Marine oil, and other prostaglandin precursor supplementation for pregnancy uncomplicated by pre-eclampsia or intrauterine growth restriction. Cochrane Database Syst Rev 3:CD003402, 2006

Manten GT, van der Hoek YY, Marko Sikkema J, et al: The role of lipoprotein (a) in pregnancies complicated by pre-eclampsia. Med Hypotheses 64:162, 2005

Martin JN, Bailey AP, Rehberg JF, et al: Thrombotic thrombocytopenic purpura in 166 pregnancies: 1955–2006. Am J Obstet Gynecol 199(2), 98, 2008

Martin JN Jr, Brewer JM, Wallace K, et al: HELLP syndrome and composite major maternal morbidity: importance of Mississippi classification System. J Matern Fetal Neonatal Med 26(12):1201, 2013

Martin JN Jr, Files JC, Blake PG, et al: Postpartum plasma exchange for atypical preeclampsia–eclampsia as HELLP (hemolysis, elevated liver enzymes, and low platelets) syndrome. Am J Obstet Gynecol 172:1107, 1995

Martin JN Jr, Owens My, Keiser SD, et al: Standardized Mississippi protocol treatment of 190 patients with HELLP syndrome: slowing disease progression and preventing new major maternal morbidity. Hypertens Pregnancy 31(1):79, 2012

Martin JN Jr, Thigpen BD, Moore RC, et al: Stroke and severe preeclampsia and eclampsia: a paradigm shift focusing on systolic blood pressure. Obstet Gynecol 105(2):246, 2005

Martin JN Jr, Thigpen BD, Rose CH, et al: Maternal benefit of high-dose intravenous corticosteroid therapy for HELLP syndrome. Am J Obstet Gynecol 189:830, 2003

Marya RK, Rathee S, Manrow M: Effect of calcium and vitamin D supplementation on toxaemia of pregnancy. Gynecol Obstet Invest 24:38, 1987

Matijevic R, Johnston T: In vivo assessment of failed trophoblastic invasion of the spiral arteries in pre-eclampsia. Br J Obstet Gynaecol 106:78, 1999

Mattar F, Sibai BM: Eclampsia: VIII. Risk factors for maternal morbidity. Am J Obstet Gynecol 182:307, 2000

Maxwell CV, Lieberman E, Norton M, et al: Relationship of twin zygosity and risk of preeclampsia. Am J Obstet Gynecol 185:819, 2001

Maynard S, Epstein FH, Karumanchi SA: Preeclampsia and angiogenic imbalance. Annu Rev Med 59:61, 2008

Maynard SE, Min J-Y, Merchan J, et al: Excess placental soluble fms-like tyrosine kinase 1 (sFlt1) may contribute to endothelial dysfunction, hypertension, and proteinuria in preeclampsia. J Clin Invest 111(5):649, 2003

McCubbin JH, Sibai BM, Abdella TN, et al: Cardiopulmonary arrest due to acute maternal hypermagnesemia. Lancet 1:1058, 1981

McDonald SD, Best C, Lam K: The recurrence risk of severe de novo preeclampsia in singleton pregnancies: a population-based cohort. BJOG 116(12):1578, 2009

McElrath TF, Hecht JL, Dammann O, et al: Pregnancy disorders that lead to delivery before the 28th week of gestation: an epidemiologic approach to classification. Am J Epidemiol 168(9):980, 2008

McMahon K, Karumanchi SA, Stillman IE, et al: Does soluble fms-like tyrosine kinase-1 regulate placental invasion? Insight from the invasive placenta. Am J Obstet Gynecol 10:66.e1, 2014

Meher S, Duely L: Rest during pregnancy for preventing pre-eclampsia and its complications in women with normal blood pressure. Cochrane Database Syst Rev 19:CD005939, 2006

Melchiorre K, Sutherland G, Sharma R, et al: Mid-gestational maternal cardiovascular profile in preterm and term pre-eclampsia: a prospective study. BJOG 120(4):496, 2013

Melchiorre K, Sutherland G, Watt-Coote I, et al: Severe myocardial impairment and chamber dysfunction in preterm preeclampsia. Hypertens Pregnancy 31(4):454, 2012

Meldrum BS: Implications for neuroprotective treatments. Prog Brain Res 135:487, 2002

Melrose EB: Maternal deaths at King Edward VIII Hospital, Durban. A review of 258 consecutive cases. S Afr Med J 65:161, 1984

Mignini LE, Latthe PM, Villar J, et al: Mapping the theories of preeclampsia: the role of homocysteine. Obstet Gynecol 105: 411, 2005

Milne F, Redman C, Walker J, et al: Assessing the onset of pre-eclampsia I the hospital day unit: summary of the pre-eclampsia guideline (PRECOG II). BMJ 339:b3129, 2009

Moodley J: Maternal deaths associated with eclampsia in South Africa: lessons to learn from the confidential enquiries into maternal deaths, 2005–2007. S Afr Med J 100(11):717, 2010

Morisaki H, Yamamoto S, Morita Y, et al: Hypermagnesemia-induced cardiopulmonary arrest before induction of anesthesia for emergency cesarean section. J Clin Anesth 12(3):224, 2000

Moroz L, Simhan H: Noninvasive hemodynamic monitoring and the phenotype of severe hypertension: a prospective cohort study. Abstract No. 635, Am J Obstet Gynecol 208(1 Suppl):S269, 2013

Morris RK, Riley RD, Doug M, et al: Diagnostic accuracy of spot urinary protein and albumin to creatinine ratios for detection of significant proteinuria or adverse pregnancy outcome in patients with suspected pre-eclampsia: a systematic review and meta-analysis. BMJ 345:e4342, 2012
Moseman CP, Shelton S: Permanent blindness as a complication of pregnancy induced hypertension. Obstet Gynecol 100:943, 2002
Mosimann B, Wagner M, Poon LC, et al: Maternal serum cytokines at 30–33 weeks in the prediction of preeclampsia. Prenat Diagn 33(9):823, 2013
Mostello D, Catlin TK, Roman L, et al: Preeclampsia in the parous woman: who is at risk? Am J Obstet Gynecol 187:425, 2002
Murphy MA, Ayazifar M: Permanent visual deficits secondary to the HELLP syndrome. J Neuroophthalmol 25(2): 122, 2005
Myatt L, Brewer AS, Langdon G, et al: Attenuation of the vasoconstrictor effects of thromboxane and endothelin by nitric oxide in the human fetal–placental circulation. Am J Obstet Gynecol 166:224, 1992
Myatt L, Clifton R, Roberts J, et al: Can changes in angiogenic biomarkers between the first and second trimesters of pregnancy predict development of pre-eclampsia in a low-risk nulliparous patient population? BJOG 120(10):1183, 2013
Myatt L, Clifton RG, Roberts JM, et al: First-trimester prediction of preeclampsia in nulliparous women at low risk. Obstet Gynecol 119(6):2012a
Myatt L, Clifton RG, Roberts JM, et al: The utility of uterine artery Doppler velocimetry in prediction of preeclampsia in a low-risk population. Obstet Gynecol 120(4):815, 2012b
Myers JE, Hart S, Armstrong S, et al: Evidence for multiple circulating factor in preeclampsia. Am J Obstet Gynecol 196(3):266.e1, 2007
Myers JE, Tuytten R, Thomas G, et al: Integrated proteomics pipeline yields novel biomarkers for predicting preeclampsia. Hypertension 61(6):1281, 2013
National High Blood Pressure Education Program: Working group report on high blood pressure in pregnancy. Am J Obstet Gynecol 183:51, 2000
National Institute for Health and Clinical Excellence: Hypertension in pregnancy: the management of hypertensive disorders during pregnancy. Clinical Guideline No. 107, August 2010
Napolitano R, Thilaganathan B: Mean, lowest, and highest pulsatility index of the uterine artery and adverse pregnancy outcome in twin pregnancies. Am J Obstet Gynecol 206(6):e8, 2012
Navaratnam K, Alfirevic Z, Baker PN: A multi-centre phase IIa clinical study of predictive testing for preeclampsia: improved pregnancy outcomes via early detection (IMPROvED). BMC Pregnancy and Childbirth, 13:226, 2013
Nayeri U, Buhimschi C, Hardy J, et al: Evaluation of "unquantifiable" urine protein species in preeclampsia (PE). Abstract No. 659, Am J Obstet Gynecol 208(1 Suppl):S278, 2013
Ndaboine EM, Kihunrwa A, Rumanyika R, et al: Maternal and perinatal outcomes among eclamptic patients admitted to Bugando Medical Centre, Mwanza, Tanzania. Afr J Reprod Health 16(1):35, 2012
Nelson DB, Yost NP, Cunningham FG: Acute fatty liver of pregnancy: clinical outcomes and expected duration of recovery. Am J Obstet Gynecol 209(5):456.e1, 2013
Nelson DB, Ziadie MS, McIntire DD, et al: Placental pathology suggesting that preeclampsia is more than one disease. Am J Obstet Gynecol 210:66.e1, 2014
Nelson KB, Grether JK: Can magnesium sulfate reduce the risk of cerebral palsy in very low birthweight infants? Pediatrics 95:263, 1995
Ness RB, Roberts JM: Heterogeneous causes constituting the single syndrome of preeclampsia: a hypothesis and its implications. Am J Obstet Gynecol 175(5):1365, 1996
Newsome LR, Bramwell RS, Curling PE: Severe preeclampsia: hemodynamic effects of lumbar epidural anesthesia. Anesth Analg 65:31, 1986
Nguyen TM, Crowther CA, Wilkinson D, et al: Magnesium sulfate for women at term for neuroprotection of the fetus. Cochrane Database Syst Rev 2:CD009395, 2013
Nilsson E, Ros HS, Cnattingius S, et al: The importance of genetic and environmental effects for pre-eclampsia and gestational hypertension: a family study. Br J Obstet Gynaecol 111:200, 2004
North RA, Taylor RS, Schellenberg J-C: Evaluation of a definition of preeclampsia. Br J Obstet Gynaecol 106:767, 1999
Obeidat B, MacDougall J, Harding K: Plasma exchange in a woman with thrombotic thrombocytopenic purpura or severe pre-eclampsia. Br J Obstet Gynaecol 109:961, 2002
O'Brien JM, Shumate SA, Satchwell SL, et al: Maternal benefit of corticosteroid therapy in patients with HELLP (hemolysis, elevated liver enzymes, and low platelet count) syndrome: impact on the rate of regional anesthesia. Am J Obstet Gynecol 186:475, 2002
Odibo AO, Rada CC, Cahill AG, et al: First-trimester serum soluble fms-like tyrosine kinase-1, free vascular endothelial growth factor, placental growth factor and uterine artery Doppler in preeclampsia. J Perinatol 2013 33(9):670, 2013
Oettle C, Hall D, Roux A, et al: Early onset severe pre-eclampsia: expectant management at a secondary hospital in close association with a tertiary institution. BJOG 112(1):84, 2005
Øian P, Maltau JM, Noddleland H, et al: Transcapillary fluid balance in preeclampsia. Br J Obstet Gynaecol 93:235, 1986
Olafsdottir AS, Skuladottir GV, Thorsdottir I, et al: Relationship between high consumption of marine fatty acids in early pregnancy and hypertensive disorders in pregnancy. BJOG 113:301, 2006
Olsen RN, Woelkers D, Dunsmoor-Su R, et al: Abnormal second-trimester serum analytes are more predictive of preterm eclampsia. Am J Obstet Gynecol 207:228.e1, 2012
Olsen SF, Secher NJ, Tabor A, et al: Randomized clinical trials of fish oil supplementation in high risk pregnancies. Br J Obstet Gynaecol 107:382, 2000
Ong SS, Moore RJ, Warren AY, et al: Myometrial and placental artery reactivity alone cannot explain reduced placental perfusion in pre-eclampsia and intrauterine growth restriction. BJOG 110(10):909, 2003
Ostchega Y, Zhang G, Sorlie P, et al: Blood pressure randomized methodology study comparing automatic oscillometric and mercury sphygmomanometer devices: National Health and Nutrition Examination Survey, 2009–2010. National Health Statistics Report 59:1, 2012
Palmer SK, Moore LG, Young DA, et al: Altered blood pressure and increased preeclampsia at high altitude (3100 meters) in Colorado. Am J Obstet Gynecol 180:1161, 1999
Papanna R, Mann LK, Kouides RW, et al: Protein/creatinine ratio in preeclampsia: a systematic review. Obstet Gynecol 112:135, 2008
Parra MC, Lees C, Mann GE, et al: Vasoactive mediator release by endothelial cells in intrauterine growth restriction and preeclampsia. Am J Obstet Gynecol 184:497, 2001
Patrelli TS, Dal'asta A, Gizzo S, et al: Calcium supplementation and prevention of preeclampsia: a meta-analysis. J Matern Fetal Neonatal Med 25(12):2570, 2012
Petrozella L, Mahendroo M, Timmons B, et al: Endothelial microparticles and the antiangiogenic state in preeclampsia and the postpartum period. Am J Obstet Gynecol 207(2):140.e20, 2012
Phelan JP, Yurth DA: Severe preeclampsia. I. Peripartum hemodynamic observations. Am J Obstet Gynecol 144(1):17, 1982
Phillips JK, Janowiak M, Badger GJ, et al: Evidence for distinct preterm and term phenotypes of preeclampsia. J Matern Fetal Neonatal Med 23(7):622, 2010
Pickles CJ, Broughton Pipkin F, Symonds EM: A randomised placebo controlled trial of labetalol in the treatment of mild to moderate pregnancy induced hypertension. Br J Obstet Gynaecol 99(12):964, 1992
Pimenta E, Ruano R, Francisco R, et al: 3D-power Doppler quantification of placental vascularity in pregnancy complicated with hypertensive disorders. Abstract No. 652, Am J Obstet Gynecol 208(1 Suppl):S275, 2013
Pisani-Conway C, Simhan H: Does abnormal hemostasis as reflected by a thromboelastogram (TEG) correlate with preeclampsia disease severity? Abstract No. 621, Am J Obstet Gynecol 208(1 Suppl):S264, 2013
Podymow T, August P: Postpartum course of gestational hypertension and preeclampsia. Hypertens Pregnancy 29(3):294, 2010
Poon LC, Kametas N, Bonino S, et al: Urine albumin concentration and albumin-to-creatinine ratio at 11(+0) to 13(+6) weeks in the prediction of pre-eclampsia. BJOG 115:866, 2008
Postma IR, Wessel I, Aarnoudse JG, et al: Neurocognitive functioning in formerly eclamptic women: sustained attention and executive functioning. Reprod Sci 16:175A, 2009
Poston L, Briley AL, Seed PT, et al: Vitamin C and vitamin E in pregnant women at risk for pre-eclampsia (VIP trial): randomized placebo-controlled trial. Lancet 367:1145, 2006
Powers RW, Bodnar LM, Ness RB, et al: Uric acid concentrations in early pregnancy among preeclamptic women with gestational hyperuricemia at delivery. Am J Obstet Gynecol 194:160.e1, 2006
Powers RW, Evans RW, Ness RB, et al: Homocysteine is increased in preeclampsia but not in gestational hypertension (Abstract #375). J Soc Gynecol Invest 7(1):(Suppl), 2000
Pritchard JA: The use of magnesium ion in the management of eclamptogenic toxemias. Surg Gynecol Obstet 100:131, 1955
Pritchard JA, Cunningham FG, Mason RA: Coagulation changes in eclampsia: their frequency and pathogenesis. Am J Obstet Gynecol 124:855, 1976
Pritchard JA, Cunningham FG, Pritchard SA: The Parkland Memorial Hospital protocol for treatment of eclampsia: evaluation of 245 cases. Am J Obstet Gynecol 148(7):951, 1984
Pritchard JA, Cunningham FG, Pritchard SA, et al: How often does maternal preeclampsia–eclampsia incite thrombocytopenia in the fetus? Obstet Gynecol 69:292, 1987
Pritchard JA, Pritchard SA: Standardized treatment of 154 consecutive cases of eclampsia. Am J Obstet Gynecol 123(5):543, 1975

Pritchard JA, Weisman R Jr, Ratnoff OD, et al: Intravascular hemolysis, thrombocytopenia and other hematologic abnormalities associated with severe toxemia of pregnancy. N Engl J Med 250:87, 1954

Raab W, Schroeder G, Wagner R, et al: Vascular reactivity and electrolytes in normal and toxemic pregnancy. J Clin Endocrinol 16:1196, 1956

Rafferty TD, Berkowitz RL: Hemodynamics in patients with severe toxemia during labor and delivery. Am J Obstet Gynecol 138:263, 1980

Raijmakers MT, Dechend R, Poston L: Oxidative stress and preeclampsia: rationale for antioxidant clinical trials. Hypertension 44:374, 2004

Rana S, Hacker MR, Modest AM, et al: Circulating angiogenic factors and risk of adverse maternal and perinatal outcomes in two pregnancies with suspected preeclampsia. Hypertension 60(2):451, 2012

Redman CW, Sargent IL, Taylor RN: Immunology of abnormal pregnancy and preeclampsia. In Taylor RN, Roberts JM, Cunningham FG (eds): Chesley's Hypertensive Disorders in Pregnancy, 4th ed. Amsterdam, Academic Press, 2014

Redman CW, Tannetta DS, Dragovic RA, et al: Review: does size matter? Placental debris and the pathophysiology of pre-eclampsia. Placenta 33(Suppl):S48, 2012

Reimer T, Rohrmann H, Stubert J, et al: Angiogenic factors and acute-phase proteins in serum samples of preeclampsia and HELLP syndrome patients: a matched-pair analysis. J Matern Fetal Neonatal Med 26(3):263, 2013

Richards A, Graham DI, Bullock MRR: Clinicopathological study of neurological complications due to hypertensive disorders of pregnancy. J Neurol Neurosurg Psychiatry 51:416, 1988

Roberge S, Giguere Y, Villa P, et al: Early administration of low-dose aspirin for the prevention of severe and mild preeclampsia: a systematic review and meta-analysis. Am J Perinatol 29(7):551, 2012

Roberts CL, Ford JB, Algert CS, et al: Population-based trends in pregnancy hypertension and pre-eclampsia: an international comparative study. BMJ Open 1(1):e000101, 2011

Roberts JM: A randomized controlled trial of antioxidant vitamins to prevent serious complications associated with pregnancy related hypertension in low risk, nulliparous women. Abstract No 8. Presented at the 29th Annual Meeting of the Society for Maternal-Fetal Medicine, January 26–31, 2009

Rogers BB, Bloom SL, Leveno KJ: Atherosis revisited: current concepts on the pathophysiology of implantation site disorders. Obstet Gynecol Surv 54:189, 1999

Roos NM, Wiegman MJ, Jansonius NM, et al: Visual disturbance in (pre) eclampsia. Obstet Gynecol Surv 67(4):242, 2012

Royal College of Obstetricians and Gynaecologists: The management of severe pre-eclampsia. RCOG Guideline 10A:1, 2006

Rumbold AR, Crowther CA, Haslam RR: Vitamins C and E and the risks of preeclampsia and perinatal complications. N Engl J Med 354:17, 2006

Sagsoz N, Kucukozkan T: The effect of treatment on endothelin-1 concentration and mean arterial pressure in preeclampsia and eclampsia. Hypertens Pregnancy 22:185, 2003

Saito Y, Tano Y: Retinal pigment epithelial lesions associated with choroidal ischemia in preeclampsia. Retina 18:103, 1998

Salinger DH, Mundle S, Regi A, et al: Magnesium sulphate for prevention of eclampsia: are intramuscular and intravenous regimens equivalent? A population pharmacokinetic study. BJOG 120(7):894, 2013

Sanchez-Ramos L, Adair CD, Todd JC, et al: Erythrocyte membrane fluidity in patients with preeclampsia and the HELLP syndrome: a preliminary study. J Matern Fetal Invest 4:237, 1994

Sarsam DS, Shamden M, Al Wazan R: Expectant versus aggressive management in severe preeclampsia remote from term. Singapore Med J 49(9):698, 2008

Saucedo M, Deneux-Tharaux C, Bouvier-Colle MH, et al: Ten years of confidential inquiries into maternal deaths in France, 1998–2007. Obstet Gynecol 122(4):752, 2013

Scardo JA, Vermillion ST, Newman RB, et al: A randomized, double-blind, hemodynamic evaluation of nifedipine and labetalol in preeclamptic hypertensive emergencies. Am J Obstet Gynecol 181:862, 1999

Schendel DE, Berg CJ, Yeargin-Allsopp M, et al: Prenatal magnesium sulfate exposure and the risk for cerebral palsy or mental retardation among very low birthweight children aged 3 to 5 years. JAMA 276:1805, 1996

Scholten RR, Hopman MT, Sweep FC, et al: Co-occurrence of cardiovascular and prothrombotic risk factors in women with a history of preeclampsia. Obstet Gynecol 121(1):97, 2013

Schutte JM, Schuitemaker NW, van Roosmalen J, et al: Substandard care in maternal mortality due to hypertensive disease in pregnancy in the Netherlands. BJOG 115(10):1322, 2008

Schwartz RB, Feske SK, Polak JF, et al: Preeclampsia-eclampsia: clinical and neuroradiographic correlates and insights into the pathogenesis of hypertensive encephalopathy. Radiology 217:371, 2000

Sciscione AC, Ivester T, Largoza M, et al: Acute pulmonary edema in pregnancy. Obstet Gynecol 101:511, 2003

Sep S, Verbeek J, Spaanderman M, et al: Clinical differences between preeclampsia and the HELLP syndrome suggest different pathogeneses. Reprod Sci 16:176A, 2009

Sergis F, Clara DM, Galbriella F, et al: Prophylaxis of recurrent preeclampsia: low molecular weight heparin plus low-dose aspirin versus low-dose aspirin alone. Hypertension Pregnancy 25:115, 2006

Shahabi A, Wilson ML, Lewinger JP, et al: Genetic admixture and risk of hypertensive disorders of pregnancy among Latinas in Los Angeles County. Epidemiology 24(2):285, 2013

Shear RM, Rinfret D, Leduc L: Should we offer expectant management in cases of severe preterm preeclampsia with fetal growth restriction? Am J Obstet Gynecol 192:1119, 2005

Sheehan HL, Lynch JB (eds): Cerebral lesions. In Pathology of Toxaemia of Pregnancy. Baltimore, Williams & Wilkins, 1973

Shekhar S, Chanderdeep S, Thakur S, et al: Oral nifedipine or intravenous labetalol for hypertensive emergency in pregnancy: a randomized controlled trial. Obstet Gynecol 122(5):1057, 2013

Sibai BM: Diagnosis and management of gestational hypertension and preeclampsia. Obstet Gynecol 102:181, 2003

Sibai BM: Diagnosis, controversies, and management of the syndrome of hemolysis, elevated liver enzymes, and low platelet count. Obstet Gynecol 103:981, 2004

Sibai BM: Diagnosis, prevention, and management of eclampsia. Obstet Gynecol 105:402, 2005

Sibai BM: Etiology and management of postpartum hypertension-preeclampsia. Am J Obstet Gynecol 206(6):470, 2012

Sibai BM: Imitators of severe preeclampsia. Obstet Gynecol 109:956, 2007a

Sibai BM, Barton JR: Expectant management of severe preeclampsia remote from term: patient selection, treatment and delivery indications. Am J Obstet Gynecol 196:514, 2007b

Sibai BM, Barton JR, Akl S, et al: A randomized prospective comparison of nifedipine and bed rest versus bed rest alone in the management of preeclampsia remote from term. Am J Obstet Gynecol 167(1):879, 1992

Sibai BM, El-Nazer A, Gonzalez-Ruiz A: Severe preeclampsia–eclampsia in young primigravid women: subsequent pregnancy outcome and remote prognosis. Am J Obstet Gynecol 155:1011, 1986

Sibai BM, Gonzalez AR, Mabie WC, et al: A comparison of labetalol plus hospitalization versus hospitalization alone in the management of preeclampsia remote from term. Obstet Gynecol 70:323, 1987a

Sibai BM, Graham JM, McCubbin JH: A comparison of intravenous and intramuscular magnesium sulfate regimens in preeclampsia. Am J Obstet Gynecol 150:728, 1984

Sibai BM, Hauth J, Caritis S, et al: Hypertensive disorders in twin versus singleton gestations. Am J Obstet Gynecol 182:938, 2000

Sibai BM, Mabie BC, Harvey CJ, et al: Pulmonary edema in severe preeclampsia–eclampsia: analysis of thirty-seven consecutive cases. Am J Obstet Gynecol 156:1174, 1987b

Sibai BM, Mercer B, Sarinoglu C: Severe preeclampsia in the second trimester: recurrence risk and long-term prognosis. Am J Obstet Gynecol 165:1408, 1991

Sibai BM, Mercer BM, Schiff E, et al: Aggressive versus expectant management of severe preeclampsia at 28 to 32 weeks' gestation: a randomized controlled trial. Am J Obstet Gynecol 171:818, 1994

Sibai BM, Ramadan MK, Chari RS, et al: Pregnancies complicated by HELLP syndrome (hemolysis, elevated liver enzymes, and low platelets): subsequent pregnancy outcome and long-term prognosis. Am J Obstet Gynecol 172:125, 1995

Sibai BM, Spinnato JA, Watson DL, et al: Eclampsia, 4. Neurological findings and future outcome. Am J Obstet Gynecol 152:184, 1985

Sibai BM, Stella CL: Diagnosis and management of atypical preeclampsia-eclampsia. Am J Obstet Gynecol 200:481.e1, 2009

Silver HM, Seebeck M, Carlson R: Comparison of total blood volume in normal, preeclamptic, and non-proteinuric gestational hypertensive pregnancy by simultaneous measurement of red blood cell and plasma volumes. Am J Obstet Gynecol 179:87, 1998

Smith GN, Pudwell J, Walker M, et al: Ten-year, thirty-year, and lifetime cardiovascular disease risk estimates following pregnancy complicated by preeclampsia. J Obstet Gynaecol Can 34(9):830, 2012

Smith GN, Walker MC, Liu A, et al: A history of preeclampsia identifies women who have underlying cardiovascular risk factors. Am J Obstet Gynecol 200:58.e1, 2009

Smith JM, Lowe RF, Fullerton J, et al: An integrative review of the side effects related to the use of magnesium sulfate for preeclampsia and eclampsia management. BMC Pregnancy Childbirth 13:34, 2013

Smyth RM, Spark P, Armstrong N, et al: Magpie Trial in the UK: methods and additional data for women and children at 2 years following pregnancy complicated by pre-eclampsia. BMC Pregnancy Childbirth 9:15, 2009

Society for Maternal-Fetal Medicine, Sibai BM: Evaluation and management of severe preeclampsia before 34 weeks' gestation. Am J Obstet Gynecol 205(3):191, 2011

Somjen G, Hilmy M, Stephen CR: Failure to anesthetize human subjects by intravenous administration of magnesium sulfate. J Pharmacol Exp Ther 154(3):652, 1966

Spaan JJ, Ekhart T, Spaanderman MEA, et al: Remote hemodynamics and renal function in formerly preeclamptic women. Obstet Gynecol 113:853, 2009

Spaan JJ, Ekhart T, Spaanderman MEA, et al: Renal function after preeclampsia: a longitudinal pilot study. Nephron Clin Pract 120(3):c156, 2012a

Spaan JJ, Sep SJS, Lopes van Balen V, et al: Metabolic syndrome as a risk factor for hypertension after preeclampsia. Obstet Gynecol 120(2 Pt 1):311, 2012b

Spargo B, McCartney CP, Winemiller R: Glomerular capillary endotheliosis in toxemia of pregnancy. Arch Pathol 68:593, 1959

Spencer J, Polavarapu S, Timms D, et al: Regional and monthly variation in rates of preeclampsia at delivery among U.S. births. Abstract No 294. Presented at the 29th Annual Meeting of the Society for Maternal-Fetal Medicine, January 26–31, 2009

Spitz B, Magness RR, Cox SM: Low-dose aspirin. I. Effect on angiotensin II pressor responses and blood prostaglandin concentrations in pregnant women sensitive to angiotensin II. Am J Obstet Gynecol 159(5):1035, 1988

Staff AC, Braekke K, Johnsen GM, et al: Circulating concentration of soluble endoglin (CD105) in fetal and maternal serum and in amniotic fluid in preeclampsia. Am J Obstet Gynecol 197(2):176.e1, 2007

Staff AC, Sibai BM, Cunningham FG: Prevention of preeclampsia and eclampsia. In Taylor RN, Roberts JM, Cunningham FG (eds): Chesley's Hypertensive Disorders in Pregnancy. Amsterdam, Academic Press, 2014

Staines-Urias E, Paez MC, Doyle P, et al: Genetic association studies in preeclampsia: systematic meta-analyses and field synopsis. Int J Epidemiol 41(6):1764, 2012

Stekkinger E, Scholten R, van der Vlugt MJ, et al: Metabolic syndrome and the risk for recurrent pre-eclampsia: a retrospective cohort study. BJOG 120(8):979, 2013

Strickland DM, Guzick DS, Cox K, et al: The relationship between abortion in the first pregnancy and the development of pregnancy-induced hypertension in the subsequent pregnancy. Am J Obstet Gynecol 154:146, 1986

Stout MJ, Scifres CM, Stamilio DM: Diagnostic utility of urine protein-to-creatinine ratio for identifying proteinuria in pregnancy. J Matern Fetal Neonatal Med 26(1):66, 2013

Stubbs TM, Lazarchick J, Horger EO III: Plasma fibronectin levels in preeclampsia: a possible biochemical marker for vascular endothelial damage. Am J Obstet Gynecol 150: 885, 1984

Sugulle M, Herse F, Hering L, et al: Cardiovascular biomarker midregional proatrial natriuretic peptide during and after preeclamptic pregnancies. Hypertension 59(3):395, 2012

Sunderji S, Sibai B, Wothe D et al: Differential diagnosis of preterm preeclampsia and hypertension using prototype automated assays for SVEGF R1 and PLGF: a prospective clinical study. Abstract No 249. Presented at the 29th Annual Meeting of the Society for Maternal-Fetal Medicine, January 26–31, 2009

Suzuki Y, Yamamoto T, Mabuchi Y, et al: Ultrastructural changes in omental resistance artery in women with preeclampsia. Am J Obstet Gynecol 189:216, 2003

Swank M, Nageotte M, Hatfield T: Necrotizing pancreatitis associated with severe preeclampsia. Obstet Gynecol 120(2 Pt 2):453, 2012

Szal SE, Croughan-Minibane MS, Kilpatrick SJ: Effect of magnesium prophylaxis and preeclampsia on the duration of labor. Am J Obstet Gynecol 180:1475, 1999

Taber EB, Tan L, Chao CR, et al: Pharmacokinetics of ionized versus total magnesium in subjects with preterm labor and preeclampsia. Am J Obstet Gynecol 186:1017, 2002

Tajik P, van der Tuuk K, Koopmans CM, et al: Should cervical favourability play a role in the decision for labour induction in gestational hypertension or mild preeclampsia at term? An exploratory analysis of the HYPITAT trial. BJOG 119(9):1123, 2012

Talledo OE, Chesley LC, Zuspan FP: Renin-angiotensin system in normal and toxemic pregnancies, 3. Differential sensitivity to angiotensin II and norepinephrine in toxemia of pregnancy. Am J Obstet Gynecol 100:218, 1968

Tan LK, de Swiet M: The management of postpartum hypertension. BJOG 109(7):733, 2002

Task Force: Hypertension in pregnancy. Report of the American College of Obstetricians and Gynecologists' Task Force on Hypertension in Pregnancy. Obstet Gynecol 122:1122, 2013

Taufield PA, Ales KL, Resnick LM, et al: Hypocalciuria in preeclampsia. N Engl J Med 316:715, 1987

Taylor RN, Roberts JM: Endothelial cell dysfunction. In Lindheimer MD, Roberts JM, Cunningham FG (eds): Chesley's Hypertensive Disorders in Pregnancy, 2nd ed. Stamford, CT, Appleton & Lange, 1999, p 395

Thangaratinam S, Ismail KMK, Sharp S, et al: Accuracy of serum uric acid in predicting complications of pre-eclampsia: a systematic review. BJOG 113: 369, 2006

Thiagarajah S, Bourgeois FJ, Harbert GM, et al: Thrombocytopenia in preeclampsia: associated abnormalities and management principles. Am J Obstet Gynecol 150:1, 1984

Thornton C, Dahlen H, Korda A, et al: The incidence of preeclampsia and eclampsia and associated maternal mortality in Australia from population-linked datasets: 2000–2008. Am J Obstet Gynecol 208(6):476.e1, 2013

Thurnau GR, Kemp DB, Jarvis A: Cerebrospinal fluid levels of magnesium in patients with preeclampsia after treatment with intravenous magnesium sulfate: a preliminary report. Am J Obstet Gynecol 157:1435, 1987

Tompkins MJ, Thiagarajah S: HELLP (hemolysis, elevated liver enzymes, and low platelet count) syndrome: the benefit of corticosteroids. Am J Obstet Gynecol 181:304, 1999

Trommer BL, Homer D, Mikhael MA: Cerebral vasospasm and eclampsia. Stroke 19:326, 1988

Trudinger BJ, Cook CM: Doppler umbilical and uterine flow waveforms in severe pregnancy hypertension. Br J Obstet Gynaecol 97:142, 1990

Tudela CM, McIntire DD, Alexander JM: Effect of maternal body mass index on serum magnesium levels given for seizure prophylaxis. Obstet Gynecol 121(2 pt 1):314, 2013

Tuffnell DJ, Lilford RJ, Buchan PC, et al: Randomized controlled trial of day care for hypertension in pregnancy. Lancet 339:224, 1992

Tun C, Quiñones JN, Kurt A, et al: Comparison of 12-hour urine protein and protein:creatinine ratio with 24-hour urine protein for the diagnosis of preeclampsia. Am J Obstet Gynecol 207(3):233.e1, 2012

Turnbull DA, Wilkinson C, Gerard K, et al: Clinical, psychosocial, and economic effects of antenatal day care for three medical complications of pregnancy: a randomized controlled trial of 395 women. Lancet 363:1104, 2004

Umans JG, Abalos E: Cunningham FG: Antihypertensive treatment. In Taylor RN, Roberts JM, Cunningham FG (eds): Chesley's Hypertensive Disorders in Pregnancy, 4th ed. Amsterdam, Academic Press, 2014

Urban G, Vergani P, Ghindini A, et al: State of the art: non-invasive ultrasound assessment of the uteroplacental circulation. Semin Perinatol 31(4), 232, 2007

Valensise H, Vasapollo B, Gagliardi G, et al: Early and late preeclampsia: two different maternal hemodynamic states in the latent phase of the disease. Hypertension 52(5):873, 2008

van der Merwe JL, Hall DR, Wright C, et al: Are early and late preeclampsia distinct subclasses of the disease—what does the placenta reveal? Hypertens Pregnancy 29(4):2010

van Veen TR, Panerai RB, Haeri S, et al: Cerebral autoregulation in normal pregnancy and preeclampsia. Obstet Gynecol 122:1064, 2013

Vatten LJ, Asvold BO, Eskild A: Angiogenic factors in maternal circulation and preeclampsia with or without fetal growth restriction. Acta Obstet Gynecol Scand 91(12):1388, 2012

Venkatesha S, Toporsian M, Lam C, et al: Soluble endoglin contributes to the pathogenesis of preeclampsia. Nat Med 12:642, 2006

Ventura SJ, Martin JA, Curtin SC, et al: Births: final data for 1998. Natl Vital Stat Rep 48(3):1, 2000

Vermillion ST, Scardo JA, Newman RB, et al: A randomized, double-blind trial of oral nifedipine and intravenous labetalol in hypertensive emergencies of pregnancy. Am J Obstet Gynecol 181:858, 1999

Vigil-De Gracia P, Ortega-Paz L: Pre-eclampsia/eclampsia and hepatic rupture. Int J Gynaecol Obstet 118(3):186, 2012

Vigil-De Gracia P, Ortega-Paz L: Retinal detachment in association with pre-eclampsia, eclampsia, and HELLP syndrome. Int J Gynaecol Obstet 114(3):223, 2011

Vigil-De Gracia P, Ruiz E, Lopez JC, et al: Management of severe hypertension in the postpartum period with intravenous hydralazine or labetalol: a randomized clinical trial. Hypertens Pregnancy 26(2):163, 2007

Vigil-De Gracia P, Tejada OR, Minaca AC, et al: Expectant management of severe preeclampsia remote from term: the MEXPRE Latin Study, a randomized multicenter clinical trial. Am J Obstet Gynecol 209:425.e1, 2013

Vikse BE, Irgens LM, Leivestad T, et al: Preeclampsia and the risk of end-stage renal disease. N Engl J Med 359:800, 2008

Villa PM, Kajantie E, Räikkönen K, et al: Aspirin in the prevention of preeclampsia in high-risk women: a randomized placebo-controlled PREDO Trial and a meta-analysis of randomized trials. BJOG 120(1):64, 2013

Villar J, Hany AA, Merialdi M, et al: World Health Organization randomized trial of calcium supplementation among low calcium intake pregnant women. Am J Obstet Gynecol 194:639, 2006

Villar J, Purwar M, Merialdi M, et al: WHO randomised trial of vitamin C & E supplementation among women at high risk for preeclampsia and nutritional deficiency. Society of Maternal-Fetal Medicine Abstract No. 8. Am J Obstet Gynecol 197:S4, 2007

Virchow R: Gesammelte Abhandlungen zur Wissenschaftlichen Medicin. Frankfurt, Meidinger Sohn, 1856, p 778

Volhard F: Die doppelseitigen haematogenen Nierenerkrankungen. Berlin, Springer, 1918

Vollaard E, Zeeman G, Alexander JA, et al: "Delta eclampsia"—a hypertensive encephalopathy of pregnancy in "normotensive" women. Abstract No. 479, Am J Obstet Gynecol 197(6 Suppl):S140, 2007

Vollebregt K, Van Leijden L, Westerhof B, et al: Arterial stiffness is higher in early pregnancy in women who will develop preeclampsia. Abstract No 712. Presented at the 29th Annual Meeting of the Society for Maternal-Fetal Medicine, January 26–31, 2009

von Dadelszen P, Firoz T, Donnay F, et al: Preeclampsia in low and middle income countries—health services lessons learned from the PRE-EMPT (PRE-eclampsia monitoring, prevention, and treatment) Project. J Obstet Gynaecol Can 34(10):917, 2012

von Dadelszen P, Magee LA: Fall in mean arterial pressure and fetal growth restriction in pregnancy hypertension: an updated metaregression analysis. J Obstet Gynaecol Can 24(12):941, 2002

von Mandach U, Lauth D, Huch R: Maternal and fetal nitric oxide production in normal and abnormal pregnancy. J Matern Fetal Neonatal Med 13:22, 2003

Wagner SJ, Craici IM, Grande JP, et al: From placenta to podocyte: vascular and podocyte pathophysiology in preeclampsia. Clin Nephrol 78(3):241, 2012

Walker JJ: Pre-eclampsia. Lancet 356:1260, 2000

Wallace DH, Leveno KJ, Cunningham FG, et al: Randomized comparison of general and regional anesthesia for cesarean delivery in pregnancies complicated by severe preeclampsia. Obstet Gynecol 86:193, 1995

Wallace K, Wells A, Bennett W: African-Americans, preeclampsia and future cardiovascular disease: is nitric oxide the missing link? Abstract No 827. Presented at the 29th Annual Meeting of the Society for Maternal-Fetal Medicine, January 26–31, 2009

Wallenburg HC, Makovitz JW, Dekker GA, et al: Low-dose aspirin prevents pregnancy-induced hypertension and preeclampsia in angiotensin-sensitive primigravidae. Lancet 327:1, 1986

Walsh SW: Plasma from preeclamptic women stimulates transendothelial migration of neutrophils. Reprod Sci 16(3):320, 2009

Wang LC, Huang CY, Want HK, et al: Magnesium sulfate and nimesulide have synergistic effects on rescuing brain damage after transient focal ischemia. J Neurotrauma 29(7):1518, 2012a

Wang Y, Gu Y, Granger DN, et al: Endothelial junctional protein redistribution and increased monolayer permeability in human umbilical vein endothelial cells isolated during preeclampsia. Am J Obstet Gynecol 186:214, 2002

Wang Y, Zhao S, Loyd, et al: Increased urinary excretion of nephrin, podocalyxin, and βig-h3 in women with preeclampsia. Am J Physiol Renal Physiol 302(9):F1084, 2012b

Ward K, Taylor RN: Genetic factors in the etiology of preeclampsia. In Taylor RN, Roberts JM, Cunningham FG (eds): Chesley's Hypertensive Disorders in Pregnancy, 4th ed. Amsterdam, Academic Press, 2014

Watt-Morse ML, Caritis SN, Kridgen PL: Magnesium sulfate is a poor inhibitor of oxytocin-induced contractility in pregnant sheep. J Matern Fetal Med 4:139, 1995

Weiner CP, Thompson LP, Liu KZ, et al: Endothelium derived relaxing factor and indomethacin-sensitive contracting factor alter arterial contractile responses to thromboxane during pregnancy. Am J Obstet Gynecol 166: 1171, 1992

Weinstein L: Syndrome of hemolysis, elevated liver enzymes and low platelet count: a severe consequence of hypertension in pregnancy. Am J Obstet Gynecol 142:159, 1982

Weinstein L: Preeclampsia-eclampsia with hemolysis, elevated liver enzymes, and thrombocytopenia. Obstet Gynecol 66:657, 1985

Wicke C, Pereira PL, Neeser E, et al: Subcapsular liver hematoma in HELLP syndrome: evaluation of diagnostic and therapeutic options—a unicenter study. Am J Obstet Gynecol 190:106, 2004

Wide-Swensson DH, Ingemarsson I, Lunell NO, et al: Calcium channel blockade (isradipine) in treatment of hypertension in pregnancy: a randomized placebo-controlled study. Am J Obstet Gynecol 173(1):872, 1995

Widmer M, Villar J, Benigni A, et al: Mapping the theories of preeclampsia and the role of angiogenic factors. Obstet Gynecol 109:168, 2007

Wiegman MJ, de Groot JC, Jansonius NM, et al: Long-term visual functioning after eclampsia. Obstet Gynecol 119(5):959, 2012

Wikström AK, Haglund B, Olovsson M, et al: The risk of maternal ischaemic heart disease after gestational hypertensive disease. BJOG 112:1486, 2005

Wikström AK, Stephansson O, Cnattingius S: Previous preeclampsia and risks of adverse outcomes in subsequent nonpreeclamptic pregnancies. Am J Obstet Gynecol 204(2):148.e1, 2011

Wilson ML, Desmond DH, Goodwin TM, et al: Transforming growth factor-3 polymorphisms are associated with preeclampsia (PE). Abstract No 47. Presented at the 29th Annual Meeting of the Society for Maternal-Fetal Medicine, January 26–31, 2009

Winkel CA, Milewich L, Parker CR Jr, et al: Conversion of plasma progesterone to deoxycorticosterone in men, nonpregnant and pregnant women, and adrenalectomized subjects. J Clin Invest 66:803, 1980

Witlin AG, Friedman SA, Egerman RS, et al: Cerebrovascular disorders complicating pregnancy beyond eclampsia. Am J Obstet Gynecol 176:1139, 1997a

Witlin AG, Friedman SA, Sibai BA: The effect of magnesium sulfate therapy on the duration of labor in women with mild preeclampsia at term: a randomized, double-blind, placebo-controlled trial. Am J Obstet Gynecol 176:623, 1997b

Worley LC, Hnat MD, Cunningham FG: Advanced extrauterine pregnancy: diagnostic and therapeutic challenges. Am J Obstet Gynecol 198(3):297.e1, 2008

Yang J, Shang J, Zhang S, et al: The role of renin-angiotensin-aldosterone system in preeclampsia: genetic polymorphisms and microRNA. J Mol Endocrinol 50(2):R53, 2013

Zeeman GG, Alexander JM, McIntire DD, et al: Homocysteine plasma concentration levels for the prediction of preeclampsia in women with chronic hypertension. Am J Obstet Gynecol 189:574, 2003

Zeeman GG, Cunningham FG, Pritchard JA: The magnitude of hemoconcentration with eclampsia. Hypertens Pregnancy 28(2):127, 2009

Zeeman GG, Fleckenstein JL, Twickler DM, et al: Cerebral infarction in eclampsia. Am J Obstet Gynecol 190:714, 2004a

Zeeman GG, Hatab M, Twickler DM: Increased large-vessel cerebral blood flow in severe preeclampsia by magnetic resonance (MR) evaluation. Presented at the 24th Annual Meeting of the Society for Maternal-Fetal Medicine, New Orleans, February 2, 2004b

Zhang C, Williams MA, King IB, et al: Vitamin C and the risk of preeclampsia—results from dietary questionnaire and plasma assay. Epidemiology 13:382, 2002

Zhang J, Klebanoff MA, Levine RJ, et al: The puzzling association between smoking and hypertension during pregnancy. Am J Obstet Gynecol 181:1407, 1999

Zhou SJ, Yelland L, McPhee AJ, et al: Fish-oil supplementation in pregnancy does not reduce the risk of gestational diabetes or preeclampsia. Am J Clin Nutr 95)6):1378, 2012a

Zhou X, Zhang GY, Wang J, et al: A novel bridge between oxidative stress and immunity: the interaction between hydrogen peroxide and human leukocyte antigen G in placental trophoblasts during preeclampsia. Am J Obstet Gynecol 206(5):447.e7, 2012b

Zilberberg E, Sivan E, Yinon Y, et al: Alterations in protein secretion in preeclampsia as a function of plurality—clinical implications. Abstract No. 623, Am J Obstet Gynecol 208(1 Suppl):S265, 2013

Zinaman M, Rubin J, Lindheimer MD: Serial plasma oncotic pressure levels and echoencephalography during and after delivery in severe preeclampsia. Lancet 1:1245, 1985

Zondervan HA, Oosting J, Smorenberg-Schoorl ME, et al: Maternal whole blood viscosity in pregnancy hypertension. Gynecol Obstet Invest 25:83, 1988

Zwart JJ, Richters A, Öry F, et al: Eclampsia in The Netherlands. Obstet Gynecol 112:820, 2008

CHAPTER 41

Obstetrical Hemorrhage

Obstetrics is a bloody business.
Dr. Jack Pritchard (1976b)

Obstetrical hemorrhage continues along with hypertension and infections as one of the infamous "triad" of causes of maternal deaths in both developed and underdeveloped countries. It is a leading reason for admission of pregnant women to intensive care units (ICUs) (Crozier, 2011; Small, 2012; Zeeman, 2003; Zwart, 2008). Hemorrhage was a direct cause of nearly 13 percent of 4693 pregnancy-related maternal deaths in the United States documented by the Pregnancy Mortality Surveillance System of the Centers for Disease Control and Prevention (Berg, 2010). Similarly, Clark and coworkers (2008) reported that 12 percent of maternal deaths recorded in the Hospital Corporation of America database were caused by hemorrhage. In developing countries, its contribution is even more striking. Indeed, hemorrhage is the single most important cause of maternal death worldwide and is responsible for half of all postpartum deaths in developing countries (Lalonde, 2006; McCormick, 2002).

GENERAL CONSIDERATIONS

The decreasing maternal mortality rate from hemorrhage in this country has been a major achievement. Decreased deaths from hemorrhage have been a major contributor to the decrease in the maternal mortality rate during the 20th century—from approximately 1000 to only 10 per 100,000 births (Hoyert, 2007). But, as discussed in Chapter 1 (p. 5), probably half of maternal deaths are not reported, and at least a third are considered preventable. It thus seems unlikely that deaths from hemorrhage have reached an irreducible minimum.

Mechanisms of Normal Hemostasis

A major concept in understanding the pathophysiology and management of obstetrical hemorrhage is the mechanism by which hemostasis is achieved after normal delivery. Recall that near term an incredible amount of blood—at least 600 mL/min—flows through the intervillous space (Pates, 2010). As described in Chapter 5 (p. 96), this prodigious flow circulates through the spiral arteries, which average 120 in number. Also recall that these vessels have no muscular layer because of their endotrophoblastic remodeling, which creates a low-pressure system. With placental separation, these vessels at the implantation site are avulsed, and hemostasis is achieved first by myometrial contraction, which compresses this formidable number of relatively large vessels (Chap. 2, p. 26).

Contractions are followed by clotting and obliteration of vessel lumens.

If after delivery, the myometrium within and adjacent to the denuded implantation site contracts vigorously, fatal hemorrhage from the placental implantation site is unlikely. *Importantly, an intact coagulation system is not necessary for postpartum hemostasis unless there are lacerations in the uterus, birth canal, or perineum.* At the same time, however, fatal postpartum hemorrhage can result from uterine atony despite normal coagulation. Adhered placental pieces or large blood clots that prevent effective myometrial contraction will serve to impair hemostasis at the implantation site.

TABLE 41-1. Calculation of Maternal Total Blood Volume

Nonpregnant blood volume[a]:

$$\frac{[\text{Height (inches)} \times 50] + [\text{Weight (pounds)} \times 25]}{2} = \text{Blood volume (mL)}$$

Pregnancy blood volume:

Average increase is 30 to 60 percent of calculated nonpregnant volume

Increases across gestational age and plateaus at approximately 34 weeks

Usually larger with low normal-range hematocrit (~30) and smaller with high normal-range hematocrit (~40)

Average increase is 40 to 80 percent with multifetal gestation

Average increase is less with preeclampsia—volumes vary inversely with severity

Postpartum blood volume with serious hemorrhage:

Assume acute return to nonpregnant total volume after fluid resuscitation

Pregnancy hypervolemia cannot be restored postpartum

[a]Formula arrived at by measuring blood volume and blood loss in more than 100 women using ^{51}Cr-labeled erythrocytes.

Modified from Hernandez, 2012.

Definition and Incidence

Traditionally, postpartum hemorrhage has been defined as the loss of 500 mL of blood or more after completion of the third stage of labor. This is problematic because almost half of all women delivered vaginally shed that amount of blood or more when losses are measured quantitatively (Pritchard, 1962). These results are depicted in Figure 41-1 and show further that approximately 5 percent of women delivering vaginally lose more than 1000 mL of blood. *These studies also showed that estimated blood loss is commonly only approximately half the actual loss.* Because of this, estimated blood loss in excess of "average" or 500 mL should alert the obstetrician to possible excessive bleeding. Calibrated delivery-drape markings improve estimation accuracy, but even this technique underestimates blood loss compared with more precise methods (Sosa, 2009; Toledo, 2007).

The blood volume of a pregnant woman with normal pregnancy-induced hypervolemia usually increases by half, but increases range from 30 to 60 percent—1500 to 2000 mL for an average-sized woman (Pritchard, 1965). The equation to calculate blood volume is shown in Table 41-1. It is axiomatic that a normal pregnant woman tolerates, without any decrease in postpartum hematocrit, blood loss at delivery that approaches the volume of blood that she added during pregnancy. Thus, if blood loss is less than the pregnancy-added volume, the hematocrit remains the same acutely and during the first several days. It then increases as nonpregnant plasma volume normalizes during the next week or so. *Whenever the postpartum hematocrit is lower than one obtained on admission for delivery, blood loss can be estimated as the sum of the calculated pregnancy-added volume plus 500 mL for each 3 volume percent decrease of the hematocrit.* Blood loss in these women can also be calculated using the formula of Hernandez and associates (2012). Briefly, these investigators used admission-to-discharge red cell volumes to compute total blood loss.

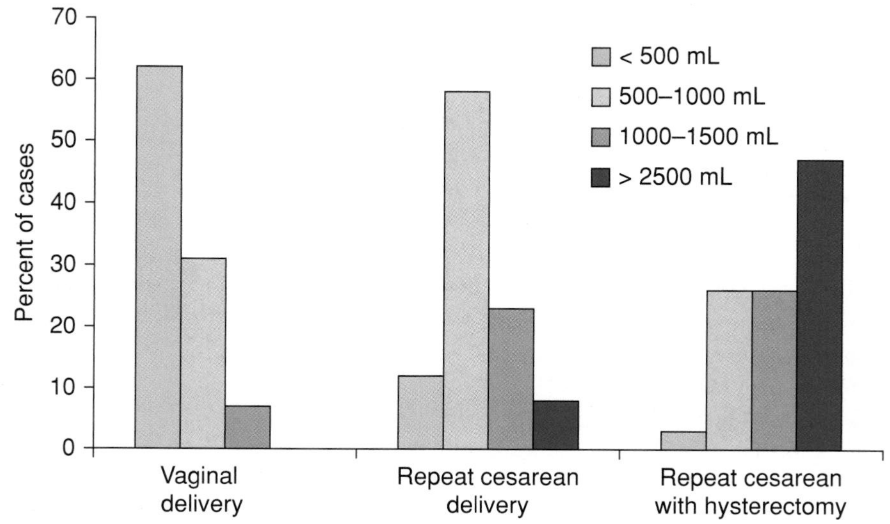

FIGURE 41-1 Blood loss associated with vaginal delivery, repeat cesarean delivery, and repeat cesarean delivery plus hysterectomy. (Data from Pritchard, 1962.)

Excessive blood loss has been estimated by several methods that include measuring loss directly, using a predetermined decline in hematocrit or hemoglobin concentration, or counting the number of women transfused. Of these, direct measurement was performed in a two-center investigation done in Argentina and Uruguay (Sosa, 2009). Specially constructed drapes were used to collect blood at vaginal delivery. These investigators reported that 10.8 percent of women had hemorrhage in excess of 500 mL, whereas 1.9 percent lost > 1000 mL. These estimates likely are too low.

Tita and colleagues (2012) used a 6-volume percent decrease in the postpartum hematocrit to define clinically significant blood loss with vaginal delivery. This decrease easily signifies greater than 1000-mL blood loss in the averaged-sized women. They documented this amount in a fourth of women, which agrees with the findings in Figure 41-1.

A final marker used to estimate the hemorrhage incidence is the transfusion rate. Because of prevailing conservative attitudes toward blood replacement, rates cited more recently are lower than transfusion rates described in older studies. In the study by Tita and colleagues (2012) cited above, more than 6 percent of women delivered vaginally underwent interventional treatment and blood transfusions. In a study of more than 66,000 women delivered at Parkland Hospital from 2002 to 2006, Hernandez and associates (2012) reported that 2.3 percent overall were given blood transfusions for hypovolemia. Half of these women had undergone cesarean delivery. Importantly, for those transfused, these investigators calculated blood loss to average approximately 3500 mL! In a recent study from Australia, 1.6 percent of women delivered in 2010 were transfused (Patterson, 2014). Last, from a registry-based Norwegian study, Skjeldestad and Øian (2012) reported that blood loss exceeded 1250 mL in 2.7 percent of women undergoing cesarean delivery.

Thus, it is apparent that significant blood loss accompanies about a fourth of vaginal deliveries. The amounts and proportions for cesarean delivery are much greater.

When audits of discharge statistics are evaluated, it is apparent that hemorrhage is also underreported. In one example, Bateman and associates (2010) queried the Nationwide Inpatient Sample for 2004 and found a 2.9-percent reported rate of postpartum hemorrhage. Similarly, using a sample of nearly 185,000 delivery outcomes from the National Hospital Discharge Summary database that represented more than 40 million deliveries, Berg and coworkers (2009) reported postpartum hemorrhage incidence of 2.0 and 2.6 percent, for two epochs. In a population-based Canadian study, the incidence of postpartum hemorrhage from atony increased from 3.6 to 4.8 percent from 2001 to 2009 (Mehrabadi, 2013). In contrast, a study encompassing 1999 to 2008 by Kramer and associates (2013) cited a rate of severe postpartum hemorrhage that increased from only 1.9 to 4.2 per 1000 births. At the same time, reported transfusion rates between 1991 and 2003 increased from only 3 to 5 per 1000 deliveries—all rather meager compared with rates in previously cited prospective studies.

TABLE 41-2. Obstetrical Hemorrhage: Causes, Predisposing Factors, and Vulnerable Patients

Abnormal Placentation
Placenta previa
Placental abruption
Placenta accreta/increta/percreta
Ectopic pregnancy
Hydatidiform mole
Injuries to the Birth Canal
Episiotomy and lacerations
Forceps or vacuum delivery
Cesarean delivery or hysterectomy
Uterine rupture
  Previously scarred uterus
  High parity
  Hyperstimulation
  Obstructed labor
  Intrauterine manipulation
  Midforceps rotation
  Breech extraction
Obstetrical Factors
Obesity
Previous postpartum hemorrhage
Early preterm pregnancy
Sepsis syndrome
Vulnerable Patients
Preeclampsia/eclampsia
Chronic renal insufficiency
Constitutionally small size
	Uterine Atony
	Uterine overdistention
	  Large fetus
	  Multiple fetuses
	  Hydramnios
	  Retained clots
	Labor induction
	Anesthesia or analgesia
	  Halogenated agents
	  Conduction analgesia with hypotension
	Labor abnormalities
	  Rapid labor
	  Prolonged labor
	  Augmented labor
	  Chorioamnionitis
	Previous uterine atony
	Coagulation Defects—Intensify Other Causes
	Massive transfusions
	Placental abruption
	Sepsis syndrome
	Severe preeclampsia syndrome
	Acute fatty liver
	Anticoagulant treatment
	Congenital coagulopathies
	Amnionic-fluid embolism
	Prolonged retention of dead fetus
	Saline-induced abortion

Predisposing Conditions

There are myriad clinical circumstances in which risks for obstetrical hemorrhage and its consequences are appreciably increased. The imposing list shown in Table 41-2 illustrates that hemorrhage can manifest at any time throughout pregnancy, delivery, and the puerperium. Thus, any description of obstetrical hemorrhage should include gestational age. Use of terms such as *third-trimester bleeding* is not recommended because of imprecision.

Importantly, inadequate obstetrical and anesthetic services in some areas contribute to maternal death from hemorrhage. This undoubtedly includes facilities in the United States. It was quantified in the United Kingdom by the 2002 Confidential Enquiry into Maternal and Child Health, which concluded that most maternal deaths from hemorrhage were associated with substandard care (Weindling, 2003). Similar experiences were reported from Japan and from the Netherlands (Nagaya, 2000; Zwart, 2008).

Timing of Hemorrhage

It is has been traditional to classify obstetrical hemorrhage as *antepartum*—such as with placenta previa or placental abruption, or as *postpartum*—commonly caused by uterine atony or genital tract lacerations. In individual women, however, these terms are nonspecific, and it is reasonable to specify the cause and gestational age as descriptors.

Antepartum Hemorrhage

Bleeding during various times in gestation may give a clue as to its cause. Many aspects of bleeding during the first half of pregnancy from abortion or ectopic pregnancy are discussed in detail in Chapters 18 and 19, respectively. Discussions that follow concern pregnancies with a viable mature living fetus. In these cases, rapid assessment should always consider the deleterious fetal effects of maternal hemorrhage.

Slight vaginal bleeding is common during active labor. This "bloody show" is the consequence of effacement and dilatation of the cervix, with tearing of small vessels. Uterine bleeding, however, coming from above the cervix, is concerning. It may follow some separation of a placenta previa implanted in the immediate vicinity of the cervical canal, or it may be from a placental abruption or uterine tear. Rarely, there may be velamentous insertion of the umbilical cord, and the involved placental vessels may overlie the cervix—*vasa previa.* Fetal hemorrhage follows laceration of these vessels at the time of membrane rupture. In many women near term, the source of uterine bleeding is not identified, symptomless bleeding ceases, and no apparent anatomical cause is found at delivery. In most of these cases, bleeding likely resulted from a slight marginal placental separation. *Despite this, any pregnancy with antepartum bleeding remains at increased risk for an adverse outcome even though bleeding has stopped and placenta previa has been excluded sonographically.*

Several reports address mid- to early third-trimester bleeding. Lipitz and colleagues (1991) reported that a fourth of 65 consecutive women with uterine bleeding between 14 and 26 weeks had placental abruption or previa, and a third of all 65 fetuses ultimately were lost. Similar outcomes were described subsequently (Ajayi, 1992; Leung, 2001). The Canadian Perinatal Network described 806 women with hemorrhage between 22 and 28 weeks' gestation (Sabourin, 2012). Placental abruption (32 percent), previa (21 percent), and cervical bleeding (6.6 percent) were the most common causes identified, and in a third, no cause was found. Of all women, 44 percent were delivered ≤ 29 weeks. Clearly, second- and third-trimester bleeding are associated with a poor pregnancy prognosis.

Postpartum Hemorrhage

In most cases, the cause of postpartum hemorrhage can and should be determined. Frequent causes are uterine atony with bleeding from the placental implantation site, genital tract trauma, or both (see Table 41-2). Postpartum hemorrhage is usually obvious. Important exceptions are unrecognized intrauterine and intravaginal blood accumulation and uterine rupture with intraperitoneal bleeding. Initial assessment should attempt to differentiate uterine atony from genital tract lacerations. Primary considerations are the predisposing risk factors shown in Table 41-2, lower genital tract examination, and uterine tone assessment. Atony is identified by a boggy, soft uterus during bimanual examination and by expression of clots and hemorrhage during uterine massage.

Persistent bleeding despite a firm, well-contracted uterus suggests that hemorrhage most likely is from lacerations. Bright red blood further suggests arterial bleeding. *To confirm that lacerations are a source of bleeding, careful inspection of the vagina, cervix, and uterus is essential.* Sometimes bleeding may be caused by both atony and trauma, especially after forceps or vacuum-assisted vaginal delivery. Importantly, if significant bleeding follows these deliveries, then the cervix and vagina are carefully examined to identify lacerations. This is easier if conduction analgesia was given. If there are no lower genital tract lacerations and the uterus is contracted, yet supracervical bleeding persists, then manual exploration of the uterus is done to exclude a uterine tear. This also is completed routinely after internal podalic version and breech extraction.

Blood Loss Estimation

Estimated blood loss—like beauty—is in the eye of the beholder.

Estimation is notoriously inaccurate, especially with excessive bleeding (p. 781). Instead of sudden massive hemorrhage, postpartum bleeding is frequently steady. If atony persists, bleeding may appear to be only moderate at any given instant but may continue until serious hypovolemia develops. Bleeding from an episiotomy or a vaginal laceration can also appear to be only minimal to moderate. However, constant seepage can lead to enormous blood loss relatively quickly. In some cases, after placental separation, blood may not escape vaginally but instead may collect within the uterine cavity, which can become distended by 1000 mL or more of blood. In others, postpartum uterine massage is applied to a roll of abdominal fat mistaken for the uterus. Thus, monitoring of the uterus immediately postpartum must not be left to an inexperienced person (Chap. 27, p. 547).

All of these factors can lead to an underappreciation of the magnitude of hemorrhage over time. The effects of hemorrhage depend to a considerable degree on the maternal nonpregnant blood volume and the corresponding degree of pregnancy-induced hypervolemia as previously discussed. For this and other reasons, hypovolemia may not be recognized until very late. *A treacherous feature of postpartum hemorrhage is the failure of the pulse and blood pressure to undergo more than moderate alterations until large amounts of blood have been lost.* The normotensive woman initially may actually become somewhat hypertensive from catecholamine release in response to hemorrhage. Moreover, women with preeclampsia may become "normotensive" despite remarkable hypovolemia.

Late Postpartum Hemorrhage

Bleeding after the first 24 hours is designated *late postpartum hemorrhage.* Such bleeding is found in up to 1 percent of women and may be serious (American College of Obstetricians and Gynecologists, 2013b). It is discussed in Chapter 36 (p. 670).

Special Considerations

In certain conditions, a pregnant woman may be particularly susceptible to hemorrhage because her blood volume expansion is less than expected. This situation is most commonly encountered in small women—even those with normal pregnancy-induced hypervolemia. Women with severe preeclampsia or eclampsia are also more vulnerable to hemorrhage because they frequently do not have a normally expanded blood volume. Specifically, Zeeman and associates (2009) documented a mean increase above nonpregnant volume of only 10 percent in *eclamptic* women (Chap. 40, p. 737). A third example is the moderate to severely curtailed pregnancy-induced volume expansion in women with chronic renal insufficiency (Chap. 53, p. 1061). *When excessive hemorrhage is suspected in*

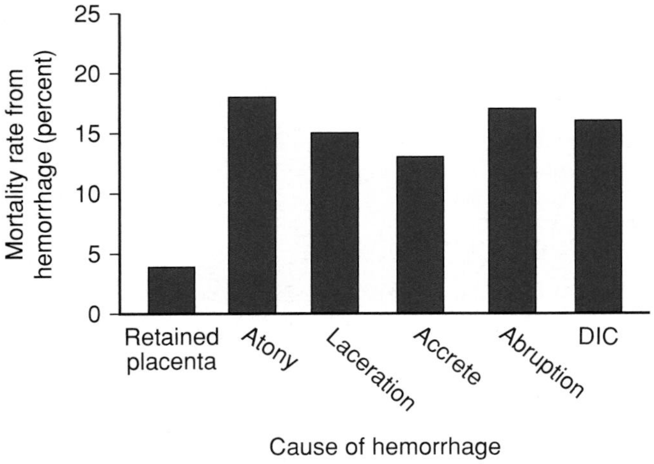

FIGURE 41-2 Contributions to maternal death from various causes of obstetrical hemorrhage. Percentages are approximations because of different classification schemata used. DIC = disseminated intravascular coagulation. (Data from Al-Zirqi, 2008; Berg, 2010; Chichakli, 1999; Zwart, 2008.)

these high-risk women, crystalloid and blood are promptly administered for suspected hypovolemia.

CAUSES OF OBSTETRICAL HEMORRHAGE

The most important causes—because of their incidence or consequence—of severe obstetrical hemorrhage and their contribution to maternal mortality rates are shown in Figure 41-2. Fatal hemorrhage is most likely in circumstances in which blood or components are not immediately available. As discussed on page 815, the ability to provide prompt resuscitation of hypovolemia and blood administration is an absolute requirement for acceptable obstetrical care.

Uterine Atony

The most frequent cause of obstetrical hemorrhage is failure of the uterus to contract sufficiently after delivery and to arrest bleeding from vessels at the placental implantation site (p. 780). That said, some bleeding is inevitable during third-stage labor as the placenta begins to separate. Blood from the implantation site may escape into the vagina immediately—the *Duncan mechanism* of placental separation, or it remains concealed behind the placenta and membranes until the placenta is delivered—the *Schultze mechanism.*

With bleeding during the third stage, the uterus should be massaged if it is not contracted firmly. After the signs of separation, placental descent is indicated by the cord becoming slack. Placental expression should be attempted by manual fundal pressure (Chap. 27, p. 546). If bleeding continues, then manual removal of the placenta may be necessary. *Separation and delivery of the placenta by cord traction, especially when the uterus is atonic, may cause uterine inversion, which is discussed on page 787.*

Third-Stage Bleeding

If significant bleeding persists after delivery of the infant and while the placenta remains partially or totally attached, then manual placental removal is indicated (Chap. 27, p. 546). For this, adequate analgesia is mandatory, and aseptic surgical technique should be used. As illustrated in Figure 41-3, the placenta is peeled off its uterine attachment by a motion similar to that used in separating the pages of a book. After its removal, trailing membranes are removed by carefully teasing them from the decidua and using ring forceps for this as necessary. Another method is to wipe out the uterine cavity with a gauze-wrapped hand.

Uterine Atony after Placental Delivery

The fundus should always be palpated following placental delivery to confirm that the uterus is well contracted. If it is not

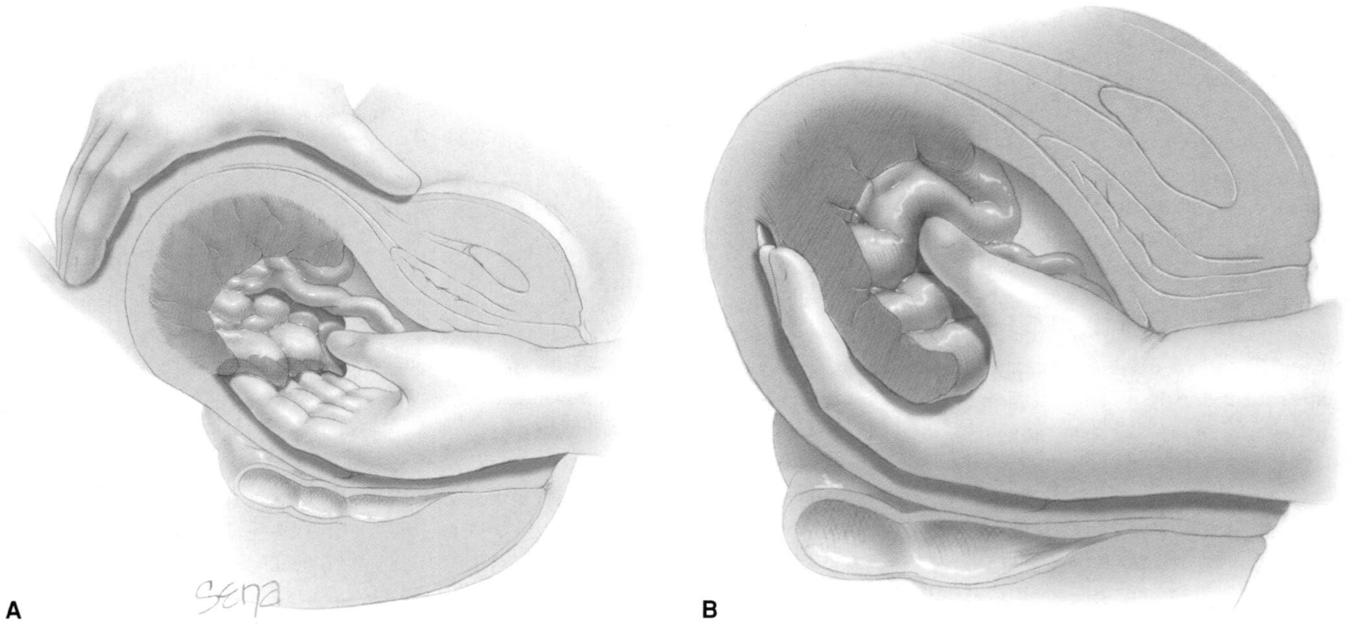

FIGURE 41-3 Manual removal of placenta. **A.** One hand grasps the fundus. The other hand is inserted into the uterine cavity, and the fingers are swept from side to side as they are advanced. **B.** When the placenta has become detached, it is grasped and removed.

firm, then vigorous fundal massage usually prevents postpartum hemorrhage from atony (Hofmeyr, 2008). Simultaneously, 20 units of oxytocin in 1000 mL of crystalloid solution will often be effective given intravenously at 10 mL/min for a dose of 200 mU/min. Higher concentrations are minimally more effective (Tita, 2012). Oxytocin should never be given as an undiluted bolus dose because serious hypotension or cardiac arrhythmias may develop.

Risk Factors

In many women, uterine atony can at least be anticipated well in advance of delivery (see Table 41-2). In one study, however, up to half of women who had atony after cesarean delivery were found to have no risk factors (Rouse, 2006). Thus, the ability to identify which individual woman will experience atony is limited. Risk factors for retained placenta are similar (Endler, 2012).

The magnitude of risk imposed by each of these factors shown in Table 41-2 varies considerably between reports. *Primiparity* has been cited as a risk factor (Driessen, 2011). *High parity* is a long-known risk factor for uterine atony. The incidence of postpartum hemorrhage was reported to increase from 0.3 percent in women of low parity to 1.9 percent with parity of 4 or greater. It was 2.7 percent with parity of 7 or greater (Babinszki, 1999). The *overdistended uterus* is prone to hypotonia after delivery, and thus women with a large fetus, multiple fetuses, or hydramnios are at greater risk. *Labor abnormalities* predispose to atony and include hyper- or hypotonic labor. Similarly, *labor induction* or *augmentation* with either prostaglandins or oxytocin is more likely to be followed by atony (Driessen, 2011). Finally, the woman who has had a *prior postpartum hemorrhage* is at risk for recurrence with a subsequent delivery.

Evaluation and Management

With immediate postpartum hemorrhage, careful inspection is done to exclude birth canal laceration. Because bleeding can be caused by retained placental fragments, inspection of the placenta after delivery should be routine. If a defect is seen, the uterus should be manually explored, and the fragment removed. Occasionally, retention of a *succenturiate lobe* may cause postpartum hemorrhage (Chap. 6, p. 117). During examination for lacerations and causes of atony, the uterus is massaged and uterotonic agents are administered.

Uterotonic Agents

There are several compounds that prompt the postpartum uterus to contract (Chap. 27, p. 547). One of these is routinely selected and given to *prevent* postpartum bleeding by ensuring uterine contractions. Most of these same agents are also used to *treat* uterine atony with bleeding. Moreover, because many trials combine results from atony prophylaxis and treatment, evaluation of these studies is problematic. For example, *oxytocin* has been used for more than 50 years, and in most cases, it is infused intravenously or given intramuscularly after placental delivery. Neither route has been shown to be superior (Oladapo, 2012). This or other uterotonins given prophylactically will prevent most cases of uterine atony.

When atony persists despite preventive measures, ergot derivatives have been used for second-line treatment. These include methylergonovine—*Methergine*—and ergonovine. Only methylergonovine is currently manufactured in the United States. Given parenterally, these drugs rapidly stimulate tetanic uterine contractions and act for approximately 45 minutes (Schimmer, 2011). A common regimen is 0.2 mg of either drug given intramuscularly. A caveat is that ergot agents, especially given intravenously, may cause dangerous hypertension, especially in women with preeclampsia. Severe hypertension is also seen with concomitant use of protease inhibitors given for human immunodeficiency viral (HIV) infection (Chap. 65, p. 1279). These adverse effects notwithstanding, it is speculative whether there are superior therapeutic effects of ergot derivatives compared with oxytocin.

In more recent years, second-line agents for atony have included the E- and F-series prostaglandins. Carboprost tromethamine— *Hemabate*—is the 15-methyl derivative of prostaglandin $F_{2\alpha}$. It was approved more than 25 years ago for uterine atony treatment in a dose of 250 μg (0.25 mg) given intramuscularly. This dose can be repeated if necessary at 15- to 90-minute intervals up to a maximum of eight doses. Oleen and Mariano (1990) reported its use for postpartum hemorrhage from 12 obstetrical units. Bleeding was controlled in 88 percent of 237 women treated. Another 7 percent required other uterotonics to control hemorrhage, and the remaining 5 percent required surgical intervention. Carboprost causes side effects in approximately 20 percent of women. These include, in descending order of frequency, diarrhea, hypertension, vomiting, fever, flushing, and tachycardia (Oleen, 1990). Another pharmacological effect is pulmonary airway and vascular constriction. Thus, carboprost should not be used for asthmatics and those with suspected amnionic-fluid embolism (p. 812). We have occasionally encountered severe hypertension with carboprost given to women with preeclampsia, and it has also been reported to cause arterial oxygen desaturation that averaged 10 percent (Hankins, 1988).

E-series prostaglandins have been used to prevent or treat atony. Dinoprostone—prostaglandin E_2—is given as a 20-mg suppository per rectum or per vaginam every 2 hours. It typically causes diarrhea, which is problematic for the rectal route, whereas vigorous vaginal bleeding may preclude its use per vaginam. Intravenous prostaglandin E_2—sulprostone—is used in Europe, but it is not available in this country (Schmitz, 2011).

Misoprostol—*Cytotec*—is a synthetic prostaglandin E_1 analogue that has also been evaluated for both prevention and treatment of atony and postpartum hemorrhage (Abdel-Aleem, 2001; O'Brien, 1998). Most studies have addressed prevention and have conflicting conclusions. In a Cochrane review, Mousa and Alfirevic (2007) reported no added benefits to misoprostol use compared with oxytocin or ergonovine. Derman and coworkers (2006) compared a 600-μg oral dose given at delivery against placebo. They found that the drug decreased hemorrhage incidence from 12 to 6 percent and that of severe hemorrhage from 1.2 to 0.2 percent. In another study, however, Gerstenfeld and Wing (2001) concluded that 400-μg misoprostol administered rectally was not more effective than intravenous oxytocin in preventing postpartum hemorrhage.

From a systematic review, Villar (2002) found that oxytocin and ergot preparations administered after delivery were more effective than misoprostol for prevention of postpartum hemorrhage (Chap. 27, p. 547).

Bleeding Unresponsive to Uterotonic Agents

Hemorrhage that persists despite uterine massage and continued uterotonin administration may be from a yet unrecognized genital tract laceration, for example, uterine rupture. Thus, if bleeding persists after initial measures for atony have been implemented, then the following management steps are performed immediately and simultaneously:

1. Begin bimanual uterine compression, which is easily done and controls most cases of continuing hemorrhage (Fig. 41-4). This technique is not simply fundal massage. The posterior uterine wall is massaged by one hand on the abdomen, while the other hand is made into a fist and placed into the vagina. This fist kneads the anterior uterine wall through the anterior vaginal wall. Concurrently, the uterus is also compressed between the two hands.
2. Immediately mobilize the emergent-care obstetrical team to the delivery room and call for whole blood or packed red cells.
3. Request urgent help from the anesthesia team.
4. Secure at least two large-bore intravenous catheters so that crystalloid with oxytocin is continued simultaneously with blood products. Insert an indwelling Foley catheter for continuous urine output monitoring.
5. Begin volume resuscitation with rapid intravenous infusion of crystalloid (p. 815).
6. With sedation, analgesia, or anesthesia established and now with optimal exposure, once again manually explore the uterine cavity for retained placental fragments and for uterine abnormalities, including lacerations or rupture.
7. Thoroughly inspect the cervix and vagina again for lacerations that may have escaped attention.
8. If the woman is still unstable or if there is persistent hemorrhage, then blood transfusions are given (p. 815).

At this juncture, after causes other than atony have been excluded and after hypovolemia is reversed, several other measures are considered if bleeding continues. Their use depends on several factors such as parity, desire for sterilization, and experience with each method.

Uterine Packing or Balloon Tamponade. Uterine packing was popular to treat refractory uterine atony during the first half of the 20th century. It subsequently fell from favor because of concerns regarding concealed bleeding and infection (Hsu, 2003). Newer techniques have been described that alleviate some of these concerns (Zelop, 2011). In one technique, the tip of a 24F Foley catheter with a 30-mL balloon is guided into the uterine cavity and filled with 60 to 80 mL of saline. The open tip permits continuous drainage of blood from the uterus. If bleeding subsides, the catheter is typically removed after 12 to 24 hours. Similar devices that have been used for tamponade include Segstaken-Blakemore and Rusch balloons and condom catheters (Georgiou, 2009; Lo, 2013a,b). Alternatively, the uterus or pelvis may be packed directly with gauze (Gilstrap, 2002).

Enthusiasm has developed for specially constructed intrauterine balloons to treat hemorrhage from uterine atony and other causes (Barbieri, 2011). A *Bakri Postpartum Balloon* (Cook Medical) or *BT-Cath* (Utah Medical Products) may be inserted and inflated to tamponade the endometrial cavity and stop bleeding (Fig. 41-5). Insertion requires two or three team members. The first performs abdominal sonography during the procedure. The second places the deflated balloon into the uterus and stabilizes it. The third member instills fluid to inflate the balloon, rapidly infusing at least 150 mL followed by further instillation over a few minutes for a total of 300 to 500 mL to arrest hemorrhage.

There have been few prospective studies with these uterine balloons, and thus data are observational (Aibar, 2013;

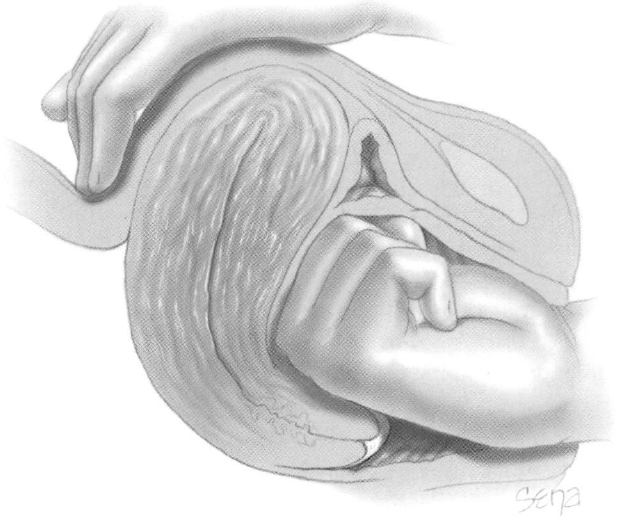

FIGURE 41-4 Bimanual compression for uterine atony. The uterus is positioned with the fist of one hand in the anterior fornix pushing against the anterior wall, which is held in place by the other hand on the abdomen. The abdominal hand is also used for uterine massage.

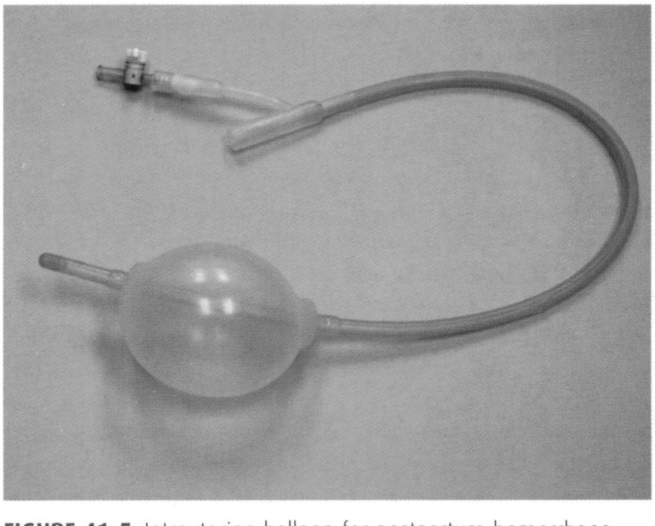

FIGURE 41-5 Intrauterine balloon for postpartum hemorrhage.

Grönvall, 2013; Laas, 2012). In all, more than 150 women were managed for postpartum hemorrhage. Perhaps a fourth were caused by uterine atony. For all causes, the success rate was noted to be approximately 85 percent. Combinations of balloon tamponade and uterine compression sutures have also been described (Diemert, 2012; Yoong, 2012). Failures for all of these require various surgical methods including hysterectomy. *Well-designed studies are needed before instituting intrauterine balloon tamponade as a second-line treatment for atony.*

Surgical Procedures. Several invasive procedures can be used to control hemorrhage from atony. These include uterine compression sutures, pelvic vessel ligation, angiographic embolization, and hysterectomy. These are discussed on page 818.

Uterine Inversion

Puerperal inversion of the uterus is considered to be one of the classic hemorrhagic disasters encountered in obstetrics. Unless promptly recognized and managed appropriately, associated bleeding often is massive. Risk factors include alone or in combination:

1. Fundal placental implantation,
2. Delayed-onset or inadequate uterine contractility after delivery of the fetus, that is, uterine atony,
3. Cord traction applied *before* placental separation, and
4. Abnormally adhered placentation such as with the accrete syndromes (p. 804).

Depending on which of these factors is contributory, the incidence and severity of uterine inversion varies, with the worst scenario being complete inversion with the uterus protruding from the birth canal as shown in Figure 41-6. There is progressive severity of inversion as shown in Figure 41-7.

The incidence of uterine inversion is variable and is usually different for vaginal and for cesarean delivery. Incidences range from approximately 1 in 2000 to 1 in 20,000 deliveries (Baskett, 2002; Ogah, 2011; Rana, 2009; Witteveen, 2013). Our experiences at Parkland Hospital comport with the higher 1:2000 incidence. This is despite our policy to discourage placental delivery by cord traction alone and before certainty of its separation. It is unknown if *active management of third-stage labor* with cord traction applied ostensibly *after* signs of placental separation increases the likelihood of uterine inversion (Deneux-Tharaux, 2013; Gülmezoglu, 2012; Peña-Marti, 2007; Prick, 2013).

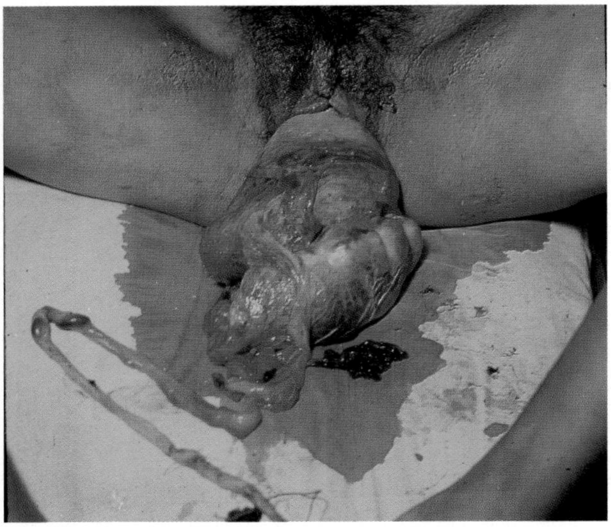

FIGURE 41-6 Maternal death from exsanguination caused by uterine inversion associated with a fundal placenta accreta during a home delivery.

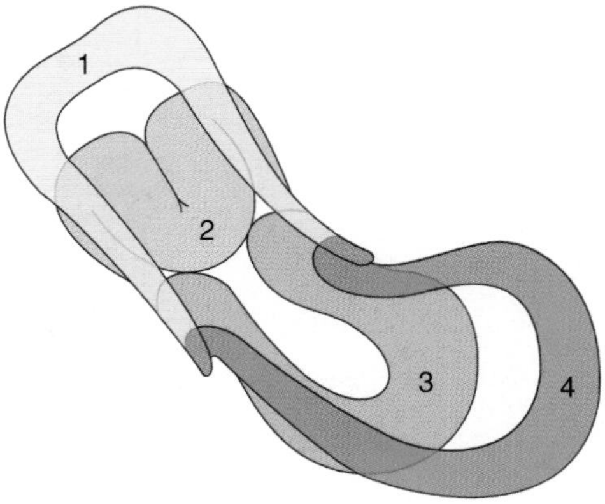

FIGURE 41-7 Progressive degrees of uterine inversion depicted. After the fundus begins and continues to invert (Nos. 1 and 2), it would not be visible externally until it was at the level of the introitus (No. 3) or completely inverted (No. 4).

Recognition and Management

Immediate recognition of uterine inversion improves the chances of a quick resolution and good outcome. That said, inexperienced attendants may have a delayed appreciation for an inverting uterus, especially if it is only partial and thus not protruding through the introitus. In these cases, continued hemorrhage likely will prompt closer examination of the birth canal. Even so, the partially inverted uterus can be mistaken for a uterine myoma, and this can be resolved by sonography (Pauleta, 2010; Rana, 2009). Many cases are associated with immediate life-threatening hemorrhage, and at least half require blood replacement (Baskett, 2002). It was previously taught that associated shock was disproportionate to blood loss because of parasympathetic stimulation from stretching pelvic tissues. This has been refuted (Watson, 1980).

Once any degree of uterine inversion is recognized, several steps must be implemented urgently and simultaneously:

1. Immediate assistance is summoned, including obstetrical and anesthesia personnel.
2. Blood is brought to the delivery suite in case it may be needed.
3. The woman is evaluated for emergency general anesthesia. Large-bore intravenous infusion systems are secured to begin rapid crystalloid infusion to treat hypovolemia while awaiting arrival of blood for transfusion.
4. If the recently inverted uterus has not contracted and retracted completely and if the placenta has already separated, then the uterus may often be replaced simply by pushing up on the

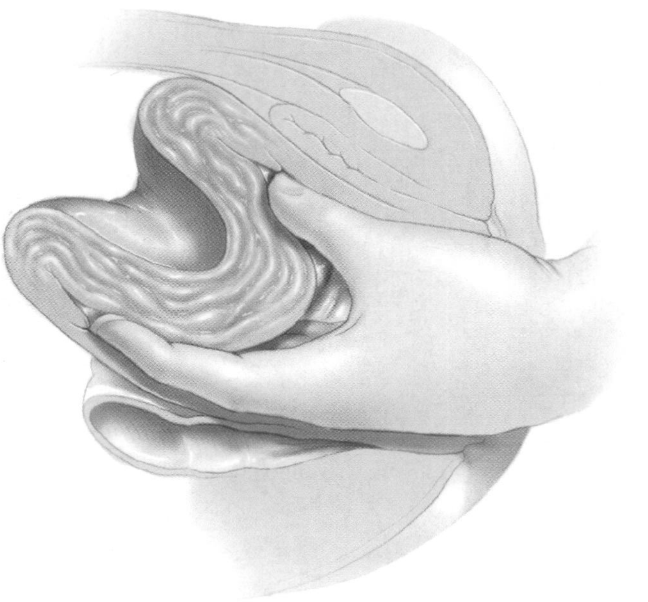

FIGURE 41-8 The incompletely inverted uterus is repositioned by using the abdominal hand for palpation of the crater-like depression while gently pushing the inverted fundus up out of the lower segment and to its normal anatomical position.

inverted fundus with the palm of the hand and fingers in the direction of the long axis of the vagina (Fig. 41-8). Some use two fingers rigidly extended to push the center of the fundus upward. *Care is taken not to apply so much pressure as to perforate the uterus with the fingertips.*

5. If the placenta is still attached, it is not removed until infusion systems are operational and a uterine relaxant drug administered. Many recommend a trial of an intravenously administered tocolytic drug such as terbutaline, magnesium sulfate, or nitroglycerin for uterine relaxation and repositioning (Hong, 2006; You, 2006). If these fail to provide sufficient relaxation, then a rapidly acting halogenated inhalational agent is administered.
6. After removing the placenta, steady pressure with the fist, palm, or fingers is applied to the inverted fundus in an attempt to push it up into and through the dilated cervix as described in Step 4.
7. Once the uterus is restored to its normal configuration, tocolysis is stopped. Oxytocin is then infused, and other uterotonics may be given as described for atony (p. 785). Meanwhile, the operator maintains the fundus in its normal anatomical position while applying bimanual compression to control further hemorrhage until the uterus is well contracted (see Fig. 41-4). The operator continues to monitor the uterus transvaginally for evidence of subsequent inversion.

Surgical Intervention

In most cases the inverted uterus can be restored to its normal position by the techniques described above. Occasionally, manual replacement fails. One cause is a dense myometrial constriction ring (Kochenour, 2002). At this point, laparotomy is imperative. The anatomical configuration found at surgery can be confusing as shown in Figure 41-9. With agents given for tocolysis, a combined effort is made to reposition the uterus by simultaneously pushing upward from below and pulling upward from above. Application of atraumatic clamps to each round ligament and upward traction may be helpful—the *Huntington procedure*. In some cases, placing a deep traction suture in the inverted fundus or grasping it with tissue forceps may be of aid. However, these may be technically difficult (Robson, 2005). If the constriction ring still prohibits repositioning, a longitudinal surgical cut—*Haultain incision*—is made posteriorly through the ring to expose the fundus and permit reinversion (Sangwan, 2009). After uterine replacement, tocolytics are stopped, oxytocin and other uterotonics are given, and the uterine incision is repaired. Risks of separation of this posterior hysterotomy incision during subsequent pregnancy, labor, and delivery are unknown.

In some cases, the uterus will again invert almost immediately after repositioning. If this is a problem, then compression sutures shown on page 819 can be used to prevent another inversion (Matsubara, 2009; Mondal, 2012). Occasionally, chronic puerperal uterine inversion may become apparent weeks after delivery.

Injuries to the Birth Canal

Childbirth is invariably associated with trauma to the birth canal, which includes the uterus and cervix, vagina, and perineum. Injuries sustained during labor and delivery range from minor mucosal tears to lacerations that create life-threatening hemorrhage or hematomas.

Vulvovaginal Lacerations

Small tears of the anterior vaginal wall near the urethra are relatively common. They are often superficial with little to no bleeding, and their repair is usually not indicated. Minor superficial perineal and vaginal lacerations occasionally require sutures for hemostasis. Those large enough to require extensive

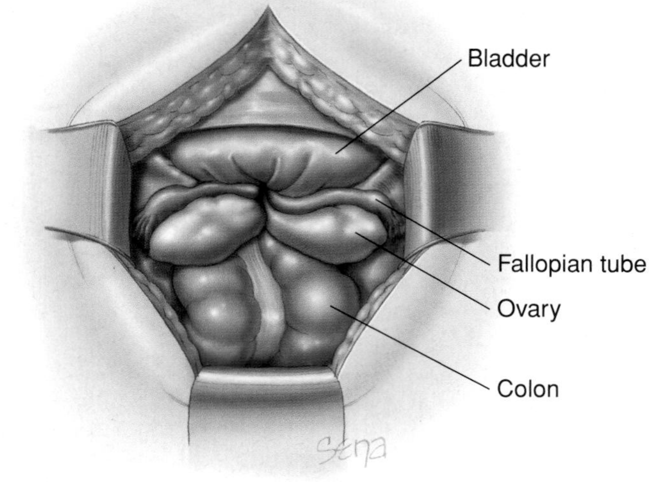

FIGURE 41-9 Surgical anatomy of a completely inverted uterus viewed from above at laparotomy. The uterine fundus is not visible and the tubes and ovaries have been drawn into the birth canal.

repair are typically associated with voiding difficulty, and an indwelling bladder catheter will obviate this.

Deeper perineal lacerations are usually accompanied by varying degrees of injury to the outer third of the vaginal vault. Some extend to involve the anal sphincter or varying depths of the vaginal walls. In more than 87,000 deliveries in the Consortium on Safe Labor database, the frequency of third- or fourth-degree perineal lacerations was 5.7 percent in nulliparas and 0.6 percent in multiparas (Landy, 2011). Bilateral vaginal lacerations are usually unequal in length, and they are separated by a tongue of vaginal tissue. Lacerations involving the middle or upper third of the vaginal vault usually are associated with injuries of the perineum or cervix. These sometimes are missed unless thorough inspection of the upper vagina and cervix is performed. Bleeding despite a firmly contracted uterus is strong evidence of genital tract laceration. Those that extend upward usually are longitudinal. They may follow spontaneous delivery but frequently result from injuries sustained during operative vaginal delivery with forceps or vacuum extractor. Most involve deeper underlying tissues and thus usually cause significant hemorrhage. Bleeding is typically controlled by appropriate suture repair.

Extensive vaginal or cervical tears should prompt a careful search for evidence of retroperitoneal hemorrhage or peritoneal perforation or hemorrhage. If this is strongly suspected, then laparotomy is considered (Rafi, 2010). Extensive vulvovaginal lacerations should also prompt intrauterine exploration for possible uterine tears or rupture. For deep vulvovaginal lacerations, suture repair is usually required, and effective analgesia or anesthesia, vigorous blood replacement, and capable assistance are mandatory. In the study reported by Melamed and colleagues (2009), 1.5 percent of women with these lacerations required blood transfusions. Repair of vulvovaginal lacerations is detailed in Chapter 27 (p. 548).

Levator Sling Injuries

The levator ani muscles, described in Chapter 2 (p. 22), are usually involved with deep vaginal vault lacerations. They also sustain stretch injuries that result from overdistention of the birth canal. Muscle fibers are torn and separated, and their diminished tone may interfere with pelvic diaphragm function to cause pelvic relaxation. If the injuries involve the pubococcygeus muscle, urinary incontinence also may result.

Cervical Lacerations

Superficial lacerations of the cervix can be seen on close inspection in more than half of all vaginal deliveries. Most of these are less than 0.5 cm and seldom require repair (Fahmy, 1991). Deeper lacerations are less frequent, but even these may be unnoticed. Due to ascertainment bias, variable incidences are described. For example, in the Consortium database, the incidence of cervical lacerations was 1.1 percent in nulliparas and 0.5 percent in multiparas (Landy, 2011). But the overall incidence reported by Melamed and coworkers (2009), in a study of more than 81,000 Israeli women, was only 0.16 percent. Parikh and associates (2007) reported a 0.2-percent incidence of lacerations that needed repair.

Cervical lacerations are not usually problematic unless they cause hemorrhage or extend to the upper third of the vagina. Rarely, the cervix may be entirely or partially avulsed from the vagina—*colporrhexis*—in the anterior, posterior, or lateral fornices. These injuries sometimes follow difficult forceps rotations or deliveries performed through an incompletely dilated cervix with the forceps blades applied over the cervix. In some women, cervical tears reach into lower uterine segment and involve the uterine artery and its major branches. They occasionally extend into the peritoneal cavity. The more severe lacerations usually manifest as external hemorrhage or as a hematoma, however, they may occasionally be unsuspected. In the large Israeli study reported by Melamed and colleagues (2009), almost 11 percent of women with a cervical laceration required blood transfusions.

Other serious cervical injuries fortunately are uncommon. In one, the edematous anterior cervical lip is caught during labor and compressed between the fetal head and maternal symphysis pubis. If this causes severe ischemia, the anterior lip may undergo necrosis and separate from the rest of the cervix. Another rare injury is when the entire vaginal portion of the cervix is avulsed. Such *annular* or *circular detachment of the cervix* is seen with difficult deliveries, especially forceps deliveries.

Diagnosis. A deep cervical tear should always be suspected in women with profuse hemorrhage during and after third-stage labor, particularly if the uterus is firmly contracted. It is reasonable to inspect the cervix routinely following major operative vaginal deliveries even if there is no third-stage bleeding. Thorough evaluation is necessary, and often the flabby cervix interferes with digital examination. The extent of the injury can be more fully appreciated with adequate exposure and visual inspection. This is best accomplished when an *assistant* applies firm downward pressure on the uterus while the operator exerts traction on the lips of the cervix with ring forceps. A second assistant can provide even better exposure with right-angle vaginal wall retractors.

Management. In general, cervical lacerations of 1 and even 2 cm are not repaired unless they are bleeding. Such tears heal rapidly and are thought to be of no significance. When healed they result in the irregular, sometime stellate appearance of the external cervical os that indicates previous delivery of a viable-size fetus.

Deep cervical tears usually require surgical repair. When the laceration is limited to the cervix or even when it extends somewhat into the vaginal fornix, satisfactory results are obtained by suturing the cervix after bringing it into view at the vulva as depicted in Figure 41-10. While cervical lacerations are repaired, associated vaginal lacerations may be tamponaded with gauze packs to arrest their bleeding. Because hemorrhage usually comes from the upper angle of the wound, the first suture using absorbable material is placed in tissue above the angle. Subsequently, either interrupted or continuous locking sutures are placed outward toward the operator. If lacerations extend to involve the lateral vaginal sulcus, then attempts to restore the normal cervical appearance may lead to subsequent stenosis.

Most cervical lacerations are successfully repaired using sutures. However, if there is uterine involvement and continued hemorrhage, some of the methods described on page 818 may

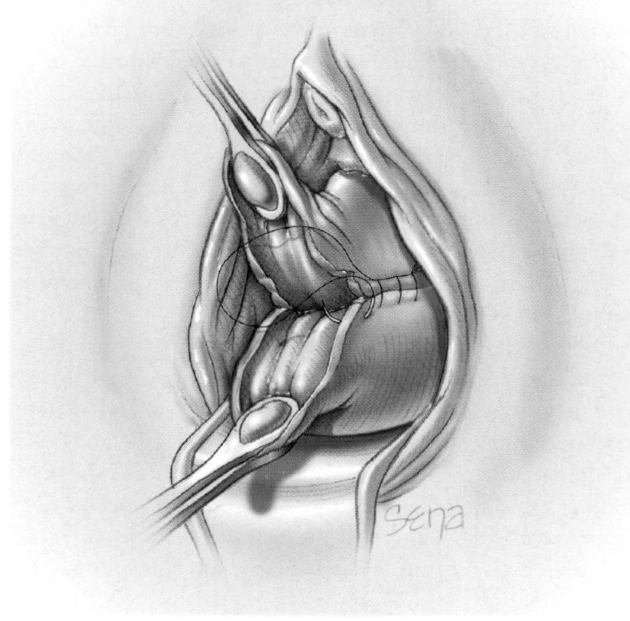

FIGURE 41-10 Repair of cervical laceration with appropriate surgical exposure. Continuous absorbable sutures are placed beginning at the upper angle of the laceration.

be necessary to obtain hemostasis. For example, Lichtenberg (2003) described successful angiographic embolization for a high cervical tear after failed surgical repair.

Puerperal Hematomas

Pelvic hematomas can have several anatomical manifestations following childbirth. They are most often associated with a laceration, episiotomy, or an operative delivery. However, they may develop following rupture of a blood vessel without associated lacerations (Nelson, 2012; Propst, 1998; Ridgway, 1995). In some cases, they are quickly apparent, but in others, hemorrhage may be delayed. Occasionally, they are associated with an underlying coagulopathy. Faulty clotting may be acquired, such as with consumptive coagulopathy from placental abruption or fatty liver failure, or may stem from a congenital bleeding disorder such as von Willebrand disease.

One classification of puerperal hematomas includes vulvar, vulvovaginal, paravaginal, and retroperitoneal hematomas. Vulvar hematomas may involve the vestibular bulb or branches of the pudendal artery, which are the inferior rectal, perineal, and clitoral arteries (Fig. 41-11). Paravaginal hematomas may involve the descending branch of the uterine artery (Zahn, 1990). In some cases, a torn vessel lies above the pelvic fascia, and a supralevator hematoma develops. These can extend into the upper portion of the vaginal canal and may almost occlude its lumen. Continued bleeding may dissect retroperitoneally to form a mass palpable above the inguinal ligament. Finally, it may even dissect up behind the ascending colon to the hepatic flexure at the lower margin of the diaphragm (Rafi, 2010).

Vulvovaginal Hematomas

These may develop rapidly and frequently cause excruciating pain, as did the one shown in Figure 41-12. If bleeding ceases, then small- to moderate-sized hematomas may be absorbed. However, we have encountered a few that rebled up to 2 weeks postpartum. In others, the tissues overlying the hematoma may rupture from pressure necrosis. At this time, profuse hemorrhage may follow, but in other cases, the hematoma drains in the form of large clots and old blood. In those that involve the paravaginal space and extend above the levator sling, retroperitoneal bleeding may be massive and occasionally fatal.

Diagnosis. A vulvar hematoma is readily diagnosed by severe perineal pain. A tense, fluctuant, and tender swelling of varying size rapidly develops and is eventually covered by discolored skin. A paravaginal hematoma may escape detection temporarily. However, symptoms of pelvic pressure, pain, or inability to void should prompt evaluation with discovery of a round, fluctuant mass encroaching on the vaginal lumen. When there is a supralevator extension, the hematoma extends upward in the paravaginal space and between the leaves of the broad ligament. The hematoma may escape detection until it can be felt on abdominal palpation or until hypovolemia develops. Imaging with sonography or computed tomographic (CT) scanning can be useful to assess hematoma location and extent. As discussed, supralevator hematomas are particularly worrisome because they can lead to hypovolemic shock and death.

Management. Vulvovaginal hematomas are managed according to their size, duration since delivery, and expansion. In general, smaller vulvar hematomas identified after the woman leaves the delivery room may be treated expectantly (Propst, 1998). But, if pain is severe or the hematoma continues to enlarge, then surgical exploration is preferable. An incision is made at the point of maximal distention, blood and clots are evacuated, and bleeding points ligated. The cavity may then be obliterated with absorbable mattress sutures. Often, no sites of bleeding are identified. Nonetheless, the evacuated hematoma cavity is surgically closed, and the vagina is packed for 12 to 24 hours. Supralevator hematomas are more difficult to treat. Although some can be evacuated by vulvar or vaginal incisions, laparotomy is advisable if there is continued hemorrhage.

Blood loss with large puerperal hematomas is nearly always considerably more than the clinical estimate. Hypovolemia is common, and transfusions are frequently required when surgical repair is necessary.

Angiographic embolization as described on page 820 has become popular for management of some puerperal hematomas. Embolization can be used primarily, or more likely secondarily, if surgical attempts at hemostasis have failed or if the hematoma is difficult to access surgically (Distefano, 2013; Ojala, 2005). The use of a Bakri balloon for a paracervical hematoma has also been described (Grönvall, 2013).

Rupture of the Uterus

Uterine rupture may be *primary*, defined as occurring in a previously intact or unscarred uterus, or may be *secondary* and

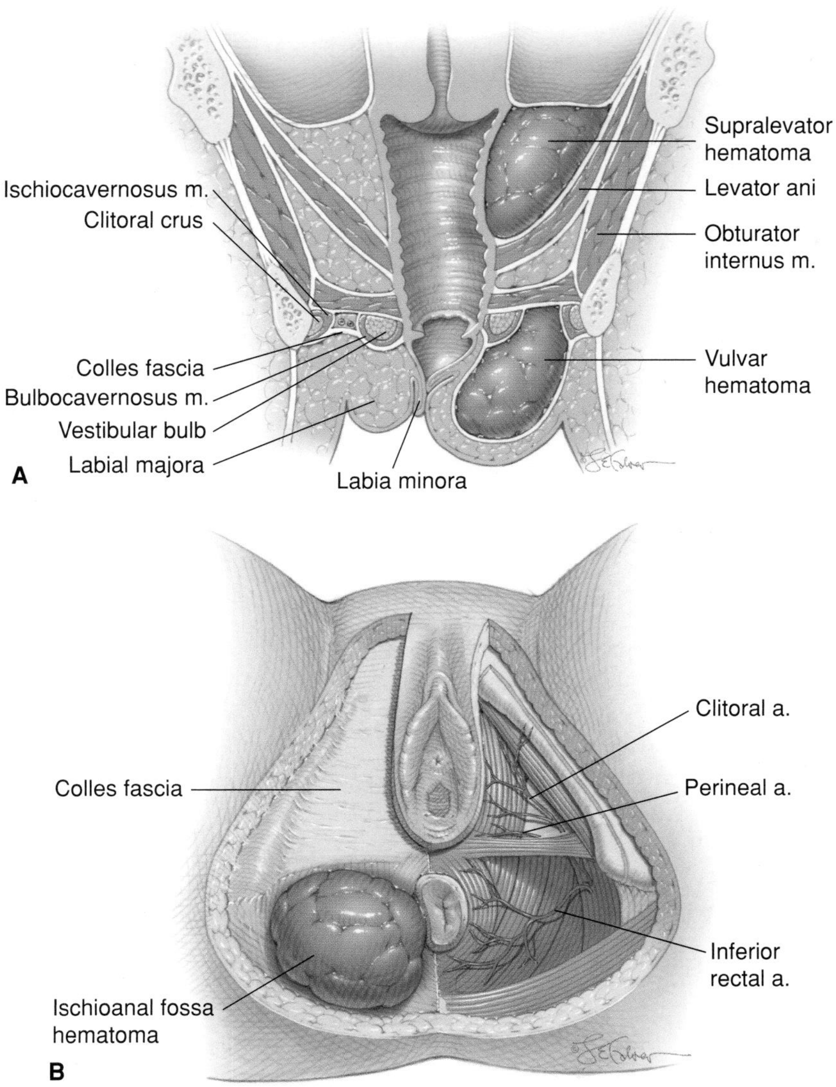

FIGURE 41-11 Schematic showing types of puerperal hematoma. **A.** Coronal view showing supralevator and anterior perineal triangle hematomas on the right. **B.** Perineal view shows anterior perineal triangle anatomy and an ischioanal fossa hematoma on the left.

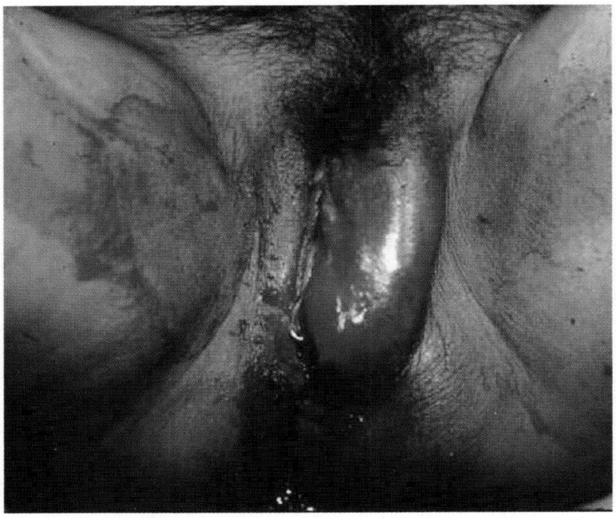

FIGURE 41-12 Left-sided anterior perineal triangle hematoma associated with a vaginal laceration following spontaneous delivery in a woman with consumptive coagulopathy from acute fatty liver of pregnancy.

associated with a preexisting myometrial incision, injury, or anomaly. Some of the etiologies associated with uterine rupture are presented in Table 41-3. Importantly, the contribution of each of these underlying causes has changed remarkably during the past 50 years. Specifically, before 1960, when the cesarean delivery rate was much lower than it is currently and when women of great parity were numerous, primary uterine rupture predominated. As the incidence of cesarean delivery increased and especially as a subsequent trial of labor in these women became prevalent through the 1990s, uterine rupture through the cesarean hysterotomy scar became preeminent. As discussed in detail in Chapter 31 (p. 617), along with diminished enthusiasm for trial of labor in women with prior cesarean delivery, the two types of rupture likely now have equivalent incidences. Indeed, in a 2006 study of 41 cases of uterine rupture from the Hospital Corporation of America, half were in women with a prior cesarean delivery (Porreco, 2009).

Predisposing Factors and Causes

In addition to the prior cesarean hysterotomy incision already discussed, risks for uterine rupture include other previous operations or manipulations that traumatize the myometrium. Examples are uterine curettage or perforation, endometrial ablation, myomectomy, or hysteroscopy (Kieser, 2002; Pelosi, 1997). In the study by Porreco and colleagues (2009) cited earlier, seven of 21 women without a prior cesarean delivery had undergone prior uterine surgery.

In developed countries, the incidence of rupture was cited by Getahun and associates (2012) as 1 in 4800 deliveries. The frequency of primary rupture approximates 1 in 10,000 to 15,000 births (Miller, 1997; Porreco, 2009). One reason is a decreased incidence of women of great parity (Maymon, 1991; Miller, 1997). Another is that excessive or inappropriate uterine stimulation with oxytocin—previously a frequent cause—has mostly disappeared. Anecdotally, however, we have encountered primary uterine rupture in a disparate number of women in whom labor was induced with prostaglandin E_1.

Pathogenesis. Rupture of the previously intact uterus during labor most often involves the thinned-out lower uterine segment. When the rent is in the immediate vicinity of the cervix, it frequently extends transversely or obliquely. When the rent is in the portion of the uterus adjacent to the broad ligament, the tear is usually longitudinal. Although these tears develop primarily in the lower uterine segment, it is not unusual for them to extend upward into the active segment or downward through the cervix and into the vagina (Fig. 41-13). In some cases, the bladder may

TABLE 41-3. Some Causes of Uterine Rupture

Preexisting Uterine Injury or Anomaly	Uterine Injury or Abnormality Incurred in Current Pregnancy
Surgery involving the myometrium:	**Before delivery:**
Cesarean delivery or hysterotomy	Persistent, intense, spontaneous contractions
Previously repaired uterine rupture	Labor stimulation—oxytocin or prostaglandins
Myomectomy incision through or to the endometrium	Intraamnionic instillation—saline or prostaglandins
Deep cornual resection of interstitial fallopian tube	Perforation by internal uterine pressure catheter
Metroplasty	External trauma—sharp or blunt
Coincidental uterine trauma:	External version
Abortion with instrumentation—sharp or suction curette, sounds	Uterine overdistention—hydramnios, multifetal pregnancy
Sharp or blunt trauma—assaults, vehicular accidents, bullets, knives	**During delivery:**
Silent rupture in previous pregnancy	Internal version second twin
Congenital:	Difficult forceps delivery
Pregnancy in undeveloped uterine horn	Rapid tumultuous labor and delivery
Defective connective tissue—Marfan or Ehlers-Danlos syndrome	Breech extraction
	Fetal anomaly distending lower segment
	Vigorous uterine pressure during delivery
	Difficult manual removal of placenta
	Acquired:
	Placental accrete syndromes
	Gestational trophoblastic neoplasia
	Adenomyosis
	Sacculation of entrapped retroverted uterus

also be lacerated (Rachagan, 1991). If the rupture is of sufficient size, the uterine contents will usually escape into the peritoneal cavity. If the presenting fetal part is firmly engaged, however, then only a portion of the fetus may be extruded from the uterus. Fetal prognosis is largely dependent on the degree of placental separation and magnitude of maternal hemorrhage and hypovolemia. In some cases, the overlying peritoneum remains intact, and this usually is accompanied by hemorrhage that extends into the broad ligament to cause a large retroperitoneal hematoma with extensive blood loss.

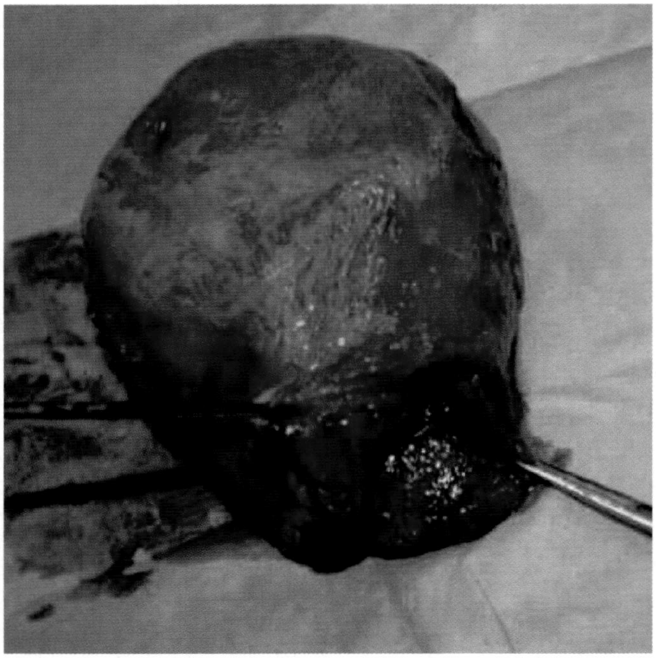

FIGURE 41-13 Supracervical hysterectomy specimen showing uterine rupture during spontaneous labor with a vertical tear at the left lateral edge of lower uterine segment.

Occasionally, there is an inherent weakness in the myometrium in which the rupture takes place. Some examples include anatomical anomalies, adenomyosis, and connective-tissue defects such as Ehlers-Danlos syndrome (Arici, 2013; Nikolaou, 2013).

Management and Outcomes. The varied clinical presentations of uterine rupture and its management are discussed in detail in Chapter 31 (p. 617).

In the most recent maternal mortality statistics from the Centers for Disease Control and Prevention, uterine rupture accounted for 14 percent of deaths caused by hemorrhage (Berg, 2010). Maternal morbidity includes hysterectomy that may be necessary to control hemorrhage. There is also considerably increased perinatal morbidity and mortality associated with uterine rupture. A major concern is that surviving infants develop severe neurological impairment (Porreco, 2009).

Traumatic Uterine Rupture

Although the distended pregnant uterus is surprisingly resistant to blunt trauma, pregnant women sustaining such trauma to the abdomen should be watched carefully for signs of a ruptured uterus (Chap. 47, p. 954). Even so, blunt trauma is more likely to cause placental abruption as described subsequently. In a study by Miller and Paul (1996), trauma accounted for only three cases of uterine rupture in more than 150 women.

Other causes of traumatic rupture that are uncommon today are those due to internal podalic version and extraction, difficult forceps delivery, breech extraction, and unusual fetal enlargement such as with hydrocephaly.

Placental Abruption

Separation of the placenta—either partially or totally—from its implantation site before delivery is described by the Latin term *abruptio placentae*. Literally translated, this refers to "rending asunder of the placenta," which denotes a sudden accident that is a clinical characteristic of most cases. In the purest sense, the cumbersome—and thus seldom used—term *premature separation of the normally implanted placenta* is most descriptive because it excludes separation of a placenta previa implanted over the internal cervical os.

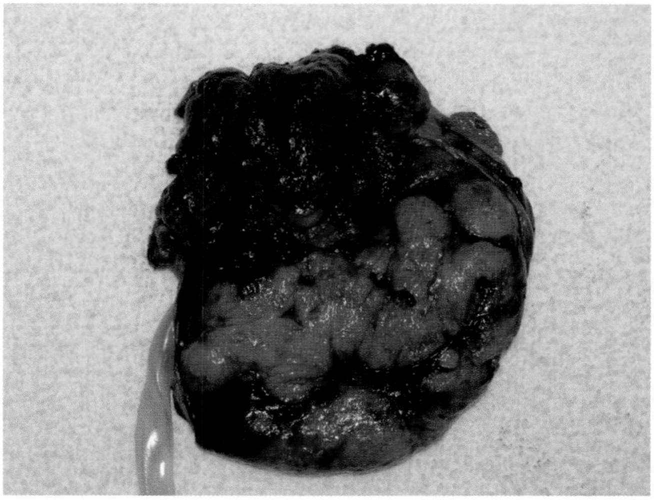

FIGURE 41-14 Partial placental abruption with a dark adhered clot.

Etiopathogenesis

Placental abruption is initiated by hemorrhage into the decidua basalis. The decidua then splits, leaving a thin layer adhered to the myometrium. Consequently, the process begins as a decidual hematoma and expands to cause separation and compression of the adjacent placenta. Inciting causes of many cases are not known, however, several have been posited. The phenomenon of impaired trophoblastic invasion with subsequent atherosis is related in some cases of preeclampsia and abruption (Brosens, 2011). Inflammation or infection may be contributory. Nath and colleagues (2007) found histological evidence of inflammation to be more common in prematurely separated placentas. *Papio* species of baboons develop abruptio placentae similar to humans, and up to half of prematurely separated placentas in these animals demonstrate neutrophilic infiltration (Schenone, 2012; Schlabritz-Loutsevich, 2013a,b).

Abruption likely begins with rupture of a decidual spiral artery to cause a retroplacental hematoma. This can expand to disrupt more vessels and extend placental separation (Fig. 6-3, p. 119). In the early stages of placental abruption, there may be no clinical symptoms. If there is no further separation, the abruption is discovered on examination of the freshly delivered placenta, as a circumscribed depression on the maternal surface. These usually measure a few centimeters in diameter and are covered by dark, clotted blood. Because several minutes are required for these anatomical changes to materialize, a very recently separated placenta may appear totally normal at delivery. Our experiences are like those of Benirschke and associates (2012) in that the "age" of the retroplacental clot cannot be determined exactly. In the example shown in Figure 41-14, a large dark clot is well formed, it has depressed the placental bulk, and it likely is at least several hours old.

Even with continued bleeding and placental separation, placental abruption can still be either *total* or *partial* (Fig. 41-15). With either, bleeding typically insinuates itself between the membranes and uterus, ultimately escaping through the cervix to cause *external hemorrhage*. Less often, the blood is retained between the detached placenta and the uterus, leading to *concealed hemorrhage* and delayed diagnosis (Chang, 2001). The delay translates into much greater maternal and fetal hazards. With concealed hemorrhage, the likelihood of consumptive coagulopathy also is greater. This is because increased pressure within the intervillous space caused by the expanding retroplacental clot forces more placental thromboplastin into the maternal circulation (p. 797).

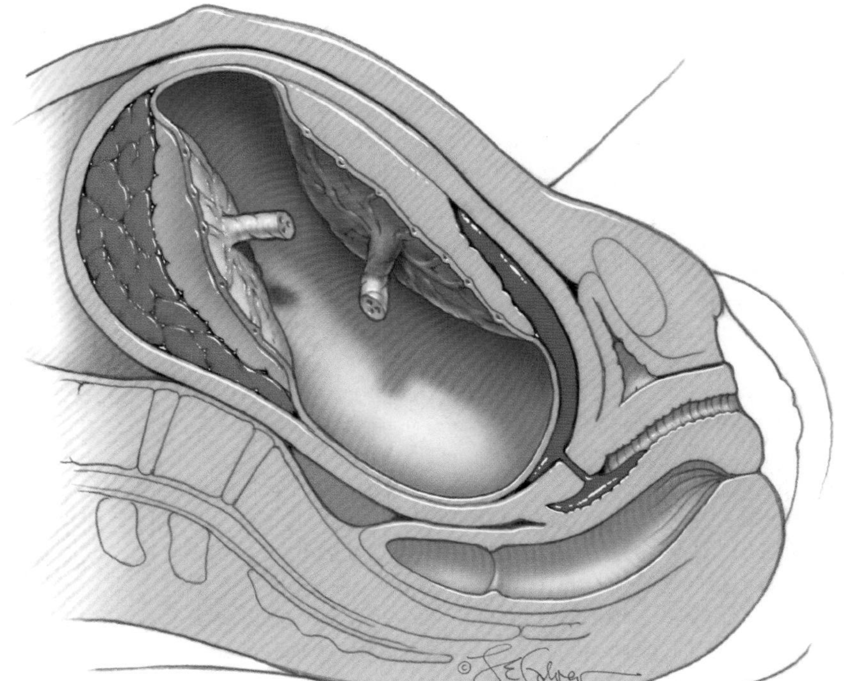

FIGURE 41-15 Schematic of placental abruption. Shown to left is a total placental abruption with concealed hemorrhage. To the right is a partial abruption with blood and clots dissecting between membranes and decidua to the internal cervical os and then externally into the vagina.

Chronic Abruption. Some cases of chronic placental separation begin early in pregnancy. Dugoff and coworkers (2004) observed an association between some abnormally elevated maternal serum aneuploidy markers and subsequent abruption. Ananth (2006) and Weiss (2004) and their associates have also correlated first- and second-trimester bleeding with third-trimester placental abruption. In some cases of a chronic abruption, subsequent oligohydramnios develops—*chronic abruption-oligohydramnios sequence—CAOS* (Elliott, 1998). Even later in pregnancy, hemorrhage with retroplacental hematoma formation is occasionally arrested completely without delivery. These women may have abnormally elevated serum levels of alpha-fetoprotein (Ngai, 2012). We documented a chronic abruption in a woman with suggestive findings by labeling her red cells with radiochromium. Her symptoms abated, and at delivery 3 weeks later, a 400-mL clot found within the uterus contained no radiochromium, whereas peripheral blood at that time did. Thus, red cells in the clot had accumulated before they were labeled with the radioisotope 3 weeks before delivery.

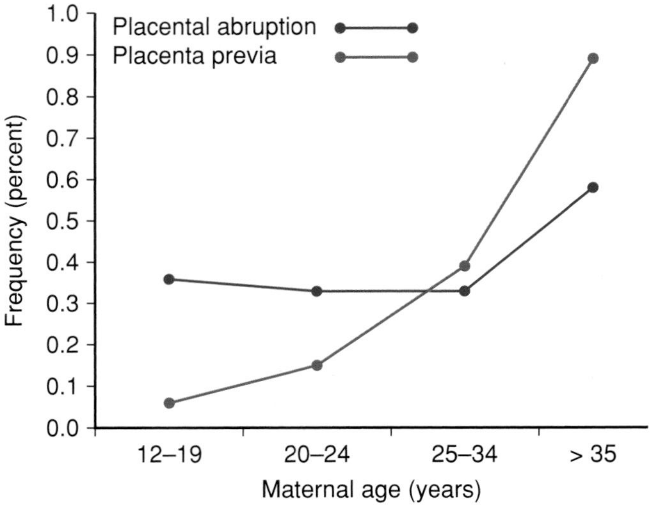

FIGURE 41-16 Frequency of placental abruption and placenta previa by maternal age in 365,700 deliveries at Parkland Hospital from 1988 through 2012. (Data courtesy of Dr. Don McIntire.)

Traumatic Abruption. External trauma—usually from motor vehicle accidents or aggravated assault—can cause placental separation. The frequency of abruption caused by trauma varies and may be dependent on whether these women are cared for in a major trauma unit. Kettel (1988) and Stafford (1988) and their coworkers have appropriately stressed that abruption can be caused by relatively minor trauma. The clinical presentation and sequelae of these abruptions are somewhat different from spontaneous cases. For example, associated fetomaternal hemorrhage, while seldom clinically significant with most spontaneous abruptions, is more common with trauma because of concomitant placental tears or "fractures" (Fig. 47-11, p. 954). Fetal bleeding that averaged 12 mL was noted in a third of women with a traumatic abruption reported by Pearlman (1990). In eight women cared for at Parkland Hospital, we found fetal-to-maternal hemorrhage of 80 to 100 mL in three of eight cases of traumatic placental abruption (Stettler, 1992). Importantly, in some cases of trauma, a nonreassuring fetal heart rate tracing may not be accompanied by other evidence of placental separation. A sinusoidal tracing is one example (Fig. 24-13, p. 482). Traumatic abruption is considered in more detail in Chapter 47 (p. 953).

Fetal-to-Maternal Hemorrhage. Most blood in the retroplacental hematoma in a nontraumatic placental abruption is maternal. This is because hemorrhage is caused by separation within the maternal decidua, and placental villi are usually initially intact. In 78 women at Parkland Hospital with a nontraumatic placental abruption, fetal-to-maternal hemorrhage was documented in only 20 percent—and all of these had < 10 mL fetal blood loss (Stettler, 1992). As discussed above, significant fetal bleeding is much more likely with a traumatic abruption that results from a concomitant placental tear.

Frequency

The reported incidence of placental abruption varies because of different criteria used. That said, its frequency averages 0.5 percent or 1 in 200 deliveries. In the National Center for Health Statistics database of 15 million deliveries, Salihu and colleagues (2005) reported an incidence of 0.6 percent or 1 in 165 births. From the National Hospital Discharge Summary database from 1999 through 2001, the incidence of placental abruption was found to be 1 percent (Ananth, 2005). From a Maternal-Fetal Medicine Units Network study of approximately 10,000 nulliparous women, the incidence was 0.6 percent (Roberts, 2010). In nearly 366,000 deliveries at Parkland Hospital from 1988 through 2012, the incidence of placental abruption averaged 0.35 percent or 1 in 290 (Fig. 41-16).

According to Ananth (2001b, 2005), the frequency of placental abruption has *increased* in this country from 0.8 percent in 1981 to 1.0 percent in 2001. Most of this increase was in black women. At Parkland Hospital, however, both the incidence and severity have *decreased*. With placental abruption *so extensive as to kill the fetus*, the incidence was 0.24 percent or 1 in 420 births from 1956 through 1967 (Pritchard, 1967). As the number of high-parity women giving birth decreased along with improved availability of prenatal care and emergency transportation, the frequency of abruption causing fetal death decreased to 0.12 percent or 1 in 830 births through 1989. Thereafter and through 2003, it decreased further to 0.06 percent or 1 in 1600, and most recently through 2012, it declined to 0.048 percent or 1 in 2060.

Perinatal Morbidity and Mortality

Major fetal congenital anomalies have an increased association with placental abruption (Riihimäki, 2013). Overall, perinatal outcomes are influenced by gestational age, and the frequency of placental abruption increases across the third trimester up to term. As seen in Figure 41-17, more than half of the placental abruptions at Parkland Hospital developed at ≥ 37 weeks. Perinatal mortality and morbidity, however, are more common with earlier abruptions. Perinatal deaths caused by abruptions can be assessed by their contribution to mortality or as an actual mortality ratio. Looked at the first way, although the

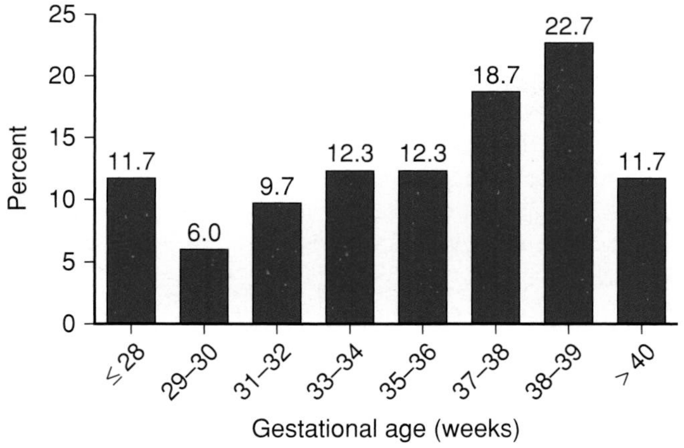

FIGURE 41-17 Frequency of placental abruption by gestational age.

rates of fetal death have declined, the contribution of abruption as a cause of stillbirths remains prominent because other causes have also decreased. For example, since the early 1990s, 10 to 12 percent of all third-trimester stillbirths at Parkland Hospital have been the consequence of placental abruption. This is similar to the rate reported by Fretts and Usher (1997) for the Royal Victoria Hospital in Montreal during the 18-year period ending in 1995 (Chap. 35, p. 662).

Looked at the other way, several investigators have documented high perinatal mortality rates caused by placental abruption. Salihu and colleagues (2005) analyzed more than 15 million singleton births in the United States between 1995 and 1998. The perinatal mortality rate associated with placental abruption was 119 per 1000 births compared with 8 per 1000 for the general obstetrical population. They emphasized that the high rate was due not just to placental abruption, but also to the associated increases in preterm delivery and fetal-growth restriction. Of the two, preterm birth has been reported to be the most important (Nath, 2008).

Perinatal morbidity—often severe—is common in survivors. An early study by Abdella and associates (1984) documented significant neurological deficits within the first year of life in 15 percent of survivors. Two subsequent studies by Matsuda and coworkers (2003, 2013) reported that 20 percent of survivors developed cerebral palsy. These observations are similar to ours from Parkland Hospital. Notably, 20 percent of liveborn neonates of women with an abruption had severe acidemia, defined by a pH < 7.0 or base deficit of ≥ 12 mmol/L. Importantly, 15 percent of liveborn neonates subsequently died.

Predisposing Factors

Demographic Factors. Several predisposing factors may increase the risk for placental abruption, and some are listed in Table 41-4. First, the incidence of abruption increases with *maternal age* (see Fig. 41-16). In the First- and Second-Trimester Evaluation of Risk (FASTER) trial, women older than 40 years were 2.3 times more likely to experience abruption compared with those 35 years or younger (Cleary-Goldman, 2005). There are conflicting data regarding women of *great parity* (Pritchard, 1991; Toohey, 1995). *Race* or ethnicity also appears to be important. In almost 366,000 deliveries at Parkland Hospital, abruption severe enough to kill the fetus was most common in African-American and white women—1 in 200—less so in Asian women—1 in 300—and least in Latin-American women—1 in 350 (Pritchard, 1991). A *familial association* was found in an analysis of a Norwegian population-based registry that included almost 378,000 sisters with more than 767,000 pregnancies (Rasmussen, 2009). If a woman had a severe abruption, then the risk for her sister was doubled, and the heritability risk was estimated to be 16 percent. The control group of their sisters-in-law had a risk similar to that for the general obstetrical population.

TABLE 41-4. Risk Factors for Placental Abruption

Risk Factor	Relative Risk
Prior abruption	10–50
Increased age and parity	1.3–2.3
Preeclampsia	2.1–4.0
Chronic hypertension	1.8–3.0
Chorioamnionitis	3.0
Preterm ruptured membranes	2.4–4.9
Multifetal gestation	2.1
Low birthweight	14.0
Hydramnios	2.0
Cigarette smoking	1.4–1.9
Thrombophilias	3–7
Cocaine use	NA
Uterine leiomyoma	NA

NA = not available.
Data from Ananth, 1999a,b, 2001b, 2004, 2007; Cleary-Goldman, 2005; Eskes, 2001; Nath, 2007, 2008.

Hypertension and Preeclampsia. Some form of hypertension is the most frequent condition associated with placental abruption. This includes gestational hypertension, preeclampsia, chronic hypertension, or a combination thereof. In the report by Pritchard and colleagues (1991) that described 408 women with placental abruption and fetal demise cared for at Parkland Hospital, hypertension was apparent in half once hypovolemia was corrected. Half of these women—a fourth of all 408—had chronic hypertension. Looked at another way, a Network study reported that 1.5 percent of pregnant women with chronic hypertension suffered placental abruption (Sibai, 1998). Risk estimates by Zetterstrom and associates (2005) included a two-fold increased incidence of abruption in women with chronic hypertension compared with normotensive women—an incidence of 1.1 versus 0.5 percent.

Chronic hypertension with superimposed preeclampsia or fetal-growth restriction confers an ever greater increased risk (Ananth, 2007). Even so, the severity of hypertension does not necessarily correlate with abruption incidence (Zetterstrom, 2005). The long-term effects of these associations are apparent from the significantly increased cardiovascular mortality risk in affected women (Pariente, 2013). Observations from the Magpie Trial Collaborative Group (2002) suggest that women with preeclampsia given magnesium sulfate may have a reduced risk for abruption.

Preterm Prematurely Ruptured Membranes. There is no doubt that there is a substantially increased risk for abruption when the membranes rupture before term. Major and colleagues (1995) reported that 5 percent of 756 women with ruptured membranes between 20 and 36 weeks developed an abruption. Kramer and coworkers (1997) found an incidence of 3.1 percent if membranes were ruptured for longer than 24 hours. Ananth and associates (2004) reported that the threefold risk of abruption with preterm rupture was further increased with infection. This same group has suggested that inflammation and infection as well as preterm delivery may be the primary causes leading to abruption (Nath, 2007, 2008).

Cigarette Smoking. Given other vascular diseases caused by smoking, it is not surprising that studies from the Collaborative Perinatal Project linked this to an increased risk for abruption (Misra, 1999; Naeye, 1980). Results of meta-analyses of 1.6 million pregnancies included a twofold risk for abruption in smokers (Ananth, 1999b). This risk increased to five- to eightfold if smokers had chronic hypertension, severe preeclampsia, or both. Similar findings have been reported by Mortensen (2001), Hogberg (2007), Kaminsky (2007), and all their coworkers.

Cocaine Abuse. Women who use cocaine can have an alarming frequency of placental abruption. Bingol and colleagues (1987) described 50 women who abused cocaine during pregnancy—eight had a stillbirth caused by placental abruption. In a systematic review, Addis and associates (2001) reported that placental abruption was more common in women who used cocaine than in those who did not.

Lupus Anticoagulant and Thrombophilias. Women affected by some of these have higher associated rates of thromboembolic disorders during pregnancy. However, the link with placental abruption is less clear (American College of Obstetricians and Gynecologists, 2012a, 2013a). Lupus anticoagulant is associated with maternal floor infarction of the placenta, but is less so with typical abruptions. There is no convincing evidence that thrombophilias—for example, factor V Leiden or prothrombin gene mutation—are associated with placental abruption. These have been reviewed by Kenny and coworkers (2014) and are discussed further in Chapters 52 (p. 1029) and 59 (p. 1174).

Uterine Leiomyomas. Especially if located near the mucosal surface behind the placental implantation site, uterine myomas can predispose to abortion or later to placental abruption (Chaps. 18, p. 360 and 63, p. 1225).

Recurrent Abruption. Because many of the predisposing factors are chronic and therefore repetitive, it would be reasonable to conclude that placental abruption would have a high recurrence rate. In fact, the woman who has suffered an abruption—especially one that caused fetal death—has an extraordinarily high risk for recurrence. In these women, Pritchard and associates (1970) identified a recurrence rate of 12 percent—and half of these caused another fetal death. Furuhashi and colleagues (2002) reported a 22-percent recurrence rate—half recurred at a gestational age 1 to 3 weeks earlier than the first abruption. Looked at a second way, Tikkanen and coworkers (2006) found that of 114 parous women who experienced an abruption, 9 percent had a prior abruption. A third perspective is provided by a population-based study of 767,000 pregnancies completed by Rasmussen and Irgens (2009). They reported a 6.5-fold increased risk for recurrence of a "mild" abruption and 11.5-fold risk for a "severe" abruption. For women who had two severe abruptions, the risk for a third was increased 50-fold.

Management of a pregnancy subsequent to an abruption is difficult because another separation may suddenly occur, even remote from term. In many of these recurrences, fetal well-being is almost always reassuring beforehand. Thus, antepartum fetal testing is usually not predictive (Toivonen, 2002).

Clinical Findings and Diagnosis

Most women with a placental abruption have sudden-onset abdominal pain, vaginal bleeding, and uterine tenderness. In a prospective study, Hurd and colleagues (1983) reported that 78 percent with placental abruption had vaginal bleeding, 66 percent had uterine tenderness or back pain, and 60 percent had a nonreassuring fetal status. Other findings included frequent contractions and persistent hypertonus. In a fifth of these women, preterm labor was diagnosed, and abruption was not suspected until fetal distress or death ensued.

Importantly, the signs and symptoms of placental abruption can vary considerably. In some women, external bleeding can be profuse, yet placental separation may not be so extensive as to compromise the fetus. In others, there may be no external bleeding, but the placenta is sufficiently sheared off that the fetus is dead—a concealed abruption. In one unusual case, a multiparous woman cared for at Parkland Hospital presented with a nosebleed. She had no abdominal or uterine pain, tenderness, or vaginal bleeding. Her fetus was dead, however, and her blood did not clot. The plasma fibrinogen level was 25 mg/dL. Labor was induced, and a total abruption was confirmed at delivery.

Differential Diagnosis. With severe placental abruption, the diagnosis generally is obvious. From the previous discussion, it follows that less severe, more common forms of abruption cannot always be recognized with certainty. Thus, the diagnosis is one of exclusion. Unfortunately, there are no laboratory tests or other diagnostic methods to accurately confirm lesser degrees of placental separation. Sonography has limited use because the placenta and fresh clots may have similar imaging characteristics. In an early study, Sholl (1987) confirmed the clinical diagnosis with sonography in only 25 percent of women. In a later study, Glantz and Purnell (2002) reported only 24-percent sensitivity in 149 consecutive women with a suspected placental abruption. *Importantly, negative findings with sonographic examination do not exclude placental abruption.* Conversely, magnetic resonance (MR) imaging is highly sensitive for placental abruption, and if knowledge of this would change management, then it should be considered (Masselli, 2011).

With abruption, intravascular coagulation is almost universal. Thus, elevated serum levels of D-dimers may be suggestive, but this has not been adequately tested. Ngai and associates

(2012) have provided preliminary data that serum levels of alpha-fetoprotein > 280 μg/L have a positive-predictive value of 97 percent.

Thus, in the woman with vaginal bleeding and a live fetus, it is often necessary to exclude placenta previa and other causes of bleeding by clinical and sonographic evaluation. It has long been taught—perhaps with some justification—that *painful* uterine bleeding signifies placental abruption, whereas *painless* uterine bleeding is indicative of placenta previa. The differential diagnosis is usually not this straightforward, and labor accompanying previa may cause pain suggestive of placental abruption. On the other hand, pain from abruption may mimic normal labor, or it may be painless, especially with a posterior placenta. At times, the cause of the vaginal bleeding remains obscure even after delivery.

Hypovolemic Shock. *Placental abruption is one of several notable obstetrical entities that may be complicated by massive and sometimes torrential hemorrhage.* Hypovolemic shock is caused by maternal blood loss. In an earlier report from Parkland Hospital, Pritchard and Brekken (1967) described 141 women with abruption so severe as to kill the fetus. Blood loss in these women often amounted to at least half of their pregnant blood volume. Importantly, massive blood loss and shock can develop with a concealed abruption. Prompt treatment of hypotension with crystalloid and blood infusion will restore vital signs to normal and reverse oliguria from inadequate renal perfusion. In the past, placental abruption was an all-too-common cause of acute kidney injury requiring dialysis (Chap. 53, p. 1063).

Consumptive Coagulopathy. Obstetrical events—mainly placental abruption and amnionic-fluid embolism—led to the initial recognition of *defibrination syndrome,* which is currently referred to as *consumptive coagulopathy* or *disseminated intravascular coagulation.* The major mechanism causing procoagulant consumption is intravascular activation of clotting. Abruption is the most common cause of clinically significant consumptive coagulopathy in obstetrics—and indeed, probably in all of medicine. There are significant amounts of procoagulants in the retroplacental clots, but these cannot account for all missing fibrinogen (Pritchard, 1967). We and others have observed that the levels of fibrin degradation products are higher in serum from peripheral blood compared with that found in serum from blood contained in the uterine cavity (Bonnar, 1969). The reverse would be anticipated in the absence of significant intravascular coagulation.

An important consequence of intravascular coagulation is the activation of plasminogen to plasmin, which lyses fibrin microemboli to maintain microcirculatory patency. With placental abruption severe enough to kill the fetus, there are always pathological levels of fibrinogen–fibrin degradation products and D-dimers in maternal serum.

Most women with placental abruption will have some degree of intravascular coagulation. However, in a third of those with an abruption severe enough to kill the fetus, the plasma fibrinogen level will be < 150 mg/dL. These clinically significant levels may cause troublesome surgical bleeding. Elevated serum levels of fibrinogen-fibrin degradation products, including D-dimers, are also found, but their quantification is not clinically useful. Serum levels of several other coagulation factors are also variably decreased. Thrombocytopenia, sometimes profound, may accompany severe hypofibrinogenemia initially and becomes common after repeated blood transfusions.

Consumptive coagulopathy is more likely with a concealed abruption because intrauterine pressure is higher, thus forcing more thromboplastin into the large veins draining the implantation site. With a partial abruption and a live fetus, severe coagulation defects are seen less commonly. Our experience has been that if serious coagulopathy develops, it is usually evident by the time abruption symptoms appear. Disseminated intravascular coagulation is discussed in more detail on page 808.

Couvelaire Uterus. At the time of cesarean delivery, it is not uncommon to find widespread extravasation of blood into the uterine musculature and beneath the serosa (Fig. 41-18). It is named after Couvelaire, who in the early 1900s termed it *uteroplacental apoplexy.* Effusions of blood are also seen beneath the tubal serosa, between the leaves of the broad ligaments, in the substance of the ovaries, and free in the peritoneal cavity. These myometrial hemorrhages seldom cause uterine atony, and alone they are not an indication for hysterectomy.

Acute Kidney Injury. Previously known as acute renal failure, acute kidney injury is a general term describing renal dysfunction from many causes (Chap. 53, p. 1063). In obstetrics, it is most commonly seen in cases of severe placental abruption in which treatment of hypovolemia is delayed or incomplete. Even whenabruption is complicated by severe intravascular

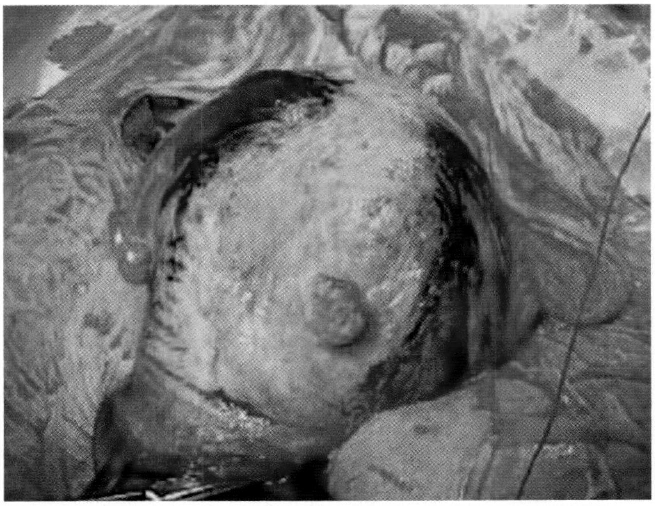

FIGURE 41-18 Couvelaire uterus from total placental abruption after cesarean delivery. Blood markedly infiltrates the myometrium to reach the serosa, especially at the cornua. It gives the myometrium a bluish-purple tone as shown. After the hysterotomy incision was closed, the uterus remained well contracted despite extensive extravasation of blood into the uterine wall. The small serosal leiomyoma seen on the lower anterior uterine surface is an incidental finding. (Courtesy of Dr. Angela Fields Walker).

coagulation, however, prompt and vigorous treatment of hemorrhage with blood and crystalloid solution usually prevents clinically significant renal dysfunction. It is unclear what contributory role abruption occupies in the increasing incidence of obstetric-related acute kidney injury in this country (Bateman, 2010; Kuklina, 2009). Undoubtedly, the risk for renal injury with abruption is magnified when preeclampsia coexists (Drakeley, 2002; Hauth, 1999). Currently, most cases of acute kidney injury are reversible and not so severe as to require dialysis. That said, irreversible *acute cortical necrosis* encountered in pregnancy is most often associated with abruption. In past years, a third of all patients admitted to renal units for chronic dialysis were women who had suffered an abruption (Grünfeld, 1987; Lindheimer, 2007).

Sheehan Syndrome. Rarely, severe intrapartum or early postpartum hemorrhage is followed by pituitary failure—*Sheehan syndrome*. The exact pathogenesis is not well understood, especially since endocrine abnormalities are infrequent even in women who suffer catastrophic hemorrhage. Findings include failure of lactation, amenorrhea, breast atrophy, loss of pubic and axillary hair, hypothyroidism, and adrenal cortical insufficiency. In some women, there may be varying degrees of anterior pituitary necrosis and impaired secretion of one or more trophic hormones (Matsuwaki, 2014; Robalo, 2012). The syndrome is discussed further in Chapter 58 (p. 1163).

Management

Treatment of the woman with a placental abruption varies depending primarily on her clinical condition, the gestational age, and the amount of associated hemorrhage. With a living viable-size fetus and with vaginal delivery not imminent, emergency cesarean delivery is chosen by most. In some women, fetal compromise will be evident (Figs. 41-19 and 41-20). When evaluating fetal status, sonographic confirmation of fetal heart activity may be necessary because sometimes an electrode applied directly to a dead fetus will provide misleading information by recording the maternal heart rate. If the fetus has died or if it is not considered mature enough to live outside the uterus, then vaginal delivery is preferable. In either case,

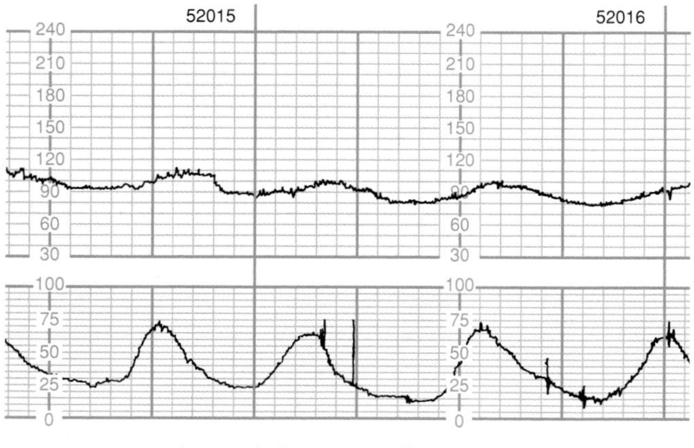

FIGURE 41-19 Placental abruption with fetal compromise. Lower panel: Uterine hypertonus with a baseline pressure of 20 to 25 mm Hg and frequent contractions peaking at approximately 75 mm Hg. Upper panel: The fetal heart rate demonstrates baseline bradycardia with repetitive late decelerations.

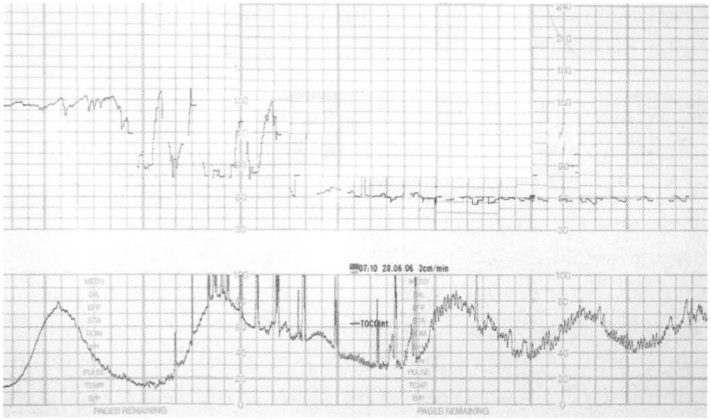

FIGURE 41-20 Intrapartum placental abruption with acute onset of fetal compromise prompted emergent cesarean delivery. An infant with 1- and 5-minute Apgar scores of 4 and 7, respectively, was delivered.

prompt and intensive resuscitation with blood plus crystalloid is begun to replace blood lost from retroplacental and external hemorrhage. These measures are lifesaving for the mother and hopefully for her fetus. If the diagnosis of abruption is uncertain and the fetus is alive and without evidence of compromise, then close observation may be warranted provided that immediate intervention is available.

A major hazard to cesarean delivery is imposed by clinically significant consumptive coagulopathy. As discussed on page 797, this likelihood is lessened if the fetus is still alive—and thus the abruption "less severe." Preparations include assessment of coagulability—especially fibrinogen content—and plans for blood and component replacement.

Cesarean Delivery. The compromised fetus is usually best served by cesarean delivery, and the speed of response is an important factor in perinatal outcomes (see Fig. 41-20). Kayani and coworkers (2003) studied this relationship in 33 singleton pregnancies with a clinically overt placental abruption and fetal bradycardia. Of the 22 neurologically intact survivors, 15 were delivered within a 20-minute decision-to-delivery interval. However, eight of 11 infants who died or developed cerebral palsy were delivered with an interval > 20 minutes.

Vaginal Delivery. If the fetus has died, then vaginal delivery is usually preferred. As reviewed on page 780, hemostasis at the placental implantation site depends primarily on myometrial contraction and not blood coagulability. Thus, after vaginal delivery, uterotonic agents and uterine massage are used to stimulate myometrial contractions. Fibers compress placental site vessels and prompt hemostasis even if coagulation is defective.

There are exceptions for which vaginal delivery may not be preferable even if the fetus is dead. For example, in some cases, hemorrhage is so brisk that it cannot be successfully managed even by vigorous blood replacement. Obstetrical complications that prohibit vaginal delivery such as a term fetus with a transverse lie are another example. Women with a prior high-risk hysterotomy incision, that is, a prior vertical or classical cesarean delivery, pose a complex situation.

Labor with extensive placental abruption tends to be rapid because the uterus is usually persistently hypertonic. This can magnify fetal compromise (see Fig. 41-19). In some cases, *baseline* intraamnionic pressures reach 50 mm Hg or higher, and rhythmic increases reach more than 100 mm Hg with contractions.

Early amniotomy has long been championed in the management of placental abruption. This ostensibly achieves better spiral artery compression that might decrease implantation site bleeding and reduce thromboplastin infusion into the maternal vascular system. Although evidence supporting this theory is lacking, membrane rupture may hasten delivery. However, if the fetus is small, the intact sac may be more efficient in promoting cervical dilatation. If rhythmic uterine contractions are not superimposed on baseline hypertonus, then oxytocin is given in standard doses. There are no data indicating that oxytocin enhances thromboplastin escape into the maternal circulation to worsen coagulopathy (Clark, 1995; Pritchard, 1967).

In the past, some had set arbitrary time limits to permit vaginal delivery. Instead, experiences indicate that maternal outcome depends on the diligence with which adequate fluid and blood replacement therapy are pursued rather than on the interval to delivery. Observations from Parkland Hospital described by Pritchard and Brekken (1967) are similar to those from the University of Virginia reported by Brame and associates (1968). Specifically, women with severe abruption who were transfused during 18 hours or more before delivery had similar outcomes to those in whom delivery was accomplished sooner.

Expectant Management with Preterm Fetus. Delaying delivery may prove beneficial when the fetus is immature. Bond and colleagues (1989) expectantly managed 43 women with placental abruption before 35 weeks' gestation, and 31 of them were given tocolytic therapy. The mean interval-to-delivery for all 43 was approximately 12 days. Cesarean delivery was performed in 75 percent, and there were no stillbirths. As discussed on page 794, women with a very early abruption frequently develop chronic abruption-oligohydramnios sequence—CAOS. In one report, Elliott and coworkers (1998) described four women with an abruption at a mean gestation of 20 weeks who developed oligohydramnios and delivered at an average gestational age of 28 weeks. In a description of 256 women with an abruption ≤ 28 weeks, Sabourin and colleagues (2012) reported that a mean of 1.6 weeks was gained. Of the group, 65 percent were delivered < 29 weeks, and half of all women underwent emergent cesarean delivery.

Unfortunately, even continuous fetal heart rate monitoring does not guarantee universally good outcomes. For example, a normal tracing may precede sudden further separation with instant fetal compromise as shown in Figure 41-20. In some of these, if the separation is sufficient, the fetus will die before it can be delivered. Tocolysis is advocated by some for suspected abruption if the fetus does not display compromise. One drawback reported in the early study by Hurd (1983) was that abruption went unrecognized for dangerously long periods if tocolysis was initiated. Subsequent studies were more optimistic and observed that tocolysis improved outcomes in a highly selected cohort of women with preterm pregnancies (Bond, 1989; Combs, 1992; Sholl, 1987). In another study, Towers and coworkers (1999) administered magnesium sulfate, terbutaline, or both to 95 of 131 women with abruption diagnosed before 36 weeks. The perinatal mortality rate was 5 percent in both groups with or without tocolysis. We are of the view that until a randomized trial is done, a clinically evident abruption contraindicates tocolytic therapy. This does not preclude magnesium sulfate given for severe gestational hypertension.

Placenta Previa

The Latin *previa* means *going before*—and in this sense, the placenta goes before the fetus into the birth canal. In obstetrics, placenta previa describes a placenta that is implanted somewhere in the lower uterine segment, either over or very near the internal cervical os. Because these anatomical relationships cannot always be precisely defined, and because they frequently change across pregnancy, terminology can sometimes be confusing.

Placental Migration

With the frequent use of sonography in obstetrics, the term *placental migration* was used to describe the apparent movement of the placenta away from the internal os (King, 1973). Obviously, the placenta does not move per se, and the mechanism of *apparent* movement is not completely understood. To begin with, *migration* is clearly a misnomer, because decidual invasion by chorionic villi on either side of the cervical os persists. Several explanations are likely additive. First, apparent movement of the low-lying placenta relative to the internal os is related to the imprecision of two-dimensional sonography in defining this relationship. Second, there is differential growth of the lower and upper uterine segments as pregnancy progresses. With greater upper uterine blood flow, placental growth more likely will be toward the fundus—*trophotropism*. Many of those placentas that "migrate" most likely never were circumferentially implanted with true villous invasion that reached the internal cervical os. *Finally, a low-lying placenta is less likely to "migrate" within a uterus with a prior cesarean hysterotomy scar.* Of interest, at the time of delivery there are an equal number of anterior and posterior placentas (Young, 2013).

Placental migration has been quantified in several studies. Sanderson and Milton (1991) studied 4300 women at midpregnancy and found that 12 percent had a low-lying placenta. Of those not covering the internal os, previa did not persist, and none subsequently had placental hemorrhage. Conversely, approximately 40 percent of placentas that covered the os at midpregnancy continued to do so until delivery. Thus, placentas that lie close to but not over the internal os up to the early third trimester are unlikely to persist as a previa by term (Dashe, 2002; Laughon, 2005; Robinson, 2012). Still, Bohrer and associates (2012) reported that a second-trimester low-lying placenta was associated with antepartum admission for hemorrhage and increased blood loss at delivery.

The likelihood that placenta previa persists after being identified sonographically at given epochs before 28 weeks' gestation is shown in Figure 41-21. Similar findings for twin

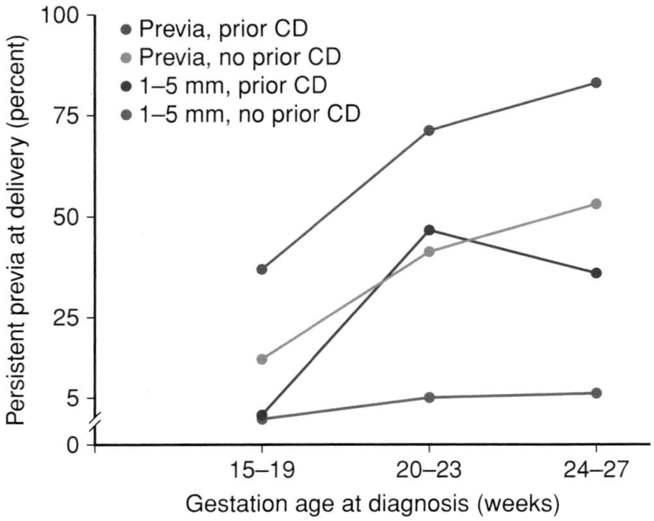

FIGURE 41-21 Likelihood of persistence of placenta previa or low-lying placenta at delivery. These are shown as a function of sonographic diagnosis at three pregnancy epochs of a previa or placental edges 1 to 5 mm from the cervical internal os. CD = cesarean delivery. (Data from Oyelese, 2006.)

pregnancies are reported until 23 weeks, after which the previa persistence rate is much higher (Kohari, 2012). A prior uterine incision also has an obvious effect. Stafford and coworkers (2010), but not Trudell and colleagues (2013), found that a previa and a third-trimester cervical length < 30 mm increased the risk for hemorrhage, uterine activity, and preterm birth. Friszer and associates (2013) showed that women admitted for bleeding had a greater chance of delivery by 7 days with the cervix < 25 mm, although Trudell and colleagues (2013) did not confirm this.

As indicated and discussed subsequently, persistent previa is more common in women who have had a prior cesarean delivery. In the absence of any other indication, sonography need not be frequently repeated simply to document placental position. Moreover, restriction of activity is not necessary unless a previa persists beyond 28 weeks or if clinical findings such as bleeding or contractions develop before this time.

Classification

Terminology for placenta previa has been confusing. In a recent Fetal Imaging Workshop sponsored by the National Institutes of Health (Dashe, 2013), the following classification was recommended:

- *Placenta previa*—the internal os is covered partially or completely by placenta. In the past, these were further classified as either total or partial previa (Figs. 41-22 and 41-23).
- *Low-lying placenta*—implantation in the lower uterine segment is such that the placental edge does not reach the internal os and remains outside a 2-cm wide perimeter around the os. A previously used term, *marginal previa,* described a placenta that was at the edge of the internal os but did not overlie it.

Clearly, the classification of some cases of previa will depend on cervical dilatation at the time of assessment (Dashe, 2013). For example, a low-lying placenta previa at 2-cm dilatation may become a partial placenta previa at 4-cm dilatation because the cervix has dilated to expose the placental edge (see Fig. 41-23). Conversely, a placenta previa that appears to be total before cervical dilatation may become partial at 4-cm dilatation because the cervical opening now extends beyond the edge of the placenta. *Digital palpation in an attempt to ascertain these changing*

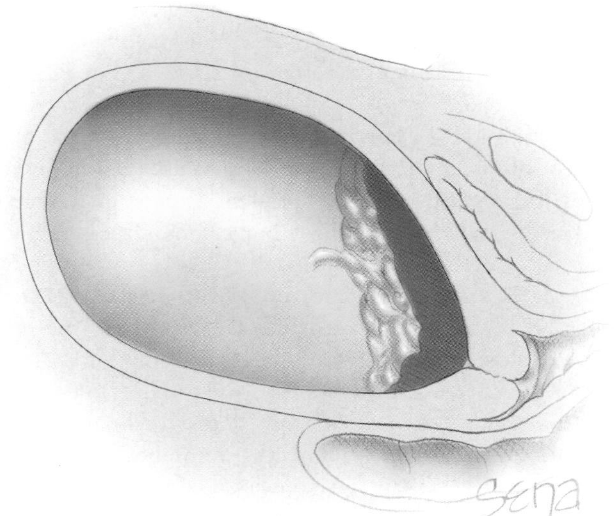

FIGURE 41-22 Total placenta previa showing that copious hemorrhage could be anticipated with any cervical dilatation.

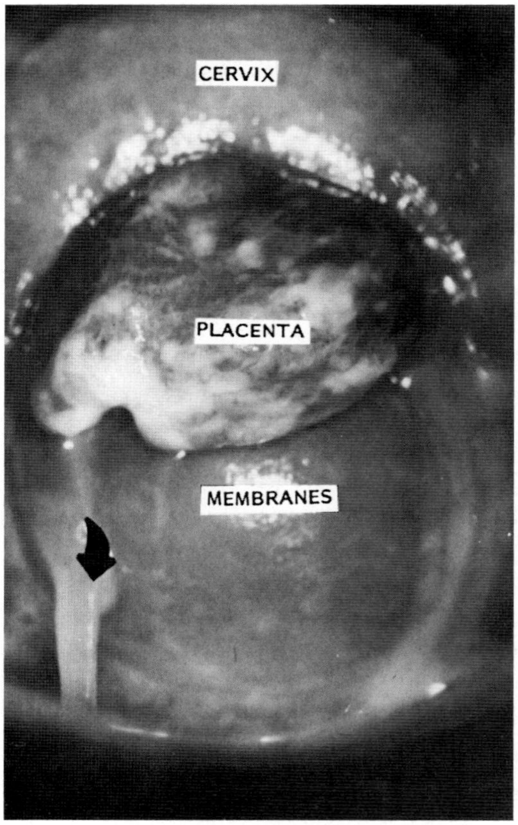

FIGURE 41-23 Second-trimester partial placenta previa. On speculum examination, the cervix is 3- to 4-cm dilated. The arrow points to mucus dripping from the cervix. (Photograph contributed by Dr. Rigoberto Santos.)

relations between the placental edge and internal os as the cervix dilates usually causes severe hemorrhage!

With both total and partial placenta previa, a certain degree of spontaneous placental separation is an inevitable consequence of lower uterine segment remodeling and cervical dilatation. Although this frequently causes bleeding, and thus technically constitutes a placental abruption, this term is usually not applied in these instances.

Somewhat but not always related is *vasa previa,* in which fetal vessels course through membranes and present at the cervical os (Bronsteen, 2013). This is discussed in Chapter 6 (p. 123).

Incidence and Associated Factors

Reported incidences for placenta previa average 0.3 percent or 1 case per 300 to 400 deliveries. It was reported to be almost 1 in 300 deliveries in the United States in 2003 (Martin, 2005). The frequency at Parkland Hospital from 1988 through 2012 was approximately 1 in 360 for nearly 366,000 births. Similar frequencies have been reported from Canada, England, and Israel, but it was only 1 in 700 deliveries from a Japanese study (Crane, 1999; Gurol-Urganci, 2011; Matsuda, 2011; Rosenberg, 2011). Except for the last study, these reported frequencies are remarkably similar considering the lack of precision in definition and classification discussed above.

Several factors increase the risk for placenta previa. One of these—multifetal gestation—seems intuitive because of the larger placental area. And indeed, the incidence of associated previa with twin pregnancy is increased by 30 to 40 percent compared with that of singletons (Ananth, 2003a; Weis, 2012). Many of the other associated factors are less intuitive.

Maternal Age. The frequency of placenta previa increases with maternal age (Biro, 2012). At Parkland Hospital, this incidence increased from a low rate of approximately 1 in 1660 for women 19 years or younger to almost 1 in 100 for women older than 35 (see Fig. 41-16). Coincidental with increasing maternal age in the United States and Australia, the overall incidence of previa has increased substantively (Frederiksen, 1999; Roberts, 2012). The FASTER Trial, which included more than 36,000 women, cited the frequency of previa to be 0.5 percent for women younger than 35 years compared with 1.1 percent in those older than 35 years (Cleary-Goldman, 2005).

Multiparity. The risk for previa increases with parity. The obvious effects of advancing maternal age and parity are confounding. Still, Babinszki and colleagues (1999) reported that the 2.2-percent incidence in women with parity of 5 or greater was increased significantly compared with that of women with lower parity.

Prior Cesarean Delivery. The cumulative risks for placenta previa that accrue with the increasing number of cesarean deliveries are extraordinary. In a Network study of 30,132 women undergoing cesarean delivery, Silver and associates (2006) reported an incidence of 1.3 percent for those with only one prior cesarean delivery, but it was 3.4 percent if there were six or more prior cesarean deliveries. In a retrospective cohort of nearly 400,000 women who were delivered of two consecutive singletons, those with a cesarean delivery for the first pregnancy had a significant 1.6-fold increased risk for previa in the second pregnancy (Gurol-Urganci, 2011). These same investigators reported a 1.5-fold increased risk from six similar population-based cohort studies. Gesteland (2004) and Gilliam (2002) and their coworkers calculated that the likelihood of previa was increased more than eightfold in women with parity greater than 4 and who had more than four prior cesarean deliveries.

Importantly, women with a prior uterine incision and placenta previa have an increased likelihood that cesarean hysterectomy will be necessary for hemostasis because of an associated accrete syndrome (p. 804). In the study by Frederiksen and colleagues (1999), 6 percent of women who had a primary cesarean delivery for previa required a hysterectomy. This rate was 25 percent for women with a previa undergoing repeat cesarean delivery.

Cigarette Smoking. The relative risk of placenta previa is increased at least twofold in women who smoke (Ananth, 2003a; Usta, 2005). It has been postulated that carbon monoxide hypoxemia causes compensatory placental hypertrophy and more surface area. Smoking may also be related to decidual vasculopathy that has been implicated in the genesis of previa.

Elevated Prenatal Screening MSAFP Levels. Women who have otherwise unexplained abnormally elevated prenatal screening levels of maternal serum alpha-fetoprotein (MSAFP) are at increased risk for previa and a host of other abnormalities as discussed on page 806. Moreover, women with a previa who also had a MSAFP level ≥ 2.0 MoM at 16 weeks' gestation were at increased risk for late-pregnancy bleeding and preterm birth. Screening with MSAFP is considered in detail in Chapter 14 (p. 284).

Clinical Features

Painless bleeding is the most characteristic event with placenta previa. Bleeding usually does not appear until near the end of the second trimester or later, but it can begin even before midpregnancy. And undoubtedly, some late abortions are caused by an abnormally located placenta. Bleeding from a previa usually begins without warning and without pain or contractions in a woman who has had an uneventful prenatal course. This so-called *sentinel bleed* is rarely so profuse as to prove fatal. Usually it ceases, only to recur. In perhaps 10 percent of women, particularly those with a placenta implanted near but not over the cervical os, there is no bleeding until labor onset. Bleeding at this time varies from slight to profuse, and it may clinically mimic placental abruption.

A specific sequence of events leads to bleeding in cases in which the placenta is located over the internal os. First, the uterine body remodels to form the lower uterine segment. With this, the internal os dilates, and some of the implanted placenta inevitably separates. Bleeding that ensues is augmented by the inherent inability of myometrial fibers in the lower uterine segment to contract and thereby constrict avulsed vessels. Similarly, bleeding from the lower segment implantation site also frequently continues after placental delivery. Last, there may be lacerations in the friable cervix and lower segment. This may be especially problematic following manual removal of a somewhat adhered placenta.

Abnormally Implanted Placenta. A frequent and serious complication associated with placenta previa arises from its abnormally firm placental attachment. This is anticipated because of poorly developed decidua that lines the lower uterine segment. Biswas and coworkers (1999) performed placental bed biopsies in 50 women with a previa and in 50 control women. Trophoblastic giant-cell infiltration of spiral arterioles—rather than endovascular trophoblast—was found in half of previa specimens. However, only 20 percent from normally implanted placentas had these changes.

Placenta accrete syndromes arise from abnormal placental implantation and adherence and are classified according to the depth of placental ingrowth into the uterine wall. These include *placenta accreta, increta,* and *percreta* (p. 804). In a study of 514 cases of previa reported by Frederiksen and associates (1999), abnormal placental attachment was identified in 7 percent. As discussed above, previa overlying a prior cesarean incision conveys a particularly high risk for accreta.

Coagulation Defects. Placenta previa is rarely complicated by coagulopathy even when there is extensive implantation site separation (Wing, 1996b). Placental thromboplastin, which incites the intravascular coagulation seen with placental abruption, is presumed to readily escape through the cervical canal rather than be forced into the maternal circulation. The paucity of large myometrial veins in this area may also be protective.

Diagnosis

Whenever there is uterine bleeding after midpregnancy, placenta previa or abruption should always be considered. In the Canadian Perinatal Network study discussed on page 783, placenta previa accounted for 21 percent of women admitted from 22 to 28 weeks' gestation with vaginal bleeding (Sabourin, 2012). Previa should not be excluded until sonographic evaluation has clearly proved its absence. Diagnosis by clinical examination is done using the *double set-up* technique because it requires that a finger be passed through the cervix and the placenta palpated. A digital examination should not be performed unless delivery is planned. *A cervical digital examination is done with the woman in an operating room and with preparations for immediate cesarean delivery. Even the gentlest examination can cause torrential hemorrhage.* Fortunately, double set-up examination is rarely necessary because placental location can almost always be ascertained sonographically.

Sonographic Placental Localization. Quick and accurate localization can be accomplished using standard sonographic techniques (Dashe, 2013). In many cases, *transabdominal sonography* is confirmatory, as shown in Figure 41-24A, and an average accuracy of 96 percent has been reported (Laing, 1996). Imprecise results may be caused by bladder distention, so doubtful cases should be confirmed after bladder emptying. Moreover, sometimes a large fundal placenta is not appreciated to extend down to the internal cervical os. *Transvaginal sonography* is safe, and the results are superior as shown in Figures 41-24B and 41-25. In a comparative study by Farine and associates (1988), the internal os was visualized in all cases using transvaginal sonography but was seen in only 70 percent using transabdominal sonography. Transperineal sonography is also accurate to localize placenta previa (Hertzberg, 1992). In a study by Rani and colleagues (2007), placenta previa was correctly identified in 69 of 70 women and was confirmed at delivery. They reported the positive-predictive value to be 98 percent, whereas the negative-predictive value was 100 percent.

Magnetic Resonance Imaging. Although several investigators have reported excellent results using MR imaging to visualize placental abnormalities, it is unlikely that this technique will replace sonography for routine evaluation anytime soon. That said, MR imaging has proved useful for evaluation of placenta accreta (p. 807).

Management of Placenta Previa

Women with a previa are managed depending on their individual clinical circumstances. The three factors that usually

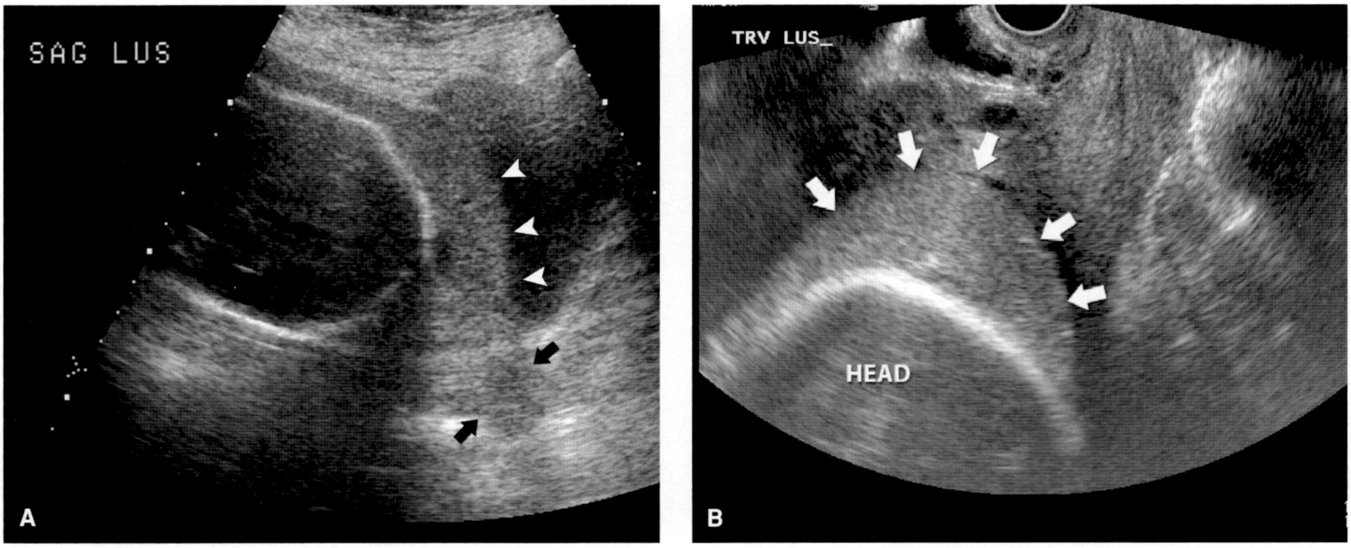

FIGURE 41-24 Total placenta previa. **A.** Transabdominal sonogram shows placenta (*white arrowheads*) covering the cervix (*black arrows*). **B.** Transvaginal sonogram shows placenta (*arrows*), lying between the cervix and fetal head.

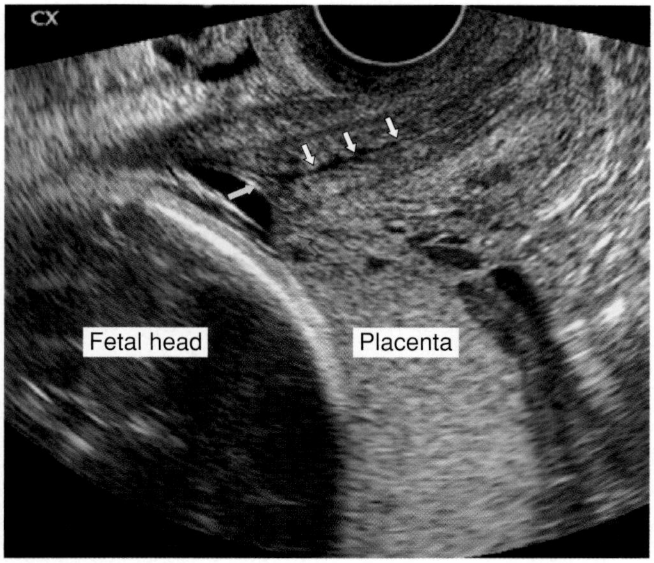

FIGURE 41-25 Transvaginal sonogram of an anterior placenta previa at 36 weeks' gestation. The placental margin (*red arrow*) extends downward toward the cervix. The internal os (*yellow arrow*) and cervical canal (*short white arrows*) are marked to show their relationship to the leading edge of the placenta.

are considered include fetal age and thus maturity; labor; and bleeding and its severity.

If the fetus is preterm and there is no persistent active bleeding, management favors close observation in an obstetrical unit. Data are sparse regarding tocolytic administration for uterine contractions. Although good randomized trials are lacking, Bose and colleagues (2011) recommend that if tocolytics are given, they be limited to 48 hours of administration. We categorically recommend against their use in this setting. After bleeding has ceased for about 2 days and the fetus is judged to be healthy, the woman can usually be discharged home. Importantly, the woman and her family must fully appreciate the possibility of recurrent bleeding and be prepared for immediate transport back to the hospital. In other cases, prolonged hospitalization may be ideal.

In properly selected patients, there appear to be no benefits to inpatient compared with outpatient management (Mouer, 1994; Neilson, 2003). In a randomized study by Wing and colleagues (1996a), no differences in maternal or fetal morbidity were noted with either management method. This trial of inpatient versus home management included 53 women who had a bleeding previa at 24 to 36 weeks' gestation. Of these 53 women, 60 percent had recurrent bleeding. Also, of all 53 women, half eventually required expeditious cesarean delivery. Home management is more economical. In one study, hospital stay length and costs for mother-infant care were reduced by half with outpatient management (Drost, 1994).

For women who are near term and who are not bleeding, plans are made for scheduled cesarean delivery. Timing is important to maximize fetal growth but to minimize the possibility of antepartum hemorrhage. A National Institutes of Health workshop concluded that women with a previa are best served by elective delivery at 36 to 37 completed weeks (Spong, 2011). With suspected placenta accrete syndromes, delivery was recommended at 34 to 35 completed weeks. At Parkland Hospital, we prefer to wait until 37 to 38 weeks before delivery (p. 807).

Delivery

Practically all women with placenta previa undergo cesarean delivery. Many surgeons recommend a vertical skin incision. Cesarean delivery is emergently performed in more than half because of hemorrhage, for which about a fourth require blood transfusion (Boyle, 2009; Sabourin, 2012). Although a low transverse hysterotomy is usually possible, this may cause fetal bleeding if there is an anterior placenta and the placenta is cut through. In such cases, fetal delivery should be expeditious. Thus, a vertical uterine incision may be preferable in some instances. That said, even when the incision extends through the placenta, maternal or fetal outcomes are rarely compromised.

Following placental removal, there may be uncontrollable hemorrhage because of poorly contracted smooth muscle of the lower uterine segment. When hemostasis at the placental implantation site cannot be obtained by pressure, the implantation site can be oversewn with 0-chromic sutures. Cho and associates (1991) described interrupted 0-chromic sutures at 1-cm intervals to form a circle around the bleeding portion of the lower segment to control hemorrhage in all eight women in whom it was employed. Huissoud and coworkers (2012) also described use of circular sutures. Kayem (2011) and Penotti (2012) and their colleagues reported that only 2 of 33 women with a previa and no accreta who had anterior-posterior uterine compression sutures required hysterectomy. Kumru and associates (2013) reported success with the Bakri balloon in 22 of 25 cases. Diemert and coworkers (2012) described good results with combined use of a Bakri balloon and compression sutures. Albayrak and colleagues (2011) described Foley balloon tamponade. Druzin (1989) proposed tightly packing the lower uterine segment with gauze, and the pack was removed transvaginally 12 hours later. Law and coworkers (2010) reported successful use of hemostatic gel. Other methods include bilateral uterine or internal iliac artery ligation as described on page 819. Finally, pelvic artery embolization as described on page 820 has also gained acceptance.

If these more conservative methods fail and bleeding is brisk, then hysterectomy is necessary. Placenta previa—especially with abnormally adhered placental variations—currently is the most frequent indication for peripartum hysterectomy at Parkland Hospital and from other reports (Wong, 2011). It is not possible to accurately estimate the impact on hysterectomy from previa alone without considering the associated accrete syndromes. *Again, for women whose placenta previa is implanted anteriorly at the site of a prior uterine incision, there is an increased likelihood of associated placenta accrete syndrome and need for hysterectomy.* In a study of 318 peripartum hysterectomies from in the United Kingdom, 40 percent were done for abnormally implanted placentation (Knight, 2007). At Parkland Hospital, 44 percent of cesarean hysterectomies were done for bleeding placenta previa or placenta accrete syndrome. In an Australian study of emergency peripartum hysterectomy, 19 percent were done for placenta previa, and another 55 percent for a morbidly adhered placenta (Awan, 2011). The technique for peripartum hysterectomy is described in Chapter 30 (p. 599).

Maternal and Perinatal Outcomes

A marked reduction in maternal mortality rates from placenta previa was achieved during the last half of the 20th century. Still, as shown in Figure 41-2, placenta previa and coexistent accrete syndromes both contribute substantively to maternal morbidity and mortality. In one review, there was a threefold increased maternal mortality ratio of 30 per 100,000 for women with previa (Oyelese, 2006). In another report of 4693 maternal deaths in the United States, placenta previa and accrete syndromes accounted for 17 percent of deaths from hemorrhage (Berg, 2010).

The report from the Consortium on Safe Labor emphasizes the ongoing perinatal morbidity with placenta previa (Lai, 2012). Preterm delivery continues to be a major cause of perinatal death (Nørgaard, 2012). For the United States in 1997, Salihu and associates (2003) reported a threefold increased neonatal mortality rate with placenta previa that was caused primarily from preterm delivery. Ananth and colleagues (2003b) reported a comparably increased risk of neonatal death even for fetuses delivered at term. This is at least partially related to fetal anomalies, which are increased two- to threefold in pregnancies with placenta previa (Crane, 1999).

The association of fetal-growth restriction with placenta previa is likely minimal after controlling for gestational age (Crane, 1999). In a population-based cohort of more than 500,000 singleton births, Ananth and associates (2001a) found that most low-birthweight infants associated with placenta previa resulted from preterm birth. Harper and coworkers (2010) reported similar findings from a cohort of nearly 58,000 women who underwent routine second-trimester sonographic evaluation at their institution.

Placenta Accrete Syndromes

These syndromes describe the abnormally implanted, invasive, or adhered placenta. Derivation of *accrete* comes from the Latin *ac-* + *crescere*—to grow from adhesion or coalescence, to adhere, or to become attached to (Benirschke, 2012). Accrete syndromes thus include any placental implantation with abnormally firm adherence to myometrium because of partial or total absence of the decidua basalis and imperfect development of the fibrinoid or *Nitabuch layer*. If the decidual spongy layer is lacking either partially or totally, then the physiological line of cleavage is absent, and some or all cotyledons are densely anchored. The surface area of the implantation site involved and the depth of trophoblastic tissue ingrowth are variable between women, but all affected placentas can potentially cause significant hemorrhage.

Accrete syndromes have evolved into one of the most serious problems in obstetrics. As subsequently discussed, the likelihood of placenta accrete syndrome is closely linked to prior uterine surgery. Thus, related to the increasing and current all-time high rate of cesarean delivery in the United States, the frequency of placenta accrete syndromes has reached seemingly epidemic proportions. And, at least until recently, there seems to be no consensus for management (Wright, 2013). To better codify some of the serious consequences associated with accrete syndromes, the American College of Obstetricians and Gynecologists (2012b) and the Society for Maternal-Fetal Medicine (2010) have taken the lead to address management problems. Accrete syndromes have also been the subject of recent reviews (Rao, 2012; Wortman, 2013a).

Etiopathogenesis

Microscopically, placental villi are anchored to muscle fibers rather than to decidual cells. Decidual deficiency then prevents normal placental separation after delivery. Intuitive thinking and now substantiated data suggest that accrete syndromes are not solely caused by an anatomical layer deficiency (Tantbirojn, 2008). Evidence indicates that the cytotrophoblasts may control decidual invasion through factors such as angiogenesis and growth expression (Cohen, 2010; Duzyj, 2013; Wehrum, 2011). Indeed, accrete syndrome tissue specimens have shown evidence for "hyperinvasiveness" compared with otherwise uncomplicated previa specimens (Pri-Paz, 2012). The distribution of large vessels is different than that seen with nonaccrete placentas (Chantraine, 2012). As described by Benirschke and colleagues (2012), there is an antecedent "constitutional endometrial defect" in most cases. The increased risk conveyed by previous uterine trauma—for example, cesarean delivery—may be partially explained by an increased vulnerability of the decidua to trophoblast invasion following incision into the decidua (Garmi, 2012).

Classification

Variants of placenta accrete syndrome are classified by the depth of trophoblastic growth (Fig. 41-26). *Placenta accreta* indicates that villi are attached to the myometrium. With *placenta increta,* villi actually invade the myometrium, and *placenta percreta* defines villi that penetrate through the myometrium and to or through the serosa. In clinical practice, these three variants are encountered in an approximate ratio of 80:15:5, respectively (Wong, 2008). In all three varieties, abnormal adherence may involve all lobules—*total placenta accreta* (Fig. 41-27). If all or part of a single lobule is abnormally attached, it is described as a *focal placenta accreta*. Histological diagnosis cannot be made from the placenta alone, and the uterus or curettings with myometrium are necessary for histopathological confirmation (Benirschke, 2012).

Incidence and Associated Conditions

The increased frequency of accrete syndromes during the past 50 years stems from the liberalized use of cesarean delivery. In 1924, Polak and Phelan presented their data from Long Island College Hospital, which had one case of placenta accreta complicating 6000 deliveries. In a 1951 review, a maternal mortality rate of up to 65 percent was cited (McKeogh, 1951). In 1971, in the 14th edition of *Williams Obstetrics*, Hellman and Pritchard described placenta accreta as the subject of case reports. In a review several years later, Breen and coworkers (1977) cited a reported average incidence of 1 in 7000 deliveries.

Since these reports, however, the incidence of accrete syndromes has increased remarkably, in direct relationship to the increasing cesarean delivery rate (Chap. 31, p. 618). The incidence of placenta accrete syndrome was cited as 1 in

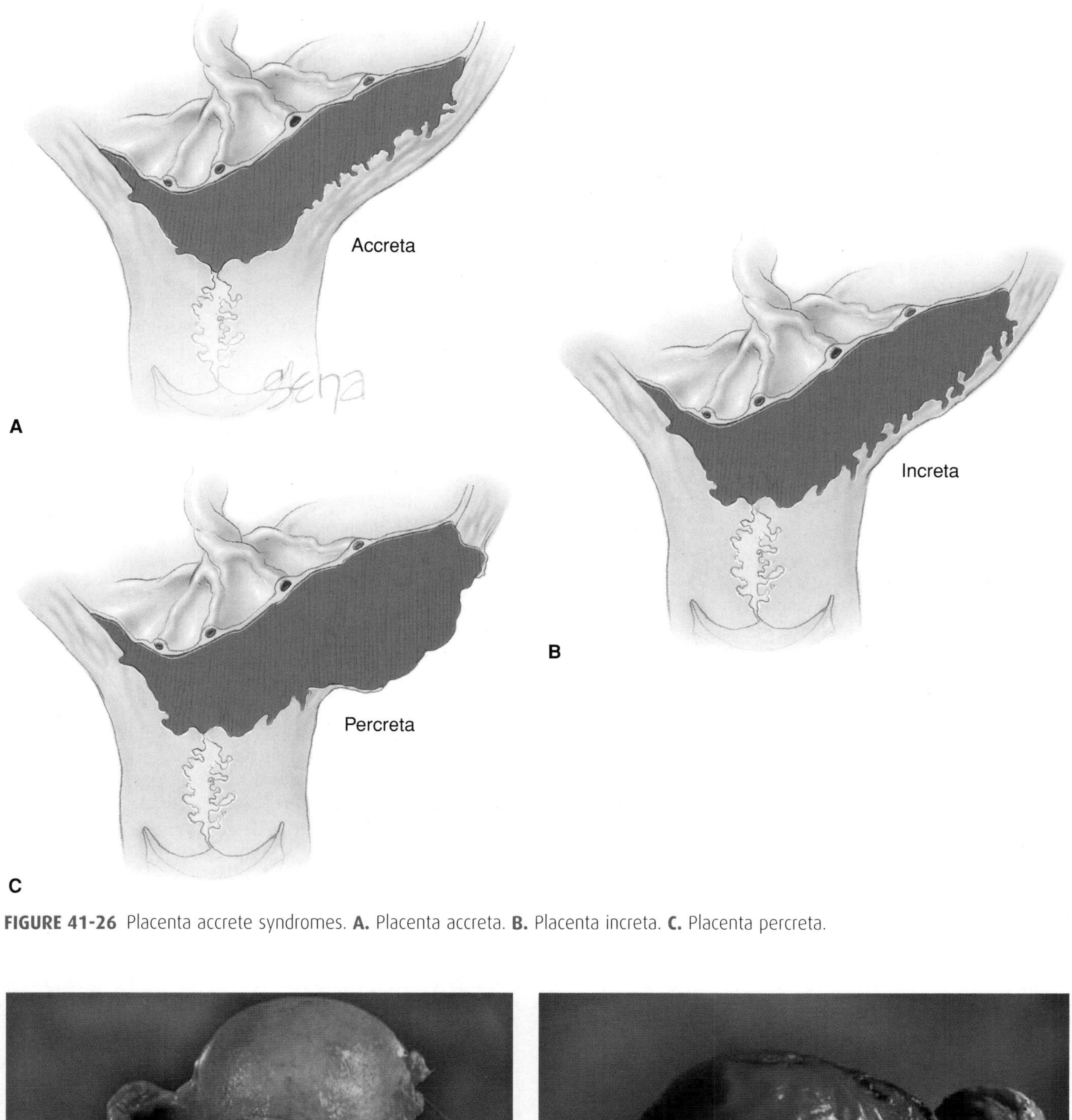

FIGURE 41-26 Placenta accrete syndromes. **A.** Placenta accreta. **B.** Placenta increta. **C.** Placenta percreta.

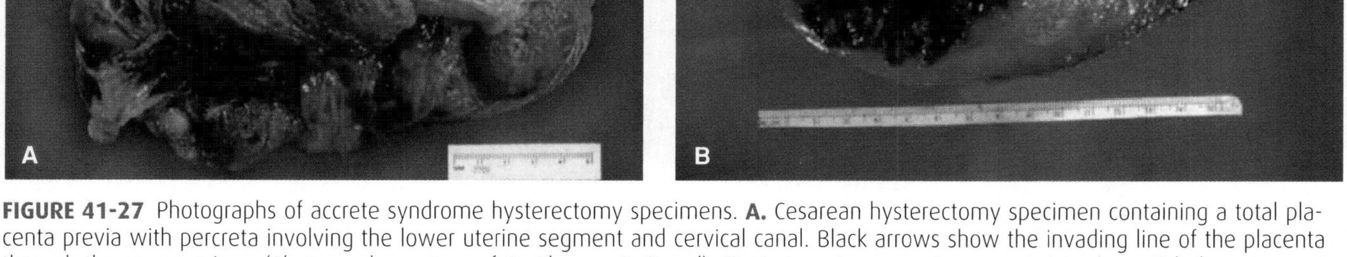

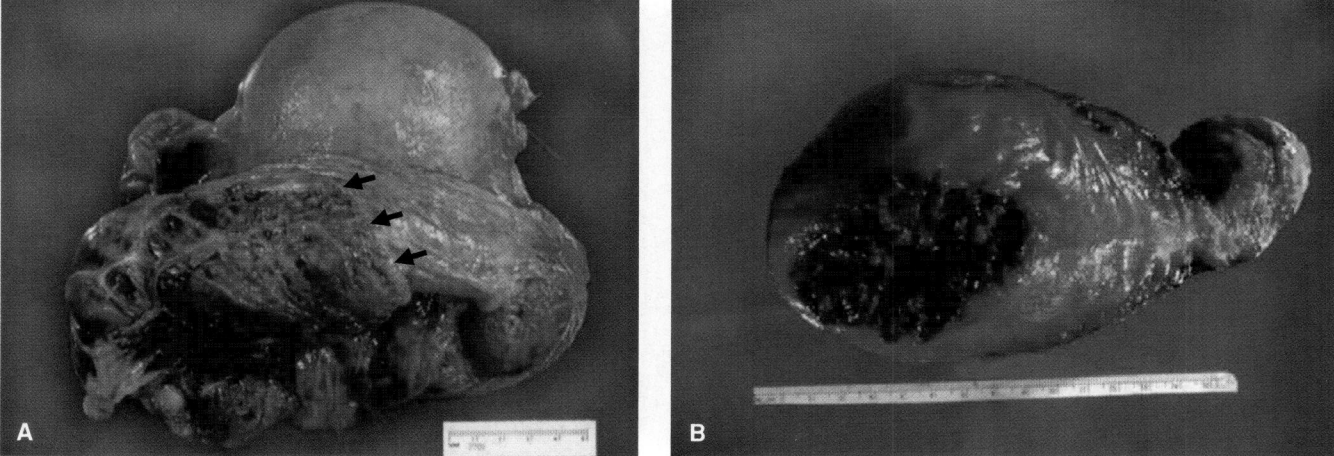

FIGURE 41-27 Photographs of accrete syndrome hysterectomy specimens. **A.** Cesarean hysterectomy specimen containing a total placenta previa with percreta involving the lower uterine segment and cervical canal. Black arrows show the invading line of the placenta through the myometrium. (Photograph courtesy of Dr. Thomas R. Dowd). **B.** Hysterectomy specimen containing a partial placenta previa with placenta percreta that invaded the lateral fundal region to cause hemoperitoneum.

2500 in the 1980s, and currently, the American College of Obstetricians and Gynecologists (2012b) cites it to be as high as 1 in 533 deliveries. Because of this increasing frequency, accrete syndromes are now one of the most serious problems in obstetrics. In addition to their significant contribution to maternal morbidity and mortality, accrete syndromes are a leading cause of intractable postpartum hemorrhage and emergency peripartum hysterectomy (Awan, 2011; Eller, 2011; Rossi, 2010). Their contribution as a cause of maternal deaths from hemorrhage is shown in Figure 41-2. *In their review of nearly 10,000 pregnancy-related maternal deaths in the United States, Berg and associates (2010) reported that 8 percent of deaths due to hemorrhage were caused by accrete syndromes.*

Risk Factors

These are similar in many aspects to those for placenta previa (p. 801). That said, the two most important risk factors are an associated previa, a prior cesarean delivery, and more likely a combination of the two. In one study, an accrete placenta more likely followed emergency compared with elective cesarean delivery (Kamara, 2013). A classical hysterotomy incision has a higher risk for a subsequent accrete placenta (Gyamfi-Bannerman, 2012). Decidual formation may be defective over a previous hysterotomy scar, and it also may follow any type of myometrial trauma such as curettage (Benirschke, 2012). Myomectomy apparently confers a low risk (Gyamfi-Bannerman, 2012). In one study, 10 percent of women with a previa had an associated accrete placenta. In another study, almost half of women with a prior cesarean delivery had myometrial fibers seen microscopically adhered to the placenta (Hardardottir, 1996; Zaki, 1998). Findings from a Maternal-Fetal Medicine Units Network study by Silver and colleagues (2006) of women with one or more prior cesarean deliveries who also had a placenta previa are shown in Figure 41-28. The astonishing increase in frequency of associated accrete syndromes is apparent.

Another risk factor became apparent with widespread use of MSAFP and human chorionic gonadotropin (hCG) screening for neural-tube defects and aneuploidies (Chap. 14, p. 285). In a study reported by Hung (1999) of more than 9300 women screened at 14 to 22 weeks, the risk for accrete syndromes was increased eightfold with MSAFP levels > 2.5 MoM, and it was increased fourfold when maternal free β-hCG levels were > 2.5 MoM.

Cesarean-Scar Pregnancy. In some women with an accrete placenta, there may be adverse outcomes before fetal viability. One presentation generally referred to as a *cesarean scar pregnancy* clinically is similar to that of an ectopic pregnancy. Its frequency has been reported to be approximately 1 in 2000 pregnancies (Ash, 2007; Rotas, 2006). Timor-Tritsch (2012) provided a scholarly review of 751 such cases, and the subject is discussed in detail in Chapter 19 (p. 391).

Clinical Presentation and Diagnosis

In cases of first- and second-trimester accrete syndromes, there is usually hemorrhage that is the consequence of coexisting placenta previa. Such bleeding will usually prompt evaluation and management. In some women who do not have an associated previa, accreta may not be identified until third-stage labor when an adhered placenta is encountered.

Ideally, abnormal placental ingrowth is identified antepartum, usually by sonography (Chantraine, 2013; Tam Tam, 2012). For gray-scale transvaginal sonography, the American College of Obstetricians and Gynecologists (2012b) cites a sensitivity of 77 to 87 percent, specificity of 96 to 98 percent, and a positive- and negative-predictive value of 65 to 93 and 98 percent, respectively. Individual studies have reported similar findings (Chalubinski, 2013; Elhawary, 2013; Maher, 2013). Although controversial, at Parkland Hospital, we have found that the addition of Doppler color flow mapping is highly predictive of myometrial invasion (Fig. 41-29). This is suspected

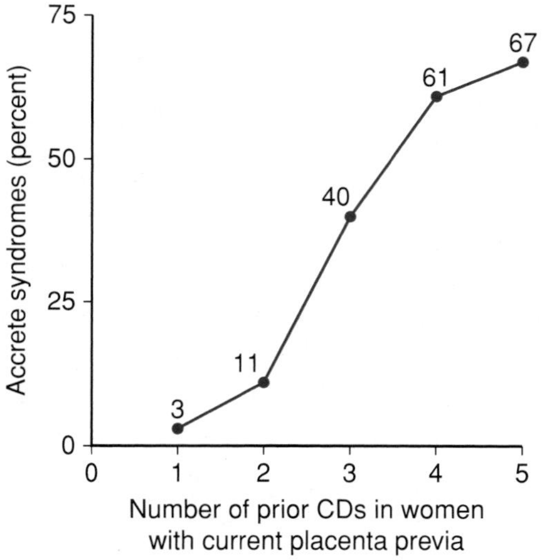

FIGURE 41-28 Frequency of accreta syndromes in women with 1 to 5 prior cesarean deliveries (CDs) now with a previa. (Data from Silver, 2006.)

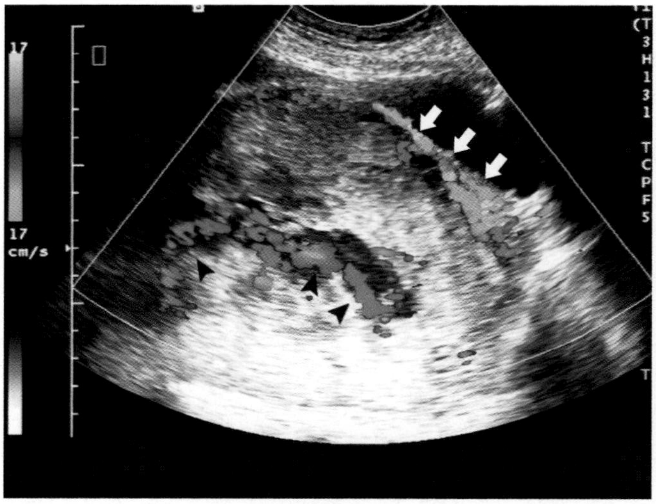

FIGURE 41-29 Transvaginal sonogram of placental invasion with accrete syndrome. Retroplacental vessels (*white arrows*) invade the myometrium and obscure the bladder-serosal interface. Abnormal intraplacental venous lakes (*black arrowheads*) are commonly seen in this setting.

if the distance between the uterine serosa-bladder wall interface and the retroplacental vessels is < 1 mm and if there are large intraplacental lacunae (Twickler, 2000). Similarly, Cali and associates (2013) reported that hypervascularity of the uterine serosa-bladder wall interface had the highest positive- and negative-predictive values for placenta percreta.

MR imaging can be used as an adjunct to sonography to define anatomy, degree of invasion, and possible ureteral or bladder involvement (Chalubinski, 2013; Palacios Jaraquemada, 2005). Lax and coworkers (2007) identified three MR imaging findings that suggested accreta. These include uterine bulging, heterogeneous signal intensity within the placenta, and dark intraplacental bands on T2-weighted imaging. Some suggest MR imaging when sonography results are inconclusive or there is a posterior previa (American College of Obstetricians and Gynecologists, 2012b; Elhawary, 2013).

Management

Preoperative assessment should begin at the time of recognition during prenatal care (Fitzpatrick, 2014; Sentilhes, 2013). A major decision concerns the ideal institution for delivery. Exigencies to be considered are appropriate surgical, anesthesia, and blood banking capabilities. An obstetrical surgeon or gynecological oncologist as well as surgical, urological, and interventional radiological consultants should all be available (Eller, 2011; Stafford, 2008). The American College of Obstetricians and Gynecologists (2012b) and the Society for Maternal-Fetal Medicine (2010) recommend planned delivery in a tertiary-care facility. In some of these, especially designed teams have been assembled and are on call (Walker, 2013). Women who refuse blood or its derivatives pose especially difficult management decisions (Barth, 2011). If possible, delivery is best scheduled for peak availability of all resources and team members. However, emergency contingent plans should also be in place.

Timing of Delivery. To accomplish scheduled surgical intervention, preterm delivery is necessary and justified given the serious adverse maternal consequences of emergency cesarean delivery. The American College of Obstetricians and Gynecologists (2012b) recommends individualization of delivery timing. It cites a decision-analysis study that justifies elective delivery without fetal lung maturity testing after 34 completed weeks (Robinson, 2010). The results of two recent surveys indicate that most practitioners do not deliver these women until 36 weeks or later (Esakoff, 2012; Wright, 2013). At Parkland Hospital, we generally schedule these procedures after 36 completed weeks but are prepared also to manage them in nonelective situations.

Preoperative Arterial Catheterization. There has been enthusiasm for placement of intraarterial catheters to mitigate blood loss and to enhance surgical visibility. Balloon-tipped catheters advanced into the internal iliac arteries are inflated after delivery to occlude pelvic blood flow to aid placental removal and hysterectomy (Ballas, 2012; Desai, 2012). Alternatively, the catheters can be used to embolize bleeding arterial sites. Others have concluded that these procedures offer borderline efficacy and have serious risks (Sentilhes, 2009; Yu, 2009). Complications have included thromboses of the common and left iliac arteries (Bishop, 2011; Greenberg, 2007). At this time, we agree with the American College of Obstetricians and Gynecologists (2012b) that a firm recommendation cannot be made for or against their use.

Cesarean Delivery and Hysterectomy. Before commencing with delivery, the risk of hysterectomy to prevent exsanguination should be estimated. Confirmation of a percreta or increta almost always mandates hysterectomy. However, some of these abnormal placentations, especially if partial, may be amenable to placental delivery with hemostatic suture placement. Because the scope of invasion may not be apparent before delivery of the fetus, we usually attempt to create a wide bladder flap *before* making the hysterotomy incision. The round ligaments are divided, and the lateral edges of the peritoneal reflection are dissected downward. If possible, these incisions are extended to encircle the entire placental implantation site that visibly occupies the prevesical space and posterior bladder wall. Following this, a classical hysterotomy incision is made to avoid the placenta and profuse hemorrhage before fetal delivery. Some advocate a transverse fundal incision if the placenta occupies the entire anterior wall (Kotsuji, 2013).

After fetal delivery, the extent of placental invasion is assessed without attempts at manual placental removal. In a report from the United Kingdom, attempts for partial or total placental removal prior to hysterectomy were associated with twice as much blood loss (Fitzpatrick, 2014). Generally speaking, with obvious percreta or increta, hysterectomy is usually the best course, and the placenta is left in situ. As discussed in Chapter 36 (p. 670), a focal partial accreta may avulse easily and later emerge as a placental polyp (Benirschke, 2012). With more extensive placental ingrowth—even with total accreta—there may be little or no bleeding until manual placental removal is attempted. Unless there is spontaneous separation with bleeding that mandates emergency hysterectomy, the operation begins after full assessment is made. With bleeding, successful treatment depends on immediate blood replacement therapy and other measures that include uterine or internal iliac artery ligation, balloon occlusion, or embolization. Various case reports have described argon beam coagulation and hemostatic combat gauze (Karam, 2003; Schmid, 2012).

Leaving the Placenta in Situ. In a few cases, after the fetus has been delivered, it may be possible to trim the umbilical cord and repair the hysterotomy incision but leave the placenta in situ. This may be wise for women in whom abnormal placentation was not suspected before cesarean delivery and in whom uterine closure stops bleeding. After this, she can be transferred to a higher-level facility for definitive management. Another consideration is the woman with a strong desire for fertility and who has received extensive counseling. In some cases, the placenta spontaneously resorbs. In others, a subsequent hysterectomy—either planned or prompted by bleeding or infection—is performed weeks postpartum when blood loss might be lessened (Hays, 2008; Kayem, 2002; Lee, 2008; Timmermans, 2007). Of 26 women treated this way, 21 percent ultimately required hysterectomy. Of the remainder, most required additional medical and surgical interventions for bleeding and infection (Bretelle, 2007). Evidence that treatment with methotrexate aids resorption is lacking. We agree with the American College of Obstetricians and Gynecologists (2012b) that this method of management is seldom indicated. For women in whom the placenta is left in situ, serial serum β-hCG measurements are not informative, and serial sonographic or MR imaging is recommended (Timmermans, 2007; Worley, 2008).

Pregnancy Outcomes

Reports describing outcomes with accrete syndromes have limited numbers of patients. That said, two large series provide data from which some basic observations can be made. First, these syndromes can have disastrous outcomes for both mother and fetus. Although the depth of placental invasion does not correspond with perinatal outcome, it is of paramount maternal significance (Seet, 2012). Shown in Table 41-5 are outcomes from three reports of women from tertiary-care hospitals and in whom the diagnosis of accrete placenta was made preoperatively. Despite these advantages, a litany of complications included hemorrhage, urinary tract injury, ICU admission, and secondary surgical procedures. These reports chronicled outcomes in a second cohort of women in whom care was not given at a tertiary-care facility or in whom the diagnosis of accrete placenta was not made until delivery, or both. In these cohorts, morbidity was higher, and there was one maternal death.

Second, in the Utah experiences, attempts at placental removal increased morbidity significantly—67 versus 36 percent—compared with no attempts at removal before hysterectomy. They also found that preoperative bilateral ureteral stenting reduced morbidity. However, no benefits accrued from internal iliac artery ligation (Eller, 2011; Po, 2012). Our management at Parkland Hospital is similar, however, the final decision for hysterectomy is not made until assessment at delivery. Also, we do not routinely perform preoperative ureteral stent placement. We have at times inserted stents transvesically if indicated intraoperatively. As discussed on page 820, preoperative arterial catheterization may be beneficial (Desai, 2012).

Subsequent Pregnancy

There is some evidence that women with accrete syndromes have an increased risks for recurrence, uterine rupture, hysterectomy, and previa (Eshkoli, 2013).

CONSUMPTIVE COAGULOPATHY

Obstetrical syndromes commonly termed *consumptive coagulopathy* or *disseminated intravascular coagulation (DIC)* were described in the 1901 report by DeLee in which "temporary hemophilia" developed with placental abruption or with a long-dead macerated fetus. In ensuing decades, similar—but frequently less intense—coagulopathic syndromes have been described for almost all areas of medicine (Levi, 2010b; Montagnana, 2010).

Disseminated Intravascular Coagulation in Pregnancy

Because of many definitions used and its variable severity, citing an accurate incidence for consumptive coagulopathy is not possible in pregnant women. For example, as will be discussed, some degree of significant coagulopathy is found with most cases of placental abruption and amnionic-fluid embolism. Other instances in which frequently occurring but insignificant degrees of coagulation activation can be found include sepsis,

TABLE 41-5. Selected Maternal Outcomes in Women with Accrete Syndromes Identified Prenatally and Delivered in Tertiary-Care Units

Outcome[a]	San Diego[b] n = 62	Utah[c] n = 60	Toronto[d] n = 33
Gestational age (wk)	33.9 ± 1.1	34 (17–41)	~ 32 (19–39)
Operating time (min)	194 ± 1.6	NS	107 (68–334)
Transfusions	~ 75%	70%	
RBC (units)	4.7 ± 2.2	≥ 4 (30%)	3.5 (0–20)
FFP (units)	4.1 ± 2.3	NS	NS
Surgical outcomes			
Bladder injury	14 (23%)	22 (37%)	10 (30%)
Ureteral injury	5 (8%)	4 (7%)	0
Postoperative			
ICU admission	43 (72%)	18 (30%)	5 (15%)
LOS (days)	7.4 ± 1.8	4 (3–13%)	5 (2–13)
Readmission	NS	7 (12%)	1 (3%)
Reoperation	NS	5 (8%)	0

[a]Outcomes shown as mean ± 1SD; as median (range); or as number (%).
[b]Data from Warshak, 2010.
[c]Data from Eller, 2011.
[d]Data from Walker, 2013.
FFP = fresh-frozen plasma; ICU = intensive care unit; LOS = length of stay; NS = not stated; RBC = red blood cells.

thrombotic microangiopathies, acute kidney injury, and preeclampsia and HELLP (hemolysis, elevated liver enzyme levels, low platelet count) syndromes (Rattray, 2012; Su, 2012). Although profound consumptive coagulopathy can be associated with fatty liver disease of pregnancy, diminished hepatic synthesis of procoagulants makes a significant contribution (Nelson, 2013).

When consumptive coagulopathy is severe, the likelihood of maternal and perinatal morbidity and mortality is increased. Rattray and colleagues (2012) described 49 cases from Nova Scotia during a 30-year period. Antecedent causes included placental abruption, obstetrical hemorrhage, preeclampsia and HELLP syndromes, acute fatty liver, sepsis, and amnionic-fluid embolism. Of these, 59 percent received blood transfusions, 18 percent underwent hysterectomy, 6 percent were dialyzed, and there were three maternal deaths. The perinatal mortality rate was 30 percent.

Pregnancy-Induced Coagulation Changes

Several changes in coagulation and fibrinolysis can be documented during normal pregnancy. Some of these include appreciable increases in the plasma concentrations of factors I (fibrinogen), VII, VIII, IX, and X. A partial list of these normal values can be found in the Appendix (p. 1288) and in Chapter 4 (p. 57). At the same time, plasminogen levels are increased considerably, but levels of plasminogen activator inhibitor-1 and -2 (PAI-1 and PAI-2) also increase. Thus, *plasmin activity* usually decreases until after delivery (Hale, 2012; Hui, 2012). The mean platelet count decreases by 10 percent during pregnancy, and there is increased platelet activation (Kenny, 2014).

The net results of these changes include increased levels of fibrinopeptide A, β-thromboglobulin, platelet factor 4, and fibrinogen-fibrin degradation products, which includes D-dimers. Along with decreased concentrations of anticoagulant protein S, hypercoagulability, and decreased fibrinolysis, there is augmented—yet compensated—intravascular coagulation that may function to maintain the uteroplacental interface.

Pathological Activation of Coagulation

Normal coagulation and fibrinolysis can be pathologically activated via two pathways. The *extrinsic pathway* is active by thromboplastin from tissue destruction, whereas the *intrinsic pathway* is initiated by collagen and other tissue components that become exposed with loss of endothelial integrity (Fig. 41-30). Tissue factor III is an integral membrane protein. It is released by endothelial cells to complex with factor VII, which in turn activates tenase (factor IX) and prothrombinase (factor X) complexes. Uncontrolled thrombin generation converts fibrinogen to fibrin, which polymerizes to deposit in small vessels of virtually every organ system. This seldom causes organ failure, because these vessels are protected by enhanced fibrinolysis stimulated by fibrin monomers released by coagulation. These monomers combine with tissue plasminogen activator and plasminogen to release plasmin, which lyses fibrinogen and fibrin monomers and polymers.

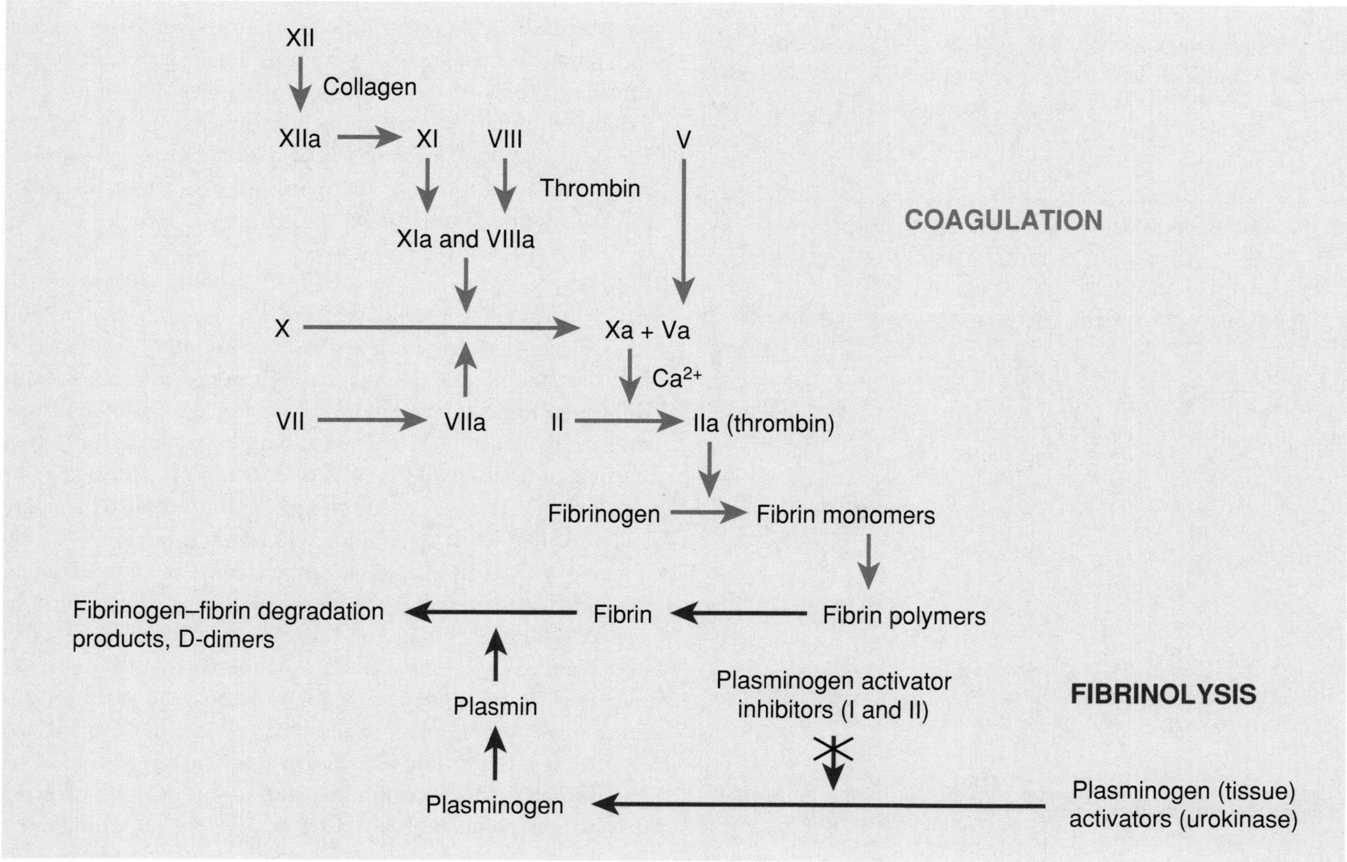

FIGURE 41-30 Mechanisms of coagulation and fibrinolysis.

The products form a series of fibrinogen-fibrin derivatives that are measured by immunoassay. These are the *fibrin degradation products* or *fibrin-split products,* which include D-*dimers* (see Fig. 41-30). There may also be evidence for *microangiopathic hemolysis* from mechanical trauma to the red cell membrane by fibrin strands in small vessels. This is likely a contributing cause of hemolysis in women with preeclampsia and HELLP syndromes (Pritchard, 1976a).

The pathologically activated cycle of coagulation and fibrinolysis becomes clinically important when coagulation factors and platelets are sufficiently depleted to cause bleeding—hence, *consumptive coagulopathy.* Several obstetrical conditions are accompanied by release of potent inciting factors for clinically significant consumptive coagulation. The best known and most common, and therefore most serious, results from thromboplastin release with placental abruption. Also, unique to obstetrics is the immediate and profound coagulation factor depletion that can follow entry of amnionic fluid into the maternal circulation. This causes activation of factor X by abundant mucin in fetal squames. Other causes include activation by release of endotoxins from gram-negative bacteria and exotoxins from gram-positive bacteria.

Diagnosis

The International Society on Thrombosis and Haemostasis has promulgated a *DIC score* to aid identification and prognosis prediction (Taylor, 2001). This algorithm, shown in Table 41-6, has not been applied in obstetrical conditions but can serve as a rough guideline to identify a pregnant woman with consumptive coagulopathy. Again, although not including obstetrical patients, the Prowess Trial evaluated 840 subjects with severe sepsis. The mortality rate increased from approximately 25 percent with a DIC score of 3 to 70 percent with a score of 7 (Dhainaut, 2004).

TABLE 41-6. Algorithm for Diagnosis of Overt Disseminated Intravascular Coagulation—"DIC Score"[a]

Factor	Score
Presence of known underlying disorder associated with DIC: no = 0; yes = 2	____
Coagulation tests:	
Platelets: > 100K = 0; < 100K = 1; < 50K = 2	____
D-dimer levels increased: no = 0; moderate = 2; strong = 3	____
PT prolongation (sec): < 3 = 0; > 3 but < 6 = 1; > 6 = 2	____
Fibrinogen (mg/dL): > 100 mg/dL = 0; < 100 mg/dL = 1	____
Total score:	
≥ 5: compatible with overt DIC	
< 5: suggestive of nonovert DIC	____

[a]From the International Society on Thrombosis and Haemostasis.
PT = prothrombin time.
Adapted from Taylor, 2001.

Evaluation and Management

Obstetrical causes of consumptive coagulopathy are almost always due to an identifiable, underlying pathological process that must be eliminated to halt ongoing defibrination. Thus, prompt identification and removal of the source of the coagulopathy is given priority. With surgical incisions or extensive lacerations accompanied by severe hemorrhage, rapid replacement of procoagulants is usually indicated. Vigorous restoration and maintenance of the circulation to treat hypovolemia cannot be overemphasized. With adequate perfusion, activated coagulation factors, fibrin, and fibrin degradation products are promptly removed by the reticuloendothelial system, along with restoration of hepatic and endothelial synthesis of procoagulants.

Some treatments for intravascular coagulation have been conceived by armchair theorists and are mentioned here only to be condemned. For example, in years past, some recommended heparin administration to block consumption of procoagulants. Others recommended epsilon-aminocaproic acid to inhibit fibrinolysis by blocking plasminogen conversion to plasmin. The dangers of giving heparin to an actively bleeding woman are obvious. Fibrinolysis inhibition is probably not quite as dangerous, but any putative benefits remain unproven.

Identification of Defective Hemostasis. *Bioassay* is an excellent method to detect or suspect clinically significant coagulopathy. *Excessive bleeding at sites of modest trauma characterizes defective hemostasis.* Examples include persistent bleeding from venipuncture sites, nicks from shaving the perineum or abdomen, trauma from bladder catheterization, and spontaneous bleeding from the gums, nose, or gastrointestinal tract. Purpuric areas at pressure sites such as sphygmomanometer cuffs or tourniquets suggest significant thrombocytopenia. As discussed, any surgical procedure provides the ultimate bioassay and elicits generalized oozing from the skin, subcutaneous and fascial tissues, the retroperitoneal space, the episiotomy, or incisions and dissections for cesarean delivery or hysterectomy.

Fibrinogen and Degradation Products. In late pregnancy, plasma fibrinogen levels typically have increased to 300 to 600 mg/dL. Even with severe consumptive coagulopathy, levels may sometimes be high enough to protect against clinically significant hypofibrinogenemia. For example, defibrination caused by a placental abruption might lower an initial fibrinogen level of 600 mg/dL to 250 mg/dL. Although this would indicate massive fibrinogen consumption, there are still adequate levels to promote clinical coagulation—usually about 150 mg/dL. If serious *hypofibrinogenemia*—less than 50 mg/dL—is present, the clot formed from whole blood in a glass tube may initially be soft but not necessarily remarkably reduced in volume. Then, over the next half hour or so, as platelet-induced clot retraction develops, the clot becomes quite small. When many of the erythrocytes are extruded, the volume of liquid in the tube clearly exceeds that of clot.

Fibrinolysis cleaves fibrin and fibrinogen into various fibrin degradation products that are detected by several sensitive test systems. There are many fragment types, and monoclonal antibodies in assay kits usually measure D-dimers specific for that assay. These values are always abnormally high with clinically significant consumptive coagulopathy. At least in obstetrical disorders, quantification has not been correlated with outcomes, although "moderate" to "strong" increases constitute part of the diagnostic algorithm shown in Table 41-6.

Thrombocytopenia

Seriously low platelet concentrations are likely if petechiae are abundant or if clotted blood fails to retract within an hour or so. Confirmation is provided by a platelet count. If there is associated severe preeclampsia syndrome, there may also be *qualitative platelet dysfunction* (Chap. 40, p. 738).

Prothrombin and Partial Thromboplastin Times

Prolongation of these standard coagulation tests may result from appreciable reductions in procoagulants essential for generating thrombin, from very low fibrinogen concentrations, or from appreciable amounts of circulating fibrinogen-fibrin degradation products. Prolongation of the prothrombin time and partial thromboplastin time need not be the consequence of consumptive coagulopathy.

Placental Abruption

This is the most common cause of severe consumptive coagulopathy in obstetrics and is discussed on page 793.

Preeclampsia Syndrome

Endothelial activation or injury is a hallmark of preeclampsia, eclampsia, and HELLP syndrome. In general, the clinical severity of preeclampsia is directly correlated with thrombocytopenia and fibrinogen-fibrin degradation products (Levi, 2010b; Kenny, 2014). That said, intravascular coagulation is seldom clinically worrisome. Delivery reverses these changes, and treatment until then is supportive. These syndromes are discussed in detail in Chapter 40.

Fetal Death and Delayed Delivery

Consumptive coagulopathy associated with prolonged retention of a dead fetus is unusual today because fetal death can be easily confirmed and there are highly effective methods for labor induction. Currently, the syndrome is only occasionally encountered when there is one dead twin fetus and an ongoing pregnancy. With singleton pregnancies, if the dead fetus is undelivered, most women enter spontaneous labor within 2 weeks. Gross disruption of maternal coagulation rarely develops before 4 weeks (Pritchard, 1959, 1973). After 1 month, however, almost a fourth will develop consumptive coagulopathy.

The pathogenesis of coagulopathy appears to be mediated by thromboplastin released by the dead fetus and the placenta (Jimenez, 1968; Lerner, 1967). Typically, the fibrinogen concentration falls during 6 weeks or more to levels that are normal for nonpregnant adults, but in some cases, this declines to < 100 mg/dL. Simultaneously, fibrin degradation product and D-dimer levels become elevated in serum, and moderate thrombocytopenia develops (Pritchard, 1973). If enough time elapses to seal the placental-decidual interface, these coagulation defects may correct spontaneously before evacuation (Pritchard, 1959).

Discordant Fetal Death in Multifetal Gestation

Obvious coagulation derangement occasionally develops in a multifetal pregnancy in which there is at least one fetal death and survival of another (Chescheir, 1988; Landy, 1989). This situation is uncommon, and in one study of 22 such pregnancies, none developed a coagulopathy (Petersen, 1999). Most cases are seen in monochorionic twins with shared circulations, which are described in Chapter 45 (p. 904). The course in such a woman cared for at Parkland Hospital is shown in Figure 41-31. In this case, the coagulopathy ceased spontaneously, and the surviving healthy twin was delivered near term. The placenta of the long-dead fetus was filled with fibrin.

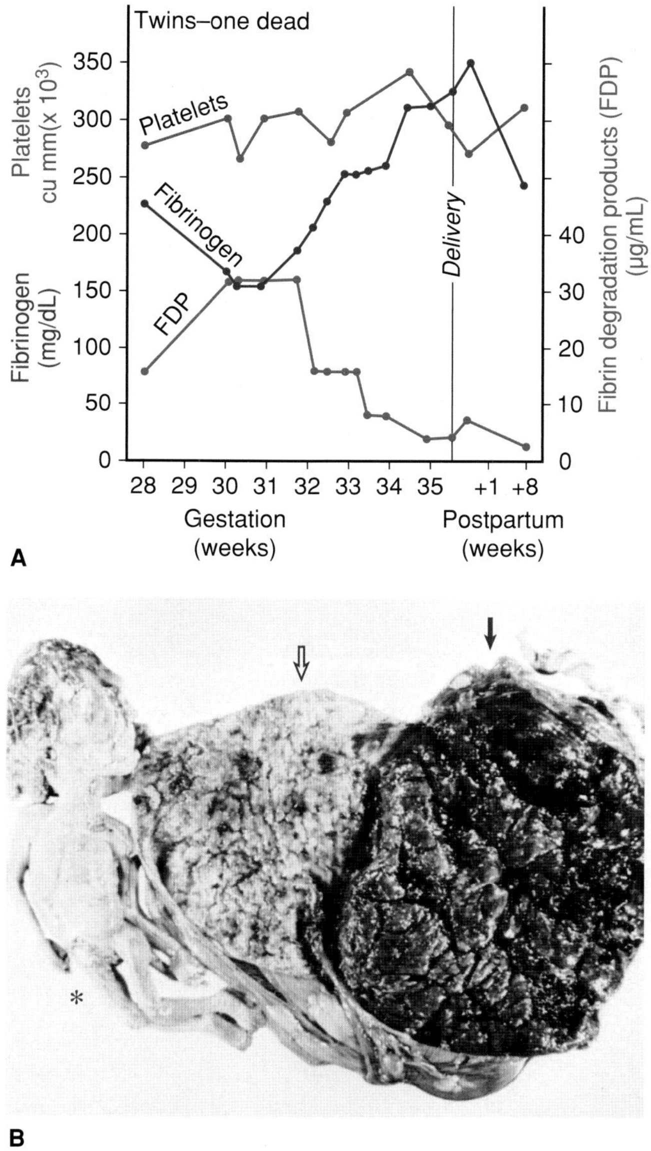

FIGURE 41-31 A. Following the confirmed death of one twin at 28 weeks' gestation, serial studies demonstrated decreasing plasma fibrinogen concentrations and elevated serum fibrin-degradation products that reached a nadir 4 weeks later. After this, fibrinogen concentrations increased and fibrin degradation product levels decreased in mirror-like fashion. **B.** When delivered at 36 weeks, the fibrin-filled placenta (*clear arrow*) of the long-dead fetus (*asterisk*) is apparent. The liveborn cotwin was healthy and had normal coagulation studies and a normal-appearing placenta (*blue arrow*).

Amnionic-Fluid Embolism

This uniquely obstetrical syndrome was described in 1941 by Steiner and Lushbaugh and became classically characterized by the abrupt onset of hypotension, hypoxia, and severe consumptive coagulopathy. Even so, amnionic-fluid embolism has great individual variation in its clinical manifestation. For example, only one of these three clinical hallmarks predominates in some affected women.

Despite variations in the reported incidence of this uncommon but extremely important complication, many reports describe a similar frequency. A study that included 3 million births in the United States cited an estimated frequency of 7.7 cases per 100,000 births (Abenhaim, 2008). The United Kingdom Obstetric Surveillance System reported an incidence of 2.0 per 100,000 births (Knight, 2010). And review of more than 4 million births in Canada yielded an incidence of 2.5 per 100,000 births (Kramer, 2012). Another review of data from five high-resource countries cites frequencies from 1.9 to 6.1 per 100,000 deliveries. The case-fatality rates in all of these studies ranged from 11 to 43 percent. From another perspective, amnionic-fluid embolism was the cause of 10 to 15 percent of all pregnancy-related deaths in the United States and Canada (Berg, 2003; 2010; Clark, 2008; Kramer, 2012).

Predisposing conditions are rapid labor, meconium-stained amnionic fluid, and tears into uterine and other large pelvic veins. Other risk factors commonly cited include older maternal age; postterm pregnancy; labor induction or augmentation; eclampsia; cesarean, forceps, or vacuum delivery; placental abruption or previa; and hydramnios (Knight, 2010, 2012; Kramer, 2012). The association of uterine hypertonus appears to be the *effect* rather than the *cause* of amnionic-fluid embolism. This is likely because uterine blood flow ceases when intrauterine pressures exceed 35 to 40 mm Hg. Thus, a hypertonic contraction would be the *least* likely circumstance for amnionic fluid and other debris to enter uterine veins (Clark, 1995). Because of this, there is also no association between this disorder and hypertonus from oxytocin.

In obvious cases of amnionic-fluid embolism, the clinical picture is unquestionably dramatic. The classic example is that of a woman in the late stages of labor or immediately postpartum who begins gasping for air and then rapidly suffers seizures or cardiorespiratory arrest complicated by massive hemorrhage from consumptive coagulopathy. It has become apparent that there is a variation in the clinical manifestations of this condition. For example, we and others have managed several women in whom otherwise uncomplicated vaginal or cesarean delivery was followed by severe acute consumptive coagulopathy without overt cardiorespiratory difficulties. In those women, consumptive coagulopathy appears to be the *forme fruste* of amnionic-fluid embolism (Kramer, 2012; Porter, 1996).

Etiopathogenesis

Some amnionic fluid commonly enters the maternal circulation at the time of normal delivery through a minor breach in the physiological barrier between maternal and fetal compartments. Thus, it is fortunate that infused amnionic fluid is generally innocuous, even in large amounts (Adamsons, 1971; Stolte, 1967). At delivery, squames, other cellular elements of fetal origin, and trophoblasts can be identified in maternal peripheral blood (Clark, 1986; Lee, 1986). These are presumed to enter venous channels from the placental implantation site or from small lacerations that inevitably develop in the lower uterine segment or cervix with delivery. Although these events are usually innocuous, amnionic fluid constituents in some women initiate a complex series of pathophysiological sequelae shown in Table 41-7. The wide range of clinical manifestations underscores the subjective nature of diagnosis of many of these women.

Considering the wide spectrum of cardiovascular pathophysiological aberrations and sometimes profound coagulopathy, one can reasonably conclude that amnionic fluid and its constituents have a multitude of actions. For example, tissue factor in amnionic fluid presumably activates factor X to incite coagulation (Ecker, 2012; Levi, 2013). Others that have been described include endothelin-1 expressed by fetal squames, phosphatidylserine expressed by amnion, and complement activators (Khong, 1998; Zhou, 2009). An anaphylactoid reaction with complement activation has been postulated because serum levels of tryptase and histamine are also elevated (Benson, 2001; Clark, 1995).

TABLE 41-7. Clinical Findings in 204 Women with Amnionic-Fluid Embolism

Clinical Findings	Clark (1995) n = 46	Weiwen (2000) n = 38	Kramer (2012) n = 120	Aggregate (%)
Hypotension	43	38	39	~60
Fetal distress	30/30	NS	NS	> 90
Pulmonary edema or ARDS	28/30	11	~44	~45
Cardiopulmonary arrest	40	38	56	~65
Cyanosis	38	38	NS	~90
Coagulopathy	38	12/16	36	~50
Dyspnea	22/45	38	~17	~75
Seizure	22	6	2	~15

Author data presents number of affected women. Denominators reflect circumstances in which the whole cohort was not evaluated for a particular finding.
ARDS = acute respiratory distress syndrome; NS = not stated.

Pathophysiology

Animal studies in primates and goats have provided important insights into central hemodynamic aberrations caused by amnionic fluid infused intravenously (Adamsons, 1971; Hankins, 1993). In general, evidence for fetal debris embolization and toxicity increases with the volume infused and the amount of meconium contamination (Hankins, 2002). If a response is evoked, its initial phase consists of pulmonary and systemic hypertension. A similar response was reported in a woman in whom transesophageal echocardiography was performed within minutes of collapse. Findings included a massively dilated akinetic right ventricle and a small, vigorously contracting, cavity-obliterated left ventricle (Stanten, 2003). Profound oxygen desaturation is often seen in the initial phase, and this is the cause of neurological injury in most survivors (Harvey, 1996). All of these observations are consistent with failure to transfer blood from the right to the left heart because of severe and unrelenting pulmonary vasoconstriction. This initial phase is probably followed by decreased systemic vascular resistance and diminished cardiac output (Clark, 1988). Women who survive beyond these first two phases invariably have a consumptive coagulopathy and usually lung and brain injury.

Postmortem Findings. Histopathological findings may be dramatic in fatal cases of amnionic-fluid embolism such as the one shown in Figure 41-32. The detection of such debris, however, may require special staining, and even then, it may not be seen. In one study, fetal elements were detected in 75 percent of autopsies and in 50 percent of specimens prepared from concentrated buffy coat aspirates taken antemortem from a pulmonary artery catheter (Clark, 1995). Several other studies, however, have demonstrated that fetal squamous cells, trophoblasts, and other debris of fetal origin may commonly be found in the central circulation of women with conditions other than amnionic-fluid embolism. Thus, the diagnosis is generally made by identifying clinically characteristic signs and symptoms and excluding other causes.

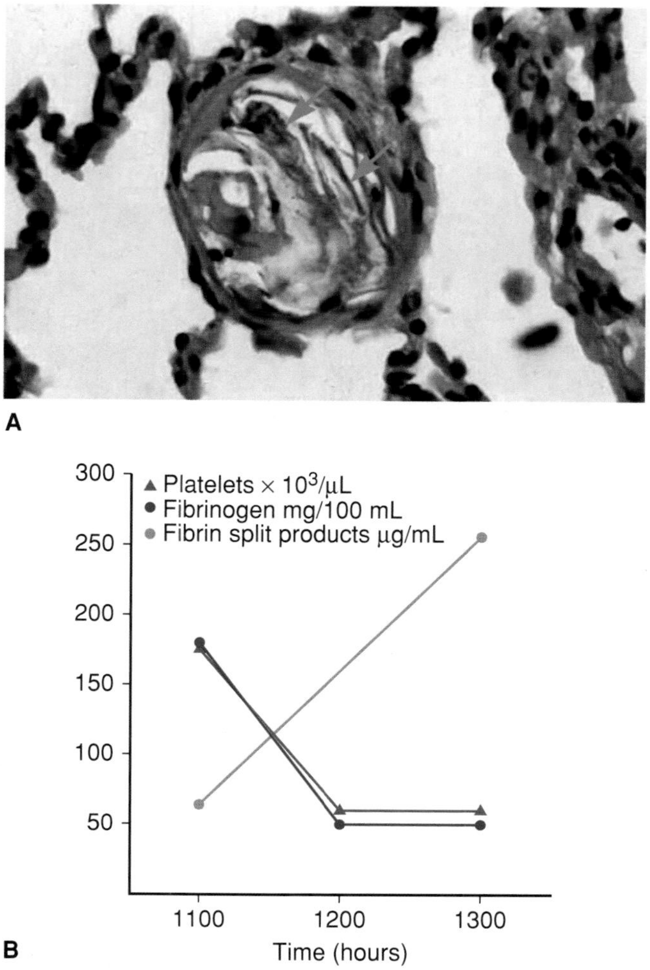

FIGURE 41-32 Fatal amnionic-fluid embolism. **A.** Lung findings at autopsy: fetal squames (*arrows*) packed into a small pulmonary artery. Most of the empty spaces within the vessel were demonstrated by special lipid stains to be filled with vernix caseosa. **B.** Laboratory findings from the same woman demonstrated acute defibrination with decreased levels of fibrinogen and platelets along with increased levels of fibrinogen-fibrin degradation products.

Management and Clinical Outcomes

Immediate resuscitative actions are necessary to interdict the high mortality rate. As discussed, the initial period of systemic and pulmonary hypertension that frequently heralds amnionic-fluid embolism is transient. Tracheal intubation, cardiopulmonary resuscitation, and other supportive measures must be instituted without delay. Treatment is directed at oxygenation and support of the failing myocardium, along with circulatory support that includes rapid blood and component replacement. That said, there are no data indicating that any type of intervention improves maternal or fetal prognosis. In undelivered women undergoing cardiopulmonary resuscitation, consideration should be given to emergency cesarean delivery to perhaps optimize these efforts and improve newborn outcome. Decision making for perimortem cesarean delivery is more complex in a woman who is hemodynamically unstable but who has not suffered cardiac arrest (Chap. 47, p. 956).

Most reports describe dismal outcomes with amnionic-fluid embolism. However, this is likely influenced by underdiagnosis and reporting biases that favor the most severe cases, which are recognized but also have the greatest mortality rates. Several reports are illustrative. From a California database of 1.1 million deliveries, there was a 60-percent mortality rate with amnionic-fluid embolism (Gilbert, 1999). In a report from the Suzhou region of China, 90 percent of mothers died (Weiwen, 2000). This latter report emphasizes that death can be amazingly rapid because 12 of the 34 women who died did so within 30 minutes. The mortality rate was less dismal in the largest study from a Canadian database. Of 120 women with an amnionic-fluid embolism, only a fourth died. In many reports, survivors commonly have profound neurological impairment. Clark (1995) observed that only 8 percent of women who lived despite cardiac arrest survived neurologically intact.

As perhaps expected, perinatal outcomes are also poor and are inversely related to the maternal cardiac arrest-to-delivery interval. Even so, neonatal survival rate is 70 percent, but unfortunately, up to half of survivors suffer residual neurological impairment. In the Canadian study, 28 percent of infants were considered to be asphyxiated at birth (Kramer, 2012).

Sepsis Syndrome

Various infections that are accompanied by endo- or exotoxin release can result in sepsis syndrome in pregnant women. Although a feature of this syndrome includes activation of coagulation, seldom does sepsis alone cause massive procoagulant consumption. *Escherichia coli* bacteremia is frequently seen with antepartum pyelonephritis and puerperal infections, however, accompanying consumptive coagulopathy is usually not severe. Some notable exceptions are septicemia associated with puerperal infection or septic abortion caused by exotoxins released from infecting organisms such as group A *Streptococcus pyogenes, Staphylococcus aureus,* or *Clostridium perfringens* or *sordellii*. Treatment of sepsis syndrome and septic shock is discussed in Chapter 47 (p. 946).

Purpura Fulminans

This severe—often lethal—form of consumptive coagulopathy is caused by microthrombi in small blood vessels leading to skin necrosis and sometimes vasculitis. Debridement of large areas of skin over the extremities and buttocks frequently requires treatment in a burn unit. Purpura fulminans usually complicates sepsis in women with heterozygous protein C deficiency and low protein C serum levels (Levi, 2010b). Recall that homozygous protein C deficiency results in fatal *neonatal purpura fulminans* (Chap. 52, p. 1031).

Abortion

Septic abortion—especially associated with the organisms discussed above—can incite coagulation and worsen hemorrhage, especially with midtrimester abortions. Indeed, sepsis syndrome accompanied by intravascular coagulation accounts for 25 percent of abortion-related deaths (Saraiya, 1999). In the past, especially with illegal abortions, infections with *Clostridium perfringens* were a frequent cause of intense intravascular hemolysis at Parkland Hospital (Pritchard, 1971). More recently, however, septic abortions from infection with *Clostridium sordellii* have emerged as important causes (Chap 18, p. 357).

Second-trimester induced abortions can stimulate intravascular coagulation even in the absence of sepsis. Ben-Ami and associates (2012) described a 1.6-percent incidence in 1249 late second-trimester pregnancies terminated by dilatation and evacuation. Two thirds were done for fetal demise, which may have been contributory to coagulopathy. Another source of intense coagulation is from instillation of hypertonic solutions to effect midtrimester abortions. These are not commonly performed currently for pregnancy terminations (Chap. 18, p. 369). The mechanism is thought to initiate coagulation by thromboplastin release into maternal circulation from placenta, fetus, and the decidua by the necrobiotic effect of the hypertonic solutions (Burkman, 1977).

MANAGEMENT OF HEMORRHAGE

One of the most crucial elements of obstetrical hemorrhage management is recognition of its severity. As discussed on page 781, visual estimation of blood loss, especially when excessive, is notoriously inaccurate, and true blood loss is often two to three times the clinical estimates. Consider also that in obstetrics, part and sometimes even all of the lost blood may be concealed. Estimation is further complicated in that peripartum hemorrhage—when most severe cases are encountered—also includes the pregnancy-induced increased blood volume. If pregnancy hypervolemia is not a factor, then following blood loss of 1000 mL, the hematocrit typically falls only 3 to 5 volume percent within an hour. The hematocrit nadir depends on the speed of resuscitation using infused intravenous crystalloids. *Recall that with abnormally increased acute blood loss, the real-time hematocrit is at its maximum whenever measured in the delivery, operating, or recovery room.*

A prudent rule is that any time blood loss is considered more than average by an experienced team member, then the hematocrit is determined and plans are made for close observation for physiological deterioration. Urine output is one of the most important "vital signs" with which to monitor the woman with obstetrical hemorrhage. Renal blood flow is especially sensitive to changes in blood volume. *Unless diuretic agents are given—and these are seldom indicated with active bleeding—accurately measured urine flow reflects renal perfusion, which in turn reflects perfusion of other vital organs.* Urine flow of at least 30 mL, and preferably 60 mL, per hour or more should be maintained. With potentially serious hemorrhage, an indwelling bladder catheter is inserted to measure hourly urine flow.

Hypovolemic Shock

Shock from hemorrhage evolves through several stages. Early in the course of massive bleeding, there are decreases in mean arterial pressure, stroke volume, cardiac output, central venous pressure, and pulmonary capillary wedge pressure. Increases in arteriovenous oxygen content difference reflect a relative increase in tissue oxygen extraction, although overall oxygen consumption falls.

Blood flow to capillary beds in various organs is controlled by arterioles. These are resistance vessels that are partially controlled by the central nervous system. However, approximately 70 percent of total blood volume is contained in venules, which are passive resistance vessels controlled by humoral factors. Catecholamine release during hemorrhage causes a generalized increase in venular tone that provides an autotransfusion from this capacitance reservoir (Barber, 1999). This is accompanied by compensatory increases in heart rate, systemic and pulmonary vascular resistance, and myocardial contractility. In addition, there is redistribution of cardiac output and blood volume by selective, centrally mediated arteriolar constriction or relaxation—*autoregulation*. Thus, although perfusion to the kidneys, splanchnic beds, muscles, skin, and uterus is diminished, relatively more blood flow is maintained to the heart, brain, and adrenal glands.

When the blood volume deficit exceeds approximately 25 percent, compensatory mechanisms usually are inadequate to maintain cardiac output and blood pressure. Importantly, additional small losses of blood will now cause rapid clinical deterioration. Following an initial increased *total oxygen extraction* by maternal tissue, maldistribution of blood flow results in *local* tissue hypoxia and metabolic acidosis. This creates a vicious cycle of vasoconstriction, organ ischemia, and cellular death. Another important clinical effect of hemorrhage is activation of lymphocytes and monocytes, which in turn cause endothelial cell activation and platelet aggregation. These cause release of vasoactive mediators with small vessel occlusion and further impairment of microcirculatory perfusion. Other common obstetrical syndromes—preeclampsia and sepsis—also lead to loss of capillary endothelial integrity, additional loss of intravascular volume into the extracellular space, and platelet aggregation (Chaps. 40, p. 734 and 47, p. 947).

The pathophysiological events just described lead to the important but often overlooked extracellular fluid and electrolyte shifts involved in both the genesis and successful treatment of hypovolemic shock. These include changes in the cellular transport of various ions such as sodium and water into skeletal muscle and potassium loss. Replacement of extracellular fluid and intravascular volume are both necessary. *Survival is enhanced in acute hemorrhagic shock if blood plus crystalloid solution is given compared with blood transfusions alone.*

Immediate Management and Resuscitation

Whenever there is suggestion of excessive blood loss in a pregnant woman, steps are simultaneously taken to identify the source of bleeding and to begin resuscitation. If she is undelivered, restoration of blood volume is beneficial to mother and fetus, and it also prepares for emergent delivery. If she is postpartum, it is essential to immediately identify uterine atony, retained placental fragments, or genital tract lacerations. At least one and preferably more large-bore intravenous infusion systems are established promptly with rapid administration of crystalloid solutions, while blood is made available. An operating room, surgical team, and anesthesia providers are assembled immediately. Specific management of hemorrhage is further dependent on its etiology. For example, antepartum bleeding from placenta previa is approached somewhat differently than that from postpartum atony.

Fluid Resuscitation

It cannot be overemphasized that treatment of serious hemorrhage demands prompt and adequate refilling of the intravascular compartment with crystalloid solutions. These rapidly equilibrate into the extravascular space, and only 20 percent of crystalloid remains intravascularly in critically ill patients after 1 hour (Zuckerbraun, 2010). Because of this, initial fluid is infused in a volume three times the estimated blood loss.

Resuscitation of hypovolemic shock with colloid versus crystalloid solutions is debated. In a Cochrane review of resuscitation of nonpregnant critically ill patients, Perel and Roberts (2007) found equivalent benefits but concluded that colloid solutions were more expensive. Similar results were found in the Saline versus Albumin Fluid Evaluation (SAFE) randomized trial of almost 7000 nonpregnant patients (Finfer, 2004). We concur with Zuckerbraun and colleagues (2010) that acute volume resuscitation is preferably done with crystalloid and blood.

Blood Replacement

There is considerable debate regarding the hematocrit level or hemoglobin concentration that mandates blood transfusion. Cardiac output does not substantively decrease until the hemoglobin concentration falls to approximately 7 g/dL or hematocrit of 20 volume percent. At this level the Society of Thoracic Surgeons (2011) recommends consideration for red-cell transfusions. Also, Military Combat Trauma Units in Iraq used a target hematocrit of 21 volume percent (Barbieri, 2007). In general, with *ongoing* obstetrical hemorrhage, we recommend rapid blood infusion when the hematocrit is < 25 volume percent. This decision is dependent on whether the fetus has been delivered, surgery is imminent or ongoing operative blood loss is expected, or acute hypoxia, vascular collapse, or other factors are present.

Scant clinical data elucidate these issues. In a study from the Canadian Critical Care Trials Group, nonpregnant patients were randomly assigned to restrictive red cell transfusions to maintain hemoglobin concentration > 7 g/dL or to liberal transfusions to maintain the hemoglobin level at 10 to 12 g/dL. The 30-day mortality rate was similar—19 versus 23 percent in the restrictive versus liberal groups, respectively (Hebert, 1999). In a subanalysis of patients who were less ill, the 30-day mortality rate was significantly lower in the restrictive group—9 versus 26 percent. In a study of women who had suffered postpartum hemorrhage and who were now isovolemic and not actively bleeding, there were no benefits of red cell transfusions when the hematocrit was between 18 and 25 volume percent (Morrison, 1991). *The number of units transfused in a given woman to reach a target hematocrit depends on her body mass and on expectations of additional blood loss.*

Blood Component Products. Contents and effects of transfusion of various blood components are shown in Table 41-8. *Compatible whole blood is ideal for treatment of hypovolemia from catastrophic hemorrhage.* It has a shelf life of 40 days, and 70 percent of the transfused red cells function for at least 24 hours following transfusion. One unit raises the hematocrit by 3 to 4 volume percent. Whole blood replaces many coagulation factors—which is important in obstetrics—especially fibrinogen—and its plasma treats hypovolemia. A collateral derivative is that women with severe hemorrhage are resuscitated with fewer blood donor exposures than with packed red cells and components (Shaz, 2009).

There are reports that support the preferable use of whole blood for massive hemorrhage, including our experiences at Parkland Hospital (Alexander, 2009; Hernandez, 2012). Of more than 66,000 deliveries, women with obstetrical hemorrhage treated with whole blood had significantly decreased incidences of renal failure, acute respiratory distress syndrome,

TABLE 41-8. Blood Products Commonly Transfused in Obstetrical Hemorrhage

Product	Volume per Unit	Contents per Unit	Effect on Hemorrhage
Whole blood	About 500 mL; Hct ~ 40 percent	RBCs, plasma, 600–700 mg fibrinogen, no platelets	Restores blood volume and fibrinogen, increases Hct 3–4 volume percent per unit
Packed RBCs	About 250–300 mL; Hct ~ 55–80 percent	RBCs, minimal fibrinogen, no platelets	Increases Hct 3–4 volume percent per unit
Fresh-frozen plasma (FFP)	About 250 mL; 30-minute thaw	Colloid, 600–700 mg fibrinogen, no platelets	Restores circulating volume and fibrinogen
Cryoprecipitate	About 15 mL, frozen	One unit ~ 200 mg fibrinogen, other clotting factors, no platelets	15–20 units or about 3–4 g will increase baseline fibrinogen ~150 mg/dL
Platelets	About 50 mL, stored at room temperature	One unit raises platelet count about 5000/μL; single-donor apheresis bag preferable	6–10 units transfused: single-donor bag preferable to raise platelets ~30,000/ μL

Hct = hematocrit; RBCs = red blood cells.

pulmonary edema, hypofibrinogenemia, ICU admissions, and maternal death compared with those given packed red cells and component therapy. Freshly donated whole blood has also been used successfully for life-threatening massive hemorrhage at combat support hospitals in Iraq (Spinella, 2008).

It is problematic that in most institutions today, whole blood is rarely available. Thus, most women with obstetrical hemorrhage and ongoing massive blood loss are given packed red cells and crystalloid in 2:1 or 3:1 proportions. In these instances, there are no data to support a 1:1 red cell:plasma transfusion ratio. Many institutions use *massive transfusion protocols* designed to anticipate all facets of obstetrical hemorrhage defined as massive. These "recipes" commonly contain a combination of red cells, plasma, cryoprecipitate, and platelets (Pacheco, 2011; Shields, 2011). If time permits, we usually prefer to await results of emergently performed hematological laboratory assessments to treat deficiencies of fibrinogen or platelets. If time does not permit this, however, the massive transfusion protocol is activated.

Dilutional Coagulopathy. A major drawback of treatment for massive hemorrhage with crystalloid solutions and packed red blood cells is depletion of platelets and clotting factors. As discussed on page 808, this can lead to a dilutional coagulopathy clinically indistinguishable from disseminated intravascular coagulation (Hossain, 2013). In some cases, impaired hemostasis further contributes to blood loss.

Thrombocytopenia is the most frequent coagulation defect found with blood loss and multiple transfusions (Counts, 1979). In addition, packed red cells have very small amounts of soluble clotting factors, and stored whole blood is deficient in platelets and in factors V, VIII, and XI. Massive replacement with red cells only and without factor replacement can also cause *hypofibrinogenemia* and prolongation of the prothrombin and partial thromboplastin times. Because many causes of obstetrical hemorrhage also cause consumptive coagulopathy, the distinction between dilutional and consumptive coagulopathy can be confusing. Fortunately, treatment for both is similar.

A few studies have assessed the relationship between massive transfusion and resultant coagulopathy in civilian trauma units and military combat hospitals (Bochicchio, 2008; Borgman, 2007; Gonzalez, 2007; Johansson, 2007). Patients undergoing massive transfusion—defined as 10 or more units of blood—had much higher survival rates as the ratio of plasma to red cell units was near 1.4, that is, one unit of plasma given for each 1.4 units of packed red cells. By way of contrast, the highest mortality group had a 1:8 ratio. *Most of these studies found that component replacement is rarely necessary with acute replacement of 5 to 10 units of packed red cells.*

From the foregoing, when red cell replacement exceeds five units or so, a reasonable practice is to evaluate the platelet count, clotting studies, and plasma fibrinogen concentration. In the woman with obstetrical hemorrhage, the platelet count should be maintained above 50,000/μL by the infusion of platelet concentrates. A fibrinogen level < 100 mg/dL or a sufficiently prolonged prothrombin or partial thromboplastin time in a woman with surgical bleeding is an indication for replacement. Fresh-frozen plasma is administered in doses of 10 to 15 mL/kg, or alternatively, cryoprecipitate is infused (see Table 41-8).

Type and Screen versus Crossmatch. A blood type and antibody screen should be performed for any woman at significant risk for hemorrhage. Screening involves mixing maternal serum with standard reagent red cells that carry antigens to which most of the common clinically significant antibodies react. Crossmatching involves the use of actual donor erythrocytes rather than the standardized red cells. Clinical results show that the type-and-screen procedure is amazingly efficient. Indeed, only 0.03 to 0.07 percent of patients identified to have no antibodies are subsequently found to have antibodies by crossmatch (Boral, 1979). *Importantly, administration of screened blood rarely results in adverse clinical sequelae.*

Packed Red Blood Cells. One unit of packed erythrocytes is derived from one unit of whole blood to have a hematocrit of 55 to 80 volume percent, depending on the length of gentle centrifugation. Thus one unit contains the same volume of erythrocytes as one whole blood unit. It will increase the hematocrit by 3 to 4 volume percent depending on patient size. *Packed red blood cell and crystalloid infusion are the mainstays of transfusion therapy for most cases of obstetrical hemorrhage.*

Platelets. With operative delivery or with lacerations, platelet transfusions are considered with ongoing obstetrical hemorrhage when the platelet count falls below 50,000/μL (Kenny, 2014). In the *nonsurgical patient*, bleeding is rarely encountered if the platelet count is 10,000/μL or higher (Murphy, 2010). The preferable source of platelets is a bag obtained by single-donor apheresis. This is the equivalent of six units from six individual donors. Depending on maternal size, each single-donor apheresis bag raises the platelet count by approximately 20,000/μL (Schlicter, 2010). If these bags are not available, then individual-donor platelet units are used. One unit contains about 5.5×10^{10} platelets, and six to eight such units are generally transfused.

Importantly, the donor plasma in platelet units must be compatible with recipient erythrocytes. Further, because some red blood cells are invariably transfused along with the platelets, only units from D-negative donors should be given to D-negative recipients. If necessary, however, adverse sequelae are unlikely. For example, transfusion of ABO-nonidentical platelets in nonpregnant patients undergoing cardiovascular surgery had no clinical effects (Lin, 2002).

Fresh-Frozen Plasma. This component is prepared by separating plasma from whole blood and then freezing it. Approximately 30 minutes are required for frozen plasma to thaw. It is a source of all stable and labile clotting factors, including fibrinogen. Thus, it is often used for treatment of women with consumptive or dilutional coagulopathy. *Plasma is not appropriate for use as a volume expander in the absence of specific clotting factor deficiencies.* It should be considered in a bleeding woman with a fibrinogen level < 100 mg/dL or with an abnormal prothrombin or partial thromboplastin time.

An alternative to frozen plasma is *liquid plasma (LQP)*. This never-frozen plasma is stored at 1 to 6°C for up to 26 days, and in vitro, it appears to be superior to thawed plasma (Matijevic, 2013).

Cryoprecipitate and Fibrinogen Concentrate. Each unit of cryoprecipitate is prepared from one unit of fresh-frozen plasma. Each 10- to 15-mL unit contains at least 200 mg of fibrinogen, factor VIII:C, factor VIII:von Willebrand factor, factor XIII, and fibronectin (American Association of Blood Banks, 2002). It is usually given as a "pool" or "bag" using an aliquot of fibrinogen concentrate taken from 8 to 120 donors. Cryoprecipitate is an ideal source of fibrinogen when levels are dangerously low and there is oozing from surgical incisions. Another alternative is virus-inactivated fibrinogen concentrate. Each gram of this raises the plasma fibrinogen level approximately 40 mg/dL (Ahmed, 2012; Kikuchi, 2013). Either is used to replace fibrinogen. However, there are no advantages to these compared with fresh-frozen plasma for general clotting factor replacement. Exceptions are general factor deficiency replacement for women in whom volume overload may be a problem—an unusual situation in obstetrics—and for those with a specific factor deficiency.

Recombinant Activated Factor VII (rFVIIa). This synthetic vitamin K-dependent protein is available as *NovoSeven.* It binds to exposed tissue factor at the site of injury to generate thrombin that activates platelets and the coagulation cascade. Since its introduction, rFVIIa has been used to help control hemorrhage from surgery, trauma, and many other causes (Mannucci, 2007). More than three fourths of Level I trauma centers include it in their massive transfusion protocols (Pacheco, 2011). It is included in the massive transfusion protocol at Parkland Hospital.

One major concern with rFVIIa use is arterial—and to a lesser degree venous—thrombosis. In a review of 35 randomized trials with nearly 4500 subjects, arterial thromboembolism developed in 55 percent (Levi, 2010a). A second concern is that it was found to be only marginally effective in most of these studies (Pacheco, 2011). In obstetrics, recombinant FVIIa has also been used to control severe hemorrhage in women with and without hemophilia (Alfirevic, 2007; Franchini, 2007). It has been used with uterine atony, lacerations, and placental abruption or previa. In approximately a third of cases, hysterectomy was required. Importantly, rFVIIa will not be effective if the plasma fibrinogen level is < 50 mg/dL or the platelet count is < 30,000/μL.

Topical Hemostatic Agents. Several agents can be used to control persistent oozing. These were recently reviewed by dos Santos and Menzin (2012). In general, these are rarely used in obstetrical hemorrhage.

Autologous Transfusion. Patient phlebotomy and autologous blood storage for transfusion has been disappointing. Exceptions are women with a rare blood type or with unusual antibodies. In one report, three fourths of women who began such a program in the third trimester donated only one unit (McVay, 1989). This is further complicated in that the need for transfusion cannot be predicted (Reyal, 2004). For these and other reasons, most have concluded that autologous transfusions are not cost effective (Etchason, 1995; Pacheco, 2011, 2013).

Cell Salvage. To accomplish autotransfusion, blood lost intraoperatively into the surgical field is aspirated and filtered. The red cells are then collected into containers with concentrations similar to packed red cells and are infused as such. Intraoperative blood salvage with reinfusion is considered to be safe in obstetrical patients (Pacheco, 2011; Rainaldi, 1998). That said, Allam and associates (2008) reported the lack of prospective trials but also found no reports of serious complications.

Complications with Transfusions. During the past several decades, substantial advances have been achieved in blood transfusion safety. Although many risks are avoided or mitigated, the most serious known risks that remain include errors leading to ABO-incompatible blood transfusion, transfusion-related acute lung injury (TRALI), and bacterial and viral transmission (Lerner, 2010).

The transfusion of an incompatible blood component may result in acute hemolysis. If severe, this can cause disseminated intravascular coagulation, acute kidney injury, and death. Preventable errors responsible for most of such reactions frequently include mislabeling of a specimen or transfusing an incorrect patient. Although the rate of such errors in the United States has been estimated to be 1 in 14,000 units, these are likely underreported (Lerner, 2010; Linden, 2001). A transfusion reaction is characterized by fever, hypotension, tachycardia, dyspnea, chest or back pain, flushing, severe anxiety, and hemoglobinuria. Immediate supportive measures include stopping the transfusion, treating hypotension and hyperkalemia, provoking diuresis, and alkalinizing the urine. Assays for urine and plasma hemoglobin concentration and an antibody screen help confirm the diagnosis.

The syndrome of *transfusion-related acute lung injury (TRALI)* can be a life-threatening complication. It is characterized by severe dyspnea, hypoxia, and noncardiogenic pulmonary edema that develop within 6 hours of transfusion (Triulzi, 2009). TRALI is estimated to complicate at least 1 in 5000 transfusions. Although the pathogenesis is incompletely understood, injury to the pulmonary capillaries may arise from anti-human leukocyte antigen (HLA) antibodies in donor plasma (Lerner, 2010; Schubert, 2013). These antibodies bind to leukocytes that aggregate in pulmonary capillaries and release inflammatory mediators. A delayed form of TRALI syndrome has been reported to have an onset 6 to 72 hours following transfusion (Marik, 2008). Management is with supportive therapy that may include mechanical ventilation (Chap. 47, p. 944).

Bacterial infection from transfusion of a contaminated blood component is unusual because bacterial growth is discouraged by refrigeration. The most often implicated contaminant of red cells include *Yersinia, Pseudomonas, Serratia, Acinetobacter,* and *Escherichia* species. The more important risk is from bacterial contamination of platelets, which are stored at room temperature. Current estimates are that 1 in 1000 to 2000 platelet units are contaminated. Death from transfusion-related sepsis is 1 per 17,000 for single-door platelets and 1 per 61,000 for apheresis-donor packs (Lerner, 2010).

Risks from many transfusion-related viral infections have been curtailed. Fortunately, the most feared infection—HIV—is the least common. With current screening methods using nucleic acid amplification, the risk of HIV or hepatitis C virus infection in screened blood is estimated to be 1 case per 1 to 2 million units transfused (Stramer, 2004). The risk for HIV-2 infection is less.

Other viral infections include *hepatitis B* transmission, which is estimated to be < 1 per 100,000 transfused units (Jackson, 2003). Choosing donors who have been vaccinated will lower this incidence. Because of its high prevalence, cytomegalovirus-infected leukocytes are necessarily often transfused. Thus, precautions are taken for immunosuppressed recipients, keeping in mind that this includes the fetus (Chap. 15, p. 310). Finally, there are slight risks for transmitting West Nile virus, human T-lymphotropic virus Type I, and parvovirus B19 (American Association of Blood Banks, 2013).

Red Cell Substitutes. Use of these artificial carriers of oxygen has been abandoned (Ness, 2007; Spiess, 2009). Three that have been studied include perfluorocarbons, liposome-encapsulated hemoglobin, and hemoglobin-based oxygen carriers.

Adjunctive Surgical Procedures to Treat Hemorrhage

Uterine Artery Ligation

Several surgical procedures may be helpful to arrest of obstetrical hemorrhage. Of these, the technique for unilateral or bilateral uterine artery ligation is used primarily for lacerations at the lateral part of a hysterotomy incision (Fig. 41-33). In our experiences, this procedure is less helpful for hemorrhage from uterine atony.

Uterine Compression Sutures. Almost 20 years ago a surgical technique to arrest hemorrhage for severe postpartum atony was introduced by B-Lynch and coworkers (1997). The procedure involves placement of a No. 2-chromic suture to compress the anterior and posterior uterine walls together. Because they give the appearance of suspenders, they are also called *braces* (Fig. 41-34). Several modifications of the B-Lynch technique have been described (Cho, 2000; Hayman, 2002; Matsubara, 2013b; Nelson, 2007). Indications vary for its application, and this will affect the success rate. For example, B-Lynch (2005) cited 948 cases with only seven failures. Conversely, Kayem and associates (2011) described 211 women in whom compression sutures were employed. The overall failure rate of 25 percent did not differ between B-Lynch sutures and their modifications. Our experiences at Parkland Hospital are not nearly so successful. The technique has been effective in perhaps half of cases in which it is used.

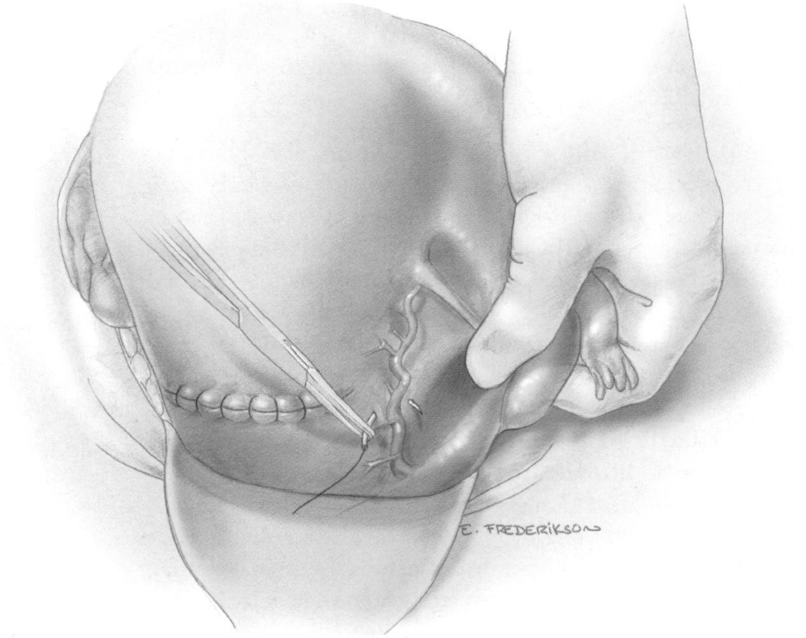

FIGURE 41-33 Uterine artery ligation. The suture goes through the lateral uterine wall anteriorly, curves around posteriorly, then re-enters anteriorly. When tied, it encompasses the uterine artery.

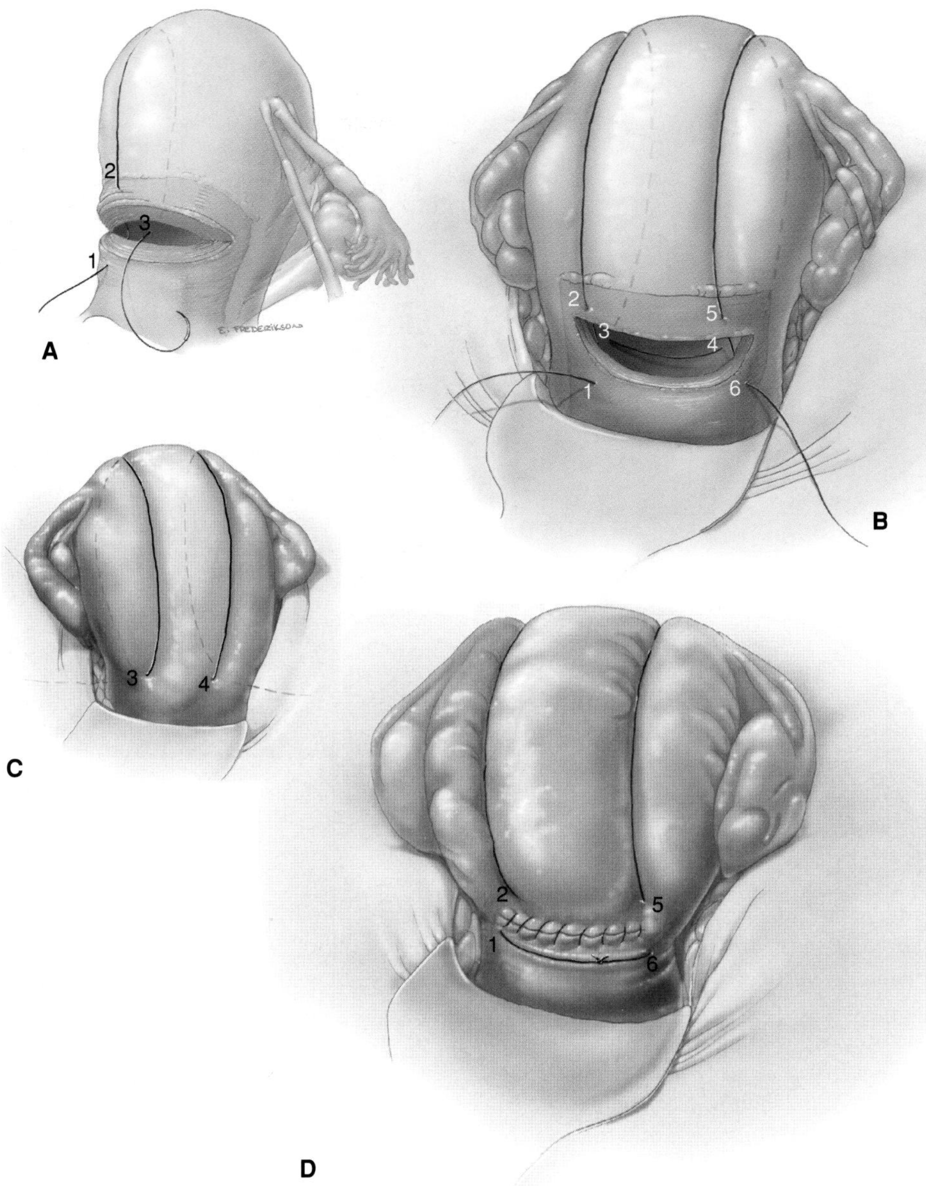

FIGURE 41-34 Uterine compression suture or "brace." The B-Lynch suture technique is illustrated from an anterior view of the uterus in Figures **A**, **B**, and **D** and a posterior view in Figure **C**. The numbers denote the sequential path of the suture and are shown in more than one figure. **Step 1.** Beginning below the incision, the needle pierces the lower uterine segment to enter the uterine cavity. **Step 2.** The needle exits the cavity above the incision. The suture then loops up and around the fundus to the posterior uterine surface. **Step 3.** The needle pierces the posterior uterine wall to reenter the uterine cavity. The suture then traverses from left to right within the cavity. **Step 4.** The needle exits the uterine cavity through the posterior uterine wall. From the back of the uterus, the suture loops up and around the fundus to the front of the uterus. **Step 5.** The needle pierces the myometrium above the incision to reenter the uterine cavity. **Step 6.** The needle exits below the incision and the sutures at points 1 and 6 are tied below the incision. The hysterotomy incision is then closed in the usual fashion.

There are complications with compression sutures, and some are unique (Matsubara, 2013b). Their precise frequency is unknown, but it is likely low. The most common involve variations of uterine ischemic necrosis with peritonitis (Gottlieb, 2008; Joshi, 2004; Ochoa, 2002; Treloar, 2006). Total uterine necrosis was described by Friederich and associates (2007) in a woman in whom B-Lynch sutures were placed along with bilateral ligation of uterine, uteroovarian, and round ligament arteries. In most cases, subsequent pregnancies are uneventful if compression sutures are placed. A few women, however, with B-Lynch or Cho sutures have been reported to have defects in the uterine wall (Akoury, 2008; An, 2013). Another long-term complication is uterine cavity synechiae, which may develop in 20 to 50 percent of these women by 3 months (Alouini, 2011; Ibrahim, 2013; Poujade, 2011).

Internal Iliac Artery Ligation

Ligation of one or both internal iliac arteries has been used for many years to reduce hemorrhage from pelvic vessels (Allahbadia, 1993; Joshi, 2007). Drawbacks are that the procedure may be technically difficult and is only successful half of the time (American College of Obstetricians and Gynecologists,

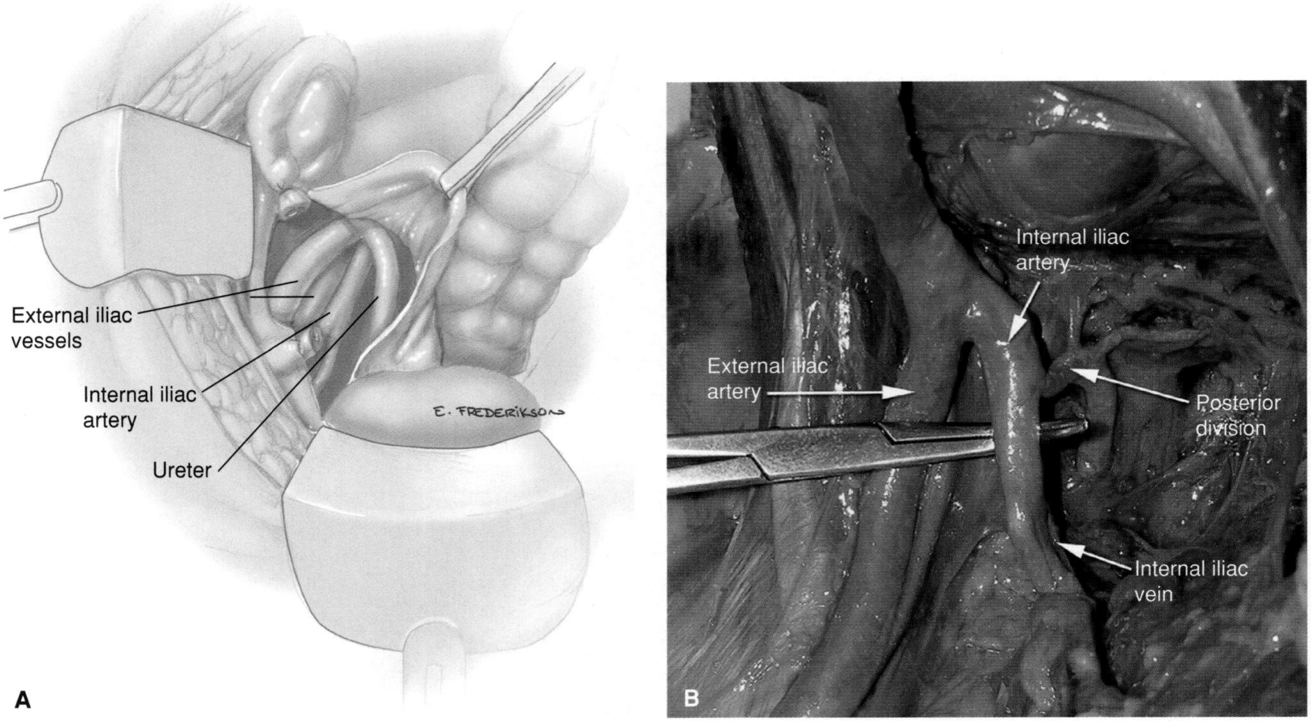

FIGURE 41-35 Ligation of the right internal iliac artery. **A.** The peritoneum covering the right iliac vessels is opened and reflected. **B.** Unembalmed cadaveric dissection shows the right-angle clamp passing underneath the anterior division of the internal iliac artery just distal to its posterior division. (Photograph contributed by Dr. Marlene Corton.)

2012b). It is not particularly helpful to abate hemorrhage with postpartum atony (Clark, 1985; Joshi, 2007).

Adequate exposure is obtained by opening the peritoneum over the common iliac artery and dissecting down to the bifurcation of the external and internal iliac arteries (Fig. 41-35). Branches distal to the external iliac arteries are palpated to verify pulsations at or below the inguinal area. Ligation of the internal iliac artery 5 cm distal to the common iliac bifurcation will usually avoid the posterior division branches (Bleich, 2007). The areolar sheath of the artery is incised longitudinally, and a right-angle clamp is carefully passed just beneath the artery from lateral to medial. Care must be taken not to perforate contiguous large veins, especially the internal iliac vein. Suture—usually nonabsorbable—is passed under the artery with a clamp, and the vessel is then securely ligated.

Following ligation, pulsations in and distal to the external iliac artery are again confirmed. If not, pulsations must be identified after arterial hypotension has been successfully treated to ensure that the artery has not been compromised. The most important mechanism of action with internal iliac artery ligation is an 85-percent reduction in pulse pressure in those arteries distal to the ligation (Burchell, 1968). This converts an arterial pressure system into one with pressures approaching those in the venous circulation. This creates vessels more amenable to hemostasis via pressure and clot formation.

Even bilateral internal iliac artery ligation does not appear to interfere with subsequent reproduction. Nizard and colleagues (2003) reported follow-up in 17 women who had bilateral artery ligation. From a total of 21 pregnancies, 13 were normal, three ended with miscarriage, three were terminated, and there were two ectopic pregnancies.

Angiographic Embolization

This tool is now used for many causes of intractable hemorrhage when surgical access is difficult. In more than 500 women reported, embolization was 90-percent effective (Bodner, 2006; Lee, 2012; Poujade, 2012; Sentilhes, 2009). Rouse (2013) recently reviewed the subject and concluded that embolization can be used to arrest refractory postpartum hemorrhage. However, the author cautioned that the procedure is less effective with placenta percreta or with concurrent coagulopathy. Other reports have been less enthusiastic, and the American College of Obstetricians and Gynecologists (2012b) describes its efficacy as "unclear." Fertility is not impaired, and many subsequent successful pregnancies have been reported (Chauleur, 2008; Fiori, 2009; Kolomeyevskaya, 2009). There are limited data describing its antepartum use. Embolization in a 20-week pregnant woman was reported for a large lower uterine segment arteriovenous malformation (Rebarber, 2009). It has also been used for renal hemorrhage (Wortman, 2013b).

Complications of embolization are relatively uncommon, but they can be severe. Uterine ischemic necrosis has been described (Coulange, 2009; Katakam, 2009; Sentilhes, 2009). Uterine infection has been reported (Nakash, 2012). Finally, Al-Thunyan and coworkers (2012) described a woman with massive buttock necrosis and paraplegia following bilateral internal iliac artery embolization.

Preoperative Pelvic Arterial Catheter Placement

There are a few instances in which massive blood loss and difficult surgical dissection is anticipated. For these, investigators have described use of balloon-tipped catheters inserted into the iliac or uterine arteries preoperatively. Catheters can then be inflated or embolization performed to mitigate heavy blood loss if it develops (Desai, 2012; Matsubara, 2013a). These techniques are used more commonly in cases of accrete syndromes (p. 804), and they have also been described for abdominal pregnancy (Chap. 19, p. 388). The reported success rates have been variable, and these techniques are not universally recommended (Angstmann, 2012; Pacheco, 2011, 2013; Zacharias, 2003). Again the American College of Obstetricians and Gynecologists (2012b) considers the use and efficacy of these techniques to be "unclear." Adverse effects are uncommon, but postoperative iliac and popliteal artery thrombosis and stenosis have been reported (Greenberg, 2007; Hoffman, 2010; Sewell, 2006).

Pelvic Umbrella Pack

The *umbrella* or *parachute pack* was described by Logothetopulos (1926) to arrest intractable pelvic hemorrhage following hysterectomy. Although seldom used today, it can be lifesaving if all other measures have failed. The pack is constructed of a sterile x-ray cassette bag that is filled with gauze rolls knotted together to provide enough volume to fill the pelvis (Fig. 41-36). The pack is introduced transabdominally with the stalk exiting the vagina. Mild traction is applied by tying the stalk to a 1-liter fluid bag, which is hung over the foot of the bed. An indwelling urinary catheter is placed to prevent urinary obstruction and to monitor urinary output. Percutaneous pelvic drains can be placed to monitor ongoing bleeding within the peritoneal cavity. Broad-spectrum antimicrobials are given, and the umbrella pack is removed vaginally after 24 hours.

Dildy and colleagues (2006) described use of the pelvic pack to arrest hemorrhage following hysterectomy in 11 women. These women were given seven to 77 units of red cells, and the pack successfully stopped bleeding in all but two women. Over the years, we have had mixed results with this technique, but we can recommend it as a "last-ditch" attempt when exsanguination is inevitable, especially in "low-resource" areas.

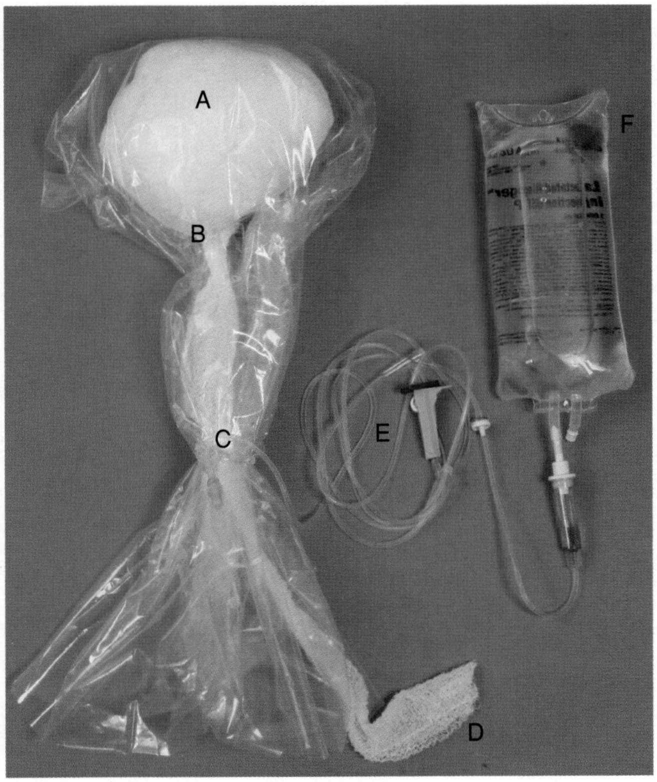

FIGURE 41-36 Assembly of a pelvic pressure pack to control hemorrhage. A sterile x-ray cassette cover drape (plastic bag) is filled with gauze rolls tied end-to-end. The length of gauze is then folded into a ball **(A)** and placed within the cassette bag in such a way that the gauze can be unwound eventually with traction on the tail **(D)**. Intravenous tubing **(E)** is tied to the exiting part of the neck **(C)** and connected to a 1-liter bag or other suitable weight **(F)**. Once in place, the gauze pack **(A)** fills the pelvis to tamponade vessels, and the narrow upper neck **(B)** passes to exit the vagina **(C)**. The IV bag is suspended off the foot of the bed to sustain pressure of the gauze pack on bleeding sites.

REFERENCES

Abdel-Aleem H, El-Nashar I, Abdel-Aleem A: Management of severe postpartum hemorrhage with misoprostol. Int J Gynaecol Obstet 72:75, 2001

Abdella TN, Sibai BM, Hays JM Jr, et al: Perinatal outcome in abruptio placentae. Obstet Gynecol 63:365, 1984

Abenhaim HA, Azoulay L, Kramer MS, et al: Incidence and risk factors of amniotic fluid embolisms: a population-based study on 3 million births in the United States. Am J Obstet Gynecol 199:49.e1, 2008

Adamsons K, Mueller-Heubach E, Myers RE: The innocuousness of amniotic fluid infusion in the pregnant rhesus monkey. Am J Obstet Gynecol 109:977, 1971

Addis A, Moretti ME, Ahmed Syed F, et al: Fetal effects of cocaine: an updated meta-analysis. Reprod Toxicol 15:341, 2001

Ahmed S, Harrity C, Johnson S, et al: The efficacy of fibrinogen concentrate compared with cryoprecipitate in major obstetric haemorrhage—an observational study. Transfus Med 22(5):344, 2012

Aibar L, Aguilar MT, Puertas A, et al: Bakri balloon for the management of postpartum hemorrhage. Acta Obstet Gynecol Scand 92(4):465, 2013

Ajayi RA, Soothill PW, Campbell S, et al: Antenatal testing to predict outcome in pregnancies with unexplained antepartum haemorrhage. BJOG 99:122, 1992

Akoury H, Sherman C: Uterine wall partial thickness necrosis following combined B-Lynch and Cho square sutures for the treatment of primary postpartum hemorrhage. J Obstet Gynaecol Can 30:421, 2008

Albayrak M, Ozdemir I, Koc O, et al: Post-partum haemorrhage from the lower uterine segment secondary to placenta previa/accreta: successful conservative management with Foley balloon tamponade. Aust N Z J Obstet Gynaecol 51(4):377, 2011

Alexander JM, Sarode R, McIntire DD, et al: Use of whole blood in the management of hypovolemia due to obstetric hemorrhage. Obstet Gynecol 113:1320, 2009

Alfirevic Z, Elbourne D, Pavord S, et al: Use of recombinant activated factor VII in primary postpartum hemorrhage: the North European Registry 2000–2004. Obstet Gynecol 110:1270, 2007

Allahbadia G: Hypogastric artery ligation: a new perspective. J Gynecol Surg 9:35, 1993

Allam J, Cox M, Yentis SM: Cell salvage in obstetrics. Int J Obstet Anesth 17(1):37, 2008

Alouini S, Coly S, Megier P, Lemaire B, et al: Multiple square sutures for postpartum hemorrhage: results and hysteroscopic assessment. Am J Obstet Gynecol 205(4):335, 2011

Al-Thunyan A, Al-Meshal O, Al-Hussainan H, et al: Buttock necrosis and paraplegia after bilateral internal iliac artery embolization for postpartum hemorrhage. Obstet Gynecol 120(2 Pt 2):468, 2012

Al-Zirqi I, Vangen S, Forsen L, et al: Prevalence and risk factors of severe obstetric haemorrhage. BJOG 115:1265, 2008

American Association of Blood Banks: Circular of information for the use of human blood and blood components. 2002. Available at: http://www.fda.gov/downloads/BiologicsBloodVaccines/GuidanceComplianceRegulatoryInformation/Guidances/Blood/ucm080296.pdf. Accessed October 13, 2013

American Association of Blood Banks: Human parvovirus B19. 2013. Available at: http://www.aabb.org/resources/bct/eid/Documents/Human-Parvovirus-B19.pdf. Accessed October 13, 2013

American College of Obstetricians and Gynecologists: Antiphospholipid syndrome. Practice Bulletin No. 132, December 2012a

American College of Obstetricians and Gynecologists: Placenta accreta. Committee Opinion No. 529, July 2012b
American College of Obstetricians and Gynecologists: Inherited thrombophilias in pregnancy. Practice Bulletin No. 138, September 2013a
American College of Obstetricians and Gynecologists: Postpartum hemorrhage. Practice Bulletin No. 76, October 2006, Reaffirmed 2013b
An GH, Ryu HM, Kim My, et al: Outcomes of subsequent pregnancies after uterine compression sutures for postpartum hemorrhage. Obstet Gynecol 122(3):565, 2013
Ananth CV, Berkowitz GS, Savitz DA, et al: Placental abruption and adverse perinatal outcomes. JAMA 282:1646, 1999a
Ananth CV, Demissie K, Smulian JC, et al: Placenta previa in singleton and twin births in the United States, 1989 through 1998: a comparison of risk factor profiles and associated conditions. Am J Obstet Gynecol 188:275, 2003a
Ananth CV, Demissie K, Smulian JC, et al: Relationship among placenta previa, fetal growth restriction, and preterm delivery: a population-based study. Obstet Gynecol 98:299, 2001a
Ananth CV, Getahun D, Peltier MR, et al: Placental abruption in term and preterm gestations. Obstet Gynecol 107:785, 2006
Ananth CV, Oyelese Y, Srinivas N, et al: Preterm premature rupture of membranes, intrauterine infection, and oligohydramnios: risk factors for placental abruption. Obstet Gynecol 104:71, 2004
Ananth CV, Oyelese Y, Yeo L, et al: Placental abruption in the United States, 1979 through 2001: temporal trends and potential determinants. Am J Obstet Gynecol 192(1):191, 2005
Ananth CV, Peltier MR, Kinzler WL, et al: Chronic hypertension and risk of placental abruption: is the association modified by ischemic placental disease? Am J Obstet Gynecol 197:273.e1, 2007
Ananth CV, Smulian JC, Demissie K, et al: Placental abruption among singleton and twin births in the United States: risk factor profiles. Am J Epidemiol 153:771, 2001b
Ananth CV, Smulian JC, Vintzileos AM: Incidence of placental abruption in relation to cigarette smoking and hypertensive disorders during pregnancy: a meta-analysis of observational studies. Obstet Gynecol 93:622, 1999b
Ananth CV, Smulian JC, Vintzileos AM: The effect of placenta previa on neonatal mortality: a population-based study in the United States, 1989 through 1997. Am J Obstet Gynecol 188:1299, 2003b
Angstmann T, Gard G, Harrington T, et al: Surgical management of placenta accreta: a cohort series and suggested approach. Am J Obstet Gynecol 202(1):38 e.1, 2012
Arici V, Corbetta R, Fossati G, et al: Acute first onset of Ehlers-Danlos syndrome type 4 with spontaneous rupture of posterior tibial artery pseudoaneurysm. Vascular 21(1):43, 2013
Ash A, Smith A, Maxwell D: Caesarean scar pregnancy. BJOG 114:253, 2007
Awan N, Bennett MJ, Walters WA: Emergency peripartum hysterectomy: a 10-year review at the Royal Hospital for Women, Sydney. Aust N Z J Obstet Gynaecol 51(3):210, 2011
Babinszki A, Kerenyi T, Torok O, et al: Perinatal outcome in grand and great-grand multiparity: effects of parity on obstetric risk factors. Am J Obstet Gynecol 181:669, 1999
Ballas J, Hull AD, Saenz, et al: Preoperative intravascular balloon catheters and surgical outcomes in pregnancies complicated by placenta accreta: a management paradox. Am J Obstet Gynecol 207(3):216.e1, 2012
Barber A, Shires GT III, Shires GT: Shock. In Schwartz SI, Shires GT, Spencer FC, et al (eds): Principles of Surgery, 7th ed. New York, McGraw-Hill, 1999, p 101
Barbieri RL: Control of massive hemorrhage: lessons from Iraq reach the U.S. labor and delivery suite. OBG Management 19:8, 2007
Barbieri RL: Have you made best use of the Bakri balloon in PPH? OBG Management 23(7):6, 2011
Barth WH Jr, Kwolek CJ, Abrams JL, et al: Case records of the Massachusetts General Hospital. Case 23–2011. A 40-year-old pregnant woman with placenta accreta who declined blood products. N Engl J Med 365(4):359, 2011
Baskett TF: Acute uterine inversion: a review of 40 cases. J Obstet Gynaecol Can 24:953, 2002
Bateman BT, Berman MF, Riley LE, et al: The epidemiology of postpartum hemorrhage in a large, nationwide sample of deliveries. Anesth Analg 110(5):1368, 2010
Ben-Ami I, Fuchs N, Schneider D, et al: Coagulopathy associated with dilation and evacuation for second-trimester abortion. Acta Obstet Gynecol Scand 91(1):10, 2012
Benirschke K, Burton, Baergen RN: Pathology of the Human Placenta, 6th ed. New York, Springer, 2012, p 204
Benson MD, Kobayashi H, Silver RK, et al: Immunologic studies in presumed amniotic fluid embolism. Obstet Gynecol 97:510, 2001
Berg CJ, Chang J, Callaghan WM, et al: Pregnancy-related mortality in the United States, 1991–1997. Obstet Gynecol 101:289, 2003
Berg CJ, Callaghan WM, Syverson C, et al: Pregnancy-related mortality in the United States, 1998–2005. Obstet Gynecol 116(6):1302, 2010
Berg CJ, MacKay AP, Qin C, et al: Overview of maternal morbidity during hospitalizations for labor and delivery in the United States. 1993–1997 and 2001–2005. Obstet Gynecol 113(5):1075, 2009
Bingol N, Fuchs M, Diaz V, et al: Teratogenicity of cocaine in humans. J Pediatr 110:93, 1987
Biro MA, Davey MA, Carolan M, et al: Advanced maternal age and obstetric morbidity for women giving birth in Victoria, Australia: a population-based study. Aust N Z J Obstet Gynaecol 52(3):229, 2012
Bishop S, Butler K, Monaghan S, et al: Multiple complications following the use of prophylactic internal iliac artery balloon catheterization in a patient with placenta percreta. Int J Obstet Anesth 20(1):70, 2011
Biswas R, Sawhney H, Dass R, et al: Histopathological study of placental bed biopsy in placenta previa. Acta Obstet Gynecol Scand 78:173, 1999
Bleich AT, Rahn DD, Wieslander CK, et al: Posterior division of the internal iliac artery: anatomic variations and clinical applications. Am J Obstet Gynecol 197:658.e1, 2007
B-Lynch C: Partial ischemic necrosis of the uterus following a uterine brace compression suture. BJOG 112:126, 2005
B-Lynch CB, Coker A, Laval AH, et al: The B-Lynch surgical technique for control of massive postpartum hemorrhage: an alternative to hysterectomy? Five cases reported. BJOG 104:372, 1997
Bochicchio GV, Napolitano L, Joshi M, et al: Outcome analysis of blood product transfusion in trauma patients: a prospective, risk-adjusted study. World J Surg 32(10):2185, 2008
Bodner LJ, Nosher JL, Grivvin C, et al: Balloon-assisted occlusion of the internal iliac arteries in patients with placenta accreta/percreta. Cardiovasc Intervent Radiol 29:354, 2006
Bohrer J, Goh W, Hirai C, et al: Obstetrical outcomes in patients with low-lying placenta in the second trimester. Abstract No. 129. Am J Obstet Gynecol 206(1):S69, 2012
Bond AL, Edersheim TG, Curry L, et al: Expectant management of abruptio placentae before 35 weeks' gestation. Am J Perinatol 6:121, 1989
Bonnar J, McNicol GP, Douglas AS: The behavior of the coagulation and fibrinolytic mechanisms in abruptio placentae. J Obstet Gynaecol Br Commonw 76:799, 1969
Boral LI, Hill SS, Apollon CJ, et al: The type and antibody screen, revisited. Am J Clin Pathol 71:578, 1979
Borgman MA, Spinella PC, Perkins JC, et al: The ratio of blood products transfused affects mortality in patients receiving massive transfusions at a combat support hospital. J Trauma 63:805, 2007
Bose DA, Assel BG, Hill JB, et al: Maintenance tocolytics for preterm symptomatic placenta previa: a review. Am J Perinatol 28(1):45, 2011
Boyle RK, Waters BA, O'Rourke PK: Blood transfusion for caesarean delivery complicated by placenta praevia. Aust N Z J Obstet Gynaecol 49(6):627, 2009
Brame RG, Harbert GM Jr, McGaughey HS Jr, et al: Maternal risk in abruption. Obstet Gynecol 31:224, 1968
Breen JL, Neubecker R, Gregori C, et al: Placenta accreta, increta, and percreta: a survey of 40 cases. Obstet Gynecol 49(1):43, 1977
Bretelle f, Courbière B, Mazouni C, et al: Management of placenta accreta: morbidity and outcome. Eur J Obstet Gynecol Reprod Biol 133(1):34, 2007
Bronsteen R, Whitten A, Balasubramanian M, et al: Vasa previa. Clinical presentations, outcomes, and implications for management. Obstet Gynecol 122(2 Pt 1):352, 2013
Brosens I, Pijnenborg R, Vercruysse L, et al: The "great obstetrical syndromes" are associated with disorders of deep placentation. Am J Obstet Gynecol 204(3):193, 2011
Burchell RC: Physiology of internal iliac artery ligation. J Obstet Gynaecol Br Commonw 75:642, 1968
Burkman RT, Bell WR, Atienza MF, et al: Coagulopathy with midtrimester induced abortion: association with hyperosmolar urea administration. Am J Obstet Gynecol 127:533, 1977
Cali G, Biambanco L, Puccio G, et al: Morbidly adherent placenta: evaluation of ultrasound diagnostic criteria and differentiation of placenta accreta from percreta. Ultrasound Obstet Gynecol 41(4):406, 2013
Chalubinski KM, Pils S, Klein K, et al: Prenatal sonography can predict the degree of placental invasion. Ultrasound Obstet Gynecol 42(5):518, 2013
Chang YL, Chang SD, Cheng PJ: Perinatal outcome in patients with placental abruption with and without antepartum hemorrhage. Int J Gynaecol Obstet 75:193, 2001
Chantraine F, Blacher S, Berndt S, et al: Abnormal vascular architecture at the placental-maternal interface in placenta increta. Am J Obstet Gynecol 207:188.e1, 2012

Chantraine F, Braun T, Gonser M, et al: Prenatal diagnosis of abnormally invasive placenta reduces maternal peripartum hemorrhage and morbidity. Acta Obstet Gynecol Scand 92(4):439, 2013
Chauleur C, Fanget C, Tourne G, et al: Serious primary post-partum hemorrhage, arterial embolization and future fertility: a retrospective study of 46 cases. Hum Reprod 23:1553, 2008
Chescheir NC, Seeds JW: Spontaneous resolution of hypofibrinogenemia associated with death of a twin in utero: a case report. Am J Obstet Gynecol 159:1183, 1988
Chichakli LO, Atrash HK, Mackay AP, et al: Pregnancy-related mortality in the United States due to hemorrhage: 1979–1992. Obstet Gynecol 94:721, 1999
Cho JH, Jun HS, Lee CN: Haemostatic suturing technique or uterine bleeding during cesarean delivery. Obstet Gynaecol 96:129, 2000
Cho JY, Kim SJ, Cha KY, et al: Interrupted circular suture: bleeding control during cesarean delivery in placenta previa accreta. Obstet Gynecol 78:876, 1991
Clark SL, Belfort MA, Dildy GA, et al: Maternal death in the 21st century: causes, prevention, and relationship to cesarean delivery. Am J Obstet Gynecol 199:36.e1, 2008
Clark SL, Cotton DB, Gonik B, et al: Central hemodynamic alterations in amniotic fluid embolism. Am J Obstet Gynecol 158:1124, 1988
Clark SL, Hankins GDV, Dudley DA, et al: Amniotic fluid embolism: analysis of the National Registry. Am J Obstet Gynecol 172:1158, 1995
Clark SL, Pavlova Z, Greenspoon J, et al: Squamous cells in the maternal pulmonary circulation. Am J Obstet Gynecol 154:104, 1986
Clark SL, Phelan JP, Yeh S-Y: Hypogastric artery ligation for obstetric hemorrhage. Obstet Gynecol 66:353, 1985
Cleary-Goldman J, Malone FD, Vidaver J, et al: Impact of maternal age on obstetric outcome. Obstet Gynecol 105:983, 2005
Cohen M, Wuillemin C, Irion O, et al: Role of decidua in trophoblastic invasion. Neuro Endocrinol Lett 31(2):193, 2010
Combs CA, Nyberg DA, Mack LA, et al: Expectant management after sonographic diagnosis of placental abruption. Am J Perinatol 9:170, 1992
Coulange L, Butori N, Loffroy R, et al: Uterine necrosis following selective embolization for postpartum hemorrhage using absorbable material. Acta Obstet Gynecol Scand 88(2):238, 2009
Counts RB, Haisch C, Simon TL, et al: Hemostasis in massively transfused trauma patients. Ann Surg 190:91, 1979
Crane JMG, Van Den Hof MC, Dodds L, et al: Neonatal outcomes with placenta previa. Obstet Gynecol 93:541, 1999
Crozier TM, Wallace EM: Obstetric admissions to an integrated general intensive care unit in a quaternary maternal facility. Aust N Z J Obstet Gynaecol 51(3):233, 2011
Dashe JS: Toward consistent terminology of placental location. Semin Perinatol 37(5):375, 2013
Dashe JS, McIntire DD, Ramus RM, et al: Persistence of placenta previa according to gestational age at ultrasound detection. Obstet Gynecol 99:692, 2002
DeLee JB: A case of fatal hemorrhagic diathesis, with premature detachment of the placenta. Am J Obstet Gynecol 44:785, 1901
Deneux-Tharaux C, Sentilhes L, Maillard F, et al: Effect of routine controlled cord traction as part of the active management of the third stage of labour on postpartum hemorrhage: multicentre randomized controlled trial (TRACOR). BMJ 346:f1541, 2013
Derman RJ, Kodkany BS, Gaudar SS, et al: Oral misoprostol in preventing postpartum haemorrhage in resource-poor communities: a randomized controlled trial. Lancet 368:1248, 2006
Desai N, Tam HT, Fleischer A: Prophylactic arterial catheterization may improve operative morbidity in suspected placenta accreta and reduce the need for hysterectomy. Am J Obstet Gynecol 206(1):S44, 2012
Dhainaut JF, Yan SB, Joyce De, et al: Treatment effects of drotrecogin alfa (activated) in patients with severe sepsis with or without overt disseminated intravascular coagulation. J Thromb Haemost 2(11):1924, 2004
Diemert A, Ortmeyer G, Hollwitz B, et al: The combination of intrauterine balloon tamponade and the B-Lynch procedure for the treatment of severe postpartum hemorrhage. Am J Obstet Gynecol 206(1):65.e1, 2012
Dildy GA, Scott AR, Saffer CS: An effective pressure pack for severe pelvic hemorrhage. Obstet Gynecol 108(5):1222, 2006
Distefano M, Casarella L, Amoroso S, et al: Selective arterial embolization as a first-line treatment for postpartum hematomas. Obstet Gynecol 121(2 Pt 2 Suppl):443, 2013
dos Santos LA, Menzin AW: Your surgical toolbox should include topical hemostatic agents—here is why. OBG Management 24(4):35, 2012
Drakeley AJ, Le Roux PA, Anthony J, et al: Acute renal failure complicating severe preeclampsia requiring admission to an obstetric intensive care unit. Am J Obstet Gynecol 186:253, 2002
Driessen M, Bouvier-Colle MH, Dupont C, et al: Postpartum hemorrhage resulting from uterine atony after vaginal delivery. Factors associated with severity. Obstet Gynecol 117(1):21, 2011
Drost S, Keil K: Expectant management of placenta previa: cost-benefit analysis of outpatient treatment. Am J Obstet Gynecol 170:1254, 1994
Druzin ML: Packing of lower uterine segment for control of postcesarean bleeding in instances of placenta previa. Surg Gynecol Obstet 169:543, 1989
Dugoff L, Hobbins JC, Malone FD, et al: First trimester maternal serum PAPPA and free-beta subunit human chorionic gonadotropin concentrations and nuchal translucency are associated with obstetric complications: a population-based screening study (The FASTER Trial). Am J Obstet Gynecol 191:1446, 2004
Duzyj C, Buhimschi I, Hardy J, et al: Decreased expression of endostatin (ES) and hypoxia-inducible factor 1α (HIF-1α) is associated with excessive trophoblast invasion and aberrant angiogenesis in placenta accreta. Abstract No. 105. Am J Obstet Gynecol 208(1):S58, 2013
Ecker JL, Solt K, Fitzsimons MG, et al: Case 40-2012—A 43-year-old woman with cardiorespiratory arrest after a cesarean section. N Engl J Med 367(26):2528, 2012
Elhawary TM, Dabees NL, Youssef MA: Diagnostic value of ultrasonography and magnetic resonance imaging in pregnant women at risk for placenta accreta. J Matern Fetal Neonatal Med 26(14):1443, 2013
Eller AG, Bennett MA, Sharshiner M, et al: Maternal morbidity in cases of placenta accreta managed by a multidisciplinary care team compared with standard obstetric care. Obstet Gynecol 117(2 Pt 1):331, 2011
Elliott JP, Gilpin B, Strong TH Jr, et al: Chronic abruption–oligohydramnios sequence. J Reprod Med 43:418, 1998
Endler M, Grünewald C, Saltvedt S: Epidemiology of retained placenta. Oxytocin as an independent risk factor. Obstet Gynecol 119(4):801, 2012
Esakoff TF, Handler SJ, Granados JM, et al: PAMUS: placenta accreta managment across the United States. J Mat Fet Neonatal Med 25:761, 2012
Eshkoli T, Weintraub AY, Sergienko R, et al: Placenta accreta: risk factors, perinatal outcomes, and consequences for subsequent births. Am J Obstet Gynecol 208(3):219.e1, 2013
Eskes TK: Clotting disorders and placental abruption: homocysteine—a new risk factor. Eur J Obstet Gynecol Reprod Biol 95:206, 2001
Etchason J, Petz L, Keeler E, et al: The cost effectiveness of preoperative autologous blood donations. N Engl J Med 332:719, 1995
Fahmy K, el-Gazar A, Sammour M, et al: Postpartum colposcopy of the cervix: injury and healing. Int J Gynaecol Obstet 34:133, 1991
Farine D, Fox HE, Jakobson S, et al: Vaginal ultrasound for diagnosis of placenta previa. Am J Obstet Gynecol 159:566, 1988
Finfer S, Bellomo R, Boyce N, et al: A comparison of albumin and saline for fluid resuscitation in the intensive care unit. N Engl J Med 350:2247, 2004
Fiori O, Deux JF, Kambale JC, et al: Impact of pelvic arterial embolization for intractable postpartum hemorrhage on fertility. Am J Obstet Gynecol 200:384.e1, 2009
Fitzpatrick K, Sellers S, Spark P, et al: The management and outcomes of placenta accreta, increta, and percreta in the UK: a population-based descriptive study. BJOG 121(1):62, 2014
Franchini M, Lippi G, Franchi M: The use of recombinant activated factor VII in obstetric and gynaecological haemorrhage. BJOG 114:8, 2007
Frederiksen MC, Glassenberg R, Stika CS: Placenta previa: a 22-year analysis. Am J Obstet Gynecol 180:1432, 1999
Fretts RC, Usher RH: Causes of fetal death in women of advanced maternal age. Obstet Gynecol 89:40, 1997
Friederich L, Roman H, Marpeau L: A dangerous development. Am J Obstet Gynecol 196:92, 2007
Friszer S, Le Ray C, Tort J, et al: Symptomatic placenta praevia: short cervix at admission is a predictive factor for delivery within 7 days. Abstract No. 158. Am J Obstet Gynecol 208(1):S78, 2013
Furuhashi M, Kurauchi O, Suganuma N: Pregnancy following placental abruption. Arch Gynecol Obstet 267:11, 2002
Garmi G, Samlim R: Epidemiology, etiology, diagnosis, and management of placenta accreta. Obstet Gynecol Int 2012:873929, 2012
Georgiou C: Balloon tamponade in the management of postpartum haemorrhage: a review. BJOG 116(6):748, 2009
Gerstenfeld TS, Wing DA: Rectal misoprostol versus intravenous oxytocin for the prevention of postpartum hemorrhage after vaginal delivery. Am J Obstet Gynecol 185:878, 2001
Gesteland K, Oshiro B, Henry E, et al: Rates of placenta previa and placental abruption in women delivered only vaginally or only by cesarean section. Abstract No. 403. J Soc Gynecol Invest 11:208A, 2004
Getahun BS, Yeshi MM, Roberts DJ: Case records of the Massachusetts General Hospital: case 34-2012: a 27-year old woman in Ethiopia with severe pain, bleeding, and shock during labor. N Engl J Med 367(19):1839, 2012

Gilbert WM, Danielsen B: Amniotic fluid embolism: decreased mortality in a population-based study. Obstet Gynecol 93:973, 1999
Gilliam M, Rosenberg D, Davis F: The likelihood of placenta previa with greater number of cesarean deliveries and higher parity. Obstet Gynecol 99:976, 2002
Gilstrap LC III: Management of postpartum hemorrhage. In Gilstrap LC III, Cunningham FG, Van Dorsten JP (eds): Operative Obstetrics, 2nd ed. New York, McGraw-Hill, 2002, p 397
Glantz C, Purnell L: Clinical utility of sonography in the diagnosis and treatment of placental abruption. J Ultrasound Med 21:837, 2002
Gonzalez EA, Moore FA, Holcomb JB, et al: Fresh frozen plasma should be given earlier to patients requiring massive transfusion. J Trauma 62:112, 2007
Gottlieb AG, Pandipati S, Davis KM, et al: Uterine necrosis. A complication of uterine compression sutures. Obstet Gynecol 112:429, 2008
Greenberg JI, Suliman A, Iranpour P, et al: Prophylactic balloon occlusion of the internal iliac arteries to treat abnormal placentation: a cautionary case. Am J Obstet Gynecol 197:470.e1, 2007
Grönvall M, Tikkanen M, Tallberg E: Use of Bakri balloon tamponade in the treatment of postpartum hemorrhage: a series of 50 cases from a tertiary teaching hospital. Acta Obstet Gynecol Scand 92(4):433, 2013
Grünfeld JP, Pertuiset N: Acute renal failure in pregnancy: 1987. Am J Kidney Dis 4:359, 1987
Gülmezoglu AM, Lumbiganon P, Landoulsi S, et al: Active management of the third stage of labor with and without controlled cord traction: a randomized, controlled, non-inferiority trial. Lancet 379(9827):1721, 2012
Gurol-Urganci I, Cromwell DA, Edozien LC, et al: Risk of placenta previa in second birth after first birth cesarean section. BMC Pregnancy Childbirth 11:95, 2011
Gyamfi-Bannerman C, Gilbert S, Landon MB, et al: Risk of uterine rupture and placenta accreta with prior uterine surgery outside of the lower segment. Obstet Gynecol 120(6):1332, 2012
Hale SA, Sobel B, Benvenuto A, et al: Coagulation and fibrinolytic system protein profiles in women with normal pregnancies and pregnancies complicated by hypertension. Pregnancy Hypertens 2(2):152, 2012
Hankins GDV, Berryman GK, Scott RT Jr, et al: Maternal arterial desaturation with 15-methyl prostaglandin F2 alpha for uterine atony. Obstet Gynecol 72:367, 1988
Hankins GDV, Snyder RR, Clark SL, et al: Acute hemodynamic and respiratory effects of amniotic fluid embolism in the pregnant goat model. Am J Obstet Gynecol 168:1113, 1993
Hankins GDV, Snyder R, Dinh T, et al: Documentation of amniotic fluid embolism via lung histopathology: fact or fiction? J Reprod Med 47:1021, 2002
Hardardottir H, Borgida AF, Sanders MM, et al: Histologic myometrial fibers adherent to the placenta: impact of method of placental removal. Am J Obstet Gynecol 174:358, 1996
Harper LM, Odibo AO, Macones GA, et al: Effect of placenta previa on fetal growth. Am J Obstet Gynecol 203(4):330.e1, 2010
Harvey C, Hankins G, Clark S: Amniotic fluid embolism and oxygen transport patterns. Am J Obstet Gynecol 174:304, 1996
Hauth JC, Cunningham FG: Preeclampsia-eclampsia. In Lindheimer ML, Roberts JM, Cunningham FG (eds): Chesley's Hypertensive Disorders in Pregnancy, 2nd ed. Stamford, CT, Appleton & Lange, 1999, p 179
Hayman RG, Arulkumaran S, Steer PJ: Uterine compression sutures: surgical management of postpartum hemorrhage. Obstet Gynecol 99:502, 2002
Hays AME, Worley KC, Roberts SR: Conservative management of placenta percreta. Experience in two cases. Obstet Gynecol 112:1, 2008
Hebert PC, Wells G, Blajchman MA, et al: A multicenter, randomized, controlled clinical trial of transfusion requirements in critical care. N Engl J Med 340:409, 1999
Hellman LM, Pritchard JA (eds): Medical and surgical illnesses during pregnancy and the puerperium. In Williams Obstetrics, 14th ed. New York, Appleton-Century-Crofts, 1971, p 763
Hernandez JS, Alexander JM, Sarode R, et al: Calculated blood loss in severe obstetric hemorrhage and its relation to body mass index. Am J Perinatol 29(7):557, 2012
Hertzberg BS, Bowie JD, Carroll BA, et al: Diagnosis of placenta previa during the third trimester: role of transperineal sonography. AJR Am J Roentgenol 159:83, 1992
Hoffman MS, Karlnoski RA, Mangar D, et al: Morbidity associated with nonemergent hysterectomy for placenta accreta. Am J Obstet Gynecol 202(6):628.e1, 2010
Hofmeyr GJ, Abdel-Aleem H, Abdel-Aleem MA: Uterine massage for preventing postpartum haemorrhage. Cochrane Database Syst Rev 7:CD006431, 2008
Hogberg V, Rasmussen S, Irgens L: The effect of smoking and hypertensive disorders on abruptio placentae in Norway 1999–2002. Acta Obstet Gynecol Scand 86:304, 2007
Hong RW, Greenfield ML, Polley LS: Nitroglycerin for uterine inversion in the absence of placental fragments. Anesth Anal 103:511, 2006
Hossain N, Paidas MJ: Disseminated intravascular coagulation. Semin Perinatol 37(4):257, 2013
Hoyert DL: Maternal mortality and related concepts. Vital Health Stat 3 33:1, 2007
Hsu S, Rodgers B, Lele A, et al: Use of packing in obstetric hemorrhage of uterine origin. J Reprod Med 48:69, 2003
Hui C, Lili M, Libin C, et al: Changes in coagulation and hemodynamics during pregnancy: a prospective longitudinal study of 58 cases. Arch Gynecol Obstet 285(5):1231, 2012
Huissoud C, Cortet M, Dubernard G, et al: A stitch in time: layers of circular sutures can staunch postpartum hemorrhage. Am J Obstet Gynecol 206:177.e1–2, 2012
Hung TH, Shau WY, Hsieh CC, et al: Risk factors for placenta accreta. Obstet Gynecol 93:545, 1999
Hurd WW, Miodovnik M, Hertzberg V, et al: Selective management of abruptio placentae: a prospective study. Obstet Gynecol 61:467, 1983
Ibrahim MI, Raafat TA, Ellaithy MI, et al: Risk of postpartum uterine synechiae following uterine compression suturing during postpartum haemorrhage. Aust N Z J Obstet Gynecol 53(1):37, 2013
Jackson BR, Busch MP, Stramer SL, et al: The cost-effectiveness of NAT for HIV, HCV, and HBV in whole-blood donations. Transfusion 43:721, 2003
Jimenez JM, Pritchard JA: Pathogenesis and treatment of coagulation defects resulting from fetal death. Obstet Gynecol 32:449, 1968
Johansson PI, Stensballe J, Rosenberg I, et al: Proactive administration of platelets and plasma for patients with a ruptured abdominal aortic aneurysm: evaluating a change in transfusion practice. Transfusion 47:593, 2007
Joshi VM, Otiv SR, Majumder R, et al: Internal iliac artery ligation for arresting postpartum haemorrhage. BJOG 114:356, 2007
Joshi VM, Shrivastava M: Partial ischemic necrosis of the uterus following a uterine brace compression suture. BJOG 111:279, 2004
Kamara M, Henderson J, Doherty D, et al: The risk of placenta accreta following primary elective caesarean delivery: a case-control study. BJOG 120(7):879, 2013
Kaminsky LM, Ananth CV, Prasad V, et al: The influence of maternal cigarette smoking on placental pathology in pregnancies complicated by abruption. Am J Obstet Gynecol 197:275.e1, 2007
Karam AK, Bristow RE, Bienstock J, et al: Argon beam coagulation facilitates management of placenta percreta with bladder invasion. Obstet Gynecol 102:555, 2003
Katakam N, Vitthala S, Sasson S, et al: Complications and failure of uterine artery embolization for intractable postpartum haemorrhage. BJOG 116(6):863, 2009
Kayani SI, Walkinshaw SA, Preston C: Pregnancy outcome in severe placental abruption. BJOG 110:679, 2003
Kayem G, Pannier E, Goffinet F, et al: Fertility after conservative treatment of placenta accreta. Fertil Steril 78:637, 2002
Kayem G, Kurinczuk JJ, Alfirevic A, et al: Uterine compression sutures for the management of severe postpartum hemorrhage. Obstet Gynecol 117(1):14, 2011
Kenny L, McCrae K, Cunningham FG: Platelets, coagulation, and the liver. In Taylor R, Roberts JM, Cunningham FG (eds) : Chesley's Hypertension in Pregnancy, 4th ed. Amsterdam, Academic Press, 2014
Kettel LM, Branch DW, Scott JR: Occult placental abruption after maternal trauma. Obstet Gynecol 71:449, 1988
Khong TY: Expression of endothelin-1 in amnionic fluid embolism and possible pathophysiological mechanism. BJOG 105(7):802, 1998
Kieser KE, Baskett TF: A 10-year population-based study of uterine rupture. Obstet Gynecol 100:749, 2002
Kikuchi M, Itakura A, Miki A, et al: Fibrinogen concentrate substitution therapy for obstetric hemorrhage complicated by coagulopathy. J Obstet Gynaecol Res 39(4):770, 2013
King DL: Placental migration demonstrated by ultrasonography. Radiology 109:167, 1973
Knight M, Berg C, Brocklehurst P, et al: Amniotic fluid embolism incidence, risk factors and outcomes: a review and recommendations. BMC Pregnancy Childbirth 12:7, 2012
Knight M, Tuffnell D, Brocklehurst P, et al: Incidence and risk factors for amniotic-fluid embolism. Obstet Gynecol 115(5):910, 2010
Knight M, UKOSS: Peripartum hysterectomy in the UK: management and outcomes of the associated haemorrhage. BJOG 114:1380, 2007
Kochenour N: Diagnosis and management of uterine inversion. In Gilstrap LG III, Cunningham FG, VanDorsten JP (eds): Operative Obstetrics. New York, McGraw-Hill, 2002, p 241
Kohari KS, Roman AS, Fox NS, et al: Persistence of placenta previa in twin gestations based on gestational age at sonographic detection. J Ultrasound Med 31(7):985, 2012

Kolomeyevskaya NV, Tanyi JL, Coleman NM, et al: Balloon tamponade of hemorrhage after uterine curettage for gestational trophoblastic disease. Obstet Gynecol 113:557, 2009

Kotsuji F, Nishihima K, Kurokawa T, et al: Transverse uterine fundal incision for placenta praevia with accreta, involving the entire anterior uterine wall: a case series. BJOG 120(9):1144, 2013

Kramer MS, Berg C, Abenhaim H, et al: Incidence, risk factors, and temporal trends in severe postpartum hemorrhage. Am J Obstet Gynecol 209(5):449.e1, 2013

Kramer MS, Rouleau J, Liu S, et al: Amniotic fluid embolism: incidence, risk factors, and impact on perinatal outcomes. BJOG 119(7):874, 2012

Kramer MS, Usher RH, Pollack R, et al: Etiologic determinants of abruptio placentae. Obstet Gynecol 89:221, 1997

Kuklina EV, Meikle SG, Jamieson DJ, et al: Severe obstetric morbidity in the United States: 1998–2005. Obstet Gynecol 113:298, 2009

Kumru P, Demirci O, Erdogdu E, et al: The Bakri balloon for the management of postpartum hemorrhage in cases with placenta previa. Eur J Obstet Gynecol Reprod Biol 167(2):167, 2013

Laas E, Bui C, Popowski T, et al: Trends in the rate of invasive procedures after the addition of the intrauterine tamponade test to a protocol for management of severe postpartum hemorrhage. Am J Obstet Gynecol 207(4):281.e1, 2012

Lai J, Caughey AB, Qidwai GI, et al: Neonatal outcomes in women with sonographically identified uterine leiomyomata. J Matern Fetal Neonatal Med 25(6):710, 2012

Laing FC: Ultrasound evaluation of obstetric problems relating to the lower uterine segment and cervix. In Fleischer AC, Manning FA, Jeanty P, et al (eds): Sonography in Obstetrics and Gynecology: Principles and Practice, 5th ed. Stamford, CT, Appleton & Lange, 1996, p 720

Lalonde A, Daviss BA, Acosta A, et al: Postpartum hemorrhage today: ICM/FIGO initiative 2004–2006. Int J Obstet Gynaecol 94:243, 2006

Landy HJ, Laughon K, Bailit JL, et al: Characteristics associated with severe perineal and cervical lacerations during vaginal delivery. Obstet Gynecol 117(3):627, 2011

Landy HJ, Weingold AB: Management of a multiple gestation complicated by an antepartum fetal demise. Obstet Gynecol Surv 44:171, 1989

Laughon SK, Wolfe HM, Visco AG: Prior cesarean and the risk for placenta previa on second-trimester ultrasonography. Obstet Gynecol 105:962, 2005

Law LW, Chor CM, Leung TY: Use of hemostatic gel in postpartum hemorrhage due to placenta previa. Obstet Gynecol 116(Suppl 2:528, 2010

Lax A, Prince MR, Mennitt KW, et al: The value of specific MRI features in the evaluation of suspected placental invasion. Magn Reson Imaging 25:87, 2007

Lee HY, Shin JH, Kim J, et al: Primary postpartum hemorrhage: outcome of pelvic arterial embolization in 251 patients at a single institution. Radiology 264(3):903, 2012

Lee PS, Bakelaar R, Fitpatrick CB, et al: Medical and surgical treatment of placenta percreta to optimize bladder preservation. Obstet Gynecol 112:421, 2008

Lee W, Ginsburg KA, Cotton DB, et al: Squamous and trophoblastic cells in the maternal pulmonary circulation identified by invasive hemodynamic monitoring during the peripartum period. Am J Obstet Gynecol 155:999, 1986

Lerner R, Margolin M, Slate WG, et al: Heparin in the treatment of hypofibrinogenemia complicating fetal death in utero. Am J Obstet Gynecol 97:373, 1967

Lerner NB, Refaai MA, Blumberg N: Red cell transfusion. In Kaushansky K, Lichtman M, Beutler K, et al (eds): Williams Hematology, 8th ed. New York, McGraw-Hill, 2010, p 2287

Leung TY, Chan LW, Tam WH, et al: Risk and prediction of preterm delivery in pregnancies complicated by antepartum hemorrhage of unknown origin before 34 weeks. Gynecol Obstet Invest 52:227, 2001

Levi M: Pathogenesis and management of peripartum coagulopathic calamities (disseminated intravascular coagulation and amniotic fluid embolism). Thromb Res 131(Suppl 1):S32, 2013

Levi M, Levy JH, Andersen HF, et al: Safety of recombinant activated factor VII in randomized clinical trials. N Engl J Med 363(19):1791, 2010a

Levi M, Seligsohn U: Disseminated intravascular coagulation. In Kaushansky K, Lichtman M, Beutler K, et al (eds): Williams Hematology, 8th ed. New York, McGraw-Hill, 2010b, p 2101

Lichtenberg ES: Angiography as treatment for a high cervical tear—a case report. J Reprod Med 48:287, 2003

Lin Y, Callum JL, Coovadia AS, et al: Transfusion of ABO-nonidentical platelets is not associated with adverse clinical outcomes in cardiovascular surgery patients. Transfusion 42:166, 2002

Linden JV, Wagner K, Voytovich AE, et al: Transfusion errors in New York State: an analysis of 10 years' experience. Transfusion 40:1207, 2001

Lindheimer MD, Conrad KP, Karumanchi SA: Renal physiology and disease in pregnancy. In Alpern R (ed): Seldin and Greisch's The Kidney. New York, Elsevier, 2007, p 2361

Lipitz S, Admon D, Menczer J, et al: Midtrimester bleeding: variables which affect the outcome of pregnancy. Gynecol Obstet Invest 32:24, 1991

Lo TK, Lau WL, Leung WC: Conservative management of placenta accreta. Abstract No. 165. Am J Obstet Gynecol 208(1):S81, 2013a

Lo TK, Lau WL, Leung WC: Use of Sengstaken tube for management of severe postpartum hemorrhage. Abstract No. 164. Am J Obstet Gynecol 208(1):S80, 2013b

Logothetopulos K: Eine absolut sichere Blutstillungsmethode bei vaginalen und abdominalen gynakologischen Operationen. Zentralbl Gynakol 50:3202, 1926

Magpie Trial Collaborative Group: Do women with preeclampsia, and their babies, benefit from magnesium sulphate? The Magpie Trial: a randomised placebo-controlled trial. Lancet 359:1877, 2002

Maher MA, Abdelaziz A, Bazeed MF: Diagnostic accuracy of ultrasound and MRI in the prenatal diagnosis of placenta accreta. Acta Obstet Gynecol Scand 92(9):1017, 2013

Major CA, deVeciana M, Lewis DF, et al: Preterm premature rupture of membranes and abruptio placentae: is there an association between these pregnancy complications? Am J Obstet Gynecol 172:672, 1995

Mannucci PM, Levi M: Prevention and treatment of major blood loss. N Engl J Med 356:2301, 2007

Marik PE, Corwin HL: Acute lung injury following blood transfusion: expanding the definition. Crit Care Med 36(11):3080, 2008

Martin JA, Hamilton BE, Sutton PD, et al: Births: final data for 2003. Natl Vital Stat Rep 54(2):1, 2005

Masselli G, Brunelli R, Di Tola M, et al: MR imaging in the evaluation of placental abruption: correlation with sonographic findings. Radiology 259(1):222, 2011

Matijevic N, Wang YW, Cotton BA, et al: Better hemostatic profiles of never-frozen liquid plasma compared with thawed fresh frozen plasma. J Trauma Acute Care Surg 74(1):84, 2013

Matsubara S, Kuwata T, Usui R, et al: Important surgical measures and techniques at cesarean hysterectomy for placenta previa accreta. Acta Obstet Gynecol Scand 92(4):372, 2013a

Matsubara S, Yano H, Ohkuchi A, et al: Uterine compression suture for postpartum hemorrhage: an overview. Acta Obstet Gynecol Scand 92(4):378, 2013b

Matsubara S, Yano H, Taneichi A, et al: Uterine compression suture against impending recurrence of uterine inversion immediately after laparotomy positioning. J Obstet Gynaecol Res 35(4):819, 2009

Matsuda Y, Hayashi K, Shiozaki A, et al: Comparison of risk factors for placental abruption and placenta previa: case-cohort study. J Obstet Gynaecol Res 37(6):538, 2011

Matsuda Y, Maeda T, Kouno S: Comparison of neonatal outcome including cerebral palsy between abruptio placentae and placenta previa. Eur J Obstet Gynecol Reprod Biol 106:125, 2003

Matsuda Y, Ogawa M, Konno J, et al: Prediction of fetal acidemia in placental abruption. BMC Pregnancy Childbirth 13:156, 2013

Matsuwaki T, Khan KN, Inoue T, et al: Evaluation of obstetrical factors related to Sheehan syndrome. J Obstet Gynaecol Res 40(1):46, 2014

Maymon R, Shulman A, Pomeranz M, et al: Uterine rupture at term pregnancy with the use of intracervical prostaglandin E2 gel for induction of labor. Am J Obstet Gynecol 165:368, 1991

McCormick ML, Sanghvi HC, McIntosh N: Preventing postpartum hemorrhage in low-resource settings. Int J Gynaecol Obstet 77:267, 2002

McKeogh RP, D'Errico E: Placenta accreta: clinical manifestations and conservative management. N Engl J Med 245(5):159, 1951

McVay PA, Hoag RW, Hoag MS, et al: Safety and use of autologous blood donation during the third trimester of pregnancy. Am J Obstet Gynecol 160:1479, 1989

Mehrabadi A, Hutcheon J, Lee L, et al: Epidemiological investigation of a temporal increase in atonic postpartum haemorrhage: a population-base retrospective cohort study. BJOG 120(7):853, 2013

Melamed N, Ben-Haroush A, Chen R, Kaplan B, et al: Intrapartum cervical lacerations: characteristics, risk factors, and effects on subsequent pregnancies. Am J Obstet Gynecol 200(4):388.e1, 2009

Miller DA, Goodwin TM, Gherman RB, et al: Intrapartum rupture of the unscarred uterus. Obstet Gynecol 89:671, 1997

Miller DA, Paul RH: Rupture of the unscarred uterus. Am J Obstet Gynecol 174:345, 1996

Misra DP, Ananth CV: Risk factor profiles of placental abruption in first and second pregnancies: heterogeneous etiologies. J Clin Epidemiol 52:453, 1999

Mondal PC, Ghosh D, Santra D, et al: Role of Hayman technique and its modification in recurrent puerperal uterine inversion. J Obstet Gynaecol Res 38(2):438, 2012

Montagnana M, Franchi M, Danese E, et al: Disseminated intravascular coagulation in obstetric and gynecologic disorders. Semin Thromb Hemost 36(4):404, 2010

Morrison JC, Martin RW, Dodson MK, et al: Blood transfusions after postpartum hemorrhage due to uterine atony. J Matern Fetal Invest 1:209, 1991
Mortensen JT, Thulstrup AM, Larsen H, et al: Smoking, sex of the offspring, and risk of placental abruption, placenta previa, and preeclampsia: a population-based cohort study. Acta Obstet Gynecol Scand 80:894, 2001
Mouer JR: Placenta previa: antepartum conservative management, inpatient versus outpatient. Am J Obstet Gynecol 170:1683, 1994
Mousa HA, Alfirevic Z: Treatment for primary postpartum haemorrhage. Cochrane Database Syst Rev 1:CD003249, 2007
Murphy M, Vassallo R: Preservation and clinical use of platelets. In Kaushansky K, Lichtman M, Beutler K, et al (eds): Williams Hematology, 8th ed. New York, McGraw-Hill, 2010, p 2301
Naeye RL: Abruptio placentae and placenta previa: frequency, perinatal mortality, and cigarette smoking. Obstet Gynecol 55:701, 1980
Nagaya K, Fetters MD, Ishikawa M, et al: Causes of maternal mortality in Japan. JAMA 283:2661, 2000
Nakash A, Tuck S, Davies N: Uterine sepsis with uterine artery embolisation in the management of obstetric bleeding. J Obstet Gynecol 32(1):26, 2012
Nath CA, Ananth CV, DeMarco C, et al: Low birthweight in relation to placental abruption and maternal thrombophilia status. Am J Obstet Gynecol 198:293.e1, 2008
Nath CA, Ananth CV, Smulian JC, et al: Histologic evidence of inflammation and risk of placental abruption. Am J Obstet Gynecol 197:319.e1, 2007
Neilson JP: Interventions for suspected placenta praevia. Cochrane Database Syst Rev 2:CD001998, 2003
Nelson DB, Yost NP, Cunningham FG: Acute fatty liver of pregnancy: clinical outcomes and expected durations of recovery. Am J Obstet Gynecol 209(5):456.e1, 2013
Nelson EL, Parker AN, Dudley DJ: Spontaneous vulvar hematoma during pregnancy: a case report. J Reprod Med 57(1–2):74, 2012
Nelson WL, O'Brien JM: The uterine sandwich for persistent uterine atony: combining the B-Lynch compression suture and an intrauterine Bakri balloon. Am J Obstet Gynecol 196(5):e9, 2007
Ness PM, Cushing M: Oxygen therapeutics: pursuit of an alternative to the donor red blood cell. Arch Pathol Lab Med 131(5):734, 2007
Ngai I, Bernstein P, Chazotte C, et al: Maternal serum alpha fetoprotein (MSAFP) and placental abruption. Abstract No. 122. Am J Obstet Gynecol 206(1):S66, 2012
Nikolaou M, Kourea HP, Antonopoulos K, et al: Spontaneous uterine rupture in a primigravid woman in the early third trimester attributed to adenomyosis: a case report and review of literature. J Obstet Gynaecol Res 39(3):727, 2013
Nizard J, Barrinque L, Frydman R, et al: Fertility and pregnancy outcomes following hypogastric artery ligation for severe post-partum haemorrhage. Hum Reprod 18:844, 2003
Nørgaard LN, Pinborg A, Lidegaard Ø, et al: A Danish national cohort study on neonatal outcome in singleton pregnancies with placenta previa. Acta Obstet Gynecol Scand 91(5):546, 2012
O'Brien P, El-Refaey H, Gordon A, et al: Rectally administered misoprostol for the treatment of postpartum hemorrhage unresponsive to oxytocin and ergometrine: a descriptive study. Obstet Gynecol 92:212, 1998
Ochoa M, Allaire AD, Stitely ML: Pyometria after hemostatic square suture technique. Obstet Gynecol 99:506, 2002
Ogah K, Munjuluri N: Complete uterine inversion after vaginal delivery. J Obstet Gynaecol 31(3):265, 2011
Ojala K, Perala J, Kariniemi J, et al: Arterial embolization and prophylactic catheterization for the treatment for severe obstetric hemorrhage. Acta Obstet Gynecol Scand 84:1075, 2005
Oladapo OT, Okusanya BO, Abalos E: Intramuscular versus intravenous prophylactic oxytocin for the third stage of labour. Cochrane Database Syst Rev 2:CD009332, 2012
Oleen MA, Mariano JP: Controlling refractory atonic postpartum hemorrhage with Hemabate sterile solution. Am J Obstet Gynecol 162:205, 1990
Oyelese Y, Smulian JC: Placenta previa, placenta accreta, and vasa previa. Obstet Gynecol 107:927, 2006
Pacheco LD, Saade GR, Constantine MM, et al: The role of massive transfusion protocols in obstetrics. Am J Perinatol 30(1):1, 2013
Pacheco LD, Saade GR, Gei AF, et al: Cutting-edge advances in the medical management of obstetrical hemorrhage. Am J Obstet Gynecol 205(6):526, 2011
Palacios Jaraquemada JM, Bruno CH: Magnetic resonance imaging in 300 cases of placenta accreta: surgical correlation of new findings. Acta Obstet Gynecol Scand 84:716, 2005
Pariente G, Shoham-Vardi I, Kessous R, et al: Placental abruption as a marker for long term cardiovascular mortality: a follow-up period of more than a decade. Am J Obstet Gynecol 208(1):S62, 2013
Parikh R, Brotzman S, Anasti JN: Cervical lacerations: some surprising facts. Am J Obstet Gynecol 196(5):e17, 2007
Pates JA, Hatab MR, McIntire DD, et al: Determining uterine blood flow in pregnancy with magnetic resonance imaging. Magn Reson Imaging 28(4):507, 2010
Patterson JA, Roberts CL, Bowen JR, et al: Blood transfusions during pregnancy, birth, and the postnatal period. Obstet Gynecol 123(1):126, 2014
Pauleta JR, Rodrigues R, Melo MA, et al: Ultrasonographic diagnosis of incomplete uterine inversion. Ultrasound Obstet Gynecol 36:260, 2010
Pearlman MD, Tintinalli JE, Lorenz RP: A prospective controlled study of outcome after trauma during pregnancy. Am J Obstet Gynecol 162:1502, 1990
Pelosi MA III, Pelosi MA: Spontaneous uterine rupture at thirty-three weeks subsequent to previous superficial laparoscopic myomectomy. Am J Obstet Gynecol 177:1547, 1997
Peña-Marti G, Coumunián-Carrasco G: Fundal pressure versus controlled cord traction as part of the active management of the third stage of labour. Cochrane Database Sys Rev 4:CD005462, 2007
Penotti M, Vercellini P, Bolis G: Compressive suture of the lower uterine segment for the treatment of postpartum hemorrhage due to complete placenta previa: a preliminary study. Gynecol Obstet Invest 73(4):314, 2012
Perel P, Roberts I: Colloids versus crystalloids for fluid resuscitation in critically ill patients. Cochrane Database Syst Rev 17:CD000567, 2007
Petersen IR, Nyholm HCJ: Multiple pregnancies with single intrauterine demise. Description of twenty-eight pregnancies. Acta Obstet Gynecol Scand 78:202, 1999
Po LK, Simons ME, Levinsky ES: Concealed postpartum hemorrhage treated with transcatheter arterial embolization. Obstet Gynecol 120(2 Pt 2):461, 2012
Porreco RP, Clark SL, Belfort MA, et al: The changing specter of uterine rupture. Am J Obstet Gynecol 200(3):269.e1, 2009
Porter TF, Clark SL, Dildy GA, et al: Isolated disseminated intravascular coagulation and amniotic fluid embolism. Am J Obstet Gynecol 174:486, 1996
Poujade O, Grossetti A, Mougel L, et al: Risk of synechiae following uterine compression sutures in the management of major postpartum haemorrhage. BJOG 118(4):433, 2011
Poujade O, Zappa M, Letendre I, et al: Predictive factors for failure of pelvic arterial embolization for postpartum hemorrhage. Int J Gynaecol Obstet 117(2):119, 2012
Prick BW, Vos AA, Hop WC, et al: The current state of active third stage management to prevent postpartum hemorrhage: a cross-sectional study. Acta Obstet Gynecol Scand 92(11):1277, 2013
Pri-Paz S, Devine PC, Miller RS, et al: Cesarean hysterectomy requiring emergent thoracotomy: a case report of a complication of placenta percreta requiring a multidisciplinary effort. J Reprod Med 57(1–2):58, 2012
Pritchard JA: Changes in the blood volume during pregnancy and delivery. Anesthesiology 26:393, 1965
Pritchard JA: Fetal death in utero. Obstet Gynecol 14:573, 1959
Pritchard JA: Haematological problems associated with delivery, placental abruption, retained dead fetus, and amniotic fluid embolism. Clin Haematol 2:563, 1973
Pritchard JA, Baldwin RM, Dickey JC, et al: Blood volume changes in pregnancy and the puerperium, 2. Red blood cell loss and changes in apparent blood volume during and following vaginal delivery, cesarean section, and cesarean section plus total hysterectomy. Am J Obstet Gynecol 84:1271, 1962
Pritchard JA, Brekken AL: Clinical and laboratory studies on severe abruptio placentae. Am J Obstet Gynecol 97:681, 1967
Pritchard JA, Cunningham FG, Mason RA: Coagulation changes in eclampsia: their frequency and pathogenesis. Am J Obstet Gynecol 124:855, 1976a
Pritchard JA, Cunningham FG, Pritchard SA, et al: On reducing the frequency of severe abruptio placentae. Am J Obstet Gynecol 165:1345, 1991
Pritchard JA, MacDonald, PC (eds): Williams Obstetrics, 15th ed. Appleton-Century-Crofts, New York, 1976b
Pritchard JA, Mason R, Corley M, et al: Genesis of severe placental abruption. Am J Obstet Gynecol 108:22, 1970
Pritchard JA, Whalley PJ: Abortion complicated by *Clostridium perfringens* infection. Am J Obstet Gynecol 111:484, 1971
Propst AM, Thorp JM Jr: Traumatic vulvar hematomas: conservative versus surgical management. South Med J 91:144, 1998
Rachagan SP, Raman S, Balasundram G, et al: Rupture of the pregnant uterus—a 21-year review. Aust N Z J Obstet Gynaecol 31:37, 1991
Rafi J, Muppala H: Retroperitoneal haematomas in obstetrics: literature review. Arch Gynecol Obstet 281(3):435, 2010
Rainaldi MP, Tazzari PL, Scagliarini G, et al: Blood salvage during caesarean section. Br J Anesth 81(5):825, 1998
Rana KA, Patel PS: Complete uterine inversion: an unusual yet crucial sonographic diagnosis. J Ultrasound Med 28(12):1719, 2009

Rani PR, Haritha PH, Gowri R: Comparative study of transperineal and transabdominal sonography in the diagnosis of placenta previa. J Obstet Gynaecol 33:134, 2007
Rao KP, Belogolovkin V, Hankowitz J, et al: Abnormal placentation: evidence-base diagnosis and management of placenta previa, placenta accreta, and vasa previa. Obstet Gynecol Surv 67(8):503, 2012
Rasmussen S, Irgens LM: Occurrence of placental abruption in relatives. BJOG 116:693, 2009
Rattray DD, O'Connell CM, Baskett TF: Acute disseminated intravascular coagulation in obstetrics: a tertiary centre population review (1980 to 2009). J Obstet Gynaecol Can 34(4):341, 2012
Rebarber A, Fox NS, Eckstein DA, et al: Successful bilateral uterine artery embolization during an ongoing pregnancy. Obstet Gynecol 113:554, 2009
Reyal F, Sibony O, Oury JF, et al: Criteria for transfusion in severe postpartum hemorrhage: analysis of practice and risk factors. Eur J Obstet Gynecol Reprod Biol 112:61, 2004
Ridgway LE: Puerperal emergency: vaginal and vulvar hematomas. Obstet Gynecol Clin North Am 22:275, 1995
Riihimäki O, Metsäranta M, Ritvanen A, et al: Increased prevalence of major congenital anomalies in births with placental abruption. Obstet Gynecol 122(2 Pt 1):268, 2013
Robalo R, Pedroso C, Agapito A, et al: Acute Sheehan's syndrome presenting as central diabetes insipidus. BMJ Case Rep Online Nov 6, 2012
Roberts CL, Algert CS, Warrendorf J, et al: Trends and recurrence of placenta previa: a population-based study. Aust N Z J Obstet Gynaecol 52(5):483, 2012
Roberts JM, Myatt L, Spong CY, et al: Vitamins C and E to prevent complications of pregnancy-associated hypertension. N Engl J Med 362(14):1282, 2010
Robinson AJ, Muller PR, Allan R, et al: Precise mid-trimester placenta localisation: does it predict adverse outcomes? Aust N Z J Obstet Gynaecol 52(2):156, 2012
Robinson CJ, Villers MS, Johnson DD, et al: Timing of elective repeat cesarean delivery at term and neonatal outcomes: a cost analysis. Am J Obstet Gynecol 202(6):632, 2010
Robson S, Adair S, Bland P: A new surgical technique for dealing with uterine inversion. Aust N Z J Obstet Gynaecol 45:250, 2005
Rosenberg T, Pariente G, Sergienko R, et al: Critical analysis of risk factors and outcome of placenta previa. Arch Gynecol Obstet 284(1):47, 2011
Rossi AC, Lee RH, Chmait RH: Emergency postpartum hysterectomy for uncontrolled postpartum bleeding: a systematic review. Obstet Gynecol 115(3):637, 2010
Rotas MA, Haberman S, Luvgur M: Cesarean scar ectopic pregnancies: etiology, diagnosis, and management. Obstet Gynecol 107:1373, 2006
Rouse DJ: Epidemiological investigation of a temporal increase in atonic postpartum haemorrhage: a population-based retrospective cohort study. Obstet Gynecol 122(3):693, 2013
Rouse DJ, MacPherson C, Landon M, et al: Blood transfusion and cesarean delivery. Obstet Gynecol 108:891, 2006
Sabourin JN, Lee T, Magee LA, et al: Indications for, timing of, and modes of delivery in a national cohort of women admitted with antepartum hemorrhage at 22+0 to 28+6 weeks' gestation. J Obstet Gynaecol Can 34(11):1043, 2012
Salihu HM, Bekan B, Aliyu MH, et al: Perinatal mortality associated with abruptio placenta in singletons and multiples. Am J Obstet Gynecol 193:198, 2005
Salihu HM, Li Q, Rouse DJ, et al: Placenta previa: neonatal death after live births in the United States. Am J Obstet Gynecol 188:1305, 2003
Sanderson DA, Milton PJD: The effectiveness of ultrasound screening at 18–20 weeks gestational age for predication of placenta previa. J Obstet Gynaecol 11:320, 1991
Sangwan N, Nanda S, Singhal S, et al: Puerperal uterine inversion associated with unicornuate uterus. Arch Gynecol Obstet 280(4):625, 2009
Saraiya M, Green CA, Berg CJ, et al: Spontaneous abortion-related deaths among women in the United States—1981–1991. Obstet Gynecol 94:172, 1999
Schenone MH, Schlabritz-Loutsevitch N, Zhang J, et al: Abruptio placentae in the baboon (*Papio* spp.). Placenta 33(4):278, 2012
Schimmer BP, Parker KL: Contraception and pharmacotherapy of obstetrical and gynecological disorders. In Brunton LL, Chabner BA, Knollmann BC (ed): Goodman and Gilman's The Pharmacological Basis of Therapeutics, 12th ed. New York, McGraw-Hill, 2011, p 1851
Schlabritz-Loutsevitch N, Hubbard G, Zhang J, et al: Recurrent abruptio placentae in a cynomolgus monkey (*Macaca fascicularis*). Placenta 34(4):388, 2013a
Schlabritz-Loutsevitch N, Schenone A, Schenone M, et al: Abruptio placentae in cynomolgus macaque (*Macaca fascicularis*). Male bias. J Med Primatol 42(4):204, 2013b
Schlicter SJ, Kaufman RM, Assmann SF, et al: Dose of prophylactic platelet transfusions and prevention of hemorrhage. N Engl J Med 362(7):600, 2010
Schmid BC, Rezniczek GA, Rolf N, et al: Postpartum hemorrhage: use of hemostatic combat gauze. Am J Obstet Gynecol 206(1):e12, 2012
Schmitz T, Tararbit K, Dupont C, et al: Prostaglandin E2 analogue sulprostone for treatment of atonic postpartum hemorrhage. Obstet Gynecol 118 (Pt 2):257, 2011
Schubert N, Berthold T, Muschter S, et al: Human neutrophil antigen-3a antibodies induce neutrophil aggregation in a plasma-free medium. Blood Transfus 11:1, 2013
Seet EL, Kay HH, Wu S, et al: Placenta accreta: depth of invasion and neonatal outcomes. J Matern Fetal Neonatal Med 25(10):2042, 2012
Sentilhes L, Goffinet F, Kayem G: Management of placenta accreta. Acta Obstet Gynecol Scand 92(10):1125, 2013
Sentilhes L, Gromez A, Clavier E, et al: Predictors of failed pelvic arterial embolization for severe postpartum hemorrhage. Obstet Gynecol 113:992, 2009
Sewell MF, Rosenblum D, Ehrenberg H: Arterial embolus during common iliac balloon catheterization at cesarean hysterectomy. Obstet Gynecol 108:746, 2006
Shaz BH, Dente CJ, Harris RS, et al: Transfusion management of trauma patients. Anesth Analg 108:1760, 2009
Shields LE, Smalarz K, Reffigee L, et al: Comprehensive maternal hemorrhage protocols improve patient safety and reduce utilization of blood products. Am J Obstet Gynecol 205:368.e1, 2011
Sholl JS: Abruptio placentae: clinical management in nonacute cases. Am J Obstet Gynecol 156:40, 1987
Sibai BM, Lindheimer M, Hauth J, et al: Risk factors for preeclampsia, abruptio placentae, and adverse neonatal outcomes among women with chronic hypertension. N Engl J Med 339:667, 1998
Silver RM, Landon MB, Rouse DJ, et al: Maternal morbidity associated with multiple repeat cesarean deliveries. Obstet Gynecol 107:1226, 2006
Skjeldestad FE, Oian P: Blood loss after cesarean delivery: a registry-based study in Norway, 1999–2008. Am J Obstet Gynecol 206(1):76.e1, 2012
Small MJ, James AH, Kershaw T, et al: Near-miss maternal mortality: cardiac dysfunction as the principal cause of obstetric intensive care admissions. Obstet Gynecol 119(2 Pt 1):250, 2012
Society for Maternal-Fetal Medicine, Belfort MA: Placenta accreta. Am J Obstet Gynecol 203(5):430, 2010
Society of Thoracic Surgeons: 2011 update to the Society of Thoracic Surgeons and the Society of Cardiovascular Anesthesiologists blood conservation clinical practice guidelines. Ann Thorac Surg 91(3):944, 2011
Sosa CG, Alathabe F, Belizan JM, et al: Risk factors for postpartum hemorrhage in vaginal deliveries in a Latin-American population. Obstet Gynecol 113:1313, 2009
Spiess BD: Perfluorocarbon emulsions as a promising technology: a review of tissue and vascular gas dynamics. J Appl Physiol 106:1444, 2009
Spinella PC, Perkins JC, Grathwohl KW, et al: Fresh whole blood transfusions in coalition military, foreign national, and enemy combatant patients during Operation Iraqi Freedom at a U.S. combat support hospital. World J Surg 32:2, 2008
Spong CY, Mercer BM, D'alton M, et al: Timing of indicated late-preterm and early-term birth. Obstet Gynecol 118 (2 Pt 1):323, 2011
Stafford I, Belfort MA: Placenta accrete, increta, and percreta: a team-based approach starts with prevention. Contemp Ob/Gyn April:77, 2008
Stafford IA, Dashe JS, Shivvers SA, et al: Ultrasonographic cervical length and risk of hemorrhage in pregnancies with placenta previa. Obstet Gynecol 116(3):595, 2010
Stafford PA, Biddinger PW, Zumwalt RE: Lethal intrauterine fetal trauma. Am J Obstet Gynecol 159:485, 1988
Stanten RD, Iverson LI, Daugharty TM, et al: Amniotic fluid embolism causing catastrophic pulmonary vasoconstriction: diagnosis by transesophageal echocardiogram and treatment by cardiopulmonary bypass. Obstet Gynecol 102:496, 2003
Steiner PE, Lushbaugh CC: Maternal pulmonary embolism by amniotic fluid. JAMA 117:1245, 1941
Stettler RW, Lutich A, Pritchard JA, et al: Traumatic placental abruption: a separation from traditional thought. Presented at the American College of Obstetricians and Gynecologists Annual Clinical Meeting, Las Vegas, April 27, 1992
Stolte L, van Kessel H, Seelen J, et al: Failure to produce the syndrome of amniotic fluid embolism by infusion of amniotic fluid and meconium into monkeys. Am J Obstet Gynecol 98:694, 1967
Stramer SL, Glynn SA, Kleinman SH, et al: Detection of HIV-I and HCV infections among antibody-negative blood donors by nucleic acid–amplification testing. N Engl J Med 351:760, 2004

Su LL, Chong YS: Massive obstetric haemorrhage with disseminated intravascular coagulopathy. Best Pract Res Clin Obstet Gynaecol 26(1):77, 2012
Tam Tam KB, Dozier J, Martin JN Jr: Approaches to reduce urinary tract injury during management of placenta accreta, increta, and percreta: a systematic review. J Maternal Fetal Neonatal Med 25(4):329, 2012
Tantbirojn P, Crum CP, Parast MM: Pathophysiology of placenta accreta: the role of decidua and extravillous trophoblast. Placenta 29(7):639, 2008
Taylor FB Jr, Toh CH, Hoots WK, et al: Towards definition, clinical and laboratory criteria, and a scoring system for disseminated intravascular coagulation. Thromb Haemost 86(5):1327, 2001
Tikkanen M, Nuutila M, Hiilesmaa V, et al: Prepregnancy risk factors for placental abruption. Acta Obstet Gynecol Scand 85:40, 2006
Timmermans S, van Hof AC, Duvekot JJ: Conservative management of abnormally invasive placentation. Obstet Gynecol Surv 62:529, 2007
Timor-Tritsch IE. Monteagudo A: Unforeseen consequences of the increasing rate of cesarean deliveries: early placenta accreta and cesarean scar pregnancy. A review. Am J Obstet Gynecol 207 (1):14, 2012
Tita ATN, Szychowski JM, Rouse DJ, et al: Higher-dose oxytocin and hemorrhage after vaginal delivery. Obstet Gynecol 119(2 Pt 1):293, 2012
Toivonen S, Heinonen S, Anttila M, et al: Reproductive risk factors, Doppler findings, and outcome of affected births in placental abruption: a population-based analysis. Am J Perinatol 19:451, 2002
Toledo P, McCarthy RJ, Hewlett BJ, et al: The accuracy of blood loss estimation after simulated vaginal delivery. Anesth Analg 105:1736, 2007
Toohey JS, Keegan KA Jr, Morgan MA, et al: The "dangerous multipara": fact or fiction? Am J Obstet Gynecol 172:683, 1995
Towers CV, Pircon RA, Heppard M: Is tocolysis safe in the management of third-trimester bleeding? Am J Obstet Gynecol 180:1572, 1999
Treloar EJ, Anderson RS, Andrews HG, et al: Uterine necrosis following B-Lynch suture for primary postpartum haemorrhage. BJOG 113:486, 2006
Triulzi DJ: Transfusion-related acute lung injury: current concepts for the clinician. Anesth Analg 108(3):770, 2009
Trudell A, Stout M, Cahill A, et al: Second trimester cervical length and persistence of placental previa in the third trimester. Abstract No. 91. Presented at the 33rd Annual Meeting of the Society for Maternal-Fetal Medicine, 11–16 February 2013
Twickler DM, Lucas MJ, Balis AB, et al: Color flow mapping for myometrial invasion in women with a prior cesarean delivery. J Matern Fetal Med 9:330, 2000
Usta IM, Hobeika EM, Abu Musa AA, et al: Placenta previa-accreta: risk factors and complications. Am J Obstet Gynecol 193:1045, 2005
Villar J, Gülmezoglu AM, Hofmeyr GJ, et al: Systematic review of randomized controlled trials of misoprostol to prevent postpartum hemorrhage. Obstet Gynecol 100:1301, 2002
Walker MG, Allent L, Windrim RC, et al: Multidisciplinary management of invasive placenta previa. J Obstet Gynaecol Can 35(5):417, 2013
Warshak CR, Ramos GA, Eskander R, et al: Effect of predelivery diagnosis in 99 consecutive cases of placenta accreta. Obstet Gynecol 115(1):65, 2010
Watson P, Besch N, Bowes WA Jr: Management of acute and subacute puerperal inversion of the uterus. Obstet Gynecol 55:12, 1980
Wehrum MJ, Buhimschi IA, Salafia C, et al: Accreta complicating complete placenta previa is characterized by reduced systemic levels of vascular endothelial growth factor and by epithelial-to-mesenchymal transition of the invasive trophoblast. Am J Obstet Gynecol 204(5):411.e1, 2011
Weindling AM: The confidential enquiry into maternal and child health (CEMACH). Arch Dis Child 88:1034, 2003
Weis MA, Harper LM, Roehl KA, et al: Natural history of placenta previa in twins. Obstet Gynecol 120(4):753, 2012
Weiss JL, Malone FD, Vidaver J, et al: Threatened abortion: a risk factor for poor pregnancy outcome, a population-based screening study. Am J Obstet Gynecol 190:745, 2004
Weiwen Y: Study of the diagnosis and management of amniotic fluid embolism: 38 cases of analysis. Obstet Gynecol 95:385, 2000
Wing DA, Paul RH, Millar LK: Management of the symptomatic placenta previa: a randomized, controlled trial of inpatient versus outpatient expectant management. Am J Obstet Gynecol 174:305, 1996a
Wing DA, Paul RH, Millar LK: The usefulness of coagulation studies and blood banking in the symptomatic placenta previa. Am J Obstet Gynecol 174:346, 1996b
Witteveen T, van Stralen G, Zwart J, et al: Puerperal uterine inversion in the Netherlands: a nationwide cohort study. Acta Obstet Gynecol Scand 92(3):334, 2013
Wong, HS, Cheung YK, Zuccollo J, et al: Evaluation of sonographic diagnostic criteria for placenta accreta. J Clin Ultrasound 36(9):551, 2008
Wong TY: Emergency peripartum hysterectomy: a 10-year review in a tertiary obstetric hospital. N Z Med J 124(1345):34, 2011
Worley KC, Hnat MD, Cunningham FG: Advanced extrauterine pregnancy: diagnostic and therapeutic challenges. Am J Obstet Gynecol 198:297.e1, 2008
Wortman AC, Alexander JM: Placenta accreta, increta, and percreta. Obstet Gynecol Clin North Am 40(1):137, 2013a
Wortman A, Miller DL, Donahue TF, et al: Embolization of renal hemorrhage in pregnancy. Obstet Gynecol 121:480, 2013b
Wright JD, Silver RM, Bonanno C, et al: Practice patterns and knowledge of obstetricians and gynecologists regarding placenta accreta. J Matern Fetal Neonatal Med 26(16):1602, 2013
Yoong W, Ridout A, Memtsa M, et al: Application of uterine compression suture in association with intrauterine balloon tamponade ("uterine sandwich") for postpartum hemorrhage. Acta Obstet Gynecol Scand 91(1):147, 2012
You WB, Zahn CM: Postpartum hemorrhage: abnormally adherent placenta, uterine inversion, and puerperal hematomas. Clin Obstet Gynecol 49:184, 2006
Young B, Nadel A, Panda B, et al: Does placenta previa location matter? Surgical morbidity associated with previa location. Abstract No. 101. Presented at the 33rd Annual Meeting of the Society for Maternal-Fetal Medicine, 11–16 February 2013
Yu PC, Ou HY, Tsang LC, et al: Prophylactic intraoperative uterine artery embolization to control hemorrhage in abnormal placentation during late gestation. Fertil Steril 91(5):1951, 2009
Zacharias N, Gei AF, Suarez V, et al: Balloon tip catheter occlusion of the hypogastric arteries for the management of placental accreta. Am J Obstet Gynecol 189:S128, 2003
Zahn CM, Yeomans ER: Postpartum hemorrhage: placenta accreta, uterine inversion and puerperal hematomas. Clin Obstet Gynecol 33:422, 1990
Zaki ZM, Bahar AM, Ali ME, et al: Risk factors and morbidity in patients with placenta previa accreta compared to placenta previa non-accreta. Acta Obstet Gynecol Scand 77:391, 1998
Zeeman GG, Cunningham FG, Pritchard JA: The magnitude of hemoconcentration with eclampsia. Hypertens Pregnancy 28(2):127, 2009
Zeeman GG, Wendel Jr GD, Cunningham FG: A blueprint for obstetric critical care. Am J Obstet Gynecol 188:532, 2003
Zelop CM: Postpartum hemorrhage. Becoming more evidence-based. Obstet Gynecol 117(1):3, 2011
Zetterstrom K, Lindeberg SN, Haglund B, et al: Maternal complications in women with chronic hypertension: a population-based cohort study. Acta Obstet Gynecol Scand 84:419, 2005
Zhou J, Liu S, Ma M, et al: Procoagulant activity and phosphatidylserine of amniotic fluid cells. Thromb Haemost 101:795, 2009
Zuckerbraun BS, Peitzman AB, Billiar TR: Shock. In Brunicardi FC, Andersen DK, Billiar TR, et al: Schwartz's Principles of Surgery, 9th ed. New York, McGraw-Hill, 2010, p 89
Zwart JJ, Richters JM, Öry F, et al: Severe maternal morbidity during pregnancy, delivery and puerperium in the Netherlands: a nationwide population-based study of 371,000 pregnancies. BJOG 115:842, 2008

CHAPTER 42

Preterm Labor

Low birthweight defines neonates who are born too small. *Preterm or premature births* are terms used to describe neonates who are born too early. With respect to gestational age, a newborn may be preterm, term, or postterm. With respect to size, a newborn may be normally grown and *appropriate for gestational age*; undersized, thus, small for gestational age; or overgrown and consequently, large for gestational age. In recent years, the term *small for gestational age* has been widely used to categorize newborns whose birthweight is usually < 10th percentile for gestational age. Other frequently used terms have included *fetal-growth restriction* or *intrauterine growth restriction*. The term *large for gestational age* has been widely used to categorize newborns whose birthweight is > 90th percentile for gestational age. The term *appropriate for gestational age* designates newborns whose weight is between the 10th and 90th percentiles.

Thus, infants born before term can be small or large for gestational age but still fit the definition of preterm. *Low birthweight* refers to neonates weighing 1500 to 2500 g; *very low birthweight* refers to those between 500 and 1500 g; and *extremely low birthweight* refers to those between 500 and 1000 g. In 1960, a neonate weighing 1000 g had a 95-percent risk of death. Today, a neonate with the same birthweight has a 95-percent chance of surviving (Ingelfinger, 2007). This remarkable improvement in survival is due to the widespread application of neonatal intensive care in the early 1970s.

DEFINITION OF PRETERM

Up until the 15th edition of this textbook (1976), a *preterm* or *premature infant* was defined by birthweight < 2500 g. Beginning with the 15th edition, preterm infants were those delivered before 37 completed weeks, that is, $\leq 36^{6/7}$ weeks. This definition, which has now been in use for almost 40 years, was first promulgated in 1976 by the World Health Organization (WHO) and the International Federation of Gynecology and Obstetrics (FIGO). This definition was based on a statistical analysis of gestational age distribution at birth (Steer, 2005). It lacks a specific functional basis and should be clearly distinguished from the concept of prematurity. Prematurity represents incomplete development of various organ systems at birth. The lungs are particularly affected, leading to the respiratory distress syndrome.

Beginning in 2005, in recognition that infants born between $34^{0/7}$ weeks and $36^{6/7}$ weeks experience morbidities and mortality characteristic of premature infants, preterm births were subdivided. Those before $33^{6/7}$ weeks are labeled—*early preterm,* and those occurring between 34 and 36 completed weeks—*late preterm.* Most recently, Spong (2013) observed, "it has become apparent that infants born between 37 weeks 0 days and 38 weeks 6 days gestation experience morbidities that are associated with prematurity compared to births at 39 weeks 0 days through 40 weeks 6 days when infant mortality is lower than at any other time in human gestation." Those births $37^{0/7}$ weeks through $38^{6/7}$ weeks are now defined as *early term* and those 39 weeks 0 days through 40 weeks 6 days are defined as *term.*

In the United States in 2011, 23,910 infants died in their first year of life (Hamilton, 2012). *Preterm birth,* defined as delivery before 37 completed weeks, has been implicated in approximately two thirds of these deaths (Mathews, 2013). As shown in Table 42-1, *late preterm births,* defined as those 34 to 36 weeks' gestation, comprised approximately 70 percent of all births before 37 completed weeks. The data in Table 42-1 suggest the possibility of redefining births attributed to short gestation to be those before 39 weeks. Surprisingly, 40 percent of live births in the United States in 2009 were associated with a shortened period of gestation when births 39 to 41 weeks are taken as the reference standard. Moreover, these 40 percent of live births with shortened gestation contributed 80 percent of the infant deaths. Another implication of these data is that only 55 percent of births in the United States occurred during the optimal 39 to 41 weeks' gestation. Put yet another way, only 55 percent of births were "normal" based on infant outcomes. Does this mean that almost half of pregnancies resulting in live births are "abnormal"? Alternatively, perhaps the adjectives "normal" and "abnormal" should be abandoned and replaced with the realization that fetal maturation in humans is a continuum that is completed later in human pregnancy than previously appreciated.

Steer (2005) observed that signs of immaturity at birth and shorter than average gestational length have an unusually high incidence in *Homo sapiens* compared with other mammals. This has been attributed to the development of a narrow pelvis for bipedal gait, coupled with evolution toward a large brain and head that is associated with language and social skill acquisition. It is hypothesized that this combination results in a relatively high incidence of obstructed labor, which favors an evolutionary trend toward shorter gestation and thus an earlier birth.

TABLE 42-1. Infant Mortality Rates in the United States in 2009

	Live Births No. (%)	Infant Deaths (per 1000 births)
Total infants	4,130,665 (100)	26,408 (6)
Gestational age at birth:		
< 34 weeks	144,961 (4)	15,000 (104)
34–36 weeks	357,345 (9)	2549 (7)
< 37 weeks	502,306 (12)	17,550 (35)
37–38 weeks	1,138,029 (28)	3521 (3)
39–41 weeks	2,256,457 (55)	4474 (2)
≥ 42 weeks	228,588 (6)	654 (3)

Adapted from Mathews, 2013.

As previously noted, if infant mortality rates are used as the outcome of interest, the data in Table 42-1 suggest that optimal pregnancy outcomes vis-à-vis prematurity are achieved at 39 weeks' gestation. Is the 39-week threshold correct for defining pathologically shortened human gestation? For example, if neonatal death is used as the outcome of interest, delivery at $38^{0/7}$ through $38^{6/7}$ weeks is equivalent to delivery at 39 weeks (McIntire, 2008). Similarly, if respiratory morbidity is used as the outcome of interest, $38^{0/7}$ through $38^{6/7}$ weeks is equivalent to 39 weeks (Consortium on Safe Labor, 2010). These examples suggest that shortened human gestation with regard to prematurity is birth before $38^{0/7}$ weeks rather than before $39^{0/7}$ weeks.

A consequence of defining optimal pregnancy outcomes to occur at 39 weeks has been the concern that some births before 39 weeks may be unnecessary, that is, intentional deliveries not based on medical indications. Indeed, Bailit (2012) observed, "The dangers of delivering a newborn before 39 weeks for nonmedical reasons have become increasingly clear." The evidence that unnecessary deliveries are occurring before 39 weeks in the United States is not robust. Martin (2009b) used birth certificate data to analyze late preterm births between 1990 and 2006. The rate of infants born late preterm increased 20 percent during this time period. Moreover, the percentage of late preterm births for which labor was induced more than doubled between 1990 and 2006, climbing from 7.5 to 17.3 percent. The percentage of late preterm births delivered by cesarean also rose substantially, from 23.5 to 34.3 percent. Such increases in obstetrical interventions inevitably raise the specter of medically unnecessary interventions.

Reddy (2009) used 2001 United States birth certificate data to examine delivery indications for late preterm birth. A total of 23 percent of late preterm births had no recorded indication for delivery. Some of the factors significantly increasing the chance of no recorded indication were older maternal age, non-Hispanic white mother, and ≥ 13 years of education. Factors such as these raised the possibility that patient factors—as opposed to medical factors—were playing a role in late preterm births without a specified medical indication in the birth certificate. But Bailit (2012) has described the complexities of ascertaining the indications for delivery.

In contrast, an analysis of the indications for delivery of 21,771 late preterm births at Parkland Hospital using a research data set showed that 99.8 percent of such births were indicated and that 80 percent were due to idiopathic preterm labor or preterm spontaneously ruptured membranes. Indeed, and as shown in Figure 42-1, medically *indicated* preterm births are largely responsible for the increase in preterm births in the United States.

Undoubtedly, unnecessary obstetrical interventions are occurring before 38 or 39 weeks' gestation, but the magnitude of this problem is unclear at this time. Caution is urged before assuming that obstetrical interventions before 38 or 39 weeks are unnecessary. For example, Koopmans and colleagues (2009) randomized women with mild preeclampsia or

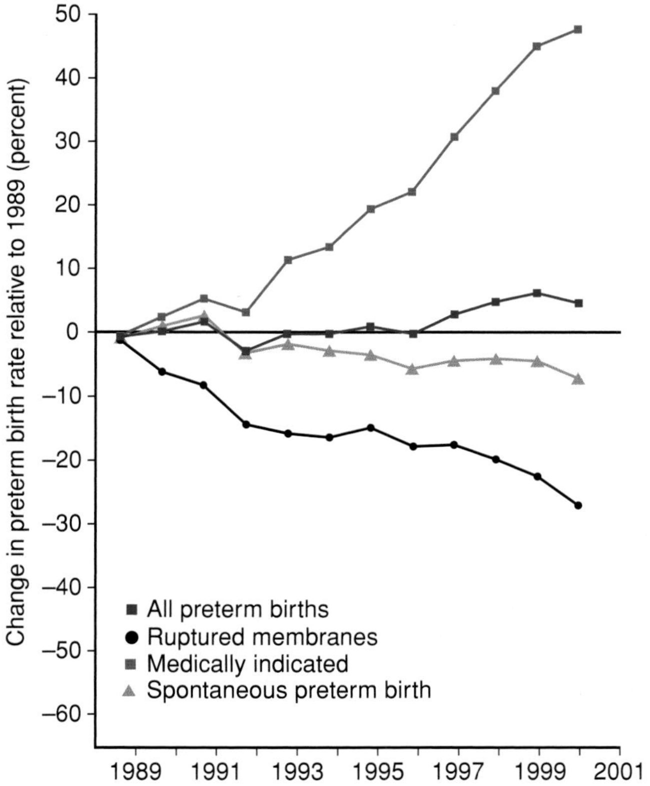

FIGURE 42-1 Rates of births < 37 weeks in the United States from 1989 to 2001. (Redrawn from Ananth, 2005, with permission.)

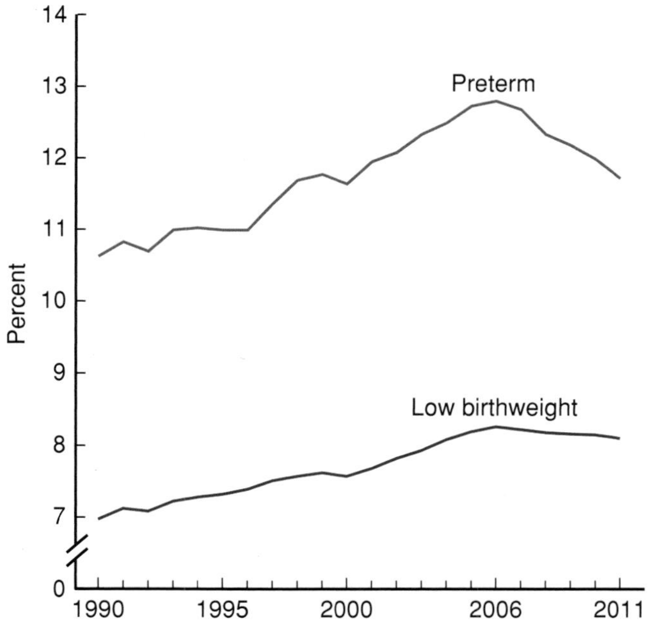

FIGURE 42-2 Preterm and low-birthweight rate: United States, final 1990 to 2010 and preliminary 2011. (Redrawn from Hamilton, 2012.)

gestational hypertension at 36 weeks' gestation to induction of labor versus expectant management. This trial showed that delivery at 37 weeks was better for women and their newborns compared with later delivery. The American College of Obstetricians and Gynecologists (2013b) also recommends caution before withholding indicated intervention.

TRENDS IN PRETERM BIRTH RATES

The percentage of preterm births increased 36 percent from 9.4 percent in 1984 to a high of 12.8 percent in 2006 (Mathews, 2013). Since 2006, however, the trend has reversed, and the percentage of preterm births declined to 11.7 percent in 2011 (Figure 42-2). This decline in the percentage of preterm births occurred for both the early—less than 34 weeks—and later preterm periods (Hamilton, 2012). Although the lowest level in more than a decade, the 2011 preterm birth rate is still higher than rates reported during the 1980s and most of the 1990s.

Is the decrease in preterm births shown in Figure 42-2 real? It could be argued that the decrease since 2006 is a result of changes in the birth certificate that is used to compute United States preterm birth rates. In 2003, a revised birth certificate intended to expand the collection of clinical information was introduced in the United States. Implementation depends on the rapidity with which the various states transitioned to the new version. For example, by 2008, the revised birth certificate had been implemented in 27 states representing 65 percent of all 2008 births (Osterman, 2011). This "trickle in" implementation coincides with the decline in preterm births shown in Figure 42-2.

Importantly, the 2003 version of the birth certificate introduced use of a clinical estimate of gestational age rather than primarily the last menstrual period, which was used in the previous 1989 version of the birth certificate. Joseph and associates (2007) noticed that preterm birth rates were much higher in the United States compared with Canada. This difference, however, was reduced when the United States rate was based on the clinical estimate of gestational age rather than menstrual dating. For example, the preterm birth rate in the United States in 2002 was 12.3 percent if computed using menstrual dating compared with 10.1 percent when a clinical estimate was used. The decrease in preterm births shown in Figure 42-2 from 12.8 percent in 2006 to 11.7 percent in 2011 is well within the range of change to be expected if the change was attributable to the method used for determining gestational age for the 2003 birth certificate.

A disturbing aspect of the trend in preterm birth rates in the United States is the persistence of racial and ethnic disparity (Fig. 42-3). Indeed, 77 percent of the race/ethnicity-related disparity in infant mortality rates in the United States in 2009 was associated with preterm birth (Mathews, 2013). Some investigators attribute this disparity to socioeconomic circumstances (Collins, 2007). Rates of preterm birth in the United States are also higher compared with those in other industrialized countries (Ananth, 2009; Joseph, 2007). For example, the preterm birth rate was 12.3 percent in the United States in 2003 compared with 7.7 percent in Canada. Indeed, similar differences have been noted in the preterm delivery rates between the United States and virtually all the other industrialized countries.

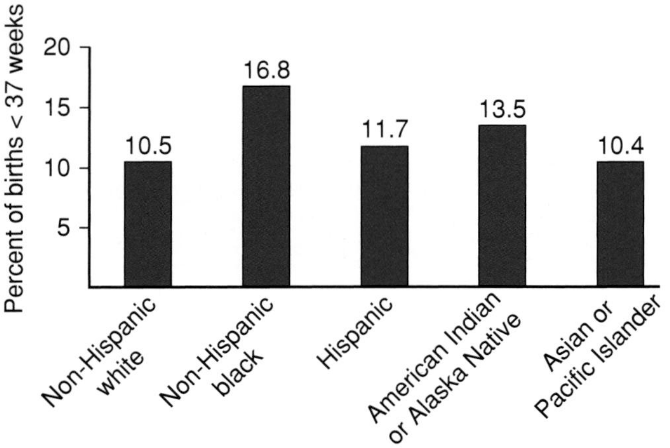

FIGURE 42-3 Preterm births in the United States in 2011 according to maternal race and ethnicity. (Redrawn from Hamilton, 2012.)

MORBIDITY IN PRETERM INFANTS

Various morbidities, largely due to organ system immaturity, are significantly increased in infants born before 37 weeks' gestation compared with those delivered at term (Table 42-2). For approximately 40 years, complications in infants born before 34 weeks have been the primary focus. Only recently (2005) have *late preterm* infants—34 to 36 weeks—gained attention because of their increased morbidity. Attention has also been given to increasingly small preterm infants—*very low birthweight* and *extremely low birthweight*. These very small infants suffer disproportionately not only the immediate complications of prematurity but also long-term sequelae such as neurodevelopmental disability. Indeed, live births once considered "abortuses" because they weighed < 500 g are now classified as live births. Indeed, there were 6331 live births between 400 and 500 g recorded in the United States in 2009 (Martin, 2011). Remarkable strides have been made in neonatal survival for infants born preterm. This is especially true for those born after 28 weeks. Shown in Figure 42-4 are survival rates for more than 18,000 infants born between 400 and 1500 g or between 22 and 32 weeks' gestation. Importantly, the results are shown as a function of both birthweight *and* gestational age. After achieving a birthweight of ≥ 1000 g or a gestational age of 28 weeks for females or 30 weeks for males, survival rates reach 95 percent.

Resources used to care for low-birthweight infants are a measure of the societal burden of preterm birth. The annual cost of preterm birth in the United States in 2006 was estimated to be $26.2 billion, or $51,000 per premature infant (Institute of Medicine, 2007). The economic consequences of preterm birth that reach beyond the newborn period into infancy, adolescence, and adulthood are difficult to estimate. However, they must be enormous when the effects of adult diseases associated with prematurity, such as hypertension and diabetes, are considered.

Mortality and Morbidity at the Extremes of Prematurity

The tremendous advances in the perinatal and neonatal care of the preterm infant have been found predominantly in those infants delivered at ≤ 33 weeks. With survival of increasingly very immature infants in the 1990s, there has been uncertainty and controversy as to the lower limit of fetal maturation compatible with extrauterine survival. This has resulted in continual reassessment of the *threshold of viability*.

TABLE 42-2. Major Short- and Long-Term Problems in Very-Low-Birthweight Infants

Organ or System	Short-Term Problems	Long-Term Problems
Pulmonary	Respiratory distress syndrome, air leak, bronchopulmonary dysplasia, apnea of prematurity	Bronchopulmonary dysplasia, reactive airway disease, asthma
Gastrointestinal or nutritional	Hyperbilirubinemia, feeding intolerance, necrotizing enterocolitis, growth failure	Failure to thrive, short-bowel syndrome, cholestasis
Immunological	Hospital-acquired infection, immune deficiency, perinatal infection	Respiratory syncytial virus infection, bronchiolitis
Central nervous system	Intraventricular hemorrhage, periventricular leukomalacia, hydrocephalus	Cerebral palsy, hydrocephalus, cerebral atrophy, neurodevelopmental delay, hearing loss
Ophthalmological	Retinopathy of prematurity	Blindness, retinal detachment, myopia, strabismus
Cardiovascular	Hypotension, patent ductus arteriosus, pulmonary hypertension	Pulmonary hypertension, hypertension in adulthood
Renal	Water and electrolyte imbalance, acid-base disturbances	Hypertension in adulthood
Hematological	Iatrogenic anemia, need for frequent transfusions, anemia of prematurity	
Endocrinological	Hypoglycemia, transiently low thyroxine levels, cortisol deficiency	Impaired glucose regulation, increased insulin resistance

Data from Eichenwald, 2008.

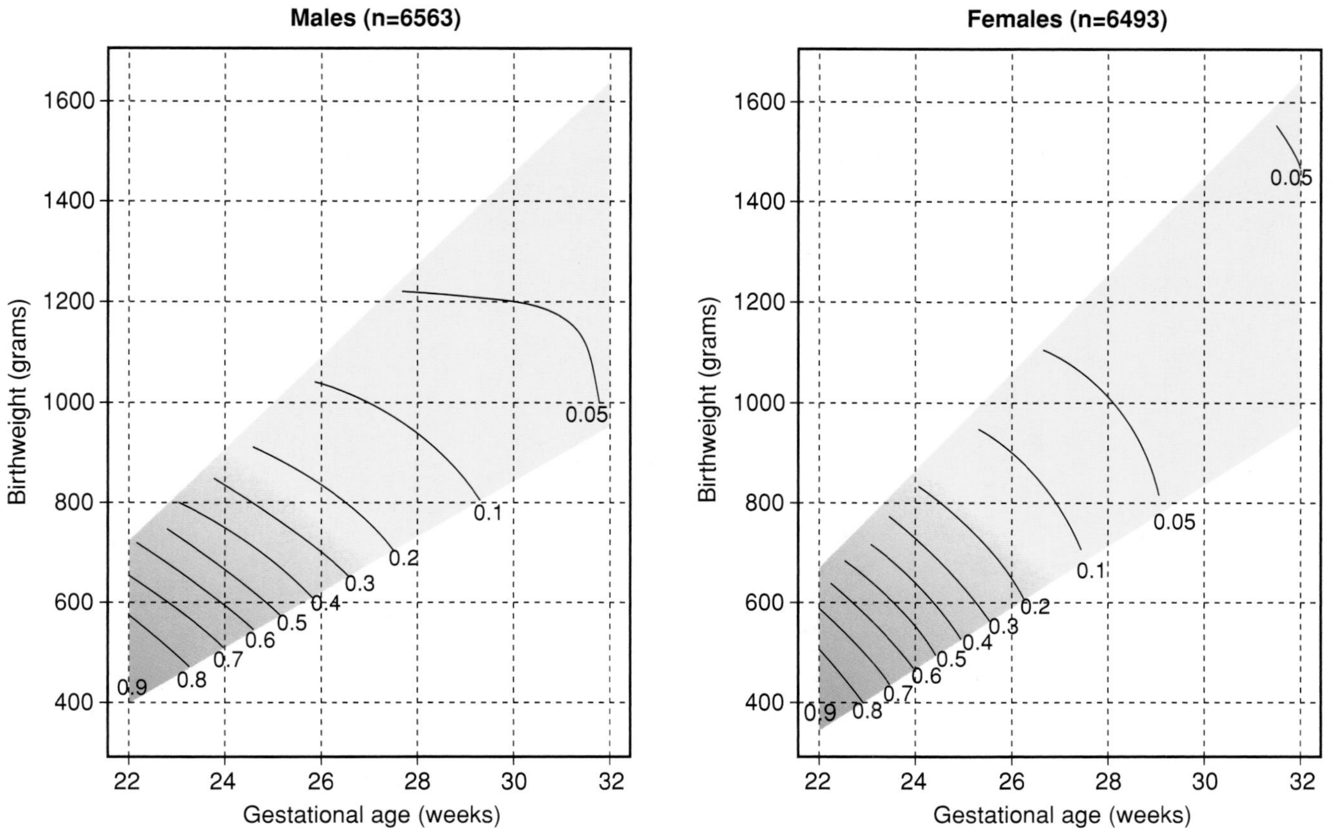

FIGURE 42-4 Mortality rates by birthweight, gestational age, and gender. The limits of the colored area indicate the upper 95th and lower 5th percentiles of birthweight for each gestational age. The curved lines indicate combinations of birthweight and gestational age with the same estimated probability of mortality from 10 to 90 percent. The gradation of color denotes the change in estimated probability of death. Green indicates infants of lower gestational age and birthweight who are more likely to die, whereas yellow indicates infants of higher gestational age and birthweight who are less likely to die. The methods used underestimate mortality rates in those at 22 and 23 weeks with a birthweight up to 600 g. (Redrawn from Fanaroff, 2007, with permission.)

Threshold of Viability

Births *before* 26 weeks are generally considered at the current threshold of viability, and these preterm infants pose various complex medical, social, and ethical considerations. For example, Sidney Miller is a child who was born at 23 weeks, weighed 615 g, and survived but developed severe physical and mental impairment (Annas, 2004). At age 7 years, she was described as a child who "could not walk, talk, feed herself, or sit up on her own...was legally blind, suffered from severe mental retardation, cerebral palsy, seizures, and spastic quadriparesis in her limbs." An important issue for her family was the need for a lifetime of medical care estimated to cost tens of millions of dollars.

Infants now considered to be at the threshold of viability are those born at 22, 23, 24, or 25 weeks (American College of Obstetricians and Gynecologists, 2012a,b). These infants have been described as fragile and vulnerable because of their immature organ systems. Moreover, they are at high risk for brain injury from hypoxic-ischemic injury and sepsis. In this setting, hypoxia and sepsis start a cascade of events that lead to brain hemorrhage, white-matter injury that causes periventricular leukomalacia, and poor subsequent brain growth eventuating in neurodevelopmental impairment (Chap. 34, p. 656). Because active brain development normally occurs throughout the second and third trimesters, those infants born at 22 to 25 weeks are believed especially vulnerable to brain injury.

Until recently, discussion of clinical management and ethical and economic considerations of extremely premature infants were hampered by data compromised by ascertainment bias (American College of Obstetricians and Gynecologists, 2012a,b). For example, the mean survival rate was 45 percent if the denominator was all live births compared with 72 percent if the denominator used was only infants admitted to neonatal intensive care (Guillen, 2011). Another source of ascertainment bias was use of multicenter datasets. There were considerable center differences in obstetrical and early neonatal interventions, particularly at 22 and 23 weeks (Stoll, 2010).

A remarkable report on infants born before 27 weeks was recently published (Serenius, 2013). This report is unique in that it details a national population-based prospective study of all infants born alive or stillborn before 27 weeks in Sweden. This country is a uniform society without extreme poverty, and antenatal care is easily accessible and used by almost 100 percent of mothers. All citizens are covered by health insurance including 480 days of parental leave after childbirth and additional benefits for severely sick children. Active perinatal care in Sweden includes early and free access to specialist perinatal care, centralization of extremely preterm births to

SECTION 11

TABLE 42-3. Outcomes at 2½ Years Corrected Age by Gestational Age at Birth in Sweden, 2004–2007

Outcome	Gestational Age (wk)					
	22	23	24	25	26	Total
Liveborn infants (No.)	51	101	144	205	206	707
Survived to 1 year (%)	10	53	67	82	85	70
Percentage with disability[a] at 2½ years corrected age:						
No disability	0	30	34	44	49	42
Mild	40	19	33	29	34	31
Moderate	20	30	21	17	10	16
Severe	40	21	13	10	7	11

[a]The overall rate of disabilities includes performance on the Bayley III assessments, mental development delay, cerebral palsy, and visual and hearing disabilities.
Adapted from Serenius, 2013.

TABLE 42-4. Survival and Disability Rates for 5736 Live Births Born between 22 and 26 Weeks' Gestation at 20 Medical Centers in the United States During 2003–2007

Outcome	Gestational Age (wk)				
	22	23	24	25	26
Liveborn infants (No.)	421	871	1370	1498	1576
Survived to discharge (%)	6	26	55	72	84
Percentage with no chronic morbidity[a]	0	8	9	20	34

[a]Morbidities included severe intraventricular hemorrhage, periventricular leukomalacia, bronchopulmonary dysplasia, necrotizing enterocolitis, infections, and retinopathy of prematurity stage ≥ 3.
Adapted from Stoll, 2010.

level III hospitals, a low threshold to provide life support at birth, and near universal admission of infants born at 23 to 26 weeks for neonatal intensive care. Thus, this report likely describes infant outcomes at the threshold of viability under optimal circumstances.

Shown in Table 42-3 are the survival and disability rates for 707 infants born alive from 22 to 26 weeks between 2004 and 2007 in Sweden. The proportion of children with mild or no disabilities increased from 40 percent at 22 weeks to 83 percent at 26 weeks. Conversely, the number of infants with moderate or severe disabilities decreased with advancing gestational age at birth. Moderate or severe disabilities were found in 31 percent of preterm boys compared with 23 percent of preterm girls. No differences in overall outcomes were noted if singletons and multiple births were compared.

The most recent report from the United States concerning survival and morbidity rates for births at 22 to 26 weeks is from the National Institute of Child Health and Human Development (NICHD) Neonatal Network. This dataset includes 5736 live births delivered between 2003 and 2007 at 20 medical centers across the United States. Rates of survival and survival without morbidity in the neonatal period are shown in Table 42-4.

Cesarean delivery at the threshold of viability is controversial. For example, if the fetus-infant is perceived to be too immature for aggressive support, then cesarean delivery for common indications such as breech presentation or nonreassuring fetal heart rate patterns might be preempted. This aside, national data clearly show a high frequency of cesarean delivery for these small infants (Fig. 42-5). Determining the optimal delivery mode for newborns at the threshold of viability is virtually impossible given that randomizing the delivery route has extreme ethical considerations. That said, retrospective, nonrandomized studies have consistently failed to document a benefit of cesarean delivery for the extremely preterm fetus (American College of Obstetricians and Gynecologists, 2012a). Reddy (2012) analyzed 2906 singleton live births between $24^{0/7}$ and $31^{6/7}$ weeks selected because they were eligible for attempted vaginal birth after excluding those cases with fetal distress, placenta previa, placental abruption, and anomalies. Attempted vaginal delivery for cephalic presenting fetuses had a high success rate (84 percent), and there was no difference in the neonatal mortality rate compared with that with planned cesarean delivery. For *breech* presentations, however, there was a threefold increased relative risk in mortality when vaginal delivery was attempted. Werner (2013) analyzed 20,231 preterm infants at 24 to 34 weeks born in New York City between 1995 and 2003. Cesarean delivery was not protective against poor outcomes such as neonatal death, intraventricular hemorrhage, seizures, respiratory distress, and subdural hemorrhage.

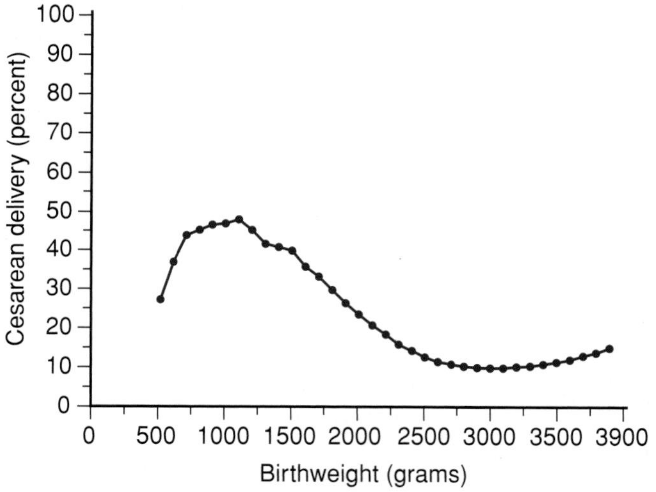

FIGURE 42-5 United States cesarean delivery rates by birthweight from 1999 to 2000. (Redrawn from Lee, 2006, with permission.)

Threshold of Viability at Parkland Hospital

Policies were developed in conjunction with the Neonatology Service. We must emphasize that the decision not to perform cesarean delivery does not necessarily imply that the fetus is "nonviable" or "written off." Neonatologists are consulted before delivery, and there is discussion of survival and morbidity with the woman and her family. A neonatologist attends each delivery and determines subsequent management.

From an obstetrical standpoint, all fetal indications for cesarean delivery in more advanced pregnancies are practiced in women at 25 weeks. Cesarean delivery is not offered for fetal indications at 23 weeks. At 24 weeks, cesarean delivery is not offered unless fetal weight is estimated at 750 g or greater. Aggressive obstetrical management is practiced in cases of growth restriction.

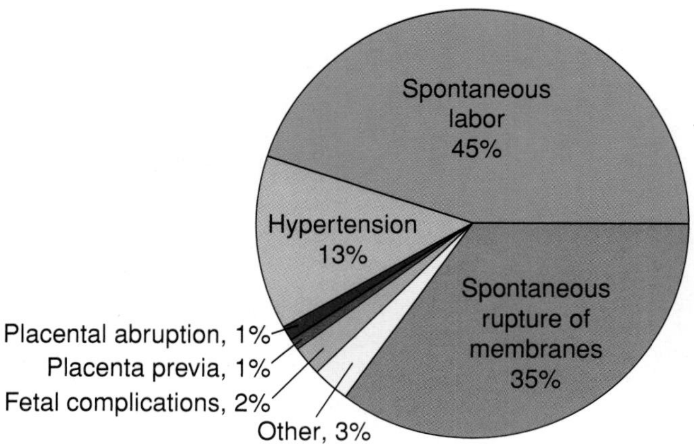

FIGURE 42-7 Obstetrical complications associated with 21,771 late preterm births at Parkland Hospital. (Adapted from McIntire, 2008.)

Late Preterm Birth

As shown in Figure 42-6, infants between 34 and 36 weeks account for more than 70 percent of all preterm births. These are the fastest increasing and largest proportion of singleton preterm births in the United States (Raju, 2006). Thus, increased attention is being given to determining optimal obstetrical and neonatal management of late preterm birth.

To estimate the risks associated with late preterm births, we analyzed neonatal mortality and morbidity rates at 34, 35, and 36 weeks compared with those of births at term between 1988 and 2005 at Parkland Hospital (McIntire, 2008). We were particularly interested in obstetrical complications during this time, because if modified, rates of late preterm birth can possibly be decreased. Approximately 3 percent of all births during the study period occurred between 24 and 32 weeks, and 9 percent were during the late preterm weeks. Thus, late preterm births accounted for three fourths of all preterm births. Approximately 80 percent of these were due to idiopathic spontaneous preterm labor or prematurely ruptured membranes (Fig. 42-7). Complications such as hypertension or placental accidents were implicated in the other 20 percent of cases.

Neonatal mortality rates were significantly increased in each late preterm week compared with those at 39 weeks as the referent and as shown in Figure 42-8. Similarly, Tomashek (2007) analyzed all United States births between 1995 and 2002 and also found higher neonatal mortality rates for late preterm infants. Importantly, indices of neonatal morbidity shown in Table 42-5 are increased in these late preterm infants born at Parkland. Fuchs (2008) reported similar results regarding respiratory morbidity in 722 infants. Specifically, the frequency of respiratory morbidity decreased by approximately 50 percent per week from 34 to 37 completed weeks. Increased rates of adverse neurodevelopment have also been found in late preterm infants compared with term newborns (Petrini, 2009).

These findings suggest that the health-care focus on prematurity should be expanded to include late preterm births. Even so, because approximately 80 percent of these women begin labor spontaneously—similar to births before 34 weeks—attempts to interrupt preterm labor have not been satisfactory. Specifically, the Institute of Medicine (2007) report, *Preterm Birth: Causes, Consequences, and Prevention*, acknowledges that treatment of preterm labor has not prevented preterm

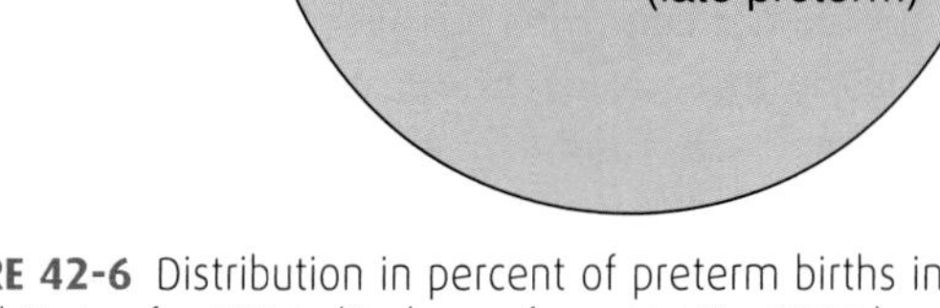

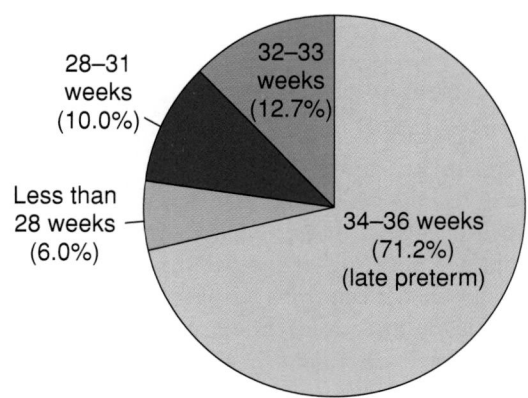

FIGURE 42-6 Distribution in percent of preterm births in the United States for 2004. (Redrawn from Martin, 2006.)

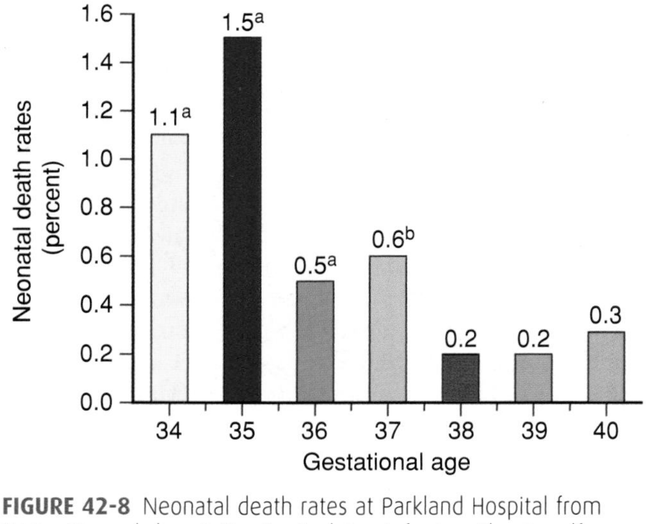

FIGURE 42-8 Neonatal death rates at Parkland Hospital from 34 to 40 weeks' gestation in singleton infants without malformations. [a]$p < .001$ compared with 39 weeks as the referent. [b]$p = .02$ compared with 39 weeks as the referent. (Redrawn from McIntire, 2008, with permission.)

TABLE 42-5. Neonatal Morbidity Rates at Parkland Hospital in Live Births Delivered Late Preterm Compared with 39 Weeks

	Preterm Births			Term Births
Morbidity[a]	34 Weeks n = 3498	35 Weeks n = 6571	36 Weeks n = 11,702	39 Weeks n = 84,747
Respiratory distress				
Ventilator	116 (3.3)[b]	109 (1.7)[b]	89 (0.8)[b]	275 (0.3)
Transient tachypnea	85 (2.4)[b]	103 (1.6)[b]	130 (1.1)[b]	34 (0.4)
Intraventricular hemorrhage				
Grades 1, 2	16 (0.5)[b]	13 (0.2)[b]	7 (0.06)[c]	13 (0.01)
Grades 3, 4	0	1 (0.02)	1 (0.01)	3 (0.004)
Sepsis				
Evaluation	1073 (31)[b]	1443 (22)[b]	1792 (15)[b]	10,588 (12)
Culture proven	18 (0.5)[b]	23 (0.4)[b]	26 (0.2)[c]	97 (0.1)
Phototherapy	13 (6.1)[b]	227 (3.5)[b]	36 (2.0)[b]	857 (1)
Necrotizing enterocolitis	3 (0.09)[b]	1 (0.02)[c]	1 (0.001)	1 (0.001)
Apgar ≤ 3 at 5 min	5 (0.1)	12 (0.2)[b]	10 (0.9)	54 (0.06)
Intubation in delivery room	49 (1.4)[b]	55 (0.8)[c]	36 (0.6)	477 (0.6)
One or more of the above	1175 (34)[b]	1565 (24)[b]	1993 (17)[b]	11,513 (14)

[a]Data presented as n (%).
[b]$p < .001$ compared with 39 weeks referent.
[c]$p < .05$ compared with 39 weeks referent.
From McIntire, 2008, with permission.

birth. Thus, we are of the view that a national strategy aimed at prevention of late preterm births is unlikely to provide discernible benefit without new developments in the prevention and management of preterm labor. In the meantime, the Maternal-Fetal Medicine Units (MFMU) Network is studying the efficacy of corticosteroids in late preterm births. The American College of Obstetricians and Gynecologists (2013b) has emphasized that intentional late preterm deliveries should occur only when an accepted maternal or fetal indication for delivery exists.

CAUSES OF PRETERM DELIVERY

There are four main direct reasons for preterm births in the United States. These include: (1) spontaneous unexplained preterm labor with intact membranes, (2) idiopathic preterm premature rupture of membranes (PPROM), (3) delivery for maternal or fetal indications, and (4) twins and higher-order multifetal births. Of all preterm births, 30 to 35 percent are indicated, 40 to 45 percent are due to spontaneous preterm labor, and 30 to 35 percent follow preterm membrane rupture (Goldenberg, 2008). Indeed, much of the increase in the singleton preterm birth rate in the United States is explained by rising numbers of indicated preterm births (Ananth, 2005).

Reasons for preterm birth have multiple, often interacting, antecedents and contributing factors. This complexity has greatly confounded efforts to prevent and manage this complication. This is particularly true for preterm ruptured membranes and spontaneous preterm labor, which together lead to 70 to 80 percent of preterm births. Last, according to data from Martin (2006), approximately one in six preterm births in the United States is from twins or higher-order multifetal pregnancies (Chap. 45, p. 891). For example, in 2004, there were 508,356 preterm births, and of these, 86,116 or 17 percent were from multifetal pregnancies. Many of these pregnancies were achieved using ovulation-inducing drugs and assisted reproductive technologies (ART).

Analogous to other complex disease processes, multiple coexistent genetic alterations and environment may lead to preterm birth (Esplin, 2005; Ward, 2008). There are polymorphisms in genes associated with inflammation and infection and in those associated with collagen turnover (Velez, 2008). Inherited mutations in genes regulating collagen assembly may predispose individuals to cervical insufficiency or prematurely ruptured membranes (Anum, 2009; Wang, 2006; Warren, 2007).

Basic Science of Spontaneous Preterm Labor

For both clinical and research purposes, pregnancies with intact fetal membranes and spontaneous preterm labor must be distinguished from those complicated by preterm prematurely ruptured membranes. Even so, those with spontaneous preterm labor do not constitute a homogeneous group characterized singularly by early initiation of parturition (American College of Obstetricians and Gynecologists, 2012b). This certainly is one reason why preventative therapies and clinical tools to assess the risks for preterm birth have been difficult to identify. Among the more common associated findings are multifetal pregnancy, intrauterine infection, bleeding, placental infarction, premature cervical dilatation, cervical insufficiency, hydramnios, uterine fundal abnormalities, and fetal anomalies. Severe maternal illness as a result of infections, autoimmune diseases, and gestational hypertension also increases preterm labor risks.

Although there are unique aspects to each cause of preterm labor, these diverse processes culminate in a common end point, which is premature cervical dilatation and effacement and premature activation of uterine contractions. It seems important to emphasize that the actual process of preterm labor should be considered a final step—one that results from progressive or acute changes that could be initiated days or even weeks before labor onset. Indeed, many forms of spontaneous preterm labor that result from premature initiation of phase 2 of parturition may be viewed in this light (Chap. 21, p. 410). Although the end result in preterm birth is the same as at term, namely cervical ripening and myometrial activation, recent studies in animal models support the idea that preterm birth is not always an acceleration of the normal process. Diverse pathways to instigate parturition exist and are dependent on the etiology of preterm birth. Identification of both common and uncommon factors has begun to explain the physiological processes of human parturition at term and preterm. Four major causes of spontaneous preterm labor include uterine distention, maternal–fetal stress, premature cervical changes, and infection.

Uterine Distention

There is no doubt that multifetal pregnancy and hydramnios lead to an increased risk of preterm birth (Chap. 45, p. 913). It is likely that early uterine distention acts to initiate expression of contraction-associated proteins (CAPs) in the myometrium. The *CAP* genes that are influenced by stretch include those coding for gap-junction proteins such as connexin 43, for oxytocin receptors, and for prostaglandin synthase (Korita, 2002; Lyall, 2002; Sooranna, 2004). Recent reports suggest that gastrin-releasing peptides (GRPs) are increased with stretch to promote myometrial contractility and that GRP antagonists can inhibit uterine contractility (Tattershell, 2012). There is also a stretch-induced potassium channel—TREK-1—that is upregulated during gestation and downregulated in labor. This pattern of expression is consistent with a potential role in uterine relaxation during pregnancy (Buxton, 2010). Expression of TREK-1 splice variants that block function of the full-length TREK-1 have been recently identified in myometrium from women with preterm labor. This further implicates a role for TREK-1 in uterine quiescence (Wu, 2012). Although these and other regulatory factors remain to be validated, it is clear that excessive uterine stretch causes premature loss of myometrial quiescence.

Excessive uterine stretch also leads to early activation of the placental–fetal endocrine cascade shown in Figure 21-17 (p. 425). The resulting early rise in maternal corticotropin-releasing hormone and estrogen levels can further enhance the expression of myometrial *CAP* genes (Warren, 1990; Wolfe, 1988). Finally, the influence of uterine stretch should be considered with regard to the cervix. For example, cervical length is an important risk factor for preterm birth in multifetal pregnancies (Goldenberg, 1996). Prematurely increased stretch and endocrine activity may initiate events that shift the timing of uterine activation, including premature cervical ripening.

Maternal–Fetal Stress

Stress is defined as a condition or adverse circumstance that disturbs the normal physiological or psychological functioning of an individual. But the complexities of measuring "stress" are what cause difficulty in defining its exact role (Lobel, 1994). That said, considerable evidence shows a correlation between some sort of maternal stress and preterm birth (Hedegaard, 1993; Hobel, 2003; Ruiz, 2003). Moreover, there is a correlation between maternal psychological stress and the placental–adrenal endocrine axis that provides a potential mechanism for stress-induced preterm birth (Lockwood, 1999; Petraglia, 2010; Wadhwa, 2001).

As discussed earlier, the last trimester is marked by rising maternal serum levels of placental-derived corticotropin-releasing hormone (CRH). This hormone works with adrenocorticotropic hormone (ACTH) to increase adult and fetal adrenal steroid hormone production, including the initiation of fetal cortisol biosynthesis. Rising levels of maternal and fetal cortisol further increase placental CRH secretion, which develops a feed-forward endocrine cascade that does not end until delivery (Fig. 21-17, p. 425). Rising levels of CRH further stimulate fetal adrenal dehydroepiandrosterone sulfate (DHEA-S) biosynthesis, which acts as substrate to increase maternal plasma estrogens, particularly estriol.

It has been hypothesized that a premature rise in cortisol and estrogens results in an early loss of uterine quiescence. A number of studies have reported that spontaneous preterm labor is associated with an early rise in maternal CRH levels and that CRH determination may be a useful biomarker for preterm birth risk assessment (Holzman, 2001; McGrath, 2002; McLean, 1995; Moawad, 2002). Because of large variations in CRH levels among pregnant women, however, a single CRH measurement has low sensitivity (Leung, 2001; McGrath, 2002). It may be that the *rate of increase* in maternal CRH levels is possibly a more accurate predictor of preterm birth. Confounding factors include CRH variability among ethnic groups. Another is that placental CRH enters the fetal circulation—albeit at lower levels than in the maternal circulation. In vitro studies have shown that CRH can directly stimulate fetal adrenal production of DHEA-S and cortisol (Parker, 1999; Smith, 1998). Thus, current studies do not support the idea that CRH levels alone have a positive-predictive value for preterm birth risk.

If preterm delivery is associated with early activation of the fetal adrenal–placental endocrine cascade, maternal estrogen levels would likely be prematurely elevated. This is indeed the case. An early rise in serum estriol concentrations is noted in women with subsequent preterm labor (Heine, 2000; McGregor, 1995). Physiologically, this premature rise in estrogen levels may alter myometrial quiescence and accelerate cervical ripening.

Taken together, these observations suggest that preterm birth is associated, in many cases, with a maternal–fetal biological stress response. The stressors that activate this cascade likely are broad, and the stress response is dependent on the stressor. For example, CRH or estriol levels are prematurely elevated in preterm birth due to infection and multifetal pregnancies but not in pregnant women with perceived stress (Gravett, 2000; Himes, 2011; Warren, 1990). Chronic, psychological stress—resulting for example from racial discrimination—appears to promote impaired cellular immune competence (Christian, 2012b). A growing body of work in the area of psychoneuroimmunology will perhaps enhance the understanding of pathways that link stress with adverse birth outcomes (Christian, 2012a).

Infection

There is great interest in the role of infection as a primary cause of preterm labor in pregnancies with intact membranes (Goncalves, 2002; Iams, 1987). In some cases, there is histological evidence of inflammation in the fetal membranes, decidua, or umbilical cord, whereas other cases are deemed "subclinical." More recently, new technologies based on genomic analysis of a mixed population of microorganisms have shown that the nonpregnant vaginal tract hosts a complex microbial community that can differ widely between women who are all healthy (Gajer, 2012; White, 2011). The application of the field of *metagenomics* to understanding microbiome complexity in term and preterm birth and to identifying microbe populations that may mediate subclinical infection holds great promise. Aagaard and coworkers (2012) used metagenomics to determine how the vaginal microbiome changes during normal pregnancy. They reported that the diversity and richness of microbes is reduced through pregnancy. Compared with nonpregnant controls, there is an increased dominance of *Lactobacillus* species. These findings lay the foundation for future studies to identify microbial populations associated with "subclinical" infection-induced preterm birth.

Current data suggest that microbial invasion of the reproductive tract is sufficient to induce infection-mediated preterm birth—more specifically, there is ongoing "subclinical" infection. However, microorganisms certainly are not ubiquitous in the amnionic fluid of all women with preterm labor, and indeed, positive cultures are found in only 10 to 40 percent (Goncalves, 2002). This minority of women with amnionic fluid bacteria are more likely to develop clinical chorioamnionitis and preterm ruptured membranes compared with women with sterile cultures. Moreover, their neonates are also more likely to have complications (Hitti, 2001). Although infection is more severe when there is clinically obvious intraamnionic infection, inflammation in the absence of detectable microorganisms is also a risk factor for a fetal inflammatory response (Lee, 2007, 2008). The earlier the onset of preterm labor, the greater the likelihood of documented infection (Goldenberg, 2000; Watts, 1992). It is enigmatic that the incidence of culture-positive amnionic fluids collected by amniocentesis during spontaneous term labor is similar to that with preterm labor (Gomez, 1994; Romero, 1993). It has been suggested that at term, amnionic fluid is infiltrated by bacteria as a consequence of labor, whereas in preterm pregnancies, bacteria represent an important cause of labor. If true, this explanation questions the contribution of fetal infection as a major cause of preterm labor and delivery.

Despite these observations, there are considerable data that associate chorioamnionitis with preterm labor (Goldenberg, 2002; Üstün, 2001). In such infections, the microbes may invade maternal tissue only and not amnionic fluid. Despite this, endotoxins can stimulate amnionic cells to secrete cytokines that enter amnionic fluid. This scenario may serve to explain the apparently contradictory observations concerning an association between amnionic fluid cytokines and preterm labor, in which microbes were not detectable in the amnionic fluid.

Sources for Intrauterine Infection. The patency of the female reproductive tract, although essential for achievement of pregnancy and delivery, is theoretically problematic during phase 1 of parturition. It has been suggested that bacteria can gain access to intrauterine tissues through: (1) transplacental transfer of maternal systemic infection, (2) retrograde flow of infection into the peritoneal cavity via the fallopian tubes, or (3) ascending infection with bacteria from the vagina and cervix. The lower pole of the fetal membrane–decidual junction is contiguous with the cervical canal orifice, which is patent to the vagina. This anatomical arrangement provides a passageway for microorganisms, and ascending infection is considered to be the most common. A thoughtful description of the potential degrees of intrauterine infection has been provided by Goncalves and associates (2002). They categorize intrauterine infection into four stages of microbial invasion that include bacterial vaginosis—stage I, decidual infection—stage II, amnionic infection—stage III, and finally, fetal systemic infection—stage IV. As expected, progression of these stages is thought to increase rates of preterm birth and neonatal morbidity.

Based on these insights, it is straightforward to construct a theory for the pathogenesis of infection-induced preterm labor. Ascending microorganisms colonize the cervix, decidua, and possibly the membranes, where they then may enter the amnionic sac. Lipopolysaccharide (LPS) or other toxins elaborated by bacteria induce immune-cell recruitment into the reproductive tract and cytokine production by immune cells and by cells within the cervix, decidua, membranes, or fetus itself. Both LPS and cytokines then provoke prostaglandin release from the membranes, decidua, or cervix. These influence both cervical ripening and loss of myometrial quiescence (Challis, 2002; Keelan, 2003; Olson, 2003). Current evidence based on animal and human studies suggests that many aspects of infection-mediated preterm birth differ from pathways that regulate term parturition (Hamilton, 2012; Holt, 2011; Shynlova, 2013a,b).

Microbes Associated with Preterm Birth. Some microorganisms—examples include *Gardnerella vaginalis, Fusobacterium, Mycoplasma hominis,* and *Ureaplasma urealyticum*—are detected more frequently than others in amnionic fluid of women with preterm labor (Gerber, 2003; Hillier, 1988; Yoon, 1998). This finding was interpreted by some as presumptive evidence that specific microorganisms are more commonly involved as pathogens in the induction of preterm labor. Another interpretation, however, is that given direct access to the membranes after cervical dilatation, selected microorganisms, such as fusobacteria, that are more capable of burrowing through these exposed tissues will do so. Fusobacteria are found in the vaginal fluid of only 9 percent of women but in 28 percent of positive amnionic fluid cultures from pregnancies with preterm labor and intact membranes (Chaim, 1992). Knowledge from metagenomic studies will better define these interactions in the future. In addition, host responses to pathogens with respect to mucosal immunity, barrier protection of cervical and vaginal epithelia, and expression of antimicrobial peptides is likely to provide insights. Specifically, the mechanisms that render some women more susceptible to infection-mediated preterm birth may be found.

Intrauterine Inflammatory Response. The initial inflammatory response elicited by bacterial toxins is mediated, in large measure, by specific receptors on mononuclear phagocytes, decidual cells, cervical epithelia, and trophoblasts. These *Toll-like receptors* represent a family that has evolved to recognize pathogen-associated molecules (Janssens, 2003). Toll-like receptors are present in the placenta on trophoblast cells, in the cervical epithelia, and on fixed and invading leukocytes (Chuang, 2000; Gonzalez, 2007; Holmlund, 2002). Loss of specific Toll-like receptors results in delayed parturition in mouse models (Montalbano, 2013).

Under the influence of ligands such as bacterial LPS, these receptors increase chemokine, cytokine, and prostaglandin release as part of an inflammatory response. One example is interleukin-1β (IL-1β), which is produced rapidly after LPS stimulation (Dinarello, 2002). This cytokine in turn acts to promote a series of responses that include: (1) increased synthesis of others, that is, IL-6, IL-8, and tumor-necrosis factor alpha (TNF-α); (2) proliferation, activation, and migration of leukocytes; (3) modifications in extracellular matrix proteins; and (4) mitogenic and cytotoxic effects such as fever and acute-phase response (El-Bastawissi, 2000). Also, IL-1 promotes prostaglandin formation in many tissues, including myometrium, decidua, and amnion (Casey, 1990). The importance of prostaglandins to infection-mediated preterm birth is supported by the observation that prostaglandin inhibitors can reduce the rate of LPS-induced preterm birth in both the mouse and nonhuman primate (Gravett, 2007; Gross, 2000). Inhibition of cyclooxygenase-2 prevents inflammation-mediated preterm labor in the mouse. And immunomodulators plus antibiotics delay preterm delivery after experimental intraamnionic infection in a nonhuman primate model. Thus, there appears to be a cascade of events once an inflammatory response is initiated that can result in preterm labor.

Origin of Cytokines. Cytokines within the normal term uterus are likely important for normal and preterm labor. The transfer of cytokines such as IL-1 from decidua across the membranes into amnionic fluid appears to be severely limited. It is reasonable that cytokines produced in maternal decidua and myometrium will have effects on that side, whereas cytokines produced in the membranes or in cells within the amnionic fluid will not be transferred to maternal tissues. The human myometrium expresses chemokine receptors that decline during labor (Hua, 2013). Macrophages are reported to infiltrate the human and rat decidua before labor onset and may be important for decidual activation (Hamilton, 2012). Still, the requirement of leukocytes for initiation of term labor in women remains inconclusive. In most cases of inflammation resulting from infection, resident and invading leukocytes produce the bulk of cytokines. Indeed, with infection, leukocytes—mainly neutrophils, macrophages, and T lymphocytes—infiltrate the cervix, lower uterine segment, fundus, and membranes at the time of labor. Thus, invading leukocytes may be the major source of cytokines in preterm labor. Along with proinflammatory cytokines, studies in women and animal models highlight the importance of the antiinflammatory limb of the immune response in parturition (Gotsch, 2008; Timmons, 2009).

Immunohistochemical studies in the term laboring uterus have shown that both invading leukocytes and certain parenchymal cells produce cytokines. These leukocytes appear to be the primary source of myometrial cytokines, including IL-1, IL-6, IL-8, and TNF-α (Young, 2002). By contrast, in the decidua, both stromal cells and leukocytes are likely to contribute because they have been shown to produce these same cytokines. In the cervix, glandular and surface epithelial cells appear to produce IL-6, IL-8, and TNF-α. Of these, IL-8 is considered a critical cytokine in cervical dilation, and it is produced in both cervical epithelial and stromal cells.

The presence of cytokines in amnionic fluid and their association with preterm labor has been well documented. But their exact cellular origin—with or without recoverable microorganisms—has not been well defined. Although the rate of IL-1 secretion from forebag decidual tissue is great, Kent (1994) found that there is negligible in vivo transfer of radiolabeled IL-1 across the membranes. Amnionic fluid IL-1 probably does not arise from amnion, fetal urine, or fetal lung secretions. It most likely is secreted by mononuclear phagocytes or neutrophils activated and recruited into the amnionic fluid. Therefore, IL-1 in amnionic fluid likely is generated in situ from newly recruited cells (Young, 2002). Thus, the amount of amnionic fluid IL-1 would be determined by the number of leukocytes recruited, their activational status, or the effect of amnionic fluid constituents on their IL-1 secretion rate.

Leukocyte infiltration may be regulated by fetal membrane synthesis of specific chemokines. In term labor, there are increased amnionic fluid concentrations of the potent chemoattractant and monocyte-macrophage activator *monocyte chemotactic protein-1 (MCP-1)*, which is also called *chemokine (C-C motif) ligand 2 (CCL2)*. As is true for prostaglandins and other cytokines, the levels of MCP-1 are much higher in the forebag compared with the upper compartment (Esplin, 2003). Levels in preterm labor were significantly higher than those found in normal term amnionic fluid (Jacobsson, 2003). MCP-1 may initiate fetal leukocyte infiltration of the placenta and membranes, and its production may act as a marker for intraamnionic infection and inflammation.

Preterm Premature Rupture of Membranes

This term defines spontaneous rupture of the fetal membranes before 37 completed weeks and *before labor onset* (American College of Obstetricians and Gynecologists, 2013d). Such rupture likely has various causes, but intrauterine infection is believed by many to be a major predisposing event (Gomez, 1997; Mercer, 2003). There are associated risk factors that include low socioeconomic status, body mass index ≤ 19.8, nutritional deficiencies, and cigarette smoking. Women with prior preterm premature rupture of membranes (PPROM) are at increased risk for recurrence during a subsequent pregnancy (Bloom, 2001). Despite these known risk factors, none is identified in most cases of preterm rupture.

Molecular Changes

Preterm membrane rupture pathogenesis may be related to increased apoptosis of membrane cellular components and to increased levels of specific proteases in membranes and amnionic fluid. Most tensile strength of the membranes is provided by the amnionic extracellular matrix and interstitial amnionic collagens—primarily type I and III—which are produced in mesenchymal cells (Casey, 1996). For that reason, collagen degradation has been a focus of research. The matrix metalloproteinase (MMP) family is involved with normal tissue remodeling and particularly with collagen degradation. The MMP-1, MMP-2, MMP-3, and MMP-9 members of this family are found in higher concentrations in amnionic fluid from pregnancies with preterm prematurely ruptured membranes (Maymon, 2000; Park, 2003; Romero, 2002). MMP activity is in part regulated by tissue inhibitors of matrix metalloproteinases—TIMPs. Several of these inhibitors are found in lower concentrations in amnionic fluid from women with ruptured membranes. Elevated MMP levels found at a time when protease inhibitor expression decreases supports further that their expression alters amnionic tensile strength. Studies of amniochorion explants have demonstrated that the expression of MMPs can be increased by treatment with IL-1, TNF-α, and IL-6 (Fortunato, 1999a,b, 2002). Recent studies by Mogami (2013) provide a mechanism by which bacterial endotoxin or TNF-α elicits release of fetal fibronectin (fFN) by amnion epithelial cells. The fFN then binds Toll-like receptor 4 in the amnion mesenchymal cells to activate signaling cascades. These result in increased prostaglandin E (PGE_2) synthesis and elevated activity of MMP-1, MP-2, and MMP-9. Increased prostaglandin levels promote cervical ripening and uterine contractions. Increased MMPs allow collagen breakdown in the fetal membranes resulting in premature rupture.

In pregnancies with PPROM, the amnion exhibits a higher degree of cell death and more apoptosis markers than that in term amnion (Arechavaleta-Velasco, 2002; Fortunato, 2003). In vitro studies indicate that apoptosis is likely regulated by bacterial endotoxin, IL-1, and TNF-α. Last, there are proteins involved in the synthesis of mature cross-linked collagen or matrix proteins that bind collagen and thereby promote tensile strength. These proteins are altered in membranes with premature rupture (Wang, 2006). Taken together, these observations suggest that many PPROM cases result from collagen degradation, altered collagen assembly, and cell death, which all lead to a weakened amnion.

Infection

Several studies have been done to ascertain the incidence of infection-induced premature membrane rupture. Bacterial cultures of amnionic fluid support a role for infection in a significant proportion. A review of 18 studies comprising almost 1500 women with PPROM found that in a third, bacteria were isolated from amnionic fluid (Goncalves, 2002). Accordingly, some have given prophylactic antimicrobial treatment to prevent premature rupture (Miyazaki, 2012; Phupong, 2012).

Overall, there is compelling evidence that infection causes a significant proportion of PPROM cases. The inflammatory response that leads to membrane weakening is currently being defined. Research is focused on mediators of this process with a goal to identify early risk markers for PPROM.

Multifetal Gestation

Twins and higher-order multifetal births account for approximately 3 percent of infants born in the United States (Martin, 2009a). The majority—95 percent—of these births are twins. Compared with 1980, the rates of multiple births increased steadily and peaked in 1998. Current rates have declined since then, but remain higher than the 1980s. The increased rate of multifetal births is due to the increased number of women having babies after the age of 30, at which time the risk to conceive multiples rises. In addition, the use of fertility treatments has contributed to the elevated rates of multifetal pregnancies. Preterm delivery continues to be the major cause of the excessive perinatal morbidity and mortality with multifetal pregnancies. The effects of uterine stretch discussed on page 837 are obvious in these pregnancies, and this likely is related to the increased incidence of preterm cervical dilatation. Many of these interrelationships are discussed in Chapter 45.

Summary of Preterm Labor Pathophysiology

Preterm labor is a pathological condition with multiple etiologies. Romero (2006) termed it the *preterm parturition syndrome*. Most research in this field has been focused on the role of infection in mediating preterm birth. It is possible that intrauterine infection causes some cases currently categorized as idiopathic spontaneous preterm labor. There are various sites for intrauterine infection—maternal, fetal, or both—and increasing evidence that the inflammatory response may have distinct and compartment-specific functions that differ between uterus, fetal membranes, and cervix in normal birth. Thus, determining the proportion of pregnancies that end prematurely because of infection is difficult.

Infection does not explain all causes of preterm birth. In recent years, our understanding of other influences on the parturition process, such as maternal nutrition before or during pregnancy, genetics, the vaginal microbiome, and dynamic regulation of the extracellular matrix, has led to new avenues of research and a broader understanding of this complicated and multifactorial process. The current and future application of genomic and bioinformatics as well as molecular and biochemical studies will shed light on pathways involved in term and preterm labor and identify processes critical to all phases of cervical remodeling and uterine function.

ANTECEDENTS AND CONTRIBUTING FACTORS

Myriad genetic and environmental factors affect the frequency of preterm labor.

Threatened Abortion

Vaginal bleeding in early pregnancy is associated with increased adverse outcomes later. Weiss (2004) reported outcomes with vaginal bleeding at 6 to 13 weeks in nearly 14,000 women. Both light and heavy bleeding were associated with subsequent preterm labor, placental abruption, and subsequent pregnancy loss before 24 weeks.

Lifestyle Factors

Cigarette smoking, inadequate maternal weight gain, and illicit drug use have important roles in both the incidence and outcome of low-birthweight neonates (Chap. 12, p. 253). Overweight and obese mothers have an elevated risk of preterm birth (Cnattingius, 2013). Other maternal factors implicated include young or advanced maternal age, poverty, short stature, and vitamin C deficiency (Casanueva, 2005; Gielchinsky, 2002; Kramer, 1995; Meis, 1995; Satin, 1994).

As discussed on page 837, psychological factors such as depression, anxiety, and chronic stress have been reported in association with preterm birth (Copper, 1996; Li, 2008; Littleton, 2007). Neggers and coworkers (2004) found a significant link between low birthweight and preterm birth in women injured by physical abuse (Chap. 47, p. 951).

Studies of work and physical activity related to preterm birth have produced conflicting results (Goldenberg, 2008). There is some evidence, however, that working long hours and hard physical labor are probably associated with increased risk of preterm birth (Luke, 1995).

Genetic Factors

The recurrent, familial, and racial nature of preterm birth has led to the suggestion that genetics may play a causal role. An accumulating literature on genetic variants buttresses this concept (Gibson, 2007; Hampton, 2006; Li, 2004; Macones, 2004). As discussed on page 839, several such studies have also implicated immunoregulatory genes in potentiating chorioamnionitis in cases of preterm delivery due to infection (Varner, 2005).

Birth Defects

In a secondary analysis of data from the First- and Second-Trimester Evaluation of Risk (FASTER) Trial, it was found that birth defects were associated with preterm birth and low birthweight (Dolan, 2007).

Periodontal Disease

Gum inflammation is a chronic anaerobic inflammation that affects as many as 50 percent of pregnant women in the United States (Goepfert, 2004). Vergnes and Sixou (2007) performed a metaanalysis of 17 studies and concluded that periodontal disease was significantly associated with preterm birth—odds ratio 2.83. The researchers concluded, however, that the data were not robust enough to recommend screening and treatment of pregnant women (Stamilio, 2007).

To better study the relationship with periodontitis, Michalowicz (2006) randomly assigned 813 pregnant women between 13 and 17 weeks' gestation who had periodontal disease to treatment during pregnancy or postpartum. They found that treatment during pregnancy improved periodontal disease and that it is safe. However, treatment failed to significantly alter preterm birth rates.

Interval between Pregnancies

Short intervals between pregnancies have been known for some time to be associated with adverse perinatal outcomes. In a metaanalysis, Conde-Agudelo and colleagues (2006) reported that intervals < 18 months and > 59 months were associated with increased risks for both preterm birth and small-for-gestational age newborns.

Prior Preterm Birth

A major risk factor for preterm labor is prior preterm delivery (Spong, 2007). Shown in Table 42-6 is the incidence of recurrent preterm birth in nearly 16,000 women delivered at Parkland Hospital. The recurrent preterm delivery risk for women whose first delivery was preterm was increased threefold compared with that of women whose first neonate was born at term. More than a third of women whose first two newborns were preterm subsequently delivered a third preterm newborn. Most—70 percent—of the recurrent births in this study occurred within 2 weeks of the gestational age of the prior preterm delivery. Importantly, the causes of prior preterm delivery also recurred.

Although women with prior preterm births are clearly at risk for recurrence, they contributed only 10 percent of the total preterm births in this study. Expressed another way, 90 percent of the preterm births at Parkland Hospital cannot be predicted based on a history of preterm birth. Extrapolating data from the 2003 revised birth certificates, it is estimated that approximately 2.5 percent of women delivered in 2004 had a history of prior preterm birth (Martin, 2007).

TABLE 42-6. Recurrent Spontaneous Preterm Births According to Prior Outcome

Birth Outcome[a]	Second Birth ≤ 34 Weeks (%)
First birth ≥ 35 weeks	5
First birth ≤ 34 weeks	16
First and second birth ≤ 34 weeks	41

[a]Data from 15,863 women delivering their first and subsequent pregnancies at Parkland Hospital.
Adapted from Bloom, 2001.

Infection

As discussed, a link between preterm birth and infection seems irrefutable. Goldenberg and coworkers (2008) have reviewed this association. Intrauterine infections are believed to trigger preterm labor by activation of the innate immune system. In this hypothesis, microorganisms elicit release of inflammatory cytokines such as interleukins and TNF-α, which in turn stimulate the production of prostaglandin and/or matrix-degrading enzymes. Prostaglandins stimulate uterine contractions, whereas degradation of extracellular matrix in the fetal membranes leads to preterm rupture of membranes. It is estimated that 25 to 40 percent of preterm births result from intrauterine infection. The basic science of preterm birth due to infection is discussed at length beginning on page 838.

In several studies, antimicrobial treatment has been given to prevent preterm labor due to microbial invasion. Based on available data, these strategies especially targeted mycoplasma species. Morency and colleagues (2007) performed a metaanalysis of 61 articles and suggested that antimicrobials given in the second trimester may prevent subsequent preterm birth. Andrews and associates (2006) reported results of a double-blind interconceptional trial in which they gave a course of azithromycin plus metronidazole every 4 months to 241 nonpregnant women whose last pregnancy resulted in spontaneous delivery before 34 weeks. Approximately 80 percent of the women with subsequent pregnancies had received study drug within 6 months of their subsequent conception. Such interconceptional antimicrobial treatment did not reduce the rate of recurrent preterm birth. Tita and coworkers (2007) performed a subgroup analysis of these same data and concluded that such use of antimicrobials may be harmful. In another study, Goldenberg and colleagues (2006) randomized 2661 women at four African sites to placebo or metronidazole plus erythromycin between 20 and 24 weeks' gestation followed by ampicillin plus metronidazole during labor. This antimicrobial regimen did not reduce the rate of preterm birth or that of histological chorioamnionitis.

Bacterial Vaginosis

In this condition, normal, hydrogen peroxide-producing, lactobacillus-predominant vaginal flora is replaced with anaerobes that include *Gardnerella vaginalis, Mobiluncus* species, and *Mycoplasma hominis* (Hillier, 1995; Nugent, 1991). Its diagnosis and management are discussed in Chapter 65 (p. 1276). Using Gram staining, relative concentrations of the bacterial morphotypes characteristic of bacterial vaginosis are determined and graded as the *Nugent score.*

Bacterial vaginosis has been associated with spontaneous abortion, preterm labor, PPROM, chorioamnionitis, and amnionic fluid infection (Hillier, 1995; Kurki, 1992; Leitich, 2003a,b). Environmental factors appear to be important in bacterial vaginosis development. Exposure to chronic stress, ethnic differences, and frequent or recent douching have all been associated with increased rates of the condition (Culhane, 2002; Ness, 2002). A gene-environment interaction has been described (Macones, 2004). Women with bacterial vaginosis and a susceptible TNF-α genotype had a ninefold increased incidence of preterm birth. From all of these studies, there seems no doubt that adverse vaginal flora is associated in some way with spontaneous preterm birth. Unfortunately, to date, screening and treatment have not been shown to prevent preterm birth. Indeed, microbial resistance or antimicrobial-induced change in the vaginal flora has been reported as a result of regimens intended to eliminate bacterial vaginosis (Beigi, 2004; Carey, 2005). Okun and associates (2005) performed a systematic review of antibiotics given for bacterial vaginosis and for *Trichomonas vaginalis.* They found no evidence to support such use for the prevention of preterm birth in either low-risk or high-risk women.

DIAGNOSIS

Preterm labor is primarily diagnosed by symptoms and physical examination. Sonography is used to identify asymptomatic cervical dilation and effacement.

Symptoms

Early differentiation between true and false labor is difficult before there is demonstrable cervical effacement and dilatation. Uterine activity alone can be misleading because of *Braxton Hicks contractions,* which are discussed in detail in Chapter 21 (p. 409). These contractions, described as irregular, nonrhythmical, and either painful or painless, can cause considerable confusion in the diagnosis of true preterm labor. Not infrequently, women who deliver before term have uterine activity that is attributed to Braxton Hicks contractions, prompting an incorrect diagnosis of false labor. Accordingly, the American Academy of Pediatrics and the American College of Obstetricians and Gynecologists (2012) define preterm labor to be regular contractions before 37 weeks that are associated with cervical change.

In addition to painful or painless uterine contractions, symptoms such as pelvic pressure, menstrual-like cramps, watery vaginal discharge, and lower back pain have been empirically associated with impending preterm birth. Such complaints are thought by some to be common in normal pregnancy and are therefore often dismissed by patients, clinicians, and nurses.

The importance of these symptoms as a harbinger of labor has been emphasized by some but not all investigators (Iams, 1990; Kragt, 1990). Iams and coworkers (1994) found that the signs and symptoms signaling preterm labor, including uterine contractions, appeared only within 24 hours of preterm labor.

Chao (2011) prospectively studied 843 women with singletons who presented to Parkland Hospital with preterm labor symptoms, between $24^{0/7}$ and $33^{6/7}$ weeks, intact membranes, and cervical dilation < 2 cm. These women underwent electronic fetal and uterine contraction monitoring for 2 hours. Those whose cervix remained < 2 cm were sent home with a diagnosis of false preterm labor. When analyzed compared with the general obstetrical population, women sent home had a similar and nonsignificant rate of birth before 34 weeks—2 versus 1 percent. However, these women had a significantly higher rate of birth between 34 and 36 weeks—5 percent compared with 2 percent. Women with cervical dilation of 1 cm at discharge were significantly more likely to deliver before 34 weeks compared with women without cervical dilatation—5 percent versus 1 percent. Importantly, almost 90 percent of the 1-cm group delivered > 21 days after the initial presentation.

Cervical Change

Dilatation

Researchers have evaluated asymptomatic cervical changes that may presage and thus predict preterm labor. Asymptomatic cervical dilatation after midpregnancy is suspected to be a risk factor for preterm delivery, although some clinicians consider it to be a normal anatomical variant. Moreover, study results have suggested that parity alone is not sufficient to explain cervical dilatation discovered early in the third trimester. Cook (1996) longitudinally evaluated cervical status with transvaginal sonography between 18 and 30 weeks in both nulliparous and parous women who all subsequently gave birth at term. Cervical length and diameter were identical in both groups throughout these critical weeks. In a study from Parkland Hospital, routine digital cervical examinations were performed between 26 and 30 weeks in 185 women. Approximately 25 percent of women whose cervix was dilated 2 or 3 cm delivered before 34 weeks. Other investigators have verified cervical dilatation as a predictor of increased preterm delivery risk (Copper, 1995; Pereira, 2007).

Although women with dilatation and effacement in the third trimester are at increased risk for preterm birth, detection does not improve pregnancy outcome. Buekens and associates (1994) randomly assigned 2719 women to undergo routine cervical examinations at each prenatal visit and compared them with 2721 women in whom serial examinations were not performed. Knowledge of antenatal cervical dilatation did not affect any pregnancy outcome related to preterm birth or the frequency of interventions for preterm labor. The investigators also reported that cervical examinations were not related to preterm membrane rupture. At this time, it seems that prenatal cervical examinations are neither beneficial nor harmful.

Length

Vaginal-probe sonographic cervical assessment has been evaluated extensively during the past two decades. When performed by trained operators, cervical length analysis using transvaginal sonography is safe, highly reproducible, and more predictive than transabdominal sonographic screening (American College of Obstetricians and Gynecologists, 2012b). Unlike the transabdominal approach, transvaginal cervical sonography is not affected by maternal obesity, cervix position, or shadowing from the fetal presenting part. Technique is important, and Yost and colleagues (1999) have cautioned that special expertise is needed. Iams and coworkers (1996) measured cervical length at approximately 24 weeks' gestation and again at 28 weeks in 2915 women not at risk for preterm birth. The mean cervical length at 24 weeks was approximately 35 mm, and those women with progressively shorter cervices experienced increased rates of preterm birth.

Until recently, routine cervical length evaluation in women at low risk was not advocated because, like other factors associated with potentially higher preterm birth risk, no effective treatments were available. Randomized trials done to investigate vaginal progesterone use in women with short cervix diagnosed during screening have stimulated consideration of whether or not such screening is warranted (Fonseca, 2007; Hassan, 2011). These trials are discussed subsequently on page 844.

Ambulatory Uterine Monitoring

An external tocodynamometer belted around the abdomen and connected to an electronic waist recorder allows a woman to ambulate while uterine activity is recorded. Results are transmitted via telephone daily. Women are educated concerning signs and symptoms of preterm labor, and clinicians are kept apprised of their progress. The 1985 approval of this monitor by the Food and Drug Administration (FDA) prompted its widespread clinical use. Subsequently, the American College of Obstetricians and Gynecologists (1995) concluded that the use of this expensive, bulky, and time-consuming system does not reduce preterm birth rates. A subsequent study by the Collaborative Home Uterine Monitoring Study Group (1995) confirmed these conclusions. And Iams and associates (2002) analyzed data from almost 35,000 hours of daily home monitoring and verified that no contraction pattern efficiently predicted preterm birth. The American College of Obstetricians and Gynecologists (2012a) does not recommend home uterine activity monitoring.

Fetal Fibronectin

This glycoprotein is produced in 20 different molecular forms by various cell types, including hepatocytes, fibroblasts, endothelial cells, and fetal amnion. Present in high concentrations in maternal blood and in amnionic fluid, it is thought to function in intercellular adhesion during implantation and in maintenance of placental adherence to uterine decidua (Leeson, 1996). Fetal fibronectin is detected in cervicovaginal secretions in women who have normal pregnancies with intact membranes at term. It appears to reflect stromal remodeling of the cervix before labor.

Lockwood (1991) reported that fibronectin detection in cervicovaginal secretions before membrane rupture was a possible marker for impending preterm labor. Fetal fibronectin is measured using an enzyme-linked immunosorbent assay, and values exceeding 50 ng/mL are considered positive. Sample contamination by amnionic fluid and maternal blood should be avoided. Interventional studies based on the use of fetal fibronectin screening in asymptomatic women have not demonstrated improved perinatal outcomes (Andrews, 2003; Grobman, 2004). The American College of Obstetricians and Gynecologists (2012b) does not recommend screening with fetal fibronectin tests.

PRETERM BIRTH PREVENTION

Prevention of preterm birth has been an elusive goal. Recent reports, however, suggest that prevention in selected populations may be achievable.

Cervical Cerclage

There are at least three circumstances when cerclage placement may be used to prevent preterm birth. Two are done prophylactically, and a third is done for treatment. The first prophylactic cerclage is used in women who have a history of recurrent midtrimester losses and who are diagnosed with cervical insufficiency (Chap. 18, p. 360). The second prophylactic cerclage is for women identified during sonographic examination to have a short cervix. The third indication is "rescue" cerclage, done emergently when cervical incompetence is recognized in women with threatened preterm labor.

For women with a short cervix detected by sonography, Berghella and colleagues (2005) reviewed several small trials of cerclage in this group and concluded that cerclage may reduce preterm birth rates in those women with a prior preterm birth. Owen (2009) randomly assigned 302 women with prior preterm birth from 16 centers with a short cervix—defined as length < 25 mm—to cerclage or no procedure. Women with a cervical length < 15 mm delivered before 35 weeks significantly less often following cerclage compared with women with no cerclage—30 versus 65 percent. This study suggests that recurrent preterm birth can be prevented in a subset of women who have a history of prior preterm births.

In a multinational study, To and associates (2004) screened 47,123 women and randomized the 253 women with cervices < 15 mm to cerclage or no cerclage. The frequency of preterm delivery < 33 weeks was not significantly different between the treatment groups. Thus, cerclage for sonographically detected *short cervix alone* has not been found to be beneficial. In contrast, women with a very short cervix, that is, < 15 mm, and a history of prior preterm birth may benefit.

Prophylaxis with Progestin Compounds

Progesterone levels in most mammals fall rapidly before the onset of labor. This is termed *progesterone withdrawal* and is considered to be a parturition-triggering event. During human parturition, however, maternal, fetal, and amnionic fluid progesterone levels remain elevated with no decline. It has been proposed that human parturition involves functional progesterone withdrawal mediated by decreased progesterone activity of progesterone receptors (Ziyan, 2010). It follows conceptually that the administration of progesterone to maintain uterine quiescence may block preterm labor. This hypothesis has stimulated several studies in the past half century.

Prior Preterm Birth and Progestin Compounds

Initial Studies

Studies in the past 15 years have included several investigations to evaluate progestin compounds given prophylactically. A pivotal study was done by the MFMU Network to evaluate prophylactic progestin treatment for women at high-risk for recurrent preterm birth (Meis, 2003). In this trial, 310 women with a prior preterm birth were randomized to receive *17-hydroxyprogesterone caproate (17-OHPC)* (Romero, 2013). Another 153 women received placebo, and these were administered as weekly intramuscular injections of either inert oil or 17-OHPC from 16 through 36 weeks' gestation. Delivery rates before 37, 35, and 32 weeks were all significantly reduced by 17-OHPC therapy. At the same time, however, similar studies of 17-OHPC in both twins and triplets done by the Network showed no improvement in preterm birth rates (Caritis, 2009; Rouse, 2007).

The 17-OHPC study by Meis and colleagues (2003) has been challenged because of the unexpectedly high preterm delivery rate in the placebo arm of the trial. Fifty-five percent delivered rather than the expected rate of 36 percent, which was derived from a pretrial cohort (Romero, 2013). The criticism is that 17-OHPC may have been shown to be effective only because the placebo group was distorted by this high 55-percent preterm delivery rate. This compared with the 36-percent rate, which was actually observed when women were treated with 17-OHPC in the trial. To further elucidate this disparity, a confirmation trial by the Network is underway.

Also in contrast to the 17-OHPC study by Meis and coworkers (2003), O'Brien and associates (2007) randomly assigned 659 women with a prior preterm birth to treatment with daily vaginal progesterone gel (90 mg) or placebo. They found no differences in preterm birth rates.

Subsequent Studies

Perhaps no other topic in contemporary obstetrics has generated as much interest and debate since the 23rd edition of *Williams Obstetrics* as has the use of progestins to prevent preterm birth. At the center of the controversy is whether or not progestins prevent preterm birth in women with a singleton pregnancy but without prior preterm birth—especially nulliparous women. If progestins are effective in women at low risk for preterm birth, this would justify sonographic screening of all pregnant women to detect short cervices (Silver, 2011).

Three randomized trials are at the center of the controversy, and these are summarized in Table 42-7. Fonseca and colleagues (2007) randomly assigned 250 women with sonographically short cervices—15 mm or less—identified during routine prenatal care. Women were given nightly 200-mg micronized progesterone vaginal capsules or placebo from 24 to 34 weeks' gestation. As shown in Table 42-7, spontaneous delivery before 34 weeks was significantly reduced by progesterone therapy. Importantly, this trial included not only nulliparous women but also those with twins or prior preterm birth.

Hassan and coworkers (2011) randomly assigned 465 women with a sonographically short cervix—10 to 20 mm—to vaginal progesterone gel, 90 mg daily or placebo. As shown in Table 42-7, this trial also included nulliparous women as well as women with prior preterm births. Unlike the Fonseca (2007) trial, however, twin gestations were excluded. This trial was performed in 44 hospitals located in 10 countries including the United States. The FDA rejected progesterone gel for use in the United States because the results did not meet the level of statistical significance required to show efficacy in the subjects recruited in this country. Neither the Fonseca (2007) nor the

TABLE 42-7. Randomized Trials of Progestin Compounds Given Prophylactically to Prevent Preterm Labor

Investigator	Women Randomized	Cervical Length[a]	Progestin Compound	Progestin vs Placebo
Fonseca (2007)	n = 250; 5% nulliparous, 10% twins, 15% prior PTB; 8 hospitals: UK, Greece, Brazil, Chile	< 15 mm	Progesterone, 200-mg vaginal capsules daily	Delivery < 34 weeks: 19% vs 34%, p = .02
Hassan (2011)	n = 465; singletons only; 55% nulliparous; 13% prior PTB; 44 hospitals in 10 countries	10–20 mm	Progesterone, 90-mg vaginal gel daily	Delivery < 33 weeks: 9% vs 16%, p = .02
Grobman (2012)	n = 657; singletons only; nulliparous only; 14 centers across US	< 30 mm	17-OHPC, 250 mg IM weekly	Delivery < 37 weeks: 25% vs 24%, p = NS

[a]Determined sonographically.
17-OHPC = 17-hydroxyprogesterone caproate; IM = intramuscularly; NS = nonsignificant; PTB = preterm birth; UK = United Kingdom; US = United States.

Hassan (2011) studies report subset analyses exclusive to nulliparas (Parry, 2012). According to Likis and colleagues (2012), the heterogeneity of these two studies that included women with varied indications for progestin treatment, combined with the fact that outcomes were not reported by risk factors such as nulliparity, makes it impossible to interpret the efficacy of progesterone for specific indications. Based on these studies, the American College of Obstetricians and Gynecologists (2012a,b) concluded that it could not "mandate universal cervical length screening in women without a prior preterm birth, but that this screening strategy may be considered."

The most recently published study that addresses use of progestins to prevent preterm birth in nulliparas included 657 randomly assigned to 17-OHPC or placebo (Grobman, 2012). This study was limited to women with singletons and sonographic cervical length < 30 mm detected between 16 and $22^{3/7}$ weeks. Treatment with 17-OHPC given weekly did not reduce the frequency of preterm birth before 37 weeks. Subgroup analyses by cervical length and gestational age at delivery are summarized in Table 42-8. Regardless of cervical length, 17-OHPC was ineffective.

Another interesting development vis-à-vis progestin therapy for preterm birth since the last edition of *Williams Obstetrics* was the marketing of 17-OHPC by KV Pharmaceuticals under the brand name *Makena*. The original retail price was $1500 per 250-mg injectable dose. Thus, a 20-week course for one woman would cost $30,000. This caused an uproar among the leadership of organizations in obstetrics and gynecology. The United States Congress became involved, and the FDA permitted continued availability of 17-hydroxyprogesterone

TABLE 42-8. Comparison of 17-OHPC versus Placebo to Prevent Preterm Birth at < 37 and < 34 Weeks

Variable	17-OHPC N = 327	Placebo N = 330	RR (95% CI)	p value[a]
Preterm birth < 37 wk:				
Cervical length, mm				.59
< 10	5/9 (56)	10/16 (63)	0.89 (0.4–1.78)	
10–20	19/50 (38)	18/40 (45)	0.84 (0.52–1.38)	
> 20	58/268 (21)	52/274 (19)	1.4 (0.82–1.52)	
Preterm birth < 34 wk:				
Cervical length, mm				.49
< 10	5/9 (56)	6/16 (38)	1.48 (0.63–3.51)	
10–20	11/50 (22)	12/40 (30)	0.73 (0.36–1.48)	
> 20	25/268 (9)	30/274 (11)	0.85 (0.52–1.41)	

[a]p value for Breslow-Day interaction term.
Data are presented as n/N (%).
CI = confidence interval; RR = relative risk; 17-OHPC = 17-hydroxyprogesterone caproate.
Data from Grobman, 2012.

compounded by pharmacies as an alternative to *Makena*. In Dallas in 2013, a 250-mg injectable dose of compounded 17-OHPC cost about \$18. KV Pharmaceuticals filed for Chapter 11 bankruptcy 4 in August 2012. The company cited that it had been unable to realize the full value of its most important drug, *Makena* (St Louis Business Journal, 2012).

So, how does the clinician reconcile the conflicting evidence as to the efficacy of progestins across the spectrum of the various specific indications? Romero and Stanczyk (2013) argue that one explanation for the conflicting evidence is that progesterone is not the same as 17-hydroxyprogesterone caproate (Figure 42-9). Progesterone is a natural steroid produced by the corpus luteum and the placenta, whereas 17-hydroxyprogesterone caproate is a synthetic steroid. These authors reviewed the basic science of natural and synthetic progestins vis-à-vis effects on the uterus and cervix in pregnant women, animals, and in vitro experiments. For example, natural progesterone suppresses myometrial contractility in strips that were obtained at cesarean delivery, whereas synthetic 17-OHPC did not. This report is an excellent source of information on the issues involved with progestin use in preterm birth.

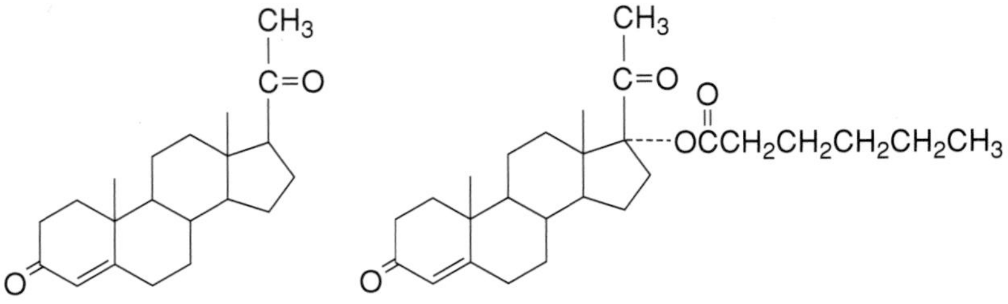

FIGURE 42-9 Chemical structure of progesterone and 17α-hydroxyprogesterone caproate.

The evidence for or against the preventive efficacy of progestins for preterm birth is clearly complex. As outlined in this section, virtually all evidence supporting use for a specific indication can be challenged in some way. Currently, at Parkland Hospital, we are prescribing weekly injections of 17-hydroxyprogesterone compounded by a local pharmacy for women with a prior preterm birth. In our view, all other indications for the use of progestin in the prevention of preterm birth are investigational.

Geographic-Based Public Health-Care Programs

A well-organized prenatal system results in a decreased preterm birth rate in high-risk indigent populations. The decreasing preterm birth rate at Parkland Hospital between 1988 and 2006 shown in Figure 42-10 coincided with a substantial increase in prenatal care utilization. In the early 1990s, a concerted effort was made to improve access to and use of prenatal care. The intention was to develop a program of seamless care beginning with enrollment during the prenatal period and extending through delivery and into the puerperium. Prenatal clinics are placed strategically throughout Dallas County to provide convenient access for indigent women. When possible, these clinics were colocated with comprehensive medical and pediatric clinics that enhance patient use. Because the entire clinic system is operated by Parkland Hospital, administrative and medical oversight is seamless. For example, prenatal protocols are used by nurse practitioners at all clinic sites to guarantee homogeneous care. Women with high-risk pregnancy complications are referred to the hospital-based central clinic system. Here, high-risk pregnancy clinics operate each weekday, with specialty clinics for women with prior preterm birth, gestational diabetes, infectious diseases, multifetal pregnancy, and hypertensive disorders. Clinics are staffed by residents and midwives supervised by maternal-fetal medicine fellows and faculty. Because Parkland Hospital has a closed medical staff, all attending physicians are employed by the University of Texas Southwestern Department of Obstetrics and Gynecology. These faculty members adhere to agreed-upon practice guidelines using an evidence-based outcomes approach. Thus, prenatal care is considered one component of a comprehensive and orchestrated public health care system that is community-based. Putting this together, we hypothesize that the decrease in preterm births experienced at our inner-city hospital was attributable to a geographically based public health-care program specifically targeting minority populations of pregnant women. A similar obstetrical care system for indigent women at the University of Alabama at Birmingham has also produced salutary results (Tita, 2011).

MANAGEMENT OF PRETERM PREMATURELY RUPTURED MEMBRANES

Methods used to diagnose ruptured membranes are detailed in Chapter 22 (p. 448). A history of vaginal leakage of fluid, either as a continuous stream or as a gush, should prompt a

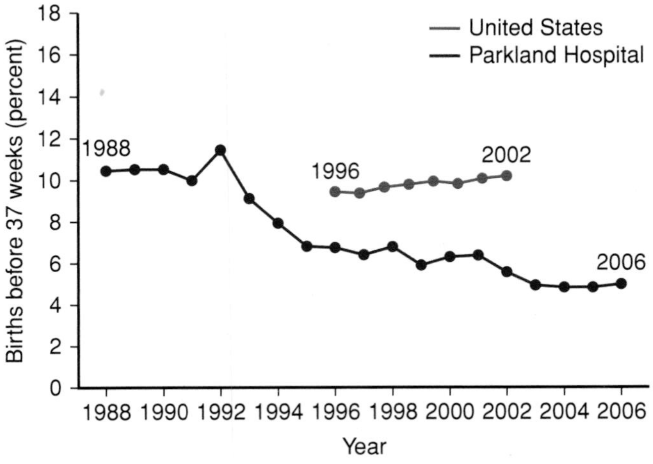

FIGURE 42-10 Percentage of births before 37 weeks' gestation at Parkland Hospital from 1988 to 2006 compared with that in the United States from 1996 to 2002. Analysis in both cohorts was limited to singleton live births ≥ 500 g who received prenatal care. (Redrawn from Leveno, 2009, with permission.)

speculum examination to visualize gross vaginal pooling of amnionic fluid, clear fluid from the cervical canal, or both. Confirmation of ruptured membranes is usually accompanied by sonographic examination to assess amnionic fluid volume, to identify the presenting part, and if not previously determined, to estimate gestational age. Amnionic fluid is slightly alkaline (pH 7.1–7.3) compared with vaginal secretions (pH 4.5–6.0). This is the basis of frequently used pH testing for ruptured membranes. Blood, semen, antiseptics, or bacterial vaginosis, however, are all also alkaline and can give false-positive results.

Natural History

Cox and associates (1988) described pregnancy outcomes of 298 consecutive women who gave birth following spontaneously ruptured membranes between 24 and 34 weeks at Parkland Hospital. Although this complication was identified in only 1.7 percent of pregnancies, it contributed to 20 percent of all perinatal deaths. By the time they presented, 75 percent of the women were already in labor, 5 percent were delivered for other complications, and another 10 percent delivered within 48 hours. In only 7 percent was delivery delayed 48 hours or more after membrane rupture. This last subgroup, however, appeared to benefit from delayed delivery because there were no neonatal deaths. This contrasted with a neonatal death rate of 80 per 1000 in preterm newborns delivered within 48 hours of membrane rupture. Nelson (1994) reported similar results.

The time from PPROM to delivery is inversely proportional to the gestational age when rupture occurs (Carroll, 1995). As shown in Figure 42-11, very few days were gained when membranes ruptured during the third trimester compared with midpregnancy.

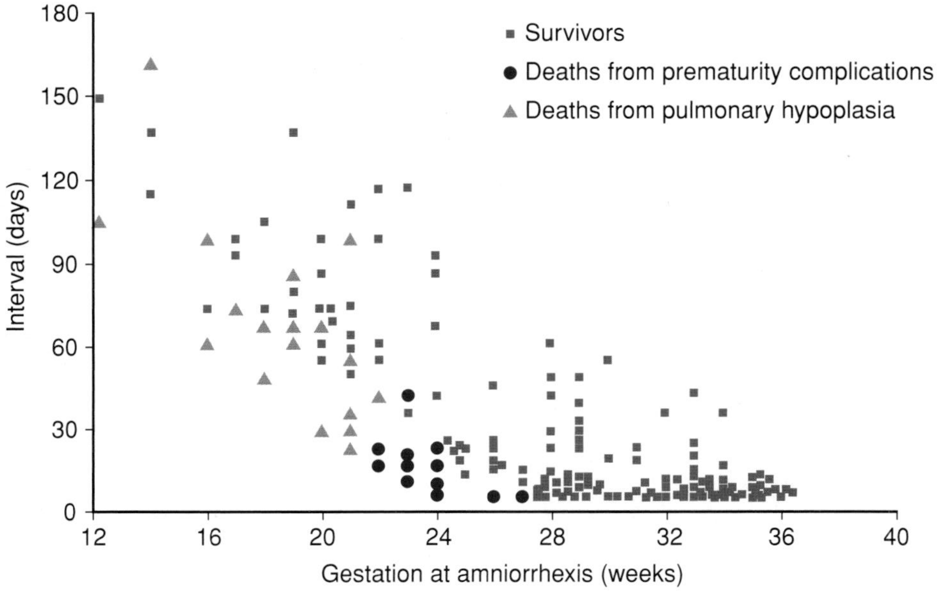

FIGURE 42-11 Relationship of time between preterm membrane rupture and delivery in 172 singleton pregnancies. (Redrawn from Carroll, 1995, with permission.)

Hospitalization

Most clinicians hospitalize women with PPROM. Concerns regarding the costs of lengthy hospitalizations are usually moot, because most women enter labor within a week or less after membrane rupture. Carlan and coworkers (1993) randomly assigned 67 women with ruptured membranes to home or hospital management. No benefits were found for hospitalization, and maternal hospital stays were reduced by 50 percent in those sent home—14 versus 7 days. Importantly, the investigators emphasized that this study was too small to conclude that home management was safe vis-à-vis umbilical cord prolapse.

Intentional Delivery

Before the mid-1970s, labor was usually induced in women with preterm ruptured membranes because of fear of sepsis. Two randomized trials compared labor induction with expectant management in such pregnancies. Mercer and associates (1993) randomly assigned 93 women with pregnancies between 32 and 36 weeks to undergo delivery or expectant management. Fetal lung maturity, as evidenced by mature surfactant profiles, was present in all cases. Intentional delivery reduced the length of maternal hospitalization and also reduced infection rates in both mothers and neonates. Cox and coworkers (1995) similarly apportioned 129 women between 30 and 34 weeks. Fetal lung maturity was not assessed. One fetal death resulted from sepsis in the pregnancies managed expectantly. Among those intentionally delivered, there were three neonatal deaths—two from sepsis and one from pulmonary hypoplasia. Thus, neither management approach proved to be superior for perinatal outcomes.

Expectant Management

Despite extensive literature concerning expectant management of PPROM, tocolysis has been used in few studies. In randomized studies, women were assigned to receive either tocolysis or expectant management. The investigators concluded that active interventions did not improve perinatal outcomes (Garite, 1981, 1987; Nelson, 1985).

Other considerations with expectant management involve the use of digital cervical examination and cerclage. Alexander and colleagues (2000) analyzed findings in women expectantly managed between 24 and 32 weeks' gestation. They compared those who had one or two digital cervical examinations with women who were not examined digitally. Women who were examined had a rupture-to-delivery interval of 3 days compared with 5 days in those who were not examined. This difference did not worsen maternal or neonatal outcomes.

There is uncertainty regarding ruptured membranes in the woman who has undergone cervical cerclage. McElrath and associates (2002) studied 114 women with cerclage in place who later had ruptured membranes before 34 weeks. They were compared with 288 controls who had not received a cerclage. Pregnancy outcomes were equivalent in both groups. As discussed in Chapter 18 (p. 363), such management is controversial.

Risks of Expectant Management

Maternal and fetal risks vary with the gestational age at membrane rupture. Morales (1993b) expectantly managed 94 singleton pregnancies with ruptured membranes before 25 weeks. The average time gained was 11 days. *Although 41 percent of infants survived to age 1 year, only 27 percent were neurologically normal.* Similar results were reported by Farooqi (1998) and Winn (2000) and their colleagues. Lieman and associates (2005) found no improved neonatal outcomes with expectant management beyond 33 weeks. In contrast, McElrath and coworkers (2003) found that prolonged latency after membrane rupture was not associated with an increased incidence of fetal neurological damage.

The volume of amnionic fluid remaining after rupture appears to have prognostic importance in pregnancies before 26 weeks. Hadi and colleagues (1994) described 178 pregnancies with ruptured membranes between 20 and 25 weeks. Forty percent of women developed oligohydramnios, defined by the absence of fluid pockets 2 cm or larger. Virtually all women with oligohydramnios delivered before 25 weeks, whereas 85 percent with adequate amnionic fluid volume were delivered in the third trimester. Carroll and coworkers (1995) observed no cases of pulmonary hypoplasia in fetuses born after membrane rupture at 24 weeks or beyond. This suggests that 23 weeks or less is the threshold for development of lung hypoplasia. Further, when contemplating early expectant management, consideration is also given to oligohydramnios and resultant limb compression deformities (Chap. 11, p. 237).

Other risk factors have also been evaluated. In neonates born to women with active herpetic lesions who were expectantly managed, the infectious morbidity risk appeared to be outweighed by risks associated with preterm delivery (Major, 2003). Lewis and associates (2007) found that expectant management of women with preterm ruptured membranes and noncephalic presentation was associated with an increased rate of umbilical cord prolapse, especially before 26 weeks.

Clinical Chorioamnionitis

Most authors report that prolonged membrane rupture is associated with increased fetal and maternal sepsis (Ho, 2003). If chorioamnionitis is diagnosed, prompt efforts to effect delivery, preferably vaginally, are initiated. Fever is the only reliable indicator for this diagnosis, and temperature of 38°C (100.4°F) or higher accompanying ruptured membranes implies infection. Maternal leukocytosis alone has not been found to be reliable. During expectant management, monitoring for sustained maternal or fetal tachycardia, for uterine tenderness, and for a malodorous vaginal discharge is warranted.

With chorioamnionitis, fetal and neonatal morbidity is substantively increased. Alexander and colleagues (1998) studied 1367 very-low-birthweight neonates delivered at Parkland Hospital. Approximately 7 percent were born to women with overt chorioamnionitis, and their outcomes were compared with similar newborns without clinical infection. Those in the infected group had a higher incidence of sepsis, respiratory distress syndrome, early-onset seizures, intraventricular hemorrhage, and periventricular leukomalacia. The investigators concluded that these very-low-birthweight neonates were vulnerable to neurological injury attributable to chorioamnionitis.

Although Locatelli and coworkers (2005) have challenged this finding, there is other evidence that very small newborns are at increased risk for sepsis. Yoon and colleagues (2000) found that intraamnionic infection in preterm neonates was related to increased rates of cerebral palsy. Petrova and associates (2001) studied more than 11 million singleton live births in the United States from 1995 to 1997. During labor, 1.6 percent of all women had fever, and this was a strong predictor of infection-related death in both term and preterm neonates. Bullard and colleagues (2002) reported similar results.

Accelerated Pulmonary Maturation

Various clinical events—some well defined—were once proposed to accelerate fetal surfactant production (Gluck, 1979). These included chronic renal or cardiovascular disease, hypertensive disorders, heroin addiction, fetal-growth restriction, placental infarction, chorioamnionitis, and preterm ruptured membranes. Although this view was widely held for many years, subsequent observations do not support this association (Hallak, 1993; Owen, 1990).

Antimicrobial Therapy

The proposed microbial pathogenesis for spontaneous preterm labor or ruptured membranes has prompted investigators to give various antimicrobials in an attempt to forestall delivery. Mercer and associates (1995) reviewed 13 randomized trials performed before 35 weeks. Metaanalysis indicated that only three of 10 outcomes were *possibly* benefited: (1) fewer women developed chorioamnionitis, (2) fewer newborns developed sepsis, and (3) pregnancy was more often prolonged 7 days in women given antimicrobials. Neonatal survival, however, was unaffected, as was the incidence of necrotizing enterocolitis, respiratory distress, or intracranial hemorrhage.

To further address this issue, the MFMU Network designed a trial to study expectant management combined with a 7-day treatment with ampicillin, amoxicillin plus erythromycin, or placebo. The women had membrane rupture between 24 and 32 weeks. Neither tocolytics nor corticosteroids were given. Antimicrobial-treated women had significantly fewer newborns with respiratory distress syndrome, necrotizing enterocolitis, and composite adverse outcomes (Mercer, 1997). The latency period was significantly longer. Specifically, 50 percent of women given an antimicrobial regimen remained undelivered after 7 days of treatment compared with only 25 percent of those given placebo. There was also significant prolongation of pregnancy at 14 and 21 days. Cervicovaginal group B streptococcal colonization did not alter these results.

More recent studies have examined the efficacy of shorter treatment lengths and other antimicrobial combinations. Three-day treatment compared with 7-day regimens using either ampicillin or ampicillin-sulbactam appeared equally effective in regard to perinatal outcomes (Lewis, 2003; Segel, 2003). Similarly, erythromycin compared with placebo offered a range of significant neonatal benefits. The amoxicillin-clavulanate regimen was not recommended, however, because of its association with an increased incidence of necrotizing enterocolitis (Kenyon, 2004).

Some predicted that prolonged antimicrobial therapy in such pregnancies might have unwanted consequences. Carroll (1996) and Mercer (1999) and their coworkers cautioned that such therapy potentially increased the risk for resistant bacteria. Stoll and associates (2002) studied 4337 neonates weighing from 400 to 1500 g and born from 1998 to 2000. Their outcomes were compared with those of 7606 neonates of similar birthweight born from 1991 to 1993. The overall rate of early-onset sepsis did not change between these two epochs. But the rate of group B streptococcal sepsis decreased from 5.9 per 1000 births in the 1991 to 1993 group to 1.7 per 1000 births in the 1998 to 2000 group. Comparing these same epochs, the rate of *Escherichia coli* sepsis increased from 3.2 to 6.8 per 1000 births. Almost 85 percent of coliform isolates from the more recent cohort were ampicillin resistant. Neonates with early-onset sepsis were more likely to die, especially if they were infected with coliforms. Kenyon and coworkers (2008a) found that antimicrobials given for women with PPROM had no effect on the health of children at age 7 years.

Corticosteroids to Accelerate Fetal Lung Maturity

The National Institutes of Health (NIH) (2000) in their Consensus Development Conference recommended a single course of antenatal corticosteroids for women with preterm membrane rupture before 32 weeks and in whom there was no evidence of chorioamnionitis. Since then, several metaanalyses have addressed this issue, and according to the American College of Obstetricians and Gynecologists (2013d), single-dose therapy is recommended from 24 to 32 weeks. There is no consensus regarding treatment between 32 and 34 weeks. Corticosteroid therapy is not recommended before 24 weeks.

Membrane Repair

Tissue sealants have been used for various purposes in medicine and have become important in maintaining surgical hemostasis and stimulating wound healing. Devlieger and colleagues (2006) have reviewed the efficacy of sealants in the repair of fetal membrane defects such as in preterm ruptured membranes.

Management Recommendations

The management scheme recommended by the American College of Obstetricians and Gynecologists (2013d) is summarized in Table 42-9. This management is similar to that practiced at Parkland Hospital.

MANAGEMENT OF PRETERM LABOR WITH INTACT MEMBRANES

Women with signs and symptoms of preterm labor with intact membranes are managed much the same as described above for

TABLE 42-9. Recommended Management of Preterm Ruptured Membranes

Gestational Age	Management
34 weeks or more	Proceed to delivery, usually by induction of labor Group B streptococcal prophylaxis is recommended
32 weeks to 33 completed weeks	Expectant management unless fetal pulmonary maturity is documented Group B streptococcal prophylaxis is recommended Corticosteroids—no consensus, but some experts recommend Antimicrobials to prolong latency if no contraindications
24 weeks to 31 completed weeks	Expectant management Group B streptococcal prophylaxis is recommended Single-course corticosteroid use is recommended Tocolytics—no consensus Antimicrobials to prolong latency if no contraindications
Before 24 weeks[a]	Patient counseling Expectant management or induction of labor Group B streptococcal prophylaxis is not recommended Corticosteroids are not recommended Antimicrobials—there are incomplete data on use in prolonging latency

[a]The combination of birthweight, gestational age, and sex provides the best estimate of chances of survival and should be considered in individual cases.

those with preterm ruptured membranes. If possible, delivery before 34 weeks is delayed. Drugs used to abate or suppress preterm uterine contractions are subsequently discussed.

Amniocentesis to Detect Infection

Several tests have been used to diagnose intraamnionic infection. Romero and coworkers (1993) evaluated the diagnostic value of amnionic fluid containing an elevated leukocyte count, a low glucose level, a high IL-6 concentration, or a positive Gram stain result in 120 women with preterm labor and intact membranes. Women with positive amnionic fluid culture results were considered infected. These investigators found that a negative Gram stain result was 99-percent specific to exclude amnionic fluid bacteria. A high IL-6 level was 82-percent sensitive for detection of amnionic fluid containing bacteria. Other investigators have also found good correlation between amnionic fluid IL-6 or leukocyte levels and chorioamnionic infection (Andrews, 1995; Yoon, 1996). Despite these correlations, amniocentesis to diagnose infection does not improve pregnancy outcomes in women with or without membrane rupture (Feinstein, 1986). The American College of Obstetricians and Gynecologists (2012a) has concluded that there is no evidence to support routine amniocentesis to identify infection.

Corticosteroids for Fetal Lung Maturation

Because glucocorticosteroids were found to accelerate lung maturation in preterm sheep fetuses, Liggins and Howie (1972) evaluated them to treat women. Corticosteroid therapy was effective in lowering the incidence of respiratory distress syndrome and neonatal mortality rates if birth was delayed for at least 24 hours after *initiation* of betamethasone. Infants exposed to corticosteroids in these early studies have now been followed to age 31 years with no ill effects detected. In 1995, an NIH Consensus Development Conference panel recommended corticosteroids for fetal lung maturation in threatened preterm birth.

In a subsequent meeting, the NIH Consensus Development Conference (2000) concluded that data were insufficient to assess corticosteroid effectiveness in pregnancies complicated by hypertension, diabetes, multifetal gestation, fetal-growth restriction, and fetal hydrops. It concluded, however, that it was reasonable to administer corticosteroids in women with these complications.

The issue of the fetal and neonatal safety with single versus repeat courses of intramuscular corticosteroids for lung maturation has been the topic of two major trials. Although both found repeated courses to be beneficial in reducing neonatal respiratory morbidity rates, the long-term consequences were much different. Specifically, Crowther and associates (2007) studied outcomes in 982 women who were given a single weekly dose of 11.4 mg of betamethasone. These investigators found no adverse effects in the infants followed to age 2 years. Wapner and colleagues (2007) studied infants born to 495 women who were randomly assigned to receive a single corticosteroid course or repeated courses that were given weekly. With each round, a 12-mg betamethasone dose was injected, followed by a second given 24 hours later. A nonsignificant rise in cerebral palsy rates was identified in infants exposed to repeated courses. The twice-as-large betamethasone dose in this study was worrisome because some experimental evidence supports the view that adverse corticosteroid effects are dose dependent. Bruschettini and coworkers (2006) studied the equivalent of 12-mg versus 6-mg betamethasone given to pregnant cats. They reported that the lower dose had less severe effects on somatic growth without affecting fetal brain cell proliferation. Stiles (2007) summarized these two human studies as "early gain, long-term questions." We agree, and at Parkland Hospital, we follow the recommendation by the American College of Obstetricians and Gynecologists (2013c) for single-course therapy.

"Rescue Therapy"

This refers to administration of a repeated corticosteroid dose when delivery becomes imminent and more than 7 days have elapsed since the initial dose. The 2000 NIH Consensus Development Conference recommended that rescue therapy should not be routinely used and that it should be reserved for clinical trials. The first randomized trial, reported by Peltoniemi and coworkers (2007), allocated 326 women to placebo or 12-mg betamethasone single-dose rescue regimens. Paradoxically, these researchers found that the rescue dose of betamethasone increased the risk of respiratory distress syndrome! In a multicenter study of 437 women < 33 weeks who were randomly assigned to rescue therapy or placebo, Kurtzman and associates (2009) reported significantly decreased rates of respiratory complications and neonatal composite morbidity with rescue corticosteroids. There were, however, no differences in perinatal mortality rates and other morbidities. In another trial, McEvoy and colleagues (2010) showed that treated infants had improved respiratory compliance.

Garite and coworkers (2009) randomly assigned 437 women with singletons or twins < 33 weeks' gestation and with intact membranes to one "rescue" course of either betamethasone or dexamethasone or placebo. These women had all previously completed a single course of corticosteroids before 30 weeks' gestation and at least 14 days before the "rescue" course. Respiratory distress syndrome developed in 41 percent of the infants given corticosteroids compared with 62 percent of those randomized to placebo. There were no differences in other morbidities attributable to prematurity. In a metaanalysis, Crowther and colleagues (2011) concluded that a single course of corticosteroids should be considered in women whose prior course was administered at least 7 days previously and were < 34 weeks' gestation. The American College of Obstetricians and Gynecologists (2012a) has taken the position that a single rescue course of antenatal corticosteroids *should be considered* in women before 34 weeks whose prior course was administered at least 7 days previously.

Choice of Corticosteroid

As summarized by Murphy (2007), there is a 10-year question as to whether betamethasone is superior to dexamethasone for fetal lung maturation. Elimian and associates (2007) randomly assigned 299 women between 24 and 33 weeks to betamethasone or dexamethasone. These two drugs were comparable in reducing rates of major neonatal morbidities in preterm infants.

Antimicrobials

As with preterm ruptured membranes, antimicrobials have been given in an attempt to arrest preterm labor. Results have been disappointing. A Cochrane metaanalysis by King and colleagues (2000) found no difference in the rates of newborn respiratory distress syndrome or sepsis between placebo- and antimicrobial-treated groups. They did find, however, increased perinatal morbidity in the antimicrobial-treated group. Kenyon (2001) reported the ORACLE Collaborative Group study of 6295 women with spontaneous preterm labor, intact membranes, but without evidence of infection. Women were randomly assigned to receive antimicrobial or placebo therapy. The primary outcomes of neonatal death, chronic lung disease, and major cerebral abnormality were similar in both groups. In his review, Goldenberg (2002) also concluded that antimicrobial treatment of women with preterm labor for the sole purpose of preventing delivery is generally not recommended. In a follow-up of the ORACLE II trial, Kenyon and associates (2008b) reported that fetal exposure to antimicrobials in this clinical setting was associated with an increased cerebral palsy rate at age 7 years compared with that of children without fetal exposure.

Bed Rest

This is one of the most often prescribed interventions during pregnancy, yet one of the least studied. Goldenberg (1994) reviewed the available literature on bed rest in pregnancy and found no evidence supporting or refuting the benefit of either bed rest or hospitalization for women with threatened preterm labor. Moreover, Sosa and colleagues (2004) searched the Cochrane Database and concluded that evidence neither supported nor refuted bed rest to prevent preterm birth.

Goulet and coworkers (2001) randomly assigned 250 Canadian women to either home care or hospitalization after treatment of an acute episode of preterm labor and also found no benefits. Yost and associates (2005) attempted a randomized study at Parkland Hospital but terminated the study after 6 years due to low recruitment. In this study, bed rest in the hospital compared with bed rest at home had no effect on pregnancy duration in women with threatened preterm labor before 34 weeks. Kovacevich and coworkers (2000) reported that bed rest for 3 days or more increased thromboembolic complications to 16 per 1000 women compared with only 1 per 1000 with normal ambulation. Promislow and colleagues (2004) observed significant bone loss in pregnant women prescribed outpatient bed rest.

Most recently there were three articles on bed rest in the journal *Obstetrics & Gynecology*. Grobman and associates (2013) found that nearly 40 percent of women enrolled in a trial to study the efficacy of 17-OHPC in those with a sonographically short cervix had some form of activity restriction. Women with activity restriction were nearly 2.5 times more likely to have a preterm birth before 34 weeks. This finding, however, may reflect ascertainment bias in that women with restricted activity may have received bed rest because they were viewed to be at more imminent risk of preterm delivery. In the same journal issue, McCall and coworkers (2013) summarized the literature on bed rest. They found insufficient evidence to support the use of bed rest and found several studies showing harm with its use. They opined that it is unethical to continue to prescribe bed rest. In an accompanying editorial, Biggio (2013) called for appropriate trials to settle these issues.

Cervical Pessaries

There is increasing interest in the use of cervical pessaries to prevent preterm birth. Silicone rings, also know as the *Arabin pessary*, are being used to support the cervix in women with a sonographically short cervix. For 385 Spanish women with cervical lengths ≤ 25 mm, Goya and colleagues (2012) provided a silicone pessary or expectant management. There was spontaneous delivery before 34 weeks' gestation in 6 percent of women in the pessary group compared with 27 percent in the expectant management group. Hui and associates (2013) randomly assigned approximately 100 women with cervices < 25 mm at 20 to 24 weeks to silicone pessaries or expectant management. The prophylactic use of silicone pessary did not reduce the rate of delivery before 34 weeks. These two studies with conflicting results are the only randomized trials to date. Currently, the MFMU Network is designing a trial to study pessary use to prevent preterm labor in twin pregnancies.

Emergency or Rescue Cerclage

There is support for the concept that cervical incompetence and preterm labor lie on a spectrum leading to preterm delivery. Consequently, investigators have evaluated cerclage performed after preterm labor begins to manifest clinically. More than 30 years ago, Harger (1983) concluded that if cervical incompetence is recognized with threatened preterm labor, then emergency cerclage can be attempted, albeit with an appreciable risk of infection and pregnancy loss. Althuisius and colleagues (2003) randomly assigned 23 women with cervical incompetence before 27 weeks to bed rest, with or without emergency McDonald cerclage. Delivery delay was significantly greater in the cerclage group compared with that assigned to bed rest alone—54 versus 24 days. Terkildsen and coworkers (2003) studied 116 women who underwent second-trimester emergency cerclage. Nulliparity, membranes extending beyond the external cervical os, and cerclage before 22 weeks were associated with a significantly decreased chance of pregnancy continuation to 28 weeks or beyond.

Tocolysis to Treat Preterm Labor

Although several drugs and other interventions have been used to prevent or inhibit preterm labor, none has been shown to be completely effective. The American College of Obstetricians and Gynecologists (2012a) has concluded that tocolytic agents do not markedly prolong gestation but may delay delivery in some women for up to 48 hours. This may allow transport to a regional obstetrical center and permit time for corticosteroid therapy. Beta-adrenergic agonists, calcium-channel blockers, or indomethacin are the recommended tocolytic agents for such short-term use—up to 48 hours. In contrast, the College has concluded that "Maintenance therapy with tocolytics is ineffective for preventing preterm birth and improving neonatal outcome and is not recommended for this purpose." Moreover, the College recommends that women with preterm contractions without cervical change, especially those with cervical dilation of less than 2 cm, generally should not be treated with tocolytics.

β-Adrenergic Receptor Agonists

Several compounds react with β-adrenergic receptors to reduce intracellular ionized calcium levels and prevent activation of myometrial contractile proteins (Chap. 21, p. 421). In the United States, ritodrine and terbutaline have been used in obstetrics, but only ritodrine had been approved for preterm labor by the FDA.

Ritodrine. According to the Federal Register, ritodrine was voluntarily withdrawn from the United States market in 2003. A discussion is included here because knowledge concerning β-mimetic drugs accrued with its use. In an early multicenter trial, neonates whose mothers were treated with ritodrine for threatened preterm labor had lower rates of preterm birth, death, and respiratory distress (Merkatz, 1980). In a randomized trial at Parkland Hospital, Leveno and associates (1986) found that intravenous drug treatment delayed delivery for 24 hours but without other benefits. Additional studies of parenteral β-agonists confirmed a delivery delay up to 48 hours (Canadian Preterm Labor Investigators Group, 1992).

Unfortunately, this delay in preterm delivery provided no fetal benefits. Macones and colleagues (1995) used metaanalysis to assess the efficacy of *oral* β-agonist therapy and found no benefits. Keirse (1995b) suggested that this brief delay may aid maternal transport to tertiary care or permit fetal lung maturation with corticosteroids. Although this intuitive reasoning is logical, there are no data to support this.

β-Agonist infusion has resulted in frequent and, at times, serious and even fatal maternal side effects. Pulmonary edema is a special concern, and its contribution to morbidity is discussed in Chapter 47 (p. 942). Tocolysis was the third most common cause of acute respiratory distress and death in pregnant women during a 14-year period in Mississippi (Perry, 1998). The cause of pulmonary edema is multifactorial. Risk factors include tocolytic therapy with β-agonists, multifetal gestation, concurrent corticosteroid therapy, tocolysis for more than 24 hours, and large intravenous crystalloid volume infusion. Because β-agonists cause retention of sodium and water, with time—usually 24 to 48 hours, these can cause volume overload (Hankins, 1988). The drugs have been implicated in increased capillary permeability, cardiac rhythm disturbances, and myocardial ischemia.

Terbutaline. This β-agonist is commonly used to forestall preterm labor. Like ritodrine, it can cause pulmonary edema (Angel, 1988). Low-dose terbutaline can be administered long-term by subcutaneous pump (Lam, 1988). Marketed between 1987 and 1993, these pumps were used in nearly 25,000 women with suspected preterm labor (Perry, 1995). Adverse reports describe a sudden maternal death and a newborn with myocardial necrosis after the mother used the pump for 12 weeks (Fletcher, 1991; Hudgens, 1993). Elliott and associates (2004) used continuous terbutaline subcutaneous infusion in 9359 patients and reported that only 12 women experienced severe adverse events—primarily pulmonary edema.

However, randomized trials have reported no benefit for terbutaline pump therapy. Wenstrom and coworkers (1997) randomly assigned 42 women with preterm labor to a terbutaline pump, to a saline pump, or to oral terbutaline. In another trial, Guinn and colleagues (1998) randomly treated 52 women with terbutaline or with saline pump therapy. Terbutaline did not significantly prolong pregnancy, prevent preterm delivery, or improve neonatal outcomes in either of these studies.

Oral terbutaline therapy to prevent preterm delivery has also not been effective (How, 1995; Parilla, 1993). In a double-blind trial, Lewis and coworkers (1996) studied 203 women with arrested preterm labor at 24 to 34 weeks. Women were randomly assigned to receive 5-mg terbutaline tablets or placebo every 4 hours. Delivery rates at 1 week were similar in both groups, as was median latency, mean gestational age at delivery, and the incidence of recurrent preterm labor. In 2011, the FDA issued a warning regarding use of terbutaline to treat preterm labor because of reports of serious maternal side effects.

Magnesium Sulfate

Ionic magnesium in a sufficiently high concentration can alter myometrial contractility. Its role is presumably that of a calcium antagonist, and when given in pharmacological doses, it may inhibit labor. Steer and Petrie (1977) concluded that intravenous magnesium sulfate—a 4-g loading dose followed by a continuous infusion of 2 g/hr—usually arrests labor. The pharmacology and toxicology of magnesium are considered in more detail in Chapter 40 (p. 759). Samol and associates (2005) reported 67 cases—8.5 percent—of pulmonary edema among 789 women given tocolysis with magnesium sulfate at their hospital.

There have been only two randomized placebo-controlled studies of tocolysis with magnesium sulfate. Cotton and colleagues (1984) compared magnesium sulfate, ritodrine, and placebo in 54 women in preterm labor. They identified few differences in outcomes. Cox and coworkers (1990) randomly assigned 156 women to receive magnesium sulfate or normal saline infusions. Magnesium-treated women and their fetuses had identical outcomes compared with those given placebo. Because of these findings, this method of tocolysis was abandoned at Parkland Hospital. Grimes (2006) reviewed this tocolytic agent and concluded it was ineffective and potentially harmful.

Recently, the FDA (2013) warned against prolonged use of magnesium sulfate given to arrest preterm labor due to bone thinning and fractures in fetuses exposed for more than 5 to 7 days. This was attributed to low calcium levels in the fetus.

Prostaglandin Inhibitors

Prostaglandins are intimately involved in contractions of normal labor (Chap. 21, p. 426). Antagonists act by inhibiting prostaglandin synthesis or by blocking their action on target organs. A group of enzymes collectively termed *prostaglandin synthase* is responsible for the conversion of free arachidonic acid to prostaglandins (Fig. 21-16, p. 422). Several drugs block this system, including acetylsalicylate and indomethacin.

Indomethacin was first used as a tocolytic for 50 women by Zuckerman and associates (1974). Studies that followed reported the efficacy of indomethacin in halting contractions and delaying preterm birth (Muench, 2003; Niebyl, 1980). Morales and coworkers (1989, 1993a), however, compared indomethacin with either ritodrine or magnesium sulfate and found no difference in their efficacy to forestall preterm delivery. Berghella and associates (2006) reviewed four trials of indomethacin given to women with sonographically short cervices and found such therapy ineffective.

Indomethacin is administered orally or rectally. A dose of 50 to 100 mg is followed at 8-hour intervals not to exceed a total 24-hour dose of 200 mg. Serum concentrations usually peak 1 to 2 hours after oral administration, whereas levels after rectal administration peak slightly earlier. Most studies have limited indomethacin use to 24 to 48 hours because of concerns for oligohydramnios, which can develop with these doses. If amnionic fluid is monitored, oligohydramnios can be detected early, and it is reversible with drug discontinuation.

Case-control studies have assessed neonatal effects of exposure to indomethacin given for preterm labor. In a study of neonates born before 30 weeks, Norton and coworkers (1993) identified necrotizing enterocolitis in 30 percent of 37 indomethacin-exposed newborns compared with 8 percent of 37 control newborns. Higher incidences of intraventricular hemorrhage and patent ductus arteriosus were also documented in the indomethacin group. The impact of treatment duration and its timing in relation to delivery were not reported. In contrast, several investigators have challenged the association between indomethacin exposure and necrotizing enterocolitis (Muench, 2001; Parilla, 2000). Finally, Gardner (1996) and Abbasi (2003) and their colleagues found no link between indomethacin use and intraventricular hemorrhage, patent ductus arteriosus, sepsis, necrotizing enterocolitis, or neonatal death.

Schmidt and associates (2001) followed 574 newborns who were randomly assigned to receive either indomethacin or placebo to prevent pulmonary hypertension from patent ductus arteriosus. The infants, who weighed 500 to 1000 g, were followed to a corrected age of 18 months. Those given indomethacin had a significantly *reduced* incidence of both patent ductus arteriosus and severe intraventricular hemorrhage. Survival without impairment, however, was similar in both groups. Peck and coworkers (2003) reported that indomethacin therapy for 7 or more days before 33 weeks does not increase the risk of neonatal or childhood medical problems. Two metaanalyses of the effects of antenatal indomethacin on neonatal outcomes had conflicting findings (Amin, 2007; Loe, 2005).

Calcium-Channel Blockers

Myometrial activity is directly related to cytoplasmic free calcium, and a reduction in its concentration inhibits contractions (Chap. 21, p. 417). Calcium-channel blockers act to inhibit, by various mechanisms, calcium entry through cell membrane channels. Although they were developed to treat hypertension, their ability to arrest preterm labor has been evaluated.

Using the Cochrane Database, Keirse (1995a) compared nifedipine and β-agonists. They concluded that although nifedipine treatment reduced births of neonates weighing < 2500 g, significantly more of these were admitted for intensive care. Other investigators have also concluded that calcium-channel blockers, especially nifedipine, are safer and more effective tocolytic agents than are β-agonists (King, 2003; Papatsonis, 1997). Lyell and colleagues (2007) randomized 192 women at 24 to 33 weeks to either magnesium sulfate or nifedipine and found no substantial differences in efficacy or adverse effects. Salim and associates (2012) randomly assigned 145 women in preterm labor between 24 and 33 weeks to nifedipine or atosiban. No clear superiority of either to delay delivery was identified, and otherwise, neonatal morbidity was equivalent. Importantly, no randomized trial has compared nifedipine to placebo for *acute tocolysis*.

The combination of nifedipine with magnesium for tocolysis is potentially dangerous. Ben-Ami (1994) and Kurtzman (1993) and their coworkers reported that nifedipine enhances the neuromuscular blocking effects of magnesium that can interfere with pulmonary and cardiac function. How and associates (2006) randomly provided 54 women between $32^{0/7}$ and $34^{6/7}$ weeks with magnesium sulfate plus nifedipine or no tocolytic and found neither benefit nor harm.

Atosiban

This nonapeptide oxytocin analogue is a competitive antagonist of oxytocin-induced contractions. Goodwin and colleagues (1995) described its pharmacokinetics in pregnant women. In randomized clinical trials, atosiban failed to improve relevant neonatal outcomes and was linked with significant neonatal morbidity (Moutquin, 2000; Romero, 2000). The FDA has denied approval of atosiban because of concerns regarding efficacy and fetal–newborn safety. Goodwin (2004) has reviewed the history of atosiban both in the United States and in Europe, where this drug is approved and widely used as a tocolytic.

Nitric Oxide Donors

These potent smooth-muscle relaxants affect the vasculature, gut, and uterus. In randomized clinical trials, nitroglycerin administered orally, transdermally, or intravenously was not effective or showed no superiority to other tocolytics. In addition, maternal hypotension was a common side effect (Bisits, 2004; Clavin, 1996; El-Sayed, 1999; Lees, 1999).

Summary of Tocolysis for Preterm Labor

In many women, tocolytics stop contractions temporarily but rarely prevent preterm birth. In a metaanalysis of tocolytic therapy, Gyetvai and associates (1999) concluded that although delivery may be delayed long enough for administration of corticosteroids, treatment does not result in improved perinatal outcome. Berkman and colleagues (2003) reviewed 60 reports and concluded that tocolytic therapy can prolong gestation, but that β-agonists are no better than other drugs and pose potential maternal danger. They also concluded that there are no benefits of maintenance tocolytic therapy.

In general, if tocolytics are given, they should be administered concomitantly with corticosteroids. The gestational age range for their use is debatable. However, because corticosteroids are not generally used after 33 weeks and because the perinatal outcomes in preterm neonates are generally good after this time, most practitioners do not recommend use of tocolytics at or after 33 weeks (Goldenberg, 2002).

Labor

Whether labor is induced or spontaneous, abnormalities of fetal heart rate and uterine contractions should be sought. We prefer continuous electronic monitoring. Fetal tachycardia, especially with ruptured membranes, is suggestive of sepsis. There is some evidence that intrapartum acidemia may intensify some of the neonatal complications usually attributed to preterm delivery. For example, Low and colleagues (1995) observed that intrapartum acidosis—umbilical artery blood pH less than 7.0—had an important role in neonatal complications (Chap. 32, p. 629). Similarly, Kimberlin and coworkers (1996) found that increasing umbilical artery blood acidemia was related to more severe respiratory disease in preterm neonates. Despite this, no effects were found in short-term neurological outcomes that included intracranial hemorrhages.

Group B streptococcal infections are common and dangerous in the preterm neonate. Accordingly, as discussed in Chapter 64 (p. 1249), prophylaxis should be provided.

Delivery

In the absence of a relaxed vaginal outlet, an episiotomy for delivery may be necessary once the fetal head reaches the perineum. Perinatal outcome data do not support routine forceps delivery to protect the "fragile" preterm fetal head. Staff proficient in resuscitative techniques commensurate with the gestational age and fully oriented to any specific problems should be present at delivery. Principles of resuscitation described in Chapter 32 are applicable. The importance of specialized personnel and facilities for preterm newborn care is underscored by the improved survival rates of these neonates when delivered in tertiary-care centers.

Prevention of Neonatal Intracranial Hemorrhage

Preterm newborns frequently have intracranial germinal matrix bleeding that can extend to more serious intraventricular hemorrhage (Chap. 34, p. 656). It was hypothesized that cesarean delivery to obviate trauma from labor and vaginal delivery might prevent these complications. This has not been validated by most subsequent studies. Malloy (1991) analyzed 1765 newborns with birthweights less than 1500 g and found that cesarean delivery did not lower the risk of mortality or intracranial hemorrhage. Anderson (1988), however, made an interesting observation regarding the role of cesarean delivery in intracranial hemorrhage prevention. These hemorrhages correlated with exposure to active-phase labor. However, they emphasized that avoidance of active-phase labor is impossible in most preterm births because decisions for delivery route are not required until active labor is firmly established.

Magnesium Sulfate for Fetal Neuroprotection

In intriguing reports, very-low-birthweight neonates whose mothers were treated with magnesium sulfate for preterm labor or preeclampsia were found to have a reduced incidence of cerebral palsy at 3 years (Grether, 2000; Nelson, 1995). Because epidemiological evidence suggested that maternal magnesium sulfate therapy had a fetal neuroprotective effect, randomized trials were designed to investigate this hypothesis. An Australian randomized trial by Crowther and coworkers (2003) included 1063 women at imminent risk of delivery before 30 weeks and who were given magnesium sulfate or placebo. These investigators showed that magnesium exposure improved some perinatal outcomes. Rates of both neonatal death and cerebral palsy were lower in the magnesium-treated group—but this study was not sufficiently powered. The multicenter French trial reported by Marret and associates (2008) had similar problems.

More convincing evidence for magnesium neuroprotection came from the NICHD MFMU Network study reported by Rouse and colleagues (2008). The *Beneficial Effects of Antenatal Magnesium Sulfate—BEAM—Study* was a placebo-controlled trial in 2241 women at imminent risk for preterm birth between 24 and 31 weeks. Almost 87 percent had preterm ruptured membranes, and almost a fifth had previously received magnesium sulfate for tocolysis. Women randomized to magnesium sulfate were given a 6-g bolus over 20 to 30 minutes followed by a maintenance infusion of 2 g per hour. Magnesium sulfate was actually infusing at the time of delivery in approximately half of the treated women. A 2-year follow-up was available for 96 percent of the children. Selected results are shown in Table 42-10. This trial can be interpreted differently depending on statistical philosophy. Some opt to interpret these findings to mean that magnesium sulfate infusion prevents cerebral palsy regardless of the gestational age at which the therapy is given. Those with a differing view conclude that this trial only supports use of magnesium sulfate for prevention of cerebral palsy before 28 weeks. What is certain, however, is that maternally administered magnesium sulfate infusions cannot be implicated in increased perinatal deaths as reported by Mittendorf (1997).

Subsequent to these studies, Doyle and associates (2009) performed a Cochrane review of the five available randomized trials to assess neuroprotective effects of magnesium sulfate. A total of 6145 infants were studied, and as expected, most came from the three larger Australian, French, and MFMU Network multicenter studies. These reviewers reported that magnesium exposure compared with no exposure significantly decreased risks for cerebral palsy, with a relative risk of 0.68. There were no significant effects on rates of pediatric mortality or other neurological impairments or disabilities. It was calculated that treatment given to 63 women would prevent one case of cerebral palsy.

There was debate regarding magnesium efficacy for neuroprotection at the 2011 annual meeting of the Society for Maternal-Fetal Medicine. Rouse (2011) spoke for the benefits of magnesium sulfate, whereas Sibai (2011) challenged that the reported benefits vis-à-vis neuroprotection were false positive due to random statistical error in the Doyle (2009) metaanalysis.

TABLE 42-10. Magnesium Sulfate for the Prevention of Cerebral Palsy[a]

	Treatment		
Perinatal Outcome[a]	Magnesium Sulfate No. (%)	Placebo No. (%)	Relative Risk (95% CI)
Infants with 2-year follow-up	1041 (100)	1095 (100)	—
Fetal or infant death	99 (9.5)	93 (8.5)	1.12 (0.85–1.47)
Moderate or severe cerebral palsy:			
Overall	20/1041 (1.9)	3/1095 (3.4)	0.55 (0.32–0.95)
< 28–31 weeks[b]	12/442 (2.7)	30/496 (6)	0.45 (0.23–0.87)
≥ 24–27 weeks[b]	8/599 (1.3)	8/599 (1.3)	1.00 (0.38–2.65)

[a]Selected results from the Beneficial Effects of Antenatal Magnesium Sulfate (BEAM) Study.
[b]Weeks' gestation at randomization.
Data from Rouse, 2008.

The American College of Obstetricians and Gynecologists (2013a) recognized that "none of the individual studies found a benefit with regard to their primary outcome." It was concluded that "Physicians electing to use magnesium sulfate for fetal neuroprotection should develop specific guidelines regarding inclusion criteria, treatment regimen. ..." Subsequently, the American College of Obstetricians and Gynecologists (2012a) issued a *Patient Safety Checklist* that could be used if magnesium sulfate is given for neuroprotection.

Because of these findings, at Parkland Hospital our policy is to provide magnesium sulfate for threatened preterm delivery from $24^{0/7}$ to $27^{6/7}$ weeks. A 6-g loading dose is followed by an infusion of 2 g per hour for at least 12 hours.

REFERENCES

Aagaard K, Riehle K, Ma J, et al: A metagenomic approach to characterization of the vaginal microbiome signature in pregnancy. PLoS One 7(6):e36466, 2012

Abbasi S, Gerdes JS, Sehdev HM, et al: Neonatal outcomes after exposure to indomethacin in utero: a retrospective case cohort study. Am J Obstet Gynecol 189:782, 2003

Alexander JM, Gilstrap LC, Cox SM, et al: Clinical chorioamnionitis and the prognosis for very low birthweight infants. Obstet Gynecol 91:725, 1998

Alexander JM, Mercer BM, Miodovnik M, et al: The impact of digital cervical examination on expectantly managed preterm ruptured membranes. Am J Obstet Gynecol 183:1003, 2000

Althuisius SM, Dekker G, Hummel P, et al: Cervical incompetence prevention randomized cerclage trial: emergency cerclage with bed rest versus bed rest alone. Am J Obstet Gynecol 189:907, 2003

American Academy of Pediatrics and the American College of Obstetricians and Gynecologists: Guidelines for Perinatal Care, 7th ed. Washington, 2012, p 158

American College of Obstetricians and Gynecologists: Preterm labor. Technical Bulletin No. 206, June 1995

American College of Obstetricians and Gynecologists: Management of preterm labor. Practice Bulletin No. 127, June 2012a

American College of Obstetricians and Gynecologists: Prediction and prevention of preterm birth. Practice Bulletin No. 130, October 2012b

American College of Obstetricians and Gynecologists: Magnesium sulfate before anticipated preterm birth for neuroprotection. Committee Opinion No. 455, March 2010, Reaffirmed 2013a

American College of Obstetricians and Gynecologists: Medically indicated late-preterm and early-term deliveries. Committee Opinion No. 560, April 2013b

American College of Obstetricians and Gynecologists: Nonmedically indicated early-term deliveries. Committee Opinion No. 561, April 2013c

American College of Obstetricians and Gynecologists: Premature rupture of membranes. Practice Bulletin No. 139, October 2013d

Amin SB, Sinkin RA, Glantz C: Metaanalysis of the effect of antenatal indomethacin on neonatal outcomes. Am J Obstet Gynecol 197:486, 2007

Ananth CV, Joseph KS, Oyelese Y, et al: Trends in preterm birth and perinatal mortality among singletons: United States, 1989 through 2000. Obstet Gynecol 105:1084, 2005

Ananth CV, Liu S, Joseph KS, et al: A comparison of foetal and infant mortality in the United States and Canada. Int J Epidemiol 38(2):480, 2009

Anderson GD, Bada HS, Sibai BM, et al: The relationship between labor and route of delivery in the preterm infant. Am J Obstet Gynecol 158:1382, 1988

Andrews WW, Goldenberg RL, Hauth JC, et al: Interconceptional antibiotics to prevent spontaneous preterm birth: a randomized clinical trial. Am J Obstet Gynecol 194:617, 2006

Andrews WW, Hauth JC, Goldenberg RL, et al: Amniotic fluid interleukin-6: correlation with upper genital tract microbial colonization and gestational age in women delivered after spontaneous labor versus indicated delivery. Am J Obstet Gynecol 173:606, 1995

Andrews WW, Sibai BM, Thom EA, et al: Randomized clinical trial of metronidazole plus erythromycin to prevent spontaneous preterm delivery in fetal fibronectin-positive women. Obstet Gynecol 101:847, 2003

Angel JL, O'Brien WF, Knuppel RA, et al: Carbohydrate intolerance in patients receiving oral tocolytics. Am J Obstet Gynecol 159:762, 1988

Annas GJ: Extremely preterm birth and parental authority to refuse treatment—the case of Sidney Miller. N Engl J Med 35:2118, 2004

Anum EA, Springel EH, Shriver MD, et al: Genetic contributions to disparities in preterm birth. Pediatr Res 65(1):1, 2009

Arechavaleta-Velasco F, Mayon-Gonzalez J, Gonzalez-Jimenez M, et al: Association of type II apoptosis and 92-kDa type IV collagenase expression in human amniochorion in prematurely ruptured membranes with tumor necrosis factor receptor-1 expression. J Soc Gynecol Investig 9:60, 2002

Bailit JL, Iams J, Silber A, et al: Changes in the indications for scheduled births to reduce nonmedically indicated deliveries occurring before 39 weeks of gestation. Obstet Gynecol 120:241, 2012

Beigi RH, Austin MN, Meyn LA, et al: Antimicrobial resistance associated with the treatment of bacterial vaginosis. Am J Obstet Gynecol 191:1124, 2004

Ben-Ami M, Giladi Y, Shalev E: The combination of magnesium sulphate and nifedipine: a cause of neuromuscular blockade. BJOG 101:262, 1994

Berghella V, Odibo AO, To MS, et al: Cerclage for short cervix on ultrasonography: meta-analysis of trials using individual patient-level data. Obstet Gynecol 106(1):181, 2005

Berghella V, Rust OA, Althuisius SM: Short cervix on ultrasound: does indomethacin prevent preterm birth? Am J Obstet Gynecol 195:809, 2006

Berkman ND, Thorp JM, Lohr KN, et al: Tocolytic treatment for the management of preterm labor: a review of the evidence. Am J Obstet Gynecol 188:1648, 2003

Biggio JR: Bed rest in pregnancy: time to put the issue to rest. Obstet Gynecol 1212(6):1158, 2013
Bisits A, Madsen G, Knox M, et al: The randomized nitric oxide tocolysis trial (RNOTT) for the treatment of preterm labor. Am J Obstet Gynecol 191:683, 2004
Bloom SL, Yost NP, McIntire DD, et al: Recurrence of preterm birth in singleton and twin pregnancies. Obstet Gynecol 98:379, 2001
Bruschettini M, van den Hove DL, Gazzolo D, et al: Lowering the dose of antenatal steroids: the effects of a single course of betamethasone on somatic growth and brain cell proliferation in the rat. Am J Obstet Gynecol 194:1341, 2006
Buekens P, Alexander S, Boutsen M, et al: Randomised controlled trial of routine cervical examinations in pregnancy. Lancet 344:841, 1994
Bullard I, Vermillion S, Soper D: Clinical intraamniotic infection and the outcome for very low birth weight neonates [Abstract]. Am J Obstet Gynecol 187:S73, 2002
Buxton IL, Singer CA, Tichenor JN: Expression of stretch-activated two-pore potassium channels in human myometrium in pregnancy and labor. PLoS One 5(8):e12372, 2010
Canadian Preterm Labor Investigators Group: Treatment of preterm labor with the beta-adrenergic agonist ritodrine. N Engl J Med 327:308, 1992
Carey JC, Klebanoff MA: Is a change in the vaginal flora associated with an increased risk of preterm birth? Am J Obstet Gynecol 192(4):1341, 2005
Caritis SN, Rouse DJ, Peaceman AM, et al: Prevention of preterm birth in triplets using 17alpha-hydroxyprogesterone caproate. Obstet Gynecol 113:285, 2009
Carlan SJ, O'Brien WF, Parsons MT, et al: Preterm premature rupture of membranes: a randomized study of home versus hospital management. Obstet Gynecol 81:61, 1993
Carroll SG, Blott M, Nicolaides KH: Preterm prelabor amniorrhexis: outcome of live births. Obstet Gynecol 86:18, 1995
Carroll SG, Papaionnou S, Ntumazah IL, et al: Lower genital tract swabs in the prediction of intrauterine infection in preterm prelabour rupture of the membranes. BJOG 103:54, 1996
Casanueva E, Ripoll C, Meza-Camacho C, et al: Possible interplay between vitamin C deficiency and prolactin in pregnant women with premature rupture of membranes: facts and hypothesis. Med Hypotheses 64:241, 2005
Casey ML, Cox SM, Word RA, et al: Cytokines and infection-induced preterm labour. Reprod Fertil Devel 2:499, 1990
Casey ML, MacDonald PC: Biomolecular mechanisms in human parturition: Activation of uterine decidua. In d'Arcangues C, Fraser IS, Newton JR, Odlind V (eds): Contraception and Mechanisms of Endometrial Bleeding. Cambridge, England, Cambridge University Press, 1990, p 501
Casey ML, MacDonald PC: Transforming growth factor-beta inhibits progesterone-induced enkephalinase expression in human endometrial stromal cells. J Clin Endocrinol Metab 81:4022, 1996
Chaim W, Mazor M: Intraamniotic infection with fusobacteria. Arch Gynecol Obstet 251:1, 1992
Challis JR, Sloboda DM, Alfaidy N, et al: Prostaglandins and mechanisms of preterm birth. Reproduction 124:1, 2002
Chao TT, Bloom SL, Mitchell JS, et al: The diagnosis and natural history of false preterm labor. Obstet Gynecol 118(6):1301, 2011
Christian LM: Psychoneuroimmunology in pregnancy: immune pathways linking stress with maternal health, adverse birth outcomes, and fetal development. Neurosci Biobehav Rev 36(1):350, 2012a
Christian LM, Iams JD, Porter K, et al: Epstein-Barr virus reactivation during pregnancy and postpartum: effects of race and racial discrimination. Brain Behav Immun 26(8), 1280, 2012b
Chuang TH, Ulevitch RJ: Cloning and characterization of a sub-family of human toll-like receptors: hTLR7, hTLR8, and hTLR9. Eur Cytokine Netw 11:372, 2000
Clavin DK, Bayhi DA, Nolan TE, et al: Comparison of intravenous magnesium sulfate and nitroglycerin for preterm labor: preliminary data. Am J Obstet Gynecol 174:307, 1996
Cnattingius S, Villamor E, Johansson S, et al: Maternal obesity and risk of preterm delivery. JAMA 309(22):2362, 2013
Collaborative Home Uterine Monitoring Study Group: A multicenter randomized controlled trial of home uterine monitoring: active versus sham device. Am J Obstet Gynecol 173:1170, 1995
Collins JW Jr, David RJ, Simon DM, et al: Preterm birth among African American and white women with a lifelong residence in high-income Chicago neighborhoods: an exploratory study. Ethn Dis 17(1):113, 2007
Conde-Agudelo A, Rosas-Bermúdez A, Kafury-Goeta AC: Birth spacing and risk of adverse perinatal outcomes: a meta-analysis. JAMA 295:1809, 2006
Consortium on Safe Labor: Respiratory morbidity in preterm births. JAMA 301(1):419, 2010
Cook CM, Ellwood DA: A longitudinal study of the cervix in pregnancy using transvaginal ultrasound. BJOG 103:16, 1996
Copper RL, Goldenberg RL, Dubard MB, et al: Cervical examination and tocodynamometry at 28 weeks' gestation: prediction of spontaneous preterm birth. Am J Obstet Gynecol 172:666, 1995
Cotton DB, Strassner HT, Hill LM, et al: Comparison between magnesium sulfate, terbutaline and a placebo for inhibition of preterm labor: a randomized study. J Reprod Med 29:92, 1984
Cox SM, Leveno KJ: Intentional delivery versus expectant management with preterm ruptured membranes at 30–34 weeks' gestation. Obstet Gynecol 86:875, 1995
Cox SM, Sherman ML, Leveno KJ: Randomized investigation of magnesium sulfate for prevention of preterm birth. Am J Obstet Gynecol 163:767, 1990
Cox SM, Williams ML, Leveno KJ: The natural history of preterm ruptured membranes: what to expect of expectant management. Obstet Gynecol 71:558, 1988
Crowther CA, Doyle LW, Haslam RR, et al: Outcomes at 2 years of age after repeat doses of antenatal corticosteroids. N Engl J Med 357:1179, 2007
Crowther CA, Hiller JE, Doyle LW, et al: Effect of magnesium sulfate given for neuroprotection before preterm birth: a randomized controlled trial. JAMA 290:2669, 2003
Crowther CA, McKinlay CJ, Middleton P, et al: Repeat doses of prenatal corticosteroids for women at risk for preterm birth for improving neonatal health outcomes. Cochran Database Syst Rev 6:CD003935, 2011
Culhane JF, Rauh V, McCollum KF, et al: Exposure to chronic stress and ethnic differences in rates of bacterial vaginosis among pregnant women. Am J Obstet Gynecol 187(5):1272, 2002
Devlieger R, Millar LK, Bryant-Greenwood G, et al: Fetal membrane healing after spontaneous and iatrogenic membrane rupture: a review of current evidence. Am J Obstet Gynecol 195:1512, 2006
Dinarello CA: The IL-1 family and inflammatory diseases. Clin Exp Rheumatol 20:S1, 2002
Dolan SM, Gross SJ, Merkatz IR, et al: The contribution of birth defects to preterm birth and low birth weight. Obstet Gynecol 110:318, 2007
Doyle LW, Crowther CA, Middleton S, et al: Magnesium sulfate for women at risk of preterm birth for neuroprotection of the fetus. Cochrane Database Syst Rev 1:CD004661, 2009
Eichenwald EC, Stark AR: Management and outcomes of very low birth weight. N Engl J Med 358(16):1700, 2008
El-Bastawissi AY, Williams MA, Riley DE, et al: Amniotic fluid interleukin-6 and preterm delivery: a review. Obstet Gynecol 95:1056, 2000
Elimian A, Garry D, Figueroa R, et al: Antenatal betamethasone compared with dexamethasone (Betacode Trial): a randomized controlled trial. Obstet Gynecol 110:26, 2007
Elliott JP, Istwan NB, Rhea D, et al: The occurrence of adverse events in women receiving continuous subcutaneous terbutaline therapy. Am J Obstet Gynecol 191:1277, 2004
El-Sayed Y, Riley ET, Holbrook RH, et al: Randomized comparison of intravenous nitroglycerin and magnesium sulfate for treatment of preterm labor. Obstet Gynecol 93:79, 1999
Esplin MS, Romero R, Chaiworapongsa T, et al: Amniotic fluid levels of immunoreactive monocyte chemotactic protein-1 increase during term parturition. J Matern Fetal Neonatal Med 14:51, 2003
Esplin MS, Varner MW: Genetic factors in preterm birth—the future. BJOG 112 Suppl 1):97, 2005
Fanaroff AA, Stoll BJ, Wright LL, et al: Trends in neonatal morbidity and mortality for very low birthweight infants. Am J Obstet Gynecol 196:e1.147, 2007
Farooqi A, Holmgren PA, Engberg S, et al: Survival and 2-year outcome with expectant management of second trimester rupture of membranes. Obstet Gynecol 92:895, 1998
Feinstein SJ, Vintzileos AM, Lodeiro JG, et al: Amniocentesis with premature rupture of membranes. Obstet Gynecol 68:147, 1986
Fletcher SE, Fyfe DA, Case CL, et al: Myocardial necrosis in a newborn after long-term maternal subcutaneous terbutaline infusion for suppression of preterm labor. Am J Obstet Gynecol 165:1401, 1991
Fonseca EB, Celik E, Para M, et al: Progesterone and the risk of preterm birth among women with a short cervix. N Engl J Med 357:462, 2007
Fortunato SJ, Menon R: IL-1 beta is a better inducer of apoptosis in human fetal membranes than IL-6. Placenta 24:922, 2003
Fortunato SJ, Menon R, Lombardi SJ: MMP/TIMP imbalance in amniotic fluid during PROM: an indirect support for endogenous pathway to membrane rupture. J Perinat Med 27:362, 1999a
Fortunato SJ, Menon R, Lombardi SJ: Role of tumor necrosis factor-alpha in the premature rupture of membranes and preterm labor pathways. Am J Obstet Gynecol 187:1159, 2002
Fortunato SJ, Menon R, Lombardi SJ: Stromelysins in placental membranes and amniotic fluid with premature rupture of membranes. Obstet Gynecol 94:435, 1999b

Fuchs K, Albright C, Scott K, et al: Obstetric factors affecting respiratory morbidity among late preterm infants. Am J Obstet Gynecol 199(6SA):S63, 2008
Gajer P, Brotman RM, Bai G, et al: Temporal dynamics of the human vaginal microbiota. Sci Transl Med 4(132):132ra52, 2012
Gardner MO, Owen J, Skelly S, et al: Preterm delivery after indomethacin: a risk factor for neonatal complications? J Reprod Med 41:903, 1996
Garite TJ, Freeman RK, Linzey EM, et al: Prospective randomized study of corticosteroids in the management of premature rupture of the membranes and the premature gestation. Am J Obstet Gynecol 141:508, 1981
Garite TJ, Keegan KA, Freeman RK, et al: A randomized trial of ritodrine tocolysis versus expectant management in patients with premature rupture of membranes at 25 to 30 weeks of gestation. Am J Obstet Gynecol 157:388, 1987
Garite TJ, Kurtzmann J, Maurel K, et al: Impact of a "rescue course" of antenatal corticosteroids: a multicenter randomized placebo-controlled trial. Am J Obstet Gynecol 200:248.e.1, 2009
Goya M, Pratcorona L, Merced C, et al: Cervical pessary in pregnant women with a short cervix (PECEP): an open-label randomised controlled trial. Lancet 379(9828):1790, 2012
Gerber S, Vial Y, Hohlfeld P, et al: Detection of *Ureaplasma urealyticum* in second-trimester amniotic fluid by polymerase chain reaction correlates with subsequent preterm labor and delivery. J Infect Dis 187:518, 2003
Gibson CS, MacLennan AH, Dekker GA, et al: Genetic polymorphisms and spontaneous preterm birth. Obstet Gynecol 109:384, 2007
Gielchinsky Y, Mankuta D, Samueloff A, et al: First pregnancy in women over 45 years of age carries increased obstetrical risk [Abstract]. Am J Obstet Gynecol 187:S87, 2002
Gluck L: Fetal lung maturity. Paper presented at the 78th Ross Conference on Pediatric Research, San Diego, May 1979
Goepfert AR, Jeffcoat MK, Andrews W, et al: Periodontal disease and upper genital tract inflammation in early spontaneous preterm birth. Obstet Gynecol 104:777, 2004
Goldenberg RL: The management of preterm labor. Obstet Gynecol 100:1020, 2002
Goldenberg RL, Cliver SP, Bronstein J, et al: Bed rest in pregnancy. Obstet Gynecol 84:131, 1994
Goldenberg RL, Culhane JF, Iams JD, et al: Preterm birth 1: epidemiology and causes of preterm birth. Lancet 371:75, 2008
Goldenberg RL, Hauth JC, Andrews WW: Intrauterine infection and preterm delivery. N Engl J Med 342:1500, 2000
Goldenberg RL, Iams JD, Miodovnik M, et al: The preterm prediction study: risk factors in twin gestations. National Institute of Child Health and Human Development Maternal-Fetal Medicine Units Network. Am J Obstet Gynecol 175:1047, 1996
Goldenberg RL, Mwatha A, Read JS, et al: The HPTN 024 Study: the efficacy of antibiotics to prevent chorioamnionitis and preterm birth. Am J Obstet Gynecol 194:650, 2006
Gomez R, Romero R, Edwin SS, et al: Pathogenesis of preterm labor and preterm premature rupture of membranes associated with intraamniotic infection. Infect Dis Clin North Am 11:135, 1997
Gomez R, Romero R, Glasasso M, et al: The value of amniotic fluid interleukin-6, white blood cell count, and gram stain in the diagnosis of microbial invasion of the amniotic cavity in patients at term. Am J Reprod Immunol 32:200, 1994
Goncalves LF, Chaiworapongsa T, Romero R: Intrauterine infection and prematurity. Ment Retard Dev Disabil Res Rev 8:3, 2002
Gonzalez JM, Xu H, Ofori E, et al: Toll-like receptors in the uterus, cervix, and placenta: is pregnancy an immunosuppressed state? Am J Obstet Gynecol 197(3):296, 2007
Goodwin TM: The Gordian knot of developing tocolytics. J Soc Gynecol Investig 11(6)339, 2004
Goodwin TM, Millar L, North L, et al: The pharmacokinetics of the oxytocin antagonist atosiban in pregnant women with preterm uterine contractions. Am J Obstet Gynecol 173:913, 1995
Gotsch F, Romero R, Kusanovic JP, et al: The anti-inflammatory limb of the immune response in preterm labor, intra-amniotic infection/inflammation, and spontaneous parturition at term: a role for interleukin-10. J Matern Fetal Neonatal Med 21(8):529, 2008
Goulet C, Gevry H, Lemay M, et al: A randomized clinical trial of care for women with preterm labour: home management versus hospital management. CMAJ 164:985, 2001
Goya M, Pratcorona L, Merced C, et al: Cervical pessary in pregnancy women with a short cervix (PECEP): an open-label randomized controlled trial. Lancet 379(9828):1800, 2012
Gravett MG, Adams KM, Sadowsky DW, et al: Immunomodulators plus antibiotics delay preterm delivery after experimental intraamniotic infection in a nonhuman primate model. Am J Obstet Gynecol 197(5):518.e1, 2007
Gravett MG, Hitti J, Hess DL, et al: Intrauterine infection and preterm delivery: evidence for activation of the fetal hypothalamic-pituitary-adrenal axis. Am J Obstet Gynecol 182:1404, 2000
Grether JK, Hoogstrate J, Walsh-Greene E, et al: Magnesium sulfate for tocolysis and risk of spastic cerebral palsy in premature children born to women without preeclampsia. Am J Obstet Gynecol 183:717, 2000
Grimes DA, Nanda K: Magnesium sulfate tocolysis: time to quit. Obstet Gynecol 108:986, 2006
Grobman WA, Gilbert SA, Iams JD, et al: Activity restriction among women with a short cervix. Obstet Gynecol 121:1181, 2013
Grobman WA, Thom EA, Spong CY, et al: 17alpha-Hydroxyprogesterone caproate to prevent prematurity in nulliparas with cervical length less than 30 mm. Am J Obstet Gynecol 207(5):390e.1, 2012
Grobman WA, Welshman EE, Calhoun EA: Does fetal fibronectin use in the diagnosis of preterm labor affect physician behavior and health care costs? A randomized trial. Am J Obstet Gynecol 191:235, 2004
Gross G, Imamura T, Vogt SK, et al: Inhibition of cyclooxygenase-2 prevents inflammation-mediated preterm labor in the mouse. Am J Physiol Regul Integr Comp Physiol 278(6):R1415, 2000
Guillen Ú, DeMauro S, Ma L, et al: Survival rates in extremely low birthweight infants depend on the denominator: avoiding potential for bias by specifying denominators. Am J Obstet Gynecol 205:328.e1, 2011
Guinn DA, Goepfert AR, Owen J, et al: Terbutaline pump maintenance therapy for prevention of preterm delivery: a double-blind trial. Am J Obstet Gynecol 179:874, 1998
Gyetvai K, Hannah ME, Hodnett ED, et al: Tocolytics for preterm labor: a systematic review. Obstet Gynecol 94:869, 1999
Hadi HA, Hodson CA, Strickland D: Premature rupture of the membranes between 20 and 25 weeks' gestation: role of amniotic fluid volume in perinatal outcome. Am J Obstet Gynecol 170:1139, 1994
Hallak M, Bottoms SF: Accelerated pulmonary maturation from preterm premature rupture of membranes: a myth. Am J Obstet Gynecol 169:1045, 1993
Hamilton S, Oomomian Y, Stephen G, et al: Macrophages infiltrate the human and rat decidua during term and preterm labor: evidence that decidual inflammation precedes labor. Biol Reprod 86(2):39, 2012
Hampton T: Genetic link found for premature birth risk. JAMA 296:1713, 2006
Hankins GD, Hauth JC, Cissik JH, et al: Effects of ritodrine hydrochloride on arteriovenous blood gas and shunt in healthy pregnant yellow baboons. Am J Obstet Gynecol 158:658, 1988
Harger JM: Cervical cerclage: patient selection, morbidity, and success rates. Clin Perinatol 10: 321, 1983
Hassan SS, Romero R, Vidyadhari D, et al: Vaginal progesterone reduces the rate of preterm birth in women with sonographic short cervix: a multicenter, randomized, double-blind, placebo-controlled trial. Ultrasound Obstet Gynecol 38:18, 2011
Hedegaard M, Henriksen TB, Sabroe S, et al: Psychological stress in pregnancy and preterm delivery. BMJ 307(6898):234, 1993
Heine RP, McGregor JA, Goodwin TM, et al: Serial salivary estriol to detect an increased risk of preterm birth. Obstet Gynecol 96:490, 2000
Hillier SL, Martius J, Krohn M, et al: A case-control study of chorioamnionic infection and histologic chorioamnionitis in prematurity. N Engl J Med 319:972, 1988
Hillier SL, Nugent RP, Eschenbach DA, et al: Association between bacterial vaginosis and preterm delivery of a low-birthweight infant. N Engl J Med 333:1737, 1995
Himes KP, Simhan HN: Plasma corticotropin-releasing hormone and cortisol concentrations and perceived stress among pregnant women with preterm and term birth. Am J Perinatol 28(6):443, 2011
Hitti J, Tarczy-Hornoch P, Murphy J, et al: Amniotic fluid infection, cytokines, and adverse outcome among infants at 34 weeks' gestation or less. Obstet Gynecol 98:1080, 2001
Ho M, Ramsey P, Brumfield C, et al: Changes in maternal and neonatal infectious morbidity as latency increases after preterm premature rupture of membranes [Abstract]. Obstet Gynecol 101:41S, 2003
Hobel C, Culhane J: Role of psychosocial and nutritional stress on poor pregnancy outcome. J Nutr 133:1709S, 2003
Holmlund U, Cabers G, Dahlfors AR, et al: Expression and regulation of the pattern recognition receptors Toll-like receptor-2 and Toll-like receptor-4 in the human placenta. Immunology 107:145, 2002
Holt R, Timmons BC, Akgul Y, et al: The molecular mechanisms of cervical ripening differ between term and preterm birth. Endocrinology 152:1036, 2011
Holzman C, Jetton J, Siler-Khodr T, et al: Second trimester corticotropin-releasing hormone levels in relation to preterm delivery and ethnicity. Obstet Gynecol 97:657, 2001
How HY, Hughes SA, Vogel RL, et al: Oral terbutaline in the outpatient management of preterm labor. Am J Obstet Gynecol 173:1518, 1995

How HY, Zafaranchi L, Stella CL, et al: Tocolysis in women with preterm labor between $32^{0/7}$ and $34^{6/7}$ weeks of gestation: a randomized controlled pilot study. Am J Obstet Gynecol 194:976, 2006
Hua R, Pease JE, Cheng W, et al: Human labour is associated with decline in myometrial chemokine receptor expression: the role of prostaglandins, oxytocin, and cytokines. Am J Reprod Immunol 69:21, 2013
Hudgens DR, Conradi SE: Sudden death associated with terbutaline sulfate administration. Am J Obstet Gynecol 169:120, 1993
Hui SYA, Chor CM, Lau TK, et al: Cerclage pessary for preventing preterm birth in women with a singleton pregnancy and a short cervix at 20 to 24 weeks: a randomized controlled trial. Am J Perinatol 30:283, 2013
Iams JD, Clapp DH, Contox DA, et al: Does extraamniotic infection cause preterm labor? Gas-liquid chromatography studies of amniotic fluid in amnionitis, preterm labor, and normal controls. Obstet Gynecol 70:365, 1987
Iams JD, Goldenberg RL, Meis PJ, et al: The length of the cervix and the risk of spontaneous premature delivery. N Engl J Med 334:567, 1996
Iams JD, Johnson FF, Parker M: A prospective evaluation of the signs and symptoms of preterm labor. Obstet Gynecol 84:227, 1994
Iams JD, Newman RB, Thom EA, et al: Frequency of uterine contractions and the risk of spontaneous preterm birth. N Engl J Med 346:250, 2002
Iams JD, Stilson R, Johnson FF, et al: Symptoms that precede preterm labor and preterm premature rupture of the membranes. Am J Obstet Gynecol 162:486, 1990
Ingelfinger JR: Prematurity and the legacy of intrauterine stress. N Engl J Med 356:2093, 2007
Institute of Medicine: Preterm Birth: Causes, Consequences, and Prevention. Washington, National Academies Press, 2007
Jacobsson B, Holst RM, Wennerholm UR, et al: Monocyte chemotactic protein-1 in cervical and amniotic fluid: relationship to microbial invasion of the amniotic cavity, intraamniotic inflammation, and preterm delivery. Am J Obstet Gynecol 189:1161, 2003
Janssens S, Beyaert R: Role of Toll-like receptors in pathogen recognition. Clin Microbiol Rev 16:637, 2003
Joseph KS, Huang L, Liu S, et al: Reconciling the high rates of preterm and postterm birth in the United States. Obstet Gynecol 109(4):813, 2007
Keelan JA, Blumenstein M, Helliwell RJ, et al: Cytokines, prostaglandins and parturition—a review. Placenta 24:S33, 2003
Keirse MJNC: Calcium antagonists vs. betamimetics in preterm labour. In Neilson JP, Crowther C, Hodnett ED, et al (eds): Pregnancy and Childbirth Module. Cochrane Database System Review Issue 2. Oxford, Update Software, 1995a
Keirse MJNC: New perspectives for the effective treatment of preterm labor. Am J Obstet Gynecol 173:618, 1995b
Kent AS, Sullivan MH, Elder MG: Transfer of cytokines through human fetal membranes. J Reprod Fertil 100:81, 1994
Kenyon S, Boulvain M, Neilson J: Antibiotics for preterm rupture of the membranes: a systematic review. Obstet Gynecol 104:1051, 2004
Kenyon S, Pike K, Jones DR, et al: Childhood outcomes after prescription of antibiotics to pregnant women with preterm rupture of the membranes: 7-year follow-up of the ORACLE I trial. Lancet 372:1310, 2008a
Kenyon S, Pike K, Jones DR, et al: Childhood outcomes after prescription of antibiotics to pregnant women with spontaneous preterm labour: 7-year follow-up of the ORACLE II trial. Lancet 372:1319, 2008b
Kenyon SL, Taylor DJ, Tarnow-Mordi, et al: Broad-spectrum antibiotics for spontaneous preterm labour: the ORACLE II randomized trial. Lancet 357:989, 2001
Kimberlin DF, Hauth JC, Goldenberg RL, et al: Relationship of acid–base status and neonatal morbidity in 1000 g infants. Am J Obstet Gynecol 174:382, 1996
King J, Flenady V: Antibiotics for preterm labour with intact membranes. Cochrane Database Syst Rev 2:CD000246, 2000
King JF, Flenady V, Papatsonis D, et al: Calcium channel blockers for inhibiting preterm labour: a systematic review of the evidence and a protocol for administration of nifedipine. Aust N Z J Obstet Gynaecol 43:192, 2003
Koopmans CM, Bijilenga D, Groen H, et al: Induction of labour versus expectant monitoring for gestation hypertension or mild pre-eclampsia after 36 weeks' gestation (HYPITAT): a multicenter, open-label randomized controlled trial. Lancet 374:979, 2009
Korita D, Sagawa N, Itoh H, et al: Cyclic mechanical stretch augments prostacyclin production in cultured human uterine myometrial cells from pregnant women: possible involvement of up-regulation of prostacyclin synthase expression. J Clin Endocrinol Metab 87:5209, 2002
Kovacevich GJ, Gaich SA, Lavin JP, et al: The prevalence of thromboembolic events among women with extended bed rest prescribed as part of the treatment for premature labor or preterm premature rupture of membranes. Am J Obstet Gynecol 182:1089, 2000
Kragt H, Keirse MJ: How accurate is a woman's diagnosis of threatened preterm delivery? BJOG 97:317, 1990
Kramer MS, Coates AL, Michoud MC, et al: Maternal anthropometry and idiopathic preterm labor. Obstet Gynecol 86:744, 1995
Kurki T, Sivonen A, Renkonen OV, et al: Bacterial vaginosis in early pregnancy and pregnancy outcome. Obstet Gynecol 80:173, 1992
Kurtzman J, Garite T, Clark R, et al: Impact of a "rescue course" of antenatal corticosteroids (ACS): a multi-center randomized placebo controlled trial. Am J Obstet Gynecol 200(3):248.e1, 2009
Kurtzman JL, Thorp JM Jr, Spielman FJ, et al: Do nifedipine and verapamil potentiate the cardiac toxicity of magnesium sulfate? Am J Perinatol 10:450, 1993
Lam F, Gill P, Smith M, et al: Use of the subcutaneous terbutaline pump for long-term tocolysis. Obstet Gynecol 72:810, 1988
Lee HC, Gould JB: Survival advantage associated with cesarean delivery in very low birth weight vertex neonates. Obstet Gynecol 107:97, 2006
Lee SE, Romero R, Jung H: The intensity of the fetal inflammatory response in intraamniotic inflammation with and without microbial invasion of the amniotic cavity. Am J Obstet Gynecol 197(3):294, 2007
Lee SE, Romero R, Park CW: The frequency and significance of intraamniotic inflammation in patients with cervical insufficiency. Am J Obstet Gynecol 198(6):633, 2008
Lees CC, Lojacono A, Thompson C, et al: Glyceryl trinitrate and ritodrine in tocolysis: an international multicenter randomized study. Obstet Gynecol 94:403, 1999
Leeson SC, Maresh MJA, Martindale EA, et al: Detection of fetal fibronectin as a predictor of preterm delivery in high risk symptomatic pregnancies. BJOG 103:48, 1996
Leitich H, Bodner-Adler B, Brunbauer M, et al: Bacterial vaginosis as a risk factor for preterm delivery: a meta-analysis. Am J Obstet Gynecol 189:139, 2003a
Leitich H, Brunbauer M, Bodner-Adler B, et al: Antibiotic treatment of bacterial vaginosis in pregnancy: a meta-analysis. Am J Obstet Gynecol 188:752, 2003b
Leung TN, Chung TK, Madsen G, et al: Rate of rise in maternal plasma corticotrophin-releasing hormone and its relation to gestational length. BJOG 108:527, 2001
Leveno KJ, Klein VR, Guzick DS, et al: Single-centre randomised trial of ritodrine hydrochloride for preterm labour. Lancet 1:1293, 1986
Leveno KJ, McIntire DD, Bloom SL, et al: Decreased preterm births in an inner-city public hospital. Obstet Gynecol 113(3):578, 2009
Lewis DF, Adair CD, Robichaux AG, et al: Antibiotic therapy in preterm premature rupture of membranes: are seven days necessary? A preliminary, randomized clinical trial. Am J Obstet Gynecol 188:1413, 2003
Lewis DF, Robichaux AG, Jaekle RK, et al: Expectant management of preterm premature rupture of membranes and nonvertex presentation: what are the risks? Am J Obstet Gynecol 196:566, 2007
Lewis R, Mercer BM, Salama M, et al: Oral terbutaline after parenteral tocolysis: a randomized, double-blind, placebo-controlled trial. Am J Obstet Gynecol 175:834, 1996
Li D, Liu L, Odouli R: Presence of depressive symptoms during early pregnancy and the risk of preterm delivery: a prospective cohort study. Hum Reprod 24:146, 2008
Li D-K, Odouli R, Liu L, et al: Transmission of parentally shared human leukocyte antigen alleles and the risk of preterm delivery. Obstet Gynecol 104:594, 2004
Lieman JM, Brumfield CG, Carlo W, et al: Preterm premature rupture of membranes: is there an optimal gestational age for delivery? Obstet Gynecol 105:12, 2005
Liggins GC, Howie RN: A controlled trial of antepartum glucocorticoid treatment for prevention of the respiratory distress syndrome in premature infants. Pediatrics 50:515, 1972
Likis FE, Velez Edwards DR, Andrews JC, et al: Progestogens for preterm birth prevention. Obstet Gynecol 120:897, 2012
Littleton HL, Breitkopf CR, Berenson AB: Correlates of anxiety symptoms during pregnancy and association with perinatal outcomes: a meta-analysis. Am J Obstet Gynecol 196:424, 2007
Lobel M: Conceptualizations, measurement, and effects of prenatal maternal stress on birth outcomes. J Behav Med 17:225, 1994
Locatelli A, Ghidini A, Paterlini G, et al: Gestational age at preterm premature rupture of membranes: a risk factor for neonatal white matter damage. Am J Obstet Gynecol 193:947, 2005
Lockwood CJ: Stress-associated preterm delivery: the role of corticotropin-releasing hormone. Am J Obstet Gynecol 180:S264, 1999
Lockwood CJ, Senyei AE, Dische MR, et al: Fetal fibronectin in cervical and vaginal secretions as a predictor of preterm delivery. N Engl J Med 325:669, 1991
Loe SM, Sanchez-Ramos L, Kaunitz AM: Assessing the neonatal safety of indomethacin tocolysis: a systematic review with meta-analysis. Obstet Gynecol 106:173, 2005

Low JA, Panagiotopoulos C, Derrick EJ: Newborn complication after intrapartum asphyxia with metabolic acidosis in the preterm fetus. Am J Obstet Gynecol 172:805, 1995
Luke B, Mamelle N, Keith L, et al: The association between occupational factors and preterm birth: a United States nurses study. Am J Obstet Gynecol 173:849, 1995
Lyall F, Lye S, Teoh T, et al: Expression of Gsalpha, connexin-43, connexin-26, and EP1, 3, and 4 receptors in myometrium of prelabor singleton versus multiple gestations and the effects of mechanical stretch and steroids on Gsalpha. J Soc Gynecol Investi 9:299, 2002
Lyell DJ, Pullen K, Campbell L, et al: Magnesium sulfate compared with nifedipine for acute tocolysis of preterm labor: a randomized controlled trial. Obstet Gynecol 1108:61, 2007
Macones GA, Berlin M, Berlin JA: Efficacy of oral beta-agonist maintenance therapy in preterm labor: a meta-analysis. Obstet Gynecol 85:313, 1995
Macones GA, Parry S, Elkousy M, et al: A polymorphism in the promoter region of TNF and bacterial vaginosis: preliminary evidence of gene-environment interaction in the etiology of spontaneous preterm birth. Am J Obstet Gynecol 190:1504, 2004
Major CA, Towers CW, Lewis DF, et al: Expectant management of preterm premature rupture of membranes complicated by active recurrent genital herpes. Am J Obstet Gynecol 188:1551, 2003
Malloy MH, Onstad L, Wright E: The effect of cesarean delivery on birth outcome in very low birth weight infants. Obstet Gynecol 77:498, 1991
Marret S, Marpeau L, Bénichou J: Benefit of magnesium sulfate given before very preterm birth to protect infant brain. Pediatrics 121(1):225, 2008
Martin JA, Hamilton BE, Sutton PD, et al: Births: final data for 2004. Natl Vital Stat Rep 55(1):1, 2006
Martin JA, Hamilton BE, Sutton PD, et al: Births: final data for 2006. Natl Vital Stat Rep 57(7):1, 2009a
Martin JA, Hamilton BE, Ventura SJ, et al: Births: final data for 2009. Natl Vital Stat Rep 60:1, 2011
Martin JA, Kirmeyer S, Osterman M, et al: Born a bit too early: recent trends in later preterm births. NCHS Data Brief 24:1, 2009b
Martin JA, Menacker F: Expanded health data from the new birth certificate, 2004. Natl Vital Stat Rep 55(12):1, 2007
Mathews TJ, MacDorman MF: Infant mortality statistics from the 2009 period linked birth/infant death data set. Natl Vital Stat Rep 61(8):1, 2013
Maymon E, Romero R, Pacora P, et al: Evidence for the participation of interstitial collagenase (matrix metalloproteinase 1) in preterm premature rupture of membranes. Am J Obstet Gynecol 183(4):914, 2000
McCall CA, Grimes DA, Drapkin Lyerly A: "Therapeutic" bed rest in pregnancy unethical and unsupported by data. Obstet Gynecol 121:1305, 2013
McElrath TF, Allred E, Leviton A: Prolonged latency after preterm premature rupture of membranes: an evaluation of histologic condition and intracranial ultrasonic abnormality in the neonate born at < 28 weeks of gestation. Am J Obstet Gynecol 189:794, 2003
McElrath TF, Norwitz ER, Lieberman ES, et al: Perinatal outcome after preterm premature rupture of membranes with in situ cervical cerclage. Am J Obstet Gynecol 187:1147, 2002
McEvoy C, Schilling D, Segel S, et al: Improved respiratory compliance in preterm infants after a single rescue course of antenatal steroids: a randomized trial. Am J Obstet Gynecol 202(6):544.e1, 2010
McGrath S, McLean M, Smith D, et al: Maternal plasma corticotropin-releasing hormone trajectories vary depending on the cause of preterm delivery. Am J Obstet Gynecol 186:257, 2002
McGrath S, Smith R: Prediction of preterm delivery using plasma corticotrophin-releasing hormone and other biochemical variables. Ann Med 34:28, 2002
McGregor JA, Jackson GM, Lachelin GC, et al: Salivary estriol as risk assessment for preterm labor: a prospective trial. Am J Obstet Gynecol 173:1337, 1995
McIntire DD, Leveno KJ: Neonatal mortality and morbidity rates in later preterm births compared with births at term. Obstet Gynecol 111:35, 2008
McLean M, Bisits A, Davies J, et al: A placental clock controlling the length of human pregnancy. Nat Med 1(5):460, 1995
Meis PJ, Klebanoff M, Thom E, et al: Prevention of recurrent preterm delivery by 17alpha-hydroxyprogesterone caproate. N Engl J Med 348:2379, 2003
Meis PJ, Michielutte R, Peters TJ, et al: Factors associated with preterm birth in Cardiff, Wales, I. Univariable and multivariable analysis. Am J Obstet Gynecol 173:590, 1995
Mercer BM: Preterm premature rupture of the membranes. Obstet Gynecol 101:178, 2003
Mercer BM, Arheart KL: Antimicrobial therapy in expectant management of preterm premature rupture of the membranes. Lancet 346:1271, 1995
Mercer BM, Carr TL, Beazley DD, et al: Antibiotic use in pregnancy and drug-resistant infant sepsis. Am J Obstet Gynecol 181:816, 1999
Mercer BM, Crocker LG, Boe NM, et al: Induction versus expectant management in premature rupture of the membranes with mature amniotic fluid at 32 to 36 weeks: a randomized trial. Am J Obstet Gynecol 169:775, 1993
Mercer BM, Miodovnik M, Thurnau GR, et al: Antibiotic therapy for reduction of infant morbidity after preterm premature rupture of the membranes. JAMA 278:989, 1997
Merkatz IR, Peter JB, Barden TP: Ritodrine hydrochloride: a betamimetic agent for use in preterm labor, II. Evidence of efficacy. Obstet Gynecol 56:7, 1980
Michalowicz BS, Hodges JS, DiAngelis AJ, et al: Treatment of periodontal disease and the risk of preterm birth. N Engl J Med 355:1885, 2006
Mittendorf R, Covert R, Boman J, et al: Is tocolytic magnesium sulfate associated with increased total paediatric mortality? Lancet 350:1517, 1997
Miyazaki K, Furuhashi M, Yoshida K, et al: Aggressive intervention of previable preterm premature rupture of membranes. Acta Obstet Gynaecol Scand 91(8):923, 2012
Moawad AH, Goldenberg RL, Mercer B, et al: The Preterm Prediction Study: the value of serum alkaline phosphatase, alpha-fetoprotein, plasma corticotropin-releasing hormone, and other serum markers for the prediction of spontaneous preterm birth. Am J Obstet Gynecol 186:990, 2002
Mogami H, Kishore AH, Shi H, et al: Fetal fibronectin signaling induces matrix metalloproteases and cyclooxygenase-2 (COX-2) in amnion cells and preterm birth in mice. J Biol Chem 288(3):1953, 2013
Montalbano AP, Hawgood S, Mendelson CR: Mice deficient in surfactant protein A (SP-A) and SP-D or in TLR2 manifest delayed parturition and decreased expression of inflammatory and contractile genes. Endocrinology 154(1):483, 2013
Morales WJ, Madhav H: Efficacy and safety of indomethacin compared with magnesium sulfate in the management of preterm labor: a randomized study. Am J Obstet Gynecol 169:97, 1993a
Morales WJ, Smith SG, Angel JL, et al: Efficacy and safety of indomethacin versus ritodrine in the management of preterm labor: a randomized study. Obstet Gynecol 74:567, 1989
Morales WJ, Talley T: Premature rupture of membranes at < 25 weeks: a management dilemma. Am J Obstet Gynecol 168:503, 1993b
Morency AM, Bujold E: The effect of second-trimester antibiotic therapy on the rate of preterm birth. J Obstet Gynaecol Can 29:35, 2007
Moutquin JM, Sherman D, Cohen H, et al: Double-blind, randomized, controlled trial of atosiban and ritodrine in the treatment of preterm labor: a multicenter effectiveness and safety study. Am J Obstet Gynecol 183:1191, 2000
Muench MV, Baschat AA, Kopelman J, et al: Indomethacin therapy initiated before 24 weeks of gestation for the prevention of preterm birth [Abstract]. Obstet Gynecol 101:65S, 2003
Muench V, Harman CR, Baschat AA, et al: Early fetal exposure to long term indomethacin therapy to prevent preterm delivery: neonatal outcome. Am J Obstet Gynecol 185:S149, 2001
Murphy KE: Betamethasone compared with dexamethasone for preterm birth: a call for trials. Obstet Gynecol 110:7, 2007
National Institutes of Health: Antenatal corticosteroids revisited: repeat courses. NIH Consens Statement 17(2):1, 2000
Neggers Y, Goldenberg R, Cliver S, et al: Effects of domestic violence on preterm birth and low birth weight. Acta Obstet Gynecol Scand 83:455, 2004
Nelson KB, Grether JK: Can magnesium sulfate reduce the risk of cerebral palsy in very-low-birthweight infants? Pediatrics 95:263, 1995
Nelson LH, Anderson RL, O'Shea M, et al: Expectant management of preterm premature rupture of the membranes. Am J Obstet Gynecol 171:350, 1994
Nelson LH, Meis PJ, Hatjis CG, et al: Premature rupture of membranes: a prospective, randomized evaluation of steroids, latent phase, and expectant management. Obstet Gynecol 66:55, 1985
Ness RB, Hillier SL, Richter HE: Douching in relation to bacterial vaginosis, lactobacilli, and facultative bacteria in the vagina. Obstet Gynecol 100:765, 2002
Niebyl JR, Blake DA, White RD, et al: The inhibition of premature labor with indomethacin. Am J Obstet Gynecol 136:1014, 1980
Norton ME, Merrill J, Cooper BA, et al: Neonatal complications after the administration of indomethacin for preterm labor. N Engl J Med 329:1602, 1993
Nugent RP, Krohn MA, Hillier SL: Reliability of diagnosing bacterial vaginosis by a standardized method of gram stain interpretation. J Clin Microbiol 29:297, 1991
O'Brien JM, Adair CD, Lewis DF, et al: Progesterone vaginal gel for the reduction of recurrent preterm birth: primary results from a randomized, double-blind, placebo-controlled trial. Ultrasound Obstet Gynecol 30:687, 2007
Okun N, Gronau KA, Hannah ME: Antibiotics for bacterial vaginosis or *Trichomonas vaginalis* in pregnancy: a systematic review. Obstet Gynecol 105:857, 2005
Olson DM, Zaragoza DB, Shallow MC: Myometrial activation and preterm labour: evidence supporting a role for the prostaglandin F receptor—a review. Placenta 24:S47, 2003

Osterman MJ, Martin JA, Mathews TJ, et al: Expanded data from the new birth certificate, 2008. Natl Vital Stat Rep 59(7):1, 2011

Owen J, Baker SL, Hauth JC, et al: Is indicated or spontaneous preterm delivery more advantageous for the fetus? Am J Obstet Gynecol 163:868, 1990

Owen J, Hankins G, Iams JD, et al: Multicenter randomized trial of cerclage for preterm birth prevention in high-risk women with shortened midtrimester cervical length. Am J Obstet Gynecol 201(4):375.e1, 2009

Park KH, Chaiworapongsa T, Kim YM, et al: Matrix metalloproteinase 3 in parturition, premature rupture of the membranes, and microbial invasion of the amniotic cavity. J Perinat Med 31:12, 2003

Parker CR Jr, Stankovic AM, Goland RS: Corticotropin-releasing hormone stimulates steroidogenesis in cultured human adrenal cells. Mol Cell Endocrinol 155:19, 1999

Papatsonis DN, Van Geijn HP, Ader HJ, et al: Nifedipine and ritodrine in the management of preterm labor: a randomized multicenter trial. Obstet Gynecol 90:230, 1997

Parilla BV, Dooley SL, Minogue JP, et al: The efficacy of oral terbutaline after intravenous tocolysis. Am J Obstet Gynecol 169:965, 1993

Parilla BV, Grobman WA, Holtzman RB, et al: Indomethacin tocolysis and risk of necrotizing enterocolitis. Obstet Gynecol 96:120, 2000

Parry S, Simhan H, Elovitz M, et al: Universal maternal cervical length screening during the second trimester: pros and cons of a strategy to identify women at risk of spontaneous preterm delivery. Am J Obstet Gynecol 207(2):101, 2012

Peck T, Lutheran G: Long-term and short-term childhood health after long-term use of indomethacin in pregnancy. Am J Obstet Gynecol 189:S168, 2003

Peltoniemi OM, Kari MA, Tammela O, et al: Randomized trial of a single repeat dose of prenatal betamethasone treatment in imminent preterm birth. Pediatrics, 119:290, 2007

Pereira L, Cotter A, Gómez R, et al: Expectant management compared with physical examination-indicated cerclage (EM-PEC) in selected women with a dilated cervix at $14^{0/7}$–$25^{6/7}$ weeks: results from the EM-PEC international cohort study. Am J Obstet Gynecol 197:483, 2007

Perry KG Jr, Martin RW, Blake PG, et al: Maternal mortality associated with adult respiratory distress syndrome. South Med J 91(5):441, 1998

Perry KG Jr, Morrison JC, Rust OA, et al: Incidence of adverse cardiopulmonary effects with low-dose continuous terbutaline infusion. Am J Obstet Gynecol 173:1273, 1995

Petraglia F, Imperatore A, Challis JRG: Neuroendocrine mechanisms in pregnancy and parturition. Endocrine Rev 31(6):783, 2010

Petrini JR, Dias T, McCormick MC, et al: Increased risk of adverse neurological development for late preterm infants. J Pediatr 154(2):169, 2009

Petrova A, Demissie K, Rhoads GG, et al: Association of maternal fever during labor with neonatal and infant morbidity and mortality. Obstet Gynecol 98:20, 2001

Phupong V, Kulmala L: Clinical course of preterm prelabor rupture of membranes in the era of prophylactic antibiotics. BMC Res Notes 5(1):515, 2012

Promislow JH, Hertz-Picciotto I, Schramm M, et al: Bed rest and other determinants of bone loss during pregnancy. Am J Obstet Gynecol 191:1077, 2004

Raju TN, Higgins RD, Stark AR, et al: Optimizing care and outcome for late-preterm (near-term) infants: a summary of the workshop sponsored by the National Institute of Child Health and Human Development. Pediatrics 118:1207, 2006

Reddy UM, Ko CW, Raju TN: Delivery indications at late-preterm gestations and infant mortality rates in the United States. Pediatrics 124(1):234, 2009

Reddy UM, Zhang J, Sun L, et al: Neonatal mortality by attempted route of delivery in early preterm birth. Am J Obstet Gynecol 207:117.e1, 2012

Romero R, Chaiworapongsa T, Espinoza J, et al: Fetal plasma MMP-9 concentrations are elevated in preterm premature rupture of the membranes. Am J Obstet Gynecol 187:1125, 2002

Romero R, Espinoza J, Kusanovic JP, et al: The preterm parturition syndrome. BJOG 3:17, 2006

Romero R, Nores J, Mazor M, et al: Microbial invasion of the amniotic cavity during term labor. Prevalence and clinical significance. J Reprod Med 38:543, 1993

Romero R, Sibai BM, Sanchez-Ramos L, et al: An oxytocin receptor antagonist (atosiban) in the treatment of preterm labor: a randomized, double-blind, placebo-controlled trial with tocolytic rescue. Am J Obstet Gynecol 182:1173, 2000

Romero R, Stanczyk FZ: Progesterone is not the same as 17α-hydroxyprogesterone caproate: implications for obstetrical practice. Am J Obstet Gynecol 208(6):421, 2013

Rouse DJ: Magnesium sulfate for fetal neuroprotection. Am J Obstet Gynecol 205(4):296, 2011

Rouse DJ, Caritis SN, Peaceman AM, et al: A trial of 17alpha-hydroxyprogesterone caproate to prevent prematurity in twins. N Engl J Med 357:454, 2007

Rouse DJ, Hirtz DG, Thom E, et al: A randomized, controlled trial of magnesium sulfate for the prevention of cerebral palsy. N Engl J Med 359:895, 2008

Ruiz RJ, Fullerton J, Dudley DJ: The interrelationship of maternal stress, endocrine factors and inflammation on gestational length. Obstet Gynecol Surv 58:415, 2003

Salim R, Garmi G, Zohar N, et al: Nifedipine compared with atosiban for treating preterm labor: a randomized controlled trial. Obstet Gynecol 120(6):1323, 2012

Samol JM, Lambers DS: Magnesium sulfate tocolysis and pulmonary edema: the drug or the vehicle? Am J Obstet Gynecol 192:1430, 2005

Satin AJ, Leveno KJ, Sherman ML, et al: Maternal youth and pregnancy outcomes: middle school versus high school age groups compared to women beyond the teen years. Am J Obstet Gynecol 171:184, 1994

Schmidt B, Davis P, Moddemann D, et al: Long-term effects of indomethacin prophylaxis in extremely-low-birth-weight infants. N Engl J Med 344:1966, 2001

Segel SY, Miles AM, Clothier B, et al: Duration of antibiotic therapy after preterm premature rupture of fetal membranes. Am J Obstet Gynecol 189:799, 2003

Serenius F, Källén K, Blennow M, et al: Neurodevelopmental outcome in extremely preterm infants at 2.5 years after active perinatal care in Sweden. JAMA 309(17):1810, 2013

Shynlova O, Nedd-Roderique T, Li Y, et al: Infiltration of myeloid cells into decidua is a critical early event in the labour cascade and post-partum uterine remodeling. J Cell Mol Med 17(2):311, 2013a

Shynlova O, Nedd-Roderique T, Li Y, et al: Myometrial immune cells contribute to term parturition, preterm labour and post-partum involution in mice. J Cell Mol Med 17(1):90, 2013b

Sibai BM: Magnesium sulfate for neuroprotection in patients at risk for early preterm delivery: not yet. Am J Obstet Gynecol 205(4):296, 2011

Silver RM, Cunningham FG: Deus ex Makena? Obstet Gynecol 117:1263, 2011

Smith R, Mesiano S, Chan EC, et al: Corticotropin-releasing hormone directly and preferentially stimulates dehydroepiandrosterone sulfate secretion by human fetal adrenal cortical cells. J Clin Endocrinol Metab 83:2916, 1998

Sooranna SR, Lee Y, Kim LU, et al: Mechanical stretch activates type 2 cyclooxygenase via activator protein-1 transcription factor in human myometrial cells. Mol Hum Reprod 10:109, 2004

Sosa C, Althabe F, Belizan J, et al: Bed rest in singleton pregnancies for preventing preterm birth. Cochrane Database Syst Rev 1:CD003581, 2004

Spong CY: Defining "term" pregnancy. Recommendations from the Defining "Term" Pregnancy Workgroup. JAMA 309(23):2445, 2013

Spong CY: Prediction and prevention of recurrent spontaneous preterm birth. Obstet Gynecol 110:405, 2007

Stamilio DM, Chang JJ, Macones GA: Periodontal disease and preterm birth: do the data have enough teeth to recommend screening and preventive treatment? Am J Obstet Gynecol 196:93, 2007

Steer CM, Petrie RH: A comparison of magnesium sulfate and alcohol for the prevention of premature labor. Am J Obstet Gynecol 129:1, 1977

Steer P: The epidemiology of preterm labour. BJOG 112(1):1, 2005

Stiles AD: Prenatal corticosteroids—early gain, long-term questions. N Engl J Med 357:1248, 2007

St Louis Business Journal: KV Pharmaceutical files for Chapter 11 bankruptcy. August 6, 2012. Available at: http://www.bizjournals.com/stlouis/morning_call/2012/08/kv-pharmaceutical-files-for-chapter-11.html. Accessed September 4, 2013

Stoll BJ, Hansen NI, Bell EF, et al: Neonatal outcomes of extremely preterm infants from the NICHD Neonatal Research Network. Pediatrics 126:443, 2010

Stoll BJ, Hansen N, Fanaroff AA, et al: Changes in pathogens causing early-onset sepsis in very-low-birth-weight infants. N Engl J Med 347:240, 2002

Tattershell M, Cordeaux Y, Charnock-Jones DS, et al: Expression of gastrin-releasing peptide is increased by prolonged stretch of human myometrium, and antagonists of its receptor inhibit contractility. J Physiol 590(Pt 9):2018, 2012

Terkildsen MFC, Parilla BV, Kumar P, et al: Factors associated with success of emergent second-trimester cerclage. Obstet Gynecol 101:565, 2003

Timmons BC, Fairhurst AM, Mahendroo MS: Temporal changes in myeloid cells in the cervix during pregnancy and parturition. J Immunol 182(5):2700, 2009

Tita A, Owen J, Cliver S, et al: Decreasing temporal trends in adjusted preterm birth among women receiving prenatal care at a university-based health system. Am J Obstet Gynecol 204:S183, 2011

Tita AT, Cliver SP, Goepfert AR, et al: Clinical trial of interconceptional antibiotics to prevent preterm birth: subgroup analyses and possible adverse antibiotic-microbial interaction. Am J Obstet Gynecol 196:367, 2007

To MS, Alfirevic Z, Heath VCF, et al: Cervical cerclage for prevention of preterm delivery in women with short cervix: randomized controlled trial. Lancet 363(9424):1849, 2004

Tomashek KM, Shapiro-Mendoza CK, Davidoff MJ, et al: Differences in mortality between late-preterm and term singleton infants in the United States, 1995–2002. J Pediatr 151:450, 2007

U.S. Food and Drug Administration: FDA drug safety communication: new warnings against use of terbutaline to treat preterm labor. February 17, 2011. Available at: http://www.fda.gov/drugs/drugsafety/ucm243539.htm. Accessed September 4, 2013

U.S. Food and Drug Administration: FDA drug safety communication: FDA recommends against prolonged use of magnesium sulfate to stop pre-term labor due to bone changes in exposed babies. May 30, 2013. Available at: http://www.fda.gov/drugs/drugsafety/ucm35333.htm. Accessed September 4, 2013

Üstün C, Kocak I, Baris S, et al: Subclinical chorioamnionitis as an etiologic factor in preterm deliveries. Int J Obstet Gynecol 72:109, 2001

Varner MW, Esplin MS: Genetic factors in preterm birth—the future. BJOG 112(Suppl 1):28, 2005

Velez DR, Fortunato SJ, Williams SM, et al: Interleukin-6 (IL-6) and receptor (IL6-R) gene haplotypes associate with amniotic fluid protein concentrations in preterm birth. Hum Mol Genet 17:1619, 2008

Vergnes J-N, Sixou M: Preterm low birthweight and maternal periodontal status: a meta-analysis. Am J Obstet Gynecol 196:135.e1, 2007

Wadhwa PD, Culhane JF, Rauh V, et al: Stress and preterm birth: neuroendocrine, immune/inflammatory, and vascular mechanisms. Matern Child Health J 5:119, 2001

Wang H, Parry S, Macones G, et al: A functional SNP in the promoter of the SERPINH1 gene increases risk of preterm premature rupture of membranes in African Americans. PNAS 103:13463, 2006

Wapner RJ, Sorokin Y, Mele L, et al: Long-term outcomes after repeat doses of antenatal corticosteroids. N Engl J Med 357:1190, 2007

Ward K: Genetic factors in common obstetric disorders. Clin Obstet Gynecol 51:74, 2008

Warren JE, Silver RM, Dalton J, et al: Collagen 1A1 and transforming growth factor-β polymorphisms in women with cervical insufficiency. Obstet Gynecol 110:619, 2007

Warren WB, Goland RS, Wardlaw SL, et al: Elevated maternal plasma corticotropin releasing hormone levels in twin gestation. J Perinat Med 18:39, 1990

Watts DH, Krohn MA, Hillier SL, et al: The association of occult amniotic fluid infection with gestational age and neonatal outcome among women in preterm labor. Obstet Gynecol 79:351, 1992

Weiss JL, Malone FD, Vidaver J, et al: Threatened abortion: a risk factor for poor pregnancy outcome, a population-based screening study. Am J Obstet Gynecol 190:745, 2004

Wenstrom K, Weiner CP, Merrill D, et al: A placebo controlled randomized trial of the terbutaline pump for prevention of preterm delivery. Am J Perinatol 14:87, 1997

Werner EF, Han CS, Savitz DA, et al: Health outcomes for vaginal compared with cesarean delivery of appropriately grown preterm neonates. Obstet Gynecol 121:1195, 2013

White BA, Creedon DJ, Nelson KE, et al: The vaginal microbiome in health and disease. Trends Endocrinol Metab 22(10):389, 2011

Winn HN, Chen M, Amon E, et al: Neonatal pulmonary hypoplasia and perinatal mortality in patients with mid-trimester rupture of amniotic membranes—a critical analysis. Am J Obstet Gynecol 182:1638, 2000

Wolfe CD, Patel SP, Linton EA, et al: Plasma corticotrophin-releasing factor (CRF) in abnormal pregnancy. BJOG 95:1003, 1988

Wu YY, Singer CA, Buxton ILO: Variants of stretch-activated two-pore potassium channel TREK-1 associated with preterm labor in humans. Biol Reprod 87(4):96, 2012

Yoon BH, Romero R, Park JS, et al: Fetal exposure to an intra-amniotic inflammation and the development of cerebral palsy at the age of three years. Am J Obstet Gynecol 182:675, 2000

Yoon BH, Romero R, Park JS, et al: Microbial invasion of the amniotic cavity with *Ureaplasma urealyticum* is associated with robust host response in fetal, amniotic, and maternal compartments. Am J Obstet Gynecol 179:1254, 1998

Yoon BH, Yang SH, Jun JK, et al: Maternal blood C-reactive protein, white blood cell count, and temperature in preterm labor: a comparison with amniotic fluid white blood cell count. Obstet Gynecol 87:231, 1996

Yost NP, Bloom SL, McIntire DD, et al: Hospitalization for women with arrested preterm labor: a randomized trial. Obstet Gynecol 106:14, 2005

Yost NP, Bloom SL, Twickler DM, et al: Pitfalls in ultrasonic cervical length measurement for predicting preterm birth. Obstet Gynecol 93:510, 1999

Young A, Thomson AJ, Ledingham M, et al: Immunolocalization of proinflammatory cytokines in myometrium, cervix, and fetal membranes during human parturition at term. Biol Reprod 66:445, 2002

Ziyan J, Huaibin R, Xiaotian M, et al: Regulation of progesterone receptor A and B expression in human preterm, term, and postterm placental villi. Acta Obstet Gynecol Scand 89(5):705, 2010

Zuckerman H, Reiss U, Rubinstein I: Inhibition of human premature labor by indomethacin. Obstet Gynecol 44:787, 1974

CHAPTER 43

Postterm Pregnancy

The adjectives *postterm, prolonged, postdates,* and *postmature* are often loosely used interchangeably to describe pregnancies that have exceeded a duration considered to be the upper limit of normal. We do not recommend use of the term *postdates* because the real issue in many postterm pregnancies is "post-*what* dates?" *Postmature* is reserved for the relatively uncommon specific clinical fetal syndrome in which the infant has recognizable clinical features indicating a pathologically prolonged pregnancy. Therefore, *postterm* or *prolonged* pregnancy is our preferred expression for an extended pregnancy.

The international definition of prolonged pregnancy, endorsed by the American College of Obstetricians and Gynecologists (2013a), is 42 completed weeks—294 days—or more from the first day of the last menstrual period. It is important to emphasize the phrase "42 completed weeks." Pregnancies between 41 weeks 1 day and 41 weeks 6 days, although in the 42nd week, do not complete 42 weeks until the seventh day has elapsed. Thus, technically speaking, prolonged pregnancy could begin either on day 294 or on day 295 following the onset of the last menses. Which is it? Day 294 or 295? We cannot resolve this question, and emphasize this dilemma only to ensure that litigators and others understand that some imprecision is inevitable when there is biological variation such as with prolonged pregnancy. Amersi and Grimes (1998) have cautioned against use of ordinal numbers such as "42nd week" because of imprecision. For example, "42nd week" refers to 41 weeks and 1 through 6 days, whereas the cardinal number "42 weeks" refers to precisely 42 completed weeks.

ESTIMATED GESTATIONAL AGE USING MENSTRUAL DATES

The definition of postterm pregnancy as one that persists for 42 weeks or more from the onset of a menstrual period assumes that the last menses was followed by ovulation 2 weeks later. That said, some pregnancies may not actually be postterm, but rather are the result of an error in gestational age estimation because of faulty menstrual date recall or delayed ovulation. Thus, there are two categories of pregnancies that reach 42 completed weeks: (1) those truly 40 weeks past conception, and (2) those of less-advanced gestation but with inaccurately estimated gestational age. Even with precisely recalled menstrual dates, there is still not precision. Specifically, Munster and associates (1992) reported that large variations in menstrual cycle lengths are common in normal women. Boyce and coworkers (1976) studied 317 French women with periconceptional basal body temperature profiles. Almost 70 percent who completed 42 postmenstrual weeks had a less-advanced gestation based on ovulation dates. These variations in the menstrual cycle may partially explain why a relatively small proportion of fetuses delivered postterm have evidence of *postmaturity syndrome*. Even so, because there is no accurate method to identify the truly prolonged pregnancy, all those judged to have reached 42 completed weeks should be managed as if abnormally prolonged. Sonographic evaluation of gestational age during pregnancy has been used to add precision. Blondel and colleagues (2002) studied 44,623 women delivered at the Royal Victoria Hospital in Montreal. Postterm pregnancy rates were analyzed according to six algorithms for gestational age based on the last menstrual period, sonographic evaluation at 16 to 18 weeks, or both. The proportion of births at 42 weeks or longer was 6.4 percent when based on the last menstrual period alone, but was 1.9 percent when based on sonographic measurements alone. Similarly, sonographic pregnancy dating at ≤ 12 weeks resulted in a 2.7-percent incidence of postterm gestation compared with 3.7 percent in a group assessed at 13 to 24 weeks (Caughey, 2008). These findings suggest that menstrual dates are frequently inaccurate in predicting postterm pregnancy. Other clinical studies confirmed these observations (Bennett, 2004; Joseph, 2007; Wingate, 2007).

INCIDENCE

From a review, the incidence of postterm pregnancy ranged from 4 to 19 percent (Divon, 2008). Using criteria that likely overestimate the incidence, approximately 6 percent of 4 million infants born in the United States during 2009 were estimated to have been delivered at 42 weeks or more (Martin, 2011). The trend toward fewer births at 42 weeks suggests earlier intervention. Specifically, in 2000, 7.2 percent of births in this country were 42 weeks or beyond compared with 5.5 percent in 2009. Zhang and colleagues (2010) studied live births in this country from 1992 through 2003 and reported dramatic increases in labor induction rates at 41 and 42 weeks' gestation (Fig. 43-1). This significantly increased use of labor induction was posited to contribute to a downward shift of the overall mean birthweight for these infants born in the United States.

There are contradictory findings concerning maternal demographic factors such as parity, prior postterm birth, socioeconomic class, and age as risks for postterm pregnancy. Olesen and associates (2006) analyzed various risk factors in 3392 participants in the 1998 to 2001 Danish Birth Cohort. Only prepregnancy body mass index (BMI) ≥ 25 and nulliparity were significantly associated with prolonged pregnancy. Caughey (2009) and Arrowsmith (2011) and their coworkers also reported similar associations.

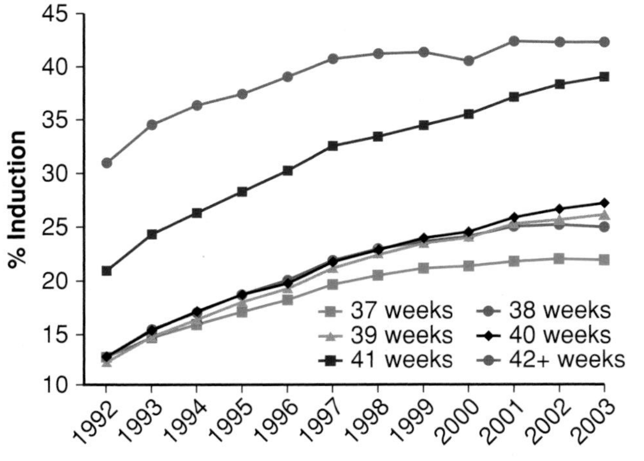

FIGURE 43-1 Rates of induction by gestational age among non-Hispanic white singleton livebirths ≥ 37 weeks from 1992 through 2003. (Redrawn from Zhang, 2010, with permission.)

The tendency for some mothers to have repeated postterm births suggests that some prolonged pregnancies are biologically determined. And Mogren and colleagues (1999) reported that prolonged pregnancy recurred across generations in Swedish women. When mother and daughter had a prolonged pregnancy, the risk for the daughter to have a subsequent postterm pregnancy was increased two- to threefold. In another Swedish study, Laursen and associates (2004) found that maternal, but not paternal, genes influenced prolonged pregnancy. As noted in Chapter 21 (p. 426), rare fetal–placental factors that have been reported as predisposing to postterm pregnancy include anencephaly, adrenal hypoplasia, and X-linked placental sulfatase deficiency (MacDonald, 1965).

PERINATAL MORTALITY

Perinatal mortality rates increase after the expected due date has passed. This is best seen when perinatal mortality rates are analyzed from times before widespread intervention for postterm pregnancies. In two large Swedish studies shown in Figure 43-2, after reaching a nadir at 39 to 40 weeks, the perinatal mortality rate increased as pregnancy exceeded 41 weeks. This trend has also been reported for the United States (MacDorman, 2009). Another study in this country of more than 2.5 million births has similar findings (Cheng, 2008). The major causes of death in these pregnancies included gestational hypertension, prolonged labor with cephalopelvic disproportion, "unexplained anoxia," and malformations. Similar outcomes were reported by Olesen and colleagues (2003) in 78,022 women with postterm pregnancies delivered before routine labor induction was adopted in Denmark. Moster and associates (2010) found increased rates of cerebral palsy in postterm births, and Yang and coworkers (2010) reported lower intelligence quotient (IQ) scores at age 6.5 years in children born ≥ 42 weeks' gestation. Conversely, autism was not associated with postterm birth (Gardener, 2011).

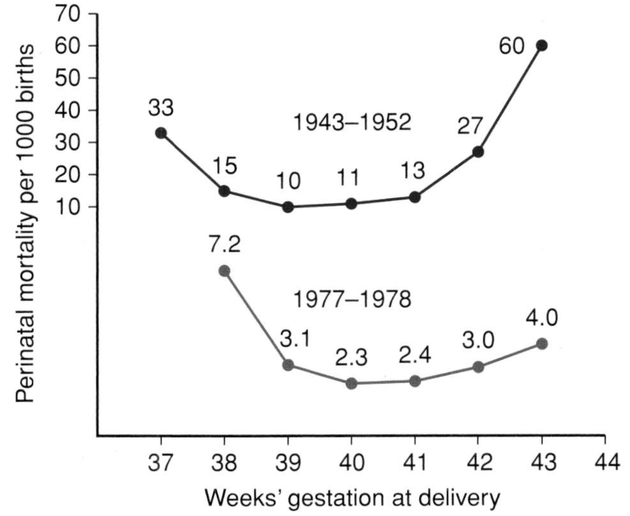

FIGURE 43-2 Perinatal mortality rates in late pregnancy according to gestational age in Sweden of all births during 1943–1952 compared with those during 1977–1978. The partially compressed scale is used for convenience in depiction. (Adapted from Bakketeig, 1991, and Lindell, 1956.)

TABLE 43-1. Pregnancy Outcomes in 56,317 Consecutive Singleton Pregnancies Delivered at or Beyond 40 Weeks at Parkland Hospital from 1988 through 1998

	Weeks' Gestation			
Outcome	40 (n = 29,136)	41 (n = 16,386)	42 (n = 10,795)	*p* value[a]
Maternal outcomes (%)				
Labor induction	2	7	35	< .001
Cesarean delivery				
Dystocia	7	6	9	< .001
Fetal distress	2	3	4	< .001
Perinatal outcomes (per 1000)				
Neonatal ICU	4	5	6	< .001
Neonatal seizures	1	1	2	.12
Stillbirth	2	1	2	.84
Neonatal death	0.2	0.2	0.6	.17

[a]*p* value is for the trend using 42 weeks as the referent.
ICU = intensive care unit.
Adapted from Alexander, 2000a.

Alexander and colleagues (2000a) reviewed 56,317 consecutive singleton pregnancies delivered at ≥ 40 weeks between 1988 and 1998 at Parkland Hospital. As shown in Table 43-1, labor was induced in 35 percent of pregnancies completing 42 weeks. The rate of cesarean delivery for dystocia and fetal distress was significantly increased at 42 weeks compared with earlier deliveries. More infants of postterm pregnancies were admitted to intensive care units. Importantly, the incidence of neonatal seizures and deaths doubled at 42 weeks. Smith (2001) has challenged analyses such as these because the population at risk for perinatal mortality in a given week consists of all ongoing pregnancies rather than just the births in a given week. Figure 43-3 shows perinatal mortality rates calculated using only births in a given week of gestation from 37 to 43 completed weeks compared with the cumulative probability—the perinatal index—of death when all ongoing pregnancies are included in the denominator. As shown, delivery at 38 weeks had the lowest risk index for perinatal death.

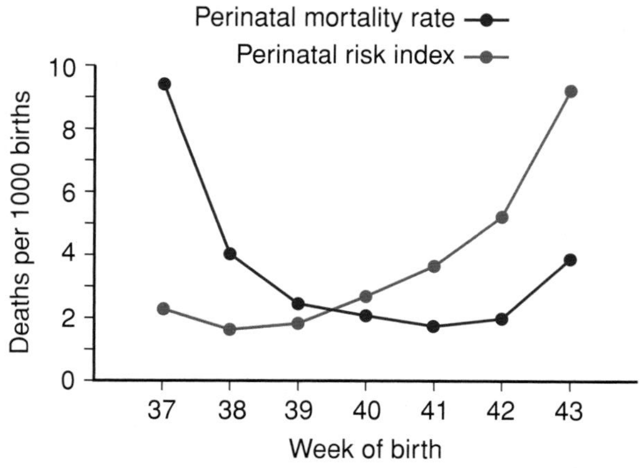

FIGURE 43-3 Perinatal mortality rate and perinatal risk index for births between 37 and 43 weeks in Scotland from 1985 through 1996. The perinatal mortality rate is the number of perinatal deaths with delivery in a given gestational week divided by the total number of births in that week multiplied by 1000. The perinatal risk index is the cumulative probability of perinatal death multiplied by 1000. (Redrawn from Smith, 2001, with permission.)

PATHOPHYSIOLOGY

Postmaturity Syndrome

The postmature infant presents a unique appearance such as shown in Figure 43-4. Features include wrinkled, patchy, peeling skin; a long, thin body suggesting wasting; and advanced maturity in that the infant is open-eyed, unusually alert, and appears old and worried. Skin wrinkling can be particularly prominent on the palms and soles. The nails are typically long. Most postmature infants are not technically growth restricted because their birthweight seldom falls below the 10th percentile for gestational age. On the other hand, severe growth restriction—which logically must have preceded completion of 42 weeks—may be present.

The incidence of postmaturity syndrome in infants at 41, 42, or 43 weeks, respectively, has not been conclusively determined. In one of the rare contemporary reports that chronicle postmaturity, Shime and colleagues (1984) found this syndrome in approximately 10 percent of pregnancies between 41 and 43 weeks. The incidence increased to 33 percent at 44 weeks. Associated oligohydramnios substantially increases the likelihood of postmaturity. Trimmer and associates (1990) reported that 88 percent of infants were postmature if there was oligohydramnios defined by a sonographic maximal vertical amnionic fluid pocket that measured ≤ 1 cm at 42 weeks.

Placental Dysfunction

Clifford (1954) proposed that the skin changes of postmaturity were due to loss of the protective effects of vernix caseosa. He also

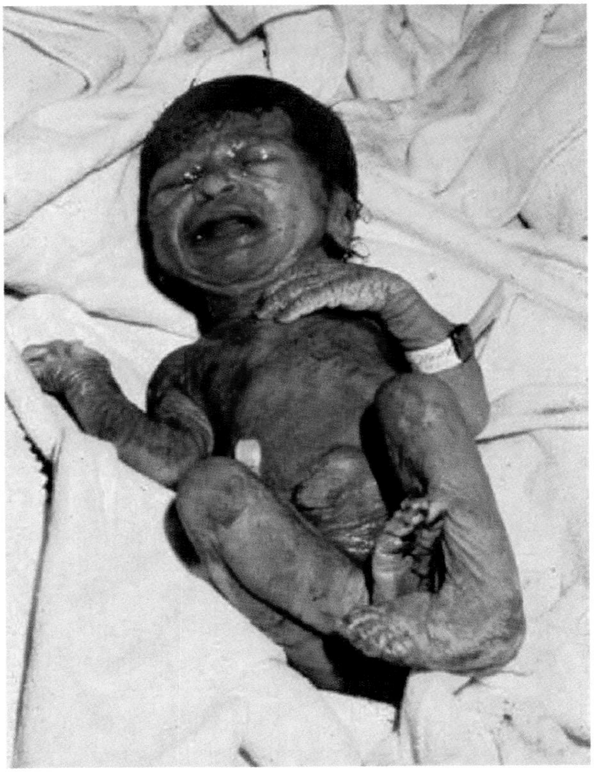

FIGURE 43-4 Postmaturity syndrome. Infant delivered at 43 weeks' gestation with thick, viscous meconium coating the desquamating skin. Note the long, thin appearance and wrinkling of the hands.

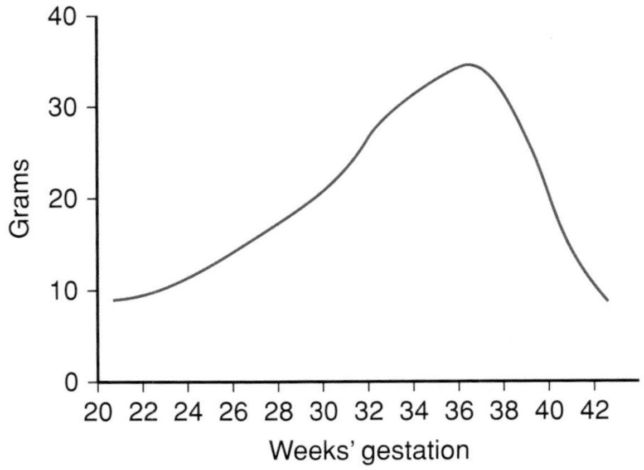

FIGURE 43-5 Mean daily fetal growth during previous week of gestation. (From Hendricks, 1964.)

attributed the postmaturity syndrome to placental senescence, although he did not find placental degeneration histologically. Still, the concept that postmaturity is due to placental insufficiency has persisted despite an absence of morphological or significant quantitative findings (Larsen, 1995; Rushton, 1991). There are findings that placental apoptosis—programmed cell death—was significantly increased at 41 to 42 completed weeks compared with that at 36 to 39 weeks (Smith, 1999). Several proapoptotic genes such as kisspeptin were shown to be upregulated in postterm placental explants compared with the same genes in term placental explants (Torricelli, 2012). The clinical significance of such apoptosis is currently unclear.

Jazayeri and coworkers (1998) investigated cord blood erythropoietin levels in 124 appropriately grown newborns delivered from 37 to 43 weeks. The only known stimulator of erythropoietin is decreased partial oxygen pressure. Thus, they sought to assess whether fetal oxygenation was compromised due to placental aging in postterm pregnancies. All women had an uncomplicated labor and delivery. These investigators reported that cord blood erythropoietin levels were significantly increased in pregnancies reaching 41 weeks or more. Although Apgar scores and acid-base studies were normal, these researchers concluded that there was decreased fetal oxygenation in some postterm gestations.

Another scenario is that the postterm fetus may continue to gain weight and thus be unusually large at birth. This at least suggests that placental function is not severely compromised. Indeed, continued fetal growth is the norm—albeit at a slower rate beginning at 37 completed weeks (Fig. 43-5). Nahum and colleagues (1995) confirmed that fetal growth continues until at least 42 weeks, however, Link and associates (2007) showed that umbilical blood flow did not increase concomitantly.

Fetal Distress and Oligohydramnios

The principal reasons for increased risks to postterm fetuses were described by Leveno and associates (1984). Both antepartum fetal jeopardy and intrapartum fetal distress were found to be the consequence of cord compression associated with oligohydramnios. In their analysis of 727 postterm pregnancies, intrapartum fetal distress detected with electronic monitoring was not associated with late decelerations characteristic of uteroplacental insufficiency. Instead, one or more prolonged decelerations such as shown in Figure 43-6 preceded three fourths of emergency cesarean deliveries for nonreassuring fetal heart rate tracings. In all but two cases, there were also variable decelerations (Fig. 43-7). Another common fetal heart rate pattern, although not ominous by itself, was the saltatory baseline shown in Figure 43-8. As described in Chapter 24 (p. 484), these findings are consistent with cord occlusion as the proximate cause of the nonreassuring tracings. Other correlates included oligohydramnios and viscous meconium. Schaffer and colleagues (2005) implicated a nuchal cord in abnormal intrapartum fetal heart rate patterns, meconium, and compromised newborn condition in prolonged pregnancies.

The volume of amnionic fluid normally continues to decrease after 38 weeks and may become problematic (Fig. 11-1, p. 233). Moreover, meconium release into an already reduced amnionic fluid volume results in thick, viscous meconium that may cause *meconium aspiration syndrome* (Chap. 33, p. 637).

Trimmer and coworkers (1990) sonographically measured hourly fetal urine production using sequential bladder volume measurements in 38 pregnancies of ≥ 42 weeks. Diminished urine production was found to be associated with oligohydramnios. They hypothesized that decreased fetal urine flow was likely the result of preexisting oligohydramnios that limited fetal swallowing. Oz and associates (2002), using Doppler waveforms, concluded that fetal renal blood flow is reduced in those postterm pregnancies complicated by oligohydramnios.

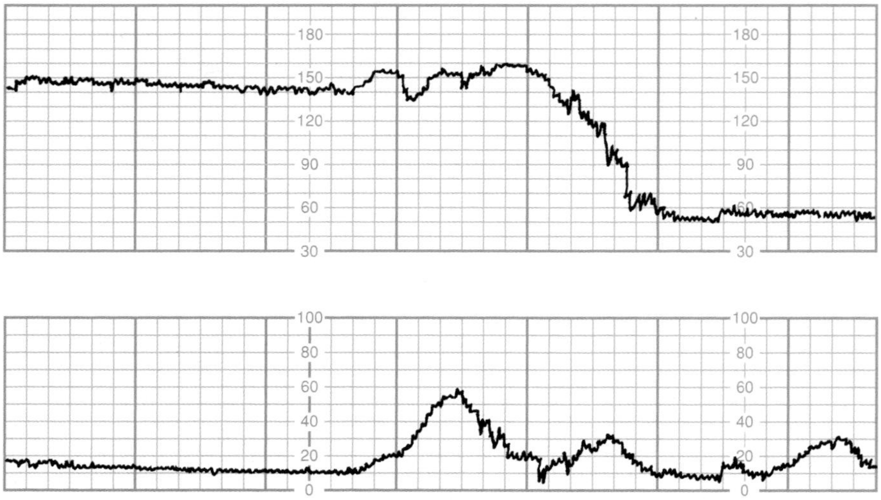

FIGURE 43-6 Prolonged fetal heart rate deceleration before emergency cesarean delivery in a postterm pregnancy with oligohydramnios. (Redrawn from Leveno, 1984, with permission.)

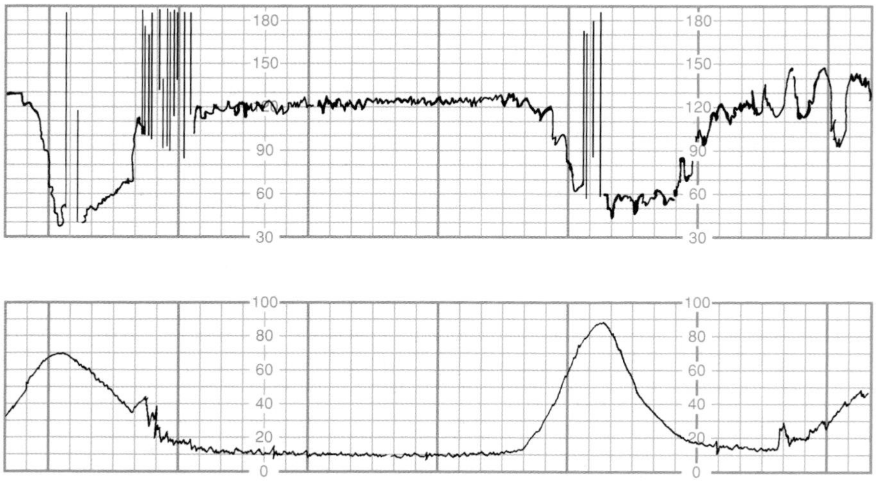

FIGURE 43-7 Severe—less than 70 bpm for 60 seconds or longer—variable decelerations in a postterm pregnancy with oligohydramnios. (Redrawn from Leveno, 1984, with permission.)

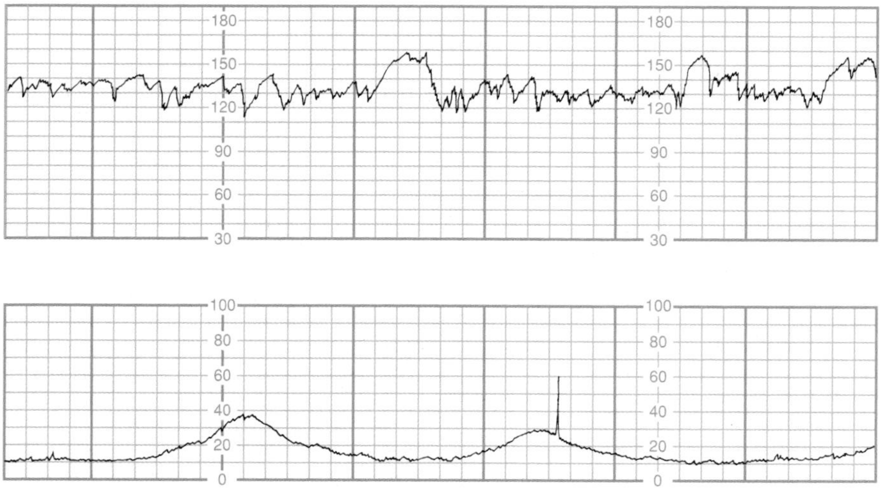

FIGURE 43-8 Saltatory baseline fetal heart rate showing oscillations exceeding 20 bpm and associated with oligohydramnios in a postterm pregnancy. (Redrawn from Leveno, 1984, with permission.)

The study mentioned above, by Link and associates (2007), showed that umbilical blood flow did not increase past term.

Fetal-Growth Restriction

It was not until the late 1990s that the clinical significance of fetal-growth restriction in the otherwise uncomplicated pregnancy became more fully appreciated. Divon (1998) and Clausson (1999) and their coworkers analyzed births between 1991 and 1995 in the National Swedish Medical Birth Registry. As shown in Table 43-2, stillbirths were more common among growth-restricted infants who were delivered after 42 weeks. Indeed, a third of postterm stillborn infants were growth restricted. During this time in Sweden, labor induction and antenatal fetal testing usually commenced at 42 weeks. In a study from Parkland Hospital, Alexander and colleagues (2000d) analyzed outcomes for 355 infants who were ≥ 42 weeks and whose birthweights were < 3rd percentile. They compared these with outcomes of 14,520 similarly aged infants above the 3rd percentile and found that morbidity and mortality rates were significantly increased in the growth-restricted infants. Notably, a fourth of all stillbirths associated with prolonged pregnancy were in this comparatively small number of growth-restricted infants.

COMPLICATIONS

Oligohydramnios

Most clinical studies support the view that diminished amnionic fluid determined by various sonographic methods identifies a postterm fetus with increased risks. Indeed, decreased amnionic fluid in any pregnancy signifies increased fetal risk (Chap. 11, p. 238). Unfortunately, lack of an exact method to define "decreased amnionic fluid" has limited investigators, and many different criteria for sonographic diagnosis have been proposed. Fischer and colleagues (1993) attempted to determine which criteria were most predictive of normal versus abnormal outcomes in postterm pregnancies. As shown in Figure 43-9, the smaller the amnionic fluid pocket, the greater the likelihood that there was clinically significant oligohydramnios. Importantly, normal

TABLE 43-2. Effects of Fetal-Growth Restriction by Gestational Age on Stillbirth Rates in 537,029 Swedish Women Delivered before and after 42 Weeks

	Pregnancy Duration	
Fetal Outcome	37–41 Weeks	≥ 42 Weeks
Births (No.)	469,056	40,973
Growth restriction[a] n (%)	10,312 (2)	1,558 (4)
Stillbirth n (per 1000)		
Appropriate growth	650 (1.4)	69 (1.8)
Growth restriction	116 (11)	23 (15)

[a]Defined as birthweight two standard deviations below mean birthweights for fetal gender and gestational age. Data from Clausson, 1999.

amnionic fluid volume did not preclude abnormal outcomes. Alfirevic and coworkers (1997) randomly assigned 500 women with postterm pregnancies to assessment using either the amnionic fluid index (AFI) or the deepest vertical pocket (Chap. 11, p. 232). They concluded that the AFI overestimated the number of abnormal outcomes in postterm pregnancies.

Regardless of the criteria used to diagnose oligohydramnios in postterm pregnancies, most investigators have found an increased incidence of some sort of "fetal distress" during labor. Thus, oligohydramnios by most definitions is a clinically meaningful finding. Conversely, reassurance of continued fetal well-being in the presence of "normal" amnionic fluid volume is tenuous. This may be related to how quickly pathological oligohydramnios develops. Although such cases are unusual,

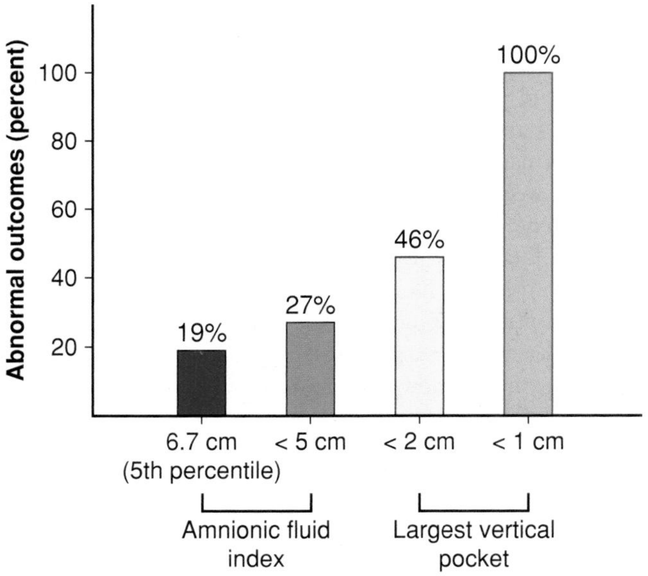

FIGURE 43-9 Comparison of the prognostic value of various sonographic estimates of amnionic fluid volume in prolonged pregnancies. Abnormal outcomes include cesarean or operative vaginal delivery for fetal jeopardy, 5-minute Apgar score ≤ 6, umbilical arterial blood pH < 7.1, or admission to the neonatal intensive care unit. (Adapted from Fischer, 1993.)

Clement and coworkers (1987) described six postterm pregnancies in which amnionic fluid volume diminished abruptly over 24 hours, and in one of these, the fetus died.

Macrosomia

The velocity of fetal weight gain peaks at approximately 37 weeks as shown in Figure 43-5. Although growth velocity slows at that time, most fetuses continue to gain weight. For example, the percentage of fetuses born in 2009 whose birthweight exceeded 4000 g was 8.2 percent at 37 to 41 weeks and increased to 11.0 percent at 42 weeks or more (Martin, 2011). However, in some studies, brachial plexus injury was not related to postterm gestation (Walsh, 2011). Intuitively at least, it seems that both maternal and fetal morbidity associated with macrosomia would be mitigated with timely induction to preempt further growth. This does not appear to be the case, however, and the American College of Obstetricians and Gynecologists (2013b) has concluded that current evidence does not support such a practice in women at term with suspected fetal macrosomia. Moreover, the College concluded that in the absence of diabetes, vaginal delivery is not contraindicated for women with an estimated fetal weight up to 5000 g. Cesarean delivery was recommended for estimated fetal weights greater than 4500 g if there is prolonged second-stage labor or arrest of descent. Obvious problems with all such recommendations are substantive variations in fetal weight estimation (Chap. 44, p. 885).

Medical or Obstetrical Complications

In the event of a medical or other obstetrical complication, it is generally not recommended that a pregnancy be allowed to continue past 42 weeks. Indeed, in many such instances, *earlier* delivery is indicated. Common examples include gestational hypertensive disorders, prior cesarean delivery, and diabetes.

MANAGEMENT

Although some form of intervention is considered to be indicated for prolonged pregnancies, the types and timing of interventions are not unanimous (Divon, 2008). The decision centers on whether labor induction is warranted or if expectant management with fetal surveillance is best. In a survey done 10 years ago, Cleary-Goldman and associates (2006) reported that 73 percent of members of the American College of Obstetricians and Gynecologists routinely induced women at 41 weeks. Most of the remainder performed twice weekly fetal testing until 42 weeks.

Prognostic Factors for Successful Induction

Unfavorable Cervix

Although all obstetricians know what an "unfavorable cervix" is, the term unfortunately defies precise objective definition. Thus, various investigators have used different criteria for studies of prolonged pregnancies. For example, Harris and coworkers (1983) defined an unfavorable cervix by a Bishop score < 7 and reported this in 92 percent of women at 42 weeks. Hannah and colleagues (1992) found that only 40 percent of 3407 women with a 41-week pregnancy had an "undilated cervix." In a study of 800 women undergoing induction for postterm pregnancy at Parkland Hospital, Alexander and associates (2000b) reported that women in whom there was no cervical dilatation had a twofold increased cesarean delivery rate for "dystocia." Yang and coworkers (2004) found that cervical length ≤ 3 cm measured with transvaginal sonography was predictive of successful induction. In a similar study, Vankayalapati and associates (2008) found that cervical length ≤ 25 mm was predictive of spontaneous labor or successful induction.

Cervical Ripening. A number of investigators have evaluated prostaglandin E_2 (PGE_2) for induction in women with an unfavorable cervix and prolonged pregnancies. The study by the National Institute of Child Health and Human Development Network of Maternal–Fetal Medicine Units (1994) found that PGE_2 gel was not more effective than placebo. Alexander and associates (2000c) treated 393 women with a postterm pregnancy with PGE_2, regardless of cervical "favorability," and reported that almost half of the 84 women with cervical dilatation of 2 to 4 cm entered labor with prostaglandin E_2 use alone. The American College of Obstetricians and Gynecologists (2011) previously concluded that PGE_2 gel could be used safely in postterm pregnancies. In another study, mifepristone was reported to increase uterine activity without uterotonic agents in women beyond 41 weeks (Fasset, 2008). Prostaglandins and other agents used for cervical ripening are discussed in Chapter 26 (p. 525).

Sweeping or stripping of the membranes to induce labor and thereby prevent postterm pregnancy was studied in 15 randomized trials during the 1990s. Boulvain and coworkers (1999) performed a metaanalysis of these and found that membrane stripping at 38 to 40 weeks decreased the frequency of postterm pregnancy. Moreover, maternal and neonatal infection rates were not increased by cervical manipulation. However, this practice did not modify the cesarean delivery risk. Since then, randomized trials by Wong (2002), Kashanian (2006), Hill (2008), and their coworkers found that sweeping membranes did not reduce the need to induce labor. Drawbacks of membrane stripping included pain, vaginal bleeding, and irregular contractions without labor.

Station of Vertex

The station of the fetal head within the pelvis is another important predictor of successful postterm pregnancy induction. Shin and colleagues (2004) studied 484 nulliparas who underwent induction after 41 weeks. The cesarean delivery rate was directly related to station. It was 6 percent if the vertex before induction was at −1 station; 20 percent at −2; 43 percent at −3; and 77 percent at −4.

Induction versus Fetal Testing

Because of marginal benefits for induction with an unfavorable cervix as discussed above, some clinicians prefer to use the alternative strategy of fetal testing beginning at 41 completed weeks. There now are several quality studies designed to resolve these important questions.

In a Canadian study, 3407 women were randomly assigned at 41 or more weeks to induction or to fetal testing (Hannah, 1992). In the surveillance group, evaluation included: (1) counting fetal movements during a 2-hour period each day, (2) nonstress testing three times weekly, and (3) amnionic fluid volume assessment two to three times weekly with pockets < 3 cm considered abnormal. Labor induction resulted in a small but significant reduction in cesarean delivery rate compared with fetal testing—21 versus 24 percent, respectively. This difference was due to fewer procedures for fetal distress. Importantly, the only two stillbirths were in the fetal testing group.

The Maternal–Fetal Medicine Network performed a randomized trial of induction versus fetal testing beginning at 41 weeks (Gardner, 1996). Fetal surveillance included nonstress testing and sonographic estimation of amnionic fluid volume performed twice weekly in 175 women. Perinatal outcomes were compared with those of 265 women also at 41 weeks randomly assigned to induction with or without cervical ripening. There were no perinatal deaths, and the cesarean delivery rate was not different between management groups. The results of this study could be used to support the validity of either of these management schemes. Similar results were subsequently reported from a Norwegian randomized trial of 508 women (Heimstad, 2007).

In an analysis of 19 trials in the Cochrane Pregnancy and Childbirth Trials Registry, Gulmezoglu and colleagues (2006) found that induction after 41 weeks was associated with fewer perinatal deaths without significantly increasing the cesarean delivery rate. In a review of two metaanalyses and a recent randomized controlled study, similar conclusions were reached (Mozurkewich, 2009).

In an attempt to "lower" the number of postterm pregnancies, Harrington and associates (2006) randomly assigned 463 women to pregnancy dating with sonography between 8 and 12 weeks versus no first-trimester sonographic evaluation. Their primary end point was the labor induction rate for prolonged pregnancy, and they found no advantages to early sonographic pregnancy dating.

At 42 weeks, labor induction has a higher cesarean delivery rate compared with spontaneous labor. From Parkland Hospital, Alexander and coworkers (2001) evaluated pregnancy outcomes in 638 such women in whom labor was induced and compared them with outcomes of 687 women with postterm pregnancies who had spontaneous labor. Cesarean delivery rates were significantly increased—19 versus 14 percent—in the induced group because of failure to progress. When these investigators corrected for risk factors, however, they concluded that intrinsic maternal factors, rather than the induction itself, led to the higher rate. These factors included nulliparity, an unfavorable cervix, and epidural analgesia.

Evidence to substantiate intervention—whether induction or fetal testing—commencing at 41 versus 42 weeks is limited. Most evidence used to justify intervention at 41 weeks is from the randomized Canadian and American investigations cited earlier. No randomized studies have specifically assessed intervention at 41 weeks versus an identical intervention used at 42 weeks. But there have been observational studies. In one, Usher and colleagues (1988) analyzed outcomes in 7663 pregnancies in women at 40, 41, or 42 weeks confirmed by early sonographic evaluation. After correction for malformations, perinatal death rates were 1.5, 0.7, and 3.0 per 1000 at 40, 41, and 42 weeks, respectively. These results could be used to challenge the concept of routine intervention at 41 instead of 42 weeks.

Management Recommendations

Because of the studies discussed above, the American College of Obstetricians and Gynecologists (2013a) defines postterm pregnancies as having completed 42 weeks. There is insufficient evidence to recommend a management strategy between 40 and 42 completed weeks. Thus, although not considered mandatory, initiation of fetal surveillance at 41 weeks is a reasonable option. After completing 42 weeks, recommendations are for either antenatal testing or labor induction. These are summarized in Figure 43-10.

At Parkland Hospital, based on results discussed above, we consider 41-week pregnancies without other complications to be normal. Thus, no interventions are practiced solely based on fetal age until 42 completed weeks. If there are complications such as hypertension, decreased fetal movement, or oligohydramnios, then labor induction is carried out. It is our view that large, randomized trials should be performed before otherwise uncomplicated 41-week gestations are routinely considered pathologically prolonged. In women in whom a *certain* gestational age is known, labor is induced at the completion of 42 weeks. Almost 90 percent of such women are induced successfully or enter labor within 2 days of induction. For those who do not deliver with the first induction, a second induction is performed within 3 days. Almost all women are delivered using this management plan, but in the unusual few who are not delivered, management decisions involve a third—or even more—induction versus cesarean delivery. Women classified as having *uncertain* postterm pregnancies are managed with weekly nonstress fetal testing and assessment of amnionic fluid volume. Women with an AFI ≤ 5 cm or with reports of diminished fetal movement undergo labor induction.

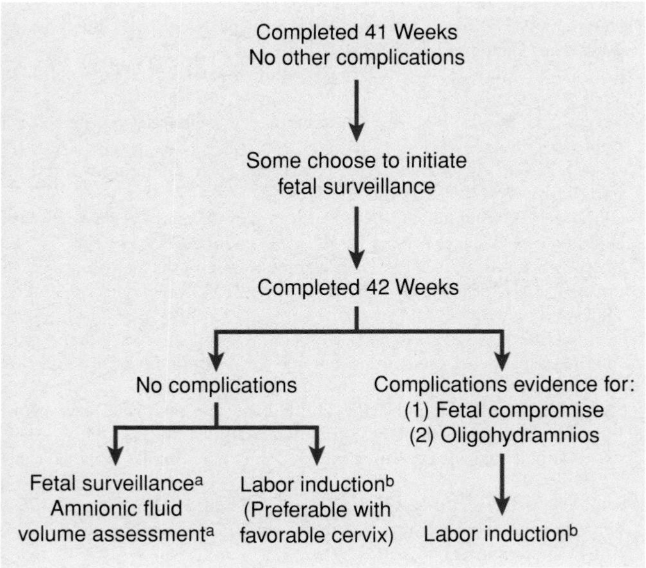

FIGURE 43-10 Management of postterm pregnancy.
[a]See text for options
[b]prostaglandins may be used for cervical ripening or induction.

INTRAPARTUM MANAGEMENT

Labor is a particularly dangerous time for the postterm fetus. Therefore, women whose pregnancies are known or suspected to be postterm should come to the hospital as soon as they suspect labor. While being evaluated for active labor, we recommend that fetal heart rate and uterine contractions be monitored electronically for variations consistent with fetal compromise.

The decision to perform amniotomy is problematic. Further reduction in fluid volume following amniotomy can certainly enhance the possibility of cord compression. Conversely, amniotomy aids identification of thick meconium, which may be dangerous to the fetus if aspirated. Also, after membrane rupture, a scalp electrode and intrauterine pressure catheter can be placed. These usually provide more precise data concerning fetal heart rate and uterine contractions.

Identification of thick meconium in the amnionic fluid is particularly worrisome. The viscosity probably signifies the lack of liquid and thus oligohydramnios. Aspiration of thick meconium may cause severe pulmonary dysfunction and neonatal death (Chap. 33, p. 637). Because of this, amnioinfusion during labor has been proposed as a way of diluting meconium to decrease the incidence of aspiration syndrome (Wenstrom, 1989). As discussed in Chapter 24 (p. 494), the benefits of amnioinfusion remain controversial. In a large randomized trial by Fraser and colleagues (2005), amnioinfusion did not reduce the risk of meconium aspiration syndrome or perinatal death. According to the American College of Obstetricians and Gynecologists (2012), amnioinfusion does not prevent meconium aspiration, however, it remains a reasonable treatment approach for repetitive variable decelerations.

The likelihood of a successful vaginal delivery is reduced appreciably for the nulliparous woman who is in early labor with thick, meconium-stained amnionic fluid. Therefore, if the woman is remote from delivery, strong consideration should be given to prompt cesarean delivery, especially when cephalopelvic disproportion is suspected or either hypotonic or hypertonic dysfunctional labor is evident. Some practitioners choose to avoid oxytocin use in these cases.

Until recently, it was taught—including at Parkland Hospital—that aspiration of meconium could be minimized but not eliminated by suctioning the pharynx as soon as the head was delivered. According to the American Academy of Pediatrics guidelines, this in no longer recommended (Perlman, 2010). The American College of Obstetricians and Gynecologists (2013c) does not recommend routine intrapartum suctioning. Alternatively, if the depressed newborn has meconium-stained fluid, then intubation is carried out. The American Academy of Pediatrics states that tracheal suctioning is neither supported nor refuted (Perlman, 2010).

REFERENCES

Alexander JM, McIntire DD, Leveno KJ: Forty weeks and beyond: pregnancy outcomes by week of gestation. Obstet Gynecol 96:291, 2000a

Alexander JM, McIntire DD, Leveno KJ: Postterm pregnancy: does induction increase cesarean rates? J Soc Gynecol Invest 7:79A, 2000b

Alexander JM, McIntire DD, Leveno KJ: Postterm pregnancy: is cervical "ripening" being used in the right patients? J Soc Gynecol Invest 7:247A, 2000c

Alexander JM, McIntire DD, Leveno KJ: The effect of fetal growth restriction on neonatal outcome in postterm pregnancy. Abstract No. 463. Am J Obstet Gynecol 182:S148, 2000d

Alexander JM, McIntire DD, Leveno KJ: Prolonged pregnancy: induction of labor and cesarean births. Obstet Gynecol 97:911, 2001

Alfirevic Z, Luckas M, Walkinshaw SA, et al: A randomized comparison between amniotic fluid index and maximum pool depth in the monitoring of postterm pregnancy. Br J Obstet Gynaecol 104:207, 1997

American College of Obstetricians and Gynecologists: Management of postterm pregnancy. Practice Bulletin No. 55, September 2004, Reaffirmed 2011

American College of Obstetricians and Gynecologists: Amnioinfusion does not prevent meconium aspiration syndrome. Committee Opinion No. 346, October 2006, Reaffirmed 2012

American College of Obstetricians and Gynecologists: Definition of term pregnancy. Committee Opinion No. 579, November 2013a

American College of Obstetricians and Gynecologists: Fetal macrosomia. Practice Bulletin No. 22, November 2000, Reaffirmed 2013b

American College of Obstetrics and Gynecologists: Management of delivery of a newborn with meconium-stained amniotic fluid. Committee Opinion No. 379, September 2007, Reaffirmed 2013c

Amersi S, Grimes DA: The case against using ordinal numbers for gestational age. Obstet Gynecol 91:623, 1998

Arrowsmith S, Wray S, Quenby S: Maternal obesity and labour complications following induction of labour in prolonged pregnancy. BJOG 118(5):578, 2011

Bakketeig LS, Bergsjø P: Post-term pregnancy: magnitude of the problem. In Chalmers I, Enkin M, Keirse M (eds): Effective Care in Pregnancy and Childbirth. Oxford, Oxford University Press, 1991, p 765

Bennett KA, Crane JM, O'Shea P, et al: First trimester ultrasound screening is effective in reducing postterm labor induction rates: a randomized controlled trial. Am J Obstet Gynecol 190:1077, 2004

Blondel B, Morin I, Platt RW, et al: Algorithms for combining menstrual and ultrasound estimates of gestational age: consequences for rates of preterm and postterm birth. Br J Obstet Gynaecol 109:718, 2002

Boulvain M, Irion O, Marcoux S, et al: Sweeping of the membranes to prevent post-term pregnancy and to induce labour: a systematic review. Br J Obstet Gynaecol 106:481, 1999

Boyce A, Magaux MJ, Schwartz D: Classical and "true" gestational post maturity. Am J Obstet Gynecol 125:911, 1976

Caughey AB, Nicholson JM, Washington AE: First- vs second-trimester ultrasound: the effect on pregnancy dating and perinatal outcomes. Am J Obstet Gynecol 198(6):703.e1, 2008

Caughey AB, Stotland NE, Washington AE, et al: Who is at risk for prolonged and postterm pregnancy? Am J Obstet Gynecol 200(6):683.e1, 2009

Cheng YW, Nicholson JM, Nakagawa S, et al: Perinatal outcomes in low-risk term pregnancies: do they differ by week of gestation? Am J Obstet Gynecol 199(4):370.e1, 2008

Clausson B, Cnattingus S, Axelsson O: Outcomes of postterm births: the role of fetal growth restriction and malformations. Obstet Gynecol 94:758, 1999

Cleary-Goldman J, Bettes B, Robinon JN, et al: Postterm pregnancy: practice patterns of contemporary obstetricians and gynecologists. Am J Perinatol 23:15, 2006

Clement D, Schifrin BS, Kates RB: Acute oligohydramnios in postdate pregnancy. Am J Obstet Gynecol 157:884, 1987

Clifford SH: Postmaturity with placental dysfunction. Clinical syndromes and pathologic findings. J Pediatr 44:1, 1954

Divon MY, Feldman-Leidner N: Postdates and antenatal testing. Semin Perinatol 32(4):295, 2008

Divon MY, Haglund B, Nisell H, et al: Fetal and neonatal mortality in the postterm pregnancy: the impact of gestational age and fetal growth restriction. Am J Obstet Gynecol 178:726, 1998

Fasset MJ, Wing DA: Uterine activity after oral mifepristone administration in human pregnancies beyond 41 weeks' gestation. Gynecol Obstet Invest 65(2):112, 2008

Fischer RL, McDonnell M, Bianculli KW, et al: Amniotic fluid volume estimation in the postdate pregnancy: a comparison of techniques. Obstet Gynecol 81:698, 1993

Fraser WD, Hofmeyr J, Lede R, et al: Amnioinfusion for the prevention of the meconium aspiration syndrome. New Engl J Med 353:909, 2005

Gardener H, Spiegelman D, Buka SL: Perinatal and neonatal risk factors for autism: a comprehensive meta-analysis. Pediatrics 128:344, 2011

Gardner M, Rouse D, Goldenberg R, et al: Cost comparison of induction of labor at 41 weeks versus expectant management in the postterm pregnancy. Am J Obstet Gynecol 174:351, 1996

Gulmezoglu AM, Crowther CA, Middleton P: Induction of labour for improving birth outcomes for women at or beyond term. Cochrane Database System Rev 4:CD004945, 2006

Hannah ME, Hannah WJ, Hellman J, et al: Induction of labor as compared with serial antenatal monitoring in post-term pregnancy. N Engl J Med 326:1587, 1992

Harrington DJ, MacKenzie IZ, Thompson K, et al: Does a first trimester data scan using crown rump length measurement reduce the rate of induction of labour for prolonged pregnancy? BJOG 113:171, 2006

Harris BA Jr, Huddleston JF, Sutliff G, et al: The unfavorable cervix in prolonged pregnancy. Obstet Gynecol 62:171, 1983

Heimstad R, Skogvoll E, Mattsson LK, et al: Induction of labor or serial antenatal fetal monitoring in postterm pregnancy: a randomized controlled trial. Obstet Gynecol 109:609, 2007

Hendricks CH: Patterns of fetal and placental growth: the second half of pregnancy. Obstet Gynecol 24:357, 1964

Hill MJ, McWilliams GC, Garcia-Sur, et al: The effect of membrane sweeping on prelabor rupture of membranes: a randomized controlled trial. Obstet Gynecol 111(6):1313, 2008

Jazayeri A, Tsibris JC, Spellacy WN: Elevated umbilical cord plasma erythropoietin levels in prolonged pregnancies. Obstet Gynecol 92:61, 1998

Joseph KS, Huang L, Liu S, et al: Reconciling the high rates of preterm and postterm birth in the United States. Obstet Gynecol 109(4):798, 2007

Kashanian M, Aktarian A, Baradaron H, et al: Effect of membrane sweeping at term pregnancy on duration of pregnancy and labor induction: a randomized trial. Gynecol Obstet Invest 62:41, 2006

Larsen LG, Clausen HV, Andersen B, et al: A stereologic study of postmature placentas fixed by dual perfusion. Am J Obstet Gynecol 172:500, 1995

Laursen M, Bille C, Olesen AW, et al: Genetic influence on prolonged gestation: a population-based Danish twin study. Am J Obstet Gynecol 190:489, 2004

Leveno KJ, Quirk JG, Cunningham FG, et al: Prolonged pregnancy, I. Observations concerning the causes of fetal distress. Am J Obstet Gynecol 150:465, 1984

Lindell A: Prolonged pregnancy. Acta Obstet Gynecol Scand 35:136, 1956

Link G, Clark KE, Lang U: Umbilical blood flow during pregnancy: evidence for decreasing placental perfusion. Am J Obstet Gynecol 196(5)489.e1, 2007

MacDonald PC, Siiteri PK: Origin of estrogen in women pregnant with an anencephalic fetus. J Clin Invest 44:465, 1965

MacDorman MF, Kirmeyer S: Fetal and perinatal mortality, United States, 2005. Natl Vital Stat Rep 57(8):1, 2009

Martin JA, Hamilton BE, Sutton PD, et al: Births: final data for 2009. Natl Vital Stat Rep 60(1):1, 2011

Mogren I, Stenlund H, Högberg U: Recurrence of prolonged pregnancy. Int J Epidemiol 28:253, 1999

Moster D, Wilcox AJ, Vollset SE, et al: Cerebral palsy among term and postterm births. JAMA 304(9):976, 2010

Mozurkewich E, Chilimigras J, Koepke E, et al: Indications for induction of labour: a best-evidence review. BJOG 116(5):626, 2009

Munster K, Schmidt L, Helm P: Length and variation in the menstrual cycle—a cross-sectional study from a Danish county. Br J Obstet Gynaecol 99:422, 1992

Nahum GG, Stanislaw H, Huffaker BJ: Fetal weight gain at term: linear with minimal dependence on maternal obesity. Am J Obstet Gynecol 172:1387, 1995

National Institute of Child Health and Human Development Network of Maternal–Fetal Medicine Units: A clinical trial of induction of labor versus expectant management in postterm pregnancy. Am J Obstet Gynecol 170:716, 1994

Olesen AW, Westergaard JG, Olsen J: Perinatal and maternal complications related to postterm delivery: a national register-based study, 1978–1993. Am J Obstet Gynecol 189:227, 2003

Olesen AW, Westergaard JG, Olsen J: Prenatal risk indicators of a prolonged pregnancy. The Danish Birth Cohort 1998–2001. Acta Obstet Gynecol Scand 85:1338, 2006

Oz AU, Holub B, Mendilcioglu I, et al: Renal artery Doppler investigation of the etiology of oligohydramnios in postterm pregnancy. Obstet Gynecol 100:715, 2002

Perlman JM, Wyllie J, Kattwinkel J, et al: Neonatal resuscitation: 2010 International Consensus on Cardiopulmonary Resuscitation and emergency Cardiovascular Care Science with Treatment Recommendations. Pediatrics 126:e1319, 2010

Rushton DI: Pathology of placenta. In Wigglesworth JS, Singer DB (eds): Textbook of Fetal and Perinatal Pathology. Boston, Blackwell, 1991, p 171

Schaffer L, Burkhardt T, Zimmerman R, et al: Nuchal cords in term and postterm deliveries—do we need to know? Obstet Gynecol 106:23, 2005

Shime J, Gare DJ, Andrews J, et al: Prolonged pregnancy: surveillance of the fetus and the neonate and the course of labor and delivery. Am J Obstet Gynecol 148:547, 1984

Shin KS, Brubaker KL, Ackerson LM: Risk of cesarean delivery in nulliparous women at greater than 41 weeks' gestational age with an unengaged vertex. Am J Obstet Gynecol 190:129, 2004

Smith GC: Life-table analysis of the risk of perinatal death at term and post term in singleton pregnancies. Am J Obstet Gynecol 184:489, 2001

Smith SC, Baker PN: Placental apoptosis is increased in postterm pregnancies. Br J Obstet Gynaecol 106:861, 1999

Torricelli M, Novembri R, Conti N, et al: Correlation with kisspeptin in postterm pregnancy and apoptosis. Reprod Sci 19(10):1133, 2012

Trimmer KJ, Leveno KJ, Peters MT, et al: Observation on the cause of oligohydramnios in prolonged pregnancy. Am J Obstet Gynecol 163:1900, 1990

Usher RH, Boyd ME, McLean FH, et al: Assessment of fetal risk in postdate pregnancies. Am J Obstet Gynecol 158:259, 1988

Vankayalapati P, Sethna F, Roberts N, et al: Ultrasound assessment of cervical length in prolonged pregnancy: prediction of spontaneous onset of labor and successful vaginal delivery. Ultrasound Obstet Gynecol 31(3):328, 2008

Walsh JM, Kandamany N, Shuibhne NN, et al: Neonatal brachial plexus injury: comparison of incidence and antecedents between 2 decades. Am J Obstet Gynecol 204:324, 2011.

Wenstrom KD, Parsons MT: The prevention of meconium aspiration in labor using amnioinfusion. Obstet Gynecol 73:647, 1989

Wingate MS, Alexander GR, Buekens, et al: Comparison of gestational age classifications: date of last menstrual period vs clinical estimate. Ann Epidemiol 17(6):425, 2007

Wong SF, Hui SK, Choi H, et al: Does sweeping of membranes beyond 40 weeks reduce the need for formal induction of labour? Br J Obstet Gynaecol 109:632, 2002

Yang S, Platt RW, Kramer MS: Variation in child cognitive ability by week of gestation among healthy term births. Am J Epidemiol 171:399, 2010

Yang SH, Roh CR, Kim JH: Transvaginal ultrasonography for cervical assessment before induction of labor. Obstet Gynecol Surv 59:577, 2004

Zhang X, Joseph KS, Kramer MS: Decreased term and postterm birthweight in the United States: impact of labor induction. Am J Obstet Gynecol 203:124.e1, 2010

CHAPTER 44

Fetal-Growth Disorders

Nearly 20 percent of the almost 4 million infants born in the United States are at the low and high extremes of fetal growth. In 2010, 8.2 percent of infants weighed < 2500 g at birth, whereas 7.6 percent weighed > 4000 g. And although most low-birthweight infants are born preterm, approximately 3 percent are term. The proportion of infants with birthweight < 2500 g has increased by more than 20 percent since 1984, and at the same time, the incidence of birthweight > 4000 g continues to decline (Martin, 2012). This shift away from the upper extreme is difficult to explain because it coincides with the epidemic prevalence of obesity (Morisaki, 2013).

FETAL GROWTH

Human fetal growth is characterized by sequential patterns of tissue and organ growth, differentiation, and maturation. However, the "obstetrical dilemma" postulates a conflict between the need to walk upright—requiring a narrow pelvis—and the need to think—requiring a large brain, and thus a large head. Some have speculated that there may be evolutionary pressure to restrict growth late in pregnancy (Dunsworth, 2012; Espinoza, 2012). Thus, the ability to *growth restrict* may be adaptive rather than pathological.

Fetal growth has been divided into three phases. The initial phase of hyperplasia occurs in the first 16 weeks and is characterized by a rapid increase in cell number. The second phase, which extends up to 32 weeks' gestation, includes both cellular hyperplasia and hypertrophy. After 32 weeks, fetal growth is by cellular hypertrophy, and it is during this phase that most fetal fat and glycogen are accumulated. The corresponding fetal-growth rates during these three phases are 5 g/day at 15 weeks' gestation, 15 to 20 g/day at 24 weeks, and 30 to 35 g/day at 34 weeks (Williams, 1982). As shown in Figure 44-1, there is considerable biological variation in the velocity of fetal growth.

Fetal development is determined by maternal provision of substrate, placental transfer of these substrates, and fetal growth potential governed by the genome. However, the precise cellular and molecular mechanisms by which normal fetal growth ensues are incompletely understood. That said, there is considerable evidence that insulin and insulin-like growth factors, particularly insulin-like growth factor-I (IGF-I), have an important role in regulation of fetal growth and weight gain (Luo, 2012; Murray, 2013). These growth factors are produced by virtually all fetal organs and are potent stimulators of cell division and differentiation.

Other hormones implicated in fetal growth have been identified in recent years, particularly hormones derived from adipose tissue. These hormones are known broadly as *adipokines* and include leptin, the protein product of the *obesity gene*. Fetal leptin concentrations increase during gestation, and they correlate with birthweight (Forhead, 2009; Karakosta, 2011). This relationship, however, is controversial in growth-restricted fetuses (Kyriakakou, 2008; Mise, 2007). Other adipokines under investigation include adiponectin, ghrelin, follistatin, resistin, visfatin, vaspin, omentin-1, apelin, and chemerin. Data for these adipokines are often conflicting, and their roles in normal and disordered fetal growth are still being elucidated (Chap. 48, p. 961).

Fetal growth is also dependent on an adequate supply of nutrients. As discussed in Chapter 4 (p. 53), glucose transfer has been extensively studied during pregnancy. Both excessive and diminished maternal glucose availability affect fetal growth. Reducing maternal glucose levels may result in a lower

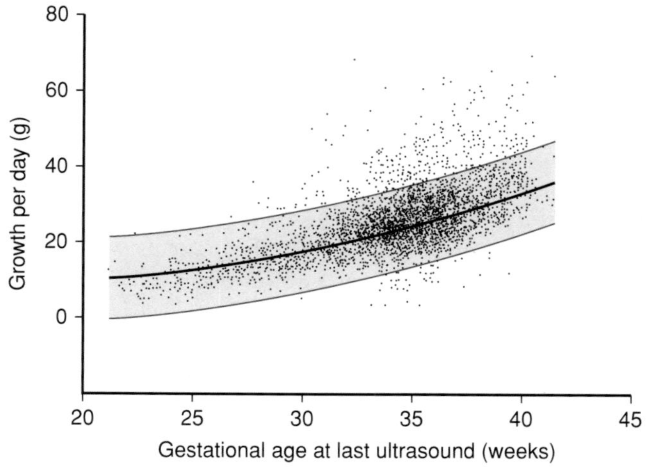

FIGURE 44-1 Increments in fetal weight gain in grams per day from 24 to 42 weeks' gestation. The black line represents the mean and the outer blue lines depict ±2 standard deviations. Data from pregnancies managed at Parkland Hospital. (Image courtesy of Dr. Don McIntire.)

birthweight. Still, growth-restricted neonates do not typically show pathologically low glucose concentrations in their cord blood (Pardi, 2006). Fetal-growth restriction in response to glucose deprivation generally results only after long-term severe maternal caloric deprivation (Lechtig, 1975).

Excessive glycemia produces macrosomia. Varying levels of glucose affect fetal growth via insulin and its associated insulin-like growth factors discussed earlier. The Hyperglycemia and Adverse Pregnancy Outcomes (HAPO) Study Cooperative Research Group (2008) found that elevated cord C-peptide levels, which reflect fetal hyperinsulinemia, have been associated with increased birthweight. This relationship was noted even in women with maternal glucose levels below the threshold for diabetes. Overgrowth does occur in the fetuses of euglycemic women. Its etiology is thus likely more complicated than a paradigm of dysregulated glucose metabolism resulting in fetal hyperinsulinemia (Catalano, 2011).

Excessive transfer of lipids to the fetus has also been postulated to result in fetal overgrowth (Higa, 2013). Free or nonesterified fatty acids in maternal plasma may be transferred to the fetus via facilitated diffusion or after liberation of fatty acids from triglycerides by trophoblastic lipases (Gil-Sánchez, 2012). Generally speaking, lipolytic activity is increased in pregnancy, and fatty acids have been reported to be increased in nonobese women during the third trimester (Diderholm, 2005). In obese women without diabetes who were fed a controlled diet, neonatal adiposity was strongly linked both with fasting triglyceride levels in early pregnancy and with free fatty acid levels at 26 to 28 weeks' gestation (Harmon, 2011). Other studies have correlated maternal triglyceride levels with birthweight in both early and late pregnancy (Di Cianni, 2005; Vrijkotte, 2011). Overgrown infants have higher placental levels of certain fatty acids, particularly omega-3, and this has been associated with increased trophoblastic lipase expression (Varastehpour, 2006). Conversely, growth restriction in the third trimester has been associated with decreased maternal lipolysis (Diderholm, 2006). This may be related to dysregulation of the triglyceride lipase gene family, which has been reported in placentas from pregnancies complicated by fetal-growth restriction (Gauster, 2007).

Amino acids undergo active transport from maternal blood to the fetus, which explains the normally higher fetal concentrations. This concentration differential is decreased in growth restriction because of lower fetal amino acid levels and higher maternal amino acid concentrations (Cetin, 1996). The etiology of this altered ratio is uncertain, but there are multiple points at which dysregulation can occur. Amino acids that reach the fetus must first cross the microvillus membrane at the maternal interface, traverse the trophoblastic cell, and finally cross the basal membrane into fetal blood (Chap. 5, p. 92). This process is incompletely understood, particularly with respect to trophoblast metabolism of amino acids and export mechanisms from the trophoblast to the fetus. Jansson and colleagues (2013) have linked expression and activity of particular amino-acid transporters at the microvillous membrane with increasing birthweight and maternal body mass index (BMI). Expression of particular amino acid efflux transporters has been positively correlated with multiple measures of fetal and neonatal growth (Cleal, 2011).

Normal Birthweight

Normative data for fetal growth based on birthweight vary with ethnicity and geographic region. For example, infants born to women who reside at high altitudes are smaller than those born at sea level. Term infants average 3400 g at sea level, 3200 g at 5000 feet, and 2900 g at 10,000 feet. Accordingly, researchers have developed fetal-growth curves using various populations and geographic locations throughout the United States (Brenner, 1976; Ott, 1993; Overpeck, 1999; Williams, 1975). Because these curves are based on specific ethnic or regional groups, they are not representative of the entire population.

To address this, data such as those shown in Table 44-1 were derived on a nationwide basis in both the United States and Canada (Alexander, 1996; Kramer, 2001). Data from more than 3.1 million mothers with singleton liveborn infants in the United States during 1991 were used to derive the growth curve by Alexander and colleagues, colored red in Figure 44-2. Also shown, the previously published regional fetal-growth curve data in general underestimated birthweights compared with national data. Importantly, there are significant ethnic and racial variations in neonatal mortality rates within the national neonatal mortality rate and within national birthweight and gestational age categories (Alexander, 1999, 2003).

The work of Alexander and associates (1996) is most accurately termed a population *reference*, rather than a *standard*. Iams (2010) emphasizes the problems that result from blending a population reference for fetal growth with a fetal-growth standard. A population reference incorporates pregnancies of varying risks, along with the resulting outcomes, both normal and abnormal. In contrast, a *standard* incorporates normal pregnancies with normal outcomes. Because population *references* include preterm births, which are more likely to be growth restricted, it has been argued that the associated birthweight data underestimate deficient fetal growth (Mayer, 2013; Zhang, 2010). That said, there is not a widely accepted *standard* for the United States.

TABLE 44-1. Smoothed Percentiles of Birthweight (g) for Gestational Age in the United States Based on 3,134,879 Singleton Live Births

	Percentile				
Age (wk)	5th	10th	50th	90th	95th
20	249	275	412	772	912
21	280	314	433	790	957
22	330	376	496	826	1023
23	385	440	582	882	1107
24	435	498	674	977	1223
25	480	558	779	1138	1397
26	529	625	899	1362	1640
27	591	702	1035	1635	1927
28	670	798	1196	1977	2237
29	772	925	1394	2361	2553
30	910	1085	1637	2710	2847
31	1088	1278	1918	2986	3108
32	1294	1495	2203	3200	3338
33	1513	1725	2458	3370	3536
34	1735	1950	2667	3502	3697
35	1950	2159	2831	3596	3812
36	2156	2354	2974	3668	3888
37	2357	2541	3117	3755	3956
38	2543	2714	3263	3867	4027
39	2685	2852	3400	3980	4107
40	2761	2929	3495	4060	4185
41	2777	2948	3527	4094	4217
42	2764	2935	3522	4098	4213
43	2741	2907	3505	4096	4178
44	2724	2885	3491	4096	4122

From Alexander, 1996, with permission.

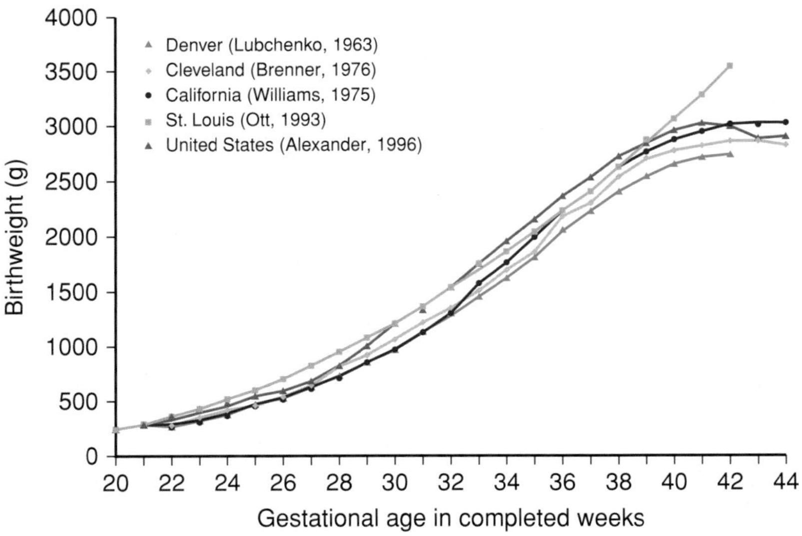

FIGURE 44-2 Comparison of fetal-growth curves for infants born in different regions of the United States and compared with those of the nation at large. (Modified from Alexander, 1996.)

Fetal Growth versus Birthweight

Most of what is known regarding normal and abnormal human fetal growth is actually based on birthweights that are assembled as references for fetal growth at particular gestational ages. This is problematic, however, because birthweight does not define the *rate* of fetal growth. Indeed, such birthweight curves reveal compromised growth only at the extreme of impaired growth. Thus, they cannot be used to identify the fetus who fails to achieve an expected size but whose birthweight is above the 10th percentile. For example, a fetus with a birthweight in the 40th percentile may not have achieved its genomic growth potential for a birthweight in the 80th percentile. The rate or *velocity* of fetal growth can be estimated by serial sonographic anthropometry. For example, Milovanovic (2012) demonstrated that the growth rate of intrinsically small-for-gestational age newborns approximates that of appropriate-for-gestational age neonates. Diminished growth velocity has been linked to perinatal morbidity and adverse postnatal metabolic changes that are independent of birthweight (Beltrand, 2008; Owen, 1997, 1998). Conversely, an excessive fetal-growth velocity, particularly of the abdominal circumference—which may be correlated with increased hepatic blood flow—is associated with an overgrown neonate. This is especially true when detected earlier in pregnancy (Ebbing, 2011; Kessler, 2011; Mulder, 2010).

FETAL-GROWTH RESTRICTION

Definition

Low-birthweight newborns who are small for gestational age are often designated as having *fetal-growth restriction.* In 1963, Lubchenco and coworkers published detailed comparisons of gestational ages with birthweights to derive norms for expected fetal size at a given gestational week. Battaglia and Lubchenco (1967) then classified *small-for-gestational-age (SGA)* neonates as those whose weights were below the 10th percentile for their gestational age. Such infants were shown to be at increased risk for neonatal death. For example, the neonatal mortality rate of SGA infants born at 38 weeks was 1 percent compared with 0.2 percent in those with appropriate birthweights.

Many infants with birthweights < 10th percentile, however, are not pathologically growth restricted, but are small simply because of normal biological factors. As many as 25 to 60 percent of SGA infants are thought to be appropriately grown when maternal ethnic group, parity, weight, and height are considered (Gardosi, 1992; Manning, 1991). These small but normal infants also do not show evidence of the postnatal metabolic derangements commonly associated with deficient fetal growth. Moreover, intrinsically SGA infants remain significantly smaller during surveillance to 2 years compared with appropriate-for-gestational age neonates, but they do not show differences in measures of metabolic risk (Milovanovic, 2012).

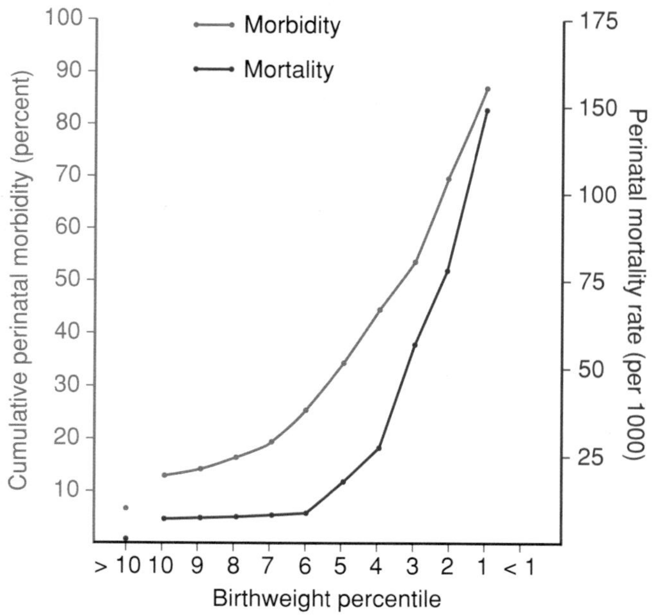

FIGURE 44-3 Relationship between birthweight percentile and perinatal mortality and morbidity rates in 1560 small-for-gestational age fetuses. A progressive increase in both mortality and morbidity rates is observed as birthweight percentile falls. (Data from Manning, 1995.)

Because of these disparities, other classifications have been developed. Seeds (1984) suggested a definition based on birthweight < 5th percentile. Usher and McLean (1969) suggested that fetal-growth standards should be based on mean weights-for-age, with normal limits defined by ±2 standard deviations. This definition would limit SGA infants to 3 percent of births instead of 10 percent. In a population-based analysis of 122,754 births at Parkland Hospital, McIntire and colleagues (1999) showed this definition to be clinically meaningful. Also, as shown in Figure 44-3, most adverse outcomes are in infants < 3rd percentile.

More recently, individual or customized fetal-growth potential has been proposed in place of a population-based cutoff. In this model, a fetus that deviates from its individual optimal size at a given gestational age is considered either overgrown or growth restricted (Bukowski, 2008). Such optimal projections are based on maternal race or ethnicity. However, the superiority of customized growth curves has not been established (Hutcheon, 2011a,b; Larkin, 2012; Zhang, 2011).

Symmetrical versus Asymmetrical Growth Restriction

Campbell and Thoms (1977) described the use of the sonographically determined *head-to-abdomen circumference ratio (HC/AC)* to differentiate growth-restricted fetuses. Those who were *symmetrical* were proportionately small, and those who were *asymmetrical* had disproportionately lagging abdominal growth. Furthermore, the onset or etiology of a particular fetal insult has been hypothetically linked to either type of growth restriction. In the instance of *symmetrical growth restriction*, an early insult could result in a relative decrease in cell number and size. For example, global insults such as from chemical exposure, viral infection, or cellular maldevelopment with aneuploidy may cause a proportionate reduction of both head and body size. *Asymmetrical growth restriction* might follow a late pregnancy insult such as placental insufficiency from hypertension. Resultant diminished glucose transfer and hepatic storage would primarily affect cell size and not number, and fetal abdominal circumference—which reflects liver size—would be reduced. Such somatic-growth restriction is proposed to result from preferential shunting of oxygen and nutrients to the brain. This allows normal brain and head growth, that is—*brain sparing*. Accordingly, the ratio of brain weight to liver weight during the last 12 weeks—usually about 3 to 1—may be increased to 5 to 1 or more in severely growth-restricted infants.

Because of brain-sparing effects, asymmetrical fetuses were thought to be preferentially protected from the full effects of growth restriction. Considerable evidence has since accrued that fetal-growth patterns are much more complex. For example, Nicolaides and coworkers (1991) observed that fetuses with aneuploidy typically had disproportionately large head sizes and thus were *asymmetrically* growth restricted, which was contrary to contemporaneous thinking. Moreover, most preterm infants with growth restriction due to preeclampsia and associated uteroplacental insufficiency were found to have more symmetrical growth impairment—again, a departure from accepted principles (Salafia, 1995).

More evidence of the complexity of growth patterns was presented by Dashe and associates (2000). These investigators analyzed 8722 consecutive liveborn singletons who had undergone sonographic examination within 4 weeks of delivery. Although only 20 percent of growth-restricted fetuses demonstrated sonographic head-to-abdomen asymmetry, these fetuses were at increased risk for intrapartum and neonatal complications. Symmetrically growth-restricted fetuses were not at increased risk for adverse outcomes compared with those appropriately grown. These investigators concluded that asymmetrical fetal-growth restriction represented significantly disordered growth, whereas symmetrical growth restriction more likely represented normal, genetically determined small stature.

Finally, data from Holland further challenge the concept of "brain sparing." Roza and associates (2008) provided surveillance of 935 Rotterdam toddlers enrolled between 2003 and 2007 in the Generation R Study. Using the Child Behavior Checklist at age 18 months, they found that infants with circulatory redistribution—*brain sparing*—had a higher incidence of behavioral problems. In another study, evidence of brain sparing was found in half of 62 growth-restricted fetuses with birthweight < 10th percentile and who showed abnormal umbilical artery Doppler flow studies (Figueras, 2011a). Compared with controls, these neonates had significantly lower neurobehavioral scores in multiple areas, suggesting profound brain injury.

Placental Abnormalities

Fetal-growth restriction was included by Brosens and colleagues (2011) as one of the "great obstetrical syndromes" associated with defects in early placentation. Rogers and coworkers (1999) had observed that implantation site disorders such as incomplete trophoblastic invasion are associated with both fetal-growth restriction and hypertensive disorders. They concluded that implantation site disorders may be both a cause and consequence of hypoperfusion at the placental site. These disorders ultimately lead to pregnancy complications such as fetal-growth restriction with or without maternal hypertension. This comports with the association of certain placental angiogenic factors with pregnancy hypertensive disorders (Chap. 40, p. 735). Thus, it may be that placentas from pregnancies complicated by hypertension elaborate these angiogenic factors in response to placental site hypoperfusion, whereas pregnancies complicated by fetal-growth restriction without hypertension do not (Jeyabalan, 2008).

Mechanisms leading to abnormal trophoblastic invasion are likely multifactorial, and both vascular and immunological etiologies have been proposed. Recently, *atrial natriuretic peptide converting enzyme*, also known as *corrin*, has been shown to play a critical role in trophoblastic invasion and remodeling of the uterine spiral arteries. These processes are impaired in corrin-deficient mice, which also develop evidence of preeclampsia. Moreover, mutations in the gene for corrin have also been reported in women with preeclampsia (Cui, 2012).

Notably, several immunological abnormalities have been associated with fetal-growth restriction. This raises the prospect of maternal rejection of the "paternal semiallograft." Rudzinski and colleagues (2013) studied C4d, a component of complement that is associated with humoral rejection of transplanted tissues. They found this to be highly associated with chronic villitis—88 percent of cases versus only 5 percent of controls—and with reduced placental weight. Greer and associates (2012) studied 10,204 placentas and reported that chronic villitis was associated with placental hypoperfusion, fetal acidemia, and fetal-growth restriction and its sequelae. Kovo and coworkers (2010) found that chronic villitis is more strongly associated with fetal-growth restriction than with preeclampsia. Redline (2007) described the findings of activated maternal lymphocytes among fetal trophoblast. However, this author notes uncertainty as to whether these pathological changes represent maternal immunological rejection.

Morbidity and Mortality

Perinatal Risk

As shown in Figure 44-3, fetal-growth restriction is associated with substantive perinatal morbidity and mortality rates. Rates of stillbirth, birth asphyxia, meconium aspiration, and neonatal hypoglycemia and hypothermia are all increased, as is the prevalence of abnormal neurological development (Jacobsson, 2008; Paz, 1995). This is true for both term and preterm growth-restricted infants (McIntire, 1999; Wu, 2006). Smulian and colleagues (2002) reported that SGA infants had a higher 1-year infant mortality rate compared with that of normally grown infants. Boulet and associates (2006) demonstrated that for a fetus at the 10th percentile, the risk of neonatal death is increased but varies with gestational age. Risk is increased threefold at 26 weeks' gestation compared with only a 1.13-fold increased risk at 40 weeks. More recently, in an analysis of 123,383 nonanomalous singleton live births, Chen and coworkers (2011) reported that SGA infants had a twofold risk for early and late neonatal death but not for postneonatal demise.

Long-Term Sequelae

Fetal Undergrowth. In his book *Fetal and Infant Origins of Adult Disease,* Barker (1992) hypothesized that adult mortality and morbidity are related to fetal and infant health. This includes both under- and overgrowth. In the context of fetal-growth restriction, there are numerous reports of a relationship between suboptimal fetal nutrition and an increased risk of subsequent adult hypertension, atherosclerosis, type 2 diabetes, and metabolic derangement (Gluckman, 2008). The degree to which low birthweight mediates adult disease is controversial. For example, it is unclear whether poor health in adulthood is mainly modulated by low birthweight, postnatal compensatory growth, or an interaction of the two (Crowther, 2008; Kerkhof, 2012; Leunissen, 2008; Nobili, 2008; Ong, 2007).

There is increasing evidence that fetal-growth restriction may affect organ development, particularly that of the heart. Individuals with low birthweight demonstrate cardiac structural changes and dysfunction persisting through childhood, adolescence, and adulthood. Crispi and coworkers (2012) studied 50 children aged between 3 and 6 years who were born small-for-gestational age at > 34 weeks and compared them with 100 normally grown children. The heart shape was altered in children born SGA. They had a more globular ventricle that resulted in systolic and diastolic dysfunction. Hietalampi and associates (2012) performed echocardiography in 418 adolescents at a mean age of 15 years and found that low birthweight was associated with increased left ventricular posterior wall thickness. Importantly, current weight and physical activity affected measurements. In another study, 102 adults previously born preterm at a mean gestational age of 30.3 weeks underwent cardiac magnetic resonance (MR) imaging. Their ventricular mass was increased compared with that of 132 adults who were delivered at term (Lewandowski, 2013). Adults previously born preterm also had persistent structural remodeling and had reduced systolic and diastolic function.

Deficient fetal growth is also associated with postnatal structural and functional renal changes. Ritz and colleagues (2011) reviewed the numerous studies associating low birthweight with disordered nephrogenesis, renal dysfunction, chronic kidney disease, and hypertension. They found that although a low nephron number is associated with hypertension in white individuals, this association does not hold true for blacks.

Fetal Overgrowth. On the other end of the spectrum, fetal overgrowth, particularly in women with diabetes and elevated cord blood levels of IGF-I, is associated with increased neonatal fat mass and morphological heart changes. Aman and coworkers (2011) reported interventricular septal hypertrophy in overgrown neonates of mothers with well-controlled diabetes in pregnancy. Garcia-Flores (2011) also reported increased fetal cardiac intraventricular septal thickness using sonography in women with well-controlled diabetes. Large-for-gestational age infants delivered of women without impaired glucose tolerance show higher insulin levels in childhood (Evagelidou, 2006). Not surprisingly, fetal overgrowth has been associated with development of the metabolic syndrome even in childhood (Boney, 2005).

Accelerated Lung Maturation

Numerous reports describe accelerated fetal pulmonary maturation in complicated pregnancies associated with growth restriction (Perelman, 1985). One possible explanation is that the fetus responds to a stressed environment by increasing adrenal glucocorticoid secretion, which leads to accelerated fetal lung maturation (Laatikainen, 1988). Although this concept pervades modern perinatal thinking, there is negligible evidence to support it.

To examine this hypothesis, Owen and associates (1990) analyzed perinatal outcomes in 178 women delivered because of hypertension. They compared these with outcomes in infants of 159 women delivered because of spontaneous preterm labor or ruptured membranes. They concluded that a "stressed" pregnancy did not confer an appreciable survival advantage. Similar findings were reported by Friedman and colleagues (1995) in women with severe preeclampsia. Two studies from Parkland Hospital also substantiate that the preterm infant accrues no apparent advantages from fetal-growth restriction (McIntire, 1999; Tyson, 1995).

Risk Factors and Etiologies

Risk factors for impaired fetal growth include potential abnormalities in the mother, fetus, and placenta. These three "compartments" are depicted in Figure 44-4. Some of these factors are known causes of fetal-growth restriction and may affect more than one compartment. For instance, infectious causes such as cytomegalovirus may affect the fetus directly. In contrast, bacterial infections such as tuberculosis may have significant maternal effects that lead to poor fetal growth. Malaria, a protozoal infection, possibly creates placental dysfunction (Umbers, 2011). Importantly, many causes of diminished fetal growth are prospectively considered risk factors, because impaired fetal growth is not consistent in all affected women.

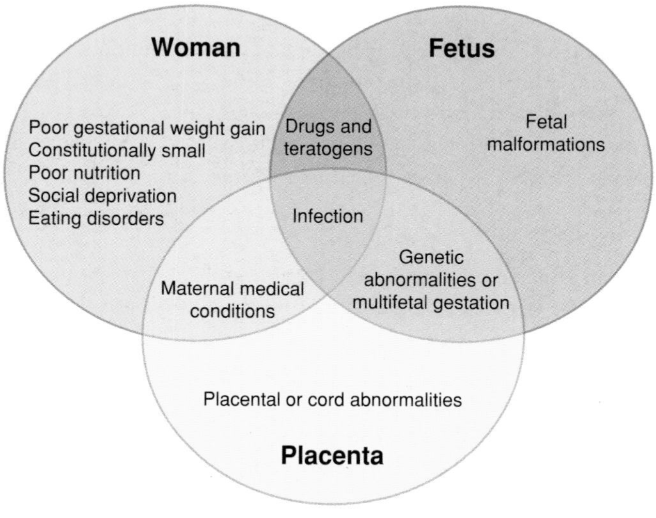

FIGURE 44-4 Risk factors and causes of impaired fetal growth centering on the mother, her fetus, and the placenta.

Constitutionally Small Mothers

It is axiomatic that small women typically have smaller newborns. If a woman begins pregnancy weighing less than 100 pounds, the risk of delivering an SGA infant is increased at least twofold (Simpson, 1975). As discussed subsequently, both prepregnancy weight and gestational weight gain modulate this risk. Durie and colleagues (2011) showed that the risk of delivering an SGA neonate was highest among underweight women who gained less weight than recommended by the Institute of Medicine (Chap. 9, p. 177). Also, both maternal and paternal size influences birthweight. In a Swedish study of 137,538 term singleton mother-father-child units, researchers estimated that the maternal and paternal birthweights explained 6 and 3 percent of variance in birthweight, respectively (Mattsson, 2013).

Gestational Weight Gain and Nutrition

In the woman of average or low BMI, poor weight gain throughout pregnancy may be associated with fetal-growth restriction (Rode, 2007). In the study by Durie cited above, gestational weight gain during the second and third trimesters that was less than that recommended by the Institute of Medicine was associated with SGA neonates in women of all weight categories except class II or III obesity. Conversely, excessive gestational weight gain was associated with an overgrown newborn in all weight categories.

As perhaps expected, eating disorders are associated with significantly increased risks of low birthweight and preterm birth (Pasternak, 2012). This is discussed further in Chapter 61 (p. 1211). Marked weight gain restriction after midpregnancy should not be encouraged even in obese women (Chap. 9, p. 177). Even so, it appears that food restriction to < 1500 kcal/day adversely affects fetal growth minimally (Lechtig, 1975). The best documented effect of famine on fetal growth was in the *Hunger Winter* of 1944 in Holland. For 6 months, the German Occupation army restricted dietary intake to 500 kcal/day for civilians, including pregnant women. This resulted in an average birthweight decline of only 250 g (Stein, 1975).

It is unclear whether undernourished women may benefit from micronutrient supplementation. In the study by the Supplementation with Multiple Micronutrients Intervention Trial (SUMMIT) Study Group (2008), almost 32,000 Indonesian women were randomized to receive micronutrient supplementation or only iron and folate tablets. Infants of those receiving the supplement had lower risks of early infant mortality and low birthweight and had improved childhood motor and cognitive abilities (Prado, 2012). Conversely, Liu and coworkers

(2013) randomized 18,775 nulliparous pregnant women to folic acid alone; folic acid and iron; or folic acid, iron, and 13 other micronutrients. Folic acid and iron with or without the additional micronutrients resulted in a 30-percent reduction in risk of third-trimester anemia. However, it did not affect other maternal or neonatal outcomes. The importance of antenatal vitamins and trace metals is further discussed in Chapter 9 (p. 179).

Social Deprivation

The effect of social deprivation on birthweight is interconnected to the influence of associated lifestyle factors such as smoking, alcohol or other substance abuse, and poor nutrition. Importantly, Coker and associates (2012) found that women screened during pregnancy for psychosocial risk factors had more appropriate interventions. These women were significantly less likely to deliver a low-birthweight infant and also had fewer preterm births and other pregnancy complications.

Women who are immigrants may be at particular risk in pregnancy. Poeran and colleagues (2013) studied 56,443 singleton pregnancies in Rotterdam between 2000 and 2007 and found that social deprivation was associated with adverse perinatal outcomes that included SGA infants among socially deprived women. However, a similar linkage was not noted in socially deprived women of non-Western origin. The effect of immigration, however, is complex and dependent on the population studied. A paradoxical relationship between pregnancy outcomes in foreign-born Latina women delivering in the United States compared with Latina women born in the United States has been described (Flores, 2012). In particular, foreign-born Latina women appear to have lower risks of preterm birth and SGA neonates.

Vascular Disease

Especially when complicated by superimposed preeclampsia, chronic vascular disease commonly causes growth restriction (Chap. 50, p. 1004). Preeclampsia may cause fetal-growth failure, which can be an indicator of its severity (Backes, 2011). In a study of more than 2000 women, vascular disease as evidenced by abnormal uterine artery Doppler velocimetry early in pregnancy was associated with increased rates of preeclampsia, SGA neonates, and delivery before 34 weeks (Groom, 2009). Roos-Hesselink and coworkers (2013) described pregnancy outcomes in women with heart disease, and only 25 of the 1321 women had ischemic heart disease, emphasizing its rareness. But these women had the worst outcomes, with significantly lower neonatal birthweights and the highest rates of preterm birth and perinatal mortality.

Renal Disease

Chronic renal insufficiency is frequently associated with underlying hypertension and vascular disease. Nephropathies are commonly accompanied by restricted fetal growth (Bramham, 2011; Cunningham, 1990; Vidaeff, 2008). These relationships are considered further in Chapter 53 (p. 1059).

Pregestational Diabetes

Fetal-growth restriction in women with diabetes may be related to congenital malformations or may follow substrate deprivation from advanced maternal vascular disease (Chap. 57, p. 1128). Also, the likelihood of restricted growth increases with development of nephropathy and proliferative retinopathy—especially in combination (Haeri, 2008). That said, the prevalence of serious vascular disease associated with diabetes in pregnancy is low, and the primary effect of overt diabetes, especially type 1, is fetal *overgrowth*. For example, Murphy and coworkers (2011) performed a prospective study of 682 consecutive pregnancies complicated by diabetes. Women with type 1 diabetes had significantly fewer of the traditional risk factors for fetal overgrowth, such as increased age, multiparity, and obesity. Yet, they were significantly more likely than women with type 2 diabetes to have a neonate weighing > 90th and 97.7th percentiles. Additionally, women with type 1 diabetes were significantly less likely to deliver an SGA newborn. Similarly, in a smaller study by Cyganek and colleagues (2011), the rate of macrosomia was higher among pregnancies complicated by type 1 diabetes. However, the rates of low birthweight were similar for those with type 1 and type 2 diabetes.

Chronic Hypoxia

Conditions associated with chronic uteroplacental hypoxia include preeclampsia, chronic hypertension, asthma, smoking, and high altitude. When exposed to a chronically hypoxic environment, some fetuses have significantly reduced birthweight. Gonzales and Tapia (2009) constructed growth charts based on 63,620 Peruvian live births between 26 and 42 weeks' gestation. They reported that mean birthweight was significantly decreased at higher altitudes compared with lower altitudes—3065 ± 475 g versus 3280 ± 525 grams. At low altitude, the rate of birthweight < 2500 g was 6.2 percent, and it was 9.2 percent at high altitude. In contrast, the rate of birthweight > 4000 g was 6.3 percent at low altitude and 1.6 percent at high altitude. As discussed in Chapter 49 (p. 985), severe hypoxia from maternal cyanotic heart disease frequently is associated with severely growth-restricted fetuses (Patton, 1990).

Anemia

In most cases, maternal anemia does not cause restricted fetal growth. Exceptions include sickle-cell disease and some other inherited anemias (Chakravarty, 2008; Tongsong, 2009). Conversely, curtailed maternal blood-volume expansion has been linked to fetal-growth restriction (Duvekot, 1995; Scholten, 2011). This is further discussed in Chapter 40 (p. 737).

Antiphospholipid Antibody Syndrome

Adverse obstetrical outcomes including fetal-growth restriction have been associated with three species of antiphospholipid antibodies: *anticardiolipin antibodies, lupus anticoagulant,* and *antibodies against beta-2-glycoprotein-I.* Mechanistically, a "two-hit" hypothesis suggests that initial endothelial damage is then followed by intervillous placental thrombosis. More specifically, oxidative damage to certain membrane proteins such as beta-2-glycoprotein I is followed by antiphospholipid antibody binding, which leads to immune complex formation and ultimately to thrombosis (Giannakopoulos, 2013). This syndrome is considered in detail in Chapters 52 (p. 1033) and

59 (p. 1173). Pregnancy outcomes in women with these antibodies may be poor and include early-onset preeclampsia and fetal demise (Levine, 2002). The primary autoantibody that predicts obstetrical antiphospholipid syndrome appears to be lupus anticoagulant (Lockshin, 2012).

Inherited Thrombophilias

Numerous investigators have evaluated the role of genetic polymorphisms in the mother or fetus and their relationship to growth restriction (Lockwood, 2002; Stonek, 2007). Most suggest that inherited thrombophilias are not a significant factor in fetal-growth restriction (Infante-Rivard, 2002; Rodger, 2008). Facco and colleagues (2009) attribute positive associations primarily to publication bias.

Infertility

Pregnancies in women with prior infertility with or without infertility treatment have an increased risk of SGA newborns (Zhu, 2007). Kondapalli and Perales-Puchalt (2013) have recently reviewed possible links between low birthweight and infertility with its various interventions. They concluded that the association remains unexplained.

Placental and Cord Abnormalities

Several placental abnormalities may cause poor fetal growth. These are discussed further throughout Chapter 6 and include chronic placental abruption, extensive infarction, chorioangioma, marginal or velamentous cord insertion, placenta previa, and umbilical artery thrombosis. Growth failure in these cases is presumed secondary to uteroplacental insufficiency.

Abnormal placental implantation leading to endothelial dysfunction may also result in limited fetal growth (Brosens, 2011). This pathology has been implicated in pregnancies complicated by preeclampsia as discussed in Chapter 40 (p. 732).

If the placenta is implanted outside the uterus, the fetus is usually growth restricted (Chap. 19, p. 388). Also, some uterine malformations have been linked to impaired fetal growth (Chap. 3, p. 40).

Multiple Fetuses

As shown in Figure 44-5, pregnancy with two or more fetuses is more likely to be complicated by diminished growth of one or more fetuses compared with that with normal singletons (Chap. 45, p. 899).

Drugs with Teratogenic and Fetal Effects

Several drugs and chemicals are capable of limiting fetal growth. Some are teratogenic and affect the fetus before organogenesis is complete. Some exert—or continue to exert—fetal effects after embryogenesis ends at 8 weeks. Many of these are considered in detail in Chapter 12, and some examples include anticonvulsants and antineoplastic agents. Some immunosuppressive drugs used for organ transplantation maintenance are also implicated in poor fetal growth (Mastrobattista, 2008). In addition, cigarette smoking, opiates and related drugs, alcohol, and cocaine may cause growth

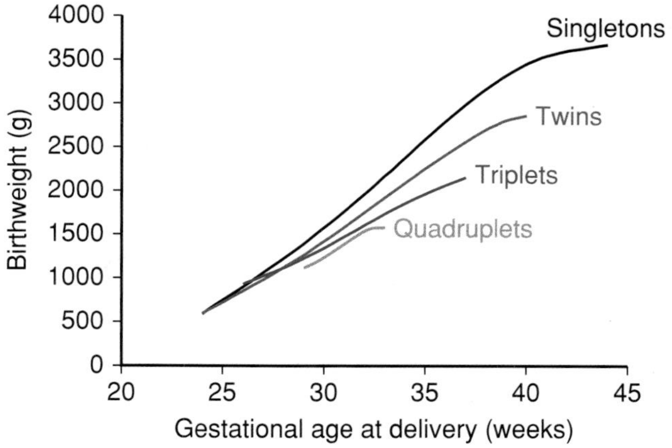

FIGURE 44-5 Birthweight and gestational age relationships in multifetal gestations delivered at Parkland Hospital without malformations. (Data courtesy of Dr. Don McIntire.)

restriction, either primarily or by decreasing maternal food intake. There is a possible link with caffeine use throughout pregnancy and fetal-growth restriction (CARE Study Group, 2008). According to the American College of Obstetricians and Gynecologists (2013c), however, this relationship remains speculative (Chap. 9, p. 187).

Maternal and Fetal Infections

Viral, bacterial, protozoan, and spirochetal infections have been implicated in up to 5 percent of fetal-growth restriction cases and are discussed throughout Chapters 64 and 65. The best known of these are *rubella* and *cytomegalovirus infection*. Both promote calcifications in the fetus that are associated with cell death, and infection earlier in pregnancy correlates with worse outcomes. Picone and associates (2013) described 238 primary cytomegalovirus infections and reported that no severe cases were observed when infection occurred after 14 weeks' gestation.

Tuberculosis and *syphilis* have both been associated with poor fetal growth. As discussed in Chapter 51 (p. 1020), both extrapulmonary and pulmonary tuberculosis have been linked with low birthweight (Jana, 1994, 1999). The etiology is uncertain. However, the adverse effect of tuberculosis on maternal health, compounded by effects of poor nutrition and poverty, is important (Jana, 2012). Congenital or transplacental tuberculosis is rare, whereas congenital syphilis is more common. Paradoxically, with syphilis, the placenta is almost always larger and heavier due to edema and perivascular inflammation. Congenital syphilis is also strongly linked with preterm birth and thus low-birthweight infants (Sheffield, 2002).

Toxoplasma gondii can also cause congenital infection, and Paquet and Yudin (2013) describe its classic association with fetal-growth restriction. Despite this, an analysis of 386 women who seroconverted during pregnancy from toxoplasma infection found no connection with low birthweight (Freeman, 2005). *Congenital malaria* has also been implicated, and malaria prophylaxis is associated with a decreased risk of low birthweight in Sub-Saharan Africa (Kayentao, 2013).

Congenital Malformations

In a study of more than 13,000 fetuses with major structural anomalies, 22 percent had accompanying growth restriction (Khoury, 1988). In their study of 115 pregnancies complicated by fetal gastroschisis, Tam Tam and coworkers (2011) identified low birthweights in 63 percent and fetal-growth restriction in 45 percent of affected newborns. As a general rule, the more severe the malformation, the more likely the fetus is to be SGA. This is especially evident in fetuses with chromosomal abnormalities or those with serious cardiovascular malformations.

Chromosomal Aneuploidies

Depending on which chromosome is redundant, there may be associated poor growth in fetuses with autosomal trisomies. For example, in *trisomy 21*, fetal-growth restriction is generally mild. By contrast, fetal growth in *trisomy 18* is virtually always significantly limited. Growth failure has been documented as early as the first trimester using crown-rump length (Baken, 2013). Bahado-Singh (1997) and Schemmer (1997) and their associates found that crown-rump length in fetuses with trisomy 18 and 13, unlike that with trisomy 21, was shorter than expected. By the second trimester, long-bone measurements typically are < 3rd percentile.

As discussed in Chapter 13 (p. 269), aneuploidic patches in the placenta—*confined placental mosaicism*—can cause placental insufficiency that may account for many previously unexplained growth-restricted fetuses (Wilkins-Haug, 2006). Although addition of an X chromosome in confined placental mosaicism can be associated with diminished fetal growth, this is not so with Klinefelter syndrome (47,XXY). Conversely, monosomy X or Turner syndrome has been associated with a low embryo volume during first-trimester sonography (Baken, 2013). This early finding manifests as growth restriction at delivery. Hagman and colleagues (2010) compared 494 children with monosomy X with normal girls and found a 6.6-fold increased risk for SGA in newborns with Turner syndrome.

First-trimester prenatal screening programs to identify women at risk for aneuploidy may incidentally identify pregnancies at risk for fetal-growth restriction unrelated to karyotype. In their analysis of 8012 women, Krantz and associates (2004) identified an increased risk for growth restriction in eukaryotic fetuses with extremely low free β-human chorionic gonadotropin (β-hCG) and pregnancy-associated plasma protein-A (PAPP-A) levels. From her review, Dugoff (2010) concluded that although most studies have found that a low PAPP-A level is strongly associated with poor fetal growth, studies of free β-hCG are conflicting. Second-trimester analytes, including elevated alpha-fetoprotein and inhibin A levels and low unconjugated serum estriol concentrations, are significantly associated with birthweight < 5th percentile. An even greater risk of poor growth has been associated with certain combinations of these analytes. Still, these markers are poor screening tools for complications such as fetal-growth restriction due to low sensitivity and positive predictive values (Dugoff, 2010). Nuchal translucency has also not been shown to be predictive of fetal-growth restriction. These markers are discussed further in Chapter 14 (p. 289).

Recognition of Fetal-Growth Restriction

Early establishment of gestational age, ascertainment of maternal weight gain, and careful measurement of uterine fundal growth throughout pregnancy will identify many cases of abnormal fetal growth in low-risk women. Risk factors, including a *previous growth-restricted fetus,* have an increased risk for recurrence of nearly 20 percent (Berghella, 2007). In women with risks, serial sonographic evaluation is considered. Although examination frequency varies depending on indications, an initial early dating examination followed by an examination at 32 to 34 weeks, or when otherwise clinically indicated, will identify many growth-restricted fetuses. Even so, *definitive diagnosis* frequently cannot be made until delivery.

Identification of the inappropriately growing fetus remains a challenge. There are, however, both simple clinical techniques and more complex technologies that may prove useful.

Uterine Fundal Height

According to a recent systematic review, insufficient evidence supports the utility of fundal height measurement to detect fetal-growth restriction (Robert Peter, 2012). Nonetheless, carefully performed serial fundal height measurements are recommended as a simple, safe, inexpensive, and reasonably accurate *screening* method to detect growth-restricted fetuses (Figueras, 2011b). As a screening tool, its principal drawback is imprecision (Jelks, 2007). For example, Sparks and coworkers (2011) reported sensitivities < 35 percent for detecting excessive or deficient fetal growth. Specificity, however, was reported to be > 90 percent.

The method used by most for fundal height measurement is described in Chapter 9 (p. 176). Between 18 and 30 weeks' gestation, the uterine fundal height in centimeters coincides within 2 weeks of gestational age. Thus, if the measurement is more than 2 to 3 cm from the expected height, inappropriate fetal growth is suspected.

Sonographic Measurements of Fetal Size

One argument in the debate regarding routine sonographic evaluation of all pregnancies is the potential for diagnosis of growth restriction. Typically, such routine screening incorporates an early initial sonographic examination—usually at 16 to 20 weeks' gestation, but increasingly in the first trimester—to establish gestational age and identify anomalies. Proponents of this view then repeat sonographic evaluation at 32 to 34 weeks to evaluate fetal growth (Chap. 10, p. 198). Although fetal-growth restriction can be detected during the first trimester, its detection using an initial sonogram from the second trimester is more likely to correspond to a birthweight that is small-for-gestational age (Baken, 2013; Mook-Kanamori, 2010; Tuuli, 2011). At Parkland Hospital, we provide midpregnancy sonographic screening examination of all pregnancies. Additional sonographic evaluations of fetal growth are performed as clinically indicated.

With sonography, the most common method for identifying poor fetal growth is estimation of weight using multiple fetal biometric measurements. Combining head, abdomen, and femur dimensions has been shown to optimize accuracy, whereas little incremental improvement is gained by adding other biometric

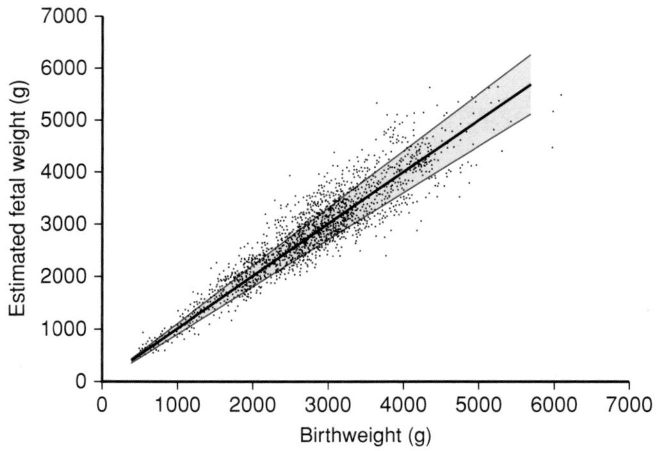

FIGURE 44-6 Correlation of sonographic fetal weight estimation using abdominal circumference (AC) and actual birthweight. Data from pregnancies managed at Parkland Hospital. (Image courtesy of Dr. Don McIntire.)

measurements (Platz, 2008). Of the dimensions, femur length measurement is technically the easiest and the most reproducible. Biparietal diameter and head circumference measurements are dependent on the plane of section and may also be affected by deformative pressures on the skull. Last, abdominal circumference measurements are more variable. However, these are most frequently abnormal with fetal-growth restriction because soft tissue predominates in this dimension (Fig. 44-6). Shown in Figure 44-7 is an example of a severely growth-restricted newborn.

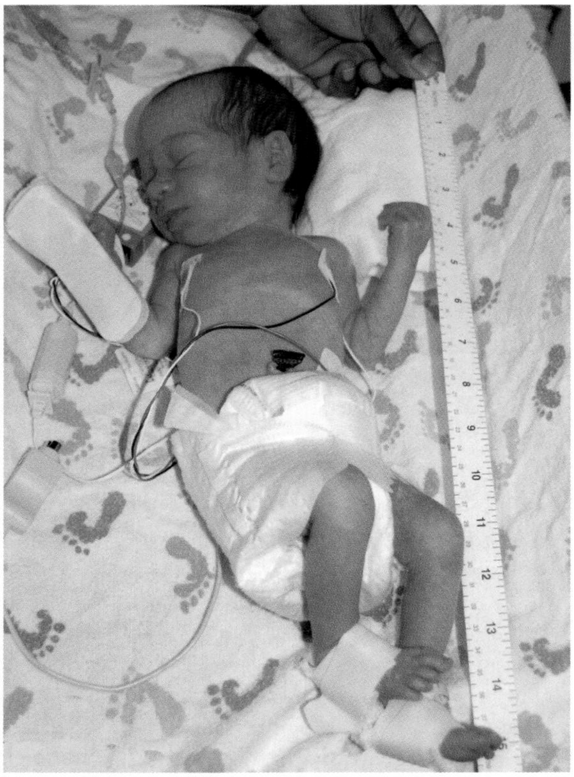

FIGURE 44-7 A 36-week newborn with severe fetal-growth restriction. (Photograph contributed by Dr. Roxane Holt.)

Some studies have reported a significant predictive value for small abdominal circumference with respect to lagging fetal growth. However, newer data indicate that abnormal Doppler velocimetry of the umbilical arteries and a combined estimated fetal weight < 3rd percentile are most strongly associated with poor obstetrical outcome (Unterscheider, 2013).

Importantly, sonographic estimates of fetal weight and actual weight may be discordant by 20 percent or more, leading to both false-positive and false-negative findings. Dashe and associates (2000) studied 8400 live births at Parkland Hospital in which fetal sonographic evaluation had been performed within 4 weeks of delivery. They reported that 30 percent of growth-restricted fetuses were not detected. In a study of 1000 high-risk fetuses, Larsen and coworkers (1992) performed serial sonographic examinations beginning at 28 weeks and then every 3 weeks subsequently. Reporting results compared with withholding results from clinicians significantly increased the diagnosis of SGA fetuses. Elective delivery rates were increased in the group whose providers received sonographic reports, but there was no overall improvement in neonatal outcomes.

Amnionic Fluid Volume Measurement

An association between pathological fetal-growth restriction and oligohydramnios has long been recognized (Chap. 11, p. 236). Chauhan and colleagues (2007) found oligohydramnios in nearly 10 percent of pregnancies suspected of growth restriction. This group of women was two times more likely to undergo cesarean delivery for nonreassuring fetal heart rate patterns. Petrozella and associates (2011) reported that decreased amnionic fluid volume between 24 and 34 weeks' gestation was significantly associated with malformations. In the absence of malformations, a birthweight < 3rd percentile was seen in 37 percent of pregnancies with oligohydramnios, in 21 percent with borderline amnionic fluid volume, but in only 4 percent with normal volumes. Hypoxia and diminished renal blood flow has been hypothesized as an explanation for oligohydramnios. However, Magann and coworkers (2011) reviewed the literature and determined that the etiology of oligohydramnios is likely more complex and possibly involves altered intramembranous absorption as well.

Doppler Velocimetry

With this technique, early changes in placenta-based growth restriction are detected in peripheral vessels such as the umbilical and middle cerebral arteries. Late changes are characterized by abnormal flow in the ductus venosus and fetal aortic and pulmonary outflow tracts and by reversal of umbilical artery flow.

Of these, abnormal umbilical artery Doppler velocimetry findings—characterized by absent or reversed end-diastolic flow—have been uniquely linked with fetal-growth restriction (Chap. 10, p. 220). These abnormalities highlight early versus severe fetal-growth restriction and represent the transition from fetal adaptation to failure. Thus, persistently absent or reversed end-diastolic flow has long been correlated with hypoxia, acidosis, and fetal death (Pardi, 1993; Woo, 1987). Umbilical artery Doppler velocimetry is considered standard in the evaluation and management of the growth-restricted fetus (Fig. 44-8). The

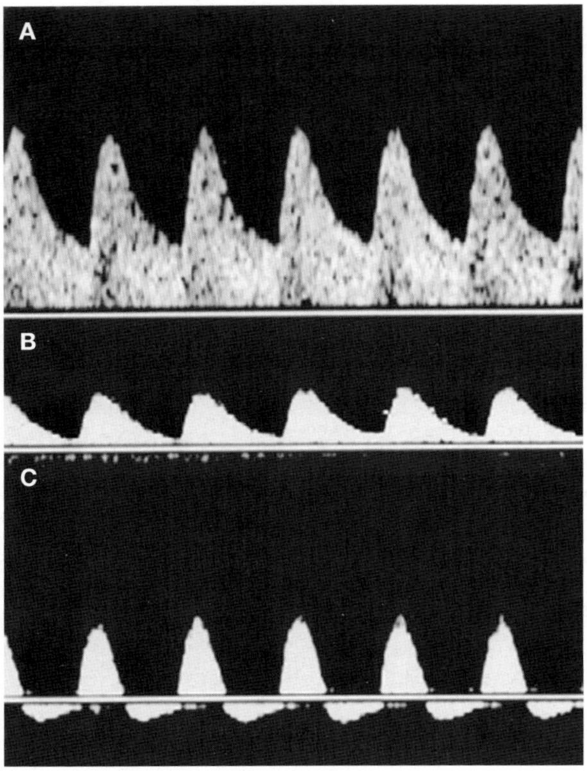

FIGURE 44-8 Umbilical arterial Doppler velocimetry studies, ranging from normal to markedly abnormal. **A.** Normal velocimetry pattern with a systolic to diastolic (S/D) ratio of < 3. **B.** The diastolic velocity approaching zero reflects increased placental vascular resistance. **C.** During diastole, arterial flow is reversed (negative S/D ratio), which is an ominous sign that may precede fetal demise.

American College of Obstetricians and Gynecologists (2013a) notes that umbilical-artery Doppler velocimetry has been shown to improve clinical outcomes. It is recommended in the management of fetal-growth restriction as an adjunct to standard surveillance techniques such as nonstress testing and biophysical profile.

As noted earlier, other Doppler assessments have been proposed but are still investigational. The ductus venosus was evaluated in a series of 604 neonates < 33 weeks who had an abdominal circumference < 5th percentile (Baschat, 2007). Investigators found that the ductus venosus Doppler parameters were the primary cardiovascular factor in predicting neonatal outcome. These late changes are felt to reflect myocardial deterioration and acidemia, which are major contributors to adverse perinatal and neurological outcome. In their longitudinal evaluation of 46 growth-restricted fetuses, Figueras and coworkers (2009) determined that Doppler flow abnormalities at the aortic valve isthmus preceded those in the ductus venosus by 1 week. Turan and associates (2008), in their evaluation of several fetal vessels, described the sequence of changes characteristic of mild placental dysfunction, progressive placental dysfunction, and severe early-onset placental dysfunction.

Prevention

Prevention of fetal-growth restriction ideally begins before conception, with optimization of maternal medical conditions, medications, and nutrition as discussed throughout Chapter 8. Smoking cessation is critical. Other risk factors should be tailored to the maternal condition, such as antimalarial prophylaxis for women living in endemic areas and correction of nutritional deficiencies. Studies have shown that treatment of mild to moderate hypertension does not reduce the incidence of growth-restricted infants (Chap. 50, p. 1005).

Accurate dating is essential during early pregnancy. Serial sonographic evaluations are typically used, but the best interval between assessments has not been clearly established. Given that a history of SGA is associated with other adverse outcomes in a subsequent pregnancy, particularly stillbirth and preterm birth, surveillance during a subsequent pregnancy may be beneficial (Gordon, 2012; Spong, 2012). According to the American College of Obstetricians and Gynecologists (2013a), if growth is normal during a pregnancy following a prior pregnancy complicated by fetal-growth restriction, Doppler velocimetry and fetal surveillance are not indicated. Prophylaxis with low-dose aspirin beginning early in gestation is not recommended because of its poor efficacy to reduce growth restriction (American College of Obstetricians and Gynecologists, 2013a; Berghella, 2007).

Management

If fetal-growth restriction is suspected, then efforts are made to confirm the diagnosis, assess fetal condition, and search for possible causes. Early-onset growth restriction is easier to recognize but presents challenging issues of management (Miller, 2008). In pregnancies in which there is a strong suspicion of fetal anomalies, patient counseling and prenatal diagnostic testing are indicated (American College of Obstetricians and Gynecologists, 2013a).

One algorithm for management is shown in Figure 44-9. In pregnancies with suspected fetal-growth restriction, antepartum fetal surveillance should include periodic Doppler velocimetry of the umbilical arteries in addition to more frequent fetal testing. At Parkland Hospital, if fetal viability has been reached, we hospitalize these women. Daily fetal heart rate tracings, weekly Doppler velocimetry, and sonographic assessment of fetal growth every 3 to 4 weeks are initiated. Other modalities of Doppler velocimetry, such as middle cerebral arteries or ductus venosus assessment, are considered experimental. The American College of Obstetricians and Gynecologists (2013a) recommends that pregnancies complicated by fetal-growth restriction and at risk for birth before 34 weeks receive antenatal corticosteroids for pulmonary maturation. According to Vidaeff and Blackwell (2011), growth-restricted fetuses may not tolerate the metabolic effects of corticosteroids in the same way as an unstressed fetus. They suggest increased surveillance during administration.

The timing of delivery is crucial, and the risks of fetal death versus the hazards of preterm delivery must be considered. Unfortunately, there are no studies that have elucidated the optimal timing of delivery. For the preterm fetus, the only randomized trial of delivery timing is the Growth Restriction Intervention Trial (GRIT) reported by Thornton and colleagues (2004). This trial was carried out in 13 European countries and

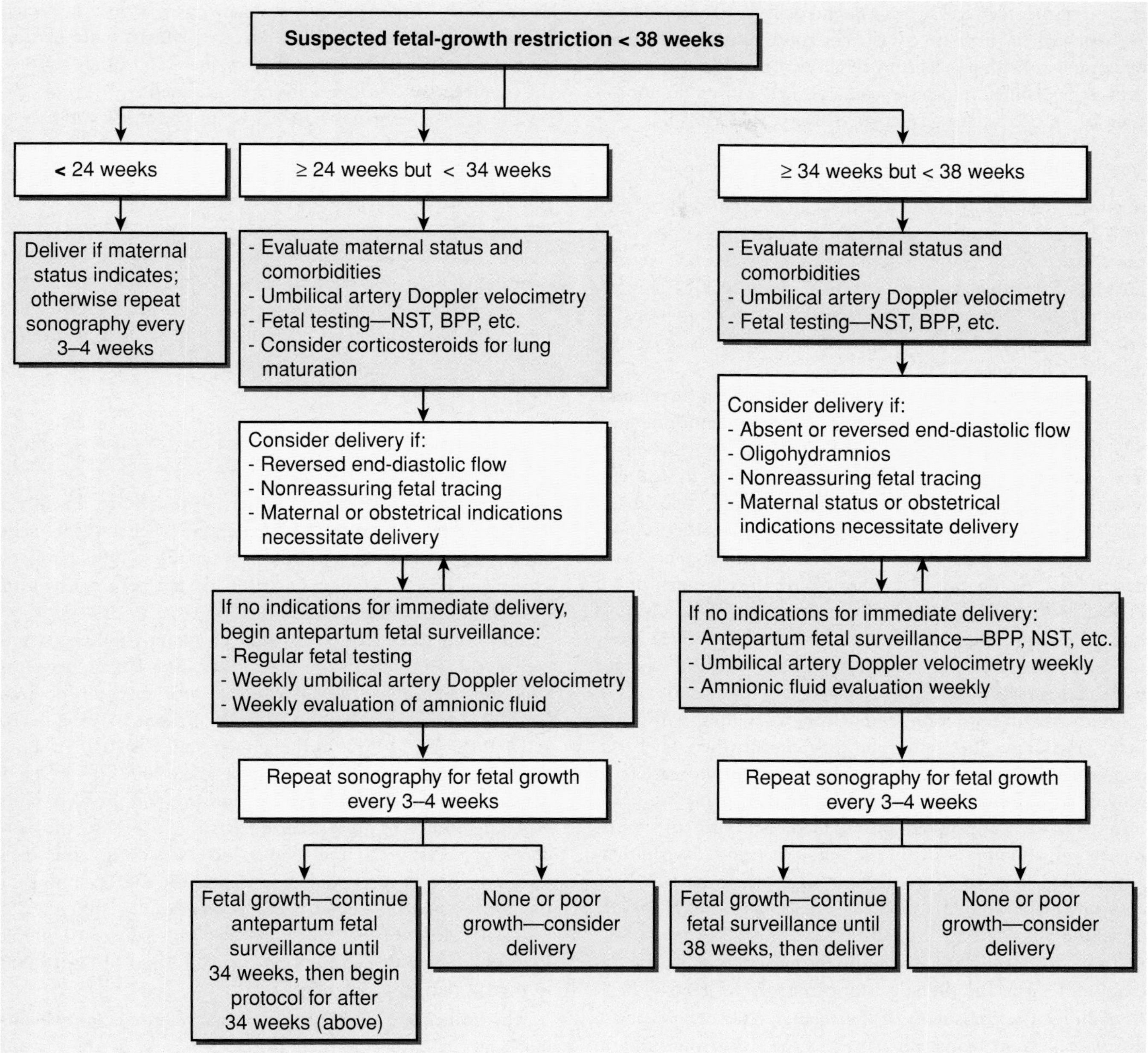

FIGURE 44-9 Algorithm for management of fetal-growth restriction at Parkland Hospital. BPP = biophysical profile; NST = nonstress test.

involved 548 women between 24 and 36 weeks' gestation with clinical uncertainty regarding delivery timing. Women were randomly assigned to immediate delivery or to delayed delivery until the situation worsened. The primary outcome was perinatal death or disability after reaching age 2 years. There were no differences in mortality rates through 2 years of age. Moreover, children aged 6 to 13 years did not show clinically significant differences between the two groups (Walker, 2011).

The DIGITAT—Disproportionate Intrauterine Growth Intervention Trial at Term—was designed to study delivery timing of growth-restricted fetuses who were 36 weeks' gestation or older. There were no differences in composite neonatal morbidity in 321 women with fetal-growth restriction and a gestational age of at least $36^{0/7}$ weeks who were randomly assigned to induction or to expectant management (Boers, 2010). Secondary analyses included assessment of neurodevelopmental and behavioral outcomes that did not differ at age 2 years (Van Wyk, 2012).

Management of the Near-Term Fetus

As shown in Figure 44-9, delivery of a suspected growth-restricted fetus with normal umbilical artery Doppler velocimetry, normal amnionic fluid volume, and reassuring fetal heart rate testing can likely be deferred until 38 weeks' gestation. Said another way, uncertainty regarding the diagnosis should preclude intervention until fetal lung maturity is assured. Expectant management can be guided using antepartum fetal surveillance techniques described in Chapter 17. Most clinicians, however, recommend delivery at 34 weeks or beyond if there is clinically significant oligohydramnios. Consensus statements by the Society of Maternal-Fetal Medicine (Spong, 2011) and the American College of Obstetricians and Gynecologists

(2013d) are similar. These recommend delivery between 34 and 37 weeks when there are concurrent conditions such as oligohydramnios. With a reassuring fetal heart rate pattern, vaginal delivery is planned. However, some of these fetuses do not tolerate labor, necessitating cesarean delivery.

Management of the Fetus Remote from Term

If growth restriction is identified in an anatomically normal fetus before 34 weeks, and amnionic fluid volume and fetal surveillance findings are normal, then observation is recommended. Screening for toxoplasmosis, cytomegalovirus infection, rubella, herpes, and other infections is recommended by some. However, we and others have not found this to be productive (Yamamoto, 2013).

As long as there is interval fetal growth and fetal surveillance test results are normal, pregnancy is allowed to continue until fetal lung maturity is reached (see Fig. 44-9). Reassessment of fetal growth is typically made no sooner than 3 to 4 weeks. Weekly assessment of umbilical artery Doppler velocimetry and amnionic fluid volume is combined with periodic nonstress testing, although the optimal frequency has not been determined. As mentioned, we hospitalize these women in our High-Risk Pregnancy Unit and monitor their fetuses daily. If interval growth, amnionic fluid volume, and umbilical artery Doppler velocimetry are normal, then the mother is discharged with intermittent outpatient surveillance.

With growth restriction remote from term, no specific treatment ameliorates the condition. For example, there is no evidence that diminished activity and bed rest result in accelerated growth or improved outcomes. Despite this, many clinicians intuitively advise a program of modified rest. Nutrient supplementation, attempts at plasma volume expansion, oxygen therapy, antihypertensive drugs, heparin, and aspirin have all been shown to be ineffective (American College of Obstetricians and Gynecologists, 2013a).

In most cases diagnosed before term, neither a precise etiology nor a specific therapy is apparent. Management decisions hinge on assessment of the relative risks of fetal death during expectant management versus the risks from preterm delivery. Although reassuring fetal testing may allow observation with continued maturation, long-term neurological outcome is a concern (Baschat, 2011; Thornton, 2004). Baschat and associates (2009) showed that neurodevelopmental outcome at 2 years in growth-restricted fetuses was best predicted by birthweight and gestational age. Doppler abnormalities are generally not associated with poor cognitive development scores among low-birthweight children delivered in the third trimester (Llurba, 2013). These findings emphasize that adverse neurodevelopmental outcomes cannot always be predicted.

Labor and Delivery

Fetal-growth restriction is commonly the result of placental insufficiency due to faulty maternal perfusion, reduction of functional placenta, or both. If present, these conditions are likely aggravated by labor. Equally important, diminished amnionic fluid volume increases the likelihood of cord compression during labor. For these reasons, a woman with a suspected growth-restricted fetus should undergo "high-risk" intrapartum monitoring (Chap. 22, p. 450). For these and other reasons, the frequency of cesarean delivery is increased.

The risk of neonatal hypoxia or meconium aspiration is also increased. Thus, care for the newborn should be provided immediately by an attendant who can skillfully clear the airway and ventilate an infant as needed (Chap. 32, p. 625). The severely growth-restricted newborn is particularly susceptible to hypothermia and may also develop other metabolic derangements such as hypoglycemia, polycythemia, and hyperviscosity. In addition, low-birthweight infants are at increased risk for motor and other neurological disabilities. Risk is greatest at the lowest extremes of birthweight (Baschat, 2007, 2009, 2011; Llurba, 2013).

FETAL OVERGROWTH

The term *macrosomia* is used rather imprecisely to describe a very large fetus or neonate. Although there is general agreement among obstetricians that newborns weighing < 4000 g are not excessively large, a similar consensus has not been reached for the definition of macrosomia.

Newborn weight rarely exceeds 11 pounds (5000 g), and excessively large infants are a curiosity. The largest newborn cited in the *Guinness Book of World Records* was a 23-lb 12-oz (10,800 g) infant boy born to a Canadian woman, Anna Bates, in 1879 (Barnes, 1957). In the United States in 2010, of more than 4 million births, 6.6 percent weighed 4000 to 4499 g; 1 percent weighed 4500 to 4999 g; and 0.1 percent were born weighing 5000 g or more (Martin, 2012). To be sure, the incidence of excessively large infants increased during the 20th century. According to Williams (1903), at the beginning of the 20th century, the incidence of birthweight > 5000 g was 1 to 2 per 10,000 births. This compares with 16 per 10,000 at Parkland Hospital from 1988 through 2008 and 11 per 10,000 in the United States in 2010.

The influence of increasing maternal obesity is overwhelming, and its association with diabetes is well known. Of Parkland mothers with infants born weighing > 5000 g, more than 15 percent were diabetic. Henriksen (2008) searched the Cochrane Database and reported that the rapid increase in the prevalence of large infants was due to maternal obesity and type 2 diabetes. Importantly however, review of data from the National Center for Health Statistics indicates that the rate of birthweight ≥ 4000 g has steadily declined more than 30 percent since 1990—from 10.9 percent to 7.6 percent in 2010 (Martin, 2012). This is discussed further in Chapters 48 (p. 967) and 57 (p. 1140).

Definition

Because there are no widely accepted and precise definitions of pathological fetal overgrowth, several terms are currently used clinically. The most common of these—*macrosomia*—is defined by birthweights that exceed certain percentiles for a given population. Another commonly used scheme is to define macrosomia by an empirical birthweight threshold.

TABLE 44-2. Birthweight Distribution of 354,509 Liveborn Infants at Parkland Hospital between 1988 and 2012

Birthweight (g)	Births		Maternal Diabetes	
	Number	Percent	Number	Percent
500–3999	322,074	90.9	13,365	4
4000–4249	19,106	5.4	1043	5
4250–4499	8391	2.4	573	7
4500–4649	3221	0.9	284	9
4750–4999	1146	0.3	134	12
5000–5249	385	0.1	57	15
5250–5499	127	0.04	31	24
5500 or more	59	0.02	14	24
Total	354,509		15,501	

Data courtesy of Dr. Don McIntire.

Birthweight Distribution

Frequently, macrosomia is defined based on mathematical distributions of birthweight. Those infants exceeding the 90th percentile for a given gestational week are usually used as the threshold for macrosomia or large-for-gestational age (LGA) birthweight. For example, the 90th percentile at 39 weeks is 4000 g. If, however, birthweights that are 2 standard deviations above the mean are used, then thresholds lie at the 97th percentile. Thus, substantially larger infants are considered macrosomic compared with those at the 90th percentile. Specifically, the birthweight threshold at 39 weeks to be macrosomic would be approximately 4500 g for the 97th percentile rather than 4000 g for the 90th percentile.

Empirical Birthweight

Newborn weight exceeding 4000 g—8 lb 13 oz—is also a frequently used threshold to define macrosomia. Others use 4250 g or even 4500 g—10 lb. As shown in Table 44-2, birthweights of 4500 g or more are uncommon. During a 30-year period at Parkland Hospital, during which there were more than 350,000 singleton births, only 1.4 percent of newborns weighed 4500 g or more. We are of the view that the upper limit of fetal growth, above which growth can be deemed abnormal, is likely two standard deviations above the mean, representing perhaps 3 percent of births. At 40 weeks, such a threshold would correspond to approximately 4500 g. The American College of Obstetricians and Gynecologists (2013b) concluded that the term *macrosomia* was an appropriate appellation for newborns who weigh 4500 g or more at birth.

Risk Factors

Some factors associated with fetal overgrowth are listed in Table 44-3. Many are interrelated and thus likely are additive. For example, advancing age is usually related to multiparity and diabetes, and obesity is obviously related to diabetes. Koyanagi and coworkers (2013) reported that the incidence of macrosomia exceeds 15 to 20 percent in Africa, Asia, and Latin America when women have diabetes, are obese, or have a postterm pregnancy. Of these, maternal diabetes is an important risk factor for fetal overgrowth (Chap. 57, p. 1129). As shown in Table 44-2, the incidence of maternal diabetes increases as birthweight > 4000 g increases. It should be emphasized, however, that maternal diabetes is associated with only a small percentage of the total number of such large infants.

TABLE 44-3. Risk Factors for Fetal Overgrowth

Obesity
Diabetes—gestational and type 2
Postterm gestation
Multiparity
Large size of parents
Advancing maternal age
Previous macrosomic infant
Racial and ethnic factors

Maternal and Perinatal Morbidity

The adverse consequences of excessive fetal growth are considerable. Neonates with a birthweight of at least 4500 g have been reported to have cesarean delivery rates exceeding 50 percent (Das, 2009; Gyurkovits, 2011; Weissmann-Brenner, 2012). The rate of shoulder dystocia has been reported to be as high as 17 percent for neonates with birthweights of at least 4500 g, and 23 percent for neonates with birthweights of at least 5000 g (Stotland, 2004). Rates of postpartum hemorrhage, perineal laceration, and maternal infection, which are related complications, are also increased in mothers delivering overgrown neonates. Maternal and neonatal outcomes by birthweight for large babies > 4000 g and delivered at Parkland Hospital are shown in Table 44-4.

Diagnosis

Because there are no current methods to estimate excessive fetal size accurately, macrosomia cannot be definitively diagnosed until delivery. Inaccuracy in clinical estimates of fetal weight by physical examination is often attributable, at least in part, to maternal obesity. Numerous attempts have been made to improve the accuracy of sonographic fetal-weight estimation. Several formulas have been proposed to calculate fetal weight using measurements of the head, femur, and abdomen. Estimates provided by these computations, although reasonably accurate for predicting the weight of small, preterm fetuses, are less valid in predicting the weight of large fetuses. Rouse and coworkers (1996) reviewed 13 studies completed between 1985 and 1995 to assess the accuracy of sonographic prediction for suspected fetal macrosomia. They found only fair sensitivity—60 percent—in the accurate diagnosis of macrosomia, but higher specificity—90 percent—in excluding excessive fetal size. Thus, sonographic estimation of fetal weight is unreliable, and its routine use to identify macrosomia is not recommended. Indeed, the findings of several studies indicate that clinical fetal-weight estimates are as reliable as, or even superior to, those made from sonographic measurements (Mattsson, 2007; Noumi, 2005; O'Reilly-Green, 2000).

TABLE 44-4. Maternal and Fetal Outcomes for 176,844 Pregnancies Delivered at Parkland Hospital from 1998 Through 2012

Outcome[a]	< 4000 g n = 187,119	4000–4499 g n = 17,750	4500–4999 g n = 2849	≥ 5000 g n = 372	*p* value
Cesarean total	46,577 (25)	5,362 (30)	1204 (42)	224 (60)	< 0.001
Scheduled	12,564 (7)	1,481 (8)	316 (11)	65 (17)	< 0.001
Dystocia	7589 (4)	1388 (8)	337 (12)	46 (12)	< 0.001
Shoulder dystocia	437 (0)	366 (2)	192 (7)	56 (15)	< 0.001
3rd- or 4th-degree laceration	7296 (4)	932 (5)	190 (7)	37 (10)	< 0.001
Labor induction	26,118 (13)	2499 (14)	420 (15)	39 (10)	0.141
Prolonged second stage	6905 (4)	899 (5)	147 (5)	14 (4)	< 0.001
Chorioamnionitis	13,448 (7)	1778 (10)	295 (10)	35 (9)	< 0.001
pH < 7.0	925 (0.5)	96 (0.6)	20 (0.7)	4 (1.1)	0.039
Apgar < 7 @ 5 minutes	1898 (1.0)	80 (0.5)	22 (0.8)	10 (2.7)	< 0.001
ICN admission	4266 (2.2)	123 (0.7)	36 (1.3)	9 (2.4)	< 0.001
Fractured clavicle	1880 (1.0)	616 (3.5)	125 (4.4)	16 (4.3)	< 0.001
Mechanical ventilation	2305 (1.2)	54 (0.3)	11 (0.4)	9 (2.4)	< 0.001
Hypoglycemia	480 (0.2)	89 (0.5)	31 (1.1)	12 (3.2)	< 0.001
Hyperbilirubinemia	5829 (3.0)	305 (1.7)	60 (2.1)	12 (3.2)	< 0.001
Erb palsy	470 (0.2)	224 (1.3)	74 (2.6)	22 (5.9)	< 0.001
Neonatal death	402 (0.2)	3 (0)	2 (0.1)	1 (0.3)	< 0.001
	176,844	16,954	2736	360	

[a]Outcome data presented as n (%).
ICN = intensive care nursery.
Data courtesy of Dr. Don McIntire.

Management

Several interventions have been proposed to interdict fetal overgrowth. Some include prophylactic labor induction for poorly defined indications such as "impending macrosomia," or elective cesarean delivery to avoid difficult delivery and shoulder dystocia. For women with diabetes in pregnancy, insulin therapy and close attention to good glycemic control reduces birthweight, but this has not consistently translated into reduced cesarean delivery rates (Crowther, 2005; Naylor, 1996). Irrespective of diabetes mellitus, fetal overgrowth among women is strongly associated with maternal obesity and excessive gestational weight gain (Durie, 2011; Johnson, 2013; Vesco, 2011). Dietary intervention to limit fetal overgrowth by curbing gestational weight gain is an active area of research. However, data to safely guide efforts to limit fetal overgrowth among at-risk women are lacking.

"Prophylactic" Labor Induction

Some clinicians have proposed labor induction when fetal macrosomia is suspected in nondiabetic women. This approach is suggested to obviate further fetal growth and thereby reduce potential delivery complications. Such prophylactic induction should theoretically reduce the risk of shoulder dystocia and cesarean delivery. Gonen and colleagues (1997) randomly assigned 273 nondiabetic women with sonographic fetal weight estimates of 4000 to 4500 g to either induction or expectant management. Labor induction did not decrease the rate of cesarean delivery or shoulder dystocia. Similar results were reported by Leaphart and associates (1997), who found that induction unnecessarily increased the cesarean delivery rate. In their systematic review of 11 studies of expectant management versus labor induction for suspected macrosomia, Sanchez-Ramos and coworkers (2002) found that labor induction results in increased cesarean delivery rates without improved perinatal outcomes.

A review of early term births indicates that elective delivery before 39 weeks' gestation does not improve maternal outcomes and is associated with worse neonatal outcomes (Wetta, 2012). We agree with the American College of Obstetricians and Gynecologists (2013b,d) that current evidence does not support a policy for early labor induction before 39 weeks' gestation or delivery for suspected macrosomia. Moreover, delivery or induction for suspected macrosomia at term is likewise not indicated.

Elective Cesarean Delivery

Rouse and colleagues (1996, 1999) analyzed the potential effects of a policy of elective cesarean delivery for sonographically diagnosed fetal macrosomia compared with standard obstetrical management. They concluded that for women who are not diabetic, a policy of elective cesarean delivery was medically and economically unsound. The American College of Obstetricians and Gynecologists (2013b) does not recommend routine cesarean delivery in women without diabetes when the estimated fetal weight is < 5000 g. Conversely, in *diabetic* women with overgrown fetuses, such a policy of elective cesarean delivery seems tenable. Conway and Langer (1998) described a protocol of routine cesarean delivery for sonographic estimates of 4250 g or greater in diabetic women. This management significantly reduced the shoulder dystocia rate from 2.4 to 1.1 percent.

Prevention of Shoulder Dystocia

With the delivery of macrosomic infants, shoulder dystocia and its attendant risks described in Chapter 27 (p. 541) are major concerns. That said, the American College of Obstetricians and Gynecologists (2012) notes that fewer than 10 percent of all shoulder dystocia cases result in a persistent brachial plexus injury, and 4 percent of these follow cesarean delivery.

It appears that planned cesarean delivery on the basis of suspected macrosomia to prevent brachial plexopathy is an unreasonable strategy in the *general population* (Chauhan, 2005). Ecker and coworkers (1997) analyzed 80 cases of brachial plexus injury in 77,616 consecutive infants born at Brigham and Women's Hospital. They concluded that an excessive number of otherwise unnecessary cesarean deliveries would be needed to prevent a single brachial plexus injury in neonates born to women without diabetes. Conversely, planned cesarean delivery may be a reasonable strategy for diabetic women with an estimated fetal weight > 4250 or > 4500 g.

In summary, when fetal overgrowth is suspected, the obstetrician naturally seeks to balance the risks to the fetus with maternal risks. Although interventions to prevent shoulder dystocia may someday prove beneficial, eliminating shoulder dystocia will likely remain an impossible goal. We agree with the American College of Obstetricians and Gynecologists that elective delivery for the fetus that is suspected to be overgrown is inadvisable, particularly before 39 weeks' gestation. Finally, we agree that elective cesarean delivery is not indicated when estimated fetal weight is < 5000 g among women without diabetes and < 4500 g among women with diabetes (American College of Obstetricians and Gynecologists, 2013b).

REFERENCES

Alexander GR, Himes JH, Kaufman RB, et al: A United States national reference for fetal growth. Obstet Gynecol 87:163, 1996

Alexander GR, Kogan M, Bader D, et al: U.S. birthweight/gestational age-specific neonatal mortality: 1995–1997 rates for whites, Hispanics and blacks. Pediatrics 111:e61, 2003

Alexander GR, Kogan MD, Himes JH, et al: Racial differences in birthweight for gestational age and infant mortality in extremely-low-risk U.S. populations. Paediatr Perinat Epidemiol 13:205, 1999

Aman J, Hansson U, Ostlund I, et al: Increased fat mass and cardiac septal hypertrophy in newborn infants of mothers with well-controlled diabetes during pregnancy. Neonatology 100(2):147, 2011

American College of Obstetricians and Gynecologists: Shoulder dystocia. Practice Bulletin No. 40, November 2002, Reaffirmed 2012

American College of Obstetricians and Gynecologists: Fetal growth restriction. Practice Bulletin No. 134, May 2013a

American College of Obstetricians and Gynecologists: Fetal macrosomia. Practice Bulletin No. 22, November 2000a, Reaffirmed 2013b

American College of Obstetricians and Gynecologists: Moderate caffeine consumption during pregnancy. Committee Opinion No. 462, August 2010, Reaffirmed 2013c

American College of Obstetricians and Gynecologists: Nonmedically indicated early-term deliveries. Committee Opinion No. 561, April 2013d

Backes CH, Markham K, Moorehead P, et al: Maternal preeclampsia and neonatal outcomes. J Pregnancy 2011:214365, 2011

Bahado-Singh RO, Lynch L, Deren O, et al: First-trimester growth restriction and fetal aneuploidy: the effect of type of aneuploidy and gestational age. Am J Obstet Gynecol 176(5):976, 1997

Baken L, van Heesch PN, Wildschut HI, et al: First-trimester crown-rump length and embryonic volume of aneuploid fetuses measured in virtual reality. Ultrasound Obstet Gynecol 41(5):521, 2013

Barker DJP (ed): Fetal and Infant Origins of Adult Disease. London, BMJ Publishing, 1992

Barnes AC: An obstetric record from the medical record. Obstet Gynecol 9(2):237, 1957

Baschat AA: Neurodevelopment following fetal growth restriction and its relationship with antepartum parameters of placental dysfunction. Ultrasound Obstet Gynecol 37(5):501, 2011

Baschat AA, Cosmi E, Bilardo CM, et al: Predictors of neonatal outcome in early-onset placental dysfunction. Obstet Gynecol 109(2, pt 1):253, 2007

Baschat AA, Viscardi RM, Hussey-Gardner B, et al: Infant neurodevelopment following fetal growth restriction: relationship with antepartum surveillance parameters. Ultrasound Obstet Gynecol 33(1):44, 2009

Battaglia FC, Lubchenco LO: A practical classification of newborn infants by weight and gestational age. J Pediatr 71(2):159, 1967

Beltrand J, Verkauskiene R, Nicolescu R, et al: Adaptive changes in neonatal hormonal and metabolic profiles induced by fetal growth restriction. J Clin Endocrinol Metab 93(10):4027, 2008

Berghella V: Prevention of recurrent fetal growth restriction. Obstet Gynecol 110(4):904, 2007

Boers KE, Vijgen SM, Bijlenga D, et al: Induction versus expectant monitoring for intrauterine growth restriction at term: randomised equivalence trial (DIGITAT). Br Med J 341:c7087, 2010

Boney CM, Verma A, Tucker R, et al: Metabolic syndrome in childhood: association with birth weight, maternal obesity, and gestational diabetes mellitus. Pediatrics 115(3):e290, 2005

Boulet SL, Alexander GR, Salihu HM, et al: Fetal growth risk curves: defining levels of fetal growth restriction by neonatal death risk. Am J Obstet Gynecol 195(6):1571; 2006

Bramham K, Briley AL, Seed PT, et al: Pregnancy outcome in women with chronic kidney disease: a prospective cohort study. Reprod Sci 18(7):623, 2011

Brenner WE, Edelman DA, Hendricks CH: A standard of fetal growth for the United States of America. Am J Obstet Gynecol 126:555, 1976

Brosens I, Pijnenborg R, Vercruysse L, et al: The "Great Obstetrical Syndromes" are associated with disorders of deep placentation. Am J Obstet Gynecol 204(3):193, 2011

Bukowski R, Uchida T, Smith GC, et al: Individualized norms of optimal fetal growth. Obstet Gynecol 111(5):1065, 2008

Campbell S, Thoms A: Ultrasound measurement of the fetal head to abdomen circumference ratio in the assessment of growth retardation. BJOG 84(3):165, 1977

CARE Study Group: Maternal caffeine intake during pregnancy and risk of fetal growth restriction: a large prospective observational study. Br Med J 337:a2332, 2008

Catalano PM, Hauguel-De Mouzon S. Is it time to revisit the Pedersen hypothesis in the face of the obesity epidemic? Am J Obstet Gynecol 204(6):479, 2011

Cetin I, Ronzoni S, Marconi AM, et al: Maternal concentrations and fetal-maternal concentration differences of plasma amino acids in normal and intrauterine growth-restricted pregnancies. Am J Obstet Gynecol 174(5): 1575, 1996

Chakravarty EF, Khanna D, Chung L: Pregnancy outcomes in systemic sclerosis, primary pulmonary hypertension, and sickle cell disease. Obstet Gynecol 111(4):927, 2008

Chauhan SP, Grobman WA, Gherman RA, et al: Suspicion and treatment of the macrosomic fetus: a review. Am J Obstet Gynecol 193(2):332, 2005

Chauhan SP, Taylor M, Shields D, et al: Intrauterine growth restriction and oligohydramnios among high risk patients. Am J Perinatol 24(4):215, 2007

Chen HY, Chauhan SP, Ward TC, et al: Aberrant fetal growth and early, late, and postneonatal mortality: an analysis of Milwaukee births, 1996–2007. Am J Obstet Gynecol l204(3):261.e1, 2011

Cleal JK, Glazier JD, Ntani G, et al: Facilitated transporters mediate net efflux of amino acids to the fetus across the basal membrane of the placental syncytiotrophoblast. J Physiol l589(Pt 4):987, 2011

Coker AL, Garcia LS, Williams CM, et al: Universal psychosocial screening and adverse pregnancy outcomes in an academic obstetric clinic. Obstet Gynecol 119(6):1180, 2012

Conway DL, Langer O: Elective delivery of infants with macrosomia in diabetic women: reduced shoulder dystocia versus increased cesarean deliveries. Am J Obstet Gynecol 178(5):922, 1998

Crispi F, Figueras F, Cruz-Lemini M, et al: Cardiovascular programming in children born small for gestational age and relationship with prenatal signs of severity. Am J Obstet Gynecol 207(2):121.e1, 2012

Crowther CA, Hiller JE, Moss JR, et al: Effect of treatment of gestational diabetes mellitus on pregnancy outcomes. N Engl J Med 352(24):2477, 2005

Crowther NJ, Cameron N, Trusler J, et al: Influence of catch-up growth on glucose tolerance and beta-cell function in 7-year-old children: results from the Birth to Twenty Study. Pediatrics 121(6):e1715, 2008

Cui Y, Wang W, Dong N, et al: Role of corin in trophoblast invasion and uterine spiral artery remodelling in pregnancy. Nature 484(7393):246, 2012

Cunningham FG, Cox SM, Harstad TW, et al: Chronic renal disease and pregnancy outcome. Am J Obstet Gynecol 163(2):453, 1990

Cyganek K, Hebda-Szydlo A, Skupien J, et al: Glycemic control and pregnancy outcomes in women with type 2 diabetes from Poland. The impact of pregnancy planning and a comparison with type 1 diabetes subjects. Endocrine 40(2):243, 2011

Das S, Irigoyen M, Patterson MB, et al: Neonatal outcomes of macrosomic births in diabetic and non-diabetic women. Arch Dis Child Fetal Neonatal Ed 94(6):F419, 2009

Dashe JS, McIntire DD, Lucas MJ, et al: Effects of symmetric and asymmetric fetal growth on pregnancy outcomes. Obstet Gynecol 96(3):321, 2000

Di Cianni G, Miccoli R, Volpe L, et al: Maternal triglyceride levels and newborn weight in pregnant women with normal glucose tolerance. Diabet Med 22(1):21, 2005

Diderholm B, Stridsberg M, Ewald U, et al: Increased lipolysis in non-obese pregnant women studied in the third trimester. BJOG 112(6):713, 2005

Diderholm B, Stridsberg M, Nordén-Lindeberg S, et al: Decreased maternal lipolysis in intrauterine growth restriction in the third trimester. BJOG 113(2):159, 2006

Dugoff L; Society for Maternal-Fetal Medicine. First- and second-trimester maternal serum markers for aneuploidy and adverse obstetric outcomes. Obstet Gynecol 115(5):1052, 2010

Dunsworth HM, Warrener AG, Deacon T, et al: Metabolic hypothesis for human altriciality. Proc Natl Acad Sci U S A 109(38):15212, 2012

Durie DE, Thornburg LL, Glantz JC: Effect of second-trimester and third-trimester rate of gestational weight gain on maternal and neonatal outcomes. Obstet Gynecol 118(3):569, 2011

Duvekot JJ, Cheriex EC, Pieters FAA, et al: Maternal volume homeostasis in early pregnancy in relation to fetal growth restriction. Obstet Gynecol 85(3):361, 1995

Ebbing C, Rasmussen S, Kiserud T: Fetal hemodynamic development in macrosomic growth. Ultrasound Obstet Gynecol 38(3):303, 2011

Ecker JL, Greenberg JA, Norwitz ER, et al: Birthweight as a predictor of brachial plexus injury. Obstet Gynecol 89(5 pt 1):643, 1997

Espinoza J: Abnormal fetal-maternal interactions: an evolutionary value? Obstet Gynecol 120(2 Pt 1):370, 2012

Evagelidou EN, Kiortsis DN, Bairaktari ET, et al: Lipid profile, glucose homeostasis, blood pressure, and obesity-anthropometric markers in macrosomic offspring of nondiabetic mothers. Diabetes Care 29(6):1197, 2006

Facco F, You W, Grobman W: Genetic thrombophilias and intrauterine growth restriction: a meta-analysis. Obstet Gynecol 113(6):1206, 2009

Figueras F, Benavides A, Del Rio M, et al: Monitoring of fetuses with intrauterine growth restriction: longitudinal changes in ductus venosus and aortic isthmus flow. Ultrasound Obstet Gynecol 33(1):39, 2009

Figueras F, Cruz-Martinez R, Sanz-Cortes M, et al: Neurobehavioral outcomes in preterm, growth-restricted infants with and without prenatal advanced signs of brain-sparing. Ultrasound Obstet Gynecol 38(3):288, 2011a

Figueras F, Gardosi J: Intrauterine growth restriction: new concepts in antenatal surveillance, diagnosis, and management. Am J Obstet Gynecol 204 (4):288, 2011b

Flores ME, Simonsen SE, Manuck TA, et al: The "Latina epidemiologic paradox": contrasting patterns of adverse birth outcomes in U.S.-born and foreign-born Latinas. Womens Health Issues 22(5):e501, 2012

Forhead AJ, Fowden AL: The hungry fetus? Role of leptin as a nutritional signal before birth. J Physiol 15;587(Pt 6):1145, 2009

Freeman K, Oakley L, Pollak A, et al: Association between congenital toxoplasmosis and preterm birth, low birthweight and small for gestational age birth. BJOG 112:31, 2005

Friedman SA, Schiff E, Kao L, et al: Neonatal outcome after preterm delivery for preeclampsia. Am J Obstet Gynecol 172(6):1785, 1995

Garcia-Flores J, Jañez M, Gonzalez MC, et al: Fetal myocardial morphological and functional changes associated with well-controlled gestational diabetes. Eur J Obstet Gynecol Reprod Biol 154(1):24, 2011

Gardosi J, Chang A, Kalyan B, et al: Customized antenatal growth charts. Lancet 339(87888):283, 1992

Gauster M, Hiden U, Blaschitz A, et al: Dysregulation of placental endothelial lipase and lipoprotein lipase in intrauterine growth-restricted pregnancies. J Clin Endocrinol Metab 92(6):2256, 2007

Giannakopoulos B, Krilis SA: The pathogenesis of the antiphospholipid syndrome. N Engl J Med 368(11):1033, 2013

Gil-Sánchez A, Koletzko B, Larqué E: Current understanding of placental fatty acid transport. Curr Opin Clin Nutr Metab Care 15(3):265, 2012

Gluckman PD, Hanson MA, Cooper C, et al: Effect of in utero and early-life conditions on adult health and disease. N Engl J Med 359(1):61, 2008

Gonen O, Rosen DJ, Dolfin Z, et al: Induction of labor versus expectant management in macrosomia: a randomized study. Obstet Gynecol 89(6):913, 1997

Gonzales GF, Tapia V: Birth weight charts for gestational age in 63,620 healthy infants born in Peruvian public hospitals at low and at high altitude. Acta Paediatr 98(3):454, 2009

Gordon A, Raynes-Greenow C, McGeechan K, et al: Stillbirth risk in a second pregnancy. Obstet Gynecol 119(3):509, 2012

Greer LG, Ziadie MS, Casey BM, et al: An immunologic basis for placental insufficiency in fetal growth restriction. Am J Perinatol 29(7):533, 2012

Groom KM, North RA, Stone PR, et al: Patterns of change in uterine artery Doppler studies between 20 and 24 weeks of gestation and pregnancy outcomes. Obstet Gynecol 113(2 pt 1):332, 2009

Gyurkovits Z, Kálló K, Bakki J, et al: Neonatal outcome of macrosomic infants: an analysis of a two-year period. Eur J Obstet Gynecol Reprod Biol 159(2):289, 2011

HAPO Study Cooperative Research Group: Hyperglycemia and adverse pregnancy outcomes. N Engl J Med 358(19):1991, 2008

Haeri S, Khoury J, Kovilam O, et al: The association of intrauterine growth abnormalities in women with type 1 diabetes mellitus complicated by vasculopathy. Am J Obstet Gynecol 199(3):278, 2008

Hagman A, Wennerholm UB, Källén K, et al: Women who gave birth to girls with Turner syndrome: maternal and neonatal characteristics. Hum Reprod 25(6):1553, 2010

Harmon KA, Gerard L, Jensen DR, et al: Continuous glucose profiles in obese and normal-weight pregnant women on a controlled diet: metabolic determinants of fetal growth. Diabetes Care 34(10):2198, 2011

Henriksen T: The macrosomic fetus: a challenge in current obstetrics. Acta Obstet Gynecol Scand 87(2):134, 2008

Hietalampi H, Pahkala K, Jokinen E, et al: Left ventricular mass and geometry in adolescence: early childhood determinants. Hypertension 60(5):1266, 2012

Higa R, Jawerbaum A: Intrauterine effects of impaired lipid homeostasis in pregnancy diseases. Curr Med Chem 20(18):2338, 2013

Hutcheon JA, Walker M, Platt RW: Assessing the value of customized birth weight percentiles. Am J Epidemiol 173(4):459, 2011a

Hutcheon JA, Zhang X, Platt RW, et al: The case against customised birthweight standards. Paediatr Perinat Epidemiol 25(1):11, 2011b

Iams JD: Small for gestational age (SGA) and fetal growth restriction (FGR). Am J Obstet Gynecol 202(6):513, 2010

Infante-Rivard C, Rivard GE, Yotov WV, et al: Absence of association of thrombophilia polymorphisms with intrauterine growth restriction. N Engl J Med 347(1):19, 2002

Jacobsson B, Ahlin K, Francis A, et al: Cerebral palsy and restricted growth status at birth: population-based case-control study. BJOG 115(10):1250, 2008

Jana N, Barik S, Arora N, et al: Tuberculosis in pregnancy: the challenges for South Asian countries. J Obstet Gynaecol Res 38(9):1125, 2012

Jana N, Vasishta K, Jindal SK, et al: Perinatal outcome in pregnancies complicated by pulmonary tuberculosis. Int J Gynaecol Obstet 44(2):119, 1994

Jana N, Vasishta K, Saha SC, et al: Obstetrical outcomes among women with extrapulmonary tuberculosis. N Engl J Med 341(9):645, 1999

Jansson N, Rosario FJ, Gaccioli F, et al: Activation of placental mTOR signaling and amino acid transporters in obese women giving birth to large babies. J Clin Endocrinol Metab 98(1):105, 2013

Jelks A, Cifuentes R, Ross MG: Clinician bias in fundal height measurement. Obstet Gynecol 110(4):892, 2007

Jeyabalan A, McGonigal S, Gilmour C, et al: Circulating and placental endoglin concentrations in pregnancies complicated by intrauterine growth restriction and preeclampsia. Placenta 29(6):555, 2008

Johnson J, Clifton RG, Roberts JM, et al: Pregnancy Outcomes with Weight Gain above or below the 2009 Institute of Medicine Guidelines. Obstet Gynecol 121(5):969, 2013

Karakosta P, Chatzi L, Plana E, et al: Leptin levels in cord blood and anthropometric measures at birth: a systematic review and meta-analysis. Paediatr Perinat Epidemiol 25(2):150, 2011

Kayentao K, Garner P, van Eijk AM, et al: Intermittent preventive therapy for malaria during pregnancy using 2 vs 3 or more doses of sulfadoxine-pyrimethamine and risk of low birth weight in Africa: systematic review and meta-analysis. JAMA 309(6):594, 2013

Kerkhof GF, Willemsen RH, Leunissen RW, et al: Health profile of young adults born preterm: negative effects of rapid weight gain in early life. J Clin Endocrinol Metab 97(12):4498, 2012

Kessler J, Rasmussen S, Godfrey K, et al: Venous liver blood flow and regulation of human fetal growth: evidence from macrosomic fetuses. Am J Obstet Gynecol 204(5):429.e1, 2011

Khoury MJ, Erickson JD, Cordero JF, et al: Congenital malformations and intrauterine growth retardation: a population study. Pediatrics 82(1):83, 1988

Kondapalli LA, Perales-Puchalt A: Low birth weight: is it related to assisted reproductive technology or underlying infertility? Fertil Steril 99(2):303, 2013

Kovo M, Schreiber L, Ben-Haroush A, et al: Placental vascular lesion differences in pregnancy-induced hypertension and normotensive fetal growth restriction. Am J Obstet Gynecol 202(6):561.e1, 2010

Koyanagi A, Zhang J, Dagvadorj A, et al: Macrosomia in 23 developing countries: an analysis of a multicountry, facility-based, cross-sectional survey. Lancet 381(9865):476, 2013

Kramer MS, Platt RW, Wen SW, et al: Fetal/Infant Health Study Group of the Canadian Perinatal Surveillance System. A new and improved population-based Canadian reference for birth weight for gestational age. Pediatrics 108(2):E35, 2001

Krantz D, Goetzl L, Simpson J, et al: Association of extreme first-trimester free human chorionic gonadotropin-β, pregnancy-associated plasma protein A, and nuchal translucency with intrauterine growth restriction and other adverse pregnancy outcomes. Am J Obstet Gynecol 191(4):1452, 2004

Kyriakakou M, Malamitisi-Puchner A, Militsi H, et al: Leptin and adiponectin concentrations in intrauterine growth restricted and appropriate for gestational age fetuses, neonates and their mothers. Eur J Endocrinol 158(3):343, 2008

Laatikainen TJ, Raisanen IJ, Salminen KR: Corticotrophin-releasing hormone in amnionic fluid during gestation and labor and in relation to fetal lung maturation. Am J Obstet Gynecol 159(4):891, 1988

Larkin JC, Hill LM, Speer PD, et al: Risk of morbid perinatal outcomes in small-for-gestational-age pregnancies: customized compared with conventional standards of fetal growth. Obstet Gynecol 119(1):21, 2012

Larsen T, Larsen JF, Petersen S, et al: Detection of small-for-gestation-age fetuses by ultrasound screening in a high risk population: a randomized controlled study. BJOG 9(6):469, 1992

Leaphart WL, Meyer MC, Capeless EL: Labor induction with a prenatal diagnosis of fetal macrosomia. J Matern Fetal Med 6(2):99, 1997

Lechtig A, Delgado H, Lasky RE, et al: Maternal nutrition and fetal growth in developing societies. Am J Dis Child 129(5):434, 1975

Leunissen RW, Kerkhof GF, Stijnen T, et al: Fat mass and apolipoprotein E genotype influence serum lipoprotein levels in early adulthood, whereas birth size does not. J Clin Endocrinol Metab 93(11):4307, 2008

Levine JS, Branch DW, Rauch J: The antiphospholipid syndrome. N Engl J Med 346(10):752, 2002

Lewandowski AJ, Augustine D, Lamata P, et al: Preterm heart in adult life: cardiovascular magnetic resonance reveals distinct differences in left ventricular mass, geometry, and function. Circulation 127(2):197, 2013

Liu JM, Mei Z, Ye R, et al: Micronutrient supplementation and pregnancy outcomes: double-blind randomized controlled trial in China. JAMA Intern Med 173(4):276, 2013

Llurba E, Baschat AA, Turan OM, et al: Childhood cognitive development after fetal growth restriction. Ultrasound Obstet Gynecol 41(4):383, 2013

Lockshin MD, Kim M, Laskin CA, et al: Prediction of adverse pregnancy outcome by the presence of lupus anticoagulant, but not anticardiolipin antibody, in patients with antiphospholipid antibodies. Arthritis Rheum 64(7):2311, 2012

Lockwood CJ: Inherited thrombophilias in pregnant patients: Detection and treatment paradigm. Obstet Gynecol 99(2):333, 2002

Lubchenco LO, Hansman C, Dressler M, et al: Intrauterine growth as estimated from liveborn birth-weight data at 24 to 42 weeks of gestation. Pediatrics 32:793, 1963

Luo ZC, Nuyt AM, Delvin E, et al: Maternal and fetal IGF-I and IGF-II levels, fetal growth, and gestational diabetes. J Clin Endocrinol Metab 97(5):1720, 2012

Magann EF, Sandlin AT, Ounpraseuth ST: Amniotic fluid and the clinical relevance of the sonographically estimated amniotic fluid volume: oligohydramnios. J Ultrasound Med 30(11):1573, 2011

Manning FA: Intrauterine growth retardation. In: Fetal Medicine. Principles and Practice. Norwalk, CT, Appleton & Lange, 1995, p 317

Manning FA, Hohler C: Intrauterine growth retardation: diagnosis, prognostication, and management based on ultrasound methods. In Fleischer AC, Romero R, Manning FA, et al (eds): The Principles and Practices of Ultrasonography in Obstetrics and Gynecology, 4th ed. Norwalk, Appleton & Lange, 1991, p 331

Martin JA, Hamilton BE, Venture SJ, et al: Births: final data for 2010. Natl Vital Stat Rep 61(1):1, 2012

Mastrobattista JM, Gomez-Lobo V, Society for Maternal-Fetal Medicine: Pregnancy after solid organ transplantation. Obstet Gynecol 112(4):919, 2008

Mattsson N, Rosendahl H, Luukkaala T: Good accuracy of ultrasound estimations of fetal weight performed by midwives. Acta Obstet Gynecol Scand 86(6):688, 2007

Mattsson K, Rylander L: Influence of maternal and paternal birthweight on offspring birthweight—a population-based intergenerational study. Paediatr Perinat Epidemiol 27(2):138, 2013

Mayer C, Joseph KS. Fetal growth: a review of terms, concepts and issues relevant to obstetrics. Ultrasound Obstet Gynecol 41(2):136, 2013

McIntire DD, Bloom SL, Casey BM, et al: Birthweight in relation to morbidity and mortality among newborn infants. N Engl J Med 340(16):1234, 1999

Miller J, Turan S, Baschat AA: Fetal growth restriction. Semin Perinatol 32(4):274, 2008

Milovanovic I, Njuieyon F, Deghmoun S, et al: Innate small babies are metabolically healthy children. J Clin Endocrinol Metab 97(12):4407, 2012

Mise H, Yura S, Itoh H, et al: The relationship between maternal plasma leptin levels and fetal growth restriction. Endocr J 54(6) 945, 2007

Mook-Kanamori DO, Steegers EA, Eilers PH, et al: Risk factors and outcomes associated with first-trimester fetal growth restriction. JAMA 303(6):527, 2010

Morisaki N, Esplin MS, Varner MW, et al: Declines in birth weight and fetal growth independent of gestational length. Obstet Gynecol 121(1):51, 2013

Mulder EJ, Koopman CM, Vermunt JK, et al: Fetal growth trajectories in Type-1 diabetic pregnancy. Ultrasound Obstet Gynecol 36(6):735, 2010

Murphy HR, Steel SA, Roland JM, et al: East Anglia Study Group for Improving Pregnancy Outcomes in Women with Diabetes (EASIPOD). Obstetric and perinatal outcomes in pregnancies complicated by Type 1 and Type 2 diabetes: influences of glycaemic control, obesity and social disadvantage. Diabet Med 28(9):1060, 2011

Murray PG, Clayton PE: Endocrine control of growth. Am J Med Genet Part C Semin Med Genet 163(2):76, 2013

Naylor CD, Sermer M, Chen E, et al: Cesarean delivery in relation to birth weight and gestational glucose tolerance: pathophysiology or practice style? Toronto Trihospital Gestational Diabetes Investigators. JAMA 275(15):1165, 1996

Nicolaides KH, Snijders RJM, Noble P: Cordocentesis in the study of growth-retarded fetuses. In Divon MY (ed): Abnormal Fetal Growth. New York, Elsevier, 1991

Nobili V, Alisi A, Panera N, et al: Low birth weight and catch-up-growth associated with metabolic syndrome: a ten year systematic review. Pediatr Endocrinol Rev. 6(2):241, 2008

Noumi G, Collado-Khoury F, Bombard A, et al: Clinical and sonographic estimation of fetal weight performed during labor by residents. Am J Obstet Gynecol. 192(5):1407, 2005

Ong KK: Catch-up growth in small for gestational age babies: good or bad? Curr Opin Endocrinol Diabetes Obes 14(1):30, 2007

O'Reilly-Green C, Divon M: Sonographic and clinical methods in the diagnosis of macrosomia. Clin Obstet Gynecol 43:309, 2000

Ott W: Intrauterine growth retardation and preterm delivery. Am J Obstet Gynecol 168:710, 1993

Overpeck MD, Hediger ML, Zhang J, et al: Birthweight for gestational age of Mexican American infants born in the United States. Obstet Gynecol 93:943, 1999

Owen J, Baker SL, Hauth JC: Is indicated or spontaneous preterm delivery more advantageous for the fetus? Am J Obstet Gynecol 163(3):868, 1990

Owen P, Harrold AJ, Farrell T: Fetal size and growth velocity in the prediction of intrapartum cesarean section for fetal distress. BJOG 104(4):445, 1997

Owen P, Khan KS: Fetal growth velocity in the prediction of intrauterine growth restriction in a low risk population. BJOG 105(5):536, 1998

Paquet C, Yudin MH: Toxoplasmosis in pregnancy: prevention, screening, and treatment. J Obstet Gynaecol Can. 35(1):78, 2013

Pardi G, Cetin I: Human fetal growth and organ development: 50 years of discoveries. Am J Obstet Gynecol 194(4):1008, 2006

Pardi G, Cetin I, Marconi AM, et al: Diagnostic value of blood sampling in fetuses with growth retardation. N Engl J Med. 328(10):692, 1993

Pasternak Y, Weintraub AY, Shoham-Vardi I, et al: Obstetric and perinatal outcomes in women with eating disorders. J Womens Health 21(1):61, 2012

Patton DE, Lee W, Cotton DB, et al: Cyanotic maternal heart disease in pregnancy. Obstet Gynecol Surv 45(9):594, 1990

Paz I, Gale R, Laor A, et al: The cognitive outcome of full-term small-for-gestational age infants at late adolescence. Obstet Gynecol 85(3):452, 1995

Perelman RH, Farrell PM, Engle MJ, et al: Development aspects of lung lipids. Annu Rev Physiol 47:803, 1985

Petrozella LN, Dashe JS, McIntire DD, et al: Clinical significance of borderline amniotic fluid index and oligohydramnios in preterm pregnancy. Obstet Gynecol 117(2 Pt 1):338, 2011

Picone O, Vauloup-Fellous C, Cordier AG, et al: A series of 238 cytomegalovirus primary infections during pregnancy: description and outcome. Prenat Diagn 2:1, 2013
Platz E, Newman R: Diagnosis of IUGR: traditional biometry. Semin Perinatol 32(3):140, 2008
Poeran J, Maas AF, Birnie E, et al: Social deprivation and adverse perinatal outcomes among Western and non-Western pregnant women in a Dutch urban population. Soc Sci Med 83:42, 2013
Prado EL, Alcock KJ, Muadz H, et al: Maternal multiple micronutrient supplements and child cognition: a randomized trial in Indonesia. Pediatrics 130(3):e536, 2012
Redline RW: Villitis of unknown etiology: noninfectious chronic villitis in the placenta. Hum Pathol 38(10):1439, 2007
Ritz E, Amann K, Koleganova N, et al: Prenatal programming—effects on blood pressure and renal function. Nat Rev Nephrol 7(3):137, 2011
Robert Peter J, Ho JJ, Valliapan J, et al: Symphysial fundal height (SFH) measurement in pregnancy for detecting abnormal fetal growth. Cochrane Database Syst Rev 7:CD008136, 2012
Rode L, Hegaard HK, Kjaergaard H, et al: Association between maternal weight gain and birth weight. Obstet Gynecol 109(6):1309, 2007
Rodger MA, Paidas M, Claire M, et al: Inherited thrombophilia and pregnancy complications revisited. Obstet Gynecol 112:320, 2008
Rogers BB, Bloom SL, Leveno KJ. Atherosis revisited: current concepts on the pathophysiology of implantation site disorders. Obstet Gynecol Surv 54(3):189, 1999
Roos-Hesselink JW, Ruys TP, Stein JI, et al: Outcome of pregnancy in patients with structural or ischaemic heart disease: results of a registry of the European Society of Cardiology. Eur Heart J 34(9):657, 2013
Rouse DJ, Owen J: Prophylactic cesarean delivery for fetal macrosomia diagnosed by means of ultrasonography—a Faustian bargain? Am J Obstet Gynecol 181:332, 1999
Rouse DJ, Owen J, Goldenberg RL, et al: The effectiveness and costs of elective cesarean delivery for fetal macrosomia diagnosed by ultrasound. JAMA 276(2):1480, 1996
Roza SJ, Steegers EA, Verburg BO, et al: What is spared by fetal brain-sparing? Fetal circulatory redistribution and behavioral problems in the general population. Am J Epidemiol 168(10):1145, 2008
Rudzinski E, Gilroy M, Newbill C, et al: Positive C4d immunostaining of placental villous syncytiotrophoblasts supports host-versus-graft rejection in villitis of unknown etiology. Pediatr Dev Pathol 16(1):7, 2013
Salafia CM, Minior VK, Pezzullo JC, et al: Intrauterine growth restriction in infants of less than 32 weeks' gestation: associated placental pathologic features. Am J Obstet Gynecol 173(4):1049, 1995
Sanchez-Ramos L, Bernstein S, Kaunitz AM: Expectant management versus labor induction for suspected fetal macrosomia: a systematic review. Obstet Gynecol 100(5 pt 1):997, 2002
Schemmer G, Wapner RJ, Johnson A, et al: First-trimester growth patterns of aneuploid fetuses. Prenat Diagn 17(2):155, 1997
Scholten RR, Sep S, Peeters L, et al: Prepregnancy low-plasma volume and predisposition to preeclampsia and fetal growth restriction. Obstet Gynecol 117(5):1085, 2011
Seeds JW: Impaired fetal growth: definition and clinical diagnosis. Obstet Gynecol 64(3):303, 1984
Sheffield JS, Sánchez PJ, Morris G, et al: Congenital syphilis after maternal treatment for syphilis during pregnancy. Am J Obstet Gynecol 186(3):569, 2002
Simpson JW, Lawless RW, Mitchell AC: Responsibility of the obstetrician to the fetus, II. Influence of prepregnancy weight and pregnancy weight gain on birth weight. Obstet Gynecol 45(4):481, 1975
Smulian JC, Ananth CV, Vintzileos AM, et al: Fetal deaths in the United States. Influence of high risk conditions and implications for management. Obstet Gynecol 100(6):1183, 2002
Sparks TN, Cheng YW, McLaughlin B, et al: Fundal height: a useful screening tool for fetal growth? J Matern Fetal Neonatal Med 24(5):708, 2011
Spong CY: Add stillbirth to the list of outcomes to worry about in a pregnant woman with a history of preterm birth or fetal growth restriction. Obstet Gynecol 119(3):495, 2012
Spong CY, Mercer BM, D'alton M, et al: Timing of indicated late-preterm and early-term birth. Obstet Gynecol 118(2 Pt 1):323, 2011
Stein Z, Susser M, Saenger G, et al: In Famine and Human Development: The Dutch Hunger Winter of 1944–1945. New York, Oxford University Press, 1975
Stonek F, Hafner E, Philipp K, et al: Methylenetetrahydrofolate reductase C677T polymorphism and pregnancy complications. Obstet Gynecol 110(2 pt 1):363, 2007
Stotland NE, Caughey AB, Breed EM, et al: Risk factors and obstetric complications associated with macrosomia. Int J Gynaecol Obstet 87(3):220, 2004
Supplementation with Multiple Micronutrients Intervention Trial (SUMMIT) Study Group: Effect of maternal multiple micronutrient supplementation on fetal loss and infant death in Indonesia: a double-blind cluster-randomized trial. Lancet 371(9608):215, 2008
Tam Tam KB, Briery C, Penman AD, et al: Fetal gastroschisis: epidemiological characteristics and pregnancy outcomes in Mississippi. Am J Perinatol 28(9):689, 2011
Thornton JG, Hornbuckle J, Vail A, et al: Infant well-being at 2 years of age in the Growth Restriction Intervention Trial (GRIT): multicenter randomized controlled trial. Lancet 364(9433):513, 2004
Tongsong T, Srisupundit K, Luewan S: Outcomes of pregnancies affected by hemoglobin H disease. Int J Gynaecol Obstet 104(3):206, 2009
Turan OM, Turan S, Gungor S, et al: Progression of Doppler abnormalities in intrauterine growth restriction. Ultrasound Obstet Gynecol 32(2):160, 2008
Tuuli MG, Cahill A, Stamilio D, et al: Comparative efficiency of measures of early fetal growth restriction for predicting adverse perinatal outcomes. Obstet Gynecol 117(6):1331, 2011
Tyson JE, Kennedy K, Broyles S, et al: The small for gestational age infant: accelerated or delayed pulmonary maturation? Increased or decreased survival? Pediatrics 95(4):534, 1995
Umbers AJ, Aitken EH, Rogerson SJ: Malaria in pregnancy: small babies, big problem. Trends Parasitol 27(4):168, 2011
Unterscheider J, Daly S, Geary MP, et al: Optimizing the definition of intrauterine growth restriction: the multicenter prospective PORTO study. Am J Obstet Gynecol 208(4):290.e1, 2013
Usher R, McLean F: Intrauterine growth of live-born Caucasian infants at sea level: standards obtained from measurements in 7 dimensions of infants born between 25 and 44 weeks' gestation. J Pediatr 74(6):901, 1969
van Wyk L, Boers KE, van der Post JA, et al: Effects on (neuro)developmental and behavioral outcome at 2 years of age of induced labor compared with expectant management in intrauterine growth-restricted infants: long-term outcomes of the DIGITAT trial. Am J Obstet Gynecol 206(5):406.e1, 2012
Varastehpour A, Radaelli T, Minium J, et al: Activation of phospholipase A2 is associated with generation of placental lipid signals and fetal obesity. J Clin Endocrinol Metab 91(1):248, 2006
Vesco KK, Sharma AJ, Dietz PM, et al: Newborn size among obese women with weight gain outside the 2009 Institute of Medicine recommendation. Obstet Gynecol 117(4):812, 2011
Vidaeff AC, Blackwell SC: Potential risks and benefits of antenatal corticosteroid therapy prior to preterm birth in pregnancies complicated by severe fetal growth restriction. Obstet Gynecol Clin North Am 38(2):205, 2011
Vidaeff AC, Yeomans ER, Ramin SM: Pregnancy in women with renal disease. Part I: general principles. Am J Perinatol 25(7):385, 2008
Vrijkotte TG, Algera SJ, Brouwer IA, et al: Maternal triglyceride levels during early pregnancy are associated with birth weight and postnatal growth. J Pediatr 159(5):736, 2011
Walker DM, Marlow N, Upstone L, et al: The Growth Restriction Intervention Trial: long-term outcomes in a randomized trial of timing of delivery in fetal growth restriction. Am J Obstet Gynecol 204(1):34.e1, 2011
Weissmann-Brenner A, Simchen MJ, Zilberberg E, et al: Maternal and neonatal outcomes of macrosomic pregnancies. Med Sci Monit 18(9):PH77, 2012
Wetta L, Tita AT: Early term births: considerations in management. Obstet Gynecol Clin North Am 39(1):89, 2012
Wilkins-Haug L, Quade B, Morton CC: Confined placental mosaicism as a risk factor among newborns with fetal growth restriction. Prenat Diagn 26(5):428, 2006
Williams JW: Obstetrics: A Text-Book for Students and Practitioners, 1st ed. New York, Appleton, 1903, p 133
Williams RL: Intrauterine growth curves. Intra- and international comparisons with different ethnic groups in California. Prev Med 4:163, 1975
Williams RL, Creasy RK, Cunningham GC, et al: Fetal growth and perinatal viability in California. Obstet Gynecol 59:624, 1982
Woo JS, Liang ST, Lo RL: Significance of an absent or reversed end diastolic flow in Doppler umbilical artery waveforms. J Ultrasound Med 6(6):291, 1987
Wu YW, Croen LA, Shah SJ, et al: Cerebral palsy in term infants. Pediatrics 118(2):690, 2006
Yamamoto R, Ishii K, Shimada M, et al: Significance of maternal screening for toxoplasmosis, rubella, cytomegalovirus and herpes simplex virus infection in cases of fetal growth restriction. J Obstet Gynaecol Res 39(3):653, 2013
Zhang J, Merialdi M, Platt LD, et al: Defining normal and abnormal fetal growth: promises and challenges. Am J Obstet Gynecol 202(6):522, 2010
Zhang J, Mikolajczyk R, Grewal J, et al: Prenatal application of the individualized fetal growth reference. Am J Epidemiol 173(5):539, 2011
Zhu JL, Obel C, Hammer Bech B, et al: Infertility, infertility treatment and fetal growth restriction. Obstet Gynecol 110(6):1326, 2007

CHAPTER 45

Multifetal Pregnancy

Multifetal pregnancies may result from two or more fertilization events, from a single fertilization followed by an "erroneous" splitting of the zygote, or from a combination of both. Such pregnancies are associated with increased risk for both mother and child, and this risk increases with the number of offspring. For example, 60 percent of twins, 90 percent of triplets, and virtually all of quadruplets are born preterm (Martin, 2012). From these observations, it is apparent that women were not intended to concurrently bear more than one offspring. And although they are often viewed as a novelty or miracle, multifetal pregnancies represent a potentially perilous journey for the mother and her unborn children.

Fueled largely by infertility therapy, both the rate and the number of twin and higher-order multifetal births have increased dramatically since 1980. Specifically, the twinning rate rose 76 percent from 18.9 to 32.1 per 1000 live births in 2009 (Martin, 2012). During the same time, the number of higher-order multifetal births increased more than 400 percent to a peak in 1998. Since then, however, evolving infertility management has resulted in decreased rates of higher-order multifetal births to its lowest level in 15 years. Specifically, the rate of triplets or more decreased by 10 percent from 153 per 100,000 births in 2009 to 138 per 100,000 births in 2010 (Martin, 2012).

The overall increase in prevalence of multifetal births is of concern because the corresponding increase in the rate of preterm birth compromises neonatal survival and increases the risk of lifelong disability. For example, in this country, about a fourth of very-low-birthweight neonates—those born weighing < 2500 g—are from multifetal gestations, and 15 percent of infants who die in the first year after birth are from multifetal pregnancies (Martin, 2012). In 2009, the infant mortality rate for multiple births was five times the rate for singletons (Mathews, 2013). A comparison of singleton and twin outcomes from infants delivered at Parkland Hospital is shown in Table 45-1. These risks are magnified further with triplets or quadruplets. In addition to these adverse outcomes, the risks for congenital malformations are increased with multifetal gestation. Importantly, this increased risk is for *each* fetus and is not simply because there are more fetuses per pregnancy.

The mother may also experience higher obstetrical morbidity and mortality rates. These also increase with the number of fetuses (Mhyre, 2012; Wen, 2004). In a study of more than 44,000 multifetal pregnancies, Walker and colleagues (2004) reported that, compared with singletons, the risks for preeclampsia, postpartum hemorrhage, and maternal death were increased twofold or more. The risk for peripartum hysterectomy is also increased, and Francois and associates (2005) reported this to

TABLE 45-1. Selected Outcomes in Singleton and Twin Pregnancies Delivered at Parkland Hospital from 2002 through 2012

Outcome	Singletons (No.)	Twins (No.)
Pregnancies	78,879	850
Births[a]	78,879	1700
Stillbirths	406 (5.1)	24 (14.1)
Neonatal deaths	253 (3.2)	38 (22.4)
Perinatal deaths	659 (8.4)	62 (36.5)
Very low birthweight (< 1500 g)	895 (1.0)	196 (11.6)

[a]Birth data are represented as number (per 1000).
Data courtesy of Dr. Don McIntire.

be threefold for twins and 24-fold for triplets or quadruplets. Finally, these mothers are at increased risk for depression compared with women with a singleton pregnancy (Choi, 2009).

MECHANISMS OF MULTIFETAL GESTATIONS

Twin fetuses usually result from fertilization of two separate ova–*dizygotic* or *fraternal twins.* Less often, twins arise from a single fertilized ovum that divides–*monozygotic* or *identical twins.* Either or both processes may be involved in the formation of higher numbers. Quadruplets, for example, may arise from as few as one to as many as four ova.

Dizygotic versus Monozygotic Twinning

Dizygotic twins are not in a strict sense true twins because they result from the maturation and fertilization of two ova during a single ovulatory cycle. Moreover, from a genetic perspective, dizygotic twins are like any other pair of siblings. On the other hand, monozygotic or identical twins, although they have virtually the same genetic heritage, are usually not identical.

As discussed subsequently, the division of one fertilized zygote into two does not necessarily result in equal sharing of protoplasmic material. Monozygotic twins may actually be discordant for genetic mutations because of a postzygotic mutation, or may have the same genetic disease but with marked variability in expression. In female fetuses, skewed lyonization can produce differential expression of X-linked traits or diseases. Furthermore, the process of monozygotic twinning is in a sense a teratogenic event, and monozygotic twins have an increased incidence of often discordant malformations (Glinianaia, 2008). For example, in a study of 926 monozygotic twins, Pettit (2013) reported a 12-fold increase in the prevalence of congenital heart defects, but 68 percent of affected infants had a normal sibling. Accordingly, dizygotic or fraternal twins of the same sex may appear more nearly identical at birth than monozygotic twins.

Genesis of Monozygotic Twins

The developmental mechanisms underlying monozygotic twinning are poorly understood. Minor trauma to the blastocyst during assisted reproductive technology (ART) may lead to the increased incidence of monozygotic twinning observed in pregnancies conceived in this manner (Wenstrom, 1993).

The outcome of the monozygotic twinning process depends on when division occurs. If zygotes divide within the first 72 hours after fertilization, two embryos, two amnions, and two chorions develop, and a diamnionic, dichorionic twin pregnancy evolves (Fig. 45-1). Two distinct placentas or a single, fused placenta may develop. If division occurs between the fourth and eighth day, a diamnionic, monochorionic twin pregnancy results. By approximately 8 days after fertilization, the chorion and the amnion have already differentiated, and division results in two embryos within a common amnionic sac, that is, a monoamnionic, monochorionic twin pregnancy. Conjoined twins result if twinning is initiated later.

It has long been accepted that monochorionicity incontrovertibly indicated monozygosity. Rarely, however, monochorionic twins may in fact be dizygotic (Hack, 2009). Mechanisms for this are speculative, but Ekelund and coworkers (2008) found in their review of 14 such cases that nearly all have been conceived after ART procedures.

Superfetation and Superfecundation

In *superfetation,* an interval as long as or longer than a menstrual cycle intervenes between fertilizations. Superfetation requires ovulation and fertilization during the course of an established pregnancy, which is theoretically possible until the uterine cavity is obliterated by fusion of the decidua capsularis to the decidua parietalis. Although known to occur in mares, superfetation is not known to occur spontaneously in humans. Lantieri and colleagues (2010) reported a case after ovarian hyperstimulation and intrauterine insemination in the presence of an undiagnosed tubal pregnancy. Most authorities believe that alleged cases of human superfetation result from markedly unequal growth and development of twin fetuses with the same gestational age.

Superfecundation refers to fertilization of two ova within the same menstrual cycle but not at the same coitus, nor necessarily by sperm from the same male. An instance of superfecundation or heteropaternity, documented by Harris (1982), is demonstrated in Figure 45-2. The mother was sexually assaulted on the 10th day of her menstrual cycle and had intercourse 1 week later with her husband. She was delivered of a black neonate whose blood type was A and a white neonate whose blood type was O. The blood type of the mother and her husband was O.

Frequency of Twinning

Dizygotic twinning is much more common than monozygous splitting of a single oocyte, and its incidence is influenced by race, heredity, maternal age, parity, and, especially, fertility treatment. By contrast, the frequency of monozygotic twin births is relatively constant worldwide—approximately one set per 250 births, and this incidence is generally independent of race, heredity, age, and parity. One exception is that zygotic splitting is increased following ART (Aston, 2008).

The "Vanishing Twin"

The incidence of twins in the first trimester is much greater than the incidence of twins at birth. Studies in which fetuses were

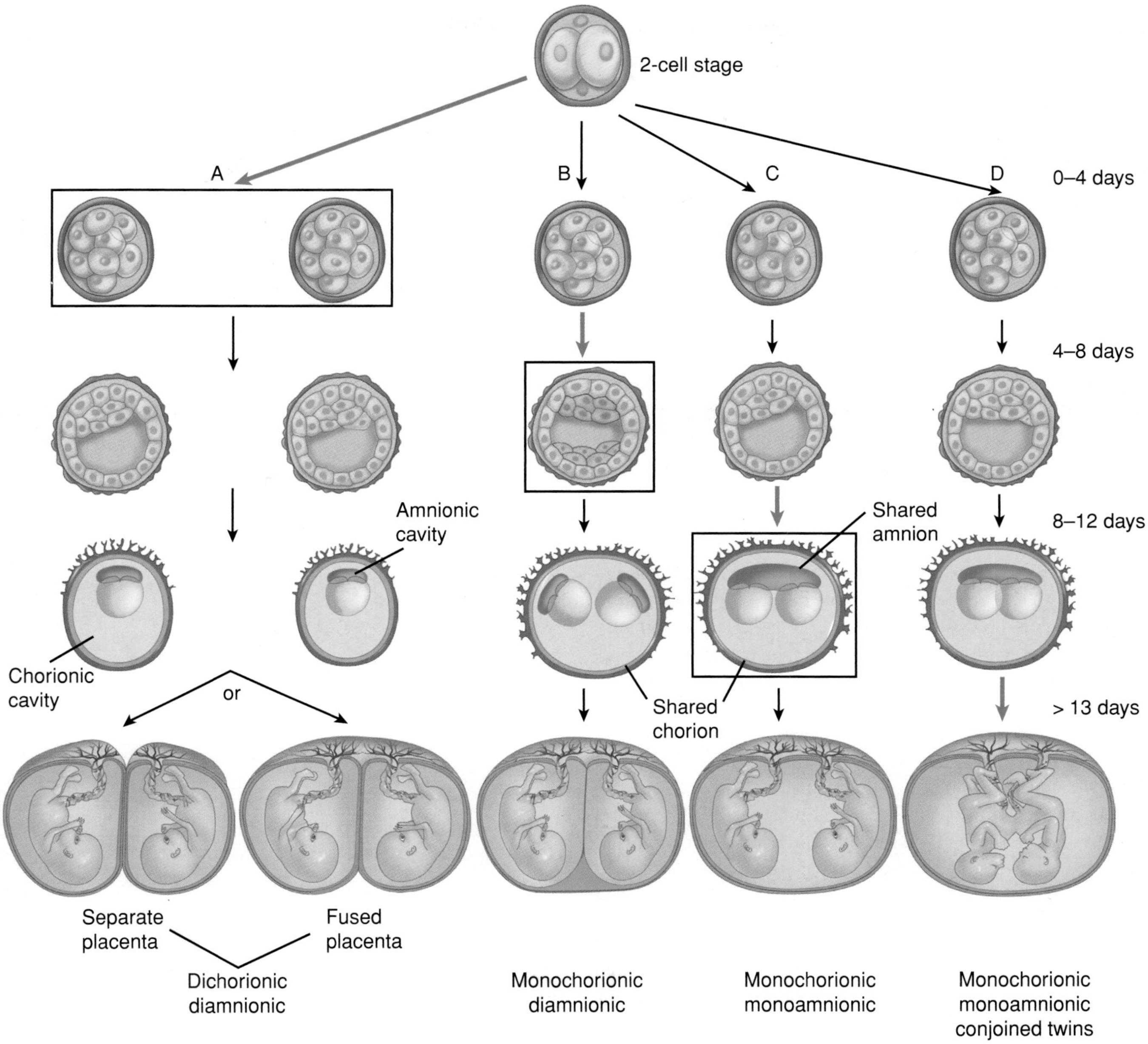

FIGURE 45-1 Mechanism of monozygotic twinning. Black boxing and blue arrows in columns A, B, and C indicate timing of division. **A.** At 0 to 4 days postfertilization, an early conceptus may divide into two. Division at this early stage creates two chorions and two amnions (dichorionic, diamnionic). Placentas may be separate or fused. **B.** Division between 4 and 8 days leads to formation of a blastocyst with two separate embryoblasts (inner cell masses). Each embryoblast will form its own amnion within a shared chorion (monochorionic, diamnionic). **C.** Between 8 and 12 days, the amnion and amnionic cavity form above the germinal disc. Embryonic division leads to two embryos with a shared amnion and shared chorion (monochorionic, monoamnionic). **D.** Differing theories explain conjoined twin development. One describes an incomplete splitting of one embryo into two. The other describes fusion of a portion of one embryo from a monozygotic pair onto the other.

evaluated with sonography in the first trimester have shown that one twin is lost or "vanishes" before the second trimester in up to 10 to 40 percent of all twin pregnancies (Brady, 2013). The incidence is higher in the setting of ART.

Monochorionic twins have a significantly greater risk of abortion than dichorionic twins (Sperling, 2006). In some cases, the entire pregnancy aborts. In many cases, however, only one fetus dies, and the remaining fetus delivers as a singleton. Undoubtedly, some threatened abortions have resulted in death and resorption of one embryo from an unrecognized twin gestation. It has been estimated that 1 in *80 births* are multifetal, whereas 1 in 8 *pregnancies* begin multifetal followed by spontaneous reduction of one or more embryos or fetuses (Corsello, 2010).

Dickey and associates (2002) described spontaneous reduction in 709 women with a multifetal pregnancy. Before 12 weeks, one or more embryos died in 36 percent of twin pregnancies, 53 percent of triplet pregnancies, and 65 percent of quadruplet pregnancies. Interestingly, pregnancy duration and birthweight were inversely related to the initial gestational sac number regardless

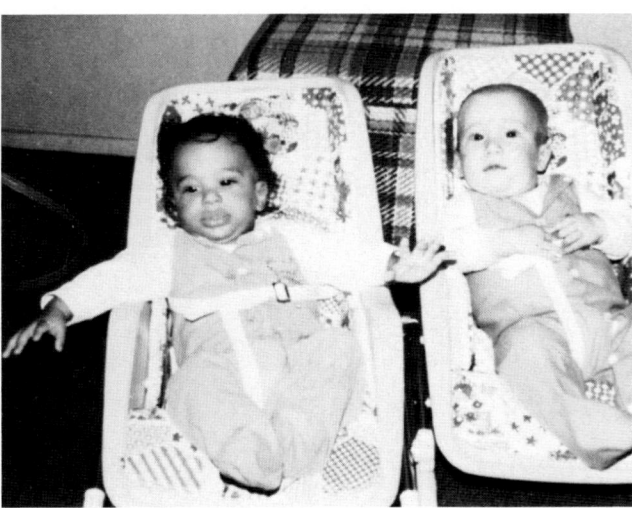

FIGURE 45-2 An example of dizygotic twin boys as the consequence of superfecundation.

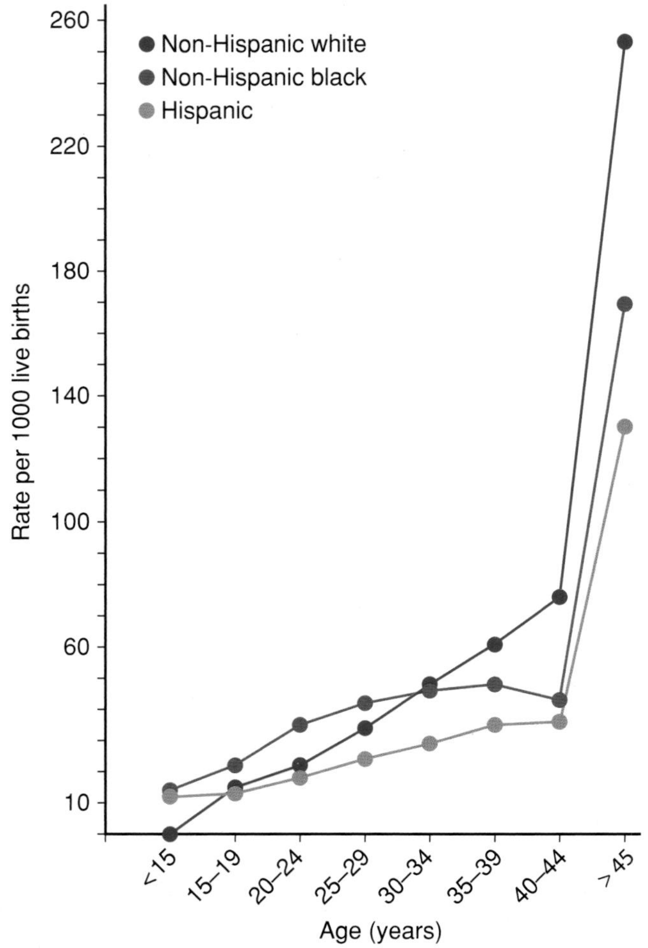

FIGURE 45-3 Multifetal birth rates in the United States according to maternal age and race, 2010. (Data from Martin, 2012.)

of the final number of fetuses at delivery. This effect was most pronounced in twins who started as quadruplets. Chasen and coworkers (2006) reported that spontaneous reduction of an in vitro fertilization (IVF) twin pregnancy to a singleton pregnancy was associated with perinatal outcomes intermediate between IVF singleton pregnancies and IVF twin pregnancies that did not undergo spontaneous reduction.

In one analysis of 41 cases of spontaneous reduction, higher values of *pregnancy-associated plasma protein A* (PAPP-A) and free β-human chorionic gonadotropin (β-hCG) were identified (Chasen, 2006). Gjerris and colleagues (2009) compared 56 cases of "vanishing twin" to 897 singletons after ART and did not identify any differences in first-trimester serum markers as long as the reduction was identified before 9 weeks. If diagnosed after 9 weeks, the serum markers were higher and less precise than in singleton ART gestations. Therefore, the diagnosis of vanishing twin should be excluded to avoid confusion during maternal serum screening for Down syndrome or neural-tube defects (Chap. 14, p. 283).

Factors That Influence Twinning

Race. The frequency of multifetal births varies significantly among different races and ethnic groups (Table 45-2). Abel and Kruger (2012) analyzed more than 8 million births in the United States between 2004 and 2008. These investigators found the highest rate of twinning in African American women (3.5 percent) and lower rates in white (3.0 percent) women. Hispanic, Asian, and Native American women had comparatively lower rates then white women. In one rural community in Nigeria, Knox and Morley (1960) found that twinning occurred once in every 20 births! These marked differences in twinning frequency may be the consequence of racial variations in levels of follicle-stimulating hormone—FSH (Nylander, 1973).

TABLE 45-2. Twinning Rates per 1000 Births by Zygosity

Country	Monozygotic	Dizygotic	Total
Nigeria	5.0	49	54
United States			
Black	4.7	11.1	15.8
White	4.2	7.1	11.3
England and Wales	3.5	8.8	12.3
India (Calcutta)	3.3	8.1	11.4
Japan	3.0	1.3	4.3

From MacGillivray, 1986, with permission.

Maternal Age. As depicted in Figure 45-3, maternal age is another important risk factor for multiple births. Dizygotic twinning frequency increases almost fourfold between the ages of 15 and 37 years (Painter, 2010). It is in this age range that maximal FSH stimulation increases the rate of multiple follicles developing (Beemsterboer, 2006). The rate of twinning also increases dramatically with advancing maternal age because the use of ART is more likely in older women (Ananth, 2012). Although paternal age has been linked to frequency of twinning, its affect is felt to be small (Abel, 2012).

Parity. Increasing parity has been shown to independently increase the incidence of twinning in all populations studied. Antsaklis and coworkers (2013) noted a progressive increase in multiparity in twinning during a 30-year period, but cautioned that some of this increase is presumably due to ART. In a two-year study from Nigeria, where such technology is not commonly available, Olusanya (2012) calculated an eightfold increase in multiple gestations when parity was 4 or less and a 20-fold increase when parity was 5 or more compared with primiparas.

Heredity. As a determinant of twinning, the family history of the mother is more important than that of the father. In a study of 4000 genealogical records, White and Wyshak (1964) found that women who themselves were a dizygotic twin gave birth to twins at a rate of 1 set per 58 births. Women who were not a twin, but whose husbands were a dizygotic twin, gave birth to twins at a rate of 1 set per 116 pregnancies. Painter and associates (2010) performed genome-wide linkage analyses on more than 500 families of mothers of dizygotic twins and identified four potential linkage peaks. The highest peak was on the long arm of chromosome 6, with other suggestive peaks on chromosomes 7, 9, and 16. That said, the contribution of these variants to the overall incidence of twinning is likely small (Hoekstra, 2008).

Nutritional Factors. In animals, litter size increases in proportion to nutritional sufficiency. Evidence from various sources indicates that this occurs in humans as well. Nylander (1971) showed a definite increasing gradient in the twinning rate related to greater nutritional status as reflected by maternal size. Taller, heavier women had a twinning rate 25 to 30 percent greater than short, nutritionally deprived women. Evidence acquired during and after World War II showed that twinning correlated more with nutrition than body size. Widespread undernourishment in Europe during those years was associated with a marked fall in the dizygotic twinning rate (Bulmer, 1959). Several investigators have reported a 40-percent increase in the prevalence of twinning among women who have taken supplementary folic acid (Ericson, 2001; Haggarty, 2006; Hasbargen, 2000). Conversely, in a systematic review, Muggli and Halliday (2007) were unable to demonstrate a significant association. Analysis of twinning rate in Texas after folic acid fortification of cereal-grain products also did not demonstrate an independent increase in twinning between 1996 and 1998 (Waller, 2003).

Pituitary Gonadotropin. The common factor linking race, age, weight, and fertility to multifetal gestation may be FSH levels (Benirschke, 1973). This theory is supported by the fact that increased fecundity and a higher rate of dizygotic twinning have been reported in women who conceive within 1 month after stopping oral contraceptives, but not during subsequent months (Rothman, 1977). This may be due to the sudden release of pituitary gonadotropin in amounts greater than usual during the first spontaneous cycle after stopping hormonal contraception. Indeed, the paradox of declining fertility but increasing twinning with advancing maternal age can be explained by an exaggerated pituitary release of FSH in response to decreased negative feedback from impending ovarian failure (Beemsterboer, 2006).

Infertility Therapy. Ovulation induction with FSH plus chorionic gonadotropin or clomiphene citrate remarkably enhances the likelihood of multiple ovulations. A mainstay of current infertility therapy and common antecedent to IVF is ovarian stimulation followed by timed intrauterine insemination. In their review of this practice, McClamrock and coworkers (2012) reported rates of twin and higher-order multifetal pregnancies as high as 28.6 percent and 9.3 percent, respectively. Rates this high remain a major concern. There are currently two ongoing multicenter trials—Assessment of Multiple Gestations from Ovarian Stimulation (AMIGOS) and Pregnancy in Polycystic Ovary Syndrome II (PPCOSII)—that are designed to provide guidance on achieving maximum pregnancy rates while minimizing multifetal gestation rates (Diamond, 2011; Legro, 2012).

In general with IVF, the greater the number of embryos that are transferred, the greater the risk of twins and multiple fetuses. In 2005, 1 percent of infants born in the United States were conceived through ART, and these infants accounted for 17 percent of multifetal births (Wright, 2008). The American Society for Reproductive Medicine (2013) recently revised their age-related guidelines on numbers of cleavage-stage embryos or blastocysts to transfer in an effort to reduce the incidence of higher-order multifetal pregnancies. For example, women younger than 35 years with a favorable prognosis should have no more than two embryos transferred. These practices have effectively lowered rates (Kulkarni, 2013).

Sex Ratios with Multiple Fetuses

In humans, as the number of fetuses per pregnancy increases, the percentage of male conceptuses decreases. Strandskov and coworkers (1946) found the percentage of males in 31 million singleton births in the United States was 51.6 percent. For twins, it was 50.9 percent; for triplets, 49.5 percent; and for quadruplets, 46.5 percent. Swedish birth data spanning 135 years reveals the number of males per 100 female infants born was 106 among singletons, 103 among twins, and 99 among triplets (Fellman, 2010). Females predominate even more in twins from late twinning events. For example, 68 percent of thoracopagus conjoined twins are female (Mutchinick, 2011). Two explanations have been offered. First, beginning in utero and extending throughout the life cycle, mortality rates are lower in females. Second, female zygotes have a greater tendency to divide.

Determination of Zygosity

Twins of opposite sex are almost always dizygotic. In rare instances, due to somatic mutations or chromosome aberrations, the karyotype or phenotype of a monozygous twin gestation can be different. Most reported cases are related to postzygotic loss of the Y chromosome in one 46,XY twin. This results in a phenotypically female twin due to Turner syndrome (45,X). Zech and colleagues (2008) reported a rare case of a 47,XXY zygote that underwent postzygotic loss of the X chromosome in some cells and loss of the Y chromosome in other cells. The phenotype of the resultant twins was one male and one female. Karyotype analyses revealed both to be 46,XX/46,XY genetic mosaics.

TABLE 45-3. Overview of the Incidence of Twin Pregnancy Zygosity and Corresponding Twin-Specific Complications

		Rates of Twin-Specific Complications in Percent			
Type of Twinning	Twins	Fetal-Growth Restriction	Preterm Delivery[a]	Placental Vascular Anastomosis	Perinatal Mortality
Dizygous	80	25	40	0	10–12
Monozygous	20	40	50		15–18
Diamnionic/dichorionic	6–7	30	40	0	18–20
Diamnionic/monochorionic	13–14	50	60	100	30–40
Monoamnionic/monochorionic	< 1	40	60–70	80–90	58–60
Conjoined	0.002 to 0.008	—	70–80	100	70–90

[a]Delivery before 37 weeks.
Modified from Manning, 1995, with permission.

The risk for twin-specific complications varies in relation to zygosity as well as *chorionicity*—the number of chorions. As shown in Table 45-3, the latter is the more important determinant. Specifically, there are increased rates of perinatal mortality and neurological injury in monochorionic diamnionic twins compared with dichorionic pairs (Hack, 2008; Lee, 2008). In their retrospective analysis of more than 2000 twins, McPherson and associates (2012) reported that the risk of fetal demise in one or both monochorionic twins was twice that in dichorionic multifetal gestations.

Sonographic Determination of Chorionicity

Chorionicity can sometimes be identified in the first trimester with sonography. Two separate placentas suggest dizygosity. In pregnancies with a single placental mass, it may be difficult to identify chorionicity. Identification of a thick dividing membrane—generally 2 mm or greater—supports a presumed diagnosis of dichorionicity. Also, the *twin peak sign* is seen by examining the point of origin of the dividing membrane on the placental surface. The peak appears as a triangular projection of placental tissue extending a short distance between the layers of the dividing membrane (Fig. 45-4).

In contrast, monochorionic pregnancies have a dividing membrane that is so thin it may not be seen until the second trimester. The membrane is generally less than 2-mm thick, and magnification reveals only two layers. The right-angle relationship between the membranes and placenta and no apparent extension of placenta between the dividing membranes is called the *T sign* (Fig. 45-5). Evaluation of the dividing membrane can establish chorionicity in more than 99 percent of pregnancies in the first trimester (Miller, 2012).

Placental Examination

A carefully performed visual examination of the placenta and membranes after delivery serves to establish zygosity and chorionicity promptly in approximately two thirds of cases. The following systematic examination is recommended. As the first neonate is delivered, one clamp is placed on a portion of its cord. Cord blood is generally not collected until after delivery of the other twin. As the second neonate is delivered, two clamps are placed on that cord. Three clamps are used to mark the cord of a third neonate, and so on as necessary. Until the delivery of the last fetus, each cord segment must remain clamped to prevent fetal hypovolemia and anemia caused by blood leaving the placenta via anastomoses and then through an unclamped cord.

The placenta should be carefully delivered to preserve the attachment of the amnion and chorion. With one common amnionic sac, or with juxtaposed amnions not separated by chorion arising between the fetuses, the fetuses are monozygotic. If adjacent amnions are separated by chorion, then the fetuses could be either dizygotic or monozygotic, but dizygosity is more common (see Figs. 45-1 and 45-6). If the neonates are of the same sex, blood typing of cord blood samples may be helpful. Different blood types confirm dizygosity, although demonstrating the same blood type in each fetus does not confirm monozygosity. For definitive diagnosis, more complicated techniques such as DNA fingerprinting can be used, but these tests are generally not performed at birth unless there is a pressing medical indication.

DIAGNOSIS OF MULTIPLE FETUSES

Clinical Evaluation

During examination, accurate fundal height measurement, described in Chapter 9 (p. 176), is essential. With multiple fetuses, uterine size is typically larger during the second trimester than expected. Rouse and associates (1993) reported fundal heights in 336 well-dated twin pregnancies. Between 20 and 30 weeks, fundal heights averaged approximately 5 cm greater than expected for singletons of the same fetal age.

In general, it is difficult to diagnose twins by palpation of fetal parts before the third trimester. Even late in pregnancy, it may be difficult to identify twins by abdominal palpation, especially if one twin overlies the other, if the woman is obese, or if there is hydramnios. Palpating two fetal heads, often in different uterine quadrants, strongly supports a twin diagnosis.

Late in the first trimester, fetal heart action may be detected with Doppler ultrasonic equipment. Thereafter, it becomes possible to identify two fetal heartbeats if their rates are clearly distinct from each other and from that of the mother. Careful examination with an aural fetal stethoscope can identify fetal heart sounds in twins as early as 18 to 20 weeks.

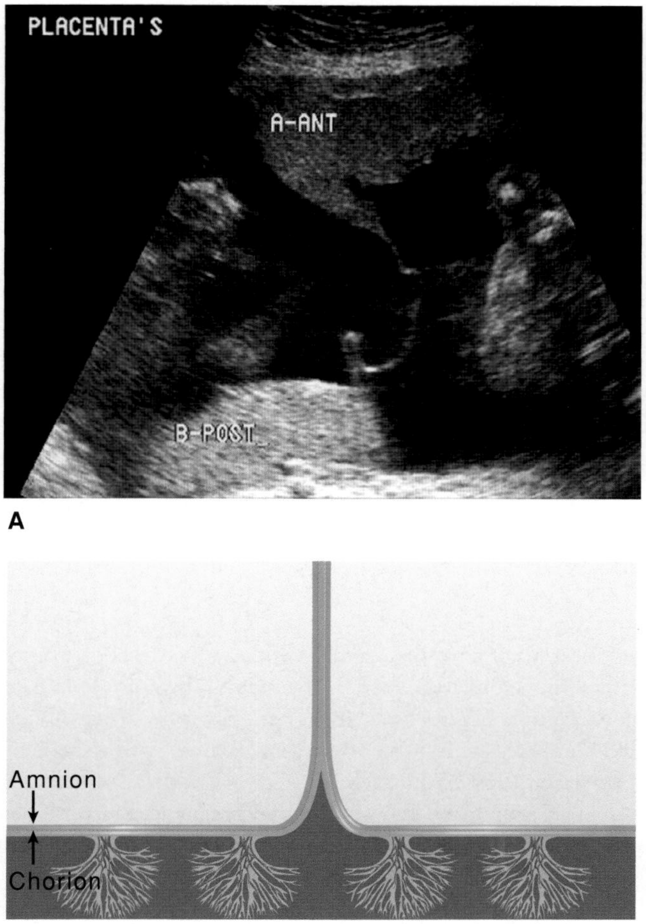

FIGURE 45-4 A. Sonographic image of the "twin-peak" sign, also termed the "lambda sign," in a 24-week gestation. At the top of this sonogram, tissue from the anterior placenta is seen extending downward between the amnion layers. This sign confirms dichorionic twinning. **B.** Schematic diagram of the "twin-peak" sign. A triangular portion of placenta is seen insinuating between the amniochorion layers.

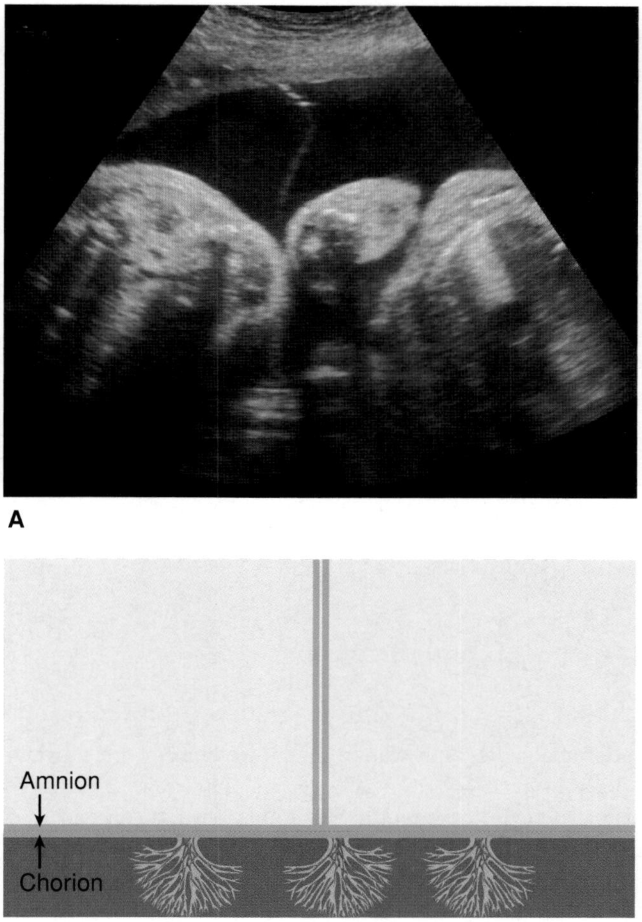

FIGURE 45-5 A. Sonographic image of the "T" sign in a monochorionic diamnionic gestation at 30 weeks. **B.** Schematic diagram of the "T" sign. Twins are separated only by a membrane created by the juxtaposed amnion of each twin. A "T" is formed at the point at which amnions meet the placenta.

Sonography

By careful sonographic examination, separate gestational sacs can be identified early in twin pregnancy (Fig. 45-7). Subsequently, each fetal head should be seen in two perpendicular planes so as not to mistake a cross section of the fetal trunk for a second fetal head. Ideally, two fetal heads or two abdomens should be seen in the same image plane, to avoid scanning the same fetus twice and interpreting it as twins. Sonographic examination should detect practically all sets of twins. Given the increased frequency of sonographic examinations during the first trimester, early detection of a twin pregnancy is common. Indeed, one argument in favor of routine first-trimester sonographic screening is earlier detection of multiple fetuses.

Higher-order multifetal gestations are more difficult to evaluate. Even in the first trimester, it can be difficult to identify the actual number of fetuses and their position. This determination is especially important if pregnancy reduction or selective termination is considered (p. 919).

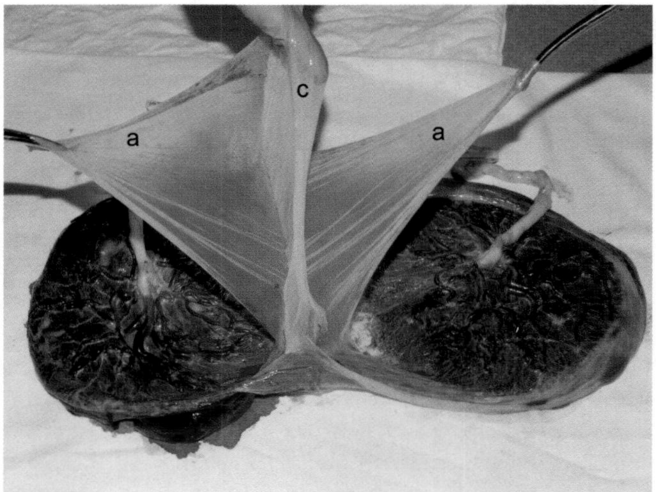

FIGURE 45-6 Dichorionic diamnionic twin placenta. The membrane partition that separated twin fetuses is elevated and consists of chorion (*c*) between two amnions (*a*).

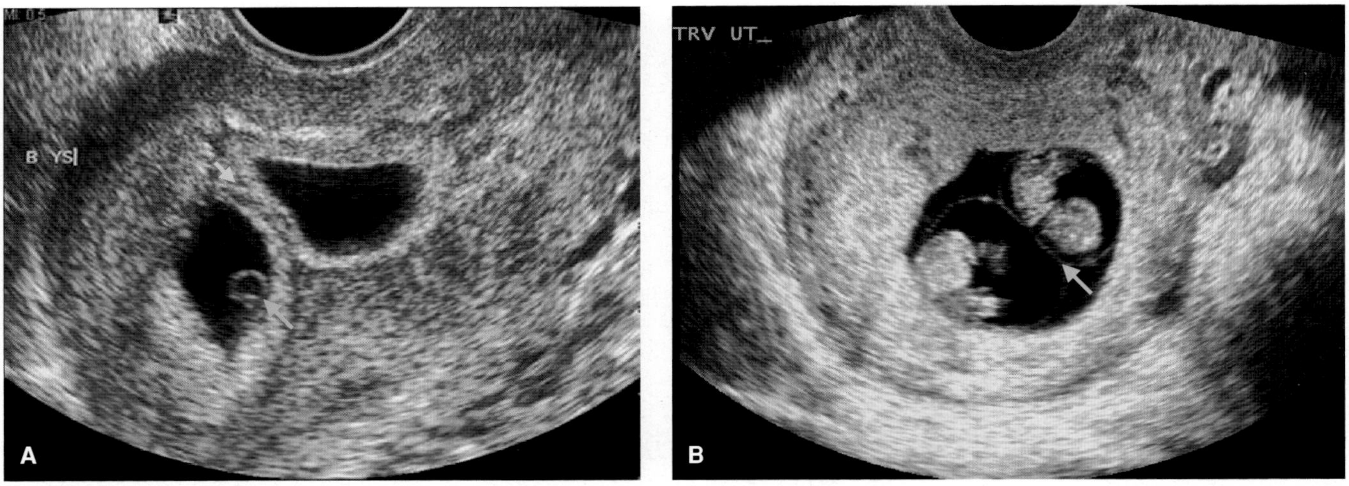

FIGURE 45-7 Sonograms of first-trimester twins. **A.** Dichorionic diamnionic twin pregnancy at 6 weeks' gestation. Note the thick dividing chorion (*yellow arrow*). One of the yolk sacs is indicated (*blue arrow*). **B.** Monochorionic diamnionic twin pregnancy at 8 weeks' gestation. Note the thin amnion encircling each embryo, resulting in a thin dividing membrane (*blue arrow*).

Other Diagnostic Aids

Radiography and Magnetic Resonance Imaging

Abdominal radiography can be used if fetal number in a higher-order multifetal gestation is uncertain. However, radiographs generally have limited utility and may lead to an incorrect diagnosis if there is hydramnios, obesity, fetal movement during the exposure, or inappropriate exposure time. Additionally, fetal skeletons before 18 weeks' gestation are insufficiently radiopaque and may be poorly seen.

Although not typically used to diagnose multifetal pregnancy, magnetic resonance (MR) imaging may help delineate complications in monochorionic twins (Hu, 2006). Bekiesinska-Figatowska and colleagues (2013) reviewed their experience with 17 complicated twin gestations evaluated by both sonographic and MR imaging. They concluded that MR imaging provides a more detailed assessment of pathology in twins and is particularly helpful in cases of conjoined twins.

Biochemical Tests

There is no biochemical test that reliably identifies multiple fetuses. Serum and urine levels of β-hCG and maternal serum alpha-fetoprotein (MSAFP) are generally higher with twins compared with singletons. However, levels may vary considerably and overlap with those of singletons.

MATERNAL ADAPTATION TO MULTIFETAL PREGNANCY

The various physiological burdens of pregnancy and the likelihood of serious maternal complications are typically greater with multiple fetuses than with a singleton. This should be considered, especially when counseling a woman whose health is compromised and in whom multifetal gestation is recognized early. Similar consideration is given to a woman who is not pregnant but is considering infertility treatment.

Beginning in the first trimester, and temporarily associated with higher serum β-hCG levels, women with multifetal gestation often have nausea and vomiting in excess of women with a singleton pregnancy. In women with multiple fetuses, blood volume expansion is greater and averages 50 to 60 percent compared with 40 to 50 percent in those with a singleton (Pritchard, 1965). Although the red cell mass also increases, it does so proportionately less in twin pregnancies. Combined with increased iron and folate requirements, this predisposes to anemia. This augmented hypervolemia teleologically offsets blood loss with vaginal delivery of twins, which is twice that with a single fetus.

Women carrying twins also have a typical pattern of arterial blood pressure change. MacDonald-Wallis and coworkers (2012) analyzed serial blood pressures in more than 13,000 singleton and twin pregnancies. As early as 8 weeks' gestation, the diastolic blood pressure in women with twins was lower than that with singleton pregnancies but generally increased to a greater degree at term. In an earlier study, Campbell (1986) demonstrated that this increase was at least 15 mm Hg in 95 percent of women with twins compared with only 54 percent of women with a singleton.

Hypervolemia along with decreased vascular resistance has an impressive affect on cardiac function. Kametas and associates (2003) assessed function in 119 women with a twin pregnancy. In these women, cardiac output was increased another 20 percent above that in women with a singleton pregnancy. Kuleva and colleagues (2011) compared serial echocardiography results in 20 women with uncomplicated twin pregnancies with those of 10 women with singletons. Similarly, they also demonstrated a greater increase in cardiac output in those with twins. Both studies found the cardiac output rise was predominantly due to greater stroke volume and to a much lesser degree due to increased heart rate. Vascular resistance was significantly lower in twin gestations throughout pregnancy compared with singleton gestations (Kuleva, 2011).

Uterine growth in a multifetal gestation is substantively greater than in a singleton pregnancy. The uterus and its nonfetal contents may achieve a volume of 10 L or more and weigh in excess of 20 pounds. Especially with monozygotic twins, excessive amounts of amnionic fluid may rapidly accumulate. In these circumstances, maternal abdominal viscera and lungs can be appreciably compressed and displaced by the expanding uterus. As a result, the size and weight of the large uterus may preclude more than a sedentary existence for these women.

If hydramnios develops, maternal renal function can become seriously impaired, most likely as the consequence of obstructive uropathy (Quigley, 1977). With severe hydramnios, therapeutic amniocentesis may provide relief for the mother, may improve obstructive uropathy, and possibly may lower the preterm delivery risk that follows preterm labor or prematurely ruptured membranes (Chap. 11, p. 236). Unfortunately, hydramnios is often characterized by acute onset remote from term and by rapid reaccumulation following amniocentesis.

PREGNANCY COMPLICATIONS

Spontaneous Abortion

Miscarriage is more likely with multiple fetuses. During a 16-year study, Joo and colleagues (2012) demonstrated that the spontaneous abortion rate per live birth in singleton pregnancies was 0.9 percent compared with 7.3 percent in multiple pregnancies. Furthermore, they found that monochorial placentation was more common in multiple gestations ending in miscarriage than in those resulting in a livebirth. Twin pregnancies achieved through ART are at increased risk for abortion compared with those conceived spontaneously (Szymusik, 2012).

Congenital Malformations

The incidence of congenital malformations is appreciably increased in multifetal gestations compared with singletons. Glinianaia and associates (2008) reported that the rate of congenital malformations was 406 per 10,000 twins versus 238 per 10,000 singletons. In this survey-based study, the malformation rate in monochorionic twins was almost twice that of dichorionic twin gestations. This increase has been attributed to the high incidence of structural defects in monozygotic twins. But from a 30-year European registry of multifetal births, Boyle and coworkers (2013) found a steady increase in structural anomalies from 1987 (2.16 percent) to 2007 (3.26 percent). During this time, the proportion of dizygotic twins increased by 30 percent, while the proportion of monozygotic twins remained stable. This higher risk of congenital malformations in dizygotic twins over time correlates with increased availability of ART. An increase in birth defects related to ART has been reported repeatedly (Talauliker, 2012).

Low Birthweight

Multifetal gestations are more likely to be low birthweight than singleton pregnancies due to restricted fetal growth and preterm delivery. From 1988 to 2012 at Parkland Hospital, data were collected from 357,205 singleton neonates without malformations and from 3714 normal twins who were both liveborn. Birthweights in twin infants closely paralleled those of singletons until 28 to 30 weeks' gestation. Thereafter, twin birthweights progressively lagged (Fig. 45-8). Beginning at 35 to 36 weeks, twin birthweights clearly diverge from those of singletons.

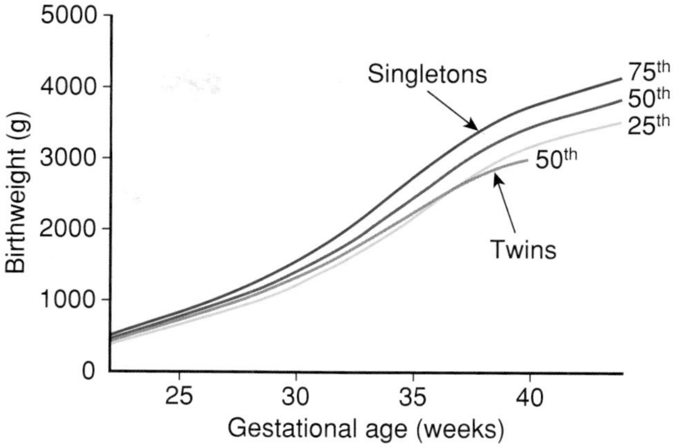

FIGURE 45-8 Birthweight percentiles (25th to 75th) for 357,205 singleton neonates compared with the 50th birthweight percentile for 3714 twins, Parkland Hospital 1988—2012. Infants with major malformations, pregnancies complicated by stillbirth, and twin gestations with > 25 percent discordance were excluded. (Data courtesy of Dr. Don McIntire.)

In general, the degree of growth restriction increases with fetal number. The caveat is that this assessment is based on growth curves established for singletons. Several authorities argue that fetal growth in twins is different from that of singleton pregnancies, and thus abnormal growth should be diagnosed only when fetal size is less than expected for *multifetal gestation.* Accordingly, twin and triplet growth curves have been developed (Kim, 2010; Odibo, 2013; Vora, 2006).

The degree of growth restriction in monozygotic twins is likely to be greater than that in dizygotic pairs (Fig. 45-9). With monochorionic embryos, allocation of blastomeres may not be equal, vascular anastomoses within the placenta may cause unequal distribution of nutrients and oxygen, and discordant structural anomalies resulting from the twinning event

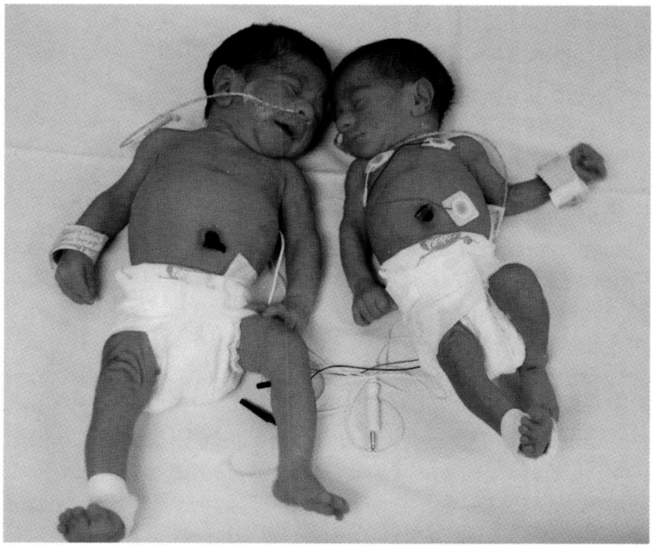

FIGURE 45-9 Marked growth discordance in monochorionic twins. (Photograph contributed by Dr. Laura Greer.)

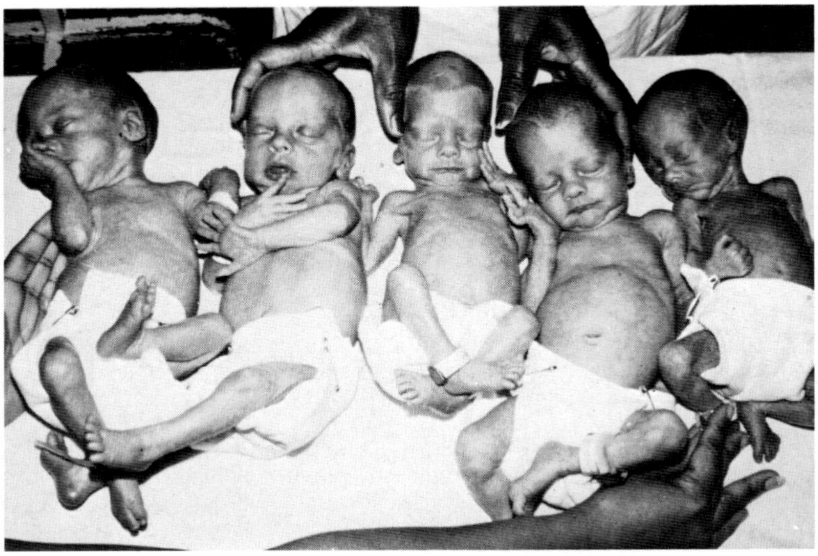

FIGURE 45-10 Davis quintuplets at 3 weeks following delivery. The first, second, and fourth newborns from the left each arose from separate ova, whereas the third and fifth neonates are from the same ovum.

itself may affect growth. For example, the quintuplets shown in Figure 45-10 represent three dizygotic and two monozygotic fetuses. When delivered at 31 weeks, the three neonates from separate ova weighed 1420, 1530, and 1440 g, whereas the two derived from the same ovum weighed 990 and 860 g.

In the third trimester, the larger fetal mass leads to accelerated placental maturation and relative placental insufficiency. In dizygotic pregnancies, marked size discordancy usually results from unequal placentation, with one placental site receiving more perfusion than the other. Size differences may also reflect different genetic fetal-growth potentials. Discordancy can also result from fetal malformations, genetic syndromes, infection, or umbilical cord abnormalities such as velamentous insertion, marginal insertion, or vasa previa (Chap. 6, p. 122).

Hypertension

Hypertensive disorders due to pregnancy are more likely to develop with multiple fetuses. The exact incidence attributable to twin gestation is difficult to determine because twin pregnancies are more likely to deliver preterm before preeclampsia can develop and because women with twin pregnancies are often older and multiparous. The incidence of pregnancy-related hypertension in women with twins is 20 percent at Parkland Hospital. In their analysis of 513 twin pregnancies > 20 weeks' gestation, Fox and coworkers (2014) also identified 20 percent of parturients with either gestational hypertension or preeclampsia. Case-control analyses suggest that prepregnancy body mass index (BMI) ≥ 30 kg/m^2 and egg donation are additional independent risk factors for preeclampsia. Gonzalez and colleagues (2012) compared 257 women with twins and gestational diabetes with 277 nondiabetic women carrying twins. These researchers found a twofold increased risk of preeclampsia in women diagnosed with gestational diabetes. Finally, in the Matched Multiple Birth Dataset for the National Center for Health Statistics, Luke and associates (2008) analyzed 316,696 twin, 12,193 triplet, and 778 quadruple pregnancies. These investigators found that the risk for pregnancy-associated hypertension was significantly increased for triplets and quadruplets (11 and 12 percent, respectively) compared with that for twins (8 percent).

These data suggest that fetal number and placental mass are involved in preeclampsia pathogenesis. Women with twin pregnancies have levels of antiangiogenic soluble fms-like tyrosine kinase-1 (sFlt-1) that are twice that of singletons. Levels are seemingly related to increased placental mass rather than primary placental pathology (Bdolah, 2008; Maynard, 2008). Rana and coworkers (2012) measured antiangiogenic sFlt-1 and proangiogenic placental growth factor (PlGF) in 79 women with twins referred for evaluation of preeclampsia. In the 58 women identified with either gestational hypertension or preeclampsia, there was a stepwise increase in sFlt-1 concentrations, decrease in PlGF levels, and increase in sFlt-1/PlGF ratios compared with normotensive twin pregnancies. With multifetal gestation, hypertension not only develops more often but also tends to develop earlier and be more severe. In the analysis of angiogenic factors mentioned above, more than one half presented before 34 weeks, and in those who did, the sFlt-1/PlGF ratio rise was more striking (Rana, 2012). This relationship is discussed in Chapter 40 (p. 735).

Preterm Birth

The duration of gestation decreases with increasing fetal number (Fig. 45-11). According to Martin and colleagues (2012), more than five of every 10 twins and nine of 10 triplets born in the United States in 2010 were delivered preterm. Delivery before term is a major reason for increased neonatal morbidity and mortality ra[illegible] in multifetal pregnancy. Prematurity is increased sixfold an[illegible] fold in twins and triplets, respectively (Giuffre, 2012). In the[illegible]eview, Chauhan and associates (2010) reported that, similar to singleton pregnancies, approximately 60 percent of preterm births in twins are indicated, about a third result from spontaneous labor, and 10 percent follow prematurely ruptured membranes. In their analysis of almost 300,000 live births in Ohio, Pakrashi and DeFranco (2013) found that the proportion of preterm birth associated with premature membrane rupture increased with gestational plurality from 13 percent with singletons to 20 percent with triplets or more.

The preterm birth rate among multifetal gestations has increased during the past two decades. In an analysis of nearly 350,000 twin births, Kogan and coworkers (2000) showed that during the 16-year period ending in 1997, the term birth rate among twins declined by 22 percent. Joseph and colleagues (2001) attributed this decline to an increased rate of indicated preterm deliveries. This trend is not necessarily negative, as it was associated with decreased perinatal morbidity and mortality

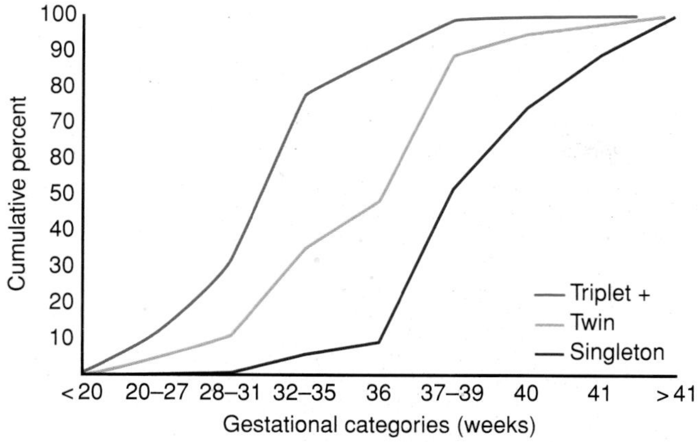

FIGURE 45-11 Cumulative percent of singleton, twin, and triplet or higher-order multifetal births according to gestational age at delivery in the United States during 1990. (From Luke, 1994, with permission.)

rates among twins that reached 34 weeks. Although the causes of preterm delivery in twins and singletons may be different, neonatal outcome is generally the same at similar gestational ages (Gardner, 1995; Kilpatrick, 1996; Ray, 2009). Importantly, outcomes for preterm twins who are markedly discordant may not be comparable with those for singletons because whatever caused the discordance may have long-lasting effects.

Prolonged Pregnancy

More than 40 years ago, Bennett and Dunn (1969) suggested that a twin pregnancy of 40 weeks or more should be considered postterm. Twin stillborn neonates delivered at 40 weeks or beyond commonly had features similar to those of postmature singletons (Chap. 43, p. 864). From an analysis of almost 300,000 twin births, Kahn and coworkers (2003) calculated that at and beyond 39 weeks, the risk of subsequent stillbirth was greater than the risk of neonatal mortality. At Parkland Hospital, twin gestations have empirically been considered to be prolonged at 40 weeks.

Long-Term Infant Development

Historically, twins have been considered cognitively delayed compared with singletons (Record, 1970; Ronalds, 2005). However, in cohort studies evaluating normal-birthweight term infants, cognitive outcomes between twins and singletons are similar (Lorenz, 2012). Christensen and associates (2006) found similar national standardized test scores in ninth grade in 3411 twins and 7796 singletons born between 1986 and 1988. In contrast, among normal-birthweight infants, the cerebral palsy risk is higher among twins and higher-order multiples. For example, the cerebral palsy rate has been reported to be 2.3 per 1000 in singletons, 12.6 per 1000 in twins, and 44.8 per 1000 in triplets (Giuffre, 2012). Much of this excess risk is thought to be related to an increased risk of fetal-growth restriction, congenital anomalies, twin-twin transfusion syndrome, and fetal demise of a cotwin (Lorenz, 2012).

UNIQUE FETAL COMPLICATIONS

Several unique and fascinating complications arise in multifetal pregnancies. These have been best described in twins but can be found in higher-order multifetal gestations. Most fetal complications due to the twinning process itself are seen with monozygotic twins. Their pathogenesis is best understood after reviewing the possibilities shown in Figure 45-1.

Monoamnionic Twins

Only about 1 percent of all monozygotic twins will share an amnionic sac (Hall, 2003). Said another way, approximately 1 in 20 monochorionic twins are monoamnionic (Lewi, 2013). This configuration is associated with a high fetal death rate from cord entanglement, congenital anomalies, preterm birth, or twin-twin-transfusion syndrome, which is described subsequently. In a comprehensive review, Allen and associates (2001) reported that monoamnionic twins diagnosed antenatally and alive at 20 weeks have approximately a 10-percent risk of subsequent fetal demise. In a Dutch report of 98 monoamnionic twin pregnancies, the perinatal mortality rate was 17 percent (Hack, 2009). Umbilical cord entanglement, a frequent cause of death, is estimated to complicate at least half of cases (Fig. 45-12). Diamnionic twins can become monoamnionic if the dividing membrane ruptures and therefore have similar associated morbidity and mortality rates.

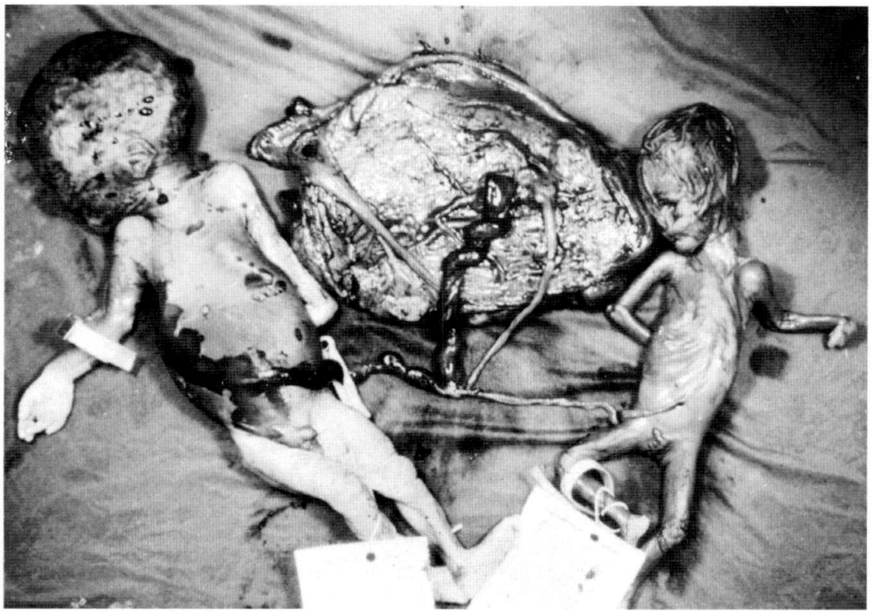

FIGURE 45-12 Monozygotic twins in a single amnionic sac. The smaller fetus apparently died first, and the second subsequently succumbed when umbilical cords entwined.

Unfortunately, there are no management methods that guarantee good outcomes for either or both twins. This is because of the unpredictability of fetal death from cord entanglement and the lack of an effective means of monitoring for it. Quinn and colleagues (2011) retrospectively evaluated the feasibility of inpatient continuous fetal heart monitoring in 17 sets of monoamnionic twins. After review of more than 10,000 hours of fetal tracing, these investigators concluded that this was possible in only 50 percent of cases. Importantly, an abnormal fetal heart rate tracing prompted delivery in only six cases. Morbid cord entanglement appears to occur early, and monoamnionic pregnancies that have successfully reached 30 to 32 weeks are at reduced risk. In the Dutch series described above, the incidence of intrauterine demise dropped from 15 percent after 20 weeks to 4 percent when gestational age exceeded 32 weeks (Hack, 2009).

Although umbilical cords frequently entangle, factors that lead to pathological umbilical vessel constriction are unknown. Color-flow Doppler sonography can be used to diagnose entanglement (Fig. 45-13). However, once identified, evidence to guide management is observational, retrospective, and subject to biased reporting. One proposed management scheme is based on a study by Heyborne and coworkers (2005), who reported no stillbirths in 43 twin pregnancies of women admitted at 26 to 27 weeks' gestation for daily fetal surveillance. Conversely, there were 13 stillbirths in 44 women who were managed as outpatients and admitted only for an obstetrical indication. Because of this report, women with monoamnionic twins are recommended to undergo 1 hour of daily fetal heart rate monitoring, either as outpatients or as inpatients, beginning at 26 to 28 weeks. With initial testing, a course of betamethasone is given to promote pulmonary maturation (Chap. 42, p. 850). If fetal testing remains reassuring, cesarean delivery is performed at 34 weeks and after a second course of betamethasone. This management scheme is used at Parkland Hospital and resulted in the successful 34-week delivery of the twins depicted in Figure 45-13.

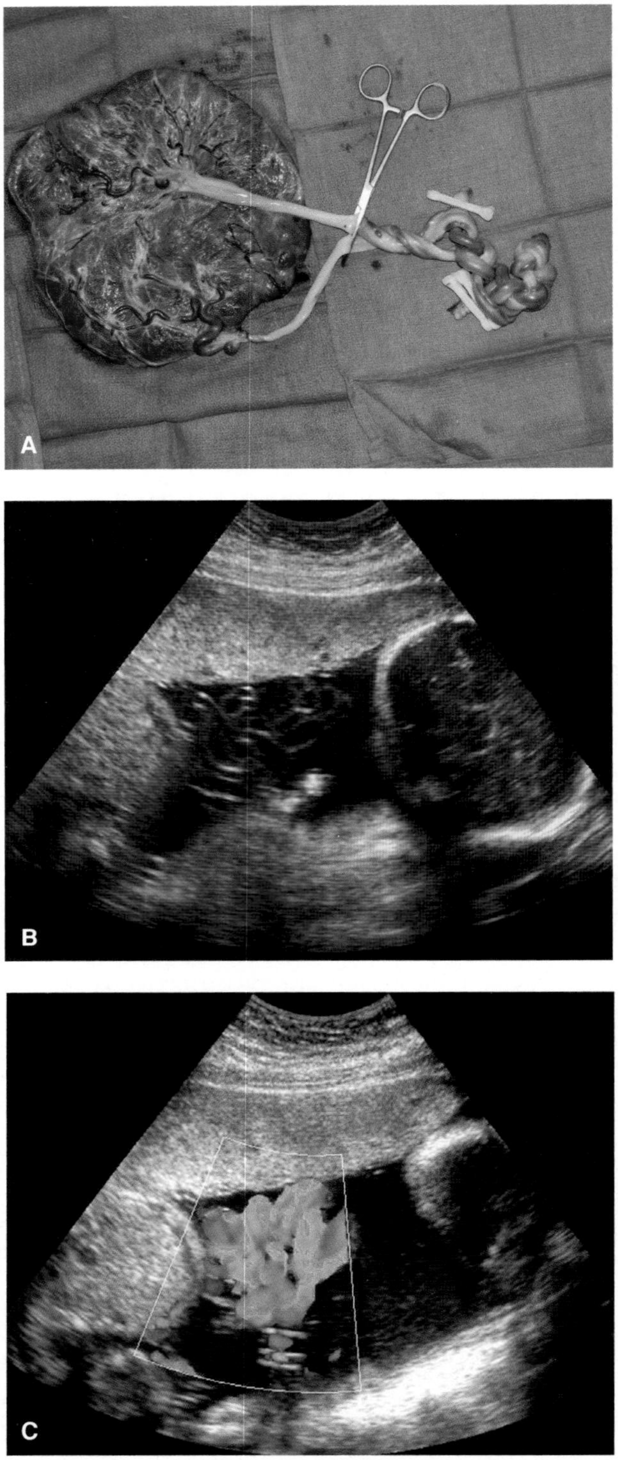

FIGURE 45-13 Monochorionic monoamnionic cord entanglement. **A.** Despite marked knotting of the cords, vigorous twins were delivered by cesarean. **B.** Preoperative sonogram of this pregnancy shows entwined cords. **C.** This finding is accentuated with application of color Doppler. (Photographs contributed by Dr. Julie Lo.)

Aberrant Twinning Mechanisms

Several aberrations in the twinning process result in a spectrum of fetal malformations. These are traditionally ascribed to incomplete splitting of an embryo into two separate twins. However, it is possible that they may result from early secondary fusion of two separate embryos. These separated embryos are either symmetrical or asymmetrical, and the spectrum of anomalies is shown in Figure 45-14.

Conjoined Twins

In the United States, united or conjoined twins have been referred to as *Siamese twins*–after Chang and Eng Bunker of Siam (Thailand), who were displayed worldwide by P. T. Barnum. Joining of the twins may begin at either pole and may produce characteristic forms depending on which body parts are joined or shared (Fig. 45-15). Of these, thoracopagus is the most common (Mutchinick, 2011). The frequency of conjoined twins is not well established. At Kandang Kerbau Hospital in Singapore, Tan and coworkers (1971) identified seven cases of conjoined twins among more than 400,000 deliveries–an incidence of 1 in 60,000.

As reviewed by McHugh and associates (2006), conjoined twins can frequently be identified using sonography at midpregnancy. This provides an opportunity for parents to decide whether to continue the pregnancy. As shown in

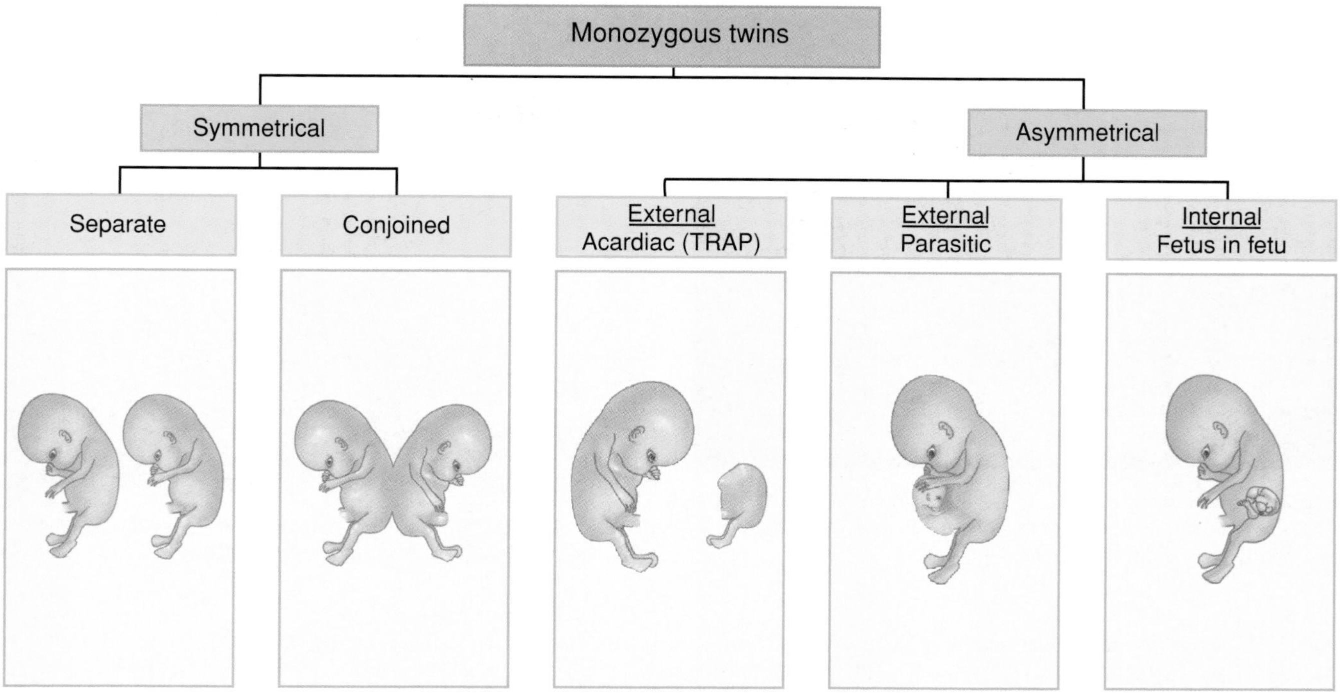

FIGURE 45-14 Possible outcomes of monozygotic twinning. The asymmetrical category contains twinning types in which one twin complement is substantially smaller and incompletely formed.

Figure 45-16, identification of cases during the first trimester is also possible. A targeted examination, including a careful evaluation of the connection and the organs involved, is necessary before counseling can be provided. As shown in Figure 45-17, MR imaging can play an important adjunctive role in clarifying shared organs. Compared with sonography, MR imaging may provide superior views, especially in later pregnancy when amnionic fluid is diminished and fetal crowding is increased (Hibbeln, 2012).

Surgical separation of an almost completely joined twin pair may be successful if essential organs are not shared (Spitz, 2003; Tannuri, 2013). Consultation with a pediatric surgeon often assists parental decision making. Conjoined twins may have discordant structural anomalies that further complicate decisions about whether to continue the pregnancy.

Viable conjoined twins should be delivered by cesarean. For the purpose of pregnancy termination, however, vaginal delivery is possible because the union is most often pliable (Fig. 45-18). Still, dystocia is common, and if the fetuses are mature, vaginal delivery may be traumatic to the uterus or cervix.

External Parasitic Twins

This is a grossly defective fetus or merely fetal parts, attached externally to a relatively normal twin. A parasitic twin usually consists of externally attached supernumerary limbs, often with some viscera. Classically, however, a functional heart or brain is absent. Attachment mirrors those sites described earlier for conjoined twins (see Fig. 45-14). Parasites are believed to result from demise of the defective twin, with its surviving tissues attached to and vascularized by its normal twin (Spencer,

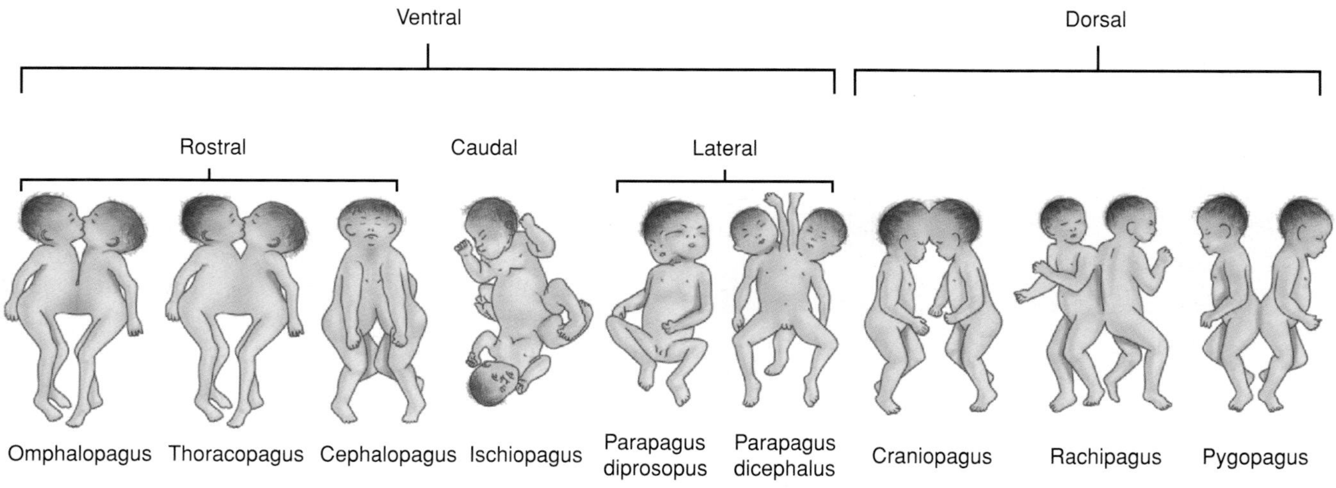

FIGURE 45-15 Types of conjoined twins. (Redrawn from Spencer, 2000.)

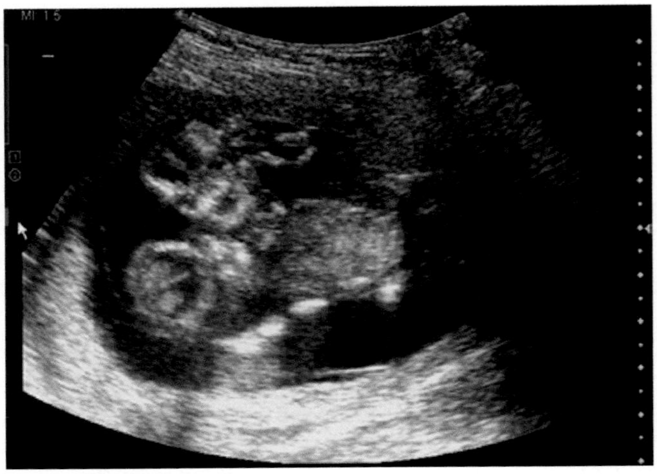

FIGURE 45-16 Sonogram of a conjoined twin pregnancy at 13 weeks' gestation. These thoracoomphalopagus twins have two heads but a shared chest and abdomen.

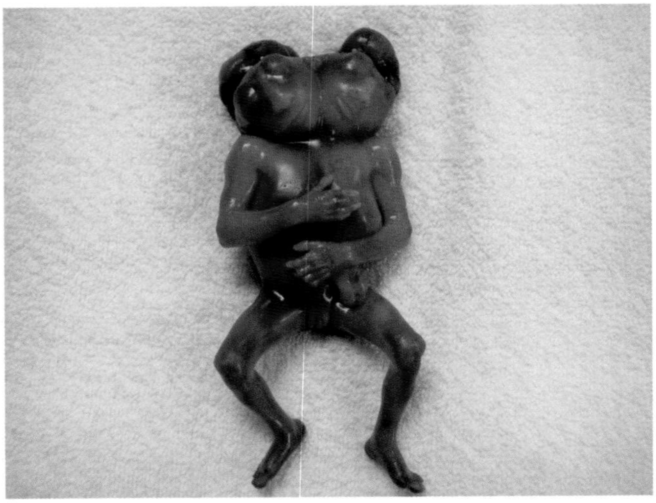

FIGURE 45-18 Conjoined twins aborted at 17 weeks' gestation. (Photograph contributed by Dr. Jonathan Willms.)

2001). In a worldwide collaborative epidemiological study, parasitic twins were found to account for 3.9 percent of all conjoined twins and to occur more frequently in male fetuses (Mutchinick, 2011).

Fetus-in-Fetu

Early in development, one embryo may be enfolded within its twin. Normal development of this rare parasitic twin usually arrests in the first trimester. As a result, normal spatial arrangement of and presence of many organs is lost. Classically, vertebral or axial bones are found in these fetiform masses, whereas heart and brain are lacking. These masses are typically supported by their host by a few large parasitic vessels (Spencer, 2000). Malignant degeneration is rare (Kaufman, 2007).

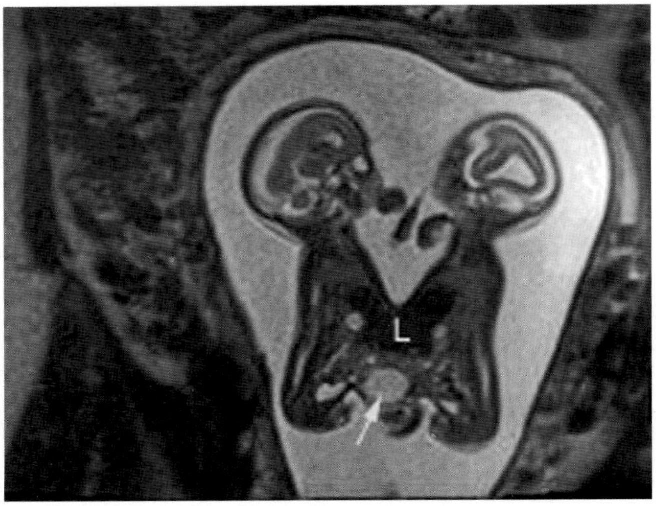

FIGURE 45-17 Magnetic resonance imaging of conjoined twins. This T2-weighted HASTE sagittal image demonstrates fusion from the level of the xiphoid process to just below the level of the umbilicus, that is, omphalopagus twins. Below the fused liver (*L*), there is a midline cystic mass (*arrow*) within the tissue connecting the twins. An omphalomesenteric cyst was favored given the location within the shared tissue. (Image contributed by Dr. April Bailey.)

Monochorionic Twins and Vascular Anastomoses

Another group of fascinating fetal syndromes can arise when monozygotic twinning results in two amnionic sacs and a common surrounding chorion. This leads to anatomical sharing of the two fetal circulations through anastomoses of placental arteries and veins. All monochorionic placentas likely share some anastomotic connections. However, there are marked variations in the number, size, and direction of these seemingly haphazard connections (Fig. 45-19). In their analyses of more than 200 monochorionic placentas, Zhao and colleagues (2013) found the median number of anastomoses to be 8 with an interquartile range of 4 to 14. With rare exceptions, anastomoses between twins are unique to monochorionic twin placentas.

Artery-to-artery anastomoses are most common and are identified on the chorionic surface of the placenta in up to 75 percent of monochorionic twin placentas. Vein-to-vein and artery-to-vein communications are each found in approximately half. One vessel may have several connections, sometimes to both arteries and veins. In contrast to these superficial vascular connections on the surface of the chorion, deep artery-to-vein communications can extend through the capillary bed of a given villus (Fig. 45-20). These deep arteriovenous anastomoses create a common villous compartment or third circulation that has been identified in approximately half of monochorionic twin placentas.

Whether these anastomoses are dangerous to either twin depends on the degree to which they are hemodynamically balanced. In those with significant pressure or flow gradients, a shunt will develop between fetuses. This chronic fetofetal transfusion may result in several clinical syndromes that include *twin-twin transfusion syndrome (TTTS), twin anemia polycythemia sequence (TAPS),* and *acardiac twinning.*

Twin-Twin Transfusion Syndrome (TTTS)

The prevalence of this condition is approximately 1 to 3 per 10,000 births (Simpson, 2013). In this syndrome, blood is

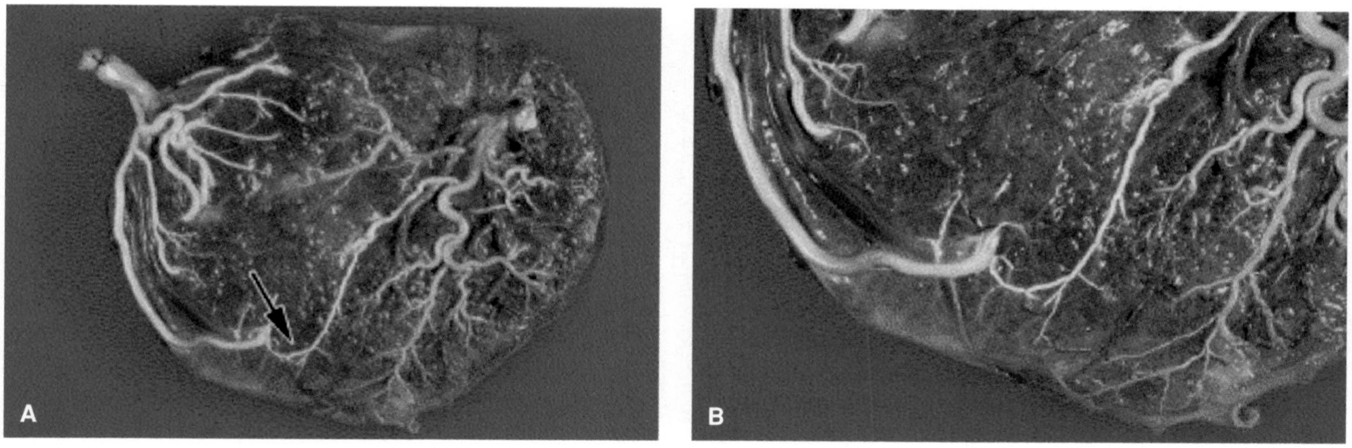

FIGURE 45-19 Shared placenta from pregnancy complicated by twin-twin transfusion syndrome. The following color code was applied for injection. Left twin: yellow = artery, blue = vein; right twin: red = artery, green = vein. **A.** Part of the arterial network of the right twin is filled with yellow dye, due to the presence of a small artery-to-artery anastomosis (*arrow*). **B.** Close-up of the lower portion of the placenta displays the yellow dye-filled anastomosis. (From De Paepe, 2005, with permission.)

transfused from a donor twin to its recipient sibling such that the donor may eventually become anemic and its growth may be restricted. In contrast, the recipient becomes polycythemic and may develop circulatory overload manifest as hydrops. The donor twin is pale, and its recipient sibling is plethoric (Fig. 45-21). Similarly, one portion of the placenta often appears pale compared with the remainder.

The recipient neonate may have circulatory overload from heart failure and severe hypervolemia and hyperviscosity. Occlusive thrombosis is another concern. Finally, polycythemia in the recipient twin may lead to severe hyperbilirubinemia and kernicterus (Chap. 33, p. 644).

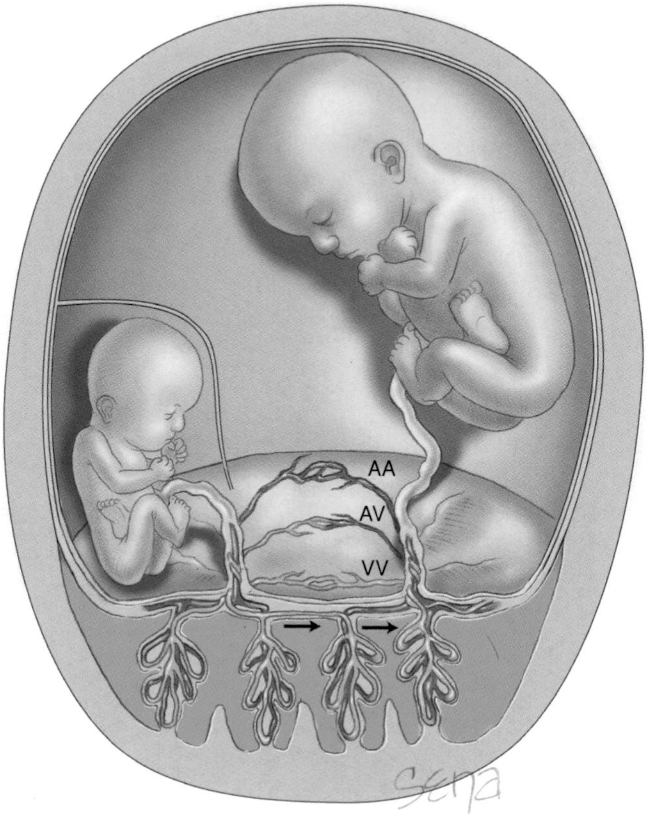

FIGURE 45-20 Anastomoses between twins may be artery-to-vein (AV), artery-to-artery (AA), or vein-to-vein (VV). Schematic representation of an AV anastomosis in twin-twin transfusion syndrome that forms a "common villous district" or "third circulation" deep within the villous tissue. Blood from a donor twin may be transferred to a recipient twin through this shared circulation. This transfer leads to a growth-restricted discordant donor twin with markedly reduced amnionic fluid, causing it to be "stuck."

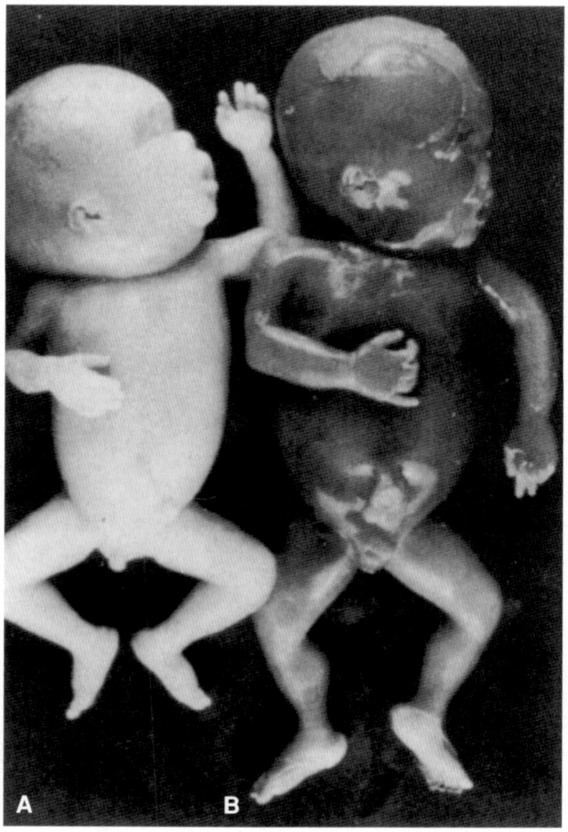

FIGURE 45-21 Twin-twin transfusion syndrome at 23 weeks. **A.** Pale donor twin (690 g) also had oligohydramnios. **B.** The plethoric recipient twin (730 g) had hydramnios. (From Mahone, 1993, with permission.)

Pathophysiology. Any of the different types of vascular anastomoses discussed before may be found with monochorionic placentas. Classically, chronic TTTS results from unidirectional flow through arteriovenous anastomoses. Deoxygenated blood from a *donor* placental artery is pumped into a cotyledon shared by the recipient (see Fig. 45-20). Once oxygen exchange is completed in the chorionic villus, the oxygenated blood leaves the cotyledon via a placental vein of the *recipient* twin. Unless compensated—typically through arterioarterial anastomoses—this unidirectional flow leads to an imbalance in blood volumes (Lewi, 2013).

Clinically important twin-twin transfusion syndrome frequently is chronic and results from significant vascular volume differences between the twins. Even so, the pathogenesis is more complex than a net transfer of red blood cells from one twin to another. Indeed, in most monochorionic twin pregnancies complicated by the syndrome, there is no difference in hemoglobin concentrations between the donor and recipient twin (Lewi, 2013).

The syndrome typically presents in midpregnancy when the donor fetus becomes oliguric from decreased renal perfusion (Simpson, 2013). This fetus develops oligohydramnios, and the recipient fetus develops severe hydramnios, presumably due to increased urine production. Virtual absence of amnionic fluid in the donor sac prevents fetal motion, giving rise to the descriptive term *stuck twin* or *polyhydramnios-oligohydramnios–syndrome—"poly-oli."* This amnionic fluid imbalance is associated with growth restriction, contractures, and pulmonary hypoplasia in the donor twin, and premature rupture of the membranes and heart failure in the recipient.

Fetal Brain Damage. Cerebral palsy, microcephaly, porencephaly, and multicystic encephalomalacia are serious complications associated with placental vascular anastomoses in multifetal gestation. The exact pathogenesis of neurological damage is not fully understood but is likely caused by ischemic necrosis leading to cavitary brain lesions (Fig. 45-22). In the donor twin, ischemia results from hypotension, anemia, or both. In the recipient, ischemia develops from blood pressure instability and episodes of severe hypotension (Lopriore, 2011). Cerebral lesions may also be due to postnatal injury associated with preterm delivery. Quarello and associates (2007) reviewed data from 315 liveborn fetuses from pregnancies with twin-twin-transfusion syndrome and reported cerebral abnormalities in 8 percent.

If one twin of an affected pregnancy dies, cerebral pathology in the survivor probably results from acute hypotension. A less likely cause is emboli of thromboplastic material originating from the dead fetus. Fusi and coworkers (1990, 1991) observed that with the death of one twin, acute twin-twin anastomotic transfusion from the high-pressure vessels of the living twin to the low-resistance vessels of the dead twin leads rapidly to hypovolemia and ischemic antenatal brain damage in the survivor. In their systematic review of 343 twin pregnancies complicated by single fetal demise, Hillman and colleagues (2011) calculated a 26-percent risk of neurodevelopmental morbidity in monochorionic twins compared with 2 percent in dichorionic twins. They also found that this morbidity was related to gestational age at the death of the cotwin. If the death occurred between 28 and 33 weeks' gestation, monochorionic twins had an almost eightfold risk of neurodevelopmental morbidity compared with dichorionic twins of the same gestational age. With fetal death after 34 weeks, the likelihood dramatically decreased—odds ratio 1.48.

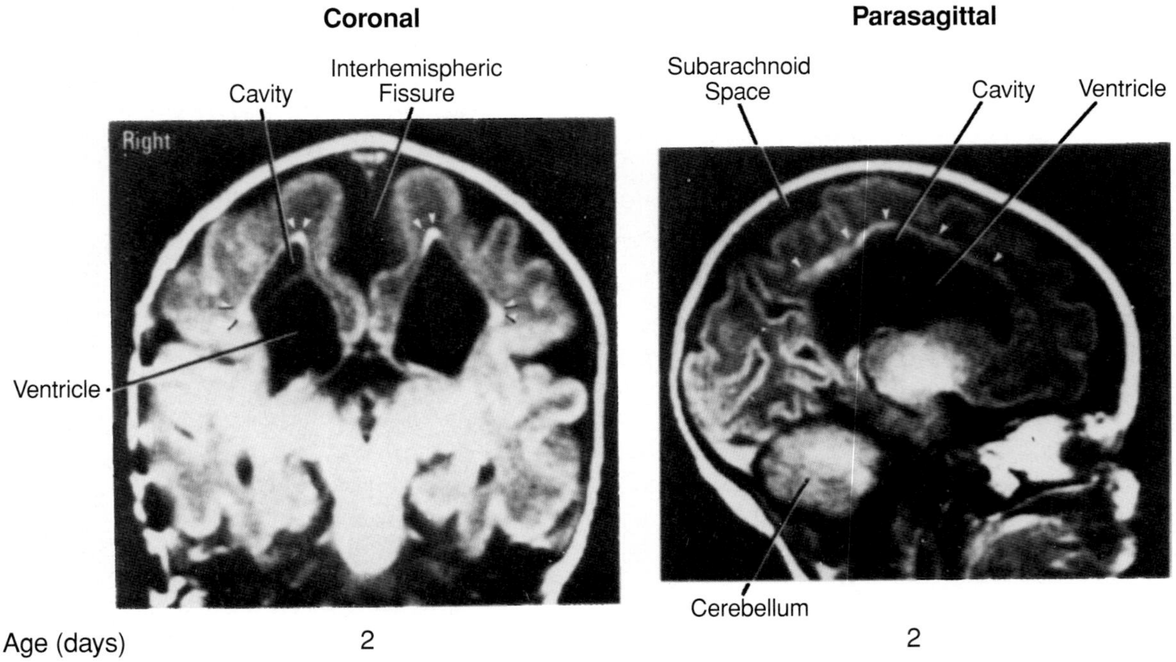

FIGURE 45-22 Cranial magnetic resonance imaging study of a diamnionic–monochorionic twin performed on day 2 of life. The subarachnoid space and lateral ventricles are markedly enlarged. There are large cavitary lesions in the white matter adjacent to the ventricles. The bright signals (*arrowheads*) in the periphery of the cavitary lesions most probably correspond to gliosis. (From Bejar, 1990, with permission.)

The acuity of hypotension following the death of one twin with twin-twin-transfusion syndrome makes successful intervention for the survivor nearly impossible. Even with delivery immediately after a cotwin demise is recognized, the hypotension that occurs at the moment of death has likely already caused irreversible brain damage (Langer, 1997; Wada, 1998).

Diagnosis. There have been dramatic changes in the criteria used to diagnose and classify varying severities of twin-twin transfusion syndrome. Previously, weight discordancy and hemoglobin differences in monochorionic twins were calculated. However, it was soon appreciated that in many cases these were late-onset findings. According to the Society for Maternal-Fetal Medicine (2013), TTTS is diagnosed based on two criteria: (1) presence of a monochorionic diamnionic pregnancy, and (2) hydramnios defined if the largest vertical pocket is > 8 cm in one twin and oligohydramnios defined if the largest vertical pocket is < 2 cm in the other twin. Only 15 percent of pregnancies complicated by lesser degrees of fluid imbalance progress to TTTS (Huber, 2006).

Once identified, TTTS is typically staged by the Quintero (1999) staging system:

- Stage I—discordant amnionic fluid volumes as described above, but urine is still visible sonographically within the bladder of the donor twin.
- Stage II—criteria of stage I, but urine is not visible within the donor bladder.
- Stage III—criteria of stage II and abnormal Doppler studies of the umbilical artery, ductus venosus, or umbilical vein.
- Stage IV—ascites or frank hydrops in either twin.
- Stage V—demise of either fetus.

In addition to these criteria, there is evidence that cardiac function of the recipient twin correlates with fetal outcome (Crombleholme, 2007). Although fetal echocardiographic findings are not part of the staging system above, many centers routinely perform fetal echocardiography for TTTS. It has been theorized that early diagnosis of cardiomyopathy in the recipient twin may identify pregnancies that would benefit from early intervention. One system for evaluating cardiac function—the *myocardial performance index (MPI)* or *Tei index*—is a Doppler index of ventricular function calculated for each ventricle (Michelfelder, 2007). Although scoring systems that include assessment of cardiac function have been developed, their usefulness in prediction of outcomes remains controversial (Simpson, 2013).

At Parkland Memorial Hospital, evaluation before and during treatment includes anatomical and neurological fetal assessment using echocardiography, MPI calculation, Doppler velocimetry, and MR imaging; genetic counseling and amniocentesis; and placental mapping.

Management and Prognosis. The prognosis for multifetal gestations complicated by TTTS is related to Quintero stage and gestational age at presentation. More than three fourths of stage I cases remain stable or regress without intervention. Conversely, outcomes in those identified at stage III or higher are much worse, and the perinatal loss rate is 70 to 100 percent without intervention (Simpson, 2013). Several therapies are currently used for TTTS, including amnioreduction, laser ablation of vascular anastomoses, selective feticide, and septostomy (intentional creation of a communication in the dividing amnionic membrane). Comparative data from randomized trials for some of these techniques are discussed below.

The Eurofetus trial included 142 women with severe TTTS diagnosed before 26 weeks. Participants were randomly assigned to laser ablation of vascular anastomoses or to serial amnioreduction (Senat, 2004). These investigators reported an increased survival rate to age 6 months for at least one twin with laser ablation compared with serial amnioreduction–76 versus 51 percent, respectively. Moreover, analyses of randomized studies confirm better neonatal outcomes with laser therapy compared with selective amnioreduction (Roberts, 2008; Rossi, 2008, 2009). In contrast, Crombleholme and associates (2007), in a randomized trial of 42 women, found equivalent rates of 30-day survival of one or both twins treated with either amnioreduction or selective fetoscopic laser ablation–75 versus 65 percent, respectively. Furthermore, evaluation of twins from the Eurofetus trial through 6 years of age did not demonstrate any additional survival benefit beyond 6 months or improved neurological outcomes in those treated with laser (Salomon, 2010).

At this time, laser ablation of anastomoses is preferred for severe TTTS (stages II-IV), although optimal therapy for stage I disease is controversial. After laser therapy, close ongoing surveillance is necessary. Robyr and colleagues (2006) reported that a fourth of 101 pregnancies treated with laser required additional invasive therapy because of either recurrent TTTS, or middle cerebral artery Doppler evidence of anemia or polycythemia. Recently, in a comparison of selective laser ablation of individual anastomoses versus ablation of the entire surface of chorionic plate along the vascular equator, Baschat and coworkers (2013) found that equatorial photocoagulation reduced the likelihood of recurrence.

Moise and associates (2005) compared amnioreduction and septostomy in a multicentered randomized trial of 73 women. Repeated procedures were performed for symptoms or if the greatest vertical pocket of amnionic fluid met the original inclusion criteria of 8 to 12 cm, depending on gestational age. Perinatal outcomes were the same in each group, with at least one survivor in 80 percent of pregnancies. The average number of additional procedures was two in each group. Much of this is moot, however, because intentional septostomy has largely been abandoned as treatment (Simpson, 2013).

Selective reduction has generally been considered if severe amnionic fluid and growth disturbances develop before 20 weeks. In such cases, both fetuses typically will die without intervention. Selection of which twin is to be terminated is based on evidence of damage to either fetus and comparison of their prognoses. Any substance injected into one twin may affect the other twin because of shared circulations. Therefore, feticidal techniques include methods to occlude the circulation of the chosen fetal umbilical vein or by umbilical cord occlusion using radiofrequency ablation, fetoscopic ligation, or coagulation with laser, monopolar, or bipolar cauterization (Challis, 1999; Chang, 2009; Donner, 1997). Even after these procedures, however, the risks to the remaining fetus are still appreciable (Rossi, 2009).

Twin Anemia Polycythemia Sequence (TAPS)

This form of chronic fetofetal transfusion is characterized by significant hemoglobin differences between donor and recipient twins *without* the discrepancies in amnionic fluid volumes typical of twin-twin-transfusion syndrome (Slaghekke, 2010). It is diagnosed antenatally by middle cerebral artery (MCA) peak systolic velocity (PSV) > 1.5 multiples of the median (MoM) in the donor and < 1.0 MoM in the recipient twin (Simpson, 2013). The spontaneous form reportedly complicates 3 to 5 percent of monochorionic pregnancies, and it occurs in up to 13 percent of pregnancies after laser photocoagulation. *Spontaneous* TAPS usually occurs after 26 weeks and *iatrogenic* TAPS develops within 5 weeks of a procedure (Lewi, 2013). Although a staging system has been proposed by Slaghekke and colleagues (2010), further studies are necessary to better understand the natural history of TAPS and its management.

Twin-Reversed Arterial Perfusion (TRAP) Sequence

Also known as an *acardiac twin*, this is a rare—1 in 35,000 births—but serious complication of monochorionic multifetal gestation. In the TRAP sequence, there is usually a normally formed donor twin that has features of heart failure and a recipient twin that lacks a heart (acardius) and other structures. It has been hypothesized that the TRAP sequence is caused by a large artery-to-artery placental shunt, often also accompanied by a vein-to-vein shunt (Fig. 45-23). Within the single, shared placenta, arterial perfusion pressure of the donor twin exceeds that in the recipient twin, who thus receives reverse blood flow of deoxygenated arterial blood from its cotwin (Lewi, 2013). This "used" arterial blood reaches the recipient twin through its umbilical arteries and preferentially goes to its iliac vessels. Thus, only the lower body is perfused, and disrupted growth and development of the upper body results. Failure of head growth is called *acardius acephalus*; a partially developed head with identifiable limbs is called *acardius myelacephalus*; and failure of any recognizable structure to form is *acardius amorphous,* which is shown in Figure 45-24 (Faye-Petersen, 2006). Because of this vascular connection, the normal donor twin must not only support its own circulation but also pump its blood through the underdeveloped acardiac recipient. This may lead to cardiomegaly and high-output heart failure in the normal twin (Fox, 2007).

Lewi and coworkers (2010) reviewed 26 cases of TRAP sequence identified in the first trimester. In one third, the pump twin died before planned intervention at 16 to 18 weeks. In more than half of all the cases, there was spontaneous cessation of flow to the acardiac twin, and such flow arrest was associated with subsequent death or neurological injury in 85 percent of the normal twins. Quintero and associates (1994, 2006) have reviewed methods of in utero treatment of acardiac twinning in which the goal is interruption of aberrant vascular communication between the twins. Of these methods, Lee (2007), Lewi (2010), Livingston (2007), and their colleagues found an approximate 90-percent survival rate following second-trimester radiofrequency ablation. This method cauterizes umbilical vessels in the malformed recipient

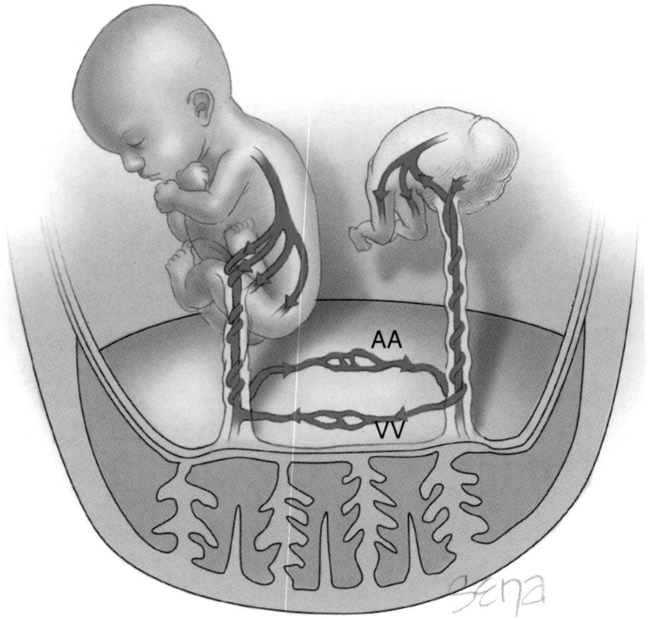

FIGURE 45-23 Twin reversed-arterial-perfusion sequence. In the TRAP sequence, there is usually a normally formed donor twin that has features of heart failure, and a recipient twin that lacks a heart. It has been hypothesized that the TRAP sequence is caused by a large artery-to-artery placental shunt, often also accompanied by a vein-to-vein shunt. Within the single, shared placenta, perfusion pressure of the donor twin overpowers that in the recipient twin, who thus receives reverse blood flow from its twin sibling. The "used" arterial blood (*colored blue*) that reaches the recipient twin preferentially goes to its iliac vessels and thus perfuses only the lower body. This disrupts growth and development of the upper body.

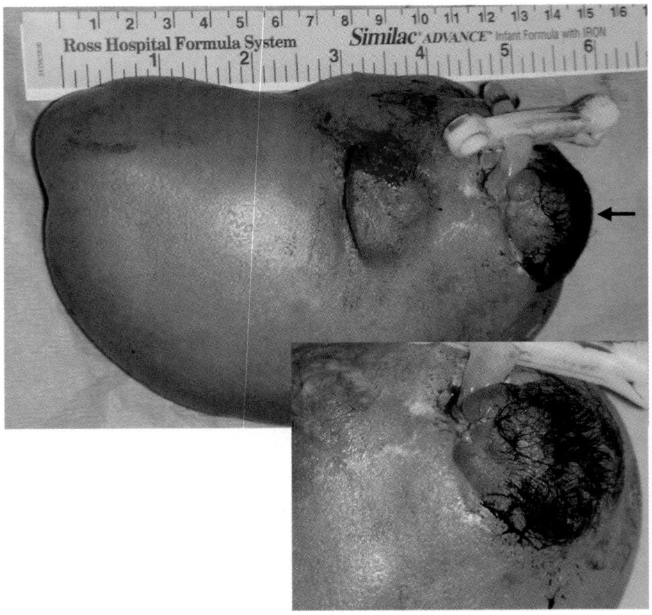

FIGURE 45-24 Photograph of an acardiac twin weighing 475 grams. The underdeveloped head is indicated by the black arrow, and its details are shown in the inset. A yellow clamp is seen on its umbilical cord. Its viable donor cotwin was delivered vaginally at 36 weeks and weighed 2325 grams. (Photograph contributed by Dr. Michael D. Hnat.)

twin to terminate blood flow from the donor. In a review of 118 complicated monochorionic twin gestations that underwent bipolar cord coagulation, Lanna and associates (2012) reported a fetal loss rate in those treated before 19 weeks of 45 percent compared with 3 percent in those treated after 19 weeks. Prompted by the high mortality rate of TRAP sequence in the first trimester, small case series of early intervention have been reported (O'Donoghue, 2008; Scheier, 2012). Importantly, efficacy and safety of intervention before fusion of the amnion and chorion has not been demonstrated convincingly (Lewi, 2013).

Complete Hydatidiform Mole with Coexisting Normal Fetus

Also termed a twin molar pregnancy, this is due to a complete diploid molar pregnancy comprising one conceptus, whereas the cotwin is a normal fetus. Reported prevalence rates range from 1 in 22,000 to 1 in 100,000 pregnancies (Dolapcioglu, 2009). It must be differentiated from a partial molar pregnancy in which an anomalous singleton fetus—usually triploid—is accompanied by molar tissue (Chap. 20, p. 398).

Optimal management is not known for this twin gestation. Diagnosis is usually made in the first half of pregnancy, and termination at that time would remove the mole but also the normal fetus. However, pregnancy progression exposes the woman to the later postpartum dangers of persistent trophoblastic disease that requires chemotherapy and may be fatal. Despite this, pregnancy continuation is increasingly being recommended in cases with a karyotypically normal and nonanomalous twin, no early preeclampsia, and declining hCG levels (Sebire, 2002).

If observation and pregnancy progression is chosen, preterm delivery is frequently required because of persistent and heavy bleeding or severe preeclampsia. Dolapcioglu and coworkers (2009) reviewed 159 reported cases and reported a live birth in 35 percent. Preeclampsia and preterm birth each developed in a third. Niemann and colleagues (2007) reported that persistent trophoblastic disease rates following such a twin gestation were not increased compared with those after a singleton complete mole.

DISCORDANT GROWTH OF TWIN FETUSES

Size inequality of twin fetuses, which can be a sign of pathological growth restriction in one fetus, is calculated using the larger twin as the index. Generally, as the weight difference within a twin pair increases, the perinatal mortality rate increases proportionately. Because the single placenta is not always equally shared in monochorionic twins, these twins have greater rates of discordant growth outside of TTTS than dichorionic twins. It develops in approximately 15 percent of twin gestations (Lewi, 2013; Miller, 2012). As discussed further in Chapter 44 (p. 879), restricted growth of one twin fetus usually develops late in the second and early third trimester. Earlier discordancy indicates higher risk for fetal demise in the smaller twin. Specifically, when discordant growth is identified before 20 weeks, fetal death occurs in about 20 percent (Lewi, 2013). Importantly, differences in crown-rump length (CRL) are associated with fetal structural and chromosomal anomalies but are not reliable predictors for birthweight discordance (Miller, 2012).

Etiopathogenesis

The cause of birthweight inequality in twin fetuses is often unclear, but the etiology in monochorionic twins likely differs from that in dichorionic twins. Discordancy in monochorionic twins is usually attributed to placental vascular anastomoses that cause hemodynamic imbalance between the twins. Reduced pressure and perfusion of the donor twin can cause diminished placental and fetal growth. Even so, unequal placental sharing is probably the most important determinant of discordant growth in monochorionic twins (Lewi, 2013). Occasionally, monochorionic twins are discordant in size because they are discordant for structural anomalies.

Discordancy in dichorionic twins may result from various factors. Dizygotic fetuses may have different genetic growth potential, especially if they are of opposite genders. Alternatively, because the placentas are separate and require more implantation space, one placenta might have a suboptimal implantation site. Bagchi and associates (2006) observed that the incidence of severe discordancy is twice as great in triplets as it is in twins. This finding lends credence to the view that in utero crowding is a factor in fetal-growth restriction. Placental pathology may play a role as well. Kent and coworkers (2012) evaluated placental abnormalities in 668 twin gestations. They observed a strong relationship between histological placental abnormalities and birthweight discordancy with associated growth restriction in dichorionic, but not monochorionic, twin pregnancies.

Diagnosis

Size discordancy between twins can be determined sonographically in several ways. One common method uses sonographic fetal biometry to compute an estimated weight for each twin (Chap. 10, p. 198). The weight of the smaller twin is then compared with that of the larger twin. Thus, percent discordancy = weight of larger twin minus weight of smaller twin, divided by weight of larger twin. Alternatively, considering that growth restriction is the primary concern and that abdominal circumference (AC) reflects fetal nutrition, some use the sonographic AC value of each twin. With these methods, some specify discordance if the AC measurements differ more than 20 mm or if the estimated fetal weight difference is 20 percent or more.

That said, several different weight disparities between twins have been used to define discordancy. Accumulated data suggest that weight discordancy greater than 25 to 30 percent most accurately predicts an adverse perinatal outcome. Hollier and coworkers (1999) retrospectively evaluated 1370 twin pairs delivered at Parkland Hospital and stratified twin weight discordancy in 5-percent increments within a range of 15 to 40 percent. They found that the incidence of respiratory distress, intraventricular hemorrhage, seizures, periventricular leukomalacia, sepsis, and necrotizing enterocolitis increased directly with the degree of weight discordancy. These conditions increased substantially if discordancy was greater than 25 percent. The relative risk of fetal death increased significantly to 5.6 if there was more than 30-percent discordancy. It increased to 18.9 if there was greater than 40-percent discordancy.

Management

Sonographic monitoring of growth within a twin pair and calculating discordancy has become a mainstay in management. Other sonographic findings, such as oligohydramnios, may be helpful in gauging fetal risk. Monochorionic twins are generally monitored more frequently. This is because their risk of death is higher—3.6 percent versus 1.1 percent—and the risk of neurological damage in the surviving twin is substantial compared with those risks in dichorionic twins (Hillman, 2011; Lee, 2008). Thorson and colleagues (2011) retrospectively analyzed 108 monochorionic twin pregnancies and found that a sonographic surveillance interval of greater than 2 weeks was associated with detection of higher-stage twin-twin transfusion syndrome. These findings have led some to recommend serial sonographic surveillance every 2 weeks in monochorionic twins (Simpson, 2013; Society for Maternal-Fetal Medicine, 2013). However, there have been no randomized trials of the optimal frequency of sonographic surveillance in monochorionic twin pregnancies. At Parkland Hospital, monochorionic twins undergo sonographic evaluation to assess interval growth every 4 weeks. Dichorionic twins are evaluated every 6 weeks. Depending on the degree of discordancy and the gestational age, fetal surveillance may be indicated, especially if one or both fetuses exhibit restricted growth. Nonstress testing, biophysical profile scores, and umbilical artery Doppler assessment have all been recommended in the management of twins, but none have been evaluated in appropriately sized prospective trials (Miller, 2012).

The American College of Obstetricians and Gynecologists (2010) recommends that antepartum testing be performed in multifetal gestations for the same indications as in singleton fetuses (Chap 17, p. 345). At Parkland Hospital, all women with twin discordance of 25 percent or greater undergo daily monitoring as an inpatient. There are limited data to establish the optimal timing of delivery of twins. Delivery is usually not prompted by size discordancy alone, except occasionally at advanced gestational ages. The Royal College of Obstetricians and Gynecologists (2008) advocates delivery by 37 weeks' gestation in monochorionic twins and by 38 weeks in dichorionic twins.

FETAL DEMISE

At any time during multifetal pregnancy, one or more fetuses may die, either simultaneously or sequentially. The causes and incidence of fetal death are related to zygosity, chorionicity, and growth concordance.

Death of One Fetus

In some pregnancies, one fetus dies remote from term, but pregnancy continues with one or more live fetuses. When this occurs early in pregnancy, it may manifest as a *vanishing twin* discussed on page 892. Fetal death in a slightly more advanced gestation may go undetected until delivery of a normal-appearing live infant along with a dead fetus that is barely identifiable. It may be compressed appreciably—*fetus compressus,* or it may be flattened remarkably through desiccation—*fetus papyraceus* (Fig. 45-25).

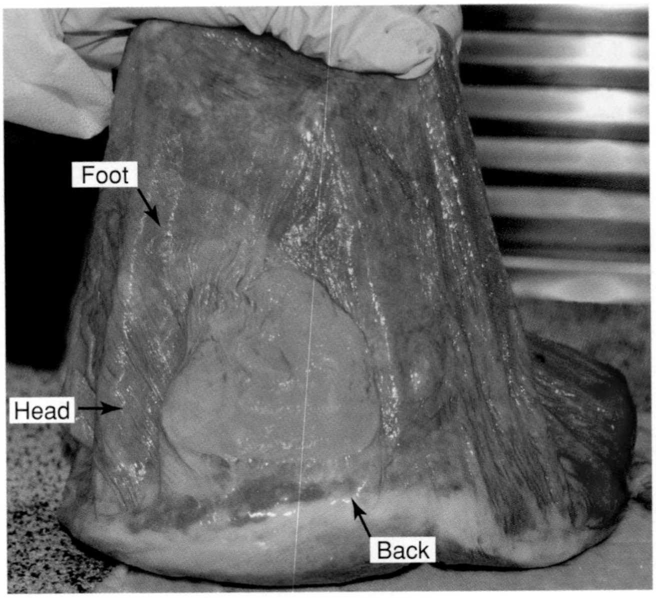

FIGURE 45-25 This fetus papyraceus is a tan ovoid mass compressed against the fetal membranes. Anatomical parts can be identified as marked. Demise of this twin had been noted during sonographic examination performed at 17 weeks' gestation. Its viable cotwin delivered at 40 weeks. (Photograph contributed by Dr. Michael V. Zaretsky.)

In a review of 9822 Japanese twin pregnancies, Morikawa and associates (2012) reported that 2.5 percent of monochorionic diamnionic twins greater than 22 weeks' gestation had a death of one or both twins compared with 1.2 percent of dichorionic twins. As shown in Figure 45-26, the risk of stillbirth is related to gestational age in all twins, but is much higher for monochorionic twin pregnancies before 32 weeks. In this same review, women with monochorionic diamnionic twins who lost one twin were 16 times more likely to experience death of the cotwin than women with dichorionic

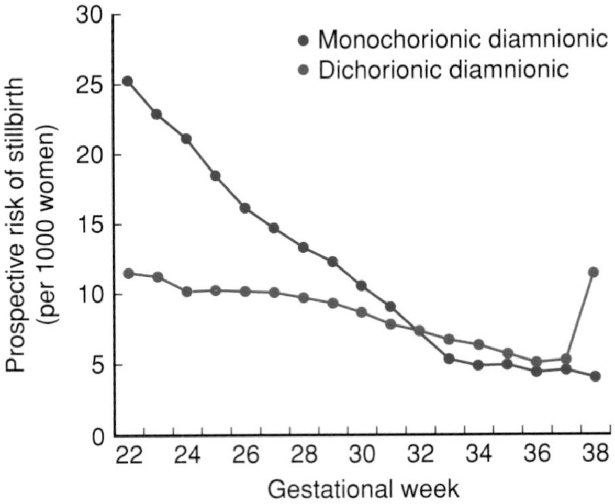

FIGURE 45-26 Prospective risk of stillbirth among women who reached a given gestational week (per 1000 women). (From Morikawa, 2012, with permission.)

twins who lost one twin (Morikawa, 2012). Similarly, in their analysis of 1094 twin pregnancies, Mahony and associates (2011) identified a threefold increased risk of death of one or both fetuses in monochorionic twins compared with dichorionic pairs. Last, in their systematic review and metaanalyses, Hillman and colleagues (2011) concluded that after one twin dies, the odds of cotwin demise was five times higher in monochorionic twins compared with dichorionic twins experiencing the same fate. Analyses of 701 triplets identified mortality rates to be 2.1 percent, 3.2 percent, and 5.3 percent in trichorionic triamnionic, dichorionic triamnionic, and monochorionic triamnionic triplets, respectively (Kawaguchi, 2013).

Other factors that affect the prognosis for the surviving twin include gestational age at the time of the demise and duration between the demise and delivery of the surviving twin. With demise of the *vanishing twin* discussed earlier, after the first trimester, the risk of death is not increased for the survivor. However, when one fetus dies in the second trimester or later, the effect of gestational age at the time of death and the mortality risk to the cotwin is less clear. In the analysis by Hillman and colleagues (2011), cotwin demise rates were unaffected regardless of whether the first death occurred at 13 to 27 weeks or at 28 to 34 weeks. In cases with the death of one twin after the first trimester, however, the odds of spontaneous and iatrogenic preterm delivery of the remaining living twin were increased (Hillman, 2011). Preterm birth was five times more likely in monochorionic twin gestations complicated by demise of one twin between 28 and 33 weeks' gestation. If the fetus died after 34 weeks, preterm delivery rates were similar.

The neurological prognosis for a surviving cotwin depends almost exclusively on chorionicity. In their comprehensive review, Ong and coworkers (2006) found an 18-percent rate of neurological abnormality in twins with monochorionic placentation compared with only 1 percent in those with dichorionic placentation. In another review, in twin pregnancies complicated by a single fetal demise before 34 weeks, a fivefold increased risk of neurodevelopmental morbidity was identified in monochorionic twins compared with dichorionic twins. If the one fetus died after 34 weeks, the likelihood of neurological deficits was essentially the same between monochorionic and dichorionic twin pregnancies (Hillman, 2011).

Later in gestation, the death of one of multiple fetuses could theoretically trigger coagulation defects in the mother. Only a few cases of maternal coagulopathy after a single fetal death in a twin pregnancy have been reported. This is probably because the surviving twin is usually delivered within a few weeks of the demise (Eddib, 2006). That said, we have observed transient, spontaneously corrected consumptive coagulopathy in multifetal gestations in which one fetus died and was retained in utero along with its surviving twin. The plasma fibrinogen concentration initially decreased but then increased spontaneously, and the level of serum fibrinogen-fibrin degradation products increased initially but then returned to normal levels. At delivery, the portions of the placenta that supplied the living fetus appeared normal. In contrast, the part that had once provided for the dead fetus was the site of massive fibrin deposition. This is further discussed and illustrated in Chapter 41 (p. 811).

Management

Decisions should be based on gestational age, the cause of death, and the risk to the surviving fetus. As mentioned previously, if the loss occurs early in the first trimester, a vanishing twin is considered harmless to the survivor. If the loss occurs after the first trimester, the risk of death or damage to the survivor is largely limited to monochorionic twin gestations. Morbidity in the monochorionic twin survivor is almost always due to vascular anastomoses, which often cause the demise of one twin followed by sudden hypotension in the other. If one fetus of a monochorionic twin gestation dies after the first trimester but before viability, pregnancy termination can be considered (Blickstein, 2013). Occasionally, death of one but not all fetuses results from a maternal complication such as diabetic ketoacidosis or severe preeclampsia with abruption. Pregnancy management is based on the diagnosis and the status of both the mother and surviving fetus. If the death of one dichorionic twin is due to a discordant congenital anomaly, its death should not affect its surviving twin.

Single fetal death during late second and early third trimester presents the greatest risk to the surviving twin. Although the risks of subsequent death or neurological damage to the survivor are comparatively increased for monochorionic twins at this gestational age, the risk of preterm birth is equally increased in mono- and dichorionic twins (Ong, 2006). Delivery generally occurs within 3 weeks of diagnosis of fetal demise, thus antenatal corticosteroids for survivor lung maturity should be considered (Blickstein, 2013). Regardless, unless there is a hostile intrauterine environment, the goal should be to prolong pregnancy.

Timing of elective delivery after conservative management of a late second or early third trimester single fetal death is a matter of debate. Dichorionic twins can probably be safely delivered at term. Monochorionic twin gestations are more difficult to manage and are often delivered between 34 and 37 weeks' gestation (Blickstein, 2013). In cases of single fetal death at term, especially when the etiology is unclear, most opt for delivery instead of expectant management.

Impending Death of One Fetus

Abnormal antepartum test results of fetal health in one twin fetus, but not the other, pose a particular dilemma. Delivery may be the best option for the compromised fetus yet may result in death from immaturity of the cotwin. If fetal lung maturity is confirmed, salvage of both the healthy fetus and its jeopardized sibling is possible. Unfortunately, ideal management if twins are immature is problematic but should be based on the chances of intact survival for both fetuses. Often the compromised fetus is severely growth restricted or anomalous. Thus, performing amniocentesis for fetal karyotyping in women of advanced maternal age carrying twin pregnancies is advantageous, even for those who would continue their pregnancies regardless of the diagnosis. Aneuploidy identification in one fetus allows rational decisions regarding interventions.

PRENATAL CARE AND ANTEPARTUM MANAGEMENT

Primary goals of prenatal management of multifetal pregnancy are to provide close observation of the mother and her fetuses to prevent or interdict complications as they develop. A major imperative is to prevent preterm delivery of markedly immature neonates. At Parkland Hospital, women with multifetal gestations are seen every 2 weeks beginning at 22 weeks' gestation, and a digital cervical examination is performed at each visit. Identification of other unique complications discussed above may also lead to interventions including early delivery. We routinely perform sonographic studies to assess fetal growth and amnionic fluid every 4 weeks in monochorionic twins or 6 weeks in dichorionic pairs.

Diet

Along with more frequent prenatal visits, it must be ensured that the maternal diet provides additional requirements for calories, protein, minerals, vitamins, and essential fatty acids. Achievement of BMI-specific weight gain goals, supplementation with macro- and micronutrients to meet the increased needs associated with a twin gestation, and carbohydrate-controlled diets have been recommended (Goodnight, 2009). The Institute of Medicine guidelines for twin pregnancy recommend a 37- to 54-lb weight gain for women with a normal BMI. In their extensive review of the topic, Goodnight and Newman (2009) recommend supplementation of micronutrients such as calcium, magnesium, zinc, and vitamins C, D, and E based on upper intake levels from the Food and Nutrition Board of the Institute of Medicine. The daily recommended increased caloric intake for women with twins is 40 to 45 kcal/kg/d, composed of 20 percent protein, 40 percent carbohydrate, and 40 percent fat divided into three meals and three snacks daily.

Surveillance of Fetal Growth and Health

Because a cornerstone of fetal assessment in twin pregnancy is identification of abnormal fetal growth or discordancy, serial sonographic examinations are usually performed throughout the third trimester. Assessment of amnionic fluid volume is also important. Associated oligohydramnios may indicate uteroplacental pathology and should prompt further evaluation of fetal well-being. That said, quantifying amnionic fluid volume in multifetal gestation is sometimes difficult. Some measure the deepest vertical pocket in each sac or assess the fluid subjectively. Measurement of the amnionic fluid index (AFI) may also be helpful. Using data from 488 diamnionic twins with birthweight between the 10th and 90th percentiles, Hill and associates (2000) described a protocol for measuring the AFI in twin gestations. Each amnionic sac was divided into quadrants that extended along a vertical, horizontal, or oblique axis. The deepest vertical pocket free of umbilical cord in each quadrant was measured. They found a slightly lower median value in twins than singletons. The AFI was highest at 26 to 28 weeks' gestation and declined until delivery. Magann and coworkers (2000) compared subjective assessment and several objective methods of assessing amnionic fluid in 23 sets of twins. They found all methods to be equally poor in predicting abnormal volumes in diamnionic twins. At Parkland Hospital, the single deepest vertical pocket is measured in each sac. A measurement < 2 cm is considered oligohydramnios and a measurement ≥ 8 cm is considered hydramnios (Hernandez, 2012).

Tests of Fetal Well-Being

As described throughout Chapter 17, there are several methods of assessing fetal health in singleton pregnancies. The nonstress test or biophysical profile is commonly used in management of twin or higher-order multifetal gestations. Because of the complex complications associated with multifetal gestations and the potential technical difficulties in differentiating fetuses during antepartum testing, the usefulness of these methods appears limited. According to DeVoe (2008), the few exclusive studies of nonstress testing in twins suggest that the method performs the same as in singleton pregnancies. Elliott and Finberg (1995) used the biophysical profile as the primary method for monitoring higher-order multifetal gestations. They reported that four of 24 monitored pregnancies had a poor outcome despite reassuring biophysical profile scores. Although biophysical testing is commonly performed in multifetal gestations, there are insufficient data to determine its efficacy (DeVoe, 2008).

In an early study of 272 twin sets, Giles and colleagues (1990) reported that availability of umbilical artery Doppler velocimetry led to a reduced perinatal mortality rate. In a later randomized trial of 526 twin pregnancies by the same group, the addition of umbilical artery Doppler velocimetry to management compared with fetal testing based on fetal-growth parameters alone resulted in no perinatal outcome improvement (Giles, 2003). Hack and associates (2008) investigated the utility of umbilical artery Doppler velocimetry in 67 uncomplicated monochorionic twin gestations. They found similar mortality rates in those with abnormal pulsatility indices of the umbilical artery compared with those with normal indices. Differences in neonatal morbidity were explained by gestational age at delivery.

All testing schemes have high false-positive rates in singletons, and data suggest that testing in multifetal gestations performs no better. In cases of abnormal testing in one twin and normal results in another, iatrogenic preterm delivery remains a major concern.

Pulmonary Maturation

According to Robinson and coworkers (2012), beyond a strategy of planned delivery of uncomplicated monochorionic twins at 38 weeks, a secondary strategy is amniocentesis to verify pulmonary maturity before delivery between 36 and 38 weeks. In cases of complicated twin gestations, amniocentesis may be performed earlier. As measured by determination of the lecithin-sphingomyelin ratio, pulmonary maturation is usually synchronous in twins (Leveno, 1984). Moreover, although this ratio usually does not exceed 2.0 until 36 weeks in singleton pregnancies, it often exceeds this value by approximately 32 weeks in multifetal pregnancies. McElrath and colleagues (2000) reported similar increased values of surfactant in twins after 31 weeks' gestation. In a comparison of respiratory morbidity in 100 twins and 241 singleton newborns delivered by cesarean before labor, Ghi and associates (2013) found less neonatal respiratory morbidity in twins, especially those delivered ≤ 37 weeks' gestation. In some cases, however, pulmonary function may be markedly different, and the smallest, most stressed twin fetus is typically more mature.

PRETERM BIRTH

Preterm labor is common in multifetal pregnancies and may complicate up to 50 percent of twin, 75 percent of triplet, and 90 percent of quadruplet pregnancies (Elliott, 2007). The proportion of preterm births in multifetal gestations, however, varies widely. For example, the preterm birth rate is 42 percent in Ireland but is 68 percent in Austria (Giuffre, 2012). These differences likely reflect different clinical approaches to management. Several techniques have been applied in attempts to prolong these pregnancies. Methods include bed rest—especially through hospitalization, prophylactic administration of β-mimetic drugs or progestins, prophylactic cervical cerclage, and pessary placement.

Prediction of Preterm Birth

A major goal of multifetal pregnancy prenatal care is accurate prediction of women likely to experience preterm delivery, with prediction followed by prevention. This has been an elusive goal, but some advances have been made. Goldenberg and coworkers (1996) prospectively screened 147 twin pregnancies for more than 50 potential preterm birth risk factors. These investigators found that cervical length and fetal fibronectin concentration in the cervical canal were predictive of preterm birth (Chap. 42, p. 843). At 24 weeks, a cervical length ≤ 25 mm was the best predictor of birth before 32 weeks. At 28 weeks, an elevated fetal fibronectin level was the best predictor. Similarly, To and associates (2006) sonographically measured cervical length in 1163 twin pregnancies at 22 to 24 weeks. Rates of preterm delivery before 32 weeks were 66 percent in those with cervical lengths of 10 mm; 24 percent for lengths of 20 mm; 12 percent for 25 mm; and only 1 percent for 40 mm. McMahon and colleagues (2002) found that women with multifetal gestations at 24 weeks who had a closed internal os on digital cervical examination, a normal cervical length by sonographic examination, and a negative fetal fibronectin test result had a *low* risk to deliver before 32 weeks. Interestingly, a closed internal os by digital examination was as predictive of early delivery as the combination of normal sonographically measured cervical length and negative fetal fibronectin test results.

In a systematic review and metaanalysis of transvaginal cervical length for the prediction of preterm birth, Conde-Agudelo and coworkers (2010) concluded that cervical length between 20 and 24 weeks was a good predictor of spontaneous preterm birth in asymptomatic women with twin pregnancies. These authors found that a cervical length ≤ 20 mm was most accurate for predicting birth < 34 weeks, with a specificity of 97 percent and positive likelihood ratio of 9.0.

Prevention of Preterm Birth

Several schemes have been evaluated to prevent preterm labor and delivery. In recent years, some have been shown to decrease the risk of preterm delivery in small subgroups of singleton pregnancies. Unfortunately, most have been disappointingly ineffective.

Bed Rest

Most evidence suggests that routine hospitalization is not beneficial in prolonging multifetal pregnancy. In a metaanalysis of seven trials of hospitalization with bed rest, Crowther and Han (2010) concluded that the practice did not reduce the risk of preterm birth or perinatal mortality. Also at Parkland Hospital, elective hospitalization was compared with outpatient management, and no advantages were found (Andrews, 1991). Importantly, however, almost half of the women required admission for specific indications such as hypertension or threatened preterm delivery.

Limited physical activity, early work leave, more frequent health care visits and sonographic examinations, and structured maternal education regarding preterm delivery risks have been advocated to reduce preterm birth rates in women with multiple fetuses. Unfortunately, there is little evidence that these measures substantially change outcome.

Prophylactic Tocolysis

Tocolytic therapy in multifetal pregnancies has not been extensively studied. In a Cochrane review of five randomized trials of prophylactic oral β-mimetic therapy that included 374 twin pregnancies, Yamasmit and coworkers (2012) concluded that treatment did not reduce the rate of twins delivering before 37 or before 34 weeks. Especially in light of the recent Food and Drug Administration warning against the use of oral terbutaline, prophylactic use of β-mimetics in multifetal gestations seems especially unwarranted.

Intramuscular Progesterone Therapy

Although somewhat effective in reducing recurrent preterm birth in women with a singleton pregnancy, weekly injections of 17α-hydroxyprogesterone caproate (17-OHPC) are not effective for multifetal gestations (Caritis, 2009; Rouse, 2007). These results were corroborated in a more recent randomized trial in 240 twin pregnancies (Combs, 2011). Moreover, women carrying twins and identified with a cervical length < 36 mm (25th percentile) did not benefit despite their increased risk for preterm birth (Durnwald, 2010). Senat and colleagues (2013) randomly assigned 165 asymptomatic women with twins and a cervical length < 25 mm to 17-OHPC and also found no reduction in delivery before 37 weeks.

Caritis and associates (2012), in an evaluation of plasma drug concentrations in a Maternal-Fetal Medicine Units (MFMU) Network trial, reported that higher concentrations of 17-OHPC were associated with earlier gestational age at delivery. They concluded that 17-OHPC may adversely lower the gestational age at delivery in women with twin gestations. When taken together, administration of intramuscular 17-OHPC to women with twin pregnancies, even to those with a shortened cervix, does not lower the preterm birth risk.

Vaginal Progesterone Therapy

Micronized progesterone administered vaginally to women with twins is of uncertain benefit. Cetingoz and coworkers (2011) gave 100 mg of micronized progesterone intravaginally daily from 24 to 34 weeks. These authors reported that this practice reduced rates of delivery before 37 weeks from 79 to 51 percent in 67 women with twins. In contrast, several studies have failed to demonstrate any preterm birth rate reduction in women receiving various formulations of vaginal progesterone. Norman and colleagues (2009) randomly assigned 494 women with twins to 10 weeks of daily 90-mg intravaginal progesterone and failed to show reduced rates of delivery before 34 weeks. In the multicenter Prevention of Preterm Delivery in Twin Gestations (PREDICT) trial, Rode and associates (2011) randomly assigned 677 women with twins to receive prophylactic, 200-mg progesterone pessaries or placebo pessaries. These investigators also failed to demonstrate a reduction in delivery rates before 34 weeks. In a subgroup analysis of this trial that included only women with a short cervix or a history of prior preterm birth, Klein and associates (2011) also did not demonstrate a benefit. At Parkland Hospital, management of women with multifetal gestations does not typically include progesterone in any formulation.

Cervical Cerclage

Prophylactic cerclage has not been shown to improve perinatal outcome in women with multifetal pregnancies. Studies have included women who were not specially selected and those who were selected because of a shortened cervix that was identified sonographically (Dor, 1982; Elimian, 1999; Newman, 2002; Rebarber, 2005). In the latter group, cerclage may actually worsen outcomes (Berghella, 2005).

Pessary

A vaginal pessary that encircles and theoretically compresses the cervix, alters the inclination of the cervical canal, and relieves direct pressure on the internal cervical os has been proposed as an alternative to cerclage. The most popular is the silicone Arabin pessary. In a study of pessary use in women with a short cervix between 18 and 22 weeks, a subgroup analysis of 23 women with twins showed a significant reduction in the delivery rate before 32 weeks compared with the rate in 23 control pregnancies (Arabin, 2003). Liem and coworkers (2013) recently reported on the open-label Pessaries in Multiple Pregnancy as a Prevention of Preterm Birth (ProTWIN) trial completed at 40 centers throughout the Netherlands. These researchers randomized 813 unselected women with twins to receive either the Arabin pessary between 12 and 20 weeks or no treatment. The pessary failed to reduce preterm birth overall but did decrease delivery rates before 32 weeks in a subset of women with a cervical length < 38 mm—29 versus 14 percent. At this time, before such treatment can be recommended, beneficial effects of pessary use in women with a short cervix need to be confirmed.

Treatment of Preterm Labor

Although many advocate their use, therapy with tocolytic agents to forestall preterm labor in multifetal pregnancy has not resulted in measurably improved neonatal outcomes (Chauhan, 2010; Gyetvai, 1999). They are similarly ineffective in singleton pregnancy as discussed in further detail in Chapter 42 (p. 851). Another caveat is that tocolytic therapy in women with a multifetal pregnancy entails higher risk than in singleton pregnancy. This is in part because of the augmented pregnancy-induced hypervolemia and its increased cardiac demands and susceptibility to iatrogenic pulmonary edema. Gabriel and colleagues (1994) compared outcomes of 26 twin and six triplet pregnancies with those of 51 singletons—all treated with a β-mimetic drug for preterm labor. Women with a multifetal gestation had significantly more cardiovascular complications—43 versus 4 percent—including three with pulmonary edema. In a recent retrospective analysis, Derbent and coworkers (2011) evaluated nifedipine tocolysis in 58 singleton and 32 twin pregnancies. These authors reported higher incidences of side effects such as maternal tachycardia in women with twins—19 versus 9 percent.

Glucocorticoids for Lung Maturation

Administration of corticosteroids to stimulate fetal lung maturation has not been well studied in multifetal gestation. However, these drugs logically should be as beneficial for multiples as they are for singletons (Roberts, 2006). Battista and colleagues (2008) compared the efficacy of betamethasone therapy in 60 preterm twin pregnancies to 60 preterm singleton pregnancies. These researchers found no differences in neonatal morbidity, including respiratory distress. Moreover, Gyamfi and associates (2010) evaluated betamethasone concentrations in maternal and umbilical cord blood in 30 singleton and 15 twin pregnancies receiving weekly antenatal corticosteroids. They found no differences in levels between twins and singletons. These treatments are discussed in Chapter 42 (p. 850). At this time, guidelines for the use of these agents are not different from those for singleton gestations (American College of Obstetricians and Gynecologists, 2010).

Preterm Premature Membrane Rupture

The frequency of preterm premature rupture of membranes (PPROM) increases with increasing plurality. In a population-based retrospective cohort study of more than 290,000 live births in Ohio, Pakrashi and coworkers (2013) reported the proportion of preterm birth complicated by premature rupture was 13.2 percent in singletons. This rate was compared with 17, 20, 20, and 100 percent in twins, triplets, quadruplets, and higher-order multiples, respectively. Multifetal gestations with PPROM are managed expectantly much like singleton pregnancies (Chap. 42, p. 846). Ehsanipoor and colleagues (2012) compared outcomes of 41 twin and 82 singleton pregnancies, both with ruptured membranes between 24 and 32 weeks. They found the median latency was overall shorter for twins—3.6 days compared with 6.2 days for singletons. This difference was significant in pregnancies after 30 weeks—1.7 days and

6.9 days. Importantly, latency beyond 7 days approximated 40 percent in both groups.

Delayed Delivery of Second Twin

Infrequently, after preterm birth of the presenting fetus, it may be advantageous for undelivered fetus(es) to remain in utero. Trivedi and Gillett (1998) reviewed the English literature and described 45 case reports of asynchronous birth in multifetal gestation. Although likely biased, those pregnancies with a surviving retained twin or triplet continued for an average of 49 days. No advantage was gained by management with tocolytics, prophylactic antimicrobials, or cerclage. In their 10-year experience, Roman and associates (2010) reported a median latency of 16 days in 13 twin and five triplet pregnancies with delivery of the first fetus between 20 and 25 weeks. Survival of the firstborn infant was 16 percent. Although 54 percent of the retained fetuses survived, only 37 percent of survivors did so without major morbidity. Livingston and coworkers (2004) described 14 pregnancies in which an active attempt was made to delay delivery of 19 fetuses after delivery of the first neonate. Only one fetus survived without major sequelae, and one mother developed sepsis syndrome with shock. Arabin and van Eyck (2009) reported better outcomes in a few of the 93 twin and 34 triplet pregnancies that qualified for delayed delivery in their center during a 17-year period.

If asynchronous birth is attempted, there must be careful evaluation for infection, abruption, and congenital anomalies. The mother must be thoroughly counseled, particularly regarding the potential for serious, life-threatening infection. The range of gestational age in which the benefits outweigh the risks for delayed delivery is likely narrow. Avoidance of delivery from 23 to 26 weeks would seem most beneficial. In our experience, good candidates for delayed delivery are rare.

LABOR AND DELIVERY

There is a litany of complications that may be encountered during labor and delivery of multiple fetuses. In addition to preterm labor and delivery as already discussed, there are increased rates of uterine contractile dysfunction, abnormal fetal presentation, umbilical cord prolapse, placenta previa, placental abruption, emergent operative delivery, and postpartum hemorrhage from uterine atony. All of these must be anticipated and thus certain precautions and special arrangements are prudent. These should include:

1. An appropriately trained obstetrical attendant should remain with the mother throughout labor. Continuous external electronic monitoring is preferable. If membranes are ruptured and the cervix dilated, the presenting fetus is monitored internally.
2. An intravenous infusion system capable of delivering fluid rapidly is established. In the absence of hemorrhage, lactated Ringer or an aqueous dextrose solution is infused at a rate of 60 to 125 mL/hr.
3. Blood for transfusion is readily available if needed.
4. An obstetrician skilled in intrauterine identification of fetal parts and in intrauterine manipulation of a fetus should be present.
5. A sonography machine is readily available to evaluate the presentation and position of the fetuses during labor and to image the remaining fetus(es) after delivery of the first.
6. An anesthesia team is immediately available in the event that emergent cesarean delivery is necessary or that intrauterine manipulation is required for vaginal delivery.
7. For each fetus, at least one attendant who is skilled in resuscitation and care of newborns and who has been appropriately informed of the case should be immediately available.
8. The delivery area should provide adequate space for the nursing, obstetrical, anesthesia, and pediatric team members to work effectively. Equipment must be on site to provide emergent anesthesia, operative intervention, and maternal and neonatal resuscitation.

Evaluation upon Admission

Fetal Presentation

In addition to the standard preparations for the conduct of labor and delivery discussed in Chapter 22, there are special considerations for women with a multifetal pregnancy. First, the positions and presentations of fetuses are best confirmed sonographically (American College of Obstetricians and Gynecologists, 2011). Although any possible combination of positions may be encountered, those most common at admission for delivery are cephalic-cephalic, cephalic-breech, and cephalic-transverse. At Parkland Hospital between 2008 and 2013, 71 percent of twin pregnancies had cephalic presentation of the first fetus at the time of admission to labor and delivery. Importantly, with perhaps the exception of cephalic–cephalic presentations, these are all unstable before and during labor and delivery. Accordingly, compound, face, brow, and footling breech presentations are relatively common, and even more so if fetuses are small, amnionic fluid is excessive, or maternal parity is high. Cord prolapse is also frequent in these circumstances.

After this initial evaluation, if active labor is confirmed, then a decision is made to attempt vaginal delivery or to proceed with cesarean delivery. The latter is chosen in many cases because of fetal presentations. Cephalic presentation of the first fetus in a laboring woman with twins may be considered for expectant management. Of the 547 women who presented like this at Parkland Hospital during 5 years, 32 percent delivered spontaneously. Nevertheless, the overall cesarean delivery rate in twin pregnancies during those years was 77 percent. Notably, 5 percent of cesareans performed were for emergent delivery of the second twin following vaginal delivery of the first twin. The desire to avoid this obstetrical dilemma has contributed to the increasing cesarean delivery rate in twin pregnancies across the United States (Antsaklis, 2013; Lee, 2011).

Labor Induction or Stimulation

According to a comparison of 891 twins with more than 100,000 singleton pregnancies included in the *Consortium of Safe Labor*, Leftwich and colleagues (2013) concluded that both nulliparas and multiparas with twins had slower progression of active labor. Women with twins required between 1 and 3 additional hours to complete first-stage labor. This was despite equivalent rates of labor induction or augmentation. Provided women with twins meet all criteria for oxytocin administration, it may be used as described in Chapter 26 (p. 529). Wolfe and associates (2013) evaluated the success of labor induction in 40 sets of twins compared with 80 singletons and found that protocols for oxytocin alone or in combination with cervical ripening can safely be used in twin gestations. Taylor and coworkers (2012) reported that 100 women with twins undergoing labor induction had similar labor lengths and cesarean delivery rates compared with those of 100 matched women with singleton pregnancies. Still, in an analysis of twin births in the United States between 1995 and 2008, Lee and colleagues (2011) reported that induction rates of twin pregnancies has decreased from a maximum of 13.8 percent in 1999 to 9.9 percent in 2008.

Analgesia and Anesthesia

During labor and delivery of multiple fetuses, decisions regarding analgesia and anesthesia may be complicated by problems imposed by preterm labor, preeclampsia, desultory labor, need for intrauterine manipulation, and postpartum uterine atony and hemorrhage.

Labor epidural analgesia is ideal because it provides excellent pain relief and can be rapidly extended cephalad if internal podalic version or cesarean delivery is required. There are special considerations for women with severe preeclampsia or with hemorrhage as discussed in their respective chapters. Because of these eventualities, most recommend that continuous epidural analgesia be performed by anesthesia personnel with special expertise in obstetrics.

If general anesthesia becomes necessary for intrauterine manipulation, then uterine relaxation can be accomplished rapidly with one of the halogenated inhalation agents discussed in Chapter 25 (p. 519). Some clinicians use intravenous or sublingual nitroglycerin to achieve uterine relaxation yet avoid the aspiration and hypoxia risks associated with general anesthetics.

Delivery Route

Regardless of fetal presentation during labor, there must be a readiness to deal with any change of fetal position during delivery and especially following delivery of the first twin. If the first fetus is nonvertex, cesarean delivery is typically performed, whereas cephalic-cephalic twins are commonly considered for vaginal delivery (Peaceman, 2009; Rossi, 2011). Importantly, when comparing neonatal outcomes among all these options, second twins at term as a group have worse composite neonatal outcomes than those of their cotwin regardless of delivery method (Smith, 2007; Thorngren-Jerneck, 2001).

Cephalic-Cephalic Presentation

If the first twin presents cephalic, delivery can usually be accomplished spontaneously or with forceps. According to D'Alton (2010), there is general consensus that a trial of labor is reasonable in women with cephalic-cephalic twins. Hogle and associates (2003) performed an extensive literature review and concluded that planned cesarean delivery does not improve neonatal outcome when both twins are cephalic. The recent randomized trial by Barrett and coworkers (2013) affirms this conclusion. Muleba and colleagues (2005) identified increased rates of respiratory distress in the second twin of preterm pairs regardless of delivery mode or corticosteroid use.

Cephalic-Noncephalic Presentation

The optimal delivery route for cephalic–noncephalic twin pairs remains controversial (D'Alton, 2010). Patient selection is crucial, and options include cesarean delivery of both twins, or less commonly, vaginal delivery with intrapartum external cephalic version of the second twin. Longer intertwin delivery time has been shown in some studies to be associated with poorer second twin outcome (Edris, 2006; Stein, 2008). Thus, breech extraction may be preferable to version. Least desirable, vaginal delivery of the first but cesarean delivery of the second twin may be required due to intrapartum complications such as umbilical cord prolapse, placental abruption, contracting cervix, and fetal distress. Most, but not all, studies show the worst composite fetal outcomes for this scenario (Alexander, 2008; Rossi, 2011; Wen, 2004).

Several reports attest to the safety of vaginal delivery of second noncephalic twins whose birthweight is > 1500 g. Recently, Fox and associates (2014) reported outcomes of 287 diamnionic twin pregnancies between 2005 and 2009. Cesarean delivery was routinely performed for all women with a noncephalic presenting twin fetus, a noncephalic second twin weighing < 1500 g, or a second twin estimated to be 20 percent larger than the presenting twin. All others without contraindications to labor were offered a vaginal delivery and were treated using a strict protocol of second-stage labor management. This included vaginal delivery of a second cephalic twin, breech extraction of a second noncephalic twin, and internal podalic version of an unengaged cephalic second twin followed by breech extraction. Of the 130 who planned a vaginal delivery, only 15 percent underwent cesarean delivery. There was no difference in the rate of 5-minute Apgar score < 7 or of umbilical arterial pH < 7.20 in second twins. The data are less informative concerning vaginal delivery of a second twin whose estimated fetal weight is < 1500 g. That said, however, comparable or even better fetal outcomes with vaginal delivery have been reported with these smaller infants compared with those who weigh > 1500 g (Caukwell, 2002; Davidson, 1992; Rydhström, 1990).

Other investigators advocate cesarean delivery for both members of a cephalic-noncephalic twin pair (Armson, 2006; Hoffmann, 2012). Yang and coworkers (2005a,b) studied 15,185 cephalic-noncephalic twin pairs. The risk of asphyxia-related neonatal deaths and morbidity was increased in the group in which both twins were delivered vaginally compared with the group in which both twins underwent cesarean delivery.

Randomized Trial of Planned Cesarean versus Vaginal Delivery. To add insight into the clinical complexities discussed above, a randomized trial was designed by the Twin Birth Study Collaborative Group from Canada. The study

TABLE 45-4. Maternal and Perinatal Outcomes of Women with a Twin Pregnancy Randomized to Planned Cesarean versus Vaginal Delivery

Outcome	Planned Cesarean Delivery	Planned Vaginal Delivery	p value
Maternal (No.)	1393	1393	
Cesarean delivery	89.9%	39.6%	
Before labor	53.8%	14.1%	
Serious morbidity	7.3%	8.5%	0.29
Death (No.)	1	1	
Hemorrhage	6.0%	7.8%	
Blood Transfusion	4.7%	5.4%	
Thromboembolism	0.4%	0.1%	
Perinatal (No.)	2783	2782	
Primary composite outcome	2.2%	1.9%	0.49
Perinatal mortality	9 per 1000	6 per 1000	
Serious morbidity	1.3%	1.3%	
Possible encephalopathy[a]	0.5%	0.4%	
Intubation	1.0%	0.6%	

[a]Includes coma; stupor; hyperalert, drowsy or lethargic; or ≥ 2 seizures.
Data from Barrett, 2013.

results described by Barrett and colleagues (2013) included 2804 women carrying a presumed diamnionic twin pregnancy with the first fetus presenting cephalic. Women were randomly assigned between 32 and 38 weeks to planned cesarean or vaginal delivery. The time from randomization to delivery—12.4 versus 13.3 days, the mean gestational age at delivery—36.7 versus 36.8 weeks, and use of regional analgesia—92 versus 87 percent was similar in both groups. Salient maternal and perinatal outcomes are shown in Table 45-4. No significant differences in outcomes were noted between the two groups of women. Although there were no increased risks to mother or fetuses with planned vaginal delivery in these circumstances, we agree with Greene (2013) that this trial will moderately affect the cesarean delivery rate of women with twins.

Breech Presentation of First Twin

Problems with the first twin presenting as a breech are similar to those encountered with a singleton breech fetus. Thus, major problems may develop if:

1. The fetus is unusually large, and the aftercoming head is larger than the birth canal.
2. The fetal body is small, and delivery of the extremities and trunk through an inadequately effaced and dilated cervix causes the relatively larger head to become trapped above the cervix. This is more likely when there is disproportion between the fetal buttocks or trunk and the head. This may be seen with preterm or growth-restricted fetuses or with a macrocephalic fetus due to hydrocephaly.
3. The umbilical cord prolapses.

If these problems are anticipated or identified, cesarean delivery is often preferred with a viable-size fetus. But even without these problems, many obstetricians perform cesarean delivery if the first twin presents as breech. This is despite data that support the safety of vaginal delivery. Specifically, Blickstein and associates (2000) reported experiences from 13 European centers with 613 twin pairs and the first twin presenting breech. Vaginal delivery was attempted in 373 of these cases and was successful in 64 percent. Cesarean delivery of the second twin was done in 2.4 percent. There was no difference in the rate of 5-minute Apgar score < 7 or of mortality in breech-presenting first twins who weighed at least 1500 g. Details of techniques for delivery of a breech presentation are described in Chapter 28 (p. 563).

Locked Twins. For twin fetuses to become locked together during delivery, the first must present as breech and the second as cephalic. As the breech of the first twin descends through the birth canal, the chin locks between the neck and chin of the second cephalic-presenting cotwin. This phenomenon is rare, and Cohen and coworkers (1965) described it only once in 817 twin gestations. Cesarean delivery should be considered when the potential for locking is identified.

Vaginal Delivery of the Second Twin

Following delivery of the first twin, the presenting part of the second twin, its size, and its relationship to the birth canal should be quickly and carefully ascertained by combined abdominal, vaginal, and at times, intrauterine examination. Sonography may be a valuable aid. If the fetal head or the breech is fixed in the birth canal, moderate fundal pressure is applied and membranes are ruptured. Immediately afterward, digital examination of the cervix is repeated to exclude cord prolapse. Labor is allowed to resume. If contractions do not begin within approximately 10 minutes, dilute oxytocin may be used to stimulate contractions.

In the past, the safest interval between delivery of the first and second twins was frequently cited as less than 30 minutes. Rayburn and colleagues (1984), and others, have shown that if continuous fetal monitoring is used, a good outcome is achieved even if this interval is longer. Several investigators have demonstrated a direct correlation between worsening umbilical cord blood gas values and increasing time between delivery of first and second twins (Leung, 2002; Stein, 2008). Gourheux and associates (2007) retrospectively reviewed delivery intervals in 239 twin gestations in France and determined that mean umbilical arterial pH was significantly lower after the interval exceeded 15 minutes. Thus, vigilant monitoring for nonreassuring fetal heart rate or bleeding is required. Hemorrhage may indicate clinically significant placental abruption.

If the occiput or breech presents immediately over the pelvic inlet, but is not fixed in the birth canal, the presenting part can often be guided into the pelvis by one hand in the vagina, while a second hand on the uterine fundus exerts moderate pressure caudally. Alternatively, with abdominal manipulation, an assistant can guide the presenting part into the pelvis. Sonography can aid guidance and allow heart rate monitoring. Intrapartum external version of a noncephalic second twin has also been described.

A presenting shoulder may be gently converted into a cephalic presentation. If the occiput or breech is not over the pelvic inlet and cannot be so positioned by gentle pressure or if appreciable uterine bleeding develops, delivery of the second twin can be problematic.

To obtain a favorable outcome, it is essential to have an obstetrician skilled in intrauterine fetal manipulation and anesthesia personnel skilled in providing anesthesia to effectively relax the uterus for vaginal delivery of a noncephalic second twin (American College of Obstetricians and Gynecologists, 2010). To take maximum advantage of the dilated cervix before the uterus contracts and the cervix retracts, delay must be avoided. Prompt cesarean delivery of the second fetus is preferred if no one present is skilled in the performance of internal podalic version or if anesthesia that will provide effective uterine relaxation is not immediately available.

Internal Podalic Version

With this maneuver, a fetus is turned to a breech presentation using the hand placed into the uterus (Fig. 45-27). The obstetrician grasps the fetal feet to then effect delivery by breech extraction. As mentioned earlier, Fox and colleagues (2010) described a strict protocol for management of the delivery of the second twin, which included internal podalic version. They reported that none of the 110 women who delivered the first twin vaginally underwent a cesarean delivery for the second twin. Chauhan and coworkers (1995) compared outcomes of 23 second twins delivered by podalic version and breech extraction with those of 21 who underwent external cephalic version. Breech extraction was considered superior to external version because less fetal distress developed. The technique of breech extraction is described in Chapter 28 (p. 567).

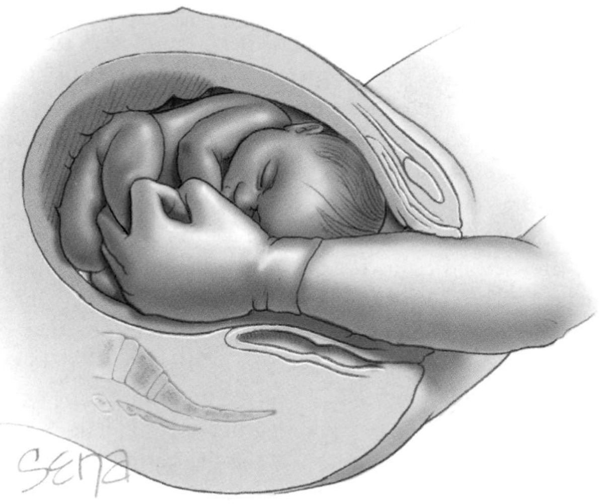

FIGURE 45-27 Internal podalic version. Upward pressure on the head by an abdominal hand is applied as downward traction is exerted on the feet.

Vaginal Birth after Cesarean Delivery

Any attempt to deliver twins vaginally in a woman who has previously undergone one or more cesarean deliveries should be carefully considered. As discussed in Chapter 31 (p. 614), some studies support the safety of attempting a vaginal birth after cesarean delivery (VBAC) for selected women with twins (Cahill, 2005; Ford, 2006; Varner, 2005). According to the American College of Obstetricians and Gynecologists (2013b), there currently is no evidence of an increased risk of uterine rupture, and women with twins and one previous cesarean delivery with a low transverse incision may be considered candidates for trial of labor. At Parkland Hospital, such women are generally offered repeat cesarean delivery.

Cesarean Delivery for Multifetal Gestation

There are several unusual intraoperative problems that can arise during cesarean delivery of twins or higher-order multiples. Supine hypotension is common, and thus these women should be positioned in a left lateral tilt to deflect uterine weight off the aorta (Chap. 4, p. 60). A low-transverse hysterotomy is preferable if the incision can be made large enough to allow atraumatic delivery of both fetuses. Piper forceps can be used if the second twin is presenting breech (Fig. 28-13, p. 568). In some cases, a vertical hysterotomy beginning as low as possible in the lower uterine segment may be advantageous. For example, if a fetus is transverse with its back down and the arms are inadvertently delivered first, it is much easier and safer to extend a vertical uterine incision upward than to extend a transverse incision laterally or to make a "T" incision vertically.

Cesarean Delivery of the Second Twin

It is not uncommon for cesarean delivery to become necessary for delivery of a second twin after the first has been delivered vaginally. As described earlier, this occurred in 32 of 770 women with twins at Parkland Hospital between 2008 and 2013. In these cases, prompt cesarean delivery is required and is frequently emergently indicated. Indications most often cited are a second fetus that is much larger than the first and is presenting breech or transverse. In other cases, the cervix promptly contracts and thickens after delivery of the first twin. This may be followed by a nonreassuring fetal status or by a cervix that fails to completely dilate again despite adequate uterine contractions.

TRIPLET OR HIGHER-ORDER GESTATION

Fetal heart rate monitoring during labor with triplet pregnancies is challenging. A scalp electrode can be attached to the presenting fetus, but it is difficult to ensure that the other two fetuses are each being monitored separately. With vaginal delivery, the first neonate is usually born with little or no manipulation. Subsequent fetuses, however, are delivered according to the presenting part. This often requires complicated obstetrical maneuvers such as total breech extraction with or without internal podalic version or even cesarean delivery. Associated with malposition of fetuses is an increased incidence of cord prolapse. Moreover, reduced placental perfusion and hemorrhage from separating placentas are more likely during delivery.

For all these reasons, many clinicians believe that pregnancies complicated by three or more fetuses are best delivered by cesarean. Vaginal delivery is reserved for those circumstances in which survival is not expected because fetuses are markedly immature or maternal complications make cesarean delivery hazardous to the mother. Others believe that vaginal delivery is safe under certain circumstances. For example, Alamia and colleagues (1998) evaluated a protocol for vaginal delivery of triplet pregnancies in which the presenting fetus was cephalic. A total of 23 sets of triplets were analyzed, and a third of these were delivered vaginally. Neonatal outcomes were the same in the vaginal and cesarean delivery groups, with no morbidity and 100-percent fetal survival. Grobman and associates (1998) and Alran and coworkers (2004) reported vaginal delivery completion rates of 88 and 84 percent, respectively, in women carrying triplets who underwent a trial of labor. Neonatal outcomes did not differ from those of a matched group of triplet pregnancies delivered by elective cesarean. Conversely, Vintzeleos and colleagues (2005) reviewed more than 7000 triplet pregnancies and found that vaginal delivery was associated with an increased perinatal mortality rate. Importantly, the overall cesarean delivery rate among triplets was 95 percent. At Parkland Hospital, triplet gestations are routinely delivered by cesarean.

SELECTIVE REDUCTION OR TERMINATION

In some cases of higher-order multifetal gestation, reduction of the fetal number to two or three improves survival of the remaining fetuses. *Selective reduction* implies early pregnancy intervention, whereas *selective termination* is performed later.

Selective Reduction

Reduction of a selected fetus or fetuses in a multichorionic multifetal gestation may be chosen as a therapeutic intervention to enhance survival of the remaining fetuses (American College of Obstetricians and Gynecologists, 2013a). There are no randomized controlled trials on the effects of such reduction. However, a metaanalysis of nonrandomized prospective studies indicates that pregnancy reduction to twins compared with expectant management is associated with lower rates of maternal complications, preterm birth, and neonatal death (Dodd, 2004, 2012). Pregnancy reduction can be performed transcervically, transvaginally, or transabdominally, but the transabdominal route is usually easiest.

Transabdominal fetal reductions are typically performed between 10 and 13 weeks. This gestational age is chosen because most spontaneous abortions have already occurred, the remaining fetuses are large enough to be evaluated sonographically, the amount of devitalized fetal tissue remaining after the procedure is small, and the risk of aborting the entire pregnancy as a result of the procedure is low. The smallest fetuses and any anomalous fetuses are chosen for reduction. Potassium chloride is then injected under sonographic guidance into the heart or thorax of each selected fetus. Care is used to not enter or traverse the sacs of fetuses selected for retention. In most cases, pregnancies are reduced to twins to increase the chances of delivering at least one viable fetus.

Evans and associates (2005) reported continued improvement in fetal outcomes with this procedure. They analyzed more than 1000 pregnancies managed in 11 centers from 1995 to 1998. The pregnancy loss rate varied from a low of 4.5 percent for triplets who were reduced to twins. The loss rate increased with each addition to the starting number of fetuses and peaked at 15 percent for six or more fetuses (Evans, 2001). Operator skill and experience are believed responsible for the low and declining rates of pregnancy loss.

Selective Termination

With the identification of multiple fetuses discordant for structural or genetic abnormalities, three options are available: abortion of all fetuses, selective termination of the abnormal fetus, or pregnancy continuation. Because anomalies are typically not discovered until the second trimester, selective termination is performed later in gestation than selective reduction and entails greater risk. This procedure is therefore usually not performed unless the anomaly is severe but not lethal. Thus, a triplet pregnancy in which one fetus has Down syndrome might be a candidate for selective termination, whereas a twin pregnancy in which one fetus has trisomy 18 might not. In some cases, termination is considered because the abnormal fetus may jeopardize the normal one. For example, pathological hydramnios in a twin with esophageal atresia could lead to preterm birth of its sibling.

Prerequisites to selective termination include a precise diagnosis for the anomalous fetus and absolute certainty of fetal location. Thus, if genetic amniocentesis is performed on a multifetal gestation, a map of the uterus with locations of all the fetuses clearly labeled should be made at the time of the diagnostic procedure. Unless a special procedure such as umbilical cord interruption is used, selective termination should be performed only in multichorionic multifetal gestations to avoid damaging the surviving fetuses (Lewi, 2006). Roman and coworkers (2010) compared 40 cases of bipolar umbilical cord coagulation with 20 cases of radiofrequency ablation for treatment of complicated monochorionic multifetal gestations at midpregnancy. They found similar survival rates of 87 and 88 percent, and a median gestational age > 36 weeks at delivery in both. Prefumo and colleagues (2013) reported their preliminary experience with microwave ablation of the umbilical cord for selective termination in two monochorionic twin pregnancies. One pregnancy aborted within 7 days, and the other resulted in a term singleton delivered at 39 weeks' gestation.

Evans and coworkers (1999) have provided the most comprehensive results to date on second-trimester selective termination for fetal abnormalities. A total of 402 cases were analyzed from eight centers worldwide. Included were 345 twin, 39 triplet, and 18 quadruplet pregnancies. Selective termination using potassium chloride resulted in delivery of a viable neonate or neonates in more than 90 percent of cases, with a mean age of 35.7 weeks at delivery. The entire pregnancy was lost in 7.1 percent of pregnancies reduced to singletons and in 13 percent of those reduced to twins. The gestational age at the time of the procedure did not appear to affect the pregnancy loss rate. Several losses occurred because the pregnancy was actually monochorionic, and potassium chloride also killed the normal fetus through placental vascular anastomoses.

Ethics

The ethical issues associated with these techniques are almost limitless. There is a beneficence-based justification for offering selective termination in cases in which continuation of the pregnancy poses a threat to the life of coexistent fetuses. The final decision to continue the pregnancy without intervention, to terminate the entire pregnancy, or to elect selective termination is solely the patient's (Chervenak, 2013). The interested reader is referred to the excellent reviews by Evans and coworkers (1996, 2004) and Simpson and Carson (1996).

Informed Consent

Before selective termination or reduction, a discussion should include the morbidity and mortality rates expected if the pregnancy is continued; the morbidity and mortality rates expected with surviving twins or triplets; and the risks of the procedure itself.

With couples seeking infertility treatment, the issue of selective reduction should ideally be discussed *before* conception. Grobman and associates (2001) reported that these couples were generally unaware of the risks associated with multifetal gestation, and they were less desirous of having a multifetal gestation once apprised of the risks.

Specific risks that are common to selective termination or reduction include:

1. Abortion of the remaining fetuses
2. Abortion of the wrong (normal) fetus(es)
3. Retention of genetic or structurally abnormal fetuses after a reduction in number
4. Damage without death to a fetus
5. Preterm labor
6. Discordant or growth-restricted fetuses
7. Maternal infection, hemorrhage, or possible disseminated intravascular coagulopathy because of retained products of conception.

The procedure should be performed by an operator skilled and experienced in sonographically guided procedures.

Psychological Reaction

Women and their spouses who elect to undergo selective termination or reduction find this decision highly stressful. Schreiner-Engel and colleagues (1995) retrospectively studied the emotional reactions of 100 women following selective reduction. Although 70 percent of the women mourned for their dead fetus(es), most grieved only for 1 month. Persistent depressive symptoms were mild, although moderately severe sadness and guilt continued for many of them. Fortunately, most were reconciled to the termination of some fetuses to preserve the lives of a remaining few. Indeed, 93 percent of the women would have made the same decision again.

REFERENCES

Abel EL, Kruger ML: Maternal and paternal age and twinning in the United States, 2004–2008. J Perinat Med 40:237, 2012

Alamia V Jr, Royek AB, Jaekle RK, et al: Preliminary experience with a prospective protocol for planned vaginal delivery of triplet gestations. Am J Obstet Gynecol 179:1133, 1998

Alexander JM, Leveno KJ, Rouse D, et al: Cesarean delivery for the second twin. Obstet Gynecol 112(4):748, 2008

Allen VM, Windrim R, Barrett J, et al: Management of monoamniotic twin pregnancies: a case series and systematic review of the literature. BJOG 108:931, 2001

Alran S, Sibony O, Luton D, et al: Maternal and neonatal outcome of 93 consecutive triplet pregnancies with 71% vaginal delivery. Acta Obstet Gynecol Scand 83:554, 2004

American College of Obstetricians and Gynecologists: Multiple gestation: complicated twin, triplet, and high-order multifetal pregnancy. Practice Bulletin No. 56, October 2004, Reaffirmed 2010

American College of Obstetricians and Gynecologists: Ultrasonography in pregnancy. Practice Bulletin No. 101, February 2009, Reaffirmed 2011

American College of Obstetricians and Gynecologists: Multifetal pregnancy reduction. Committee Opinion No. 553, February 2013a

American College of Obstetricians and Gynecologists: Vaginal birth after previous cesarean delivery. Practice Bulletin No. 115, August 2010, Reaffirmed 2013b

American Society for Reproductive Medicine and Society for Assisted Reproductive Technology: Criteria for number of embryos to transfer: a committee opinion. Fertil Steril 99(1):44, 2013

Ananth CV, Chauhan SP: Epidemiology of twinning in developed countries. Semin Perinatol 36:156, 2012

Andrews WW, Leveno KJ, Sherman ML, et al: Elective hospitalization in the management of twin pregnancies. Obstet Gynecol 77:826, 1991

Antsaklis A, Fotodotis M, Sindos, M, et al: Trends in twin pregnancies and mode of delivery during the last 30 years: inconsistency between guidelines and clinical practice. J Perinat Med 41(4):355, 2013

Arabin B, Halbesma JR, Vork F, et al: Is treatment with vaginal pessaries an option in patients with a sonographically detected short cervix? J Perinat Med 31:122, 2003

Arabin B, van Eyck J: Delayed-interval delivery in twin and triplet pregnancies: 17 years of experience in 1 perinatal center. Am J Obstet Gynecol 200(2):154.e1, 2009

Armson BA, O'Connell C, Persad V, et al: Determinants of perinatal mortality and serious neonatal morbidity in the second twin. Obstet Gynecol 108 (3 Pt 1):556, 2006

Aston K, Peterson C, Carrell D: Monozygotic twinning associated with assisted reproductive technologies: a review. Reproduction 136(4):377, 2008

Bagchi S, Salihu HM: Birth weight discordance in multiple gestations: occurrence and outcomes. J Obstet Gynaecol 26(4):291, 2006

Barrett JFR, Hannah ME, Hutton EK, et al: A randomized trial of planned cesarean or vaginal delivery for twin pregnancy. N Engl J Med 369:1295, 2013

Baschat AA, Barber J, Pedersen N, et al: Outcome after fetoscopic selective laser ablation of placental anastomoses vs equatorial laser dichorionization for the treatment of twin-to-twin transfusion syndrome. Am J Obstet Gynecol 209:1.e1, 2013

Battista L, Winovitch KC, Rumney PJ, et al: A case-control comparison of the effectiveness of betamethasone to prevent neonatal morbidity and mortality in preterm twin and singleton pregnancies. Am J Perinat 25(7):449, 2008

Bdolah Y, Lam C, Rajakumar A, et al: Twin pregnancy and the risk of preeclampsia: bigger placenta or relative ischemia? Am J Obstet Gynecol 198: 438.e1, 2008

Beemsterboer SN, Homburg R, Gorter NA, et al: The paradox of declining fertility but increasing twinning rates with advancing maternal age. Hum Reprod 21:1531, 2006

Bejar R, Vigliocco G, Gramajo H, et al: Antenatal origin of neurological damage in newborn infants. 2. Multiple gestations. Am J Obstet Gynecol 162:1230, 1990

Bekiesinka-Figatowska M, Herman-Sucharska I, Romaniuk-Doroszewska A, et al: Diagnostic problems in case of twin pregnancies: US vs MRI study. J Perinat Med 41(5):535, 2013

Benirschke K, Kim CK: Multiple pregnancy. N Engl J Med 288:1276, 1973

Bennett D, Dunn LC: Genetical and embryological comparisons of semilethal t-alleles from wild mouse populations. Genetics 61:411, 1969

Berghella V, Odibo AO, To MS, et al: Cerclage for short cervix on ultrasonography: meta-analysis of trials using individual patient-level data. Obstet Gynecol 106(1):181, 2005
Blickstein I, Goldman RD, Kupferminc M: Delivery of breech first twins: a multicenter retrospective study. Obstet Gynecol 95:37, 2000
Blickstein I, Perlman S: Single fetal death in twin gestations. J Perinat Med 41:65, 2013
Boyle B, McConkey R, Garne E, et al: Trends in the prevalence, risk and pregnancy outcome of multiple births with congenital anomaly: a registry-based study in 14 European countries 1984–2007. BJOG 120:707, 2013
Brady PC, Correia KF, Missmer SA, et al: Early β-human chorionic gonadotropin trends in vanishing twin pregnancies. Fertil Steril 100(1):116, 2013
Bulmer MG: The effect of parental age, parity, and duration of marriage on the twinning rate. Hum Genet 23:454, 1959
Cahill A, Stamilio DM, Paré E, et al: Vaginal birth after cesarean (VBAC) attempt in twin pregnancies: is it safe? Am J Obstet Gynecol 193:1050, 2005
Campbell DM: Maternal adaptation in twin pregnancy. Semin Perinatol 10: 14, 1986
Caritis SN, Rouse DJ, Peaceman AM, et al: Prevention of preterm birth in triplets using 17alpha-hydroxyprogesterone caproate: a randomized controlled trial. Obstet Gynecol 113(2 Pt 1):285, 2009
Caritis SN, Simhan H, Zhao Y, et al: Relationship between 17-hydroxyprogesterone caproate concentrations and gestational age at delivery in twin gestation. Am J Obstet Gynecol 207:396.e1, 2012
Caukwell S, Murphy DJ: The effect of mode of delivery and gestational age on neonatal outcome of the non-cephalic-presenting second twin. Am J Obstet Gynecol 187:1356, 2002
Cetingoz E, Cam C, Sakalh M, et al: Progesterone effects on preterm birth in high-risk pregnancies: a randomized placebo-controlled trial. Arch Gynecol Obstet 283:423, 2011
Challis D, Gratacos E, Deprest JA: Cord occlusion techniques for selective termination in monochorionic twins. J Perinat Med 27:327, 1999
Chang E, Park M, Kim Y, et al: A case of successful selective abortion using radio-frequency ablation in twin pregnancy suffering from severe twin to twin transfusion syndrome. J Korean Med Sci 24:513, 2009
Chasen ST, Luo G, Perni SC, et al: Are in vitro fertilization pregnancies with early spontaneous reduction high risk? Am J Obstet Gynecol 195:814, 2006
Chauhan SP, Roberts WE, McLaren RA, et al: Delivery of the nonvertex second twin: breech extraction versus external cephalic version. Am J Obstet Gynecol 173:1015, 1995
Chauhan SP, Scardo JA, Hayes E, et al: Twins: prevalence, problems, and preterm births. Am J Obstet Gynecol 203(4):305, 2010
Chervenak FA, McCullough LB: Ethical challenges in the management of multiple pregnancies: the professional responsibility model of perinatal ethics. J Perinat Med 41:61, 2013
Choi Y, Bishai D, Minkovitz CS: Multiple births are a risk factor for postpartum maternal depressive symptoms. Pediatrics 123(4):1147, 2009
Christensen K, Petersen I, Skytthe A, et al: Comparison of academic performance of twins and singletons in adolescence: follow-up study. BMJ 333:1095, 2006
Cohen M, Kohl SG, Rosenthal AH: Fetal interlocking complicating twin gestation. Am J Obstet Gynecol 91:407, 1965
Combs CA, Garite T, Maurel K, et al: 17-Hydroxyprogesterone caproate for twin pregnancy: a double-blind, randomized clinical trial. Am J Obstet Gynecol 204(3):221.e1, 2011
Conde-Agudelo A, Romero R, Hassan SS, et al: Transvaginal sonographic cervical length for the prediction of spontaneous preterm birth in twin pregnancies: a systematic review and metaanalysis. Am J Obstet Gynecol 203:128.e1, 2010
Corsello G, Piro E: The world of twins: an update. J Matern Fetal Neonatal Med 23(S3):59, 2010
Crombleholme TM, Shera D, Lee H, et al: A prospective, randomized, multicenter trial of amnioreduction vs selective fetoscopic laser photocoagulation for the treatment of severe twin-twin transfusion syndrome. Am J Obstet Gynecol 197:396.e1, 2007
Crowther CA, Han S: Hospitalization and bed rest for multiple pregnancy. Cochrane Database Syst Rev 7:CD000110, 2010
D'Alton ME: Delivery of the second twin. Obstet Gynecol 115(2):221, 2010
Davidson L, Easterling TR, Jackson JC, et al: Breech extraction of low-birthweight second twins. Am J Obstet Gynecol 166:497, 1992
De Paepe ME, DeKoninck P, Friedman RM: Vascular distribution patterns in monochorionic twin placentas. Placenta 26(6):471, 2005
Derbent A, Simavli S, Gumus I, et al: Nifedipine for the treatment of preterm labor in twin and singleton pregnancies. Arch Gynecol Obstet 284:821, 2011
DeVoe LD: Antenatal fetal assessment: multifetal gestation—an overview. Semin Perinatol 32:281, 2008
Diamond MP, Mitwally M, Casper R, et al: Estimating rates of multiple gestation pregnancies: sample size calculation from the assessment of multiple intrauterine gestations from ovarian stimulation (AMIGOS) trial. Contemp Clin Trials 32:902, 2011
Dickey RP, Taylor SN, Lu PY, et al: Spontaneous reduction of multiple pregnancy: incidence and effect on outcome. Am J Obstet Gynecol 186:77, 2002
Dodd J, Crowther C: Multifetal pregnancy reduction of triplet and higher-order multiple pregnancies to twins. Fertil Steril 81(5):1420, 2004
Dodd JM, Crowther CA: Reduction of the number of fetuses for women with a multiple pregnancy. Cochran Database Syst Rev 10:CD003932, 2012
Dolapcioglu K, Gungoren A, Hakverdi S, et al: Twin pregnancy with a complete hydatidiform mole and co-existent live fetus: two case reports and review of the literature. Arch Gynecol Obstet 279:431, 2009
Donner C, Shahabi S, Thomas D, et al: Selective feticide by embolization in twin-twin transfusion syndrome. A report of two cases. J Reprod Med 42: 747, 1997
Dor J, Shalev J, Mashiach S, et al: Elective cervical suture of twin pregnancies diagnosed ultrasonically in the first trimester following induced ovulation. Gynecol Obstet Invest 13:55, 1982
Durnwald CP, Momirova V, Rouse DJ, et al: Second trimester cervical length and risk of preterm birth in women with twin gestations treated with 17-α hydroxyprogesterone caproate. J Matern Fetal Neonatal Med 23(12):1360, 2010
Eddib A, Rodgers B, Lawler J, et al: Monochorionic pseudomonoamniotic twin pregnancy with fetal demise of one twin and development of maternal consumptive coagulopathy. Ultrasound Obstet Gynecol 28:735, 2006
Edris F, Oppenheimer L, Yang Q, et al: Relationship between intertwin delivery interval and metabolic acidosis in the second twin. Am J Perinatol 23(8):481, 2006
Ehsanipoor R, Arora N, Lagrew DC, et al: Twin versus singleton pregnancies complicated by preterm premature rupture of membranes. J Matern Fetal Neonatal Med 25(6):658, 2012
Ekelund CK, Skibsted L, Sogaard K, et al: Dizygotic monochorionic twin pregnancy conceived following intracytoplasmic sperm injection treatment and complicated by twin-twin transfusion syndrome and blood chimerism. Ultrasound Obstet Gynecol 32:282, 2008
Elimian A, Figueroa R, Nigam S, et al: Perinatal outcome of triplet gestation: does prophylactic cerclage make a difference? J Matern Fetal Neonatal Med 8:119, 1999
Elliott JP: Preterm labor in twins and high-order multiples. Clin Perinatol 34:599, 2007
Elliott JP, Finberg HJ: Biophysical profile testing as an indicator of fetal well-being in high-order multiple gestations. Am J Obstet Gynecol 172:508, 1995
Ericson A, Källén B, Aberg A: Use of multivitamins and folic acid in early pregnancy and multiple births in Sweden. Twin Res 4(2):63, 2001
Evans MI, Berkowitz RL, Wapner RJ, et al: Improvement in outcomes of multifetal pregnancy reduction with increased experience. Am J Obstet Gynecol 184:97, 2001
Evans MI, Ciorica D, Britt DW, et al: Update on selective reduction. Prenat Diagn 25:807, 2005
Evans MI, Goldberg JD, Horenstein J, et al: Elective termination for structural, chromosomal, and mendelian anomalies: international experience. Am J Obstet Gynecol 181:893, 1999
Evans MI, Johnson MP, Quintero RA, et al: Ethical issues surrounding multifetal pregnancy reduction and selective termination. Clin Perinatol 23:437, 1996
Evans MI, Kaufman MI, Urban AJ, et al: Fetal reduction from twins to a singleton: a reasonable consideration? Obstet Gynecol 104:1423, 2004
Faye-Petersen OM, Heller DS, Joshi VV: Handbook of Placental Pathology, 2nd ed, London, Taylor & Francis, 2006
Fellman J, Eriksson AW: Secondary sex ratio in multiple births. Twin Res Hum Genet 13(1):101, 2010
Ford AA, Bateman BT, Simpson LL: Vaginal birth after cesarean delivery in twin gestations: a large, nationwide sample of deliveries. Am J Obstet Gynecol 195:1138, 2006
Fox H, Sebire NJ: Pathology of the Placenta, 3rd ed. Philadelphia, Saunders, 2007
Fox NS, Roman AS, Saltzman DH, et al: Risk factors for preeclampsia in twin pregnancies. Am J Perinatol 31(2):163, 2014
Fox NS, Silverstein M, Bender S, et al: Active second-stage management in twin pregnancies undergoing planned vaginal delivery in a U.S. population. Obstet Gynecol 115:229, 2010
Francois K, Ortiz J, Harris C, et al: Is peripartum hysterectomy more common in multiple gestations? Obstet Gynecol 105:1369, 2005
Fusi L, Gordon H: Twin pregnancy complicated by single intrauterine death. Problems and outcome with conservative management. BJOG 97:511, 1990
Fusi L, McParland P, Fisk N, et al: Acute twin-twin transfusion: a possible mechanism for brain-damaged survivors after intrauterine death of a monochorionic twin. Obstet Gynecol 78:517, 1991

Gabriel R, Harika G, Saniez D, et al: Prolonged intravenous ritodrine therapy: a comparison between multiple and singleton pregnancies. Eur J Obstet Gynecol Reprod Biol 57:65, 1994
Gardner MO, Goldenberg RL, Cliver SP, et al: The origin and outcome of preterm twin pregnancies. Obstet Gynecol 85:553, 1995
Ghi T, Nanni M, Pierantoni L, et al: Neonatal respiratory morbidity in twins versus singletons after elective prelabor caesarean section. Eur J Obstet Gynecol Reprod Biol 166:156, 2013
Giles W, Bisits A, O'Callaghan S, et al: The Doppler assessment in multiple pregnancy randomized controlled trial of ultrasound biometry versus umbilical artery Doppler ultrasound and biometry in twin pregnancy. BJOG 110:593, 2003
Giles WB, Trudinger BJ, Cook CM, et al: Doppler umbilical artery studies in the twin-twin transfusion syndrome. Obstet Gynecol 76(6):1097, 1990
Giuffre M, Piro E, Corsello G: Prematurity and twinning. J Matern Fetal Neonatal Med 25(53):6, 2012
Gjerris AC, Loft A, Pinborg A, et al: The effect of a "vanishing twin" on biochemical and ultrasound first trimester screening markers for Down's syndrome in pregnancies conceived by assisted reproductive technology. Hum Reprod 24(1):55, 2009
Glinianaia SV, Rankin J, Wright C: Congenital anomalies in twins: a register-based study. Hum Reprod 23:1306, 2008
Goldenberg RL, Iams JD, Miodovnik M, et al: The preterm prediction study: risk factors in twin gestations. Am J Obstet Gynecol 175:1047, 1996
Gonzalez NL, Goya M, Bellart J, et al: Obstetric and perinatal outcome in women with twin pregnancy and gestational diabetes. J Matern Fetal Neonatal Med 25(7):1084, 2012
Goodnight W, Newman R: Optimal nutrition for improved twin pregnancy outcome. Obstet Gynecol 114:1121, 2009
Gourheux N, Deruelle P, Houfflin-Debarge V, et al: Twin-to-twin delivery interval: is a time limit justified? Gynecol Obstet Fertil 35(10):982, 2007
Greene MF: Comment on: A randomized trial of planned cesarean or vaginal delivery for twin pregnancy. N Engl J Med 369(14):1365, 2013
Grobman WA, Milad MP, Stout J, et al: Patient perceptions of multiple gestations: an assessment of knowledge and risk aversion. Am J Obstet Gynecol 185:920, 2001
Grobman WA, Peaceman AM, Haney EI, et al: Neonatal outcomes in triplet gestations after a trial of labor. Am J Obstet Gynecol 179:942, 1998
Gyamfi C, Mele L, Wapner R, et al: The effect of plurality and obesity on betamethasone concentrations in women at risk for preterm delivery. Am J Obstet Gynecol 203:219.e1, 2010
Gyetvai K, Hannah ME, Hodnett ED, et al: Tocolytics for preterm labor: a systematic review. Obstet Gynecol 94:869, 1999
Hack KE, Derks JB, Elias SG, et al: Increased perinatal mortality and morbidity in monochorionic versus dichorionic twin pregnancies: clinical implications of a large Dutch cohort study. BJOG 115:58, 2008
Hack KE, Derks JB, Schaap AH: Placental characteristics of monoamniotic twin pregnancies in relation to perinatal outcome. Obstet Gynecol 113(2 Pt 1):353, 2009
Haggarty P, McCallum H, McBain H, et al: Effect of B vitamins and genetics on success of in-vitro fertilization: prospective cohort study. Lancet 367(9521):1513, 2006
Hall JG: Twinning. Lancet 362:735, 2003
Harris DW: Superfecundation: letter. J Reprod Med 27:39, 1982
Hasbargen U, Lohse P, Thaler CJ: The number of dichorionic twin pregnancies is reduced by the common MTHFR 677C—>T mutation. Hum Reprod 15(12):2659, 2000
Hernandez JS, Twickler DM, McIntire DD, et al: Hydramnios in twin gestations. Obstet Gynecol 120(4):759, 2012
Heyborne KD, Porreco RP, Garite TJ, et al: Improved perinatal survival of monoamniotic twins with intensive inpatient monitoring. Am J Obstet Gynecol 192(1):96, 2005
Hibbeln JF, Shors SM, Byrd Se: MRI: is there a role in obstetrics? Clin Obstet Gynecol 55(1):352, 2012
Hill LM, Krohn M, Lazebnik N, et al: The amniotic fluid index in normal twin pregnancies. Am J Obstet Gynecol 182(4):950, 2000
Hillman SC, Morris RK, Kilby MD: Co-twin prognosis after single fetal death. A systematic review and meta-analysis. Obstet Gynecol 118(4):928, 2011
Hoekstra C, Zhao ZZ, Lambalk CB, et al: Dizygotic twinning. Hum Reprod Update 14:37, 2008
Hoffmann E, Oldenburg A, Rode L, et al: Twin births: cesarean section or vaginal delivery? Acta Obstet Gynecol Scand 91(4):463, 2012
Hogle KL, Hutton EK, McBrien KA, et al: Cesarean delivery for twins: a systematic review and meta-analysis. Am J Obstet Gynecol 188:220, 2003
Hollier LM, McIntire DD, Leveno KJ: Outcome of twin pregnancies according to intrapair birth weight differences. Obstet Gynecol 94:1006, 1999
Hu LS, Caire J, Twickler DM: MR findings of complicated multifetal gestations. Pediatr Radiol 36:76, 2006
Huber A, Diehl W, Zikulnig L, et al: Perinatal outcome in monochorionic twin pregnancies complicated by amniotic fluid discordance without severe twin-twin transfusion syndrome. Ultrasound Obstet Gynecol 27:45, 2006
Joo JG, Csaba A, Szigeti Z, et al: Spontaneous abortion in multiple pregnancy: focus on fetal pathology. Pathol Res Pract 208:458, 2012
Joseph KS, Allen AC, Dodds L, et al: Causes and consequences of recent increases in preterm birth among twins. Obstet Gynecol 98:57, 2001
Kahn B, Lumey LH, Zybert PA, et al: Prospective risk of fetal death in singleton, twin, and triplet gestations: implications for practice. Obstet Gynecol 102:685, 2003
Kametas NA, McAuliffe F, Krampl E, et al: Maternal cardiac function in twin pregnancy. Obstet Gynecol 102:806, 2003
Kaufman D, Du L, Velcek F, et al: Fetus-in-fetu. J Am Coll Surg 205(2):378, 2007
Kawaguchi H, Ishii K, Yamamoto R, et al: Perinatal death of triplet pregnancies by chorionicity. Am J Obstet Gynecol 209(1):36.e1, 2013
Kent EM, Breathnach FM, Gillan JE, et al: Placental pathology, birthweight discordance, and growth restriction in twin pregnancy: results of the ESPRIT Study. Am J Obstet 207(3):220.e1, 2012
Kilpatrick SJ, Jackson R, Croughan-Minihane MS: Perinatal mortality in twins and singletons matched for gestational age at delivery at > or = 30 weeks. Am J Obstet Gynecol 174:66, 1996
Kim JH, Park SW, Lee JJ: Birth weight reference for triples in Korea. J Korean Med Sci 25:900, 2010
Klein K, Mailath-Pokorny M, Elhenicky M, et al: Mean, lowest, and highest pulsatility index of the uterine artery and adverse pregnancy outcome in twin pregnancies. Am J Obstet Gynecol 205:549 e1, 2011
Knox G, Morley D: Twinning in Yoruba women. J Obstet Gynaecol Br Emp 67:981, 1960
Kogan MD, Alexander GR, Kotelchuck M: Trends in twin birth outcomes and prenatal care utilization in the United States, 1981–1997. JAMA 283:335, 2000
Kuleva M, Youssef A, Maroni E, et al: Maternal cardiac function in normal twin pregnancy: a longitudinal study. Ultrasound Obstet Gynecol 38:575, 2011
Kulkarni AD, Jamieson DJ, Jones HW Jr, et al: Fertility treatments and multiple births in the United States. N Engl J Med 369(23):2218, 2013
Langer B, Boudier E, Gasser B, et al: Antenatal diagnosis of brain damage in the survivor after the second trimester death of a monochorionic monoamniotic co-twin: case report and literature review. Fetal Diagn Ther 12:286, 1997
Lanna MM, Rustico MA, Dell'Avanzo M, et al: Bipolar cord coagulation for selective deicide in complicated monochorionic twin pregnancies: 118 consecutive cases at a single center. Ultrasound Obstet Gynecol 39:407, 2012
Lantieri T, Revelli A, Gaglioti P, et al: Superfetation after ovulation induction and intrauterine insemination performed during an unknown ectopic pregnancy. Reprod Biomed Online 20(5):664, 2010
Lee H, Wagner AJ, Sy E, et al: Efficacy of radiofrequency ablation for twin-reversed arterial perfusion sequence. Am J Obstet Gynecol 196:459.e1, 2007
Lee HC, Gould JB, Boscardin WJ, et al: Trends in cesarean delivery for twin births in the United State 1995–2008. Obstet Gynecol 118(5):1095, 2011
Lee YM, Wylie BJ, Simpson LL, et al: Twin chorionicity and the risk of stillbirth. Obstet Gynecol 111:301, 2008
Leftwich HK, Zaki MN, Wilkins I, et al: Labor patterns in twin gestations. Am J Obstet Gynecol 209(3):254.e1, 2013
Legro RS, Kunselman AR, Brzyski RG, et al: The pregnancy in polycystic ovary syndrome II (PPCOS II) trial: rationale and design of a double-blind randomized trial of clomiphene citrate and letrozole for the treatment of infertility in women with polycystic ovary syndrome. Contemp Clin Trials 33:470, 2012
Leung TY, Tam WH, Leung TN, et al: Effect of twin-to-twin delivery interval on umbilical cord blood gas in the second twins. BJOG 109(1):63, 2002
Leveno KJ, Quirk JG, Whalley PJ, et al: Fetal lung maturation in twin gestation. Am J Obstet Gynecol 148:405, 1984
Lewi L, Deprest J, Hecher K: The vascular anastomoses in monochorionic twin pregnancies and their clinical consequences. Am J Obstet Gynecol 208(1):19, 2013
Lewi L, Gratacos E, Ortibus E, et al: Pregnancy and infant outcome of 80 consecutive cord coagulations in complicated monochorionic multiple pregnancies. Am J Obstet Gynecol 194(3):782, 2006
Lewi L, Valencia C, Gonzalez E, et al: The outcome of twin reversed arterial perfusion sequence diagnosed in the first trimester. Am J Obstet Gynecol 293(3):213.e1, 2010
Liem S, Schuit E, Hegerman M, et al: Cervical pessaries for prevention of preterm birth in women with a multiple pregnancy (ProTWIN): a multicenter, open-label randomised controlled trial. Lancet 382(9901):1341, 2013
Livingston JC, Lim FY, Polzin W, et al: Intrafetal radiofrequency ablation for twin reversed arterial perfusion (TRAP): a single-center experience. Am J Obstet Gynecol 197:399.e1, 2007

Livingston JC, Livingston LW, Ramsey R, et al: Second-trimester asynchronous multifetal delivery results in poor perinatal outcome. Obstet Gynecol 103:77, 2004

Lopriore E, Oepkes D: Neonatal morbidity in twin-twin transfusion syndrome. Early Hum Dev 87:595, 2011

Lorenz JM: Neurodevelopmental outcomes of twins. Semin Perinatol 36(3): 201, 2012

Luke B: The changing pattern of multiple births in the United States: maternal and infant characteristics, 1973 and 1990. Obstet Gynecol 84:101, 1994

Luke B, Brown MB: Maternal morbidity and infant death in twin vs triplet and quadruplet pregnancies. Am J Obstet Gynecol 198:401.e1, 2008

MacDonald-Wallis C, Lawlor DA, Fraser A, et al: Blood pressure change in normotensive, gestational hypertensive, preeclamptic, and essential hypertensive pregnancies. Hypertension 59:1241, 2012

MacGillivray I: Epidemiology of twin pregnancy. Semin Perinatol 10:4, 1986

Magann EF, Chauhan SP, Whitworth NS, et al: Determination of amniotic fluid volume in twin pregnancies: ultrasonographic evaluation versus operator estimation. Am J Obstet Gynecol 182:1606, 2000

Mahone PR, Sherer DM, Abramowicz JS, et al: Twin-twin transfusion syndrome: rapid development of severe hydrops of the donor following selective feticide of the hydropic recipient. Am J Obstet Gynecol 169:166, 1993

Mahony BS, Mulcahy C, McCauliffe F, et al: Fetal death in twins. Acta Obstet Gynecol Scand 90(11):1274, 2011

Manning FA (ed): Fetal biophysical profile scoring. In Fetal Medicine: Principles and Practices. Norwalk, Appleton & Lange, 1995, p 288

Martin JA, Hamilton BE, Ventura SJ, et al: Births: final data for 2010. Natl Vital Stat Rep 61(1):1, 2012

Mathews TH, MacDorman MF: Infant mortality statistics from the 2009 period linked birth/infant death data set. Natl Vital Stat Rep 61(8):1, 2013

Maynard SE, Moore Simas TA, Solitro MJ, et al: Circulating angiogenic factors in singleton vs multiple gestation pregnancies. Am J Obstet 198:200.e1, 2008

McClamrock HD, Jones HW, Adashi EY: Ovarian stimulation and intrauterine insemination at the quarter centennial: implications for the multiple births epidemic. Fertil Steril 97(4):802, 2012

McElrath TF, Norwitz ER, Robinson JN, et al: Differences in TDx fetal lung maturity assay values between twin and singleton pregnancies. Am J Obstet Gynecol 182:1110, 2000

McHugh K, Kiely EM, Spitz L: Imaging of conjoined twins. Pediatr Radiol 36:899, 2006

McMahon KS, Neerhof MG, Haney EI, et al: Prematurity in multiple gestations: identification of patients who are at low risk. Am J Obstet Gynecol 186:1137, 2002

McPherson JA, Odibo o, Shanks AL, et al: Impact of chorionicity on risk and timing of intrauterine fetal demise in twin pregnancies. Am J Obstet Gynecol 207:190.e1, 2012

Mhyre JM: Maternal mortality. Curr Opin Anesthesiol 25:277, 2012

Michelfelder E, Gottliebson W, Border W, et al: Early manifestations and spectrum of recipient twin cardiomyopathy in twin-twin transfusion syndrome: relation to Quintero stage. Ultrasound Obstet Gynecol 30:965, 2007

Miller J, Chauhan SP, Abuhamad AZ: Discordant twins: diagnosis, evaluation and management. Am J Obstet Gynecol 206(1):10, 2012

Moise KJ, Dorman K, Lamvu G, et al: A randomized trial of amnioreduction versus septostomy in the treatment of twin-twin transfusion syndrome. Am J Obstet Gynecol 193:701, 2005

Morikawa M, Yamada T, Yamada T, et al: Prospective risk of stillbirth: monochorionic diamniotic twins vs dichorionic twins. J Perinat Med 40:245, 2012

Muggli EE, Halliday JL: Folic acid and risk of twinning: a systematic review of the recent literature, July 1994 to July 2006. MJA 186(5):243, 2007

Muleba N, Dashe N, Yost D, et al: Respiratory morbidity among second-born twins. Presented at the 25th Annual Meeting of the Society for Maternal Fetal Medicine, Reno, Nevada, February 7–12, 2005

Mutchinick OM, Luna-Munoz L, Amar E, et al: Conjoined twins: a worldwide collaborative epidemiological study of the international clearinghouse for birth defects surveillance and research. Am J Med Genet C Semin Med Genet 15;157C(4):274, 2011

Newman RB, Krombach S, Myers MC, et al: Effect of cerclage on obstetrical outcome in twin gestations with a shortened cervical length. Am J Obstet Gynecol 186:634, 2002

Niemann I, Sunde L, Petersen LK: Evaluation of the risk of persistent trophoblastic disease after twin pregnancy with diploid hydatidiform mole and coexisting normal fetus. Am J Obstet Gynecol 197:45.e1, 2007

Norman JE, Mackenzie F, Owen P, et al: Progesterone for the prevention of preterm birth in twin pregnancy (STOPPIT): a randomised, double-blind, placebo-controlled study and meta-analysis. Lancet 373:2034, 2009

Nylander PP: Biosocial aspects of multiple births. J Biosoc Sci 3:29, 1971

Nylander PP: Serum levels of gonadotropins in relation to multiple pregnancy in Nigeria. BJOG 80:651, 1973

Odibo AO, Cahill AG, Goetzinger KR, et al: Customized growth charts for twin gestations to optimize identification of small-for-gestational age fetuses at risk of intrauterine fetal death. Ultrasound Obstet Gynecol 41:637, 2013

O'Donoghue KO, Barlgye O, Pasquini L: Interstitial laser therapy for fetal reduction in monochorionic multiple pregnancy: loss rate and association with aplasia cutis congenita. Prenat Diagn 28:535, 2008

Olusanya BO, Solanke OA: Perinatal correlates of delayed childbearing in a developing country. Arch Gynecol Obstet 285(4):951, 2012

Ong SS, Zamora J, Khan KS, et al: Prognosis for the co-twin following single-twin death: a systematic review. BJOG 113:992, 2006

Painter JN, Willemsen G, Nyholt D, et al: A genome wide linkage scan for dizygotic twinning in 525 families of mothers of dizygotic twins. Human Reprod 25(6):1569, 2010

Pakrashi T, Defranco EA: The relative proportion of preterm births complicated by premature rupture of membranes in multifetal gestations: a population-based study. Am J Perinatol 30:69, 2013

Peaceman AM, Kuo L, Feinglass J: Infant morbidity and mortality associated with vaginal delivery in twin gestations. Am J Obstet Gynecol 200(4):462.e1, 2009

Pettit KE, Merchant M, Machin GA, et al: Congenital heart defects in a large, unselected cohort of monochorionic twins. J Perinatol 33:467, 2013

Prefumo F, Cabassa P, Fichera A, et al: Preliminary experience with microwave ablation for selective feticide in monochorionic twin pregnancies. Ultrasound Obstet Gynecol 41:469, 2013

Pritchard JA: Changes in blood volume during pregnancy. Anesthesiology 26: 393, 1965

Quarello E, Molho M, Ville Y: Incidence, mechanisms, and patterns of fetal cerebral lesions in twin-to-twin transfusion syndrome. J Matern Fetal Neonatal Med 20:589, 2007

Quigley MM, Cruikshank DP: Polyhydramnios and acute renal failure. J Reprod Med 19:92, 1977

Quinn KH, Cao CT, Lacoursiere Y, et al: Monoamniotic twin pregnancy: continuous inpatient electronic fetal monitoring—an impossible goal? Am J Obstet Gynecol 204:161, 2011

Quintero RA, Chmait RH, Murakoshi T, et al: Surgical management of twin reversed arterial perfusion sequence. Am J Obstet Gynecol 194:982, 2006

Quintero RA, Morales WJ, Allen MH, et al: Staging of twin-twin transfusion syndrome. J Perinatol 19:550, 1999

Quintero RA, Reich H, Puder KS, et al: Brief report: umbilical-cord ligation in an acardiac twin by fetoscopy at 19 weeks gestation. N Engl J Med 330:469, 1994

Rana S, Hacker MR, Modest AM, et al: Circulating angiogenic factors and risk of adverse maternal and perinatal outcomes in twin pregnancies with suspected preeclampsia novelty and significance. Hypertension 60:451, 2012

Ray B, Platt MP: Mortality of twin and singleton livebirths under 30 weeks' gestation: a population-based study. Arch Dis Child Fetal Neonatal Ed 94(2):F140, 2009

Rayburn WF, Lavin JP Jr, Miodovnik M, et al: Multiple gestation: time interval between delivery of the first and second twins. Obstet Gynecol 63:502, 1984

Rebarber A, Roman AS, Istwan N, et al: Prophylactic cerclage in the management of triplet pregnancies. Am J Obstet Gynecol 193:1193, 2005

Record RG, McKeown T, Edwards JH: An investigation of the difference in measured intelligence between twins and single births. Ann Hum Genet 34(1):11, 1970

Roberts D, Dalziel S: Antenatal corticosteroids for accelerating fetal lung maturation for women at risk of preterm birth. Cochrane Database Syst Rev 3:CD004454, 2006

Roberts D, Gates S, Kilby M, et al: Interventions for twin-twin transfusion syndrome: a Cochrane review. Ultrasound Obstet Gynecol 31:701, 2008

Robinson BK, Miller RS, D'Alton ME, et al: Effectiveness of timing strategies for delivery of monochorionic diamniotic twins. Am J Obstet Gynecol 207:53, 2012

Robyr R, Lewi L, Salomon LJ, et al: Prevalence and management of late fetal complications following successful selective laser coagulation of chorionic plate anastomoses in twin-to-twin transfusion syndrome. Am J Obstet Gynecol 194:796, 2006

Rode L, Klein K, Nicolaides KH, et al: Prevention of preterm delivery in twin gestations (PREDICT): a multicenter, randomized, placebo-controlled trial on the effect of vaginal micronized progesterone. Ultrasound Obstet Gynecol 38:272, 2011

Roman A, Papanna R, Johnson A, et al: Selective reduction in complicated monochorionic pregnancies: radiofrequency ablation vs bipolar cord coagulation. Ultrasound Obstet Gynecol 36:37, 2010

Ronalds, GA, De Stavola BL, Leon DA: The cognitive cost of being a twin: evidence from comparisons within families in the Aberdeen children of the 1950s cohort study. BMJ 331(7528):1306, 2005

Rossi AC, D'Addario V: Laser therapy and serial amnioreduction as treatment for twin-twin transfusion syndrome: a metaanalysis and review of literature. Am J Obstet Gynecol 198:147, 2008

Rossi AC, D'Addario V: Umbilical cord occlusion for selective feticide in complicated monochorionic twins: a systematic review of literature. Am J Obstet Gynecol 200(2):123, 2009

Rossi AC, Mullin PM, Chmait RH: Neonatal outcomes of twins according to birth order, presentation and mode of delivery: a systematic review and meta-analysis. BJOG 118(5):523, 2011

Rothman KJ: Fetal loss, twinning and birthweight after oral contraceptive use. N Engl J Med 297:468, 1977

Rouse DJ, Caritis SN, Peaceman AM, et al: A trial of 17alpha-hydroxyprogesterone caproate to prevent prematurity in twins. N Engl J Med 357:454, 2007

Rouse DJ, Skopec GS, Zlatnik FJ: Fundal height as a predictor of preterm twin delivery. Obstet Gynecol 81:211, 1993

Royal College of Obstetricians and Gynaecologists: Management of monochorionic twin pregnancy. Green-Top Guideline No. 51, December 2008

Rydhström H: Prognosis for twins with birthweight < 1,500 g: the impact of cesarean section in relation to fetal presentation. Am J Obstet Gynecol 163:528, 1990

Salomon LJ, Örtqviast L, Aegerter P, et al: Long-term developmental follow-up of infants who participated in a randomized clinical trial of amniocentesis vs laser photocoagulation for the treatment of twin-to-twin transfusion syndrome. Am J Obstet Gynecol 203(5):444.e1, 2010

Scheier M, Molina F: Outcome of twin reversed arterial perfusion sequence following treatment with interstitial laser: a retrospective study. Fetal Diagn Ther 31:35, 2012

Schreiner-Engel P, Walther VN, Mindes J, et al: First-trimester multifetal pregnancy reduction: acute and persistent psychologic reactions. Am J Obstet Gynecol 172:544, 1995

Sebire NJ, Foskett M, Paradinas FJ, et al: Outcome of twin pregnancies with complete hydatidiform mole and healthy co-twin. Lancet 359:2165, 2002

Senat MV, Deprest J, Boulvain M, et al: Endoscopic laser surgery versus serial amnioreduction for severe twin-to-twin transfusion syndrome. N Engl J Med 351:136, 2004

Senat MV, Porcher R, Winer N, et al: Prevention of preterm delivery by 17alpha-hydroxyprogesterone caproate in asymptomatic twin pregnancies with a short cervix: a randomized controlled trial. Am J Obstet Gynecol 208(3):194.e1, 2013

Simpson JL, Carson SA: Multifetal reduction in high-order gestations: a nonelective procedure? J Soc Gynecol Invest 3:1, 1996

Simpson LL: Ultrasound in twins: dichorionic and monochorionic. Semin Perinatol 37(5):348, 2013

Slaghekke F, Kist WJ, Oepkes D, et al: Twin anemia-polycythemia sequence: diagnostic criteria, classification, perinatal management and outcome. Fetal Diagn Ther 27(4):181, 2010

Smith GC, Fleming KM, White IR: Birth order of twins and risk of perinatal death related to delivery in England, Northern Ireland, and Wales, 1994–2003: retrospective cohort study. BMJ 334(7593):576, 2007

Society for Maternal-Fetal Medicine, Simpson LL: Twin-twin transfusion syndrome. Am J Obstet Gynecol 208(1):3, 2013

Spencer R: Theoretical and analytical embryology of conjoined twins: part I: embryogenesis. Clin Anat 13:36, 2000

Spencer R: Parasitic conjoined twins: external, internal (fetuses in fetu and teratomas), and detached (acardiacs). Clin Anat 14:428, 2001

Sperling L, Kiil C, Larsen LU, et al: Naturally conceived twins with monochorionic placentation have the highest risk of fetal loss. Ultrasound Obstet Gynecol 28:644, 2006

Spitz L, Kiely EM: Conjoined twins. JAMA 289:1307, 2003

Stein W, Misselwitz B, Schmidt S: Twin-to-twin delivery time interval: influencing factors and effect on short term outcome of the second twin. Acta Obstet Gynecol Scand 87(3):346, 2008

Strandskov HH, Edelen EW, Siemens GJ: Analysis of the sex ratios among single and plural births in the total white and colored U.S. populations. Am J Phys Anthropol 4:491, 1946

Szymusik I, Kosinska-Kaczynska K, Bomba-Opon D, et al: IVG versus spontaneous twin pregnancies—which are at higher risk of complications? J Matern Fetal Neonatal Med 25(12):2725, 2012

Talauliker VS, Arulkumaran S: Reproductive outcomes after assisted conception. Obstet Gynecol Surv 67(9):566, 2012

Tan KL, Goon SM, Salmon Y, et al: Conjoined twins. Acta Obstet Gynecol Scand 50:373, 1971

Tannuri A, Batatinha J, Velhote M, et al: Conjoined twins—twenty years' experience at a reference center in Brazil. Clinics 68(3):371, 2013

Taylor M, Rebarber A, Saltzman DH, et al: Induction of labor in twin compared with singleton pregnancies. Obstet Gynecol 120(2):297, 2012

Thorngren-Jerneck K, Herbst A: Low 5-minute Apgar score: a population-based register study of 1 million term births. Obstet Gynecol 98(1):65, 2001

Thorson HL, Ramaeker DM, Emery ST: Optimal interval for ultrasound surveillance in monochorionic twin gestations. Obstet Gynecol 117(1):131, 2011

To MS, Fonseca EB, Molina FS, et al: Maternal characteristics and cervical length in the prediction of spontaneous early preterm delivery in twins. Am J Obstet Gynecol 194(5):1360, 2006

Trivedi AN, Gillett WR: The retained twin/triplet following a preterm delivery–an analysis of the literature. Aust N Z J Obstet Gynaecol 38:461, 1998

Varner MW, Leindecker S, Spong CY, et al: The Maternal-Fetal Medicine Unit Cesarean Registry: trial of labor with a twin gestation. Am J Obstet Gynecol 193:135, 2005

Vintzileos AM, Ananth CV, Kontopoulos E, et al: Mode of delivery and risk of stillbirth and infant mortality in triplet gestations: United States, 1995 through 1998. Am J Obstet Gynecol 192:464, 2005

Vora NL, Ruthazer R, House M, et al: Triplet ultrasound growth parameters. Obstet Gynecol 107:694, 2006

Wada H, Nunogami K, Wada T, et al: Diffuse brain damage caused by acute twin-twin transfusion during late pregnancy. Acta Paediatr Jpn 40:370, 1998

Walker MC, Murphy KE, Pan S, et al: Adverse maternal outcomes in multifetal pregnancies. BJOG 111:1294, 2004

Waller DK, Tita TN, Annegers JF: Rates of twinning before and after fortification of foods in the U.S. with folic acid, Texas, 1996 to 1998. Paediatr Perinat Epidemiol 17(4):378, 2003

Wen SW, Demissie K, Yang Q, et al: Maternal morbidity and obstetric complications in triplet pregnancies and quadruplet and higher-order multiple pregnancies. Am J Obstet Gynecol 191:254, 2004

Wenstrom KD, Syrop CH, Hammitt DG, et al: Increased risk of monochorionic twinning associated with assisted reproduction. Fertil Steril 60:510, 1993

White C, Wyshak G: Inheritance in human dizygotic twinning. N Engl J Med 271:1003, 1964

Wright VC, Chang J, Jeng G, et al: Assisted reproductive technology surveillance–United States, 2005. MMWR 57(5):1, 2008

Wolfe MD, de la Torre L, Moore LE, et al: Is the protocol for induction of labor in singletons applicable to twin gestations? J Reprod Med 58(304):137, 2013

Yamasmit W, Chaithongwongwatthana S, Tolosa JE, et al: Prophylactic oral betamimetics for reducing preterm birth in women with a twin pregnancy. Cochrane Database Syst Rev 3:CD004733, 2005

Yang Q, Wen SW, Chen Y, et al: Occurrence and clinical predictors of operative delivery for the vertex second twin after normal vaginal delivery of the first twin. Am J Obstet Gynecol 192(1):178, 2005a

Yang Q, Wen SW, Chen Y, et al: Neonatal death and morbidity in vertex-nonvertex second twins according to mode of delivery and birth weight. Am J Obstet Gynecol 192(3):840, 2005b

Zech NH, Wisser J, Natalucci G, et al: Monochorionic-diamniotic twins discordant in gender form a naturally conceived pregnancy through postzygotic sex chromosome loss in a 47,XXY zygote. Prenat Diagn 28:759, 2008

Zhao DP, de Villiers SF, Slaghekke F, et al: Prevalence, size, number and localization of vascular anastomoses in monochorionic placentas. Placenta 34:589, 2013

SECTION 12
MEDICAL AND SURGICAL COMPLICATIONS

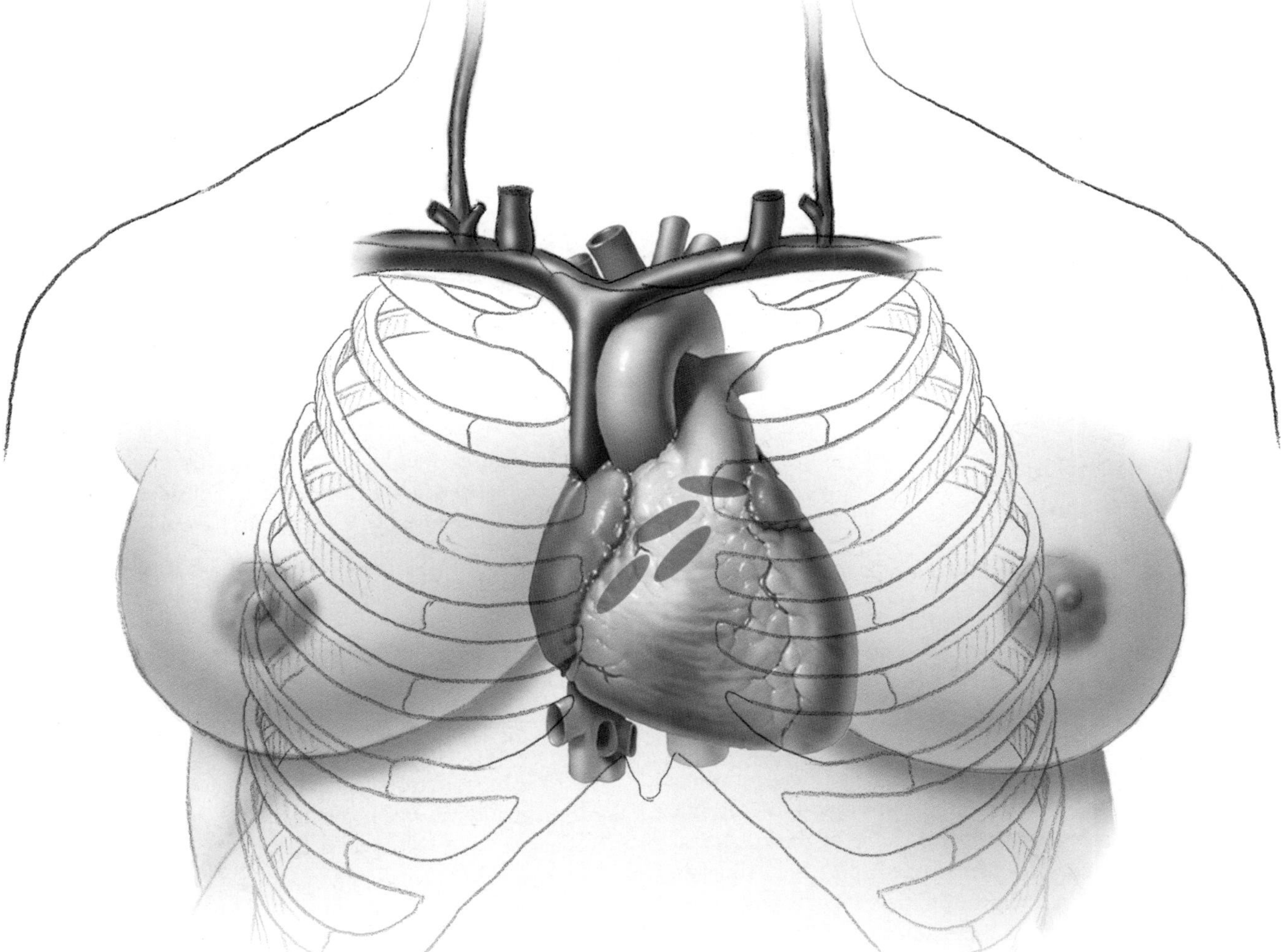

CHAPTER 46

General Considerations and Maternal Evaluation

Never penalize a woman because she is pregnant. Pregnant women are susceptible to any of the medical and surgical disorders that can affect childbearing-aged women. Some of these, especially those that are chronic, more often precede pregnancy. But, they as well as others can acutely complicate an otherwise normal pregnancy. It is difficult to accurately quantify nonobstetrical disorders that complicate pregnancy, however, some estimates can be made. For example, one managed-care population had an overall antenatal hospitalization rate of 10.1 per 100 deliveries (Gazmararian, 2002). Of these, approximately a third were for nonobstetrical conditions that included renal, pulmonary, and infectious diseases. In another study from the 2002 Nationwide Inpatient Sample, the injury hospitalization rate was found to be 4.1 women per 1000 deliveries (Kuo, 2007). Approximately 1 in every 635 pregnant women will undergo a nonobstetrical surgical procedure (Corneille, 2010; Kizer, 2011).

Many of these nonobstetrical disorders are within the purview of the obstetrician. Some, however, will warrant consultation, and still others require a multidisciplinary team. The latter may include maternal-fetal medicine specialists, internists and medical subspecialists, surgeons, anesthesiologists, and numerous other disciplines (American College of Obstetricians and Gynecologists, 2013). In these latter situations, obstetricians should have a working knowledge of the wide range of medical disorders common to childbearing-aged women. At the same time, nonobstetricians who help care for these women and their unborn fetuses should be familiar with pregnancy-induced physiological changes and special fetal considerations. Many of these normal pregnancy perturbations have clinically significant effects on various diseases and cause seemingly aberrant changes in routine laboratory values.

It should be axiomatic that a woman should never be penalized because she is pregnant. To ensure this, a number of questions should be addressed:

- What management plan would be recommended if the woman was not pregnant?
- If the proposed management is different because the woman is pregnant, can this be justified?
- What are the risks versus benefits to the mother and her fetus, and are they counter to each other?
- Can an individualized management plan be devised that balances the benefits versus risks of any alterations?

Such an approach should allow individualization of care for women with most medical and surgical disorders complicating pregnancy. Moreover, it may be especially helpful for consideration by nonobstetrical consultants.

MATERNAL PHYSIOLOGY AND LABORATORY VALUES

Pregnancy induces physiological changes in virtually all organ systems. Some are profound and may amplify or obfuscate evaluation of coexisting conditions. Coincidentally, results of numerous laboratory tests are altered, and some values would, in the nonpregnant woman, be considered abnormal. Conversely, some may appear to be within a normal range but are decidedly abnormal for the pregnant woman. The wide range of pregnancy effects on normal physiology and laboratory values are discussed in the chapters that follow as well as throughout Chapter 4 and the Appendix.

MEDICATIONS DURING PREGNANCY

It is indeed fortunate that most medications necessary to treat the most frequently encountered illnesses complicating pregnancy can be given with relative safety. That said, there are notable exceptions, which are considered in Chapter 12.

SURGICAL PROCEDURES DURING PREGNANCY

The risk of an adverse pregnancy outcome is not appreciably increased in most women who undergo an uncomplicated surgical procedure. With complications, however, risks likely will be increased. For example, perforative appendicitis with feculent peritonitis has significant maternal and perinatal morbidity and mortality rates even if surgical and anesthetic techniques are flawless. Conversely, procedure-related complications may adversely affect outcomes. For example, a woman who has uncomplicated removal of an inflamed appendix may suffer aspiration of acidic gastric contents at the time of tracheal intubation or extubation. Still, compared with nonpregnant women undergoing similar procedures, pregnant women do not appear to have excessive complications (Silvestri, 2011).

Effect of Surgery and Anesthesia on Pregnancy Outcome

The most extensive data regarding anesthetic and surgical risks to pregnancy are from the Swedish Birth Registry as described by Mazze and Källén (1989). The effects on pregnancy outcomes of 5405 nonobstetrical surgical procedures performed in 720,000 pregnant women from 1973 to 1981 were analyzed. General anesthesia was used for approximately half of these procedures and commonly involved nitrous oxide supplemented by another inhalation agent or intravenous medications. These procedures were performed in 41 percent of women in the first trimester, 35 percent in the second, and 24 percent in the third. The distribution by the type of procedure is shown in Figure 46-1. Overall, 25 percent were abdominal operations and 20 percent were gynecological or urological procedures. Laparoscopy was the most frequently performed operation, and appendectomy was the most common second-trimester procedure.

Perinatal Outcomes

Excessive perinatal morbidity associated with nonobstetrical surgery is attributable in many cases to the disease itself rather than to adverse effects of surgery and anesthesia. The Swedish Birth Registry again provides valuable data as shown in Table 46-1 (Mazze, 1989). The incidence of neonates with congenital malformations or those stillborn was not significantly different from that of nonexposed control newborns. There were, however, significantly increased incidences of low birthweight, preterm birth, and neonatal death in infants born to women who had undergone surgery. Increased neonatal deaths were largely due to preterm birth. These investigators concluded that these adverse outcomes likely were due to a synergistic effect of the illness in concert with the surgical procedures. In another study, there was an increased preterm delivery rate in 235 women undergoing adnexal mass surgery (Hong, 2006).

In a follow-up study of the Swedish database, Källén and Mazze (1990) scrutinized 572 operations performed at 4 to 5 weeks' gestation and reported a nonsignificant relationship with increased neural-tube defect rates. In a similar study from a Hungarian database, Czeizel and colleagues (1998) found no evidence that anesthetic agents were teratogenic. In a review, Kuczkowski (2006) concluded that there is no robust evidence that anesthetic agents are harmful to the fetus.

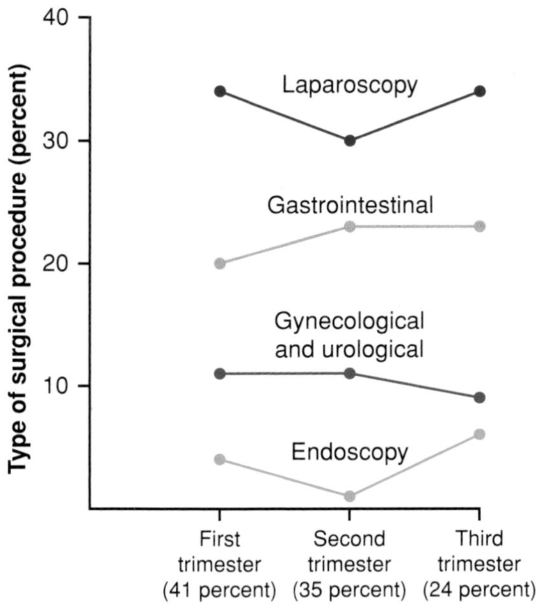

FIGURE 46-1 Proportions of surgical procedures by trimester in 3615 women. (Data from Mazze, 1989.)

TABLE 46-1. Birth Outcomes in 5405 Pregnant Women Undergoing Nonobstetrical Surgery

Outcome	Rate	*p* value[a]
Major malformation	1.9%	NS
Stillbirth	7 per 1000	NS
Neonatal death by 7 days	10.5 per 1000	< 0.05
Preterm < 37 wk	7.5%	< 0.05
Birthweight < 1500 g	1.2%	< 0.05
Birthweight < 2500 g	6.6%	< 0.05

[a]Compared with 720,000 pregnancies in women without surgery.
NS = not significant.
Data from Mazze, 1989.

LAPAROSCOPIC SURGERY DURING PREGNANCY

Laparoscopy has become the most common first-trimester procedure used for diagnosis and management of several surgical disorders (Kuczkowski, 2007). In addition to management of ectopic pregnancy (Chap. 19, p. 385), it is used preferentially during most of pregnancy for exploration and treatment of adnexal masses (Chap. 63, p. 1226), for appendectomy (Chap. 54, p. 1079), and for cholecystectomy (Chap. 55, p. 1096). In 2011, the Guidelines Committee of the Society of American Gastrointestinal and Endoscopic Surgeons (SAGES) updated its recommendations concerning laparoscopy use in pregnant women. Some of these guidelines are listed in Table 46-2.

Information regarding surgical approach selection in pregnant women comes from the American College of Surgeons database (Silvestri, 2011). During the 5-year period ending in 2009, almost 1300 pregnant women who had undergone either appendectomy or cholecystectomy were studied. Open appendectomy was performed in 36 percent of 857 pregnant women compared with only 17 percent of those not pregnant. Of those undergoing cholecystectomy, an open procedure was used in 10 percent of 436 pregnant women compared with 5 percent of nonpregnant women.

There are no randomized trials comparing laparoscopic with open surgery, however, most reviews report equally satisfactory outcomes (Bunyavejchevin, 2013; Fatum, 2001; Lachman, 1999). The most frequently performed procedures were cholecystectomy, adnexal surgery, and appendectomy. Laparoscopic adnexal mass surgery in pregnancy is preferred, and its relative safety is attested to by several investigators (Biscette, 2011; Hoover, 2011; Koo, 2011, 2012). At first, 26 to 28 weeks became the upper gestational-age limit recommended, but as experience has continued to accrue, many now describe laparoscopic surgery performed in the third trimester (Donkervoort, 2011; Kizer, 2011). In one report of 59 pregnant women undergoing laparoscopic cholecystectomy or appendectomy, a third were > 26 weeks pregnant (Rollins, 2004). There were no serious adverse sequelae to these procedures. There are now reports of laparoscopic splenectomy, adrenalectomy, and nephrectomy done in pregnant women (Aubrey-Bassier, 2012; Gernsheimer, 2007; Kosaka, 2006; Miller, 2012; Stroup, 2007).

TABLE 46-2. Some Guidelines for the Performance of Laparoscopic Surgery in Pregnancy

Indications—same as for nonpregnant women
Adnexal mass excision
Investigation of acute abdominal processes
Appendectomy, cholecystectomy, nephrectomy, adrenalectomy, splenectomy
Timing—all trimesters
Technique
Position: left lateral recumbent
Entry: open technique, careful Veress needle, or optical trocar; fundal height may alter insertion site selection
Trocars: direct visualization for placement; fundal height may alter insertion site selection
CO_2 insufflation pressures: 10–15 mm Hg
Monitoring: capnography intraoperatively, FHR assessment pre- and postoperatively
Perioperative pneumatic compression devices and early postoperative ambulation

CO_2 = carbon dioxide; FHR = fetal heart rate.
Summarized from Pearl, 2011.

Hemodynamic Effects

Abdominal insufflation for laparoscopy causes hemodynamic changes that are similar in pregnant and nonpregnant women, and these are summarized in Table 46-3. Reedy and associates (1995) studied baboons at the human equivalent of 22 to 26 weeks' gestation. There were no substantive physiological changes with 10 mm Hg insufflation pressures, but 20 mm Hg caused significant maternal cardiovascular and respiratory changes after 20 minutes. These included increased respiratory rate, respiratory acidosis, diminished cardiac output, and increased pulmonary artery and capillary wedge pressures.

In women, cardiorespiratory changes are generally not severe if insufflation pressures are kept below 20 mm Hg. With noninvasive hemodynamic monitoring in women at midpregnancy, the cardiac index decreased 26 percent by 5 minutes of insufflation and 21 percent by 15 minutes (Steinbrook, 2001). Despite this, mean arterial pressures, systemic vascular resistance, and heart rate did not change significantly.

Perinatal Outcomes

Because precise effects of laparoscopy in the human fetus are unknown, animal studies are informative. In early studies of pregnant ewes, various investigators reported that uteroplacental blood flow decreased when intraperitoneal insufflation pressure exceeded 15 mm Hg (Barnard, 1995; Hunter, 1995). This was the result of decreased perfusion pressure and increased placental vessel resistance (see Table 46-3). The previously cited baboon studies by Reedy and coworkers (1995) produced similar findings. Since then, other studies in sheep have corroborated these observations (O'Rourke, 2006; Reynolds, 2003).

Pregnancy outcomes in women are limited to observations. Reedy and colleagues (1997) used the updated Swedish Birth Registry database to analyze a 20-year period and more than 2 million deliveries. There were 2181 laparoscopic procedures, most of which were performed during the first trimester. Perinatal outcomes for these women were compared with those of all women in the database as well as those undergoing open surgical procedures. These investigators confirmed the earlier findings of an increased risk of low birthweight, preterm delivery, and fetal-growth restriction in pregnancies of women in both operative groups compared with controls. There were no differences, however, when outcomes of women undergoing laparoscopy versus laparotomy were compared. Similar findings were reported from an observational study of 262 women undergoing surgery for an adnexal mass (Koo, 2012).

Technique

Preparation for laparoscopy differs little from that used for laparotomy. Bowel cleansing empties the large intestine and may aid

TABLE 46-3. Physiological Effects of CO_2 Insufflation of the Peritoneal Cavity

System	Effects[a]	Mechanisms	Possible Maternal-Fetal Effects
Respiratory	P_{CO_2} increases, pH decreases	CO_2 absorption	Hypercarbia, acidosis
Cardiovascular	Increased—heart rate; systemic vascular resistance; pulmonary, central venous, and mean arterial pressures	Hypercarbia and increased intraabdominal pressure	Uteroplacental hypoperfusion—possible fetal hypoxia, acidosis, and hypoperfusion[b]
	Decreased—cardiac output	Decreased venous return	
Blood flow	Decreased splanchnic flow with hypoperfusion of liver, kidneys, and gastrointestinal organs	Increased intraabdominal pressure	As above
	Decreased venous return from lower extremities	Increased intraabdominal pressure	As above
	Increased cerebral blood flow	Hypercarbia possibly from shunting due to splanchnic tamponade	Increased CSF pressure[b]

[a]Effects intensified when insufflation pressure > 20 mm Hg in baboons (Reedy, 1995).
[b]Data primarily from animal studies.
CO_2 = carbon dioxide; CSF = cerebrospinal fluid; P_{CO_2} = partial pressure of CO_2.
Data from O'Rourke, 2006; Reynolds, 2003.

visualization. Nasogastric or orogastric decompression reduces the risk of stomach trocar puncture and aspiration. Aortocaval compression is avoided by a left-lateral tilt. Positioning of the lower extremities in boot-type stirrups maintains access to the vagina for fetal sonographic assessment or *manual* uterine displacement. Vaginally placed instruments that enter the cervix or uterus for uterine manipulation should not be used during pregnancy.

Most reports describe the use of general anesthesia after tracheal intubation with monitoring of end-tidal carbon dioxide—$EtCO_2$ (Hong, 2006; Ribic-Pucelj, 2007). With controlled ventilation, $EtCO_2$ is maintained at 30 to 35 mm Hg.

Beyond the first trimester, technical modifications of standard pelvic laparoscopic entry are required to avoid uterine puncture or laceration. Many recommend *open entry* techniques to avoid perforations of the uterus, pelvic vessels, and adnexa (Kizer, 2011; Koo, 2012). The abdomen is incised at or above the umbilicus, and the peritoneal cavity entered under direct visualization. At this point, the cannula is then connected to the insufflation system, and a 12-mm Hg pneumoperitoneum is created. The initial insufflation should be conducted slowly to allow for prompt assessment and reversal of any untoward pressure-related effects. Gas leakage around the cannula is managed by tightening the surrounding skin with a towel clamp. Insertion of secondary trocars into the abdomen is most safely performed under direct laparoscopic visual observation through the primary port. Single-port surgery has also been described (Dursun, 2013).

In more advanced pregnancies, direct entry through a left upper quadrant port in the midclavicular line, 2 cm beneath the costal margin, has been described (Donkervoort, 2011; Stepp, 2004). Known as Palmer point, this entry site is used in gynecological laparoscopy because visceroparietal adhesions uncommonly form here (Vilos, 2007).

Gasless Laparoscopy

This is a less commonly used alternative approach that uses a rod with intraabdominal fan-blade-shaped retractors. When opened, these allow the abdominal wall to be lifted upward. It avoids the typical laparoscopic cardiovascular changes because the pneumoperitoneum is created by retraction rather than insufflation (Phupong, 2007).

Complications

Risks inherent to any abdominal endoscopy are possibly increased slightly during pregnancy. The obvious unique complication is perforation of the pregnant uterus with either a trocar or Veress needle (Azevedo, 2009; Kizer, 2011). That said, reported complications are infrequent (Fatum, 2001; Joumblat, 2012; Koo, 2012). After a Cochrane database review, it was determined that randomized trials would be necessary to deduce comparative benefits and risks of laparoscopy versus laparotomy during pregnancy (Bunyavejchevin, 2013). Pragmatically, this seems unfeasible, and common sense should dictate the approach used.

IMAGING TECHNIQUES

Imaging modalities that are used as adjuncts for diagnosis and therapy during pregnancy include sonography, radiography, and magnetic resonance (MR) imaging. Of these, radiography is the most problematic. Inevitably, some radiographic procedures are performed before recognition of early pregnancy, usually because of trauma or serious illness. Fortunately, most diagnostic radiographic procedures are associated with minimal fetal risks. As with drugs and medications, however, these procedures may lead to litigation if there is an adverse pregnancy outcome. And x-ray exposure may lead to a needless therapeutic abortion because of patient or physician anxiety.

Beginning 2007, the American College of Radiology (ACR) has addressed the growing concern of radiation dose in all fields of medicine. Some of the goals were to limit exposure through radiation safety practices and promote lifelong accumulated records of exposures in any given patient (Amis, 2007). Task Force recommendations included additional considerations for special radiosensitive populations, such as children and pregnant and potentially pregnant women. The Task Force also suggested that the College should encourage radiologists to record all ionizing radiation times and exposures, compare them with benchmarks, and evaluate outliers as part of ongoing quality assurance programs. At the present time at Parkland Hospital, special recommendations are made for the pregnant woman. Radiation exposure values and duration are recorded in high-exposure areas such as computed tomography (CT) and fluoroscopy. Moreover, quality assurance mechanisms are in place to monitor these parameters.

An excellent review of ionizing radiation exposure during pregnancy was performed following the recent Fukushima nuclear plant disaster in Japan (Groen, 2012). This review reinforced considerations during pregnancy that are discussed subsequently.

Ionizing Radiation

The term *radiation* is poorly understood. Literally, it refers to energy transmission and thus is often applied not only to x-rays, but also to microwaves, ultrasound, diathermy, and radio waves. Of these, x-rays and gamma rays have short wavelengths with very high energy and are ionizing radiation forms. The other four energy forms have rather long wavelengths and low energy (Brent, 1999b, 2009).

The biological effects of x-rays are caused by an electrochemical reaction that can damage tissue. According to Brent (1999a, 2009), x- and gamma-radiation at high doses can create two types of biological effects and reproductive risks in the fetus:

1. *Deterministic effects*—these may cause congenital malformations, fetal-growth restriction, mental retardation, and abortion. Although controversial, this so-called NOAEL—No Observed Adverse Effect Level—suggests that there is a threshold dose (0.05 gray or 5 rad) below which there is no risk. It also suggests that the threshold for gross fetal malformations is more likely to be 0.2 gray (20 rad).
2. *Stochastic effects*—these are randomly determined probabilities, which may cause genetic diseases and carcinogenesis. In this case, cancer risk is increased, and hypothetically, at even very low doses.

In this sense, ionizing radiation refers to waves or particles—photons—of significant energy that can change the structure of molecules such as those in DNA, or that can create free radicals or ions capable of causing tissue damage (Hall, 1991; National Research Council, 1990). Methods of measuring the effects of x-rays are summarized in Table 46-4. The standard terms used are *exposure* (in air), *dose* (to tissue), and *relative effective dose* (to tissue). In the range of energies for diagnostic x-rays, the dose is now expressed in grays (Gy), and the relative effective dose is now expressed in sieverts (Sv). These can be used interchangeably. For consistency, all doses discussed subsequently are expressed in contemporaneously used units of gray (1 Gy = 100 rad) or sievert (1 Sv = 100 rem). To convert, 1 Sv = 100 rem = 100 rad.

TABLE 46-4. Some Measures of Ionizing Radiation

Exposure	Number of ions produced by x-rays per kg of air Unit: roentgen (R)
Dose	Amount of energy deposited per kg of tissue Modern unit: gray (Gy) (1 Gy = 100 rad) Traditional unit: rad
Relative effective dose	Amount of energy deposited per kg of tissue normalized for biological effectiveness Modern unit: sievert (Sv) (1 Sv = 100 rem) Traditional unit: rem

X-Ray Dosimetry

When calculating the ionizing radiation dose, such as that from x-rays, several factors to be considered include: (1) type of study, (2) type and age of equipment, (3) distance of target organ from radiation source, (4) thickness of the body part penetrated, and (5) method or technique used for the study (Wagner, 1997).

Estimates of dose to the uterus and embryo for various frequently used radiographic examinations are summarized in Table 46-5. Studies of maternal body parts farthest from the uterus, such as the head, result in a very small dose of radiation scatter to the embryo or fetus. The size of the woman, radiographic technique, and equipment performance are variable factors. Thus, data in the table serve only as guidelines. When the radiation dose for a specific individual is required, a medical physicist should be consulted. Brent (2009) recommends consulting the Health Physics Society website (www.hps.org) to view some examples of questions and answers posed by patients exposed to radiation.

Deterministic Effects of Ionizing Radiation

One potential harmful effect of radiation exposure is deterministic, which may result in abortion, growth restriction, congenital malformations, microcephaly, or mental retardation. These deterministic effects are threshold effects, and the level below which they are induced is the NOAEL (Brent, 2009).

The harmful deterministic effects of ionizing radiation have been extensively studied for cell damage with resultant embryogenesis dysfunction. These have been assessed in animal models, as well as in Japanese atomic bomb survivors and the Oxford Survey of Childhood Cancers (Sorahan, 1995). Additional sources have confirmed previous observations and provided more information (Groen, 2012). One is the 2003 International Commission on Radiological Protection publication, which describes biological fetal effects from prenatal irradiation. Another is the Biological Effects of Ionizing Radiation—BEIR VII Phase 2 report of the National Research

TABLE 46-5. Dose to the Uterus for Common Radiological Procedures

Study	View	Dose[a] per View (mGy)	No. Films[b]	Dose (mGy)
Skull[c]	AP, PA, Lat	< 0.0001	4.1	< 0.0005
Chest	AP, PA[c], Lat[d]	< 0.0001–0.0008	1.5	0.0002–0.0007
Mammogram[d]	CC, Lat	< 0.0003–0.0005	4.0	0.0007–0.002
Lumbosacral spine[e]	AP, Lat	1.14–2.2	3.4	1.76–3.6
Abdomen[e]	AP		1.0	0.8–1.63
Intravenous pyelogram[e]	3 views		5.5	6.9–14
Hip[b] (single)	AP	0.7–1.4		
	Lat	0.18–0.51	2.0	1–2

[a]Calculated for x-ray beams with half-value layers ranging from 2 to 4 mm aluminum equivalent using the methodology of Rosenstein, 1988.
[b]Based on data and methods reported by Laws, 1978.
[c]Entrance exposure data from Conway, 1989.
[d]Estimates based on compilation of above data.
[e]Based on NEXT data reported in National Council on Radiation Protection and Measurements, 1989.
AP = anterior-posterior; CC = cranial-caudal; Lat = lateral; PA = posterior-anterior.

Council (2006), which discusses health risks from exposure to low levels of ionizing radiation.

Animal Studies

In the mouse model, the lethality risk is highest during the preimplantation period—up to 10 days postconception. This is likely due to blastomere destruction caused by chromosomal damage (Hall, 1991). The NOAEL for lethality is 0.15 to 0.2 Gy. Genomic instability can be induced in some mouse models at levels of 0.5 Gy (50 rad), which greatly exceeds levels with diagnostic studies (International Commission on Radiological Protection, 2003).

During organogenesis, high-dose radiation—1 gray or 100 rad—is more likely to cause malformations and growth restriction and less likely to have lethal effects in the mouse. Acute low-dose ionizing radiation appears to have no deleterious effects (Howell, 2013). Studies of brain development suggest that there are effects on neuronal development and a window of cortical sensitivity in early and midfetal periods. During this, the threshold ranges from 0.1 to 0.3 Gy or 10 to 30 rad (International Commission on Radiological Protection, 2003).

Human Data

Data on adverse human effects of high-dose ionizing radiation have most often been derived from atomic bomb survivors from Hiroshima and Nagasaki (Greskovich, 2000; Otake, 1987). The International Commission on Radiological Protection (2003) confirmed initial studies showing that the increased risk of severe mental retardation was greatest between 8 and 15 weeks (Fig. 46-2). There may be a lower-threshold dose of 0.3 Gy—30 rad—a range similar to the window of cortical sensitivity in the mouse model discussed above. The mean decrease in intelligence quotient (IQ) scores was 25 points per Gy or 100 rad. There appears to be linear dose response, but it is not clear whether there is a threshold dose. Most estimates err on the conservative side by assuming a linear nonthreshold hypothesis. From their review, Strzelczyk and coworkers (2007) conclude that limitations of epidemiological studies at low-level exposures, along with new radiobiological findings, challenge the hypothesis that any amount of radiation causes

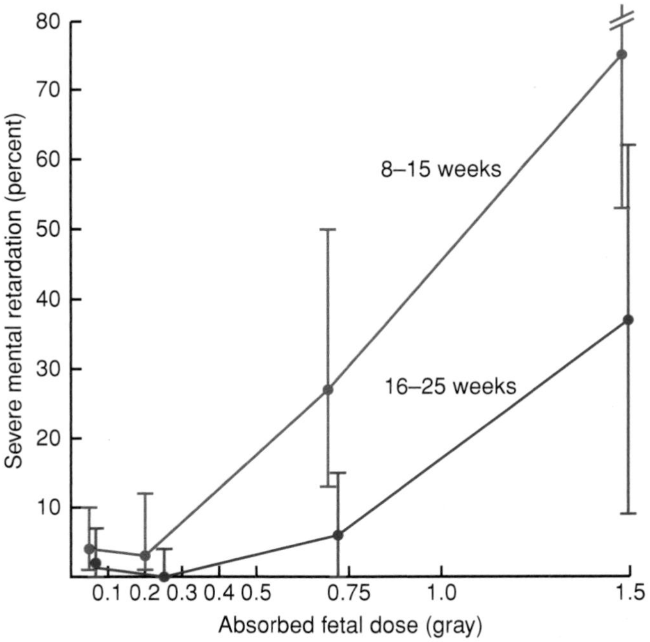

FIGURE 46-2 Follow-up of subjects from Hiroshima and Nagasaki after the atomic bomb explosion in 1945. Subsequent severe mental retardation caused by exposure to ionizing in utero radiation at two gestational age epochs to 1 Gy, that is, 100 rad. Mean values and 90-percent confidence levels are estimated from dosimetry calculated by two methods—T65DR and D586—used by the Radiation Effects Research Foundation of the Japanese Ministry of Health and National Academy of Sciences of the United States. (Data from Otake, 1987, with permission.)

adverse effects. In one such study describing fetuses exposed to low radiation doses, Choi and colleagues (2012) did not find an increased risk for congenital anomalies.

Finally, there is no documented increased risk of mental retardation in humans less than 8 weeks' or greater than 25 weeks' gestation, even with doses exceeding 0.5 Gy or 50 rad (Committee on Biological Effects, BEIR V, 1990; International Commission on Radiological Protection, 2003).

There are reports that have described high-dose radiation used to treat women for malignancy, menorrhagia, and uterine myomas. Dekaban (1968) described 22 infants with microcephaly, mental retardation, or both following exposure in the first half of pregnancy to an estimated 2.5 Gy or 250 rad. Malformations in other organs were not found unless they were accompanied by microcephaly, eye abnormalities, or growth restriction (Brent, 1999b).

The implications of these findings seem straightforward. From 8 to 15 weeks, the embryo is most susceptible to radiation-induced mental retardation. It has not been resolved whether this is a threshold or nonthreshold linear function of dose. The Committee on Biological Effects (1990) estimates the risk of severe mental retardation to be as low as 4 percent for 0.1 Gy (10 rad) and as high as 60 percent for 1.5 Gy (150 rad). But recall that these doses are 2 to 100 times higher than those considered maximal from diagnostic radiation. Importantly, cumulative doses from multiple procedures may reach the harmful range, especially at 8 to 15 weeks. At 16 to 25 weeks, the risk is less. And again, there is no proven risk before 8 weeks or after 25 weeks.

Embryo-fetal risks from low-dose diagnostic radiation appear to be minimal. Current evidence suggests that there are no increased risks for malformations, growth restriction, or abortion from a radiation dose of less than 0.05 Gy (5 rad). Indeed, Brent (2009) concluded that gross congenital malformations would not be increased with exposure to less than 0.2 Gy (20 rad). Because diagnostic x-rays seldom exceed 0.1 Gy (10 rad), Strzelczyk and associates (2007) concluded that these procedures are unlikely to cause deterministic effects. As emphasized by Groen and coworkers (2012), 0.1 Gy is the radiation equivalent to that from more than 1000 chest x-rays!

Stochastic Effects of Ionizing Radiation

This refers to random, presumably unpredictable oncogenic or mutagenic effects of radiation exposure. They concern associations between fetal diagnostic radiation exposure and increased risk of childhood cancers or genetic diseases. According to Doll and Wakeford (1997), as well as the National Research Council (2006) BEIR VII Phase 2 report, excess cancers can result from in utero exposure to doses as low as 0.01 Sv or 1 rad. Stated another way by Hurwitz and colleagues (2006), the estimated risk of childhood cancer following fetal exposure to 0.03 Gy or 3 rad doubles the background risk of 1 in 600 to that of 2 in 600.

In one report, in utero radiation exposure was determined for 10 solid cancers in adults from age 17 to 45 years. There was a dose-response relationship as previously noted at the 0.1 Sv or 10 rem threshold. Intriguingly, nine of 10 cancers were found in females (National Research Council, 2006). These likely are associated with a complex series of interactions between DNA and ionizing radiation. They also make it more problematic to predict cancer risk from low-dose radiation of less than 0.1 Sv or 10 rem. Importantly, below doses of 0.1 to 0.2 Sv, there is no convincing evidence of a carcinogenic effect (Brent, 2009; Preston, 2008; Strzelczyk, 2007).

Therapeutic Radiation

In an earlier report, the Radiation Therapy Committee Task Group of the American Association of Physics in Medicine found that approximately 4000 pregnant women annually undergo cancer therapy in the United States (Stovall, 1995). Their recommendations, however, stand to date. The Task Group emphasizes careful individualization of radiotherapy for the pregnant woman (Chap. 63, p. 1220). For example, in some cases, shielding of the fetus and other safeguards can be employed (Fenig, 2001; Nuyttens, 2002). In other instances, the fetus will be exposed to dangerous radiation doses, and a carefully designed plan must be improvised (Prado, 2000). One example is the model to estimate the fetal dose with maternal brain radiotherapy, and another is the model to calculate the fetal dose with tangential breast irradiation (Mazonakis, 1999, 2003). The impact of radiotherapy on future fertility and pregnancy outcomes was reviewed by Wo and Viswanathan (2009) and others, and this is discussed in detail in Chapter 63 (p. 1220).

Diagnostic Radiation

To estimate fetal risk, approximate x-ray dosimetry must be known. According to the American College of Radiology no single diagnostic procedure results in a radiation dose significant enough to threaten embryo-fetal well-being (Hall, 1991).

Radiographs

Dosimetry for standard radiographs is presented in Table 46-5. In pregnancy, the AP-view chest radiograph is the most commonly used study, and fetal exposure is exceptionally small—0.0007 Gy or 0.07 mrad. With one abdominal radiograph, because the embryo or fetus is directly in the x-ray beam, the dose is higher—0.001 Gy or 100 mrad. The standard intravenous pyelogram may exceed 0.005 Gy or 500 mrad because of several films. The one-shot pyelogram described in Chapter 53 (p. 1056) is useful when urolithiasis or other causes of obstruction are suspected but unproven by sonography. Most "trauma series," such as radiographs of an extremity, skull, or rib series, deliver low doses because of the fetal distance from the target area.

Fetal indications for radiographic studies are limited. In some countries, x-ray pelvimetry is done for a breech presentation (Chap. 28, p. 562).

Fluoroscopy and Angiography

Dosimetry calculations are much more difficult with these procedures because of variations in the number of radiographs obtained, total fluoroscopy time, and fluoroscopy

TABLE 46-6. Estimated X-Ray Doses to the Uterus/Embryo from Common Fluoroscopic Procedures

Procedure	Dose to Uterus (mGy)	Fluoroscopic Exposure in Seconds (SD)
Cerebral angiography[a]	< 0.1	—
Cardiac angiography[b,c]	0.65	223 (± 118)
Single-vessel PTCA[b,c]	0.60	1023 (± 952)
Double-vessel PTCA[b,c]	0.90	1186 (± 593)
Upper gastrointestinal series[d]	0.56	136
Barium swallow[b,e]	0.06	192
Barium enema[b,f,g]	20–40	289–311

[a]Wagner, 1997.
[b]Calculations based on data of Gorson, 1984.
[c]Finci, 1987.
[d]Suleiman, 1991.
[e]Based on female data from Rowley, 1987.
[f]Assumes embryo in radiation field for entire examination.
[g]Bednarek, 1983.
PTCA = percutaneous transluminal coronary angioplasty; SD = standard deviation.

time in which the fetus is in the radiation field. As shown in Table 46-6, the range is variable. The Food and Drug Administration limits the exposure rate for conventional fluoroscopy such as barium studies, however, special-purpose systems such as angiography units have the potential for much higher exposure.

Endoscopy is the preferred method of gastrointestinal tract evaluation in pregnancy (Chap. 54, p. 1069). Occasionally, an upper gastrointestinal series or barium enema may be performed before a pregnancy is recognized. Most would likely be done during preimplantation or early organogenesis.

Angiography and vascular embolization may occasionally be necessary for serious maternal disorders, especially renal disease, and for trauma (Wortman, 2013). As before, the greater the distance from the embryo or fetus, the less the exposure and risk.

Computed Tomography

This is usually performed by obtaining a spiral of 360-degree images that are postprocessed in multiple planes. Of these, the axial image remains the most commonly obtained. Multidetector CT (MDCT) images are now standard for common clinical indications. The most recent detectors have 16 or 64 channels, and MDCT protocols may result in increased dosimetry compared with traditional CT imaging. A number of imaging parameters have an effect on exposure (Brenner, 2007). These include pitch, kilovoltage, tube current, collimation, number of slices, tube rotation, and total acquisition time. If a study is performed with and without contrast, the dose is doubled because twice as many images are obtained. Fetal exposure is also dependent on factors such as maternal size as well as fetal size and position. And as with plain radiography, the closer the target area is to the fetus, the greater the delivered dose.

TABLE 46-7. Estimated Radiation Dosimetry with 16-Channel Multidetector Computed-Tomographic (MDCT) Imaging Protocols

Protocol	Dosimetry (mGy) Preimplantation	Dosimetry (mGy) 3 Months' Gestation
Pulmonary embolism	0.20–0.47	0.61–0.66
Renal stone	8–12	4–7
Appendix	15–17	20–40

Data from Hurwitz, 2006.

Cranial CT scanning is the most commonly requested study in pregnant women. It is used in women with neurological disorders as discussed in Chapter 60 (p. 1187) and with eclampsia as noted in Chapter 40 (p. 744). Nonenhanced CT scanning is commonly used to detect acute hemorrhage within the epidural, subdural, or subarachnoid spaces. Because of the distance from the fetus, radiation dosage is negligible (Goldberg-Stein, 2012).

Abdominal procedures are more problematic. Hurwitz and associates (2006) employed a 16-MDCT to calculate fetal exposure at 0 and 3 months' gestation using a phantom model (Table 46-7). Calculations were made for three commonly requested procedures in pregnant women. The pulmonary embolism protocol has the same dosimetry exposure as the ventilation-perfusion (V/Q) lung scan discussed below. Because of the pitch used, the appendicitis protocol has the highest radiation exposure, however, it is very useful clinically (Fig. 46-3). Using a similar protocol in 67 women with suspected appendicitis, Lazarus and coworkers (2007) reported sensitivity of 92 percent, specificity of 99 percent, and a negative-predictive value of 99 percent. Here dosimetry was markedly decreased compared with standard appendiceal imaging because of a different pitch. For suspected urolithiasis, the MDCT-scan

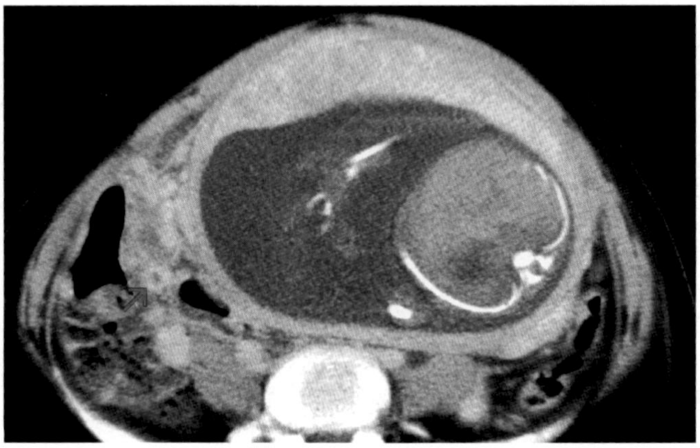

FIGURE 46-3 Computed-tomographic protocol for appendix shows an enlarged, enhancing—and thus inflamed—appendix (*arrow*) next to the 25-week pregnancy. (Image contributed by Dr. Jeffrey H. Pruitt.)

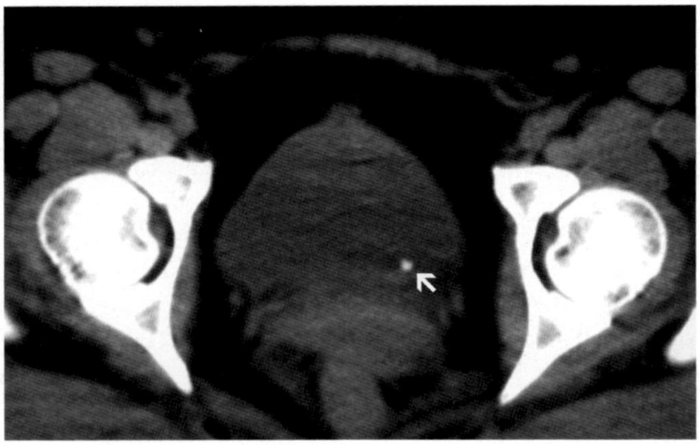

FIGURE 46-4 Computed-tomographic protocol imaging for urolithiasis disclosed a renal stone in the distal ureter (*arrow*) at its junction with the bladder. (Image contributed by Dr. Jeffrey H. Pruitt.)

protocol shown in Figure 46-4 is used if sonography is nondiagnostic. Using a similar protocol, White and colleagues (2007) identified urolithiasis in 13 of 20 women at an average of 26.5 weeks. Finally, and as discussed in Chapter 47 (p. 954), abdominal tomography should be performed if indicated in the pregnant woman with severe trauma.

Most experience with chest CT-scanning is with suspected pulmonary embolism. The most recent recommendations for its use in pregnancy from the Prospective Investigation of Pulmonary Embolism Diagnosis—PIOPED—II investigators were summarized by Stein and associates (2007). They found that pulmonary scintigraphy—the V/Q scan—was recommended for pregnant women by 70 percent of radiologists and chest CT angiography by 30 percent. And scintigraphy is still recommended by the American Thoracic Society in pregnant women with a normal chest x-ray (Leung, 2012). But most agree that MDCT angiography has improved accuracy because of increasingly faster acquisition times. Others have reported a higher use rate for CT angiography and emphasize that dosimetry is similar to that with V/Q scintigraphy (Brenner, 2007; Hurwitz, 2006; Matthews, 2006). At Parkland and UT Southwestern University Hospitals, we prefer MDCT scanning initially for suspected pulmonary embolism (Chap. 52, p. 1042).

CT pelvimetry is used by some before attempting breech vaginal delivery (Chap. 28, p. 562). The fetal dose approaches 0.015 Gy or 1.5 rad, but use of a low-exposure technique may reduce this to 0.0025 Gy or 0.25 rad.

Nuclear Medicine Studies

These studies are performed by "tagging" a radioactive element to a carrier that can be injected, inhaled, or swallowed. For example, the radioisotope technetium-99m may be tagged to red blood cells, sulfur colloid, or pertechnetate. The method used to tag the agent determines fetal radiation exposure. The amount of placental transfer is obviously important, but so is renal clearance because of fetal proximity to the maternal bladder. Measurement of radioactive technetium is based on its decay, and the units used are the curie (Ci) or the becquerel (Bq). Dosimetry is usually expressed in millicuries (mCi). As shown in Table 46-4, the effective tissue dose is expressed in sievert units (Sv) with conversion as discussed: 1 Sv = 100 rem = 100 rad.

Depending on the physical and biochemical properties of a radioisotope, an average fetal exposure can be calculated (Wagner, 1997; Zanzonico, 2000). Commonly used radiopharmaceuticals and estimated absorbed fetal doses are given in Table 46-8. The radionuclide dose should be kept as low as possible (Adelstein, 1999). Exposures vary with gestational age and are greatest earlier in pregnancy for most radiopharmaceuticals. One exception is the later effect of iodine-131 on the fetal thyroid (Wagner, 1997). The International Commission on Radiological Protection (2001) has compiled dose coefficients for radionuclides. Stather and coworkers (2002) detailed the biokinetic and dosimetric models used by the Commission to estimate fetal radiation doses from maternal radionuclide exposure.

As discussed above, MDCT-angiography is being used preferentially for suspected pulmonary embolism during pregnancy. Until recently, the imaging modality was the ventilation-perfusion lung scan in this setting. It is used if CT angiography is nondiagnostic (Chap. 52, p. 1043). Perfusion is measured with injected ^{99}Tc-macroaggregated albumin, and ventilation is measured with inhaled xenon-127 or xenon-133. Fetal exposure with either is negligible (Chan, 2002; Mountford, 1997).

Thyroid scanning with iodine-123 or iodine-131 seldom is indicated in pregnancy. With trace doses used, however, fetal risk is minimal. Importantly, therapeutic radioiodine in doses to treat Graves disease or thyroid cancer may cause fetal thyroid ablation and cretinism.

The sentinel lymphoscintigram, which uses ^{99m}Tc-sulfur colloid to detect the axillary lymph node most likely to have metastases from breast cancer, is a commonly used preoperative study in nonpregnant women (Newman, 2007; Spanheimer, 2009; Wang, 2007). As shown in Table 46-8, the calculated dose is approximately 0.014 mSv or 1.4 mrad, which should not preclude its use during pregnancy.

SONOGRAPHY

Of all of the major advances in obstetrics, the development of sonography for study of the fetus and mother certainly is one of the greater achievements. The technique has become virtually indispensable in everyday practice. The wide range of clinical uses of sonography in pregnancy is further discussed in Chapter 10 and in most other sections of this book.

MAGNETIC RESONANCE IMAGING

Magnetic resonance technology does not use ionizing radiation, and its application is cited throughout this book. Advantages include high soft-tissue contrast, ability to characterize tissue, and acquisition of images in any plane—particularly axial, sagittal, and coronal. An entire section in Chapter 10 (p. 222) is devoted to mechanisms that generate MR images.

Safety

The most recent update of the Blue Ribbon Panel on MR safety of the American College of Radiology was summarized

TABLE 46-8. Radiopharmaceuticals Used in Nuclear Medicine Studies

Study	Estimated Activity Administered per Examination (mCi)[a]	Weeks' Gestation[b]	Dose to Uterus/ Embryo (mSv)[c]
Brain	20 mCi ^{99m}Tc DTPA	< 12	8.8
		12	7[c]
Hepatobiliary	5 mCi ^{99m}Tc sulfur colloid	12	0.45
	5 mCi ^{99m}Tc HIDA		1.5
Bone	20 mCi ^{99m}Tc phosphate	< 12	4.6
Pulmonary			
Perfusion	3 mCi ^{99m}Tc-macroaggregated albumin	Any	0.45–0.57 (combined)
Ventilation	10 mCi ^{133}Xe gas		
Renal	20 mCi ^{99m}Tc DTPA	< 12	8.8
Abscess or tumor	3 mCi ^{67}Ga citrate	< 12	7.5
Cardiovascular	20 mCi ^{99m}Tc-labeled red blood cells	< 12	5
	3 mCi ^{210}Tl chloride	< 12	11
		12	6.4
		24	5.2
		36	3
Thyroid	5 mCi $^{99m}TcO_4$	< 8	2.4
	0.3 mCi ^{123}I (whole body)[d]	1.5–6	0.10
	0.1 mCi ^{131}I		
	Whole body	2–6	0.15
	Whole body	7–9	0.88
	Whole body	12–13	1.6
	Whole body	20	3
	Thyroid-fetal	11	720
	Thyroid-fetal	12–13	1300
	Thyroid-fetal	20	5900
Sentinel lymphoscintigram	5 mCi ^{99m}Tc sulfur colloid (1–3 mCi)		5

[a]mCi = millicuries. To convert to mrad, multiply by 100.
[b]Exposures are generally greater prior to 12 weeks compared with increasing gestational ages.
[c]Some measurements account for placental transfer.
[d]The uptake and exposure of ^{131}I increases with gestational age.
DPTA = diethylenetriaminepentaacetic acid; Ga = gallium; HIDA = hepatobiliary iminodiacetic acid; I = iodine; mCi = millicurie; mSv = millisievert; Tc = technetium; TcO_4 = pertechnetate; Tl = thallium.
Data from Adelstein, 1999; Schwartz, 2003; Stather, 2002; Wagner, 1997; Zanzonico, 2000.

by Kanal and colleagues (2007). The panel concluded that there are no reported harmful human effects from MR imaging. Chew and associates (2001) found no differences in blastocyst formation exposure of early murine embryos to MR imaging with 1.5 T strength. Vadeyar and coworkers (2000) noted no demonstrable fetal heart rate pattern changes during MR imaging in women. Chung (2002) has reviewed these safety issues.

Contraindications to MR imaging include internal cardiac pacemakers, neurostimulators, implanted defibrillators and infusion pumps, cochlear implants, shrapnel or other metal in biologically sensitive areas, some intracranial aneurysm clips, and any metallic foreign body in the eye. Of more than 51,000 nonpregnant patients scheduled for MR imaging, Dewey and colleagues (2007) found that only 0.4 percent had an absolute contraindication to the procedure.

Contrast Agents

Several elemental gadolinium chelates are used to create paramagnetic contrast. Some are gadopentetate, gadodiamide, gadoteridol, and gadoterate. These cross the placenta and are found in amnionic fluid. In doses approximately 10 times the human dose, gadopentetate caused slight developmental delay in rabbit fetuses. There is little experience with gadolinium in humans

(Wang, 2012). In one study, De Santis and associates (2007) described 26 women given a gadolinium derivative in the first trimester without adverse fetal effects. Currently, according to Briggs and coworkers (2011), as well as the Panel, these contrast agents are not recommended unless there are overwhelming benefits.

Maternal Indications

In some cases, MR imaging may be complementary to CT, and in others, MR imaging is preferable. Maternal central nervous system abnormalities, such as brain tumors or spinal trauma, are more clearly seen with MR imaging. As discussed in Chapter 40 (p. 743), MR imaging has provided valuable insights into the pathophysiology of eclampsia and to calculate cerebrovascular blood flow in preeclampsia (Twickler, 2007; Zeeman, 2003, 2004a,b, 2009). It is invaluable in the diagnosis of neurological emergencies (Edlow, 2013). MR imaging is a superb technique to evaluate the maternal abdomen and retroperitoneal space. It is chosen by many to determine the degree and extent of placenta accreta and its variants in women who have had a prior cesarean delivery (Chap. 41, p. 806). It has been employed for detection and localization of adrenal tumors, renal lesions, gastrointestinal lesions, and pelvic masses in pregnancy. It has particular value in evaluating neoplasms of the chest, abdomen, and pelvis in pregnancy (Boyd, 2012; Oto, 2007; Tica, 2013). MR urography has been used successfully for renal urolithiasis (Mullins, 2012). MR imaging may be selected to confirm pelvic and vena caval thrombosis—a common source of pulmonary embolism in pregnant women (Fig. 46-5). As discussed in Chapter 37 (p. 688), CT and MR imaging is useful for evaluation of puerperal infections, but MR imaging provides better visualization of the bladder flap area following cesarean delivery (Brown, 1999; Twickler, 1997). MR imaging now includes evaluation of right lower quadrant pain in pregnancy, specifically appendicitis (Baron, 2012; Dewhurst, 2013; Pedrosa, 2007, 2009). Investigators have also found other disorders of the gastrointestinal tract to be easily diagnosed with MR imaging (Chap. 54, p. 1069).

Fetal Indications

Fetal MR imaging provides a complement to sonography (De Wilde, 2005; Laifer-Narin, 2007; Sandrasegaran, 2006). According to Zaretsky and colleagues (2003a), MR imaging can be used to image almost all elements of the standard fetal anatomical survey. The most frequent fetal indications for MR imaging are evaluation of complex abnormalities of the brain, chest, and genitourinary system. Bauer (2009), Reichel (2003), Twickler (2002), Weisz (2009), and their associates have validated its use for fetal central nervous system anomalies and biometry (Fig. 46-6). Caire and coworkers (2003) reported its merits for fetal genitourinary anomalies. Hawkins and colleagues (2008) described MR imaging in 21 fetuses with renal anomalies and oligohydramnios. Zaretsky and associates (2003b) noted that fetal-weight estimation was more accurate using MR imaging than with sonography. Fast-acquisition sequencing has solved problems with fetal movement to improve imaging. The technique is termed *HASTE*—*H*alf-Fourier *A*cquisition *S*ingle slow *T*urbo spin *E*cho, or *SSFSE*—*Single* *S*hot *F*ast *S*pin *E*cho. A more extensive discussion of fetal indications and findings of MR imaging are discussed in Chapter 10 and throughout this book.

GUIDELINES FOR DIAGNOSTIC IMAGING DURING PREGNANCY

The American College of Obstetricians and Gynecologists (2009) has reviewed the effects of radiographic, sonographic, and magnetic-resonance exposure during pregnancy. Its suggested guidelines are shown in Table 46-9.

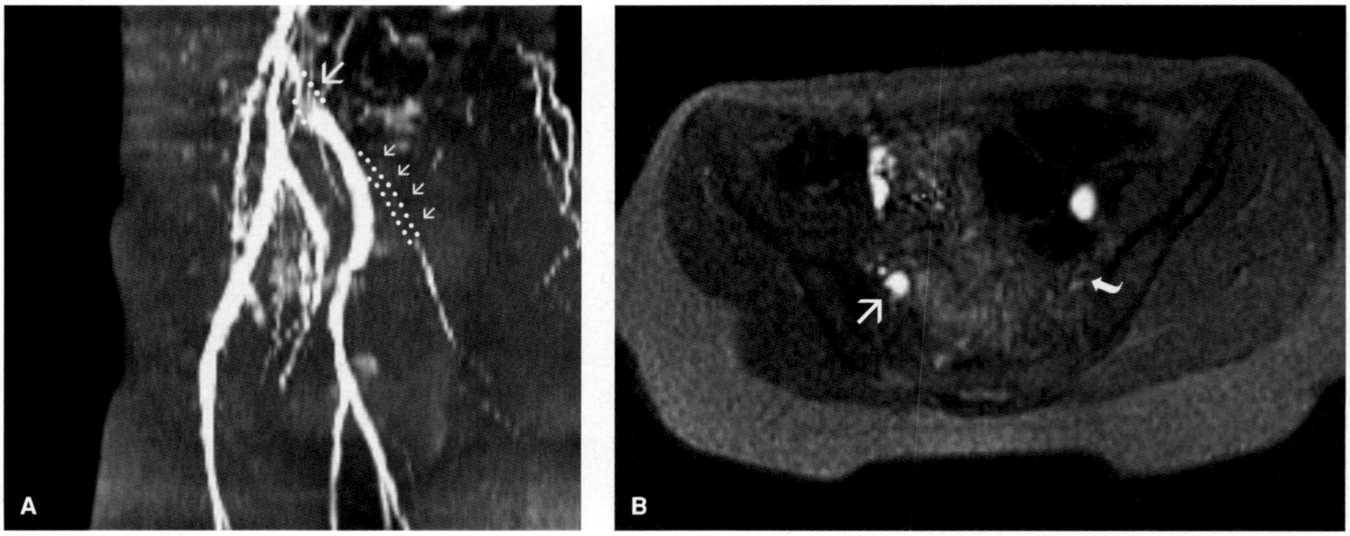

FIGURE 46-5 Magnetic-resonance images of a pelvic vein thrombosis in a 15-week pregnant woman who presented with left leg pain but no symptoms of a pulmonary embolus. **A.** Reconstructed magnetic resonance venogram demonstrates partial chronic occlusion of the left common iliac vein (*large arrow*) and thrombosis and complete occlusion of the left internal iliac vein (*small arrows*). **B.** From the axial images, there is normal flow in the right (*arrow*) and no flow in the left internal iliac vein (*curved arrow*). (Image contributed by Dr. R. Douglas Sims.)

TABLE 46-9. Guidelines for Diagnostic Imaging During Pregnancy

1. Women should be counseled that x-ray exposure from a single diagnostic procedure does not result in harmful fetal effects. Specifically, exposure to less than 5 rads has not been associated with an increase in fetal anomalies or pregnancy loss.
2. Concern about possible effects of high-dose ionizing radiation exposure should not prevent medically indicated diagnostic x-ray procedures from being performed on a pregnant woman. During pregnancy, other imaging procedures not associated with ionizing radiation, e.g., ultrasonography, and MRI, should be considered instead of x-rays when appropriate.
3. Ultrasonography and MRI are not associated with known adverse fetal effects.
4. Consultation with an expert in dosimetry calculation may be helpful in calculating estimated fetal dose when multiple diagnostic x-rays are performed on a pregnant patient.
5. The use of radioactive isotopes of iodine is contraindicated for therapeutic use during pregnancy.
6. Radiopaque and paramagnetic contrast agents are unlikely to cause harm and may be of diagnostic benefit, but these agents should be used during pregnancy only if the potential benefit justifies the potential risk to the fetus.

Summarized from the American College of Obstetricians and Gynecologists, 2009.

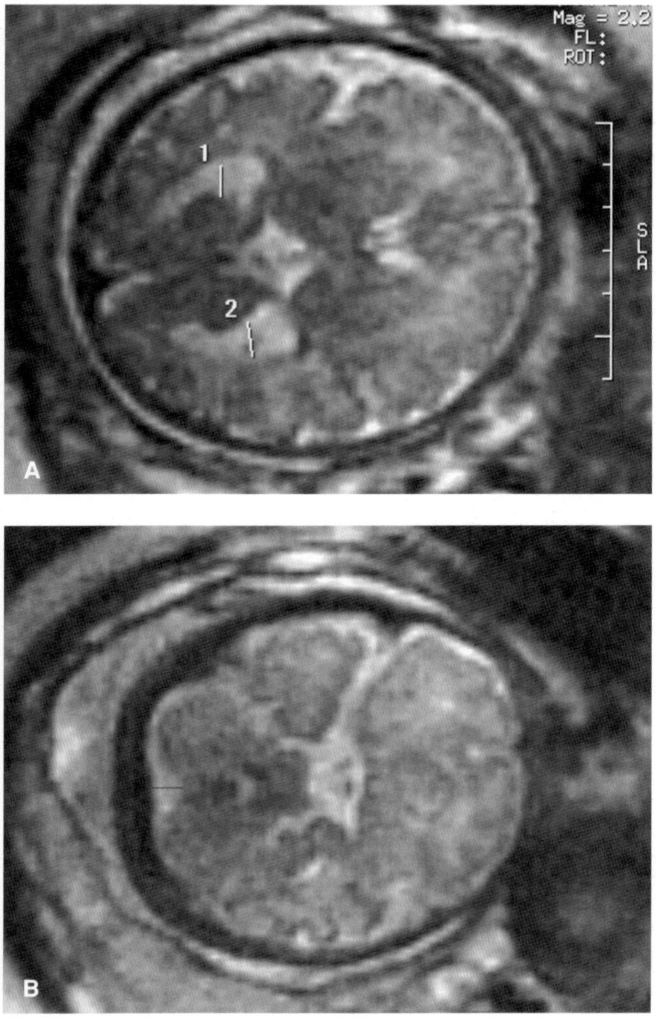

FIGURE 46-6 Magnetic-resonance images of the brain of a 35-week fetus. **A.** Axial images show the normal frontal horns, cavum septum pellucidum, and cerebellum. **B.** Sagittal images demonstrate the normal corpus callosum, brainstem, and vermis.

REFERENCES

Adelstein SJ: Administered radionuclides in pregnancy. Teratology 59:236, 1999

American College of Obstetricians and Gynecologists: Guidelines for diagnostic imaging during pregnancy. Committee Opinion No. 299, September 2004, Reaffirmed 2009

American College of Obstetricians and Gynecologists: Nonobstetric surgery in pregnancy. Committee Opinion No. 474, February 2011, Reaffirmed 2013

Amis ES Jr, Butler PF, Applegate KE, et al: American College of Radiology white paper on radiation dose in medicine. J Am Coll Radiol 4(5):272, 2007

Aubrey-Bassler FK, Sowers N: 613 cases of splenic rupture without risk factors or previously diagnosed disease: A systematic review. EMC Emerg Med 12(1):11, 2012

Azevedo JL, Azevedo OC, Miyahira SA, et al: Injuries caused by Veress needle insertion for creation of pneumoperitoneum: a systematic literature review. Surg Endosc 23(7):1428, 2009

Barnard JM, Chaffin D, Droste S, et al: Fetal response to carbon dioxide pneumoperitoneum in the pregnant ewe. Obstet Gynecol 85:669, 1995

Baron KT, Arleo EK, Robinson C, et al: Comparing the diagnostic performance of MRI versus CT in the evaluation of acute nontraumatic abdominal pain during pregnancy. Emerg Radiol 19(6):519, 2012

Bauer S, Mirza F, Pri-Paz S, et al: Dandy-Walker malformations: a comparison of prenatal ultrasound and magnetic resonance imaging. Abstract No. 396 Presented at the 29th Annual Meeting of the Society for Maternal-Fetal Medicine. 26–31 January 2009

Bednarek DR, Rudin S, Wong, et al: Reduction of fluoroscopic exposure for the air-contrast barium enema. Br J Radiol 56:823, 1983

Biscette S, Yoost J, Hertweck P, et al: Laparoscopy in pregnancy and the pediatric patient. Obstet Gynecol Clin North Am 38(4):757, 2011

Boyd CA, Benarroch-Gampel J, Kilic G, et al: Pancreatic neoplasms in pregnancy: diagnosis, complications, and management. J Gastrointest Surg 16(5):1064, 2012

Brenner DJ, Hall JH, Phil D: Computed tomography—an increasing source of radiation exposure. N Engl J Med 357:2277, 2007

Brent RL: Developmental and reproductive risks of radiological procedures utilizing ionizing radiation during pregnancy. Proceedings No. 21 in Radiation Protection in Medicine: Contemporary Issues. Proceedings of the Thirty-Fifth Annual Meeting of the National Council on Radiation Protection and Measurements. Arlington, VA, 7–8 April , 1999a

Brent RL: Saving lives and changing family histories: appropriate counseling of pregnant women and men and women of reproductive age, concerning risk of diagnostic radiation exposure during and before pregnancy. Am J Obstet Gynecol 200(1):4, 2009

Brent RL: Utilization of developmental basic science principles in the evaluation of reproductive risks from pre- and postconception environmental radiation exposures. Teratology 59:182, 1999b

Briggs GG, Freeman RK, Yaffe SJ: Drugs in Pregnancy and Lactation, 8th ed. Philadelphia, Lippincott Williams & Wilkins, 2011

Brown CE, Stettler RW, Twickler D, et al. Puerperal septic pelvic thrombophlebitis: incidence and response to heparin therapy. Am J Obstet Gynecol 181:143, 1999

Bunyavejchevin S, Phupong V: Laparoscopic surgery for presumed benign ovarian tumor during pregnancy. Cochrane Database Syst Rev 1:CD005459, 2013

Caire JT, Ramus RM, Magee KP, et al: MRI of fetal genitourinary anomalies. AJR Am J Roentgenol 181:1381, 2003

Chan WS, Ray JG, Murray S, et al: Suspected pulmonary embolism in pregnancy. Arch Intern Med 152:1170, 2002

Chew S, Ahmadi A, Goh PS, et al: The effects of 1.5T magnetic resonance imaging on early murine in-vitro embryo development. J Magn Reson Imaging 13:417, 2001

Choi JS, Han JY, Ahn HK, et al: Fetal and neonatal outcomes in first-trimester pregnant women exposed to abdominal or lumbar radiodiagnostic procedures without administration of radionucleotides. Intern Med J 43(5):513, 2013

Chung SM: Safety issues in magnetic resonance imaging. J Neuroophthalmol 22:35, 2002

Committee on Biological Effects of Ionizing Radiation, National Research Council: Other somatic and fetal effects. In BEIR V: Effects of Exposure to Low Levels of Ionizing Radiation. Washington, National Academy Press, 1990

Conway BJ: Nationwide evaluation of x-ray trends: tabulation and graphical summary of surveys 1984 through 1987. Frankfort, Conference of Radiation Control Program Directors, 1989

Corneille MG, Gallup TM, Bening T, et al: The use of laparoscopic surgery in pregnancy: evaluation of safety and efficacy. Am J Surg 200:363, 2010

Czeizel AE, Pataki T, Rockenbauer M: Reproductive outcome after exposure to surgery under anesthesia during pregnancy. Arch Gynecol Obstet 261:193, 1998

Dekaban AS: Abnormalities in children exposed to x-irradiation during various stages of gestation: tentative timetable of radiation injury to the human fetus. J Nucl Med 9:471, 1968

De Santis M, Straface G, Cavaliere AF, et al: Gadolinium periconceptional exposure: pregnancy and neonatal outcome. Acta Obstet Gynecol Scand 86:99, 2007

Dewey M, Schink T, Dewey CF: Frequency of referral of patients with safety-related contraindications to magnetic resonance imaging. Eur J Radiol 63(1):124, 2007

Dewhurst C, Beddy P, Pedrosa I: MRI evaluation of acute appendicitis in pregnancy. J Magn Reson Imaging 37(3):566, 2013

De Wilde JP, Rivers AW, Price DL: A review of the current use of magnetic resonance imaging in pregnancy and safety implications for the fetus. Prog Biophys Mol Biol 87:335, 2005

Doll R, Wakeford R: Risk of childhood cancer from fetal irradiation. Br J Radiol 70:130, 1997

Donkervoort SC, Boerma D: Suspicion of acute appendicitis in the third trimester of pregnancy: pros and cons of a laparoscopic procedure. JSLS 15(3):379, 2011

Dursun P, Gülümser C, Cağlar M, et al: Laparoendoscopic single-site surgery for acute adnexal pathology during pregnancy: preliminary experience. J Matern Fetal Neonatal Med 26(13):1282, 2013

Edlow JA, Caplan LR, O'Brien K, et al: Diagnosis of acute neurological emergencies in pregnant and postpartum women. Lancet Neurol 12(2):175, 2013

Fatum M, Rojansky N: Laparoscopic surgery during pregnancy. Obstet Gynecol Surv 56:50, 2001

Fenig E, Mishaeli M, Kalish Y, et al: Pregnancy and radiation. Cancer Treat Rev 27:1, 2001

Finci L, Meier B, Steffenino G, et al: Radiation exposure during diagnostic catheterization and single- and double-vessel percutaneous transluminal coronary angioplasty. Am J Cardiol 60:1401, 1987

Gazmararian JA, Petersen R, Jamieson DJ, et al: Hospitalizations during pregnancy among managed care enrollees. Obstet Gynecol 100:94, 2002

Gernsheimer T, McCrae KR: Immune thrombocytopenic purpura in pregnancy. Curr Opin Hematol 14:574, 2007

Goldberg-Stein SA, Liu B, Hahn PF, et al: Radiation dose management: part 2, estimating fetal radiation risk from CT during pregnancy. AJR Am J Roentgenol 198(4):W352, 2012

Gorson RO, Lassen M, Rosenstein M: Patient dosimetry in diagnostic radiology. In Waggener RG, Kereiakes JG, Shalek R (eds): Handbook of Medical Physics, Vol II. Boca Raton, CRC Press, 1984

Greskovich JF, Macklis RM: Radiation therapy in pregnancy: risk calculation and risk minimization. Semin Oncol 27:633, 2000

Groen RS, Bae JY, Lim KJ: Fear of the unknown: ionizing radiation exposure during pregnancy. Am J Obstet Gynecol 206(6):456, 2012

Hall EJ: Scientific view of low-level radiation risks. RadioGraphics 11:509, 1991

Hawkins JS, Dashe JS, Twickler DM: Magnetic resonance imaging diagnosis of severe fetal renal anomalies. Am J Obstet Gynecol 198:328.e1, 2008

Hong JY: Adnexal mass surgery and anesthesia during pregnancy: a 10-year retrospective review. Intl J Obstet Anesth 15:212, 2006

Hoover K, Jenkins TR: Evaluation and management of adnexal mass in pregnancy. Am J Obstet Gynecol 205(2):97, 2011

Howell EK, Gaschak SP, Griffith KD: Radioadaptive response following in utero low-dose irradiation. Radiat Res 179(1):29, 2013

Hunter JG, Swanstrom L, Thornburg K: Carbon dioxide pneumoperitoneum induces fetal acidosis in a pregnant ewe model. Surg Endosc 9:272, 1995

Hurwitz LM, Yoshizumi T, Reiman RE, et al: Radiation dose to the fetus from body MDCT during early gestation. Am J Roentgenol 186:871, 2006

International Commission on Radiological Protection: Biological effects after prenatal irradiation (embryo and fetus). IRCP Publication 90. Ann IRCP: September/December 2003

International Commission on Radiological Protection: Doses to the embryo and fetus from intakes of radionuclides by the mother. Ann ICRP 31:19, 2001

Joumblat N, Grubbs B, Chmait RH: Incidental fetoscopy during laparoscopy in pregnancy: management of perforation of the gravid uterus. Surg Laparosc Endosc Percutan Tech 22(2):e76, 2012

Källén B, Mazze RI: Neural tube defects and first trimester operations. Teratology 41:717, 1990

Kanal E, Barkovich AJ, Bell C, et al: ACR guidance document for safe MR practices: 2007. Am J Roentgenol 188:1, 2007

Kizer NT, Powell MA: Surgery in the pregnant patient. Clin Obstet Gynecol 54(4):2011

Koo YJ, Kim HJ, Lim KT, et al: Laparotomy versus laparoscopy for the treatment of adnexal masses during pregnancy. Aust N Z J Obstet Gynaecol 52(1):34, 2012

Koo YJ Lee JE, Lim KT, et al: A 10-year experience of laparoscopic surgery for adnexal masses during pregnancy. Int J Gynaecol Obstet 113(1):36, 2011

Kosaka K, Onoda N, Ishikawa T, et al: Laparoscopic adrenalectomy on a patient with primary aldosteronism during pregnancy. Endo J 53:461, 2006

Kuczkowski KM: Laparoscopic procedures during pregnancy and the risks of anesthesia: what does an obstetrician need to know? Arch Gynecol Obstet March 13, 2007

Kuczkowski KM: The safety of anaesthetics in pregnant women. Expert Opin Surg Saf 5:251, 2006

Kuo C, Jamieson DJ, McPheeters ML, et al: Injury hospitalizations of pregnant women in the United States, 2002. Am J Obstet Gynecol 196:161, 2007

Lachman E, Schienfeld A, Voss E, et al: Pregnancy and laparoscopic surgery. J Am Assoc Gynecol Laparosc 6:347, 1999

Laifer-Narin S, Budorick NE, Simpson LL, et al: Fetal magnetic resonance imaging: a review. Curr Opin Obstet Gynecol 19:151, 2007

Laws PW, Rosenstein M: A somatic index for diagnostic radiology. Health Phys 35:629, 1978

Lazarus E, Mayo-Smith WW, Mainiero MB, et al: CT in the evaluation of nontraumatic abdominal pain in pregnant women. Radiology 244:784, 2007

Leung AN, Bull TM, Jaeschke R, et al: American Thoracic Society documents: an official American Thoracic Society/Society of Thoracic Radiology Clinical Practice Guidelines—Evaluation of suspected Pulmonary Embolism in Pregnancy. Radiology 262(2):635, 2012

Matthews S: Imaging pulmonary embolism in pregnancy: What is the most appropriate imaging protocol? B J Radiol 79(941):441, 2006

Mazonakis M, Damilakis J, Varveris H, et al: A method of estimating fetal dose during brain radiation therapy. Int J Radiat Oncol Biol Phys 44:455, 1999

Mazonakis M, Varveris H, Damilakis J, et al: Radiation dose to conceptus resulting from tangential breast irradiation. Int J Radiat Oncol Biol Phys 55:386, 2003

Mazze RI, Källén B: Reproductive outcome after anesthesia and operation during pregnancy: a registry study of 5405 cases. Am J Obstet Gynecol 161:1178, 1989

Miller MA, Mazzaglia PJ, Larson L, et al: Laparoscopic adrenalectomy for phaeochromocytoma in a twin gestation. J Obstet Gynaecol 32(2):186, 2012

Mountford PJ: Risk assessment of the nuclear medicine patient. Br J Radiol 100:671, 1997

Mullins JK, Semins MJ, Hayams ES, et al: Half Fourier single-shot turbo-echo magnetic resonance urography for the evaluation of suspected renal colic in pregnancy. Urology 79(6):1252, 2012

National Council on Radiation Protection and Measurements: Medical X-ray, electron beam and gamma-ray protection for energies up to 50 MeV. Report No. 102, Bethesda, 1989

National Research Council: Health effects of exposure to low levels of ionizing radiation BEIR V. Committee on the Biological Effects of Ionizing Radiations. Board on Radiation Effects Research Commission on Life Sciences. National Academy Press, Washington, 1990

National Research Council: Health risks from exposure to low levels of ionizing radiation BEIR VII Phase 2. Committee to assess health risks from exposure to low levels of ionizing radiation. Board on Radiation Effects Research Division on Earth and Life Studies. National Academies Press, Washington, 2006

Newman EA, Newman LA: Lymphatic mapping techniques and sentinel lymph node biopsy in breast cancer. Surg Clin North Am 87:353, 2007

Nuyttens JJ, Prado KL, Jenrette JM, et al: Fetal dose during radiotherapy: clinical implementation and review of the literature. Cancer Radiother 6:352, 2002

O'Rourke N, Kodali BS: Laparoscopic surgery during pregnancy. Curr Opin Anaesthesiol 19:254, 2006

Otake M, Yoshimaru H, Schull WJ: Severe mental retardation among the prenatally exposed survivors of the atomic bombing of Hiroshima and Nagasaki: a comparison of the old and new dosimetry systems. Radiation Effects Research Foundation, Technical Report No. 16–87, 1987

Oto A, Ernst R, Jesse MK, et al: Magnetic resonance imaging of the chest, abdomen, and pelvis in the evaluation of pregnant patients with neoplasms. Am J Perinatol 24:243, 2007

Pearl J, Price R, Richardson W, et al: Guidelines for diagnosis, treatment, and use of laparoscopy for surgical problems during pregnancy. Surg Endosc 25(11):3479, 2011

Pedrosa I, Lafornara M, Pandharipande PV, et al: Pregnant patients suspected of having acute appendicitis: effect of MR imaging on negative laparotomy rate and appendiceal rate. Radiology 250(3):749, 2009

Pedrosa I, Zeikus EA, Deborah L, et al: MR imaging of acute right lower quadrant pain in pregnant and nonpregnant patients. RadioGraphics 27:721, 2007

Phupong V, Bunyavejchewin S: Gasless laparoscopic surgery for ovarian cyst in a second trimester pregnant patient with a ventricular septal defect. Surg Laparosc Endosc Percutan Tech 17:565, 2007

Prado KL, Nelson SJ, Nuyttens JJ, et al: Clinical implementation of the AAPM Task Group 36 recommendations on fetal dose from radiotherapy with photon beams: a head and neck irradiation case report. J Appl Clin Med Phys 1:1–7, 2000

Preston DL, Cullings H, Suyama A, et al: Solid cancer incidence in atomic bomb survivors exposed in utero or as young children. J Natl Cancer Inst 100:428, 2008

Reedy MB, Galan HL, Bean-Lijewski JD, et al: Maternal and fetal effects of laparoscopic insufflation in the gravid baboon. J Am Assoc Gynecol Laparosc 2:399, 1995

Reedy MB, Källén B, Kuehl TJ: Laparoscopy during pregnancy: a study of five fetal outcome parameters with use of the Swedish Health Registry. Am J Obstet Gynecol 177:673, 1997

Reichel TF, Ramus RM, Caire JT, et al: Fetal central nervous system biometry on MR imaging. AJR Am J Roentgenol 180:1155, 2003

Reynolds JD, Booth JV, de la Fuente S, et al: A review of laparoscopy for nonobstetric-related surgery during pregnancy. Curr Surg 60:164, 2003

Ribic-Pucelj M, Kobal B, Peternelj-Marinsek S: Surgical treatment of adnexal masses in pregnancy: indications, surgical approach and pregnancy outcome. J Reprod Med 52:273, 2007

Rollins MD, Chan KJ, Price RR: Laparoscopy for appendicitis and cholelithiasis during pregnancy. Surg Endosc 18:237, 2004

Rosenstein M: Handbook of selected tissue doses for projections common in diagnostic radiology. Rockville, MD, Department of Health and Human Services, Food and Drug Administration. DHHS Pub No. (FDA) 89:8031, 1988

Rowley KA, Hill SJ, Watkins RA, et al: An investigation into the levels of radiation exposure in diagnostic examinations involving fluoroscopy. Br J Radiol 60:167, 1987

Sandrasegaran K, Lall CG, Aisen AA: Fetal magnetic resonance imaging. Curr Opin Obstet Gynecol 18:605, 2006

Schwartz JL, Mozurkewich EL, Johnson TM: Current management of patients with melanoma who are pregnant, want to get pregnant, or do not want to get pregnant. Cancer 97:2130, 2003

Silvestri MT, Pettker CM, Brousseau EC, et al: Morbidity of appendectomy and cholecystectomy in pregnant and nonpregnant women. Obstet Gynecol 118(6):1261, 2011

Sorahan T, Lancashire RJ, Temperton DH, et al: Childhood cancer and paternal exposure to ionizing radiation: a second report from the Oxford Survey of Childhood Cancers. Am J Ind Med 28(1):71, 1995

Spanheimer PM, Graham MM, Sugg SL, et al: Measurement of uterine radiation exposure from lymphoscintigraphy indicates safety of sentinel lymph node biopsy during pregnancy. Ann Surg Oncol 16(5):1143, 2009

Stather JW, Phipps AW, Harrison JD, et al: Dose coefficients for the embryo and fetus following intakes of radionuclides by the mother. J Radiol Prot 22:1, 2002

Stein, PD, Woodard PK, Weg JG, et al: Diagnostic pathways in acute pulmonary embolism: recommendations of the PIOPED II investigators. Radiology 242(1):15, 2007

Steinbrook RA, Bhavani-Shankar K: Hemodynamics during laparoscopic surgery in pregnancy. Anesth Analg 93:1570, 2001

Stepp K, Falcone T: Laparoscopy in the second trimester of pregnancy. Obstet Gynecol Clin North Am 31:485, 2004

Stovall M, Blackwell CR, Cundif J, et al: Fetal dose from radiotherapy with photon beams: report of AAPM Radiation Therapy Committee Task Group No. 36. Med Phys 22:63, 1995

Stroup SP, Altamar HO, L'Esperance JO, et al: Retroperitoneoscopic radical nephrectomy for renal-cell carcinoma during twin pregnancy. J Endourol 21:735, 2007

Strzelczyk, J, Damilakis J, Marx MV, et al: Facts and controversies about radiation exposure, part 2: low-level exposures and cancer risk. J Am Coll Radiol 4:32, 2007

Suleiman OH, Anderson J, Jones B, et al: Tissue doses in the upper gastrointestinal examination. Radiology 178(3):653, 1991

Tica AA, Tica OS, Saftoiu A, et al: Large pancreatic mucinous cystic neoplasm during pregnancy: what should be done? Gynecol Obstet Invest 75(2):132, 2013

Twickler DM, Cunningham FG: Central nervous system findings in preeclampsia and eclampsia. In Lyall F, Belfort M (eds): Pre-eclampsia—Etiology, and Clinical Practice. Cambridge, Cambridge University Press, 2007, p 424

Twickler DM, Reichel T, McIntire DD, et al: Fetal central nervous system ventricle and cisterna magna measurements by magnetic resonance imaging. Am J Obstet Gynecol 187:927, 2002

Twickler DM, Setiawan AT, Evans R, et al: Imaging of puerperal septic thrombophlebitis: a prospective comparison of MR imaging, CT, and sonography. AJR Am J Roentgenol 169:1039, 1997

Vadeyar SH, Moore RJ, Strachan BK, et al: Effect of fetal magnetic resonance imaging on fetal heart rate patterns. Am J Obstet Gynecol 182:666, 2000

Vilos GA, Ternamian A, Dempster J, et al: Laparoscopic entry: a review of techniques, technologies, and complications. J Obstet Gynaecol Can 29:433, 2007

Wagner LK, Lester RG, Saldana LR: Exposure of the Pregnant Patient to Diagnostic Radiation. Philadelphia, Medical Physics Publishing, 1997

Wang L, Yu JM, Wang YS, et al: Preoperative lymphoscintigraphy predicts the successful identification but is not necessary in sentinel lymph nodes biopsy in breast cancer. Ann Surg Oncol 14(8):2215, 2007

Wang PI, Chong ST, Kielar AZ, et al: Imaging of pregnant and lactating patients: part 1, evidence-based review and recommendations. AJR Am J Roentgenol 198 (4):778, 2012

Weisz B, Hoffman C, Chayenn B, et al: Diffusion MRI findings in monochorionic twin pregnancies after intrauterine fetal death. Abstract No. 399 Presented at the 29th Annual Meeting of the Society for Maternal-Fetal Medicine. 26–31 January 2009

White WM, Zite NB, Gash J, et al: Low-dose computer tomography for the evaluation of flank pain in the pregnant population. J Endourol 21:1255, 2007

Wo JY, Viswanathan AN: Impact of radiotherapy on fertility, pregnancy, and neonatal outcomes in female cancer patients. Int J Radiat Oncol Biol Phys 73(5):1304, 2009

Wortman A, Miller DL, Donahue TF, et al: Embolization of renal hemorrhage in pregnancy. Obstet Gynecol 121(Pt 2 Suppl 1):480, 2013

Zanzonico PB: Internal radionuclide radiation dosimetry: a review of basic concepts and recent developments. J Nucl Med 41:297, 2000

Zaretsky M, McIntire D, Twickler DM: Feasibility of the fetal anatomic and maternal pelvic survey by magnetic resonance imaging at term. Am J Obstet Gynecol 189:997, 2003a

Zaretsky M, Reichel TF, McIntire DD, et al: Comparison of magnetic resonance imaging to ultrasound in the estimation of birth weight at term. Am J Obstet Gynecol 189:1017, 2003b

Zeeman GG, Cipolla MJ, Cunningham FG: Cerebrovascular (patho)physiology in preeclampsia. In Lindheimer MD, Roberts JM, Cunningham FG (eds): Chesley's Hypertensive Disorders in Pregnancy, 3rd ed. New York, Elsevier, 2009, p 229

Zeeman GG, Fleckenstein JL, Twickler DM, et al: Cerebral infarction in eclampsia. Am J Obstet Gynecol 190:714, 2004a

Zeeman G, Hatab M, Twickler D: Increased large vessel cerebral blood flow in severe preeclampsia by magnetic resonance evaluation. Am J Obstet Gynecol 191:2148, 2004b

Zeeman GG, Hatab M, Twickler D: Maternal cerebral blood flow changes in pregnancy. Am J Obstet Gynecol 189:968, 2003

CHAPTER 47

Critical Care and Trauma

An endless number of medical, surgical, and obstetrical complications may be encountered in pregnancy or the puerperium. Those that are more complex and life threatening can be particularly challenging, especially when a multidisciplinary team is necessary for optimal care. It is axiomatic that obstetricians and other members of the health-care team have a working knowledge of the unique considerations for pregnant women. Some of those discussed in Chapter 46 include pregnancy-induced physiological changes, alterations in normal laboratory values, and finally and importantly, consideration for the second patient—the fetus. Because these severely ill women are usually young and in good health, their prognosis is generally better than that of many other patients admitted to intensive care units.

OBSTETRICAL INTENSIVE CARE

In the United States each year, 1 to 3 percent of pregnant women require critical care services, and the risk of death during such admission ranges from 2 to 11 percent (American Academy of Pediatrics and the American College of Obstetricians and Gynecologists, 2012). Those with pregnancy-associated complications—especially hemorrhage and hypertension—have the greatest need for intensive care (Baskett, 2009; Kuklina, 2009; Madan, 2008). That said, many antepartum admissions are for nonobstetrical reasons, and in our experiences from Parkland Hospital, these include diabetes, pneumonia or asthma, heart disease, chronic hypertension, pyelonephritis, or thyrotoxicosis (Zeeman, 2006). In addition to antenatal treatment, intrapartum and postpartum critical care for hypertensive disorders, hemorrhage, sepsis, or cardiopulmonary complications may be required for many. In instances of life-threatening hemorrhage, surgical procedures may be necessary, and close proximity to a delivery-operating room is paramount. For women who are undelivered, fetal well-being is also better served by this close proximity.

Organization of Critical Care

The concept and development of critical care for all aspects of medicine and surgery began in the 1960s. The National Institutes of Health held a Consensus Conference (1983) and the Society of Critical Care Medicine (1988, 1999) subsequently established guidelines for intensive care units (ICUs). Especially pertinent to obstetrics, costly ICUs prompted evolution of a step-down *intermediate care unit.* These units were designed for patients who did not require intensive care, but who needed a higher level of care than that provided on a general ward. The American College of Critical Care Medicine and the Society of Critical Care Medicine (1998) published guidelines for these units (Table 47-1).

Obstetrical Critical Care

Although the evolution of critical care for obstetrical patients has generally followed developments described above, there are no specific guidelines. Most hospitals employ a blend of these concepts, and in general, units can be divided into three types.

1. Medical or Surgical ICU—in most hospitals, severely ill women are transferred to a unit operated by medical and

TABLE 47-1. Guidelines for Conditions That Could Qualify for Intermediate Care

Cardiac: evaluation for possible infarction, stable infarction, stable arrhythmias, mild-to-moderate congestive heart failure, hypertensive urgency without end-organ damage
Pulmonary: stable patients for weaning and chronic ventilation, patients with potential for respiratory failure who are otherwise stable
Neurological: stable central nervous system, neuromuscular, or neurosurgical conditions that require close monitoring
Drug overdose: hemodynamically stable
Gastrointestinal: stable bleeding, liver failure with stable vital signs
Endocrine: diabetic ketoacidosis, thyrotoxicosis that requires frequent monitoring
Surgical: postoperative from major procedures or complications that require close monitoring
Miscellaneous: early sepsis, patients who require closely titrated intravenous fluids, pregnant women with severe preeclampsia or other medical problems

From Nasraway, 1998.

TABLE 47-2. Comparison of Acuity of Patient Mix for Obstetrical Critical Care Shown in Percent

Factor	Intermediate Care Unit (n = 483)[a]	Medical-Surgical ICU (n = 564)[b]
Stage		
Antepartum	20	30
Postpartum	80	70
Indication[c]		
Hypertension	45	40
Hemorrhage	18	19
Cardiopulmonary	12	18
Sepsis	5	9
Pregnancy-Related Mortality	0.2	7

[a]Data from Zeeman, 2003.
[b]Data from Baskett, 2009; Keizer, 2006; Small, 2012; Stevens, 2006; Vasquez, 2007.
[c]Columns of indications do not total 100 percent because some diagnoses are not listed.

surgical "intensivists." Admissions or transfers to these units are situation-specific and based on the acuity of care needed and on the ability of the facility to provide it. For example, in most institutions, pregnant women who require ventilatory support, invasive monitoring, or pharmacological support of circulation are transferred to an ICU. Another example is the neurological ICU (Sheth, 2012). A review of more than 25 tertiary-care referral institutions indicated that approximately 0.5 percent of obstetrical patients are transferred to these types of ICUs (Zeeman, 2006).

2. Obstetrical Intermediate Care Unit—sometimes referred to as a High-Dependency Care Unit (HDU)—an example of this system is the one at Parkland Hospital. Located within the labor and delivery unit, it has designated rooms and experienced personnel. The two-tiered system incorporates the guidelines for intermediate and intensive care. Care is provided by maternal-fetal medicine specialists and nurses with experience in critical care obstetrics. As needed, this team is expanded to include other obstetricians and anesthesiologists, gynecological oncologists, pulmonologists, cardiologists, surgeons, and other medical and surgical subspecialists. Many tertiary-care centers have developed similar intermediate care units and use selected triage to ICUs. Guidelines for such transfers must follow the federal Emergency Medical Treatment and Labor Act (EMTALA) guidelines. According to the American Academy of Pediatrics and the American College of Obstetricians and Gynecologists (2012), the minimal monitoring required for a critically ill patient during transport includes continuous pulse oximetry, electrocardiography, and regular assessment of vital signs. All critically ill patients must have secure venous access before transfer. Those who are mechanically ventilated must have their endotracheal tube position confirmed and secured before transfer. Left uterine displacement and supplemental oxygen should be applied routinely during transport of antepartum patients. The utility of continuous fetal heart rate or tocodynamic monitoring is unproven, therefore, its use should be individualized.
3. Obstetrical Intensive Care Unit—these units are full-care ICUs as described above, but are operated by obstetrical and anesthesia personnel in the labor and delivery unit. Very few units have these capabilities (Zeeman, 2003, 2006).

For smaller hospitals, transfer to a medical or surgical ICU may be preferable, and sometimes transfer to another hospital is necessary. As discussed, indications for admission to these various types of critical care units are highly variable. Shown in Table 47-2 are some examples. The American College of Obstetricians and Gynecologists (2011a) has summarized critical obstetrical care implementation depending on hospital size and technical facilities. Somewhat related, the concept has been explored of a *medical emergency team—MET*—for rapid response to emergent obstetrical situations (Gosman, 2008).

Pulmonary Artery Catheter

Data obtained during pregnancy with the pulmonary artery catheter (PAC) have contributed immensely to the understanding of normal pregnancy hemodynamics and pathophysiology of common obstetrical conditions. These include preeclampsia-eclampsia, acute respiratory distress syndrome

(ARDS), and amnionic-fluid embolism (Clark, 1988, 1995, 1997; Cunningham, 1986, 1987; Hankins, 1984, 1985). Because of these studies, most have concluded that such monitoring is seldom necessary (American College of Obstetricians and Gynecologists, 2013; Dennis, 2012).

In nonobstetrical patients, randomized trials of nearly 5000 subjects have shown no benefits with pulmonary artery catheter monitoring (Harvey, 2005; Richard, 2003; Sandham, 2003). A randomized trial by the National Heart, Lung, and Blood Institute (2006b) assessed catheter-guided therapy in 1000 patients with ARDS. Invasive monitoring did not improve outcomes and had more complications. According to a recent Cochrane Database review, there have been no randomized trials using this for preeclampsia management (Li, 2012). Overall mechanisms, benefits, and risks were reviewed by Vincent (2011).

Hemodynamic Changes in Pregnancy

Formulas for deriving some hemodynamic parameters are shown in Table 47-3. These measurements can be corrected for body size by dividing by body surface area (BSA) to obtain *index values*. Normal values for nonpregnant adults are used but with the caveat that these may not necessarily reflect changes induced by more "passive" uteroplacental perfusion (Van Hook, 1997).

In a landmark investigation, Clark and colleagues (1989) used pulmonary artery catheterization to obtain cardiovascular measurements in healthy pregnant women and again in these same women when nonpregnant. These values are shown in Chapter 4 (Table 4-4, p. 60) and are also plotted on a *ventricular function curve* (Fig. 4-9, p. 59). Because increased blood volume and cardiac output are compensated by decreased vascular resistance and increased pulse rate, ventricular performance remains within the normal range at term. A working knowledge of these changes is paramount to understanding the pathophysiology of pregnancy complications discussed later in this chapter and throughout the book.

ACUTE PULMONARY EDEMA

The incidence of pulmonary edema complicating pregnancy averages 1 in 500 to 1000 deliveries at tertiary referral centers. The two general causes are: (1) *cardiogenic*—hydrostatic edema caused by high pulmonary capillary hydraulic pressures and (2) *noncardiogenic*—permeability edema caused by capillary endothelial and alveolar epithelial damage. In pregnancy, noncardiogenic pulmonary edema is more common. Taken in toto, studies in pregnant women indicate that more than half who develop pulmonary edema have some degree of sepsis syndrome in conjunction with tocolysis, severe preeclampsia, or obstetrical hemorrhage combined with vigorous fluid therapy (Thornton, 2011). To categorize these differences, Dennis and Solnordal (2012) proposed a classification to include those women who are normotensive or hypotensive versus those with hypertension.

Although cardiogenic pulmonary edema is less frequent, common precipitating causes include resuscitation for hemorrhage and vigorous treatment of preterm labor. The causes in 51 women with pulmonary edema were cardiac failure, tocolytic therapy, iatrogenic fluid overload, or preeclampsia, approximately a fourth each (Sciscione, 2003). In another study, more than half of cases were associated with preeclampsia, and there was equal distribution of the other three causes (Hough, 2007). Although used less commonly today, tocolytic therapy with β-mimetic drugs at one time was the cause of up to 40 percent of pulmonary edema cases (DiFederico, 1998; Jenkins, 2003).

Noncardiogenic Increased Permeability Edema

Endothelial activation is the common denominator that is associated with preeclampsia, sepsis syndrome, and acute hemorrhage—or frequently combinations thereof—and they are the most common predisposing factors to pulmonary edema (Table 47-4). As discussed, these clinical scenarios are often

TABLE 47-3. Formulas for Deriving Various Cardiopulmonary Parameters

Mean arterial pressure (MAP) (mm Hg) = [SBP + 2 (DBP)] ÷ 3
Cardiac output (CO) (L/min) = heart rate × stroke volume
Stroke volume (SV) (mL/beat) = CO/HR
Stroke index (SI) (mL/beat/m^2) = stroke volume/BSA
Cardiac index (CI) (L/min/m^2) = CO/BSA
Systemic vascular resistance (SVR) (dynes × sec × cm^{-5}) = [(MAP − CVP)/CO] × 80
Pulmonary vascular resistance (PVR) (dynes × sec × cm^{-5}) = [(MPAP − PCWP)/CO] × 80

BSA = body surface area (m^2); CO = cardiac output (L/min); CVP = central venous pressure (mm Hg); DBP = diastolic blood pressure; HR = heart rate (beats/min); MAP = mean systemic arterial pressure (mm Hg); MPAP = mean pulmonary artery pressure (mm Hg); PCWP = pulmonary capillary wedge pressure (mm Hg); SBP = systolic blood pressure.

TABLE 47-4. Some Causes and Associated Factors for Pulmonary Edema in Pregnancy

Noncardiogenic permeability edema—endothelial activation with capillary-alveolar leakage:
- Preeclampsia syndrome
- Acute hemorrhage
- Sepsis syndrome
- Tocolytic therapy—β-mimetics, $MgSO_4$
- Aspiration pneumonitis
- Vigorous intravenous fluid therapy

Cardiogenic pulmonary edema—myocardial failure with hydrostatic edema from excessive pulmonary capillary pressure:
- Hypertensive cardiomyopathy
- Obesity—adipositas cordis
- Left-sided valvular disease
- Vigorous intravenous fluid therapy

associated with corticosteroids given to hasten fetal lung maturation along with vigorous fluid replacement and tocolytic therapy (Thornton, 2011). Although parenteral β-agonists are undisputedly linked to pulmonary edema, indictment of magnesium sulfate is less convincing. In one study in which pulmonary edema developed in 8 percent of nearly 800 women given magnesium sulfate for preterm labor, half of these were also given terbutaline (Samol, 2005). In our extensive experiences at Parkland Hospital with the use of magnesium sulfate for neuroprophylaxis for severe preeclampsia, we remain dubious that magnesium per se causes pulmonary edema. Similar conclusions were reached following a review by Martin and Foley (2006).

Cardiogenic Hydrostatic Edema

Ventricular failure causing pulmonary edema in pregnancy is usually associated with some form of gestational hypertension. Although it can be due to congenital or acquired anatomical defects, diastolic dysfunction is frequently from chronic hypertension, obesity, or both (Jessup, 2003; Kenchaiah, 2002). In these women, acute systolic hypertension exacerbates diastolic dysfunction and causes pulmonary edema (Dennis, 2012; Gandhi, 2001). Of note, concentric and eccentric hypertrophy is two- to threefold more common in black women compared with white women (Drazner, 2005).

Despite an underlying cardiomyopathy, heart failure is commonly precipitated by preeclampsia, hypertension, hemorrhage and anemia, and puerperal sepsis (Cunningham, 1986; Sibai, 1987). In many of these, when echocardiography is done later, systolic function is normal as measured by ejection fraction, but evidence for diastolic dysfunction can often be found (Aurigemma, 2004). The use of *brain natriuretic peptide (BNP)* has not been evaluated extensively in pregnancy (Chap. 4, p. 61 and Appendix, p. 1291). This neurohormone is secreted from ventricle myocytes and fibroblasts with distention seen in heart failure. In nonpregnant patients, values < 100 pg/mL have an excellent negative-predictive value, and levels > 500 pg/mL have an excellent positive-predictive value. It is problematic that levels frequently are 100 to 500 pg/mL, and thus nondiagnostic (Ware, 2005). Values for N-terminal BNP and atrial natriuretic peptide (ANP) are both elevated with preeclampsia (Tihtonen, 2007).

Management

Acute pulmonary edema requires emergency management. Furosemide is given in 20- to 40-mg intravenous doses along with therapy to control dangerous hypertension. Further treatment depends on whether a woman is ante- or postpartum and whether the fetus is alive or not. A live fetus prohibits the use of cardioactive drugs that might lower peripheral resistance and in turn severely diminish uteroplacental circulation. The cause of cardiogenic failure is determined by echocardiography, which will help direct further therapy. Acute pulmonary edema is not, per se, an indication for emergency cesarean delivery. Indeed, in most cases, these women are better served by vaginal delivery.

ACUTE RESPIRATORY DISTRESS SYNDROME

Acute lung injury that causes a form of severe permeability pulmonary edema and respiratory failure is termed acute respiratory distress syndrome (ARDS). This is a pathophysiological continuum from mild pulmonary insufficiency to dependence on high inspired oxygen concentrations and mechanical ventilation. Because there are no uniform criteria for its diagnosis, the incidence is variably reported. One review computed it to be 1 in 3000 to 6000 deliveries, and this comports with our experiences at Parkland Hospital (Catanzarite, 2001). In its most extreme form requiring ventilatory support, there is an associated mortality rate of 45 percent. This rate can be as high as 90 percent if caused or complicated by sepsis (Phua, 2009). Although they are younger and usually healthier than the overall population, pregnant women still have mortality rates of 25 to 40 percent (Catanzarite, 2001; Cole, 2005). Finally, if ARDS develops antepartum, there is a correspondingly high perinatal mortality rate.

Definitions

Physiological criteria required for diagnosis of acute respiratory distress syndrome are study dependent. In general, less precise terms are used for clinical care. Most investigators have defined ARDS as radiographically documented pulmonary infiltrates, a ratio of arterial oxygen tension to the fraction of inspired oxygen (Pao_2:Fio_2) < 200, and no evidence of heart failure (Mallampalli, 2010). Recently, the international consensus-revised *Berlin Definition* was reported by the ARDS Definition Task Force (2012). It describes categories of mild (200 mm Hg < $Pao_2/Fio_2 \leq$ 300 mm Hg); moderate (100 mm Hg < $Pao_2/Fio_2 \leq$ 200 mm Hg); and severe ($Pao_2/Fio_2 \leq$ 100 mm Hg). To date, for most interventional studies, however, a working diagnosis of *acute lung injury* is made when the Pao_2:Fio_2 ratio is < 300 along with dyspnea, tachypnea, oxygen desaturation, and radiographic pulmonary infiltrates (Wheeler, 2007).

Etiopathogenesis

ARDS is a pathophysiological description that begins with acute lung injury from various causes. Several disorders have been implicated as causes of acute pulmonary injury and permeability edema during pregnancy (Table 47-5). Although many are coincidental, some are more common in pregnant women. For example, in nonpregnant patients, sepsis and diffuse infectious pneumonia are the two most common single-agent causes and together account for 60 percent of cases. In pregnancy, however, pyelonephritis, chorioamnionitis, and puerperal pelvic infection are the most frequent causes of sepsis. As discussed previously, severe preeclampsia and obstetrical hemorrhage are also commonly associated with permeability edema. Importantly, more than half of pregnant women with acute respiratory distress syndrome have some combination of sepsis, shock, trauma, and fluid overload. With acute hemorrhage, the contribution of *transfusion-related acute lung injury (TRALI)* is unclear in obstetrical patients (Kopko, 2002). This entity is discussed further in Chapter 41 (p. 818).

TABLE 47-5. Some Causes of Acute Lung Injury and Respiratory Failure in Pregnant Women

Pneumonia—bacterial, viral, aspiration
Sepsis syndrome—chorioamnionitis, pyelonephritis, puerperal infection, septic abortion
Hemorrhage—shock, massive transfusion, transfusion-related acute lung injury (TRALI)
Preeclampsia syndrome
Tocolytic therapy
Embolism—amnionic fluid, trophoblastic disease, air, fat
Connective-tissue disease
Substance abuse
Irritant inhalation and burns
Pancreatitis
Drug overdose
Fetal surgery
Trauma
Sickle-cell disease
Miliary tuberculosis

From Catanzarite, 2001; Cole, 2005; Golombeck, 2006; Jenkins, 2003; Lapinsky, 2005; Martin, 2006; Oram, 2007; Sheffield, 2005; Sibai, 2014; Zeeman, 2003, 2006.

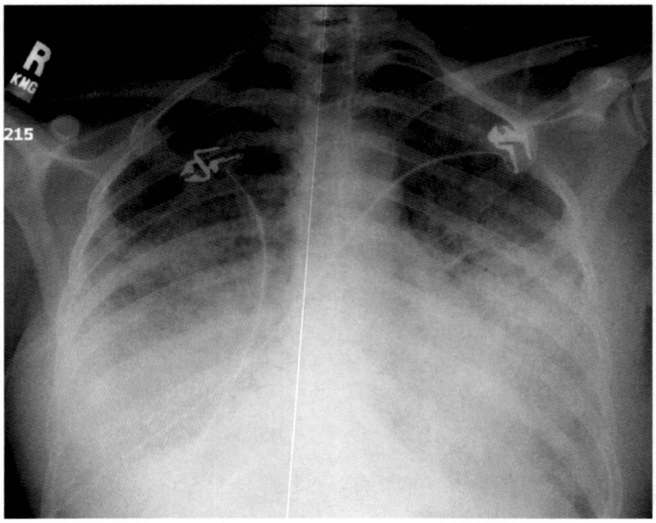

FIGURE 47-1 Anteroposterior chest radiograph of a second-trimester pregnant woman with marked bilateral parenchymal and pleural opacification secondary to acute respiratory distress syndrome (ARDS).

Endothelial injury in the lung capillaries releases cytokines that recruit neutrophils to the site of inflammation. Here, they elaborate more cytokines to worsen tissue injury. There are three stages of ARDS development. First, the *exudative phase* follows widespread injury to microvascular endothelium, including the pulmonary vasculature, and there is also alveolar epithelial injury. These result in increased pulmonary capillary permeability, surfactant loss or inactivation, diminished lung volume, and vascular shunting with resultant arterial hypoxemia. Next, the *fibroproliferative phase* usually begins 3 to 4 days later and lasts up to day 21. Last, the *fibrotic phase* results from healing, and despite this, the long-term prognosis for pulmonary function is surprisingly good (Herridge, 2003; Levy, 2012).

Clinical Course

With pulmonary injury, the clinical condition depends largely on the insult magnitude, the ability to compensate for it, and the disease stage. For example, soon after the initial injury, there commonly are no physical findings except perhaps hyperventilation. And at first, arterial oxygenation usually is adequate. Pregnancy-induced mild metabolic alkalosis may be accentuated by hyperventilation. With worsening, clinical and radiological evidence for pulmonary edema, decreased lung compliance, and increased intrapulmonary blood shunting become apparent. Progressive alveolar and interstitial edema develop with extravasation of inflammatory cells and erythrocytes.

Ideally, pulmonary injury is identified at this early stage, and specific therapy is directed at the insult if possible. Further progression to acute respiratory failure is characterized by marked dyspnea, tachypnea, and hypoxemia. Additional lung volume loss results in worsening of pulmonary compliance and increased shunting. There are now diffuse abnormalities by auscultation, and a chest radiograph characteristically demonstrates bilateral lung involvement (Fig. 47-1). At this phase, the injury ordinarily would be lethal in the absence of high inspired-oxygen concentrations and positive airway pressure by mask or by intubation. When shunting exceeds 30 percent, severe refractory hypoxemia develops along with metabolic and respiratory acidosis that can result in myocardial irritability, dysfunction, and cardiac arrest.

Management

In cases of severe acute lung injury, attempts are made to provide adequate oxygenation of peripheral tissues while ensuring that therapeutic maneuvers do not further aggravate lung injury. At least intuitively, increasing oxygen delivery should produce a corresponding increase in tissue uptake, but this is difficult to measure (Evans, 1999). Support of systemic perfusion with intravenous crystalloid and blood is imperative. As discussed on page 941, the trial conducted by the National Heart, Lung, and Blood Institute (2006b) showed that pulmonary artery catheterization did not improve outcomes. Because sepsis is commonplace in lung injury, vigorous antimicrobial therapy is given for infection, along with debridement of necrotic tissues. Oxygen delivery can be greatly improved by correction of anemia—each gram of hemoglobin carries 1.25 mL of oxygen when 90-percent saturated. By comparison, increasing the arterial Po_2 from 100 to 200 mm Hg results in the transport of only 0.1 mL of additional oxygen for each 100 mL of blood.

Reasonable goals in caring for the woman with severe lung injury are to attain a Pao_2 of 60 mm Hg or 90-percent saturation at an inspired oxygen content of < 50 percent and with positive end-expiratory pressures < 15 mm Hg. With regard to the pregnancy, it remains controversial whether delivery of the fetus improves maternal oxygenation (Cole, 2005; Mallampalli, 2010).

Mechanical Ventilation

Positive pressure ventilation by face mask may be effective in some women in early stages of pulmonary insufficiency (Roy, 2007). In an attempt to maximize the fetal environment, early intubation is preferred in the pregnant woman if respiratory failure is more likely than not, and especially if it appears imminent. There are many successful formulas for mechanical ventilation management (Levy, 2012). High-frequency oscillation ventilation (HFOV) has not been shown effective in ARDS (Ferguson, 2013; Slutsky, 2013; Young, 2013). Adjustments are made to obtain a $Pao_2 > 60$ mm Hg or a hemoglobin saturation of ≥ 90 percent and a $Paco_2$ of 35 to 45 mm Hg. Lower levels for Pao_2 should be avoided, because placental perfusion may be impaired (Levinson, 1974).

For women who require ventilation for any length of time, the maternal mortality rate is approximately 20 percent. In a study of 51 such women, of whom almost half had severe preeclampsia, most required intubation postpartum. Eleven were delivered while being ventilated, and another six were discharged undelivered (Jenkins, 2003). There were two maternal deaths, including a woman who died as a complication of tocolytic treatment. In two other reports, maternal mortality rates were 17 and 25 percent (Chen, 2003; Schneider, 2003). None of these investigators concluded that delivery improved maternal outcome.

Positive End-Expiratory Pressure. With severe lung injury and high intrapulmonary shunt fractions, it may not be possible to provide adequate oxygenation with usual ventilatory pressures, even with 100-percent oxygen. Positive end-expiratory pressure is usually successful in decreasing the shunt by recruiting collapsed alveoli. At low levels of 5 to 15 mm Hg, positive pressure can typically be used safely. At higher levels, impaired right-sided venous return can result in decreased cardiac output, decreased uteroplacental perfusion, alveolar overdistention, falling compliance, and barotrauma (Slutsky, 2013).

Extracorporeal Membrane Oxygenation

As discussed in Chapter 33 (p. 638), extracorporeal membrane oxygenation (ECMO) has been successfully used for neonatal meconium aspiration syndrome. Preliminary observation suggests that it may be useful in adults (Brodie, 2011; Levy, 2012; Peek, 2009). ECMO has been used in pregnant women. In one study, 12 women with influenza-induced lung failure were treated with ECMO, and of four maternal deaths, three were due to anticoagulation-related hemorrhage (Nair, 2011). In other reports, ECMO was used to allow time for lung healing in five pregnant women, and the duration of support in the four survivors was 2 to 28 days (Cunningham, 2006). Technical aspects of ECMO were recently reviewed by Brodie and Bacchetta (2011).

Fetal Oxygenation

The propensity of the hemoglobin molecule to release oxygen is described by the *oxyhemoglobin dissociation curve* (Fig. 47-2). For clinical purposes, the curve can be divided into an upper oxygen association curve representing the alveolar-capillary environment and a lower oxygen dissociation portion representing the tissue-capillary environment. Shifts of the curve have their greatest impact at the steep portion because they affect oxygen delivery. A rightward shift is associated with decreased hemoglobin affinity for oxygen and hence increased tissue-capillary oxygen interchange. Rightward shifts are produced by hypercapnia, metabolic acidosis, fever, and increased 2,3-diphosphoglycerate levels. During pregnancy, the erythrocyte concentration of 2,3-diphosphoglycerate is increased by approximately 30 percent. This favors oxygen delivery to both the fetus and maternal peripheral tissues (Rorth, 1971).

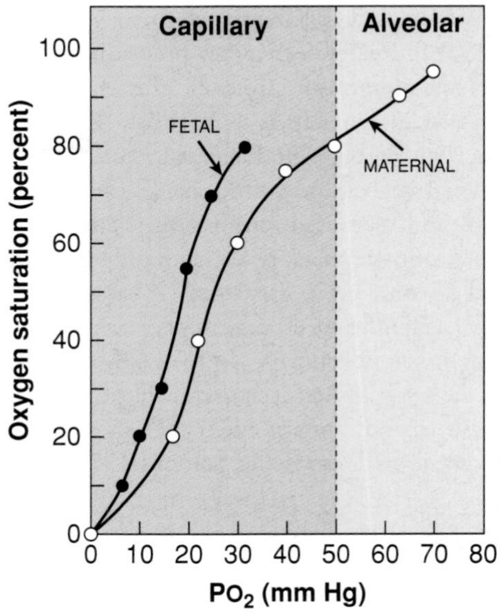

FIGURE 47-2 Oxyhemoglobin dissociation curve. With higher oxygen tension (Pao_2) in the pulmonary alveoli, adult hemoglobin is maximally saturated compared with that at the lower oxygen tension in the tissue capillaries. Note that at any given oxygen tension, fetal hemoglobin carries more oxygen than adult hemoglobin, as indicated by percent saturation.

Fetal hemoglobin has a higher oxygen affinity than adult hemoglobin. As seen in Figure 47-2, its curve is positioned to the left of the adult curve. To achieve 50-percent hemoglobin saturation in the mother, the Pao_2 must be 27 mm Hg compared with only 19 mm Hg in the fetus. Under normal physiological conditions, the fetus is constantly on the dissociation, or tissue, portion of the curve. Even with severe maternal lung disease and very low Pao_2 levels, oxygen displacement to fetal tissues is favored. Another example of this comes from pregnant women who live at high altitudes, where despite a maternal Pao_2 of only 60 mm Hg, the fetal Pao_2 is equivalent to that of fetuses at sea level (Subrevilla, 1971).

Intravenous Fluids

Although mortality outcomes are similar, conservative versus liberal fluid management is associated with fewer days of mechanical ventilation (Wiedemann, 2006). There are some pregnancy-induced physiological changes that predispose to a greater risk of permeability edema from vigorous fluid therapy. Colloid oncotic pressure (COP) is determined by serum albumin concentration—1 g/dL exerts approximately 6 mm Hg pressure. As discussed in Chapter 4 (p. 67), serum albumin concentrations normally decrease in pregnancy. This results in a decline in oncotic pressure from 28 mm Hg in the nonpregnant woman to 23 mm Hg at term and to 17 mm Hg in the puerperium (Benedetti, 1979; Dennis, 2012). With preeclampsia, endothelial activation with leakage causes extravascular albumin loss and decreased serum albumin levels. As a result in these cases, oncotic pressure averages only 16 mm Hg antepartum and 14 mm Hg postpartum (Zinaman, 1985). These changes have a significant clinical impact on the *colloid oncotic pressure/wedge pressure gradient.* Normally, this gradient exceeds 8 mm Hg, however, when it is 4 mm Hg or less, there is an increased risk for pulmonary edema. These associations were recently reviewed by Dennis and Solnordal (2012).

Other Therapy

There were no benefits from *artificial* or *replacement surfactant therapy* in 725 nonpregnant patients with sepsis-induced lung failure (Anzueto, 1996). Although inhalation of *nitric oxide* was found to cause early improvement, mortality rates were unchanged in two studies (Taylor, 2004; Wheeler, 2007). In a trial conducted by the National Heart, Lung, and Blood Institute (2006a), *prolonged methylprednisolone* therapy did not reduce mortality rates.

Long-Term Outcomes

There are no long-term follow-up studies of pregnant women who recover from respiratory distress syndrome. In nonpregnant subjects, there are significant risks for impaired global cognitive function at 3 and 12 months (Pandharipande, 2013). Data from nonpregnant patients indicate a 1- to 2-year hiatus before basic normal activity is restored in all. In a 5-year follow-up study, Herridge and associates (2011) reported normal lung function but significant exercise limitation, physical and psychological sequelae, decreased physical quality of life, and increased costs and use of health-care services.

SEPSIS SYNDROME

Sepsis is derived from the ancient Greek *sepein,* "to rot." The sepsis syndrome is induced by a systemic inflammatory response to bacteria or viruses or their by-products such as endotoxins or exotoxins. The severity of the syndrome is a continuum or spectrum (Fig. 47-3). Infections that most commonly cause the sepsis syndrome in obstetrics are pyelonephritis (Chap. 53, p. 1054), chorioamnionitis and puerperal sepsis (Chap. 37, p. 683), septic abortion (Chap. 18, p. 356), and necrotizing fasciitis (Chap. 37, p. 686). The mortality rate in nonpregnant patients is 20 to 35 percent with severe sepsis and 40 to 60 percent with septic shock (Angus, 2013; Munford, 2012). Mabie and coworkers (1997) reported a 28-percent mortality rate in 18 pregnant women with sepsis and shock. That said, the maternal mortality risk from sepsis is significantly underestimated (Acosta, 2013).

Etiopathogenesis

Most of what is known concerning sepsis pathogenesis comes from study of lipopolysaccharide—LPS or endotoxin (Munford, 2012). The lipid A moiety is bound by mononuclear blood cells, becomes internalized, and stimulates release of mediators and a series of complex downstream perturbations. Clinical aspects of the sepsis syndrome are manifest when cytokines are released that have endocrine, paracrine, and autocrine effects (Angus, 2013).

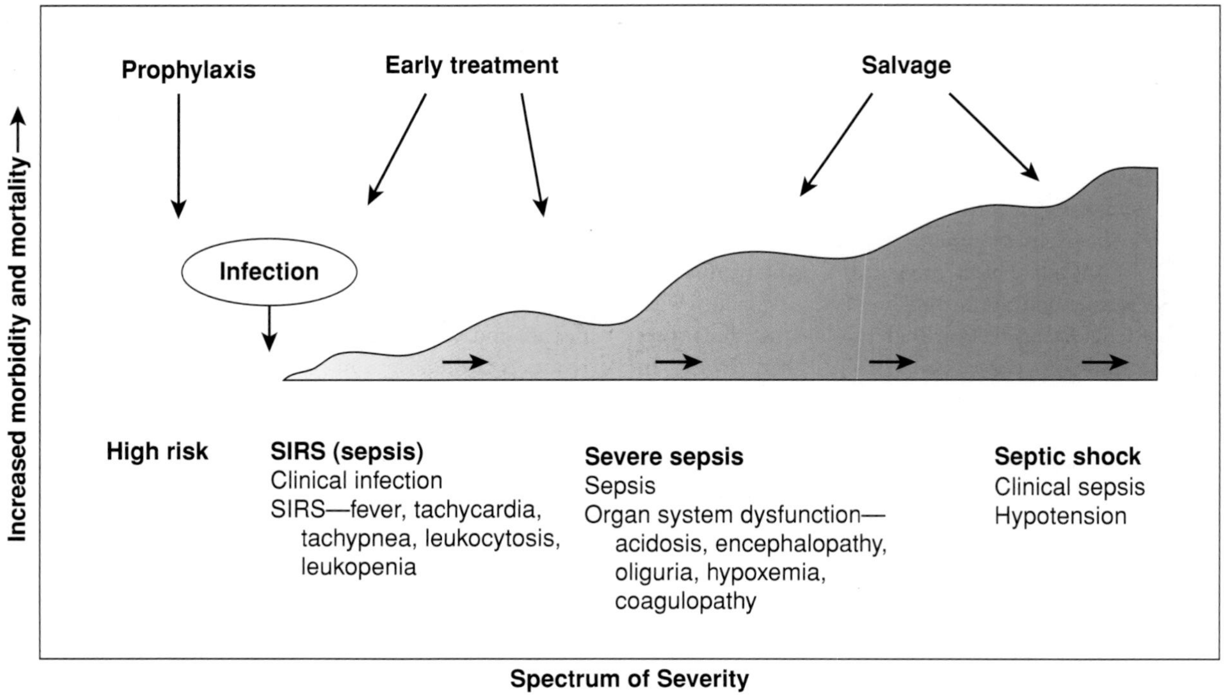

FIGURE 47-3 The sepsis syndrome begins with a systemic inflammatory response syndrome (SIRS) in response to infection that may progress to septic shock.

Although the sepsis syndrome in obstetrics may be caused by several pathogens, most cases represent a small group. For example, pyelonephritis complicating pregnancy caused by *Escherichia coli* and *Klebsiella* species commonly is associated with bacteremia and sepsis syndrome (Cunningham, 1987; Mabie, 1997). And although pelvic infections are usually polymicrobial, bacteria that cause severe sepsis syndrome are frequently endotoxin-producing Enterobacteriaceae, most commonly *E coli.* Other pelvic pathogens are aerobic and anaerobic streptococci, *Bacteroides* species, and *Clostridium* species. Some strains of group A β-hemolytic streptococci and *Staphylococcus aureus*—including community-acquired methicillin-resistant strains (CA-MRSA)—produce a superantigen that activates T cells to rapidly cause all features of the sepsis syndrome—*toxic shock syndrome* (Moellering, 2011; Soper, 2011). This is discussed further in Chapter 37 (p. 690).

There are also potent bacterial *exotoxins* that can cause severe sepsis syndrome. Examples include exotoxins from *Clostridium perfringens*, toxic-shock-syndrome toxin-1 (TSST-1) from *S aureus*, and toxic shock-like exotoxin from group A β-hemolytic streptococci (Daif, 2009; Soper, 2011). These last exotoxins cause rapid and extensive tissue necrosis and gangrene, especially of the postpartum uterus, and may cause profound cardiovascular collapse and maternal death (Nathan, 1993; Sugiyama, 2010). In a review discussed subsequently, the maternal mortality rate from these infections was 58 percent (Yamada, 2010).

Thus, the sepsis syndrome begins with an inflammatory response that is directed against microbial endotoxins and exotoxins (Angus, 2013). CD4 T cells and leukocytes are stimulated to produce proinflammatory compounds that include tumor necrosis factor-α (TNF-α), several interleukins, other cytokines, proteases, oxidants, and bradykinin that result in a "cytokine storm" (Que, 2005; Russell, 2006). Many other cellular reactions then follow that include stimulation of pro- and antiinflammatory compounds, procoagulant activity, gene activation, receptor regulation, and immune suppression (Filbin, 2009; Moellering, 2011). It is also likely that IL-6 mediates myocardial suppression (Pathan, 2004).

The pathophysiological response to this cascade is selective vasodilation with maldistribution of blood flow. Leukocyte and platelet aggregation cause capillary plugging. Worsening endothelial injury causes profound permeability capillary leakage and interstitial fluid accumulation (Fig. 47-4). Depending on the degree of injury and inflammatory response, there is a pathophysiological and clinical continuum as depicted in Figure 47-3. The clinical syndrome begins with subtle signs of sepsis from infection and terminates with *septic shock,* which is defined by hypotension unresponsive to intravenous hydration. In its early stages, clinical shock results primarily from decreased systemic vascular resistance that is not compensated fully by increased cardiac output. Hypoperfusion results in lactic acidosis, decreased tissue oxygen extraction, and end-organ dysfunction that includes acute lung and kidney injury.

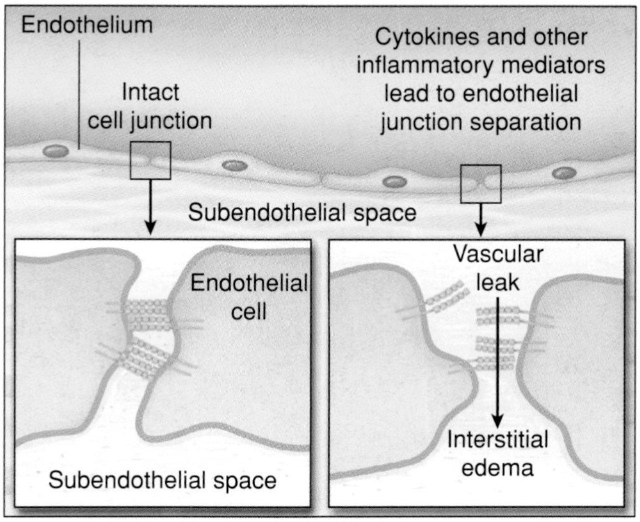

FIGURE 47-4 Endothelial permeability. The normal interendothelial interface is shown in the left inset. Cytokines and other inflammatory mediators disassemble the cellular junctions, resulting in microvascular leaks (*right*). (Modified from Lee, 2010.)

Clinical Manifestations

The sepsis syndrome has myriad clinical manifestations that, at least in part, are dependent on the specific invading microorganism and its particular endo- or exotoxins. Some of the general effects of LPS are as follows:

1. Central nervous system: confusion, somnolence, coma, combativeness, fever, or hypoxemia
2. Cardiovascular: tachycardia, hypotension
3. Pulmonary: tachypnea, arteriovenous shunting with dysoxia and hypoxemia, exudative infiltrates from endothelial-alveolar damage, pulmonary hypertension
4. Gastrointestinal: gastroenteritis—nausea, vomiting, and diarrhea; hepatocellular necrosis—jaundice, hyperglycemia
5. Renal: prerenal oliguria, acute kidney injury
6. Hematological: leukocytosis or leukopenia, thrombocytopenia, activation of coagulation with disseminated intravascular coagulation
7. Cutaneous: acrocyanosis, erythroderma, bullae, digital gangrene.

Thus, although capillary leakage initially causes hypovolemia, if intravenous crystalloid is given at this point, then sepsis hemodynamically can be described as a high cardiac output, low systemic vascular resistance condition (Fig. 47-5). Concomitantly, pulmonary hypertension develops, and despite the high cardiac output, severe sepsis likely also causes myocardial depression (Ognibene, 1988). This is often referred to as the *warm phase* of septic shock. These findings are the most common cardiovascular manifestations of early sepsis, but they can be accompanied by some of the other clinical or laboratory aberrations listed above.

The response to initial intravenous hydration may be prognostic. Most pregnant women who have early sepsis show a salutary response with crystalloid and antimicrobial therapy, and if indicated, debridement of infected tissue. Conversely, if hypotension is not corrected following vigorous fluid infusion, then the prognosis is more guarded. At this juncture, if there also is no response to β-adrenergic inotropic agents, this indicates severe and unresponsive extracellular fluid

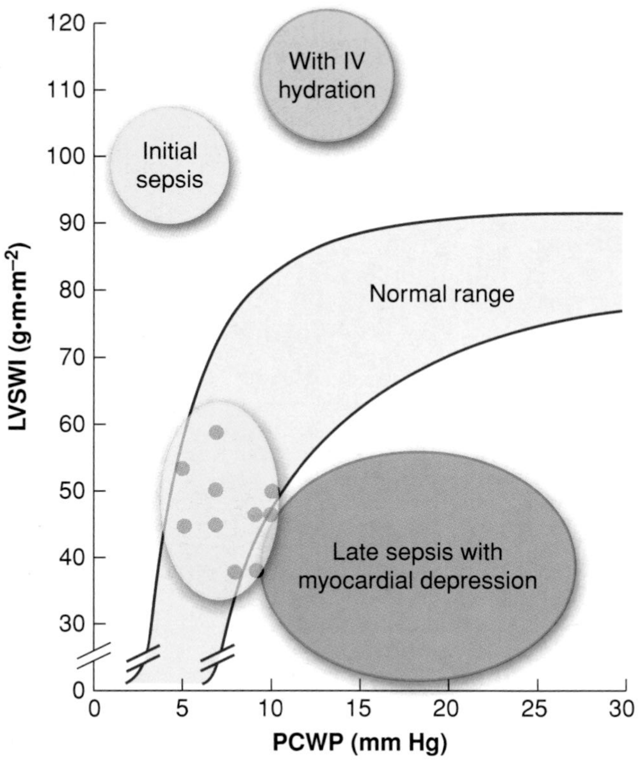

FIGURE 47-5 Hemodynamic effects of sepsis syndrome. Values for normal women at term are shown by dots. With early sepsis, there is high cardiac output and low vascular resistance. With fluid resuscitation, cardiac output increases even more, but so does capillary hydraulic pressure. With continued sepsis, there may be myocardial depression to further increase capillary hydraulic pressure. Decreased plasma oncotic pressure (serum albumin [g] × 6 mm Hg) contributes to interstitial lung fluid and endo/epithelial leak causes alveolar flooding. LVSWI = left ventricular stroke work index; PCWP = pulmonary capillary wedge pressure.

extravasation with vascular insufficiency, overwhelming myocardial depression, or both. Oliguria and continued peripheral vasoconstriction characterize a secondary, *cold phase* of septic shock that is rarely survived. Another poor prognostic sign is continued renal, pulmonary, and cerebral dysfunction once hypotension has been corrected (Angus, 2013). The average risk of death increases by 15 to 20 percent with failure of each organ system. With three systems, mortality rates are 70 percent (Martin, 2003; Wheeler, 1999).

Management

In 2004 an internationally directed consensus effort was launched as the *Surviving Sepsis Campaign* (Dellinger, 2008). The cornerstone of management is *early goal-directed management,* and it stresses prompt recognition of serious bacterial infection and close monitoring of vital signs and urine flow. Institution of this protocol has improved survival rates (Angus, 2013; Barochia, 2010).

An algorithm for management of sepsis syndrome is shown in Figure 47-6. The three basic steps are performed as simultaneously as possible and include evaluation of the sepsis source and its sequelae, cardiopulmonary function assessment, and immediate management. The most important step in sepsis management is rapid infusion of 2 L and sometimes as many as 4 to 6 L of crystalloid fluids to restore renal perfusion in severely affected women (Vincent, 2013). Simultaneously, appropriately chosen broad-spectrum antimicrobials are begun. There is hemoconcentration because of the capillary leak. Thus, if anemia coexists with severe sepsis, then blood is given along with crystalloid to maintain the hematocrit at approximately 30 percent (Munford, 2012; Rivers, 2001). The use of colloid solution such as hetastarch is controversial, and we as well as others do not recommend its use (Angus, 2013; Ware, 2000). Indeed, a recent Scandinavian randomized trial comparing hydroxyethyl starch and Ringer acetate reported a higher mortality rate with the starch solution (Perner, 2012). Another recent study found equivalent results with 6-percent hydroxyethyl starch compared with normal saline (Myburgh, 2012). In vasopressor-dependent shock, some recommend albumin infusions (Angus, 2013; Vincent, 2013).

Aggressive volume replacement ideally is promptly followed by urinary output of at least 30 and preferably 50 mL/hr, as well as other indicators of improved perfusion. If not, then consideration is given for vasoactive drug therapy. Mortality rates are high when sepsis is further complicated by respiratory or renal failure. With severe sepsis, damage to pulmonary capillary endothelium and alveolar epithelium causes alveolar flooding and pulmonary edema. This may occur even with low or normal pulmonary capillary wedge pressures, as with the acute respiratory distress syndrome discussed on page 943 and depicted in Figure 47-1.

Broad-spectrum antimicrobials are chosen empirically based on the source of infection. They are given promptly in maximal doses after appropriate cultures are taken of blood, urine, or exudates not contaminated by normal flora. In severe sepsis, appropriate empirical coverage results in better survival rates (Barochia, 2010; MacArthur, 2004). Acute pyelonephritis is usually caused by Enterobacteriaceae as discussed in Chapter 53 (p. 1054). For pelvic infections, empirical coverage with regimens such as ampicillin plus gentamicin plus clindamycin generally suffices (Chap. 37, p. 685). Associated incisional and other soft-tissue infections are increasingly likely to be caused by methicillin-resistant *S aureus*, thus vancomycin therapy is added (Klevens, 2007; Rotas, 2007). With a septic abortion, a Gram-stained smear may be helpful in identifying *Clostridium perfringens* or group A streptococcal organisms. This is also true for deep fascial infections.

Surgical Treatment

Continuing sepsis may prove fatal, and debridement of necrotic tissue or drainage of purulent material is crucial (Angus, 2013; Mabie, 1997). In obstetrics, the major causes of sepsis are infected abortion, pyelonephritis, and puerperal pelvic infections that include infection of perineal lacerations or of hysterotomy or laparotomy incisions. With an infected abortion, uterine contents must be removed promptly by curettage as described in Chapter 18 (p. 356). Hysterectomy is seldom indicated unless gangrene has resulted.

For women with pyelonephritis, continuing sepsis should prompt a search for obstruction caused by calculi or by a perinephric or intrarenal phlegmon or abscess. Renal sonography or "one-shot" pyelography may be used to diagnose obstruction

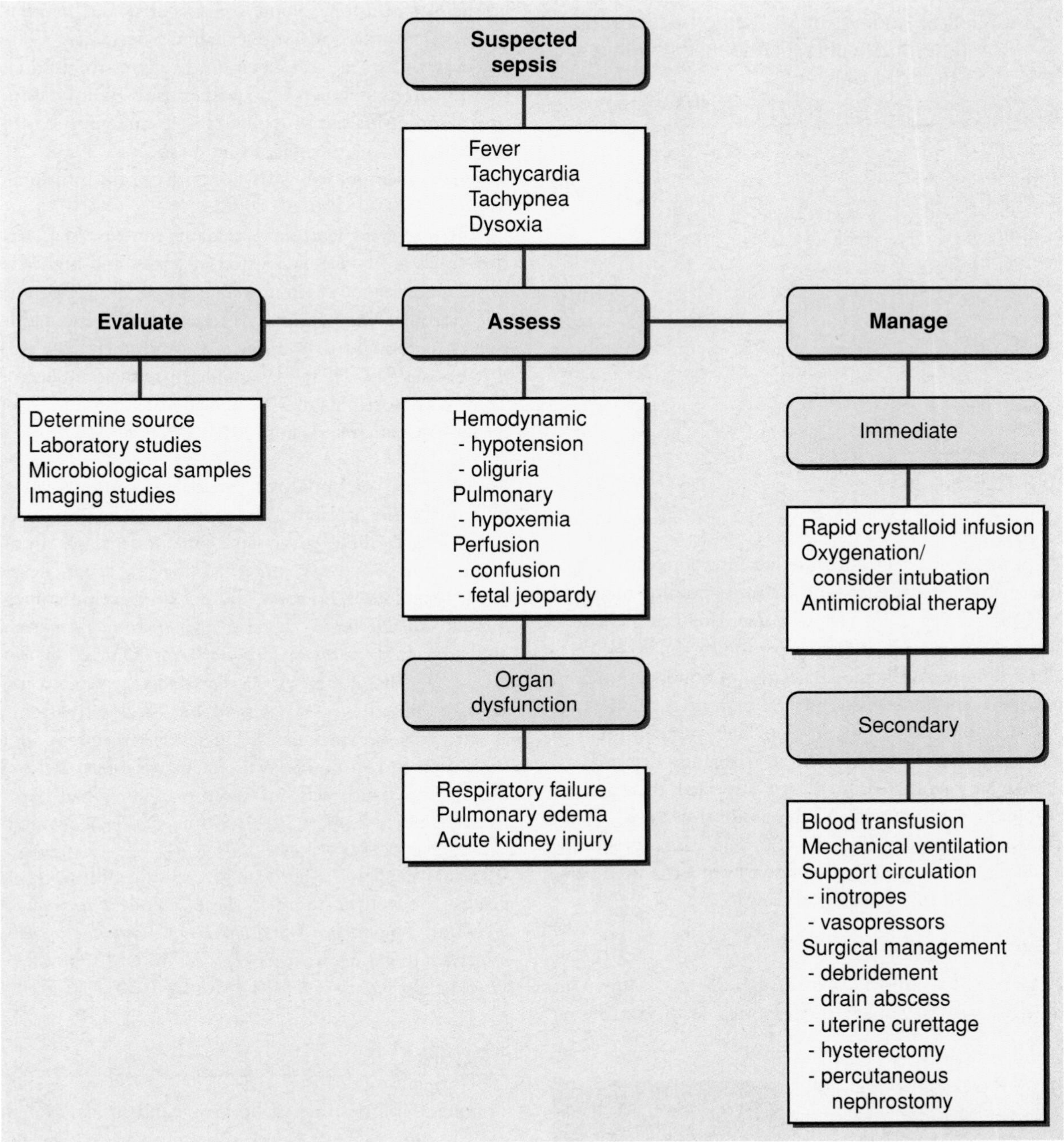

FIGURE 47-6 Algorithm for evaluation and management of sepsis syndrome. Rapid and aggressive implementation is paramount for success. The three steps—Evaluate, Assess, and Manage—are carried out as simultaneously as possible.

and calculi. Computed tomography (CT) may be helpful to identify a phlegmon or abscess. With obstruction, ureteral catheterization, percutaneous nephrostomy, or flank exploration may be lifesaving (Chap. 53, p. 1057).

Most cases of puerperal pelvic sepsis are clinically manifested in the first several days postpartum, and intravenous antimicrobial therapy without tissue debridement is generally curative. There are several exceptions. First is massive uterine myonecrosis caused by group A β-hemolytic streptococcal or clostridial infections (Soper, 2011; Sugiyama, 2010; Yamada, 2010). Those with early-onset disease have presenting findings listed in Table 47-6. The mortality rate in these women with gangrene as shown in Figure 47-7 is high, and prompt hysterectomy may be lifesaving (Mabie, 1997; Nathan, 1993). Group A β-hemolytic streptococci and clostridial colonization or infection also cause toxic-shock syndrome without obvious gangrene as reviewed by Mason and Aronoff (2012). These are due to either streptococcal toxic-shock syndrome-like toxin or clostridial exotoxin that evolved from *S aureus* (Chap. 37, p. 690). In many of these cases, there is bacteremia and widespread tissue invasion, but an intact uterus and abdominal incisions. If uterine necrosis can be excluded—usually by CT scanning—then in our experiences, as well as in others, hysterectomy may not be necessary (Soper, 2011). Still, these infections are highly lethal (Yamada, 2010).

A second exception is necrotizing fasciitis of the episiotomy site or abdominal surgical incision. As described by Gallup and coworkers (2002), these infections are a surgical emergency and are aggressively managed as discussed in Chapter 37 (p. 686).

TABLE 47-6. Clinical Findings in 55 Women with Group A β-Hemolytic Infection Manifest within 12 Hours of Delivery

Finding	Frequency (%)
Multiparous	83
Third-trimester	90
Flu-like symptoms	
High fever	94
Upper respiratory	40
Gastrointestinal	49
Uterine hypertonus	73
Early-onset shock	91
Mortality	
Maternal	58
Perinatal	66

Data from Yamada, 2010.

Third, persistent or aggressive uterine infection with necrosis, uterine incision dehiscence, and severe peritonitis may lead to sepsis (Chap. 37, p. 688). Thus, women following cesarean delivery who are suspected of having peritonitis should be carefully evaluated for uterine incisional necrosis or bowel perforation. These infections tend to be less aggressive than necrotizing group A streptococcal infections and develop later postpartum. CT imaging of the abdomen and pelvis can frequently determine if either of these has eventuated. If either is suspected, then prompt surgical exploration is indicated. With incisional necrosis, hysterectomy is usually necessary (Fig. 37-4, p. 688). Last, peritonitis and sepsis much less commonly may result from a ruptured parametrial, intraabdominal, or ovarian abscess (Chap. 37, p. 687).

Adjunctive Therapy

Vasoactive Drugs and Corticosteroids. As shown in Figure 47-6, a septic woman is supported with continuing crystalloid infusion, blood transfusions, and ventilation. In some cases, other measures may be necessary. Of options, vasoactive drugs are not given unless aggressive fluid treatment fails to correct hypotension and perfusion abnormalities. First-line vasopressors are norepinephrine, epinephrine, dopamine, dobutamine, or phenylephrine (Vincent, 2013). Low-dose vasopressin combined with norepinephrine infusion did not improve survival (Russell, 2008).

The use of corticosteroids remains controversial. Serum cortisol levels are typically elevated in sepsis, and higher levels are associated with increased mortality rates (Sam, 2004). Some but not all studies show a salutary effect of corticosteroid administration. It is thought that *critical illness-related corticosteroid insufficiency—CIRCI*—may play a role in recalcitrant hypotension. Thus, corticosteroids may be considered for use in vasopressor-dependent patients (Angus, 2013; Dellinger, 2008).

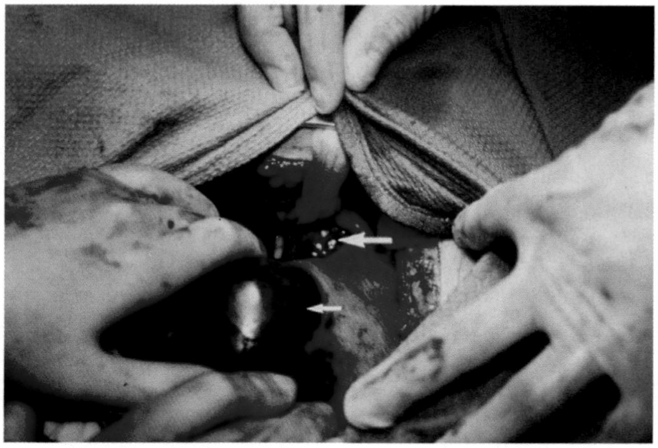

FIGURE 47-7 A fatal case of group A β-hemolytic *Streptococcus pyogenes* puerperal infection following an uncomplicated vaginal delivery at term. The infection caused uterine gangrene and overwhelming sepsis syndrome. Arrows point to overtly "ballooned-out" black gangrenous areas of the postpartum uterus at the time of laparotomy for hysterectomy.

Coagulopathy. Endotoxin stimulates endothelial cells to upregulate tissue factor and thus procoagulant production (Chap. 41, p. 808). At the same time, it decreases the anticoagulant action of activated protein C. Several agents developed to block coagulation, however, did not improve outcomes—some include *antithrombin III, platelet-activating factor antagonist,* and *tissue factor pathway inhibitor* (Abraham, 2003; Suffredini, 2011; Warren, 2001). A 10-year dalliance with recombinant activated protein C—*drotrecogin alfa*—followed after results of an early trial were promising. However, subsequent randomized trials have shown no survival benefits (Ranieri, 2012; Wenzel, 2012). Experience with its use in pregnancy had been limited to case reports (Eppert, 2011; Gupta, 2011; Medve, 2005).

Other Therapies. There are several other therapies that have proven ineffective. Some of these include *antiendotoxin antibody* and *E5 murine monoclonal IgM antiendotoxin antibody; anticytokine antibodies* to *IL-1*, *TNF-α,* and *bradykinin;* and a *nitric oxide synthase inhibitor* (Munford, 2012; Russell, 2006).

TRAUMA

Traumatic injuries such as homicide and similar violent events are a leading cause of death in young women. Depending on definitions used, up to 20 percent of pregnant women suffer physical trauma (American College of Obstetricians and Gynecologists, 2010; Romero, 2012). Injury-related deaths are the most commonly identified nonobstetrical cause of maternal mortality (Brown, 2009; Horon, 2001). In a California study of 4.8 million pregnancies, almost 1 in 350 women were hospitalized for injuries from assaults (El Kady, 2005). In an audit from Parkland Hospital, motor vehicle accidents and falls accounted for 85 percent of injuries sustained by 1682 pregnant women (Hawkins, 2007). Homicides and suicides are also a major cause of pregnancy-associated deaths (Lin, 2011; Shadigian, 2005). From the National Violent Death Reporting System, Palladino and colleagues (2011) found that there were 2.0 pregnancy-associated suicides per 100,000 live births. The rate was 2.9 per 100,000 for pregnancy-associated homicides. And interrelated, intimate partner violence may be linked to these suicides (Martin, 2007).

Blunt Trauma

Physical Abuse—Intimate Partner Violence

According to the United States Department of Justice (2013), women aged 16 to 24 years have the highest per capita rates of intimate partner violence—19.4 per 1000. As many as 10 million women each year are physically assaulted, sexually assaulted, or stalked by an intimate partner (Centers for Disease Control and Prevention, 2013a). One goal in violence prevention for Healthy People 2010 was the reduction of physical abuse directed at women by male partners. The Pregnancy Risk Assessment Monitoring Systems—PRAMS—report showed some improvement in these areas (Suellentrop, 2006).

Even more appalling is that physical violence directed at women continues during pregnancy. Most data have been accrued by public institutions, and abuse rates range from 1 to 20 percent during pregnancy (American College of Obstetricians and Gynecologists, 2011b). In Phoenix, more than 13 percent of women who enrolled for prenatal services had a history of physical or sexual abuse (Coonrod, 2007). Abuse is linked to poverty, poor education, and use of tobacco, alcohol, and illicit drugs (Centers for Disease Control and Prevention, 2008). Unfortunately, abused women tend to remain with their abusers, and the major risk factor for intimate partner homicide is prior domestic violence (Campbell, 2007). Finally, women seeking pregnancy termination have a higher incidence of intimate partner violence (Bourassa, 2007).

The woman who is physically abused tends to present late, if at all, for prenatal care. In the study cited above, pregnant women hospitalized in California as a result of assault had significantly increased perinatal morbidity rates (El Kady, 2005). Immediate sequelae included uterine rupture, preterm delivery, and maternal and perinatal death. Subsequent outcomes included increased rates of placental abruption, preterm and low-birthweight infants, and other adverse outcomes. Silverman and associates (2006) reported similar results from PRAMS, which included more than 118,000 pregnancies in 26 states. Others have cited increased preterm birth and depression (Rodriguez, 2008).

Preventatively, the American Academy of Pediatrics and the American College of Obstetricians and Gynecologists (2012) recommend universal screening for intimate partner violence at the initial prenatal visit, during each trimester, and again at the postpartum visit (Chap. 9, p. 174). Others recommend a case-finding approach based on clinical suspicion (Robertson-Blackmore, 2013; Wathen, 2003).

Sexual Assault

According to the Centers for Disease Control and Prevention (2012), 20 percent of adult women will be sexually assaulted sometime during their lives. More than 90 percent of the nearly 200,000 rape victims in the United States in 2006 were women; 80 percent were younger than 30 years; and 44 percent were younger than 18. Satin and coworkers (1992) reviewed more than 5700 female sexual assault victims in Dallas County and reported that 2 percent were pregnant. Associated physical trauma is common (Sugar, 2004). From a forensic standpoint, evidence collection protocol is not altered (Linden, 2011).

In addition to attention to physical injuries, exposure to sexually transmitted diseases must be considered. The Centers for Disease Control and Prevention (2010) recommends antimicrobial prophylaxis against gonorrhea, chlamydial infection, and trichomoniasis (Table 47-7). If the woman is not pregnant, another very important aspect is emergency contraception, as recommended by the American College of Obstetricians and Gynecologists (2012) and discussed in detail in Chapter 38 (p. 714).

The importance of psychological counseling for the rape victim and her family cannot be overemphasized. There is a 30- to 35-percent lifetime risk each for posttraumatic stress disorder, major depression, and suicide contemplation (Linden, 2011).

Automobile Accidents

At least 3 percent of pregnant women are involved in motor vehicle accidents each year in the United States. Using data from PRAMS, Sirin and colleagues (2007) estimated that 92,500 pregnant women are injured annually. Motor-vehicle crashes are the most common causes of serious, life-threatening, or fatal blunt trauma during pregnancy (Brown, 2009; Luley, 2013; Patteson, 2007; Vladutiu, 2013). Mattox and Goetzl (2005) report these accidents to be the leading cause of traumatic fetal deaths as well, and this was also true for Parkland Hospital (Hawkins, 2007). As with all motor vehicle crashes, alcohol use is commonly associated. But sadly, as many as half of accidents occur without seat-belt use, and many of these deaths would likely be preventable by the three-point restraints shown in Figure 47-8 (Klinich, 2008; Luley, 2013; Metz, 2006). Seat belts prevent contact with the steering wheel, and they reduce abdominal impact pressure (Motozawa, 2010).

Original concerns regarding injuries caused by airbag deployment have been somewhat allayed (Matsushita, 2014). One study included 30 such women from 20 to 37 weeks' gestation whose airbag deployed in accidents with a median speed of 35 mph (Metz, 2006). A third were not using seat belts, and there was one fetal death from the single case of placental abruption. Almost 75 percent had contractions, half had abdominal pain, and in 20 percent, there were abnormal fetal heart rate tracings. In a retrospective cohort study that included 2207 pregnant women in crashes with airbag deployment, perinatal outcomes were not clinically different from 1141 controls without airbags (Schiff, 2010). Importantly, 96 percent of both groups used seat belts.

Other Blunt Trauma

Some other common causes of blunt trauma are falls and aggravated assaults. In the California review reported by El Kady and associates (2005), intentionally inflicted injuries were present in approximately a third of pregnant women who were hospitalized for trauma. Less common are blast or crush injury (Sela, 2008). With blunt trauma, there can be serious intraabdominal injuries. Even so, bowel injuries are less frequent because of the protective effect of a large uterus. Still, diaphragmatic, splenic, liver, and kidney injuries may also be sustained. Particularly worrisome is the specter of amnionic-fluid embolism, which has been reported with even mild trauma (Ellingsen, 2007;

TABLE 47-7. Guidelines for Prophylaxis against Sexually Transmitted Disease in Victims of Sexual Assault

Prophylaxis Against	Regimen	Alternative
Neisseria gonorrhoeae	Ceftriaxone 125 mg IM single dose ***plus*** Azithromycin 1 g orally single dose	Cefixime 400 mg orally single dose ***plus*** Azithromycin 1 g orally single dose ***or*** Azithromycin 2 g orally single dose
Chlamydia trachomatis	Azithromycin 1 g orally single dose[a] ***or*** Amoxicillin 500 mg orally three times daily for 7 days	Erythromycin-base 500 mg orally four times daily for 7 days ***or*** Levofloxacin 500 mg orally once daily for 7 days ***or*** Ofloxacin 300 mg orally twice daily for 7 days
Bacterial vaginosis	Metronidazole 2 g orally in a single dose ***or*** Metronidazole 500 mg orally twice daily for 7 days	Metronidazole gel 0.75%, 5 g intravaginally daily for 5 days ***or*** Clindamycin cream 2%, 5 g intravaginally daily for 7 days
Trichomonas vaginalis	Metronidazole 2 g orally single dose ***or*** Tinidazole 2 g orally single dose[b]	Metronidazole 500 mg orally twice daily for 7 days
Hepatitis B (HBV)	If not previously vaccinated, give first dose HBV vaccine, repeat at 1–2 and 4–6 months	
Human immunodeficiency virus (HIV)	Consider retroviral prophylaxis if risk for HIV exposure is high	

[a]For nonpregnant women, doxycycline, 100 mg orally twice daily for 7 days, can be given instead.
[b]Pregnancy category C.
From Centers for Disease Control and Prevention, 2010, 2012.

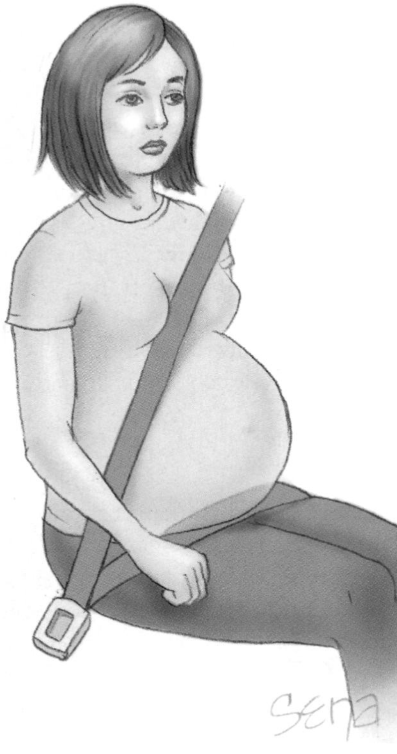

FIGURE 47-8 Illustration showing correct use of three-point automobile restraint. The upper belt is *above* the uterus, and the lower belt fits snugly across the upper thighs and well *below* the uterus.

Pluymakers, 2007). Retroperitoneal hemorrhage is possibly more common than in nonpregnant women (Takehana, 2011).

Orthopedic injuries are also encountered with some regularity (Desai, 2007). From the Parkland Hospital trauma unit, 6 percent of 1682 pregnant women evaluated had orthopedic injuries. This subset was also at increased risk for placental abruption, preterm delivery, and perinatal mortality (Cannada, 2008). In a review of 101 pelvic fractures during pregnancy, there was a 9-percent maternal and 35-percent fetal mortality rate (Leggon, 2002). In another study of pelvic and acetabular fractures during 15 pregnancies, there was one maternal death, and four of 16 fetuses died (Almog, 2007). Finally, head trauma and neurosurgical care raise unique issues (Qaiser, 2007).

Fetal Injury and Death

Perinatal death rates increase with the severity of maternal injuries. Fetal death is more likely with direct fetoplacental injury, maternal shock, pelvic fracture, maternal head injury, or hypoxia (Ikossi, 2005; Pearlman, 2008). Motor vehicle accidents caused 82 percent of fetal deaths from trauma. Death was caused by placental injury in half, and by uterine rupture in 4 percent (Weiss, 2001). Patteson and coworkers (2007) reported similar findings.

Although uncommon, fetal skull and brain injuries are more likely if the head is engaged and the maternal pelvis is fractured (Palmer, 1994). Conversely, fetal head injuries,

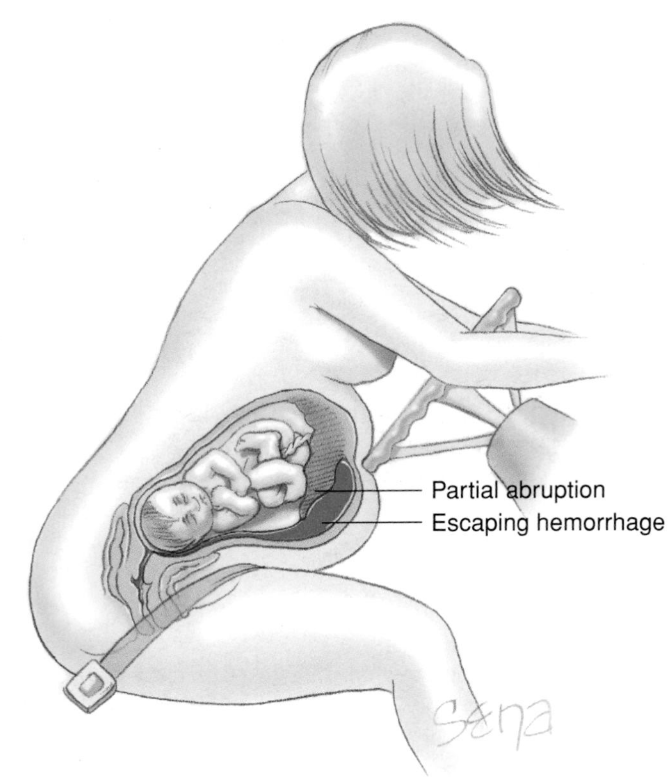

FIGURE 47-9 Acute deceleration injury occurs when the elastic uterus meets the steering wheel. As the uterus stretches, the inelastic placenta shears from the decidua basalis. Intrauterine pressures as high as 550 mm Hg are generated.

presumably from a contrecoup effect, may be sustained in unengaged vertex or nonvertex presentations. Fetal skull fractures are rare and best seen using CT imaging (Sadro, 2012). Sequelae include intracranial hemorrhage (Green-Thompson, 2005). A newborn with paraplegia and contractures associated with a motor vehicle accident sustained several months before birth was described by Weyerts and colleagues (1992). Other injuries have included fetal decapitation or incomplete midabdominal fetal transection at midpregnancy (Rowe, 1996; Weir, 2008).

Placental Injuries—Abruption or Tear

Catastrophic events that occur with blunt trauma include placental injuries—abruption or placental tear or "fracture"—and uterine rupture (Fig. 47-9 and 47-10). Placental separation from trauma is likely caused by deformation of the elastic myometrium around the relatively inelastic placenta (Crosby, 1968). This may result from a deceleration injury as the large uterus meets the immovable steering wheel or seat belt. Some degree of abruption complicates 1 to 6 percent of "minor" injuries and up to 50 percent of "major" injuries (Pearlman, 1990; Schiff, 2002). Abruption was found to be more likely if vehicle speed exceeded 30 mph (Reis, 2000).

Clinical findings with traumatic abruption may be similar to those for spontaneous placental abruption (Chap. 41, p. 796). Kettel and coworkers (1988) emphasized that traumatic abruption may be occult and unaccompanied by uterine pain, tenderness, or bleeding. Stettler and associates (1992) reviewed our experiences with 13 such women at Parkland Hospital. Of these, 11 had uterine tenderness, but only five had vaginal bleeding. Because traumatic abruption is more likely to be concealed and generate higher intrauterine pressures, associated coagulopathy is more likely than with nontraumatic abruption. Partial separation may also generate uterine activity as described more fully on page 955. Other features are evidence of fetal compromise such as fetal tachycardia, late decelerations, and acidosis and fetal death.

If there is considerable abdominal force associated with trauma, then the placenta can be torn, or "fractured" (see Fig. 47-10). If so, then life-threatening fetal hemorrhage may be encountered either into the amnionic sac or by fetomaternal hemorrhage (Pritchard, 1991). The tear is linear or stellate such as shown in Figure 47-11 and is caused by rapid deformation and reformation. Especially if there is ABO compatibility, fetomaternal hemorrhage is quantified using a

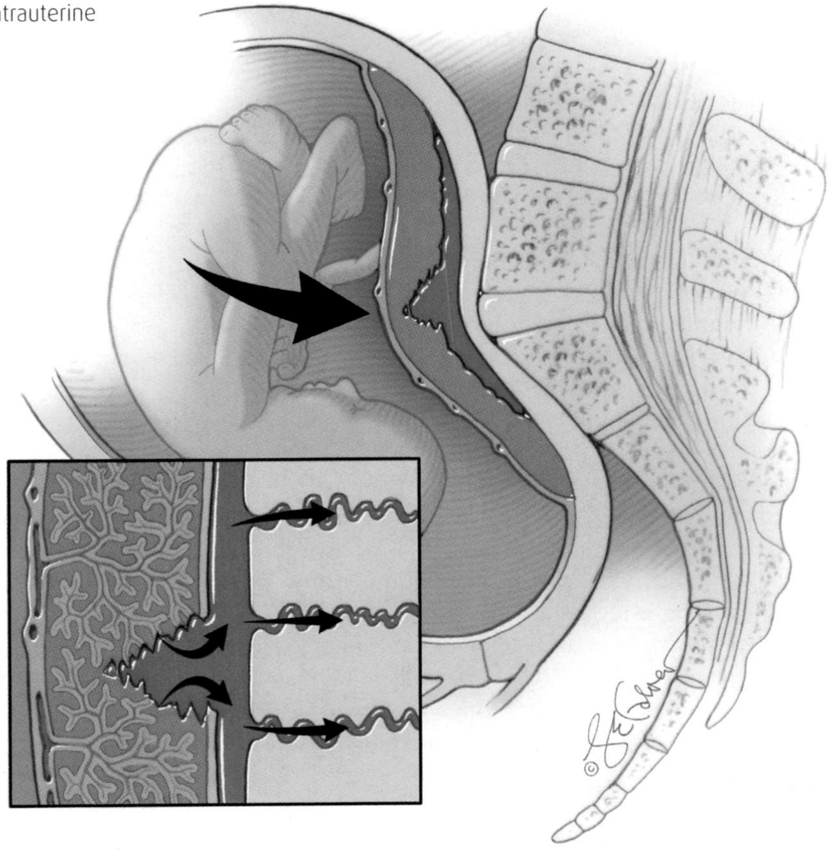

FIGURE 47-10 Mechanism of placental tear or "fracture" caused by a deformation-reformation injury. Placental abruption is seen as blood collecting in the retroplacental space. **Inset**. From here, blood can be forced into placental bed venules and enter maternal circulation. Such maternofetal hemorrhage may be identified with Kleihauer-Betke testing.

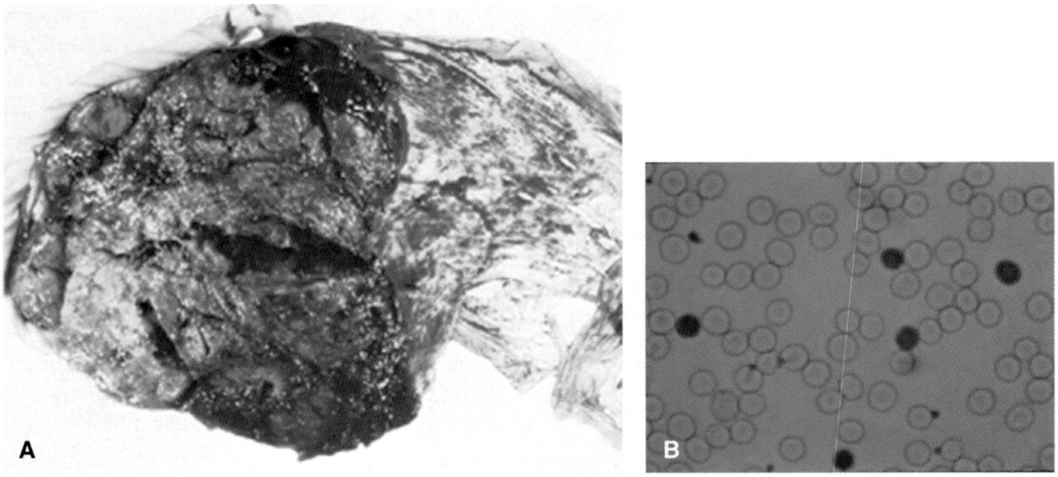

FIGURE 47-11 A. Partial placental abruption in which the adherent blood clot has been removed. Note the laceration of the placenta (*arrow*), which caused fetal death from massive fetomaternal hemorrhage. **B.** Kleihauer-Betke stain of a peripheral smear of maternal blood. The dark cells that constituted 4.5 percent of red blood cells are fetal in origin, whereas the empty cells are maternal.

Kleihauer-Betke stain of maternal blood (see Fig. 47-11). A small amount of fetal-maternal bleeding has been described in up to a third of trauma cases, and in 90 percent of these, the volume is < 15 mL (Goodwin, 1990; Pearlman, 1990). Nontraumatic placental abruption is much less often associated with significant fetomaternal hemorrhage because there usually is only minimal fetal bleeding into the intervillous space. With traumatic abruption, however, massive fetomaternal hemorrhage may coexist (Stettler, 1992). In one study there was a 20-fold risk of associated uterine contractions and preterm labor if there is evidence for a fetomaternal bleed (Muench, 2004).

Uterine Rupture

Blunt trauma results in uterine rupture in < 1 percent of severe cases (American College of Obstetricians and Gynecologists, 2010). Rupture is more likely in a previously scarred uterus and is usually associated with a direct impact of substantial force. Decelerative forces following a 25-mph collision can generate up to 500 mm Hg of intrauterine pressure in a properly restrained woman (Crosby, 1968). Clinical findings may be identical to those for placental abruption with an intact uterus, and maternal and fetal deterioration are soon inevitable. Pearlman and Cunningham (1996) described uterine fundal "blowout" with fetal decapitation in a 20-week pregnancy following a high-speed collision. Similarly, Weir and colleagues (2008) described supracervical uterine avulsion and fetal transection at 22 weeks. CT scanning may be useful to diagnose uterine rupture with a dead fetus or placental separation (Kopelman, 2013; Manriquez, 2010; Sadro, 2012; Takehana, 2011).

Penetrating Trauma

In a study of 321 pregnant women with abdominal trauma, Petrone (2011) reported a 9-percent incidence of penetrating injuries—77 percent were gunshot wounds and 23 percent were stab wounds. The incidence of maternal visceral injury with penetrating trauma is only 15 to 40 percent compared with 80 to 90 percent in nonpregnant individuals (Stone, 1999). When the uterus sustains penetrating wounds, the fetus is more likely than the mother to be seriously injured. Indeed, although the fetus sustains injury in two thirds of cases with penetrating uterine injuries, maternal visceral injuries are seen in only 20 percent. Still, their seriousness is underscored in that maternal-fetal mortality rates are significantly higher than those seen with blunt abdominal injuries in pregnancy. Specifically, maternal mortality was 7 versus 2 percent, and fetal mortality was 73 versus 10 percent, respectively.

Management of Trauma

Maternal and fetal outcomes are directly related to the severity of injury. That said, commonly used methods of severity scoring do not take into account significant morbidity and mortality rates related to placental abruption and thus to pregnancy outcomes. In a study of 582 pregnant women hospitalized for injuries, the injury severity score did not accurately predict adverse pregnancy outcomes (Schiff, 2005). Importantly, relatively minor injuries were associated with preterm labor and placental abruption. Others have reached similar conclusions (Biester, 1997; Ikossi, 2005). In a study of 317 pregnant women at 24 weeks' gestation or more who had "minor trauma," 14 percent had clinically significant uterine contractions requiring extended fetal evaluation past 4 hours (Cahill, 2008).

With few exceptions, treatment priorities in injured pregnant women are directed as they would be in nonpregnant patients (Barraco, 2010; Mirza, 2010). Primary goals are evaluation and stabilization of maternal injuries. Attention to fetal assessment during the acute evaluation may divert attention from life-threatening maternal injuries (American College of Obstetricians and Gynecologists, 2010; Brown, 2009). Basic rules of resuscitation include ventilation, arrest of hemorrhage, and treatment of hypovolemia with crystalloid and blood products. Importantly, the large uterus is positioned off the great vessels to diminish its affect on vessel compression and decreased cardiac output.

Following emergency resuscitation, evaluation is continued for fractures, internal injuries, bleeding sites, and placental, uterine, and fetal trauma. Radiography is not proscribed, but special attention is given to indications. One report observed that pregnant trauma victims had less radiation exposure than nonpregnant controls (Ylagan, 2008). Brown and colleagues (2005) advocated screening abdominal sonography followed by CT scanning for positive sonographic findings. Procedures used include the FAST scan—focused assessment with sonography for trauma. This is a 5-minute, four- to six-view imaging study that evaluates perihepatic, perisplenic, pelvic, and pericardial views (Rose, 2004). In general, if fluid is seen in any of these views, then the volume is > 500 mL. However, this amount has not been corroborated for pregnancy. In some cases, open peritoneal lavage may be informative (Tsuei, 2006).

Penetrating injuries in most cases must be evaluated using radiography. Because clinical response to peritoneal irritation is blunted during pregnancy, an aggressive approach to exploratory laparotomy is pursued. Whereas exploration is mandatory for abdominal gunshot wounds, some clinicians advocate close observation for selected stab wounds. Diagnostic laparoscopy has also been used (Chap. 46, p. 928).

Cesarean Delivery

The necessity for cesarean delivery of a live fetus depends on several factors. Laparotomy itself is not an indication for hysterotomy. Some considerations include gestational age, fetal condition, extent of uterine injury, and whether the large uterus hinders adequate treatment or evaluation of other intraabdominal injuries (Tsuei, 2006).

Electronic Monitoring

As for many other acute or chronic maternal conditions, fetal well-being may reflect the status of the mother. Thus, fetal monitoring is another "vital sign" that helps to evaluate the extent of maternal injuries. Even if the mother is stable, electronic monitoring may suggest placental abruption. In a study by Pearlman and coworkers (1990), no woman had an abruption if uterine contractions were less often than every 10 minutes within the 4 hours after trauma was sustained. Almost 20 percent of women who had contractions more frequently than every 10 minutes in the first 4 hours had an associated placental abruption. In these cases, abnormal tracings were common and included fetal tachycardia and late decelerations. Conversely, no adverse outcomes were reported in women who had normal monitor tracings (Connolly, 1997). Importantly, if tocolytics are used for these contractions, they may obfuscate findings, and we do not recommend them.

Because placental abruption usually develops early following trauma, fetal monitoring is begun as soon as the mother is stabilized. The ideal duration of posttrauma monitoring is not precisely known. From data cited above, observation for 4 hours is reasonable with a normal tracing and no other sentinel findings such as contractions, uterine tenderness, or bleeding. Certainly, monitoring should be continued as long as there are uterine contractions, nonreassuring fetal heart patterns, vaginal bleeding, uterine tenderness or irritability, serious maternal injury, or ruptured membranes (American College of Obstetricians and Gynecologists, 2010). In rare cases, placental abruption has developed days after trauma (Higgins, 1984).

Fetal-Maternal Hemorrhage

It is unclear whether routine use of the Kleihauer-Betke or an equivalent test in pregnant trauma victims might modify adverse outcomes associated with fetal anemia, cardiac arrhythmias, and death (Pak, 1998). In a retrospective review of 125 pregnant women with blunt injuries, the Kleihauer-Betke test was reported to have a sensitivity of 56 percent, a specificity of 71 percent, and an accuracy of 27 percent (Towery, 1993). These investigators concluded that the test was of little value during acute trauma management. They also concluded that electronic fetal monitoring or sonography or both were more useful in detecting fetal or pregnancy-associated complications than the Kleihauer-Betke test. Others have reached similar conclusions, although a positive test with fetal cells of 0.1 percent was predictive of uterine contractions or preterm labor (Connolly, 1997; Muench, 2003, 2004).

For the woman who is D-negative, administration of anti-D immunoglobulin should be considered. This may be omitted if a test for fetal bleeding is negative. Even with anti-D immunoglobulin, alloimmunization may still develop if the fetal-maternal hemorrhage exceeds 15 mL of fetal cells (Chap. 15, p. 311).

Another important aspect of care for the pregnant trauma patient is to ensure that her tetanus immunization is current. When indicated, a dose of tetanus toxoid, reduced diphtheria toxoid, and acellular pertussis vaccine (Tdap) is preferred for its neonatal pertussis immunity benefits described in Chapter 9 (p. 184) (Centers for Disease Control and Prevention, 2013b). If unavailable, tetanus toxoid (TT) or tetanus and diphtheria toxoids (Td) are suitable alternatives.

THERMAL INJURY

Treatment of burned pregnant women is similar to that for nonpregnant patients (Pacheco, 2005). With treatment, it is generally agreed that pregnancy does not alter maternal outcome from thermal injury compared with that of nonpregnant women of similar age. As perhaps expected, maternal and fetal survival parallels the percentage of burned surface area. Karimi and colleagues (2009) reported higher mortality rates for both with suicidal attempts and with inhalational injuries. The composite mortality for more than 200 women from six studies increased in a linear fashion as the percent body-surface area burned increased (Fig. 47-12). For 20-, 40-, and 60-percent burns, the maternal mortality rates were approximately 4, 30, and 93 percent, respectively. The corresponding fetal mortality rates were 20, 48, and 96 percent, respectively. With severe burns, the woman usually enters labor spontaneously within a few days to a week and often delivers a stillborn. Contributory factors are hypovolemia, pulmonary injury, septicemia, and the intensely catabolic state associated with these burns (Radosevich, 2013).

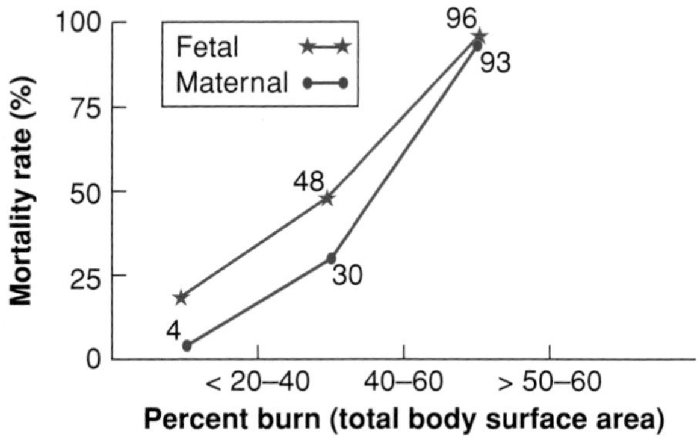

FIGURE 47-12 Maternal and fetal mortality rates by burn severity in 211 women. (Data from Akhtar, 1994; Amy, 1985; Mabrouk, 1977; Maghsoudi, 2006; Rayburn, 1984; Rode, 1990.)

Following serious abdominal burns, skin contractures that develop may be painful during a subsequent pregnancy and may even require surgical decompression and split-skin autografts (Matthews, 1982; Widgerow, 1991). In a follow-up study of seven women with severe circumferential truncal burns sustained at a mean age of 7.7 years, all of 14 subsequent pregnancies were delivered at term without major complications (McCauley, 1991). Loss or distortion of nipples may cause problems in breast feeding (Fig. 47-13). Interestingly, normal abdominal tissue expansion due to pregnancy appears to be an excellent source for obtaining skin grafts postpartum to correct scar deformities at other body sites (Del Frari, 2004).

Electrical and Lightning Injuries

Earlier case reports suggested a high fetal mortality rate with electric shock (Fatovich, 1993). In a prospective cohort study, however, Einarson and coworkers (1997) showed similar perinatal outcomes in 31 injured women compared with those of noninjured controls. They concluded that traditional 110-volt North American electrical current likely is less dangerous than 220-volt currents available in Europe. A woman with iliofemoral thrombosis at 29 weeks' gestation that *may* have been related to a mild electrical shock at 22 weeks was described (Sozen, 2004). Thermal burns may be extensive and require expert wound care.

The pathophysiological effects of lightning injuries can be devastating. García Gutiérrez and associates (2005) reviewed 12 case reports of injuries during pregnancy and added their own.

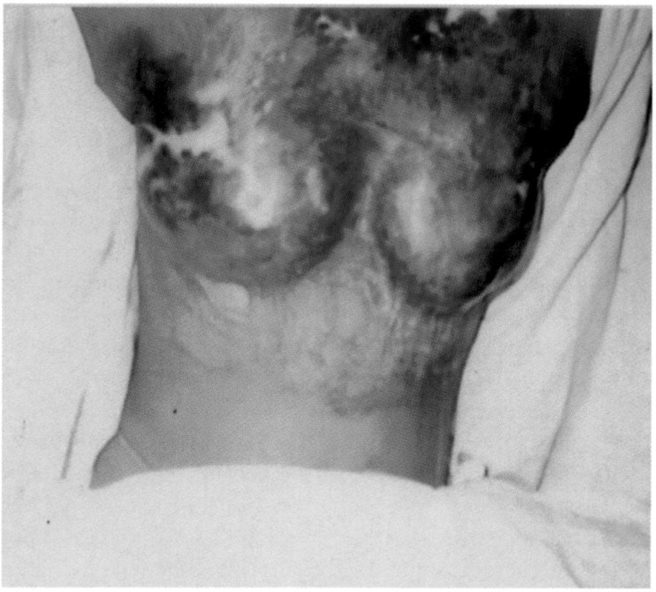

FIGURE 47-13 This 22-year-old nullipara sustained severe burns at age 12 years, and massive scarring followed. Both breasts were replaced by scar tissue. Following delivery, a few drops of colostrum were expressed from the left nipple, but no breast engorgement was noted. (Photograph contributed by Drs. A. R. Mahale and A. P. Sakhare, Maharashtra, India.)

CARDIOPULMONARY RESUSCITATION

Cardiac arrest is rare during pregnancy. General topics regarding planning and equipment have been reviewed by the American College of Obstetricians and Gynecologists (2011a). There are special considerations for cardiopulmonary resuscitation (CPR) conducted in the second half of pregnancy, and these are outlined in the American Heart Association 2010 guidelines (Vanden Hoek, 2010). The committee acknowledges the following as standards for critically ill pregnant women: (1) relieve possible vena caval compression by left lateral uterine displacement, (2) administer 100-percent oxygen, (3) establish intravenous access above the diaphragm, (4) assess for hypotension that warrants therapy, which is defined as systolic blood pressure < 100 mmHg or < 80 percent of baseline, and (5) review possible causes of critical illness and treat conditions as early as possible.

In nonpregnant women, external chest compression results in a cardiac output approximately 30 percent of normal. In late pregnancy, this may be even less with CPR because of uterine aortocaval compression (Clark, 1997). Thus, it is paramount to accompany other resuscitative efforts with uterine displacement. Displacement can be accomplished by tilting the operating table laterally, by placing a wedge under the right hip—an example is the Cardiff resuscitation wedge, or by pushing the uterus to the left manually (Rees, 1988). If no equipment is available, such as in an out-of-hospital arrest, an individual may kneel on the floor with the maternal back on his or her thighs to form a "human wedge" (Whitty, 2002).

Cesarean Delivery

During maternal resuscitation, because of pregnancy-induced hindrances on CPR efforts, emergent *perimortem cesarean delivery* for fetal salvage and improved maternal resuscitation may be considered (Vanden Hoek, 2010). Some have stated that cesarean delivery is indicated with 4 to 5 minutes of beginning CPR if the fetus is viable (Moise, 1997). There is an undeniably inverse correlation between neurologically intact neonatal survival and the cardiac arrest-to-delivery interval in women delivered by perimortem cesarean (Katz, 2012). Specifically, of newborns delivered within 5 minutes of arrest, 98 percent are neurologically intact; within 6 to 15 minutes, 83 percent are intact; within 16 to 25 minutes, 33 percent are intact; and within 26 to 35 minutes, only 25 percent are intact (Clark, 1997). This, coupled with some evidence that delivery *may* also enhance maternal resuscitation, has led the American College of Obstetricians and Gynecologists

(2011a) to recommend *consideration* for cesarean delivery within 4 minutes of cardiac arrest in these cases.

This serious and sometimes contentious issue is far from evidence based. To wit, Katz and associates (2005) reviewed 38 perimortem cesarean deliveries with a "large selection bias." They concluded that these reports supported—but "fell far from proving"—that perimortem cesarean delivery within 4 minutes of maternal cardiac arrest improves maternal and fetal outcomes. Even so, as emphasized by Clark and coworkers (1997), and in our experiences, these goals rarely can be met in actual practice. For example, most cases of cardiac arrest occur in uncontrolled circumstances, and thus, the time to CPR initiation alone would exceed the first 5 minutes. Thus "crash" cesarean delivery would supersede resuscitative efforts, be necessarily done without appropriate anesthesia or surgical equipment, and more likely than not, would lead to maternal death. Moreover, the distinction between a perimortem versus postmortem cesarean operation is imperative (Katz, 2012). Last, in the balance, any choice *may* favor survival of the mother over the fetus, or vice versa, and thus there are immediate unresolvable ethical concerns. Katz (2012) has recently provided a scholarly review of perimortem cesarean delivery.

Maternal Brain Death

Occasionally, a pregnant woman with a supposedly healthy intact fetus will be kept on somatic support to await fetal viability or maturity. This is discussed in Chapter 60 (p. 1199).

Envenomation

According to their review, Brown and colleagues (2013) reported that clinically significant envenomations in pregnant women are from snakes, spiders, scorpions, jellyfish, and hymenoptera such as bees, wasps, hornets, and ants. Adverse outcomes are related to maternal effects. They conclude that limited evidence supports the use of a venom-specific approach that includes symptomatic care, antivenom administration when appropriate, anaphylaxis treatment, and fetal assessment.

REFERENCES

Abraham E, Reinhart K, Opal S, et al: Efficacy and safety of tifacogin (recombinant tissue factor pathway inhibitor) in severe sepsis: a randomized controlled trial. JAMA 290:238, 2003

Acosta CD, Knight M: Sepsis and maternal mortality. Curr Opin Obstet Gynecol 25(2):109, 2013

Akhtar MA, Mulawkar PM, Kulkarni HR: Burns in pregnancy: effect on maternal and fetal outcomes. Burns 20:351, 1994

Almog G, Liebergall M, Tsafrir A, et al: Management of pelvic fractures during pregnancy. Am J Orthop 36:E153, 2007

American Academy of Pediatrics and American College of Obstetricians and Gynecologists: Guidelines for Perinatal Care, 7th ed. Washington, 2012

American College of Critical Care Medicine and the Society of Critical Care Medicine: Guidelines on admission and discharge for adult intermediate care units. Crit Care Med 26:607, 1998

American College of Obstetricians and Gynecologists: Obstetric aspects of trauma management. Practice Bulletin No. 251, September 1998, Reaffirmed 2010

American College of Obstetricians and Gynecologists: Critical care in pregnancy. Practice Bulletin No. 100, February 2009, Reaffirmed 2011a

American College of Obstetricians and Gynecologists: Sexual assault. Committee Opinion No. 499, August 2011b

American College of Obstetricians and Gynecologists: Access to emergency contraception. Committee Opinion No. 542, November 2012

American College of Obstetricians and Gynecologists: Hypertension in pregnancy: report of the American College of Obstetricians and Gynecologists' task force on hypertension in pregnancy. Executive summary. Obstet Gynecol 122:1122, 2013

Amy BW, McManus WF, Goodwin CW, et al: Thermal injury in the pregnant patient. Surg Gynecol Obstet 161:209, 1985

Angus DC, van der Poll T: Severe sepsis and septic shock. N Engl J Med 369:840, 2013

Anzueto A, Baughman RP, Guntupalli KK, et al: Aerosolized surfactant in adults with sepsis-induced acute respiratory distress syndrome. N Engl J Med 334:1417, 1996

Aurigemma GP, Gaasch WH: Diastolic heart failure. N Engl J Med 351:1097, 2004

Barochia AV, Cui X, Vitberg D, et al: Bundled care for septic shock: an analysis of clinical trials. Crit Care Med 38(2):668, 2010

Barraco RD, Chiu WC, Clancy TV, et al: Practice management guidelines for the diagnosis and management of injury in the pregnant patient: the EAST Practice Management Guidelines Work Group. J Trauma 69(1):211, 2010

Baskett TF, O'Connell CM: Maternal critical care in obstetrics. J Obstet Gynaecol Can 31(3):218, 2009

Benedetti TJ, Carlson RW: Studies of colloid osmotic pressure in pregnancy-induced hypertension. Am J Obstet Gynecol 135:308, 1979

Biester EM, Tomich PG, Esposito TJ, et al: Trauma in pregnancy: Normal Revised Trauma Score in relation to other markers of maternofetal status—preliminary study. Am J Obstet Gynecol 176:1206, 1997

Bourassa D, Bérubé J: The prevalence of intimate partner violence among women and teenagers seeking abortion compared with those continuing pregnancy. J Obstet Gynaecol Can 29:415, 2007

Brodie D, Bacchetta M: Extracorporeal membrane oxygenation for ARDS in adults. N Engl J Med 365(20):1905, 2011

Brown HL: Trauma in pregnancy. Obstet Gynecol 114(1):147, 2009

Brown MA, Sirlin CB, Farahmand N, et al: Screening sonography in pregnant patients with blunt abdominal trauma. J Ultrasound Med 24:175, 2005

Brown SA, Seifert SA, Rayburn WF: Management of envenomations during pregnancy. Clin Toxicol (Phila.) 51:3, 2013

Cahill AG, Bastek JA, Stamilio DM. et al: Minor trauma in pregnancy—is the evaluation unwarranted? Am J Obstet Gynecol 198:208.e1, 2008

Campbell JC, Glass N, Sharps PW, et al: Intimate partner homicide: review and implications of research and policy. Trauma Violence Abuse 8:246, 2007

Cannada LK, Hawkins JS, Casey BM, et al: Outcomes in pregnant trauma patients with orthopedic injuries. Submitted for Fall Meeting of American Academy of Orthopaedic Surgeons; Dallas, TX, October 2008

Catanzarite V, Willms D, Wong D, et al: Acute respiratory distress syndrome in pregnancy and the puerperium: causes, courses, and outcomes. Obstet Gynecol 97:760, 2001

Centers for Disease Control and Prevention: Adverse health conditions and health risk behaviors associated with intimate partner violence—United States, 2005. MMWR 57(5):113, 2008

Centers for Disease Control and Prevention: Sexually Transmitted Diseases Treatment Guidelines. MMWR 59(12):91, 2010

Centers for Disease Control and Prevention: The National Intimate Partner and Sexual Violence Survey. 2013a. Available at: cdc.gov/violenceprevention/nisvs. Accessed July 28, 2013

Centers for Disease Control and Prevention: Update to CDC's Sexually Transmitted Diseases Treatment Guidelines, 2010: oral cephalosporins no longer a recommended treatment for gonococcal infections. MMWR 61(31):590, 2012

Centers for Disease Control and Prevention: Updated recommendations for use of tetanus toxoid, reduced diphtheria toxoid, and acellular pertussis vaccine (Tdap) in pregnant women—Advisory Committee on Immunization Practices (ACIP), 2012. MMWR 62(7):131, 2013b

Chen CY, Chen CP, Wang KG, et al: Factors implicated in the outcome of pregnancies complicated by acute respiratory failure. J Reprod Med 48:641, 2003

Clark SL, Cotton DB: Clinical indications for pulmonary artery catheterization in the patient with severe preeclampsia. Am J Obstet Gynecol 158:453, 1988

Clark SL, Cotton DB, Hankins GDV, et al: Critical Care Obstetrics, 3rd ed. Boston, Blackwell Science, 1997

Clark SL, Cotton DB, Lee W, et al: Central hemodynamic assessment of normal term pregnancy. Am J Obstet Gynecol 161:1439, 1989

Clark SL, Hankins GD, Dudley DA, et al: Amniotic fluid embolism: analysis of a national registry. Am J Obstet Gynecol 172:1158, 1995

Cole DE, Taylor TL, McCullough DM, et al: Acute respiratory distress syndrome in pregnancy. Crit Care Med 33:S269, 2005

Connolly AM, Katz VL, Bash KL, et al: Trauma and pregnancy. Am J Perinatol 14:331, 1997
Coonrod DV, Bay RC, Mills TE, et al: Asymptomatic bacteriuria and intimate partner violence in pregnant women. Am J Obstet Gynecol 196:581.e1, 2007
Crosby WM, Snyder RG, Snow CC, et al: Impact injuries in pregnancy, 1. Experimental studies. Am J Obstet Gynecol 101:100, 1968
Cunningham FG, Lucas MJ, Hankins GD: Pulmonary injury complicating antepartum pyelonephritis. Am J Obstet Gynecol 156:797, 1987
Cunningham FG, Pritchard JA, Hankins GDV, et al: Peripartum heart failure: a specific pregnancy-induced cardiomyopathy or the consequence of coincidental compounding cardiovascular events? Obstet Gynecol 67:157, 1986
Cunningham JA, Devine PC, Jelic S: Extracorporeal membrane oxygenation in pregnancy. Obstet Gynecol 108:792, 2006
Daif JL, Levie M, Chudnoff S, et al: Group A *Streptococcus* causing necrotizing fasciitis and toxic shock syndrome after medical termination of pregnancy. Obstet Gynecol 113:504, 2009
Del Frari B, Pulzl P, Schoeller T, et al: Pregnancy as a tissue expander in the correction of a scar deformity. Am J Obstet Gynecol 190:579, 2004
Dellinger RP, Levy MM, Carlet JM, et al: Surviving Sepsis Campaign: international guidelines for management of severe sepsis and septic shock: 2008. Crit Care Med 36(1):296, 2008
Dennis AT, Solnordal CB: Acute pulmonary oedema in pregnant women. Anaesthesia 67(6):646, 2012
Desai P, Suk M: Orthopedic trauma in pregnancy. Am J Orthop 36:E160, 2007
DiFederico EM, Burlingame JM, Kilpatrick SJ, et al: Pulmonary edema in obstetric patients is rapidly resolved except in the presence of infection or of nitroglycerine tocolysis after open fetal surgery. Am J Obstet Gynecol 179:925, 1998
Drazner MH, Dries Dl, Peshock RM, et al: Left ventricular hypertrophy is more prevalent in blacks than whites in the general population. The Dallas Heart Study. Hypertension 45:124, 2005
Einarson A, Bailey B, Inocencion G, et al: Accidental electric shock in pregnancy: a prospective cohort study. Am J Obstet Gynecol 176:678, 1997
El Kady D, Gilbert WM, Xing G, et al: Maternal and neonatal outcomes of assaults during pregnancy. Obstet Gynecol 105:357, 2005
Ellingsen CL, Eggebo TM, Lexow K: Amniotic fluid embolism after blunt abdominal trauma. Resuscitation 75(1):180, 2007
Eppert HD, Goddard KB, King CL: Successful treatment with drotrecogin alfa (activated) in a pregnant patient with severe sepsis. Pharmacotherapy 31(3):333, 2011
Evans TW, Smithies M: ABC of intensive care. Organ dysfunction. BMJ 318:1606, 1999
Fatovich DM: Electric shock in pregnancy. J Emerg Med 11:175, 1993
Ferguson ND, Cook DJ, Guyatt GH, et al: High-frequency oscillation in early acute respiratory distress syndrome. N Engl J Med 368(9):795, 2013
Filbin MR, Ring DC, Wessels MR, et al: Case 2–2009: a 25-year-old man with pain and swelling of the right hand and hypotension. N Engl J Med 360:281, 2009
Gallup DG, Freedman MA, Meguiar RV, et al: Necrotizing fasciitis in gynecologic and obstetric patients: a surgical emergency. Am J Obstet Gynecol 187:305, 2002
Gandhi SK, Powers JC, Nomeir A-M, et al: The pathogenesis of acute pulmonary edema associated with hypertension. N Engl J Med 344:17, 2001
García Gutiérrez JJ, Meléndez J, Torrero JV, et al: Lightning injuries in a pregnant woman: a case report and review of the literature. Burns 31:1045, 2005
Golombeck K, Ball RH, Lee H, et al: Maternal morbidity after maternal-fetal surgery. Am J Obstet Gynecol 194:834, 2006
Goodwin TM, Breen MT: Pregnancy outcome and fetomaternal hemorrhage after noncatastrophic trauma. Am J Obstet Gynecol 162:665, 1990
Gosman GG, Baldisseri MR, Stein KL, et al: Introduction of an obstetrics-specific medical emergency team for obstetric crises: implementation and experience. Am J Obstet Gynecol 198:367.e1, 2008
Green-Thompson R, Moodley J: In-utero intracranial haemorrhage probably secondary to domestic violence: case report and literature review. J Obstet Gynaecol 25:816, 2005
Gupta R, Strickland KM, Mertz HL: Successful treatment of severe sepsis with recombinant activated protein C during the third trimester of pregnancy. Obstet Gynecol 118(2 Pt 2):492, 2011
Hankins GD, Wendel GD, Cunningham FG, et al: Longitudinal evaluation of hemodynamic changes in eclampsia. Am J Obstet Gynecol 150:506, 1984
Hankins GD, Wendel GD, Leveno KJ, et al: Myocardial infarction during pregnancy. A review. Obstet Gynecol 65:139, 1985
Harvey S, Harrison DA, Singer M, et al: Assessment of the clinical effectiveness of pulmonary artery catheters in management of patients in intensive care (PAC-Man): a randomized controlled trial. Lancet 366:472, 2005
Hawkins JS, Casey BM, Minei J, et al: Outcomes after trauma in pregnancy. Am J Obstet Gynecol 197:S92, 2007
Herridge MS, Cheung AM, Tansey CM, et al: One-year outcomes in survivors of the acute respiratory distress syndrome. N Engl J Med 348:683, 2003
Herridge MS, Tansey CM, Matté A, et al: Functional disability 5 years after acute respiratory distress syndrome. N Engl J Med 364(14):1293, 2011
Higgins SD, Garite TJ: Late abruptio placentae in trauma patients: implications for monitoring. Obstet Gynecol 63:10S, 1984
Horon IL, Cheng D: Enhanced surveillance for pregnancy-associated mortality—Maryland, 1993–1998. JAMA 285:1455, 2001
Hough ME, Katz V: Pulmonary edema a case series in a community hospital. Obstet Gynecol 109:115S, 2007
Ikossi DG, Lazar AA, Morabito D, et al: Profile of mothers at risk: an analysis of injury and pregnancy loss in 1,195 trauma patients. J Am Coll Surg 200:49, 2005
Jenkins TM, Troiano NH, Graves CR, et al: Mechanical ventilation in an obstetric population: characteristics and delivery rates. Am J Obstet Gynecol 188:439, 2003
Jessup M, Brozena S: Heart failure. N Engl J Med 348:2007, 2003
Karimi H, Momeni M, Momeni M, et al: Burn injuries during pregnancy in Iran. Int J Gynaecol Obstet 104(2):132, 2009
Katz V, Balderston K, DeFreest M: Perimortem cesarean delivery: were our assumptions correct? Am J Obstet Gynecol 192:1916, 2005
Katz VL: Perimortem cesarean delivery: its role in maternal mortality. Semin Perinatol 36(1):68, 2012
Keizer JL, Zwart JJ, Meerman RH, et al: Obstetric intensive care admission: a 12-year review in a tertiary care centre. Eur J Obstet Gynecol Reprod Biol 128:152, 2006
Kenchaiah S, Evans JC, Levy D, et al: Obesity and the risk of heart failure. N Engl J Med 347:305, 2002
Kettel LM, Branch DW, Scott JR: Occult placental abruption after maternal trauma. Obstet Gynecol 71:449, 1988
Klevens RM, Morrison MA, Nadle J, et al: Invasive methicillin-resistant *Staphylococcus aureus* infections in the United States. JAMA 298 (15):1763, 2007
Klinich KD, Flannagan CA, Rupp JD, et al: Fetal outcome in motor-vehicle crashes: effects of crash characteristics and maternal restraint. Am J Obstet Gynecol 198(4):450.e1, 2008
Kopelman TR, Manriquez NE, Gridley M, et al: The ability of computed tomography to diagnose placental abruption in the trauma patient. J Trauma Acute Care Surgery 74(1):236, 2013
Kopko PM, Marshall CS, MacKenzie MR, et al: Transfusion-related acute lung injury: report of a clinical look-back investigation. JAMA 287:1968, 2002
Kuklina EV, Meikle SF, Jamieson DJ, et al: Severe obstetric morbidity in the United States: 1996–2006. Obstet Gynecol 113:293, 2009
Lapinsky SE: Cardiopulmonary complications of pregnancy. Crit Care Med 33:1616, 2005
Lee WL, Slutsky AS: Sepsis and endothelial permeability. N Engl J Med 363(7):689, 2010
Leggon RE, Wood GC, Indeck MC: Pelvic fractures in pregnancy: factors influencing maternal and fetal outcomes. J Trauma 53:796, 2002
Levinson G, Shnider SM, DeLorimier AA, et al: Effects of maternal hyperventilation on uterine blood flow and fetal oxygenation and acid-base status. Anesthesiology 40:340, 1974
Levy BD, Choi AMK: Acute respiratory distress syndrome. In Longo D, Fauci A, Kasper D, et al (eds): Harrison's Principles of Internal Medicine, 18th ed. New York, McGraw Hill, 2012, p 2205
Li YH, Novikova N: Pulmonary artery flow catheters for directing management in pre-eclampsia. Cochrane Database Syst Rev 6:CD008882, 2012
Lin P, Gill JR: Homicides of pregnant women. Am J Forensic Med Pathol 32(2):161, 2011
Linden JA: Care of the adult patient after sexual assault. N Engl J Med 365(9):834, 2011
Luley T, Fitzpatrick CB, Grotegut CA, et al: Perinatal implications of motor vehicle accident trauma during pregnancy: identifying populations at risk. Am J Obstet Gynecol 208:466.e1–5, 2013
Mabie WC, Barton JR, Sibai BM: Septic shock in pregnancy. Obstet Gynecol 90:553, 1997
Mabrouk AR, el-Feky AEH: Burns during pregnancy: a gloomy outcome. Burns 23:596, 1997
MacArthur RD, Miller M, Albertson T, et al: Adequacy of early empiric antibiotic treatment and survival in severe sepsis: experience from the MONARCS trial. Clin Infect Dis 38:284, 2004
Madan I, Puri I, Jain NJ, et al: Intensive care unit admissions among pregnant patients. Presented at the 56th Annual Clinical Meeting of the American College of Obstetricians and Gynecologists, New Orleans, LA, May 2008.
Maghsoudi H, Samnia R, Garadaghi A, et al: Burns in pregnancy. Burns 32:246, 2006

Mallampalli A, Hanania A, Guntupalli KK: Acute lung injury and acute respiratory distress syndrome. In Belfort MA, Saade GR, Foley MR, et al (eds): Critical Care Obstetrics, 5th ed. Wiley-Blackwell, 2010, p 338
Manriquez M, Srinivas G, Bollepalli S, et al: Is computed tomography a reliable diagnostic modality in detecting placental injuries in the setting of acute trauma? Am J Obstet Gynecol 202(6):611.e1, 2010
Martin GS, Mannino DM, Eaton S, et al: The epidemiology of sepsis in the United States from 1979 through 2000. N Engl J Med 348:1546, 2003
Martin SL, Macy RJ, Sullivan K, et al: Pregnancy-associated violent deaths: the role of intimate partner violence. Trauma Violence Abuse 8:135, 2007
Martin SR, Foley MR: Intensive care in obstetrics: an evidence-based review. Am J Obstet Gynecol 195:673, 2006
Mason KL, Aronoff DM: Postpartum group A *Streptococcus* sepsis and maternal immunology. Am J Reprod Immunol 67(2):91, 2012
Matsushita H, Harada A, Sato T, et al: Fetal intracranial injuries following motor vehicle accidents with airbag deployment. J Obstet Gynaecol Res 40(2):599, 2014
Matthews RN: Old burns and pregnancy. Br J Obstet Gynaecol 89:610, 1982
Mattox KL, Goetzl L: Trauma in pregnancy. Crit Care Med 33:S385, 2005
McCauley RL, Stenberg BA, Phillips LG, et al: Long-term assessment of the effects of circumferential truncal burns in pediatric patients on subsequent pregnancies. J Burn Care Rehabil 12:51, 1991
Medve L, Csitári IK, Molnár Z, et al: Recombinant human activated protein C treatment of septic shock syndrome in a patient at 18th week of gestation: a case report. Am J Obstet Gynecol 193:864, 2005
Metz TD, Abbott JT: Uterine trauma in pregnancy after motor vehicle crashes with airbag deployment: a 30-case series. J Trauma 61:658, 2006
Mirza FG, Devine PC, Gaddipati S: Trauma in pregnancy: a systematic approach. Am J Perinatol 27(7):579, 2010
Moellering RC Jr, Abbott GF, Ferraro MJ: Case 2–2011: a 30-year-old woman with shock after treatment for a furuncle. N Engl J Med 364(3):266, 2011
Moise KJ Jr, Belfort MA: Damage control for the obstetric patient. Surg Clin North Am 77:835, 1997
Motozawa y, Hitosugi M, Abe T, et al: Effects of seat belts worn by pregnant drivers during low-impact collisions. Am J Obstet Gynecol 203(1):62.e1, 2010
Muench M, Baschat A, Kush M, et al: Maternal fetal hemorrhage of greater than or equal to 0.1 percent predicts preterm labor in blunt maternal trauma. Am J Obstet Gynecol 189:S119, 2003
Muench MV, Baschat AA, Reddy UM, et al: Kleihauer-Betke testing is important in all cases of maternal trauma. J Trauma 57:1094, 2004
Munford RS: Severe sepsis and septic shock: introduction. In Longo DL, Fauci AS, Kasper DL, et al (eds): Harrison's Principles of Internal Medicine, 18th ed. New York, McGraw Hill, 2012, p 2223
Myburgh JA, Finfer S, Bellomo R, et al: Hydroxyethyl starch or saline for fluid resuscitation in intensive care. N Engl J Med 367(20):1901, 2012
Nair P, Davies AR, Beca J, et al: Extracorporeal membrane oxygenation for severe ARDS in pregnant and postpartum women during the 2009 H1N1 pandemic. Intensive Care Med 37(4):648, 2011
Nasraway SA, Cohen IL, Dennis RC, et al: Guidelines on admission and discharge for adult intermediate care units. Crit Care Med 26(3):607, 1998
Nathan L, Peters MT, Ahmed AM, et al: The return of life-threatening puerperal sepsis caused by group A streptococci. Am J Obstet Gynecol 169:571, 1993
National Heart, Lung, and Blood Institute Acute Respiratory Distress Syndrome (ARDS) Clinical Trials Network: Efficacy and safety of corticosteroids for persistent acute respiratory distress syndrome. N Engl J Med 354:1671, 2006a
National Heart, Lung, and Blood Institute Acute Respiratory Distress Syndrome (ARDS) Clinical Trials Network: Pulmonary-artery versus central venous catheter to guide treatment of acute lung injury. N Engl J Med 354:2213, 2006b
National Institutes of Health: Critical Care Medicine Consensus Conference. JAMA 250:798, 1983
Ognibene FP, Parker MM, Natanson C, et al: Depressed left ventricular performance. Response to volume infusion in patients with sepsis and septic shock. Chest 93:903, 1988
Oram MP, Seal P, McKinstry CE: Severe acute respiratory distress syndrome in pregnancy. Caesarean section in the second trimester to improve maternal ventilation. Anaesth Intensive Care 35(6):975, 2007
Pacheco LD, Gei AF, VanHook JW, et al: Burns in pregnancy. Obstet Gynecol 106:1210, 2005
Pak LL, Reece EA, Chan L: Is adverse pregnancy outcome predictable after blunt abdominal trauma? Am J Obstet Gynecol 179:1140, 1998
Palladino CL, Singh V, Campbell J, et al: Homicide and suicide during the perinatal period. Obstet Gynecol 118(5):1056, 2011
Palmer JD, Sparrow OC: Extradural haematoma following intrauterine trauma. Injury 25:671, 1994
Pandharipande PP, Girad TD, Jackson A, et al: Long-term cognitive impairment after critical illness. N Engl J Med 369:1306, 2013
Pathan N, Hemingway CA, Alizadeh AA, et al: Role of interleukin 6 in myocardial dysfunction of meningococcal septic shock. Lancet 363:203, 2004
Patteson SK, Snider CC, Meyer DS, et al: The consequences of high-risk behaviors: trauma during pregnancy. J Trauma 62:1015, 2007
Pearlman MD, Cunningham FG: Trauma in pregnancy. In Cunningham FG, MacDonald PC, Gant NF, Leveno KJ, Gilstrap LC (eds): Williams Obstetrics, 19th ed. Supplement No. 21, October/November 1996
Pearlman MD, Klinch KD, Flannagan CAC: Fetal outcome in motor-vehicle crashes: effects of crash characteristics and maternal restraint. Am J Obstet Gynecol, 198(4):450.e1, 2008
Pearlman MD, Tintinalli JE, Lorenz RP: A prospective controlled study of outcome after trauma during pregnancy. Am J Obstet Gynecol 162:1502, 1990
Peek GJ, Mugford M, Tiruvoipati R, et al: Efficacy and economic assessment of conventional ventilatory support versus extracorporeal membrane oxygenation for severe adult respiratory failure (CESAR): a multicenter randomized controlled trial. Lancet 374(9698):1351, 2009
Perner A, Naase N, Guttormsen, et al: Hydroxyethyl starch 130/0.4 versus Ringer's acetate in severe sepsis. N Engl J Med 367(2):124, 2012
Petrone P, Talving P, Browder T, et al: Abdominal injuries in pregnancy: a 155-month study at two level 1 trauma centers. Injury 42(1):47, 2011
Phua J, Badia JR, Adhikari NK, et al: Has mortality from acute respiratory stress syndrome decreased over time? A systematic review. Am J Respir Crit Care Med 179(3):220, 2009
Pluymakers C, De Weerdt A, Jacquemyn Y, et al: Amniotic fluid embolism after surgical trauma: two case reports and review of the literature. Resuscitation 72(2):324, 2007
Pritchard JA, Cunningham G, Pritchard SA, et al: On reducing the frequency of severe abruptio placentae. Am J Obstet Gynecol 165:1345, 1991
Qaiser R, Black P: Neurosurgery in pregnancy. Semin Neurol 27:476, 2007
Que YA, Haefliger JA, Piroth L, et al: Fibrinogen and fibronectin binding cooperate for valve infection and invasion in *Staphylococcus aureus* experimental endocarditis. J Experimental Med 20:1627, 2005
Radosevich MA, Finegold H, Goldfarb W, et al: Anesthetic management of the pregnant burn patient: excision and grafting to emergency cesarean section. J Clin Anesth 25:582, 2013
Ranieri VM, Thompson BT, Barie PS, et al: Drotrecogin alfa (activated) in adults with septic shock. N Engl J Med 366(22):2055, 2012
Rayburn W, Smith B, Feller I, et al: Major burns during pregnancy: effects on fetal well being. Surg Gynecol Obstet 63:392, 1984
Rees GA, Willis BA: Resuscitation in late pregnancy. Anaesthesia 43(5):347, 1988
Reis PM, Sander CM, Pearlman MD: Abruptio placentae after auto accidents. A case control study. J Reprod Med 45:6, 2000
Richard C, Warszawski J, Anguel N, et al: Early use of the pulmonary artery catheter and outcomes in patients with shock and acute respiratory distress syndrome. JAMA 290:2713, 2003
Rivers E, Nguyen B, Havstad S, et al: Early goal-directed therapy in the treatment of severe sepsis and septic shock. N Engl J Med 345:1368, 2001
Robertson-Blackmore E, Putnam FW, Rubinow DR, et al: Antecedent trauma exposure and risk of depression in the perinatal period. J Clin Psychiatry 74:e942, 2013
Rode H, Millar AJ, Cywes S, et al: Thermal injury in pregnancy—the neglected tragedy. S Afr Med J 77:346, 1990
Rodriguez MA, Heilemann MV, Fielder E, et al: Intimate partner violence, depression, and PTSD among pregnant Latina women. Ann Fam Med 6:44, 2008
Romero VC, Pearlman M: Maternal mortality due to trauma. Semin Perinatol 36(1):60, 2012
Rorth M, Bille-Brahe NE: 2,3-Diphosphoglycerate and creatine in the red cells during pregnancy. Scand J Clin Lab Invest 28:271, 1971
Rose JS: Ultrasound in abdominal trauma. Emerg Med Clin North Am 22(3):581, 2004
Rotas M, McCalla S, Liu C, et al: Methicillin-resistant *Staphylococcus aureus* necrotizing pneumonia arising from an infected episiotomy site. Obstet Gynecol 109:533, 2007
Rowe TF, Lafayette S, Cox S: An unusual fetal complication of traumatic uterine rupture. J Emerg Med 14:173, 1996
Roy B, Cordova FC, Travaline JM, et al: Full face mask for noninvasive positive-pressure ventilation in patients with acute respiratory failure. JAOA 107(4):148, 2007
Russell JA: Management of sepsis. N Engl J Med 355:1699, 2006
Russell JA, Walley KR, Singer J, et al: Vasopressin versus norepinephrine infusion in patients with septic shock. N Engl J Med 358:877, 2008
Sadro CT, Zins AM, Debiec K, et al: Case report: lethal fetal head injury and placental abruption in a pregnant trauma patient. Emerg Radiol 19(2):175, 2012

Sam S, Corbridge TC, Mokhlesi B: Cortisol levels and mortality in sepsis. Clin Endocrinol (Oxf) 60:29, 2004
Samol JM, Lambers DS: Magnesium sulfate tocolysis and pulmonary edema: the drug or the vehicle? Am J Obstet Gynecol 192:1430, 2005
Sandham JD, Hull RD, Brant RF, et al: A randomized, controlled trial of the use of pulmonary-artery catheters in high-risk surgical patients. N Engl J Med 348:5, 2003
Satin AJ, Ramin JM, Paicurich J, et al: The prevalence of sexual assault: a survey of 2404 puerperal women. Am J Obstet Gynecol 167:973, 1992
Schiff MA, Holt VL: Pregnancy outcomes following hospitalization for motor vehicle crashes in Washington State from 1989 to 2001. Am J Epidemiol 161:503, 2005
Schiff MA, Holt VL, Daling JR: Maternal and infant outcomes after injury during pregnancy in Washington state from 1989 to 1997. J Trauma 53:939, 2002
Schiff MA, Mack CD, Kaufman RP, et al: The effect of air bags on pregnancy outcomes in Washington state: 2002–2005. Obstet Gynecol 115(1):85, 2010
Schneider MB, Ivester TS, Mabie WC, et al: Maternal and fetal outcomes in women requiring antepartum mechanical ventilation. Obstet Gynecol [abstract] 101:69S, 2003
Sciscione A, Invester T, Largoza M, et al: Acute pulmonary edema in pregnancy. Obstet Gynecol 101:511, 2003
Sela HY, Shveiky D, Laufer N, et al: Pregnant women injured in terror-related multiple casualty incidents: injuries and outcomes. J Trauma 64(3):727, 2008
Shadigian EM, Bauer ST: Pregnancy-associated death: a qualitative systematic review of homicide and suicide. Obstet Gynecol Surv 60:183, 2005
Sheffield JS, Cunningham FG: Urinary tract infection in women. Obstet Gynecol 106:1085, 2005
Sheth SS, Sheth KN: Treatment of neurocritical care emergencies in pregnancy. Curr Treat Options Neurol 14:197, 2012
Sibai BM, Mabie BC, Harvey CJ, et al: Pulmonary edema in severe preeclampsia–eclampsia: analysis of thirty-seven consecutive cases. Am J Obstet Gynecol 156:1174, 1987
Sibai BM, Viteri OA: Diabetic ketoacidosis in pregnancy. Obstet Gynecol 123:167, 2014
Silverman JG, Decker MR, Reed E, et al: Intimate partner violence victimization prior to and during pregnancy among women residing in 26 U.S. states: associations with maternal and neonatal death. Am J Obstet Gynecol 195:140, 2006
Sirin H, Weiss HB, Sauber-Schatz EK, et al: Seat belt use, counseling and motor-vehicle injury during pregnancy: Results from a multi-state population-based survey. Matern Child Health J 11:505, 2007
Slutsky AD, Ranieri VM: Ventilator-induced lung injury. N Engl J Med 369:2126, 2013
Small MK, James AH, Kershaw T, et al: Near-miss maternal mortality: cardiac dysfunction as the principal cause of obstetric intensive care unit admissions. Obstet Gynecol 119(2 pt 1):250, 2012
Society of Critical Care Medicine: Guidelines for intensive care unit admission, discharge, and triage. Crit Care Med 27(3):633, 1999
Society of Critical Care Medicine: Recommendations for intensive care unit admission and discharge criteria. Crit Care Med 16(8):807, 1988
Soper DE, Lee SI, Kim JY, et al: Case 35–2011: a 33-year-old woman with postpartum leukocytosis and gram-positive bacteremia. N Engl J Med 365(20:1916, 2011
Sozen I, Nesin N: Accidental electric shock in pregnancy and antenatal occurrence of maternal deep vein thrombosis. A case report. J Reprod Med 49:58, 2004
Stettler RW, Lutich A, Pritchard JA, et al: Traumatic placental abruption: a separation from traditional thought. Presented at the annual clinical meeting of the American College of Obstetricians and Gynecologists, Las Vegas, May 1992
Stevens TA, Carroll MA, Promecene PA, et al: Utility of acute physiology, age, and chronic health evaluation (APACHE III) score in maternal admissions to the intensive care unit. Am J Obstet Gynecol 194:e13, 2006
Stone IK: Trauma in the obstetric patient. Obstet Gynecol Clin North Am 26:459, 1999
Subrevilla LA, Cassinelli MT, Carcelen A, et al: Human fetal and maternal oxygen tension and acid-base status during delivery at high altitude. Am J Obstet Gynecol 111:1111, 1971
Suellentrop K, Morrow B, Williams L, et al: Monitoring progress toward achieving maternal and infant Healthy People 2010 objectives—19 states, Pregnancy Risk Assessment Monitoring System (PRAMS), 2000–2003. MMWR 55(9):1, 2006
Suffredini AF, Munford RS: Novel therapies for septic shock over the past 4 decades. JAMA 306(2):194, 2011
Sugar NF, Fine DN, Eckert LO: Physical injury after sexual assault: findings of a large case series. Am J Obstet Gynecol 190:71, 2004
Sugiyama T, Kobayashi T, Nagao K, et al: Group A streptococcal toxic shock syndrome with extremely aggressive course in the third trimester. J Obstet Gynaecol Res 36(4):852, 2010
Takehana CS, Kang YS: Acute traumatic gonadal vein rupture in a pregnant patient involved in a major motor vehicle collision. Emerg Radiol 18(4):349, 2011
Taylor RW, Zimmerman JL, Dellinger RP, et al: Inhaled Nitric Oxide in ARDS Study Group: low-dose inhaled nitric oxide in patients with acute lung injury: a randomized controlled trial. JAMA 291:1603, 2004
The ARDS Definition Task Force: Acute respiratory distress syndrome. The Berlin Definition. JAMA 307(23):2526, 2012
Thornton CE, von Dadelszen P, Makris A, et al: Acute pulmonary oedema as a complication of hypertension during pregnancy. Hypertens Pregnancy 30(2):169, 2011
Tihtonen KM, Kööbi, T, Vuolteenaho O, et al: Natriuretic peptides and hemodynamics in preeclampsia. Am J Obstet Gynecol 196:328, 2007
Towery R, English TP, Wisner D: Evaluation of pregnant women after blunt injury. J Trauma 35:731, 1993
Tsuei BJ: Assessment of the pregnant trauma patient. Injury Int J Care Injured 37:367, 2006
United States Department of Justice: Office of Justice Programs. www.ncjrs.gov/pdffiles1/nij/183781.pdf. Accessed May 7, 2013
Vanden Hoek TL, Morrison LJ, Shuster M, et al: Part 12: cardiac arrest in special situations: 2010 American Heart Association guidelines for cardiopulmonary resuscitation and emergency cardiovascular care. Circulation 122:S829, 2010
Van Hook JW, Hankins GDV: Invasive hemodynamic monitoring. Prim Care Update Ob/Gyn 4:39, 1997
Vasquez DN, Estenssoror E, Canales HS, et al: Clinical characteristics and outcomes of obstetric patients requiring ICU admission. Chest 131(3):718, 2007
Vincent JL, De Backer D: Circulatory shock. N Engl J Med 369:1726, 2013
Vincent JL, Rhodes W, Perel A, et al: Clinical review: update on hemodynamic monitoring–a consensus of 16. Critical Care 15:229, 2011
Vladutiu CJ, Marshall SW, Poole C, et al: Adverse pregnancy outcomes following motor vehicle crashes. Am J Prev Med 45:629, 2013
Ware LB, Matthay MA: Acute pulmonary edema. N Engl J Med 353:2788, 2005
Ware LB, Matthay MA: The acute respiratory distress syndrome. N Engl J Med 342:1334, 2000
Warren BL, Eid A, Singer P, et al: Caring for the critically ill patient: high-dose antithrombin III in severe sepsis: a randomized controlled trial. JAMA 286:1869, 2001
Wathen CN, MacMillan HL: Interventions for violence against women: scientific review. JAMA 289:589, 2003
Weir LF, Pierce BT, Vazquez JO: Complete fetal transection after a motor vehicle collision. Obstet Gynecol 111(2):530, 2008
Weiss HB, Songer TJ, Fabio A: Fetal deaths related to maternal injury. JAMA 286:1863, 2001
Wenzel RP, Edmond MB: Septic shock—evaluating another failed treatment. N Engl J Med 366(22):2122, 2012
Weyerts LK, Jones MC, James HE: Paraplegia and congenital contractures as a consequence of intrauterine trauma. Am J Med Genet 43:751, 1992
Wheeler AP, Bernard GR: Acute lung injury and the acute respiratory distress syndrome: a clinical review. Lancet 369:1553, 2007
Wheeler AP, Bernard GR: Treating patients with severe sepsis. N Engl J Med 340:207, 1999
Whitty JE: Maternal cardiac arrest in pregnancy. Clin Obstet Gynecol 45:377, 2002
Wiedemann HP, Wheeler AP, Bernard GR, et al: Comparison of two fluid-management strategies in acute lung injury. N Engl J Med 354(24):2213, 2006
Widgerow AD, Ford TD, Botha M: Burn contracture preventing uterine expansion. Ann Plast Surg 27:269, 1991
Yamada T, Yamada T, Yamamura MK, et al: Invasive group A streptococcal infection in pregnancy. J Infect 60(6):417, 2010
Ylagan MV, Trivedi N, Basu T, et al: Radiation exposure in the pregnant trauma patient: implications for fetal risk counseling. Abstract No. 320. Am J Obstet Gynecol 199(6):S100, 2008
Young D, Lamb SE, Shah S, et al: High-frequency oscillation for acute respiratory distress syndrome. N Engl J Med 368(9):806, 2013
Zeeman GG: Obstetric critical care: a blueprint for improved outcomes. Crit Care Med 34:S208, 2006
Zeeman GG, Wendel GD Jr, Cunningham FG: A blueprint for obstetric critical care. Am J Obstet Gynecol 188:532, 2003
Zinaman M, Rubin J, Lindheimer MD: Serial plasma oncotic pressure levels and echoencephalography during and after delivery in severe preeclampsia. Lancet 1:1245, 1985

CHAPTER 48

Obesity

Excessive weight is a major health problem in the United States and other affluent societies. For a number of years, obesity was said to be *epidemic*—strictly defined, this implies a *temporary* widespread outbreak of greatly increased frequency and severity. Unfortunately, obesity more correctly is *endemic*—a condition that is habitually present. By 1991, approximately a third of adults in the United States were overweight, and thus a stated goal of *Healthy People 2000* was to reduce the prevalence of overweight people to 20 percent or less by the end of the 20th century (Public Health Service, 1990). Not only was this goal not achieved, but by 2000, more than half of the population was overweight. In 2010, a third of all adults were obese (Ogden, 2012).

The adverse health aspects of obesity are staggering. Obesity-related diseases include diabetes, heart disease, hypertension, stroke, and osteoarthritis. Obese women who become pregnant—and their fetuses—are predisposed to various serious pregnancy-related complications. Moreover, long-term maternal and fetal effects include significant and increased morbidity and mortality rates.

GENERAL CONSIDERATIONS

Definitions

A number of systems have been used to define and classify obesity. The *body mass index* (*BMI*), also known as the *Quetelet index*, is currently most often used. The BMI is calculated as weight in kilograms divided by the square of the height in meters (kg/m^2). Calculated BMI values are available in various chart and graphic forms, such as the one shown in Figure 48-1. The National Institutes of Health (2000) classifies adults according to BMI as follows: *normal* (18.5 to 24.9 kg/m^2); *overweight* (25 to 29.9 kg/m^2); and *obese* (≥ 30 kg/m^2). Obesity is further divided into: *class 1* (30 to 34.9 kg/m^2); *class 2* (35 to 39.9 kg/m^2); and *class 3* (≥ 40 kg/m^2).

Prevalence

By 2000, 28 percent of men and 33 percent of women were obese (Ogden, 2012). For the period 2009 to 2010, among men and women these percentages were almost identical at approximately 35 percent. Shown in Figure 48-2 are the prevalences of obesity among girls and women. Obesity increases with age as well as with ethnic minority, and almost 60 percent of black women were obese in 2010. This is also true among indigent individuals (Drewnowski, 2004).

Adipose Tissue as an Organ System

Fat tissue is much more complex than its energy storage function. Many cell types in fat tissue communicate with all other tissues via endocrine and paracrine factors—*adipokines*, or *adipocytokines*. Some of those with metabolic functions include adiponectin, leptin, tumor necrosis factor-α (TNF-α), interleukin 6 (IL-6), resistin, visfatin, apelin, vascular endothelium growth factor (VEGF), lipoprotein lipase, and insulin-like growth factor (Briana, 2009; Scherer, 2006). A principal adipokine is adiponectin, which is a 30-kDa protein. It enhances insulin sensitivity, blocks hepatic release of glucose, and has cardioprotective effects on circulating plasma lipids. An adiponectin deficit leads to diabetes, hypertension, endothelial cell activation, and cardiovascular disease.

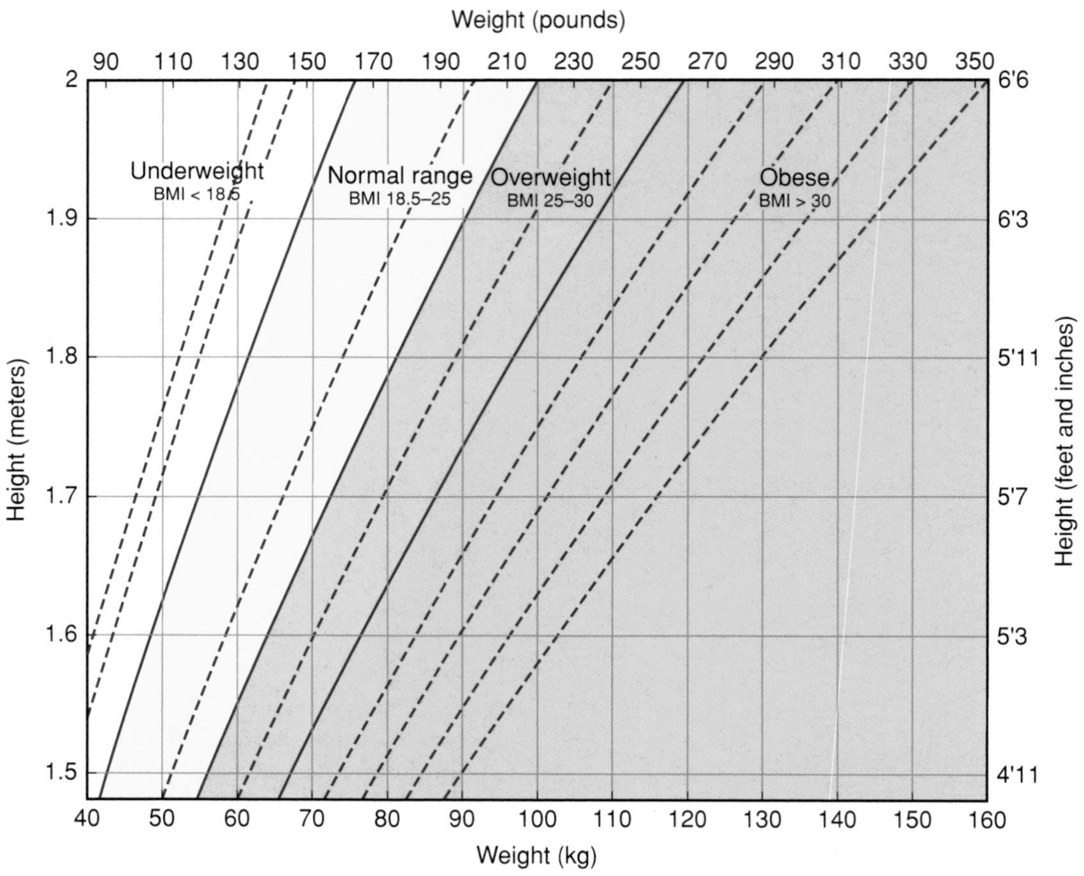

FIGURE 48-1 Chart for estimating body mass index (BMI). To find the BMI category for a particular subject, locate the point at which the height and weight intersect.

Adipocytokines in Pregnancy

Cytokines that result in insulin resistance—leptin, resistin, TNF-α, and IL-6—are increased during pregnancy. Indeed, these may be the primary stimulant of insulin resistance. Secretion of the remaining adipokines is either unchanged or decreased. Specific patterns have been variously described with gestational diabetes, preeclampsia, and fetal-growth restriction (Briana, 2009). In a longitudinal study of 55 pregnant women, Meyer and associates (2013) confirmed that higher BMIs are associated with lower adiponectin but higher leptin levels.

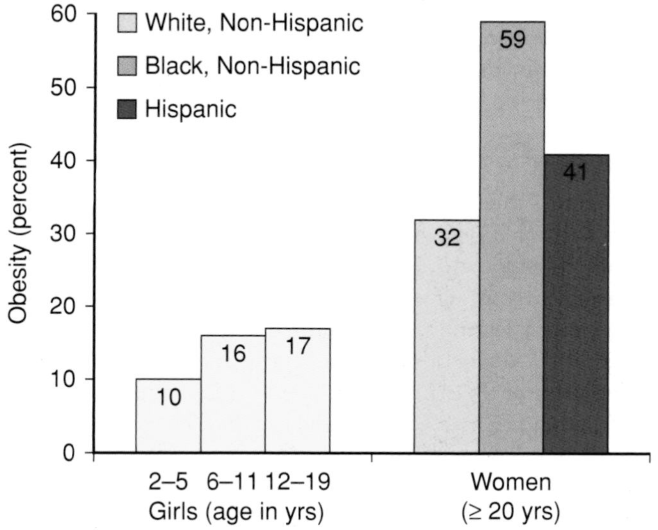

FIGURE 48-2 Prevalence of obesity in girls and women in the United States for 2009–2010. (Data from Flegal, 2012; Ogden, 2012.)

Metabolic Syndrome

Given its multifaceted endocrine and paracrine functions, it is not surprising that excessive fat tissue is detrimental (Cornier, 2011). One major drawback is that obesity interacts with inherited factors to cause *insulin resistance* and in some cases, the metabolic syndrome. This resistance is characterized by impaired glucose metabolism and a predisposition to type 2 diabetes. Insulin resistance also causes several subclinical abnormalities that predispose to cardiovascular disease and accelerate its onset. The most important among these are type 2 diabetes, dyslipidemia, and hypertension, which define the metabolic syndrome.

Criteria used by the National Institutes of Health (2001) to define the metabolic syndrome are shown in Table 48-1. Virtually all obese women with hypertension demonstrate elevated plasma insulin levels. These are even higher in women with excessive fat in the abdomen—an apple shape—compared with those whose fat is in the hips and thighs—a pear shape (American College of Obstetricians and Gynecologists, 2003).

Prevalence

Ford and colleagues (2002) did a follow-up study of men and women enrolled in the Third National Health and Nutrition

TABLE 48-1. Criteria for Diagnosis of the Metabolic Syndrome

Patients with three or more of the following:
Waist circumference: > 88 cm (34.7 in) in women; > 102 cm (40.2 in) in men
Hypertriglyceridemia: ≥ 150 mg/dL
High-density lipoprotein (HDL): < 50 mg/dL in women; < 40 mg/dL in men
High blood pressure: ≥ 130/85 mm Hg[a]
High fasting glucose: ≥ 110 mg/dL[a]

[a]Those with normal values while taking medications are considered to meet these criteria.
From National Institutes of Health, 2001.

Survey (NHANES III). They found an overall prevalence of the metabolic syndrome in 24 percent of women and 22 percent of men. As expected, prevalence increased with age. For women, prevalence was approximately 6 percent in those 20 to 29 years; 14 percent in those 30 to 39 years; 20 percent in those 40 to 49 years; and 30 percent for women older than 50 years. Jordan and colleagues (2012) reported similar figures in adults in New York City in 2004.

Nonalcoholic Fatty Liver Disease (NAFLD)

Generally speaking, visceral adiposity correlates with hepatic fat content (Cornier, 2011). With obesity, excessive fat accumulates in the liver—*hepatic steatosis*. Specifically, in persons with the metabolic syndrome, steatosis can progress to nonalcoholic steatohepatitis (NASH) and cirrhosis. Indeed, a fourth of cases of chronic liver disease in Western countries are caused by nonalcoholic fatty liver disease (NAFLD) (Targher, 2010). Moreover, NAFLD either is a marker for cardiovascular disease or is involved in its pathogenesis. This may be related to an inherited prothrombotic state (Verrijken, 2014).

Pregnancy

Experience with NAFLD in pregnancy is limited (Page, 2011). It also appears that the increased insulin resistance it imposes causes excess gestational diabetes (Forbes, 2011). In addition, insulin resistance mobilizes free fatty acids to increase their plasma levels. In nonpregnant adults, hepatic fat content normally is 1 to 5 percent of liver mass, however, this has not been studied in pregnant women (Browning, 2004). However, Meyer and associates (2013) found that overweight and obese gravidas had a higher proportion of low-density lipoprotein III (LDL-III) compared with that of normal-weight women. LDL-III predominance is a hallmark of ectopic liver fat accumulation that is typical of NAFLD. At Parkland Hospital, with increasing frequency we are encountering obese women who have NAFLD with evidence of steatohepatitis manifest by elevated serum hepatic aminotransferase levels. In some cases, liver biopsy is necessary to exclude other causes.

MORBIDITY AND MORTALITY ASSOCIATED WITH OBESITY

Obese individuals are at increased risk for an imposing number of complications (Table 48-2). The direct link between obesity and type 2 diabetes mellitus is well known. Ninety percent of type 2 diabetes cases are attributable to excess weight, and 75 percent of these diabetics have the metabolic syndrome (Hossain, 2007). Heart disease due to obesity—*adipositas cordis*—is caused by hypertension, hypervolemia, and dyslipidemia. Higher rates of abnormal left ventricular function, heart failure, myocardial infarction, and stroke have been noted (Chinali, 2004; Kenchaiah, 2002; Targher, 2010).

TABLE 48-2. Long-Term Complications of Obesity

Disorder	Possible Cause(s)
Type 2 diabetes mellitus	Insulin resistance
Hypertension	Increased blood volume and cardiac output
Coronary heart disease	Hypertension, dyslipidemia, type 2 diabetes
Cardiomyopathy	Eccentric left ventricular hypertrophy
Sleep apnea/pulmonary dysfunction	Pharyngeal fat deposition
Ischemic stroke	Atherosclerosis, decreased cerebral blood flow
Gallbladder disease	Hyperlipidemia
Liver disease—nonalcoholic steatohepatitis (NASH)	Increased visceral adiposity, elevated serum free fatty acids, hyperinsulinemia
Osteoarthritis	Stress on weight-bearing joints
Subfertility	Hyperinsulinemia
Cancer—endometrium, colon, breast	Hyperestrogenemia
Deep-vein thrombosis	Endothelial inflammation
Carpal tunnel syndrome	
Poor wound healing	

From Calle, 2003, 2005; Chinali, 2004; de Gonzalez, 2010; Flegal, 2007; Kenchaiah, 2002; National Task Force on the Prevention and Treatment of Obesity, 2000; Ninomiya, 2004; Targher, 2010.

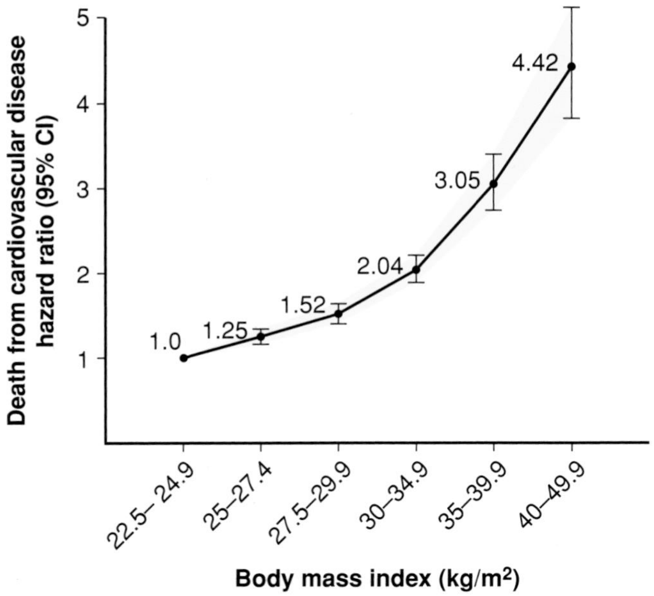

FIGURE 48-3 Estimated hazard ratios (95% CI) for death due to cardiovascular disease according to body mass index among 1.46 million white adult men and women. (Data from de Gonzalez, 2010.)

Excessive weight is associated with increased rates of early mortality, as shown by Peeters (2003) and Fontaine (2003) and their colleagues in follow-up studies from both the Framingham Heart Study and the NHANES III cohort. Mortality results from pooled data from 19 prospective studies are shown in Figure 48-3. In these and other studies, mortality risk from cardiovascular disease and cancer increased directly with increasing BMI.

TREATMENT OF OBESITY

Weight loss is tremendously difficult for obese individuals. If achieved, long-term maintenance poses equivalent or even more daunting difficulties. Even the most legitimate nonsurgical methods are fraught with frequent failure. If they are successful, slow and inexorable return to preintervention weight usually follows (Yanovski, 2005). Successful weight loss approaches include behavioral, pharmacological, and surgical techniques or a combination of these methods (Eckel, 2008; Zimmet, 2012). As such, obstetrician-gynecologists are encouraged to aid assessment and management of obesity in adult women. Weight loss and lifestyle changes have been shown to reduce the associated metabolic syndrome (Crist, 2012). When used in conjunction with bariatric surgery, there is improved glucose control with type 2 diabetes (Mingrone, 2012; Schauer, 2012).

PREGNANCY AND OBESITY

Obese women unequivocally have reproductive disadvantages. This translates into difficulty in achieving pregnancy, early and recurrent pregnancy loss, preterm delivery, and a myriad increased obstetrical, medical, and surgical complications with pregnancy, labor, delivery, and the puerperium (American College of Obstetricians and Gynecologists, 2013a). Obesity in pregnancy is also associated with increased health-care utilization and costs (Pauli, 2013). Finally, infants—and later, adults—of obese mothers have correspondingly increased rates of morbidity, mortality, and obesity (Reynolds, 2013).

Obesity results in subfertility due to increased insulin resistance as in polycystic ovarian syndrome. Leptin dysregulation also results in loss of gonadotropin secretory rhythms (Maguire, 2012). Impaired fecundity has been linked to women with a BMI > 30 kg/m^2 (Neill, 2001). In 6500 in vitro fertilization-intracytoplasmic sperm injection cycles, Bellver and associates (2010) found that implantation, pregnancy, and livebirth rates were progressively and significantly reduced with each unit of maternal BMI. As discussed in Chapter 8 (p. 157), obesity is associated with increased risk of first-trimester and recurrent miscarriage (Lashen, 2004; Metwally, 2008). In the many overweight and obese women who achieve pregnancy, there is a litany of increased and interrelated adverse perinatal outcomes that are discussed subsequently.

Prevalence

As expected from reviewing Figure 48-2, obesity complicating pregnancy has increased substantially in this country. Before adoption of the BMI, investigators used various definitions of obesity to assess risks during pregnancy. For example, in an earlier study from the University of Alabama at Birmingham, four definitions were used, but regardless of how obesity was defined, all groups showed at least twofold increases in prevalence during the 20-year period (Lu, 2001). Equivalent findings were reported from a 15-year study done in Cleveland (Ehrenberg, 2002). Our experience at Parkland Hospital is similar, as shown in the three epochs depicted in Figure 48-4.

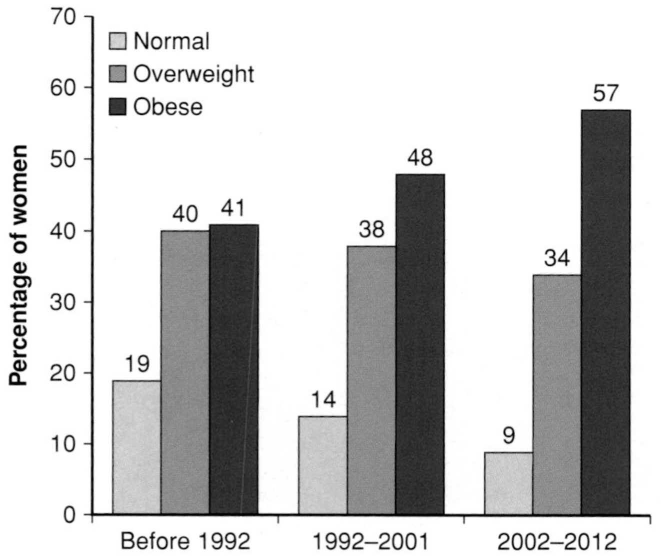

FIGURE 48-4 Increasing prevalence of obesity during three epochs in pregnant women classified at the time of their first prenatal visit at Parkland Hospital. (Data courtesy of Dr. Don McIntire.)

Maternal Weight Gain and Energy Requirement

The Institute of Medicine (2009) updated its previous comprehensive reviews of maternal weight gain determinants in relation to biological, metabolic, and social predictors. Its recommended weight gains for various BMI categories are shown in Table 9-5 (p. 177). For overweight women, weight gain of 15 to 25 pounds is recommended. For obese women, the Institute recommends a gain of 11 to 20 pounds. This is because fat deposition is greater in women with high BMIs, and thus, energy costs are significantly lower (Butte, 2004). Kinoshita and Itoh (2006) found that during the third trimester, increases were predominantly in visceral fat. Despite these stores, maternal catabolism is—at least intuitively—not good for fetal growth and development. The American College of Obstetricians and Gynecologists (2013c) has endorsed these Institute guidelines.

These Institute guidelines for obese women have some, although minimal, foundation in scientific evidence (Rasmussen, 2010). In a study of 2080 obese women, there was no advantage to weight gain > 20 pounds (Vesco, 2011). However, Chu and coworkers (2009) reported in the United States in 2004 to 2005 that 40 percent of normal-weight and 60 percent of overweight women gained excessive weight during pregnancy. The Maternal-Fetal Medicine Units Network arrived at similar conclusions. Seventy-five percent of nearly 8300 nulliparas gained more weight than the Institute recommendations (Johnson, 2013). Additionally, women who gained more than the recommended amount had excessive postpartum weight gain at 3, 8, and 15 years after delivery (Nehring, 2011; Rooney, 2002).

Maternal Morbidity

Some of the excess perinatal morbidity due to obesity is listed in Table 48-3. In studies, various definitions of obesity in pregnant women have included 150 percent of ideal body weight, BMI > 35 kg/m^2, BMI > 40 kg/m^2, BMI > 50 kg/m^2, and > 150 pounds over ideal body weight (Cedergren, 2004; Crane, 2013; Denison, 2008; Kabiru, 2004; Kumari, 2001; Stamilio, 2013). In one study, Weiss and colleagues (2004) reported similar adverse outcomes and maternal morbidity in a prospective multicenter study of more than 16,000 women from the FASTER trial (First- and Second-Trimester Evaluation of Risk). As shown in Figures 48-5 and 48-6, especially striking are the marked increases in gestational diabetes and hypertension. Lipkind and associates (2013) showed obesity to be an independent risk factor for "near-miss" maternal morbidity (Chap. 1, p. 6).

Not shown in Figure 48-5 are the cesarean delivery rates. These were 33.8 percent for obese and 47.4 percent for morbidly obese women compared with only 20.7 percent for the normal-weight control group (Weiss, 2004). Similar results were subsequently described by Garabedian and coworkers (2011). Haeri and colleagues (2009) also found increased rates of cesarean delivery and gestational diabetes in obese adolescents. More worrisome is that obese women also have increased rates of *emergency* cesarean delivery (Lynch, 2008; Poobalan, 2009). Finally, wound infections are more common. Alanis and associates (2010) reported this complication in 30 percent in women whose BMI was > 50 kg/m^2.

There are also reports of increased adverse pregnancy outcomes in overweight women whose BMI is 25 to 29.9 kg/m^2 (Hall, 2005). Shown in Table 48-3 were results of two studies that included more than 285,000 singleton pregnancies.

TABLE 48-3. Adverse Pregnancy Effects in Overweight and Obese Women

Complication	Prevalence (%) in Women with Normal BMI 20–24.9 n = 176,923	Increased Complications (Odds Ratio[a]) Overweight BMI 25–29.9 n = 79,014	Obese BMI > 30 n = 31,276
Gestational diabetes	0.8	1.7–3.5	3.0–3.6
Preeclampsia	0.7	1.5–1.9	2.1
Postterm pregnancy	0.13	1.2[b]	1.7
Emergency cesarean delivery	7.8	1.3–1.4	1.7–1.8
Elective cesarean delivery	4.0	1.2	1.3–1.4
Postpartum hemorrhage	10.4	1.04–1.2	1.0–1.4
Pelvic infection	0.7	1.2	1.3
Urinary tract infection	0.7	1.2	1.4
Wound infection	0.4	1.3	2.2
Fetal macrosomia	9.0	1.6	2.4
Stillbirth	0.4	1.4	1.4–1.6
Thrombosis	—	1.6	0.97[b]

[a]Odds ratios (99% CI) are significant except when denoted.
[b]Not significantly different.
BMI = body mass index.
Data from Ovesen, 2011; Sebire, 2001.

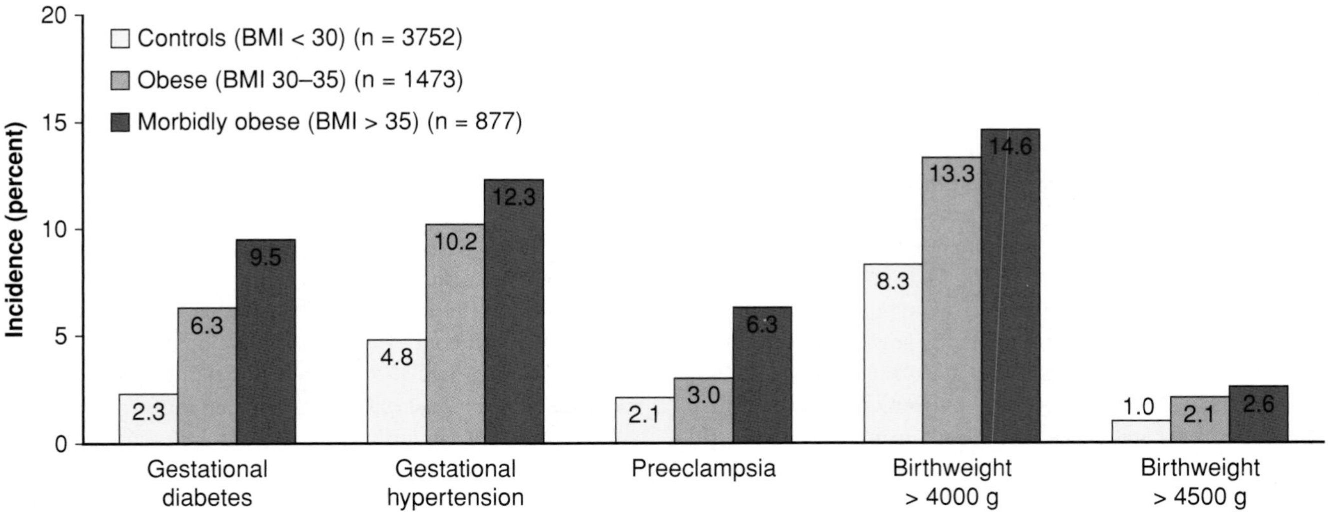

FIGURE 48-5 Incidence of selected pregnancy outcomes in 16,102 women enrolled in the FASTER (First- and Second-Trimester Evaluation of Risk) trial according to body mass index (BMI) status. (Data from Weiss, 2004.)

Although not as magnified as in the obese cohort, almost all complications are significantly increased in overweight women compared with those whose BMI is normal.

Obesity is detrimental to the accuracy of obstetrical ultrasound examination (Weichert, 2011). Other morbidity includes a higher incidence of failed trial of labor with a prior cesarean delivery (Bujold, 2005; Goodall, 2005; Hibbard, 2006; Robinson, 2005). Obesity and hypertension are common cofactors in causing peripartum heart failure (Cunningham, 1986, 2012). And, obese women present anesthesia challenges that include difficult epidural and spinal analgesia placement and complications from failed or difficult intubations (Hood, 1993; Mace, 2011). Second-trimester dilatation and evacuation was reported to take longer and be more difficult in women whose BMI was 30 kg/m^2 or greater (Dark, 2002).

Obese women are less likely to breast feed than normal-weight women (Li, 2003). They also have greater weight retention 1 year after delivery (Catalano, 2007; National Research Council and Institute of Medicine, 2007; Rode, 2005). Finally, there is evidence that quality-of-life measures are negatively affected by obesity during pregnancy (Amador, 2008). LaCoursiere and Varner (2009) found that postpartum depression was significantly increased in obese women in relation to the degree of obesity—class 1, 23 percent; class 2, 32 percent; and class 3, 40 percent.

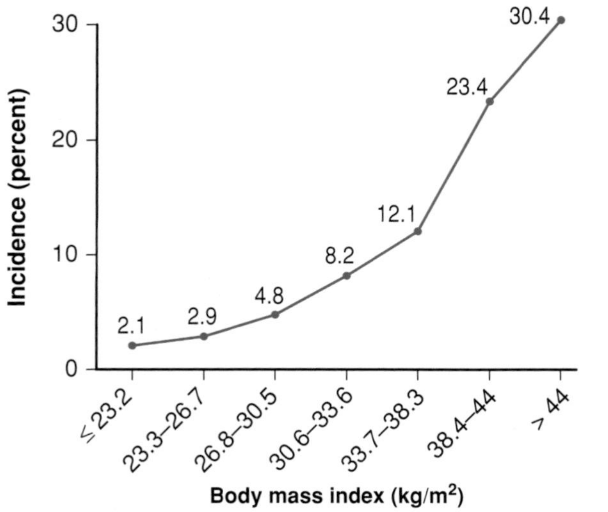

FIGURE 48-6 Frequency of preeclampsia according to body mass index. (Data from the Hyperglycemia and Adverse Pregnancy Outcome [HAPO] Study Cooperative Research Group, 2010.)

Gestational Diabetes

Obesity and gestational diabetes are inextricably linked. Their coexistence with and adverse effects on pregnancy outcomes are discussed in Chapter 57 (p. 1139).

Preeclampsia

There is no doubt that obesity is a consistent risk factor for preeclampsia (see Fig. 48-6). In a review of studies that included more than 1.4 million women, O'Brien and associates (2003) found that the preeclampsia risk doubled with each 5 to 7 kg/m^2 increase in prepregnancy BMI. In The Hyperglycemia and Adverse Pregnancy Outcome (HAPO) study (2010), the incidence of preeclampsia increased almost geometrically with each BMI category. Obesity and the metabolic syndrome discussed on page 962 are characterized by insulin resistance causing low-grade inflammation and endothelial activation (Catalano, 2010). These have a central and integral role in development of preeclampsia as discussed in Chapter 40 (p. 733). Wolf and colleagues (2001) linked these two conditions, and Ramsay and coworkers (2002) confirmed that obese pregnant women had significantly elevated serum levels of IL-6 and C-reactive protein and impaired endothelial function. Obese gravidas were found to have significantly higher levels of triglycerides, very-low-density lipoprotein cholesterol, insulin, and leptin compared with normal-weight pregnant woman.

Contraception

Most studies report that oral contraceptive failure is more likely in overweight women. This is discussed in detail in Chapter 38 (p. 695).

Perinatal Mortality

Stillbirths are more prevalent as the degree of obesity increases (see Table 48-3). Indeed, in a review of almost 100 population-based studies, Flenady and associates (2011) found that obesity was the highest ranking modifiable risk factor for stillbirth. Chronic hypertension with superimposed preeclampsia associated with obesity is one cause of excessive stillbirths. An increased incidence of otherwise inexplicable late-pregnancy stillbirths and early neonatal deaths is also associated with obesity (Cnattingius, 1998; Stephansson, 2001; Waldenström, 2014; Yao, 2014). In one metaanalysis, there was a 1.5-fold increased risk for stillbirth in overweight and a 2.1-fold risk in obese women (Chu, 2007). A Scottish study of more than 186,000 nulliparas described an almost fourfold increased stillbirth rate in women with a BMI ≥ 35 kg/m^2 compared with women of normal size (Denison, 2008). Increased prepregnancy weight was the factor most strongly associated with unexplained fetal deaths even after adjusting for maternal age and excluding women with diabetes and hypertensive disorders (Huang, 2000; Nohr, 2005; Ovesen, 2011).

Perinatal Morbidity

Both fetal and neonatal complications are increased in obese women. The Atlantic Birth Defects Risk Factor Surveillance Study found a two- to threefold increased incidence in various anomalies in obese women (Watkins, 2003). Rasmussen and coworkers (2008) performed a metaanalysis and found 1.2-, 1.7-, and 3.1-fold increased risks for neural-tube defects in overweight, obese, and severely obese women, respectively. Another metaanalysis found that maternal obesity was significantly associated with an increased risk of a wide range of anomalies (Stothard, 2009). The National Birth Defect Prevention Study reported a correlation between BMI and congenital heart defects (Gilboa, 2010). According to Biggio and colleagues (2010), however, this may be related to diabetes as a cofactor. Already mentioned is concern for unreliable fetal anatomy sonographic screening in obese women (Dashe, 2009; Thornburg, 2009; Weichert, 2011).

Two important and interrelated cofactors that contribute to excessive rates of perinatal morbidity are chronic hypertension and diabetes mellitus, both of which are associated with obesity. Affected women have increased rates of preterm delivery and fetal-growth restriction (McDonald, 2010; Waldenström, 2014; Wang, 2011). As discussed above, pregestational diabetes increases the birth defect rate, and gestational diabetes is complicated by excessive numbers of large-for-gestational age and macrosomic fetuses (Chap. 44, p. 884).

Even without diabetes, the prevalence of macrosomic newborns is increased in obese women (Cedergren, 2004; Ovesen, 2011). The group from MetroHealth Medical Center in Cleveland has conducted studies of prepregnancy obesity, gestational weight gain, and prepregnancy and gestational diabetes and their relationship to newborn weight and fat mass (Catalano, 2005, 2007; Ehrenberg, 2004; Sewell, 2006). Although each of these variables was found to be associated with larger and more corpulent newborns, prepregnancy BMI had the strongest influence on the prevalence of macrosomic neonates. They attributed this increased prevalence of macrosomic infants to the marked frequency of overweight or obese women in pregnancy—47 percent—rather than the 4 percent of pregnant women with diabetes. More recently, Edlow and associates (2013) have shown that genes expressed in the adult metabolic syndrome may be initiated in the fetus.

Morbidity in Children Born to Obese Women

It appears that obese women beget obese children, who themselves become obese adults. Whitaker (2004) studied low-income children in the Special Supplemental Food Program for Women, Infants, and Children (WIC) and found a linear association between early pregnancy maternal BMI and prevalence of overweight children at 2, 3, and 4 years. Schack-Nielson and associates (2005) reported a direct association between maternal, newborn, and childhood BMI. This association strengthened as offspring progressed to adulthood. Catalano and coworkers (2005) studied offspring at a median age of 7 years and found a direct association with maternal prepregnancy obesity and childhood obesity. They also reported associations with central obesity, elevated systolic blood pressure, increased insulin resistance, and decreased high-density lipoprotein (HDL) cholesterol levels—all elements of the metabolic syndrome. In their analysis of 28,540 women, Reynolds and associates (2013) found increased rates of cardiovascular disease and all-cause mortality in offspring of overweight and obese mothers. Boney and colleagues (2005) studied offspring of women with or without gestational diabetes. They observed that children who were large for gestational age at birth and whose mothers were either obese or had gestational diabetes had significantly increased risks for developing metabolic syndrome.

It also appears that excessive maternal weight gain in pregnancy may predict adulthood obesity in their offspring. Schack-Nielsen and associates (2005) found a linear association of maternal weight gain with the subsequent BMI in their children. Analyzing data from Project Viva, Oken (2006) confirmed this. However, not all studies concur. In their analysis of children in the WIC program cited above, Whitaker and associates (2004) found no obvious linear association between gestational weight gain and childhood obesity. This is also discussed in some detail in Chapter 44 (p. 876).

Fetal Programming and Childhood Morbidity

Epidemiological studies have addressed the association of childhood, adolescent, and even adult adverse health outcomes in relation to the fetal environment. Adverse outcomes include obesity, diabetes, hypertension, and the metabolic syndrome. Variables studied have included maternal prepregnancy BMI, obesity, gestational weight gain, and pregestational or gestational diabetes. The most robust evidence suggests a direct association between children born to women who had prepregnancy obesity or gestational diabetes and being overweight in childhood and adulthood.

The potential biological causes and mechanisms of these associations are not clear. Elucidation is limited by insufficient data on potential maternal and genetic predisposing factors and on the environment of the infant and child in relation to diet and activity. The science of *epigenetics* has provided some support for the possibility that perturbations of the maternal-fetal environment can adversely alter postdelivery events (Aagard-Tillery, 2006). Perhaps more likely are contributions of the maternal-child environment subsequent to birth (Gluck, 2009). These and other factors regarding fetal programming are discussed in Chapter 44 (p. 876).

Antepartum Management

Dietary Intervention in Pregnancy

Weight reduction is not advisable during pregnancy (Catalano, 2013). As noted, recommended weight gain in obese women is 11 to 20 pounds, and several dietary interventions to limit weight gain to these targets have been reported. These include lifestyle interventions and physical activity (Petrella, 2013). Reviews by Quinlivan (2011) and Tanentsapf (2011) found that randomized trials generally reported successful results with intervention. On the other hand, in many other studies, either these have been unsuccessful or the results were insufficient to permit a conclusion (Campbell, 2011; Dodd, 2010; Guelinckx, 2010; Nascimento, 2011; Ronnberg, 2010). Special attention to psychological aspects of pregnancy has been recommended by some (Skouteris, 2010).

Prenatal Care

Close prenatal surveillance detects most early signs of diabetes or hypertension. Standard screening tests for fetal anomalies are sufficient, while being mindful of sonographic limitations for detection of fetal anomalies. Accurate assessment of fetal growth usually requires serial sonography. Antepartum and intrapartum external fetal heart rate monitoring are likewise more difficult, and sometimes these are even impossible.

Surgical and Anesthetic Concerns

Evaluation by the anesthesia team is performed at a prenatal visit or on arrival at the labor unit (American College of Obstetricians and Gynecologists, 2013b). Anesthetic risks and complications faced by obese women are discussed in Chapter 25 (p. 505). Special attention is given to complications that might arise during labor and delivery. Vricella and coworkers (2010) reported the following frequencies of anesthetic complications in 142 morbidly obese women at cesarean delivery. These included technical problems with regional analgesia—up to 6 percent; use of general anesthesia—6 percent; hypotension—3 percent; and overall anesthetic complications of 8.4 percent.

For cesarean delivery, forethought is given to optimal placement and type of abdominal incision to allow access to the fetus and to effect the best wound closure with the least intervening tissue (Alexander, 2006). One technique is shown in Figure 48-7. Others prefer a transverse abdominal incision (Alanis, 2010). Individual differences in maternal body habitus preclude naming any one approach as superior (Gilstrap, 2002; McLean, 2012). Although some have reported similar wound complications with either incision, others reported a fourfold wound complication rate when a vertical abdominal incision was compared with a transverse incision—31 versus 8 percent (Houston, 2000; Thornburg, 2012; Wall, 2003). Finally, a mid-abdomen transverse incision has been advocated by some (Tixier, 2009).

Attention to closure of the subcutaneous layer is important. Chelmow and associates (2004) performed a metaanalysis

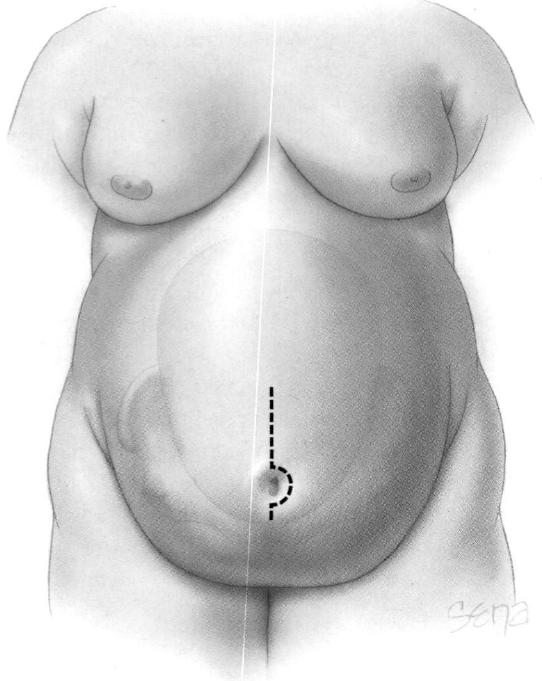

A

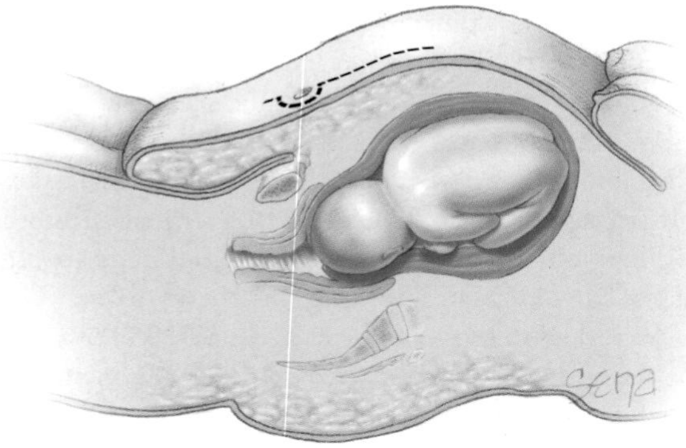

B

FIGURE 48-7 Abdominal incision for the obese woman. **A.** Frontal view. The dotted line indicates an appropriate skin incision for abdominal entry relative to the panniculus. As shown by the uterus in the background, selection of this periumbilical site permits access to the lower uterine segment. **B.** Sagittal view.

of subcutaneous closure in 887 women undergoing cesarean delivery whose wound thickness was greater than 2 centimeters. Subcutaneous closure resulted in a modest but significant 6-percent decrease in wound disruption. The frequency of abdominal wound infections is directly related to BMI (Norman, 2013). Comorbid diabetes apparently increases this risk (Leth, 2011). Several reports describe a wound complication rate of 15 to 45 percent. Alanis and colleagues (2010) reported a 30-percent rate in 194 women whose BMI was > 50 kg/m^2. Of these, 90-percent were wound disruptions to the fascia, but there was only one evisceration. As indicated above, the transverse abdominal incision had fewer complications. Walsh and coworkers (2009) have reviewed the prevention and management of surgical site infections in morbidly obese women.

To lower thromboembolic complications, graduated compression stockings, hydration, and early mobilization after cesarean delivery in obese women are recommended by the American College of Obstetricians and Gynecologists (2013a). Some also recommend "mini-dose" heparin prophylaxis, but we do not routinely use this (Chap. 52, p. 1044).

Bariatric Surgery

Several surgical procedures have been designed to treat morbid obesity either by decreasing gastric volume—*restrictive*, or by bypassing gastrointestinal absorption—*restrictive malabsorptive* (Adams, 2007; Kushner, 2012). In nonpregnant patients, these procedures have been shown to improve or resolve diabetes, hyperlipidemia, hypertension, and obstructive sleep apnea (Buchwald, 2007; Mingrone, 2012; Schauer, 2012).

Pregnancy

Because of these successes, bariatric surgery currently has become popular, and many women are becoming pregnant following weight-reduction surgery (Abodeely, 2008). Several observational studies have reported improved fertility rates and reduced risks of obstetrical complications in women following bariatric surgery and compared with morbidly obese controls (Alatishe, 2013; Guelinckx, 2009; Kjaer, 2013a; Lesko, 2012; Tan, 2012). The largest of these studies is from the Swedish Birth Register, which included 681 women with a pregnancy following bariatric surgery (Josefsson, 2011). Despite surgical treatments, half of these women were still obese by the time of their first pregnancy following bypass, however, the proportion with morbid obesity was smaller. The frequency of large-for-gestational age infants decreased from 9.1 to 3.2 percent and that of small-for-gestational age neonates *increased* from 2.1 to 5.6 percent. In a recent systematic review, Kjaer and Nilas (2013b) reported a decreased risk after bariatric surgery for diabetes, preeclampsia, and large-for-gestational age infants. Most studies confirmed a higher risk for small-for-gestational age fetuses.

Restrictive Procedures

The prototypical vertical banded gastroplasty has been largely replaced by the laparoscopic adjustable silicone gastric banding (LASGB) operation. With the two approved LASGB procedures—*LAPBAND* and *REALIZE,* an adjustable band is placed 2 cm below the gastroesophageal junction to create a small pouch. The pouch size is controlled by a saline reservoir in the band. Salutary effects on pregnancy outcomes involve before-and-after cohorts as well as pregnancies in postsurgical women compared with obese, nonsurgical controls (Vrebosch, 2012). In a report by Dixon and colleagues (2005), pregnancy outcomes were compared with their preprocedural outcomes and with a matched cohort of obese women. Following banding, the incidences of gestational hypertension—10 versus 45 percent—and gestational diabetes—6 versus 15 percent—were significantly lower compared with their preprocedural pregnancies. Incidences in banded patients were also significantly lower than those in the obese cohort, whose rates for hypertension were 38 percent, and for diabetes, 19 percent. The results from these and other studies are shown in Table 48-4.

TABLE 48-4. Pregnancy Outcomes Following Gastric Banding Surgery and Roux-en-Y Gastric Bypass

Outcome[a]	Gastric Banding[b] (n = 258)	Roux-en-Y Gastric Bypass[c] (n = 236)
Hypertension	8%	6%
Gestational diabetes	12%	4%
Cesarean delivery	25%	23%
Mean birthweight	3000 g	3300 g
Small for gestational age	10%	17%
Stillbirth	4/1000	6/1000

[a]Data not reported identically—frequencies are approximations.
[b]Data from Bar-Zohar, 2006; Dixon, 2001; Ducarme, 2013; Martin, 2000; Skull, 2004.
[c]From review by Abodeely, 2008.

Reported complications have been few and include excessive nausea and vomiting that abated with band adjustment (Martin, 2000). Rarely, women may have band slippage associated with hyperemesis or with advancing gestation (Pilone, 2012; Suffee, 2012). One newborn died after fetal cerebral hemorrhage developed from vitamin K deficiency associated with band slippage (Van Mieghem, 2008).

Restrictive Malabsorptive Procedures

There are three procedures to accomplish gastric restriction and selective malabsorption. The most commonly used is the laparoscopically performed *Roux-en-Y gastric bypass* and *biliopancreatic diversion with duodenal switch.* With the Roux-en-Y procedure, the proximal stomach is completely transected to leave a 30-mL pouch. A gastroenterotomy is then created by connecting the proximal end of the distal jejunum to the pouch. A Roux-en-Y enteroenterostomy is also completed 60 cm distal to this gastrojejunostomy to allow drainage of the unused stomach and proximal small intestine.

As with other bariatric procedures, pregnancy outcomes are changed remarkably following Roux-en-Y bypass (Wittgrove, 1998). As shown in Table 48-4, rates of hypertension, gestational diabetes, and fetal macrosomia are reduced. Serious complications are uncommon. Intussusception and small bowel obstruction develop from internal herniation, and maternal deaths from herniation and obstruction have been reported (Kakarla, 2005; Moore, 2004; Renault, 2012; Wax, 2007). Bowel obstruction is notoriously difficult to diagnose, and Wax and associates (2013) caution for a high index of suspicion.

Recommendations

The American College of Obstetricians and Gynecologists (2013a) recommends that women who have undergone bariatric surgery be assessed for vitamin and nutritional sufficiency. When indicated, vitamin B_{12} and D, folic acid, and calcium supplementation are given. Vitamin A deficiency has also been reported (Chagas, 2013). Women with a gastric band should be monitored by their bariatric team during pregnancy because adjustments of the band may be necessary. Finally, special vigilance is appropriate for signs of intestinal obstruction.

REFERENCES

Aagard-Tillery K, Holland W, McKnight R, et al: Fetal origins of disease: essential nutrient supplementation prevents adult metabolic disease in a transgenerational model of IUGR. Am J Obstet Gynecol 195:S3, 2006

Abodeely A, Roye GD, Harrington DT, et al: Pregnancy outcomes after bariatric surgery: maternal, fetal, and infant implications. Surg Obes Relat Dis 4(3):464, 2008

Adams TD, Gress RE, Smith SC, et al: Long-term mortality after gastric bypass surgery. N Engl J Med 357(8):753, 2007

Alanis MC, Villers S, Law TL, et al: Complications of cesarean delivery in the massively obese parturient. Am J Obstet Gynecol 203:271.e1, 2010

Alatishe A, Ammori BJ, New JP, et al: Bariatric surgery in women of childbearing age. QJM 106(8):717, 2013

Alexander CI, Liston WA: Operating on the obese woman—a review. BJOG 113(10):1167, 2006

Amador N, Juárez JM, Guizar JM, et al: Quality of life in obese pregnant women: a longitudinal study. Am J Obstet Gynecol 198:203.e1, 2008

American College of Obstetricians and Gynecologists: Weight control: assessment and management. Clinical Updates in Women's Health Care. Vol II, No. 3, 2003

American College of Obstetricians and Gynecologists: Obesity in pregnancy. Committee Opinion No. 549, January 2013a

American College of Obstetricians and Gynecologists: Obstetric analgesia and anesthesia. Practice Bulletin No. 36, July 2002, Reaffirmed 2013b

American College of Obstetricians and Gynecologists: Weight gain during pregnancy. Committee Opinion No. 548, January 2013c

Bar-Zohar D, Azem F, Klausner J, et al: Pregnancy after laparoscopic adjustable gastric banding: perinatal outcome is favorable also for women with relatively high gestational weight gain. Surg Endosc 20(10):1580, 2006

Bellver J, Ayllón Y, Verrando M, et al: Female obesity impairs in vitro fertilization outcome without affecting embryo quality. Fertil Steril 93(2):447, 2010

Biggio JR Jr, Chapman V, Neely C, et al: Fetal anomalies in obese women: the contribution of diabetes. Obstet Gynecol 115:290, 2010

Boney CM, Verma A, Tucker R, et al: Metabolic syndrome in childhood: association with birth weight, maternal obesity, and gestational diabetes mellitus. Pediatrics 115:e290, 2005

Briana DD, Malamitsi-Puchner A: Adipocytokines in normal and complicated pregnancies. Reprod Sci 16(10):921, 2009

Browning JD, Szczepaniak LS, Dobbins R, et al: Prevalence of hepatic steatosis in an urban population in the United States: impact of ethnicity. Hepatology 40:1387, 2004

Buchwald H, Estok R. Fahrbach K, et al: Trends in mortality in bariatric surgery: a systematic review and meta-analysis. Surgery 142(4):621, 2007

Bujold E, Hammoud A, Schild C, et al: The role of maternal body mass index in outcomes of vaginal births after cesarean. Am J Obstet Gynecol 193(4):1517, 2005

Butte NF, Wong WW, Treuth MS, et al: Energy requirements during pregnancy based on total energy expenditure and energy deposition. Am J Clin Nutr 79:1078, 2004

Calle EE, Rodriguez C, Walker-Thurmond K, et al: Overweight, obesity, and mortality from cancer in a prospectively studied cohort of U.S. adults. N Engl J Med 348:1625, 2003

Calle EE, Teras LR, Thun MJ: Obesity and mortality. N Engl J Med 353:20, 2005

Campbell F, Johnson M, Messina J, et al: Behavioural interventions for weight management in pregnancy: a systematic review of quantitative and qualitative data. BMC Public Health 11:491, 2011

Catalano P: Weight loss in overweight and obese pregnant women (OW/OB): what is the effect on fetal growth? Abstract No. 349. Am J Obstet Gynecol 208(1):S155, 2013

Catalano P, Farrell K, Presley L, et al: Long-term follow-up of infants of women with normal glucose tolerance (NGT) and gestational diabetes (GDM): risk factors for obesity and components of the metabolic syndrome in childhood. Am J Obstet Gynecol 193:S3, 2005

Catalano PM: Management of obesity in pregnancy. Obstet Gynecol 109:419, 2007

Catalano PM: Obesity, insulin resistance, and pregnancy outcome. Reproduction 140(3):365, 2010

Cedergren MI: Maternal morbid obesity and the risk of adverse pregnancy outcome. Obstet Gynecol. 103:219, 2004

Chagas CB, Saunders C, Pereira S, et al: Vitamin A deficiency in pregnancy: perspectives after bariatric surgery. Obes Surg 23(2):249, 2013

Chelmow D, Rodriquez EJ, Sabatini MM: Suture closure of subcutaneous fat and wound disruption after cesarean delivery: a meta-analysis. Obstet Gynecol 103:974, 2004

Chinali M, Devereux RB, Howard BV, et al: Comparison of cardiac structure and function in American Indians with and without the metabolic syndrome (the Strong Heart Study). Am J Cardiol 93:40, 2004

Chu SY, Callaghan WM, Bish CL, et al: Gestational weight gain by body mass index among US women delivering live births, 2004–2005: fueling future obesity. Am J Obstet Gynecol 200:271.e1, 2009

Chu SY, Kim SY, Lau J, et al: Maternal obesity and risk of stillbirth: a metaanalysis. Am J Obstet Gynecol 197(3):223, 2007

Cnattingius S, Bergstrom R, Lipworth L, et al: Prepregnancy weight and the risk of adverse pregnancy outcomes. N Engl J Med 338: 147, 1998

Cornier MA, Després JP, Davis N, et al: Assessing adiposity: a scientific statement from the American Heart Association. Circulation 124:00, 2011

Crane J, Murphy P, Burrage L, et al: Maternal and perinatal complications of super-obesity (BMI at least 50.00 kg/m^2). Abstract No. 669. Am J Obstet Gynecol 208(1):S282, 2013

Crist LA, Champagne CM, Corsino L, et al: Influence of change in aerobic fitness and weight on prevalence of metabolic syndrome. Prev Chronic Dis 9:E68, 2012

Cunningham FG: Peripartum cardiomyopathy: we've come a long way, but. . . . Obstet Gynecol 120(5):992, 2012

Cunningham FG, Pritchard JA, Hankins GVD, et al: Idiopathic cardiomyopathy or compounding cardiovascular events? Obstet Gynecol 67:157, 1986

Dark AC, Miller L, Kothenbeutel RL, et al: Obesity and second-trimester abortion by dilation and evacuation. J Reprod Med 47:226, 2002

Dashe JS, McIntire DD, Twickler DM: Effect of maternal obesity on the ultrasound detection of anomalous fetuses. Obstet Gynecol 113:1, 2009

De Gonzalez AB, Hartge P, Cherhan JR, et al: Body mass index and mortality among 1.46 million white adults. N Engl J Med 363:23, 2010

Denison FC, Price J, Graham C, et al: Maternal obesity, length of gestation, risk of postdates pregnancy and spontaneous onset of labour at term. BJOG 115(6):720, 2008

Dixon JB, Dixon ME, O'Brien PE: Birth outcomes in obese women after laparoscopic adjustable gastric banding. Obstet Gynecol 106:965, 2005

Dixon JB, Dixon ME, O'Brien PE: Pregnancy after Lap-Band surgery: management of the band to achieve healthy weight outcomes. Obes Surg 11:59, 2001

Dodd JM, Grivell RM, Crowther CA, et al: Antenatal interventions for overweight or obese pregnant women: a systematic review of randomised trials. BJOG 117(11):1316, 2010

Drewnowski A, Specter SE: Poverty and obesity: the role of energy density and energy costs. Am J Clin Nutr 79:6, 2004

Ducarme G, Parisio L, Santulli P, et al: Neonatal outcomes in pregnancies after bariatric surgery: a retrospective multi-centric cohort study in three French referral centers. J Matern Fetal Neonatal Med 26(3):275, 2013

Eckel RH: Nonsurgical management of obesity in adults. N Engl J Med 358:1941, 2008

Edlow A, Neeta V, Hui L, et al: Antenatal origins of metabolic syndrome in fetuses of obese women. Abstract No. 4. Am J Obstet Gynecol 208(1):S3, 2013

Ehrenberg HM, Dierker L, Milluzzi C, et al: Prevalence of maternal obesity in an urban center. Am J Obstet Gynecol 187:1189, 2002

Ehrenberg HM, Mercer BM, Catalano PM: The influence of obesity and diabetes on the prevalence of macrosomia. Am J Obstet Gynecol 191:964, 2004

Flegal KM, Carroll MD, Kit BK, Ogden CL: Prevalence of obesity and trends in body mass index among US adults, 1999–2000. JAMA 307(5):491, 2012

Flegal KM, Graubard BI, Williamson DF, et al: Cause-specific excess deaths associated with underweight, overweight, and obesity. JAMA 298:2028, 2007

Flenady V, Koopmans L, Middleton P, et al: Major risk factors for stillbirth in high-income countries: a systematic review and meta-analysis. Lancet 377(9774):1331, 2011

Fontaine KR, Redden DT, Wang C, et al: Years of life lost due to obesity. JAMA 289:187, 2003

Forbes S, Taylor-Robinson SD, Patel N, et al: Increased prevalence of nonalcoholic fatty liver disease in European women with a history of gestational diabetes. Diabetologia 54(3):641, 2011

Ford ES, Giles WH, Dietz WH: Prevalence of the metabolic syndrome among U.S. adults. Findings from the Third National Health and Nutrition Examination Survey. JAMA 287:356, 2002

Garabedian MJ, Williams CM, Pearce CF, et al: Extreme morbid obesity and labor outcome in nulliparous women at term. Am J Perinatol 28(9):729, 2011

Gilboa SM, Correa A, Botto LD, et al: Association between prepregnancy body mass index and congenital heart defects. Am J Obstet Gynecol 202(1):51.e1, 2010

Gilstrap LC, Cunningham FG, Van Dorsten JP (eds): Anatomy, incisions, and closures. In Operative Obstetrics, 2nd ed. New York, McGraw-Hill, 2002, p 55
Gluck ME, Venti CA, Lindsay RS, et al: Maternal influence, not diabetic intrauterine environment, predicts children's energy intake. Obesity 17:772, 2009
Goodall PT, Ahn JT, Chapa JB, et al: Obesity as a risk factor for failed trial of labor in patients with previous cesarean delivery. Am J Obstet Gynecol 192:1423, 2005
Guelinckx I, Devlieger R, Mullie P, et al: Effect of lifestyle intervention on dietary habits, physical activity, and gestational weight gain in obese pregnant women: a randomized controlled trial. Am J Clin Nutr 91(2):373, 2010
Guelinckx I, Devlieger R, Vansant G: Reproductive outcome after bariatric surgery: a critical review. Hum Reprod Update 15(2):189, 2009
Haeri S, Guichard I, Baker AM, et al: The effect of teenage maternal obesity on perinatal outcomes. Obstet Gynecol 113:300, 2009
Hall LF, Neubert AG: Obesity and pregnancy. Obstet Gynecol Surv 60(4):253, 2005
Hibbard JU, Gilbert S, Landon MB, et al: Trial of labor or repeat cesarean delivery in women with morbid obesity and previous cesarean delivery. Obstet Gynecol 108(1):125, 2006
Hood DD, Dewan DM: Anesthetic and obstetric outcome in morbidly obese parturients. Anesthesiology 79:1210, 1993
Hossain P, Kawar B, El Nahas M: Obesity and diabetes in the developing world—a growing challenge. N Engl J Med 356(9):973, 2007
Houston MC, Raynor BD: Postoperative morbidity in the morbidly obese parturient woman: supraumbilical and low transverse abdominal approaches. Am J Obstet Gynecol 182(5):1033, 2000
Huang DY, Usher RH, Kramer MS, et al: Determinants of unexplained antepartum fetal deaths. Obstet Gynecol 95:215, 2000
Institute of Medicine: The development of DRIs 1994–2004: lessons learned and new challenges. Workshop summary. November 30, 2007
Institute of Medicine: Weight gain during pregnancy: reexamining the guidelines. National Academy of Sciences. 28 May 2009
Johnson J, Clifton RB, Roberts JM, et al: Pregnancy outcomes with weight gain above or below the 2009 Institute of Medicine guidelines. Obstet Gynecol 121:969, 2013
Jordan HT, Tabaei BP, Nash D, et al: Metabolic syndrome among adults in New York City, 2004 New York City Health and Nutrition Examination Survey. Prev Chronic Dis 9:E04, 2012
Josefsson A, Blomberg M, Bladh M, et al: Bariatric surgery in a national cohort of women: sociodemographics and obstetric outcomes. Am J Obstet Gynecol 205(5):206.e1, 2011
Kabiru W, Raynor BD: Obstetric outcomes associated with increase in BMI category during pregnancy. Am J Obstet Gynecol 191:928, 2004
Kakarla N, Dailey C, Marino T, et al: Pregnancy after gastric bypass surgery and internal hernia formation. Obstet Gynecol 105(5, Part 2):1195, 2005
Kenchaiah S, Evans JC, Levy D, et al: Obesity and the risk of heart failure. N Engl J Med 347:305, 2002
Kinoshita T, Itoh M: Longitudinal variance of fat mass deposition during pregnancy evaluated by ultrasonography: the ratio of visceral fat to subcutaneous fat in the abdomen. Gynecol Obstet Invest 61:115, 2006
Kjaer MM, Lauenborg J, Breum BM, et al: The risk of adverse pregnancy outcome after bariatric surgery: a nationwide register-based matched cohort study. Am J Obstet Gynecol 208(6):464.e1, 2013a
Kjaer MM, Nilas L: Pregnancy after bariatric surgery—a review of benefits and risks. Acta Obstet Gynecol Scand 92(3):264, 2013b
Kumari AS: Pregnancy outcome in women with morbid obesity. Int J Gynaecol Obstet 73:101, 2001
Kushner RF: Evaluation and management of obesity. In Longo DL, Fauci AS, Kasper DL, et al (eds): Harrison's Principles of Internal Medicine, 18th ed. McGraw-Hill, New York, 2012, p. 629
LaCoursiere Y, Varner M: The association between prepregnancy obesity and postpartum depression, supported by NIH grant R03-HD-048865. Abstract No. 92. Presented at the 29th Annual Meeting of the Society for Maternal-Fetal Medicine. 26–31 January 2009
Lashen H, Fear K, Sturdee DW: Obesity is associated with increased risk of first trimester and recurrent miscarriage: matched case-control study. Hum Reprod 19:1644, 2004
Lesko J, Peaceman A: Pregnancy outcomes in women after bariatric surgery compared with obese and morbidly obese controls. Obstet Gynecol 119(3):547, 2012
Leth RA, Uldbjerg N, Norgaard M, et al: Obesity, diabetes, and the risk of infections diagnosed in hospital and post-discharge infections after cesarean section: a prospective cohort study. Acta Obstet Gynecol Scand 90(5):501, 2011
Li R, Jewell S, Grummer-Strawn L: Maternal obesity and breast-feeding practices. Am J Clin Nutr 77:931, 2003
Lipkind H, Campbell K, Savitz D, et al: Obesity as an independent risk factor for severe maternal morbidity ("near miss") during delivery hospitalization. Abstract No. 666. Am J Obstet Gynecol 208(1):S281, 2013
Lu GC, Rouse DJ, DuBard M, et al: The effect of the increasing prevalence of maternal obesity on perinatal morbidity. Am J Obstet Gynecol 185(4):845, 2001
Lynch CM, Sexton DJ, Hession M, et al: Obesity and mode of delivery in primigravid and multigravid women. Am J Perinatol 25(3):163, 2008
McDonald SD, Han Z, Mulla S, et al: Overweight and obesity in mothers and risk of preterm birth and low birth weight infants: systematic review and meta-analyses. BMJ 341:c3428, 2010
Mace HS, Paech MJ, McDonnell NJ: Obesity and obstetric anaesthesia. Anaesth Intensive Care 39(4):559, 2011
Maguire M, Lungu A, Gorden P, et al: Pregnancy in women with congenital generalized lipodystrophy. Leptin's vital role in reproduction. Obstet Gynecol 119(2 Pt 2):452, 2012
Martin LF, Finigan KM, Nolan TE: Pregnancy after adjustable gastric banding. Obstet Gynecol 95:927, 2000
McLean M, Hines R, Polinkovsky M, et al: Type of skin incision and wound complications in the obese parturient. Am J Perinatol 29(4):301, 2012
Metwally M, Ong KJ, Ledger WL, et al: Does high body mass index increase the risk of miscarriage after spontaneous and assisted conception? A meta-analysis of the evidence. Fertil Steril 88:446, 2008
Meyer BJ, Stewart FM, Brown EA, et al: Maternal obesity is associated with the formation of small dense LDL and hypoadiponectinemia in the third trimester. J Clin Endocrinol Metab 98(2):643, 2013
Mingrone G, Panunzi s, De Gaetano A, et al: Bariatric surgery versus conventional medical therapy for Type 2 diabetes. N Engl J Med 366(17):1577, 2012
Moore KA, Ouyang DW, Whang EE: Maternal and fetal deaths after gastric bypass surgery for morbid obesity. N Engl J Med 351:721, 2004
Nascimento SL, Surita FG, Parpinelli MÂ, et al: The effect of an antenatal exercise programme on maternal/perinatal outcomes and quality of life in overweight and obese women: a randomised clinical trial. BJOG 118(12):1455, 2011
National Institutes of Health: The practical guide: identification, evaluation, and treatment of overweight and obesity in adults. NIH Publication 00-4084. Bethesda, National Institutes of Health, 2000
National Institutes of Health: Third report of the National Cholesterol Education Program Expert Panel on detection, evaluation, and treatment of high blood cholesterol in adults (Adult Treatment Panel III), NIH Publication 01-3670. Bethesda, National Institutes of Health, 2001
National Research Council and Institute of Medicine: Influence of pregnancy weight on maternal and child health. Workshop report. Committee on the Impact of Pregnancy Weight on Maternal and Child Health. Board on Children, Youth, and Families, Division of Behavioral and Social Sciences and Education and Food and Nutrition Board, Institute of Medicine. Washington, The National Academies Press, 2007
National Task Force on the Prevention and Treatment of Obesity: Overweight, obesity, and health risk. Arch Intern Med 160:898, 2000
Nehring I, Schmoll S, Beyerlein A, et al: Gestational weight gain and long-term postpartum weight retention: a meta-analysis. Am J Clin Nutr 94(5):1225, 2011
Neill AM, Nelson-Piercy C: Hazards of assisted conception in women with severe medical disease. Hum Fertil (Camb) 4:239, 2001
Ninomiya JK, L'Italien G, Criqui MH, et al: Association of the metabolic syndrome with history of myocardial infarction and stroke in the Third National Health and Nutrition Examination Survey. Circulation 109:42, 2004
Nohr EA, Bech BH, Davies MJ, et al: Pregnancy obesity and fetal death: a study within the Danish National Birth Cohort. Obstet Gynecol 106:250, 2005
Norman S, Verticchio J, Odibo A: The effects of degree of obesity on risk for post-cesarean wound complication. Abstract No. 157. Am J Obstet Gynecol 208(1):S78, 2013
O'Brien TE, Ray JG, Chan WS: Maternal body mass index and the risk of preeclampsia: a systematic overview. Epidemiology 14:368, 2003
Ogden CL, Carroll MD, Kit BK, et al: Prevalence of obesity in the United States, 2009–2010. NCHS data brief No. 82, Hyattsville, National Center for Health Statistics, 2012
Oken E: Maternal weight and gestational weight gain as predictors of long-term off-spring growth and health. Presentation at the Workshop on the Impact of Pregnancy Weight on Maternal and Child Health, May 30, Washington, 2006
Ovesen P, Rasmussen S, Kesmodel U: Effect of prepregnancy maternal overweight and obesity on pregnancy outcome. Obstet Gynecol 118(2 Pt 2):305, 2011
Page LM, Girling JC: A novel cause for abnormal liver function tests in pregnancy and the puerperium: non-alcoholic fatty liver disease. BJOG 118(12):1532, 2011

Pauli J, Zhu Junjia, Repke J, et al: Health care utilization during pregnancy: the impact of pre-pregnancy body mass index. Abstract No. 344. Am J Obstet Gynecol 208(1):S153, 2013
Peeters A, Barendregt JJ, Willekens F, et al: Obesity in adulthood and its consequences for life expectancy: a life-table analysis. Ann Intern Med 138:24, 2003
Petrella E, Facchinetti F, Bertarini V, et al: Occurrence of pregnancy complications in women with BMI > 25 submitted to a healthy lifestyle and eating habits program. Abstract No. 55. Am J Obstet Gynecol 208(1):S33, 2013
Pilone V, Di Micco R, Monda A, et al: LAGB in pregnancy: slippage after hyperemesis gravidarum. Report of a case. Ann Ital Chir 83(5):429, 2012
Poobalan AS, Aucott LS, Gurung T, et al: Obesity as an independent risk factor for elective and emergency caesarean delivery in nulliparous women—systematic review and meta-analysis of cohort studies. Obes Rev 10:28, 2009
Public Health Service: Healthy People 2000: National Health Promotion and Disease Prevention Objectives. Washington, U.S. Department of Health and Human Services, Public Health Service, DHHS Publication No. (PHS) 90–50212, 1990
Quinlivan JA, Julania S, Lam L: Antenatal dietary interventions in obese pregnant women to restrict gestational weight gain to Institute of Medicine recommendations. Obstet Gynecol 118(6):1395, 2011
Ramsay JE, Ferrell WR, Crawford L, et al: Maternal obesity is associated with dysregulation of metabolic, vascular, and inflammatory pathways. J Clin Endocrinol Metab 87:4231, 2002
Rasmussen KM, Abrams B, Bodnar LM, et al: Recommendations for weight gain during pregnancy in the context of the obesity epidemic. Obstet Gynecol 116(5):1191, 2010
Rasmussen SA, Chu SY, Kim SY, et al: Maternal obesity and risk of neural tube defects: a metaanalysis. Am J Obstet Gynecol 198(6):611, 2008
Renault K, Gyrtrup HJ, Damgaard K, et al: Pregnant women with fatal complication after laparoscopic Roux-en-Y gastric bypass. Acta Obstet Gynecol Scand 91(7):873, 2012
Reynolds RM, Allan KM, Raja EA, et al: Maternal obesity during pregnancy and premature mortality from cardiovascular event in adult offspring: follow-up of 1 323 275 person years. BMJ 347:f4539, 2013
Robinson HE, O'Connell CM, Joseph KS, et al: Maternal outcomes in pregnancies complicated by obesity. Obstet Gynecol 106(6):1357, 2005
Rode L, Nilas L, Wøjdemann K, et al: Obesity-related complications in Danish single cephalic term pregnancies. Obstet Gynecol 105:537, 2005
Ronnberg AK, Nilsson K: Interventions during pregnancy to reduce excessive gestational weight gain: a systematic review assessing current clinical evidence using the Grading of Recommendations, Assessment, Development and Evaluation (GRADE) system. BJOG 117(11):1327, 2010
Rooney BL, Schauberger CW: Excess pregnancy weight gain and long-term obesity: one decade later. Obstet Gynecol 100:245, 2002
Schack-Nielsen L, Mortensen EL, Sorensen TIA: High maternal pregnancy weight gain is associated with an increased risk of obesity in childhood and adulthood independent of maternal BMI. Pediatric Res 58:1020, 2005
Schauer PR, Kashyap SR, Wolski K, et al: Bariatric surgery versus intensive medical therapy in obese patients with diabetes. N Engl J Med 366(17):1567, 2012
Scherer PE, Williams S, Fogliano M, et al: A novel serum protein similar to C1q, produced exclusively in adipocytes. J Biol Chem 270:26746, 2006
Sebire NJ, Jolly M, Harris JP, et al: Maternal obesity and pregnancy outcome: a study of 287,213 pregnancies in London. Int J Obes Relat Metab Disord 25:1175, 2001
Sewell MF, Huston-Presley L, Super DM, et al: Increased neonatal fat mass, not lean body mass, is associated with maternal obesity. Am J Obstet Gynecol 195:1100, 2006
Skouteris H, Hartley-Clark L, McCabe M, et al: Preventing excessive gestational weight gain: a systematic review of interventions. Obes Rev 11(11):757, 2010
Skull AJ, Slater GH, Duncombe JE, et al: Laparoscopic adjustable banding in pregnancy: safety, patient tolerance and effect on obesity-related pregnancy outcomes. Obes Surg 14:230, 2004
Stamilio D, Stout M, Macones G, et al: Post-cesarean maternal complications in patients with extreme obesity. Abstract No. 754. Am J Obstet Gynecol 208(1):S317, 2013
Stephansson O, Dickman PW, Johansson A, et al: Maternal weight, pregnancy weight gain, and the risk of antepartum stillbirth. Am J Obstet Gynecol 184:463, 2001
Stothard KJ, Tennant PW, Bell R, et al: Maternal overweight and obesity and the risk of congenital anomalies: a systematic review and meta-analysis. JAMA 301:636, 2009
Suffee MT, Poncelet C, Barrat C: Gastric band slippage at 30 weeks' gestation: diagnosis and laparoscopic management. Surg Obes Relat Dis 8(3):366, 2012
Tan O, Carr BR: The impact of bariatric surgery on obesity-related infertility and in vitro fertilization outcomes. Semin Reprod Med 30(6):517, 2012
Tanentsapf I, Heitmann BL, Adegboye AR: Systematic review of clinical trials of dietary interventions to prevent excessive weight gain during pregnancy among normal weight, overweight and obese women. BMC Pregnancy Childbirth 11:81, 2011
Targher G, Day CP, Bonora E: Risk of cardiovascular disease in patients with nonalcoholic fatty liver disease. N Engl J Med 363(14):1341, 2010
The Hyperglycemia and Adverse Pregnancy Outcome (HAPO) Study Cooperative Research Group: Hyperglycemia and Adverse Pregnancy Outcome (HAPO) Study: preeclampsia. Am J Obstet Gynecol 202:255.e1, 2010
Thornburg L, Mulconry M, Grace M, et al: Nuchal translucency measurements in the obese gravida. Abstract No. 456. Presented at the 29th Annual Meeting of the Society for Maternal-Fetal Medicine. January 26–31, 2009
Thornburg LL, Linder MA, Durie DE, et al: Risk factors for wound complications in morbidly obese women undergoing primary cesarean delivery. J Matern Fetal Neonatal Med 25(9):1544, 2012
Tixier H, Thouvenot S, Coulange L, et al: Cesarean section in morbidly obese women: supra or subumbilical transverse incision? Acta Obstet Gynecol Scand 88(9):1049, 2009
Van Mieghem T, Van Schoubroeck D, Depiere M, et al: Fetal cerebral hemorrhage caused by vitamin K deficiency after complicated bariatric surgery. Obstet Gynecol 112:434, 2008
Verrijken A, Mertens FS, Prawitt J, et al: Prothrombotic factors in histologically proven nonalcoholic fatty liver disease and nonalcoholic steatohepatitis. Hepatology 59:121, 2014
Vesco K, Sharma A, Dietz P, et al: Newborn size among obese women with weight gain outside the 2009 Institute of Medicine recommendation. Obstet Gynecol 117(4):812, 2011
Vrebosch L, Bel S, Vansant G et al: Maternal and neonatal outcome after laparoscopic adjustable gastric banding: a systematic review. Obes Surg 22(10):1568, 2012
Vricella LK, Louis JM, Mercer BM, et al: Anesthesia complications during scheduled cesarean delivery for morbidly obese women. Am J Obstet Gynecol 203(3):276.e1, 2010
Waldenström U, Aasheim V, Nilson ABV, et al: Adverse pregnancy outcomes related to advanced maternal age compared with smoking and being overweight. Obstet Gynecol 123:104, 2014
Wall PD, Deucy EE, Glantz JC, et al: Vertical skin incisions and wound complications in the obese parturient. Obstet Gynecol 102:952, 2003
Walsh C, Scaife C, Hopf H: Prevention and management of surgical site infection in morbidly obese women. Obstet Gynecol 113:411, 2009
Wang T, Zhang J, Lu X, et al: Maternal early pregnancy body mass index and risk of preterm birth. Arch Gynecol Obstet 284(4):813, 2011
Watkins ML, Rasmussen SA, Honein MA, et al: Maternal obesity and risk for birth defects. Pediatrics 111:1152, 2003
Wax JF, Pinette MG, Cartin A: Roux-en-Y gastric bypass-associated bowel obstruction complicating pregnancy–an obstetrician's map to the clinical minefield. Am J Obstet Gynecol 208(4):265, 2013
Wax JR, Wolff R, Cobean R, et al: Intussusception complicating pregnancy following laparoscopy Roux-en-Y gastric bypass. Obes Surg 17(7):977, 2007
Weichert J, Hartge DR: Obstetrical sonography in obese women: a review. J Clin Ultrasound 39(4):209, 2011
Weiss JL, Malon FD, Emig D, et al: Obesity, obstetric complications and cesarean delivery rate—a population based screening study. FASTER Research Consortium. Am J Obstet Gynecol 190:1091, 2004
Whitaker RC: Predicting preschooler obesity at birth: the role of maternal obesity in early pregnancy. Pediatrics 114:e29, 2004
Wittgrove AC, Jester L, Wittgrove P, et al: Pregnancy following gastric bypass for morbid obesity. Obes Surg 8:461, 1998
Wolf M, Kettyle E, Sandler L, et al: Obesity and preeclampsia: the potential role of inflammation. Obstet Gynecol 98:757, 2001
Yao R, Ananth C, Park B, et al: Obesity and the risk of still birth: a population-based cohort study. Am J Obstet Gynecol 210:S31, 2014
Yanovski SZ: Pharmacotherapy for obesity—promise and uncertainty. N Engl J Med 353(20):2187, 2005
Zimmet P, Alberti KGMM: Surgery or medical therapy for obese patients with Type 2 diabetes? N Engl J Med 366(17):1635, 2012

CHAPTER 49

Cardiovascular Disorders

Heart disease complicates more than 1 percent of all pregnancies and is now the leading cause of indirect maternal deaths—accounting for 20 percent of all cases (Simpson, 2012). In an analysis of maternal mortality in the United States between 1987 and 2005, the causes previously responsible for most maternal deaths—hemorrhage and hypertensive disorders—had progressively decreased rates, whereas deaths attributable to cardiovascular diseases had the greatest percentage increase (Berg, 2010). Similarly, in the United Kingdom, the rate of maternal mortality due to cardiac disease increased from 1.65 to 2.31 per 100,000 births between 1997–1999 and 2006–2008 (Centre for Maternal and Child Enquiries, 2011). Cardiovascular diseases also account for significant maternal morbidity and are a leading cause of obstetrical intensive care unit admissions (Small, 2012).

The increasing prevalence of cardiovascular diseases complicating pregnancy is likely due to a number of causes, including higher rates of obesity, hypertension, and diabetes. Indeed, according to the United States National Center for Health Statistics, almost half of adults aged 20 and older have at least one risk factor for cardiovascular disease (Fryar, 2012). And as shown in Figure 49-1, the prevalence of these risk factors among reproductive-aged women is dramatic. Other related factors include delayed childbearing. From 1970 to 2006 the proportion of first births to women aged 35 years or older increased nearly eightfold (Mathews, 2009). Finally, as discussed subsequently, an increasing number of patients with congenital heart disease are now becoming pregnant.

PHYSIOLOGICAL CONSIDERATIONS IN PREGNANCY

Cardiovascular Physiology

The marked pregnancy-induced anatomical and functional changes in cardiac physiology can have a profound effect on underlying heart disease (Chap. 4, p. 58). Some of these changes are listed in Table 49-1. Importantly, cardiac output increases approximately 40 percent during pregnancy. Almost half of this total increase takes place by 8 weeks and is maximal by midpregnancy (Capeless, 1989). The early increase stems from augmented stroke volume that results from decreased vascular resistance. Later in pregnancy, resting pulse and stroke volume increase even more because of increased end-diastolic ventricular volume that results from pregnancy hypervolemia. This along with an increase in heart rate translates to increased cardiac output that continues to rise across pregnancy to average 40 percent higher at term.

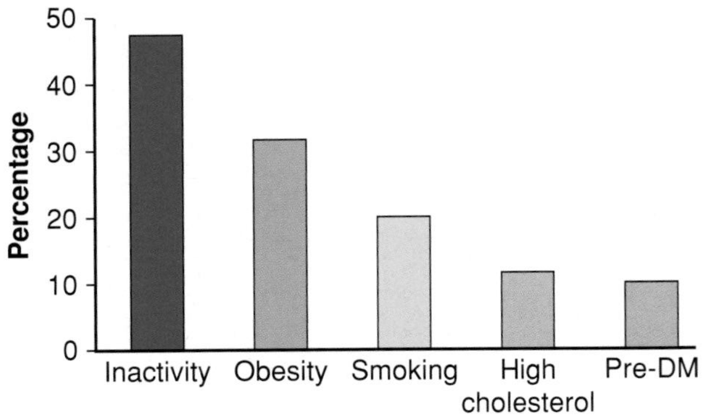

FIGURE 49-1 Prevalence of risk factors for cardiovascular disease among reproductive-aged women. DM = diabetes mellitus. (From Centers for Disease Control and Prevention, 2011.)

These changes are even more profound in multifetal pregnancy (Kametas, 2003; Kuleva, 2011).

An important study by Clark and colleagues (1989) contributed greatly to the understanding of cardiovascular physiology during pregnancy. Using right-sided heart catheterization, hemodynamic function was measured in 10 healthy primigravid volunteers, and pregnancy values were compared with those measured again at 12 weeks postpartum. As shown in Table 49-1, the cardiac output near term in the lateral recumbent position increased 43 percent. Systemic and pulmonary vascular resistances were concomitantly decreased. Importantly, intrinsic left ventricular contractility did not change. Thus, normal left ventricular function is maintained during pregnancy, that is, pregnancy is not characterized by hyperdynamic function or a high cardiac-output state.

Women with underlying cardiac disease may not always accommodate these changes, and ventricular dysfunction leads to cardiogenic heart failure. A few women with severe cardiac dysfunction may experience evidence of heart failure before midpregnancy. In others, heart failure may develop after 28 weeks when pregnancy-induced hypervolemia and cardiac output reach their maximum. In most, however, heart failure develops peripartum when labor, delivery, and a number of common obstetrical conditions add undue cardiac burdens. Some of these include preeclampsia, hemorrhage and anemia, and sepsis syndrome. In a report of 542 women with heart disease, eight of 10 maternal deaths were during the puerperium (Etheridge, 1977).

TABLE 49-1. Hemodynamic Changes in 10 Normal Pregnant Women at Term Compared with Repeat Values Obtained 12 Weeks Postpartum

Parameter	Change (%)
Cardiac output	+43
Heart rate	+17
Left ventricular stroke work index	+17
Vascular resistance	
Systemic	−21
Pulmonary	−34
Mean arterial pressure	+4
Colloid osmotic pressure	−14

Data from Clark, 1989.

Ventricular Function in Pregnancy

Ventricular volumes increase to accommodate pregnancy-induced hypervolemia. This is reflected by increasing end-systolic as well as end-diastolic dimensions. At the same time, however, there is no change in septal thickness or in ejection fraction. This is because these changes are accompanied by substantive ventricular remodeling—*plasticity*—which is characterized by eccentric expansion of left-ventricular mass that averages 30 to 35 percent near term. All of these adaptations return to prepregnancy values within a few months postpartum.

Certainly for clinical purposes, ventricular function during pregnancy is normal as estimated by the *Braunwald ventricular function* graph depicted in Figure 4-9 (p. 59). For given filling pressures, there is appropriate cardiac output so that cardiac function during pregnancy is eudynamic. Despite these findings, it remains controversial whether myocardial function per se is normal, enhanced, or depressed. Myocardial performance is measured by preload, afterload, contractility, and heart rate. Because these depend on ventricular geometry, they can only be measured indirectly (Savu, 2012). In nonpregnant subjects with a normal heart who sustain a high-output state, the left ventricle undergoes *longitudinal remodeling,* and echocardiographic functional indices of its deformation provide normal values. In pregnancy, there instead appears to be *spherical remodeling*, and these calculated indices that measure longitudinal deformation are depressed. Thus, these normal indices are likely inaccurate when used to assess function in pregnant women because they do not take into account the spherical eccentric hypertrophy characteristic of normal pregnancy.

DIAGNOSIS OF HEART DISEASE

The physiological adaptations of normal pregnancy can induce symptoms and alter clinical findings that may confound the diagnosis of heart disease. For example, in normal pregnancy, functional systolic heart murmurs are common; respiratory effort is accentuated and at times suggests dyspnea; edema in the lower extremities after midpregnancy is common; and fatigue and exercise intolerance develop in most women. Some systolic flow murmurs may be loud, and normal changes in the various heart sounds depicted in Figure 49-2 may suggest cardiac disease.

Clinical findings that may suggest heart disease are listed in Table 49-2. Pregnant women with none of these rarely have serious heart disease. As an interesting aside, Melchiorre and associates (2011) found that the prevalence of previously undiagnosed maternal cardiac structural abnormalities is significantly increased in women with high midtrimester uterine artery Doppler resistance indices (Chap. 17, p. 345).

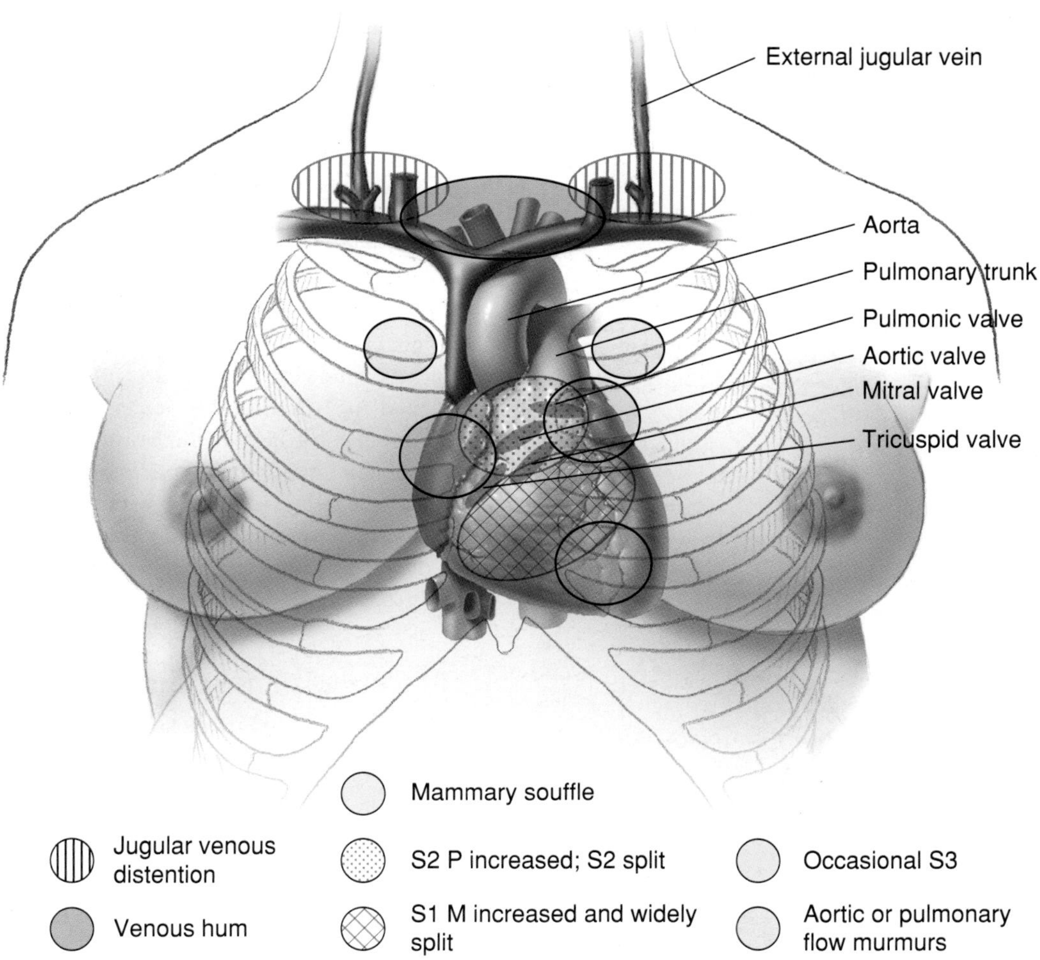

FIGURE 49-2 Normal cardiac examination findings in the pregnant woman. S_1 = first sound; M_1 = mitral first sound; S_2 = second sound; P_2 = pulmonary second sound. (From Gei, 2001; Hytten, 1991.)

TABLE 49-2. Clinical Indicators of Heart Disease During Pregnancy

Symptoms
- Progressive dyspnea or orthopnea
- Nocturnal cough
- Hemoptysis
- Syncope
- Chest pain

Clinical Findings
- Cyanosis
- Clubbing of fingers
- Persistent neck vein distention
- Systolic murmur grade 3/6 or greater
- Diastolic murmur
- Cardiomegaly
- Persistent arrhythmia
- Persistent split second sound
- Criteria for pulmonary hypertension

Diagnostic Studies

In most women, noninvasive cardiovascular studies such as electrocardiography, chest radiography, and echocardiography will provide data necessary for evaluation. In some situations, such as complex congenital heart disease, transesophageal echocardiography may be useful. Albumin or red cells tagged with technicium-99m are rarely needed during pregnancy to evaluate ventricular function. That said, the estimated fetal radiation exposure from nuclear medicine studies of myocardial perfusion are calculated to range between 5 and 17 mGy depending on the technique employed (Colletti, 2013). If indicated, cardiac catheterization can be performed with limited fluoroscopy time. During coronary angiography, the mean radiation exposure to the unshielded abdomen is 1.5 mGy, and less than 20 percent of this reaches the fetus because of tissue attenuation (European Society of Cardiology, 2011). Shielding the fetus from direct radiation and shortening the fluoroscopic time help to minimize radiation exposure. In women with clear indications, any minimal theoretical fetal risk is outweighed by maternal benefits (Chap. 46, p. 932).

Electrocardiography

As the diaphragm is elevated in advancing pregnancy, there is an average 15-degree left-axis deviation in the electrocardiogram (ECG), and mild ST changes may be seen in the inferior leads. Atrial and ventricular premature contractions are relatively frequent (Carruth, 1981). Pregnancy does not alter voltage findings.

Chest Radiography

Anteroposterior (AP) and lateral chest radiographs are useful, and when a lead apron shield is used, fetal radiation exposure is minimal (Chap. 46, p. 931). Gross cardiomegaly can usually be excluded, but slight heart enlargement cannot be detected accurately because the heart silhouette normally is larger in pregnancy. This is accentuated further with a portable AP chest radiograph.

Echocardiography

Widespread use of echocardiography has allowed accurate diagnosis of most heart diseases during pregnancy. It allows noninvasive evaluation of structural and functional cardiac factors. Some normal pregnancy-induced changes include slightly but significantly increased tricuspid regurgitation, left atrial end-diastolic dimension, and left ventricular mass. Savu (2012) and Vitarelli (2011) and their coworkers have provided normal morphological and functional echocardiographic parameters for pregnancy, which are listed in the Appendix (p. 1293).

Classification of Functional Heart Disease

There is no clinically applicable test for accurately measuring functional cardiac capacity. The clinical classification of the New York Heart Association (NYHA) was first published in 1928, and it was revised for the eighth time in 1979. This classification is based on past and present disability and is uninfluenced by physical signs:

- Class I. *Uncompromised—no limitation of physical activity:* These women do not have symptoms of cardiac insufficiency or experience anginal pain.
- Class II. *Slight limitation of physical activity:* These women are comfortable at rest, but if ordinary physical activity is undertaken, discomfort in the form of excessive fatigue, palpitation, dyspnea, or anginal pain results.
- Class III. *Marked limitation of physical activity:* These women are comfortable at rest, but less than ordinary activity causes excessive fatigue, palpitation, dyspnea, or anginal pain.
- Class IV. *Severely compromised—inability to perform any physical activity without discomfort*: Symptoms of cardiac insufficiency or angina may develop even at rest. If any physical activity is undertaken, discomfort is increased.

Siu and associates (2001b) expanded the NYHA classification and developed a scoring system for predicting cardiac complications during pregnancy. The system is based on a prospective analysis of 562 consecutive pregnant women with heart disease during 617 pregnancies in 13 Canadian teaching hospitals. Predictors of cardiac complications included the following: (1) prior heart failure, transient ischemic attack, arrhythmia, or stroke; (2) baseline NYHA class III or IV or cyanosis; (3) left-sided obstruction defined as mitral valve area < 2 cm^2, aortic valve area < 1.5 cm^2, or peak left ventricular outflow tract gradient > 30 mm Hg by echocardiography; (4) ejection fraction less than 40 percent. The risk of pulmonary edema, sustained arrhythmia, stroke, cardiac arrest, or cardiac death was substantially increased with one of these factors and even more so with two or more.

At least two studies have been conducted using these latter risk criteria. Khairy and colleagues (2006) reviewed 90 pregnancies in 53 women with congenital heart disease at Brigham and Women's Hospital. There were no maternal deaths, and heart failure and symptomatic arrhythmias developed in 16.7 and 2.8 percent of the women, respectively. Similar to the Canadian study cited above, the most important predictors of complications were prior congestive heart failure, depressed ejection fraction, and smoking. In a German study that also used these predefined risk predictors, they were found to be accurate in assessing most cardiac outcomes (Stangl, 2008).

Preconceptional Counseling

Women with severe heart disease will benefit immensely from counseling before undertaking pregnancy, and they usually are referred for maternal-fetal medicine or cardiology consultation (Clark, 2012; Seshadri, 2012).

Maternal mortality rates generally vary directly with functional classification, and this relationship may change as pregnancy progresses. In the Canadian study, Siu and colleagues (2001b) observed significant worsening of NYHA class in 4.4 percent of 579 pregnancies in which the baseline class was I or II. Their experiences, however, as well as those of McFaul and coworkers (1988), were that there were no maternal deaths in 1041 women with class I or II disease. As described later, some women have life-threatening cardiac abnormalities that can be reversed by corrective surgery, and subsequent pregnancy becomes less dangerous. In other cases, such as women with mechanical valves taking warfarin, fetal considerations predominate.

The World Health Organization Risk Classification of Cardiovascular Disease and Pregnancy is useful for assessing maternal risk associated with various cardiovascular conditions and for preconceptional counseling and planning (Thorne, 2006). Maternal risk is divided among four progressively worsening classes as shown in Table 49-3. Its use has been recommended by the European Society of Cardiology (2011).

Congenital Heart Disease in Offspring

Many congenital heart lesions appear to be inherited as polygenic characteristics, which are discussed in Chapter 13 (p. 274). Because of this, some women with congenital heart lesions give birth to similarly affected infants, the risk of which varies widely as shown in Table 49-4. Environmental factors are also important. One example is a study from Tibet in which the prevalence of fetal heart disease was increased among women living at higher altitudes (> 3600 meters) and was presumably due to lower oxygen concentrations (Chen, 2008).

TABLE 49-3. World Health Organization (WHO) Risk Classification of Cardiovascular Disease and Pregnancy

Risk Category	Associated Conditions
WHO 1—Risk no higher than general population	Uncomplicated, small, or mild: Pulmonary stenosis Ventricular septal defect Patent ductus arteriosus Mitral valve prolapse with no more than trivial mitral regurgitation Successfully repaired simple lesions: Ostium secundum atrial septal defect Ventricular septal defect Patent ductus arteriosus Total anomalous pulmonary venous drainage Isolated ventricular extrasystoles and atrial ectopic beats
WHO 2—Small increase in risk of maternal mortality and morbidity	If otherwise uncomplicated: Unoperated atrial septal defect Repaired Fallot tetralogy Most arrhythmias
WHO 2 or 3—depends on individual case	Mild left ventricular impairment Hypertrophic cardiomyopathy Native or tissue valvular heart disease not considered WHO 4 Marfan syndrome without aortic dilation Heart transplantation
WHO 3—Significantly increased risk of maternal mortality or expert cardiac and obstetrical care required	Mechanical valve Systemic right ventricle—congenitally corrected transposition, simple transposition post-Mustard or -Senning repair Post-Fontan operation Cyanotic heart disease Other complex congenital heart disease
WHO 4—Very high risk of maternal mortality or severe morbidity; pregnancy contraindicated and termination discussed	Pulmonary arterial hypertension Severe systemic ventricular dysfunction (NYHA III-IV or LVEF < 30%) Previous peripartum cardiomyopathy with any residual impairment of left ventricular function Severe left heart obstruction Marfan syndrome with aorta dilated > 40 mm

Modified from Thorne, 2006.

TABLE 49-4. Risks for Fetal Heart Lesions Related to Affected Family Members

	Congenital Heart Disease in Fetus (%)		
Cardiac Lesion	Previous Sibling Affected	Father Affected	Mother Affected
Marfan syndrome	NS	50	50
Aortic stenosis	2	3	15–18
Pulmonary stenosis	2	2	6–7
Ventricular septal defect	3	2	10–16
Atrial septal defect	2.5	1.5	5–11
Patent ductus arteriosus	3	2.5	4
Coarctation of the aorta	NS	NS	14
Fallot tetralogy	2.5	1.5	2–3

NS = not stated.
Data from Lupton, 2002.

PERIPARTUM MANAGEMENT CONSIDERATIONS

In most instances, management involves a team approach with an obstetrician, cardiologist, anesthesiologist, and other specialists as needed. With complex lesions or with women who are especially at risk, evaluation by a multidisciplinary team is recommended early in pregnancy. During consultation, cardiovascular changes likely to be poorly tolerated by an individual woman are identified, and plans are formulated to minimize these. In some, pregnancy termination may be advisable. Maxwell (2010) has provided an in-depth checklist that considers detailed management options. The four changes that affect management that are emphasized by the American College of Obstetricians and Gynecologists (1992) include decreased vascular resistance, increased blood volume and cardiac output and their fluctuations peripartum, and hypercoagulability. Within this framework, both prognosis and management are influenced by the type and severity of the specific lesion and by the patient's functional classification.

With rare exceptions, women in NYHA class I and most in class II negotiate pregnancy without morbidity. Special attention should be directed toward both prevention and early recognition of heart failure as discussed on page 990. Infection with sepsis syndrome is an important factor in precipitating cardiac failure. Moreover, bacterial endocarditis is a deadly complication of valvular heart disease (p. 990). Each woman should receive instructions to avoid contact with persons who have respiratory infections, including the common cold, and to report at once any evidence for infection. Pneumococcal and influenza vaccines are recommended.

Cigarette smoking is prohibited, because of both its cardiac effects and its propensity to cause upper respiratory infections. Illicit drug use may be particularly harmful, an example being the cardiovascular effects of cocaine or amphetamines. In addition, intravenous drug use increases the risk of infective endocarditis.

Fortunately, cases of NYHA class III and IV are uncommon today. In the Canadian study, only 3 percent of approximately 600 pregnancies were complicated by NYHA class III heart disease, and no women had class IV when first seen (Siu, 2001b). In a Turkish study, 8 percent of pregnancies in women with cardiac diseases were NYHA class III or IV (Madazli, 2010). An important question in these women is whether pregnancy should be undertaken. If women make that choice, they must understand the risks, and they are encouraged to be compliant with planned care. In some, prolonged hospitalization or bed rest is often necessary with continued pregnancy.

Labor and Delivery

In general, vaginal delivery is preferred, and labor induction is usually safe (Oron, 2004). Cesarean delivery is limited to obstetrical indications, and considerations are given for the specific cardiac lesion, overall maternal condition, and availability of experienced anesthesia personnel and general support facilities. Some of these women tolerate major surgical procedures poorly and are best delivered in a unit experienced with management of complicated cardiac disease. In some women, pulmonary artery catheterization may be indicated for hemodynamic monitoring (Chap. 47, p. 941). In our experiences, however, invasive monitoring is rarely indicated.

Based on her review, Simpson (2012) recommends cesarean delivery for women with the following: (1) dilated aortic root > 4 cm or aortic aneurysm; (2) acute severe congestive heart failure; (3) recent myocardial infarction; (4) severe symptomatic aortic stenosis; (5) warfarin administration within 2 weeks of delivery; and (6) need for emergency valve replacement immediately after delivery. Although we agree with most of these, we have some caveats. For example, we prefer aggressive medical stabilization of pulmonary edema followed by vaginal delivery if possible. Also, warfarin anticoagulation can be reversed with vitamin K, plasma, or prothrombin concentrates.

During labor, the mother with significant heart disease should be kept in a semirecumbent position with lateral tilt. Vital signs are taken frequently between contractions. Increases in pulse rate much above 100 bpm or respiratory rate above 24 per minute, particularly when associated with dyspnea, may suggest impending ventricular failure. If there is any evidence of cardiac decompensation, intensive medical management must be instituted immediately. It is essential to remember that delivery itself does not necessarily improve the maternal condition and in fact, may worsen it. Moreover, emergency operative delivery may be particularly hazardous. Clearly, both maternal and fetal status must be considered in the decision to hasten delivery under these circumstances.

Analgesia and Anesthesia

Relief from pain and apprehension is important. Although intravenous analgesics provide satisfactory pain relief for some women, continuous epidural analgesia is recommended for most. The major problem with conduction analgesia is maternal hypotension (Chap. 25, p. 514). This is especially dangerous in women with intracardiac shunts in whom flow may be reversed. Blood passes from right to left within the heart or aorta and thereby bypasses the lungs. Hypotension can also be life-threatening if there is pulmonary arterial hypertension or aortic stenosis because ventricular output is dependent on adequate preload. In women with these conditions, narcotic conduction analgesia or general anesthesia may be preferable.

For vaginal delivery in women with only mild cardiovascular compromise, epidural analgesia given with intravenous sedation often suffices. This has been shown to minimize intrapartum cardiac output fluctuations and allows forceps or vacuum-assisted delivery. Subarachnoid blockade is not generally recommended in women with significant heart disease. For cesarean delivery, epidural analgesia is preferred by most clinicians with caveats for its use with pulmonary arterial hypertension (p. 987). Finally, general endotracheal anesthesia with thiopental, succinylcholine, nitrous oxide, and at least 30-percent oxygen has also proved satisfactory.

Intrapartum Heart Failure

Cardiovascular decompensation during labor may manifest as pulmonary edema with hypoxia or as hypotension, or both. The proper therapeutic approach depends on the specific hemodynamic status and the underlying cardiac lesion. For example, decompensated mitral stenosis with pulmonary edema due to fluid overload is often best approached with aggressive diuresis. If precipitated by tachycardia, heart rate control with β-blocking agents is preferred. Conversely, the same treatment in a woman suffering decompensation and hypotension due to aortic stenosis could prove fatal. Unless the underlying pathophysiology is understood and the cause of the decompensation is clear, empirical therapy may be hazardous. Heart failure is discussed in more detail on page 990.

Puerperium

Women who have shown little or no evidence of cardiac compromise during pregnancy, labor, or delivery may still decompensate postpartum when fluid mobilization into the intravascular compartment and reduction of peripheral vascular resistance place higher demands on myocardial performance. Therefore, it is important that meticulous care be continued into the puerperium (Keizer, 2006; Zeeman, 2006).

Postpartum hemorrhage, anemia, infection, and thromboembolism are much more serious complications with heart disease. Indeed, these factors often act in concert to precipitate postpartum heart failure (Cunningham, 1986). In addition to increased cardiac work, many of these—for example, sepsis and severe preeclampsia—cause or worsen pulmonary edema because of endothelial activation and capillary-alveolar leakage (Chap. 47, p. 947).

Sterilization and Contraception

If indicated, tubal sterilization is performed at cesarean delivery. If it is to be performed after vaginal delivery, the procedure can be delayed up to several days to ensure that the mother has become hemodynamically near normal and that she is afebrile, not anemic, and ambulating normally. Other women are given detailed contraceptive advice. Special considerations for contraception in women with various cardiac disorders are discussed in some of the following sections and in Table 38-3 (p. 698).

SURGICALLY CORRECTED HEART DISEASE

Most clinically significant congenital heart lesions are repaired during childhood. Examples of those frequently not diagnosed until adulthood include atrial septal defects, pulmonic stenosis, bicuspid aortic valve, and aortic coarctation (Brickner, 2000). In some cases, the defect is mild and surgery is not required. In others, a significant structural anomaly is amenable to surgical correction. With successful repair, many women attempt pregnancy. In some instances, surgical corrections have been performed during pregnancy.

Valve Replacement before Pregnancy

Numerous reports describe subsequent pregnancy outcomes in women who have a prosthetic mitral or aortic valve. The type of valve is paramount, and pregnancy is undertaken only after serious consideration in women with a prosthetic mechanical valve. This is because anticoagulation is requisite, and at least when not pregnant, warfarin is necessary. As shown in Table 49-5, a number of serious complications can develop with mechanical valves. Both thromboembolisms involving the prosthesis and hemorrhage from anticoagulation are of extreme concern. This is in addition to deterioration in cardiac function. Overall, the maternal mortality rate is 3 to 4 percent with mechanical valves, and fetal loss is common.

Porcine tissue valves are much safer during pregnancy, primarily because thrombosis is rare and anticoagulation is not required (see Table 49-5). Despite this, valvular dysfunction with cardiac deterioration or failure is common and develops in 5 to 25 percent of involved pregnancies. Another drawback is that bioprostheses are not as durable as mechanical ones, and valve replacement longevity averages 10 to 15 years. Based on their longitudinal study of 100 reproductive-aged women with a biological heart valve prosthesis, Cleuziou and colleagues (2010) concluded that pregnancy does not accelerate the risk for replacement.

TABLE 49-5. Outcomes Reported Since 1990 in Pregnancies Complicated by a Heart-Valve Replacement

Type of Valve	Total	Complications[a] Maternal	Perinatal
Mechanical	567[b]	38 thromboses 17 emboli 19 hemorrhages 14 deaths	107 miscarriages/ abortions 37 stillbirths
Porcine	265[c]	32 valve failures or deterioration	9 abortions 3 stillbirths

[a]Numbers estimated in some because definitions are not consistent.
[b]Data from Cotrufo, 2002; Hanania, 1994; Kawamata, 2007; Nassar, 2004; Sadler, 2000; Sbarouni, 1994; Suri, 1999, 2011.
[c]Data from Hanania, 1994; Lee, 1994; Sadler, 2000; Sbarouni, 1994.

Anticoagulation

This is critical for women with mechanical prosthetic valves. Unfortunately, warfarin is the most effective anticoagulant for preventing maternal thromboembolic complications but causes significant fetal morbidity and mortality. Anticoagulation with heparin is less hazardous for the fetus, however, the risk of maternal thromboembolic complications is much higher (McLintock, 2011).

As noted, warfarin, despite its effective anticoagulation, is teratogenic and causes miscarriage, stillbirths, and fetal malformations (Chap. 12, p. 252). In one study of 71 pregnancies in women given warfarin throughout pregnancy, the rates of miscarriage were 32 percent; stillbirth, 7 percent; and embryopathy, 6 percent (Cotrufo, 2002). The risk was highest when the mean daily dose of warfarin exceeded 5 mg. From a systematic review, Chan and coworkers (2000) concluded that the best maternal outcomes were achieved with warfarin anticoagulation but with a 6.4-percent embryopathy rate. And although heparin substituted before 12 weeks' gestation eliminated embryopathy, thromboembolic complications during that time were increased significantly.

In examining heparin, anticoagulation for mechanical valves using low-dose unfractionated heparin is definitely inadequate and has a high associated maternal mortality rate (Chan, 2000; Iturbe-Alessio, 1986). Even *full* anticoagulation with either unfractionated heparin (UFH) or one of the low-molecular-weight heparins (LMWH) is associated with valvular thrombosis (Leyh, 2002, 2003; Rowan, 2001). Thus, many authorities recommend warfarin. However, the American College of Chest Physicians has recommended use of any of several regimens that include adjusted-dose UFH or LMWH heparin given throughout pregnancy as subsequently discussed (Bates, 2012).

Recommendations for Anticoagulation. A number of different treatment options—none of which are completely ideal—have been proposed and are principally based on

TABLE 49-6. American College of Chest Physicians Guidelines for Anticoagulation of Pregnant Women with Mechanical Prosthetic Valves

Any one of the following anticoagulant regimens is recommended:
Adjusted-dose LMWH twice daily throughout pregnancy. The doses should be adjusted to achieve the manufacturer's peak anti-Xa level 4 hours after subcutaneous injection
Adjusted-dose UFH administered every 12 hours throughout pregnancy. The doses should be adjusted to keep the midinterval aPTT at least twice control or attain an anti-Xa level of 0.35 to 0.70 U/mL
LMWH or UFH as above until 13 weeks' gestation, then warfarin substitution until close to delivery when LMWH or UFH is resumed
In women judged to be at very high risk of thromboembolism and in whom concerns exist about the efficacy and safety of LMWH or UFH as dosed above—some examples include older-generation prosthesis in the mitral position or history of thromboembolism—warfarin treatment is suggested throughout pregnancy with replacement by UFH or LMWH (as above) close to delivery. In addition, low-dose aspirin—75 to 100 mg daily—should be orally administered

aPTT = activated partial thromboplastin time; LMWH = low-molecular-weight heparin; UFH = unfractionated heparin.
Adapted from Bates, 2012.

consensus opinion. For this reason, they differ and allow more than one scheme. For example, and as shown in Table 49-6, the most recent guidelines of the American College of Chest Physicians for the management of pregnant women with mechanical prosthetic valves offer several different treatment options.

Heparin is discontinued just before delivery. If delivery supervenes while the anticoagulant is still effective, and extensive bleeding is encountered, then protamine sulfate is given intravenously. Anticoagulant therapy with warfarin or heparin may be restarted 6 hours following vaginal delivery, usually with no problems. Following cesarean delivery, full anticoagulation is withheld, but the duration is not exactly known. The American College of Obstetricians and Gynecologists (2011b) advises resuming unfractionated or low-molecular-weight heparin 6 to 12 hours after cesarean delivery. It is our practice, however, to wait at least 24 hours, and preferably 48 hours, following a major surgical procedure.

Because warfarin, low-molecular-weight heparin, and unfractionated heparin do not accumulate in breast milk, they do not induce an anticoagulant effect in the infant. Therefore, these anticoagulants are compatible with breast feeding (American College of Obstetricians and Gynecologists, 2011b).

Contraception

Because of their possible thrombogenic action, estrogen-progestin oral contraceptives are relatively contraindicated in women with prosthetic valves. Because these women are generally fully anticoagulated, however, any increased risk is speculative. Contraceptive options are discussed in Chapters 38 and 39. Sterilization should be considered because of the serious pregnancy risks faced by women with significant heart disease.

Cardiac Surgery During Pregnancy

Although usually postponed until after delivery, valve replacement or other cardiac surgery during pregnancy may be lifesaving. Several reviews confirm that such surgery is associated with major maternal and fetal morbidity and mortality. Sutton and associates (2005) found that maternal mortality rates with cardiopulmonary bypass are between 1.5 and 5 percent. Although these are similar to those for nonpregnant women, the fetal mortality rate approaches 20 percent. In a longitudinal study from the Mayo Clinic, John and coworkers (2011) reported the outcomes of 21 pregnant women who underwent cardiothoracic surgery requiring cardiopulmonary bypass between 1976 and 2009. The procedures included eight aortic valve replacements, six mitral valve repairs or replacements, two myxoma excisions, two aortic aneurysm repairs, one patent foramen ovale closure, one prosthetic aortic valve thrombectomy, and one septal myectomy. Median cardiopulmonary bypass time was 53 minutes, with a range of 16 to 185 minutes. One woman died two days after surgery, and three other deaths occurred 2, 10, and 19 years postoperatively. Three fetuses died, and 52 percent delivered before 36 weeks. To optimize outcomes, Chandrasekhar and coworkers (2009) recommend the following: surgery done electively when possible, pump flow rate maintained > 2.5 L/min/m^2, normothermic perfusion pressure > 70 mm Hg, pulsatile flow used, and hematocrit kept > 28 percent.

Mitral Valvotomy During Pregnancy

Tight mitral stenosis that requires intervention during pregnancy was previously treated by closed mitral valvotomy (Pavankumar, 1988). More recently, however, percutaneous transcatheter balloon dilatation of the mitral valve has largely replaced surgical valvotomy during pregnancy (Fawzy, 2007). Rahimtoola (2006) summarized outcomes of 36 women—25 of whom were NYHA class III or IV—who underwent balloon commissurotomy at an average gestational age of 26 weeks. Surgery was successful in 35 women, and left atrial and pulmonary artery pressures were reduced as the mitral valve area was increased from 0.74 to 1.59 cm^2. Esteves and associates (2006) described similarly good outcomes in 71 pregnant women with tight mitral stenosis and heart failure who underwent percutaneous valvuloplasty. At delivery, 98 percent were either NYHA class I or II. At a mean of 44 months, the total event-free maternal survival rate was 54 percent, however, eight women required another surgical intervention. The 66 infants who were delivered at term all had normal growth and development.

Pregnancy after Heart Transplantation

The first successful pregnancy in a heart-transplant recipient was reported 25 years ago by Löwenstein and associates (1988). Since that time, more than 50 pregnancies in heart-transplant recipients have been described. Key (1989) and Kim (1996) and their colleagues provide detailed data to show that the transplanted heart responds normally to pregnancy-induced changes. Despite this, complications are common during pregnancy (Dashe, 1998).

Armenti (2002) from the National Transplantation Pregnancy Registry and Miniero (2004), each with their coworkers, described outcomes of 53 pregnancies in 37 heart recipients. Almost half developed hypertension, and 22 percent suffered at least one rejection episode during pregnancy. They were delivered—usually by cesarean—at a mean of 37 to 38 weeks. Three fourths of infants were liveborn. At follow-up, at least five women had died more than 2 years postpartum. From Scandinavia, Estensen and associates (2011) detailed the outcomes of 19 women who had received a heart transplant and six who received both a heart and lung transplant. These 25 women had 42 pregnancies, and there were no maternal deaths. Major complications included two rejections during the early puerperium, two cases of renal failure, and 11 spontaneous abortions. Five women died 2 to 12 years after delivery. Ethical considerations of counseling and caring for such women related to pregnancy were summarized by Ross (2006).

VALVULAR HEART DISEASE

Rheumatic fever is uncommon in the United States because of less crowded living conditions, availability of penicillin, and evolution of nonrheumatogenic streptococcal strains. Still, it remains the chief cause of serious mitral valvular disease (Roeder, 2011).

Mitral Stenosis

Rheumatic endocarditis causes most mitral stenosis lesions. The normal mitral valve surface area is 4.0 cm^2, and when stenosis narrows this to < 2.5 cm^2, symptoms usually develop (Desai, 2000). The contracted valve impedes blood flow from the left atrium to the ventricle. The most prominent complaint is dyspnea due to pulmonary venous hypertension and edema. Fatigue, palpitations, cough, and hemoptysis are also common.

With more severe stenosis, the left atrium dilates, left atrial pressure is chronically elevated, and significant passive pulmonary hypertension develops (Table 49-7). These women have a relatively fixed cardiac output, and thus the increased preload of normal pregnancy, as well as other factors that increase cardiac output, may cause ventricular failure and pulmonary edema. Indeed, a fourth of women with mitral stenosis have cardiac failure for the first time during pregnancy (Caulin-Glaser, 1999). Because the murmur may not be heard in some women, this clinical picture at term may be confused with idiopathic peripartum cardiomyopathy (Cunningham, 1986, 2012).

Also with significant stenosis, tachycardia shortens ventricular diastolic filling time and increases the mitral gradient. This raises left atrial as well as pulmonary venous and capillary pressures and may result in pulmonary edema. Thus, sinus tachycardia is often treated prophylactically with β-blocking agents. Atrial tachyarrhythmias, including fibrillation, are common in mitral stenosis and are treated aggressively. Atrial fibrillation also predisposes to mural thrombus formation and cerebrovascular embolization that can cause stroke (Chap. 60, p. 1192). Atrial thrombosis can develop despite a sinus rhythm, and

TABLE 49-7. Major Cardiac Valve Disorders

Type	Cause	Pathophysiology	Pregnancy
Mitral stenosis	Rheumatic valvulitis	LA dilation and passive pulmonary hypertension Atrial fibrillation	Heart failure from fluid overload, tachycardia
Mitral insufficiency	Rheumatic valvulitis Mitral-valve prolapse LV dilatation	LV dilatation and eccentric hypertrophy	Ventricular function improves with afterload decrease
Aortic stenosis	Congenital bicuspid valve	LV concentric hypertrophy, decreased cardiac output	Moderate stenosis is tolerated; severe is life-threatening with decreased preload, e.g., obstetrical hemorrhage or regional analgesia
Aortic insufficiency	Rheumatic valvulitis Connective-tissue disease Congenital	LV hypertrophy and dilatation	Ventricular function improves with afterload decrease
Pulmonary stenosis	Rheumatic valvulitis Congenital	Severe stenosis associated with RA and RV enlargement	Mild stenosis usually well tolerated; severe stenosis associated with right heart failure and atrial arrhythmias

LA = left atrium; LV = left ventricle; RA = right atrium; RV = right ventricle.

Hameed (2005) reported three such women. One suffered an embolic stroke, and another had pulmonary edema causing maternal hypoxemia leading to fetal encephalopathy.

Pregnancy Outcomes

In general, complications are directly associated with the degree of valvular stenosis. Recall that investigators from the large Canadian study found that women with a mitral-valve area < 2 cm^2 were at greatest risk. In another study, Hameed (2001) described 46 pregnant women with mitral stenosis—43 percent developed heart failure and 20 percent developed arrhythmias. Fetal-growth restriction was more common in those women with a mitral valve area < 1.0 cm^2.

Prognosis is also related to maternal functional capacity. Among 486 pregnancies complicated by rheumatic heart disease—predominantly mitral stenosis—Sawhney (2003) reported that eight of 10 maternal deaths were in women in NYHA classes III or IV.

Management

Limited physical activity is generally recommended in women with mitral stenosis. If symptoms of pulmonary congestion develop, activity is further reduced, dietary sodium is restricted, and diuretics are given (Siva, 2005). A β-blocker drug is usually given to slow the ventricular response to activity (Maxwell, 2010). If new-onset atrial fibrillation develops, intravenous verapamil, 5 to 10 mg, is given, or electrocardioversion is performed. For chronic fibrillation, digoxin, a β-blocker, or a calcium-channel blocker is given to slow ventricular response. Therapeutic anticoagulation with heparin is indicated with persistent fibrillation. Some recommend heparin anticoagulation for those with severe stenosis even if there is a sinus rhythm (Hameed, 2005).

Labor and delivery are particularly stressful for women with symptomatic mitral stenosis. Uterine contractions increase cardiac output by increasing circulating blood volume. Pain, exertion, and anxiety cause tachycardia with possible rate-related heart failure. Epidural analgesia for labor is ideal, but with strict attention to avoid fluid overload. Abrupt increases in preload may increase pulmonary capillary wedge pressure and cause pulmonary edema. The effects of labor on pulmonary pressures in women with mitral stenosis are shown in Figure 49-3. Wedge pressures increase most immediately postpartum. Clark and colleagues (1985) hypothesize that this is likely due to loss of the low-resistance placental circulation along with the venous "autotransfusion" from a now-empty uterus and from the lower extremities and pelvis.

Most consider vaginal delivery to be preferable in women with mitral stenosis. Elective induction is reasonable so that labor and delivery are attended by a scheduled, experienced team. With severe stenosis and chronic heart failure, insertion of a pulmonary artery catheter may help guide management.

Mitral Insufficiency

A trivial degree of mitral insufficiency is found in most normal patients (Maxwell, 2010). But if there is improper coaptation of mitral valve leaflets during systole, abnormal degrees of

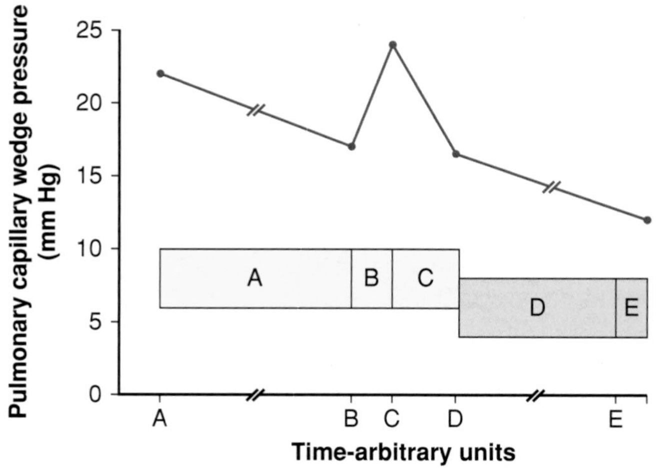

FIGURE 49-3 Mean pulmonary capillary wedge pressure measurements (*red graph line*) in eight women with mitral valve stenosis. Shaded yellow and blue boxes are mean (± 1 SD) pressures in nonlaboring normal women at term. **A.** First-stage labor. **B.** Second-stage labor 15 to 30 minutes before delivery. **C.** Postpartum 5 to 15 minutes. **D.** Postpartum 4 to 6 hours. **E.** Postpartum 18 to 24 hours. (Data from Clark, 1985, 1989.)

mitral regurgitation may develop. This is eventually followed by left ventricular dilatation and eccentric hypertrophy (see Table 49-7). Chronic mitral regurgitation has a number of causes, including rheumatic fever, mitral valve prolapse, or left ventricular dilatation of any etiology—for example, dilated cardiomyopathy. Less common causes include a calcified mitral annulus, possibly some appetite suppressants, and in older women, ischemic heart disease. Mitral valve vegetations—*Libman-Sacks endocarditis*—are relatively common in women with antiphospholipid antibodies (Roldan, 1996; Shroff, 2012). These sometimes coexist with systemic lupus erythematosus (Chap. 59, p. 1170). In contrast, acute mitral insufficiency is caused by chordae tendineae rupture, papillary muscle infarction, or leaflet perforation from infective endocarditis.

In nonpregnant patients, symptoms from mitral valve incompetence are rare, and valve replacement is seldom indicated unless infective endocarditis develops. Likewise, mitral regurgitation is well tolerated during pregnancy, probably because decreased systemic vascular resistance results in less regurgitation. Heart failure only rarely develops during pregnancy, and occasionally tachyarrhythmias require treatment.

Mitral Valve Prolapse

This diagnosis implies the presence of a pathological connective tissue disorder—often termed *myxomatous degeneration*—which may involve the valve leaflets themselves, the annulus, or the chordae tendineae. Mitral insufficiency may develop. Most women with mitral valve prolapse are asymptomatic and are diagnosed by routine examination or while undergoing echocardiography. The small percentage of women with symptoms have anxiety, palpitations, atypical chest pain, dyspnea with exertion, and syncope (Guy, 2012).

Pregnant women with mitral valve prolapse rarely have cardiac complications. Hypervolemia may even improve alignment of the mitral valve, and women without pathological myxomatous change generally have excellent pregnancy outcomes (Leśniak-Sobelga, 2004; Rayburn, 1987). In a study of 3100 women in the Taiwanese Birth Registry with mitral valve prolapse, however, the preterm birth rate was 1.2 times higher than among controls (Chen, 2011).

For women who are symptomatic, β-blocking drugs are given to decrease sympathetic tone, relieve chest pain and palpitations, and reduce the risk of life-threatening arrhythmias. According to the American College of Obstetricians and Gynecologists (2011a), mitral valve prolapse is not considered an indication for infective endocarditis prophylaxis.

Aortic Stenosis

Usually a disease of aging, aortic stenosis in women younger than 30 years is most likely due to a congenital lesion. This stenosis is less common since the decline in incidences of rheumatic diseases, and the most frequent cause in this country is a bicuspid valve (Friedman, 2008). A normal aortic valve has an area of 3 to 4 cm^2, with a pressure gradient of less than 5 mm Hg. If the valve area is < 1 cm^2, there is severe obstruction to flow and a progressive pressure overload on the left ventricle (Carabello, 2002; Roeder, 2011). Concentric left ventricular hypertrophy follows, and if severe, end-diastolic pressures become elevated, ejection fraction declines, and cardiac output is reduced (see Table 49-7). Characteristic clinical manifestations develop late and include chest pain, syncope, heart failure, and sudden death from arrhythmias. Life expectancy averages only 5 years after exertional chest pain develops, and valve replacement is indicated for symptomatic patients.

Pregnancy

Clinically significant aortic stenosis is infrequent during pregnancy. Mild to moderate degrees of stenosis are well tolerated, however, severe disease is life threatening. The principal underlying hemodynamic problem is the fixed cardiac output associated with severe stenosis. During pregnancy, a number of events acutely decrease preload further and thus aggravate the fixed cardiac output. These include vena caval occlusion, regional analgesia, and hemorrhage. Importantly, these also decrease cardiac, cerebral, and uterine perfusion. It follows that severe aortic stenosis may be extremely dangerous during pregnancy. From the large Canadian multicenter study cited above, there were increased complications if the aortic valve area was < 1.5 cm^2 (Siu, 2001b). And in the report by Hameed and associates (2001) described earlier, the maternal mortality rate with aortic stenosis was 8 percent. Women with valve gradients exceeding 100 mm Hg appear to be at greatest risk.

Management

For the asymptomatic woman with aortic stenosis, no treatment except close observation is required. Management of the symptomatic woman includes strict limitation of activity and prompt treatment of infections. If symptoms persist despite bed rest, valve replacement or valvotomy using cardiopulmonary bypass must be considered. In general, balloon valvotomy for aortic valve disease is avoided because of serious complications, which exceed 10 percent. These include stroke, aortic rupture, aortic valve insufficiency, and death (Reich, 2004). In rare cases, it may be preferable to perform valve replacement during pregnancy (Datt, 2010).

For women with critical aortic stenosis, intensive monitoring during labor is important. Pulmonary artery catheterization may be helpful because of the narrow margin separating fluid overload from hypovolemia. Women with aortic stenosis are dependent on adequate end-diastolic ventricular filling pressures to maintain cardiac output and systemic perfusion. Abrupt decreases in end-diastolic volume may result in hypotension, syncope, myocardial infarction, and sudden death. Thus, the management key is avoidance of decreased ventricular preload and the maintenance of cardiac output. During labor and delivery, such women should be managed on the "wet" side, maintaining a margin of safety in intravascular volume in anticipation of possible hemorrhage. In women with a competent mitral valve, pulmonary edema is rare, even with moderate volume overload.

During labor, narcotic epidural analgesia seems ideal, thus avoiding potentially hazardous hypotension, which may be encountered with standard conduction analgesia techniques. Easterling and coworkers (1988) studied the effects of epidural analgesia in five women with severe stenosis and demonstrated immediate and profound effects of decreased filling pressures. Xia and associates (2006) emphasize slow administration of dilute local anesthetic agents into the epidural space. Forceps or vacuum delivery is used for standard obstetrical indications in hemodynamically stable women. Late cardiac events include pulmonary edema, arrhythmias, cardiac interventions, and death, which were identified within 1 year of delivery in 70 pregnancies (Tzemos, 2009).

Aortic Insufficiency

Aortic valve regurgitation or insufficiency allows diastolic flow of blood from the aorta back into the left ventricle. Frequent causes of abnormal insufficiency are rheumatic fever, connective-tissue abnormalities, and congenital lesions. With Marfan syndrome, the aortic root may dilate, resulting in regurgitation. Acute insufficiency may develop with bacterial endocarditis or aortic dissection. Aortic and mitral valve insufficiency have been linked to the appetite suppressants fenfluramine and dexfenfluramine and to the ergot-derived dopamine agonists cabergoline and pergolide (Gardin, 2000; Schade, 2007; Zanettini, 2007). With chronic insufficiency, left ventricular hypertrophy and dilatation develop and are followed by slow-onset fatigue, dyspnea, and edema, although rapid deterioration usually follows (see Table 49-7).

Aortic insufficiency is generally well tolerated during pregnancy. Like mitral valve incompetence, diminished vascular resistance is thought to improve hemodynamic function. If symptoms of heart failure develop, diuretics are given and bed rest is encouraged.

Pulmonic Stenosis

The pulmonary valve is affected by rheumatic fever far less often than the other valves. Instead, pulmonic stenosis is usually congenital and also may be associated with Fallot tetralogy or Noonan syndrome. The clinical diagnosis is typically identified by auscultating a systolic ejection murmur over the pulmonary area that is louder during inspiration.

Increased hemodynamic burdens of pregnancy can precipitate right-sided heart failure or atrial arrhythmias in women with severe stenosis. Surgical correction ideally is done before pregnancy, but if symptoms progress, a balloon angioplasty may be necessary antepartum (Maxwell, 2010; Siu, 2001a). In a study of 81 pregnancies in 51 Dutch women with pulmonic stenosis, cardiac complications were infrequent (Drenthen, 2006). NYHA classification worsened in two women, and nine experienced palpitations or arrhythmias. No changes in pulmonary valvular function or other adverse cardiac events were reported. However, noncardiac complications were increased—17 percent had preterm delivery; 15 percent had hypertension; and 4 percent developed thromboembolism. Interestingly, two of the offspring were diagnosed with pulmonic stenosis, and another had complete transposition and anencephaly.

CONGENITAL HEART DISEASE

The incidence of congenital heart disease in the United States is approximately 8 per 1000 liveborn infants. Approximately a third of these have critical disease that requires cardiac catheterization or surgery during the first year of life. Others require surgery in childhood, and it is currently estimated that there are nearly 1 million adults in this country with congenital heart disease (Bashore, 2007).

According to an analysis from the Nationwide Inpatient Sample discharge database, more than 30,000 women admitted for delivery between 1998 and 2007 had congenital heart disease—a rate of 71.6 per 100,000 deliveries (Opotowsky, 2012). After statistical adjustments, women with congenital heart disease were found to be eight times more likely to sustain an adverse cardiovascular event that included death, heart failure, arrhythmia, and cerebrovascular or embolic event. Of these, arrhythmia was the most common, and the rate of maternal death was approximately 1.5 per 1000. Thompson and coworkers (2014) found similar risks.

Septal Defects

Atrial Septal Defects

After bicuspid aortic valve, these are the most frequently encountered adult congenital cardiac lesions. Indeed, a fourth of all adults have a patent foramen ovale (Kizer, 2005). Most are asymptomatic until the third or fourth decade. The secundum-type defect accounts for 70 percent, and associated mitral valve myxomatous abnormalities with prolapse are common. Most recommend repair if discovered in adulthood. Pregnancy is well tolerated unless pulmonary hypertension has developed, but this is uncommon (Maxwell, 2010; Zuber, 1999). Treatment is indicated for congestive heart failure or an arrhythmia. Based on their review, Aliaga and associates (2003) concluded that the risk of endocarditis with an atrial septal defect is negligible.

With the potential to shunt blood from right to left, a *paradoxical embolism,* that is, entry of a venous thrombus through the septal defect and into the systemic arterial circulation, is possible and may cause an embolic stroke (Chap. 60, p. 1192). Erkut and associates (2006) described a woman who developed an entrapped thrombus in a patent foramen ovale postpartum. In asymptomatic women, thromboembolism prophylaxis is problematic, and recommendations include either observation or antiplatelet therapy such as low-dose aspirin (Kizer, 2005; Maxwell, 2010). Compression stockings and prophylactic heparin for a pregnant woman with a septal defect and concurrent immobility or other risk factors for thromboembolism have also been recommended (Head, 2005).

Ventricular Septal Defects

These lesions close spontaneously during childhood in 90 percent of cases. Most defects are paramembranous, and physiological derangements are related to lesion size. In general, if the defect is less than 1.25 cm^2, pulmonary hypertension and heart failure do not develop. If the effective defect size exceeds that of the aortic valve orifice, symptoms rapidly develop. For these reasons, most children undergo surgical repair before pulmonary hypertension develops. Adults with unrepaired large defects develop left ventricular failure and pulmonary hypertension and have a high incidence of bacterial endocarditis (Brickner, 2000; Maxwell, 2010).

Pregnancy is well tolerated with small to moderate left-to-right shunts. If pulmonary arterial pressures reach systemic levels, however, there is reversal or bidirectional flow—*Eisenmenger syndrome* (p. 985). When this develops, the maternal mortality rate is significantly increased, and thus, pregnancy is not generally advisable. Bacterial endocarditis is more common with unrepaired defects, and antimicrobial prophylaxis is often required (p. 991). As shown in Table 49-4, up to 15 percent of offspring born to these women also have a ventricular septal defect.

Atrioventricular Septal Defects

These account for approximately 3 percent of all congenital cardiac malformations and are distinct from isolated atrial or ventricular septal defects. An atrioventricular (AV) septal defect is characterized by a common, ovoid AV junction. This defect is associated with aneuploidy, Eisenmenger syndrome, and other malformations, but still, some of these women become pregnant. Compared with simple septal defects, complications are more frequent during pregnancy. In a review of 48 pregnancies in 29 such women, complications included persistent deterioration of NYHA class in 23 percent, significant arrhythmias in 19 percent, and heart failure in 2 percent (Drenthen, 2005b). Congenital heart disease was identified in 15 percent of the offspring.

Persistent (Patent) Ductus Arteriosus

The ductus connects the proximal left pulmonary artery to the descending aorta just distal to the left subclavian artery. Functional closure of the ductus from vasoconstriction occurs shortly after term birth (Akintunde, 2011). The physiological consequences of persistence of this structure are related to its size. Most significant lesions are repaired in childhood, but for individuals who do not undergo repair, the mortality rate is high after the fifth decade (Brickner, 2000). In some younger women with an unrepaired ductus during pregnancy, however, pulmonary hypertension, heart failure, or cyanosis will develop if systemic blood pressure falls and leads to shunt reversal of blood from the pulmonary artery into the aorta (Maxwell, 2010). A sudden blood pressure decline at delivery—such as with conduction analgesia or hemorrhage—may lead to fatal collapse. Therefore, hypotension should be avoided whenever possible and treated vigorously if it develops. Prophylaxis for bacterial endocarditis may be indicated at delivery for unrepaired defects (p. 991). As shown in Table 49-4, the incidence of inheritance is approximately 4 percent.

Cyanotic Heart Disease

When congenital heart lesions are associated with right-to-left shunting of blood past the pulmonary capillary bed, cyanosis develops. The classic and most commonly encountered lesion in adults and during pregnancy is the *Fallot tetralogy* (Maxwell, 2010). It is characterized by a large ventricular septal defect, pulmonary stenosis, right ventricular hypertrophy, and an overriding aorta that receives blood from both the right and left ventricles. The magnitude of the shunt varies inversely with systemic vascular resistance. Hence, during pregnancy, when peripheral resistance decreases, the shunt increases and cyanosis worsens. Women who have undergone repair and who do not have a recurrence of cyanosis do well in pregnancy.

Some women with *Ebstein anomaly* with a malpositioned, malformed tricuspid valve may reach reproductive age. Right ventricular failure from volume overload and appearance or worsening of cyanosis are common during pregnancy. In the absence of cyanosis, these women usually tolerate pregnancy well.

Women with cyanotic heart disease generally do poorly during pregnancy. With uncorrected Fallot tetralogy, for example, maternal mortality rates approach 10 percent. Moreover, any disease complicated by severe maternal hypoxemia is likely to lead to miscarriage, preterm delivery, or fetal death. There is a relationship between chronic hypoxemia, polycythemia, and pregnancy outcome. When hypoxemia is intense enough to stimulate a rise in hematocrit above 65 percent, pregnancy wastage is virtually 100 percent.

Pregnancy after Surgical Repair

Some of the more complex lesions cannot be successfully repaired. But with satisfactory surgical correction of cyanotic lesions before pregnancy, maternal and fetal outcomes are much improved (Maxwell, 2010).

Fallot Tetralogy. Balci (2011) and Kamiya (2012) and their associates described a total of 197 pregnancies in 99 women with surgically corrected Fallot tetralogy. Pregnancy was usually well tolerated, and there were no maternal deaths. Still, almost 9 percent of pregnancies were complicated by adverse cardiac events including new onset or worsening of arrhythmias and heart failure. For women with a pulmonary valve replacement, Oosterhof and coworkers (2006) reported that pregnancy did not adversely affect graft function.

Transposition of the Great Vessels. Pregnancy following surgical correction of transposition also has risks. Canobbio (2006) and Drenthen (2005a), each with their colleagues, described outcomes of 119 pregnancies in 68 women—90 percent had a Mustard procedure and 10 percent a Senning procedure. During pregnancy, a fourth had arrhythmias. Twelve percent developed heart failure, and one of these patients subsequently required cardiac transplantation. One woman died suddenly a month after delivery, and another died 4 years later. A third of the newborns were delivered preterm, but no infant had heart disease. In a more recent study, Metz and associates (2011) reported that five of 14 pregnancies resulting in live births were complicated by symptomatic intracardiac baffle obstruction, which required postpartum stenting. In review, baffles are surgically constructed conduits that redirect anomalous cardiac blood flow and are integral to initial transposition correction.

Successful—although eventful—pregnancies in women with previously repaired *truncus arteriosus* and *double-outlet right ventricle* have also been described (Drenthen, 2008; Hoendermis, 2008).

Single Functional Ventricle. Feinstein and associates (2012) recently reviewed the remarkably improved treatments for patients with *hypoplastic left heart syndrome*. Almost 70 percent of these women are now expected to survive into adulthood and frequently become pregnant. Those who have undergone a *Fontan repair* are at particularly high risk for complications, which include atrial arrhythmias and peripartum heart failure (Nitsche, 2009). In a report of four pregnancies post-Fontan repair, there were no maternal deaths, but complications were frequent (Hoare, 2001). All were delivered preterm, two had supraventricular arrhythmias, and two developed ventricular failure. Similarly high complication rates were described by Jain and coworkers (2011) in 15 women with a systemic right ventricle, that is, one in which the right ventricle rather than the left pumps blood to the support systemic circulation.

Eisenmenger Syndrome

This describes secondary pulmonary hypertension that develops from any cardiac lesion. The syndrome develops when pulmonary vascular resistance exceeds systemic resistance and leads to concomitant right-to-left shunting. The most common underlying defects are atrial or ventricular septal defects and persistent ductus arteriosus (Fig. 49-4). Patients are asymptomatic for years, but eventually pulmonary hypertension becomes severe enough to cause right-to-left shunting, and few persons survive into the fifth decade (Makaryus, 2006; Maxwell, 2010).

The prognosis for pregnancy depends on the severity of pulmonary hypertension but survival has improved during the past 50 years. Women with Eisenmenger syndrome tolerate

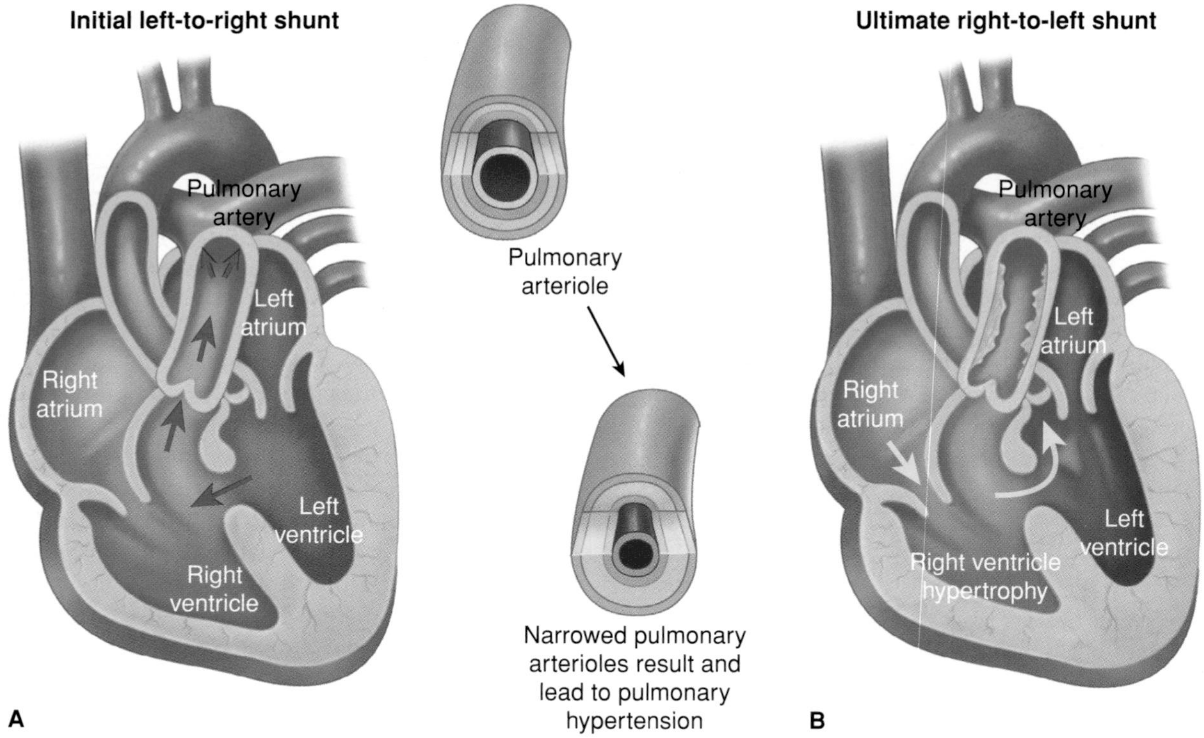

FIGURE 49-4 Eisenmenger syndrome due to a ventricular septal defect (VSD). **A.** Substantial left-to-right shunting through the VSD leads to morphological changes in the smaller pulmonary arteries and arterioles. Specifically, medial hypertrophy, intimal cellular proliferations, and fibrosis lead to narrowing or closure of the vessel lumen. These vascular changes create pulmonary hypertension and a resultant reversal of the intracardiac shunt **(B)**. With sustained pulmonary hypertension, extensive atherosclerosis and calcification often develop in the large pulmonary arteries. Although a VSD is shown here, Eisenmenger syndrome may also develop in association with a large atrial septal defect or patent ductus arteriosus.

hypotension poorly, and the cause of death usually is right ventricular failure with cardiogenic shock. Management is discussed subsequently. In a review of 44 cases through 1978, maternal and perinatal mortality rates approximated 50 percent (Gleicher, 1979). In a later review of 73 pregnancies, Weiss and coworkers (1998) cited a 36-percent maternal death rate. Three of 26 deaths were antepartum, and the remainder died intrapartum or within a month of delivery. In a more recent study of 13 pregnant women, there was one maternal death 17 days after delivery, and there were five perinatal deaths (Wang, 2011).

PULMONARY HYPERTENSION

Normal resting mean pulmonary artery pressure is 12 to 16 mm Hg. In the study by Clark and colleagues (1989), pulmonary vascular resistance in late pregnancy was approximately 80 dyn/sec/cm^{-5}, which was 34-percent less than the nonpregnant value of 120 dyne/sec/cm^{-5}. *Pulmonary hypertension* is a hemodynamic observation and not a diagnosis and is defined in nonpregnant individuals as a mean pulmonary pressure > 25 mm Hg.

The World Health Organization classification shown in Table 49-8 has been adopted by the American College of Cardiology and the American Heart Association (McLaughlin, 2009). There are important prognostic and therapeutic distinctions between group I pulmonary hypertension and the other groups. Group I indicates that a specific disease affects pulmonary arterioles. It includes idiopathic or primary pulmonary arterial hypertension as well as those cases secondary to a known cause such as connective-tissue disease. Approximately a third of women with scleroderma and 10 percent with systemic lupus erythematosus have pulmonary hypertension (Rich, 2005). Other causes in young women are sickle-cell disease and thyrotoxicosis (Sheffield, 2004). Another is plexogenic pulmonary arteriopathy associated with cirrhosis and portal hypertension, and this has been reported to cause a maternal death (Sigel, 2007).

Group II disorders are the most commonly encountered in pregnant women. These are secondary to pulmonary *venous* hypertension caused by left-sided atrial, ventricular, or valvular disorders. A typical example is mitral stenosis discussed on page 981. In contrast, groups III through V are seen infrequently in young otherwise healthy women.

Diagnosis

Symptoms may be vague, and dyspnea with exertion is the most common. With group II disorders, orthopnea and nocturnal dyspnea are also usually present. Angina and syncope occur when right ventricular output is fixed, and they suggest advanced disease. Chest radiography commonly shows enlarged pulmonary hilar arteries and attenuated peripheral markings. It also may disclose parenchymal causes of hypertension. Although cardiac catheterization remains the standard criterion

TABLE 49-8. World Health Organization Classification of Some Causes of Pulmonary Hypertension

I	**Pulmonary arterial hypertension**
	Idiopathic—previously "primary" pulmonary hypertension
	Familial—chromosome 2 gene in TGF superfamily
	Associated with: collagen-vascular disorders, congenital left-to-right cardiac shunts, HIV infection, thyrotoxicosis, sickle hemoglobinopathies, antiphospholipid antibody syndrome, diet drugs, portal hypertension
	Persistent pulmonary hypertension of the newborn
	Other
II	**Pulmonary hypertension with left-sided heart disease**
	Left-sided atrial or ventricular disease
	Left-sided valvular disease
III	**Pulmonary hypertension associated with lung disease**
	Chronic obstructive pulmonary disease
	Interstitial lung disease
	Other
IV	**Pulmonary hypertension due to chronic thromboembolic disease**
V	**Miscellaneous**

HIV = human immunodeficiency virus; TGF = transforming growth factor.
Adapted from Simmoneau, 2004.

for the measurement of pulmonary artery pressures, noninvasive echocardiography is often used to provide an estimate. In 33 pregnant women who underwent both echocardiography and cardiac catheterization, pulmonary artery pressures were significantly overestimated by echocardiography in a third of cases (Penning, 2001).

Prognosis

Longevity depends on the severity and cause of pulmonary hypertension at discovery. For example, although invariably fatal, idiopathic pulmonary hypertension has a 3-year survival rate of 60 percent, whereas that due to collagen-vascular diseases has only a 35-percent rate (McLaughlin, 2004). Some disorders respond to pulmonary vasodilators, calcium-channel blockers, prostacyclin analogues, or endothelin-receptor blockers, all which may improve quality of life. The prostacyclin analogues epoprostenol and treprostinil significantly lower pulmonary vascular resistance but must be given parenterally (Humbert, 2004; Roeleveld, 2004). Preconceptional counseling is imperative as emphasized by Easterling and associates (1999).

Pulmonary Hypertension and Pregnancy

The maternal mortality rate is appreciable, but this is especially so with idiopathic pulmonary hypertension. In the past, there were frequently poor distinctions in identifying both causes and severity of hypertension. Thus, although most severe cases of idiopathic pulmonary arterial hypertension had the worst prognosis, it was erroneously assumed that all types of pulmonary hypertension were equally dangerous. With widespread use of echocardiography, less-severe lesions with a better prognosis are now separable. Curry (2012) and Weiss (1998) and their colleagues reviewed 36 cases of pulmonary hypertension in pregnancy and found an approximate 30-percent mortality rate. Bédard and coworkers (2009) reported that mortality statistics improved during the decade ending in 2007 compared with those for the decade ending in 1996. Mortality rates were 25 and 38 percent, respectively. Importantly, almost 80 percent of the deaths were during the first month postpartum.

Pregnancy is contraindicated with severe disease, especially those with pulmonary arterial changes—most cases in group I. With milder disease from other causes—group II being the most common—the prognosis is much better. With the more frequent use of echocardiography and pulmonary artery catheterization in young women with heart disease, we have identified women with mild to moderate pulmonary hypertension who tolerate pregnancy, labor, and delivery well. One example described by Sheffield and Cunningham (2004) is that of pulmonary hypertension that develops with thyrotoxicosis but is reversible with treatment (Chap. 58, p. 1151). Similarly, Boggess and colleagues (1995) described nine women with interstitial and restrictive lung disease with varying degrees of pulmonary hypertension, and all tolerated pregnancy reasonably well.

Management

Treatment of symptomatic pregnant women includes activity limitation and avoidance of the supine position in late pregnancy. Diuretics, supplemental oxygen, and vasodilator drugs are standard therapy for symptoms. Some recommend anticoagulation (Hsu, 2011; Larson, 2010). In addition, there are many reports describing the successful use of intravenous pulmonary artery vasodilators in both singleton and twin gestations (Badalian, 2000; Easterling, 1999; Garabedian, 2010). Prostacyclin analogues that can be administered parenterally include epoprostenol and treprostinil, whereas iloprost is inhaled. There are reports of successful use of each in pregnant women, but data are insufficient to prefer one over another. Inhaled nitric oxide is also an option that has been employed in cases of acute cardiopulmonary decompensation during pregnancy or the puerperium (Lane, 2011).

Labor and Delivery

These women are at greatest risk during labor and delivery when there is diminished venous return and decreased right ventricular filling—both associated with most maternal deaths. To avoid hypotension, assiduous attention is given to epidural analgesia induction and to blood loss prevention and treatment at delivery. Parneix and coworkers (2009) describe low-dose spinal-epidural analgesia for cesarean delivery. Women with group I severe hypertension have been delivered successfully while using either inhaled nitric oxide or iloprost (Lam, 2001; Weiss, 2000).

CARDIOMYOPATHIES

The American Heart Association defines cardiomyopathies as a heterogeneous group of myocardial diseases associated with mechanical and/or electrical dysfunction. Affected women usually—but not invariably—have inappropriate ventricular hypertrophy or dilatation. Cardiomyopathies are due to various causes that frequently are genetic (Maron, 2006). In general, and as shown in Table 49-9, cardiomyopathies may be divided into two major groups:

- *Primary*—cardiomyopathies solely or predominantly confined to heart muscle—examples include hypertrophic cardiomyopathy, dilated cardiomyopathies, and peripartum cardiomyopathy.
- *Secondary*—cardiomyopathies due to generalized systemic disorders that produce pathological myocardial involvement—examples are diabetes, lupus, and thyroid disorders.

Hypertrophic Cardiomyopathy

Epidemiological studies suggest that the disorder is common, affecting approximately 1 in 500 adults (Maron, 2004). The condition—characterized by cardiac hypertrophy, myocyte disarray, and interstitial fibrosis—is caused by mutations in any one of more than a dozen genes that encode cardiac sarcomere proteins. Inheritance is autosomal dominant, and genetic screening is complex and not currently clinically available (Osio, 2007; Spirito, 2006). The myocardial muscle abnormality is characterized by left ventricular myocardial hypertrophy with a pressure gradient to left ventricular outflow. Diagnosis is established by echocardiographic identification of a hypertrophied and nondilated left ventricle in the absence of other cardiovascular conditions.

Most affected women are asymptomatic, but dyspnea, anginal or atypical chest pain, syncope, and arrhythmias may develop. Complex arrhythmias may progress to sudden death, which is the most common form of death. Asymptomatic patients with runs of ventricular tachycardia are especially prone to sudden death. Symptoms are usually worsened by exercise.

TABLE 49-9. Some Primary and Secondary Causes of Cardiomyopathy

Primary Causes
Genetic—hypertrophic cardiomyopathy, arrhythmogenic right ventricular dysplasia, left ventricular noncompaction, glycogen storage diseases, conduction system disease, mitochondrial myopathies, ion-channelopathies
Mixed—predominantly nongenetic—dilated and restrictive cardiomyopathy
Acquired—myocarditis, stress (takotsubo), peripartum cardiomyopathy
Secondary Causes
Infiltrative—amyloidosis, Gaucher disease, Hurler and Hunter diseases
Storage—hemochromatosis
Toxicity—drugs, heavy metals
Endomyocardial—hypereosinophilic syndrome
Granulomatous—sarcoidosis
Endocrine—diabetes mellitus, thyroid dysfunction
Cardiofacial—Noonan syndrome
Neuromuscular/neurological—Friedrich ataxia, neurofibromatosis
Autoimmune—systemic lupus erythematosus, scleroderma

Adapted from Maron, 2006.

Pregnancy

Although limited reports suggest that pregnancy is well tolerated, adverse cardiac events are common. Thaman and coworkers (2003) reviewed 271 pregnancies in 127 affected women. Although there were no maternal deaths, more than a fourth had at least one adverse cardiac symptom—including dyspnea, chest pain, or palpitations. Singla and associates (2011) described a pregnant patient with undiagnosed hypertrophic cardiomyopathy who presented with preeclampsia and an acute myocardial infarction.

Management is similar to that for aortic stenosis. Strenuous exercise is prohibited during pregnancy. Abrupt positional changes are avoided to prevent reflex vasodilation and decreased preload. Likewise, drugs that evoke diuresis or diminish vascular resistance are generally not used. If symptoms develop, especially angina, β-adrenergic or calcium-channel blocking drugs are given. The delivery route is determined by obstetrical indications. Choice of anesthesia is controversial, and in the opinion of some authors, general anesthesia is considered safest (Pitton, 2007). Infants rarely demonstrate inherited lesions at birth.

Dilated Cardiomyopathy

This is characterized by left and/or right ventricular enlargement and reduced systolic function in the absence of coronary, valvular, congenital, or systemic disease known to cause myocardial dysfunction. Although there are many known causes of dilated cardiomyopathy—both inherited and acquired, the etiology remains undefined in approximately half of cases (Stergiopoulos, 2011). Some cases are result from viral infections, including myocarditis and human immunodeficiency virus (Barbaro, 1998; Felker, 2000). Other causes, which are potentially reversible, include alcoholism, cocaine abuse, and thyroid disease. Watkins and colleagues (2011) reviewed the many complex genetic mutations associated with inherited forms of dilated cardiomyopathy.

Peripartum Cardiomyopathy

This disorder is very similar to other forms of nonischemic dilated cardiomyopathy except for its unique relationship with pregnancy (Pyatt, 2011). Currently, it is a diagnosis of exclusion following a concurrent evaluation for peripartum heart failure. Although the term peripartum cardiomyopathy has been used widely, at least until recently, there was little evidence to

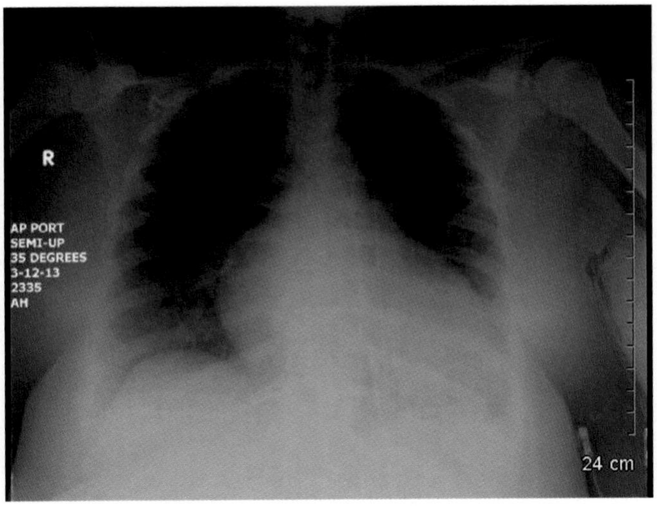

FIGURE 49-5 Peripartum cardiomyopathy with mild pulmonary edema. Anterior-posterior projection chest radiograph of a woman with an abnormally enlarged heart and mild perihilar opacification consistent with dilated cardiomyopathy.

support a unique pregnancy-induced cardiomyopathy. Pearson (2000) reported findings of a workshop of the National Heart, Lung, and Blood Institute and the Office of Rare Diseases that established the following diagnostic criteria:

1. Development of cardiac failure in the last month of pregnancy or within 5 months after delivery,
2. Absence of an identifiable cause for the cardiac failure,
3. Absence of recognizable heart disease prior to the last month of pregnancy, and
4. Left ventricular systolic dysfunction demonstrated by classic echocardiographic criteria, such as depressed ejection fraction or fractional shortening along with a dilated left ventricle (Fig. 49-5).

The etiology of peripartum cardiomyopathy remains unknown, and many potential causes—including viral myocarditis, abnormal immune response to pregnancy, abnormal response to the increased hemodynamic burden of pregnancy, hormonal interactions, malnutrition, inflammation, and apoptosis—have been proposed but not proven (Elkayam, 2011). Another theory suggests that oxidative stress during late pregnancy leads to the proteolytic cleavage of prolactin (Hilfiker-Kleiner, 2007). The resulting 16-kDa prolactin fragment has been found to be cardiotoxic and can impair the metabolism and contractility of cardiomyocytes. Based on this proposed mechanism, bromocriptine therapy has been suggested because it inhibits prolactin secretion (Chap. 36, p. 673). Indeed, there has been at least one preliminary study in which bromocriptine improved recovery of affected women (Sliwa, 2010).

Another intriguing mechanism to explain the etiology of peripartum cardiomyopathy was described by Patten (2012). It links peripartum cardiomyopathy to preeclampsia syndrome. This is biologically plausible given that hypertensive disorders frequently coexist with peripartum cardiomyopathy (Cunningham, 2012; Fong, 2014; Gunderson, 2011). These investigators showed that antiangiogenic factors—already known to be associated with preeclampsia—can induce peripartum cardiomyopathy in susceptible mice. Thus, they posit peripartum cardiomyopathy to be a vascular disease precipitated by antiangiogenic factors that act in a host made susceptible because of insufficient proangiogenic factors.

In the absence of a proven etiology, the diagnosis of peripartum cardiomyopathy currently requires that other causes of cardiac dysfunction be excluded. Bültmann and coworkers (2005) studied endomyocardial biopsy specimens from 26 women with peripartum cardiomyopathy and reported that more than half had histological evidence of "borderline myocarditis." They noted viral genomic material for parvovirus B19, human herpesvirus 6, Epstein-Barr virus, and cytomegalovirus. They attributed these findings to reactivation of latent viral infection that triggered an autoimmune response. Another report described 28 women at Parkland Hospital who had peripartum heart failure of obscure etiology who were initially thought to have idiopathic peripartum cardiomyopathy (Cunningham, 1986). In 21 of these, heart failure was found to be caused by hypertensive heart disease, clinically silent mitral stenosis, obesity, or viral myocarditis. Particularly important were the silent cardiomyopathic effects that even intermediate-duration chronic hypertension may have on ventricular function.

After exclusion of an underlying cause for heart failure, the default diagnosis is idiopathic or peripartum cardiomyopathy. Thus, its incidence is highly dependent on the diligence of the search for a cause. Because of this, the cited incidence varies from approximately 1 in 2500 to 1 in 15,000 births. In a review of the National Hospital Discharge Survey database of 3.6 million births, a prevalence of 1 in 3200 births was computed (Mielniczuk, 2006). Two other large population-based studies cited a frequency of 1 in 2000 to 2800 (Gunderson, 2011; Harper, 2012). In an earlier study from Parkland Hospital, we identified idiopathic cardiomyopathy in only approximately 1 in 15,000 deliveries—an incidence similar to that of idiopathic cardiomyopathy in young nonpregnant women (Cunningham, 1986).

Prognosis. The distinction between heart failure from an identifiable cause and peripartum cardiomyopathy is of obstetrical importance. Women with a true cardiomyopathy do not fare well overall as a group, and their immediate and 1-year mortality rate is 2 to 15 percent (Harper, 2012; Mielniczuk, 2006). Approximately 50 percent of women suffering from peripartum cardiomyopathy recover baseline ventricular function within 6 months of delivery, but in those with persistent cardiac failure, the mortality rate approaches 85 percent over 5 years (Moioli, 2010).

A study from India described the outcomes of 36 women with peripartum cardiomyopathy (Mandal, 2011). Five women died either from heart failure or cerebrovascular accident. Of six women who had a subsequent pregnancy, one woman died and two developed heart failure. In a follow-up study from Haiti, Fett and coworkers (2009) performed echocardiography every 6 months in 116 women with peripartum cardiomyopathy. Only 28 percent of these women recovered a left ventricular ejection fraction > 0.51, and in three fourths of these, this level was not attained until after a year. With a mean follow-up of 39 months, de Souza and colleagues (2001) reported that 18 percent of 44 such women had died from end-stage heart failure. Similar long-term outcomes were assessed by a survey of members of the American College of Cardiology (Elkayam, 2001). Respondents reported that a return to normal ventricular function does not guarantee a problem-free pregnancy, and that if another pregnancy is undertaken in women with an ejection fraction persistently < 0.5, it should be with great trepidation.

Other Primary Causes of Cardiomyopathy

Arrhythmogenic Right Ventricular Dysplasia

This unique cardiomyopathy is defined histologically by progressive replacement of right ventricular myocardium with adipose and fibrous tissue. As described on page 992, this disorder predisposes to ventricular tachyarrhythmias. It has an estimated prevalence is 1 in 5000 and is a cause of sudden death, particularly in younger people (Elliott, 2008). The additional risk of pregnancy in women with arrhythmogenic right ventricular cardiomyopathy is unknown. However, based on a systematic review, Krul and associates (2011) advise against pregnancy.

Restrictive Cardiomyopathy

This inherited cardiomyopathy is probably the least common type. It is characterized by a ventricular filling pattern in which increased myocardial stiffness causes ventricular pressure to rise precipitously with only a small increase in volume (Elliott, 2008). Due to the severe clinical course in nonpregnant patients and the poor prognosis in general, pregnancy is not advised (Krul, 2011).

HEART FAILURE

Regardless of the underlying condition that causes cardiac dysfunction, women who develop peripartum heart failure almost always have obstetrical complications that either contribute to or precipitate heart failure. For example, preeclampsia is common and may precipitate afterload failure. High-output states caused by hemorrhage and acute anemia increase cardiac workload and magnify the physiological effects of compromised ventricular function. Similarly, infection and sepsis syndrome increase cardiac output and oxygen utilization tremendously, and sepsis can depress myocardial function (Chap. 47, p. 948).

As described in Chapter 50 (p. 1003), in many populations, chronic hypertension with superimposed preeclampsia is the most frequent cause of heart failure in pregnant women. Many of these women have concentric left ventricular hypertrophy. In some, mild antecedent undiagnosed hypertension causes covert cardiomyopathy, and when superimposed preeclampsia develops, together they may cause otherwise inexplicable peripartum heart failure. As discussed throughout Chapter 48 (p. 963), obesity is a common cofactor with chronic hypertension, and it leads to eccentric ventricular hypertrophy. In the Framingham Heart Study, obesity alone was associated with a doubling of the heart failure risk in nonpregnant individuals (Kenchaiah, 2002).

Diagnosis

Congestive heart failure can have a gradual onset or may present as acute "flash" pulmonary edema. The first warning sign is likely to be persistent basilar rales, frequently accompanied by a nocturnal cough (Jessup, 2003). A sudden decline in the ability to complete usual duties, increased dyspnea on exertion, and/or attacks of smothering with cough are symptoms of serious heart failure. Clinical findings may include hemoptysis, progressive edema, tachypnea, and tachycardia. Dyspnea is universal, and other symptoms include orthopnea, palpitations, and substernal chest pain (Sheffield, 1999). Hallmark findings usually include cardiomegaly and pulmonary edema (see Fig. 49-5). Acutely, there is usually systolic failure, and echocardiographic findings include an ejection fraction < 0.45 or a fractional shortening < 30 percent, or both, and an end-diastolic dimension > 2.7 cm/m^2 (Hibbard, 1999). Coincidental diastolic failure may also be found, depending on the underlying cause.

Management

Pulmonary edema from heart failure usually responds promptly with diuretic administration to reduce preload. Hypertension is common, and afterload reduction is accomplished with hydralazine or another vasodilator. Because of marked fetal effects, angiotensin-converting enzyme inhibitors are withheld until the woman is delivered (Chap. 12, p. 247). With chronic heart failure, there is a high incidence of associated thromboembolism, and thus prophylactic heparin is often recommended.

Left ventricular assist devices (LVADs) are employed more frequently for acute and chronic heart failure treatment. However, there are only a few reports describing their use during pregnancy (LaRue, 2011; Sims, 2011). *Extracorporeal membrane oxygenation (ECMO)* was reported to be lifesaving in a woman with fulminating cardiomyopathy (Smith, 2009).

INFECTIVE ENDOCARDITIS

Bacterial infection of a heart valve involves cardiac endothelium and usually results in valvular vegetations. In this country, those at greatest risk are women with congenital heart lesions, intravenous drug use, degenerative valve disease, and intracardiac devices (Karchmer, 2012). *Subacute bacterial endocarditis* usually is due to a low-virulence bacterial infection superimposed on an underlying structural lesion. These are usually native valve infections. Organisms that cause indolent endocarditis are most often viridans-group streptococci or *Staphylococcus* or *Enterococcus* species. Among intravenous drug abusers and those with catheter-related infections, *Staphylococcus aureus* is the predominant organism. *Staphylococcus epidermidis* frequently causes prosthetic valve infections. *Streptococcus pneumoniae* and *Neisseria gonorrhoeae* may occasionally cause acute, fulminating disease. Antepartum endocarditis has also been described with *Neisseria sicca* and *Neisseria mucosa*, the latter causing maternal death (Cox, 1988; Deger, 1992). Only a few cases of group B streptococcal endocarditis have been described (Kangavari, 2000). Endocarditis due to *Escherichia coli* following cesarean delivery was described in an otherwise healthy young woman (Kulaš, 2006).

Diagnosis

Endocarditis symptoms are variable and often develop insidiously. Fever, often with chills, is seen in 80 to 90 percent of cases, a murmur is heard in 80 to 85 percent, and anorexia, fatigue, and other constitutional symptoms are common. The illness is frequently described as "flulike" (Karchmer, 2012). Other findings are anemia, proteinuria, and manifestations of embolic lesions, including petechiae, focal neurological manifestations, chest or abdominal pain, and ischemia in an extremity. In some cases, heart failure develops. Symptoms may persist for several weeks before the diagnosis is found, and a high index of suspicion is necessary.

Diagnosis is made using the *Duke criteria,* which include positive blood cultures for typical organisms and evidence of endocardial involvement (Hoen, 2013; Pierce, 2012). Echocardiography may be diagnostic, but lesions < 2 mm in diameter or those on the tricuspid valve may be missed. If uncertain, transesophageal echocardiography (TEE) is accurate and informative. Importantly, a negative echocardiographic study does not exclude endocarditis.

TABLE 49-10. Antibiotic Prophylaxis for Infective Endocarditis in High-Risk Patients

ACOG (2011a):
Standard (IV): ampicillin 2 g or cefazolin or ceftriaxone 1 g
Penicillin-allergic (IV): cefazolin or ceftriaxone 1 g or clindamycin 600 mg
Oral: amoxicillin 2 g
American Heart Association (Wilson, 2007):
Standard: ampicillin 2 g IV or IM or amoxicillin 2 g PO
Penicillin-allergic: clarithromycin or azithromycin 500 mg PO; cephalexin 500 mg PO; clindamycin 600 mg PO, IV, or IM; or cefazolin or ceftriaxone 1 g IV or IM

ACOG = American College of Obstetricians and Gynecologists; IM = intramuscular; IV = intravenous; PO = orally.

Management

Treatment is primarily medical with appropriate timing of surgical intervention if necessary. Knowledge of the infecting organism and its sensitivities is imperative for sensible antimicrobial selection. Guidelines for appropriate antibiotic treatment are published by professional societies and are updated regularly (Hoen, 2013). Most streptococci are sensitive to penicillin G, ceftriaxone, or vancomycin given intravenously for 4 to 6 weeks, along with gentamicin for 2 to 4 weeks. Complicated infections are treated longer, and women allergic to penicillin are either desensitized or given intravenous ceftriaxone or vancomycin for 4 weeks. Staphylococci, enterococci, and other organisms are treated according to microbial sensitivity for 4 to 6 weeks (Darouiche, 2004; Karchmer, 2012). Prosthetic valve infections are usually treated for 6 weeks. Recalcitrant bacteremia and heart failure due to valvular dysfunction are but a few reasons that persistent valvular infection may require replacement.

Endocarditis in Pregnancy

Infective endocarditis is uncommon during pregnancy and the puerperium. Treatment is the same as that described above. During a 7-year period, the incidence of endocarditis at Parkland Hospital was approximately 1 in 16,000 births, and two of seven women died (Cox, 1988). From their reviews, Seaworth (1986) and Cox (1989) cited a maternal mortality rate of 25 to 35 percent.

Endocarditis Prophylaxis

For years, patients with real or imagined heart valve problems were given periprocedural antibiotic prophylaxis for endocarditis. This was despite the questioned efficacy of antimicrobial prophylaxis. Currently, however, recommendations are more stringent. The American Heart Association recommends prophylaxis for dental procedures in those with prosthetic valves; prior endocarditis; unrepaired or incompletely repaired cyanotic heart defects or during the 6 months following complete repair; and valvulopathy after heart transplantation (Wilson, 2007). In agreement with this, the American College of Obstetricians and Gynecologists (2011a) does not recommend endocarditis prophylaxis for either vaginal or cesarean delivery in the absence of pelvic infection. Exceptions are the small subset of patients cited above. Women at highest risk for endocarditis are those with cyanotic cardiac disease, prosthetic valves, or both.

When indicated, and for women not already receiving intrapartum antimicrobial therapy for another indication that would also provide coverage against endocarditis, prophylactic regimens are shown in Table 49-10. These are administered as close to 30 to 60 minutes before the anticipated delivery time as is feasible. Despite these new recommendations, prophylaxis is still overused, likely because of prior liberal recommendations. In a study from one institution, only six of 50 women who received antibiotics for endocarditis prophylaxis were judged to have an appropriate indication (Pocock, 2006).

ARRHYTHMIAS

Both preexisting and new-onset cardiac arrhythmias are often encountered during pregnancy, labor, delivery, and the puerperium (Gowda, 2003). In a study of 73 women with a history of supraventricular tachycardia, paroxysmal atrial flutter or fibrillation, or ventricular tachycardia, recurrence rates during pregnancy were 50, 52, and 27 percent, respectively (Silversides, 2006). The mechanism(s) responsible for the increased incidence of arrhythmias during pregnancy are not well elucidated. According to Eghbali and associates (2006), adaptive electric cardiac remodeling of potassium-channel genes may be important. Perhaps the normal but mild hypokalemia of pregnancy and/or the physiological increase in heart rate serves to induce arrhythmias (Chap. 4, p. 58). Alternatively, detection of arrhythmias may be increased because of the frequent visits typical of normal prenatal care.

Bradyarrhythmias

Slow heart rhythms, including complete heart block, are compatible with a successful pregnancy outcome. Some women with complete heart block have syncope during labor and delivery, and occasionally temporary cardiac pacing is necessary (Hidaka, 2006). In our experiences, as well as those of Hidaka (2011) and Jaffe (1987) and their associates, women with permanent artificial pacemakers usually tolerate pregnancy well. With fixed-rate devices, cardiac output apparently is increased by augmented stroke volume.

Supraventricular Tachycardias

The most common arrhythmia seen in reproductive-aged women is *paroxysmal supraventricular tachycardia* (Robins, 2004). If diagnosed when nonpregnant, approximately a third of women have an occurrence during pregnancy (Maxwell, 2010). Conversely, rarely do *atrial fibrillation* and *atrial flutter* present for the first time during pregnancy. Indeed, new-onset atrial fibrillation should prompt a search for underlying etiologies including cardiac anomalies, hyperthyroidism, pulmonary embolism, drug toxicity, and electrolyte disturbances (DiCarlo-Meacham, 2011). Major complications include embolic stroke, and when associated with mitral stenosis, pulmonary edema may develop in later pregnancy if the ventricular rate is increased.

Treatment of supraventricular tachycardias include vagal maneuvers—Valsalva, carotid sinus massage, bearing down, and immersion of the face in ice water—which serve to increase vagal tone and block the atrioventricular node (Link, 2012). Intravenous adenosine is a very short-acting endogenous nucleotide that also blocks atrioventricular nodal conduction. Our experiences are similar to those of others in that adenosine is safe and effective for cardioversion in hemodynamically stable pregnant women (Maxwell, 2010; Robins, 2004). Transient fetal bradycardia has been described with adenosine (Dunn, 2000).

Electrical cardioversion with standard energy settings is not contraindicated in pregnancy, but vigilance is important. Barnes and associates (2002) described a case in which direct current cardioversion led directly to a sustained uterine contraction and fetal bradycardia. If cardioversion fails or is unsafe because of concurrent thrombus, then long-term anticoagulation and heart rate control with medication are necessary (DiCarlo-Meacham, 2011).

Pregnancy may predispose otherwise asymptomatic women with *Wolff-Parkinson-White (WPW) syndrome* to exhibit arrhythmias (Maxwell, 2010). In a study of 25 women who had supraventricular tachycardia diagnosed before pregnancy, three of 12 women with WPW syndrome and six of 13 without the condition developed supraventricular tachycardia during pregnancy. In some patients, accessory pathway ablation may be indicated (Pappone, 2003). For this, the typical fluoroscopic procedure-related fetal radiation dose is < 1 cGy (Damilakis, 2001).

Ventricular Tachycardia

This form of arrhythmia is uncommon in healthy young women without underlying heart disease. Brodsky and associates (1992) described seven pregnant women with new-onset ventricular tachycardia and reviewed 23 reports. Most of these women were not found to have structural heart disease. In 14 cases, tachycardia was precipitated by physical exercise or psychological stress. Abnormalities found included two cases of myocardial infarction, two of prolonged QT interval, and anesthesia-provoked tachycardia in another. They concluded that pregnancy events precipitated the tachycardia and recommended β-blocker therapy for control. As previously discussed, arrhythmogenic right ventricular dysplasia will result occasionally in ventricular tachyarrhythmias (Lee, 2006). If unstable, emergency cardioversion is indicated, and standard adult energy settings are adequate (Jeejeebhoy, 2011; Nanson, 2001).

Prolonged QT-Interval

This conduction anomaly may predispose individuals to a potentially fatal ventricular arrhythmia known as *torsades de pointes* (Roden, 2008). Two studies involving a combined total of 502 pregnant women with *long QT syndrome* both reported a significant increase in cardiac events postpartum but not during pregnancy (Rashba, 1998; Seth, 2007). It was hypothesized that the normal increase in heart rate during pregnancy may be partially protective. Paradoxically, β-blocker therapy has been shown to decrease the risk of torsades de pointes in patients with long QT syndrome and should be continued during pregnancy and postpartum (Gowda, 2003; Seth, 2007). Importantly, many medications, including some used during pregnancy such as azithromycin, erythromycin, and clarithromycin, may predispose to QT prolongation (Al-Khatib, 2003; Ray, 2012; Roden, 2004).

DISEASES OF THE AORTA

Aortic Dissection

Marfan syndrome and coarctation are two aortic diseases that place the pregnant woman at increased risk for aortic dissection. Indeed, half of cases in young women are related to pregnancy (O'Gara, 2004). Other risk factors are bicuspid aortic valve and Turner or Noonan syndrome. Pepin and colleagues (2000) also reported a high rate of aortic dissection or rupture in patients with Ehlers-Danlos syndrome (Chap. 59, p. 1181). Although the mechanism(s) involved are unclear, the initiating event is a tear in the aorta's intima layer, followed by hemorrhage into the media layer, and finally rupture.

In most cases, aortic dissection presents with severe chest pain described as ripping, tearing, or stabbing. Diminution or loss of peripheral pulses in conjunction with a recently acquired aortic insufficiency murmur is an important physical finding. The differential diagnosis of aortic dissection includes myocardial infarction, pulmonary embolism, pneumothorax, and aortic valve rupture as well as obstetrical catastrophes, especially placental abruption and uterine rupture (Lang, 1991).

More than 90 percent of patients with aortic dissection have an abnormal chest radiograph. Aortic angiography is the most definitive method for confirming the diagnosis. However, noninvasive imaging—sonography, computed tomography, and magnetic resonance (MR) imaging—is used more frequently. The urgency of the clinical situation frequently dictates which procedure is best.

Initial medical treatment is given to lower blood pressure. Proximal dissections most often need to be resected, and the aortic valve replaced if necessary. Distal dissections are more complex, and many may be treated medically. Survival in nonpregnant patients is not improved by elective repair of abdominal aortic aneurysms smaller than 5.5 cm (Lederle, 2002).

Marfan Syndrome

This autosomal dominant disorder has a high degree of penetrance. The incidence is 2 to 3 per 10,000 individuals and is without racial or ethnic predilection (Ammash, 2008). Prenatal diagnosis is usually possible using linkage analysis (Chap. 13, p. 277). The syndrome is due to abnormal *fibrillin*—a constituent of elastin—caused by any of dozens of mutations in the *FBN1* gene located on chromosome 15q21 (Biggin, 2004). Thus, Marfan syndrome is a connective-tissue disorder characterized by generalized tissue weakness that can result in dangerous cardiovascular complications. Because all tissues are involved, other defects are frequent and include joint laxity and scoliosis. Progressive aortic dilatation causes aortic valve insufficiency, and there may be infective endocarditis and mitral valve prolapse with insufficiency. Aortic dilatation and dissecting aneurysm are the most serious abnormalities. Early death is due either to valvular insufficiency and heart failure or to a dissecting aneurysm.

Effect of Pregnancy on Marfan Syndrome

In the past, case reports reflected biased outcomes, and the maternal mortality rate was inaccurately magnified (Elkayam, 1995). In a prospective evaluation of 21 women during 45 pregnancies cared for at the Johns Hopkins Hospital, only two had dissection, and one died postpartum from graft infection (Rossiter, 1995). Although there were no maternal deaths among 14 women followed by Rahman and coworkers (2003), two required surgical correction of an aortic aneurysm. These investigators concluded that aortic dilatation > 40 mm or mitral valve dysfunction are high-risk factors for life-threatening cardiovascular complications during pregnancy. Conversely, women with minimal or no dilatation, and those with normal cardiac function by echocardiography, are counseled regarding the small but serious potential risk of aortic dissection.

The aortic root usually measures approximately 2 cm, and during normal pregnancy, it increases slightly (Easterling, 1991). With Marfan syndrome, if aortic root dilatation reaches 4 cm, then dissection is more likely. If dilatation reaches 5 to 6 cm, then elective surgery should be considered before pregnancy (Gott, 1999; Williams, 2002). Prophylactic β-blocker therapy has become the standard medical approach for pregnant women with Marfan syndrome because it reduces hemodynamic stress on the ascending aorta and slows the rate of dilation (Simpson, 2012). Vaginal delivery with regional analgesia and an assisted second stage seem safe for women with an aortic root diameter < 4 cm.

When the aortic root measures 4 to 5 cm or greater, elective cesarean delivery is recommended with consideration of postpartum replacement of the proximal aorta with a prosthetic graft (Simpson, 2012). Successful aortic root replacement during pregnancy has been described, but the surgery has also been associated with fetal hypoxic-ischemic cerebral damage (Mul, 1998; Seeburger, 2007). There are a number of case reports describing emergency cesarean deliveries in women with acute type A dissection that was repaired successfully at the time of delivery (Guo, 2011; Haas, 2011; Papatsonis, 2009).

Perinatal Outcomes

Obstetrical outcomes of 63 women with Marfan syndrome with a total of 142 pregnancies were reviewed by Meijboom and coworkers (2006). Of 111 women delivered after 20 weeks, 15 percent had preterm delivery, and 5 percent had preterm prematurely ruptured membranes. There were eight perinatal deaths, and half of the neonate survivors were subsequently diagnosed with Marfan syndrome.

Aortic Coarctation

This is a relatively rare lesion often accompanied by abnormalities of other large arteries. A fourth of affected patients have a bicuspid aortic valve, and another 10 percent have cerebral artery aneurysms. Other associated lesions are persistent ductus arteriosus, septal defects, and Turner syndrome. The collateral circulation arising above the coarctation remodels and expands, often to a striking extent, to cause localized erosion of rib margins by hypertrophied intercostal arteries. Typical findings include hypertension in the upper extremities but normal or reduced pressures in the lower extremities. Several authors have described diagnosis during pregnancy using MR imaging (Dizon-Townson, 1995; Sherer, 2002; Zwiers, 2006).

Effect of Pregnancy on Coarctation

Major complications include congestive heart failure after longstanding severe hypertension, bacterial endocarditis of the bicuspid aortic valve, and aortic rupture. Because hypertension may worsen in pregnancy, antihypertensive therapy using β-blocking drugs is usually required. Aortic rupture is more likely late in pregnancy or early postpartum. Cerebral hemorrhage from *circle of Willis aneurysms* may also develop. Beauchesne and associates (2001) described the outcomes of 188 pregnancies from the Mayo Clinic. A third had hypertension that was related to significant coarctation gradients, and one woman died from dissection at 36 weeks. Using the United States Nationwide Inpatient Sample between 1998 and 2007, Krieger and colleagues (2011) studied nearly 700 deliveries among women with coarctation. Hypertensive complications of pregnancy were increased three- to fourfold in women with coarctation. Importantly, almost 5 percent of women with coarctation had an adverse cardiovascular outcome—maternal death, heart failure, arrhythmia, cerebrovascular or other embolic event—compared with 0.3 percent of controls. A total of 41 percent of women with coarctation underwent cesarean delivery compared with 26 percent of controls.

Congestive heart failure demands vigorous efforts to improve cardiac function and may warrant pregnancy interruption. Some authors have recommended that resection of the coarctation be undertaken during pregnancy to protect against the possibility of a dissecting aneurysm and aortic rupture. This poses significant risk, especially for the fetus, because all the collaterals must be clamped for variable periods.

Some authors recommend cesarean delivery to prevent transient blood pressure elevations that might lead to rupture of the aorta or coexisting cerebral aneurysms. Available evidence, however, suggests that cesarean delivery should be limited to obstetrical indications.

ISCHEMIC HEART DISEASE

United States statistics indicate that the mortality rate from coronary heart disease among all women aged 35 to 44 years has been increasing by an average of 1.3 percent per year since 1997 (Ford, 2007). Still, *coronary artery disease* and *myocardial infarction* are rare complications of pregnancy. In a review of California hospital discharge records between 1991 and 2000, Ladner and associates (2005) reported myocardial infarction in 2.7 per 100,000 deliveries. James and coworkers (2006) used the Nationwide Inpatient Sample database and reported acute myocardial infarction in 6.2 per 100,000 deliveries. In Canadian hospitals between 1970 and 1998, MacArthur and colleagues (2006) reported the incidence of peripartum myocardial ischemia to be 1.1 per 100,000 deliveries.

Pregnant women with coronary artery disease commonly have classic risk factors such as diabetes, smoking, hypertension, hyperlipidemia, and obesity (James, 2006). As an aside, a large, prospective population-based study from Germany found that women who had experienced recurrent spontaneous abortions or stillbirths were also at a substantially higher risk of myocardial infarction later in life (Kharazmi, 2011). Although the reason(s) for this association were not specifically studied, there are a number of conditions—such as certain thrombophilias—which are associated with both (Chap. 59, p. 1173).

Bagg and colleagues (1999) reviewed the course of 22 diabetic pregnant women with White class H ischemic heart disease (Chap. 57, p. 1126). These and other authors documented unusually high mortality rates in those who suffered myocardial infarction (Pombar, 1995; Reece, 1986). Coronary artery occlusion in two pregnant smokers with hypercholesterolemia has been described following a routine intramuscular injection of 0.5-mg ergometrine (Mousa, 2000; Sutaria, 2000). Finally, Schulte-Sasse (2000) described myocardial ischemia associated with prostaglandin E_1 vaginal suppositories for labor induction.

Diagnosis during pregnancy is not different from the nonpregnant patient. Measurement of serum levels of the cardiac-specific contractile protein *troponin I* provides an accurate diagnosis (Shade, 2002). Troponin I was reported by Shivvers and colleagues (1999) to be undetectable near term (Appendix, p. 1291). Koscica and colleagues (2002) found that levels do not increase following either vaginal or cesarean delivery. Importantly, however, levels of troponin I are higher in preeclamptic women than in normotensive controls (Atalay, 2005; Yang, 2006).

Pregnancy with Prior Ischemic Heart Disease

The advisability of pregnancy after a myocardial infarction is unclear. Ischemic heart disease is characteristically progressive, and because it is usually associated with hypertension or diabetes, pregnancy in most of these women seems inadvisable. Vinatier and associates (1994) reviewed 30 pregnancies in women who had sustained an *infarction remote from pregnancy*. Although none of these women died, four had congestive heart failure and four had worsening angina during pregnancy. Pombar and coworkers (1995) reviewed outcomes of women with diabetes-associated ischemic heart disease and infarction. Three had undergone coronary artery bypass grafting before pregnancy. Of 17 women, eight died during pregnancy. Certainly, pregnancy increases cardiac workload, and all of these investigators concluded that ventricular performance should be assessed using ventriculography, radionuclide studies, echocardiography, or coronary angiography before conception. If there is no significant ventricular dysfunction, pregnancy will likely be tolerated.

For the woman who becomes pregnant before these studies are performed, echocardiography should be done. Exercise tolerance testing may be indicated, and radionuclide ventriculography results in minimal radiation exposure for the fetus (Chap. 46, p. 932). Zaidi and associates (2008) described the use of serial T2-weighted cardiovascular MR imaging in a woman who suffered a myocardial infarction during the first trimester to better define the extent and severity of infarction.

Myocardial Infarction During Pregnancy

The mortality rate with myocardial infarction in pregnancy is increased compared with age-matched nonpregnant women. Hankins and coworkers (1985) reviewed 68 cases and reported an overall maternal mortality rate of approximately 35 percent. Hands and colleagues (1990) found an overall mortality rate of 30 percent, and this was highest in the third trimester. Later studies are more reassuring. In a Nationwide Inpatient Sample study totaling 859 pregnancies complicated by acute infarction during 2000 to 2002, there was a 5.1-percent death rate (James, 2006). Women who sustain an infarction less than 2 weeks before delivery are at especially high risk of death due to the increased myocardial demand during labor or delivery (Esplin, 1999).

Treatment is similar to that for nonpregnant patients (Maxwell, 2010; Roth, 2008). Acute management includes administration of oxygen, nitroglycerin, low-dose aspirin, heparin, and β-blocking drugs with close blood pressure monitoring. Lidocaine is used to suppress malignant arrhythmias and calcium-channel blockers or β-blockers are given if indicated. *Tissue plasminogen activator* has been used in pregnant women, but only those remote from delivery because of hemorrhage. In some women, invasive or surgical procedures may be indicated because of acute or unrelenting disease. A number of reports describe successful percutaneous transluminal coronary angioplasty and stent placement during pregnancy (Balmain, 2007; Duarte, 2011; Dwyer, 2005). Cardiopulmonary resuscitation may be required, and maternal and perinatal effects are discussed in Chapter 47 (p. 956).

If the infarct has healed sufficiently, cesarean delivery is reserved for obstetrical indications, and epidural analgesia is ideal for labor (Esplin, 1999).

REFERENCES

Akintunde AA, Opadijo OG: Case report of a 26-year-old primigravida with patent ductus arteriosus (PDA) in heart failure. Afr Health Sci 11:138, 2011

Aliaga L, Santiago FM, Marti J, et al: Right-sided endocarditis complicating an atrial septal defect. Am J Med Sci 325:282, 2003

Al-Khatib SM, LaPointe NM, Kramer JM, et al: What clinicians should know about the QT interval. JAMA 289:2120, 2003

American College of Obstetricians and Gynecologists: Cardiac disease in pregnancy. Technical Bulletin No. 168, June 1992

American College of Obstetricians and Gynecologists: Use of prophylactic antibiotics in labor and delivery. Practice Bulletin No. 120, June 2011a

American College of Obstetricians and Gynecologists: Thromboembolism in pregnancy. Practice Bulletin No. 123, September 2011b

Ammash NM, Sundt TM, Connolly HM: Marfan syndrome—diagnosis and management. Curr Probl Cardiol 33:7, 2008

Armenti VT, Radomski JS, Moritz MJ, et al: Report from the National Transplantation Pregnancy Registry (NTPR): outcomes of pregnancy after transplantation. In Cecka JM, Terasaki PI (eds): Clin Transpl 121:30, 2002

Atalay C, Erden G, Turhan T, et al: The effect of magnesium sulfate treatment on serum cardiac troponin I levels in preeclamptic women. Acta Obstet Gynecol Scand 84:617, 2005

Badalian SS, Silverman RK, Aubry RH, et al: Twin pregnancy in a woman on long-term epoprostenol therapy for primary pulmonary hypertension: a case report. J Reprod Med 45:149, 2000

Bagg W, Henley PG, Macpherson P, et al: Pregnancy in women with diabetes and ischemic heart disease. Aust N Z J Obstet Gynaecol 39:99, 1999

Balci A, Drenthen W, Mulder BJ, et al: Pregnancy in women with corrected tetralogy of Fallot: occurrence and predictors of adverse events. Am Heart J 161:307, 2011

Balmain S, McCullough CT, Love C, et al: Acute myocardial infarction during pregnancy successfully treated with primary percutaneous coronary intervention. Intl J Cardiol 116:e85, 2007

Barbaro G, di Lorenzo G, Grisorio B, et al: Incidence of dilated cardiomyopathy and detection of HIV in myocardial cells of HIV-positive patients. N Engl J Med 339:1093, 1998

Barnes EJ, Eben F, Patterson D: Direct current cardioversion during pregnancy should be performed with facilities available for fetal monitoring and emergency caesarean section. Br J Obstet Gynaecol 109:1406, 2002

Bashore TM: Adult congenital heart disease: right ventricular outflow tract lesions. Circulation 115:1933, 2007

Bates SM, Greer IA, Middleldorp S, et al: VTE, thrombophilia, antithrombotic therapy, and pregnancy. Chest 141:e691S, 2012

Beauchesne LM, Connolly HM, Ammash NM, et al: Coarctation of the aorta: outcome of pregnancy. J Am Coll Cardiol 38:1728, 2001

Bédard E, Dimopoulos K, Gatzoulis MA: Has there been any progress made on pulmonary outcomes among women with pulmonary arterial hypertension? Eur Heart J 30:256, 2009

Berg CJ, Callaghan WM, Syverson C, et al: Pregnancy-related mortality in the United States, 1998 to 2005. Obstet Gynecol 116:1302, 2010

Biggin A, Holman K, Brett M, et al: Detection of thirty novel FBN1 mutations in patients with Marfan syndrome or a related fibrillinopathy. Hum Mutat 23:99, 2004

Boggess KA, Easterling TR, Raghu G: Management and outcome of pregnant women with interstitial and restrictive lung disease. Am J Obstet Gynecol 173:1007, 1995

Brickner ME, Hillis LD, Lange RA: Congenital heart disease in adults. First of two parts. N Engl J Med 342:256, 2000

Brodsky M, Doria R, Allen B, et al: New-onset ventricular tachycardia during pregnancy. Am Heart J 123:933, 1992

Bültmann BD, Klingel K, Näbauer M, et al: High prevalence of viral genomes and inflammation in peripartum cardiomyopathy. Am J Obstet Gynecol 193:363, 2005

Canobbio MM, Morris CD, Graham TP, et al: Pregnancy outcomes after atrial repair for transposition of the great arteries. Am J Cardiol 98:668, 2006

Capeless EL, Clapp JF: Cardiovascular changes in early phase of pregnancy. Am J Obstet Gynecol 161:1449, 1989

Carabello BA: Aortic stenosis. N Engl J Med 346:677, 2002

Carruth JE, Mirvis SB, Brogan DR, et al: The electrocardiogram in normal pregnancy. Am Heart J 102:1075, 1981

Caulin-Glaser T, Setaro JF: Pregnancy and cardiovascular disease. In Burrow GN, Duffy TP (eds): Medical Complications During Pregnancy, 5th ed. Philadelphia, Saunders, 1999, p 111

Centers for Disease Control and Prevention: Preventing and managing chronic disease to improve the health of women and infants. 2011. Available at: http://www.cdc.gov/reproductivehealth/WomensRH/ChronicDiseaseandReproductiveHealth.htm. Accessed February 18, 2013

Centre for Maternal and Child Enquiries (CMACE): Saving mothers' lives: reviewing maternal deaths to make motherhood safer. 2006–08. The Eighth Report on Confidential Enquiries into Maternal Deaths in the United Kingdom. BJOG 118(1):1, 2011

Chan WS, Anand S, Ginsberg JS: Anticoagulation of pregnant women with mechanical heart valves: a systematic review of the literature. Arch Intern Med 160:191, 2000

Chandrasekhar S, Cook CR, Collard CD: Cardiac surgery in the parturient. Anesth Analg 108:777, 2009

Chen CH, Huang MC, Liu HC, et al: Increased risk of preterm birth among women with mitral valve prolapse: a nationwide, population-based study. Ann Epidemiol 21:391, 2011

Chen QH, Wang XQ, Qi SG: Cross-sectional study of congenital heart disease among Tibetan children aged from 4 to 18 years at different altitudes in Qinghai Province. Chin Med J 121:2469, 2008

Clark SL, Cotton DB, Lee W, et al: Central hemodynamic assessment of normal term pregnancy. Am J Obstet Gynecol 161:1439, 1989

Clark SL, Hankins GD: Preventing maternal death: 10 clinical diamonds. Obstet Gynecol 119:360, 2012

Clark SL, Phelan JP, Greenspoon J, et al: Labor and delivery in the presence of mitral stenosis: central hemodynamic observations. Am J Obstet Gynecol 152:984, 1985

Cleuziou J, Hörer J, Kaemmerer H, et al: Pregnancy does not accelerate biological valve degeneration. Int J Cardiol 145:418, 2010

Colletti PM, Lee KH, Elkayam U: Cardiovascular imaging of the pregnant patient. AJR Am J Roentgenol 200(3):515, 2013

Cotrufo M, De Feo M, De Santo LS, et al: Risk of warfarin during pregnancy with mechanical valve prostheses. Obstet Gynecol 99:35, 2002

Cox SM, Hankins GDV, Leveno KJ, et al: Bacterial endocarditis: a serious pregnancy complication. J Reprod Med 33:671, 1988

Cox SM, Leveno KJ: Pregnancy complicated by bacterial endocarditis. Clin Obstet Gynecol 32:48, 1989

Cunningham FG: Peripartum cardiomyopathy: we've come a long way, but. . . . Obstet Gynecol 120:992, 2012

Cunningham FG, Pritchard JA, Hankins GDV, et al: Peripartum heart failure: idiopathic cardiomyopathy or compounding cardiovascular events? Obstet Gynecol 67:157, 1986

Curry RA, Fletcher C, Gelson E, et al: Pulmonary hypertension and pregnancy—a review of 12 pregnancies in nine women. BJOG 119:752, 2012

Damilakis J, Theocharopoulos N, Perisinakis K, et al: Conceptus radiation dose and risk from cardiac catheter ablation procedures. Circulation 104:893, 2001

Darouiche RO: Treatment of infections associated with surgical implants. N Engl J Med 350:1422, 2004

Dashe JS, Ramin KD, Ramin SM: Pregnancy following cardiac transplantation. Prim Care Update Ob Gyns 5:257, 1998

Datt V, Tempe DK, Virmani S, et al: Anesthetic management for emergency cesarean section and aortic valve replacement in a parturient with severe bicuspid aortic valve stenosis and congestive heart failure. Ann Card Anaesth 13:64, 2010

Deger R, Ludmir J: *Neisseria sicca* endocarditis complicating pregnancy. J Reprod Med 37:473, 1992

Desai DK, Adanlawo M, Naidoo DP, et al: Mitral stenosis in pregnancy: a four-year experience at King Edward VIII Hospital, Durban, South Africa. Br J Obstet Gynaecol 107:953, 2000

de Souza JL Jr, Frimm CD, Nastari L, et al: Left ventricular function after a new pregnancy in patients with peripartum cardiomyopathy. J Card Fail 7:30, 2001

DiCarlo-Meacham LT, Dahlke LC: Atrial fibrillation in pregnancy. Obstet Gynecol 117:389, 2011

Dizon-Townson D, Magee KP, Twickler DM, et al: Coarctation of the abdominal aorta in pregnancy: diagnosis by magnetic resonance imaging. Obstet Gynecol 85:817, 1995

Drenthen W, Pieper PG, Ploeg M, et al: Risk of complications during pregnancy after Senning or Mustard (atrial) repair of complete transposition of the great arteries. Eur Heart J 26:2588, 2005a

Drenthen W, Pieper PG, Roos-Hesselink JW, et al: Non-cardiac complications during pregnancy in women with isolated congenital pulmonary valvar stenosis. Heart 92:1838, 2006

Drenthen W, Pieper PG, van der Tuuk K, et al: Cardiac complications relating to pregnancy and recurrence of disease in the offspring of women with atrioventricular septal defects. Eur Heart J 26:2581, 2005b
Drenthen W, Pieper PG, van der Tuuk K, et al: Fertility, pregnancy and delivery in women after biventricular repair for double outlet right ventricle. Cardiology 109:105, 2008
Duarte FP, O'Neill P, Centeno MJ, et al: Myocardial infarction in the 31st week of pregnancy—case report. Rev Bras Anesthesiol 61:225, 2011
Dunn JS Jr, Brost BC: Fetal bradycardia after IV adenosine for maternal PSVT. Am J Emerg Med 18:234, 2000
Dwyer BK, Taylor L, Fuller A, et al: Percutaneous transluminal coronary angioplasty and stent placement in pregnancy. Obstet Gynecol 106:1162, 2005
Easterling TR, Benedetti TJ, Schmucker BC, et al: Maternal hemodynamics and aortic diameter in normal and hypertensive pregnancies. Obstet Gynecol 78:1073, 1991
Easterling TR, Chadwick HS, Otto CM, et al: Aortic stenosis in pregnancy. Obstet Gynecol 72:113, 1988
Easterling TR, Ralph DD, Schmucker BC: Pulmonary hypertension in pregnancy: treatment with pulmonary vasodilators. Obstet Gynecol 93:494, 1999
Eghbali M, Wang Y, Toro L, et al: Heart hypertrophy during pregnancy: a better functioning heart? Trends Cardiovasc Med 16:285, 2006
Elkayam U: Clinical characteristics of peripartum cardiomyopathy in the United States: diagnosis, prognosis, and management. J Am Coll Cardiol 58:659, 2011
Elkayam U, Ostrzega E, Shotan A, et al: Cardiovascular problems in pregnant women with Marfan syndrome. Ann Intern Med 123:117, 1995
Elkayam U, Tummala PP, Rao K, et al: Maternal and fetal outcomes of subsequent pregnancies in women with peripartum cardiomyopathy. N Engl J Med 344:1567, 2001
Elliott P, Andersson B, Arbustini E, et al: Classification of the cardiomyopathies: a position statement from the European Society of Cardiology working group on myocardial and pericardial diseases. Euro Heart J 29:270, 2008
Erkut B, Kocak H, Becit N, et al: Massive pulmonary embolism complicated by a patent foramen ovale with straddling thrombus: report of a case. Surg Today 36:528, 2006
Esplin S, Clark SL: Ischemic heart disease and myocardial infarction during pregnancy. Contemp Ob/Gyn 44:27, 1999
Estensen M, Gude E, Ekmehag B, et al: Pregnancy in heart- and heart/lung recipients can be problematic. Scand Cardiovasc J 45:349, 2011
Esteves CA, Munoz JS, Braga S, et al: Immediate and long-term follow-up of percutaneous balloon mitral valvuloplasty in pregnant patients with rheumatic mitral stenosis. Am J Cardiol 98:812, 2006
Etheridge MJ, Pepperell RJ: Heart disease and pregnancy at the Royal Women's Hospital. Med J Aust 2:277, 1977
European Society of Cardiology: ESC guidelines on the management of cardiovascular diseases during pregnancy. Eur Heart J 32:3147, 2011
Fawzy ME: Percutaneous mitral balloon valvotomy. Catheter Cardiovasc Interv 69:313, 2007
Feinstein JA, Benson W, Dubin AM, et al: Hypoplastic left heart syndrome: current considerations and expectations. J Am Coll Cardiol 59:S1, 2012
Felker GM, Thompson RE, Hare JM, et al: Underlying causes and long-term survival in patients with initially unexplained cardiomyopathy. N Engl J Med 342:1077, 2000
Fett JD, Sannon H, Thélisma E, et al: Recovery from severe heart failure following peripartum cardiomyopathy. Int J Obstet Gynecol 104:125, 2009
Fong A, Lovell S, Gabby L, et al: Peripartum cardiomyopathy: demographics, antenatal factors, and a strong association with hypertensive disorders. Am J Obstet Gynecol 210:S254, 2014
Ford ES, Capewell S: Coronary heart disease mortality among young adults in the U.S. from 1980 through 2002. J Am Coll Cardiol 50:2128, 2007
Friedman T, Mani A, Elefteriades JA: Bicuspid aortic valve: clinical approach and scientific review of a common clinical entity. Expert Rev Cardiovasc Ther 6:235, 2008
Fryar CD, Chen T, Li X: Prevalence of uncontrolled risk factors for cardiovascular disease: United States, 1999–2010. NCHS Data Brief 103:1, 2012
Garabedian MJ, Hansen WF, Gianferrari EA, et al: Epoprostenol treatment for idiopathic pulmonary arterial hypertension in pregnancy. J Perinatol 30:628, 2010
Gardin J, Schumacher D, Constantine G, et al: Valvular abnormalities and cardiovascular status following exposure to dexfenfluramine or phentermine/fenfluramine. JAMA 283:1703, 2000
Gei AF, Hankins GD: Cardiac disease and pregnancy. Obstet Gynecol Clin North Am 28:465, 2001
Gleicher N, Midwall J, Hochberger D, et al: Eisenmenger's syndrome and pregnancy. Obstet Gynecol Surv 34:721, 1979
Gott VL, Greene PS, Alejo DE, et al: Replacement of the aortic root in patients with Marfan's syndrome. N Engl J Med 340:1307, 1999
Gowda RM, Khan IA, Mehta NJ, et al: Cardiac arrhythmias in pregnancy: clinical and therapeutic considerations. Int J Cardiol 88:129, 2003
Gunderson EP, Croen LA, Chiang V, et al: Epidemiology of peripartum cardiomyopathy: incidence, predictors, and outcomes. Obstet Gynecol 118:583, 2011
Guo C, Xu D, Wang C: Successful treatment for acute aortic dissection in pregnancy—Bentall procedure concomitant with cesarean section. J Cardiothorac Surg 6:139, 2011
Guy TS, Hill AC: Mitral valve prolapse. Annu Rev Med 63:277, 2012
Haas S, Trepte C, Rybczynski M, et al: Type A aortic dissection during late pregnancy in a patient with Marfan syndrome. Can J Anesth/J Can Anesth 58:1024, 2011
Hameed A, Akhter M, Bitar F, et al: Left atrial thrombosis in pregnant women with mitral stenosis and sinus rhythm. Am J Obstet Gynecol 193:501, 2005
Hameed A, Karaalp IS, Tummala PP, et al: The effect of valvular heart disease on maternal and fetal outcome of pregnancy. J Am Coll Cardiol 37:893, 2001
Hanania G, Thomas D, Michel PL, et al: Pregnancy and prosthetic heart valves: a French cooperative retrospective study of 155 cases. Eur Heart J 15:1651, 1994
Hands ME, Johnson MD, Saltzman DH, et al: The cardiac, obstetric, and anesthetic management of pregnancy complicated by acute myocardial infarction. J Clin Anesth 2:258, 1990
Hankins GD, Wendel GD Jr, Leveno KJ, et al: Myocardial infarction during pregnancy: a review. Obstet Gynecol 65:138, 1985
Harper MA, Meyer RE, Berg CJ: Peripartum cardiomyopathy: population-based birth prevalence and 7-year mortality. Obstet Gynecol 120:1013, 2012
Head CEG, Thorne SA: Congenital heart disease in pregnancy. Postgrad Med J 81:292, 2005
Hibbard JU, Lindheimer M, Lang RM: A modified definition for peripartum cardiomyopathy and prognosis based on echocardiography. Obstet Gynecol 94:311, 1999
Hidaka N, Chiba Y, Fukushima K, et al: Pregnant women with complete atrioventricular block: perinatal risks and review of management. Pacing Clin Electrophysiol 34:1161, 2011
Hidaka N, Chiba Y, Kurita T, et al: Is intrapartum temporary pacing required for women with complete atrioventricular block? An analysis of seven cases. BJOG 113:605, 2006
Hilfiker-Kleiner D, Kaminski K, Podewski E, et al: A cathepsin D-cleaved 16kDa form of prolactin mediates postpartum cardiomyopathy. Cell 128:589, 2007
Hoare JV, Radford D: Pregnancy after Fontan repair of complex congenital heart disease. Aust N Z J Obstet Gynaecol 41:464, 2001
Hoen B, Duval X: Infective endocarditis. N Engl J Med 369(8):785, 2013
Hoendermis ES, Drenthen W, Sollie KM, et al: Severe pregnancy-induced deterioration of truncal valve regurgitation in an adolescent patient with repaired truncus arteriosus. Cardiology 109:177, 2008
Hsu CH, Maitland MG, Glassner C, et al: The management of pregnancy and pregnancy-related medical conditions in pulmonary arterial hypertension patients. Int J Clin Pract 65:6, 2011
Humbert M, Sitbon O, Simonneau G: Treatment of pulmonary arterial hypertension. N Engl J Med 351:1425, 2004
Hytten FE, Chamberlain G: Clinical Physiology in Obstetrics. Oxford, Blackwell, 1991
Iturbe-Alessio I, Fonseca MDC, Mutchinik O, et al: Risks of anticoagulant therapy in pregnant women with artificial heart valves. N Engl J Med 315:1390, 1986
Jaffe R, Gruber A, Fejgin M, et al: Pregnancy with an artificial pacemaker. Obstet Gynecol Surv 42:137, 1987
Jain VD, Moghbeli N, Webb G, et al: Pregnancy in women with congenital heart disease: the impact of a systemic right ventricle. Congenit Heart Dis 6:147, 2011
James AH, Jamison MG, Biswas MS, et al: Acute myocardial infarction in pregnancy: a United States population-base study. Circulation 113:1564, 2006
Jeejeebhoy FM, Zelop CM, Windrim R, et al: Management of cardiac arrest in pregnancy: a systematic review. Resuscitation 82:801, 2011
Jessup M, Brozena S: Heart failure. N Engl J Med 348:2007, 2003
John AS, Gurley F, Schaff HV, et al: Cardiopulmonary bypass during pregnancy. Ann Thorac Surg 91:1191, 2011
Kametas NA, McAuliffe F, Krampl E, et al: Maternal cardiac function in twin pregnancy. Obstet Gynecol 102:806, 2003
Kamiya CA, Iwamiya T, Neki R, et al: Outcome of pregnancy and effects on the right heart in women with repaired tetralogy of Fallot. Circ J 76:957, 2012
Kangavari S, Collins J, Cercek B, et al: Tricuspid valve group B streptococcal endocarditis after an elective termination of pregnancy. Clin Cardiol 23:301, 2000
Karchmer AW: Infective Endocarditis. In Longo DL, Fauci AS, Kasper DL, et al (eds): Harrison's Principles of Internal Medicine, 18th ed. New York, McGraw-Hill, 2012, p 1052

Kawamata K, Neki R, Yamanaka K, et al: Risks and pregnancy outcome in women with prosthetic mechanical heart valve replacement. Circ J 71:211, 2007

Keizer JL, Zwart JJ, Meerman RH, et al: Obstetric intensive care admission: a 12-year review in a tertiary care centre. Eur J Obstet Gynecol Reprod Biol 128:152, 2006

Kenchaiah S, Evans JC, Levy D, et al: Obesity and the risk of heart failure. N Engl J Med 347:305, 2002

Key TC, Resnik R, Dittrich HC, et al: Successful pregnancy after cardiac transplantation. Am J Obstet Gynecol 160:367, 1989

Khairy P, Ouyang DW, Fernandes SM, et al: Pregnancy outcomes in women with congenital heart disease. Circulation 113:517, 2006

Kharazmi E, Dossus L, Rohrmann S, et al: Pregnancy loss and risk of cardiovascular disease: a prospective population-based cohort study (EPIC-Heidelberg). Heart 97:49, 2011

Kim KM, Sukhani R, Slogoff S, et al: Central hemodynamic changes associated with pregnancy in a long-term cardiac transplant recipient. Am J Obstet Gynecol 174:1651, 1996

Kizer JR, Devereux RB: Patent foramen ovale in young adults with unexplained stroke. N Engl J Med 353:2361, 2005

Koscica KL, Anyaogu C, Bebbington M, et al: Maternal levels of troponin I in patients undergoing vaginal and cesarean delivery. Obstet Gynecol 99:83S, 2002

Krieger EV, Landzberg MJ, Economy KE, et al: Comparison of risk of hypertensive complications of pregnancy among women with versus without coarctation of the aorta. Am J Cardiol 107:1529, 2011

Krul SP, van der Smag JJ, van den Berg MP, et al: Systematic review of pregnancy in women with inherited cardiomyopathies. Euro J Heart Failure 13:584, 2011

Kulaš T, Habek D: Infective puerperal endocarditis caused by *Escherichia coli*. J Perinat Med 34:342, 2006

Kuleva M, Youssef A, Maroni E, et al: Maternal cardiac function in normal twin pregnancy: a longitudinal study. Ultrasound Obstet Gynecol 38:575, 2011

Ladner HE, Danielser B, Gilbert WM: Acute myocardial infarction in pregnancy and the puerperium: a population-based study. Obstet Gynecol 105:480, 2005

Lam GK, Stafford RE, Thorp J, et al: Inhaled nitric oxide for primary pulmonary hypertension in pregnancy. Obstet Gynecol 98:895, 2001

Lane CR, Trow TK: Pregnancy and pulmonary hypertension: Clin Chest Med 32:165, 2011

Lang RM, Borow KM: Heart disease. In Barron WM, Lindheimer MD (eds): Medical Disorders During Pregnancy. St Louis, Mosby Yearbook, 1991, p 148

Larson L, Mehta N, Paglia MJ, et al: Pulmonary disease in pregnancy. In Powrie RO, Greene MF, Camann W (eds): de Swiet's Medical Disorders in Obstetric Practice, 5th ed. Wiley-Blackwell, Oxford, 2010, p 1

LaRue S, Shanks A, Wang IW, et al: Left ventricular assist device in pregnancy. Obstet Gynecol 118:426, 2011

Lederle FA, Wilson SE, Johnson GR, et al: Immediate repair compared with surveillance of small abdominal aortic aneurysms. N Engl J Med 346:1437, 2002

Lee CN, Wu CC, Lin PY, et al: Pregnancy following cardiac prosthetic valve replacement. Obstet Gynecol 83:353, 1994

Lee LC, Bathgate SL, Macri CJ: Arrhythmogenic right ventricular dysplasia in pregnancy. A case report. J Reprod Med 51:725, 2006

Leśniak-Sobelga A, Tracz W, Kostkiewicz M, et al: Clinical and echocardiographic assessment of pregnant women with valvular heart disease—maternal and fetal outcome. Intl J Cardiol 94:15, 2004

Leyh RG, Fischer S, Ruhparwar A, et al: Anticoagulation for prosthetic heart valves during pregnancy: is low-molecular-weight heparin an alternative? Eur J Cardiothorac Surg 21:577, 2002

Leyh RG, Fischer S, Ruhparwar A, et al: Anticoagulation therapy in pregnant women with mechanical valves. Arch Gynecol Obstet 268:1, 2003

Link MS: Evaluation and initial treatment of supraventricular tachycardia. N Engl J Med 367:1438, 2012

Löwenstein BR, Vain NW, Perrone SV, et al: Successful pregnancy and vaginal delivery after heart transplantation. Am J Obstet Gynecol 158:589, 1988

Lupton M, Oteng-Ntim E, Ayida G, et al: Cardiac disease in pregnancy. Curr Opin Obstet Gynecol 14:137, 2002

MacArthur A, Cook L, Pollard JK, et al: Peripartum myocardial ischemia: a review of Canadian deliveries from 1970 to 1998. Am J Obstet Gynecol 194:1027, 2006

Madazli R, Şal V, Çift T, et al: Pregnancy outcomes in women with heart disease. Arch Gynecol Obstet 281:29, 2010

Makaryus AN, Forouzesh A, Johnson M: Pregnancy in the patient with Eisenmenger's syndrome. Mount Sinai J Med 73:1033, 2006

Mandal D, Mandal S, Mukherjee D, et al: Pregnancy and subsequent pregnancy outcomes in peripartum cardiomyopathy. J Obstet Gynaecol Res 37:222, 2011

Maron BJ: Hypertrophic cardiomyopathy: an important global disease. Am J Med 116:63, 2004

Maron BJ, Towbin JA, Thiene G, et al: Contemporary definitions and classification of the cardiomyopathies an American Heart Association Scientific Statement from the Council on Clinical Cardiology, Heart Failure and Transplantation Committee; Quality of Care and Outcomes Research and Functional Genomics and Translational Biology Interdisciplinary Working Groups; and Council on Epidemiology and Prevention. Circulation 113:1807, 2006

Mathews TJ, Hamilton B: Delayed childbearing: more women are having their first child later in life. NCHS Data Brief, No 21. Hyattsville, National Center for Health Statistics, 2009

Maxwell C, Poppas A, Sermer M, et al: Heart disease in pregnancy. In Powrie C, Greene MF, Camann W (eds): de Swiet's Medical Disorders, 5th ed. Wiley-Blackwell, Oxford, 2010, p 118

McFaul PB, Dornan JC, Lamki H, et al: Pregnancy complicated by maternal heart disease: a review of 519 women. Br J Obstet Gynaecol 95:861, 1988

McLaughlin VV, Archer SL, Badesch DB, et al: ACCF/AHA 2009 expert consensus document on pulmonary hypertension: a report of the American College of Cardiology Foundation Task Force on expert consensus documents and the American Heart Association: developed in collaboration with the American College of Chest Physicians, American Thoracic Society, Inc., and the Pulmonary Hypertension Association. Circulation 119:2250, 2009

McLaughlin VV, Presberg KW, Doyle RL, et al: Prognosis of pulmonary arterial hypertension: ACCP evidence-based clinical practice guidelines. Chest 126:78S, 2004

McLintock C: Anticoagulant therapy in pregnant women with mechanical prosthetic heart valves: no easy option. Thrombosis Research 127:556, 2011

Meijboom LJ, Drenthen W, Pieper PG, et al: Obstetric complications in Marfan syndrome. Intl J Cardiol 110:53, 2006

Melchiorre K, Sutherland GR, Libertati M, et al: Prevalence of maternal cardiac defects in women with high-resistance uterine artery Doppler indices. Ultrasound Obstet Gynecol 37:310, 2011

Metz TD, Jackson M, Yetman AT: Pregnancy outcomes in women who have undergone an atrial switch repair for congenital d-transposition of the great arteries. Am J Obstet Gynecol 205:273.e1, 2011

Mielniczuk LM, Williams K, Davis DR, et al: Peripartum cardiomyopathy: frequency of peripartum cardiomyopathy. Am J Cardiol 97:1765, 2006

Miniero R, Tardivo I, Centofanti P, et al: Pregnancy in heart transplant recipients. J Heart Lung Transplant 23:898, 2004

Moioli M, Mendada, MV, Bentivoglio G, et al: Peripartum cardiomyopathy. Arch Gynecol Obstet 281:183, 2010

Mousa HA, McKinley CA, Thong J: Acute postpartum myocardial infarction after ergometrine administration in a woman with familial hypercholesterolaemia. Br J Obstet Gynaecol 107:939, 2000

Mul TFM, van Herwerden LA, Cohen-Overbeek TE, et al: Hypoxic–ischemic fetal insult resulting from maternal aortic root replacement, with normal fetal heart rate at term. Am J Obstet Gynecol 179:825, 1998

Nanson J, Elcock D, Williams M, et al: Do physiological changes in pregnancy change defibrillation energy requirements? Br J Anaesth 87:237, 2001

Nassar AH, Hobeika EM, Abd Essamad HM, et al: Pregnancy outcome in women with prosthetic heart valves. Am J Obstet Gynecol 191:1009, 2004

Nitsche JF, Phillips SD, Rose CH, et al: Pregnancy and delivery in patients with Fontan circulation. A case report and review of obstetric management. Obstet Gynecol Surv 64:607, 2009

O'Gara PT, Greenfield AJ, Afridi NA, et al: Case 12-2004: a 38-year-old woman with acute onset of pain in the chest. N Engl J Med 350:16, 2004

Oosterhof T, Meijboom FJ, Vliegen HW, et al: Long-term follow-up of homograft function after pulmonary valve replacement in patients with tetralogy of Fallot. Eur Heart J 27:1478, 2006

Opotowsky AR, Siddiqi OK, D'Souza B, et al: Maternal cardiovascular events during childbirth among women with congenital heart disease. Heart 98:145, 2012

Oron G, Hirsch R, Ben-Haroush A, et al: Pregnancy outcome in women with heart disease undergoing induction of labour. BJOG 111:669, 2004

Osio A, Tan L, Chen SN, et al: Myozenin 2 is a novel gene for human hypertrophic cardiomyopathy. Circ Res 100:766, 2007

Papatsonis DNM, Heetkamp A, van den Hombergh C, et al: Acute type A aortic dissection complicating pregnancy at 32 weeks: surgical repair after cesarean section. Am J Perinatol 26:153, 2009

Pappone C, Santinelli V, Manguso F, et al: A randomized study of prophylactic catheter ablation in asymptomatic patients with the Wolff-Parkinson-White syndrome. N Engl J Med 349:1803, 2003

Parneix M, Fanou L, Morau E, et al: Low-dose combined spinal-epidural anaesthesia for caesarean section in a patient with Eisenmenger's syndrome. Int J Obstet Anesth 18:81, 2009

Patten IS, Rana S, Shahul S, et al: Cardiac angiogenic imbalance leads to peripartum cardiomyopathy. Nature 485:333, 2012
Pavankumar P, Venugopal P, Kaul U, et al: Closed mitral valvotomy during pregnancy: a 20 year experience. Scand J Thorac Cardiovasc Surg 22:11, 1988
Pearson GD, Veille JC, Rahimtoola S, et al: Peripartum cardiomyopathy. National Heart, Lung, and Blood Institute and Office of Rare Diseases (National Institutes of Health) workshop recommendations and review. JAMA 283:1183, 2000
Penning S, Robinson KD, Major CA, et al: A comparison of echocardiography and pulmonary artery catheterization for evaluation of pulmonary artery pressures in pregnant patients with suspected pulmonary hypertension. Am J Obstet Gynecol 184:1568, 2001
Pepin M, Schwarze U, Superti-Furga A, et al: Clinical and genetic features of Ehlers–Danlos syndrome type IV, the vascular type. N Engl J Med 342:673, 2000
Pierce D, Calkins BC, Thornton K: Infectious endocarditis: diagnosis and treatment. Am Fam Physician 85:981, 2012
Pitton MA, Petolillo M, Munegato E, et al: Hypertrophic obstructive cardiomyopathy and pregnancy: anesthesiological observations and clinical series. Minerva Anestesiol 73:313, 2007
Pocock SB, Chen KT: Inappropriate use of antibiotic prophylaxis to prevent infective endocarditis in obstetric patients. Obstet Gynecol 108:280, 2006
Pombar X, Strassner HT, Fenner PC: Pregnancy in a woman with class H diabetes mellitus and previous coronary artery bypass graft: a case report and review of the literature. Obstet Gynecol 85:825, 1995
Pyatt JR, Dubey G: Peripartum cardiomyopathy: current understanding, comprehensive management review and new developments. Postgrad Med J 87:34, 2011
Rahimtoola SH: The year in valvular heart disease. J Am Coll Cardiol 47:427, 2006
Rahman J, Rahman FZ, Rahman W, et al: Obstetric and gynecologic complications in women with Marfan syndrome. J Reprod Med 48:723, 2003
Rashba EJ, Zareba W, Moss AJ, et al: Influence of pregnancy on the risk for cardiac events in patients with hereditary long QT syndrome. Circulation 97:451, 1998
Ray WA, Murray KT, Hall K, et al: Azithromycin and the risk of cardiovascular death. N Engl J Med 366:1881, 2012
Rayburn WF, LeMire MS, Bird JL, et al: Mitral valve prolapse: echocardiographic changes during pregnancy. J Reprod Med 32:185, 1987
Reece EA, Egan JFX, Coustan DR, et al: Coronary artery disease in diabetic pregnancies. Am J Obstet Gynecol 154:150, 1986
Reich O, Tax P, Marek J, et al: Long term results of percutaneous balloon valvoplasty of congenital aortic stenosis: independent predictors of outcome. Heart 90:70, 2004
Rich S, McLaughlin VV: Pulmonary hypertension. In Zipes DP (ed): Braunwald's Heart Disease: A Textbook of Cardiovascular Medicine, 7th ed. Philadelphia, Saunders, 2005, p 1817
Robins K, Lyons G: Supraventricular tachycardia in pregnancy. Br J Anaesth 92:140, 2004
Roden DM: Drug-induced prolongation of the QT interval. N Engl J Med 350:1013, 2004
Roden DM: Long-QT syndrome. N Engl J Med 358:169, 2008
Roeder HA, Kuller JA, Barker PC, et al: Maternal valvular heart disease in pregnancy. Obstet Gynecol Surv 66:561, 2011
Roeleveld RJ, Vonk-Noordegraaf A, Marcus JT, et al: Effects of epoprostenol on right ventricular hypertrophy and dilatation in pulmonary hypertension. Chest 125:572, 2004
Roldan CA, Shively BK, Crawford MH: An echocardiographic study of valvular heart disease associated with systemic lupus erythematosus. N Engl J Med 335:1424, 1996
Ross LF: Ethical considerations related to pregnancy in transplant recipients. N Engl J Med 354:1313, 2006
Rossiter JP, Repke JT, Morales AJ, et al: A prospective longitudinal evaluation of pregnancy in the Marfan syndrome. Am J Obstet Gynecol 173:1599, 1995
Roth A, Elkayam U: Acute myocardial infarction associated with pregnancy. J Am Coll Cardiol 52:171, 2008
Rowan JA, McCowan LM, Raudkivi PJ, et al: Enoxaparin treatment in women with mechanical heart valves during pregnancy. Am J Obstet Gynecol 185:633, 2001
Sadler L, McCowan L, White H, et al: Pregnancy outcomes and cardiac complications in women with mechanical, bioprosthetic and homograft valves. Br J Obstet Gynaecol 107:245, 2000
Savu O, Jurcuţ R, Giuşcă S, et al: Morphological and functional adaptation of the maternal heart during pregnancy. Circ Cardiovasc Imaging 5:289, 2012
Sawhney H, Aggarwal N, Suri V, et al: Maternal and perinatal outcome in rheumatic heart disease. Int J Gynaecol Obstet 80:9, 2003
Sbarouni E, Oakley CM: Outcome of pregnancy in women with valve prostheses. Br Heart J 71:196, 1994
Schade R, Andersohn F, Suissa S, et al: Dopamine agonists and the risk of cardiac-valve regurgitation. N Engl J Med 356:29, 2007
Schulte-Sasse U: Life threatening myocardial ischaemia associated with the use of prostaglandin E_1 to induce abortion. Br J Obstet Gynaecol 107:700, 2000
Seaworth BJ, Durack DT: Infective endocarditis in obstetric and gynecologic practice. Am J Obstet Gynecol 154:180, 1986
Seeburger J, Wilhelm-Mohr F, Falk V: Acute type A dissection at 17 weeks of gestation in a Marfan patient. Ann Thorac Surg 83:674, 2007
Seshadri S, Oakeshott P, Nelson-Piercy C, et al: Prepregnancy care. BMJ 344:34, 2012
Seth R, Moss AJ, McNitt S, et al: Long QT syndrome and pregnancy. J Am Coll Cardiol 49:1092, 2007
Shade GH Jr, Ross G, Bever FN, et al: Troponin I in the diagnosis of acute myocardial infarction in pregnancy, labor, and postpartum. Am J Obstet Gynecol 187:1719, 2002
Sheffield JS, Cunningham FG: Diagnosing and managing peripartum cardiomyopathy. Contemp Ob/Gyn 44:74, 1999
Sheffield JS, Cunningham FG: Thyrotoxicosis and heart failure that complicate pregnancy. Am J Obstet Gynecol 190:211, 2004
Sherer DM: Coarctation of the descending thoracic aorta diagnosed during pregnancy. Obstet Gynecol 100:1094, 2002
Shivvers SA, Wians FH Jr, Keffer JH, et al: Maternal cardiac troponin I levels during normal labor and delivery. Am J Obstet Gynecol 180:122, 1999
Shroff H, Benenstein R, Freedberg R, et al: Mitral valve Libman-Sacks endocarditis visualized by real time three-dimensional transesophageal echocardiography. Echocardiography 29:E100, 2012
Sigel CS, Harper TC, Thorne LB: Postpartum sudden death from pulmonary hypertension in the setting of portal hypertension. Obstet Gynecol 110:501, 2007
Silversides CK, Harris L, Haberer K, et al: Recurrence rates of arrhythmias during pregnancy in women with previous tachyarrhythmia and impact on fetal and neonatal outcomes. Am J Cardiol 97:1206, 2006
Simmoneau G, Galie N, Rubin LJ, et al: Clinical classification of pulmonary hypertension. J Am Coll Cardiol 43:55, 2004
Simpson LL: Maternal cardiac disease: update for the clinician. Obstet Gynecol 119:345, 2012
Sims DB, Vink J, Uriel N, et al: A successful pregnancy during mechanical circulatory device support. J Heart Lung Transplant 30:1065, 2011
Singla A, Lipshultz SE, Fisher S: Mid-ventricular obstructive hypertrophic cardiomyopathy during pregnancy complicated by preeclampsia and acute myocardial infarction: a case report. Congenit Heart Dis 6:257, 2011
Siu SC, Colman JM: Congenital heart disease: heart disease and pregnancy. Heart 85:710, 2001a
Siu SC, Sermer M, Colman JM, et al: Prospective multicenter study of pregnancy outcomes in women with heart disease. Circulation 104:515, 2001b
Siva A, Shah AM: Moderate mitral stenosis in pregnancy: the haemodynamic impact of diuresis. Heart 91:e3, 2005
Sliwa K, Blauwet L, Tibazarwa K, et al: Evaluation of bromocriptine in the treatment of acute severe peripartum cardiomyopathy: a proof-of-concept pilot study. Circulation 121:1465, 2010
Small MJ, James AH, Kershaw T, et al: Near-miss maternal mortality: cardiac dysfunction as the principal cause of obstetric intensive care unit admissions. Obstet Gynecol 119:250, 2012
Smith IJ, Gillham MJ: Fulminant peripartum cardiomyopathy rescue with extracorporeal membranous oxygenation. Int J Obstet Anesth 18:186, 2009
Spirito P, Autore C: Management of hypertrophic cardiomyopathy. BMJ 332:1251, 2006
Stangl V, Schad J, Gossing G, et al: Maternal heart disease and pregnancy outcome: a single-centre experience. Eur J Heart Fail 10:855, 2008
Stergiopoulos K, Shiang E, Bench T: Pregnancy in patients with pre-existing cardiomyopathies. J Am Coll Cardiol 58:337, 2011
Suri V, Keepanasseril A, Aggarwal N, et al: Mechanical valve prosthesis and anticoagulation regimens in pregnancy: a tertiary centre experience. Eur J Obstet Gynecol Reprod Biol 159:320, 2011
Suri V, Sawhney H, Vasishta K, et al: Pregnancy following cardiac valve replacement surgery. Int J Gynaecol Obstet 64:239, 1999
Sutaria N, O'Toole L, Northridge D: Postpartum acute MI following routine ergometrine administration treated successfully by primary PTCA. Heart 83:97, 2000
Sutton SW, Duncan MA, Chase VA, et al: Cardiopulmonary bypass and mitral valve replacement during pregnancy. Perfusion 20:359, 2005
Thaman R, Varnava A, Hamid MS, et al: Pregnancy related complications in women with hypertrophic cardiomyopathy. Heart 89:752, 2003
Thompson J, Kuklina E, Bateman B, et al: Medical and pregnancy complications among women with congenital heart disease at delivery. Am J Obstet Gynecol 210:S43, 2014

Thorne S, MacGregor A, Nelson-Piercy C: Risks of contraception and pregnancy in heart disease. Heart 92:1520, 2006

Tzemos N, Silversides CK, Colman JM, et al: Late cardiac outcomes after pregnancy in women with congenital aortic stenosis. Am Heart J 157:474, 2009

Vinatier D, Virelizier S, Depret-Mosser S, et al: Pregnancy after myocardial infarction. Eur J Obstet Gynecol Reprod Biol 56:89, 1994

Vitarelli A, Capotosto L: Role of echocardiography in the assessment and management of adult congenital heart disease in pregnancy. Int J Cardiovasc Imaging 27:843, 2011

Wang H, Zhang W, Liu T: Experience of managing pregnant women with Eisenmenger's syndrome: maternal and fetal outcome in 13 cases. J Obstet Gynaecol Res 37:64, 2011

Watkins H, Ashrafian H, Redwood C: Inherited cardiomyopathies. N Engl J Med 364:1643, 2011

Weiss BM, Maggiorini M, Jenni R, et al: Pregnant patient with primary pulmonary hypertension: inhaled pulmonary vasodilators and epidural anesthesia for cesarean delivery. Anesthesiology 92:1191, 2000

Weiss BM, Zemp L, Seifert B, et al: Outcome of pulmonary vascular disease in pregnancy: a systematic overview from 1978 through 1996. J Am Coll Cardiol 31:1650, 1998

Williams A, Child A, Rowntree J, et al: Marfan's syndrome: successful pregnancy after aortic root and arch replacement. Br J Obstet Gynaecol 109:1187, 2002

Wilson W, Taubert KA, Gewitz M, et al: Prevention of infective endocarditis. Guidelines from the American Heart Association. Circulation 116:1736, 2007

Xia VW, Messerlian AK, Mackley J, et al: Successful epidural anesthesia for cesarean section in a parturient with severe aortic stenosis and a recent history of pulmonary edema—a case report. J Clin Anesth 18:142, 2006

Yang X, Wang H, Wang Z, et al: Alteration and significance of serum cardiac troponin I and cystatin C in preeclampsia (Letter). Clin Chim Acta 374:168, 2006

Zaidi AN, Raman SV, Cook SC: Acute myocardial infarction in early pregnancy: definition of myocardium at risk with noncontrast T2-weighted cardiac magnetic resonance. Am J Obstet Gynecol 198(3):e9, 2008

Zanettini R, Antonini A, Gatto G, et al: Valvular heart disease and the use of dopamine agonists for Parkinson's disease. N Engl J Med 356:39, 2007

Zeeman GG: Obstetric critical care: a blueprint for improved outcomes. Crit Care Med 34:S208, 2006

Zuber M, Gautschi N, Oechslin E, et al: Outcome of pregnancy in women with congenital shunt lesions. Heart 81:271, 1999

Zwiers WJ, Blodgett TM, Vallejo MC, et al: Successful vaginal delivery for a parturient with complete aortic coarctation. J Clin Anesth 18:300, 2006

CHAPTER 50

Chronic Hypertension

Chronic hypertension is one of the most common serious complications encountered during pregnancy. This is not surprising because, according to the National Health and Nutrition Examination Survey (NHANES) from the Centers for Disease Control and Prevention (2011), the average prevalence of hypertension in women aged 18 to 39 years is approximately 7 percent. The incidence of chronic hypertension in pregnancy is variable depending on population vicissitudes. In a study of more than 56 million deliveries from the Nationwide Patient Sample, 1.8 percent of births in 2007 and 2008 were in women with chronic hypertension (Bateman, 2012). The incidence was 1.0 percent in more than 530,000 singleton pregnancies in California in 2006 (Yanit, 2012). And according to the American College of Obstetricians and Gynecologists (2012), the incidence may be up 5 percent. Despite this substantive prevalence, optimal management has not been well studied. It is known that chronic hypertension usually improves during early pregnancy. This is followed by variable behavior later in pregnancy and importantly, by its unpredictable development of superimposed preeclampsia, which carries increased risks for maternal and perinatal morbidity and mortality.

GENERAL CONSIDERATIONS

To define chronic hypertension, first, the range of normal blood pressure levels must be established. This is not a simple task because, like all polygenic-determined biological variants, blood pressure norms differ between populations. And, within these norms, there are wide variations between individuals. Moreover, these are also greatly influenced by numerous epigenetic factors. For example, blood pressure not only varies between races and gender, but the pressures—especially systolic—increase directly with increasing age and weight. Pragmatically then, normal adults have a wide range of blood pressures, but so do those with chronic hypertension.

After these variables are acknowledged, an important consideration for any population is the attendant risks of chronic hypertension. There is an increasing incremental rate of cardiovascular, cerebrovascular, and renal disease that follows increasing levels of both diastolic and systolic pressures (Kotchen, 2012).

Definition and Classification

For the foregoing reasons, it seems logical that chronic hypertension would be defined as some level of sustained blood pressure that is associated with an increase in acute or long-term adverse effects. For many years in the United States, these values were based primarily on actuarial tables constructed using data derived from white adult males and compiled by life insurance companies. These "norms" disregarded interrelated factors such as ethnicity and gender as well as other important covariants. The importance of race, for example, was emphasized by

TABLE 50-1. Eighth Joint National Committee (JNC 8)—2014 Chronic Hypertension Guidelines and Recommendations

Evidence-based recommendations from randomized controlled trials
Definitions hypertension and prehypertension not addressed
Lifestyle modifications endorsed from the Lifestyle Work Group (Eckel, 2013)
Recommend selection among four specific medication classes: angiotensin-converting enzyme inhibitors (ACE-I), angiotensin-receptor blockers (ARB), calcium-channel blockers, or diuretics:
General population < 60 years old—initiate pharmacological therapy to lower diastolic pressure ≤ 90 mm Hg and systolic pressure ≤ 140 mm Hg
Diabetics—lower pressure < 140/90 mm Hg
Chronic kidney disease—lower pressure < 140/90 mm Hg. Also add ACE-I or ARB to improve outcomes
General nonblack population—initial therapy should include thiazide-type diuretic, calcium-channel blocker, ACE-I, or ARB
General black population—primary antihypertensive therapy should include thiazide-type diuretic or calcium-channel blocker
Assess monthly, and after 1 month, if goals not met, then increase primary drug dose or add second drug. If no response, increase either or add third drug; then if no response, refer to hypertension specialist

Summarized from James, 2013.

Kotchen (2012), who cites statistics derived from 65 million American adults. In this study, the incidence of hypertension—defined as blood pressure > 140/90 mm Hg—was 34 percent in blacks, 29 percent in whites, and 21 percent in Mexican Americans.

For many years, guidelines for diagnosis, classification, and management of chronic hypertension have been promulgated by the Joint National Committee. In 2008, the National Heart Lung and Blood Institute discontinued these guidelines, and the Joint National Committee 8 (JNC 8) was instead asked to provide an evidence-based review (James, 2013). Findings pertinent to caring for young women with chronic hypertension are summarized in Table 50-1.

Treatment and Benefits for Nonpregnant Adults

There are proven benefits that accrue with treatment of otherwise normal adults who have sustained hypertension. A myriad studies evaluating many combinations of antihypertensive therapy have been conducted with salutary results. Some of these include the ACCORD, ASCOT, ACCOMPLISH, ALLHAT, SPRINT, TOHMS, TROPHY, and VALUE studies. Importantly, these trials evaluated monotherapy versus combination therapeutic regimens as well as ethnospecific benefits. Most evaluated cardiovascular outcomes, but many also confirmed risk reduction in cerebrovascular accidents, renal insufficiency, and overall mortality rates. Because of these incontrovertible benefits, the JNC 8 recommends the treatment outlined in Table 50-1.

Thus, even for mildly elevated blood pressures cited in Table 50-1, interventions to reduce pressure are beneficial. Moreover, it is clear that antihypertensive therapy in nonpregnant reproductive-aged women with sustained diastolic pressures ≥ 90 mm Hg would be considered standard. Not clear from these observations, however, is what constitutes the best management for the woman being treated who contemplates pregnancy, or the best management of the woman undergoing treatment who becomes pregnant, or the woman who is first identified to have chronic hypertension during pregnancy (August, 2014). In these and similar women, the benefits and safety of instituting antihypertensive therapy are less clear, as subsequently discussed.

Preconceptional Counseling

Women with chronic hypertension should ideally be counseled before pregnancy. The duration of hypertension, degree of blood-pressure control, and current therapy are ascertained. Home measurement devices should be checked for accuracy. Those who require multiple medications for control or those who are poorly controlled are also at increased risk for adverse pregnancy outcomes. General health, daily activities, and dietary habits are also assessed as shown in Table 50-2.

In those with hypertension for more than 5 years or in diabetic women, cardiovascular and renal function should be assessed (August, 2014; Gainer, 2005). Women with evidence for organ dysfunction or those with prior adverse events such as cerebrovascular accident, arrhythmias, ventricular failure, or myocardial infarction are at markedly increased risk for a recurrence or worsening during pregnancy. Renal function is assessed by serum creatinine measurement, and proteinuria is quantified if the urine spot protein/creatinine ratio is abnormally high (Hladunewich, 2011). The Working Group Report on High Blood Pressure in Pregnancy (2000) of the National Heart, Lung, and Blood Institute concluded that the risks of fetal loss and accelerated deterioration of renal disease are increased if serum creatinine level is above 1.4 mg/dL (Chap. 53, p. 1061).

Although pregnancy is considered by many to be contraindicated in women with severe, poorly controlled hypertension, there is not a consensus regarding this. Certainly, pregnancy

TABLE 50-2. Lifestyle Modifications for Hypertensive Patients—American Heart Association and American College of Cardiology

Consume a dietary pattern that emphasizes intake of vegetables, fruits, and whole grains; includes low-fat dairy products, poultry, fish, legumes, nontropical vegetable oils, and nuts; limits sweets and red meats—e.g. DASH dietary pattern, USDA Food Pattern, or the AHA Diet
Lower sodium intake—consume no more than 2400 mg sodium/day; 1500 mg/day desirable
Engage in aerobic physical activity three to four sessions per week, lasting on average 40 minutes per session, and involving moderate-to-vigorous intensity physical activity

AHA = American Heart Association; DASH = Dietary Approaches to Stop Hypertension; USDA = United States Department of Agriculture.

Summarized from Eckel, 2013.

is at least relatively contraindicated in women who maintain persistent diastolic pressures of ≥ 110 mm Hg despite therapy, who require multiple antihypertensives, or who have a serum creatinine > 2 mg/dL. Even stronger contraindications include prior cerebrovascular accident, myocardial infarction, or cardiac failure.

DIAGNOSIS AND EVALUATION IN PREGNANCY

Classification of the hypertensive disorders complicating pregnancy is discussed in Chapter 40 (p. 728). Women are diagnosed with chronic hypertension if it is documented to precede pregnancy or if hypertension is identified before 20 weeks' gestation. In some women without overt chronic hypertension, there is a history of repeated pregnancies complicated by gestational hypertension with or without the preeclampsia syndrome. Each is a risk marker for latent chronic hypertension, and this is especially so for preeclampsia, especially early-onset preeclampsia. In many ways, gestational hypertension is analogous to gestational diabetes in that such women have a *chronic hypertensive diathesis*, in which heredity plays a major role (Chap. 40, p. 769).

Although uncommon, secondary causes of hypertension are always a possibility in these women. Thus, consideration is given to an underlying pheochromocytoma, connective-tissue disease, Cushing syndrome, chronic renal disease, and myriad other causes. That said, most pregnant women with antecedent hypertension will have uncomplicated disease. As discussed above, some women—especially those with long-term or untreated hypertension—have complications that increase the risk of adverse pregnancy events. Thus, if not already accomplished, assessment during pregnancy is done for the cardiovascular system, the kidneys, and the cerebrovascular circulation.

Associated Risk Factors

Several factors increase the likelihood that pregnant women will have chronic hypertension. Three of those most frequently cited are ethnicity, obesity, and diabetes. As previously discussed, chronic hypertension has a population incidence that is highest in black and lower in white and Mexican-American women (Kotchen, 2012). Related to this, hundreds of blood pressure-related phenotypes and genomic regions have been identified, including candidate genes for preeclampsia and chronic hypertension (Cowley, 2006; Lévesque, 2004).

The *metabolic syndrome* with superimposed preeclampsia is a risk marker for persistent hypertension postpartum (Spaan, 2012). This is not surprising because obesity may increase the prevalence of hypertension tenfold, and it is an important factor predisposing to chronic hypertension (Chap. 48, p. 963). In addition, obese women are more likely to develop superimposed preeclampsia. Diabetes is also prevalent in chronically hypertensive women, and its interplay with obesity and preeclampsia is overwhelming. In the study of more than 56 million births cited above, the most common comorbidities associated with chronic hypertension were pregestational diabetes—6.6 percent, thyroid disorders—4.1 percent, and collagen-vascular disease—0.6 percent (Bateman, 2012). Similar comorbidities were described by Cruz and associates (2011).

Effects of Pregnancy on Chronic Hypertension

Blood pressure falls in early pregnancy in most women with chronic hypertension. It rises again during the third trimester (Fig. 50-1). According to studies by Tihtonen and coworkers

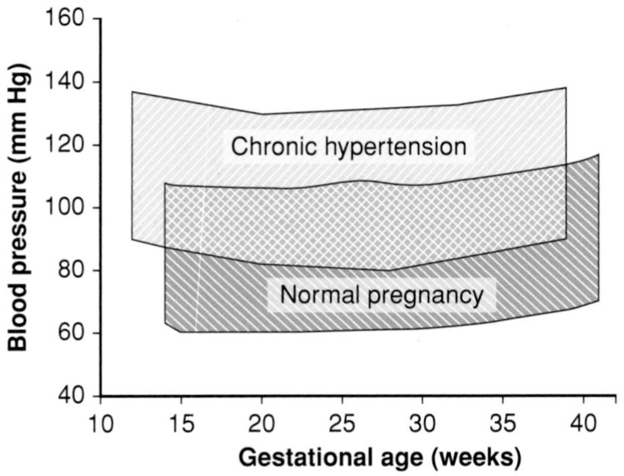

FIGURE 50-1 Mean systolic and diastolic blood pressures across pregnancy in 107 untreated chronically hypertensive women (*yellow*) compared with blood pressures across pregnancy in 4589 healthy nulliparous women (*blue*). (Data from August, 2014; Levine, 1997; Sibai, 1990a.)

(2007), women with chronic hypertension have persistently elevated vascular resistance and possibly a reduced intravascular volume increase. There is no doubt that adverse outcomes in these women are dependent largely on whether superimposed preeclampsia develops. This may be related to observations reported by Hibbard and colleagues (2005, 2014) that arterial mechanical properties are most marked in women with superimposed preeclampsia.

ADVERSE PREGNANCY EFFECTS

Chronic hypertension is associated with several adverse maternal and perinatal outcomes listed in Table 50-3. The recurring theme is that these are directly related to severity and duration of hypertension before pregnancy and whether superimposed preeclampsia develops, especially early in gestation. In women with mild chronic hypertension, outcomes are also related to blood pressure levels during pregnancy (Ankumah, 2013).

Maternal Morbidity and Mortality

Most women whose hypertension is well controlled with monotherapy before pregnancy will do well. Even these women, however, are at increased risk for adverse outcomes. Complications are more likely with severe baseline hypertension and especially with documented end-organ damage (Czeizel, 2011; Odibo, 2013). In a study of pregnancy outcomes in nearly 30,000 chronically hypertensive women, Gilbert and associates (2007) reported markedly increased maternal morbidity including stroke, pulmonary edema, and renal failure. These observations were verified in the report from the Nationwide Patient Sample of more than 56 million deliveries by Bateman and colleagues (2012). Complications of hypertension included stroke—2.7 per 1000, acute renal failure—5.9 per 1000, pulmonary edema—1.5 per 1000, mechanical ventilation—3.8 per 1000, and in-house maternal mortality—0.4 per 1000. The contribution of hypertension to pregnancy-related strokes is discussed in Chapter 60 (p. 1191) and to hypertensive and idiopathic peripartum hypertensive cardiomyopathy in Chapter 49 (p. 988).

TABLE 50-3. Some Adverse Effects of Chronic Hypertension on Maternal and Perinatal Outcomes

Maternal	Perinatal
Superimposed preeclampsia	Fetal death
HELLP syndrome	Growth restriction
Stroke	Preterm delivery
Acute kidney injury	Neonatal death
Heart failure	Neonatal morbidity
Hypertensive cardiomyopathy	
Myocardial infarction	
Placental abruption	
Maternal death	

HELLP = hemolysis, elevated liver enzyme levels, low platelet count.

Pregnancy-aggravated hypertension may be due to gestational hypertension or to superimposed preeclampsia. In either instance, blood pressures can be dangerously elevated. As emphasized by Clark and Hankins (2012), systolic pressure ≥ 160 mm Hg or diastolic pressure ≥ 110 mm Hg will rapidly cause renal or cardiopulmonary dysfunction or cerebral hemorrhage. With superimposed severe preeclampsia or eclampsia, the maternal prognosis is poor unless the pregnancy is ended. Placental abruption is a common and serious complication (Chap. 41, p. 793). In addition to hypertensive heart failure mentioned above, aortic dissection has been described by Weissman-Brenner and coworkers (2004) and is discussed in Chapter 49 (p. 992).

Chronic hypertension has been associated with a fivefold risk for maternal death (Gilbert, 2007). This is emphasized by the report by Berg (2010) describing 4693 pregnancy-related deaths in the United States from 1998 through 2005. Hypertensive disorders, including chronic hypertension and preeclampsia syndrome, accounted for 12.3 percent of these deaths. Undoubtedly related were other causes of death such as cardiovascular conditions—12.4 percent, cerebrovascular conditions—6.3 percent, and cardiomyopathy—11.5 percent. Moodley (2007) reported similar findings with 3406 maternal deaths from South Africa. Interestingly, Sibai and associates (2011) reported that chronically hypertensive women with a history of preeclampsia were not at higher risk for complications compared with hypertensive women without such a history.

Superimposed Preeclampsia

Because there is no precise definition of superimposed preeclampsia in women with chronic hypertension, the reported incidence is variable. The risk is directly related to the severity of baseline hypertension. In a Maternal-Fetal Medicine Units Network trial, Caritis and coworkers (1998) identified superimposed preeclampsia in 25 percent. It was 29 percent in the California database study cited above (Yanit, 2012). According to the American College of Obstetricians and Gynecologists (2012), mild chronic hypertension has a 20-percent incidence for superimposed preeclampsia, whereas with severe hypertension, it is 50 percent. August and colleagues (2014) posit that this predilection may be because of similarities of genetic, biochemical, and metabolic abnormalities. In the study cited above, a history of superimposed preeclampsia did not increase the risk for recurrence, however, it was a marker for increased preterm delivery (Sibai, 2011).

Thus far, prognostic and predictive tests for superimposed preeclampsia have been disappointing when used clinically (American College of Obstetricians and Gynecologists, 2012; Conde-Agudelo, 2014; Zeeman, 2003). For example, Di Lorenzo and colleagues (2012) studied serum markers for Down syndrome and reported a sensitivity of 60 percent with a 20-percent false-positive rate. Similar results were found using antiangiogenic factors to discriminate among chronic hypertension, gestational hypertension, and preeclampsia (Sibai, 2008; Woolcock, 2008). According to Elovitz and coworkers (2013), microRNA assays may prove valuable as predictors of pregnancy-associated hypertension. This subject is discussed further in Chapter 40 (p. 747).

Prevention of Superimposed Preeclampsia

Trials of various substances to prevent preeclampsia in women with chronic hypertension have generally been disappointing. Low-dose aspirin has been evaluated most frequently. In the Network study by Caritis and associates (1998) cited above, the incidence of superimposed preeclampsia, fetal-growth restriction, or both was similar in women given low-dose aspirin or placebo. That said, Duley (2007) and Meads (2008) and their colleagues performed Cochrane reviews and found that low-dose aspirin was beneficial in some high-risk women. Minimal benefits were also found from a metaanalysis (Askie, 2007). To the contrary, however, the PARIS Collaborative Group (2007) reviewed individual data from 33,897 pregnant women enrolled in 33 randomized trials of low-dose aspirin and reported that women with chronic hypertension derived no benefits.

Spinnato and coworkers (2007) randomly assigned 311 women with chronic hypertension to antioxidant treatment with vitamins C and E or to a placebo. A similar number in both groups developed preeclampsia—17 versus 20 percent, respectively.

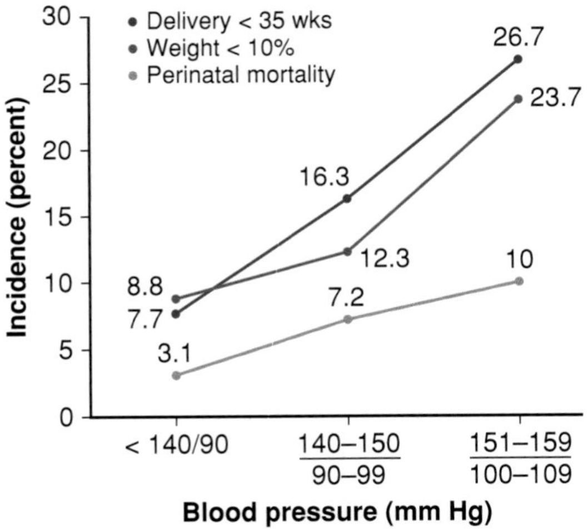

FIGURE 50-2 Perinatal outcomes in 759 women with midrange chronic hypertension enrolled in a Maternal-Fetal Medicine Units Network study (Ankumah, 2013).

Placental Abruption

There seems to be no doubt that chronic hypertension increases the risk two- to threefold for premature placental separation (American College of Obstetricians and Gynecologists, 2012). As discussed in Chapter 41 (p. 793), the overall risk is one in 200 to 300 pregnancies, and this is increased to 1 in 60 to 120 pregnancies in women with chronic hypertension (Ananth, 2007; Cruz, 2011; Madi, 2012; Tuuli, 2011). This risk is increased further if the woman smokes or if she develops superimposed preeclampsia. The risk is highest with severe hypertension, and Vigil-De Gracia and colleagues (2004) reported it to be 8.4 percent. Most abruptions are in women with worsening gestational hypertension or superimposed preeclampsia. From the Norwegian Birth Registry, supplemental folic acid slightly decreased the abruption incidence in women with chronic hypertension (Nilsen, 2008).

Perinatal Morbidity and Mortality

From the foregoing, it is not surprising that almost all adverse perinatal outcomes are increased in women with chronic hypertension. Some of those from a Network study are shown in Figure 50-2. The increasing incremental adverse effects of rising blood pressure levels are apparent. Interestingly, Bánhidy and colleagues (2011) have provided data suggesting that severe hypertension may be associated with fetal esophageal atresia or stenosis. As expected, for the entire group of women, those who developed preeclampsia had substantially increased adverse outcome rates compared with those without preeclampsia.

The stillbirth frequency is substantively greater in most reports (Chap. 35, p. 663). In the Nationwide Patient Sample study, the stillbirth rate was 15.1 per 1000 births (Bateman, 2012). This is similar to the frequency of 18 per 1000 from a Norwegian study (Ahmad, 2012). The rate was increased two- to threefold in the California database study by Yanit and associates (2012).

Low-birthweight infants are common and due to preterm delivery, fetal-growth restriction, or both. In the California study, a fourth of fetuses were delivered preterm (Yanit, 2012). This and other studies attest to the increased risk for fetal-growth restriction, and the incidence averages 20 percent. Zetterström and coworkers (2006) reported a 2.4-fold risk for fetal-growth restriction in 2754 chronically hypertensive Swedish women compared with the risk in normotensive women. Broekhuijsen and associates (2012) found a 1.3-fold increased risk for 1609 Dutch nulliparas with chronic hypertension compared with that in normotensive controls. Fetal-growth dysfunction is more likely in the chronically hypertensive women who develop superimposed preeclampsia. In one study, Chappell and colleagues (2008) reported an almost 50-percent incidence of growth-restricted fetuses born to women with superimposed preeclampsia compared with only 21 percent in women without preeclampsia. Because worsening hypertension frequently mandates preterm delivery, neonates born to these women have a correspondingly high rate of intensive-care nursery admission.

All of these aforementioned adverse perinatal effects of chronic hypertension contribute to the increased perinatal mortality rate, which is three- to fourfold higher in pregnancies complicated by chronic hypertension compared with those of normotensive women (American College of Obstetricians and Gynecologists, 2012). In the Network study shown in Figure 50-2, the perinatal death rate was 31 per 1000 with mild hypertension, 72 per 1000 with moderate disease, and 100 per 1000 in women with severe chronic hypertension. Again as expected, the highest rates are in women who develop superimposed preeclampsia, for whom the risk doubled from 4 to 8 percent. And, if diabetes coexists with chronic hypertension, then preterm delivery, fetal-growth restriction, and perinatal mortality rates are increased even more (Gonzalez-Gonzalez, 2008; Yanit, 2012).

MANAGEMENT DURING PREGNANCY

The diagnosis of chronic hypertension in pregnancy should be confirmed. For example, Brown and associates (2005) reported "white-coat" hypertension in a third of 241 women diagnosed in early pregnancy. Within this third, pregnancy outcomes were good, and only 8 percent developed preeclampsia.

Management goals for chronic hypertension include reductions of adverse maternal or perinatal outcomes just discussed. Treatment is targeted to prevent moderate or severe hypertension and to delay or ameliorate pregnancy-aggravated hypertension. To some extent, these goals can be achieved pharmacologically. Blood-pressure self-monitoring is encouraged, but for accuracy, automated devices must be properly calibrated (Brown, 2004; Staessen, 2004). Personal health modification includes dietary counseling and reduction of behaviors such as tobacco, alcohol, cocaine, or other substance abuse (see Table 50-2).

Blood Pressure Control

Women with *severe hypertension* must be treated for maternal neuro-, cardio-, and renoprotection regardless of pregnancy status (American College of Obstetricians and Gynecologists, 2012). This includes women with prior adverse outcomes such as cerebrovascular events, myocardial infarction, and cardiac or renal dysfunction. We agree with the philosophy of beginning antihypertensive treatment in otherwise healthy pregnant women with persistent systolic pressures > 150 mm Hg or diastolic pressures of 95 to 100 mm Hg or greater (August, 2014; Working Group Report, 2000). With end-organ dysfunction, treatment of diastolic pressures ≥ 90 mm Hg is reasonable to mitigate further organ damage.

There are only sparse data indicating salutary effects on pregnancy outcomes with simply lowering blood pressure. These studies are relatively small and have widely varying inclusion and outcome criteria. In a Cochrane review of 46 of these studies that included a total of 4282 women, Abalos and coworkers (2007) confirmed that the risk for severe hypertension was lowered with therapy. There were, however, no differences in the frequencies of superimposed preeclampsia, eclampsia, abruption, preterm birth, fetal-growth restriction, or perinatal or maternal mortality. These studies do attest to the apparent safety of antihypertensive therapy except for angiotensin-converting enzyme (ACE) inhibitors and angiotensin-receptor blockers (Chap. 12, p. 247). As emphasized by the Working Group Report (2000), there is a need for further trials in chronically hypertensive women.

"Tight Control"

During the past decade, the concept of *tight control* of blood pressure has been espoused as a means of optimizing maternal and perinatal outcomes. Such control is compared with that of glycemic control for management of the pregnant diabetic. In one study, El Guindy and Nabhan (2008) randomly assigned 125 pregnant women with mild chronic hypertension or gestational hypertension to rigid versus less strict blood pressure control. More women in the latter group developed severe hypertension, they had more hospital admissions, and they were delivered of infants at a lower mean gestational age than the tight-control group. Other than these preliminary observations, there are limited data concerning this type of treatment.

Antihypertensive Drugs

As concluded by the American College of Obstetricians and Gynecologists (2012), treatment during pregnancy has included every drug class, but there still is limited information regarding safety and efficacy (Czeizel, 2011; Podymow, 2011). Although many studies indicate increased perinatal adverse effects in treated women, it is still not known whether this is due to cause or effect (Orbach, 2013). The following summary of antihypertensive drugs is abstracted from several sources, including the *2014 Physicians' Desk Reference.* Many of these drugs are also discussed throughout Chapter 12 (p. 247) and have been recently reviewed by Umans and associates (2014).

Diuretics

Thiazide diuretics are sulfonamides, and these were the first drug group used to successfully treat chronic hypertension (Beyer, 1982). These agents and loop-acting diuretics such as furosemide are commonly used in nonpregnant hypertensives. In the short term, they provide sodium and water diuresis with volume depletion. But with time, there is *sodium escape,* and volume depletion is corrected. Some aspect of lowered peripheral vascular resistance likely contributes to their effectiveness in reducing long-term morbidity (Umans, 2014; Williams, 2001).

Thiazide drugs may be mildly diabetogenic, and expected volume expansion may be curtailed in pregnant women. Sibai and colleagues (1984) showed that plasma volume expanded only about 20 percent over time in hypertensive pregnant women who continued diuretic therapy compared with a 50-percent expansion in women who discontinued treatment. Although perinatal outcomes were similar in these women, such concerns have led to practices of withholding diuretics as first-line therapy, particularly after 20 weeks (Working Group Report, 2000). Even so, in a Cochrane review, Churchill and associates (2007) reported no differences in perinatal outcomes in 1836 nonhypertensive women randomly assigned to a thiazide diuretic or placebo for primary preeclampsia prevention. Overall, thiazide diuretics are considered safe in pregnancy (Briggs, 2011; Umans, 2014).

Adrenergic-Blocking Agents

This was the second class of effective antihypertensives. *Peripherally* acting β-adrenergic receptor blockers cause a generalized decrease in sympathetic tone. Examples are propranolol, metoprolol, and atenolol. Labetalol is a commonly used α/β-adrenergic blocker. Some adrenergic-blocking drugs act *centrally* by reducing sympathetic outflow to effect a generalized decreased vascular tone. Some of these are clonidine and α-methyldopa. The drugs most frequently used in pregnancy to treat hypertension are methyldopa or a β- or α/β-receptor blocking agent.

Vasodilators

Hydralazine relaxes arterial smooth muscle and has been used parenterally for decades to safely treat severe peripartum hypertension (Chap. 40, p. 767). Oral hydralazine monotherapy for chronic hypertension is not generally used because of its weak antihypertensive effects and resultant tachycardia. It may be an effective adjunct for long-term use with other antihypertensives, especially if there is chronic renal insufficiency. In the study by Su and coworkers (2013), vasodilator treatment of chronically hypertensive women was associated with a twofold increase in low-birthweight and growth-restricted neonates.

Calcium-Channel Blocking Agents

These drugs are divided into three subclasses based on their modification of calcium entry into cells and interference with binding sites on voltage-dependent calcium channels. Common agents include nifedipine—a dihydropyridine, and verapamil—a phenylalkyl amine derivative. These agents have negative inotropic effects and thus can worsen ventricular dysfunction and congestive heart failure. Theoretically, they may potentiate the actions of magnesium sulfate that is given for eclampsia neuroprophylaxis. There is minimal published experience with these agents during pregnancy (Abalos, 2007). That said, calcium-channel blockers appear to be safe for therapy for chronic hypertension (Briggs, 2011; Podymow, 2011; Umans, 2014).

The safety of acute peripartum nifedipine treatment has been questioned. The drug is used by some for rapid control of severe peripartum hypertension, and it is also widely used for tocolysis in preterm labor (Chap. 42, p. 853). Nifedipine for tocolysis should not be combined with intravenous β-agonists (Oei, 2006). Adverse outcomes reported in women given nifedipine for tocolysis or severe gestational hypertension include myocardial infarction and pulmonary edema (Abbas, 2006; Bal, 2004; Oei, 1999; Verhaert, 2004). Severe maternal hypotension with resultant fetal compromise necessitating cesarean delivery and fetal death have also been reported (Johnson, 2005; Kandysamy, 2005; van Veen, 2005).

Angiotensin-Converting Enzyme Inhibitors

These drugs inhibit the conversion of angiotensin-I to the potent vasoconstrictor angiotensin-II. They can cause severe fetal malformations when given in the second and third trimesters. These include hypocalvaria and renal dysfunction (Chap. 12, p. 247). Some preliminary studies have also suggested teratogenic effects, and because of this, they are not recommended during pregnancy (Briggs, 2011; Podymow, 2011).

Angiotensin-receptor blockers act in a similar manner. But, instead of blocking the production of angiotensin-II, they inhibit binding to its receptor. They are presumed to have the same fetal effects as ACE inhibitors and thus are also contraindicated.

Antihypertensive Treatment in Pregnancy

As discussed, continuation of prepregnancy antihypertensive treatment when women become pregnant is debated. Although blood-pressure reduction is certainly beneficial to the mother long term, it at least theoretically can decrease uteroplacental perfusion. According to older observational reports, in general, most pregnancy outcomes in women with mild to moderate hypertension were good without treatment and unless superimposed preeclampsia developed (Chesley, 1978; Umans, 2014).

There are no large randomized trials to settle the questions surrounding empirical treatment. Abalos and associates (2007) performed a Cochrane database review of 46 small trials enrolling a total of 4282 women. These studies varied widely in definitions of hypertension severity, use of placebos, gestational age at entry, and the type of drug(s) used. The salient results are shown in Table 50-4. These led the investigators to conclude again that treatment reliably lowered risk for severe hypertension during pregnancy.

TABLE 50-4. Comparison of Pregnancy Outcomes in Women with and without Antepartum Treatment for Mild to Moderate Chronic Hypertension

Outcome	Studies (Subjects)	RR (95% CI)[a]
Severe hypertension	19 (2409)	0.50 [0.41, 0.61]
Preeclampsia	22 (2702)	0.97 [0.83, 1.13]
SGA infants	9 (904)	1.38 [0.99, 1.92]
Perinatal mortality	26 (3081)	0.73 [0.50, 1.08]
Delivery < 37 weeks	14 (1992)	1.02 [0.89, 1.16]

[a]Pertains to those receiving treatment.
SGA = small-for-gestational age.
Includes only studies in which β-blocking drugs were given.
Data from a Cochrane database review by Abalos, 2007.

This Cochrane review does raise concern for fetal-growth restriction with β-blocking drugs. It is not resolved, however, because diminished placental perfusion secondary to lowered maternal blood pressure is confounded by the fact that worsening blood pressure itself is associated with abnormal fetal growth. Some also posit that the drugs have a direct fetal action (Umans, 2014). In two of the larger randomized trials, however, the incidence of growth restriction was not altered in women randomly assigned to treatment (Gruppo di Studio Ipertensione in Gravidanza, 1998; Sibai, 1990a).

Severe Chronic Hypertension

Most data suggest that the prognosis for pregnancy outcome with chronic hypertension is dependent on the severity of disease antedating pregnancy. This may be related to findings that many women with severe hypertension have renal disease—as either cause or effect (Cunningham, 1990). One report by Sibai and coworkers (1986) described outcomes from 44 pregnancies in women whose blood pressure at 6 to 11 weeks was ≥ 170/110 mm Hg. All were given oral treatment with α-methyldopa and hydralazine to maintain pressures < 160/110 mm Hg. If dangerous hypertension developed, then the woman was hospitalized and treated with parenteral hydralazine. Of the 44 pregnancies, superimposed preeclampsia developed in half, and all adverse perinatal outcomes were in this group. Moreover, all neonates of women in the latter group were delivered preterm, nearly 80 percent were also growth restricted, and they had a 48-percent perinatal mortality rate. Conversely, those women with severe chronic hypertension who did not develop superimposed preeclampsia had reasonably good outcomes. There were no perinatal deaths, and only 5 percent of fetuses were growth restricted.

Recommendations for Therapy in Pregnancy

The Working Group on High Blood Pressure in Pregnancy (2000) concluded that there were limited data from which to draw conclusions concerning any decision to treat mild chronic hypertension in pregnancy. As discussed on page 1005, the Group did recommend empirical therapy in women whose blood pressures exceed threshold levels of 150 to 160 mm Hg systolic or 100 to 110 mm Hg diastolic or in women with target-organ damage such as left ventricular hypertrophy or renal insufficiency. They also concluded that early treatment of hypertension would probably reduce subsequent hospitalization rates during pregnancy.

Some women will have persistently worrisome hypertension despite usual therapy (Samuel, 2011; Sibai, 1990a). In these women, primary attention is given to the likelihood of pregnancy-aggravated hypertension, with or without superimposed preeclampsia. Other possibilities include inaccurate blood-pressure measurements, suboptimal treatment, and antagonizing substances (Moser, 2006). Causes reported in nonpregnant cohorts were nonsteroidal antiinflammatory drugs including cyclooxygenase-2 inhibitors and alcohol consumption (Sowers, 2005; Xin, 2001).

Pregnancy-Aggravated Hypertension or Superimposed Preeclampsia

As discussed, the incidence of superimposed preeclampsia for women with chronic hypertension varies depending on the study population and hypertension severity. A reasonable average is 20 to 30 percent. The incidence of superimposed preeclampsia may be underreported if the diagnosis is based solely on urine protein dipstick testing (Gangaram, 2005; Lai, 2006). Importantly, in approximately half of chronically hypertensive women, superimposed preeclampsia develops before 37 weeks (Chappell, 2008).

The diagnosis may be difficult to make, especially in women with hypertension who have underlying renal disease with chronic proteinuria (Cunningham, 1990). As discussed in Chapter 40 (p. 730), conditions that support the diagnosis of superimposed preeclampsia include worsening hypertension, new-onset proteinuria, neurological symptoms such as severe headaches and visual disturbances, generalized edema, oliguria, and certainly, convulsions or pulmonary edema. Supporting laboratory abnormalities are increasing serum creatinine levels, thrombocytopenia, serum hepatic transaminase elevations, or the triad of HELLP—hemolysis, elevated liver enzyme levels, low platelet count—syndrome. For women with chronic hypertension and superimposed preeclampsia with severe features, magnesium sulfate for maternal neuroprophylaxis is recommended (American College of Obstetricians and Gynecologists, 2013).

Some pregnant women with chronic hypertension have worsening hypertension with no other findings of superimposed preeclampsia. This is most commonly encountered near the end of the second trimester. In the absence of other supporting criteria for superimposed preeclampsia, including fetal-growth restriction or decreased amnionic fluid volume, this likely represents the higher end of the normal blood-pressure curve shown in Figure 50-1. In such women, if preeclampsia can be reasonably excluded, then it is reasonable to begin or to increase the dose of antihypertensive therapy.

Fetal Assessment

Women with well-controlled chronic hypertension and who have no complicating factors can generally be expected to have a good pregnancy outcome. Because even those with mild hypertension have an increased risk of superimposed preeclampsia and fetal-growth restriction, serial antepartum assessment of fetal well-being is recommended by many. That said, according to the American College of Obstetricians and Gynecologists (2012), with the exception of sonographic fetal-growth monitoring, there are no conclusive data to address either benefit or harm associated with various antepartum surveillance strategies.

Expectant Management

Given that half of these women develop superimposed preeclampsia before term, considerations for expectant management may be reasonable in some cases. In a study from Magee-Women's Hospital, 41 carefully selected women with a median gestational age of 31.6 weeks were expectantly managed (Samuel, 2011). Despite liberal criteria to mandate delivery, 17 percent developed either placental abruption or pulmonary edema. The latency period was extended by a mean of 9.7 days, and there were no perinatal deaths. These investigators recommended randomized trials to study expectant management.

Delivery

For chronically hypertensive women who have complications such as fetal-growth restriction or superimposed preeclampsia, the decision to deliver is made by clinical judgment. The route of delivery is dictated by obstetrical factors. Certainly, most women with superimposed severe preeclampsia are better delivered even when there is a markedly preterm pregnancy. These women are at increased risk for placental abruption, cerebral hemorrhage, and peripartum heart failure (Cunningham, 1986, 2005; Martin, 2005).

For women with mild to moderate chronic hypertension who continue to have an uncomplicated pregnancy, there are at least two options for timing of delivery (American College of Obstetricians and Gynecologists, 2012). The first is delivery at term, that is, ≥ 39 completed weeks. Another option is from consensus committee findings by Spong and associates (2011), which recommend consideration for delivery at 38 to 39 weeks, that is, ≥ 37 completed weeks. A trial of labor induction is preferable, and many of these women respond favorably and will be delivered vaginally (Alexander, 1999; Atkinson, 1995).

Intrapartum Consideration

For women with severe preeclampsia, peripartum management is the same as described in Chapter 40 (p. 761). Epidural analgesia for labor and delivery is optimal with the caveat that it is not given to treat hypertension (Lucas, 2001). That said, women with severe superimposed preeclampsia are more sensitive to the acute hypotensive effects of epidural analgesia (Vricella, 2012). Magnesium sulfate neuroprophylaxis is initiated for prevention of eclampsia (Alexander, 2006). Severe hypertension—diastolic blood pressure ≥ 110 mm Hg or systolic pressure ≥ 160 mm Hg—is treated with either intravenous hydralazine or labetalol. Some prefer to treat women with a diastolic pressure of 100 to 105 mm Hg. Vigil-De Gracia and colleagues (2006) randomized 200 women to intravenous hydralazine or labetalol to acutely lower severe high blood pressure in pregnancy. Outcomes were similar except for significantly more maternal palpitations and tachycardia with hydralazine and significantly more neonatal hypotension and bradycardia with labetalol.

Postpartum Hypertension

In most respects, postpartum observation, prevention, and management of adverse complications are similar in women with severe chronic hypertension and in those with severe preeclampsia–eclampsia (Chap. 40, p. 767). For persistent severe hypertension, consideration is given for a cause such as pheochromocytoma or Cushing disease (Sibai, 2012). And because of chronic end-organ damage, certain complications are more common. These include cerebral or pulmonary edema, heart failure, renal dysfunction, or cerebral hemorrhage, especially within the first 48 hours after delivery (Martin, 2005; Sibai, 1990b). These frequently are preceded by sudden increases—"spikes"—of mean arterial blood pressure, especially the systolic component (Cunningham, 2000, 2005).

Following delivery, as maternal peripheral resistance increases, left ventricular workload also increases. This rise is further aggravated by appreciable and pathological amounts of interstitial fluid that are mobilized to be excreted as endothelial damage from preeclampsia resolves. In these women, sudden hypertension—either moderate or severe—exacerbates diastolic dysfunction, causes systolic dysfunction, and leads to pulmonary edema (Cunningham, 1986; Gandhi, 2001). Prompt hypertension control, along with furosemide-evoked diuresis, usually quickly resolves pulmonary edema. It is possible in many women to forestall this by the administration of intravenous furosemide to augment the normal postpartum diuresis. Daily weights are helpful in this regard. On average, a woman should weigh 15 pounds less immediately after delivery. Excessive extracellular fluid can be estimated by subtracting the postpartum weight from the predelivery weight—if not determined on hospital admission, the weight at the last prenatal visit provides a relatively accurate estimate. In one study, 20-mg oral furosemide given daily to postpartum women with severe preeclampsia aided blood-pressure control (Ascarelli, 2005).

Contraception

Women with chronic hypertension have special considerations for contraceptive and sterilization choices. These are discussed in detail throughout Chapters 38 and 39. These women are also at ultimate high risk for lifetime cardiovascular complications, especially when accompanied by diabetes, obesity, and the metabolic syndrome.

REFERENCES

Abalos E, Duley L, Steyn DW, et al: Antihypertensive drug therapy for mild to moderate hypertension during pregnancy. Cochrane Database Syst Rev 1:CD002252, 2007

Abbas OM, Nassar AH, Kanj N, et al: Acute pulmonary edema during tocolytic therapy with nifedipine. Am J Obstet Gynecol 195(4):e3, 2006

Ahmad AS, Samuelsen SO: Hypertensive disorders in pregnancy and fetal death at different gestational lengths: a population study of 2,121,371 pregnancies. BJOG 119(12):1521, 2012

Alexander JM, Bloom SL, McIntire DD, et al: Severe preeclampsia and the very low birth weight infant: is induction of labor harmful? Obstet Gynecol 93:485, 1999

Alexander JM, McIntire DD, Leveno KJ, et al: Selective magnesium sulfate prophylaxis for the prevention of eclampsia in women with gestational hypertension. Obstet Gynecol 108(4):826, 2006

American College of Obstetricians and Gynecologists: Chronic hypertension in pregnancy. Practice Bulletin No. 125, February 2012

American College of Obstetricians and Gynecologists: Hypertension in pregnancy. Report of the American College of Obstetricians and Gynecologists' Task Force on Hypertension in Pregnancy. Obstet Gynecol 122:1122, 2013

Ananth CV, Peltier MR, Kinzler WL, et al: Chronic hypertension and risk of placental abruption: is the association modified by ischemic placental disease? Am J Obstet Gynecol 197(3):273.e1, 2007

Ankumah NA, Tita A, Cantu J, et al: Pregnancy outcome vary by blood pressure level in women with mild-range chronic hypertension. Abstract No. 614. Am J Obstet Gynecol 208(1):S261, 2013

Ascarelli MH, Johnson V, McCreary H, et al: Postpartum preeclampsia management with furosemide: a randomized clinical trial. Obstet Gynecol 105(1):29, 2005

Askie LM, Duley L, Henderson-Smart DJ, et al: Antiplatelet agents for prevention of pre-eclampsia: a meta-analysis of individual patient data. Lancet 369(9575):1791, 2007

Atkinson MW, Guinn D, Owen J, et al: Does magnesium sulfate affect the length of labor induction in women with pregnancy-associated hypertension? Am J Obstet Gynecol 173(4):1219, 1995

August P, Jeyabalan A, Roberts JM: Chronic hypertension in pregnancy. In Taylor RN, Roberts JM, Cunningham FG (eds) Chesley's Hypertensive Disorders in Pregnancy. Amsterdam, Academic Press, 2014

Bal L, Thierry S, Brocas E, et al: Pulmonary edema induced by calcium-channel blockade for tocolysis. Anesth Analg 99(3):910, 2004

Bánhidy F, Ács N, Puhó EH, et al: Chronic hypertension with related drug treatment of pregnant women and congenital abnormalities in their offspring: a population-based study. Hypertens Res 34(2):257, 2011

Bateman BT, Bansil P, Hernandez-Diaz S, et al: Prevalence, trends, and outcomes of chronic hypertension: a nationwide sample of delivery admissions. Am J Obstet Gynecol 206(2):134.e1, 2012

Berg CJ, Callaghan WM, Syverson C, et al: Pregnancy-related mortality in the United States, 1998 to 2005. Obstet Gynecol 116(6):1302, 2010

Beyer KH: Chlorothiazide. J Clin Pharmacol 13:15, 1982

Briggs GG, Freeman RK, Yaffe SJ: Drugs in Pregnancy and Lactation, 9th ed. Philadelphia, Lippincott Williams & Wilkins, 2011

Broekhuijsen K, Langeveld J, van den Berg P, et al: Maternal and neonatal outcomes in pregnancy in women with chronic hypertension. Am J Obstet Gynecol 206:S344, 2012

Brown MA, Mangos G, Homer C: The natural history of white coat hypertension during pregnancy. Br J Obstet Gynaecol 112:601, 2005

Brown M, McHugh L, Mangos G, et al: Automated self-initiated blood pressure or 24-hour ambulatory blood pressure monitoring in pregnancy? Br J Obstet Gynaecol 111:38, 2004

Caritis S, Sibai B, Hauth J, et al: Low-dose aspirin to prevent preeclampsia in women at high risk. N Engl J Med 338(11):701, 1998

Centers for Disease Control and Prevention: Vital signs: prevalence, treatment, and control of hypertension—United States, 1999–2002 and 2005–2008. MMWR 60(4):1, 2011

Chappell LC, Enye S, Seed P, et al: Adverse perinatal outcomes and risk factors for preeclampsia in women with chronic hypertension: a prospective study. Hypertension 51(4):1002, 2008

Chesley LC: Superimposed preeclampsia or eclampsia. In Chesley LC (ed): Hypertensive Disorders in Pregnancy. New York, Appleton-Century-Crofts, 1978, pp 14, 302, 482

Churchill D, Beevers GD, Meher S, et al: Diuretics for preventing pre-eclampsia. Cochrane Database Syst Rev 1:CD004451, 2007

Clark, SL, Hankins GDV: Preventing maternal death. 10 clinical diamonds. Obstet Gynecol 119(2):360, 2012

Conde-Agudelo A, Romero R, Roberts JM: Tests to predict preeclampsia. In Taylor RN, Roberts JM, Cunningham FG (eds): Chesley's Hypertensive Disorders in Pregnancy, 4th ed. Amsterdam, Academic Press, 2014

Cowley AW Jr: The genetic dissection of essential hypertension. Nat Rev Genet 7:829, 2006

Cruz MO, Gao W, Hibbard JU: Obstetrical and perinatal outcomes among women with gestational hypertension, mild preeclampsia, and mild chronic hypertension. Am J Obstet Gynecol 205:260.e1, 2011

Cunningham FG: Severe preeclampsia and eclampsia: systolic hypertension is also important. Obstet Gynecol 105:237, 2005

Cunningham FG, Cox SM, Harstad TW, et al: Chronic renal disease and pregnancy outcome. Am J Obstet Gynecol 163:453, 1990

Cunningham FG, Pritchard JA, Hankins GDN, et al: Idiopathic cardiomyopathy or compounding cardiovascular events? Obstet Gynecol 67:157, 1986

Cunningham FG, Twickler D: Cerebral edema complicating eclampsia. Am J Obstet Gynecol 182(1):94, 2000

Czeizel AE, Bánhidy F: Chronic hypertension in pregnancy. Curr Opin Obstet Gynecol 23(2):76, 2011

Di Lorenzo G, Ceccarello M, Cecotti V, et al: First trimester maternal serum PIGF, free β-hCG, PAPP-A, PP-13, uterine artery Doppler and maternal history for the prediction of preeclampsia. Placenta 33(6):495, 2012

Duley L, Henderson-Smart DJ, Meher S, et al: Antiplatelet agents for preventing pre-eclampsia and its complications. Cochrane Database Syst Rev 2:CD004659, 2007

Eckel RH, Jakicic JM, Ard JD, et al: 2013 AHA/ACC guidelines on lifestyle management to reduce cardiovascular risk: a report of the American College of Cardiology/American Heart Association task force on practice guidelines. Circulation 2013

El Guindy AA, Nabhan AF: A randomized trial of tight vs. less tight control of mild essential and gestational hypertension in pregnancy. J Perinat Med 36(5):413, 2008

Elovitz M, Anton Lauren, Bastek J, et al: MicroRNA 210 levels in the first and second trimester of pregnancy are accurate predictors of pregnancy related hypertension. Abstract No. 647. Am J Obstet Gynecol 208:S273, 2013

Gainer J, Alexander J, McIntire D, et al: Maternal echocardiogram findings in pregnant patients with chronic hypertension. Presented at the 25th Annual Meeting of the Society for Maternal-Fetal Medicine, Reno, Nevada, February 7–12, 2005

Gandhi SK, Powers JC, Nomeir A, et al: The pathogenesis of acute pulmonary edema associated with hypertension. N Engl J Med 344(1):17, 2001

Gangaram R, Ojwang PJ, Moodley J, et al: The accuracy of urine dipsticks as a screening test for proteinuria in hypertensive disorders of pregnancy. Hypertens Pregnancy 24(2):117, 2005

Gilbert WM, Young AL, Danielsen B: Pregnancy-outcomes in women with chronic hypertension: a population-based study. J Reprod Med 52(11):1046, 2007

Gonzalez-Gonzalez NL, Ramirez O, Mozas J, et al: Factors influencing pregnancy outcomes in women with type 2 versus type 1 diabetes mellitus. Acta Obstet Gynecol Scand. 87(1):43, 2008

Gruppo di Studio Ipertensione in Gravidanza: Nifedipine versus expectant management in mild to moderate hypertension in pregnancy. Br J Obstet Gynaecol 105(7):718, 1998

Hibbard JU, Korcarz CE, Nendaz GG, et al: The arterial system in pre-eclampsia and chronic hypertension with superimposed pre-eclampsia. BJOG 112(7):897, 2005

Hibbard JU, Shroff S, Cunningham FG: Cardiovascular alterations in pregnancy and preeclampsia. In Taylor RN, Roberts JM, Cunningham FG (eds): Chesley's Hypertensive Disorders in Pregnancy. Amsterdam, Academic Press, 2014

Hladunewich MA, Schaefer F: Proteinuria in special populations: pregnant women and children. Adv Chronic Kidney Dis 18(4):267, 2011

James PA, Oparil S, Carter BL, et al: 2014 evidence-based guidelines for the management of high blood pressure in adults. Report from the panel members appointed to the eighth Joint National Committee (JNC 8). JAMA December 18, 2013 [Epub ahead of print]

Johnson KA, Mason GC: Severe hypotension and fetal death due to tocolysis with nifedipine. BJOG 112(11):1583, 2005

Kandysamy V, Thomson AJ: Severe hypotension and fetal death due to tocolysis with nifedipine. BJOG 112(11):1583, 2005

Kotchen TA: Antihypertensive therapy-associated hypokalemia and hyperkalemia. Hypertension 59(5):906, 2012

Lai J, Tan J, Moore T, et al: Comparing urine dipstick to protein/creatinine ratio in the setting of suspected preeclampsia. Am J Obstet Gynecol 195:S148, 2006

Lévesque S, Moutquin JM, Lindsay C, et al: Implication of an AGT haplotype in a multigene association study with pregnancy hypertension. Hypertension 43(11):71, 2004

Levine RJ, Hauth JC, Curet LB, et al: Trial of calcium to prevent preeclampsia. N Engl J Med 337(2):69, 1997

Lucas MJ, Sharma SK, McIntire DD, et al: A randomized trial of labor analgesia in women with pregnancy-induced hypertension. Am J Obstet Gynecol 185(4):970, 2001

Madi JM, Araújo BF, Zatti H, et al: Chronic hypertension and pregnancy at a tertiary-care and university hospital. Hypertens Pregnancy 31(3):350, 2012

Martin JN Jr, Thigpen BD, Moore RC, et al: Stroke and severe preeclampsia and eclampsia: a paradigm shift focusing on systolic blood pressure. Obstet Gynecol 105(2):246, 2005

Meads CA, Cnossen JS, Meher S, et al: Methods of prediction and prevention of pre-eclampsia: systematic reviews of accuracy and effectiveness literature with economic modelling. Health Technol Assess 12(6):1, 2008

Moodley J: Maternal deaths due to hypertensive disorders in pregnancy: Saving Mothers report 2002–2004. Cardiovasc J Afr 18:358, 2007

Moser M, Setaro JF: Resistant or difficult-to-control hypertension. N Engl J Med 355:385, 2006

Nilsen RM, Vollset SE, Rasmussen SA, et al: Folic acid and multivitamin supplement use and risk of placental abruption: a population-based registry study. Am J Epidemiol 167(7):867, 2008

Odibo I, Zilberman D, Apuzzio J, et al: Utility of posterior and septal wall thickness in predicting adverse pregnancy outcomes in patients with chronic hypertension. Abstract No. 624. Am J Obstet Gynecol 208:S265, 2013

Oei SG: Calcium channel blockers for tocolysis: a review of their role and safety following reports of serious adverse events. Eur J Obstet Gynecol Repro Biol 126(2):137, 2006

Oei SG, Oei SK, Brolmann HA: Myocardial infarction during nifedipine therapy for preterm labour. N Engl J Med 340(2):154, 1999

Orbach H, Matok I, Gorodischer R, et al: Hypertension and antihypertensive drugs in pregnancy and perinatal outcomes. Am J Obstet Gynecol 208(4):301.e1, 2013

PARIS: Perinatal Anteplatelet Review of International Studies (PARIS) Collaborative Group: Antiplatelet agents prevent pre-eclampsia, and its consequences: an individual patient data review. Lancet, 369:1791, 2007

Physicians' Desk Reference, 66th ed. Montvale, Thomson PDR, 2014

Podymow T, August P: Antihypertensive drugs in pregnancy. Semin Nephrol 31(1):70, 2011

Samuel A, Lin C, Parviainen K, et al: Expectant management of preeclampsia superimposed on chronic hypertension. J Matern Fetal Neonatal Med 24(7):907, 2011

Sibai BM: Etiology and management of postpartum hypertension-preeclampsia. Am J Obstet Gynecol 206(6):470, 2012

Sibai BM, Anderson GD: Pregnancy outcome of intensive therapy in severe hypertension in first trimester. Obstet Gynecol 67(4):517, 1986

Sibai BM, Grossman RA, Grossman HG: Effects of diuretics on plasma volume in pregnancies with long-term hypertension. Am J Obstet Gynecol 150(7):831, 1984

Sibai BM, Koch MA, Freire S, et al: The impact of prior preeclampsia on the risk of superimposed preeclampsia and other adverse pregnancy outcomes in patients with chronic hypertension. Am J Obstet Gynecol 204(4):345.e1, 2011

Sibai BM, Koch MA, Freire S, et al: Serum inhibin A and angiogenic factor levels in pregnancies with previous preeclampsia and/or chronic hypertension: are they useful markers for prediction of subsequent preeclampsia? Am J Obstet Gynecol 199(3):268.e1, 2008

Sibai BM, Mabie WC, Shamsa F, et al: A comparison of no medication versus methyldopa or labetalol in chronic hypertension during pregnancy. Am J Obstet Gynecol 162(4):960, 1990a

Sibai BM, Villar MA, Mabie BC: Acute renal failure in hypertensive disorders of pregnancy. Pregnancy outcome and remote prognosis in thirty-one consecutive cases. Am J Obstet Gynecol 162(3):777, 1990b

Sowers JR, White WB, Pitt B, et al: The effects of cyclooxygenase-2 inhibitors and nonsteroidal anti-inflammatory therapy on 24-hour blood pressure in patients with hypertension, osteoarthritis, and type 2 diabetes mellitus. Arch Intern Med 165(2):161, 2005

Spaan JJ, Sep SJ, van Balen VL, et al: Metabolic syndrome as a risk factor for hypertension after preeclampsia. Obstet Gynecol 120(2 Pt 1):311, 2012

Spinnato JA 2nd, Freire S, Pinto E Silva JL, et al: Antioxidant therapy to prevent preeclampsia: a randomized controlled trial. Obstet Gynecol 110(6):1311, 2007

Staessen JA, Den Hond E, Celis H, et al: Antihypertensive treatment based on blood pressure measurement at home or in the physician's office: a randomized controlled trial. JAMA 291(8):955, 2004

Su CY, Lin HC, Cheng HC, et al: Pregnancy outcomes of anti-hypertensives for women with chronic hypertension: a population-based study. PLoS One 8(2):e53844, 2013

Tihtonen K, Kööbi T, Huhtala H, et al: Hemodynamic adaptation during pregnancy in chronic hypertension. Hypertens Pregnancy 26(3):315, 2007

Tuuli MG, Rampersad R, Stamilio D, et al: Perinatal outcomes in women with preeclampsia and superimposed preeclampsia: do they differ? Am J Obstet Gynecol 204(6):508.e1, 2011

Umans JG, Abalos E, Cunningham FG: Antihypertensive treatment. In Taylor RN, Roberts JM, Cunningham FG (eds): Chesley's Hypertensive Disorders in Pregnancy, 4th ed. Amsterdam, Academic Press, 2014

van Veen AJ, Pelinck MJ, van Pampus MG, et al: Severe hypotension and fetal death due to tocolysis with nifedipine. BJOG 112(4):509, 2005

Verhaert D, Van Acker R: Acute myocardial infarction during pregnancy. Acta Cardiol 59(3):331, 2004

Vigil-De Gracia P, Lasso M, Montufar-Rueda C: Perinatal outcome in women with severe chronic hypertension during the second half of pregnancy. Int J Gynaecol Obstet 85(2):139, 2004

Vigil-De Gracia P, Lasso M, Ruiz E, et al: Severe hypertension in pregnancy: hydralazine or labetalol a randomized clinical trial. Eur J Obstet Gynecol Repro Biol 128(1–2):157, 2006

Vricella LK, Louis JM, Mercer BM, et al: Epidural-associated hypotension is more common among severely preeclamptic patients in labor. Am J Obstet Gynecol 207(4):335.e1, 2012

Weissman-Brenner A, Schoen R, Divon MY: Aortic dissection in pregnancy. Obstet Gynecol 103:1110, 2004

Williams GH: Hypertensive vascular disease. In Braunwald E, Fauci AS, Kasper DL, et al (eds): Harrison's Principles of Internal Medicine, 15th ed. New York, McGraw-Hill, 2001, p 1421

Woolcock J, Hennessy A, Xu B, et al: Soluble Flt-1 as a diagnostic marker of preeclampsia. Aust N Z J Obstet Gynaecol 48(1):64, 2008

Working Group Report on High Blood Pressure in Pregnancy: Report of the National High Blood Pressure Education Program Working Group on High Blood Pressure in Pregnancy. Am J Obstet Gynecol 183:S1, 2000

Xin X, He J, Frontini MG, et al: Effects of alcohol reduction on blood pressure: a meta-analysis of randomized controlled trials. Hypertension 38(5):1112, 2001

Yanit KE, Snowden JM, Cheng YW, et al: The impact of chronic hypertension and pregestational diabetes on pregnancy outcomes. Am J Obstet Gynecol 207(4):333.e1, 2012

Zeeman GG, McIntire DD, Twickler DM: Maternal and fetal artery Doppler findings in women with chronic hypertension who subsequently develop superimposed preeclampsia. J Matern Fetal Neonatal Med 14(5):318, 2003

Zetterström K, Lindeberg SN, Haglund B, et al: Chronic hypertension as a risk factor for offspring to be born small for gestational age. Acta Obstet Gynecol Scand 85(9):1046, 2006

CHAPTER 51

Pulmonary Disorders

Acute and chronic pulmonary disorders are frequently encountered during pregnancy. Chronic asthma or an acute exacerbation is the most common and affects up to 4 percent of pregnant women. These disorders along with community-acquired pneumonia accounted for almost 10 percent of nonobstetrical hospitalizations in one managed care plan (Gazmararian, 2002). Pneumonia is also a frequent complication requiring readmission postpartum (Belfort, 2010). These and other pulmonary disorders are superimposed on several important pregnancy-induced changes of ventilatory physiology. For example, pregnant women, especially those in the last trimester, do not appear to tolerate severe acute pneumonitis as evidenced by the disparate number of maternal deaths during the 1918 and 1957 influenza pandemics.

The important and sometimes marked changes in the respiratory system induced by pregnancy are reviewed in Chapter 4 (p. 62), and values for associated tests can be found in the Appendix (p. 1292). Lung volumes and capacities that are measured directly to assess pulmonary pathophysiology may be significantly altered. In turn, these change gas concentrations and acid-base values in blood. Some of the physiological alterations induced by pregnancy were summarized by Wise and associates (2006):

1. *Vital capacity* and *inspiratory capacity* increase by approximately 20 percent by late pregnancy.
2. *Expiratory reserve volume* decreases from 1300 mL to approximately 1100 mL.
3. *Tidal volume* increases approximately 40 percent as a result of respiratory stimulation by progesterone.
4. *Minute ventilation* increases 30 to 40 percent due to increased tidal volume. As a result, arterial Po_2 increases from 100 to 105 mm Hg.
5. Increasing metabolic demands cause a 30-percent increase in *carbon dioxide production*, but because of its concomitantly increased diffusion capacity along with hyperventilation, the arterial Pco_2 decreases from 40 to 32 mm Hg.
6. *Residual volume* decreases approximately 20 percent from 1500 mL to approximately 1200 mL.
7. *Chest wall compliance* is reduced by a third by the expanding uterus and increased abdominal pressure, which causes a 10- to 25-percent decrease in *functional residual capacity*—the sum of expiratory reserve and residual volumes.

The end result of these pregnancy-induced changes is substantively increased ventilation due to deeper but not more frequent breathing. These are thought to be stimulated by basal oxygen consumption as it increases incrementally from 20 to 40 mL/min in the second half of pregnancy.

ASTHMA

Asthma is seen frequently in young women and therefore often complicates pregnancy. Asthma prevalence increased steadily in many countries beginning in the mid-1970s but may have plateaued in the United States, with a prevalence in adults of approximately 10 percent (Barnes, 2012; Centers for Disease Control and Prevention, 2010c). The estimated asthma prevalence during pregnancy ranges between 4 and 8 percent, and this appears to be increasing (Kwon, 2006; Namazy, 2005). Finally, evidence is accruing that fetal as well as neonatal environmental exposures may contribute to the origins of asthma in certain individuals (Harding, 2012; Henderson, 2012).

Pathophysiology

Asthma is a chronic inflammatory airway syndrome with a major hereditary component. Increased airway responsiveness and persistent subacute inflammation have been associated with genes on chromosomes 5q that include cytokine gene clusters, β-adrenergic and glucocorticoid receptor genes, and the T-cell antigen receptor gene (Barnes, 2012). Asthma is heterogeneous, and there inevitably is an *environmental allergic stimulant* such as influenza or cigarette smoke in susceptible individuals (Bel, 2013).

The hallmarks of asthma are reversible airway obstruction from bronchial smooth muscle contraction, vascular congestion, tenacious mucus, and mucosal edema. There is mucosal infiltration with eosinophils, mast cells, and T lymphocytes that causes airway inflammation and increased responsiveness to numerous stimuli including irritants, viral infections, aspirin, cold air, and exercise. Several inflammatory mediators produced by these and other cells include histamine, leukotrienes, prostaglandins, cytokines, and many others. IgE also plays a central role in pathophysiology (Strunk, 2006). *Because F-series prostaglandins and ergonovine exacerbate asthma, these commonly used obstetrical drugs should be avoided if possible.*

Clinical Course

Asthma findings range from mild wheezing to severe bronchoconstriction, which obstructs airways and decreases airflow. These reduce the forced expiratory volume in 1 second

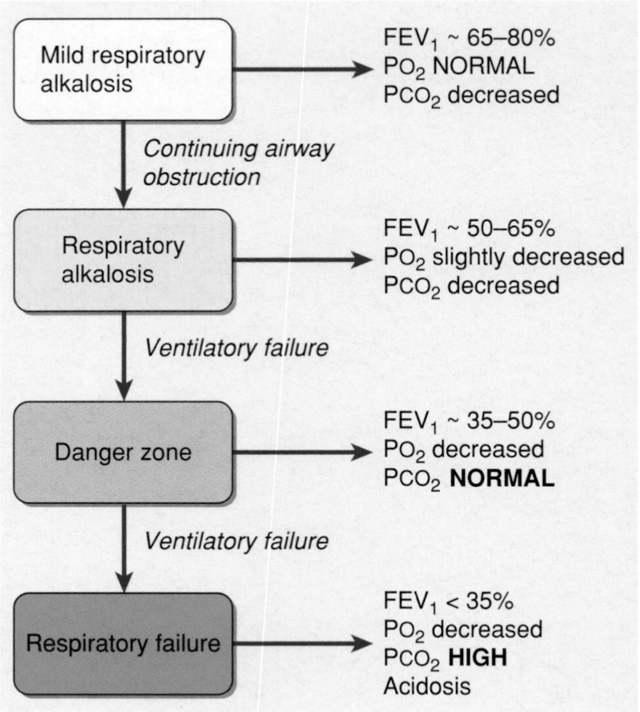

FIGURE 51-1 Clinical stages of asthma. FEV_1 = forced expiratory volume in 1 second.

(FEV_1)/forced vital capacity (FVC) ratio and the peak expiratory flow (PEF). The work of breathing progressively increases, and patients note chest tightness, wheezing, or breathlessness. Subsequent alterations in oxygenation primarily reflect ventilation–perfusion mismatching, because the distribution of airway narrowing is uneven.

Varied manifestations of asthma have led to a simple classification that considers severity as well as onset and duration of symptoms (Table 51-1). With persistent or worsening bronchial obstruction, stages progress as shown in Figure 51-1. Hypoxia initially is well augmented by hyperventilation, which

TABLE 51-1. Classification of Asthma Severity

	Severity			
		Persistent		
Component	Intermittent	Mild	Moderate	Severe
Symptoms	≤ 2 day/wk	> 2 day/wk, not daily	Daily	Throughout day
Nocturnal awakenings	≤ 2×/mo	3–4×/mo	> 1/wk, not nightly	Often 7×/wk
Short-acting β-agonist for symptoms	≤ 2 day/wk	≥ 2 day/wk, but not > 1×/day	Daily	Several times daily
Interference with normal activity	None	Minor limitation	Some limitation	Extremely limited
Lung function	Normal between exacerbations			
• FEV_1	> 80% predicted	≥ 80% predicted	60–80% predicted	< 60% predicted
• FEV_1/FVC	Normal	Normal	Reduced 5%	Reduced > 5%

FEV = forced expiratory volume; FVC = forced vital capacity.
From National Heart, Lung, and Blood Institute, 2007.

maintains arterial Po_2 within a normal range while causing the Pco_2 to decrease with resultant respiratory alkalosis. As airway narrowing worsens, ventilation–perfusion defects increase, and arterial hypoxemia ensues. With severe obstruction, ventilation becomes impaired as fatigue causes early CO_2 retention. Because of hyperventilation, this may only be seen initially as an arterial Pco_2 returning to the normal range. With continuing obstruction, respiratory failure follows from fatigue.

Although these changes are generally reversible and well tolerated by the healthy nonpregnant individual, even early asthma stages may be dangerous for the pregnant woman and her fetus. This is because smaller functional residual capacity and increased pulmonary shunting render the woman more susceptible to hypoxia and hypoxemia.

Effects of Pregnancy on Asthma

There is no evidence that pregnancy has a predictable effect on underlying asthma. In their review of six prospective studies of more than 2000 pregnant women, Gluck and Gluck (2006) reported that approximately a third each improved, remained unchanged, or clearly worsened. Exacerbations are more common with severe disease (Ali, 2013). In a study by Schatz and associates (2003), baseline severity correlated with asthma morbidity during pregnancy. With mild disease, 13 percent of women had an exacerbation and 2.3 percent required admission; with moderate disease, these numbers were 26 and 7 percent; and for severe asthma, 52 and 27 percent. Others have reported similar observations (Charlton, 2013; Hendler, 2006; Murphy, 2005). Carroll and colleagues (2005) reported disparate morbidity in black compared with white women.

Some women have asthma exacerbations during labor and delivery. Up to 20 percent of women with mild or moderate asthma have been reported to have an intrapartum exacerbation (Schatz, 2003). Conversely, Wendel and associates (1996) reported exacerbations at the time of delivery in only 1 percent of women. Mabie and coworkers (1992) reported an 18-fold increased exacerbation risk following cesarean versus vaginal delivery.

Pregnancy Outcome

Women with asthma have had improved pregnancy outcomes during the past 20 years. From his review, Dombrowski (2006) concluded that, unless disease is severe, pregnancy outcomes are generally excellent. The incidence of spontaneous abortion in women with asthma may be slightly increased (Blais, 2013). Maternal and perinatal outcomes for nearly 30,000 pregnancies in asthmatic women are shown in Table 51-2. Findings are not consistent among these studies. For example, in some, but not all, incidences of preeclampsia, preterm labor, growth-restricted infants, and perinatal mortality are slightly increased (Murphy, 2011). Another report cited a small rise in the incidence of placental abruption and in preterm rupture of membranes (Getahun, 2006, 2007). But, in a European report of 37,585 pregnancies of women with asthma, the risks for most obstetrical complications were not increased (Tata, 2007). In the Canadian study in which inhaled-corticosteroid dosage was quantified, Cossette and coworkers (2013) found a nonsignificant trend between perinatal complications and increasing dosage. They concluded that low to moderate doses were not associated with perinatal risks and noted that more data were needed regarding higher doses.

Thus, there appears to be significantly increased morbidity linked to severe disease, poor control, or both. In the study by the Maternal-Fetal Medicine Units (MFMU) Network, delivery before 37 weeks' gestation was not increased among the 1687 pregnancies of asthmatics compared with those of 881 controls (Dombrowski, 2004a). But for women with severe asthma, the rate was increased approximately twofold. In a prospective evaluation of 656 asthmatic pregnant women and 1052 pregnant controls, Triche and coworkers (2004) found that women with moderate to severe asthma, regardless of treatment, are at increased risk of preeclampsia. Finally, the MFMU Network study suggests a direct relationship of baseline pregnancy forced expiratory volume at 1 second (FEV_1) with birthweight and an inverse relationship with rates of gestational hypertension and preterm delivery (Schatz, 2006).

Life-threatening complications from status asthmaticus include muscle fatigue with respiratory arrest, pneumothorax, pneumomediastinum, acute cor pulmonale, and cardiac arrhythmias.

TABLE 51-2. Maternal and Perinatal Outcomes in Pregnancies Complicated by Asthma

		Perinatal Outcomes (%)		
Study	No.	Gestational Hypertension[a]	Growth Restriction	Preterm Delivery
Liu (2001)	2193	13	12	10
Ramsey (2003)	1381	NS	1.7	Not ↑[b]
Dombrowski (2004a)	1739	12.2[b]	7.1[b]	16[b]
Mendola (2013)	17,044	10.2[c]	NS	14.8[c]
Cossette (2013)	7376	NS	13.5[c]	9.5[c]
Approximate average	29,733	~ 11	~ 11	~ 13

[a]Includes preeclampsia syndromes.
[b]Incidence not significantly different compared with control group or general obstetrical population.
[c]Incidence significantly greater than control group or general obstetrical population.
NS = not stated.

Maternal and perinatal mortality rates are substantively increased when mechanical ventilation is required.

Fetal Effects

With reasonable asthma control, perinatal outcomes are generally good. For example, in the MFMU Network study cited above, there were no significant adverse neonatal sequelae from asthma (Dombrowski, 2004a). The caveat is that severe asthma was uncommon in this closely monitored group. When respiratory alkalosis develops, both animal and human studies suggest that fetal hypoxemia develops well before the alkalosis compromises maternal oxygenation (Rolston, 1974). It is hypothesized that the fetus is jeopardized by decreased uterine blood flow, decreased maternal venous return, and an alkaline-induced leftward shift of the oxyhemoglobin dissociation curve.

The fetal response to maternal hypoxemia is decreased umbilical blood flow, increased systemic and pulmonary vascular resistance, and decreased cardiac output. Observations by Bracken and colleagues (2003) confirm that the incidence of fetal-growth restriction increases with asthma severity. The realization that the fetus may be seriously compromised as asthma severity increases underscores the need for aggressive management. Monitoring the fetal response is, in effect, an indicator of maternal status.

Possible teratogenic or adverse fetal effects of drugs given to control asthma have been a concern. Fortunately, considerable data have accrued with no evidence that commonly used antiasthmatic drugs are harmful (Blais, 2007; Källén, 2007; Namazy, 2006). Thus, it is worrisome that Enriquez and coworkers (2006) reported a 13- to 54-percent patient-generated decrease in β-agonist and corticosteroid use between 5 and 13 weeks' gestation.

Clinical Evaluation

The subjective severity of asthma frequently does not correlate with objective measures of airway function or ventilation. Although clinical examination can also be an inaccurate predictor, useful clinical signs include labored breathing, tachycardia, pulsus paradoxus, prolonged expiration, and use of accessory muscles. Signs of a potentially fatal attack include central cyanosis and altered consciousness.

Arterial blood gas analysis provides objective assessment of maternal oxygenation, ventilation, and acid-base status. With this information, the severity of an acute attack can be assessed (see Fig. 51-1). That said, in a prospective evaluation, Wendel and associates (1996) found that *routine* arterial blood gas analysis did not help to manage most pregnant women who required admission for asthma control. If used, the results must be interpreted in relation to normal values for pregnancy. For example, a $Pco_2 > 35$ mm Hg with a $pH < 7.35$ is consistent with hyperventilation and CO_2 retention in a pregnant woman.

Pulmonary function testing should be routine in the management of chronic and acute asthma. Sequential measurement of the FEV_1 or the *peak expiratory flow rate—PEFR*—are the best measures of severity. An FEV_1 less than 1 L, or less than 20 percent of predicted value, correlates with severe disease defined by hypoxia, poor response to therapy, and a high relapse rate. The PEFR correlates well with the FEV_1, and it can be measured reliably with inexpensive portable meters. Each woman determines her own baseline when asymptomatic—*personal best*—to compare with values when symptomatic. The PEFR does not change during the course of normal pregnancy (Brancazio, 1997).

Management of Chronic Asthma

The management guidelines of the Working Group on Asthma and Pregnancy include:

1. Patient education—general asthma management and its effect on pregnancy
2. Environmental precipitating factors—avoidance or control. Viral infections—including the common cold—are frequent triggering events (Murphy, 2013).
3. Objective assessment of pulmonary function and fetal well-being—monitor with PEFR or FEV_1
4. Pharmacological therapy—in appropriate combinations and doses to provide baseline control and treat exacerbations. Compliance may be a problem, and periodic medication reviews are helpful (Sawicki, 2012).

In general, women with moderate to severe asthma should measure and record either their FEV_1 or PEFR twice daily. The FEV_1 ideally is > 80 percent of predicted. For PEFR, predicted values range from 380 to 550 L/min. Each woman has her own baseline value, and therapeutic adjustments can be made using this (American College of Obstetricians and Gynecologists, 2012; Rey, 2007).

Treatment depends on disease severity. Although β-agonists help to abate bronchospasm, corticosteroids treat the inflammatory component. Regimens recommended for outpatient management are listed in Figure 51-2. For mild asthma, inhaled *β-agonists* as needed are usually sufficient. For persistent asthma, *inhaled corticosteroids* are administered every 3 to 4 hours. The goal is to reduce the use of β-agonists for symptomatic relief. A case-control study from Canada with a cohort of more than 15,600 nonpregnant women with asthma showed that inhaled corticosteroids reduced hospitalizations by 80 percent (Blais, 1998). And Wendel and colleagues (1996) achieved

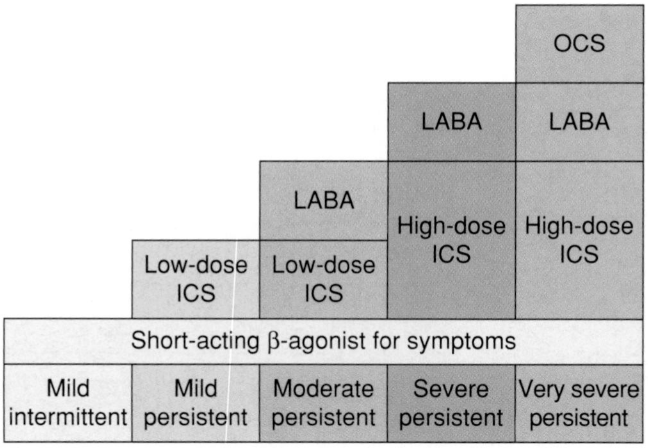

FIGURE 51-2 Stepwise approach to asthma treatment. ICS = inhaled corticosteroids; LABA = long-acting β-agonists; OCS = oral corticosteroids. (Modified from Barnes, 2012.)

a 55-percent reduction in readmissions for severe exacerbations in pregnant asthmatics given maintenance inhaled corticosteroids along with β-agonist therapy.

Theophylline is a methylxanthine, and its various salts are bronchodilators and possibly antiinflammatory agents. They have been used less frequently since inhaled corticosteroids became available. Some theophylline derivatives are considered useful for oral maintenance therapy if the initial response to inhaled corticosteroids and β-agonists is not optimal. Dombrowski and associates (2004b) conducted a randomized trial with nearly 400 pregnant women with moderate asthma. Oral theophylline was compared with inhaled beclomethasone for maintenance. In both groups, approximately 20 percent had exacerbations. Women taking theophylline had a significantly higher discontinuation rate because of side effects. Pregnancy outcomes were similar in the two groups.

Antileukotrienes inhibit leukotriene synthesis and include *zileuton, zafirlukast,* and *montelukast.* These drugs are given orally or by inhalation for prevention, but they are not effective for acute disease. For maintenance, they are used in conjunction with inhaled corticosteroids to allow minimal dosing. Approximately half of asthmatics will improve with these drugs (McFadden, 2005). They are not as effective as inhaled corticosteroids (Fanta, 2009). Finally, there is little experience with their use in pregnancy (Bakhireva, 2007).

Cromones include *cromolyn* and *nedocromil,* which inhibit mast cell degranulation. They are ineffective for acute asthma and are taken chronically for prevention. They are not as effective as inhaled corticosteroids and are used primarily to treat childhood asthma.

Management of Acute Asthma

Treatment of acute asthma during pregnancy is similar to that for the nonpregnant asthmatic (Barnes, 2012). However, the threshold for hospitalization is significantly lowered. Intravenous hydration may help clear pulmonary secretions, and supplemental oxygen is given by mask. The therapeutic aim is to maintain the $Po_2 > 60$ mm Hg, and preferably normal, along with 95-percent oxygen saturation. Baseline pulmonary function testing includes FEV_1 or PEFR. Continuous pulse oximetry and electronic fetal monitoring, depending on gestational age, may provide useful information.

First-line therapy for acute asthma includes a *β-adrenergic agonist,* such as terbutaline, albuterol, isoetharine, epinephrine, isoproterenol, or metaproterenol, which is given subcutaneously, taken orally, or inhaled. These drugs bind to specific cell-surface receptors and activate adenylyl cyclase to increase intracellular cyclic AMP and modulate bronchial smooth muscle relaxation. Long-acting preparations are used for outpatient therapy.

If not previously given for maintenance, inhaled corticosteroids are commenced along with intensive β-agonist therapy. For severe exacerbations, magnesium sulfate may prove efficacious. *Corticosteroids should be given early to all patients with severe acute asthma.* Unless there is a timely response to bronchodilator and inhaled corticosteroid therapy, oral or parenteral corticosteroids are given (Lazarus, 2010). Intravenous methylprednisolone, 40 to 60 mg, every 6 hours for four doses is commonly used. Equipotent doses of hydrocortisone by infusion or prednisone orally can be given instead. *Because their onset of action is several hours, corticosteroids are given initially along with β-agonists for acute asthma.*

Further management depends on the response to therapy. If initial therapy with β-agonists is associated with improvement of FEV_1 or PEFR to above 70 percent of baseline, then discharge can be considered. Some women may benefit from observation. Alternatively, for the woman with obvious respiratory distress, or if the FEV_1 or PEFR is < 70 percent of predicted after three doses of β-agonist, admission is likely advisable (Lazarus, 2010). Intensive therapy includes inhaled β-agonists, intravenous corticosteroids, and close observation for worsening respiratory distress or fatigue in breathing (Wendel, 1996). The woman is cared for in the delivery unit or an intermediate or intensive care unit (ICU) (Dombrowski, 2006; Zeeman, 2003).

Status Asthmaticus and Respiratory Failure

Severe asthma of any type not responding after 30 to 60 minutes of intensive therapy is termed status asthmaticus. Braman and Kaemmerlen (1990) have shown that management of nonpregnant patients with status asthmaticus in an intensive care setting results in a good outcome in most cases. Consideration should be given to early intubation when maternal respiratory status worsens despite aggressive treatment (see Fig. 51-1). Fatigue, carbon dioxide retention, and hypoxemia are indications for mechanical ventilation. Lo and colleagues (2013) have described a woman with status asthmaticus in whom cesarean delivery was necessary to effect ventilation. Andrews (2013) cautioned that such clinical situations are uncommon.

Labor and Delivery

For the laboring asthmatic, maintenance medications are continued through delivery. Stress-dose corticosteroids are administered to any woman given systemic corticosteroid therapy within the preceding 4 weeks. The usual dose is 100 mg of hydrocortisone given intravenously every 8 hours during labor and for 24 hours after delivery. The PEFR or FEV_1 should be determined on admission, and serial measurements are taken if symptoms develop.

Oxytocin or prostaglandins E_1 or E_2 are used for cervical ripening and induction. A nonhistamine-releasing narcotic such as fentanyl may be preferable to meperidine for labor, and epidural analgesia is ideal. For surgical delivery, conduction analgesia is preferred because tracheal intubation can trigger severe bronchospasm. Postpartum hemorrhage is treated with oxytocin or prostaglandin E_2. *Prostaglandin $F_{2\alpha}$ or ergotamine derivatives are contraindicated because they may cause significant bronchospasm.*

ACUTE BRONCHITIS

Infection of the large airways is manifest by cough without pneumonitis. It is common in adults, especially in winter months. Infections are usually caused by viruses, and of these, influenza A and B, parainfluenza, respiratory syncytial, coronavirus, adenovirus, and rhinovirus are frequent isolates (Wenzel, 2006). Bacterial agents causing community-acquired pneumonia are rarely implicated. The cough of acute bronchitis persists for 10 to 20 days (mean 18 days) and occasionally lasts for a month or longer. According to the 2006 guidelines of the American College of Chest Physicians, routine antibiotic treatment is not justified (Braman, 2006). Influenza bronchitis is managed as discussed below.

PNEUMONIA

According to Anand and Kollef (2009), current classification includes several types of pneumonia. *Community-acquired pneumonia (CAP)* is typically encountered in otherwise healthy young women, including during pregnancy. *Health-care-associated pneumonia (HCAP)* develops in patients in outpatient care facilities and more closely resembles *hospital-acquired pneumonia (HAP)*. Other types are *nursing home-acquired pneumonia (NHAO)* and *ventilator-associated pneumonia (VAP)*.

Community-acquired pneumonia in pregnant women is relatively common and is caused by several bacterial or viral pathogens (Brito, 2011; Sheffield, 2009). Gazmararian and coworkers (2002) reported that pneumonia accounts for 4.2 percent of antepartum admissions for nonobstetrical complications. Pneumonia is also a frequent indication for postpartum readmission (Belfort, 2010). During influenza season, admission rates for respiratory illnesses double compared with rates in the remaining months (Cox, 2006). Mortality from pneumonia is infrequent in young women, but during pregnancy severe pneumonitis with appreciable loss of ventilatory capacity is not as well tolerated (Rogers, 2010). This generalization seems to hold true regardless of the pneumonia etiology. Hypoxemia and acidosis are also poorly tolerated by the fetus and frequently stimulate preterm labor after midpregnancy. Because many cases of pneumonia follow viral upper respiratory illnesses, worsening or persistence of symptoms may represent developing pneumonia. *Any pregnant woman suspected of having pneumonia should undergo chest radiography.*

Bacterial Pneumonia

Many bacteria that cause community-acquired pneumonia, such as *Streptococcus pneumoniae*, are part of the normal resident flora (Bogaert, 2004). Some factors that perturb the symbiotic relationship between colonizing bacteria and mucosal phagocytic defenses include acquisition of a virulent strain or bacterial infections following a viral infection. Cigarette smoking and chronic bronchitis favor colonization with *S pneumoniae*, *Haemophilus influenzae*, and *Legionella* species. Other risk factors include asthma, binge drinking, and human immunodeficiency virus (HIV) infection (Goodnight, 2005; Sheffield, 2009).

Incidence and Causes

Pregnancy itself does not predispose to pneumonia. Jin and colleagues (2003) reported the antepartum hospitalization rate for pneumonia in Alberta, Canada, to be 1.5 per 1000 deliveries—almost identical to the rate of 1.47 per 1000 for nonpregnant women. Likewise, Yost and associates (2000) reported an incidence of 1.5 per 1000 for pneumonia complicating 75,000 pregnancies cared for at Parkland Hospital. More than half of adult pneumonias are bacterial, and *S pneumoniae* is the most common cause. Lim and coworkers (2001) studied 267 nonpregnant inpatients with pneumonia and identified a causative agent in 75 percent—*S pneumoniae* in 37 percent; influenza A, 14 percent; *Chlamydophila pneumoniae*, 10 percent; *H influenzae*, 5 percent; and *Mycoplasma pneumoniae* and *Legionella pneumophila*, 2 percent each. More recently, community-acquired methicillin-resistant *Staphylococcus aureus* (CA-MRSA) has emerged as the second most common pathogen in nonpregnant adults (Moran, 2013). These staphylococci may cause necrotizing pneumonia (Mandell, 2012; Rotas, 2007).

Diagnosis

Typical symptoms include cough, dyspnea, sputum production, and pleuritic chest pain. Mild upper respiratory symptoms and malaise usually precede these symptoms, and mild leukocytosis is usually present. Chest radiography is essential for diagnosis but does not accurately predict the etiology (Fig. 51-3). The responsible pathogen is identified in fewer than half of cases. According to the Infectious Diseases Society of America (IDSA) and the American Thoracic Society (ATS), tests to identify a specific agent are optional. Thus, sputum cultures, serological testing, cold agglutinin identification, and tests for bacterial antigens are not recommended. At Parkland Hospital, the one exception to this is rapid serological testing for influenza A and B (Sheffield, 2009).

Management

Although many otherwise healthy young adults can be safely treated as outpatients, at Parkland Hospital we hospitalize all pregnant women with radiographically proven pneumonia. For some, outpatient therapy or 23-hour observation is reasonable with optimal follow-up. Risk factors shown in Table 51-3 should prompt hospitalization.

With severe disease, admission to an ICU or intermediate care unit is advisable. Approximately 20 percent of pregnant

TABLE 51-3. Criteria for Severe Community-Acquired Pneumonia[a]

Respiratory rate ≥ 30/min
Pao_2/Fio_2 ratio ≤ 250
Multilobular infiltrates
Confusion/disorientation
Uremia
Leukopenia—WBC < 4000/μL
Thrombocytopenia—platelets < 100,000/μL
Hypothermia—core temperature < 36°C
Hypotension requiring aggressive fluid resuscitation

[a]Criteria of the Infectious Diseases Society of America/American Thoracic Society.
WBC = white blood cell.
Adapted from Mandell, 2007.

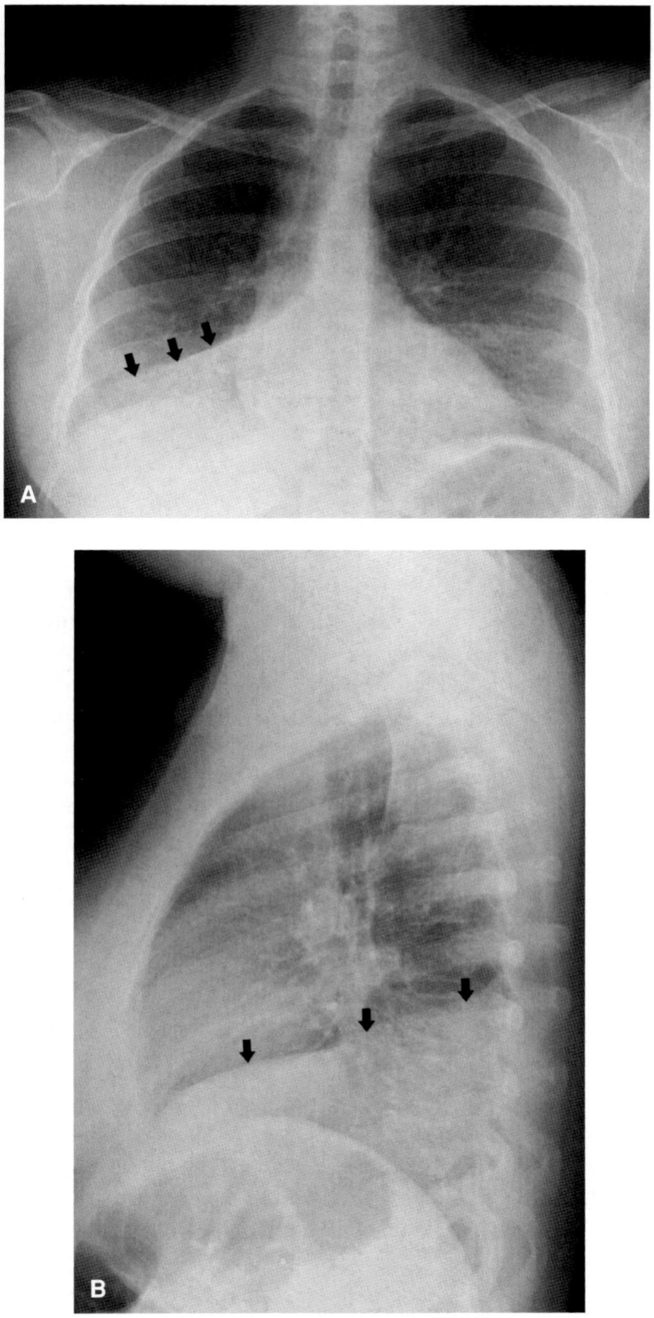

FIGURE 51-3 Chest radiographs in a pregnant woman with right lower lobe pneumonia. **A.** Complete opacification of the right lower lobe (*arrows*) is consistent with the clinical suspicion of pneumonia. **B.** Opacification (*arrows*) is also seen on the lateral projection.

women admitted to Parkland Hospital for pneumonia require this level of care (Zeeman, 2003). Severe pneumonia is a relatively common cause of acute respiratory distress syndrome during pregnancy, and mechanical ventilation may become necessary. Indeed, of the 51 pregnant women who required mechanical ventilation in the review by Jenkins and coworkers (2003), 12 percent had pneumonia.

Antimicrobial treatment is empirical (Mandell, 2012). Because most adult pneumonias are caused by pneumococci, mycoplasma, or chlamydophila, monotherapy initially is with a macrolide—azithromycin, clarithromycin, or erythromycin. Yost and colleagues (2000) reported that erythromycin monotherapy, given intravenously and then orally, was effective in all but one of 99 pregnant women with uncomplicated pneumonia.

For women with severe disease according to criteria in Table 51-3, Mandell and associates (2007) summarized IDSA/ATS guidelines, which call for either: (1) a respiratory fluoroquinolone—levofloxacin, moxifloxacin, or gemifloxacin; or (2) a macrolide plus a β-lactam—high-dose amoxicillin or amoxicillin-clavulanate, which are preferred β-lactams. β-lactam alternatives include ceftriaxone, cefpodoxime, or cefuroxime. In areas in which there is "high-level" resistance of pneumococcal isolates to macrolides, these latter regimens are preferred. The teratogenicity risk of fluoroquinolones is low, and these should be given if indicated (Briggs, 2011). If community-acquired methicillin-resistant *S aureus* is suspected, then vancomycin or linezolid are added (Mandell, 2012; Sheffield, 2009). At this time, such therapy is empirical, and there are no tested regimens against CA-MRSA (Moran, 2013).

Clinical improvement is usually evident in 48 to 72 hours with resolution of fever in 2 to 4 days. Radiographic abnormalities may take up to 6 weeks to completely resolve (Torres, 2008). Worsening disease is a poor prognostic feature, and follow-up radiography is recommended if fever persists. Even with improvement, however, approximately 20 percent of women develop a pleural effusion. Pneumonia treatment is recommended for a minimum of 5 days. Treatment failure may occur in up to 15 percent of cases, and a wider antimicrobial regimen and more extensive diagnostic testing are warranted in these cases.

Pregnancy Outcome with Pneumonia

During the preantimicrobial era, as many as a third of pregnant women with pneumonia died (Finland, 1939). Although much improved, maternal and perinatal mortality rates both remain formidable. In five studies published after 1990, the maternal mortality rate was 0.8 percent of 632 women. Importantly, almost 7 percent of the women required intubation and mechanical ventilation.

Prematurely ruptured membranes and preterm delivery are frequent complications and have been reported in up to a third of cases (Getahun, 2007; Shariatzadeh, 2006). Likely related are older studies reporting a twofold increase in low-birthweight infants (Sheffield, 2009). In a more recent population-based study from Taiwan of nearly 219,000 births, there were significantly increased incidences of preterm and growth-restricted infants as well as preeclampsia and cesarean delivery (Chen, 2012).

Prevention

Pneumococcal vaccine is 60- to 70-percent protective against its 23 included serotypes. Its use has been shown to decrease emergence of drug-resistant pneumococci (Kyaw, 2006). The vaccine is not recommended for otherwise healthy pregnant women (American College of Obstetricians and Gynecologists, 2013). It is recommended for those who are immunocompromised, including those with HIV infection; significant smoking history; diabetes; cardiac, pulmonary, or renal disease; and asplenia, such as with sickle-cell disease (Table 9-9, p. 185). Protection against pneumococcal infection in women with chronic diseases may be less efficacious than in healthy patients (Moberley, 2013).

Influenza Pneumonia

Clinical Presentation

Influenza A and B are RNA viruses that cause respiratory infection, including pneumonitis. Influenza pneumonia can be serious, and it is epidemic in the winter months. The virus is spread by aerosolized droplets and quickly infects ciliated columnar epithelium, alveolar cells, mucus gland cells, and macrophages. Disease onset is 1 to 4 days following exposure (Longman, 2007). In most healthy adults, infection is self-limited.

Pneumonia is the most frequent complication of influenza, and it is difficult to distinguish from bacterial pneumonia. According to the Centers for Disease Control and Prevention (2010a), infected pregnant women are more likely to be hospitalized as well as admitted to an ICU. At Parkland Hospital during the 2003 to 2004 influenza season, pneumonia developed in 12 percent of pregnant women with influenza (Rogers, 2010). The 2009 influenza pandemic with the H1N1 strain was particularly severe. In a Maternal-Fetal Medicine Units Network study, 10 percent of pregnant or postpartum women admitted with H1N1 influenza were cared for in an ICU, and 11 percent of these ICU patients died (Varner, 2011). Risk factors included late pregnancy, smoking, and chronic hypertension. In California, 22 percent of H1N1-infected women required intensive care, and a third of these died.

Primary influenza pneumonitis is the most severe and is characterized by sparse sputum production and radiographic interstitial infiltrates. More commonly, secondary pneumonia develops from bacterial superinfection by streptococci or staphylococci after 2 to 3 days of initial clinical improvement. The Centers for Disease Control and Prevention (2007b) reported several cases in which CA-MRSA caused influenza-associated pneumonitis with a case-fatality rate of 25 percent. Other possible adverse effects of influenza A and B on pregnancy outcome are discussed in Chapter 64 (p. 1241).

Management

Supportive treatment with antipyretics and bed rest is recommended for uncomplicated influenza. Early antiviral treatment has been shown to be effective (Jamieson, 2011). As discussed, influenza hospitalizations for those with advanced pregnancy are increased compared with nonpregnant women (Dodds, 2007; Schanzer, 2007). Rapid resistance of influenza A (H3N2) strains to amantadine or rimantadine in 2005 prompted the Centers for Disease Control and Prevention (2006) to recommend against their use. Instead, neuraminidase inhibitors were given within 2 days of symptom onset for chemoprophylaxis and treatment of influenza A and B (Chap. 64, p. 1242). The drugs interfere with release of progeny virus from infected host cells and thus prevent infection of new host cells (Moscona, 2005). Oseltamivir is given orally, 75 mg twice daily, or zanamivir is given by inhalation, 10 mg twice daily. Recommended treatment duration with either is 5 days. The drugs shorten the course of illness by 1 to 2 days, and they may reduce the risk for pneumonitis (Jamieson, 2011). Our practice is to treat all pregnant women with influenza whether or not pneumonitis is identified. There are few data regarding use of these agents in pregnant women, but the drugs were not teratogenic in animal studies and are considered low risk (Briggs, 2011).

Other concerns for viral resistance are for avian H5N1 and H7N9 strains isolated in Southeast Asia. These are candidate viruses for an influenza pandemic with a projected mortality rate that exceeds 50 percent (Beigi, 2007; World Health Organization, 2008). Currently, international efforts are being made to produce a vaccine effective against both strains.

Preventively, vaccination for influenza A is recommended and is discussed in detail in Chapter 64 (p. 1242). Prenatal vaccination also affords protection for a third of infants for at least 6 months (Zaman, 2008). During the 2012–2013 flu season, the Centers for Disease Control and Prevention (2013b) reported that only half of pregnant women received the vaccine.

Varicella Pneumonia

Infection with varicella-zoster virus—chicken pox—results in pneumonitis in 5 percent of pregnant women (Harger, 2002). Diagnosis and management are considered in Chapter 64 (p. 1240).

Fungal and Parasitic Pneumonia

Pneumocystis Pneumonia

Fungal and parasitic pulmonary infections are usually of greatest consequence in immunocompromised hosts, especially in women with acquired immunodeficiency syndrome (AIDS). Of these, lung infection with *Pneumocystis jiroveci*, formerly called *Pneumocystis carinii*, is a common complication in women with AIDS. The opportunistic fungus causes interstitial pneumonia characterized by dry cough, tachypnea, dyspnea, and diffuse radiographic infiltrates. Although this organism can be identified by sputum culture, bronchoscopy with lavage or biopsy may be necessary.

In a report from the AIDS Clinical Trials Centers, Stratton and colleagues (1992) described pneumocystis pneumonia as the most frequent HIV-related disorder in pregnant women. Ahmad and coworkers (2001) reviewed 22 cases during pregnancy and cited a 50-percent mortality rate. Treatment is with trimethoprim-sulfamethoxazole or the more toxic pentamidine (Walzer, 2005). Experience with dapsone or atovaquone is limited. In some cases, tracheal intubation and mechanical ventilation may be required.

As prophylaxis, several international health agencies recommend one double-strength trimethoprim-sulfamethoxazole tablet orally daily for certain HIV-infected pregnant women. These include women with $CD4^+$ T-lymphocyte counts

< 200/μL, those whose CD4⁺ T lymphocytes constitute less than 14 percent, or if there is an AIDS-defining illness, particularly oropharyngeal candidiasis (Centers for Disease Control and Prevention, 2013a; Forna, 2006).

Fungal Pneumonia

Any of a number of fungi can cause pneumonia. In pregnancy, this is usually seen in women with HIV infection or who are otherwise immunocompromised. Infection is usually mild and self-limited. It is characterized initially by cough and fever, and dissemination is infrequent.

Histoplasmosis and *blastomycosis* do not appear to be more common or more severe during pregnancy. Data concerning *coccidioidomycosis* are conflicting (Bercovitch, 2011; Patel, 2013). In a case-control study from an endemic area, Rosenstein and coworkers (2001) reported that pregnancy was a significant risk factor for disseminated disease. In another study, however, Caldwell and coworkers (2000) identified 32 serologically confirmed cases during pregnancy and documented dissemination in only three cases. Arsura (1998) and Caldwell (2000) and their associates reported that pregnant women with symptomatic infection had a better overall prognosis if there was associated *erythema nodosum*. Crum and Ballon-Landa (2006) reviewed 80 cases of coccidioidomycosis complicating pregnancy. Almost all women diagnosed in the third trimester had disseminated disease. Although the overall maternal mortality rate was 40 percent, it was only 20 percent for 29 cases reported since 1973. Spinello (2007) and Bercovitch (2011), with their associates, have provided reviews of coccidioidomycosis in pregnancy.

Most cases of *cryptococcosis* reported during pregnancy have been reported to manifest as meningitis. Ely and colleagues (1998) described four otherwise healthy pregnant women with cryptococcal pneumonia. Diagnosis is difficult because clinical presentation is similar to that of other community-acquired pneumonias.

The 2007 IDSA/ATS guidelines recommend itraconazole as preferred therapy for disseminated fungal infections (Mandell, 2007). Pregnant women have also been given intravenous *amphotericin B* or *ketoconazole* (Hooper, 2007; Paranyuk, 2006). Amphotericin B has been used extensively in pregnancy with no embryo-fetal effects. Because of evidence that fluconazole, itraconazole, and ketoconazole may be embryotoxic in large doses in early pregnancy, Briggs and associates (2011) recommend that first-trimester use should be avoided if possible.

Three echinocandin derivatives—*caspofungin*, *micafungin*, and *anidulafungin*—are effective for invasive candidiasis (Medical Letter, 2006; Reboli, 2007). They are embryotoxic and teratogenic in laboratory animals and use in human pregnancies has not been reported (Briggs, 2011).

Severe Acute Respiratory Syndrome (SARS)

This coronaviral respiratory infection was first identified in China in 2002, but no new cases have been reported since 2005. It caused atypical pneumonitis with a case-fatality rate of approximately 10 percent (Dolin, 2012). SARS in pregnancy had a case-fatality rate of up to 25 percent (Lam, 2004; Longman, 2007; Wong, 2004). Ng and coworkers (2006) reported that the placentas from 7 of 19 cases showed abnormal intervillous or subchorionic fibrin deposition in three, and extensive fetal thrombotic vasculopathy in two.

TUBERCULOSIS

Although tuberculosis is still a major worldwide concern, it is uncommon in the United States. The incidence of *active tuberculosis* in this country has plateaued since 2000 (Raviglione, 2012). More than half of active cases are in immigrants (Centers for Disease Control and Prevention, 2009b). Persons born in the United States have newly acquired infection, whereas foreign-born persons usually have reactivation of latent infection. In this country, tuberculosis is a disease of the elderly, the urban poor, minority groups—especially black Americans, and patients with HIV infection (Raviglione, 2012).

Infection is via inhalation of *Mycobacterium tuberculosis*, which incites a granulomatous pulmonary reaction. In more than 90 percent of patients, infection is contained and is dormant for long periods (Zumla, 2013). In some patients, especially those who are immunocompromised or who have other diseases, tuberculosis becomes reactivated to cause clinical disease. Manifestations usually include cough with minimal sputum production, low-grade fever, hemoptysis, and weight loss. Various infiltrative patterns are seen on chest radiograph, and there may be associated cavitation or mediastinal lymphadenopathy. Acid-fast bacilli are seen on stained smears of sputum in approximately two thirds of culture-positive patients. Forms of extrapulmonary tuberculosis include lymphadenitis, pleural, genitourinary, skeletal, meningeal, gastrointestinal, and miliary or disseminated (Raviglione, 2012).

Treatment

Cure rates with 6-month short-course *directly observed therapy*—DOT—approach 90 percent for new infections. Resistance to antituberculosis drugs was first manifest in the United States in the early 1990s following the epidemic from 1985 through 1992 (Centers for Disease Control and Prevention, 2007a). Strains of *multidrug-resistant tuberculosis* (*MDR-TB*) increased rapidly as tuberculosis incidence fell during the 1990s. Because of this, the Centers for Disease Control and Prevention (2003) now recommends a multidrug regimen for initial empirical treatment of patients with symptomatic tuberculosis. Isoniazid, rifampin, pyrazinamide, and ethambutol are given until susceptibility studies are performed. Other second-line drugs may need to be added. Drug susceptibility is performed on all first isolates.

In 2005, there was a worldwide emergence of *extensively drug-resistant tuberculosis*—*XDR-TB*. This is defined as resistance in vitro to at least the first-line drugs isoniazid and rifampin as well as to three or more of the six main classes of second-line drugs—aminoglycosides, polypeptides, fluoroquinolones, thioamides, cycloserine, and *para*-aminosalicylic acid (Centers for Disease Control and Prevention,

2009a). Like their predecessor MDR-TB, these extensively resistant strains predominate in foreign-born persons (Tino, 2007).

Tuberculosis and Pregnancy

The considerable influx of women into the United States from Asia, Africa, Mexico, and Central America has been accompanied by an increased frequency of tuberculosis in pregnant women. Sackoff and coworkers (2006) reported positive-tuberculin tests in half of 678 foreign-born women attending perinatal clinics in New York City. Almost 60 percent were newly diagnosed. Pillay and colleagues (2004) stress the prevalence of tuberculosis in HIV-positive pregnant women. Margono and coworkers (1994) reported that for two New York City hospitals, more than half of pregnant women with active tuberculosis were HIV positive. At Jackson Memorial Hospital in Miami, Schulte and associates (2002) reported that 21 percent of 207 HIV-infected pregnant women had a positive skin test result. Recall also that silent endometrial tuberculosis can cause tubal infertility (Levison, 2010).

Without antituberculosis therapy, active tuberculosis appears to have adverse effects on pregnancy (Anderson, 1997; Mnyani, 2011). Contemporaneous experiences are few, however, because antitubercular therapy has diminished the frequency of severe disease. Outcomes are dependent on the site of infection and timing of diagnosis in relation to delivery. Jana and colleagues (1994) from India and Figueroa-Damian and Arrendondo-Garcia (1998) from Mexico City reported that active pulmonary tuberculosis was associated with increased incidences of preterm delivery, low-birthweight and growth-restricted infants, and perinatal mortality. From her review, Efferen (2007) cited twofold increased rates of low-birthweight and preterm infants as well as preeclampsia. The perinatal mortality rate was increased almost tenfold. Adverse outcomes correlate with late diagnosis, incomplete or irregular treatment, and advanced pulmonary lesions. From Taiwan, 761 pregnant women diagnosed with tuberculosis had a higher incidence of low-birthweight and growth-restricted infants (Lin, 2010).

Extrapulmonary tuberculosis is less common. Jana and coworkers (1999) reported outcomes in 33 pregnant women with renal, intestinal, and skeletal tuberculosis, and a third had low-birthweight newborns. Llewelyn and associates (2000) reported that nine of 13 pregnant women with extrapulmonary disease had delayed diagnoses. Prevost and Fung Kee Fung (1999) reviewed 56 cases of tuberculous meningitis in which a third of mothers died. Spinal tuberculosis may cause paraplegia, but vertebral fusion may prevent it from becoming permanent (Badve, 2011; Nanda, 2002). Other presentations include widespread intraperitoneal tuberculosis simulating ovarian carcinomatosis and degenerating leiomyoma, and hyperemesis gravidarum from tubercular meningitis (Kutlu, 2007; Moore, 2008; Sherer, 2005).

Diagnosis

There are two types of tests to detect latent or active tuberculosis. One is the time-honored *tuberculin skin test (TST),* and the others are *interferon-gamma release assays (IGRAs),* which are becoming preferred (Horsburgh, 2011). IGRAs are blood tests that measure interferon-gamma release in response to antigens present in *M tuberculosis*, but not bacille Calmette-Guérin (BCG) vaccine (Ernst, 2007; Levison, 2010). The Centers for Disease Control and Prevention (2005b, 2010b) recommend either skin testing or IGRA testing of pregnant women who are in any of the high-risk groups shown in Table 51-4. For those who received BCG vaccination, IGRA testing is used (Mazurek, 2010).

TABLE 51-4. Groups at High Risk for Having Latent Tuberculosis Infection

Health-care workers
Contact with infectious person(s)
Foreign-born
HIV-infected
Working or living in homeless shelters
Alcoholics
Illicit drug use
Detainees and prisoners

HIV = human immunodeficiency virus.
From the Centers for Disease Control and Prevention, 2005a.

For skin testing, the preferred antigen is purified protein derivative (PPD) of intermediate strength of 5 tuberculin units. If the intracutaneously applied test result is negative, no further evaluation is needed. A positive skin test result measures ≥ 5 mm in diameter and requires evaluation for active disease, including a chest radiograph (Centers for Disease Control and Prevention, 2005a, 2010b). It also may be interpreted according to risk factors proposed by the American Thoracic Society/Centers for Disease Control and Prevention (1990). For *very high-risk* patients—that is, those who are HIV-positive, those with abnormal chest radiography, or those who have a recent contact with an active case—5 mm or greater is considered a reason to treat. For those at *high risk*—foreign-born individuals, intravenous drug users who are HIV-negative, low-income populations, or those with medical conditions that increase the risk for tuberculosis—10 mm or greater is considered treatable. For persons with none of these risk factors, 15 mm or greater is defined as requiring treatment.

There are two IGRAs available: *QuantiFERON-TB Gold* and *T-SPOT.TB* tests are recommended by the Centers for Disease Control and Prevention (2005a,b) for the same indications as skin testing. These tests have not been evaluated as extensively as tuberculin skin testing. Lalvani (2007) reviewed them and found them to be useful in identifying patients with latent tuberculosis and at risk for progression to active disease. Kowada (2014) concluded that these tests are cost effective.

Essential laboratory methods for detection or verification of infection—both active and latent—include microscopy, culture, nucleic acid amplification assay, and drug-susceptibility testing (Centers for Disease Control and Prevention, 2009a, 2010b).

Treatment

Latent Infection. Different schemes are recommended for latent and active tuberculosis. In nonpregnant tuberculin-positive patients who are younger than 35 years and who have no evidence of active disease, isoniazid, 300 mg orally daily, is given for 9 months. Isoniazid has been used for decades, and it is considered safe in pregnancy (Briggs, 2011; Taylor, 2013). Compliance is a major problem, and Sackoff (2006) and Cruz (2005) and their associates reported a disappointing 10-percent treatment completion. One obvious disconnect is that care for tuberculosis is given in health systems different from prenatal care (Zenner, 2012). These observations are important because most recommend that isoniazid therapy be delayed until after delivery. Because of possibly increased isoniazid-induced hepatitis risk in postpartum women, some recommend withholding treatment until 3 to 6 months after delivery. That said, neither method is as effective as antepartum treatment to prevent active infection. Boggess and colleagues (2000) reported that only 42 percent of 167 tuberculin-positive asymptomatic women delivered at San Francisco General Hospital completed 6-month therapy that was not given until the first postpartum visit.

There are exceptions to delayed treatment in pregnancy. Known recent skin-test convertors are treated antepartum because the incidence of active infection is 5 percent in the first year (Zumla, 2013). Skin-test-positive women exposed to active infection are treated because the incidence of infection is 0.5 percent per year.

HIV-positive women are treated because they have an approximate 10-percent annual risk of active disease. Treatment of these women is of special concern if there is antiretroviral naiveté. In these circumstances, beginning concomitant therapy with antituberculosis and antiretroviral therapy can cause the *immune reconstitution inflammatory syndrome (IRIS)* with toxic drug effects (Török, 2011). Recent studies, however, support earlier administration of highly active antiretroviral therapy (HAART)—within 2 to 4 weeks—after beginning antituberculosis therapy (Blanc, 2011; Havlir, 2011; Karim, 2011).

Active Infection. Recommended initial treatment for active tuberculosis in pregnant patients is a four-drug regimen with isoniazid, rifampin, ethambutol, and pyrazinamide, along with pyridoxine. In the first 2-month phase, all four drugs are given—*bactericidal phase*. This is followed by a 4-month phase of isoniazid and rifampin—*continuation phase* (Raviglione, 2012; Zumla, 2013). Reports of MDR-TB during pregnancy are few, and Lessnau and Qarah (2003) and Shin and coworkers (2003) have reviewed treatment options. Breast feeding is not prohibited during antituberculous therapy.

As discussed above, beginning concomitant antituberculosis and antiretroviral therapy may cause the immune reconstitution inflammatory syndrome, and risks versus benefits are assessed. Also, for HIV-infected women, rifampin or rifabutin use may be contraindicated if certain protease inhibitors or nonnucleoside reverse transcriptase inhibitors are being administered. If there is resistance to rifabutin or rifampin, then pyrazinamide therapy is given. Of the second-line regimens, the aminoglycosides—streptomycin, kanamycin, amikacin, and capreomycin—are ototoxic to the fetus and are contraindicated (Briggs, 2011).

Neonatal Tuberculosis. Tubercular bacillemia can infect the placenta, but it is uncommon that the fetus becomes infected—*congenital tuberculosis*. The term also applies to newborns who are infected by aspiration of infected secretions at delivery. Each route of infection constitutes approximately half of the cases. A rare case of congenital tuberculosis caused by in vitro fertilization (IVF) was reported (Doudier, 2008). Neonatal tuberculosis simulates other congenital infections and manifests with hepatosplenomegaly, respiratory distress, fever, and lymphadenopathy (Smith, 2002).

Cantwell and associates (1994) reviewed 29 cases of congenital tuberculosis reported since 1980. Only 12 of the mothers had active infection, and tuberculosis was frequently demonstrated by postpartum endometrial biopsy. Adhikari and colleagues (1997) described 11 South African postpartum women whose endometrial biopsy was culture-positive. Six of their neonates had congenital tuberculosis.

Neonatal infection is unlikely if the mother with active disease has been treated before delivery or if her sputum culture is negative. Because the newborn is susceptible to tuberculosis, most authors recommend isolation from the mother suspected of having active disease. If untreated, the risk of disease in the infant born to a woman with active infection is 50 percent in the first year (Jacobs, 1988).

SARCOIDOSIS

Sarcoidosis is a chronic, multisystem disease of unknown etiology characterized by an accumulation of T lymphocytes and phagocytes within noncaseating granulomas (Baughman, 2012). Predisposition to the disease is genetically determined and characterized by an exaggerated response of helper T lymphocytes to environmental triggers (Moller, 2007; Spagnolo, 2007). Pulmonary involvement is most common, followed by skin, eyes, and lymph nodes. The prevalence of sarcoid in the United States is 20 to 60 per 100,000, with equal sex distribution, but it is 3 to 17 times more common for black compared with white persons (Baughman, 2012). Most patients are between 20 and 40 years. Clinical presentation varies, but more than half of patients have dyspnea and a dry cough without constitutional symptoms that develop insidiously over months. Disease onset is abrupt in about 25 percent of patients, and 10 to 20 percent are asymptomatic at discovery.

Pulmonary symptoms are dominant, and more than 90 percent of patients have an abnormal chest radiograph at some point (Lynch, 2007). *Interstitial pneumonitis* is the hallmark of pulmonary involvement. Approximately 50 percent of affected patients develop permanent radiological changes. *Lymphadenopathy*, especially of the mediastinum, is present in 75 to 90 percent of cases, and 25 percent have *uveitis*. A fourth have skin involvement, usually manifest as *erythema nodosum*. In women, sarcoid causes about 10 percent of cases of erythema nodosum (Acosta, 2013; Mert, 2007). Finally, any other organ system may be involved. Confirmation of the diagnosis is with biopsy, and because the lung may be the only obviously involved organ, tissue acquisition is often difficult.

The overall prognosis for sarcoidosis is good, and it resolves without treatment in 50 percent of patients. Still, there is diminished quality of life (de Vries, 2007). In the other 50 percent, permanent organ dysfunction, albeit mild and nonprogressive, persists. About 10 percent die because of their disease.

Glucocorticoids are the most widely used treatment, and methotrexate is second-line medication. Permanent organ derangement is seldom reversed by their use (Paramothayan, 2002). Thus, the decision to treat is based on symptoms, physical findings, chest radiograph, and pulmonary function tests. Unless respiratory symptoms are prominent, therapy is usually withheld for a several-month observation period. If inflammation does not subside, then prednisone, 1 mg/kg, is given daily for 4 to 6 weeks (Baughman, 2012). For those with an inadequate response, cytotoxic agents or cytokine modulators may be indicated.

Sarcoidosis and Pregnancy

Because sarcoidosis is uncommon and is frequently benign, it is not often seen in pregnancy. De Regt (1987) described 14 cases in 20,000 pregnancies during a 12-year period—almost 1 in 1500. Although sarcoidosis seldom affects pregnancy adversely, serious complications such as meningitis, heart failure, and neurosarcoidosis have been described (Cardonick, 2000; Maisel, 1996; Seballos, 1994).

In general, perinatal outcomes are unaffected by sarcoidosis. Selroos (1990) reviewed 655 patients with sarcoidosis referred to the Mjölbolsta Hospital District in Finland. Of 252 women between 18 and 50 years, 15 percent had sarcoidosis during pregnancy or within 1 year postpartum. There was no evidence for disease progression in the 26 pregnancies in women with active disease. Three aborted spontaneously, and the other 23 women were delivered at term. In 18 pregnancies in 12 women with inactive disease, pregnancy outcomes were good. Agha and coworkers (1982) reported similar experiences with 35 pregnancies at the University of Michigan.

Active sarcoidosis is treated using the same guidelines as for the woman who is not pregnant. Severe disease warrants serial determination of pulmonary function. Symptomatic uveitis, constitutional symptoms, and pulmonary symptoms are treated with prednisone, 1 mg/kg orally per day.

CYSTIC FIBROSIS

One of the most common fatal genetic disorders in whites, cystic fibrosis is caused by one of more than 1500 mutations in a 230-kb gene on the long arm of chromosome 7 that encodes an amino acid polypeptide (Boucher, 2012). This peptide functions as a chloride channel and is termed the *cystic fibrosis transmembrane conductance regulator (CFTR)*. There is a wide phenotypic variation, even among homozygotes for the common ΔF508 mutation (Rowntree, 2003). This is discussed in greater detail in Chapter 14 (p. 295). Approximately 20 percent of affected individuals are diagnosed shortly after birth because of *meconium peritonitis* (Boucher, 2012). Currently, nearly 80 percent of females with cystic fibrosis now survive to adulthood, and their median survival is about 30 years (Gillet, 2002).

Pathophysiology

Mutations in the chloride channel cause altered epithelial cell membrane transport of electrolytes. This affects all organs that express CFTR—secretory cells, sinuses, lung, pancreas, liver, and reproductive tract. Disease severity depends on which two alleles are inherited, and homozygosity for ΔF508 is one of the most severe (McKone, 2003).

Exocrine gland ductal obstruction develops from thick, viscid secretions (Rowe, 2005). In the lung, submucosal glandular ducts are affected. Eccrine sweat gland abnormalities are the basis for the diagnostic *sweat test*, characterized by elevated sodium, potassium, and chloride levels in sweat.

Lung involvement is commonplace and is frequently the cause of death. Bronchial gland hypertrophy with mucous plugging and small-airway obstruction leads to subsequent infection that ultimately causes chronic bronchitis and bronchiectasis. For complex and not completely explicable reasons, chronic inflammation from *Pseudomonas aeruginosa* occurs in more than 90 percent of patients. *S aureus, H influenzae,* and *Burkholderia cepacia* are recovered in a minority (Rowe, 2005). Colonization with the last has been reported to signify a worse prognosis, especially in pregnancy (Gillet, 2002). Acute and chronic parenchymal inflammation ultimately causes extensive fibrosis, and along with airway obstruction, there is a ventilation–perfusion mismatch. Pulmonary insufficiency is the end result. Lung or heart–lung transplantation has a 5-year survival rate of 33 percent (Aurora, 1999). A few women have successfully undergone pregnancy following lung transplantation (Kruszka, 2002; Shaner, 2012).

Preconceptional Counseling

Women with cystic fibrosis are subfertile because of tenacious cervical mucus. Males have oligospermia or aspermia from vas deferens obstruction, and 98 percent are infertile (Ahmad, 2013). Despite this, the North American Cystic Fibrosis Foundation estimates that 4 percent of affected women become pregnant every year (Edenborough, 1995). The endometrium and tubes express some CFTR but are functionally normal, and the ovaries do not express the *CFTR* gene (Edenborough, 2001). Both intrauterine insemination and IVF have been used successfully in affected women (Rodgers, 2000). Several ethical considerations of undertaking pregnancy by these women were reviewed by Wexler and colleagues (2007). For male infertility, Sobczyńska-Tomaszewska and associates (2006) have emphasized the importance of molecular diagnosis.

Screening

The American College of Obstetricians and Gynecologists (2011) recommends that carrier screening be offered to at-risk couples. This is discussed in detail in Chapter 14 (p. 295). The Centers for Disease Control and Prevention also added cystic fibrosis to newborn screening programs (Comeau, 2007). This is discussed also in Chapter 32 (p. 632) and was the subject of a Cochrane Database review (Southern, 2009).

Pregnancy with Cystic Fibrosis

Pregnancy outcome is inversely related to severity of lung dysfunction. Severe chronic lung disease, hypoxia, and frequent infections may prove deleterious. At least in the past, *cor pulmonale* was common, but even that does not preclude successful pregnancy (Cameron, 2005). In some women, *pancreatic dysfunction* may cause poor maternal nutrition. Normal pregnancy-induced insulin resistance frequently results in gestational diabetes after midpregnancy (Hardin, 2005; McMullen, 2006). In one study of 48 pregnancies, half had pancreatic insufficiency and a third required insulin (Thorpe-Beeson, 2013). Diabetes is most frequent with the ΔF508 homozygous mutation (Giacobbe, 2012).

Cystic fibrosis per se is not affected by pregnancy (Schechter, 2013). Early reports of a deleterious effect on the course of cystic fibrosis were related to severe disease (Olson, 1997). An important factor to be considered in childbearing is the long-term prognosis for the mother. When matched with nonpregnant women by disease severity, recent reports indicate no deleterious effects on long-term survival (McMullen, 2006; Schechter, 2013).

Management

Prepregnancy counseling is imperative. Women who choose to become pregnant should have close surveillance for development of superimposed infection, diabetes, and heart failure. They are followed closely with serial pulmonary function testing, for management as well as for prognosis. When the FEV_1 is at least 70 percent, women usually tolerate pregnancy well. Emphasis is placed on postural drainage, bronchodilator therapy, and infection control.

β-Adrenergic bronchodilators help control airway constriction. Inhaled recombinant human deoxyribonuclease I improves lung function by reducing sputum viscosity (Boucher, 2012). Inhaled 7-percent saline has been shown to produce short- and long-term benefits (Donaldson, 2006; Elkins, 2006). Nutritional status is assessed and appropriate dietary counseling given. Pancreatic insufficiency is treated with replacement of oral pancreatic enzyme.

Infection is heralded by increasing cough and mucus production. Oral semisynthetic penicillins or cephalosporins usually suffice to treat staphylococcal infections. *Pseudomonas* infection is most problematic in adults. Inhaled tobramycin and colistin have been used successfully to control this organism (Boucher, 2012; Ratjen, 2003).

Immediate hospitalization and aggressive therapy are warranted for serious pulmonary infections. The threshold for hospitalization with other complications is low. For labor and delivery, epidural analgesia is recommended.

Pregnancy Outcome

When Cohen and coworkers (1980) conducted the first major survey of cystic fibrosis centers, severity was assessed by the *Schwachman-Kulezycki* or *Taussig* scores based on radiological and clinical criteria. Although pregnancy outcomes were not disastrous, 18 percent of 129 women died within 2 years of giving birth. In a later review through 1991, Kent and Farquharson (1993) described similar outcomes in 215 pregnancies in 160 women.

More recent reports describe better outcomes, but there still are serious complications. Disease severity is now quantified by pulmonary function studies, which are the best predictor of pregnancy and long-term maternal outcome. Edenborough and colleagues (2000) reported 69 pregnancies from 11 cystic fibrosis centers in the United Kingdom. If prepregnancy FEV_1 was < 60 percent of predicted, there was substantive risk for preterm delivery, respiratory complications, and death of the mother within a few years of childbirth. Thorpe-Beeson and associates (2013) reported similar findings.

Fitzsimmons and coworkers (1996) performed a case-control study of 258 women with cystic fibrosis who had a live birth. The 889 matched controls were women with cystic fibrosis who had not been pregnant. Pregnancy had no effect on worsening of any serious complications, and 8 percent in both groups had died by 2 years. Gillet and colleagues (2002) reported 75 pregnancies from the French Cystic Fibrosis Registry. Almost 20 percent of infants were delivered preterm, and 30 percent had growth restriction. The one maternal death was due to *Pseudomonas* sepsis in a woman whose prepregnancy FEV_1 was 60 percent. Long-term, however, 17 percent of women died and four infants had confirmed cystic fibrosis. Likewise, in the study by Thorpe-Beeson (2013) cited above, four of eight women whose FEV_1 was < 40 to 50 percent died from 2 to 8 years after delivery.

Lung Transplantation

Cystic fibrosis is a common antecedent disease leading to lung transplantation. Gyi and coworkers (2006) reviewed 10 pregnancies in such women and reported nine liveborn infants. Maternal outcomes were less favorable—three developed rejection during pregnancy, and all three had progressively declining pulmonary function and died of chronic rejection by 38 months after delivery.

CARBON MONOXIDE POISONING

Carbon monoxide is a ubiquitous gas, and most nonsmoking adults have a carbon monoxyhemoglobin saturation of 1 to 3 percent. In cigarette smokers, levels may be as high as 5 to 10 percent. Carbon monoxide is the most frequent cause of poisoning worldwide (Stoller, 2007). Toxic levels are often encountered in inadequately ventilated areas warmed by space heaters.

Carbon monoxide is particularly toxic because it is odorless and tasteless and has a high affinity for hemoglobin binding. Thus, it displaces oxygen and impedes its transfer with resultant hypoxia. Besides acute sequelae including death and anoxic encephalopathy, cognitive defects develop in as many as half of patients following loss of consciousness or in those with carbon monoxide levels > 25 percent (Weaver, 2002). Hypoxic brain damage has a predilection for the cerebral cortex and white matter and for the basal ganglia (Lo, 2007; Prockop, 2007).

Pregnancy and Carbon Monoxide Poisoning

Through several physiological alterations, the rate of endogenous carbon monoxide production almost doubles in normal pregnancy (Longo, 1977). Although the pregnant woman is not more susceptible to carbon monoxide poisoning, the fetus does not tolerate excessive exposure. With chronic exposure, maternal symptoms usually appear when the carboxyhemoglobin concentration is 5 to 20 percent. Symptoms include headache, weakness, dizziness, physical and visual impairment, palpitations, and nausea and vomiting. With acute exposure, concentrations of 30 to 50 percent produce symptoms of impending cardiovascular collapse. Levels > 50 percent may be fatal for the mother.

Because hemoglobin F has an even higher affinity for carbon monoxide, fetal carboxyhemoglobin levels are 10 to 15 percent higher than those in the mother. This may be due to facilitated diffusion (Longo, 1977). Importantly, the half-life of carboxyhemoglobin is 2 hours in the mother but 7 hours in the fetus. Because carbon monoxide is bound so tightly to hemoglobin F, the fetus may be hypoxic even before maternal carbon monoxide levels are appreciably elevated. Several anomalies are associated with embryonic exposure, and anoxic encephalopathy is the primary sequela of later fetal exposure (Alehan, 2007; Aubard, 2000).

Treatment

For all victims, treatment of carbon monoxide poisoning is supportive along with immediate administration of 100-percent inspired oxygen. Indications for hyperbaric oxygen treatment in nonpregnant individuals are unclear (Kao, 2005). Weaver and associates (2002) reported that hyperbaric oxygen treatment minimized the incidence of cognitive defects in adults at both 6 weeks and 1 year compared with that with normobaric oxygen. Hyperbaric oxygen is generally recommended in pregnancy if there has been "significant" carbon monoxide exposure (Aubard, 2000; Ernst, 1998). The problem is how to define significant exposure. Although maternal carbon monoxide levels are not accurately predictive of those in the fetus, some clinicians recommend hyperbaric therapy if maternal levels exceed 15 to 20 percent. With fetal heart rate pattern evaluation, Towers and Corcoran (2009) described affected fetuses to have an elevated baseline, diminished variability, and absent accelerations and decelerations. Treatment of the affected newborn with hyperbaric oxygen is also controversial (Bar, 2007).

Elkharrat and colleagues (1991) reported successful hyperbaric treatments in 44 pregnant women. Silverman and Montano (1997) reported successful management of a woman whose abnormal neurological and cardiopulmonary findings abated in a parallel fashion with resolution of associated fetal heart rate variable decelerations. Greingor and coworkers (2001) used 2.5-atm hyperbaric 100-percent oxygen for 90 minutes in a 21-week pregnant woman who was delivered of a healthy infant at term. According to the Divers Alert Network—DAN (2013)—at Duke University, there are 700 chambers in North and Central America and the Caribbean. Consultation from DAN is available at 919-684-9111.

REFERENCES

Acosta KA, Haver MC, Kelly B: Etiology and therapeutic management of erythema nodosum during pregnancy: an update. Am J Clin Dermatol 14(3):215, 2013

Adhikari M, Pillay T, Pillay DG: Tuberculosis in the newborn: an emerging disease. Pediatr Infect Dis J 16:1108, 1997

Agha FP, Vade A, Amendola MA, et al: Effects of pregnancy on sarcoidosis. Surg Gynecol Obstet 155:817, 1982

Ahmad A, Ahmed A, Patrizio P: Cystic fibrosis and fertility. Curr Opin Obstet Gynecol 25(3):167, 2013

Ahmad H, Mehta NJ, Manikal VM, et al: *Pneumocystis carinii* pneumonia in pregnancy. Chest 120:666, 2001

Alehan F, Erol I, Onay OS: Cerebral palsy due to nonlethal maternal carbon monoxide intoxication. Birth Defects Res A Clin Mol Teratol 79(8):614, 2007

Ali Z, Ulrik CS: Incidence and risk factors for exacerbations of asthma during pregnancy. J Asthma Allergy 6:53, 2013

American College of Obstetricians and Gynecologists: Asthma in Pregnancy. Practice Bulletin No. 90, February 2008, Reaffirmed 2012

American College of Obstetricians and Gynecologists: Update on carrier screening for cystic fibrosis. Committee Opinion No. 486, April 2011

American College of Obstetricians and Gynecologists: Integrating immunizations into practice. Committee Opinion No. 558, April 2013

American Thoracic Society/Centers for Disease Control and Prevention: Diagnostic standards and classification of tuberculosis. Am Rev Respir Dis 142: 725, 1990

Anand N, Kollef MH: The alphabet soup of pneumonia: CAP, HAP, HCAP, NHAP, and VAP. Semin Respir Crit Care Med 30(1):3, 2009

Anderson GD: Tuberculosis in pregnancy. Semin Perinatol 21:328, 1997

Andrews WW: Cesarean delivery for refractory status asthmaticus. Obstet Gynecol 121:417, 2013

Arsura EL, Kilgore WB, Ratnayake SN: Erythema nodosum in pregnant patients with coccidioidomycosis. Clin Infect Dis 27:1201, 1998

Aubard Y, Magne I: Carbon monoxide poisoning in pregnancy. Br J Obstet Gynaecol 107:833, 2000

Aurora P, Whitehead B, Wade A, et al: Lung transplantation and life extension in children with cystic fibrosis. Lancet 354:1594, 1999

Badve SA, Ghate SD, Badve MS, et al: Tuberculosis of spine with neurological deficit in advanced pregnancy: a report of three cases. Spine J 11(1):e9, 2011

Bakhireva LN, Jones KL, Schatz M, et al: Safety of leukotriene receptor antagonists in pregnancy. J Allergy Clin Immunol 119 (3):618, 2007

Bar R, Cohen M, Bentur Y, et al: Pre-labor exposure to carbon monoxide: should the neonate be treated with hyperbaric oxygenation? Clin Toxicol 45(5):579, 2007

Barnes PJ: Asthma. In Longo D, Fauci A, Kasper D, et al (eds): Harrison's Principles of Internal Medicine, 18th ed. New York, McGraw-Hill, 2012, p 2102

Baughman RP, Lower EE: Sarcoidosis. In Longo DL, Fauci AS, Kasper DL, et al (eds): Harrison's Principles of Internal Medicine, 18th ed. New York, McGraw-Hill, 2012, p 2805

Beigi RH: Pandemic influenza and pregnancy. Obstet Gynecol 109:1193, 2007

Bel EH: Mild asthma. N Engl J Med 369(6):549, 2013

Belfort MA, Clark SL, Saade GR, et al: Hospital readmission after delivery: evidence for an increased incidence of nonurogenital infection in the immediate postpartum period. Am J Obstet Gynecol 202:35.e1, 2010

Bercovitch RS, Catanzaro A, Schwartz BS, et al: Coccidioidomycosis during pregnancy: a review and recommendations for management. Clin Infect Dis 53(4):363, 2011

Blais L, Beauchesne MF, Malo RE, et al: Use of inhaled corticosteroids during the first trimester of pregnancy and the risk of congenital malformations among women with asthma. Thorax 62(4):320, 2007

Blais L, Kettani FZ, Forget A: Relationship between maternal asthma, its severity and control and abortion. Hum Reprod 28(4):908, 2013

Blais L, Suissa S, Boivin JF, et al: First treatment with inhaled corticosteroids and the prevention of admissions to hospital for asthma. Thorax 53:1025, 1998

Blanc FX, Sok T, Laureillard D, et al: Earlier versus later start of antiretroviral therapy in HIV-infected adults with tuberculosis. N Engl J Med 365(16):1471, 2011

Bogaert D, De Groot R, Hermans PW: *Streptococcus pneumoniae* colonisation: the key to pneumococcal disease. Lancet Infect Dis 4:144, 2004

Boggess KA, Myers ER, Hamilton CD: Antepartum or postpartum isoniazid treatment of latent tuberculosis infection. Obstet Gynecol 96:747, 2000

Boucher RC: Cystic Fibrosis. In Longo DL, Fauci AS, Kasper DL, et al (eds): Harrison's Principles of Internal Medicine, 18th ed. New York, McGraw-Hill, 2012, p 2805

Bracken MB, Triche EW, Belanger K, et al: Asthma symptoms, severity, and drug therapy: a prospective study of effects on 2205 pregnancies. Obstet Gynecol 102:739, 2003

Braman SS: Chronic cough due to acute bronchitis: ACCP evidence-based clinical practice guidelines. Chest 129:95S, 2006

Braman SS, Kaemmerlen JT: Intensive care of status asthmaticus. A 10-year experience. JAMA 264:366, 1990

Brancazio LR, Laifer SA, Schwartz T: Peak expiratory flow rate in normal pregnancy. Obstet Gynecol 89:383, 1997
Briggs GG, Freeman RK, Yaffe SJ (eds): Drugs in Pregnancy and Lactation, 9th ed. Baltimore, Williams & Wilkins, 2011
Brito V, Niederman MS: Pneumonia complicating pregnancy. Clin Chest Med 32:121, 2011
Caldwell JW, Asura EL, Kilgore WB, et al: Coccidioidomycosis in pregnancy during an epidemic in California. Obstet Gynecol 95:236, 2000
Cameron AJ, Skinner TA: Management of a parturient with respiratory failure secondary to cystic fibrosis. Anaesthesia 60:77, 2005
Cantwell MF, Shehab ZM, Costello AM, et al: Congenital tuberculosis. N Engl J Med 330:1051, 1994
Cardonick EH, Naktin J, Berghella V: Neurosarcoidosis diagnosed during pregnancy by thoracoscopic lymph node biopsy. J Reprod Med 45:585, 2000
Carroll KN, Griffin MR, Gebretsadik T, et al: Racial differences in asthma morbidity during pregnancy. Obstet Gynecol 106(1):66, 2005
Centers for Disease Control and Prevention: Treatment of tuberculosis. American Thoracic Society, CDC, and Infection Disease Society of America. MMWR 52(11):1, 2003
Centers for Disease Control and Prevention: Controlling tuberculosis in the United States. Recommendations from the American Thoracic Society, CDC, and the Infectious Disease Society of America. MMWR 54(12):1, 2005a
Centers for Disease Control and Prevention: Guidelines for using the QuantiFERON-TB gold test for detecting *Mycobacterium tuberculosis* infection, United States. MMWR 54(15):29, 2005b
Centers for Disease Control and Prevention: Prevention and control of influenza. Recommendations of the Advisory Committee on Immunization Practices (ACIP). MMWR 55(10):1, 2006
Centers for Disease Control and Prevention: Extensively drug-resistant tuberculosis—United States, 1993–2006. MMWR 56(11):250, 2007a
Centers for Disease Control and Prevention: Severe methicillin-resistant *Staphylococcus aureus* community-acquired pneumonia associated with influenza—Louisiana and Georgia—December 2006–January 2007. MMWR 56(14):325, 2007b
Centers for Disease Control and Prevention: Plan to combat extensively drug-resistant tuberculosis. MMWR 58(3):1, 2009a
Centers for Disease Control and Prevention: Trends in tuberculosis–United States, 2008. MMWR 58(10):1, 2009b
Centers for Disease Control and Prevention: 2009 pandemic influenza A (H1N1) in pregnant women requiring intensive care—New York City, 2009. MMWR 59(11):321, 2010a
Centers for Disease Control and Prevention: Decrease in reported tuberculosis cases—United States, 2009. MMWR 59(10):289, 2010b
Centers for Disease Control and Prevention: National Center for Health E-Stat: asthma prevalence, health care use and morbidity: United States, 2003–05. 2010c. Available at: http://www.cdc.gov/nchs/data/hestat/asthma03-05/asthma03-05.htm. Accessed August 13, 2013
Centers for Disease Control and Prevention: Guidelines for prevention and treatment of opportunistic infections in HIV-infected adults and adolescents, June 17, 2013. Available at: http://aidsinfo.nih.gov/contentfiles/Adult_OI.pdf. Accessed August 13, 2013a
Centers for Disease Control and Prevention: Influenza vaccination coverage among pregnant women–United States, 2012–2013 influenza season. MMWR 62:787, 2013b
Charlton RA, Hutchison A, Davis KJ, et al: Asthma management in pregnancy. PLoS One 8(4):e60247, 2013
Chen YH, Keller J, Wang IT, et al: Pneumonia and pregnancy outcomes: a nationwide population-base study. Am J Obstet Gynecol 207:288.e1, 2012
Cohen LF, di Sant Agnese PA, Friedlander J: Cystic fibrosis and pregnancy: a national survey. Lancet 2:842, 1980
Comeau AM, Accurso FJ, White TB, et al: Guidelines for implementation of cystic fibrosis newborn screening programs: Cystic Fibrosis Foundation workshop report. Pediatrics 119:e495, 2007
Cossette B, Forget A, Beauchesne MF: Impact of maternal use of asthma-controller therapy on perinatal outcomes. Thorax 68:724, 2013
Cox S, Posner SF, McPheeters M, et al: Hospitalizations with respiratory illness among pregnant women during influenza season. 107:1315, 2006
Crum NF, Ballon-Landa G: Coccidioidomycosis in pregnancy: case report and review of the literature. Am J Med 119:993, 2006
Cruz CA, Caughey AB, Jasmer R: Postpartum follow-up of a positive purified protein derivative (PPD) among an indigent population. Am J Obstet Gynecol 192:1455, 2005
de Regt RH: Sarcoidosis and pregnancy. Obstet Gynecol 70:369, 1987
de Vries J, Drent M: Quality of life and health status in sarcoidosis: a review. Semin Respir Crit Care Med 28:121, 2007
Divers Alert Network: Chamber location and availability. Available at: http://www.diversalertnetwork.org/medical. Accessed July 29, 2013
Dodds L, McNeil SA, Fell DB, et al: Impact of influenza exposure on rates of hospital admissions and physician visits because of respiratory illness among pregnant women. CMAJ 17:463, 2007
Dolin R: Common viral respiratory infections. In Longo D, Fauci A, Kasper D, et al (eds): Harrison's Principles of Internal Medicine, 18th ed. New York, McGraw-Hill, 2012, p 1485
Dombrowski MP: Asthma and pregnancy. Obstet Gynecol 108:667, 2006
Dombrowski MP, Schatz M, Wise R, et al: Asthma during pregnancy. Obstet Gynecol 103:5, 2004a
Dombrowski MP, Schatz M, Wise R, et al: Randomized trial of inhaled beclomethasone dipropionate versus theophylline for moderate asthma during pregnancy. Am J Obstet Gynecol 190:737, 2004b
Donaldson SH, Bennett WD, Zeman KL, et al: Mucus clearance and lung function in cystic fibrosis with hypertonic saline. N Engl J Med 354:241, 2006
Doudier B, Mosnier E, Rovery C, et al: Congenital tuberculosis after in vitro fertilization. Pediatr Infect Dis J 28:277, 2008
Edenborough FP: Women with cystic fibrosis and their potential for reproduction. Thorax 56:648, 2001
Edenborough FP, Mackenzie WE, Stableforth DE: The outcome of 72 pregnancies in 55 women with cystic fibrosis in the United Kingdom 1977–1996. Br J Obstet Gynaecol 107:254, 2000
Edenborough FP, Stableforth DE, Webb AK, et al: The outcome of pregnancy in cystic fibrosis. Thorax 50:170, 1995
Efferen LS: Tuberculosis and pregnancy. Curr Opin Pulm Med 13:205, 2007
Elkharrat D, Raphael JC, Korach JM, et al: Acute carbon monoxide intoxication and hyperbaric oxygen in pregnancy. Intensive Care Med 17:289, 1991
Elkins MR, Robinson M, Rose BR, et al: A controlled trial of long-term inhaled hypertonic saline in patients with cystic fibrosis. N Engl J Med 354:229, 2006
Ely EW, Peacock JE, Haponik EF, et al: Cryptococcal pneumonia complicating pregnancy. Medicine 77:153, 1998
Enriquez R, Pingsheng W, Griffin MR, et al: Cessation of asthma medication in early pregnancy. Am J Obstet Gynecol 195:149, 2006
Ernst A, Zibrak JD: Carbon monoxide poisoning. N Engl J Med 339:1603, 1998
Ernst JD, Trevejo-Nuñez G, Banaiee N: Genomics and the evolution, pathogenesis, and diagnosis of tuberculosis. J Clin Invest 117:1738, 2007
Fanta CH: Asthma. N Engl J Med 360:1002, 2009
Figueroa-Damian R, Arrendondo-Garcia JL: Pregnancy and tuberculosis: influence of treatment on perinatal outcome. Am J Perinatol 15:303, 1998
Finland M, Dublin TD: Pneumococcic pneumonias complicating pregnancy and the puerperium. JAMA 112:1027, 1939
Fitzsimmons SC, Fitzpatrick S, Thompson D, et al: A longitudinal study of the effects of pregnancy on 325 women with cystic fibrosis. Pediatr Pulmonol 113:99, 1996
Forna F, McConnell M, Kitabire FN: Systematic review of the safety of trimethoprim-sulfamethoxazole for prophylaxis in HIV-infected pregnant women: implications for resource-limited settings. AIDS Rev 8:24, 2006
Gazmararian JA, Petersen R, Jamieson DJ, et al: Hospitalizations during pregnancy among managed care enrollees. Obstet Gynecol 100:94, 2002
Getahun D, Ananth CV, Oyelese MR: Acute and chronic respiratory diseases in pregnancy: associations with spontaneous premature rupture of membranes. J Matern Fetal Neonatal Med 20(9):669, 2007
Getahun D, Ananth CV, Peltier MR: Acute and chronic respiratory disease in pregnancy: association with placental abruption. Am J Obstet Gynecol 195:1180, 2006
Giacobbe LE, Nguyen RH, Aguilera MN, et al: Effect of maternal cystic fibrosis genotype on diabetes in pregnancy. Obstet Gynecol 120(6):1394, 2012
Gillet D, de Brackeleer M, Bellis G, et al: Cystic fibrosis and pregnancy. Report from French data (1980–1999). Br J Obstet Gynaecol 109:912, 2002
Gluck JC, Gluck PA: The effect of pregnancy on the course of asthma. Immunol Allergy Clin North Am 26:63, 2006
Goodnight WH, Soper DE: Pneumonia in pregnancy. Crit Care Med 33(10):S390, 2005
Greingor JL, Tosi JM, Ruhlmann S, et al: Acute carbon monoxide intoxication during pregnancy. One case report and review of the literature. Emerg Med J 18:399, 2001
Gyi KM, Hodson ME, Yacoub MY: Pregnancy in cystic fibrosis lung transplant recipients: case series and review. J Cyst Fibros 5(3):171, 2006
Hardin DS, Rice J, Cohen RC, et al: The metabolic effects of pregnancy in cystic fibrosis. Obstet Gynecol 106(2):367, 2005
Harding R, Maritz G: Maternal and fetal origins of lung disease in childhood. Semin Fetal Neonatal Med 17(2):67, 2012

Harger JH, Ernest JM, Thurnau GR, et al: Risk factors and outcome of varicella-zoster virus pneumonia in pregnant women. J Infect Dis 185:422, 2002
Havlir DV, Kendall MA, Ive P, et al: Timing of antiretroviral therapy for HIV-1 infection and tuberculosis. N Engl J Med 365(16):1482, 2011
Henderson AJ, Warner JO: Fetal origins of asthma. Semin Fetal Neonatal Med 17(2):82, 2012
Hendler I, Schatz M, Momirova V, et al: Association of obesity with pulmonary and nonpulmonary complications of pregnancy in asthmatic women. Obstet Gynecol 108(1):77, 2006
Hooper JE, Lu Q, Pepkowitz SH: Disseminated coccidioidomycosis in pregnancy. Arch Pathol Lab Med 131:652, 2007
Horsburgh CR Jr, Rubin EJ: Latent tuberculosis infection in the United States. N Engl J Med 364:15:1441, 2011
Jacobs RF, Abernathy RS: Management of tuberculosis in pregnancy and the newborn. Clin Perinatol 15:305, 1988
Jamieson DJ, Rasmussen SA, Uyeki TM, et al: Pandemic influenza and pregnancy revisited: lessons learned from 2009 pandemic influenza A (H1N1). Am J Obstet Gynecol 204(6 Suppl 1):S1, 2011
Jana N, Vasishta K, Jindal SK, et al: Perinatal outcome in pregnancies complicated by pulmonary tuberculosis. Int J Gynecol Obstet 44:119, 1994
Jana N, Vasishta K, Saha SC, et al: Obstetrical outcomes among women with extrapulmonary tuberculosis. N Engl J Med 341:645, 1999
Jenkins TM, Troiano NH, Grave CR, et al: Mechanical ventilation in an obstetric population: characteristics and delivery rates. Am J Obstet Gynecol 188:549, 2003
Jin Y, Carriere KC, Marrie TJ, et al: The effects of community-acquired pneumonia during pregnancy ending with a live birth. Am J Obstet Gynecol 188:800, 2003
Källén B, Otterblad Olausson PO: Use of anti-asthmatic drugs during pregnancy. 2. Infant characteristics excluding congenital malformations. Eur J Clin Pharmacol 63(4):375, 2007
Kao LW, Nañagas KA: Carbon monoxide poisoning. Med Clin North Am 89(6):1161, 2005
Karim SSA, Naidoo K, Grobler A, et al: Integration of antiretroviral therapy with tuberculosis treatment. N Engl J Med 365(16):1492, 2011
Kent NE, Farquharson DF: Cystic fibrosis in pregnancy. Can Med Assoc J 149: 809, 1993
Kowada A: Cost effectiveness of interferon-gamma release assay for TB screening of HIV positive pregnant women in low TB incidence countries. J Infect 688:32, 2014
Kruszka SJ, Gherman RB: Successful pregnancy outcome in a lung transplant recipient with tacrolimus immunosuppression. A case report. J Reprod Med 47:60, 2002
Kutlu T, Tugrul S, Aydin A, et al: Tuberculosis meningitis in pregnancy presenting as hyperemesis gravidarum. J Matern Fetal Neonatal Med 20:357, 2007
Kwon HL, Triche EW, Belander K, et al: The epidemiology of asthma during pregnancy: prevalence, diagnosis, and symptoms. Immunol Allergy Clin North Am 26:29, 2006
Kyaw MH, Lynfield R, Schaffner W, et al: Effect of introduction of the pneumococcal conjugate vaccine on drug-resistant *Streptococcus pneumoniae*. N Engl J Med 354:1455, 2006
Lalvani A: Diagnosing tuberculosis infection in the 21st century: new tools to tackle an old enemy. Chest 131:1898, 2007
Lam CM, Wong SF, Leung TN, et al: A case-controlled study comparing clinical course and outcomes of pregnant and non-pregnant women with severe acute respiratory syndrome. BJOG 111:771, 2004
Lazarus SC: Emergency treatment of asthma. N Engl J Med 363(8):755, 2010
Lessnau KD, Qarah S: Multidrug-resistant tuberculosis in pregnancy: case report and review of the literature. Chest 123:953, 2003
Levison JH, Barbieri RL, Katx JT, et al: Hard to conceive. N Engl J Med 363(10):965, 2010
Lim WS, Macfarlane JT, Boswell TC, et al: Study of community acquired pneumonia etiology (SCAPA) in adults admitted to hospital: implications for management guidelines. Thorax 56:296, 2001
Lin HC, Lin HC, Chen SF: Increased risk of low birthweight and small for gestational age infants among women with tuberculosis. BJOG 117(5):585, 2010
Liu S, Wen SW, Demissie K, et al: Maternal asthma and pregnancy outcomes: a retrospective cohort study. Am J Obstet Gynecol 184:90, 2001
Llewelyn M, Cropley I, Wilkinson RJ, et al: Tuberculosis diagnosed during pregnancy: a prospective study from London. Thorax 55:129, 2000
Lo CP, Chen SY, Lee KW, et al: Brain injury after acute carbon monoxide poisoning: early and late complications. AJR Am J Roentgenol 189(4):W205, 2007
Lo JO, Boltax J, Metz TD: Cesarean delivery for life-threatening status asthmaticus. Obstet Gynecol 121(2 Pt 2 Suppl 1):422, 2013
Longman RE, Johnson TRB: Viral respiratory disease in pregnancy. Curr Opin Obstet Gynecol 18:120, 2007
Longo L: The biologic effects of carbon monoxide on the pregnant woman, fetus and newborn infant. Am J Obstet Gynecol 129:69, 1977
Lynch III JP, Ma YL, Koss MN, et al: Pulmonary sarcoidosis. Semin Respir Crit Care Med 28:53, 2007
Mabie WC, Barton JR, Wasserstrum N, et al: Clinical observations on asthma in pregnancy. J Matern Fetal Med 1:45, 1992
Maisel JA, Lynam T: Unexpected sudden death in a young pregnant woman: unusual presentation of neurosarcoidosis. Ann Emerg Med 28:94, 1996
Mandell LA, Wunderink R: Pneumonia. In Longo D, Fauci A, Kasper D, et al (eds): Harrison's Principles of Internal Medicine, 18th ed. New York, McGraw-Hill, 2012, p 2130
Mandell LA, Wunderink RG, Anzueto A, et al: Infectious Diseases Society of America/American Thoracic Society consensus guidelines on the management of community-acquired pneumonia in adults. Clin Infect Dis 44:S27, 2007
Margono F, Mroueh J, Garely A, et al: Resurgence of active tuberculosis among pregnant women. Obstet Gynecol 83:911, 1994
Mazurek GH, Vernon A, LoBue P, et al: Updated guidelines for using interferon gamma release assays to detect *Mycobacterium tuberculosis* infection, United States, 2010. MMWR Recomm Rep 59(RR-5):2, 2010
McFadden ER: Asthma. In Kasper DL, Fauci AS, Longo DL, et al (eds): Harrison's Principles of Internal Medicine, 16th ed. New York, McGraw-Hill, 2005, p 1508
McKone EF, Emerson SS, Edwards KL, et al: Effect of genotype on phenotype and mortality in cystic fibrosis: a retrospective cohort study. Lancet 361:1671, 2003
McMullen AH, Past DJ, Frederick PD: Impact of pregnancy on women with cystic fibrosis. Chest 129(3):706, 2006
Medical Letter: Anidulafungin (Eraxis) for candida infections. 48:1235, 2006
Mendola P, Laughon SK, Männistö TI, et al: Obstetric complications among US women with asthma. Am J Obstet Gynecol 208(2):127.e1, 2013
Mert A, Kumbasar H, Ozaras R, et al: Erythema nodosum: an evaluation of 100 cases. Clin Exp Rheumatol 25:563, 2007
Mnyani CN, McIntyre JA: Tuberculosis in pregnancy. BJOG 118(2):226, 2011
Moberley S, Holden J, Tatham DP, et al: Vaccines for preventing pneumococcal infection in adults. Cochrane Database Syst Rev 1:CD000422, 2013
Moller DR: Potential etiologic agents in sarcoidosis. Proc Am Thorac Soc 4:465, 2007
Moore AR, Rogers FM, Dietrick D, et al: Extrapulmonary tuberculosis in pregnancy masquerading as a degenerating leiomyoma. Obstet Gynecol 111(2): 551, 2008
Moran GJ, Rothman RE, Volturo GA: Emergency management of community-acquired bacterial pneumonia: what is new since the 2007 Infectious Diseases Society of America/American Thoracic Society guidelines. Am J Obstet Gynecol 31:602, 2013
Moscona A: Neuraminidase inhibitors for influenza. N Engl J Med 353(13): 1363, 2005
Murphy VE, Gibson P, Talbot P, et al: Severe asthma exacerbations during pregnancy. Obstet Gynecol 106(5):1046, 2005
Murphy VE, Namazy JA, Powell H, et al: A meta-analysis of adverse perinatal outcomes in women with asthma. BJOG 118:1314, 2011
Murphy VE, Powell H, Wark PA: A prospective study of respiratory viral infection in pregnant women with and without asthma. Chest 144(2):420, 2013
Namazy JA, Schatz M: Current guidelines for the management of asthma during pregnancy. Immunol Allergy Clin North Am 26:93, 2006
Namazy JA, Schatz M: Pregnancy and asthma: recent developments. Curr Opin Pulm Med 11:56, 2005
Nanda S, Agarwal U, Sangwan K: Complete resolution of cervical spinal tuberculosis with paraplegia in pregnancy. Acta Obstet Gynecol Scand 81:569, 2002
National Heart, Lung, and Blood Institute: National Asthma Education and Prevention Program. Expert panel report 3: guidelines for the diagnosis and management of asthma, 2007. Available at: www.nhlbli.nih.gov/guidelines/asthma/index.htm. Accessed August 13, 2013
Ng WF, Wong SF, Lam A, et al: The placentas of patients with severe acute respiratory syndrome: a pathophysiological evaluation. Pathology 38:210, 2006
Olson GL: Cystic fibrosis in pregnancy. Semin Perinatol 21:307, 1997
Paramothayan S, Jones PW: Corticosteroid therapy in pulmonary sarcoidosis. A systematic review. JAMA 287:1301, 2002
Paranyuk Y, Levine G, Figueroa R: Candida septicemia in a pregnant woman with hyperemesis receiving parenteral nutrition. Obstet Gynecol 107:535, 2006
Patel S, Lee RH: The case of the sinister spores: the patient was hospitalized for a menacing infection in the second trimester of pregnancy. Am J Obstet Gynecol 208(5):417.e1, 2013

Pillay T, Khan M, Moodley J, et al: Perinatal tuberculosis and HIV-1: considerations for resource-limited settings. Lancet Infect Dis 4:155, 2004
Prevost MR, Fung Kee Fung KM: Tuberculous meningitis in pregnancy—implications for mother and fetus: case report and literature review. J Matern Fetal Med 8:289, 1999
Prockop LD, Chichkova RI: Carbon monoxide intoxication: an updated review. J Neurol Sci 262(1–2):122, 2007
Ramsey PS, Maddox DE, Ramin KD, et al: Asthma: Impact on maternal morbidity and adverse perinatal outcome [Abstract]. Obstet Gynecol 101:40S, 2003
Raviglione MC, O'Brien RJ: Tuberculosis. In Longo D, Fauci A, Kasper D, et al (eds): Harrison's Principles of Internal Medicine, 18th ed. New York, McGraw-Hill, 2012, p 1340
Ratjen F, Döring G: Cystic fibrosis. Lancet 361:681, 2003
Reboli AC, Rotstein C, Pappas PG, et al: Anidulafungin versus fluconazole for invasive candidiasis. N Engl J Med 356:2472, 2007
Rey E, Boulet LP: Asthma in pregnancy. BMJ 334:582, 2007
Rodgers HC, Knox AJ, Toplis PH, et al: Successful pregnancy and birth after IVF in a woman with cystic fibrosis. Human Reprod 15:2152, 2000
Rogers VL, Sheffield JS, Roberts SW, et al: Presentation of seasonal influenza A in pregnancy: 2003–2004 influenza season. Obstet Gynecol 115(5):924, 2010
Rolston DH, Shnider SM, de Lorimer AA: Uterine blood flow and fetal acid–base changes after bicarbonate administration to the pregnant ewe. Anesthesiology 40:348, 1974
Rosenstein NE, Emery KW, Werner SB, et al: Risk factors for severe pulmonary and disseminated coccidioidomycosis: Kern County, California, 1995–1996. Clin Infect Dis 32:708, 2001
Rotas M, McCalla S, Liu C, et al: Methicillin-resistant *Staphylococcus aureus* necrotizing pneumonia arising from an infected episiotomy site. Obstet Gynecol 109(2):533, 2007
Rowe SM, Miller S, Sorscher EJ: Cystic fibrosis. N Engl J Med 353:1992, 2005
Rowntree RK, Harris A: The phenotypic consequences of *CFTR* mutations. Ann Hum Genet 67(5):471, 2003
Sackoff JE, Pfieffer MR, Driver CR, et al: Tuberculosis prevention for non-U.S.-born pregnant women. Am J Obstet Gynecol 194:451, 2006
Sawicki E, Stewart K, Wong S: Management of asthma by pregnant women attending an Australian maternity hospital. Aust N Z J Obstet Gynecol 52(2):183, 2012
Schanzer DL, Langley JM, Tam TW: Influenza-attributed hospitalization rates among pregnant women in Canada 1994–2000. J Obstet Gynaecol Can 29:622, 2007
Schatz M, Dombrowski MP, Wise R, et al: Asthma morbidity during pregnancy can be predicted by severity classification. J Allergy Clin Immunol 112:283, 2003
Schatz M, Dombrowski MP, Wise R, et al: Spirometry is related to perinatal outcomes in pregnant women with asthma. Am J Obstet Gynecol 194:120, 2006
Schechter MS, Quittner AL, Konstan MW, et al: Long-term effects of pregnancy and motherhood on disease outcomes of women with cystic fibrosis. Ann Am Thorac Soc 10(3):213, 2013
Schulte JM, Bryan P, Dodds S, et al: Tuberculosis skin testing among HIV-infected pregnant women in Miami, 1995 to 1996. J Perinatol 22:159, 2002
Seballos RJ, Mendel SG, Mirmiran-Yazdy A, et al: Sarcoid cardiomyopathy precipitated by pregnancy with cocaine complications. Chest 105:303, 1994
Selroos O: Sarcoidosis and pregnancy: a review with results of a retrospective survey. J Intern Med 227:221, 1990
Shaner J, Coscia LA, Constantinescu S, et al: Pregnancy after lung transplant. Prog Transplant 22(2):134, 2012
Shariatzadeh MR, Marrie TJ: Pneumonia during pregnancy. Am J Med 119:872, 2006
Sheffield JS, Cunningham FG: Management of community-acquired pneumonia in pregnancy. Obstet Gynecol 114(4):915, 2009
Sherer DM, Osho, JA, Zinn H, et al: Peripartum disseminated extrapulmonary tuberculosis simulating ovarian carcinoma. Am J Perinatol 22:383, 2005
Shin S, Guerra D, Rich M, et al: Treatment of multidrug-resistant tuberculosis during pregnancy: a report of 7 cases. Clin Infect Dis 36:996, 2003
Silverman RK, Montano J: Hyperbaric oxygen treatment during pregnancy in acute carbon monoxide poisoning. A case report. J Reprod Med 42:309, 1997
Smith KC: Congenital tuberculosis: A rare manifestation of a common infection. Curr Opin Infect Dis 15:269, 2002
Sobczyńska-Tomaszewska A, Bak D, Wolski JK, et al: Molecular analysis of defects in the *CFTR* gene and *AZF* locus of the Y chromosome in male infertility. J Reprod Med 51(2):120, 2006
Southern KW, Mérelle MM, Dankert-Roelse JE, et al: Newborn screening for cystic fibrosis. Cochrane Database Syst Rev 1:CD001402, 2009
Spagnolo P, du Bois RM: Genetics of sarcoidosis. Clin Dermatol 25:242, 2007
Spinello IM, Johnson RH, Baqi S: Coccidioidomycosis and pregnancy: a review. Ann N Y Acad Sci 1111:358, 2007
Stoller KP: Hyperbaric oxygen and carbon monoxide poisoning: a critical review. Neurol Res 29(2):146, 2007
Stratton P, Mofenson LM, Willoughby AD: Human immunodeficiency virus infection in pregnant women under care at AIDS Clinical Trials Centers in the United States. Obstet Gynecol 79:364, 1992
Strunk RC, Bloomberg GR: Omalizumab for asthma. N Engl J Med 354(24):2689, 2006
Tata LJ, Lewis SA, McKeever TM, et al: A comprehensive analysis of adverse obstetric and pediatric complications in women with asthma. Am J Respir Crit Care Med 175:991, 2007
Taylor AW, Mosimaneotsile B, Mathebula U, et al: Pregnancy outcomes in HIV-infected women receiving long-term isoniazid prophylaxis for tuberculosis and antiretroviral therapy. Infect Dis Obstet Gynecol 2013:195637, 2013
Thorpe-Beeson JG, Madge S, Gyi K, et al: The outcome of pregnancies in women with cystic fibrosis—single centre experience 1998–2011. BJOG 120(3):354, 2013
Tino G, Ware LB, Moss M: Clinical Year in Review IV: chronic obstructive pulmonary disease, nonpulmonary critical care, diagnostic imaging, and mycobacterial disease. Proc Am Thorac Soc 4(6):494, 2007
Török ME, Farrar JJ, et al: When to start antiretroviral therapy in HIV-associated tuberculosis. N Engl J Med 365(16):1538, 2011
Torres A, Menéndez R: Hospital admission in community-acquired pneumonia [Spanish]. Med Clin (Barc) 131(6):216, 2008
Towers CV, Corcoran VA: Influence of carbon monoxide poisoning on the fetal heart monitor tracing: a report of 3 cases. J Reprod Med 54(3):184, 2009
Triche EW, Saftlas AF, Belanger K, et al: Association of asthma diagnosis, severity, symptoms, and treatment with risk of preeclampsia. Obstet Gynecol 104:585, 2004
Varner MW, rice MM, Anderson B, et al: Influenza-like illness in hospitalized pregnant and postpartum women during the 2009–20120 H1N1 pandemic. Obstet Gynecol 118(3), 2011
Walzer PD: Pneumocystis infection. In Kasper DL, Fauci AS, Longo DL, et al (eds): Harrison's Principles of Internal Medicine, 16th ed. New York, McGraw-Hill, 2005, p 1194
Weaver LK, Hopkins RO, Chan KJ, et al: Hyperbaric oxygen for acute carbon monoxide poisoning. N Engl J Med 347:1057, 2002
Wendel PJ, Ramin SM, Hamm CB, et al: Asthma treatment in pregnancy: a randomized controlled study. Am J Obstet Gynecol 175:150, 1996
Wenzel RP, Fowler AA 3rd: Acute bronchitis. N Engl J Med 355:2125, 2006
Wexler ID, Johnnesson M, Edenborough FP, et al: Pregnancy and chronic progressive pulmonary disease. Am J Respir Crit Care Med 175:330, 2007
Wise RA, Polito AJ, Krishnan V: Respiratory physiologic changes in pregnancy. Immunol Allergy Clin North Am 26:1, 2006
Wong SF, Chow KM, Leung TN, et al: Pregnancy and perinatal outcomes of women with severe acute respiratory syndrome. Am J Obstet Gynecol 191:292, 2004
World Health Organization: Update on avian influenza A (H5N1) virus infection in humans. N Engl J Med 358:261, 2008
Yost NP, Bloom SL, Richey SD, et al: An appraisal of treatment guidelines for antepartum community-acquired pneumonia. Am J Obstet Gynecol 183:131, 2000
Zaman K, Roy E, Arifeen SE, et al: Effectiveness of maternal influenza immunization in mothers and infants. N Engl J Med 359(15):1555, 2008
Zeeman GG, Wendel GD, Cunningham FG: A blueprint for obstetrical critical care. Am J Obstet Gynecol 188:532, 2003
Zenner D, Kruijshaar ME, Andrews N, et al: Risk of tuberculosis in pregnancy: a national, primary care-based cohort and self-controlled case series study. Am J Respir Crit Care Med 185(7):779, 2012
Zumla A, Raviglione M, Hafner R, et al: Tuberculosis. N Engl J Med 368:745, 2013

CHAPTER 52

Thromboembolic Disorders

The risk of venous thrombosis and pulmonary embolism in otherwise healthy women is considered highest during pregnancy and the puerperium. Indeed, in a recent study from the United Kingdom of nearly 1 million reproductive-aged women, the risks of venous thromboembolism for those during the third trimester and the first 6 weeks postpartum were calculated to be six and 22 times higher, respectively, than for nonpregnant women (Sultan, 2011). The incidence of all thromboembolic events averages approximately 1 per 1000 pregnancies, and about an equal number are identified antepartum and in the puerperium. In a study from Norway of more than 600,000 pregnancies, Jacobsen and colleagues (2008) reported that deep-vein thrombosis alone was more frequent antepartum, whereas pulmonary embolism was more common in the first 6 weeks postpartum.

Venous thromboembolism frequency during the puerperium has decreased remarkably as early ambulation has become more widely practiced. Even so, the thromboembolism rate has increased significantly during the past two decades (Callaghan, 2012). Although this increase may reflect the higher sensitivities of newer diagnostic modalities, pulmonary embolism still remains a leading cause of maternal death in the United States (Table 1-3, p. 6) (O'Connor, 2011). Specifically, Berg and associates (2010) reported that approximately 10 percent of pregnancy-related maternal deaths in the United States between 1998 and 2005 were caused by thrombotic pulmonary embolism.

PATHOPHYSIOLOGY

Rudolf Virchow (1856) postulated that stasis, local trauma to the vessel wall, and hypercoagulability predisposed to venous thrombosis development. The risk for each of these increases during normal pregnancy. For example, compression of the pelvic veins and inferior vena cava by the enlarging uterus renders the lower extremity venous system particularly vulnerable to stasis. From their review, Marik and Plante (2008) cite a 50-percent reduction in venous flow velocity in the legs that lasts from the early third trimester until 6 weeks postpartum. This stasis is the most constant predisposing risk factor for venous thrombosis. Venous stasis and delivery may also contribute to endothelial cell injury. Last, as listed in the Appendix (p. 1288), marked increases in the synthesis of most clotting factors during pregnancy favor coagulation.

Risk factors for developing thromboembolism during pregnancy are shown in Table 52-1. The most important of these is a personal history of thrombosis. Indeed, 15 to 25 percent of all venous thromboembolism cases during pregnancy are recurrent events (American College of Obstetricians and Gynecologists, 2011). The magnitude of other risk factors was estimated by James and coworkers (2006) using data from the Agency for Healthcare Research and Quality of all hospital discharges during 2000 and 2001. They identified the diagnosis of venous thromboembolism in 7177 women during pregnancy and 7158 during the postpartum period. Calculated risks for

TABLE 52-1. Some Risk Factors Associated with an Increased Risk for Thromboembolism

Risk Factor[a]	Chapter Referral
Obstetrical	
Cesarean delivery	30
Diabetes	57
Hemorrhage and anemia	41
Hyperemesis	54
Immobility—prolonged bed rest	—
Multifetal gestation	45
Multiparity	
Preeclampsia	40
Puerperal infection	37
General	
Age 35 years or older	8
Cancer	63
Connective-tissue disease	59
Dehydration	54
Immobility—long-distance travel	8
Infection and inflammatory disease	37
Myeloproliferative disease	56
Nephrotic syndrome	53
Obesity	48
Oral contraceptive use	38
Orthopedic surgery	46
Paraplegia	60
Prior thromboembolism	52
Sickle-cell disease	56
Smoking	8
Thrombophilia	52

[a]Risk factors are listed alphabetically.

thromboembolism were approximately doubled in women with multifetal gestation, anemia, hyperemesis, hemorrhage, and cesarean delivery. The risk was even greater in pregnancies complicated by postpartum infection. In a more recent nested case-control study of nearly 100,000 women with 10-year follow-up, Waldman and colleagues (2013) found that the risk of venous thromboembolism was slightly higher in women with advanced maternal age and approximately doubled in women with great parity, a hypertensive disorder, cesarean delivery, or obesity. Risks were significantly greater among women who had a stillbirth or who underwent peripartum hysterectomy. At Parkland Hospital, the risk of postpartum thromboembolism most recently is approximately 1 in 5350 deliveries, with all of these risk factors confirmed.

The likelihood of developing a thrombosis during pregnancy is especially increased in women with certain genetic risk factors. Indeed—and likely related—after personal history of thrombosis, the next most important individual risk factor is thrombophilia. An estimated 20 to 50 percent of women who develop a venous thrombosis during pregnancy or postpartum have an identifiable underlying genetic disorder (American College of Obstetricians and Gynecologists, 2011).

THROMBOPHILIAS

Several important regulatory proteins act as inhibitors in the coagulation cascade. Normal values for many of these proteins during pregnancy are found in the Appendix (p. 1288). Inherited or acquired deficiencies of these inhibitory proteins are collectively referred to as *thrombophilias*. These can lead to hypercoagulability and recurrent venous thromboembolism. Although these disorders are collectively present in about 15 percent of white European populations, they are responsible for approximately 50 percent of all thromboembolic events during pregnancy (Lockwood, 2002; Pierangeli, 2011). Some aspects of the more common inherited thrombophilias are summarized in Table 52-2 and Figure 52-1.

Inherited Thrombophilias

Patients with inherited thrombophilic disorders often have a family history of thrombosis. Inherited thrombophilias are also found in up to half of all patients who present with venous thromboembolism before the age of 45 years, particularly in those whose event occurred in the absence of well-recognized risk factors, such as surgery or immobilization,

TABLE 52-2. Inherited Thrombophilias and Their Association with Venous Thromboembolism (VTE) in Pregnancy

	Prevalence in General Population (%)	VTE Risk per Pregnancy (No History) (%)	VTE Risk per Pregnancy (Prior VTE) (%)	All VTE (%)
Factor V Leiden heterozygote	1–15	0.5–1.2	10	40
Factor V Leiden homozygote	< 1	4	17	2
Prothrombin gene heterozygote	2–5	< 0.5	> 10	17
Prothrombin gene homozygote	< 1	2–4	> 17	0.5
Factor V Leiden/prothrombin double heterozygote	0.01	4–5	> 20	1–3
Antithrombin III activity (< 60%)	0.02	3–7	40	1
Protein C activity (< 50%)	0.2–0.4	0.1–0.8	4–17	14
Protein S free antigen (< 55%)	0.03–0.13	0.1	0–22	3

Adapted from the American College of Obstetricians and Gynecologists, 2013.

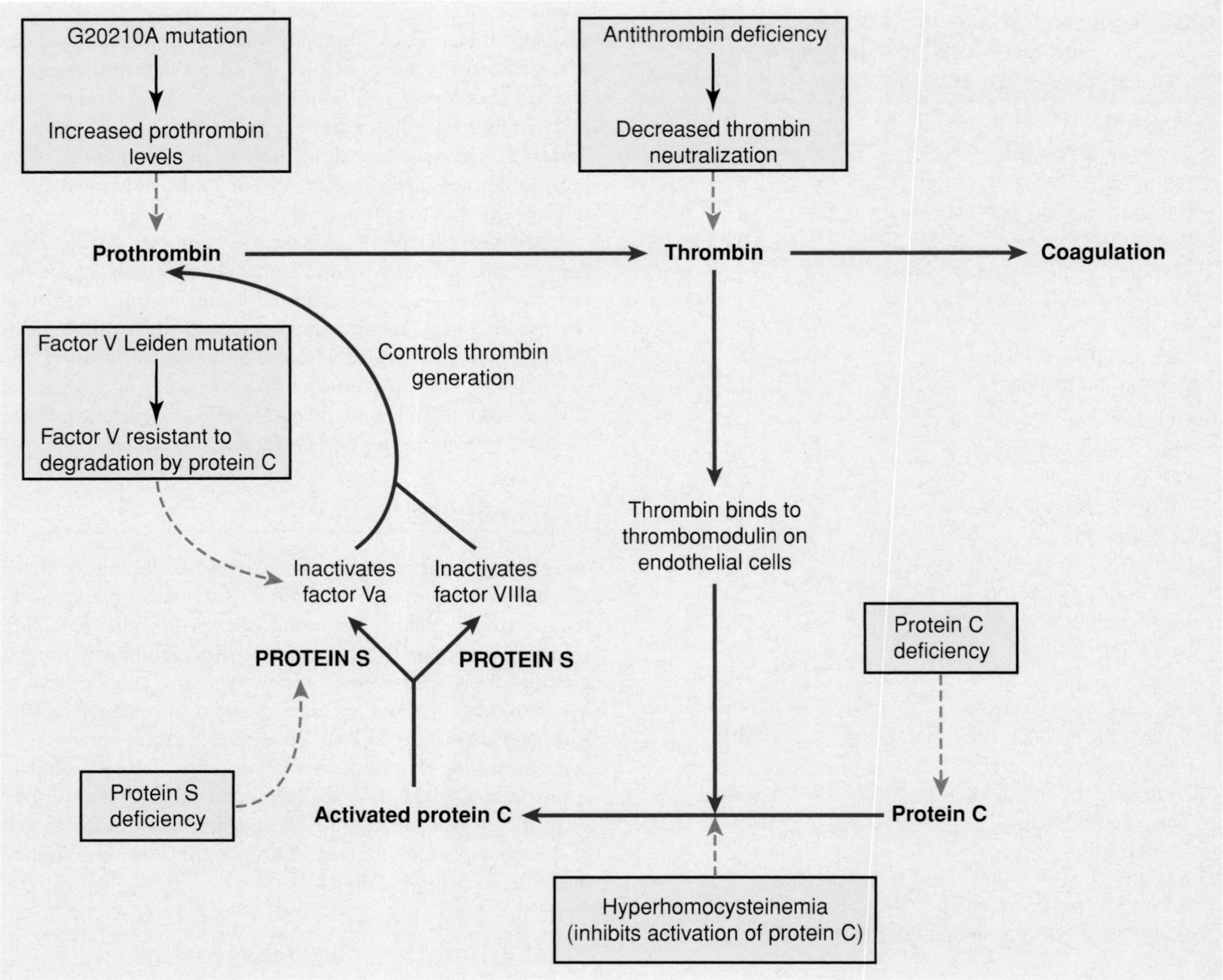

FIGURE 52-1 Overview of the inherited thrombophilias and their effect(s) on the coagulation cascade. (Adapted from Seligsohn, 2001.)

or with minimal provocation such as after a long-distance flight or after taking estrogens. Of greatest significance is a family history of sudden death due to pulmonary embolism or a history of multiple family members requiring long-term anticoagulation therapy because of recurrent thrombosis (Anderson, 2011).

Antithrombin Deficiency

Synthesized in the liver, antithrombin is one of the most important inhibitors of thrombin in clot formation. Antithrombin functions as a natural anticoagulant by binding and inactivating thrombin and the activated coagulation factors IXa, Xa, XIa, and XIIa (Franchini, 2006). Of note, the rate of antithrombin interaction with its target proteases is accelerated by heparin (Anderson, 2011). Antithrombin deficiency may result from hundreds of different mutations that are almost always autosomal dominant. Type I deficiency is the result of reduced synthesis of biologically normal antithrombin, and type II deficiency is characterized by normal levels of antithrombin with reduced functional activity (Anderson, 2011). Homozygous antithrombin deficiency is lethal (Katz, 2002).

Antithrombin deficiency is rare—it affects approximately 1 in 2000 to 5000 individuals, and it is the most thrombogenic of the heritable coagulopathies. Indeed, the thrombosis risk during pregnancy among antithrombin-deficient women without a personal or family history is 3 to 7 percent, and it is 11 to 40 percent with such a history (Lockwood, 2012). Specifically, those affected have approximately a 50-percent lifetime risk of venous thromboembolism.

Sabadell and associates (2010) studied the outcomes of 18 pregnancies complicated by antithrombin deficiency. Twelve of these were treated with low-molecular-weight heparin, and six were not treated because antithrombin deficiency had not yet been diagnosed. Three of the untreated patients suffered a thromboembolic episode compared with none in the treated group. Untreated women also had a 50-percent risk of stillbirth and fetal-growth restriction. By comparison, none of the treated women had a stillbirth, and approximately a fourth developed fetal-growth restriction. Seguin and coworkers (1994) reviewed the outcomes of 23 newborns with antithrombin deficiency and described 11 cases of thrombosis and 10 deaths.

Given such risk, affected women are treated during pregnancy with heparin regardless of whether they have had a prior thrombosis. When anticoagulation is necessarily withheld, such as during surgery or delivery, Paidas and colleagues (2013) found that treatment with recombinant human antithrombin protected against venous thromboembolism development in 21 patients with hereditary antithrombin deficiency. Sharpe and associates (2011) described successful use of antithrombin concentrate infusions plus therapeutic anticoagulation in a pregnant woman with antithrombin deficiency who developed a thrombosis during the third trimester despite therapeutic doses of low-molecular-weight heparin.

Protein C Deficiency

When thrombin is bound to thrombomodulin on endothelial cells of small vessels, its procoagulant activities are neutralized. This binding also activates protein C, a natural anticoagulant that in the presence of protein S controls thrombin generation, in part, by inactivating factors Va and VIIIa (see Fig. 52-1). Activated protein C also inhibits the synthesis of plasminogen-activator inhibitor 1 (p. 1032).

Protein C activity is largely unchanged in pregnancy (Appendix, p. 1288). Based on their study of 440 healthy women, however, Said and associates (2010b) found that protein C activity increases modestly but significantly throughout the first half of pregnancy. These investigators speculated that this increase may play a role in maintaining early pregnancy through both anticoagulant and inflammatory regulatory pathways.

More than 100 different autosomal dominant mutations for the protein C gene have been described. The prevalence of protein C deficiency is 2 to 3 per 1000, but many of these individuals do not have a thrombosis history because the phenotypic expression is highly variable (Anderson, 2011). These prevalence estimates correspond with functional activity threshold values of 50 to 60 percent, which are used by most laboratories and which are associated with a six- to 12-fold increased risk for venous thromboembolism (Lockwood, 2012).

Protein S Deficiency

This circulating anticoagulant is activated by protein C, which enhances its capacity to inactiviate factors Va and VIIIa (see Fig. 52-1). Protein S deficiency may be caused by more than 100 different mutations, with an aggregate prevalence of approximately 2 per 1000 (Lockwood, 2012). Protein S deficiency may be measured by antigenically determined free, functional, and total S levels. All three decline substantively during normal gestation, thus the diagnosis in pregnant women—as well as in those taking certain oral contraceptives—is difficult (Archer, 1999). If screening during pregnancy is necessary, threshold values for free protein S antigen levels in the second and third trimesters have been identified at less than 30 percent and less than 24 percent, respectively. Among those with a positive family history, the venous thromboembolism risk in pregnancy has been reported to be 6 to 7 percent (American College of Obstetricians and Gynecologists, 2013).

Conard and coworkers (1990) described thrombosis in 5 of 29 pregnant women with protein S deficiency. One woman had a cerebral vein thrombosis. Similarly, Burneo and colleagues (2002) reported maternal cerebral vein thrombosis at 14 weeks' gestation. Neonatal homozygous protein C or S deficiency is usually associated with a severe clinical phenotype known as purpura fulminans. This is characterized by extensive thromboses in the microcirculation soon after birth leading to skin necrosis (Salonvaara, 2004).

Activated Protein C Resistance—Factor V Leiden Mutation

The most prevalent of the known thrombophilia syndromes, this condition is characterized by resistance of plasma to the anticoagulant effects of activated protein C. A number of mutations have been described, but the most common is the factor V Leiden mutation, which was named after the city in which it was described. This missense mutation in the factor V gene results from a substitution of glutamine for arginine at position 506 in the factor V polypeptide, which gains resistance to degradation by activated protein C. The unimpeded abnormal factor V protein retains its procoagulant activity and predisposes to thrombosis (see Fig. 52-1).

Heterozygous inheritance for factor V Leiden is the most common heritable thrombophilia. It is found in 3 to 15 percent of select European populations and 3 percent of African Americans, but it is virtually absent in African blacks and Asians (Lockwood, 2012). As shown in Table 52-2, women who are heterozygous for factor V Leiden account for approximately 40 percent of venous thromboembolism cases during pregnancy. However, the actual risk among pregnant women who are heterozygous and who do not have a personal history or a first-degree relative with a thrombotic episode before age 50 years is 5 to 12 per 1000. In contrast, this risk increases to at least 10 percent among women with a personal or family history. Pregnant women who are homozygous without a personal or family history have a 1- to 4-percent risk for venous thromboembolism, whereas those with such a history have an approximately 17-percent risk (American College of Obstetricians and Gynecologists, 2013).

As described later (p. 1034), diagnosis during pregnancy is performed by DNA analysis for the mutant factor V gene. This is because bioassay is confounded by the fact that resistance is normally increased after early pregnancy because of alterations in other coagulation proteins (Walker, 1997). Of note, activated protein C resistance can also be caused by antiphospholipid syndrome, which is described later (p. 1033) and also detailed in Chapter 59 (p. 1173) (Eldor, 2001; Saenz, 2011).

To assess the prognostic significance of maternal factor V Leiden mutation during pregnancy, Kjellberg and colleagues (2010) compared the outcomes of 491 carriers with 1055 controls. All three of the thromboembolic events occurred among the carriers. But, there were no differences in preterm birth, birthweight, or hypertensive complications between the two groups. Similarly, Hammerová and coworkers (2011) found that adverse pregnancy events were not increased among women with heterozygous mutations. In a meticulously executed prospective observational study of approximately 5000 women conducted by the Maternal-Fetal Medicine Units Network, Dizon-Townson and associates (2005) found that the heterozygous mutant gene incidence was 2.7 percent. Of three pulmonary emboli and one deep-vein thrombosis cases—a rate of 0.8 per 1000 pregnancies—none were among these carriers. There was no increased risk of preeclampsia, placental abruption, fetal-growth restriction, or pregnancy loss in heterozygous women. The investigators concluded that universal prenatal screening for the Leiden mutation and prophylaxis for carriers without a prior venous thromboembolism is not indicated. Finally, Clark and colleagues (2002) concluded that such routine prenatal screening was not cost effective.

Prothrombin G20210A Mutation

This missense mutation in the prothrombin gene leads to excessive accumulation of prothrombin, which then may be converted to thrombin. As with factor V Leiden, a personal history or a family history of venous thromboembolism in a first-degree relative before age 50 years increases the risk of venous thromboembolism during pregnancy (see Table 52-2). For a heterozygous carrier with such a history, the risk exceeds 10 percent. Without such a history, heterozygous carriers of the mutation have less than a 1-percent risk of venous thromboembolism during pregnancy (American College of Obstetricians and Gynecologists, 2013).

Homozygous patients or those who coinherit a G20210A mutation with a factor V Leiden mutation have an even greater thromboembolism risk. Stefano and associates (1999) performed a retrospective cohort study of 624 nonpregnant patients with one prior episode of deep-vein thrombosis. They found that those doubly heterozygous individuals had a 2.6-fold increased risk of recurrence relative to those with the heterozygous Leiden mutation alone. They concluded that carriers with both mutations are candidates for lifelong anticoagulation after a first thrombotic episode.

In a secondary analysis of the Maternal-Fetal Medicine Units Network study described earlier, Silver and coworkers (2010) tested nearly 4200 women for the prothrombin G20210A mutation. A total of 157—or 3.8 percent—of the women carried the mutation, and only one of these was homozygous. Carriers had similar rates of pregnancy loss, preeclampsia, growth restriction, and placental abruption compared with noncarriers. The three thromboembolic events occurred in women who tested negative for the mutation.

Hyperhomocysteinemia

The most common cause of elevated homocysteine is the C667T thermolabile mutation of the enzyme 5, 10-methylenetetrahydrofolate reductase (MTHFR). Inheritance is autosomal recessive. Elevated homocysteine levels may also result from deficiency of one of several enzymes involved in methionine metabolism and from correctible nutritional deficiencies of folic acid, vitamin B_6, or vitamin B_{12} (Hague, 2003; McDonald, 2001). During normal pregnancy, mean homocysteine plasma concentrations are decreased (López-Quesada, 2003; McDonald, 2001). Thus, to make a diagnosis during pregnancy, Lockwood (2002) recommends a fasting threshold of > 12 μmol/L to define hyperhomocysteinemia.

Although hyperhomocysteinemia was previously reported to be a modest risk factor for venous thromboembolism, more recent data indicate that an elevated homocysteine level is actually a weak risk factor (American College of Obstetricians and Gynecologists, 2013). In an interesting metaanalysis, den Heijer and colleagues (2005) found that international studies of MTHFR polymorphisms were collectively associated with slightly increased significant risks for thrombosis—odds ratios 1.15 to 1.6. In contrast, studies conducted in North America collectively demonstrated no such association. The authors speculated that folic acid supplementation could explain the difference. Recall that folic acid serves as a cofactor in the remethylation reaction of homocysteine to methionine. Similarly, the American College of Chest Physicians concluded that the lack of an association with thromboembolism could reflect the physiological reductions in homocysteine levels associated with pregnancy and the effects of widespread prenatal folic acid supplementation (Bates, 2012).

In a follow-up study of 167 women who developed a venous thromboembolism during pregnancy and 128 controls, Kovac and associates (2010) found no difference in the prevalence of MTHFR C677T homozygosity between the two groups. The American College of Obstetricians and Gynecologists (2013) has concluded that there is insufficient evidence to support assessment of MTHFR polymorphisms or measurement of fasting homocysteine levels in the evaluation for venous thromboembolism.

Other Thrombophilia Mutations

A number of potentially thrombophilic polymorphisms are being discovered at an ever-increasing rate. Unfortunately, information regarding the prognostic significance of such newly discovered mutations is limited. For example, protein Z is a vitamin K-dependent protein that serves as a cofactor in factor Xa inactivation. Studies in nonpregnant patients have found that low protein Z levels are associated with an increased thromboembolism risk (Santacroce, 2006). Similarly, plasminogen activator inhibitor type 1 (PAI-1) is an important regulator of fibrinolysis. Certain polymorphisms in the gene promoter have been associated with small increased venous thromboembolism risks. These thrombophilias and others, including alternative mutations in the factor V gene and activity-enhancing mutations in various clotting factor genes, appear to exert little independent risk for venous thromboembolism. And although they may exacerbate risk among patients when coinherited with other thrombophilias, the American College of Obstetricians and Gynecologists (2013) has concluded that there is insufficient evidence to recommend screening.

As an interesting aside, Galanaud and coworkers (2010) hypothesized that a paternal thrombophilia could increase the risk of a maternal thromboembolism. Specifically, these investigators found that a paternal thrombophilia—the PROCR 6936G allele—affects the endothelial protein C receptor. This receptor is expressed by villous trophoblast and thus is exposed to maternal blood. Although this research is preliminary, it could help explain the pathogenesis of recurrent idiopathic thromboses in pregnant women.

Acquired Thrombophilias

Some examples of acquired hypercoagulable states include antiphospholipid syndrome (Chap. 59, p. 1173), heparin-induced thrombocytopenia (p. 1040), and cancer (Chap. 63, p. 1219).

Antiphospholipid Antibodies

These autoantibodies are detected in approximately 2 percent of patients who have nontraumatic venous thrombosis. The antibodies are directed against cardiolipin(s) or against phospholipid-binding proteins such as β_2-glycoprotein I. They are commonly—but not always—found in patients with systemic lupus erythematosus and are described in detail in Chapter 59 (p. 1169). Women with moderate-to-high levels of these antibodies may have antiphospholipid syndrome, which, as summarized by the American College of Obstetricians and Gynecologists (2012), is defined by a number of clinical features. In addition to vascular thromboses, these include: (1) at least one otherwise unexplained fetal death at or beyond 10 weeks; (2) at least one preterm birth before 34 weeks because of eclampsia, severe preeclampsia, or placental insufficiency; or (3) at least three unexplained consecutive spontaneous abortions before 10 weeks.

In these women, thromboembolism—either venous or arterial—most commonly involves the lower extremities. Importantly, the syndrome should also be considered in women with thromboses in unusual sites, such as the portal, mesenteric, splenic, subclavian, axillary, and cerebral veins. Antiphospholipid antibodies predispose to arterial thromboses, which may also occur in relatively unusual locations, such as the retinal, subclavian, brachial, or digital arteries. The thrombotic mechanisms associated with antiphospholipid syndrome have recently been reviewed by Giannakopoulos and Krilis (2013).

The thrombosis risk increases significantly during pregnancy in women with antiphospholipid syndrome. Indeed, up to 25 percent of thrombotic events in women with antiphospholipid syndrome occur during pregnancy or in the puerperium. Looking at this a different way, women with antiphospholipid syndrome have a 5- to 12-percent risk of thrombosis during pregnancy or the puerperium (American College of Obstetricians and Gynecologists, 2012).

Thrombophilias and Pregnancy Complications

Attention has been directed toward possible relationships between inherited thrombophilias and pregnancy complications other than thromboses. Summarized in Table 52-3 are

TABLE 52-3. Obstetrical Complications Associated with Thrombophilias

Type of Thrombophilia	Early Loss	Recurrent First-Trimester Loss	Nonrecurrent Second-Trimester Loss	Late Loss	Preeclampsia	Placental Abruption	Fetal-Growth Restriction
Factor V Leiden (homozygous)	**2.71 (1.32–5.58)**	—[a]	—[a]	1.98 (0.40–9.69)	1.87 (0.44–7.88)	8.43 (0.41–171.20)	4.64 (0.19–115.68)
Factor V Leiden (heterozygous)	**1.68 (1.09–2.58)**	**1.91 (1.01–3.61)**[a]	**4.12 (1.91–8.81)**[a]	**2.06 (1.10–3.86)**	**2.19 (1.46–3.27)**	**4.70 (1.13–19.59)**	2.68 (0.59–12.13)
Prothrombin gene mutation (heterozygous)	**2.49 (1.24–5.00)**	**2.70 (1.37–5.34)**	**8.60 (2.18–33.95)**	**2.66 (1.28–5.53)**	**2.54 (1.52–4.23)**	**7.71 (3.01–19.76)**	2.92 (0.62–13.70)
MTHFR C677T (homozygous)	1.40 (0.77–2.55)	0.86 (0.44–1.69)	NA	1.31 (0.89–1.91)	**1.37 (1.07–1.76)**	1.47 (0.40–5.35)	1.24 (0.84–1.82)
Antithrombin deficiency	0.88 (0.17–4.48)	NA	NA	7.63 (0.30–196.36)	3.89 (0.16–97.19)	1.08 (0.06–18.12)	NA
Protein C deficiency	2.29 (0.20–26.43)	NA	NA	3.05 (0.24–38.51)	5.15 (0.26–102.22)	5.93 (0.23–151.58)	NA
Protein S deficiency	3.55 (0.35–35.72)	NA	NA	**20.09 (3.70–109.15)**	2.83 (0.76–10.57)	2.11 (0.47–9.34)	NA
Anticardiolipin antibodies	**3.40 (1.33–8.68)**	**5.05 (1.82–14.01)**	NA	**3.30 (1.62–6.70)**	**2.73 (1.65–4.51)**	1.42 (0.42–4.77)	**6.91 (2.70–17.68)**
Lupus anticoagulants (nonspecific inhibitor)	**2.97 (1.03–9.76)**	NA	**14.28 (4.72–43.20)**	2.38 (0.81–6.98)	1.45 (0.70–4.61)	NA	NA
Hyper-homocysteinemia	**6.25 (1.37–28.42)**	**4.21 (1.28–13.87)**	NA	0.98 (0.17–5.55)	**3.49 (1.21–10.11)**	2.40 (0.36–15.89)	NA

[a]Homozygous and heterozygous carriers were grouped together; it is not possible to extract data for each state.
Data are presented as odds ratio (OR [95% CI]) and are derived from Robertson, 2005. Bolded numbers are statistically significant.
MTHFR = methylene tetrahydrofolate reductase variant; NA = not available.
From Bates, 2012.

the findings of 25 studies systematically reviewed by Robertson and associates (2005). These were incorporated into the most recent recommendations of the American College of Chest Physicians (Bates, 2012). Importantly, the considerable heterogeneity and wide confidence intervals illustrate the uncertainty of these associations.

More recent investigations continue to underscore the heterogeneity of results. For example, Kahn and coworkers (2009) found no increased risk for early-onset or severe preeclampsia in women with factor V Leiden mutation, prothrombin G20210A mutation, MTHFR C677T polymorphism, or hyperhomocysteinemia. Said and associates (2010a) prospectively screened more than 2000 healthy nulliparous women for factor V Leiden, prothrombin gene mutation, MTHFR C677T, MTHFR A1298C, and thrombomodulin polymorphism. Women who carried the prothrombin gene mutation had a 3.6-fold increased risk of adverse pregnancy outcome, including severe preeclampsia, fetal-growth restriction, placental abruption, or stillbirth. But, none of the other polymorphisms conferred an increased risk of these adverse outcomes. Moreover, this group of investigators found no association between the PAI-1 4G/5G polymorphism and adverse pregnancy outcome (Said, 2012). Similarly, based on their prospective study of 750 pregnancies complicated by stillbirth, Korteweg and colleagues (2010) concluded that routine thrombophilia testing after fetal death is inadvisable.

Because of uncertainties associated with the magnitude of risk as well as any benefits of prophylaxis given to prevent pregnancy complications in women with heritable thrombophilias, it remains unproven that screening is in the best interest of these women. The American College of Obstetricians and Gynecologists (2013) has concluded that a definitive causal link cannot be made between inherited thrombophilias and adverse pregnancy outcomes. Similarly, the American College of Chest Physicians recently concluded that it was unclear whether screening for inherited thrombophilias is prudent in women with pregnancy complications (Bates, 2012). In contrast, and as shown in Table 52-3 and detailed in Chapter 59 (p. 1174), the association between antiphospholipid syndrome and adverse pregnancy outcomes—including fetal loss, recurrent pregnancy loss, and preeclampsia—is much stronger.

Thrombophilia Screening

Given the high incidence of thrombophilia in the population and the low incidence of venous thromboembolism, universal screening during pregnancy is not cost effective (Carbone, 2010). Thus, a selective screening strategy is required. The American Academy of Pediatrics and the American College of Obstetricians and Gynecologists (2012) recommend that thrombophilia screening be considered in the following clinical circumstances: (1) a personal history of venous thromboembolism that was associated with a nonrecurrent risk factor such as fractures, surgery, and/or prolonged immobilization; and (2) a first-degree relative (parent or sibling) with a history of high-risk thrombophilia or venous thromboembolism before age 50 years in the absence of other risk factors.

As described earlier, the American College of Obstetricians and Gynecologists (2013) has concluded that testing for inherited thrombophilias in women who have experienced recurrent fetal loss or placental abruption is not recommended because there is insufficient clinical evidence that antepartum heparin prophylaxis prevents recurrence. Similarly, testing is not recommended for women with a history of fetal-growth restriction or preeclampsia. The American College of Chest Physicians also recommends against screening women with prior pregnancy complications (Bates, 2012). As discussed in Chapter 59, however, screening for antiphospholipid antibodies may be appropriate in women who have experienced a fetal loss.

Screening Tests

Methods of screening for the more common inherited thrombophilias are shown in Table 52-4. Whenever possible, laboratory testing should be performed at least 6 weeks after the

TABLE 52-4. Inherited Thrombophilia Testing

Thrombophilia	Testing Method	Is Testing Reliable During Pregnancy?	Is Testing Reliable During Acute Thrombosis?	Is Testing Reliable with Anticoagulation?
Factor V Leiden mutation	Activated protein C resistance assay (second generation)	Yes	Yes	No
	If abnormal: DNA analysis	Yes	Yes	Yes
Prothrombin gene mutation G20210A	DNA analysis	Yes	Yes	Yes
Protein C deficiency	Protein C activity (< 60%)	Yes	No	No
Protein S deficiency	Functional assay (< 55%)	No[a]	No	No
Antithrombin deficiency	Antithrombin activity (< 60%)	Yes	No	No

[a]In nonpregnant patients, protein S deficiency should be assessed initially by performing a functional assay. A value < 55 percent should be followed with measurement of free protein S levels. A free protein S antigen value < 55 percent is consistent with protein S deficiency. If screening in pregnancy is necessary, threshold values for free protein S antigen levels in the second and third trimesters have been identified at < 30 percent and < 24 percent, respectively.
Adapted from the American College of Obstetricians and Gynecologists, 2013.

thrombotic event, while the patient is not pregnant, and when she is not receiving anticoagulation or hormonal therapy. Because of the lack of association between methylenetetrahydrofolate reductase (MTHFR) gene mutations—the most common cause of hyperhomocysteinemia—and adverse pregnancy outcomes, screening with fasting homocysteine levels or MTHFR mutation analyses is not recommended (American College of Obstetricians and Gynecologists, 2013).

DEEP-VEIN THROMBOSIS

Clinical Presentation

During pregnancy, most venous thromboses are confined to the deep veins of the lower extremity. Approximately 70 percent of cases are located in the iliofemoral veins without involvement of the calf veins. Isolated iliac vein and calf vein thromboses occur in approximately 17 and 6 percent of cases, respectively (Chan, 2010).

The signs and symptoms vary greatly and depend on the degree of occlusion and the intensity of the inflammatory response. Most cases during pregnancy are left sided. Ginsberg and coworkers (1992) reported that 58 of 60 antepartum women—97 percent—had left leg thromboses. Blanco-Molina and coworkers (2007) reported left-leg involvement in 78 percent. Our experiences at Parkland Hospital are similar—approximately 90 percent of lower extremity thromboses involved the left leg. Greer (2003) hypothesizes that this results from compression of the left iliac vein by the right iliac and ovarian artery, both of which cross the vein only on the left side. Yet, as described in Chapter 53 (p. 1051), the ureter is compressed more on the right side!

Classic thrombosis involving the lower extremity is abrupt in onset, and there is pain and edema of the leg and thigh. The thrombus typically involves much of the deep-venous system to the iliofemoral region. Occasionally, reflex arterial spasm causes a pale, cool extremity with diminished pulsations. Conversely, there may be appreciable clot, yet little pain, heat, or swelling. Importantly, calf pain, either spontaneous or in response to squeezing or to Achilles tendon stretching—*Homans sign*—may be caused by a strained muscle or contusion. Between 30 and 60 percent of women with a confirmed lower-extremity acute deep-vein thrombosis have an asymptomatic pulmonary embolism (p. 1041).

Diagnosis

Clinical diagnosis of deep-vein thrombosis is difficult, and thus other methods are imperative for confirmation. In one study of pregnant women, the clinical diagnosis was confirmed in only 10 percent (Hull, 1990). Shown in Figure 52-2 is one diagnostic algorithm recommended by the American College of Chest Physicians that can be used for evaluation of pregnant women (Guyatt, 2012). With a few modifications, we follow a similar evaluation at Parkland Hospital.

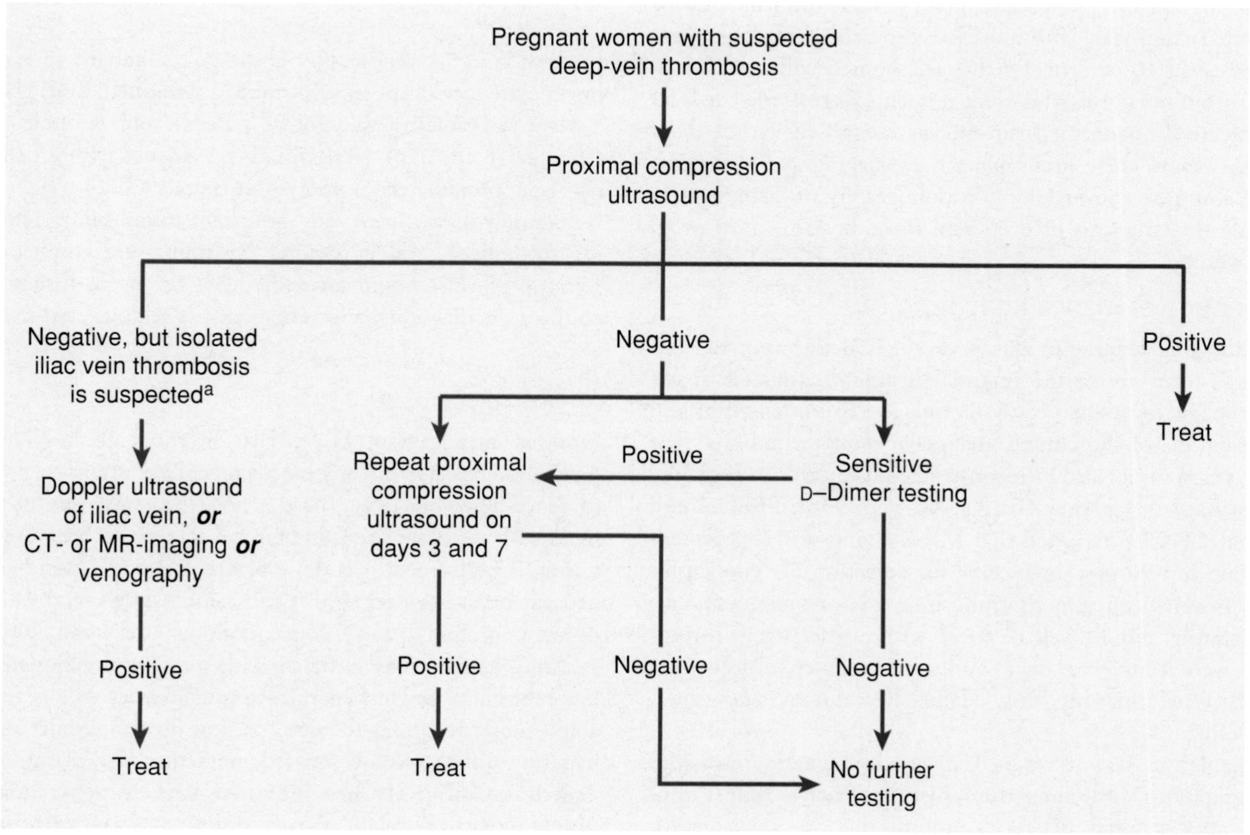

FIGURE 52-2 Algorithm for evaluation of suspected deep-vein thrombosis in pregnancy. CT = computed tomography; MR = magnetic resonance. (Adapted from the American College of Chest Physicians, Guyatt, 2012.) [a]Signs and symptoms include swelling of the entire leg, with or without flank, buttock, or back pain.

Compression Ultrasonography

In pregnant women with suspected deep-vein thrombosis, the American Academy of Pediatrics and the American College of Obstetricians and Gynecologists (2012) recommend compression ultrasonography of the proximal veins as the initial diagnostic test. According to the American College of Chest Physicians, this noninvasive technique is currently the most-used first-line test to detect deep-vein thrombosis (Guyatt, 2012). The diagnosis is based on the noncompressibility and typical echoarchitecture of a thrombosed vein.

For *nonpregnant* patients with suspected thrombosis, the safety of withholding anticoagulation has been established for those who have normal serial compression examinations over a week (Birdwell, 1998; Heijboer, 1993). Specifically, isolated calf thromboses that extend into the proximal veins in about a fourth of patients will do so within 1 to 2 weeks of presentation. Moreover, these are usually detected by serial ultrasonographic compression.

In *pregnant* women, the important caveat is that normal findings with venous ultrasonography results do not always exclude a pulmonary embolism. This is because the thrombosis may have already embolized or because it arose from iliac or other deep-pelvic veins, which are less accessible to ultrasound evaluation (Goldhaber, 2004). Thrombosis associated with pulmonary embolism during pregnancy frequently originates in the iliac veins. Although serial investigations are recommended by many, Le Gal and colleagues (2012) recently studied the use of nonserial proximal and distal compression ultrasonography in 226 pregnant and postpartum women with suspected deep-vein thrombosis. Deep-vein thrombosis was diagnosed in 10 percent. Of the 177 women without a deep-vein thrombosis and who were not anticoagulated, two had an objectively confirmed thrombosis diagnosed within three months. Thus, these preliminary data suggest that a negative single complete compression ultrasonography study may safely exclude the diagnosis of deep-vein thrombosis in most pregnant women.

Magnetic Resonance Imaging

This imaging technique allows excellent delineation of anatomical detail above the inguinal ligament. Thus, in many cases, magnetic resonance (MR) imaging is immensely useful for diagnosis of iliofemoral and pelvic vein thrombosis. The venous system can also be reconstructed using MR venography as discussed in Chapter 46 (Fig. 46-5, p. 936). Erdman and associates (1990) reported that MR imaging was 100-percent sensitive and 90-percent specific for detection of venographically proven deep-vein thrombosis in nonpregnant patients. Importantly, almost half of those without deep-vein thrombosis were found to have nonthrombotic conditions that included cellulitis, myositis, edema, hematomas, and superficial phlebitis.

Khalil and coworkers (2012) used magnetic resonance venography to study the natural history of pelvic vein thrombosis after vaginal delivery. Among the 30 *asymptomatic* patients who were all within four days of delivery, 30 percent had a definitive thrombosis in either the iliac or ovarian veins, and another 37 percent had a suspected thrombosis. Our experience with hundreds of postpartum MR scans does not support these findings. Thus, although the clinical significance of their findings is uncertain, it seems clear that some degree of pelvic vein intraluminal filling defect may be a normal finding.

D-Dimer Screening Tests

These specific fibrin degradation products are generated when fibrinolysin degrades fibrin, as occurs in thromboembolism (Chap. 41, p. 809). Their measurement is frequently incorporated into diagnostic algorithms for venous thromboembolism in nonpregnant patients (Kelly, 2002; Wells, 2003). Screening with the D-dimer test in pregnancy, however, is problematic for a number of reasons. As shown in the Appendix (p. 1288), depending on assay sensitivity, D-dimer serum levels increase with gestational age along with substantively elevated plasma fibrinogen concentrations (McCrae, 2014). Levels are also affected by multifetal gestation and cesarean delivery (Morikawa, 2011). In a serial study of 50 healthy women, Kline and colleagues (2005) found that D-dimer levels increased progressively during pregnancy. Also, 22 percent of women in midpregnancy and no women in the third trimester had a D-dimer concentration below 0.50 mg/L—a conventional threshold used to exclude thromboembolism. D-Dimer concentrations can also be elevated in certain pregnancy complications such as placental abruption, preeclampsia, and sepsis syndrome. For these reasons, their use during pregnancy remains uncertain, but a negative D-dimer test should be considered reassuring (Lockwood, 2012; Marik, 2008).

Venography

Invasive contrast venography is the gold standard to exclude lower extremity deep-vein thrombosis (Chunilal, 2001). It has a negative-predictive value of 98 percent, and as discussed in Chapter 46 (p. 932), fetal radiation exposure without shielding is approximately 3 mGy (Nijkeuter, 2006). That said, venography is associated with significant complications, including thrombosis, and it is time consuming and cumbersome. Because of this, noninvasive methods are used primarily to confirm the diagnosis, and venography is seldom used today.

Management

Optimal management of venous thromboembolism during pregnancy has not undergone major clinical study to provide evidence-based practices. There is, however, consensus for treatment with anticoagulation and limited activity. If thrombophilia testing is performed, it is done before anticoagulation because heparin induces a decline in antithrombin levels, and warfarin decreases protein C and S concentrations (Lockwood, 2002).

Anticoagulation is initiated with either unfractionated or low-molecular-weight heparin. Although either type is acceptable, most recommend one of the low-molecular-weight heparins. In its recently revised guidelines, for example, the American College of Chest Physicians suggests preferential use of low-molecular-weight heparin during pregnancy because of better bioavailability, longer plasma half-life, more predictable dose response, reduced risks of osteoporosis and thrombocytopenia, and less frequent dosing (Bates, 2012).

During pregnancy, heparin therapy is continued, and for postpartum women, anticoagulation is begun simultaneously with warfarin. Recall that pulmonary embolism develops in as many as 60 percent of patients with untreated venous thrombosis, and anticoagulation decreases this risk to less than 5 percent. In nonpregnant patients, the mortality rate is approximately 1 percent (Douketis, 1998; Pollack, 2011).

Over several days, leg pain dissipates. After symptoms have abated, graded ambulation should be started. Elastic stockings are fitted, and anticoagulation is continued. Recovery to this stage usually takes 7 to 10 days. Graduated compression stockings should be continued for 2 years after the diagnosis to reduce the incidence of postthrombotic syndrome (Brandjes, 1997). This syndrome can include chronic leg paresthesias or pain, intractable edema, skin changes, and leg ulcers.

Unfractionated Heparin

This agent should be considered for the initial treatment of thromboembolism and in situations in which delivery, surgery, or thrombolysis may be necessary (p. 1039) (American College of Obstetricians and Gynecologists, 2011). Unfractionated heparin (UFH) can be administered by one of two alternatives: (1) initial intravenous therapy followed by adjusted-dose subcutaneous UFH given every 12 hours; or (2) twice-daily, adjusted dose subcutaneous UFH with doses adjusted to prolong the activated partial thromboplastin time (aPTT) into the therapeutic range 6 hours postinjection (Bates, 2012). As shown in Table 52-5, the therapeutic dose for subcutaneous UFH is usually 10,000 units or more every 12 hours.

For intravenous therapy, there are a number of acceptable protocols. In general, UFH is initiated with a bolus intravenous dose of 70 to 100 U/kg, about 5000 to 10,000 U, followed by continuous intravenous infusions beginning at 1000 U/hr or 15 to 20 U/kg/hr, titrated to achieve an aPTT of 1.5 to 2.5 times control values (Brown, 2010). Intravenous anticoagulation should be maintained for at least 5 to 7 days, after which treatment is converted to subcutaneous heparin to maintain the aPTT to at least 1.5 to 2.5 times control throughout the dosing interval. For women with antiphospholipid syndrome, aPTT does not accurately assess heparin anticoagulation, and thus anti-factor Xa levels are preferred.

TABLE 52-5. Anticoagulation Regimen Definitions

Anticoagulation Regimen	Definition
Prophylactic LMWH*	Enoxaparin, 40 mg SC once daily Dalteparin, 5,000 units SC once daily Tinzaparin, 4,500 units SC once daily
Therapeutic LMWH†	Enoxaparin, 1 mg/kg every 12 hours Dalteparin, 200 units/kg once daily Tinzaparin, 175 units/kg once daily Dalteparin, 100 units/kg every 12 hours May target an anti-Xa level in the therapeutic range of 0.6–1.0 units/mL for twice daily regimen; slightly higher doses may be needed for a once-daily regimen.
Minidose prophylactic UFH	UFH, 5,000 units SC every 12 hours
Prophylactic UFH	UFH, 5,000–10,000 units SC every 12 hours UFH, 5,000–7,500 units SC every 12 hours in first trimester UFH 7,500–10,000 units SC every 12 hours in the second trimester UFH, 10,000 units SC every 12 hours in the third trimester, unless the aPTT is elevated
Therapeutic UFH†	UFH, 10,000 units or more SC every 12 hours in doses adjusted to target aPTT in the therapeutic range (1.5–2.5) 6 hours after injection
Postpartum anticoagulation	Prophylactic LMWH/UFH for 4–6 weeks or vitamin K antagonists for 4–6 weeks with a target INR of 2.0–3.0, with initial UFH or LMWH therapy overlap until the INR is 2.0 or more for 2 days
Surveillance	Clinical vigilance and appropriate objective investigation of women with symptoms suspicious of deep vein thrombosis or pulmonary embolism

Abbreviations: aPTT, activated partial thromboplastin time; INR, international normalized ratio; LMWH, low molecular weight heparin; SC, subcutaneously; UFH, unfractionated heparin.

*Although at extremes of body weight, modification of dose may be required.

†Also referred to as weight adjusted, full treatment dose.

From Inherited thrombophilias in pregnancy. Practice Bulletin No. 138. American College of Obstetricians and Gynecologists. Obstet Gynecol 2013;122:706–17.

The duration of full anticoagulation varies, and there are no studies that have defined the optimal duration for pregnancy-related thromboembolism. In nonpregnant patients with venous thromboembolism, evidence supports a minimum treatment duration of 3 months (Kearon, 2012). For pregnant patients, the American College of Chest Physicians recommends anticoagulation throughout pregnancy and postpartum for a minimum total duration of 3 months (Bates, 2012). Lockwood (2012) recommends that full anticoagulation be continued for at least 20 weeks followed by prophylactic doses if the woman is still pregnant. Prophylactic doses of subcutaneous unfractionated heparin can range from 5000 to 10,000 units every 12 hours titrated to maintain an anti-factor Xa level of 0.1 to 0.2 units, measured 6 hours after the last injection. If the venous thromboembolism occurs during the postpartum period, Lockwood (2012) recommends a minimum of 6 months of anticoagulation treatment.

Low-Molecular-Weight Heparin

This is a family of derivatives of unfractionated heparin, and their molecular weights average 4000 to 5000 daltons compared with 12,000 to 16,000 daltons for conventional heparin. None of these heparins cross the placenta, and all exert their anticoagulant activity by activating antithrombin. The primary difference is their relative inhibitory activity against factor Xa and thrombin (Garcia, 2008). Specifically, unfractionated heparin has equivalent activity against factor Xa and thrombin, but low-molecular-weight heparins (LMWH) have greater activity against factor Xa than thrombin. They also have a more predictable anticoagulant response and fewer bleeding complications than unfractionated heparin because of their better bioavailability, longer half-life, dose-independent clearance, and decreased interference with platelets (Tapson, 2008). These LMWH compounds are cleared by the kidneys and must be used cautiously when there is renal dysfunction.

A number of studies have shown that venous thromboembolism is treated effectively with LMWH (Quinlan, 2004; Tapson, 2008). Using serial venograms, Breddin and associates (2001) observed that these compounds were more effective than UFH in reducing thrombus size without increasing mortality rates or major bleeding complications. Several different treatment regimens using adjusted-dose LMWH for treatment of acute venous thromboembolism are recommended by the American College of Obstetricians and Gynecologists (2011) and are listed in Table 52-5.

Pharmacokinetics in Pregnancy

Low-molecular-weight heparins available for use in pregnancy include enoxaparin, tinzaparin, and dalteparin. Enoxaparin (Lovenox) pharmacokinetics were studied by Rodie and coworkers (2002) in 36 women with venous thromboembolism during pregnancy or immediately postpartum. The dose was approximately 1 mg/kg given twice daily based on early pregnancy weight. Treatment was monitored by peak anti-factor Xa activity 3 hours postinjection, with a target therapeutic range of 0.4–1.0 U/mL. In 33 women, enoxaparin provided satisfactory anticoagulation. In the other three women, dose reduction was necessary. None developed recurrent thromboembolism or bleeding complications. Smith and colleagues (2004) reported similar results with tinzaparin (Innohep) given as a once-daily 50 U/kg dose. They found that a dosage of 75 to 175 U/kg/day was necessary to achieve peak anti-factor Xa levels of 0.1 to 1.0 U/mL.

Dalteparin (Fragmin) pharmacokinetics were studied by Barbour (2004) and Jacobsen (2003) and their associates in longitudinal studies of 13 and 20 pregnant women, respectively. Both groups of investigators concluded that conventional starting doses of dalteparin—100 U/kg every 12 hours—were likely insufficient to maintain full anticoagulation and that slightly higher doses than that shown in Table 52-5 may be required. As an aside, several groups of investigators have found in preliminary studies that dalteparin use is associated with shorter labors (Ekman-Ordeberg, 2010; Isma, 2010). If these observations are verified, then the mechanism of action may involve increased cytokine secretion as in vitro studies suggest.

Dosing and Monitoring

Standard prophylactic and therapeutic dosages recommended by the American College of Obstetricians and Gynecologists (2011) for various LMWHs are listed in Table 52-5. Whether such dosages require adjustments during the course of pregnancy is controversial (Cutts, 2013). Some suggest periodic measurement of anti-factor Xa levels 4 to 6 hours after an injection with dose adjustment to maintain a therapeutic level. According to Bates and coworkers (2012), large studies using clinical end points that demonstrate an optimal therapeutic range or that show dose adjustments increase therapy safety or efficacy are lacking. Moreover, assay measurement accuracy and reliability are uncertain; correlations with bleeding and recurrence risks are lacking; and assay costs are high. Accordingly, the American College of Chest Physicians has concluded that routine monitoring with anti-Xa levels is difficult to justify.

Safety in Pregnancy

Early reviews by Sanson (1999) and Lepercq (2001), each with their colleagues, concluded that low-molecular-weight heparins were safe and effective. Despite this, in 2002, the manufacturer of Lovenox warned that its use in pregnancy had been associated with congenital anomalies and an increased risk of hemorrhage. After its own extensive review, the American College of Obstetricians and Gynecologists (2002) concluded that these risks were rare, that their incidence was not higher than expected, and that no cause-and-effect relationship had been established. It further concluded that enoxaparin and dalteparin could be given safely during pregnancy, and subsequent reports have continued to confirm their safety (Andersen, 2010; Bates, 2012; Deruelle, 2007; Galambosi, 2012).

Nelson-Piercy and coworkers (2011) assessed the safety profile of tinzaparin through a comprehensive study of 1267 pregnant women treated at 28 participating hospitals in

North America and Europe. There were no maternal deaths or complications from regional analgesia. Although thrombocytopenia developed in 1.8 percent, there were no cases of heparin-induced thrombocytopenia (p. 1040). The allergy incidence was 1.3 percent. Osteoporotic fractures in three women (0.2 percent) were judged to be related to tinzaparin (p. 1038). A total of 43 women (3.4 percent) required medical intervention for bleeding. Of the 15 stillbirths, four were judged as possibly being related to tinzaparin use. But, none of the neonatal deaths or congenital abnormalities was attributed to tinzaparin. The authors concluded that tinzaparin during pregnancy was safe for mother and fetus.

Like unfractionated heparin, LMWHs are safe during breast feeding. Although there may be detectable levels of these drugs in breast milk, the bioavailability when ingested orally is poor, and there is no anticoagulant effect in the infant (Lim, 2010).

Caveats are that LMWHs should be avoided in women with renal failure (Krivak, 2007). Moreover, when given within 2 hours of cesarean delivery, these agents increase the risk of wound hematoma (van Wijk, 2002). Lee and Goodwin (2006) described development of a massive subchorionic hematoma associated with enoxaparin use. Forsnes and associates (2009) reported a woman who developed a spontaneous thoracolumbar epidural hematoma that required surgical drainage.

Labor and Delivery

Women receiving either therapeutic or prophylactic anticoagulation should be converted from LMWH to the shorter half-life UFH in the last month of pregnancy or sooner if delivery appears imminent. The purpose of conversion to UFH has less to do with any risk of maternal bleeding at the time of delivery, but rather with neuraxial blockade complicated by an epidural or spinal hematoma (Chap. 25, p. 516). The American College of Chest Physicians recommends that women scheduled for a planned delivery who are receiving twice-daily adjusted-dose subcutaneous UFH or LMWH discontinue their heparin 24 hours before labor induction or cesarean delivery. Patients receiving once-daily LMWH should take only 50 percent of their normal dose on the morning of the day before delivery (Bates, 2012). The American College of Obstetricians and Gynecologists (2013) advises that adjusted-dose subcutaneous LMWH or UFH can be discontinued 24 to 36 hours before an induction of labor or scheduled cesarean delivery. The American Society of Regional Anesthesia and Pain Medicine advises withholding neuraxial blockade for 10 to 12 hours after the last prophylactic dose of LMWH or 24 hours after the last therapeutic dose (Horlocker, 2010).

If a woman begins labor while taking UFH, clearance can be verified by an aPTT. Reversal of heparin with protamine sulfate is rarely required and is not indicated with a prophylactic dose of heparin (p. 1044). For women in whom anticoagulation therapy has temporarily been discontinued, pneumatic compression devices are recommended (American College of Obstetricians and Gynecologists, 2011).

Anticoagulation with Warfarin Compounds

Warfarin derivatives are generally contraindicated because they readily cross the placenta and may cause fetal death and malformations from hemorrhages (Chap. 12, p. 252). Like UFH and LMWH, however, they do not accumulate in breast milk and do not induce an anticoagulant effect in the infant and are thus safe during breast feeding.

Postpartum venous thrombosis is usually treated with intravenous heparin and oral warfarin initiated simultaneously. The initial dose of warfarin is usually 5 to 10 mg for the first 2 days. Subsequent doses are titrated to achieve an international normalized ratio (INR) of 2 to 3. To avoid paradoxical thrombosis and skin necrosis from the early anti-protein C effect of warfarin, these women are maintained on therapeutic doses of UFH or LMWH for 5 days and until the INR is in a therapeutic range (2.0–3.0) for 2 consecutive days (American College of Obstetricians and Gynecologists, 2013; Stewart, 2010). Warfarin skin necrosis has been described in a postpartum patient with protein S deficiency (Cheng, 1997).

Treatment in the puerperium may require larger doses of anticoagulant. Brooks and colleagues (2002) compared anticoagulation in postpartum women with that of age-matched nonpregnant controls. The former required a significantly larger median total dose of warfarin—45 versus 24 mg—and a longer time—7 versus 4 days—to achieve the target INR. Moreover, the mean maintenance dose was slightly higher in postpartum women compared with that in the control group—4.9 versus 4.3 mg.

Newer Agents

Several oral anticoagulants have recently become available. These inhibit thrombin—dabigatran, or factor Xa—rivaroxaban and apixaban. Preliminary studies in nonpregnant patients have been very promising (Cohen, 2013; Schulman, 2013). In one study of nearly 2500 nonpregnant subjects, anticoagulation with apixaban significantly reduced the risk of recurrent venous thromboembolism without increasing major bleeding complications (Agnelli, 2013). Currently, there are no studies of these newer agents during pregnancy, and thus the human reproductive risks are unknown (Bates, 2012).

Complications of Anticoagulation

Three significant complications associated with anticoagulation are hemorrhage, thrombocytopenia, and osteoporosis. The latter two are unique to heparin, and their risk may be reduced with low-molecular-weight heparins. The most serious complication is hemorrhage, which is more likely if there has been recent surgery or lacerations. Troublesome bleeding also is more likely if the heparin dosage is excessive. Unfortunately, management schemes using laboratory testing to identify when a heparin dosage is sufficient to inhibit further thrombosis, yet not cause serious hemorrhage, have been discouraging.

Heparin-Induced Thrombocytopenia

There are two types—the most common is a nonimmune, benign, reversible thrombocytopenia that develops within the first few days of therapy and resolves in approximately 5 days without therapy cessation. The second is the severe form of heparin-induced thrombocytopenia (HIT), which results from an immune reaction involving IgG antibodies directed against complexes of platelet factor 4 and heparin. When severe, HIT paradoxically causes thrombosis, which is the most common presentation.

The incidence of HIT is approximately 3 to 5 percent in nonpregnant individuals. Interestingly, however, Fausett and coworkers (2001) reported no cases among 244 heparin-treated pregnant women compared with 10 among 244 nonpregnant patients. Accordingly, the American College of Chest Physicians estimates that the incidence of HIT in obstetrical patients is less than 0.1 percent (Linkins, 2012). In the latest guidelines, moreover, the American College of Chest Physicians recommends against platelet count monitoring when the risk of HIT is considered to be less than 1 percent. In others, they suggest monitoring every 2 or 3 days from day 4 until day 14 (Linkins, 2012). Kelton and colleagues (2013) have recently provided a scholarly review of HIT.

Management

When HIT is diagnosed, heparin therapy is stopped and alternative anticoagulation initiated. LMWH may not be entirely safe because it has some cross reactivity with unfractionated heparin. The American College of Chest Physicians recommends danaparoid—a sulfated glycosaminoglycan heparinoid (Bates, 2012; Linkins, 2012). In a review of nearly 50 pregnant women with either HIT or a skin rash, Lindhoff-Last and associates (2005) concluded that danaparoid—available only from Canada—was a reasonable alternative. However, they reported two fatal maternal hemorrhages and three fetal deaths. Magnani (2010) reviewed 30 case reports of pregnant women treated with danaparoid. Although it was effective, two patients died related to bleeding, three patients suffered nonfatal major bleeds, and three women developed thromboembolic events unresponsive to danaparoid.

Other agents are fondaparinux and argatroban (Kelton, 2013; Linkins, 2012). Argatroban is a direct thrombin inhibitor available in this country to treat HIT (Chapman, 2008; Tapson, 2008). Fondaparinux is a pentasaccharide factor Xa inhibitor that is also used for HIT (Kelton, 2013). Successful use in pregnancy has been reported (Knol, 2010; Mazzolai, 2006). Tanimura and coworkers (2012) successfully used argatroban, and later fondaparinux, to manage HIT in a pregnant woman with hereditary antithrombin deficiency. Interestingly, heparin-dependent antibodies do not invariably reappear with subsequent heparin use (Warkentin, 2001).

Heparin-Induced Osteoporosis

Bone loss may develop with long-term heparin administration—usually 6 months or longer—and is more prevalent in cigarette smokers (Chap. 58, p. 1159). UFH can cause osteopenia, and this is less likely with LMWH (Deruelle, 2007). Women treated with any heparin should be encouraged to take a daily 1500-mg calcium supplement (Cunningham, 2005; Lockwood, 2012). In one study, Rodger and colleagues (2007) found that long-term use for a mean of 212 days with dalteparin was not associated with a significant decrease in bone mineral density.

Anticoagulation and Abortion

The treatment of deep-vein thrombosis with heparin does not preclude pregnancy termination by careful curettage. After the products are removed without trauma to the reproductive tract, full-dose heparin can be restarted in several hours.

Anticoagulation and Delivery

The effects of heparin on blood loss at delivery depend on several variables: (1) dose, route, and timing of administration; (2) number and depth of incisions and lacerations; (3) intensity of postpartum myometrial contractions; and (4) presence of other coagulation defects. Blood loss should not be greatly increased with vaginal delivery if the episiotomy—if any—is modest in depth, there are no lacerations, and the uterus promptly contracts. Unfortunately, such ideal circumstances do not always prevail. For example, Mueller and Lebherz (1969) described 10 women with antepartum thrombophlebitis treated with heparin. Three women who continued to receive heparin during labor and delivery bled remarkably and developed large hematomas. Thus, heparin therapy generally is stopped during labor and delivery. The American Academy of Pediatrics and the American College of Obstetricians and Gynecologists (2012) recommend restarting UFH or LMWH no sooner than 4 to 6 hours after vaginal delivery or 6 to 12 hours after cesarean delivery. It is our practice, however, to wait at least 24 hours if there are significant lacerations or following a major surgical procedure.

Slow intravenous administration of protamine sulfate generally reverses the effect of heparin promptly and effectively. It should not be given in excess of the amount needed to neutralize the heparin, because it also has an anticoagulant effect. Serious bleeding may occur when heparin in usual therapeutic doses is administered to a woman who has undergone cesarean delivery within the previous 24 to 48 hours.

SUPERFICIAL VENOUS THROMBOPHLEBITIS

Thrombosis limited strictly to the superficial veins of the saphenous system is treated with analgesia, elastic support, heat, and rest. If it does not soon subside or if deep-vein involvement is suspected, appropriate diagnostic measures are performed. Heparin is given if deep-vein involvement is confirmed. Superficial thrombophlebitis is typically seen in association with varicosities or as a sequela to an indwelling intravenous catheter.

PULMONARY EMBOLISM

Although it causes approximately 10 percent of maternal deaths, pulmonary embolism is relatively uncommon during pregnancy and the puerperium. The incidence averages

1 in 7000 pregnancies. There is an almost equal prevalence for antepartum and postpartum embolism, but those developing postpartum have a higher mortality rate. According to Marik and Plante (2008), 70 percent of women presenting with a pulmonary embolism have associated clinical evidence of deep-vein thrombosis. And recall that between 30 and 60 percent of women with a deep-vein thrombosis will have a coexisting silent pulmonary embolism.

Clinical Presentation

Findings from the international cooperative pulmonary embolism registry were reported by Goldhaber and colleagues (1999). During a 2-year period, almost 2500 nonpregnant patients with a proven pulmonary embolism were enrolled. Symptoms included dyspnea in 82 percent, chest pain in 49 percent, cough in 20 percent, syncope in 14 percent, and hemoptysis in 7 percent. Pollack and coworkers (2011) presented results from a similar study of 1880 nonpregnant patients who presented to an emergency room and were found to have a proven pulmonary embolism. Half had dyspnea at rest, 40 percent had pleuritic chest pain, 27 percent had dyspnea with exertion, and 25 percent had coughing. Other predominant clinical findings typically included tachypnea, apprehension, and tachycardia. In some cases, there was an accentuated pulmonic closure sound, rales, and/or friction rub.

Right axis deviation and T-wave inversion in the anterior chest leads may be evident on the electrocardiogram. In at least half, chest radiography is normal. But, there is atelectasis, an infiltrate, or an effusion each in 14 percent of nonpregnant patients (Pollack, 2011). There also may be loss of vascular markings in the lung region supplied by the obstructed artery. Although most women are hypoxemic, a normal arterial blood gas analysis does not exclude pulmonary embolism. Approximately a third of young patients have po_2 values > 80 mm Hg. In contrast, the alveolar-arterial oxygen tension difference is a more useful indicator of disease. More than 86 percent of patients with acute pulmonary embolism will have an alveolar-arterial difference of > 20 mm Hg (Lockwood, 2012). Even with massive pulmonary embolism, signs, symptoms, and laboratory data to support the diagnosis may be deceptively nonspecific.

Massive Pulmonary Embolism

This is defined as embolism causing hemodynamic instability (Tapson, 2008). Acute mechanical obstruction of the pulmonary vasculature causes increased vascular resistance and pulmonary hypertension followed by acute right ventricular dilatation. In otherwise healthy patients, significant pulmonary hypertension does not develop until 60 to 75 percent of the pulmonary vascular tree is occluded (Guyton, 1954). Moreover, circulatory collapse requires 75- to 80-percent obstruction. This is depicted schematically in Figure 52-3 and emphasizes that most acutely symptomatic emboli are large and likely a saddle embolism. These are suspected when the pulmonary artery pressure is substantively increased as estimated by echocardiography.

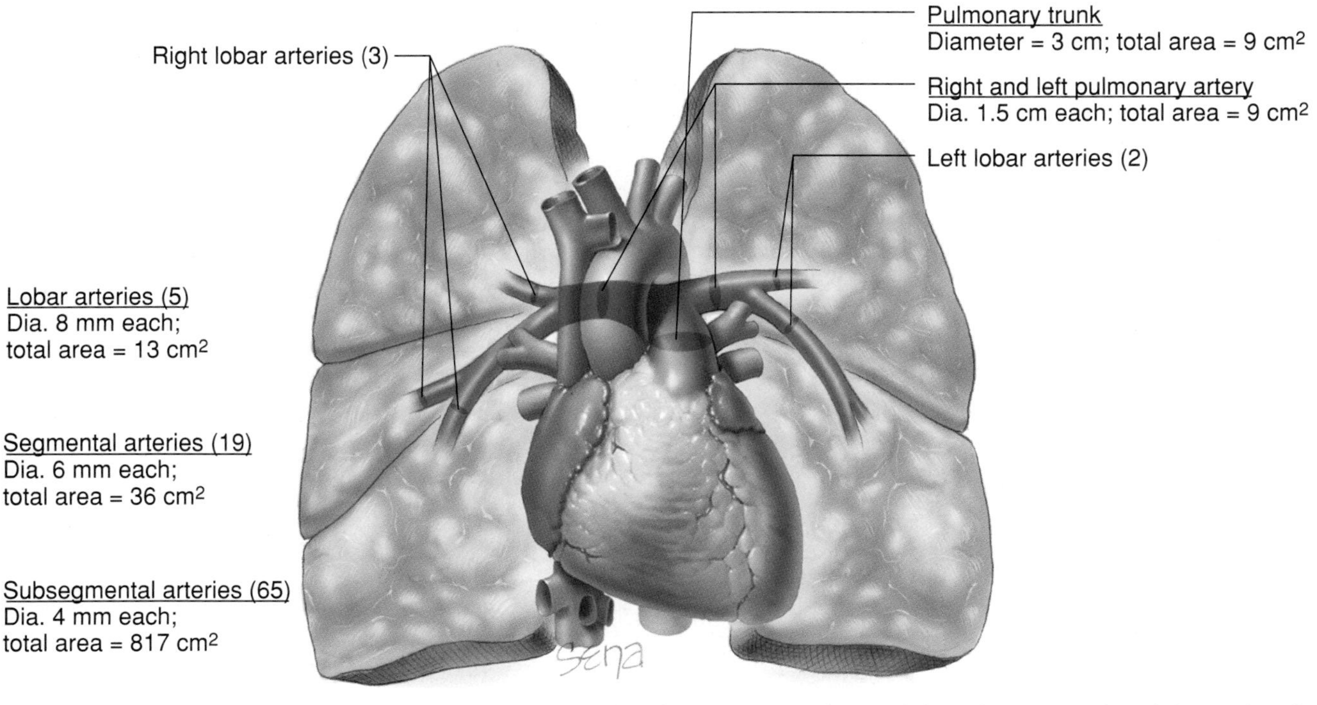

FIGURE 52-3 Schematic of pulmonary arterial circulation. Note that the cross-sectional area of the pulmonary trunk and the combined pulmonary arteries is 9 cm^2. A large saddle embolism could occlude 50 to 90 percent of the pulmonary tree, causing hemodynamic instability. As the arteries give off distal branches, the total surface area rapidly increases, that is, 13 cm^2 for the combined five lobar arteries, 36 cm^2 for the combined 19 segmental arteries, and more than 800 cm^2 for the total 65 subsegmental arterial branches. Thus, hemodynamic instability is less likely with emboli past the lobar arteries. (Data from Singhal, 1973.)

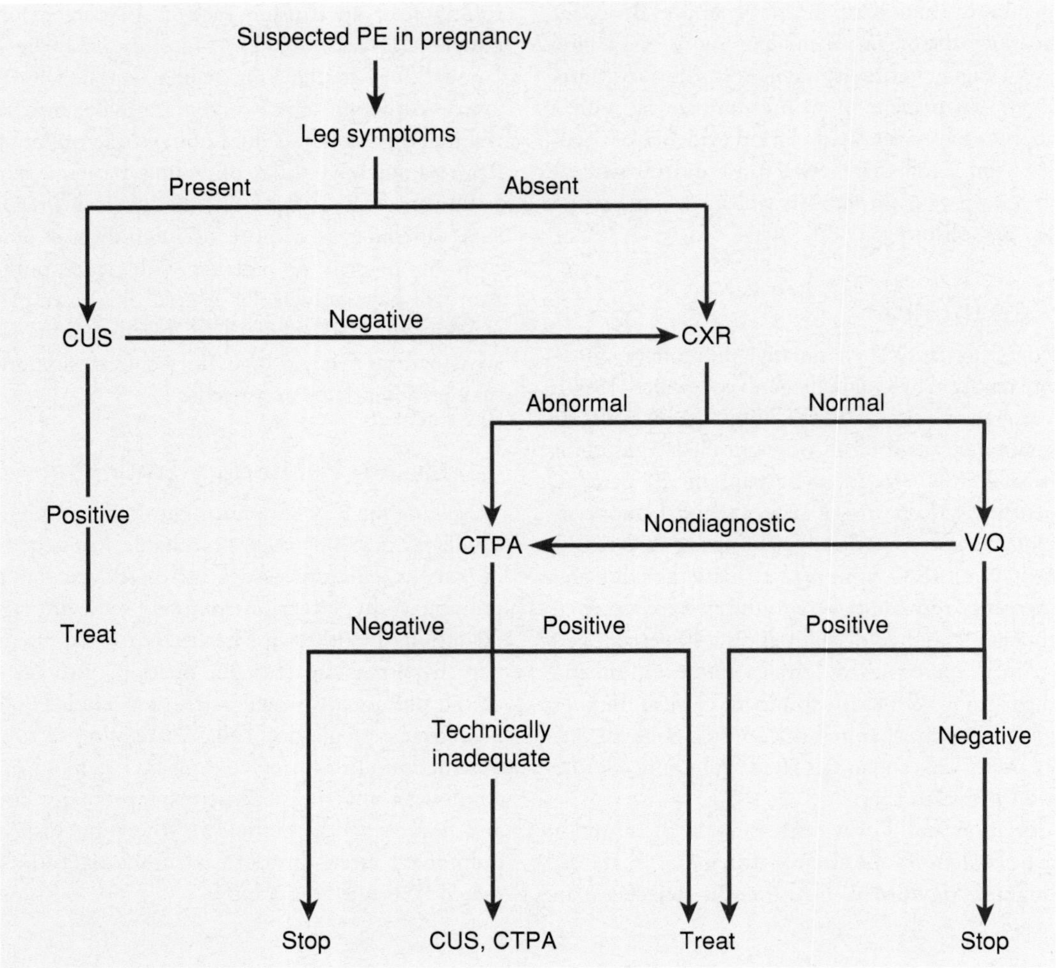

FIGURE 52-4 The American Thoracic Society and Society of Thoracic Radiology diagnostic algorithm for suspected pulmonary embolism during pregnancy. CTPA = computed tomographic pulmonary angiography; CUS = compression ultrasonography; CXR = chest x-ray; PE = pulmonary embolism; V/Q = ventilation/perfusion scintigraphy. (Redrawn from Leung, 2011, with permission.)

If there is evidence of right ventricular dysfunction, the mortality rate approaches 25 percent, compared with 1 percent without such dysfunction (Kinane, 2008). It is important in these cases to infuse crystalloids carefully and to support blood pressure with vasopressors. Oxygen treatment, endotracheal intubation, and mechanical ventilation are completed preparatory to thrombolysis, filter placement, or embolectomy (Tapson, 2008).

Diagnosis

In most cases, recognition of a pulmonary embolism requires a high index of suspicion that prompts objective evaluation. In 2011, the American Thoracic Society and the Society of Thoracic Radiology developed an algorithm—shown in Figure 52-4—for the diagnosis of pulmonary embolism during pregnancy (Leung, 2011). In addition to compression ultrasonography, which was previously discussed (p. 1036), the algorithm includes computed-tomographic pulmonary angiography (CTPA) and ventilation-perfusion scintigraphy.

Computed-Tomographic Pulmonary Angiography

Multidetector computed tomography with pulmonary angiography is currently the most commonly employed technique used for pulmonary embolism diagnosis in nonpregnant patients (Bourjeily, 2012; Pollack, 2011). The technique is described further in Chapter 46 (p. 934), and an imaging example is shown in Figure 52-5.

There is some controversy regarding the best imaging method to be used in pregnancy. The American College of Radiology has concluded CTPA to be the most accurate. With a normal chest radiograph, however, the perfusion scan alone with radioisotopes is similarly accurate, and the ventilation scan can be omitted. And because pregnant women frequently have an accompanying normal chest radiograph, the British Society of Haemostasis and Thrombosis recommends the perfusion scan as the initial preferred procedure (Cutts, 2013). Finally, the estimated breast dose of 10 to 70 mGy attributable to CTPA far exceeds that of approximately 0.5 mGy with lung scintigraphy (Cutts, 2013; Revel, 2011).

In a prospective study of 102 consecutive nonpregnant patients with suspected pulmonary embolism who underwent

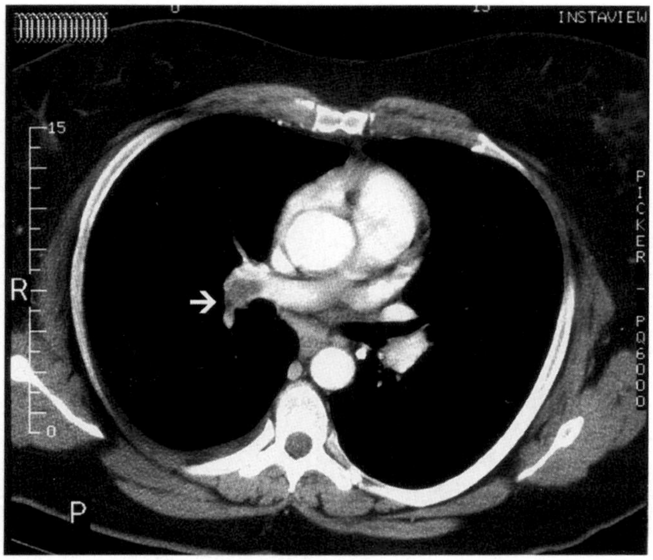

FIGURE 52-5 Axial image of the chest from a four-channel multidetector spiral computed tomographic scan performed after administration of intravenous contrast. There is enhancement of the pulmonary artery with a large thrombus on the right (*arrow*) consistent with pulmonary embolism. (Image contributed by Dr. Michael Landay.)

TABLE 52-6. Estimated Mean Fetal Radiation Dosimetry from Ventilation-Perfusion (V/Q) Lung Scanning Compared with 4-Channel Multidetector Spiral Computed Tomography (CT) Scanning

Pregnancy Duration	V/Q Scintigraphy		Spiral CT Scanning	
	mGy	mrem	mGy	mrem
Early	0.46	46	0.04	4
First trimester	0.46	46	0.04	4
Second trimester	0.57	57	0.11	11
Third trimester[a]	0.45	45	0.31	31

[a]In late pregnancy, the maximum exposure with spiral CT scanning may exceed the estimated mean by a factor of 5 to 7 due to increased proximity of the fetus to the primary beam.

Data courtesy of Dr. Jon Anderson.

CTPA, Kavanagh and coworkers (2004) found that during a mean surveillance period of 9 months, only one patient had a false-negative scan. Bourjeily and colleagues (2012) performed a similar follow-up study of 318 pregnant women who had a negative CTPA performed for a suspected pulmonary embolism. All were seen 3 months following their initial presentation or at 6 weeks postpartum. None of these women were subsequently diagnosed with a venous thromboembolism.

Although CTPA has many advantages, we have found that the better resolution allows detection of previously inaccessible smaller distal emboli that have uncertain clinical significance. Similar observations have been reported by Anderson (2007) and Hall (2009) and all their associates. Others have found that the hyperdynamic circulation and increased plasma volume associated with pregnancy lead to a higher number of nondiagnostic studies compared with nonpregnant patients (Ridge, 2011; Scarsbrook, 2006).

Ventilation-Perfusion Scintigraphy—Lung Scan

This technique is used less commonly in the United States. It involves a small dose of radiotracer such as intravenously administered technetium-99m–macroaggregated albumin. As shown in Table 52-6, there is negligible fetal radiation exposure. The scan may not provide a definite diagnosis because many other conditions—for example, pneumonia or local bronchospasm—can cause perfusion defects. Ventilation scans with inhaled xenon-133 or technetium-99m were added to perfusion scans to detect abnormal areas of ventilation in areas with normal perfusion such as with pneumonia or hypoventilation. The method is not precise, and although ventilation scanning increased the probability of an accurate diagnosis with large perfusion defects and ventilation mismatches, normal V/Q scan findings do not exclude pulmonary embolism. Chan and coworkers (2002) found that a fourth of V/Q scans in pregnant women were nondiagnostic. In these instances, CTPA is preferred.

Revel and colleagues (2011) retrospectively compared the performance of lung scintigraphy and CTPA in 137 pregnant women with suspected pulmonary embolism. They found that the two modalities had comparable performance, and no significant differences between the proportions of positive, negative, or indeterminate results were found. Specifically, the proportion of indeterminate results for both was approximately 20 percent. By way of comparison, about a fourth of the nonpregnant population has indeterminate studies. The investigators attributed this difference to the younger age of the pregnant patients.

Magnetic Resonance Angiography

Although this technique has a high sensitivity for detection of central pulmonary emboli, the sensitivity for detection of subsegmental emboli is less precise (Scarsbrook, 2006). In a study of 141 nonpregnant patients with suspected pulmonary embolism, Oudkerk and associates (2002) performed magnetic resonance angiography (MRA) before conventional angiography. Approximately a third of patients were found to have an embolus. And, the sensitivity of MRA for isolated subsegmental, segmental, and central or lobar pulmonary embolism was 40, 84, and 100 percent, respectively. There are no reports specifically involving MRA during pregnancy.

Intravascular Pulmonary Angiography

This requires catheterization of the right side of the heart and is considered the reference test for pulmonary embolism. With newer generation multidetector CT scanners, however, the role of invasive pulmonary angiography has been questioned (Kuriakose, 2010). Other detractions are that it is time consuming, uncomfortable, and associated with dye-induced allergy and renal failure. Indeed, the procedure-related mortality rate is approximately 1 in 200 (Stein,

1992). It is reserved for confirmation when less invasive tests are equivocal.

Management

Immediate treatment for pulmonary embolism is full anticoagulation similar to that for deep-vein thrombosis as discussed on page 1036. A number of complementary procedures may be indicated.

Vena Caval Filters

The woman who has very recently suffered a pulmonary embolism and who must undergo cesarean delivery presents a particularly serious problem. Reversal of anticoagulation may be followed by another embolus, and surgery while fully anticoagulated frequently results in life-threatening hemorrhage or troublesome hematomas. In these, placement of a vena caval filter should be considered before surgery (Marik, 2008). Although an uncommon occurrence, we have had good outcomes at Parkland Hospital with placement of a short-term filter. Routine filter placement has no added advantage to heparin given alone (Decousus, 1998). In the very infrequent circumstances in which heparin therapy fails to prevent recurrent pulmonary embolism from the pelvis or legs, or when embolism develops from these sites despite heparin treatment, a vena caval filter may be indicated. Such filters can also be used with massive emboli in patients who are not candidates for thrombolysis (Deshpande, 2002). The device may be inserted through either the jugular or femoral vein and can be inserted during labor (Jamjute, 2006).

Retrievable filters may be used as short-term protection against embolism. These may be removed before they become endothelialized, or they can be left in place permanently (Tapson, 2008). Liu and colleagues (2012) describe the successful use of retrievable filters placed on the day of cesarean delivery in 15 women with deep-vein thrombosis and then removed 1 to 2 weeks later.

Thrombolysis

Compared with heparin, thrombolytic agents provide more rapid lysis of pulmonary clots and improvement of pulmonary hypertension (Tapson, 2008). Konstantinides and coworkers (2002) studied 256 nonpregnant patients receiving heparin for an acute submassive pulmonary embolism. They also were assigned randomly to a placebo or the recombinant tissue plasminogen activator alteplase. Those given the placebo had a threefold increased risk of death or treatment escalation compared with those given alteplase. Agnelli and associates (2002) performed a metaanalysis of nine randomized trials involving 461 nonpregnant patients. They reported that the risk of recurrence or death was significantly lower in patients given thrombolytic agents and heparin compared with those given heparin alone—10 versus 17 percent. Importantly, however, there were five—2 percent—fatal bleeding episodes in the thrombolysis group and none in the heparin-only group.

There are a few cases reports of thrombolysis during pregnancy. In their review, Leonhardt and colleagues (2006) identified 28 reports of thrombolytic therapy using tissue plasminogen activator during pregnancy. Ten of these cases were for thromboembolism. Complication rates were similar compared with reports from nonpregnant patients, and the authors concluded that such therapy should not be withheld during pregnancy if indicated. More recent reports of the successful use of thrombolysis for massive pulmonary embolism in five pregnant patients support this conclusion (Fașullo, 2011; Holden, 2011; Lonjaret, 2011). Our anecdotal experiences with these drugs also have been favorable. Tissue plasminogen activator does not cross the placenta.

Embolectomy

Surgical embolectomy is uncommonly indicated with use of thrombolysis and filters. Published experience with emergency embolectomy during pregnancy is limited to case reports such as those by Funakoshi (2004) and Taniguchi (2008) and their coworkers. Based on their review, Ahearn and associates (2002) found that although the operative risk to the mother is reasonable, the stillbirth rate is 20 to 40 percent.

THROMBOPROPHYLAXIS

Most recommendations regarding thromboprophylaxis during pregnancy stem from consensus guidelines, and thus not are all congruent. Okoroh and colleagues (2012) performed a systematic review of evidence-based guidelines for thromboprophylaxis published between 2000 and 2011. From the nine separate guidelines, they concluded that "there is a lack of overall agreement about which groups of women should be offered thromboprophylaxis during or after pregnancy or offered testing for thrombophilias." The confusion that has ensued has provided fertile ground for the plaintiff bar to plow. Cleary-Goldman and associates (2007) surveyed 151 fellows of the American College of Obstetricians and Gynecologists and reported that intervention without a firm indication is common. Table 52-7 and 52-8 list several consensus recommendations for thromboprophylaxis. In some cases, more than one option is listed, thus illustrating the confusion that currently reigns.

In general, and as shown in Table 52-8, either antepartum surveillance or heparin prophylaxis is recommended for women without a recurrent risk factor, including no known thrombophilia. The study by Tengborn and coworkers (1989), however, suggested that such management may not be effective. They reported outcomes in 87 pregnant Swedish women who had prior thromboembolic disease and were not tested for thrombophilias. Despite heparin prophylaxis, which was usually 5000 U twice daily, three of 20—or 15 percent—of women developed antepartum recurrence compared with eight of 67—or 12 percent—of women not given heparin.

Brill-Edwards and colleagues (2000) prospectively studied 125 pregnant women with a single prior venous thromboembolism. Antepartum heparin was not given, but anticoagulant therapy was given for 4 to 6 weeks postpartum. A total of six women had a recurrent venous thrombosis—three antepartum and three postpartum. There were no recurrences in the 44 women without a known thrombophilia or whose prior thrombosis was associated with a temporary risk factor.

TABLE 52-7. American College of Chest Physicians Recommendations for Thromboprophylaxis Following Cesarean Delivery

Major Risk Factors	Minor Risk Factors
Immobility (strict antepartum bed rest for ≥ 1 week)	Body mass index > 30 kg/m^2
Postpartum hemorrhage ≥ 1 L with surgery	Multifetal pregnancy
Previous venous thromboembolism	Postpartum hemorrhage > 1 L
Thrombophilia	Smoking > 10 cigarettes/day
Antithrombin deficiency	Fetal-growth restriction (gestational age + sex-adjusted birthweight < 25th percentile)
Factor V Leiden (homozygous or heterozygous)	Thrombophilia
Prothrombin G20210A (homozygous or heterozygous)	Protein C deficiency
Medical conditions	Protein S deficiency
Systemic lupus erythematosus	Preeclampsia
Heart disease	
Sickle-cell disease	
Blood transfusion	
Postpartum infection	
Concurrent malignancy	

If no risk factors, recommend early mobilization.
If one major or two minor risk factors, recommend prophylactic low-molecular-weight heparin or mechanical prophylaxis (elastic stockings or intermittent pneumatic compression) in those with contraindications to anticoagulants while in the hospital.
If at higher risk, recommend low-molecular weight heparin plus mechanical prophylaxis.
If significant risk factors persist following delivery, prophylaxis should be extended for up to 6 weeks postpartum.
Adapted from Bates, 2012.

These findings imply that prophylactic heparin may not be required for these two groups of women. In contrast, women with a prior thrombosis in association with a thrombophilia or in the absence of a temporary risk factor generally should be given both antepartum and postpartum prophylaxis (see Table 52-8).

De Stefano and coworkers (2006) studied 1104 women who had a first-episode venous thromboembolism before the age of 40 years. After excluding those with antiphospholipid antibodies, 88 women were identified who subsequently had a total of 155 pregnancies and who were not given antithrombotic prophylaxis. There were 19 women—22 percent—who had a subsequent pregnancy- or puerperium-related venous thromboembolism. Of 20 women whose original thrombosis was associated with a transient risk factor—not including pregnancy or oral contraceptive use—there were no recurrences during pregnancy, but two during the puerperium. Like the findings by Brill-Edwards and associates (2000), these data suggest that for women with a prior venous thromboembolism, antithrombotic prophylaxis during pregnancy could be tailored according to the circumstances of the original event. It is emphasized that more data are needed.

Our practice at Parkland Hospital for many years for women with a history of prior thromboembolism was to administer subcutaneous unfractionated heparin, 5000 to 7500 units two to three times daily. With this regimen, the recurrence of documented deep-vein thrombosis embolization was rare. Beginning approximately 10 years ago, we have successfully used 40 mg enoxaparin given subcutaneously daily.

Cesarean Delivery

For many years in the United States, thromboprophylaxis for women undergoing cesarean delivery was not widely employed. In a survey of 157 members of the Society for Maternal-Fetal Medicine, for example, Casele and Grobman (2007) found that only 8 percent of respondents routinely used thromboprophylaxis—defined as compression boots, stockings, or heparin—for women undergoing cesarean delivery. Friedman and colleagues (2013) found that the rate of postcesarean prophylaxis increased from 8 percent in 2003 to 41 percent in 2010. The risk for deep-vein thrombosis and especially for fatal thromboembolism is increased manyfold in women following cesarean compared with vaginal delivery. When considering that a third of women giving birth in the United States yearly undergo cesarean delivery, it is easily understandable that pulmonary embolism is a major cause of maternal mortality (Chap. 1, p. 5).

For these reasons, the American College of Obstetricians and Gynecologists (2011) recently has recommended placement of pneumatic compression devices before cesarean delivery for all women not already receiving thromboprophylaxis. For patients undergoing cesarean delivery with additional risk factors for thromboembolism, both pneumatic compression devices and unfractionated or low-molecular-weight heparin may be recommended. Cesarean delivery in an emergency setting should not be delayed because of the time necessary to implement thromboprophylaxis. The American College of Chest Physicians recommends the risk-adjusted approach to thromboprophylaxis shown in Table 52-7 (Bates, 2012).

TABLE 52-8. Some Recommendations for Thromboprophylaxis during Pregnancy

Clinical Scenario	Pregnancy		Postpartum	
	ACOG[a]	ACCP[b]	ACOG[a]	ACCP[b]
Prior single VTE				
Risk factor no longer present	Surveillance only	Surveillance only	Postpartum anticoagulation[c] "Surveillance only acknowledged by some experts."	Prophylactic or intermediate-dose LMWH ***or*** warfarin target INR 2.0–3.0 × 6 weeks
Pregnancy- or estrogen-related or no known association (idiopathic) ***and*** not receiving long-term therapy	Prophylactic UFH or LMWH ***or*** "Surveillance only acknowledged by some experts"	Prophylactic or intermediate-dose LMWH	Postpartum anticoagulation[c]	Prophylactic or intermediate-dose LMWH ***or*** warfarin target INR 2.0–3.0 × 6 weeks
Receiving long-term warfarin	NSS	Adjusted-dose LMWH ***or*** 75% of a therapeutic dose of LMWH	NSS	Resume long-term anticoagulation
Associated with a high-risk thrombophilia[d] ***and*** not receiving long-term anticoagulation or an affected first-degree relative	Prophylactic, intermediate-, or adjusted-dose LMWH or UFH	NSS	Postpartum anticoagulation[c] ***or*** intermediate- or adjusted-dose LMWH or UFH × 6 weeks[c]	Prophylactic or intermediate-dose LMWH ***or*** warfarin target INR 2.0–3.0 × 6 weeks
Associated with a low-risk thrombophilia[e] and not receiving treatment	Prophylactic or intermediate-dose LMWH or UFH ***or*** surveillance only	NSS	Postpartum anticoagulation[c] ***or*** intermediate-dose LMWH or UFH	Prophylactic or intermediate-dose LMWH ***or*** warfarin target INR 2.0–3.0 × 6 weeks
Two or more prior VTEs with or without thrombophilia				
Not receiving long-term therapy	Prophylactic or therapeutic-dose UFH or LMWH	NSS	Postpartum anticoagulation[c] ***or*** therapeutic-dose LMWH or UFH × 6 weeks	Prophylactic or intermediate-dose LMWH ***or*** warfarin target INR 2.0–3.0 × 6 weeks
Receiving long-term anticoagulation	Therapeutic-dose LMWH or UFH	Adjusted-dose LMWH ***or*** 75% of a therapeutic dose of LMWH	Resumption of long-term anticoagulation	Resumption of long-term anticoagulation
No prior VTE				
High-risk thrombophilia[d]	Surveillance only ***or*** prophylactic or intermediate-dose LMWH or UFH	Prophylactic or intermediate-dose LMWH	Postpartum anticoagulation[c]	Intermediate-dose LMWH ***or*** warfarin target INR 2.0–3.0 × 6 weeks
Positive family history VTE ***and*** homozygous factor V Leiden or prothrombin 20210A mutation	NSS	Prophylactic or intermediate-dose LMWH	NSS	Prophylactic or intermediate-dose LMWH ***or*** warfarin target INR 2.0–3.0 × 6 weeks

TABLE 52-8. Continued

Clinical Scenario	Pregnancy		Postpartum	
	ACOG[a]	ACCP[b]	ACOG[a]	ACCP[b]
Negative family history VTE and homozygous factor V Leiden or prothrombin 20210A mutation	Surveillance only ***or*** prophylactic LMWH or UFH	Surveillance only	Postpartum anticoagulation[c]	Prophylactic- or intermediate-dose LMWH ***or*** warfarin target INR 2.0–3.0 × 6 weeks
Positive family history VTE and low-risk thrombophilias[e]	Surveillance only	Surveillance only	Postparum anticoagulation[c] ***or*** intermediate-dose LMWH or UFH	Prophylactic or intermediate-dose LMWH ***or*** in women not protein C or S deficient, warfarin target INR 2.0–3.0
Low-risk thrombophilia[e]	Surveillance only	Surveillance only if no family history	Surveillance only; postpartum anticoagulation with additional risk factors[f]	Surveillance only if no family history
Antiphospholipid antibodies				
History of VTE	Prophylactic anticoagulation with UFH or LMWH (?plus low-dose aspirin)	NSS	Prophylactic anticoagulation[c]; referral to specialist[g]	NSS
No prior VTE	Surveillance only ***or*** prophylactic LMWH or UFH ***or*** prophylactic LMWH or UFH plus low-dose aspirin if prior recurrent pregnancy loss or stillbirth	Prophylactic- or intermediate-dose UFH ***or*** prophylactic-dose LMWH, both given with 75–100 mg/day aspirin[h]	Prophylactic heparin plus low-dose aspirin × 6 weeks if prior recurrent pregnancy loss or stillbirth[g]	NSS

[a]American College of Obstetricians and Gynecologists, 2012, 2013.
[b]American College of Chest Physicians (Bates, 2012).
[c]Postpartum treatment levels should be ≥ antepartum treatment.
[d]Antithrombin deficiency; doubly heterozygous or homozygous for prothrombin 20210A and factor V Leiden.
[e]Heterozygous factor V Leiden or prothrombin 20210A; protein S or C deficiency.
[f]First-degree relative with VTE at < 50 years; other major thrombotic risk factors, e.g., obesity, prolonged immobility.
[g]Women with antiphospholipid syndrome should not use estrogen-containing contraceptives.
[h]Treatment is recommended if the diagnosis of antiphospholipid syndrome is based on three or more prior pregnancy losses.
LMWH = low-molecular-weight heparin; NSS = not specifically stated; UFH = unfractionated heparin; VTE = venous thromboembolism.
Prophylactic, intermediate-, and adjusted-dose regimens are listed in Table 52-5 (p. 1037).

Prolonged Antepartum Bed Rest

There are no recommendations concerning thromboprophylaxis for women placed on bed rest for a number of obstetrical indications. This danger is possibly mitigated because strict bed rest is seldom indicated or enforced. In the survey cited above by Casele and Grobman (2007), 25 percent of maternal-fetal medicine specialists routinely use some form of thromboprophylaxis for women on bed rest > 72 hours. It seems reasonable to consider such measures if additional risk factors are identified, for example, obesity or diabetes.

REFERENCES

Agnelli G, Becattini C, Kirschstein T: Thrombolysis vs heparin in the treatment of pulmonary embolism. Arch Intern Med 162: 2537, 2002

Agnelli G, Buller HR, Cohen A, et al: Apixaban for extended treatment of venous thromboembolism. N Engl J Med 368:699, 2013

Ahearn GS, Hadjiliadis D, Govert JA, et al: Massive pulmonary embolism during pregnancy successfully treated with recombinant tissue plasminogen activator. Arch Intern Med 162:1221, 2002

American Academy of Pediatrics and American College of Obstetricians and Gynecologists: Guidelines for Perinatal Care, 7th ed., 2012

American College of Obstetricians and Gynecologists: Safety of Lovenox in pregnancy. Committee Opinion No. 276, October 2002

American College of Obstetricians and Gynecologists: Thromboembolism in pregnancy. Practice Bulletin No. 123, September 2011

American College of Obstetricians and Gynecologists: Antiphospholipid syndrome. Practice Bulletin No. 132, December 2012

American College of Obstetricians and Gynecologists: Inherited thrombophilias in pregnancy. Practice Bulletin No. 138, September 2013

Andersen AS, Berthelsen JG, Bergholt T: Venous thromboembolism in pregnancy: prophylaxis and treatment with low molecular weight heparin. cta Obstet Gynecol 89:15, 2010

Anderson DR, Kahn SR, Rodger MA, et al: Computed tomographic pulmonary angiography vs ventilation-perfusion lung scanning in patients with suspected pulmonary embolism: a randomized controlled trial. JAMA 298:2743, 2007

Anderson JA, Weitz JI: Hypercoagulable states. Crit Care Clin 27:933, 2011

Archer DF, Mammen EF, Grubb GS: The effects of a low-dose monophasic preparation of levonorgestrel and ethinyl estradiol on coagulation and other hemostatic factors. Am J Obstet Gynecol 181:S63, 1999

Barbour LA, Oja JL, Schultz LK: A prospective trial that demonstrates that dalteparin requirements increase in pregnancy to maintain therapeutic levels of anticoagulation. Am J Obstet Gynecol 191:1024, 2004

Bates SM, Greer IA, Middledorp S, et al: VTE, thrombophilia, antithrombotic therapy, and pregnancy. Chest 141:e691S, 2012

Berg CJ, Callaghan WM, Syverson C, et al: Pregnancy-related mortality in the United States, 1998 to 2005. Obstet Gynecol 116:1302, 2010

Birdwell BG, Raskob GE, Whitsett TL, et al: The clinical validity of normal compression ultrasonography in outpatients suspected of having deep venous thrombosis. Ann Intern Med 128:1, 1998

Blanco-Molina A, Trujillo-Santos J, Criado J, et al: Venous thromboembolism during pregnancy or postpartum: findings from the RIETE Registry. Thromb Haemost 97:186, 2007

Bourjeily G, Khalil H, Raker C, et al: Outcomes of negative multidetector computed tomography with pulmonary angiography in pregnant women suspected of pulmonary embolism. Lung 190:105, 2012

Brandjes DP, Buller HR, Heijboer H, et al: Randomised trial of effect of compression stockings in patients with symptomatic proximal-vein thrombosis. Lancet 349:759, 1997

Breddin HK, Hach-Wunderle V, Nakov R, et al: Effects of a low-molecular-weight heparin on thrombus regression and recurrent thromboembolism in patients with DVT. N Engl J Med 344:626, 2001

Brill-Edwards P, Ginsberg JS, Gent M, et al: Safety of withholding heparin in pregnant women with a history of venous thromboembolism. N Engl J Med 343:1439, 2000

Brooks C, Rutherford JM, Gould J, et al: Warfarin dosage in postpartum women: a case-control study. Br J Obstet Gynaecol 109:187, 2002

Brown HL, Hiett AK: Deep vein thrombosis and pulmonary embolism in pregnancy: diagnosis, complications, and management. Clin Obstet Gynecol 53:345, 2010

Burneo JG, Elias SB, Barkley GL: Cerebral venous thrombosis due to protein S deficiency in pregnancy. Lancet 359:892, 2002

Callaghan WM, Creanga AA, Kuklina EV: Severe maternal morbidity among delivery and postpartum hospitalizations in the United States. Obstet Gynecol 120:1029, 2012

Carbone JF, Rampersad R: Prenatal screening for thrombophilias: indications and controversies. Clin Lab Med 30:747, 2010

Casele HL, Grobman WA: Management of thromboprophylaxis during pregnancy among specialists in maternal—fetal medicine. J Reprod Med 52:1085, 2007

Chan WS, Ray JG, Murray S, et al: Suspected pulmonary embolism in pregnancy. Arch Intern Med 162:1170, 2002

Chan WS, Spencer FA, Ginsberg JS: Anatomic distribution of deep vein thrombosis in pregnancy. CMAJ 182:657, 2010

Chapman ML, Martinez-Borges AR, Mertz HL: Lepirudin for treatment of acute thrombosis during pregnancy. Obstet Gynecol 112:432, 2008

Cheng A, Scheinfeld NS, McDowell B, et al: Warfarin skin necrosis in a postpartum woman with protein S deficiency. Obstet Gynecol 90:671, 1997

Chunilal SD, Ginsberg JS: Advances in the diagnosis of venous thromboembolism—a multimodal approach. J Thromb Thrombolysis 12:53, 2001

Clark P, Twaddle S, Walker ID, et al: Cost-effectiveness of screening for the factor V Leiden mutation in pregnant women. Lancet 359:1919, 2002

Cleary-Goldman J, Bettes B, Robinson JN, et al: Thrombophilia and the obstetric patient. Obstet Gynecol 110:669, 2007

Cohen AT, Spiro TE, Büller HR, et al: Rivaroxaban for thromboprophylaxis in acutely ill medical patients. N Engl J Med 368:513, 2013

Conard J, Horellou MH, Van Dreden P, et al: Thrombosis and pregnancy in congenital deficiencies in AT III, protein C or protein S: study of 78 women. Thromb Haemost 63:319, 1990

Cunningham FG: Screening for osteoporosis. N Engl J Med 353:1975, 2005

Cutts BA, Dasgupta D, Hunt BJ: New directions in the diagnosis and treatment of pulmonary embolism in pregnancy. Am J Obstet Gynecol 208(2):102, 2013

Decousus H, Leizorovicz A, Parent F, et al: A clinical trial of vena caval filters in the prevention of pulmonary embolism in patients with proximal deep-vein thrombosis. N Engl J Med 338:409, 1998

Den Heijer M, Lewington S, Clarke R: Homocysteine, MTHRF and risk of venous thrombosis: a meta-analysis of published epidemiological studies. Thromb Haemost 3:292, 2005

Deruelle P, Coulon C: The use of low-molecular-weight heparins in pregnancy—how safe are they? Curr Opin Obstet Gynecol 19:573, 2007

Deshpande KS, Hatem C, Karwa M, et al: The use of inferior vena cava filter as a treatment modality for massive pulmonary embolism. A case series and review of pathophysiology. Respir Med 96:984, 2002

De Stefano V, Martinelli I, Rossi E, et al: The risk of recurrent venous thromboembolism in pregnancy and puerperium without antithrombotic prophylaxis. Br J Haematol 135:386, 2006

Dizon-Townson D, Miller C, Sibai B, et al: The relationship of the Factor V Leiden mutation and pregnancy outcomes for mother and fetus. Obstet Gynecol 106:517, 2005

Douketis JD, Kearon C, Bates S, et al: Risk of fatal pulmonary embolism in patients with treated venous thromboembolism. JAMA 279:458, 1998

Ekman-Ordeberg G, Åkerud A, Dubicke A, et al: Does low molecular weight heparin shorten term labor? Acta Obstet Gynecol Scand 89:147, 2010

Eldor A: Thrombophilia, thrombosis and pregnancy. Thromb Haemost 86: 104, 2001

Erdman WA, Jayson HT, Redman HC, et al: Deep venous thrombosis of extremities: role of MR imaging in the diagnosis. Radiology 174:425, 1990

Fasullo S, Scalzo S, Maringhini G, et al: Thrombolysis for massive pulmonary embolism in pregnancy: a case report. Am J Emerg Med 29:698.e1, 2011

Fausett MB, Vogtlander M, Lee RM, et al: Heparin-induced thrombocytopenia is rare in pregnancy. Am J Obstet Gynecol 185:148, 2001

Forsnes E, Occhino A, Acosta R: Spontaneous spinal epidural hematoma in pregnancy associated with low molecular weight heparin. Obstet Gynecol 113:532, 2009

Franchini M, Veneri D, Salvagno GL, et al: Inherited thrombophilia. Crit Rev Clin Lab Sci 43:249, 2006

Friedman AM, Ananth CV, Lu YS: Underuse of postcesarean thromboembolism prophylaxis. Obstet Gynecol 122(6):1197, 2013

Funakoshi Y, Kato M, Kuratani T, et al: Successful treatment of massive pulmonary embolism in the 38th week of pregnancy. Ann Thorac Surg 77:694, 2004

Galambosi PJ, Kaaja RJ, Stefanovic V, et al: Safety of low-molecular-weight heparin during pregnancy: a retrospective controlled cohort study. Eur J Obstet Gynecol Reprod Bio 163:154, 2012

Galanaud JP, Cochery-Nouvellon E, Alonso S, et al: Paternal endothelial protein C receptor 219Gly variant as a mild and limited risk factor for deep vein thrombosis during pregnancy. J Thromb Haemost 8:707, 2010

Garcia DA, Spyropoulos AC: Update in the treatment of venous thromboembolism. Semin Respir Crit Care Med 29:40, 2008

Giannakopoulos B, Krilis SA: The pathogenesis of the antiphospholipid syndrome. N Engl J Med 368(11):1033, 2013

Ginsberg JS, Brill-Edwards P, Burrows RF, et al: Venous thrombosis during pregnancy: leg and trimester of presentation. Thromb Haemost 67:519, 1992

Goldhaber SZ, Tapson VF, DVT FREE Steering Committee: A prospective registry of 5,451 patients with ultrasound-confirmed deep vein thrombosis. Am J Cardiol 93:259, 2004

Goldhaber SZ, Visani L, De Rosa M: Acute pulmonary embolism: Clinical outcomes in the International Cooperative Pulmonary Embolism Registry (ICOPER). Lancet 353:1386, 1999

Greer IA: Prevention and management of venous thromboembolism in pregnancy. Clin Chest Med 24:123, 2003
Guyatt GH, Akl EA, Crowther M, et al: Executive summary: Antithrombotic therapy and prevention of thrombosis, 9th ed: American College of Chest Physicians evidence-based clinical practice guidelines. Chest 141:7S, 2012
Guyton AC, Lindsey AW, Gilluly JJ: The limits of right ventricular compensation following acute increase in pulmonary circulatory resistance. Circ Res 2:326, 1954
Hague WM: Homocysteine and pregnancy. Best Pract Res Clin Obstet Gynaecol 17:459, 2003
Hall WB, Truitt SG, Scheunemann LP, et al: The prevalence of clinically relevant incidental findings on chest computed tomographic angiograms ordered to diagnose pulmonary embolism. Arch Intern Med 169:1961, 2009
Hammerová L, Chabada J, Drobný A, et al: Factor V Leiden mutation and its impact on pregnancy complications. Acta Med 54:117, 2011
Heijboer H, Buller HR, Lensing AW, et al: A comparison of real-time compression ultrasonography with impedance plethysmography for the diagnosis of deep-vein thrombosis in symptomatic outpatients. N Engl J Med 329:1365, 1993
Holden EL, Ranu H, Sheth A, et al: Thrombolysis for massive pulmonary embolism in pregnancy—a report of three cases and follow up over a two year period. Thromb Res 127:58, 2011
Horlocker TT, Wedel DJ, Rowlingson JC, et al: Executive summary: Regional anesthesia in the patient receiving antithrombotic or thrombolytic therapy: American Society of Regional Anesthesia and Pain Medicine evidence-based guideline, 3rd ed. Reg Anesth Pain Med 35:102, 2010
Hull RD, Raskob GF, Carter CJ: Serial IPG in pregnancy patients with clinically suspected DVT: clinical validity of negative findings. Ann Intern Med 112:663, 1990
Isma N, Svensson PJ, Lindblad B, et al: The effect of low molecular weight heparin (dalteparin) on duration and initiation of labour. J Thromb Thrombolysis 30:149, 2010
Jacobsen AF, Qvigstad E, Sandset, PM: Low molecular weight heparin (dalteparin) for the treatment of venous thromboembolism in pregnancy. BJOG 110:139, 2003
Jacobsen AF, Skjeldstad FE, Sandset PM: Incidence and risk patterns of venous thromboembolism in pregnancy and puerperium—a register-based case-control study. Am J Obstet Gynecol 198:233.e1, 2008
James AH, Jamison MG, Brancazio LR, et al: Venous thromboembolism during pregnancy and the postpartum period: incidence, risk factors, and mortality. Am J Obstet Gynecol 194:1311, 2006
Jamjute P, Reed N, Hinwood D: Use of inferior vena cava filters in thromboembolic disease during labor: case report with a literature review. J Matern Fetal Neonatal Med 19:741, 2006
Kahn SR, Platt R, McNamara H, et al: Inherited thrombophilia and preeclampsia within a multicenter cohort: the Montreal Preeclampsia Study. Am J Obstet Gynecol 200:151.e1, 2009
Katz VL: Detecting thrombophilia in OB/GYN patients. Contemp Ob/Gyn, October 2002
Kavanagh EC, O'Hare A, Hargaden G, et al: Risk of pulmonary embolism after negative MDCT pulmonary angiography findings. AJR Am J Roentgenol 182:499, 2004
Kearon C, Akl EA Comerota AJ, et al: Antithrombotic therapy for VTE disease: antithrombotic therapy and prevention of thrombosis, 9th ed: American College of Chest Physicians evidence-based clinical practice guidelines. Chest 141:e419S, 2012
Kelly J, Hunt BJ: Role of D-dimers in diagnosis of venous thromboembolism. Lancet 359:456, 2002
Kelton JG, Arnold DM, Bates SM: Nonheparin anticoagulants for heparin-induced thrombocytopenia. N Engl J Med 368:737, 2013
Khalil H, Avruck L, Olivier A, et al: The natural history of pelvic vein thrombosis on magnetic resonance venography after vaginal delivery. Am J Obstet Gynecol 206:356.e1, 2012
Kinane TB, Grabowski EF, Sharma A, et al: Case 7-2008: a 17-year-old girl with chest pain and hemoptysis. N Engl J Med 358:941, 2008
Kjellberg U, van Rooijen M, Bremme K, et al: Factor V Leiden mutation and pregnancy-related complications. Am J Obstet Gynecol 203:469.e1, 2010
Kline JA, Williams GW, Hernandez-Nino J: D-Dimer concentrations in normal pregnancy: new diagnostic thresholds are needed. Clin Chem 51:825, 2005
Knol HM, Schultinge L, Erwich JJ, et al: Fondaparinux as an alternative anticoagulant therapy during pregnancy. J Thromb Haemost 8:1876, 2010
Konstantinides S, Geibel A, Heusel G, et al: Heparin plus alteplase compared with heparin alone in patients with submassive pulmonary embolism. N Engl J Med 347:1143, 2002
Korteweg FJ, Erwich JJ, Folkeringa N, et al: Prevalence of parental thrombophilic defects after fetal death and relation to cause. Obstet Gynecol 116:355, 2010
Kovac M, Mitic G, Mikovic Z, et al: Thrombophilia in women with pregnancy-associated complications: fetal loss and pregnancy-related venous thromboembolism. Gynecol Obstet Invest 69:223, 2010
Krivak TC, Zorn KK: Venous thromboembolism in obstetrics and gynecology. Obstet Gynecol 109:761, 2007
Kuriakose J, Patel S: Acute pulmonary embolism. Radiol Clin North Am 48:31, 2010
Lee RH, Goodwin TM: Massive subchorionic hematoma associated with enoxaparin. Obstet Gynecol 108:787, 2006
Le Gal G, Kercret G, Yahmed KB, et al: Diagnostic value of single complete compression ultrasonography in pregnant and postpartum women with suspected deep vein thrombosis: prospective study. BMJ 344:e2635, 2012
Leonhardt G, Gaul C, Nietsch HH, et al: Thrombolytic therapy in pregnancy. J Thromb Thrombolysis 21:271, 2006
Lepercq J, Conard J, Borel-Derlon A, et al: Venous thromboembolism during pregnancy: a retrospective study of enoxaparin safety in 624 pregnancies. Br J Obstet Gynaecol 108:1134, 2001
Leung AN, Bull TM, Jaeschke R, et al: An official American Thoracic Society/Society of Thoracic Radiology Clinical Practice Guideline: evaluation of suspected pulmonary embolism in pregnancy. Am J Respir Crit Care Med 184:1200, 2011
Lim W: Using low molecular weight heparin in special patient populations. J Thromb Thrombolysis 29:233, 2010
Lindhoff-Last E, Kreutzenbeck HJ, Magnani HN: Treatment of 51 pregnancies with danaparoid because of heparin intolerance. Thromb Haemost 93:63, 2005
Linkins L-A, Dans AL, Moores LK, et al: Treatment and prevention of heparin-induced thrombocytopenia. Chest 141:e495S, 2012
Liu Y, Sun Y, Zhang S, et al: Placement of a retrievable inferior vena cava filter for deep venous thrombosis in term pregnancy. J Vasc Surg 55:1042, 2012
Lockwood C: Thrombosis, thrombophilia, and thromboembolism: clinical updates in women's health care. American College of Obstetricians and Gynecologists Vol. VI, No. 4, October 2007, Reaffirmed 2012
Lockwood CJ: Inherited thrombophilias in pregnant patients: detection and treatment paradigm. Obstet Gynecol 99:333, 2002
Lonjaret L, Lairez O, Galinier M: Thrombolysis by recombinant tissue plasminogen activator during pregnancy: a case of massive pulmonary embolism. Am J Emerg Med 29:694.e1, 2011
López-Quesada E, Vilaseca MA, Lailla JM: Plasma total homocysteine in uncomplicated pregnancy and in preeclampsia. Eur J Obstet Gynecol Reprod Biol 108:45, 2003
Magnani HN: An analysis of clinical outcomes of 91 pregnancies in 83 women treated with danaparoid (Orgaran). Thromb Res 125:297, 2010
Marik PE, Plante LA: Venous thromboembolic disease and pregnancy. N Engl J Med 359:2025, 2008
Mazzolai L, Hohlfeld P, Spertini F, et al: Fondaparinux is a safe alternative in case of heparin intolerance during pregnancy. Blood 108:1569, 2006
McCrae KR, Kenny L, Cunningham FG: Platelets, coagulation, and the liver. In Taylor RN, Roberts JM, Cunningham FG (eds): Chesley's Hypertensive Disorders in Pregnancy, 4th ed. Amsterdam, Academic Press, 2014
McDonald SD, Walker MC: Homocysteine levels in pregnant women who smoke cigarettes. Med Hypotheses 57:792, 2001
Morikawa M, Yamada T, Yamada T, et al: Changes in D-dimer levels after cesarean section in women with singleton and twin pregnancies. Thromb Res 128:e33, 2011
Mueller MJ, Lebherz TB: Antepartum thrombophlebitis. Obstet Gynecol 34:867, 1969
Nelson-Piercy C, Powrie R, Borg J-Y, et al: Tinzaparin use in pregnancy: an international, retrospective study of the safety and efficacy profile. Eur J Obstet Gynecol Reprod Biol 159:293, 2011
Nijkeuter M, Ginsberg JS, Huisman MV: Diagnosis of deep vein thrombosis and pulmonary embolism in pregnancy: a systematic review. J Thromb Haemost 4:496, 2006
O'Connor DJ, Scher LA, Gargiulo NJ, III, et al: Incidence and characteristics of venous thromboembolic disease during pregnancy and the postnatal period: a contemporary series. Ann Vasc Surg 25:9, 2011
Okoroh E, Azonobi I, Grosse S, et al: Prevention of venous thromboembolism in pregnancy. J Women Health 21:611, 2012
Oudkerk M, van Beek JR, Wielopolski P, et al: Comparison of contrast-enhanced magnetic resonance angiography and conventional pulmonary angiography for the diagnosis of pulmonary embolism: a prospective study. Lancet 359:1643, 2002

Paidas M, Triche E, James A, et al: Recombinant human antithrombin (rhAT) for prevention of venous thromboembolism (VTE) in pregnant patients with hereditary antithrombin deficiency (HD). Am J Obstet Gynecol 208:S234, 2013
Pierangeli SS, Leader B, Barilaro G, et al: Acquired and inherited thrombophilia disorders in pregnancy. Obstet Gynecol Clin North Am 38:271, 2011
Pollack CV, Schreiber D, Goldhaber SZ, et al: Clinical characteristics, management, and outcomes of patients diagnosed with acute pulmonary embolism in the emergency department. JACC 57:700, 2011
Quinlan DJ, McQuillan A, Eikelboom JW: Low-molecular-weight heparin compared with intravenous unfractionated heparin for treatment of pulmonary embolism: a meta-analysis of randomized, controlled trials. Ann Intern Med 140:143, 2004
Revel M-P, Cohen S, Sanchez O, et al: Pulmonary embolism during pregnancy: diagnosis with lung scintigraphy or CT angiography? Radiology 258:590, 2011
Ridge CA, Mhuircheartaigh JN, Dodd JD, et al: Pulmonary CT angiography protocol adapted to the hemodynamic effects of pregnancy. AJR Am J Roentgenol 197:1058, 2011
Robertson L, Wu O, Langhorne P, et al: Thrombophilia in pregnancy: a systematic review. Br J Haematol 132:171, 2005
Rodger MA, Kahn SR, Cranney A, et al: Long-term dalteparin in pregnancy not associated with a decrease in bone mineral density: substudy of a randomized controlled trial. J Thromb Haemost 5:1600, 2007
Rodie VA, Thomson AJ, Stewart FM, et al: Low molecular weight heparin for the treatment of venous thromboembolism in pregnancy: a case series. Br J Obstet Gynaecol 109:1020, 2002
Sabadell J, Casellas M, Alijotas-Reig J, et al: Inherited antithrombin deficiency and pregnancy: maternal and fetal outcomes. Eur J Obstet Gynecol Reprod Biol 149:47, 2010
Saenz AJ, Johnson NV, Van Cott, EM: Acquired activated protein C resistance cause by lupus anticoagulants. Am J Clin Pathol 136:344, 2011
Said JM, Higgins JR, Moses EK, et al: Inherited thrombophilia polymorphisms and pregnancy outcomes in nulliparous women. Obstet Gynecol 115:5, 2010a
Said JM, Ignjatovic V, Monagle PT, et al: Altered reference ranges for protein C and protein S during early pregnancy: implications for the diagnosis of protein C and protein S deficiency during pregnancy. Thromb Haemost 103:984, 2010b
Said JM, Tsui R, Borg AJ, et al: The PAI-1 4G/5G polymorphism is not associated with an increased risk of adverse pregnancy outcome in asymptomatic nulliparous women. J Thromb Haemost 10:881, 2012
Salonvaara M, Kuismanen K, Mononen T, et al: Diagnosis and treatment of a newborn with homozygous protein C deficiency. Acta Paediatr 93:137, 2004
Sanson BJ, Lensing AW, Prins MH, et al: Safety of low-molecular-weight heparin in pregnancy: a systematic review. Thromb Haemost 81:668, 1999
Santacroce R, Sarno M, Cappucci F, et al: Low protein Z levels and risk of occurrence of deep vein thrombosis. J Thromb Haemost 4:2417, 2006
Scarsbrook AF, Evans AL, Owen AR, et al: Diagnosis of suspected venous thromboembolic disease in pregnancy. Clin Radiol 61:1, 2006
Schulman S, Kearon C, Kakkar AK, et al: Extended use of dabigatran, warfarin, or placebo in venous thromboembolism. N Engl J Med 368:709, 2013
Seguin J, Weatherstone K, Nankervis C: Inherited antithrombin III deficiency in the neonate. Arch Pediatr Adolesc Med 148:389, 1994
Seligsohn U, Lubetsky A: Genetic susceptibility to venous thrombosis. N Engl J Med 344:1222, 2001
Sharpe CJ, Crowther MA, Webert KE, et al: Cerebral venous thrombosis during pregnancy in the setting of type I antithrombin deficiency: case report and literature review. Transf Med Rev 25:61, 2011
Silver RM, Zhao Y, Spong CY, et al: Prothrombin gene G20210A mutation and obstetric complications. Obstet Gynecol 115:14, 2010
Singhal S, Henderson R, Horsfield K, et al: Morphometry of the human pulmonary arterial tree. Circ Res 33:190, 1973
Smith MP, Norris LA, Steer PJ, et al: Tinzaparin sodium for thrombosis treatment and prevention during pregnancy. Am J Obstet Gynecol 190:495, 2004
Stefano VD, Martinelli I, Mannucci PM, et al: The risk of recurrent deep venous thrombosis among heterozygous carriers of both factor V Leiden and the G20210A prothrombin mutation. N Engl J Med 341:801, 1999
Stein PD, Athanasoulis C, Alavi A, et al: Complications and validity of pulmonary angiography in acute pulmonary embolism. Circulation 85:462, 1992
Stewart A: Warfarin-induced skin necrosis treated with protein C concentrate (human). Am J Health-Syst Pharm 67:901, 2010
Sultan AA, West J, Tata LJ, et al: Risk of first venous thromboembolism in and around pregnancy: a population-based cohort study. Br J Haematol 156:366, 2011
Taniguchi S, Fukuda I, Minakawa M, et al: Emergency pulmonary embolectomy during the second trimester of pregnancy: report of a case. Surg Today 38:59, 2008
Tanimura K, Ebina Y, Sonoyama A, et al: Argatroban therapy for heparin-induced thrombocytopenia during pregnancy in a woman with hereditary antithrombin deficiency. J Obstet Gynaecol Res 38:749, 2012
Tapson VF: Acute pulmonary embolism. N Engl J Med 358:1037, 2008
Tengborn L, Bergqvist D, Matzsch T, et al: Recurrent thromboembolism in pregnancy and puerperium: is there a need for thromboprophylaxis? Am J Obstet Gynecol 160:90, 1989
van Wijk FH, Wolf H, Piek JM, et al: Administration of low molecular weight heparin within two hours before caesarean section increases the risk of wound haematoma. Br J Obstet Gynaecol 109:955, 2002
Virchow R: Gesammelte Abhandlungen zur wissenschaftlichen Medizin. Frankfurt: Medinger Sohn & Co., 1856, p 219
Waldman M, Sheiner E, Vardi IS: Can we profile patients at risk for thromboembolic events after delivery: a decade of follow up. Am J Obstet Gynecol 208:S234, 2013
Walker MC, Garner PR, Keely EJ, et al: Changes in activated protein C resistance during normal pregnancy. Am J Obstet Gynecol 177:162, 1997
Warkentin TE, Kelton JG: Temporal aspects of heparin-induced thrombocytopenia. N Engl J Med 344:1286, 2001
Wells PS, Anderson DR, Rodger M, et al: Evaluation of D-dimer in the diagnosis of suspected deep-vein thrombosis. N Engl J Med 349:1227, 2003

CHAPTER 53

Renal and Urinary Tract Disorders

Renal and urinary tract disorders are commonly encountered in pregnancy. Some precede pregnancy—one example being nephrolithiasis. In some women, pregnancy-induced changes may predispose to development or worsening of urinary tract disorders—an example is the markedly increased risk for pyelonephritis. Finally, there may be renal pathology unique to pregnancy such as preeclampsia. With good prenatal care, however, most women with these disorders will likely have no long-term sequelae.

PREGNANCY-INDUCED URINARY TRACT CHANGES

Significant changes in both structure and function that take place in the urinary tract during normal pregnancy are discussed in Chapter 4 (p. 63). The kidneys become larger, and as shown in Figure 53-1, dilatation of the renal calyces and ureters can be striking. Some dilatation develops before 14 weeks and likely is due to progesterone-induced relaxation of the muscularis. More marked dilatation is apparent beginning in midpregnancy because of ureteral compression, especially on the right side (Faúndes, 1998). There is also some *vesicoureteral reflux* during pregnancy. An important consequence of these physiological changes is an increased risk of upper urinary infection, and occasionally erroneous interpretation of studies done to evaluate obstruction.

Evidence of functional renal hypertrophy becomes apparent very soon after conception. Glomeruli are larger, although cell numbers do not increase (Strevens, 2003). Pregnancy-induced intrarenal vasodilatation—both afferent and efferent resistance decreases—leads to increased effective renal plasma flow and glomerular filtration (Helal, 2012; Hussein, 2014). By 12 weeks' gestation, the glomerular filtration rate is already increased 20 percent above nonpregnant values (Hladunewich, 2004). Ultimately, plasma flow and glomerular filtration increase by 40 and 65 percent, respectively. Consequently, serum concentrations of creatinine and urea decrease substantively across pregnancy, and values within a nonpregnant normal range may be abnormal for pregnancy (Appendix, p. 1289). Other alterations include those related to maintaining normal acid-base homeostasis, osmoregulation, and fluid and electrolyte retention.

Assessment of Renal Function During Pregnancy

The *urinalysis* is essentially unchanged during pregnancy, except for occasional glucosuria. Although *protein excretion* normally is increased, it seldom reaches levels that are detected by usual screening methods. As discussed in Chapter 4 (p. 65), Higby and colleagues (1994) reported 24-hour protein excretion to be 115 mg with a 95-percent confidence level of 260 mg/day. There were no significant differences by trimester. Albumin constitutes only a small part of total protein excretion and ranges from 5 to 30 mg/day. From their review, Airoldi and Weinstein (2007) concluded that proteinuria must exceed 300 mg/day to be considered abnormal. Many consider 500 mg/day to be important with gestational hypertension. Quantification

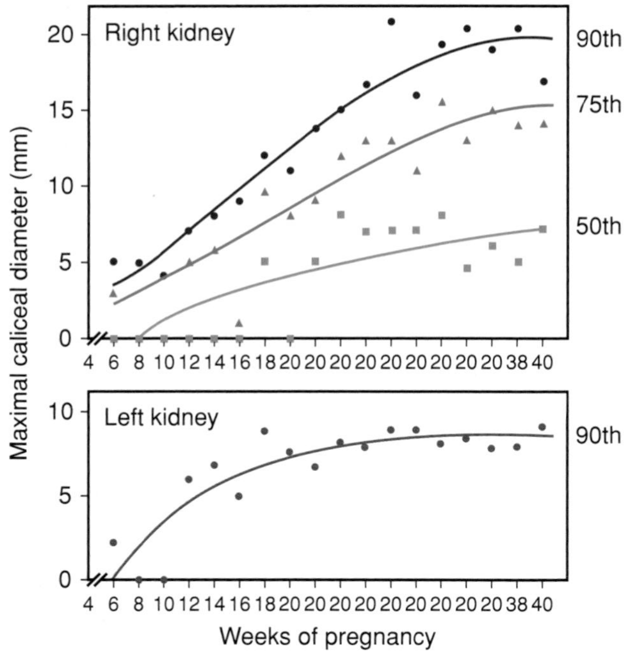

FIGURE 53-1 The 50th, 75th, and 90th percentiles for maternal renal caliceal diameters measured using sonography in 1395 pregnant women from 4 to 42 weeks. (Redrawn from Faúndes, 1998.)

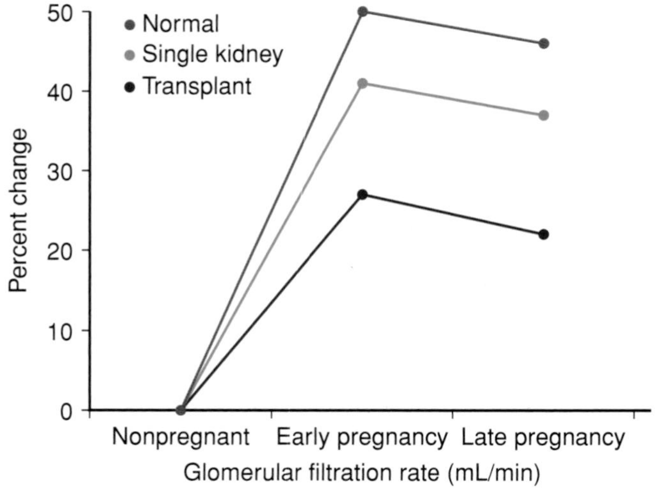

FIGURE 53-2 Increased glomerular filtration rate in early pregnancy in normal women, those stable after unilateral nephrectomy, and those with a successful renal transplant. (Data from Newcastle-upon-Tyne, 1974–2006, courtesy of Dr. John Davison.)

of urinary albumin-to-creatinine ratio (ACR) in a spot urine sample—ideally from a first-morning void—is helpful in estimating a 24-hour albumin excretion rate (AER), in which ACR (mg/g) approximates AER (mg/24 h). Some laboratories measure total proteins instead of albumin.

Stehman-Breen and associates (2002) found that 3 percent of 4589 nulliparas had *idiopathic hematuria*, defined as 1+ or greater blood on urine dipstick when screened before 20 weeks. They also reported that these women had a twofold risk of developing preeclampsia. In another study of 1000 women screened during pregnancy, Brown and coworkers (2005) reported a 15-percent incidence of dipstick hematuria. Most women had trace levels of hematuria, and the false-positive rate was 40 percent.

If the serum creatinine level in pregnancy persistently exceeds 0.9 mg/dL (75 μmol/L), then intrinsic renal disease should be suspected. In these cases, some determine the creatinine clearance as an estimate of the glomerular filtration rate. *Sonography* provides imaging of renal size, relative consistency, and elements of obstruction (see Fig. 53-1). Full-sequence *intravenous pyelography* is not done routinely, but injection of contrast media with one or two abdominal radiographs may be indicated by the clinical situation (Chap. 46, p. 931). The usual clinical indications for *cystoscopy* are followed. There is an approximate 5-percent complication rate of *ureteroscopy* done for stone removal during pregnancy (Johnson, 2012; Semins, 2009). Magnetic resonance (MR) imaging of renal masses has been shown to have excellent results (Putra, 2009).

Although *renal biopsy* is relatively safely performed during pregnancy, it usually is postponed unless results may change therapy. From a review of 243 biopsies in pregnant women, the incidence of complications was 7 percent—this compares with 1 percent in postpartum women (Piccoli, 2013). Lindheimer and colleagues (2007a) recommend its consideration for rapid deterioration of renal function with no obvious cause or for symptomatic nephrotic syndrome. We and others have found biopsy helpful in selected cases to direct management (Chen, 2001; Piccoli, 2013). Strevens and associates (2003) performed renal biopsy in 12 *normal* pregnant volunteers and reported that five had slight to moderate glomerular endotheliosis. In contrast, all 27 women with proteinuric hypertension had endotheliosis, and in all but one, it was moderate to severe.

Pregnancy after Unilateral Nephrectomy

After removal of one kidney, and if the remaining kidney is normal, there is hypertrophy of renal function. In addition, with pregnancy, the surviving kidney undergoes further hypertrophy of function (Fig. 53-2). Because of this, women with one normal kidney most often have no difficulty in pregnancy (Baylis, 1991). Thorough functional evaluation of the remaining kidney is essential. Finally, there are no long-term adverse consequences of kidney donation done before pregnancy (Ibrahim, 2009).

URINARY TRACT INFECTIONS

These are the most common bacterial infections during pregnancy. Although *asymptomatic bacteriuria* is the most common, symptomatic infection includes *cystitis*, or it may involve the renal calyces, pelvis, and parenchyma—*pyelonephritis*.

Organisms that cause urinary infections are those from the normal perineal flora. Approximately 90 percent of *Escherichia coli* strains that cause nonobstructive pyelonephritis have *adhesins* such as P- and S-fimbriae. These are cell-surface protein structures that enhance bacterial adherence and thereby, virulence (Foxman, 2010; Hooton, 2012). These adhesins promote binding to vaginal and uroepithelial cells through expression of the *PapG* gene that encodes the

P-fimbriae tip and by production of toxins and other virulence factors (Spurbeck, 2011).

Data suggest that pregnant women have more severe sequelae from urosepsis. The T-helper cell—Th1/Th2 ratio—reversal of normal pregnancy is discussed in Chapter 4 (p. 56). There are also various perturbations of cytokine expression that have been reported (Chaemsaithong, 2013). And maternal deaths have been attributed to *E coli* bearing Dr^{+} and P adhesins (Sledzińska, 2011). But even if pregnancy itself does not enhance these virulence factors, urinary stasis, vesicoureteral reflux, and diabetes predispose to symptomatic upper urinary infections (Czaja, 2009; Twickler, 1994).

In the puerperium, there are several risk factors that predispose a woman to urinary infections. Bladder sensitivity to intravesical fluid tension is often decreased as a consequence of labor trauma or conduction analgesia (Chap. 36, p. 676). Sensation of bladder distention can also be diminished by discomfort caused by an episiotomy, periurethral lacerations, or vaginal wall hematomas. Normal postpartum diuresis may worsen bladder overdistention, and catheterization to relieve retention commonly leads to urinary infection. Postpartum pyelonephritis is treated in the same manner as antepartum renal infections (McDonnold, 2012).

Asymptomatic Bacteriuria

This refers to persistent, actively multiplying bacteria within the urinary tract in asymptomatic women. Its prevalence in nonpregnant women is 5 to 6 percent and depends on parity, race, and socioeconomic status (Hooton, 2000). The highest incidence is in African-American multiparas with sickle-cell trait, and the lowest incidence is in affluent white women of low parity. Asymptomatic infection is also more common in diabetics (Schneeberger, 2014). Because in most women there is recurrent or persistent bacteriuria, it frequently is discovered during prenatal care. The incidence during pregnancy is similar to that in nonpregnant women and varies from 2 to 7 percent.

Bacteriuria is typically present at the first prenatal visit. An initial positive urine culture result prompts treatment, after which, fewer than 1 percent of women develop a urinary tract infection (Whalley, 1967). A clean-voided specimen containing more than 100,000 organisms/mL is diagnostic. It may be prudent to treat when lower concentrations are identified, because pyelonephritis develops in some women despite colony counts of only 20,000 to 50,000 organisms/mL (Lucas, 1993).

Significance

If asymptomatic bacteriuria is not treated, approximately 25 percent of infected women will develop symptomatic infection during pregnancy. Eradication of bacteriuria with antimicrobial agents prevents most of these. The American Academy of Pediatrics and the American College of Obstetricians and Gynecologists (2012), as well as a U.S. Preventive Services Task Force (2008), recommend screening for bacteriuria at the first prenatal visit (Chap. 9, p. 174). Standard urine cultures may not be cost effective when the prevalence is low. However, less expensive screening tests such as the leukocyte esterase-nitrite dipstick are when the prevalence is 2 percent or less (Rouse, 1995). Because of a high prevalence—5 to 8 percent—at Parkland Hospital, culture screening is done in most women. Susceptibility determination is not necessary because initial treatment is empirical (Hooton, 2012). Also, a dipstick culture technique has excellent positive- and negative-predictive values (Mignini, 2009). With this, a special agar-coated dipstick is first placed into urine and then also serves as the culture plate.

In some, but not all studies, covert bacteriuria has been associated with preterm or low-birthweight infants (Kass, 1962). It is even more controversial whether eradication of bacteriuria decreases these complications. Evaluating a cohort of 25,746 mother-infant pairs, Schieve and coworkers (1994) reported urinary tract infection to be associated with increased risks for low-birthweight infants, preterm delivery, pregnancy-associated hypertension, and anemia. These findings vary from those of Gilstrap and colleagues (1981b) and Whalley (1967). In most studies, asymptomatic infection is not evaluated separately from acute renal infection (Banhidy, 2007). A Cochrane database review by Vasquez and Abalos (2011) found that benefits of treatment for asymptomatic bacteria are limited to the reduction of the incidence of pyelonephritis.

Treatment

Bacteriuria responds to empirical treatment with any of several antimicrobial regimens listed in Table 53-1. Although selection can be based on in vitro susceptibilities, in our extensive

TABLE 53-1. Oral Antimicrobial Agents Used for Treatment of Pregnant Women with Asymptomatic Bacteriuria

Single-dose treatment
Amoxicillin, 3 g
Ampicillin, 2 g
Cephalosporin, 2 g
Nitrofurantoin, 200 mg
Trimethoprim-sulfamethoxazole, 320/1600 mg
3-day course
Amoxicillin, 500 mg three times daily
Ampicillin, 250 mg four times daily
Cephalosporin, 250 mg four times daily
Ciprofloxacin, 250 mg twice daily
Levofloxacin, 250 or 500 mg daily
Nitrofurantoin, 50 to 100 mg four times daily or 100 mg twice daily
Trimethoprim-sulfamethoxazole, 160/800 mg two times daily
Other
Nitrofurantoin, 100 mg four times daily for 10 days
Nitrofurantoin, 100 mg twice daily for 5 to 7 days
Nitrofurantoin, 100 mg at bedtime for 10 days
Treatment failures
Nitrofurantoin, 100 mg four times daily for 21 days
Suppression for bacterial persistence or recurrence
Nitrofurantoin, 100 mg at bedtime for pregnancy remainder

experience, empirical oral treatment for 10 days with nitrofurantoin macrocrystals, 100 mg at bedtime, is usually effective. Lumbiganon and associates (2009) reported satisfactory results with a 7-day oral course of nitrofurantoin, 100 mg given twice daily. Single-dose antimicrobial therapy has also been used with success for bacteriuria. The important caveat is that, regardless of regimen given, the recurrence rate is approximately 30 percent. This may indicate covert upper tract infection and the need for longer therapy.

Periodic surveillance is necessary to prevent recurrent urinary infections (Schneeberger, 2012). For recurrent bacteriuria, we have had success with nitrofurantoin, 100 mg orally at bedtime for 21 days (Lucas, 1994). For women with persistent or frequent bacteriuria recurrences, suppressive therapy for the remainder of pregnancy can be given. We routinely use nitrofurantoin, 100 mg orally at bedtime. This drug may rarely cause an acute pulmonary reaction that dissipates on its withdrawal (Boggess, 1996).

Cystitis and Urethritis

Lower urinary infection during pregnancy may develop without antecedent covert bacteriuria (Harris, 1981). Cystitis is characterized by dysuria, urgency, and frequency, but with few associated systemic findings. Pyuria and bacteriuria are usually found. Microscopic hematuria is common, and occasionally there is gross hematuria from hemorrhagic cystitis (Fakhoury, 1994). Although cystitis is usually uncomplicated, the upper urinary tract may become involved by ascending infection. Almost 40 percent of pregnant women with acute pyelonephritis have preceding symptoms of lower tract infection (Gilstrap, 1981a).

Women with cystitis respond readily to any of several regimens. Most of the three-day regimens listed in Table 53-1 are usually 90-percent effective (Fihn, 2003). Single-dose therapy is less effective, and if it is used, concomitant pyelonephritis must be confidently excluded.

Lower urinary tract symptoms with pyuria accompanied by a sterile urine culture may be from urethritis caused by *Chlamydia trachomatis*. Mucopurulent cervicitis usually coexists, and azithromycin therapy is effective. (Chap. 65, p. 1270)

Acute Pyelonephritis

Renal infection is the most common serious medical complication of pregnancy. In a study of the 2006 Nationwide Inpatient Sample by Jolley and coworkers (2012), there were nearly 29,000 hospitalizations for acute pyelonephritis. Rates were highest for adolescents at 17.5 per 1000 and for Hispanic women at 10.1 per 1000. In another study of more than 70,000 pregnancies in a managed care organization, Gazmararian and colleagues (2002) reported that 3.5 percent of antepartum admissions were for urinary infections. The potential seriousness is underscored by the observations of Snyder and associates (2013) that pyelonephritis was the leading cause of septic shock during pregnancy. And in a 2-year audit of admissions to the Parkland Hospital Obstetrical Intensive Care Unit, 12 percent of antepartum admissions were for sepsis syndrome caused by pyelonephritis (Zeeman, 2003). There is also concern that urosepsis may be related to an increased incidence of cerebral palsy in preterm infants (Jacobsson, 2002). Fortunately, there appear to be no serious long-term maternal sequelae (Raz, 2003).

Clinical Findings

Renal infection develops more frequently in the second trimester, and nulliparity and young age are associated risk factors (Hill, 2005). Pyelonephritis is unilateral and right-sided in more than half of cases, and it is bilateral in a fourth. There is usually a rather abrupt onset with fever, shaking chills, and aching pain in one or both lumbar regions. Anorexia, nausea, and vomiting may worsen dehydration. Tenderness usually can be elicited by percussion in one or both costovertebral angles. The urinary sediment contains many leukocytes, frequently in clumps, and numerous bacteria. Bacteremia is demonstrated in 15 to 20 percent of these women. *E coli* is isolated from urine or blood in 70 to 80 percent of infections, *Klebsiella pneumoniae* in 3 to 5 percent, *Enterobacter* or *Proteus* species in 3 to 5 percent, and gram-positive organisms, including group B *Streptococcus* and *S aureus*, in up to 10 percent of cases (Hill, 2005; Wing, 2000). The differential diagnosis includes, among others, labor, chorioamnionitis, appendicitis, placental abruption, or infarcted leiomyoma. Evidence of the sepsis syndrome is common, and this is discussed in detail in Chapter 47 (p. 946).

Plasma creatinine is monitored because early studies reported that 20 percent of pregnant women developed renal dysfunction. More recent findings, however, show this to be only 5 percent if aggressive fluid resuscitation is provided (Hill, 2005). Follow-up studies have demonstrated that this endotoxin-induced damage is reversible in the long term. Varying degrees of respiratory insufficiency from endotoxin-induced alveolar injury are manifest in up to 10 percent of women and may result in frank pulmonary edema (Cunningham, 1987; Sheffield, 2005; Snyder, 2013). In some cases, pulmonary injury may be so severe that it causes *acute respiratory distress syndrome (ARDS)* (Fig. 53-3).

Uterine activity from endotoxin is common and is related to fever severity (Graham, 1993). In the study by Millar and coworkers (2003), women with pyelonephritis averaged 5 contractions per hour at admission, and this decreased to 2 per hour within 6 hours of intravenous fluid and antimicrobial administration. As discussed in Chapter 47 (p. 942), β-agonist therapy for tocolysis increases the likelihood of respiratory insufficiency from permeability edema because of the sodium- and fluid-retaining properties of those agents (Lamont, 2000). The incidence of pulmonary edema in women with pyelonephritis who were given β-agonists was reported to be 8 percent—a fourfold increase over that expected (Towers, 1991).

Endotoxin-induced *hemolysis* is common, and approximately a third of patients with pyelonephritis develop anemia (Cox, 1991). With recovery, hemoglobin regeneration is normal because acute infection does not affect erythropoietin production (Cavenee, 1994).

Management

One scheme for management of acute pyelonephritis is shown in Table 53-2. Although we routinely obtain urine and blood

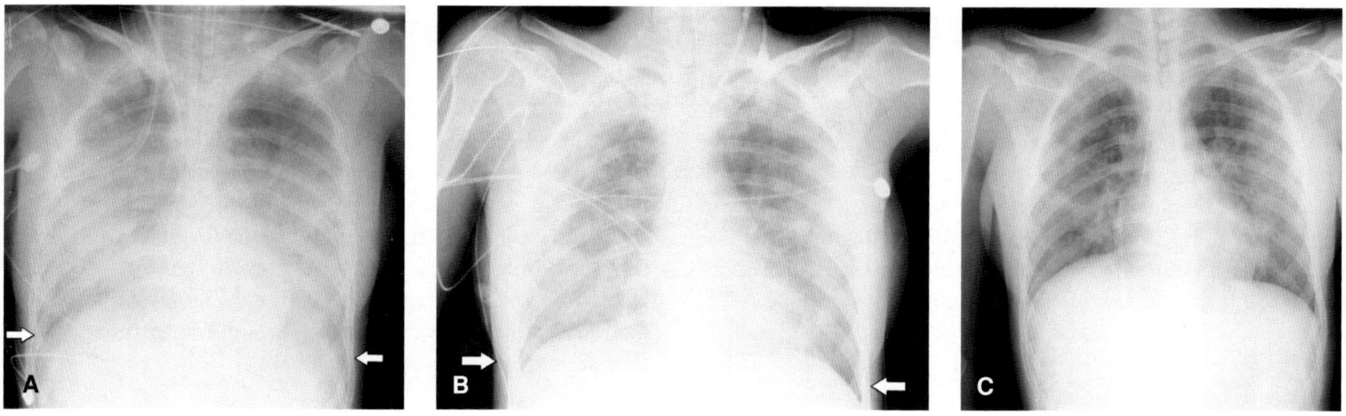

FIGURE 53-3 A series of anterior-posterior projection chest radiographs of improving acute respiratory distress syndrome (ARDS) in a second-trimester pregnant woman with severe pyelonephritis. **A.** An extensive infiltrative process and complete obliteration of the diaphragm (*white arrows*) is seen. **B.** Improved aeration of lung fields bilaterally is noted as pleural disease resolves (*arrows*). **C.** Markedly improved visualization of the lungs fields with residual platelike atelectasis and normal appearance of the diaphragm.

cultures, prospective trials show them to be of limited clinical utility (Wing, 2000). *Intravenous hydration to ensure adequate urinary output is the cornerstone of treatment.* Antimicrobials are also begun promptly with the caveat that they may initially worsen endotoxemia from bacterial lysis. Ongoing surveillance for worsening of sepsis syndrome is monitored by serial determinations of urinary output, blood pressure, pulse, temperature, and oxygen saturation. High fever should be lowered with a cooling blanket or acetaminophen. This is especially important in early pregnancy because of possible teratogenic effects of hyperthermia (Chap. 14, p. 284).

Antimicrobial therapy usually is empirical, and ampicillin plus gentamicin; cefazolin or ceftriaxone; or an extended-spectrum antibiotic were all 95-percent effective in randomized trials (Sanchez-Ramos, 1995; Wing, 1998, 2000). Fewer than half of *E coli* strains are sensitive to ampicillin in vitro, but cephalosporins and gentamicin generally have excellent activity.

TABLE 53-2. Management of the Pregnant Woman with Acute Pyelonephritis

Hospitalize patient
Obtain urine and blood cultures
Evaluate hemogram, serum creatinine, and electrolytes
Monitor vital signs frequently, including urinary output—consider indwelling catheter
Establish urinary output ≥ 50 mL/hr with intravenous crystalloid solution
Administer intravenous antimicrobial therapy (see text)
Obtain chest radiograph if there is dyspnea or tachypnea
Repeat hematology and chemistry studies in 48 hours
Change to oral antimicrobials when afebrile
Discharge when afebrile 24 hours, consider antimicrobial therapy for 7 to 10 days
Repeat urine culture 1 to 2 weeks after antimicrobial therapy completed

Modified from Lucas, 1994; Sheffield, 2005.

Serum creatinine is monitored if nephrotoxic drugs are given. Initial treatment at Parkland Hospital is ampicillin plus gentamicin. Some recommend suitable substitutes if bacterial studies show in vitro resistance. With any of the regimens discussed, response is usually prompt, and 95 percent of women are afebrile by 72 hours (Hill, 2005; Sheffield, 2005; Wing, 2000). After discharge, most recommend oral therapy for a total of 7 to 14 days (Hooton, 2012).

Persistent Infection. Generally, intravenous hydration and antimicrobial therapy are followed by stepwise defervescence of approximately 1°F per day. With persistent spiking fever or lack of clinical improvement by 48 to 72 hours, urinary tract obstruction or another complication or both are considered. Renal sonography is recommended to search for obstruction manifest by abnormal ureteral or pyelocaliceal dilatation (Seidman, 1998). Although most women with continuing infection have no evidence of obstruction, some are found to have calculi. Although renal sonography will detect hydronephrosis, stones are not always seen in pregnancy (Butler, 2000; Maikranz, 1987). If stones are strongly suspected despite a nondiagnostic sonographic examination, a plain abdominal radiograph will identify nearly 90 percent. Another option is the modified *one-shot intravenous pyelogram*—a single radiograph obtained 30 minutes after contrast injection—which usually provides adequate imaging (Butler, 2000).

In some women, MR imaging may disclose the cause of persistent infection (Spencer, 2004). Even without urinary obstruction, persistent infection can be due to an intrarenal or perinephric abscess or phlegmon (Cox, 1988; Rafi, 2012). Obstruction relief is important, and one method is cystoscopic placement of a double-J ureteral stent (Rodriguez, 1988). Because these stents are usually left in place until after delivery, they frequently become encrusted and require replacement. We have found that percutaneous nephrostomy is preferable because the stents are more easily replaced. Finally, surgical removal of stones may be required in some women (p. 1057).

Outpatient Management of Pyelonephritis. Outpatient management is an option for nonpregnant women with uncomplicated pyelonephritis (Hooton, 2012). Wing and associates (1999) have described outpatient management in 92 pregnant women who were first given in-hospital intramuscular ceftriaxone, two 1-g doses 24 hours apart. At this point, one third of the group was considered suitable for outpatient therapy, and these women were randomized either to discharge and oral antimicrobials or to continued hospitalization with intravenous therapy. A third of the outpatient management group was unable to adhere to the treatment regimen and was admitted. These findings suggest that outpatient management is applicable to very few pregnant women.

Surveillance

Recurrent infection—either covert or symptomatic—is common and develops in 30 to 40 percent of women following completion of treatment for pyelonephritis (Cunningham, 1973). Unless other measures are taken to ensure urine sterility, nitrofurantoin, 100 mg orally at bedtime given for the remainder of the pregnancy, reduces bacteriuria recurrence (Van Dorsten, 1987).

Reflux Nephropathy

Vesicoureteral reflux in early childhood can cause recurrent urinary tract infections, and thus, subsequent chronic interstitial nephritis was attributed to *chronic pyelonephritis*. Moreover, it was also found that high-pressure sterile reflux impaired normal renal growth. Combined, this leads to patchy interstitial scarring, tubular atrophy, and loss of nephron mass and is termed *reflux nephropathy*. In adults, long-term complications include hypertension, which may be severe if there is demonstrable renal damage (Diamond, 2012; Köhler, 2003).

Perhaps half of women with reflux nephropathy were treated during childhood for renal infections. Of these, many also had surgical correction of reflux as children, and these commonly have bacteriuria when pregnant (Mor, 2003). In the other half of women with reflux nephropathy, there is no clear history of recurrent cystitis, acute pyelonephritis, or obstructive disease (Diamond, 2012). Reports describing 939 pregnancies in 379 women with reflux nephropathy indicate that impaired renal function and bilateral renal scarring were associated with increased maternal complications (El-Khatib, 1994; Jungers, 1996; Köhler, 2003). Chronic renal disease and pregnancy outcome is discussed further on page 1061.

NEPHROLITHIASIS

Kidney stones develop in 7 percent of women during their lifetime with an average age of onset in the third decade (Asplin, 2012). Calcium salts make up approximately 80 percent of stones, and up to half of affected women have polygenic *familial idiopathic hypercalciuria* (Worcester, 2010). Hyperparathyroidism should be excluded. Although calcium oxalate stones in young nonpregnant women are most common, most stones in pregnancy—65 to 75 percent—are calcium phosphate or hydroxyapatite (Ross, 2008; Tan, 2013). Patients who have a stone typically form another stone every 2 to 3 years.

Contrary to past teachings, a low-calcium diet *promotes* stone formation. Prevention of recurrences with hydration and a diet low in sodium and protein is currently recommended (Asplin, 2012). Thiazide diuretics also diminish stone formation. In general, obstruction, infection, intractable pain, and heavy bleeding are indications for stone removal. Removal by a flexible basket via cystoscopy, although used less often than in the past, is still a reasonable consideration for pregnant women. In nonpregnant patients, stone destruction by *lithotripsy* is preferred to surgical therapy in most cases. There is limited information on the use of these procedures during pregnancy, and they are not generally recommended.

Stone Disease During Pregnancy

The incidence of stone disease complicating pregnancy has been reported with widespread variability. At the low end, Butler and colleagues (2000) found the incidence to be 0.3 admissions per 1000 pregnancies in more than 186,000 deliveries at Parkland Hospital. In an Israeli population-based study, the incidence in nearly 220,000 pregnancies was 0.8 per 1000 (Rosenberg, 2011). In a population-based study from Washington state, Swartz and coworkers (2007) reported an incidence of 1.7 per 1000 pregnancies. Bladder stones are rare, but recurrent infection and labor obstructed by stones have been reported (Ait Benkaddour, 2006; Ruan, 2011).

Data are conflicting whether women with kidney stones have an increased risk for low-birthweight and preterm infants. The case-control study by Swartz and colleagues (2007) of 2239 women with nephrolithiasis reported excessive preterm delivery—10.6 versus 6.4 percent—compared with normal controls. The more recent nationwide population-based case-control study from Taiwan also reported 20- to 40-percent increases in low-birthweight and preterm births (Chung, 2013). To the contrary, a case-control study from Hungary reported that pregnancy outcomes, including preterm delivery, were similar in women with stones and normal controls (Banhidy, 2007). Comparable conclusions were drawn from the Israeli population-based study noted earlier (Rosenberg, 2011).

Diagnosis

There is some evidence that pregnant women may have fewer symptoms with stone passage because of urinary tract dilatation (Hendricks, 1991; Tan, 2013). That said, more than 90 percent of pregnant women with nephrolithiasis present with pain. Gross hematuria is less common than in nonpregnant women and was reported to be a presenting symptom in 23 percent of women described by Butler and associates (2000). In another study, however, Lewis and coworkers (2003) found that only 2 percent had hematuria. Sonography is usually selected to visualize stones, but as discussed above, many are not detected because hydronephrosis may obscure findings (McAleer, 2004). If there is abnormal dilatation without stone visualization, then the one-shot pyelogram may be useful. Transabdominal color Doppler sonography to detect presence or absence of ureteral "jets" of urine into the bladder has been used to exclude obstruction (Asrat, 1998).

Helical computed tomography (CT) scanning is the imaging method of choice for nonpregnant individuals, however, it is avoided during pregnancy if possible (Brown, 2010). If it is used, the slices can be tailored as needed (Chap. 46, p. 934). For pregnant women, White and colleagues (2007) recommend unenhanced helical CT and cite an average fetal radiation dose to be 7 mGy. These exigencies have led some to recommend MR imaging as the second-line test following nondiagnostic sonography (Masselli, 2013).

Management

Treatment depends on symptoms and gestational age (Semins, 2013). Intravenous hydration and analgesics are given. In half of women with symptomatic stones, infection will be identified, and this is treated vigorously. Although calculi infrequently cause symptomatic obstruction during pregnancy, persistent pyelonephritis should prompt a search for obstruction due to nephrolithiasis.

Approximately 65 to 80 percent of symptomatic women will have improvement with conservative therapy, and the stone usually passes spontaneously (Tan, 2013). Others require an invasive procedure such as ureteral stenting, ureteroscopy, percutaneous nephrostomy, transurethral laser lithotripsy, or basket extraction (Butler, 2000; Semins, 2010). The need for fluoroscopy limits the utility of percutaneous nephrolithotomy (Toth, 2005). In the case-control study cited above by Swartz and associates (2007), there were 623 procedures performed in 2239 symptomatic pregnant women, but less than 2 percent required surgical exploration.

As noted earlier, extracorporeal shock-wave lithotripsy is contraindicated in pregnancy. Watterson and coworkers (2002) described successful transurethral holmium:YAG laser lithotripsy in nine of 10 women. Semins and Matlaga (2010) found that ureteroscopic removal is also safe in pregnancy.

PREGNANCY AFTER RENAL TRANSPLANTATION

In 2013, there were approximately 97,000 registrants on the waiting list for renal transplantations through the Organ Procurement and Transplantation Network—OPTN (2013). The 1-year graft survival rate is 95 percent for grafts from living donors and 89 percent from deceased donors (Carpenter, 2008). Survival rates approximately doubled between 1988 and 1996, due in large part to the introduction of cyclosporine and muromonab-CD3 (OKT3 monoclonal antibody) to prevent and treat organ rejection. Since then, mycophenolate mofetil and tacrolimus have further reduced acute rejection episodes, however, the former is considered teratogenic (Briggs, 2011). In the report from the National Transplant Pregnancy Registry, 23 percent of fetuses exposed to mycophenolate had birth defects (Coscia, 2010). Importantly, resumption of renal function after transplantation promptly restores fertility in reproductive-aged women (Hladunewich, 2011; Lessan-Pezeshki, 2004). More than half of transplant recipients reported that they were not counseled regarding contraception (French, 2013).

Pregnancy Outcomes

Coscia and coworkers (2010) reviewed the outcomes of 2000 pregnancies in transplant recipients as reported to the National Transplantation Pregnancy Registry. Most were treated with cyclosporine and tacrolimus, and approximately 75 percent of pregnancies resulted in a live birth. Similar outcomes were described for the Australian and New Zealand Transplant Registry by Wyld and associates (2013). Bramham and colleagues (2013) identified 105 pregnancies in renal transplant recipients and the United Kingdom Obstetric Surveillance System (UKOSS). Excluding nine abortions, there was only one perinatal death and 97 living children. Half were delivered before 37 weeks' gestation, but only 9 percent before 32 weeks. Half were born weighing < 2500 g, and a fourth were growth restricted. Importantly, the incidence of fetal malformations was not increased, except in those who took mycophenolate mofetil (Coscia, 2010). Twin pregnancy has also been described following renal transplantation (Gizzo, 2014).

The incidence of preeclampsia is high in all transplant recipients (Brosens, 2013). In the UK National Cohort Study reported by Bramham and associates (2013), the incidence of preeclampsia was 22 percent. From their review, Josephson and McKay (2011) cite an incidence of a third of pregnancies but question the validity of this frequency. Importantly, in some cases, rejection is difficult to distinguish from preeclampsia. That said, the incidence of rejection episodes approximates only 2 percent (Bramham, 2013). Viral infections—especially polyomavirus hominis 1, also called BK virus, infections—are frequent. Also, gestational diabetes is found in approximately 5 percent. Both are likely related to immunosuppression therapy. Similar outcomes have been reported by several other investigators (Al Duraihimh, 2008; Cruz Lemini, 2007; Ghafari, 2008; Gutierrez, 2005).

Lindheimer (2007a) and Josephson (2011) and their coworkers recommend that women who have undergone transplantation satisfy several requisites before attempting pregnancy. First, women should be in good general health for at least 1 to 2 years after transplantation. Also, there should be stable renal function without severe renal insufficiency—serum creatinine < 2 mg/dL and preferably < 1.5 mg/dL—and < 500 mg/day proteinuria. Evidence for graft rejection should be absent for 6 months, and pyelocalyceal distention by urography should not be apparent. Moreover, hypertension should be absent or well controlled. And last, no teratogenic drugs are being given, and drug therapy is reduced to maintenance levels.

Cyclosporine or tacrolimus is given routinely to renal transplantation recipients (Jain, 2004). Cyclosporine blood levels decline during pregnancy, although this was not reported to be associated with rejection episodes (Thomas, 1997). Unfortunately, these agents are nephrotoxic and also may cause renal hypertension. In fact, they likely contribute substantively to chronic renal disease that develops in 10 to 20 percent of patients with nonrenal solid-organ transplantation (Goes, 2007).

Concern persists regarding the possible late effects in offspring subjected to immunosuppressive therapy in utero. These include malignancy, germ cell dysfunction, and malformations in the children of the offspring. In addition, cyclosporine is secreted in breast milk, and in at least one instance, it produced therapeutic serum levels in the nursing child (Moretti, 2003).

Finally, although pregnancy-induced renal hyperfiltration theoretically may impair long-term graft survival, Sturgiss and

Davison (1995) found no evidence for this in a case-control study of 34 allograft recipients followed for a mean of 15 years.

Management

Close surveillance is necessary. Covert bacteriuria is treated, and if it is recurrent, suppressive treatment is given for the remainder of the pregnancy. Serial hepatic enzyme concentrations and blood counts are monitored for toxic effects of azathioprine and cyclosporine. Some recommend measurement of serum cyclosporine levels. Gestational diabetes is more common if corticosteroids are taken, and overt diabetes must be excluded with glucose tolerance testing done at approximately 26 weeks' gestation. Surveillance for opportunistic infections from herpesvirus, cytomegalovirus, and toxoplasmosis is important because these infections are common. Some recommend surveillance for BK virus in women known to be infected (Josephson, 2011). Treatment is problematic.

Renal function is monitored, and as shown in Figure 53-2, the glomerular filtration rate usually increases 20 to 25 percent. If a significant rise in the serum creatinine level is detected, then its cause must be determined. Possibilities include acute rejection, cyclosporine toxicity, preeclampsia, infection, and urinary tract obstruction. Evidence of pyelonephritis or graft rejection should prompt admission for aggressive management. Imaging studies and kidney biopsy may be indicated. The woman is carefully monitored for development or worsening of underlying hypertension, and especially superimposed preeclampsia. Management of hypertension during pregnancy is the same as for patients without a transplant.

Because of increased incidences of fetal-growth restriction and preterm delivery, vigilant fetal surveillance is indicated (Chaps. 42, p. 842 and 44, p. 880). Although cesarean delivery is reserved for obstetrical indications, occasionally the transplanted kidney obstructs labor. In all women with a renal transplant, the cesarean delivery rate exceeds 60 percent (Bramham, 2013; Rocha, 2013).

POLYCYSTIC KIDNEY DISEASE

This usually autosomally dominant systemic disease primarily affects the kidneys. Its basic pathophysiology is one of a *ciliopathy* (Hildebrandt, 2011). The disease is found in 1 in 800 live births and causes approximately 5 to 10 percent of end-stage renal disease in the United States (Bargman, 2012). Although genetically heterogeneous, almost 85 percent of cases are due to *PKD1* gene mutations on chromosome 16, and the other 15 percent to *PKD2* mutations on chromosome 4 (Salant, 2012). Prenatal diagnosis is available if the mutation has been identified in a family member or if linkage has been established in the family.

Renal complications are more common in men than in women, and symptoms usually appear in the third or fourth decade. Flank pain, hematuria, proteinuria, abdominal masses, and associated calculi and infection are common findings. Hypertension develops in 75 percent, and progression to renal failure is a major problem. Superimposed acute renal failure may also develop from infection or obstruction from ureteral angulation by cyst displacement.

Other organs are commonly involved. Hepatic involvement is more common and more aggressive in women than in men (Chapman, 2003). Asymptomatic *hepatic cysts* coexist in a third of patients with polycystic kidneys. Approximately 10 percent of patients with polycystic kidney disease die from rupture of an associated *intracranial berry aneurysm*. Up to a fourth of patients have *cardiac valvular lesions*, with mitral valve prolapse and mitral, aortic, and tricuspid valvular incompetence.

Pregnancy Outcomes

The prognosis for pregnancy in women with polycystic kidney disease depends on the degree of associated hypertension and renal insufficiency. Urinary tract infections are common. Chapman and coworkers (1994) compared pregnancy outcomes in 235 affected women who had 605 pregnancies with those of 108 unaffected family members who had 244 pregnancies. Composite perinatal complication rates were similar—33 versus 26 percent—but hypertension, including preeclampsia, was more common in women with polycystic kidneys. Pregnancy does not seem to accelerate the natural disease course (Lindheimer, 2007b).

GLOMERULAR DISEASES

The glomerulus and its capillaries are subject to numerous and various conditions and agents that can lead to acute and chronic diseases. Glomerular damage can be caused by several agents such as toxins or infections or from systemic disorders such as hypertension or diabetes. It may also be idiopathic. When there is capillary inflammation, the process is termed *glomerulonephritis*, and in many of these cases, an autoimmune process is involved. Glomerular disease or glomerulonephritis may result from a single stimulus such as that following group A streptococcal infections. However, it may be a manifestation of a multisystem disease such as systemic lupus erythematosus or diabetes (Sethi, 2012).

Persistent glomerulonephritis eventually leads to renal functional decline. Progression is variable and often does not become apparent until chronic renal insufficiency is diagnosed as discussed on page 1060. Lewis and Neilsen (2012) group glomerular injuries into six syndromes based on clinical patterns (Table 53-3). Some underlying disorders—examples include infections, vasculitides, and diabetes—can result in one clinical pattern in different individuals. Finally, within each of these categories, there are disorders encountered in young women, and thus, these may antedate or first manifest during pregnancy.

Acute Nephritic Syndromes

Acute glomerulonephritis may result from any of several causes (see Table 53-3). The clinical presentation usually includes hypertension, hematuria, red-cell casts, pyuria, and proteinuria. Varying degrees of renal insufficiency and salt and water retention result in edema, hypertension, and circulatory congestion (Lewis, 2012). The prognosis and treatment of nephritic syndromes depends on their etiology. Some recede spontaneously or with treatment. However, in some patients, *rapidly progressive glomerulonephritis* leads to end-stage renal failure, whereas in others, *chronic glomerulonephritis* develops with slowly progressive renal disease.

TABLE 53-3. Patterns of Clinical Glomerulonephritis

Acute Nephritic Syndromes: poststreptococcal, infective endocarditis, SLE, antiglomerular basement membrane disease, IgA nephropathy, ANCA vasculitis, Henoch-Schönlein purpura, cryoglobulinemia, membranoproliferative and mesangioproliferative glomerulonephritis
Pulmonary-Renal Syndromes: Goodpasture, ANCA vasculitis, Henoch-Schönlein purpura, cryoglobulinemia
Nephrotic Syndromes: minimal change disease, focal segmental glomerulosclerosis, membranous glomerulonephritis, diabetes, amyloidosis, others
Basement Membrane Syndromes: anti-GBM disease, others
Glomerular Vascular Syndromes: atherosclerosis, chronic hypertension, sickle-cell disease, thrombotic microangiopathies, antiphospholipid antibody syndrome, ANCA vasculitis, others
Infectious Disease-Associated Syndromes: poststreptococcal, infective endocarditis, HIV, HBV, HCV, syphilis, others

ANCA = antineutrophilic cytoplasmic antibodies; anti-GBM = anti-glomerular basement membrane; HBV = hepatitis B virus; HCV = hepatitis C virus; HIV = human immunodeficiency virus; IgA = immunoglobulin A; SLE = systemic lupus erythematosus.
Adapted from Lewis, 2012.

The prototype is *acute poststreptococcal glomerulonephritis,* which is historically interesting because it was confused with eclampsia until the mid-1800s. *IgA nephropathy,* also known as *Berger disease,* is the most common form of acute glomerulonephritis worldwide (Wyatt, 2013). The isolated form occurs sporadically, and it may be related to *Henoch-Schönlein purpura* as the systemic form (Donadio, 2002). Isolated nephritis may be due to antiglomerular basement membrane (GBM) antibodies. These may also involve the lungs to manifest as a pulmonary-renal syndrome with alveolar hemorrhage, which is termed *Goodpasture syndrome* (Bazari, 2012; Vasilou, 2005).

Pregnancy

Acute nephritic syndromes during pregnancy can be difficult to differentiate from severe preeclampsia or eclampsia. One example is systemic lupus erythematosus with a flare during the second half of pregnancy (Bramham, 2012; Zhao, 2013). In some cases, renal biopsy may be necessary to determine etiology as well as to direct management (Lindheimer, 2007a; Ramin, 2006). This is discussed further in Chapter 59 (p. 1170).

Whatever the underlying etiology, acute glomerulonephritis has profound effects on pregnancy outcome. In an older study, Packham and coworkers (1989) described 395 pregnancies in 238 women with *primary* glomerulonephritis diagnosed before pregnancy. The most common lesions on biopsy were membranous glomerulonephritis, IgA glomerulonephritis, and diffuse mesangial glomerulonephritis. Although most of these women had normal renal function, half developed hypertension, a fourth were delivered preterm, and the perinatal mortality rate after 28 weeks' gestation was 80 per 1000. As expected, the worst perinatal outcomes were in women with impaired renal function, early or severe hypertension, and nephrotic-range proteinuria.

Similar outcomes have been reported for pregnancies in women with IgA nephropathy. From their review of more than 300 such pregnancies, Lindheimer and colleagues (2000) concluded that pregnancy outcome was related to the degree of renal insufficiency and hypertension. Ronkainen and associates (2006) followed a cohort of children with IgA nephritis for an average of 19 years. They described 22 pregnancies of which half were complicated by hypertension and a third were delivered preterm.

Nephrotic Syndromes

Heavy proteinuria is the hallmark of the nephrotic syndromes, which may be caused by several primary and secondary kidney disorders. These can cause immunological- or toxic-mediated injury with glomerular capillary wall breakdown that allows excessive filtration of plasma proteins. In addition to heavy urine protein excretion, the syndrome is characterized by hypoalbuminemia, hypercholesterolemia, and edema. There frequently is hypertension, and along with albumin nephrotoxicity, renal insufficiency eventually develops.

Some of the more common causes of the nephrotic syndrome are shown in Table 53-4. In most cases, renal biopsy will disclose microscopic abnormalities that may help direct treatment, which depends on etiology. Edema is problematic, especially during pregnancy (Jakobi, 1995). Normal amounts of dietary protein of high biological value are encouraged—indeed, high-protein diets increase proteinuria. The incidence of thromboembolism is increased and varies with the severity of hypertension, proteinuria, and renal insufficiency (Stratta, 2006). Although both arterial and venous thromboses may develop, renal vein thrombosis is particularly worrisome. The value, if any, of prophylactic anticoagulation is unclear. Some cases of nephrosis from primary glomerular disease respond to glucocorticosteroids and other immunosuppressants or cytotoxic drug therapy. In most of those cases caused by infection or drugs, proteinuria recedes when the underlying cause is corrected.

Pregnancy

Maternal and perinatal outcomes in women with the nephrotic syndromes depend on its underlying cause and severity. Whenever possible, these should be ascertained, and renal biopsy may be indicated to determine if there is a treatment-responsive

TABLE 53-4. Causes of the Nephrotic Syndrome in Adults and Percentage of Attributable Cases

Minimal change disease (MCD) (10–15%): primary idiopathic (most cases), drug-induced (NSAIDs), allergies, viral infections
Focal segmental glomerulosclerosis (FSGS) (35%): viruses, hypertension, reflux nephropathy, sickle-cell disease
Membranous glomerulonephritis (30%): idiopathic (most cases), malignancy, infection, connective-tissue diseases
Diabetic nephropathy: most common cause of ESRD
Amyloidosis

ESRD = end-stage renal disease; NSAIDs = nonsteroidal antiinflammatory drugs.
Adapted from Lewis, 2012.

etiology. Half of women with nephrotic-range proteinuria will have rise in daily protein excretion as pregnancy progresses (Packham, 1989). In women with nephrosis cared for at Parkland Hospital, we reported that two thirds had protein excretion that exceeded 3 g/day (Stettler, 1992). At the same time, however, if these women had only mild degrees of renal dysfunction, they had normally augmented glomerular filtration across pregnancy (Cunningham, 1990).

Management of edema during pregnancy can be particularly challenging as it is intensified by normally increasing hydrostatic pressure in the lower extremities. In some women, massive vulvar edema may develop as described by Jakobi and coworkers (1995) in diabetic women. Massive vulvar edema associated with the nephrotic syndrome caused by secondary syphilis is shown in Figure 53-4. Another major problem is that up to half of these women have chronic hypertension that may require treatment (Chap. 50, p. 1005). In these, as well as in previously normotensive women, preeclampsia is common and often develops early in pregnancy.

Most women with nephrotic syndromes who do not have severe hypertension or renal insufficiency will have successful pregnancy outcomes. Conversely, if there is renal insufficiency, moderate to severe hypertension, or both, the prognosis is much worse. Our experiences from women with 65 pregnancies cared for at Parkland Hospital noted that there are frequent complications (Stettler, 1992). Protein excretion during pregnancy averaged 4 g daily, and a third of the women had classic nephrotic syndrome. There was some degree of renal insufficiency in 75 percent, chronic hypertension in 40 percent, and persistent anemia in 25 percent. Importantly, preeclampsia developed in 60 percent, and 45 percent had preterm deliveries. Even so, after excluding abortions, 53 of 57 infants were born alive. Stratta and associates (2006) reported fetal-growth restriction in a third of these women.

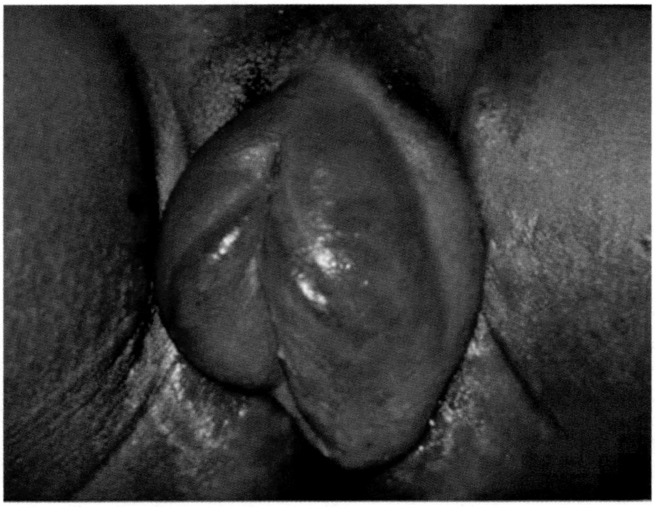

FIGURE 53-4 Massive vulvar edema in a pregnant woman with the nephrotic syndrome due to secondary syphilis. (Photograph contributed by Dr. George Wendel, Jr.)

Long-Term Outcomes

Women identified to have nephrotic syndromes either before or during pregnancy are at risk for serious long-term adverse outcomes. In women cared for at Parkland Hospital cited in the report above, all 21 women who subsequently underwent renal biopsy had abnormal histological findings (Stettler, 1992). At least 20 percent of women followed for 10 years progressed to end-stage renal failure. Similarly, Chen and colleagues (2001) reported short-term outcomes in 15 women with nephrotic syndromes in whom they had performed renal biopsy during pregnancy. By 2 years, three of these women had died, three had developed chronic renal failure, and two had progressed to end-stage renal disease. In the report by Imbasciati and coworkers (2007), women whose serum creatinine level was > 1.4 mg/dL and whose 24-hour protein excretion exceeded 1 g/day had the shortest renal survival times following pregnancy.

CHRONIC RENAL DISEASE

This describes a pathophysiological process that can progress to end-stage renal disease. The National Kidney Foundation describes six stages of chronic kidney disease defined by decreasing glomerular filtration rate (GFR). It progresses from stage 0—GFR > 90 mL/min/1.73 m^2 to stage 5—GFR < 15 mL/min/1.73 m^2. There are a number of diseases that result in progressively declining renal function, and many result from one of the glomerular diseases that were discussed earlier. Those that most commonly lead to end-stage disease requiring dialysis and kidney transplantation and their approximate percentages include: diabetes, 33 percent; hypertension, 25 percent; glomerulonephritis, 20 percent; and polycystic kidney disease, 15 percent (Abboud, 2010; Bargman, 2012).

Most reproductive-aged women with these diseases have varying degrees of renal insufficiency, proteinuria, or both. To counsel regarding fertility and pregnancy outcome, the degree of renal functional impairment and of associated hypertension are assessed. Successful pregnancy outcome in general may be more related to these two factors than to the specific underlying renal disorder. A general prognosis can be estimated by considering women with chronic renal disease in arbitrary categories of renal function (Davison, 2011). These include normal or *mild impairment*—defined as a serum creatinine < 1.5 mg/dL; *moderate impairment*—defined as a serum creatinine 1.5 to 3.0 mg/dL; and *severe renal insufficiency*—defined as a serum creatinine > 3.0 mg/dL. Although some have suggested adopting the classification of the National Kidney Foundation, others recommend using the older categories (Davison, 2011; Piccoli, 2010a, 2011). Thus, the obstetrician must be familiar with both.

Pregnancy and Chronic Renal Disease

Most women have relatively mild renal insufficiency, and its severity along with any underlying hypertension is prognostic of pregnancy outcome. Renal disease with comorbidities secondary to a systemic disorder—for example, diabetes or systemic lupus erythematosus—portends a worse prognosis (Davison, 2011; Fischer, 2004). For all women with chronic renal disease, the incidences of hypertension and preeclampsia, preterm and growth-restricted infants, and other problems are high. Despite these, the National High Blood Pressure Education Program Working Group (2000) has concluded that the prognosis has substantively improved since the 1980s. This has subsequently been verified by several reviews (Davison, 2011; Nevis, 2011; Ramin, 2006).

Loss of renal tissue is associated with compensatory intrarenal vasodilation and hypertrophy of the surviving nephrons. The resultant hyperperfusion and hyperfiltration eventually damage surviving nephrons to cause *nephrosclerosis* and worsening renal function. With mild renal insufficiency, pregnancy causes greater augmentation of renal plasma flow and glomerular filtration (Baylis, 2003; Helal, 2012). With progressively declining renal function, there is little, if any, augmented renal plasma flow. In one study, only half of women with moderate renal insufficiency demonstrated pregnancy-augmented glomerular filtration, and women with severe disease had no increase (Cunningham, 1990).

Importantly, chronic renal insufficiency also curtails normal pregnancy-induced hypervolemia. Blood volume expansion during pregnancy is related to disease severity and correlates inversely with serum creatinine concentration. As shown in Figure 53-5, women with mild to moderate renal dysfunction have normal blood volume expansion that averages 55 percent. With severe renal insufficiency, however, volume expansion averages only 25 percent, which is similar to that seen with hemoconcentration from eclampsia. In addition, these women have variable degrees of chronic anemia due to intrinsic renal disease.

Renal Disease with Preserved Function

In some women, although glomerular disease has not yet caused renal dysfunction, there is still an increased incidence of pregnancy complications. As shown in Table 53-5, these complications are less frequent than in cohorts of women with moderate and severe renal insufficiency. Two studies illustrate this. In one, Surian and colleagues (1984) described outcomes in 123 pregnancies in women with biopsy-proven glomerular disease. Although only a few of these women had renal dysfunction, 40 percent developed obstetrical or renal complications. In another study, Packham and coworkers (1989) described outcomes in 395 pregnancies in women with preexisting

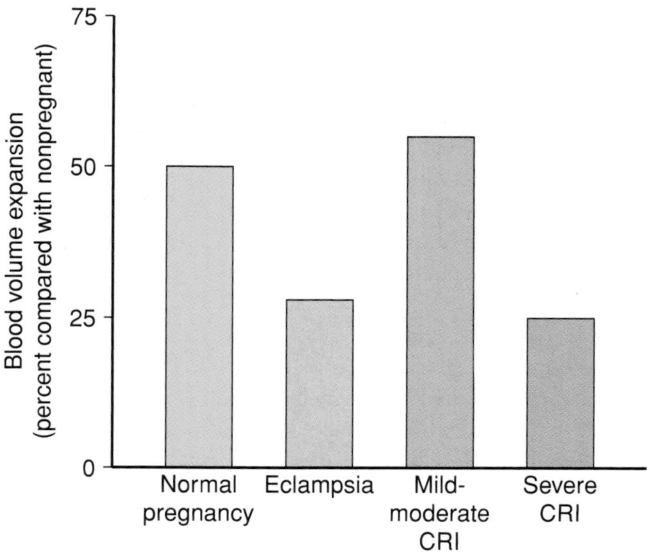

FIGURE 53-5 Blood volume expansion in 44 normally pregnant women at term compared with 29 who had eclampsia; 10 with moderate chronic renal insufficiency (CRI)—serum creatinine 1.5 to 2.9 mg/dL; and four with severe CRI—serum creatinine ≥ 3.0 mg/dL. (Data from Zeeman, 2009; Cunningham, 1990.)

TABLE 53-5. Complications (%) Associated with Chronic Renal Disease During Pregnancy

		Renal Insufficiency	
Complication	Preserved Function	Moderate and Severe	Severe
Chronic hypertension	25	30–70	50
Gestational hypertension	20–50	30–50	75
Worsening renal function	8–15	20–43	35
Permanent dysfunction	4–5	10–20	35
Preterm delivery	7	30–60	73
Fetal-growth restriction	8–14	30–38	57
Perinatal mortality	5–14	4–7	0

Data from Alsuwaida, 2011; Cunningham, 1990; Farwell, 2013; Imbasciati, 2007; Maruotti, 2012; Nevis, 2011; Packham, 1989; Piccoli, 2010a, 2011; Stettler, 1992; Surian, 1984; Trevisan, 2004.

glomerulonephritis and minimal renal insufficiency. Impaired renal function developed in 15 percent of these women during pregnancy, and 60 percent had worsening proteinuria. Only 12 percent had antecedent chronic hypertension, however, more than half of the 395 pregnancies were complicated by hypertension. The perinatal mortality rate was 140 per 1000, but even without early-onset or severe hypertension or nephrotic-range proteinuria, the rate was 50 per 1000. Importantly, in 5 percent, worsening renal function was permanent.

Chronic Renal Insufficiency

As indicated, pregnancy complication rates are greater in women with chronic kidney disease who also have renal insufficiency compared with women with preserved renal function. Furthermore, adverse outcomes are generally directly related to the degree of renal impairment. Of the more recent reports shown in Table 53-5, outcomes of women with moderate versus severe renal insufficiency are usually not separated. That said, Piccoli and associates (2010a) described 91 pregnancies complicated by stage 1 chronic kidney disease. Primarily because of hypertension, 33 percent were delivered preterm, and 13 percent had fetal-growth restriction. Alsuwaida and colleagues (2011) reported similar observations.

Other investigators have described pregnancies complicated by moderate or severe renal insufficiency (Cunningham, 1990; Imbasciati, 2007; Jones, 1996). Despite a high incidence of chronic hypertension, anemia, preeclampsia, preterm delivery, and fetal-growth restriction, perinatal outcomes were generally acceptable. As shown in Figure 53-6, fetal growth is frequently impaired and related to renal dysfunction severity.

Management

There are several important aspects of prenatal care for women with chronic renal disease. Frequent monitoring of blood pressure is paramount, and serum creatinine levels and 24-hour protein excretion are quantified as indicated. Bacteriuria is treated to decrease the risk of pyelonephritis and further nephron loss.

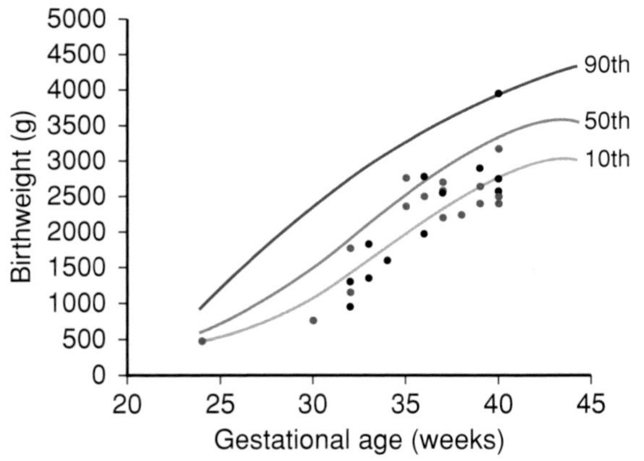

FIGURE 53-6 Birthweight percentiles of infants born to 29 women at Parkland Hospital with mild to moderate renal insufficiency—serum creatinine 1.4–2.4 mg/dL (*black points*) and severe renal insufficiency—serum creatinine ≥ 2.5 mg/dL (*red points*). (Data from Cunningham, 1990; Stettler, 1992. Growth curves are those reported by Alexander, 1996.)

Protein-restricted diets are not recommended (Lindheimer, 2000; Ruggenenti, 2001). In some women with anemia from chronic renal insufficiency, a response is seen with recombinant erythropoietin. However, hypertension is a common side effect. Serial sonography is performed to follow fetal growth (Chap. 44, p. 880). The differentiation between worsening hypertension and superimposed preeclampsia is problematic. Preliminary data indicate that the angiogenic biomarkers placental growth factor (PlGF) and its soluble receptor (sFlt-1) may be useful to separate chronic from gestational hypertension. This is described in Chapter 40 (p. 747).

Long-Term Effects

In some women, pregnancy may accelerate chronic renal disease progression by increasing hyperfiltration and glomerular pressure to worsen nephrosclerosis (Baylis, 2003; Helal, 2012). Women with more severe renal insufficiency have increased susceptibility. For example, Jungers and associates (1995) reported few long-term pregnancy-related adverse effects in 360 women with chronic glomerulonephritis and antecedent normal renal function. In women with severe chronic renal insufficiency, however, renal insufficiency may become worse during pregnancy (Abe, 1991; Jones, 1996). In the study by Imbasciati and coworkers (2007), worsening renal function was more likely in women who had a serum creatinine ≥ 1.4 mg/dL and > 1 g/day protein excretion.

As noted, progression is common for many women with chronic renal disorders. At 1 year after pregnancy, Jones and Hayslett (1996) reported that 10 percent of the women had developed end-stage renal failure—stage 5 chronic kidney disease. In a study from Parkland Hospital, we found that 20 percent of pregnant women with moderate to severe insufficiency had developed end-stage renal failure by a mean of 4 years (Cunningham, 1990). Similar findings in women with a median follow-up of 3 years were described by Imbasciati and colleagues (2007). By this time, end-stage disease was apparent in 30 percent of women whose serum creatinine was ≥ 1.4 mg/dL and who had proteinuria > 1 g/day. Chronic proteinuria is also a marker for subsequent development of renal failure. In another report from Parkland Hospital, we found that 20 percent of women with chronic proteinuria discovered during pregnancy progressed to end-stage renal failure within several years (Stettler, 1992).

Dialysis During Pregnancy

Significantly impaired renal function is accompanied by subfertility that may be corrected with chronic renal replacement therapy—either hemodialysis or peritoneal dialysis (Hladunewich, 2011; Shahir, 2013). Not unexpectedly, these pregnancies can be complicated. Chou and associates (2008) reviewed 131 cases reported since 1990. They found that mean fetal birthweight was higher in women who conceived while undergoing dialysis—1530 g versus 1245 g in women who conceived before starting dialysis. This was also true for 77 pregnancies reported to the Australian and New Zealand Dialysis and Transplantation Registry (Jesudason, 2014). Similar outcomes from several reports since 1999 are shown in Table 53-6.

TABLE 53-6. Pregnancy Outcomes in 156 Women Undergoing Dialysis During Pregnancy

Study (Year)	Pregnancies			Pregnancy Outcomes (%)			
	N	Delivery (wk)	Birthweight (g)	Hypertension	Hydramnios	Perinatal Mortality	Surviving Infants
Toma (1999)	54	31.9	1545	35	44	33	67
Chao (2002)	13	32	1540	72	46	31	69
Tan (2006)	11	31	1390	36	18	18	82
Chou (2008)	13	30.8	1510	57	71	50	50
Luders (2010)	52	32.7	1555	67	40	13	87
Shahir (2013)	13	NS	2130	19[a]	14	22	78
Jesudason (2014)	77	33.8	1750	NS	NS	20	80
Approximate averages	233	~32	~1600	~45–5	~44	~20–5	~80

[a]Preeclampsia only.
NS = not stated.

These reports described similar outcomes with either hemodialysis or peritoneal dialysis. Thus, for the woman already undergoing either method, it seems reasonable to continue that method with consideration for its increasing frequency. In the woman who has never been dialyzed, the threshold for initiation during pregnancy is unclear. Lindheimer and colleagues (2007a) recommend initiation when serum creatinine levels are between 5 and 7 mg/dL. Because it is imperative to avoid abrupt volume changes that cause hypotension, dialysis frequency may be extended to five to six times weekly (Reddy, 2007).

Hladunewich and coworkers (2011) recommend attention to certain protocols that include replacement of substances lost through dialysis. Multivitamin doses are doubled, and calcium and iron salts are provided along with sufficient dietary protein and calories. Chronic anemia is treated with erythropoietin. To meet pregnancy changes, extra calcium is added to the dialysate along with less bicarbonate.

Maternal complications are common and include severe hypertension, placental abruption, heart failure, and sepsis. Piccoli and associates (2010b) reviewed reported outcomes in 90 pregnancies in 78 women. They found that these studies were heterogeneous for definitions; types of dialysis, frequency, and prescription; and perinatal outcomes. Although they were encouraged by their findings, they described high incidences of maternal hypertension and anemia, preterm and growth-restricted infants, stillbirths, and hydramnios.

ACUTE KIDNEY INJURY

Previously termed *acute renal failure,* acute kidney injury is now used to describe sudden impairment of kidney function with retention of nitrogenous and other waste products normally excreted by the kidneys (American Society of Nephrology, 2005; Waikar, 2012). Acute kidney injury has become less common today. For example, in a 6-year period the overall incidence at the Mayo Clinic was 0.4 percent (Gurrieri, 2012). Although the incidence of acute kidney injury in pregnancy has decreased substantially, it still occasionally causes significant obstetrical morbidity, and women who require acute dialysis have increased mortality rates (Kuklina, 2009; Singri, 2003). Outcomes are available from four older studies comprising a total of 266 women with renal failure (Drakeley, 2002; Nzerue, 1998; Sibai, 1990; Turney, 1989). Approximately 70 percent had preeclampsia, 50 percent had obstetrical hemorrhage, and 30 percent had a placental abruption. Almost 20 percent required dialysis, and the maternal mortality rate in these was approximately 15 percent.

Obstetrical cases of acute kidney injury that require dialysis have become less common today. That said, acute renal ischemia is still commonly associated with severe preeclampsia and hemorrhage (Gurrieri, 2012). Particularly contributory are HELLP syndrome and placental abruption (Audibert, 1996; Drakely, 2002). Septicemia is another common comorbidity, especially in resource-poor countries (Acharya, 2013; Srinil, 2011; Zeeman, 2003). Acute kidney injury is also common in women with acute fatty liver of pregnancy (Sibai, 2007). Nelson and colleagues (2013) reported some degree of renal insufficiency in virtually all of 52 such women cared for at Parkland Hospital (Chap. 55, p. 1087). Another woman from Parkland Hospital developed acute kidney injury from dehydration caused by severe hyperemesis gravidarum at 15 weeks (Hill, 2002). Her serum creatinine level peaked at 10.7 mg/dL, and she required hemodialysis for 5 days. Other causes that are discussed further in Chapter 56 (p. 1116) include thrombotic microcoagulopathies (Ganesan, 2011).

Diagnosis and Management

In most women, renal failure develops postpartum, thus management is usually not complicated by fetal considerations. An acute increase in serum creatinine is most often due to renal ischemia (Abuelo, 2007). Oliguria is an important sign of acutely impaired renal function. In obstetrical cases, both prerenal and intrarenal factors are commonly operative. For example, with total placental abruption, severe hypovolemia is common from massive hemorrhage, and frequently associated preeclampsia causes preexistent renal ischemia.

When azotemia is evident and severe oliguria persists, some form of renal replacement treatment is indicated, and hemofiltration or dialysis is initiated before marked deterioration occurs. Hemodynamic measurements are normalized. Medication dose adjustments are imperative, and magnesium sulfate is a prominent example (Singri, 2003; Waikar, 2012). Early dialysis appears to reduce the mortality rate appreciably and may enhance the extent of renal function recovery. With time, renal function usually returns to normal or near normal.

Prevention

Acute kidney injury in obstetrics is most often due to acute blood loss, especially that associated with preeclampsia. Thus, it may often be prevented by the following means:

1. Prompt and vigorous volume replacement with crystalloid solutions and blood in instances of massive hemorrhage, such as in placental abruption, placenta previa, uterine rupture, and postpartum uterine atony (Chap. 41, p. 814).
2. Delivery or termination of pregnancies complicated by severe preeclampsia or eclampsia, and careful blood transfusion if loss is more than average (Chap. 40, p. 766).
3. Close observation for early signs of sepsis syndrome and shock in women with pyelonephritis, septic abortion, chorioamnionitis, or sepsis from other pelvic infections (Chap. 47, p. 946).
4. Avoidance of loop diuretics to treat oliguria before ensuring that blood volume and cardiac output are adequate for renal perfusion.
5. Judicious use of vasoconstrictor drugs to treat hypotension, and only after it has been determined that pathological vasodilatation is the cause.

Irreversible ischemic renal failure caused by *acute cortical necrosis* has become exceedingly uncommon in obstetrics. Before widespread availability of dialysis, it complicated a fourth of obstetrical renal failure cases (Grünfeld, 1987; Turney, 1989). Most cases followed placental abruption, preeclampsia-eclampsia, and endotoxin-induced shock. Once common with septic abortion, this is a rare cause in this country today (Lim, 2011; Srinil, 2011). Histologically, the lesion appears to result from thrombosis of segments of the renal vascular system. The lesions may be focal, patchy, confluent, or gross. Clinically, renal cortical necrosis follows the course of acute renal failure, and its differentiation from acute tubular necrosis is not possible during the early phase. The prognosis depends on the extent of the necrosis. Recovery of function is variable, and stable renal insufficiency may result (Lindheimer, 2007a).

Obstructive Renal Failure

Rarely, bilateral ureteral compression by a very large pregnant uterus is greatly exaggerated. Resultant ureteral obstruction in turn, may cause severe oliguria and azotemia. An extreme example is shown in Figure 53-7. Brandes and Fritsche (1991) reviewed 13 cases that were the consequence of a markedly overdistended uterus. They described a woman with twins who developed anuria and a serum creatinine level of 12.2 mg/dL at 34 weeks' gestation. After amniotomy, urine flow resumed at 500 mL/hr and was followed by a rapid decline in serum creatinine levels to normal range. Eckford and Gingell (1991) described 10 women in whom ureteral obstruction was relieved by stenting. The stents were left in place for a mean of 15.5 weeks and removed 4 to 6 weeks postpartum. Sadan and coworkers (1994) reported a similar experience in eight such women who underwent stent placement at a mean of 29 weeks for moderate to severe hydronephrosis. The stents remained in situ for a mean of 9 weeks, during which time renal function remained normal.

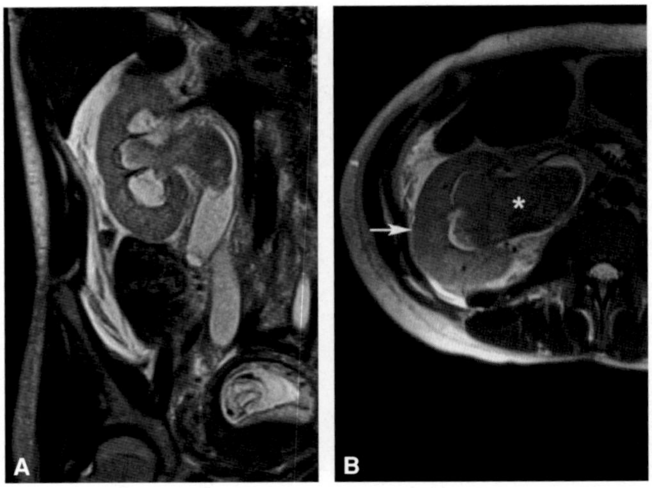

FIGURE 53-7 A. Magnetic resonance image in a coronal plane of a pregnant woman with unilateral hydronephrosis caused by ureteral obstruction. The serum creatinine was 8 mg/dL and decreased to 0.8 mg/dL after a percutaneous nephrostomy tube was placed. **B.** Left kidney (*arrow*) and associated hydronephrosis (*asterisk*) are again noted in this axial plane image.

We have observed this phenomenon on several occasions (Satin, 1993). Partial ureteral obstruction may be accompanied by fluid retention and significant hypertension. When the obstructive uropathy is relieved, diuresis ensues and hypertension dissipates. In one woman with massive hydramnios (9.4 L) and an anencephalic fetus, amniocentesis and removal of some of the amnionic fluid was followed promptly by diuresis, a decline in the plasma creatinine concentration, and improvement of hypertension. In our experience, women with previous urinary tract surgery for reflux are more likely to have such obstructions.

LOWER GENITAL TRACT LESIONS

Urethral Diverticulum

Infrequently complicating pregnancy, this type of diverticulum is thought to originate from an enlarging paraurethral gland abscess that ruptures into the urethral lumen. As infection clears, the remaining dilated diverticular sac and its ostium into the urethra persist. Urine collecting within and dribbling from the sac, pain, palpable mass, and recurrent urinary infections may be associated findings. In general, a diverticulum is managed expectantly during pregnancy. Rarely, drainage may be necessary, or surgery required (Iyer, 2013). If additional antepartum evaluation is needed, MR imaging is preferred for its superior soft tissue resolution and ability to define complex diverticula (Dwarkasing, 2011; Pathi, 2013).

Genital Tract Fistulas

Fistulas found during pregnancy likely existed previously, but in rare cases, they form during pregnancy. In developed countries, *vesicovaginal fistula* following a McDonald cerclage has been reported (Massengill, 2012). These fistulas may also form with prolonged obstructed labor that is more commonly seen in resource-poor countries. In these cases, the genital tract is compressed between the fetal head and bony pelvis. Brief pressure is not significant, but prolonged pressure leads to tissue necrosis with subsequent fistula formation (Wall, 2012). *Vesicouterine fistulas* that developed after prior cesarean delivery have been described (DiMarco, 2012; Manjunatha, 2012). Rarely, *vesicocervical fistula* may follow cesarean delivery or may form if the anterior cervical lip is compressed against the symphysis pubis (Dudderidge, 2005).

REFERENCES

Abboud H, Henrich WL: Stage IV chronic kidney disease. N Engl J Med 362(1):56, 2010

Abe S: An overview of pregnancy in women with underlying renal disease. Am J Kidney Dis 17:112, 1991

Abuelo JG: Normotensive ischemic acute renal failure. N Engl J Med 357:797, 2007

Acharya A, Santos J, Linde B, et al: Acute kidney injury in pregnancy–current status. Adv Chronic Kidney Dis 20:215, 2013

Airoldi J, Weinstein L: Clinical significance of proteinuria in pregnancy. Obstet Gynecol Surv 62(2):117, 2007

Ait Benkaddour Y, Aboulfalah A, Abbassi H: Bladder stone: uncommon cause of mechanical dystocia. Arch Gynecol Obstet 274(5):323, 2006

Al Duraihimh H, Ghamdi G, Moussa D, et al: Outcome of 234 pregnancies in 140 renal transplant recipients from five Middle Eastern countries. Transplantation 85:840, 2008

Alexander GR, Himes JH, Kaufman RB, et al: A United States national reference for fetal growth. Obstet Gynecol 87:163, 1996

Alsuwaida A, Mousa D, Al-Harbi A, et al: Impact of early chronic kidney disease on maternal and fetal outcomes of pregnancy. J Matern Fetal Neonatal Med 24(12):1432, 2011

American Academy of Pediatrics and American College of Obstetricians and Gynecologists: Guidelines for perinatal care, 7th ed. Washington, 2012, p 113

American Society of Nephrology: American Society of Nephrology Renal Research Report. J Am Soc Nephrol 16:1886, 2005

Asplin JR, Coe FL, Favus MJ: Nephrolithiasis. In Longo DL, Fauci AS, Kasper DL, et al (eds): Harrison's Principles of Internal Medicine, 18th ed. New York, McGraw-Hill, 2012, p 2382

Asrat T, Roossin M, Miller EI: Ultrasonographic detection of ureteral jets in normal pregnancy. Am J Obstet Gynecol 178:1194, 1998

Audibert F, Friedman SA, Frangieh AY, et al: Diagnostic criteria for HELLP syndrome: tedious or "helpful"? Am J Obstet Gynecol 174:454, 1996

Banhidy F, Acs N, Puho EH, et al: Pregnancy complications and birth outcomes of pregnant women with urinary tract infections and related drug treatments. Scand J Infect Dis 39:390, 2007

Bargman JM, Shorecki K: Chronic kidney disease. In Longo DL, Fauci AS, Kasper DL, et al (eds): Harrison's Principles of Internal Medicine, 18th ed. New York, McGraw-Hill, 2012, p. 2308

Baylis C: Impact of pregnancy on underlying renal disease. Adv Ren Replace Ther 10:31, 2003

Baylis C, Davison J: The urinary system. In Hytten F, Chamberlain G (eds): Clinical Physiology in Obstetrics, 2nd ed. London, Blackwell, 1991, p 245

Bazari H, Guimaraes AR, Kushner YB: Case 20–2012: A 77-year-old man with leg edema, hematuria, and acute renal failure. N Engl J Med 366(26):2503, 2012

Boggess KA, Benedetti TJ, Raghu G: Nitrofurantoin-induced pulmonary toxicity during pregnancy: a report of a case and review of the literature. Obstet Gynecol Surv 41:367, 1996

Bramham K, Nelson-Piercy C, Gao H, et al: Pregnancy in renal transplant recipients: a UK National Cohort Study. Clin J Am Soc Nephrol 8(2):290, 2013

Bramham K, Soh MC, Nelson-Piercy C: Pregnancy and renal outcomes in lupus nephritis: an update and guide to management. Lupus 21(12):1271, 2012

Brandes JC, Fritsche C: Obstructive acute renal failure by a gravid uterus: a case report and review. Am J Kidney Dis 18:398, 1991

Briggs GG, Freeman RK, Yaffe SJ: Drugs in Pregnancy and Lactation, 8th ed. Philadelphia, Lippincott Williams & Wilkins, 2011

Brosens I, Pijnenborg R, Benagiano G: Risk of obstetrical complications in organ transplant recipient pregnancies. Transplantation 96(3):227, 2013

Brown MA, Holt JL, Mangos GK, et al: Microscopic hematuria in pregnancy: relevance to pregnancy outcome. Am J Kidney Dis 45:667, 2005

Brown MA, Mangos GJ, Peek M: Renal disease in pregnancy. In De Swiet M (ed): Medical Disorders in Obstetric Practice, 4th ed. Oxford, Wiley-Blackwell, 2010, p 182

Butler EL, Cox SM, Eberts E, et al: Symptomatic nephrolithiasis complicating pregnancy. Obstet Gynecol 96:753, 2000

Carpenter CB, Milford EL, Sayegh MH: Transplantation in the treatment of renal failure. In Harrison's Principles of Internal Medicine, 17th ed. New York, McGraw-Hill, 2008, p 1776

Cavenee MR, Cox SM, Mason R, et al: Erythropoietin in pregnancies complicated by pyelonephritis. Obstet Gynecol 84:252, 1994

Chaemsaithong P, Romero R. Korzeniewski SJ, et al: Soluble TRAIL in normal pregnancy and acute pyelonephritis: a potential explanation for the susceptibility of pregnant women to microbial products and infection. J Matern Fetal Neonatal Med 26(16):1568, 2013

Chao AS, Huang JY, Lien R, et al: Pregnancy in women who undergo long-term hemodialysis. Am J Obstet Gynecol 187(1):152, 2002

Chapman AB: Cystic disease in women: clinical characteristics and medical management. Adv Ren Replace Ther 10:24, 2003

Chapman AB, Johnson AM, Gabow PA: Pregnancy outcome and its relationship to progression of renal failure in autosomal dominant polycystic kidney disease. J Am Soc Nephrol 5:1178, 1994

Chen HH, Lin HC, Yeh JC, et al: Renal biopsy in pregnancies complicated by undetermined renal disease. Acta Obstet Gynecol Scand 80:888, 2001

Chou CY, Ting IW, Lin TH, et al: Pregnancy in patients on chronic dialysis: a single center experience and combined analysis of reported results. Eur J Obstet Gynecol Reprod Biol 136:165, 2008

Chung SD, Chen YH, Keller JJ, et al: Urinary calculi increased the risk for adverse pregnancy outcomes: a nationwide study. Acta Obstet Gynecol Scand 921:69, 2013

Coscia LA, Constantinescu S, Moritz MJ, et al: Report from the National Transplantation Pregnancy Registry (NTPR): outcomes of pregnancy after transplantation. Clin Transpl 65, 2010

Cox SM, Cunningham FG: Acute focal pyelonephritis (lobar nephronia) complicating pregnancy. Obstet Gynecol 71:510, 1988

Cox SM, Shelburne P, Mason R, et al: Mechanisms of hemolysis and anemia associated with acute antepartum pyelonephritis. Am J Obstet Gynecol 164:587, 1991

Cruz Lemini MC, Ibarguengoitia Ochoa F, Villanueva Gonzalez MA: Perinatal outcome following renal transplantation. Int J Gynaecol Obstet 95:76, 2007

Cunningham FG, Cox SM, Harstad TW, et al: Chronic renal disease and pregnancy outcome. Am J Obstet Gynecol 163:453, 1990

Cunningham FG, Lucas MJ, Hankins GCV: Pulmonary injury complicating antepartum pyelonephritis. Am J Obstet Gynecol 156:797, 1987

Cunningham FG, Morris GB, Mickal A: Acute pyelonephritis of pregnancy: a clinical review. Obstet Gynecol 42:112, 1973

Czaja CA, Rutledge BN, Cleary PA, et al: Urinary tract infections in women with type 1 diabetes mellitus: survey of female participants in the epidemiology of diabetes interventions and complications study cohort. J Urol 181(3):1129, 2009

Davison JM, Lindheimer MD: Pregnancy and chronic kidney disease. Semin Nephrol 31(1):86, 2011

Diamond DA, Mattoo TK: Endoscopic treatment of primary vesicoureteral reflux. N Engl J Med 366(13):1218, 2012

DiMarco CS, DiMarco DS, Klingele CJ, et al: Vesicouterine fistula: a review of eight cases. Int Urogynecol J Pelvic Floor Dysfunct 17(4):395, 2006

Donadio JV, Grande JP: IgA nephropathy. N Engl J Med 347:738, 2002

Drakeley AJ, Le Roux PA, Anthony J, et al: Acute renal failure complicating severe preeclampsia requiring admission to an obstetric intensive care unit. Am J Obstet Gynecol 186:253, 2002

Dudderidge TJ, Haynes SV, Davies AJ, et al: Vesicocervical fistula: rare complication of cesarean section demonstrated by magnetic resonance imaging. 65(1):174, 2005

Dwarkasing RS, Dinkelaar W, Hop WC, et al: MRI evaluation of urethral diverticula and differential diagnosis in symptomatic women. AJR 197(3):676, 2011

Eckford SD, Gingell JC: Ureteric obstruction in pregnancy—diagnosis and management. Br J Obstet Gynaecol 98:1137, 1991

El-Khatib M, Packham DK, Becker GJ, et al: Pregnancy-related complications in women with reflux nephropathy. Clin Nephrol 41:50, 1994

Fakhoury GF, Daikoku NH, Parikh AR: Management of severe hemorrhagic cystitis in pregnancy: a report of two cases. J Reprod Med 39:485, 1994

Farwell J, Emerson J, Wyatt S, et al: Outcomes of pregnancies complicated by chronic kidney disease. Abstract No. 346, Am J Obstet Gynecol 208 (1 Suppl):S153, 2013

Faúndes A, Bricola-Filho M, Pinto e Silva JC: Dilatation of the urinary tract during pregnancy: proposal of a curve of maximal caliceal diameter by gestational age. Am J Obstet Gynecol 178:1082, 1998

Fihn SD: Acute uncomplicated urinary tract infection in women. N Engl J Med 349:259, 2003

Fischer MJ, Lehnerz SD, Hebert JR, et al: Kidney disease is an independent risk factor for adverse fetal and maternal outcomes in pregnancy. Am J Kidney Dis 43:415, 2004

Foxman B: The epidemiology of urinary tract infection. Nat Rev Urol 7(12):653, 2010

French VA, Davis, JB, Savies HS, et al: Contraception and fertility awareness among women with solid organ transplants. Obstet Gynecol 122:809, 2013

Ganesan C, Maynard SE: Acute kidney injury in pregnancy: the thrombotic microangiopathies. J Nephrol 24(5):554, 2011

Gazmararian JA, Petersen R, Jamieson DJ, et al: Hospitalizations during pregnancy among managed care enrollees. Obstet Gynecol 100:94, 2002

Ghafari A, Sanadgol H: Pregnancy after renal transplantation: ten-year single-center experience. Transplant Proc 40:251, 2008

Gilstrap LC III, Cunningham FG, Whalley PJ: Acute pyelonephritis in pregnancy: an anterospective study. Obstet Gynecol 57:409, 1981a

Gilstrap LC III, Leveno KJ, Cunningham FG, et al: Renal infection and pregnancy outcome. Am J Obstet Gynecol 141:708, 1981b

Gizzo S, Noventa M, Saccardi C, et al: Twin pregnancy after kidney transplantation: what's on? A case report and review of the literature. J Matern Fetal Neonatal Med February 3, 2014 [Epub ahead of print]

Goes NB, Calvin RB: Case 12–2007: A 56-year-old woman with renal failure after heart–lung transplantation. N Engl J Med 356:1657, 2007

Graham JM, Oshiro BT, Blanco JD, et al: Uterine contractions after antibiotic therapy for pyelonephritis in pregnancy. Am J Obstet Gynecol 168:577, 1993

Grünfeld JP, Pertuiset N: Acute renal failure in pregnancy: 1987. Am J Kidney Dis 9:359, 1987

Gurrieri C, Garovic VD, Gullo A, et al: Kidney injury during pregnancy: associated comorbid conditions and outcomes. Arch Gynecol Obstet 286(3):567, 2012

Gutierrez MJ, Acebedo-Ribo M, Garcia-Donaire JA, et al: Pregnancy in renal transplant recipients. Transplant Proc 37:3721, 2005

Harris RE, Gilstrap LC III: Cystitis during pregnancy: a distinct clinical entity. Obstet Gynecol 57:578, 1981

Helal I, Fick-Brosnahan GM, Reed-Gitomer B, et al: Glomerular hyperfiltration: definitions, mechanisms, and clinical implications. Nat Rev Nephrol 8:293, 2012

Hendricks SK, Ross SO, Krieger JN: An algorithm for diagnosis and therapy of management and complications of urolithiasis during pregnancy. Surg Gynecol Obstet 172:49, 1991

Higby K, Suiter CR, Phelps JY, et al: Normal values of urinary albumin and total protein excretion during pregnancy. Am J Obstet Gynecol 171:984, 1994

Hildebrandt F, Benzing T, Katsanis N: Ciliopathies. N Engl J Med 364(16):1533, 2011

Hill JB, Sheffield JS, McIntire DD, et al: Acute pyelonephritis in pregnancy. Obstet Gynecol 105:38, 2005

Hill JB, Yost NP, Wendel GD Jr: Acute renal failure in association with severe hyperemesis gravidarum. Obstet Gynecol 100:1119, 2002

Hladunewich M, Herca AE, Keunen J, et al: Pregnancy in end stage renal disease. Semin Dial 24(6):634, 2011

Hladunewich MA, Lafayette RA, Derby GC, et al: The dynamics of glomerular filtration in the puerperium. Am J Physiol Renal Physiol 286:F496, 2004

Hooton TM: Uncomplicated urinary tract infection. N Engl J Med 366(11):1028, 2012

Hooton TM, Scholes D, Stapleton AE, et al: A prospective study of asymptomatic bacteriuria in sexually active young women. N Engl J Med 343:992, 2000

Hussein W, Lafayette RA: Renal function in normal and disordered pregnancy. Curr Opin Nephrol Hypertens 23:46, 2014

Ibrahim HN, Foley R, Tan L, et al: Long-term consequences of kidney donation. N Engl J Med 360:459, 2009

Imbasciati E, Gregorini G, Cabiddu G, et al: Pregnancy in CKD stages 3 to 5: fetal and maternal outcomes. Am J Kidney Dis 49:753, 2007

Iyer S, Minassian VA: Resection of urethral diverticulum in pregnancy. Obstet Gynecol 122(2 Pt 2):467, 2013

Jacobsson B, Hagberg G, Hagberg B, et al: Cerebral palsy in preterm infants: a population-based case-control study of antenatal and intrapartal risk factors. Acta Paediatr 91:946, 2002

Jain AB, Shapiro R, Scantlebury VP, et al: Pregnancy after kidney and kidney-pancreas transplantation under tacrolimus: a single center's experience. Transplantation 77:897, 2004

Jakobi P, Friedman M, Goldstein I, et al: Massive vulvar edema in pregnancy: a case report. J Reprod Med 40:479, 1995

Jesudason S, Grace BS, McDonald SP: Pregnancy outcomes according to dialysis commencing before or after contraception in women with ESRD. Clin J Am Soc Nephrol 9:143, 2014

Jolley JA, Kim S, Wing DA: Acute pyelonephritis and associated complications during pregnancy in 2006 in US hospitals. J Matern Fetal Neonatal Med 25(12):2494, 2012

Johnson EB, Krambeck AE, White WM, et al: Obstetric complications of ureteroscopy during pregnancy. J Urol 188(1):151, 2012

Jones DC, Hayslett JP: Outcome of pregnancy in women with moderate or severe renal insufficiency. N Engl J Med 335:226, 1996

Josephson MA, McKay DB: Pregnancy and kidney transplantation. Semin Nephrol 31(1):100, 2011

Jungers P, Houillier P, Chauveau D, et al: Pregnancy in women with reflux nephropathy. Kidney Int 50:593, 1996

Jungers P, Houillier P, Forget D, et al: Influence of pregnancy on the course of primary chronic glomerulonephritis. Lancet 346:1122, 1995

Kass EH: Pyelonephritis and bacteriuria. Ann Intern Med 56:46, 1962

Köhler JR, Tencer J, Thysell H, et al: Long-term effects of reflux nephropathy on blood pressure and renal function in adults. Nephron Clin Pract 93:c35, 2003

Kuklina EV, Meikle SF, Jamieson DJ, et al: Severe obstetric morbidity in the United States: 1998–2005. Obstet Gynecol 113:293, 2009

Lamont RF: The pathophysiology of pulmonary edema with the use of beta-agonists. Br J Obstet Gynaecol 107:439, 2000

Lessan-Pezeshki M, Ghazizadeh S, Khatami MR, et al: Fertility and contraceptive issues after kidney transplantation in women. Transplant Proc 36:1405, 2004

Lewis DF, Robichaux AG III, Jaekle RK, et al: Urolithiasis in pregnancy: diagnosis, management and pregnancy outcome. J Reprod Med 48:28, 2003

Lewis JB, Neilsen EG: Glomerular diseases. In Harrison's Principles of Internal Medicine, 18th ed. New York, McGraw-Hill, 2012, p 2334

Lim LM, Tsai KB, Hwang DY, et al: Anuric acute renal failure after elective abortion. Inter Med 50(16):1715, 2011

Lindheimer MD, Conrad KP, Karumanchi SA: Renal physiology and diseases in pregnancy. In Alpern R, Hebert S (eds): Seldin and Giebisch's The Kidney, Elsevier, 2007a, p 2339

Lindheimer MD, Davison JM: Pregnancy and CKD: Any progress? Am J Kidney Dis 49:729, 2007b

Lindheimer MD, Grünfeld JP, Davison JM: Renal disorders. In Barron WM, Lindheimer MD (eds): Medical Disorders During Pregnancy, 3rd ed. St. Louis, Mosby, 2000, p 39

Lucas MJ, Cunningham FG: Urinary infection in pregnancy. Clin Obstet Gynecol 36:855, 1993

Lucas MJ, Cunningham FG: Urinary tract infections complicating pregnancy. Williams Obstetrics, 19th ed. (Suppl 5). Norwalk, Appleton & Lange, February/March 1994

Luders C, Martins MC, Titak SM, et al: Obstetric outcome in pregnancy women on long-term dialysis: a case series. Am J Kidney Dis 56(1):77, 2010

Lumbiganon P, Villar J, Laopaiboon M, et al: One-day compared with 7-day nitrofurantoin for asymptomatic bacteriuria in pregnancy. Obstet Gynecol 113:339, 2009

Maikranz P, Coe FL, Parks J, et al: Nephrolithiasis in pregnancy. Am J Kidney Dis 9:354, 1987

Manjunatha YC, Sonwalkar P: Spontaneous antepartum vesicouterine fistula causing severe oligohydramnios in a patient with a previous cesarean delivery. J Ultrasound Med 31(8):1294, 2012

Maruotti GM, Sarno L, Napolitano R, et al: Preeclampsia in women with chronic kidney disease. J Matern Fetal Neonatal Med 25(8):1367, 2012

Masselli G, Derme M, Laghi F, et al: Imaging of stone disease in pregnancy. Abdom Imaging 38(6):1409, 2013

Massengill JC, Baker TM, Von Pechmann WS, et al: Commonalities of cerclage-related genitourinary fistulas. Female Pelvic Med Reconstr Surg 18(6):362, 2012

McAleer SJ, Loughlin KR: Nephrolithiasis and pregnancy. Curr Opin Urol 14:123, 2004

McDonnold M, Friedman A, Raker C, et al: Is postpartum pyelonephritis associated with the same maternal morbidity as antepartum pyelonephritis? J Matern Fetal Neonatal Med 25(9):1709, 2012

Mignini L, Carroli G, Abalos E, et al: Accuracy of diagnostic tests to detect asymptomatic bacteriuria during pregnancy. Obstet Gynecol 113(1):346, 2009

Millar LK, DeBuque L, Wing DA: Uterine contraction frequency during treatment of pyelonephritis in pregnancy and subsequent risk of preterm birth. J Perinat Med 31:41, 2003

Mor Y, Leibovitch I, Zalts R, et al: Analysis of the long-term outcome of surgically corrected vesicoureteric reflux. BJU Int 92:97, 2003

Moretti ME, Sgro M, Johnson DW, et al: Cyclosporine excretion into breast milk. Transplantation 75:2144, 2003

National High Blood Pressure Education Program Working Group on High Blood Pressure in Pregnancy: Report of the National High Blood Pressure Education Program Working Group on High Blood Pressure in Pregnancy. Am J Obstet Gynecol 183:S1, 2000

Nelson DB, Yost NP, Cunningham FG: Acute fatty liver of pregnancy: clinical outcomes and expected durations of recovery. Am J Obstet Gynecol 209(5):456.e1, 2013

Nevis IF, Reitsma A, Dominic A, et al: Pregnancy outcomes in women with chronic kidney disease: a systematic review. Clin J Am Soc Nephrol 6:2587, 2011

Nzerue CM, Hewan-Lowe K, Nwawka C: Acute renal failure in pregnancy: a review of clinical outcomes at an inner city hospital from 1986–1996. J Natl Med Assoc 90:486, 1998

Organ Procurement and Transplantation Network. Data. 2013. Available at: http://optn.transplant.hrsa.gov/data. Accessed August 24, 2013

Packham DK, North RA, Fairley KF, et al: Primary glomerulonephritis and pregnancy. Q J Med 71:537, 1989

Pathi SD, Rahn DD, Sailors JL, et al: Utility of clinical parameters, cystourethroscopy, and magnetic resonance imaging in the preoperative diagnosis of urethral diverticula. Int Urogynecol J 24(2):319, 2013

Piccoli GB, Attini R, Vasario E, et al: Pregnancy and chronic kidney disease: a challenge in all CKD stages. Clin J Am Soc Nephrol 5:844, 2010a

Piccoli GB, Conijn A, Attini R, et al: Pregnancy in chronic kidney disease: need for a common language. J Nephrol 24(03)282, 2011

Piccoli GB, Conijn A, Consiglio V, et al: Pregnancy in dialysis patients: is the evidence strong enough to lead us to change our counseling policy? Clin J Am Soc Nephrol 5:62, 2010b

Piccoli GB, Daidola G, Attini R, et al: Kidney biopsy in pregnancy: evidence for counseling? A systematic narrative review. BJOG 120(4):412, 2013

Putra LGJ, Minor TX, Bolton DM, et al: Improved assessment of renal lesions in pregnancy with magnetic resonance imaging. Urology 74:535, 2009

Rafi J, Smith RB: Acute lobar nephronia in pregnancy: a rarely reported entity in obstetric renal medicine. Arch Gynecol Obstet 286(3):797, 2012

Ramin SM, Vidaeff AC, Yeomans ER, et al: Chronic renal disease in pregnancy. Obstet Gynecol 108(6):1531, 2006

Raz R, Sakran W, Chazan B, et al: Long-term follow-up of women hospitalized for acute pyelonephritis. Clin Infect Dis 37:1014, 2003

Reddy SS, Holley JL: Management of the pregnant chronic dialysis patient. Adv Chronic Kidney Dis 14:146, 2007

Rocha A, Cardoso A, Malheiro J, et al: Pregnancy after kidney transplantation: graft, mother, and newborn complications. Transplant Proc 45(3):1088, 2013

Rodriguez PN, Klein AS: Management of urolithiasis during pregnancy. Surg Gynecol Obstet 166:103, 1988

Ronkainen J, Ala-Houhala M, Autio-Harmainen H, et al: Long-term outcome 19 years after childhood IgA nephritis: a retrospective cohort study. Pediatr Nephrol 21:1266, 2006

Rosenberg E, Sergienko R, Abu-Ghanem S: Nephrolithiasis during pregnancy: characteristics, complications, and pregnancy outcome. World J Urol 29(6):743, 2011

Ross AE, Handa S, Lingeman JE, et al: Kidney stones during pregnancy: an investigation into stone composition. Urol Res 36:99, 2008

Rouse DJ, Andrews WW, Goldenberg RL, et al: Screening and treatment of asymptomatic bacteriuria of pregnancy to prevent pyelonephritis. A cost-effectiveness and cost benefit analysis. Obstet Gynecol 86:119, 1995

Ruan JM, Adams SR, Carpinito G, et al: Bladder calculus presenting as recurrent urinary tract infections: a late complication of cervical cerclage placement: a case report. J Reprod Med 56(3–4):172, 2011

Ruggenenti P, Schieppati A, Remuzzi G: Progression, remission, regression of chronic renal diseases. Lancet 357:1601, 2001

Sadan O, Berar M, Sagiv R, et al: Ureteric stent in severe hydronephrosis of pregnancy. Eur J Obstet Gynecol Reprod Biol 56:79, 1994

Salant DJ, Patel PS: Polycystic kidney disease and other inherited tubular disorders. In Harrison's Principles of Internal Medicine, 18th ed. New York, McGraw-Hill, 2012, p 2355

Sanchez-Ramos L, McAlpine KJ, Adair CD, et al: Pyelonephritis in pregnancy: once a day ceftriaxone versus multiple doses of cefazolin. A randomized double-blind trial. Am J Obstet Gynecol 172:129, 1995

Satin AJ, Seiken GL, Cunningham FG: Reversible hypertension in pregnancy caused by obstructive uropathy. Obstet Gynecol 81:823, 1993

Schieve LA, Handler A, Hershow R, et al: Urinary tract infection during pregnancy: its association with maternal morbidity and perinatal outcome. Am J Public Health 84:405, 1994

Schneeberger C, Geerlings SE, Middleton P, et al: Interventions for preventing recurrent urinary tract infection during pregnancy. Cochrane Database Syst Rev 11:CD009279, 2012

Schneeberger C, Kazemier BM, Geerlins SE: Asymptomatic bacteriuria and urinary tract infections in special patient groups: women with diabetes mellitus and pregnant women. Curr Opin Infect Dis 27:106, 2014

Seidman DS, Soriano D, Dulitzki M, et al: Role of renal ultrasonography in the management of pyelonephritis in pregnant women. J Perinatol 18:98, 1998

Semins MJ, Matlaga BR: Management of stone disease in pregnancy. Curr Opin Urol 20(2):174, 2010

Semins MJ, Matlaga BR: Management of urolithiasis in pregnancy. Int J Womens Health 5:590, 2013

Semins MJ, Trock BJ, Matlaga BR: The safety of ureteroscopy during pregnancy: a systematic review and meta-analysis. J Urol 181(1):139, 2009

Sethi S, Fervenza FC: Membranoproliferative glomerulonephritis—a new look at an old entity. N Engl J Med 366(12):1119, 2012

Shahir AK, Briggs N, Katsoulis J, et al: An observational outcomes study from 1966–2008, examining pregnancy and neonatal outcomes from dialysed women using data from the ANZDATA Registry. Nephrology 18(4):276, 2013

Sheffield JS, Cunningham FG: Urinary tract infection in women. Obstet Gynecol 106:1085, 2005

Sibai BM: Imitators of severe preeclampsia. Obstet Gynecol 109:956, 2007

Sibai BM, Villar MA, Mabie BC: Acute renal failure in hypertensive disorders of pregnancy. Pregnancy outcome and remote prognosis in thirty-one consecutive cases. Am J Obstet Gynecol 162(3):777, 1990

Singri N, Ahya SN, Levin ML: Acute renal failure. JAMA 289:747, 2003

Sledzińska A, Mielech A, Krawczyk B, et al: Fatal sepsis in a pregnant woman with pyelonephritis caused by *Escherichia coli* bearing Dr and P adhesions: diagnosis based on postmortem strain genotyping. BJOG 118(2):266, 2011

Snyder CC, Barton JR, Habli M, et al: Severe sepsis and septic shock in pregnancy: indications for delivery and maternal and perinatal outcomes. J Matern Fetal Neonatal Med 26(5):503, 2013

Spencer JA, Chahal R, Kelly A, et al: Evaluation of painful hydronephrosis in pregnancy: magnetic resonance urographic patterns in physiological dilatation versus calculous obstruction. J Urol 171:256, 2004

Spurbeck RR, Stapleton AE, Johnson JR, et al: Fimbrial profiles predict virulence of uropathogenic *Escherichia coli* strains: contribution of ygi and yad fimbriae. Infect Immun 79(12):4753, 2011

Srinil S, Panaput T: Acute kidney injury complicating septic unsafe abortion: clinical course and treatment outcomes of 44 cases. J Obstet Gynaecol Res 37(11):1525, 2011

Stehman-Breen CO, Levine RJ, Qian C, et al: Increased risk of preeclampsia among nulliparous pregnant women with idiopathic hematuria. Am J Obstet Gynecol 187:703, 2002

Stettler RW, Cunningham FG: Natural history of chronic proteinuria complicating pregnancy. Am J Obstet Gynecol 167:1219, 1992

Stratta P, Canavese C, Quaglia M: Pregnancy in patients with kidney disease. Nephrol 19:135, 2006

Strevens H, Wide-Swensson D, Hansen A, et al: Glomerular endotheliosis in normal pregnancy and pre-eclampsia. Br J Obstet Gynaecol 110:831, 2003

Sturgiss SN, Davison JM: Effect of pregnancy on long-term function of renal allografts. Am J Kidney Dis 26:54, 1995

Surian M, Imbasciati E, Cosci P, et al: Glomerular disease and pregnancy: a study of 123 pregnancies in patients with primary and secondary glomerular diseases. Nephron 36:101, 1984

Swartz MA, Lydon-Rochelle MT, Simon D, et al: Admission for nephrolithiasis in pregnancy and risk of adverse birth outcomes. Obstet Gynecol 109(5):1099, 2007

Tan LK, Kanagalingam D, Tan HK, et al: Obstetric outcomes in women with end-stage renal failure requiring renal dialysis. Int J Gynaecol Obstet 94:17, 2006

Tan YK, Cha DY, Gupta M: Management of stones in abnormal situations. Urol Clin North Am 0(1):79, 2013

Thomas AG, Burrows L, Knight R, et al: The effect of pregnancy on cyclosporine levels in renal allograft patients. Obstet Gynecol 90:916, 1997

Toma H, Tanabe K, Tokumoto T, et al: Pregnancy in women receiving renal dialysis or transplantation in Japan: a nationwide survey. Nephrol Dial Transplant 14(6):1511, 1999

Toth C, Toth G, Varga A, et al: Percutaneous nephrolithotomy in early pregnancy. Int Urol Nephrol 37:1, 2005

Towers CV, Kaminskas CM, Garite TJ, et al: Pulmonary injury associated with antepartum pyelonephritis: can patients at risk be identified? Am J Obstet Gynecol 164:974, 1991
Trevisan G, Ramos JG, Martins-Costa S, et al: Pregnancy in patients with chronic renal insufficiency at Hospital de Clinicas of Porto Alegre, Brazil. Ren Fail 26:29, 2004
Turney JH, Ellis CM, Parsons FM: Obstetric acute renal failure 1956–1987. Br J Obstet Gynaecol 96:679, 1989
Twickler DM, Lucas MJ, Bowe L, et al: Ultrasonographic evaluation of central and end-organ hemodynamics in antepartum pyelonephritis. Am J Obstet Gynecol 170:814, 1994
U.S. Preventive Services Task Force. Screening for asymptomatic bacteriuria in adults. Reaffirmation recommendation statement. 2008. Available at: http://www.uspreventiveservicestaskforce.org/uspstf08/asymptbact/asbactrs.htm. Accessed August 25, 2013
Van Dorsten JP, Lenke RR, Schifrin BS: Pyelonephritis in pregnancy: the role of in-hospital management and nitrofurantoin suppression. J Reprod Med 32:897, 1987
Vasilou DM, Maxwell C, Prakesykumar S, et al: Goodpasture syndrome in a pregnant woman. Obstet Gynecol 106:1196, 2005
Vasquez JC, Abalos E: Treatments for symptomatic urinary tract infections during pregnancy. Cochrane Database Syst Rev 19(1): CD002256, 2011
Waikar SS, Bonventure JV: Acute kidney injury. In Harrison's Principles of Internal Medicine, 18th ed. New York, McGraw-Hill, 2012, p 2293
Wall LL: Preventing obstetric fistulas in low-resource countries: insights from a Haddon matrix. Obstet Gynecol Surv 67(2):111, 2012
Watterson JD, Girvan AR, Beiko DT, et al: Management strategy for ureteral calculi in pregnancy. Urology 60:383, 2002
Whalley PJ: Bacteriuria of pregnancy. Am J Obstet Gynecol 97:723, 1967
White WM, Zite NB, Gash J, et al: Low-dose computed tomography for the evaluation of flank pain in the pregnant population. J Endourol 21(11):1255, 2007
Wing DA, Hendershott CM, Debuque L, et al: A randomized trial of three antibiotic regimens for the treatment of pyelonephritis in pregnancy. Am J Obstet Gynecol 92:249, 1998
Wing DA, Hendershott CM, Debuque L, et al: Outpatient treatment of acute pyelonephritis in pregnancy after 24 weeks. Obstet Gynecol 94:683, 1999
Wing DA, Park AS, DeBuque L, et al: Limited clinical utility of blood and urine cultures in the treatment of acute pyelonephritis during pregnancy. Am J Obstet Gynecol 182:1437, 2000
Worcester EM, Coe FL: Calcium kidney stones. N Engl J Med 363(10):954, 2010
Wyld ML, Clayton PA, Jesudason S, et al: Pregnancy outcomes for kidney transplant recipients. Am J Transplant 13:3173, 2013
Wyatt RJ, Julian BA: IgA nephropathy. N Engl J Med 368(25):2402, 2013
Zeeman GG, Cunningham FG, Pritchard JA: The magnitude of hemoconcentration with eclampsia. Hypertens Pregnancy 28:127, 2009
Zeeman GG, Wendel GD Jr, Cunningham FG: A blueprint for obstetric critical care. Am J Obstet Gynecol 188:532, 2003
Zhao C, Zhao J, Huang Y, et al: New-onset systemic lupus erythematosus during pregnancy. Clin Rheumatol 32(6):815, 2013

CHAPTER 54

Gastrointestinal Disorders

During normal pregnancy, the gastrointestinal tract and its appendages undergo remarkable anatomical, physiological, and functional changes. These changes, which are discussed in detail in Chapter 4 (p. 66), can appreciably alter clinical findings normally relied on for diagnosis and treatment of gastrointestinal disorders. Moreover, as pregnancy progresses, gastrointestinal symptoms become more difficult to assess. Physical findings are often obscured by a large uterus that displaces abdominal organs and can alter the location and intensity of pain and tenderness.

GENERAL CONSIDERATIONS

Diagnostic Techniques

Endoscopy

Various methods can evaluate the gastrointestinal tract during pregnancy without reliance on x-ray techniques. Fiberoptic endoscopic instruments have revolutionized diagnosis and management of most gastrointestinal conditions, and these are particularly well suited for pregnancy. With endoscopy, the esophagus, stomach, duodenum, and colon can be inspected (Cappell, 2006, 2011). The proximal jejunum can also be studied, and the ampulla of Vater cannulated to perform *endoscopic retrograde cholangiopancreatography—ERCP* (Fogel, 2014; Kamani, 2012; Tang, 2009). Experience in pregnancy with *videocapsule endoscopy* for small-bowel evaluation is limited (Storch, 2006).

Upper gastrointestinal endoscopy is used for management as well as diagnosis of several problems. Common bile duct exploration and drainage are used for choledocholithiasis as described in Chapter 55 (p. 1096). It is also used for sclerotherapy as well as placement of *percutaneous endoscopic gastrostomy (PEG)* tubes. A number of concise reviews have been provided (Cappell, 2011; Fogel, 2014; Gilinsky, 2006).

Flexible sigmoidoscopy can be used safely in pregnant women (Siddiqui, 2006). In nonpregnant patients, *colonoscopy* is indispensible for viewing the entire colon and distal ileum for diagnosis and management of inflammatory bowel disease. Except for the midtrimester, reports of colonoscopy during pregnancy are limited, but preliminary results indicate that it should be performed if indicated (Cappell, 2010, 2011). Bowel preparation is completed using polyethylene glycol electrolyte or sodium phosphate solutions. With these, serious maternal dehydration that may cause diminished uteroplacental perfusion should be avoided.

Noninvasive Imaging Techniques

The obvious ideal technique for gastrointestinal evaluation during pregnancy is abdominal sonography. Because computed tomography (CT) use is limited in pregnancy due to radiation exposure, magnetic resonance (MR) imaging is now commonly used to evaluate the abdomen and retroperitoneal space (Khandelwal, 2013). One example is magnetic-resonance cholangiopancreatography—MRCP (Oto, 2009). These and other imaging modalities, and their safe use in pregnancy, are considered in more detail in Chapter 46 (p. 933).

Laparotomy and Laparoscopy

Surgery is lifesaving for certain gastrointestinal conditions—perforative appendicitis being the most common example. From the Swedish Registry database through 1981, abdominal exploration by laparotomy or laparoscopy was performed in 1331 of 720,000 pregnancies—approximately 1 in every 500 (Mazze, 1989). A similar incidence of 1 in 635 in nearly 50,000 pregnancies was described by Kort (1993). In both studies, the most common indications for surgery were appendicitis, an adnexal mass, and cholecystitis.

Laparoscopic procedures have replaced traditional surgical techniques for many abdominal disorders during pregnancy (Carter, 2004). In an updated report from the Swedish Registry database, there were 2181 pregnant women who underwent laparoscopy and 1522 who had laparotomy for nonobstetrical indications (Reedy, 1997). Use of these procedures was similar to their first study—approximately 1 in every 800 pregnancies. Both approaches were used usually before 20 weeks, and they were found to be safe. Long-term surveillance studies also suggest no deleterious effects for mother or fetus (Rizzo, 2003).

The most common nongynecological laparoscopic procedures performed during pregnancy are cholecystectomy and appendectomy (Fatum, 2001; Rollins, 2004). For more details and for descriptions of surgical technique, see Chapter 46 (p. 928) as well as *Operative Obstetrics*, 2nd edition (Gilstrap, 2002). Guidelines for diagnosis, treatment, and use of laparoscopy for surgical problems during pregnancy have been provided by the Society of American Gastrointestinal and Endoscopic Surgeons (Pearl, 2011).

Nutritional Support

Specialized nutritional support can be delivered *enterally*, usually via nasogastric tube feedings, or *parenterally* with nutrition given by venous catheter access, either peripherally or centrally.

When possible, enteral alimentation is preferable because it has fewer serious complications (Bistrian, 2012; Hamaoui, 2003). In obstetrical patients, very few conditions prohibit enteral nutrition as a first effort to prevent catabolism. Even in extreme cases, such as recalcitrant hyperemesis gravidarum, percutaneous endoscopic gastrostomy with a jejunal port—PEG (J) tube—has been described (Saha, 2009).

The purpose of *parenteral feeding*, or *hyperalimentation*, is to provide nutrition when the intestinal tract must be kept quiescent. Central venous access is necessary for total parenteral nutrition because its hyperosmolarity requires rapid dilution in a high-flow vascular system. These solutions provide 24 to 40 kcal/kg/day, principally as a hypertonic glucose solution.

There have been a variety of conditions for which total parenteral nutrition has been employed during pregnancy (Table 54-1). Gastrointestinal disorders are the most common indication, and in the many studies cited, feeding duration averaged 33 days. It is imperative to emphasize that complications of parenteral nutrition are frequent, and they may be severe (Guglielmi, 2006). In an early report of 26 pregnancies, a 50-percent rate of complications, which included pneumothorax, hemothorax, and brachial plexus injury, was described (Russo-Stieglitz, 1999).

TABLE 54-1. Some Conditions Treated with Enteral or Parenteral Nutrition During Pregnancy[a]

Achalasia
Anorexia nervosa
Appendiceal rupture
Bowel obstruction
Burns
Cholecystitis
Crohn disease
Diabetic gastropathy
Esophageal injury
Hyperemesis gravidarum
Jejunoileal bypass
Malignancies
Pancreatitis
Preeclampsia syndrome
Preterm labor/ruptured membranes
Short gut syndrome
Stroke

[a]Risk are listed alphabetically.
From Folk, 2004; Guglielmi, 2006; Ogura, 2003; Russo-Stieglitz, 1999; Saha, 2009; Spiliopoulos, 2013.

The most frequent serious complication is catheter sepsis, and Folk (2004) reported a 25-percent incidence in 27 women with hyperemesis gravidarum. Although bacterial sepsis is most common, *Candida* septicemia has been described (Paranyuk, 2006). The Centers for Disease Control and Prevention (2002) has published detailed guidelines to prevent catheter-related sepsis, and these have served to lessen the dangers of serious infections. Perinatal complications are uncommon, however, fetal subdural hematoma caused by maternal vitamin K deficiency has been described (Sakai, 2003).

There is also appreciable morbidity from long-term use of a *peripherally inserted central catheter (PICC)*. Ogura (2003) reported infection with long-term access in 31 of 52 pregnant women. Holmgren (2008) reported complications in 21 of 33 women in whom a PICC line was placed for hyperemesis. Infections were the most common, and half of infected women also had bacteremia. From a review of 48 reports of nonpregnant adults, Turcotte and associates (2006) concluded that there were no advantages to peripherally placed catheters compared with centrally placed ones. Still, it seems reasonable for short-term nutrition—weeks— that PICC placement has a greater benefit-versus-risk ratio (Bistrian, 2012).

DISORDERS OF THE UPPER GASTROINTESTINAL TRACT

Hyperemesis Gravidarum

Mild to moderate nausea and vomiting are especially common in pregnant women until approximately 16 weeks (Chap. 9,

p. 187). In a small proportion of these, however, it is severe and unresponsive to simple dietary modification and antiemetics. In an attempt to quantify nausea and vomiting severity, Lacasse and colleagues (2008) have proposed a *pregnancy-unique quantification of emesis and nausea (PUQE) scoring index.* Severe unrelenting nausea and vomiting—hyperemesis gravidarum—is defined variably as being sufficiently severe to produce weight loss, dehydration, ketosis, alkalosis from loss of hydrochloric acid, and hypokalemia. Acidosis develops from partial starvation. In some women, transient hepatic dysfunction develops, and there is accumulation of biliary sludge (Matsubara, 2012). Other causes should be considered because hyperemesis gravidarum is a diagnosis of exclusion (Benson, 2013).

Study criteria have not been homogeneous, thus reports of population incidences vary. There does, however, appear to be an ethnic or familial predilection (Grjibovski, 2008). In population-based studies from California and Nova Scotia, the hospitalization rate for hyperemesis gravidarum was 0.5 to 0.8 percent (Bailit, 2005; Fell, 2006). Up to 20 percent of those hospitalized in a previous pregnancy for hyperemesis will again require hospitalization (Dodds, 2006; Trogstad, 2005). In general, obese women are less likely to be hospitalized for this (Cedergren, 2008).

The etiopathogenesis of hyperemesis gravidarum is likely multifactorial and certainly is enigmatic. It appears to be related to high or rapidly rising serum levels of pregnancy-related hormones. Putative culprits include human chorionic gonadotropin (hCG), estrogens, progesterone, leptin, placental growth hormone, prolactin, thyroxine, and adrenocortical hormones (Verberg, 2005). More recently implicated are other hormones that include ghrelins, leptin, nesfatin-1, and PYY-3 (Albayrak, 2013; Gungor, 2013).

Superimposed on this hormonal cornucopia are an imposing number of biological and environmental factors. Moreover, in some but not all severe cases, interrelated psychological components play a major role (Buckwalter, 2002; Christodoulou-Smith, 2011; McCarthy, 2011). Other factors that increase the risk for admission include hyperthyroidism, previous molar pregnancy, diabetes, gastrointestinal illnesses, some restrictive diets, and asthma and other allergic disorders (Fell, 2006; Mullin, 2012). The vestibular system has been implicated (Goodwin, 2008). An association of *Helicobacter pylori* infection has also been proposed, but evidence is not conclusive (Goldberg, 2007). And for unknown reasons—perhaps estrogen-related—a female fetus increases the risk by 1.5-fold (Schiff, 2004; Tan, 2006; Veenendaal, 2011). Finally, Bolin and coworkers (2013) reported an association between hyperemesis gravidarum and preterm labor, placental abruption, and preeclampsia.

Complications

Vomiting may be prolonged, frequent, and severe, and a list of potentially fatal complications is given in Table 54-2. Various degrees of acute kidney injury from dehydration are encountered (Nwoko, 2012). We have cared for a number of women with markedly impaired renal function. The extreme example was a woman who required 5 days of dialysis when her serum creatinine level rose to 10.7 mg/dL (Hill, 2002). Complications from continuous retching include a Mallory-Weiss tear, such as that shown in Figure 54-1. Others are pneumothorax, pneumomediastinum, diaphragmatic rupture, and gastroesophageal rupture, which is Boerhaave syndrome (Chen, 2012; Schwartz, 1994; Yamamoto, 2001).

TABLE 54-2. Some Life-Threatening Complications of Recalcitrant Hyperemesis Gravidarum

Acute kidney injury—may require dialysis
Depression—cause versus effect?
Diaphragmatic rupture
Esophageal rupture—Boerhaave syndrome
Hypoprothrombinemia—vitamin K deficiency
Hyperalimentation complications
Mallory-Weiss tears—bleeding, pneumothorax, pneumomediastinum, pneumopericardium
Wernicke encephalopathy—thiamine deficiency

In more severe cases, plasma zinc levels are increased, copper levels decreased, and magnesium levels unchanged (Dokmeci, 2004). At least two serious vitamin deficiencies have been reported with hyperemesis in pregnancy. *Wernicke encephalopathy* from thiamine deficiency has been reported with increasing frequency (Di Gangi, 2012; Palacios-Marqués, 2012). In a review of 49 such cases, Chiossi (2006) reported that only half had the triad of confusion, ocular findings, and ataxia. With this encephalopathy, an abnormal electroencephalogram (EEG) may be seen, and usually there are MR imaging findings (Vaknin, 2006; Zara, 2012). At least three maternal deaths have been described, and long-term sequelae include blindness, convulsions, and coma (Selitsky, 2006). Last, *vitamin K deficiency* has been reported to cause maternal coagulopathy and fetal intracranial hemorrhage (Kawamura, 2008; Robinson, 1998; Sakai, 2003).

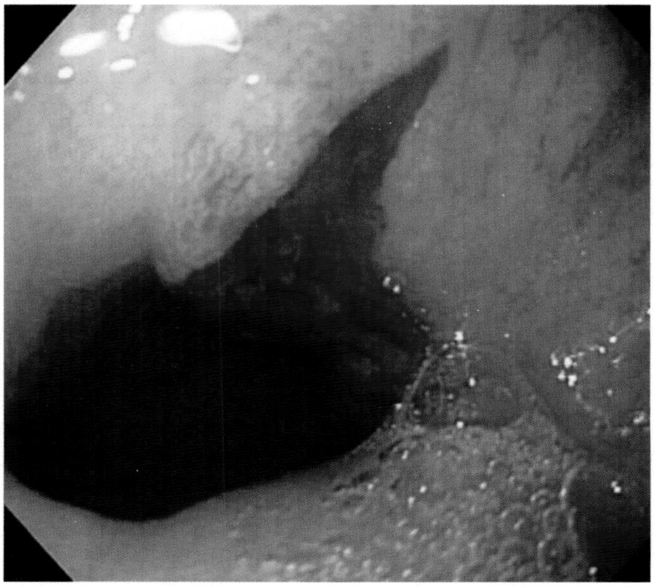

FIGURE 54-1 Endoscopic view of Mallory-Weiss tear. (From Song, 2012, with permission.)

Management

One algorithm for management of nausea and vomiting of pregnancy is shown in Figure 54-2. A Cochrane review reported a salutary effect from several antiemetics given orally or by rectal suppository as first-line agents (Jewell, 2000). The Food and Drug Administration (2013) recently approved Diclegis—a combination of doxylamine-pyridoxine—for morning sickness. When simple measures fail, intravenous Ringer lactate or normal saline solutions are given to correct dehydration, ketonemia, electrolyte deficits, and acid-base imbalances. There are no benefits to using 5-percent dextrose along with crystalloids (Tan, 2013). Thiamine, 100 mg, is given to prevent Wernicke encephalopathy (Niebyl, 2010).

If vomiting persists after rehydration and failed outpatient management, hospitalization is recommended (American College of Obstetricians and Gynecologists, 2013). Antiemetics such as promethazine, prochlorperazine, chlorpromazine, or metoclopramide are given parenterally. There is little evidence that treatment with *glucocorticosteroids* is effective. Two small trials found no benefits of *methylprednisolone* compared with placebo, but the corticosteroid-treated group had significantly fewer readmissions (Duggar, 2001; Safari, 1998). In another study from Parkland Hospital, Yost (2003) compared placebo with intravenous methylprednisolone plus two different tapered oral steroid regimens. They noted that a third in each group required readmission. In a study reported by Bondok (2006), pulsed hydrocortisone therapy was superior to metoclopramide to reduce vomiting and readmissions. *Serotonin antagonists* are most effective for controlling chemotherapy-induced nausea and vomiting (Hesketh, 2008). But when used for hyperemesis gravidarum, *ondansetron* was not superior to promethazine (Sullivan, 1996). Serotonin antagonist use in pregnancy is limited, but these drugs appear to be safe (Briggs, 2011).

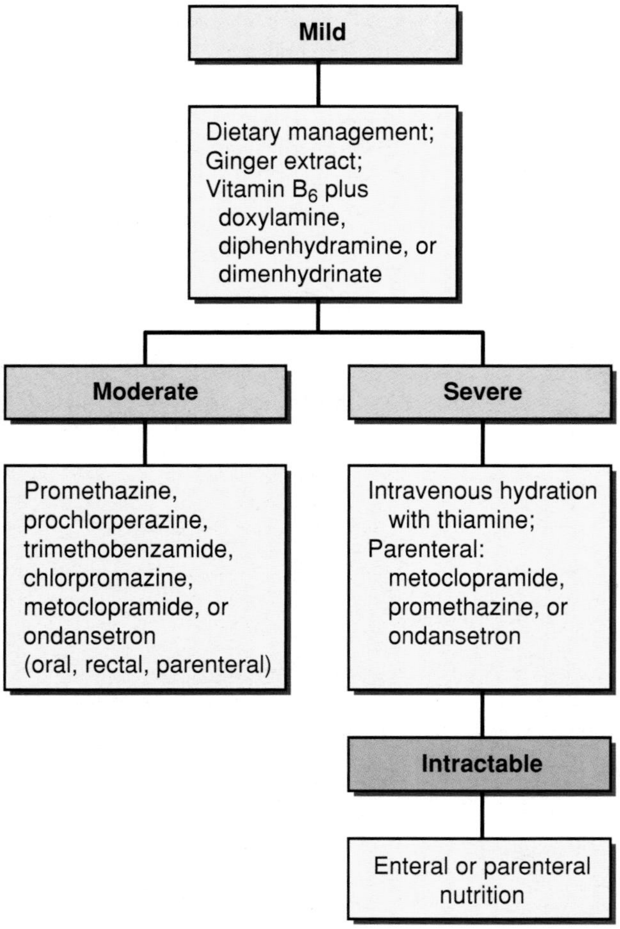

FIGURE 54-2 Algorithm for outpatient and inpatient management of hyperemesis gravidarum.

With persistent vomiting after hospitalization, appropriate steps should be taken to exclude possible underlying diseases as a cause of hyperemesis. In one study, endoscopy did not change management in 49 women (Debby, 2008). Other potential causes include gastroenteritis, cholecystitis, pancreatitis, hepatitis, peptic ulcer, and pyelonephritis. In addition, severe preeclampsia and fatty liver are more likely after midpregnancy. And although clinical thyrotoxicosis has been implicated as a cause of hyperemesis, it is more likely that abnormally elevated serum thyroxine levels are a surrogate for higher-than-average serum hCG levels (Chap. 5, p. 103). This was termed "chemical hyperthyroidism" by Tan (2002). And of interest, Panesar and associates (2006) showed that a cohort of women with hyperemesis had lower serum thyrotropin levels. In our experiences, serum free thyroxine levels normalize quickly with hydration.

With treatment, most women will have a salutary response and may be sent home with antiemetic therapy. Their readmission rate is 25 to 35 percent in most prospective studies. If associated psychiatric and social factors contribute to the illness, the woman usually improves remarkably while hospitalized (Swallow, 2004). That said, symptoms may relapse in these women, and some go on to develop *posttraumatic stress syndrome* (Christodoulou-Smith, 2011; McCarthy, 2011). For some women, hyperemesis can be an indication for elective termination (Poursharif, 2007).

In the small percentage of women who continue to have recalcitrant vomiting, consideration is given for enteral nutrition. Vaisman (2004) described successful use of nasojejunal feeding for up to 21 days in 11 such women. Use of sonography to confirm correct placement of the tube has been described (Swartzlander, 2013). Percutaneous endoscopic gastrostomy with a jejunal port has also been reported (Saha, 2009; Schrag, 2007).

In our experiences, only a very few women will require parenteral nutrition (Yost, 2003). In a study of 166 women, Folk (2004) reported that 16 percent had central venous access established for nutrition. The litany of complications included line sepsis in 25 percent and thrombosis and infective endocarditis in one woman each.

Gastroesophageal Reflux Disease (GERD)

Reflux disease is seen in up to 15 percent of nonpregnant individuals (Kahrilas, 2012). Heartburn, or *pyrosis*, is especially common in late pregnancy, and it appears at some point in 50 to 80 percent of pregnancies (Mehta, 2010). The retrosternal burning sensation is caused by esophagitis from gastroesophageal reflux related to relaxation of the lower esophageal sphincter (Hytten, 1991). According to Costigan and colleagues (2006), common folklore is confirmed in that women with excessive heartburn do give birth to infants with more hair! Long-term complications are chronic esophagitis and adenocarcinoma.

Reflux symptoms usually respond to tobacco and alcohol abstinence, small meals, head of the bed elevation, and avoidance of postprandial recumbency and "trigger" foods. Oral antacids are first-line therapy. If severe symptoms persist, sucralfate is given with an H_2-receptor antagonist such as *cimetidine* or *ranitidine*. If these are not successful, commonly used proton-pump inhibitors such as *omeprazole* or *pantoprazole* are also safe for use in pregnancy (Briggs, 2011; Mahadevan, 2006b). If there is still no relief, then endoscopy should be considered. *Misoprostol* is contraindicated because it stimulates labor (Chap. 26, p. 529).

For medical treatment failures in nonpregnant patients, surgical fundoplication is performed (Kahrilas, 2012). Although the procedure was not done during pregnancy, Biertho (2006) described 25 women who had undergone laparoscopic Nissen fundoplication before pregnancy. Only 20 percent had reflux symptoms during pregnancy.

Hiatal Hernia

The older literature is informative regarding hiatal hernias in pregnancy. Upper gastrointestinal radiographs performed in 195 women in late pregnancy showed that 20 percent of 116 multiparas and 5 percent of 79 nulliparas had a hiatal hernia (Rigler, 1935). Of 10 women studied postpartum, hernia persisted in three at 1 to 18 months.

The relationship of hiatal hernia with reflux esophagitis, and thus symptoms, is not clear. One study demonstrated no relationship between reflux and hernia and showed that the lower esophageal sphincter functioned effectively even when displaced intrathoracically (Cohen, 1971). Nevertheless, during pregnancy, these hiatal hernias may cause vomiting, epigastric pain, and bleeding from ulceration. Schwentner (2011) reported severe herniation requiring surgical repair in a woman with a 12-week gestation. Curran (1999) described a 30-week pregnancy complicated by gastric outlet obstruction from a paraesophageal hernia.

Diaphragmatic Hernia

These are caused by herniations of abdominal contents through either the foramen of Bochdalek or that of Morgagni. Fortunately, they rarely complicate pregnancy. Kurzel and associates (1988) reviewed the outcomes of 18 pregnant women with such a hernia and who developed acute obstruction. Because the maternal mortality rate was 45 percent, they recommend repair during pregnancy even if a woman is asymptomatic. Herniation has been reported in one pregnant woman from a previous traumatic diaphragmatic defect and in another who had antireflux surgery in early pregnancy (Brygger, 2013; Flick, 1999). Several case reports also describe spontaneous diaphragmatic rupture from increased intraabdominal pressure during delivery (Chen, 2012; Ortega-Carnicer, 1998; Sharifah, 2003).

Achalasia

A rare disorder, achalasia is a motility disorder in which the lower esophageal sphincter does not relax properly with swallowing. There is also nonperistaltic contraction activity of the esophageal muscularis to cause symptoms (Kahrilas, 2012; Khudyak, 2006). The defect is caused by inflammatory destruction of the myenteric (Auerbach) plexus within smooth muscle of the lower esophagus and its sphincter. Postganglionic cholinergic neurons are unaffected, thus, there is unopposed sphincter stimulation. Symptoms are dysphagia, chest pain, and regurgitation. Barium swallow radiography demonstrates *bird beak* or *ace of spades* narrowing at the distal esophagus. Endoscopy is performed to exclude gastric carcinoma, and manometry is confirmatory. If dilatation of the esophagus and medical therapy does not provide relief, myotomy is considered (Torquati, 2006).

During pregnancy, normal relaxation of the lower esophageal sphincter in those with achalasia theoretically should not occur. Even so, in most women, pregnancy does not seem to worsen achalasia. One report of 20 affected pregnant women found no excessive reflux esophagitis (Mayberry, 1987). Khudyak and coworkers (2006) reviewed 35 cases and described most women as symptom free, although esophageal dilatation was needed in a few. A maternal death at 24 weeks associated with perforation of a 14-cm diameter megaesophagus has been reported (Fassina, 1995).

Management of achalasia includes soft diet and anticholinergic drugs. With persistent symptoms, other options include nitrates, calcium-channel antagonists, and botulinum toxin A injected locally (Khudyak, 2006; Wataganara, 2009). Balloon dilatation of the sphincter may be necessary, and 85 percent of nonpregnant patients respond to this. Satin (1992) and Fiest (1993) and their associates reported successful use of pneumatic dilatation in pregnancy. *One caveat is that esophageal perforation is a serious complication of dilatation.* Spiliopoulos and colleagues (2013) described a 29-week pregnant woman with achalasia treated for 10 weeks with parenteral nutrition with surgical correction done postpartum.

Peptic Ulcer

Erosive ulcer disease more often involves the duodenum rather than the stomach in young women. Gastroduodenal ulcers in nonpregnant women may be caused by chronic gastritis from *H pylori,* or they develop from use of aspirin or other nonsteroidal antiinflammatory drugs. Neither is common in pregnancy (McKenna, 2003; Weyermann, 2003). Acid secretion is also important, and thus underlies the efficacy of antisecretory agents (Suerbaum, 2002). Gastroprotection during pregnancy is probably due to reduced gastric acid secretion, decreased motility, and considerably increased mucus secretion (Hytten, 1991). Despite this, ulcer disease may be underdiagnosed because of frequent treatment for reflux esophagitis (Cappell, 1998; Mehta, 2010). In the past 45 years at Parkland Hospital, during which time we have cared for more than 500,000 pregnant women, we have encountered very few who had symptomatic ulcer disease. Before appropriate therapy was commonplace, Clark (1953) studied 313 pregnancies in 118 women with proven ulcer disease. They noted a clear remission during pregnancy in almost 90 percent. However, benefits were short lived. Symptoms recurred in more than half by 3 months postpartum and in almost all by 2 years.

Antacids are first-line therapy, and H_2-receptor blockers or proton-pump inhibitors are safely prescribed for those who do not respond (Briggs, 2011; Diav-Citrin, 2005; Mahadevan, 2006b). *Sucralfate* is the aluminum salt of sulfated sucrose that inhibits pepsin. It provides a protective coating at the ulcer base. Approximately 10 percent of the aluminum salt is absorbed, and it is considered safe for pregnant women (Briggs, 2011).

With active ulcers, a search for *H pylori* is undertaken. Diagnostic aids include the urea breath test, serological testing, or endoscopic biopsy. If any of these are positive, antimicrobial therapy is indicated. There are several effective oral treatment regimens that do not include tetracycline and that can be used during pregnancy. These 14-day regimens include amoxicillin, 1000 mg twice daily along with clarithromycin, 500 mg twice daily; or metronidazole, 500 mg twice daily (Dzieniszewski, 2006; Mehta, 2010).

Upper Gastrointestinal Bleeding

In some women, persistent vomiting is accompanied by worrisome upper gastrointestinal bleeding. Occasionally, there is a bleeding peptic ulceration, however, most of these women have small linear mucosal tears near the gastroesophageal junction—*Mallory-Weiss tears*, as shown in Figure 54-1. Bleeding usually responds promptly to conservative measures, including iced saline irrigations, topical antacids, and intravenously administered H_2-blockers or proton-pump inhibitors. Transfusions may be needed, and if there is persistent bleeding, then endoscopy may be indicated (O'Mahony, 2007). With persistent retching, the less common, but more serious, esophageal rupture—*Boerhaave syndrome*—may develop from greatly increased esophageal pressure.

DISORDERS OF THE SMALL BOWEL AND COLON

The small bowel has diminished motility during pregnancy. Using a nonabsorbable carbohydrate, Lawson (1985) showed that small bowel mean transit times were 99, 125, and 137 minutes in each trimester, compared with 75 minutes when nonpregnant. In a study cited by Everson (1992), mean transit time for a mercury-filled balloon from the stomach to the cecum was 58 hours in term pregnant women compared with 52 hours in nonpregnant women.

Muscular relaxation of the colon is accompanied by increased absorption of water and sodium that predisposes to constipation. This complaint is reported by almost 40 percent of women at some time during pregnancy (Everson, 1992). Such symptoms are usually only mildly bothersome, and preventive measures include a high-fiber diet and bulk-forming laxatives. Wald (2003) has reviewed treatment options. We have encountered several pregnant women who developed megacolon from impacted stool. These women almost invariably had chronically abused stimulatory laxatives.

Acute Diarrhea

Most cases of acute diarrhea are caused by infectious agents. The large variety of viruses, bacteria, helminths, and protozoa that cause diarrhea in adults inevitably also afflict pregnant women. Some of these are discussed in Chapter 64. Evaluation of acute diarrhea depends on its severity and duration. According to Camilleri and Murray (2012), some indications for evaluation include profuse diarrhea with dehydration, grossly bloody stools, fever ≥ 38.5°C, duration of > 48 hours without improvement, recent antimicrobial use, immunocompromise, and new community outbreaks. Cases of moderately severe diarrhea with fecal leukocytes or gross blood may best be treated with empirical antibiotics rather than evaluation. Some features of the more common acute diarrheal syndromes are shown in Table 54-3.

The mainstay of treatment is intravenous hydration using normal saline or Ringer lactate with potassium supplementation in amounts to restore maternal blood volume and to ensure uteroplacental perfusion. Vital signs and urine output are monitored for signs of sepsis syndrome. For moderately severe nonfebrile illness without bloody diarrhea, antimobility agents such as loperamide may be useful. Bismuth subsalicylate may also alleviate symptoms.

Judicious use of antimicrobial agents is warranted. For moderate to severely ill women, some recommend empirical treatment with ciprofloxacin, 500 mg twice daily for 3 to 5 days.

TABLE 54-3. Causative Agents and Clinical Features of Common Acute, Infectious Diarrheal Syndromes

Agents	Incubation	Emesis	Pain	Fever	Diarrhea
Toxin-producers (*Staphylococcus, Clostridium perfringens*, enterotoxigenic *E coli*)	1–72 hr	3–4+	1–2+	0–1+	3–4+, watery
Enteroadherent (*E coli, Giardia*, helminths)	1–8 day	0–1+	1–3+	0–2+	1–2+, watery, mushy
Cytotoxin producers (*C difficile*, hemorrhagic *E coli*)	1–3 day	0–1+	3–4+	1–2+	1–3+, watery, then bloody
Inflammatory					
Minimal (rotavirus, norovirus)	1–3 day	1–3+	2–3+	3–4+	1–3+, watery
Variable (*Salmonella, Campylobacter, Vibrio, Yersinia*)	1–11 day	0–3+	2–4+	3–4+	1–4+, watery or bloody
Severe (*Shigella, E coli, Entamoeba histolytica*)	1–8 day	0–1+	3–4+	3–4+	1–2+, bloody

C difficile = Clostridium difficile; E coli = Escherichia coli.
Adapted from Camilleri, 2012.

TABLE 54-4. Some Shared and Differentiating Characteristics of Inflammatory Bowel Disease

	Ulcerative Colitis	Crohn Disease
	Shared Characteristics	
Hereditary	More than 100 disease-associated genetic loci–a third shared; Jewish predominance; familial in 5–10% of cases; Turner syndrome; immune dysregulation	
Other	Chronic and intermittent with exacerbations and remissions; arthritis, erythema nodosum; uveitis	
	Differentiating Characteristics	
Major symptoms	Diarrhea, tenesmus, rectal bleeding, cramping pain; chronic, intermittent	Fibrostenotic–recurrent RLQ colicky pain; fever Fistulizing–cutaneous, bladder, interenteric
Bowel involvement	Mucosa and submucosa of large bowel; usually begins at rectum (40% proctitis only)	Deep layers small and large bowel; commonly transmural; discontinuous involvement; strictures and fistulas
Endoscopy	Granular and friable erythematous mucosa; rectal involvement	Patchy; rectum spared; perianal involvement
Serum antibodies	Antineutrophil cytoplasmic (pANCA) ~ 70%	Anti-*S cerevisiae* ~ 50%
Complications	Toxic megacolon; strictures; arthritis; cancer (3–5%)	Fistulas; arthritis; toxic megacolon
Management	Medical; proctocolectomy curative	Medical; segmental and fistula resection

RLQ = right lower quadrant.
From Friedman, 2012; Lichtenstein, 2009; Podolsky, 2002.

Specific pathogens are treated as needed when identified. Syndromes for which treatment is usually unnecessary include those caused by *Escherichia coli*, staphylococcus, *Bacillus cereus*, and Norwalk-like virus. Severe illness caused by *Salmonella* is treated with trimethoprim-sulfamethoxazole or azithromycin; *Campylobacter* with azithromycin; *Clostridium difficile* with oral metronidazole or vancomycin; and *Giardia* and *Entamoeba histolytica* with metronidazole (Mehta, 2010).

Inflammatory Bowel Disease

The two presumably noninfectious forms of intestinal inflammation are ulcerative colitis and Crohn disease. Differentiation between the two is important because treatment differs. That said, they both share common factors, and sometimes are indistinguishable if Crohn disease involves the colon. The salient clinical and laboratory features shown in Table 54-4 permit a reasonably confident diagnostic differentiation in most cases. The etiopathogenesis of both disorders is enigmatic, but there is genetic predisposition toward either. Inflammation is thought to result from dysregulated mucosal immune function in response to normal bacterial flora, with or without an autoimmune component (Friedman, 2012).

Ulcerative Colitis

This is a mucosal disorder with inflammation confined to the superficial luminal layers of the colon. It typically begins at the rectum and extends proximally for a variable distance. In approximately 40 percent, disease is confined to the rectum and rectosigmoid, and 20 percent have pancolitis. Endoscopic findings include mucosal granularity and friability that is interspersed with mucosal ulcerations and a mucopurulent exudate (Fig. 54-3).

Major symptoms of ulcerative colitis include diarrhea, rectal bleeding, tenesmus, and abdominal cramps. The disease can be acute or intermittent and is characterized by exacerbations and remissions. For unknown reasons, prior appendectomy protects

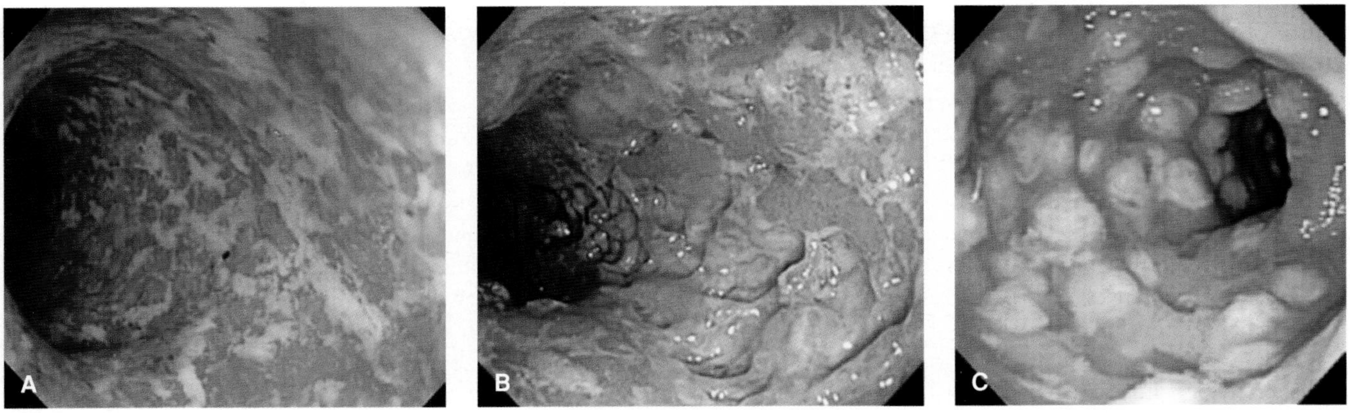

FIGURE 54-3 Causes of colitis. **A.** Chronic ulcerative colitis with diffuse ulcerations and exudates. **B.** Crohn colitis with deep ulcers. **C.** Pseudomembranous colitis with yellow pseudomembranes. (From Song, 2012, with permission.)

against development of ulcerative colitis (Friedman, 2012; Selby, 2002). *Toxic megacolon* and catastrophic hemorrhage are particularly dangerous complications that may necessitate colectomy. *Extraintestinal manifestations* include arthritis, uveitis, and erythema nodosum. Another serious problem is that the risk of colon cancer approaches 1 percent per year. With either ulcerative colitis or Crohn disease, there is also concern for possible increased risks for thromboembolism (Kappelman, 2011; Novacek, 2010).

Crohn Disease

Also known as regional enteritis, Crohn ileitis, and granulomatous colitis, Crohn disease has more protean manifestations than ulcerative colitis. It involves not only the bowel mucosa but also the deeper layers, and sometimes there is transmural involvement. Lesions can be seen throughout the entire gastrointestinal tract, from the mouth to the anus (Friedman, 2012). It is typically segmental. Approximately 30 percent of patients have small-bowel involvement, 25 percent have isolated colonic involvement, and 40 percent have both, usually with the terminal ileum and colon involved. Perirectal fistulas and abscesses develop in a third of those with colonic involvement.

Symptoms depend on which bowel segment(s) is involved. Thus, complaints may include right-sided lower cramping abdominal pain, diarrhea, weight loss, low-grade fever, and obstructive symptoms. The disease is chronic with exacerbations and remissions, and importantly, it cannot be cured medically or surgically (Lichtenstein, 2009). Approximately a third of patients require surgery within the first year after diagnosis, and thereafter, 5 percent per year. Reactive arthritis is common, and the gastrointestinal cancer risk, although not as great as with ulcerative colitis, is increased substantially.

Inflammatory Bowel Disease and Fertility

Subfertility is commonly linked to chronic medical disease. That said, Mahadevan (2006a) cited a normal fertility rate for inflammatory bowel disease unless severe disease warranted surgery. Alstead (2003) reported that decreased female fertility from active Crohn disease returned to normal with remission. For women requiring surgical resection, laparoscopic anastomosis has a higher subsequent fertility rate (Beyer-Berjot, 2013). Even though fertility is improved after colectomy, up to half of women will still be infertile (Bartels, 2012; Waljee, 2006). Subfertility may also be partially due to sulfasalazine, which causes reversible sperm abnormalities (Feagins, 2009).

Inflammatory Bowel Disease and Pregnancy

Because ulcerative colitis and Crohn disease are relatively common in young women, they are encountered with some frequency in pregnancy. In this regard, a few generalizations can be made. The consensus is that pregnancy does not increase the likelihood of an inflammatory bowel disease flare. To the contrary, in a 10-year surveillance of women in the European Collaborative on Inflammatory Bowel Disease, the likelihood of a flare during pregnancy was decreased compared with the preconceptional rate (Riis, 2006). This diminished rate persisted for years after pregnancy and was attributed to close attention and monitoring of enrolled women.

Although most of those with quiescent disease in early pregnancy uncommonly have relapses, when a flare develops, it may be severe. Conversely, active disease in early pregnancy increases the likelihood of poor pregnancy outcome. In general, most usual treatment regimens may be continued during pregnancy. If needed to direct management, diagnostic evaluations should be undertaken, and if indicated, surgery should be performed. For women who successfully complete pregnancy, half experience improvement in their health-related quality of life (Ananthakrishnan, 2012).

At first glance, it appears that adverse pregnancy outcomes are increased with inflammatory bowel disease (Bush, 2004; Cornish, 2012; Elbaz, 2005; Mahadevan, 2005). Initially, this was attributed to the fact that most studies included women with either form of disease. Specifically, Crohn disease was noted to be linked to excessive morbidity (Dominitz, 2002; Stephansson, 2010). But, according to Reddy (2008) as well as others, these adverse outcomes were in women with severe disease and multiple recurrences. Indeed, in the prospective *European case-control ECCO-EpiCom study* of 332 pregnant women with inflammatory disease, Bortoli and coworkers (2011) found similar outcomes in women with ulcerative colitis or Crohn disease compared with normally pregnant women. Importantly, even reports of adverse outcomes found that perinatal mortality rates are not appreciably increased.

Ulcerative Colitis and Pregnancy. Pregnancy has no significant effects on ulcerative colitis. In a metaanalysis of 755 pregnancies, Fonager (1998) reported that ulcerative colitis quiescent at conception worsened in approximately a third of pregnancies. In women with active disease at the time of conception, approximately 45 percent worsened, 25 percent remained unchanged, and only 25 percent improved. These observations are similar to those previously described in an extensive review by Miller (1986) and a report from Oron and colleagues (2012).

Calcium supplementation is provided for osteoporosis. Folic acid is given in high doses to counteract the antifolate actions of sulfasalazine. Flares may be caused by psychogenic stress, and reassurance is important. Management for colitis for the most part is the same as for nonpregnancy. Treatment of active colitis, as well as maintenance therapy, is with drugs that deliver 5-aminosalicyclic acid (5-ASA) or mesalamine. *Sulfasalazine* is the prototype, and its 5-ASA moiety inhibits prostaglandin synthase in colonic mucosa. Others include olsalazine (Dipentum) and coated 5-ASA derivatives (Asacol, Pentasa, Lialda). Glucocorticoids are given orally, parenterally, or by enema for more severe disease that does not respond to 5-ASA. Recalcitrant disease is managed with immunomodulating drugs, including *azathioprine*, *6-mercaptopurine*, or *cyclosporine*, which appear relatively safe in pregnancy (Briggs, 2011; Moskovitz, 2004). Importantly, *methotrexate* is contraindicated in pregnancy. High-dose intravenous cyclosporine may be beneficial for severely ill patients and used in lieu of colectomy. Parenteral nutrition is occasionally necessary for women with prolonged exacerbations.

Colorectal endoscopy is performed as indicated (Katz, 2002). During pregnancy, colectomy and ostomy creation for fulminant colitis may be needed as a lifesaving measure, and it has been described during each trimester. Dozois (2006) reviewed 42 such cases and found that, in general, outcomes have been good in recent reports. Most women underwent partial or complete colectomy, but Ooi and colleagues (2003) described decompression colostomy with ileostomy in a 10- and a 16-week pregnancy.

More commonly for nonpregnant women undergoing proctocolectomy for ulcerative colitis, an ileal pouch is constructed and an anal anastomosis completed. For women with this procedure performed before pregnancy, sexual function and fertility are improved (Cornish, 2007). Disadvantages include frequent bowel movements, fecal incontinence that includes nocturnal soilage in almost half of patients, and pouchitis. *Pouchitis* is an inflammatory condition of the ileoanal pouch, probably due to bacterial proliferation, stasis, and endotoxin release. It usually responds to cephalosporins or metronidazole. Although these disadvantages temporarily worsen during pregnancy, they typically abate postpartum. In one rare case, adhesions to the growing uterus led to ileal pouch perforation (Aouthmany, 2004).

Women who have had a prior proctocolectomy and ileal pouch–anal anastomosis can safely deliver vaginally (Ravid, 2002). Hahnloser (2004) reviewed routes of delivery in women with 235 pregnancies before and 232 pregnancies after ileoanal pouch surgery. Functional outcomes were similar, and it was concluded that cesarean delivery should be reserved for obstetrical indications. Postcesarean delivery ileoanal pouch obstruction has been described (Malecki, 2010).

As previously discussed, ulcerative colitis likely has minimal adverse effects on pregnancy outcome. Modigliani (2000) reviewed perinatal outcomes in 2398 pregnancies and reported them to be not substantively different from those in the general obstetrical population. Specifically, the incidences of spontaneous abortion, preterm delivery, and stillbirth were remarkably low. In a population-based cohort study of 107 women from Washington state, perinatal outcomes, with two exceptions, were similar to those of 1308 normal pregnancies (Dominitz, 2002). One exception was an inexplicably increased incidence of congenital malformations, and the other was a cesarean delivery rate that was increased from 20 to 29 percent compared with normal controls. The previously described ECCO-EpiCom study reported similar outcomes in 187 women with ulcerative colitis compared with their normal controls (Bortoli, 2011). There are smaller studies in which the risks for preterm birth and low birthweight are increased (Emerson, 2013).

Crohn Disease and Pregnancy. In general, Crohn disease activity during pregnancy is related to its status around the time of conception. In a cohort study of 279 pregnancies, for 186 women whose disease was inactive at conception, a fourth relapsed during pregnancy (Fonager, 1998). In 93 with active disease at conception, however, two thirds either remained active or worsened. Miller (1986) had described similar findings from his earlier review as did Oron and associates (2012).

Calcium and folic acid supplementation are given as for ulcerative colitis. There is no regimen that is universally effective for maintenance during asymptomatic periods. *Sulfasalazine* is effective for some, but the newer 5-ASA formulations are better tolerated. As a class, they appear to be safe in pregnancy (Briggs, 2011; Rahimi, 2008). *Prednisone* therapy may control moderate to severe flares but is less effective for small-bowel involvement. Immunomodulators such as *azathioprine*, *6-mercaptopurine*, and *cyclosporine* are used for active disease and for maintenance and appear relatively safe during pregnancy (Briggs, 2011; Moskovitz, 2004; Prefontaine, 2009). As discussed in Chapter 12 (p. 248), methotrexate, mycophenolate mofetil, and mycophenolic acid are contraindicated in pregnancy (Briggs, 2011; Food and Drug Administration, 2008). Anti-tumor necrosis factor (TNF)-α antibodies, which include *infliximab, adalimumab*, and *certolizumab*, are also effective for active Crohn disease and maintenance (Casanova, 2013; Colombel, 2010; Cominelli, 2013; Friedman, 2012; Sandborn, 2007; Schreiber, 2007). This class of immunomodulators is considered safe in pregnancy, but data are limited (Katz, 2004; Roux, 2007; Schnitzler, 2011). Parenteral hyperalimentation has been used successfully during severe recurrences (Russo-Stieglitz, 1999).

Endoscopy or conservative surgery is indicated for complications. Patients with small-bowel involvement more likely will require surgery for complications that include fistulas, strictures, abscesses, and intractable disease. An abdominal surgical procedure was required during 5 percent of pregnancies described by Woolfson (1990). Those with an ileal loop colostomy may have significant problems as discussed below. Women with a perianal fistula—unless these are rectovaginal—usually can undergo vaginal delivery without complications (Forsnes, 1999; Takahashi, 2007).

As discussed, there seems to be a greater likelihood that Crohn disease may be associated with adverse pregnancy outcomes compared with ulcerative colitis (Stephansson, 2010). Outcomes are probably related to disease activities. For example, based on a 20-year review, Korelitz (1998) concluded that perinatal outcomes were generally good with quiescent disease. That said, in a case-control Danish study, Norgård (2007) reported a twofold risk of preterm births. Dominitz (2002) reported a two- to threefold increase in preterm delivery, low birthweight, fetal-growth restriction, and cesarean delivery in 149 women with Crohn disease. Recall, however, that the prospective ECCO-EpiCom study found outcomes to be similar to those for normal pregnancies.

Ostomy and Pregnancy

A colostomy or an ileostomy can be problematic during pregnancy because of its location (Hux, 2010). In a report of 82 pregnancies in 66 women with an ostomy, *stomal dysfunction* was common, but it responded to conservative management in all cases (Gopal, 1985). Surgical intervention was necessary, however, in three of six women who developed *bowel obstruction* and in another four with *ileostomy prolapse*—almost 10 percent overall. In this older study, only a third of 82 women underwent cesarean delivery, but Takahashi (2007) described six of seven cesarean deliveries in women with Crohn disease and a stoma. Fortunately, Farouk and coworkers (2000) reported that pregnancy did not worsen long-term ostomy function.

Intestinal Obstruction

The incidence of bowel obstruction is not increased during pregnancy, although it generally is more difficult to diagnose. Meyerson (1995) reported a 20-year incidence of 1 in 17,000 deliveries at two Detroit hospitals. In one study, adhesive disease leading to small bowel obstruction was the second most common cause of an acute abdomen in pregnancy following appendicitis—15 versus 30 percent, respectively (Unal, 2011). As shown in Table 54-5, approximately half of cases are due to adhesions from previous pelvic surgery that includes cesarean delivery (Al-Sunaidi, 2006; Andolf, 2010; Lyell, 2011). Another 25 percent of bowel obstruction is caused by volvulus—sigmoid, cecal, or small bowel. These have been reported in late pregnancy or early puerperium (Alshawi, 2005; Biswas, 2006; Lal, 2006). Wax and colleagues (2013) described small bowel obstruction in pregnancy following the currently popular Roux-en-Y gastric bypass. Intussusception is occasionally encountered (Gould, 2008; Harma, 2011). Bowel obstruction subsequent to colorectal surgery for cancer was increased threefold in women who had open versus laparoscopic surgery (Haggar, 2013).

Most cases of intestinal obstruction during pregnancy result from pressure of the growing uterus on intestinal adhesions. According to Davis and Bohon (1983), this more likely occurs: (1) around midpregnancy, when the uterus becomes an abdominal organ; (2) in the third trimester, when the fetal head descends; or (3) immediately postpartum, when there is an acute change in uterine size. Perdue (1992) reported that 98 percent of pregnant women had either continuous or colicky abdominal pain, and 80 percent had nausea and vomiting. Abdominal tenderness was found in 70 percent, and abnormal bowel sounds noted in only 55 percent. Plain abdominal radiographs following soluble contrast showed evidence of obstruction in 90 percent of women. Plain radiographs, however, are less accurate for diagnosing small-bowel obstruction, and we and others have found that CT and MR imaging can be diagnostic (Biswas, 2006; Essilfie, 2007; McKenna, 2007). Colonoscopy can be both diagnostic and therapeutic for colonic volvulus (Dray, 2012; Khan, 2012).

TABLE 54-5. Causes of Intestinal Obstruction During Pregnancy and the Puerperium

Cause of Obstruction	Percent
Adhesions:	~ 60
1st and 2nd trimester ~ 30%	
3rd trimester ~ 5%	
Postpartum ~ 25%	
Volvulus:	~ 25
Midgut ~ 2%	
Cecal ~ 5%	
Sigmoid ~ 10%	
Intussusception	~ 5
Hernia, carcinoma, other	~ 5

Data from Connolly, 1995; Khan, 2012; Redlich, 2007.

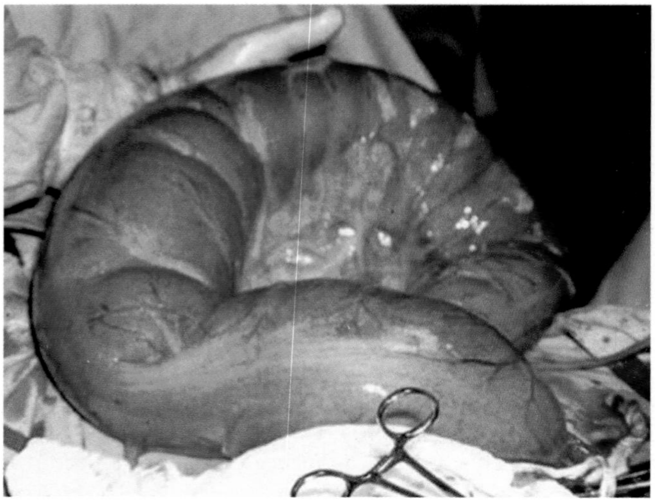

FIGURE 54-4 Massively dilated colon in a pregnant woman with colonic volvulus. (Courtesy of Dr. Lowell Davis.)

During pregnancy, mortality rates with obstruction can be excessive because of difficult and thus delayed diagnosis, reluctance to operate during pregnancy, and the need for emergency surgery (Firstenberg, 1998; Shui, 2011). In an older report of 66 pregnancies, Perdue and associates (1992) described a 6-percent maternal mortality rate and 26-percent fetal mortality rate. Two of the four women who died were in late pregnancy, and they had sigmoid or cecal volvulus caused by adhesions. Perforation from massive bowel dilation such as that shown in Figure 54-4 causes severe sepsis syndrome.

Colonic Pseudo-obstruction

Also known as *Ogilvie syndrome,* pseudo-obstruction is caused by adynamic colonic ileus. It is characterized by massive abdominal distention with cecal and right-hemicolon dilatation. Approximately 10 percent of all cases are associated with pregnancy. The syndrome usually develops postpartum—most commonly after cesarean delivery—but it has been reported antepartum (Tung, 2008). Although this is unusual, the large bowel may rupture (Singh, 2005). Treatment with an intravenous infusion of neostigmine, 2 mg, usually results in prompt decompression (Ponec, 1999). In some cases, colonoscopic decompression is performed, but laparotomy is done for perforation (De Giorgio, 2009; Rawlings, 2010).

Appendicitis

Suspected appendicitis is one of the most common indications for abdominal exploration during pregnancy. The frequency for *suspected* appendicitis approximated 1 in 1000 women in the Swedish registry of 720,000 pregnancies (Mazze, 1991). Disease was confirmed in 65 percent for an incidence of approximately 1 in 1500 births. Inexplicably, the incidence was much lower in the Danish registry of more than 320,000 pregnancies—the confirmed appendicitis rate was only 1 per 5500 pregnancies (Hée, 1999).

It is repeatedly—and appropriately—emphasized that pregnancy makes the diagnosis of appendicitis more difficult. Nausea and vomiting accompany normal pregnancy, but also, as the uterus enlarges, the appendix commonly moves upward and outward from the right-lower quadrant (Baer, 1932; Pates, 2009). Another often-stated reason for late diagnosis is that some degree of leukocytosis accompanies normal pregnancy. For these and other reasons, pregnant women—especially those late in gestation—frequently do not have clinical findings "typical" for appendicitis. Thus, it commonly is confused with cholecystitis, preterm labor, pyelonephritis, renal colic, placental abruption, or uterine leiomyoma degeneration.

Most reports indicate increasing morbidity and mortality rates with increasing gestational age. And as the appendix is progressively deflected upward by the growing uterus, omental containment of infection becomes increasingly unlikely. It is indisputable that appendiceal perforation is more common during later pregnancy. In the studies by Andersson (2001) and Ueberrueck (2004), the incidence of perforation was approximately 8, 12, and 20 percent in successive trimesters.

Diagnosis

Persistent abdominal pain and tenderness are the most reproducible findings. Right-lower quadrant pain is the most frequent, although pain migrates upward with appendiceal displacement (Mourad, 2000). For evaluation, sonographic abdominal imaging is reasonable in suspected appendicitis, even if to exclude an obstetrical cause of right-lower quadrant pain (Butala, 2010). That said, *graded compression sonography* is difficult because of cecal displacement and uterine imposition (Pedrosa, 2009). *Appendiceal computed tomography* is more sensitive and accurate than sonography to confirm suspected appendicitis (Gearhart, 2008; Katz, 2012; Raman, 2008). Specific views can be designed to decrease fetal radiation exposure (Chap. 46, p. 933). In one study, the negative appendectomy rate was 54 percent with clinical diagnosis alone, but only 8 percent if sonography and CT scanning were used (Wallace, 2008). *MR imaging* may be preferable, and as shown in Figure 54-5, we and others have had good results with its use (Dewhurst, 2013; Israel, 2008). One metaanalysis cited positive- and negative-predictive values of 90 and 99.5 percent, respectively (Blumenfeld, 2011). Using a decision-analysis model, CT and MR imaging were found to be cost effective (Kastenberg, 2013).

Management

When appendicitis is suspected, treatment is prompt surgical exploration. Although diagnostic errors may lead to removal of a normal appendix, surgical evaluation is preferable to postponed intervention and generalized peritonitis. In earlier reports, the diagnosis was verified in only 60 to 70 percent of pregnant women. However, as indicated above, with CT and MR imaging, these figures have improved (Blumenfeld, 2011; Wallace, 2008). Importantly, the accuracy of diagnosis is inversely proportional to gestational age (Mazze, 1991).

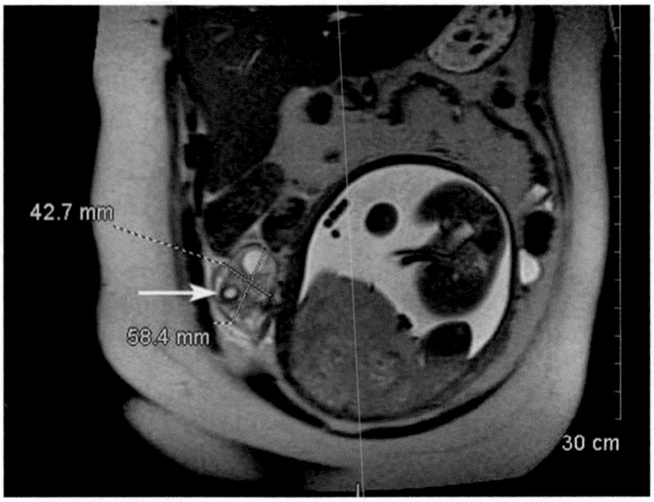

FIGURE 54-5 Anterior-posterior magnetic resonance image of a periappendiceal abscess in a midtrimester pregnancy. The abscess is approximately 5 × 6 cm, and the appendiceal lumen (*arrow*) is visible within the right-lower quadrant mass.

Laparoscopy is almost always used to treat suspected appendicitis during the first two trimesters. There were similar perinatal outcomes reported from the Swedish database of nearly 2000 laparoscopic appendectomies compared with those of more than 1500 open laparotomies done before 20 weeks (Reedy, 1997). Conversely, from their review, Wilasrusmee and coworkers (2012) reported a higher fetal loss with laparoscopy. It has evolved that in many centers, laparoscopic appendectomy is performed in most cases during the third trimester (Barnes, 2004; Donkervoort, 2011). This is sanctioned and encouraged by the Society of American Gastrointestinal and Endoscopic Surgeons (Pearl, 2011; Soper, 2011). Some are of the opinion that laparoscopic surgery in pregnancy after 26 to 28 weeks should be performed only by the most experienced endoscopic surgeons (Parangi, 2007).

Before exploration, intravenous antimicrobial therapy is begun, usually with a second-generation cephalosporin or third-generation penicillin. Unless there is gangrene, perforation, or a periappendiceal phlegmon, antimicrobial therapy can usually be discontinued after surgery. Without generalized peritonitis, the prognosis is excellent. Seldom is cesarean delivery indicated at the time of appendectomy. Uterine contractions are common, and although some clinicians recommend tocolytic agents, we do not. De Veciana (1994) reported that tocolytic use substantially increased the risk for pulmonary-permeability edema caused by sepsis syndrome (Chap. 47, p. 947).

Pregnancy Outcomes

Appendicitis increases the likelihood of abortion or preterm labor, especially if there is peritonitis. In two studies, spontaneous labor after 23 weeks ensued with greater frequency following surgery for appendicitis compared with surgery for other indications (Cohen-Kerem, 2005; Mazze, 1991). In one study, the fetal loss rate was 22 percent if surgery was performed after 23 weeks. There are at least two large population-based studies that attest to the adverse outcomes from appendicitis in pregnancy. From the California Inpatient File of 3133 pregnant women undergoing surgery for suspected appendicitis, the fetal loss rate was 23 percent, and it was doubled—6 versus 11 percent—with simple versus complicated disease (McGory, 2007). A nationwide study from Taiwan found that there were 1.5- to twofold increased risks for low birthweight and preterm delivery when outcomes in 908 women with acute appendicitis were compared with those of controls (Wei, 2012).

Long-term complications are not common. The possible link between sepsis and neonatal neurological injury has not been verified (Mays, 1995). Finally, appendicitis during pregnancy does not appear to be associated with subsequent infertility (Viktrup, 1998).

Postpartum Acute Appendicitis

Although new-onset appendicitis during the immediate puerperium is uncommon, in some women it is undiagnosed before delivery. Appendicitis in these women often stimulated labor and when the large uterus rapidly empties, walled-off infection may be disrupted to result in an acute surgical abdomen. In some cases, acute appendicitis or a periappendiceal abscess or phlegmon may be found at the time of cesarean delivery or puerperal tubal ligation (see Fig. 54-5). It is important to remember that puerperal pelvic infections typically do not cause peritonitis.

REFERENCES

Albayrak M, Karatas A, Demiraran Y, et al: Ghrelin, acylated ghrelin, leptin, and PYY-3 levels in hyperemesis gravidarum. J Matern Fetal Neonatal Med 26(9):866, 2013

Alshawi JS: Recurrent sigmoid volvulus in pregnancy: report of a case and review of the literature. Dis Colon Rectum 48:1811, 2005

Alstead EM, Nelson-Piercy C: Inflammatory bowel disease in pregnancy. Gut 52:159, 2003

Al-Sunaidi M, Tulandi T: Adhesion-related bowel obstruction after hysterectomy for benign conditions. Obstet Gynecol 108:1162, 2006

American College of Obstetricians and Gynecologists: Nausea and vomiting of pregnancy. Practice Bulletin No. 52, April 2013

Ananthakrishnan AN, Zadvornova Y, Naik AS, et al: Impact of pregnancy on health-related quality of life of patients with inflammatory bowel disease. J Dig Dis 13(9):472, 2012

Andersson RE, Lambe M: Incidence of appendicitis during pregnancy. Int J Epidemiol 30:1281, 2001

Andolf E, Thorsell M, Käkkén K: Cesarean delivery and risk for postoperative adhesions and intestinal obstruction: a nested case-control study of the Swedish Medical Birth Registry. Am J Obstet Gynecol 203(4):406, 2010

Aouthmany A, Horattas MC: Ileal pouch perforation in pregnancy: report of a case and review of the literature. Dis Colon Rectum 47:243, 2004

Baer JL, Reis RA, Arens RA: Appendicitis in pregnancy with changes in position and axis of normal appendix in pregnancy. JAMA 98:1359, 1932

Bailit JL: Hyperemesis gravidarum: epidemiologic findings from a large cohort. Am J Obstet Gynecol 193:811, 2005

Barnes SL, Shane MD, Schoemann MB, et al: Laparoscopic appendectomy after 30 weeks pregnancy: report of two cases and description of technique. Am Surg 70:733, 2004

Bartels SA, D'Hoore A, Cuesta MA, et al: Significantly increased pregnancy rates after laparoscopic restorative proctocolectomy: a cross-sectional study. Ann Surg 256(6):1045, 2012

Benson BC, Guinto RE, Parks JR: Primary hyperparathyroidism mimicking hyperemesis gravidarum. Hawaii J Med Public Health 72(1):11, 2013

Beyer-Berjot L, Maggiori L, Birnbaum D, et al: A total laparoscopic approach reduces the infertility rate after ileal pouch-anal anastomosis: a 2-center study. Ann Surg 258(2):275, 2013

Biertho L, Sebajang H, Bamehriz F, et al: Effect of pregnancy on effectiveness of laparoscopic Nissen fundoplication. Surg Endosc 20:385, 2006

Bistrian BR, Driscoll DF: Enteral and parenteral nutrition therapy. In Longo DL, Fauci AS, Kasper DL, et al (eds): Harrison's Principles of Internal Medicine, 18th ed. New York, McGraw-Hill, 2012, p 612

Biswas S, Gray KD, Cotton BA: Intestinal obstruction in pregnancy: a case of small bowel volvulus and review of the literature. Am Surg 72:1218, 2006

Blumenfeld YJ, Wong AE, Jafari A, et al: MR imaging in cases of antenatal suspected appendicitis—a meta-analysis. J Matern Fetal Neonatal Med 24(3):485, 2011

Bolin M, Akerud H, Cnattingius S, et al: Hyperemesis gravidarum and risks of placental dysfunction disorders: a population-based cohort study. BJOG 120(5):541, 2013

Bondok RS, Sharnouby NM, Eid HE, et al: Pulsed steroid therapy is an effective treatment for intractable hyperemesis gravidarum. Crit Care Med 34:2781, 2006

Bortoli A, Pedersen N, Duricova D, et al: Pregnancy outcome in inflammatory bowel disease: prospective European case-control ECCO-Epicom study, 2003–2006. Aliment Pharmacol Ther 34(7):724, 2011

Briggs GG, Freeman RK, Yaffee SJ: Drugs in Pregnancy and Lactation, 9th ed. Baltimore, Williams & Wilkins, 2011

Brygger L, Fristrup CW, Harbo FS, et al: Acute gastric incarceration from thoracic herniation in pregnancy following laparoscopic antireflux surgery. BMJ Case Rep pii: bcr2012008391, 2013

Buckwalter JG, Simpson SW: Psychological factors in the etiology and treatment of severe nausea and vomiting in pregnancy. Am J Obstet Gynecol 186:S210, 2002

Bush MC, Patel S, Lapinski RH, et al: Perinatal outcomes in inflammatory bowel disease. J Matern Fetal Neonatal Med 15:237, 2004

Butala P, Greenstein AJ, Sur MD, et al: Surgical management of acute right lower-quadrant pain in pregnancy: a prospective cohort study. J Am Coll Surg 211(4):491, 2010

Camilleri M, Murray JA: Diarrhea and constipation. In Longo DL, Fauci AS, Kasper DL, et al (eds): Harrison's Principles of Internal Medicine, 18th ed. New York, McGraw-Hill, 2012, p 308

Cappell MS: Risks versus benefits of gastrointestinal endoscopy during pregnancy. Nat Rev Gastroenterol Hepatol 8(11):610, 2011

Cappell MS: Sedation and analgesia for gastrointestinal endoscopy during pregnancy. Gastrointest Endosc Clin North Am 16:1, 2006

Cappell MS, Fox SR, Gorrepati N: Safety and efficacy of colonoscopy during pregnancy: an analysis of pregnancy outcome in 20 patients. J Reprod Med 55(3–4):115, 2010

Cappell MS, Garcia A: Gastric and duodenal ulcers during pregnancy. Gastroenterol Clin North Am 27:169, 1998

Carter JF, Soper DE: Operative laparoscopy in pregnancy. J Soc Laparoendosc Surg 8:57, 2004

Casanova MJ, Chaparro M, Doménech E, et al: Safety of thiopurines and anti-TNF-α drugs during pregnancy in patients with inflammatory bowel disease. Am J Gastroenterol 108(3):433, 2013

Cedergren M, Brynhildsen, Josefsson A, et al: Hyperemesis gravidarum that requires hospitalization and the use of antiemetic drugs in relation to maternal body composition. Am J Obstet Gynecol 198:412.e1, 2008

Centers for Disease Control and Prevention: Guidelines for the prevention of intravascular catheter-related infections. MMWR 51(10):1, 2002

Chen X, Yang X, Cheng W: Diaphragmatic tear in pregnancy induced by intractable vomiting: a case report and review of the literature. J Matern Fetal Neonatal Med 25(9):1822, 2012

Chiossi G, Neri I, Cavazzuti M, et al: Hyperemesis gravidarum complicated by Wernicke encephalopathy: background, case report, and review of the literature. Obstet Gynecol Surv 61:255, 2006

Christodoulou-Smith J, Gold JI, Romero R, et al: Posttraumatic stress symptoms following pregnancy complicated by hyperemesis gravidarum. J Matern Fetal Neonatal Med 24(11):1307, 2011

Clark DH: Peptic ulcer in women. BMJ 1:1254, 1953

Cohen S, Harris LD: Does hiatus hernia affect competence of the gastroesophageal sphincter? N Engl J Med 284(19):1053, 1971

Cohen-Kerem R, Railton C, Oren D, et al: Pregnancy outcome following nonobstetric surgical intervention. Am J Surg 190:467, 2005

Colombel JF, Sanborn WJ, Reinisch W, et al: Infliximab, azathioprine, or combination therapy for Crohn's disease. N Engl J Med 362(15):1383, 2010

Cominelli F: Inhibition of leukocyte trafficking in inflammatory bowel disease. N Engl J Med 369(8):775, 2013

Connolly MM, Unti JA, Nora PF: Bowel obstruction in pregnancy. Surg Clin North Am 75:101, 1995

Cornish J, Wooding K, Tan E, et al: Study of sexual, urinary, and fecal function in females following restorative proctocolectomy. Inflamm Bowel Dis 18(9):1601, 2012

Cornish JA, Tan E, Teare J, et al: The effect of restorative proctocolectomy on sexual function, urinary function, fertility, pregnancy and delivery: a systematic review. Dis Colon Rectum 50:1128, 2007

Costigan KA, Sipsma HL, DiPietro JA: Pregnancy folklore revisited: the case of heartburn and hair. Birth 33:311, 2006

Curran D, Lorenz R, Czako P: Gastric outlet obstruction at 30 weeks' gestation. Obstet Gynecol 93:851, 1999
Davis MR, Bohon CJ: Intestinal obstruction in pregnancy. Clin Obstet Gynecol 26:832, 1983
Debby A, Golan A, Sadan O, et al: Clinical utility of esophagogastroduodenoscopy in the management of recurrent and intractable vomiting in pregnancy. J Reprod Med 53:347, 2008
De Giorgio R, Knowles CH: Acute colonic pseudo-obstruction. Br J Surg 96(3):229, 2009
de Veciana M, Towers CV, Major CA, et al: Pulmonary injury associated with appendicitis in pregnancy: who is at risk? Am J Obstet Gynecol 171(4):1008, 1994
Dewhurst C, Beddy P, Pedrosa I: MRI evaluation of acute appendicitis in pregnancy. J Magn Reson Imaging 37(3):566, 2013
Diav-Citrin O, Arnon J, Shechtman S, et al: The safety of proton pump inhibitors in pregnancy: a multicentre prospective controlled study. Aliment Pharmacol Ther 21:269, 2005
Di Gangi S, Gizzo S, Patrelli TS, et al: Wernicke's encephalopathy complicating hyperemesis gravidarum: from the background to the present. J Matern Fetal Neonatal Med 25(8):1499, 2012
Dodds L, Fell DB, Joseph KS, et al: Outcomes of pregnancies complicated by hyperemesis gravidarum. Obstet Gynecol 107:285, 2006
Dokmeci F, Engin-Ustun Y, Ustun Y, et al: Trace element status in plasma and erythrocytes in hyperemesis gravidarum. J Reprod Med 49:200, 2004
Dominitz JA, Young JC, Boyko EJ: Outcomes of infants born to mothers with inflammatory bowel disease: a population-based cohort study. Am J Gastroenterol 97:641, 2002
Donkervoort SC, Boerma D: Suspicion of acute appendicitis in the third trimester of pregnancy: pros and cons of a laparoscopic procedure. JSLS 15(3):379, 2011
Dozois EJ, Wolff BG, Tremaine WJ, et al: Maternal and fetal outcome after colectomy for fulminant ulcerative colitis during pregnancy: case series and literature review. Dis Colon Rectum 49:64, 2006
Dray X, Hamzi L, Lo Dico R, et al: Endoscopic reduction of a volvulus of the sigmoid colon in a pregnancy woman. Dig Liver Dis 44(5):447, 2012
Duggar CR, Carlan SJ: The efficacy of methylprednisolone in the treatment of hyperemesis gravidarum: a randomized double-blind controlled study [Abstract]. Obstet Gynecol 97:45S, 2001
Dzieniszewski J, Jarosz M: Guidelines in the medical treatment of *Helicobacter pylori* infection. J Physiol Pharmacol 57(Suppl 3):143, 2006
Elbaz G, Fich A, Levy A: Inflammatory bowel disease and preterm pregnancy. Int J Gynecol Obstet 90:193, 2005
Emerson J, Allen A, Page J, et al: Ulcerative colitis in pregnancy. Abstract No. 171, Am J Obstet Gynecol 208(1 Suppl):S83, 2013
Essilfie P, Hussain M, Stokes IM: Small bowel infarction secondary to volvulus during pregnancy: a case report. J Reprod Med 52:553, 2007
Everson GT: Gastrointestinal motility in pregnancy. Gastroenterol Clin North Am 21:751, 1992
Farouk R, Pemberton JH, Wolff BG, et al: Functional outcomes after ileal pouch–anal anastomosis for chronic ulcerative colitis. Ann Surg 231:919, 2000
Fassina G, Osculati A: Achalasia and sudden death: a case report. Forensic Sci Int 75:133, 1995
Fatum M, Rojansky N: Laparoscopic surgery during pregnancy. Obstet Gynecol Surv 56:50, 2001
Feagins LA, Kane SV: Sexual and reproductive issues for men with inflammatory bowel disease. Am J Gastroenterol 104(3):768, 2009
Fell DB, Dodds L, Joseph KS, et al: Risk factors for hyperemesis gravidarum requiring hospital admission during pregnancy. Obstet Gynecol 107:277, 2006
Fiest TC, Foong A, Chokhavatia S: Successful balloon dilation of achalasia during pregnancy. Gastrointest Endosc 39:810, 1993
Firstenberg MS, Malangoni MA: Gastrointestinal surgery during pregnancy. Gastroenterol Clin North Am 27:73, 1998
Flick RP, Bofill JA, King JC: Pregnancy complicated by traumatic diaphragmatic rupture. A case report. J Reprod Med 44:127, 1999
Fogel EL, Sherman S: ERCP for gallstone pancreatitis. N Engl J Med 370:150, 2014
Folk JJ, Leslie-Brown HF, Nosovitch JT, et al: Hyperemesis gravidarum: Outcomes and complications with and without total parenteral nutrition. J Reprod Med 49:497, 2004
Fonager K, Sorensen HT, Olsen J, et al: Pregnancy outcome for women with Crohn's disease: a follow-up study based on linkage between national registries. Am J Gastroenterol 93:2426, 1998
Food and Drug Administration: FDA news release. FDA approves Diclegis for pregnant women experiencing nausea and vomiting. 2013. Available at: http://www.fda.gov/NewsEvents/Newsroom/PressAnnouncements/ucm347087.htm. Accessed January 17, 2014
Food and Drug Administration: Information for Healthcare Professionals: Mycophenolate Mofetil (marketed as CellCept) and Mycophenolic Acid (marketed as Myfortic), 2008. Available at: http://www.fda.gov/drugs/drugsafety/postmarketdrugsafetyinformationforpatientsandproviders/ucm124776.htm. Accessed May 14, 2013
Forsnes EV, Eggleston MK, Heaton JO: Enterovesical fistula complicating pregnancy: a case report. J Reprod Med 44:297, 1999
Friedman S, Blumberg RS: Inflammatory bowel disease. In Longo DL, Fauci AS, Kasper DL, et al (eds): Harrison's Principles of Internal Medicine, 18th ed. New York, McGraw-Hill, 2012, p 2477
Gearhart SL, Silen W: Acute appendicitis and peritonitis. In Fauci AS, Braunwald E, Kasper DL, et al (eds): Harrison's Principles of Internal Medicine, 17th ed. New York, McGraw-Hill, 2008, p 1914
Gilinsky NH, Muthunayagam N: Gastrointestinal endoscopy in pregnant and lactating women: emerging standard of care to guide decision-making. Obstet Gynecol Surv 61:791, 2006
Gilstrap LC, Van Dorsten PV, Cunningham FG (eds): Diagnostic and operative laparoscopy. In Operative Obstetrics, 2nd ed. New York, McGraw-Hill, 2002, p 453
Goldberg D, Szilagyi A, Graves L: Hyperemesis gravidarum and *Helicobacter pylori* infection. Obstet Gynecol 110:695, 2007
Goodwin TM, Nwankwo OA, O'Leary LD, et al: The first demonstration that a subset of women with hyperemesis gravidarum has abnormalities in the vestibuloocular reflex pathway. Am J Obstet Gynecol 199:417.e1, 2008
Gopal KA, Amshel AL, Shonberg IL, et al: Ostomy and pregnancy. Dis Colon Rectum 28:912, 1985
Gould CH, Maybee GJ, Leininger B, et al: Primary intussusception in pregnancy: a case report. J Reprod Med 53:703, 2008
Grjibovski AM, Vikanes A, Stoltenberg C, et al: Consanguinity and the risk of hyperemesis gravidarum in Norway. Acta Obstet Gynecol Scand 87:20, 2008
Guglielmi FW, Baggio-Bertinet D, Federico A, et al: Total parenteral nutrition-related gastroenterological complications. Digest Liver Dis 38:623, 2006
Gungor S, Gurates B, Aydin S, et al: Ghrelins, obestatin, nesfatin-1 and leptin levels in pregnant women with and without hyperemesis gravidarum. Clin Biochem 46(9):828, 2013
Haggar F, Pereira G, Preen D, et al: Maternal and neonatal outcomes in pregnancies following colorectal cancer. Surg Endosc 27(7):2327, 2013
Hahnloser D, Pemberton JH, Wolff BG, et al: Pregnancy and delivery before and after ileal pouch-anal anastomosis for inflammatory bowel disease: immediate and long-term consequences and outcomes. Dis Colon Rectum 47:1127, 2004
Hamaoui E, Hamaoui M: Nutritional assessment and support during pregnancy. Gastroenterol Clin North Am 32:59, 2003
Harma M, Harma MI, Karadeniz G, et al: Idiopathic ileoileal invagination two days after cesarean section. J Obstet Gynaecol Res 37(2):160, 2011
Hée P, Viktrup L: The diagnosis of appendicitis during pregnancy and maternal and fetal outcome after appendectomy. Int J Gynaecol Obstet 65:129, 1999
Hesketh PJ: Chemotherapy-induced nausea and vomiting. N Engl J Med 358: 2482, 2008
Hill JB, Yost NP, Wendel GW Jr: Acute renal failure in association with severe hyperemesis gravidarum. Obstet Gynecol 100:1119, 2002
Holmgren C, Aagaard-Tillery KM, Silver RM, et al: Hyperemesis in pregnancy: an evaluation of treatment strategies with maternal and neonatal outcomes. Am J Obstet Gynecol 198:56.e1, 2008
Hux C: Ostomy and pregnancy. Ostomy Wound Manage 56(1):48, 2010
Hytten FE: The alimentary system. In Hytten F, Chamberlain G (eds): Clinical Physiology in Obstetrics. London, Blackwell, 1991, p 137
Israel GM, Malguira N, McCarthy S, et al: MRI vs. ultrasound for suspected appendicitis during pregnancy. J Magn Reson Imaging 28:428, 2008
Jewell D, Young G: Interventions for nausea and vomiting in early pregnancy. Cochrane Database Syst Rev 2: CD000145, 2000
Kahrilas PJ, Hirano I: Diseases of the esophagus. In Longo DL, Fauci AS, Kasper DL, et al (eds): Harrison's Principles of Internal Medicine, 18th ed. New York, McGraw-Hill, 2012, p 2427
Kamani L, Mahmood S, Faisal N: Therapeutic endoscopic retrograde cholangiopancreatography without ultrasound or fluoroscopy in pregnancy. Endoscopy 44(Suppl 2):E196, 2012
Kappelman MD, Horvath-Puho E, Sandler RS, et al: Thromboembolic risk among Danish children and adults with inflammatory bowel diseases: a population-based nationwide study. Gut 60(7):937, 2011
Kastenberg ZJ, Hurley MP, Luan A, et al: Cost-effectiveness of preoperative imaging ultrasonography in the second or third trimester of pregnancy. Obstet Gynecol 122:821, 2013
Katz DS, Klein MA, Ganson G, et al: Imaging of abdominal pain in pregnancy. Radiol Clin North Am 50(1):149, 2012
Katz JA: Endoscopy in the pregnant patient with inflammatory bowel disease. Gastrointest Endosc Clin North Am 12:635, 2002

Katz JA, Antonio C, Keenan GF, et al: Outcome pregnancy in women receiving infliximab for the treatment of Crohn's disease and rheumatoid arthritis. Am J Gastroenterol 99:2385, 2004
Kawamura Y, Kawamata K, Shinya M, et al: Vitamin K deficiency in hyperemesis gravidarum as a potential cause of fetal intracranial hemorrhage and hydrocephalus. Prenat Diagn 28:59, 2008
Khan MR, Ur Rehman S: Sigmoid volvulus in pregnancy and puerperium: a surgical and obstetric catastrophe. Report of a case and review of the world literature. World J Emerg Surg 7(1):10, 2012
Khandelwal A, Fasih N, Kielar A: Imaging of the acute abdomen in pregnancy. Radiol Clin North Am 51:1005, 2013
Khudyak V, Lysy J, Mankuta D: Achalasia in pregnancy. Obstet Gynecol Surv 61:207, 2006
Korelitz BI: Inflammatory bowel disease and pregnancy. Gastroenterol Clin North Am 27:214, 1998
Kort B, Katz VL, Watson MJ: The effect of nonobstetric operation during pregnancy. Surg Gynecol Obstet 177:371, 1993
Kurzel RB, Naunheim KS, Schwartz RA: Repair of symptomatic diaphragmatic hernia during pregnancy. Obstet Gynecol 71:869, 1988
Lacasse A, Rey E, Ferreira E, et al: Validity of a modified Pregnancy-Unique Quantification of Emesis and Nausea (PUQE) scoring index to assess severity of nausea and vomiting of pregnancy. Am J Obstet Gynecol 198:71.e1, 2008
Lal SK, Morgenstern R, Vinjirayer EP, et al: Sigmoid volvulus: an update. Gastrointest Endosc Clin North Am 16:175, 2006
Lawson M, Kern F, Everson GT: Gastrointestinal transit time in human pregnancy: prolongation in the second and third trimesters followed by postpartum normalization. Gastroenterology 89:996, 1985
Lichtenstein GC, Hanauer SB, Sandborn WJ, et al: Management of Crohn's disease in adults. Am J Gastroenterol 104(2):465, 2009
Lyell DJ: Adhesions and perioperative complications of repeat cesarean delivery. Am J Obstet Gynecol 205(6 Suppl):S11, 2011
Mahadevan U: Fertility and pregnancy in the patient with inflammatory bowel disease. Gut 55:1198, 2006a
Mahadevan U, Kane S: American Gastroenterological Association Institute technical review on the use of gastrointestinal medications in pregnancy. Gastroenterology 131(1):283, 2006b
Mahadevan US, Sandborn W, Hakimian S: Pregnancy outcomes in women with inflammatory bowel disease: a population based cohort study. Gastroenterology 128(Suppl 2):A322, 2005
Malecki EA, Skagen CL, Frick TJ, et al: Ileoanal pouch inlet obstruction following cesarean section. Am J Gastroenterol 105(8):1906, 2010
Matsubara S, Kuwata T, Kamozawa C, et al: Connection between hyperemesis gravidarum, jaundice or liver dysfunction, and biliary sludge. J Obstet Gynaecol Res 38(2):446, 2012
Mayberry JF, Atkinson M: Achalasia and pregnancy. Br J Obstet Gynaecol 94:855, 1987
Mays J, Verma U, Klein S, et al: Acute appendicitis in pregnancy and the occurrence of major intraventricular hemorrhage and periventricular leukomalacia. Obstet Gynecol 86:650, 1995
Mazze RI, Källén B: Appendectomy during pregnancy: a Swedish registry study of 778 cases. Obstet Gynecol 77:835, 1991
Mazze RI, Källén B: Reproductive outcome after anesthesia and operation during pregnancy: a registry study of 5405 cases. Am J Obstet Gynecol 161:1178, 1989
McCarthy FP, Khashan AS, North RA, et al: A prospective cohort study investigating associations between hyperemesis gravidarum and cognitive, behavioural and emotional well-being in pregnancy. PLoS One 6(11):e27678, 2011
McGory ML, Zingmond DS, Tillou A, et al: Negative appendectomy in pregnant women is associated with a substantial risk of fetal loss. J Am Coll Surg 205:534, 2007
McKenna D, Watson P, Dornan J: *Helicobacter pylori* infection and dyspepsia in pregnancy. Obstet Gynecol 102:845, 2003
McKenna DA, Meehan CP, Alhajeri AN, et al: The use of MRI to demonstrate small bowel obstruction during pregnancy. Br J Radiol 80:e11, 2007
Mehta N, Saha S, Chien EKS, et al: Disorders of the gastrointestinal tract in pregnancy. In Powrie R, Greene M, Camann W (eds): de Swiet's Medical Disorders in Obstetric Practice, 5th ed. New Jersey, Wiley-Blackwell, 2010, p 256
Meyerson S, Holtz T, Ehrinpresis M, et al: Small bowel obstruction in pregnancy. Am J Gastroenterol 90:299, 1995
Miller JP: Inflammatory bowel disease in pregnancy: a review. J R Soc Med 79:221, 1986
Modigliani RM: Gastrointestinal and pancreatic disease. In Barron WM, Lindheimer MD, Davison JM (eds): Medical Disorders of Pregnancy, 3rd ed. St. Louis, Mosby, 2000, p 316
Moskovitz DN, Bodian C, Chapman ML, et al: The effect on the fetus of medications used to treat pregnant inflammatory bowel-disease patients. Am J Gastroenterol 99:656, 2004
Mourad J, Elliott JP, Erickson L, et al: Appendicitis in pregnancy: new information that contradicts long-held clinical beliefs. Am J Obstet Gynecol 185:1027, 2000
Mullin PM, Ching C, Schoenberg R, et al: Risk factors, treatments, and outcomes associated with prolonged hyperemesis gravidarum. J Matern Fetal Neonatal Med 25(6):632, 2012
Niebyl JR: Nausea and vomiting in pregnancy. N Engl J Med 363(16):1544, 2010
Norgård B, Hundborg HH, Jacobsen BA, et al: Disease activity in pregnant women with Crohn's disease and birth outcomes: a regional Danish cohort study. Am J Gastroenterol 102:1947, 2007
Novacek G, Weltermann A, Sobala A, et al: Inflammatory bowel disease is a risk factor for recurrent venous thromboembolism. Gastroenterology 139(3):779, 2010
Nwoko R, Plecas D, Garovic VD: Acute kidney injury in the pregnant patient. Clin Nephrol 78(6):478, 2012
Ogura JM, Francois KE, Perlow JH, et al: Complications associated with peripherally inserted central catheter use during pregnancy. Am J Obstet Gynecol 188:1223, 2003
O'Mahony S: Endoscopy in pregnancy. Best Pract Res Clin Gastroenterol 21:893, 2007
Ooi BS, Remzi FH, Fazio VW: Turnbull-blowhole colostomy for toxic ulcerative colitis in pregnancy: report of two cases. Dis Colon Rectum 46:111, 2003
Oron G, Yogev Y, Shkolnik S, et al: Inflammatory bowel disease: risk factors for adverse pregnancy outcome and the impact of maternal weight gain. J Matern Fetal Neonatal Med 25(112):2256, 2012
Ortega-Carnicer J, Ambrós A, Alcazar R: Obstructive shock due to labor-related diaphragmatic hernia. Crit Care Med 26:616, 1998
Oto A, Ernst R, Ghulmiyyah L, et al: The role of MR cholangiopancreatography in the evaluation of pregnant patients with acute pancreaticobiliary disease. Br J Radiol 82(976):279, 2009
Palacios-Marqués A, Delgado-Garcia S, Martín-Bayón T, et al: Wernicke's encephalopathy induced by hyperemesis gravidarum. BMJ Case Rep Jun 8, 2012
Panesar NS, Chan KW, Li CY, et al: Status of anti-thyroid peroxidase during normal pregnancy and in patients with hyperemesis gravidarum. Thyroid 16:481, 2006
Parangi S, Levine D, Henry A, et al: Surgical gastrointestinal disorders during pregnancy. Am J Surg 193:223, 2007
Paranyuk Y, Levin G, Figueroa R: Candida septicemia in a pregnant woman with hyperemesis receiving parenteral nutrition. Obstet Gynecol 107:535, 2006
Pates JA, Avendanio TC, Zaretsky MV, et al: The appendix in pregnancy: confirming historical observations with a contemporary modality. Obstet Gynecol 114(4):805, 2009
Pearl J, Price R, Richardson W: SAGES' guidelines for diagnosis, treatment, and use of laparoscopy for surgical problems during pregnancy. Surg Endosc 25:1927, 2011
Pedrosa I, Lafornara M, Pandharipande PV, et al: Pregnant patients suspected of having acute appendicitis: effect of MR imaging on negative laparotomy rate and appendiceal perforation rate. Radiology 250(3):749, 2009
Perdue PW, Johnson HW Jr, Stafford PW: Intestinal obstruction complicating pregnancy. Am J Surg 164:384, 1992
Podolsky DK: Inflammatory bowel disease. N Engl J Med 347(6):417, 2002
Ponec RJ, Saunders MD, Kimmey MB: Neostigmine for the treatment of acute colonic pseudo-obstruction. N Engl J Med 341:137, 1999
Poursharif B, Korst LM, Macgibbon KW, et al: Elective pregnancy termination in a large cohort of women with hyperemesis gravidarum. Contraception 76:451, 2007
Prefontaine E, Sutherland LR, Macdonald JK, et al: Azathioprine or 6-mercaptopurine for maintenance of remission in Crohn's disease. Cochrane Database Syst Rev 1:CD000067, 2009
Rahimi R, Nikfar S, Rezaie A, et al: Pregnancy outcome in women with inflammatory bowel disease following exposure to 5-aminosalicylic acid drugs: a meta-analysis. Reprod Toxicol 25:271, 2008
Raman SS, Osuagwu FC, Kadell B, et al: Effect of CE on false positive diagnosis of appendicitis and perforation. N Engl J Med 358:972, 2008
Ravid A, Richard CS, Spencer LM, et al: Pregnancy, delivery, and pouch function after ileal pouch-anal anastomosis for ulcerative colitis. Dis Colon Rectum 45:1283, 2002
Rawlings C: Management of postcaesarian Ogilvie's syndrome and their subsequent outcomes. Aust N Z J Obstet Gynaecol 50(6):573, 2010
Reddy D, Murphy SJ, Kane SV, et al: Relapses of inflammatory bowel disease during pregnancy: in-hospital management and birth outcomes. Am J Gastroenterol 103:1203, 2008
Reedy MB, Källén B, Kuehl TJ: Laparoscopy during pregnancy: a study of five fetal outcome parameters with use of the Swedish Health Registry. Am J Obstet Gynecol 177:673, 1997

Redlich A, Rickes S, Costa SD, et al: Small bowel obstruction in pregnancy. Arch Gynecol Obstet 275(5):381, 2007
Rigler LG, Eneboe JB: Incidence of hiatus hernia in pregnant women and its significance. J Thorac Surg 4:262, 1935
Riis L, Vind I, Politi P, et al: Does pregnancy change the disease course? A study in a European cohort of patients with inflammatory bowel disease. Am J Gastroenterol 101:1539, 2006
Rizzo AG: Laparoscopic surgery in pregnancy: long-term follow-up. J Laparoendosco Adv Surg Tech A 13:11, 2003
Robinson JN, Banerjee R, Thiet MP: Coagulopathy secondary to vitamin K deficiency in hyperemesis gravidarum. Obstet Gynecol 92:673, 1998
Rollins MD, Chan KJ, Price RR: Laparoscopy for appendicitis and cholelithiasis during pregnancy: a new standard of care. Surg Endosc 18:237, 2004
Roux CH, Brocq O, Breuil V, et al: Pregnancy in rheumatology patients exposed to anti-tumour necrosis factor (TNF)-α therapy. Rheumatology 46:695, 2007
Russo-Stieglitz KE, Levine AB, Wagner BA, et al: Pregnancy outcome in patients requiring parenteral nutrition. J Matern Fetal Med 8:164, 1999
Safari HR, Fassett MJ, Souter IC, et al: The efficacy of methylprednisolone in the treatment of hyperemesis gravidarum: a randomized, double-blind, controlled study. Am J Obstet Gynecol 179:921, 1998
Saha S, Loranger D, Pricolo V, et al: Geeding jejunostomy for the treatment of sever hyperemesis gravidarum: a case series. JPEN J Parenter Enteral Nutr 33(5):529, 2009
Sakai M, Yoneda S, Sasaki Y, et al: Maternal total parenteral nutrition and fetal subdural hematoma. Obstet Gynecol 101:1142, 2003
Sandborn WJ, Feagan BG, Stoinov S, et al: Certolizumab pegol for the treatment of Crohn's disease. N Engl J Med 357:228, 2007
Satin AJ, Twickler D, Gilstrap LC: Esophageal achalasia in late pregnancy. Obstet Gynecol 79:812, 1992
Schiff MA, Reed SD, Daling JR: The sex ratio of pregnancies complicated by hospitalisation for hyperemesis gravidarum. Br J Obstet Gynaecol 111:27, 2004
Schnitzler F, Fidder H, Ferrante M, et al: Outcome of pregnancy in women with inflammatory bowel disease treated with antitumor necrosis factor therapy. Inflamm Bowel Dis 17(9):1846, 2011
Schrag SP, Sharma R, Jaik NP, et al: Complications related to percutaneous endoscopic gastrostomy (PEG) tubes: a comprehensive clinical review. J Gastrointest Liver Dis 16:407, 2007
Schreiber S, Khaliq-Kareemi M, Lawrance IC, et al: Maintenance therapy with certolizumab pegol for Crohn's disease. N Engl J Med 357:239, 2007
Schwartz M, Rossoff L: Pneumomediastinum and bilateral pneumothoraces in a patient with hyperemesis gravidarum. Chest 106:1904, 1994
Schwentner L, Wulff C, Kreienberg R, et al: Exacerbation of a maternal hiatus hernia in early pregnancy presenting with symptoms of hyperemesis gravidarum: case report and review of the literature. Arch Gynecol Obstet 283(3):409, 2011
Selby WS, Griffin S, Abraham N, et al: Appendectomy protects against the development of ulcerative colitis but does not affect its course. Am J Gastroenterol 97:2834, 2002
Selitsky T, Chandra P, Schiavello HJ: Wernicke's encephalopathy with hyperemesis and ketoacidosis. Obstet Gynecol 107:486, 2006
Sharifah H, Naidu A, Vimal K: Diaphragmatic hernia: an unusual cause of postpartum collapse. Br J Obstet Gynaecol 110:701, 2003
Shui LH, Rafi J, Corder A, et al: Mid-gut volvulus and mesenteric vessel thrombosis in pregnancy: case report and literature review. Arch Gynecol Obstet 283 (Suppl 1):39, 2011
Siddiqui U, Denise-Proctor D: Flexible sigmoidoscopy and colonoscopy during pregnancy. Gastrointest Endosc Clin North Am 16:59, 2006
Singh S, Nadgir A, Bryan RM: Post-cesarean section acute colonic pseudo-obstruction with spontaneous perforation. Int J Gynaecol Obstet 89:144, 2005
Song LMWK, Topazian M: Gastrointestinal endoscopy. In Longo DL, Fauci AS, Kasper DL, et al (eds): Harrison's Principles of Internal Medicine, 18th ed. New York, McGraw-Hill, 2012, p 2409
Soper NJ: SAGES' guidelines for diagnosis, treatment, and use of laparoscopy for surgical problems during pregnancy. Surg Endosc 25:3477, 2011
Spiliopoulos D, Spiliopoulos M, Awala A: Esophageal achalasia: an uncommon complication during pregnancy treated conservatively. Case Rep Obstet Gynecol 2013(639698):1, 2013
Stephansson O, Larsson H, Pedersen L, et al: Crohn's disease is a risk factor for preterm birth. Clin Gastroenterol Hepatol 8(6):509, 2010
Storch I, Barkin JS: Contraindications to capsule endoscopy: do any still exist? Gastrointest Endosc Clin North Am 16:329, 2006
Suerbaum S, Michetti P: *Helicobacter pylori* infection. N Engl J Med 347:1175, 2002
Sullivan CA, Johnson CA, Roach H, et al: A pilot study of intravenous ondansetron for hyperemesis gravidarum. Am J Obstet Gynecol 174:1565, 1996
Swallow BL, Lindow SW, Masson EA, et al: Psychological health in early pregnancy: relationship with nausea and vomiting. J Obstet Gynaecol 24:28, 2004
Swartzlander TK, Carlan SJ, Locksmith G, et al: Sonographic confirmation of the correct placement of a nasoenteral tube in a women with hyperemesis gravidarum: case report. J Clin Ultrasound 41(Suppl 1):18, 2013
Takahashi K, Funayama Y, Fukushima K, et al: Pregnancy and delivery in patients with enterostomy due to anorectal complications from Crohn's disease. Int J Colorectal Dis 22:313, 2007
Tan JY, Loh KC, Yeo GS, et al: Transient hyperthyroidism of hyperemesis gravidarum. Br J Obstet Gynaecol 109:683, 2002
Tan PC, Jacob R, Quek KF, et al: The fetal sex ratio and metabolic, biochemical, haematological and clinical indicators of severity of hyperemesis gravidarum. BJOG 113:733, 2006
Tan PC, Norazilah MJ, Omar SZ: Dextrose saline compared with normal saline rehydration of hyperemesis gravidarum: a randomized controlled trial. Obstet Gynecol 121(2 Pt1):291, 2013
Tang SJ, Mayo MJ, Rodriguez-Frias E, et al: Safety and utility of ERCP during pregnancy. Gastrointest Endosc 69(3Pt 1):453, 2009
Torquati A, Lutfi R, Khaitan L, et al: Heller myotomy vs Heller myotomy plus Dor fundoplication: cost-utility analysis of a randomized trial. Surg Endosc 20:389, 2006
Trogstad LI, Stoltenberg C, Magnus P, et al: Recurrence risk in hyperemesis gravidarum. BJOG 112:1641, 2005
Tung CS, Zighelboim I, Gardner MO: Acute colonic pseudoobstruction complicating twin pregnancy. J Reprod Med 53:52, 2008
Turcotte S, Dubé S, Beauchamp G: Peripherally inserted central venous catheters are not superior to central venous catheters in the acute care of surgical patients on the ward. World J Surg 30:1603, 2006
Ueberrueck T, Koch A, Meyer L, et al: Ninety-four appendectomies for suspected acute appendicitis during pregnancy. World J Surg 28:508, 2004
Unal A, Sayherman SE, Ozel L, et al: Acute abdomen in pregnancy requiring surgical management: a 20-case series. Eur J Obstet Gynecol Reprod Biol 159(1):87, 2011
Vaisman N, Kaidar R, Levin I, et al: Nasojejunal feeding in hyperemesis gravidarum—a preliminary study. Clin Nutr 23:53, 2004
Vaknin Z, Halperin R, Schneider D, et al: Hyperemesis gravidarum and nonspecific abnormal EEG findings. J Reprod Med 51:623, 2006
Veenendaal MV, van Abeelen AF, Painter RC, et al: Consequences of hyperemesis gravidarum for offspring: a systematic review and meta-analysis. BJOG 118(11):1302, 2011
Verberg MF, Gillott JD, Fardan NA, et al: Hyperemesis gravidarum, a literature review. Hum Reprod Update 11:527, 2005
Viktrup L, Hée P: Fertility and long-term complications four to nine years after appendectomy during pregnancy. Acta Obstet Gynecol Scand 77:746, 1998
Wald A: Constipation, diarrhea, and symptomatic hemorrhoids during pregnancy. Gastroenterol Clin North Am 32:309, 2003
Waljee A, Waljee J, Morris AM, et al: Threefold increased risk of infertility: a meta-analysis of infertility after ileal pouch anal anastomosis in ulcerative colitis. Gut 55:1575, 2006
Wallace CA, Petrov MS, Soybel DI, et al: Influence of imaging on the negative appendectomy rate in pregnancy. J Gastrointest Surg 12:46, 2008
Wataganara T, Leelakusolvong S, Sunsaneevithayakul P, et al: Treatment of severe achalasia during pregnancy with esophagoscopic injection of botulinum toxin A: a case report. J Perinatol 29(9):637, 2009
Wax JR, Pinette MG, Cartin A: Roux-en-Y gastric bypass-associated bowel obstruction complicating pregnancy—an obstetrician's map to the clinical minefield. Am J Obstet Gynecol 208(4):265, 2013
Wei PL, Keller JJ, Liang HH, et al: Acute appendicitis and adverse pregnancy outcomes: a nationwide population-based study. J Gastrointest Surg 16(6):1204, 2012
Weyermann M, Brenner H, Adler G, et al: *Helicobacter pylori* infection and the occurrence and severity of gastrointestinal symptoms during pregnancy. Am J Obstet Gynecol 189:526, 2003
Wilasrusmee C Sukrat B, McEvoy M, et al: Systematic review and meta-analysis of safety laparoscopic versus open appendicectomy for suspected appendicitis in pregnancy. Br J Surg 99(11):1470, 2012
Woolfson K, Cohen Z, McLeod RS: Crohn's disease and pregnancy. Dis Colon Rectum 33:869, 1990
Yamamoto T, Suzuki Y, Kojima K, et al: Pneumomediastinum secondary to hyperemesis gravidarum during early pregnancy. Acta Obstet Gynecol Scand 80:1143, 2001
Yost NP, McIntire DD, Wians FH Jr, et al: A randomized, placebo-controlled trial of corticosteroids for hyperemesis due to pregnancy. Obstet Gynecol 102:1250, 2003
Zara G, Codemo V, Palmieri A, et al: Neurological complications in hyperemesis gravidarum. Neurol Sci 33(1):133, 2012

CHAPTER 55

Hepatic, Biliary, and Pancreatic Disorders

Disorders of the liver, gallbladder, and pancreas together comprise a formidable list of complications that may arise in pregnancy from preexisting conditions or from some that are unique to pregnancy. The relationships of several of these with pregnancy can be fascinating, intriguing, and challenging.

HEPATIC DISORDERS

It is customary to divide liver diseases complicating pregnancy into three general categories. The first includes those specifically related to pregnancy that resolve either spontaneously or following delivery. Examples are hepatic dysfunction from hyperemesis gravidarum, intrahepatic cholestasis, acute fatty liver, and hepatocellular damage with preeclampsia—the *HELLP syndrome*—hemolysis, elevated serum liver aminotransferase levels, and low platelet counts (Mufti, 2012; Reau, 2014). The second category includes acute hepatic disorders that are coincidental to pregnancy, such as acute viral hepatitis. The third category includes chronic liver diseases that predate pregnancy, such as chronic hepatitis, cirrhosis, or esophageal varices.

There are several pregnancy-induced physiological changes that induce appreciable liver-related clinical and laboratory manifestations (Chap. 4, p. 67, and Appendix, p. 1289). Findings such as elevated serum alkaline phosphatase levels, palmar erythema, and spider angiomas, which might suggest liver disease, are commonly found during normal pregnancy. Metabolism is also affected, due to altered expression of the cytochrome P450 system that is mediated by higher levels of estrogen, progesterone, and other hormones. For example, in pregnancy, hepatic CYP1A2 expression is decreased, whereas that of CYP2D6 and CYP3A4 is increased. Importantly, cytochrome enzymes are expressed in many organs besides the liver, most notably the placenta. The net effect is complex and likely influenced by gestational age and organ of expression (Isoherranen, 2013). Despite all of these functional changes, no major hepatic histological changes are induced by normal pregnancy.

Hyperemesis Gravidarum

Pernicious nausea and vomiting of pregnancy may involve the liver. There may be mild hyperbilirubinemia with serum aminotransferase levels elevated in up to half of women hospitalized. However, these levels seldom exceed 200 U/L (Table 55-1). Liver biopsy may show minimal fatty changes. Hyperemesis gravidarum is discussed in detail in Chapter 54 (p. 1070).

Intrahepatic Cholestasis of Pregnancy

This disorder also has been referred to as recurrent jaundice of pregnancy, cholestatic hepatosis, and icterus gravidarum. It is characterized clinically by pruritus, icterus, or both. It may be more common in multifetal pregnancy, and there is a significant

TABLE 55-1. Clinical and Laboratory Findings with Acute Liver Diseases in Pregnancy

			Hepatic		Renal	Hematological and Coagulation					
Disorder	Onset in Pregnancy	Clinical Findings	AST (U/L)	Bili (mg/dL)	Cr (mg/dL)	Hct	Plat	Fib	DD	PT	Hemolysis
Hyperemesis	Early	Severe N&V	NL–300	NL–4	↑	↑↑	NL	NL	NL	NL	No
Cholestasis	Late	Pruritus, jaundice	NL–200	1–5	NL	NL	NL	NL	NL	NL	No
Fatty liver	Late	Moderate N&V, ± HTN, liver failure	200–800	4–10	↑↑↑	↑↑↑	↓↓	↓↓↓	↑	↑↑	↑↑↑
Preeclampsia	Mid to late	HA, HTN	NL–300	1–4	↑	↑	↓↓	NL	↑	NL	↑–↑↑
Hepatitis	Variable	Jaundice	2000+	5–20	NL	↑	↓	NL	NL	↑	No

↑ = increased levels; ↓ = decreased levels; AST = aspartate aminotransferase; Bili = bilirubin; Cr = creatinine; DD = D-dimers; Fib = fibrinogen; HA = headache; Hct = hematocrit; HTN = hypertension; N&V = nausea and vomiting; NL = normal; Plat = platelets; PT = prothrombin time.

genetic influence (Lausman, 2008; Webb, 2014). Because of this, the incidence of the disorder varies by population. For example, cholestasis is uncommon in North America, with an overall incidence of approximately 1 in 500 to 1000 pregnancies, but is as high as 5.6 percent among Latina women in Los Angeles (Lee, 2006). In Israel, the incidence reported by Sheiner and associates (2006) is approximately 1 in 400. In Sweden, it is 1.5 percent, and in Chile, it is 4 percent (Glantz, 2004; Lee, 2006; Reyes, 1997).

Pathogenesis

The cause of obstetrical cholestasis is unknown. Both increases and decreases in sex steroid levels have been implicated, but current research centers on the numerous mutations that have been identified in the many genes that control hepatocellular transport systems. One example involves mutations of the *ABCB4* gene, which encodes multidrug resistance protein 3 (MDR3) associated with *progressive familial intrahepatic cholestasis,* as well as a bile salt export pump encoded by *ABCB11* (Anzivino, 2013; Davit-Spraul, 2010, 2012; Dixon, 2014). Other potential gene products of interest include the Farnesoid X receptor and transporting ATPase encoded by *ATP8B1* (Davit-Spraul, 2012; Müllenbach, 2005). Some drugs that similarly decrease canalicular transport of bile acids aggravate the disorder. For example, we have encountered impressive cholestatic jaundice in pregnant women taking azathioprine following renal transplantation.

Whatever the inciting cause(s), bile acids are cleared incompletely and accumulate in plasma. Hyperbilirubinemia results from retention of conjugated pigment, but total plasma concentrations rarely exceed 4 to 5 mg/dL. Alkaline phosphatase is usually elevated even more so than in normal pregnancy. Serum aminotransferase levels are normal to moderately elevated but seldom exceed 250 U/L (see Table 55-1). Liver biopsy shows mild cholestasis with bile plugs in the hepatocytes and canaliculi of the centrilobular regions, but without inflammation or necrosis. These changes disappear after delivery but often recur in subsequent pregnancies or with estrogen-containing contraceptives.

Clinical Presentation

Pruritus develops in late pregnancy, although it occasionally manifests earlier. There are no constitutional symptoms, and generalized pruritus shows predilection for the soles. Skin changes are limited to excoriations from scratching. Biochemical tests may be abnormal at presentation, but pruritus may precede laboratory findings by several weeks. Approximately 10 percent of women have jaundice.

With normal liver enzymes, the differential diagnosis of pruritus includes other skin disorders (Chap. 62, p. 1214). Findings are unlikely to be due to preeclamptic liver disease if there are no blood pressure changes or proteinuria. Sonography may be warranted to exclude cholelithiasis and biliary obstruction. *Acute* viral hepatitis is an unlikely diagnosis because of the usually low serum aminotransferase levels seen with cholestasis. Conversely, *chronic hepatitis C* is associated with a significantly increased risk of cholestasis, which may be as high as 20-fold among women who are hepatitis C RNA positive (Marschall, 2013; Paternoster, 2002).

Management

Pruritus may be troublesome and is thought to result from elevated serum bile salt concentrations. *Antihistamines* and *topical emollients* may provide some relief. Although cholestyramine has been reported to be effective, this compound also causes further decreased absorption of fat-soluble vitamins, which may lead to vitamin K deficiency. Fetal coagulopathy may develop, and there are reports of intracranial hemorrhage and stillbirth (Matos, 1997; Sadler, 1995).

A recent metaanalysis suggests that *ursodeoxycholic acid* relieves pruritus, lowers bile acid and serum enzyme levels, and may reduce certain neonatal complications such as preterm birth, fetal distress, respiratory distress syndrome, and neonatal intensive care unit (NICU) admission (Bacq, 2012). Lucangioli and colleagues (2009) documented an especially profound decrease in serum lithocholic acid levels. Kondrackiene and associates (2005) randomly assigned 84 symptomatic women to receive either ursodeoxycholic acid (8 to 10 mg/kg/d) or cholestyramine (8 g/d). They reported superior relief with ursodeoxycholic acid—67 versus 19 percent, respectively. Similarly, Glantz and coworkers (2005) found superior benefits to women randomly assigned to ursodeoxycholic acid versus dexamethasone. The American College of Obstetricians and Gynecologists (2012a) has concluded that ursodeoxycholic acid both relieves pruritus and improves fetal outcomes, although evidence for the latter is not compelling.

Cholestasis and Pregnancy Outcomes

Earlier reports described excessive adverse pregnancy outcomes in women with cholestatic jaundice. Data accrued during the past two decades are ambiguous concerning increased perinatal mortality rates and whether close fetal surveillance is preventative. A review of a few studies illustrates this. Glantz and colleagues (2004) described outcomes in 693 Swedish women. Perinatal mortality rates were slightly increased, but death was limited to infants of mothers with severe disease characterized by total bile acid levels ≥ 40 μmol/L. Sheiner and coworkers (2006) described no differences in perinatal outcomes in 376 affected pregnancies compared with their overall obstetrical population. There was, however, a significant increase in labor inductions and cesarean deliveries in affected women. Lee and associates (2009) described two cases of sudden fetal death not predicted by nonstress testing. Rook and colleagues (2012) reported outcomes of 101 affected women in Northern California. Although there were no term fetal demises, 87 percent of women underwent labor induction, ostensibly to avoid adverse outcomes. Nonetheless, neonatal complications occurred in a third of the pregnancies, particularly respiratory distress, fetal distress, and meconium-stained amnionic fluid, all of which were reported more frequently with higher total bile acid levels. Finally, Wikström Shemer and coworkers (2013) reported outcomes for a population-based Swedish study of 5477 pregnancies complicated by intrahepatic cholestasis of pregnancy among 1,213,668 singleton deliveries. The authors reported novel associations of cholestasis with preeclampsia and gestational diabetes. Although neonates were more likely to have a low 5-minute Apgar score and to be large for gestational age, there was no increased risk of stillbirth. Importantly, the pregnancies were actively managed to avoid stillbirths, and this was reflected in the higher induction and preterm birth rates. Many recommend early delivery by labor induction to avoid stillbirth.

An intriguing finding indicates that bile acids may cause fetal death. Strehlow and associates (2010) reported that the PR interval on fetal echocardiography was significantly prolonged in women with intrahepatic cholestasis. Gorelik and colleagues (2006) suggest that bile acids may cause fetal cardiac arrest after entering cardiomyocytes in abnormal amounts. Using fetal myocyte cultures, they showed expression of several genes that may play a role in bile transport.

Acute Fatty Liver of Pregnancy

The most common cause of acute liver failure during pregnancy is acute fatty liver—also called *acute fatty metamorphosis* or *acute yellow atrophy*. In its worst form, the incidence probably approximates 1 in 10,000 pregnancies (Nelson, 2013). Fatty liver recurring in subsequent pregnancy is uncommon, but a few cases have been described (Usta, 1994).

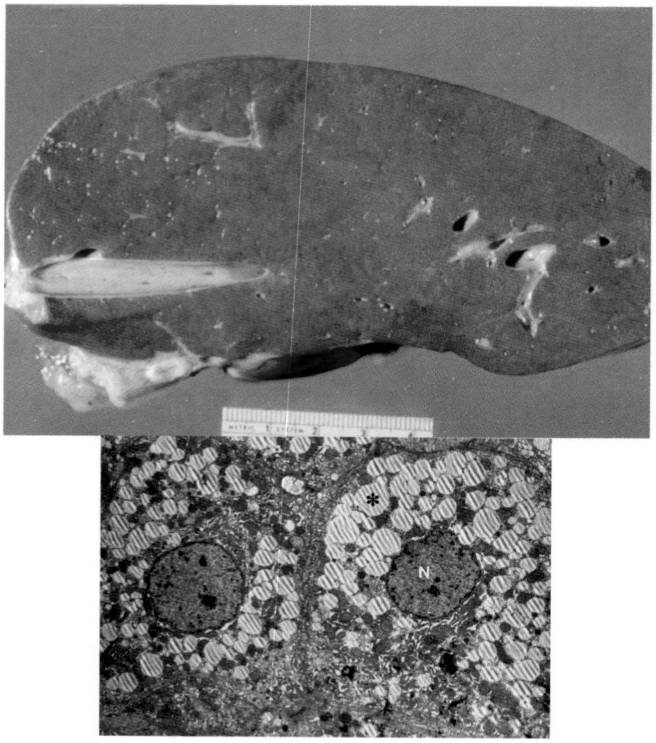

FIGURE 55-1 Acute fatty liver of pregnancy. Cross section of the liver from a woman who died as the result of pulmonary aspiration and respiratory failure. The liver has a greasy yellow appearance, which was present throughout the entire specimen. Inset: Electron photomicrograph of two swollen hepatocytes containing numerous microvesicular fat droplets (*). The nuclei (N) remain centered within the cells, in contrast to the case with macrovesicular fat deposition. (Photograph contributed by Dr. Don Wheeler.)

Fatty liver is characterized by accumulation of microvesicular fat that literally "crowds out" normal hepatocytic function (Fig. 55-1). Grossly, the liver is small, soft, yellow, and greasy.

Etiopathogenesis

Although much has been learned about this disorder, interpretation of conflicting data has led to incomplete but intriguing observations. For example, some if not most cases of maternal fatty liver are associated with recessively inherited mitochondrial abnormalities of fatty acid oxidation. These are similar to those in children with Reye-like syndromes. Several mutations have been described for the mitochondrial trifunctional protein enzyme complex that catalyzes the last oxidative steps in the pathway. The most common are the G1528C and E474Q mutations of the gene on chromosome 2 that code for long-chain-3-hydroxyacyl-CoA-dehydrogenase—known as LCHAD. There are other mutations for medium-dehydrogenase—MCHAD, as well as carnitine palmitoyltransferase 1 (CPT1) deficiency (Santos, 2007; Ylitalo, 2005).

Sims and coworkers (1995) observed that some *homozygous* LCHAD-deficient children with Reye-like syndromes had *heterozygous* mothers with fatty liver. This was also seen in women with a compound heterozygous fetus. Although some conclude that *only* heterozygous LCHAD-deficient mothers are at risk when their fetus is homozygous, this is not always true (Baskin, 2010).

There is a controversial association between fatty acid β-oxidation enzyme defects and severe preeclampsia—especially in women with HELLP syndrome (Chap. 40, p. 742). Most of these observations have been arrived at by retrospectively studying mothers delivered of a child who later developed Reye-like syndrome. For example, Browning and coworkers (2006) performed a case-control study of 50 mothers of children with a fatty-acid oxidation defect and 1250 mothers of matched control infants. During their pregnancy, 16 percent of mothers with an affected child developed liver problems compared with only 0.9 percent of control women. Problems included HELLP syndrome in 12 percent and fatty liver in 4 percent. Despite these findings, the clinical, biochemical, and histopathological findings are sufficiently disparate to suggest that severe preeclampsia, with or without HELLP syndrome, and fatty liver are distinct syndromes (American College of Obstetricians and Gynecologists, 2012a; Sibai, 2007).

Clinical and Laboratory Findings

Acute fatty liver almost always manifests late in pregnancy. Nelson and colleagues (2013) described 51 such women at Parkland Hospital with a mean gestational age of 37 weeks—range 31.7 to 40.9. Almost 20 percent were delivered at 34 weeks' gestation or earlier. Of these 51 women, 41 percent were nulliparous, and two thirds carried a male fetus. Ten to 20 percent of cases are in women with a multifetal gestation (Fesenmeier, 2005; Vigil-De Gracia, 2011).

Fatty liver has a clinical spectrum of severity. In the worst cases, symptoms usually develop over several days. Persistent nausea and vomiting are major complaints, and there are varying degrees of malaise, anorexia, epigastric pain, and progressive jaundice. Perhaps half of affected women have hypertension, proteinuria, and edema, alone or in combination—signs suggestive of preeclampsia. As shown in Tables 55-1 and 55-2, there are variable degrees of moderate to severe liver dysfunction manifest by hypofibrinogenemia, hypoalbuminemia, hypocholesterolemia, and prolonged clotting times. Serum bilirubin levels usually are < 10 mg/dL, and serum aminotransferase levels are modestly elevated and usually < 1000 U/L.

In almost all severe cases, there is profound endothelial cell activation with capillary leakage causing hemoconcentration, acute kidney injury, ascites, and sometimes pulmonary permeability edema (Bernal, 2013). With severe hemoconcentration, uteroplacental perfusion is reduced and this, along with maternal acidosis, can cause fetal death even before presentation for care. Maternal and fetal acidemia is also related to a high incidence of fetal jeopardy with a concordantly high cesarean delivery rate.

Hemolysis can be severe and evidenced by leukocytosis, nucleated red cells, mild to moderate thrombocytopenia, and elevated serum levels of lactic acid dehydrogenase (LDH). Because of hemoconcentration, however, the hematocrit is often within the normal range. The peripheral blood smear demonstrates echinocytosis, and it has been suggested that hemolysis is caused by the effects of hypocholesterolemia on erythrocyte membranes (Cunningham, 1985).

Various liver imaging techniques have been used to confirm the diagnosis, however, none are particularly reliable. Specifically, Castro and associates (1996) reported poor sensitivity for confirmation by sonography—three of 11 patients, computed tomography (CT)—five of 10, and magnetic resonance (MR) imaging—none of five. Similarly, in a prospective evaluation of the Swansea criteria proposed by Ch'ng and coworkers (2002), only a quarter of women had classic sonographic findings such as maternal ascites or an echogenic hepatic appearance (Knight, 2008). Our experiences are similar (Nelson, 2013).

The syndrome typically continues to worsen after diagnosis. Hypoglycemia is common, and obvious hepatic encephalopathy, severe coagulopathy, and some degree of renal failure each develop in approximately half of women. Fortunately, delivery arrests liver function deterioration.

We have encountered several women with a *forme fruste* of this disorder. Clinical involvement is relatively minor and laboratory aberrations—usually only hemolysis and decreased plasma fibrinogen—herald the syndrome. Thus, the spectrum of liver involvement varies from milder cases that go unnoticed or are attributed to preeclampsia, to overt hepatic failure with encephalopathy.

TABLE 55-2. Laboratory Findings in 137 Women with Acute Fatty Liver of Pregnancy

		Most Abnormal Laboratory Values Mean ± 1 SD (range)[a]			
Series	No.	Fibrinogen (mg/dL)	Platelets (10^3/μL)	Creatinine (mg/dL)	AST (U/L)
Castro (1996)	28	125 (32–446)	113 (11–186)	2.5 (1.1–5.2)	210 (45–1200)
Pereira (1997)	32	ND	123 (26–262)	2.7 (1.1–8.4)	99 (25–911)
Vigil-De Gracia (2001)	10	136 ± 120	76 ± 50	ND	444 ± 358
Fesenmeier (2005)	16	ND	88 (22–226)	3.3 (0.5–8.6)	692 (122–3195)
Nelson (2013)[b]	51	147 ± 96 (27–400)	99 ± 68 (9–385)	2.0 ± 0.8 (0.7–5.0)	449 ± 375(53–2245)
Estimated average		140	105	2.5	330

[a]Fibrinogen and platelet values listed reflect the nadir for each patient, whereas creatinine and AST values reflect peak values for each patient.
[b]Extended data courtesy of Dr. David Nelson.
AST = aspartate aminotransferase; ND = not done.

Coagulopathy. The degree of clotting dysfunction is also variable and can be serious and life threatening, especially if operative delivery is undertaken. Coagulopathy is caused by diminished hepatic procoagulant synthesis, although there is also some evidence for increased consumption with disseminated intravascular coagulation. As shown in Table 55-2, hypofibrinogenemia sometimes is profound. Of 51 women with fatty liver cared for at Parkland Hospital, almost a third had a plasma fibrinogen nadir < 100 mg/dL (Nelson, 2013). Modest elevations of serum D-dimers or fibrin split product levels indicate an element of consumptive coagulopathy. Although usually modest, occasionally there is profound thrombocytopenia (Table 55-2). Among the 51 women from Parkland Hospital, 20 percent had platelet counts < 100,000/μL and 10 percent had platelet counts < 50,000/μL (Nelson, 2013).

Management

Intensive supportive care and good obstetrical management are essential. In some cases, the fetus may be already dead when the diagnosis is made, and the route of delivery is less problematic. Often, viable fetuses tolerate labor poorly. Because significant procrastination in effecting delivery may increase maternal and fetal risks, we prefer a trial of labor induction with close fetal surveillance. Although some recommend cesarean delivery to hasten hepatic healing, this increases maternal risk when there is severe coagulopathy. Nonetheless, cesarean delivery is common, and rates approach 90 percent. Transfusions with whole blood or packed red cells, along with fresh-frozen plasma, cryoprecipitate, and platelets, are usually necessary if surgery is performed or if obstetrical lacerations complicate vaginal delivery (Chap. 41, p. 815).

Hepatic dysfunction resolves postpartum. It usually normalizes within a week, and in the interim, intensive medical support may be required. There are two associated conditions that may develop around this time. Perhaps a fourth of women have evidence for *transient diabetes insipidus.* This presumably is due to elevated vasopressinase concentrations caused by diminished hepatic production of its inactivating enzyme. Finally, *acute pancreatitis* develops in approximately 20 percent.

With supportive care, recovery usually is complete. Maternal deaths are caused by sepsis, hemorrhage, aspiration, renal failure, pancreatitis, and gastrointestinal bleeding. There were two maternal deaths in the series of 51 women at Parkland Hospital. One was an encephalopathic woman who aspirated before intubation during transfer to Parkland Hospital. The other was in a woman with massive liver failure and nonresponsive hypotension (Nelson, 2013). In some centers, other measures have included plasma exchange and even liver transplantation (Fesenmeier, 2005; Franco, 2000; Martin, 2008).

Maternal and Perinatal Outcomes

Although maternal mortality rates with acute fatty liver of pregnancy have approached 75 percent in the past, the contemporaneous outlook is much better. From his review, Sibai (2007) cites an average mortality rate of 7 percent. He also cited a 70-percent preterm delivery rate and a perinatal mortality rate of approximately 15 percent, which in the past was nearly 90 percent. At Parkland Hospital, the maternal and perinatal mortality rates during the past four decades have been 4 percent and 12 percent, respectively (Nelson, 2013).

Preeclampsia Syndrome

Hepatic involvement is relatively common in women with severe preeclampsia and eclampsia (see Table 55-1). These changes are discussed in detail in Chapter 40 (p. 741).

Viral Hepatitis

Although most viral hepatitis syndromes are asymptomatic, during the past 25 years, acute symptomatic infections have become even less common in the United States (Centers for Disease Control and Prevention, 2008). There are at least five distinct types of viral hepatitis: A (HAV), B (HBV), D (HDV) caused by the hepatitis B-associated delta agent, C (HCV), and E (HEV). The clinical presentation is similar in all, and although the viruses themselves probably are not hepatotoxic, the immunological response to them causes hepatocellular necrosis (Dienstag, 2012a,b). Asymptomatic chronic viral hepatitis remains the leading cause of liver cancer and the most frequent reason for liver transplantation.

Acute Hepatitis

As discussed above, acute infections are most often subclinical and *anicteric.* When they are clinically apparent, nausea and vomiting, headache, and malaise may precede jaundice by 1 to 2 weeks. Low-grade fever is more common with hepatitis A. By the time jaundice develops, symptoms are usually improving. Serum aminotransferase levels vary, and their peaks do not correspond with disease severity (see Table 55-1). Peak levels that range from 400 to 4000 U/L are usually reached by the time jaundice develops. Serum bilirubin typically continues to rise, despite falling aminotransferase levels, and peaks at 5 to 20 mg/dL.

Any evidence for severe disease should prompt hospitalization. These include incessant nausea and vomiting, prolonged prothrombin time, low serum albumin level, hypoglycemia, high serum bilirubin level, or central nervous system symptoms. In most cases, however, there is complete clinical and biochemical recovery within 1 to 2 months in all cases of hepatitis A, in most cases of hepatitis B, but in only a small proportion of cases of hepatitis C.

When patients are hospitalized, their feces, secretions, bedpans, and other articles in contact with the intestinal tract should be handled with glove-protected hands. Extra precautions, such as double gloving during delivery and surgical procedures, are recommended. Due to significant exposure of health-care personnel to hepatitis B, the Centers for Disease Control and Prevention (CDC) recommend active and passive vaccination. There is no vaccine for hepatitis C, so recommendations are for postexposure serosurveillance only.

Acute hepatitis has a case-fatality rate of 0.1 percent. For patients ill enough to be hospitalized, it is as high as 1 percent. Most fatalities are due to *fulminant hepatic necrosis,* which in later pregnancy may resemble acute fatty liver. In these cases, hepatic encephalopathy is the usual presentation, and the mortality rate is 80 percent. Approximately half of patients with fulminant disease have hepatitis B infection, and co-infection with the delta agent is common.

Chronic Hepatitis

The Centers for Disease Control and Prevention (2012) estimates that 4.4 million Americans are living with chronic viral hepatitis. By far, the most frequent complication of hepatitis B and C is subsequent development of chronic hepatitis, which is usually diagnosed serologically (Table 55-3). Chronic infection follows acute hepatitis B in approximately 5 to 10 percent of cases in adults. Most become asymptomatic carriers, but a small percentage have low-grade chronic persistent hepatitis or chronic active hepatitis with or without cirrhosis. With acute hepatitis C, however, chronic hepatitis develops in most patients. With persistently abnormal biochemical tests, liver biopsy usually discloses active inflammation, continuing necrosis, and fibrosis that may lead to cirrhosis. Chronic hepatitis is classified by cause; grade, defined by histological activity; and stage, which is the degree of progression (Dienstag, 2012b). In these cases, there is evidence that a cellular immune reaction is interactive with a genetic predisposition.

Although most chronically infected persons are asymptomatic, approximately 20 percent develop cirrhosis within 10 to 20 years (Dienstag, 2012b). When present, symptoms are nonspecific and usually include fatigue. Diagnosis can be confirmed by liver biopsy, however, treatment is usually given to patients after serological or virological diagnosis. In some patients, cirrhosis with liver failure or bleeding varices may be the presenting findings. The management of chronic hepatitis B and hepatitis C is discussed in their respective sections.

Chronic Hepatitis and Pregnancy. Most young women with chronic hepatitis either are asymptomatic or have only mild liver disease. For seropositive asymptomatic women, there usually are no problems with pregnancy. With *symptomatic* chronic active hepatitis, pregnancy outcome depends primarily on disease and fibrosis intensity, and especially on the presence of portal hypertension. The few women whom we have managed have done well, but their long-term prognosis is poor. Accordingly, they should be counseled regarding possible liver transplantation as well as abortion and sterilization options.

Hepatitis A

Because of vaccination programs, the incidence of hepatitis A has decreased 95 percent since 1995. In 2010, the rate was 0.6 per 100,000 individuals—the lowest rate ever reported in the United States (Centers for Disease Control and Prevention, 2012). This 27-nm RNA picornavirus is transmitted by the fecal–oral route, usually by ingestion of contaminated food or water. The incubation period is approximately 4 weeks. Individuals shed virus in their feces, and during the relatively brief period of viremia, their blood is also infectious. Signs and symptoms are often nonspecific and usually mild, although jaundice develops in most patients. Symptoms usually last less than 2 months, although 10 to 15 percent of patients may remain symptomatic or relapse for up to 6 months (Dienstag, 2012a). Early serological detection is by identification of IgM anti-HAV antibody that may persist for several months. During convalescence, IgG antibody predominates, and it persists and provides subsequent immunity. There is no chronic stage of hepatitis A.

Management of hepatitis A in pregnant women consists of a balanced diet and diminished physical activity. Women with less severe illness may be managed as outpatients. In developed countries, the effects of hepatitis A on pregnancy outcomes are not dramatic (American College of Obstetricians and Gynecologists, 2012a,b). Both perinatal and maternal mortality rates, however, are substantively increased in resource-poor countries. There is no evidence that hepatitis A virus is teratogenic, and transmission to the fetus is negligible. Preterm birth may be increased, and neonatal cholestasis has been reported (Urganci, 2003). Although hepatitis A RNA has been isolated in breast milk, no cases of neonatal hepatitis A have been reported secondary to breast feeding (Daudi, 2012).

Preventatively, vaccination during childhood with formalin-inactivated hepatitis viral vaccine is more than 90-percent effective. HAV vaccination is recommended by the American College

TABLE 55-3. Simplified Diagnostic Approach in Patients with Hepatitis

	Serological Test			
Diagnosis	HBsAg	IgM Anti-HAV	IgM Anti-HBc	Anti-HCV
Acute hepatitis A	–	+	–	–
Acute hepatitis B	+	–	+	–
Chronic hepatitis B	+	–	–	–
Acute hepatitis A with chronic B	+	+	–	–
Acute hepatitis A and B	+	+	+	
Acute hepatitis C	–	–	–	+

HAV = hepatitis A virus; HBc = hepatitis B core; HBsAg = hepatitis B surface antigen; HCV = hepatitis C virus.
From the Centers for Disease Control and Prevention, 2010; Dienstag, 2012a.

of Obstetricians and Gynecologists (2012b) and the Centers for Disease Control and Prevention (2010) for high-risk adults, a category that includes behavioral and occupational populations and travelers to high-risk countries. These countries are listed by the Centers for Disease Control and Prevention in the 2014 CDC Health Information for International Travel "yellow book," which is available at: http://wwwnc.cdc.gov/travel/yellowbook/2014/table-of-contents.

Passive immunization for the pregnant woman recently exposed by close personal or sexual contact with a person with hepatitis A is provided by a 0.02 mL/kg dose of immune globulin (Centers for Disease Control and Prevention, 2010). Victor and colleagues (2007) reported that a single dose of HAV vaccine given in the usual dosage within 2 weeks of exposure to exposed persons was as effective as immune serum globulin to prevent hepatitis A. In both groups, HAV developed in 3 to 4 percent.

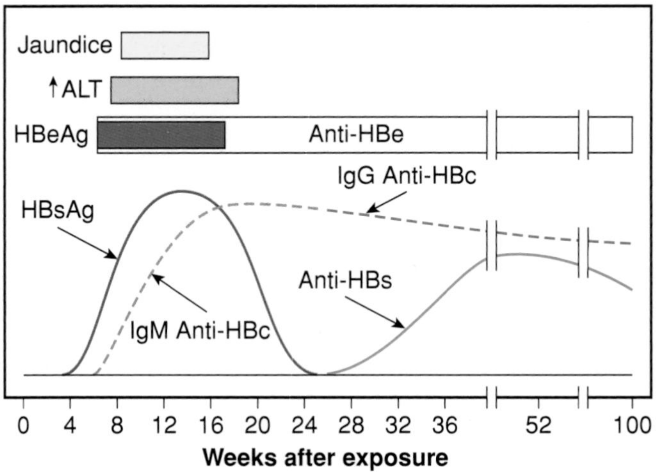

FIGURE 55-2 Sequence of various antigens and antibodies in acute hepatitis B. ALT = alanine aminotransferase; anti-HBc = antibody to hepatitis B core antigen; anti-HBe = antibody to hepatitis B e antigen; anti-HBs = antibody to hepatitis B surface antigen; HBeAg = hepatitis B e antigen; HBsAg = hepatitis B surface antigen. (Redrawn from Dienstag, 2012a.)

Hepatitis B

This is a double-stranded DNA virus of the Hepadnaviridae family. It is found worldwide and is endemic in Africa, Central and Southeast Asia, China, Eastern Europe, the Middle East, and certain areas of South America, with prevalence rates as high as 5 to 20 percent. The World Health Organization (2009) estimates that more than two billion people worldwide are infected with HBV, and of these, 370 million have chronic infection. The Centers for Disease Control and Prevention (2012) estimated that there were 43,000 acute hepatitis B cases in the United States in 2010—a decline of more than 80 percent since vaccination was introduced in the 1980s. The World Health Organization considers hepatitis B to be second only to tobacco among human carcinogens.

The hepatitis B virus is transmitted by exposure to blood or body fluids from infected individuals. In endemic countries, vertical transmission, that is, from mother to fetus or newborn, accounts for at least 35 to 50 percent of chronic HBV infections. In low-prevalence countries such as the United States, which has a prevalence < 2 percent, the more frequent mode of HBV transmission is via sexual transmission or sharing of contaminated needles. HBV can be transmitted by any body fluid, but exposure to virus-laden serum is the most efficient.

Acute hepatitis B develops after an incubation period of 30 to 180 days with a mean of 8 to 12 weeks. At least half of acute infections are asymptomatic. If symptoms are present, they are usually mild and include anorexia, nausea, vomiting, fever, abdominal pain, and jaundice. Acute HBV accounts for half of cases of fulminant hepatitis. Complete resolution of symptoms occurs within 3 to 4 months in more than 90 percent of patients. Figure 55-2 details the sequence of the various HBV antigens and antibodies in acute infection. The first serological marker to be detected is the hepatitis B surface antigen (HBsAg), often preceding the increase in aminotransferase levels. As HBsAg disappears, antibodies to the surface antigen develop (anti-HBs), marking complete resolution of disease. Hepatitis B core antigen is an intracellular antigen and not detectable in serum. However, anti-HBc is detectable within weeks of HBsAg appearance. The hepatitis Be antigen (HBeAg) is present during times of high viral replication and often correlates with detectable HBV DNA. After acute hepatitis, approximately 90 percent of adult persons recover completely. The 10 percent who remain chronically infected are considered to have chronic hepatitis B.

Chronic HBV infection is often asymptomatic but may be clinically suggested by persistent anorexia, weight loss, fatigue, and hepatosplenomegaly. Extrahepatic manifestations may include arthritis, generalized vasculitis, glomerulonephritis, pericarditis, myocarditis, transverse myelitis, and peripheral neuropathy. One risk factor for chronic disease is age at acquisition—more than 90 percent in newborns, 50 percent in young children, and less than 10 percent in immunocompetent adults. Another risk is an immunocompromised state such as those with human immunodeficiency virus (HIV) infection, transplant recipients, or persons receiving chemotherapy. Chronically infected persons may be asymptomatic carriers or have chronic disease with or without cirrhosis. Patients with chronic disease have persistent HBsAg serum positivity. The patients with evidence of high viral replication—HBV DNA with or without HBeAg, have the highest likelihood of developing cirrhosis and hepatocellular carcinoma. HBV DNA has been found to be the best correlate of liver injury and disease progression risk.

Pregnancy

Hepatitis B infection is not a cause of excessive maternal morbidity and mortality. It is often asymptomatic and found only on routine prenatal screening (Connell, 2011; Stewart, 2013). A review of the National Inpatient Sample (NIS) Agency for Healthcare Research and Quality reported a modest increase in preterm birth rates in HBV-positive mothers but no effect on fetal-growth restriction or preeclampsia rates (Reddick, 2011). Others have shown similar results (Connell, 2011; Safir, 2010). Transplacental viral infection is uncommon, and Towers and associates (2001) reported that viral DNA is rarely found in amnionic fluid or cord blood. Interestingly, HBV DNA has been found in the ovaries of HBV-positive pregnant women, and the highest levels were found in women who transmitted HBV to their fetuses (Hu, 2012; Lou, 2010; Yu, 2012).

In the absence of HBV immunoprophylaxis, 10 to 20 percent of women positive for HBsAg transmit viral infection to their infant. This rate increases to almost 90 percent if the mother is HBsAg and HBeAg positive. Immunoprophylaxis and hepatitis B vaccine given to infants born to HBV-infected mothers has decreased transmission dramatically and prevented approximately 90 percent of infections (Smith, 2012). But, women with high HBV vital loads—106 to 108 copies/mL, or those who are HBeAg positive, still have a least a 10-percent vertical transmission rate, regardless of immunoprophylaxis.

To decrease vertical transmission in women at highest risk because of high HBV DNA levels, some have recommended antiviral therapy. Lamivudine, a cytidine nucleoside analogue, has been found to significantly decrease the risk of fetal HBV infection in women with high HBV viral loads (Dusheiko, 2012; Giles, 2011; Han, 2011; Shi, 2010; Xu, 2009). Safety data in early pregnancy, although limited, are promising (Yi, 2012; Yu, 2012). Early reports of two other antiviral medications, telbivudine and tenofovir, for use in pregnancy also show promise (Deng, 2012; Han, 2011; Liu, 2013; Pan, 2012a,b). Hepatitis B immunoglobulin (HBIG) given antepartum to women at highest risk of transmission has also been shown to be effective in decreasing transmission rates (Shi, 2010). Antiviral therapy or HBIG has been shown to be cost-effective in recent analyses (Nayeri, 2012).

Infants born to seropositive mothers are given HBIG very soon after birth. This is accompanied by the first of a three-dose hepatitis B recombinant vaccine. Hill and colleagues (2002) applied this strategy in 369 infants and reported that the 2.4-percent transmission rate was not increased with breast feeding if vaccination was completed. Although virus is present in breast milk, the incidence of transmission is not lowered by formula feeding (Shi, 2011). The American Academy of Pediatrics does not consider maternal HBV infection a contraindication to breast feeding.

For high-risk mothers who are seronegative, hepatitis B vaccine can be given during pregnancy. The efficacy has been shown to be similar to that for nonpregnant adults, with overall seroconversion rates approaching 95 percent after three doses (Stewart, 2013). The traditional vaccination schedule of 0, 1, and 6 months may be difficult to complete during a pregnancy, and compliance rates decline after delivery. Sheffield and coworkers (2006) reported that the three-dose regimen given prenatally—initially and at 1 and 4 months—resulted in seroconversion rates of 56, 77, and 90 percent, respectively, This regimen was noted to be easily be completed during routine prenatal care.

Hepatitis D

Also called *delta hepatitis*, this is a defective RNA virus that is a hybrid particle with an HBsAg coat and a delta core. The virus must co-infect with hepatitis B either simultaneously or secondarily. It cannot persist in serum longer than hepatitis B virus. Transmission is similar to hepatitis B. Chronic co-infection with B and D hepatitis is more severe and accelerated than with HBV alone, and up to 75 percent of affected patients develop cirrhosis. HDV infection is detected by the presence of anti-HDV and HDV DNA. Neonatal transmission is unusual as neonatal HBV vaccination usually prevents delta hepatitis.

Hepatitis C

This is a single-stranded RNA virus of the family Flaviviridae. There are at least six major genotypes—type 1 accounts for 70 percent of HCV infections in the United States. Transmission occurs via blood and body fluids, although sexual transmission is inefficient. Up to a third of anti-HCV positive persons have no identifiable risk factors (Dienstag, 2012b). Screening for HCV is recommended for HIV-infected individuals, persons with injection drug use, hemodialysis patients, children born to mothers with HCV, persons exposed to HCV-positive blood or body fluids, persons with unexplained elevations in aminotransferase values, and recipients of blood or transplants before July 1992. Prenatal screening has been recommended in high-risk women, and in the United States, seroprevalence rates as high as 1 to 2.4 percent have been reported (American College of Obstetricians and Gynecologists, 2012b; Arshad, 2011; Connell, 2011). It is higher in women who are HIV positive, and Santiago-Munoz and associates (2005) found that 6.3 percent of HIV-infected pregnant women at Parkland Hospital were co-infected with hepatitis B or C.

Acute HCV infection is usually asymptomatic or with mild symptoms. Only 10 to 15 percent develop jaundice. The incubation period ranges from 15 to 160 days with a mean of 7 weeks. Aminotransferase levels are elevated episodically during the acute infection. Hepatitis C RNA testing is now considered the "gold standard" for the diagnosis of HCV—levels may be detected even before aminotransferase elevations and the development of anti-HCV. Anti-HCV antibody is not detected for an average of 15 weeks and in some cases as long as a year (Dienstag, 2012a).

As many as 80 to 90 percent of patients with acute HCV will be chronically infected. Although most remain asymptomatic, approximately 20 to 30 percent progress to cirrhosis within 20 to 30 years. Aminotransferase values fluctuate, and HCV RNA levels vary over time. Liver biopsy reveals chronic disease and fibrosis in up to 50 percent, however, these findings are often mild. Overall, the long-term prognosis for most patients is excellent.

As expected, most pregnant women diagnosed with HCV have chronic disease. HCV infection was initially thought to have limited pregnancy effects. However, more recent reports have chronicled modestly increased fetal risks for low birthweight, NICU admission, preterm delivery, and mechanical ventilation (Berkley, 2008; Pergam, 2008; Reddick, 2011). In some women, these adverse outcomes may have been influenced by concurrent high-risk behaviors associated with HCV infection.

The primary adverse perinatal outcome is vertical transmission of HCV infection to the fetus-infant. This is higher in mothers with viremia (Indolfi, 2014; Joshi, 2010). From their review, Airoldi and Berghella (2006) cited a rate of 1 to

3 percent in HCV-positive, RNA-negative women compared with 4 to 6 percent in those who were RNA-positive. In a report from Dublin, McMenamin and colleagues (2008) described transmission rates in 545 HCV-positive women. They found a 7.1-percent vertical transmission rate in RNA-positive women compared with none in those who were RNA-negative. Some have found an even greater risk when the mother is co-infected with HIV (Ferrero, 2003). Approximately two thirds of prenatal transmission occurs peripartum. HCV genotype, invasive prenatal procedures, breast feeding, and delivery mode are not associated with mother-to-child transmission (Babik, 2011; Cottrell, 2013; Ghamar Chehreh, 2011; López, 2010). That said, invasive procedures such as internal electronic fetal heart rate monitoring should be avoided. HCV infection is not a contraindication to breast feeding.

There is currently no licensed vaccine for HCV prevention. The chronic HCV infection treatment has traditionally included alpha interferon (standard and pegylated), alone or in combination with ribavirin. This regimen is contraindicated in pregnancy because of the teratogenic potential of ribavirin in animals (Joshi, 2010). The initial 5-year review of the Ribavirin Pregnancy Registry found no evidence for human teratogenicity. However, the registry has enrolled fewer than half of the necessary numbers to allow a conclusive statement to be made (Roberts, 2010). The development and study of direct acting and host-targeted antiviral drugs in the past decade has shown great promise for the management of chronic hepatitis C (Liang, 2013; Lok, 2012; Poordad, 2013). Current interferon-free, ribavirin-free regimens are being evaluated, although no data are available for pregnant women.

Hepatitis E

This water-borne RNA virus usually is enterically transmitted by contaminated water supplies. Hepatitis E is probably the most common cause of acute hepatitis (Hoofnagle, 2012). It causes epidemic outbreaks in third-world countries with substantial morbidity and mortality rates. Pregnant women have a higher case-fatality rate than nonpregnant individuals. Rein and coworkers (2012) suggested a 20-percent mortality rate using modeling estimates from the developing world. Fulminant hepatitis, although rare overall, is more common in pregnant women and contributes to the increased mortality rates (Labrique, 2012; Mehta, 2012).

Higher hepatitis E viral loads and increased cytokine secretion in pregnant compared with nonpregnant women may be factors in the development of fulminant hepatitis (Borkakoti, 2013; Salam, 2013). Recombinant HEV vaccine efficacy is reported to be > 90 percent, and preliminary data from inadvertently vaccinated pregnant women have shown no adverse maternal or fetal events. Even so, there is no currently available Food and Drug Administration (FDA)-approved vaccine (Labrique, 2012; Wedemeyer, 2012; Wu, 2012).

Hepatitis G

This blood-borne infection with a flavivirus-like RNA virus does not actually cause hepatitis (Dienstag, 2012a). Its seroprevalence ranges from 0.08 to 5 percent, and there is currently no recommended treatment aside from basic blood and body fluid precautions. Infant transmission has been described (Feucht, 1996; Inaba, 1997).

Autoimmune Hepatitis

This is a generally progressive chronic hepatitis that is important to distinguish from chronic viral hepatitis because treatments are markedly different. According to Krawitt (2006), an environmental agent—a virus or drug—triggers events that mediate T cells to destroy liver antigens in genetically susceptible patients. Type 1 hepatitis is more common and is characterized by multiple autoimmune antibodies such as antinuclear antibodies (ANA) as well as certain human leukocyte genes. Treatment employs corticosteroids, alone or combined with azathioprine (Gossard, 2012). In some patients, cirrhosis or hepatocellular carcinoma develops.

As with other autoimmune disorders, chronic autoimmune hepatitis is more common in women and frequently coexists with thyroiditis, ulcerative colitis, type 1 diabetes, and rheumatoid arthritis. Hepatitis is usually subclinical, but exacerbations can cause fatigue and malaise that can be debilitating.

In general, pregnancy outcomes of women with autoimmune hepatitis are poor, but the prognosis is good with well-controlled disease (Uribe, 2006). In one study, Schramm and colleagues (2006) described 42 pregnancies in 22 German women with autoimmune hepatitis. A fifth had a flare antepartum, and half had a flare postpartum. One woman underwent liver transplantation at 18 weeks' gestation, and another died of sepsis at 19 weeks. In their 38-year review, Candia and associates (2005) found 101 pregnancies in 58 women. They reported that preeclampsia developed in approximately a fourth, and there were two maternal deaths. Westbrook and coworkers (2012) reported the outcomes of 81 pregnancies in 53 women. Flares occurred in a third of the women. There were more common in those not taking medication and those with active disease in the year before conception. Only a minority—20 of 81—were not taking medications. Maternal and fetal complications were higher among women with cirrhosis, particularly with respect to the risks of death or need for liver transplantation during the pregnancy or within 12 months postpartum.

Nonalcoholic Fatty Liver Disease

Steatohepatitis is an increasingly recognized condition that may occasionally progress to hepatic cirrhosis. As a macrovesicular fatty liver condition, it resembles alcohol-induced liver injury but is seen without alcohol abuse. Obesity, type 2 diabetes, and hyperlipidemia—*syndrome X*—frequently coexist and likely are etiological agents or "triggers" (McCullough, 2006). Nonalcoholic fatty liver disease (NAFLD) is common in obese persons, and as many as 50 percent of the morbidly obese are affected (Chap. 48, p. 963). Moreover, half of persons with type 2 diabetes have NAFLD. Browning and associates (2004) used magnetic resonance spectroscopy to determine the prevalence of NAFLD in Dallas County and found that approximately a third of adults were affected. This varied by ethnicity, with 45 percent of Hispanics, 33 percent of whites, and 24 percent of blacks being affected. Most people—80 percent—found to have steatosis had normal liver enzymes. Welsh and colleagues (2013) showed that nonalcoholic fatty liver disease among adolescents increased from 3.9 to 10.7 percent between 1988 to 1994 and 2007 to 2010. The risk increased with age, body mass index, male gender, and Mexican American race. And half of obese male adolescents are affected.

There is a continuum or spectrum of liver damage in which fatty liver progresses to *nonalcoholic steatohepatitis—NASH,* and then *hepatic fibrosis* develops that may progress to cirrhosis (Levene, 2012). Still, in most persons, the disease is usually asymptomatic, and it is a frequent explanation for elevated aminotransferase levels found in blood donors and other routine screening testing. Indeed, it is the cause of elevated asymptomatic aminotransferase levels in up to 90 percent of cases in which other liver disease is excluded. It also is the most common cause of abnormal liver tests among adults in this country. Currently, weight loss along with diabetes and dyslipidemia control is the only recommended treatment.

Pregnancy

Fatty liver infiltration is probably much more common than realized in obese and diabetic pregnant women. During the past decade, we encountered an increasing number of pregnant women with these disorders. Once severe liver injury, that is, acute fatty liver of pregnancy, was excluded, gravidas with fatty liver infiltration had no adverse outcomes relative to liver involvement. Page and Girling (2011) reported five women who had mild liver enzyme abnormalities after exclusion of other obstetrical and nonobstetrical etiologies. Four women had steatosis diagnosed by sonography, and a fifth woman without sonographic abnormalities had biopsy-confirmed steatosis postpartum. Forbes and colleagues (2011) studied women with and without a history of gestational diabetes who had nondiabetic glucose tolerance testing postpartum. Although body mass index did not differ significantly, women with a history of gestational diabetes were more than twice as likely to have NAFLD diagnosed sonographically, and this correlated with increased dyslipidemia and measures of insulin resistance. As the obesity endemic worsens, any adverse effects of this liver disorder on pregnancy outcome should become apparent.

Cirrhosis

Irreversible chronic liver injury with extensive fibrosis and regenerative nodules is the final common pathway for several disorders. *Laënnec cirrhosis* from chronic alcohol exposure is the most frequent cause in the general population. But in young women—including pregnant women—most cases are caused by *postnecrotic cirrhosis* from chronic hepatitis B and C. Many cases of *cryptogenic cirrhosis* are now known to be caused by nonalcoholic fatty liver disease (Dienstag, 2012b). Clinical manifestations of cirrhosis include jaundice, edema, coagulopathy, metabolic abnormalities, and portal hypertension with gastroesophageal varices and splenomegaly. The incidence of deep-vein thromboembolism is increased (Søgaard, 2009). The prognosis is poor, and 75 percent have progressive disease that leads to death in 1 to 5 years.

Cirrhosis and Pregnancy

Women with symptomatic cirrhosis frequently are infertile. Those who become pregnant generally have poor outcomes. Common complications include transient hepatic failure, variceal hemorrhage, preterm delivery, fetal-growth restriction, and maternal death (Tan, 2008). Outcomes are generally worse if there are coexisting esophageal varices.

Another potentially fatal complication of cirrhosis arises from associated splenic artery aneurysms. Up to 20 percent of ruptures occur during pregnancy, and 70 percent of these rupture in the third trimester (Tan, 2008). In a review of 32 cases of these aneurysms, Ha and coworkers (2009) found that the mean diameter was 2.25 cm, and in half of cases, the diameter was < 2 cm. The maternal mortality rate of 22 percent was likely related to the emergent diagnosis of these cases, as almost all were diagnosed at the time of rupture.

Portal Hypertension and Esophageal Varices

Approximately half of esophageal varices cases in pregnant women are caused by either cirrhosis or extrahepatic portal vein obstruction, which leads to portal system hypertension. Some cases of extrahepatic hypertension develop following portal vein thrombosis associated with one of the *thrombophilia syndromes* (Chap. 52, p. 1029). Others follow thrombosis from umbilical vein catheterization when the woman was a neonate, especially if she was born preterm.

With either intrahepatic or extrahepatic resistance to flow, portal vein pressure rises from its normal range of 5 to 10 mm Hg, and values may exceed 30 mm Hg. Collateral circulation develops that carries portal blood to the systemic circulation. Drainage is via the gastric, intercostal, and other veins to the esophageal system, where varices develop. Bleeding is usually from varices near the gastroesophageal junction, and hemorrhage can be torrential. Bleeding during pregnancy from varices occurs in a third to half of affected women and is the major cause of maternal mortality (Tan, 2008).

Maternal prognosis is largely dependent on whether there is variceal hemorrhage. Mortality rates are higher if varices are associated with cirrhosis compared with rates for varices without cirrhosis—18 versus 2 percent, respectively. Perinatal mortality rates are high in women with varices and are worse if cirrhosis caused the varices.

Management

Treatment is the same as for nonpregnant patients. Preventatively, all patients with cirrhosis, including pregnant women, should undergo screening endoscopy for identification of variceal dilatation (Tan, 2008). Beta-blocking drugs such as propranolol are given to reduce portal pressure and hence the bleeding risk (Groszmann, 2005).

For acute bleeding, endoscopic band ligation is preferred to sclerotherapy, as it avoids any potential risks of injecting sclerotherapeutic chemicals (Tan, 2008). Zeeman and Moise (1999) described a pregnant woman who underwent *prophylactic* banding at 15, 26, and 31 weeks' gestation to prevent bleeding. Acute medical management for bleeding varices verified by endoscopy includes intravenous vasopressin or octreotide and somatostatin (Chung, 2005). *Balloon tamponade* using a triple-lumen tube placed into the esophagus and stomach to compress bleeding varices can be lifesaving if endoscopy is not available. The interventional radiology procedure—*transjugular intrahepatic portosystemic stent shunting (TIPSS)*—can also control bleeding from gastric varices that is unresponsive to other measures (Khan, 2006; Tan, 2008). TIPSS can be done electively in patients with previous variceal hemorrhage.

Acute Acetaminophen Overdose

Nonsteroidal antiinflammatory drugs (NSAIDs) are often used in suicide attempts. In a study from Denmark, Flint and associates (2002) reported that more than half of such attempts by 122 pregnant women were with either acetaminophen or aspirin. In the United States, acetaminophen is much more commonly used during pregnancy, and overdose may lead to hepatocellular necrosis and acute liver failure (Lee, 2008). Massive necrosis causes a *cytokine storm* and multiorgan dysfunction. Early symptoms of overdose are nausea, vomiting, diaphoresis, malaise, and pallor. After a latent period of 24 to 48 hours, liver failure ensues and usually begins to resolve in 5 days. In a prospective Danish study, only 35 percent of patients who were treated for fulminant hepatic failure spontaneously recovered before being listed for liver transplantation (Schmidt, 2007).

The antidote is *N-acetylcysteine,* which must be given promptly. The drug is thought to act by increasing glutathione levels, which aid metabolism of the toxic metabolite, *N*-acetyl-*para*-benzoquinoneimine. The need for treatment is based on projections of possible plasma hepatotoxic levels as a function of the time from acute ingestion. Many poison control centers use the nomogram established by Rumack and Matthew (1975). A plasma level is measured 4 hours after ingestion, and if the level is > 120 μg/mL, treatment is given. If plasma determinations are not available, empirical treatment is given if the ingested amount exceeded 7.5 g. An oral loading dose of 140 mg/kg of *N*-acetylcysteine is followed by 17 maintenance doses of 70 mg/kg every 4 hours for 72 hours of total treatment time. Both the oral and an equally efficacious intravenous dosing regimen have been recently reviewed by Hodgman and Garrard (2012). Although the drug reaches therapeutic concentrations in the fetus, any protective effects are unknown (Heard, 2008).

After 14 weeks, the fetus has some cytochrome P450 activity necessary for metabolism of acetaminophen to the toxic metabolite. Riggs and colleagues (1989) reported follow-up data from the Rocky Mountain Poison and Drug Center in 60 such women. The likelihood of maternal and fetal survival was better if the antidote was given soon after overdose. At least one 33-week fetus appears to have died as a direct result of hepatotoxicity 2 days after maternal ingestion. In another case, Wang and associates (1997) confirmed acetaminophen placental transfer with maternal and cord blood levels that measured 41 μg/mL. Both mother and infant died from hepatorenal failure.

Focal Nodular Hyperplasia

This is considered a benign lesion of the liver, characterized in most cases by a well-delineated accumulation of normal but disordered hepatocytes that surround a central stellate scar. These usually can be differentiated from hepatic adenomas by MR and CT imaging. Except in the rare situation of unremitting pain, surgery is rarely indicated, and most women remain asymptomatic during pregnancy. Rifai and coworkers (2013) reviewed 20 cases at a single center in Germany. None of the women had complications during pregnancy, and tumor size did not vary significantly before, during, or after pregnancy. Three women had 20-percent tumor growth; in 10 patients, the tumor decreased in size; and the remaining seven were unchanged across pregnancy. Ramirez-Fuentes and associates (2013) studied 44 lesions in 30 women, who each had a minimum of two MR imaging studies 12 months apart. They reported that 80 percent of the lesions were unchanged in size, and most of the remainder decreased in size. They concluded that changes in size were unrelated to pregnancy, oral contraceptive use, or menopause. As noted in Chapter 38 (p. 709), this lesion is not a contraindication to estrogen-containing contraceptives.

Hepatic Adenoma

This benign neoplasm has a significant risk of rupture-associated hemorrhage, particularly in pregnancy. As discussed above, adenomas can usually be differentiated from focal nodular hyperplasia by MR or CT imaging. Adenomas have a 9:1 predominance among women and are strongly linked with combination oral contraceptive use. The risk of rupture increases with lesion size, and surgery is generally recommended for tumors measuring > 5 cm. From their review, Cobey and Salem (2004) found 27 cases in pregnancy, 23 of which became apparent in the third trimester and puerperium. They found no cases of hemorrhage when the tumor size was < 6.5 cm. In their review, 16 of 27 (60 percent) women with an adenoma presented with tumor rupture that resulted in seven maternal deaths and six fetal deaths. Of note, 13 of 27 women presented within 2 months postpartum, and in half, hemorrhage heralded rupture. Santambrogio and coworkers (2009) provided a case report of a woman with a 12-cm adenoma that ruptured shortly after emergent cesarean for placental abruption and that ultimately prompted liver transplantation.

Liver Transplantation

According to the Organ Procurement and Transplantation Network (2012), liver transplant patients comprise nearly 18 percent of all proposed waiting organ recipients. Approximately a fourth of these are women of childbearing age. The first human liver transplant was performed 50 years ago, and a recent literature review cited 450 pregnancies in 306 women who had undergone transplantation (Deshpande, 2012). Although their livebirth rate of 80 percent and miscarriage rates compared favorably with those of the general population, there were significantly increased risks of preeclampsia, cesarean delivery, and preterm birth. A fourth of pregnancies were complicated by

TABLE 55-4. Pregnancy Complications (%) in 558 Pregnancies after Liver Transplantation

Series	No.	Preeclampsia/ Hypertension	Cesarean Delivery	Rejection	Live Birth
Jain (2003)	49	2–8	45	24	100
Nagy (2003)	38	21	46	17	63
Christopher (2006)	71	13–28	28	17	70
Sibanda (2007)	18	NA	63	NA	61
Coscia (2010)	281	22–33	32	6	75
Jabiry-Zieniewicz (2011)	39	8–26	79	8	100
Blume (2013)	62	6	30	13	77
Weighted Average:	558	16–28	38	10	78

NA = not available.

hypertension, approximately a third resulted in preterm birth, and in 10 percent, there was one or more rejection episodes (Table 55-4). Importantly, 4 percent of mothers had died within a year after delivery, but this rate is comparable with nonpregnant liver transplantation patients.

In pregnant women who have undergone transplantation, close surveillance is mandatory to detect hypertension, renal dysfunction, preeclampsia, and graft rejection. Management considerations, including immunosuppressive therapy, were reviewed by Mastrobattista and Gomez-Lobo (2008) and by McKay and Josephson (2006). Because of increased metabolic clearance, serum levels of some antirejection drugs should be determined. Ethical considerations of pregnancy in transplant recipients were reviewed earlier by Ross (2006).

GALLBLADDER DISORDERS

Cholelithiasis and Cholecystitis

In the United States, 20 percent of women older than 40 years have gallstones. Most stones contain cholesterol, and its oversecretion into bile is thought to be a major factor in stone formation. Biliary sludge, which may increase during pregnancy, is an important precursor to gallstone formation. The incidence of sonographically identified asymptomatic gallstones in more than 1500 pregnant or postpartum women was 2.5 to 10 percent (Maringhini, 1993; Valdivieso, 1993). Moreover, the cumulative risk of all patients with silent gallstones to require surgery for symptoms or complications is 10 percent at 5 years, 15 percent at 10 years, and 18 percent at 15 years (Greenberger, 2008). For these reasons, prophylactic cholecystectomy is not warranted for *asymptomatic* stones. For *symptomatic* gallstone disease, nonsurgical approaches have been used and include oral bile acid therapy with ursodeoxycholic acid and extracorporeal shock wave lithotripsy. There is no experience with these during pregnancy.

Acute cholecystitis usually develops when there is obstruction of the cystic duct. Bacterial infection plays a role in 50 to 85 percent of cases. In more than half of patients with acute cholecystitis, a history of previous right upper quadrant pain from cholelithiasis is elicited. With acute disease, pain is accompanied by anorexia, nausea and vomiting, low-grade fever, and mild leukocytosis. As shown in Figure 55-3, sonography can be used to see stones as small as 2 mm, and false-positive and false-negative rates are 2 to 4 percent (Greenberger, 2008).

Symptomatic gallbladder disorders in young women include acute cholecystitis, biliary colic, and acute pancreatitis. Rarely, a gallbladder undergoes torsion or a neoplasm is found (Kleiss, 2003; Wiseman, 2008). In most symptomatic patients, cholecystectomy is warranted. Although acute cholecystitis responds to medical therapy, contemporary consensus is that early cholecystectomy is indicated (Greenberger, 2008). In acute cases, medical therapy consists of intravenous fluids, antimicrobials, analgesics, and in some instances, nasogastric suction, before surgical therapy. Laparoscopic cholecystectomy has become the preferred treatment for most patients.

Gallbladder Disease During Pregnancy

The incidence of cholecystitis during pregnancy is reported to be approximately 1 in 1000. There is no doubt that pregnancy is "lithogenic." After the first trimester, the gallbladder fasting volume as well as the residual volume after postprandial emptying are doubled. Incomplete emptying may result in retention

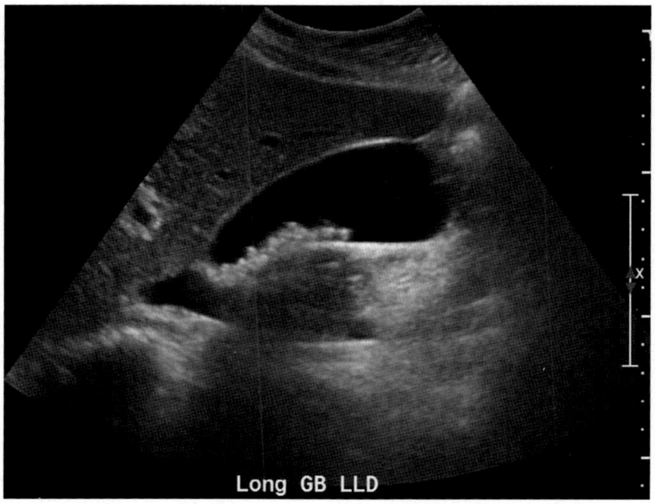

FIGURE 55-3 This sonogram shows multiple hyperechoic gallstones filling an anechoic gallbladder.

of cholesterol crystals, a prerequisite for cholesterol gallstones. Maringhini and colleagues (1993) showed that the incidence of biliary sludge—which can be a forerunner to gallstones—and gallstones in pregnancy are 31 and 2 percent, respectively. Ko and colleagues (2014), however, cited a combined incidence to be lower at about 5 percent. Postpartum, there is frequently regression of sludge, and occasionally gallstones will resorb. Still, after delivery, hospitalization for gallbladder disease within a year remains relatively common. Ko (2006) studied Washington state discharge databases and documented that 0.5 percent of postpartum women were hospitalized within a year for various conditions. Of these 6211 women, 76 had uncomplicated cholecystitis, and 55 underwent cholecystectomy.

Medical versus Surgical Management

Acute cholecystitis during pregnancy or the puerperium is usually associated with gallstones or biliary sludge. Symptomatic cholecystitis is initially managed in a manner similar to that for nonpregnant women. In the past, most favored medical therapy. However, the recurrence rate during the same pregnancy is high, and 25 to 50 percent of women ultimately required cholecystectomy for persistent symptoms. Moreover, if cholecystitis recurs later in gestation, preterm labor is more likely and cholecystectomy technically more difficult.

For these reasons, operative and endoscopic interventions are increasingly favored over conservative measures. Othman and coworkers (2012) showed that women managed conservatively had more pain, more recurrent visits to the emergency department, more hospitalizations, and a higher rate of cesarean delivery. Dhupar and associates (2010) reported more complications with conservative management of gallbladder disease compared with laparoscopic cholecystectomy in pregnancy. These included multiple admissions, prolonged total parenteral nutrition, and unplanned labor induction for worsening gallbladder symptoms.

Cholecystectomy was performed safely in all trimesters. Only one of 19 patients who underwent laparoscopic cholecystectomy had a complication, which did not require further surgery. Date and coworkers (2008) reviewed the literature and found no increased risk of preterm birth or fetal demise for operative compared with conservative management. There was, however, a significantly higher rate of fetal death from gallstone pancreatitis when women were managed conservatively compared with surgical management. There were no perinatal deaths in 20 women undergoing cholecystectomy and in nine undergoing endoscopic retrograde cholangiopancreatography. Management at Parkland Hospital has evolved to a more aggressive surgical approach, especially if there is concomitant biliary pancreatitis as subsequently discussed. During the past two decades, laparoscopic cholecystectomy has evolved as the favored surgical approach and is discussed in Chapter 46 (p. 928).

Endoscopic Retrograde Cholangiopancreatography

Relief from symptomatic biliary duct gallstones during pregnancy has been greatly aided by use of endoscopic retrograde cholangiopancreatography—ERCP (Fogel, 2014; Menees, 2006). The procedure is performed if there is suspected or proven common duct obstruction, usually from stones. Approximately 10 percent of patients with symptomatic stone disease have common duct stones (Greenberger, 2008). ERCP can be modified in many cases so that radiation exposure from fluoroscopy is avoided (Shelton, 2008; Simmons, 2004).

Tang and associates (2009) reported results from 68 ERCP procedures performed in 65 pregnant women at Parkland Hospital. All but two women had gallstones, and sphincterotomy was performed in all but one woman. Common-duct stones were identified in half of these 65 women, and in all but one, the stones were successfully removed. A biliary stent was placed in 22 percent and removed after delivery. Complications were minimal, and post-ERCP pancreatitis developed in 16 percent. Pregnancy outcomes were not different than for the general obstetrical population. As a less invasive approach, magnetic resonance cholangiopancreatography (MRCP) has been reported to have utility in pregnancy, particularly with otherwise unexplained biliary duct dilatation identified sonographically (Oto, 2009). Use of MRCP in this situation identified the cause of the biliary ductal dilatation in four cases and excluded obstructive pathology in the remaining four cases.

PANCREATIC DISORDERS

Pancreatitis

Acute pancreatic inflammation is triggered by activation of pancreatic trypsinogen followed by autodigestion. It is characterized by cellular membrane disruption and proteolysis, edema, hemorrhage, and necrosis (Fogel, 2014; Whitcomb, 2006). Approximately 20 percent have severe pancreatitis, and mortality rates in these patients reach up to 25 percent (Swaroop, 2004).

In nonpregnant patients, acute pancreatitis is almost equally associated with gallstones and alcohol abuse. During pregnancy, however, cholelithiasis is almost always the predisposing condition. Other causes are hyperlipidemias, usually hypertriglyceridemia; hyperparathyroidism; congenital ductal anomalies; and rarely autoimmune pancreatitis (Crisan, 2008; Finkelberg, 2006). Nonbiliary pancreatitis occasionally develops postoperatively, or it is associated with trauma, drugs, or some viral infections. Certain metabolic conditions, including acute fatty liver of pregnancy and familial hypertriglyceridemia, also predispose to pancreatitis (Nelson, 2013). Acute and chronic pancreatitis have been linked to the more than 1000 mutations of the cystic fibrosis transmembrane conductance regulator gene (Rowntree, 2003).

At Parkland Hospital, with a large Mexican American population, acute pancreatitis complicated approximately 1 in 3300 pregnancies (Ramin, 1995). At Brigham and Women's Hospital, with a more diversely ethnic population, Hernandez and colleagues (2007) reported an incidence of 1 in 4450. In a multiple-institution Midwestern three-state review of more than 305,000 pregnancies, Eddy and associates (2008) found the incidence of acute pancreatitis to be 1 in 3450.

Diagnosis

Acute pancreatitis is characterized by mild to incapacitating epigastric pain, nausea and vomiting, and abdominal distention.

TABLE 55-5. Laboratory Values in 173 Pregnant Women with Acute Pancreatitis

Test	Mean	Range	Normal
Serum amylase (IU/L)	1980	111–8917	28–100
Serum lipase (IU/L)	3076	36–41,824	7–59
Total bilirubin (mg/dL)	1.7	0.1–8.71	0.2–1.3
Aspartate transferase (U/L)	115	11–1113	10–35
Leukocytes (per μL)	10,700	1000–27,200	3900–10,700

From Ramin, 1995; Tang, 2010; Turhan, 2010.

Patients are usually in distress and have low-grade fever, tachycardia, hypotension, and abdominal tenderness. As many as 10 percent have systemic inflammatory response syndrome, which causes endothelial activation and can lead to *acute respiratory distress syndrome* (Chap. 47, p. 943).

Laboratory confirmation is from serum amylase levels three times upper normal values. As shown in Table 55-5, the mean amylase value was approximately 2000 IU/L in 173 pregnant women with pancreatitis, and the mean lipase value approximated 3000 IU/L. *Importantly, there is no correlation between the degree of enzyme elevation and disease severity.* Indeed, by 48 to 72 hours, amylase levels may return to normal despite other evidence for continuing pancreatitis. Serum lipase activity is also increased and usually remains elevated with continued inflammation. There is usually leukocytosis, and 25 percent of patients have hypocalcemia. Elevated serum bilirubin and aspartate aminotransferase levels may signify gallstone disease.

Several prognostic factors may be used to predict disease severity (Whitcomb, 2006). Some of these are respiratory failure, shock, need for massive colloid replacement, hypocalcemia < 8 mg/dL, and dark hemorrhagic fluid removed with paracentesis. If three of the first four features are documented, survival is only 30 percent.

Management

Medical treatment is the same as that for nonpregnant patients and includes analgesics, intravenous hydration, and measures to decrease pancreatic secretion by interdiction of oral intake. Other than supportive therapy, no particular treatment schemes have improved outcomes (Whitcomb, 2006). In the series by Ramin and colleagues (1995), all 43 affected pregnant women responded to conservative treatment and were hospitalized for a mean of 8.5 days. Nasogastric suction does not improve outcomes of mild to moderate disease, but enteral feeding may be helpful once pain improves and associated ileus resolves. Although we try to avoid parenteral nutrition, in 65 women with acute pancreatitis described by Eddy and coworkers (2008), a fourth had total parenteral nutrition. If there is bacterial superinfection of necrotizing pancreatitis, then antimicrobials are indicated. If common duct stones are found, then ERCP is indicated (Fogel, 2014). For pregnant patients with gallstone pancreatitis, ERCP for removal of common duct stones and papillotomy has been used successfully (Simmons, 2004; Tang, 2009). Cholecystectomy should be considered after inflammation subsides if there is gallbladder disease. Hernandez and associates (2007) reported that half of such women who did not undergo cholecystectomy had recurrent pancreatitis during the same pregnancy. Severe necrotizing pancreatitis can be life threatening, and laparotomy for debridement and drainage may be required (Gosnell, 2001; Robertson, 2006).

Pregnancy outcomes appear to be related to acute pancreatitis severity. Eddy and associates (2008) reported a 30-percent preterm delivery rate, and 11 percent were delivered before 35 weeks' gestation. There were two pancreatitis-related deaths. Importantly, almost a third of 73 women had recurrent pancreatitis during pregnancy.

Pancreatic Transplantation

According to the United Network for Organ Sharing, the 5-year graft survival for pancreatic transplantation is 80 percent. Because there is improved survival when a combined pancreas and kidney are grafted for those with type 1 diabetes and renal failure, most transplants include both organs.

Mastrobattista and Gomez-Lobo (2008) reported results from the National Transplantation Pregnancy Registry. Of 44 pregnancies in 73 women following pancreas-kidney transplantation, outcomes have been encouraging, and vaginal delivery has been described. Although the incidence of hypertension, preeclampsia, preterm delivery, and fetal-growth restriction was high, there was only one perinatal death. There were four rejection episodes during pregnancy, which were treated successfully.

Pancreatic islet autotransplantation may be performed to prevent diabetes following pancreatectomy, and at least three successful pregnancies have been described (Jung, 2007).

REFERENCES

Airoldi J, Berghella V: Hepatitis C and pregnancy. Obstet Gynecol Surv 61:666, 2006

American College of Obstetricians and Gynecologists: Upper gastrointestinal tract, biliary, and pancreatic disorders. Clinical Updates in Women's Health Care, Vol. XI, No. 4, 2012a

American College of Obstetricians and Gynecologists: Viral hepatitis in pregnancy. Practice Bulletin No. 86, October 2007, Reaffirmed 2012b

Anzivino C, Odoardi MR, Meschiari E, et al: ABCB4 and ABCB11 mutations in intrahepatic cholestasis of pregnancy in an Italian population. Dig Liver Dis 45(3):226, 2013

Arshad M, El-Kamary SS, Jhaveri R: Hepatitis C virus infection during pregnancy and the newborn period—are they opportunities for treatment? J Viral Hepat 18(4):229, 2011

Babik JM, Cohan D, Monto A, et al: The human fetal immune response to hepatitis C virus exposure in utero. J Infect Dis 203(2):196, 2011

Bacq Y, Sentilhes L, Reyes HB, et al: Efficacy of ursodeoxycholic acid in treating intrahepatic cholestasis of pregnancy: a meta-analysis. Gastroenterology 143(6):1492, 2012

Baskin B, Geraghty M, Ray PN: Paternal isodisomy of chromosome 2 as a cause of long chain 3-hydroxyacyl-CoA dehydrogenase (LCHAD) deficiency. Am J Med Genet A 152A(7):1808, 2010

Berkley EMF, Leslie KK, Arora S, et al: Chronic hepatitis C in pregnancy. Am J Obstet Gynecol 112(2 Pt 1):304, 2008

Bernal W, Wendon J: Acute liver failure. N Engl J Med 369(26):2525, 2013

Blume C, Sensoy A, Gross MM, et al: A comparison of the outcome of pregnancies after liver and kidney transplantation. Transplantation 95(1):222, 2013
Borkakoti J, Hazam RK, Mohammad A, et al: Does high viral load of hepatitis E virus influence the severity and prognosis of acute liver failure during pregnancy? J Med Virol 85(4):620, 2013
Browning JD, Szczepaniak LS, Dobbins R, et al: Prevalence of hepatic steatosis in an urban population in the United States: impact of ethnicity. Hepatology 40(6):1387, 2004
Browning MF, Levy HL, Wilkins-Haug LE, et al: Fetal fatty acid oxidation defects and maternal liver disease in pregnancy. Obstet Gynecol 107:115, 2006
Candia L, Marquez J, Espinoza LR: Autoimmune hepatitis and pregnancy: a rheumatologist's dilemma. Semin Arthritis Rheum 35:49, 2005
Castro MA, Ouzounian JG, Colletti PM, et al: Radiologic studies in acute fatty liver of pregnancy. A review of the literature and 19 new cases. J Reprod Med 41:839, 1996
Centers for Disease Control and Prevention: Surveillance for acute viral hepatitis—United States, 2006. MMWR 57(2):1, 2008
Centers for Disease Control and Prevention: Sexually transmitted diseases guidelines, 2010. MMWR 59(1):1, 2010
Centers for Disease Control and Prevention: Viral Hepatitis Surveillance United States, 2010. August 20, 2012. Available at: http://www.cdc.gov/hepatitis/Statistics/2010Surveillance/. Accessed August 14, 2013
Ch'ng CL, Morgan M, Hainsworth I, et al: Prospective study of liver dysfunction in pregnancy in Southwest Wales. Gut 51(6):876, 2002
Christopher V, Al-Chalabi T, Richardson PD, et al: Pregnancy outcome after liver transplantation: a single-center experience of 71 pregnancies in 45 recipients. Liver Transpl 12:1037, 2006
Chung RT, Podolsky DK: Cirrhosis and its complications. In Kasper DL, Braunwald E, Fauci AS, et al (eds): Harrison's Principles of Internal Medicine, 16th ed. New York, McGraw-Hill, 2005, p 1858
Cobey FC, Salem RR: A review of liver masses in pregnancy and a proposed algorithm for their diagnosis and management. Am J Surg 187(2):181, 2004
Connell LE, Salihu HM, Salemi JL, et al: Maternal hepatitis B and hepatitis C carrier status and perinatal outcomes. Liver Int 31(8):1163, 2011
Coscia LA, Constantinescu S, Moritz MJ, et al: Report from the National Transplantation Pregnancy Registry (NTPR): outcomes of pregnancy after transplantation. Clin Transpl 2010:65
Cottrell EB, Chou R, Wasson N, et al: Reducing risk for mother-to-infant transmission of hepatitis C virus: a systematic review of the U.S. Preventive Services Task Force. Ann Intern Med 158(2):109, 2013
Crisan LS, Steidl ET, Rivera-Alsina ME: Acute hyperlipidemic pancreatitis in pregnancy. Am J Obstet Gynecol 198(5):e57, 2008
Cunningham FG, Lowe TW, Guss S, et al: Erythrocyte morphology in women with severe preeclampsia and eclampsia. Am J Obstet Gynecol 153:358, 1985
Date RS, Kaushal M, Ramesh A: A review of the management of gallstone disease and its complications in pregnancy. Am J Surg 196(4):599, 2008
Daudi N, Shouval D, Stein-Zamir C, et al: Breastmilk hepatitis A virus DNA in nursing mothers with acute hepatitis A virus infection. Breastfeed Med 7:313, 2012
Davit-Spraul A, Gonzales E, Baussan C, et al: The spectrum of liver diseases related to ABCB4 gene mutations: pathophysiology and clinical aspects. Semin Liver Dis 30(2):134, 2010
Davit-Spraul A, Gonzales E, Jacquemin E: NR1H4 analysis in patients with progressive familial intrahepatic cholestasis, drug-induced cholestasis or intrahepatic cholestasis of pregnancy unrelated to ATP8B1, ABCB11 and ABCB4 mutations. Clin Res Hepatol Gastroenterol 36(6):569, 2012
Deng M, Zhou X, Gao S, et al: The effects of telbivudine in late pregnancy to prevent intrauterine transmission of the hepatitis B virus: a systematic review and meta-analysis. Virol J 9:185, 2012
Deshpande NA, James NT, Kucirka LM, et al: Pregnancy outcomes of liver transplant recipients: a systematic review and meta-analysis. Liver Transpl 18(6):621, 2012
Dhupar R, Smaldone GM, Hamad GG. Is there a benefit to delaying cholecystectomy for symptomatic gallbladder disease during pregnancy? Surg Endosc 24(1):108, 2010
Dienstag JL: Acute viral hepatitis. In Longo DL, Fauci AS, Kasper DL, et al (eds) Harrison's Principles of Internal Medicine, 18th ed. New York, McGraw-Hill, 2012a
Dienstag JL: Chronic hepatitis. In Longo DL, Fauci AS, Kasper DL, et al (eds) Harrison's Principles of Internal Medicine, 18th ed. New York, McGraw-Hill, 2012b
Dixon PH, Wadsworth CA, Chambers J, et al: A comprehensive analysis of common genetic variation around six candidate loci for intrahepatic cholestasis of pregnancy. Am J Gastroenterol 109:76, 2014
Dusheiko G: Interruption of mother-to-infant transmission of hepatitis B: time to include selective antiviral prophylaxis? Lancet 379(9830):2019, 2012
Eddy JJ, Gideonsen MD, Song JY, et al: Pancreatitis in pregnancy. Obstet Gynecol 112:1075, 2008
Ferrero S, Lungaro P, Bruzzone BM, et al: Prospective study of mother-to-infant transmission of hepatitis C virus: a 10-year survey (1990–2000). Acta Obstet Gynecol Scand 82:229, 2003
Fesenmeier MF, Coppage KH, Lambers DS, et al: Acute fatty liver of pregnancy in 3 tertiary care centers. Am J Obstet Gynecol 192:1416, 2005
Feucht HH, Zollner B, Polywka S, et al: Vertical transmission of hepatitis G. Lancet 347:615, 1996
Finkelberg DL, Sahani D, Deshpande V, et al: Autoimmune pancreatitis. N Engl J Med 355:2670, 2006
Flint C, Larsen H, Nielsen GL, et al: Pregnancy outcome after suicide attempt by drug use: a Danish population-based study. Acta Obstet Gynecol Scand 81:516, 2002
Fogel EL, Sherman S: ERCP for gallstone pancreatitis. N Engl J Med 370:150, 2014
Forbes S, Taylor-Robinson SD, Patel N, et al: Increased prevalence of non-alcoholic fatty liver disease in European women with a history of gestational diabetes. Diabetologia 54(3):641, 2011
Franco J, Newcomer J, Adams M, et al: Auxiliary liver transplant in acute fatty liver of pregnancy. Obstet Gynecol 95:1042, 2000
Ghamar Chehreh ME, Tabatabaei SV, Khazanehdari S, et al: Effect of cesarean section on the risk of perinatal transmission of hepatitis C virus from HCV-RNA+/HIV–mothers: a meta-analysis. Arch Gynecol Obstet 283(2):255, 2011
Giles M, Visvanathan K, Sasadeusz J: Antiviral therapy for hepatitis B infection during pregnancy and breastfeeding. Antivir Ther 16(5):621, 2011
Glantz A, Marschall H, Lammert F, et al: Intrahepatic Cholestasis of pregnancy: a randomized controlled trial comparing dexamethasone and ursodeoxycholic acid. Hepatology 42:1399, 2005
Glantz A, Marschall H, Mattsson L: Intrahepatic cholestasis of pregnancy: relationships between bile acid levels and fetal complication rates. Hepatology 40:467, 2004
Gorelik J, Patel P, Ng'andwe C, et al: Genes encoding bile acid, phospholipid and anion transporters are expressed in a human fetal cardiomyocyte culture. BJOG 113:552, 2006
Gosnell FE, O'Neill BB, Harris HW: Necrotizing pancreatitis during pregnancy: a rare case and review of the literature. J Gastrointest Surg 5:371, 2001
Gossard AA, Lindor KD: Autoimmune hepatitis: a review. J Gastroenterol 47(5):498, 2012
Greenberger NJ, Paumgartner G: Diseases of the gallbladder and bile ducts. In Fauci AS, Braunwald E, Kasper DL, et al (eds): Harrison's Principles of Internal Medicine, 17th ed. New York, McGraw-Hill, 2008, p 1991
Groszmann RJ, Garcia-Tsao G, Bosch J, et al: Beta-blockers to prevent gastroesophageal varices in patients with cirrhosis. N Engl J Med 353:2254, 2005
Ha JF, Phillips M, Faulkner K: Splenic artery aneurysm rupture in pregnancy. Eur J Obstet Gynecol Reprod Biol 146(2):133, 2009
Han L, Zhang HW, Xie JX, et al: A meta-analysis of lamivudine for interruption of mother-to-child transmission of hepatitis B virus. World J Gastroenterol 17(38):4321, 2011
Heard KJ: Acetylcysteine for acetaminophen poisoning. N Engl J Med 359: 285, 2008
Hernandez A, Petrov MS, Brooks DC, et al: Acute pancreatitis and pregnancy: a 10-year single center experience. J Gastrointest Surg 11:1623, 2007
Hill JB, Sheffield JS, Kim MJ, et al: Risk of hepatitis B transmission in breast-fed infants of chronic hepatitis B carriers. Obstet Gynecol 99(6):1049, 2002
Hodgman MJ, Garrard AR: A review of acetaminophen poisoning. Crit Care Clin 28(4):499, 2012
Hoofnagle JH, Nelson KE, Purcell RH: Hepatitis E. N Engl J Med 367:13, 2012
Hu Y, Zhang S, Luo C, et al: Gaps in the prevention of perinatal transmission of hepatitis B virus between recommendations and routine practices in a highly endemic region: a provincial population-base study in China. BMC Infect Dis 12:221, 2012
Inaba N, Okajima Y, Kang XS, et al: Maternal–infant transmission of hepatitis G virus. Am J Obstet Gynecol 177:1537, 1997
Indolfi G, Azzari C, Resti M: Hepatitis: immunoregulation in pregnancy and perinatal transmission of HCV. Nat Rev Gastroenterol Hepatol 11:6, 2014
Isoherranen N, Thummel KE: Drug metabolism and transport during pregnancy: how does drug disposition change during pregnancy and what are the mechanisms that cause such changes? Drug Metab Dispos 41(2):256, 2013
Jabiry-Zieniewicz Z, Szpotanska-Sikorska M, Pietrzak B, et al: Pregnancy outcomes among female recipients after liver transplantation: further experience. Transplant Proc 43(8):3043, 2011

Jain AB, Reyes J, Marcos A, et al: Pregnancy after liver transplantation with tacrolimus immunosuppression: a single center's experience update at 13 years. Transplantation 76(5):827, 2003
Joshi D, James A, Quaglia A, et al: Liver disease in pregnancy. Lancet 375(9714):594, 2010
Jung HS, Choi SH, Noh JH, et al: Healthy twin birth after autologous islet transplantation in a pancreatectomized patient due to a benign tumor. Transplant Proc 39(5):1723, 2007
Khan S, Tudur Smith C, Williamson P, et al: Portosystemic shunts versus endoscopic therapy for variceal rebleeding in patients with cirrhosis. Cochrane Database Syst Rev 4:CD000553, 2006
Kleiss K, Choy-Hee L, Fogle R, et al: Torsion of the gallbladder in pregnancy: a case report. J Reprod Med 48:206, 2003
Knight M, Nelson-Piercy C, Kurinczuk JJ, et al: A prospective national study of acute fatty liver of pregnancy in the UK. Gut 57(7):951, 2008
Ko CW: Risk factors for gallstone-related hospitalization during pregnancy and the postpartum. Am J Gastroenterol 101(10):2263, 2006
Ko CW, Napolitano PG, Lee SP, et al: Physical activity, maternal metabolic measures, and the incidence of gallbladder sludge or stones during pregnancy: a randomized trial. Am J Perinatol 31:39, 2014
Kondrackiene J, Beuers U, Kupcinskas L: Efficacy and safety of ursodeoxycholic acid versus cholestyramine in intrahepatic cholestasis of pregnancy. Gastroenterology 129:894, 2005
Krawitt EL: Autoimmune hepatitis. N Engl J Med 354:54, 2006
Labrique AB, Sikder SS, Krain LJ, et al: Hepatitis E, a vaccine-preventable cause of maternal deaths. Emerg Infect Dis 18(9):1401, 2012
Lausman AY, Al-Yaseen E, Sam E, et al: Intrahepatic cholestasis of pregnancy in women with a multiple pregnancy: an analysis of risks and pregnancy outcomes. J Obstet Gynaecol Can 30(11):1008, 2008
Lee RH, Goodwin TM, Greenspoon J, et al: The prevalence of intrahepatic cholestasis of pregnancy in a primarily Latina Los Angeles population. J Perinatol 26(9):527, 2006
Lee RH, Incerpi MH, Miller DA, et al: Sudden death in intrahepatic cholestasis of pregnancy. Obstet Gynecol 113(2):528, 2009
Lee WM, Squires RH Jr, Nyberg SL, et al: Acute liver failure: Summary of a workshop. Hepatology 47:1401, 2008
Levene AP, Goldin RD: The epidemiology, pathogenesis and histopathology of fatty liver disease. Histopathology 61(2):141, 2012
Liang TJ, Ghany MG: Current and future therapies for hepatitis C virus infection. N Engl J Med 368(20):1907, 2013
Liu M, Cai H, Yi W: Safety of telbivudine treatment for chronic hepatitis B for the entire pregnancy. J Viral Hepat 20(Suppl 1):65, 2013
Lok AS, Gardiner DF, Lawitz E, et al: Preliminary study of two antiviral agents for hepatitis C genotype 1. N Engl J Med 366(3):216, 2012
López M, Coll O: Chronic viral infections and invasive procedures: risk of vertical transmission and current recommendations. Fetal Diagn Ther 28(1):1, 2010
Lou H, Ding W, Dong M, et al: The presence of hepatitis B surface antigen in the ova of pregnant women and its relationship with intra-uterine infection by hepatitis B virus. J Int Med Res 38(1):214, 2010
Lucangioli SE, Castaño G, Contin MD, et al: Lithocholic acid as a biomarker of intrahepatic cholestasis of pregnancy during ursodeoxycholic acid treatment. Ann Clin Biochem 46(1):44, 2009
Maringhini A, Ciambra M, Baccelliere P, et al: Biliary sludge and gallstones in pregnancy: incidence, risk factors, and natural history. Ann Intern Med 119(2):116, 1993
Marschall HU, Shemer EW, Ludvigsson JF, et al: Intrahepatic cholestasis of pregnancy and associated hepatobiliary disease: a population based cohort study. Hepatology 58(4):1385, 2013
Martin JN Jr, Briery CM, Rose CH, et al: Postpartum plasma exchange as adjunctive therapy for severe acute fatty liver of pregnancy. J Clin Apher 23(4):138, 2008
Mastrobattista JM, Gomez-Lobo V: Pregnancy after solid organ transplantation. Obstet Gynecol 112:919, 2008
Matos A, Bernardes J, Ayres-de-Campos D, et al: Antepartum fetal cerebral hemorrhage not predicted by current surveillance methods in cholestasis of pregnancy. Obstet Gynecol 89:803, 1997
McCullough AJ: Thiazolidinediones for nonalcoholic steatohepatitis—promising but not ready for prime time. N Engl J Med 355:2361, 2006
McKay DB, Josephson MA: Pregnancy in recipients of solid organs—Effects on mother and child. N Engl J Med 354:1281, 2006
McMenamin MB, Jackson AD, Lambert J, et al: Obstetric management of hepatitis C-positive mothers: analysis of vertical transmission in 559 mother-infant pairs. Am J Obstet Gynecol 199:315.e1, 2008
Mehta S, Singla A, Rajaram S: Prognostic factors for fulminant viral hepatitis in pregnancy. Int J Gynaecol Obstet 118(2):172, 2012
Menees S, Elta G: Endoscopic retrograde cholangiopancreatography during pregnancy. Gastrointest Endoscopy Clin North Am 16:41, 2006
Mufti AR, Reau N: Liver disease in pregnancy. Clin Liver Dis 16(2):247, 2012
Müllenbach R, Bennett A, Tetlow N, et al: ATP8B1 mutations in British cases with intrahepatic cholestasis of pregnancy. Gut 54(6):829, 2005
Nagy S, Bush MC, Berkowitz R, et al: Pregnancy outcome in liver transplant recipients. Obstet Gynecol 102(1):121, 2003
Nayeri UA, Werner EF, Han CS, et al: Antenatal lamivudine to reduce perinatal hepatitis B transmission: a cost-effectiveness analysis. Am J Obstet Gynecol 207(3):231.e1, 2012
Nelson DB, Yost NP, Cunningham FG: Acute fatty liver of pregnancy: clinical outcomes and expected durations of recovery. Am J Obstet Gynecol 209(5):456.e1, 2013
Organ Procurement and Transplantation Network: 2011 Annual data report. 2012. Available at: http://srtr.transplant.hrsa.gov/annual_reports/2011/default.aspx. Accessed August 16,2013
Othman MO, Stone E, Hashimi M, et al: Conservative management of cholelithiasis and its complications in pregnancy is associated with recurrent symptoms and more emergency department visits. Gastrointest Endosc 76(3):564, 2012
Oto A, Ernst R, Ghulmiyyah L, et al: The role of MR cholangiopancreatography in the evaluation of pregnant patients with acute pancreaticobiliary disease. Br J Radiol 82(976):279, 2009
Page L, Girling J: A novel cause for abnormal liver function tests in pregnancy and the puerperium: non-alcoholic fatty liver disease. BJOG 118(12):1532, 2011
Pan CQ, Han GR, Jiang HX, et al: Telbivudine prevents vertical transmission from HBeAg-positive women with chronic hepatitis B. Clin Gastroenterol Hepatol 10(5):520, 2012a
Pan CQ, Mi LJ, Bunchorntavakul C, et al: Tenofovir disoproxil fumarate for prevention of vertical transmission of hepatitis B virus infection by highly viremic pregnant women: a case series. Dig Dis Sci 57(9):2423, 2012b
Paternoster DM, Fabris F, Palù G, et al: Intra-hepatic cholestasis of pregnancy in hepatitis C virus infection. Acta Obstet Gynecol Scand 81:99, 2002
Pereira SP, O'Donohue J, Wendon J, et al: Maternal and perinatal outcome in severe pregnancy-related liver disease. Hepatology 26:1258, 1997
Pergam SA, Wang CC, Gardella CM, et al: Pregnancy complications associated with hepatitis C: data from a 2003–2005 Washington state birth cohort. Am J Obstet Gynecol 199:38.e1, 2008
Poordad F, Lawitz E, Kowdley KV, et al: Exploratory study of oral combination antiviral therapy for hepatitis C. N Engl J Med 368:1, 2013
Ramin KD, Ramin SM, Richey SD, et al: Acute pancreatitis in pregnancy. Am J Obstet Gynecol 173:187, 1995
Ramírez-Fuentes C, Martí-Bonmatí L, Torregrosa A, et al: Variations in the size of focal nodular hyperplasia on magnetic resonance imaging. Radiologia 55(6):499, 2013
Reau N: Finding the needle in the haystack: predicting mortality in pregnancy-related liver disease. Clin Gastroenterol Hepatol 12:114, 2014
Reddick KLB, Jhaveri R, Gandhi M, et al: Pregnancy outcomes associated with viral hepatitis. J Viral Hepat 18(7):e394, 2011
Rein DB, Stevens GA, Theaker J, et al: The global burden of hepatitis E virus genotypes 1 and 2 in 2005. Hepatology 55(4):988, 2012
Reyes H: Intrahepatic cholestasis. A puzzling disorder of pregnancy. J Gastroenterol Hepatol 12:211, 1997
Rifai K, Mix H, Krusche S, et al: No evidence of substantial growth progression or complications of large focal nodular hyperplasia during pregnancy. Scand J Gastroenterol 48(1):88, 2013
Riggs BS, Bronstein AC, Kulig K, et al: Acute acetaminophen overdose during pregnancy. Obstet Gynecol 74:247, 1989
Roberts SS, Miller RK, Jones JK, et al: The Ribavirin Pregnancy Registry: findings after 5 years of enrollment, 2003–2009. Birth Defects Res A Clin Mol Teratol 88(7):551, 2010
Robertson KW, Stewart IS, Imrie CW: Severe acute pancreatitis and pregnancy. Pancreatology 6:309, 2006
Rook M, Vargas J, Caughey A, et al: Fetal outcomes in pregnancies complicated by intrahepatic cholestasis of pregnancy in a Northern California cohort. PLoS One 7(3):e28343, 2012
Ross LF: Ethical considerations related to pregnancy in transplant recipients. N Engl J Med 354:1313, 2006
Rowntree RK, Harris A: The phenotypic consequences of CFTR mutations. Ann Hum Genet 67:471, 2003
Rumack BH, Matthew H: Acetaminophen poisoning and toxicity. Pediatrics 55:871, 1975
Sadler LC, Lane M, North R: Severe fetal intracranial haemorrhage during treatment with cholestyramine for intrahepatic cholestasis of pregnancy. Br J Obstet Gynaecol 102:169, 1995
Safir A, Levy A, Sikuler E, et al: Maternal hepatitis B virus or hepatitis C virus carrier status as an independent risk factor for adverse perinatal outcome. Liver Int 30(5):765, 2010

Salam GD, Kumar A, Kar P, et al: Serum tumor necrosis factor-alpha level in hepatitis E virus-related acute viral hepatitis and fulminant hepatic failure in pregnant women. Hepatol Res 43(8):826, 2013
Santambrogio R, Marconi AM, Ceretti AP, et al: Liver transplantation for spontaneous intrapartum rupture of a hepatic adenoma. Obstet Gynecol 113(2 Pt 2):508, 2009
Santiago-Munoz P, Roberts S, Sheffield J, et al: Prevalence of hepatitis B and C in pregnant women who are infected with human immunodeficiency virus. Am J Obstet Gynecol 193:1270, 2005
Santos L, Patterson A, Moreea SM, et al: Acute liver failure in pregnancy associated with maternal MCAD deficiency. J Inherit Metab Dis 30(1):103, 2007
Schmidt LE, Larsen FS: MELD score as a predictor of liver failure and death in patients with acetaminophen-induced liver injury. Hepatology 45(3):789, 2007
Schramm C, Herkel J, Beuers U, et al: Pregnancy in autoimmune hepatitis: Outcome and risk factors. Am J Gastroenterol 101:556, 2006
Sheffield J, Roberts S, Laibl V, et al: The efficacy of an accelerated hepatitis B vaccination program during pregnancy [Abstract No. 212]. Am J Obstet Gynecol 195:S73, 2006
Sheiner E, Ohel I, Levy A, et al: Pregnancy outcome in women with pruritus gravidarum. J Reprod Med 51:394, 2006
Shelton J, Linder JD, Rivera-Alsina ME, et al: Commitment, confirmation, and clearance: new techniques for nonradiation ERCP during pregnancy (with videos). Gastrointest Endosc 67:364, 2008
Shi Z, Tang Y, Wang H, et al: Breastfeeding of newborns by mothers carrying hepatitis B virus: a meta-analysis and systematic review. Arch Pediatr Adolesc Med 165(9):837, 2011
Shi Z, Yang Y, Ma L, et al: Lamivudine in late pregnancy to interrupt in utero transmission of hepatitis B virus. A systematic review and meta-analysis. Obstet Gynecol 116(1):147, 2010
Sibai BM: Imitators of severe preeclampsia. Obstet Gynecol 109:956, 2007
Sibanda N, Briggs JD, Davison JM, et al: Pregnancy after organ transplantation: a report from the UK Transplant pregnancy registry. Transplantation 83:1301, 2007
Simmons DC, Tarnasky PR, Rivera-Alsina ME, et al: Endoscopic retrograde cholangiopancreatography (ERCP) in pregnancy without the use of radiation. Am J Obstet Gynecol 190:1467, 2004
Sims HF, Brackett JC, Powell CK, et al: The molecular basis of pediatric long chain 3-hydroxyacyl-CoA dehydrogenase deficiency associated with maternal acute fatty liver of pregnancy. Proc Natl Acad Sci U S A 92:841, 1995
Smith EA, Jacques-Carroll L, Walker TY, et al: The National Perinatal Hepatitis B Prevention Program, 1994–2008. Pediatrics 129(4):609, 2012
Søgaard KK, Horváth-Puhó E, Grønback H, et al: Risk of venous thromboembolism in patients with liver disease: a nationwide population-based case-control study. Am J Gastroenterol 104(1):96, 2009
Stewart RD, Sheffield JS: Hepatitis B vaccination in pregnancy in the United States. Vaccines 1(2):167, 2013
Strehlow SL, Pathak B, Goodwin TM, et al: The mechanical PR interval in fetuses of women with intrahepatic cholestasis of pregnancy. Am J Obstet Gynecol 203(5):455.e1, 2010
Swaroop VS, Chari ST, Clain JE: Severe acute pancreatitis. JAMA 291:2865, 2004
Tan J, Surti B, Saab S: Pregnancy and cirrhosis. Liver Transpl 14(8):1081, 2008
Tang S, Mayo MJ, Rodriguez-Frias E, et al: Safety and utility of ERCP during pregnancy. Gastrointest Endosc 69:453, 2009
Tang SJ, Rodriguez-Frias E, Singh S, et al: Acute pancreatitis during pregnancy. Clin Gastroenterol Hepatol 8(1):85, 2010
Towers CV, Asrat T, Rumney P: The presence of hepatitis B surface antigen and deoxyribonucleic acid in amniotic fluid and cord blood. Am J Obstet Gynecol 184:1514, 2001
Turhan AN, Gönenç M, Kapan S, et al: Acute biliary pancreatitis related with pregnancy: a 5-year single center experience. Ulus Travma Acil Cerrahi Derg 16(2):160, 2010
Urganci N, Arapoglu M, Akyildiz B, et al: Neonatal cholestasis resulting from vertical transmission of hepatitis A infection. Pediatr Infect Dis J 22(4):381, 2003
Uribe M, Chavez-Tapia NC, Mendez-Sanchez N: Pregnancy and autoimmune hepatitis. Ann Hepatol 5(3):187, 2006
Usta IM, Barton JR, Amon EA, et al: Acute fatty liver of pregnancy: an experience in the diagnosis and management of fourteen cases. Am J Obstet Gynecol 171:1342, 1994
Valdivieso V, Covarrubias C, Siegel F, et al: Pregnancy and cholelithiasis: pathogenesis and natural course of gallstones diagnosed in early puerperium. Hepatology 17:1, 1993
Victor JC, Monto AS, Surdina TY, et al: Hepatitis A vaccine versus immune globulin for postexposure prophylaxis. N Engl J Med 357:1685, 2007
Vigil-De Gracia P, Lavergne JA: Acute fatty liver of pregnancy. Int J Gynaecol Obstet 72(2):193, 2001
Vigil-de Gracia P, Montufar-Rueda C: Acute fatty liver of pregnancy: diagnosis, treatment, and outcome based on 35 consecutive cases. J Matern Fetal Neonatal Med 24(9):1143, 2011
Wang PH, Yang MJ, Lee WL, et al: Acetaminophen poisoning in late pregnancy. A case report. J Reprod Med 42:367, 1997
Webb GJ, Elsharkawy AM, Hirschfield G: Editorial: the etiology of intrahepatic cholestasis of pregnancy: towards solving a monkey puzzle. Am J Gastroenterol 109:85, 2014
Wedemeyer H, Pischke S, Manns MP: Pathogenesis and treatment of hepatitis E virus infection. Gastroenterology 142(6):1388, 2012
Welsh JA, Karpen S, Vos MB: Increasing prevalence of nonalcoholic fatty liver disease among United States adolescents, 1988–1994 to 2007–2010. J Pediatr 162(3):496.e1, 2013
Westbrook RH, Yeoman AD, Kriese S, et al: Outcomes of pregnancy in women with autoimmune hepatitis. J Autoimmun 38(2–3):J239, 2012
Whitcomb DC: Acute pancreatitis. N Engl J Med 354:2142, 2006
Wikström Shemer E, Marschall HU, Ludvigsson JF, et al: Intrahepatic cholestasis of pregnancy and associated adverse pregnancy and fetal outcomes: a 12-year population-based cohort study. BJOG 120(6):717, 2013
Wiseman JE, Yamamoto M, Nguyen TD, et al: Cystic pancreatic neoplasm in pregnancy: a case report and review of the literature. Arch Surg 143(1):84, 2008
World Health Organization: Weekly epidemiological Record 84(40):405, 2009
Wu T, Zhu FC, Huang SJ, et al: Safety of the hepatitis E vaccine for pregnant women: a preliminary analysis. Hepatology 55(6):2038, 2012
Xu WM, Cui YT, Wang L, et al: Lamivudine in late pregnancy to prevent perinatal transmission of hepatitis B virus infection: a multicentre, randomized, double-blind, placebo-controlled study. J Viral Hepat 16(2):94, 2009
Yi W, Liu M, Cai HD: Safety of lamivudine treatment for hepatitis B in early pregnancy. World J Gastroenterol 18(45):6645, 2012
Ylitalo K, Vänttinen T, Halmesmäki E, et al: Serious pregnancy complications in a patient with previously undiagnosed carnitine palmitoyltransferase 1 deficiency. Am J Obstet Gynecol 192:2060, 2005
Yu M, Jiang Q, Ji Y, et al: The efficacy and safety of antiviral therapy with lamivudine to stop the vertical transmission of hepatitis B virus. Eur J Clin Microbiol Infect Dis 31(9):2211, 2012
Zeeman GG, Moise KJ: Prophylactic banding of severe esophageal varices associated with liver cirrhosis in pregnancy. Obstet Gynecol 94:842, 1999

CHAPTER 56

Hematological Disorders

Pregnant women are susceptible to hematological abnormalities that may affect any woman of childbearing age. These include chronic disorders such as hereditary anemias, immunological thrombocytopenia, and malignancies such as leukemias and lymphomas. Other disorders arise during pregnancy because of pregnancy-induced demands. Two examples are iron deficiency and megaloblastic anemias. Pregnancy may also unmask underlying hematological disorders such as compensated hemolytic anemias caused by hemoglobinopathies or red cell membrane defects. Finally, any hematological disease may first arise during pregnancy. Importantly, pregnancy induces physiological changes that often confuse the diagnosis of these hematological disorders and assessment of their treatment. Several pregnancy-induced hematological changes are discussed in detail in Chapter 4 (p. 55).

ANEMIAS

Extensive hematological measurements have been made in healthy nonpregnant women. Concentrations of many cellular elements that are normal during pregnancy are listed in the Appendix (p. 1287). The Centers for Disease Control and Prevention (CDC) (1998) defined anemia in iron-supplemented pregnant women using a cutoff of the 5th percentile—11 g/dL in the first and third trimesters, and 10.5 g/dL in the second trimester (Fig. 56-1). An ongoing study of 278 women is currently evaluating the accuracy of an erythrogram and serum ferritin levels for anemia diagnosis and prediction of responsiveness to oral iron (Bresani, 2013).

The modest fall in hemoglobin levels during pregnancy is caused by a relatively greater expansion of plasma volume compared with the increase in red cell volume (Chap. 4, p. 55). The disproportion between the rates at which plasma and erythrocytes are added to the maternal circulation is greatest during the second trimester. Late in pregnancy, plasma expansion essentially ceases, while hemoglobin mass continues to increase.

General Considerations

The causes of anemia in pregnancy and their frequency are dependent on multiple factors such as geography, ethnicity, nutritional status, preexisting iron status, and prenatal iron supplementation. Other factors are socioeconomic, and anemia is more prevalent among indigent women (American College of Obstetricians and Gynecologists, 2013a). Approximately 25 percent of almost 48,000 Israeli pregnant women had a hemoglobin level < 10 g/dL (Kessous, 2013). Ren and colleagues (2007) found that 22 percent of 88,149 Chinese women were anemic in the first trimester. Of 1000 Indian women, half were anemic at some point, and 40 percent were throughout pregnancy (Kumar, 2013). The importance of

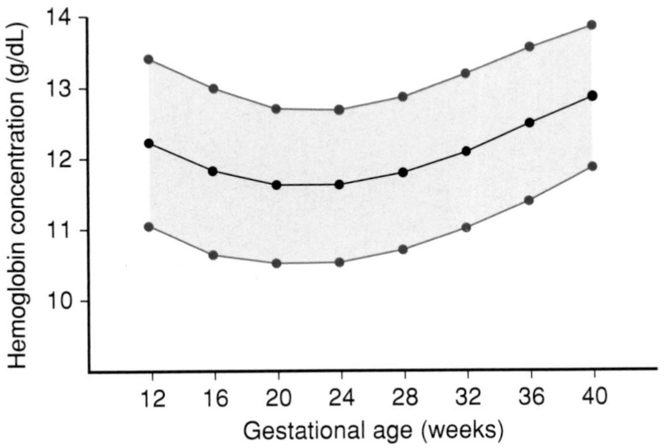

FIGURE 56-1 Mean hemoglobin concentrations (*black line*) and 5th and 95th percentiles (*blue lines*) for healthy pregnant women taking iron supplements. (Data from the Centers for Disease Control and Prevention, 1989.)

prenatal iron therapy is illustrated by the study of Taylor and associates (1982), who reported that hemoglobin levels at term averaged 12.7 g/dL among women who took supplemental iron compared with 11.2 g/dL for those who did not. Bodnar and coworkers (2001) studied a cohort of 59,248 pregnancies and found a postpartum anemia prevalence of 27 percent that correlated both with prenatal anemia and hemorrhage at delivery.

The etiologies of the more common anemias encountered in pregnancy are listed in Table 56-1. The specific cause of anemia is important when evaluating effects on pregnancy outcome. For example, maternal and perinatal outcomes are seldom affected by moderate iron deficiency anemia, yet they are altered markedly in women with sickle-cell anemia.

Effects on Pregnancy Outcomes

Most studies of anemia during pregnancy describe large populations. As indicated, these likely deal with nutritional anemias, specifically those due to iron deficiency. Klebanoff and associates (1991) studied nearly 27,000 women and found a slightly increased risk of preterm birth with midtrimester anemia. Ren and colleagues (2007) found that a low first-trimester hemoglobin concentration increased the risk of low birthweight, preterm birth, and small-for-gestational age infants. In a study from Tanzania, Kidanto and coworkers (2009) reported that the incidence of preterm delivery and low birthweight was increased as the severity of anemia increased. They did not, however, take into account the cause(s) of anemia, which was diagnosed in almost 80 percent of their obstetrical population. Kumar and colleagues (2013) studied 1000 Indian women and also found that second- and third-trimester anemia was associated with preterm birth and low birthweight. Chang and associates (2013) followed 850 children born to women classified as iron deficient in the third trimester. Children without iron supplementation had lower mental development at 12, 18, and 24 months of age, suggesting that prenatal iron deficiency is associated with mental development. Tran and associates (2014) reported similar findings from a Vietnamese study.

TABLE 56-1. Causes of Anemia During Pregnancy

Acquired
Iron deficiency anemia
Anemia caused by acute blood loss
Anemia of inflammation or malignancy
Megaloblastic anemia
Acquired hemolytic anemia
Aplastic or hypoplastic anemia
Hereditary
Thalassemias
Sickle-cell hemoglobinopathies
Other hemoglobinopathies
Hereditary hemolytic anemias

A seemingly paradoxical finding is that healthy pregnant women with a higher hemoglobin concentration are also at increased risk for adverse perinatal outcomes (von Tempelhoff, 2008). This may result from lower than average plasma volume expansion of pregnancy concurrent with normal red cell mass increase. Murphy and coworkers (1986) described more than 54,000 singleton pregnancies in the Cardiff Birth Survey and reported excessive perinatal morbidity with *high* maternal hemoglobin concentrations. Scanlon and associates (2000) studied the relationship between maternal hemoglobin levels and preterm or growth-restricted infants in 173,031 pregnancies. Women whose hemoglobin concentration was three standard deviations *above* the mean at 12 or 18 weeks' gestation had 1.3- to 1.8-fold increases in the incidence of fetal-growth restriction. These findings have led some to the illogical conclusion that withholding iron supplementation to cause iron deficiency anemia will improve pregnancy outcomes (Ziaei, 2007).

Iron Deficiency Anemia

The two most common causes of anemia during pregnancy and the puerperium are iron deficiency and acute blood loss. The CDC (1989) estimated that as many as 8 million American women of childbearing age were iron deficient. In a study of more than 1300 women, 21 percent had third-trimester anemia with 16 percent due to iron deficiency anemia (Vandevijvere, 2013). In a typical singleton gestation, the maternal need for iron averages close to 1000 mg. Of this, 300 mg is for the fetus and placenta; 500 mg for maternal hemoglobin mass expansion; and 200 mg that is shed normally through the gut, urine, and skin. The total amount of 1000 mg considerably exceeds the iron stores of most women and results in iron deficiency anemia unless iron supplementation is given.

Iron deficiency is often manifested by an appreciable drop in hemoglobin concentration. In the third trimester, additional iron is needed to augment maternal hemoglobin and for transport to the fetus. Because the amount of iron diverted to the fetus is similar in a normal and in an iron-deficient mother, the newborn infant of a severely anemic mother does not suffer from iron deficiency anemia. As discussed in Chapter 33 (p. 643), neonatal iron stores are related to maternal iron status and to timing of cord clamping.

Diagnosis

Classic morphological evidence of iron deficiency anemia—erythrocyte hypochromia and microcytosis—is less prominent in the pregnant woman compared with that in the nonpregnant woman. Moderate iron deficiency anemia during pregnancy usually is not accompanied by obvious morphological changes in erythrocytes. Serum ferritin levels, however, are lower than normal, and there is no stainable bone marrow iron. Iron deficiency anemia during pregnancy is the consequence primarily of expansion of plasma volume without normal expansion of maternal hemoglobin mass.

The initial evaluation of a pregnant woman with moderate anemia should include measurements of hemoglobin, hematocrit, and red cell indices; careful examination of a peripheral blood smear; a sickle-cell preparation if the woman is of African origin; and measurement of serum iron or ferritin levels, or both. Expected values in pregnancy are found in the Appendix (p. 1287). Serum ferritin levels normally decline during pregnancy (Goldenberg, 1996). Levels less than 10 to 15 mg/L confirm iron deficiency anemia (American College of Obstetricians and Gynecologists, 2013a). Pragmatically, the diagnosis of iron deficiency in moderately anemic pregnant women usually is presumptive and based largely on exclusion.

When pregnant women with moderate iron deficiency anemia are given adequate iron therapy, a hematological response is detected by an elevated reticulocyte count. The rate of increase of hemoglobin concentration or hematocrit is typically slower than in nonpregnant women due to the increasing and larger blood volumes during pregnancy.

Treatment

Regardless of anemia status, daily oral supplementation with 30 to 60 mg of elemental iron and 400 μg of folic acid is recommended in pregnancy (Peña-Rosas, 2012; World Health Organization, 2012). Anemia resolution and restitution of iron stores can be accomplished with simple iron compounds—ferrous sulfate, fumarate, or gluconate—that provide about 200 mg daily of *elemental iron*. If a woman cannot or will not take oral iron preparations, then parenteral therapy is given. Although both are administered intravenously, ferrous sucrose has been shown to be safer than iron-dextran (American College of Obstetricians and Gynecologists, 2013a). There are equivalent increases in hemoglobin levels in women treated with either oral or parenteral iron therapy (Bayouneu, 2002; Sharma, 2004).

Anemia from Acute Blood Loss

In early pregnancy, anemia caused by acute blood loss is common with abortion, ectopic pregnancy, and hydatidiform mole. Anemia is much more common postpartum from obstetrical hemorrhage. Massive hemorrhage demands immediate treatment as described in Chapter 41 (p. 814). If a moderately anemic woman—defined by a hemoglobin value of approximately 7 g/dL—is hemodynamically stable, is able to ambulate without adverse symptoms, and is not septic, then blood transfusions are not indicated. Instead, iron therapy is given for at least 3 months (Krafft, 2005). In a randomized trial, Van Wyck and colleagues (2007) reported that intravenous ferric carboxymaltose given weekly was as effective as thrice-daily oral ferrous sulfate tablets for hemoglobin regeneration for postpartum anemia.

Anemia Associated with Chronic Disease

Weakness, weight loss, and pallor have been recognized since antiquity as characteristics of chronic disease. Various disorders, such as chronic renal failure, cancer and chemotherapy, human immunodeficiency virus (HIV) infection, and chronic inflammation, result in moderate and sometimes severe anemia, usually with slightly hypochromic and microcytic erythrocytes. It is the second most common form of anemia worldwide (Weiss, 2005).

In nonpregnant patients with chronic inflammatory diseases, the hemoglobin concentration is rarely < 7 g/dL; bone marrow cellular morphology is not altered; and serum iron concentrations are decreased. However, ferritin levels usually are elevated. The low levels of iron are mediated by *hepcidin*, a polypeptide produced in the liver that participates in iron balance and transport (Weiss, 2005). These anemias share similar features that include alterations in reticuloendothelial function, iron metabolism, and decreased erythropoiesis (Cullis, 2013).

Pregnancy

Women with chronic disorders may develop anemia for the first time during pregnancy. In those with preexisting anemia, it may be intensified as plasma volume expands disproportionately to red cell mass expansion. Causes include chronic renal insufficiency, inflammatory bowel disease, and connective-tissue disorders. Others are granulomatous infections, malignant neoplasms, rheumatoid arthritis, and chronic suppurative conditions.

Of these, chronic renal insufficiency is the most common disorder that we have encountered as a cause of anemia during pregnancy. Some cases are accompanied by erythropoietin deficiency. As discussed in Chapter 53 (p. 1060), during pregnancy in women with mild chronic renal insufficiency, the degree of red cell mass expansion is inversely related to renal impairment. At the same time, plasma volume expansion usually is normal, and thus anemia is intensified (Cunningham, 1990). Anemia often accompanies acute pyelonephritis but is due to acute endotoxin-mediated erythrocyte destruction. With normal erythropoietin production, red cell mass is restored as pregnancy progresses (Cavenee, 1994; Dotters-Katz, 2013).

Treatment

Adequate iron stores must be ensured. *Recombinant erythropoietin* has been used successfully to treat chronic anemia (Weiss, 2005). In pregnancies complicated by chronic renal insufficiency, recombinant erythropoietin is usually considered when the hematocrit approximates 20 percent (Ramin, 2006). Cyganek and coworkers (2011) described good results in five pregnant renal transplant recipients treated with human recombinant erythropoietin. One worrisome side effect is hypertension, which is already prevalent in women with renal disease. In addition, Casadevall and colleagues (2002) reported pure red cell aplasia and antierythropoietin antibodies in 13 nonpregnant patients given recombinant human erythropoietin. Numerous additional cases have been reported. However, because of changes in manufacturing and new regulations, it is an infrequent toxicity today (McKoy, 2008).

Megaloblastic Anemia

These anemias are characterized by blood and bone-marrow abnormalities from impaired DNA synthesis. Worldwide, the prevalence of megaloblastic anemia during pregnancy varies considerably. In the United States, it is rare.

Folic Acid Deficiency

In the United States, megaloblastic anemia beginning during pregnancy almost always results from folic acid deficiency. In the past, this condition was referred to as *pernicious anemia of pregnancy*. It usually is found in women who do not consume fresh green leafy vegetables, legumes, or animal protein. As folate deficiency and anemia worsen, anorexia often becomes intense and further aggravates the dietary deficiency. In some instances, excessive ethanol ingestion either causes or contributes to folate deficiency.

In nonpregnant women, the folic acid requirement is 50 to 100 μg/day. During pregnancy, requirements are increased, and 400 μg/day is recommended (Chap. 9, p. 181). The earliest biochemical evidence is low plasma folic acid concentrations (Appendix, p. 1287). Early morphological changes usually include neutrophils that are hypersegmented and newly formed erythrocytes that are macrocytic. With preexisting iron deficiency, macrocytic erythrocytes cannot be detected by measurement of the mean corpuscular volume. Careful examination of a peripheral blood smear, however, usually demonstrates some macrocytes. As the anemia becomes more intense, peripheral nucleated erythrocytes appear, and bone marrow examination discloses megaloblastic erythropoiesis. Anemia may then become severe, and thrombocytopenia, leukopenia, or both may develop. The fetus and placenta extract folate from maternal circulation so effectively that the fetus is not anemic despite severe maternal anemia. There have been instances in which newborn hemoglobin levels were 18 g/dL or more, whereas maternal values were as low as 3.6 g/dL (Pritchard, 1970). A Cochrane review by Lassi and associates (2013) evaluated the effectiveness of oral prenatal folic acid supplementation alone or with other micronutrients versus no folic acid. There was no conclusive evidence of supplement benefit for pregnancy outcomes that included preterm birth and perinatal mortality. There was, however, increased mean birthweight and a significant reduction in the incidence of megaloblastic anemia.

Treatment. Folic acid is given along with iron, and a nutritious diet is encouraged. As little as 1 mg of folic acid administered orally once daily produces a striking hematological response. By 4 to 7 days after beginning folic acid treatment, the reticulocyte count is increased, and leukopenia and thrombocytopenia are corrected.

Prevention. A diet sufficient in folic acid prevents megaloblastic anemia. The role of folate deficiency in the genesis of neural-tube defects has been well studied (Chap. 14, p. 283). Since the early 1990s, nutritional experts and the American College of Obstetricians and Gynecologists (2013c) have recommended that all women of childbearing age consume at least 400 μg of folic acid daily. More folic acid is given in circumstances in which requirements are increased. These include multifetal pregnancy, hemolytic anemia, Crohn disease, alcoholism, and inflammatory skin disorders. There is evidence that women who previously have had infants with neural-tube defects have a lower recurrence rate if a daily 4-mg folic acid supplement is given preconceptionally and throughout early pregnancy.

Vitamin B_{12} Deficiency

During pregnancy, vitamin B_{12} levels are lower than nonpregnant values because of decreased levels of binding proteins that include haptocorrin—transcobalamins I and III—and transcobalamin II (Morkbak, 2007). During pregnancy, megaloblastic anemia is rare from deficiency of vitamin B_{12}, that is, cyanocobalamin. The typical example is *Addisonian pernicious anemia,* which results from absent intrinsic factor that is requisite for dietary vitamin B_{12} absorption. This autoimmune disorder usually has its onset after age 40 years (Stabler, 2013).

In our limited experience, vitamin B_{12} deficiency in pregnancy is more likely encountered following gastric resection. Those who have undergone total gastrectomy require 1000 μg of vitamin B_{12} given intramuscularly each month. Those with a partial gastrectomy usually do not need supplementation, but adequate serum vitamin B_{12} levels should be ensured during pregnancy (Appendix, p. 1290). Other causes of megaloblastic anemia from vitamin B_{12} deficiency include Crohn disease, ileal resection, and bacterial overgrowth in the small bowel (Stabler, 2013).

Hemolytic Anemia

There are several conditions in which accelerated erythrocyte destruction is stimulated by a congenital red cell abnormality or by antibodies directed against red cell membrane proteins. The cause may also go unproven. In some cases, hemolysis may be the primary disorder—some examples include sickle-cell disease and hereditary spherocytosis. In other cases, hemolysis develops secondary to an underlying disorder—examples include lupus erythematosus and the preeclampsia syndrome.

Autoimmune Hemolysis

The cause of aberrant antibody production in this uncommon condition is unknown. Typically, both the direct and indirect antiglobulin (Coombs) tests are positive. Anemias caused by these factors may be due to warm-active autoantibodies (80 to 90 percent), cold-active antibodies, or a combination. These syndromes also may be classified as primary (idiopathic) or secondary due to underlying diseases or other factors. Examples of the latter include lymphomas and leukemias, connective-tissue diseases, infections, chronic inflammatory diseases, and drug-induced antibodies (Provan, 2000). *Cold-agglutinin disease* may be induced by infectious etiologies such as *Mycoplasma pneumoniae* or Epstein-Barr viral mononucleosis (Dhingra, 2007). Hemolysis and positive antiglobulin test results may be the consequence of either IgM or IgG antierythrocyte antibodies. Spherocytosis and reticulocytosis are characteristic of the peripheral blood smear. When there is concomitant thrombocytopenia, it is termed *Evans syndrome* (Wright, 2013).

During pregnancy, there may be marked acceleration of hemolysis. This usually responds to glucocorticoids, and treatment is given with prednisone, 1 mg/kg given orally each day, or its equivalent. Coincidental thrombocytopenia usually is corrected by therapy. Transfusion of red cells is complicated by antierythrocyte antibodies, but warming the donor cells to body temperature may decrease their destruction by cold agglutinins.

Drug-Induced Hemolysis

These hemolytic anemias must be differentiated from other causes of autoimmune hemolysis. In most cases, hemolysis is mild, it resolves with drug withdrawal, and recurrence is prevented by avoidance of the drug. One mechanism is by hemolysis induced through drug-mediated immunological injury to red cells. The drug may act as a high-affinity hapten when bound to a red cell protein to which antidrug antibodies attach—for example, IgM antipenicillin or anticephalosporin antibodies. Some other drugs act as low-affinity haptens and adhere to cell membrane proteins—examples include probenecid, quinidine, rifampin, and thiopental. A more common mechanism for drug-induced hemolysis is related to a congenital erythrocyte enzymatic defect. An example is *glucose-6-phosphate dehydrogenase (G6PD) deficiency*, which is common in African American women (p. 1106).

Drug-induced hemolysis is usually chronic and mild to moderate, but occasionally there is severe acute hemolysis. For example, Garratty and coworkers (1999) described seven women with severe Coombs-positive hemolysis stimulated by cefotetan given as prophylaxis for obstetrical procedures. Alpha-methyldopa can cause similar hemolysis (Grigoriadis, 2013). Moreover, maternal hemolysis has been reported after intravenous immune globulin (IVIG) given for fetal and neonatal alloimmune thrombocytopenia (Rink, 2013). As treatment, response to glucocorticoids may be suboptimal, but withdrawal of the offending drug frequently halts the hemolysis.

Pregnancy-Induced Hemolysis

In some cases, unexplained severe hemolytic anemia develops during early pregnancy and resolves within months postpartum. There is no evidence of an immune mechanism or intraerythrocytic or extraerythrocytic defects (Starksen, 1983). Because the fetus-infant also may demonstrate transient hemolysis, an immunological cause is suspected. Maternal corticosteroid treatment is often—but not always—effective (Kumar, 2001). We have cared for a woman who during each pregnancy developed intense severe hemolysis with anemia that was controlled by prednisone. Her fetuses were not affected, and in all instances, hemolysis abated spontaneously after delivery.

Paroxysmal Nocturnal Hemoglobinuria

Although commonly regarded as a hemolytic anemia, this hemopoietic stem cell disorder is characterized by formation of defective platelets, granulocytes, and erythrocytes. Paroxysmal nocturnal hemoglobinuria is acquired and arises from one abnormal clone of cells, much like a neoplasm (Nguyen, 2006). One mutated X-linked gene responsible for this condition is termed *PIG-A* because it codes for phosphatidylinositol glycan protein A. Resultant abnormal anchor proteins of the erythrocyte and granulocyte membrane make these cells unusually susceptible to lysis by complement (Provan, 2000). The most serious complication is thrombosis, which is heightened in the hypercoagulable state of pregnancy.

Chronic hemolysis has an insidious onset, and its severity ranges from mild to lethal. Hemoglobinuria develops at irregular intervals and is not necessarily nocturnal. Hemolysis may be initiated by transfusions, infections, or surgery. Almost 40 percent of patients suffer venous thromboses and may also experience renal failure, hypertension, and Budd-Chiari syndrome. Because of the thrombotic risk, prophylactic anticoagulation is recommended (Parker, 2005). Median survival after diagnosis is 10 years, and bone marrow transplantation is the definitive treatment. Successful treatment of nonpregnant patients has been reported with eculizumab, an antibody that inhibits complement activation (Hillmen, 2006; Parker, 2009). Kelly and colleagues (2010) described seven pregnant women exposed to eculizumab with successful outcomes.

During pregnancy, paroxysmal nocturnal hemoglobinuria can be serious and unpredictable. Complications have been reported in up to three fourths of affected women, and the maternal mortality rate is 10 to 20 percent (De Gramont, 1987). Complications more often develop postpartum, and half of affected women develop venous thrombosis during the puerperium (Fieni, 2006; Greene, 1983; Ray, 2000). In one report of 27 pregnancies in 22 women, the maternal mortality rate was 8 percent and related to postpartum thrombosis (de Guibert, 2011).

Severe Preeclampsia and Eclampsia

Fragmentation or microangiopathic hemolysis with thrombocytopenia is relatively common with severe preeclampsia and eclampsia (Kenny, 2014; Pritchard, 1976). Mild degrees are likely present in most cases of severe preeclampsia and may be referred to as *HELLP syndrome*—hemolysis, elevated liver enzymes, and low platelet count (Chap. 40, p. 742).

Acute Fatty Liver of Pregnancy

This syndrome is associated with moderate to severe hemolytic anemia (Nelson, 2013). It is discussed further in Chapter 55 (p. 1086).

Bacterial Toxins

The most fulminant acquired hemolytic anemia encountered during pregnancy is caused by the exotoxin of *Clostridium perfringens* or by group A β-hemolytic streptococcus (Chap. 47, p. 949). Endotoxin of gram-negative bacteria, that is, lipopolysaccharide—especially with bacteremia from severe pyelonephritis—may be accompanied by hemolysis and mild to moderate anemia (Cox, 1991).

Inherited Erythrocyte Membrane Defects

The normal erythrocyte is a biconcave disc. Its shape allows numerous cycles of reversible deformations as the erythrocyte withstands arterial shearing forces and negotiates through splenic slits half the width of its cross-sectional diameter. Several genes encode expression of erythrocyte structural membrane proteins or intraerythrocytic enzymes. Various mutations of these genes may result in inherited membrane defects or enzyme deficiencies that destabilize the lipid bilayer. The loss of lipids from the erythrocyte membrane causes a surface area deficiency and poorly deformable cells that undergo hemolysis. Anemia severity depends on the degree of rigidity or decreased distensibility. Erythrocyte morphology similarly is dependent on these factors, and these disorders are usually named after the most dominant red-cell shape characteristic of the disorder. Three examples are *hereditary spherocytosis, pyropoikilocytosis,* and *ovalocytosis.*

Hereditary Spherocytosis. Hemolytic anemias that comprise this group of inherited membrane defects are probably the most common identified in pregnant women. Mutations are usually an autosomally dominant, variably penetrant *spectrin* deficiency. Others are autosomally recessive or de novo gene mutations that result from deficiency of *ankyrin, protein 4.2, moderate band 3,* or combinations of these (Gallagher, 2010; Yawata, 2000). Clinically, varying degrees of anemia and jaundice result from hemolysis. Diagnosis is confirmed by identification of spherocytes on peripheral smear, reticulocytosis, and increased osmotic fragility (Fig. 56-2).

Spherocytic anemias may be associated with the so-called *crisis* that is characterized by severe anemia from accelerated hemolysis, and it develops in patients with an enlarged spleen. Infection can also accelerate hemolysis or suppress erythropoiesis to worsen anemia. An example of the latter is infection with parvovirus B19 (Chap. 64, p. 1244). In severe cases, splenectomy reduces hemolysis, anemia, and jaundice.

Pregnancy. In general, women with inherited red-cell membrane defects do well during pregnancy. Folic acid supplementation is given to sustain erythropoiesis. Pregnancy outcomes in women with hereditary spherocytosis cared for at Parkland Hospital were reported by Maberry and associates (1992). Twenty-three women with 50 pregnancies were described. In late pregnancy, these women had hematocrits ranging from 23 to 41 volume percent—mean 31. Their reticulocyte count ranged from 1 to 23 percent. Eight women miscarried. Four of 42 infants were born preterm, but none were growth restricted. Infection in four women intensified hemolysis, and three of these required transfusions. Similar results were reported by Pajor and coworkers (1993) in 19 pregnancies in eight women.

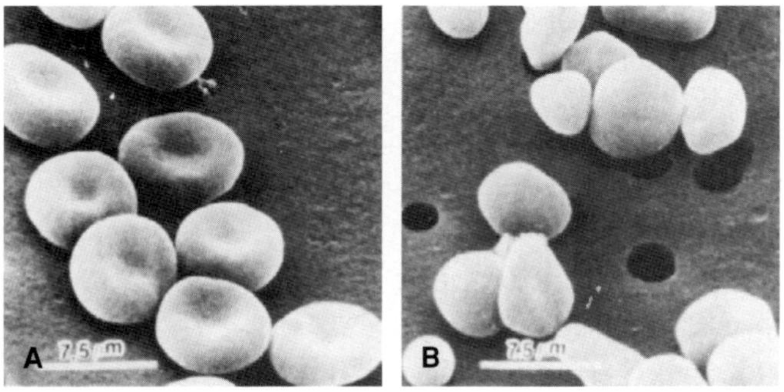

FIGURE 56-2 Scanning electron micrograph showing **(A)** normal-appearing erythrocytes from a heterozygous carrier of recessive spherocytosis, and **(B)** from her daughter, a homozygote with severe anemia. (From Agre, 1989, with permission.)

Because these disorders are inherited, the newborn may be affected. Celkan and Alhaj (2008) report prenatal diagnosis via cordocentesis at 18 weeks' gestation and testing for osmotic fragility. Those with hereditary spherocytosis may manifest hyperbilirubinemia and anemia shortly after birth.

Erythrocyte Enzyme Deficiencies

An intraerythrocytic deficiency of enzymes that permit anaerobic glucose metabolism may cause *hereditary nonspherocytic anemia.* Most of these mutations are autosomal recessive traits, and *pyruvate kinase deficiency* is probably the most clinically significant. Another is X-linked *glucose-6-phosphate dehydrogenase (G6PD) deficiency* (Puig, 2013). Other rare enzyme abnormalities may cause varying degrees of chronic hemolysis. As discussed on page 1105, most episodes of severe anemia with enzyme deficiencies are induced by drugs or infections. During pregnancy, oxidant drugs are avoided, infections are treated promptly, and iron and folic acid are given.

Pyruvate kinase deficiency is associated with variable anemia and hypertensive complications (Wax, 2007). Due to recurrent transfusions in homozygous carriers, iron overload is frequent, and associated myocardial dysfunction should be monitored (Dolan, 2002). The fetus that is homozygous for this mutation may develop *hydrops fetalis* from anemia and heart failure (Chap. 15, p. 315). Gilsanz and colleagues (1993) used funipuncture to diagnose fetal anemia and pyruvate kinase deficiency.

Glucose-6-phosphate dehydrogenase deficiency is complex because there are more than 400 known enzyme variants. The most common are caused by a base substitution that leads to an amino acid replacement and a broad range of phenotypic severity (Beutler, 1991; Puig, 2013)). In the homozygous or A variant, both X chromosomes are affected, and erythrocytes are markedly deficient in G6PD activity. Approximately 2 percent of African American women are affected. The heterozygous variant that is found in 10 to 15 percent of African American women may confer some degree of protection against malaria (Mockenhaupt, 2003). In both instances, random X-chromosome inactivation—*lyonization*—results in a variable deficiency of enzyme activity.

During pregnancy, infections or drugs can induce hemolysis in both heterozygous and homozygous women, and the severity is related to enzyme activity. Anemia is usually episodic, although some variants induce chronic nonspherocytic hemolysis. Because young erythrocytes contain more enzyme activity than older erythrocytes, in the absence of bone marrow depression, anemia ultimately stabilizes and is corrected soon after the inciting cause is eliminated. Newborn screening for G6PD deficiency is not recommended by the American College of Medical Genetics (2013) as discussed in Chapter 32 (Table 32-3, p. 632).

Aplastic and Hypoplastic Anemia

Although rarely encountered during pregnancy, aplastic anemia is a grave complication. It is characterized by pancytopenia and markedly hypocellular bone marrow (Young, 2008). There are multiple etiologies, and at least one is linked to autoimmune diseases (Stalder, 2009). The inciting cause can be identified in approximately a third of cases. These include drugs and other chemicals, infection, irradiation, leukemia, immunological disorders, and inherited conditions such as *Fanconi anemia* and *Diamond-Blackfan syndrome* (Green, 2009; Lipton, 2009). The functional defect appears to be a marked decrease in committed marrow stem cells.

Hematopoietic stem-cell transplantation is optimal therapy in a young patient (Young, 2008). Immunosuppressive therapy is given. In some nonresponders, *eltrombopag* has been used successfully (Olnes, 2012). Definitive treatment is bone marrow transplantation, and approximately three fourths of patients have a good response with long-term survival when treated with antithymocyte globulin and cyclosporine (Rosenfeld, 2003). There is a potential for transplantation with umbilical cord blood-derived stem cells (Moise, 2005; Pinto, 2008). Previous blood transfusions and even pregnancy enhance the risk of graft rejection, which is the most common serious complication, causing two thirds of deaths within the first 2 years (Socié, 1999).

Pregnancy

Hypoplastic or aplastic anemia complicating pregnancy is rare. In most cases, the diagnosis precedes conception, or the condition develops during pregnancy as a chance occurrence. That said, there are a few well-documented cases of *pregnancy-induced hypoplastic anemia* (Bourantas, 1997; Choudhry, 2002). We have cared for a few such women in whom hypoplastic anemia was first identified during a pregnancy. Anemia and other cytopenias improved or remitted following delivery or pregnancy termination. In some cases, recurrence in a subsequent pregnancy was documented.

Diamond-Blackfan anemia is a rare form of pure red-cell hypoplasia, and approximately 40 percent are familial and have autosomal dominant inheritance (Orfali, 2004). There is usually a good response to glucocorticoid therapy. However, continuous treatment is necessary, and most become at least partially transfusion dependent (Vlachos, 2008). In 64 pregnancies complicated by this syndrome, Faivre and associates (2006) reported that two thirds had complications related to placental vascular etiologies that included miscarriage, preeclampsia, preterm birth, stillbirth, or growth-restricted newborn.

Gaucher disease is an autosomally recessive lysosomal enzyme deficiency characterized by deficient *acid β-glucosidase* activity. It involves multiple systems, including bone marrow. Affected women have anemia and thrombocytopenia that is usually worsened by pregnancy (Granovsky-Grisaru, 1995). Elstein and colleagues (1997) described six pregnant women whose disease improved when they were given *alglucerase* enzyme replacement. Imiglucerase therapy, which is human recombinant enzyme replacement therapy, has been available since 1994. European guidelines recommend treatment in pregnancy, whereas the Food and Drug Administration states it may be given in pregnancy with "clear indications" (Granovsky-Grisaru, 2011).

The major risks to pregnant woman with hypoplastic anemia are hemorrhage and infection. Management depends on gestational age, disease severity, and whether treatment has been given. Supportive care includes continuous infection surveillance and prompt antimicrobial therapy. Granulocyte transfusions are given only during infections. Red cells are transfused to improve symptomatic anemia and routinely to maintain the hematocrit at or above 20 volume percent. Platelet transfusions may be needed to control hemorrhage. Even when thrombocytopenia is intense, the risk of severe hemorrhage can be minimized by vaginal rather than cesarean delivery. Maternal mortality rates reported since 1960 have averaged nearly 50 percent (Choudhry, 2002). Better outcomes are reported with more recent series (Kwon, 2006).

Pregnancy after Bone Marrow Transplantation

There have been several reports of successful pregnancies in women who have undergone bone marrow transplantation (Borgna-Pignatti, 1996; Eliyahu, 1994). In their review, Sanders and coworkers (1996) reported 72 pregnancies in 41 women who had undergone transplantation. In the 52 pregnancies resulting in a liveborn infant, almost half were complicated by preterm delivery or hypertension. Our experiences with a few of these women indicate that they have normal pregnancy-augmented erythropoiesis and total blood volume expansion.

POLYCYTHEMIAS

Secondary Polycythemia

Excessive erythrocytosis during pregnancy is usually related to chronic hypoxia from maternal congenital cardiac disease or a chronic pulmonary disorder. Unusually heavy cigarette smoking can cause polycythemia. We have encountered otherwise healthy pregnant women who were heavy smokers, had chronic bronchitis, and had hematocrits ranging from 55 to 60 volume percent! Brewer and colleagues (1992) described a woman with persistent erythrocytosis associated with a placental site tumor. If polycythemia is severe, the probability of a successful pregnancy outcome is low.

Polycythemia Vera

This is a primary myeloproliferative hemopoietic stem cell disorder characterized by excessive proliferation of erythroid, myeloid, and megakaryocytic precursors. It is uncommon and likely an acquired genetic disorder of stem cells (Spivak, 2008). Virtually all patients have either a *JAK2*V617F or a *JAK2* exon 12 gene mutation (Harrison, 2009). Serum erythropoietin level measurement is helpful to differentiate polycythemia vera—low values—from secondary erythrocytosis—high values. Symptoms are related to increased blood viscosity, and thrombotic complications are common. Fetal loss has been reported to be high in women with polycythemia vera, and pregnancy outcome may be improved with aspirin therapy (Griesshammer, 2006; Robinson, 2005; Tefferi, 2000).

HEMOGLOBINOPATHIES

Sickle-Cell Hemoglobinopathies

Hemoglobin A is the most common hemoglobin tetramer and consists of two α- and two β-chains. In contrast, sickle hemoglobin (hemoglobin S) originates from a single β-chain substitution of glutamic acid by valine, which stems from an A-for-T substitution at codon 6 of the β-globin gene. Hemoglobinopathies that can result in clinical features of the *sickle-cell syndrome* include sickle-cell anemia—Hb SS; sickle cell-hemoglobin C disease—Hb SC; sickle cell-β-thalassemia disease—either Hb S/B^0 or Hb S/B^+; and sickle-cell E disease—Hb SE (Stuart, 2004). All are also associated with increased maternal and perinatal morbidity and mortality.

Inheritance

Sickle-cell anemia originates from the inheritance of the gene for S hemoglobin from each parent. In the United States, 1 of 12 African Americans has sickle-cell trait, which results from inheritance of one gene for hemoglobin S and one for normal hemoglobin A. The computed incidence of sickle-cell anemia among African Americans is 1 in 576 (1/12 × 1/12 × 1/4 = 1/576). But, the disease is less common in adults and therefore during pregnancy because of earlier mortality, especially during early childhood.

Hemoglobin C originates from a single β-chain substitution of glutamic acid by lysine at codon 6 of the β-globin gene. Approximately 1 in 40 African Americans has the gene for hemoglobin C. Thus, the theoretical incidence for coinheritance of the gene for hemoglobin S and an allelic gene for hemoglobin C in an African American child is about 1 in 2000 (1/12 × 1/40 × 1/4). β-Thalassemia minor is approximately 1 in 40, thus S-β-thalassemia also is found in approximately 1 in 2000 (1/12 × 1/40 × 1/4).

Pathophysiology

Red cells with hemoglobin S undergo sickling when they are deoxygenated, and the hemoglobin aggregates. Constant sickling and unsickling cause membrane damage, and the cell may become irreversibly sickled. Events that slow erythrocyte transit through the microcirculation contribute to vasoocclusion. These include endothelial cell adhesion, erythrocytic dehydration, and vasomotor dysregulation. Clinically, the hallmarks of sickling episodes are periods during which there is ischemia and infarction in various organs. These produce clinical symptoms, predominately pain, which is often severe—the *sickle-cell crisis*. There may be aplastic, megaloblastic, sequestration, and hemolytic crises.

Chronic and acute changes from sickling include bony abnormalities such as osteonecrosis of femoral and humeral heads, renal medullary damage, autosplenectomy in homozygous SS patients and splenomegaly in other variants, hepatomegaly, ventricular hypertrophy, pulmonary infarctions, pulmonary hypertension, cerebrovascular accidents, leg ulcers, and a propensity for infection and sepsis (Driscoll, 2003; Gladwin, 2004; Stuart, 2004). Of increasing importance is acquisition of pulmonary hypertension, which can be demonstrated in 20 percent of adults with SS hemoglobin (Gladwin, 2008). Depending on its severity, this complication increases the relative risk for death from four- to 11-fold. Another emerging problem with improved survival is chronic sickle-cell disease nephropathy (Maigne, 2010). The median age at death for women is 48 years. Even so, Serjeant and associates (2009) described a cohort of 102 patients followed since birth in which 40 were still alive at 60 to 87 years!

Treatment

Good supportive care is essential to prevent mortality in patients with sickle-cell syndromes. Specific therapies are evolving, and many are still experimental (Stuart, 2004). One treatment is hemoglobin F induction given for both sickling and thalassemia syndromes. These drugs stimulate gamma-chain synthesis. This increases hemoglobin F (fetal hemoglobin), which inhibits hemoglobin S polymerization. One inducing agent, *hydroxyurea,* when given to patients with moderate to severe disease, increases hemoglobin F production and mitigates erythrocyte membrane damage. This reduces the number of clinical sickling episodes (Platt, 2008). It is not known yet if hydroxyurea increases long-term patient survival (Brawley, 2008). Hydroxyurea is teratogenic in animals, although a preliminary 17-year surveillance of antenatally exposed children was reassuring (Ballas, 2009; Briggs, 2011; Italia, 2010).

Various forms of hemopoietic cell transplantation are emerging as "cures" for sickle-cell syndromes and severe thalassemias (Hsieh, 2009). Oringanje and coworkers (2009) performed a Cochrane Review and found that only observational studies have been reported. *Bone marrow transplantation,* as discussed on page 1107, has 5-year survival rates that exceed 90 percent (Dalle, 2013). *Cord-blood stem-cell transplantation* from related donors has also shown great promise (Shenoy, 2013). One intriguing treatment uses cells taken for prenatal diagnosis from a fetus destined to have sickle-cell anemia. Research suggests these cells can be conditioned to produce hemoglobin A and used for replacement after birth (Ye, 2009).

Pregnancy and Sickle-Cell Syndromes

Pregnancy is a serious burden to women with any of the major sickle hemoglobinopathies, particularly those with hemoglobin SS disease. Two large studies define this relationship. The first, by Villers and colleagues (2008), included 17,952 births delivered of women with sickle-cell syndromes from 2000 through 2003. The second study, by Chakravarty and associates (2008), was from 2002 through 2004 and included 4352 pregnancies. A more recent cohort study of 1526 women was reported by Boulet and coworkers (2013). Common obstetrical and medical complications and their relative risks from these studies are shown in Table 56-2. Added to these are findings of Chakravarty and associates (2008), who reported significantly increased risks for renal failure, gestational hypertension, and fetal-growth restriction.

Maternal morbidity common in pregnancy includes ischemic necrosis of multiple organs, especially bone marrow, that causes episodes of severe pain. Pyelonephritis, pneumonia, and other pulmonary complications are frequent. The *acute chest syndrome* is manifest by the radiological appearance of a new pulmonary infiltrate accompanied by fever and respiratory symptoms. There are four precipitants of this—infection, marrow emboli, thromboembolism, and atelectasis (Medoff, 2005). Of these, infection causes approximately half of cases and results from typical bacteria and viruses. When the chest syndrome develops, the mean duration of hospitalization is 10.5 days. Mechanical ventilation is required in approximately 15 percent, and the mortality rate is about 3 percent (Gladwin, 2008).

TABLE 56-2. Increased Rates for Maternal Complications in Pregnancies Complicated by Sickle-Cell Syndromes

Complications	OR or PR	*p* value
Preexisting Medical Disorders		
Cardiomyopathy	3.7	< .001
Pulmonary hypertension	6.3	< .001
Renal failure	3.5–6.4	< .05
Pregnancy Complications		
Cerebral vein thrombosis	4.9–7.9	< .05
Pneumonia	9.8–17	< .001
Pyelonephritis	1.3–2.1	< .05
Deep-vein thrombosis	2.5–7.8	< .001
Pulmonary embolism	1.7–10.3	< .05
Sepsis syndrome	5.3–6.8	< .001
Delivery Complications		
Gestational hypertension/ preeclampsia	1.2	.01
Eclampsia	2.3–3.2	< .05
Placental abruption	1.1–1.6	< .05
Preterm delivery	1.4	< .001
Fetal-growth restriction	2.2	< .001

OR = odds ratios; PR = prevalence ratio.
Data from Boulet, 2013; Villers, 2008.

TABLE 56-3. Perinatal Outcomes in Women with Hemoglobin SS and SC Disease

		Perinatal Outcomes (%)			
Study	**Number**[a]	**FGR**	**SB**	**ND**	**PMR**
Sun (2001)					
SS Hgb	69	45	4	7	11
SC Hgb	58	21	2	0	2
Serjeant (2004, 2005)[b]					
SS Hgb	54	42	11	1.9	12.9
SC Hgb	70	NS	3	1.4	4.4
Thame (2007)[b]					
SS Hgb	126	33	10	1.6	11.6
Total/Weighted Average	377	~35	6.4	2.3	8.7

[a]Excludes spontaneous and induced abortions.
[b]Study periods overlap and may contain some duplicated pregnancy outcomes.
FGR = fetal-growth restriction; ND = neonatal death; NS = not stated; PMR = perinatal mortality rate; SB = stillborn.

Despite these complications, the maternal mortality rate has decreased. And although improved, perinatal morbidity and mortality rates remain formidable (Yu, 2009). Some perinatal outcomes reported since 2000 are shown in Table 56-3. In addition to increased risks for preterm birth shown in Table 56-2, the frequency of fetal-growth restriction and perinatal mortality are daunting.

Hemoglobin SC

In nonpregnant women, morbidity and mortality rates from SC disease are appreciably lower than those from sickle-cell anemia. Indeed, fewer than half of women with SC disease have symptoms before pregnancy. In our experiences, affected pregnant and puerperal women suffer attacks of severe bone pain and episodes of pulmonary infarction and embolization—acute chest syndrome—more commonly compared with when they are not pregnant (Cunningham, 1983). It is arguable whether SC disease has a maternal mortality rate equivalent to that of hemoglobin SS disease (Pritchard, 1973; Serjeant, 2005). In the reports shown in Table 56-3, the perinatal mortality rate is somewhat greater than that of the general obstetrical population, but nowhere as great as with sickle-cell anemia (Tita, 2007).

Management During Pregnancy

Women with sickle-cell hemoglobinopathies require close prenatal observation. These women maintain hemoglobin mass by intense hemopoiesis to compensate for the markedly shortened erythrocyte life span. Thus, any factor that impairs erythropoiesis or increases red cell destruction or both aggravates the anemia. Prenatal folic acid supplementation with 4 mg daily is needed to support the rapid red blood cell turnover (American College of Obstetricians and Gynecologists, 2013b).

One danger is that a symptomatic woman may categorically be considered to be suffering from a sickle-cell crisis. As a result, serious obstetrical or medical problems that cause pain, anemia, or both may be overlooked. Some examples are ectopic pregnancy, placental abruption, pyelonephritis, or appendicitis. Thus, the term "sickle-cell crisis" importantly should be applied only after all other possible causes of pain or fever or worsening anemia have been excluded. Pain with sickle-cell syndromes is caused by intense sequestration of sickled erythrocytes and infarction in various organs. These episodes may develop acutely, especially late in pregnancy, during labor and delivery, and early in the puerperium. Because bone marrow is frequently involved, intense bone pain is common.

A system for care of these women has been appropriately stressed by Rees and colleagues (2003). Marti-Carvajal and coworkers (2009) performed a Cochrane review and reported that no randomized trials have evaluated treatment during pregnancy. At minimum, intravenous fluids are given and opioids administered promptly for severe pain. Oxygen via nasal cannula may decrease the intensity of sickling at the capillary level. We have found that red cell transfusions after the onset of severe pain do not dramatically improve the intensity of the current pain crisis and may not shorten its duration. Conversely, as discussed later, prophylactic transfusions almost always prevent further vasoocclusive episodes and pain crises. Recent reports suggest benefits from epidural analgesia used for severe sickle-cell crisis in nonlaboring obstetrical patients (Verstraete, 2012; Winder, 2011).

During the past few years, we have encountered several affected women who apparently are habituated to narcotics given chronically to alleviate sickle-cell pain. It is problematic that such women complain of "sickling pain" even when they have effectively undergone exchange transfusion with normal AA-hemoglobin-containing donor red cells.

Rates of covert bacteriuria and acute pyelonephritis are increased substantively, and screening and treatment for bacteriuria are essential. If pyelonephritis develops, sickle cells are extremely susceptible to bacterial endotoxin, which can cause dramatic and rapid red cell destruction while simultaneously suppressing erythropoiesis. Pneumonia, especially due to *Streptococcus pneumoniae,* is common. The CDC (2013a) recommends the following vaccines for those with sickle-cell disease and all asplenic patients: polyvalent pneumococcal, *Haemophilus influenzae* type B, and meningococcal vaccines.

Pulmonary complications are often encountered. *Acute chest syndrome* is characterized by pleuritic chest pain, fever, cough, lung infiltrates, and hypoxia, and usually also by bone and joint pain (Vichinsky, 2000). The spectrum of its pathology includes infection, infarction, pulmonary sequestration, and fat embolization from bone marrow. At least for nonpregnant adults, some recommend rapid simple or exchange transfusions to remove the "trigger" for acute chest syndromes (Gladwin, 2008). In a cohort study of nonpregnant patients, Turner and colleagues (2009) reported that there were no increased benefits of exchange versus simple transfusions, and the former were associated with fourfold increased blood usage. Recurrent episodes of acute chest syndrome may lead to restrictive chronic lung disease or arteriolar vasculopathy and pulmonary hypertension.

Pregnant women with sickle-cell anemia usually have some degree of *cardiac dysfunction* from ventricular hypertrophy. There is increased preload, decreased afterload, normal ejection fraction, and a high cardiac output. Chronic hypertension worsens this pattern (Gandhi, 2000). During pregnancy, the basal hemodynamic state characterized by high cardiac output and increased blood volume is augmented (Veille, 1994). Although most women tolerate pregnancy without problems, complications such as severe preeclampsia or serious infections may result in ventricular failure (Cunningham, 1986). As discussed in Chapter 49 (p. 986), heart failure caused by pulmonary hypertension must also be considered (Chakravarty, 2008; Stuart, 2004).

In the review of 4352 pregnancies in women with sickle-cell syndromes noted earlier, Chakravarty and associates (2008) reported significantly increased pregnancy complications compared with the total population of 11.2 million women. Compared with controls, women with sickling disorders had a 63-percent rate of nondelivery-related admissions. They had a 1.8-fold increased incidence of hypertensive disorders—19 percent; a 2.9-fold increased rate of fetal-growth restriction—6 percent; and a 1.7-fold increased cesarean delivery rate—45 percent.

Prophylactic Red Cell Transfusions. There are several clinical situations for which prophylactic transfusions have been shown to decrease morbidity from sickle-cell syndromes. For example, chronic transfusion therapy prevents strokes in high-risk children. However, there are no randomized trials of such therapy to prevent pulmonary hypertension and chronic sickle-cell lung disease (Cho, 2014). Preoperative transfusions improved some postoperative outcomes (Howard, 2013). During pregnancy, the most dramatic impact of prophylactic transfusions has been on maternal morbidity. In an observational 10-year prospective study at Parkland Hospital, we offered prophylactic transfusions to all pregnant women with sickle-cell syndromes. Transfusions were given throughout pregnancy to maintain the hematocrit above 25 volume percent and the portion of hemoglobin S below 60 percent (Cunningham, 1979). There was minimal maternal morbidity, and erythropoiesis suppression was not problematic. Their outcomes were compared with historical controls who were not routinely transfused. Morbidity and hospitalizations were significantly reduced in the transfused group (Cunningham, 1983). Others have reported similar data (Grossetti, 2009; Howard, 1995). Still, adverse perinatal outcomes are prevalent (Ngô, 2010).

In a multicenter trial, Koshy and coworkers (1988) randomly assigned 72 pregnant women with sickle-cell syndrome to prophylactic or indicated transfusions. They reported a significant decline in the incidence of painful sickle-cell crises with prophylactic transfusions but no differences in perinatal outcomes. Because of risks inherent with blood administration, they concluded that prophylactic transfusions were not necessary.

There is no doubt that morbidity from multiple transfusions is significant. Up to 10 percent of women had a delayed hemolytic transfusion reaction, and infections are major concerns (Garratty, 1997). From our experiences from Parkland Hospital cited above, we found the incidence of red cell alloimmunization to be 3 percent per unit of blood transfused (Cox, 1988). Similarly, in 12 studies reviewed by Garratty (1997), alloimmunization developed in a fourth of women undergoing chronic transfusions. According to Kacker and colleagues (2014), it not cost effective to extensively match blood donors for these women. Finally, although worrisome, we found no evidence of transfusional iron overload, hemochromatosis, or chronic hepatitis in liver biopsies performed in 40 women transfused during pregnancy (Yeomans, 1990).

Because of what some consider marginal benefits, routine prophylactic transfusions during pregnancy remain controversial (American College of Obstetricians and Gynecologists, 2013b). Similar conclusions were reached after a Cochrane Database analysis (Okusayna, 2013). Current consensus is that their use should be individualized. For example, some clinicians recommend prophylactic transfusions for women with either frequent vasoocclusive episodes or poor obstetrical outcomes (Castro, 2003).

Fetal Assessment. Because of the high incidence of fetal-growth restriction and perinatal mortality, serial fetal assessment is necessary. According to the American College of Obstetricians and Gynecologists (2013b), a plan for serial sonographic examinations and antepartum fetal surveillance is reasonable. Anyaegbunam and colleagues (1991) evaluated fetal well-being during 39 sickling crises in 24 women. Almost 60 percent had nonreactive stress tests, which became reactive with crisis resolution, and all had an increased uterine artery systolic-diastolic (S/D) ratio. At the same time, there were no changes in umbilical artery S/D ratios (Chap. 10, p. 219). These investigators concluded that transient effects of sickle-cell crisis do not compromise umbilical, and hence fetal, blood flow. At Parkland Hospital, we serially assess these women with sonography for fetal growth and amnionic fluid volume changes. Nonstress or contraction stress tests are not done routinely unless complications such as fetal-growth restriction develop or fetal movement is reported to be diminished.

Labor and Delivery. Management is essentially identical to that for women with cardiac disease (Chap. 49, p. 978). Women should be kept comfortable but not oversedated. Labor epidural analgesia is ideal, and conduction analgesia seems preferable for operative delivery (Camous, 2008). Compatible blood should be available. If a difficult vaginal or cesarean delivery is contemplated, and the hematocrit is < 20 volume percent, then packed erythrocyte transfusions are administered. There is no categorical contraindication to vaginal delivery, and cesarean delivery is reserved for obstetrical indications (Rogers, 2010). Circulatory overload and pulmonary edema from ventricular failure should be avoided.

Contraception and Sterilization

Because of chronic debility, complications caused by pregnancy, and the predictably shortened life span of women with sickle-cell anemia, contraception and possibly sterilization are important considerations. Many clinicians do not recommend combined hormonal pills because of potential adverse vascular and thrombotic effects. After a systematic review, however, it was concluded that there was no increase in complications with their use in women with sickle-cell syndromes (Haddad, 2012). The CDC (2013b) regards the contraceptive pill, patch, and ring along with the copper intrauterine device (IUD) as having "advantages that generally outweigh theoretical or proven risks." All progestin-only methods may be used without restrictions. Because progesterone has been long known to prevent painful sickle-cell crises, low-dose oral progestins or progesterone injections or implants seem ideal. In one study, de Abood and associates (1997) reported significantly fewer and less intense pain crises in women given depot medroxyprogesterone intramuscularly.

Sickle-Cell Trait

The heterozygous inheritance of the gene for hemoglobin S results in sickle-cell trait, or AS hemoglobin. Hemoglobin A is most abundant, and the amount of hemoglobin S averages approximately 30 percent in each red cell. The frequency of sickle-cell trait among African Americans averages 8 percent. There is evidence that carriers have occasional hematuria, renal papillary necrosis, and hyposthenuria (Tsaras, 2009). And although controversial, we believe that sickle-cell trait is not associated with increased rates of abortion, perinatal mortality, low birthweight, or pregnancy-induced hypertension (Pritchard, 1973; Tita, 2007; Tuck, 1983). One unquestioned relationship is the twofold increased incidence of asymptomatic bacteriuria and urinary infection. Sickle-cell trait therefore should not be considered a deterrent to pregnancy on the basis of increased maternal risks.

Preliminary findings from a cohort study by Austin and coworkers (2009) suggested that African American women with sickle trait may have a higher incidence of venous thromboembolism when using hormonal contraceptives compared with women without the trait. However, more data are needed before these effective contraceptive methods are withheld from trait-positive women.

Inheritance is a concern for the infant of a mother with sickle-cell trait whenever the father carries a gene for abnormal hemoglobins that include S, C, and D or for β-thalassemia trait. Prenatal diagnosis through amniocentesis, chorionic villus sampling (CVS), or preimplantation genetic evaluation is available (Chap. 14, p. 297).

Hemoglobin C and C-β-Thalassemia

Approximately 2 percent of African Americans are heterozygous for hemoglobin C, but even if homozygous, hemoglobin C is innocuous (Nagel, 2003). Neither cause severe anemia or adverse pregnancy outcomes. However, when coinherited with sickle-cell trait, hemoglobin SC is the second most common serious sickle-cell syndrome.

Pregnancy and homozygous hemoglobin CC disease or hemoglobin C-β-thalassemia are relatively benign associations. Maberry and colleagues (1990) reported our experiences from Parkland Hospital as shown in Table 56-4. Other than mild to moderate anemia, pregnancy outcomes were not different compared with those of the general obstetrical population. When severe anemia is identified, iron or folic acid deficiency or some other superimposed cause should be suspected. Supplementation with folic acid and iron is indicated.

Hemoglobin E

Although it is uncommon in the United States, hemoglobin E is the second most frequent hemoglobin variant worldwide. Hemoglobin E results from a single β-chain substitution of lysine for glutamic acid at codon 26. The hemoglobin is particularly susceptible to oxidative stress. The heterozygous E trait is common in Southeast Asia. Hurst and coworkers (1983) identified homozygous hemoglobin E, hemoglobin E plus β-thalassemia, or hemoglobin E trait in 36 percent of Cambodians and 25 percent of Laotians. In addition, α- and β-thalassemia traits were prevalent in all groups.

Homozygous hemoglobin EE is associated with little or no anemia, hypochromia, marked microcytosis, or erythrocyte

TABLE 56-4. Outcomes in 72 Pregnancies Complicated by Hemoglobin CC and C-β-Thalassemia

	Hemoglobin CC	C-β-Thalassemia
Women (No.)	15	5
Pregnancies (No.)	49	23
Hematocrit (range)	27 (21–23)	30 (28–33)
Birthweight (g)		
Mean	2990	2960
Range	1145–4770	2320–3980
Perinatal deaths	1	2
Surviving infants	42	20

Data from Maberry, 1990.

targeting. In our limited experience, pregnant women do not appear to be at increased risk. Conversely, doubly heterozygous hemoglobin E-β-thalassemia is a common cause of childhood anemia in Southeast Asia (Fucharoen, 2000). In a cohort study of 54 women with singleton pregnancies, Luewan and associates (2009) reported a threefold increased risk of preterm birth and fetal-growth restriction in affected women. It is unclear if hemoglobin SE disease is as ominous during pregnancy as hemoglobin SC or S-β-thalassemia disease (Ramahi, 1988).

Hemoglobinopathy in the Newborn

Infants with homozygous SS, SC, and CC disease can be identified accurately at birth by cord blood electrophoresis. The United States Preventive Services Task Force recommends that all newborn infants be tested for sickle-cell disease (Lin, 2007). In most states, such screening is mandated by law and performed routinely (Chap. 32, p. 632). Screening for sickle hemoglobinopathies leads to clearly decreased mortality rates in children with sickle-cell disease identified at birth.

Prenatal Diagnosis

There are many tests to detect sickle-cell disease prenatally. Most are DNA based and use CVS samples or amnionic fluid specimens (American College of Obstetricians and Gynecologists, 2013b). Several mutations that encode hemoglobin S and other abnormal hemoglobins can be detected by targeted mutation analysis as well as polymerase chain reaction-based techniques (Chap. 13, p. 277).

THALASSEMIA SYNDROMES

Hundreds of mutations have been described for genes that control production of the normal hemoglobins. Some of these mutations impair synthesis of one or more of the normal globin peptide chains and may result in a clinical syndrome characterized by varying degrees of ineffective erythropoiesis, hemolysis, and anemia. Thalassemias are classified according to the globin chain that is deficient. The two major forms involve impaired production or instability of α-peptide chains—causing α-thalassemia, or of β-chains—causing β-thalassemia. These may form from point mutations, deletions, or translocations involving the α- or non-α-globin gene. The estimated prevalence for thalassemia trait is 16 percent in Southern European, 10 percent in Thai, and 3 to 8 percent in Indian and Chinese populations (Leung, 2012).

Alpha Thalassemias

Because there are four α-globin genes, the inheritance of α-thalassemia is more complicated than for β-thalassemia (Weatherall, 2010). Possible genotypes and phenotypes arising from these mutations are shown in Table 56-5. For each, a close correlation has been established between clinical severity and the degree of α-globin chains synthesis impairment. In most populations, the α-globin chain "cluster" or gene loci are doubled on chromosome 16. Thus, the normal genotype for diploid cells can be expressed as αα/αα. There are two main groups of α-thalassemia determinants: α^0-thalassemia is characterized by the deletion of both loci from one chromosome (−−/αα), whereas α^+-thalassemia is characterized by the loss of a single locus from one allele (−α/αα heterozygote) or a loss from each allele alleles (−α/−α homozygote).

There are two major phenotypes. The deletion of all four α-globin chain genes (−−/−−) characterizes *homozygous* α-thalassemia. Because α-chains are contained in fetal hemoglobin, the fetus is affected. With none of the four genes expressed, there are no α-globin chains, and instead, hemoglobin Bart (γ_4) and hemoglobin H (β_4) are formed as abnormal tetramers (Chap. 7, p. 137).

Frequency

The relative frequency of α-thalassemia minor, hemoglobin H disease, and hemoglobin Bart disease varies remarkably among racial groups. All of these variants are encountered in Asians. In those of African descent, although α-thalassemia minor has a frequency of approximately 2 percent, hemoglobin H disease is rare and hemoglobin Bart disease is unreported. This is because Asians usually have α^0-thalassemia minor inherited with both gene deletions typically from the same chromosome (−−/αα), whereas blacks usually have a^+-thalassemia minor in which one gene is deleted from each chromosome (−α/−α). The α-thalassemia syndromes appear sporadically in other

TABLE 56-5. Genotypes and Phenotypes of α-Thalassemia Syndromes

Genotype	Genotype	Phenotype
Normal	αα/αα	Normal
α^+-Thalassemia heterozygote	−α/αα αα/−α	Normal; silent carrier
α^+-Thalassemia homozygote[a] α^0-Thalassemia heterozygote[b]	−α/−α −−/αα	α-Thalassemia minor—mild hypochromic microcytic anemia
Compound heterozygous α^0/α^+	−−/−α	Hgb H (β^4) with moderate to severe hemolytic anemia
Homozygous α-thalassemia	−−/−−	Hgb Bart (γ^4) disease, hydrops fetalis

[a]More common in African Americans.
[b]More common in Asian Americans.

racial and ethnic groups. Diagnosis of β-thalassemia minor and α-thalassemia major in the fetus can be accomplished by DNA analysis using molecular techniques (American College of Obstetricians and Gynecologists, 2013b). Fetal diagnosis of hemoglobin Bart has been described using capillary electrophoresis or high-performance liquid chromatography (HPLC) techniques (Sirichotiyakul, 2009; Srivorakun, 2009). Molecular genetic testing for *HBA1* and *HBA2* identifies 90 percent of deletions and 10 percent of point mutations in affected individuals (Galanello, 2011b).

Pregnancy

Important obstetrical aspects of some α-thalassemia syndromes depend on the number of gene deletions in a given woman. The silent carrier state with one gene deletion is of no consequence. Deletion of two genes resulting in *α-thalassemia minor* is characterized by minimal to moderate hypochromic microcytic anemia. This is due to either the α^0- or the α^+-thalassemia trait, and thus genotypes may be –α/–α or – –/αα. Differentiation is possible only by DNA analysis (Weatherall, 2000a,b). Because there are no other clinical abnormalities with either α-thalassemia minor, it often goes unrecognized and is usually of no maternal consequence. The fetus with these forms of thalassemia minor will have hemoglobin Bart at birth, but as its levels drop, it is not replaced by hemoglobin H. Red cells are hypochromic and microcytic, and the hemoglobin concentration is normal to slightly depressed.

Hemoglobin H disease (β_4) results from the compound heterozygous state for α^0- plus α^+-thalassemia with deletion of three of four alpha genes (– –/–α). With only one functional α-globin gene per diploid genome, the newborn will have abnormal red cells containing a mixture of hemoglobin Bart (γ_4), hemoglobin H (β_4), and hemoglobin A. The neonate appears normal but soon develops hemolytic anemia as most of the hemoglobin Bart is replaced by hemoglobin H. Anemia is moderate to severe, and it usually worsens during pregnancy.

Inheritance of all four abnormal alpha genes causes homozygous α-thalassemia with predominant production of hemoglobin Bart, which has an appreciably increased affinity for oxygen. This is incompatible with extended survival, and stillbirths caused by the homozygous condition are especially common in Southeast Asia. Hsieh and colleagues (1989) reported that blood obtained by funipuncture from 20 hydropic fetuses contained 65 to 98 percent Bart hemoglobin. Either these fetuses are stillborn, or they die very soon after birth and have the typical features of nonimmune hydrops fetalis shown in Figure 16-4 (p. 330).

Lam and associates (1999) reported that sonographic measurement of the fetal cardiothoracic ratio at 12 to 13 weeks' gestation was 100-percent sensitive and specific for identifying affected fetuses. Sonographic evaluation of the myocardial performance index—the *Tei index*—in the first half of pregnancy has been evaluated. Changes predating hydrops are seen in affected fetuses (Luewan, 2013). Severe anemia can be detected using Doppler velocimetry of the middle cerebral artery (Chap. 10, p. 221). Although a successful case of hemopoietic cell transplantation with a fetal "cure" has been described, this remains experimental (Galanello, 2011a; Yi, 2009).

Beta Thalassemias

The β-thalassemias are the consequences of impaired β-globin chain production or α-chain instability. Genes that encode control of β-globin synthesis are in the δγβ-gene "cluster" located on chromosome 11 (Fig. 7-10, p. 138). More than 150 point mutations in the β-globin gene have been described (Weatherall, 2010). Most are single-nucleotide substitutions that produce transcriptional or translational defects, RNA splicing or modification, or frameshifts that result in highly unstable hemoglobins. Thus, deletional and nondeletional mutations affect β-globin RNA. In β-thalassemia, there is decreased β-chain production, and excess α-chains precipitate to cause cell membrane damage. Other forms of β-thalassemias are caused by α-chain instability (Kihm, 2002). Because of the variety of genetic defects and their combinations with genes that code for globin chain synthesis, these are collectively referred to as thalassemia syndromes (Weatherall, 2010).

The heterozygous trait is *β-thalassemia minor*, and those most commonly encountered have elevated hemoglobin A_2 levels. This hemoglobin is composed of two α- and two δ-globin chains, and concentrations are usually more than 3.5 percent. Hemoglobin F—composed of two α- and two γ-globin chains—also usually has increased concentrations of more than 2 percent. Some patients with heterozygous β-thalassemia minor do not have anemia, and others have mild to moderate anemia characterized by hypochromia and microcytosis.

Homozygous β-thalassemia—also called *β-thalassemia major* or *Cooley anemia*—is a serious and frequently fatal disorder. There is intense hemolysis and severe anemia. Many patients become transfusion dependent, and the subsequent iron load, along with abnormally increased gastrointestinal iron absorption, leads to hemochromatosis, which is fatal in many cases. A heterozygous form of β-thalassemia that clinically manifests as *thalassemia intermedia* produces moderate anemia.

Pregnancy

There are few problems that arise during pregnancy in women with β-thalassemia minor who have mild anemia. Iron and folate supplements are given. In some women, anemia will worsen because normal plasma volume expansion may be accompanied by slightly subnormal erythropoiesis.

Thalassemia major and some of the other severe forms were uncommonly encountered during pregnancy before the advent of transfusion and iron chelation therapy. With such management, there were 63 pregnancies reported without serious complications (Aessopos, 1999; Daskalakis, 1998; Kumar, 1997). Pregnancy is considered advisable if there is normal maternal cardiac function. Transfusions are given throughout pregnancy to maintain the hemoglobin concentration at 10 g/dL. This is coupled with surveillance of fetal growth (American College of Obstetricians and Gynecologists, 2013b; Sheiner, 2004).

Prenatal Diagnosis

Because β-thalassemia major is caused by numerous mutations, prenatal diagnosis is difficult. For a given individual, targeted mutation analysis is done that requires prior identification of that familial mutation. These are done using CVS and other techniques discussed in Chapter 14 (p. 300). Noninvasive testing of circulating fetal nucleic acids in maternal plasma for the diagnosis of β-thalassemia has been described (Galbiati, 2012; Leung, 2012).

PLATELET DISORDERS

Thrombocytopenia

Various platelet abnormalities may precede pregnancy, may develop during pregnancy coincidentally, or may be induced by pregnancy. Abnormally low platelet counts are relatively common in the pregnant woman and have various causes. These disorders may be inherited or idiopathic, acute or chronic in onset, and either primary or associated with other disorders. For example, thrombocytopenia in obstetrics is seen often with severe preeclampsia syndrome; massive hemorrhage with transfusions; consumptive coagulopathy from placental abruption, sepsis syndrome, or amnionic-fluid embolism; hemolytic anemias; systemic lupus erythematosus and antiphospholipid antibody syndrome; or hypoplastic or aplastic anemia. Other causes include viral infections, exposure to various drugs, and allergic reactions (Aster, 2007; Diz-Küçükkāya, 2010). Thrombocytopenia defined as < 150,000/μL platelets occurs in 6 to 15 percent of pregnant women, and 75 percent of these cases stem from gestational thrombocytopenia (Boehlen, 2006).

Burrows and Kelton (1993) reported that 6.6 percent of 15,471 pregnant women had a platelet count < 150,000/μL, and in 1.2 percent, it was < 100,000/μL. They reported that almost 75 percent of 1027 women whose platelet counts were < 150,000/μL were found to have normal-variant incidental thrombocytopenia. Of the remainder, 21 percent had a hypertensive disorder of pregnancy, and 4 percent had an immunological disorder. A platelet count of < 80,000/μL should trigger an evaluation for etiologies other than incidental or gestational thrombocytopenia, which is unlikely to have a platelet count of < 50,000/μL (Gernsheimer, 2013).

Gestational Thrombocytopenia

Normal pregnancy may be accompanied by a physiological decrease in platelet concentration (Appendix, p. 1287). This is usually evident in the third trimester and is thought to be predominantly due to hemodilution. However, the increased splenic mass characteristic of normal pregnancy may be contributory (Maymon, 2006). Most evidence shows that platelet life span is unchanged in normal pregnancy (Kenny, 2014). Thus, some degree of *gestational thrombocytopenia* is considered normal. Obviously, the definition used for thrombocytopenia is important. In their review, Rouse and coworkers (1998) cited an incidence of 4 to 7 percent for gestational thrombocytopenia, defined by platelet counts < 150,000/μL.

Inherited Thrombocytopenias

The *Bernard-Soulier syndrome* is characterized by lack of platelet membrane glycoprotein (GPIb/IX), which causes severe dysfunction. Maternal antibodies against fetal GPIb/IX antigen can cause alloimmune fetal thrombocytopenia. Peng and colleagues (1991) described an affected woman who during four pregnancies had episodes of postpartum hemorrhage, gastrointestinal hemorrhage, and fetal thrombocytopenia. Fujimori and associates (1999) described a similarly affected woman whose neonate died from thrombocytopenic intracranial hemorrhage. A systematic review of 30 pregnancies in 18 women reported a 33-percent rate of primary postpartum hemorrhage, and half of women with bleeding required blood transfusion. The reviewers also noted six cases of neonatal alloimmune thrombocytopenia and two perinatal deaths (Peitsidis, 2010). Close monitoring through pregnancy and 6 weeks postpartum is critical due to the possibility of life-threatening hemorrhage (Prabu, 2006).

Chatwani and coworkers (1992) reported a woman with autosomally dominant *May-Hegglin anomaly* whose infant was not affected. This condition is characterized by thrombocytopenia, giant platelets, and leukocyte inclusions. Urato and Repke (1998) also described such a woman who was delivered vaginally. Despite a platelet count of 16,000/μL, she did not bleed excessively. The neonate inherited the anomaly, but also had no bleeding despite a platelet count of 35,000/μL. Fayyad and colleagues (2002) managed three pregnancies in a woman with May-Hegglin anomaly. In the first, the mother had a term cesarean delivery of an unaffected infant; in the second, she had a fetal demise with multiple placental infarcts; and in the third, she received low-dose aspirin (75 mg/d) and gave birth to an unaffected infant.

Immune Thrombocytopenic Purpura

The primary form—also termed *idiopathic thrombocytopenic purpura (ITP)*—is usually caused by a cluster of IgG antibodies directed against one or more platelet glycoproteins (Schwartz, 2007). Antibody-coated platelets are destroyed prematurely in the reticuloendothelial system, especially the spleen. Although this is not proven, the disorder is probably mediated by autoantibodies directed at platelet-associated immunoglobulins—PAIgG, PAIgM, and PAIgA. In adults, ITP most often is a chronic disease that rarely resolves spontaneously.

Secondary forms of chronic thrombocytopenia appear in association with systemic lupus erythematosus, lymphomas, leukemias, and several systemic diseases. Approximately 2 percent of thrombocytopenic patients have positive serological tests for lupus, and in some cases there are high levels of anticardiolipin antibodies. Perhaps 10 percent of HIV-positive patients will have associated thrombocytopenia (Scaradavou, 2002).

Diagnosis and Management. Only a few adults with primary ITP recover spontaneously, and for those who do not, platelet counts usually range from 10,000 to 100,000/μL (George, 2010). There is no irrefutable evidence that pregnancy increases the risk of relapse in women with previously diagnosed ITP or worsens thrombocytopenia in women with active disease. That said, it is certainly not unusual for women who have been in clinical remission for several years to have recurrent thrombocytopenia during pregnancy. Although this may be from closer surveillance, hyperestrogenemia has also been suggested as a cause.

Therapy is considered if the platelet count is less than 30,000 to 50,000/μL (George, 2010). Primary treatment includes IVIG or corticosteroids (Neunert, 2011). Prednisone, 1 mg/kg daily, is given to suppress the phagocytic activity of the splenic monocyte-macrophage system. IVIG given in a total dose of 2 g/kg during 2 to 5 days is also usually effective.

In pregnant women with no response to corticosteroid or IVIG therapy, open or laparoscopic splenectomy may be effective. In late pregnancy, surgery is technically more difficult, and cesarean delivery may be necessary for exposure. Intravenous anti-D IgG, 50 to 75 μg/kg, has been described for treatment of resistant ITP in D-positive patients with a spleen (Konkle, 2008). There usually is improvement by 1 to 3 days, with a peak at approximately 8 days (Sieunarine, 2007). Cytotoxic agents are typically avoided in pregnancy due to teratogenicity risks. Azathioprine and rituximab, however, which are used in nonpregnant ITP, have been used for other conditions in pregnancy. Finally, the thrombopoietin agonist *romiplostim* has improved responses (Imbach, 2011; Kuter, 2010).

Fetal and Neonatal Effects. Platelet-associated IgG antibodies cross the placenta and may cause thrombocytopenia in the fetus-neonate. Fetal death from hemorrhage occurs occasionally (Webert, 2003). The severely thrombocytopenic fetus is at increased risk for intracranial hemorrhage with labor and delivery. This fortunately is unusual. Payne and associates (1997) reviewed studies of maternal ITP published since 1973 and added their experiences with 55 cases. Of 601 newborns, 12 percent had severe thrombocytopenia defined as a platelet count < 50,000/μL. Six infants had intracranial hemorrhage, and in three, their initial platelet count was > 50,000/μL. This is consistent with a study of 127 pregnancies in women with ITP in which 10 to 15 percent of neonates were found to have transient ITP (Koyama, 2012).

Considerable attention has been directed at identifying the fetus with potentially dangerous thrombocytopenia. All investigators have concurred that there is not a strong correlation between fetal and maternal platelet counts (George, 2009; Payne, 1997). Because of this, there have been attempts to quantify the relationships among maternal IgG free platelet antibody levels, platelet-associated antibody levels, and fetal platelet count. Again, however, there is little concurrence with these.

Investigators have also examined the association between the specific maternal cause of thrombocytopenia and risk of a thrombocytopenic fetus. Four causes investigated include gestational thrombocytopenia, hypertension-associated thrombocytopenia, ITP, and alloimmune thrombocytopenia. Burrows and Kelton (1993) reported neonatal umbilical cord platelet counts of < 50,000/μL in 19 of 15,932 consecutive newborns (0.12 percent). Of all of these pregnancies, only one of 756 mothers with gestational thrombocytopenia had an affected infant. Of 1414 hypertensive women with thrombocytopenia, five infants had thrombocytopenia. In contrast, of 46 mothers with ITP, four infants had thrombocytopenia. Finally, alloimmune thrombocytopenia was associated with profound thrombocytopenia and cord platelet counts < 20,000/μL. One of these fetuses died, and two others had intracranial hemorrhage.

Detection of Fetal Thrombocytopenia. Because there are no clinical characteristics or laboratory tests that accurately predict fetal platelet count, direct fetal blood sampling is necessary. Scott and coworkers (1983) obtained intrapartum scalp blood samples and recommended cesarean delivery for fetuses with platelet counts < 50,000/μL. Daffos and colleagues (1985) reported that percutaneous umbilical cord blood sampling (PUBS) had a high complication rate (Chap. 14, p. 300). Conversely, using PUBS, Berry and associates (1997) reported no complications but found a high negative predictive value of low platelet counts. Payne and coworkers (1997) summarized six studies in which fetal blood sampling was done for platelet estimation. Of the total of 195 fetuses, severe neonatal thrombocytopenia—defined as < 50,000/μL—was found in 7 percent. However, there were serious complications from cordocentesis in 4.6 percent. Because of the low incidence of severe neonatal thrombocytopenia and morbidity, fetal platelet determinations and cesarean delivery are not recommended for women with ITP (Neunert, 2011).

Neonatal Alloimmune Thrombocytopenia (NAIT). Disparity between maternal and fetal platelet antigens can stimulate maternal production of antiplatelet antibodies. Such platelet alloimmunization is identical to that caused by red cell antigens (Chap. 15, p. 313).

Thrombocytosis

Also called *thrombocythemia*, thrombocytosis generally is defined as persistent platelet counts > 450,000/μL. Common causes of *secondary* or *reactive thrombocytosis* are iron deficiency, infection, inflammatory diseases, and malignant tumors (Deutsch, 2013). Platelet counts seldom exceed 800,000/μL in these secondary disorders, and prognosis depends on the underlying disease. On the other hand, *primary* or *essential thrombocytosis* accounts for most cases in which platelet counts exceed 1 million/μL. It is a clonal disorder frequently due to an acquired mutation in the *JAK2* gene (Beer, 2010). Thrombocytosis usually is asymptomatic, but arterial and venous thromboses may develop (Rabinerson, 2007). These cases must be differentiated from the *sticky platelet syndrome,* which is also associated with thromboses (Rac, 2011). Cortelazzo and colleagues (1995) reported that myelosuppression with hydroxyurea for nonpregnant patients with essential thrombocytosis decreased thrombotic episodes from 24 to 4 percent compared with rates in untreated controls.

Normal pregnancies have been described in women whose mean platelet counts were > 1.25 million/μL (Beard, 1991; Randi, 1994). Others report more adverse outcomes. Niittyvuopio and associates (2004) described 40 pregnancies in 16 women with essential thrombocythemia. Almost half had a spontaneous abortion, fetal demise, or preeclampsia. In 63 pregnancies in 36 women cared for at the Mayo Clinic, a third had a spontaneous miscarriage, but other pregnancy complications were uncommon (Gangat, 2009). In this observational study, aspirin therapy was associated with a significantly lower abortion rate than that in untreated women—1 versus 75 percent, respectively.

Suggested treatments for thrombocytosis during pregnancy include aspirin, low-molecular-weight heparin, and interferon-α (Finazzi, 2012). Interferon-α therapy during pregnancy was successful in 11 women in the review by Delage and coworkers (1996). One of these women had transient blindness at midpregnancy when her platelet count was 2.3 million/μL. Thrombocytapheresis and interferon-α were used to maintain platelet counts at approximately 1 million/μL until delivery.

Thrombotic Microangiopathies

Although not a proven primary platelet disorder, there almost always is some degree of thrombocytopenia with the thrombotic microangiopathies. Their similarities to the HELLP syndrome allude to their obstetrical ramifications (George, 2013). Moschcowitz (1925) originally described *thrombotic thrombocytopenic purpura (TTP)* by the pentad of thrombocytopenia, fever, neurological abnormalities, renal impairment, and hemolytic anemia. Gasser and colleagues (1955) later described the similar *hemolytic uremic syndrome (HUS)*, which had more profound renal involvement and fewer neurological aberrations. Scully and associates (2012) provided guidelines for the diagnosis and management of thrombotic microangiopathic hemolytic anemias. The syndromes have an incidence of 2 to 6 per million persons per year (Miller, 2004).

Etiopathogenesis

Different causes likely account for the variable findings within these syndromes. Clinically, however, they frequently are indistinguishable in adults. Most cases of TTP are thought to be caused by a plasma deficiency of or antibodies to a von Willebrand factor-cleaving protease termed *ADAMTS-13 (ADAM metallopeptidase with thrombospondin type 1 motif, 13)* (Ganesan, 2011; Sadler, 2010). Conversely, HUS is usually due to endothelial damage incited by viral or bacterial infections and is seen primarily in children (Ardissino, 2013; George, 2013).

The general consensus is that intravascular platelet aggregation stimulates a cascade of events leading to end-organ failure. Although there is endothelial activation and damage, it is unclear whether this is a consequence or a cause. Elevated levels of unusually large multimers of von Willebrand factor are identified with active TTP. The *ADAMTS13* gene encodes the endothelium-derived protease responsible for cleaving von Willebrand factor—vWF (Sadler, 2010). Defects in this gene result in various clinical presentations of thrombotic microangiopathy (Camilleri, 2007; Moake, 2002, 2004). In another scheme, antibodies raised against ADAMTS-13 neutralize its action to cleave vWF multimers during an acute episode. The end result is microthrombi of hyaline material consisting of platelets and small amounts of fibrin develop within arterioles and capillaries. When sufficient in number or size, these aggregates produce ischemia or infarctions in various organs.

Clinical and Laboratory Manifestations

Thrombotic microangiopathies are characterized by thrombocytopenia, fragmentation hemolysis, and variable organ dysfunction. Neurological symptoms develop in up to 50 percent and include headache, altered consciousness, convulsions, fever, or stroke. Because renal involvement is common, TTP and HUS are difficult to separate clinically. Renal failure is thought to be more severe with the HUS, and in half of the cases, dialysis is required.

Thrombocytopenia is usually severe, but fortunately, even with very low platelet counts, spontaneous severe hemorrhage is uncommon. Microangiopathic hemolysis is associated with moderate to marked anemia, and erythrocyte transfusions are frequently necessary. The blood smear is characterized by erythrocyte fragmentation with schizocytosis. Reticulocytes and nucleated red blood cells are increased, lactate dehydrogenase (LDH) levels are high, and haptoglobin concentrations are decreased. Consumptive coagulopathy, although common, is usually subtle and clinically insignificant.

Treatment

The cornerstone of treatment is plasmapheresis with fresh-frozen plasma replacement. Plasma exchange removes inhibitors and replaces the ADAMTS-13 enzyme (George, 2010; Michael, 2009; Sadler, 2010). This has remarkably improved outcomes with these formerly fatal syndromes. Red cell transfusions are imperative for life-threatening anemia. If there are neurological abnormalities or rapid clinical deterioration, then plasmapheresis and plasma exchange can be performed twice daily. These are usually continued until the platelet count is > 150,000/μL. Unfortunately, relapses are common (Sadler, 2010). Additionally, there may be long-term sequelae such as renal impairment (Dashe, 1998).

Pregnancy

As shown in the Appendix (p. 1288), ADAMTS-13 enzyme activity decreases across pregnancy by as much as 50 percent (Sánchez-Luceros, 2004). Levels are decreased even further with the preeclampsia syndrome (Chap. 40, p. 731). This is consonant with prevailing opinions that TTP is more commonly seen during pregnancy. The Parkland Hospital experiences were described by Dashe and coworkers (1998), who identified 11 pregnancies complicated by these syndromes among nearly 275,000 obstetrical patients—a frequency of 1 in 25,000.

It seems likely that the disparately higher incidence in pregnancy reported by others is because of inclusion of women with severe preeclampsia and eclampsia (Hsu, 1995; Magann, 1994). There are differences that allow appropriate diagnosis (Table 56-6). For example, moderate to severe hemolysis is a rather constant feature of thrombotic microangiopathies. This is seldom severe with the preeclampsia syndrome, even when complicated by HELLP syndrome (Chap. 40, p. 742). And, although there is deposition of hyaline microthrombi within the liver with thrombotic microangiopathy, hepatocellular necrosis with elevated serum hepatic aminotransferase levels characteristic of preeclampsia is not a common feature (Ganesan, 2011; Sadler, 2010). Importantly, whereas delivery is imperative to reverse the preeclampsia syndrome in women with the HELLP syndrome, there is no evidence that thrombotic microangiopathy is improved by delivery (Dashe, 1998; Letsky, 2000). Finally, microangiopathic syndromes are usually recurrent and unassociated with pregnancy. For example, seven of 11 women described by Dashe and colleagues (1998) had recurrent disease either when not pregnant or within the first trimester of a subsequent pregnancy. George (2009) reported recurrent TTP in only five of 36 subsequent pregnancies.

Unless the diagnosis is unequivocally one of these thrombotic microangiopathies, rather than severe preeclampsia, the response to pregnancy termination should be evaluated before resorting to plasmapheresis and exchange transfusion, massive-dose glucocorticoid therapy, or other therapy. Unfortunately, recall that determination of ADAMTS-13 enzyme activity may

TABLE 56-6. Some Differential Factors between HELLP Syndrome and Thrombotic Microangiopathies[a]

	HELLP Syndrome	Thrombotic Microangiopathies
Thrombocytopenia	Mild/Mod.	Mod./severe
Microangiopathic hemolysis (schizocytosis)	Mild	Severe
ADAMTS13 def.	Mild/Mod.	Severe
DIC	Mild	Mild
Transaminitis (AST, ALT)	Mod./severe	None/mild
Treatment	Delivery	Plasmapheresis

[a]Includes thrombotic thrombocytopenia purpura (TTP) and hemolytic uremic syndrome (HUS).
ADAMTS13 = ADAM metallopeptidase with thrombospondin type 1 motif, 13; AST = aspartate aminotransferase; ALT = alanine aminotransferase; def. = deficiency; DIC = disseminated intravascular coagulation; HELLP = hemolysis, elevated liver enzymes, and low platelets; Mod. = moderate.

be difficult to interpret if not within the already lower range for normal pregnancy. With HELLP syndrome, enzyme activity levels are much lower and similar to those reported with microangiopathies (Franchini, 2007). It cannot be overemphasized that plasmapheresis is not indicated for preeclampsia-eclampsia complicated by hemolysis and thrombocytopenia.

During the past two decades, and coincidental with plasmapheresis and plasma exchange, maternal survival rates from thrombotic microangiopathy have improved dramatically (Dashe, 1998). Although previously fatal in up to half of mothers, with such treatment, Egerman and coworkers (1996) reported two maternal and three fetal deaths in 11 pregnancies. Hunt and associates (2013) reported that TTP accounted for 1 percent of maternal deaths in the United Kingdom from 2003 to 2008. Finally, a case of sudden maternal death from TTP has been described (Yamamoto, 2013).

Long-Term Prognosis

Women who are diagnosed with thrombotic microangiopathy during pregnancy are at risk for serious long-term complications. The Parkland experiences included a mean 9-year surveillance period (Dashe, 1998). These women had multiple recurrences; renal disease requiring dialysis, transplantation, or both; severe hypertension; and transfusion-acquired infectious diseases. Two women died remote from pregnancy—one from dialysis complications and one from transfusion-acquired HIV infection. Similar observations were reported by Egerman and colleagues (1996).

There have been reports of persistent cognitive defects and physical disabilities in nonpregnant women who have recovered from thrombotic microangiopathies (Kennedy, 2009; Lewis, 2009). Interestingly, these cognitive defects are very similar to those found in long-term surveillance studies of women who had eclampsia. Aukes (2009, 2012) and Wiegman (2012) and their associates from The Netherlands have documented cognitive and visual defects years following an eclamptic episode as further discussed in Chapter 40 (p. 770).

INHERITED COAGULATION DEFECTS

Hemophilias A and B

Obstetrical hemorrhage may infrequently be the consequence of an inherited defect of a protein that controls coagulation. As examples, both types of hemophilia may be involved. These are dependent on plasma factor levels and are categorized as mild—levels of 6 to 30 percent; moderate—2 to 5 percent; or severe—less than 1 percent (Mannucci, 2001).

Hemophilia A is an X-linked recessively transmitted disease characterized by a marked deficiency of small component antihemophilic factor (factor VIII). It is rare among women compared with men, in whom the heterozygous state is responsible for the disease. Heterozygous women have diminished factor VIII levels, but almost invariably, the homozygous state is the requisite for hemophilia A. In a few instances, it appears in women spontaneously from a newly mutant gene. Pregnancy-associated acquired hemophilia A from antibodies may result in severe morbidity from bleeding (Tengborn, 2012).

Christmas disease or *hemophilia B* is caused by severe deficiency of factor IX and has genetic and clinical features similar to those of hemophilia A.

Pregnancy

The obstetrical bleeding risk with these is directly related to factor VIII or factor IX levels. Affected women have a range of activity that is determined by random X-chromosome inactivation—lyonization—although activity is expected to average 50 percent (Letsky, 2000). If levels fall below 10 to 20 percent, there is a risk of hemorrhage. If levels fall to near zero, the risks are substantial. Pregnancy does afford some protection, however, because both of these clotting factors increase appreciably during normal pregnancy (Appendix, p. 1288). Treatment with desmopressin may also stimulate factor VIII release. Risks are further reduced by avoiding lacerations, minimizing episiotomy use, and maximizing postpartum uterine contractions. Operative vaginal deliveries should be avoided (Ljung, 1994).

There are few published experiences during pregnancy in women with hemophilia complications. Kadir and coworkers (1997) reported that 20 percent of carriers had postpartum hemorrhage, and in two, it was massive. Guy and associates (1992) reviewed five pregnancies in women with hemophilia B, and in all, outcomes were favorable. They recommended factor IX administration if levels are below 10 percent. Desmopressin has been shown in selected cases to reduce obstetrical bleeding complications (Trigg, 2012).

If a male fetus has hemophilia, the risk of hemorrhage increases after delivery in the neonate. This is especially true if circumcision is attempted.

Inheritance

If a mother has hemophilia A or B, all of her sons will have the disease, and all of her daughters will be carriers. If she is a carrier, half of her sons will inherit the disease, and half of her daughters will be carriers. Prenatal diagnosis of hemophilia is possible in some families using CVS (Chap. 14, p. 300). Preimplantation genetic diagnosis for hemophilia was reviewed by Lavery (2009).

Factor VIII or IX Inhibitors

Rarely, antibodies directed against factor VIII or IX are acquired and may lead to life-threatening hemorrhage. Patients with hemophilia A or B, because of prior treatment with factor VIII or IX, more commonly develop such antibodies. In contrast, acquisition of these antibodies in nonhemophiliacs is extraordinary. That said, this phenomenon has been identified rarely in women during the puerperium (Santoro, 2009). The prominent clinical feature is severe, protracted, repetitive hemorrhage from the reproductive tract starting a week or so after an apparently uncomplicated delivery (Reece, 1988). The activated partial thromboplastin time is markedly prolonged. Treatment has included multiple transfusions of whole blood and plasma; huge doses of cryoprecipitate; large volumes of an admixture of activated coagulation factors, including porcine factor VIII; immunosuppressive therapy; and attempts at various surgical procedures, especially curettage and hysterectomy. Another treatment involves bypassing factor VIII or IX by the use of activated forms of factors VII, IX, and X. A recombinant activated factor VII (NovoSeven) stops bleeding in up to 75 percent of patients with these inhibitors (Mannucci, 2001). As discussed in Chapter 41 (p. 817), NovoSeven has also been used in nonhemophiliac patients in cases of intractable obstetrical hemorrhage caused by uterine atony and by dilutional effects of multiple transfusions.

Von Willebrand Disease

There are at least 20 heterogeneous clinical disorders involving aberrations of factor VIII complex and platelet dysfunction—collectively termed *von Willebrand disease (vWD)*. These abnormalities are the most commonly inherited bleeding disorders, and their prevalence is as high as 1 to 2 percent (Mannucci, 2004; Pacheco, 2010). Most von Willebrand variants are inherited as autosomal dominant traits, and types I and II are the most common. Type III, which is the most severe, is a recessive trait (Nichols, 2008).

Although far less common than inherited von Willebrand disease, acquired disorders have been described. These are stimulated by underlying conditions such as benign and malignant hematological diseases, solid tumors, autoimmune disorders, and medications such as ciprofloxacin (Shau, 2002). Although most cases of acquired vWD develop after age 50 years, some have been reported in pregnant women (Lipkind, 2005).

Pathogenesis

The *von Willebrand factor* is a series of large plasma multimeric glycoproteins that form part of the factor VIII complex. It is essential for normal platelet adhesion to subendothelial collagen and formation of a primary hemostatic plug at the site of blood vessel injury. It also plays a major role in stabilizing the coagulant properties of factor VIII. The procoagulant component is the antihemophilic factor or factor VIII, which is a glycoprotein synthesized by the liver. Conversely, von Willebrand precursor, which is present in platelets and plasma, is synthesized by endothelium and megakaryocytes under the control of autosomal genes on chromosome 12. The von Willebrand factor antigen (vWF:Ag) is the antigenic determinant measured by immunoassays.

Clinical Presentation

Symptomatic patients usually present with bleeding suggestive of a chronic coagulation disorder. The classic autosomal dominant form usually causes symptoms in the heterozygous state. The less common but clinically more severe autosomal recessive form is manifest when inherited from both parents, who typically demonstrate little or no disease. Type I, which accounts for 75 percent of von Willebrand variants, is characterized by easy bruising; epistaxis; mucosal hemorrhage; and excessive bleeding with trauma, including surgery. Its laboratory features are usually a prolonged bleeding time, prolonged partial thromboplastin time, decreased vWF antigen levels, decreased factor VIII immunological and coagulation-promoting activity, and inability of platelets from an affected person to react to various stimuli.

Pregnancy

During normal pregnancy, maternal levels of both factor VIII and vWF antigen increase substantively (Appendix, p. 1288). Because of this, pregnant women with vWD often develop normal levels of factor VIII coagulant activity and vWF antigen, although the bleeding time still may be prolonged. If factor VIII activity is very low or if there is bleeding, treatment is recommended. Desmopressin by infusion may transiently increase factor VIII and vWF levels, especially in patients with type I disease (Kujovich, 2005; Mannucci, 2004). With significant bleeding, 15 or 20 units of cryoprecipitate are given every 12 hours. Alternatively, factor VIII concentrates may be given that contain high-molecular-weight vWF multimers (Alfanate, Hemate-P). These concentrates are highly purified and are heat treated to destroy HIV. Lubetsky and colleagues (1999) described continuous infusion with Hemate-P in a woman during a vaginal delivery. According to Chi and coworkers (2009), conduction analgesia can be given safely if coagulation defects have normalized or if hemostatic agents are given prophylactically.

Pregnancy outcomes in women with von Willebrand disease are generally good, but postpartum hemorrhage is encountered in up to 50 percent of cases. Of 38 cases summarized by Conti and associates (1986), bleeding was reported with abortion, with delivery, or in the puerperium in a fourth. Greer and colleagues (1991) noted that eight of 14 pregnancies were complicated by postpartum hemorrhage. Kadir and coworkers (1998) reported their experiences with 84 pregnancies. They described a 20-percent incidence of immediate postpartum hemorrhage and another 20-percent incidence of late hemorrhage. Most cases were associated with low vWF levels in untreated women, and none given treatment peripartum had hemorrhage. In our experiences, levels of coagulant factors within the normal range do not always protect against such bleeding.

Inheritance

Although most patients with von Willebrand disease have heterozygous variants and associated minor bleeding complications, the disease can be severe. Moreover, homozygous offspring develop a serious clotting dysfunction. CVS with DNA analysis to detect the missing genes has been described. Some authorities recommend cesarean delivery to avoid trauma to a possibly affected fetus if the mother has severe disease.

Other Factor Deficiencies

In general, the activity of most procoagulant factors increases across pregnancy (Appendix, p. 1288). In addition to the hemophilias, there are other inherited deficiencies of these factors that may cause a coagulopathy.

Factor VII deficiency is a rare autosomal recessive disorder. Levels of this factor normally increase during pregnancy, but these may rise only mildly in women with factor VII deficiency (Fadel, 1989). A systematic review of 94 births found no difference in postpartum hemorrhage rates with or without prophylaxis with recombinant factor VIIa (Baumann Kreuziger, 2013).

Factor X or *Stuart-Prower factor* deficiency is rare and is inherited as an autosomal recessive trait. Factor X levels typically rise by 50 percent during normal pregnancy. Konje and colleagues (1994) described a woman who had 2-percent factor activity. She was given prophylactic treatment with plasma-derived factor X, which raised her plasma levels to 37 percent. Despite this, she suffered an intrapartum placental abruption. Bofill and coworkers (1996) gave intrapartum fresh-frozen plasma to a woman with less than 1-percent factor X activity. She delivered spontaneously without incident. Beksaç and associates (2010) described a woman with severe factor X deficiency who was successfully managed with prophylactic prothrombin complex concentrate. Nance and colleagues (2012) reported on 24 pregnancies, of which 18 resulted in a healthy baby. However, the authors found a 2.5-fold increased risk of preterm birth.

Factor XI—plasma thromboplastin antecedent—deficiency is inherited as an autosomal trait. It is manifest as severe disease in homozygotes but only as a minor defect in heterozygotes. It is most prevalent in Ashkenazi Jews and is rarely seen in pregnancy. Musclow and coworkers (1987) reported 41 deliveries in 17 affected women, and none required transfusion. They also described a woman who developed a spontaneous hemarthrosis at 39 weeks. Kadir and associates (1998) analyzed 29 pregnancies in 11 affected women. None of these had factor XI level increases; 15 percent had immediate postpartum hemorrhage; and another 25 percent had delayed hemorrhage. In 105 pregnancies from 33 affected women, Myers and colleagues (2007) reported an uneventful pregnancy and delivery in 70 percent. They recommended peripartum treatment with factor XI concentrate if cesarean delivery is performed and advised against epidural analgesia unless factor XI is given. From their review, Martin-Salces and associates (2010) found that there was poor correlation between factor XI levels and bleeding in women with severe deficiency.

Factor XII deficiency is another autosomal recessive disorder that rarely complicates pregnancy. An increased incidence of thromboembolism is encountered in nonpregnant patients with this deficiency. Lao and coworkers (1991) reported an affected pregnant woman in whom placental abruption developed at 26 weeks' gestation.

Factor XIII deficiency is an autosomal recessive trait and may be associated with maternal intracranial hemorrhage (Letsky, 2000). In their review, Kadir and associates (2009) cited an increased risk of recurrent miscarriage and placental abruption. It has also been reported to cause umbilical cord bleeding (Odame, 2014). Treatment is fresh frozen plasma. Naderi and colleagues (2012) described 17 successful pregnancies in women receiving weekly prophylaxis with FXIII concentrate.

Fibrinogen abnormalities—either qualitative or quantitative—also may cause coagulation abnormalities. Autosomally inherited abnormalities usually involve the formation of a functionally defective fibrinogen—commonly referred to as *dysfibrinogenemia* (Edwards, 2000). Familial *hypofibrinogenemia* and sometimes *afibrinogenemia* are infrequent recessive disorders. In some cases, both are found—*hypodysfibrinogenemia* (Deering, 2003). Our experience suggests that hypofibrinogenemia represents a heterozygous autosomal dominant state. Typically, the thrombin-clottable protein level in these patients ranges from 80 to 110 mg/dL when nonpregnant, and this increases by 40 or 50 percent in normal pregnancy. Those pregnancy complications that give rise to acquired hypofibrinogenemia, for example, placental abruption, are more common with fibrinogen deficiency. Trehan and Fergusson (1991) and Funai and coworkers (1997) described successful outcomes in two affected women in whom fibrinogen or plasma infusions were given weekly or biweekly throughout pregnancy.

Conduction Analgesia with Bleeding Disorders

Most serious bleeding disorders would logically preclude the use of epidural or spinal analgesia for labor or delivery. If the bleeding disorder is controlled, however, conduction analgesia may be considered. Chi and colleagues (2009) reviewed intrapartum outcomes in 80 pregnancies in 63 women with an inherited bleeding disorder. These included those with factor XI deficiency, hemophilia carrier status, von Willebrand disease, platelet disorders, or a deficiency of factor VII, XI, or X. Regional block was used in 41. Of these, 35 had spontaneously normalized hemostatic dysfunction, and others were given prophylactic replacement therapy. The reviewers encountered no unusual complications and concluded that such practices were safe. Singh and associates (2009) reviewed 13 women with factor XI deficiency. Nine received neuraxial analgesia without complications, but only after fresh-frozen plasma was given to most to correct the activated partial thromboplastin time.

THROMBOPHILIAS

Several important regulatory proteins inhibit clotting. There are physiological antithrombotic proteins that act as inhibitors at strategic sites in the coagulation cascade to maintain blood fluidity. Inherited deficiencies of these inhibitory proteins are caused by gene mutations. Because they may be associated with recurrent thromboembolism, they are collectively referred to as *thrombophilias*. Because these deficiencies may be associated with thromboembolism, they are discussed in Chapter 52 (p. 1029), and they have been recently reviewed by the American College of Obstetricians and Gynecologists (2013d).

REFERENCES

Aessopos A, Karabatsos F, Farmakis D, et al: Pregnancy in patients with well-treated β-thalassemia: outcome for mothers and newborn infants. Am J Obstet Gynecol 180:360, 1999

Agre P: Hereditary spherocytosis. JAMA 262:2887, 1989

American College of Medical Genetics: Recommended uniform screening panel core conditions. 2013. Available at: http://www.hrsa.gov/advisorycommittees/mchbadvisory/heritabledisorders/recommendedpanel/uniformscreeningpanel.pdf. Accessed September 19, 2013

American College of Obstetricians and Gynecologists: Anemia in pregnancy. Committee Opinion No. 95, July 2008, Reaffirmed 2013a

American College of Obstetricians and Gynecologists: Hemoglobinopathies in pregnancy. Practice Bulletin No. 78, January 2007, Reaffirmed 2013b

American College of Obstetricians and Gynecologists: Neural tube defects. Practice Bulletin No. 44, July 2003, Reaffirmed 2013c

American College of Obstetricians and Gynecologists: Inherited thrombophilias in pregnancy. Practice Bulletin No. 138, September 2013d

Anyaegbunam A, Morel MIG, Merkatz IR: Antepartum fetal surveillance tests during sickle cell crisis. Am J Obstet Gynecol 165:1081, 1991

Ardissino G, Ossola MW, Baffero GM, et al: Eculizumab for atypical hemolytic uremic syndrome in pregnancy. Obstet Gynecol 122(2):487, 2013

Aster RH, Bougie DW: Drug-induced immune thrombocytopenia. N Engl J Med 357:580, 2007

Aukes AM, de Groot JC, Aarnoudse JG, et al: Brain lesions several years after eclampsia. Am J Obstet Gynecol 200:504.e1, 2009

Aukes AM, de Groot JC, Wiegman MJ, et al: Long-term cerebral imaging after preeclampsia. BJOG 119(9):1117, 2012

Austin H, Lally C, Benson JM, et al: Hormonal contraception, sickle cell trait, and risk for venous thromboembolism among African American women. Am J Obstet Gynecol 200(6):620.e1, 2009

Ballas SK, McCarthy WF, Guo N, et al: Multicenter study of hydroxyurea in sickle cell anemia. Exposure to hydroxyurea and pregnancy outcomes in patients with sickle cell anemia. J Natl Med Assoc 101(10):1046, 2009

Baumann Kreuziger LM, Morton CT, Reding MT: Is prophylaxis required for delivery in women with factor VII deficiency? Haemophilia 19(6):827, 2013

Bayouneu F, Subiran-Buisset C, Baka NE, et al: Iron therapy in iron deficiency anemia in pregnancy: intravenous route versus oral route. Am J Obstet Gynecol 186:518, 2002

Beard J, Hillmen P, Anderson CC, et al: Primary thrombocythaemia in pregnancy. Br J Haematol 77:371, 1991

Beer PA, Green AR: Essential thrombocythemia. In Kaushansky K, Lichtman MA, Beutler E, et al (eds): Williams Hematology, 8th ed. New York, McGraw-Hill, 2010, p 1237

Beksaç MS, Atak Z, Ozlü T: Severe factor X deficiency in a twin pregnancy. Arch Gynecol Obstet 281(1):151, 2010

Berry SM, Leonardi MR, Wolfe HM, et al: Maternal thrombocytopenia. Predicting neonatal thrombocytopenia with cordocentesis. J Reprod Med 42:276, 1997

Beutler E: Glucose-6-phosphate dehydrogenase deficiency. N Engl J Med 324:169, 1991

Bodnar LM, Scanlon KS, Freedman DS, et al: High prevalence of postpartum anemia among low-income women in the United States. Am J Obstet Gynecol 185:438, 2001

Boehlen F: Thrombocytopenia during pregnancy. Importance, diagnosis and management. Hamostaseologie 26:72, 2006

Bofill JA, Young RA, Perry KG Jr: Successful pregnancy in a woman with severe factor X deficiency. Obstet Gynecol 88:723, 1996

Borgna-Pignatti C, Marradi P, Rugolotto S, et al: Successful pregnancy after bone marrow transplantation for thalassaemia. Bone Marrow Transplant 18:235, 1996

Boulet SL, Okoroh EM, Azonobi I, et al: Sickle cell disease in pregnancy: maternal complications in a Medicaid-enrolled population. Matern Child Health J 17(2):200, 2013

Bourantas K, Makrydimas G, Georgiou I, et al: Aplastic anemia: report of a case with recurrent episodes in consecutive pregnancies. J Reprod Med 42:672, 1997

Brawley OW, Cornell LJ, Edwards LR, et al: National Institutes of Health Consensus Development Conference Statement: Hydroxyurea treatment for sickle cell disease. Ann Intern Med 148:1, 2008

Bresani CC, Braga MC, Felisberto DF, et al: Accuracy of erythrogram and serum ferritin for the maternal anemia diagnosis (AMA): a phase 3 diagnostic study on prediction of the therapeutic responsiveness to oral iron in pregnancy. BMC Pregnancy Childbirth 13:13, 2013

Brewer CA, Adelson MD, Elder RC: Erythrocytosis associated with a placental-site trophoblastic tumor. Obstet Gynecol 79:846, 1992

Briggs GG, Freeman RK, Yaffe SJ: Drugs in Pregnancy and Lactation, 8th ed. Philadelphia, Lippincott, Williams & Wilkins, 2011

Burrows RF, Kelton JG: Fetal thrombocytopenia and its relation to maternal thrombocytopenia. N Engl J Med 329:1463, 1993

Camilleri RS, Cohen H, Mackie I, et al: Prevalence of the ADAMTS13 missense mutation R1060W in late onset adult thrombotic thrombocytopenic purpura. J Thromb Haemost 6(2):331, 2007

Camous J, N'da A, Etienne-Julan M, et al: Anesthetic management of pregnant women with sickle cell diseases—effect on postnatal sickling complications. Can J Anaesth 55:276, 2008

Casadevall N, Nataraf J, Viron B, et al: Pure red-cell aplasia and antierythropoietin antibodies in patients treated with recombinant erythropoietin. N Engl J Med 346:469, 2002

Castro O, Hogue M, Brown BD: Pulmonary hypertension in sickle cell disease: cardiac catheterization results and survival. Blood 101:4, 2003

Cavenee MR, Cox SM, Mason R, et al: Erythropoietin in pregnancies complicated by pyelonephritis. Obstet Gynecol 84:252, 1994

Celkan T, Alhaj S: Prenatal diagnosis of hereditary spherocytosis with osmotic fragility test. Indian Pediatr 45(1):63, 2008

Centers for Disease Control and Prevention: CDC criteria for anemia in children and childbearing-aged women. MMWR 38:400, 1989

Centers for Disease Control and Prevention: Recommendations to prevent and control iron deficiency in the United States. MMWR 47:1, 1998

Centers for Disease Control and Prevention: Recommended adult immunization schedule-2013a. Available at: http://www.cdc.gov/vaccines/schedules/downloads/adult/adult-schedule.pdf. Accessed September 19, 2013

Centers for Disease Control and Prevention: U.S. selected practice recommendations for contraceptive use, 2013b. Available at: http://www.cdc.gov/mmwr/pdf/rr/rr6205.pdf. Accessed September 19, 2013

Chakravarty EF, Khanna D, Chung L: Pregnancy outcomes in systemic sclerosis, primary pulmonary hypertension, and sickle cell disease. Obstet Gynecol 111:927, 2008

Chang S, Zeng L, Brouwer ID, t al: Effect of iron deficiency anemia in pregnancy on child mental development in rural China. Pediatrics 131(3):e755, 2013

Chatwani A, Bruder N, Shapiro T, et al: May–Hegglin anomaly: a rare case of maternal thrombocytopenia in pregnancy. Am J Obstet Gynecol 166:143, 1992

Chi C, Lee CA, England A, et al: Obstetric analgesia and anaesthesia in women with inherited bleeding disorders. Thromb Haemost 101(6):1104, 2009

Cho G, Hambleton IR: Regular long-term red blood cell transfusions for managing chronic chest complications in sickle cell disease. Cochrane Database Syst Rev 1:CD008360, 2014

Choudhry VP, Gupta S, Gupta M, et al: Pregnancy associated aplastic anemia—a series of 10 cases with review of literature. Hematology 7(4):233, 2002

Conti M, Mari D, Conti E, et al: Pregnancy in women with different types of von Willebrand disease. Obstet Gynecol 68:282, 1986

Cortelazzo S, Finazzi G, Ruggeri M, et al: Hydroxyurea for patients with essential thrombocythemia and a high risk of thrombosis. N Engl J Med 332:1132, 1995

Cox JV, Steane E, Cunningham G, et al: Risk of alloimmunization and delayed hemolytic transfusion reactions in patients with sickle cell disease. Arch Intern Med 148:2485, 1988

Cox SM, Shelburne P, Mason R, et al: Mechanisms of hemolysis and anemia associated with acute antepartum pyelonephritis. Am J Obstet Gynecol 164:587, 1991

Cullis J: Anaemia of chronic disease. Clin Med 13(2):193, 2013

Cunningham FG, Cox SM, Harstad TW, et al: Chronic renal disease and pregnancy outcome. Am J Obstet Gynecol 163:453, 1990

Cunningham FG, Pritchard JA: Prophylactic transfusions of normal red blood cells during pregnancies complicated by sickle cell hemoglobinopathies. Am J Obstet Gynecol 135:994, 1979

Cunningham FG, Pritchard JA, Hankins GDV, et al: Idiopathic cardiomyopathy or compounding cardiovascular events. Obstet Gynecol 67:157, 1986
Cunningham FG, Pritchard JA, Mason R: Pregnancy and sickle hemoglobinopathy: results with and without prophylactic transfusions. Obstet Gynecol 62:419, 1983
Cyganek A, Pietrzak B, Kociszewska-Najman B, et al: Anemia treatment with erythropoietin in pregnant renal recipients. Transplant Proc 43(8):2970, 2011
Daffos F, Capella-Pavlovsky M, Forestier F: Fetal blood sampling during pregnancy with the use of a needle guided by ultrasound: a study of 606 consecutive cases. Am J Obstet Gynecol 153:655, 1985
Dalle JH: Hematopoietic stem cell transplantation in SCD. C R Biol 336(3):148, 2013
Dashe JS, Ramin SM, Cunningham FG: The long-term consequences of thrombotic microangiopathy (thrombotic thrombocytopenic purpura and hemolytic uremic syndrome) in pregnancy. Obstet Gynecol 91:662, 1998
Daskalakis GJ, Papageorgiou IS, Antsaklis AJ, et al: Pregnancy and homozygous beta thalassaemia major. Br J Obstet Gynaecol 105:1028, 1998
de Abood M, de Castillo Z, Guerrero F, et al: Effect of Depo-Provera or Microgynon on the painful crises of sickle cell anemia patients. Contraception 56:313, 1997
Deering SH, Landy HL, Tchabo N, et al: Hypodysfibrinogenemia during pregnancy, labor, and delivery. Obstet Gynecol 101:1092, 2003
De Gramont A, Krulik M, Debray J: Paroxysmal nocturnal haemoglobinuria and pregnancy. Lancet 1:868, 1987
de Guibert S, Peffault de Latour R, et al: Paroxysmal nocturnal hemoglobinuria and pregnancy before the eculizumab era: the French experience. Haematologica 96(9):1276, 2011
Delage R, Demers C, Cantin G, et al: Treatment of essential thrombocythemia during pregnancy with interferon-α. Obstet Gynecol 87:814, 1996
Deutsch VR, Tomer A: Advances in megakaryocytopoiesis and thrombopoiesis: from bench to bedside. Br J Haematol 161(6):778, 2013
Dhingra S, Wiener JJ, Jackson H: Management of cold agglutinin-immune hemolytic anemia in pregnancy. Obstet Gynecol 110:485, 2007
Diz-Küçükkāya R, Chen J, Geddis A, et al: Thrombocytopenia. In Kaushansky K, Lichtman MA, Beutler E, et al (eds): Williams Hematology, 8th ed. New York, McGraw-Hill, 2010, p 891
Dolan LM, Ryan M, Moohan J: Pyruvate kinase deficiency in pregnancy complicated by iron overload. Br J Obstet Gynaecol 109:844, 2002
Dotters-Katz SK, Grotegut CA, Heine RP: The effects of anemia on pregnancy outcome with pyelonephritis. Inf Dis Obstet Gynecol Nov 27, 2013 [Epub ahead of print]
Driscoll MC, Hurlet A, Styles L, et al: Stroke risk in siblings with sickle cell anemia. Blood 101:2401, 2003
Edwards RZ, Rijhsinghani A: Dysfibrinogenemia and placental abruption. Obstet Gynecol 95:1043, 2000
Egerman RS, Witlin AG, Friedman SA, et al: Thrombotic thrombocytopenic purpura and hemolytic uremic syndrome in pregnancy: review of 11 cases. Am J Obstet Gynecol 195:950, 1996
Eliyahu S, Shalev E: A successful pregnancy after bone marrow transplantation for severe aplastic anaemia with pretransplant conditioning of total lymph-node irradiation and cyclophosphamide. Br J Haematol 86:649, 1994
Elstein D, Granovsky-Grisaru S, Rabinowitz R, et al: Use of enzyme replacement therapy for Gaucher disease during pregnancy. Am J Obstet Gynecol 177:1509, 1997
Fadel HE, Krauss JS: Factor VII deficiency and pregnancy. Obstet Gynecol 73:453, 1989
Faivre L, Meerpohl J, Da Costa L, et al: High-risk pregnancies in Diamond-Blackfan anemia: a survey of 64 pregnancies from the French and German registries. Haematologica 91:530, 2006
Fayyad AM, Brummitt DR, Barker HF, et al: May-Hegglin anomaly: the role of aspirin in the treatment of this rare platelet disorder in pregnancy. Br J Obstet Gynaecol 109:223, 2002
Fieni S, Bonfanti L, Gramellini D, et al: Clinical management of paroxysmal nocturnal hemoglobinuria in pregnancy: a case report and updated review. Obstet Gynecol Surv 61:593, 2006
Finazzi G: How to manage essential thrombocythemia. Leukemia 26(5):875, 2012
Franchini M, Montagnana M, Targher G, et al: Reduced von Willebrand factor-cleaving protease levels in secondary thrombotic microangiopathies and other diseases. Semin Thromb Hemost 33(8):787, 2007
Fucharoen S, Winichagoon P: Clinical and hematologic aspects of hemoglobin E beta-thalassemia. Curr Opin Hematol 7:106, 2000
Fujimori K, Ohto H, Honda S, et al: Antepartum diagnosis of fetal intracranial hemorrhage due to maternal Bernard–Soulier syndrome. Obstet Gynecol 94:817, 1999
Funai EF, Klein SA, Lockwood CJ: Successful pregnancy outcome in a patient with both congenital hypofibrinogenemia and protein S deficiency. Obstet Gynecol 90:858, 1997
Galanello R, Cao A: Alpha-thalassemia. In Pagon RA, Bird TD, Dolan CR, et al (eds): GeneReviews. Seattle, University of Washington, 2011a
Galanello R, Cao A: Gene test review. Alpha-thalassemia. Genet Med 13(2):83, 2011b
Galbiati S, Brisci A, Damin F, et al: Fetal DNA in maternal plasma: a noninvasive tool for prenatal diagnosis of beta-thalassemia. Expert Opin Biol Ther 12(Suppl 1):S181, 2012
Gallagher PG: The red blood cell membrane and its disorders: hereditary spherocytosis, elliptocytosis, and related diseases. In Kaushansky K, Lichtman MA, Beutler E, et al (eds): Williams Hematology, 8th ed. New York, McGraw-Hill, 2010, p 617
Gandhi SK, Powers JC, Nomeir A-M, et al: The pathogenesis of acute pulmonary edema associated with hypertension. N Engl J Med 344:17, 2000
Ganesan C, Maynard SE: Acute kidney injury in pregnancy: the thrombotic microangiopathies. J Nephrol 24(5):554, 2011
Gangat N, Wolanskij AP, Schwager S, et al: Predictors of pregnancy outcomes in essential thrombocythemia: a single institution study of 63 pregnancies. Eur J Haematol 82(5):350, 2009
Garratty G: Severe reactions associated with transfusion of patients with sickle cell disease. Transfusion 37:357, 1997
Garratty G, Leger RM, Arndt PA: Severe immune hemolytic anemia associated with prophylactic use of cefotetan in obstetric and gynecologic procedures. Am J Obstet Gynecol 181:103, 1999
Gasser C, Gautier E, Steck A, et al: Haemolytisch-uramisch Syndrome: bilaterale Nierenrindennekrosen bei akuten erworbenin haemolytischen Anamien. Schweiz Med Wochenschr 85:905, 1955
George JN: How I treat patients with thrombotic thrombocytopenic purpura: 2010. Blood 116(20):4060, 2010
George JN: The thrombotic thrombocytopenic purpura and hemolytic uremic syndromes: overview of pathogenesis (experience of The Oklahoma TTP-HUS Registry, 1989–2007). Kidney Int 75(112):S8, 2009
George JN, Charania RS: Evaluation of patients with microangiopathic hemolytic anemia and thrombocytopenia. Semin Thromb Hemost 39(2):153, 2013
Gernsheimer T, James AH, Stasi R: How I treat thrombocytopenia in pregnancy. Blood 121(1):38, 2013
Gilsanz F, Vega MA, Gomez-Castillo E, et al: Fetal anaemia due to pyruvate kinase deficiency. Arch Dis Child 69:523, 1993
Gladwin MT, Sachdev V, Jison ML, et al: Pulmonary hypertension as a risk factor for death in patients with sickle cell disease. N Engl J Med 350:886, 2004
Gladwin MT, Vichinsky E: Pulmonary complications of sickle cell disease. N Engl J Med 359:2254, 2008
Goldenberg RL, Tamura T, DuBard M, et al: Plasma ferritin and pregnancy outcome. Am J Obstet Gynecol 175:1356, 1996
Granovsky-Grisaru S, Aboulafia Y, Diamant YZ, et al: Gynecologic and obstetric aspects of Gaucher's disease: a survey of 53 patients. Am J Obstet Gynecol 172:1284, 1995
Granovsky-Grisaru S, Belmatoug N, vom Dahl S, et al: The management of pregnancy in Gaucher disease. Eur J Obstet Gynecol Reprod Biol 156(1):3, 2011
Green AM, Kupfer GM: Fanconi anemia. Hematol Oncol Clin North Am 23(2):193, 2009
Greene MF, Frigoletto FD Jr, Claster SZ, et al: Pregnancy and paroxysmal nocturnal hemoglobinuria: report of a case and review of the literature. Obstet Gynecol Surv 38:591, 1983
Greer IA, Lowe GDO, Walker JJ, et al: Haemorrhagic problems in obstetrics and gynaecology in patients with congenital coagulopathies. Br J Obstet Gynaecol 98:909, 1991
Griesshammer M, Struve S, Harrison CM: Essential thrombocythemia/polycythemia vera and pregnancy: the need for an observational study in Europe. Semin Thromb Hemost 32:422, 2006
Grigoriadis C, Tympa A, Liapis A, et al: Alpha-methyldopa-induced autoimmune hemolytic anemia in the third trimester of pregnancy. Case Rep Obstet Gynecol Sept 23, 2013 [Epub ahead of print]
Grossetti E, Carles G, El Guindi W, et al: Selective prophylactic transfusion in sickle cell disease. Acta Obstet Gynecol 88:1090, 2009
Guy GP, Baxi LV, Hurlet-Jensen A, et al: An unusual complication in a gravida with factor IX deficiency: case report with review of the literature. Obstet Gynecol 80:502, 1992
Haddad LB, Curtis KM, Legardy-Williams JK, et al: Contraception for individuals with sickle cell disease: a systematic review of the literature. Contraception 85(6):527, 2012
Harrison C: Do we know more about essential thrombocythemia because of JAK2V617F? Curr Hematol Malig Rep 4(1):25, 2009
Hillmen P, Young NS, Schubert J, et al: The complement inhibitor eculizumab in paroxysmal nocturnal hemoglobinuria. N Engl J Med 355:1233, 2006
Howard J, Malfroy M, Llewelyn C, et al: The transfusion alternatives preoperatively in sickle cell disease (TAPS) study: a randomised, controlled, multicentre clinical trial. Lancet 381(9870):930, 2013

Howard RJ, Tuck SM, Pearson TC: Pregnancy in sickle cell disease in the UK: results of a multicentre survey of the effect of prophylactic blood transfusion on maternal and fetal outcome. Br J Obstet Gynaecol 102:947, 1995
Hsieh FJ, Chang FM, Ko TM, et al: The antenatal blood gas and acid–base status of normal fetuses and hydropic fetuses with Bart hemoglobinopathy. Obstet Gynecol 74:722, 1989
Hsieh MM, Kang EM, Fitzhugh CD, et al: Allogenic hematopoietic stem-cell transplantation for sickle cell disease. N Engl J Med 361(24):2309, 2009
Hsu HW, Belfort MA, Vernino S, et al: Postpartum thrombotic thrombocytopenic purpura complicated by Budd–Chiari syndrome. Obstet Gynecol 85:839, 1995
Hunt BJ, Thomas-Dewing RR, Bramham K, et al: Preventing maternal deaths due to acquired thrombotic thrombocytopenic purpura. J Obstet Gynaecol Res 39(1):347, 2013
Hurst D, Little B, Kleman KM, et al: Anemia and hemoglobinopathies in Southeast Asian refugee children. J Pediatric 102:692, 1983
Imbach P, Crowther M: Thrombopoietin-receptor agonists for primary immune thrombocytopenia. N Engl J Med 365(8):734, 2011
Italia KY, Jijina FF, Chandrakala S, et al: Exposure to hydroxyurea during pregnancy in sickle-beta thalassemia: a report of 2 cases. J Clin Pharmacol 50(2):231, 2010
Kacker S, Ness PM, Savage WJ, et al: Cost-effectiveness of prospective red blood cell antigen matching to prevent alloimmunization among sickle cell patients. Transfusion 54:86, 2014
Kadir R, Chi C, Bolton-Maggs P: Pregnancy and rare bleeding disorders. Haemophilia 15(5):990, 2009
Kadir RA, Economides DL, Braithwaite J, et al: The obstetric experience of carriers of haemophilia. Br J Obstet Gynaecol 104:803, 1997
Kadir RA, Lee CA, Sabin CA, et al: Pregnancy in women with von Willebrand's disease or factor XI deficiency. Br J Obstet Gynaecol 105:314, 1998
Kelly R, Arnold L, Richards S, et al: The management of pregnancy in paroxysmal nocturnal haemoglobinuria on long term eculizumab. Br J Haematol 149(3):446, 2010
Kennedy AS, Lewis QF, Scott JG, et al: Cognitive deficits after recovery from thrombotic thrombocytopenic purpura. Transfusion 49(6):1092, 2009
Kenny L, McCrae K, Cunningham FG: Platelets, coagulation, and the liver. In Taylor RN, Roberts JM, Cunningham FG (eds): Chesley's Hypertensive Disorders in Pregnancy. Elsevier, Amsterdam, 2014
Kessous R, Pariente G, Shoham-Vardi I, et al: Anemia during pregnancy as a marker for long-term cardiovascular morbidity: a decade of follow up. Abstract No. 677, Am J Obstet Gynecol 208(1):S285, 2013
Kidanto HL, Mogren I, Lindmark G, et al: Risks for preterm delivery and low birth weight are independently increased by severity of maternal anaemia. S Afr Med J 99(2):98, 2009
Kihm AJ, Kong Y, Hong W, et al: An abundant erythroid protein that stabilizes free alpha-haemoglobin. Nature 417(6890):758, 2002
Klebanoff MA, Shiono PH, Selby JV, et al: Anemia and spontaneous preterm birth. Am J Obstet Gynecol 164:59, 1991
Konje JC, Murphy P, de Chazal R, et al: Severe factor X deficiency and successful pregnancy. Br J Obstet Gynaecol 101:910, 1994
Konkle BA: Disorder of platelets and vessel wall. In Fauci AS, Braunwald E, Kasper DL, et al (eds): Harrison's Principles of Internal Medicine, 17th ed. New York, McGraw-Hill, 2008, p 718
Koshy M, Burd L, Wallace D, et al: Prophylactic red-cell transfusions in pregnant patients with sickle cell disease: a randomized cooperative study. N Engl J Med 319:1447, 1988
Koyama S, Tomimatsu T, Kanagawa T, et al: Reliable predictors of neonatal immune thrombocytopenia in pregnant women with idiopathic thrombocytopenic purpura. Am J Hematol 87(1):15, 2012
Krafft A, Perewusnyk G, Hänseler E, et al: Effect of postpartum iron supplementation on red cell and iron parameters in non-anaemic iron-deficient women: a randomized placebo-controlled study. BJOG 112:445, 2005
Kujovich JL: Von Willebrand disease and pregnancy. J Thromb Haemost 3:246, 2005
Kumar KJ, Asha N, Murthy DS, et al: Maternal anemia in various trimesters and its effect on newborn weight and maturity: an observational study. Int J Prev Med 4(2):193, 2013
Kumar R, Advani AR, Sharan J, et al: Pregnancy induced hemolytic anemia: an unexplained entity. Ann Hematol 80:623, 2001
Kumar RM, Rizk DEE, Khuranna A: β-Thalassemia major and successful pregnancy. J Reprod Med 42:294, 1997
Kuter DJ, Rummel M, Boccia R, et al: Romioplostim or standard of care in patients with immune thrombocytopenia. N Engl J Med 363(20):1889, 2010
Kwon JY, Lee Y, Shin JC, et al: Supportive management of pregnancy-associated aplastic anemia. Int J Gynecol Obstet 95:115, 2006
Lam YH, Tang MHY, Lee CP, et al: Prenatal ultrasonographic prediction of homozygous type 1 alpha-thalassemia at 12 to 13 weeks of gestation. Am J Obstet Gynecol 180:148, 1999
Lao TT, Lewinsky RM, Ohlsson A, et al: Factor XII deficiency and pregnancy. Obstet Gynecol 78:491, 1991
Lassi ZS, Salam RA, Haider BA, et al: Folic acid supplementation during pregnancy for maternal health and pregnancy outcomes. Cochrane Database Syst Rev 3:CD006896, 2013
Lavery S: Preimplantation genetic diagnosis of haemophilia. Br J Haematol 144(3):303, 2009
Letsky EA: Hematologic disorders. In Barron WM, Lindheimer MD (eds): Medical Disorders During Pregnancy, 3rd ed. St. Louis, Mosby, 2000, p 267
Leung TY, Lao TT: Thalassaemia in pregnancy. Best Pract Res Clin Obstet Gynaecol 26(1):37, 2012
Lewis QF, Lanneau MS, Mathias SD, et al: Long-term deficits in health-related quality of life after recovery from thrombotic thrombocytopenia purpura. Transfusion 49(1):118, 2009
Lin K, Barton MB: Screening for hemoglobinopathies in newborns: reaffirmation update for the U.S. Preventative Task Force. AHRQ Publication No 07-05104-EF-1, 2007
Lipkind HS, Kurtis JD, Powrie R, et al: Acquired von Willebrand disease: management of labor and delivery with intravenous dexamethasone, continuous factor concentrate, and immunoglobulin infusion. Am J Obstet Gynecol 192:2067, 2005
Lipton JM, Ellis SR: Diamond-Blackfan anemia: diagnosis, treatment, and molecular pathogenesis. Hematol Oncol Clin North Am 23(2):261, 2009
Ljung R, Lindgren AC, Petrini P, et al: Normal vaginal delivery is to be recommended for haemophilia carrier gravidae. Acta Paediatr 83(6):609, 1994
Lubetsky A, Schulman S, Varon D, et al: Safety and efficacy of continuous infusion of a combined factor VIII–von Willebrand factor (vWF) concentrate (Haemate-P) in patients with von Willebrand disease. Thromb Haemost 81:229, 1999
Luewan S, Srisupundit K, Tongsong T: Outcomes of pregnancies complicated by beta-thalassemia/hemoglobin E disease. Int J Gynaecol Obstet 104(3):203, 2009
Luewan S, Tongprasert F, Srisupundit K, et al: Fetal myocardial performance (Tei) index in fetal hemoglobin Bart's disease. Ultraschall Med 34(4):355, 2013
Maberry MC, Mason RA, Cunningham FG, et al: Pregnancy complicated by hemoglobin CC and C–beta-thalassemia disease. Obstet Gynecol 76:324, 1990
Maberry MC, Mason RA, Cunningham FG, et al: Pregnancy complicated by hereditary spherocytosis. Obstet Gynecol 79:735, 1992
Magann EF, Bass D, Chauhan SP, et al: Antepartum corticosteroids: disease stabilization in patients with the syndrome of hemolysis, elevated liver enzymes, and low platelets (HELLP). Am J Obstet Gynecol 171:1148, 1994
Maigne G, Ferlicot S, Galacteros F, et al: Glomerular lesions in patients with sickle cell disease. Medicine 89(1):18, 2010
Mannucci PM: Treatment of von Willebrand's Disease. N Engl J Med 351: 683, 2004
Mannucci PM, Tuddenham EGD: The hemophilias—from royal genes to gene therapy. N Engl J Med 344:1773, 2001
Marti-Carvajal AJ, Peña-Marti GE, Comunián-Carrasco G, et al: Interventions for treating painful sickle cell crisis during pregnancy. Cochrane Database Syst Rev 1:CD006786, 2009
Martin-Salces M, Jimenez-Yuste V, Alvarez MT, et al: Factor XI deficiency: review and management in pregnant women. Clin Appl Thromb Hemost 16(2):209, 2010
Maymon R, Strauss S, Vaknin Z, et al: Normal sonographic values of maternal spleen size throughout pregnancy. Ultrasound Med Biol 32(12):1827, 2006
McKoy JM, Stonecash RE, Cournoyer D, et al: Epoetin-associated pure red cell aplasia: past, present, and future considerations. Transfusion 48(8):1754, 2008
Medoff BD, Shepard JO, Smith RN, et al: Case 17–2005: a 22-year-old woman with back and leg pain and respiratory failure. N Engl J Med 352:2425, 2005
Michael M, Elliott EJ, Ridley GF, et al: Interventions for haemolytic uraemic syndrome and thrombotic thrombocytopenic purpura. Cochrane Database Sys Rev 1:CDE003595, 2009
Miller DP, Kaye JA, Shea K, et al: Incidence of thrombotic thrombocytopenic purpura/hemolytic uremic syndrome. Epidemiology 15:208, 2004
Moake JL: Thrombotic microangiopathies. N Engl J Med 347:589, 2002
Moake JL: Von Willebrand factor, ADAMTS-13, and thrombotic thrombocytopenic purpura. Semin Hematol 41:4, 2004
Mockenhaupt FP, Mandelkow J, Till H, et al: Reduced prevalence of *Plasmodium falciparum* infection and of concomitant anaemia in pregnant women with heterozygous G6PD deficiency. Trop Med Int Health 8:118, 2003
Moise KJ Jr: Umbilical cord stem cells. Obstet Gynecol 106:1393, 2005

Morkbak AL, Hvas AM, Milman N, et al: Holotranscobalamin remains unchanged during pregnancy. Longitudinal changes of cobalamins and their binding proteins during pregnancy and postpartum. Haematologica 92:1711, 2007

Moschcowitz E: An acute febrile pleiochromic anemia with hyaline thrombosis of the terminal arterioles and capillaries. Arch Intern Med 36:89, 1925

Murphy JF, O'Riordan J, Newcombe RG, et al: Relation of haemoglobin levels in first and second trimester to outcome of pregnancy. Lancet 1:992, 1986

Musclow CE, Goldenberg H, Bernstein EP, et al: Factor XI deficiency presenting as hemarthrosis during pregnancy. Am J Obstet Gynecol 157:178, 1987

Myers B, Pavorod S, Kean L, et al: Pregnancy outcome in Factor XI deficiency: incidence of miscarriage, antenatal and postnatal haemorrhage in 33 women with Factor XI deficiency. BJOG 114:643, 2007

Naderi M, Eshghi P, Cohan N, et al: Successful delivery in patients with FXIII deficiency receiving prophylaxis: report of 17 cases in Iran. Haemophilia 18(5):773, 2012

Nagel RL, Fabry ME, Steinberg MH: The paradox of hemoglobin SC disease. Blood Rev 17(3):167, 2003

Nance D, Josephson NC, Paulyson-Nunez K, et al: Factor X deficiency and pregnancy: preconception counselling and therapeutic options. Haemophilia 18(3):e277, 2012

Nelson DB, Yost NP, Cunningham FG: Acute fatty liver of pregnancy: clinical outcomes and expected duration of recovery. Am J Obstet Gynecol 209:1.e1, 2013

Neunert C. Lim W, Crowther M, et al: The American Society of Hematology 2011 evidence-based practice guideline for immune thrombocytopenia. Blood 117(16):4190, 2011

Nichols WL, Hultin MB, James AH, et al: von Willebrand disease (VWD): evidence-based diagnosis and management guidelines, the National Heart, Lung, and Blood Institute (NHLBI) Expert Panel report (USA). Haemophilia 14(2):171, 2008

Niittyvuopio R, Juvonen E, Kaaja R, et al: Pregnancy in essential thrombocythaemia: experience with 40 pregnancies. Eur J Haematol 73:431, 2004

Ngô C, Kayem G, Habibi A, et al: Pregnancy in sickle cell disease: maternal and fetal outcomes in a population receiving prophylactic partial exchange transfusions. Eur J Obstet Gynecol Reprod Biol 152(2):138, 2010

Nguyen JS, Marinopoulos SS, Ashar BH, et al: More than meets the eye. N Engl J Med 355:1048, 2006

Odame JE, Chan AK, Breakey VR: Factor XIII deficiency management: a review of the literature. Blood Coag Fibrinolysis Jan 7, 2014 [Epub ahead of print]

Okusayna BO, Oladapo OT: Prophylactic versus selective blood transfusion for sickle cell disease in pregnancy. Cochrane Database Syst 12:CD01378, 2013

Olnes MJ, Scheinberg P, Calvo KR, et al: Eltrombopag and improved hematopoiesis in refractory aplastic anemia. N Engl J Med 367(1):11, 2012

Orfali KA, Ohene-Abuakwa Y, Ball SE: Diamond Blackfan anaemia in the UK: clinical and genetic heterogeneity. Br J Haematol 125(2):243, 2004

Oringanje C, Nemecek E, Oniyangi O: Hematopoietic stem cell transplantation for children with sickle cell disease. Cochrane Database Syst Rev 1:CD007001, 2009

Pacheco LD, Constantine MM, Saade GR: von Willebrand disease and pregnancy: a practical approach for the diagnosis and treatment. Am J Obstet Gynecol 203(3):194, 2010

Pajor A, Lehoczky D, Szakács Z: Pregnancy and hereditary spherocytosis. Arch Gynecol Obstet 253:37, 1993

Parker C: Eculizumab for paroxysmal nocturnal haemoglobinuria. Lancet 373(9665):759, 2009

Parker C, Omine M, Richards S, et al: Diagnosis and management of paroxysmal nocturnal hemoglobinuria. Blood 106:3699, 2005

Payne SD, Resnik R, Moore TR, et al: Maternal characteristics and risk of severe neonatal thrombocytopenia and intracranial hemorrhage in pregnancies complicated by autoimmune thrombocytopenia. Am J Obstet Gynecol 177(1):149, 1997

Peitsidis P, Datta T, Pafilis I, et al: Bernard-Soulier syndrome in pregnancy: a systematic review. Haemophilia 16(4):584, 2010

Peña-Rosas JP, De-Regil LM, Dowswell T, et al: Daily oral iron supplementation during pregnancy. Cochrane Database Syst Rev 12:CD004736, 2012

Peng TC, Kickler TS, Bell WR, et al: Obstetric complications in a patient with Bernard–Soulier syndrome. Am J Obstet Gynecol 165:425, 1991

Pinto FO, Roberts I: Cord blood stem cell transplantation for haemoglobinopathies. Br J Haematol 141(3):309, 2008

Platt OS: Hydroxyurea for the treatment of sickle cell anemia. N Engl J Med 358:1362, 2008

Prabu P, Parapia LA: Bernard-Soulier syndrome in pregnancy. Clin Lab Haem 28:198, 2006

Pritchard JA, Cunningham FG, Mason RA: Coagulation changes in eclampsia: their frequency and pathogenesis. Am J Obstet Gynecol 124:855, 1976

Pritchard JA, Scott DE: Iron demands in pregnancy. In Hallberg L, Harwerth HG, Vanotti A (eds): Iron Deficiency Pathogenesis, Clinical Aspects, Therapy. New York, Academic Press, 1970

Pritchard JA, Scott DE, Whalley PJ, et al: The effects of maternal sickle cell hemoglobinopathies and sickle cell trait on reproductive performance. Am J Obstet Gynecol 117:662, 1973

Provan D, Weatherall D: Red cells II: acquired anaemias and polycythaemia. Lancet 355:1260, 2000

Puig A, Dighe AS: Case 20-2013: a 29-year-old man with anemia and jaundice. N Engl J Med 368(26):2502, 2013

Rabinerson D, Fradin Z, Zeidman A, et al: Vulvar hematoma after cunnilingus in a teenager with essential thrombocythemia: a case report. J Reprod Med 52:458, 2007

Rac MWF, Crawford NM, Worley KC: Extensive thrombosis and first-trimester pregnancy loss caused by sticky platelet syndrome. Obstet Gynecol 117(2 part 2):501, 2011

Ramahi AJ, Lewkow LM, Dombrowski MP, et al: Sickle cell E hemoglobinopathy and pregnancy. Obstet Gynecol 71:493, 1988

Ramin SM, Vidaeff AC, Yeomans ER, et al: Chronic renal disease in pregnancy. Obstet Gynecol 108:1531, 2006

Randi ML, Barbone E, Rossi C, et al: Essential thrombocythemia and pregnancy. A report of six normal pregnancies in five untreated patients. Obstet Gynecol 83:915, 1994

Ray JG, Burrows RF, Ginsberg JS, et al: Paroxysmal nocturnal hemoglobinuria and the risk of venous thrombosis: review and recommendations for management of the pregnant and nonpregnant patient. Haemostasis 30(3):103, 2000

Reece EA, Coustan DR, Hayslett JP, et al: Diabetic nephropathy: pregnancy performance and fetomaternal outcome. Am J Obstet Gynecol 159:56, 1988

Rees DC, Olujohungbe AD, Parker NE, et al: Guidelines for the management of the acute painful crisis in sickle cell disease. Br J Haematol 120:744, 2003

Ren A, Wang J, Ye RW, et al: Low first-trimester hemoglobin and low birth weight, preterm birth and small for gestational age newborns. Int J Gynaecol Obstet 98:124, 2007

Rink BD, Gonik B, Chmait RH, et al: Maternal hemolysis after intravenous immunoglobulin treatment in fetal and neonatal alloimmune thrombocytopenia. Obstet Gynecol 121(2 Pt 2 Suppl 1):471, 2013

Robinson S, Bewley S, Hunt BJ, et al: The management and outcome of 18 pregnancies in women with polycythemia vera. Haematol 90: 1477, 2005

Rogers DT, Molokie R: Sickle cell disease in pregnancy. Obstet Gynecol Clin North Am 37(2):223, 2010

Rosenfeld S, Follmann D, Nunez O, et al: Antithymocyte globulin and cyclosporine for severe aplastic anemia: association between hematologic response and long-term outcome. JAMA 289:1130, 2003

Rouse DJ, Owen J, Goldenberg RL: Routine maternal platelet count: an assessment of a technologically driven screening practice. Am J Obstet Gynecol 179:573, 1998

Sadler JE, Ponca M: Antibody-mediated thrombotic disorders: thrombotic disorders: thrombotic thrombocytopenic purpura and heparin-induced thrombocytopenia. In Kaushansky K, Lichtman MA, Beutler E, et al (eds): Williams Hematology, 8th ed. New York, McGraw-Hill, 2010, p 2163

Sánchez-Luceros A, Farias CE, Amaral MM, et al: von Willebrand factor-cleaving protease (ADAMTS13) activity in normal non-pregnant women, pregnant and post-delivery women. Thromb Haemost 92(6):1320, 2004

Sanders JE, Hawley J, Levy W, et al: Pregnancies following high-dose cyclophosphamide with or without high-dose busulfan or total body irradiation and bone marrow transplantation. Blood 87:3045, 1996

Santoro RC, Prejanò S: Postpartum-acquired haemophilia A: a description of three cases and literature review. Blood Coagul Fibrinolysis 20(6):461, 2009

Scanlon KS, Yip R, Schieve LA, et al: High and low hemoglobin levels during pregnancy: differential risk for preterm birth and small for gestational age. Obstet Gynecol 96:741, 2000

Scaradavou A: HIV-related thrombocytopenia. Blood Rev 16:73, 2002

Schwartz RS: Immune thrombocytopenic purpura—from agony to agonist. N Engl J Med 357:2299, 2007

Scott JR, Rote NS, Cruikshank DP: Antiplatelet antibodies and platelet counts in pregnancies complicated by autoimmune thrombocytopenic purpura. Am J Obstet Gynecol 145:932, 1983

Scully M, Hunt BJ, Benjamin S, et al: British Committee for Standards in Haematology. Guidelines on the diagnosis and management of thrombotic thrombocytopenic purpura and other thrombotic microangiopathies. Br J Haematol 158(3):323, 2012

Serjeant GR, Hambleton I, Thame M: Fecundity and pregnancy outcome in a cohort with sickle cell-haemoglobin C disease followed from birth. BJOG 112:1308, 2005

Serjeant GR, Loy LL, Crowther M, et al: Outcome of pregnancy in homozygous sickle cell disease. Obstet Gynecol 103:1278, 2004

Serjeant GR, Serjeant BE, Mason KP, et al: The changing face of homozygous sickle cell disease: 102 patients over 60 years. Int J Lab Hematol 31(6):585, 2009

Sharma JB, Jain S, Mallika V, et al: A prospective, partially randomized study of pregnancy outcomes and hematologic responses to oral and intramuscular iron treatment in moderately anemic pregnant women. Am J Clin Nutr 79:116, 2004

Shau WY, Hsieh CC, Hsieh TT, et al: Factors associated with endometrial bleeding in continuous hormone replacement therapy. Menopause 9:188, 2002

Sheiner E, Levy A, Yerushalmi R, et al: Beta-thalassemia minor during pregnancy. Obstet Gynecol 103:1273, 2004

Shenoy S: Umbilical cord blood: an evolving stem cell source for sickle cell disease transplants. Stem Cells Transl Med 2(5):337, 2013

Sieunarine K, Shapiro S, Al Obaidi MJ, et al: Intravenous anti-D immunoglobulin in the treatment of resistant immune thrombocytopenic purpura in pregnancy. BJOG 114(4):505, 2007

Singh A, Harnett MJ, Connors JM, et al: Factor XI deficiency and obstetrical anesthesia. Anesth Analg 108:1882, 2009

Sirichotiyakul S, Saetung R, Sanguansermsri T: Prenatal diagnosis of beta-thalassemia/Hb E by hemoglobin typing compared to DNA analysis. Hemoglobin 33(1):17, 2009

Socié G, Stone JV, Wingard JR, et al: Long-term survival and late deaths after allogeneic bone marrow transplantation. N Engl J Med 341:14, 1999

Spivak JL: Polycythemia vera and other myeloproliferative diseases. In Fauci AS, Braunwald E, Kasper DL, et al (eds): Harrison's Principles of Internal Medicine, 17th ed. New York, McGraw-Hill, 2008, p 671

Srivorakun H, Fucharoen G, Sae-Ung N, et al: Analysis of fetal blood using capillary electrophoresis system: a simple method for prenatal diagnosis of severe thalassemia diseases. Eur J Haematol 83(1):79, 2009

Stabler SP: Vitamin B_{12} deficiency. N Engl J Med 368(2):149, 2013

Stalder MP, Rovó A, Halter J, et al: Aplastic anemia and concomitant autoimmune diseases. Ann Hematol 88(7):659, 2009

Starksen NF, Bell WR, Kickler TS: Unexplained hemolytic anemia associated with pregnancy. Am J Obstet Gynecol 146:617, 1983

Stuart MJ, Nagel RL: Sickle-cell disease. Lancet 364:1343, 2004

Sun PM, Wilburn W, Raynor D, et al: Sickle cell disease in pregnancy: twenty years of experience at Grady Memorial Hospital, Atlanta, Georgia. Am J Obstet Gynecol 184:1127, 2001

Taylor DJ, Mallen C, McDougal N, et al: Effect of iron supplementation on serum ferritin levels during and after pregnancy. Br J Obstet Gynaecol 89:1011, 1982

Tefferi A, Soldberg LA, Silverstein MN: A clinical update in polycythemia vera and essential thrombocythemia. Am J Med 109:141, 2000

Tengborn L, Baudo F, Huth-Kühne A, et al: Pregnancy-associated acquired haemophilia A: results from the European Acquired Haemophilia (EACH2) registry. BJOG 119(12):1529, 2012

Thame M, Lewis J, Trotman H, et al: The mechanisms of low birth weight in infants of mothers with homozygous sickle cell disease. Pediatrics 120:e677, 2007

Tita ATN, Biggio JR, Chapman V, et al: Perinatal and maternal outcomes in women with sickle or hemoglobin C trait. Obstet Gynecol 110:1113, 2007

Tran TD, Tran T, Simpson JA, et al: Infant motor development in rural Vietnam and intrauterine exposures to anaemia, iron deficiency and common mental disorders: a prospective community-based study. BMC Pregnancy Childbirth 14:8, 2014

Trehan AK, Fergusson ILC: Congenital afibrinogenaemia and successful pregnancy outcome. Case report. Br J Obstet Gynaecol 98:722, 1991

Trigg DE, Stergiotou I, Peitsidis P, et al: A systematic review: the use of desmopressin for treatment and prophylaxis of bleeding disorders in pregnancy. Haemophilia 18(1):25, 2012

Tsaras G, Owusu-Ansah, Boateng FO, et al: Complications associated with sickle cell trait: a brief narrative review. Am J Med 122(6):507, 2009

Tuck SM, Studd JWW, White JM: Pregnancy in women with sickle cell trait. Br J Obstet Gynaecol 90:108, 1983

Turner JM, Kaplan JB, Cohen HW, et al: Exchange versus simple transfusion for acute chest syndrome in sickle cell anemia adults. Transfusion 49(5):863, 2009

Urato AC, Repke JT: May-Hegglin anomaly: a case of vaginal delivery when both mother and fetus are affected. Am J Obstet Gynecol 179:260, 1998

Vandevijvere S, Amsalkhir S, Oyen HV, et al: Iron status and its determinants in a nationally representative sample of pregnant women. J Acad Nutr Diet 113(5):659, 2013

Van Wyck DB, Martens MG, Seid MH, et al: Intravenous ferric carboxymaltose compared with oral iron in the treatment of postpartum anemia: a randomized controlled trial. Obstet Gynecol 110:267, 2007

Veille J, Hanson R: Left ventricular systolic and diastolic function in pregnant patients with sickle cell disease. Am J Obstet Gynecol 170:107, 1994

Verstraete S, Verstraete R: Successful epidural analgesia for a vaso-occlusive crisis of sickle cell disease during pregnancy: a case report. J Anesth 26(5):783, 2012

Vichinsky EP, Neumayr LD, Earles AN, et al: Causes and outcomes of the acute chest syndrome in sickle cell disease. N Engl J Med 342:1855, 2000

Villers MS, Jamison MG, De Castro LM, et al: Morbidity associated with sickle cell disease in pregnancy. Am J Obstet Gynecol 199:125.e1, 2008

Vlachos A, Ball S, Dahl N, et al: Diagnosing and treating Diamond Blackfan anaemia: results of an international clinical consensus conference. Br J Haematol 142(6):859, 2008

von Tempelhoff GF, Heilmann L, Rudig L, et al: Mean maternal second-trimester hemoglobin concentration and outcome of pregnancy: a population based study. Clin Appl Thromb/Hemost 14:19, 2008

Wax JR, Pinette MG, Cartin A, et al: Pyruvate kinase deficiency complicating pregnancy. Obstet Gynecol 109:553, 2007

Weatherall D: The thalassemias: disorders of globin chain synthesis. In Kaushansky K, Lichtman MA, Beutler E, et al (eds): Williams Hematology, 8th ed. New York, McGraw-Hill, 2010, p 675

Weatherall DJ: Single gene disorders or complex traits: lessons from the thalassemias and other monogenic diseases. BMJ 321:1117, 2000a

Weatherall DJ, Provan AB: Red cell I: inherited anaemias. Lancet 355:1169, 2000b

Webert KE, Mittal R, Sigouin C, et al: A retrospective 11-year analysis of obstetric patients with idiopathic thrombocytopenic purpura. Blood 102:4306, 2003

Weiss G, Goodnough LT: Anemia of chronic disease. N Engl J Med 352:1011, 2005

Wiegman MF, DeGroot JC, Jansonius NM, et al: Long-term visual functioning after eclampsia. Obstet Gynecol 119(5):959, 2012

Winder AD, Johnson S, Murphy J, et al: Epidural analgesia for treatment of a sickle cell crisis during pregnancy. Obstet Gynecol 118(2 Pt 2):495, 2011

Wright DE, Rosovsky RP, Platt MY: Case 36-2013: a 38-year-old woman with anemia and thrombocytopenia. N Engl J Med 369:21, 2013

World Health Organization (Geneva): Guideline: Daily iron and folic acid supplementation in pregnant women. 2012. Available at: http://www.who.int/nutrition/publications/micronutrients/guidelines/daily_ifa_supp_pregnant_women/en/. Accessed September 19, 2013

Yamamoto T, Fujimura Y, Emoto Y, et al: Autopsy case of sudden maternal death from thrombotic thrombocytopenic purpura. J Obstet Gynaecol Res 39(1):351, 2013

Yawata Y, Kanzaki A, Yawata A, et al: Characteristic features of the genotype and phenotype of hereditary spherocytosis in the Japanese population. Int J Hematol 71:118, 2000

Ye L, Chang JC, Lin C, et al: Induced pluripotent stem cells offer new approach to therapy in thalassemia and sickle cell anemia and option in prenatal diagnosis in genetic diseases. Proc Natl Acad Sci U S A 16(24):9826, 2009

Yeomans E, Lowe TW, Eigenbrodt EH, et al: Liver histopathologic findings in women with sickle cell disease given prophylactic transfusion during pregnancy. Am J Obstet Gynecol 163:958, 1990

Yi JS, Moertel CL, Baker KS: Homozygous alpha-thalassemia treated with intrauterine transfusions and unrelated donor hematopoietic cell transplantation. J Pediatr 154:766, 2009

Young NS: Aplastic anemia. In Fauci AS, Braunwald E, Kasper DL, et al (eds): Harrison's Principles of Internal Medicine, 17th ed. New York, McGraw-Hill, 2008, p 663

Yu CKH, Stasiowska E, Stephens A, et al: Outcome of pregnancy in sickle cell disease patients attending a combined obstetric and haematology clinic. J Obstet Gynaecol 29(6):512, 2009

Ziaei S, Norrozi M, Faghihzadeh S, et al: A randomized placebo-controlled trial to determine the effect of iron supplementation on pregnancy outcome in pregnant women with haemoglobin ≥ 13.2 g/dl. BJOG 114:684, 2007

CHAPTER 57

Diabetes Mellitus

According to the National Center for Health Statistics (2013), the number of adults diagnosed with diabetes in the United States has tripled from 6.9 million in 1991 to 20.9 million in 2011. Astoundingly, the Centers for Disease Control and Prevention (2010) have estimated that the number of Americans with diabetes will range from 1 in 3 to 1 in 5 by 2050. Reasons for this rise include an aging population more likely to develop type 2 diabetes, increases in minority groups at particular risk for type 2 diabetes, and dramatic increases in obesity—also referred to as diabesity. This term reflects the strong relationship of diabetes with the current obesity epidemic in the United States and underlines the critical need for diet and lifestyle interventions to change the trajectory of both.

There is keen interest in events that precede diabetes, and this includes the uterine environment, where early imprinting is believed to have effects later in life (Saudek, 2002). For example, in utero exposure to maternal hyperglycemia leads to fetal hyperinsulinemia, causing an increase in fetal fat cells. This leads to obesity and insulin resistance in childhood (Feig, 2002). This in turn leads to impaired glucose tolerance and diabetes in adulthood. This cycle of fetal exposure to diabetes leading to childhood obesity and glucose intolerance has been reported in Pima Indians and a heterogeneous Chicago population (Silverman, 1995).

TYPES OF DIABETES

In nonpregnant individuals, the type of diabetes is based on its presumed etiopathogenesis and its pathophysiological manifestations. Absolute insulin deficiency characterizes *type 1 diabetes*. In contrast, defective insulin secretion, insulin resistance, or increased glucose production characterizes *type 2 diabetes* (Table 57-1). Both types are generally preceded by a period of abnormal glucose homeostasis. The terms insulin-dependent diabetes mellitus (IDDM) and noninsulin-dependent diabetes mellitus (NIDDM) are now obsolete. Pancreatic β-cell destruction can begin at any age, but type 1 diabetes is clinically apparent most often before age 30. Type 2 diabetes usually develops with advancing age but is increasingly identified in younger obese adolescents.

Classification During Pregnancy

Diabetes is the most common medical complication of pregnancy. Women can be separated into those who were known to have diabetes before pregnancy—*pregestational* or *overt*, and those diagnosed during pregnancy—*gestational diabetes*. The incidence of diabetes complicating pregnancy increased approximately 40 percent between 1989 and 2004 (Getahun, 2008). In 2006, slightly more than 179,000—4.2 percent—of American women had pregnancies coexistent with some form of diabetes (Martin, 2009). African American, Native

TABLE 57-1. Etiological Classification of Diabetes Mellitus

Type 1: β-Cell destruction, usually absolute insulin deficiency
- Immune-mediated
- Idiopathic

Type 2: Ranges from predominantly insulin resistance to predominantly an insulin secretory defect with insulin resistance

Other types
- Genetic mutations of β-cell function—MODY 1–6, others
- Genetic defects in insulin action
- Genetic syndromes—Down, Klinefelter, Turner
- Diseases of the exocrine pancreas—pancreatitis, cystic fibrosis
- Endocrinopathies—Cushing syndrome, pheochromocytoma, others
- Drug or chemical induced—glucocorticosteroids, thiazides, β-adrenergic agonists, others
- Infections—congenital rubella, cytomegalovirus, coxsackievirus

Gestational diabetes

MODY = maturity-onset diabetes of the young.
Modified from Powers, 2012.

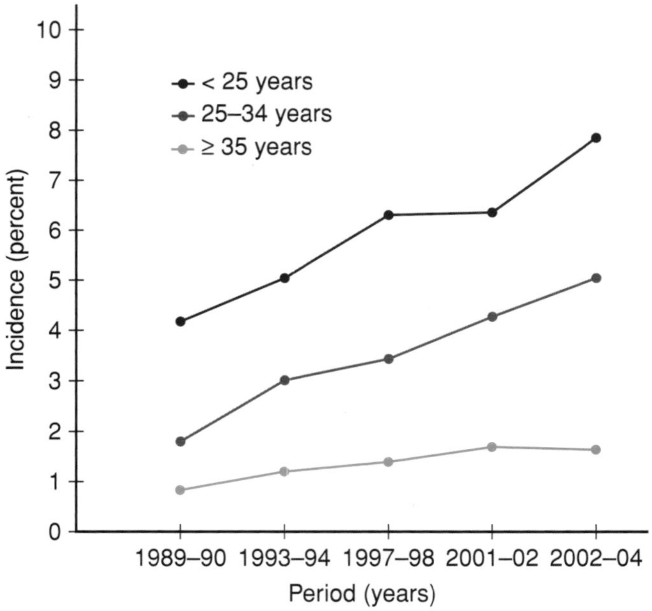

FIGURE 57-1 Age-specific incidence of gestational diabetes from National Hospital Discharge Survey Data of nearly 59 million births in the United States from 1989 to 2004. (Redrawn from Getahun, 2008.)

American, Asian, and Hispanic women are at higher risk for gestational diabetes compared with white women (Ferrara, 2007). The increasing incidence of gestational diabetes during the past 15 years, shown in Figure 57-1, is reminiscent of similar statistics for obesity (Chap. 48, p. 961).

White Classification in Pregnancy

Until the mid-1990s, the classification by Priscilla White for diabetic pregnant women was the linchpin of management. Today, the White classification is used less frequently, but its role remains important. And because most currently cited literature contains data from these older classifications, the one previously recommended by the American College of Obstetricians and Gynecologists (1986) is provided in Table 57-2.

Beginning several years ago, the American College of Obstetricians and Gynecologists (2012, 2013) no longer recommended the White classification. Instead, the current focus is whether diabetes antedates pregnancy or is first diagnosed during pregnancy. Many now recommend adoption of the classification proposed by the American Diabetes Association (ADA), as shown in Table 57-3.

TABLE 57-2. Classification Scheme Used from 1986 through 1994 for Diabetes Complicating Pregnancy

		Plasma Glucose Level		
Class	Onset	Fasting	2-Hour Postprandial	Therapy
A_1	Gestational	< 105 mg/dL	< 120 mg/dL	Diet
A_2	Gestational	> 105 mg/dL	> 120 mg/dL	Insulin
Class	**Age of Onset (yr)**	**Duration (yr)**	**Vascular Disease**	**Therapy**
B	Over 20	< 10	None	Insulin
C	10 to 19	10 to 19	None	Insulin
D	Before 10	> 20	Benign retinopathy	Insulin
F	Any	Any	Nephropathy[a]	Insulin
R	Any	Any	Proliferative retinopathy	Insulin
H	Any	Any	Heart	Insulin

[a]When diagnosed during pregnancy: proteinuria ≥ 500 mg/24 hr before 20 weeks' gestation.

TABLE 57-3. Proposed Classification System for Diabetes in Pregnancy

Gestational diabetes: diabetes diagnosed during pregnancy that is not clearly overt (type 1 or type 2) diabetes

Type 1 Diabetes:	**Type 2 Diabetes:**
Diabetes resulting from β-cell destruction, usually leading to absolute insulin deficiency	Diabetes from inadequate insulin secretion in the face of increased insulin resistance
a. Without vascular complications	a. Without vascular complications
b. With vascular complications (specify which)	b. With vascular complications (specify which)

Other types of diabetes: genetic in origin, associated with pancreatic disease, drug-induced, or chemically induced

Data from American Diabetes Association, 2012.

PREGESTATIONAL DIABETES

The increasing prevalence of type 2 diabetes in general, and in younger people in particular, has led to an increasing number of affected pregnancies (Ferrara, 2007). In Los Angeles County, Baraban and coworkers (2008) reported that the age-adjusted prevalence tripled from 14.5 cases per 1000 women in 1991 to 47.9 cases per 1000 in 2003. Thus, the number of pregnant women with diabetes that was undiagnosed before pregnancy is increasing. Many women found to have gestational diabetes are likely to have type 2 diabetes that has previously gone undiagnosed (Feig, 2002). In fact, 5 to 10 percent of women with gestational diabetes are found to have diabetes immediately after pregnancy.

Diagnosis

Women with high plasma glucose levels, glucosuria, and ketoacidosis present no problem in diagnosis. Similarly, women with a random plasma glucose level > 200 mg/dL plus classic signs and symptoms such as polydipsia, polyuria, and unexplained weight loss or those with a fasting glucose level exceeding 125 mg/dL are considered by the ADA (2012) to have overt diabetes. Women with only minimal metabolic derangement may be more difficult to identify. To diagnose overt diabetes in pregnancy, The International Association of Diabetes and Pregnancy Study Groups (IADPSG) Consensus Panel (2010) recommends threshold values for fasting or random plasma glucose and glycosylated hemoglobin (A_{1c}) levels at prenatal care initiation (Table 57-4). There was no consensus on whether such testing should be universal or limited to those women classified as high risk. Regardless, the tentative diagnosis of overt diabetes during pregnancy based on these thresholds should be confirmed postpartum. Risk factors for impaired carbohydrate metabolism in pregnant women include a strong familial history of diabetes, prior delivery of a large newborn, persistent glucosuria, or unexplained fetal losses.

Impact on Pregnancy

With pregestational—or overt—diabetes, the embryo, fetus, and mother frequently experience serious complications directly attributable to diabetes. The likelihood of successful outcomes with overt diabetes is related somewhat to the degree of glycemic control, but more importantly, to the degree of underlying cardiovascular or renal disease. Thus, advancing stages of the White classification, seen in Table 57-2, are inversely related to favorable pregnancy outcomes. As an example shown in Table 57-5, data from Yang and associates (2006) chronicles the deleterious pregnancy outcomes of overt

TABLE 57-4. Diagnosis of Overt Diabetes in Pregnancy[a]

Measure of Glycemia	Threshold
Fasting plasma glucose	At least 7.0 mmol/L (126 mg/dL)
Hemoglobin A_{1c}	At least 6.5%
Random plasma glucose	At least 11.1 mmol/L (200 mg/dL) plus confirmation

[a]Apply to women without known diabetes antedating pregnancy. The decision to perform blood testing for evaluation of glycemia on all pregnant women or only on women with characteristics indicating a high risk for diabetes is based on the background frequency of abnormal glucose metabolism in the population and on local circumstances.

Modified from International Association of Diabetes and Pregnancy Study Groups Consensus Panel, 2010.

TABLE 57-5. Pregnancy Outcomes of Births in Nova Scotia from 1988 to 2002 in Women with and without Pregestational Diabetes

Factor	Diabetic (n = 516) %	Nondiabetic (n = 150,598) %	*p* value
Gestational hypertension	28	9	< .001
Preterm birth	28	5	< .001
Macrosomia	45	13	< .001
Fetal-growth restriction	5	10	< .001
Stillbirth	1.0	0.4	.06
Perinatal death	1.7	0.6	.004

Adapted from Yang, 2006.

diabetes. These maternal and fetal complications are described in the following sections.

Fetal Effects

Spontaneous Abortion. Several studies have shown that early miscarriage is associated with poor glycemic control. In 215 women with type 1 diabetes enrolled for prenatal care before 9 weeks' gestation, 24 percent had an early pregnancy loss (Rosenn, 1994). Only those whose initial glycohemoglobin A_{1c} concentrations were > 12 percent or whose preprandial glucose concentrations were persistently > 120 mg/dL were at increased risk. In another analysis of 127 Spanish women with pregestational diabetes, poor glycemic control, defined by glycohemoglobin A_{1c} concentrations > 7 percent, was associated with a threefold increase in the spontaneous abortion rate (Galindo, 2006).

Preterm Delivery. Overt diabetes is an undisputed risk factor for preterm birth. Eidem and associates (2011) analyzed 1307 births in women with pregestational type 1 diabetes from the Norwegian Medical Birth Registry. More than 26 percent were delivered preterm compared with 6.8 percent in the general obstetrical population. Moreover, almost 60 percent were indicated preterm births, that is, due to obstetrical or medical complications. In the Canadian study shown in Table 57-5, the incidence of preterm birth was 28 percent—a fivefold increase compared with that of their normal population.

Malformations. The incidence of major malformations in women with type 1 diabetes is doubled and approximates 5 percent (Eidem, 2010; Sheffield, 2002). These account for almost half of perinatal deaths in diabetic pregnancies. A twofold increased risk of major congenital defects in Norwegian women with pregestational type 1 diabetes included cardiovascular malformations that accounted for more than half of the anomalies (Table 57-6). In the National Birth Defects Prevention Study, the risk of an isolated cardiac defect was fourfold higher in women with pregestational diabetes compared with the twofold increased risk of noncardiac defects (Correa, 2008). The caudal regression

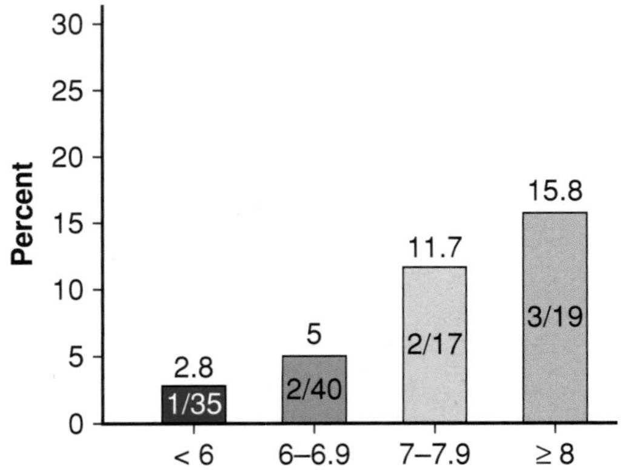

FIGURE 57-2 The frequency of major congenital malformations in newborns of women with pregestational diabetes stratified by hemoglobin A_{1c} levels at first prenatal visit. (Data from Galindo, 2006.)

sequence is a rare malformation frequently associated with maternal diabetes (Garne, 2012).

Poorly controlled diabetes, both preconceptionally and early in pregnancy, is thought to underlie this increased severe-malformation risk. As shown in Figure 57-2, Galindo and colleagues (2006) demonstrated a clear correlation between increased maternal glycohemoglobin A_{1c} at first prenatal visit and major malformations. Eriksson (2009) concluded that the etiology was multifactorial. At least three interrelated molecular chain reactions have been linked to maternal hyperglycemia

TABLE 57-6. Congenital Anomalies in Fetuses of 91 Women with Type 1 Diabetes between 1999 and 2004 in Norway

Organ System	Babies Affected n (%)
Cardiovascular	47 (52)
Musculoskeletal	11 (12)
Urogenital	8 (9)
CNS	4 (4)
Gastrointestinal	2 (2)
Chromosomal	3 (3)
Others	9 (10)
Multiorgan	7 (8)

CNS = central nervous system.
Data from Eidem, 2010.

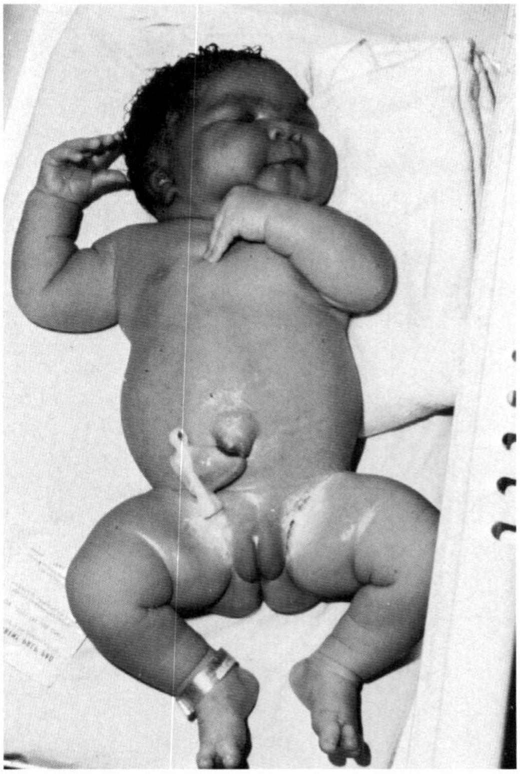

FIGURE 57-3 This 6050-g macrosomic infant was born to a woman with diabetes.

and can potentially explain the mechanism behind poor glycemic control and increased risk for major malformations (Reece, 2012). These include alterations in cellular lipid metabolism, excess production of toxic superoxide radicals, and activation of programmed cell death. For example, Morgan and associates (2008) demonstrated that hyperglycemia-induced oxidative stress inhibited migration of cardiac neural-crest cells in embryos of diabetic mice.

Altered Fetal Growth. Diminished growth may result from congenital malformations or from substrate deprivation due to advanced maternal vascular disease. However, fetal overgrowth is more typical of pregestational diabetes. Maternal hyperglycemia prompts fetal hyperinsulinemia, particularly during the second half of gestation. This in turn stimulates excessive somatic growth or macrosomia. Except for the brain, most fetal organs are affected by the macrosomia that characterizes the fetus of a diabetic woman. Such infants are described as being anthropometrically different from other large-for-gestational age (LGA) infants (Durnwald, 2004; McFarland, 2000). Specifically, those whose mothers are diabetic have excessive fat deposition on the shoulders and trunk, which predisposes to shoulder dystocia or cesarean delivery (Fig. 57-3).

The incidence of macrosomia rises significantly when mean maternal blood glucose concentrations chronically exceed 130 mg/dL (Hay, 2012). Hammoud and coworkers (2013) reported that the macrosomia rates for Nordic women with type 1, type 2, or gestational diabetes were 35 percent, 28 percent, and 24 percent, respectively. As shown in Figure 57-4, the birthweight distribution of neonates of diabetic mothers is skewed toward consistently heavier birthweights compared with that of normal pregnancies.

In the study by Hammoud and colleagues (2013), fetal growth profiles from 897 sonographic examinations in 244 women with diabetes were compared with 843 examinations in 145 control women. The abdominal circumference evolved differently in the diabetic groups. Analysis of head circumference/abdominal circumference (HC/AC) ratios shows that this disproportionate growth occurs mainly in diabetic pregnancies that ultimately yield macrosomic newborns (Fig. 57-5). These findings comport with the observation that virtually all neonates of diabetic mothers are growth promoted. Ben-Haroush and associates (2007) analyzed fetal sonographic measurements between 29 and 34 weeks' gestation in 423 diabetic pregnancies and found that accelerated fetal growth was particularly evident in women with poor glycemic control.

Unexplained Fetal Demise. The risk of fetal death is three to four times higher in women with type 1 diabetes compared with that of the general obstetrical population (Eidem, 2011). Stillbirth without an identifiable cause is a phenomenon relatively limited to pregnancies complicated by overt diabetes. These stillbirths are "unexplained" because common factors such as obvious placental insufficiency, abruption, fetal-growth restriction, or oligohydramnios are not identified. These infants are typically LGA and die before labor, usually after 35 weeks' gestation or later (Garner, 1995).

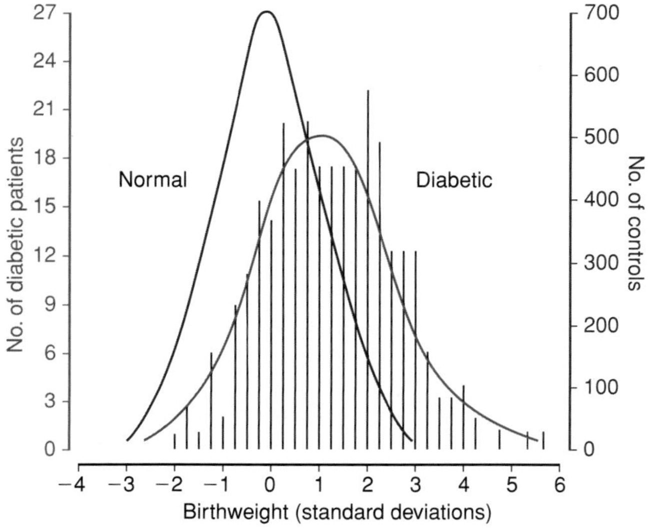

FIGURE 57-4 Distribution of birthweight standard deviation from the normal mean for gestational age in 280 infants of diabetic mothers and in 3959 infants of nondiabetic mothers. (From Bradley, 1988, with permission.)

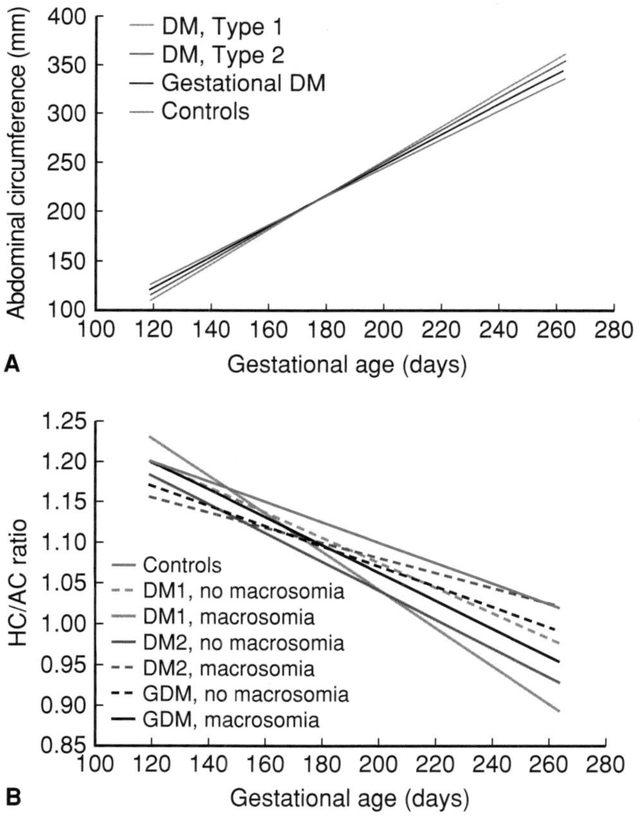

FIGURE 57-5 Comparison of sonographic fetal anatomic measurements by gestational age and subdivided according to presence or absence of macrosomia among women with various types of diabetes types and controls. **A.** Abdominal circumference measurements. **B.** Head circumference (HC)/Abdominal circumference (AC) ratio. DM = diabetes mellitus; GDM = gestational diabetes mellitus. (Redrawn from Hammoud, 2013, with permission.)

These unexplained stillbirths are associated with poor glycemic control. Lauenborg and coworkers (2003) identified suboptimal glycemic control in two thirds of unexplained stillbirths between 1990 and 2000. Also, fetuses of diabetic mothers often have elevated lactic acid levels. Salvesen and colleagues (1992, 1993) analyzed fetal blood samples and reported that mean umbilical venous blood pH was lower in diabetic pregnancies and was significantly related to fetal insulin levels. Such findings support the hypothesis that hyperglycemia-mediated chronic aberrations in oxygen and fetal metabolite transport may underlie these unexplained fetal deaths (Pedersen, 1977). However, the exact mechanisms by which uncontrolled hyperglycemia leads to elevated lactic acid levels and fetal acidosis remain unclear.

Explicable stillbirths due to placental insufficiency also occur with increased frequency in women with overt diabetes, usually in association with severe preeclampsia. In a retrospective analysis of more than 500,000 singleton deliveries, Yanit and associates (2012) found that the fetal death risk was sevenfold higher in women with hypertension and pregestational diabetes compared with the threefold increased risk associated with diabetes alone. Stillbirth is also increased in women with advanced diabetes and vascular complications. Maternal ketoacidosis can also cause fetal death.

Hydramnios. Diabetic pregnancies are often complicated by excess amnionic fluid. According to Idris and coworkers (2010), 18 percent of 314 women with pregestational diabetes were identified with hydramnios, defined as an amnionic fluid index (AFI) greater than 24 cm in the third trimester. A likely—albeit unproven—explanation is that fetal hyperglycemia causes polyuria (Chap. 11, p. 234). In a study from Parkland Hospital, Dashe and colleagues (2000) found that the AFI parallels the amnionic fluid glucose level among women with diabetes. This finding suggests that the hydramnios associated with diabetes is a result of increased amnionic fluid glucose concentration. Further support for this hypothesis was provided by Vink and associates (2006), who linked poor maternal glucose control to macrosomia and hydramnios. In their retrospective analysis of diabetic pregnancies, Idris and coworkers (2010) also found that women with elevated glycohemoglobin A_{1c} values in the third trimester were more likely to have hydramnios.

Neonatal Effects. Before tests of fetal health and maturity became available, delivery before term was deliberately selected for women with diabetes to avoid unexplained fetal death. Although this practice has been abandoned, there is still an increased frequency of preterm delivery in women with diabetes. Most are due to advanced diabetes with superimposed preeclampsia. Thankfully, modern neonatal care has largely eliminated neonatal deaths due to immaturity. Conversely, neonatal *morbidity* due to preterm birth continues to be a serious consequence.

Respiratory Distress Syndrome. Historically, newborns of diabetic mothers were thought to be at increased risk for respiratory distress from delayed lung maturation. Subsequent observations challenged this concept, and gestational age rather than overt diabetes is likely the most significant factor associated with respiratory distress syndrome. Indeed, in their analysis of 19,399 very-low-birthweight neonates delivered between 24 and 33 weeks' gestation, Bental and colleagues (2011) were unable to demonstrate an increased rate of respiratory distress syndrome in newborns of diabetic mothers. This is discussed further in Chapter 33 (p. 637).

Hypoglycemia. Newborns of a diabetic mother experience a rapid drop in plasma glucose concentration after delivery. This is attributed to hyperplasia of the fetal β-islet cells induced by chronic maternal hyperglycemia. Low glucose concentrations—defined as < 45 mg/dL—are particularly common in newborns of women with unstable glucose concentrations during labor (Persson, 2009). In a recent analysis of prenatal outcomes during a 20-year period in Finnish women with type 1 diabetes, the incidence of neonatal hypoglycemia declined significantly over time (Klemetti, 2012). The authors attributed this to frequent blood glucose measurements and active early feeding practices in such neonates. Prompt recognition and treatment of the hypoglycemic newborn minimizes adverse sequelae.

Hypocalcemia. Defined as a total serum calcium concentration < 8 mg/dL in term newborns, hypocalcemia is one of the potential metabolic derangements in neonates of diabetic mothers. Its cause has not been explained. Theories include aberrations in magnesium–calcium economy, asphyxia, and preterm birth. In a randomized study by DeMarini and associates (1994), 137 pregnant women with type 1 diabetes were managed with strict versus customary glucose control. Almost a third of neonates in the customary control group developed hypocalcemia compared with only 18 percent of those in the strict control group.

Hyperbilirubinemia and Polycythemia. The pathogenesis of hyperbilirubinemia in neonates of diabetic mothers is uncertain. A major contributing factor is newborn polycythemia, which increases the bilirubin load (Chap. 33, p. 643). Polycythemia is thought to be a fetal response to relative hypoxia. According to Hay (2012), the sources of this fetal hypoxia are hyperglycemia-mediated increases in maternal affinity for oxygen and fetal oxygen consumption. Together with insulin-like growth factors, this hypoxia leads to increased fetal erythropoietin levels and red cell production. Venous hematocrits of 65 to 70 volume percent have been observed in up to 40 percent of these newborns (Salvesen, 1992). Renal vein thrombosis is reported to result from polycythemia.

Cardiomyopathy. Infants of diabetic pregnancies may have hypertrophic cardiomyopathy that primarily affects the interventricular septum (Rolo, 2011). In severe cases, this cardiomyopathy may lead to obstructive cardiac failure. Russell and coworkers (2008) performed serial echocardiograms on fetuses of 26 women with pregestational diabetes. In the first trimester, fetal diastolic dysfunction was evident compared with that of nondiabetic controls. In the third trimester, the fetal interventricular septum and right ventricular wall were thicker in fetuses of diabetic mothers. The authors concluded that cardiac dysfunction precedes these structural changes. Fortunately, most affected newborns are asymptomatic following birth, and hypertrophy resolves in the months after delivery. Relief from maternal hyperglycemia is presumed to promote this resolution (Hornberger, 2006). Conversely, fetal cardiomyopathy may progress to adult cardiac disease.

Long-Term Cognitive Development. Intrauterine metabolic conditions have long been linked to neurodevelopment in offspring. This may also be true in children of diabetic mothers. Despite rigorous antepartum management, Rizzo and colleagues (1995) found numerous correlations between maternal glycemia and intellectual performance in children up to age 11 years in 139 offspring of diabetic women. In a study of more than 700,000 Swedish-born men, the intelligence quotient of those whose mothers had diabetes during pregnancy averaged 1 to 2 points lower (Fraser, 2014). DeBoer and associates (2005) demonstrated impaired memory performance in infants of diabetic mothers at age 1 year. Finally, results from the Childhood Autism Risks from Genetics and the Environment (CHARGE) study indicated that autism spectrum disorders or developmental delay were more common in children of diabetic women (Krakowiak, 2012). Although interpreting effects of the intrauterine environment on neurodevelopment is certainly confounded by postnatal events, emerging data at least support a link between maternal diabetes, glycemic control, and neurocognitive outcome.

Inheritance of Diabetes. The risk of developing type 1 diabetes if either parent is affected is 3 to 4 percent. Type 2 diabetes has a much stronger genetic component. If both parents have type 2 diabetes, the risk of developing it approaches 40 percent. McKinney and coworkers (1999) studied 196 children with type 1 diabetes and found that older maternal age and maternal type 1 diabetes are important risk factors. Plagemann and colleagues (2002) have implicated breast feeding by diabetic mothers in the genesis of childhood diabetes. Conversely, breast feeding has also been associated with a reduced risk of type 2 diabetes (Owen, 2006). The Trial to Reduce Insulin-dependent Diabetes Mellitus in the Genetically At Risk (TRIGR) was designed to analyze hydrolyzed formula use, rather than breast milk, to reduce rates of type 1 diabetes in at-risk children by age 10. This study will be complete in 2017 (Knip, 2011).

Maternal Effects

Diabetes and pregnancy interact significantly such that maternal welfare can be seriously jeopardized. With the possible exception of diabetic retinopathy, however, the long-term course of diabetes is not affected by pregnancy.

Maternal death is uncommon, but rates in women with diabetes are still increased. In an analysis of 972 women with type 1 diabetes, Leinonen and associates (2001) reported a maternal mortality rate of 0.5 percent. Deaths resulted from diabetic ketoacidosis, hypoglycemia, hypertension, and infection. Especially morbid is ischemic heart disease. Pombar and coworkers (1995) reviewed 17 women with coronary artery disease—class H diabetes—and reported that only half survived pregnancy.

Preeclampsia. Hypertension that is induced or exacerbated by pregnancy is the complication that most often forces preterm delivery in diabetic women. The incidence of chronic and gestational hypertension—and especially preeclampsia—is remarkably increased in diabetic mothers. In the study cited earlier by Yanit and colleagues (2012), preeclampsia developed three to four times more often in women with overt diabetes. Moreover, those diabetics with coexistent chronic hypertension were almost 12 times more likely to develop preeclampsia. Special risk factors for preeclampsia include any vascular complication and preexisting proteinuria, with or without chronic hypertension. As shown in Figure 57-6, women with type 1 diabetes who are in more advanced White classes of overt diabetes increasingly developed preeclampsia. This increasing risk with duration of diabetes may be related to oxidative stress, which plays a key role in the pathogenesis of diabetic complications and preeclampsia. With this in mind, the Diabetes and Preeclampsia Intervention Trial (DAPIT) randomly assigned 762 women with type 1 diabetes to antioxidant vitamin C and E supplementation or placebo in the first half of pregnancy (McCance, 2010). There were no differences in preeclampsia rates except in a few women with a low antioxidant status at baseline. Temple and coworkers (2006) prospectively studied hemoglobin A_{1c} levels at 24 weeks' gestation in 290 women with type 1 diabetes and found that preeclampsia was related to glucose control. Management of preeclampsia is discussed in Chapter 40 (p. 749).

Diabetic Nephropathy. Diabetes is the leading cause of end-stage renal disease in the United States (Chap. 53, p. 1060). Clinically detectable nephropathy begins with microalbuminuria—30 to 300 mg/24 hours. This may manifest as early as 5 years after diabetes onset. Macroalbuminuria—more than 300 mg/24 hours—develops in patients destined to have end-stage renal disease. Hypertension almost invariably develops during this period, and renal failure ensues typically in the next 5 to 10 years. The incidence of overt proteinuria is nearly 30 percent in individuals with type 1 diabetes and ranges

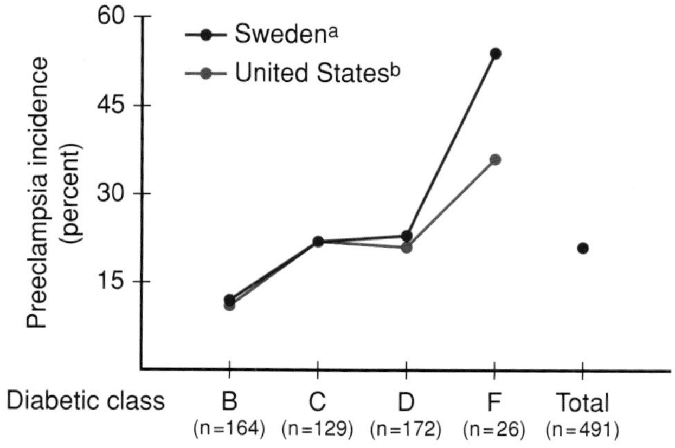

FIGURE 57-6 Incidence of preeclampsia in 491 type 1 diabetic women in Sweden and the United States. (Data from Hanson[a], 1993; Sibai[b], 2000.)

from 4 to 20 percent in those with type 2 diabetes (Reutens, 2013). Progression from microalbuminuria is not inexorable, and regression is common. Presumably from improved glucose control, the incidence of nephropathy in individuals with type 1 diabetes has declined in the past few decades. Investigators for the Diabetes Control and Complications Trial (2002) reported that there was a 25-percent decrease in the rate of nephropathy for each 10-percent decrease in hemoglobin A_{1c} levels.

Approximately 5 percent of pregnant women with diabetes already have renal involvement. Approximately 40 percent of these will develop preeclampsia (Vidaeff, 2008). High rates are also illustrated in Figure 57-6. However, this may not be the case with microproteinuria. In one analysis of 460 women, How and colleagues (2004) found no association between preeclampsia and microproteinuria. Nevertheless, they found that chronic hypertension with overt diabetic nephropathy increased the risk of preeclampsia to 60 percent.

In general, pregnancy does not appear to worsen diabetic nephropathy. In their prospective study of 43 women with diabetes, Young and associates (2012) could not demonstrate diabetic nephropathy progression through 12 months after delivery. Most of these women had only mild renal impairment. Conversely, pregnancy in women with moderate to severe renal impairment may accelerate progression of their disease (Vidaeff, 2008). As in women with glomerulopathies, hypertension or substantial proteinuria before or during pregnancy is a major predictive factor for progression to renal failure in women with diabetic nephropathy (Chap. 53, p. 1062).

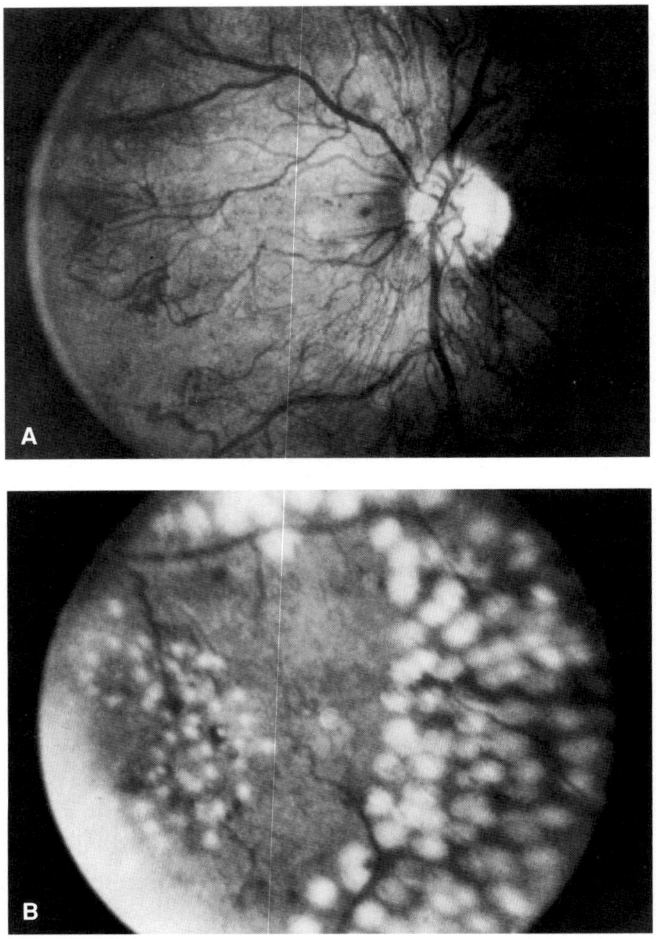

FIGURE 57-7 Retinal photographs from a 30-year-old diabetic woman. **A.** Optic nerve head showing severe proliferative retinopathy characterized by extensive networks of new vessels surrounding the optic disc. **B.** A portion of the acute photocoagulation full "scatter" pattern following argon laser treatment. (From Elman, 1990, with permission.)

Diabetic Retinopathy. Retinal vasculopathy is a highly specific complication of both type 1 and type 2 diabetes. In the United States, diabetic retinopathy is the most important cause of visual impairment in persons younger than age 60 years (Frank, 2004). The first and most common visible lesions are small microaneurysms followed by blot hemorrhages that form when erythrocytes escape from the aneurysms. These areas leak serous fluid that creates hard exudates. Such features are termed *benign* or *background* or *nonproliferative retinopathy*. With increasingly severe retinopathy, the abnormal vessels of background eye disease become occluded, leading to retinal ischemia and infarctions that appear as *cotton wool exudates.* These are considered *preproliferative retinopathy.* In response to ischemia, there is neovascularization on the retinal surface and out into the vitreous cavity. Vision is obscured when there is hemorrhage. Laser photocoagulation before hemorrhage, as shown in Figure 57-7, reduces the rate of visual loss progression and blindness by half. The procedure is performed during pregnancy when indicated.

Vestgaard and coworkers (2010) reported that almost two thirds of 102 pregnant women with type 1 diabetes examined by 8 weeks' gestation had background retinal changes, proliferative retinopathy, or macular edema. A fourth of these women developed progression of retinopathy in at least one eye. The same group of investigators evaluated 80 type 2 diabetics and identified retinopathy, mostly mild, in 14 percent during early pregnancy. Progression was identified in only 14 percent (Rasmussen, 2010). This complication is believed to be a rare example of a long-term adverse effect of pregnancy. However, in a prospective postpartum 5-year surveillance of 59 type 1 diabetic women, Arun and Taylor (2008) found that baseline retinopathy was the only independent risk factor for progression.

Other risk factors that have been associated with progression of retinopathy include hypertension, higher levels of insulin-like growth factor-I, and macular edema identified in early pregnancy (Bargiota, 2011; Mathiesen, 2012; Ringholm, 2011; Vestgaard, 2010). The National Institute for Health and Clinical Excellence (2008) established guidelines recommending that pregnant women with preexisting diabetes should routinely be offered retinal assessment after the first prenatal visit. Currently, most agree that laser photocoagulation and good glycemic control during pregnancy minimize the potential for deleterious effects of pregnancy.

Ironically, "acute" rigorous metabolic control during pregnancy has been linked to acute worsening of retinopathy. In a study of 201 women with retinopathy, McElvy and associates (2001) found that almost 30 percent suffered eye disease progression during pregnancy despite intensive glucose control. That said, Wang and coworkers (1993) have observed that retinopathy worsened during the critical months of rigorous glucose control, but long term, deterioration of eye disease slowed. In their study mentioned above, Arun and Taylor (2008) found that only four women required laser photocoagulation during pregnancy, and none required laser in the next 5 years.

Diabetic Neuropathy. Peripheral symmetrical sensorimotor diabetic neuropathy is uncommon in pregnant women. But a form of this, known as *diabetic gastropathy*, is troublesome during pregnancy. It causes nausea and vomiting, nutritional problems, and difficulty with glucose control. Women with gastroparesis should be advised that this complication is associated with a high risk of morbidity and poor perinatal outcome (Kitzmiller, 2008). Treatment with metoclopramide and H_2-receptor antagonists is sometimes successful. *Hyperemesis gravidarum* is further discussed in Chapter 54 (p. 1070).

Diabetic Ketoacidosis. This serious complication develops in approximately 1 percent of diabetic pregnancies (Hawthorne, 2011). It is most often encountered in women with type 1 diabetes. It is increasingly being reported in women with type 2 or even those with gestational diabetes (Sibai, 2014). Diabetic ketoacidosis (DKA) may develop with hyperemesis gravidarum, β-mimetic drugs given for tocolysis, infection, and corticosteroids given to induce fetal lung maturation. DKA results from an insulin deficiency combined with an excess in counter-regulatory hormones such as glucagon. This leads to gluconeogenesis and ketone body formation. The ketone body β-hydroxybutyrate is synthesized at a much greater rate than acetoacetate, which is preferentially detected by commonly used ketosis detection methodologies. Therefore, serum or plasma assays for β-hydroxybutyrate more accurately reflect true ketone body levels.

The incidence of fetal loss can be as high as 20 percent with DKA. Noncompliance is a prominent factor, and this and ketoacidosis were historically considered prognostically bad signs in pregnancy (Pedersen, 1974). Pregnant women usually develop ketoacidosis at lower blood glucose thresholds than when nonpregnant. In a study from China, the mean glucose level for pregnant women with DKA was 293 mg/dL compared with 495 mg/dL for nonpregnant women (Guo, 2008). Chico and associates (2008) reported ketoacidosis in a pregnant woman whose plasma glucose was only 87 mg/dL.

One management protocol for diabetic ketoacidosis is shown in Table 57-7. An important cornerstone of management is vigorous rehydration with crystalloid solutions of normal saline or Ringer lactate.

Infections. Almost all types of infections are increased in diabetic pregnancies. Stamler and coworkers (1990) reported that almost 80 percent of women with type 1 diabetes develop at least one infection during pregnancy compared with only 25 percent in those without diabetes. Common infections include *Candida* vulvovaginitis, urinary and respiratory tract

TABLE 57-7. Protocol Recommended by the American College of Obstetricians and Gynecologists (2012) for Management of Diabetic Ketoacidosis During Pregnancy

Laboratory assessment
Obtain arterial blood gases to document degree of acidosis present; measure glucose, ketones, and electrolyte levels at 1- to 2-hour intervals
Insulin
Low-dose, intravenous
Loading dose: 0.2–0.4 U/kg
Maintenance: 2–10 U/hr
Fluids
Isotonic sodium chloride
Total replacement in first 12 hours of 4–6 L
1 L in first hour
500–1000 mL/hr for 2–4 hours
250 mL/hr until 80 percent replaced
Glucose
Begin 5-percent dextrose in normal saline when glucose plasma level reaches 250 mg/dL (14 mmol/L)
Potassium
If initially normal or reduced, an infusion rate up to 15–20 mEq/hr may be required; if elevated, wait until levels decrease into the normal range, then add to intravenous solution in a concentration of 20–30 mEq/L
Bicarbonate
Add one ampule (44 mEq) to 1 L of 0.45 normal saline if pH is < 7.1

From Landon, 2007, with permission.

infections, and puerperal pelvic sepsis. In their population-based study of almost 200,000 pregnancies, Sheiner and colleagues (2009) found a twofold increased risk of asymptomatic bacteruria in women with diabetes. Similarly, Alvarez and associates (2010) reported positive urine cultures in a fourth of diabetic women compared with 10 percent of nondiabetic pregnant women. In a 2-year analysis of pyelonephritis at Parkland Hospital, 5 percent of women with diabetes developed pyelonephritis compared with 1.3 percent of the non-diabetic population (Hill, 2005). Fortunately, these latter infections can be minimized by screening and eradication of asymptomatic bacteriuria (Chap. 53, p. 1053). Takoudes and colleagues (2004) found that pregestational diabetes is associated with a two- to threefold increase in wound complications after cesarean delivery.

Management of Diabetes in Pregnancy

Because of the relationship between pregnancy complications and maternal glycemic control, efforts to achieve glucose targets are typically more aggressive during pregnancy. Management preferably should begin before pregnancy and include specific goals during each trimester.

Preconceptional Care

To minimize early pregnancy loss and congenital malformations in offspring of diabetic mothers, optimal medical care and education are recommended before conception (Chap. 8, p. 157). Unfortunately, nearly half of pregnancies in the United States are unplanned, and many diabetic women frequently begin pregnancy with suboptimal glucose control (Finer, 2011; Kim, 2005).

The ADA has defined optimal preconceptional glucose control using insulin to include self-monitored preprandial glucose levels of 70 to 100 mg/dL, peak postprandial values of 100 to 129 mg/dL, and mean daily glucose concentrations < 110 mg/dL (Kitzmiller, 2008). Glycosylated hemoglobin measurement, which reflects an average of circulating glucose for the past 4 to 8 weeks, is useful to assess early metabolic control. The ADA (2012) defines optimal values to be < 7 percent. In their prospective population-based study of 933 pregnant women with type 1 diabetes, Jensen and colleagues (2010) found the risk of congenital malformations was not demonstrably higher with glycosylated hemoglobin levels < 6.9 percent compared with that in more than 70,000 nondiabetic controls. They also identified a substantial fourfold increased risk for malformations at levels > 10 percent.

If indicated, evaluation and treatment for diabetic complications such as retinopathy or nephropathy should also be instituted before pregnancy. Finally, folate, 400 μg/day orally is given periconceptionally and during early pregnancy to decrease the risk of neural-tube defects.

First Trimester

Careful monitoring of glucose control is essential. For this reason, many clinicians hospitalize overtly diabetic women during early pregnancy to initiate an individualized glucose control program and offer education. It also provides an opportunity to assess the extent of diabetic vascular complications and precisely establish gestational age.

TABLE 57-8. Action Profiles of Commonly Used Insulins

Insulin Type	Onset	Peak (hr)	Duration (hr)
Short-acting (SC)			
Lispro	< 15 min	0.5–1.5	3–4
Glulisine	< 15 min	0.5–1.5	3–4
Aspart	< 15 min	0.5–1.5	3–4
Regular	30–60 min	2–3	4–6
Long-acting (SC)			
Detemir	1–4 hr	Minimal[a]	Up to 24
Glargine	1–4 hr	Minimal[a]	Up to 24
NPH	1–4 hr	6–10	10–16

[a]Minimal peak activity.
NPH = neutral protamine Hagedorn; SC = subcutaneous.
Modified from Powers, 2012.

Insulin Treatment

The overtly diabetic pregnant woman is best treated with insulin. Although oral hypoglycemic agents have been used successfully for gestational diabetes (p. 1141), these agents are not currently recommended for overt diabetes except for limited and individualized use (American College of Obstetricians and Gynecologists, 2012). Maternal glycemic control can usually be achieved with multiple daily insulin injections and adjustment of dietary intake. The action profiles of commonly used short- and long-term insulins are shown in Table 57-8.

Subcutaneous insulin infusion by a calibrated pump may be used during pregnancy. However, as demonstrated in a Cochrane Database review by Farrar and associates (2007), there is scarce robust evidence for specific salutary pregnancy effects. In a metaanalysis of six small randomized trials comparing insulin pumps to multiple daily injections of insulin, there were no significant differences in LGA birthweight, maternal hypoglycemia, or retinopathy progression (Mukhopadhyay, 2007). Notably, more women using insulin pumps developed ketoacidosis. Roeder and colleagues (2012) noted with insulin pump use in women with type 1 diabetes that total daily doses declined in the first trimester but later increased by more than threefold. Postprandial glucose excursions accounted for most increases. Women who use an insulin pump must be highly motivated and compliant to minimize the risk of nocturnal hypoglycemia (Gabbe, 2003).

Monitoring. Self-monitoring of capillary glucose levels using a glucometer is recommended because this involves the woman in her own care. Glucose goals recommended during pregnancy are shown in Table 57-9. Advances in noninvasive glucose monitoring will undoubtedly render intermittent capillary glucose monitoring obsolete. Subcutaneous continuous glucose monitoring devices reveal that pregnant women with

TABLE 57-9. Self-Monitored Capillary Blood Glucose Goals

Specimen	Level (mg/dL)
Fasting	≤ 95
Premeal	≤ 100
1-hr postprandial	≤ 140
2-hr postprandial	≤ 120
0200–0600	≥ 60
Mean (average)	100
Hemoglobin A_{1c}	≤ 6%

diabetes experience significant periods of daytime hyperglycemia and nocturnal hypoglycemia that are undetected by traditional monitoring (Combs, 2012). In one randomized trial of 71 women, those with periodic supplemental access to continuous glucose data had lower glycosylated hemoglobin levels—5.8 versus 6.4 percent—and delivered fewer overgrown newborns (Murphy, 2008). To date however, there have been no trials evaluating the impact of *personal* continuous monitoring devices that give immediate feedback to pregnant women. Such glucose monitoring systems, coupled with a continuous insulin pump, offer the potential of an "artificial pancreas" to avoid undetected hypo- or hyperglycemia during pregnancy.

Diet. Nutritional planning includes appropriate weight gain through carbohydrate and caloric modifications based on height, weight, and degree of glucose intolerance (American Diabetes Association, 2012; Bantle, 2008). The mix of carbohydrate, protein, and fat is adjusted to meet the metabolic goals and individual patient preferences, but a 175-g minimum of carbohydrate per day should be provided. Carbohydrate should be distributed throughout the day in three small- to moderate-sized meals and two to four snacks (Bantle, 2008). Weight loss is not recommended, but modest caloric restriction may be appropriate for overweight or obese women. An ideal dietary composition is 55 percent carbohydrate, 20 percent protein, and 25 percent fat, of which < 10 percent is saturated fat.

Hypoglycemia. Diabetes tends to be unstable in the first trimester. Hellmuth and associates (2000) reported that 37 percent of 43 women with type 1 diabetes had maternal hypoglycemia during the first trimester, and the average duration was more than 2 hours. Similarly, Chen and coworkers (2007) identified hypoglycemic events—blood glucose < 40 mg/dL—in 37 of 60 women with type 1 diabetes. A fourth of these were considered severe because the women were unable to treat their own symptoms. Rosenn and colleagues (1994) noted that maternal hypoglycemia had a peak incidence between 10 and 15 weeks' gestation. Caution is recommended when attempting euglycemia in women with recurrent episodes of hypoglycemia.

We have reported that good pregnancy outcomes can be achieved in women with mean preprandial plasma glucose values up to 143 mg/dL (Leveno, 1979). In women with diabetes who are not pregnant, the Diabetes Control and Complications Trial Research Group (1993) found that similar glucose values delayed and slowed diabetic retinopathy, nephropathy, and neuropathy. Thus, women with overt diabetes who have glucose values considerably above those defined as normal both during and after pregnancy can expect good outcomes.

Second Trimester

Maternal serum alpha-fetoprotein determination at 16 to 20 weeks' gestation is used in association with targeted sonographic examination at 18 to 20 weeks to detect neural-tube defects and other anomalies (Chap. 14, p. 284). Maternal alpha-fetoprotein levels may be lower in diabetic pregnancies, and interpretation is altered accordingly. Because the incidence of congenital cardiac anomalies is five times greater in mothers with diabetes, fetal echocardiography is an important part of second-trimester sonographic evaluation (Fouda, 2013). Despite advances in ultrasound technology, however, Dashe and associates (2009) cautioned that detection of fetal anomalies in obese diabetic women is more difficult than in similarly sized women without diabetes.

Regarding second-trimester glucose control, euglycemia with self-monitoring continues to be the goal in management. After the first-trimester instability, a stable period ensues. This is followed by an increased insulin requirement. Recall that Roeder and coworkers (2012) identified a threefold increase in total daily insulin after the first trimester in women using an insulin pump. This is due to the increased peripheral resistance to insulin described in Chapter 4 (p. 53).

Third Trimester and Delivery

During the last several decades, the threat of late-pregnancy fetal death in women with diabetes has prompted recommendations for various fetal surveillance programs beginning in the third trimester. Such protocols include fetal movement counting, periodic fetal heart rate monitoring, intermittent biophysical profile evaluation, and contraction stress testing (Chap. 17, p. 335). None of these techniques has been subjected to prospective randomized clinical trials, and their primary value seems related to their low false-negative rates. The American College of Obstetricians and Gynecologists (2012) suggests initiating such testing at 32 to 34 weeks' gestation.

At Parkland Hospital, women with diabetes are seen in a specialized obstetrical complications clinic every 2 weeks. During these visits, glycemic control is evaluated and insulin adjusted. They are routinely instructed to perform fetal kick counts beginning early in the third trimester. At 34 weeks, admission is offered to all insulin-treated women. While in the hospital, they continue daily fetal movement counts and undergo fetal heart rate monitoring three times a week. Delivery is planned for 38 weeks.

Labor induction may be attempted when the fetus is not excessively large and the cervix is considered favorable (Chap. 26, p. 523). Cesarean delivery at or near term has frequently been used to avoid traumatic birth of a large infant in a woman with diabetes. In women with more advanced diabetes, especially those with vascular disease, the reduced likelihood of successful labor induction remote from term has also contributed to an

TABLE 57-10. Insulin Management During Labor and Delivery

- Usual dose of intermediate-acting insulin is given at bedtime.
- Morning dose of insulin is withheld.
- Intravenous infusion of normal saline is begun.
- Once active labor begins or glucose levels decrease to < 70 mg/dL, the infusion is changed from saline to 5-percent dextrose and delivered at a rate of 100–150 mL/hr (2.5 mg/kg/min) to achieve a glucose level of approximately 100 mg/dL.
- Glucose levels are checked hourly using a bedside meter allowing for adjustment in the insulin or glucose infusion rate.
- Regular (short-acting) insulin is administered by intravenous infusion at a rate of 1.25 U/hr if glucose levels exceed 100 mg/dL.

Data from Coustan DR. Delivery: timing, mode, and management. In: Reece EA, Coustan DR, Gabbe SG, editors. Diabetes in women: adolescence, pregnancy, and menopause. 3rd ed. Philadelphia (PA): Lippincott Williams & Wilkins; 2004; and Jovanovic L, Peterson CM. Management of the pregnant, insulin-dependent diabetic woman. Diabetes Care 1980;3:63–8. From Pregestational diabetes mellitus. ACOG Practice Bulletin No. 60. American College of Obstetricians and Gynecologists. Obstet Gynecol 2005;105:675–85; reaffirmed 2012.

increased cesarean delivery rate. In a nested case-control study of 209 women with type 1 diabetes, Lepercq and colleagues (2010) reported a 70-percent cesarean delivery rate overall. Two thirds of these were delivered without labor. Both maternal body mass index (BMI) > 25 kg/m^2 and low Bishop score were independently associated with cesarean delivery for those in labor. In another study, a glycohemoglobin level > 6.4 percent at delivery was independently associated with urgent cesarean delivery. This suggests that tighter glycemic control during the third trimester might reduce late fetal compromise and cesarean delivery for fetal indications (Miailhe, 2013). The cesarean delivery rate for women with overt diabetes has remained at approximately 80 percent for the past 35 years at Parkland Hospital.

Reducing or withholding the dose of long-acting insulin given on the day of delivery is recommended. Regular insulin should be used to meet most or all of the insulin needs of the mother during this time, because insulin requirements typically drop markedly after delivery. We have found that continuous insulin infusion by calibrated intravenous pump is most satisfactory (Table 57-10). Throughout labor and after delivery, the woman should be adequately hydrated intravenously and given glucose in sufficient amounts to maintain normoglycemia. Capillary or plasma glucose levels should be checked frequently, especially during active labor, and regular insulin should be administered accordingly.

Puerperium

Often, women may require virtually no insulin for the first 24 hours or so postpartum. Subsequently, insulin requirements may fluctuate markedly during the next few days. Infection must be promptly detected and treated.

Counseling in the puerperium should include a discussion of birth control. Available options are discussed in Chapter 38 (p. 695). Effective contraception is especially important in women with overt diabetes to allow optimal glucose control before subsequent conceptions.

GESTATIONAL DIABETES

In the United States, 5 to 6 percent of pregnancies—almost 250,000 women—are affected annually by various forms of gestational diabetes. Worldwide, its prevalence differs according to race, ethnicity, age, and body composition and by screening and diagnostic criteria. There continue to be several controversies pertaining to the diagnosis and treatment of gestational diabetes. Accordingly, a National Institutes of Health (NIH) Consensus Development Conference (2013) was convened. Coincidental with publication of the Conference findings, the American College of Obstetricians and Gynecologists (2013) also updated its recommendations. These two authoritative sources provide an up-to-date analysis of the issues surrounding this diagnosis and bolster the approach to identifying and treating women with gestational diabetes, as described subsequently.

The word *gestational* implies that diabetes is induced by pregnancy—ostensibly because of exaggerated physiological changes in glucose metabolism (Chap. 4, p. 53). Gestational diabetes is defined as carbohydrate intolerance of variable severity with onset or first recognition during pregnancy (American College of Obstetricians and Gynecologists, 2013). This definition applies whether or not insulin is used for treatment and undoubtedly includes some women with previously unrecognized overt diabetes. In their analysis of more than 1500 nonpregnant adults as part of National Health and Nutrition Examinations Survey (NHANES) IV, Karve and Hayward (2010) estimated that only 4.8 percent of individuals with impaired fasting glucose or glucose intolerance were aware of their diagnosis.

Use of the term *gestational diabetes* has been encouraged to communicate the need for increased surveillance and to stimulate women to seek further testing postpartum. The most important perinatal correlate is excessive fetal growth, which may result in both maternal and fetal birth trauma. The likelihood of fetal death with appropriately treated gestational diabetes is not different from that in the general population. Importantly, more than half of women with gestational diabetes ultimately develop overt diabetes in the ensuing 20 years. And, as discussed on page 1125, evidence is mounting for long-range complications that include obesity and diabetes in their offspring.

Screening and Diagnosis

Despite more than 40 years of research, there is still no agreement regarding optimal gestational diabetes screening. The difficulty in achieving consensus is underscored by the controversy following publication of the single-step approach espoused by

TABLE 57-11. Threshold Values for Diagnosis of Gestational Diabetes

Plasma Glucose	Glucose Concentration Threshold[a]		Above Threshold (%) Cumulative
	mmol/L	mg/dL	
Fasting	5.1	92	8.3
1-hr OGTT	10.0	180	14.0
2-hr OGTT	8.5	153	16.1[b]

[a]One or more of these values from a 75-g OGTT must be equaled or exceeded for the diagnosis of gestational diabetes.
[b]In addition, 1.7% of participants in the initial cohort were unblinded because of fasting plasma glucose levels > 5.8 mmol/L (105 mg/dL) or 2-hr OGTT values > 11.1 mmol/L (200 mg/dL), bringing the total to 17.8%.
OGTT = oral glucose tolerance test.

the IADPSG Consensus Panel (2010) (Table 57-11). This strategy was greatly influenced by results of the Hypoglycemia and Pregnancy Outcomes (HAPO) Study described later. Although the ADA adopted this new scheme, the American College of Obstetricians and Gynecologists (2013) declined to endorse the single 75-gram oral glucose tolerance test. Instead, the College continues to recommend a two-step approach to screen and diagnose gestational diabetes. Similarly, the NIH Consensus Development Conference in 2013 concluded that evidence is insufficient to adopt a one-step approach.

The recommended two-step approach begins with either universal or risk-based selective screening using a 50-g, 1-hour oral glucose challenge test. Participants in the Fifth International Workshop Conferences on Gestational Diabetes endorsed use of *selective screening* criteria shown in Table 57-12. *Universal screening* is also acceptable. Gabbe and associates (2004) surveyed practicing obstetricians and reported that 96 percent used universal screening. Screening should be performed between 24 and 28 weeks' gestation in those women not known to have glucose intolerance earlier in pregnancy. This *50-g screening test* is followed by a *diagnostic 100-g, 3-hour oral glucose tolerance test (OGTT)* if screening results meet or exceed a predetermined plasma glucose concentration.

For the 50-g screen, the plasma glucose level is measured 1 hour after a 50-g oral glucose load without regard to the time of day or time of last meal. In a recent review, the pooled sensitivity for a threshold of 140 mg/dL ranged from 74 to 83 percent depending on 100-g thresholds used for diagnosis (van Leeuwen, 2012). Sensitivity estimates for a 50-g screen threshold of 135 mg/dL improved only slightly to 78 to 85 percent. Importantly, specificity dropped from a range of 72 to 85 percent for 140 mg/dL to 65 to 81 percent for a threshold of 135 mg/dL. That said, the American College of Obstetricians and Gynecologists (2013) recommends using either 135 or 140 mg/dL as the 50-g screen threshold. At Parkland Hospital, we continue to use 140 mg/dL.

TABLE 57-12. Fifth International Workshop-Conference on Gestational Diabetes: Recommended Screening Strategy Based on Risk Assessment for Detecting Gestational Diabetes (GDM)

GDM risk assessment: should be ascertained at the first prenatal visit

Low Risk: Blood glucose testing not routinely required if all the following are present:
- Member of an ethnic group with a low prevalence of GDM
- No known diabetes in first-degree relatives
- Age < 25 years
- Weight normal before pregnancy
- Weight normal at birth
- No history of abnormal glucose metabolism
- No history of poor obstetrical outcome

Average Risk: Perform blood glucose testing at 24 to 28 weeks using either:
- Two-step procedure: 50-g oral glucose challenge test (GCT), followed by a diagnostic 100-g OGTT for those meeting the threshold value in the GCT
- One-step procedure: diagnostic 100-g OGTT performed on all subjects

High Risk: Perform blood glucose testing as soon as feasible, using the procedures described above, if one or more of these are present:
- Severe obesity
- Strong family history of type 2 diabetes
- Previous history of GDM, impaired glucose metabolism, or glucosuria
- If GDM is not diagnosed, blood glucose testing should be repeated at 24 to 28 weeks' gestation or at any time symptoms or signs suggest hyperglycemia

OGTT = oral glucose tolerance test.
Modified from Metzger, 2007.

TABLE 57-13. Fifth International Workshop Conference on Gestational Diabetes: Diagnostic Criteria of Gestational Diabetes by Oral Glucose Tolerance Testing

	Oral Glucose Load[a]			
Time	100-g Glucose[b]		75-g Glucose[b]	
Fasting	95 mg/dL	5.3 mmol/L	95 mg/dL	5.3 mmol/L
1-hr	180 mg/dL	10.0 mmol/L	180 mg/dL	10.0 mmol/L
2-hr	155 mg/dL	8.6 mmol/L	155 mg/dL	8.6 mmol/L
3-hr	140 mg/dL	7.8 mmol/L	—	—

[a]The test should be performed in the morning after an overnight fast of at least 8 hr but not more than 14 hr and after at least 3 days of unrestricted diet (≥ 150 g/d) and physical activity. The subject should remain seated and should not smoke during the test.
[b]Two or more of the venous plasma glucose concentrations listed must be met or exceeded for a positive diagnosis.
Data from Metzger, 2007.

Justification for screening and treatment of women with gestational diabetes was strengthened by the study by Crowther and coworkers (2005). They assigned 1000 women with gestational diabetes between 24 and 34 weeks' gestation to receive dietary advice with blood glucose monitoring plus insulin therapy—the intervention group—or to undergo routine prenatal care. Women were diagnosed as having gestational diabetes if their blood glucose was < 100 mg/dL after an overnight fast and was between 140 and 198 mg/dL 2 hours after ingesting a 75-g glucose solution. Women in the intervention group had a significantly reduced risk of a composite adverse outcome that included perinatal death, shoulder dystocia, fetal bone fracture, and fetal nerve palsy. Macrosomia defined by birthweight ≥ 4000 g complicated 10 percent of deliveries in the intervention group compared with 21 percent in the routine prenatal care group. Cesarean delivery rates were almost identical in the two study groups.

Slightly different results were reported by the Maternal-Fetal Medicine Units Network randomized trial of 958 women (Landon, 2009). Dietary counseling plus glucose monitoring was compared with standard obstetrical care in women with mild gestational diabetes to reduce perinatal morbidity rates. Mild gestational diabetes was identified in women with fasting glucose levels < 95 mg/dL. They reported no differences in rates of composite morbidity that included stillbirth; neonatal hypoglycemia, hyperinsulinemia, and hyperbilirubinemia; and birth trauma. Importantly, secondary analyses demonstrated a 50-percent reduction in macrosomia, fewer cesarean deliveries, and a significant decrease in shoulder dystocia rates—1.5 versus 4 percent—in treated versus control women.

Based largely on these two studies, the U.S. Preventive Services Task Force (2013) now recommends universal screening in low-risk women after 24 weeks' gestation. However, the Task Force concluded that evidence is insufficient to assess the balance of benefits versus harms of screening before 24 weeks. From the foregoing, there obviously is not international agreement as to the optimal glucose tolerance test to identify gestational diabetes. The World Health Organization (1998) and now the American Diabetes Association (2013) recommend the 75-g 2-hour oral glucose tolerance test. In the United States, however, the 100-g, 3-hour OGTT test performed after an overnight fast is recommended by the American College of Obstetricians and Gynecologists (2013). Criteria for interpretation of the 100-g diagnostic glucose tolerance test are shown in Table 57-13. Also shown are the criteria for the 75-g test most often used outside the United States.

The Hyperglycemia and Adverse Pregnancy Outcome (HAPO) Study

This was a 7-year international epidemiological study of 23,325 pregnant women at 15 centers in nine countries (HAPO Study Cooperative Research Group, 2008). The investigation analyzed the association of various levels of glucose intolerance during the third trimester with adverse infant outcomes in women with gestational diabetes. Between 24 and 32 weeks' gestation, the general population of pregnant women underwent 75-g oral glucose tolerance testing after overnight fasting. Blood glucose levels were measured fasting and then 1 and 2 hours after glucose ingestion. Caregivers were blinded to results except for women whose glucose levels exceeded values that required treatment and removal from the study. Glucose values at each of these three time posts were stratified into seven categories (Fig. 57-8). Values were then correlated with rates for birthweight > 90th percentile (LGA), primary cesarean delivery, clinical neonatal hypoglycemia, and cord-serum C-peptide levels > 90th percentile. C-peptide is a measurable by-product created during insulin production. Odds of each outcome were calculated using the lowest category—for example, fasting plasma glucose < 75 mg/dL—as the referent group. Their findings in general supported the supposition that increasing plasma glucose levels at each epoch were associated with increasing adverse outcomes.

In an editorial accompanying publication of the HAPO trial, Ecker and Greene (2008) posed the question: "Given

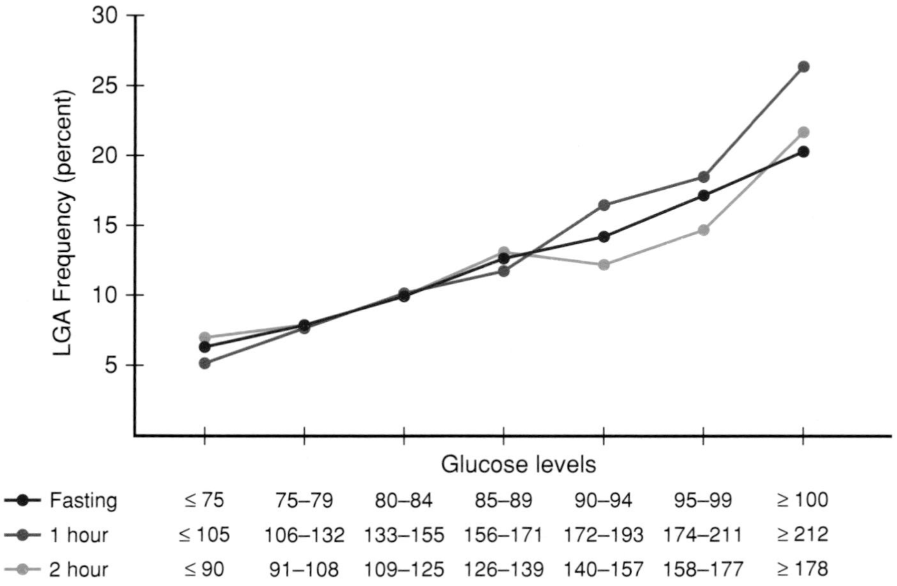

FIGURE 57-8 Hyperglycemia and Adverse Pregnancy Outcome (HAPO) Study. The frequency of newborn birthweight ≥ 90th percentile for gestational age plotted against glucose levels (mg/dL) fasting and at 1- and 2-hr intervals following a 75-g oral glucose load. LGA = large for gestational age. (Adapted from The HAPO Study Cooperative Research Group, 2008.)

the results of the HAPO study, should we lower our threshold for the diagnosis and treatment of gestational diabetes?" It was adjudged that it will be difficult to show that treating lesser degrees of carbohydrate intolerance—as suggested in the HAPO study—would provide any meaningful improvements in clinical outcomes. Thus Ecker and Greene (2008) concluded, and we agree, that changes in criteria are not justified until clinical trials prove benefits. Most recently, this position was endorsed by the 2013 NIH Consensus Development Conference.

International Association of Diabetes and Pregnancy Study Group

The IADPSG sponsored a workshop conference on the diagnosis and classification of gestational diabetes in 2008. After reviewing the results of the HAPO study, a panel was appointed to develop recommendations for the diagnosis and classification of hyperglycemia during pregnancy. This panel allowed for the diagnosis of overt diabetes during pregnancy as shown in Table 57-4. It also recommended a single-step approach to the diagnosis of gestational diabetes using the 75-g, 2-hour OGTT. Thresholds for fasting, 1-, and 2-hour values based on mean glucose concentrations from the entire HAPO study cohort were considered. These thresholds were derived using an arbitrary 1.75 odds ratio of outcomes such as LGA birthweight and cord serum C-peptide levels > 90th percentile. Only one of these thresholds would need to be met or exceeded to make the diagnosis of gestational diabetes (see Table 57-11).

It is estimated that implementation of these recommendations would increase the prevalence of gestational diabetes in the United States to 17.8 percent! Said another way, the number of women with mild gestational diabetes would increase almost threefold with no evidence of treatment benefit (Cundy, 2012). Despite these significant drawbacks, the ADA (2013) recommended adopting this new approach based on benefits inferred from trials in women identified using a two-step approach described on page 1138 (Crowther, 2005; Landon, 2009).

National Institutes of Health Consensus Development Conference on Diagnosing Gestational Diabetes Mellitus

Prompted by the IADPSG recommendations (2010) and their adoption by the ADA (2013), an NIH Consensus Development Conference (2013) was convened. This conference included input from a multidisciplinary planning committee, a systematic evidence review by the Agency for Healthcare Research and Quality (AHRQ) Evidence-Based Practice Center, expert testimony, and a nonbiased panel to produce the overall report. The panel concluded that there were potential benefits to worldwide standardization. However, it found insufficient evidence to adopt a one-step diagnostic process such as the one proposed by the IADPSG. Moreover, as mentioned previously, after consideration of these findings, the American College of Obstetricians and Gynecologists (2013) continues to recommend a two-step screening and diagnostic approach to gestational diabetes diagnosis. It noted no significant improvements in maternal or perinatal outcomes that would offset the tripling of gestational diabetes incidence that would derive from the one-step approach. We applaud this decision.

Maternal and Fetal Effects

Adverse consequences of gestational diabetes differ from those of pregestational diabetes. Unlike in women with overt diabetes, rates of fetal anomalies do not appear to be substantially increased (Sheffield, 2002). In a study of more than 1 million women from the Swedish Medical Birth Registry, major malformation rates were marginally increased—2.3 versus 1.8 percent (Fadl, 2010). The stillbirth rate was not increased in this study or in an analysis of 130 perinatal deaths in the HAPO study (2008). In contrast, and not unexpectedly, women with *elevated* fasting glucose levels have increased rates of unexplained stillbirths similar to women with overt diabetes. The ADA (2003) concluded that fasting hyperglycemia > 105 mg/dL may be associated with an increased risk of fetal death during the final 4 to 8 weeks. This increasing risk with progressive maternal hyperglycemia prompted the IADPSG (2010) to emphasize the importance of identifying women with evidence of preexisting diabetes early in pregnancy (see Table 57-4). Similar to women with overt diabetes, adverse maternal effects associated with gestational diabetes include an increased frequency of hypertension and cesarean delivery.

Fetal Macrosomia

The primary effect attributed to gestational diabetes is excessive fetal size or macrosomia that is variably defined and discussed further in Chapter 44 (p. 884). Maternal hyperglycemia prompts fetal hyperinsulinemia, particularly during the second half of pregnancy. This in turn stimulates excessive somatic growth. The perinatal goal is to avoid difficult delivery from macrosomia and concomitant birth trauma associated with shoulder dystocia. In a retrospective analysis of more than 80,000 vaginal deliveries in Chinese women, Cheng and associates (2013) calculated a 76-fold increased risk for shoulder dystocia in newborns weighing ≥ 4200 g compared with the risk in those weighing < 3500 g. Importantly, however, the odds ratio for shoulder dystocia in women with diabetes was less than 2. Although gestational diabetes is certainly a risk factor, it accounts for only a small number of pregnancies complicated by shoulder dystocia.

The excessive shoulder and trunk fat that commonly characterizes the macrosomic infant of a diabetic mother theoretically predisposes such infants to shoulder dystocia or cesarean delivery (Durnwald, 2004; McFarland, 2000). Landon and colleagues (2011) identified shoulder dystocia in approximately 4 percent of women with mild gestational diabetes compared with < 1 percent of women with a 50-g glucose screen result < 120 mg/dL. In a prospective study of fetal adipose measurements, however, Buhling and coworkers (2012) demonstrated no differences between measurements in 630 offspring of women with gestational diabetes and 142 without diabetes. The authors attributed this negative finding to successful treatment of gestational diabetes.

There is extensive evidence that insulin-like growth factors also play a role fetal-growth regulation (Chap. 44, p. 872). These proinsulin-like polypeptides are produced by virtually all fetal organs and are potent stimulators of cell differentiation and division. Luo and coworkers (2012) reported that insulin-like growth factor-I strongly correlated with birthweight. The HAPO study investigators also reported dramatic increases of cord-serum C-peptide levels with increasing maternal glucose levels following a 75-g OGTT. C-peptide levels > 90th percentile were found in almost a third of newborns in the highest glucose categories. Other factors implicated in macrosomia include epidermal growth factor, fibroblast growth factor, platelet-derived growth factor, leptin, and adiponectin (Grissa, 2011; Loukovaara, 2004; Mazaki-Tovi, 2005).

Neonatal Hypoglycemia

Neonatal hyperinsulinemia may provoke hypoglycemia within minutes of birth. The incidence varies depending on the threshold definition. Cornblath and associates (2000) established a threshold of 35 mg/dL in term newborns. An NIH workshop conference on neonatal hypoglycemia supported use of such operational thresholds but cautioned that these are not strictly evidence-based (Hay, 2009). Newborns described by the HAPO study (2008) had an incidence of clinical neonatal hypoglycemia that increased with increasing maternal OGTT values defined in Figure 57-8. The frequency varied from 1 to 2 percent, but it was as high as 4.6 percent in women with fasting glucose levels ≥ 100 mg/dL. Likewise, cord-blood insulin levels are related to maternal glucose control (Leipold, 2004).

Maternal Obesity

In women with gestational diabetes, maternal BMI is an independent and more substantial risk factor for fetal macrosomia than is glucose intolerance (Ehrenberg, 2004; Mission, 2013). Stuebe and colleagues (2012) completed a secondary analysis of women with either untreated mild gestational diabetes or normal glucose tolerance testing results. They found that higher BMI levels were associated with increasing birthweight, regardless of glucose levels. Also, maternal obesity is an important confounding factor in the diagnosis of gestational diabetes. In their metaanalysis, Torloni and coworkers (2009) estimated that the gestational diabetes prevalence increases by approximately 1 percent for every 1 kg/m^2 increase in BMI. Weight distribution also seems to play a role because the risk of gestational diabetes is increased with truncal obesity. Suresh and colleagues (2012) verified that increased maternal abdominal subcutaneous fat thickness as measured by sonography at 18 to 22 weeks' gestation correlated with BMI and was a better predictor of gestational diabetes. Martin and associates (2009) reported similar findings for sonographically measured maternal visceral adipose depth. Importantly, excessive gestational weight gain is commonly identified in women with gestational diabetes and also confers an additive risk for fetal macrosomia (Egan, 2014).

Management

Women with gestational diabetes can be divided into two functional classes using fasting glucose levels. Pharmacological methods are usually recommended if diet modification does not consistently maintain the fasting plasma glucose levels < 95 mg/dL or the 2-hour postprandial plasma glucose < 120 mg/dL (American College of Obstetricians and Gynecologists, 2013). Whether pharmacological treatment should be used in women with lesser degrees of fasting hyperglycemia—105 mg/dL or less before dietary intervention—is unclear. There have been no controlled trials to identify ideal glucose targets for fetal risk prevention. On the other hand, the HAPO study (2008) did demonstrate increased fetal risk at glucose levels below the threshold used for diagnosis of diabetes. The Fifth International Workshop Conference recommended that fasting capillary glucose levels be kept ≤ 95 mg/dL (Metzger, 2007).

In a systematic review, Hartling and colleagues (2013) concluded that treating gestational diabetes resulted in a significantly lower incidence of preeclampsia, shoulder dystocia, and macrosomia. For example, the calculated risk ratio for delivering an infant > 4000 g after treatment was 0.50. These investigators caution that the attributed risk for these outcomes is low, especially when glucose values are only moderately elevated. Importantly, they were unable to demonstrate an effect on neonatal hypoglycemia or future metabolic outcomes in the offspring.

Diabetic Diet

As discussed previously, reports by Crowther (2005) and Landon (2009) and their colleagues describe the benefits of dietary counseling and monitoring in women with gestational diabetes. The ADA recommends individualized nutritional counseling based on height and weight (Bantle, 2008). Nutritional instructions generally include a carbohydrate-controlled diet sufficient to maintain normoglycemia and avoid ketosis. On average, this includes a daily caloric intake of 30 to 35 kcal/kg. Moreno-Castilla and associates (2013) randomly assigned 152 women with gestational diabetes to either a 40- or a 55-percent daily carbohydrate diet and found no difference in insulin levels and pregnancy outcomes. The American College of Obstetricians and Gynecologists (2013) suggests that carbohydrate intake be limited to 40 percent of total calories. The remaining calories are apportioned to give 20 percent as protein and 40 percent as fat.

Although the most appropriate diet for women with gestational diabetes has not been established, the ADA (2003) has suggested that obese women with a BMI > 30 kg/m^2 may benefit from a 30-percent caloric restriction, which approximates 25 kcal/kg/d. This should be monitored with weekly assessment for ketonuria, which has been linked with impaired psychomotor development in offspring (Rizzo, 1995; Scholte, 2012). That said, Most and Langer (2012) found that insulin was necessary to reduce excess birthweight in offspring of obese women with gestational diabetes.

Exercise

The American College of Obstetricians and Gynecologists (2009) reviewed three randomized trials of exercise in women with gestational diabetes (Avery, 1997; Bung, 1993; Jovanovic-Peterson, 1989). The results suggest that exercise improved cardiorespiratory fitness without improving pregnancy outcome. Importantly, these trials were small and had limited power to show improvement in outcomes. Dempsey and coworkers (2004) found that physical activity during pregnancy reduced the risk of gestational diabetes. Brankston and associates (2004) reported that resistance exercise diminished the need for insulin therapy in overweight women with gestational diabetes. Conversely, Stafne and colleagues (2012), in a randomized controlled trial in 855 women, observed that a 1-week exercise program during the second half of pregnancy did not prevent gestational diabetes or improve insulin resistance. Importantly, the average BMI at enrollment was 24.8 ± 3.2. The American College of Obstetricians and Gynecologists (2013) recommends a moderate exercise program as part of the treatment plan for women with gestational diabetes.

Glucose Monitoring

Hawkins and colleagues (2008) compared outcomes in 315 women with diet-treated gestational diabetes who used personal glucose monitors with those of 615 gestational diabetics who were also diet-treated but who underwent intermittent fasting glucose evaluation during semi-weekly obstetrical visits. Women using daily blood-glucose self-monitoring had significantly fewer macrosomic infants and gained less weight after diagnosis than women evaluated during clinic visits only. These findings support the common practice of blood-glucose self-monitors for women with diet-treated gestational diabetes.

Postprandial surveillance for gestational diabetes has been shown to be superior to preprandial surveillance. DeVeciana and coworkers (1995) studied 66 pregnant women with gestational diabetes in whom insulin was initiated for fasting hyperglycemia. The women were randomly assigned to glucose surveillance using either preprandial or 1-hour postprandial capillary blood-glucose concentrations. Postprandial surveillance was shown to be superior in that blood-glucose control was significantly improved and was associated with fewer cases of neonatal hypoglycemia—3 versus 21 percent; less macrosomia—12 versus 42 percent; and fewer cesarean deliveries for dystocia—24 versus 39 percent. At Parkland Hospital, we were unable to demonstrate similar findings when we reviewed the impact of changing to postprandial monitoring in women with diet-treated gestational diabetes. We did, however, demonstrate a significant reduction in maternal weight gain per week—0.63 lb/week to 0.45 lb/week—in women managed with a postprandial monitoring schema. The American College of Obstetricians and Gynecologists (2013) recommends four-times daily glucose monitoring performed fasting and either 1 or 2 hours after each meal.

Insulin Treatment

Historically, insulin has been considered standard therapy in women with gestational diabetes when target glucose levels cannot be consistently achieved through nutrition and exercise. It does not cross the placenta, and tight glycemic control can typically be achieved. In a report prepared for the AHRQ, Nicholson and associates (2009) were unable to determine a threshold above which insulin should be initiated. Pharmacological therapy—in this case insulin—is typically added if fasting levels persistently exceed 95 mg/dL in women with gestational diabetes. The American College of Obstetricians and Gynecologists (2013) also recommends that insulin be considered in women with 1-hour postprandial levels that persistently exceed 140 mg/dL or those with 2-hour levels above 120 mg/dL. Importantly, all of these thresholds are extrapolated from recommendations for managing women with overt diabetes.

If insulin is initiated, the starting dose is typically 0.7–1.0 units/kg/day given in divided doses (American College of Obstetricians and Gynecologists, 2013). A combination of intermediate-acting and short-acting insulin may be used, and dose adjustments are based on glucose levels at particular times of the day. At Parkland Hospital, insulin instruction for these women is accomplished either in a specialized outpatient clinic or during a short hospital stay. As shown in Table 57-8, insulin analogues such as insulin aspart and insulin lispro have a more rapid onset of action than regular insulin and theoretically could be helpful in postprandial glucose management. Experience with these analogues with gestational diabetes is limited, and Singh and coworkers (2008) were unable to demonstrate a benefit compared with conventional insulins.

Oral Hypoglycemic Agents

Several studies have attested to the safety and efficacy of gestational diabetes treatment with either glyburide (Micronase) or metformin (Glucophage) (Langer, 2000; Nicholson, 2009;

Rowan, 2008). In one study, Langer and colleagues (2000, 2005) randomly assigned 404 women to insulin or glyburide therapy. Near normoglycemic levels were achieved with either regimen, and there were no apparent neonatal complications attributable to glyburide. In a follow-up study, Conway and coworkers (2004) reported that women with fasting glucose levels > 110 mg/dL did not adequately respond to glyburide therapy. Similar results were reported by Chmait (2004) and Kahn (2006) and their associates. At one time, glyburide was thought not to cross the placenta. However, Hebert and colleagues (2008, 2009) sampled 20 paired maternal-cord specimens and found the latter to have glyburide concentrations approximately half that of maternal levels.

Metformin treatment for polycystic ovarian disease throughout pregnancy reduced the incidence of gestational diabetes (Glueck, 2004). Because metformin crosses to the fetus, there was reticence to use it in pregnant women (Harborne, 2003). Subsequent studies have helped allay these concerns. Rowan and associates (2008) randomly assigned 751 women with gestational diabetes to metformin or insulin treatment. The primary outcome was a composite of neonatal hypoglycemia, respiratory distress syndrome, phototherapy, birth trauma, 5-minute Apgar score ≤ 7, and preterm birth. Similarities in the composite outcome between metformin and insulin led investigators to conclude that metformin was not associated with adverse perinatal outcomes. It is noteworthy that 46 percent of women in the metformin trial required supplemental insulin compared with only 4 percent of women treated with glyburide (Langer, 2000).

In their systematic review and metaanalysis of oral hypoglycemic agents for gestational diabetes, Nicholson and coworkers (2009) found no evidence of increased adverse maternal or neonatal outcomes with glyburide or metformin compared with insulin. Moore and associates (2010) randomly assigned 149 women with gestational diabetes who did not achieve glycemic control on diet therapy to either glyburide or metformin treatment. More than a third of women in the metformin group required supplemental insulin compared with 16 percent of those treated with glyburide.

Oral hypoglycemic agents are being increasingly used for gestational diabetes, although they have not been approved by the Food and Drug Administration for this indication. A survey of almost 1400 fellows of the American College of Obstetricians and Gynecologists found that 13 percent of respondents were using glyburide as first-line therapy for diet failure in women with gestational diabetes (Gabbe, 2004). The American College of Obstetricians and Gynecologists (2013) acknowledges that both glyburide and metformin are appropriate, as is insulin, for first-line glycemic control in women with gestational diabetes. Because long-term outcomes have not been studied, the committee recommends appropriate counseling when hypoglycemic agents are used.

Obstetrical Management

In general, for women with gestational diabetes who do not require insulin, early delivery or other interventions are seldom required. There is no consensus regarding the value or timing of antepartum fetal testing. It is typically reserved for women with pregestational diabetes because of the increased stillbirth risk. The American College of Obstetricians and Gynecologists (2013) endorses fetal surveillance in women with gestational diabetes and poor glycemic control. At Parkland Hospital, women with gestational diabetes are routinely instructed to perform daily fetal kick counts in the third trimester (Chap. 17, p. 335). Insulin-treated women are offered inpatient admission after 34 weeks' gestation, and fetal heart rate monitoring is performed three times each week.

Women with gestational diabetes and adequate glycemic control are managed expectantly. Elective labor induction to prevent shoulder dystocia compared with spontaneous labor remains controversial. One randomized trial evaluated induction at 38 weeks in 200 women with insulin-treated diabetes—187 of whom had gestational diabetes. Investigators reported a significantly lower proportion of newborns with a birthweight > 90th percentile in the active induction group—10 versus 23 percent (Kjos, 1993). However, there were no differences in rates of cesarean delivery or shoulder dystocia or in neonatal outcomes. Witkop and colleagues (2009) performed a systematic review and concluded that, in the aggregate, a reduction in fetal macrosomia is likely in women with gestational diabetes who undergo an elective labor induction at term. They also found a limited ability to draw definite conclusions based on available evidence. The American College of Obstetricians and Gynecologists (2013) also has concluded that no evidence-based recommendation can be made regarding delivery timing in women with gestational diabetes. To study this, a large multicenter trial (NCT01058772) expected to enroll 1760 women with gestational diabetes is currently recruiting participants (Maso, 2011).

Elective cesarean delivery to avoid brachial plexus injuries in overgrown fetuses is also an important issue. The American College of Obstetricians and Gynecologists (2013) has suggested that cesarean delivery should be considered in women with gestational diabetes whose fetuses have a sonographically estimated weight ≥ 4500 g. From their systematic review, Garabedian and coworkers (2010) estimated that as many as 588 cesarean deliveries in women with gestational diabetes and an estimated fetal weight of ≥ 4500 g would be necessary to avoid one case of permanent brachial plexus palsy. Effects of such a policy were retrospectively analyzed by Gonen and associates (2000) in a general obstetrical population of more than 16,000 women. Elective cesarean delivery had no significant effect on the incidence of brachial plexus injury.

Postpartum Evaluation

Recommendations for postpartum evaluation are based on the 50-percent likelihood of women with gestational diabetes developing overt diabetes within 20 years (O'Sullivan, 1982). The Fifth International Workshop Conference on Gestational Diabetes recommended that women diagnosed with gestational diabetes undergo evaluation with a 75-g oral glucose tolerance test at 6 to 12 weeks postpartum and other intervals thereafter (Metzger, 2007). These recommendations are shown in Table 57-14 along with the classification scheme of the ADA

TABLE 57-14. Fifth International Workshop-Conference: Metabolic Assessments Recommended after Pregnancy with Gestational Diabetes

Time	Test	Purpose
Postdelivery (1–3 d)	Fasting or random plasma glucose	Detect persistent, overt diabetes
Early postpartum (6–12 wk)	75-g, 2-hr OGTT	Postpartum classification of glucose metabolism
1-yr postpartum	75-g, 2-hr OGTT	Assess glucose metabolism
Annually	Fasting plasma glucose	Assess glucose metabolism
Triannually	75-g, 2-hr OGTT	Assess glucose metabolism
Prepregnancy	75-g, 2-hr OGTT	Classify glucose metabolism
Classification of the American Diabetes Association (2013)		
Normal Values	**Impaired Fasting Glucose or Impaired Glucose Tolerance**	**Diabetes Mellitus**
Fasting < 100 mg/dL	100–125 mg/dL	≥ 126 mg/dL
2 hr < 140 mg/dL	2 hr ≥ 140–199 mg/dL	2 hr ≥ 200 mg/dL
Hemoglobin A_{1c} < 5.7%	5.7–6.4%	≥ 6.5%

OGTT = oral glucose tolerance test.
From American Diabetes Association, 2013; Metzger, 2007.

(2013). Hunt and colleagues (2010) reviewed performance rates of postpartum glucose screening and found that anywhere between 23 and 58 percent of women actually undergo 75-g glucose testing. The American College of Obstetricians and Gynecologists (2013) recommends either a fasting glucose or the 75-g, 2-hour OGTT for the diagnosis of overt diabetes. The ADA (2011) recommends testing at least every 3 years in women with a history of gestational diabetes but normal postpartum glucose screening.

Women with a history of gestational diabetes are also at risk for cardiovascular complications associated with dyslipidemia, hypertension, and abdominal obesity—the *metabolic syndrome* (Chap. 48, p. 962). In a study of 47,909 parous women, Kessous and coworkers (2013) evaluated subsequent hospitalizations due to cardiovascular morbidity. They found that almost 5000 women with gestational diabetes were 2.6 times more likely to be hospitalized for cardiovascular morbidity. Shah and coworkers (2008) also documented excessive cardiovascular disease by 10 years in women with gestational diabetes. Akinci and associates (2009) reported that a fasting glucose level ≥ 100 mg/dL in the index OGTT was an independent predictor of the metabolic syndrome.

Recurrent Gestational Diabetes

In subsequent pregnancies, recurrence was documented in 40 percent of 344 primiparous women with gestational diabetes (Holmes, 2010). Obese women were more likely to have impaired glucose tolerance in subsequent pregnancies. Thus, lifestyle behavioral changes, including weight control and exercise between pregnancies, likely would prevent gestational diabetes recurrence (Kim, 2008). Ehrlich and colleagues (2011) found that the loss of at least two BMI units was associated with a lower risk of gestational diabetes in women who were overweight or obese in the first pregnancy. Getahun and coworkers (2010) found that only 4.2 percent of women without gestational diabetes in their first pregnancy were diagnosed with gestational diabetes when screened in a second pregnancy. This compared with 41.3 percent in women with a history of gestational diabetes.

Contraception

Low-dose hormonal contraceptives may be used safely by women with recent gestational diabetes (Chap. 38, p. 709). The rate of subsequent diabetes in oral contraceptive users is not significantly different from that in those who did not use hormonal contraception (Kerlan, 2010). Importantly, comorbid obesity, hypertension, or dyslipidemia should direct the choice for contraception toward a method without potential cardiovascular consequences. In these instances, the intrauterine device is a good alternative.

REFERENCES

Akinci B, Celtik A, Yener S, et al: Prediction of developing metabolic syndrome after gestational diabetes mellitus. Fertil Steril 93(4):1248, 2010

Alvarez JR, Fechner AJ, Williams SF, et al: Asymptomatic bacteriuria in pregestational diabetic pregnancies and the role of group B streptococcus. Am J Perinat 27(3):231, 2010

American College of Obstetricians and Gynecologists: Management of diabetes mellitus in pregnancy. Technical Bulletin No. 92, May 1986

American College of Obstetricians and Gynecologists: Exercise during pregnancy and the postpartum period. Committee Opinion No. 267, January 2009

American College of Obstetricians and Gynecologists: Pregestational diabetes mellitus. Practice Bulletin No. 60, 2005, Reaffirmed 2012

American College of Obstetricians and Gynecologists: Gestational diabetes mellitus. Practice Bulletin No. 137, August 2013

American Diabetes Association: Gestational diabetes mellitus. Diabetes Care 26:S103, 2003

American Diabetes Association: Standards of medical care in diabetes—2011. Diabetes Care 34(1 Suppl):S11, 2011

American Diabetes Association: Standards of medical care in diabetes—2012. Diabetes Care 35(1 Suppl):S11, 2012

American Diabetes Association: Standards of medical care in diabetes—2013. Diabetes Care 36(suppl 1):S11, 2013

Arun CS, Taylor R: Influence of pregnancy on long-term progression of retinopathy in patients with type 1 diabetes. Diabetologia 51:1041, 2008

Avery MD, Leon AS, Kopher RA: Effects of a partially home-based exercise program for women with gestational diabetes. Obstet Gynecol 89:10, 1997

Bantle JP, Wylie-Rosett J, Albright AL, et al: Nutrition recommendations and interventions for diabetes. Diabetes Care 31(1 Suppl):S61, 2008

Baraban E, McCoy L, Simon P: Increasing prevalence of gestational diabetes and pregnancy-related hypertension in Los Angeles County, California, 1991–2003. Prev Chronic Dis 5:A77, 2008

Bargiota A, Kotoula M, Tsironi E, et al: Diabetic papillopathy in pregnancy. Obstet Gynecol 118:457, 2011

Ben-Haroush A, Chen R, Hadar E, et al: Accuracy of a single fetal weight estimation at 29–34 weeks in diabetic pregnancies: can it predict large-for-gestational-age infants at term? Am J Obstet Gynecol 197:497, 2007

Bental Y, Reichman B, Shiff Y, et al: Impact of maternal diabetes mellitus on mortality and morbidity of preterm infants (24–33 weeks gestation). Pediatrics 128:e848, 2011

Bradley RJ, Nicolaides KH, Brudenell JM: Are all infants of diabetic mothers "macrosomic"? BMJ 297:1583, 1988

Brankston GH, Mitchell BF, Ryan EA, et al: Resistance exercise decreases the need for insulin in overweight women with gestational diabetes mellitus. Am J Obstet Gynecol 190:188, 2004

Buhling KJ, Doll I, Siebert G, et al: Relationship between sonographically estimated fetal subcutaneous adipose tissue measurements and neonatal skinfold measurements. Ultrasound Obstet Gynecol 39:558, 2012

Bung P, Bung C, Artal R, et al: Therapeutic exercise for insulin-requiring gestational diabetes: effects on the fetus—results of a randomized prospective longitudinal study. J Perinat Med 21:125, 1993

Centers for Disease Control and Prevention: Press release: number of Americans with diabetes projected to double or triple by 2050. October 22, 2010. Available at: http:/www.cdc.gov/media/pressrel/2010/r101022.html. Accessed October 5, 2013

Chen R, Ben-Haroush A, Weissmann-Brenner A, et al: Level of glycemic control and pregnancy outcome in type q diabetes: a comparison between multiple daily insulin injections and continuous subcutaneous insulin infusions. Am J Obstet Gynecol 197:404e.1, 2007

Cheng YKY, Lao TT, Sahota DS, et al: Use of birth weight threshold for macrosomia to identify fetuses at risk of shoulder dystocia among Chinese populations. Int J Gynecol Obstet 120:249, 2013

Chico M, Levine SN, Lewis DF: Normoglycemic diabetic ketoacidosis in pregnancy. J Perinatol 28:310, 2008

Chmait R, Dinise T, Moore T: Prospective observational study to establish predictors of glyburide success in women with gestational diabetes mellitus. J Perinatol 24:617, 2004

Combs CA: Continuous glucose monitoring and insulin pump therapy for diabetes in pregnancy. J Matern Fetal Neonatal Med 25(10):2025, 2012

Conway DL, Gonzales O, Skiver D: Use of glyburide for the treatment of gestational diabetes: the San Antonio experience. J Matern Fetal Neonatal Med 15:51, 2004

Cornblath M, Hawdon JM, Williams AF, et al: Controversies regarding definition of neonatal hypoglycemia: suggested operational thresholds. Pediatrics 105:1141, 2000

Correa A, Gilboa SM, Besser LM, et al: Diabetes mellitus and birth defects. Am J Obstet Gynecol 199:237.e1, 2008

Crowther CA, Hiller JE, Moss JR, et al: Effect of treatment of gestational diabetes mellitus on pregnancy outcomes. N Engl J Med 352:2477, 2005

Cundy T: Proposed new diagnostic criteria for gestational diabetes—a pause for thought? Diabet Med 29(2):176, 2012

Dashe JS, McIntire DD, Twickler DM: Effect of maternal obesity on the ultrasound detection of anomalous fetuses. Obstet Gynecol 113(5):1001, 2009

Dashe JS, Nathan L, McIntire DD, et al: Correlation between amniotic fluid glucose concentration and amniotic fluid volume in pregnancy complicated by diabetes. Am J Obstet Gynecol 182:901, 2000

DeBoer T, Wewerka S, Bauer PJ, et al: Explicit memory performance in infants of diabetic mothers at 1 year of age. Dev Med Child Neurol 47:525, 2005

DeMarini S, Mimouni F, Tsang RC, et al: Impact of metabolic control of diabetes during pregnancy on neonatal hypocalcemia: a randomized study. Obstet Gynecol 83:918, 1994

Dempsey JC, Sorensen TK, Williams MA, et al: Prospective study of gestational diabetes mellitus in relation to maternal recreational physical activity before and during pregnancy. Am J Epidemiol 159:663, 2004

DeVeciana M, Major CA, Morgan M, et al: Postprandial versus preprandial blood glucose monitoring in women with gestational diabetes mellitus requiring insulin therapy. N Engl J Med 333:1237, 1995

Diabetes Control and Complications Trial: Effect of intensive therapy on the microvascular complications of type 1 diabetes mellitus. JAMA 287(19):2563, 2002

Diabetes Control and Complications Trial Research Group: The effect of intensive treatment of diabetes on the development and progression of long-term complications in insulin-dependent diabetes mellitus. N Engl J Med 329:977, 1993

Durnwald C, Huston-Presley L, Amini S, et al: Evaluation of body composition of large-for-gestational-age infants of women with gestational diabetes mellitus compared with women with normal glucose levels. Am J Obstet Gynecol 191:804, 2004

Ecker JL, Greene MF: Gestational diabetes—setting limits, exploring treatment. N Engl J Med 358(19):2061, 2008

Egan AM, Dennedy MC, Al-Ramli W: ATLANTIC-DIP: Excessive gestational weight gain and pregnancy outcomes in women with gestational or pregestational diabetes mellitus. J Clin Endocrinol Metab 99(1):212, 2014

Ehrenberg HM, Mercer BM, Catalano PM: The influence of obesity and diabetes on the prevalence of macrosomia. Am J Obstet Gynecol 191:964, 2004

Ehrlich SF, Hedderson MM, Feng J, et al: Change in body mass index between pregnancies and the risk of gestational diabetes in a second pregnancy. Obstet Gynecol 117(6):1323, 2011

Eidem I, Stene LC, Henriksen T, et al: Congenital anomalies in newborns of women with type 1 diabetes: nationwide population-based study in Norway, 1999–2004. Acta Obstet Gynecol Scand 89(11):1403, 2010

Eidem I, Vangen S, Hanssen KF, et al: Perinatal and infant mortality in term and preterm births among women with type 1 diabetes. Diabetologia 54(11):2771, 2011

Elman KD, Welch RA, Frank RN, et al: Diabetic retinopathy in pregnancy: a review. Obstet Gynecol 75:119, 1990

Eriksson UJ: Congenital anomalies in diabetic pregnancy. Semin Fetal Neonatal Med 14(2):85, 2009

Fadl HE, Ostlund KM, Magnusont AFK, et al: Maternal and neonatal outcomes and time trends of gestational diabetes mellitus in Sweden from 1991 to 2003. Diabet Med 27:436, 2010

Farrar D, Tufnell DJ, West J: Continuous subcutaneous insulin infusion versus multiple daily injections of insulin for pregnant women with diabetes. Cochrane Database Syst Rev 3:CD005542, 2007

Feig DS, Palda VA: Type 2 diabetes in pregnancy: a growing concern. Lancet 359:1690, 2002

Ferrara A: Increasing prevalence of gestational diabetes. Diabetes Care 30:S141, 2007

Finer LB, Zolna MR: Unintended pregnancy in the United States: incidence and disparities, 2006. Contraception 84:478, 2011

Fouda UM, Abou ElKassem MM, Hefny SM, et al: Role of fetal echocardiography in the evaluation of structure and function of fetal heart in diabetic pregnancies. J Matern Fetal Neonatal Med 26(6):571, 2013

Frank RN: Diabetic retinopathy. N Engl J Med 350:48, 2004

Fraser A, Almqvist C, Larsson H: Maternal diabetes in pregnancy and offspring cognitive ability: sibling study with 723,775 men from 579,857 families. Diabetologia 57(1):102, 2014

Gabbe S, Gregory R, Power M, et al: Management of diabetes mellitus by obstetricians-gynecologists. Obstet Gynecol 103:1229, 2004

Gabbe SG, Graves CR: Management of diabetes mellitus complicating pregnancy. Obstet Gynecol 102:857, 2003

Galindo A, Burguillo AG, Azriel S, et al: Outcome of fetuses in women with pregestational diabetes mellitus. J Perinat Med 34(4):323, 2006

Garne E, Loane M, Dolk H, et al: Spectrum of congenital anomalies in pregnancies withy pregestational diabetes. Birth Defects Res A Clin Mol Teratol 94(3):134, 2012

Garner PR: Type 1 diabetes and pregnancy. Lancet 346:966, 1995

Garabedian C, Deruelle P: Delivery (timing, route, peripartum glycemic control) in women with gestational diabetes mellitus. Diabetes Metab 36:515, 2010

Getahun D, Fassett MJ, Jacobsen SJ: Gestational diabetes: risk of recurrence in subsequent pregnancies. Am J Obstet Gynecol 203:467, 2010

Getahun D, Nath C, Ananth CV, et al: Gestational diabetes in the United States: temporal trends 1989 through 2004. Am J Obstet Gynecol 198:525.e1, 2008

Glueck CJ, Goldenberg N, Wang P, et al: Metformin during pregnancy reduces insulin, insulin resistance, insulin secretion, weight, testosterone and development of gestational diabetes: prospective longitudinal assessment of women with polycystic ovary syndrome from preconception throughout pregnancy. Hum Reprod 19:510, 2004

Gonen R, Bader D, Ajami M: Effects of policy of elective cesarean delivery in cases of suspected fetal macrosomia on the incidence of brachial plexus injury and the rate of cesarean delivery. Am J Obstet Gynecol 183:1296, 2000

Grissa O, Yessoufou A, Mrisak I, et al: Growth factor concentrations and their placental mRNA expression are modulated in gestational diabetes mellitus: possible interactions with macrosomia. BMC Pregnancy Childbirth 10:7, 2010

Guo RX, Yang LZ, Li LX, et al: Diabetic ketoacidosis in pregnancy tends to occur at lower blood glucose levels: case-control study and a case report of euglycemic diabetic ketoacidosis in pregnancy. J Obstet Gynaecol Res 34(3):324, 2008

Hammoud NM, Visser GHA, Peterst SAE, et al: Fetal growth profiles of macrosomic and non-macrosomic infants of women with pregestational or gestational diabetes. Ultrasound Obstet Gynecol 41(4):390, 2013

Hanson U, Persson B: Outcome of pregnancies complicated by type 1 insulin-dependent diabetes in Sweden: acute pregnancy complications, neonatal mortality and morbidity. Am J Perinatol 10:330, 1993

HAPO Study Cooperative Research Group: Hyperglycemia and adverse pregnancy outcomes. N Engl J Med 358:2061, 2008

Harborne L, Fleming R, Lyall H, et al: Descriptive review of the evidence for the use of metformin in polycystic ovary syndrome. Lancet 361:1894, 2003

Hartling L, Dryden DM, Guthrie A, et al: Benefits and harms of treating gestational diabetes mellitus: a systematic review and meta-analysis for the U.S. Preventive Services Task Force and the National Institutes of Health Office of Medical Applications of Research. Ann Intern Med 159(2):123, 2013

Hawkins JS, Lo JY, Casey BM, et al: Diet-treated gestational diabetes: comparison of early versus routine diagnosis. Am J Obstet Gynecol, 198:287, 2008

Hawthorne G: Maternal complications in diabetic pregnancy. Best Pract Res Clin Obstet Gynaecol 25(1):77, 2011

Hay WW: Care of the infant of the diabetic mother. Curr Diab Rep 12:4, 2012

Hay WW, Raju TNK, Higgins RD, et al: Knowledge gaps and research needs for understanding and treating neonatal hypoglycemia: workshop report from Eunice Kennedy Shriver National Institute of Child Health and Human Development. J Pediatrics 155(5):612, 2009

Hebert MF, Naraharisetti SB, Krudys KM, et al: Are we optimizing gestational diabetes treatment with glyburide? The pharmacologic basis for better clinical practice. Clin Pharmacol Ther 85(6):607, 2009

Hebert MF, Naraharisetti SB, Ma X, et al: Are we guessing glyburide dosage in the treatment of gestational diabetes (GDM)? The pharmacological evidence for better clinical practice. Am J Obstet Gynecol 197:S25, 2008

Hellmuth E, Damm P, Molsted-Pedersen L, et al: Prevalence of nocturnal hypoglycemia in first trimester of pregnancy in patients with insulin treated diabetes mellitus. Acta Obstet Gynecol Scand 79:958, 2000

Hill JB, Sheffield JS, McIntire DD, et al: Acute pyelonephritis in pregnancy. Am J Obstet Gynecol 105(1):18, 2005

Holmes HJ, Casey BM, Lo JY, et al: Likelihood of diabetes recurrence in women with mild gestational diabetes (GDM). Am J Obstet Gynecol 189 (6):161, 2003

Hornberger LK: Maternal diabetes and the fetal heart. Heart 92:1019, 2006

How HY, Sibai B, Lindheimer M, et al: Is early-pregnancy proteinuria associated with an increased rate of preeclampsia in women with pregestational diabetes mellitus? Am J Obstet Gynecol 190:775, 2004

Hunt KJ, Logan SL, Conway DL, et al: Postpartum screening following GDM: how well are we doing? Curr Diab Rep 10:235, 2010

Idris N, Wong SF, Thomae M, et al: Influence of polyhydramnios on perinatal outcome in pregestational diabetic pregnancies. Ultrasound Obstet Gynecol 36(3):338, 2010

International Association of Diabetes and Pregnancy Study Groups Consensus Panel: Recommendations on the diagnosis and classification of hyperglycemia in pregnancy. Diabetes Care 33(3), 2010

Jensen DM, Damm P, Ovesen P, et al: Microalbuminuria, preeclampsia, and preterm delivery in pregnant women with type 1 diabetes. Diabetes Care 33:90, 2010

Jovanovic-Peterson L, Durak EP, Peterson CM: Randomized trial of diet versus diet plus cardiovascular conditioning on glucose levels in gestational diabetes. Am J Obstet Gynecol 161:415, 1989

Kahn BF, Davies JK, Lynch AM, et al: Predictors of glyburide failure in the treatment of gestational diabetes. Obstet Gynecol 107:1303, 2006

Karve A, Hayward RA: Prevalence, diagnosis, and treatment of impaired fasting glucose and impaired glucose tolerance in nondiabetic U.S. adults. Diabetes Care 33:2355, 2010

Kerlan V: Postpartum and contraception in women after gestational diabetes. Diabetes Metab 36:566, 2010

Kessous R, Shoham-Vardi I, Pariente G, et al: An association between gestational diabetes mellitus and long-term maternal cardiovascular morbidity. Heart 99:1118, 2013

Kim C, Cheng YJ, Beckles GL: Cardiovascular disease risk profiles in women with histories of gestational diabetes but without current diabetes. Obstet Gynecol 112(4):875, 2008

Kim C, Ferrara A, McEwen LN, et al: Preconception care in managed care: the translating research into action for diabetes study. Am J Obstet Gynecol 192:227, 2005

Kitzmiller JL, Block JM, Brown FM, et al: Managing preexisting diabetes for pregnancy. Diabetes Care 31(5):1060, 2008

Kjos SL, Henry OA, Montoro M, et al: Insulin-requiring diabetes in pregnancy: a randomized trial of active induction of labor and expectant management. Am J Obstet Gynecol 169:611, 1993

Klemetti M, Nuutila M, Tikkanen M, et al: Trends in maternal BMI, glycaemic control and perinatal outcome among type 1 diabetic pregnant women in 1989–2008. Diabetologia 55:2327, 2012

Knip M, Virtanen SM, Becker D, et al: Early feeding and risk of type 1 diabetes: experiences from the trial to reduce insulin-dependent diabetes mellitus in the genetically at risk (TRIGR). Am J Clin Nutr 94(Suppl 1):1814S, 2011

Krakowiak P, Walker CK, Bremer AA, et al: Maternal metabolic conditions and risk for autism and other neurodevelopmental disorders. Pediatrics 129:e1121, 2012

Landon MB, Catalano PM, Gabbe SG: Diabetes mellitus complicating pregnancy. In Gabbe SG, Niebyl JR, Simpson JL, et al (eds): Obstetrics: Normal and Problem Pregnancies, 5th ed. Philadelphia, Churchill Livingstone, 2007, p 997

Landon MB, Mele L, Spong CY, et al: The relationship between maternal glycemia and perinatal outcome. Obstet Gynecol 117(2):218, 2011

Landon MB, Spong CY, Thom E, et al: A multicenter, randomized treatment trial of mild gestational diabetes. N Engl J Med 361(14):1339, 2009

Langer O, Conway DL, Berkus MD, et al: A comparison of glyburide and insulin in women with gestational diabetes mellitus. N Engl J Med 343:1134, 2000

Langer O, Yogev Y, Xenakis EMJ, et al: Insulin and glyburide therapy: dosage, severity level of gestational diabetes, and pregnancy outcome. Am J Obstet Gynecol 192:134, 2005

Lauenborg J, Mathiesen E, Ovesen P, et al: Audit on stillbirths in women with pregestational type 1 diabetes. Diabetes Care 26(5):1385, 2003

Leinonen PJ, Hiilesmaa VK, Kaaja RJ: Maternal mortality in type 1 diabetes. Diabetes Care 24(8):1501, 2001

Leipold H, Kautzsky-willer, Ozbal A, et al: Fetal hyperinsulinism and maternal one-hour post load plasma glucose level. Obstet Gynecol 104:1301, 2004

Lepercq J, Le Meaux JP, Agman A, et al: Factors associated with cesarean delivery in nulliparous women with type 1 diabetes. Obstet Gynecol 115(5):1014, 2010

Leveno KJ, Hauth JC, Gilstrap LC III, et al: Appraisal of "rigid" blood glucose control during pregnancy in the overtly diabetic woman. Am J Obstet Gynecol 135:853, 1979

Loukovaara M, Leinonen P, Teramo K, et al: Diabetic pregnancy associated with increased epidermal growth factor in cord serum at term. Obstet Gynecol 103:240, 2004

Luo ZC, Nuyt AM, Delvin E, et al: Maternal and fetal IGF-1 and IGF-11 levels, fetal growth, and gestational diabetes. J Clin Endocrinol Metab 97:1720, 2012

Martin JA, Hamilton BE, Sutton PD, et al: Births: final data for 2006. Natl Vital Stat Rep 57 (7):1, 2009

Maso G, Alberico S, Wisenfeld U, et al: GINEXMAL RCT: induction of labour versus expectant management in gestational diabetes pregnancies. BMC Pregnancy Childbirth 11:31, 2011

Mathiesen ER, Ringholm L, Feldt-Rasmussen B, et al: Obstetric nephrology: pregnancy in women with diabetic nephropathy–the role of antihypertensive treatment. Clin J Am Soc Nephrol 7:2081, 2012

Mazaki-Tovi S, Kanety H, Pariente C, et al: Cord blood adiponectinin large-for-gestational age newborns. Am J Obstet Gynecol 193:1238, 2005

McCance DR, Holmes VA, Maresh MJA, et al: Vitamins C and E for prevention of preeclampsia in women with type 1 diabetes (DAPIT): a randomised placebo-controlled trial. Lancet 376:259, 2010

McElvy SS, Demarini S, Miodovnik M, et al: Fetal weight and progression of diabetic retinopathy. Obstet Gynecol 97:587, 2001

McFarland MB, Langer O, Fazioni E, et al: Anthropometric and body composition differences in large-for-gestational age, but not appropriate-for-gestational age infants of mothers with and without diabetes mellitus. J Soc Gynecol Investig 7:231, 2000

McKinney PA, Parslow R, Gurney KA, et al: Perinatal and neonatal determinants of childhood type 1 diabetes: a case-control study in Yorkshire, U.K. Diabetes Care 22:928, 1999

Metzger BE, Buchanan TA, Coustan DR, et al: Summary and recommendations of the Fifth International Workshop-Conference on Gestational Diabetes. Diabetes Care 30(Suppl 2):S251, 2007

Miailhe G, Le Ray C, Timsit J, et al: Factors associated with urgent cesarean delivery in women with type 1 diabetes mellitus. Obstet Gynecol 121:983, 2013

Mission JF, Marshall NE, Caughey AB: Obesity in pregnancy: a big problem and getting bigger. Obstet Gynecol Sur 88(5):389, 2013

Moore LE, Clokey D, Rappaport VJ: Metformin compared with glyburide in gestational diabetes. Obstet Gynecol 115(1):55, 2010

Moreno-Castilla C, Hernandez M, Bergua M, et al: Low-carbohydrate diet for the treatment of gestational diabetes mellitus. Diabetes Care 36:2233, 2013

Morgan SC, Relaix F, Sandell LL, et al: Oxidative stress during diabetic pregnancy disrupts cardiac neural crest migration and causes outflow tract defects. Birth Defects Res A Clin Mol Teratol 82:452, 2008

Mukhopadhyay A, Farrell T, Fraser RB, et al: Continuous subcutaneous insulin infusion vs intensive conventional insulin therapy in pregnant diabetic women: a systematic review and meta-analysis of randomized, controlled trials. Am J Obstet Gynecol 197(5):447, 2007

Murphy HR, Rayman G, Lewis K, et al: Effectiveness of continuous glucose monitoring in pregnant women with diabetes: randomised clinical trial. BMJ 337:a1680, 2008

Most O, Langer O: Gestational diabetes: maternal weight gain in relation to fetal growth, treatment modality, BMI and glycemic control. J Matern Fetal Med 25(11):2458, 2012

National Center for Health Statistics: Gestational diabetes. Available at: http://www.cdc.gov/nchs. Accessed October 8, 2013

National Institutes of Health: NIH Consensus Development Conference on Diagnosing Gestational Diabetes Mellitus. 2013. Available at: http://prevention.nih.gov/cdp/conferences/2013/gdm/files/Gestational_Diabetes_Mellitus508.pdf. Accessed October 8, 2013

National Institute for Health and Clinical Excellence: Diabetes in pregnancy. Management of diabetes and its complications from pre-conception to the postnatal period. Clinical Guideline No. 63, July 2008

Nicholson W, Bolen S, Witkop CT, et al: Benefits and risks of oral diabetes agents compared with insulin in women with gestational diabetes. Obstet Gynecol 113(1):193, 2009

O'Sullivan JB: Body weight and subsequent diabetes mellitus. JAMA 248:949, 1982

Owen CG, Martin RM, Whincup PH, et al: Does breastfeeding influence risk of type 2 diabetes in later life? A quantitative analysis of published evidence. Am J Clin Nutr 84:1043, 2006

Pedersen J: The Pregnant Diabetic and Her Newborn, 2nd ed. Baltimore, Williams & Wilkins, 1977, p 211

Pedersen J, Mølsted-Pedersen L, Andersen B: Assessors of fetal perinatal mortality in diabetic pregnancy. Analysis of 1332 pregnancies in the Copenhagen series, 1946–1972. Diabetes 23:302, 1974

Persson M, Norman M, Hanson U: Obstetric and perinatal outcomes in type I diabetic pregnancies. Diabetes Care 32:2005, 2009

Plagemann A, Franke K, Harder T, et al: Long-term impact of neonatal breastfeeding on bodyweight and glucose tolerance in children of diabetic mothers. Diabetes Care 25:16, 2002

Pombar X, Strassner HT, Fenner PC: Pregnancy in a woman with class H diabetes mellitus and previous coronary artery bypass graft: a case report and review of the literature. Obstet Gynecol 85:825, 1995

Powers AC: Diabetes mellitus. In: Longo DL, Fauci AS, Kaspar DL, et al (eds): Harrison's Principles of Internal Medicine, 18th ed. McGraw Hill, New York, 2012, p 2968

Rasmussen KL, Laugesen CS, Ringholm L, et al: Progression of diabetic retinopathy during pregnancy in women with type 2 diabetes. Diabetologia 53:1076, 2010

Reece EA: Diabetes-induced birth defects: what do we know? What can we do? Curr Diab Rep 12:24, 2012

Reutens AT: Epidemiology of diabetic kidney disease. Med Clin North Am 97:1, 2013

Ringholm L, Vestgaard M, Laugesen CS, et al: Pregnancy-induced increase in circulating IGF-1 is associated with progression of diabetic retinopathy in women with type 1 diabetes. Growth Horm IGF Res 21:25, 2011

Rizzo TA, Dooley SL, Metzger BE, et al: Prenatal and perinatal influences on long-term psychomotor development in offspring of diabetic mothers. Am J Obstet Gynecol 173:1753, 1995

Roeder HA, Moore TR, Ramos GA: Insulin pump dosing across gestation in women with well-controlled type 1 diabetes mellitus. Am J Obstet Gynecol 207:324.e1, 2012

Rolo LC, Nardozza LMM, Junior EA, et al: Reference curve of the fetal ventricular septum area by the STIC method: preliminary study. Arq Bras Cardiol 96(5):386, 2011

Rosenn B, Miodovnik M, Combs CA, et al: Glycemic thresholds for spontaneous abortion and congenital malformations in insulin-dependent diabetes mellitus. Obstet Gynecol 84:515, 1994

Rowan JA, Hague WM, Wanzhen G, et al: Metformin versus insulin for the treatment of gestational diabetes. N Engl J Med 358:2003, 2008

Russell NE, Foley M, Kinsley BT, et al: Effect of pregestational diabetes mellitus on fetal cardiac function and structure. Am J Obstet Gynecol 199:312.e1, 2008

Salvesen DR, Brudenell MJ, Nicolaides KH: Fetal polycythemia and thrombocytopenia in pregnancies complicated by maternal diabetes mellitus. Am J Obstet Gynecol 166:1287, 1992

Salvesen DR, Brudenell MJ, Snijders JM, et al: Fetal plasma erythropoietin in pregnancies complicated by maternal diabetes mellitus. Am J Obstet Gynecol 168:88, 1993

Saudek CD: Progress and promise of diabetes research. JAMA 287:2582, 2002

Scholte JBJ, Boer WE: A case of nondiabetic ketoacidosis in third term twin pregnancy. J Clin Endocrinol Metab 97:3021, 2012

Shah BR, Retnakaran R, Booth GL: Increased risk of cardiovascular disease in young women following gestational diabetes. Diabetes Care 31(8):1668, 2008

Sheffield JS, Butler-Koster EL, Casey BM, et al: Maternal diabetes mellitus and infant malformations. Obstet Gynecol 100:925, 2002

Sheiner E, Mazor-Drey E, Levy A: Asymptomatic bacteriuria during pregnancy. J Matern Fetal Neonatal Med 22(5):423, 2009

Sibai BM, Caritis S, Hauth J, et al: Risks of preeclampsia and adverse neonatal outcomes among women with pregestational diabetes mellitus. Am J Obstet Gynecol 182:364, 2000

Sibai BM, Viteri OA: Diabetic ketoacidosis in pregnancy. Obstet Gynecol 123(1):167, 2014

Silverman BL, Metzger BI, Cho NH, et al: Fetal hyperinsulinism and impaired glucose intolerance in adolescent offspring of diabetic mothers. Diabetes Care 18:611, 1995

Singh, SR, Ahmad F, Lai A, et al: Efficacy and safety of insulin analogues for the management of diabetes mellitus: a meta-analysis. CMAJ 180(4):385, 2009

Stafne SN, Salvesen KA, Romundstad PR, et al: Regular exercise during pregnancy to prevent gestational diabetes. Obstet Gynecol 119(1):29, 2012

Stamler EF, Cruz ML, Mimouni F, et al: High infectious morbidity in pregnant women with insulin-dependent diabetes: an understated complication. Am J Obstet Gynecol 163:1217, 1990

Stuebe AM, Landon MB, Lai Y, et al: Maternal BMI, glucose tolerance, and adverse pregnancy outcomes. Am J Obstet Gynecol 207:62.e.1, 2012

Suresh A, Liu A, Poulton A, et al: Comparison of maternal abdominal subcutaneous fat thickness and body mass index as markers for pregnancy outcomes: a stratified cohort study. Aust N Z J Obstet Gynecol 52:420, 2012

Takoudes TC, Weitzen S, Slocum J, et al: Risk of cesarean wound complications in diabetic gestations. Am J Obstet Gynecol 191:958, 2004

Temple RC, Aldridge V, Stanley K, et al: Glycaemic control throughout pregnancy and risk of pre-eclampsia in women with type 1 diabetes. BJOG 113:1329, 2006

Torloni MR, Betran AP, Horta BL, et al: Prepregnancy BMI and the risk of gestational diabetes: a systematic review of the literature with meta-analysis. Obes Rev 10:194, 2009

U.S. Preventive Services Task Force: Screening for gestational diabetes mellitus: U.S. Preventive Services Task Force draft recommendation statement. Available at: http://www.uspreventiveservicestaskforce.org/draftrec2.htm. Accessed October 8, 2013

Van Leeuwen M, Louwerse MD, Opmeer BC, et al: Glucose challenge test for detecting gestational diabetes mellitus: a systematic review. BJOG 119(4):393, 2012

Vestgaard M, Ringholm L, Laugesen CS, et al: Pregnancy-induced sight-threatening diabetic retinopathy in women with type 1 diabetes. Diabet Med 27:431, 2010

Vidaeff AC, Yeomans ER, Ramin SM: Pregnancy in women with renal disease. Part II: specific underlying renal conditions. Am J Perinatol 25:399, 2008

Vink JY, Poggi SH, Ghidini A: Amniotic fluid index and birth weight: is there a relationship in diabetics with poor glycemic control? Am J Obstet Gynecol 195:848, 2006

Wang PH, Lau J, Chalmers TC: Meta-analysis of effects of intensive blood-glucose control on late complications of type 1 diabetes. Lancet 341:1306, 1993

White P: Classification of obstetric diabetes. Am J Obstet Gynecol 130:228, 1978

Witkop CT, Neale D, Wilson LM, et al: Active compared with expectant delivery management in women with gestational diabetes. Obstet Gynecol 113(1):206, 2009

World Health Organization: Definition, diagnosis and classification of diabetes mellitus and its complications. Part 1: diagnosis and classification of diabetes mellitus, provisional report of a WHO consultation. Diabet Med 15:539, 1998

Yang J, Cummings EA, O'Connell C, et al: Fetal and neonatal outcomes of diabetic pregnancies. Obstet Gynecol 108:644, 2006

Yanit KE, Snowden JM, Cheng YW, et al: The impact of chronic hypertension and pregestational diabetes on pregnancy outcomes. Am J Obstet Gynecol 207:333, 2012

Young EC, Pires M, Marques L, et al: Effects of pregnancy on the onset and progression of diabetic nephropathy and of diabetic nephropathy on pregnancy outcomes. Diabetes Metab Syndr 5:137, 2012

CHAPTER 58

Endocrine Disorders

There are no endocrine disorders that are unique to pregnancy. However, endocrinopathies seem particularly closely related to pregnancy due to their proclivity for hormone secretion. Indeed, some hormones are secreted in prodigious quantities. This is probably best illustrated by placental lactogen in diabetes, the most common endocrinopathy encountered in pregnancy (Chap. 57, p. 1125). Pregnancy is also interrelated with some endocrinopathies that are at least partially due to autoimmune dysregulation. Clinical manifestations of this result from complex interplay among genetic, environmental, and endogenous factors that activate the immune system against targeted cells within endocrine organs. An extraordinary example of these interactions comes from studies that implicate maternal organ engraftment by fetal cells that were transferred during pregnancy. These cells later provoke antibody production, tissue destruction, and autoimmune endocrinopathies.

THYROID DISORDERS

Taken in aggregate, these are common in young women and thus frequently managed in pregnancy. There is an intimate relationship between maternal and fetal thyroid function, and drugs that affect the maternal thyroid also affect the fetal gland. Moreover, thyroid autoantibodies have been associated with increased early pregnancy wastage, and uncontrolled thyrotoxicosis and untreated hypothyroidism are both associated with adverse pregnancy outcomes. Finally, there is evidence that autoimmune thyroid disorder severity may be ameliorated during pregnancy, only to be exacerbated postpartum.

Thyroid Physiology and Pregnancy

Maternal thyroid changes are substantial, and normally altered gland structure and function are sometimes confused with thyroid abnormalities. These alterations are discussed in detail in Chapter 4 (p. 68), and normal hormone level values are found in the Appendix (p. 1290). First, maternal serum concentrations of thyroid-binding globulin are increased concomitantly with total or bound thyroid hormone levels (Fig. 4-17, p. 69). Second, *thyrotropin,* also called *thyroid-stimulating hormone (TSH),* currently plays a central role in screening and diagnosis of many thyroid disorders. Serum TSH levels in early pregnancy decline because of weak TSH-receptor stimulation from massive quantities of human chorionic gonadotropin (hCG) secreted by placental trophoblast. Because TSH does not cross the placenta, it has no direct fetal effects. During the first 12 weeks of gestation, when hCG serum levels are maximal, thyroid hormone secretion is stimulated. The resulting increased serum free thyroxine levels act to suppress hypothalamic *thyrotropin-releasing hormone (TRH)* and in turn limit pituitary TSH secretion (Fig. 58-1). Accordingly, TRH is undetectable in maternal serum. Conversely, beginning at midpregnancy,

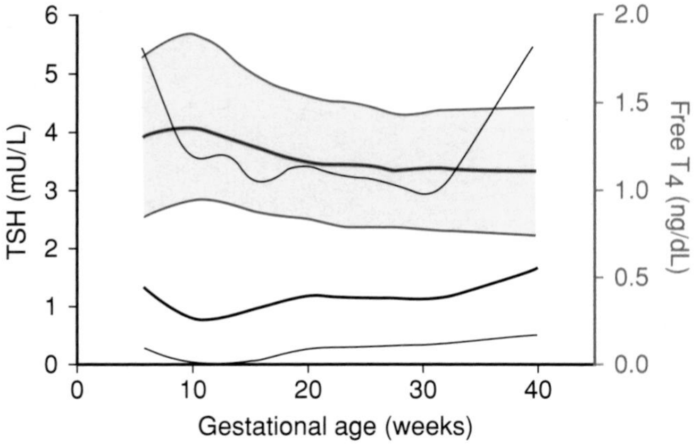

FIGURE 58-1 Gestational age-specific values for serum thyroid-stimulating hormone (TSH) levels (*black lines*) and free thyroxine (T_4) levels (*blue lines*). Data were derived from 17,298 women tested during pregnancy. For each color, the dark solid lines represent the 50th percentile, whereas the upper and lower light lines represent the 2.5th and 97.5th percentiles, respectively. (Data from Casey, 2005; Dashe, 2005.)

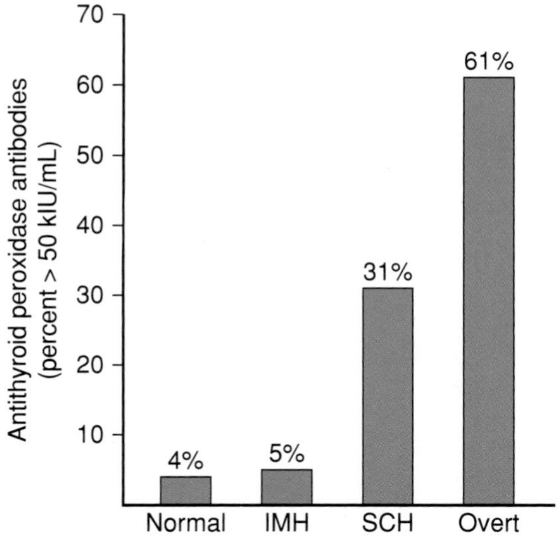

FIGURE 58-2 Incidence in percent of antithyroid peroxidase antibodies in 16,407 women who are normal or euthyroid, in 233 with isolated maternal hypothyroxinemia (IMH), in 598 with subclinical hypothyroidism (SCH), and in 134 with overt hypothyroidism. (Data from Casey, 2007).

TRH becomes detectable in fetal serum, but levels are static and do not increase with advancing gestation.

Throughout pregnancy, maternal thyroxine is transferred to the fetus (Calvo, 2002). Maternal thyroxine is important for normal fetal brain development, especially before development of fetal thyroid gland function (Bernal, 2007). And even though the fetal gland begins concentrating iodine and synthesizing thyroid hormone after 12 weeks' gestation, maternal thyroxine contribution remains important. In fact, maternal sources account for 30 percent of thyroxine in fetal serum at term (Thorpe-Beeston, 1991; Vulsma, 1989). Developmental risks associated with maternal hypothyroidism after midpregnancy, however, remain poorly understood (Morreale de Escobar, 2004).

Autoimmunity and Thyroid Disease

Most thyroid disorders are inextricably linked to autoantibodies against various cell components. Several of these antibodies variably stimulate thyroid function, block function, or cause thyroid inflammation that may lead to follicular cell destruction. Often, these effects overlap or even coexist.

Thyroid-stimulating autoantibodies, also called *thyroid-stimulating immunoglobulins (TSIs)*, bind to the TSH receptor and activate it, causing thyroid hyperfunction and growth. Although these antibodies are identified in most patients with classic Graves disease, simultaneous production of *thyroid-stimulating blocking antibodies* may blunt this effect (Weetman, 2000). *Thyroid peroxidase (TPO)* is a thyroid gland enzyme that normally functions in the production of thyroid hormones. *Thyroid peroxidase antibodies*, previously called *thyroid microsomal autoantibodies*, are directed against TPO and have been identified in 5 to 15 percent of all pregnant women (Fig. 58-2) (Abbassi-Ghanavati, 2010; Kuijpens, 2001). These antibodies have been associated in some studies with early pregnancy loss and preterm birth (Abramson, 2001; Negro, 2006; Thangaratinam, 2011). Conversely, in a study with more than 1000 TPO antibody-positive pregnant women, there was no increased risk for preterm birth, however, there was an increased risk for placental abruption (Abbassi-Ghanavati, 2010). These women are also at high risk for postpartum thyroid dysfunction and at lifelong risk for permanent thyroid failure (Premawardhana, 2000; Stagnaro-Green, 2011b).

Fetal Microchimerism

Autoimmune thyroid disease is much more common in women than in men. One intriguing explanation for this disparity is fetal-to-maternal cell trafficking (Greer, 2011). When fetal lymphocytes enter the maternal circulation, they can live for more than 20 years. Stem cell interchange also occurs with engraftment in several maternal tissues including the thyroid (Bianchi, 2003; Khosrotehrani, 2004). A high prevalence of Y-chromosome-positive cells has been identified using fluorescence in situ hybridization (FISH) in thyroid glands of women with Hashimoto thyroiditis—60 percent, or Graves disease—40 percent (Renné, 2004). In another study of women giving birth to a male fetus, Lepez and colleagues (2011) identified significantly more circulating male mononuclear cells in those with Hashimoto thyroiditis.

Hyperthyroidism

The incidence of thyrotoxicosis or hyperthyroidism in pregnancy is varied and complicates between 2 and 17 per 1000 births when gestational-age appropriate TSH threshold values are used (Table 58-1). Because normal pregnancy simulates some clinical findings similar to thyroxine (T_4) excess, clinically mild thyrotoxicosis may be difficult to diagnose. Suggestive findings include tachycardia that exceeds that usually seen with normal pregnancy, thyromegaly, exophthalmos, and failure to gain weight despite adequate food intake. Laboratory confirmation is by a markedly depressed TSH level along with an elevated

TABLE 58-1. Incidence of Overt Hyperthyroidism in Pregnancy

Study	Country	Overt Hypothyroidism
Wang (2011)[a]	China	1%
Vaidya (2007)[a]	United Kingdom	0.7%
Lazarus (2007)[b]	United Kingdom	1.7%
Casey (2006b)[c]	United States	0.4%

[a]Screened in the first trimester.
[b]Screened at 9–15 weeks.
[c]Screened at < 20 weeks.

serum free T_4 (fT_4) level. Rarely, hyperthyroidism is caused by abnormally high serum triiodothyronine (T_3) levels—so-called *T_3-toxicosis.*

Thyrotoxicosis and Pregnancy

The overwhelming cause of thyrotoxicosis in pregnancy is *Graves disease*, an organ-specific autoimmune process associated with thyroid-stimulating TSH-receptor antibodies as previously discussed. Because these antibodies are specific to Graves hyperthyroidism, such assays have been proposed for diagnosis, management, and prognosis in pregnancies complicated by hyperthyroidism (Barbesino, 2013). At Parkland Hospital, these receptor antibody assays are generally reserved for cases in which fetal thyrotoxicosis is suspected. With Graves disease, during the course of pregnancy, hyperthyroid symptoms may initially worsen because of chorionic gonadotropin stimulation, but then subsequently diminish with decreases in receptor antibody titers in the second half of pregnancy (Mestman, 2012; Stagnaro-Green, 2011a). Amino and coworkers (2003) have found that levels of blocking antibodies are also decreased during pregnancy.

Treatment. Thyrotoxicosis during pregnancy can nearly always be controlled by thionamide drugs. *Propylthiouracil (PTU)* has been historically preferred because it partially inhibits the conversion of T_4 to T_3 and crosses the placenta less readily than *methimazole.* The latter has also been associated with a rare methimazole embryopathy characterized by *esophageal* or *choanal atresia* as well as *aplasia cutis*, a congenital skin defect. Yoshihara and associates (2012) analyzed more than 5000 Japanese women with first-trimester hyperthyroidism and found a twofold increased risk of major fetal malformations in pregnancies exposed to methimazole compared with the risk from PTU. Specifically, seven of nine cases with aplasia cutis and the only case of esophageal atresia were in the group of methimazole-exposed infants.

Until recently, PTU has been the preferred thionamide in the United States (Brent, 2008). In 2009, however, the Food and Drug Administration issued a safety alert on PTU-associated hepatotoxicity. This warning prompted the American Thyroid Association and the American Association of Clinical Endocrinologists (2011) to recommend PTU therapy during the first trimester followed by methimazole beginning in the second trimester. The obvious disadvantage is that this might lead to poorly controlled thyroid function. Accordingly, at Parkland Hospital we continue to prescribe PTU treatment throughout pregnancy.

Transient leukopenia can be documented in up to 10 percent of women taking antithyroid drugs, but this does not require therapy cessation. In 0.3 to 0.4 percent, however, *agranulocytosis* develops suddenly and mandates drug discontinuance. It is not dose related, and because of its acute onset, serial leukocyte counts during therapy are not helpful. Thus, if fever or sore throat develops, women are instructed to discontinue medication immediately and report for a complete blood count (Brent, 2008).

As mentioned above, hepatotoxicity is another potentially serious side effect that develops in 0.1 to 0.2 percent. Serial measurement of hepatic enzymes has not been shown to prevent fulminant PTU-related hepatotoxicity. Also, approximately 20 percent of patients treated with PTU develop *antineutrophil cytoplasmic antibodies (ANCA).* However, only a small percentage of these subsequently develop serious vasculitis (Helfgott, 2002; Kimura, 2013). Finally, although thionamides have the potential to cause fetal complications, these are uncommon. In some cases, thionamides may even be therapeutic, because TSH-receptor antibodies cross the placenta and can stimulate the fetal thyroid gland to cause thyrotoxicosis and goiter.

The initial thionamide dose is empirical. For nonpregnant patients, the American Thyroid Association recommends that methimazole be used at an initial higher daily dose of 10 to 20 mg orally followed by a lower maintenance dose of 5 to 10 mg. If PTU is selected, a dose of 50 to 150 mg orally three times daily may be initiated depending on clinical severity (Bahn, 2011). At Parkland Hospital, we usually initially give 300 or 450 mg of PTU daily in three divided doses for pregnant women. Occasionally, daily doses of 600 mg are necessary. As discussed, we generally do not transition women to methimazole during the second trimester. The goal is treatment with the lowest possible thionamide dose to maintain thyroid hormone levels slightly above or in the high normal range while TSH levels remains suppressed (Bahn, 2011). Serum free T_4 concentrations are measured every 4 to 6 weeks (National Academy of Clinical Biochemistry, 2002).

Subtotal thyroidectomy can be performed after thyrotoxicosis is medically controlled. This seldom is done during pregnancy but may be appropriate for the very few women who cannot adhere to medical treatment or in whom drug therapy proves toxic (Davison, 2001; Stagnaro-Green, 2012a). Surgery is best accomplished in the second trimester. Potential drawbacks of thyroidectomy during pregnancy include inadvertent resection of parathyroid glands and injury to the recurrent laryngeal nerve (Fitzpatrick, 2010).

Thyroid ablation with therapeutic radioactive iodine is contraindicated during pregnancy. These doses may also cause fetal thyroid gland destruction. Thus, when given unintentionally, many clinicians recommend abortion. Any exposed fetus must be carefully evaluated, and the incidence of fetal hypothyroidism depends on gestational age and radioiodine dose (Berlin, 2001). Tran and colleagues (2010) describe a case in which a relatively high dose (19.8 mCi) of radioiodine early in the first trimester resulted in a normal euthyroid male infant assessed at 6 months. The authors hypothesized that the exposure occurred well before thyroid embryogenesis. There is no evidence that radioiodine given before pregnancy causes fetal anomalies if enough time has passed to allow radiation effects to dissipate and if the woman is euthyroid (Ayala, 1998). The International Commission on Radiological Protection has recommended that women avoid pregnancy for 6 months after radioablative therapy (Brent, 2008). Moreover, during lactation, the breast also concentrates a substantial amount of iodide. This may pose neonatal risk due to ^{131}I-containing milk ingestion and maternal risk from significant breast irradiation. To limit maternal exposure and her cancer risks, a delay of 3 months between lactation and ablation will more reliably ensure complete breast involution (Sisson, 2011).

Pregnancy Outcome. Women with thyrotoxicosis have pregnancy outcomes that largely depend on whether metabolic control is achieved. For example, as discussed in Chapter 18 (p. 353), excess thyroxine may cause miscarriage (Anselmo, 2004). In untreated women or in those who remain hyperthyroid despite therapy, there is a higher incidence of preeclampsia, heart failure, and adverse perinatal outcomes (Table 58-2). A prospective cohort study from China reported that women with clinical hyperthyroidism had a 12-fold increased risk of delivering an infant with hearing loss (Su, 2011). Perinatal mortality rates varied from 6 to 12 percent in several studies.

Fetal and Neonatal Effects

In most cases, the perinate is euthyroid. In some, however, hyper- or hypothyroidism can develop with or without a goiter (Fig. 58-3). Clinical hyperthyroidism develops in approximately 1 percent of neonates born to women with Graves disease (Barbesino, 2013; Fitzpatrick, 2010; Luton, 2005). If fetal thyroid disease is suspected, nomograms are available for

TABLE 58-2. Pregnancy Outcomes in 239 Women with Overt Thyrotoxicosis

Factor	Treated and Euthyroid[a] n = 149	Uncontrolled Thyrotoxicosis[a] n = 90
Maternal outcome		
Preeclampsia	17 (11%)	15 (17%)
Heart failure	1	7 (8%)
Death	0	1
Perinatal outcome		
Preterm delivery	12 (8%)	29 (32%)
Growth restriction	11 (7%)	15 (17%)
Stillbirth	0/59	6/33 (18%)
Thyrotoxicosis	1	2
Hypothyroidism	4	0
Goiter	2	0

[a]Data presented as n (%).
Data from Davis, 1989; Kriplani, 1994; Millar, 1994.

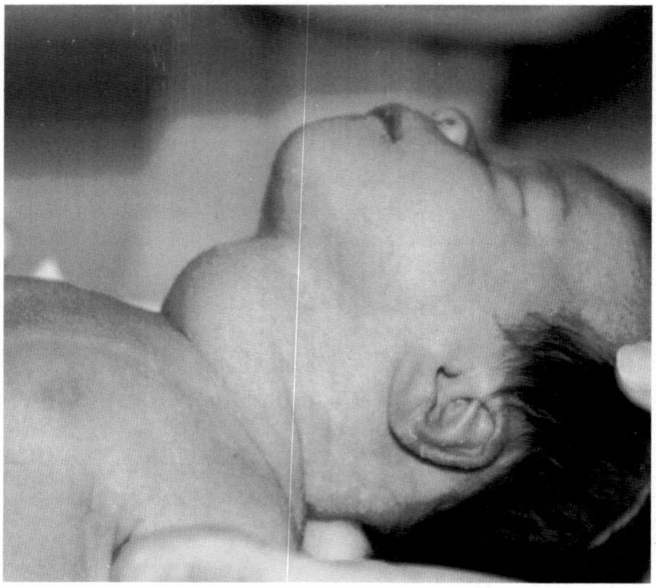

FIGURE 58-3 Term neonate delivered of a woman with a 3-year history of thyrotoxicosis that recurred at 26 weeks' gestation. The mother was given methimazole 30 mg orally daily and was euthyroid at delivery. Laboratory studies showed that the infant was hypothyroid.

sonographically measured thyroid volume (Gietka-Czernel, 2012; Ranzini, 2001).

The fetus or neonate who was exposed to excessive maternal thyroxine may have any of several clinical presentations. First, *goitrous thyrotoxicosis* is caused by placental transfer of thyroid-stimulating immunoglobulins. *Nonimmune hydrops* and fetal demise have been reported with fetal thyrotoxicosis (Nachum, 2003; Stulberg, 2000). The best predictor of perinatal thyrotoxicosis is presence of thyroid-stimulating TSH-receptor antibodies in women with Graves disease. This is especially true if their levels are more than threefold higher than the upper normal limit (Barbesino, 2013). In a study of 72 pregnant women with Graves disease, Luton and associates (2005) reported that none of the fetuses in 31 low-risk mothers had a goiter, and all were euthyroid at delivery. Low risk was defined by no antithyroid medications during the third trimester or absence of antithyroid antibodies. Conversely, in a group of 41 women who either were taking antithyroid medication at delivery or had thyroid receptor antibodies, 11 fetuses—27 percent—had sonographic evidence of a goiter at 32 weeks' gestation. Seven of these 11 were determined to be hypothyroid, and the remaining fetuses were hyperthyroid. In response to such results, the American Thyroid Association and American Association of Clinical Endocrinologists (2011) recommend routine evaluation of TSH-receptor antibodies between 22 and 26 weeks' gestation in women with Graves disease. The American College of Obstetricians and Gynecologists (2013), however, does not recommend such testing because management is rarely changed by the results. If the fetus is thyrotoxic, treatment is by adjustment of maternal thionamide drugs even though maternal thyroid function may be within the targeted range (Duncombe, 2001; Mestman, 2012). Occasionally, neonatal thyrotoxicosis may also require short-course antithyroid drug treatment.

A second presentation is *goitrous hypothyroidism* caused by fetal exposure to maternally administered thionamides (see Fig. 58-3). Although there are theoretical neurological implications, reports of adverse fetal effects seem to have been exaggerated. Available data indicate that thionamides carry an extremely small risk for causing neonatal hypothyroidism (Momotani, 1997; O'Doherty, 1999). For example, of the 239 treated thyrotoxic women shown in Table 58-1, there was evidence of hypothyroidism in only four infants despite relatively high maternal PTU doses. Furthermore, at least four long-term studies report no abnormal intellectual and physical development of these children (Mestman, 1998). If hypothyroidism is identified, the fetus can be treated by a reduced maternal antithyroid medication dose and injection of intraamnionic thyroxine if necessary.

A third presentation, *nongoitrous hypothyroidism,* may develop from transplacental passage of maternal TSH-receptor blocking antibodies (Fitzpatrick, 2010; Gallagher, 2001). And finally, *fetal thyrotoxicosis* after maternal thyroid gland ablation, usually with ^{131}I radioiodine, may result from transplacental thyroid-stimulating antibodies. In the previously described case of early fetal exposure to radioiodine, neonatal thyroid studies indicated transient hyperthyroidism from maternal transfer of stimulating antibodies (Tran, 2010).

Fetal Diagnosis. Evaluation of fetal thyroid function is somewhat controversial. Although fetal thyroid sonographic assessment has been reported in women taking thionamide drugs or those with thyroid-stimulating antibodies, most investigators do not currently recommend this routinely (Cohen, 2003; Luton, 2005). Kilpatrick (2003) recommends umbilical blood sampling and fetal antibody testing only if the mother has previously undergone radioiodine ablation. Because fetal hyper- or hypothyroidism may cause hydrops, growth restriction, goiter, or tachycardia, fetal blood sampling may be appropriate if these are identified (Brand, 2005). The Endocrine Society Clinical Practice Guidelines recommend umbilical blood sampling only when the diagnosis of fetal thyroid disease cannot be reasonably ascertained based on clinical and sonographic data (Garber, 2012). Diagnosis and treatment are considered further in Chapter 16 (p. 324).

Thyroid Storm and Heart Failure

Both are acute and life-threatening in pregnancy. Thyroid storm is a hypermetabolic state and is rare in pregnancy. In contrast, pulmonary hypertension and heart failure from cardiomyopathy caused by the profound myocardial effects of thyroxine is common in pregnant women (Sheffield, 2004). As shown in Table 58-2, heart failure developed in 8 percent of 90 women with uncontrolled thyrotoxicosis. In these women, cardiomyopathy is characterized by a high-output state, which may lead to a dilated cardiomyopathy (Fadel, 2000; Klein, 1998). The pregnant woman with thyrotoxicosis has minimal cardiac reserve, and decompensation is usually precipitated by preeclampsia, anemia, sepsis, or a combination of these. Fortunately, thyroxine-induced cardiomyopathy and pulmonary hypertension are frequently reversible (Sheffield, 2004; Siu, 2007; Vydt, 2006).

Management. Treatment for thyroid storm or heart failure is similar and should be carried out in an intensive care area that may include special-care units within labor and delivery (Fitzpatrick, 2010; Zeeman, 2003). Shown in Figure 58-4 is our stepwise approach to medical management of thyroid storm or thyrotoxic heart failure. An hour or two after initial thionamide administration, iodide is given to inhibit thyroidal release of T_3 and T_4. It can be given intravenously as sodium iodide or orally as either saturated solution of potassium iodide (SSKI) or Lugol solution. With a history of iodine-induced anaphylaxis, lithium carbonate, 300 mg every 6 hours, is given instead. Most authorities recommend dexamethasone, 2 mg intravenously every 6 hours for four doses, to further block peripheral conversion of T_4 to T_3. If a β-blocker drug is given to control tachycardia, its effect on heart failure must be considered. Propranolol, labetalol, and esmolol have all been used successfully. Coexisting severe preeclampsia, infection, or anemia should be aggressively managed before delivery is considered.

Hyperemesis Gravidarum and Gestational Transient Thyrotoxicosis

Transient biochemical features of hyperthyroidism may be observed in 2 to 15 percent of women in early pregnancy (Fitzpatrick, 2010). Many women with hyperemesis gravidarum have abnormally high serum thyroxine levels and low TSH levels (Chap. 54, p. 1070). This results from TSH-receptor stimulation from massive—but normal for pregnancy—concentrations of hCG. This transient condition is also termed *gestational transient thyrotoxicosis.* Even if associated with hyperemesis, antithyroid drugs are not warranted (American College of Obstetricians and Gynecologists, 2013). Serum thyroxine and TSH values become more normal by midpregnancy (Fitzpatrick, 2010).

Thyrotoxicosis and Gestational Trophoblastic Disease

The prevalence of increased thyroxine levels in women with molar pregnancy has been reported to be between 25 and 65 percent (Hershman, 2004). As discussed, abnormally high hCG levels lead to overstimulation of the TSH receptor. Because these tumors are now usually diagnosed early, clinically apparent hyperthyroidism has become less common. With definitive treatment, serum free-T_4 levels usually normalize rapidly in parallel with the decline in hCG concentrations. This is discussed further in Chapter 20 (p. 399).

Subclinical Hyperthyroidism

Third-generation TSH assays with an analytical sensitivity of 0.002 mU/mL permit identification of subclinical thyroid disorders. These biochemically defined extremes usually represent normal biological variations but may herald the earliest stages of thyroid dysfunction. *Subclinical hyperthyroidism* is characterized by an abnormally low serum TSH concentration in concert with thyroxine hormone levels within the normal reference range (Surks, 2004). Long-term effects of persistent subclinical thyrotoxicosis include osteoporosis,

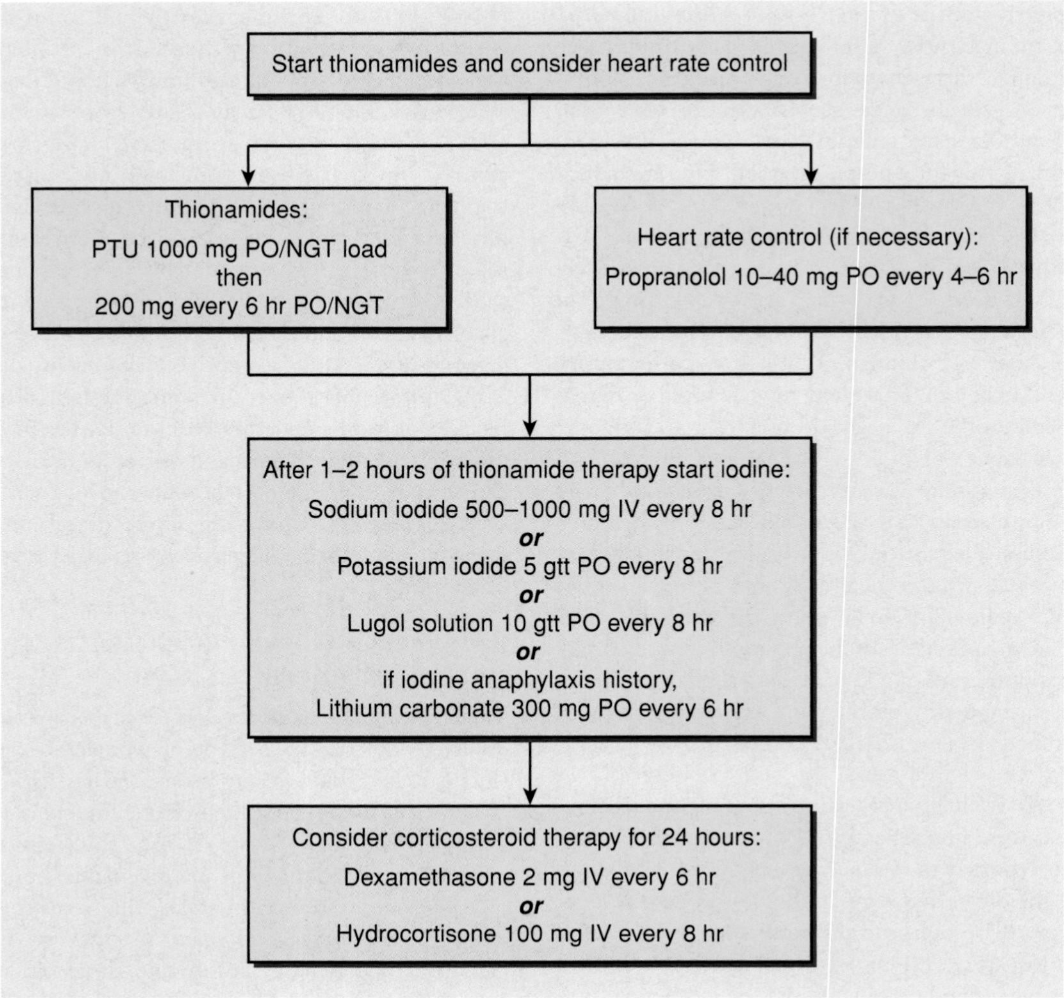

FIGURE 58-4 One management method for thyroid storm or thyrotoxic heart failure. gtt = drops; NGT = nasogastric tube; PO = orally.

cardiovascular morbidity, and progression to overt thyrotoxicosis or thyroid failure. Casey and Leveno (2006b) identified subclinical hyperthyroidism in 1.7 percent of pregnant women. Importantly, these investigators showed that subclinical hyperthyroidism was not associated with adverse pregnancy outcomes. In separate retrospective analyses of almost 25,000 women who underwent thyroid screening throughout pregnancy, Wilson and colleagues (2012) and Tudela and coworkers (2012) confirmed no relationship between subclinical hyperthyroidism and preeclampsia or gestational diabetes.

The American Thyroid Association and American Association of Clinical Endocrinologists guidelines recommend consideration for treatment of subclinical hyperthyroidism in individuals 65 years or older and in postmenopausal women to improve cardiovascular health and bone mineral density. There is, however, no convincing evidence that subclinical hyperthyroidism should be treated in younger nonpregnant individuals. Thus, treatment seems especially unwarranted in pregnancy because antithyroid drugs may affect the fetus. Women identified with subclinical hyperthyroidism may benefit from periodic surveillance, and approximately half eventually have normal TSH concentrations.

Hypothyroidism

Overt or symptomatic hypothyroidism, as shown in Table 58-3, has been reported to complicate between 2 and 10 pregnancies per 1000. It is characterized by insidious nonspecific clinical findings that include fatigue, constipation, cold intolerance, muscle cramps, and weight gain. A pathologically enlarged thyroid gland depends on the etiology

TABLE 58-3. Frequency of Overt Hypothyroidism in Pregnancy

Study	Country	Overt Hypothyroidism
Wang (2011)[a]	China	0.3%
Cleary-Goldman (2008)[a]	United States	0.3%
Vaidya (2007)[a]	United Kingdom	1.0%
Casey (2005)[b]	United States	0.2%

[a]Screened during first trimester.
[b]Screened at < 20 weeks' gestation.

of hypothyroidism and is more likely in women in areas of endemic iodine deficiency or those with Hashimoto thyroiditis. Other findings include edema, dry skin, hair loss, and prolonged relaxation phase of deep tendon reflexes. *Clinical* or *overt hypothyroidism* is confirmed when an abnormally high serum TSH level is accompanied by an abnormally low thyroxine level. *Subclinical hypothyroidism* is defined by an elevated serum TSH level and *normal* serum thyroxine concentration (Surks, 2004). Included in the spectrum of subclinical thyroid disease are asymptomatic individuals with measurable antithyroid peroxidase or antithyroglobulin antibodies. Euthyroid autoimmune thyroid disease represents a new investigative frontier in screening and treatment of thyroid dysfunction during pregnancy.

TABLE 58-4. Pregnancy Complications in 440 Women with Hypothyroidism

	Hypothyroidism (%)	
Complications	Overt n = 112	Subclinical n = 328
Preeclampsia	32	8
Placental abruption	8	1
Cardiac dysfunction	3	2
Birthweight < 2000 g[a,b]	33	32
Stillbirths[c]	9	3[c]

[a]Preterm or term deliveries were the only outcomes reported by Abalovich, 2002.
[b]Low birthweight and stillbirth were outcomes reported by Su, 2011.
[c]One infant died from syphilis.
Data from Abalovich, 2002; Davis, 1988; Leung, 1993; Männistö, 2009; Su, 2011.

Overt Hypothyroidism and Pregnancy

The most common cause of hypothyroidism in pregnancy is Hashimoto thyroiditis, characterized by glandular destruction from autoantibodies, particularly antithyroid peroxidase antibodies. Clinical identification of hypothyroidism is especially difficult during pregnancy because many of the signs or symptoms are also common to pregnancy itself. Thyroid analyte testing should be performed on symptomatic women or those with a history of thyroid disease (American College of Obstetricians and Gynecologists, 2013). As discussed in Chapter 18 (p. 353), *severe hypothyroidism* during pregnancy is uncommon, probably because it is often associated with infertility and increased spontaneous abortion rates (Abalovich, 2002; De Groot, 2012). Even women with treated hypothyroidism undergoing in vitro fertilization have a significantly decreased chance of achieving pregnancy (Scoccia, 2012).

Treatment. The American Thyroid Association and American Association of Clinical Endocrinologists (2011) recommend replacement therapy for hypothyroidism beginning with levothyroxine in doses of 1 to 2 μg/kg/day or approximately 100 μg daily. Women who are athyreotic after thyroidectomy or radioiodine therapy may require higher doses. Surveillance is with TSH levels measured at 4- to 6-week intervals, and the thyroxine dose is adjusted by 25- to 50-μg increments until TSH values become normal. Pregnancy is associated with an increased thyroxine requirement in approximately a third of supplemented women (Abalovich, 2010; Alexander, 2004). Because a similar increased requirement is seen in women with postmenopausal hypothyroidism after estrogen replacement, the increased demand in pregnancy is believed to be related to increased estrogen production (Arafah, 2001).

Increased thyroxine requirements begin as early as 5 weeks. In a randomized trial that provided an increased levothyroxine dose at pregnancy confirmation in 60 mothers, Yassa and coworkers (2010) found that a 29- to 43-percent increase in the weekly dose maintained serum TSH values < 5.0 mU/L during the first trimester in all women. Importantly, however, this increase caused TSH suppression in more than a third of women. Significant hypothyroidism may develop early in women without thyroid reserve such as those with a previous thyroidectomy, those with prior radioiodine ablation, or those undergoing assisted reproductive techniques (Alexander, 2004; Loh, 2009; Rotondi, 2004). Anticipatory 25-percent increases in thyroxine replacement at pregnancy confirmation will reduce this likelihood. All other women with hypothyroidism should undergo TSH testing at initiation of prenatal care.

Pregnancy Outcome with Overt Hypothyroidism. Observational studies, although limited, indicate that there are excessive adverse perinatal outcomes associated with overt thyroxine deficiency (Table 58-4). With appropriate replacement therapy, however, adverse effects are not increased in most reports (Matalon, 2006; Tan, 2006; Wolfberg, 2005). In one dissenting study, however, there was an increased risk for some pregnancy complications even in women taking replacement therapy (Wikner, 2008). Most experts agree that adequate hormone replacement during pregnancy minimizes the risk of adverse outcomes and most complications (Abalovich, 2002; Fitzpatrick, 2010).

Fetal and Neonatal Effects. There is no doubt that maternal and fetal thyroid abnormalities are related. In both, thyroid function is dependent on adequate iodide intake, and its deficiency early in pregnancy can cause both maternal and fetal hypothyroidism. And as discussed, maternal TSH-receptor-blocking antibodies can cross the placenta and cause fetal thyroid dysfunction. Rovelli and colleagues (2010) evaluated 129 neonates born to women with autoimmune thyroiditis. They found that 28 percent had an elevated TSH level on the third or fourth day of life, and 47 percent of these had TPO antibodies on day 15. Still, autoantibodies were undetectable at 6 months of age. It seems paradoxical that despite these transient laboratory findings in the *neonate*, TPO and antithyroglobulin (TG) antibodies have little or no effect on *fetal* thyroid function (Fisher, 1997). Indeed, prevalence of fetal hypothyroidism in women with Hashimoto thyroiditis is estimated to be only 1 in 180,000 neonates (Brown, 1996).

Subclinical Hypothyroidism

This thyroid condition is common in women, but its incidence can be variable depending on age, race, dietary iodine intake, and serum TSH thresholds used to establish the diagnosis (Cooper, 2012). According to Fitzpatrick and Russell (2010), its prevalence in pregnancy has been estimated to be between 2 and 5 percent. In two large studies totaling more than 25,000 pregnant women screened in the first half of pregnancy, subclinical hypothyroidism was identified in 2.3 percent of women (Casey, 2005; Cleary-Goldman, 2008). The rate of progression to overt thyroid failure is affected by TSH level, age, other disorders such as diabetes, and presence and concentration of antithyroid antibodies. Diez and Iglesias (2004) prospectively followed 93 nonpregnant women with subclinical hypothyroidism for 5 years and reported that in a third, TSH values became normal. In the other two thirds, those women whose TSH levels were 10 to 15 mU/L developed overt disease at a rate of 19 per 100 patient-years. Those women whose TSH levels were < 10 mU/L developed overt hypothyroidism at a rate of 2 per 100 patient-years. The U.S. Preventative Services Task Force on screening for subclinical hypothyroidism also reported that nearly all patients who develop overt hypothyroidism within 5 years have an initial TSH level > 10 mU/L (Helfand, 2004; Karmisholt, 2008). In a 20-year follow-up study of 5805 women who were screened in early pregnancy, only 3 percent developed thyroid disease. Of the 224 women identified with subclinical hypothyroidism during pregnancy, 36 (17 percent) developed thyroid disease in the next 20 years, and most of these had either TPO or TG antibodies during pregnancy (Männistö, 2010). Consequently, the likelihood of progression to overt hypothyroidism *during* pregnancy in otherwise healthy women with subclinical hypothyroidism seems unlikely.

Subclinical Hypothyroidism and Pregnancy

Observational studies spanning almost 25 years and shown in Table 58-4 suggest that subclinical hypothyroidism is likely associated with some adverse pregnancy outcomes. In 1999, interest was heightened by two studies that suggested that undiagnosed maternal thyroid hypofunction may impair fetal neuropsychological development. In one study, Pop and associates (1999) described 22 women who had free T_4 levels < 10th percentile in early pregnancy whose offspring were at increased risk for impaired psychomotor development. In the other study, Haddow and coworkers (1999) retrospectively evaluated children born to 48 untreated women whose serum TSH values were > 98th percentile. Some had diminished school performance, reading recognition, and intelligent quotient (IQ) scores. Although described as "subclinically hypothyroid," these women had an abnormally low mean serum free thyroxine level, and thus, many had overt hypothyroidism.

To further evaluate any adverse effects, Casey and colleagues (2005) identified subclinical hypothyroidism in 2.3 percent of 17,298 women screened before midpregnancy. As shown in Table 58-5, these women had higher incidences of preterm birth, placental abruption, and admission of infants to the intensive care nursery compared with euthyroid women. In the study of 10,990 participants in the First- and Second-Trimester Evaluation of Risk (FASTER) Trial, Cleary-Goldman and associates (2008) did not find such a link with these adverse obstetrical outcomes.

In a study of 24,883 women screened throughout pregnancy, Wilson and coworkers (2012) found that women identified with subclinical hypothyroidism had an almost twofold increased risk of severe preeclampsia. The authors hypothesized that this was related to endothelial cell dysfunction that has been linked to subclinical hypothyroidism in older patients. In their analysis of the same cohort, Tudela and associates (2012) identified a consistent relationship between increasing TSH level and risk for gestational diabetes. More specifically, 6.3 percent of women with subclinical hypothyroidism were diagnosed with gestational diabetes compared with 4.2 percent in euthyroid women. Nelson and colleagues (2014) evaluated 230 women diagnosed with subclinical hypothyroidism during a prior pregnancy. These women were at increased risk for

TABLE 58-5. Pregnancy Outcomes in Women with Untreated Subclinical Hypothyroidism and Isolated Maternal Hypothyroxinemia Compared with Euthyroid Pregnant Women

Outcome	Euthyroid n = 16,011	Subclinical Hypothyroidism n = 598	*p* value	Isolated Hypothyroxinemia n = 233	*p* value
Hypertension (%)	9	9	0.68	11	0.53
Placental abruption (%)	0.3	1.0	0.03	0.4	0.75
Gestational age delivered (%)					
≤ 36 weeks	6.0	7.0	0.09	6.0	0.84
≤ 34 weeks	2.5	4.3	0.005	2.0	0.44
≤ 32 weeks	1.0	2.2	0.13	1.0	0.47
RDS/ventilator (%)	1.5	2.5	0.05	1.3	0.78
Neonatal intensive care (%)	2.2	4.0	0.005	1.3	0.32

RDS = respiratory distress syndrome.
Data from Casey, 2007.

diabetes and stillbirth in subsequent pregnancies. Although these findings are intriguing, there is currently no evidence that identification and treatment of subclinical hypothyroidism during pregnancy improves these outcomes.

TSH Level Screening in Pregnancy. Because of the findings from the 1999 studies cited above, some professional organizations recommend routine prenatal screening and treatment for subclinical hypothyroidism (Gharib, 2005). The American College of Obstetricians and Gynecologists (2013) has reaffirmed that although observational data were consistent with the *possibility* that subclinical hypothyroidism was associated with adverse neuropsychological development, there have been no interventional trials to demonstrate improvement. The College thus has consistently recommended against implementation of screening until further studies are done to validate or refute these findings (American College of Obstetricians and Gynecologists, 2012).

Lazarus and colleagues (2012) reported the findings of the international multicenter Controlled Antenatal Thyroid Screening (CATS) study of thyroid screening and treatment of subclinical hypothyroidism and isolated maternal hypothyroxinemia during pregnancy. The primary outcome was offspring IQ scores at 3 years of age. Cognitive function in the children was not improved with screening and treatment. A second comparable study is being conducted by the Maternal-Fetal Medicine Units Network, and the results are anticipated in 2016.

Consequent to the Lazarus study, clinical practice guidelines from the Endocrine Society, The American Thyroid Association, and the American Association of Clinical Endocrinologists now uniformly recommend screening only those at increased risk during pregnancy (De Groot, 2012; Garber, 2012). Furthermore, previous cost-effectiveness analyses that favored a universal screening strategy are no longer valid since they were based on assumptions of improved neurodevelopmental outcomes in offspring (Dosiou, 2008; Thung, 2009).

Isolated Maternal Hypothyroxinemia

Women with low serum free T_4 values but a normal range TSH level are considered to have *isolated maternal hypothyroxinemia*. This was identified by Casey and colleagues (2007) in 1.3 percent of more than 17,000 pregnant women screened at Parkland Hospital before 20 weeks. Cleary-Goldman and associates (2008) found a 2.1-percent incidence in the FASTER Trial cohort described earlier. As discussed previously, offspring of women with isolated hypothyroxinemia have been reported to have neurodevelopmental difficulties at age 3 weeks, 10 months, and 2 years (Kooistra, 2006; Pop, 1999, 2003). These findings have not stimulated recommendations for prenatal serum thyroxine screening. Importantly, free T_4 estimates by currently available immunoassays may not be accurate during pregnancy because of sensitivity to alterations in binding proteins (Lee, 2009).

In a study of 233 women with isolated maternal hypothyroxinemia, Casey and colleagues (2007) reported that there were no increased adverse perinatal outcomes compared with those of euthyroid women (see Table 58-5). And, as shown in Figure 58-2, unlike subclinical hypothyroidism, these women had a low prevalence of antithyroid antibodies. The only other finding was from Cleary-Goldman and coworkers (2008), who reported a twofold incidence of fetal macrosomia. Taken together, these findings indicate that isolated maternal hypothyroxinemia has no apparent serious adverse effects on pregnancy outcome. Finally, the aforementioned CATS study did not find improved neurodevelopmental outcomes in women with isolated hypothyroxinemia who were then treated with thyroxine (Lazarus, 2012). Because of this, routine screening for isolated hypothyroxinemia is not recommended.

Euthyroid Autoimmune Thyroid Disease

Autoantibodies to TPO and TG have been identified in 6 to 20 percent of reproductive-aged women (Thangaratinam, 2011). Most who test positive for such antibodies, however, are euthyroid. That said, such women are at a two- to fivefold increased risk for early pregnancy loss (Stagnaro-Green, 2004; Thangaratinam, 2011). The presence of thyroid antibodies has also been associated with preterm birth (Stagnaro-Green, 2009). In a randomized treatment trial of 115 euthyroid women with TPO antibodies, Negro and coworkers (2006) reported that treatment with levothyroxine astoundingly reduced the preterm birth rate from 22 to 7 percent. Contrarily, Abbassi-Ghanavati and associates (2010) evaluated pregnancy outcomes in more than 1000 untreated women with TPO antibodies and did not find an increased risk for preterm birth compared with the risk in 16,000 euthyroid women without antibodies. These investigators, however, found a threefold increased risk of placental abruption in these women. As with nonpregnant subjects with TPO antibodies, these women are also at increased risk for progression of thyroid disease and postpartum thyroiditis (Stagnaro-Green, 2012a).

This group of euthyroid women with abnormally high thyroid autoantibody levels represents a new focus of thyroid research. Dosiou and colleagues (2012) performed a cost-effectiveness analysis of universal screening for autoimmune thyroid disease during pregnancy. Their results favored universal screening. There is, however, a paucity of studies that show benefit to identifying and treating euthyroid women with thyroid autoantibodies. Thus, calls for routine antibody screening seem premature. Currently, universal screening for the thyroid autoantibodies is not recommended by any professional organizations (De Groot, 2012; Stagnaro-Green, 2011a, 2012a).

Iodine Deficiency

Decreasing iodide fortification of table salt and bread products in the United States during the past 25 years has led to occasional iodide deficiency (Caldwell, 2005; Hollowell, 1998). Importantly, the most recent National Health and Nutrition Examination survey indicated that, overall, the United States population remains iodine sufficient (Caldwell, 2011). Even so, experts agree that iodine nutrition in vulnerable populations such as pregnant women requires continued monitoring.

In 2011 the Office of Dietary Supplements of the National Institutes of Health sponsored a workshop to prioritize iodine research. Participants emphasized the decline in median urinary iodine to 125 μg/L in pregnant women and the serious potential impact on the developing fetus (Swanson, 2012).

Dietary iodine requirements are increased during pregnancy due to increased thyroid hormone production, increased renal losses, and fetal iodine requirements. Adequate iodine is requisite for fetal neurological development beginning soon after conception, and abnormalities are dependent on the degree of deficiency. The World Health Organization (WHO) has estimated that at least 50 million people worldwide have varying degrees of preventable brain damage due to iodine deficiency (Brundtland, 2002). Although it is doubtful that *mild deficiency* causes intellectual impairment, supplementation does prevent fetal goiter (Stagnaro-Green, 2012b). *Severe deficiency*, on the other hand, is frequently associated with damage typically encountered with *endemic cretinism* (Delange, 2001). It is presumed that *moderate deficiency* has intermediate and variable effects. Berbel and associates (2009) began daily supplementation in more than 300 pregnant women with moderate deficiency at three time periods—4 to 6 weeks, 12 to 14 weeks, and after delivery. They found improved neurobehavioral development scores in offspring of women supplemented with 200 μg potassium iodide very early in pregnancy. Similarly, Velasco and coworkers (2009) found improved Bayley Psychomotor Development scores in offspring of women supplemented with 300 μg of iodide in the first trimester. In contrast, Murcia and colleagues (2011) identified lower psychomotor scores in 1-year-old infants whose mothers reported daily supplementation of more than 150 μg. There are two ongoing randomized controlled trials of iodine supplementation in mildly to moderately iodine-deficient pregnant women in India and Thailand. These studies should provide needed answers as to whether iodine supplementation in these women is beneficial (Pearce, 2013).

The Institute of Medicine (2001) recommends daily iodine intake during pregnancy of 220 μg/day, and 290 μg/day for lactating women (Chap. 9, p. 180). The Endocrine Society (De Groot, 2012) recommends an average iodine intake of 150 μg per day in childbearing-aged women, and this should be increased to 250 μg during pregnancy and breast feeding. The American Thyroid Association has recommended that 150 μg of iodine be added to prenatal vitamins to achieve this average daily intake (Becker, 2006). According to Leung and coworkers (2011), however, only 51 percent of the prenatal multivitamins in the United States contain iodine. It has even been suggested that because most cases of maternal hypothyroxinemia worldwide are related to relative iodine deficiency, supplementation may obviate the need to consider thyroxine treatment in such women (Gyamfi, 2009).

On the other hand, experts caution against oversupplementation. Teng and associates (2006) contend that excessive iodine intake—defined as > 300 μg/day—may lead to subclinical hypothyroidism and autoimmune thyroiditis. And the Endocrine Society, in accordance with the WHO, advises against exceeding twice the daily recommended intake of iodine, or 500 μg/day (De Groot, 2012; Leung, 2011).

Congenital Hypothyroidism

Because the clinical diagnosis of hypothyroidism in neonates is usually missed, universal newborn screening was introduced in 1974 and is now required by law in all states. Congenital hypothyroidism develops in approximately 1 in 3000 newborns and is one of the most preventable causes of mental retardation (LaFranchi, 2011). Developmental disorders of the thyroid gland such as agenesis and hypoplasia account for 80 to 90 percent of these cases (LaFranchi, 2011; Topaloglu, 2006). The exact underlying etiology of thyroid dysgenesis remains unknown. The remaining primary congenital hypothyroidism cases are caused by hereditary defects in thyroid hormone production. The list of identified gene mutations that cause hypothyroidism continues to grow rapidly (Moreno, 2008).

Early and aggressive thyroxine replacement is critical for infants with congenital hypothyroidism. Still, some infants identified by screening programs with severe congenital hypothyroidism who were treated promptly will exhibit cognitive deficits into adolescence (Song, 2001). Therefore, in addition to timing of treatment, the severity of congenital hypothyroidism is an important factor in long-term cognitive outcomes (Kempers, 2006). Accordingly, in infants with screening results suggestive of severe hypothyroidism, therapy should be started immediately without waiting for confirmatory results (Abduljabbar, 2012). Olivieri and colleagues (2002) reported that 8 percent of 1420 infants with congenital hypothyroidism also had other major congenital malformations.

Postpartum Thyroiditis

Transient autoimmune thyroiditis is consistently found in approximately 5 to 10 percent of women during the first year after childbirth (Amino, 2000; Stagnaro-Green, 2011b, 2012a). Postpartum thyroid dysfunction with an onset within 12 months includes hyperthyroidism, hypothyroidism, or both. The propensity for thyroiditis antedates pregnancy and is directly related to increasing serum levels of thyroid autoantibodies. Up to 50 percent of women who are thyroid-antibody positive in the first trimester will develop postpartum thyroiditis (Stagnaro-Green, 2012a). In a Dutch study of 82 women with type 1 diabetes, postpartum thyroiditis developed in 16 percent and was threefold higher than in the general population (Gallas, 2002). Importantly, 46 percent of those identified with overt postpartum thyroiditis had TPO antibodies in the first trimester.

Clinical Manifestations

In clinical practice, postpartum thyroiditis is diagnosed infrequently because it typically develops months after delivery and causes vague and nonspecific symptoms that often are thought to be stresses of motherhood (Stagnaro-Green, 2004). The clinical presentation varies, and classically there are two recognized clinical phases that may develop in succession. The first and earliest is *destruction-induced thyrotoxicosis* with symptoms from excessive release of hormone from glandular disruption. The onset is abrupt, and a small, painless goiter is commonly found. Although there may be many symptoms, only fatigue and palpitations are more frequent in thyrotoxic women compared with normal controls. This thyrotoxic phase usually lasts only a few months. Thionamides are ineffective, and if symptoms are severe, a β-blocker agent may be given. The second and usually later phase is clinical *hypothyroidism* from thyroiditis between 4 and 8 months postpartum. Thyromegaly and other symptoms are common and more prominent than during the thyrotoxic phase. Thyroxine replacement with 25 to 75 μg/day is typically given for 6 to 12 months.

Stagnaro-Green and associates (2011b) reported postpartum follow-up from 4562 Italian pregnant women who had been screened for thyroid disease in pregnancy. Serum TSH and anti-TPO antibody levels were measured again at 6 and 12 months. Overall, two thirds of 169 women (3.9 percent) with postpartum thyroiditis were identified to have hypothyroidism only. The other third were diagnosed with hyperthyroidism, but only 14 percent of all women demonstrated the "classic" biphasic progression described above. These findings are consistent with data compiled from 20 other studies between 1982 and 2008 (Stagnaro-Green, 2012a).

Importantly, women who experience either type of postpartum thyroiditis have an approximately 30-percent risk of eventually developing permanent hypothyroidism, and the annual progression rate is 3.6 percent (Lucas, 2005; Muller, 2001; Premawardhana, 2000). Women at increased risk for developing hypothyroidism are those with higher titers of thyroid antibodies and higher TSH levels during the initial hypothyroid phase. Others may develop subclinical disease, but half of those with thyroiditis who are positive for TPO antibodies develop permanent hypothyroidism by 6 to 7 years (Stagnaro-Green, 2012a).

An association between postpartum thyroiditis and postpartum depression has been proposed but remains unresolved. Lucas and coworkers (2001) found a 1.7-percent incidence of postpartum depression at 6 months in women with thyroiditis as well as in controls. Pederson and colleagues (2007) found a significant correlation between abnormal scores on the Edinburgh Postnatal Depression Scale and total thyroxine values in the low normal range during pregnancy in 31 women. Similarly unsettled is the link between depression and thyroid antibodies. Kuijpens and associates (2001) reported that TPO antibodies were a marker for postpartum depression in euthyroid women. In a randomized trial, Harris and coworkers (2002) reported no difference in postpartum depression in 342 women with TPO antibodies who were given either levothyroxine or placebo.

Nodular Thyroid Disease

Thyroid nodules can be found in 1 to 2 percent of reproductive-aged women (Fitzpatrick, 2010). Management of a palpable thyroid nodule during pregnancy depends on gestational age and mass size. Small nodules detected by sensitive sonographic methods are more common during pregnancy in some populations. For example, Kung and associates (2002) used high-resolution sonography and found that 15 percent of Chinese women had nodules larger than 2 mm in diameter. Almost half were multiple, and the nodules usually enlarged modestly across pregnancy and did not regress postpartum. Biopsy of those > 5 mm^3 that persisted at 3 months usually showed nodular hyperplasia, and none was malignant. In some studies, however, up to 40 percent of solitary nodules were malignant (Doherty, 1995; Rosen, 1986). Even so, most were low-grade neoplasms.

Evaluation of thyroid nodules during pregnancy should be similar to that for nonpregnant patients. As discussed in Chapter 46 (p. 934), most recommend against *radioiodine scanning* in pregnancy despite the fact that tracer doses used are associated with minimal fetal irradiation (Popoveniuc, 2012). *Sonographic* examination reliably detects nodules larger than 0.5 cm, and their solid or cystic structure also is determined. According to the American Association of Clinical Endocrinologists, sonographic characteristics associated with malignancy include hypoechogenic pattern, irregular margins, and microcalcifications (Gharib, 2005). *Fine-needle aspiration (FNA)* is an excellent assessment method, and histological tumor markers and immunostaining are reliable to evaluate for malignancy (Bartolazzi, 2001; Hegedüs, 2004). If the FNA biopsy shows a follicular lesion, surgery may be deferred until after delivery.

Evaluation of thyroid cancer involves a multidisciplinary approach (American College of Obstetricians and Gynecologists, 2013). Most thyroid carcinomas are well differentiated and pursue an indolent course. When thyroid malignancy is diagnosed during the first or second trimester, thyroidectomy may be performed before the third trimester (Chap. 63, p. 1231). In women without evidence of an aggressive thyroid cancer, or in those diagnosed in the third trimester, surgical treatment can be deferred to the immediate postpartum period (Gharib, 2010).

PARATHYROID DISEASES

The function of *parathyroid hormone (PTH)* is to maintain extracellular fluid calcium concentration. This 115-amino acid hormone acts directly on bone and kidney and indirectly on small intestine through its effects on synthesis of vitamin D (1,25[OH_2]-D) to increase serum calcium. Secretion is regulated by serum ionized calcium concentration through a negative feedback system. *Calcitonin* is a potent parathyroid hormone that acts as a physiological parathyroid hormone antagonist. The interrelationships between these hormones, calcium metabolism, and *PTH-related protein* produced by fetal tissue are discussed in Chapter 4 (p. 70).

Fetal calcium needs—300 mg/day in late pregnancy and a total of 30 g—as well as increased renal calcium loss from augmented glomerular filtration, substantively increase maternal calcium demands. Pregnancy is associated with a twofold rise in serum concentrations of 1,25-dihydroxyvitamin D, which increases gastrointestinal calcium absorption. The effectuating hormone is probably of placental and decidual origin because maternal PTH levels are low normal or decreased during pregnancy (Cooper, 2011; Molitch, 2000). Total serum calcium levels decline with serum albumin concentrations, but ionized calcium levels remain unchanged. Vargas Zapata (2004), and others, have suggested a role for insulin-like growth factor-1

(IGF-1) in maternal calcium homeostasis and bone turnover, especially in mothers with low calcium intake.

Hyperparathyroidism

Hypercalcemia is caused by hyperparathyroidism or cancer in 90 percent of cases. Primary hyperparathyroidism is reported most often in women older than 50 (Miller, 2008). Because many automated laboratory systems include serum calcium measurement, hyperparathyroidism has changed from being a condition defined by symptoms to one that is discovered on routine screening (Pallan, 2012). It has a reported prevalence of 2 to 3 per 1000 women, but some have estimated the rate to be as high as 14 per 1000 when asymptomatic cases are included (Farford, 2007; Schnatz, 2005). Almost 80 percent are caused by a solitary adenoma, and another 15 percent by hyperfunction of all four glands. In the remainder, a malignancy and the cause of increased serum calcium levels are obvious. Of note, PTH produced by tumors is not identical to the natural hormone and may not be detected by routine assays.

In most patients, the serum calcium level is only elevated to within 1 to 1.5 mg/dL above the upper normal limit. This may help to explain why only 20 percent of those who have abnormally elevated levels are symptomatic (Bilezikian, 2004). In a fourth, however, symptoms become apparent when the serum calcium level continues to rise. *Hypercalcemic crisis* manifests as stupor, nausea, vomiting, weakness, fatigue, and dehydration.

All women with symptomatic hyperparathyroidism should be surgically treated. Guidelines for management in nonpregnant patients were revised after the Third International Workshop on the Management of Asymptomatic Primary Hyperparathyroidism (Bilezikian, 2009). Indications for parathyroidectomy include a serum calcium level 1.0 mg/dL above the upper normal range, a calculated creatinine clearance less than 60 mL/min, reduced bone density, or age < 50 years. Those not meeting these criteria should undergo annual calcium and creatinine level measurement and bone density assessment every 1 to 2 years (Pallan, 2012).

Hyperparathyroidism in Pregnancy

In their review, Schnatz and Thaxton (2005) found fewer than 200 reported cases complicating pregnancy. As in nonpregnant patients, hyperparathyroidism is usually caused by a parathyroid adenoma. Gravidas with ectopic parathyroid hormone production and rare cases of parathyroid carcinoma have been reported (Montoro, 2000). Symptoms include hyperemesis, generalized weakness, renal calculi, and psychiatric disorders. Occasionally, pancreatitis is the presenting finding (Cooper, 2011; Dahan, 2001).

Pregnancy theoretically improves hyperparathyroidism because of significant calcium shunting to the fetus and augmented renal excretion (Power, 1999). When the "protective effects" of pregnancy are withdrawn, however, there is significant danger of postpartum hypercalcemic crisis. This life-threatening complication can be seen with serum calcium levels greater than 14 mg/dL and is characterized by nausea, vomiting, tremors, dehydration, and mental status changes (Malekar-Raikar, 2011). Early reports described excessive stillbirths and preterm deliveries in pregnancies complicated by hyperparathyroidism (Shangold, 1982). More recent reports, however, described lower rates of stillbirth, neonatal death, and neonatal tetany (Kovacs, 2011). Other fetal complications include miscarriage, fetal-growth restriction, and low birthweight (Chamarthi, 2011). Schnatz (2005) reported a 25-percent incidence of preeclampsia.

Management in Pregnancy. Surgical removal of a symptomatic parathyroid adenoma is preferable. This should prevent fetal and neonatal morbidities, as well as postpartum parathyroid crises (Kovacs, 2011). Elective neck exploration during pregnancy is usually well tolerated, even in the third trimester (Graham, 1998; Kort, 1999; Schnatz, 2005). In one woman, a mediastinal adenoma was removed at 23 weeks (Rooney, 1998).

None of the three International Workshop Conferences on Asymptomatic Hyperparathyroidism have addressed its management during pregnancy (Bilezikian, 2009). Medical management may be appropriate in asymptomatic pregnant women with mild hypercalcemia. If so, patients are carefully monitored in the postpartum period for hypercalcemic crisis (Kovacs, 2011). Initial medical management might include *calcitonin* to decrease skeletal calcium release, or oral phosphate, 1 to 1.5 g daily in divided doses to bind excess calcium. For women with dangerously elevated serum calcium levels or those who are mentally obtunded with *hypercalcemic crisis*, emergency treatment is instituted. Diuresis with intravenous normal saline is begun so that urine flow exceeds 150 mL/hr. *Furosemide* is given in conventional doses to block tubular calcium reabsorption. Importantly, hypokalemia and hypomagnesemia should be prevented. Adjunctive therapy includes *mithramycin,* which inhibits bone resorption.

Neonatal Effects. Normally, cord blood calcium levels are higher than maternal levels (Chap. 7, p. 135). With maternal hyperparathyroidism, abnormally elevated maternal and thence fetal levels further suppress fetal parathyroid function. Because of this, after birth, there is a rapidly decreasing newborn calcium level, and 15 to 25 percent of these infants develop severe hypocalcemia with or without tetany (Molitch, 2000). Neonatal hypoparathyroidism caused by maternal hyperparathyroidism is usually transient and should be treated with calcium and calcitriol. Calcitriol will not be effective in preterm infants, however, because the intestinal vitamin D receptor is not sufficiently expressed (Kovacs, 2011). Neonatal tetany or seizures should stimulate an evaluation for maternal hyperparathyroidism (Beattie, 2000; Ip, 2003; Jaafar, 2004).

Hypoparathyroidism

The most common cause of hypocalcemia is hypoparathyroidism that usually follows parathyroid or thyroid surgery. Hypoparathyroidism is estimated to follow up to 7 percent of total thyroidectomies (Shoback, 2008). It is rare and characterized by facial muscle spasms, muscle cramps, and paresthesias of the lips, tongue, fingers, and feet. This can progress to tetany and seizures. Chronically, hypocalcemic pregnant women may also have a fetus with skeletal demineralization resulting in multiple bone fractures in the neonatal period (Alikasifoglu, 2005).

Maternal treatment includes 1,25-dihydroxyvitamin D_3 (calcitriol), dihydrotachysterol, or large vitamin D doses of 50,000 to 150,000 U/day; calcium gluconate or calcium lactate in doses of 3 to 5 g/day; and a low-phosphate diet. The therapeutic challenge in women with known hypoparathyroidism is management of blood calcium levels. The goal during pregnancy is maintenance of the corrected calcium level in the low normal range. It is possible that the increased calcium absorption typical of pregnancy will result in lower calcium requirements or that the fetal demand for calcium will result in increased need. Since both scenarios are possible, it is best to carefully monitor the corrected serum calcium on a frequent, perhaps monthly, basis throughout pregnancy (Cooper, 2011; Kovacs, 2011). The fetal risks from large doses of vitamin D have not been established.

Pregnancy-Associated Osteoporosis

Even with remarkably increased calcium requirements, it is uncertain whether pregnancy causes osteopenia in most women (Kaur, 2003; To, 2003). In one study of 200 pregnant women in which bone mass was measured using quantitative ultrasonometry of the calcaneus, Kraemer and colleagues (2011) demonstrated a decline in bone density during pregnancy. Women who breast fed, carried twin pregnancies, or had a low body mass index (BMI) were at higher risk of bone loss. From their review, Thomas and Weisman (2006) cite a 3- to 4-percent average reduction in bone-mineral density during pregnancy. Lactation also represents a period of negative calcium balance that is corrected through maternal skeletal resorption. Feigenberg and coworkers (2008) found cortical bone mass reductions using ultrasound in young primiparas in the puerperium compared with nulligravid controls. Rarely, some women develop idiopathic osteoporosis while pregnant or lactating. Its incidence is estimated to be 4 per million women (Hellmeyer, 2007).

The most common symptom of osteoporosis is back pain in late pregnancy or postpartum. Other symptoms are hip pain, either unilateral or bilateral, and difficulty in weight bearing until nearly immobilized (Maliha, 2012). In more than half of women, no apparent reason for osteopenia is found. Some known causes include heparin, prolonged bed rest, and corticosteroid therapy (Cunningham, 2005; von Mandach, 2003). In a few cases, overt hyperparathyroidism or thyrotoxicosis eventually develops.

Treatment is problematical and includes calcium and vitamin D supplementation as well as standard pain management. Shown in Figure 58-5 is a hip radiograph from a woman treated at Parkland Hospital during the third trimester for transient osteoporosis of pregnancy.

For women with pregnancy-associated osteopenia, long-term surveillance indicates that although bone density improves, these women and their offspring may have chronic osteopenia (Carbone, 1995). There is an ongoing randomized, placebo-controlled trial of vitamin D supplementation in pregnant women to determine its effect on neonatal bone mineral content as assessed by dual-energy x-ray absorptiometry (DEXA) (Harvey, 2012).

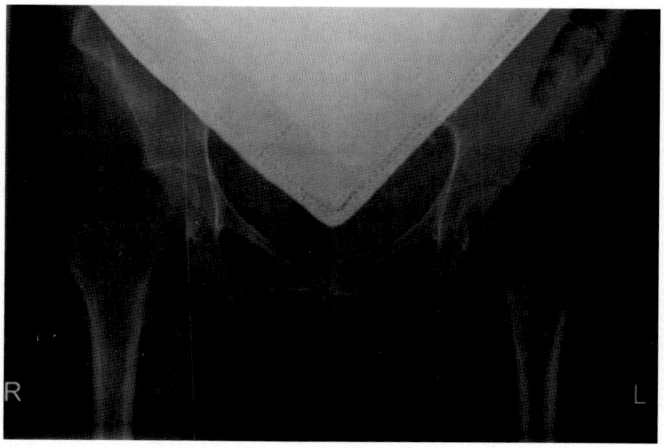

FIGURE 58-5 Anteroposterior plain radiograph with abdominal shielding of a 25-year-old patient's hips at 26-weeks' gestation. She complained of left hip and knee pain and progressive weakness. Her transient osteoporosis of the left femur responded over 3 months to physical therapy combined with vitamin D and calcium supplementation.

ADRENAL GLAND DISORDERS

Pregnancy has profound effects on adrenal cortical secretion and its control or stimulation. These interrelationships were reviewed by Lekarev and New (2011) and are discussed in detail in Chapter 4 (p. 70).

Pheochromocytoma

These tumors are clinically uncommon and complicate approximately 1 per 10,000 pregnancies. Notably, they are found in 0.1 percent of hypertensive patients (Abdelmannan, 2011). However, they are more commonly found at autopsy with infrequent clinical recognition. Pheochromocytomas are chromaffin tumors that secrete catecholamines and usually are located in the adrenal medulla, although 10 percent are located in sympathetic ganglia. They are called the *10-percent tumor* because approximately 10 percent are bilateral, 10 percent are extraadrenal, and 10 percent are malignant. These tumors can be associated with medullary thyroid carcinoma and hyperparathyroidism in some of the autosomally dominant or recessive *multiple endocrine neoplasia syndromes*, as well as in neurofibromatosis and von Hippel-Lindau disease.

Symptoms are usually paroxysmal and manifest as hypertensive crisis, seizure disorders, or anxiety attacks. Hypertension is sustained in 60 percent of patients, but half of these also have paroxysmal crises. Other symptoms during paroxysmal attacks are headaches, profuse sweating, palpitations, chest pain, nausea and vomiting, and pallor or flushing.

The standard screening test is quantification of catecholamine metabolites in a 24-hour urine specimen (Abdelmannan, 2011). Diagnosis is established by measurement of a 24-hour

TABLE 58-6. Outcomes of Pregnancies Complicated by Pheochromocytoma and Reported in Three Contiguous Epochs

Factor	Incidence (%)		
	1980–87 Harper (1989) n = 48	1988–97 Ahlawat (1999) n = 42	1998–2008 Sarathi (2010) n = 60
Diagnosis			
Antepartum	51	83	70
Postpartum	36	14	23
Autopsy	12	2	7
Maternal death	16	4	12
Fetal wastage	26	11	17

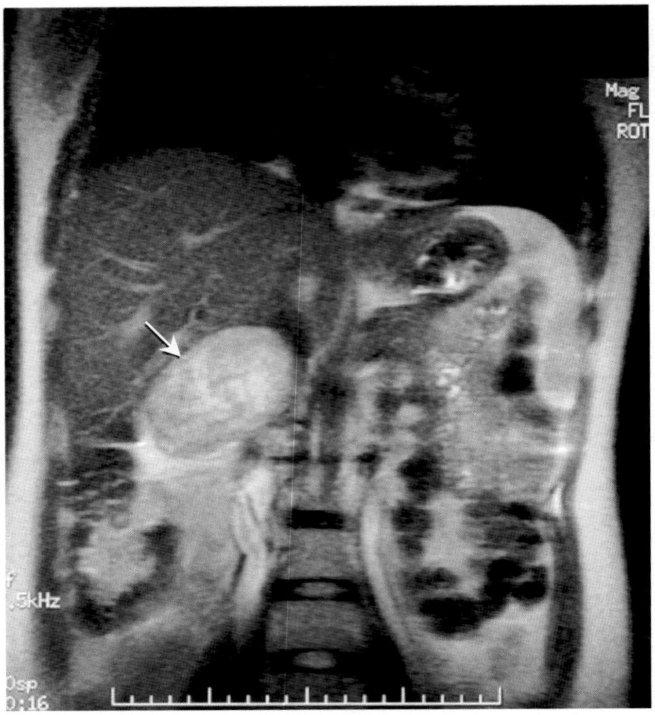

FIGURE 58-6 Coronal magnetic resonance image taken in a 32-week pregnant woman shows a right-sided pheochromocytoma (*arrow*) and its position relative to the liver above it.

urine collection with at least two of three assays for free catecholamines, metanephrines, or vanillylmandelic acid (VMA). Determination of plasma catecholamine levels may be accurate but is associated with technical difficulties (Conlin, 2001; Lenders, 2002). Boyle and colleagues (2007) determined that measurement of urinary free metanephrine was superior to assessment of a VMA or urinary or plasma catecholamine level. In nonpregnant patients, adrenal localization is usually successful with either computed tomography (CT) or magnetic resonance (MR) imaging. For most cases, preferred treatment is laparoscopic adrenalectomy (Lal, 2003).

Pheochromocytoma Complicating Pregnancy

These tumors are rare but result in dangerous pregnancy complications. Geelhoed (1983) provided an earlier review of 89 cases in which 43 mothers died. Maternal death was much more common if the tumor was not diagnosed antepartum—58 versus 18 percent. As seen in Table 58-6, maternal mortality rates are now lower but still formidable. In their review of 60 cases, Sarathi and associates (2010) confirmed that antepartum diagnosis is the most important determinant of maternal mortality risk. Maternal death was rare if the diagnosis is made antepartum.

Diagnosis of pheochromocytoma in pregnancy is similar to that for nonpregnant patients. MR imaging is the preferred imaging technique because it almost always locates adrenal and extraadrenal pheochromocytomas (Fig. 58-6) (Manger, 2005). In many cases, the principal challenge is to differentiate preeclampsia from the hypertensive crisis caused by pheochromocytoma. Desai and coworkers (2009) describe a woman who was initially treated for severe preeclampsia, suffered an intrapartum fetal death, and was then treated for presumed peripartum cardiomyopathy. When she returned 1 week later with paroxysmal hypertension, pheochromocytoma was diagnosed and her blood pressure and ventricular function returned to normal after tumor resection. Grimbert and colleagues (1999) diagnosed two pheochromocytomas during 56 pregnancies in 30 women with von Hippel-Lindau disease.

Management

Immediate control of hypertension and symptoms with an α-adrenergic blocker such as *phenoxybenzamine* is imperative. The dose is 10 to 30 mg, two to four times daily. After α-blockade is achieved, β-blockers may be given for tachycardia. In many cases, surgical exploration and tumor removal are performed during pregnancy, preferably during the second trimester (Dong, 2014; Miller, 2005). Successful laparoscopic removal of adrenal tumors has become the norm (Junglee, 2007; Kim, 2006; Miller, 2012; Zuluaga-Gómez, 2012). If diagnosed later in pregnancy, either planned cesarean delivery with tumor excision or postpartum resection is appropriate.

Recurrent tumors are troublesome, and even with good blood pressure control, dangerous peripartum hypertension may develop. We have cared for three women in whom recurrent pheochromocytoma was identified during pregnancy. Hypertension was managed with phenoxybenzamine in all three. Two infants were healthy, but a third was stillborn in a mother with a massive tumor burden who was receiving phenoxybenzamine, 100 mg daily. In all three women, tumor was resected postpartum.

Cushing Syndrome

This syndrome is rare and has an annual incidence of 2 to 3 per million. The female:male ratio is 3:1 (Steffenson, 2010). Most cases are iatrogenic from long-term corticosteroid treatment. However, endogenous Cushing syndrome is typically due to *Cushing disease*, which is bilateral adrenal hyperplasia stimulated by corticotropin-producing pituitary adenomas. Most are small microadenomas < 1 cm, and half measure ≤ 5 mm. Rarely, abnormal secretion of hypothalamic corticotropin-releasing factor may cause corticotropic hyperplasia. Such hyperplasia may also be caused by nonendocrine tumors that produce polypeptides similar to either corticotropin-releasing factor or corticotropin. Less than a fourth of cases of Cushing syndrome are corticotropin independent, and most of these are caused by an adrenal adenoma. Tumors are usually bilateral, and half are malignant. Occasionally, associated androgen excess may lead to severe virilization (Danilowicz, 2002).

The typical cushingoid body habitus is caused by adipose tissue deposition that characteristically results in *moon facies,* a *buffalo hump,* and *truncal obesity.* Fatigability and weakness, hypertension, hirsutism, and amenorrhea are each encountered in 75 to 85 percent of nonpregnant patients (Hatipoglu, 2012; Williams, 2001). Personality changes, easy bruisability, and cutaneous striae are common. Up to 60 percent may have impaired glucose tolerance. Diagnosis is verified by elevated plasma cortisol levels that cannot be suppressed by dexamethasone or by elevated 24-hour urine free cortisol excretion (Boscaro, 2001). Neither test is totally accurate, and both are more difficult to interpret in obese patients. CT and MR imaging are used to localize pituitary and adrenal tumors or hyperplasia.

TABLE 58-7. Maternal and Perinatal Complications in Pregnancies Complicated by Cushing Syndrome

Complication	Approximate Incidence (%)
Maternal	
Hypertension	68
Diabetes	25
Preeclampsia	15
Osteoporosis/fracture	5
Psychiatric disorders	4
Cardiac failure	3
Mortality	2
Perinatal	
Fetal-growth restriction	21
Preterm delivery	43
Stillbirth	6
Neonatal death	2

Data from Lindsay, 2005.

Cushing Syndrome and Pregnancy

Because most women have corticotropin-dependent Cushing syndrome, associated androgen excess may cause anovulation, and pregnancy is rare. In their review, Lekarev and New (2011) identified fewer than 140 reported cases of Cushing syndrome in pregnancy. These differ compared with nonpregnant women in that half are caused by corticotropin-independent adrenal adenomas (Abdelmannan, 2011; Klibanski, 2006). Approximately 30 percent of cases are from a pituitary adenoma, and 10 percent from adrenal carcinomas (Lekarev, 2011; Lindsay, 2005). All reports stress difficulties in diagnosis because of pregnancy-induced increases in plasma cortisol, corticotropin, and corticotropin-releasing factor levels. Measurement of 24-hour urinary free cortisol excretion is recommended, with consideration for normal elevation in pregnancy.

Pregnancy outcomes in women with Cushing syndrome are listed in Table 58-7. Heart failure is common during pregnancy and is a major cause of maternal mortality (Buescher, 1992). Hypercortisolism in pregnancy may also cause poor wound healing, osteoporotic fracture, and psychiatric complications (Kamoun, 2014).

Long-term medical therapy for Cushing syndrome usually is ineffective, and definitive therapy is resection of the pituitary or adrenal adenoma or bilateral adrenalectomy for hyperplasia (Lekarev, 2011; Motivala, 2011). During pregnancy, management of hypertension in mild cases may suffice until delivery. In their review, Lindsay and associates (2005) described primary medical therapy in 20 women with Cushing syndrome. Most were successfully treated with *metyrapone* as an interim treatment until definitive surgery after delivery. A few cases were treated with oral *ketoconazole.* However, because this drug also blocks testicular steroidogenesis, treatment during pregnancy with a male fetus is worrisome. *Mifepristone,* the norethindrone derivative used for abortion and labor induction, has shown promise for treating Cushing disease but should not be used in pregnancy for obvious reasons. If necessary, pituitary adenomas can be treated by transsphenoidal resection (Boscaro, 2001; Lindsay, 2005). Unilateral adrenalectomy has been safely performed in the early third trimester and can also be curative (Abdelmannan, 2011).

Adrenal Insufficiency—Addison Disease

Primary adrenocortical insufficiency is rare because more than 90 percent of total gland volume must be destroyed for symptoms to develop. *Autoimmune adrenalitis* is the most common cause in the developed world, but tuberculosis is a more frequent etiology in resource-poor countries (Kamoun, 2014). There is an increased incidence of concurrent Hashimoto thyroiditis, premature ovarian failure, type 1 diabetes, and Graves disease. These *polyglandular autoimmune syndromes* also include pernicious anemia, vitiligo, alopecia, nontropical sprue, and myasthenia gravis.

Untreated adrenal hypofunction frequently causes infertility, but with replacement therapy, ovulation is restored. The incidence of primary adrenal insufficiency has been cited as being as high as 1 in 3000 births in Norway (Lekarev, 2011). If untreated, symptoms often include weakness, fatigue, nausea and vomiting, and weight loss (Mestman, 2002). Because serum cortisol levels are increased during pregnancy, the finding of a low value should prompt an adrenocorticotropic hormone (ACTH) stimulation test to document the lack of response to infused corticotropin (Salvatori, 2005).

In a large Swedish cohort study, 1188 women with Addison disease were compared with more than 11,000 age-matched controls who delivered between 1973 and 2006. Women diagnosed with adrenal insufficiency within 3 years of delivery were twice as likely to deliver preterm, were three times more likely to deliver a low-birthweight infant, and were more likely to undergo cesarean delivery (Björnsdottir, 2010). Most pregnant women with Addison disease are already taking cortisone-like drugs. These should be continued and women observed for evidence of either inadequate or excessive corticosteroid replacement. During labor, delivery, and postpartum, or after a surgical procedure, corticosteroid replacement must be increased appreciably to approximate the normal adrenal response—so-called *stress doses.* Hydrocortisone, 100 mg, is usually given intravenously every 8 hours. It is important that shock from causes other than adrenocortical insufficiency—for example, hemorrhage or sepsis—be recognized and treated promptly.

Primary Aldosteronism

Hyperaldosteronism is caused by an adrenal aldosteronoma in approximately 75 percent of cases. Idiopathic bilateral adrenal hyperplasia comprise the remainder, except for rare cases of adrenal carcinoma (Abdelmannan, 2011; Ganguly, 1998). Findings include hypertension, hypokalemia, and muscle weakness. High serum or urine levels of aldosterone confirm the diagnosis.

In normal pregnancy, as discussed in Chapter 4 (p. 61), progesterone blocks aldosterone action, and thus there are very high levels of aldosterone (Appendix, p. 1290). Accordingly, the diagnosis of hyperaldosteronism during pregnancy can be difficult. Since renin levels are suppressed in pregnant women with hyperaldosteronism, a plasma aldosterone-to-renin activity ratio may be helpful for diagnosis (Kamoun, 2014). Medical management includes potassium supplementation and antihypertensive therapy. In many cases, hypertension responds to *spironolactone,* but β-blockers or calcium-channel blockers may be preferred because of the potential fetal antiandrogenic effects of spironolactone. Mascetti and coworkers (2011) reported successful use of *amiloride* in a pregnant woman. Use of *eplerenone,* a mineralocorticoid receptor antagonist, has also been reported (Cabassi, 2012). Tumor resection is curative, and laparoscopic adrenalectomy has been shown to be safe (Kamoun, 2014; Kosaka, 2006; Miller, 2012).

PITUITARY DISORDERS

There is impressive pituitary enlargement during pregnancy, predominately from lactotrophic cellular hyperplasia induced by estrogen stimulation (Chap. 4, p. 67).

Prolactinomas

These adenomas are found often in nonpregnant women since the advent of widely available serum prolactin assays. Serum levels less than 25 pg/mL are considered normal in nonpregnant women (Motivala, 2011). Adenoma symptoms and findings include amenorrhea, galactorrhea, and hyperprolactinemia. Tumors are classified arbitrarily by their size measured by CT or MR imaging. A microadenoma is ≤ 10 mm, and a macroadenoma is > 10 mm. Treatment for microadenomas is usually with bromocriptine, a dopamine agonist and powerful prolactin inhibitor, which frequently restores ovulation. For suprasellar macroadenomas, most recommend surgical resection before pregnancy is attempted (Schlechte, 2007).

In a pooled analysis of more than 500 pregnant women with prolactinomas, only 1.4 percent with *microadenomas* developed symptomatic enlargement during pregnancy (Molitch, 2003). Symptomatic enlargement of *macroadenomas,* however, is more frequent and was found in 26 percent of 84 pregnant women included in this analysis. Schlechte (2007) also reported that 15 to 35 percent of suprasellar macroadenomas have tumor enlargement that causes visual disturbances, headaches, and diabetes insipidus.

Gillam and colleagues (2006) recommend that pregnant women with microadenomas be queried regularly for headaches and visual symptoms. Those with macroadenomas should be followed more closely and have visual field testing during each trimester. CT or MR imaging is recommended only if symptoms develop. Serial serum prolactin levels are of little use because of normal increases during pregnancy (Appendix, p. 1291). Symptomatic tumor enlargement should be treated immediately with a dopamine antagonist such as bromocriptine or cabergoline. The safety of bromocriptine in pregnancy is well established. It is less well known for cabergoline, which is increasingly used in nonpregnant women because it is better tolerated and more effective. It is generally considered safe for use in pregnancy (Briggs, 2011). Lebbe and colleagues (2010) described 100 pregnancies exposed to cabergoline and found no adverse effects. Similar findings were reported in 85 exposed Japanese pregnant women (Ono, 2010). Surgery is recommended for women with no response, and Gondim and associates (2003) have described transnasal transseptal endoscopic resection.

Acromegaly

This is caused by excessive growth hormone, usually from an acidophilic or a chromophobic pituitary adenoma. In normal pregnancy, pituitary growth hormone levels decrease as placental epitopes are secreted. Diagnosis is confirmed by the failure of an oral glucose tolerance test to suppress pituitary growth hormone (Melmed, 2006). There have been fewer than 100 cases of acromegaly reported during pregnancy (Motivala, 2011). Pregnancy is probably rare in women with acromegaly, because half are hyperprolactinemic and anovulatory. In a recent report describing 46 pregnant women with acromegaly, Caron and coworkers (2010) concluded that such women were at marginally increased risk for gestational diabetes and hypertension.

Management is similar to that for prolactinomas, with close monitoring for symptoms of tumor enlargement. Dopamine agonist therapy is not as effective as it is for prolactinomas. And transsphenoidal resection, generally considered first-line treatment outside of pregnancy, may be necessary for symptomatic tumor enlargement during pregnancy (Motivala, 2011). Guven and associates (2006) reported a case of pituitary apoplexy necessitating emergent transsphenoidal adenoma resection and cesarean delivery at 34 weeks. Successful treatment of pregnant women with the somatostatin-receptor ligand *octreotide* and with the GH analogue *pegvisomant* has also been reported (Brian, 2007; Herman-Bonert, 1998; Neal, 2000).

Diabetes Insipidus

The vasopressin deficiency evident in diabetes insipidus is usually due to a hypothalamic or pituitary stalk disorder rather than to a pituitary lesion (Lamberts, 1998). True diabetes insipidus is a rare complication of pregnancy.

Therapy for diabetes insipidus is intranasal administration of a synthetic analogue of vasopressin, *desmopressin,* which is 1-deamino-8-d-arginine vasopressin (DDAVP). Ray (1998) reviewed 53 cases in which DDAVP was used during pregnancy with no adverse sequelae. Most women require increased doses during pregnancy because of an increased metabolic clearance rate stimulated by placental vasopressinase (Lindheimer, 1994). By this same mechanism, *subclinical diabetes insipidus* may become symptomatic or cases of *transient diabetes insipidus* may be encountered during pregnancy (Brewster, 2005; Wallia, 2013). The prevalence of vasopressinase-induced diabetes insipidus is estimated at 2 to 4 per 100,000 pregnancies (Wallia, 2013).

In our experiences, as described in Chapter 55 (p. 1086), transient secondary diabetes insipidus is more likely encountered with *acute fatty liver of pregnancy* (Nelson, 2013). This probably is due to altered vasopressinase clearance because of hepatic dysfunction.

Sheehan Syndrome

Sheehan (1937) reported that pituitary ischemia and necrosis associated with obstetrical blood loss could result in hypopituitarism. With modern methods of hemorrhagic shock treatment, Sheehan syndrome is now seldom encountered (Feinberg, 2005; Tessnow, 2010). An example is shown in Figure 58-7.

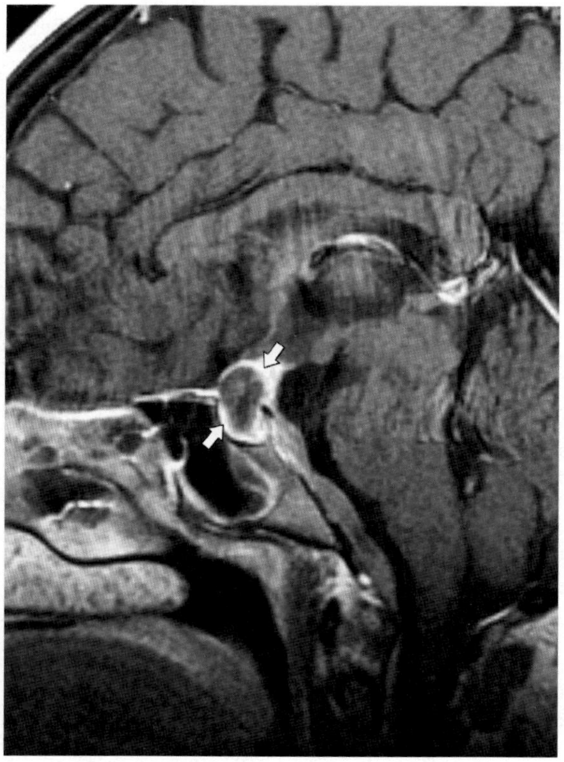

FIGURE 58-7 Sheehan syndrome in a 23-year-old primipara who had major postpartum hemorrhage and hypotension intraoperatively during cesarean delivery. Magnetic resonance imaging was obtained because she failed to lactate, and her serum prolactin level was 18 ng/mL. This sagittal magnetic resonance image shows a large pituitary gland mass (*arrows*) consistent with hemorrhage. Subsequent imaging showed complete hematoma involution, and replacement therapy was not required.

Affected women may have persistent hypotension, tachycardia, hypoglycemia, and lactation failure. Because deficiencies of some or all pituitary responsive hormones may develop after the initial insult, Sheehan syndrome can be heterogenous and may not be identified for years (Tessnow, 2010). In one cohort study of 60 women from Costa Rica with Sheehan syndrome, the average time to diagnosis was 13 years (Gei-Guardia, 2011). Because adrenal insufficiency is the most life-threatening complication, adrenal function should be immediately assessed in any woman suspected of having Sheehan syndrome. After glucocorticoid replacement, subsequent analyses and replacement of thyroid, gonadal, and growth hormones should be considered (Gei-Guardia, 2011; Tessnow, 2010).

Lymphocytic Hypophysitis

This autoimmune pituitary disorder is characterized by massive infiltration by lymphocytes and plasma cells with parenchymal destruction of the gland. Most cases are temporally linked to pregnancy (Caturegli, 2005; Foyouzi, 2011; Madsen, 2000). There are varying degrees of hypopituitarism or symptoms of mass effect, including headaches and visual field defects. A sellar mass is seen with CT or MR imaging. A mass accompanied by a modestly elevated serum prolactin level—usually < 100 pg/mL—suggests lymphocytic hypophysitis. In contrast, levels > 200 pg/mL are encountered with a prolactinoma. The etiology is unknown, but nearly 30 percent have a history of coexisting autoimmune diseases including Hashimoto thyroiditis, Addison disease, type 1 diabetes, and pernicious anemia. Treatment is with hormone replacement and because the disease may be self-limited, a careful withdrawal of hormone replacement should be attempted after inflammation resolution (Foyouzi, 2011; Gagneja, 1999). Surgery during pregnancy is warranted only in cases of severe chiasmal compression unresponsive to corticosteroid therapy (Lee, 2003).

REFERENCES

Abalovich M, Alcaraz G, Kleiman-Rubinsztein J, et al: The relationship of preconception thyrotropin levels to requirements for increasing the levothyroxine dose during pregnancy in women with primary hypothyroidism. Thyroid 20(10):1175, 2010

Abalovich M, Gutierrez S, Alcaraz G, et al: Overt and subclinical hypothyroidism complicating pregnancy. Thyroid 12:63, 2002

Abbassi-Ghanavati M, Casey B, Spong C, et al: Pregnancy outcomes in women with thyroid peroxidase antibodies. Obstet Gynecol 116(2, Pt 1):381, 2010

Abdelmannan D, Aron D: Adrenal disorders in pregnancy. Endocrinol Metab Clin North Am 40:779, 2011

Abduljabbar M, Affi A: Congenital hypothyroidism. J Pediatr Endocrinol Metab 25(1–2):13, 2012

Abramson J, Stagnaro-Green A: Thyroid antibodies and fetal loss: an evolving story. Thyroid 11:57, 2001

Ahlawat SK, Jain S, Kumari S, et al: Pheochromocytoma associated with pregnancy: case report and review of the literature. Obstet Gynecol Surv 54:728, 1999

Alexander EK, Marquesee E, Lawrence J, et al: Timing and magnitude of increases in levothyroxine requirements during pregnancy in women with hypothyroidism. N Engl J Med 351:241, 2004

Alikasifoglu A, Gonc EN, Yalcin E, et al: Neonatal hyperparathyroidism due to maternal hypoparathyroidism and vitamin D deficiency: a cause of multiple bone fractures. Clin Pediatr 44:267, 2005

American College of Obstetricians and Gynecologists: Subclinical hypothyroidism in pregnancy. Committee Opinion No. 381, October 2007, Reaffirmed 2012

American College of Obstetricians and Gynecologists: Thyroid disease in pregnancy. Practice Bulletin No. 37, August 2002, Reaffirmed 2013
American Thyroid Association and American Association of Clinical Endocrinologists: Hyperthyroidism and other causes of thyrotoxicosis: management guidelines of the American Thyroid Association and American Association of Clinical Endocrinologists. Endocr Pract 17(3):456, 2011
Amino N, Izumi Y, Hidaka Y, et al: No increase of blocking type anti-thyrotropin receptor antibodies during pregnancy in patients with Graves' disease. J Clin Endocrinol Metab 88(12):5871, 2003
Amino N, Tada H, Hidaka Y, et al: Postpartum autoimmune thyroid syndrome. Endocr J 47:645, 2000
Anselmo J, Cao D, Karrison T, et al: Fetal loss associated with excess thyroid hormone exposure. JAMA 292:691, 2004
Arafah BM: Increased need for thyroxine in women with hypothyroidism during estrogen therapy. N Engl J Med 344:1743, 2001
Ayala C, Navarro E, Rodríguez JR, et al: Conception after iodine-131 therapy for differentiated thyroid cancer. Thyroid 8:1009, 1998
Bahn RS, Burch HB, Cooper DS, et al: Hyperthyroidism and other causes of thyrotoxicosis: management guidelines of the American Thyroid Association and American Association of Clinical Endocrinologists. Endocr Pract 17(3):456, 2011
Barbesino G, Tomer Y: Clinical utility of TSH receptor antibodies. J Clin Endocrinol Metab 98(6):2247, 2013
Bartolazzi A, Gasbarri A, Papotti M, et al: Application of an immunodiagnostic method for improving reoperative diagnosis of nodular thyroid lesions. Lancet 357:1644, 2001
Beattie GC, Ravi NR, Lewis M, et al: Rare presentation of maternal primary hyperparathyroidism. BMJ 321:223, 2000
Becker DV, Braverman LE, Delange F, et al: Iodine supplementation for pregnancy and lactation—United States and Canada: recommendations of the American Thyroid Association. Thyroid 16:949, 2006
Berbel P. Mestre JL, Santamaria A, et al: Delayed neurobehavioral development in children born to pregnant women with mild hypothyroxinemia during the first month of gestation: the importance of early iodine supplementation. Thyroid 19:511, 2009
Berlin L: Malpractice issues in radiology: iodine-131 and the pregnant patient. AJR 176:869, 2001
Bernal J: Thyroid hormone receptors in brain development and function. Nat Clin Pract Endocrinol Metab 3(3):249, 2007
Bianchi DW, Romero R: Biological implications of bi-directional fetomaternal cell trafficking summary of a National Institute of Child Health and Human Development-sponsored conference. J Matern Fetal Neonatal Med 14:123, 2003
Bilezikian JP, Khan AA, Potts JT Jr: Guidelines for the management of asymptomatic primary hyperparathyroidism: summary statement of the Third International Workshop. J Clin Endocrinol Metab 94(2):335, 2009
Bilezikian JP, Silverberg SJ: Asymptomatic primary hyperparathyroidism. N Engl J Med 350:1746, 2004
Björnsdottir S, Cnattingius S, Brandt L, et al: Addison's disease in women is a risk factor for an adverse pregnancy outcome. J Clin Endocrinol Metab 95(12):5249, 2010
Boscaro M, Barzon L, Fallo F, et al: Cushing's syndrome. Lancet 357:783, 2001
Boyle JG, Davidson DF, Perry CG, et al: Comparison of diagnostic accuracy of urinary free metanephrines, vanillyl mandelic acid, and catecholamines and plasma catecholamines for diagnosis of pheochromocytoma. J Clin Endocrinol Metab 92:4602, 2007
Brand F, Liegeois P, Langer B: One case of fetal and neonatal variable thyroid dysfunction in the context of Graves' disease. Fetal Diagn Ther 20:12, 2005
Brent GA: Graves' disease. N Engl J Med 358:2594, 2008
Brewster UC, Hayslett JP: Diabetes insipidus in the third trimester of pregnancy. Obstet Gynecol 105:1173, 2005
Brian SR, Bidlingmaier M, Wajnrajch MP, et al: Treatment of acromegaly with pegvisomant during pregnancy: maternal and fetal effects. J Clin Endocrinol Metab 92:3374, 2007
Briggs GG, Freeman RK, Yaffe SJ (eds): Drugs in Pregnancy and Lactation, 9th ed. Philadelphia, Lippincott Williams & Wilkins, 2011
Brown RS, Bellisario RL, Botero D, et al: Incidence of transient congenital hypothyroidism due to maternal thyrotropin receptor-blocking antibodies in over one million babies. J Clin Endocrinol Metab 81:1147, 1996
Brundtland GH: United Nations General Assembly Special Session on Children. Sustained elimination of iodine deficiency disorders. World Health Organization, 2002. Available at: http://www.who.int/director-general/speeches/2002/english/20020508_UNGASSSustainedeliminationofIodineDeficiencyDisorders.html. Accessed August 1, 2013
Buescher MA, McClamrock HD, Adashi EY: Cushing syndrome in pregnancy. Obstet Gynecol 79:130, 1992
Cabassi A, Rocco R, Berretta R, et al: Eplerenone use in primary aldosteronism during pregnancy. Hypertension 59(2):e18, 2012
Caldwell KL, Jones R, Hollowell JG: Urinary Iodine Concentration: United States National Health and Nutrition Examination Survey 1001–2002. Thyroid 15(7):692, 2005
Caldwell KL, Makhmudov A, Ely E, et al: Iodine status of the U.S. population, national health and nutrition examination survey, 2005–2006 and 2007–2008. Thyroid 21(4):419, 2011
Calvo RM, Jauniaux E, Gulbis B, et al: Fetal tissues are exposed to biologically relevant free thyroxine concentrations during early phases of development. J Clin Endocrinol Metab 87:1768, 2002
Carbone LD, Palmieri GMA, Graves SC, et al: Osteoporosis of pregnancy: long-term follow-up of patient and their offspring. Obstet Gynecol 86:664, 1995
Caron P, Broussaud S, Bertherat J, et al: Acromegaly and pregnancy: a retrospective multicenter study of 59 pregnancies in 46 women. J Clin Endocrinol Metab 95(10):4680, 2010
Casey BM: Subclinical hypothyroidism and pregnancy. Obstet Gynecol Survey 61(6):415, 2006a
Casey BM, Dashe JS, Spong CY, et al: Perinatal significance of isolated maternal hypothyroxinemia identified in the first half of pregnancy. Obstet Gynecol 109:1129, 2007
Casey BM, Dashe JS, Wells CE, et al: Subclinical hypothyroidism pregnancy outcomes. Obstet Gynecol 105:38, 2005
Casey BM, Leveno KJ: Thyroid disease in pregnancy. Obstet Gynecol 108: 1283, 2006b
Caturegli P, Newschaffer C, Olivi A, et al: Autoimmune hypophysitis. Endocr Rev 26(5):599, 2005
Chamarthi B, Greene M, Dluhy R: A problem in gestation. N Engl J Med 365(9):843, 2011
Cleary-Goldman J, Malone FD, Lambert-Messerlian G, et al: Maternal thyroid hypofunction and pregnancy outcome. Obstet Gynecol 112(1):85, 2008
Cohen O, Pinhas-Hamiel O, Sivian E, et al: Serial in utero ultrasonographic measurements of the fetal thyroid: a new complementary tool in the management of maternal hyperthyroidism in pregnancy. Prenat Diagn 23:740, 2003
Conlin PR: Case 13-2001. Case records of the Massachusetts General Hospital. N Engl J Med 344:1314, 2001
Cooper D, Biondi B: Subclinical thyroid disease. Lancet 379:1172, 2012
Cooper MS: Disorders of calcium metabolism and parathyroid disease. Best Pract Res Clin Endocrinol Metabol 25:975, 2011
Cunningham FG: Screening for osteoporosis. N Engl J Med 353:1975, 2005
Dahan M, Chang RJ: Pancreatitis secondary to hyperparathyroidism during pregnancy. Obstet Gynecol 98:923, 2001
Danilowicz K, Albiger N, Vanegas M, et al: Androgen-secreting adrenal adenomas. Obstet Gynecol 100:1099, 2002
Dashe JS, Casey BM, Wells CE, et al: Thyroid-stimulating hormone in singleton and twin pregnancy: importance of gestational age-specific reference ranges. Obstet Gynecol 107(1):205, 2005
Davis LE, Leveno KL, Cunningham FG: Hypothyroidism complicating pregnancy. Obstet Gynecol 72:108–112, 1988
Davis LE, Lucas MJ, Hankins GDV, et al: Thyrotoxicosis complicating pregnancy. Am J Obstet Gynecol 160:63, 1989
Davison S, Lennard TWJ, Davison J, et al: Management of a pregnant patient with Graves' disease complicated by thionamide-induced neutropenia in the first trimester. Clin Endocrin 54:559, 2001
De Groot L, Abalovich M, Alexander EK, et al: Management of thyroid dysfunction during pregnancy and postpartum: an Endocrine Society clinical practice guideline. J Clin Endocrinol Metab 97(8):2543, 2012
Delange F: Iodine deficiency as a cause of brain damage. Postgrad Med J 77:217, 2001
Desai A, Chutkow W, Edelman E, et al: A crisis in late pregnancy. N Engl J Med 361(23):2271, 2009
Diez JJ, Iglesias P: Spontaneous subclinical hypothyroidism in patients older than 55 years: an analysis of natural course and risk factors for the development of overt thyroid failure. J Clin Endocrinol Metab 89:4890, 2004
Doherty CM, Shindo ML, Rice DH, et al: Management of thyroid nodules during pregnancy. Laryngoscope 105:251, 1995
Dong D, Li H: Diagnosis and treatment of pheochromocytoma during pregnancy. J Matern Fetal Neonatal Med Jan 8, 2014 [Epub ahead of print]
Dosiou C, Barnes J, Schwartz A, et al: Cost-effectiveness of universal and risk-based screening for autoimmune thyroid disease in pregnant women. J Clin Endocrinol Metab 97(5):1536, 2012
Dosiou C, Sanders GC, Araki SS, et al: Screening pregnant women for autoimmune thyroid disease: a cost-effectiveness analysis. Eur J Endocrinol 158(6):841, 2008
Duncombe GJ, Dickinson JE: Fetal thyrotoxicosis after maternal thyroidectomy. Aust N Z J Obstet Gynaecol 41: 2:224, 2001
Fadel BM, Ellahham S, Ringel MD, et al: Hyperthyroid heart disease. Clin Cardiol 23:402, 2000

Farford B, Presutti RJ, Moraghan TJ: Nonsurgical management of primary hyperparathyroidism. Mayo Clin Proc 82:351, 2007
Feigenberg T, Ben-Shushan A, Daka K, et al: Ultrasound-diagnosed puerperal osteopenia in young primiparas. J Reprod Med 53(4):287, 2008
Feinberg EC, Molitch ME, Endres LK, et al: The incidence of Sheehan's syndrome after obstetric hemorrhage. Fertil Steril 84:975, 2005
Fisher DA: Fetal thyroid function: Diagnosis and management of fetal thyroid disorders. Clin Obstet Gynecol 40:16, 1997
Fitzpatrick D, Russell M: Diagnosis and management of thyroid disease in pregnancy. Obstet Gynecol Clin North Am 37:173, 2010
Foyouzi N: Lymphocytic adenohypophysitis. Obstet Gynecol Surv 66(2):109, 2011
Gagneja H, Arafah B, Taylor HC: Histologically proven lymphocytic hypophysitis: spontaneous resolution and subsequent pregnancy. Mayo Clin Proc 74:150, 1999
Gallagher MP, Schachner HC, Levine LS, et al: Neonatal thyroid enlargement associated with propylthiouracil therapy of Graves' diseases during pregnancy: a problem revisited. J Pediatr 139:896, 2001
Gallas PRJ, Stolk RP, Bakker K, et al: Thyroid function during pregnancy and in the first postpartum year in women with diabetes mellitus type 1. Eur J Endocrinol 147(4):443, 2002
Ganguly A: Primary aldosteronism. N Engl J Med 339:1828, 1998
Garber JR, Cobin RH, Gharib H, et al: Clinical practice guidelines for hypothyroidism in adults: cosponsored by the American Association of Clinical Endocrinologists and the American Thyroid Association. Thyroid 22(12):1200, 2012
Geelhoed GW: Surgery of the endocrine glands in pregnancy. Clin Obstet Gynecol 26:865, 1983
Gei-Guardia O, Soto-Herrera E, Gei-Brealey A, et al: Sheehan syndrome in Costa Rica: clinical experience with 60 cases. Endocr Pract 17(3):337, 2011
Gharib H, Papini E, Paschke R, et al: American Association of Clinical Endocrinologists, Associazione Medici Endocrinologi, and European Thyroid Association medical guidelines for clinical practice for the diagnosis and management of thyroid nodules: executive summary of recommendations. J Endocrinol Invest 33(5):287, 2010
Gharib H, Tuttle RM, Baskin HJ, et al: Subclinical thyroid dysfunction: a joint statement on management from the American Association of Clinical Endocrinologists, the American Thyroid Association, and The Endocrine Society. J Clin Endocrinol Metab 90:581, 2005
Gietka-Czernel M, Debska M, Kretowicz P, et al: Fetal thyroid in two-dimensional ultrasonography: nomograms according to gestational age and biparietal diameter. Eur J Obstet Gynecol Reprod Biol 162(2):131, 2012
Gillam MP, Molitch ME, Lombardi G, et al: Advances in the treatment of prolactinomas. Endocr Rev 27:485, 2006
Gondim J, Ramos JF, Pinheiro I, et al: Minimally invasive pituitary surgery in a hemorrhagic necrosis adenoma during pregnancy. Minim Invasive Neurosurg 46(3):173, 2003
Graham EM, Freedman LJ, Forouzan I: Intrauterine growth retardation in a woman with primary hyperparathyroidism. J Reprod Med 43:451, 1998
Greer LG, Casey BM, Halvorson LM, et al: Antithyroid antibodies and parity: further evidence for microchimerism in autoimmune thyroid disease. Am J Obstet Gynecol 205(5):471, 2011
Grimbert P, Chauveau D, Richard S, et al: Pregnancy in von Hippel–Lindau disease. Am J Obstet Gynecol 180:110, 1999
Guven S, Durukan T, Berker M, et al: A case of acromegaly in pregnancy: concomitant transsphenoidal adenomectomy and cesarean section. J Matern Fetal Neonatal Med 19:69, 2006
Gyamfi C, Wapner RJ, D'Alton ME: Thyroid dysfunction in pregnancy. The basic science and clinical evidence surrounding the controversy in management. Obstet Gynecol 113:702, 2009
Haddow JE, Palomaki GE, Allan WC, et al: Maternal thyroid deficiency during pregnancy and subsequent neuropsychological development of the child. N Engl J Med 341:549, 1999
Harper MA, Murnaghan GA, Kennedy L, et al: Pheochromocytoma in pregnancy. Five cases and a review of the literature. Br J Obstet Gynaecol 96:594, 1989
Harris B, Oretti R, Lazarus J, et al: Randomised trial of thyroxine to prevent postnatal depression in thyroid-antibody-positive women. Br J Psychiatry 180:327, 2002
Harvey N, Javaid K, Bishop N, et al: MAVIDOS maternal vitamin D osteoporosis study: study protocol for a randomized controlled trial. The MAVIDOS study group. Trials 13:13, 2012
Hatipoglu B: Cushing's syndrome. J Surg Oncol 106(5):565, 2012
Hegedüs L: The thyroid nodule. N Engl J Med 351:1764, 2004
Helfand M: Screening for subclinical thyroid dysfunction in nonpregnant adults: a summary of the evidence for the U.S. Preventive Services Task Force. Ann Intern Med 140:128, 2004
Helfgott SM: Weekly clinicopathological exercises: Case 21-2002. N Engl J Med 347:122, 2002
Hellmeyer L, Kühnert M, Ziller V, et al: The use of I.V. bisphosphonate in pregnancy-associated osteoporosis—case study. Exp Clin Endocrinol Diabetes 115:139, 2007
Herman-Bonert V, Seliverstov M, Melmed S: Pregnancy in acromegaly: successful therapeutic outcome. J Clin Endocrinol Metab 83:727, 1998
Hershman J: Physiological and pathological aspects of the effect of human chorionic gonadotropin on the thyroid. Best Pract Res Clin Endocrinol Metab 18(2):249, 2004
Hollowell JG, Staehling NW, Hannon WH, et al: Iodine nutrition in the United States. Trends and public health implications: iodine excretion data from National Health and Nutrition Examination Surveys I and III (1971–1974 and 1988–1994). J Clin Endocrinol Metab 83:3401, 1998
Institute of Medicine: Dietary Reference Intakes for vitamin A, vitamin K, arsenic, boron, chromium, copper, iodine, manganese, molybdenum, nickel, silicon, vanadium, and zinc. Washington, National Academies Press, 2001
Ip P: Neonatal convulsion revealing maternal hyperparathyroidism: an unusual case of late neonatal hypoparathyroidism. Arch Gynecol Obstet 268:227, 2003
Jaafar R, Boo NY, Rasat R, et al: Neonatal seizures due to maternal primary hyperparathyroidism. Letters to the Editor. J Paediatr Child Health 40:329, 2004
Junglee N, Harries SE, Davies N, et al: Pheochromocytoma in pregnancy: when is operative intervention indicated? J Womens Health 16:1362, 2007
Kamoun M, Mnif M, Charfi N, et al: Adrenal diseases during pregnancy: pathophysiology, diagnosis and management strategies. Am J Med Sci 347(1):64, 2014
Karmisholt J, Andersen S, Laurberg P: Variation in thyroid function tests in patients with stable untreated subclinical hypothyroidism. Thyroid 18(3): 303, 2008
Kaur M, Pearson D, Godber I, et al: Longitudinal changes in bone mineral density during normal pregnancy. Bone 32:449, 2003
Kempers MJE, van der Sluijs Veer, Nijhuis-van der Sanden MWG, et al: Intellectual and motor development of young adults with congenital hypothyroidism diagnosed by neonatal screening. J Clin Endocrinol Metab 91:418, 2006
Khosrotehrani K, Johnson KL, Cha DH, et al: Transfer of fetal cells with multilineage potential to maternal tissue. JAMA 292:75, 2004
Kilpatrick S: Umbilical blood sampling in women with thyroid disease in pregnancy: is it necessary? Am J Obstet Gynecol 189:1, 2003
Kim PTW, Kreisman SH, Vaughn R, et al: Laparoscopic adrenalectomy for pheochromocytoma in pregnancy. Can J Surg 49:62, 2006
Kimura M, Seki T, Ozawa H, et al: The onset of antineutrophil cytoplasmic antibody-associated vasculitis immediately after methimazole was switched to propylthiouracil in a woman with Graves' disease who wished to become pregnant. Endocr J 60(3):383, 2013
Klein I, Ojamaa K: Thyrotoxicosis and the heart. Endocrinol Metab Clin North Am 27:51, 1998
Klibanski A, Stephen AE, Green MF, et al: Case records of the Massachusetts General Hospital. Case 36–2006, A 35-year-old pregnant woman with new hypertension. N Engl J Med 355:2237, 2006
Kooistra L, Crawford S, van Baar AL, et al: Neonatal effects of maternal hypothyroxinemia during early pregnancy. Pediatrics 117:161, 2006
Kort KC, Schiller HJ, Numann PJ: Hyperparathyroidism and pregnancy. Am J Surg 177:66, 1999
Kosaka K, Onoda N, Ishikawa T, et al: Laparoscopic adrenalectomy on a patient with primary aldosteronism during pregnancy. Endocr J 53:461, 2006
Kovacs CS: Calcium and bone metabolism disorders during pregnancy and lactation. Endocrinol Metab Clin North Am 40:795, 2011
Kraemer B, Schneider S, Rothmund R, et al: Influence of pregnancy on bone density: a risk factor for osteoporosis? Measurements of the calcaneus by ultrasonometry. Arch Gynecol Obstet 285:907, 2011
Kriplani A, Buckshee K, Bhargava VL, et al: Maternal and perinatal outcome in thyrotoxicosis complicating pregnancy. Eur J Obstet Gynecol Reprod Biol 54:159, 1994
Kuijpens JL, Vader HL, Drexhage HA, et al: Thyroid peroxidase antibodies during gestation are a marker for subsequent depression postpartum. Eur J Endocrinol 145:579, 2001
Kung AWC, Chau MT, LAO TT, et al: The effect of pregnancy on thyroid nodule formation. J Clin Endocrinol Metab 87:1010, 2002
LaFranchi, SH: Approach to the diagnosis and treatment of neonatal hypothyroidism. J Clin Endocrinol Metab 96(10):2959, 2011
Lal G, Duh QY: Laparoscopic adrenalectomy—indications and technique. Surg Oncol 12:105, 2003
Lamberts SWJ, de Herder WW, van der Lely AJ: Pituitary insufficiency. Lancet 352:127, 1998

Lazarus J, Kaklamanou K: Significance of low thyroid-stimulating hormone in pregnancy. Curr Opin Endocrinol Diabetes Obes 14:389, 2007
Lazarus JH, Bestwick JP, Channon S, et al: Antenatal thyroid screening and childhood cognitive function. N Engl J Med 366(6):493, 2012
Lebbe M, Hubinot C, Bernard P, et al: Outcome of 100 pregnancies initiated under treatment with cabergoline in hyperprolactinaemic women. Clin Endocrinol 73:236, 2010
Lee MS, Pless M: Apoplectic lymphocytic hypophysitis: case report. J Neurosurg 98:183, 2003
Lee RH, Spencer CA, Mestman JH, et al: Free T_4 immunoassays are flawed during pregnancy. Am J Obstet Gynecol 200:260.e1, 2009
Lekarev O, New MI: Adrenal disease in pregnancy. Best Pract Res Clin Endocrinol Metab 25(6):959, 2011
Lenders JWM, Pacak K, Walther MM, et al: Biochemical diagnosis of pheochromocytoma: which test is best? JAMA 287:1427, 2002
Lepez T, Vandewoesttyne M, Hussain S, et al: Fetal microchimeric cells in blood of women with an autoimmune thyroid disease. PLoS One 6(12):1, 2011
Leung AM, Pearce EN, Braverman LE: Iodine nutrition in pregnancy and lactation. Endocrinol Metab Clin North Am 40:765, 2011
Leung AS, Millar LE, Koonings PP, et al: Perinatal outcome in hypothyroid pregnancies. Obstet Gynecol 81:349, 1993
Lindheimer MD, Barron WM: Water metabolism and vasopressin secretion during pregnancy. Baillieres Clin Obstet Gynaecol 8:311, 1994
Lindsay JR, Jonklaas J, Oldfield EH, et al: Cushing's syndrome during pregnancy: personal experience and review of literature. J Clin Endocrinol Metab 90:3077, 2005
Loh JA, Wartofsky L, Jonklaas J, et al: The magnitude of increased levothyroxine requirements in hypothyroid pregnant women depends upon the etiology of the hypothyroidism. Thyroid 19(3):269, 2009
Lucas A, Pizarro E, Granada ML, et al: Postpartum thyroid dysfunction and postpartum depression: are they two linked disorders? Clin Endocrinol 55:809, 2001
Lucas A, Pizarro E, Granada ML, et al: Postpartum thyroiditis: epidemiology and clinical evolution in a nonselected population. Thyroid 10:71, 2000
Luton D, Le Gac I, Vuillard E, et al: Management of Graves' disease during pregnancy: the key role of fetal thyroid gland monitoring. J Clin Endocrinol Metab 90:6093, 2005
Madsen JR: Case records of the Massachusetts General Hospital: Case 34-2000. N Engl J Med 343:1399, 2000
Malekar-Raikar S, Sinnott B: Primary hyperparathyroidism in pregnancy—a rare case of life-threatening hypercalcemia: case report and literature review. Case Rep Endocrinol 2011:520516, 2011
Maliha G, Morgan J, Varhas M: Transient osteoporosis of pregnancy. Int J Care Injured 43:1237, 2012
Manger WM: The vagaries of pheochromocytomas. Am J Hypertens 18:1266, 2005
Männistö, T, Vääräsmäki M, Pouta A, et al: Perinatal outcome of children born to mothers with thyroid dysfunction or antibodies: a prospective population-based cohort study. J Clin Endocrinol Metab 94:772, 2009
Männistö, T, Vääräsmäki M, Pouta A, et al: Thyroid dysfunction and autoantibodies during pregnancy as predictive factors of pregnancy complications and maternal morbidity in later life. J Clin Endocrinol Metab 95:1084, 2010
Mascetti L, Bettinelli A, Simonetti GD, et al: Pregnancy in inherited hypokalemic salt-losing renal tubular disorder. Obstet Gynecol 117(2 Pt 2):512, 2011
Matalon S, Sheiner E, Levy A, et al: Relationship of treated maternal hypothyroidism and perinatal outcome. J Reprod Med 51:59, 2006
Melmed S: Acromegaly. N Engl J Med 355(24):2558, 2006
Mestman JH: Endocrine diseases in pregnancy. In Gabbe S, Niebyl JR, Simpson JL (eds): Obstetrics: Normal and Problem Pregnancies, 4th ed. New York, Churchill Livingstone, 2002, p 1117
Mestman JH: Hyperthyroidism in pregnancy. Curr Opin Endocrinol Diabetes Obes 19:394, 2012
Mestman JH: Hyperthyroidism in pregnancy. Endocrinol Metab Clin North Am 27:127, 1998
Millar LK, Wing DA, Leung AS, et al: Low birth weight and preeclampsia in pregnancies complicated by hyperthyroidism. Obstet Gynecol 84:946, 1994
Miller BS, Dimick J, Wainess R, et al: Age- and sex-related incidence of surgically treated primary hyperparathyroidism. World J Surg 32:795, 2008
Miller C, Bernet V, Elkas JC, et al: Conservative management of extra-adrenal pheochromocytoma during pregnancy. Obstet Gynecol 105:1185, 2005
Miller MA, Mazzaglia PJ, Larson L, et al: Laparoscopic adrenalectomy for pheochromocytoma in a twin gestation. J Obstet Gynecol 32(2):186, 2012
Molitch ME: Pituitary, thyroid, adrenal, and parathyroid disorders. In Barron WM, Lindheimer MD (eds): Medical Disorders During Pregnancy, 3rd ed. St. Louis, Mosby, 2000, p 101
Molitch ME: Pituitary tumors and pregnancy. Growth Horm IGF Res 13(Suppl A):S38, 2003
Momotani N, Noh JH, Ishikawa N, et al: Effects of propylthiouracil and methimazole on fetal thyroid status in mothers with Graves' hyperthyroidism. J Clin Endocrinol Metab 82:3633, 1997
Montoro MN, Paler RJ, Goodwin TM, et al: Parathyroid carcinoma during pregnancy. Obstet Gynecol 96: 841, 2000
Moreno JC, Klootwijk W, van Toor H, et al: Mutations in the iodotyrosine deiodinase gene and hypothyroidism. N Engl J Med 358(17):1811, 2008
Morreale de Escobar G, Obregon MJ, Escobar Del Rey F: Role of thyroid hormone during early brain development. Eur J Endocrinol 151:U25, 2004
Motivala S, Gologorsky Y, Kostandinov J, et al: Pituitary disorders during pregnancy. Endocrinol Metab Clin North Am 40:827, 2011
Muller AF, Drexhage HA, Berghout A: Postpartum thyroiditis and autoimmune thyroiditis in women of childbearing age: recent insights and consequences for antenatal and postnatal care. Endocr Rev 22:605, 2001
Murcia M, Rebagliato M, Iniguez C, et al: Effect of iodine supplementation during pregnancy on infant neurodevelopment at 1 year of age. Am J Epidemiol 173:804, 2011
Nachum Z, Rakover Y, Weiner E, Shalev E: Graves' disease in pregnancy: Prospective evaluation of a selective invasive treatment protocol. Am J Obstet Gynecol 189:159, 2003
National Academy of Clinical Biochemistry: NACB: laboratory support for the diagnosis and monitoring of thyroid disease. Washington, National Academy of Clinical Biochemistry, 2002, p 125
Neal JM: Successful pregnancy in a woman with acromegaly treated with octreotide: case report. Endocr Pract 6:148, 2000
Negro T, Formoso G, Mangieri T, et al: Levothyroxine treatment in euthyroid pregnant women with autoimmune thyroid disease: effects on obstetrical complications. J Clin Endocrinol Metab 91(7):2587, 2006
Nelson DB, Casey BM, McIntire DD, et al: Subsequent pregnancy outcomes in women previously diagnosed with subclinical hypothyroidism. Am J Perinatol 31(1):77, 2014
Nelson DB, Yost NP, Cunningham FG: Acute fatty liver of pregnancy: clinical outcomes and expected durations of recovery. Am J Obstet Gynecol 209(5):456.e1, 2013
O'Doherty MJ, McElhatton PR, Thomas SHL: Treating thyrotoxicosis in pregnant or potentially pregnant women. BMJ 318:5, 1999
Olivieri A, Stazi MA, Mastroiacovo P, et al: A population-based study on the frequency of additional congenital malformations in infants with congenital hypothyroidism: data from the Italian Registry for Congenital hypothyroidism (1991–1998). J Clin Endocrinol Metab 87:557, 2002
Ono M, Miki N, Amano K, et al: Individualized high-dose cabergoline therapy for hyperprolactinemic infertility in women with micro-and macroprolactinomas. J Clin Endocrinol Metab 95(6):2672, 2010
Pallan S, Rahman M, Khan A: Diagnosis and management of primary hyperparathyroidism. BMJ 344:e1013, 2012
Pearce EN: Monitoring and effects of iodine deficiency in pregnancy: still an unsolved problem? Eur J Clin Nutr 67(5):481, 2013
Pederson CA, Johnson JL, Silva S, et al: Antenatal thyroid correlates of postpartum depression. Psychoneuroendocrinology 32:235, 2007
Pop VJ, Brouwers EP, Vader HL, et al: Maternal hypothyroxinemia during early pregnancy and subsequent child development: a 3-year follow-up study. Clin Endocrinol 59:282, 2003
Pop VJ, Kujipens JL, van Baar AL, et al: Low maternal free thyroxine concentrations during early pregnancy are associated with impaired psychomotor development in infancy. Clin Endocrinol 50:149, 1999
Popoveniuc G, Jonklaas J: Thyroid nodules. Med Clin North Am 96:329, 2012
Power ML, Heaney RP, Kalkwarf HJ, et al: The role of calcium in health and disease. Am J Obstet Gynecol 181:1560, 1999
Premawardhana LD, Parkes AB, Ammari F, et al: Postpartum thyroiditis and long-term thyroid status: prognostic influence of thyroid peroxidase antibodies and ultrasound echogenicity. J Clin Endocrinol Metab 85:71, 2000
Ranzini AC, Ananth CV, Smulian JC, et al: Ultrasonography of the fetal thyroid: nomograms based on biparietal diameter and gestational age. J Ultrasound Med 20:613, 2001
Ray JG: DDAVP use during pregnancy: an analysis of its safety for mother and child. Obstet Gynecol Surv 53:450, 1998
Renné C, Lopez ER, Steimle-Grauer SA, et al: Thyroid fetal male microchimerisms in mothers with thyroid disorders: presence of Y-chromosomal immunofluorescence in thyroid-infiltrating lymphocytes is more prevalent in Hashimoto's thyroiditis and Graves' disease than in follicular adenomas. J Clin Endocrinol Metab 89:5810, 2004
Rooney DP, Traub AI, Russell CFJ, et al: Cure of hyperparathyroidism in pregnancy by sternotomy and removal of a mediastinal parathyroid adenoma. Postgrad Med J 74:233, 1998

Rosen IB, Walfish PG: Pregnancy as a predisposing factor in thyroid neoplasia. Arch Surg 121:1287, 1986

Rotondi M, Mazziotti G, Sorvillo F, et al: Effects of increased thyroxine dosage pre-conception on thyroid function during early pregnancy. Eur J Endocrinol 151:695, 2004

Rovelli R, Vigone M, Giovanettoni C, et al: Newborns of mothers affected by autoimmune thyroiditis: the importance of thyroid function monitoring in the first months of life. Ital J Pediatr 36:24, 2010

Salvatori R: Adrenal insufficiency. JAMA 294:2481, 2005

Sarathi V, Lila A, Bandgar T, et al: Pheochromocytoma and pregnancy: a rare but dangerous combination. Endocr Pract 16(2):300, 2010

Schlechte JA: Long-term management of prolactinomas. J Clin Endocrinol Metab 92:2861, 2007

Schnatz PF, Thaxton S: Parathyroidectomy in the third trimester of pregnancy. Obstet Gynecol Surv 60:672, 2005

Scoccia B, Demir H, Kang Y, et al: *In vitro* fertilization pregnancy rates in levothyroxine-treated women with hypothyroidism compared to women without thyroid dysfunction disorders. Thyroid 22(6):631, 2012

Shangold MM, Dor N, Welt SI, et al: Hyperparathyroidism and pregnancy: a review. Obstet Gynecol Surv 37:217, 1982

Sheehan HL: Post-partum necrosis of the anterior pituitary. J Path Bact 45:189, 1937

Sheffield JS, Cunningham FG: Thyrotoxicosis and heart failure that complicate pregnancy, Am J Obstet Gynecol 190:211, 2004

Shoback D: Hypoparathyroidism. N Engl J Med 359:391, 2008

Siu CW, Zhang XH, Yung C, et al: Hemodynamic changes in hyperthyroidism-related pulmonary hypertension: A prospective echocardiographic study. J Clin Endocrinol Metab 92:1736, 2007

Song SI, Daneman D, Rovet J: The influence of etiology and treatment factors on intellectual outcome in congenital hypothyroidism. J Dev Behav Pediatr 22:376, 2001

Stagnaro-Green A: Maternal thyroid disease and preterm delivery. J Clin Endocrinol Metab 94:21, 2009

Stagnaro-Green A: Overt hyperthyroidism and hypothyroidism during pregnancy. Clin Obstet Gynecol 54(3):478, 2011a

Stagnaro-Green A, Glinoer D: Thyroid autoimmunity and the risk of miscarriage. Baillieres Best Pract Res Clin Endocrinol Metab 18:167, 2004

Stagnaro-Green A, Pearce E: Thyroid disorders in pregnancy. Nat Rev Endocrinol 8:650, 2012a

Stagnaro-Green A, Schwartz A, Gismondi R, et al: High rate of persistent hypothyroidism in a large-scale prospective study of postpartum thyroiditis in southern Italy. J Clin Endocrinol Metab 96(3):652, 2011b

Stagnaro-Green A, Sullivan S, Pearch EN: Iodine supplementation during pregnancy and lactation. JAMA 308(23):2463, 2012b

Steffensen C, Bak AM, Rubeck KZ, et al: Epidemiology of Cushing's syndrome. Neuroendocrinology 92 Suppl 1:1, 2010

Stulberg RA, Davies GAL: Maternal thyrotoxicosis and fetal nonimmune hydrops. Obstet Gynecol 95:1036, 2000

Su PY, Huang K, Hao JH, et al: Maternal thyroid function in the first twenty weeks of pregnancy and subsequent fetal and infant development: a prospective population-based cohort study in China. J Clin Endocrinol Metab 96(10):3234, 2011

Surks MI, Ortiz E, Daniels GH, et al: Subclinical thyroid disease: scientific review and guidelines for diagnosis and management. JAMA (291)2:228, 2004

Swanson CA, Zimmerman MB, Skeaff S, et al: Summary of an NIH workshop to identify research needs to improve the monitoring of iodine status in the United States and to inform the DRI1–3. J Nutr 142:1175S, 2012

Tan TO, Cheng YW, Caughey AB: Are women who are treated for hypothyroidism at risk for pregnancy complications? Am J Obstet Gynecol 194:e1, 2006

Teng W, Shan Z, Teng X, et al: Effect of iodine intake on thyroid diseases in China. N Engl J Med 354:2783, 2006

Tessnow A, Wilson J: The changing face of Sheehan's syndrome. Am J Med Sci 340(5):402, 2010

Thangaratinam S, Tan A, Knox E, et al: Association between thyroid autoantibodies and miscarriage and preterm birth: meta-analysis of evidence. BMJ 342:d2616, 2011

Thomas M, Weisman SM: Calcium supplementation during pregnancy and lactation: effects on the mother and the fetus. Am J Obstet Gynecol 194:937, 2006

Thorpe-Beeston JG, Nicolaides KH, Snijders RJM, et al: Thyroid function in small for gestational age fetuses. Obstet Gynecol 77:701, 1991

Thung SF, Funai EF, Grobman WA: The cost-effectiveness of universal screening in pregnancy for subclinical hypothyroidism. Am J Obstet Gynecol 200(3):267.e1, 2009

To WW, Wong MW, Leung TW: Relationship between bone mineral density changes in pregnancy and maternal and pregnancy characteristics: a longitudinal study. Acta Obstet Gynecol Scand 82:820, 2003

Topaloglu AK: Athyreosis, dysgenesis, and dyshormonogenesis in congenital hypothyroidism. Pediatr Endocrinol Rev 3:498, 2006

Tran P, DeSimone S, Barrett M, et al: I-131 treatment of Graves' disease in an unsuspected first trimester pregnancy; the potential for adverse effects on the fetus and a review of the current guidelines for pregnancy screening. Int J Pediatr Endocrinol 2010:858359, 2010

Tudela CM, Casey BM, McIntire DD, et al: Relationship of subclinical thyroid disease to the incidence of gestational diabetes. Obstet Gynecol 119(5):983, 2012

Vaidya B, Anthony S, Bilous M, et al: Detection of thyroid dysfunction in early pregnancy: universal screening or targeted high-risk case finding? J Clin Endocrinol Metab 92(1):203, 2007

Vargas Zapata CL, Donangelo CM, Woodhouse LR, et al: Calcium homeostasis during pregnancy and lactation in Brazilian women with low calcium intakes: a longitudinal study. Am J Clin Nutr 80:417, 2004

Velasco I, Carreira M, Santiago P, et al: Effect of iodine prophylaxis during pregnancy on neurocognitive development of children during the first two years of life. J Clin Endocrinol Metab 94:3234, 2009

von Mandach U, Aebersold F, Huch R, et al: Short-term low-dose heparin plus bedrest impairs bone metabolism in pregnant women. Eur J Obstet Gynecol Reprod Biol 106:25, 2003

Vulsma T, Gons M, De Vijilder JJM: Maternal–fetal transfer of thyroxine in congenital hypothyroidism due to a total organification defect or thyroid agenesis. N Engl J Med 321:13, 1989

Vydt T, Verhelst J, De Keulenaer G: Cardiomyopathy and thyrotoxicosis: tachycardiomyopathy or thyrotoxic cardiomyopathy? Acta Cardiol 61:115, 2006

Wallia A, Bizhanova A, Huang W, et al: Acute diabetes insipidus mediated by vasopressinase after placental abruption. J Clin Endocrinol Metab 98:881, 2013

Wang W, Teng W, Shan Z, et al: The prevalence of thyroid disorders during early pregnancy in China: the benefits of universal screening in the first trimester of pregnancy. Eur J Endocrinol 164(2):263, 2011

Weetman AP: Graves' disease. N Engl J Med 343:1236, 2000

Wikner BN, Sparre LS, Stiller CO, et al: Maternal use of thyroid hormones in pregnancy and neonatal outcome. Acta Obstet Gynecol Scand 87(6):617, 2008

Williams DH, Dluhy RG: Diseases of the adrenal cortex. In Braunwald E, Fauci AS, Kasper DL, et al (eds): Harrison's Principles of Internal Medicine, 15th ed. New York, McGraw-Hill, 2001, p 2084

Wilson KL, Casey BM, McIntire DD, et al: Diagnosis of subclinical hypothyroidism early in pregnancy is a risk factor for the development of severe preeclampsia. Clin Thyroidol 24(5):15, 2012

Wolfberg AJ, Lee-Parritz A, Peller AJ, et al: Obstetric and neonatal outcomes associated with maternal hypothyroid disease. J Maternal Fetal Neonatal Med 17(1):35, 2005

Yassa L, Marqusee E, Fawcett R, et al: Thyroid hormone early adjustment in pregnancy (the THERAPY) trial. J Clin Endocrinol Metab 95(7):3234, 2010

Yoshihara A, Noh JY, Yamaguchi T, et al: Treatment of Graves disease with antithyroid drugs in the first trimester of pregnancy and the prevalence of congenital malformation. J Clin Endocrinol Metab 97:2396, 2012

Zeeman GG, Wendel G, Cunningham FG: A blueprint for obstetric critical care. Am J Obstet Gynecol 188:532, 2003

Zuluaga-Gómez A, Arrabal-Polo MÁ, Arrabal-Martin M, et al: Management of pheochromocytoma during pregnancy: laparoscopic adrenalectomy. Am Surg 78(3):E156, 2012

CHAPTER 59

Connective-Tissue Disorders

Connective-tissue disorders, which are also termed collagen-vascular disorders, have two basic underlying causes. First are the *autoantibody-mediated immune-complex diseases* in which connective-tissue damage is caused by deposition of immune complexes in specific organ(s) or tissue sites. Because these are manifest by sterile inflammation—predominately of the skin, joints, blood vessels, and kidneys—they are referred to as rheumatic diseases. Many of these immune-complex diseases are more prevalent in women, for example, systemic lupus erythematosus (SLE), rheumatoid arthritis, and a host of vasculitis syndromes. Second are the *inherited disorders* of bone, skin, cartilage, blood vessels, and basement membranes. Some examples include Marfan syndrome, osteogenesis imperfecta, and Ehlers-Danlos syndrome.

IMMUNE-MEDIATED CONNECTIVE-TISSUE DISEASES

These disorders can be separated into those associated with and those without autoantibody formation. So-called *rheumatoid factor (RF)* is an autoantibody found in many autoimmune inflammatory conditions such as SLE, rheumatoid arthritis, systemic sclerosis (scleroderma), mixed connective-tissue disease, dermatomyositis, polymyositis, and various vasculitis syndromes. The *RF-seronegative spondyloarthropathies* are strongly associated with expression of the HLA-B27 antigen and include ankylosing spondylitis, psoriatic arthritis, Reiter disease, and other arthritis syndromes.

Pregnancy may mitigate activity in some of these syndromes as a result of the immunosuppression that also allows successful engraftment of fetal and placental tissues. These changes are discussed in detail in Chapters 4 and 5 (p. 56). One example is pregnancy-induced predominance of T2 helper cells compared with cytokine-producing T1 helper cells (Keeling, 2009). Pregnancy hormones alter immune cells, for example, estrogens upregulate and androgens downregulate T-cell response, and progesterone is immunosuppressive (Cutolo, 2006; Häupl, 2008a; Robinson, 2012).

Some immune-mediated diseases may either be caused or activated as a result of previous pregnancies. To explain, fetal cells and free fetal DNA are detectable in maternal blood beginning early in pregnancy (Simpson, 2013; Sitar, 2005; Waldorf, 2008). *Fetal cell microchimerism* is the persistence of fetal cells in the maternal circulation and organs following pregnancy. These persistent fetal cells may stimulate autoantibodies, or they may become engrafted in maternal tissues. This raises the possibility that fetal cell microchimerism is related to the predilection of autoimmune disorders for women (Adams, 2004; Lissauer, 2009). Evidence for this includes findings of fetal stem cells engrafted in maternal tissues in women with autoimmune thyroiditis and systemic sclerosis (Jimenez, 2005; Srivatsa, 2001). Such microchimerism has also been described in women with SLE and those with rheumatoid arthritis-associated HLA alleles (Johnson, 2001; Lee, 2010; Rak, 2009a). Similarly, engrafted maternal cells may provoke autoimmune conditions in a woman's offspring (Ye, 2012). Perhaps related, women with SLE have a 0.6 male:female offspring ratio suggesting excessive male fetal loss in these women (Aggarwal, 2013).

TABLE 59-1. Some Autoantibodies Produced in Patients with Systemic Lupus Erythematosus (SLE)

Antibody	Prevalence (%)	Clinical Associations
Antinuclear (ANA)	84–98	Best screening test, multiple antibodies; a second negative test makes SLE unlikely
Anti-double-stranded (ds)-DNA	62–70	High titers SLE-specific; may correlate with disease activity, nephritis, and vasculitis
Anti-Sm (Smith)	25–38	Specific for SLE
Anti-RNP	33–40	Not SLE-specific, high titers associated with rheumatic syndromes
Anti-Ro (SS-A)	30–49	Not SLE-specific; associated with Sjögren syndrome, predisposes to cutaneous lupus, neonatal lupus with heart block, reduced risk of nephritis
Anti-La (SS-B)	10–35	Associated with anti-Ro; possible decreased nephritis risk
Antihistone	70	Common in drug-induced lupus (95%)
Antiphospholipid	21–50	Lupus anticoagulant and anticardiolipin antibodies associated with thrombosis, fetal loss, thrombocytopenia, valvular heart disease; false-positive test for syphilis
Anti-erythrocyte	60	Small number develop hemolysis
Antiplatelet	30	Thrombocytopenia in 15%; poor clinical test

Data from Arbuckle, 2003; Hahn, 2012.

Systemic Lupus Erythematosus

Lupus is a heterogeneous autoimmune disease with a complex pathogenesis that results in interactions between susceptibility genes and environmental factors (Hahn, 2012; Tsokos, 2011). Immune system abnormalities include overactive B lymphocytes that are responsible for autoantibody production. These result in tissue and cellular damage when autoantibodies or immune complexes are directed at one or more cellular nuclear components (Tsokos, 2011). In addition, immunosuppression is impaired, including regulatory T-cell function (Tower, 2013). Some autoantibodies produced in patients with lupus are shown in Table 59-1.

Almost 90 percent of lupus cases are in women, and its prevalence in those of childbearing age is approximately 1 in 500 (Lockshin, 2000). Accordingly, the disease is encountered relatively frequently during pregnancy. The 10-year survival rate is 70 to 90 percent (Hahn, 2012; Tsokos, 2011). Infection, lupus flares, end-organ failure, hypertension, stroke, and cardiovascular disease account for most deaths.

Genetic influences are implicated by a higher concordance with monozygotic compared with dizygotic twins—25 versus 2 percent, respectively. Moreover, there is a 10-percent frequency in patients with one affected family member. The relative risk of disease is increased if there is inheritance of the "autoimmunity gene" on chromosome 16 that predisposes to SLE, rheumatoid arthritis, Crohn disease, and psoriasis (Hahn, 2012). Susceptibility genes such as *HLA-A1, B8, DR3, DRB1*, and *TET3* explain only a portion of the genetic heritability (Hom, 2008; Tsokos, 2011; Yang, 2013).

Clinical Manifestations and Diagnosis

Lupus is notoriously variable in its presentation, course, and outcome (Table 59-2). Findings may be confined initially to one organ system, and others become involved later. Or,

TABLE 59-2. Clinical Manifestations of Systemic Lupus Erythematosus

Organ System	Clinical Manifestations	Percent
Systemic	Fatigue, malaise, fever, weight loss	95
Musculoskeletal	Arthralgias, myalgias, polyarthritis, myopathy	95
Hematological	Anemia, hemolysis, leukopenia, thrombocytopenia, lupus anticoagulant, splenomegaly	85
Cutaneous	Malar (butterfly) rash, discoid rash, photosensitivity, oral ulcers, alopecia, skin rashes	80
Neurological	Cognitive dysfunction, mood disorder, headache, seizures	60
Cardiopulmonary	Pleuritis, pericarditis, myocarditis, endocarditis, pneumonitis, pulmonary hypertension	60
Renal	Proteinuria, casts, nephrotic syndrome, renal failure	30–50
Gastrointestinal	Nausea, pain, diarrhea, abnormal liver enzyme levels	40
Vascular	Thrombosis: venous (10%), arterial (5%)	15
Ocular	Conjunctivitis	15

Modified from Hahn, 2012.

the disease may first manifest with multisystem involvement. Common findings are malaise, fever, arthritis, rash, pleuropericarditis, photosensitivity, anemia, and cognitive dysfunction. At least half of patients have renal involvement. There is evidence that lupus is associated with decline in attention, memory, and reasoning (Kozora, 2008). Although *Libman-Sacks endocarditis* was described with lupus, it is likely due to presence of subsequently discussed anticardiolipin antibodies (Hojnik, 1996).

Identification of antinuclear antibodies (ANA) is the best screening test. However, a positive result is not specific for lupus. For example, low titers are found in normal individuals, other autoimmune diseases, acute viral infections, and chronic inflammatory processes. Several drugs can also cause a positive reaction. Antibodies to double-stranded DNA (dsDNA) and to Smith (Sm) antigens are relatively specific for lupus, whereas other antibodies are not (see Table 59-1). Although hundreds of autoantibodies have been described in SLE, only a few have been shown to participate in tissue injury (Sherer, 2004; Tsokos, 2011). Microarray profiles are being developed for customized and more accurate SLE diagnoses (Lin, 2013; Yeste, 2013).

Anemia develops frequently, and there may be leukopenia and thrombocytopenia. Proteinuria and casts are found in the half of patients with glomerular lesions. Lupus nephritis can also cause renal insufficiency, which is more common if there are antiphospholipid antibodies (Moroni, 2004). Other laboratory findings include false-positive syphilis serology, prolonged partial thromboplastin time, and higher rheumatoid factor levels. Elevated serum D-dimer levels often follow a flare or infection, but unexplained persistent elevations are associated with a high risk for thrombosis (Wu, 2008).

The diagnostic criteria for SLE are listed in Table 59-3. If any four or more of these 11 criteria are present, serially or simultaneously, the diagnosis of lupus is made.

Importantly, numerous drugs can induce a lupus-like syndrome. These include procainamide, quinidine, hydralazine, α-methyldopa, phenytoin, and phenobarbital. Drug-induced lupus is rarely associated with glomerulonephritis and usually regresses when the medication is discontinued (Rubin, 1997).

TABLE 59-3. Criteria of the American Rheumatism Association for Systemic Lupus Erythematosus (SLE)

Criteria[a]	Comments
Malar rash	Malar erythema
Discoid rash	Erythematous patches, scaling, follicular plugging
Photosensitivity	Exposure to UV light causes rash
Oral ulcers	Usually painless oral and nasopharyngeal ulcers
Arthritis	Nonerosive involving two or more peripheral joints with tenderness, swelling, or effusion
Serositis	Pleuritis or pericarditis
Renal	Proteinuria greater than 0.5 g/day or > 3+ dipstick, or cellular casts
Neurological	Seizures or psychosis without other cause
Hematological	Hemolytic anemia, leukopenia, lymphopenia, or thrombocytopenia
Autoantibodies	Anti-dsDNA or anti-Sm antibodies, or false-positive VDRL, abnormal level of IgM or IgG anticardiolipin antibodies, or lupus anticoagulant
ANA	Abnormally elevated ANA titers

[a]If four or more criteria are present at any time during disease course, SLE can be diagnosed with 75-percent specificity and 95-percent sensitivity.
ANA = antinuclear antibodies; dsDNA = double-stranded DNA; Sm = Smith; UV = ultraviolet; VDRL = Venereal Disease Research Laboratory.
Modified from Hahn, 2012; Hochberg, 1997; Tan, 1982.

Lupus and Pregnancy

Of nearly 16.7 million pregnancies in the United States from 2000 to 2003, 13,555 were complicated by lupus—an incidence of approximately 1 in 1250 pregnancies (Clowse, 2008). During the past several decades, pregnancy outcomes in women with SLE have improved remarkably. Important factors for pregnancy outcome include whether disease is active at the beginning of pregnancy, age and parity, coexistence of other medical or obstetrical disorders, and whether antiphospholipid antibodies are detected (p. 1173). There is evidence that newly diagnosed lupus during pregnancy tends to be severe (Zhao, 2013).

During pregnancy, lupus improves in a third of women, remains unchanged in a third, and worsens in the remaining third. Thus, in any given pregnancy, the clinical condition can worsen or *flare* without warning (Khamashta, 1997). Petri (1998) reported a 7-percent risk of major morbidity during pregnancy. Women who have confined cutaneous lupus do not usually have adverse outcomes (Hamed, 2013). Frequent complications in a cohort of 13,555 women with SLE during pregnancy are shown in Table 59-4. The maternal mortality and severe morbidity rate was 325 per 100,000. In a review of 13 studies with 17 maternal deaths attributable to SLE and lupus nephritis, all occurred in those with active disease (Ritchie, 2012).

From the foregoing, it is certain that lupus can be life threatening for both mother and fetus. Generally speaking, pregnancy outcome is best in those women in whom: (1) lupus activity has been quiescent for at least 6 months before conception; (2) there is no lupus nephritis manifest by proteinuria or renal dysfunction; (3) there is no evidence of the antiphospholipid antibody syndrome or lupus anticoagulant; and (4) superimposed preeclampsia does not develop (Peart, 2014; Stojan, 2012).

Lupus Nephritis. Active nephritis has been associated with particularly bad pregnancy outcomes, although these have improved remarkably during the past 30 years (Moroni, 2005; Stojan, 2012). Women with renal disease have a high incidence

TABLE 59-4. Complications in 13,555 Pregnancies in Women with Systemic Lupus Erythematosus

Complications	Percent
Comorbid illness	
Pregestational diabetes	5.6
Thrombophilia	4.0
Hypertension	3.9
Renal failure	0.2
Pulmonary hypertension	0.2
Pregnancy complications	
Preeclampsia	22.5
Preterm labor	20.8
Fetal-growth restriction	5.6
Eclampsia	0.5
Medical complications	
Anemia	12.6
Thrombocytopenia	4.3
Thrombotic—stroke, pulmonary embolism, deep-vein thrombosis	1.7
Infections—pneumonia, sepsis syndrome	2.2
Maternal morbidity-mortality rate	325/100,000

Data from Clowse, 2008.

of gestational hypertension and preeclampsia. However, if their disease remains in remission, they usually have good pregnancy outcomes (Huong, 2001; Moroni, 2002). Of the 125 pregnancies reported by Lockshin (1989), 63 percent of women with preexisting renal disease developed preeclampsia compared with only 14 percent of those without underlying renal disease. Moroni and Ponticelli (2005) reviewed results from a total of 309 pregnancies complicated by established lupus nephritis. Of these, 30 percent suffered a flare, and 40 percent of these had associated renal insufficiency. The maternal mortality rate was 1.3 percent.

In two studies describing pregnancy outcomes in women with lupus nephritis, Wagner and coworkers (2009) compared outcomes of 58 women cared for during 90 pregnancies at the Mayo Clinic. Active nephritis was associated with a significantly higher incidence of maternal complications compared with women without nephritis—57 versus 11 percent. Quiescent nephritis had a nonsignificant effect on preeclampsia rates compared with lupus patients without renal impairment. The fetal death rate with active maternal nephritis was 35 percent compared with 9 percent in those with quiescent nephritis. In another study, Imbasciati and associates (2009) described outcomes in 113 pregnancies in 81 women with known lupus nephritis. During a third of pregnancies, there was a renal flare. After excluding nine miscarriages, of the 104 remaining pregnancies, a third were delivered preterm, a third of infants weighed < 2500 g, and the perinatal mortality rate was 6 percent.

Most recommend continuation of immunosuppressive therapy for nephritis during pregnancy. It is not clear whether the dose should be increased peripartum. Although it is often stated that this is the time that activation or exacerbations are most likely to develop, the evidence is not conclusive.

Lupus versus Preeclampsia-Eclampsia. Chronic hypertension complicates up to 30 percent of pregnancies in women with SLE (Egerman, 2005). And as discussed, preeclampsia is common, and superimposed preeclampsia is encountered even more often in those with nephritis or antiphospholipid antibodies (Bertsias, 2008). It may be difficult, if not impossible to differentiate lupus nephropathy from severe preeclampsia if the kidney is the only involved organ (Petri, 2007). Central nervous system involvement with lupus may culminate in convulsions similar to those of eclampsia. Thrombocytopenia, with or without hemolysis, may further confuse the diagnosis because of its similarity to the hemolysis, elevated liver enzymes, low platelet count (HELLP) syndrome. Management is identical to that for preeclampsia-eclampsia, described in Chapter 40 (p. 749).

Management During Pregnancy

Lupus management consists primarily of monitoring maternal clinical and laboratory conditions as well as fetal well-being (Lateef, 2012). Pregnancy-induced thrombocytopenia and proteinuria resemble lupus disease activity, and the identification of a lupus flare is confounded by the increase in facial and palmar erythema of normal pregnancy (Lockshin, 2003). Some authorities have advocated a number of numerical scales to emphasize ongoing disease activity. Components are weighted for severity, both with the SLE-Pregnancy Disease Activity Index (SLEPDAI) and with the Lupus Activity Index (Buyon, 1999; Ruiz-Irastorza, 2004). We have not found these to be useful.

Lupus activity monitoring and identification of lupus flares by various laboratory techniques has been recommended. The sedimentation rate may be misleading because of pregnancy-induced hyperfibrinogenemia. Serum complement levels are also normally increased in pregnancy (Chap. 4, p. 56 and Appendix, p. 1291). And, although falling or low levels of complement components C_3, C_4, and CH_{50} are more likely to be associated with active disease, higher levels provide no assurance against disease activation. Our experiences, as well as those of Varner and colleagues (1983) and Lockshin and Druzin (1995), are that there is no correlation between clinical manifestations of disease and complement levels.

Serial hematological studies may detect changes in disease activity. Hemolysis is characterized by a positive Coombs test, anemia, reticulocytosis, and unconjugated hyperbilirubinemia. Thrombocytopenia, leukopenia, or both may develop. According to Lockshin and Druzin (1995), chronic thrombocytopenia in early pregnancy may be due to antiphospholipid antibodies. Later, thrombocytopenia may indicate preeclampsia.

Serum aminotransferase activity reflects hepatic involvement, as does a rise in serum bilirubin levels. Azathioprine therapy also may induce enzyme elevations. Urine is tested frequently to detect new-onset or worsening proteinuria. Overt proteinuria that persists is an ominous sign, even more so if accompanied by other evidence of the nephrotic syndrome or abnormal serum creatinine levels.

The fetus should be closely observed for adverse effects such as growth restriction and oligohydramnios. Many recommend screening for anti-SS-A (anti-Ro) and anti-SS-B (anti-La) antibodies, because of associated fetal complications described subsequently. As discussed in Chapter 17 (p. 335), antepartum fetal surveillance is done as outlined by the American College of Obstetricians and Gynecologists (2012a). Unless hypertension develops or there is evidence of fetal compromise or growth restriction, pregnancy is allowed to progress to term. Peripartum corticosteroids in "stress doses" are given to women who are taking these drugs or who recently have done so.

Pharmacological Treatment. There is no cure, and complete remissions are rare. Approximately a fourth of women have mild disease, which is not life threatening, but may be disabling because of pain and fatigue. Arthralgia and serositis can be managed by occasional doses of nonsteroidal antiinflammatory drugs (NSAIDs). However, chronic or large intermittent dosing is avoided due to pregnancy side effects with these drugs described in Chapter 12 (p. 247) (Briggs, 2011). Low-dose aspirin can be used throughout gestation. Severe disease is managed with corticosteroids such as prednisone, 1 to 2 mg/kg orally per day. After the disease is controlled, this dose is tapered to a daily morning dose of 10 to 15 mg. Corticosteroid therapy can result in the development of gestational diabetes.

Immunosuppressive agents such as azathioprine are beneficial in controlling active disease (Contreras, 2004; Hahn, 2012). In nonpregnant patients, these are usually reserved for lupus nephritis or disease that is corticosteroid resistant. Azathioprine has a good safety record during pregnancy (Fischer-Betz, 2013; Petri, 2007). Its recommended daily oral dose is 2 to 3 mg/kg. According to Buhimschi and Weiner (2009), cyclophosphamide is teratogenic, and although not usually recommended during pregnancy, severe disease may be treated after 12 weeks' gestation. As discussed in Chapter 12 (p. 250), medications to be avoided include mycophenolate mofetil and methotrexate (Anderka, 2009; Briggs, 2011; Food and Drug Administration, 2008). In some situations, mycophenolate is the only treatment that achieves disease stability. In these cases, counseling regarding fetal risks is essential (Bramham, 2012).

Antimalarials help control skin disease. Although these agents cross the placenta, hydroxychloroquine has not been associated with congenital malformations. Because of the long half-life of antimalarials and because discontinuing therapy can precipitate a lupus flare, most recommend their continuation during pregnancy (Borden, 2001; Harris, 2002). Levy and associates (2001) randomly assigned 20 pregnant women to receive hydroxychloroquine or placebo and reported improved SLEPDAI scores with hydroxychloroquine.

When severe disease supervenes—usually a lupus flare—high-dose glucocorticoid therapy is given. Petri (2007) recommends pulse therapy consisting of methylprednisolone, 1000 mg given intravenously over 90 minutes daily for 3 days, then a return to maintenance doses if possible.

Perinatal Mortality and Morbidity

Adverse perinatal outcomes are increased significantly in pregnancies complicated by lupus. These include preterm delivery, fetal-growth restriction, stillbirths, and neonatal lupus syndrome (Madazli, 2014). Outcomes are worse with a lupus flare, significant proteinuria, or renal impairment, and with chronic hypertension, preeclampsia, or both (Aggarwal, 1999; Bramham, 2012; Scott, 2002; Wagner, 2009). The observations of Lee and coworkers (2009) are worrisome. In a mouse SLE model, they showed that autoantibodies directed against the *N*-methyl-D-aspartate neuroreceptor caused fetal neurotoxicity. This suggests an underlying etiology for the CNS manifestations and learning disorders in children of affected mothers. Ongoing work on anti-dsDNA antibodies has identified peptides that can protect target organs from antibody-mediated damage (Diamond, 2011).

The reasons at least partially responsible for adverse fetal consequences include decidual vasculopathy with placental infarction and decreased perfusion (Hanly, 1988; Lubbe, 1984). Placental pathology is discussed in more detail in Chapter 6 (p. 119).

Neonatal Lupus Syndrome. This unusual constellation is characterized by newborn skin lesions—lupus dermatitis; a variable number of hematological and systemic derangements; and occasionally congenital heart block (Boh, 2004; Lee, 2009). Although usually associated with anti-SS-A and -SS-B antibodies, McGeachy and Lam (2009) described an affected infant in whom only anti-ribonucleoprotein (RNP) antibodies were found. Thrombocytopenia and hepatic involvement are seen in 5 to 10 percent of affected infants. One report suggests that neonatal lupus may appear up to 4 weeks after birth (Stirnemann, 2002). Lockshin and colleagues (1988) prospectively followed 91 infants born to women with lupus. Eight were possibly affected—four had definite neonatal lupus and four had possible disease. Clinical manifestations, which include cutaneous lupus, thrombocytopenia, and autoimmune hemolysis, are transient and clear within a few months (Lee, 1984). This may not be so for congenital heart block. In subsequent offspring, the recurrence risk for neonatal lupus is up to 25 percent (Julkunen, 1993).

Congenital Heart Block. Fetal and neonatal heart block results from diffuse myocarditis and fibrosis in the region between the atrioventricular (AV) node and bundle of His. Buyon and associates (1993) reported that congenital heart block developed almost exclusively in fetuses of women with antibodies to the SS-A or SS-B antigens. These antibodies may also cause otherwise unexplained stillbirths (Ottaviani, 2004). Even in the presence of such antibodies, however, the incidence of myocarditis is only 2 to 3 percent but increases to 20 percent with a prior affected child (Bramham, 2012; Lockshin, 1988). Fetal cardiac monitoring should be performed between 18 and 26 weeks' gestation in pregnancies with either of these antibodies. The cardiac lesion is permanent, and a pacemaker is generally necessary. Long-term prognosis is poor. Of 325 infants with cardiac neonatal lupus, nearly 20 percent died, and of these, a third were stillborn (Izmirly, 2011).

Maternal administration of corticosteroids, plasma exchange, or intravenous immunoglobulin have not been found to reduce the risk of congenital heart block. Corticosteroid therapy to treat fetal heart block has not been subjected to randomized trials. There is some evidence that early treatment may mitigate fetal myocarditis. Shinohara and coworkers (1999) reported no heart block in 26 neonates whose mothers received corticosteroids before 16 weeks' gestation as part of SLE maintenance therapy. By contrast, 15 of 61 neonates with heart block were born to women in whom corticosteroid therapy was begun after 16 weeks for SLE exacerbation. Rein and colleagues (2009) followed 70 fetuses prospectively of mothers positive for anti-SS-A or -SS-B antibodies with serial fetal kinetocardiography (FKCG) to measure AV conduction time. In six fetuses, first-degree heart block developed at 21 to 34 weeks, and maternal dexamethasone treatment was associated with normalization of AV conduction in all within 3 to 14 days. There were no recurrences, and the infants all were well at a median follow-up of 4 years. However, as noted in Chapter 16 (p. 322), corticosteroids may be less effective for higher degrees of heart block. Moreover, potential benefit should be weighed against the risks of chronic corticosteroid treatment, including impaired fetal growth (Friedman, 2009).

Long-Term Prognosis and Contraception

In general, women with lupus and chronic vascular or renal disease may limit family size because of morbidity associated with the disease as well as increased adverse perinatal outcomes. Two large multicenter clinical trials have shown that combination oral contraceptives (COCs) did not increase the incidence of lupus flares (Petri, 2005; Sánchez-Guerrero, 2005). Still, the American College of Obstetricians and Gynecologists (2013) recommends that COC use be avoided in women who have nephritis, antiphospholipid antibodies, or vascular disease. Progestin-only implants and injections provide effective contraception with no known effects on lupus flares (Chabbert-Buffet, 2010). Concerns that intrauterine device (IUD) use and immunosuppressive therapy lead to increased infection rates in these patients are not evidenced-based. Tubal sterilization may be advantageous and is performed with greatest safety postpartum or whenever the disease is quiescent. These options are discussed in further detail in Chapters 38 and 39.

Antiphospholipid Antibody Syndrome

Phospholipids are the main lipid constituents of cell and organelle membranes. There are proteins in plasma that associate noncovalently with these phospholipids. Antiphospholipid antibodies are directed against these phospholipids or phospholipid-binding proteins (Erkan, 2011; Giannakopoulos, 2013; Tsokos, 2011). This antibody group may be of IgG, IgM, and IgA classes, alone or in combination. Antiphospholipid antibodies are most common with lupus and other connective-tissue disorders, although a small proportion of otherwise normal women and men are found to have these antibodies in various forms.

The stimulus for autoantibody production is unclear, but it possibly is due to a preceding infection. The pathophysiology encountered in the *antiphospholipid antibody syndrome*—variably referred to as APAS or APS—is mediated by one or more of the following: (1) activation of various procoagulants, (2) inactivation of natural anticoagulants, (3) complement activation, and (4) inhibition of syncytiotrophoblast differentiation (Moutsopoulos, 2012; Tsokos, 2011). Clinically, these result in arterial or venous thromboses or pregnancy morbidity, and virtually every organ system may be involved as shown in Table 59-5.

Central nervous system involvement is one of the most prominent clinical manifestations. In addition to cerebrovascular arterial and venous thrombotic events, there may be psychiatric features and even multiple sclerosis (Binder, 2010; Sanna, 2003). Renovascular involvement may lead to renal failure that may be difficult to differentiate from lupus nephritis (D'Cruz, 2009). Peripheral and visceral thromboses are also a feature. For example, Ahmed and associates (2009) reported a postpartum woman who developed spontaneous cecal perforation associated with a mesenteric vessel infarction. As discussed in Chapter 18 (p. 359), antiphospholipid antibodies have been associated with excessive pregnancy loss (Branch, 2010). These and other detrimental effects on pregnancy outcomes are discussed subsequently.

A small proportion of these patients develop the *catastrophic antiphospholipid antibody syndrome—CAPS*. This is defined as a rapidly progressive thromboembolic disorder simultaneously involving three or more organ systems or tissues (Moutsopoulos, 2012).

Specific Antiphospholipid Antibodies

Several autoantibodies have been described that are directed against a specific phospholipid or phospholipid-binding protein. First, *β_2-glycoprotein I*—also known as apolipoprotein H—is a phospholipid-binding plasma protein that inhibits prothrombinase activity within platelets and inhibits

TABLE 59-5. Some Clinical Features of Antiphospholipid Antibody Syndrome

Venous thrombosis—thromboembolism, thrombophlebitis, livedo reticularis
Arterial thrombosis—stroke, transient ischemic attack, Libman-Sacks cardiac vegetations, myocardial ischemia, distal extremity and visceral thrombosis and gangrene
Hematological—thrombocytopenia, autoimmune hemolytic anemia
Other—neurological manifestations, migraine headaches, epilepsy; renal artery, vein, or glomerular thrombosis; arthritis and arthralgia
Pregnancy—preeclampsia syndrome, recurrent miscarriage, fetal death

Data from Giannakopoulos, 2013; Moutsopoulos, 2012.

ADP-induced platelet aggregation (Giannakopoulos, 2013; Shi, 1993). Thus, its normal action is to inhibit procoagulant binding and thereby prevent coagulation cascade activation. Logically, antibodies directed against β_2-glycoprotein I would inhibit its anticoagulant activity and promote thrombosis. This is important from an obstetrical viewpoint because β_2-glycoprotein I is expressed in high concentrations on the syncytiotrophoblastic surface. Complement activation may contribute to it pathogenesis (Avalos, 2009; Tsokos, 2011). Teleologically, this seems appropriate because the decidua intuitively should be a critical area to prevent coagulation that might result in intervillous space thrombosis. Another possibility is that β_2-glycoprotein I may be involved in implantation, and it may result in pregnancy loss via an inflammatory mechanism (Iwasawa, 2012; Meroni, 2011).

Second, *lupus anticoagulant (LAC)* is a heterogeneous group of antibodies directed also against phospholipid-binding proteins. LAC induces prolongation in vitro of the prothrombin, partial thromboplastin, and Russell viper venom times (Feinstein, 1972). Thus, paradoxically, this so-called anticoagulant is actually powerfully thrombotic in vivo.

Last, there are *anticardiolipin antibodies (ACAs)*. These are directed against one of the many phospholipid cardiolipins found in mitochondrial membranes and platelets.

Antibodies against Natural Anticoagulants

Antiphospholipid antibodies have also been described that are directed against the natural anticoagulant proteins C and S (Robertson, 2006). Another is directed against the anticoagulant protein annexin V, which is expressed in high concentrations by the syncytiotrophoblast (Chamley, 1999; Giannakopoulos, 2013). That said, criteria to diagnosis antiphospholipid-antibody syndrome require testing for elevated levels of the following antiphospholipid antibodies: LAC, ACA, and anti-β_2 glycoprotein I. Testing for other antibodies is not recommended (American College of Obstetricians and Gynecologists, 2012b).

Antiphospholipid Antibody Syndrome Diagnosis

Clinical classification criteria shown in Table 59-5 provide indications for testing. By international consensus, the syndrome is diagnosed based on laboratory and clinical criteria (Miyakis, 2006). First, one of two clinical criteria—which are vascular thrombosis or certain pregnancy morbidity—must be present. In addition, at least one laboratory criterion that includes LAC activity or medium- to high-positive levels of specific IgG- or IgM-ACAs must be confirmed on two occasions 12 weeks apart.

Tests for LAC are nonspecific coagulation tests. The *partial thromboplastin time* is generally prolonged because the anticoagulant interferes with conversion of prothrombin to thrombin in vitro. Tests considered more specific are the *dilute Russell viper venom test* and the *platelet neutralization procedure*. There is currently disagreement as to which of these two is best for screening. If either is positive, then identification of LAC is confirmed.

Branch and Khamashta (2003) recommend conservative interpretation of results based on repeated tests from a reliable laboratory that are consistent with each clinical case. Only approximately 20 percent of patients with APS have a positive LAC reaction alone. Thus, anticardiolipin enzyme-linked immunosorbent assay (ELISA) testing should also be performed. Many laboratories have a premade panel to use for APS testing.

Efforts have been made to standardize ACA assays by using ELISA. Values are reported in units and expressed as *negative, low-positive, medium-positive,* or *high-positive* (Harris, 1987a,b). Despite this, these assays remain without international standardization (Adams, 2013; Branch, 2003; Capuano, 2007). Interlaboratory variation can be large, and agreement between commercial kits is poor.

Pregnancy and Antiphospholipid Antibodies

Nonspecific low levels of antiphospholipid antibodies are identified in approximately 5 percent of normal adults (Branch, 2010). When Lockwood and coworkers (1989) first studied 737 normal pregnant women, they reported that 0.3 percent had lupus anticoagulant and 2.2 percent had elevated concentrations of either IgM or IgG anticardiolipin antibodies. Later studies confirmed this, and taken together, they totaled almost 4000 normal pregnancies with an average prevalence for APAs of 4.7 percent. This is the same as for normal nonpregnant individuals (Harris, 1991; Pattison, 1993; Yasuda, 1995).

In women with high levels of ACAs, and especially when lupus anticoagulant is identified, there are increased risks for decidual vasculopathy, placental infarction, fetal-growth restriction, early-onset preeclampsia, and recurrent fetal death. Some of these women, like those with lupus, also have a high incidence of venous and arterial thromboses, cerebral thrombosis, hemolytic anemia, thrombocytopenia, and pulmonary hypertension (American College of Obstetricians and Gynecologists, 2012b; Clowse, 2008). In 191 LAC-negative women with antiphospholipid-antibody syndrome, women with antibodies to cardiolipin and β_2-glycoprotein I had significantly higher miscarriage rates than if either one alone was positive (Liu, 2013).

Pregnancy Pathophysiology. It is not precisely known how these antibodies cause damage, but it is likely that their actions are multifactorial (Tsokos, 2011). Platelets may be damaged directly by antiphospholipid antibody or indirectly by binding β_2-glycoprotein I, which causes platelets to be susceptible to aggregation (Chamley, 1999; Giannakopoulos, 2013). Rand and colleagues (1997a,b, 1998) propose that phospholipid-containing endothelial cell or syncytiotrophoblast membranes may be damaged directly by the antiphospholipid antibody or indirectly by antibody binding to either β_2-glycoprotein I or annexin V. This prevents the cell membranes from protecting the syncytiotrophoblast and endothelium. It results in exposure of basement membrane to which damaged platelets can adhere and form a thrombus (Lubbe, 1984).

Pierro and associates (1999) reported that antiphospholipid antibodies decreased decidual production of the vasodilating prostaglandin E_2. Decreased protein C or S activity and increased prothrombin activation may also be contributory (Ogunyemi, 2002; Zangari, 1997). Amengual and coworkers (2003) presented evidence that thrombosis with APS is due to activation of the tissue factor pathway. Finally, uncontrolled placental complement activation by antiphospholipid antibodies may play a role in fetal loss and growth restriction (Holers, 2002).

Complications from APS cannot be completely explained by thrombosis alone. Animal models suggest that these are due to inflammation rather than thrombosis (Cohen, 2011). Some investigators theorize that APS-associated clotting is triggered by a "second hit" from innate inflammatory immune responses and recommend antiinflammatory agents (Meroni, 2011).

Adverse Pregnancy Outcomes. Antiphospholipid antibodies are associated with increased rates of fetal wastage (Chap. 18, p. 359). In most early reports, however, women were included *because* they had had repeated adverse outcomes. Both are common—recall that the incidence of antiphospholipid antibodies in the general obstetrical population is about 5 percent and early pregnancy loss approximates 20 percent. Accordingly, data currently are too limited to allow precise conclusions to be drawn concerning the impact of these antibodies on adverse pregnancy outcomes. Fetal deaths, however, are more characteristic with APS than are first-trimester miscarriages (Oshiro, 1996; Roque, 2001). It has also been shown that women with higher antibody titers have worse outcomes compared with those with low titers (Nodler, 2009; Simchen, 2009).

Looking at the issue another way, the frequency of antiphospholipid antibodies may be increased with associated adverse obstetrical outcomes. Polzin and colleagues (1991) identified antiphospholipid antibodies in a fourth of 37 women with growth-restricted fetuses, however, none had evidence for lupus anticoagulant. Approximately a third of women with APS will develop preeclampsia during pregnancy (Clark, 2007b). Moodley and associates (1995) found antiphospholipid antibodies in 11 percent of 34 women with severe preeclampsia before 30 weeks.

When otherwise unexplained fetal deaths are examined, the data are mixed. Haddow and coworkers (1991) measured ACAs in 309 pregnancies with fetal death and found no differences compared with those in 618 normal pregnancies. In women with a history of recurrent pregnancy loss, those with antiphospholipid antibodies had a higher rate of preterm delivery (Clark, 2007a). In a case-control study of 582 stillbirths and 1547 live births, Silver and colleagues (2013) found a three- to fivefold increased risk for stillbirth in women with elevated anticardiolipin and anti-β_2-glycoprotein I levels. Due to the risk of fetal-growth abnormalities and stillbirth, serial sonographic assessment of fetal growth and antepartum testing in the third trimester are recommended by the American College of Obstetricians and Gynecologists (2012b).

Treatment in Pregnancy. Because of the heterogeneity of studies, current treatment recommendations for women with antiphospholipid antibodies can be confusing (Branch, 2003; Robertson, 2006). As discussed, antiphospholipid antibodies that bind to immunoglobulins G, M, and A are semiquantified, and GPL, MPL, and APL binding units are expressed as negative, low-positive, medium-positive, or high-positive (American College of Obstetricians and Gynecologists, 2012b). Of the three, higher titers for GPL and MPL anticardiolipin antibodies are clinically important, whereas low-positive titers are of questionable clinical significance. And *any titer* of APL antibodies has no known relevance at this time.

As discussed in Chapter 52 (p. 1033), women with prior thromboembolic events who have antiphospholipid antibodies are at risk for recurrence in subsequent pregnancies. For these women, prophylactic anticoagulation with heparin throughout pregnancy and for 6 weeks postpartum with either heparin or warfarin is recommended (American College of Obstetricians and Gynecologists, 2012b). For those without history of thromboembolic events, recommendations for management from the American College of Obstetricians and Gynecologists (2012b) and the American College of Chest Physicians (Bates, 2012) are varied and listed in Table 52-8 (p. 1046). Some acceptable schemes include close antepartum observation with or without prophylactic or intermediate-dose heparin, and some form of postpartum anticoagulation for 4 to 6 weeks.

Recent trials have caused the need for heparin to be questioned in women with antibodies but no history of thrombosis (Branch, 2010). Although this is less clear, some recommend that women be treated if they have medium- or high-positive ACA titers or LAC activity and a previous second- or third-trimester fetal death not attributable to other causes (Dizon-Townson, 1998; Lockshin, 1995). Some report that women with recurrent early pregnancy loss and medium- or high-positive titers of antibodies may benefit from therapy (Robertson, 2006). Some individual agents are now considered for pregnant women with antiphospholipid antibody syndrome who have no prior thromboembolic event. These agents are described in the following paragraphs.

Aspirin, given in doses of 60 to 80 mg orally daily, blocks the conversion of arachidonic acid to thromboxane A_2 while sparing prostacyclin production. This reduces synthesis of thromboxane A_2, which usually causes platelet aggregation and vasoconstriction, and simultaneously spares prostacyclin, which normally has the opposite effect. There appear to be no major side effects from low-dose aspirin other than a slight risk of small-vessel bleeding during surgical procedures. Low-dose aspirin does not appear to reduce adverse pregnancy outcomes in antiphospholipid antibody-positive women without the complete syndrome (Del Ross, 2013).

Unfractionated heparin is given subcutaneously in dosages of 5000 to 10,000 units every 12 hours. Some prefer low-molecular-weight heparin, such as 40 mg enoxaparin once daily, because of its ease of administration and smaller risk of osteoporosis and heparin-induced thrombocytopenia (Kwak-Kim, 2013). With therapeutic dosing, some recommend measurement of heparin levels because clotting tests may be altered by lupus anticoagulant (Cowchock, 1998). The rationale for heparin therapy is to prevent venous and arterial thrombotic episodes. Heparin therapy also prevents thrombosis in the microcirculation, including the decidual-trophoblastic interface (Toglia, 1996). As discussed, heparin binds to β_2-glycoprotein I, which coats the syncytiotrophoblast. This prevents binding of anticardiolipin and anti-β_2-glycoprotein I antibodies to their surfaces, which likely prevents cellular damage (Chamley, 1999; Tsokos, 2011). Heparin also binds to antiphospholipid antibodies in vitro and likely in vivo. It is problematic that heparin therapy is associated with a number of complications that include bleeding, thrombocytopenia, osteopenia, and osteoporosis. A detailed description of the use of various heparins and their doses and adverse effects is found in Chapter 52 (p. 1037).

Glucocorticosteroids generally should not be used with *primary APS*—that is, without an associated connective-tissue disorder. For women with lupus or those being treated for APS who develop lupus, corticosteroid therapy is indicated (Carbone, 1999). In such cases of *secondary APS* seen with lupus, the dose of prednisone should be maintained at the lowest effective level to prevent flares.

Immunoglobulin therapy is controversial and has usually been reserved for women with either overt disease or heparin-induced thrombocytopenia, or both (Alijotas-Reig, 2013). It is used when other first-line therapies have failed, especially in the setting of preeclampsia and fetal-growth restriction (Cowchock, 1996, 1998; Heilmann, 2003; Silver, 1997). Intravenous immunoglobulin (IVIG) is administered in doses of 0.4 g/kg daily for 5 days—total dose of 2 g/kg. This is repeated monthly, or it is given as a single dose of 1 g/kg each month. Treatment is expensive, and at $75 per gram, one course for a 70-kg woman costs more than $10,000. A Cochrane review of seven trials found no improvement in the livebirth rate for immunotherapy given to women with recurrent pregnancy loss (Porter, 2006). Xiao and associates (2013) studied prednisone and aspirin in 87 patients compared with prednisone, aspirin, low-molecular-weight heparin, and IVIG in 42 women with antiphospholipid antibody syndrome. They reported livebirth rates of 84 and 98 percent and obstetrical morbidity rates of 23 and 7 percent, respectively. We are of the view that randomized trials are needed before there is widespread application of this expensive and cumbersome therapy.

Immunosuppression has not been well evaluated, but azathioprine and cyclosporine do not appear to improve standard therapies (Silver, 1997). As mentioned with lupus on page 1172, methotrexate, cyclophosphamide, and mycophenolate mofetil are contraindicated because of teratogenic potential (Briggs, 2011; Buhimschi, 2009). Hydroxychloroquine therapy may be beneficial with APS (Albert, 2014).

Aspirin plus heparin is the most efficacious regimen (de Jesus, 2014). Low-dose unfractionated heparin—7500 to 10,000 units is used subcutaneously twice daily. Concurrently, low-dose aspirin—60 to 80 mg orally once daily—is given. Although typically given in addition to heparin in women with a prior thromboembolic event, the benefit of aspirin is unclear (American College of Obstetricians and Gynecologists, 2012b; Bouvier, 2014).

Treatment Efficacy. Fetal loss is common in women with antiphospholipid antibodies if untreated (Branch, 1992; Rai, 1995). Even with treatment, recurrent fetal loss rates remain at 20 to 30 percent (Branch, 2003; Empson, 2005; Ernest, 2011). Importantly, some women with lupus and antiphospholipid antibodies have normal pregnancy outcomes without treatment. Again, it is emphasized that women with lupus anticoagulant and prior bad pregnancy outcomes have had liveborns without treatment (Trudinger, 1988).

In a manner similar to neonatal lupus syndrome (p. 1172), up to 30 percent of neonates demonstrate passively acquired antiphospholipid antibodies, and thus there is concern for their adverse effects. For example, Tincani and coworkers (2009) found increased learning disabilities in these children. Simchen and colleagues (2009) reported a fourfold increased risk for perinatal strokes. Of 141 infants followed in a European registry, the rate of preterm birth was 16 percent; low birthweight, 17 percent; and behavioral abnormalities in 4 percent of the children. There were no cases of neonatal thrombosis (Motta, 2010).

Rheumatoid Arthritis

This is a chronic multisystem disease of unknown cause with an immunologically mediated pathogenesis. Infiltrating T cells secrete cytokines that mediate inflammation and systemic symptoms. Its worldwide prevalence is 0.5 to 1 percent, women are affected three times more often than men, and peak onset is from 25 to 55 years (Shah, 2012). The cardinal feature is inflammatory synovitis that usually involves the peripheral joints. The disease has a propensity for cartilage destruction, bony erosions, and joint deformities. Criteria for classification are shown in Table 59-6, and a score of 6 or greater fulfills the requirements for definitive diagnosis.

There is a genetic predisposition, and heritability is estimated at 15 to 30 percent (McInnes, 2011). Genome-wide associated studies have identified more than 30 loci involved in rheumatoid arthritis pathogenesis (Kurkó, 2013). There is an association with the class II major histocompatibility complex molecule HLA-DR4 and HLA-DRB1 alleles (McInnes, 2011; Shah, 2012). In addition, there is a genetic component to joint destruction in rheumatoid arthritis, as alterations in the *IL2RA* gene are associated with less destructive disease (Knevel, 2013). Cigarette smoking appears to increase the risk of rheumatoid arthritis (Papadopoulos, 2005). As discussed subsequently, a protective effect of pregnancy has been reported for development of rheumatoid arthritis, and this may be related to HLA-disparate fetal microchimerism (Guthrie, 2010; Hazes, 1990).

Clinical Manifestations

Rheumatoid arthritis is a chronic polyarthritis with symptoms of synovitis, fatigue, anorexia, weakness, weight loss, depression, and vague musculoskeletal symptoms. The hands, wrists, knees, and feet are commonly involved. Pain, aggravated by movement, is accompanied by swelling and tenderness. Extraarticular manifestations include rheumatoid nodules, vasculitis, and pleuropulmonary symptoms. The American College of Rheumatology criteria for rheumatoid arthritis diagnosis have been revised and are shown in Table 59-6 (Aletaha, 2010). The revision focuses on features at earlier stages to permit earlier therapy initiation with a goal of preventing or decreasing long-term sequelae.

Management

Treatment is directed at pain relief, inflammation reduction, protection of articular structures, and preservation of function.

TABLE 59-6. Criteria for Classification of Rheumatoid Arthritis

Factor	Criteria	Score
Joint involvement	1 large—shoulder, elbow, hip, knee, ankle	0
	2–10 large	1
	1–3 small—MCP, PIP, thumb IP, MTP, wrists	2
	4–10 small	3
	> 10—at least 1 small	5
Serological testing	Negative RF and negative ACPA	0
	Low-positive RF or anti-CCP	2
	High-positive RF or anti-CCP	3
Acute-phase reactants	Normal CRP and ESR	0
	Abnormal CRP or ESR	1
Duration of symptoms	Less than 6 weeks	0
	6 weeks or longer	1

ACPA = anti-citrullinated protein antibody; CCP = cyclic citrullinated peptides; CRP = C-reactive protein; ESR = erythrocyte sedimentation rate; IP = interphalangeal joint; MCP = metacarpophalangeal joint; MTP = metatarsophalangeal joint; PIP = proximal interphalangeal joint; RF = rheumatoid factor.
Criteria established in collaboration with the American College of Rheumatology and the European League Against Rheumatism. A score ≥ 6 fulfills criteria for diagnosis.
Modified from Aletaha, 2010.

Physical and occupational therapy and self-management instructions are essential. Although aspirin and other NSAIDs are the cornerstone of symptomatic therapy, they do not retard disease progression. Conventional NSAIDs nonspecifically inhibit both cyclooxygenase-1 (COX-1)—an enzyme critical to normal platelet function, and COX-2—an enzyme that mediates inflammatory response mechanisms. Gastritis with acute bleeding is an unwanted side effect common to conventional NSAIDs. Specific COX-2 inhibitors have been used to avert this complication. However, there are now concerns that their long-term use is associated with increased risk for myocardial infarction, stroke, and heart failure (Solomon, 2005). A systematic review by Adams and colleagues (2012) identified two studies of women treated for inflammatory arthritis. They reported a higher rate of cardiac malformations in infants exposed to NSAIDs in the first trimester. In addition, NSAIDs are associated with early spontaneous abortions, ductus constriction, and neonatal pulmonary hypertension (Briggs, 2011). Thus, risks versus benefits of these medications must be considered.

Glucocorticoid therapy may be added to NSAIDs. Of these, prednisone, 7.5 mg orally daily for the first 2 years of active disease, substantively reduces progressive joint erosions (Kirwan, 1995). Although corticosteroids are usually avoided if possible, low-dose therapy is used by some along with salicylates.

Because NSAIDs and glucocorticoids are primarily for symptomatic relief, the American College of Rheumatology (2012) recommends disease-modifying antirheumatic drugs (DMARDs). These have the potential to reduce or prevent joint damage and are given within 3 months of diagnosis. There are several DMARDs, and many have considerable toxicity. For example, methotrexate and leflunomide are teratogenic (Briggs, 2011). Sulfasalazine and hydroxychloroquine are safe for use in pregnancy (Partlett, 2011; Raza, 2010). These, combined with COX-2 inhibitors and with relatively low-dose prednisone—7.5 to 20 mg daily—for flares are often all the pharmacotherapy needed. Azathioprine treatment may be used if immunosuppressive drugs are warranted. From their review, Kuriya and associates (2011) found that a fourth of women with rheumatoid arthritis took a DMARD within 6 months of conception. During pregnancy, 4 percent of 393 pregnant women were given a category D or X medication. Methotrexate was the most common—2.9 percent. These authors advocate continued efforts to counsel women and their physicians regarding potential risks of many rheumatoid arthritis therapies during pregnancy.

Cytokine inhibitors, which include etanercept (Enbrel), adalimumab (Humira), and infliximab (Remicade), are also being used (McInnes, 2011). The newer immune-targeted drugs for rheumatoid arthritis have shown great promise. But, their use in pregnancy is limited, and fetal safety issues are a concern (Makol, 2011; Ojeda-Uribe, 2013). In the review by Kuriya and coworkers (2011) discussed earlier, 13 percent of 393 women were given a biological cytokine-inhibiting DMARD—primarily etanercept. Experience with these agents in pregnancy has been accruing (Verstappen, 2011). Berthelot and colleagues (2009) found more than 300 reported cases in their review and noted no fetal effects from exposure. Patients considered for etanercept treatment can be entered into a registry at 877-311-8972. There is also little known regarding pregnancy effects of the interleukin-1 receptor antagonist, anakinra (Kineret), and the antagonist to the B-cell CD20 antigen, rituximab (Rituxan).

Other drugs used less frequently include penicillamine, gold salts, minocycline, and cyclosporine. Orthopedic surgery for joint deformities, including replacement, is frequently performed outside of pregnancy.

Pregnancy and Rheumatoid Arthritis

Up to 90 percent of women with rheumatoid arthritis will experience improvement during pregnancy (de Man, 2008). Animal studies suggest this may be due to regulatory T-cell alterations. Transfer of regulatory T cells from pregnant mice conferred protection to those not pregnant (Munoz-Suano, 2012). That said, some women develop disease during pregnancy, and others become worse (Nelson, 1997).

A downside to this respite during pregnancy is that postpartum exacerbation is common (Østensen, 2007). This may be due to alterations in innate immunity postpartum (Häupl, 2008b). Barrett and coworkers (2000a) reported that a postpartum flare was more common if women were breast feeding. These same investigators performed a prospective United Kingdom study involving 140 women with rheumatoid arthritis (Barrett, 2000b). During 1 to 6 months postpartum, there was only a modest fall in objective disease activity, and only 16 percent had complete remission. At least 25 percent had substantive levels of disability. They observed that although overall disease actually did not exacerbate postpartum, the mean number of inflamed joints increased significantly.

There are some studies that report a protective effect of pregnancy for women developing subsequent new-onset rheumatoid arthritis. Silman and associates (1992) performed a case-control study of 88 affected women. They found that although there was a protective effect of pregnancy in the long term, the likelihood of new-onset rheumatoid arthritis was increased sixfold during the first 3 postpartum months. Pikwer and colleagues (2009) reported a significant reduction in the risk of subsequent arthritis in women who breast fed longer than 12 months.

As an explanation for these findings, and as discussed previously, sex hormones supposedly interfere with a number of putative processes involved in arthritis pathogenesis, including immunoregulation and interactions with the cytokine system (Häupl, 2008a,b). First, Unger and associates (1983) reported that amelioration of rheumatoid arthritis correlated with serum levels of *pregnancy-associated* α_2*-glycoprotein.* This compound has immunosuppressive properties. Second, Nelson and coworkers (1993) reported that amelioration of disease was associated with a disparity in HLA class II antigens between mother and fetus. They suggested that the maternal immune response to paternal HLA antigens may play a role in pregnancy-induced remission of arthritis. In addition to monocyte activations, there also may be T-lymphocyte activation (Förger, 2008).

Juvenile Rheumatoid Arthritis

This is a group of diseases that are the most frequent cause of chronic arthritis in children. They persist into adulthood. Østensen (1991) reviewed outcomes of 76 pregnancies in 51 affected Norwegian women. Pregnancy had no effects on presentation of disease, but disease activity usually became quiescent or remained so during pregnancy. Postpartum flares were common as was discussed for rheumatoid arthritis. Joint deformities often developed in these women, and 15 of 20 cesarean deliveries were done for contracted pelves or joint prostheses. These observations are supported by the summary of similar results in 39 Polish women with juvenile rheumatoid arthritis (Musiej-Nowakowska, 1999).

Perinatal Outcome. There are no obvious adverse effects of rheumatoid arthritis on pregnancy outcome, but an increased risk for preterm birth is debated (Klipple, 1989; Langen, 2014; Wallenius, 2011). In a population-based cohort study, Skomsvoll and associates (2002) reported that women with rheumatic disease with two previous poor pregnancy outcomes were at high risk for recurrent adverse outcomes. Kaplan (1986) reported that women who later develop the disease had a prior higher-than-expected incidence of spontaneous abortion. However, Nelson and colleagues (1992) did not corroborate this.

Management During Pregnancy. Treatment of symptomatic women during pregnancy is with aspirin and NSAIDs. These are used with appropriate concerns for first-trimester effects, impaired hemostasis, prolonged gestation, premature ductus arteriosus closure, and persistent pulmonary circulation (Chap. 12, p. 247) (Briggs, 2011). Low-dose corticosteroids are also prescribed as indicated. Gold compounds have been administered in pregnancy. Of 14 women experiencing 20 pregnancies on gold therapy, 75 percent delivered healthy liveborn neonates (Almarzouqi, 2007).

Immunosuppressive therapy with azathioprine, cyclophosphamide, or methotrexate is not routinely used during pregnancy. Of these, only azathioprine should be considered during early pregnancy because the other agents are teratogenic (Briggs, 2011; Buhimschi, 2009). As noted earlier, DMARDs including sulfasalazine and hydroxychloroquine are acceptable for use in pregnancy.

If the cervical spine is involved, particular attention is warranted during pregnancy. Subluxation is common, and pregnancy, at least theoretically, predisposes to this because of joint laxity (Chap. 4, p. 71). Importantly, there are anesthesia concerns regarding endotracheal intubation.

Following pregnancy, contraceptive counseling may include combination oral contraceptives. These are a logical choice because of their effectiveness and their potential to improve disease (Bijlsma, 1992; Farr, 2010). That said, all methods of contraception are appropriate.

Systemic Sclerosis—Scleroderma

This is a chronic multisystem disorder of unknown etiology. It is characterized by microvascular damage, immune system activation leading to inflammation, and excessive deposition of collagen in the skin and often in the lungs, heart, gastrointestinal tract, and kidneys. It is uncommon, displays a 3-to-1 female dominance, and typically affects those aged 30 to 50 years.

This strong prevalence of scleroderma in women and its increased incidence in the years following childbirth contribute to the hypothesis that *microchimerism* is involved as discussed on page 1168 (Lambert, 2010). Artlett and coworkers (1998) demonstrated Y-chromosomal DNA in almost half of women with systemic sclerosis compared with only 4 percent of controls. Rak and colleagues (2009b) identified male microchimerism in peripheral blood mononuclear cells more frequently in women with limited versus diffuse scleroderma—20 versus 5 percent.

Clinical Course

The hallmark is overproduction of normal collagen. In the more benign form—*limited cutaneous systemic sclerosis*—progression is slow. With *diffuse cutaneous systemic sclerosis*, skin thickening progresses rapidly, and skin fibrosis is followed by gastrointestinal tract fibrosis, especially the distal esophagus (Varga, 2012). Pulmonary interstitial fibrosis along with vascular changes may cause pulmonary hypertension. Antinuclear antibodies are found in 95 percent of patients, and immunoincompetence often develops.

Frequent symptoms are Raynaud phenomenon, which includes cold-induced episodic digital ischemia in 95 percent, as well as swelling of the distal extremities and face. Half of patients have symptoms from esophageal involvement, especially fullness and epigastric burning pain. Pulmonary involvement is common and causes dyspnea. The 10-year cumulative survival rate is 70 percent in those with pulmonary fibrosis, and pulmonary arterial hypertension is the main causes of death (Joven, 2010; Ranque, 2010). Women with limited cutaneous disease such as the *CREST syndrome—calcinosis, Raynaud phenomenon, esophageal involvement, sclerodactyly, and telangiectasia*—have milder disease.

Overlap syndrome refers to the presence of systemic sclerosis with features of other connective-tissue disorders. *Mixed-connective-tissue disease* is a term used for the syndrome involving features of lupus, systemic sclerosis, polymyositis, rheumatoid arthritis, and high titers of anti-RNP antibodies (see Table 59-1). The disorder is also termed *undifferentiated connective-tissue disease* (Spinillo, 2008).

Although systemic sclerosis cannot be cured, treatment directed at end-organ involvement can relieve symptoms and improve function (Varga, 2012). Hydroxychloroquine and low-dose corticosteroids are helpful, and intravenous immunoglobulin may be indicated for pericarditis and hemolytic anemia. Renal involvement and hypertension are common. At times, angiotensin-converting enzyme (ACE) inhibitors may be required for blood pressure control despite their known teratogenicity (Buhimschi, 2009). *Scleroderma renal crisis* develops in up to a fourth of these patients and is characterized by obliterative vasculopathy of the renal cortical arteries. This results in renal failure and malignant hypertension. Interstitial restrictive lung disease is common and frequently becomes life threatening. Associated pulmonary hypertension is usually fatal. Cyclophosphamide provides some improvement (Tashkin, 2006).

Pregnancy and Systemic Sclerosis

The prevalence of scleroderma in pregnancy is estimated from a study of nearly 11.2 million pregnant women registered in the Nationwide Inpatient Sample. In this study, Chakravarty and associates (2008) reported that 504 women suffered from systemic sclerosis—a prevalence of approximately 1 in 22,000 pregnancies. These women usually have stable disease during gestation if their baseline function is good. As perhaps expected, dysphagia and reflux esophagitis are aggravated by pregnancy (Steen, 1999). Dysphagia results from loss of esophageal motility due to neuromuscular dysfunction. A decrease in amplitude or disappearance of peristaltic waves in the lower two thirds of the esophagus is seen using manometry. Symptomatic treatment for reflux is described in Chapter 54 (p. 1072). Women with renal insufficiency and malignant hypertension have an increased incidence of superimposed preeclampsia. In the presence of rapidly worsening renal or cardiac disease, pregnancy termination should be considered. As discussed, renal crisis is life threatening and is treated with ACE inhibitors, but it does not improve with delivery (Gayed, 2007). Pulmonary hypertension usually contraindicates pregnancy (Chap. 49, p. 987).

Vaginal delivery may be anticipated, unless the soft tissue thickening wrought by scleroderma produces dystocia requiring cesarean delivery. Tracheal intubation for general anesthesia has special concerns because of limited ability of these women to open their mouths widely (Black, 1989). Because of esophageal dysfunction, aspiration is also more likely, and epidural analgesia is preferable.

Pregnancy Outcomes

Maternal and fetal outcomes are related to the severity of underlying disease. Steen and colleagues (1989, 1999) described pregnancies in 214 women with systemic sclerosis—45 percent had diffuse disease. Major complications included renal crisis in three women and increased rates of preterm birth. Chung and coworkers (2006) also reported increased rates of preterm delivery, fetal-growth restriction, and perinatal mortality. A multicenter study of 109 pregnancies from 25 centers reported higher rates of preterm delivery, fetal-growth restriction, and very-low-birthweight infants (Taraboreli, 2012). These are likely related to placental abnormalities that include decidual vasculopathy, acute atherosis, and infarcts. These reduce placental blood flow and are found in many cases (Doss, 1998; Papakonstantinou, 2007).

Contraception

Scleroderma may be associated with subfertility (Bernatsky, 2008; Lambe, 2004). For women who do not choose pregnancy, several reversible contraceptive methods are acceptable. However, hormonal agents, especially combination oral contraceptives, probably should not be used, especially in women with pulmonary, cardiac, or renal involvement. Due to the often unrelenting progression of systemic sclerosis, permanent sterilization should also be considered.

Vasculitis Syndromes

Inflammation and damage to blood vessels may be primary or due to another disease. Most cases are presumed to be caused by immune-complex deposition (Langford, 2012). Primary causes include polyarteritis nodosa, Wegener granulomatosis, Churg-Strauss syndrome, temporal or giant cell arteritis, Takayasu arteritis, Henoch-Schönlein purpura, Behçet syndrome, and cutaneous or hypersensitivity arteritis (Goodman, 2014). Some of these syndromes have antibodies directed against proteins in the cytoplasmic granules of leukocytes—*antineutrophil cytoplasmic antibodies—ANCA*. Their role in vasculitis is unclear, and disease activity is not related to increasing titers.

Polyarteritis Nodosa

This necrotizing vasculitis of small and medium-sized arteries is characterized clinically by myalgia, neuropathy, gastrointestinal disorders, hypertension, and renal disease (Goodman, 2014). Approximately a third of cases are associated with hepatitis B antigenemia (Langford, 2012).

Symptoms are nonspecific and vague. Fever, weight loss, and malaise are present in more than half of cases. Renal failure, hypertension, and arthralgias are common. Diagnosis is made by biopsy, and treatment consists of high-dose prednisone plus cyclophosphamide. Vasculitis due to hepatitis B antigenemia responds to antivirals, glucocorticoids, and plasma exchange (Chap. 55, p. 1090).

There have been only a few reports of documented cases of polyarteritis nodosa associated with pregnancy. Even without definitive data, active arteritis in pregnancy is associated with high mortality rates. Owen and Hauth (1989) reviewed the courses of 12 such pregnant women. In seven, polyarteritis first manifested during pregnancy, and it was rapidly fatal by 6 weeks postpartum. The diagnosis was not made until autopsy in six of the seven women. Four women continued pregnancy, which resulted in one stillborn and three successful outcomes.

Wegener Granulomatosis

This is a necrotizing granulomatous vasculitis of the upper and lower respiratory tract and kidney. Disease frequently includes sinusitis and nasal disease—90 percent; pulmonary infiltrates, cavities, or nodules—85 percent; glomerulonephritis—75 percent; and musculoskeletal lesions—65 percent (Sneller, 1995). At least 90 percent have polyangiitis (Langford, 2012). It is uncommon and usually encountered after 50 years of age. Koukoura and associates (2008) reviewed 36 cases reported in association with pregnancy. In another report, a woman with Wegener disease developed thrombotic microangiopathy associated renal impairment at 32 weeks. A second woman had pneumonitis, but pregnancy did not appear to affect disease activity (Pagnoux, 2011). Because subglottic stenosis is found in up to a fourth, the anesthesia team should be consulted during pregnancy (Engel, 2011; Kayatas, 2012).

Corticosteroids are standard treatment, but azathioprine, cyclosporine, and intravenous immunoglobulin may also be used. For severe disease in the late second or third trimester, cyclophosphamide in combination with prednisolone seems acceptable.

Takayasu Arteritis

Also called *pulseless disease,* this syndrome is most prevalent in young women. It is a chronic inflammatory arteritis affecting large vessels (Goodman, 2014). Unlike *temporal arteritis,* which develops almost exclusively after age 55, the onset of Takayasu arteritis is almost always before age 40. It is associated with abnormal angiography of the upper aorta and its main branches and with upper extremity vascular impairment. Death usually results from congestive heart failure or cerebrovascular events. Computed tomography or magnetic resonance angiography can detect this disorder before the development of severe vascular compromise (Numano, 1999). Takayasu arteritis may respond symptomatically to corticosteroid therapy, however, it is not curative. Selection of surgical bypass or angioplasty has improved survival rates.

Severe renovascular hypertension, cardiac involvement, or pulmonary hypertension worsen pregnancy prognosis. Hypertension is relatively common and should be carefully controlled. Blood pressure is measured in the lower extremity. Overall, the prognosis for pregnancy is good (de Jesús, 2012; Hernández-Pacheco, 2011; Hidaka, 2012; Johnston, 2002; Kraemer, 2008; Mandal, 2012). When the abdominal aorta is involved, however, pregnancy outcome may be disastrous (Sharma, 2000). Vaginal delivery is preferred, and epidural analgesia has been advocated for labor and delivery (Langford, 2002).

Other Vasculitides

Vasculitis caused by *Henoch-Schönlein purpura* is uncommon after childhood. Tayabali and associates (2012) reviewed 20 pregnancies complicated by this vasculitis and described cutaneous lesions in three fourths. Approximately half had arthralgias. Jadaon and colleagues (2005) described 135 pregnancies in 31 women with *Behçet disease* compared with matched nonaffected controls. Although there were no deleterious effects of pregnancy on the underlying disease, the miscarriage rate was significantly increased threefold. Hwang and coworkers (2009) described necrotizing villitis and decidual vasculitis in a placenta from a first-trimester pregnancy termination and another from a term delivery. *Churg-Strauss vasculitis* is rare in pregnancy. Hot and associates (2007) described a pregnant woman who responded to intravenous immune globulin therapy. Corradi and associates (2009) described an affected 35-year-old woman at term whose necrotizing vasculitis involved the heart, and she subsequently underwent cardiac transplantation.

INFLAMMATORY MYOPATHIES

This is the largest group of acquired and potentially treatable causes of skeletal muscle weakness. That said, these disorders have a prevalence of 1 in 100,000 persons (Dalakas, 2012). There are three major groups: polymyositis, dermatomyositis, and inclusion-body myositis, which all present with progressive asymmetrical muscle weakness. They have a variable association with connective-tissue diseases, malignancy, drugs, systemic autoimmune disease such as Crohn disease, and viral, bacterial, and parasitic infections.

Polymyositis is a subacute inflammatory myopathy that is frequently associated with one of the autoimmune connective-tissue disorders. *Dermatomyositis* manifests as a characteristic rash accompanying or preceding weakness. Laboratory findings include elevated muscle enzyme levels in serum and an abnormal electromyogram. Confirmation is by biopsy, which shows perivascular and perimysial inflammatory infiltrates, vasculitis, and muscle fiber degeneration. It usually develops alone but can overlap with scleroderma or mixed connective-tissue disease.

Prevailing theories suggest that the syndromes are caused by viral infections, autoimmune disorders, or both. *Importantly, approximately 15 percent of adults who develop dermatomyositis have an associated malignant tumor.* The timing of myositis and tumor appearance may be separated by several years. The most common sites of associated cancer are breast, lung, stomach, and ovary. The disease usually responds to high-dose corticosteroid therapy, immunosuppressive drugs such as azathioprine or methotrexate, or IVIG (Dalakas, 2012; Williams, 2007). Linardaki and colleagues (2011) report successful treatment with IVIG and corticosteroids in pregnancy.

Experiences in pregnancy are garnered mostly from case series and reviews. Gutierrez and coworkers (1984) reviewed outcomes in 10 pregnancies among seven women with active disease. They reported three abortions, three perinatal deaths, and five preterm deliveries. Rosenzweig and colleagues (1989) reviewed 24 pregnancy outcomes in 18 women with primary polymyositis-dermatomyositis. In 12, the diagnosis preceded pregnancy. Of these, a fourth had an exacerbation in the second or third trimester. Excluding abortions, there were two perinatal deaths and two growth-restricted neonates. In the other 12 in whom disease became manifest first during pregnancy, outcomes were even less favorable. Excluding abortions, half of the eight pregnancies resulted in perinatal death, and one woman died postpartum. Ohno (1992) and Papapetropoulos (1998) and their coworkers described similar cases. From their review, Doria and associates (2004) concluded that pregnancy outcome was related to disease activity and that new-onset disease was particularly aggressive.

HEREDITARY CONNECTIVE-TISSUE DISORDERS

Numerous inherited mutations involve genes that encode for structural proteins of bone, skin, cartilage, blood vessels, and basement membranes. Although connective tissues contain many complex macromolecules such as elastin and more than 30 proteoglycans, the most common constituents are fibrillar collagen types I, II, and III. Various mutations, some recessively and some dominantly inherited, result in clinical syndromes that include Marfan and Ehlers-Danlos syndromes, osteogenesis imperfecta, chondrodysplasias, and epidermolysis bulla. Of concern during pregnancy is the predilection for these disorders to result in aortic aneurysms (Schoenhoff, 2013).

Marfan Syndrome

This is a common autosomal dominant connective-tissue disorder that has a prevalence of 1 in 3000 to 5000 (Prockop, 2012). Marfan syndrome affects both sexes equally. It is caused by a mutation of the fibrillin-1 (*FBN1*) gene on the long arm of chromosome 15 (Loeys, 2002). The *FBN1* gene has a high mutation rate, and there are many mild, subclinical cases. In severe disease, there is degeneration of the elastic lamina in the media of the aorta. This weakness predisposes to aortic dilatation or dissecting aneurysm, which appears more commonly during pregnancy (Bloom, 2010; Curry, 2014; Savi, 2007). Marfan syndrome complicating pregnancy is discussed in detail in Chapter 49 (p. 993).

Ehlers–Danlos Syndrome

This disease is characterized by various connective tissue changes, including skin hyperelasticity. In the more severe types, there is a strong tendency for rupture of any of several arteries to cause either stroke or bleeding. Rupture of the colon or uterus has been described. There are several types of disease based on skin, joint, or other tissue involvement. Some are autosomal dominant, some recessive, and some X-linked (Solomons, 2013). Their aggregate prevalence is approximately 1 in 5000 births (Prockop, 2012). Types I, II, and III are autosomally dominant, and each accounts for about 30 percent of cases. Type IV is uncommon but is known to predispose to preterm delivery, maternal great-vessel rupture, postpartum bleeding, and uterine rupture (Pepin, 2000). In most, the underlying molecular defect is one of collagen or procollagen.

In general, women with Ehlers-Danlos syndrome have an increased frequency of preterm rupture of membranes, preterm delivery, and antepartum and postpartum hemorrhage (Volkov, 2006). Several cases of spontaneous uterine rupture have been described (Bloom, 2010; Rudd, 1983; Walsh, 2007). Tissue fragility makes episiotomy repair and cesarean delivery difficult. Sorokin and colleagues (1994) surveyed female members of the Ehlers-Danlos National Foundation. They reported a stillbirth rate of 3 percent, a preterm delivery rate of 23 percent, and a cesarean delivery rate of 8 percent. Fifteen percent had problematic postpartum bleeding. A maternal and fetal death from spontaneous rupture of the right iliac artery was described by Esaka and coworkers (2009). Finally, Bar-Yosef and associates (2008) described a newborn with multiple congenital skull fractures and intracranial hemorrhage caused by Ehlers-Danlos type VIIC.

Osteogenesis Imperfecta

This disorder is characterized by very low bone mass resulting in brittle bones. Affected patients often have blue sclerae, hearing loss, a history of multiple fractures, and dental abnormalities. There are seven subtypes that range from severe to mild clinical disease. Subtypes show differing genetic inheritance and include autosomal dominant, autosomal recessive, and sporadic patterns. Type I is the mildest form, whereas type II is typically lethal in utero (Prockop, 2012). There are well-characterized gene mutations coding for type I procollagen. These are associated with the specific subtypes. For example, the typical mutation with type I is a premature stop codon in the *COL1A1* gene (Sykes, 1990). Osteogenesis imperfecta has a prevalence of 1 in 30,000 births for type I and 1 in 60,000 for type II.

Women with osteogenesis imperfecta, most commonly type I, may have successful pregnancies (Lyra, 2010). That said, there are several risks in pregnancy, including fractures, complications related to scoliosis with restrictive lung disease, micrognathia, brittle teeth, an unstable cervical spine, uterine rupture, and cephalopelvic disproportion. These women may also have hyperthyroidism and valvular heart disease. It is not unusual for affected women to enter pregnancy having had 20 to 30 prior fractures. Most women with this skeletal disorder require minimal treatment other than management of the fractures and consideration of bisphosphonates to decrease bone loss. The anesthesia team should be consulted during pregnancy regarding plans for delivery (Murray, 2010).

Depending on the type of osteogenesis imperfecta, the fetus may be affected and may also suffer fractures in utero or during delivery (Chap. 10, p. 217). Prenatal diagnosis is available in many situations, if desired.

REFERENCES

Adams K, Bombardier C, van der Heijde DM: Safety of pain therapy during pregnancy and lactation in patients with inflammatory arthritis: a systematic literature review. J Rheumatol Suppl 90:59, 2012

Adams KM, Nelson JL: Microchimerism: An investigative frontier in autoimmunity and transplantation. JAMA 291:1127, 2004

Adams M: Measurement of lupus anticoagulants: an update on quality in laboratory testing. Semin Thromb Hemost 39(3):267, 2013

Aggarwal N, Sawhney H, Vasishta K, et al: Pregnancy in patients with systemic lupus erythematosus. Aust N Z J Obstet Gynaecol 39:28, 1999

Aggarwal R, Sestak AL, Chakravarty EF, et al: Excess female siblings and male fetal loss in families with systemic lupus erythematosus. J Rheumatol 40(4):430, 2013

Ahmed K, Darakhshan A, Au E, et al: Postpartum spontaneous colonic perforation due to antiphospholipid syndrome. World J Gastroenterol 15(4):502, 2009

Albert CR, Schlesinger WJ, Viall CA, et al: Effect of hydroxychloroquine on antiphospholipid antibody-induced changes in first trimester trophoblast function. Am J Reprod Immunol 71:154, 2014

Aletaha D, Neogi T, Silman AJ, et al: 2010 rheumatoid arthritis classification criteria: an American College of Rheumatology/European League Against Rheumatism collaborative initiative. Ann Rheum Dis 69(9):1580, 2010

Alijotas-Reig J: Treatment of refractory obstetric antiphospholipid syndrome: the state of the art and new trends in the therapeutic management. Lupus 22(1):6, 2013

Almarzouqi M, Scarsbrook D, Klinkhoff A: Gold therapy in women planning pregnancy: outcomes in one center. J Rheumatol 34:1827, 2007

Amengual O, Atsumi T, Khamashta MA: Tissue factor in antiphospholipid syndrome: shifting the focus from coagulation to endothelium. Rheumatology 42:1029, 2003

American College of Obstetricians and Gynecologists: Antepartum fetal surveillance. Practice Bulletin No. 9, October 1999, Reaffirmed 2012a

American College of Obstetricians and Gynecologists: Antiphospholipid syndrome. Practice Bulletin No. 132, December 2012b

American College of Obstetricians and Gynecologists: Use of hormonal contraception in women with coexisting medical conditions. Practice Bulletin No. 73, June 2006, Reaffirmed 2013

American College of Rheumatology: Guidelines for the management of rheumatoid arthritis. Arthritis Rheum 46(2):328, 2002

Anderka MT, Lin AE, Abuelo DN: Reviewing the evidence for mycophenolate mofetil as a new teratogen: case report and review of the literature. Am J Med Genet A 149A(6):1241, 2009

Arbuckle MF, McClain MT, Rubertone MV, et al: Development of autoantibodies before the clinical onset of systemic lupus erythematosus. N Engl J Med 349:1526, 2003

Artlett CM, Smith B, Jimenez SA: Identification of fetal DNA and cells in skin lesions from women with systemic sclerosis. N Engl J Med 338:1186, 1998

Avalos I, Tsokos GC: The role of complement in the antiphospholipid syndrome-associated pathology. Clin Rev Allergy Immunol 34(2–3):141, 2009

Barrett JH, Brennan P, Fiddler M, et al: Breast-feeding and postpartum relapse in women with rheumatoid and inflammatory arthritis. Arthritis Rheum 43:1010, 2000a

Barrett JH, Brennan P, Fiddler M, et al: Does rheumatoid arthritis remit during pregnancy and relapse postpartum? Results from a nationwide study in the United Kingdom performed prospectively from late pregnancy. Arthritis Rheum 42:1219, 2000b

Bar-Yosef O, Polak-Charcon S, Hoffman C, et al: Multiple congenital skull fractures as a presentation of Ehlers-Danlos syndrome type VIIC. Am J Med Genet A 146A:3054, 2008

Bates SM, Greer IA, Middledorp S, et al: VTE, thrombophilia, antithrombotic therapy, and pregnancy. Chest 141(2 Suppl):e691S, 2012

Bernatsky S, Hudson M, Pope J, et al: Assessment of reproductive history in systemic sclerosis. Arthritis Rheum 59:1661, 2008

Berthelot JM, De Bandt M, Goupille P, et al: Exposition to anti-TNF drugs during pregnancy: outcome of 15 cases and review of the literature. Joint Bone Spine 76(1):28, 2009

Bertsias G, Ionnidis JPA, Boletis J, et al: EULAR recommendations for the management of systemic lupus erythematosus (SLE). Ann Rheum Dis 67(2):195, 2008

Bijlsma JWJ, Van Den Brink HR: Estrogens and rheumatoid arthritis. Am J Reprod Immunol 28:231, 1992

Binder WD, Traum AZ, Makar RS, et al: Case 37-2010: a 16-year-old girl with confusion, anemia, and thrombocytopenia. N Engl J Med 363(24):2352, 2010

Black CM, Stevens WM: Scleroderma. Rheum Dis Clin North Am 15:193, 1989

Bloom SL, Uppot R, Roberts DJ: Case records of the Massachusetts General Hospital. Case 32-2010. A pregnant woman with abdominal pain and fluid in the peritoneal cavity. N Engl J Med 363(17):1657, 2010

Boh EE: Neonatal lupus erythematosus. Clin Dermatol 22:125, 2004

Borden M, Parke A: Antimalarial drugs in systemic lupus erythematosus. Drug Saf 24:1055, 2001

Bouvier S, Cochery-Nouvellon E, Lavigne-Lissalde G, et al: Comparative incidence of pregnancy outcomes in treated obstetric antiphospholipid syndrome: the NOH-APS observational study. Blood 123:404, 2014

Bramham K, Soh MC, Nelson-Piercy C: Pregnancy and renal outcomes in lupus nephritis: an update and guide to management. Lupus 21(12):1271, 2012

Branch DW, Gibson M, Silver RM: Recurrent miscarriage. N Engl J Med 363:18, 2010

Branch DW, Khamashta M: Antiphospholipid syndrome: obstetric diagnosis, management, and controversies. Obstet Gynecol 101:1333, 2003

Branch DW, Silver RM, Blackwell JL, et al: Outcome of treated pregnancies in women with antiphospholipid syndrome: an update of the Utah experience. Obstet Gynecol 80:614, 1992

Briggs GG, Freeman RK, Sumner J, et al (eds): Drugs in Pregnancy and Lactation: a Reference Guide to Fetal and Neonatal Risk. 9th ed. Philadelphia, Lippincott Williams & Wilkins, 2011

Buhimschi CS, Weiner CP: Medications in pregnancy and lactation. Part 1. Teratol Obstet Gynecol 113:166, 2009

Buyon J, Kalunian K, Ramsey-Goldman R, et al: Assessing disease activity in SLE patients during pregnancy. Lupus 8:677, 1999

Buyon JP, Winchester RJ, Slade SG, et al: Identification of mothers at risk for congenital heart block and other neonatal lupus syndromes in their children. Comparison of enzyme-linked immunoabsorbent assay and immunoblot for measurement of anti SSA/Ro and anti SSB/La antibodies. Arthritis Rheum 36:1263, 1993

Capuano F, Grasso V, Belforte L, et al: Development of automated assays for anticardiolipin antibodies determination: addressing antigen and standardization issues. Ann N Y Acad Sci 1109:493, 2007

Carbone J, Orera M, Rodriguez-Mahou M, et al: Immunological abnormalities in primary APS evolving into SLE: 6 years' follow-up in women with repeated pregnancy loss. Lupus 8:274, 1999

Chabbert-Buffet N, Amoura Z, Scarabin PY, et al: Pregnane progestin contraception in systemic lupus erythematosus: a longitudinal study of 187 patients. Contraception 83(3):229, 2011

Chakravarty EF, Khanna D, Chung L: Pregnancy outcomes in systemic sclerosis, primary pulmonary hypertension, and sickle cell disease. Obstet Gynecol 111(4):927, 2008

Chamley LW, Duncalf AM, Konarkowska B, et al: Conformationally altered beta(2)-glycoprotein I is the antigen for anti-cardiolipin autoantibodies. Clin Exp Immunol 115:571, 1999

Chung L, Flyckt RL, Colon I, et al: Outcome of pregnancies complicated by systemic sclerosis and mixed connective tissue disease. Lupus 15:595, 2006

Clark CA, Spitzer KA, Crowther MA, et al: Incidence of postpartum thrombosis and preterm delivery in women with antiphospholipid antibodies and recurrent pregnancy loss. J Rheumatol 34:992, 2007a

Clark EAS, Silver RM, Branch DW: Do antiphospholipid antibodies cause preeclampsia and HELLP syndrome? Curr Rheum Rep 9:219, 2007b

Clowse ME, Jamison M, Myers E, et al: A national study of the complications of lupus in pregnancy. Am J Obstet Gynecol 199:127.e1, 2008

Cohen D, Buurma A, Goemaere NN, et al: Classical complement activation as a footprint for murine and human antiphospholipid antibody-induced fetal loss. J Pathol 225(4):502, 2011

Contreras G, Pardo V, Leclercq B, et al: Sequential therapies for proliferative lupus nephritis. N Engl J Med 350:971, 2004

Corradi D, Maestri R, Facchetti F: Postpartum Churg-Strauss syndrome with severe cardiac involvement: description of a case and review of the literature. Clin Rheumatol 28(6):739, 2009

Cowchock S: Prevention of fetal death in the antiphospholipid antibody syndrome. Lupus 5:467, 1996

Cowchock S: Treatment of antiphospholipid syndrome in pregnancy. Lupus 7:S95, 1998

Curry R, Gelson E, Swan L, et al: Marfan syndrome and pregnancy: maternal and neonatal outcomes. BJOG January 13, 2014 [Epub ahead of print]

Cutolo M, Capellino S, Sulli A, et al: Estrogens and autoimmune diseases. Ann N Y Acad Sci 1089:538, 2006

Dalakas MC: Polymyositis, dermatomyositis, and inclusion body myositis. In Longo DL, Fauci AS, Kasper DL, et al (eds): Harrison's Principles of Internal Medicine, 18th ed. New York, McGraw-Hill, 2012, p 3508

D'Cruz D: Renal manifestations of the antiphospholipid syndrome. Curr Rheumatol Rep 11(1):52, 2009

de Man YA, Dolhain RJ, van de Geijn FE, et al: Disease activity of rheumatoid arthritis during pregnancy: results from a nationwide prospective study. Arthritis Rheum 59:1241, 2008 de Jesús GR, d'Oliveira IC, dos Santos FC, et al: Pregnancy may aggravate arterial hypertension in women with Takayasu arteritis. Isr Med Assoc J 14(12):724, 2012

de Jesus GR, Rodrigues G, de Jesus NR, et al: Pregnancy morbidity in antiphospholipid syndrome: what is the impact of treatment? Curr Rheumatol Rep 16:403, 2014

Del Ross T, Ruffatti A, Wisentin MS, et al: Treatment of 139 pregnancies in antiphospholipid-positive women not fulfilling criteria for antiphospholipid syndrome: a retrospective study. J Rheumatol 40(4):425, 2013

Diamond B, Bloom O, Al Abed Y, et al: Moving towards a cure: blocking pathogenic antibodies in systemic lupus erythematosus. J Intern Med 269(1):36, 2011

Dizon-Townson D, Branch DW: Anticoagulant treatment during pregnancy: an update. Semin Thromb Hemost 24:55S, 1998

Doria A, Iaccarino L, Ghirardello A, et al: Pregnancy in rare autoimmune rheumatic diseases: UCTD, MCTD, myositis, systemic vasculitis and Behçet disease. Lupus 13:690, 2004

Doss BJ, Jacques SM, Mayes MD, et al: Maternal scleroderma: placental findings and perinatal outcome. Hum Pathol 29(12):1524, 1998

Egerman RS, Ramsey RD, Kao LW, et al: Hypertensive disease in pregnancies complicated by systemic lupus erythematosus. Am J Obstet Gynecol 193:1676, 2005

Empson M, Lassere M, Craig J, et al: Prevention of recurrent miscarriage for women with antiphospholipid antibody or lupus anticoagulant. Cochrane Database Syst Rev 2:CD002859, 2005

Engel NM, Gramke HF, Peeters L, et al: Combined spinal-epidural anaesthesia for a woman with Wegener's granulomatosis with subglottic stenosis. Int J Obstet Anesth 20(1):94, 2011

Erkan D, Derksen R, Levy R, et al: Antiphospholipid Syndrome Clinical Research Task Force report. Lupus 20(2):219, 2011

Ernest JM, Marshburn PB, Kutteh WH: Obstetric antiphospholipid syndrome: an update on pathophysiology and management. Semin Reprod Med 29:522, 2011

Esaka EJ, Golde SH, Stever MR, et al: A maternal and perinatal mortality in pregnancy complicated by the kyphoscoliotic form of Ehlers-Danlos syndrome. Obstet Gynecol 113(2):515, 2009

Farr SL, Folger SG, Paulen ME, et al: Safety of contraceptive methods for women with rheumatoid arthritis: a systematic review. Contraception 82(1):64, 2010

Feinstein DI, Rapaport SI: Acquired inhibitors of blood coagulation. In Spaet TH (ed): Progress in Hemostasis and Thrombosis, Vol 1. New York, Grune & Stratton, 1972, p 75

Fischer-Betz R, Specker C, Brinks R, et al: Low risk of renal flares and negative outcomes in women with lupus nephritis conceiving after switching from mycophenolate mofetil to azathioprine. Rheumatology (Oxford) 52(6):1070, 2013

Food and Drug Administration: FDA Alert: inosine monophosphate dehydrogenase inhibitors (IMPDH) immunosuppressants. May 16, 2008. Available at: http://www.fda.gov/drugs/drugsafety/postmarketdrugsafetyinformationforpatientsandproviders/ucm124776.htm. Accessed June 15, 2013

Förger F, Marcoli N, Gadola S, et al: Pregnancy induces numerical and functional changes of CD4 + CD25 high regulatory T cells in patients with rheumatoid arthritis. Ann Rheum Dis 67(7):984, 2008

Friedman DM, Kim MY, Copel JA, et al: Prospective evaluation of fetuses with autoimmune associated congenital heart block followed in the PR interval and dexamethasone evaluation (PRIDE) study. Am J Cardiol 103(8):1102, 2009

Gayed M, Gordon C: Pregnancy and rheumatic diseases. Rheumatology 46: 1634, 2007

Giannakopoulos B, Krilis SA: The pathogenesis of the antiphospholipid syndrome. N Engl J Med 368:1033, 2013

Goodman R, Dellaripa PF, Miller AL, et al: An unusual case of abdominal pain. N Engl J Med 370:70, 2014

Guthrie KA, Dugowson CE, Voigt LF, et al: Does pregnancy provide vaccine-like protection against rheumatoid arthritis? Arthritis Rheum 62(7):1842, 2010

Gutierrez G, Dagnino R, Mintz G: Polymyositis/dermatomyositis and pregnancy. Arthritis Rheum 27:291, 1984

Haddow JE, Rote NS, Dostaljohnson D, et al: Lack of an association between late fetal death and antiphospholipid antibody measurements in the 2nd trimester. Am J Obstet Gynecol 165:1308, 1991

Hahn BH: Systemic Lupus Erythematosus. In Longo DL, Fauci AS, Kasper DL, et al, (eds): Harrison's Principles of Internal Medicine, 18th ed. New York, McGraw-Hill, 2012

Hamed HO, Ahmed SR, Alzolibani A, et al: Does cutaneous lupus erythematosus have more favorable pregnancy outcomes than systemic disease? A two-center study. Acta Obstet Gynecol Scand 92(8):934, 2013

Hanly JG, Gladman DD, Rose TH, et al: Lupus pregnancy: a prospective study of placental changes. Arthritis Rheum 31:358, 1988

Harris EN: Antirheumatic drugs in pregnancy. Lupus 11:683, 2002

Harris EN, Gharavi AE, Patel SP, et al: Evaluation of the anti-cardiolipin antibody test: report of an international workshop. Clin Exp Immunol 68:215, 1987a

Harris EN, Hughes GRV: Standardizing the anticardiolipin antibody-test. Lancet 1:277, 1987b

Harris EN, Spinnato JA: Should anticardiolipin tests be performed in otherwise healthy pregnant women? Am J Obstet Gynecol 165:1272, 1991

Häupl T, Østensen M, Grützkau A, et al: Interaction between rheumatoid arthritis and pregnancy: correlation of molecular data with clinical disease activity measures. Rheumatology (Oxford) 47(Supp l):19, 2008a

Häupl T, Østensen M, Grützkau A, et al: Reactivation of rheumatoid arthritis after pregnancy: increased phagocyte and recurring lymphocyte gene activity. Arthritis Rheum 58(10):2981, 2008b

Hazes JMW, Dijkmans BAC, Vandenbroucke JP, et al: Pregnancy and the risk of developing rheumatoid arthritis. Arthritis Rheum 33:1770, 1990

Heilmann L, von Tempelhoff GF, Pollow K: Antiphospholipid syndrome in obstetrics. Clin Appl Thromb Hemost 9:143, 2003

Hernández-Pacheco JA, Estrada-Altamirano A, Valenzuela-Jirón A, et al: Takayasu's arteritis in pregnancy: report of seven cases. Ginecol Obstet Mex 79(3):143, 2011

Hidaka N, Yamanaka Y, Fujita Y, et al: Clinical manifestations of pregnancy in patients with Takayasu arteritis: experience from a single tertiary center. Arch Gynecol Obstet 285(2):377, 2012

Hochberg MC: Updating the American College of Rheumatology revised criteria for the classification of systemic lupus erythematosus. Arthritis Rheum 40:1725, 1997

Hojnik M, George J, Ziporen L, et al: Heart valve involvement (Libman–Sacks endocarditis) in the antiphospholipid syndrome. Circulation 93:1579, 1996

Holers VM, Girardi G, Mo L, et al: Complement C3 activation is required for antiphospholipid antibody-induced fetal loss. J Exp Med 195:211, 2002

Hom G, Graham RR, Modrek B, et al: Association of systemic lupus erythematosus with C8orf13—BLK and ITGAM—ITGAX. N Engl J Med 358:900, 2008

Hot A, Perard L, Coppere B, et al: Marked improvement of Churg-Strauss vasculitis with intravenous gamma globulins during pregnancy. Clin Rheumatol 26(12):2149, 2007

Huong DLT, Wechsler B, Vauthier-Brouzes D, et al: Pregnancy in past or present lupus nephritis: a study of 32 pregnancies from a single centre. Ann Rheum Dis 60:599, 2001

Hwang I, Lee CK, Yoo B, et al: Necrotizing villitis and decidual vasculitis in the placentas of mothers with Behçet disease. Hum Pathol 40(1):135, 2009

Imbasciati E, Tincani A, Gregorini G, et al: Pregnancy in women with preexisting lupus nephritis: predictors of fetal and maternal outcome. Nephrol Dial Transplant 24(2):519, 2009

Iwasawa Y, Kawana K, Fujii T, et al: A possible coagulation-independent mechanism for pregnancy loss involving β(2) glycoprotein 1-dependent antiphospholipid antibodies and CD1d. Am J Reprod Immunol 67(1):54, 2012

Izmirly PM, Saxena AM, Kim MY, et al: Maternal and fetal factors associated with mortality and morbidity in a multi–racial/ethnic registry of anti-SSA/Ro–associated cardiac neonatal lupus. Circulation 124:1927, 2011

Jadaon J, Shushan A, Ezra Y, et al: Behçet's disease and pregnancy. Acta Obstet Gynecol Scand 84:939, 2005

Jimenez SA, Artlett CM: Microchimerism and systemic sclerosis. Curr Opin Rheumatol 17:86, 2005

Johnson KL, McAlindon TE, Mulcahy E, et al: Microchimerism in a female patient with systemic lupus erythematosus. Arthritis Rheum 44:2107, 2001

Johnston SL, Lock RJ, Gompels MM: Takayasu arteritis: a review. J Clin Pathol 55:481, 2002

Joven BE, Almodovar R, Carmona L, et al: Survival, causes of death, and risk factors associated with mortality in Spanish systemic sclerosis patients: results from a single university hospital. Semin Arthritis Rheum 39(4):285, 2010

Julkunen H, Kurki P, Kaaja R, et al: Isolated congenital heart block. Long-term outcome of mothers and characterization of the immune response to SS-A/Ro and to SS-B/La. Arthritis Rheum 36(11):1588, 1993

Kaplan D: Fetal wastage in patients with rheumatoid arthritis. J Rheumatol 13:875, 1986

Kayatas S, Asoglu MR, Selcuk S, et al: Pregnancy in a patient with Wegener's granulomatosis: a case report. Bull NYU Hosp Jt Dis 70(2):127, 2012

Keeling SO, Oswald AE: Pregnancy and rheumatic disease: "By the book" or "by the doc." Clin Rheumatol 28(1):1, 2009

Khamashta MA, Ruiz-Irastorza G, Hughes GRV: Systemic lupus erythematosus flares during pregnancy. Rheum Dis Clin North Am 23:15, 1997

Kirwan JR, The Arthritis and Rheumatism Council Low-Dose Glucocorticoid Study Group: The effect of glucocorticoids on joint destruction in rheumatoid arthritis. N Engl J Med 333(3):142, 1995

Klipple GL, Cecere FA: Rheumatoid arthritis and pregnancy. Rheum Dis Clin North Am 15:213, 1989

Knevel R, de Rooy DP, Zhernakova A, et al: Association of variants in IL2RA with progression of joint destruction in rheumatoid arthritis. Arthritis Rheum 65(7):1684, 2013

Koukoura O, Mantas N, Linardakis H, et al: Successful term pregnancy in a patient with Wegener's granulomatosis: case report and literature review. Fertil Steril 89:457.e1, 2008

Kozora E, Arciniegas DB, Filley CM, et al: Cognitive and neurologic status in patients with systemic lupus erythematosus without major neuropsychiatric syndromes. Arthritis Rheum 59:1639, 2008

Kraemer B, Abele H, Hahn M, et al: A successful pregnancy in a patient with Takayasu's arteritis. Hypertens Pregnancy 27(3):247, 2008

Kuriya B, Hernández-Díaz S, Liu J, et al: Patterns of medication use during pregnancy in rheumatoid arthritis. Arthritis Care Res (Hoboken) 63(5):721, 2011

Kurkó J, Besenyei T, Laki J, et al: Genetics of rheumatoid arthritis—a comprehensive review. Clin Rev Allergy Immunol 45(2):170, 2013

Kwak-Kim J, Agcaoili MSL, Aleta L, et al: Management of women with recurrent pregnancy losses and antiphospholipid antibody syndrome. Am J Reprod Immunol 69(6):596, 2013

Lambe M, Bjornadal L, Neregard P, et al: Childbearing and the risk of scleroderma: a population-based study in Sweden. Am J Epidemiol 159:162, 2004

Lambert NC: Microchimerism in scleroderma: ten years later. Rev Med Interne 31(7):523, 2010

Langen ES, Chakravarty EF, Liaquat M, et al: High rate of preterm birth in pregnancies complicated by rheumatoid arthritis. Am J Perinatol 31(1):9, 2014

Langford C, Kerr G: Pregnancy in vasculitis. Curr Opin Rheumatol 14:36, 2002

Langford CA, Fauci AS: The vasculitis syndromes. In Longo DL, Fauci AS, Kasper DL, et al (eds): Harrison's Principles of Internal Medicine, 18th ed. New York, McGraw-Hill, 2012

Lateef A, Petri M: Management of pregnancy in systemic lupus erythematosus. Nat Rev Rheumatol 8(12):710, 2012

Lee ES, Bou-Gharios G, Seppanen E, et al: Fetal stem cell microchimerism: natural-born healers or killers? Mol Hum Reprod 16(11):869, 2010

Lee LA, Weston WL: New findings in neonatal lupus syndrome. Am J Dis Child 138:233, 1984

Lee JY, Huerta PT, Zhang J, et al: Neurotoxic autoantibodies mediate congenital cortical impairment of offspring in maternal lupus. Nat Med 15(1):91, 2009

Levy RA, Vilela VS, Cataldo MJ, et al: Hydroxychloroquine (HCQ) in lupus pregnancy: double-blind and placebo-controlled study. Lupus 10:401, 2001

Lin MW, Ho JW, Harrison LC, et al: An antibody-based leukocyte-capture microarray for the diagnosis of systemic lupus erythematosus. PLoS One 8(3):e58199, 2013

Linardaki G, Cherouvim E, Goni G, et al: Intravenous immunoglobulin treatment for pregnancy-associated dermatomyositis. Rheumatol Int 31(1):113, 2011

Lissauer DM, Piper KP, Moss PA, et al: Fetal microchimerism: the cellular and immunological legacy of pregnancy. Expert Rev Mol Med 11:e33, 2009

Liu XL, Xiao J, Zhu F: Anti-β2 glycoprotein I antibodies and pregnancy outcome in antiphospholipid syndrome. Acta Obstet Gynecol Scand 92(2):234, 2013

Lockshin MD: Pregnancy does not cause systemic lupus erythematosus to worsen. Arthritis Rheum 32:665, 1989

Lockshin M, Sammaritano L: Lupus pregnancy. Autoimmunity 36:33, 2003

Lockshin MD, Bonfa E, Elkon K, et al: Neonatal lupus risk to newborns of mothers with systemic lupus erythematosus. Arthritis Rheum 31:697, 1988

Lockshin MD, Druzin ML: Rheumatic disease. In Barron WM, Lindheimer JD (eds): Medical Disorders During Pregnancy, 2nd ed. St. Louis, Mosby, 1995, p 307

Lockshin MD, Sammaritano LR: Rheumatic disease. In Barron WM, Lindheimer MD (eds): Medical Disorders During Pregnancy, 3rd ed. St. Louis, Mosby, 2000, p 355

Lockwood CJ, Romero R, Feinberg RF, et al: The prevalence and biologic significance of lupus anticoagulant and anticardiolipin antibodies in a general obstetric population. Am J Obstet Gynecol 161:369, 1989

Loeys B, Nuytinck L, Van Acker P, et al: Strategies for prenatal and preimplantation genetic diagnosis in Marfan syndrome (MFS). Prenat Diagn 22:22, 2002

Lubbe WF, Liggins GC: The lupus-anticoagulant: clinical and obstetric complications. NZ Med J 97:398, 1984

Lyra TG, Pinto VA, Ivo FA, et al: Osteogenesis imperfecta in pregnancy. Case report. Rev Bras Anestesiol 60(3):321, 2010

Madazli R, Yuksel MA, Oncul M, et al: Obstetric outcomes and prognostic factors of lupus pregnancies. Arch Gynecol Obstet 289:49, 2014

Makol A, Wright K, Amin S: Rheumatoid arthritis and pregnancy: safety considerations in pharmacological management. Drugs 71(15):1973, 2011

Mandal D, Mandal S, Dattaray C, et al: Takayasu arteritis in pregnancy: an analysis from eastern India. Arch Gynecol Obstet 285(3):567, 2012

McGeachy C, Lam J: Anti-RNP neonatal lupus in a female newborn. Lupus 18(2):172, 2009

McInnes IB, Schett G: The pathogenesis of rheumatoid arthritis. N Engl J Med 365(23):2205, 2011

Meroni PL, Borghi MO, Raschi E, et al: Pathogenesis of antiphospholipid syndrome: understanding the antibodies. Nat Rev Rheumatol 7(6):330, 2011

Miyakis S, Lockshin MD, Atsumi T, et al: International consensus statement on an update of the classification criteria for definite antiphospholipid syndrome (APS). J Thromb Haemost 4:295, 2006

Moodley J, Ramphal SR, Duursma J, et al: Antiphospholipid antibodies in eclampsia. Hypertens Pregnancy 14:179, 1995

Moroni G, Ponticelli C: Pregnancy after lupus nephritis. Lupus 14:89, 2005

Moroni G, Quaglini S, Banfi G, et al: Pregnancy in lupus nephritis. Am J Kidney Dis 40:713, 2002

Moroni G, Ventura D, Riva P, et al: Antiphospholipid antibodies are associated with an increased risk for chronic renal insufficiency in patients with lupus nephritis. Am J Kidney Dis 43:28, 2004

Motta M, Lachassinne E, Boffa MC, et al: European registry of infants born to mothers with antiphospholipid syndrome: preliminary results. Minerva Pediatr 62(3 Suppl 1):25, 2010

Moutsopoulos HM, Vlachoylannopoulos PG: Antiphospholipid antibody syndrome. In Longo DL, Fauci AS, Kasper DL, et al (eds): Harrison's Principles of Internal Medicine, 18th ed. New York, McGraw-Hill, 2012, p 2736

Munoz-Suano A, Kallikourdis M, Sarris M, e al: Regulatory T cells protect from autoimmune arthritis during pregnancy. J Autoimmun 38(2–3):J103, 2012

Murray S, Shamsuddin W, Russell R: Sequential combined spinal-epidural for caesarean delivery in osteogenesis imperfecta. Int J Obstet Anesth 19(1):127, 2010

Musiej-Nowakowska E, Ploski R: Pregnancy and early onset pauciarticular juvenile chronic arthritis. Ann Rheum Dis 58:475, 1999

Nelson JL, Hughes KA, Smith AG, et al: Maternal–fetal disparity in HLA class II alloantigens and the pregnancy-induced amelioration of rheumatoid arthritis. N Engl J Med 329:466, 1993

Nelson JL, Østensen M: Pregnancy and rheumatoid arthritis. Rheum Dis Clin North Am 23:195, 1997

Nelson JL, Voigt LF, Koepsell TD, et al: Pregnancy outcome in women with rheumatoid arthritis before disease onset. J Rheumatol 19:18, 1992

Nodler J, Moolamalla SR, Ledger EM, et al: Elevated antiphospholipid antibody titers and adverse pregnancy outcomes: analysis of a population-based hospital dataset. BMC Pregnancy Childbirth 9(1):11, 2009

Numano F, Kobayashi Y: Takayasu arteritis—beyond pulselessness. Intern Med 38:226, 1999

Ogunyemi D, Ku W, Arkel Y: The association between inherited thrombophilia, antiphospholipid antibodies and lipoprotein A levels with obstetrical complications in pregnancy. J Thromb Thrombolysis 14:157, 2002

Ohno T, Imai A, Tamaya T: Successful outcomes of pregnancy complicated with dermatomyositis. Gynecol Obstet Invest 33:187, 1992

Ojeda-Uribe M, Afif N, Dahan E, et al: Exposure to abatacept or rituximab in the first trimester of pregnancy in three women with autoimmune diseases. Clin Rheumatol 32(5):695, 2013

Oshiro BT, Silver RM, Scott JR, et al: Antiphospholipid antibodies and fetal death. Obstet Gynecol 87:489, 1996

Østensen M: Pregnancy in patients with a history of juvenile rheumatoid arthritis. Arthritis Rheum 34:881, 1991

Østensen M, Villiger PM: The remission of rheumatoid arthritis during pregnancy. Semin Immunopathol 29:185, 2007

Ottaviani G, Lavezzi AM, Rossi L, et al: Sudden unexpected death of a term fetus in an anticardiolipin-positive mother. Am J Perinatol 21:79, 2004

Owen J, Hauth JC: Polyarteritis nodosa in pregnancy: a case report and brief literature review. Am J Obstet Gynecol 160:606, 1989

Pagnoux C, Le Guern V, Goffinet F, et al: Pregnancies in systemic necrotizing vasculitides: report on 12 women and their 20 pregnancies. Rheumatology (Oxford) 50(5):953, 2011

Papadopoulos NG, Alamanos Y, Voulgari PV, et al: Does cigarette smoking influence disease expression, activity and severity in early rheumatoid arthritis patients? Clin Exp Rheumatol 23(6):861, 2005

Papakonstantinou K, Hasiakos D, Kondi-Paphiti A: Clinicopathology of maternal scleroderma. Int J Gynaecol Obstet 99(3):248, 2007

Papapetropoulos T, Kanellakopoulou N, Tsibri E, et al: Polymyositis and pregnancy: report of a case with three pregnancies. J Neurol Neurosurg Psychiatry 64:406, 1998

Partlett R, Roussou E: The treatment of rheumatoid arthritis during pregnancy. Rheumatol Int 31(4):445, 2011
Pattison NS, Chamley LW, McKay EJ, et al: Antiphospholipid antibodies in pregnancy—prevalence and clinical associations. Br J Obstet Gynecol 100:909, 1993
Peart E, Clowse ME: Systemic lupus erythematosus and pregnancy outcomes: an update and review of the literature. Curr Opin Rheumatol January 10, 2014 [Epub ahead of print]
Pepin M, Schwarze U, Superti-Furga A, et al: Clinical and genetic features of Ehlers-Danlos syndrome type IV, the vascular type. N Engl J Med 342:673, 2000
Petri M: Pregnancy in SLE. Baillières Clin Rheumatol 12:449, 1998
Petri M, Kim MY, Kalunian KC, et al: Combined oral contraceptives in women with systemic lupus erythematosus. N Engl J Med 353:2550, 2005
Petri M, The Hopkins Lupus Pregnancy Center: Ten key issues in management. Rheum Dis Clin North Am 33:227, 2007
Pierro E, Cirino G, Bucci MR, et al: Antiphospholipid antibodies inhibit prostaglandin release by decidual cells of early pregnancy: possible involvement of extracellular secretory phospholipase A2. Fertil Steril 71:342, 1999
Pikwer M, Bergström U, Nilsson JA, et al: Breast feeding, but not use of oral contraceptives, is associated with a reduced risk of rheumatoid arthritis. Ann Rheum Dis 68(4):526, 2009
Polzin WJ, Kopelman JN, Robinson RD, et al: The association of antiphospholipid antibodies with pregnancies complicated by fetal growth restriction. Obstet Gynecol 78:1108, 1991
Porter TF, LaCoursiere Y, Scott JR: Immunotherapy for recurrent miscarriage. Cochrane Database Syst Rev 2:CD000112, 2006
Prockop DJ, Bateman JF: Heritable disorders of connective tissue. In Longo DL, Fauci AS, Kasper DL, et al (eds): Harrison's Principles of Internal Medicine, 18th ed. New York, McGraw-Hill, 2012
Rai RS, Clifford K, Cohen H, et al: High prospective fetal loss rate in untreated pregnancies of women with recurrent miscarriage and antiphospholipid antibodies. Hum Reprod 10:3301, 1995
Rak JM, Maestroni L, Balandraud C, et al: Transfer of the shared epitope through microchimerism in women with rheumatoid arthritis. Arthritis Rheum 60(1):73, 2009a
Rak JM, Pagni PP, Tiev K, et al: Male microchimerism and HLA compatibility in French women with scleroderma: a different profile in limited and diffuse subset. Rheumatology 48(4):363, 2009b
Rand JH, Wu XX, Andree HAM, et al: Antiphospholipid antibodies accelerate plasma coagulation by inhibiting annexin-V binding to phospholipids: a "lupus procoagulant" phenomenon. Blood 92:1652, 1998
Rand JH, Wu XX, Andree HAM, et al: Pregnancy loss in the antiphospholipid antibody syndrome—a possible thrombogenic mechanism. N Engl J Med 337:154, 1997a
Rand JH, Wu XX, Guller S, et al: Antiphospholipid immunoglobulin G antibodies reduce annexin-V levels on syncytiotrophoblast apical membranes and in culture media of placental villi. Am J Obstet Gynecol 177:918, 1997b
Ranque B, Mouthon L: Geoepidemiology of systemic sclerosis. Autoimmun Rev 9(5):A311, 2010
Raza SH, Pattanaik D, Egerman RS: Painful, swollen hands in a young woman. Obstet Gynecol 116(4):983, 2010
Rein AJ, Mevorach D, Perles Z, et al: Early diagnosis and treatment of atrioventricular block in the fetus exposed to maternal anti-SSA/Ro-SSB/La antibodies: a prospective, observational, fetal kinetocardiogram-based study. Circulation 119(14):1867, 2009
Ritchie J, Smyth A, Tower C, et al: Maternal deaths in women with lupus nephritis: a review of published evidence. Lupus 21(5):534, 2012
Robertson B, Greaves M: Antiphospholipid syndrome: An evolving story. Blood Reviews 20:201, 2006
Robinson DP, Klein SL: Pregnancy and pregnancy-associated hormones alter immune responses and disease pathogenesis. Horm Behav 62(3):263, 2012
Roque H, Paidas M, Rebarber A, et al: Maternal thrombophilia is associated with second- and third-trimester fetal death. Am J Obstet Gynecol 184:S27, 2001
Rosenzweig BA, Rotmensch S, Binette SP, et al: Primary idiopathic polymyositis and dermatomyositis complicating pregnancy: diagnosis and management. Obstet Gynecol Surv 44:162, 1989
Rubin RL: Drug induced lupus. In Wallace DJ, Hahn BH (eds): Dubois' Lupus Erythematosus, 5th ed. Baltimore, Williams & Wilkins, 1997, p 871
Rudd NL, Nimrod C, Holbrook KA, et al: Pregnancy complications in type IV Ehlers-Danlos Syndrome. Lancet 1(8314–5):50, 1983
Ruiz-Irastorza G, Khamashta MA, Gordon C, et al: Measuring systemic lupus erythematosus activity during pregnancy: validation of the lupus activity index in pregnancy scale. Arthritis Rheum 51:78, 2004
Sánchez-Guerrero J, Uribe AG, Jiménez-Santana L, et al: A trial of contraceptive methods in women with systemic lupus erythematosus. N Engl J Med 353:2539, 2005
Sanna G, Bertolaccini ML, Cuadrado MJ: Central nervous system involvement in the antiphospholipid (Hughes) syndrome. Rheumatology 42:200, 2003
Savi C, Villa L, Civardi L, et al: Two consecutive cases of type A aortic dissection after delivery. Minerva Anestesiol 73:381, 2007
Schoenhoff F, Schmidli J, Czerny M, et al: Management of aortic aneurysms in patients with connective tissue disease. J Cardiovasc Surg 54(1 suppl 1):125, 2013
Scott JR: Risks to the children born to mothers with autoimmune diseases. Lupus 11:655, 2002
Shah A, St. Clair EW: Rheumatoid arthritis. In Longo DL, Fauci AS, Kasper DL, et al (eds): Harrison's Principles of Internal Medicine, 18th ed. New York, McGraw-Hill, 2012, p 2738
Sharma BK, Jain S, Vasishta K: Outcome of pregnancy in Takayasu arteritis. Int J Cardiol 75:S159, 2000
Sherer Y, Gorstein A, Fritzler MJ, et al: Autoantibody explosion in systemic lupus erythematosus: more than 100 different antibodies found in SLE patients. Semin Arthritis Rheum 34(2):501, 2004
Shi W, Chong BH, Hogg PJ, et al: Anticardiolipin antibodies block the inhibition by β_2 glycoprotein I of the factor Xa generating activity of platelets. Thromb Haemost 70:342, 1993
Shinohara K, Miyagawa S, Fujita T, et al: Neonatal lupus erythematosus: results of maternal corticosteroid therapy. Obstet Gynecol 93:952, 1999
Silman A, Kay A, Brennan P: Timing of pregnancy in relation to the onset of rheumatoid arthritis. Arthritis Rheum 35:152, 1992
Silver RM, Branch DW: Autoimmune diseases in pregnancy: systemic lupus erythematosus and antiphospholipid syndrome. Clin Perinatol 24:91, 1997
Silver RM, Parker CB, Reddy UM, et al: Antiphospholipid antibodies in stillbirth. Obstet Gynecol 122(3):641, 2013
Simchen MJ, Goldstein G, Lubetsky A, et al: Factor V Leiden and antiphospholipid antibodies in either mothers or infants increase the risk for perinatal arterial ischemic stroke. Stroke 40(1):65, 2009
Simpson JL: Cell-free fetal DNA and maternal serum analytes for monitoring embryonic and fetal status. Fertil Steril 99(4):1124, 2013
Sitar G, Brambati B, Baldi M, et al: The use of non-physiological conditions to isolate fetal cells from maternal blood. Exp Cell Res 302:153, 2005
Skomsvoll JF, Baste V, Irgens LM, et al: The recurrence risk of adverse outcome in the second pregnancy in women with rheumatic disease. Obstet Gynecol 100:1196, 2002
Sneller MC: Wegener's granulomatosis. JAMA 273:1288, 1995
Solomon SD, McMurray JJ, Pfeffer MA, et al: Cardiovascular risk associated with celecoxib in a clinical trial for colorectal adenoma prevention. N Engl J Med 352(11):1071, 2005
Solomons J, Coucke P, Symoens S, et al: Dermatosparaxis (Ehlers-Danlos Type VIIC): prenatal diagnosis following a previous pregnancy with unexpected skull fractures at delivery. Am J Med Genet A 161(5):1122, 2013
Sorokin Y, Johnson MP, Rogowski N, et al: Obstetric and gynecologic dysfunction in the Ehlers–Danlos syndrome. J Reprod Med 39:281, 1994
Spinillo A, Veneventi F, Epis OM, et al: The effect of newly diagnosed undifferentiated connective tissue disease on pregnancy outcome. Am J Obstet Gynecol 199(6):632.e1, 2008
Srivatsa B, Srivatsa S, Johnson K, et al: Microchimerism of presumed fetal origin in thyroid specimens from women: a case-control study. Lancet 358:2034, 2001
Steen VD: Pregnancy in women with systemic sclerosis. Obstet Gynecol 94:15, 1999
Steen VD, Conte C, Day N, et al: Pregnancy in women with systemic sclerosis. Arthritis Rheum 32:151, 1989
Stirnemann J, Fain O, Lachassinne E, et al: Neonatal lupus erythematosus. Presse Med 31(30):1407, 2002
Stojan G, Baer AN: Flares of systemic lupus erythematosus during pregnancy and the puerperium: prevention, diagnosis and management. Expert Rev Clin Immunol 8(5):439, 2012
Sykes B, Ogilvie D, Wordsworth P, et al: Consistent linkage of dominantly inherited osteogenesis imperfecta to the type I collagen loci: COL1A1 and COL1A2. Am J Hum Genet 46(2):293, 1990
Tan EM, Cohen AS, Fries JF, et al: The 1982 revised criteria for the classification of systemic lupus erythematosus. Arthritis Rheum 25(11):127, 1982
Taraborelli M, Ramoni V, Brucato A, et al: Brief report: successful pregnancies but a higher risk of preterm births in patients with systemic sclerosis: an Italian multicenter study. Arthritis Rheum 64(6):1970, 2012
Tashkin DP, Elashoff R, Clements PJ, et al: Cyclophosphamide versus placebo in scleroderma lung disease. N Engl J Med 354:2655, 2006
Tayabali S, Andersen K, Yoong W: Diagnosis and management of Henoch-Schönlein purpura in pregnancy: a review of the literature. Arch Gynecol Obstet 286(4):825, 2012
Tincani A, Rebaioli CB, Andreoli L, et al: Neonatal effects of maternal antiphospholipid syndrome. Curr Rheumatol Rep 11(1):70, 2009

Toglia MR, Weg JG: Venous thromboembolism during pregnancy. N Engl J Med 335:108, 1996
Tower C, Mathen S, Crocker I, et al: Regulatory T cells in systemic lupus erythematosus and pregnancy. Am J Reprod Immunol 69(6):588, 2013
Trudinger BJ, Stewart GJ, Cook C, et al: Monitoring lupus anticoagulant-positive pregnancies with umbilical artery flow velocity waveforms. Obstet Gynecol 72:215, 1988
Tsokos GC: Systemic lupus erythematosus. N Engl J Med 365(22):2110, 2011
Unger A, Kay A, Griffin AJ, et al: Disease activity and pregnancy associated β_2-glycoprotein in rheumatoid arthritis. BMJ 286:750, 1983
Vargas J: Systemic sclerosis (scleroderma) and related disorders. In Longo DL, Fauci AS, Kasper DL, et al (eds): Harrison's Principles of Internal Medicine, 18th ed. New York, McGraw-Hill, 2012, p 2757
Varner MW, Meehan RT, Syrop CH, et al: Pregnancy in patients with systemic lupus erythematosus. Am J Obstet Gynecol 145:1025, 1983
Verstappen SM, King Y, Watson KD, et al: Anti-TNF therapies and pregnancy: outcome of 130 pregnancies in the British Society for Rheumatology Biologics Register. Ann Rheum Dis 70(5):823, 2011
Volkov N, Nisenblat V, Ohel G, et al: Ehlers-Danlos syndrome: insight on obstetric aspects. Obstet Gynecol Surv 62:51, 2006
Wagner S, Craici I, Reed D, et al: Maternal and foetal outcomes in pregnant patients with active lupus nephritis. Lupus 18(4)342, 2009
Waldorf KM, Nelson JL: Autoimmune disease during pregnancy and the microchimerism legacy of pregnancy. Immunol Invest 37:631, 2008
Wallenius M, Skomsvoll JF, Irgens LM, et al: Pregnancy and delivery in women with chronic inflammatory arthritides with a specific focus on first birth. Arthritis Rheum 63(6):1534, 2011
Walsh CA, Reardon W, Foley ME: Unexplained prelabor uterine rupture in a term primigravida. Obstet Gynecol 109:455, 2007
Williams L, Chang PY, Park E, et al: Successful treatment of dermatomyositis during pregnancy with intravenous immunoglobulin monotherapy. Obstet Gynecol 109:561, 2007
Wu H, Birmingham DJ, Rovin B, et al: D-Dimer level and the risk for thrombosis in systemic lupus erythematosus. Clin J Am Soc Nephrol 3:1628, 2008
Xiao J, Xiong J, Zhu F, et al: Effect of prednisone, aspirin, low molecular weight heparin and intravenous immunoglobulin on outcome of pregnancy in women with antiphospholipid syndrome. Exp Ther Med 5(1):287, 2013
Yang W, Tang H, Zhang Y, et al: Meta-analysis followed by replication identifies loci in or near CDKN1B, TET3, CD80, DRAM1, and ARID5B as associated with systemic lupus erythematosus in Asians. Am J Hum Genet 92(1):41, 2013
Yasuda M, Takakuwa K, Okinaga A, et al: Prospective studies of the association between anticardiolipin antibody and outcome of pregnancy. Obstet Gynecol 86:555, 1995
Ye Y, van Zyl B, Varsani H, et al: Maternal microchimerism in muscle biopsies from children with juvenile dermatomyositis. Rheumatology (Oxford) 51(6):987, 2012
Yeste A, Quintana FJ: Antigen microarrays for the study of autoimmune diseases. Clin Chem 59(7):1036, 2013
Zangari M, Lockwood CJ, Scher J, et al: Prothrombin activation fragment (F1.2) is increased in pregnant patients with antiphospholipid antibodies. Thromb Res 85:177, 1997
Zhao C, Zhao J, Huang Y, et al: New-onset systemic lupus erythematosus during pregnancy. Clin Rheumatol 32(6):815, 2013

CHAPTER 60

Neurological Disorders

A number of neurological diseases are relatively common in women of childbearing age. In the past, some of these may have precluded pregnancy, however, few do so now. Most of those encountered during pregnancy are the same as for nonpregnant women. That said, there are a few neurological disorders that may be seen more frequently in pregnant women. Some examples are Bell palsy, specific types of strokes, and benign intracranial hypertension or pseudotumor cerebri. Neurovascular disorders are an important cause of maternal mortality and accounted for 10 percent of maternal deaths in the United States from 1998 through 2005 (Berg, 2010b).

Because many neurological disorders are chronic, they frequently precede pregnancy. Although most women with chronic neurological disease who become pregnant will have successful outcomes, some of these disorders have specific risks with which clinicians should be familiar. Conversely, some women will have new-onset neurological symptoms during pregnancy, and these frequently must be distinguished from other pregnancy complications. Psychiatric disorders may also manifest with cognitive and neuromuscular abnormalities, and they should be considered in the evaluation.

CENTRAL NERVOUS SYSTEM IMAGING

Computed tomography (CT) and magnetic resonance (MR) imaging have opened new vistas for the diagnosis, classification, and management of many neurological and psychiatric disorders. As discussed in Chapter 46 (p. 933), these cranial imaging methods can be used safely during pregnancy. CT scanning is commonly used whenever rapid diagnosis is necessary and is excellent for detecting recent hemorrhage (Smith, 2012). Because it does not use radiation, MR imaging is often preferred. It is particularly helpful to diagnose demyelinating diseases, screen for arteriovenous malformations, evaluate congenital and developmental nervous system abnormalities, identify posterior fossa lesions, and diagnose spinal cord diseases (Gjelsteen, 2008). Whenever either test is done, the woman should be positioned in a left lateral tilt with a wedge under one hip to prevent hypotension as well as to diminish aortic pulsations, which may degrade the image.

Cerebral angiography with contrast injection, usually via the femoral artery, is a valuable adjunct to the diagnosis and treatment of some cerebrovascular diseases. Fluoroscopy delivers more radiation but can be performed with abdominal shielding. Positron emission tomography (PET) and functional MRI (fMRI) have not been evaluated for use in pregnant patients (Chiapparini, 2010).

HEADACHE

The National Health Interview Survey is provided by the Centers for Disease Control and Prevention (Pleis, 2010). In the 2009 survey, a fifth of all women aged 18 to 44 years reported a severe headache or migraine within the past 3 months, and headache

TABLE 60-1. Classification of Headache[a]

Primary
Tension-type (69%)
Migraine (16%)
Cluster and other trigeminal autonomic cephalgias (< 1%)
Other
Secondary
Systemic infection (63%)
Head or neck trauma (4%)
Cranial or cervical vascular disorders
Intracranial nonvascular
Substance use or withdrawal
Disorders of homeostasis
Head and neck disorders
Psychiatric disorders

[a]Percentages in parentheses are estimated frequencies. Data from Goadsby, 2012. Adapted from the International Headache Society, 2004.

was the most common neurological complaint during pregnancy. Smitherman and coworkers (2013) found that 26 percent of nonpregnant women in this age group were similarly affected. Interestingly, Aegidius and colleagues (2009) reported an overall decrease in prevalence of all headache types during pregnancy in nulliparas, especially during the third trimester. The classification of headaches by the International Headache Society (2004) is shown in Table 60-1. Primary headaches are more common in pregnant women than those with secondary causes (Digre, 2013). Migraine headaches are those most likely to be affected by the hormonal changes of pregnancy (Torelli, 2010).

Tension-Type Headache

These are most common, and characteristic features include muscle tightness and mild to moderate pain that can persist for hours in the back of the neck and head. There are no associated neurological disturbances or nausea. The pain usually responds to rest, massage, application of heat or ice, antiinflammatory medications, or mild tranquilizers.

Migraine Headache

These headaches have a 1-year prevalence in all women of approximately 15 percent, and thus they are frequently encountered during pregnancy. The term *migraine* describes a periodic, sometimes incapacitating neurological disorder characterized by episodic attacks of severe headache and autonomic nervous system dysfunction (Goadsby, 2012). The International Headache Society (2004) classifies three migraine types based on the presence or absence of an aura as well as chronicity:

1. *Migraine without aura*—was formerly termed common migraine—and is characterized by a unilateral throbbing headache, nausea and vomiting, or photophobia.
2. *Migraine with aura*—formerly termed classic migraine—has similar symptoms preceded by premonitory neurological phenomena such as visual scotoma or hallucinations. A third of patients have this type of migraine, which sometimes can be averted if medication is taken at the first premonitory sign.
3. *Chronic migraine* is defined by a migraine headache occurring at least 15 days each month for more than 3 months.

Migraines may begin in childhood, peak in adolescence, and tend to diminish in both frequency and severity with advancing years. According to Lipton and associates (2007), their annual prevalence is 17 percent in women and 6 percent in men. Another 5 percent of women have *probable migraine,* that is, they have all criteria but one (Silberstein, 2007). Migraines are especially common in young women and have been linked to hormone levels (Torelli, 2010).

The exact pathophysiology of migraines is uncertain, but they occur when neuronal dysfunction leads to decreased cortical blood flow, activation of vascular and meningeal nociceptors, and stimulation of trigeminal sensory neurons (Brandes, 2007; D'Andrea, 2010). A predilection for the posterior circulation has been described by Kruit and coworkers (2004). Migraines—especially those with aura in young women—are associated with increased risk for ischemic strokes as discussed on page 1191. The risk is greater in those who smoke or use combination oral contraceptives.

Migraine in Pregnancy

The prevalence of migraine headaches in the first trimester is 2 percent (Chen, 1994). Prospective as well as observational studies have shown that most migraineurs have improvement during pregnancy (Adeney, 2006; Menon, 2008; Torelli, 2010). Still, migraines—usually those with an aura—occasionally appear for the first time during pregnancy. Pregnant women with preexisting migraine symptoms may have other symptoms suggestive of a more serious disorder, and new neurological symptoms should prompt a complete evaluation (Detsky, 2006; Heaney, 2010).

Although conventional thinking has been that migraine headaches do not pose increased maternal or fetal risks, several recent studies have refuted this (Allais, 2010). For example, women with severe migraines in the first 8 weeks may be at slightly increased risk for a fetus with limb-reduction defects (Banhidy, 2006). Preeclampsia and other cardiovascular morbidities are also increased (Facchinetti, 2009; Sanchez, 2008; Schürks, 2009). In a case-control study of nearly 18.5 million pregnancy-related discharges from 2000 through 2003, Bushnell and coworkers (2009) identified an incidence of migraine discharge codes of 185 per 100,000. Associated diagnoses and increased significant risks were found for migraines and stroke—15.8-fold; myocardial infarction—4.9; heart disease—2.1; venous thromboembolism—2.4; and preeclampsia/gestational hypertension—2.3-fold.

Management

Data are limited regarding nonpharmacological management in pregnancy such as biofeedback techniques, acupuncture, and transcranial magnetic stimulation (Airola, 2010; Dodick, 2010). Effective pharmacological interventions include nonsteroidal antiinflammatory drugs, and most migraine headaches respond to simple analgesics such as ibuprofen or acetaminophen, especially if given early. Because of patient idiosyncrasies, multitarget drug therapy is necessary in most cases for migraine relief (Gonzalez-Hernandez, 2014). Severe headaches should be treated aggressively with intravenous hydration and parenteral antiemetics and opioids. Although intravenous magnesium sulfate has gained favor in the past few years, a recent metaanalysis reported no beneficial effects (Choi, 2014). Ergotamine derivatives are potent vasoconstrictors that should be avoided in pregnancy (Briggs, 2011).

Triptans are serotonin 5-$HT_{1B/2D}$-receptor agonists that effectively relieve headaches by causing intracranial vasoconstriction (Contag, 2010). They also relieve nausea and vomiting and greatly reduce the need for analgesics. They can be given orally, by injection, as a rectal suppository, or as a nasal spray. The greatest experience is with sumatriptan (Imitrex), and although not studied extensively in pregnancy, it appears to be safe (Briggs, 2011; Nezvalová-Henriksen, 2010).

For women with frequent migraine headaches, oral prophylactic therapy is warranted. Amitriptyline (Elavil), 10 to 150 mg daily; propranolol (Inderal), 20 to 80 mg three times daily; or metoprolol (Lopressor, Toprol), 50 to 100 mg twice daily, is safe in pregnancy and has been used with success (Contag, 2010; Lucas, 2009; Marcus, 2007).

Cluster Headaches

This rare primary headache disorder is characterized by severe unilateral lancinating pain radiating to the face and orbit, lasting 15 to 180 minutes, and occurring with autonomic symptoms and agitation. Pregnancy does not affect symptom severity. Affected women should avoid tobacco and alcohol. Acute management includes 100-percent oxygen therapy and sumatriptan given as a 6-mg dose subcutaneously (Calhoun, 2010; Francis, 2010). If recurrent, prophylaxis is administered using a calcium-channel blocking agent.

SEIZURE DISORDERS

The Centers for Disease Control and Prevention reported that the prevalence of epilepsy in adults in 2005 was 1.65 percent (Kobau, 2008). There are 1.1 million American women of childbearing age who are affected. After headaches, seizures are the next most prevalent neurological condition encountered in pregnant women, and they complicate 1 in 200 pregnancies (Brodie, 1996; Yerby, 1994). Importantly, epilepsy accounted for 13 percent of maternal deaths in the United Kingdom for the 2005 to 2007 triennium (Lewis, 2007). Seizure disorders are also associated with altered fetal development, and they can adversely affect other pregnancy outcomes. The teratogenic effects of several anticonvulsant medications are unquestioned. The American Academy of Neurology and the American Epilepsy Society have developed guidelines regarding treatment in pregnant women, which are discussed subsequently (Harden, 2009a–c).

Pathophysiology

A seizure is defined as a paroxysmal disorder of the central nervous system characterized by an abnormal neuronal discharge with or without loss of consciousness. Epilepsy encompasses different syndromes whose cardinal feature is a predisposition to recurrent unprovoked seizures. The International League Against Epilepsy Commission on Classification and Terminology recently updated its terminologies for seizures (Berg, 2010a, 2011; Shorvon, 2011). This new classification schema is under development, and for now, most adults can be said to have either focal or generalized seizures.

Focal Seizures

These originate in one localized brain area and affect a correspondingly localized area of neurological function. They are believed to result from trauma, abscess, tumor, or perinatal factors, although a specific lesion is rarely demonstrated. *Focal seizures without dyscognitive features* start in one region of the body and progress toward other ipsilateral areas of the body, producing tonic and then clonic movements. Simple seizures can affect sensory function or produce autonomic dysfunction or psychological changes. Cognitive function is not impaired, and recovery is rapid. *Focal seizures with dyscognitive features* are often preceded by an aura and followed by impaired awareness manifested by sudden behavioral arrest or motionless stare. Involuntary movements such as picking motions or lip smacking are common.

Generalized Seizures

These involve both brain hemispheres and may be preceded by an aura before an abrupt loss of consciousness. There is a strong hereditary component. In *generalized tonic-clonic seizures*, loss of consciousness is followed by tonic contraction of the muscles and rigid posturing, and then by clonic contractions of all extremities while the muscles gradually relax. Return to consciousness is gradual, and the patient may remain confused and disoriented for several hours. *Absence* seizures—also called *petit mal seizures*—are a form of generalized epilepsy that involve a brief loss of consciousness without muscle activity and are characterized by immediate recovery of consciousness and orientation.

Causes of Seizure

Some identifiable causes of convulsive disorders in young adults include head trauma, alcohol- and other drug-induced withdrawals, cerebral infections, brain tumors, biochemical abnormalities, and arteriovenous malformations. A search for these is prudent with a new-onset seizure disorder in a pregnant woman. The diagnosis of idiopathic epilepsy is one of exclusion.

Preconceptional Counseling

Women with epilepsy should undergo education and counseling before pregnancy (Chap. 8, p. 158). Folic acid supplementation with 0.4 mg per day is begun at least 1 month before conception. The dose is increased to 4 mg when the woman taking antiepileptic medication becomes pregnant. These medications are assessed and adjusted with a goal of monotherapy using the least teratogenic medication. If this is not feasible, then attempts are made to reduce the number of medications used and to use them at the lowest effective dose (Dunlop, 2008). Medication withdrawal should be considered if a woman is seizure free for 2 years or more.

Epilepsy During Pregnancy

The major pregnancy-related risks to women with epilepsy are increased seizure rates with attendant mortality risks and fetal malformations. Seizure control is the main priority. Earlier studies described worsening seizure activity during pregnancy, however, this is not as common nowadays because of more effective drugs. Contemporary studies cite increased seizure activity in only 20 to 30 percent of pregnant women (Mawer, 2010; Vajda, 2008; Viinikainen, 2006). Women who are seizure free for at least 9 months before conception will likely remain so during pregnancy (Harden, 2009b).

Increased seizure frequency is often associated with decreased and thus subtherapeutic anticonvulsant serum levels, a lower seizure threshold, or both. An impressive number of pregnancy-associated alterations can result in subtherapeutic serum levels. These include nausea and vomiting, decreased gastrointestinal motility, antacid use that diminishes drug absorption, pregnancy hypervolemia offset by protein binding, induction of hepatic enzymes such as cytochrome oxidases, placental enzymes that metabolize drugs, and increased glomerular filtration that hastens drug clearance. Importantly, some women discontinue medication because of teratogenicity concerns. Finally, the seizure threshold can be affected by pregnancy-related sleep deprivation as well as hyperventilation and pain during labor.

Pregnancy Complications

Women with epilepsy have a small increased risk of some pregnancy complications (Borthen, 2011; Harden, 2009b). A population-based study from Iceland found that epileptic women had a twofold increased cesarean delivery rate (Olafsson, 1998). In a cohort study from Montreal, Richmond and coworkers (2004) reported an increased incidence of nonproteinuric hypertension and labor induction. From a Swedish study of 1207 epileptic women, Pilo and colleagues (2006) reported a 1.5-fold increased incidence of cesarean delivery, preeclampsia, and postpartum hemorrhage. Postpartum depression rates have also been reported to be increased in epileptic women (Turner, 2009). Finally, children of epileptic mothers have a 10-percent risk of developing a seizure disorder.

Embryo-Fetal Malformations

For years, it was difficult to separate effects of epilepsy versus its therapy as the primary cause of fetal malformations. As discussed in Chapter 8 (p. 158), it is now believed that untreated epilepsy is not associated with an increased fetal malformation rate (Thomas, 2008; Viinikainen, 2006). That said, the fetus of an epileptic mother who takes certain anticonvulsant medications has an indisputably increased risk for congenital malformations. Moreover, monotherapy is associated with a lower birth defect rate compared with multiagent therapy. Thus, if necessary, increasing monotherapy dosage is at least initially preferable to adding another agent (Buhimschi, 2009).

Specific drugs, when given alone, increase the malformation rate (Chap. 12, p. 246). Some of these are listed in Table 60-2. Phenytoin and phenobarbital increase the major malformation

TABLE 60-2. Teratogenic Effects of Common Anticonvulsant Medications

Drug (Brand Name)	Abnormalities Described	Affected	Embryo-Fetal Risk[a]
Valproate (Depakote)	Neural-tube defects, clefts, cardiac anomalies; associated developmental delay	10% with monotherapy; higher with polytherapy	Yes
Phenytoin (Dilantin)	Fetal hydantoin syndrome—craniofacial anomalies, fingernail hypoplasia, growth deficiency, developmental delay, cardiac anomalies, clefts	5–11%	Yes
Carbamazepine; oxcarbazepine (Tegretol; Trileptal)	Fetal hydantoin syndrome, as above; spina bifida	1–2%	Yes
Phenobarbital	Clefts, cardiac anomalies, urinary tract malformations	10–20%	Suggested
Lamotrigine (Lamictal)	Increased risk for clefts (Registry data)	Up to 1% (4- to 10-fold higher than expected)	Suggested
Topiramate (Topamax)	Clefts	2–3% (15- to 20-fold higher than expected)	Suggested
Levetiracetam (Keppra)	Theoretical—skeletal abnormalities; impaired growth in animals	Preliminary observations	Suggested

[a]Risk categories from Briggs, 2011; Holmes, 2008; Hunt, 2008; Meador, 2009; Morrow, 2006; U.S. Food and Drug Administration (2011).

rate two- to threefold above baseline (Perucca, 2005; Thomas, 2008). A particularly potent teratogen is valproate, which has a dose-dependent effect and increases the malformation risk four- to eightfold (Eadie, 2008; Klein, 2014; Wyszynski, 2005). In general, with polytherapy, the risk increases with each drug added. At least at this time, the newer antiepileptic medications are reported to have no associations with a markedly increased risk of major birth defects (Molgaard-Nielson, 2011).

Management in Pregnancy

The major goal is seizure prevention. To accomplish this, treatment for nausea and vomiting is provided, seizure-provoking stimuli are avoided, and medication compliance is emphasized. The fewest necessary anticonvulsants are given at the lowest dosage effective for seizure control. Although some providers routinely monitor serum drug levels during pregnancy, these concentrations may be unreliable because of altered protein binding. Free or unbound drug levels, although perhaps more accurate, are not widely available. Importantly, there is no evidence that such monitoring improves seizure control (Adab, 2006). For these reasons, drug levels may be informative if measured following seizures or if noncompliance is suspected. Some of the newer agents such as lamotrigine and oxcarbazepine may be more amenable to serum drug level monitoring (Harden, 2009a; Pennell, 2008).

For women taking anticonvulsant drugs, a targeted sonographic examination at midpregnancy is recommended by some to search for anomalies (Chap. 10, p. 197). Testing to assess fetal well-being is generally not indicated for women with uncomplicated epilepsy.

Breast Feeding and Contraception

There are limited available data regarding the safety of breast feeding with the various anticonvulsant medications. That said, no obvious deleterious effects, such as long-term cognitive issues, have been reported (Briggs, 2011; Harden, 2009c). Some of the anticonvulsant agents are associated with increased oral contraceptive failures. Thus, other more reliable methods should be considered (Chap 38, p. 696).

CEREBROVASCULAR DISEASES

Abnormalities of the cerebrovascular circulation include strokes—both ischemic and hemorrhagic, as well as anatomical anomalies, such as arteriovenous malformations and aneurysms. The current endemic of obesity in this country, along with concomitant increases in heart disease, hypertension, and diabetes, has also resulted in increased stroke prevalence (Centers for Disease Control and Prevention, 2012). Women have a higher lifetime risk of stroke than men as well as higher associated mortality rates (Martínez-Sánchez, 2011; Roger, 2012). Moreover, pregnancy increases the immediate and lifetime risk of both ischemic and hemorrhagic stroke (Jamieson, 2010; Jung, 2010).

Stroke is relatively uncommon in pregnant women, but it contributes disparately to maternal mortality rates. Reported incidences of strokes in pregnancy range from 1.5 to 71 per 100,000 pregnancies (James, 2005; Kuklina, 2011; Scott, 2012). The incidence is increasing as measured by pregnancy-related hospitalizations for stroke (Callaghan, 2008; Kuklina, 2011). Importantly, most are associated with hypertensive disorders or heart disease. Almost 9 percent of the pregnancy-related mortality rate in the United States is due to cerebrovascular accidents, with a third being associated with preeclampsia (Berg, 2010b).

Risk Factors

Most strokes in pregnancy manifest either during labor and delivery or in the puerperium. In a study of 2850 pregnancy-related strokes, approximately 10 percent developed antepartum, 40 percent intrapartum, and almost 50 percent postpartum (James, 2005). Several risk factors—unrelated and related to pregnancy—have been reported from studies that included more than 10 million pregnancies. These include older age; migraines, hypertension, obesity, and diabetes; cardiac disorders such as endocarditis, valvular prostheses, and patent foramen ovale; and smoking. Those related to pregnancy include hypertensive disorders, gestational diabetes, obstetrical hemorrhage, and cesarean delivery. By far, the most common risk factors are pregnancy-associated hypertensive disorders. As noted, one third of strokes are associated with gestational hypertension, and there is a three- to eightfold increased risk of stroke in hypertensive compared with normotensive women (Scott, 2012; Wang, 2011). Women with preeclampsia undergoing general anesthesia may be at higher risk of stroke compared with those given neuraxial anesthesia (Huang, 2010). Another risk factor for peripartum stroke is cesarean delivery, which increases the risk 1.5-fold compared with vaginal delivery (Lin, 2008).

Pregnancy-induced effects on cerebrovascular hemodynamics are unclear as related to risk for stroke. Although cerebral blood flow *decreased* by 20 percent from midpregnancy until term, importantly, it *increased* significantly with gestational hypertension (Zeeman, 2003, 2004b). Such hyperperfusion would at least intuitively be dangerous in women with certain vascular anomalies.

Ischemic Stroke

Acute occlusion or embolization of an intracranial blood vessel causes cerebral ischemia, which may result in death of brain tissue (Fig. 60-1). The more common associated conditions and etiologies of ischemic stroke are shown in Table 60-3. A transient ischemic attack (TIA) is caused by reversible ischemia, and symptoms usually last less than 24 hours. Patients with a stroke usually have a sudden onset of severe headache, hemiplegia or other neurological deficits, or occasionally, seizures. Focal neurological symptoms accompanied by an aura usually signify a first-episode migraine (Liberman, 2008).

Evaluation of an ischemic stroke includes echocardiography and cranial imaging with CT, MR, or angiography. Serum lipids are measured with the caveat that their values are distorted by normal pregnancy (Appendix, p. 1291). Antiphospholipid antibodies and lupus anticoagulant are sought—these cause up to a third of ischemic strokes in otherwise healthy young women (Chap. 59, p. 1173). Also, tests for sickle-cell syndromes are completed when indicated. With a thorough evaluation, most causes can be identified, although treatment is not always available. Some of these include cardiac-associated embolism, vasculitis, or vasculopathy such as Moyamoya disease (Ishimori, 2006; Miyakoshi, 2009; Simolke, 1991).

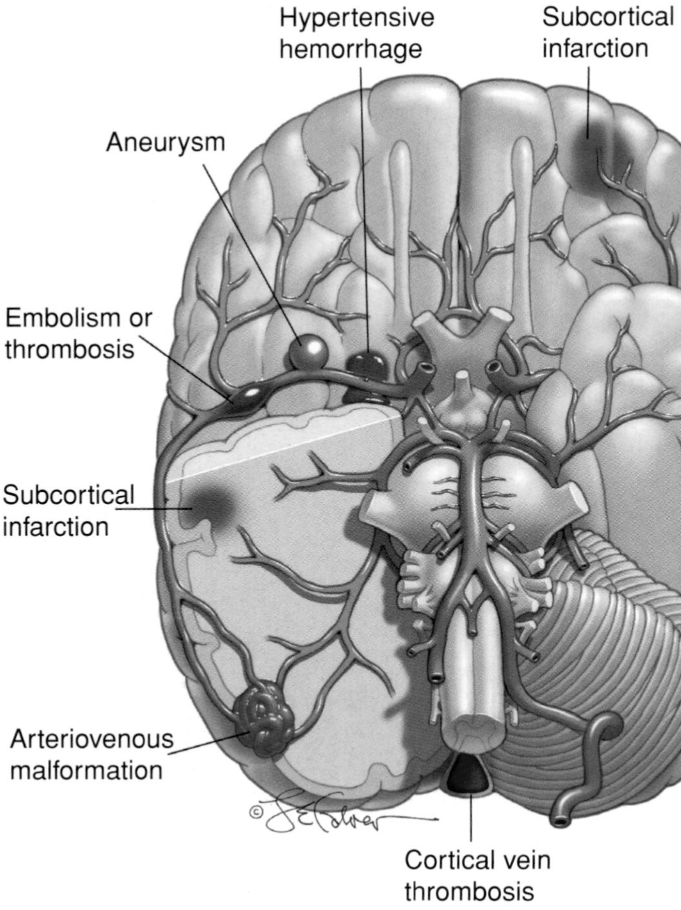

FIGURE 60-1 Illustrations of a brain showing various types of strokes seen in pregnancy: (1) subcortical infarction (preeclampsia), (2) hypertensive hemorrhage, (3) aneurysm, (4) embolism or thrombosis in middle cerebral artery, (5) arteriovenous malformation, and (6) cortical vein thrombosis.

TABLE 60-3. Some Associated Disorders or Causes of Ischemic and Hemorrhagic Strokes During Pregnancy or the Puerperium

Ischemic Stroke	Hemorrhagic Stroke
Preeclampsia syndrome	Chronic hypertension
Arterial thrombosis	Preeclampsia syndrome
Venous thrombosis	Arteriovenous malformation
Lupus anticoagulant	Saccular aneurysm
Antiphospholipid antibodies	Angioma
Thrombophilias	Cocaine, methamphetamines
Migraine induced	Vasculopathy
Paradoxical embolus	
Cardioembolic	
Sickle hemoglobinopathy	
Arterial dissection	
Vasculitis	
Moyamoya disease	
Cocaine, amphetamines	

From Smith, 2012; Yager, 2012.

Preeclampsia Syndrome

In reproductive-age women, a significant proportion of pregnancy-related ischemic strokes are caused by gestational hypertension and preeclampsia syndrome (Jeng, 2004). As shown in Figure 60-1, areas of subcortical perivascular edema and petechial hemorrhage may progress to cerebral infarction (Aukes, 2007, 2009; Zeeman, 2004a). Although these are usually clinically manifest by an eclamptic convulsion, a few women will suffer a symptomatic stroke from a larger cortical infarction (Chap. 40, p. 742).

Other conditions with findings similar to preeclampsia include *thrombotic microangiopathies* (Chap. 56, p. 1116) and the *reversible cerebral vasoconstriction syndrome* (Chap. 40, p. 743). The latter, which is also termed *postpartum angiopathy*, can cause extensive cerebral edema with necrosis as well as widespread infarction with areas of hemorrhage (Katz, 2014; Ramnarayan, 2009; Singhal, 2009).

Cerebral Embolism

These strokes usually involve the middle cerebral artery (see Fig. 60-1). They are more common during the latter half of pregnancy or early puerperium (Lynch, 2001). The diagnosis can be made with confidence only after thrombosis and hemorrhage have been excluded. The diagnosis is more certain if an embolic source is identified. Hemorrhage may be more difficult to exclude because embolization and thrombosis are both followed by hemorrhagic infarction. Paradoxical embolism is an uncommon cause, even considering that more than a fourth of adults have a patent foramen ovale through which right-sided venous thromboemboli are deported (Kizer, 2005; Scott, 2012). Foraminal closure may not improve outcomes in these patients, however, this procedure has been performed during pregnancy (Dark, 2011; Furlan, 2012). Assorted cardioembolic causes of stroke include arrhythmias—especially atrial fibrillation, valvular lesions, mitral valve prolapse, mural thrombus, infective endocarditis, and peripartum cardiomyopathy.

Management of embolic stroke in pregnancy consists of supportive measures and antiplatelet therapy. Thrombolytic therapy and anticoagulation are controversial issues at this time (Kizer, 2005; Li, 2012).

Cerebral Artery Thrombosis

Most thrombotic strokes affect older individuals and are caused by atherosclerosis, especially of the internal carotid artery. Many are preceded by one or more transient ischemic attacks. Thrombolytic therapy with *recombinant tissue plasminogen activator—rt-PA* or *alteplase* is recommended within the first 3-hour window if there is measurable neurological deficit and if neuroimaging has excluded hemorrhage. This can be used in pregnancy. A principal risk is hemorrhagic transformation of an ischemic stroke in approximately 5 percent of treated patients (van der Worp, 2007).

Cerebral Venous Thrombosis

In a 10-center study in the United States, 7 percent of cerebral venous thromboses were associated with pregnancy (Wasay, 2008). Even so, pregnancy-associated cerebral venous thrombosis is rare in developed countries, and reported incidences range from 1 in 11,000 to 1 in 45,000 pregnancies (Lanska, 1997; Simolke, 1991). In the Nationwide Inpatient Sample of more than 8 million deliveries, James and associates (2005) observed that venous thrombosis caused only 2 percent of pregnancy-related strokes (Saposnik, 2011). There are numerous predisposing causes, and the greatest risk is in late pregnancy and the puerperium.

Thrombosis of the lateral or superior sagittal venous sinus usually occurs in the puerperium and often in association with preeclampsia, sepsis, or thrombophilia (see Fig. 60-1). It is more common in patients with inherited thrombophilias, lupus anticoagulant, or antiphospholipid antibodies (Chaps. 52, p. 1029 and 59, p. 1173). Headache is the most common presenting symptom, neurological deficits are common, and up to a third of patients have convulsions (Wasay, 2008). Diagnosis is with MR venography (Saposnik, 2011).

Management includes anticonvulsants for seizures, and although heparinization is recommended by most, its efficacy is controversial (de Freitas, 2008; Saposnik, 2011; Smith, 2012). Antimicrobials are given if there is septic thrombophlebitis, and fibrinolytic therapy is reserved for those women failing systemic anticoagulation. The prognosis for venous thrombosis in pregnancy is better than in nonpregnant subjects, and mortality rates are less than 10 percent (McCaulley, 2011). The recurrence rate is 1 to 2 percent during a subsequent pregnancy (Mehraein, 2003).

Recurrence Risk of Ischemic Stroke

Women with previous ischemic stroke have a low risk for recurrence during a subsequent pregnancy unless a specific, persistent cause is identified. Lamy and colleagues (2000) followed 37 women who had an ischemic stroke during pregnancy or the puerperium, and none of their 24 subsequent pregnancies was complicated by another stroke. In another study of 23 women who had prepregnancy strokes from a variety of causes, there were 35 subsequent pregnancies without a stroke recurrence (Coppage, 2004). Finally, in a follow-up study of 1770 nonpregnant women with antiphospholipid-related ischemic stroke, investigators reported no difference in the recurrence risk as long as preventative treatment was given with warfarin or aspirin (Levine, 2004). In another study of nonpregnant subjects, low-dose aspirin following venous thromboembolism decreased the risk of a subsequent stroke (Brighton, 2012).

Currently, there are no firm guidelines regarding prophylaxis in pregnant women with a stroke history (Helms, 2009). The American Heart Association stresses the importance of controlling risk factors such as hypertension and diabetes (Furie, 2011). Women with antiphospholipid antibody syndrome or certain cardiac conditions should be considered for prophylactic anticoagulation as discussed in Chapters 49 (p. 979) and 59 (p. 1175).

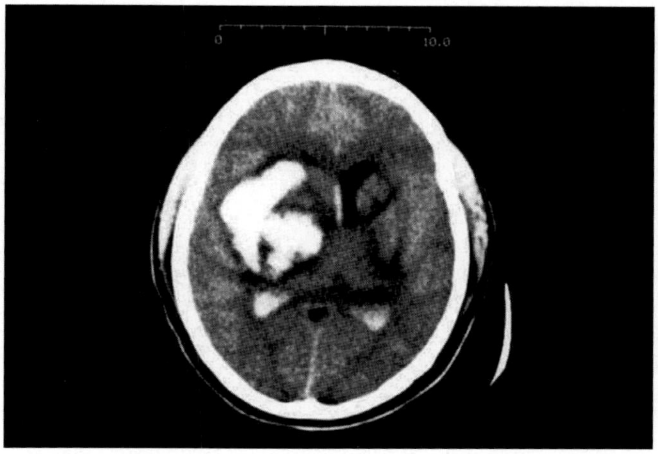

FIGURE 60-2 Large intracerebral hemorrhage caused by hypertensive stroke.

Hemorrhagic Stroke

The two distinct categories of spontaneous intracranial bleeding are intracerebral and subarachnoid hemorrhage. The symptoms of a hemorrhagic stroke are similar to those of an ischemic stroke. Their differentiation is only possible with CT or MR imaging (Morgenstern, 2010).

Intracerebral Hemorrhage

Bleeding into the brain parenchyma most commonly is caused by spontaneous rupture of small vessels previously damaged by chronic hypertension as depicted in Figure 60-1 (Qureshi, 2001; Takebayashi, 1983). Thus, pregnancy-associated hemorrhagic strokes such as the one shown in Figure 60-2 are often associated with chronic hypertension and superimposed preeclampsia (Cunningham, 2005; Martin, 2005). Because of its location, this type of hemorrhage has much higher morbidity and mortality rates than does subarachnoid hemorrhage (Morgenstern, 2010). Chronic hypertension is uniquely associated with *Charcot-Bouchard microaneurysms* of the penetrating branches of the middle cerebral artery. Pressure-induced rupture causes bleeding in the putamen, thalamus, adjacent white matter, pons, and cerebellum. In the 28 women described by Martin and associates (2005), half died and most survivors had permanent disabilities. This cautions for the importance of proper management for gestational hypertension—especially systolic hypertension—to prevent cerebrovascular pathology (Chap. 40, p. 761).

Subarachnoid Hemorrhage

In a study of 639 cases of pregnancy-related subarachnoid hemorrhage from the Nationwide Inpatient Sample, the incidence was 5.8 per 100,000 pregnancies, with half being postpartum (Bateman, 2012). These bleeds are more likely caused by an underlying cerebrovascular malformation in an otherwise normal patient (see Fig. 60-1). Ruptured saccular or "berry" aneurysms cause 80 percent of all subarachnoid hemorrhages. The remaining cases are caused by a ruptured arteriovenous malformation, coagulopathy, angiopathy, venous thrombosis, infection, drug abuse, tumors, or trauma. Such cases are uncommon, and a ruptured aneurysm or angioma or bleeding from a vascular malformation has an incidence of 1 in 75,000 pregnancies. Although this frequency is not different from that in the general population, the mortality rate during pregnancy is reported to be as high as 35 percent.

Intracranial Aneurysm. Approximately 2 to 5 percent of adults have this lesion (see Fig. 60-1). Fortunately, only a small percentage rupture—approximately 0.1 percent for aneurysms < 10 mm and 1 percent for those > 10 mm (Smith, 2008). Most aneurysms identified during pregnancy arise from the circle of Willis, and 20 percent are multiple (Stoodley, 1998). Pregnancy does not increase the risk for aneurysmal rupture. However, because of their high prevalence, they are more likely to cause subarachnoid bleeding than other causes (Hirsch, 2009; Tiel Groenestege, 2009). Aneurysms are more likely to bleed during the second half of pregnancy—only approximately 20 percent bleed during the first half (Dias, 1990).

The cardinal symptom of a subarachnoid hemorrhage from an aneurysm rupture is sudden severe headache, accompanied by visual changes, cranial nerve abnormalities, focal neurological deficits, and altered consciousness. Patients typically have signs of meningeal irritation, nausea and vomiting, tachycardia, transient hypertension, low-grade fever, leukocytosis, and proteinuria. Prompt diagnosis and treatment may prevent potentially lethal complications. The American Heart Association recommends noncontrast cranial CT imaging as the first diagnostic test, although MR imaging may be superior (Chalela, 2007; Connolly, 2012).

Treatment includes bed rest, analgesia, and sedation, with neurological monitoring and strict blood pressure control. Repair of a potentially accessible aneurysm during pregnancy depends in part on the recurrent hemorrhage risk versus surgical risks. At least in nonpregnant patients, the risk of subsequent bleeding with conservative treatment is 20 to 30 percent for the first month and then 3 percent per year. The risk of rebleeding is highest within the first 24 hours, and recurrent hemorrhage leads to death in 70 percent.

Early repair is done by surgical clipping of the aneurysm or by endovascular coil placement completed using fluoroscopic angiography yet attempting to limit radiation exposure. For women remote from term, repair without hypotensive anesthesia seems optimal. For women near term, cesarean delivery followed by aneurysm repair is a consideration, and we have successfully done this in several cases. For aneurysms repaired either before or during pregnancy, most allow vaginal delivery if remote from aneurysmal repair. A problem is what defines "remote," and although some recommend 2 months, the time for complete healing is unknown. For women who survive subarachnoid hemorrhage, but in whom surgical repair is not done, we agree with Cartlidge (2000) and recommend against bearing down—put another way, we favor cesarean delivery.

Arteriovenous Malformations. These are congenital focal abnormal conglomerations of dilated arteries and veins with subarteriolar disorganization (see Fig. 60-1). They lack capillaries and have resultant arteriovenous shunting. Although unclear, the risk of bleeding may increase with gestational age. When arteriovenous malformations (AVMs) bleed, half do so into the subarachnoid space, whereas half are intraparenchymal with subarachnoid extension (Smith, 2008). They are uncommon and are estimated to occur in 0.01 percent of the general population. Bleeding does not appear to be more likely during pregnancy (Finnerty, 1999; Horton, 1990). AVMs are correspondingly rare during pregnancy, and in the study from Parkland Hospital, there was only one AVM in nearly 90,000 deliveries (Simolke, 1991).

Treatment of AVMs in nonpregnant patients is largely individualized. There is no consensus whether all those that are accessible should be resected. It also depends on whether the lesion is symptomatic or an incidental finding; its anatomy and size; presence of associated aneurysm, which is found in up to 60 percent; and especially, whether or not the lesion has bled. After hemorrhage, the risk of recurrent bleeding in unrepaired lesions is 6 to 20 percent within the first year, and 2 to 4 percent per year thereafter (Friedlander, 2007; Smith, 2008). The mortality rate with a bleeding AVM is 10 to 20 percent. In pregnancy, the decision to operate is usually based on neurosurgical considerations, and Friedlander (2007) recommends strong consideration for treatment if bleeding occurs. Because of the high risk of recurrent hemorrhage from an unresected or inoperable lesion, we favor cesarean delivery. An unusual case of spontaneous regression of a cerebral AVM has been described (Couldwell, 2011).

DEMYELINATING OR DEGENERATIVE DISEASES

The *demyelinating diseases* are neurological disorders characterized by immune-mediated focal or patchy destruction of myelin sheaths accompanied by an inflammatory response. The *degenerative diseases* are multifactorial and are characterized by progressive neuronal death.

Multiple Sclerosis

In the United States, multiple sclerosis (MS) is second only to trauma as a cause of neurological disability in middle adulthood (Hauser, 2012b). Because the disease affects women twice as often as men and usually begins in the 20s and 30s, women of reproductive age are most susceptible. The familial recurrence rate of MS is 15 percent, and the incidence in offspring is increased 15-fold.

The demyelinating characteristic of this disorder results from predominately T cell-mediated autoimmune destruction of oligodendrocytes that synthesize myelin. There is a genetic susceptibility and likely an environmental trigger such as exposure to certain bacteria and viruses, for example, *Chlamydophila pneumoniae,* human herpesvirus 6, or Epstein-Barr virus (Frohman, 2006; Goodin, 2009).

There are four clinical types of multiple sclerosis (Hauser, 2012b):

1. *Relapsing-remitting MS* accounts for initial presentation in 85 percent of affected individuals. It is characterized by unpredictable recurrent episodes of focal or multifocal

neurological dysfunction usually followed by full recovery. Over time, however, relapses lead to persistent deficits.

2. *Secondary progressive MS* disease is relapsing-remitting disease that begins to pursue a progressive downhill course after each relapse. It is likely that all patients eventually develop this type.
3. *Primary progressive MS* accounts for 15 percent of cases. It is characterized by gradual progression of disability from the time of initial diagnosis.
4. *Progressive-relapsing MS* refers to primary progressive MS with apparent relapses.

Classic findings of MS include sensory loss, visual symptoms from optic neuritis, weakness, paresthesias, and a host of other neurological symptoms. Almost 75 percent of women with isolated optic neuritis develop multiple sclerosis within 15 years. Clinical diagnosis is confirmed by MR imaging and cerebrospinal fluid analysis. In greater than 95 percent of cases, MR imaging shows characteristic multifocal white matter plaques that represent discrete areas of demyelination such as shown in Figure 60-3. Their appearance and extent are less helpful for treatment response. Similarly, Kuhle and colleagues (2007) reported that identification of serum antibodies against myelin oligodendrocyte glycoprotein and myelin basic protein are not predictive of recurrent disease activity.

Effects of Pregnancy on MS

The *PR*egnancy *In Multiple Sclerosis*—*PRIMS*—study is a European prospective multicenter study in which 254 pregnancies were described (Vukusic, 2006). A principal finding was a confirmed 70-percent reduction in relapse risk during pregnancy, but with a significantly increased relapse rate postpartum. This may be related to increased pregnancy-induced numbers of T-helper lymphocytes with an increased T2/T1 ratio (Airas, 2008). In a metaanalysis of women with more than 1200 pregnancies complicated by multiple sclerosis, their relapse rate was 0.4 per year before pregnancy; 0.26 per year during pregnancy; and this increased to 0.7 per year after delivery (Finkelsztejn, 2011). Factors associated with postpartum relapse include a high relapse rate before pregnancy, relapses during pregnancy, and a high MS disability score (Portaccio, 2014; Vukusic, 2006). Breast feeding has no apparent effect on postpartum relapses (Airas, 2010; Portaccio, 2011).

Effects of MS on Pregnancy

There are usually no adverse effects on pregnancy outcome with uncomplicated disease. Some women may become fatigued more easily, those with bladder dysfunction are predisposed to urinary infection, and women with spinal lesions at or above T_6 are at risk for autonomic dysreflexia. Dahl and coworkers (2006) described 449 such pregnancies, and they reported a higher labor induction rate and longer second-stage labor. The increased induction rate as well as elective operations contributed to the overall increased cesarean delivery rate. They also reported outcomes in 649 affected women and described a lower mean birthweight but similar perinatal mortality rate compared with that of controls (Dahl, 2005). Other studies have corroborated that MS does not significantly affect obstetrical and neonatal outcomes (Finkelsztejn, 2011).

Management During Pregnancy and the Puerperium

Goals are to arrest acute or initial attacks, employ disease-modifying agents, and provide symptomatic relief. Some treatments may need to be modified during pregnancy. Acute or initial attacks are treated with high-dose intravenous methylprednisolone—500 to 1000 mg daily for 3 to 5 days, followed by oral prednisone for 2 weeks. Plasma exchange may be considered. Symptomatic relief can be provided by analgesics; carbamazepine, phenytoin, or amitriptyline for neurogenic pain; baclofen (Lioresal, Kemstro) for spasticity; α_2-adrenergic

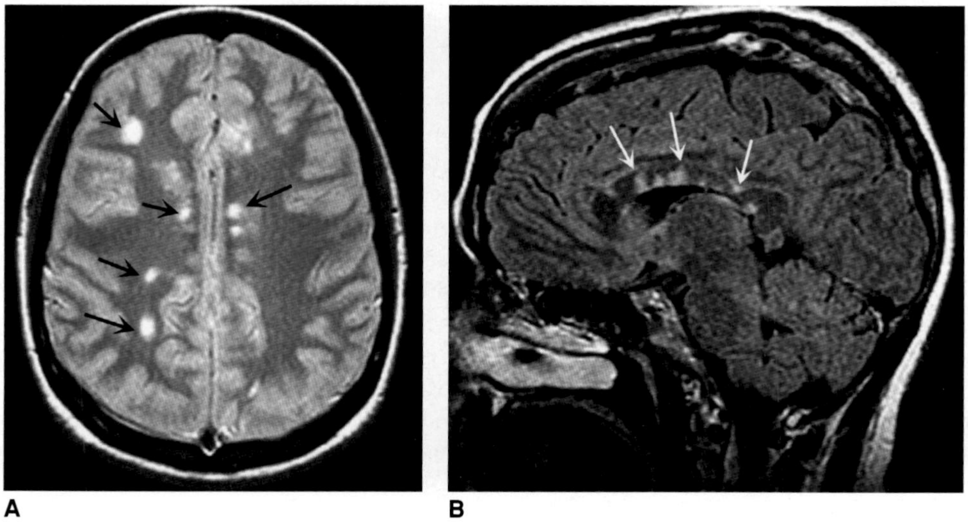

FIGURE 60-3 Magnetic resonance cranial images from a woman with multiple sclerosis. **A.** T2-weighted axial image shows bright signal abnormalities in white matter, typical for multiple sclerosis. **B.** Sagittal T2-FLAIR image shows hyperintense areas within the corpus callosum that are representative of demyelination in multiple sclerosis. (From Hauser, 2012b, with permission.)

blockade for bladder neck relaxation; and cholinergic and anticholinergic drugs to stimulate or inhibit bladder contractions.

Several disease-modifying therapies can be used for relapsing multiple sclerosis or exacerbations. Examples include interferons β1a (Rebif) and β1b (Betaseron) and glatiramer acetate (Copaxone), which have been shown to decrease relapse rates by a third (Rudick, 2011). Data concerning safety in pregnancy are limited but overall reassuring (Amato, 2010; Salminen, 2010). Clinical trials with natalizumab (Tysabri), an alpha 4 integrin antagonist—especially when combined with interferon β1a—significantly reduced MS clinical relapse rates (Polman, 2006; Rudick, 2006). In a review of 35 pregnancies, early pregnancy drug exposure did not worsen outcomes (Hellwig, 2011). Because of limited data, however, women are currently advised to stop the drug 3 months before conception. Fingolimad (Gilenya) is a new oral medication, and pregnancy safety data are unavailable (Briggs, 2011).

Prevention of relapses postpartum is afforded by treatment with intravenous immune globulin (IVIG) given in a dose of 0.4 g/kg daily for 5 days during weeks 1, 6, and 12 (Argyriou, 2008). The Prevention of Postpartum Relapses with Progestin and Estradiol in Multiple Sclerosis (POPART'MUS) trial is a multicenter randomized controlled trial currently enrolling patients (Vukusic, 2009).

Huntington Disease

This adult-onset neurodegenerative disease results from an autosomal dominant expanded CAG trinucleotide repeat within the Huntington gene on chromosome 4. It is characterized by a combination of choreoathetotic movements, progressive dementia, and psychiatric manifestations. Because the mean age of onset is 40 years, Huntington disease rarely complicates pregnancy. Prenatal diagnosis is discussed in Chapter 14 (p. 297). However, prenatal screening is controversial because this usually is a late-onset adult disease. Thus, extensive pretest counseling is imperative (Novak, 2010).

Myasthenia Gravis

This autoimmune-mediated neuromuscular disorder affects approximately 1 in 7500 persons. It is more common in women, and its incidence peaks in their 20s and 30s. The etiology is unknown, but genetic factors likely play a role. Most patients demonstrate antibodies to the acetylcholine receptor, although 10 to 20 percent are seronegative. The latter often have antibodies to muscle-specific tyrosine kinase (MuSK) that regulates assembly of the acetylcholine receptor subunits at the neuromuscular junction (Cavalcante, 2011; Pal, 2011).

Cardinal features of MG are weakness and easy fatigability of facial, oropharyngeal, extraocular, and limb muscles. Deep tendon reflexes are preserved. Cranial muscles are involved early and disparately, and diplopia and ptosis are common. Facial muscle weakness causes difficulty in smiling, chewing, and speaking. In 85 percent of patients, the weakness becomes generalized. Other autoimmune diseases may coexist, and hypothyroidism should be excluded. The clinical course is marked by exacerbations and remissions, especially when it first becomes clinically apparent. Remissions are not always complete and are seldom permanent. Systemic diseases, concurrent infections, and even emotional upset may precipitate exacerbations, of which there are three types:

1. *Myasthenic crises*—characterized by severe muscle weakness, inability to swallow, and respiratory muscle paralysis.
2. *Refractory crises*—characterized by the same symptoms but unresponsive to the usual therapy.
3. *Cholinergic crises*—excessive cholinergic medication leads to nausea, vomiting, muscle weakness, abdominal pain, and diarrhea.

All three of these can be life threatening, but a refractory crisis is a medical emergency. Those with bulbar myasthenia are at particular risk because they may be unable to swallow or even ask for help.

Management

Myasthenia is manageable but not curable. Thymectomy is generally recommended for long-term benefits in the 75 percent of patients who have thymic hyperplasia or a thymoma seen with CT or MR imaging (Drachman, 2012; Nam, 2011). Anticholinesterase medications such as pyridostigmine (Mestinon), an analogue of neostigmine, improve symptoms by impeding acetylcholine degradation. They seldom produce normal muscle function. Ironically, overdose is manifest by increased weakness—the cholinergic crisis—that may be difficult to differentiate from myasthenic symptoms. Most of those refractory to anticholinesterase therapy respond to immunosuppressive therapy with glucocorticoids, azathioprine, methotrexate, cyclosporine, and mycophenolate mofetil. Tacrolimus, an immunosuppressant used in organ transplantation, and rituximab, a chimeric monoclonal antibody, are currently being evaluated (Ibrahim, 2010; Maddison, 2011; Yoshikawa, 2011). Cyclophosphamide is reserved for severe, generalized refractory cases. When short-term, rapid clinical improvement is needed—such as for a surgical procedure or a myasthenic crisis—high-dose immunoglobulin G or plasma exchange is usually effective (Barth, 2011; Cortese, 2011; Mandawat, 2010).

Myasthenia and Pregnancy

Because the greatest period of risk is within the first year following diagnosis, it seems reasonable to postpone pregnancy until there is sustained improvement. Antepartum management of myasthenia includes close observation with liberal rest and prompt treatment of infections (Heaney, 2010; Kalidindi, 2007). Women in remission who become pregnant while taking corticosteroids or azathioprine should continue these. Thymectomy has been successfully performed during pregnancy in refractory cases (Ip, 1986). Acute onset of myasthenia or its exacerbation demands prompt hospitalization and supportive care. Plasmapheresis and high-dose immunoglobulin therapy should be used for emergency situations (Drachman, 2012).

Although pregnancy does not appear to affect the overall course of MG, fatigue common to most pregnancies may be exacerbated, and the expanding uterus may compromise respiration. During pregnancy, maternal hypotension or hypovolemia are avoided. The clinical course of MG during pregnancy is unpredictable, and frequent hospitalizations are the norm. Up to a third of women have worsening MG during pregnancy, with exacerbations occurring equally in all three trimesters (Djelmis, 2002; Podciechowski, 2005).

Myasthenia gravis has no significant adverse effects on pregnancy outcomes (Wen, 2009). Preeclampsia is a concern because magnesium sulfate may precipitate a severe myasthenic crisis (Hamaoui, 2009; Heaney, 2010). Although phenytoin use is also problematic in this regard, its adverse effects are less troublesome, and thus many choose it for neuroprophylaxis in MG patients with severe preeclampsia. Because smooth muscle is unaffected, most women have normal labor. Oxytocin is given for the usual indications, and cesarean delivery reserved for obstetrical indications. Because narcotics may cause respiratory depression, close observation and respiratory support are essential during labor and delivery. Curariform drugs should be avoided—examples include magnesium sulfate discussed above, muscle relaxants used with general anesthesia, and aminoglycosides. Neuraxial analgesia is accomplished with amide-type local agents. Regional analgesia is preferred unless there is significant bulbar involvement or respiratory compromise (Almeida, 2010; Blichfeldt-Lauridsen, 2012). During second-stage labor, some women may have impaired voluntary expulsive efforts that may warrant operative vaginal delivery.

Neonatal Effects

As discussed above, 80 percent of mothers with myasthenia gravis have anti-acetylcholine-receptor IgG antibodies. These and anti-MuSK antibodies are transported transplacentally, and the fetus can be affected to cause hydramnios (Heaney, 2010). Similarly, 10 to 20 percent of neonates manifest MG symptoms (Murray, 2010; Niks, 2008). Transient symptoms usually include a feeble cry, poor suckling, and respiratory distress. Symptoms usually respond to cholinesterase inhibitors and resolve within a few weeks.

NEUROPATHIES

Peripheral neuropathy is a general term used to describe disorders of peripheral nerve(s) of any cause. Because neuropathy can result from a variety of sources, its discovery should prompt a search for an etiology. *Polyneuropathies* can be either axonal or demyelinating as well as acute, subacute, or chronic (Chaudhry, 2008). They are often associated with systemic diseases such as diabetes, with drug or environmental toxin exposure, or with genetic diseases.

Mononeuropathies are relatively common in pregnancy, and they signify focal involvement of a single nerve trunk and imply local causation such as trauma, compression, or entrapment. Traumatic pudendal, obturator, femoral, and common fibular mononeuropathies are usually caused by childbirth and are discussed in Chapter 36 (p. 676).

Guillain-Barré Syndrome

In 75 percent of cases, this acute demyelinating polyradiculoneuropathy has clinical or serological evidence for an acute infection. Commonly associated are infection with *Campylobacter jejuni*, cytomegalovirus, and Epstein-Barr virus; surgical procedures; and immunizations (Haber, 2009; Hauser, 2012a). Guillain-Barré syndrome (GBS) is thought to be immune-mediated from antibodies formed against nonself antigens. Demyelination causes sensory and motor conduction blockade, and recovery occurs with remyelination in most cases.

Clinical features include areflexic paralysis—usually ascending—with or without sensory disturbances. Autonomic dysfunction is common. The full syndrome develops over 1 to 3 weeks. Management is supportive, but in the worsening phase, patients should be hospitalized because at least a third will need ventilatory assistance. Intravenous high-dose immunoglobulin (IVIG) or plasmapheresis is beneficial if begun within 1 to 2 weeks of motor symptoms, however, neither decreases mortality rates (Cortese, 2011; Gwathmey, 2011; Hughes, 2011). Although most patients recover fully within several months to a year, up to 20 percent are severely disabled, and 5 percent die, despite treatment (Yuki, 2012). Some manifest as *chronic inflammatory demyelinating polyneuropathy,* and our experiences indicate that it may be relatively common in these young women.

Pregnancy

Guillain-Barré syndrome is not more common in pregnancy, although inconclusive data suggest rates are increased in the puerperium (Cheng, 1998). Its clinical course in pregnancy is the same as for nonpregnant individuals, and after an insidious onset, paresis and paralysis most often continue to ascend to cause ventilatory weakness. Hurley and colleagues (1991) reported that a third of pregnant women required ventilatory support, with a mortality rate of 13 percent. The acute syndrome is treated with either high-dose IVIG or plasmapheresis (Chan, 2004; Yuki, 2012).

Bell Palsy

This disfiguring palsy is usually a mononeuropathic acute facial paralysis that is relatively common in reproductive-aged women (Fig. 60-4). It has a female predominance, and pregnant women

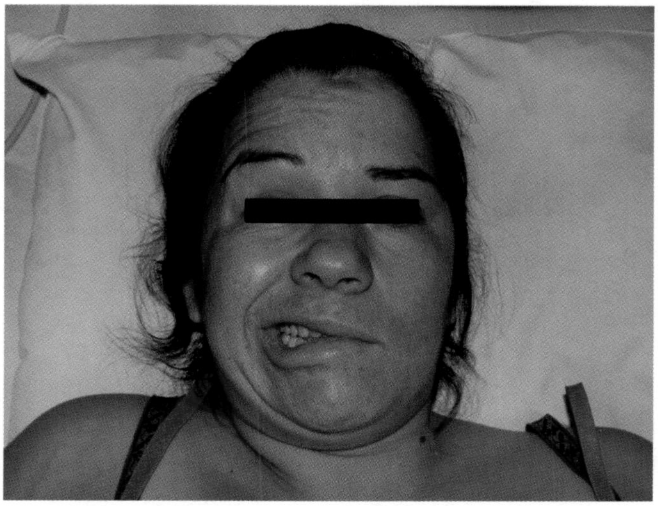

FIGURE 60-4 Bell facial nerve palsy developing on the day of delivery after a cesarean for dichorionic twins. This woman was treated with prednisone and antiviral medication, and the palsy had almost resolved 3 weeks postpartum.

are at a fourfold risk compared with nonpregnant women (Cohen, 2000; Heaney, 2010). The disease is characterized by facial nerve inflammation and often is associated with reactivation of herpes virus or herpes zoster virus.

Bell palsy usually has an abrupt and painful onset with maximum weakness by 48 hours. In some cases, hyperacusis and loss of taste accompany paralysis (Beal, 2012). Management includes supportive care with facial muscle massage and eye protection against corneal lacerations from drying. There is general consensus that prednisone, 1 mg per kg given orally daily for 5 days, will result in improved outcomes and a shortened recovery period (Salinas, 2010; Sullivan, 2007). It is controversial if addition of an antiviral medication will improve these outcomes (de Almeida, 2009; Lockhart, 2009; Quant, 2009).

Pregnancy

It is unclear if pregnancy alters the prognosis for spontaneous facial palsy recovery. Gillman and colleagues (2002) found that only half of pregnant women recovered to a satisfactory level after 1 year—this compared with approximately 80 percent of nonpregnant women and men. Some prognostic markers for incomplete recovery are bilateral palsy, recurrence in a subsequent pregnancy, greater percentage of nerve function loss, and a faster rate of loss (Cohen, 2000; Gilden, 2004). Corticosteroid therapy given early in the course of the disease significantly improves outcomes. Other than a fivefold increased rate for gestational hypertension or preeclampsia, women with Bell palsy do not have increased adverse pregnancy outcomes (Katz, 2011; Shmorgun, 2002).

Carpal Tunnel Syndrome

This syndrome results from compression of the median nerve and is the most frequent mononeuropathy in pregnancy (Padua, 2010). Symptoms include burning, numbness, or tingling along the inner half of one or both hands. Also, wrist pain and numbness extend into the forearm and sometimes into the shoulder (Katz, 2002). Symptoms are bilateral in 80 percent of pregnant women, and 10 percent have evidence for severe denervation (Seror, 1998). Differential diagnosis includes cervical radiculopathy of C_6–C_7 and de Quervain tendonitis, which is caused by swelling of the conjoined tendons and their sheaths near the distal radius. Nerve conduction studies may be helpful (Alfonso, 2010).

Pregnancy

The reported incidence is 7 to 43 percent and varies greatly because the range of symptoms is marked (Finsen, 2006; Padua, 2010). Symptomatic treatment with a splint applied to the slightly flexed wrist during sleep relieves pressure and usually provides relief. Although symptoms typically are self-limited, occasionally surgical decompression and corticosteroid injections are necessary (Keith, 2009; Shi, 2011). Symptoms may persist in more than half of patients at one year and in a third at 3 years (Padua, 2010).

SPINAL-CORD INJURY

According to the National Spinal Cord Injury Statistical Center (2012), there are approximately 12,000 spinal cord injuries each year. At least half affect reproductive-age individuals, with a male-to-female predominance of 4 to 1. The severity of cord injury determines the short- and long-term prognosis as well as that for pregnancy. Incomplete neurological lesions are associated with at least some sensory and/or motor function below the level of injury, whereas there is none with complete cord transection. Many women develop sexual function alteration and transient hypothalamic pituitary hypogonadism, however, pregnancy is not uncommon if menstruation resumes (Bughi, 2008).

Women with spinal cord injury have an increased frequency of pregnancy complications that include preterm and low-birthweight infants. Most have asymptomatic bacteriuria with sporadic symptomatic urinary infections. Bowel dysfunction causes constipation in more than half, and anemia and pressure-necrosis skin lesions are also common. There are two serious and life-threatening complications with spinal cord injuries:

1. If the cord is transected above T_{10}, the cough reflex is impaired, respiratory function may be compromised, and pneumonitis from covert aspiration can be serious. Pulmonary function tests are considered, and some women may need ventilatory support in late pregnancy or in labor.
2. Women with lesions above T_5–T_6 are at risk for *autonomic dysreflexia*. With this, stimuli from structures innervated below the level of the spinal lesion results in massive disordered sympathetic stimulation. Abrupt catecholamine release can cause vasoconstriction with severe hypertension and symptoms that include throbbing headaches, facial flushing, sweating, bradycardia, tachycardia, arrhythmias, and respiratory distress. Dysreflexia can be precipitated by a variety of stimuli, such as urethral catheterization; bladder distention from retention; rectal or cervical distention with digital examinations; uterine contractions and cervical dilatation; or any other pelvic structure manipulation (American College of Obstetricians and Gynecologists, 2005; Krassioukov, 2009). In one report, 12 of 15 women at risk for autonomic dysreflexia suffered at least one episode during pregnancy (Westgren, 1993).

Because uterine contractions are not affected by spinal cord lesions, labor is usually easy—even precipitous, and comparatively painless. If the lesion is below T_{12}, uterine contractions are felt normally. For lesions above T_{12}, the risk of out-of-hospital delivery is substantial and can be minimized by teaching women to palpate for uterine contractions. This is especially important because up to 20 percent of women deliver preterm (Westgren, 1993). Some recommend tocodynamometry and weekly cervical examinations beginning at 28 to 30 weeks. Another reasonable option that we frequently employ at Parkland Hospital is elective hospitalization after 36 to 37 weeks (Hughes, 1991).

Spinal or epidural analgesia extending to T_{10} prevents autonomic dysreflexia and should be instituted at the start of labor. If there are severe symptoms before epidural placement, steps are taken to abolish the provoking stimulus. A parenteral antihypertensive agent such as hydralazine or labetalol is given. Labor and vaginal delivery with epidural or spinal analgesia are preferable and will minimize autonomic dysreflexia (Kuczkowski, 2006). Operative vaginal delivery is frequently necessary.

IDIOPATHIC INTRACRANIAL HYPERTENSION

Also known as *pseudotumor cerebri* or *benign intracranial hypertension*, this disorder is characterized by increased intracranial pressure without hydrocephalus. The cause is unknown, but it may be the result of either overproduction or underabsorption of cerebrospinal fluid. Symptoms include headache in at least 90 percent of cases, visual disturbances such as loss of a visual field or central visual acuity in 70 percent, and commonly occurring papilledema that may be sight-threatening (Evans, 2000; Heaney, 2010). Other complaints are stiff neck, back pain, pulsatile tinnitus, cranial nerve palsies such as facial palsy, ataxia, or paresthesias. The syndrome is commonly found in young women and is prevalent in those who are obese, who recently gained weight, or both (Fraser, 2011). Along with symptoms, other criteria for diagnosis include elevated intracranial pressure > 250 mm H_2O, normal cerebrospinal fluid (CSF) composition, normal cranial CT or MR imaging findings, and no evidence for systemic disease (International Headache Society, 2005).

Idiopathic intracranial hypertension is usually self-limited. Visual defects can be prevented by lowering the cerebrospinal fluid pressure. Drugs given to lower pressure include acetazolamide (Diamox) to reduce fluid production, furosemide (Lasix), or topiramate (Topamax). Corticosteroids are now rarely used. Surgical intervention is occasionally necessary and is accomplished by either lumboperitoneal shunting of spinal fluid or optic nerve sheath fenestration.

Effects of Pregnancy

It is controversial if pregnancy is a risk factor for idiopathic intracranial hypertension. Certainly, symptoms may first appear in pregnancy, and women previously diagnosed may become symptomatic. These usually develop by midpregnancy, tend to be self-limited, and usually resolve postpartum.

There is general agreement that pregnancy does not alter management. Some recommend serial visual field testing to prevent permanent vision loss. In a report of 16 pregnant women, visual field loss developed in four, and it became permanent in one (Huna-Baron, 2002). Visual field loss is often coincident with the development of papilledema, for which acetazolamide is given. Lee and associates (2005) reported successful treatment of 12 pregnant women. Although outmoded for treatment of nonpregnant individuals, repeated lumbar punctures are generally successful in providing temporary relief throughout pregnancy. In some pregnant women, surgical therapy becomes necessary, and we and others have had promising results with optic nerve sheath fenestration (Thambisetty, 2007).

Pregnancy complications are likely due to associated obesity and not to intracranial hypertension. In a review of 54 pregnancies, there were no excessive adverse perinatal outcomes (Katz, 1989). The route of delivery depends on obstetrical indications, and conduction analgesia is safe (Aly, 2007; Karmaniolou, 2011).

MATERNAL VENTRICULAR SHUNTS

Pregnancies in women with previously placed ventricular shunts for obstructive hydrocephalus usually have satisfactory outcomes (Landwehr, 1994). Shunts may be ventriculoperitoneal, ventriculoatrial, or ventriculopleural. Partial obstruction of a shunt is common, especially late in pregnancy (Schiza, 2012). In one report of 17 such pregnancies, neurological complications were reported in 13 (Wisoff, 1991). Findings included headaches in 60 percent, nausea and vomiting in 35 percent, lethargy in 30 percent, and ataxia or gaze paresis, each in 20 percent. Most symptoms respond to conservative management. However, if CT scanning during symptom evaluation discloses acute hydrocephaly, then the shunt is tapped or pumped several times daily. In some cases, surgical revision is necessary and may be emergently required (Murakami, 2010).

Another shunting procedure involves placement of an endoscopic third ventriculostomy for hydrocephalus in children or adults (de Ribaupierre, 2007). One report described successful results in five pregnant women who underwent successful ventriculostomy placement (Riffaud, 2006). In a review, reproductive function and miscarriage rates were found to significantly worsen in these women (Bedaiwy, 2008).

Vaginal delivery is preferred in women with shunts, and unless there is a meningomyelocele, conduction analgesia is permitted. Antimicrobial prophylaxis is indicated if the peritoneal cavity is entered for cesarean delivery or tubal sterilization.

MATERNAL BRAIN DEATH

Brain death is rare in obstetrics. Life-support systems and parenteral alimentation for up to 15 weeks have been described while awaiting delivery (Hussein, 2006; Powner, 2003; Souza, 2006). Some women were treated with aggressive tocolysis and antimicrobial therapy. Chiossi and coworkers (2006) reviewed outcomes in 17 women with persistent vegetative state who were given various levels of support. At least five died after delivery, and most of the remainder continued to be in the vegetative state. There are no published reports of neurological recovery with a diagnosis of brain death using the uniform Determination of Death Act definition (Wijdicks, 2010). The ethical, financial, and legal implications, both civil and criminal, that arise from attempting or not attempting such care are profound (Farragher, 2005; Feldman, 2000). In some women, perimortem cesarean delivery is performed as discussed in Chapter 47 (p. 956).

REFERENCES

Adab N: Therapeutic monitoring of antiepileptic drugs during pregnancy and in the postpartum period: is it useful? CNS Drugs 20:791, 2006

Adeney KL, Williams MA: Migraine headaches and preeclampsia: an epidemiologic review. Headache 46:794, 2006

Aegidius K, Anker-Zwart J, Hagen K, et al: The effect of pregnancy and parity on headache prevalence: the head-HUNT study. Headache 49:851, 2009

Airas L, Jalkanen A, Alanen A, et al: Breast-feeding, postpartum and prepregnancy disease activity in multiple sclerosis. Neurology 75:474, 2010

Airas L, Saraste M, Rinta S, et al: Immunoregulatory factors in multiple sclerosis patients during and after pregnancy: relevance of natural killer cells. Clin Exp Immunol 151:235, 2008

Airola G, Allais G, Castagnoli I, et al: Non-pharmacological management of migraine during pregnancy. Neurol Sci 31(1):S63, 2010
Alfonso C, Jann S, Massa R, et al: Diagnosis, treatment and follow-up of the carpal tunnel syndrome: a review. Neurol Sci 31:243, 2010
Allais G, Castagnoli Gabellari I, Borgogno P, et al: The risks of women with migraine during pregnancy. Neurol Sci 31(Suppl 1):S59, 2010
Almeida C, Coutinho E, Moreira D, et al: Myasthenia gravis and pregnancy: anaesthetic management—a series of cases. Eur J Anaesthesiol 27:985, 2010
Aly EE, Lawther BK: Anaesthetic management of uncontrolled idiopathic intracranial hypertension during labour and delivery using an intrathecal catheter. Anaesthesia 62:178, 2007
Amato MP, Portaccio E, Ghezzi A, et al: Pregnancy and fetal outcomes after interferon-beta exposure in multiple sclerosis. Neurology 75:1794, 2010
American College of Obstetricians and Gynecologists: Obstetric management of patients with spinal cord injuries. Committee Opinion No. 275, September 2002, Reaffirmed 2005
Argyriou AA, Makris N: Multiple sclerosis and reproductive risks in women. Reprod Sci 15(8):755, 2008
Aukes AM, de Groot JC, Aarnoudse JG, et al: Brain lesions several years after eclampsia. Am J Obstet Gynecol 200(5):504.e1, 2009
Aukes AM, Wessel I, Dubois AM, et al: Self-reported cognitive functioning in formerly eclamptic women. Am J Obstet Gynecol 197:365.e1, 2007
Banhidy F, Acs N, Horvath-Puho E, et al: Maternal severe migraine and risk of congenital limb deficiencies. Birth Defects Res A Clin Mol Teratol 76:592, 2006
Barth D, Nouri M, Ng E, et al: Comparison of IVIg and PLEX in patients with myasthenia gravis. Neurology 76:2017, 2011
Bateman BT, Olbrecht VA, Berman MF, et al: Peripartum subarachnoid hemorrhage. Anesthesiology 116:242, 2012
Beal MF, Hauser SL: Trigeminal neuralgia, Bell's palsy, and other cranial nerve disorders. In Longo DL, Fauci AS, Kasper DL, et al (eds): Harrison's Principles of Internal Medicine, 18th ed. McGraw-Hill, New York, 2012, p 3362
Bedaiwy MA, Fathalla MM, Shaaban OM, et al: Reproductive implications of endoscopic third ventriculostomy for the treatment of hydrocephalus. Eur J Obstet Gynecol Reprod Biol 140(1):55, 2008
Berg AT, Berkovic SF, Brodie MJ, et al: Revised terminology and concepts for organization of seizures and epilepsies: report of the ILAE Commission on Classification and Terminology, 2005–2009. Epilepsia 51:676, 2010a
Berg AT, Scheffer IE: New concepts in classification of the epilepsies: entering the 21st century. Epilepsia 52(6):1058, 2011
Berg CJ, Callaghan WM, Syverson C: Pregnancy-related mortality in the United States, 1998 to 2005. Obstet Gynecol 116:1302, 2010b
Blichfeldt-Lauridsen L, Hansen BD: Anesthesia and myasthenia gravis. Acta Anaesthesiol Scand 56(1):17, 2012
Borthen I, Eide MG, Daltveit AK, et al: Obstetric outcome in women with epilepsy: a hospital-based, retrospective study. BJOG 118(8):956, 2011
Brandes JL, Kudrow D, Stark SR, et al: Sumatriptan-naproxen for acute treatment of migraine. JAMA 297:1443, 2007
Briggs GG, Freeman RK, Yaffe SJ: Drugs in Pregnancy and Lactation, 9th ed. Philadelphia, Lippincott Williams & Wilkins, 2011
Brighton TA, Eikelboom JW, Mann K, et al: Low-dose aspirin for preventing recurrent venous thromboembolism. N Engl J Med 367:1979, 2012
Brodie MJ, Dichter MA: Antiepileptic drugs. N Engl J Med 334:168, 1996
Bughi S, Shaw SJ, Mahmood G, et al: Amenorrhea, pregnancy, and pregnancy outcomes in women following spinal cord injury: a retrospective cross-sectional study. Endocr Pract 14(4):437, 2008
Buhimschi CS, Weiner CP: Medication in pregnancy and lactation: part 1. Teratology. Obstet Gynecol 113:166, 2009
Bushnell CD, Jamison M, James AH: Migraines during pregnancy linked to stroke and vascular diseases: US population based case-control study. BMJ 338:b664, 2009
Calhoun AH, Peterlin BL: Treatment of cluster headache in pregnancy and lactation. Curr Pain Headache Rep 14:164, 2010
Callaghan WM, MacKay AP, Berg CJ: Identification of severe maternal morbidity during delivery hospitalizations, United States, 1991–2003. Am J Obstet Gynecol 199:133.e1, 2008
Cartlidge NEF: Neurologic disorders. In Barron WM, Lindheimer MD (eds): Medical Disorders During Pregnancy, 3rd ed. St. Louis, Mosby, 2000, p 516
Cavalcante P, Le Panse R, Berrih-Aknin S, et al: The thymus in myasthenia gravis: site of "innate autoimmunity"? Muscle Nerve 44(4):467, 2011
Centers for Disease Control and Prevention: Prevalence of stroke–United States, 2006–2010, MMWR 61:379, 2012
Chalela JA, Kidwell CS, Nentwich LM, et al: Magnetic resonance imaging and computed tomography in emergency assessment of patients with suspected acute stroke: a prospective comparison. Lancet 369:293, 2007
Chan LY, Tsui MH, Leung TN: Guillain-Barré syndrome in pregnancy. Acta Obstet Gynecol Scand 83:319, 2004
Chaudhry V: Peripheral neuropathy. In Fauci AS, Braunwald E, Kasper DL, et al (eds): Harrison's Principles of Internal Medicine, 17th ed. McGraw-Hill, New York, 2008, p 2651
Chen TC, Leviton A: Headache recurrence in pregnant women with migraine. Headache 34:107, 1994
Cheng Q, Jiang GX, Fredrikson S, et al: Increased incidence of Guillain-Barré syndrome postpartum. Epidemiology 9:601, 1998
Chiapparini L, Ferraro S, Grazzi L: Neuroimaging in chronic migraine. Neurol Sci 31(Suppl 1):S19, 2010
Chiossi G, Novic K, Celebrezze JU, et al: Successful neonatal outcome in 2 cases of maternal persistent vegetative state treated in a labor and delivery suite. Am J Obstet Gynecol 195:316, 2006
Choi H, Parman N: The use of intravenous magnesium sulphate for acute migraine: meta-analysis of randomized controlled trials. Eur J Emerg Med 21:2, 2014
Cohen Y, Lavie O, Granoxsky-Grisaru S, et al: Bell palsy complicating pregnancy: a review. Obstet Gynecol Surv 55:184, 2000
Connolly ES JR, Rabinstein AA, Carhuapoma JR: Guidelines for the management of aneurismal subarachnoid hemorrhage: a guideline for healthcare professionals from the American Heart Association/American Stroke Association. Stroke 43:1711, 2012
Contag SA, Bushnell C: Contemporary management of migraine disorders in pregnancy. Curr Opin Obstet Gynecol 22:437, 2010
Coppage KH, Hinton AC, Moldenhauer J, et al: Maternal and perinatal outcome in women with a history of stroke. Am J Obstet Gynecol 190:1331, 2004
Cortese I, Chaudhry V, So YT, et al: Evidence-based guideline update: plasmapheresis in neurologic disorders. Neurology 76:294, 2011
Couldwell SM, Kraus KL, Couldwell WT: Regression of cerebral arteriovenous malformation in the puerperium. Acta Neurochir 153:359, 2011
Cunningham FG: Severe preeclampsia and eclampsia: systolic hypertension is also important. Obstet Gynecol 105:237, 2005
D'Andrea G, Leon A: Pathogenesis of migraine: from neurotransmitters to neuromodulators and beyond. Neurol Sci 31(Supp 1):S1, 2010
Dahl J, Myhr KM, Daltveit AK, et al: Planned vaginal births in women with multiple sclerosis: delivery and birth outcome. Acta Neurol Scand Suppl 183:51, 2006
Dahl J, Myhr KM, Daltveit AK, et al: Pregnancy, delivery, and birth outcome in women with multiple sclerosis. Neurology 65:1961, 2005
Dark L, Loiselle A, Hatton R, et al: Stroke during pregnancy: therapeutic options and role of percutaneous device closure. Heart Lung Circ 20:538, 2011
De Almeida JR, Khabori MA, Guyatt GH, et al: Combined corticosteroid and antiviral treatment for Bell palsy. JAMA 302(9):985, 2009
De Freitas GR, Bogousslavsky J: Risk factors of cerebral vein and sinus thrombosis. Front Neurol Neurosci 23:23, 2008
De Ribaupierre S, Rilliet B, Vernet O, et al: Third ventriculostomy vs ventriculoperitoneal shunt in pediatric obstructive hydrocephalus: results from a Swiss series and literature review. Childs Nerv Syst 23:527, 2007
Detsky ME, McDonald DR, Baerlocher MO: Does this patient with headache have a migraine or need neuroimaging? JAMA 296(10):1274, 2006
Dias MS, Sekhar LN: Intracranial hemorrhage from aneurysms and arteriovenous malformations during pregnancy and the puerperium. Neurosurgery 27:855, 1990
Digre KB: Headaches during pregnancy. Clin Obstet Gynecol 56:317, 2013
Djelmis J, Sostarko M, Mayer D, et al: Myasthenia gravis in pregnancy: report on 69 cases. Eur J Obstet Gynecol Reprod Biol 104:21, 2002
Dodick DW, Schembri CT, Helmuth M, et al: Transcranial magnetic stimulation for migraine: a safety review. Headache 50:1153, 2010
Drachman DB: Myasthenia gravis and other diseases of the neuromuscular junction. In Longo DL, Fauci AS, Kasper DL, et al (eds): Harrison's Principles of Internal Medicine, 18th ed. McGraw-Hill, New York, 2012, p 3480
Dunlop AL, Jack BW, Bottalico JN, et al: The clinical content of preconception care: women with chronic medical conditions. Am J Obstet Gynecol 199(6B):S310, 2008
Eadie MJ: Antiepileptic drugs as human teratogens. Expert Opin Drug Saf 7:195, 2008
Evans RW, Friedman DI: Expert opinion: the management of pseudotumor cerebri during pregnancy. Headache 40:495, 2000
Facchinetti F, Allais G, Nappi RE: Migraine is a risk factor for hypertensive disorders in pregnancy: a prospective cohort study. Cephalagia 29(3):286, 2009
Farragher RA, Laffey JG: Maternal brain death and somatic support. Neurocrit Care 3:99, 2005
Feldman DM, Borgida AF, Rodis JF, et al: Irreversible maternal brain injury during pregnancy: a case report and review of the literature. Obstet Gynecol Surv 55:708, 2000

Finkelsztejn A, Brooks JBB, Paschoal FM Jr, et al: What can we really tell women with multiple sclerosis regarding pregnancy? A systemic review and meta-analysis of the literature. BJOG 118:790, 2011

Finnerty JJ, Chisholm CA, Chapple H, et al: Cerebral arteriovenous malformation in pregnancy: presentation and neurologic, obstetric, and ethical significance. Am J Obstet Gynecol 181:296, 1999

Finsen V, Zeitlmann H: Carpal tunnel syndrome during pregnancy. Scand J Plast Reconstr Hand Surg 40:41, 2006

Francis GJ, Becker WJ, Pringsheim TM: Acute and preventive pharmacologic treatment of cluster headache. Neurology 75:463, 2010

Fraser C, Plant GT: The syndrome of pseudotumour cerebri and idiopathic intracranial hypertension. Curr Opin Neurol 24:12, 2011

Friedlander RM: Arteriovenous malformations of the brain. N Engl J Med 356(26):2704, 2007

Frohman EM, Racke MK, Raine CS: Multiple sclerosis—the plaque and its pathogenesis. N Engl J Med 354:942, 2006

Furie KL, Kasner SE, Adams RJ, et al: Guidelines for the prevention of stroke in patients with stroke or transient ischemic attack: a guideline for healthcare professionals from the American Heart Association/American Stroke Association. Stroke 42:227, 2011

Furlan AJ, Reisman M, Massaro J, et al: Closure or medical therapy for cryptogenic stroke with patient foramen ovale. N Engl J Med 366:991, 2012

Gilden DH: Bell's palsy. N Engl J Med 351:1323, 2004

Gillman GS, Schaitkin BM, May M, et al: Bell's palsy in pregnancy: a study of recovery outcomes. Otolaryngol Head Neck Surg 126:26, 2002

Gjelsteen AC, Ching BH, Meyermann MW: CT, MRI, PET, PET/CT, and ultrasound in the evaluation of obstetric and gynecologic patients. Surg Clin North Am 88:361, 2008

Goadsby PJ, Raskin NH: Headache. In Longo DL, Fauci AS, Kasper DL, et al (eds): Harrison's Principles of Internal Medicine, 18th ed. McGraw-Hill, New York, 2012, p 112

Gonzalez-Hernandez A, Condes-Lara M: The multitarget drug approach in migraine treatment: the new challenge to conquer. Headache 64:197, 2014

Goodin DS: The causal cascade to multiple sclerosis: a model for MS pathogenesis. PLoS One 4(2):e4565, 2009

Gwathmey K, Balogun RA, Burns T: Neurologic indications for therapeutic plasma exchange: an update. J Clin Apheresis 26:261, 2011

Haber P, Sejvar J, Mikaeloff Y, et al: Vaccines and Guillain-Barré syndrome. Drug Saf 32(4):309, 2009

Hamaoui A, Mercado R: Association of preeclampsia and myasthenia: a case report. J Reprod Med 54(9):587, 2009

Harden CL, Hopp J, Ting TY, et al: Practice parameter update: management issues for women with epilepsy—focus on pregnancy (an evidence-based review): obstetrical complications and change in seizure frequency. Neurology 73(2):126, 2009a

Harden CL, Meador KJ, Pennell PB, et al: Practice parameter update: management issues for women with epilepsy—focus on pregnancy (an evidence-based review): teratogenesis and perinatal outcomes. Neurology 73(2):133, 2009b

Harden CL, Pennell PB, Koppel BS, et al: Practice parameter update: management issues for women with epilepsy—focus on pregnancy (an evidence-based review): vitamin K, folic acid, blood levels, and breastfeeding. Neurology 73(2):142, 2009c

Hauser SL, Amato AA: Guillain-Barré and other immune-mediated neuropathies. In Longo DL, Fauci AS, Kasper DL, et al (eds): Harrison's Principles of Internal Medicine, 18th ed. McGraw-Hill, New York, 2012a, p 3474

Hauser SL, Goodin DS: Multiple Sclerosis and other demyelinating diseases. In Longo DL, Fauci AS, Kasper DL, et al (eds): Harrison's Principles of Internal Medicine, 18th ed. McGraw-Hill, New York, 2012b, p 3395

Heaney DC, Williams DJ, O'Brien PO: Neurology. In Powrie R, Greene M, Camann W (eds): de Swiet's Medical Disorders in Obstetric Practice, 5th ed. Wiley-Blackwell, Oxford, 2010, p 371

Hellwig K, Haghikia A, Gold R. Pregnancy and natalizumab: results of an observational study in 35 accidental pregnancies during natalizumab treatment. Mult Scler 17:958, 2011

Helms AK, Drogan O, Kittner SJ: First trimester stroke prophylaxis in pregnant women with a history of stroke. Stroke 40(4):1158, 2009

Hirsch KG, Froehler MT, Huang J, et al: Occurrence of perimesencephalic subarachnoid hemorrhage during pregnancy. Neurocrit Care 10(3):339, 2009

Holmes LB, Baldwin EJ, Smith CR, et al: Increased frequency of isolated cleft palate in infants exposed to lamotrigine during pregnancy. Neurology 70(22 Pt 2):2152, 2008

Horton JC, Chambers WA, Lyons SL, et al: Pregnancy and the risk of hemorrhage from cerebral arteriovenous malformations. Neurosurgery 27(6):867, 1990

Huang CJ, Fan YC, Tsai PS: Differential impacts of modes of anaesthesia on the risk of stroke among preeclamptic women who undergo Caesarean delivery: a population-based study. BJA 105(6):818, 2010

Hughes RA, Pritchard J, Hadden RD: Pharmacological treatment other than corticosteroids, intravenous immunoglobulin and plasma exchange for Guillain-Barré syndrome. Cochrane Database Syst Rev 3:CD008630, 2011

Hughes SJ, Short DJ, Usherwood MM, et al: Management of the pregnant women with spinal cord injuries. Br J Obstet Gynaecol 98:513, 1991

Huna-Baron R, Kupersmith MJ: Idiopathic intracranial hypertension in pregnancy. J Neurol 249(8):1078, 2002

Hunt S, Russell A, Smithson WH, et al: Topiramate in pregnancy: preliminary experience from the UK Epilepsy and Pregnancy Register. Neurology 71(4):272, 2008

Hurley TJ, Brunson AD, Archer RL, et al: Landry Guillain-Barré Strohl syndrome in pregnancy: report of three cases treated with plasmapheresis. Obstet Gynecol 78:482, 1991

Hussein IY, Govenden V, Grant JM, et al: Prolongation of pregnancy in a woman who sustained brain death at 26 weeks of gestation. BJOG 113:120, 2006

Ibrahim H, Dimachkie MM, Shaibani A: A review: the use of rituximab in neuromuscular diseases. J Clin Neuromusc Dis 12:91, 2010

International Headache Society: The International Classification of Headache Disorders, 2nd ed. Cephalalgia 24:1, 2004

International Headache Society: The International Classification of Headache Disorders, 2nd ed.—revision of criteria for 8.2 Medication-overuse headache. Cephalalgia 25:460, 2005

Ip MSM, So SY, Lam WK, et al: Thymectomy in myasthenia gravis during pregnancy. Postgrad Med J 62:473, 1986

Ishimori ML, Cohen SN, Hallegue DS, et al: Ischemic stroke in a postpartum patient: understanding the epidemiology, pathogenesis, and outcome of Moyamoya disease. Semin Arthritis Rheum 35:250, 2006

James AH, Bushnell CD, Jamison MG, et al: Incidence and risk factors for stroke in pregnancy and the puerperium. Obstet Gynecol 106:509, 2005

Jamieson DG, Skliut M: Stroke in women: what is different? Curr Atheroscler Rep 12:236, 2010

Jeng JS, Tang SC, Yip PK: Stroke in women of reproductive age: comparison between stroke related and unrelated to pregnancy. J Neurol Sci 221:25, 2004

Jung SY, Bae HJ, Park BJ, et al: Parity and risk of hemorrhagic strokes. Neurology 74:1424, 2010

Kalidindi M, Ganpot S, Tahmesebi F, et al: Myasthenia gravis and pregnancy. J Obstet Gynaecol 27:30, 2007

Karmaniolou I, Petropoulos G, Theodoraki K: Management of idiopathic intracranial hypertension in parturients: anesthetic considerations. Can J Anesth 58:650, 2011

Katz A, Sergienko R, Dior U, et al: Bell's palsy during pregnancy: is it associated with adverse perinatal outcome? Laryngoscope 121:1395, 2011

Katz BS, Fugate JE, Ameriso SF, et al: Clinical worsening in reversible vasoconstriction syndrome. JAMA Neurol 71:68, 2014

Katz JN, Simmons BP: Carpal tunnel syndrome. N Engl J Med 346: 1807, 2002

Katz VL, Peterson R, Cefalo RC: Pseudotumor cerebri and pregnancy. Am J Perinatol 6:442, 1989

Keith MW, Masear V, Amadio PC, et al: Treatment of carpal tunnel syndrome. J Am Acad Orthop Surg 17:397, 2009

Kizer JR, Devereux RB: Patient foramen ovale in young adults with unexplained stroke. N Engl J Med 353:2361, 2005

Klein P, Mathews GC: Antiepileptic drugs and neurocognitive development. Neurology January 8, 2014 [Epub ahead of print]

Kobau R, Zahran H, Thurman DJ, et al: Epilepsy surveillance among adults—19 states, behavioral risk factor surveillance system, 2005. MMWR 57:1, 2008

Krassioukov A, Warburton DE, Teasell R, et al: A systematic review of the management of autonomic dysreflexia after spinal cord injury. Arch Phys Med Rehabil 90:682, 2009

Kruit MC, van Buchem MA, Hofman PA, et al: Migraine as a risk factor for subclinical brain lesions. JAMA 291:427, 2004

Kuczkowski KM: Labor analgesia for the parturient with spinal cord injury: what does an obstetrician need to know? Arch Gynecol Obstet 274:108, 2006

Kuhle J, Pohl C, Mehling M, et al: Lack of association between antimyelin antibodies and progression to multiple sclerosis. N Engl J Med 356:371, 2007

Kuklina EV, Tong X, Bansil P, et al: Trends in pregnancy hospitalizations that included a stroke in the United States from 1994 to 2007. Stroke 42:2564, 2011

Lamy C, Hamon JB, Coste J, et al: Ischemic stroke in young women. Neurology 55:269, 2000

Landwehr JB, Isada NB, Pryde PG, et al: Maternal neurosurgical shunts and pregnancy outcome. Obstet Gynecol 83:134, 1994

Lanska DJ, Kryscio RJ: Peripartum stroke and intracranial venous thrombosis in the National Hospital Discharge Survey. Obstet Gynecol 89:413, 1997

Lee AG, Pless M, Falardeau J, et al: The use of acetazolamide in idiopathic intracranial hypertension during pregnancy. Am J Ophthalmol 139:855, 2005

Levine SR, Brey RL, Tilley BC, et al: Antiphospholipid antibodies and subsequent thrombo-occlusive events in patients with ischemic stroke. JAMA 291:576, 2004

Lewis G: Saving mothers' lives: reviewing maternal deaths to make motherhood safer—2003–2005. Confidential Enquiries into Maternal and Child Health, London, 2007

Li Y, Margraf J, Kluck B, et al: Thrombolytic therapy for ischemic stroke secondary to paradoxical embolism in pregnancy. Neurologist 18:44, 2012

Liberman A, Karussis D, Ben-Hur T, et al: Natural course and pathogenesis of transient focal neurologic symptoms during pregnancy. Arch Neurol 65:218, 2008

Lin SY, Hu CJ, Lin HC: Increased risk of stroke in patients who undergo cesarean section delivery: a nationwide population-based study. Am J Obstet Gynecol 198:391.e1, 2008

Lipton RB, Bigal ME, Diamond M, et al: Migraine prevalence, disease burden, and the need for preventive therapy. Neurology 68:343, 2007

Lockhart P, Daly F, Pitkethly M, et al: Antiviral treatment for Bell's palsy (idiopathic facial paralysis). Cochrane Database Syst Rev 4:CD001869, 2009

Lucas S. Medication use in the treatment of migraine during pregnancy and lactation. Curr Pain Headache Rep 13:392, 2009

Lynch JK, Nelson KB: Epidemiology of perinatal stroke. Curr Opin Pediatr 13:499, 2001

Maddison P, McConville J, Farrugia ME, et al: The use of rituximab in myasthenia gravis and Lambert-Eaton myasthenic syndrome. J Neurol Neurosurg Psychiatry 82(6):671, 2011

Mandawat A, Kaminski HJ, Cutter G, et al: Comparative analysis of therapeutic options used for myasthenia gravis. Ann Neurol 68:797, 2010

Marcus DA: Headache in pregnancy. Curr Treat Options Neurol 9:23, 2007

Martin JN Jr, Thigpen BD, Moore RC, et al: Stroke and severe preeclampsia and eclampsia: a paradigm shift focusing on systolic blood pressure. Obstet Gynecol 105:246, 2005

Martínez-Sánchez P, Fuentes B, Fernández-Domínguez J, et al: Young women have poorer outcomes than men after stroke. Cerebrovasc Dis 31:455, 2011

Mawer G, Briggs M, Baker GA, et al: Pregnancy with epilepsy: obstetric and neonatal outcome of a controlled study. Seizure 19(2):112, 2010

McCaulley JA, Pates JA: Postpartum cerebral venous thrombosis. Obstet Gynecol 118:423, 2011

Mehraein S, Ortwein H, Busch M, et al: Risk of recurrence of cerebral venous and sinus thrombosis during subsequent pregnancy and puerperium. J Neurol Neurosurg Psychiatry 74:814, 2003

Menon R, Bushnell CD: Headache and pregnancy. Neurologist 14:108, 2008

Miyakoshi K, Matsuoka M, Yasutomi D, et al: Moyamoya-disease-related ischemic stroke in the postpartum period. J Obstet Gynaecol Res 35(5):974, 2009

Molgaard-Nielsen D, Hviid A: Newer-generation antiepileptic drugs and the risk of major birth defects. JAMA 305(19):1996, 2011

Morgenstern LB, Hemphill III JC, Anderson C, et al: Guidelines for the management of spontaneous intracerebral hemorrhage: a guideline for healthcare professionals from the American Heart Association/American Stroke Association. Stroke 41:2108, 2010

Morrow J, Russell A, Guthrie E, et al: Malformation risks of antiepileptic drugs in pregnancy: a prospective study from the UK Epilepsy and Pregnancy Register. J Neurol Neurosurg Psychiatry77(2):193, 2006

Murakami M, Morine M, Iwasa T, et al: Management of maternal hydrocephalus requires replacement of ventriculoperitoneal shunt with ventriculoatrial shunt: a case report. Arch Gynecol Obstet 282:339, 2010

Murray EL, Kedar S, Vedanarayanan VV: Transmission of maternal muscle-specific tyrosine kinase (MuSK) to offspring: report of two cases. J Clin Neuromusc Dis 12:76, 2010

Nam TS, Lee SH, Kim BC, et al: Clinical characteristics and predictive factors of myasthenic crisis after thymectomy. J Clin Neurosci 18(9):1185, 2011

National Spinal Cord Injury Statistical Center: Spinal cord injury facts and figures at a glance. 2012. Available at: https://www.nscisc.uab.edu. Accessed February 9, 2012

Nezvalová-Henriksen K, Spigset O, Nordeng H: Triptan exposure during pregnancy and the risk of major congenital malformations and adverse pregnancy outcomes: results from the Norwegian Mother and Child Cohort Study. Headache 50:563, 2010

Niks EH, Verrips A, Semmekrot BA, et al: A transient neonatal myasthenic syndrome with anti-MuSK antibodies. Neurol 70(14):1215, 2008

Novak MJ, Tabrizi SJ: Huntington's disease. BMJ 340:c3109, 2010

Olafsson E, Hallgrimsson JT, Hauser WA, et al: Pregnancies of women with epilepsy: a population-based study in Iceland. Epilepsia 39:887, 1998

Padua L, Di Pasquale A, Pazzaglia C, et al: Systematic review of pregnancy-related carpal tunnel syndrome. Muscle Nerve 42:697, 2010

Pal J, Rozsa C, Komoly S, et al: Clinical and biological heterogeneity of autoimmune myasthenia gravis. J Neuroimmunol 231:43, 2011

Pennell PB, Peng L, Newport DJ, et al: Lamotrigine in pregnancy. Clearance, therapeutic drug monitoring, and seizure frequency. Neurology 70(22 pt 2):2130, 2008

Perucca E: Birth defects after prenatal exposure to antiepileptic drugs. Lancet Neurol 4:781, 2005

Pilo C, Wide K, Winbladh B: Pregnancy, delivery, and neonatal complications after treatment with antiepileptic drugs. Acta Obstet Gynecol 85:643, 2006

Pleis JR, Ward BW, Lucas JW: Summary health statistics for U.S. adults: National Health Interview Survey, 2009. Vital Health Stat 10(249):1, 2010

Podciechowski L, Brocka-Nitecka U, Dabrowska K, et al: Pregnancy complicated by myasthenia gravis—twelve years experience. Neuro Endocrinol Lett 26:603, 2005

Polman CH, O'Connor PW, Havrdova E, et al: A randomized, placebo-controlled trial of natalizumab for relapsing multiple sclerosis. N Engl J Med 354:899, 2006

Portaccio E, Ghezzi A, Hakiki B, et al: Breastfeeding is not related to postpartum relapses in multiple sclerosis. Neurology 77:145, 2011

Portaccio E, Ghezzi A, Hakiki B, et al: Postpartum relapses increase the disability progression in multiple sclerosis: the role of disease modifying drugs. J Neurol Neurosurg Psychiatry January 8, 2014 [Epub ahead of print]

Powner DJ, Bernstein IM: Extended somatic support in pregnant women after brain death. Crit Care Med 31:1241, 2003

Quant EC, Jeste SS, Muni RH, et al: The benefits of steroids versus steroids plus antivirals for treatment of Bell's palsy: a meta-analysis. BMJ 339:b3354, 2009

Qureshi AI, Tuhrim S, Broderick JP, et al: Spontaneous intracerebral hemorrhage. N Engl J Med 344:1450, 2001

Ramnarayan R, Sriganesh J: Postpartum cerebral angiopathy mimicking hypertensive putaminal hematoma: a case report. Hypertens Pregnancy 28(1)34, 2009

Richmond JR, Krishnamoorthy P, Andermann E, et al: Epilepsy and pregnancy: an obstetric perspective. Am J Obstet Gynecol 190:371, 2004

Riffaud L, Ferre JC, Carsin-Nicol B, et al: Endoscopic third ventriculostomy for the treatment of obstructive hydrocephalus during pregnancy. Obstet Gynecol 108:801, 2006

Roger VL, Go AS, Lloyd-Jones DM, et al: Heart disease and stroke statistics—2012 update: a report from the American Heart Association. Circulation 125:e2, 2012

Rudick RA, Goelz SE: Beta-interferon for multiple sclerosis. Exp Cell Res 317:1301, 2011

Rudick RA, Stuart WH, Calabresi PA, et al: Natalizumab plus interferon beta-1a for relapsing multiple sclerosis. N Engl J Med 354:911, 2006

Salinas RA, Alvarez G, Daly F, et al: Corticosteroids for Bell's palsy (idiopathic facial paralysis). Cochrane Database Syst Rev. 3:CD001942, 2010

Salminen HJ, Leggett H, Boggild M: Glatiramer acetate exposure in pregnancy: preliminary safety and birth outcomes. J Neurol 257:2020, 2010

Sanchez SE, Qui C, Williams MA, et al: Headaches and migraines are associated with an increased risk of preeclampsia in Peruvian women. Am J Hypertens 21(3):360, 2008

Saposnik G, Barinagarrementeria F, Brown RD, et al: Diagnosis and management of cerebral venous thrombosis: a statement for healthcare professionals from the American Heart Association/American Stroke Association. Stroke 42:1158, 2011

Schiza S, Starnatakis E, Panagopoulou A, et al: Management of pregnancy and delivery of a patient with malfunctioning ventriculoperitoneal shunt. J Obstet Gynaecol 32(1):6, 2012

Schürks M, Rist PM, Bigal ME, et al: Migraines and cardiovascular disease: systemic review and meta analyses. BMJ 339:b3914, 2009

Scott CA, Bewley S, Rudd A: Incidence, risk factors, management, and outcomes of stroke in pregnancy. Obstet Gynecol 120:318, 2012

Seror P: Pregnancy-related carpal tunnel syndrome. J Hand Surg Br 23:98, 1998

Shi Q, MacDermid JC: Is surgical intervention more effective than non-surgical treatment for carpal tunnel syndrome? A systemic review. J Orthop Surg 6:17, 2011

Shorvon SD: The etiologic classification of epilepsy. Epilepsia 52(6):1052, 2011

Shmorgun D, Chan WS, Ray JG: Association between Bell's palsy in pregnancy and pre-eclampsia. QJM 95:359, 2002

Silberstein S, Loder E, Diamond S, et al: Probable migraine in the United States: results of the American Migraine Prevalence and Prevention (AMPP) Study. Cephalalgia 27(3):220, 2007

Simolke GA, Cox SM, Cunningham FG: Cerebrovascular accident complicating pregnancy and the puerperium. Obstet Gynecol 78:37, 1991

Singhal AB, Kimberly WT, Schaefer PW, et al: Case 8—2009—a 36-year-old woman with headache, hypertension, and seizure 2 weeks postpartum. N Engl J Med 360(11):1126, 2009

Smith WS, English JD, Johnston C: Cerebrovascular diseases. In Fauci AS, Braunwald E, Kasper DL, et al (eds): Harrison's Principles of Internal Medicine, 17th ed. McGraw-Hill, New York, 2008, p 2513

Smith WS, English JD, Johnston C: Cerebrovascular diseases. In Longo DL, Fauci AS, Kasper DL, et al (eds): Harrison's Principles of Internal Medicine, 18th ed. McGraw-Hill, New York, 2012, p 3270

Smitherman TA, Burch R, Sheikh H, et al: The prevalence, impact, and treatment of migraine and severe headaches in the United States: a review of statistics from national surveillance studies. Headache 53(3):427, 2013

Souza JP, Oliveira-Neto A, Surita FG, et al: The prolongation of somatic support in a pregnant woman with brain-death: a case report. Reprod Health 27:3, 2006

Stoodley MA, Macdonald RL, Weir BK: Pregnancy and intracranial aneurysms. Neurosurg Clin North Am 9:549, 1998

Sullivan FM, Swan IR, Donnan PT, et al: Early treatment with prednisolone or acyclovir in Bell's palsy. N Engl J Med 357:1598, 2007

Takebayashi S, Kaneko M: Electron microscopic studies of ruptured arteries in hypertensive intracerebral hemorrhage. Stroke 14:28, 1983

Thambisetty M, Lavin PJ, Newman NJ, et al: Fulminant idiopathic intracranial hypertension. Neurology 68:229, 2007

Thomas SV, Ajaykumar B, Sindhu K, et al: Cardiac malformations are increased in infants of mothers with epilepsy. Pediatr Cardiol 29:604, 2008

Tiel Groenestege AT, Rinkel GJ, van der Bom JG, et al: The risk of aneurysmal subarachnoid hemorrhage during pregnancy, delivery, and the puerperium in the Utrecht population: case-crossover study and standardized incidence ratio estimation. Stroke 40(4):1148, 2009

Torelli P, Allais G, Manzoni GC: Clinical review of headache in pregnancy. Neurol Sci 31(Suppl 1):S55, 2010

Turner K, Piazzini A, Franza A, et al: Epilepsy and postpartum depression. Epilepsia 50(1):24, 2009

U.S. Food and Drug Administration: FDA drug safety communication: risk of oral clefts in children born to mothers taking Topamax (topiramate). 2011. Available at: http://www.fda.gov/drugs/drugsafety/ucm245085.htm. Accessed January 11, 2014

Vajda FJ, Hitchcock A, Graham J, et al: Seizure control in antiepileptic drug-treated pregnancy. Epilepsia 49(1):172, 2008

van der Worp HB, van Gijn J: Acute ischemic stroke. N Engl J Med 357(6):572, 2007

Viinikainen K, Heinonen S, Eriksson K, et al: Community-based, prospective, controlled study of obstetric and neonatal outcome of 179 pregnancies in women with epilepsy. Epilepsia 47:186, 2006

Vukusic S, Confavreux C: Pregnancy and multiple sclerosis: the children of PRIMS. Clin Neurol Neurosurg 108:266, 2006

Vukusic S, Ionescu I, El-Etr M: The prevention of post-partum relapses with progestin and estradiol in multiple sclerosis (POPART'MUS) trial: rational, objectives and state of advancement. J Neurol Sci 286(1):114, 2009

Wang IK, Chang SN, Liao CC, et al: Hypertensive disorders in pregnancy and preterm delivery and subsequent stroke in Asian women: a retrospective cohort study. Stroke 42:716, 2011

Wasay M, Bakshi R, Bobustuc G, et al: Cerebral venous thrombosis: analysis of a multicenter cohort from the United States. J Stroke Cerebrovasc Dis 17:49, 2008

Wen JC, Liu TC, Chen YH, et al: No increased risk of adverse pregnancy outcomes for women with myasthenia gravis: a nationwide population-based study. Eur J Neurol 16:889, 2009

Westgren N, Hultling C, Levi R, et al: Pregnancy and delivery in women with a trauma spinal cord injury in Sweden, 1980–1991. Obstet Gynecol 81:926, 1993

Wijdicks EFM, Varelas PN, Gronseth GS, et al: Evidence-based guideline update: determining brain death in adults. Neurology 74:1911, 2010

Wisoff JH, Kratzert KJ, Handwerker SM, et al: Pregnancy in patients with cerebrospinal fluid shunts: report of a series and review of the literature. Neurosurgery 29:827, 1991

Wyszynski DF, Nambisan M, Surve T, et al: Increased rate of major malformations in offspring exposed to valproate during pregnancy. Neurology 64:961, 2005

Yager PH, Singhal AB, Nogueira RG: Case 31-2012: an 18-year-old-man with blurred vision, dysarthria, and ataxia. N Engl J Med 367:1450, 2012

Yerby MS: Pregnancy, teratogenesis, and epilepsy. Neurol Clin 12:749, 1994

Yoshikawa H, Kiuchi T, Salda T, et al: Randomised, double-blind, placebo-controlled study of tacrolimus in myasthenia gravis. J Neurol Neurosurg Psychiatry 82(9):970, 2011

Yuki N, Hartung HP: Guillain-Barré syndrome. N Engl J Med 366:2294, 2012

Zeeman GG, Fleckenstein JL, Twickler DM, et al: Cerebral infarction in eclampsia. Am J Obstet Gynecol 190:714, 2004a

Zeeman GG, Hatab M, Twickler DM: Increased cerebral blood flow in preeclampsia with magnetic resonance imaging. Am J Obstet Gynecol 191:1425, 2004b

Zeeman GG, Hatab M, Twickler DM: Maternal cerebral blood flow changes in pregnancy. Am J Obstet Gynecol 189:968, 2003

CHAPTER 61

Psychiatric Disorders

Pregnancy and the puerperium are at times sufficiently stressful to provoke mental illness. Such illness may represent recurrence or exacerbation of a preexisting psychiatric disorder, or may signal the onset of a new disorder. Psychiatric disorders during pregnancy have been associated with less prenatal care, substance abuse, poor obstetrical and infant outcomes, and a higher risk of postpartum psychiatric illness (Frieder, 2008). Of pregnant women identified with psychiatric disorders, Andersson and colleagues (2003) in one Swedish study reported that more than 80 percent had a mood disorder. According to the Agency for Healthcare Research and Quality, the period prevalence of any depressive disorder during pregnancy in the United States is 18 percent (Yonkers, 2011). Unfortunately, most pregnant women with depressive disorders are not treated. In the Swedish study mentioned above, only 5 percent of women identified with psychiatric disorders received some form of treatment.

Suicide is the fifth leading cause of death in the United States among women during the perinatal period, and major depression is among the strongest predictors of suicidal ideation (Melville, 2010). In both the United Kingdom and Australia, psychiatric illness is a leading cause of mortality for late maternal deaths—those between 43 and 365 days postpartum (Austin, 2007). Suicide by violent means was responsible for 65 percent of these. In a 10-year case-control analysis of Washington state hospitalizations, Comtois and associates (2008) studied 355 women with a postpartum suicide attempt. Significant risk factors and their associated rates included prior hospitalization for a psychiatric diagnosis—27-fold, and for substance abuse—sixfold. These rates were further increased if there were multiple hospitalizations.

PSYCHOLOGICAL ADJUSTMENTS TO PREGNANCY

Biochemical factors—including hormonal effects—and life stressors can markedly influence mental illness. Thus, intuitively, pregnancy exacerbates some coexisting mental disorders. Indeed, pregnancy-related shifts in sex steroids and monoamine neurotransmitter levels; dysfunction of the hypothalamic-pituitary-adrenal axis; thyroid dysfunction; and alterations in immune response are all associated with an increased risk for mood disorders (Yonkers, 2011). These changes, coupled with evidence of familiality of depression, suggest that there may be a subgroup of women at risk for developing a unipolar major depressive disorder during pregnancy.

Women respond in a variety of ways to stressors of pregnancy, and some express persistent concerns regarding fetal health, child care, lifestyle changes, or fear of childbirth pain. Anxiety, sleep disorders, and functional impairment are common (Morewitz, 2003; Romero, 2014; Vythilingum, 2008). According to Littleton and coworkers (2007), however, anxiety symptoms in pregnancy are associated with psychosocial variables similar to those for nonpregnant women. The level of perceived stress is significantly higher for women whose fetus is at high risk for a malformation, for those with preterm labor or delivery, and for those with other medical complications (Alder, 2007; Ross, 2006). Hippman (2009) screened 81 women for depression who had an increased risk for a fetus with aneuploidy. Half of these women had a positive depression screening score, whereas only 2.4 percent of those with a normal pregnancy did so.

A number of steps can be taken to diminish psychological stress in the event of a poor obstetrical outcome. For example, following a stillbirth, Gold (2007) encouraged parental contact with the newborn and provision of photographs and other infant memorabilia. Addressing associated sleep disorders also seems reasonable (Romero, 2014).

The Puerperium

The puerperium is a particularly stressful time and carries as increased risk for mental illness. Up to 15 percent of women develop a nonpsychotic postpartum depressive disorder within 6 months of delivery (Tam, 2007; Yonkers, 2011). A few have a more severe, psychotic illness following delivery, and half of these have a bipolar disorder (Yonkers, 2011). Depressive disorders are more likely in women with obstetrical complications such as severe preeclampsia or fetal-growth restriction, especially if associated with early delivery. However, among women with a history of bipolar disorder, these factors do not seem to play as great a role in the development of mania or depression (Yonkers, 2011).

Maternity Blues

Also called *postpartum blues,* this is a time-limited period of heightened emotional reactivity experienced by half of women within approximately the first week after parturition. Prevalence estimates for the blues range from 26 to 84 percent depending on criteria used for diagnosis (O'Hara, 2014). This emotional state generally peaks on the fourth or fifth postpartum day and normalizes by day 10 (O'Keane, 2011). The predominant mood is happiness. However, affected mothers are more emotionally labile, and insomnia, weepiness, depression, anxiety, poor concentration, irritability, and affective lability may be noted. Mothers may be transiently tearful for several hours and then recover completely, only to be tearful again the next day. Supportive treatment is indicated, and sufferers can be reassured that the dysphoria is transient and most likely due to biochemical changes. They should be monitored for development of depression and other severe psychiatric disturbances.

Prenatal Evaluation

Screening for mental illness is generally done at the first prenatal visit. Factors include a search for psychiatric disorders, including hospitalizations, outpatient care, prior or current use of psychoactive medications, and current symptoms. Risk factors should be evaluated—for example, a prior personal or family history of depression conveys a significant risk for depression. Women with a history of sexual, physical, or verbal abuse; substance abuse; and personality disorders are also at greater risk for depression (Akman, 2007; Tam, 2007). Smoking and nicotine dependence have been associated with an increase in rates of *all* mental disorders in pregnancy (Goodwin, 2007). Finally, because eating disorders may be exacerbated by pregnancy, affected women should be followed closely.

According to the American College of Obstetricians and Gynecologists (2012a), there is currently insufficient evidence to make a firm recommendation for routine depression screening, either during or after pregnancy. At Parkland Hospital, all women are asked about depression and domestic violence at their first prenatal visit. They are also screened again during their first postpartum visit using the Edinburgh Postnatal Depression Scale (EPDS). In an analysis of more than 17,000 of these questionnaires, 6 percent had scores that indicated either minor or major depressive symptoms. Twelve of these 1106 women also had thoughts of self-harm (Nelson, 2013).

Treatment Considerations

A large number of psychotropic medications may be used for management of the myriad mental disorders encountered in pregnancy. For treatment options that include psychosocial and psychological interventions, treatment decisions are ideally shared between patients and their health-care providers. Women taking psychotropic medication should be informed of likely side effects. Many of these drugs are discussed in Chapter 12 as well as by the American College of Obstetricians and Gynecologists (2012b). Additionally, these drugs are discussed subsequently in this chapter. Babbitt (2014) and Pozzi (2014) and their colleagues have recently reviewed principles of antenatal and intrapartum care of women with major mental disorders.

Pregnancy Outcomes

There are only a few reports of psychiatric disorders and pregnancy outcomes. Some, but not all, link maternal psychiatric illness with untoward outcomes such as preterm birth, low birthweight, and perinatal mortality (Schneid-Kofman, 2008; Steinberg, 2014; Yonkers, 2009). In a population-based cohort of more than 500,000 California births, Kelly and colleagues (2002) assessed the perinatal effects of a psychiatric diagnosis that included all International Classification of Diseases 9th Edition Clinical Modification (ICD-9-CM) diagnostic codes. Women with these diagnoses had up to a threefold increased incidence of a very-low- or low-birthweight neonate or preterm delivery. In another study of more than 1100 women enrolled in a Healthy Start initiative, women with depression were found to be 1.5 times more likely to be delivered early compared with nondepressed women. Conversely, Littleton and associates (2007) reviewed 50 studies and concluded that anxiety symptoms—a common comorbidity in depression—had no adverse effect on outcomes.

CLASSIFICATION OF MENTAL DISORDERS

The *Diagnostic and Statistical Manual-V* is the most recent version by the American Psychiatric Association (2013). Its purpose is to assist in the classification of mental disorders, and it specifies criteria for each diagnosis. Shown in Table 61-1 are 12-month prevalences of mental disorders for adults.

TABLE 61-1. The 12-Month Prevalence of Mental Disorders in Adults in the United States

Disorder[a]	1-Year Prevalence (%)	Adults Affected[b]	Lifetime Prevalence (%)	Comments
All disorders	26.2	58 million	—	1 in 4 adults affected annually
Mood disorders—all		21 million	20.8	Median onset age 30 years
Major depression	6.7	15 million	—	Leading cause of disability in the United States; high suicide rate
Dysthymia	1.5	3.3 million	—	Chronic, mild depression
Bipolar disorder	2.6	5.7 million	3.9	Manic-depressive illness
Suicide	—	32,400	—	90% have mental disorder; depression most common
Schizophrenia	1.1	18 million		Men = women; onset women 20s or early 30s
Anxiety disorder—all	18	40 million		Frequent co-occurrence with depression or substance abuse
Panic	2.7			
Obsessive-compulsive	1			
Posttraumatic stress	3.5			
Generalized anxiety	3.1			
Social phobias	6.8			
Eating disorders				Adolescent and adult females—85–95%
Anorexia nervosa		—	2–3	Mortality rate 0.56% per year
Bulimia nervosa		—	2–3	
Binge eating—6 months	2–5		—	

[a]Based on Diagnostic and Statistical Manual-IV-R (DSM-IV-R) of the American Psychiatric Association, 2000b.
[b]Based on 2004 census data.
From the National Institute of Mental Health, 2006, 2010.

Depressive Disorders

According to the National Institute of Mental Health (2010), the lifetime prevalence of depressive disorders in the United States is 21 percent. Women are 50 percent more likely than men to experience a major mood disorder during their lifetime. Historically, these include major depression—a unipolar disorder—and manic-depression—a bipolar disorder with both manic and depressive episodes. It also includes dysthymia, which is chronic, mild depression. When concurrent with medical complications such as diabetes, heart disease, and asthma, major mood disorders worsen medical outcomes, and as a group, contribute to two thirds of all suicides (Yonkers, 2011).

Major Depression

This is the most common depressive disorder, and an estimated 12 million women each year in the United States are affected (Mental Health America, 2013a). The lifetime prevalence is 17 percent, but only half ever seek care. The diagnosis is arrived at by identifying symptoms listed in Table 61-2.

Major depression is multifactorial and prompted by genetic and environmental factors. First-degree relatives have a 25-percent risk, and female relatives are at even higher risk. One genome-wide linkage analysis of more than 1200 mothers suggests that variation in chromosomes 1 and 9 increases susceptibility to postpartum mood symptoms (Mahon, 2009). Families of affected individuals also often have members with alcohol

TABLE 61-2. Symptoms of Depressive Illness[a]

Persistent sad, anxious, or "empty" feelings
Feelings of hopelessness and/or pessimism
Feelings of guilt, worthlessness, and/or helplessness
Irritability, restlessness
Loss of interest in activities or hobbies once pleasurable, including sex
Fatigue and decreased energy
Difficulty concentrating, remembering detail, and making decisions
Insomnia, early-morning wakefulness, or excessive sleeping
Overeating or appetite loss
Thoughts of suicide, suicide attempts
Persistent aches or pains, headaches, cramps, or digestive problems that do not ease even with treatment

[a]Not all patients experience the same symptoms, and their severity, frequency, and duration will vary among individuals.
From the National Institute of Mental Health, 2010.

abuse and anxiety disorders. Provocative conditions leading to depression include life events that prompt grief reactions, substance abuse, use of certain medications, and other medical disorders. Although life events can trigger depression, genes influence the response to life events, making the distinction between genetic and environmental factors difficult.

Pregnancy

It is unquestionable that pregnancy is a major life stressor that can precipitate or exacerbate depressive tendencies. In addition, there are likely various pregnancy-induced effects. Hormones certainly affect mood as evidenced by premenstrual syndrome and menopausal depression. Estrogen has been implicated in increased serotonin synthesis, decreased serotonin breakdown, and serotonin receptor modulation (Deecher, 2008). Concordantly, women who experience postpartum depression often have higher predelivery serum estrogen and progesterone levels and experience a greater decline postpartum (Ahokas, 1999).

Dennis and associates (2007) queried the Cochrane Database and reported the prevalence of antenatal depression to average 11 percent. Melville and coworkers (2010) found it in nearly 10 percent of more than 1800 women enrolled for prenatal care at a single university obstetrical clinic. Others have reported the incidence to be much higher (Lee, 2007; Westdahl, 2007). In another report, Luke and colleagues (2009) found major depressive symptoms in 25 percent of pregnant African American women. Hayes and associates (2012) reported that 13 percent of pregnant women in the Tennessee Medicaid program filled an antidepressant prescription either before or during pregnancy. In another report of almost 119,000 pregnancies in seven health plans, Andrade and coworkers (2008) found that only 6.6 percent received antidepressants at any time during pregnancy. These findings support to the notion that only half of pregnant women with depression receive treatment.

Postpartum depression—major or minor—develops in 10 to 20 percent of parturients (Centers for Disease Control and Prevention, 2008; Mental Health America, 2013b). Available data indicate that unipolar major depression may be slightly more prevalent during the puerperium than among women in the general population (Yonkers, 2011). In addition to antenatal depression, postpartum depression has been associated with young maternal age, unmarried status, smoking or drinking, substance abuse, hyperemesis gravidarum, preterm birth, and high utilization of sick leave during pregnancy (Endres, 2013; Lee, 2007; Marcus, 2009).

Depression is frequently recurrent. At least 60 percent of women taking antidepressant medication before pregnancy have symptoms during pregnancy. According to Hayes and colleagues (2012), approximately three fourths of women taking antidepressants before pregnancy stopped taking them before or during the first trimester. For those who discontinue treatment, almost 70 percent have a relapse compared with 25 percent who continue therapy. Up to 70 percent of women with previous postpartum depression have a subsequent episode. Women with both prior puerperal depression and a current episode of "maternity blues" are at inordinately high risk for major depression. Indeed, the need for postpartum depression help was the fourth most common challenge identified at 2 to 9 months postpartum by the Pregnancy Risk Assessment Monitoring System—PRAMS (Kanotra, 2007).

Postpartum depression is generally underrecognized and undertreated. Major depression during pregnancy or after delivery can have devastating consequences for affected women, their children, and families. Among new mothers, one of the most significant contributions to their mortality rate is suicide, which is most common among women with mental illness (Koren, 2012; Palladino, 2011). If left untreated, up to 25 percent of women with postpartum depression will be depressed 1 year later. As the duration of depression increases, so too do the number of sequelae and their severity. In addition, maternal depression during the first weeks and months after delivery can lead to insecure attachment and later behavioral problems in the child.

Treatment

Antidepressant medications, along with some form of psychotherapy, are indicated for severe depression during pregnancy or the puerperium (American College of Obstetricians and Gynecologists, 2012b). Shown in Figure 61-1 is one algorithm regarding initiation of treatment of mood disorders and management with a mental health professional. In women with severe depression a selective serotonin-reuptake inhibitor—SSRI—should be tried initially (Table 61-3). Tricyclic antidepressants and monoamine oxidase inhibitors are infrequently used in contemporary practice. If depressive symptoms improve during a 6-week trial, the medication should be continued for a minimum of 6 months to prevent relapse (Wisner, 2002). If the response is suboptimal or a relapse occurs, another SSRI is substituted, or psychiatric referral is considered. Mozurkewich and associates (2013) reported no salutary effects of docosahexaenoic acid (DHA) to prevent perinatal depression.

Importantly, in a recent metaanalysis by Huang and colleagues (2014), women using antidepressants during pregnancy were found to be at increased risk for preterm birth and low-birthweight neonates. Nevertheless, in their review of antidepressant medication use in pregnancy, Ray and Stowe (2014) concluded that the relative reproductive safety data is reassuring and that antidepressants remain a viable treatment option.

Recurrence some time after medication is discontinued develops in 50 to 85 percent of women with an initial postpartum depressive episode. Women with a history of more than one depressive episode are at greater risk (American Psychiatric Association, 2000a). Surveillance should include monitoring for thoughts of suicide or infanticide, emergence of psychosis, and response to therapy. For some women, the course of illness is severe enough to warrant hospitalization.

Fetal Effects of Therapy

Some known and possible fetal and neonatal effects of treatment are listed in Table 61-3. Studies implicating SSRIs with an increased teratogenic risk for fetal cardiac defects were

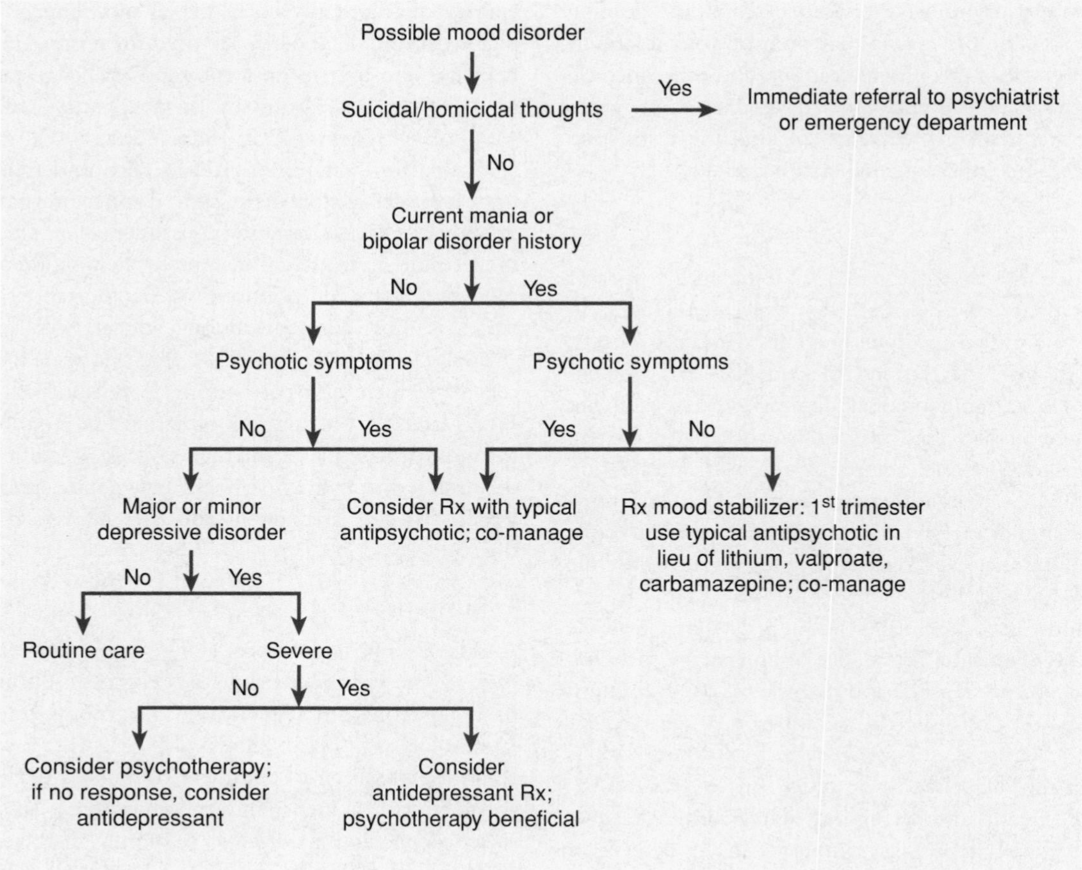

FIGURE 61-1 Treatment algorithm of pregnant women with mood disorders. (Modified from Yonkers, 2011.)

TABLE 61-3. Some Drugs Used for Treatment of Major Mental Disorders in Pregnancy

Indication of Class	Examples	Comments
Antidepressants		
SSRIs[a]	Citalopram, fluoxetine, paroxetine, sertraline	*Possible* link with heart defects; neonatal withdrawal syndrome; *possible* persistent pulmonary hypertension[a]; paroxetine use avoided by some
Others	Bupropion, duloxetine, nefazodone, venlafaxine	
Tricyclics	Amitriptyline, desipramine, doxepin, imipramine, nortriptyline	Not commonly used currently; no evidence of teratogenicity
Antipsychotics		
Typical	Chlorpromazine, fluphenazine, haloperidol, thiothixene	
Atypical	Aripiprazole, clozapine, olanzapine, risperidone, ziprasidone	
Bipolar Disorders		
Lithium[a]	Lithium carbonate	Tx manic episodes; teratogen—heart defects, viz., Ebstein anomaly; few data after 12 wks
Valproic acid[b]		
Carbamazepine[b]		
Antipsychotics	See above	

[a]Chapter 12 (p. 250). [b]Chapter 60 (p. 1190).
SSRI = selective serotonin-reuptake inhibitor; Tx = treat.
Data from American College of Obstetricians and Gynecologists, 2012b; Briggs, 2011; Buhimschi, 2009; Physicians' Desk Reference, 2012.

isolated to paroxetine and were most consistent for ventricular septal defects (VSDs). It is estimated that the risk is no greater than 1 in 200 exposed infants (Koren, 2012). Nevertheless, the American College of Obstetricians and Gynecologists (2012b) has recommended that paroxetine be avoided in women who are either pregnant or planning pregnancy. Fetal echocardiography should be considered in women exposed to paroxetine in the first trimester.

In a case-control study, there was a sixfold increased risk of persistent pulmonary hypertension of the newborn (PPHN) in infants exposed to SSRIs after 20 weeks (Chambers, 2006). This translates to an overall risk of pulmonary hypertension that would be less than 1 in 100 exposed infants (Koren, 2012). In contrast, a population-based cohort study of 1.6 million pregnancies from Nordic countries identified a twofold increased risk in exposed neonates. It was estimated that this yields an attributable risk of 2 per 1000 births (Kieler, 2012). This marginally increased risk must be weighed against the risk associated with discontinuing or tapering medication during pregnancy.

Women who abruptly discontinue either serotonin- or norepinephrine-reuptake inhibitor therapy typically experience some form of withdrawal. Not surprisingly, up to 30 percent of exposed neonates may also exhibit withdrawal symptoms. Symptoms are similar to opioid withdrawal, but typically are less severe. This condition—*neonatal behavioral syndrome*—is self-limited, and the newborn rarely remains in the nursery more than 5 days. (Koren, 2009). Currently, convincing evidence of long-term neurobehavioral effects of fetal exposure to these medications is lacking (Koren, 2012).

Some psychotropic medications pass into breast milk. However, in most cases, levels are very low or undetectable. Importantly, the average amount of drug detected in breast milk is higher with fluoxetine than most other reuptake inhibitors (National Library of Medicine, 2012). Adverse effects include transient irritability, sleep disturbances, and colic. Agents with lower excretion into breast milk may therefore be preferred.

Electroconvulsive Therapy

This form of depression treatment is occasionally necessary during pregnancy for women with major mood disorders unresponsive to pharmacotherapy. With proper preparation, the risks to both mother and fetus appear to be reasonable (Pinette, 2007). O'Reardon and coworkers (2011) reported a woman who underwent 18 electroconvulsive therapy (ECT) sessions during the second and third trimesters. She was delivered of a normal child without evidence of developmental delay up to 18 months of age. That said, adverse maternal and perinatal outcomes have been described from complications of convulsive therapy. Balki and associates (2006) reported a pregnancy in which fetal brain damage likely was caused by sustained maternal hypotension associated with treatment of status epilepticus stimulated by electroshock.

Women undergoing ECT should be fasting for at least 6 hours. They should be given a rapid-acting antacid before the procedure, and their airway should be protected to decrease the likelihood of aspiration. A wedge should be placed under the right hip to prevent sudden maternal hypotension from aortocaval compression. Other important preparatory steps include cervical assessment, discontinuation of nonessential anticholinergic medication, uterine and fetal heart rate monitoring, and intravenous hydration. During the procedure, excessive hyperventilation should be avoided. In most cases, maternal and fetal heart rate and maternal blood pressure and oxygen saturation remain normal throughout the procedure.

There have been at least two reviews of ECT outcomes in pregnancy. In the earlier one, Miller (1994) found 300 cases and reported complications in 10 percent. These included fetal arrhythmias, vaginal bleeding, abdominal pain, and self-limited contractions. Women not adequately prepared had increased risks for aspiration, aortocaval compression, and respiratory alkalosis. In the more recent review, Andersen and Ryan (2009) described 339 cases, undoubtedly with some homology with the earlier study. In most cases, ECT therapy was done to treat depression, and it was 78-percent effective. They reported a 5-percent maternal ECT-related complication rate and a 3-percent associated perinatal complication rate that included two fetal deaths. For all of these reasons, we agree with Richards (2007) that ECT in pregnancy is not "low risk" and that it should be reserved for women whose depression is recalcitrant to intensive pharmacotherapy.

Bipolar and Related Disorders

According to the National Institute of Mental Health (2010), the lifetime prevalence for manic-depression illness is 3.9 percent. There is no difference in the prevalence of bipolar disorder between pregnant women and nonpregnant reproductive-aged women (Yonkers, 2011). It has a strong genetic component and has been linked to possible mutations on chromosomes 16 and 8 (Jones, 2007). The risk that monozygotic twins are both affected is 40 to 70 percent, and the risk for first-degree relatives is 5 to 10 percent (Muller-Oerlinghausen, 2002). Periods of depression last at least 2 weeks. At other times, there are manic episodes, distinct periods during which there is an abnormally raised, expansive, or irritable mood. Potential organic causes of mania include substance abuse, hyperthyroidism, and central nervous system tumors. Importantly, however, pregnancy frequently prompts medication discontinuation, and this translates to a twofold increased risk for relapse during pregnancy (Viguera, 2007). Up to 20 percent of patients with manic-depression illness commit suicide.

Typical therapy for bipolar disorder includes mood stabilizers such as lithium, valproic acid, and carbamazepine, as well as antipsychotic medications (see Table 61-3). As depicted in Figure 61-1, treatment of bipolar disorder in pregnancy is complex and should be co-managed with a psychiatrist. Treatment decisions include risks versus benefits of using mood stabilizers, some of which are teratogenic. For example, lithium has been linked to Ebstein anomaly in exposed infants (Chap. 12, p. 250). More recent data, however, suggest a lower risk of cardiac malformations than previously indicated (Reprotox, 2012). Nevertheless, fetal echocardiography is recommended by many for exposed fetuses. There is some limited evidence suggesting that lithium in breast milk can adversely affect the infant when its elimination is impaired as in dehydration or immaturity (Davanzo, 2011). Lithium use in mothers with a healthy term fetus, however, is considered moderately safe. A more detailed discussion of other mood stabilizers and antipsychotic medications side effects can be found in Chapter 12 (p. 250).

Postpartum Psychosis

This severe mental disorder is usually a bipolar disorder, but it may be due to major depression (American Psychiatric Association, 2013). Its incidence is estimated to be 1 in every 1000 deliveries, and it is more common in primiparas, especially those with obstetrical complications (Bergink, 2011; Blackmore, 2006). In most cases, illness manifests within 2 weeks of delivery. In a case-control study of postpartum women with their first lifetime episode of psychosis, the median onset of psychiatric symptoms was 8 days after delivery, and the median duration of the episode was 40 days (Bergink, 2011).

The most important risk factor for postpartum psychosis is a history of bipolar disease. These women typically exhibit symptoms sooner—1 to 2 days after delivery (Heron, 2007, 2008). Manic symptoms include feeling excited, elated, "high"; not needing sleep or unable to sleep; feeling active or energetic; and feeling "chatty." Affected women have signs of confusion and disorientation but may also have episodes of lucidity. Because those with underlying disease have a 10- to 15-fold risk for recurrence postpartum, close monitoring is imperative. Postpartum psychosis has a 50-percent recurrence risk in the next pregnancy. As a result, Bergink and colleagues (2012) recommend initiating lithium therapy immediately postpartum in women with a history of postpartum psychosis.

The clinical course of bipolar illness with postpartum psychosis is comparable with that for nonpregnant women. Patients usually require hospitalization, pharmacological treatment, and long-term psychiatric care. Psychotic women may have delusions leading to thoughts of self-harm or harm to their infants. Unlike women with nonpsychotic depression, these women commit infanticide, albeit uncommonly (Kim, 2008). In most instances, women with postpartum psychosis ultimately develop relapsing, chronic psychotic manic-depression.

Anxiety Disorders

These relatively common disorders–18 percent prevalence overall–include panic attack, panic disorder, social anxiety disorder, specific phobia, separation anxiety disorder, and generalized anxiety disorder. All are characterized by irrational fear, tension, and worry, which are accompanied by physiological changes such as trembling, nausea, hot or cold flashes, dizziness, dyspnea, insomnia, and frequent urination (Schneier, 2006). They are treated with psychotherapy and medication, including selective serotonin-reuptake inhibitors, tricyclic antidepressants, monoamine oxide inhibitors, and others.

Pregnancy

Despite their relative high prevalence in childbearing-aged women as shown in Table 61-1, little specific attention has been directed to anxiety disorders in pregnancy. Most reports conclude that there is no difference in rates in between pregnant and nonpregnant women. One recent analysis of 268 pregnant women with generalized anxiety disorder demonstrated that both symptoms and severity of anxiety decrease across pregnancy (Buist, 2011). Older studies indicate increased risks for adverse pregnancy outcomes with some of these disorders (American College of Obstetricians and Gynecologists, 2012b).

From their review, Ross and McLean (2006) concluded that some of the anxiety disorders may have important maternal-fetal implications. Some have been linked to preterm birth and fetal-growth restriction as well as poor neurobehavioral development (Van den Bergh, 2005). Children with a history of in utero exposure to maternal anxiety are felt to be at increased risk for a variety of neuropsychiatric conditions such as attention deficit/hyperactivity disorder (ADHD). Hunter and coworkers (2012) analyzed infants of 60 mothers with an anxiety disorder and found that auditory sensory gating—a reflection of inhibitory neurotransmission—was impaired, particularly in offspring of untreated women. Conversely, Littleton and associates (2007) found no excessive adverse pregnancy outcomes with "anxiety symptoms." One important exception is their link with postpartum depression (Vythilingum, 2008).

Treatment

Mood and anxiety disorders coexist in more than half of women identified with either diagnosis (Frieder, 2008). Anxiety disorders can be effectively treated during pregnancy with psychotherapy, cognitive behavioral therapy, or medications. Antidepressants listed in Table 61-3 are often the first line of pharmacotherapy. Benzodiazepines are also commonly used to treat anxiety or panic disorders before and during pregnancy. Earlier case-control studies linked use of these central nervous system depressants to an increased risk for cleft lip and palate. However, a recent metaanalysis that included more than 1 million exposed pregnancies did not identify a teratogenic risk (Enato, 2011). Benzodiazepines, especially when taken during the third trimester, can cause neonatal withdrawal syndrome, which persists for days to weeks after delivery.

Schizophrenia Spectrum Disorders

This major form of mental illness affects 1.1 percent of adults (see Table 61-1). Schizophrenia spectrum disorders are defined by abnormalities in one or more of the following domains: delusions, hallucinations, disorganized thinking, grossly disorganized or abnormal motor behavior, and negative symptoms. Brain-scanning techniques such as positron-emission tomography (PET) and functional magnetic resonance imaging (fMRI) have shown that schizophrenia is a degenerative brain disorder. Subtle anatomical abnormalities are present early in life and worsen with time.

Schizophrenia has a major genetic component , and there is a 50-percent concordance in monozygotic twins. If one parent has schizophrenia, the risk to offspring is 5 to 10 percent. Some data, including a strong association between schizophrenia and the velocardiofacial syndrome, suggest that associated genes are located on chromosome 22q11 (Murphy, 2002).

But sophisticated gene mapping studies have shown clearly that schizophrenia is not related to a single gene or mutation. Instead, there are multiple DNA variants that likely interact to lead to schizophrenia (Kukshal, 2012). Other putative risk factors for subsequent schizophrenia in an exposed fetus include maternal iron deficiency anemia, diabetes, and acute maternal stress (Insel, 2008; Malaspina, 2008; Van Lieshout, 2008). These remain unproven, as does the association with maternal influenza A (Chap. 64, p. 1241).

Signs of illness begin approximately at age 20 years, and commonly, work and psychosocial functioning deteriorate over time. Women have a slightly later onset than men and are less susceptible to autism and other neurodevelopmental abnormalities. Thus, many investigators theorize that estrogen is protective. Affected women may marry and become pregnant before symptoms manifest. With appropriate treatment, patients may experience a decrease or cessation of symptoms. Within 5 years from the first signs of illness, 60 percent have social recovery, 50 percent are employed, 30 percent are mentally handicapped, and 10 percent require continued hospitalization (American Psychiatric Association, 2013).

Pregnancy

There has been an apparent increase in relative fertility in schizophrenic women (Solari, 2009). Most studies have not found adverse maternal outcomes, although researchers in a Swedish study noted increased risks of low birthweight, fetal-growth restriction, and preterm delivery (Bennedsen, 1999). In an Australian study of more than 3000 pregnancies in schizophrenic women, Jablensky and colleagues (2005) reported that placental abruption was increased threefold and "fetal distress"—vaguely defined—was increased 1.4-fold.

Treatment

Because schizophrenia has a high recurrence if medications are discontinued, it is advisable to continue therapy during pregnancy. After 40 years of use, there is no evidence that conventional or "typical" antipsychotic drugs listed in Table 61-3 cause adverse fetal or maternal sequelae (McKenna, 2005; Robinson, 2012; Yaeger, 2006). Because less is known about "atypical" antipsychotics, the American College of Obstetricians and Gynecologists (2012b) recommends against their routine use in pregnant and breast-feeding women. In response to adverse event reports, the Food and Drug Administration (2011) issued a safety communication alerting health-care providers concerning some antipsychotic medications. These have been associated with neonatal extrapyramidal and withdrawal symptoms similar to the neonatal behavioral syndrome seen in those exposed to selective serotonin-reuptake inhibitors.

Feeding and Eating Disorders

These severe disturbances in eating behavior largely affect adolescent females and young adults with a lifetime prevalence of 2 to 3 percent each (see Table 61-1). They include *anorexia nervosa*, in which the patient refuses to maintain minimally normal body weight. With *bulimia nervosa*, there usually is binge eating followed by purging or by excessive fasting to maintain normal body weight (Zerbe, 2008). Bulik and coworkers (2009) studied pregnancy outcomes in almost 36,000 Norwegian women screened for eating disorders. Approximately 0.1 percent—1 in 1025—had anorexia nervosa; 0.85 percent—1 in 120—had bulimia nervosa; and 5.1 percent reported a binge-eating disorder—a 6-percent pregnancy prevalence similar to the 6-month prevalence for nonpregnant individuals (see Table 61-1). The last subtype had a higher risk for large-for-gestational age infants with a concomitantly increased cesarean delivery rate. All eating disorders begin with the desire to be slim, and women with chronic eating disorders may migrate between subtypes (Andersen, 2009).

Pregnancy

As discussed in Chapter 18 (p. 352), there is an increased risk for pregnancy complications with both eating disorders, but especially in women with bulimia nervosa (Andersen, 2009; Hoffman, 2011; Sollid, 2004). Generally, eating disorder symptoms improve during pregnancy, and remission rates may reach 75 percent. In contrast, what may appear as a typical case of hyperemesis gravidarum could actually be a new or relapsing case of bulimia nervosa or of anorexia nervosa, binge-purge type (Torgerson, 2008). As perhaps expected, anorexia is associated with low-birthweight infants (Micali, 2007). Additional risks associated with eating disorders include poor wound healing and difficulties with breast feeding (Andersen, 2009). At a minimum, closely monitoring gestational weight gain in women with a suspected history of an eating disorder seems prudent.

Personality Disorders

These disorders are characterized by the chronic use of certain coping mechanisms in an inappropriate, stereotyped, and maladaptive manner. They are rigid and unyielding personality traits. The American Psychiatric Association (2013) recognizes three clusters of personality disorders:

1. Paranoid, schizoid, and schizotypal personality disorders, which are characterized by oddness or eccentricity.
2. Histrionic, narcissistic, antisocial, and borderline disorders, which are all characterized by dramatic presentations along with self-centeredness and erratic behavior.
3. Avoidant, dependent, compulsive, and passive-aggressive personalities, which are characterized by underlying fear and anxiety.

Genetic and environmental factors are important in the genesis of these disorders, whose prevalence may be as high as 20 percent. Although management is through psychotherapy, most affected individuals do not recognize their problem, and thus only 20 percent seek help. In an observational study of 202 women with borderline personality disorder, De Genna and associates (2012) demonstrated that such women become pregnant during the most severe trajectory of their illness. They are at increased risk for teen and unintended pregnancies, however, it was not a risk factor for elective or spontaneous abortion.

Pregnancy

Personality disorders during pregnancy are probably no different than in nonpregnant women. Management of women with some of these disorders may be vexing. Akman and colleagues (2007) reported that avoidant, dependent, and obsessive-compulsive disorders are associated with an excessive prevalence of postpartum major depression. Magnusson and associates (2007) found a link between some *personality traits*—not disorders—and excessive alcohol consumption, but not necessarily addiction or dependence. Conroy and coworkers (2010) found that a mother's ability to care for her newborn was obviously impaired only when a personality disorder was coupled with depression.

REFERENCES

Ahokas A, Kaukoranta J, Aito M: Effect of oestradiol on postpartum depression. Psychopharmacology 146:108, 1999

Akman C, Uguz F, Kaya N: Postpartum-onset major depression is associated with personality disorders. Compr Psychiatry 48:343, 2007

Alder J, Fink N, Bitzer J, et al: Depression and anxiety during pregnancy: a risk factor for obstetric, fetal and neonatal outcome? A critical review of the literature. J Matern Fetal Neonatal Med 20:189, 2007

American College of Obstetricians and Gynecologists: Screening for depression during and after pregnancy. Committee Opinion No. 453, November 2010, Reaffirmed 2012a

American College of Obstetricians and Gynecologists: Use of psychiatric medication during pregnancy and lactation. Practice Bulletin No. 92. April 2008, Reaffirmed 2012b

American Psychiatric Association: Guidelines for the treatment of patients with major depressive disorder (Revision). Am J Psychiatry 157:1, 2000a

American Psychiatric Association: The Diagnostic and Statistical Manual of Mental Disorders, 4th ed, Text Revision (DSM-IV-TR). Washington, DC, 2000b

American Psychiatric Association (2013). The Diagnostic and Statistical Manual of Mental Disorders, 5th ed (DSM-V). Arlington, American Psychiatric Publishing, 2013

Andersen AE, Ryan GL: Eating disorders in the obstetric and gynecologic patient population. Obstet Gynecol 114:1353, 2009

Andersson L, Sundström-Poromaa I, Bixo M, et al: Point prevalence of psychiatric disorders during the second trimester of pregnancy: a population-based study. Am J Obstet Gynecol 189:148, 2003

Andrade SE, Raebel MA, Brown J, et al: Use of antidepressant medications during pregnancy: a multisite study. Am J Obstet Gynecol 198:194 e.1, 2008

Austin MP, Kildea S, Sullivan E: Maternal mortality and psychiatric morbidity in the perinatal period: challenges and opportunities for prevention in the Australian setting. MJA 186:364, 2007

Babbitt KE, Bailey KJ, Coverdale JH, et al: Professionally responsible intrapartum management of patients with major mental disorders. Am J Obstet Gynecol 210: 27, 2014

Balki M, Castro C, Ananthanarayan C: Status epilepticus after electroconvulsive therapy in a pregnant patient. Int J Obstet Anest 15:325, 2006

Bennedsen BE, Mortensen PB, Olesen Av, et al: Preterm birth and intra-uterine growth retardation among children of women with schizophrenia. Br J Psychiatry 175:239, 1999

Bergink V, van den Berg L, Koorengevel KM, et al: First-onset psychosis occurring in the postpartum period: a prospective cohort study. J Clin Psychiatry 72(11):1531, 2011

Bergink V, Bouvy PF, Vervoort JSP, et al: Prevention of postpartum psychosis and mania in women at high risk. Am J Psychiatry 169:609, 2012

Blackmore ER, Jones I, Doshi M, et al: Obstetric variables associated with bipolar affective puerperal psychosis. Br J Psychiatry 188:32, 2006

Briggs GG, Freeman RK, Yaffe SJ: Drugs in Pregnancy and Lactation, 9th ed. Philadelphia, Lippincott Williams & Wilkins, 2011

Buhimschi CS, Weiner CP: Medication in pregnancy and lactation: Part 1. Teratology. Obstet Gynecol 113:166, 2009

Buist A, Gotman N, Yonkers KA: Generalized anxiety disorder: course and risk factors in pregnancy. J Affective Dis 131(1–3):277, 2011

Bulik CM, Von Holle A, Siega-Riz AM, et al: Birth outcomes in women with eating disorders in the Norwegian mother and child cohort (MoBa). Int J Eat Disord 42(1):9, 2009

Centers for Disease Control and Prevention: Prevalence of self-reported postpartum depressive symptoms—17 states, 2004–2005. MMWR 57(14):361, 2008

Chambers CD, Hernandez-Diaz S, Van Martin LJ, et al: Selective serotonin-reuptake inhibitors and risk of persistent pulmonary hypertension of the newborn. N Engl J Med 354(6):579, 2006

Comtois KA, Schiff MA, Grossman DC: Psychiatric risk factors associated with postpartum suicide attempt in Washington state, 1992–2001. Am J Obstet Gynecol 199:120.e1, 2008

Conroy S, Marks MN, Schacht R, et al: The impact of maternal depression and personality disorder on early infant care. Soc Psychiatry Epidemiol 45(3):285, 2010

Davanzo R, Copertino M, De Cunto A, et al: Antidepressant drugs and breastfeeding: a review of the literature. Breastfeeding Med 6(2):89, 2011

De Genna NM, Feske U, Larkby C, et al: Pregnancies, abortions, and births among women with and without borderline personality disorder. Women's Health Issues 22(4):e371, 2012

Deecher D, Andree TH, Sloan D, et al: From menarche to menopause: exploring the underlying biology of depression in women experiencing hormonal changes. Psychoneuroendocrinology 33:3, 2008

Dennis CL, Ross LE, Grigoriadis S: Psychosocial and psychological interventions for treating antenatal depression. Cochrane Database Syst Rev 3:CD006309, 2007

Enato E: The fetal safety of benzodiazepines: an updated meta-analysis. J Obstet Gynaecol Can 33(4):319, 2011

Endres L, Straub H, Plunkett B, et al: Postpartum depression signals ongoing health risks. Abstract No. 673, Am J Obstet Gynecol 208(1 Suppl):S283, 2013

Food and Drug Administration: Antipsychotic drug labels updated on use during pregnancy and risk of abnormal muscle movements and withdrawal symptoms in newborns, 2011. Available at: http://www.fda.gov/Drugs/DrugSafety/ucm243903.htm. Accessed April 1, 2012

Frieder A, Dunlop AI, Culpepper L, et al: The clinical content of preconception care: women with psychiatric conditions. Am J Obstet Gynecol 199:S328, 2008

Gold KJ, Dalton VK, Schwenk TL: Hospital care for parents after perinatal death. Obstet Gynecol 109:1156, 2007

Goodwin RD, Keyes K, Simuro N: Mental disorders and nicotine dependence among pregnant women in the United States. Obstet Gynecol 109:875, 2007

Hayes RM, Wu P, Shelton RC, et al: Maternal antidepressant use and adverse outcomes: a cohort study of 228,876 pregnancies. Am J Obstet Gynecol 207:49.e1, 2012

Heron J, Blackmore ER, McGuinnes M, et al: No "latent period" in the onset of bipolar affective puerperal psychosis. Arch Womens Ment Health 10:79, 2007

Heron J, McGuinness M, Blackmore ER, et al: Early postpartum symptoms in puerperal psychosis. BJOG 115(3):348, 2008

Hippman C, Oberlander TG, Honer WG, et al: Depression during pregnancy: the potential impact of increased risk for fetal aneuploidy on maternal mood. Clin Genet 75(1):30, 2009

Hoffman ER, Zerwas SC, Bulik CM: Reproductive issues in anorexia nervosa. Obstet Gynecol 6:403, 2011

Huang H, Coleman S, Bridge JA, et al: A meta-analysis of the relationship between antidepressant use in pregnancy and the risk of preterm birth and low birth weight. Gen Hosp Psychiatry 36(1):13, 2014

Hunter SK, Mendoza J, D'Anna K: Antidepressants may mitigate the effects of prenatal maternal anxiety on infant auditory sensory gating. Am J Psychiatry 169: 616, 2012

Insel BJ, Schaefer CA, McKeague IW, et al: Maternal iron deficiency and the risk of schizophrenia in offspring. Arch Gen Psychiatry 65(10):1136, 2008

Jablensky AV, Morgan V, Zubrick SR, et al: Pregnancy, delivery, and neonatal complications in a population cohort of women with schizophrenia and major affective disorders. Am J Psychiatry 162:79, 2005

Jones I, Hamshere M, Nangle JM, et al: Bipolar affective puerperal psychosis: genome-wide significant evidence for linkage to chromosome 16. Am J Psychiatry 164:999, 2007

Kanotra S, D'Angelo D, Phares TM, et al: Challenges faced by new mothers in the early postpartum period: an analysis of comment data from the 2000 Pregnancy Risk Assessment Monitoring System (PRAMS) Survey. Matern Child Health J 11(6):549, 2007

Kelly RH, Russo J, Holt VL, et al: Psychiatric and substance use disorders as risk factors for low birth weight and preterm delivery. Obstet Gynecol 100:297, 2002

Kieler H, Artama M, Engeland A, et al: Selective serotonin reuptake inhibitors during pregnancy and risk of persistent pulmonary hypertension in the newborn: population based cohort study from the five Nordic countries. BMJ 344:d8012, 2012

Kim JH, Choi SS, Ha K: A closer look at depression in mothers who kill their children: is it unipolar or bipolar depression? J Clin Psychiatry 69(10):1625, 2008

Koren G, Finkelstein Y, Matsui D, et al: Diagnosis and management of poor neonatal adaptation syndrome in newborns exposed in utero to selective serotonin/norepinephrine reuptake inhibitors. J Obstet Gynaecol Can 31(4):348, 2009
Koren G, Nordeng H: Antidepressant use during pregnancy: the benefit-risk ratio. Am J Obstet Gynecol 207:157, 2012
Kukshal P, Thelma BK, Nimgaonkar VL, et al: Genetics of schizophrenia from a clinical perspective. Int Rev Psychiatry 24(5):393, 2012
Lee AM, Lam SK, Lau SM, et al: Prevalence, course, and risk factors for antenatal anxiety and depression. Obstet Gynecol 110:1102, 2007
Littleton HL, Breitkopf CR, Berenson AB: Correlates of anxiety symptoms during pregnancy and association with perinatal outcomes: a meta-analysis. Am J Obstet Gynecol 424, May 2007
Luke S, Salhu HM, Alio AP, et al: Risk factors for major antenatal depression among low-income African American women. J Women's Health 18:1841, 2009
Magnusson Å, Göransson M, Heilig M: Hazardous alcohol users during pregnancy: psychiatric health and personality traits. Drug Alcohol Depend 89:275, 2007
Mahon P, Payne JL, MacKinnon DF, et al: Genome-wide linkage and follow-up association study of postpartum mood symptoms. Am J Psychiatry 166:1229, 2009
Malaspina D, Corcoran C, Kleinhaus KR, et al: Acute maternal stress in pregnancy and schizophrenia in offspring: a cohort prospective. BMC Psychiatry 8:71, 2008
Marcus SM: Depression during pregnancy: rates, risks and consequences—Motherisk Update 2008. Can J Clin Pharmacol 16(1):e15, 2009
McKenna K, Koren G, Tetelbaum M, et al: Pregnancy outcome of women using atypical antipsychotic drugs: a prospective comparative study. J Clin Psychiatry 66:444, 2005
Melville JL, Gavin A, Guo Y, et al: Depressive disorders during pregnancy. Obstet Gynecol 116:1064, 2010
Mental Health America: Depression in women. 2013a. Available at: http://mentalhealthamerica.net/index.cfm?objectid=C7DF952E-1372-4D20-C8A3DDCD5459D07B. Accessed May 14, 2013
Mental Health America: Postpartum disorders. 2013b. Available at: http://www.mentalhealthamerica.net/go/postpartum www.mentalhealthamerica.net. Accessed May 14, 2013
Micali N, Simonoff E, Treasure J: Risk of major adverse perinatal outcomes in women with eating disorders. Br J Psychiatry 190:255, 2007
Miller LJ: Use of electroconvulsive therapy during pregnancy. Hosp Community Psychiatry 45:444, 1994
Morewitz SJ: Feelings of anxiety and functional impairment during pregnancy. Obstet Gynecol 101:109S, 2003
Mozurkewich E, Clinton C, Chilimigras J, et al: The Mother's, Omega-3 & Mental Health Study: a double-blind, randomized controlled trial. Abstract No. 29, Am J Obstet Gynecol 208(1 Suppl):S19, 2013
Muller-Oerlinghausen B, Berghofer A, Bauer M: Bipolar disorder. Lancet 359:241, 2002
Murphy KC: Schizophrenia and velocardiofacial syndrome. Lancet 359(9304):426, 2002
National Institute of Mental Health: The numbers count: mental disorders in America. NIH Publication No. 06-4584, 2006
National Institute of Mental Health: Spotlight on postpartum depression. 2010. Available at: http://www.nimh.nih.gov/about/director/2010/spotlight-on-postpartum-depression.shtml. Accessed May 14, 2013
National Library of Medicine: Drugs and Lactation Database (LactMed): fluoxetine. 2012. Available at: http://toxnet.nlm.nih.gov/cgi-bin/sis/search/f?./temp/~eNg5Oo:1. Accessed May 14, 2013
Nelson DB, Freeman MP, Johnson NL, et al: A prospective study of postpartum depression in 17648 parturients. J Matern Fetal Neonatal Med 26(12):1156, 2013
O'Hara MW, Wisner KL: Perinatal mental illness: definition, description and aetiology. Best Pract Res Clin Obstet Gynaecol 28(1):3, 2014
O'Keane V, Lightman S, Patrick K, et al: Changes in the maternal hypothalamic-pituitary-adrenal axis during the early puerperium may be related to the postpartum blues. J Neuroendocrinol 23(11):1149, 2011
O'Reardon JP, Cristancho MA, von Andreae CV, et al: Acute and maintenance electroconvulsive therapy for treatment of severe major depression during the second and third trimesters of pregnancy with infant follow-up to 18 months. J ECT 27(1):e23, 2011
Palladino CL, Singh V, Campbell H, et al: Homicide and suicide during the perinatal period: findings from the National Violent Death Reporting System. Obstet Gynecol 118(5):1056, 2011
Physicians' Desk Reference, 62nd ed. Toronto, Thomson Corp, 2012
Pinette MG, Santarpio C, Wax JR, et al: Electroconvulsive therapy in pregnancy. Obstet Gynecol 110:465, 2007
Pozzi RA, Yee LM, Brown K, et al: Pregnancy in the severely mentally ill patient as an opportunity for global coordination of care. Am J Obstet Gynecol 210:32, 2014
Ray S, Stowe ZN: The use of antidepressant medication in pregnancy. Best Pract Res Clin Obstet Gynaecol 28(1):71, 2014
Reprotox-Micromedex 2.0: Lithium. Available at: http://www.micromedexsolutions.com. Accessed April 10, 2013
Richards DS: Is electroconvulsive therapy in pregnancy safe? Obstet Gynecol 110:451, 2007
Robinson GE: Treatment of schizophrenia in pregnancy and postpartum. J Popul Ther Clin Pharmacol 19(3):e380, 2012
Romero R, Badr MS: A role for sleep disorders in pregnancy complications: challenges and opportunities. Am J Obstet Gynecol 210:3, 2014
Ross LE, McLean LM: Anxiety disorders during pregnancy and the postpartum period: a systematic review. J Clin Psychiatry 67:1285, 2006
Schneid-Kofman N, Sheiner E, Levy A: Psychiatric illness and adverse pregnancy outcome. Int J Gynaecol Obstet 101(1):53, 2008
Schneier FR: Clinical practice. Social anxiety disorder. N Engl J Med 355(10):1029, 2006
Solari H, Dickson KE, Miller L: Understanding and treating women with schizophrenia during pregnancy and postpartum—Motherisk Update 2008. Can J Clin Pharmacol 16(1):e32, 2009
Sollid CP, Wisborg K, Hjort J, et al: Eating disorder that was diagnosed before pregnancy and pregnancy outcome. Am J Obstet Gynecol 190:206, 2004
Steinberg JR, McCulloch CE, Adler NE: Abortion and mental health: findings from the National Comorbidity Survey Replication. Obstet Gynecol 123:263, 2014
Tam WH, Chung T: Psychosomatic disorders in pregnancy. Curr Opin Obstet Gynecol 19:126, 2007
Torgerson L, Von Holle A, Reichborn-Kjennerud T, et al: Nausea and vomiting of pregnancy in women with bulimia nervosa and eating disorders not otherwise specified. Int J Eat Disord 41:722, 2008
Van Lieshout RJ, Voruganti LP: Diabetes mellitus during pregnancy and increased risk of schizophrenia in offspring: a review of the evidence and putative mechanisms. J Psychiatry Neurosci 33(5):395, 2008
Van den Bergh BRH, Mulder EJH, Mennes M, et al: Antenatal maternal anxiety and stress and the neurobehavioural development of the fetus and child: links and possible mechanisms. A review. Neurosci Biobehav Rev 29(2):237, 2005
Viguera AC, Whitfield T, Baldessarini RJ, et al: Risk of recurrence in women with bipolar disorder during pregnancy: prospective study of mood stabilizer discontinuation. Am J Psychiatry 164(12):1817, 2007
Vythilingum B: Anxiety disorders in pregnancy. Curr Psychiatry Rep 10(4):331, 2008
Westdahl C, Milan S, Magriples U, et al: Social support and social conflict as predictors of prenatal depression. Obstet Gynecol 110:134, 2007
Wisner KL, Parry BL, Piontek CM: Postpartum depression. N Engl J Med 347:194, 2002
Yaeger D, Smith HG, Altshuler LL: Atypical antipsychotics in the treatment of schizophrenia during pregnancy and the postpartum. Am J Psychiatry 163:2064, 2006
Yonkers KA, Vigod S, Ross LE: Diagnosis, pathophysiology, and management of mood disorders in pregnant and postpartum women. Obstet Gynecol 117:961, 2011
Yonkers KA, Wisner KL, Stewart DE, et al: The management of depression during pregnancy: a report from the American Psychiatric Association and the American College of Obstetricians and Gynecologists. Obstet Gynecol 114:703, 2009
Zerbe KJ, Rosenberg J: Eating disorders. Clinical Updates in Women's Health Care. American College of Obstetricians and Gynecologists, Vol VII, No. 1, January 2008

CHAPTER 62

Dermatological Disorders

Normal physiological changes of pregnancy include alterations to skin, hair, and nails as discussed in Chapter 4 (p. 51). In addition, several dermatoses are seen only in pregnancy. Finally, it is axiomatic that skin diseases that affect childbearing-age women are commonly encountered in pregnancy.

PREGNANCY-SPECIFIC DERMATOSES

Four dermatoses considered unique to pregnancy include intrahepatic cholestasis of pregnancy, pruritic urticarial papules and plaques of pregnancy (PUPPP), atopic eruption of pregnancy (AEP), and pemphigoid gestationis (Table 62-1). As a group, these are diagnosed in up to 5 percent of pregnancies with the following relative occurrences: intrahepatic cholestasis 1 in 100; PUPPP, 1 in 130 to 350; atopic eruptions, 1 in 300 to 450, and pemphigoid, 1 in 50,000 (Chander, 2011). Their gross appearance may be similar to each other or to other skin disorders, and pruritus is a common feature of all four. Only intrahepatic cholestasis and pemphigoid gestationis have been linked with adverse fetal outcomes.

Intrahepatic Cholestasis of Pregnancy

Previously termed pruritus gravidarum and in contrast to the other pregnancy-specific dermatoses, intrahepatic cholestasis of pregnancy generally has no primary skin lesions. Rarely, a rash preceded pruritus (Chao, 2011). Pruritus is associated with abnormally elevated serum bile acid levels, and hepatic aminotransferase levels may also be mildly increased. Adverse fetal affects have been linked to this condition, and it is discussed in detail in Chapter 55 (p. 1084).

Pemphigoid Gestationis

This rare autoimmune bullous disease is notable for its maternal and fetal effects. Initially, pruritic papules and urticarial plaques form and are then followed in most cases after 1 to 2 weeks by vesicles or bullae. Lesions are frequently distributed periumbilically, and they often develop on other skin surfaces with sparing of mucous membranes, scalp, and face (Fig. 62-1).

Previously termed *herpes gestationis*, pemphigoid gestationis is not related to the herpesvirus. It is a result of a primary reaction between maternal immunoglobulin G (IgG) antibodies directed against collagen XVII found in the basement membrane of skin as well as amnionic epithelium (Kelly, 1988; Shimanovich, 2002). Collagen XVII is also termed bullous pemphigoid 180 (BP 180). Autoantibody binding to collagen XVII, either in the amnion or in the skin, activates complement to promote eosinophil chemotaxis to the antigen-antibody complexes on the basement membrane. Eosinophilic degranulation damages the dermal-epidermal junction with blister formation (Engineer, 2000).

Pregnancy

In most cases, pemphigoid gestationis develops during a first pregnancy, and it may rarely be associated with gestational trophoblastic disease (Takatsuka, 2012). Most subsequent pregnancies are also affected and usually earlier and more severely. Whites have a higher incidence, and other autoimmune diseases are common in affected women (Shornick, 1984, 1992).

Pemphigoid gestationis usually begins during the second or third trimester. The disease course is frequently marked by antepartum exacerbations and remissions and by intrapartum flares (Shornick, 1998). It is possible that there is an association

TABLE 62-1. Pregnancy-specific Dermatoses

Disorder	Frequency	Characteristic Lesion	Adverse Pregnancy Effects	Treatment
Cholestasis of pregnancy	Common	No primary lesions, secondary excoriations from scratching	Increased perinatal morbidity	Antipruritics, cholestyramine, ursodeoxycholic acid
Pruritic urticarial papules and plaques of pregnancy (PUPPP)	Common	Erythematous pruritic papules or plaques; patchy or generalized on abdomen, thighs, buttocks, especially within striae, but with umbilical sparing	None	
Atopic eruptions of pregnancy (AEP)			None	
Eczema of pregnancy	Common	Dry, red scaly patches on extremity flexures, neck, face		Antipruritics, emollients, topical corticosteroids, oral steroids if severe
Prurigo of pregnancy	Common	1–5 mm pruritic red papules on extensor surfaces, trunk		
Pruritic folliculitis of pregnancy	Rare	Small red papules, sterile pustules on trunk		
Pemphigoid gestationis	Rare	Erythematous pruritic papules, plaques, vesicles, and bullae; abdomen often with umbilical involvement, extremities	Preterm birth, fetal-growth restriction, transient neonatal lesions	

of pemphigoid gestationis with preterm birth and fetal-growth restriction, especially with early-onset disease and with blistering (Chi, 2009). These theoretically may result from mild placental insufficiency stemming from IgG and complement deposition along the amnionic basement membrane (Huilaja, 2013). Because of this, antepartum surveillance of affected pregnancies may be prudent.

In approximately 10 percent of neonates, IgG antibodies passively transferred from the mother will cause similar skin lesions in the newborn (Erickson, 2002). These eruptions require only wound care and clear spontaneously within a few weeks as the passively acquired IgG levels decrease.

Slowly following delivery, maternal lesions resolve without scarring, and most women are disease-free after 6 months (Jenkins, 1999). In some, however, resolution is protracted, and disease may be exacerbated during menses or by oral contraceptives (Semkova, 2009).

Diagnosis and Treatment

Before bullae form, these lesions may resemble PUPPP (p. 1216). Other diagnoses include pustular psoriasis of pregnancy, dermatitis herpetiformis, erythema multiforme, linear IgA bullous dermatosis, urticaria, allergic contact dermatitis, bullous pemphigoid, and atopic eruptions of pregnancy (Lipozenčić, 2012). Drug-induced blistering syndromes must also be excluded, as some are life-threatening. Examples include Stevens-Johnson syndrome and toxic epidermal necrolysis (Stern, 2012).

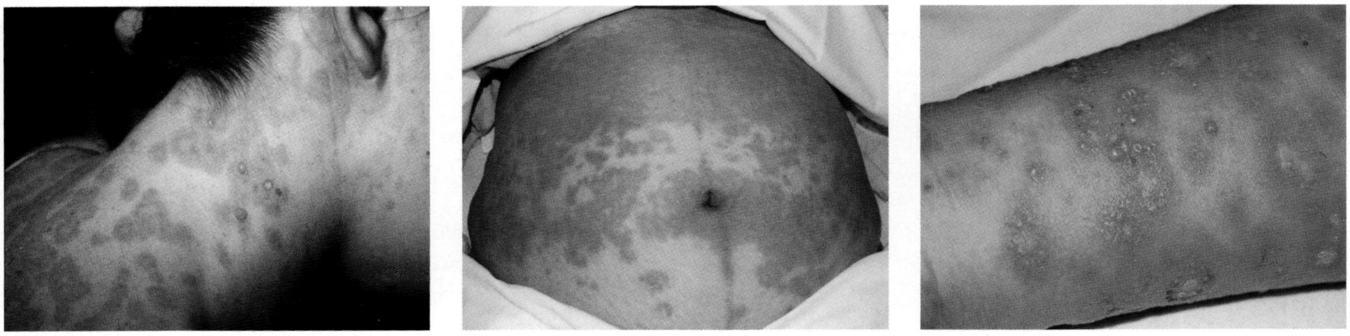

A B C

FIGURE 62-1 Pemphigoid gestationis. **A.** Bullae commonly develop within erythematous plaques. (Photograph contributed by Dr. Amit Pandya.) **B.** Abdominal lesions classically involve the umbilicus. **C.** Lesions on the wrist and forearm are shown here. (Photographs contributed by Dr. Kara Ehlers.)

Skin biopsy and serum antibody assays may be informative (Semkova, 2009). Immunofluorescent skin tissue staining is the gold standard, and C3 complement and sometimes IgG are seen deposited along the basement membrane between the epidermis and the dermis (Katz, 1976). Also, in many cases, circulating IgG antibodies against collagen XVII may be detected in patient serum (Powell, 2005; Sitaru, 2004).

Pruritus can be severe. Early in its course, topical high-potency corticosteroids and oral antihistamines may be effective. Oral prednisone, 0.5 to 1 mg/kg daily gradually tapered to a maintenance dose, may be needed for relief and also inhibition of new lesions. Plasmapheresis or high-dose intravenous immunoglobulin (IVIG) therapy has been used in intractable cases (Gan, 2012; Van de Wiel, 1980).

Pruritic Urticarial Papules and Plaques of Pregnancy (PUPPP)

This relatively common pregnancy-specific dermatosis is characterized by its intensely pruritic 1- to 2-mm erythematous papules that coalesce to form urticarial plaques and by its benign effects on pregnancy (Rudolph, 2005). Its cause is unknown, but it is not an autoimmune dermatosis. Also known as polymorphic eruption of pregnancy, PUPPP usually appears late in pregnancy, but 15 percent begin postpartum (Buccolo, 2005). The rash affects the abdomen and proximal thighs in 97 percent of women (Fig. 62-2). Lesions often initially form within striae but show periumbilical sparing. Rarely, the face, palms, and soles may be involved (High, 2005). It is more frequently seen in white and nulliparous women, those with multifetal gestation, and those carrying a male fetus (Regnier, 2008). It seldom recurs in subsequent pregnancies (Ahmadi, 2005).

Diagnosis and Treatment

PUPPP may be compared with a number of skin eruptions. Some include contact dermatitis, drug eruption, viral exanthem, insect bites, scabies infestation, pityriasis rosea, and the other pregnancy-specific dermatoses. It also may appear similar to early pemphigoid gestationis that has not yet blistered. In unclear cases, skin biopsy and negative serum collagen XVII antibody levels help to differentiate the two. Pruritus will usually respond to treatment with oral antihistamines, skin emollients, and topical corticosteroids. A small number of women will need systemic corticosteroids to relieve severe itching (Scheinfeld, 2008).

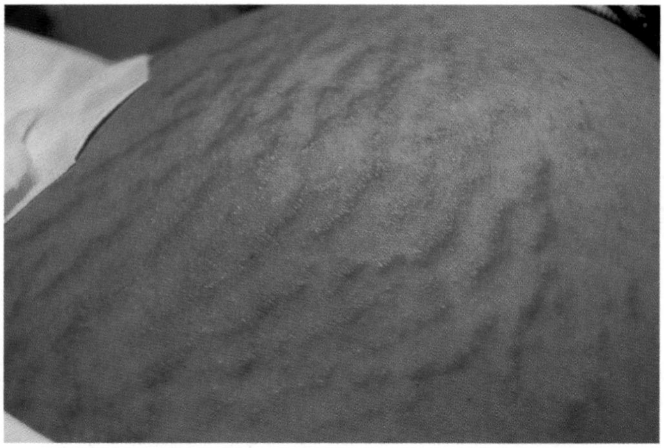

FIGURE 62-2 Pruritic urticarial papules and plaques of pregnancy (PUPPP) shows small papules within abdominal striae.

PUPPP usually resolves within several days following delivery and leaves no scarring. In 15 to 20 percent of women, however, symptoms persist for 2 to 4 weeks postpartum (Vaughan Jones, 1999).

Atopic Eruption of Pregnancy (AEP)

This umbrella term is thought by some authorities, but not all, to encompass three conditions previously considered separate: eczema in pregnancy, prurigo of pregnancy, and pruritic folliculitis of pregnancy (Ambros-Rudolph, 2006; Cohen, 2007; Ingber, 2010). Two thirds of women with AEP have widespread eczematous changes, whereas the other third have papular lesions. As a group, these pose no adverse risk to the fetus. Diagnosis is greatly aided by a history of atopy and by rash characteristics.

Eczema in pregnancy has the appearance of traditional eczema but with a pregnancy onset. It is the most common pregnancy-specific dermatosis, and affected skin shows dry, thickened, scaly, red patches involving extremity flexures, nipples, neck, and face. In contrast, *prurigo of pregnancy*, also known as prurigo gestationis, is characterized by 5- to 10-mm, itchy, erythematous papules or nodules commonly found on the extensor surfaces and trunk. Last, *pruritic folliculitis of pregnancy* is rare and notable for small, erythematous follicular papules and sterile pustules predominantly on the trunk. Onset for all is during the second or third trimester, although eczema in pregnancy may develop earlier than the other two. All lesions commonly resolve with delivery, but may persist for up to 3 months postpartum. Recurrence with subsequent pregnancies is variable but common.

Diagnosis is one of exclusion. Serum bile acid levels are elevated to concentrations expected for normal pregnancy, and aminotransferase levels are normal. Serology specific for pemphigoid gestationis is negative. Many women with eczema of pregnancy have elevated serum IgE levels, which are not seen with the two other AEP dermatoses (Ambros-Rudolph, 2011).

For all three manifestations, skin lesions and pruritus are usually controlled with low- or moderate-potency topical corticosteroids and oral antihistamines. For severe eczema, second-line agents include short-course ultrapotent topical corticosteroids. However, oral corticosteroids, narrow-band ultraviolet B, or cyclosporine are occasionally required (Koutroulis, 2011).

DERMATOLOGICAL CONDITIONS NOT SPECIFIC TO PREGNANCY

Any chronic dermatological disorders can complicate pregnancy. *Acne* is unpredictably affected by pregnancy and if necessary, is treated with benzoyl peroxide, azelaic acid, or topical erythromycin, which are category B drugs (Krautheim, 2003). Topical retinoids, which include tretinoin, adapalene, and tazarotene, also appear safe, but are probably best avoided during pregnancy, especially during the first trimester (Akhavan, 2003). If topical antibiotics are required, benzoyl peroxide plus erythromycin is advocated to minimize *Propionibacterium acnes* drug resistance (Strauss, 2007; Thiboutot, 2009). With topical salicylic acid, systemic absorption is variable, and efforts to minimize absorption are encouraged (Lam, 2008).

Psoriasis also has a variable course during pregnancy, however, postpartum flares are common with nonsevere disease (Oumeish, 2006). Emollients and low- or moderate-potency topical corticosteroids are given initially. Anthralin and ultraviolet B phototherapy can also be used (Weatherhead, 2007). In resistant cases, restrained use of topical preparations such as high-potency or ultrapotent corticosteroids, calcipotriene, and coal tar appear to be safe in the second and third trimesters, and cyclosporine also may be used (Rosmarin, 2010; Ryan, 2010). With severe disease, a small increased risk for low-birthweight neonates has been shown by some (Lima, 2012; Yang, 2011). Also, in general, psoriatic patients have higher associated rates of depression (Rieder, 2012).

Psoriasis is most commonly of the chronic plaque variety. In contrast, with *generalized pustular psoriasis of pregnancy*—formerly called impetigo herpetiformis—severe systemic symptoms may develop. This rare pustular form has erythematous, sometimes pruritic, plaques ringed by sterile pustules that enlarge and then crust. Lesions initially involve intertriginous areas but may spread to the torso, extremities, and oral mucosa. Constitutional symptoms are common. For accurate diagnosis, skin biopsy is typically required (Roth, 2011). Extensive lesions can lead to sepsis from secondary infection and to massive fluid loss with hypovolemia and placental insufficiency. Treatment is with systemic corticosteroids along with antimicrobials for secondary infection, and cyclosporine is used in refractory cases (Geraghty, 2011; Huang, 2011). Pustular psoriasis typically resolves quickly in the puerperium, but recurrences have been reported in subsequent pregnancies and with menstruation or oral contraceptive use.

Erythema nodosum is a cutaneous reaction associated with numerous disorders that include pregnancy, but typically it is caused by infections, sarcoidosis, drugs, Behçet's syndrome, inflammatory bowel disease, or a malignancy (Mert, 2007; Papagrigoraki, 2010). Characteristically, 1- to 5-cm tender, red, warm nodules and plaques develop rapidly on the extensor surface of the legs and arms. Within a few days, lesions flatten and undergo the color evolution of a bruise—from dark red and purple to yellow green. Constitutional symptoms may also be present (Requena, 2007). Initial evaluation and treatment focuses on the underlying etiology.

Pyogenic granuloma are frequently seen in pregnancy. This is a lobular capillary hemangioma commonly forming on the mouth or hand in response to low-grade local irritation or traumatic injury (Fig. 62-3). They grow quickly and bleed with minimal provocation. Active bleeding can be controlled with pressure and application of a silver nitrate stick or Monsel paste (ferric subsulfate). These growths often resolve within months postpartum. But with symptomatic or postpartum lesions, or with unclear diagnosis, excision can be done using suture and scalpel, electrosurgical curettage, laser photocoagulation, or cryotherapy. Oral lesions are best referred to oral health-care specialists.

Rosacea fulminans—also known as pyoderma faciale—is characterized by facial pustules and coalescing draining sinuses.

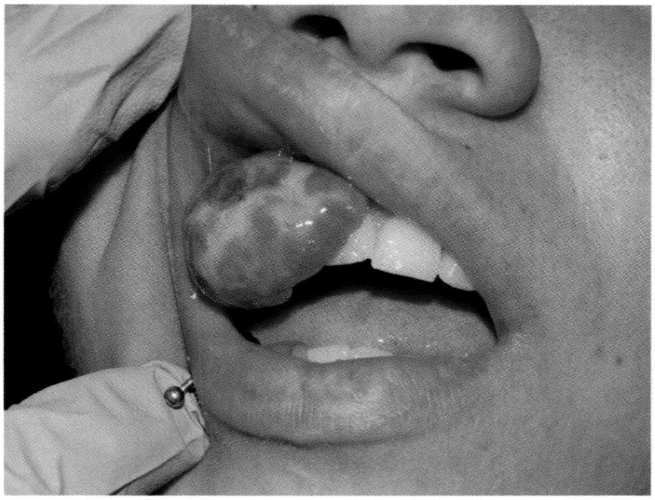

FIGURE 62-3 Pyogenic granuloma is characterized grossly by a lobulated red growth on a pedunculated or sessile base. (Photograph contributed by Dr. Abel Moron.)

It may rarely complicate pregnancy. Topical or oral antimicrobials are primary treatment, although surgical drainage and corticosteroids have also been used (Fuentelsaz, 2011; Jarrett, 2010). *Hidradenitis suppurativa* has been said to improve with pregnancy, but in our experiences, it is not appreciably changed. Oral antimicrobials or clindamycin gel are initial choices. *Neurofibromatosis* lesions may increase in size and number as a result of pregnancy. Other skin conditions that are discussed include hirsutism and melanoma (Chap. 63, p 1233), cutaneous lupus (Chap. 59, p. 1169), and skin lesions seen with infections (Chaps. 64 and 65, p. 1239).

DERMATOLOGICAL TREATMENT

Local skin care, oral antihistamines, and topical corticosteroids are commonly used for many dermatoses. Oral antihistamines are given for pruritus. Suitable options include first-generation agents such as diphenhydramine (Benadryl), 25 to 50 mg every 6 hours, or chlorpheniramine (Chlor-Trimeton), 4 mg every 6 hours. Second-generation agents—loratadine (Claritin) 10 mg daily and cetirizine (Zyrtec) 5 or 10 mg daily—may produce less sedation and are also pregnancy category B.

Hundreds of topical corticosteroid preparations are available, and in the United States, these are categorized by potency into seven groups. For initial treatment of dermatological disorders, low- or moderate-potency agents are preferred. Low-potency agents include those in groups 6 and 7, such as 1-percent hydrocortisone or 0.05-percent desonide (DesOwen). Moderate-potency drugs are in groups 5, 4, and 3—such as 0.1-percent triamcinolone acetonide (Aristocort) or 0.1-percent mometasone furoate (Elocon). High-potency medications are in group 2, such as 0.05-percent betamethasone diproprionate (Diprolene). Ultrapotent agents in group 1, such as 0.05-percent clobetasol propionate (Temovate), are best reserved for refractory disorders and used for only 2 to 4 weeks on small surface areas.

Mild and moderate strengths are not associated with adverse pregnancy outcomes, whereas high- and ultrapotent agents pose a small risk for fetal-growth restriction if used long-term. Even then, this risk is less than that with systemic corticosteroids (Chi, 2011). Importantly, with any topical agent, factors that increase systemic absorption include a large surface area treated, compromised epidermal barrier, occlusive dressings, prolonged treatment duration, and coadministration of topical agents that increase absorption.

With some severe skin diseases, systemic immune modulating agents, such as corticosteroids and cyclosporine, may be required. Although these are not contraindicated in pregnancy, their risks must be balanced against therapeutic benefits. Of these, cyclosporine is not recommended with breast feeding (Rosmarin, 2010). Bacterial infections are a potential secondary complication of skin disorders and are treated promptly with oral antimicrobial agents with gram-positive coverage. Therapeutic agents to be avoided during pregnancy include methotrexate, psoralen plus ultraviolet A, biological agents, mycophenolate mofetil, and systemic retinoids (Lam, 2008). These are discussed in more detail in Chapter 12 (p. 250).

REFERENCES

Ahmadi S, Powell FC: Pruritic urticarial papules and plaques of pregnancy: current status. Australas J Dermatol 46(2):53, 2005

Akhavan A, Bershad S: Topical acne drugs: review of clinical properties, systemic exposure, and safety. Am J Clin Dermatol 4(7):473, 2003

Ambros-Rudolph CM: Dermatoses of pregnancy—clues to diagnosis, fetal risk and therapy. Ann Dermatol 23(3):265, 2011

Ambros-Rudolph CM, Müllegger RR, Vaughan-Jones SA, et al: The specific dermatoses of pregnancy revisited and reclassified: results of a retrospective two-center study on 505 pregnant patients. J Am Acad Dermatol 54:395, 2006

Buccolo LS, Viera AJ: Pruritic urticarial papules and plaques of pregnancy presenting in the postpartum period: a case report. J Reprod Med 50:61, 2005

Chander R, Garg T, Kakkar S, et al: Specific pregnancy dermatoses in 1430 females from Northern India. J Dermatol Case Rep 5(4):69, 2011

Chao TT, Sheffield JS: Primary dermatologic findings with early-onset intrahepatic cholestasis of pregnancy. Obstet Gynecol 117:456, 2011

Chi CC, Kirtschig G, Aberer W, et al: Evidence-based (S3) guideline on topical corticosteroids in pregnancy. Br J Dermatol 165(5):943, 2011

Chi CC, Wang SH, Charles-Holmes R, et al: Pemphigoid gestationis: early onset and blister formations are associated with adverse pregnancy outcomes. Br J Dermatol 160(6):1222, 2009

Cohen LM, Kroumpouzos G: Pruritic dermatoses of pregnancy: to lump or to split? J Am Acad Dermatol 56:708, 2007

Engineer L, Bhol K, Ahmed AR: Pemphigoid gestationis: a review. Am J Obstet Gynecol 183(2):483, 2000

Erickson NI, Ellis RL: Neonatal rash due to herpes gestationis. N Engl J Med 347(9):660, 2002

Fuentelsaz V, Ara M, Corredera C, et al: Rosacea fulminans in pregnancy: successful treatment with azithromycin. Clin Exp Dermatol 36(6):674, 2011

Gan DC, Welsh B, Webster M: Successful treatment of a severe persistent case of pemphigoid gestationis with antepartum and postpartum intravenous immunoglobulin followed by azathioprine. Australas J Dermatol 53(1):66, 2012

Geraghty LN, Pomeranz MK: Physiologic changes and dermatoses of pregnancy. Int J Dermatol 50(7):771, 2011

Griffith WF, Werner CL: Benign disorders of the lower reproductive tract. In Hoffman BL, Schorge JO, Schaffer JI, et al (eds), Williams Gynecology, 2nd ed. New York, McGraw-Hill, 2012, p 115

High WA, Hoang MP, Miller MD: Pruritic urticarial papules and plaques of pregnancy with unusual and extensive palmoplantar involvement. Obstet Gynecol 105:1261, 2005

Huang YH, Chen YP, Liang CC, et al: Impetigo herpetiformis with gestational hypertension: a case report and literature review. Dermatology 222(3):221, 2011

Huilaja L, Mäkikallio K, Sormunen R, et al: Gestational pemphigoid: placental morphology and function. Acta Derm Venereol 93(1):33, 2013

Ingber A: Atopic eruption of pregnancy. J Eur Acad Dermatol Venereol 24(8):974, 2010

Jarrett R, Gonsalves R, Anstey AV: Differing obstetric outcomes of rosacea fulminans in pregnancy: report of three cases with review of pathogenesis and management. Clin Exp Dermatol 35(8):888, 2010

Jenkins RE, Hern S, Black MM: Clinical features and management of 87 patients with pemphigoid gestationis. Clin Exp Dermatol 24(4):255, 1999

Katz SI, Hertz KC, Yaoita H: Herpes gestationis. Immunopathology and characterization of the HG factor. J Clin Invest 57(6):1434, 1976

Kelly SE, Bhogal BS, Wojnarowska F, et al: Expression of a pemphigoid gestationis-related antigen by human placenta. Br J Dermatol 118:605, 1988

Koutroulis I, Papoutsis J, Kroumpouzos G: Atopic dermatitis in pregnancy: current status and challenges. Obstet Gynecol Surv 66(10):654, 2011

Krautheim A, Gollnick H: Transdermal penetration of topical drugs used in the treatment of acne. Clin Pharmacokinet 42(14):1287, 2003

Lam J, Polifka JE, Dohil MA: Safety of dermatologic drugs used in pregnant patients with psoriasis and other inflammatory skin diseases. J Am Acad Dermatol 59(2):295, 2008

Lima XT, Janakiraman V, Hughes MD, et al: The impact of psoriasis on pregnancy outcomes. J Invest Dermatol 132(1):85, 2012

Lipozenčić J, Ljubojevic S, Bukvić-Mokos Z: Pemphigoid gestationis. Clin Dermatol 30(1):51, 2012

Mert A, Kumbasar H, Ozaras R, et al: Erythema nodosum: an evaluation of 100 cases. Clin Exp Rheumatol 25(4):563, 2007

Oumeish OY, Al-Fouzan AW: Miscellaneous diseases affected by pregnancy. Clin Dermatol 24:113, 2006

Papagrigoraki A, Gisondi P, Rosina P, et al: Erythema nodosum: etiological factors and relapses in a retrospective cohort study. Eur J Dermatol 20(6):773, 2010

Powell AM, Sakuma-Oyama Y, Oyama N, et al: Usefulness of BP180 NC16a enzyme-linked immunosorbent assay in the serodiagnosis of pemphigoid gestationis and in differentiating between pemphigoid gestationis and pruritic urticarial papules and plaques of pregnancy. Arch Dermatol 141(6):705, 2005

Regnier S, Fermand V, Levy P, et al: A case-control study of polymorphic eruption of pregnancy. J Am Acad Dermatol 58 (1):63, 2008

Requena L, Sánchez YE: Erythema nodosum. Semin Cutan Med Surg 26(2):114, 2007

Rieder E, Tausk F: Psoriasis, a model of dermatologic psychosomatic disease: psychiatric implications and treatments. Int J Dermatol 51(1):12, 2012

Rosmarin DM, Lebwohl M, Elewski BE, et al: Cyclosporine and psoriasis: 2008 National Psoriasis Foundation Consensus Conference. J Am Acad Dermatol 62(5):838, 2010

Roth MM: Pregnancy dermatoses: diagnosis, management, and controversies. Am J Clin Dermatol 12(1):25, 2011

Rudolph CM, Al-Fares S, Vaughan-Jones SA, et al: Polymorphic eruption of pregnancy: clinicopathology and potential trigger factors in 181 patients. Br J Dermatol 154:54, 2005

Ryan C, Amor KT, Menter A: The use of cyclosporine in dermatology: part II. J Am Acad Dermatol 63(6):949, 2010

Scheinfeld N: Pruritic urticarial papules and plaques of pregnancy wholly abated with one week twice daily application of fluticasone propionate lotion: a case report and review of the literature. Dermatol Online 14(11):4, 2008

Semkova K, Black M: Pemphigoid gestationis: current insights into pathogenesis and treatment. Eur J Obstet Gynecol Reprod Biol 145(2):138, 2009

Shimanovich I, Skrobek C, Rose C, et al: Pemphigoid gestationis with predominant involvement of oral mucous membranes and IgA autoantibodies targeting the C-terminus of BP180. J Am Acad Dermatol 47:780, 2002

Shornick JK: Dermatoses of pregnancy. Semin Cutan Med Surg 17:172, 1998

Shornick JK, Black MM: Fetal risks in herpes gestationis. J Am Acad Dermatol 26:63, 1992

Shornick JK, Meek TJ, Nesbitt LT, et al: Herpes gestationis in blacks. Arch Dermatol 120(4):511, 1984

Sitaru C, Powell J, Messer G, et al: Immunoblotting and enzyme-linked immunosorbent assay for the diagnosis of pemphigoid gestationis. Obstet Gynecol 103(4):757, 2004

Stern RS: Exanthematous drug eruptions. N Engl J Med 366:2492, 2012

Strauss JS, Krowchuk DP, Leyden JJ, et al: Guidelines of care for acne vulgaris management. J Am Acad Dermatol 56(4):651, 2007

Takatsuka Y, Komine M, Ohtsuki M: Pemphigoid gestationis with a complete hydatidiform mole. J Dermatol 39(5):474, 2012

Thiboutot D, Gollnick H, Bettoli V, et al: New insights into the management of acne: an update from the Global Alliance to Improve Outcomes in Acne group. J Am Acad Dermatol 60(5 Suppl):S1, 2009

Van de Wiel A, Hart HC, Flinterman J, et al: Plasma exchange in herpes gestationis. BMJ 281:1041, 1980

Vaughan Jones SA, Hern S, Nelson-Piercy C, et al: A prospective study of 200 women with dermatoses of pregnancy correlating clinical findings with hormonal and immunopathological profiles. Br J Dermatol 141:71, 1999

Weatherhead S, Robson SC, Reynolds NJ: Management of psoriasis in pregnancy. BMJ 334(7605):1218, 2007

Yang YW, Chen CS, Chen YH, et al: Psoriasis and pregnancy outcomes: a nationwide population-based study. J Am Acad Dermatol 64(1):71, 2011

CHAPTER 63

Neoplastic Disorders

Neoplasms are commonly found in pregnant women. Although most are benign, if a malignancy complicates pregnancy, then usual management schemes become problematic. Uterine leiomyomas and ovarian cysts are the most frequently encountered benign neoplasms during pregnancy. Malignancies have an incidence of approximately 1 per 1000 pregnancies (Brewer, 2011). One third are diagnosed prenatally and the others within 12 months of delivery. Some of the more common cancers found in pregnant women are shown in Figure 63-1. Of these, the three most common are breast—1 per 5000 pregnancies, thyroid—1 per 7000, and cervical—1 per 8500 (Smith, 2003). These, along with lymphoma and melanoma, account for 65 percent of cancer cases in pregnancy (Eibye, 2013).

PRINCIPLES OF CANCER THERAPY RELATED TO PREGNANCY

Management of the pregnant woman with cancer poses unique problems related to fetal concerns. Because of these, treatment must be individualized. Considerations include the type and stage of cancer and the desire for pregnancy continuation with the inherent risks associated with modifying or delaying treatment.

Surgery

Operative procedures indicated for cancer include those for diagnosis, staging, or therapy. Fortunately, most procedures that do not interfere with the reproductive tract are well tolerated by both mother and fetus (Chap. 46, p. 927). Although many procedures have classically been deferred until after 12 to 14 weeks' gestation to minimize abortion risks, this probably is not necessary. We are of the opinion that surgery should be performed regardless of gestational age if maternal well-being is imperiled.

Both pregnancy and malignancy are risk factors for venous thromboembolism. There are no guidelines specific for thromboprophylaxis in pregnant women undergoing surgical procedures for cancer. Thus, depending on the complexity of the planned procedure, it seems reasonable to use mechanical prophylaxis compression or pneumatic stockings, low-molecular-weight heparin, or both (Chap. 52, p. 1044). There are general evidenced-based practice guidelines available from the American College of Chest Physicians (Guyatt, 2012).

Diagnostic Imaging

Sonography is a preferred imaging tool during pregnancy when appropriate. In addition, according to the American College of Obstetricians and Gynecologists (2009), most diagnostic radiographic procedures have very low x-ray exposure and should not be delayed if they would directly affect therapy (Chap. 46, p. 932). Computed tomography is useful for imaging extraabdominal tumors, and abdominal shielding usually helps to decrease fetal exposure. Routine magnetic resonance (MR) imaging use is not recommended, and if needed, is used preferentially after the first trimester.

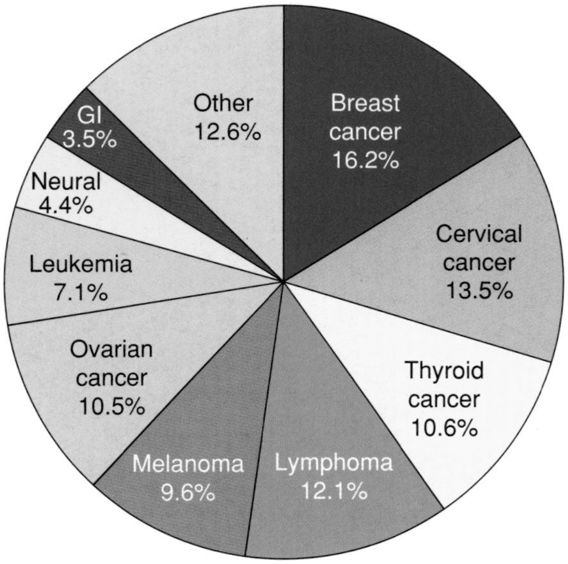

FIGURE 63-1 Proportion of malignancies during pregnancy and within 12 months of delivery in 4.85 million women from the California Cancer Registry. GI = gastrointestinal. (Data from Smith, 2003.)

Gadolinium contrast administered with MR imaging crosses the placenta, resulting in high fetal concentrations. It should not be used in the first trimester and should be used later in pregnancy only when the benefits overwhelmingly outweigh the risks (Kanal, 2007). Some radioisotopes are relatively safe, but positron emission tomography (PET) scanning is usually not performed during pregnancy. Moreover, ^{18}F-FDG (fludeoxyglucose) is concentrated in both breast tissue and milk. Thus, in the puerperium, breast feeding should be discontinued for 72 hours following a procedure (Rizack, 2009).

Radiation Therapy

Therapeutic radiation often results in significant fetal exposure depending on the dose, tumor location, and field size. The most susceptible period is organogenesis, although there is no gestational age considered safe for therapeutic radiation exposure. Adverse effects include cell death, carcinogenesis, and mutagenic changes in future generations (Brent, 1999; Hall, 1991). Characteristic fetal effects are microcephaly and mental retardation, and even late exposure can cause growth restriction and brain damage. Thus, radiotherapy to the maternal abdomen is contraindicated. With some head and neck cancers, however, radiotherapy to supradiaphragmatic areas can be used relatively safely with abdominal shielding. In others, such as breast cancer, significant scatter doses can accrue to the fetus.

Chemotherapy

Various antineoplastic drugs may be given for primary treatment or for adjunctive therapy. Although chemotherapy often improves long-term maternal outcomes, many are reluctant to employ it during pregnancy. As discussed in Chapter 12 (p. 248), fetal concerns include malformations, growth restriction, mental retardation, and the risk of future malignancies. Risks are dependent primarily on fetal age at exposure, and most agents are potentially detrimental given in the first trimester during organogenesis. Indeed, embryonic exposure to cytotoxic drugs may cause major malformations in up to 20 percent of cases (Pavlidis, 2011).

After organogenesis, most antineoplastic drugs are without immediate obvious adverse sequelae (Abdel-Hady, 2012; Cardonick, 2004). Similarly, late mutagenic effects appear limited. Children born to 68 women receiving chemotherapy and who were assessed at 18 months had no excessive adverse effects to their central nervous system, heart, or hearing or to their general health or growth (Amant, 2012b).

Although not always practicable, some recommend that chemotherapy be withheld in the 3 weeks before expected delivery because neutropenia or pancytopenia might cause undue risk for maternal infection or hemorrhage. Another concern is that neonatal hepatic and renal clearance of chemotherapy metabolites is limited (Ko, 2011). For these reasons, chemotherapy is also contraindicated with breast feeding.

Molecular Therapy

Drugs designed to stimulate hemopoiesis are commonly used with cancer treatments. Some of these include the granulocyte colony-stimulating factors filgrastim (Neupogen) and pegfilgrastim (Neulasta). If required in pregnancy, limited data support the safety of these factors (Dale, 2003). Red blood cells can be stimulated by erythropoietin alfa (Procrit), which likely is also safe in pregnancy (Briggs, 2011).

Immunotherapy

Hybridized monoclonal antibodies directed against tumor-specific antigens are designed to treat an ever-increasing list of malignant neoplasms. Some of these drugs are described in the discussion of tumors for which they are used. Little is known regarding their fetal effects, but concerns for teratogenicity by tyrosine kinase inhibitors—for example, imatinib (Gleevec)—have been raised (Ali, 2009).

Fertility and Pregnancy after Cancer Therapy

The number of cancer survivors continues to increase. From the Childhood Cancer Survival Study (CCSS), a fourth of survivors have significant morbidity at 25 years (Diller, 2011). One is that subsequent fertility may be diminished after chemotherapy or radiotherapy, and couples should be counseled regarding potential risks (American Society for Reproductive Medicine, 2013). Guidelines for this counseling have been developed by the American Society of Clinical Oncology (Loren, 2013).

Embryo cryopreservation is standard and widely available, however, other methods are considered investigational and limited to referral centers. Some are oocyte or ovarian cryopreservation, preradiotherapy ovarian transposition, and/or ovarian suppression with gonadotropin-releasing hormone agonists before therapy. Educational materials concerning these methods have been provided by a National Institutes of Health (NIH) interdisciplinary group—the Oncofertility Consortium (Woodruff, 2010). This is available online at: http://oncofertility.northwestern.edu.

Not surprisingly, abdominopelvic radiation impairs subsequent reproductive function (Wo, 2009). Data from the CCSS are informative for women who conceive following cancer therapy. Since the database was established in 1994, 4029 pregnancies have been reported in 1953 women. A number of reports have described increased adverse pregnancy outcomes by type of cancer treatment given. For example, fetuses born to women who had undergone prior pelvic radiation were more likely to have a birthweight < 2500 g (Green, 2002; Robison, 2005). There was a higher rate of preterm birth in cancer survivors—especially those given pelvic radiotherapy—compared with their siblings (Signorello, 2006). In another study of 917 pregnancies, cancer survivors had slightly higher rates of preterm birth and postpartum hemorrhage (Clark, 2007). In yet another study of 1657 women from the CCSS, Signorello and colleagues (2010) reported that uterine or ovarian irradiation significantly increased the risk of stillbirth and neonatal death. One possible explanation for adverse reproductive effects is that radiotherapy, but not chemotherapy, at a young age irreversibly reduces the uterine volume in survivors (Larsen, 2004). Perhaps the most reassuring findings from all of these studies are that fetuses of women who were treated in childhood with radiotherapy did not have significantly increased risks for congenital malformations (Lawrenz, 2012; Winther, 2009).

Placental Metastases

Tumors infrequently metastasize to the placenta. The most common types are malignant melanomas, leukemias, lymphomas, and breast cancer (Al-Adnani, 2007). Placentas from pregnancies in these and all other women with a malignancy should be sent for histological evaluation. Because tumor cells are usually confined within the intervillous spaces, fetal metastases are infrequent. Melanoma is the most common example, and typically fetal metastases are found in the liver or subcutaneous tissue with an 80-percent associated mortality rate (Alexander, 2003; Altman, 2003; Gottschalk, 2009).

REPRODUCTIVE TRACT NEOPLASMS

Benign neoplasms are common in the female reproductive tract and include leiomyomas, ovarian neoplasms, and endocervical polyps. Malignancies of these organs are the most frequent cancers encountered in pregnant women, and of these, cervical cancers make up the majority (Fig. 63-2).

Cervix

Endocervical Polyp

A number of benign, premalignant, and malignant cervical neoplasms are frequently recognized during pregnancy. Endocervical polyps are overgrowths of benign endocervical stroma covered by epithelium. If asymptomatic, these polyps

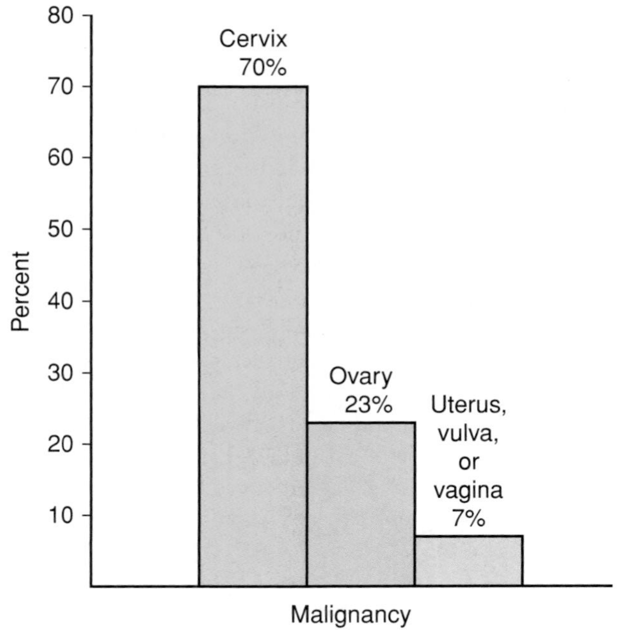

FIGURE 63-2 Frequency of reproductive-tract malignancies in 844 pregnant women. (Data from Haas, 1984; Lutz, 1977; Smith, 2003.)

are usually seen at the time of the initial pelvic examination, although they can cause bleeding at any time. They typically appear as single, red, smooth, elongated fleshy masses of variable size that extend outward from the endocervical canal. Typically benign, they can however be a source of Pap smear results describing atypical glandular cells of undetermined significance—AGUS. And although malignant transformation in these growths is uncommon, polypoid cervical cancers can mimic these (Chin, 2002; Younis, 2010). Thus, most recommend their removal and evaluation. Polyps with a slender stalk are removed by grasping the tumor with ring or polyp forceps. It is then twisted repeatedly about its base to strangulate feeding vessels. With repeated twisting, the base narrows and avulses. Monsel solution, which is ferric subsulfate, can be applied with pressure to the stalk stub for hemostasis. A thick-pedicle polyp may sometimes warrant surgical excision.

Epithelial Neoplasia

Pregnancy provides an opportune time to screen for premalignant and malignant cervical epithelial neoplasia, especially in women without regular access to health care. With prenatal Pap smear screening, the pregnancy status is noted on the requisition form because interpretation may be hindered by pregnancy-associated physiological changes (Connor, 1998). Some changes include glandular epithelial hyperplasia, Arias-Stella reaction, and presence of decidual cells.

Screening guidelines also applicable in pregnant women were updated in 2012 by the American Society for Colposcopy and Cervical Pathology (ASCCP). These include: (1) no screening until age 21, (2) cytology alone every 3 years in those aged 21 to 29 years, and (3) in those older than 30, human papillomavirus (HPV) *and* cytology co-testing every 5 years, or cytology alone every 3 years. Importantly, these broad guidelines do not cover women in high-risk populations who may need more intensive screening. Examples include diethylstilbestrol (DES)-exposed women, cervical cancer survivors, and the immunocompromised (Saslow, 2012).

Oncogenic Human Papillomaviruses. Certain serovars of HPV are associated with high-grade intraepithelial lesions and invasive cancer. Some of these high-risk viruses—HPV types 16, 18, 31, 35, 45, 51, 52, and 56—may have an increased incidence in pregnant compared with nonpregnant women (Fife, 1996). Cotesting for such high-risk serotypes at the time of the Pap test is now incorporated into the recent screening guidelines for women 30 years and older. Cells can be collected directly into liquid-based cytology medium, namely, PreservCyt Solution of the ThinPrep Pap Test. Additionally, the cobas HPV Test and Digene HC2 HPV DNA test also allow collection into a specific collection medium if traditional cytology is performed.

HPV Vaccination. The clear link between HPV infection and cervical neoplasia has prompted development of two Food and Drug Administration-approved vaccines. These are available for girls and women aged 9 to 26 years. The quadrivalent HPV-6/11/16/18 vaccine (Gardasil) and the bivalent HPV-16/18 vaccine (Cervarix) decrease the incidence of high-grade dysplasia, and thus, cervical carcinoma (American College of Obstetricians and Gynecologists, 2012b; FUTURE II Study Group, 2007; Paavonen, 2009).

Vaccination is not recommended during pregnancy, and contraception during the series is recommended by the American College of Obstetricians and Gynecologists (2010) and the Centers for Disease Control and Prevention (2010). That said, both vaccines are considered safe and are not associated with higher rates of adverse pregnancy outcomes if conception occurs during the series (Dana, 2009; Descamps, 2009; Garland, 2009). Completion of the series should be delayed until after delivery. Both of these inactivated vaccines can be given postpartum in a typical regimen of three doses, with injections given at 0, at 1 to 2, and at 6 months. The vaccines are safe for use in breast-feeding women.

Abnormal Cytological Results. The incidence of abnormal cervical cytology during pregnancy is at least as high as that reported for nonpregnant women. Abnormal cytological findings and their suggested management according to consensus guidelines are summarized in Table 63-1. Many of these cytological abnormalities should prompt colposcopy to exclude invasive cancer. Accordingly, lesions suspicious for high-grade disease or cancer should undergo biopsy (American College of Obstetricians and Gynecologists, 2013a). These may actively bleed because of hyperemia, but this can be stopped with Monsel paste and pressure, silver nitrate application, vaginal packing, or suture.

Unsatisfactory colposcopic evaluation is less common during pregnancy because the transformation zone is better exposed due to cervical eversion. With unsatisfactory visualization, colposcopy is repeated in 6 to 8 weeks, during which time the squamocolumnar junction will further evert (Randall, 2009). Once satisfactory examination is possible and advanced disease is excluded, additional colposcopic and cytological

TABLE 63-1. American Society for Colposcopy and Cervical Pathology (ASCCP) Guidelines for Initial Management of Epithelial Cell Abnormalities in Pregnancy

Abnormality	Adults	Adolescents[a]
ASC-US		Repeat cytology 6 wk pp
HPV positive	Colposcopy 6 wk pp	
HPV negative	Repeat cytology 6 wk pp	
HPV unknown	Repeat cytology 6 wk pp	
LSIL	Colposcopy during pregnancy (preferred) May defer until 6 wk pp	Repeat cytology 6 wk pp
ASC-H HSIL SCCA AGC AIS adenoCA	Colposcopy during pregnancy[b]	

[a]Adolescents = < 21 years.
[b]Endocervical curettage and endometrial sampling are contraindicated in pregnancy.
adenoCA = adenocarcinoma; AGC = atypical glandular cells; AIS = adenocarcinoma in situ; ASC-H = atypical squamous cells, cannot exclude high-grade squamous intraepithelial lesion; ASC-US = atypical squamous cells of undetermined significance; HPV = human papillomavirus; HSIL = high-grade squamous intraepithelial lesion; LSIL = low-grade squamous intraepithelial lesion; SCCA = squamous cell carcinoma.
Adapted from Wright, 2007a; American College of Obstetricians and Gynecologists, 2013a.
Table summary courtesy of Drs. Claudia L. Werner and William F. Griffith.

examinations during pregnancy are not encouraged. After delivery, repeat cytology and colposcopy should generally be delayed for at least 6 weeks to allow reparative healing.

Cervical Intraepithelial Neoplasia. Women with histologically confirmed intraepithelial neoplasia during pregnancy may be allowed to deliver vaginally, with further evaluation planned after delivery. For those with cervical intraepithelial neoplasia (CIN) 1, the recommended management is reevaluation postpartum. For those with CIN 2 or 3 in which invasive disease has been excluded, or with advanced pregnancy, repeat colposcopic and cytological evaluations are performed at intervals no more frequent than 12 weeks. Repeat biopsy is recommended if appearance of the lesion worsens or if cytology suggests invasive cancer. Alternatively, deferring reevaluation until at least 6 weeks postpartum is acceptable (Wright, 2007b).

Regression of CIN lesions is common during pregnancy or postpartum. In a study of 1079 pregnant women with cervical dysplasia in which biopsy correlated with colposcopic findings, 61 percent reverted to normal postpartum (Fader, 2010). In another study, Yost and colleagues (1999) reported postpartum regression in 70 percent of women with CIN 2 and CIN 3 lesions. And although 7 percent of women with CIN 2 lesions progressed to CIN 3, none progressed to invasive carcinoma. In another study of 77 women with carcinoma in situ (CIS) diagnosed during pregnancy, a third had postpartum regression, two thirds had persistent CIS, and only two women had microinvasive cancer on cone biopsy after delivery (Ackermann, 2006).

Adenocarcinoma in situ (AIS) is managed similarly to CIN 3 (Dunton, 2008). Thus, unless invasive cancer is identified, treatment of AIS is not recommended until 6 weeks postpartum (Wright, 2007b).

Cervical Conization. If invasive epithelial lesions are suspected, conization is indicated and may be done with loop electrosurgical excisional procedure (LEEP) or by cold knife conization. If possible, conization is avoided in pregnancy because of increased risks for abortion, membrane rupture, hemorrhage, and preterm delivery. The epithelium and underlying stroma within the endocervical canal cannot be extensively excised without the risk of membrane rupture. Residual disease is common. Of 376 conization procedures during pregnancy, Hacker and colleagues (1982) found residual neoplasia in 43 percent of subsequent specimens. In addition, nearly 10 percent of 180 pregnant women required transfusion after conization (Averette, 1970).

Women with CIN treated *before* pregnancy may encounter pregnancy complications. Cicatricial cervical stenosis is uncommon, but it may follow cervical trauma from conization, the loop electrosurgical excision procedure (LEEP), and laser surgery. Cervical stenosis almost always yields during labor. A so-called conglutinated cervix may undergo almost complete effacement without dilation, with the presenting part separated from the vagina by only a thin layer of cervical tissue. Dilatation usually promptly follows pressure with a fingertip, although manual dilatation or cruciate incisions may be required.

For decades, cold-knife conization has been associated with cervical incompetence and preterm birth. However, the relationship between preterm birth and LEEP continues to be debated, with some studies showing increased risk, but others not (Castanon, 2012; Jakobsson, 2009; Samson, 2005; Werner, 2010). An important study confounder is the increased risk of preterm birth in women with CIN compared with the general population even if they have not undergone an excisional procedure (Bruinsma, 2007; Shanbhag, 2009).

Invasive Cervical Cancer

The incidence of invasive cervical carcinoma has dramatically declined and approximates 1 in 8500 pregnancies in the United States (Pettersson, 2010; Smith, 2003). The diagnosis is confirmed with biopsies taken during colposcopy, with conization, or from a grossly abnormal lesion. Of the histological types, squamous cell carcinomas comprises 75 percent of all cervical cancers, whereas adenocarcinomas account for 20 to 25 percent. Cancers may appear as exophytic or endophytic growth; as a polypoid mass, papillary tissue, or barrel-shaped cervix; as a cervical ulceration or granular mass; or as necrotic tissue. A watery, purulent, foul, or bloody discharge may also be present. Biopsy with Tischler forceps is warranted for suspicious lesions.

Cervical cancer is staged clinically, and 70 percent of cases that are diagnosed in pregnancy are stage I (Morice, 2012). Physiological pregnancy changes may impede accurate staging, and the extent of cancer is more likely to be underestimated in pregnant women (Oto, 2007). Specifically, induration of the broad ligament base, which characterizes tumor spread beyond the cervix, may be less prominent due to cervical, paracervical, and parametrial pregnancy-induced softening. Staging is modified and typically incorporates findings from pelvic examination and from renal sonography, chest radiography, cystoscopy, proctoscopy, and perhaps cone biopsy. Although MR imaging is not formally considered for clinical staging, it can be used without gadolinium contrast, ideally after the first trimester, to ascertain disease involvement of the urinary tract and lymph nodes (Fig. 63-3).

Management and Prognosis. Treatment of cervical cancer in pregnant women is individualized and depends on the clinical stage, fetal age, and individual desire to continue pregnancy (Hunter, 2008). Stage IA1 is termed microinvasive disease and describes lesions with deepest invasion ≤ 3 mm and widest lateral extension ≤ 7 mm (FIGO Committee on Gynecologic Oncology, 2009b). If diagnosed by cone biopsy, treatment follows guidelines similar to those for intraepithelial disease. In general, continuation of pregnancy and vaginal delivery are considered safe, and definitive therapy is reserved until 6 weeks postpartum.

Truly invasive cancer demands relatively prompt therapy. During the first half of pregnancy, immediate treatment is advised by most, but this depends on the decision whether to continue pregnancy. With diagnosis during the latter half of pregnancy, most agree that pregnancy can safely be continued not only until fetal viability is reached, but also until fetal lung

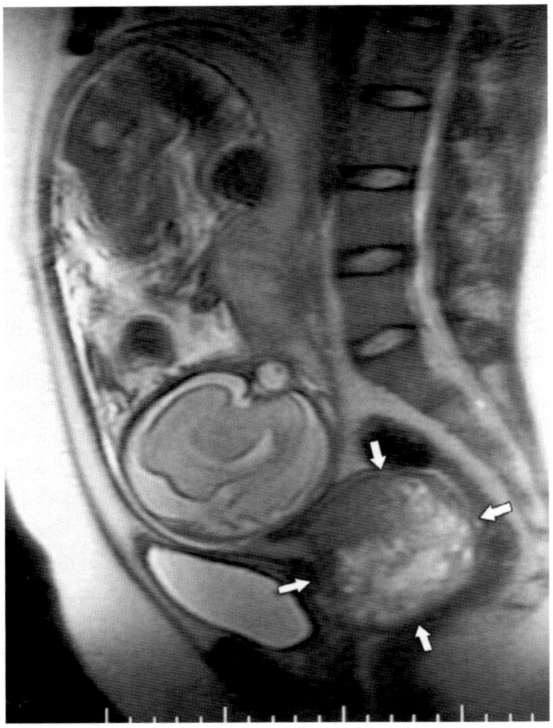

FIGURE 63-3 Sagittal T-2 weighted magnetic resonance image of a gravid uterus at 32 weeks' gestation with a large cervical carcinoma (*arrows*).

maturity is attained (Greer, 1989). In two studies with a total of 40 women past 20 weeks with either stage I or stage IIA carcinoma, it was concluded that delayed treatment was reasonable in women without bulky lesions (Takushi, 2002; van Vliet, 1998). Another option is to complete staging using laparoscopic lymphadenectomy and to delay treatment if metastases are excluded (Alouini, 2008; Favero, 2010). In a recent metaanalysis, neoadjuvant chemotherapy with platinum derivatives was found to be promising for treatment in pregnancy (Zagouri, 2013).

Although surgical therapy and radiation are equally effective, radical hysterectomy plus pelvic lymphadenectomy is the preferred treatment for invasive carcinoma in most women with stage I and early stage IIA lesions (American College of Obstetricians and Gynecologists, 2010a). Before 20 weeks, hysterectomy is usually performed with the fetus in situ. In later pregnancy, however, hysterotomy is often performed first. Radiotherapy for cervical cancer destroys ovarian and possibly sexual function, and frequently causes intestinal and urinary tract injury. In 49 women with pregnancy-associated stage IB cancer, there was a 30-percent severe complication rate from radiotherapy compared with only 7 percent with surgery (Nisker, 1983).

Although less commonly selected, fertility-preserving procedures for early-stage cervical cancers have been investigated. Ungár and colleagues (2006) performed abdominal radical trachelectomy before 20 weeks for stage IB1 carcinoma in five pregnant women. Yahata and associates (2008) treated four women at 16 to 23 weeks for stage IA1 adenocarcinoma with laser conization, and all delivered at term. Van Calsteren and coworkers (2008) reported similar success in a woman at 8 weeks with stage IB2 adenocarcinoma.

Radiotherapy is given for more advanced-stage cancer. External beam radiation is given for treatment early in pregnancy, and then if spontaneous abortion does not ensue, curettage is performed. During the second trimester, spontaneous abortion may not promptly occur and may necessitate hysterotomy in up to a fourth of cases.

Stage-for-stage, the survival rate for invasive cervical carcinoma is similar in pregnant and nonpregnant women (Sood, 1998). In a case-control study of 44 women with pregnancy-associated cervical cancer, the overall 5-year survival rate was approximately 80 percent in both pregnant women and nonpregnant controls (Van der Vange, 1995).

Delivery. Any adverse prognostic effects that vaginal delivery through a cancerous cervix might have are unknown. For this reason, the mode of delivery is controversial, especially for small, early-stage lesions. In some cases of bulky or friable lesions, there may be significant hemorrhage with vaginal delivery. Also, recurrences in the episiotomy scar, which result from tumor cells apparently "seeding" the episiotomy, have been reported (Goldman, 2003). Thus, most favor cesarean delivery and use a classical hysterotomy incision to avoid the risk of cutting through tumor.

Pregnancy after Radical Trachelectomy. There is growing experience with pregnancy in women who have previously undergone fertility-sparing radical trachelectomy for stage IB1 and IB2 cervical cancer before conception. During the typically vaginal procedure, the cervix is amputated at the level of the internal os, and a permanent-suture cerclage is placed around the isthmus for support in future pregnancies. The uterine isthmus is then reconstructed to the vagina. Because of the permanent cerclage, a classical cesarean incision is required for delivery.

Shepherd and colleagues (2006) presented outcomes for 123 such women cared for at their institution. Of 63 women who attempted pregnancy, 19 had 28 live births. All had classical cesarean deliveries, and a fourth were before 32 weeks. Similar findings were reported by Kim (2012) and Park (2014) and their colleagues.

Uterus

Leiomyomas

Also known as myomas and somewhat erroneously called *fibroids*, uterine leiomyomas are common benign smooth muscle tumors. Their incidence during pregnancy is approximately 2 percent, and the cited range depends on the frequency of routine sonography and population characteristics (Qidwai, 2006; Stout, 2010). For example, in a study of 4271 women, Laughlin and coworkers (2009) reported that first-trimester leiomyoma prevalence was highest in black women—18 percent—and lowest in whites—8 percent.

Leiomyomas vary in location and may develop as submucous, subserosal, or intramural growths. Less frequently, these develop in the cervix or broad ligament. Some become parasitic and their blood supply is derived from adjacent structures such as the highly vascularized omentum. In the rare manifestation of leiomyomatosis peritonealis disseminata, numerous

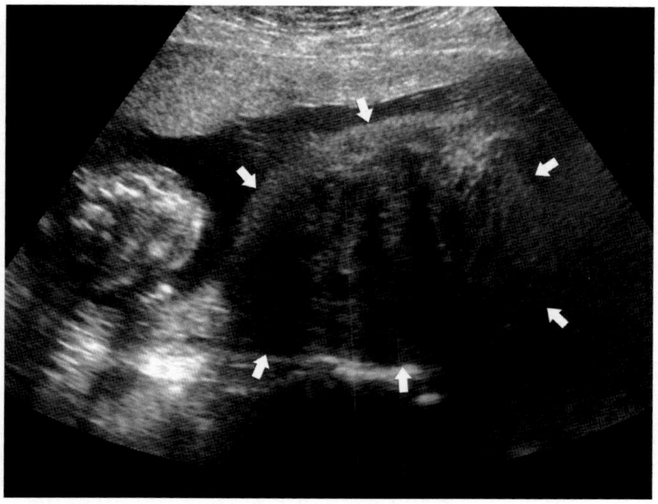

FIGURE 63-4 Sonogram of a pregnant uterus with a large uterine leiomyoma. The heterogeneous mass (*arrows*) lies beside the fetus (seen in cross section) and has the classic appearance of a leiomyoma in pregnancy. The placenta is located anteriorly, and the mass originates from the posterior lower uterine segment and occupies more than half of the total uterine volume.

subperitoneal benign smooth muscle tumors may appear similar to disseminated carcinomatosis. The tumors are likely caused by estrogen stimulation of multicentric subcoelomic mesenchymal cells to become smooth-muscle cells (Bulun, 2013). In their review of 45 cases, Lashgari and colleagues (1994) found that half were discovered during pregnancy. Often, these tumors regress after pregnancy.

The stimulatory effects of pregnancy on myoma growth are unpredictable and can be impressive. These tumors respond differently in individual women and may grow, regress, or remain unchanged in size during pregnancy (Laughlin, 2009; Neiger, 2006).

Especially during pregnancy, myomas can be confused with other adnexal masses, and sonographic imaging is indispensable (Fig. 63-4). In women in whom sonographic findings are unclear, MR imaging performed after the first trimester may be necessary (Torashima, 1997). Once diagnosed, leiomyomas do not require surveillance with serial sonography unless associated complications are anticipated.

Symptoms. Most leiomyomas are asymptomatic, but acute or chronic pain or pressure may develop. For chronic pain secondary to large tumor size, nonnarcotic analgesic drugs may be given. More acutely, in some cases, myomas outgrow their blood supply and hemorrhagic infarction follows, which is termed red or carneous degeneration. Clinically, there is acute focal abdominal pain and tenderness, and sometimes a low-grade fever and leukocytosis is noted. As such, tumor degeneration may be difficult to differentiate from appendicitis, placental abruption, ureteral stone, or pyelonephritis. Sonographic imaging may be helpful, but close observation is requisite because an infarcted myoma is essentially a diagnosis of exclusion. In some women, preterm labor is stimulated by associated inflammation.

Treatment is analgesic medications, and most often, symptoms abate within a few days. If further treatment is given to forestall preterm labor, then close observation to exclude a septic cause is imperative. Although surgery is rarely necessary during pregnancy, myomectomy in highly selected cases has resulted in good outcomes (Celik, 2002; De Carolis, 2001). Most of 23 reported women were 14 to 20 weeks, and in almost half, surgery was performed because of pain. In some, an intramural leiomyoma was in contact with the implantation site. Except for one loss immediately following surgery at 19 weeks, most underwent cesarean delivery later at term.

Occasionally, pedunculated subserosal myomas will undergo torsion with subsequent painful necrosis. In such cases, laparoscopy or laparotomy can be used to ligate the stalk and resect the necrotic tumor. That said, we are of the opinion that surgery should be limited to tumors with a discrete pedicle that can be easily clamped and ligated.

Pregnancy Complications. Myomas are associated with a number of complications including preterm labor, placental abruption, fetal malpresentation, obstructed labor, cesarean delivery, and postpartum hemorrhage (Klatsky, 2008; Qidwai, 2006; Sheiner, 2004). In a review of pregnancy outcomes in 2065 women with leiomyomas, Coronado and coworkers (2000) reported that placental abruption and breech presentation were each increased fourfold; first-trimester bleeding and dysfunctional labor, twofold; and cesarean delivery, sixfold. Salvador and associates (2002) reported an eightfold increased second-trimester abortion risk in these women but found that genetic amniocentesis did not increase this risk.

The two factors most important in determining morbidity in pregnancy are leiomyoma size and location (Shavell, 2012). The proximity of myomas to the placental implantation site is also a factor. Specifically, abortion, preterm labor, placental abruption, and postpartum hemorrhage all are increased if the placenta is adjacent to or implanted over a leiomyoma. Tumors in the cervix or lower uterine segment may obstruct labor, as did the one shown in Figure 63-5. Despite these complications,

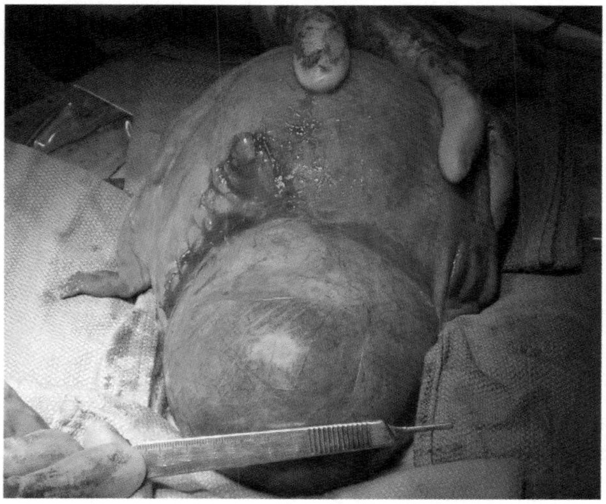

FIGURE 63-5 Cesarean delivery performed because of a large leiomyoma in the lower uterine segment. A classical vertical uterine incision, seen to the left of the myoma, was required for delivery of the fetus.

Qidwai and colleagues (2006) reported a 70-percent vaginal delivery rate in women in whom myomas were ≥ 10 cm. These data argue against empirical cesarean delivery for leiomyomas, and we allow a trial of labor unless myomas clearly obstruct the birth canal. If cesarean delivery is indicated, myomas are generally left alone unless they cause recalcitrant bleeding. An important caveat is that cesarean hysterectomy may be technically difficult because of lateral ureteral displacement by the tumors.

Bleeding due to myomas may develop during pregnancy from any of several factors. Especially common is bleeding with miscarriage, preterm labor, or placenta previa and abruption. Much less frequently, bleeding may result from a submucous myoma that has prolapsed from the uterus and into the cervix or vagina. In these unusual cases, although heavy or persistent bleeding may require earlier intervention, the stalk can be ligated vaginally near term if accessible to avoid tumor avulsion during delivery.

Fortunately, myomas rarely become infected (Genta, 2001). This is most frequent postpartum, especially if the tumor is located immediately adjacent to the implantation site (Lin, 2002). They also may become infected with an associated septic abortion and myoma perforation by a sound, dilator, or curette.

Fertility Considerations. Despite the relatively high prevalence of myomas in young women, it is not clear whether they diminish fertility, other than by possibly causing miscarriage as discussed in Chapter 18 (p. 359). In a review of 11 studies, Pritts (2001) concluded that submucous myomas did significantly affect fertility. He also found that hysteroscopic myomectomy improved infertility and early miscarriage rates in these women. Infertility-related myomas in other locations may require laparoscopy or laparotomy for excision.

Some of these methods of treatment for infertility may affect successful pregnancies. For example, after myomectomy, there is concern for uterine rupture before and during labor (American College of Obstetricians and Gynecologists, 2012a). Management is individualized, and review of the prior operative report is prudent. If resection resulted in a defect into or immediately adjacent to the endometrial cavity, then cesarean delivery is usually done before labor begins.

Although less effective than surgery, uterine artery embolization of myomas has also been used to treat infertility or myoma symptoms (Mara, 2008). Women so treated have increased rates of miscarriage, cesarean delivery, and postpartum hemorrhage (Homer, 2010). At this time, the Society of Interventional Radiology (Stokes, 2010) considers myoma embolization relatively contraindicated in women who plan future pregnancies.

Endometriosis and Adenomyosis

Rarely do endometriomas cause problems in pregnancy. If they are identified sonographically, they can be resected if cesarean delivery is performed. With vaginal delivery, endometriotic tumors or cysts may be removed after the puerperium or followed clinically depending on symptoms and cyst characteristics (Levine, 2010). Occasionally, endometriosis can develop after delivery from endometrial implants within abdominal incisions made at cesarean delivery or within episiotomy scars (Bumpers, 2002).

Adenomyosis is traditionally found in older women. Its acquisition may be at least partially related to disruption of the endometrial-myometrial border during sharp curettage for abortion (Curtis, 2002). Although problems during pregnancy are rare, in an 80-year review, Azziz (1986) reported concurrent adenomyosis to be associated with uterine rupture, ectopic pregnancy, uterine atony, and placenta previa.

Endometrial Carcinoma

This estrogen-dependent neoplasia is usually found in women older than 40 years. Thus, it is seen only rarely with pregnancy. Hannuna and colleagues (2009) found 27 cases that were identified during pregnancy or within the first 4 months postpartum. Most were found in first-trimester curettage specimens.

These are usually early-stage well-differentiated adenocarcinomas for which treatment consists primarily of total abdominal hysterectomy and bilateral salpingo-oophorectomy. Much less commonly, to preserve future fertility, curettage with or without postprocedural progestational therapy has been used for the rare patient with cancer identified in a miscarriage curettage specimen (Schammel, 1998).

Many more studies describe a conservative approach for well-selected *nonpregnant* women diagnosed with endometrial cancer who wish to preserve fertility. In one study of 13 women treated with progestins for early-stage well-differentiated adenocarcinoma, nine had liveborn infants, and four of six women with a recurrence responded to another course of therapy (Gotlieb, 2003). Similar outcomes were described in 12 women by Niwa and associates (2005) and in 21 women by Signorelli and coworkers (2009). Despite these acceptable pregnancy rates, recurrences and death have been reported, and conservative management is not considered standard (Erkanli, 2010).

Ovary

Ovarian masses found during pregnancy are relatively common, and the reported incidences are population- and investigation-dependent. Factors include whether studies are referral or primary care sources, the frequency of prenatal sonography, and what size constitutes a "mass." It is thus not surprising that the incidence has been reported as 1 in 100 to 1 in 2000 pregnancies (Whitecar, 1999; Zanetta, 2003). Of ovarian malignancies, the absolute incidence in the California Cancer Registry was 1 in 19,000 pregnancies (Smith, 2003).

The most frequent types of ovarian masses are corpus luteum cysts, endometriomas, benign cystadenomas, and mature cystic teratomas, colloquially termed dermoids. Because pregnant women are usually young, malignant tumors and those of low malignant potential are proportionately uncommon and vary from 4 to 13 percent (Hoffman, 2007; Sherard, 2003). Our experiences from Parkland Hospital are similar to those reported by Leiserowitz and colleagues (2006), who found that 1 percent of 9375 ovarian masses were frankly malignant and that another 1 percent was of low malignant potential.

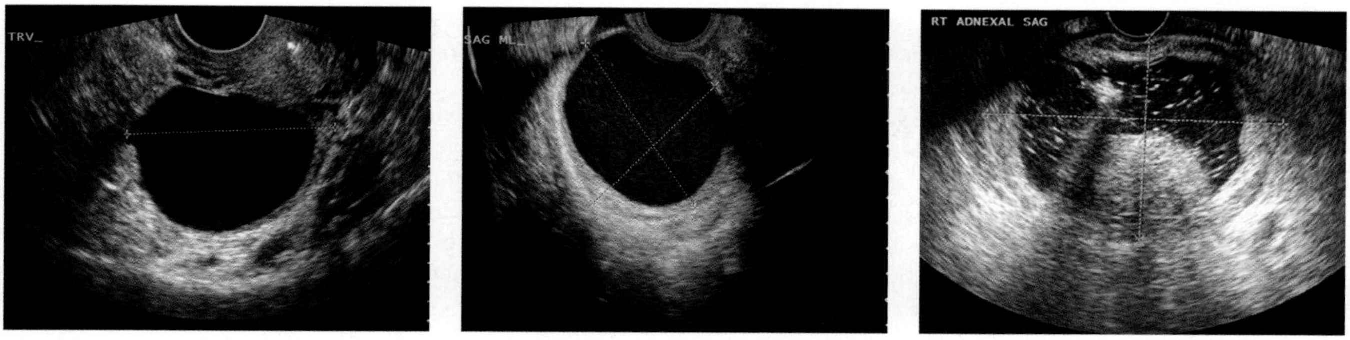

A B C

FIGURE 63-6 Sonographic characteristics of common adnexal masses in pregnancy. **A.** A simple anechoic cyst with smooth walls is characteristic of a physiological corpus luteum cyst or benign cystadenoma. **B.** Cystic structure with diffuse internal low-level echoes suggestive of an endometrioma or hemorrhagic corpus luteum. **C.** Mature cystic teratoma appears as an adnexal cyst (*marked by calipers*) with accentuated lines and dots that represent hair in both longitudinal and transverse planes. At the central inferior aspect of this cyst, a mural nodule—Rokitansky protuberance—is seen. These typically rounded protuberances range in size from 1 to 4 cm, they are predominantly hyperechoic, and they create an acute angle with the cyst wall. Although not seen here, fat-fluid levels are often identified with cystic teratomas. (Image contributed by Dr. Elysia Moschos.)

Most ovarian masses are asymptomatic in pregnant women. Some cause pressure or chronic pain, and acute abdominal pain may be due to torsion, rupture, or hemorrhage. Seldom is blood loss significant enough to cause hypovolemia.

Sonography

Many ovarian masses are detected during routine prenatal sonography or during imaging done for other indications, including evaluation of symptoms. The typical sonographic appearance of these masses is shown in Figure 63-6. In some instances, MR imaging can be used to evaluate complicated anatomy (American College of Obstetricians and Gynecologists, 2013b).

Tumor Markers

Cancer antigen 125 (CA125) levels are frequently elevated with ovarian malignancy. Importantly, concentrations in early pregnancy and early puerperium are normally elevated, possibly from the decidua (Aslam, 2000; Haga, 1986; Spitzer, 1998). From the second trimester until term, levels are not normally higher than those in the nonpregnant woman (Appendix, p. 1289). Other tumor markers that have not been proven for diagnosis or posttreatment surveillance in pregnancy include OVA1, human chorionic gonadotropin (hCG), alpha-fetoprotein, and inhibins A and B (Liu, 2011). Of these, OVA1 is a biomarker blood test that measures five analytes, one of which is CA125.

Complications

The two most common complications of any ovarian mass are torsion and hemorrhage. Torsion usually causes acute constant or episodic lower abdominal pain that frequently is accompanied by nausea and vomiting. Sonography often aids the diagnosis. With color Doppler, presence of an ovarian mass with absent flow strongly correlates with torsion. However, minimal or early twisting may compromise only venous flow, thus leaving arterial supply intact. If torsion is suspected, laparoscopy or laparotomy is warranted. Contrary to prior teaching, adnexectomy is generally unnecessary to avoid clot release, thus, most recommend attempts at untwisting (McGovern, 1999; Zweizig, 1993). With a salvageable ovary, within minutes, congestion is relieved, and ovarian volume and cyanosis diminish. If cyanosis persists, however, then removal of the infarcted adnexa is typically indicated.

If the adnexa is healthy, there are options. First, neoplasms are resected. However, ovarian cystectomy in an ischemic, edematous ovary may be technically difficult, and adnexectomy may be necessary. Second, unilateral or bilateral oophoropexy has been described to minimize the risk of repeated torsion (Djavadian, 2004; Germain, 1996). Techniques described include shortening of the uteroovarian ligament or fixing the uteroovarian ligament to the posterior uterus, the lateral pelvic wall, or the round ligament (Fuchs, 2010; Weitzman, 2008).

The most common case of ovarian hemorrhage follows rupture of a corpus luteum cyst. If the diagnosis is certain and symptoms abate, then observation and surveillance is usually sufficient. Concern for ongoing bleeding will typically prompt surgical evaluation. If the corpus luteum is removed before 10 weeks' gestation, progestational support is recommended to maintain the pregnancy. Suitable regimens include: (1) micronized progesterone (Prometrium) 200 or 300 mg orally once daily; (2) 8-percent progesterone vaginal gel (Crinone) one premeasured applicator vaginally daily plus micronized progesterone 100 or 200 mg orally once daily; or (3) intramuscular 17-hydroxyprogesterone caproate, 150 mg. For the last, if given between 8 and 10 weeks' gestation, only one injection is required immediately after surgery. If the corpus luteum is excised between 6 and 8 weeks' gestation, then two additional doses should be given 1 and 2 weeks after the first.

Management of an Asymptomatic Adnexal Mass

Because most of these are incidental findings, management considerations include whether resection is necessary and its timing. A cystic benign-appearing mass that is < 5 cm often requires no additional antepartum surveillance. Early in pregnancy, this is likely a corpus luteum cyst, which typically resolves by the early second trimester. For cysts ≥ 10 cm, because of the substantial risk of malignancy, torsion, or labor obstruction, surgical removal is reasonable. Tumors between 5 and 10 cm should be carefully evaluated by sonography along with color Doppler and possibly MR imaging. If they have a simple cystic appearance, these cysts can be managed expectantly with sonographic surveillance (Schmeler, 2005; Zanetta, 2003). Resection is done if cysts grow, begin to display malignant qualities, or becomes symptomatic. However, if there are sonographic characteristics that suggest a cancer—thick septa, nodules, papillary excrescences, or solid components—then immediate resection is indicated (Caspi, 2000; Fleischer, 1990). Approximately 1 in 1000 pregnant women undergoes surgical exploration for an adnexal mass (Boulay, 1998). In general, we plan resection at 14 to 20 weeks because most masses that will regress will have done so by this time. Those with classic findings of endometrioma or mature cystic teratoma may be resected postpartum or during cesarean for obstetrical indications. Importantly, in any instance in which cancer is strongly suspected, the American College of Obstetricians and Gynecologists (2011) recommends consultation with a gynecologic oncologist.

Pregnancy-Related Ovarian Tumors

A group of adnexal masses result directly from the stimulating effects of various pregnancy hormones on ovarian stroma. These include pregnancy luteoma, hyperreactio luteinalis, and ovarian hyperstimulation syndrome.

Pregnancy Luteoma. These are rare, benign, ovarian neoplasms that are thought to arise from luteinized stromal cells and that classically cause elevated testosterone levels (Irving, 2011). Up to 25 percent of affected women will be virilized, and of these affected women, approximately half of their female fetuses will have some degree of virilization. Fortunately, most mothers and their fetuses are unaffected by the hyperandrogenemia because the placenta rapidly converts androgens to estrogens (Kaňová, 2011).

In some cases, an adnexal mass along with maternal virilization will prompt sonography and measurement of testosterone and CA125 levels. Luteomas range in size from microscopic to greater than 20 cm. They appear as solid tumors, may be multiple or bilateral, and may be complex because of hemorrhagic areas (Choi, 2000). Concerns for malignancy may be further investigated by MR imaging (Kao, 2005; Tannus, 2009).

Total testosterone levels are increased, but with the caveat that levels in normal pregnancy can be substantially elevated (Appendix, p. 1291). Levels of CA125 antigen tumor marker are normal with a pregnancy luteoma, and significantly elevated levels indicate another cause. Differential diagnoses are primary ovarian cancer or metastatic disease and include granulosa cell tumors, thecomas, Sertoli-Leydig cell tumors, Leydig cell tumors, stromal hyperthecosis, and hyperreactio luteinalis.

Generally, luteomas do not require surgical intervention unless there is torsion, rupture, or hemorrhage (Masarie, 2010). These tumors spontaneously regress during the first few months postpartum, and androgen levels drop precipitously during the first 2 weeks following delivery (Wang, 2005). Lactation may be delayed a week or so by hyperandrogenemia (Clement, 1993; Dahl, 2008). Recurrence in subsequent pregnancies is rare.

Hyperreactio Luteinalis. In this condition, one or both ovaries develop multiple large theca-lutein cysts, typically after the first trimester. Cysts are caused by luteinization of the follicular theca interna layer, and most are in response to stimulation by exceptionally high hCG levels (Russell, 2009). For this reason, they are more common with gestational trophoblastic disease, twins, fetal hydrops, and other conditions with increased placental mass. Similar to luteoma, maternal virilization develops in approximately a third of women, but there have been no reports of fetal virilization (Kaňová, 2011).

These ovarian tumors appear sonographically to have a "spoke wheel" pattern (Fig. 20-3, p. 399). If the diagnosis is confident, and unless complicated by torsion or hemorrhage, surgical intervention is not required. These masses resolve after delivery.

Ovarian Hyperstimulation Syndrome. This rare event is typified by multiple ovarian follicular cysts accompanied by increased capillary permeability. It most often is a complication of ovulation-induction therapy for infertility, although it rarely may develop in an otherwise normal pregnancy. Its etiopathogenesis is thought to involve hCG stimulation of vascular endothelial growth factor (VEGF) expression in granulosa-lutein cells (Soares, 2008). This causes increased vascular permeability that can lead to hypovolemia with ascites, pleural or pericardial effusion, acute kidney injury, and hypercoagulability. There is a clinical spectrum with symptoms that may include abdominal distention, rapid weight gain, dyspnea, and progressive hypovolemia. Serious complications are renal dysfunction, adult respiratory distress syndrome, ovarian rupture with hemorrhage, and thromboembolism.

Although most cases of ovarian hyperstimulation are associated with in vitro fertilization, increasing hCG levels from pregnancy can worsen the syndrome (Chen, 2012). Detailed guidelines for management have been outlined by the American Society for Reproductive Medicine (2008). Treatment is primarily supportive with attention to maintaining vascular volume and thromboprophylaxis.

Ovarian Cancer

Malignancies of the ovary are most common in older women and are the leading cause of death in all women from genital-tract cancers (American Cancer Society, 2012). That said, the incidence of ovarian malignancy during pregnancy ranges from 1 in 20,000 to 50,000 births (Palmer, 2009; Eibye, 2013; Smith, 2003). Fortunately, 75 percent of these found in pregnancy are early-stage malignancies with a 5-year survival rate between 70 and 90 percent (Brewer, 2011). The types of malignancy are also markedly different in pregnant women compared with those in older women. In pregnant women, these are, in decreasing order of frequency, germ cell and sex cord-stromal tumors, low malignant potential tumors, and last, epithelial tumors (Morice, 2012).

Pregnancy apparently does not alter the prognosis of most ovarian malignancies. Management is similar to that for nonpregnant women, with the usual proviso that it may be modified depending on gestational age. Thus, if frozen section histopathological analysis verifies malignancy, then surgical staging is done with careful inspection of all accessible peritoneal and visceral surfaces (Giuntoli, 2006; Yazigi, 1988). Peritoneal washings are taken for cytology; biopsies are taken from the diaphragmatic surface and peritoneum; omentectomy is done; and biopsies are taken from pelvic and infrarenal para-aortic lymph nodes. Depending on the uterine size, some of these components, especially lymphadenectomy, may not be technically feasible.

If there is advanced disease, bilateral adnexectomy and omentectomy will decrease most tumor burden. In early pregnancy, hysterectomy and aggressive surgical debulking procedures may be elected. In other cases, minimal debulking as described is done and the operation terminated. In some cases of aggressive or large-volume disease, chemotherapy can be given during pregnancy while awaiting pulmonary maturation. As discussed on page 1227, monitoring maternal CA125 serum levels during chemotherapy is not accurate in pregnancy (Aslam, 2000; Morice, 2012).

Adnexal Cysts

Paratubal and paroovarian cysts are either distended remnants of the paramesonephric ducts or are mesothelial inclusion cysts. Although most are ≤ 3 cm, they occasionally attain worrisome dimensions (Genadry, 1977). Their reported incidence is influenced by size, but one autopsy series in nonpregnant women cited this to be 5 percent (Dorum, 2005). The most common paramesonephric cyst is the hydatid of Morgagni, which is pedunculated and typically dangles from one of the fimbria. These cysts infrequently cause complications and are most commonly identified at the time of cesarean delivery or puerperal sterilization, at which time they can simply be drained or excised. Neoplastic paraovarian cysts are rare, histologically resemble tumors of ovarian origin, and rarely are of borderline potential or frankly malignant (Honore, 1980; Korbin, 1998).

Vulva and Vagina

Preinvasive Disease

In young women, vulvar intraepithelial neoplasia (VIN) and vaginal intraepithelial neoplasia (VAIN) are seen more often than invasive disease and are commonly associated with HPV infection. As with cervical neoplasia, these premalignant conditions are treated after the puerperium.

Squamous Cell Carcinoma

Cancer of the vulva or vagina is generally a malignancy of older women, and thus, these are rarely associated with pregnancy. Even so, any suspicious lesions should be biopsied. Treatment is individualized according to the clinical stage and depth of invasion. In a review of 23 cases, investigators concluded that radical surgery for stage I disease was feasible during pregnancy—including in the last trimester (Heller, 2000). We and others question the necessity of resection in late pregnancy in that definitive therapy can often be delayed because of vulvar cancer's typical slow progression (Anderson, 2001). It appears that vaginal delivery is not contraindicated if vulvar and inguinal incisions are well healed.

Vulvar sarcoma, vulvar melanoma, and vaginal malignancies are rare in pregnancy and are the subjects of case reports (Alexander, 2004; Kuller, 1990; Matsuo, 2009).

BREAST CARCINOMA

The incidence of breast cancer is age dependent, however, because of its overall high frequency in women, it is relatively common in young women. Recall from Figure 63-1 that breast malignancies are the most frequent cancer found in pregnant women. And, as more women choose to delay childbearing, the frequency of associated breast cancer is certain to increase (Amant, 2012a). As an example, postponed childbearing was considered partially responsible for the increase in pregnancy-associated breast cancer in Sweden from 16 to 37 percent during the 40-year period from 1963 to 2002 (Andersson, 2009). Similar findings have been reported from Denmark (Eibye, 2013).

Risk Factors

Some, but not all, studies suggest that women with a family history of breast cancer—especially those with *BRCA1* and *BRCA2* breast cancer gene mutations—are more likely to develop breast malignancy during pregnancy (Johannsson, 1998; Shen, 1999; Wohlfahrt, 2002). However, although there is a definitely increased long-term risk with *BRCA1* and *BRCA2* mutations, it may be that parity modifies this risk. Specifically, parous women older than 40 years with these mutations have a significantly lower cancer risk than nulliparas with these mutations (Andrieu, 2006; Antoniou, 2006). Women with *BRCA1* and *BRCA2* gene mutations who undergo induced abortion or those who breast feed do not have an increased risk of breast cancer (Beral, 2004; Friedman, 2006). Moreover, Jernström and associates (2004) found that breast feeding actually conveyed a protective effect against this cancer in those with *BRCA1* gene mutation, but not in those with *BRCA2* mutations. Of other congenital risks, it is controversial whether diethylstilbestrol exposure in utero is associated with an increased breast cancer risk (Hoover, 2011; Larson, 2006; Titus-Ernstoff, 2006).

Diagnosis

More than 90 percent of pregnant women with breast cancer have a palpable mass, and greater than 80 percent are self-reported (Brewer, 2011). There are usually slight delays in clinical assessment, diagnostic procedures, and treatment of pregnant women with breast tumors (Berry, 1999). This can partially be attributed to increased pregnancy-induced breast tissue that obscures masses.

Evaluation of pregnant women with a breast mass should not differ from that for nonpregnant women. Thus, any suspicious breast mass should be pursued to diagnosis. Pragmatically, a palpable discrete mass can be biopsied or excised. If imaging is desirable to distinguish between a solid mass and a cystic lesion, then sonography has high sensitivity and specificity (Navrozoglou, 2008). Mammography is appropriate if indicated, and the fetal radiation risk is negligible with appropriate shielding. Fetal exposure is only 0.04 mGy for the typical mammogram study. But, because breast tissue is denser in pregnancy, mammography has a false-negative rate of 35 to 40 percent (Woo, 2003). If the decision to biopsy is uncertain, then MR imaging may be used (Amant, 2010). With such techniques, masses can usually be described as either solid or cystic.

Cystic breast lesions are simple, complicated, or complex (Berg, 2003). Simple cysts do not require special management or monitoring, but they may be aspirated if symptomatic. Complicated cysts show internal echoes during sonography, and they sometimes are indistinguishable from solid masses. These are typically aspirated, and if the sonographic abnormality does not resolve completely, a core-needle biopsy is usually performed. Complex cysts have septa or intracystic masses seen on sonographic evaluation. Because some forms of breast cancer may be complex cysts, excision is usually recommended.

For solid breast masses, evaluation is with the triple test, that is, clinical examination, imaging, and needle biopsy. If all three suggest a benign lesion or if all three suggest a breast cancer, the test is said to be concordant. A concordant benign triple test is > 99-percent accurate, and breast lumps in this category can be followed by clinical examination alone. Fortunately, most masses in pregnancy have these three reassuring features. To the contrary, however, if any of the three assessments is suggestive of malignancy, then the mass should be excised regardless of the other two findings.

Management

Once breast cancer is diagnosed, a limited search of the most common metastatic sites is completed. For most women, this includes a chest radiograph, liver sonography, and skeletal MR imaging (Amant, 2012a).

Treatment of breast cancer is by a multidisciplinary team that includes an obstetrician, surgeon, and medical oncologist. Desires for pregnancy continuation are addressed up front. Data indicate that pregnancy interruption does not influence the course or prognosis of breast cancer (Cardonick, 2010). With pregnancy continuation, treatment in general is similar to that for nonpregnant women. However, chemotherapy and surgery are delayed to the second trimester, and adjuvant radiotherapy is withheld until after delivery (Brewer, 2011).

Surgical treatment may be definitive. In the absence of metastatic disease, either a wide excision or a modified or total mastectomy—each with axillary node staging—can be performed (Rosenkranz, 2006; Woo, 2003). Staging by sentinel lymph node biopsy and lymphoscintigraphy with technetium-99m is safe. Although often administered concurrently with lymphoscintigraphy, isosulfan blue and methylene blue dyes are pregnancy class C drugs, and some recommend that they be avoided (Mondi, 2007; Spanheimer, 2009). Breast reconstruction, if desired, is typically delayed until after delivery (Viswanathan, 2011).

Chemotherapy is usually given with either positive- or negative-node breast cancers. In premenopausal women, survival is improved even if lymph nodes are cancer free. For node-positive disease, multiagent chemotherapy is begun if delivery is not anticipated within several weeks. Drug classes are alkylating agents, anthracyclines, antimetabolites, and taxanes (Lippman, 2012). Cyclophosphamide, doxorubicin, methotrexate, and 5-fluorouracil are currently in use (García-Manero, 2009). After the first trimester, methotrexate can be substituted for doxorubicin. If an anthracycline-based agent such as doxorubicin is used, pretherapy maternal echocardiography is performed because of associated cardiotoxicity (Brewer, 2011). In 22 pregnant women treated with modified radical mastectomy that was followed by chemotherapy in most, Berry and colleagues (1999) reported minimal fetal risks. Moreover, Hahn and coworkers (2006) reported good short-term outcomes for the offspring of 57 women treated during pregnancy with multiagent chemotherapy for breast cancer.

Immunotherapy for breast cancers has become commonplace. Trastuzumab (Herceptin) is a monoclonal antibody to the HER2/neu receptor, which is found in approximately a third of invasive breast cancers (Hudis, 2007). The drug is used more commonly as adjunctive therapy for early disease in HER2/neu-positive tumors but is not recommended in pregnancy (Amant, 2010). This is because HER2/neu is strongly expressed in fetal renal epithelium, and trastuzumab has been linked with miscarriage, with fetal renal failure and related oligohydramnios, and with neonatal deaths from preterm birth (Azim, 2010). For these reasons, highly effective contraception is used during and for 6 months following trastuzumab treatment. For women who conceive after only brief exposure, fetal renal effects appear to be reversible, and short-term neonatal outcomes have been normal with no congenital anomalies reported (Azim, 2012).

Prognosis

The effects of pregnancy on the course of breast cancer and its prognosis are complex. There is no doubt that breast cancer is more aggressive in younger women, but whether it is more aggressive during pregnancy in these same women is debatable. Clinically, most studies indicate little difference in overall survival rates with pregnancy-associated breast cancer compared with similarly aged and staged nonpregnant women (Beadle, 2009). There have been other reports of worse overall survival rates with pregnancy-associated breast cancer (Rodriguez, 2008). These investigators did both conclude, however, that later disease stages are more prevalent in pregnant women.

Thus, it appears that because breast cancer is usually found at a more advanced stage in pregnant women, overall prognosis is diminished. In an earlier review, Jacob and Stringer (1990) reported that approximately 30 percent of pregnant women had stage I disease, 30 percent had stage II, and 40 percent had stages III or IV. In addition, the aggregate of studies published after 1990 indicate that up to 60 percent of pregnant women have concomitant axillary node involvement at diagnosis. And although, stage for stage, the 5-year survival rate is comparable in pregnant and nonpregnant women, the more advanced stages that are typical of pregnant women worsen their prognosis (King, 1985; Nugent, 1985; Zemlickis, 1992).

Pregnancy Following Breast Cancer

After breast cancer treatment, chemotherapy will render some women infertile, and options for childbearing are limited (Kim, 2011). For those who became pregnant, there appear to be no adverse effects on long-term maternal survival rates (Averette, 1999; Velentgas, 1999). Moreover, a metaanalysis of 10 studies found that for women with early breast cancer, pregnancy that occurs 10 months after diagnosis may, in fact, have a survival benefit (Valachis, 2010). There are also no data indicating that lactation adversely affects the course of previously diagnosed breast cancer. Also, lactation and breast feeding are possible after conservative surgery and radiation of the treated breast (Higgins, 1994).

Recommendations for subsequent pregnancies in women successfully treated for breast malignancy are based on several factors that include consideration for the recurrence risk. Simply because recurrences are more common soon after treatment, it seems reasonable to advise a delay of 2 to 3 years for observation. Hormonal contraceptive methods are contraindicated, and a copper-containing intrauterine device is an excellent long-acting reversible method for many. Even with contraceptive failure, women who conceive do not appear to have diminished survival (Ives, 2006). It is reassuring that women who undertake pregnancy after breast cancer treatment overall have good outcomes (Langagergaard, 2006). Of particular concern is that women treated with tamoxifen are at risk for several months after its discontinuation for having an infant with congenital anomalies. This is because of its extremely long half-life, and thus delaying conception is recommended for at least 2 months after its completion (Braems, 2011).

THYROID CANCER

Various thyroid gland malignancies constitute the most common endocrine cancers. Because most of these originate within discrete nodules, their evaluation is important. This typically includes sonography and measurement of serum thyroid-stimulating hormone (TSH) and free thyroxine levels. Fine-needle aspiration is indicated for any suspicious nodule (Yazbeck, 2012).

With a diagnosis of thyroid malignancy, pregnancy termination is not necessary (Alves, 2011). Primary therapy is total thyroidectomy performed ideally during the second trimester. Postoperatively, replacement thyroxine is given to maintain serum TSH levels between 0.1 and 0.5 mIU/L (Abalovich, 2007). Most thyroid cancers are well differentiated and follow an indolent course. Thus, delayed surgical treatment does not usually alter outcome (Yazbeck, 2012). If surgical therapy is postponed until after pregnancy, thyroxine is given to suppress any growth stimulus of TSH on tumor cells (Pacini, 2012).

In some types of thyroid malignancies, primary or postoperative treatment is given with radioiodine. This is contraindicated in both pregnancy and lactation. Transplacental iodine-131 is avidly trapped by the fetal thyroid gland to cause hypothyroidism (Chap. 58, p. 1149). During lactation, the breast also concentrates a substantial amount of iodide. This may pose neonatal risk due to ^{131}I-containing milk ingestion and maternal risk from significant breast irradiation. To limit maternal exposure, a delay of 3 months between lactation and ablation will more reliably ensure complete breast involution (Sisson, 2011). Last, pregnancy should be avoided for 6 months to 1 year in women with thyroid cancer who receive ^{131}I doses. This time ensures thyroid function stability and confirms thyroid cancer remission (Abalovich, 2007).

LYMPHOID CELL MALIGNANCIES

Hematological malignancies comprise 10 to 20 percent of cancers in pregnancy (Cohen, 2011; Eibye, 2013; Smith, 2003). Some of these present as leukemia involving bone marrow and blood. Others are solid lymphomas, which may be of B- or T-cell origin.

Hodgkin Disease

This lymphoma is probably B-cell derived and is cytologically distinguished from other lymphomas by Reed–Sternberg cells. It is the most common malignant lymphoma in women of childbearing age. In a population-based review of approximately 4 million pregnancies, Smith and associates (2003) reported that Hodgkin lymphoma complicated only 1 in 34,000 live births. Our experiences are similar during the past 40 years at Parkland Hospital with nearly 500,000 births.

In more than 70 percent of Hodgkin disease cases, there is painless enlargement of lymph nodes above the diaphragm—the axillary, cervical, or submandibular chains. Approximately one third of patients have symptoms including fever, night sweats, malaise, weight loss, and pruritus. Diagnosis is by histological examination of involved nodes (Longo, 2012).

Staging and Treatment

The Ann Arbor staging system, shown in Table 63-2, is used for Hodgkin and other lymphomas. Recent studies have used

TABLE 63-2. Ann Arbor Staging System for Hodgkin and Other Lymphomas

Stage	Findings
I	Involvement in a single lymph node region or lymphoid site—e.g., spleen or thymus
II	Involvement of two or more lymph node groups on the same side of the diaphragm—the mediastinum is a single site
III	Involvement of lymph nodes on both sides of the diaphragm
IV	Extralymphatic involvement—e.g., liver or bone marrow

Substage A = no symptoms; substage B = fever, sweats, or weight loss; substage E = extralymphatic involvement excluding liver and bone marrow.

CHAPTER 63

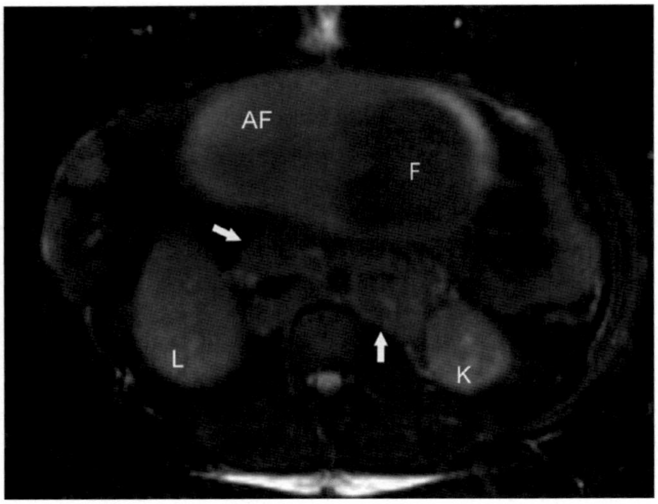

FIGURE 63-7 Hodgkin lymphoma. Magnetic resonance imaging for staging shows an axial T2-weighted image taken from the midabdomen that demonstrates bilateral paraaortic adenopathy (*arrows*). Amnionic fluid (*AF*), fetal abdomen (*F*), maternal right inferior liver (*L*), and maternal left kidney (*K*) are seen. (Image contributed by Dr. Desiree Morgan.)

risk categories—high, low, and very low—however, these are not succinctly defined (Armitage, 2010). Pregnancy limits the use of some radiographic studies for staging, but at minimum, chest radiography, abdominal imaging with sonography or MR imaging, and bone marrow biopsy are completed (Williams, 2001). MR imaging is excellent for evaluating thoracic and abdominal paraaortic lymph nodes (Fig. 63-7) (Brenner, 2012).

The current trend for nonpregnant individuals is to administer chemotherapy for all stages of Hodgkin disease. In pregnancy, for early-stage disease in the first trimester, options include observation until after 12 weeks, single-agent vinblastine until the second trimester, pregnancy termination followed by multiagent chemotherapy, or radiotherapy alone for isolated neck or axillary sites (El-Hemaidi, 2012; Rizack, 2009).

For advanced-stage disease, chemotherapy is recommended regardless of gestational age. Before 20 weeks, therapeutic abortion is a consideration, but if termination is unacceptable, then treatment with vinblastine followed by multiagent therapy in the second trimester can be used (Pereg, 2007). For most advanced-stage disease after the first trimester, cycles of doxorubicin, bleomycin, vinblastine, and dacarbadine (ABVD) are given, and radiotherapy can be added postpartum (Cohen, 2011). In general, postponement of therapy until fetal maturity is achieved seems justifiable only when the diagnosis is made late in pregnancy (Shulman, 2008). Importantly, in our experiences, pregnant women with Hodgkin disease—even after they are "cured"—are inordinately susceptible to infection and sepsis. Active antineoplastic therapy increases this vulnerability.

Prognosis

The overall prognosis with Hodgkin lymphoma is good, and survival rates exceed 70 percent. Pregnancy does not adversely affect the course or survival rate of women with this lymphoma (Brenner, 2012; Pavlidis, 2002). Moreover, adverse perinatal outcomes do not appear to be increased (Langagergaard, 2008). Finally, neither chemotherapy after the first trimester nor mediastinal and neck irradiation had reported adverse fetal effects (Jacobs, 1981).

The long-term prognosis for women with Hodgkin disease is encouraging. Horning and coworkers (1981) reported that half of women resumed normal menses after chemotherapy and that there were no birth defects in 24 neonates subsequently born to these women. Long-term complications of lymphoma treatment include secondary leukemia in those treated with chemotherapy, secondary breast cancer in those treated with radiotherapy, and myocardial damage and infarction, pulmonary fibrosis, hypothyroidism, and marrow suppression (Longo, 2012).

Non-Hodgkin Lymphomas

Although usually B-cell tumors, non-Hodgkin can also be T-cell or natural killer (NK)-cell neoplasms. Their biology, classification, and treatment are complex (Longo, 2012; O'Gara, 2009). For example, they are associated with viral infections, and indeed, their incidence has risen sharply at least partly because 5 to 10 percent of HIV-infected persons develop lymphoma. Other associated viruses include Epstein-Barr virus, hepatitis C virus, and human herpes virus 8. Some of these lymphomas are quite aggressive, and survival varies with the type of cell line involved.

Non-Hodgkin lymphomas are uncommon during pregnancy, and only approximately 100 cases have been reported (Brenner, 2012). They are staged according to the Ann Arbor system shown in Table 63-2. If diagnosed in the first trimester, pregnancy termination followed by multiagent chemotherapy is recommended for all but indolent or very early disease. These less aggressive forms may either be observed or be temporized with focal supradiaphragmatic radiotherapy, with full treatment after entering the second trimester. If one of these lymphomas is diagnosed after the first trimester, chemotherapy and immunotherapy with rituximab (Rituxan) are given (Cohen, 2011; Rizack, 2009). In a report describing follow-up at 6 to 29 years in 55 individuals whose mothers were given chemotherapy during pregnancy, there were no congenital, neurological, or psychological abnormalities (Avilés, 2001). Furthermore, these exposed persons had no cancers, including leukemia.

Burkitt lymphoma is an aggressive B-cell tumor associated with Epstein-Barr virus infection. Prognosis is poor, and treatment is given with multiagent chemotherapy. In a review of 19 women whose pregnancies were complicated by this lymphoma, 17 died within a year of diagnosis (Barnes, 1998).

Leukemias

In general, these malignancies arise either from lymphoid tissues—lymphoblastic or lymphocytic leukemias, or from bone marrow—myeloid leukemias. They can be acute or chronic. Although adult leukemias are more prevalent after age 40, they still are among the most common malignancies of young women. Leukemia was diagnosed in 1 in 40,000 pregnancies reported to the California Cancer Registry (Smith, 2003). In a review of 350 reports of pregnancy complicated by leukemia, of 72 cases reported from 1975 until 1988, 44 had acute myelogenous leukemia; 20 had acute lymphocytic leukemia; and eight had one of the chronic leukemias (Caligiuri, 1989). The last are uncommon in young women, and chronic hairy-cell leukemia has been reported in only six pregnancies (Stiles, 1998).

Acute leukemias almost always cause marked peripheral blood count abnormalities, and frequently there is an elevated white blood cell count with readily recognizable circulating blast cells. The diagnosis is made from bone marrow biopsy.

Currently, with contemporary therapy, remission during pregnancy is common, compared with almost 100-percent mortality before 1970. The goal of remission is aggressively pursued with multiagent chemotherapy. There is no evidence that pregnancy termination further improves the prognosis, however, abortion is a consideration in early pregnancy to avoid potential chemotherapy teratogenesis. One example is treatment of acute promyelocytic leukemia with all-*trans*-retinoic acid, also known as tretinoin (Carradice, 2002; Celo, 1994). This is a potent teratogen that causes retinoic acid syndrome (Chap. 12, p. 251). In other cases, pregnancy termination before viability may simplify management of the acutely ill woman.

Other than these caveats, treatment of pregnant women with leukemia is similar to that for nonpregnant women. After induction chemotherapy, postremission maintenance therapy is mandatory to prevent a relapse, which is usually then treated with stem-cell transplantation (Wetzler, 2012). If allogeneic stem-cell transplantation is indicated, early delivery is considered. With some chronic leukemias, it may be possible to delay therapy until after delivery (Fey, 2008). As with lymphoma, infection and hemorrhage are significant complications that should be anticipated in women with active disease. Puerperal infection is particularly problematic.

There are few contemporaneous studies of leukemia treated during pregnancy. In an earlier review of 58 cases, Reynoso and colleagues (1987) reported that 75 percent were diagnosed after the first trimester. Half were acute myelogenous leukemia, which had a remission rate of 75 percent with chemotherapy. Only 40 percent of these pregnancies resulted in liveborn infants. Preterm delivery and stillbirth rates were also reported to be increased (Caligiuri, 1989).

MALIGNANT MELANOMA

These malignant tumors most frequently originate in the skin from a preexisting nevus and its pigment-producing melanocytes. Melanomas should be suspected in pigmented lesions with changes in contour, surface elevation, discoloration, itching, bleeding, or ulceration, which should prompt biopsy. They are most common in light-skinned whites and develop relatively frequently in women of childbearing age. They sometimes are first diagnosed during pregnancy, and the reported incidence ranges widely from 0.03 to 2.8 per 1000 live births (Eibye, 2013; Smith, 2003; Wong, 1990). This is likely because many are treated on an outpatient basis, and thus they are not entered into a tumor registry. As noted on page 1221, malignant melanoma is one of the tumors that is known to metastasize to the placenta and fetus. Placental evaluation for metastasis should be performed after delivery.

Staging and Treatment

Staging is clinical as follows: stage I is a melanoma with no palpable lymph nodes; in stage II, lymph nodes are palpable; and in stage III, there are distant metastases. For patients with stage I, tumor thickness is the single most important predictor of survival. The Clark classification includes five levels of involvement by depth into the epidermis, dermis, and subcutaneous fat. The Breslow scale measures tumor thickness and size, in addition to depth of invasion.

Primary surgical treatment for melanoma is determined by the stage and includes wide local resection, sometimes with extensive regional lymph node dissection. Schwartz and associates (2003) recommend sentinel lymph node mapping and biopsy using ^{99m}Tc-sulfur colloid, which has a calculated fetal dose of 0.014 mSv or 0.014 mGy. Routine regional node dissection reportedly improves survival in nonpregnant patients with microscopic metastases (Cascinelli, 1998). For pregnant patients, an algorithm has been proposed that begins with resection of the primary tumor under local anesthesia and postpones sentinel lymph node biopsy until after delivery (Broer, 2012). Although prophylactic chemotherapy or immunotherapy is usually avoided during pregnancy, it may be given if indicated by tumor stage and maternal prognosis. In most cases of distant metastatic melanoma, treatment is at best palliative. At this time, the role of estrogen receptor-β in melanoma progression is under investigation, and it may be a target for therapeutic intervention (de Giorgi, 2011).

Prognosis

Stage-for-stage, survival is equivalent between pregnant and nonpregnant women. Therapeutic abortion does not appear to improve survival. Clinical stage is the strongest determinant of survival, and women with deep cutaneous invasion or regional node involvement have the worst prognosis (Dipaola, 1997; Kjems, 1993; Lens, 2008). Approximately 60 percent of recurrences will manifest within 2 years, and 90 percent by 5 years. Thus, most recommend that pregnancy be avoided for 3 to 5 years after surgical resection. Interim contraception can include combination oral contraceptives, as they do not appear to have adverse effects (Gandini, 2011). Related, subsequent pregnancies in women with localized melanoma do not appear to adversely affect cancer survival rates (Driscoll, 2009).

GASTROINTESTINAL TRACT CANCER

Colorectal Cancer

Malignancies of the colon and rectum are the third most frequent in women of all age groups in the United States (American Cancer Society, 2012). Even so, colorectal tumors seldom complicate pregnancy because they are uncommon before age 40. Smith and colleagues (2003) reported an approximate incidence of 1 per 150,000 deliveries in the California Cancer Registry. It was about 1 per 35,000 births in the Danish Registry (Eibye, 2013). The majority—80 percent—of colorectal carcinomas in pregnant women arise from the rectum. In one review, there were only 41 reported cases in pregnancy with cancer above the peritoneal reflection (Chan, 1999).

The most frequent symptoms of colorectal cancer are abdominal pain, distention, nausea and vomiting, constipation, and rectal bleeding. The diagnosis may be delayed because many of these symptoms are common in pregnancy. Certainly, if symptoms suggestive of colon disease persist, digital rectal examination, stool tests for occult blood, and flexible sigmoidoscopy or colonoscopy should be done.

Treatment of colon cancer in pregnant women follows the same general guidelines as for nonpregnant women. Without evidence of metastatic disease, surgical resection is preferred, but most pregnant women have advanced lesions (Walsh, 1998). During the first half of pregnancy, hysterectomy is not necessary to perform colon or rectal resection, and thus, therapeutic abortion is not mandated. During later pregnancy, therapy may be delayed until fetal maturation, however, hemorrhage, obstruction, or perforation may force surgical intervention (Minter, 2005). Vaginal delivery is usually avoided because lower rectal lesions may cause dystocia, or delivery may cause tumor hemorrhage.

There is no evidence that pregnancy influences the course of colorectal cancer, and the prognosis appears to be similar to that for identical stages in nonpregnant patients (Dahling, 2009). Carcinoembryonic antigen (CEA) is a tumor marker for colon cancer, and although it may be elevated during normal pregnancy, baseline values may be useful to monitor disease (Minter, 2005).

Other Gastrointestinal Neoplasms

Gastric cancer is rarely associated with pregnancy, and most reported cases are from Japan. Hirabayashi and associates (1987) reviewed outcomes in 60 pregnant women during a 70-year period from 1916 to 1985. Delayed diagnosis during pregnancy is common, and the prognosis is consistently poor (Lee, 2009). It is axiomatic that persistent unexplained upper gastrointestinal symptoms should be evaluated by endoscopy.

With Zollinger–Ellison syndrome, tumors typically found in the duodenum or pancreas secrete excess gastrin. This leads to increased stomach acid production and gastric ulceration. Most tumors are slow growing, and thus, the primary goal in pregnancy is control of acid secretion. Some advise surgical resection before pregnancy (Stewart, 1997). In pregnant women with metastatic disease or in those with previously undiagnosed tumors, antacids and antisecretory treatment with histamine H_2-receptor antagonists or proton-pump inhibitors usually controls acid secretion.

MISCELLANEOUS TUMORS

Various other neoplasms have been reported in pregnancy and are usually the subject of case reports. Examples include carcinoid tumors, which are usually of gastrointestinal origin (Durkin, 1983). Both pancreatic and hepatocellular cancer are rare during pregnancy (Kakoza, 2009; Marinoni, 2006; Papoutsis, 2012; Perera, 2011). Bladerston and coworkers (1998) described a massive intrahepatic cholangiocarcinoma masquerading as HELLP (hemolysis, elevated liver enzymes, and low platelet count) syndrome. Gastrointestinal cancers during pregnancy are often discovered because of ovarian metastases—Krukenberg tumors—which have a bleak prognosis (Glišić, 2006). Central nervous system benign and malignant neoplasms had a reported frequency of 1 in 10,000 to 28,000 (Eibye, 2013; Smith, 2003). Bladder and urachal duct carcinoma have been rarely reported coincident with pregnancy (McNally, 2013; Yeaton-Massey, 2013). Finally, bone and vaginal tumors have been described (ElNaggar, 2012; Kathiresan, 2011).

REFERENCES

Abalovich M, Amino N, Barbour LA, et al: 2007 management of thyroid dysfunction during pregnancy and postpartum: an Endocrine Society Clinical Practice Guideline. J Clin Endocrinol Metab 92:S1, 2007

Abdel-Hady ES, Hemida RA, Gamal A, et al: Cancer during pregnancy: perinatal outcome after in utero exposure to chemotherapy. Arch Gynecol Obstet 286(2):283, 2012

Ackermann S, Gehrsitz C, Mehihorn G, et al: Management and course of histologically verified cervical carcinoma *in situ* during pregnancy. Acta Obstet Gynecol Scand 85:1134, 2006

Al-Adnani M, Kiho L, Scheimberg I: Maternal pancreatic carcinoma metastatic to the placenta: a case report and literature review. Pediatr Dev Pathol 10:61, 2007

Alexander A, Harris RM, Grossman D, et al: Vulvar melanoma: diffuse melanosis and metastases to the placenta. J Am Acad Dermatol 50(20):293, 2004

Alexander A, Samlowski WE, Grossman D, et al: Metastatic melanoma in pregnancy: risk of transplacental metastases in the infant. J Clin Oncol 21:2179, 2003

Ali R, Ozkalemkas F, Kimya Y, et al: Imatinib use during pregnancy and breast feeding: a case report and review of the literature. Arch Gynecol Obstet 280:169, 2009

Alouini S, Rida K, Mathevet P: Cervical cancer complicating pregnancy: implications of laparoscopic lymphadenectomy. Gynecol Oncol 108(3):472, 2008

Altman JF, Lowe L, Redman B, et al: Placental metastasis of maternal melanoma. J Am Acad Dermatol 49:1150, 2003

Alves GV, Santin AP, Furlanetto TW: Prognosis of thyroid cancer related to pregnancy: a systematic review. J Thyroid Res 2011:1, 2011

Amant F, Deckers S, Van Calsteren K, et al: Breast cancer in pregnancy: recommendations of an international consensus meeting. Eur J Cancer 46(18):3158, 2010

Amant F, Loibl S, Neven P, et al: Breast cancer in pregnancy. Lancet 379:570, 2012a

Amant F, Van Calsteren K, Halaska MJ: Long-term cognitive and cardiac outcomes after prenatal exposure to chemotherapy in children aged 18 months or older: an observational study. Lancet Oncol, 13(3):256, 2012b

American Cancer Society: Cancer Facts & Figures 2012. Available at: http://www.cancer.org/acs/groups/content/@epidemiologysurveilance/documents/document/acspc-031941.pdf. Accessed June 14, 2012

American College of Obstetricians and Gynecologists: Guidelines for diagnostic imaging during pregnancy. Committee Opinion No. 299, September 2004, Reaffirmed 2009

American College of Obstetricians and Gynecologists: Human papillomavirus vaccination. Committee Opinion No. 467, September 2010

American College of Obstetricians and Gynecologists: The role of the obstetrician-gynecologist in the early detection of epithelial ovarian cancer. Committee Opinion No. 477, March 2011

American College of Obstetricians and Gynecologists: Alternatives to hysterectomy in the management of leiomyomas. Practice Bulletin No. 96, August 2008, Reaffirmed 2012a

American College of Obstetricians and Gynecologists: Screening for cervical cancer. Practice Bulletin No. 109, November 2012b

American College of Obstetricians and Gynecologists: Management of abnormal cervical cancer screening test results and cervical cancer precursors. Practice Bulletin No. 140, December 2013a

American College of Obstetricians and Gynecologists: Management of adnexal masses. Practice Bulletin No. 83, July 2007, Reaffirmed 2013b

American Society for Reproductive Medicine: Fertility preservation and reproduction in patients facing gonadotoxic therapies: a committee opinion. Fertil Steril 100(5):1224, 2013

American Society for Reproductive Medicine: Ovarian hyperstimulation syndrome. Fertil Steril 90(5 Suppl):S188, 2008

Anderson ML, Mari G, Schwartz PE: Gynecologic malignancies in pregnancy. In Barnea ER, Jauniaux E, Schwartz PE (eds): Cancer and Pregnancy. London, Springer, 2001, p 33

Andersson TM, Johansson AL, Hsieh CC et al: Increasing incidence of pregnancy-associated breast cancer in Sweden. Obstet Gynecol 114:568, 2009

Andrieu N, Goldgar DE, Easton DF, et al: Pregnancies, breast-feeding, and breast cancer risk in the International BRCA1/2 Carrier Cohort Study (IBCCS). J Natl Cancer Inst 98:535, 2006

Antoniou AC, Shenton A, Maher ER, et al: Parity and breast cancer risk among BRCA1 and BRCA2. Breast Cancer Res 8:R72, 2006

Armitage J: Early-stage Hodgkin's lymphoma. N Engl J Med 363:653, 2010

Aslam N, Ong C, Woelfer B, et al: Serum CA125 at 11–14 weeks of gestation in women with morphologically normal ovaries. Br J Obstet Gynaecol 107:689, 2000

Averette HE, Mirhashemi R, Moffat FL: Pregnancy after breast carcinoma: the ultimate medical challenge. Cancer 85:2301, 1999

Averette HE, Nasser N, Yankow SL, et al: Cervical conization in pregnancy: analysis of 180 operations. Am J Obstet Gynecol 106:543, 1970

Avilés A, Neri N: Hematological malignancies and pregnancy: a final report of 84 children who received chemotherapy in utero. Clin Lymphoma 2(3):173, 2001

Azim HA Jr, Azim H, Peccatori FA: Treatment of cancer during pregnancy with monoclonal antibodies: a real challenge. Expert Rev Clin Immunol 6(6):821, 2010

Azim HA Jr, Metzger-Filho O, deAzambuja E, et al: Pregnancy occurring during or following adjuvant trastuzumab in patients enrolled in the HERA trial (BIG 01-01). Breast Cancer Res Treat 133(1)387, 2012

Azziz R: Adenomyosis in pregnancy: a review. J Reprod Med 31:223, 1986

Barnes MN, Barrett JC, Kimberlin DF, et al: Burkitt lymphoma in pregnancy. Obstet Gynecol 92:675, 1998

Beadle BM, Woodward WA, Middleton LP, et al: The impact of pregnancy on breast cancer outcomes in women < or = 35 years. Cancer 115(6):1174, 2009

Beral V, Bull D, Doll R, et al: Breast cancer and abortion: collaborative reanalysis of data from 53 epidemiological studies, including 83,000 women with breast cancer from 16 countries. Lancet 363:1007, 2004

Berg WA, Campassi CI, Loffe OB: Cystic lesions of the breast: sonographic-pathologic correlation. Radiology 227:183, 2003

Berry DL, Theriault RL, Holmes FA, et al: Management of breast cancer during pregnancy using a standardized protocol. J Clin Oncol 17:855, 1999

Bladerston KD, Tewari K, Azizi F, et al: Intrahepatic cholangiocarcinoma masquerading as the HELLP syndrome (hemolysis, elevated liver enzymes, and low platelet count) in pregnancy: case report. Am J Obstet Gynecol 179:823, 1998

Boulay R, Podczaski E: Ovarian cancer complicating pregnancy. Obstet Gynecol Clin North Am 25:3856, 1998

Braems G, Denys H, DeWever O, et al: Use of tamoxifen before and during pregnancy. Oncologist 16(11):1547, 2011

Brenner B, Avivi I, Lishner M: Haematological cancers in pregnancy. Lancet 379:580, 2012

Brent RL: Utilization of developmental basic science principles in the evaluation of reproductive risks from pre- and postconception environmental radiation exposures. Teratology 59:182, 1999

Brewer M, Kueck An, Runowicz CD: Chemotherapy in pregnancy. Clin Obstet Gynecol 54:602, 2011

Briggs GC, Freeman RK, Yaffee SJ (eds): Drugs in Pregnancy and Lactation: a Reference Guide to Fetal and Neonatal Risk, 9th ed. Philadelphia, Lippincott Williams & Wilkins, 2011, p 499

Broer N, Buonocore S, Goldberg C: A proposal for the timing of management of patients with melanoma presenting during pregnancy. J Surg Oncol 106(1):36, 2012

Bruinsma F, Lumley J, Tan J, et al: Precancerous changes in the cervix and risk of subsequent preterm birth. BJOG 114:70, 2007

Bulun SE: Uterine fibroids. N Engl J Med 369:1344, 2013

Bumpers HL, Butler KL, Best IM: Endometrioma of the abdominal wall. Am J Obstet Gynecol 187:1709, 2002

Caligiuri MA, Mayer RJ: Pregnancy and leukemia. Semin Oncol 16:388, 1989

Cardonick E, Dougherty R, Grana G et al: Breast cancer during pregnancy: maternal and fetal outcomes. Cancer 16:76, 2010

Cardonick E, Iacobucci A: Use of chemotherapy during human pregnancy. Lancet Oncol 5:283, 2004

Carradice D, Austin N, Bayston K, et al: Successful treatment of acute promyelocytic leukaemia during pregnancy. Clin Lab Haematol 24:307, 2002

Cascinelli N, Morabito A, Santinami M, et al: Immediate or delayed dissection of regional nodes in patients with melanoma of the trunk: a randomized trial. Lancet 351:793, 1998

Caspi B, Levi R, Appelman Z, et al: Conservative management of ovarian cystic teratoma during pregnancy and labor. Am J Obstet Gynecol 182:503, 2000

Castanon A, Brocklehurst P, Evans H, et al: Risk of preterm birth after treatment for cervical intraepithelial neoplasia among women attending colposcopy in England: retrospective-prospective cohort study. BMJ 345:e5174, 2012

Celik C, Acar A, Cicek N, et al: Can myomectomy be performed during pregnancy? Gynecol Obstet Invest 53:79, 2002

Celo JS, Kim HC, Houlihan C, et al: Acute promyelocytic leukemia in pregnancy: all-trans retinoic acid as a newer therapeutic option. Obstet Gynecol 83:808, 1994

Centers for Disease Control and Prevention: FDA licensure of bivalent human papillomavirus vaccine (HPV2, Cervarix) for use in females and updated HPV vaccination recommendations from the Advisory Committee on Immunization Practices (ACIP). MMWR 59:626, 2010

Chan YM, Ngai SW, Lao TT: Colon cancer in pregnancy. A case report. J Reprod Med 44:733, 1999

Chen CD, Chen SU, Yang YS: Prevention and management of ovarian hyperstimulation syndrome. Best Pract Res Clin Obstet Gynaecol 26(6):817, 2012

Chin N, Platt AB, Nuovo GJ: Squamous intraepithelial lesions arising in benign endocervical polyps: a report of 9 cases with correlation to the Pap smears, HPV analysis, and immunoprofile. Int J Gynecol Pathol 27(4):582, 2008

Choi JR, Levine D, Finberg H: Luteoma of pregnancy: sonographic findings in two cases. J Ultrasound Med 19(12):877, 2000

Clark H, Kurinczuk JJ, Lee AJ, et al: Obstetric outcomes in cancer survivors. Obstet Gynecol 110(4):849, 2007

Clement PB: Tumor-like lesions of the ovary associated with pregnancy. Int J Gynecol Pathol 12(2):108, 1993

Cohen JB, Blum KA: Evaluation and management of lymphoma and leukemia in pregnancy. Clin Obstet Gynecol 54:556, 2011

Connor JP: Noninvasive cervical cancer complicating pregnancy. Obstet Gynecol Clin North Am 25:331, 1998

Coronado GD, Marshall LM, Schwartz SM: Complications in pregnancy, labor, and delivery with uterine leiomyomas: a population-based study. Obstet Gynecol 95:764, 2000

Curtis KM, Hillis SD, Marchbanks PA, et al: Disruption of the endometrial-myometrial border during pregnancy as a risk factor for adenomyosis. Am J Obstet Gynecol 187(3):543, 2002

Dahl SK, Thomas MA, Williams DB, et al: Maternal virilization due to luteoma associated with delayed lactation. Fertil Steril 90(5):2006.e17, 2008

Dahling MT, Xing G, Cress R, et al: Pregnancy-associated colon and rectal cancer: perinatal and cancer outcomes. J Matern Fetal Neonatal Med 22(3):204, 2009

Dale DC, Cottle TE, Fier CJ, et al: Severe chronic neutropenia: treatment and follow-up of patients in the Severe Chronic Neutropenia International Registry. Am J Hematol 72(2):82, 2003

Dana A, Buchanan KM, Goss MA, et al: Pregnancy outcomes from the pregnancy registry of a human papillomavirus type 6/11/16/18 vaccine. Obstet Gynecol 2009 114(6):1170, 2009

De Carolis S, Fatigante G, Ferrazzani S, et al: Uterine myomectomy in pregnant women. Fetal Diagn Ther 16:116, 2001

de Giorgi V, Gori A, Grazzini M, et al: Estrogens, estrogen receptors and melanoma. Expert Rev Anticancer Ther 11:739, 2011

Descamps D, Hardt K, Spiessens B, et al: Safety of human papillomavirus (HPV)-16/18 AS04-adjuvanted vaccine for cervical cancer prevention: a pooled analysis of 11 clinical trials. Hum Vaccin 5(5):332, 2009

Diller L: Adult primary care after childhood acute lymphoblastic leukemia. N Engl J Med 365:1417, 2011

Dipaola RS, Goodin S, Ratzell M, et al: Chemotherapy for metastatic melanoma during pregnancy. Gynecol Oncol 66:526, 1997

Djavadian D, Braendle W, Jaenicke F: Laparoscopic oophoropexy for the treatment of recurrent torsion of the adnexa in pregnancy: case report and review. Fertil Steril 82(4):933, 2004

Dorum A, Blom GP, Ekerhovd E, et al: Prevalence and histologic diagnosis of adnexal cysts in postmenopausal women: an autopsy study. Am J Obstet Gynecol 192(1):48, 2005

Driscoll MS, Grant-Kels JM: Nevi and melanoma in the pregnant woman. Clin Dermatol 27(1):116, 2009

Dunton CJ: Management of atypical glandular cells and adenocarcinoma in situ. Obstet Gynecol Clin North Am 35(4):623, 2008

Durkin JW Jr: Carcinoid tumor and pregnancy. Am J Obstet Gynecol 145:757, 1983

Eibye S, Kjaer SK, Mellemkjaer L: Incidence of pregnancy-associated cancer in Denmark, 1977–2006. Obstet Gynecol 122:608, 2013

El-Hemaidi I, Robinson SE: Management of haematological malignancy in pregnancy. Best Pract Res Clin Obstet Gynaecol 26(1):149, 2012

ElNaggar A, Patil A, Singh K, et al: Neuroendocrine carcinoma of the vagina in pregnancy. Obstet Gynecol 119:445, 2012

Erkanli S, Ayhan A: Fertility-sparing therapy in young women with endometrial cancer: 2010 update. Int J Gyn Cancer 20:1170, 2010
Fader AN, Alward EK, Niederhauser A, et al: Cervical dysplasia in pregnancy: a multi-institutional evaluation. Am J Obstet Gynecol 203:113, 2010
Favero G, Chiantera V, Oleszczuk A, et al: Invasive cervical cancer during pregnancy: laparoscopic nodal evaluation before oncologic treatment delay. Gynecol Oncol 118:123, 2010
Fey MF, Surbek D: Leukaemia and pregnancy. Recent Results Cancer Res 178:97, 2008
Fife KH, Katz BP, Roush J, et al: Cancer-associated human papillomavirus types are selectively increased in the cervix of women in the first trimester of pregnancy. Am J Obstet Gynecol 174:1487, 1996
FIGO Committee on Gynecologic Oncology: Current FIGO staging for cancer of the vagina, fallopian tube, ovary, and gestational trophoblastic neoplasia. Int J Gynaecol Obstet 105(1):3, 2009a
FIGO Committee on Gynecologic Oncology: Revised FIGO staging for carcinoma of the vulva, cervix, and endometrium. Int J Gynaecol Obstet 105:103, 2009b
Fleischer AC, Dinesh MS, Entman SS: Sonographic evaluation of maternal disorders during pregnancy. Radiol Clin North Am 28:51, 1990
Friedman E, Kotsopoulos J, Lubinski J, et al: Spontaneous and therapeutic abortions and the risk of breast cancer among BRCA mutation carriers. Breast Cancer Res 8:R15, 2006
Fuchs N, Smorgick N, Tovbin Y, et al: Oophoropexy to prevent adnexal torsion: how, when, and for whom? J Minim Invasive Gynecol 17(2):205, 2010
FUTURE II Study Group: Quadrivalent vaccine against human papillomavirus to prevent high-grade cervical lesions. N Engl J Med 356:1915, 2007
Gandini S, Iodice S, Koomen E, et al: Hormonal and reproductive factors in relation to melanoma in women: current review and meta-analysis. Eur J Cancer 47(17):2607, 2011
García-Manero M, Royo MP, Espinos J, et al: Pregnancy associated breast cancer. Eur J Surg Oncol 35(2):215, 2009
Garland SM, Ault KA, Gall SA, et al: Pregnancy and infant outcomes in the clinical trials of a human papillomavirus type 6/11/16/18 vaccine: a combined analysis of five randomized controlled trials. Obstet Gynecol 114(6):1179, 2009
Genadry R, Parmley T, Woodruff JD: The origin and clinical behavior of the parovarian tumor. Am J Obstet Gynecol 129(8):873, 1977
Genta PR, Dias ML, Janiszewski TA, et al: *Streptococcus agalactiae* endocarditis and giant pyomyoma simulating ovarian cancer. South Med J 94:508, 2001
Germain M, Rarick T, Robins E: Management of intermittent ovarian torsion by laparoscopic oophoropexy. Obstet Gynecol 88(4 Pt 2):715, 1996
Giuntoli RL II, Vang RS, Bristow RE: Evaluation and management of adnexal masses during pregnancy. Clin Obstet Gynecol 49(3):492, 2006
Glišić A, Atanacković J: Krukenberg tumor in pregnancy. The lethal outcome. Pathol Oncol Res 12(2):108, 2006
Goldman NA, Goldberg GL: Late recurrence of squamous cell cervical cancer in an episiotomy site after vaginal delivery. Obstet Gynecol 101:1127, 2003
Gotlieb WH, Beiner ME, Shalmon B, et al: Outcome of fertility-sparing treatment with progestins in young patients with endometrial cancer. Obstet Gynecol 102:718, 2003
Gottschalk N, Jacobs VR, Hein R, et al: Advanced metastatic melanoma during pregnancy: a multidisciplinary challenge. Onkologie 32:748, 2009
Green DM, Whitton JA, Stovall M, et al: Pregnancy outcome of female survivors of childhood cancer: a report from the Childhood Cancer Survivor Study. Am J Obstet Gynecol 187:1070, 2002
Greer BE, Easterling TR, McLennan DA, et al: Fetal and maternal considerations in the management of stage I-B cervical cancer during pregnancy. Gynecol Oncol 34:61, 1989
Griffith WF, Werner CL: Benign disorders of the lower reproductive tract. In Hoffman BL, Schorge JO, Schaffer JI, et al (eds): Williams Gynecology, 2nd ed. New York, McGraw-Hill, 2012, p 110
Guyatt GH, Akl EA, Crowther M, et al: Executive summary: Antithrombotic Therapy and Prevention of Thrombosis, 9th ed: American College of Chest Physicians Evidence-Based Clinical Practice Guidelines. Chest 141(2 Suppl): 7S, 2012
Haas JF: Pregnancy in association with newly diagnosed cancer: a population-based epidemiologic assessment. Int J Cancer 34:229, 1984
Hacker NF, Berek JS, Lagasse LD, et al: Carcinoma of the cervix associated with pregnancy. Obstet Gynecol 59:735, 1982
Haga Y, Sakamoto K, Egami H, et al: Evaluation of serum CA125 values in healthy individuals and pregnant women. Am J Med Sci 292(1):25, 1986
Hahn KM, Johnson PH, Gordon N, et al: Treatment of pregnant breast cancer patients and outcomes of children exposed to chemotherapy in utero. Cancer 107:1219, 2006
Hall EJ: Scientific view of low-level radiation risks. Radiographics 11:509, 1991
Hannuna KY, Putignani L, Silvestri E, et al: Incidental endometrial adenocarcinoma in early pregnancy: a case report and review of the literature. Int J Gynecol Cancer 19(9):1580, 2009
Heinzman AB: Pelvic mass. In Hoffman BL, Schorge JO, Schaffer JI, et al (eds): Williams Gynecology, 2nd ed. New York, McGraw-Hill, 2012, p 246
Heller DS, Cracchiolo B, Hameed M, et al: Pregnancy-associated invasive squamous cell carcinoma of the vulva in a 28-year-old, HIV-negative woman: a case report. J Reprod Med 45:659, 2000
Higgins S, Haffty BG: Pregnancy and lactation after breast-conserving therapy for early stage breast cancer. Cancer 73:2175, 1994
Hirabayashi M, Ueo H, Okudaira Y, et al: Early gastric cancer and a concomitant pregnancy. Am Surg 53:730, 1987
Hoffman MS, Sayer RA: A guide to management: adnexal masses in pregnancy. OBG Management 19(3):27, 2007
Homer H, Saridogan E: Uterine artery embolization for fibroids is associated with an increased risk of miscarriage. Fertil Steril 94(1):324, 2010
Honore LH, O'Hara KE: Serous papillary neoplasms arising in paramesonephric parovarian cysts. A report of eight cases. Acta Obstet Gynecol Scand 59(6):525, 1980
Hoover RN, Hyer M, Pfeiffer RM, et al: Adverse health outcomes in women exposed in utero to diethylstilbestrol. N Engl J Med 365:1304, 2011
Horning SJ, Hoppe RT, Kaplan HS, et al: Female reproductive potential after treatment for Hodgkin's disease. N Engl J Med 304:1377, 1981
Hudis CA: Trastuzumab—mechanism of action and use in clinical practice. N Engl J Med 357:39, 2007
Hunter MI, Tewari KS, Monk BJ: Cervical neoplasia in pregnancy. Part 2: current treatment of invasive disease. Am J Obstet Gynecol 199(1):10, 2008
Irving JA, Clement PB: Nonneoplastic lesions of the ovary. In Kurman RJ, Ellenson LH, Ronnett BM (eds): Blaustein's Pathology of the Female Genital Tract, 6th ed. New York, Springer, 2011, p 606
Ives A, Saunders C, Bulsara M, et al: Pregnancy after breast cancer: population based study. BMJ 334:194, 2006
Jacobs C, Donaldson SS, Rosenberg SA, et al: Management of the pregnant patient with Hodgkin's disease. Ann Intern Med 95:669, 1981
Jacob JH, Stringer CA: Diagnosis and management of cancer during pregnancy. Semin Perinatol 14:79, 1990
Jakobsson M, Gissler M, Paavonen J, et al: Loop electrosurgical excision procedure and the risk for preterm birth. Obstet Gynecol 114:504, 2009
Jernström H, Lubinski J, Lynch HT, et al: Breast-feeding and the risk of breast cancer in BRCA1 and BRCA2 mutation carriers. J Natl Cancer Inst 96(14):1094, 2004
Johannsson O, Loman N, Borg A, et al: Pregnancy-associated breast cancer in BRCA1 and BRCA2 germ-line mutation carriers. Lancet 352:1359, 1998
Kakoza RM, Vollmer CM Jr, Stuart KE, et al: Pancreatic adenocarcinoma in the pregnant patient: a case report and literature review. J Gastrointest Surg 13(3):535, 2009
Kanal E, Barkovich AJ, Bell C, et al: ACR guidance document for safe MR practices: 2007. AJR Am J Roentgenol 188(6):1447, 2007
Kaňová N, Bičíková M: Hyperandrogenic states in pregnancy. Physiol Res 60(2):243, 2011
Kao HW, Wu CJ, Chung KT, et al: MR imaging of pregnancy luteoma: a case report and correlation with the clinical features. Korean J Radiol 6(1):44, 2005
Kathiresan AS, Johnson JN, Hood BJ, et al: Giant cell bone tumor of the thoracic spine presenting in late pregnancy. Obstet Gynecol 118(2 Pt 2):428, 2011
Kim CH, Abu-Rustum NR, Chi DS, et al: Reproductive outcomes of patients undergoing radical trachelectomy for early-stage cervical cancer. Gynecol Oncol 125(3):585, 2012
Kim SS, Klemp J, Fabian C: Breast cancer and fertility preservation. Fertil Steril 95(5):1535, 2011
King RM, Welch JS, Martin JK Jr, et al: Carcinoma of the breast associated with pregnancy. Surg Gynecol Obstet 160:228, 1985
Kjems E, Krag C: Melanoma and pregnancy. Acta Oncol 32:371, 1993
Klatsky PC, Tran ND, Caughey AB, et al: Fibroids and reproductive outcomes: a systematic literature review from conception to delivery. Am J Obstet Gynecol 198(4):357, 2008
Ko EM, Van Le L: Chemotherapy for gynecologic cancers occurring during pregnancy. Obstet Gynecol Surv 66(5):291, 2011
Korbin CD, Brown DL, Welch WR: Paraovarian cystadenomas and cystadenofibromas: sonographic characteristics in 14 cases. Radiology 208(2):459, 1998
Kuller JA, Zucker PK, Peng TC: Vulvar leiomyosarcoma in pregnancy. Am J Obstet Gynecol 162:164, 1990
Langagergaard V, Gislum M, Skriver MV, et al: Birth outcome in women with breast cancer. Br J Cancer 94:142, 2006

Langagergaard V, Horvath-Puho E, Norgaard M, et al: Hodgkin's disease and birth outcome: a Danish nationwide cohort study. Br J Cancer 98(1):183, 2008

Larsen EC, Schmiegelow K, Rechnitzer C, et al: Radiotherapy at a young age reduces uterine volume of childhood cancer survivors. Acta Obstet Gynecol Scand 83:96, 2004

Larson PS, Ungarelli RA, de Las Morenas A, et al: In utero exposure to diethylstilbestrol (DES) does not increase genomic instability in normal or neoplastic breast epithelium. Cancer 107(9):212, 2006

Lashgari M, Behmaram B, Ellis M: Leiomyomatosis peritonealis disseminata: a report of two cases. J Reprod Med 39:652, 1994

Laughlin SK, Baird DD, Savitz DA, et al: Prevalence of uterine leiomyomas in the first trimester of pregnancy: an ultrasound-screening study. Obstet Gynecol 113(3):630, 2009

Lawrenz B, Henes M, Neunhoeffer E, et al: Pregnancy after successful cancer treatment: what needs to be considered? Onkologie 35:128, 2012

Lee HJ, Lee IK, Kim JW, et al: Clinical characteristics of gastric cancer associated with pregnancy. Dig Surg 26(1):31, 2009

Leiserowitz GS, Xing G, Cress R, et al: Adnexal masses in pregnancy: how often are they malignant? Gynecol Oncol 101:315, 2006

Lens M, Bataille V: Melanoma in relation to reproductive and hormonal factors in women: current review on controversial issues. Cancer Causes Control 19(5):437, 2008

Levine D, Brown DL, Andreotti RF, et al: Management of asymptomatic ovarian and other adnexal cysts imaged at US: Society of Radiologists in Ultrasound Consensus Conference Statement. Radiology 256(3):943, 2010

Lin YH, Hwang JL, Huang LW, et al: Pyomyoma after a cesarean section. Acta Obstet Gynecol Scand 81:571, 2002

Lippman ME: Breast Cancer. In Longo DL, Fauci AS, Kasper DL, et al (eds): Harrison's Principles of Internal Medicine, 18th ed. New York, McGraw-Hill, 2012, p 754

Liu J, Zanotti K: Management of the adnexal mass. Obstet Gynecol 117:1413, 2011

Longo DL: Malignancies of lymphoid cells. In Longo DL, Fauci AS, Kasper DL, et al (eds): Harrison's Principles of Internal Medicine, 18th ed. New York, McGraw-Hill, 2012, p 919

Loren AW, Mangu PB, Beck LN, et al: Fertility preservation for patients with cancer: American Society of Clinical Oncology clinical practice guideline update. J Clin Oncol 31(19):2500, 2013

Lutz MH, Underwood PB Jr, Rozier JC, et al: Genital malignancy in pregnancy. Am J Obstet Gynecol 129:536, 1977

Mara M, Maskova J, Fucikova Z, et al: Midterm clinical and first reproductive results of a randomized controlled trial comparing uterine fibroid embolization and myomectomy. Cardiovasc Intervent Radiol 31(1):73, 2008

Marinoni, E, Di Netta T, Caramanico L, et al: Metastatic pancreatic cancer in late pregnancy: a case report and review of the literature. J Matern Fetal Neonatal Med 19(4):247, 2006

Masarie K, Katz V, Balderston K: Pregnancy luteomas: clinical presentations and management strategies. Obstet Gynecol Surv 65(9):575, 2010

Matsuo K, Eno ML, Im DD, et al: Pregnancy and genital sarcoma: a systematic review of the literature. Am J Perinatol 26(7):507, 2009

McGovern PG, Noah R, Koenigsberg R, et al: Adnexal torsion and pulmonary embolism: case report and review of the literature. Obstet Gynecol Surv 54(9):601, 1999

McNally L, Osmundson S, Barth R, et al: Urachal duct carcinoma complicating pregnancy. Obstet Gynecol 122:469, 2013

Minter A, Malik R, Ledbetter L, et al: Colon cancer in pregnancy. Cancer Control 12(3):196, 2005

Mondi MM, Cuenca RE, Ollila DW, et al: Sentinel lymph node biopsy during pregnancy: initial clinical experience. Ann Surg Oncol 14(1):218, 2007

Morice P, Uzan C, Gouy S, et al: Gynaecological cancers in pregnancy. Lancet 379:558, 2012

Navrozoglou I, Vrekoussis T, Kontostolis E et al: Breast cancer during pregnancy: a mini-review. Eur J Surg Oncol 34:837, 2008

Neiger R, Sonek JD, Croom CS, et al: Pregnancy-related changes in the size of uterine leiomyomas. J Reprod Med 51:671, 2006

Nisker JA, Shubat M: Stage IB cervical carcinoma and pregnancy: report of 49 cases. Am J Obstet Gynecol 145:203, 1983

Niwa K, Tagami K, Lian Z, et al: Outcome of fertility-preserving treatment in young women with endometrial carcinomas. Br J Obstet Gynaecol 112:317, 2005

Nugent P, O'Connell TX: Breast cancer and pregnancy. Arch Surg 120:1221, 1985

O'Gara P, Shepard J, Yared K, et al: Case 39-2009L: a 28-year-old pregnant woman with acute cardiac failure. N Engl J Med 361:2462, 2009

Oto A, Ernst R, Jesse MK, et al: Magnetic resonance imaging of the chest, abdomen, and pelvis in the evaluation of pregnant patients with neoplasms. Am J Perinatol 24(4):243, 2007

Paavonen J, Naud P, Salmerón J, et al: Efficacy of human papillomavirus (HPV)-16/18 AS04-adjuvanted vaccine against cervical infection and precancer caused by oncogenic HPV types (PATRICIA): final analysis of a double-blind, randomised study in young women. Lancet 374(9686):301, 2009

Pacini F, Castagna MG: Approach to and treatment of differentiated thyroid carcinoma. Med Clin North Am 96(2):369, 2012

Palmer J, Vatish M, Tidy J: Epithelial ovarian cancer in pregnancy: a review of the literature. BJOG 116:480, 2009

Papoutsis D, Sindos M, Papantoniou N, et al: Management options and prognosis of pancreatic adenocarcinoma at 16 weeks' gestation: a case report. J Reprod Med 57:167, 2012

Park JY, Kim DY, Suh DS, et al: Reproductive outcomes after laparoscopic radical trachelectomy for early-stage cervical cancer. J Gynecol Oncol 25:9, 2014

Pavlidis N: Cancer and pregnancy: what should we know about the management with systemic treatment of pregnant women with cancer? Eur J Cancer 47 Suppl 3:S348, 2011

Pavlidis NA: Coexistence of pregnancy and malignancy. Oncologist 7:279, 2002

Pereg D, Koren G, Lishner M: The treatment of Hodgkin's and non-Hodgkin's lymphoma in pregnancy. Haematologica 92(9):1230, 2007

Perera D, Kandavar R, Palacios E: Pancreatic adenocarcinoma presenting as acute pancreatitis during pregnancy: clinical and radiologic manifestations. J La State Med Soc 163:114, 2011

Pettersson BF, Andersson S, Hellman K, et al: Invasive carcinoma of the uterine cervix associated with pregnancy: 90 years of experience. Cancer 116:2343, 2010

Pritts EA: Fibroids and infertility: a systematic review of the evidence. Obstet Gynecol Surv 56:483, 2001

Qidwai II, Caughey AB, Jacoby AF: Obstetric outcomes in women with sonographically identified uterine leiomyomata. Obstet Gynecol 107:376, 2006

Randall ME, Michael H, Long H III, et al: Uterine cervix. In Barakat RR, Markman M, Randall ME (eds): Principles and Practice of Gynecologic Oncology, 5th ed. Philadelphia, Lippincott Williams & Wilkins, 2009, p 647

Reynoso EE, Shepherd FA, Messner HA, et al: Acute leukemia during pregnancy: the Toronto Leukemia Study Group experience with long-term follow-up of children exposed in utero to chemotherapeutic agents. J Clin Oncol 5:1098, 1987

Richardson DL: Cervical cancer. In Hoffman BL, Schorge JO, Schaffer JI, et al (eds): Williams Gynecology, 2nd ed. New York, McGraw-Hill, 2012, p 769

Rizack T, Mega A, Legare R, et al: Management of hematological malignancies during pregnancy. Am J Hematol 84(12):830, 2009

Robison LL, Green DM, Hudson M, et al: Long-term outcomes of adult survivors of childhood cancer. Results from the Childhood Cancer Survivor Study. Cancer Suppl 104(11):2557, 2005

Rodriguez AO, Chew H, Cress R, et al: Evidence of poorer survival in pregnancy-associated breast cancer. Obstet Gynecol 112(1):71, 2008

Rosenkranz KM, Lucci A: Surgical treatment of pregnancy associated breast cancer. Breast Dis 23:87, 2006

Russell P, Robboy SJ: Ovarian cysts, tumor-like, iatrogenic and miscellaneous conditions. In Robboy SJ, Mutter GL, Prat J, et al (eds): Robboy's Pathology of the Female Reproductive Tract, 2nd ed. London, Churchill Livingstone, 2009, p 577

Salvador E, Bienstock J, Blakemore KJ, et al: Leiomyomata uteri, genetic amniocentesis, and the risk of second-trimester spontaneous abortion. Am J Obstet Gynecol 186:913, 2002

Samson SL, Bentley JR, Fahey TJ, et al: The effect of loop electrosurgical excision procedure on future pregnancy outcome. Obstet Gynecol 105:325, 2005

Saslow D, Solomon D, Lawson HW, et al: American Cancer Society, American Society for Colposcopy and Cervical Pathology, and American Society for Clinical Pathology screening guidelines for the prevention and early detection of cervical cancer. Am J Clin Pathol 137(4):516, 2012

Schammel DP, Mittal KR, Kaplan K, et al: Endometrial adenocarcinoma associated with intrauterine pregnancy: a report of five cases and a review of the literature. Int J Gynecol Pathol 17:327, 1998

Schmeler KM, Mayo-Smith WW, Peipert JF, et al: Adnexal masses in pregnancy: surgery compared with observation. Obstet Gynecol 105:1098, 2005

Schwartz JL, Mozurkewich EL, Johnson TM: Current management of patients with melanoma who are pregnant, want to get pregnant, or do not want to get pregnant. Cancer 97(9):2130, 2003

Shanbhag S, Clark H, Timmaraju V, et al: Pregnancy outcome after treatment for cervical intraepithelial neoplasia. Obstet Gynecol 114:727, 2009

Shavell VI, Thakur M, Sawant A, et al: Adverse obstetric outcomes associated with sonographically identified large uterine fibroids. Fertil Steril 97(1):107, 2012

Sheiner E, Bashiri A, Levy A, et al: Obstetric characteristics and perinatal outcome of pregnancies with uterine leiomyomas. Obstet Gynecol Surv 59:647, 2004

Shen T, Vortmeyer AO, Zhuang Z, et al: High frequency of allelic loss of BRCA2 gene in pregnancy-associated breast carcinoma. J Natl Cancer Inst 91:1686, 1999
Shepherd JH, Spencer C, Herod J, et al: Radical vaginal trachelectomy as a fertility-sparing procedure in women with early-stage cervical cancer—cumulative pregnancy rate in a series of 123 women. Br J Obstet Gynaecol 113:719, 2006
Sherard GB III, Hodson CA, Williams HJ, et al: Adnexal masses and pregnancy: a 12-year experience. Am J Obstet Gynecol 189:358, 2003
Shulman LN, Hitt RA, Ferry JA: Case records of the Massachusetts General Hospital. Case 4-2008. A 33-year-old pregnant woman with swelling of the left breast and shortness of breath. N Engl J Med 358(5):513, 2008
Signorelli M, Caspani G, Bonazzi C, et al: Fertility-sparing treatment in young women with endometrial cancer or atypical complex hyperplasia: a prospective single-institution experience of 21 cases. BJOG 116(1):114, 2009
Signorello LB, Cohen SS, Bosetti C, et al: Female survivors of childhood cancer: preterm birth and low birth weight among their children. J Natl Cancer Inst 98:1453, 2006
Signorello LB, Mulvihill JJ, Green DM, et al: Stillbirth and neonatal death in relation to radiation exposure before conception: a retrospective cohort study. Lancet 376:624, 2010
Silverberg SG, Kurman RJ, Nogales F, et al: Tumors of the Uterine Corpus [Epithelial tumors and related lesions]. In Tavassoli FA, Devilee P (eds): World Health Organization Classification of Tumours. 2003, p 221
Sisson JC, Freitas J, McDougall IR, et al: Radiation safety in the treatment of patients with thyroid diseases by radioiodine 131I: practice recommendations of the American Thyroid Association. Thyroid 21(4):335, 2011
Smith LH, Danielsen B, Allen ME, et al: Cancer associated with obstetric delivery: results of linkage with the California cancer registry. Am J Obstet Gynecol 189:1128, 2003
Soares SR, Gómez R, Simón C, et al: Targeting the vascular endothelial growth factor system to prevent ovarian hyperstimulation syndrome. Hum Reprod Update 14(4):321, 2008
Sood AK, Sorosky JI: Invasive cervical cancer complicating pregnancy: how to manage the dilemma? Obstet Gynecol Clin North Am 25:343, 1998
Spanheimer PM, Graham MM, Sugg SL, et al: Measurement of uterine radiation exposure from lymphoscintigraphy indicates safety of sentinel lymph node biopsy during pregnancy. Ann Surg Oncol 16(5):1143, 2009
Spitzer M, Kaushal N, Benjamin F: Maternal CA-125 levels in pregnancy and the puerperium. J Reprod Med 43:387, 1998
Stewart CA, Termanini B, Sutliff VE, et al: Management of the Zollinger–Ellison syndrome in pregnancy. Am J Obstet Gynecol 176:224, 1997
Stiles GM, Stanco LM, Saven A, et al: Splenectomy for hairy cell leukemia in pregnancy. J Perinatol 18:200, 1998
Stokes LS, Wallace MJ, Godwin RB, et al: Quality improvement guidelines for uterine artery embolization for symptomatic leiomyomas. J Vasc Interv Radiol 21(8):1153, 2010
Stout MJ, Odibo AO, Graseck AS, et a: Leiomyomas at routine second-trimester ultrasound examination and adverse obstetric outcomes. Obstet Gynecol 116(5):1056, 2010
Takushi M, Moromizato H, Sakumoto K, et al: Management of invasive carcinoma of the uterine cervix associated with pregnancy: outcome of intentional delay in treatment. Gynecol Oncol 87:185, 2002
Tannus JF, Hertzberg BS, Haystead CM, et al: Unilateral luteoma of pregnancy mimicking a malignant ovarian mass on magnetic resonance and ultrasound. J Magn Reson Imaging 29(3):713, 2009
Tavassoli FA, Devilee P: Tumours of the ovary and peritoneum. In World Health Organization Classification of Tumours: Pathology and Genetics of Tumours of the Breast and Female Genital Organs. Lyon, International Agency for Research on Cancer, 2003, p 114
Titus-Ernstoff L, Troisi R, Hatch EE, et al: Mortality in women given diethylstilbestrol during pregnancy. Br J Cancer 95:107, 2006
Torashima M, Yamashita Y, Hatanaka Y, et al: Invasive adenocarcinoma of the uterine cervix: MR imaging. Comp Med Imaging Graph 21(4):253, 1997
Ungár L, Smith JR, Pálfavli L, et al: Abdominal radical trachelectomy during pregnancy to preserve pregnancy and fertility. Obstet Gynecol 108:811, 2006
Valachis A, Tsali L, Pesce LL, et al: Safety of pregnancy after primary breast carcinoma in young women: a meta-analysis to overcome bias of healthy mother effect studies. Obstet Gynecol Surv 65:786, 2010
Van Calsteren K, Hanssens M, Moerman P, et al: Successful conservative treatment of endocervical adenocarcinoma stage Ib1 diagnosed early in pregnancy. Acta Obstet Gynecol Scand 87(2):250, 2008
van der Vange N, Weverling GJ, Ketting BW, et al: The prognosis of cervical cancer associated with pregnancy: a matched cohort study. Obstet Gynecol 85:1022, 1995
van Vliet W, van Loon AJ, ten Hoor KA, et al: Cervical carcinoma during pregnancy: outcome of planned delay in treatment. Eur J Obstet Gynecol Reprod Biol 79:153, 1998
Velentgas P, Daling JR, Malone KE, et al: Pregnancy after breast carcinoma: outcomes and influence on mortality. Cancer 85:2424, 1999
Viswanathan S, Ramaswamy B: Pregnancy-associated breast cancer. Clin Obstet Gynecol 54(4):546, 2011
Walsh C, Fazio VW: Cancer of the colon, rectum, and anus during pregnancy. The surgeon's perspective. Gastroenterol Clin North Am 27:257, 1998
Wang YC, Su HY, Liu JY, et al: Maternal and female fetal virilization caused by pregnancy luteomas. Fertil Steril 84:509.e15, 2005
Werner CL, Lo JY, Heffernan, et al: Loop electrosurgical excision procedure and risk of preterm birth. Obstet Gynecol 115:605, 2010
Weitzman VN, DiLuigi AJ, Maier DB, et al: Prevention of recurrent adnexal torsion. Fertil Steril 90(5):2018.e1, 2008
Wetzler M, Byrd JC, Bloomfield CD: Acute and chronic myeloid leukemia. In Kasper DL, Brauward E, Fauci AS, et al (eds): Harrison's Principles of Internal Medicine, 18th ed. New York, McGraw-Hill, 2012, p 905
Whitecar MP, Turner S, Higby MK: Adnexal masses in pregnancy: a review of 130 cases undergoing surgical management. Am J Obstet Gynecol 181:19, 1999
Williams SF, Schilsky RL: Neoplastic disorders. In Barron WM, Lindheimer MD (eds): Medical Disorders During Pregnancy, 3rd ed. St. Louis, Mosby, 2001, p 392
Winther JF, Boice JD Jr, Frederiksen K, et al: Radiotherapy for childhood cancer and risk for congenital malformations in offspring: a population-based cohort study. Clin Genet 75(1):50, 2009
Wo JY, Viswanathan AN: Impact of radiotherapy on fertility, pregnancy, and neonatal outcome in female cancer patients. Int J Radiat Oncol Biol Phys 73(5):1304, 2009
Wohlfahrt J, Olsen JH, Melby M: Breast cancer risk after childbirth in young women with family history. Cancer Causes Control 13:169, 2002
Wong DJ, Strassner HT: Melanoma in pregnancy: a literature review. Clin Obstet Gynecol 33:782, 1990
Woo JC, Yu T, Hurd TC: Breast cancer in pregnancy. Arch Surg 138:91, 2003
Woodruff TK: The Oncofertility Consortium—addressing fertility in young people with cancer. Nat Rev Clin Oncol 7(8):466, 2010
Wright TC Jr, Massad S, Dunton CJ, et al: 2006 consensus guidelines for the management of women with abnormal cervical cancer screening tests. Am J Obstet Gynecol 197(4):346, 2007a
Wright TC Jr, Massad S, Dunton CJ, et al: 2006 consensus guidelines for the management of women with cervical intraepithelial neoplasia or adenocarcinoma in situ. Am J Obstet Gynecol 197(4):340, 2007b
Yahata T, Numata M, Kashima K, et al: Conservative treatment of stage IA1 adenocarcinoma of the cervix during pregnancy. Gynecol Oncol 109(1):49, 2008
Yazbeck CF, Sullivan SD. Thyroid disorders during pregnancy. Med Clin No America 96:235, 2012
Yazigi R, Sandstad J, Munoz AK: Primary staging in ovarian tumors of low malignant potential. Gynecol Oncol 31:402, 1988
Yeaton-Massey A, Brookfield KF, Aziz N, et al: Maternal bladder cancer diagnosed at routine first-trimester obstetric ultrasound examination. Obstet Gynecol 122:464, 2013
Yost NP, Santoso JT, McIntire DD, et al: Postpartum regression rates of antepartum cervical intraepithelial neoplasia II and III lesions. Obstet Gynecol 93:359, 1999
Younis MT, Iram S, Anwar B, et al: Women with asymptomatic cervical polyps may not need to see a gynaecologist or have them removed: an observational retrospective study of 1126 cases. Eur J Obstet Gynecol Reprod Biol 150(2):190, 2010
Zagouri F, Sergentanis TN, Chrysikos D, et al: Platinum derivatives during pregnancy in cervical cancer: a systematic review and meta-analysis. Obstet Gynecol 121:337, 2013
Zanetta G, Mariani E, Lissoni A, et al: A prospective study of the role of ultrasound in the management of adnexal masses in pregnancy. Br J Obstet Gynaecol 110:578, 2003
Zemlickis D, Lishner M, Degendorfer P, et al: Maternal and fetal outcome after breast cancer in pregnancy. Am J Obstet Gynecol 166:781, 1992
Zweizig S, Perron J, Grubb D, et al: Conservative management of adnexal torsion. Am J Obstet Gynecol 168(6 Pt 1):1791, 1993

CHAPTER 64

Infectious Diseases

Infections have historically been a major cause of maternal and fetal morbidity and mortality worldwide, and they remain so in the 21st century. The unique maternal-fetal vascular connection in some cases serves to protect the fetus from infectious agents, whereas in other instances it provides a conduit for their transmission to the fetus. Maternal serological status, gestational age at the time infection is acquired, the mode of acquisition, and the immunological status of both the mother and her fetus all influence disease outcome.

MATERNAL AND FETAL IMMUNOLOGY

Pregnancy-Induced Immunological Changes

Even after intensive study, many of the maternal immunological adaptations to pregnancy are not well elucidated. It is known that pregnancy is associated with an increase in CD4-positive T cells secreting Th2-type cytokines—for example interleukins 4, 5, 10, and 13. Th1-type cytokine production—for example, interferon gamma and interleukin 2—appears to be somewhat suppressed, leading to a *Th2 bias* in pregnancy. This bias affects the ability to rapidly eliminate certain intracellular pathogens during pregnancy, although the clinical implications of this suppression are unknown (Jamieson, 2006a; Raghupathy, 2001; Svensson-Arvelund, 2014). Importantly, the Th2 humoral immune response remains intact.

Fetal and Newborn Immunology

The active immunological capacity of the fetus and neonate is compromised compared with that of older children and adults. That said, fetal cell-mediated and humoral immunity begin to develop by 9 to 15 weeks' gestation (Warner, 2010). The primary fetal response to infection is immunoglobulin M (IgM). Passive immunity is provided by IgG transferred across the placenta. By 16 weeks, this transfer begins to increase rapidly, and by 26 weeks, fetal concentrations are equivalent to those of the mother. After birth, breast feeding is protective against some infections, although this protection begins to decline at 2 months of age. Current World Health Organization (2013) recommendations are to exclusively breast feed for the first 6 months of life with partial breast feeding until 2 years of age.

Vertical transmission refers to passage from the mother to her fetus of an infectious agent through the placenta, during labor or delivery, or by breast feeding. Thus, preterm rupture of membranes, prolonged labor, and obstetrical manipulations may increase the risk of neonatal infection. Those occurring less than 72 hours after delivery are usually caused by bacteria acquired in utero or during delivery, whereas infections after that time most likely were acquired afterward. Table 64-1 details specific infections by mode and timing of acquisition.

Neonatal infection, especially in its early stages, may be difficult to diagnose because neonates often fail to express classic clinical signs. If the fetus was infected in utero, there may be depression and acidosis at birth for no apparent reason. The neonate may suck poorly, vomit, or show abdominal

TABLE 64-1. Specific Causes of Some Fetal and Neonatal Infections

Intrauterine
Transplacental
Viruses: varicella-zoster, coxsackie, human parvovirus B19, rubella, cytomegalovirus, HIV
Bacteria: *Listeria*, syphilis, *Borrelia*
Protozoa: toxoplasmosis, malaria
Ascending infection
Bacteria: group B streptococcus, coliforms
Viruses: HSV
Intrapartum
Maternal exposure
Bacteria: gonorrhea, chlamydia, group B streptococcus, tuberculosis, mycoplasmas
Viruses: HSV, HPV, HIV, hepatitis B, hepatitis C
External contamination
Bacteria: staphylococcus, coliforms
Viruses: HSV, varicella zoster
Neonatal
Human transmission: staphylococcus, HSV
Respirators and catheters: staphylococcus, coliforms

HIV = human immunodeficiency virus; HPV = human papillomavirus; HSV = herpes simplex virus.

distention. Respiratory insufficiency may develop, which may present similarly to idiopathic respiratory distress syndrome. The neonate may be lethargic or jittery. The response to sepsis may be hypothermia rather than hyperthermia, and the total leukocyte and neutrophil counts may be depressed.

VIRAL INFECTIONS

Varicella-Zoster Virus

Several viruses that infect the mother can also cause devastating fetal infections. Varicella-zoster virus (VZV) is a double-stranded DNA herpes virus acquired predominately during childhood, and 95 percent of adults have serological evidence of immunity (Plourd, 2005). The incidence of adult varicella infections declined by 74 percent after the introduction of varicella vaccination, probably secondary to herd immunity (Marin, 2008). This has resulted in a decrease in maternal and fetal varicella infections (Khandaker, 2011). Primary infection—*varicella* or *chicken pox*—is transmitted by direct contact with an infected individual, although respiratory transmission has been reported. The incubation period is 10 to 21 days, and a nonimmune woman has a 60- to 95-percent risk of becoming infected after exposure (Whitley, 2012). She is then contagious from 1 day before the onset of the rash until the lesions are crusted over.

Maternal Infection

Primary varicella infection presents with a 1- to 2-day flu-like prodrome, which is followed by pruritic vesicular lesions that crust over in 3 to 7 days. Infection tends to be more severe in adults, and a quarter of varicella deaths are within the 5 percent of nonimmune adults (Centers for Disease Control and Prevention, 2007).

Mortality is predominately due to varicella pneumonia, which is thought to be more severe during adulthood and particularly in pregnancy. Between 5 and 20 percent of infected pregnant women developed pneumonitis (Centers for Disease Control and Prevention, 2007; Harger, 2002). Risk factors for VZV pneumonia include smoking and having more than 100 cutaneous lesions. Maternal mortality rates with pneumonia have decreased to 1 to 2 percent (Chandra, 1998). Symptoms of pneumonia usually appear 3 to 5 days into the course of illness. It is characterized by fever, tachypnea, dry cough, dyspnea, and pleuritic pain. Nodular infiltrates are similar to other viral pneumonias (Chap. 51, p. 1018). Although resolution of pneumonitis parallels that of skin lesions, fever and compromised pulmonary function may persist for weeks.

If primary varicella infection is reactivated years later, it causes *herpes zoster* or *shingles* (Whitley, 2012). This presents as a unilateral dermatomal vesicular eruption associated with severe pain. Zoster does not appear to be more frequent or severe in pregnant women. Enders and associates (1994) reviewed 366 cases during pregnancy and found little evidence that zoster causes congenital malformations. Zoster is contagious if blisters are broken, although less so than primary varicella infection.

Fetal and Neonatal Infection

In women with chicken pox during the first half of pregnancy, the fetus may develop congenital varicella syndrome. Some features include chorioretinitis, microphthalmia, cerebral cortical atrophy, growth restriction, hydronephrosis, limb hypoplasia, and cicatricial skin lesions as shown in Figure 64-1 (Auriti, 2009). Enders and coworkers (1994) evaluated 1373 pregnant women with varicella infection. When maternal infection developed before 13 weeks, only two of 472 pregnancies—0.4 percent—had neonates with congenital varicella.

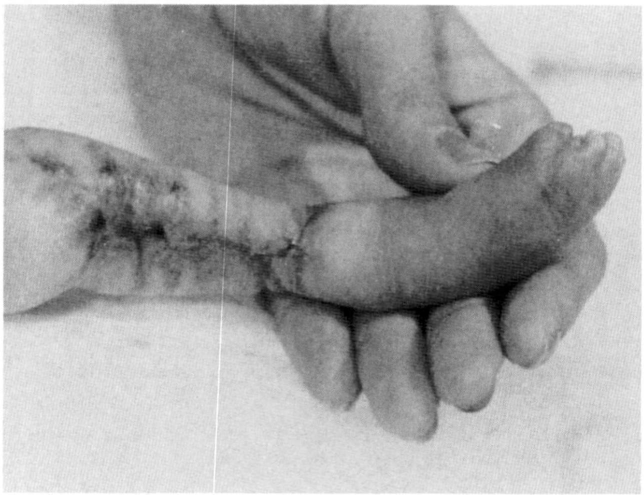

FIGURE 64-1 Atrophy of the lower extremity with bony defects and scarring in a fetus infected during the first trimester by varicella. (From Paryani, 1986, with permission.)

The highest risk was between 13 and 20 weeks, during which time seven of 351 exposed fetuses—2 percent—had evidence of congenital varicella. After 20 weeks' gestation, the researchers found no clinical evidence of congenital infection. Thus, congenital infections, particularly after 20 weeks, are uncommon. Subsequent sporadic reports have described central nervous system abnormalities and skin lesions in fetuses who developed congenital varicella in weeks 21 to 28 of gestation (Lamont, 2011b; Marin, 2007).

If the fetus or neonate is exposed to active infection just before or during delivery, and therefore before maternal antibody has been formed, then there is a serious threat to newborns. Attack rates range from 25 to 50 percent, and mortality rates approach 30 percent. In some instances, neonates develop disseminated visceral and central nervous system disease, which is commonly fatal. For this reason, varicella-zoster immune globulin should be administered to neonates born to mothers who have clinical evidence of varicella 5 days before and up to 2 days after delivery.

Diagnosis

Maternal varicella infection is usually diagnosed clinically. The virus may also be isolated by scraping the vesicle base during primary infection and performing a Tzanck smear, tissue culture, or direct fluorescent antibody testing. Also, available nucleic acid amplification tests (NAATs) are very sensitive. Congenital varicella may be diagnosed using NAAT analysis of amnionic fluid, although a positive result does not correlate well with the development of congenital infection (Mendelson, 2006). A detailed anatomical sonographic evaluation performed at least 5 weeks after maternal infection may disclose abnormalities, but the sensitivity is low (Mandelbrot, 2012).

Management

Maternal Viral Exposure. There are several aspects of maternal varicella virus exposure and infection in pregnancy that affect management. Because most adults are VZV seropositive, exposed pregnant women with a negative history for chicken pox should undergo VZV serologic testing. At least 70 percent of these women will be seropositive, and thus immune. Exposed pregnant women who are susceptible should be given VariZIG, a recently approved varicella zoster immune globulin. Although best given within 96 hours of exposure, its use is approved for up to 10 days to prevent or attenuate varicella infection (Centers for Disease Control and Prevention, 2012a, 2013h).

Maternal Infection. *Any patient diagnosed with primary varicella infection should be isolated from pregnant women.* Because pneumonia often presents with few symptoms, a chest radiograph is recommended by many. Most women require only supportive care, but those who require intravenous (IV) fluids and especially those with pneumonia are hospitalized. Intravenous acyclovir therapy is given to women requiring hospitalization—500 mg/m^2 or 10 to 15 mg/kg every 8 hours.

Vaccination. An attenuated live-virus vaccine—*Varivax*—was approved in 1995. Two doses, given 4 to 8 weeks apart, are recommended for adolescents and adults with no history of varicella. This results in 98-percent seroconversion (Centers for Disease Control and Prevention, 2007). Importantly, vaccine-induced immunity diminishes over time, and the breakthrough infection rate approximates 5 percent at 10 years (Chaves, 2007). *The vaccine is not recommended for pregnant women or for those who may become pregnant within a month following each vaccine dose.* That said, a registry of 981 vaccine-exposed pregnancies reports no cases of congenital varicella syndrome or other congenital associated malformations (Wilson, 2008). The attenuated vaccine virus is not secreted in breast milk. Thus, postpartum vaccination should not be delayed because of breast feeding (American College of Obstetricians and Gynecologists, 2013a; Bohlke, 2003).

Influenza

These respiratory infections are caused by members of the family Orthomyxoviridae. *Influenza A* and *B* form one genus of these RNA viruses, and both cause epidemic human disease. Influenza A viruses are subclassified further by hemagglutinin (H) and neuraminidase (N) surface antigens. Influenza outbreaks occur annually, and the most recent epidemic was in 2013–2014 caused by an influenza A/H_1N_1 strain.

Maternal and Fetal Infection

Maternal influenza is characterized by fever, dry cough, and systemic symptoms. Infection usually is not life-threatening in otherwise healthy adults, but pregnant women appear to be more susceptible to serious complications, particularly pulmonary involvement (Cox, 2006; Neuzil, 1998; Rasmussen, 2012). In early 2003, widespread influenza A infection affected pregnant women. At Parkland Hospital, more than 100 women were hospitalized for this infection, and 12 percent had pulmonary infiltrates seen radiographically (Rogers, 2010).

There is no firm evidence that influenza A virus causes congenital malformations (Irving, 2000; Saxén, 1990). Conversely, Lynberg and colleagues (1994) reported increased neural-tube defects in neonates born to women with influenza early in pregnancy, but this was possibly associated with hyperthermia (Chap. 12, p. 284). Viremia is infrequent, and transplacental passage is rare (Rasmussen, 2012). Stillbirth, preterm delivery, and first-trimester abortion have all been reported, usually correlated to severity of maternal infection (Centers for Disease Control and Prevention, 2011; Pierce, 2011; Yates, 2010).

Influenza may be detected in nasopharyngeal swabs using viral antigen rapid detection assays (Table 64-2). Reverse transcriptase–polymerase chain reaction (RT-PCR) is the more sensitive and specific test, although not commercially available in many hospitals (Dolin, 2012). In contrast, rapid influenza diagnostic tests (RIDTs) are least indicative, with sensitivities of 40 to 70 percent. In the Parkland Hospital emergency room, immunofluorescent antibody assays are used. Nasopharyngeal specimens are collected as early as possible after symptom onset to maximize influenza testing sensitivity. Importantly, decisions to administer antiviral medications for

TABLE 64-2. Outpatient Influenza A and B Virus Testing Methods

Method[a]	Test Time
Viral cell culture	3–10 d
Rapid cell culture	1–3 d
Direct (DFA) or indirect (IFA) fluorescent antibody assay	1–4 hr
RT-PCR and other molecular assays	1–6 hr
Rapid influenza diagnostic tests	< 30 min

[a]Nasopharyngeal or throat swab.
RT-PCR = reverse transcription-polymerase chain reaction.
Abbreviated from Centers for Disease Control and Prevention, 2013f.

influenza treatment or chemoprophylaxis should be based on clinical symptoms and epidemiological factors. Moreover, the start of therapy should not be delayed pending testing results (Centers for Disease Control and Prevention, 2013f).

Management

Two classes of antiviral medications are currently available. *Neuraminidase inhibitors* are highly effective for the treatment of early influenza A and B. These include *oseltamivir* (Tamiflu), which is taken orally for treatment and for chemoprophylaxis, and *zanamivir* (Relenza), which is inhaled for treatment. *Peramivir* is an investigational drug administered intravenously.

The *adamantanes* include amantadine and rimantadine, which were used for years for treatment and chemoprophylaxis of influenza A. In 2005, influenza A resistance to adamantine was reported to be > 90 percent in the United States, and thus, adamantane use is not currently recommended. It is possible that these drugs may again be effective for subsequently mutated strains.

There is limited experience with all five of these antiviral agents in pregnant women. They are Food and Drug Administration category C drugs, used when the potential benefits outweigh the risks. At Parkland Hospital, we recommend starting oseltamivir treatment within 48 hours of symptom onset—75 mg orally twice daily for 5 days. Prophylaxis with oseltamivir, 75 mg orally once daily for 10 days, is also recommended for significant exposures. Antibacterial medications should be added when a secondary bacterial pneumonia is suspected (Chap. 51, p. 1016).

Vaccination

Effective vaccines are formulated annually. Vaccination against influenza throughout the influenza season, but optimally in October or November, is recommended by the Centers for Disease Control and Prevention (CDC) (2013e) and the American College of Obstetricians and Gynecologists (2010) for all women who will be pregnant during the influenza season. This is especially important for those affected by chronic medical disorders such as diabetes, heart disease, asthma, or human immunodeficiency virus (HIV) infection (Jamieson, 2012). Inactivated vaccine prevents clinical illness in 70 to 90 percent of healthy adults. Importantly, there is no evidence of teratogenicity or other adverse maternal or fetal events (Conlin, 2013; Kharbanda, 2013; Munoz, 2012; Nordin, 2013; Sheffield, 2012). Moreover, several studies have found decreased rates of influenza in infants up to 6 months of age whose mothers were vaccinated during pregnancy (Steinhoff, 2012; Zaman, 2008). Immunogenicity of the trivalent inactivated seasonal influenza vaccine in pregnant women is similar to that in the nonpregnant individual (Sperling, 2012). A live attenuated influenza virus vaccine is available for intranasal use but is not recommended for pregnant women.

Mumps

This uncommon adult infection is caused by an RNA paramyxovirus. Because of childhood immunization, up to 90 percent of adults are seropositive (Rubin, 2012). The virus primarily infects the salivary glands, and hence its name—mumps—is derived from Latin, "to grimace." Infection also may involve the gonads, meninges, pancreas, and other organs. It is transmitted by direct contact with respiratory secretions, saliva, or through fomites. Treatment is symptomatic, and mumps during pregnancy is no more severe than in nonpregnant adults.

Women who develop mumps in the first trimester may have an increased risk of spontaneous abortion. Infection in pregnancy is not associated with congenital malformations, and fetal infection is rare (McLean, 2013).

The live attenuated Jeryl-Lynn vaccine strain is part of the MMR vaccine—measles, mumps, and rubella—and is contraindicated in pregnancy according to the CDC (McLean, 2013). No malformations attributable to MMR vaccination in pregnancy have been reported, but pregnancy should be avoided for 30 days after mumps vaccination. The vaccine may be given to susceptible women postpartum, and breast feeding is not a contraindication.

Rubeola (Measles)

Measles is caused by a highly contagious RNA virus of the family Paramyxoviridae that only infects humans. Annual outbreaks occur in late winter and early spring, transmission is primarily by respiratory droplets, and the secondary attack rate among contacts exceeds 90 percent (Moss, 2012). Infection is characterized by fever, coryza, conjunctivitis, and cough. The characteristic erythematous maculopapular rash develops on the face and neck and then spreads to the back, trunk, and extremities. *Koplik spots* are small white lesions with surrounding erythema found within the oral cavity. Diagnosis is most commonly performed by serology, although RT-PCR tests are available. Treatment is supportive.

Pregnant women without evidence of measles immunity should be administered intravenous immune globulin (IVIG), 400 mg/kg within 6 days of a measles exposure (McLean, 2013). Active vaccination is not performed during pregnancy. However, susceptible women can be vaccinated routinely postpartum, and breast feeding is not contraindicated (Ohji, 2009).

The virus does not appear to be teratogenic (Siegel, 1973). However, an increased frequency of abortion, preterm delivery, and low-birthweight neonates is noted with maternal measles (American Academy of Pediatrics, 2006; Siegel, 1966). If a woman develops measles shortly before birth, there is considerable risk of serious infection developing in the neonate, especially in a preterm neonate.

Rubella—German Measles

This RNA togavirus typically causes infections of minor importance in the absence of pregnancy. *Rubella infection in the first trimester, however, poses significant risk for abortion and severe congenital malformations.* Transmission occurs via nasopharyngeal secretions, and the transmission rate is 80 percent to susceptible individuals. The peak incidence is late winter and spring.

Maternal rubella infection is usually a mild, febrile illness with a generalized maculopapular rash beginning on the face and spreading to the trunk and extremities. Other symptoms may include arthralgias or arthritis, head and neck lymphadenopathy, and conjunctivitis. The incubation period is 12 to 23 days. Viremia usually precedes clinical signs by about a week, and adults are infectious during viremia and through 5 to 7 days of the rash. Up to half of maternal infections are subclinical despite viremia that may cause devastating fetal infection (McLean, 2013; Zimmerman, 2012).

Diagnosis

Rubella may be isolated from the urine, blood, nasopharynx, and cerebrospinal fluid for up to 2 weeks after rash onset. The diagnosis is usually made, however, with serological analysis. Specific IgM antibody can be detected using enzyme-linked immunoassay from 4 to 5 days after onset of clinical disease, but it can persist for up to 6 weeks after appearance of the rash (Zimmerman, 2012). Importantly, rubella reinfection can give rise to transient low levels of IgM. Serum IgG antibody titers peak 1 to 2 weeks after rash onset. This rapid antibody response may complicate serodiagnosis unless samples are initially collected within a few days after the onset of the rash. If, for example, the first specimen was obtained 10 days after the rash, detection of IgG antibodies would fail to differentiate between very recent disease and preexisting immunity to rubella. IgG avidity testing is performed concomitant with the serological tests above. High-avidity IgG antibodies indicate an infection at least 2 months in the past.

Fetal Effects

Rubella is one of the most complete teratogens, and sequelae of fetal infection are worst during organogenesis (Adams Waldorf, 2013). Pregnant women with rubella infection and a rash during the first 12 weeks of gestation have a fetus with congenital infection in up to 90 percent of cases (Miller, 1982; Zimmerman, 2012). At 13 to 14 weeks' gestation, this incidence was 54 percent, and by the end of the second trimester, it was 25 percent. Defects are rare after 20 weeks (Miller, 1982). According to Reef and colleagues (2000), congenital rubella syndrome includes one or more of the following:

- Eye defects—cataracts and congenital glaucoma
- Congenital heart defects—patent ductus arteriosus and pulmonary artery stenosis
- Sensorineural deafness—the most common single defect
- Central nervous system defects—microcephaly, developmental delay, mental retardation, and meningoencephalitis
- Pigmentary retinopathy
- Neonatal purpura
- Hepatosplenomegaly and jaundice
- Radiolucent bone disease

Neonates born with congenital rubella may shed the virus for many months and thus be a threat to other infants and to susceptible adults who contact them.

The *extended rubella syndrome*, with progressive panencephalitis and type 1 diabetes, may not develop clinically until the second or third decade of life. As many as a third of neonates who are asymptomatic at birth may manifest such developmental injury (Webster, 1998).

Management and Prevention

There is no specific treatment for rubella. Droplet precautions for 7 days after the onset of the rash are recommended. Primary prevention relies on comprehensive vaccination programs (Coonrod, 2008). Although large epidemics of rubella have virtually disappeared in the United States because of immunization, up to 10 percent of women in the United States are susceptible (Zimmerman, 2012). Cluster outbreaks during the 1990s mainly involved persons born outside the United States, as congenital rubella is still common in developing nations (Banatvala, 2004; Reef, 2002).

To eradicate rubella and prevent congenital rubella syndrome completely, a comprehensive approach is recommended for immunizing the adult population (McLean, 2013). MMR vaccine should be offered to nonpregnant women of childbearing age who do not have evidence of immunity whenever they make contact with the health-care system. Vaccination of all susceptible hospital personnel who might be exposed to patients with rubella or who might have contact with pregnant women is important. Rubella vaccination should be avoided 1 month before or during pregnancy because the vaccine contains attenuated live virus. Although there is a small overall theoretical risk of up to 2.6 percent, there is no observed evidence that the vaccine induces malformations (Badilla, 2007; McLean, 2013). MMR vaccination is not an indication for pregnancy termination. Prenatal serological screening for rubella is indicated for all pregnant women. Women found to be nonimmune should be offered the MMR vaccine postpartum.

Despite native or vaccine-induced immunity, subclinical rubella maternal *reinfection* may develop during outbreaks. And although fetal infection can rarely occur, no adverse fetal effects have been described.

Respiratory Viruses

More than 200 antigenically distinct respiratory viruses cause the common cold, pharyngitis, laryngitis, bronchitis, and pneumonia.

CHAPTER 64

Rhinovirus, coronavirus, and adenovirus are major causes of the common cold. The RNA-containing rhinovirus and coronavirus usually produce a trivial, self-limited illness characterized by rhinorrhea, sneezing, and congestion. The DNA-containing adenovirus is more likely to produce cough and lower respiratory tract involvement, including pneumonia.

Teratogenic effects of respiratory viruses are controversial. Women with a common cold had a four- to fivefold increased risk of fetal anencephaly in a 393-woman cohort in the Finnish Register of Congenital Malformations (Kurppa, 1991). In another population study, Shaw and coworkers (1998) analyzed California births from 1989 to 1991 and concluded that low attributable risks for neural-tube defects were associated with many illnesses in early pregnancy. Recently, amnionic fluid viral PCR studies were performed in 1191 women undergoing amniocentesis for fetal karyotyping. Viral PCR was positive in 6.5 percent, with adenovirus being the virus most frequently identified. There was an association with fetal-growth restriction, nonimmune hydrops, foot/hand abnormalities, and neural-tube defects (Adams, 2012).

Adenoviral infection is a known cause of childhood myocarditis. Towbin (1994) and Forsnes (1998) used PCR tests to identify and link adenovirus to fetal myocarditis and nonimmune hydrops.

Hantaviruses

These RNA viruses are members of the family Bunyaviridae. They are associated with a rodent reservoir, and transmission involves inhalation of virus excreted in rodent urine and feces. An outbreak in the Western United States occurred in 1993 due to Sin Nombre virus. The resulting Hantavirus pulmonary syndrome was characterized by severe adult respiratory distress syndrome with a case-fatality rate of 30 to 40 percent (Peters, 2012). Several outbreaks since then have occurred, the most recent in 2012.

Hantaviruses are a heterogenous group of viruses with low and variable rates of transplacental transmission. Howard and associates (1999) reported the syndrome to cause maternal death, fetal demise, and preterm birth. They found no evidence of vertical transmission of the Sin Nombre virus. However, vertical transmission occurred inconsistently in association with hemorrhagic fever and renal syndrome caused by another Hantavirus species, the Hantaan virus.

Enteroviruses

These viruses are a major subgroup of RNA picornaviruses that include poliovirus, coxsackievirus, and echovirus. They are trophic for intestinal epithelium but can also cause widespread maternal, fetal, and neonatal infections that may include the central nervous system, skin, heart, and lungs. Most maternal infections are subclinical yet can be fatal to the fetus-neonate (Goldenberg, 2003; Tassin, 2014). Hepatitis A is an enterovirus that is discussed in Chapter 55 (p. 1089).

Coxsackievirus

Infections with coxsackievirus group A and B are usually asymptomatic. Symptomatic infections—usually with group B—include aseptic meningitis, polio-like illness, hand foot and mouth disease, rashes, respiratory disease, pleuritis, pericarditis, and myocarditis. No treatment or vaccination is available (Cohen, 2012). Coxsackievirus may be transmitted by maternal secretions to the fetus at delivery in up to half of mothers who seroconverted during pregnancy (Modlin, 1988). Transplacental passage has also been reported (Ornoy, 2006).

Congenital malformations may be increased slightly in pregnant women who had serological evidence of coxsackievirus (Brown, 1972). Viremia can cause fetal hepatitis, skin lesions, myocarditis, and encephalomyelitis, all of which may be fatal. Koro'lkova and colleagues (1989) have also described cardiac anomalies. There is evidence of increased low-birthweight, preterm, and small-for-gestational-age newborns (Chen, 2010). Finally, a rare association between maternal coxsackievirus infection and insulin-dependent diabetes in offspring has been reported (Dahlquist, 1996; Hyoti, 1995; Viskari, 2012).

Poliovirus

Most of these highly contagious but rare infections are subclinical or mild. The virus is trophic for the central nervous system, and it can cause paralytic poliomyelitis (Cohen, 2012). Siegel (1955) demonstrated that pregnant women not only were more susceptible to polio but also had a higher death rate. Perinatal transmission has been observed, especially when maternal infection developed in the third trimester (Bates, 1955). Inactivated subcutaneous polio vaccine is recommended for susceptible pregnant women who must travel to endemic areas or are placed in other high-risk situations. Live oral polio vaccine has been used for mass vaccination during pregnancy without harmful fetal effects (Harjulehto, 1989).

Parvovirus

Human parvovirus B19 causes *erythema infectiosum*, or *fifth disease*. The B19 virus is a small, single-stranded DNA virus that replicates in rapidly proliferating cells such as erythroblast precursors (Brown, 2012). This can lead to anemia, which is its primary fetal effect. Only individuals with the erythrocyte globoside membrane P antigen are susceptible. In women with severe hemolytic anemia—for example, sickle-cell disease—parvovirus infection may cause an aplastic crisis.

The main mode of parvovirus transmission is respiratory or hand-to-mouth contact, and the infection is common in spring months. The maternal infection rate is highest in women with school-aged children and in day-care workers but not usually in schoolteachers. Viremia develops 4 to 14 days after exposure. By adulthood, only 40 percent of women are susceptible. The annual seroconversion rate is 1 to 2 percent but is greater than 10 percent during epidemic periods (Brown, 2012). Secondary attack rates approach 50 percent.

Maternal Infection

In 20 to 30 percent of adults, infection is asymptomatic. Fever, headache, and flu-like symptoms may begin in the last few days of the viremic phase. Several days later, a bright red rash with erythroderma affects the face and gives a slapped-cheek appearance. The rash becomes lacelike and spreads to the trunk and extremities. Adults often have milder rashes and develop symmetrical polyarthralgia that may persist several weeks. There is no evidence that parvovirus infection is altered by pregnancy (Valeur-Jensen, 1999). With recovery, there is production of IgM antibody 7 to 10 days postinfection, and this persists for 3 to 4 months. Several days after IgM is produced, IgG antibody is detectable and persists for life with natural immunity.

Fetal Infection

There is vertical transmission to the fetus in up to a third of maternal parvovirus infections (Bonvicini, 2011; de Jong, 2011; Lamont, 2011a). Fetal infection has been associated with abortion, nonimmune hydrops, and stillbirth (Enders, 2010; Lassen, 2012; McClure, 2009). In a review of 1089 cases of maternal B19 infection from nine studies, Crane (2002) reported an overall fetal loss rate of 10 percent. It was 15 percent for infections before 20 weeks but was only 2.3 percent after 20 weeks. Its role in later unexplained stillbirths is unclear because most data are from retrospective cohorts with incomplete maternal and fetal histological evaluations (Norbeck, 2002; Skjöldebrand-Sparre, 2000; Tolfvenstam, 2001). Currently, there are no data to support evaluating asymptomatic mothers and stillborn fetuses for parvovirus infection.

Parvovirus is the most frequent infectious cause of nonimmune hydrops in autopsied fetuses (Rogers, 1999). That said, this complication develops only in approximately 1 percent of infected women and usually is caused by infection in the first half of gestation (Crane, 2002; Enders, 2004; Puccetti, 2012).

Yaegashi (2000) has extensively investigated the development and pathophysiology of parvovirus B19 fetal hydrops. At least 85 percent of cases of fetal infection developed within 10 weeks of maternal infection, and the mean interval was 6 to 7 weeks. More than 80 percent of hydrops cases were found in the second trimester, with a mean gestational age of 22 to 23 weeks. The critical period for maternal infection leading to fetal hydrops was estimated to be between 13 and 16 weeks—coincidental with the period in which fetal hepatic hemopoiesis is greatest.

Diagnosis and Management

An algorithm for diagnosis of maternal parvoviral infection is illustrated in Figure 64-2. Diagnosis is generally made by maternal serological testing for specific IgG and IgM antibodies (Bonvicini, 2011; Butchko, 2004; Enders, 2006). Viral DNA may be detectable by PCR in maternal serum during the prodrome and persist for months to years after infection. Fetal infection is diagnosed by detection of B19 viral DNA in amnionic fluid or IgM antibodies in fetal serum obtained by cordocentesis (de Jong, 2011; Weiffenbach, 2012). Fetal and maternal viral loads do not predict fetal morbidity and mortality (de Haan, 2007).

Most cases of parvovirus-associated hydrops develop in the first 10 weeks after infection (Enders, 2004). Thus, serial sonography every 2 weeks should be performed in women with recent infection (see Fig. 64-2). Middle cerebral artery (MCA) Doppler interrogation can also be used to predict fetal anemia (Chap. 10, p. 221). Elevated peak systolic velocity values in the fetal MCA accurately predict fetal anemia (Chauvet, 2011; Cosmi, 2002; Delle Chiaie, 2001). Fetal blood sampling is warranted with hydrops to assess the degree of fetal anemia. Fetal myocarditis may induce hydrops with less severe anemia.

Depending on gestational age, fetal transfusion for hydrops may improve outcome in some cases (Enders, 2004; Schild, 1999; von Kaisenberg, 2001). Mortality rates as high as 30 percent have been reported in hydropic fetuses without transfusions. With transfusion, 94 percent of hydrops cases resolve within 6 to 12 weeks, and the overall mortality rate is < 10 percent. Most fetuses require only one transfusion because hemopoiesis resumes as infection resolves. The technique for fetal transfusion is described in Chapter 14 (p. 300).

Long-Term Prognosis

Reports describing neurodevelopmental outcomes in fetuses transfused for B19 infection-induced anemia are conflicting. Nagel and colleagues (2007) reviewed 25 transfusions in 24 hydropic fetuses. There was abnormal neurodevelopment in five of 16 survivors—32 percent—at 6 months to 8 years. Outcomes were not related to severity of fetal anemia or acidemia, and these investigators hypothesized that the infection itself induced cerebral damage. De Jong (2012) described long-term neurodevelopmental outcomes in 28 children treated with intrauterine transfusion. At a median age of 5 years, 11 percent had neurodevelopmental impairment. Conversely, Dembinski (2003) followed 20 children for a mean of 52 months after transfusion. They found no significant neurodevelopmental delay despite severe fetal anemia.

Prevention

There is currently no approved vaccine for human parvovirus B19, and there is no evidence that antiviral treatment prevents maternal or fetal infection (Broliden, 2006). Decisions to avoid higher-risk work settings are complex and require assessment of exposure risks. Pregnant women should be counseled that risks for infection approximate 5 percent for casual, infrequent contact; 20 percent for intense, prolonged work exposure such as for teachers; and 50 percent for close, frequent interaction such as in the home. Workers at day-care centers and schools need not avoid infected children because infectivity is greatest before clinical illness. Finally, infected children do not require isolation.

Cytomegalovirus

This ubiquitous DNA herpes virus eventually infects most humans. Cytomegalovirus (CMV) is the most common perinatal infection in the developed world. Specifically, some evidence of fetal infection is found in 0.2 to 2.5 percent of all neonates (Kenneson, 2007). The virus is secreted into all body fluids, and person-to-person contact with viral-laden saliva, semen, urine, blood, and nasopharyngeal and cervical secretions can transmit infection. The fetus may become infected by transplacental viremia, or the neonate is infected at delivery or during breast feeding. Moreover, acquisition

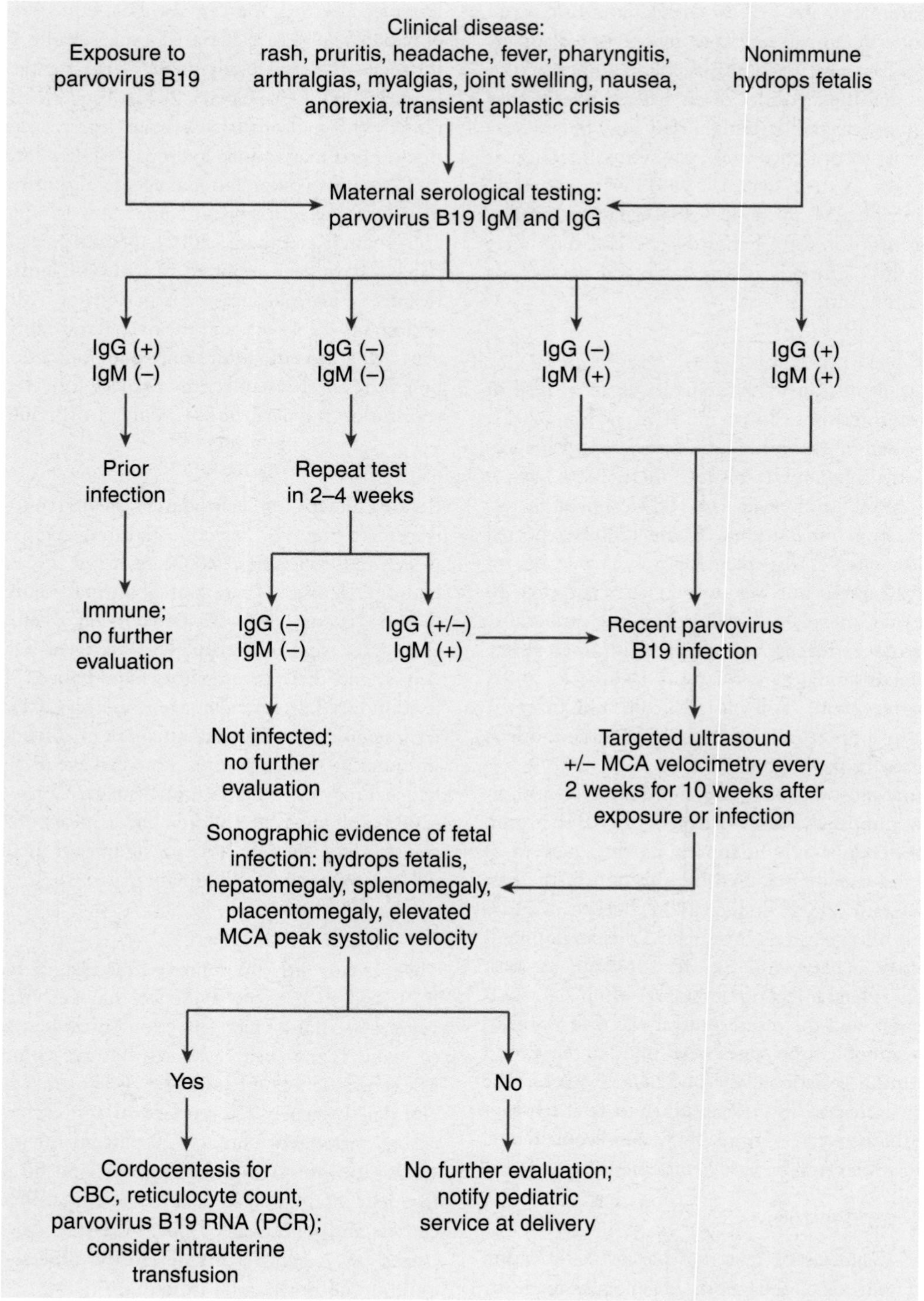

FIGURE 64-2 Algorithm for evaluation and management of human parvovirus B19 infection in pregnancy. CBC = complete blood count; IgG = immunoglobulin G; IgM = immunoglobulin M; MCA = middle cerebral artery; PCR = polymerase chain reaction; RNA = ribonucleic acid.

continues to accrue. Day-care centers, for example, are a frequent source, and by 2 to 3 years of age, many children have infected one another and may transmit infection to their parents (Demmler, 1991; Pass, 1991). Revello and coworkers (2008) reported that amniocentesis in women whose blood is positive for CMV DNA does not result in iatrogenic fetal transmission.

Up to 85 percent of women from lower socioeconomic backgrounds are seropositive by the time of pregnancy, whereas only half of women in higher income groups are immune. Following primary CMV infection, and in a manner similar to other herpes virus infections, the virus becomes latent with periodic reactivation characterized by viral shedding. This occurs despite high serum levels of anti-CMV IgG antibody. These antibodies do not prevent maternal recurrence, reactivation, or reinfection, nor do they totally mitigate fetal or neonatal infection.

Women who are seronegative before pregnancy but who develop primary CMV infection during pregnancy are at

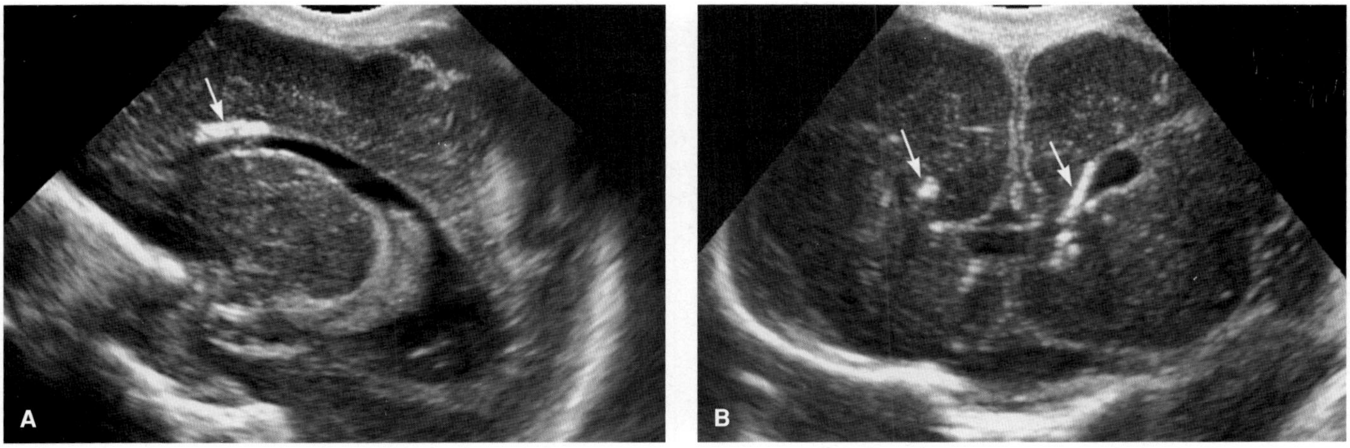

FIGURE 64-3 Sagittal **(A)** and coronal **(B)** cranial sonograms from a neonate with congenital cytomegalovirus infection. The arrows indicate periventricular calcifications.

greatest risk to have an infected fetus. It is estimated that 25 percent of congenital CMV infections in the United States are from primary maternal infection (Wang, 2011). Because most CMV infections are clinically silent, they are detected by seroconversion, and this may be as high as 1 to 7 percent (Hyde, 2010).

Maternal Infection

Pregnancy does not increase the risk or severity of maternal CMV infection. Most infections are asymptomatic, but 10 to 15 percent of infected adults have a mononucleosis-like syndrome characterized by fever, pharyngitis, lymphadenopathy, and polyarthritis. Immunocompromised women may develop myocarditis, pneumonitis, hepatitis, retinitis, gastroenteritis, or meningoencephalitis. Nigro and associates (2003) reported that most women in a cohort with primary infection had elevated serum aminotransferases or lymphocytosis. Reactivation disease usually is asymptomatic, although viral shedding is common.

Primary maternal CMV infection is transmitted to the fetus in approximately 40 percent of cases and can cause severe morbidity (Fowler, 1992; Liesnard, 2000). In contrast, recurrent maternal infection infects the fetus in only 0.15 to 1 percent of cases. A review of nine studies of CMV vertical transmission rates reported first-trimester transmission in 36 percent, second-trimester in 40 percent, and third-trimester in 65 percent (Picone, 2013). Naturally acquired immunity during pregnancy results in a 70-percent risk reduction of congenital CMV infection in future pregnancies (Fowler, 2003). However, as noted earlier, maternal immunity does not prevent recurrences, and maternal antibodies do not prevent fetal infection. Also, some seropositive women can be reinfected with a different viral strain that can cause fetal infection and symptomatic congenital disease (Ross, 2011).

Fetal Infection

When a newborn has apparent sequelae of in utero-acquired CMV infection, it is referred to as *symptomatic CMV infection*. Congenital infection is a syndrome that may include growth restriction, microcephaly, intracranial calcifications, chorioretinitis, mental and motor retardation, sensorineural deficits, hepatosplenomegaly, jaundice, hemolytic anemia, and thrombocytopenic purpura (Fig. 64-3). The pathogenesis of these outcomes has been reviewed by Cheeran and colleagues (2009). Of the estimated 40,000 infected neonates born each year, only 5 to 10 percent demonstrate this syndrome (Fowler, 1992). Thus, most infected infants are asymptomatic at birth, but some develop late-onset sequelae. They may include hearing loss, neurological deficits, chorioretinitis, psychomotor retardation, and learning disabilities.

Prenatal Diagnosis

Routine prenatal CMV serological screening is currently not recommended. Pregnant women should be tested for CMV if they present with a mononucleosis-like illness or if congenital infection is suspected based on abnormal sonographic findings. Primary infection is diagnosed using CMV-specific IgG testing of paired acute and convalescent sera. CMV IgM does not accurately reflect timing of seroconversion because IgM antibody levels may be elevated for more than a year (Stagno, 1985). Moreover, CMV IgM may be found with reactivation disease or reinfection with a new strain. Thus, specific CMV IgG avidity testing is valuable in confirming primary CMV infection (Fig. 64-4). High anti-CMV IgG avidity indicates primary maternal infection > 6 months before testing (Kanengisser-Pines, 2009). Finally, viral culture may be useful, although a minimum of 21 days is required before culture findings are considered negative.

Several fetal abnormalities associated with CMV infection may be seen with sonography, computed tomography, or magnetic resonance imaging. In some cases, they are found at the time of routine prenatal sonographic screening, but in others they are part of a specific evaluation in women with CMV infection. Findings include microcephaly, ventriculomegaly, and cerebral calcifications; ascites, hepatomegaly, splenomegaly, and hyperechoic bowel; hydrops; and oligohydramnios (Malinger, 2003). Abnormal sonographic findings seen in combination with positive findings in fetal blood or amnionic fluid are predictive of an approximate 75-percent risk of symptomatic congenital infection (Enders, 2001).

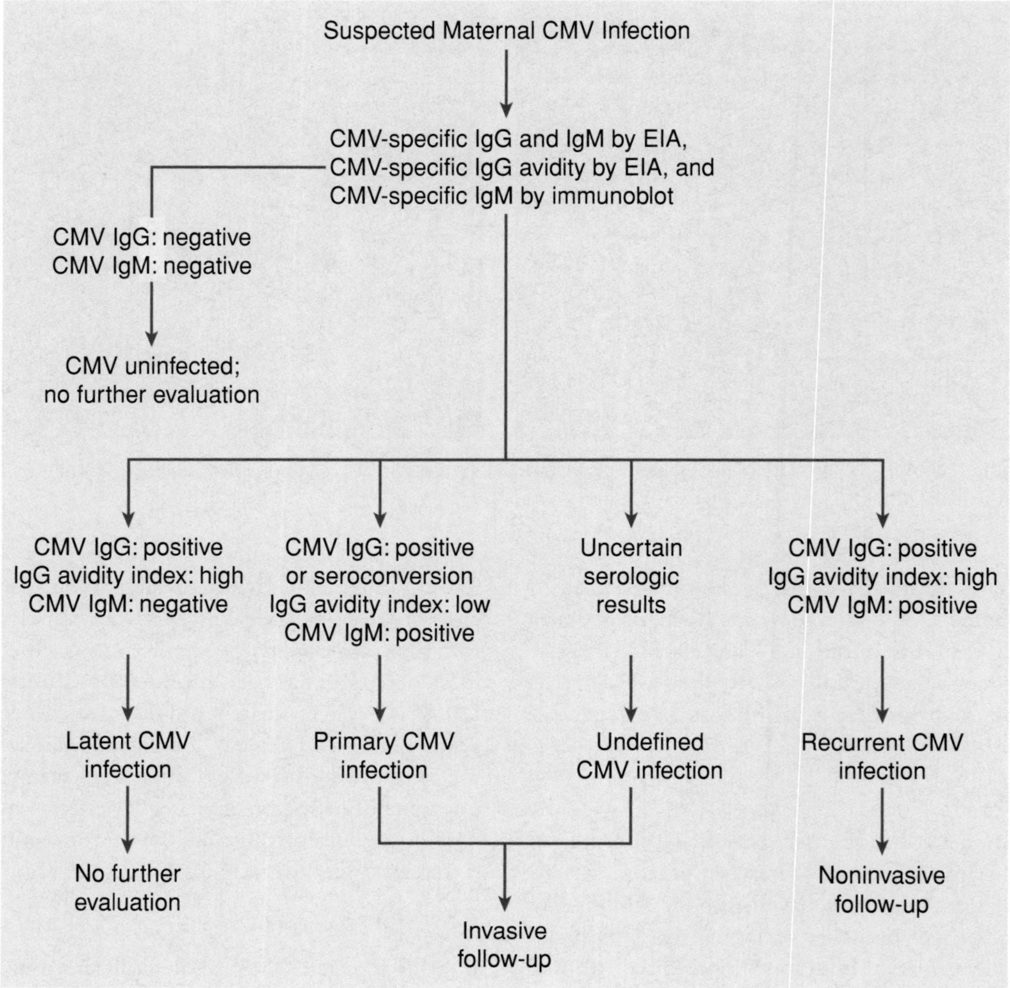

FIGURE 64-4 Algorithm for evaluation of suspected maternal primary cytomegalovirus (CMV) infection in pregnancy. EIA = enzyme immunoassay; IgG = immunoglobulin G; IgM = immunoglobulin M.

CMV nucleic acid amplification testing of amnionic fluid is considered the gold standard for the diagnosis of fetal infection. Sensitivities range from 70 to 99 percent and depend on amniocentesis timing (Nigro, 2005; Revello, 2004). Sensitivity is highest when amniocentesis is performed at least 6 weeks after maternal infection and after 21 weeks (Azam, 2001; Guerra, 2000). A negative amnionic fluid PCR does not exclude fetal infection and may need to be repeated if suspicion for fetal infection is high.

Management and Prevention

The management of the immunocompetent pregnant woman with primary or recurrent CMV is limited to symptomatic treatment. If recent primary CMV infection is confirmed, amnionic fluid analysis should be offered. Counseling regarding fetal outcome depends on the gestation age during which primary infection is documented. Even with the high infection rate with primary infection in the first half of pregnancy, most fetuses develop normally. However, pregnancy termination may be an option for some.

Kimberlin (2003) showed that intravenous ganciclovir administered for 6 weeks to neonates with symptomatic central nervous system disease prevents hearing deterioration at 6 months and possibly later. Conversely, antiviral chemotherapy given antepartum does not avert in utero CMV transmission. Passive immunization with CMV-specific hyperimmune globulin lowers the risk of congenital CMV infection when given to pregnant women with primary disease (Nigro, 2005, 2012; Visentin, 2012). Further clinical trials are necessary before this becomes standard treatment (McCarthy, 2011).

There is no CMV vaccine. Prevention of congenital infection relies on avoiding maternal primary infection, especially in early pregnancy. Basic measures such as good hygiene and hand washing have been promoted, particularly for women with toddlers in day-care settings (Fowler, 2000). Although there may be sexual transmission from infected partners, there are no data on the efficacy of preventive strategies.

BACTERIAL INFECTIONS

Group A Streptococcus

Infections caused by *Streptococcus pyogenes* are important in pregnant women. It is the most frequent bacterial cause of acute pharyngitis and is associated with several systemic and cutaneous infections. *S pyogenes* produces numerous toxins and enzymes responsible for the local and systemic toxicity associated with this organism. Pyrogenic exotoxin-producing strains are usually associated with severe disease (Mason, 2012; Wessels, 2012). In most cases, streptococcal pharyngitis, scarlet fever, and erysipelas are not life threatening. Treatment, usually with penicillin, is similar in pregnant and nonpregnant women (Shulman, 2012).

In the United States, *Streptococcus pyogenes* infrequently causes puerperal infection. Still, it remains the most common cause of severe maternal postpartum infection and death worldwide, and the incidence of these infections is increasing (Deutscher, 2011; Hamilton, 2013; Mason, 2012; Wessels, 2012). Puerperal infections are discussed in detail in Chapter 37 (p. 682). The early 1990s saw the rise of streptococcal toxic shock syndrome, manifested by hypotension, fever, and evidence of multiorgan failure with associated bacteremia. The case-fatality rate approximates 30 percent, and morbidity and mortality rates are improved with early recognition. Treatment includes clindamycin or penicillin therapy and often surgical debridement (Hamilton, 2013). No vaccine for group A streptococcus is commercially available.

Group B Streptococcus

Streptococcus agalactiae is a group B organism that can be found to colonize the gastrointestinal and genitourinary tract in 20 to 30 percent of pregnant women. Throughout pregnancy, group B *Streptococcus* (GBS) is isolated in a transient, intermittent, or chronic fashion. Although the organism is most likely always present in these same women, their isolation is not always homologous.

Maternal and Perinatal Infection

The spectrum of maternal and fetal GBS ranges from asymptomatic colonization to septicemia. *Streptococcus agalactiae* has been implicated in adverse pregnancy outcomes, including preterm labor, prematurely ruptured membranes, clinical and subclinical chorioamnionitis, and fetal infections. GBS can also cause maternal bacteriuria, pyelonephritis, osteomyelitis, postpartum mastitis, and puerperal infections. It remains the leading infectious cause of morbidity and mortality among infants in the United States (Centers for Disease Control and Prevention, 2010; Schrag, 2003; Wessels, 2012).

Neonatal sepsis has received the most attention due to its devastating consequences and available effective preventative measures. Infection < 7 days after birth is defined as *early-onset disease* and is seen in 0.24/1000 live births (Centers for Disease Control and Prevention, 2013a). Many investigators use a threshold of < 72 hours of life as most compatible with intrapartum acquisition of disease (Pulver, 2009; Wendel, 2002). We and others have also encountered several unexpected intrapartum stillbirths from GBS infections. Tudela and associates (2012) recently reported that newborns with early-onset GBS infection often had clinical evidence of fetal infection during labor or at delivery.

In many neonates, septicemia involves signs of serious illness that usually develop within 6 to 12 hours of birth. These include respiratory distress, apnea, and hypotension. At the outset, therefore, neonatal infection must be differentiated from respiratory distress syndrome caused by insufficient surfactant production of the preterm neonate (Chap. 34, p. 653). The mortality rate with early-onset disease has declined to approximately 4 percent, and preterm newborns are disparately affected.

Late-onset disease caused by GBS is noted in 0.32 per 1000 live births and usually manifests as meningitis 1 week to 3 months after birth (Centers for Disease Control and Prevention, 2013a). The mortality rate, although appreciable, is less for late-onset meningitis than for early-onset sepsis. Unfortunately, it is not uncommon for surviving infants of both early- and late-onset disease to exhibit devastating neurological sequelae.

Prophylaxis for Perinatal Infections

As GBS neonatal infections evolved beginning in the 1970s and before widespread intrapartum chemoprophylaxis, rates of early-onset sepsis ranged from 2 to 3 per 1000 live births. In 2002, the Centers for Disease Control and Prevention, the American College of Obstetricians and Gynecologists, and the American Academy of Pediatrics revised guidelines for perinatal prevention of GBS disease. They recommended universal rectovaginal culture screening for GBS at 35 to 37 weeks' gestation followed by intrapartum antibiotic prophylaxis for women identified to be carriers. Subsequent to implementation of these guidelines, the incidence of early-onset GBS neonatal sepsis has decreased to 0.24 cases per 1000 live births by 2012 (Centers for Disease Control and Prevention, 2013a). These guidelines were updated for early-onset GBS infection in 2010. They expanded laboratory identification criteria for GBS; updated algorithms for screening and intrapartum chemoprophylaxis for women with preterm prematurely ruptured membranes, preterm labor, or penicillin allergy; and described new dosing for penicillin G chemoprophylaxis.

Thus, during the past three decades, several strategies have been proposed to prevent perinatal acquisition of GBS infections (Ohlsson, 2013). These strategies have not been compared in randomized trials and are either culture-based or risk-based guidelines as subsequently discussed.

Culture-Based Prevention. The 2010 Centers for Disease Control and Prevention GBS Guidelines recommend a culture-based approach as shown in Figure 64-5. Such a protocol was also adopted by the American College of Obstetricians and Gynecologists (2013c). This approach is designed to identify women who should be given intrapartum antimicrobial prophylaxis. Women are screened for GBS colonization at 35 to 37 weeks' gestation, and intrapartum antimicrobials are given to women with rectovaginal GBS-positive cultures. Selective enrichment broth followed by subculture improves detection. In addition, more rapid techniques such as DNA probes and nucleic acid amplification tests are being developed (Chan, 2006; Helali, 2012). A previous sibling with GBS invasive disease and identification of GBS bacteriuria in the current pregnancy are also considered indications for prophylaxis.

Risk-Based Prevention. A risk-based approach is recommended for women in labor and whose GBS culture results

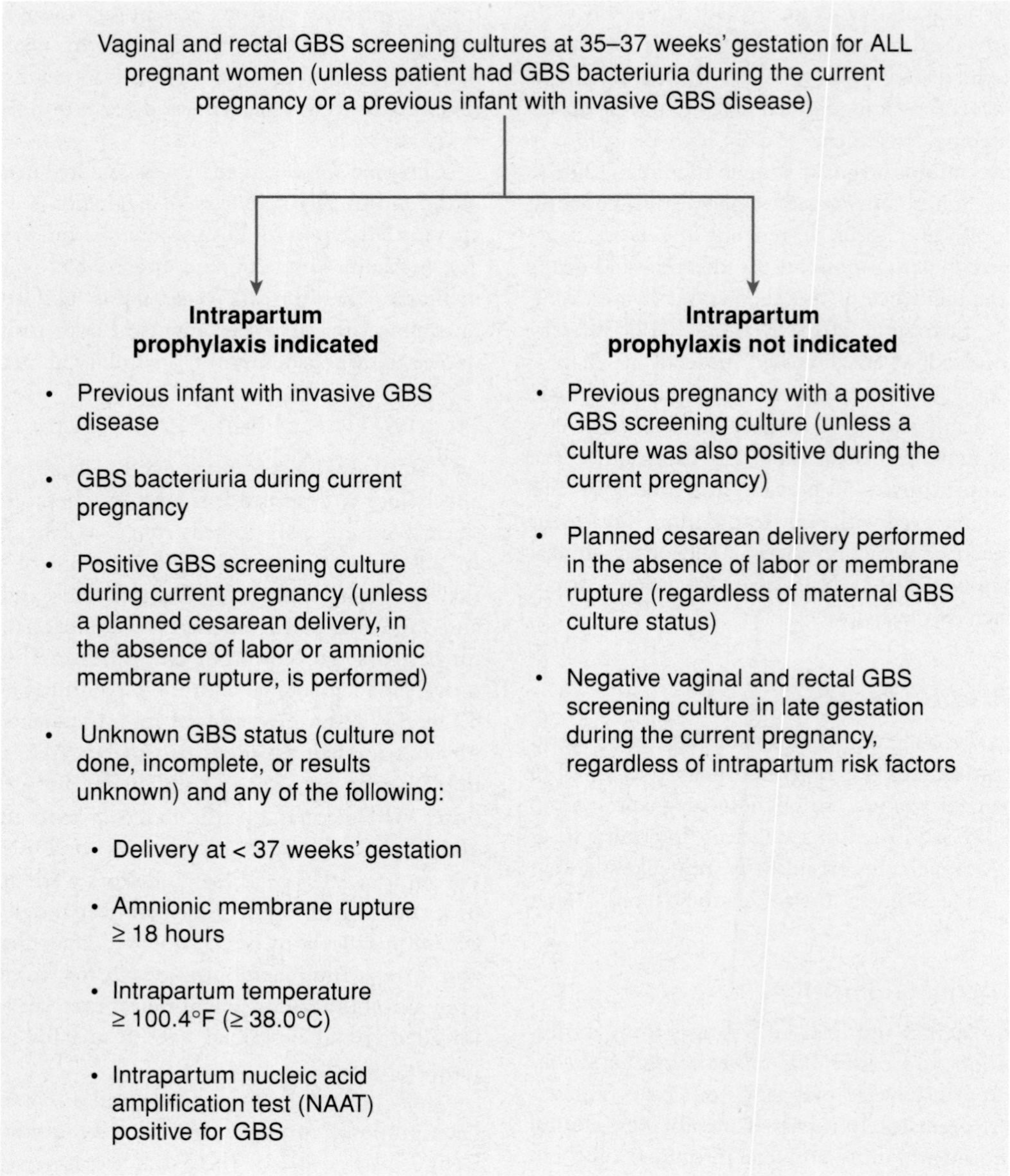

Vaginal and rectal GBS screening cultures at 35–37 weeks' gestation for ALL pregnant women (unless patient had GBS bacteriuria during the current pregnancy or a previous infant with invasive GBS disease)
Intrapartum prophylaxis indicated
• Previous infant with invasive GBS disease
• GBS bacteriuria during current pregnancy
• Positive GBS screening culture during current pregnancy (unless a planned cesarean delivery, in the absence of labor or amnionic membrane rupture, is performed)
• Unknown GBS status (culture not done, incomplete, or results unknown) and any of the following:
• Delivery at < 37 weeks' gestation
• Amnionic membrane rupture ≥ 18 hours
• Intrapartum temperature ≥ 100.4°F (≥ 38.0°C)
• Intrapartum nucleic acid amplification test (NAAT) positive for GBS
Intrapartum prophylaxis not indicated
• Previous pregnancy with a positive GBS screening culture (unless a culture was also positive during the current pregnancy)
• Planned cesarean delivery performed in the absence of labor or membrane rupture (regardless of maternal GBS culture status)
• Negative vaginal and rectal GBS screening culture in late gestation during the current pregnancy, regardless of intrapartum risk factors

FIGURE 64-5 Indications for intrapartum prophylaxis to prevent perinatal group B streptococcal (GBS) disease under a universal prenatal screening strategy based on combined vaginal and rectal cultures obtained at 35 to 37 weeks' gestation. (From Centers for Disease Control and Prevention, 2010.)

are not known. This approach relies on risk factors associated with intrapartum GBS transmission. Intrapartum chemoprophylaxis is given to women who have any of the following: delivery < 37 weeks, ruptured membranes ≥ 18 hours, or intrapartum temperature ≥ 100.4°F (≥ 38.0°C). Women with GBS during the current pregnancy and women with a prior infant with invasive early-onset GBS disease are also given chemoprophylaxis.

At Parkland Hospital in 1995—and prior to consensus guidelines—we adopted the risk-based approach for intrapartum treatment of women at high risk. In addition, all term neonates who were not given intrapartum prophylaxis were treated in the delivery room with aqueous penicillin G, 50,000 to 60,000 units intramuscularly. Rates of early-onset GBS infection and sepsis and of non-GBS sepsis decreased to 0.4–0.66 per 1000 live births (Wendel, 2002). Non-GBS early-onset sepsis was identified in 0.24 per 1000 live births, and this was stable during the past two decades (Stafford, 2012). Thus, this approach has results similar to those reported by the Centers for Disease Control and Prevention (2010) for culture-based prevention.

Intrapartum Antimicrobial Prophylaxis

Prophylaxis administered 4 or more hours before delivery is highly effective (Fairlie, 2013). Regardless of screening method, penicillin remains the first-line agent for prophylaxis, and ampicillin is an acceptable alternative (Table 64-3). Women with a penicillin allergy and no history of anaphylaxis should be given cefazolin. Those at high risk for anaphylaxis should have antimicrobial susceptibility testing performed to

TABLE 64-3. Regimens for Intrapartum Antimicrobial Prophylaxis for Perinatal GBS Disease

Regimen	Treatment
Recommended	Penicillin G, 5 million units IV initial dose, then 2.5 to 3.0 million units IV every 4 hours until delivery
Alternative	Ampicillin, 2 g IV initial dose, then 1 g IV every 4 hours or 2 g every 6 hours until delivery
Penicillin allergic	
Patients **not** at high risk for anaphylaxis	Cefazolin, 2 g IV initial dose, then 1 g IV every 8 hours until delivery
Patients at high risk for anaphylaxis and with GBS susceptible to clindamycin	Clindamycin, 900 mg IV every 8 hours until delivery
Patients at high risk for anaphylaxis and with GBS resistant to clindamycin or susceptibility unknown	Vancomycin, 1 g IV every 12 hours until delivery

GBS = group B *Streptococcus*; IV = intravenous.
Adapted from the Centers for Disease Control and Prevention, 2010.

exclude clindamycin resistance. Clindamycin-sensitive but erythromycin-resistant isolates should have a D-zone test performed to assess for inducible clindamycin resistance. If clindamycin resistance is confirmed, vancomycin should be administered. *Erythromycin is no longer used for penicillin-allergic patients.*

Further recommendations for management of spontaneous preterm labor, threatened preterm delivery, or preterm prematurely ruptured membranes are shown in Figure 64-6. Women undergoing cesarean delivery before labor onset with intact membranes do not need intrapartum GBS chemoprophylaxis, regardless of GBS colonization status or gestational age.

Methicillin-Resistant *Staphylococcus Aureus*

Staphylococcus aureus is a pyogenic gram-positive organism and is considered the most virulent of the staphylococcal species. It primarily colonizes the nares, skin, genital tissues, and oropharynx. Approximately 20 percent of normal individuals are persistent carriers, 30 to 60 percent are intermittent carriers, and 20 to 50 percent are noncarriers (Gorwitz, 2008). Colonization

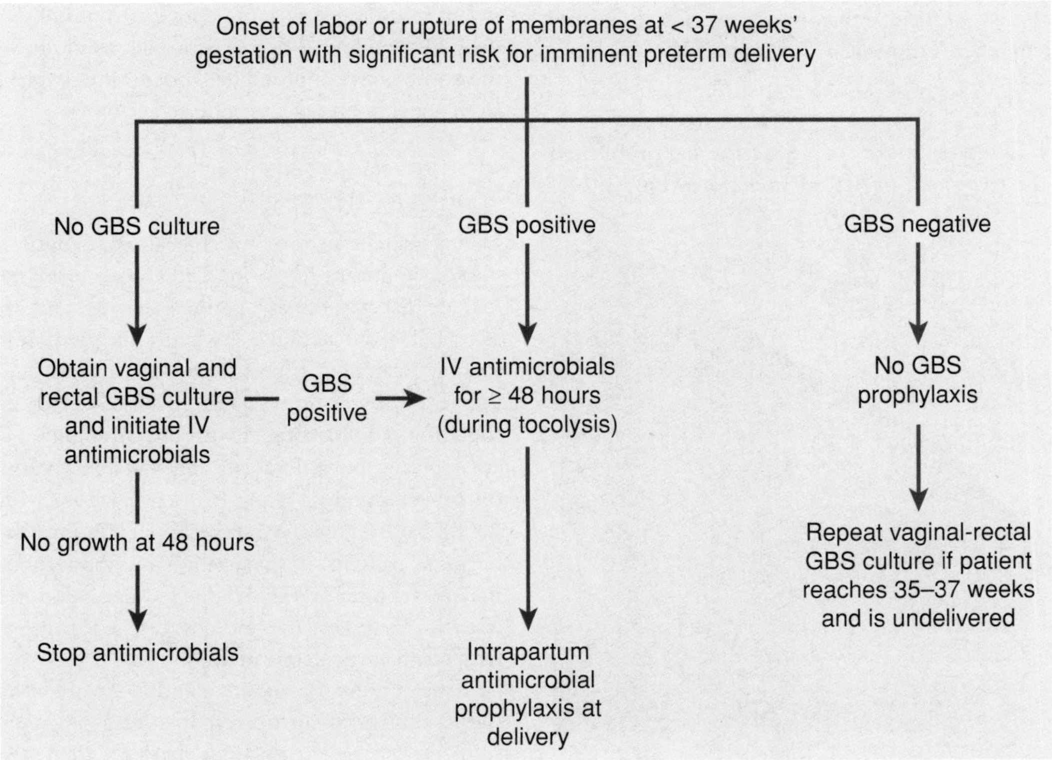

FIGURE 64-6 Sample algorithm for prophylaxis for women with group B streptococcal (GBS) disease and threatened preterm delivery. This algorithm is not an exclusive course of management, and variations that incorporate individual circumstances or institutional preferences may be appropriate. IV = intravenous. (Adapted from Centers for Disease Control and Prevention, 2010.)

is considered the greatest risk factor for infection (Sheffield, 2013). Methicillin-resistant *S aureus* (MRSA) colonizes only 2 percent of people but is a significant contributor to the health-care burden (Gorwitz, 2008). MRSA infections are associated with increased cost and higher mortality rates compared with those by methicillin-sensitive *S aureus* (MSSA) (Beigi, 2009; Butterly, 2010; Klevens, 2007).

Community-associated MRSA (CA-MRSA) is diagnosed when identified in an outpatient setting or within 48 hours of hospitalization in a person without traditional risk factors. The latter include prior MRSA infection, hospitalization, dialysis or surgery within the past year, and indwelling catheters or devices. Hospital-associated MRSA (HA-MRSA) infections are nosocomial. Most cases of MRSA in pregnant women are CA-MRSA.

MRSA and Pregnancy

Anovaginal colonization with *S aureus* is identified in 10 to 25 percent of obstetrical patients (Andrews, 2008; Creech, 2010; Top, 2010). MRSA has been isolated in 0.5 to 3.5 percent of these women. Skin and soft tissue infections are the most common presentation of MRSA in pregnant women (Fig. 64-7). Mastitis has been reported in up to a fourth of cases of MRSA complicating pregnancy (Laibl, 2005; Lee, 2010; Reddy, 2007). Perineal abscesses, wound infections at sites such as abdominal and episiotomy incisions, and chorioamnionitis are also associated with MRSA (Lareau, 2010; Pimentel, 2009; Rotas, 2007; Thurman, 2008). An increase in CA-MRSA infections has been reported in neonatal intensive care units and newborn nurseries. In these settings, infection is frequently associated with maternal and health-care worker MRSA skin infections and infected breast milk. Vertical transmission appears to be rare (Huang, 2009; Jimenez-Truque, 2012; Pinter, 2009).

Management

The Infectious Diseases Society of America has published guidelines for the treatment of MRSA infections (Liu, 2011).

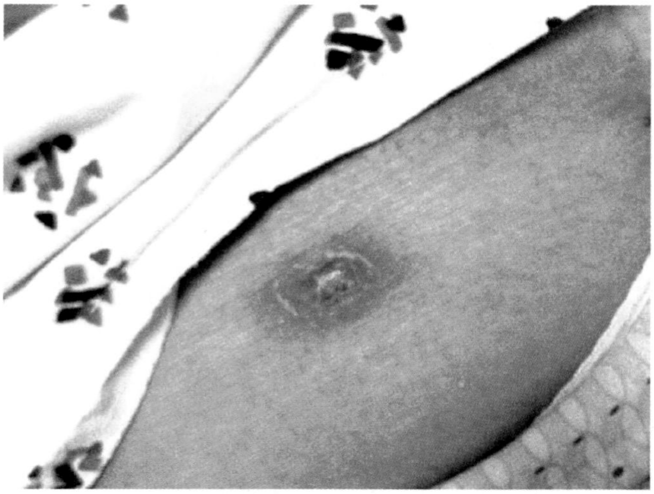

FIGURE 64-7 Typical presentation of a skin lesion caused by infection with community-acquired methicillin-resistant *Staphylococcus aureus* (CA-MRSA). Patients often present with what they describe as an infected spider bite.

Uncomplicated superficial infections are managed by drainage and local wound care. The benefits of antibiotic treatment in this setting are unproven, and most studies have not shown improved outcomes with the addition of MRSA-appropriate antibiotics (Forcade, 2012; Laibl, 2005). Severe superficial infections, especially those that fail to respond to local care or those in patients with medical comorbidities, should be treated with MRSA-appropriate antibiotics. Purulent cellulitis should be treated empirically for CA-MRSA until culture results are available.

Most CA-MRSA strains are sensitive to trimethoprim-sulfamethoxazole. If clindamycin treatment is considered, inducible resistance must be excluded by a D-zone test for erythromycin-resistant, clindamycin-sensitive isolates. Rifampin rapidly develops resistance and should not be used for monotherapy. Linezolid, although effective against MRSA, is expensive, and there is little information regarding its use in pregnancy. Doxycycline, minocycline, and tetracycline, although effective for MRSA infections, should not be used in pregnancy. Vancomycin remains the first-line therapy for inpatient MRSA infections.

The control and prevention of HA-MRSA and CA-MRSA rely on appropriate hand hygiene and prevention of skin-to-skin contact or contact with wound dressings. Decolonization should be considered only in cases in which a patient develops recurrent superficial infections despite optimal hygiene measures or if ongoing transmission occurs among household or close contacts (Liu, 2011). Decolonization measures include nasal treatment with mupirocin, chlorhexidine gluconate baths, and oral rifampin therapy. Routine decolonization has not been shown to be effective in the obstetrical population. For women with culture-proven CA-MRSA infection during pregnancy, we add single-dose vancomycin to routine β-lactam perioperative prophylaxis for cesarean deliveries and fourth-degree perineal lacerations. Breast feeding in these women is not prohibited, but optimal hygiene and attention to minor skin breaks is encouraged.

Vulvar Abscess

Labia majora infections, which begin as cellulitis, have the potential for significant expansion and abscess formation. Risk factors include diabetes, obesity, perineal shaving, and immunosuppression. For early cellulitis, sitz baths and oral antibiotics are reasonable treatment. If present, a small abscess can be incised and drained, wound cultures obtained, abscess cavity packed, and surrounding cellulitis treated with oral antibiotics. These infections are typically polymicrobial, and suitable broad-spectrum antimicrobials are given along with coverage for MRSA (Thurman, 2008). For severe infections, especially in immunosuppressed or pregnant patients, hospitalization and intravenous antimicrobial therapy are often warranted due to increased risks for necrotizing fasciitis. Large abscesses are best drained in the operating room with adequate analgesia or anesthesia.

Cysts of the Bartholin gland duct are usually unilateral, sterile, and need no treatment during pregnancy. If a cyst is sufficiently large to obstruct delivery, then needle aspiration is an appropriate temporary measure. With gland duct infection, a localized unilateral vulvar bulge, tenderness, and erythema are present. Treatment is given with broad-spectrum antimicrobials, and drainage is established. In addition to obtaining wound cultures, testing is done for *Neisseria gonorrhoeae* and *Chlamydia trachomatis.* For a small abscess, incision and placement of a Word catheter may be suitable. For larger abscesses with extensive cellulitis, drainage is best performed in the operating room. In these cases, the incised edges of the abscess cavity may be marsupialized.

Occasionally, abscesses of the periurethral glands develop. The largest of these, the Skene gland, may require drainage and broad-spectrum antimicrobial treatment if there is suppuration.

Listeriosis

Listeria monocytogenes is an uncommon but probably underdiagnosed cause of neonatal sepsis. This facultative intracellular gram-positive bacillus can be isolated from the feces of 1 to 5 percent of adults. Nearly all cases of listeriosis are thought to be food-borne (Silk, 2013). Outbreaks have been caused by raw vegetables, coleslaw, apple cider, melons, milk, fresh Mexican-style cheese, smoked fish, and processed foods, such as pâté, hummus, wieners, and sliced deli meats (Cartwright, 2013; Centers for Disease Control and Prevention, 2013i; Janakiraman, 2008; Varma, 2007; Voetsch, 2007).

Listerial infections are more common in the very old or young, pregnant women, and immunocompromised patients. The incidence of such infections appears to be increasing in several countries worldwide (Allenberger, 2010; Cartwright, 2013; Goulet, 2012). In 1651 cases reported in 2009 to 2011, the Centers for Disease Control and Prevention found that 14 percent were in pregnant women (Silk, 2013). And in a recent review, pregnant women had a significantly higher rate for listeriosis compared with nonpregnant reproductive-aged women (Pouillot, 2012). It is unclear why pregnant women still account for a significant number of these reported cases. One hypothesis is that pregnant women are susceptible because of decreased cell-mediated immunity (Baud, 2011; Jamieson, 2006b; Wing, 2002). Another is that placental trophoblasts are susceptible to invasion by *Listeria monocytogenes* (Le Monnier, 2007).

Maternal and Fetal Infection

Listeriosis during pregnancy may be asymptomatic or may cause a febrile illness that is confused with influenza, pyelonephritis, or meningitis (Centers for Disease Control and Prevention, 2013i; Mylonakis, 2002). The diagnosis usually is not apparent until blood cultures are reported as positive. Occult or clinical infection also may stimulate labor (Boucher, 1986). Discolored, brownish, or meconium-stained amnionic fluid is common with fetal infection, even preterm gestations.

In 2011, a listerial outbreak associated with cantaloupes resulted in 147 infected individuals (Centers for Disease Control and Prevention, 2012b). Seven of these infections were related to pregnancy—four in pregnant women and three in newborns. Maternal listeriosis causes fetal infection that characteristically produces disseminated granulomatous lesions with *microabscesses* (Topalovski, 1993). Chorioamnionitis is common with maternal infection, and placental lesions include multiple, well-demarcated macroabscesses. Early- and late-onset neonatal infections are similar to GBS sepsis. In a review of 222 cases by Mylonakis (2002), infection resulted in abortion or stillbirth in 20 percent, and neonatal sepsis developed in 68 percent of surviving newborns. Voetsch (2007) detailed similar findings. A stillbirth caused by listeriosis is shown in Figure 64-8.

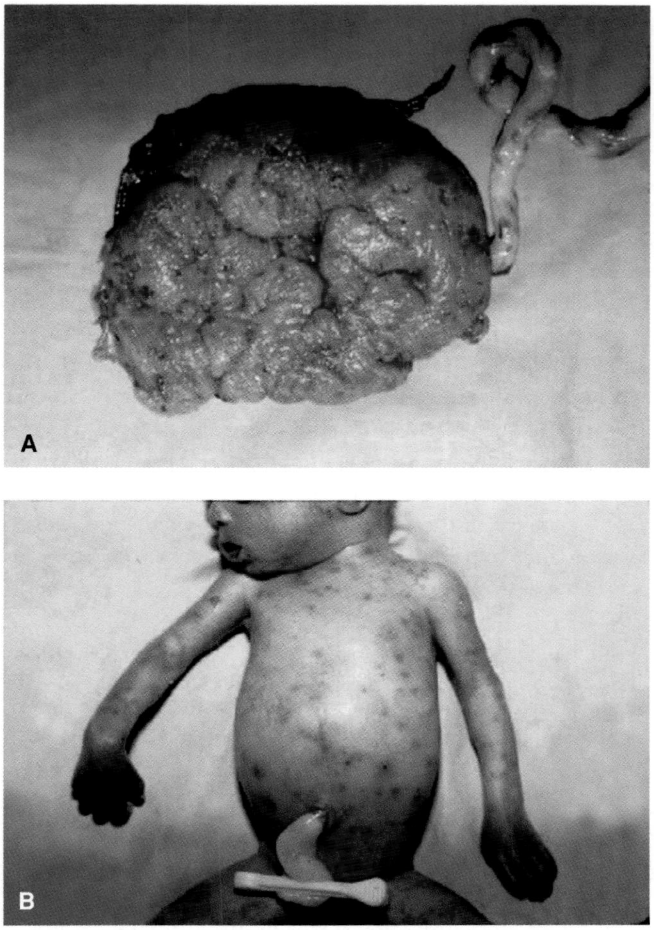

FIGURE 64-8 The pale placenta **(A)** and stillborn infant **(B)** resulted from maternal listeriosis.

Treatment with ampicillin plus gentamicin is usually recommended because of synergism against *Listeria* species. Trimethoprim-sulfamethoxazole can be given to penicillin-allergic women. Maternal treatment in most cases is also effective for fetal infection (Chan, 2013). No vaccine is available, and prevention is by washing raw vegetables and cooking all raw food (Goulet, 2012; Silk, 2012). Pregnant women should also avoid the implicated foods listed previously.

Salmonellosis

Infections from *Salmonella* species continue to be a major and increasing cause of food-borne illness (Peques, 2012). Six serotypes account for most cases in the United States, including *Salmonella* subtypes *typhimurium* and *enteritidis.* Non-typhoid *Salmonella* gastroenteritis is contracted through contaminated food. Symptoms including nonbloody diarrhea, abdominal pain, fever, chills, nausea, and vomiting begin 6 to 48 hours after exposure. Diagnosis is made by stool studies. Intravenous crystalloid is given for rehydration. Antimicrobials are not given in uncomplicated infections because they do not commonly shorten illness and may prolong the convalescent carrier state. If gastroenteritis is complicated by bacteremia, antimicrobials are given as discussed below. Rare case reports have linked *Salmonella* bacteremia with abortion (Coughlin, 2002).

Typhoid fever caused by *Salmonella typhi* remains a global health problem, although it is uncommon in the United States. Infection is spread by oral ingestion of contaminated food, water, or milk. In pregnant women, the disease is more likely to be encountered during epidemics or in those with HIV infection (Hedriana, 1995). In former years, antepartum typhoid fever resulted in abortion, preterm labor, and maternal or fetal death (Dildy, 1990).

Fluoroquinolones and third-generation cephalosporins are the preferred treatment. For enteric (typhoid) fever, antimicrobial susceptibility testing is important because of the development of drug-resistant strains (Peques, 2012). Typhoid vaccines appear to exert no harmful effects when administered to pregnant women and should be given in an epidemic or before travel to endemic areas.

Shigellosis

Bacillary dysentery caused by *Shigella* is a relatively common, highly contagious cause of inflammatory exudative diarrhea in adults. Shigellosis is more common in children attending day-care centers and is transmitted via the fecal-oral route. Clinical manifestations range from mild diarrhea to severe dysentery, bloody stools, abdominal cramping, tenesmus, fever, and systemic toxicity.

Although shigellosis may be self-limited, careful attention to treatment of dehydration is essential in severe cases. We have cared for pregnant women in whom secretory diarrhea exceeded 10 L/day! Antimicrobial therapy is imperative, and effective treatment during pregnancy includes fluoroquinolones, ceftriaxone, or azithromycin. Antimicrobial resistance is rapidly emerging, and antibiotic susceptibility testing can help guide appropriate therapy (Centers for Disease Control and Prevention, 2013c).

Hansen Disease

Also known as leprosy, this chronic infection is caused by *Mycobacterium leprae* and is rare in the United States (United States Department of Health and Human Services, 2011). Diagnosis is confirmed by PCR. Multidrug therapy with dapsone, rifampin, and clofazimine is recommended for treatment and is generally safe during pregnancy (Britton, 2004). Duncan (1980) reported an excessive incidence of low-birthweight newborns among infected women. The placenta is not involved, and neonatal infection apparently is acquired from skin-to-skin or droplet transmission (Böddinghaus, 2007; Duncan, 1984). Vertical transmission is common in untreated mothers (Moschella, 2004).

Lyme Disease

Caused by the spirochete *Borrelia burgdorferi*, Lyme disease is the most commonly reported vector-borne illness in the United States (Centers for Disease Control and Prevention, 2012c). Lyme borreliosis follows tick bites of the genus *Ixodes*. Early infection causes a distinctive local skin lesion, *erythema migrans*, which may be accompanied by a flu-like syndrome and regional adenopathy. If untreated, disseminated infection follows in days to weeks. Multisystem involvement is frequent, but skin lesions, arthralgia and myalgia, carditis, and meningitis predominate. If still untreated after several weeks to months, late or persistent infection manifests in perhaps half of patients. Native immunity is acquired, and the disease enters a chronic phase. Although some patients remain asymptomatic, others in the chronic phase develop various skin, joint, or neurological manifestations (Wormser, 2006). Although relapses were initially considered common, recent clinical and epidemiological evidence suggests that most cases of recurrent erythema migrans occurring after appropriate antimicrobial therapy are actually new infections (Nadelman, 2012).

Clinical diagnosis is important because serological and PCR testing has many pitfalls (Schoen, 2013). IgM and IgG serological testing is recommended in early infection and is followed by Western blotting for confirmation. Ideally, acute and convalescent serological evaluation is completed if possible. The false-positive and -negative rates are high, and more accurate tests are being developed (Radolf, 2012; Schoen, 2013; Steere, 2012).

Treatment and Prevention

Optimal treatment of Lyme disease was reviewed by Wormser (2006) for the Infectious Diseases Society of America. For early infection, treatment with doxycycline, amoxicillin, or cefuroxime is recommended for 14 days, although doxycycline is usually avoided in pregnancy. A 14- to 28-day course of IV ceftriaxone, cefotaxime, or penicillin G is given for complicated early infections that include meningitis, carditis, or disseminated infections. Chronic arthritis and post-Lyme disease syndrome are treated with prolonged oral or IV regimens, however, symptoms respond poorly to treatment (Steere, 2012).

No vaccine is commercially available. Avoiding areas with endemic Lyme disease and improving tick control in those areas is the most effective prevention. Self-examination with removal of unengorged ticks within 36 hours of attachment reduces infection risk (Hayes, 2003). For tick bites recognized within 72 hours, a single 200-mg oral dose of doxycycline may reduce infection development.

There are several reports of Lyme disease in pregnancy, although large series are lacking. Transplacental transmission has been confirmed, but no congenital effects of maternal borreliosis have been conclusively identified (Elliott, 2001; Maraspin, 2011; Walsh, 2006). Prompt treatment of maternal early infection should prevent most adverse pregnancy outcomes (Mylonas, 2011).

Tuberculosis

Diagnosis and management of tuberculosis during pregnancy is discussed in detail in Chapter 51 (p. 1019).

PROTOZOAL INFECTIONS

Toxoplasmosis

The obligate intracellular parasite *Toxoplasma gondii* has a life cycle with two distinct stages (Kim, 2012). The *feline* stage takes place in the cat—the definitive host—and its prey. Unsporulated oocysts are secreted in feces. In the *nonfeline* stage, tissue cysts containing bradyzoites or oocysts are ingested by the intermediate host, including humans. Gastric acid digests the cysts to release bradyzoites, which infect small-intestinal epithelium. Here, they are transformed into rapidly dividing tachyzoites, which can infect all cells within the host mammal. Humoral and cell-mediated immune defenses eliminate most of these, but tissue cysts develop. Their lifelong persistence is the chronic form of toxoplasmosis.

Human infection is acquired by eating raw or undercooked meat infected with tissue cysts or by contact with oocysts from cat feces in contaminated litter, soil, or water. Prior infection is confirmed by serological testing, and its prevalence depends on geographic locale and parasite genotype. In the United States, there is a 5 to 30 percent seroprevalence in persons aged 10 to 19 years, and this can exceed 60 percent after age 50 (Kim, 2012). Thus, a significant segment of pregnant women in this country are susceptible to infection. The incidence of prenatal infection resulting in birth of a newborn with congenital toxoplasmosis has been estimated to vary from 0.8 per 10,000 live births in the United States to 10 per 10,000 in France (Dubey, 2000). Between 400 and 4000 cases of congenital toxoplasmosis are diagnosed annually in the United States. Globally, it is estimated that a third of the population has been exposed to this parasite (Verma, 2012).

Maternal and Fetal Infection

Most acute maternal infections in Europe and North America are subclinical and are detected only by prenatal or newborn serological screening. In some cases, maternal symptoms may include fatigue, fever, headache, muscle pain, and sometimes a maculopapular rash and posterior cervical lymphadenopathy. In immunocompetent adults, initial infection confers immunity, and prepregnancy infection nearly eliminates any risk of vertical transmission. Infection in immunocompromised women, however, may be severe, and reactivation may cause encephalitis, retinochoroiditis, or mass lesions. Maternal infection is associated with a fourfold increased preterm delivery rate before 37 weeks (Freeman, 2005). Even so, growth restriction is not increased. Toxoplasmosis serotype NE-II is most commonly associated with preterm birth and severe neonatal infection (McLeod, 2012).

The incidence and severity of fetal toxoplasmosis infection depend on gestational age at the time of maternal infection. Risks for fetal infection increase with pregnancy duration (Fig. 64-9). A metaanalysis estimated the risk to be 15 percent at 13 weeks, 44 percent at 26 weeks, and 71 percent at 36 weeks (SYROCOT Study Group, 2007). Conversely, the severity of fetal infection is much greater in early pregnancy, and these fetuses are much more likely to have clinical findings of infection.

Importantly, most infected fetuses are born without obvious stigmata of toxoplasmosis. Clinically affected neonates usually have generalized disease expressed as low birthweight, hepatosplenomegaly, jaundice, and anemia. Some primarily have neurological disease with intracranial calcifications and with hydrocephaly or microcephaly. Many eventually develop chorioretinitis and exhibit learning disabilities. This classic triad—chorioretinitis, intracranial calcifications, and hydrocephalus—is often accompanied by convulsions. Infected neonates with clinical signs are at risk for long-term complications.

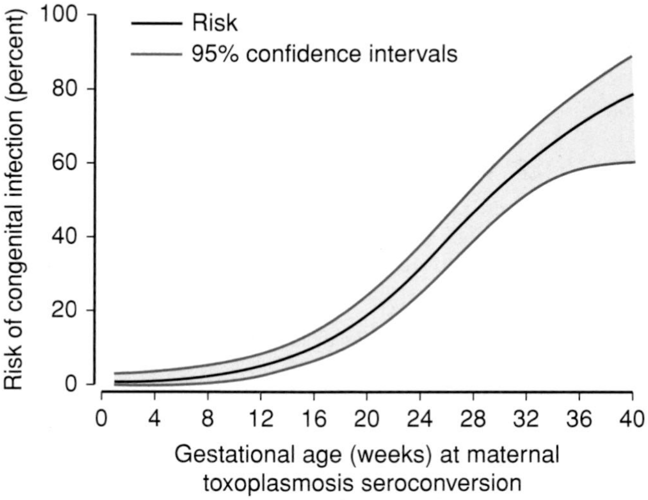

FIGURE 64-9 Risk of congenital toxoplasmosis infection by gestational age at maternal seroconversion. (From Dunn, 1999, with permission.)

Screening and Diagnosis

The American Academy of Pediatrics and the American College of Obstetricians and Gynecologists (2012) do not recommend prenatal screening for toxoplasmosis in areas of low prevalence, including the United States. In areas of high toxoplasmosis prevalence—for example, France and Austria—routine screening has resulted in diminished congenital disease (Wallon, 2013). With IgG antibody confirmed before pregnancy, there is no risk for a congenitally infected fetus (Montoya, 2004). Screening should be performed in immunocompromised pregnant women, regardless of country of residence.

Pregnant women suspected of having toxoplasmosis should be tested. The parasite is rarely detected in tissue or body fluids. Anti-toxoplasma IgG develops within 2 to 3 weeks after infection, peaks at 1 to 2 months, and usually persists for life—sometimes in high titers. Although IgM antibodies appear by 10 days after infection and usually become negative within 3 to 4 months, they may remain detectable for years. Thus, IgM antibodies should not be used alone to diagnose acute toxoplasmosis. IgA and IgE antibodies are also useful in diagnosing acute infection. Best results are obtained with the Toxoplasma Serologic Profile performed at the Palo Alto Medical Foundation Research Institute (www.toxolab@pamf.org). Toxoplasma IgG avidity increases with time. Thus, if a high-avidity IgG result is found, infection in the preceding 3 to 5 months is excluded. Multiple commercial avidity tests are now available that provide a 100-percent positive-predictive value of high avidity confirming latent infection (Villard, 2013). PCR testing has a high sensitivity and specificity.

Prenatal diagnosis of toxoplasmosis is performed using DNA amplification techniques and sonographic evaluation. PCR of amnionic fluid or fetal blood has improved sensitivity compared with standard isolation techniques (Sterkers, 2012). The sensitivity varies with gestational age, and it is lowest at

< 18 weeks (Montoya, 2008). Sonographic evidence of intracranial calcifications, hydrocephaly, liver calcifications, ascites, placental thickening, hyperechoic bowel, and growth restriction has been used prenatally to help confirm diagnosis.

Management

No randomized clinical trials have been performed to assess the benefit and efficacy of treatment to decrease the risk for congenital infection. A systematic review of data from 1438 treated pregnancies found weak evidence for early treatment to reduce congenital toxoplasmosis risks (SYROCOT Study Group, 2007). Treatment has been associated with a reduction in rates of serious neurological sequelae and neonatal demise (Cortina-Borja, 2010).

Prenatal treatment is based on two regimens—spiramycin alone or a pyrimethamine–sulfonamide combination with folinic acid. These two regimens have also been used consecutively (Hotop, 2012). Little evidence supports the use of a specific regimen. That said, most experts will use spiramycin in women with acute infection early in pregnancy. Pyrimethamine–sulfadiazine with folinic acid is selected for maternal infection after 18 weeks or if fetal infection is suspected.

Prevention

There is no vaccine for toxoplasmosis, so avoidance of infection is necessary if congenital infection is to be prevented. Efforts include: (1) cooking meat to safe temperatures; (2) peeling or thoroughly washing fruits and vegetables; (3) cleaning all food preparation surfaces and utensils that have contacted raw meat, poultry, seafood, or unwashed fruits and vegetables; (4) wearing gloves when changing cat litter, or else delegating this duty; and (5) avoiding feeding cats raw or undercooked meat and keeping cats indoors. Although these preventive steps are recommended, there are no data to support their effectiveness (Di Mario, 2009). Vaccine development is actively being pursued (Verma, 2012).

Malaria

Malaria remains a global health crisis. In 2010, there were an estimated 219 million cases and 655,000 deaths, mainly in sub-Saharan Africa (Chico, 2012; World Health Organization, 2011). Malaria has been effectively eradicated in Europe and in most of North America, and worldwide mortality rates have fallen more than 25 percent. In the United States, most cases of malaria are imported—some in returning military personnel (Centers for Disease Control and Prevention, 2013j). Transmitted by infected *Anopheles* mosquitoes, five species of *Plasmodium* cause human disease—*falciparum, vivax, ovale, malariae,* and *knowlesi* (White, 2012).

Maternal and Fetal Infection

Clinical findings are fever, chills, and flu-like symptoms including headaches, myalgia, and malaise, which may occur at intervals. Symptoms are less severe with recurrences. Malaria may be associated with anemia and jaundice, and *falciparum* infections may cause kidney failure, coma, and death. That said, many otherwise healthy but infected adults in endemic areas are asymptomatic. Pregnant women, although often asymptomatic, are said to be more likely to develop traditional symptoms (Desai, 2007).

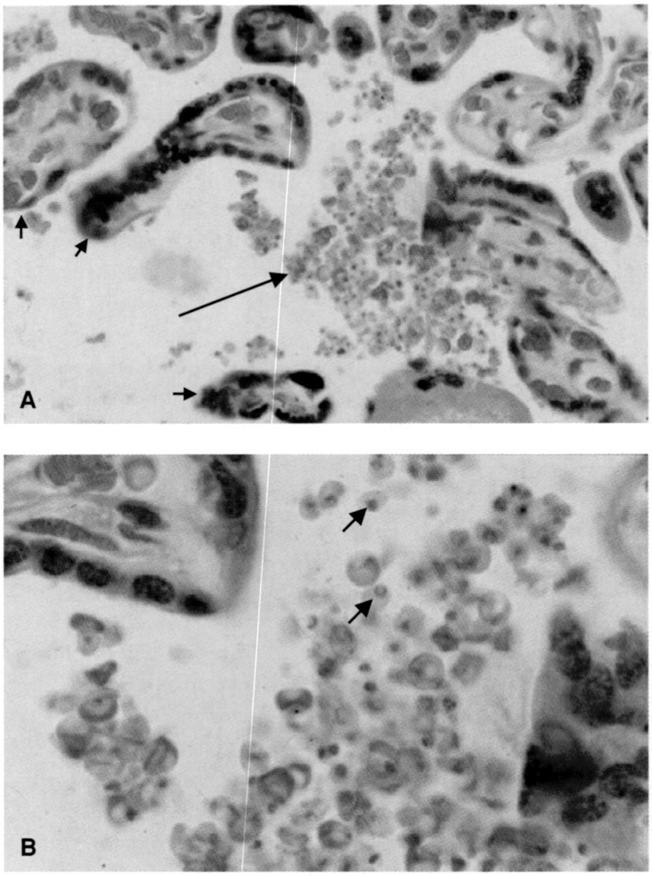

FIGURE 64-10 Photomicrograph of placental malaria. **A.** Multiple infected red blood cells (*long black arrow*) are seen in the intervillous space of this placenta. Multiple villi cut in cross section are shown, and three are highlighted (*short arrows*). **B.** Increased magnification of image **(A).** Multiple infected erythrocytes are seen, and two are identified (*arrows*).

Malarial infections during pregnancy—whether symptomatic or asymptomatic—are associated with increased rates of perinatal morbidity and mortality (Menéndez, 2007; Nosten, 2007; Rogerson, 2007). Adverse outcomes include stillbirth, preterm birth, low birthweight, and maternal anemia. The latter two are documented most frequently (Machado Filho, 2014; McClure, 2013). Maternal infection is associated with 14 percent of low-birthweight newborns worldwide (Eisele, 2012). These adverse perinatal outcomes correlate with high levels of placental parasitemia (Rogerson, 2007). The latter occurs when parasitized erythrocytes, monocytes, and macrophages accumulate in the vascular areas of the placenta (Fig. 64-10). Infections with *P falciparum* are the worst, and early infection increases the risk for abortion (Desai, 2007). The incidence of malaria increases significantly in the latter two trimesters and postpartum (Diagne, 2000). Overall, congenital malaria occurs in < 5 percent of neonates born to infected mothers.

Diagnosis

Identification of parasites by microscopical evaluation of a thick and thin blood smear remains the gold standard for diagnosis.

In women with low parasite densities, however, the sensitivity of microscopy is poor. Malaria-specific antigens are now being used for rapid diagnostic testing. Not only is their sensitivity still an issue in pregnancy, but these tests are not routinely available (Fowkes, 2012; Kashif, 2013; White, 2012).

Management

The most frequently used antimalarial drugs are not contraindicated in pregnancy. The World Health Organization recommends all infected patients living in or traveling from endemic areas be treated with an artemisinin-based regimen for uncomplicated falciparum malaria. Little is known about these regimens in pregnancy (Mutabinqwa, 2013). The Centers for Disease Control and Prevention (2013g) recommends using atovaquone-proguanil or artemether-lumefantrine only if other treatment options are not available or tolerated.

The Centers for Disease Control and Prevention (2013g) recommends that pregnant women diagnosed with uncomplicated malaria caused by *P vivax, P malariae, P ovale,* and chloroquine-sensitive *P falciparum* should be treated with chloroquine or hydroxychloroquine. For women infected with chloroquine-resistant *P falciparum*, mefloquine or quinine sulfate with clindamycin should be used. Chloroquine-resistant *P vivax* should be treated with mefloquine. Chloroquine-sensitive *P vivax* or *P ovale* should be treated with chloroquine throughout pregnancy and then primaquine postpartum. Treatment regimens for uncomplicated and severe malarial infections in pregnancy are detailed at: www.cdc.gov/malaria/diagnosis_treatment/clinicians3.html. The CDC also maintains a malaria hotline for treatment recommendations (770-488-7788).

The World Health Organization (2011) allows for the use of intermittent preventative therapy during pregnancy. This consists of at least two treatment doses of sulfadoxine-pyrimethamine in the second and third trimesters. The rationale is that each dose will clear placental asymptomatic infections and provide up to 6 weeks of posttreatment prophylaxis. This ideally will decrease the rate of low-birthweight newborns in endemic areas (Harrington, 2013). A recent metaanalysis supported the use of at least three doses of intermittent preventative therapy to improve birthweight and decrease placental and maternal malarial infection at delivery (Kayentao, 2013).

Resistance to all the antimalarial drugs has been reported, including the recently added artemisinin. The World Health Organization recommends routine monitoring of antimalarial drug resistance and tailoring medication regimens.

Prevention and Chemoprophylaxis

Malaria control and prevention relies on chemoprophylaxis when traveling to or living in endemic areas. Vector control is also important. Insecticide-treated netting, pyrethroid insecticides, and *N,N*-diethyl-*m*-toluamide (DEET)-based insect repellent decrease malarial rates in endemic areas. These are well tolerated in pregnancy (Menéndez, 2007). If travel is necessary, chemoprophylaxis is recommended.

Chloroquine and hydroxychloroquine prophylaxis is safe and well tolerated in pregnancy. It decreases placental infection from 20 percent to 4 percent in asymptomatic infected women in areas without chloroquine resistance (Cot, 1992). For travelers to areas with chloroquine-resistant *P falciparum*, mefloquine remains the only chemoprophylaxis recommended. Primaquine and doxycycline are contraindicated in pregnancy, and there are insufficient data on atovaquone/proguanil to recommend them at this time. Likewise, amodiaquine is used in Africa, but data are limited in pregnant women. The latest chemoprophylaxis regimens for pregnancy can be obtained from the Centers for Disease Control and Prevention *Travelers' Health* website at: http://www.cdc.gov/travel. The Centers also publish *Health Information for International Travel* (The Yellow Book) at: www.cdc.gov/yellowbook.

Amebiasis

Most persons infected with *Entamoeba histolytica* are asymptomatic. Amebic dysentery, however, may take a fulminant course during pregnancy, with fever, abdominal pain, and bloody stools. Prognosis is worse if complicated by a hepatic abscess. Diagnosis is made by identifying *E histolytica* cysts or trophozoites within a stool sample. Therapy is similar to that for the nonpregnant woman, and metronidazole or tinidazole is the preferred drug for amebic colitis and invasive disease. Noninvasive infections may be treated with paromomycin (Stanley, 2012).

MYCOTIC INFECTIONS

Disseminated fungal infection—usually pneumonitis—during pregnancy is uncommon with coccidiomycosis, blastomycosis, cryptococcosis, or histoplasmosis. Their identification and management are considered in Chapter 51 (p. 1019).

EMERGING INFECTIONS

These are collectively defined as infectious diseases that have newly appeared or increased in incidence or geographic spread (Jamieson, 2006a,b; Theiler, 2008). At this time, emerging infections include West Nile virus, coronavirus, and several influenza A strains. They also include many bioterrorism agents.

West Nile Virus

This mosquito-borne RNA flavivirus is a human neuropathogen. Since 1999, the reported numbers of human and animal infections have increased, and the geographical range of disease activity has expanded. The year 2012 was the second worst outbreak of total cases in the United States (Centers for Disease Control and Prevention, 2013b). West Nile viral infections are typically acquired through mosquito bites in late summer or perhaps through blood transfusion (Harrington, 2003). The incubation period is 2 to 14 days, and most persons have mild or no symptoms. Fewer than 1 percent of infected adults develop meningoencephalitis or acute flaccid paralysis (Granwehr, 2004). Presenting symptoms may include fever, mental status changes, muscle weakness, and coma (Chapa, 2003; Stewart, 2013).

Diagnosis of West Nile infection is based on clinical symptoms and the detection of viral IgG and IgM in serum and IgM in cerebrospinal fluid. There is no known effective antiviral treatment, and management is supportive. The primary strategy for preventing exposure in pregnancy is the use of insect repellant containing DEET. This is considered safe for use around pregnant women (Koren, 2003). Avoiding outdoor activity and stagnant water and wearing protective clothing are also recommended.

Adverse effects of West Nile viremia on pregnancy are unclear. Animal data suggest that embryos are susceptible, and a case report of human fetal infection at 27 weeks described chorioretinitis and severe temporal and occipital lobe leukomalacia (Alpert, 2003; Julander, 2006). Of 77 maternal infections initially reported to the West Nile Virus Pregnancy Registry, there were four miscarriages, two elective abortions, and 72 live births, of which 6 percent were preterm (O'Leary, 2006). Three of these 72 newborns were shown to have West Nile infection, and it could not be established conclusively that infection was acquired congenitally. Of three major malformations *possibly* associated with viral infection, none was definitively confirmed. Similar conclusions were reached by Pridjian and colleagues (2014), who analyzed data from the Centers for Disease Control and Prevention West Nile Virus Registry. Transmission of West Nile virus through breast feeding is rare (Hinckley, 2007).

Coronavirus Infections

Coronaviruses are single-stranded RNA viruses that are prevalent worldwide. They are associated with 10 to 35 percent of common colds, usually in the fall, winter, and early spring. In 2002, an especially virulent strain of coronavirus—*severe acute respiratory syndrome (SARS–CoV)* was first noted in China. It rapidly spread throughout Asia, Europe, and North and South America. Transmission is through droplets or contact with infected secretions, fluids, and wastes. The incubation period is 2 to 16 days, and there appears to be a triphasic pattern to its clinical progression. The first week is characterized by prodromal symptoms of fever, myalgias, headache, and diarrhea. During the second week, patients may suffer recurrent fever, watery diarrhea, and a dry nonproductive cough with mild dyspnea. These are coincident with IgG seroconversion and a declining viral load. Progression at this stage is thought to be due to an overexuberant host immune response. The third, and at times, lethal phase—seen in about 20 percent of patients—is progression to SARS (Christian, 2004; Peiris, 2003a,b). Radiographic lung findings include ground-glass opacities and airspace consolidations that can rapidly progress within 1 to 2 days. The case-fatality rate approached 10 percent in the nonpregnant population and was as high as 25 percent in pregnant women (Lam, 2004; Wong, 2004). Although there have been no confirmed cases since 2004, the Centers for Disease Control and Prevention (2013d) now lists SARS-CoV as a "select agent" that has the potential to pose a severe threat to public health and safety. Another novel coronavirus infecting humans with a high case-fatality rate was detected in the Middle East in 2012 (MERS-CoV).

TRAVEL PRECAUTIONS DURING PREGNANCY

Pregnant travelers face obstetrical risks, general medical risks, and potentially hazardous destination risks. The International Society for Tropical Medicines has comprehensive information available at: http://www.istm.org. Also, the Centers for Disease Control and Prevention have extensive travel information regarding pregnancy and breast feeding at its websites listed on page 1257.

BIOTERRORISM

Bioterrorism involves the deliberate release of bacteria, viruses, or other infectious agents to cause illness or death. These natural agents are often altered to increase their infectivity or their resistance to medical therapy. Clinicians should be alert for significant increases in the number of persons with febrile illnesses accompanied by respiratory symptoms or with rashes not easily associated with common illnesses. Clinicians are urged to contact their state health department or the Centers for Disease Control and Prevention for contemporary information and recommendations. The American College of Obstetricians and Gynecologists (2013b) has recently addressed disaster preparedness for obstetricians. It provides both general considerations and recommendations for hospital preparedness and obstetrics-specific recommendations.

Smallpox

The variola virus is considered a serious weapon because of high transmission and overall 30-percent case-fatality rate. The last case of smallpox in the United States was reported in 1949, and worldwide it was reported in Somalia in 1977. Transmission occurs with prolonged contact with infected persons, infected body fluids, or contaminated objects such as clothing. Smallpox presents with an acute-onset fever that is followed by a rash with firm, deep-seated vesicles or pustules. Nishiura (2006) and Suarez and Hankins (2002) have reviewed the severe perinatal and maternal morbidity and mortality caused by smallpox. The case-fatality rate of smallpox in pregnancy is 61 percent if the pregnant woman is unvaccinated. There is a significant increase in stillbirth, abortion, preterm labor and delivery, and neonatal demise in pregnancies complicated by smallpox infection.

Because the smallpox vaccine currently available is made with live vaccinia virus, pregnancy should be delayed for 4 weeks in recipients. It is generally not given to pregnant women because of the risk of fetal vaccinia, a rare but serious complication. Inadvertent smallpox vaccination during pregnancy has not, however, been associated with fetal malformations or preterm birth. Moreover, no cases of fetal vaccinia have been reported with second-generation smallpox vaccine exposure (Ryan, 2008a,b). The Smallpox Vaccine in Pregnancy Registry remains active, and vaccinated women are still being enrolled.

Anthrax

Bacillus anthracis is a gram-positive, spore-forming, aerobic bacterium. It can cause three main types of clinical anthrax: inhalational, cutaneous, and gastrointestinal (Holty, 2006;

Swartz, 2001; Sweeney, 2011). The bioterrorist anthrax attacks of 2001 involved inhalational anthrax (Inglesby, 2002). Spores are inhaled and deposited in the alveoli. They are engulfed by macrophages and germinate in mediastinal lymph nodes. The incubation period is usually less than 1 week but may be as long as 2 months. Initial symptoms are nonspecific and include low-grade fever, nonproductive cough, malaise, and myalgias. Within 1 to 5 days of symptom onset, the second stage is heralded by the abrupt onset of severe respiratory distress and high fevers. Mediastinitis and hemorrhagic thoracic lymphadenitis are common, and there is a widened mediastinum on chest radiograph. Case-fatality rates with inhalational anthrax are high, even with aggressive antibiotic and supportive therapy (Dixon, 1999; Holty, 2006).

Anthrax affecting pregnant women and its treatment were recently reviewed by Meaney-Delman and coworkers (2012, 2013). They reported data on 20 pregnant and postpartum women. The overall mortality rate was 80 percent, with a 60-percent fetal or neonatal loss rate. Of note, most cases were published before the advent of antibiotics.

Regimens for postexposure anthrax prophylaxis are given for 2 months. The American College of Obstetricians and Gynecologists (2009) and the Centers for Disease Control and Prevention (Wright, 2010) recommend that asymptomatic pregnant and lactating women with documented exposure to *B anthracis* be given postexposure prophylaxis with ciprofloxacin, 500 mg orally twice daily for 60 days. Amoxicillin, 500 mg orally three times daily, can be substituted if the strain is proven sensitive. In the case of ciprofloxacin allergy and either penicillin allergy or resistance, doxycycline, 100 mg orally twice daily, is given for 60 days. Risks from anthrax far outweigh any fetal risks from doxycycline (Meaney-Delman, 2013).

The anthrax vaccine (AVA) is an inactivated, cell-free product that requires five injections over 18 months. Vaccination is generally avoided in pregnancy because there are limited safety data. Reports of inadvertent vaccination of pregnant women with AVA have not found a significant increase in fetal malformations or miscarriage rates (Ryan, 2008c; Wiesen, 2002). Anthrax vaccine is an essential adjunct to postexposure antimicrobial prophylaxis, even in pregnancy (Wright, 2010).

Other Bioterrorism Agents

Other category A bioterrorism agents include *Francisella tularensis*—tularemia, *Clostridium botulinum*—botulism, *Yersinia pestis*—plague, and viral hemorrhagic fevers—for example, Ebola, Marburg, Lassa, and Machupo. Multiple agents are also listed as category B and C. The guidelines for these biological agents are evolving and are detailed at the Centers for Disease Control and Prevention Bioterrorism website: http://www.emergency.cdc.gov/agent/agentlist-category.

REFERENCES

Adams LL, Gungor S, Turan S, et al: When are amniotic fluid viral PCR studies indicated in prenatal diagnosis? Prenat Diagn 32(1):88, 2012

Adams Waldorf KM, McAdams RM: Influence of infection during pregnancy on fetal development. Reproduction 146(5):R151, 2013

Allenberger F, Wagner M: Listeriosis: a resurgent foodborne infection. Clin Microbiol Infect 16:16, 2010

Alpert SG, Fergerson J, Noël L-P: Intrauterine West Nile virus: ocular and systemic findings. Am J Ophthalmol 136:722, 2003

American Academy of Pediatrics: Measles. In Pickering IK (ed): Red Book: 2006 Report of the Committee on Infections Diseases, 27th ed. Elk Grove Village, American Academy of Pediatrics, 2006, p 441

American Academy of Pediatrics and The American College of Obstetricians and Gynecologists: Guidelines for Prenatal Care, 7th ed. Washington, 2012, p 434

American College of Obstetricians and Gynecologists: Management of asymptomatic pregnant or lactating women exposed to anthrax. Committee Opinion No. 268, February 2002, Reaffirmed 2009

American College of Obstetricians and Gynecologists: Influenza vaccination during pregnancy. Committee Opinion No. 468, October 2010

American College of Obstetricians and Gynecologists: Integrating immunizations into practice. Committee Opinion No. 558, April 2013a

American College of Obstetricians and Gynecologists: Hospital disaster preparedness for obstetricians and facilities providing maternity care. Committee Opinion No. 555, March 2013b

American College of Obstetricians and Gynecologists: Prevention of early-onset group B streptococcal disease in newborns. Committee Opinion No. 485, April 2011, Reaffirmed 2013c

Andrews WW, Schelonka R, Waites K, et al: Genital tract methicillin-resistant *Staphylococcus aureus*. Obstet Gynecol 111:113, 2008

Auriti C, Piersigilli F, De Gasperis MR, et al: Congenital varicella syndrome: still a problem? Fetal Diagn Ther 25(2):224, 2009

Azam AZ, Vial Y, Fawer CL, et al: Prenatal diagnosis of congenital cytomegalovirus infection. Obstet Gynecol 97:443, 2001

Badilla X, Morice A, Avila-Aguero ML, et al: Fetal risk associated with rubella vaccination during pregnancy. Pediatr Infect Dis J 26(9):830, 2007

Banatvala JE, Brown DW: Rubella. Lancet 363:1127, 2004

Bates T: Poliomyelitis in pregnancy, fetus and newborn. Am J Dis Child 90:189, 1955

Baud D, Greub G: Intracellular bacteria and adverse pregnancy outcomes. Clin Microbiol Infect 17:1312, 2011

Beigi RH, Bunge K, Song Y, et al: Epidemiologic and economic effect of methicillin-resistant *Staphylococcus aureus* in obstetrics. Obstet Gynecol 113(5):983, 2009

Böddinghaus BK, Ludwig RJ, Kaufmann R, et al: Leprosy in a pregnant woman. Infection 35:37, 2007

Bohlke K, Galil K, Jackson LA, et al: Postpartum varicella vaccination: is the vaccination virus excreted in breast milk? Obstet Gynecol 102:970, 2003

Bonvicini F, Puccetti C, Salfi NC, et al: Gestational and fetal outcomes in B19 maternal infection: a problem of diagnosis. J Clin Microbiol 49(10):3514, 2011

Boucher M, Yonekura ML: Perinatal listeriosis (early onset): correlation of antenatal manifestations and neonatal outcome. Obstet Gynecol 68:593, 1986

Britton WJ, Lockwood DN: Leprosy. Lancet 363:1209, 2004

Broliden K, Tolevenstam T, Norbeck O: Clinical aspects of parvovirus B19 infection. J Intern Med 260:285, 2006

Brown GC, Karunas RS: Relationship of congenital anomalies and maternal infection with selected enteroviruses. Am J Epidemiol 95:207, 1972

Brown KE: Chapter 184. Parvovirus infections. In Longo DL, Fauci AS, Kasper DL, et al (eds): Harrison's Principles of Internal Medicine, 18th ed. New York, McGraw-Hill, 2012

Butchko AR, Jordan JA: Comparison of three commercially available serologic assays used to detect human parvovirus B19-specific immunoglobulin M (IgM) and IgG antibodies in sera of pregnant women. J Clinic Microbiol 42:3191, 2004

Butterly A, Schmidt U, Wiener-Kronish J: Methicillin-resistant *Staphylococcus aureus* colonization, its relationship to nosocomial infection, and efficacy of control methods. Anesthesiology 113:1453, 2010

Cartwright EJ, Jackson KA, Johnson SD, et al: Listeriosis outbreaks and associated food vehicles, United States, 1998–2008. Emerg Infect Dis 19:1, 2013

Centers for Disease Control and Prevention: Prevention of varicella. Recommendations of the Advisory Committee on Immunization Practices (ACIP). MMWR 56(4):1, 2007

Centers for Disease Control and Prevention: Prevention of perinatal group B streptococci disease. Revised guidelines from the CDC. MMWR 59(10):1, 2010

Centers for Disease Control and Prevention: Maternal and infant outcomes among severely ill pregnant and postpartum women with 2009 pandemic influenza A (H1N1)—United States, April 2009-August 2010. MMWR 60(35):1193, 2011

Centers for Disease Control and Prevention: FDA approval of an extended period for administering VariZIG for postexposure prophylaxis of varicella. MMWR 61(12):212, 2012a

Centers for Disease Control and Prevention: Multistate outbreak of listeriosis linked to whole cantaloupes from Jensen Farms, Colorado. Final Update August 27, 2012b. Available at: http://www.cdc.gov/listeria/outbreaks/cantaloupes-jensen-farms. Accessed October 21, 2013

Centers for Disease Control and Prevention: Summary of notifiable diseases–United States, 2010. MMWR 59(53):1, 2012c

Centers for Disease Control and Prevention: Active Bacterial Core Surveillance Report, Emerging Infections Program Network, Group B *Streptococcus*, 2012. 2013a. Available at: http://www.cdc.gov/abcs/reports-findings/survreports/gbs12.pdf. Accessed October 21, 2013

Centers for Disease Control and Prevention: Final 2012 West Nile virus update. 2013b. Available at: http://www.cdc.gov/ncidod/dvbid/westnile. Accessed October 21, 2013

Centers for Disease Control and Prevention: National Center for Emerging and Zoonotic Infectious Diseases: shigellosis. 2013c. Available at: http://www.cdc.gov/nczved/divisions/dfbmd/diseases/shigellosis/#threat. Accessed October 21, 2013

Centers for Disease Control and Prevention. Novel coronavirus 2012–2013. 2013d. Available at: http://www.cdc.gov/coronavirus/ncv. Accessed October 21, 2013

Centers for Disease Control and Prevention: Prevention and control of seasonal influenza with vaccines: recommendations of the Advisory Committee on Immunization Practices—United States, 2013–2014. MMWR 62(7):1, 2013e

Centers for Disease Control and Prevention: Seasonal influenza (flu): guidance for clinicians on the use of rapid influenza diagnostic tests. 2013f. Available at: http://www.cdc.gov/flu/professionals/diagnosis/clinician_guidance_ridt.htm. Accessed October 21, 2013

Centers for Disease Control and Prevention: Treatment of malaria: guidelines for clinicians (United States). Part 3: Alternatives for pregnant women and treatment of severe malaria. 2013g. Available at: http://www.cdc.gov/malaria/diagnosis_treatment/clinicians3.html. Accessed October 21, 2013

Centers for Disease Control and Prevention: Updated recommendations for use of VariZIG–United States, 2013. MMWR 62(28):574, 2013h

Centers for Disease Control and Prevention: Vital signs: listeria illnesses, deaths, and outbreaks–United States, 2009–2011. MMWR 62(22):148, 2013i

Centers for Disease Control and Prevention: Malaria surveillance—United States, 2011. MMWR 62:1, 2013j

Chan BT, Hohmann E, Barshak MB, et al: Treatment of listeriosis in first trimester of pregnancy. Emerg Infect Dis 19:839, 2013

Chan KL, Levi K, Towner KJ, et al: Evaluation of the sensitivity of a rapid polymerase chain reaction for detection of group B streptococcus. J Obstet Gynaecol 26:402, 2006

Chandra PC, Patel H, Schiavello HJ, et al: Successful pregnancy outcome after complicated varicella pneumonia. Obstet Gynecol 92:680, 1998

Chapa JB, Ahn JT, DiGiovanni LM, et al: West Nile virus encephalitis during pregnancy. Obstet Gynecol 102:229, 2003

Chauvet A, Dewilde A, Thomas D, et al: Ultrasound diagnosis, management and prognosis in a consecutive series of 27 cases of fetal hydrops following maternal parvovirus B19 infection. Fetal Diagn Ther 30(1):41, 2011

Chaves SS, Gargiullo P, Zhang JX, et al: Loss of vaccine-induced immunity to varicella over time. N Engl J Med 356:1121, 2007

Cheeran MC, Lokensgard JR, Schleiss MR: Neuropathogenesis of congenital cytomegalovirus infection: disease mechanisms and prospects for intervention. Clin Microbiol Rev 22(1):99, 2009

Chen YH, Lin HC, Lin HC: Increased risk of adverse pregnancy outcomes among women affected by herpangina. Am J Obstet Gynecol 203(1):49.e1, 2010

Chico RM, Mayaud P, Ariti C, et al: Prevalence of malaria and sexually transmitted and reproductive tract infections in pregnancy in sub-Saharan Africa. JAMA 307(19):2079, 2012

Christian MD, Poutanen SM, Loutfy MR, et al: Severe acute respiratory syndrome. Clin Infect Dis 38:1420, 2004

Cohen JI: Enteroviruses and Reoviruses. In Longo DL, Fauci AS, Kasper DL, et al (eds): Harrison's Principles of Internal Medicine, 18th ed. New York, McGraw-Hill, 2012

Conlin AM, Bukowinski AT, Sevick CJ, et al: Safety of the pandemic H1N1 influenza vaccine among pregnant U.S. military women and their newborns. Obstet Gynecol 121(3):511, 2013

Coonrod DV, Jack BW, Boggess KA, et al: The clinical content of preconception care: infectious diseases in preconception care. Am J Obstet Gynecol 199(6 Suppl 2):S290, 2008

Cortina-Borja, M Tan HK, Wallon M, et al: Prenatal treatment for serious neurological sequelae of congenital toxoplasmosis: an observational prospective cohort study. PLoS Med 7(10):1, 2010

Cosmi E, Mari G, Delle Chiaie L, et al: Noninvasive diagnosis by Doppler ultrasonography of fetal anemia resulting from parvovirus infection. Am J Obstet Gynecol 187:1290, 2002

Cot M, Roisin A, Barro D, et al: Effect of chloroquine chemoprophylaxis during pregnancy on birth weight: results of a randomized trial. Am J Trop Med Hyg 46:21, 1992

Coughlin LB, McGuigan J, Haddad NG, et al: *Salmonella* sepsis and miscarriage. Clin Microbiol Infect 9:866, 2002

Cox S, Posner SF, McPheeters M, et al: Hospitalizations with respiratory illness among pregnant women during influenza season. Obstet Gynecol 107:1315, 2006

Crane J: Parvovirus B19 infection in pregnancy. J Obstet Gynaecol Can 24:727, 2002

Creech CB, Litzner B, Talbot TR, et al: Frequency of detection of methicillin-resistant *Staphylococcus aureus* from rectovaginal swabs in pregnant women. Am J Infect Control 38:72, 2010

Dahlquist G, Frisk G, Ivarsson SA, et al: Indications that maternal coxsackie B virus infection during pregnancy is a risk factor for childhood-onset IDDM. Diabetologia 38:1371, 1996

de Haan TR, Beersman MF, Oepkes D, et al: Parvovirus B19 infection in pregnancy: maternal and fetal viral load measurements related to clinical parameters. Prenat Diagn 27:46, 2007

de Jong EP, Lindenburg IT, van Klink JM, et al: Intrauterine transfusion for parvovirus B19 infection: long-term neurodevelopmental outcome. Am J Obstet Gynecol 206:204.e1, 2012

de Jong EP, Walther FJ, Kroes AC, et al: Parvovirus B19 infection in pregnancy: new insights and management. Prenat Diagn 31(5):419, 2011

Delle Chiaie L, Buck G, Grab D, et al: Prediction of fetal anemia with Doppler measurement of the middle cerebral artery peak systolic velocity in pregnancies complicated by maternal blood group alloimmunization or parvovirus B19 infection. Ultrasound Obstet Gynecol 18:232, 2001

Dembinski J, Eis-Hübinger AM, Maar J, et al: Long term follow up of serostatus after maternofetal parvovirus B19 infection. Arch Dis Child 88:219, 2003

Demmler GJ: Summary of a workshop on surveillance for congenital cytomegalovirus disease. Rev Infect Dis 13:315, 1991

Desai M, O ter Kuile F, Nosten F, et al: Epidemiology and burden of malaria in pregnancy. Lancet Infect Dis 7:93, 2007

Deutscher M, Lewis M, Zell ER, et al: Incidence and severity of invasive *Streptococcus pneumoniae*, Group A *Streptococcus*, and Group B *Streptococcus* infections among pregnant and postpartum women. Clin Infect Dis 53:114, 2011

Diagne N, Rogier C, Sokhna CS, et al: Increased susceptibility to malaria during the early postpartum period. N Engl J Med 343:598, 2000

Dildy GA III, Martens MG, Faro S, et al: Typhoid fever in pregnancy: a case report. J Reprod Med 35:273, 1990

Di Mario S, Basevi V, Gagliotti C, et al: Prenatal education for congenital toxoplasmosis. Cochrane Database Syst Rev 1:CD006171, 2009

Dixon TC, Meselson M, Guillemin J, et al: Anthrax. N Engl J Med 341:815, 1999

Dolin R: Influenza. In Longo DL, Fauci AS, Kasper DL, et al (eds): Harrison's Principles of Internal Medicine, 18th ed. New York, McGraw-Hill, 2012

Dubey JP: Sources of *Toxoplasma gondii* infection in pregnancy. Until rates of congenital toxoplasmosis fall, control measures are essential. BMJ 321:127, 2000

Duncan ME: Babies of mothers with leprosy have small placentae, low birth weights and grow slowly. BJOG 87:461, 1980

Duncan ME, Fox H, Harkness RA, et al: The placenta in leprosy. Placenta 5:189, 1984

Dunn D, Wallon M, Peyron F et al: Mother-to-child transmission of toxoplasmosis: risk estimates for clinical counseling. Lancet 353: 1829, 1999

Eisele TP, Larsen DA, Anglewicz PA, et al: Malaria prevention in pregnancy, birthweight, and neonatal mortality: a meta-analysis of 32 national cross-sectional datasets in Africa. Lancet Infect Dis 12:942, 2012

Elliott DJ, Eppes SC, Klein JD: Teratogen update: Lyme disease. Teratology 64:276, 2001

Enders G, Bäder U, Lindemann L, et al: Prenatal diagnosis of congenital cytomegalovirus infection in 189 pregnancies with known outcome. Prenat Diagn 21:362, 2001

Enders G, Miller E, Cradock-Watson J, et al: Consequences of varicella and herpes zoster in pregnancy: prospective study of 1739 cases. Lancet 343:1548, 1994

Enders M, Klingel K, Weidner A, et al: Risk of fetal hydrops and non-hydropic late intrauterine fetal death after gestational parvovirus B19 infection. J Clin Virol 49(3):163, 2010

Enders M, Schalasta G, Baisch C, et al: Human parvovirus B19 infection during pregnancy—value of modern molecular and serological diagnostics. J Clin Virol 35:400, 2006

Enders M, Weidner A, Zoellner I, et al: Fetal morbidity and mortality after acute human parvovirus B19 infection in pregnancy: prospective evaluation of 1018 cases. Prenat Diagn 24:513, 2004

Fairlie T, Zell ER, Schrag S: Effectiveness of intrapartum antibiotic prophylaxis for prevention of early-onset Group B streptococcal disease. Obstet Gynecol 121(3):570, 2013

Forcade NA, Wiederhold NP, Ryan L, et al: Antibacterials as adjuncts to incision and drainage for adults with purulent methicillin-resistant *Staphylococcus aureus* (MRSA) skin infections. Drugs 72:339, 2012

Forsnes EV, Eggleston MK, Wax JR: Differential transmission of adenovirus in a twin pregnancy. Obstet Gynecol 91:817, 1998

Fowkes FJI, McGready R, Cross NJ, et al: New insights into acquisition, boosting, and longevity of immunity to malaria in pregnant women. J Infect Dis 206:1612, 2012

Fowler KB, Stagno S, Pass RF: Maternal immunity and prevention of congenital cytomegalovirus infection. JAMA 289:1008, 2003

Fowler KB, Stagno S, Pass RF, et al: The outcome of congenital cytomegalovirus infection in relation to maternal antibody status. N Engl J Med 326:663, 1992

Fowler SL: A light in the darkness: predicting outcomes for congenital cytomegalovirus infections. J Pediatr 137:4, 2000

Freeman K, Oakley L, Pollak A, et al: Association between congenital toxoplasmosis and preterm birth, low birthweight and small for gestational age birth. BJOG 112:31, 2005

Goldenberg RL, Thompson C: The infectious origins of stillbirth. Am J Obstet Gynecol 189:861, 2003

Gorwitz RJ, Kruszon-Moran D, McAllister SK: Changes in the prevalence of nasal colonization with *Staphylococcus aureus* in the United States, 2001–2004. J Infect Dis 197:1226, 2008

Goulet V, Hebert M, Hedberg C, et al: Incidence of listeriosis and related mortality among groups at risk of acquiring listeriosis. Clin Infect Dis 54(5):652, 2012

Granwehr BP, Lillibridge KM, Higgs S, et al: West Nile virus: where are we now? Lancet Infect Dis 4:547, 2004

Guerra B, Lazzarotto T, Quarta S, et al: Prenatal diagnosis of symptomatic congenital cytomegalovirus infection. Am J Obstet Gynecol 183:476, 2000

Hamilton SM, Stevens DL, Bryant AE: Pregnancy-related Group A streptococcal infections: temporal relationship between bacterial acquisition, infection onset, clinical findings, and outcome. Clin Infect Dis 57:870, 2013

Harger JH, Ernest JM, Thurnau GR, et al: Risk factors and outcome of varicella-zoster virus pneumonia. J Infect Dis 185:422, 2002

Harjulehto T, Aro T, Hovi T, et al: Congenital malformations and oral poliovirus vaccination during pregnancy. Lancet 1:771, 1989

Harrington T, Kuehnert MJ, Lanciotti RS, et al: West Nile virus infection transmitted by blood transfusion. Transfusion 43:1018, 2003

Harrington WE, Morrison R, Fried M, et al: Intermittent preventive treatment in pregnant women is associated with increased risk of severe malaria in their offspring. PLoS One 8(2):e56183, 2013

Hayes EB, Piesman J: How can we prevent Lyme disease? N Engl J Med 348: 2424, 2003

Hedriana HL, Mitchell JL, Williams SB: *Salmonella typhi* chorioamnionitis in a human immunodeficiency virus–infected pregnant woman. J Reprod Med 40:157, 1995

Helali NE, Giovangrandi Y, Guyot K, et al: Cost and effectiveness of intrapartum Group B streptococcus polymerase chain reaction screening for term deliveries. Obstet Gynecol 119(4):822, 2012

Hinckley AF, O'Leary DR, Hayes EB: Transmission of West Nile virus through breast milk seems to be rare. Pediatrics 119:e666, 2007

Holty JE, Bravata DM, Liu H, et al: Systemic review: a century of inhalational anthrax cases from 1900 to 2005. Ann Intern Med 144:270, 2006

Hotop A, Hlobil H, Gross U: Efficacy of rapid treatment initiation following primary *Toxoplasma gondii* infection during pregnancy. Clin Infect Dis 54(11):1545, 2012

Howard MJ, Doyle TJ, Koster FT, et al: Hantavirus pulmonary syndrome in pregnancy. Clin Infect Dis 29:1538, 1999

Huang YC, Chao AS, Chang YJ, et al: Association of *Staphylococcus aureus* colonization in parturient mothers and their babies. Pediatr Infect Dis J 28:742, 2009

Hyde TB, Schmid DS, Cannon MJ: Cytomegalovirus seroconversion rates and risk factors: implications for congenital CMV. Rev Med Virol 20:311, 2010

Hyoti H, Hiltunen M, Knik M, et al: Childhood diabetes in Finland (DiMe) study group: a prospective study of the role of Coxsackie B and other enterovirus infections in the pathogenesis of IDDM. Diabetes 44:652, 1995

Inglesby TV, O'Toole T, Henderson DA, et al: Anthrax as a biological weapon, 2002. JAMA 287:2236, 2002

Irving WL, James DK, Stephenson T, et al: Influenza virus infection in the second and third trimesters of pregnancy: a clinical and seroepidemiological study. BJOG 107:1282, 2000

Jamieson DJ, Kissin DM, Bridges CB, et al: Benefits of influenza vaccination during pregnancy for pregnant women. Am J Obstet Gynecol 207 (3 Suppl):S17, 2012

Jamieson DJ, Ellis JE, Jernigan DB, et al: Emerging infectious disease outbreaks: old lessons and new challenges for obstetrician-gynecologists. Am J Obstet Gynecol 194:1546, 2006a

Jamieson DJ, Theiler RN, Rasmussen SA: Emerging infections and pregnancy. Emerg Infect Dis 12:1638, 2006b

Janakiraman V: Listeriosis in pregnancy: diagnosis, treatment, and prevention. Rev Obstet Gynecol 1(4):179, 2008

Jimenez-Truque N, Tedeschi S, Saye EJ, et al: Relationship between maternal and neonatal *Staphylococcus aureus* colonization. Pediatrics 129:e1252, 2012

Julander JG, Winger QA, Rickords LF, et al: West Nile virus infection of the placenta. Virology 347:175. 2006

Kanengisser-Pines B, Hazan Y, Pines G, et al: High cytomegalovirus IgG avidity is a reliable indicator of past infection in patients with positive IgM detected during the first trimester of pregnancy. J Perinat Med 37:15, 2009

Kashif AH, Adam GK, Mohmmed AA, et al: Reliability of rapid diagnostic test for diagnosing peripheral and placental malaria in an area of unstable malaria transmission in Eastern Sudan. Diagn Pathol 8:59, 2013

Kayentao K, Garner P, van Eijk AM, et al: Intermittent preventive therapy for malaria during pregnancy using 2 vs 3 or more doses of sulfadoxine-pyrimethamine and risk of low birth weight in Africa. JAMA 309(6):594, 2013

Kenneson A, Cannon MJ: Review and meta-analysis of the epidemiology of congenital cytomegalovirus (CMV) infection. Rev Med Virol 17:253, 2007

Khandaker G, Marshall H, Peadon E, et al: Congenital and neonatal varicella: impact of the national varicella vaccination programme in Australia. Arch Dis Child 96(5):453, 2011

Kharbanda EO, Vazquez-Benitez G, Lipkind H, et al: Inactivated influenza vaccine during pregnancy and risks for adverse obstetric events. Obstet Gynecol 122(3):659, 2013

Kim K, Kasper LH: Toxoplasma Infections. In Longo DL, Fauci AS, Kasper DL, et al (eds): Harrison's Principles of Internal Medicine, 18th ed. New York, McGraw-Hill, 2012

Kimberlin DW, Lin CY, Sanchez PJ, et al: Effect of ganciclovir therapy on hearing in symptomatic congenital cytomegalovirus disease involving the central nervous system: a randomized, controlled trial. J Pediatr 143:16, 2003

Klevens RM, Morrison MA, Nadle J, et al: Active bacterial core surveillance (ABCs) MRSA investigators: invasive methicillin-resistant *Staphylococcus aureus* infections in the United States. JAMA 298:1763, 2007

Koren G, Matsui D, Bailey B: DEET-based insect repellents: safety implications for children and pregnant and lactating women. CMAJ 169:209, 2003

Koro'lkova EL, Lozovskaia LS, Tadtaeva LI, et al: The role of prenatal coxsackie virus infection in the etiology of congenital heart defects in children. Kardiologiia 29:68, 1989

Kurppa K, Holmberg PC, Kuosma E, et al: Anencephaly and maternal common cold. Teratology 44:51, 1991

Laibl VR, Sheffield JS, Roberts S, et al: Clinical presentation of community-acquired methicillin-resistant *Staphylococcus aureus* in pregnancy. Obstet Gynecol 106:461, 2005

Lam CM, Wong SF, Leung TN, et al: A case-controlled study comparing clinical course and outcomes of pregnant and non-pregnant women with severe acute respiratory syndrome. BJOG 111:771, 2004

Lamont RF, Sobel JD, Vaisbuch E, et al: Parvovirus B19 infection in human pregnancy. BJOG 118(2):175, 2011a

Lamont RF, Sobel JD, Carrington D, et al: Varicella-zoster virus (chickenpox) infection in pregnancy. BJOG 118:1155, 2011b

Lareau SM, Meyn L, Beigi RH: Methicillin-resistant *Staphylococcus aureus* as the most common cause of perineal abscesses. Infect Dis Clin Pract 18:258, 2010

Lassen J, Jensen AK, Bager P, et al: Parvovirus B19 infection in the first trimester of pregnancy and risk of fetal loss: a population-based case-control study. Am J Epidemiol 176(9):803, 2012

Le Monnier A, Autret N, Join-Lambert OF, et al: ActA is required for crossing of the fetoplacental barrier by *Listeria monocytogenes*. Infect Immun 75:950, 2007

Lee IW, Kang L, Hsu HP, et al: Puerperal mastitis requiring hospitalization during a nine-year period. Am J Obstet Gynecol 203:332.e1, 2010

Liesnard C, Donner C, Brancart F, et al: Prenatal diagnosis of congenital cytomegalovirus infection: prospective study of 237 pregnancies at risk. Obstet Gynecol 95:881, 2000

Liu C, Bayer A, Cosgrove SE, et al: Clinical practice guidelines by the Infectious Diseases Society of America for the treatment of methicillin-resistant *Staphylococcus aureus* infections in adults and children. Clin Infect Dis 52:e18, 2011

Lynberg MC, Khoury MJ, Lu X, et al: Maternal flu, fever, and the risk of neural tube defects: a population-based case-control study. Am J Epidemiol 140:244, 1994

Machado Filho AC, da Costa EP, da Costa EP, et al: Effects of vivax malaria acquired before 20 weeks of pregnancy on subsequent changes in fetal growth. Am J Trop Med Hyg January 13, 2014 [Epub ahead of print]

Malinger G, Lev D, Zahalka N, et al: Fetal cytomegalovirus infection of the brain: the spectrum of sonographic findings. AJNR Am J Neuroradiol 24:28, 2003

Mandelbrot L: Fetal varicella–diagnosis, management, and outcome. Prenat Diagn 32(6):511, 2012

Maraspin V, Ružić-Sabljić E, Pleterski-Rigler D, et al: Pregnant women with erythema migrans and isolation of borreliae from blood: course and outcome after treatment with ceftriaxone. Diagn Microbiol Infect Dis 71(4):446, 2011

Marin M, Güris D, Chaves SS, et al: Prevention of varicella: recommendations of the Advisory Committee on Immunization Practices (ACIP). MMWR 56(4):1, 2007

Marin M, Watson TL, Chaves SS, et al: Varicella among adults: data from an active surveillance project, 1995–2005. J Infect Dis 197(Suppl 2):S94, 2008

Mason KL, Aronoff DM: Postpartum group A streptococcus sepsis and maternal immunology. Am J Reprod Immunol 67:91, 2012

McCarthy FP, Giles ML, Rowlands S, et al: Antenatal interventions for preventing the transmission of cytomegalovirus (CMV) from the mother to fetus during pregnancy and adverse outcomes in the congenitally infected infant. Cochrane Database Syst Rev 3:CD008371, 2011

McClure EM, Goldenberg RL, Dent AE, et al: A systematic review of the impact of malaria prevention in pregnancy on low birth weight and maternal anemia. Int J Gynaecol Obstet 121:103, 2013

McClure EM, Goldenberg RL: Infection and stillbirth. Semin Fetal Neonatal Med 14(4):182, 2009

McLean HQ, Fiebelkorn AP, Temte JL, et al: Prevention of measles, rubella, congenital rubella syndrome, and mumps, 2013: summary recommendations of the Advisory Committee on Immunization Practices (ACIP). MMWR Recomm Rep 62(4):1, 2013

McLeod R, Boyer KM, Lee D, et al: Prematurity and severity are associated with Toxoplasma gondii alleles (NCCCTS, 1981–2009). Clin Infect Dis 54(11):1595, 2012

Meaney-Delman D, Rasmussen SA, Beigi RH, et al: Prophylaxis and treatment of anthrax in pregnant women. Obstet Gynecol 122(4):885, 2013

Meaney-Delman D, Zotti ME, Rasmussen SA, et al: Anthrax cases in pregnant and postpartum women. Obstet Gynecol 120(6):1439, 2012

Mendelson E, Aboundy Y, Smetana Z, et al: Laboratory assessment and diagnosis of congenital viral infections: rubella, cytomegalovirus (CMV), varicella-zoster virus (VZV), herpes simplex virus (HSV), parvovirus B19 and human immunodeficiency virus (HIV). Reprod Toxicol 21:350, 2006

Menéndez C, D'Alessandro U, ter Kuile FO: Reducing the burden of malaria in pregnancy by preventive strategies. Lancet Infect Dis 7:126, 2007

Miller E, Cradock-Watson JE, Pollock TM: Consequences of confirmed maternal rubella at successive stages of pregnancy. Lancet 2:781, 1982

Modlin F: Perinatal echovirus and group B coxsackievirus infections. Clin Perinatol 15:233, 1988

Montoya JG, Remington JS: Management of *Toxoplasma gondii* infection during pregnancy. Clin Infect Dis 47:554, 2008

Montoya JG, Liesenfeld O: Toxoplasmosis. Lancet 363:1965, 2004

Moschella SL: An update on the diagnosis and treatment of leprosy. J Am Acad Dermatol 51:417, 2004

Moss WJ: Measles (rubeola). In Longo DL, Fauci AS, Kasper DL, et al. (eds): Harrison's Principles of Internal Medicine, 18th ed. New York, McGraw-Hill, 2012

Munoz FM: Safety of influenza vaccines in pregnant women. Am J Obstet Gynecol 207(3 Suppl):S33, 2012

Mutabinqwa TK, Adam I: Use of artemether-lumefantrine to treat malaria during pregnancy: what do we know and need to know? Expert Rev Anti Infect Ther 11(2):125, 2013

Mylonakis E, Paliou M, Hohmann EL, et al: Listeriosis during pregnancy. Medicine 81:260, 2002

Mylonas I: Borreliosis during pregnancy: a risk for the unborn child? Vector Borne Zoonotic Dis 11(7):891, 2011

Nadelman RB, Hanincová K, Mukherjee P, et al: Differentiation of reinfection from relapse in recurrent Lyme disease. N Engl J Med 367(20):1883, 2012

Nagel HT, de Haan TR, Vandenbussche FP, et al: Long-term outcome after fetal transfusion for hydrops associated with parvovirus B19 infection. Obstet Gynecol 109(1):42, 2007

Neuzil KM, Reed GW, Mitchel EF, et al: Impact of influenza on acute cardiopulmonary hospitalizations in pregnant women. Am J Epidemiol 148:1094, 1998

Nigro G, Adler SP, La Torre R, et al: Passive immunization during pregnancy for congenital cytomegalovirus infection. N Engl J Med 353:1350, 2005

Nigro G, Adler SP, Parruti G, et al: Immunoglobulin therapy of fetal cytomegalovirus infection occurring in the first half of pregnancy—a case-control study of the outcome in children. J Infect Dis 205:215, 2012

Nigro G, Anceschi MM, Cosmi EV, et al: Clinical manifestations and abnormal laboratory findings in pregnant women with primary cytomegalovirus infection. BJOG 110:572, 2003

Nishiura H: Smallpox during pregnancy and maternal outcomes. Emerg Infect Dis 12:1119, 2006

Norbeck O, Papadogiannakis N, Petersson K, et al: Revised clinical presentation of parvovirus B19–associated intrauterine fetal death. Clin Infect Dis 35:1032, 2002

Nordin JD, Kharbanda EO, Benitez GV, et al: Maternal safety of trivalent inactivated influenza vaccine in pregnant women. Obstet Gynecol 121(3):519, 2013

Nosten F, McGready R, Mutabingwa T: Case management of malaria in pregnancy. Lancet Infect Dis 7:118, 2007

Ohji G, Satoh H, Satoh H, et al: Congenital measles caused by transplacental infection. Pediatr Infect Dis J 28(2):166, 2009

Ohlsson A, Shah VS: Intrapartum antibiotics for known maternal group B streptococcal colonization. Cochrane Database Syst Rev 1:CD007467, 2013

O'Leary DR, Kuhn S, Kniss KL, et al: Birth outcomes following West Nile virus infection of pregnant women in the United States: 2003–2004. Pediatrics 117:e537, 2006

Ornoy A, Tenenbaum A: Pregnancy outcome following infections by coxsackie, echo, measles, mumps, hepatitis, polio and encephalitis viruses. Reprod Toxicol 21:446, 2006

Paryani SG, Arvin AM: Intrauterine infection with varicella zoster virus after maternal varicella. N Engl J Med 314:1542, 1986

Pass RF: Day-care centers and the spread of cytomegalovirus and parvovirus B19. Pediatr Ann 20:419, 1991

Peiris JS, Chu CM, Cheng VC, et al: Clinical progression and viral load in a community outbreak of coronavirus-associated SARS pneumonia: a prospective study. Lancet 361:1767, 2003a

Peiris JS, Yeun KY, Osterhaus AD, et al: The severe acute respiratory syndrome. N Engl J Med 349:2431, 2003b

Peques DA, Miller SI: Salmonellosis. In Longo DL, Fauci AS, Kasper DL, et al (eds): Harrison's Principles of Internal Medicine, 18th ed. New York, McGraw-Hill, 2012

Peters CJ: Infections caused by arthropod- and rodent-borne viruses. In Longo DL, Fauci AS, Kasper DL, et al (eds): Harrison's Principles of Internal Medicine, 18th ed. New York, McGraw-Hill, 2012

Picone O, Vauloup-Fellous C, Cordier AG, et al: A series of 238 cytomegalovirus primary infections during pregnancy: description and outcome. Prenat Diagn 33:751, 2013

Pierce M, Kurinczuk JJ, Spark P, et al: Perinatal outcomes after maternal 2009/H1N1 infection: national cohort study. BMJ 342:d3214, 2011

Pimentel JD, Meier FA, Samuel LP: Chorioamnionitis and neonatal sepsis from community-acquired MRSA. Emerg Infect Dis 15:2069, 2009

Pinter DM, Mandel J, Hulten KG, et al: Maternal-infant perinatal transmission of methicillin-resistant and methicillin-sensitive *Staphylococcus aureus*. Am J Perinatol 26:145, 2009

Plourd DM, Austin K: Correlation of a reported history of chickenpox with seropositive immunity in pregnant women. J Reprod Med 50:779, 2005

Pouillot R, Hoelzer K, Jackson KA, et al: Relative risk of listeriosis in foodborne diseases active surveillance network (FoodNet) sites according to age, pregnancy, and ethnicity. Clin Infect Dis 54(Suppl 5):S405, 2012

Pridjian G, Sirois P, McRae R, et al: A prospective studfy of pregnancy and newborn outcomes in mothers with West Nile virus (WNV) illness during pregnancy. Am J Obstet Gynecol 210:S197, 2014

Puccetti C, Contoli M, Bonvicini F, et al: Parvovirus B19 in pregnancy: possible consequences of vertical transmission. Prenat Diagn 32(9):897, 2012

Pulver LS, Hopfenbeck MM, Young PC, et al: Continued early onset group B streptococcal infections in the era of intrapartum prophylaxis. J Perinatol 29:20, 2009

Radolf JD, Caimano MJ, Stevenson B, et al: Of ticks, mice and men: understanding the dual-host lifestyle of Lyme disease spirochaetes. Nat Rev Microbiol 10(2):87, 2012

Raghupathy R: Pregnancy: success and failure within the Th1/Th2/Th3 paradigm. Semin Immunol 13:219, 2001

Rasmussen SA, Jamieson DJ, Uyeki TM: Effects of influenza on pregnant women and infants. Am J Obstet Gynecol 207(3 Suppl):S3, 2012

Reddy P, Qi C, Zembower T, et al: Postpartum mastitis and community-acquired methicillin-resistant *Staphylococcus aureus*. Emerg Infect Dis 13: 298, 2007

Reef SE, Frey TK, Theal K, et al: The changing epidemiology of rubella in the 1990s: on the verge of elimination and new challenges for control and prevention. JAMA 287:464, 2002

Reef SE, Plotkin S, Cordero JS, et al: Preparing for elimination of congenital rubella syndrome (CRS): summary of a workshop on CRS elimination in the United States. Clin Infect Dis 31:85, 2000

Revello MG, Gerna G: Pathogenesis and prenatal diagnosis of human cytomegalovirus infection. J Clin Virol 29:71, 2004

Revello MG, Furione M, Zavattoni M, et al: Human cytomegalovirus (HCMV) DNAemia in the mother at amniocentesis as a risk factor for iatrogenic HCMF infection of the fetus. J Infect Dis 197:593, 2008

Rogers BB: Parvovirus B19: twenty-five years in perspective. Pediatr Dev Pathol 2:296, 1999

Rogers VL, Sheffield JS, Roberts SW, et al: Presentation of seasonal influenza A in pregnancy: 2003–2004 influenza season. Obstet Gynecol 115(5):924, 2010

Rogerson SJ, Hviid L, Duffy PE, et al: Malaria in pregnancy: pathogenesis and immunity. Lancet Infect Dis 7:105, 2007

Ross SA, Novak Z, Pati S, et al: Mixed infection and strain diversity in congenital cytomegalovirus infection. J Infect Dis 204:1003, 2011

Rotas M, McCalla S, Liu C, et al: Methicillin-resistant *Staphylococcus aureus* necrotizing pneumonia arising from an infected episiotomy site. Obstet Gynecol 109:533, 2007

Rubin S, Carbone KM: Mumps. In Longo DL, Fauci AS, Kasper DL, et al. (eds): Harrison's Principles of Internal Medicine, 18th ed. New York, McGraw-Hill, 2012

Ryan MA, Gumbs GR, Conlin AS, et al: Evaluation of preterm births and birth defects in liveborn infants of US military women who received smallpox vaccine. Birth Defects Res A Clin Mol Teratol 82(7):533, 2008a

Ryan MA, Seward JF: Pregnancy, birth and infant health outcomes from the National Smallpox Vaccine in Pregnancy Registry, 2003–2006. Clin Infect Dis 46(Suppl 3):S221, 2008b

Ryan MA, Smith TC, Sevick CJ: Birth defects among infants born to women who received anthrax vaccine in pregnancy. Am J Epidemiol 168:434, 2008c

Saxén L, Holmberg PC, Kurppa K, et al: Influenza epidemics and anencephaly. Am J Public Health 80:473, 1990

Schild RL, Bald R, Plath H, et al: Intrauterine management of fetal parvovirus B19 infection. Ultrasound Obstet Gynecol 13:151, 1999

Schoen RT: Editorial comment: better laboratory testing for Lyme disease: no more Western blot. Clin Infect Dis 57(3):341, 2013

Schrag SJ, Arnold KE, Mohle-Boetani JC, et al: Prenatal screening for infectious diseases and opportunities for prevention. Obstet Gynecol 102:753, 2003

Shaw GM, Todoroff K, Velie EM, et al: Maternal illness, including fever, and medication use as risk factors for neural tube defects. Teratology 57:1, 1998

Sheffield JS: Methicillin-resistant *Staphylococcus aureus* in obstetrics. Am J Perinatol 30(2):125, 2013

Sheffield JS, Greer LG, Rogers VL, et al: Effect of influenza vaccination in the first trimester of pregnancy. Obstet Gynecol 120(3):532, 2012

Shulman ST, Bisno AL, Clegg HW, et al: Clinical practice guideline for the diagnosis and management of group A streptococcal pharyngitis: 2012 update by the Infectious Diseases Society of America. Clin Infect Dis 55(10):1279, 2012

Siegel M: Congenital malformations following chickenpox, measles, mumps, and hepatitis: results of a cohort study. JAMA 226:1521, 1973

Siegel M, Fuerst HT: Low birth weight and maternal virus diseases: a prospective study of rubella, measles, mumps, chickenpox, and hepatitis. JAMA 197:88, 1966

Siegel M, Goldberg M: Incidence of poliomyelitis in pregnancy. N Engl J Med 253:841, 1955

Silk BJ, Date KA, Jackson KA, et al: Invasive listeriosis in the Foodborne Diseases Active Surveillance Network (FoodNet), 2004–2009: further targeted prevention needed for higher-risk groups. Clin Infect Dis 54(Suppl 5): S396, 2012

Silk BJ, Mahon BE, Griffin PM, et al: Vital signs: *Listeria* illness, deaths, and outbreaks—United States, 2009–2011. MMWR 62(22):448, 2013

Skjöldebrand-Sparre L, Tolfvenstam T, Papadogiannakis N, et al: Parvovirus B19 infection: association of third-trimester intrauterine fetal death. BJOG 107:476, 2000

Sperling RS, Engel SM, Wallenstein S, et al: Immunogenicity of trivalent inactivated influenza vaccination received during pregnancy or postpartum. Obstet Gynecol 119(3):631, 2012

Stafford IA, Stewart RD, Sheffield JS, et al: Efficacy of maternal and neonatal chemoprophylaxis for early-onset group B streptococcal disease. Obstet Gynecol 120(1):123, 2012

Stagno S, Tinker MK, Elrod C, et al: Immunoglobulin M antibodies detected by enzyme-linked immunosorbent assay and radioimmunoassay in the diagnosis of cytomegalovirus infections in pregnant women and newborn infants. J Clin Microbiol 21(6):930, 1985

Stanley SL: Amebiasis and infection with free-living amebas. In Longo DL, Fauci AS, Kasper DL, et al (eds): Harrison's Principles of Internal Medicine, 18th ed. New York, McGraw-Hill, 2012

Steere AC: Lyme borreliosis. In Longo DL, Fauci AS, Kasper DL, et al (eds): Harrison's Principles of Internal Medicine, 18th ed. New York, McGraw-Hill, 2012

Steinhoff MC, Omer SB: A review of fetal and infant protection associated with antenatal influenza immunization. Am J Obstet Gynecol 207(3 Suppl): S21, 2012

Sterkers Y, Pratlong F, Albaba S, et al: Novel interpretation of molecular diagnosis of congenital toxoplasmosis according to gestational age at the time of maternal infection. J Clin Microbiol 50(12):3944, 2012

Stewart RD, Bryant SN, Sheffield JS: West Nile virus infection in pregnancy. Case report. Infect Dis 2013:351872, 2013

Suarez VR, Hankins GDV: Smallpox and pregnancy: from eradicated disease to bioterrorist threat. Obstet Gynecol 100:87, 2002

Svensson-Arvelund J, Ernerudh J, Buse E, et al: The placenta in toxicology. Part II: systemic and local immune adaptations in pregnancy. Toxicol Pathol 42(2):327, 2014

Swartz MN: Recognition and management of anthrax—an update. N Engl J Med 345:1621, 2001

Sweeney DA, Hicks CW, Cui X, et al: Anthrax infection. Am J Respir Crit Care Med 184:1333, 2011

SYROCOT (Systematic Review on Congenital Toxoplasmosis) Study Group: Effectiveness of prenatal treatment for congenital toxoplasmosis: a meta-analysis of individual patients' data. Lancet 369:115, 2007

Tassin M, Martinovic J, Mirand A, et al: A case of congenital echovirus 11 infection acquired early in pregnancy. J Clin Virol 59:71, 2014

Theiler RN, Rasmussen SA, Treadwell TA, et al: Emerging and zoonotic infections in women. Infect Dis Clin North Am 22:755, 2008

Thurman AR, Satterfield RM, Soper DE: Methicillin-resistant *Staphylococcus aureus* as a common cause of vulvar abscesses. Obstet Gynecol 112:538, 2008

Tolfvenstam T, Papadogiannakis N, Norbeck O, et al: Frequency of human parvovirus B19 infection in intrauterine fetal death. Lancet 357:1494, 2001

Top KA, Huard RC, Fox Z, et al: Trends in methicillin-resistant *Staphylococcus aureus* anovaginal colonization in pregnant women in 2005 versus 2009. J Clin Microbiol 48:3675, 2010

Topalovski M, Yang SS, Boonpasat Y: Listeriosis of the placenta: clinicopathologic study of seven cases. Am J Obstet Gynecol 169:616, 1993

Towbin JA, Griffin LD, Martin AB, et al: Intrauterine adenoviral myocarditis presenting as nonimmune hydrops fetalis: diagnosis by polymerase chain reaction. Pediatr Infect Dis J 13:144, 1994

Tudela CM, Stewart RD, Roberts SW, et al: Intrapartum evidence of early-onset group B streptococcus. Obstet Gynecol 119(3):626, 2012

United States Department of Health and Human Services: A summary of Hansen's disease in the United States, 2009. May 2011. Available at: http://www.hrsa.gov/hansensdisease/pdfs/hansens2009report.pdf. Accessed October 21, 2013

Valeur-Jensen AK, Pedersen CB, Westergaard T, et al: Risk factors for parvovirus B19 infection in pregnancy. JAMA 281:1099, 1999

Varma JK, Samuel MC, Marcus R, et al: *Listeria monocytogenes* infection from foods prepared in a commercial establishment: a case-control study of potential sources of sporadic illness in the United States. Clin Infect Dis 44:521, 2007

Verma R, Khanna P: Development of *Toxoplasma gondii* vaccine: a global challenge. Hum Vaccin Immunother 9(2):291, 2012

Villard O, Breit L, Cimon B, et al: Comparison of four commercially available avidity tests for *Toxoplasma gondii*-specific IgG antibodies. Clin Vaccine Immunol 20(2):197, 2013

Visentin S, Manara R, Milanese L, et al: Early primary cytomegalovirus infection in pregnancy: maternal hyperimmunoglobulin therapy improves outcomes among infants at 1 year of age. Clin Infect Dis 55(4):497, 2012

Viskari H, Knip M, Tauriainen S, et al: Maternal enterovirus infection as a risk factor for type 1 diabetes in the exposed offspring. Diabetes Care 35(6):1328, 2012

Voetsch AC, Angulo FJ, Jones TF, et al: Reduction in the incidence of invasive listeriosis in foodborne diseases active surveillance network sites, 1996–2003. Clin Infect Dis 44:513, 2007

von Kaisenberg CS, Jonat W: Fetal parvovirus B19 infection. Ultrasound Obstet Gynecol 18:280, 2001
Wallon M, Peyron F, Cornu C, et al: Congenital toxoplasma infection: monthly prenatal screening decreases transmission rate and improves clinical outcome at age 3 years. Clin Infect Dis 56(9):1223, 2013
Walsh CA, Mayer EQ, Baxi LV: Lyme disease in pregnancy: case report and review of the literature. Obstet Gynecol Surv 62:41, 2006
Wang C, Zhang X, Bialek S, et al: Attribution of congenital cytomegalovirus infection to primary versus non-primary maternal infection. Clin Infect Dis 52:e11, 2011
Warner MJ, Ozanne SE: Mechanisms involved in the developmental programming of adulthood disease. Biochem J 427:333, 2010
Webster WS: Teratogen update: congenital rubella. Teratology 58:13, 1998
Weiffenbach J, Bald R, Gloning KP, et al: Serological and virological analysis of maternal and fetal blood samples in prenatal human parvovirus B19 infection. J Infect Dis 205(5):782, 2012
Wendel GD Jr, Leveno KJ, Sánchez PJ, et al: Prevention of neonatal group B streptococcal disease: a combined intrapartum and neonatal protocol. Am J Obstet Gynecol 186:618, 2002
Wessels MR: Streptococcal infections. In Longo DL, Fauci AS, Kasper DL, et al (eds): Harrison's Principles of Internal Medicine, 18th ed. New York, McGraw-Hill, 2012
White NJ, Breman JG, Osler W: Malaria. In Longo DL, Fauci AS, Kasper DL, et al (eds): Harrison's Principles of Internal Medicine, 18th ed. New York, McGraw-Hill, 2012
Whitley RJ: Varicella-Zoster virus infections. In Longo DL, Fauci AS, Kasper DL, et al (eds): Harrison's Principles of Internal Medicine, 18th ed. New York, McGraw-Hill, 2012
Wiesen AR, Littell CT: Relationship between pre-pregnancy anthrax vaccination and pregnancy and birth outcomes among U.S. army women. JAMA 287:1556, 2002
Wilson E, Goss MA, Marin M, et al: Varicella vaccine exposure during pregnancy: data from 10 years of the pregnancy registry. J Infect Dis 197(Suppl 2): S178, 2008
Wing EJ, Gregory SH: *Listeria monocytogenes*: clinical and experimental update. J Infect Dis 185:S18, 2002
Wong SF, Chow KM, Leung TN, et al: Pregnancy and perinatal outcomes of women with severe acute respiratory syndrome. Am J Obstet Gynecol 191:292, 2004
World Health Organization: Long term effects of breastfeeding: a systematic review, 2013. Available at: http://www.who.int/maternal_child_adolescent/documents/breastfeeding_long_term_effects. Accessed October 21, 2013
World Health Organization: World malaria report 2011. Available at: http://www.who.int/malaria/world_malaria_report_2011. Accessed October 21, 2013
Wormser GP, Dattwyler RJ, Shapiro ED, et al: The clinical assessment, treatment, and prevention of Lyme disease, human granulocytic anaplasmosis, and babesiosis: clinical practice guidelines by the Infectious Diseases Society of America. Clin Infect Dis 43:1089, 2006
Wright JG, Quinn CP, Shadomy S, et al: Use of anthrax vaccine in the United States: recommendations of the Advisory Committee on Immunization Practices (ACIP), 2009. MMWR Recomm Rep 59(6):1, 2010
Yaegashi N: Pathogenesis of nonimmune hydrops fetalis caused by intrauterine B19 infection. Tohoku J Exp Med 190:65, 2000
Yates L, Pierce M, Stephens S, et al: Influenza A/H1N1 in pregnancy: an investigation of the characteristics and management of affected women and the relationship to pregnancy outcomes for mother and infant. Health Technol Assess 14:109, 2010
Zaman K, Roy E, Arifeen SE, et al: Effectiveness of maternal influenza immunization in mothers and infants. N Engl J Med 359(15):1555, 2008
Zimmerman LA, Reef SE: Rubella (German measles). In: Longo DL, Fauci AS, Kasper DL, et al (eds): Harrison's Principles of Internal Medicine, 18th ed. New York, McGraw-Hill, 2012

CHAPTER 65

Sexually Transmitted Infections

Sexually transmitted infections or diseases are among the most common of all infectious diseases encountered during pregnancy. Because they may be injurious to both mother and fetus, they should be aggressively sought and treated. Importantly, education, screening, treatment, and prevention are essential components of prenatal care (American Academy of Pediatrics and American College of Obstetricians and Gynecologists, 2012). Sexually transmitted infections (STIs) that affect pregnant women and potentially affect the fetus include syphilis, gonorrhea, trichomoniasis, and chlamydia, hepatitis B, human immunodeficiency virus (HIV), herpes simplex virus-1 and -2 (HSV-1, -2), and human papillomavirus (HPV) infections. Recommended therapy for most adhere to guidelines provided by the Centers for Disease Control and Prevention (CDC)(2010b). Treatment of most STIs is clearly associated with improved pregnancy outcome and prevention of perinatal mortality (Goldenberg, 2003, 2008; Ishaque, 2011; Koumans, 2012).

SYPHILIS

Despite the availability of adequate therapy for almost 70 years, syphilis remains a major issue for both mother and fetus. Syphilis rates reached an all-time low in 2000. But from 2001 through 2009 for the United States, there was a steady increase in primary and secondary syphilis rates, which then leveled in 2010 and 2011 (Centers for Disease Control and Prevention, 2013b). The primary and secondary syphilis rate among women in 2012 was 0.9 case per 100,000 persons, which is a 9-percent decrease from 2010. Congenital syphilis rates also decreased in 2012, mirroring the decline in primary and secondary syphilis rates among women since 2008. However, syphilis remains a significant global health problem, with many countries reporting high numbers of new infections (Lukehart, 2012).

Pathogenesis and Transmission

The causative agent for syphilis is *Treponema pallidum.* Minute abrasions on the vaginal mucosa provide an entry portal for the spirochete, and cervical eversion, hyperemia, and friability increase the transmission risk. Spirochetes replicate and then disseminate through lymphatic channels within hours to days. The incubation period averages 3 weeks—3 to 90 days—depending on host factors and inoculum size. The early stages of syphilis include primary, secondary, and early latent syphilis. These are associated with the highest spirochete loads and transmission rates of up to 30 to 50 percent. In late-stage disease, transmission rates are much lower because of smaller inoculum sizes.

The fetus acquires syphilis by several routes. Spirochetes readily cross the placenta to cause congenital infection. Because of immune incompetence prior to midpregnancy, the fetus generally does not manifest the immunological inflammatory response characteristic of clinical disease before this time (Silverstein, 1962). Although transplacental transmission is the most common route, neonatal infection may follow after contact with spirochetes through lesions at delivery or across the placental membranes. Increased maternal syphilis rates have been linked to substance abuse, especially crack cocaine; inadequate prenatal care and screening; and treatment failures and reinfection (Johnson, 2007; Lago, 2004; Trepka, 2006; Warner, 2001; Wilson, 2007). A report from Maricopa County, Arizona, also cited minority race or ethnicity as a risk factor (Kirkcaldy, 2011).

Clinical Manifestations

Maternal syphilis can cause preterm labor, fetal death, fetal-growth restriction, and neonatal infection (Krakauer, 2012; Saloojee, 2004). Any stage of maternal syphilis may result in fetal infection, but risk is directly related to maternal spirochete load (Fiumara, 1952; Golden, 2003). Maternal syphilis is staged according to clinical features and disease duration:

1. *Primary syphilis* is diagnosed by the characteristic chancre, which develops at the inoculation site. It is usually painless, with a raised, red, firm border and a smooth base (Fig. 65-1). Nonsuppurative lymphadenopathy may develop. A chancre will usually resolve spontaneously in 2 to 8 weeks, even if untreated. Multiple lesions may be found, predominantly in HIV-1 co-infected women.
2. *Secondary syphilis* is diagnosed when the spirochete is disseminated and affects multiple organ systems. Manifestations develop 4 to 10 weeks after the chancre appears and include dermatological abnormalities in up to 90 percent of women. A diffuse macular rash, plantar and palmar targetlike lesions, patchy alopecia, and mucous patches may be seen (Figs. 65-2 and 65-3). Condylomata lata are flesh-colored papules and nodules found on the perineum and perianal area. They are teeming with spirochetes and are highly infectious. Most women with secondary syphilis will also express constitutional symptoms such as fever, malaise, anorexia, headache, myalgias, and arthralgias. Up to 40 percent will have cerebrospinal fluid abnormalities, although only 1 to 2 percent will develop clinically apparent aseptic meningitis. Hepatitis, nephropathy, ocular changes, anterior uveitis, and periostitis may also develop.

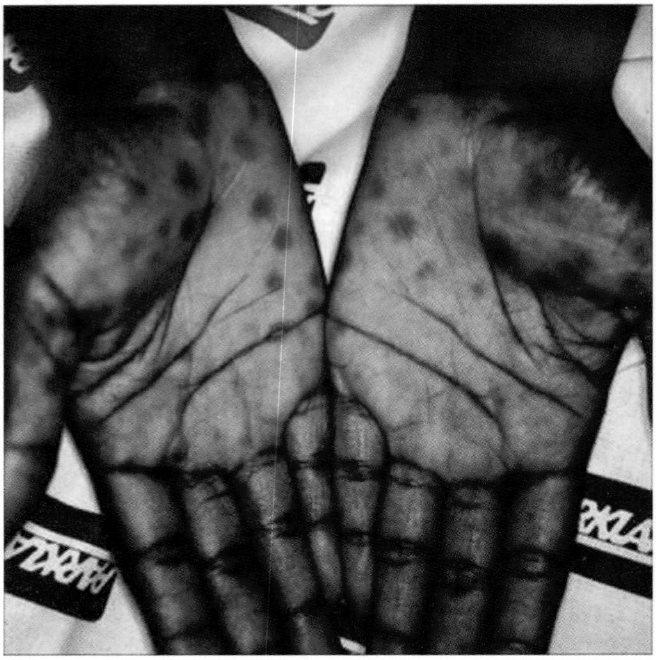

FIGURE 65-2 Target lesions on the palms of a pregnant woman with secondary syphilis.

3. *Latent syphilis* develops when primary or secondary syphilis is not treated. It is characterized by reactive serological testing, but resolved clinical manifestations. *Early latent syphilis* is latent disease acquired within the preceding 12 months. Disease diagnosed beyond 12 months is either *late latent syphilis* or *latent syphilis of unknown duration.*
4. *Tertiary* or *late syphilis* is a slowly progressive disease affecting any organ system but is rarely seen in reproductive-aged women.

As noted, congenital infection is uncommon before 18 weeks. Once fetal syphilis develops, however, it manifests as a continuum of involvement. Fetal hepatic abnormalities are followed by anemia and thrombocytopenia, then ascites and

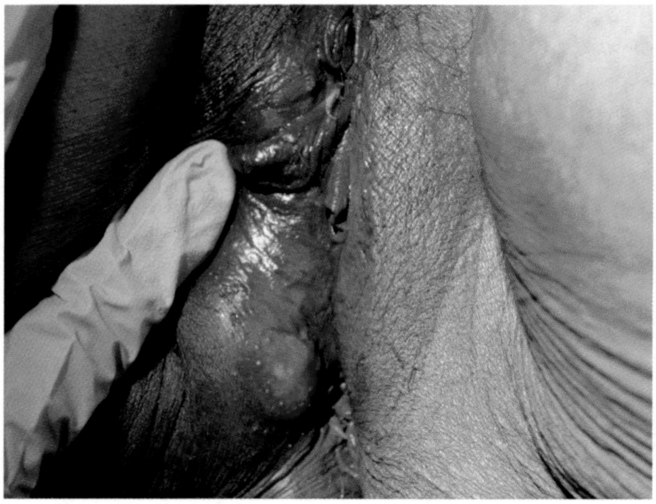

FIGURE 65-1 Primary syphilis. Photograph of a chancre with a raised, firm border and smooth, red base.

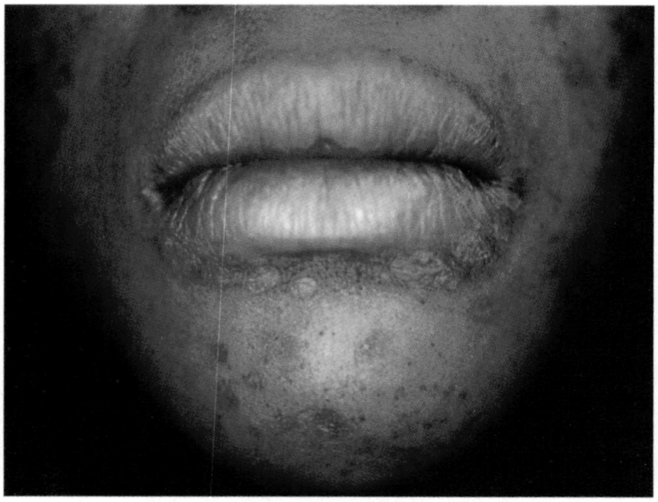

FIGURE 65-3 Mucous patches around the mouth of a pregnant woman with secondary syphilis.

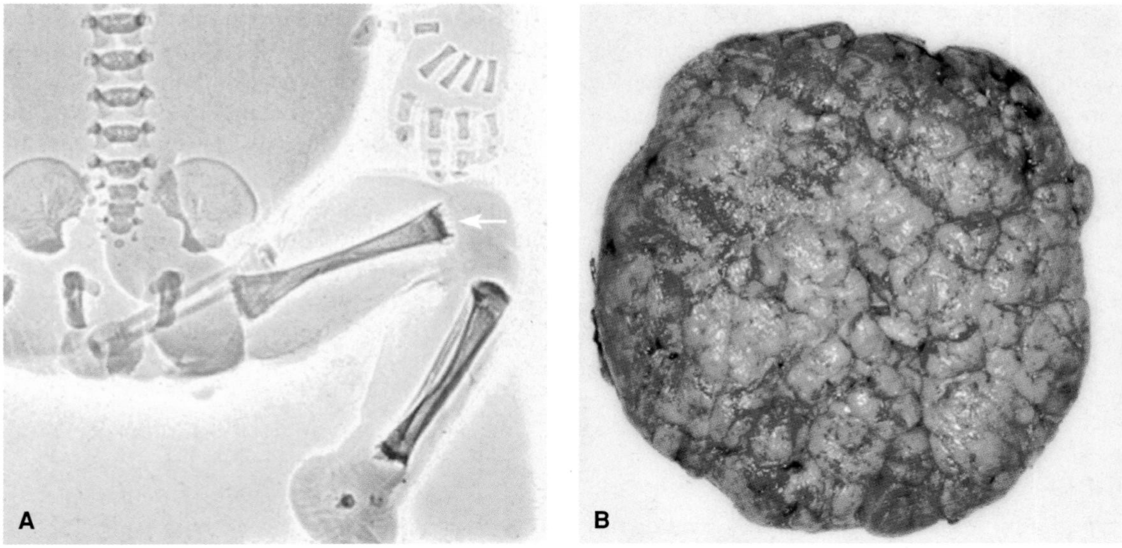

FIGURE 65-4 Congenital syphilis. **A.** Fetogram of a stillborn infant infected with syphilis showing the "moth-eaten" appearance of the femurs (*arrow*). **B.** Enlarged hydropic placenta of a syphilis-infected neonate.

hydrops (Hollier, 2001). Stillbirth remains a major complication (Di Mario, 2007; Hawkes, 2011; Rac, 2014b). The newborn may have jaundice with petechiae or purpuric skin lesions, lymphadenopathy, rhinitis, pneumonia, myocarditis, nephrosis, or long-bone involvement.

With syphilitic infection, the placenta becomes large and pale (Fig. 65-4). Microscopically, villi lose their characteristic arborization and become thicker and clubbed (Kapur, 2004). Sheffield and colleagues (2002c) described such large villi in more than 60 percent of syphilitic placentas. Blood vessels markedly diminish in number, and in advanced cases, they almost entirely disappear as a result of endarteritis and stromal cell proliferation. Likely related, Lucas and coworkers (1991) demonstrated increased vascular resistance in uterine and umbilical arteries of infected pregnancies. In a study of 25 untreated women, Schwartz and associates (1995) reported that necrotizing funisitis was present in a third. Spirochetes were detected in almost 90 percent using silver and immunofluorescent staining.

Diagnosis

The United States Preventative Services Task Force has reaffirmed its recommendation that clinicians screen all pregnant women for syphilis to treat and prevent congenital infection (Wolff, 2009). Testing is now required by law in all states and should be performed at the first prenatal visit. In populations in which the prevalence of syphilis is high, serological testing should be performed in the third trimester and again at delivery (Centers for Disease Control and Prevention, 2010b).

Treponema pallidum cannot be cultured from clinical specimens. Definitive diagnosis of early-stage lesions is made using dark-field examination and direct immunofluorescent antibody staining of lesion exudates (Centers for Disease Control and Prevention, 2010b). In asymptomatic patients or for screening purposes, serological testing is used. There are two types. The first type is nontreponemal testing that includes the Venereal Disease Research Laboratory (VDRL) and the rapid plasma reagin (RPR). These tests are quantified and expressed as titers. Because titers reflect disease activity, they increase during early syphilis and often exceed levels of 1:32 in secondary syphilis. Following treatment of primary and secondary syphilis, serological testing at 3 to 6 months usually confirms a fourfold drop in VDRL or RPR titers (Rac, 2014a). Those with treatment failure or reinfection may lack this decline. Because VDRL titers do not correspond directly to RPR titers, consistent use of the same test for surveillance is recommended.

The other type of testing is treponemal-specific and includes the fluorescent treponemal-antibody absorption tests (FTA-ABS), the microhemagglutination assay for antibodies to *T pallidum* (MHA-TP), or the *Treponema pallidum* passive particle agglutination (TP-PA) test. These treponemal-specific tests generally remain positive throughout life.

Each of the serological tests has limitations including false-positive results. Traditionally, nontreponemal tests have been used for screening in the United States, and results are then confirmed by a specific treponemal test. Several laboratories have recently implemented a reverse screening algorithm, that is, screening with a treponemal test (Binnicker, 2012; Park, 2011). Both approaches are effective if appropriate screening, follow-up, and treatment are implemented. Patel and colleagues (2012) described missed opportunities for preventing and treating congenital syphilis in New York City. They found that 63 percent of mothers with newborns diagnosed with congenital syphilis had a missed opportunity for prevention. Most of these did not receive serological testing.

Rapid syphilis testing for "point of care" diagnosis is currently being developed and may be useful in settings with limited prenatal care (Centers for Disease Control and Prevention, 2010b; Greer, 2008). Treponemal immunochromatographic strip (ICS) tests and enzyme immunoassays (EIAs) are increasingly being used for screening and confirmatory testing (Henrich, 2011; Lukehart, 2012).

The prenatal diagnosis of congenital syphilis is difficult because an infected fetus often has a normal sonographic examination. Some findings, however, may be suggestive or even diagnostic—hydrops fetalis, ascites, hepatomegaly, placental thickening, elevated middle cerebral artery Doppler velocimetry measurements, and hydramnios all suggest infection (Rac, 2014b). Polymerase chain reaction (PCR) is specific for detection of *T pallidum* in amnionic fluid, and treponemal DNA has been found in 40 percent of pregnancies infected before 20 weeks (Nathan, 1997; Wendel, 1991). Fetal syphilis has also been verified by amnionic fluid dark-field examination or rabbit infectivity testing in 64 percent of a cohort of women with untreated syphilis (Hollier, 2001). Although prenatal diagnosis can be made by funipuncture or amniocentesis, its clinical utility is not clear.

Treatment

Syphilis therapy during pregnancy is given to eradicate maternal infection and to prevent or treat congenital syphilis. Parenteral penicillin G remains the preferred treatment for all stages of syphilis during pregnancy. Currently recommended treatment guidelines are shown in Table 65-1 and are the same as for nonpregnant adults. For pregnant women, authorities recommend that a second dose of benzathine penicillin G be given 1 week after the initial dose.

In retrospective analyses, benzathine penicillin G has been shown to be highly effective for early maternal infection. In a study of 340 pregnant women so treated, Alexander and associates (1999) reported six cases—1.8 percent—of congenital syphilis. Four of these six neonates were from a group of 75 women with secondary syphilis. The other two were identified in those delivered from a group of 102 women with early latent syphilis. Congenital syphilis was generally confined to neonates of women treated after 26 weeks and is likely related to the duration and severity of fetal infection. Sheffield and coworkers (2002b) reported that high maternal serological titers, preterm delivery, and delivery shortly after antepartum therapy are all risks for failure of maternal treatment to prevent neonatal infection. There are no proven alternatives to penicillin therapy during pregnancy. Erythromycin and azithromycin may be curative for the mother, but because of limited transplacental passage, these drugs do not prevent all congenital disease (Berman, 2004; Centers for Disease Control and Prevention, 2010b; Wendel, 1988; Zhou, 2007). In several countries, macrolide resistant strains of *T pallidum* are now prevalent (Stamm, 2010). Cephalosporins may prove useful, but data are limited (Augenbraun, 1999, 2002; Zhou, 2007). Tetracyclines, including doxycycline, are effective for treatment of syphilis in the nonpregnant woman. These are generally not recommended during pregnancy, however, because of the risk of yellow-brown discoloration of fetal deciduous teeth (Chap. 12, p. 248).

Penicillin Allergy

Women with a history of penicillin allergy should have either a oral stepwise penicillin dose challenge or skin testing performed to confirm the risk of immunoglobulin E (IgE)-mediated anaphylaxis. If confirmed, penicillin desensitization is recommended, as shown in Table 65-2, and then followed by benzathine penicillin G treatment (Chisholm, 1997; Wendel, 1985).

In most women with primary syphilis and approximately half with secondary infection, penicillin treatment causes a *Jarisch-Herxheimer reaction*. Uterine contractions frequently develop with this reaction and may be accompanied by decreased fetal movement and late fetal heart rate decelerations (Klein, 1990). In a study of 50 pregnant women who received benzathine penicillin for syphilis, Myles and colleagues (1998) reported a 40-percent incidence of a Jarisch-Herxheimer reaction. Of the 31 women monitored electronically, 42 percent developed regular uterine contractions with a median onset of 10 hours, and 39 percent developed variable decelerations with a median onset of 8 hours. All contractions resolved within 24 hours of therapy. Lucas and associates (1991) used Doppler velocimetry and demonstrated acutely increased vascular resistance during this time. Beta-lactam antibiotics for group B streptococcus intrapartum prophylaxis can also trigger this reaction in a woman with untreated syphilis (Rac, 2010).

All women with syphilis should be offered counseling and testing for HIV (Koumans, 2000). For women with concomitant HIV infection, the Centers for Disease Control and

TABLE 65-1. Recommended Treatment for Pregnant Women with Syphilis

Category	Treatment
Early syphilis[a]	Benzathine penicillin G, 2.4 million units intramuscularly as a single injection—some recommend a second dose 1 week later
More than 1-year duration[b]	Benzathine penicillin G, 2.4 million units intramuscularly weekly for three doses
Neurosyphilis[c]	Aqueous crystalline penicillin G, 3–4 million units intravenously every 4 hours for 10–14 days *or* Aqueous procaine penicillin, 2.4 million units intramuscularly daily, plus probenecid 500 mg orally four times daily, both for 10–14 days

[a]Primary, secondary, and latent syphilis of less than 1-year duration.
[b]Latent syphilis of unknown or more than 1-year duration; tertiary syphilis.
[c]Some recommend benzathine penicillin, 2.4 million units intramuscularly after completion of the neurosyphilis treatment regimens.
From the Centers for Disease Control and Prevention, 2010b.

TABLE 65-2. Penicillin Allergy—Oral Desensitization Protocol for Patients with a Positive Skin Test

Penicillin V Suspension Dose[a]	Amount[b] (units/mL)	mL	Units	Cumulative Dose (units)
1	1000	0.1	100	100
2	1000	0.2	200	300
3	1000	0.4	400	700
4	1000	0.8	800	1500
5	1000	1.6	1600	3100
6	1000	3.2	3200	6300
7	1000	6.4	6400	12,700
8	10,000	1.2	12,000	24,700
9	10,000	2.4	24,000	48,700
10	10,000	4.8	48,000	96,700
11	80,000	1.0	80,000	176,700
12	80,000	2.0	160,000	336,700
13	80,000	4.0	320,000	656,700
14	80,000	8.0	640,000	1,296,700

[a]Interval between doses: 15 minutes. Elapsed time: 3 hours and 45 minutes. Cumulative dose: 1.3 million units. Observation period: 30 minutes before parenteral administration of penicillin.
[b]The specific amount of drug was diluted in approximately 30 mL of water and administered orally.
From Wendel, 1985, with permission.

Prevention (2010b) recommend the same treatment as for HIV-negative persons. Clinical and serological surveillance to detect treatment failures is also recommended at 3, 6, 9, 12, and 24 months in HIV-positive patients.

GONORRHEA

Gonorrhea remains the second most commonly reported notifiable disease in the United States. The incidence of gonorrhea in the United States for 2012 was 107.5 cases per 100,000 persons, which is an increase of 4 percent since 2011 (Centers for Disease Control and Prevention, 2013b). The highest rates in women of any ethnicity were in the groups aged 20 to 24 years (578.5) and 15 to 19 years (521.2). Its prevalence in prenatal clinics in 2011 among women aged 15 to 24 years was 0.8 percent, although inner-city STI clinics have reported a prenatal prevalence of 5 to 10 percent (Berggren, 2011; Johnson, 2007). Risk factors include single marital status, adolescence, poverty, drug abuse, prostitution, other STIs, and lack of prenatal care (Berggren, 2011; Gorgos, 2011). Gonococcal infection is also a marker for concomitant chlamydial infection in up to 40 percent of infected women (Christmas, 1989; Miller, 2004). In most pregnant women, gonococcal infection is limited to the lower genital tract—the cervix, urethra, and periurethral and vestibular glands. Acute salpingitis is rare in pregnancy, but pregnant women account for a disproportionate number of disseminated gonococcal infections (Bleich, 2012; Ross, 1996; Yip, 1993).

Gonococcal infection may have deleterious effects in any trimester. There is an association between untreated gonococcal cervicitis and septic abortion as well as infection after voluntary abortion (Burkman, 1976). Preterm delivery, prematurely ruptured membranes, chorioamnionitis, and postpartum infection are reported to be more common in women infected with *Neisseria gonorrhoeae* (Alger, 1988; Johnson, 2011). Bleich and coworkers (2012) reviewed outcomes of 32 pregnant women admitted to Parkland Hospital for disseminated gonococcal infection. Although all the women promptly responded to appropriate antimicrobial therapy, one stillbirth was attributed to gonococcal sepsis.

Screening and Treatment

The U.S. Preventative Services Task Force recommends gonorrhea screening for all sexually active women, including pregnant women, if they are at increased risk (Meyers, 2008). Risk factors include age < 25 years, prior gonococcal infection, other STIs, prostitution, new or multiple sexual partners, drug use, and inconsistent condom use. For women who test positive, screening for syphilis, *Chlamydia trachomatis,* and HIV should precede treatment, if possible. If chlamydial testing is unavailable, presumptive therapy is given. Screening for gonorrhea in women is by culture or nucleic acid amplification tests (NAATs). Rapid tests for gonorrhea, although available, do not yet reach the sensitivity or specificity of culture or NAAT (Greer, 2008).

Gonorrhea treatment has evolved during the past decade due to the ability of *N gonorrhoeae* to rapidly develop antimicrobial resistance (Centers for Disease Control and Prevention, 2011b,c; Dionne-Odom, 2011; Ram, 2012; Unemo, 2011). Rapid development of fluoroquinolone resistance caused the CDC to remove that therapeutic class from its treatment guidelines in 2007. The Gonococcal Isolate Surveillance Project, a national sentinel surveillance system established to monitor trends in gonococcal antimicrobial resistance, has reported decreasing susceptibility to cephalosporins. This is the one remaining class of antimicrobial agents currently recommended for gonorrhea treatment (Bolan, 2012; Centers for Disease Control and Prevention, 2010b, 2012). This global public health threat has led the CDC in 2012 to change the gonorrhea treatment recommendations.

Listed in Table 65-3 are the updated recommendations for treatment of uncomplicated gonococcal infection during pregnancy. The increased ceftriaxone dose of 250 mg should be given along with 1 gram of azithromycin. The latter provides

TABLE 65-3. Treatment of Uncomplicated Gonococcal Infections During Pregnancy

Ceftriaxone, 250 mg intramuscularly as a single dose
plus
Azithromycin, 1 gram orally as a single dose

From the Centers for Disease Control and Prevention, 2010b.

another drug with a different mechanism of action against *N gonorrhoeae* and treats chlamydial co-infections. Cefixime tablets should be reserved for situations that preclude ceftriaxone treatment. If they are used, a test-of-cure should be performed 1 week after treatment. Azithromycin, 2 grams orally as a single dose, can be used in cephalosporin-allergic women. However, this treatment should be limited due to emerging macrolide resistance (Centers for Disease Control and Prevention, 2011c). Treatment is also recommended for sexual contacts. A test-of-cure is unnecessary if symptoms resolve, but because gonococcal reinfection is common, a second screening in late pregnancy should be considered for women treated earlier (Blatt, 2012).

Disseminated Gonococcal Infections (DGI)

Gonococcal bacteremia may cause disseminated infections that manifest as petechial or pustular skin lesions, arthralgias, septic arthritis, or tenosynovitis. For treatment, the Centers for Disease Control and Prevention (2010b) has recommended ceftriaxone, 1000 mg intramuscularly or intravenously (IV) every 24 hours. Treatment should be continued for 24 to 48 hours after improvement, and therapy is then changed to an oral agent to complete 1 week of therapy. Prompt recognition and antimicrobial treatment will usually result in favorable outcomes in pregnancy (Bleich, 2012). Meningitis and endocarditis rarely complicate pregnancy, but they may be fatal (Bataskov, 1991; Burgis, 2006; Ram, 2012). For gonococcal *endocarditis*, ceftriaxone 1000 to 2000 mg IV every 12 hours should be continued for at least 4 weeks, and for *meningitis*, 10 to 14 days (Centers for Disease Control and Prevention, 2010b).

CHLAMYDIAL INFECTIONS

Chlamydia trachomatis is an obligate intracellular bacterium that has several serotypes, including those that cause lymphogranuloma venereum. The most commonly encountered strains are those that attach only to columnar or transitional cell epithelium and cause cervical infection. It is the most commonly reported infectious disease in the United States, with 1.4 million cases reported in 2012. It is estimated, however, that there are approximately 2.8 million new cases annually, although most are undiagnosed (Centers for Disease Control and Prevention, 2008). In 2012, the incidence of chlamydial infection among women was 2½ times greater than among men. Selective prenatal screening clinics in 2011 reported a median chlamydial infection rate of 7.7 percent (Centers for Disease Control and Prevention, 2013b).

Although most pregnant women have asymptomatic infection, a third have urethral syndrome, urethritis, or Bartholin gland infection (Peipert, 2003). Mucopurulent cervicitis may be due to chlamydial or gonococcal infection or both. It may also represent normal, hormonally stimulated endocervical glands with abundant mucus production. Other chlamydial infections not usually seen in pregnancy are endometritis, salpingitis, peritonitis, reactive arthritis, and Reiter syndrome.

The role of chlamydial infection in pregnancy complications remains controversial. A few studies have reported a direct association between *C trachomatis* and miscarriage, whereas most show no correlation (Baud, 2011; Coste, 1991; Paukku, 1999; Sugiura-Ogasawara, 2005). It is disputed whether untreated cervical infection increases the risk of preterm delivery, preterm ruptured membranes, and perinatal mortality (Andrews, 2000, 2006; Baud, 2008; Blas, 2007; Silva, 2011). Johnson and colleagues (2011) reported a twofold risk for low-birthweight infants.

Chlamydial infection has not been associated with an increased risk of chorioamnionitis or with pelvic infection after cesarean delivery (Blanco, 1985; Gibbs, 1987). Conversely, delayed postpartum uterine infection has been described by Hoyme and associates (1986). The syndrome, which develops 2 to 3 weeks postpartum, is distinct from early postpartum metritis. It is characterized by vaginal bleeding or discharge, low-grade fever, lower abdominal pain, and uterine tenderness.

There is vertical transmission to 30 to 50 percent of neonates delivered vaginally from infected women. Perinatal transmission to newborns can cause pneumonia. Moreover, *C trachomatis* is the most commonly identifiable infectious cause of ophthalmia neonatorum (Chap. 32, p. 631).

Screening and Treatment

Prenatal screening for *C trachomatis* is a complex issue, although there is little evidence for its effectiveness in asymptomatic women who are not in high-risk groups (Kohl, 2003; Meyers, 2007; Peipert, 2003). Identification and treatment of asymptomatic infected women may prevent neonatal infections, but evidence of adverse pregnancy outcome prevention is lacking. Currently, the U.S. Preventive Services Task Force (2007) and the CDC recommend prenatal screening at the first prenatal visit for women at increased risk for chlamydial infection, and again during the third trimester if high-risk behavior continues. In a systematic review of repeat chlamydial infection among women, Hosenfeld and coworkers (2009) reported a reinfection rate of 14 percent, and most recurred within the first 8 to 10 months. Interestingly, in another study, Sheffield and colleagues (2005) found that almost half of pregnant women with asymptomatic cervical chlamydia underwent spontaneous resolution of infection.

Diagnosis is made predominantly by culture or NAAT. Cultures are more expensive and less accurate than newer NAATs, including PCR (Greer, 2008). Roberts and associates (2011) evaluated nucleic acid amplification testing of urine compared with cervical secretions in more than 2000 pregnant women and found them to be equivalent.

Currently recommended treatment regimens for chlamydial infections are shown in Table 65-4. Azithromycin is first-line treatment and has been found to be safe and effective in pregnancy. The fluoroquinolones and doxycycline are avoided in pregnancy, as is erythromycin estolate because of drug-related hepatotoxicity. Repeat chlamydial testing 3 to 4 weeks after completion of therapy is recommended.

TABLE 65-4. Treatment of *Chlamydia trachomatis* Infections During Pregnancy

Regimen	Drug and Dosage
Preferred choice	Azithromycin, 1000 mg orally as a single dose
	or
	Amoxicillin, 500 mg orally three times daily for 7 days
Alternatives	Erythromycin base, 500 mg orally four times daily for 7 days
	or
	Erythromycin ethylsuccinate, 800 mg orally four times daily for 7 days
	or
	Erythromycin base, 250 mg orally four times daily for 14 days
	or
	Erythromycin ethylsuccinate, 400 mg orally four times daily for 14 days

From the Centers for Disease Control and Prevention, 2010b.

Lymphogranuloma Venereum

L_1, L_2, and L_3 serovars of *C trachomatis* cause *lymphogranuloma venereum (LGV)*. The primary genital infection is transient and seldom recognized. Inguinal adenitis may develop and at times lead to suppuration. It may be confused with chancroid. Ultimately, the lymphatics of the lower genital tract and perirectal tissues may be involved. Here, sclerosis and fibrosis can cause vulvar elephantiasis and severe rectal stricture. Fistula formation involving the rectum, perineum, and vulva also may evolve.

For treatment during pregnancy, erythromycin base, 500 mg orally four times daily, is given for 21 days (Centers for Disease Control and Prevention, 2010b). Although data regarding efficacy are scarce, some authorities recommend azithromycin, 1000 mg orally weekly for 3 weeks.

HERPES SIMPLEX VIRUS

Genital herpes simplex virus infection is one of the most common sexually transmitted diseases according to the Centers for Disease Control and Prevention (2010a,b). An estimated 50 million adolescents and adults are currently affected. In 2012, there were 228,000 initial office visits for genital herpes (Centers for Disease Control and Prevention, 2013b). Although most women are unaware of their infection, approximately one in six has serological evidence for HSV-2 infection. This incidence is as high as one in two for non-Hispanic black pregnant women (Corey, 2012). As most cases of HSV are transmitted by persons who are asymptomatic or unaware of their disease, herpes infections have become a major public health concern. It is estimated that 0.5 to 2 percent of pregnant women acquire HSV-1 or -2 during pregnancy (Brown, 1997).

Pathogenesis and Transmission

Two types of HSV have been distinguished based on immunological and clinical differences. Type 1 is responsible for most nongenital infections. However, more than half of new cases of genital herpes in adolescents and young adults are caused by HSV-1 infection. This is thought to be due to an increase in oral-genital sexual practices (Mertz, 2003; Pena, 2010; Roberts, 2003). Type 2 HSV is recovered almost exclusively from the genital tract and is usually transmitted by sexual contact. Most recurrences—greater than 90 percent—are secondary to HSV-2. There is a large amount of DNA sequence homology between the two viruses, and prior infection with one type attenuates a primary infection with the other type.

Neonatal transmission is by three routes: (1) intrauterine in 5 percent, (2) peripartum in 85 percent, or (3) postnatal in 10 percent (Kimberlin, 2004b). The fetus becomes infected by virus shed from the cervix or lower genital tract. It either invades the uterus following membrane rupture or is transmitted by contact with the fetus at delivery. The overall transmission rate is 1 in 3200 to 1 in 30,000 births depending on the population studied (Corey, 2012; Mahnert, 2007; Whitley, 2007). Neonatal herpes is caused by both HSV-1 and HSV-2, although HSV-2 infection predominates. Most infected infants are born to mothers with no reported history of HSV infection (Gardella, 2010).

The risk of neonatal infection correlates with the presence of HSV in the genital tract, the HSV type, invasive obstetrical procedures, and stage of maternal infection (Brown, 2005, 2007). Infants born to women who acquire genital HSV near the time of delivery have a 30- to 50-percent risk of infection. This is attributed to higher viral loads and the lack of transplacental protective antibodies (Brown, 1997; Brown, 2000). Women with recurrent HSV have less than a 1-percent risk of neonatal infection (Pasternak, 2010; Prober, 1987).

Clinical Manifestations

Once transmitted by genital-genital or oral-genital contact, HSV-1 or -2 replicates at the entry site. Following mucocutaneous infection, the virus moves retrograde along sensory nerves. It then remains latent in cranial nerves or dorsal spinal ganglia. HSV infections may be categorized into three groups:

1. *First episode primary infection* describes cases in which HSV-1 or -2 is isolated from genital secretions in the absence of HSV-1 or -2 antibodies. Only a third of newly acquired HSV-2 genital infections are symptomatic (Langenberg,

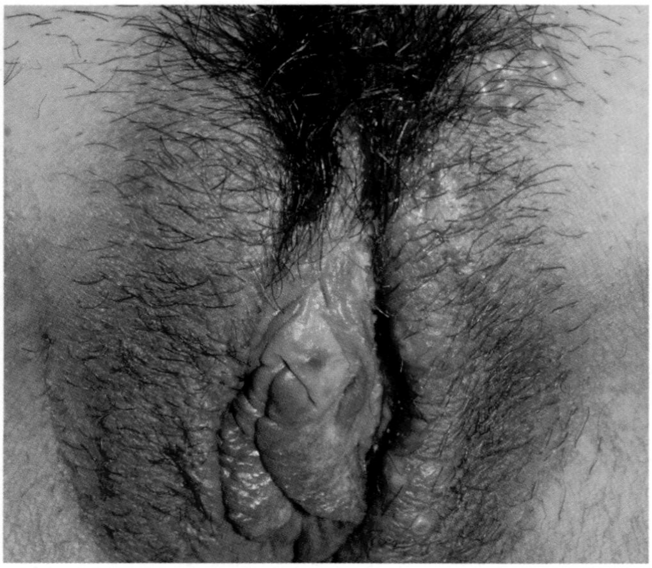

FIGURE 65-5 First-episode primary genital herpes simplex virus infection. On the left labium majora and mons, both vesicles and ulcers are seen.

1999). The typical incubation period of 6 to 8 days (range 1 to 26 days) may be followed by a "classic presentation." This is characterized by a papular eruption with itching or tingling, which then becomes painful and vesicular. Multiple vulvar and perineal lesions may coalesce, and inguinal adenopathy may be severe (Fig. 65-5). Transient systemic influenza-like symptoms are common and are presumably caused by viremia. Hepatitis, encephalitis, or pneumonia may develop, although disseminated disease is rare. Cervical involvement is common, but it may be inapparent clinically. Some cases are severe enough to require hospitalization. In 2 to 4 weeks, all signs and symptoms of infection disappear. Many women do not present with the typical lesions—instead, a pruritic or painful abraded area or knife-slit may be present. The incidence of asymptomatic primary infections may be as high as 80 percent (Centers for Disease Control and Prevention, 2010a,b).

2. *First episode nonprimary infection* is diagnosed when HSV is isolated in women who have only the other serum HSV-type antibody present. For example, HSV-2 is isolated from genital secretions in women already expressing serum HSV-1 antibodies. In general, these infections are characterized by fewer lesions, fewer systemic manifestations, less pain, and briefer duration of lesions and viral shedding. This is likely because of some immunity from cross-reacting antibodies, for example, from childhood-acquired HSV-1 infection. In many cases, it may be impossible to differentiate clinically between the two types of first infection. Thus, serological confirmation may be beneficial.
3. *Reactivation disease* is characterized by isolation of HSV-1 or -2 from the genital tract in women with the same serotype antibodies. During the latency period, in which viral particles reside in nerve ganglia, reactivation is common and mediated through variable but poorly understood stimuli. Reactivation is termed *recurrent infection* and results in herpes-virus shedding. Most recurrent genital herpes is caused by type 2 virus (Centers for Disease Control and Prevention, 2010a,b; Corey, 2012). These lesions generally are fewer in number, are less tender, and shed virus for shorter periods—2 to 5 days—than those of primary infection. Typically, they recur at the same sites. Recurrences are most common in the first year after initial infection, and rates slowly decline over several years.

Asymptomatic viral shedding is defined by HSV as detected by culture or PCR in the absence of clinical findings. Most infected women shed virus intermittently, and most HSV transmission to a partner occurs during periods of asymptomatic viral shedding. Gardella and coworkers (2005) reported an HSV culture-positive rate of 0.5 percent and a PCR-positive rate of 2.7 percent in asymptomatic women presenting for delivery. More data are needed to determine the effect of asymptomatic shedding on neonatal transmission.

Most primary and first-episode infections in early pregnancy are probably not associated with an increased rate of spontaneous abortion or stillbirth (Eskild, 2002). In their review, Fagnant and Monif (1989) found only 15 cases of congenital herpetic infection that were acquired during early pregnancy. Brown and Baker (1989) reported that late-pregnancy primary infection may be associated with preterm labor and fetal-growth restriction.

Newborn infection may manifest in a number of ways. Infection may be localized to the skin, eye, or mouth—SEM disease—in about 40 percent of cases. Central nervous system disease with encephalitis is seen in 30 percent of cases. Disseminated disease as shown in Figure 65-6 with involvement of multiple major organs is found in 32 percent. Localized infection is usually associated with a good outcome. Conversely, even with acyclovir treatment, disseminated infection has a mortality rate of nearly 30 percent (Corey, 2009; Kimberlin, 2004a,b, 2011). Importantly, serious developmental and central nervous system morbidity is seen in 20 to 50 percent of survivors with disseminated or cerebral infection.

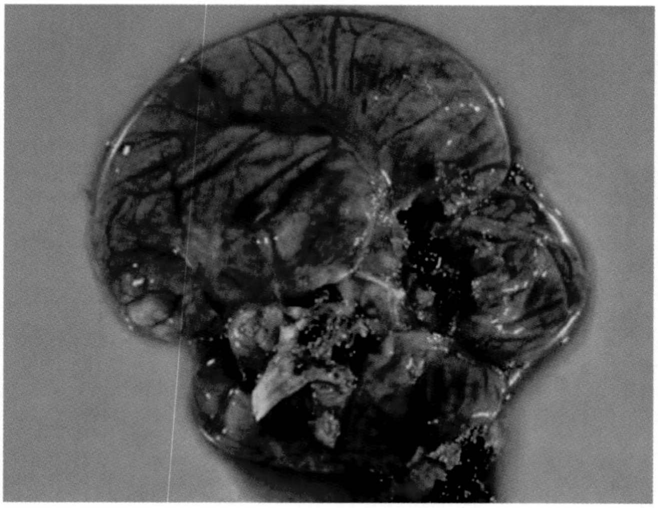

FIGURE 65-6 Cross-section showing necrotic brain tissue from a newborn who died from disseminated herpesvirus infection.

Diagnosis

According to the Centers for Disease Control and Prevention (2010a), clinical diagnosis of genital herpes is both insensitive and nonspecific and should be confirmed by laboratory testing. HSV tests available are either virological or type-specific serological tests.

Virological tests are performed on a specimen from a mucocutaneous lesion. Cell culture and PCR are the preferred tests. The sensitivity of HSV isolation is relatively low for viral culture as vesicular lesions ulcerate and then crust. Viral isolation results sometimes are not available for 1 to 2 weeks. PCR assays are more sensitive, the results generally are available in 1 to 2 days, and specimen handling is easier. The major limitation of PCR is cost and laboratory availability. The PCR assay is the preferred test for HSV detection in spinal fluid. Regardless of the test performed, HSV viral type should be differentiated because HSV type influences counseling and long-term prognosis. *A negative culture or PCR result does not exclude infection.* False-positive results are rare.

Several serological assay systems are available to detect antibody to HSV glycoproteins G1 and G2 (Anzivino, 2009; Centers for Disease Control and Prevention, 2010a). These proteins evoke type-specific antibody responses to HSV-1 and HSV-2 infection, respectively, and they reliably differentiate the two. This permits confirmation of clinical infection and identification of asymptomatic carriers. The Food and Drug Administration (FDA) has approved type-specific tests that are enzyme-linked immunosorbent assay (ELISA) or blot-style tests. Providers should request type-specific glycoprotein G-based assays when serology is being performed. Sensitivity approaches 90 to 100 percent and specificity 99 to 100 percent (Wald, 2002). IgG antibodies usually are detected 1 to 2 weeks after a primary infection. IgM antibody detection is not a useful test.

Point-of-care testing is being increasingly requested by practitioners to help guide management intrapartum or near delivery. There are type-specific serological tests available that use capillary blood or serum. Sensitivity varies from 80 to 98 percent with specificity ≥ 96 percent. False-positive and false-negative results may occur. Real-time quantitative PCR of genital tract secretions has recently been developed by Gardella and colleagues (2010). They reported sensitivity of 99.6 percent and specificity of 96.7 percent with a turnaround time of 2 hours. These features would prove valuable to guide clinical decision making at delivery.

Routine serological screening for herpes in pregnancy is not recommended by the American College of Obstetricians and Gynecologists (2012) due to cost and limited data on efficacy in reducing the incidence of neonatal herpes. Cost-decision analysis for prenatal type-specific antibody screening and suppressive therapy for partners has been found to be unacceptably expensive (Barnabas, 2002; Rouse, 2000; Thung, 2005). In contrast, it was found to be potentially cost-effective by Baker and associates (2004). Cleary and coworkers (2005) calculated that universal prenatal screening would reduce rates of perinatal death and severe sequelae from neonatal HSV. But they also found that it would require treatment of 3849 women to prevent one case of neonatal death or disease with severe sequelae. Universal screening would identify previously undiagnosed women who could then be counseled regarding safe practices and antepartum antiviral suppression, but a concrete benefit remains unproven.

Management

Antiviral therapy with acyclovir, famciclovir, or valacyclovir has been used for treatment of first-episode genital herpes in nonpregnant patients. Oral or parenteral preparations attenuate clinical infection and the viral shedding duration. Suppressive therapy has also been given to limit recurrent infections and to reduce heterosexual transmission (Corey, 2004, 2012). For intense discomfort, oral analgesics and topical anesthetics may provide some relief, and urinary retention is treated with an indwelling bladder catheter. Acyclovir appears to be safe for use in pregnant women (Briggs, 2011; Stone, 2004). The manufacturers of acyclovir and valacyclovir, in cooperation with the Centers for Disease Control and Prevention, maintained a registry of outcomes following exposure to these drugs during pregnancy through 1999. More than 700 neonates exposed during the first trimester were evaluated, and no increased adverse effects were found (Stone, 2004). At this time, there are insufficient data with famciclovir exposure, although a pregnancy registry is being maintained (1-888-669-6682).

Women with a primary outbreak during pregnancy may be given antiviral therapy to attenuate and decrease the duration of symptoms and viral shedding (Table 65-5). Women with HIV co-infection may require a longer duration of treatment. Those with severe or disseminated HSV are given IV acyclovir, 5 to 10 mg/kg, every 8 hours for 2 to 7 days until clinically improved. This is followed by oral antiviral therapy to complete at least 10 days of total therapy (Centers for Disease Control and Prevention, 2010b). Recurrent HSV infections during pregnancy are treated for symptomatic relief only (see Table 65-5). Acyclovir resistance has been reported, predominantly with HSV-2 and in immunocompromised patients (Corey, 2012).

Peripartum Shedding Prophylaxis

Several studies have shown that acyclovir or valacyclovir suppression initiated at 36 weeks' gestation will decrease the number of HSV outbreaks at term, thus decreasing the need for cesarean delivery (Hollier, 2008). Such suppressive therapy will also decrease viral shedding defined by both culture and PCR techniques (Scott, 2002; Sheffield, 2006; Watts, 2003). A systematic review of studies of acyclovir prophylaxis given from 36 weeks to delivery was reported by Sheffield and colleagues (2003). They found that delivery suppressive therapy was associated with significantly decreased rates of clinical HSV recurrence, cesarean deliveries for HSV recurrences, total HSV detection, and asymptomatic shedding. Subsequent studies using valacyclovir suppression have shown similar results (Andrews, 2006; Sheffield, 2006). Because of these studies, the American College of Obstetricians and Gynecologists (2012) recommends viral therapy at or beyond 36 weeks for women

TABLE 65-5. Antiviral Medications for Herpesvirus Infection in Pregnancy

Indication	Pregnancy Recommendation
Primary or first episode infection	Acyclovir, 400 mg orally three times daily for 7–10 days *or* Valacyclovir, 1 g orally twice daily for 7–10 days
Symptomatic recurrent infection (episodic therapy)	Acyclovir, 400 mg orally three times daily for 5 days *or* Acyclovir, 800 mg orally twice daily for 5 days *or* Valacyclovir, 500 mg orally twice daily for 3 days *or* Valacyclovir, 1 g orally once daily for 5 days
Daily suppression	Acyclovir, 400 mg orally three times daily from 36 weeks until delivery *or* Valacyclovir, 500 mg orally twice daily from 36 weeks until delivery

Adapted from the Centers for Disease Control and Prevention, 2010b.

who have any recurrence during pregnancy. It is unclear whether suppression is needed for women with outbreaks before but not during pregnancy. There have been several case reports of atypical neonatal herpes disease following maternal antiviral suppression. Thus, suppression does not prevent all cases of neonatal disease (Pinninti, 2012).

On presentation for delivery, a woman with a history of HSV should be questioned regarding prodromal symptoms such as vulvar burning or itching. A careful examination of the vulva, vagina, and cervix should be performed, and suspicious lesions should be cultured or PCR tested. Currently, there is no approved point-of-care test to guide management. Cesarean delivery is indicated for women with active genital lesions or prodromal symptoms (American College of Obstetricians and Gynecologists, 2012). Of note, 10 to 15 percent of neonates with HSV are born to women undergoing cesarean delivery. Cesarean delivery is not recommended for women with a history of HSV infection but no active genital disease at the time of delivery. Moreover, an active lesion in a nongenital area is not an indication for cesarean delivery. Instead, an occlusive dressing is placed, and vaginal delivery is allowed.

There is no evidence that external lesions cause ascending fetal infection with preterm ruptured membranes. Major and associates (2003) described expectant management of preterm premature membrane rupture in 29 women < 31 weeks. There were no cases of neonatal HSV, and the maximum infection risk was calculated to be 10 percent. Antiviral treatment use in this setting is reasonable, but of unproven efficacy. For women with a clinical recurrence at delivery, there is not an absolute duration of membrane rupture beyond which the fetus would not benefit from cesarean delivery (American College of Obstetricians and Gynecologists, 2013). Women with active HSV may breast feed if there are no active HSV breast lesions. Strict hand washing is advised. Valacyclovir and acyclovir may be used during breast feeding, as drug concentrations in breast milk are low. One study found the acyclovir concentration to be only 2 percent of that used for therapeutic dosing of the neonate (Sheffield, 2002a).

Other antiviral agents are under development. One is *pritelivir*, a viral helicase-primase complex that reduces HSV-2 shedding (Wald, 2014). Also, HSV-2 vaccine development is currently being aggressively pursued. Two glycoprotein D-based subunit vaccine trials have shown benefit in discordant couples by decreasing HSV-2 acquisition (Stanberry, 2002). Interestingly, a recent randomized controlled trial of a newer glycoprotein D-based HSV-2 vaccine showed it to be effective in women in preventing HSV-1, but not HSV-2, genital disease (Belshe, 2012). Further research is needed to better understand these challenging and contradictory results (Johnson, 2011).

CHANCROID

Haemophilus ducreyi can cause painful, nonindurated genital ulcers termed soft chancres that at times are accompanied by painful suppurative inguinal lymphadenopathy. Although common in some developing countries, it had become rare in the United States by the 1970s. There was an increase in the late 1980s, but only fifteen cases were reported in the United States in 2012. This marked decrease likely represents a true decline as well as diagnostic difficulties that led to underdiagnosis (Centers for Disease Control and Prevention, 2013b). Importantly, the ulcerative lesion is a high-risk cofactor for HIV transmission.

Diagnosis by culture is difficult because appropriate media are not widely available. Instead, clinical diagnosis is made when typical painful genital ulcer(s) are dark-field negative for spirochetes and herpes-virus test results are negative. No FDA-cleared PCR test is yet available. Recommended treatment in pregnancy is azithromycin, 1 g orally as a single dose; erythromycin base, 500 mg orally three times daily for 7 days; or ceftriaxone, 250 mg in a single intramuscular dose (Centers for Disease Control and Prevention, 2010b).

HUMAN PAPILLOMAVIRUS

Human papillomavirus (HPV) is one of the most common sexually transmitted infections, and more than 40 types infect the genital tract. Most reproductive-aged women become infected within a few years of becoming sexually active, although most infections are asymptomatic and transient. Oncogenic or high-risk HPV types 16 and 18 are associated with dysplasia and are discussed in Chapter 63 (p. 1222). Mucocutaneous external genital warts termed condyloma acuminata are usually caused by HPV types 6 and 11 but may also be caused by intermediate- and high-oncogenic-risk HPV.

The National Health and Nutrition Examination Survey (NHANES) 2003 to 2006 reported an overall HPV prevalence of 43 percent in females aged 14 to 59 years (Hariri, 2011). A 27-percent seroprevalence was also reported for subjects 18 through 25 years in the National Longitudinal Study of Adolescent Health (Manhart, 2006). Similar rates of HPV positivity have been reported for pregnant women (Aydin, 2010; Gajewska, 2005; Hernandez-Giron, 2005; Rama, 2010). Prevalence is highest in younger age groups.

External Genital Warts—Condyloma Acuminata

For unknown reasons, genital warts frequently increase in number and size during pregnancy. Acceleration of viral replication by the physiological changes of pregnancy might explain perineal lesion growth and progression of some to cervical neoplasm (Fife, 1999; Rando, 1989). These lesions may sometimes grow to fill the vagina or cover the perineum, thus making vaginal delivery or episiotomy difficult (Fig. 65-7). Because HPV infection may be subclinical and multifocal, most women with vulvar lesions also have cervical infection, and vice versa (Ault, 2003; Kroupis, 2011; Reichman, 2012).

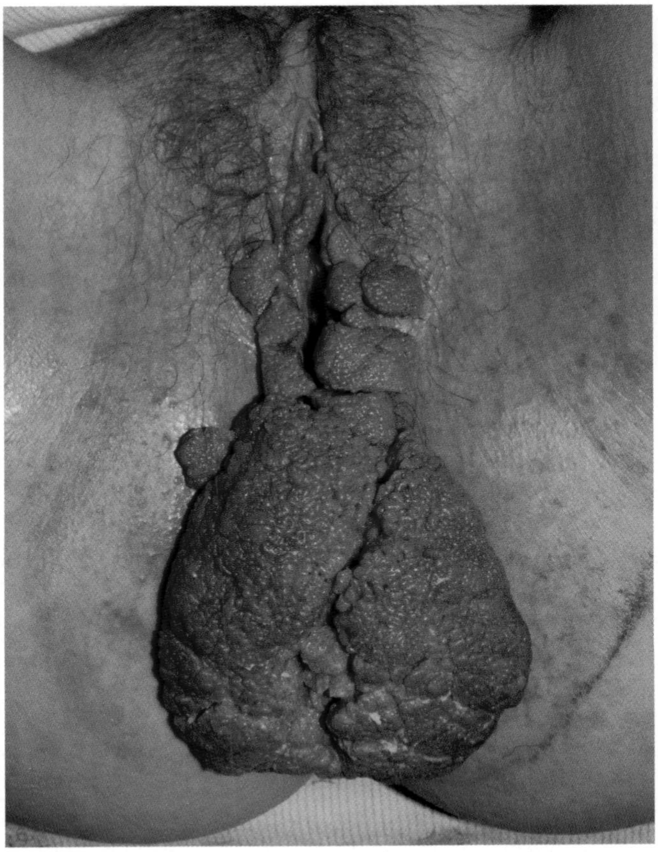

FIGURE 65-7 Extensive external genital warts in a postpartum woman.

Treatment

There may be an incomplete response to treatment during pregnancy, but lesions commonly improve or regress rapidly following delivery. Consequently, wart eradication during pregnancy is usually not necessary. Therapy is directed toward minimizing treatment toxicity to the mother and fetus and debulking symptomatic genital warts. There are several agents available, but pregnancy limits their use. There is no definitive evidence that any one of the subsequently discussed treatments is superior to another (Centers for Disease Control and Prevention, 2010b; Wiley, 2002).

Trichloroacetic or bichloracetic acid, 80- to 90-percent solution, applied topically once a week, is an effective regimen for external warts. Some prefer *cryotherapy, laser ablation*, or *surgical excision* (Arena, 2001; Centers for Disease Control and Prevention, 2010b). Agents not recommended in pregnancy because of concerns for maternal and fetal safety include podophyllin resin, podofilox 0.5-percent solution or gel, imiquimod 5-percent cream, interferon therapy, and sinecatechins.

Neonatal Infection

Juvenile-onset recurrent respiratory papillomatosis is a rare, benign neoplasm of the larynx. It can cause hoarseness and respiratory distress in children and is often due to HPV types 6 or 11. In some cases, maternal genital HPV infection is associated with laryngeal papillomatosis, but studies differ in their findings of neonatal transmission rates. Although some have reported rates as high as 50 percent, it is likely that these findings are from maternal contamination or transient HPV infection (Campisi, 2010; Winer, 2004). A Danish population-based study indicated a neonatal transmission risk of 7 per 1000 infected women (Silverberg, 2003). Prolonged rupture of membranes was associated with a twofold increased risk, but risk was not associated with delivery mode. This low transmission risk has been confirmed in subsequent studies (Heim, 2007; Smith, 2004). Finally, long-term follow-up studies are consistent with a very low vertical transmission risk (Manns, 1999; Smith, 2004). The benefit of cesarean delivery to decrease transmission risk is unknown, and thus it is currently not recommended solely to prevent HPV transmission (Centers for Disease Control and Prevention, 2010b). HPV vaccination may decrease the rate over time (Hawkes, 2008; Kim, 2008).

Immunization

Two HPV inactivated vaccines are currently licensed in the United States. These are a quadrivalent vaccine (Gardasil) containing HPV types 6, 11, 16, and 18 and a bivalent vaccine (Cervarix) containing HPV types 16 and 18. The vaccines are both a three-dose series and are licensed for females and males aged ≤ 26 years. They are effective for males (Giuliano, 2011).

The vaccines are not recommended for pregnant women, however, inadvertent exposures do occur. Garland and coworkers (2009) analyzed data on these exposures from five Phase III clinical trials of Gardasil. They found no adverse pregnancy outcomes associated with the vaccine. Wacholder and associates (2010) pooled data from two multicenter Phase III trials and found no association between HPV vaccination and miscarriage risk. Postlicensure surveillance is ongoing using a manufacturer pregnancy registry (American College of Obstetricians and Gynecologists, 2010a). Women who are breast feeding may receive the vaccine. If a woman is found to be pregnant after starting the vaccination series, the remaining doses should be delayed until after delivery.

VAGINITIS

Pregnant women commonly develop increased vaginal discharge, which in many instances is not pathological (Chap. 4, p. 50). The vaginal microbial flora provides protection against vaginal infection. Elucidation of the composition and function of the normal vaginal microflora is currently underway with the human microbiome project (Lamont, 2011).

Bacterial Vaginosis

Not an infection in the ordinary sense, bacterial vaginosis (BV) is a maldistribution of normal vaginal flora. Numbers of lactobacilli are decreased, and overrepresented species are anaerobic bacteria that include *Gardnerella vaginalis, Mobiluncus,* and some *Bacteroides* species. As many as 30 percent of childbearing-aged women have bacterial vaginosis (Allsworth, 2007; Koumans, 2007; Simhan, 2008). Vitamin D deficiency has been identified as a risk factor for vaginosis in pregnancy. Moreover, douching, multiple partners, young age, smoking, and black race are associated with vaginosis in both pregnant and nonpregnant women (Bodnar, 2009; Desseauve, 2012; Hensel, 2011). In pregnancy, it is associated with preterm birth, early and late miscarriage, low birthweight, and increased neonatal morbidity (Goldenberg, 2008; Laxmi, 2012). Treatment is reserved for symptomatic women, who usually complain of a fishy-smelling discharge. Preferred treatment is metronidazole, 500 mg twice daily orally for 7 days; 250 mg three times daily orally for 7 days; or clindamycin 300 mg orally twice daily for 7 days (Centers for Disease Control and Prevention, 2010b). Unfortunately, although eradication is possible, treatment does not reduce preterm birth rates, and routine screening is not recommended (McDonald, 2007).

Trichomoniasis

Trichomonas vaginalis can be identified during prenatal examination in up to 20 percent of women. Symptomatic vaginitis is much less prevalent, and it is characterized by foamy leukorrhea, pruritus, and irritation. Trichomonads are seen readily in fresh vaginal secretions as flagellated, pear-shaped, motile organisms that are somewhat larger than leukocytes.

Metronidazole, administered orally in a single 2-g dose, is effective in eradicating *T vaginalis* (Centers for Disease Control and Prevention, 2010b). It may be used at any gestational age—multiple studies have not shown an association between metronidazole use in any trimester of pregnancy and neonatal effects, including malformations (Briggs, 2011). Some studies have linked trichomonal infection with preterm birth, however, treatment has not decreased this risk (Gulmezoglu, 2011; Wendel, 2007). Thus, screening and treatment of asymptomatic women is not recommended during pregnancy.

Candidiasis

Candida albicans or other *Candida* species can be identified by culture from the vagina during pregnancy in approximately 25 percent of women. Asymptomatic colonization requires no treatment. However, the organism may sometimes cause an extremely profuse, irritating discharge associated with a pruritic, tender, edematous vulva. Effective treatment is given with a number of azole creams that include 2-percent butoconazole, 1-percent clotrimazole, 2-percent miconazole, and 0.4- or 0.8-percent terconazole applied for 7 days (Centers for Disease Control and Prevention, 2010b). Topical treatment is recommended, but as described in Chapter 12 (p. 247), oral azoles are generally considered safe (Pitsouni, 2008). In some women, infection is likely to recur and require repeated treatment during pregnancy. In these cases, symptomatic infection usually subsides after pregnancy (Sobel, 2007).

HUMAN IMMUNODEFICIENCY VIRUS

Acquired immunodeficiency syndrome (AIDS) was first described in 1981, and it is currently one of the worst global health pandemics in recorded history. Worldwide, it was estimated in 2012 that there were 35.3 million infected persons with HIV/AIDS; 2.3 million new cases of HIV infection; and 1.6 million HIV-related deaths (UNAIDS, 2013). In the United States through 2011, the Centers for Disease Control and Prevention (2013a) estimated that there were more than 1.1 million infected individuals and more than 636,000 deaths (Centers for Disease Control and Prevention, 2013a). In 2010, women accounted for 20 percent of all HIV/AIDS cases among adults and adolescents, most of which resulted from heterosexual contact. Comparing 2008 with 2011, HIV incidence decreased in women, primarily black/African American women and women acquiring HIV through heterosexual contact.

The estimated number of perinatally acquired AIDS cases has decreased dramatically during the past two decades (Fig. 65-8). This is predominantly due to the implementation of prenatal HIV testing and antiviral therapy given to the pregnant woman and then to her neonate (De Cock, 2012). In addition, *highly active antiretroviral therapy (HAART)* has led to an increasing number of people living with chronic HIV infection and thus the associated comorbidities also affecting pregnancy (Fenton, 2007).

Etiopathogenesis

Causative agents of AIDS are RNA retroviruses termed *human immunodeficiency viruses, HIV-1* and *HIV-2.* Most cases worldwide are caused by HIV-1 infection. Transmission is

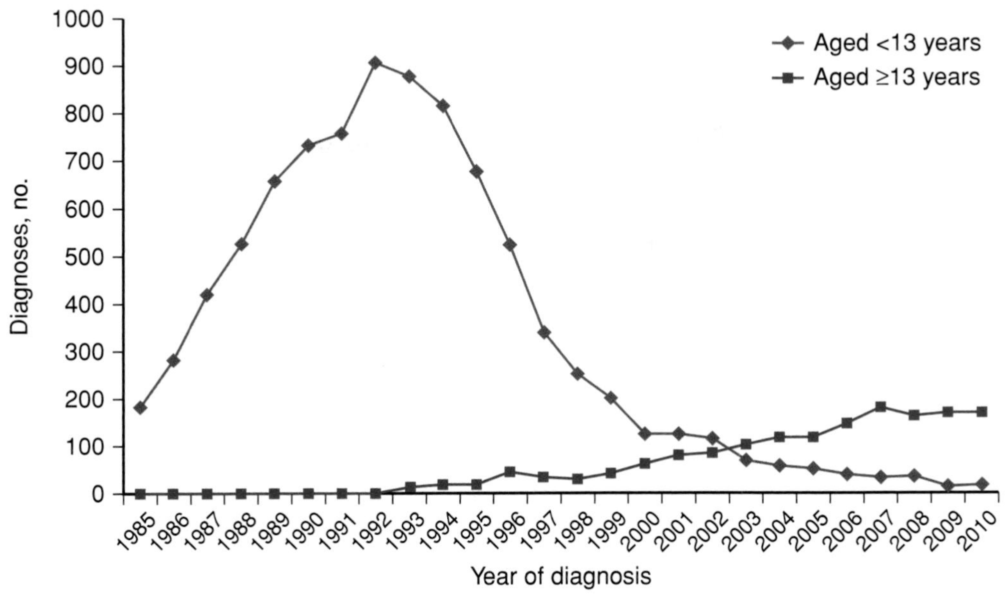

FIGURE 65-8 Estimated number of perinatally acquired AIDS cases by year of diagnosis, 1985 to 2010, in the United States and dependent areas. (Data from the Centers for Disease Control and Prevention, 2011a.)

similar to hepatitis B virus, and sexual intercourse is the major mode. The virus also is transmitted by blood or blood-contaminated products, and infected mothers may infect their fetuses perinatally or by their breast milk. The primary determinant of HIV-1 transmission is the plasma HIV-1 viral load.

The common denominator of clinical illness with AIDS is profound immunodeficiency that gives rise to various opportunistic infections and neoplasms. Sexual transmission occurs when mucosal dendritic cells bind to the HIV envelope glycoprotein gp120. These dendritic cells then present the viral particle to thymus-derived lymphocytes, that is, T lymphocytes. These lymphocytes are defined phenotypically by the cluster of differentiation 4 (CD4) glycoprotein surface antigens. The CD4 site serves as a receptor for the virus. Coreceptors are necessary for viral entry into the cell, and two chemokine receptors—CCR5 and CXCR4—are the most frequently identified (Fauci, 2012; Sheffield, 2007). The CCR5 coreceptor is found on the cell surface of CD4 positive ($CD4^+$) cells in high progesterone states such as pregnancy, possibly aiding viral entry (Sheffield, 2009).

After initial infection, the level of viremia usually decreases to a set point, and patients with the highest viral burden at this time progress more rapidly to AIDS and death (Fauci, 2007, 2012). And as shown in Figure 65-9, viral burden and neonatal infection incidence are directly related. Over time, the number of T cells drops insidiously and progressively, resulting eventually in profound immunosuppression. Although it is thought that pregnancy has minimal effects on $CD4^+$ T-cell counts and HIV RNA levels, the latter are often higher 6 months postpartum than during pregnancy. Higher levels of inflammatory cytokines and a decrease in regulatory T cells in late pregnancy may contribute to maternal and fetal morbidity (Richardson, 2011).

Clinical Manifestations

The incubation period from exposure to clinical disease is days to weeks, and the average is 3 to 6 weeks. Acute HIV infection is similar to many other viral syndromes and usually lasts less than 10 days. Common symptoms include fever and night sweats, fatigue, rash, headache, lymphadenopathy, pharyngitis, myalgias, arthralgias, nausea, vomiting, and diarrhea. After symptoms abate, the set point of chronic viremia is established. The progression from asymptomatic viremia to AIDS has a median time of approximately 10 years (Fauci, 2008). Route of infection, the pathogenicity of the infecting viral strain, the initial viral inoculum, and the immunological status of the host all affect the rapidity of progression.

Several clinical and laboratory manifestations will herald disease progression. Generalized lymphadenopathy, oral hairy leukoplakia, aphthous ulcers, and thrombocytopenia are common. A number of opportunistic infections associated with

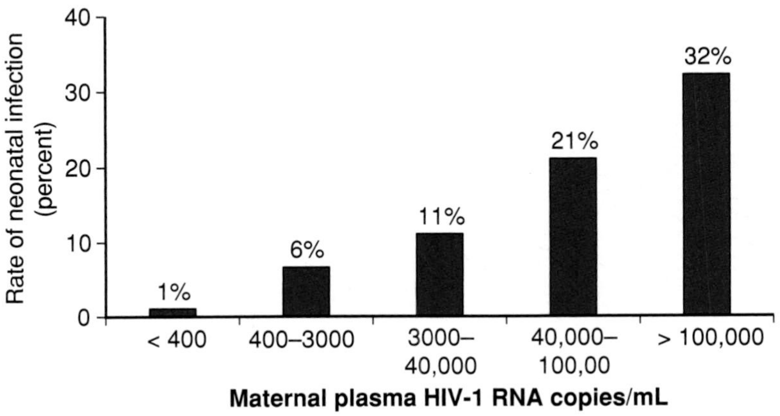

FIGURE 65-9 Incidence of perinatal human immunodeficiency virus (HIV) infection plotted against plasma HIV-1 RNA levels in 1542 neonates born to mothers in the Women and Infants Transmission Study. (Data from Cooper, 2002.)

AIDS include esophageal or pulmonary candidiasis; persistent herpes simplex or zoster lesions; condyloma acuminata; pulmonary tuberculosis; cytomegaloviral pneumonia, retinitis, or gastrointestinal disease; molluscum contagiosum; *Pneumocystis jiroveci* pneumonia; toxoplasmosis; and others. Neurological disease is common, and approximately half of patients have central nervous system symptoms. A $CD4^+$ count < $200/mm^3$ is also considered definitive for the diagnosis of AIDS.

There are unique gynecological issues for women with HIV, such as menstrual abnormalities, contraceptive needs, and genital neoplasia, that are discussed in *Williams Gynecology*, 2nd edition (Werner, 2012). Some of these as well as other STIs may persist into pregnancy (Cejtin, 2003; Stuart, 2005). Repeated pregnancy has no significant effect on the clinical or immunological course of viral infection (Minkoff, 2003).

Prenatal HIV Screening

The Centers for Disease Control and Prevention (2006, 2010a), The American Academy of Pediatrics and the American College of Obstetricians and Gynecologists (2011), and the United States Preventive Services Task Force (2012) recommend prenatal HIV screening using an *opt-out approach*. This means that the woman is notified that HIV testing is included in a comprehensive set of antenatal tests, but that testing may be declined. Women are given information regarding HIV but are not required to sign a specific consent. Through the use of such *opt-out* strategies, HIV testing rates have increased. Each provider should be aware of specific state laws concerning screening.

In areas in which the incidence of HIV or AIDS is 1 per 1000 person-years or greater, or in women at high risk for acquiring HIV during pregnancy, repeat testing in the third trimester is recommended (American College of Obstetricians and Gynecologists, 2011). High-risk factors include injection drug use, prostitution, a suspected or known HIV-infected sexual partner, multiple sexual partners, or a diagnosis of another sexually transmitted disease. Several states also recommend or require HIV testing at delivery.

Screening is performed using an enzyme-linked immunoassay with a sensitivity > 99.5 percent. A positive test is confirmed with either a Western blot or immunofluorescence assay (IFA), both of which have high specificity. According to the Centers for Disease Control and Prevention (2001), antibody can be detected in most patients within 1 month of infection, and thus, antibody serotesting may not exclude early infection. For acute primary HIV infection, identification of viral p24 core antigen or viral RNA or DNA is possible. False-positive confirmatory results are rare (Centers for Disease Control and Prevention, 2010b).

Women with limited prenatal care or with undocumented HIV status at delivery should have a "rapid" HIV test performed. These tests can detect HIV antibody in 60 minutes or less and have sensitivities and specificities comparable with those of conventional ELISAs (Chetty, 2012). A negative rapid test result does not need to be confirmed. However, in a woman exposed to HIV within the last 3 months, repeat testing is recommended. A positive rapid test result should be confirmed with a Western blot or IFA test. As shown in Table 65-6, peripartum and neonatal interventions to reduce perinatal transmission are based on the initial rapid testing results, and this can be discontinued if the confirmatory test is negative (American College of Obstetricians and Gynecologists, 2011; Centers for Disease Control and Prevention, 2010b). A detailed list of the rapid HIV tests currently available in the United States can be found at http://www.cdc.gov/hiv/topics/testing/resources/factsheets/rt-lab.htm (Centers for Disease Control and Prevention, 2007). The Mother-Infant Rapid Intervention at Delivery (MIRIAD) multicenter study indicated that rapid HIV testing can be used to identify infected women so that peripartum antiretroviral prophylaxis can be administered to mother and infant (Bulterys, 2004).

Maternal and Perinatal Transmission

Transplacental HIV transmission can occur early, and the virus has even been identified in specimens from elective abortion (Lewis, 1990). In most cases, however, mother-to-child transmission at the time of delivery is the most common cause of pediatric HIV infections. Between 15 and 40 percent of neonates born to non–breast-feeding, untreated, HIV-infected mothers are infected. Kourtis and colleagues (2001) have proposed a model for estimation of the temporal distribution of

TABLE 65-6. Strategy for Rapid Human Immunodeficiency Virus (HIV) Testing of Pregnant Women in Labor

If the rapid HIV test result in labor and delivery is positive, the obstetrical provider should take the following steps:

1. Tell the woman she may have HIV infection and that her neonate also may be exposed
2. Explain that the rapid test result is preliminary and that false-positive results are possible
3. Assure the woman that a second test is being performed to confirm the positive rapid test result
4. To reduce the risk of transmission to the infant, immediate initiation of antiretroviral prophylaxis should be recommended without waiting for the results of the confirmatory test
5. Once the woman gives birth, discontinue maternal antiretroviral therapy pending receipt of confirmatory test results
6. Tell the women that she should postpone breast feeding until the confirmatory result is available because she should not breast feed if she is infected with HIV
7. Inform pediatric care providers (depending on state requirements) of positive maternal test results so that they may institute the appropriate neonatal prophylaxis

Summarized from American College of Obstetricians and Gynecologists, 2011.

vertical transmission. They estimate that 20 percent of transmission occurs before 36 weeks' gestation, 50 percent in the days before delivery, and 30 percent intrapartum. Transmission rates for breast feeding may be as high as 30 to 40 percent and are associated with systemic HIV viral burden (Kourtis, 2006, 2007a; Slyker, 2012). Vertical transmission is more common with preterm births, especially with prolonged membrane rupture. Analyzing data from the Perinatal AIDS Collaborative Transmission Study, Kuhn and coworkers (1999) reported a nearly fourfold increased risk with preterm delivery. Although an increased risk of perinatal transmission has been associated with membrane rupture in the past, recent analyses in the setting of combination antiviral therapy have not found this to be a risk factor with an HIV viral load < 1000 copies/mL (Cotter, 2012).

In nonpregnant individuals, there is an association between concomitant STIs and horizontal HIV transmission. There is also evidence that vertical perinatal transmission may be increased with STIs (Schulte, 2001; Watts, 2012). Women with maternal HSV-2 antibody have a significant 50-percent increased risk of intrapartum HIV-1 maternal-to-child transmission (Cowan, 2008). They attributed up to 25 percent of vertical transmission to maternal HSV-2 co-infection. Elevated cytokine and chemokine levels in the placenta, reflecting inflammation, are associated with in utero transmission (Kumar, 2012). A recent Cochrane analysis, however, has failed to show that sexually transmitted infection control is an effective HIV prevention strategy (Ng, 2011).

Perinatal HIV transmission is most accurately correlated with maternal plasma HIV RNA burden (Panel on Treatment of HIV-Infected Pregnant Women and Prevention of Perinatal Transmission, 2012; Watts, 2002). As shown in Figure 65-9, cohort neonatal infection was 1 percent with < 400 copies/mL, and it was > 30 percent when maternal viral RNA levels were > 100,000 copies/mL. *Transmission of HIV infection, however, has been observed at all HIV RNA levels, including those that were nondetectable by current assays.* This may be attributed to discordance between the viral load in plasma and that in the genital secretions. Because of these findings, the viral load should not be used to determine whether to initiate antiretroviral therapy in pregnancy.

Preconceptional Counseling

Effective contraception should be discussed if pregnancy is undesired. Certain antiviral medications decrease hormonal contraception efficacy and are discussed in Chapter 38 (p. 708). Recommendations are also available at http://AIDSinfo.nih.gov and are updated frequently as new data become available. Counseling also includes education for decreasing high-risk sexual behaviors to prevent transmission and to decrease the acquisition of other sexually transmitted diseases. Currently used antiretroviral medications are reviewed to avoid those with high teratogenic potential should the woman become pregnant. A specific example is efavirenz, which has significant teratogenic effects on primate fetuses (Panel on Antiretroviral Guidelines for Adults and Adolescents, 2013). Preference should also include those that decrease HIV RNA viral load effectively before pregnancy.

Management During Pregnancy

These women need special attention and are seen in consultation by physicians with special interest in this field. At Parkland Hospital, the initial assessment of an HIV-infected pregnant woman includes:

- Standard prenatal laboratory surveys that include serum creatinine, hemogram, and bacteriuria screening (Chap. 9, p. 171)
- Plasma HIV RNA quantification—"viral load," $CD4^+$ T-lymphocyte count, and antiretroviral resistance testing
- Serum hepatic aminotransferase levels
- HSV-1 and -2, cytomegalovirus, toxoplasmosis, and hepatitis C serology screening
- Baseline chest radiograph
- Tuberculosis skin testing—purified protein derivative (PPD) or interferon-gamma release assay
- Evaluation of need for pneumococcal, hepatitis B, hepatitis A, Tdap, and influenza vaccines
- Sonographic evaluation to establish gestational age.

Antiretroviral Therapy

Treatment is recommended for all HIV-infected pregnant women. This may be a departure for those not receiving treatment when nonpregnant because they did not meet certain criteria. Treatment reduces the risk of perinatal transmission regardless of $CD4^+$ T-cell count or HIV RNA level. Antiretroviral therapy is complicated, and pregnancy only adds to the complexity. In general, HAART is begun if the woman is not already receiving one of the regimens. Antiretroviral agents are grouped into several classes and used to design antiretroviral regimens (Table 65-7). The 2012 Panel on Treatment of HIV-Infected Pregnant Women and Prevention of Perinatal Transmission classify each agent into five use categories: preferred, alternative, use in special circumstances, not recommended, and insufficient data to recommend use. The woman is counseled regarding risks and benefits of antiretroviral agents to make an informed decision as to her treatment regimen. Regardless of what regimen is begun, adherence is important because the risk of viral drug resistance is lessened.

The Panel on Treatment of HIV-Infected Pregnant Women and Prevention of Perinatal Transmission (2012) has issued guidelines that detail management of different scenarios during pregnancy (Table 65-8). Women already taking HAART at pregnancy onset are encouraged to continue the regimen if there is adequate viral suppression. The neural-tube defect risk associated with efavirenz is restricted to the first 6 weeks of pregnancy. Thus, efavirenz can be continued if the woman presents after this time and if adequate virological suppression is documented. Until recently, addition of zidovudine to all regimens was recommended. Currently, however, in women with adequate viremia suppression with a regimen not containing zidovudine, continuation of the current regimen is appropriate. Zidovudine is given intravenously during labor and delivery to women with an HIV RNA viral load > 400 copies/mL or who have an unknown viral load near delivery (Panel on Treatment of HIV-Infected Pregnant Women and Prevention of Perinatal

TABLE 65-7. Classes of Antiretroviral Drugs

Drug Class	Category[a]
Nucleoside/Nucleotide Reverse Transcriptase Inhibitors	
Lamivudine	Preferred
Zidovudine	Preferred
Abacavir	Alternative
Emtricitabine	Alternative
Tenofovir	Alternative
Didanosine	Special circumstances
Stavudine	Special circumstances
Non-nucleoside Reverse Transcriptase Inhibitors	
Nevirapine	Preferred
Efavirenz	Special circumstances
Etravirine	Insufficient data[b]
Rilpivirine	Insufficient data[b]
Protease Inhibitors	
Ritonavir	Preferred
Atazanavir	Preferred
Lopinavir/ritonavir	Preferred
Saquinavir	Alternative
Darunavir	Alternative
Indinavir	Special circumstances
Nelfinavir	Special circumstances
Fosamprenavir	Special circumstances
Tipranavir	Special circumstances
Entry Inhibitors	
Enfuvirtide	Insufficient data[b]
Maraviroc	Insufficient data[b]
Integrase Inhibitors	
Raltegravir	Special circumstances

[a]Panel on Treatment of HIV-Infected Pregnant Women and Prevention of Perinatal Transmission, 2012.
[b]Insufficient data to recommend use.

Transmission, 2012). A 2 mg/kg load is infused over 1 hour followed by zidovudine 1 mg/kg/hr until delivery.

Women who have never received antiretroviral therapy—*antiretroviral naïve*—fall into two categories. First, women who meet the criteria for antiretroviral therapy initiation in nonpregnant adults are given HAART regardless of trimester. Because of an increased risk of hepatotoxicity, *nevirapine* is reserved for women with a CD4⁺ cell count < 250 cells/mm^3. In general, the starting HAART regimen is two nucleoside reverse transcriptase inhibitors (NRTIs) plus a non-nucleoside reverse transcriptase inhibitor (NNRTI) or protease inhibitor(s). At Parkland Hospital as of 2014, our standard regimen in treatment-naïve women is lopinavir/ritonavir—formulated as *Kaletra*—plus zidovudine/lamivudine—formulated as *Combivir*. The lopinavir/ritonavir regimen should be increased in the late second and third trimester. Atazanavir, another protease inhibitor, is also now listed as a preferred agent and can be used in place of lopinavir/ritonavir. If used, it is combined with low-dose ritonavir boosting.

The second category contains treatment-naïve HIV-infected pregnant women who do not meet nonpregnant adult indications for antiretroviral therapy. These women are counseled regarding the benefits of initiating therapy to prevent perinatal viral transmission. Because of potential teratogenic effects, women may delay therapy until the second trimester. That said, however, earlier initiation may be more effective in reducing perinatal transmission (Panel on Treatment of HIV-Infected Pregnant Women and Prevention of Perinatal Transmission, 2012; Read, 2012).

Women who have previously received antiretroviral therapy but are currently not taking medications should undergo HIV resistance testing because antiretroviral use increases their risk of drug resistance. Regimens may then be tailored based on prior medication use and response as well as current resistance patterns. The final group includes women who present in labor and who are taking no medications. These women are given intravenous zidovudine intrapartum (see Table 59-8). The National Perinatal HIV Hotline (1–888–448–8765) is a federally funded service that provides free consultation to providers.

Laboratory Assessment

CD4$^+$ T-lymphocyte count, HIV RNA viral load measurement, complete blood count, and liver function tests are done 4 weeks after beginning or changing therapy to assess response and exclude toxicity. Thereafter, HIV RNA viral loads are measured monthly until RNA levels are undetectable. CD4 T-lymphocyte and HIV RNA levels can then be measured every trimester. If the HIV RNA viral load increases or does not decrease appropriately, then medication compliance and antiretroviral drug resistance are assessed. Poor adherence to therapy is a significant problem in pregnancy.

Although there was an association of early studies with glucose intolerance and protease inhibitor use, this has not been corroborated (Hitti, 2007; Tang, 2006). Standard serum glucose screening should be performed at 24 to 28 weeks unless indicated earlier. In addition, careful surveillance is important for interactions between antiretroviral drugs as well as therapies for opportunistic infection, hepatitis B and C, and tuberculosis (Panel on Treatment of HIV-Infected Pregnant Women and Prevention of Perinatal Transmission, 2012; Piscitelli, 2001).

Complications of HIV Infection

Management of some HIV complications may be altered by pregnancy. If the CD4$^+$ T-cell count is < 200/mm^3, primary prophylaxis for *Pneumocystis jiroveci* (formerly *P carinii)* pneumonia is recommended with sulfamethoxazole-trimethoprim or dapsone. Pneumonitis is treated with oral or IV sulfamethoxazole-trimethoprim or dapsone-trimethoprim. Other symptomatic opportunistic infections that may develop are from latent or newly acquired toxoplasmosis, herpes virus, mycobacteria, and candida. The National Institutes of Health, Centers for Disease Control and Prevention, and Infectious Diseases Society of America (2013) have published guidelines for prevention and treatment of opportunistic infections. Maternal HIV infection has also been associated with fetal-growth restriction, preeclampsia, and preterm membrane rupture (Ndirangu, 2012; Rollins, 2007; Suy, 2006).

TABLE 65-8. Recommendations for Antiviral Drug Use During Pregnancy

Clinical Scenario	Recommendations
HIV-infected woman taking antiretroviral therapy who becomes pregnant	Continue current medication if viral suppression adequate and patient tolerating If virus detectable, order HIV antiretroviral drug-resistance testing If first trimester, continue medications; if stopped, stop all medications and then reinitiate in the second trimester Start IV ZDV in labor if HIV RNA level > 400 copies/mL or unknown near delivery
HIV-infected woman who is antiretroviral naïve	Order HIV antiretroviral drug-resistance testing Initiate HAART: - Avoid efavirenz in the early first trimester - Use one or more NRTIs—ZDV, lamivudine, emtricitabine, tenofovir, or abacavir—if feasible - Avoid nevirapine in women with a $CD4^+$ count > 250 cells/mm^3 HAART should be initiated as early as possible for maternal indications; if high CD4 T-lymphocyte count and low HIV RNA level, can consider delaying initiation of HAART until the second trimester Start IV ZDV in labor if HIV RNA level > 400 copies/mL or unknown near delivery
HIV-infected woman previously taking antiretroviral medications but not on medications currently	Order HIV antiretroviral drug-resistance testing Initiate HAART with regimen based on prior therapy history and resistance testing Avoid efavirenz in the early first trimester Use one or more NRTIs—ZDV, lamivudine, emtricitabine, tenofovir, or abacavir—if feasible Avoid nevirapine in women with a $CD4^+$ count > 250 cells/mm^3 Start IV ZDV in labor if HIV RNA level > 400 copies/mL or unknown near delivery
HIV-infected woman on no antiretroviral medication who presents in labor	Order initial HIV laboratory assessment (p. 1279) Start IV ZDV during labor—2 mg/kg IV load over 1 hour, then 1 mg/kg/hr until delivery

CD4 = cluster of differentiation 4; HAART = highly active antiretroviral therapy; HIV = human immunodeficiency virus; IV = intravenous; NRTIs = nucleoside reverse transcriptase inhibitors; ZDV = zidovudine.
Adapted from the Panel on Treatment of HIV-Infected Pregnant Women and Prevention of Perinatal Transmission, 2012.

Perinatal Outcomes

Even with treatment, the incidence of perinatal complications in HIV-infected women is increased, although the newer drug regimens may diminish these rates. Multiple studies reviewed in the 2012 Perinatal Treatment Guidelines address the association of antiretroviral medications with preterm delivery. Most of those have shown a small but significantly increased risk. Kourtis and colleagues (2007b) performed a metaanalysis of 14 European and U.S. studies and found no overall greater risk for preterm delivery. They did find, however, that women taking regimens that included a protease inhibitor had a small increased risk—1.3-fold—that was nevertheless significant. Antiretroviral medication use in the second half of pregnancy was shown by Lopez and associates (2012) to increase iatrogenic preterm birth but did not affect spontaneous preterm birth rates. This slightly increased frequency of preterm birth clearly is outweighed by the benefits of decreasing perinatal HIV transmission.

Medication Toxicity

At least two follow-up studies of children from the Pediatric AIDS Clinical Trial Group (PACTG) 076 Study found no adverse effects at 18 months and up to a mean of 5.6 years after zidovudine exposure (Culnane, 1999; Sperling, 1998). Prenatal exposure to HAART may increase the risk for neonatal neutropenia and anemia, although no long-term hematological or hepatic toxicities have been documented (Bae, 2008; Dryden-Peterson, 2011). Preliminary data also show a possible effect on infant mitochondrial DNA proliferation and/or expression with maternal antiretroviral drug treatment (Cote, 2008; Hernandez, 2012; Jitratkosol, 2012). For these reasons, long-term follow-up is recommended for all infants exposed in utero to antiviral medications.

Prenatal HIV Transmission

Maternal HAART treatment along with intrapartum zidovudine prophylaxis has dramatically reduced the perinatal HIV transmission risk from approximately 25 percent to 2 percent or less. HAART during pregnancy was reported to be associated with a decreased incidence of placental villitis, which may partially account for the lower HIV transmission rate in treated women (Stewart, 2014a). Optimal management of labor is uncertain, but if labor is progressing with intact membranes, artificial rupture and invasive fetal monitoring are avoided. Labor augmentation is used when needed to shorten the interval to delivery to further decrease the transmission risk. Operative delivery with forceps or vacuum extractor is avoided if possible. Postpartum hemorrhage is managed with oxytocin and prostaglandin analogues. Methergine and other ergot alkaloids adversely interact with reverse transcriptase and protease inhibitors to cause severe vasoconstriction.

Cesarean delivery has been recommended to decrease HIV prenatal transmission. An earlier metaanalysis of 15 prospective cohort studies by the International Perinatal HIV Group (1999) included 8533 mother-neonate pairs. Vertical HIV transmission was shown to be reduced by about half when cesarean was compared with vaginal delivery. When antiretroviral therapy was given in the prenatal, intrapartum, and neonatal periods along with cesarean delivery, the likelihood of neonatal transmission was reduced by 87 percent compared with vaginal delivery and without antiretroviral therapy. The European Mode of Delivery Collaboration (1999) has reported similar findings.

Based on these observations, the American College of Obstetricians and Gynecologists (2010b) concluded that scheduled cesarean delivery should be discussed and recommended for HIV-infected women whose HIV-1 RNA load exceeds 1000 copies/mL. Scheduled delivery is recommended at 38 weeks' gestation in these women. Although data are insufficient to estimate such benefits for women whose HIV RNA levels are < 1000 copies/mL, it is unlikely that scheduled cesarean delivery would confer additional risk reduction if the woman has been taking antiviral therapy (Jamieson, 2007; Read, 2005). If cesarean delivery is performed for obstetrical indications, it should be performed at 39 weeks with standard perioperative antimicrobials for prophylaxis. HIV-infected women undergoing a scheduled cesarean delivery should be given IV zidovudine as a loading dose followed by 2 more hours of continuous maintenance therapy—a total of 3 hours of infused zidovudine.

Breast Feeding

Vertical transmission is increased by breast feeding, and it generally is not recommended for HIV-positive women in the United States (Panel on Treatment of HIV-Infected Pregnant Women and Prevention of Perinatal Transmission, 2012; Read, 2003). The probability of HIV transmission per liter of breast milk ingested is estimated to be similar in magnitude to heterosexual transmission with unsafe sex in adults (Richardson, 2003). As with other exposures, risk is related to the maternal HIV RNA level, HIV disease status, breast health, and duration of breast feeding (De Cock, 2000; John-Stewart, 2004). Most transmission occurs in the first 6 months, and as many as two thirds of infections in breast-fed infants are from breast milk. In the Petra Study Team (2002) from Africa, the prophylactic benefits of short-course perinatal antiviral regimens were diminished considerably by 18 months of age due to breast feeding. The World Health Organization (2010) has recommended exclusive breast feeding the first 6 months of life for infants of women living in developing countries in which infectious diseases and malnutrition are the primary causes of infant deaths. Breast feeding can be continued for 12 months until a nutritionally adequate diet is available.

Postpartum Management

Many otherwise healthy women with normal $CD4^+$ T-cell counts and low HIV RNA levels may discontinue treatment after delivery and be closely monitored according to adult guidelines. The exception is the woman who plans another pregnancy in the near future. Stewart and colleagues (2014b) showed that interpregnancy viral load suppression is associated with less vertical transmission in a subsequent pregnancy. Psychosocial support is essential during this time, especially while awaiting diagnostic testing for pediatric infection. Contraceptive needs are complex and also may entail condoms in discordantly infected couples. As discussed in Chapter 38 (p. 708), antiretroviral drugs may affect oral contraceptive hormone levels and possibly of injectable agents (Stuart, 2012). Intrauterine devices may be an acceptable choice in some women with normal immunocompetence and a low risk for STIs. The Centers for Disease Control and Prevention has recently revised the recommendations for the use of hormonal contraception among women at high risk for HIV infection or infected with HIV (Tepper, 2012). It reaffirmed prior recommendations that hormonal contraception use is safe for these women and that condom use should be encouraged regardless of contraceptive method.

REFERENCES

Alexander JM, Sheffield JS, Sanchez PJ, et al: Efficacy of treatment for syphilis in pregnancy. Obstet Gynecol 93:5, 1999

Alger LS, Lovchik JC, Hebel JR, et al: The association of *Chlamydia trachomatis, Neisseria gonorrhoeae*, and group B streptococci with preterm rupture of the membranes and pregnancy outcome. Am J Obstet Gynecol 159:397, 1988

Allsworth JE, Peipert JF: Prevalence of bacterial vaginosis: 2001–2004 National Health and Nutrition Examination Survey data. Obstet Gynecol 109(1):114, 2007

American Academy of Pediatrics and American College of Obstetricians and Gynecologists. Guidelines for Perinatal Care, 7th ed. Washington, 2012

American Academy of Pediatrics and American College of Obstetricians and Gynecologists: Joint statement of ACOG/AAP on human immunodeficiency virus screening. College Statement of Policy. May 1999; Reaffirmed 2011

American College of Obstetricians and Gynecologists: Human papillomavirus vaccination. Committee Opinion No. 467, September 2010a

American College of Obstetricians and Gynecologists: Scheduled cesarean delivery and the prevention of vertical transmission of HIV infection. Committee Opinion No. 234, May 2000. Reaffirmed 2010b

American College of Obstetricians and Gynecologists: Prenatal and perinatal human immunodeficiency virus testing: expanded recommendations. Committee Opinion No. 418, September 2008, Reaffirmed 2011

American College of Obstetricians and Gynecologists: Management of herpes in pregnancy. Practice Bulletin No. 82, June 2007, Reaffirmed 2012

American College of Obstetricians and Gynecologists: Premature rupture of membranes. Practice Bulletin No. 139, October 2013

Andrews WW, Goldenberg RL, Mercer B, et al: The Preterm Prediction Study: association of second-trimester genitourinary chlamydia infection with subsequent spontaneous preterm birth. Am J Obstet Gynecol 183:662, 2000

Andrews WW, Klebanoff MA, Thom EA, et al: Midpregnancy genitourinary tract infection with *Chlamydia trachomatis*: association with subsequent preterm delivery in women with bacterial vaginosis and *Trichomonas vaginalis*. Am J Obstet Gynecol 194:493, 2006

Anzivino E, Fioriti D, Mischitelli M, et al: Herpes simplex virus infection in pregnancy and in neonate: status of art of epidemiology, diagnosis, therapy and prevention. Virol J 6:40, 2009

Arena S, Marconi M, Frega A, et al: Pregnancy and condyloma. Evaluation about therapeutic effectiveness of laser CO_2 on 115 pregnant women. Minerva Ginecol 53:389, 2001

Augenbraun M, Workowski K: Ceftriaxone therapy for syphilis: report from the Emerging Infections Network. Clin Infect Dis 29:1337, 1999

Augenbraun MH: Treatment of syphilis 2001: nonpregnant adults. Clin Infect Dis 35:S187, 2002

Ault K: Human papillomavirus infections: diagnosis, treatment and hope for a vaccine. Obstet Gynecol Clin North Am 30:809, 2003

Aydin Y, Atis A, Tutuman T, et al: Prevalence of human papilloma virus infection in pregnant Turkish women compared with non-pregnant women. Eur J Gynaecol Oncol 31(1):72, 2010

Bae WH, Wester C, Smeaton LM, et al: Hematologic and hepatic toxicities associated with antenatal and postnatal exposure to maternal highly active antiretroviral therapy among infants. AIDS 22:1633, 2008

Baker D, Brown Z, Hollier LM, et al: Cost-effectiveness of herpes simplex virus type 2 serologic testing and antiviral therapy in pregnancy. Am J Obstet Gynecol 191:2074, 2004

Barnabas RV, Carabin H, Garnett GP: The potential role of suppressive therapy for sex partners in the prevention of neonatal herpes: a health economic analysis. Sex Transm Infect 78:425, 2002

Bataskov KL, Hariharan S, Horowitz MD, et al: Gonococcal endocarditis complicating pregnancy: a case report and literature review. Obstet Gynecol 78:494, 1991

Baud D, Goy G, Jaton K, et al: Role of *Chlamydia trachomatis* in miscarriage. Emerg Infect Dis 17(9):1630, 2011

Baud D, Regan L, Greub G: Emerging role of *Chlamydia* and *Chlamydia*-like organisms in adverse pregnancy outcomes. Curr Opin Infect Dis 21:70, 2008

Belshe RB, Leone PA, Bernstein DI, et al: Efficacy results of a trial of a herpes simplex vaccine. N Engl J Med 366(1):34, 2012

Berggren EK, Patchen L: Prevalence of *Chlamydia trachomatis* and *Neisseria gonorrhoeae* and repeat infection among pregnant urban adolescents. Sex Transm Dis 38(3):172, 2011

Berman SM: Maternal syphilis: pathophysiology and treatment. Bull World Health Organ 82:433, 2004

Binnicker MJ: Which algorithm should be used to screen for syphilis? Curr Opin Infect Dis 25(1):79, 2012

Blanco JD, Diaz KC, Lipscomb KA, et al: *Chlamydia trachomatis* isolation in patients with endometritis after cesarean section. Am J Obstet Gynecol 152:278, 1985

Blas MM, Canchihuaman FA, Alva IE, et al: Pregnancy outcomes in women infected with *Chlamydia trachomatis*: a population-based cohort study in Washington state. Sex Transm Infect 83:314, 2007

Blatt AJ, Lieberman JM, Hoover DR, et al: Chlamydial and gonococcal testing during pregnancy in the United States. Am J Obstet Gynecol 207(1):55.e1, 2012

Bleich AT, Sheffield JS, Wendel GD, et al: Disseminated gonococcal infection in women. Obstet Gynecol 119(3)597, 2012

Bodnar LM, Krohn MA, Simhan HN: Maternal vitamin D deficiency is associated with bacterial vaginosis in the first trimester of pregnancy. J Nutr 139:1157, 2009

Bolan GA, Sparling PF, Wasserheit JN: The emerging threat of untreatable gonococcal infection. N Engl J Med 366(6):485, 2012

Briggs GS, Freeman RK, Yaffe SJ (eds): Drugs in Pregnancy and Lactation: a Reference Guide to Fetal and Neonatal Risk, 9th ed. Philadelphia, Lippincott Williams & Wilkins, 2011

Brown EL, Gardella C, Malm G, et al: Effect of maternal herpes simplex virus (HSV) serostatus and HSV type on risk of neonatal herpes. Acta Obstet Gynecol 86:523, 2007

Brown ZA: HSV-2 specific serology should be offered routinely to antenatal patients. Rev Med Virol 10(3):141, 2000

Brown ZA, Baker DA: Acyclovir therapy during pregnancy. Obstet Gynecol 73:526, 1989

Brown ZA, Gardella C, Wald A, et al: Genital herpes complicating pregnancy. Obstet Gynecol 106:845, 2005

Brown ZA, Selke SA, Zeh J, et al: Acquisition of herpes simplex virus during pregnancy. N Engl J Med 337:509, 1997

Bulterys M, Jamieson DJ, O'Sullivan MJ, et al: Rapid HIV-1 testing during labor: a multicenter study. JAMA 292:219, 2004

Burgis JT, Nawaz III H: Disseminated gonococcal infection in pregnancy presenting as meningitis and dermatitis. Obstet Gynecol 108:798, 2006

Burkman RT, Tonascia JA, Atienza MF, et al: Untreated endocervical gonorrhea and endometritis following elective abortion. Am J Obstet Gynecol 126:648, 1976

Campisi P, Hawkes M. Simpson K, et al: The epidemiology of juvenile onset recurrent respiratory papillomatosis derived from a population level national database. Laryngoscope 120(6):1233, 2010

Cejtin HE: Gynecologic issues in the HIV-infected woman. Obstet Gynecol Clin North Am 30:711, 2003

Centers for Disease Control and Prevention: Revised guidelines for HIV counseling and testing. MMWR 50(19):1, 2001

Centers for Disease Control and Prevention: Revised recommendations for HIV testing of adults, adolescents, and pregnant women in health-care settings. MMWR 55(14):1, 2006

Centers for Disease Control and Prevention: General and laboratory considerations: rapid HIV tests currently available in the United States. 2007. Available at: http://www.cdc.gov/hiv/topics/testing/resources/factsheets/rt-lab.htm. Accessed June 3, 2013

Centers for Disease Control and Prevention: Sexually transmitted disease surveillance 2006 supplement, *Chlamydia* Prevalence Monitoring Project annual report 2006. May 2008. Available at: http://www.cdc.gov/std/chlamydia2006/CTSurvSupp2006Complete.pdf. Accessed June 3, 2013

Centers for Disease Control and Prevention: Seroprevalence of herpes simplex virus type 2 among persons aged 14–49—United States, 2005–2008. MMWR 59(15):456, 2010a

Centers for Disease Control and Prevention: Sexually transmitted disease treatment guidelines, 2010. MMWR 59(12):12, 2010b

Centers for Disease Control and Prevention: AIDS surveillance trends, slide set. 2011a. Available at: http://www.cdc.gov/hiv/pdf/statistics_surveillance_2010aidstrends.pdf. Accessed June 3, 2013

Centers for Disease Control and Prevention: Cephalosporin susceptibility among *Neisseria gonorrhoeae* isolates–United States, 2000–2010. MMWR 60(26):873, 2011b

Centers for Disease Control and Prevention: *Neisseria gonorrhoeae* with reduced susceptibility to azithromycin—San Diego County, California, 2009. MMWR 60(18):579, 2011c

Centers for Disease Control and Prevention: Update to CDC's sexually transmitted diseases treatment guidelines, 2010: oral cephalosporins no longer a recommended treatment for gonococcal infections. MMWR 61(31):590, 2012

Centers of Disease Control and Prevention: HIV in the United States: At a glance. 2013a. Available at: www.cdc.gov/hiv/statistics/basics/ataglance.html. Accessed January 11, 2014

Centers for Disease Control and Prevention: Sexually Transmitted Disease Surveillance 2012. December 2013b. Available at: http://www.cdc.gov/std/stats11/Surv2011.pdf. Accessed January 10, 2014

Chetty V, Moodley D, Chuturgoon A: Evaluation of a 4th generation rapid HIV test for earlier and reliable detection of HIV infection in pregnancy. J Clin Virol 54:180, 2012

Chisholm CA, Katz VL, McDonald TL, et al: Penicillin desensitization in the treatment of syphilis during pregnancy. Am J Perinatol 14:553, 1997

Christmas JT, Wendel GD, Bawdon RE, et al: Concomitant infection with *Neisseria gonorrhoeae* and *Chlamydia trachomatis* in pregnancy. Obstet Gynecol 74:295, 1989

Cleary KL, Oare E, Stamilio D, et al: Type-specific screening for asymptomatic herpes infection in pregnancy: a decision analysis. BJOG 112:731, 2005

Cooper ER, Charurat M, Mofenson L, et al: Combination antiretroviral strategies for the treatment of pregnant HIV-1-infected women and prevention of perinatal HIV-1 transmission. J Acquir Immune Defic Syndr 29:484, 2002

Corey L: Herpes simplex virus infections. In Longo DL, Fauci AS, Kasper DL, et al (eds): Harrison's Principles of Internal Medicine, 18th ed. New York, McGraw-Hill, 2012

Corey L, Wald A: Maternal and neonatal herpes simplex virus infections. N Engl J Med 361(14:1376, 2009

Corey L, Wald A, Patel R, et al: Once-daily valacyclovir to reduce the risk of transmission of genital herpes. N Engl J Med 350:11, 2004

Coste J, Job-Spira N, Fernandez H: Risk factors for spontaneous abortion: a case-control study in France. Hum Reprod 6:1332, 1991

Cote HC, Raboud J, Bitnun A, et al: Perinatal exposure to antiretroviral therapy is associated with increased blood mitochondrial DNA levels and decreased mitochondrial gene expression in infants. J Infect Dis 198:851, 2008

Cotter AM, Brookfield KF, Duthely LM, et al: Duration of membrane rupture and risk of perinatal transmission of HIV-1 in the era of combination antiretroviral therapy. Am J Obstet Gynecol 207:482.e1, 2012

Cowan FM, Humphrey JH, Ntozini R, et al: Maternal herpes simplex virus type 2 infection, syphilis and risk of intra-partum transmission of HIV-1: results of a case control study. AIDS 22(2):193, 2008

Culnane M, Fowler M, Lee SS, et al: Lack of long-term effects of in utero exposure to zidovudine among uninfected children born to HIV-infected women. Pediatric AIDS Clinical Trials Group Protocol 219/076 Teams. JAMA 281(2):151, 1999

De Cock KM, Fowler MG, Mercier E, et al: Prevention of mother-to-child HIV transmission in resource-poor countries. JAMA 283:1175, 2000

De Cock KM, Jaffe HW, Curran JW: The evolving epidemiology of HIV/AIDS. AIDS 26(10):1205, 2012

Desseauve D, Chantrel J, Fruchart A, et al: Prevalence and risk factors of bacterial vaginosis during the first trimester of pregnancy in a large French population-based study. Eur J Obstet Gynecol Reprod Biol 163(1):30, 2012

Di Mario S, Say L, Lincetto O: Risk factors for stillbirth in developing countries: a systematic review of the literature. Sex Transm Dis 34:S11, 2007

Dionne-Odom JD, Tambe P, Yee E, et al: Antimicrobial resistant gonorrhea in Atlanta: 1988–2006. Sex Transm Dis 38(8):780, 2011

Dryden-Peterson S, Shapiro RL, Hughes MD, et al: Increased risk of severe infant anemia after exposure to maternal HAART, Botswana. J Acquir Immune Defic Syndr 56(5):428, 2011

Eskild A, Jeansson S, Stray-Pedersen B, et al: Herpes simplex virus type-2 infection in pregnancy. No risk of fetal death: results from a nested case-control study within 35,940 women. Br J Obstet Gynaecol 109:1030, 2002

European Mode of Delivery Collaboration: Elective caesarean-section versus vaginal delivery in prevention of vertical HIV-1 transmission: a randomized clinical trial. Lancet 353(1):1035, 1999

Fagnant RJ, Monif GRG: How rare is congenital herpes simplex? A literature review. J Reprod Med 34:417, 1989

Fauci AS: Pathogenesis of HIV disease: opportunities for new prevention interventions. Clin Infect Dis 45:S206, 2007

Fauci AS, Lane HC: Human immunodeficiency virus disease: AIDS and related disorders: introduction. In Fauci AS, Braunwald E, Kasper DL, et al (eds): Harrison's Principles of Internal Medicine, 17th ed. New York, McGraw-Hill, 2008, p 1137

Fauci AS, Lane HC: Human immunodeficiency virus disease: AIDS and related disorders. In Longo DL, Fauci AS, Kasper DL, et al (eds): Harrison's Principles of Internal Medicine, 18th ed. New York, McGraw-Hill, 2012

Fenton KA: Changing epidemiology of HIV/AIDS in the United States: implications for enhancing and promoting HIV testing strategies. Clin Infect Dis 45:S213, 2007

Fife KH, Katz BP, Brizendine EJ, et al: Cervical human papillomavirus deoxyribonucleic acid persists throughout pregnancy and decreases in the postpartum period. Am J Obstet Gynecol 180:1110, 1999

Fiumara NJ, Fleming WL, Downing JG, et al: The incidence of prenatal syphilis at the Boston City Hospital. N Engl J Med 247:48, 1952

Gajewska M, Marianowski L, Wielgos M, et al: The occurrence of genital types of human papillomavirus in normal pregnancy and in pregnant women with pregestational insulin dependent diabetes mellitus. Neuroendocrinol Lett 26:766, 2005

Gardella C, Brown ZA, Wald A, et al: Poor correlation between genital lesions and detection of herpes simplex virus in women in labor. Obstet Gynecol 106:268, 2005

Gardella C, Huang ML, Wald A, et al: Rapid polymerase chain reaction assay to detect herpes simplex virus in the genital tract of women in labor. Obstet Gynecol 115(6):1209, 2010

Garland SM, Ault KA, Gall SA, et al: Pregnancy and infant outcomes in the clinical trials of a human papillomavirus type 6/11/16 vaccine. Obstet Gynecol 114(6):1179, 2009

Gibbs RS, Schachter J: Chlamydial serology in patients with intra-amniotic infection and controls. Sex Transm Dis 14:213, 1987

Giuliano AR, Palefsky JM, Goldstone S, et al: Efficacy of quadrivalent HPV vaccine against HPV infection and disease in males. N Engl J Med 364(5):401, 2011

Golden MR, Marra CM, Holmes KK: Update on syphilis: resurgence of an old problem. JAMA 290:1510, 2003

Goldenberg RL, Culhane JF, Iams JD, et al: Epidemiology and causes of preterm birth. Lancet 371:75, 2008

Goldenberg RL, Thompson C: The infectious origins of stillbirth. Am J Obstet Gynecol 189:861, 2003

Gorgos L, Newman L, Satterwhite C, et al: Gonorrhoea positivity among women aged 15–24 years in the USA, 2005–2007. Sex Transm Infect 87:202, 2011

Greer L, Wendel GD: Rapid diagnostic methods in sexually transmitted infections. Infect Dis Clin North Am 22:601, 2008

Gulmezoglu Am, Azhar M: Interventions for trichomoniasis in pregnancy. Cochrane Database Syst Rev 5:CD000220, 2011

Hariri S, Unger ER, Sternberg M, et al: Prevalence of genital human papillomavirus among females in the United States, the National Health and Nutrition Examination Survey, 2003–2006. J Infect Dis 204(4):566, 2011

Hawkes M, Campisi P, Zafar R, et al: Time course of juvenile onset recurrent respiratory papillomatosis caused by human papillomavirus. Pediatr Infect Dis J 27(2):149, 2008

Hawkes S, Matin N, Broutet N, et al: Effectiveness of interventions to improve screening for syphilis in pregnancy: a systematic review and meta-analysis. Lancet Infect Dis 11:684, 2011

Heim K, Hudelist G, Geier A, et al: Type-specific antiviral antibodies to genital human papillomavirus types in mothers and newborns. Reprod Sci 14:806, 2007

Henrich TJ, Yawetz S: Impact of age, gender, and pregnancy on syphilis screening using the Captia Syphilis-G assay. Sex Transm Dis 38(12):1126, 2011

Hensel KJ, Randis TM, Gelber SE, et al: Pregnancy-specific association of vitamin D deficiency and bacterial vaginosis. Am J Obstet Gynecol 204(1):41.e1, 2011

Hernandez S, Moren C, Lopez M, et al: Perinatal outcomes, mitochondrial toxicity and apoptosis in HIV-treated pregnant women and in-utero-exposed newborn. AIDS 26(4):419, 2012

Hernandez-Giron C, Smith JS, Lorincz A, et al: High-risk human papillomavirus detection and related risk factors among pregnant and nonpregnant women in Mexico. Sex Transm Dis 32:613, 2005

Hitti J, Andersen J, McComsey G, et al: Protease inhibitor-based antiretroviral therapy and glucose tolerance in pregnancy: AIDS Clinical Trials Group A5084. Am J Obstet Gynecol 196(4):331.e1, 2007

Hollier LM, Harstad TW, Sanchez PJ, et al: Fetal syphilis: clinical and laboratory characteristics. Obstet Gynecol 97:947, 2001

Hollier LM, Wendel GD: Third-trimester antiviral prophylaxis for preventing maternal genital herpes simplex virus (HSV) recurrences and neonatal infection. Cochrane Database Syst Rev 1:CD004946, 2008

Hosenfeld CB, Workowski KA, Berman S, et al: Repeat infection with *Chlamydia* and gonorrhea among females: a systematic review of the literature. Sex Transm Dis 36(8):478, 2009

Hoyme UB, Kiviat N, Eschenbach DA: The microbiology and treatment of late postpartum endometritis. Obstet Gynecol 68:226, 1986

International Perinatal HIV Group: The mode of delivery and the risk of vertical transmission of human immunodeficiency virus type 1: a meta-analysis of 15 prospective cohort studies. N Engl J Med 340:977, 1999

Ishaque S, Yakoob MY, Imdad A, et al: Effectiveness of interventions to screen and manage infections during pregnancy on reducing stillbirths: a review. BMC Public Health 11(3):53, 2011

Jamieson DJ, Read JS, Kourtis AP, et al: Cesarean delivery for HIV-infected women: recommendations and controversies. Am J Obstet Gynecol 197:S96, 2007

Jitratkosol MH, Sattha B, Maan EJ, et al: Blood mitochondrial DNA mutations in HIV-infected women and their infants exposed to HAART during pregnancy. AIDS 26(6):675, 2012

Johnson HL, Erbelding EJ, Zenilman JM, et al: Sexually transmitted diseases and risk behaviors among pregnant women attending inner city public sexually transmitted diseases clinics in Baltimore, MD, 1996–2002. Sex Transm Dis 34:991, 2007

Johnson HL, Ghanem KG, Zenilman JM, et al: Sexually transmitted infections and adverse pregnancy outcomes among women attending inner city public sexually transmitted diseases clinics. Sex Transm Dis 38(3):167, 2011

John-Stewart G, Mbori-Ngacha D, Ekpini R, et al: Breastfeeding and transmission of HIV-1. J Acquir Immune Defic Syndr 35:196, 2004

Kapur P, Rakheja D, Gomez AM, et al: Characterization of inflammation in syphilitic villitis and in villitis of unknown etiology. Pediatr Dev Pathol 7:453, 2004

Kim JJ, Goldie SJ: Health and economic implications of HPV vaccination in the United States. N Engl J Med 359:821, 2008

Kimberlin DW: Neonatal herpes simplex infection. Clin Microbiol Rev 17:1, 2004a

Kimberlin DW, Rouse DJ: Genital herpes. N Engl J Med 350:1970, 2004b

Kimberlin DW, Whitley RJ, Wan W, et al: Oral acyclovir suppression and neurodevelopment after neonatal herpes. N Engl J Med 365(14):1284, 2011

Kirkcaldy RD, Su JR, Taylor MM, et al: Epidemiology of syphilis among Hispanic women and associations with congenital syphilis, Maricopa County, Arizona. Sex Transm Dis 38(7):598, 2011

Klein VR, Cox SM, Mitchell MD, et al: The Jarisch–Herxheimer reaction complicating syphilotherapy in pregnancy. Obstet Gynecol 75:375, 1990

Kohl KS, Markowitz LE, Koumans EH: Developments in the screening for *Chlamydia trachomatis*: a review. Obstet Gynecol Clin North Am 30:637, 2003

Koumans EH, Rosen J, van Dyke K, et al: Prevention of mother-to-child transmission of infections during pregnancy: implementation of recommended interventions, United States, 2003–2004. Am J Obstet Gynecol 206:158.e1, 2012

Koumans EH, Sternberg M, Bruce C, et al: The prevalence of bacterial vaginosis in the United States, 2001–2004: associations with symptoms, sexual behaviors, and reproductive health. Sex Transm Dis 34:864, 2007

Koumans EH, Sternberg M, Gwinn M, et al: Geographic variation of HIV infection in childbearing women with syphilis in the United States. AIDS 14:279, 2000

Kourtis AP, Bulterys M, Nesheim SR, et al: Understanding the timing of HIV transmission from mother to infant. JAMA 285:709, 2001

Kourtis AP, Jamieson DJ, de Vincenzi I, et al: Prevention of human immunodeficiency virus-1 transmission to the infant through breastfeeding: new developments. Am J Obstet Gynecol 197:S113, 2007a

Kourtis AP, Lee FK, Abrams EJ, et al: Mother-to-child transmission of HIV-1: timing and implications for prevention. Lancet Infect Dis 6:726, 2006

Kourtis AP, Schmid CH, Jamieson DJ, et al: Use of antiretroviral therapy in pregnant HIV-infected women and the risk of premature delivery: a meta-analysis. AIDS 21:607, 2007b

Krakauer Y, Pariente G, Sergienko R, et al: Perinatal outcome in cases of latent syphilis during pregnancy. Int J Gynaecol Obstet 118(1):15, 2012

Kroupis C, Vourlidis N: Human papilloma virus (HPV) molecular diagnostics. Clin Chem Lab Med 49(11):1783, 2011

Kuhn L, Steketee RW, Weedon J, et al: Distinct risk factors for intrauterine and intrapartum human immunodeficiency virus transmission and consequences for disease progression in infected children. Perinatal AIDS Collaborative Transmission Study. J Infect Dis 179:52, 1999

Kumar SB, Rice CD, Milner DA, et al: Elevated cytokine and chemokine levels in the placenta are associated with in-utero HIV-1 mother-to-child transmission. AIDS 26(6):685, 2012

Lago EG, Rodrigues LC, Fiori RM, et al: Identification of two distinct profiles of maternal characteristics associated with risk. Sex Transm Dis 31:33, 2004

Lamont RF, Sobel JD, Akins RA, et al: The vaginal microbiome: new information about genital tract flora using molecular based techniques. BJOG 118(5):533, 2011

Langenberg AGM, Corey L, Ashley RL, et al: A prospective study of new infections with herpes simplex virus type 1 and type 2. N Engl J Med 341:1432, 1999

Laxmi U, Agrawal S, Raghunandan C, et al: Association of bacterial vaginosis with adverse fetomaternal outcome in women with spontaneous preterm labor: a prospective cohort study. J Matern Fetal Neonatal Med 25(1):64, 2012

Lewis SH, Reynolds-Kohler C, Fox HE, et al: HIV-1 in trophoblastic and villous Hofbauer cells, and haematological precursors in eight-week fetuses. Lancet 335:565, 1990

Lopez M, Figueras F, Hernandez S, et al: Association of HIV-infection with spontaneous and iatrogenic preterm delivery: effect of HAART. AIDS 26: 37, 2012

Lucas MJ, Theriot SK, Wendel GD: Doppler systolic–diastolic ratios in pregnancies complicated by syphilis. Obstet Gynecol 77:217, 1991

Lukehart SA: Syphilis. In Longo DL, Fauci AS, Kasper DL, et al (eds): Harrison's Principles of Internal Medicine, 18th ed. New York, McGraw-Hill, 2012

Mahnert N, Roberts SW, Laibl VR, et al: The incidence of neonatal herpes infection. Am J Obstet Gynecol 196:e55, 2007

Major CA, Towers CV, Lewis DF, et al: Expectant management of preterm rupture of membranes complicated by active recurrent genital herpes. Am J Obstet Gynecol 188:1551, 2003

Manhart LE, Holmes KK, Koutsky LA, et al: Human papillomavirus infection among sexually active young women in the United States: implications for developing a vaccination strategy. Sex Transm Dis 33:502, 2006

Manns A, Strickler HD, Wiktor SZ, et al: Low incidence of human papillomavirus type 16 antibody seroconversion in young children. Pediatr Infect Dis J 18:833, 1999

McDonald HM, Broclehurst P, Gordon A: Antibiotics for treating bacterial vaginosis in pregnancy. Cochrane Database Syst Rev 1:CD000262, 2007

Mertz GJ, Rosenthal SL, Stanberry LR: Is herpes simplex virus type 1 (HSV-1) now more common than HSV-2 in first episodes of genital herpes? Sex Transm Dis 30:801, 2003

Meyers D, Wolff T, Gregory K, et al: USPSTF recommendations for STI screening. Am Fam Physician 77:819, 2008

Meyers DS, Halvorson H, Luckhaupt S: Screening for chlamydial infection: an evidence update for the U.S. Preventive Services Task Force. Ann Intern Med 147:134, 2007

Miller WC, Ford CA, Morris M, et al: Prevalence of chlamydial and gonococcal infections among young adults in the United States. JAMA 291:2229, 2004

Minkoff HL, Hershow R, Watts H, et al: The relationship of pregnancy to human immunodeficiency virus disease progression. Am J Obstet Gynecol 189:552, 2003

Myles TD, Elam G, Park-Hwang E, et al: The Jarisch–Herxheimer reaction and fetal monitoring changes in pregnant women treated for syphilis. Obstet Gynecol 92:859, 1998

Nathan L, Bohman VR, Sanchez PJ, et al: In utero infection with *Treponema pallidum* in early pregnancy. Prenat Diagn 17:119, 1997

National Institutes of Health, the Centers for Disease Control and Prevention, and the HIV Medicine Association of the Infectious Diseases Society of America: Guidelines for prevention and treatment of opportunistic infections in HIV-infected adults and adolescents. May 7, 2013. Available at: http://aidsinfo.nih.gov/contentfiles/Adult_OI.pdf. Accessed June 3, 2013

Ndirangu J, Newell ML, Bland RM, et al: Maternal HIV infection associated with small-for-gestational age infants but not preterm births: evidence from rural South Africa. Hum Reprod 27(6)1846, 2012

Ng BE, Butler LM, Horvath T, et al: Population-based biomedical sexually transmitted infection control interventions for reducing HIV infection. Cochrane Database Syst Rev 3:CD001220, 2011

Panel on Antiretroviral Guidelines for Adults and Adolescents: Guidelines for the use of antiretroviral agents in HIV-1-infected adults and adolescents. Department of Health and Human Services, February 12, 2013. Available at: http://www.aidsinfo.nih.gov/ContentFiles/AdultandAdolescentGL.pdf. Accessed June 4, 2013

Panel on Treatment of HIV-Infected Pregnant Women and Prevention of Perinatal Transmission. Recommendations for use of antiretroviral drugs in pregnant HIV-1-infected women for maternal health and interventions to reduce perinatal HIV transmission in the United States. July 31, 2012. Available at: http://aidsinfo.nih.gov/contentfiles/lvguidelines/PerinatalGL.pdf. Accessed June 3, 2013

Park IU, Chow JM, Bolan G, et al: Screening for syphilis with the treponemal immunoassay: analysis of discordant serology results and implications for clinical management. J Infect Dis 204:1297, 2011

Pasternak B, Hiviid A: Use of acyclovir, valacyclovir, and famciclovir in the first trimester of pregnancy and the risk of birth defect. JAMA 304(8):859, 2010

Patel SJ, Klinger EJ, O'Toole D, et al: Missed opportunities for preventing congenital syphilis infection in New York City. Obstet Gynecol 120(4)882, 2012

Paukku M, Tulppala M, Puolakkainen M, et al: Lack of association between serum antibodies to *Chlamydia trachomatis* and a history of recurrent pregnancy loss. Fertil Steril 72:427, 1999

Peipert JF: Clinical practice: genital chlamydial infections. N Engl J Med 18: 349, 2003

Pena K, Adelson M, Mordechai E, et al: Genital herpes simplex virus type 1 in women: detection in cervicovaginal specimens from gynecologic practices in the United States. J Clin Microbiol 48(1):150, 2010

Petra Study Team: Efficacy of three short-course regimens of zidovudine and lamivudine in preventing early and late transmission of HIV-1 from mother to child in Tanzania, South Africa and Uganda (Petra study): a randomized, double-blind, placebo-controlled trial. Lancet 359:1178, 2002

Pinninti SG, Angara R, Feja KN, et al: Neonatal herpes disease following maternal antenatal antiviral suppressive therapy: a multicenter case series. J Pediatr 161(1):134, 2012

Piscitelli SC, Gallicano KD: Interactions among drugs for HIV and opportunistic infections. N Engl J Med 344:984, 2001

Pitsouni E, Iavazzo C, Falagas ME: Itraconazole vs fluconazole for the treatment of uncomplicated acute vaginal and vulvovaginal candidiasis in nonpregnant women: a metaanalysis of randomized controlled trials. Am J Obstet Gynecol 198:153, 2008

Prober CG, Sullender WM, Yasukawa LL, et al: Low risk of herpes simplex virus infections in neonates exposed to the virus at the time of vaginal delivery to mothers with recurrent genital herpes simplex virus infections. N Engl J Med 316:240, 1987

Rac M, Bryant S, Cantey J, et al: Maternal titers after adequate syphilotherapy during pregnancy. Am J Obstet Gynecol 210:S233, 2014a

Rac M, Bryant S, Cantey J, et al: Progression of ultrasound findings of fetal syphilis following maternal treatment. Am J Obstet Gynecol 210:S26, 2014b

Rac M, Greer LG, Wendel GD: Jarisch-Herxheimer reaction triggered by group B streptococcus intrapartum antibiotic prophylaxis. Obstet Gynecol 116(Suppl 2):552, 2010

Ram S, Rice PA: Gonococcal infections. In Longo DL, Fauci AS, et al (eds): Harrison's Principles of Internal Medicine, 18th ed. New York, McGraw-Hill, 2012

Rama CH, Villa LL, Pagliusi S, et al: Seroprevalence of human papillomavirus 6, 11, 16, and 18 in young primiparous women in Sao Paulo, Brazil. Int J Gynecol Cancer 20(8):1405, 2010

Rando RF, Lindheim S, Hasty L, et al: Increased frequency of detection of human papillomavirus deoxyribonucleic acid in exfoliated cervical cells during pregnancy. Am J Obstet Gynecol 161:50, 1989

Read JS, Committee on Pediatric AIDS: Human milk, breastfeeding, and transmission of human immunodeficiency virus type 1 in the United States. Pediatrics 112:1196, 2003

Read JS, Newell MK: Efficacy and safety of cesarean delivery for prevention of mother-to-child transmission of HIV-1. Cochrane Database Syst Rev 4:CD005479, 2005

Read PJ, Mandalia S, Khan P, et al: When should HAART be initiated in pregnancy to achieve an undetectable HIV viral load by delivery? AIDS 26:1095, 2012

Reichman RC: Human papillomavirus infections. In Longo DL, Fauci AS, Kasper DL, et al (eds): Harrison's Principles of Internal Medicine, 18th ed. New York, McGraw-Hill, 2012

Richardson BA, John-Stewart GC, Hughes JP, et al: Breast milk infectivity in human immunodeficiency virus type 1-infected mothers. J Infect Dis 187:736, 2003

Richardson K, Weinberg A: Dynamics of regulatory T-cells during pregnancy: effect of HIV infection and correlations with other immune parameters. PLoS One 6(11):e28172, 2011

Roberts CW, Pfister JR, Spear SJ: Increasing proportion of herpes simplex virus type 1 as a cause of genital herpes infection in college students. Sex Transm Dis 30:797, 2003

Roberts SW, Sheffield JS, McIntire DD, et al: Urine screening for *Chlamydia trachomatis* during pregnancy. Obstet Gynecol 117(4):883, 2011

Rollins NC, Coovadia HM, Bland RM, et al: Pregnancy outcomes in HIV-infected and uninfected women in rural and urban South Africa. Acquir Immune Defic Syndr 44:321, 2007

Ross JDC: Systemic gonococcal infection. Genitourin Med 72:404, 1996

Rouse DJ, Stringer JS: An appraisal of screening for maternal type-specific herpes simplex virus antibodies to prevent neonatal herpes. Am J Obstet Gynecol 183:400, 2000

Saloojee H, Velaphi S, Goga Y, et al: The prevention and management of congenital syphilis: an overview and recommendations. Bull World Health Organ 82:424, 2004
Schulte JM, Burkham S, Hamaker D, et al: Syphilis among HIV-infected mothers and their infants in Texas from 1988 to 1994. Sex Transm Dis 28:316, 2001
Schwartz DA, Larsen SA, Beck-Sague C, et al: Pathology of the umbilical cord in congenital syphilis: analysis of 25 specimens using histochemistry and immunofluorescent antibody to *Treponema pallidum*. Hum Pathol 26:784, 1995
Scott LL, Hollier LM, McIntire D, et al: Acyclovir suppression to prevent recurrent genital herpes at delivery. Infect Dis Obstet Gynecol 10:71, 2002
Sheffield JS, Andrews WW, Klebanoff MA, et al: Spontaneous resolution of asymptomatic *Chlamydia trachomatis* in pregnancy. Obstet Gynecol 105:557, 2005
Sheffield JS, Fish DN, Hollier LM, et al: Acyclovir concentrations in human breast milk after valacyclovir administration. Am J Obstet Gynecol 186:100, 2002a
Sheffield JS, Hill JB, Hollier LM, et al: Valacyclovir prophylaxis to prevent recurrent herpes at delivery: a randomized clinical trial. Obstet Gynecol 108:141, 2006
Sheffield JS, Hollier LM, Hill JB, et al: Acyclovir prophylaxis to prevent herpes simplex virus recurrence at delivery: a systematic review. Obstet Gynecol 102:1396, 2003
Sheffield JS, Sanchez PJ, Morris G, et al: Congenital syphilis after maternal treatment for syphilis during pregnancy. Am J Obstet Gynecol 186:569, 2002b
Sheffield JS, Sanchez PJ, Wendel GD Jr, et al: Placental histopathology of congenital syphilis. Obstet Gynecol 100:126, 2002c
Sheffield JS, Wendel GD Jr, McIntire DD, et al: Effect of genital ulcer disease on HIV-1 coreceptor expression in the female genital tract. J Infect Dis 196:1509, 2007
Sheffield JS, Wendel GD Jr, McIntire DD, et al: The effect of progesterone levels and pregnancy on HIV-1 coreceptor expression. Reprod Sci 16:20, 2009
Silva MJ, Florencio GL, Gabiatti JR, et al: Perinatal morbidity and mortality associated with chlamydial infection: a meta-analysis study. Braz J Infect Dis 15(6):533, 2011
Silverberg MJ, Thorsen P, Lindeberg H, et al: Condyloma in pregnancy is strongly predictive of juvenile-onset recurrent respiratory papillomatosis. Obstet Gynecol 101:645, 2003
Silverstein AM: Congenital syphilis and the timing of immunogenesis in the human fetus. Nature 194:196, 1962
Simhan HN, Bodnar LM, Krohn MA: Paternal race and bacterial vaginosis during the first trimester of pregnancy. Am J Obstet Gynecol 198:196.e1, 2008
Slyker JA, Chung MH, Lehman DA, et al: Incidence and correlates of HIV-1 RNA detection in the breast milk of women receiving HAART for the prevention of HIV-1 transmission. PLoS ONE 7(1):e29777, 2012
Smith EM, Ritchie JM, Yankowitz J, et al: Human papillomavirus prevalence and types in newborns and parents. Sex Transm Dis 31:57, 2004
Sobel JD: Vulvovaginal candidosis. Lancet 369:1961, 2007
Sperling RS, Shapiro DE, McSherry GD, et al: Safety of the maternal–infant zidovudine regimen utilized in the Pediatric AIDS Clinical Trial Group 076 Study. AIDS 12:1805, 1998
Stamm LV: Global challenge of antibiotic-resistant *Treponema pallidum*. Antimicrob Agents Chemother 54(2):583, 2010
Stanberry LR, Spruance SL, Cunningham AL, et al: Glycoprotein-D-adjuvant vaccine to prevent genital herpes. N Engl J Med 347:1652, 2002
Stewart R, Duryea E, Wells CE, et al: The influence of pre-pregnancy antiretroviral therapy on placental pathology in HIV infected pregnancies. Am J Obstet Gynecol 210:S258, 2014a
Stewart R, Wells CE, Roberts S, et al: Benefit of inter-pregnancy HIV viral load suppression on subsequent maternal and infant outcomes. Am J Obstet Gynecol 210:S14, 2014b
Stone KM, Reiff-Eldridge R, White AD, et al: Pregnancy outcomes following systemic prenatal acyclovir exposure: conclusions from the International Acyclovir Pregnancy Registry, 1984–1999. Birth Defects Res A Clin Mol Teratol 70:201, 2004
Stuart GS, Castano PM, Sheffield JS, et al: Postpartum sterilization choices made by HIV-infected women. Infect Dis Obstet Gynecol 13:217, 2005
Stuart GS, Cunningham FG: Contraception and sterilization. In Hoffman BH, Schorge JO, Schaffer JI, et al (eds): Williams Gynecology, 2nd ed. New York, McGraw-Hill, 2012
Sugiura-Ogasawara M, Ozaki Y, Nakanishi T, et al: Pregnancy outcome in recurrent aborters is not influenced by *Chlamydia* IgA and/or G. Am J Reprod Immunol 53:50, 2005
Suy A, Martinez E, Coll O, et al: Increased risk of preeclampsia and fetal death in HIV-infected pregnant women receiving highly active antiretroviral therapy. AIDS 20:59, 2006
Tang JH, Sheffield JS, Grimes J, et al: Effect of protease inhibitor therapy on glucose intolerance in pregnancy. Obstet Gynecol 107:1, 2006
Tepper NK, Curtis KM, Jamieson DJ, et al: Update to CDC's U.S. Medical Eligibility Criteria for Contraceptive Use, 2010: revised recommendations for the use of hormonal contraception among women at high risk for HIV infection or infected with HIV. MMWR 61(24):449, 2012
Thung SF, Grobman WA: The cost-effectiveness of routine antenatal screening for maternal herpes simplex virus-1 and -2 antibodies. Am J Obstet Gynecol 192:483, 2005
Trepka MJ, Bloom SA, Zhang G, et al: Inadequate syphilis screening among women with prenatal care in a community with a high syphilis incidence. Sex Transm Dis 33:670, 2006
Unemo M, Shafer WM: Antibiotic resistance in *Neisseria gonorrhoeae*: origin, evolution, and lessons learned for the future. Ann N Y Acad Sci 1230:E19, 2011
UNAIDS: Global Report: UNAIDS report on the global AIDS epidemic. Available at: http://unaids.org/en/media/unaids/contentassets/documents/epidemiology/2013/gr2013/UNAIDS_Global_Report_2013_en.pdf. Accessed January 11, 2014
U.S. Preventive Services Task Force: Screening for chlamydial infection: a focused evidence update for the U.S. Preventive Services Task Force. Evidence synthesis No. 48, Rockville, Agency for Healthcare Research and Quality. AHRQ publication No. 07–15101-EF-1, June 2007
U.S. Preventive Services Task Force: Screening for HIV in Pregnant Women. Systematic Review to Update the 2005 U.S. Preventive Services Task Force Recommendation. 2012. Available at: http://www.uspreventiveservicestaskforce.org/uspstf13/hiv/hivpregart.htm. Accessed December 31, 2013
Wacholder S, Chen BE, Wilcox A, et al: Risk of miscarriage with bivalent vaccine against human papillomavirus (HPV) types 16 and 18 pooled analysis of two randomized controlled trials. BMJ 340:c712, 2010
Wald A, Ashley-Morrow R: Serological testing for herpes simplex virus (HSV)-1 and HSV-2 infection. Clin Infect Dis 35:S173, 2002
Wald A, Corey L, Timmler B, et al: Helicase-primase inhibitor pritelivir for HSV-2 infection. N Engl J Med 370:201, 2014
Warner L, Rohcat RW, Fichtner RR, et al: Missed opportunities for congenital syphilis prevention in an urban southeastern hospital. Sex Transm Dis 28:92, 2001
Watts D: Mother to child transmission of HIV—another complication of bacterial vaginosis? J Acquir Immune Defic Syndr 60(3), 2012
Watts DH: Management of human immunodeficiency virus infection in pregnancy. N Engl J Med 346:1879, 2002
Watts DH, Brown ZA, Money D, et al: A double-blind, randomized, placebo-controlled trial of acyclovir in late pregnancy for the reduction of herpes simplex virus shedding and cesarean delivery. Am J Obstet Gynecol 188:836, 2003
Wendel GD Jr: Gestational and congenital syphilis. Clin Perinatol 15:287, 1988
Wendel GD Jr, Sanchez PJ, Peters MT, et al: Identification of *Treponema pallidum* in amniotic fluid and fetal blood from pregnancies complicated by congenital syphilis. Obstet Gynecol 78:890, 1991
Wendel GD Jr, Stark BJ, Jamison RB, et al: Penicillin allergy and desensitization in serious infections during pregnancy. N Engl J Med 312:1229, 1985
Wendel KA, Workowski KA: Trichomoniasis: challenges to appropriate management. Clin Infect Dis 44:S123, 2007
Werner CL, Griffith WF: Preinvasive lesions of the lower genital tract. In Hoffman BL, Schorge JO, Schaffer JI, et al (eds): Williams Gynecology, 2nd ed. New York, McGraw-Hill, 2012, p 762
Whitley R, Davis EA, Suppapanya N: Incidence of neonatal herpes simplex virus infections in a managed-care population. Sex Transm Dis 34:704, 2007
Wiley DJ, Douglas J, Beutner K, et al: External genital warts: diagnosis, treatment and prevention. Clin Infect Dis 35:S210, 2002
Wilson EK, Gavin NI, Adams EK, et al: Patterns in prenatal syphilis screening among Florida Medicaid enrollees. Sex Transm Dis 34:378, 2007
Winer RL, Koutsky LA: Delivering reassurance to parents: perinatal human papillomavirus transmission is rare. Sex Transm Dis 31:63, 2004
Wolff T, Shelton E, Sessions C, et al: Screening for syphilis infection in pregnant women: evidence for the U.S. Preventive Services Task Force Reaffirmation Recommendation Statement. Ann Intern Med 150(10):710, 2009
World Health Organization: Guidelines on HIV and infant feeding. Principles and recommendations for infant feeding in the context of HIV and a summary of evidence. Geneva, WHO Press, 2010
Yip L, Sweeny PJ, Bock BF: Acute suppurative salpingitis with concomitant intrauterine pregnancy. Am J Emerg Med 11:476, 1993
Zhou P, Qian Y, Xu J, et al: Occurrence of congenital syphilis after maternal treatment with azithromycin during pregnancy. Sex Transm Dis 34:472, 2007

APPENDIX

APPENDIX I. Serum and Blood Constituents

HEMATOLOGY

	Nonpregnant Adult[a]	1st Trimester	2nd Trimester	3rd Trimester	References
Erythropoietin[b] (U/L)	4–27	12–25	8–67	14–222	7, 10, 47
Ferritin[b] (ng/mL)	10–150[d]	6–130	2–230	0–116	7, 10, 39, 42, 45, 47, 62, 70
Folate, red blood cell (ng/mL)	150–450	137–589	94–828	109–663	45, 46, 72
Folate, serum (ng/mL)	5.4–18.0	2.6–15.0	0.8–24.0	1.4–20.7	7, 43, 45, 46, 53, 58, 72
Haptoglobin (mg/mL)	25–250	130 ± 43	115 ± 50	135 ± 65	26A
Hemoglobin[b] (g/dL)	12–15.8[d]	11.6–13.9	9.7–14.8	9.5–15.0	10, 45, 47, 58, 62
Hematocrit[b] (%)	35.4–44.4	31.0–41.0	30.0–39.0	28.0–40.0	6, 7, 10, 42, 45 58, 66
Iron, total binding capacity (TIBC)[b] (μg/dL)	251–406	278–403	Not reported	359–609	62
Iron, serum[b] (μg/dL)	41–141	72–143	44–178	30–193	10, 62
Mean corpuscular hemoglobin (MCH) (pg/cell)	27–32	30–32	30–33	29–32	42
Mean corpuscular volume (MCV) (xm³)	79–93	81–96	82–97	81–99	6, 42, 45, 58
Platelet (×10⁹/L)	165–415	174–391	155–409	146–429	4, 6, 16, 42, 45
Mean platelet volume (MPV) (μm³)	6.4–11.0	7.7–10.3	7.8–10.2	8.2–10.4	42
Red blood cell count (RBC) (×10⁶/mm³)	4.00–5.20[d]	3.42–4.55	2.81–4.49	2.71–4.43	6, 42, 45, 58
Red cell distribution width (RDW) (%)	< 14.5	12.5–14.1	13.4–13.6	12.7–15.3	42
White blood cell count (WBC) (×10³/mm³)	3.5–9.1	5.7–13.6	5.6–14.8	5.9–16.9	6, 9, 42, 45, 58
Neutrophils (×10³/mm³)	1.4–4.6	3.6–10.1	3.8–12.3	3.9–13.1	4, 6, 9, 42
Lymphocytes (×10³/mm³)	0.7–4.6	1.1–3.6	0.9–3.9	1.0–3.6	4, 6, 9, 42
Monocytes (×10³/mm³)	0.1–0.7	0.1–1.1	0.1–1.1	0.1–1.4	6, 9, 42
Eosinophils (×10³/mm³)	0–0.6	0–0.6	0–0.6	0–0.6	6, 9
Basophils (×10³/mm³)	0–0.2	0–0.1	0–0.1	0–0.1	6, 9
Transferrin (mg/dL)	200–400[c]	254–344	220–441	288–530	39, 42
Transferrin, saturation without iron (%)	22–46[b]	Not reported	10–44	5–37	47
Transferrin, saturation with iron (%)	22–46[b]	Not reported	18–92	9–98	47

COAGULATION

	Nonpregnant Adult[a]	1st Trimester	2nd Trimester	3rd Trimester	References
Antithrombin III, functional (%)	70–130	89–114	78–126	82–116	15, 16, 39A
D-Dimer (μg/mL)	0.22–0.74	0.05–0.95	0.32–1.29	0.13–1.7	16, 25, 25C, 35, 39A,41A, 51
Factor V (%)	50–150	75–95	72–96	60–88	40
Factor VII (%)	50–150	100–146	95–153	149–2110	16
Factor VIII (%)	50–150	90–210	97–312	143–353	16, 40
Factor IX (%)	50–150	103–172	154–217	164–235	16
Factor XI (%)	50–150	80–127	82–144	65–123	16
Factor XII (%)	50–150	78–124	90–151	129–194	16
Fibrinogen (mg/dL)	233–496	244–510	291–538	301–696	16, 25, 25C, 39A, 41A, 42, 51
Fibronectin (mg/L)	290 ± 85	377 ± 309	315 ± 295	334 ± 257	27A
Homocysteine (μmol/L)	4.4–10.8	3.34–11	2.0–26.9	3.2–21.4	43, 45, 46, 53, 72
International normalized ratio (INR)	0.9–1.04[g]	0.86–1.08	0.83–1.02	0.80–1.09	15, 41A
Partial thromboplastin time, activated (aPTT) (sec)	26.3–39.4	23.0–38.9	22.9–38.1	22.6–35.0	15, 16, 41A, 42
Prothrombin time (PT) (sec)	12.7–15.4	9.7–13.5	9.5–13.4	9.6–12.9	16, 41A, 42
Protein C, functional (%)	70–130	78–121	83–133	67–135	15, 24, 40
Protein S, total (%)	70–140	39–105	27–101	33–101	16, 24, 40
Protein S, free (%)	70–140	34–133	19–113	20–65	24, 40
Protein S, functional activity (%)	65–140	57–95	42–68	16–42	40
Thrombin time (TT) (sec)	17.7 ± 2.8	16.1 ± 1.5	15.4 ± 2.7	16.5 ± 2.4	27A
Thrombomodulin (ng/mL)	2.7 ± 3.1	4.3 ± 1.3	4.2 ± 1.2	3.6 ± 1.3	27A
Tissue plasminogen activator (ng/mL)	1.6–13[h]	1.8–6.0	2.36–6.6	3.34–9.20	15, 16, 25C
Tissue plasminogen activator inhibitor-1 (ng/mL)	4–43	16–33	36–55	67–92	16, 25C
von Willebrand disease					
von Willebrand factor antigen (%)	75–125	62–318	90–247	84–422	39A, 44A, 73
ADAMTS-13, von Willebrand cleaving protease (%)	40–170[i]	40–160	22–135	38–105	39A, 44A

BLOOD CHEMICAL CONSTITUTENTS

	Nonpregnant Adult[a]	1st Trimester	2nd Trimester	3rd Trimester	References
Alanine aminotransferase (ALT) (U/L)	7–41	3–30	2–33	2–25	5, 39, 42, 70
Albumin (g/dL)	4.1–5.3[d]	3.1–5.1	2.6–4.5	2.3–4.2	3, 5, 26, 29, 39, 42, 72
Alkaline phosphatase (U/L)	33–96	17–88	25–126	38–229	3, 5, 39, 42, 70
Alpha-1 antitrypsin (mg/dL)	100–200	225–323	273–391	327–487	42
Alpha-fetoprotein (ng/mL)	—	—	~130–400	~130–590	39B
Ammonia (μM)	31 ± 3.2	—	—	27.3 ± 1.6	31A
Amylase (U/L)	20–96	24–83	16–73	15–81	32, 39, 42, 68
Anion gap (mmol/L)	7–16	13–17	12–16	12–16	42
Aspartate aminotransferase (AST) (U/L)	12–38	3–23	3–33	4–32	5, 39, 42, 70
Bicarbonate (mmol/L)	22–30	20–24	20–24	20–24	42
Bilirubin, total (mg/dL)	0.3–1.3	0.1–0.4	0.1–0.8	0.1–1.1	5, 39
Bilirubin, unconjugated (mg/dL)	0.2–0.9	0.1–0.5	0.1–0.4	0.1–0.5	5, 42
Bilirubin, conjugated (mg/dL)	0.1–0.4	0–0.1	0–0.1	0–0.1	5
Bile acids (μmol/L)	0.3–4.8[j]	0–4.9	0–9.1	0–11.3	5, 14
CA-125 (μg/mL)	7.2–27	2.2–268	12–25.1	16.8–43.8	3A, 30A, 67A
Calcium, ionized (mg/dL)	4.5–5.3	4.5–5.1	4.4–5.0	4.4–5.3	26, 42, 48, 56
Calcium, total (mg/dL)	8.7–10.2	8.8–10.6	8.2–9.0	8.2–9.7	3, 29, 39, 42, 48, 56, 63
Ceruloplasmin (mg/dL)	25–63	30–49	40–53	43–78	42, 44
Chloride (mEq/L)	102–109	101–105	97–109	97–109	20, 39, 42
Creatinine (mg/dL)	0.5–0.9[d]	0.4–0.7	0.4–0.8	0.4–0.9	39, 42, 45
Gamma-glutamyl transpeptidase (GGT) (U/L)	9–58	2–23	4–22	3–26	5, 42, 39, 70
Lactate dehydrogenase (U/L)	115–221	78–433	80–447	82–524	42, 29, 39, 70
Lipase (U/L)	3–43	21–76	26–100	41–112	32
Magnesium (mg/dL)	1.5–2.3	1.6–2.2	1.5–2.2	1.1–2.2	3, 26, 29, 39, 42, 48, 63
Osmolality (mOsm/kg H_2O)	275–295	275–280	276–289	278–280	17, 63
Phosphate (mg/dL)	2.5–4.3	3.1–4.6	2.5–4.6	2.8–4.6	3, 26, 33, 39, 42
Potassium (mEq/L)	3.5–5.0	3.6–5.0	3.3–5.0	3.3–5.1	20, 26, 29, 39, 42, 63, 66
Prealbumin (mg/dL)	17–34	15–27	20–27	14–23	42
Protein, total (g/dL)	6.7–8.6	6.2–7.6	5.7–6.9	5.6–6.7	26, 29, 42
Sodium (mEq/L)	136–146	133–148	129–148	130–148	17, 26, 29, 39, 42, 63, 66
Urea nitrogen (mg/dL)	7–20	7–12	3–13	3–11	20, 39, 42
Uric acid (mg/dL)	2.5–5.6[d]	2.0–4.2	2.4–4.9	3.1–6.3	17, 39, 42

APPENDIX

METABOLIC AND ENDOCRINE TESTS

	Nonpregnant Adult[a]	1st Trimester	2nd Trimester	3rd Trimester	References
Aldosterone (ng/dL)	2–9	6–104	9–104	15–101	21, 34, 69
Angiotensin-converting enzyme (ACE) (U/L)	9–67	1–38	1–36	1–39	20, 54
Cortisol (μg/dL)	0–25	7–19	10–42	12–50	42, 69
Hemoglobin A_{1c} (%)	4–6	4–6	4–6	4–7	48, 49, 59
Parathyroid hormone (pg/mL)	8–51	10–15	18–25	9–26	3
Parathyroid hormone-related protein (pmol/L)	< 1.3[e]	0.7–0.9	1.8–2.2	2.5–2.8	3
Renin, plasma activity (ng/mL/hr)	0.3–9.0[e]	Not reported	7.5–54.0	5.9–58.8	20, 34
Thyroid stimulating hormone (TSH) (μIU/mL)	0.34–4.25	0.60–3.40	0.37–3.60	0.38–4.04	39, 42, 57
Thyroxine-binding globulin (mg/dL)	1.3–3.0	1.8–3.2	2.8–4.0	2.6–4.2	42
Thyroxine, free (fT_4) (ng/dL)	0.8–1.7	0.8–1.2	0.6–1.0	0.5–0.8	42, 57
Thyroxine, total (T_4) (μg/dL)	5.4–11.7	6.5–10.1	7.5–10.3	6.3–9.7	29, 42
Triiodothyronine, free (fT_3) (pg/mL)	2.4–4.2	4.1–4.4	4.0–4.2	Not reported	57
Triiodothyronine, total (T_3) (ng/dL)	77–135	97–149	117–169	123–162	42

VITAMINS AND MINERALS

	Nonpregnant Adult[a]	1st Trimester	2nd Trimester	3rd Trimester	References
Copper (μg/dL)	70–140	112–199	165–221	130–240	2, 30, 42
Selenium (μg/L)	63–160	116–146	75–145	71–133	2, 42
Vitamin A (retinol) (μg/dL)	20–100	32–47	35–44	29–42	42
Vitamin B_{12} (pg/mL)	279–966	118–438	130–656	99–526	45, 72
Vitamin C (ascorbic acid) (mg/dL)	0.4–1.0	Not reported	Not reported	0.9–1.3	64
Vitamin D, 1,25-dihydroxy (pg/mL)	25–45	20–65	72–160	60–119	3, 48
Vitamin D, 24,25-dihydroxy (ng/mL)	0.5–5.0[e]	1.2–1.8	1.1–1.5	0.7–0.9	60
Vitamin D, 25-hydroxy (ng/mL)	14–80	18–27	10–22	10–18	3, 60
Vitamin E (α-tocopherol) (μg/mL)	5–18	7–13	10–16	13–23	42
Zinc (μg/dL)	75–120	57–88	51–80	50–77	2, 42, 58

AUTOIMMUNE AND INFLAMMATORY MEDIATORS

	Nonpregnant Adult[a]	1st Trimester	2nd Trimester	3rd Trimester	References
C3 complement (mg/dL)	83–177	62–98	73–103	77–111	42
C4 complement (mg/dL)	16–47	18–36	18–34	22–32	42
C-reactive protein (CRP) (mg/L)	0.2–3.0	Not reported	0.4–20.3	0.4–8.1	28
Erythrocyte sedimentation rate (ESR) (mm/hr)	0–20[d]	4–57	7–47	13–70	71
IgA (mg/dL)	70–350	95–243	99–237	112–250	42
IgG (mg/dL)	700–1700	981–1267	813–1131	678–990	42
IgM (mg/dL)	50–300	78–232	74–218	85–269	42

SEX HORMONES

	Nonpregnant Adult[a]	1st Trimester	2nd Trimester	3rd Trimester	References
Dehydroepiandrosterone sulfate (DHEAS) (μmol/L)	1.3–6.8[e]	2.0–16.5	0.9–7.8	0.8–6.5	52
Estradiol (pg/mL)	< 20–443[d,f]	188–2497	1278–7192	6137–3460	13, 52
Progesterone (ng/mL)	< 1–20[d]	8–48		99–342	13, 52
Prolactin (ng/mL)	0–20[d]	36–213	110–330	137–372	3, 13, 38, 49
Sex hormone binding globulin (nmol/L)	18–114[d]	39–131	214–717	216–724	1, 52
Testosterone (ng/dL)	6–86[d]	25.7–211.4	34.3–242.9	62.9–308.6	52
17-Hydroxyprogesterone (nmol/L)	0.6–10.6[d,e]	5.2–28.5	5.2–28.5	15.5–84	52

LIPIDS

	Nonpregnant Adult[a]	1st Trimester	2nd Trimester	3rd Trimester	References
Cholesterol, total (mg/dL)	< 200	141–210	176–299	219–349	8, 18, 31, 42
HDL-cholesterol (mg/dL)	40–60	40–78	52–87	48–87	8, 18, 31, 42, 55
LDL-cholesterol (mg/dL)	< 100	60–153	77–184	101–224	8, 18, 31, 42, 55
VLDL-cholesterol (mg/dL)	6–40[e]	10–18	13–23	21–36	31
Triglycerides (mg/dL)	< 150	40–159	75–382	131–453	8, 18, 31, 39, 42, 55
Apolipoprotein A-I (mg/dL)	119–240	111–150	142–253	145–262	18, 39, 49
Apolipoprotein B (mg/dL)	52–163	58–81	66–188	85–238	18, 39, 49

CARDIAC

	Nonpregnant Adult[a]	1st Trimester	2nd Trimester	3rd Trimester	References
Atrial natriuretic peptide (ANP) (pg/mL)	Not reported	Not reported	28.1–70.1	Not reported	11
B-type natriuretic peptide (BNP) (pg/mL)	22 ± 10	22 ± 10	32 ± 15	31 ± 21	12A
Creatine kinase (U/L)	39–238[d]	27–83	25–75	13–101	41, 42
Creatine kinase-MB (U/L)	< 6[k]	Not reported	Not reported	1.8–2.4	41
NT-pro-BNP (pg/mL)	50 ± 26	60 ± 45	60 ± 40	43 ± 34	12A
Troponin I (ng/mL)	0–0.08	Not reported	Not reported	0–0.064 (intrapartum)	36, 65

APPENDIX

BLOOD GAS

	Nonpregnant Adult[a]	1st Trimester	2nd Trimester	3rd Trimester	References
Bicarbonate (HCO_3^-) (mEq/L)	22–26	Not reported	Not reported	16–22	23
Pco_2 (mm Hg)	38–42	Not reported	Not reported	25–33	23
Po_2 (mm Hg)	90–100	93–100	90–98	92–107	23, 67
pH	7.38–7.42 (arterial)	7.36–7.52 (venous)	7.40–7.52 (venous)	7.41–7.53 (venous) 7.39–7.45 (arterial)	23, 26

RENAL FUNCTION TESTS

	Nonpregnant Adult[a]	1st Trimester	2nd Trimester	3rd Trimester	References
Effective renal plasma flow (mL/min)	492–696[d,e]	696–985	612–1170	595–945	19, 22
Glomerular filtration rate (GFR) (mL/min)	106–132[d]	131–166	135–170	117–182	19, 22, 50
Filtration fraction (%)	16.9–24.7[l]	14.7–21.6	14.3–21.9	17.1–25.1	19, 22, 50
Osmolarity, urine (mOsm/kg)	500–800	326–975	278–1066	238–1034	61
24-hr albumin excretion (mg/24 hr)	< 30	5–15	4–18	3–22	27, 61
24-hr calcium excretion (mmol/24 hr)	< 7.5[e]	1.6–5.2	0.3–6.9	0.8–4.2	66
24-hr creatinine clearance (mL/min)	91–130	69–140	55–136	50–166	22, 66
24-hr creatinine excretion (mmol/24 hr)	8.8–14[e]	10.6–11.6	10.3–11.5	10.2–11.4	61
24-hr potassium excretion (mmol/24 hr)	25–100[e]	17–33	10–38	11–35	66
24-hr protein excretion (mg/24 hr)	< 150	19–141	47–186	46–185	27
24-hr sodium excretion (mmol/24 hr)	100–260[e]	53–215	34–213	37–149	17, 66

[a]Unless otherwise specified, all normal reference values are from the seventeenth edition of *Harrison's Principles of Internal Medicine* (37).
[b]Range includes references with and without iron supplementation.
[c]Reference values are from *Laboratory Reference Handbook*, Pathology Department, Parkland Hospital, 2005.
[d]Normal reference range is specific range for females.
[e]Reference values are from the 15th edition of *Harrison's Principles of Internal Medicine* (12).
[f]Range is for premenopausal females and varies by menstrual cycle phase.
[g]Reference values are from Cerneca et al: Coagulation and fibrinolysis changes in normal pregnancy increased levels of procoagulants and reduced levels of inhibitors during pregnancy induce a hypercoagulable state, combined with a reactive fibrinolysis (15).
[h]Reference values are from Cerneca et al and Choi et al: Tissue plasminogen activator levels change with plasma fibrinogen concentrations during pregnancy (15, 16).
[i]Reference values are from Mannucci et al: Changes in health and disease of the metalloprotease that cleaves von Willebrand factor (44A).
[j]Reference values are from Bacq et al: Liver function tests in normal pregnancy: a prospective study of 102 pregnant women and 102 matched controls (5).
[k]Reference values are from Leiserowitz et al: Creatine kinase and its MB isoenzyme in the third trimester and the peripartum period (41).
[l]Reference values are from Dunlop: Serial changes in renal haemodynamics during normal human pregnancy (19).
Appendix courtesy of Dr. Mina Abbassi-Ghanavati and Dr. Laura G. Greer.

APPENDIX II. Maternal Echocardiographic Measurements

Left Ventricle	Pregnancy			
	1st Trimester	2nd Trimester	3rd Trimester	Postpartum
Geometry				
IVS_d (mm)	7.3 ± 1.0	7.4 ± 1.1	7.8 ± 1.2	7.1 ± 0.9
LVEDD (mm)	45–47.8	47–48.9	47–49.6	46–48.8
LVESD (mm)	28–30	29–30.1	30–30.8	28–30.6
PW_d	6.3 ± 0.7	6.6 ± 0.7	6.9 ± 1.0	6.1 ± 0.6
RWT	0.26–0.36	0.27–0.37	0.28–0.38	0.25–0.35
LV mass (g)	111–121	121–135	136–151	114–119
LV mass (g/m^2)	66 ± 13	70 ± 12	76 ± 16	67 ± 11
Systolic function				
FS (%)	37-38	76-78	80-85	67-69
SW thickening (%)	47 ± 17	53 ± 16	51 ± 15	54 ± 19
PW thickening (%)	66 ± 16	72 ± 16	74 ± 16	71 ± 14
VCFC (circ/sec)	1.15–0.3	1.18–0.16	1.18–0.12	1.18–0.12
ESS (g/cm^2)	59 ± 9	53 ± 11	52 ± 11	66 ± 12
Diastolic function				
Heart rate	75–76	76–78	80–85	67–69
Mitral E wave (m/sec)	0.85 ± 0.13	0.84 ± 0.16	0.77 ± 0.15	0.77 ± 0.11
Mitral A wave (m/sec)	0.5 ± 0.09	0.5 ± 0.1	0.55 ± 0.1	0.46 ± 0.1
Deceleration time (ms)	176 ± 44	188 ± 40	193 ± 33	201 ± 48
IVRT (ms)	90 ±19	79 ± 18	72 ± 16	69 ± 10
E wave duration (ms)	263 ± 50	276 ± 43	282 ± 37	288 ± 48
E and A wave duration (ms)	454 ± 121	412 ± 79	375 ± 63	523 ± 88

Values are ranges or means ± SD.
Circ = circumference; d = diastolic; ESS = end-systolic wall stress; FS = fractional shortening; IVRT = isovolumic relaxation time; IVS_d = interventricular septum–diastole; LV = left ventricle; LVEDD = left ventricular end-diastolic dimension; LVESD = left ventricular end-systolic dimension; PW = posterior wall; RWT = relative wall thickening; SW = septal wall; VCFC = rate-adjusted mean velocity of circumferential fiber thickening.
Data from Savu (62A) and Vitarelli (71A).

APPENDIX III. Fetal Sonographic Measurements

TABLE III-1. Mean Gestational Sac Diameter and Crown-Rump Length and Corresponding Menstrual Age

Menstrual Age (day)	Menstrual Age (wk)	Gestational Sac Size (mm)	Crown-Rump Length (cm)
30	4.3		
32	4.6	3	
34	4.9	5	
36	5.1	6	
38	5.4	8	
40	5.7	10	0.2
42	6.0	12	0.35
44	6.3	14	0.5
46	6.6	16	0.7
48	6.9	18	0.9
50	7.1	20	1.0
52	7.4	22	1.2
54	7.7	24	1.4
56	8.0	26	1.6
58	8.3	27	1.8
60	8.6	29	2.0
62	8.9	31	2.2
64	9.1	33	2.4
66	9.4	35	2.6
68	9.7	37	2.9
70	10.0	39	3.1
72	10.3	41	3.4
74	10.6	43	3.7
76	10.9	45	4.0
78	11.1	47	4.2
80	11.4	49	4.6
82	11.7	51	5.0
84	12.0	53	5.4

Adapted from Nyberg, 2003 (51A),with permission.

TABLE III-2. Mean Gestational Age Percentiles Corresponding to Crown-Rump Length (CRL) Measurements

CRL (mm)	Gestational Age (wk) Percentile 5th	50th	95th	CRL (mm)	Gestational Age (wk) Percentile 5th	50th	95th
10	6 + 5	7 + 3	8	30	9 + 5	10 + 2	11
11	6 + 6	7 + 4	8 + 2	31	9 + 5	10 + 3	11 + 1
12	7 + 1	7 + 5	8 + 3	32	9 + 6	10 + 4	11 + 2
13	7 + 2	8	8 + 4	33	10	10 + 5	11 + 2
14	7 + 3	8 + 4	8 + 6	34	10 + 1	10 + 6	11 + 3
15	7 + 4	8 + 2	9	35	10 + 2	10 + 6	11 + 4
16	7 + 5	8 + 3	9 + 1	36	10 + 2	11	11 + 5
17	8	8 + 4	9 + 2	37	10 + 3	11 + 1	11 + 6
18	8 + 1	8 + 5	9 + 3	38	10 + 4	11 + 2	11 + 6
19	8 + 2	8 + 6	9 + 4	39	10 + 5	11 + 2	12
20	8 + 3	9	9 + 5	40	10 + 5	11 + 3	12 + 1
21	8 + 4	9 + 1	9 + 6	41	10 + 6	11 + 4	12 + 1
22	8 + 5	9 + 2	10	42	11	11 + 4	12 + 2
23	8 + 6	9 + 3	10 + 1	43	11	11 + 5	12 + 3
24	8 + 6	9 + 4	10 + 2	44	11 + 1	11 + 6	12 + 3
25	9	9 + 5	10 + 3	45	11 + 2	11 + 6	12 + 4
26	9 + 1	9 + 6	10 + 4	46	11 + 2	12	12 + 5
27	9 + 2	10	10 + 5	47	11 + 3	12 + 1	12 + 5
28	9 + 3	10 + 1	10 + 5	48	11 + 4	12 + 1	12 + 6
29	9 + 4	10 + 2	10 + 6	49	11 + 4	11 + 2	13

TABLE III-3. Fetal Weight Percentiles According to Gestational Age

Gestational Age (wk)	Fetal Weight Percentiles (g)				
	3rd	10th	50th	90th	97th
10	26	29	35	41	44
11	34	37	45	53	56
12	43	48	58	68	73
13	54	61	73	85	92
14	69	77	93	109	117
15	87	97	117	137	147
16	109	121	146	171	183
17	135	150	181	212	227
18	166	185	223	261	280
19	204	227	273	319	342
20	247	275	331	387	415
21	298	331	399	467	500
22	357	397	478	559	599
23	424	472	568	664	712
24	500	556	670	784	840
25	586	652	785	918	984
26	681	758	913	1068	1145
27	787	876	1055	1234	1323
28	903	1005	1210	1415	1517
29	1029	1145	1379	1613	1729
30	1163	1294	1559	1824	1955
31	1306	1454	1751	2048	2196
32	1457	1621	1953	2285	2449
33	1613	1795	2162	2529	2711
34	1773	1973	2377	2781	2981
35	1936	2154	2595	3026	3254
36	2098	2335	2813	3291	3528
37	2259	2514	3028	3542	3797
38	2414	2687	3236	3785	4058
39	2563	2852	3435	4018	4307
40	2700	3004	3619	4234	4538
41	2825	3144	3787	4430	4749
42	2935	3266	3934	4602	4933

From Hadlock, 1991 (25B), with permission.

TABLE III-4. Smoothed Birth Weight Percentiles for Twins with Dichorionic Placentation

	Smoothed Birth Weight Percentiles				
GA (wk)	5th	10th	50th	90th	95th
23	477	513	632	757	801
24	538	578	712	853	903
25	606	652	803	962	1018
26	684	735	906	1085	1148
27	771	829	1021	1223	1294
28	870	935	1152	1379	1459
29	980	1054	1298	1554	1645
30	1102	1186	1460	1748	1850
31	1235	1328	1635	1958	2072
32	1374	1477	1819	2179	2306
33	1515	1630	2007	2403	2543
34	1653	1778	2190	2622	2775
35	1781	1916	2359	2825	2989
36	1892	2035	2506	3001	3176
37	1989	2139	2634	3155	3339
38	2079	2236	2753	3297	3489
39	2167	2331	2870	3437	3637
40	2258	2428	2990	3581	3790
41	2352	2530	3115	3731	3948

GA = gestational age.
From Ananth, 1998 (2A), with permission

TABLE III-5. Smoothed Birth Weight Percentiles for Twins with Monochorionic Placentation

	Smoothed Birth Weight Percentiles				
GA (wk)	5th	10th	50th	90th	95th
23	392	431	533	648	683
24	456	501	620	753	794
25	530	582	720	875	922
26	615	676	836	1017	1072
27	713	784	970	1178	1242
28	823	904	1119	1360	1433
29	944	1037	1282	1559	1643
30	1072	1178	1457	1771	1867
31	1204	1323	1637	1990	2097
32	1335	1467	1814	2205	2325
33	1457	1601	1980	2407	2537
34	1562	1716	2123	2580	2720
35	1646	1808	2237	2719	2866
36	1728	1899	2349	2855	3009
37	1831	2012	2489	3025	3189
38	1957	2150	2660	3233	3408
39	2100	2307	2854	3469	3657
40	2255	2478	3065	3726	3927
41	2422	2661	3292	4001	4217

From Ananth, 1998 (2A), with permission

TABLE III-6. Fetal Thoracic Circumference Measurements (cm) According to Gestational Age

Gestational Age (wk)	No.	Predictive Percentiles 2.5	5	10	25	50	75	90	95	97.5
16	6	5.9	6.4	7.0	8.0	9.1	10.3	11.3	11.9	12.4
17	22	6.8	7.3	7.9	8.9	10.0	11.2	12.2	12.8	13.3
18	31	7.7	8.2	8.8	9.8	11.0	12.1	13.1	13.7	14.2
19	21	8.6	9.1	9.7	10.7	11.9	13.0	14.0	14.6	15.1
20	20	9.6	10.0	10.6	11.7	12.8	13.9	15.0	15.5	16.0
21	30	10.4	11.0	11.6	12.6	13.7	14.8	15.8	16.4	16.9
22	18	11.3	11.9	12.5	13.5	14.6	15.7	16.7	17.3	17.8
23	21	12.2	12.8	13.4	14.4	15.5	16.6	17.6	18.2	18.8
24	27	13.2	13.7	14.3	15.3	16.4	17.5	18.5	19.1	19.7
25	20	14.1	14.6	15.2	16.2	17.3	18.4	19.4	20.0	20.6
26	25	15.0	15.5	16.1	17.1	18.2	19.3	20.3	21.0	21.5
27	24	15.9	16.4	17.0	18.0	19.1	20.2	21.3	21.9	22.4
28	24	16.8	17.3	17.9	18.9	20.0	21.2	22.2	22.8	23.3
29	24	17.7	18.2	18.8	19.8	21.0	22.1	23.1	23.7	24.2
30	27	18.6	19.1	19.7	20.7	21.9	23.0	24.0	24.6	25.1
31	24	19.5	20.0	20.6	21.6	22.8	23.9	24.9	25.5	26.0
32	28	20.4	20.9	21.5	22.6	23.7	24.8	25.8	26.4	26.9
33	27	21.3	21.8	22.5	23.5	24.6	25.7	26.7	27.3	27.8
34	25	22.2	22.8	23.4	24.4	25.5	26.6	27.6	28.2	28.7
35	20	23.1	23.7	24.3	25.3	26.4	27.5	28.5	29.1	29.6
36	23	24.0	24.6	25.2	26.2	27.3	28.4	29.4	30.0	30.6
37	22	24.8	25.5	26.1	27.1	28.2	29.3	30.3	30.9	31.5
38	21	25.9	26.4	27.0	28.0	29.1	30.2	31.2	31.9	32.4
39	7	26.8	27.3	27.9	28.9	30.0	31.1	32.2	32.8	33.3
40	6	27.7	28.2	28.8	29.8	30.9	32.1	33.1	33.7	34.2

Adapted from Chitkara, 1987 (15A), with permission.

TABLE III-7. Length of Fetal Long Bones (mm) According to Gestational Age

	Humerus Percentile			Ulna Percentile			Radius Percentile			Femur Percentile			Tibia Percentile			Fibula Percentile		
Week	**5**	**50**	**95**	**5**	**50**	**95**	**5**	**15**	**95**	**5**	**50**	**95**	**5**	**50**	**95**	**5**	**50**	**95**
15	11	18	26	10	16	22	12	15	19	11	19	26	5	16	27	10	14	18
16	12	21	25	8	19	24	9	18	21	13	22	24	7	19	25	6	17	22
17	19	24	29	11	21	32	11	20	29	20	25	29	15	22	29	7	19	31
18	18	27	30	13	24	30	14	22	26	19	28	31	14	24	29	10	22	28
19	22	29	36	20	26	32	20	24	29	23	31	38	19	27	35	18	24	30
20	23	32	36	21	29	32	21	27	28	22	33	39	19	29	35	18	27	30
21	28	34	40	25	31	36	25	29	32	27	36	45	24	32	39	24	29	34
22	28	36	40	24	33	37	24	31	34	29	39	44	25	34	39	21	31	37
23	32	38	45	27	35	43	26	32	39	35	41	48	30	36	43	23	33	44
24	31	41	46	29	37	41	27	34	38	34	44	49	28	39	45	26	35	41
25	35	43	51	34	39	44	31	36	40	38	46	54	31	41	50	33	37	42
26	36	45	49	34	41	44	30	37	41	39	49	53	33	43	49	32	39	43
27	42	46	51	37	43	48	33	39	45	45	51	57	39	45	51	35	41	47
28	41	48	52	37	44	48	33	40	45	45	53	57	38	47	52	36	43	47
29	44	50	56	40	46	51	36	42	47	49	56	62	40	49	57	40	45	50
30	44	52	56	38	47	54	34	43	49	49	58	62	41	51	56	38	47	52
31	47	53	59	39	49	59	34	44	53	53	60	67	46	52	58	40	48	57
32	47	55	59	40	50	58	37	45	51	53	62	67	46	54	59	40	50	56
33	5	56	62	43	52	60	41	46	51	56	64	71	49	56	62	43	51	59
34	50	57	62	44	53	59	39	47	53	57	65	70	47	57	64	46	52	56
35	52	58	65	47	54	61	38	48	57	61	67	73	48	59	69	51	54	57
36	53	60	63	47	55	61	41	48	54	61	69	74	49	60	68	51	55	56
37	57	61	64	49	56	62	45	49	53	64	71	77	52	61	71	55	56	58
38	55	61	66	48	57	63	45	49	53	62	72	79	54	62	69	54	57	59
39	56	62	69	49	57	66	46	50	54	64	74	83	58	64	69	55	58	62
40	56	63	69	50	58	65	46	50	54	66	75	81	58	65	69	54	59	62

Adapted from Jeanty, 1983 (30B), with permission.

TABLE III-8. Ocular Parameters According to Gestational Age

	Binocular Distance (mm)			Interocular Distance (mm)			Ocular Diameter (mm)		
Age (wk)	5th	50th	95th	5th	50th	95th	5th	50th	95th
15	15	22	30	6	10	14	4	6	9
16	17	25	32	6	10	15	5	7	9
17	19	27	34	6	11	15	5	8	10
18	22	29	37	7	11	16	6	9	11
19	24	31	39	7	12	16	7	9	12
20	26	33	41	8	12	17	8	10	13
21	28	35	43	8	13	17	8	11	13
22	30	37	44	9	13	18	9	12	14
23	31	39	46	9	14	18	10	12	15
24	33	41	48	10	14	19	10	13	15
25	35	42	50	10	15	19	11	13	16
26	36	44	51	11	15	20	12	14	16
27	38	45	53	11	16	20	12	14	17
28	39	47	54	12	16	21	13	15	17
29	41	48	56	12	17	21	13	15	18
30	42	50	57	13	17	22	14	16	18
31	43	51	58	13	18	22	14	16	19
32	45	52	60	14	18	23	14	17	19
33	46	53	61	14	19	23	15	17	19
34	47	54	62	15	19	24	15	17	20
35	48	55	63	15	20	24	15	18	20
36	49	56	64	16	20	25	16	18	20
37	50	57	65	16	21	25	1	18	21
38	50	58	65	17	21	26	16	18	21
39	51	59	66	17	22	26	16	19	21
40	52	59	67	18	22	26	16	19	21

Adapted from Romero, 1988 (61A), with permission.

TABLE III-9. Transverse Cerebellar Diameter Measurements According to Gestational Age

Gestational Age (wk)	Cerebellum Diameter (mm)				
	10	25	50	75	90
15	10	12	14	15	16
16	14	16	16	16	17
17	16	16	17	17	18
18	17	17	18	18	19
19	18	18	19	19	22
20	18	19	19	20	22
21	19	20	22	23	24
22	21	23	23	24	24
23	22	23	24	25	26
24	22	24	25	27	28
25	23	21.5	28	28	29
26	25	28	29	30	32
27	26	28.5	30	31	32
28	27	30	31	32	34
29	29	32	34	36	38
30	31	32	35	37	40
31	32	35	38	39	43
32	33	36	38	40	42
33	32	36	40	43	44
34	33	38	40	41	44
35	31	37	40.5	43	47
36	36	29	43	52	55
37	37	37	45	52	55
38	40	40	48.5	52	55
39	52	52	52	55	55

Adapted from Goldstein, 1987 (25A), with permission.

APPENDIX

TABLE III-10. Reference Values for Umbilical Artery Doppler Indices

GA (wk)	5th Percentile Resistive Index	5th Percentile Systolic/ Diastolic Ratio	50th Percentile Resistive Index	50th Percentile Systolic/ Diastolic Ratio	95th Percentile Resistive Index	95th Percentile Systolic/ Diastolic Ratio
16	0.70	3.39	0.80	5.12	0.90	10.50
17	0.69	3.27	0.79	4.86	0.89	9.46
18	0.68	3.16	0.78	4.63	0.88	8.61
19	0.67	3.06	0.77	4.41	0.87	7.90
20	0.66	2.97	0.76	4.22	0.86	7.30
21	0.65	2.88	0.75	4.04	0.85	6.78
22	0.64	2.79	0.74	3.88	0.84	6.33
23	0.63	2.71	0.73	3.73	0.83	5.94
24	0.62	2.64	0.72	3.59	0.82	5.59
25	0.61	2.57	0.71	3.46	0.81	5.28
26	0.60	2.50	0.70	3.34	0.80	5.01
27	0.59	2.44	0.69	3.22	0.79	4.76
28	0.58	2.38	0.68	3.12	0.78	4.53
29	0.57	2.32	0.67	3.02	0.77	4.33
30	0.56	2.26	0.66	2.93	0.76	4.14
31	0.55	2.21	0.65	2.84	0.75	3.97
32	0.54	2.16	0.64	2.76	0.74	3.81
33	0.53	2.11	0.63	2.68	0.73	3.66
34	0.52	2.07	0.62	2.61	0.72	3.53
35	0.51	2.03	0.61	2.54	0.71	3.40
36	0.50	1.98	0.60	2.47	0.70	3.29
37	0.49	1.94	0.59	2.41	0.69	3.18
38	0.47	1.90	0.57	2.35	0.67	3.08
39	0.46	1.87	0.56	2.30	0.66	2.98
40	0.45	1.83	0.55	2.24	0.65	2.89
41	0.44	1.80	0.54	2.19	0.64	2.81
42	0.43	1.76	0.53	2.14	0.63	2.73

GA = gestational age.
Adapted from Kofinas, 1992 (35A), with permission.

APPENDIX REFERENCES

1. Acromite MT, Mantzoros CS, Leach RE, et al: Androgens in preeclampsia. Am J Obstet Gynecol 180:60, 1999
2. Álvarez SI, Castañón SG, Ruata MLC, et al: Updating of normal levels of copper, zinc and selenium in serum of pregnant women. J Trace Elem Med Biol 21(S1):49, 2007

2A. Ananth CV, Vintzileos, Shen-Schwarz S, et al: Standards of birth weight in twin gestations. Obstet Gynecol 91:917, 1998

3. Ardawi MSM, Nasrat HAN, BA'Aqueel HS: Calcium-regulating hormones and parathyroid hormone-related peptide in normal human pregnancy and postpartum: a longitudinal study. Eur J Endocrinol 137:402, 1997

3A. Aslam N, Ong C, Woelfer B, et al: Serum CA 125 at 11–14 weeks of gestation in women with morphologically normal ovaries. BJOG 107(5): 689, 2000

4. Aziz Karim S, Khurshid M, Rizvi JH, et al: Platelets and leucocyte counts in pregnancy. J Pak Med Assoc 42:86, 1992
5. Bacq Y, Zarka O, Bréchot JF, et al: Liver function tests in normal pregnancy: a prospective study of 102 pregnant women and 102 matched controls. Hepatology 23:1030, 1996
6. Balloch AJ, Cauchi MN: Reference ranges for haematology parameters in pregnancy derived from patient populations. Clin Lab Haematol 15:7, 1993
7. Beguin Y, Lipscei G, Thourmsin H, et al: Blunted erythropoietin production and decreased erythropoiesis in early pregnancy. Blood 78(1):89, 1991
8. Belo L, Caslake M, Gaffney D, et al: Changes in LDL size and HDL concentration in normal and preeclamptic pregnancies. Atherosclerosis 162:425, 2002
9. Belo L, Santos-Silva A, Rocha S, et al: Fluctuations in C-reactive protein concentration and neutrophil activation during normal human pregnancy. Eur J Obstet Gynecol Reprod Biol 123:46, 2005
10. Bianco I, Mastropietro F, D'Aseri C, et al: Serum levels of erythropoietin and soluble transferrin receptor during pregnancy in non-β-thalassemic and β-thalassemic women. Haematologica 85:902, 2000
11. Borghi CB, Esposti DD, Immordino V, et al: Relationship of systemic hemodynamics, left ventricular structure and function, and plasma natriuretic peptide concentrations during pregnancy complicated by preeclampsia. Am J Obstet Gynecol 183:140, 2000
12. Braunwald E, Fauci AS, Kasper DL, et al (eds): Appendices. In Harrison's Principles of Internal Medicine, 15th ed. New York, McGraw-Hill, 2001, p A-1

12A. Burlingame J, Hyeong JA, Tang WHW: Changes in cardiovascular biomarkers throughout pregnancy and the remote postpartum period. Am J Obstet Gynecol 208:S97, 2013

13. Carranza-Lira S, Hernández F, Sánchez M, et al: Prolactin secretion in molar and normal pregnancy. Int J Gynaecol Obstet 60:137, 1998
14. Carter J: Serum bile acids in normal pregnancy. BJOG 98:540, 1991
15. Cerneca F, Ricci G, Simeone R, et al: Coagulation and fibrinolysis changes in normal pregnancy increased levels of procoagulants and reduced levels of inhibitors during pregnancy induce a hypercoagulable state, combined with a reactive fibrinolysis. Eur J Obstet Gynecol Reprod Biol 73:31, 1997
15A. Chitkara J, Rosenberg J, Chervenak FA, et al: Prenatal sonographic assessment of the fetal thorax: normal values. Am J Obstet Gynecol 156:1069, 1987
16. Choi JW, Pai SH: Tissue plasminogen activator levels change with plasma fibrinogen concentrations during pregnancy. Ann Hematol 81:611, 2002
17. Davison JB, Vallotton MB, Lindheimer MD: Plasma osmolality and urinary concentration and dilution during and after pregnancy: evidence that lateral recumbency inhibits maximal urinary concentrating ability. BJOG 88:472, 1981
18. Desoye G, Schweditsch MO, Pfeiffer KP, et al: Correlation of hormones with lipid and lipoprotein levels during normal pregnancy and postpartum. J Clin Endocrinol Metab 64:704, 1987
19. Dunlop W: Serial changes in renal haemodynamics during normal human pregnancy. BJOG 88:1, 1981
20. Dux S, Yaron A, Carmel A, et al: Renin, aldosterone, and serum-converting enzyme activity during normal and hypertensive pregnancy. Gynecol Obstet Invest 17:252, 1984
21. Elsheikh A, Creatsas G, Mastorakos G, et al: The renin-aldosterone system during normal and hypertensive pregnancy. Arch Gynecol Obstet 264:182, 2001
22. Ezimokhai M, Davison JM, Philips PR, et al: Non-postural serial changes in renal function during the third trimester of normal human pregnancy. BJOG 88:465, 1981
23. Fadel HE, Northrop G, Misenhimer HR, et al: Acid-base determinations in amniotic fluid and blood of normal late pregnancy. Obstet Gynecol 53:99, 1979
24. Faught W, Garner P, Jones G, et al: Changes in protein C and protein S levels in normal pregnancy. Am J Obstet Gynecol 172:147, 1995
25. Francalanci I, Comeglio P, Liotta AA, et al: D-Dimer concentrations during normal pregnancy, as measured by ELISA. Thromb Res 78:399, 1995
25A. Goldstein I, Reece A, Pilu, et al: Cerebellar measurements with ultrasonography in the evaluation of fetal growth and development. Am J Obstet Gynecol 156:1065, 1987
25B. Hadlock FP, Harrist RB, Marinez-Poyer J: In utero analysis of fetal growth: a sonographic weight standard. Radiology 181:129, 1991.
25C. Hale SA, Sobel B, Benvenuto A, et al: Coagulation and fibrinolytic system protein profiles in women with normal pregnancies and pregnancies complicated by hypertension. Pregnancy Hypertens 2(2):152, 2012
26. Handwerker SM, Altura BT, Altura BM: Serum ionized magnesium and other electrolytes in the antenatal period of human pregnancy. J Am Coll Nutr 15:36, 1996
26A. Haram K, Augensen K, Elsayed S: Serum protein pattern in normal pregnancy with special reference to acute phase reactants. BJOG 90(2):139, 1983
27. Higby K, Suiter CR, Phelps JY, et al: Normal values of urinary albumin and total protein excretion during pregnancy. Am J Obstet Gynecol 171:984, 1994
27A. Hui C, Lili M, Libin C, et al: Changes in coagulation and hemodynamics during pregnancy: a prospective longitudinal study of 58 cases. Arch Gynecol Obstet 285:1231, 2012
28. Hwang HS, Kwon JY, Kim MA, et al: Maternal serum highly sensitive C-reactive protein in normal pregnancy and pre-eclampsia. Int J Gynecol Obstet 98:105, 2007
29. Hytten FE, Lind T: Diagnostic Indices in Pregnancy. Summit, CIBA-GEIGY Corporation, 1975
30. Ilhan N, Ilhan N, Simsek M: The changes of trace elements, malondialdehyde levels and superoxide dismutase activities in pregnancy with or without preeclampsia. Clin Biochem 35:393, 2002
30A. Jacobs IJ, Fay TN, Stabile I, et al: The distribution of CA 125 in the reproductive tract of pregnant and non-pregnant women. BJOG 95(11):1190, 1988
30B. Jeanty P: Fetal limb biometry. Radiology 147:602, 1983
31. Jimenez DM, Pocovi M, Ramon-Cajal J, et al: Longitudinal study of plasma lipids and lipoprotein cholesterol in normal pregnancy and puerperium. Gynecol Obstet Invest 25:158, 1988
31A. Jóźwik M, Jóźwik M, Pietrzycki, et al: Maternal and fetal blood ammonia concentrations in normal term human pregnancies. Biol Neonate 87:38, 2005
32. Karsenti D, Bacq Y, Bréchot JF, et al: Serum amylase and lipase activities in normal pregnancy: a prospective case-control study. Am J Gastroenterol 96:697, 2001
33. Kato T, Seki K, Matsui H, et al: Monomeric calcitonin in pregnant women and in cord blood. Obstet Gynecol 92:241, 1998
34. Kim EH, Lim JH, Kim YH, et al: The relationship between aldosterone to renin ratio and RI value of the uterine artery in the preeclamptic patient vs. normal pregnancy. Yonsei Med J 49(1):138, 2008
35. Kline JA, Williams GW, Hernandez-Nino J: D-Dimer concentrations in normal pregnancy: new diagnostic thresholds are needed. Clin Chem 51:825, 2005
35A. Kofinas AD, Espeland MA, Penry M, et al: Uteroplacental Doppler flow velocimetry waveform indices in normal pregnancy: a statistical exercise and the development of appropriate references values. Am J Perinatol 9:94, 1992
36. Koscica KL, Bebbington M, Bernstein PS: Are maternal serum troponin I levels affected by vaginal or cesarean delivery? Am J Perinatol 21(1):31, 2004
38. Larrea F, Méndez I, Parra A: Serum pattern of different molecular forms of prolactin during normal human pregnancy. Hum Reprod 8:1617, 1993
39. Larsson A, Palm M, Hansson L-O, et al: Reference values for clinical chemistry tests during normal pregnancy. BJOG 115:874, 2008
39A. Lattuada A, Rossi E, Calzarossa C, et al: Mild to moderate reduction of a von Willebrand factor cleaving protease (ADAMTS-13) in pregnant women with HELLP microangiopathic syndrome. Haematologica 88(9): 1029, 2003
39B. Leek AE, Ruoss CF, Kitau MG, et al: Maternal plasma alphafetoprotein levels in the second half of normal pregnancy: relationship to fetal weight, and maternal age and parity. BJOG 82:669, 1975
40. Lefkowitz JB, Clarke SH, Barbour LA: Comparison of protein S functional and antigenic assays in normal pregnancy. Am J Obstet Gynecol 175:657, 1996
41. Leiserowitz GS, Evans AT, Samuels SJ, et al: Creatine kinase and its MB isoenzyme in the third trimester and the peripartum period. J Reprod Med 37:910, 1992
41A. Liu XH, Jiang YM, Shi H, et al: Prospective, sequential, longitudinal study of coagulation changes during pregnancy in Chinese women. Int J Gynaecol Obstet 105(3):240, 2009
42. Lockitch G: Handbook of Diagnostic Biochemistry and Hematology in Normal Pregnancy. Boca Raton, CRC Press, 1993
43. López-Quesada E, Vilaseca MA, Lailla JM: Plasma total homocysteine in uncomplicated pregnancy and in preeclampsia. Eur J Obstet Gynecol Reprod Biol 108:45, 2003
44. Louro MO, Cocho JA, Tutor JC: Assessment of copper status in pregnancy by means of determining the specific oxidase activity of ceruloplasmin. Clin Chim Acta 312:123, 2001
44A. Mannucci PM, Canciani MT, Forza I, et al: Changes in health and disease of the metalloprotease that cleaves von Willebrand factor. Blood 98(9): 2730, 2001
45. Milman N, Bergholt T, Byg KE, et al: Reference intervals for haematological variables during normal pregnancy and postpartum in 434 healthy Danish women. Eur J Haematol 79:39, 2007
46. Milman N, Byg KE, Hvas AM, et al: Erythrocyte folate, plasma folate and plasma homocysteine during normal pregnancy and postpartum: a longitudinal study comprising 404 Danish women. Eur J Haematol 76:200, 2006
47. Milman N, Graudal N, Nielsen OJ: Serum erythropoietin during normal pregnancy: relationship to hemoglobin and iron status markers and impact of iron supplementation in a longitudinal, placebo-controlled study on 118 women. Int J Hematol 66:159, 1997
48. Mimouni F, Tsang RC, Hertzbert VS, et al: Parathyroid hormone and calcitriol changes in normal and insulin-dependent diabetic pregnancies. Obstet Gynecol 74:49, 1989
49. Montelongo A, Lasunción MA, Pallardo LF, et al: Longitudinal study of plasma lipoproteins and hormones during pregnancy in normal and diabetic women. Diabetes 41:1651, 1992
50. Moran P, Baylis PH, Lindheimer, et al: Glomerular ultrafiltration in normal and preeclamptic pregnancy. J Am Soc Nephrol 14:648, 2003
51. Morse M: Establishing a normal range for D-dimer levels through pregnancy to aid in the diagnosis of pulmonary embolism and deep vein thrombosis. J Thromb Haemost 2:1202, 2004
51A. Nyberg DA, McGahan JP, Pretorius DH, et al (eds): Diagnostic Imaging of Fetal Anomalies, 2nd ed. Philadelphia, Lippincott Williams & Wilkins, 2003, p 1015
52. O'Leary P, Boyne P, Flett P, et al: Longitudinal assessment of changes in reproductive hormones during normal pregnancy. Clin Chem 35(5):667, 1991
53. Özerol E, Özerol I, Gökdeniz R, et al: Effect of smoking on serum concentrations of total homocysteine, folate, vitamin B_{12}, and nitric oxide in pregnancy: a preliminary study. Fetal Diagn Ther 19:145, 2004
54. Parente JV, Franco JG, Greene LJ, et al: Angiotensin-converting enzyme: serum levels during normal pregnancy. Am J Obstet Gynecol 135:586, 1979
55. Piechota W, Staszewski A: Reference ranges of lipids and apolipoproteins in pregnancy. Eur J Obstet Gynecol Reprod Biol 45:27, 1992
56. Pitkin RM, Gebhardt MP: Serum calcium concentrations in human pregnancy. Am J Obstet Gynecol 127:775, 1977

APPENDIX

57. Price A, Obel O, Cresswell J, et al: Comparison of thyroid function in pregnant and non-pregnant Asian and western Caucasian women. Clin Chim Acta 208:91, 2001
58. Qvist I, Abdulla M, Jägerstad M, et al: Iron, zinc and folate status during pregnancy and two months after delivery. Acta Obstet Gynecol Scand 65:15, 1986
59. Radder JK, Van Roosmalen J: HbA1c in healthy, pregnant women. Neth J Med 63:256, 2005
60. Reiter EO, Braunstein GD, Vargas A, et al: Changes in 25-hydroxyvitamin D and 24,25-dihydroxyvitamin D during pregnancy. Am J Obstet Gynecol 135:227, 1979
61. Risberg A, Larsson A, Olsson K, et al: Relationship between urinary albumin and albumin/creatinine ratio during normal pregnancy and pre-eclampsia. Scand J Clin Lab Invest 64:17, 2004
61A. Romero R, Pilu G, Jeanty P, et al: Prenatal diagnosis of congenital anomalies. Norwalk, Appleton & Lange, 1988, p 83
62. Romslo I, Haram K, Sagen N, et al: Iron requirement in normal pregnancy as assessed by serum ferritin, serum transferrin saturation and erythrocyte protoporphyrin determinations. BJOG 90:101, 1983
62A. Savu O, Jurcuţ R, Giuşcă S, et al: Morphological and functional adaptation of the maternal heart during pregnancy. Circ Cardiovasc Imaging 5:289, 2012
63. Shakhmatova EI, Osipova NA, Natochin YV: Changes in osmolality and blood serum ion concentrations in pregnancy. Hum Physiol 26:92, 2000
64. Sharma SC, Sabra A, Molloy A, et al: Comparison of blood levels of histamine and total ascorbic acid in pre-eclampsia with normal pregnancy. Hum Nutr Clin Nutr 38C:3, 1984
65. Shivvers SA, Wians FH, Keffer JH, et al: Maternal cardiac troponin I levels during labor and delivery. Am J Obstet Gynecol 180:122, 1999
66. Singh HJ, Mohammad NH, Nila A: Serum calcium and parathormone during normal pregnancy in Malay women. J Matern Fetal Med 8:95, 1999
67. Spiropoulos K, Prodromaki E, Tsapanos V: Effect of body position on Pao_2 and $Paco_2$ during pregnancy. Gynecol Obstet Invest 58:22, 2004
67A. Spitzer M, Kaushal N, Benjamin F: Maternal CA-125 levels in pregnancy and the puerperium. J Reprod Med 43(4):387, 1998
68. Strickland DM, Hauth JC, Widish J, et al: Amylase and isoamylase activities in serum of pregnant women. Obstet Gynecol 63:389, 1984
69. Suri D, Moran J, Hibbard JU, et al: Assessment of adrenal reserve in pregnancy: defining the normal response to the adrenocorticotropin stimulation test. J Clin Endocrinol Metab 91:3866, 2006
70. Van Buul EJA, Steegers EAP, Jongsma HW, et al: Haematological and biochemical profile of uncomplicated pregnancy in nulliparous women: a longitudinal study. Neth J Med 46:73, 1995
71. van den Broek NR, Letsky EA: Pregnancy and the erythrocyte sedimentation rate. BJOG 108:1164, 2001
71A. Vitarelli A, Capotosto L: Role of echocardiography in the assessment and management of adult congenital heart disease in pregnancy. Int J Cardiovasc Imaging 27(6):843, 2011
72. Walker MC, Smith GN, Perkins SL, et al: Changes in homocysteine levels during normal pregnancy. Am J Obstet Gynecol 180:660, 1999
73. Wickström K, Edelstam G, Löwbeer CH, et al: Reference intervals for plasma levels of fibronectin, von Willebrand factor, free protein S and antithrombin during third-trimester pregnancy. Scand J Clin Lab Invest 64:31, 2004

INDEX

Note: Page numbers followed by *f* indicates for figure and *t* for tables respectively.